Cardiac Electrophysiology

From Cell to Bedside

Seventh Edition

Douglas P. Zipes, MD

Distinguished Professor, Emeritus Professor of Medicine, Pharmacology, and Toxicology, Emeritus Director, Division of Cardiology and the Krannert Institute of Cardiology, Indiana University School of Medicine; Editor-in-Chief, PracticeUpdate/Cardiology, Editor-in-Chief, Trends in Cardiovascular Medicine, Indianapolis, IN, United States

José Jalife, MD

Cyrus and Jane Farrehi Professor of Cardiovascular Research, Department of Internal Medicine; Professor, Department of Molecular and Integrative Physiology; Co-Director, Center for Arrhythmia Research, University of Michigan, Ann Arbor, MI, United States; Senior Investigator, Fundación Centro Nacional de Investigaciones Cardiovasculares (CNIC), Madrid, Spain

William G. Stevenson, MD

Director, Cardiac Arrhythmia Program, Cardiovascular Division, Brigham and Women's Hospital; Professor of Medicine, Harvard Medical School, Boston, MA, United States

ELSEVIER

ELSEVIER

1600 John F. Kennedy Blvd.
Ste 1800
Philadelphia, PA 19103-2899

CARDIAC ELECTROPHYSIOLOGY: FROM CELL TO BEDSIDE,
SEVENTH EDITION

ISBN: 978-0-323-44733-1

Previous editions copyrighted 2014, 2009, 2004, 2000, 1995, 1990.

Library of Congress Cataloging-in-Publication Data

Names: Zipes, Douglas P., editor. | Jalife, José, editor. | Stevenson,
    William G. (William Gregory), editor.
Title: Cardiac electrophysiology : from cell to bedside / [edited by] Douglas
    P. Zipes, José Jalife, William G. Stevenson.
Other titles: Cardiac electrophysiology (Zipes)
Description: Seventh edition. | Philadelphia, PA : Elsevier, [2018] |
    Includes bibliographical references and index.
Identifiers: LCCN 2017013656 | ISBN 9780323447331 (hardcover : alk. paper)
Subjects: | MESH: Arrhythmias, Cardiac | Heart--physiology |
    Electrophysiologic Techniques, Cardiac | Cardiac Electrophysiology--methods
Classification: LCC RC685.A65 | NLM WG 330 | DDC 616.1/28--dc23 LC record available at
https://lccn.loc.gov/2017013656

Executive Content Strategist: Dolores Meloni
Content Development Manager: Lucia Gunzel
Publishing Services Manager: Catherine Jackson
Book Production Specialist: Kristine Feeherty
Design Direction: Amy Buxton

Printed in China

Last digit is the print number: 9 8 7 6 5 4 3 2 1

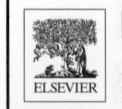

CONTRIBUTORS

Philip Aagaard, MD, PhD
Department of Cardiovascular Medicine, Heart and Vascular Institute, Cleveland Clinic Foundation, Cleveland, OH, United States
Chapter 124: Catheter Ablation: Clinical Aspects

Dominic James Abrams, MD, MRCP
Director, Inherited Cardiac Arrhythmia Program, Department of Cardiology, Boston Children's Hospital, Boston, MA, United States
Chapter 74: Atrial Tachycardia in Adults With Congenital Heart Disease

Hugues Abriel, MD, PhD
Professor of Molecular Medicine, Managing Director, Institute of Biochemistry and Molecular Medicine, University of Bern, Bern, Switzerland
Chapter 18: Microdomain Interactions of Macromolecular Complexes and Regulation of the Sodium Channel $Na_v1.5$

Wayne O. Adkisson, MD
Assistant Professor, Division of Cardiovascular Medicine, University of Minnesota Medical Center, Minneapolis, MN, United States
Chapter 67: Head-up Tilt Table Testing

Esperanza Agullo-Pascual, PhD
Postdoctoral Fellow, Leon H. Charney Division of Cardiology, New York University School of Medicine, New York, NY, United States
Chapter 22: The Intercalated Disc: A Molecular Network That Integrates Electrical Coupling, Intercellular Adhesion, and Cell Excitability

Francisco J. Alvarado, PharmD
Graduate Student, Department of Molecular and Integrative Physiology, University of Michigan, Ann Arbor, MI, United States
Chapter 53: Inheritable Phenotypes Associated With Altered Intracellular Calcium Regulation

Ahmad S. Amin, MD, PhD
Department of Clinical and Experimental Cardiology, Heart Centre, Academic Medical Center, University of Amsterdam, Amsterdam, The Netherlands
Chapter 52: Inheritable Potassium Channel Diseases

Charles Antzelevitch, PhD
Executive Director, Cardiovascular Research, Lankenau Institute for Medical Research; Director of Research, Lankenau Heart Institute, Wynnewood, PA, United States
Chapter 51: Genetic, Ionic, and Cellular Mechanisms Underlying the J Wave Syndromes

Justus M.B. Anumonwo, PhD
Department of Internal Medicine and of Molecular and Integrative Physiology, University of Michigan, Ann Arbor, MI, United States
Chapter 4: Structural and Molecular Bases of Cardiac Inward Rectifier Potassium Channel Function

Luciana Armaganijan, MD, MHS, PhD
Cardiologist Specialized in Electrophysiology, Dante Pazzanese Institute of Cardiology, São Paulo, Brazil
Chapter 115: Prevention of Stroke in Atrial Fibrillation: Warfarin and New Oral Anticoagulants

Arash Arya, MD
Department of Electrophysiology, Heart Centre, University of Leipzig, Leipzig, Germany
Chapter 85: Ventricular Tachycardia in Patients With Dilated Cardiomyopathy

Samuel Asirvatham, MD
Consultant, Department of Cardiovascular Diseases, Consultant, Department of Pediatrics and Adolescent Medicine, Mayo Clinic College of Medicine, Rochester, MN, United States
Chapter 61: Electroanatomical Mapping for Arrhythmias

Felipe Atienza, MD, PhD
Associate Professor of Medicine, School of Medicine, Universidad Complutense de Madrid; Senior Electrophysiologist, Department of Cardiology, Hospital General Universitario Gregorio Marañón, Madrid, Spain
Chapter 46: Body Surface Frequency–Phase Mapping of Atrial Fibrillation

Peter H. Backx, DVM, PhD
Professor of Biology, York University, Toronto, ON, Canada
Chapter 3: Voltage-Gated Potassium Channels

Lisa M. Ballou, PhD
Research Assistant Professor, Department of Physiology and Biophysics, Stony Brook University Medical Center, Stony Brook, NY, United States
Chapter 11: Inhibition of Phosphoinositide 3-Kinase and Acquired Long QT Syndrome

Elise Balse, PhD
UPMC Univ Paris 6, INSERM UMR1166, Sorbonne University, Faculty of Medicine Pitié-Salpêtrière, Paris, France
Chapter 20: Macromolecular Complexes and Cardiac Potassium Channels

Sujata Balulad, MD
Helmsley Electrophysiology Center, Mount Sinai Medical Center, New York, NY, United States
Chapter 138: Renal Sympathetic Denervation

Andrea Barbuti, PhD
Associate Professor, Department of Biosciences, Università degli Studi di Milano, Milan, Italy
Chapter 25: Stem Cell–Derived Sinoatrial-Like Cardiomyocytes as a Novel Pharmacological Tool

Gust H. Bardy, MD
Clinical Professor of Medicine, University of Washington School of Medicine, Seattle Institute for Cardiac Research, Seattle, WA, United States
Chapter 118: Subcutaneous Implantable Cardioverter Defibrillators

Guillaume Bassil, MD
New York-Presbyterian Hospital/Weill Cornell Medical College, New York, NY, United States
Chapter 39: Pulmonary Vein Ganglia and the Neural Regulation of the Heart Rate

David G. Benditt, MD
Professor, Division of Cardiovascular Medicine, University of Minnesota Medical Center, Minneapolis, MN, United States
Chapter 67: Head-up Tilt Table Testing

Omer Berenfeld, PhD
Associate Professor, Internal Medicine and Biomedical Engineering, University of Michigan, Ann Arbor, MI, United States
Chapter 35: Computational Approaches for Accurate Rotor Localization in the Human Atria

Donald M. Bers, PhD
Distinguished Professor and Chair, Department of Pharmacology, University of California Davis, Davis, CA, United States
Chapter 16: Excitation–Contraction Coupling

Ofer Binah, PhD
Professor, The Ruth and Bruce Rappaport Faculty of Medicine, Technion—Israel Institute of Technology, Haifa, Israel
Chapter 26: Gene Therapy and Biological Pacing

Frank Bogun, MD
Associate Professor of Internal Medicine, University of Michigan Medical School, Ann Arbor, MI, United States
Chapter 80: Premature Ventricular Complexes

Rossana Bongianino, MSc
Molecular Cardiology Labotaries, ICS Maugeri, IRCCS, Pavia, Italy
Chapter 56: Gene Therapy to Treat Cardiac Arrhythmias

Noel G. Boyle, MD, PhD
UCLA Cardiac Arrhythmia Center, David Geffen School of Medicine, UCLA Health System, Los Angeles, CA, United States
Chapter 123: Catheter Ablation: Technical Aspects

Patrick M. Boyle, PhD
Assistant Research Professor of Biomedical Engineering, Johns Hopkins University, Baltimore, MD, United States
Chapter 36: Modeling the Aging Heart

Günter Breithardt, MD
Professor Emeritus of Medicine and Cardiology, Department of Cardiovascular Medicine, University Hospital Münster, Münster, Germany
Chapter 101: Drug-Induced Ventricular Tachycardia

Marisa Brini, PhD
Department of Biology, University of Padova, Padova, Italy
Chapter 5: Mammalian Calcium Pumps in Health and Disease

Peter R. Brink, PhD
Distinguished Service Professor, Emeritus, Department of Physiology and Biophysics, Stony Brook University, Stony Brook, NY, United States
Chapter 15: Biophysical Properties of Gap Junctions
Chapter 26: Gene Therapy and Biological Pacing

Pedro Brugada, Prof., Dr.
Chairman, Cardiovascular Division, UZ Brussel—VUB, Brussels, Belgium
Chapter 92: Brugada Syndrome

Eric Buch, MD
Member, Cardiology, Adult Cardiac Catheterization Laboratory, Holter Laboratory, Pacemaker/ICD Clinic, UCLA Cardiac Arrhythmia Center, David Geffen School of Medicine, UCLA Health System, Los Angeles, CA, United States
Chapter 123: Catheter Ablation: Technical Aspects

Feliksas F. Bukauskas, PhD, Dr. Habil
Professor, Dominick P. Purpura Department of Neuroscience, Albert Einstein College of Medicine, Bronx, NY, United States; Institute of Cardiology, Lithuanian University of Health Sciences, 50009 Kaunas, Lithuania
Chapter 8: Molecular Organization, Gating, and Function of Connexin-Based Gap Junction Channels and Hemichannels

Hugh Calkins, MD
Director of the Arrhythmia Service, the Clinical Electrophysiology Laboratory, and the Arrhythmogenic Right Ventricular Dysplasia Program at Johns Hopkins, Baltimore, MD, United States
Chapter 87: Ventricular Tachycardias in Arrhythmogenic Right Ventricular Dysplasia/Cardiomyopathy

David J. Callans, MD
Associate Director of Electrophysiology, Penn Medicine, University of Pennsylvania, Philadelphia, PA, United States
Chapter 64: Intracardiac Echocardiography for Electrophysiology

Sean M. Caples, DO, MSc
Consultant, Pulmonary and Critical Care Medicine, Mayo Clinic, Rochester, MN, United States
Chapter 110: Sleep-Disordered Breathing and Arrhythmias

Ernesto Carafoli, MD
Venetian Institute for Molecular Medicine, Padova, Italy
Chapter 5: Mammalian Calcium Pumps in Health and Disease

William A. Catterall, PhD
Professor and Chair, Department of Pharmacology, University of Washington, Seattle, WA, United States
Chapter 1: Voltage-Gated Sodium Channels and Electrical Excitability of the Heart

Marina Cerrone, MD
Research Assistant Professor, Leon H. Charney Division of
    Cardiology, New York University School of Medicine, New
    York University School of Medicine, New York, NY, United
    States
*Chapter 22: The Intercalated Disc: A Molecular Network
    That Integrates Electrical Coupling, Intercellular
    Adhesion, and Cell Excitability*

Arnaud Chaumeil, MD
Department of Cardiology, Centre Hospitalier Universitaire de
    Bordeaux, Bordeaux, France
Chapter 128: Epicardial Approach in Electrophysiology

Caressa Chen, BS
Stanford Cardiovascular Institute, School of Medicine, Stanford
    University, Stanford, CA, United States
Chapter 30: Cardiac Remodeling and Regeneration

Lan S. Chen, MD
Professor of Clinical Neurology, Department of Neurology, Riley
    Hospital for Children, Indiana University, Indianapolis, IN
Chapter 40: Neural Activity and Atrial Tachyarrhythmias

Peng-Sheng Chen, MD
Medtronic Zipes Chair of Cardiology; Director, Krannert Insti-
    tute of Cardiology; Chief, Division of Cardiology, Depart-
    ment of Medicine, Indiana University School of Medicine,
    Indianapolis, IN, United States
Chapter 40: Neural Activity and Atrial Tachyarrhythmias

Jianding Cheng, MD, PhD
Department of Forensic Pathology, Zhongshan School of Medi-
    cine, Sun Yat-sen University, Guangzhou, Guangdong, China;
    Division of Cardiovascular Medicine, Department of Medi-
    cine, University of Wisconsin, Madison, WI, United States
Chapter 98: Sudden Infant Death Syndrome

Nipavan Chiamvimonvat, MD
Roger Tatarian Endowed Professor of Cardiovascular Medicine,
    Department of Internal Medicine, University of California
    Davis, Davis; Staff Cardiologist, Department of Veterans
    Affairs, Northern California Health Care System, Mather,
    CA, United States
*Chapter 24: Feedback Mechanisms for Cardiac-Specific
    MicroRNAs and cAMP Signaling in Electrical Remodeling*

David J. Christini, PhD
Professor, Department of Medicine, Division of Cardiology,
    Weill Cornell Medicine, New York, NY, United States
*Chapter 32: Global Optimization Approaches to Generate
    Dynamically Robust Electrophysiological Models*

Aman Chugh, MD
Associate Professor of Internal Medicine, University of Michi-
    gan Medical School, Ann Arbor, MI, United States
*Chapter 77: Preexcitation, Atrioventricular Reentry, and
    Variants*

Andreu M. Climent, PhD
Hospital General Universitario Gregorio Marañon, Department
    of Cardiology, Instituto de Investigación Sanitaria Gregorio
    Marañon, Madrid, Spain
*Chapter 46: Body Surface Frequency–Phase Mapping of
    Atrial Fibrillation*

Ira S. Cohen, MD, PhD
Leading Professor, Department of Physiology and Biophysics,
    Stony Brook University Medical Center, Stony Brook, NY,
    United States
*Chapter 11: Inhibition of Phosphoinositide 3-Kinase and
    Acquired Long QT Syndrome*
Chapter 26: Gene Therapy and Biological Pacing

Stuart J. Connolly, MD
Professor, Department of Medicine, McMaster University,
    Hamilton, Ontario, Canada
*Chapter 115: Prevention of Stroke in Atrial Fibrillation:
    Warfarin and New Oral Anticoagulants*

Lebron Cooper, MD
Professor and Chair, Department of Anesthesiology, University
    of Tennessee Health Science Center College of Medicine,
    Memphis, TN, United States
*Chapter 132: Anesthesiology Considerations for the
    Electrophysiology Laboratory*

Eric M. Crespo, MD
Director of the Interventional Electrophysiology Laboratory,
    Hartford Hospital, Hartford, CT
Chapter 65: Exercise-Induced Arrhythmias

Lia Crotti, MD, PhD
Assistant Professor, Molecular Medicine, University of Pavia, Pavia;
    Vice-Director, Center for Cardiac Arrhythmias of Genetic
    Origin, IRCCS Istituto Auxologico Italiano, Milano, Italy
Chapter 93: Long and Short QT Syndromes

Thomas A. Csepe, BSc
Department of Physiology & Cell Biology and Davis Heart &
    Lung Research Institute, The Ohio State University Wexner
    Medical Center, Columbus, OH, United States
*Chapter 28: Mechanisms of Normal and Dysfunctional
    Sinoatrial Nodal Excitability and Propagation*

Frank Cuoco, MD, MBA, MS
Associate Professor of Medicine, Division of Cardiology,
    Director, Cardiac Electrophysiology, Medical University
    of South Carolina, Charleston, SC, United States
*Chapter 121: Newer Applications of Cardiac Pacemakers
    and Extracardiac Stimulation*

Anne B. Curtis, MD
SUNY Distinguished Professor, Charles and Mary Bauer
    Professor and Chair, Department of Medicine, University at
    Buffalo, Buffalo, NY, United States
Chapter 107: Sex Differences in Arrhythmias

Ralph J. Damiano, Jr., MD
Evarts A. Graham Professor and Chief, Division of Cardiotho-
    racic Surgery, Washington University School of Medicine,
    St. Louis, MO, United States
*Chapter 133: Surgery for Atrial Fibrillation and Other
    Supraventricular Tachycardias*

Dawood Darbar, MD
Chief and Professor of Medicine and Pharmacology, University
    of Illinois at Chicago, Chicago, IL, United States
Chapter 112: Standard Antiarrhythmic Drugs

Mithilesh K. Das, MD
Professor of Clinical Medicine, Cardiology/Medicine, Krannert
    Institute of Cardiology, Indianapolis, IN, United States
Chapter 59: Assessment of the Patient With a Cardiac
    Arrhythmia
Chapter 60: Differential Diagnosis of Narrow and Wide
    Complex Tachycardias

Andre d'Avila, MD, PhD
Director, Cardiac Arrhythmia Service, Hospital Cardiologico,
    Florianopolis, Santa Catarina, Brazil
Chapter 138: Renal Sympathetic Denervation

Mario Delmar, MD, PhD
Patricia and Robert Martinsen Professor of Cardiology,
    Professor of Medicine and Professor of Cell Biology, Leon
    H. Charney Division of Cardiology, New York University
    School of Medicine, New York, NY, United States
Chapter 22: The Intercalated Disc: A Molecular Network
    That Integrates Electrical Coupling, Intercellular
    Adhesion, and Cell Excitability

Eva Delpón, PhD
Professor, Department of Pharmacology, School of Medicine,
    Complutense University of Madrid, CIBERCV, Madrid,
    Spain
Chapter 21: Reciprocity of Cardiac Sodium and
    Potassium Channels in the Control of Excitability and
    Arrhythmias
Chapter 54: Pharmacological Bases of Antiarrhythmic
    Therapy

Marco Denegri, PhD
Molecular Cardiology Labotatories, ICS Maugeri, IRCCS,
    Pavia, Italy
Chapter 56: Gene Therapy to Treat Cardiac Arrhythmias

Arnaud Denis, MD
Centre Hospitalier Universitaire de Bordeaux, Hôpital Cardi-
    ologique du Haut Lévêque, Bordeaux, France
Chapter 125: Ablation for Atrial Fibrillation

Nicolas Derval, MD
Centre Hospitalier Universitaire de Bordeaux, Hôpital Cardi-
    ologique du Haut Lévêque, Bordeaux, France
Chapter 125: Ablation for Atrial Fibrillation

Isabelle Deschênes, PhD
Professor of Medicine, Physiology and Biophysics, and Bio-
    medical Engineering, Case Western Reserve University;
    Director, Heart and Vascular Research Center, MetroHealth
    Medical Center, Cleveland, OH, United States
Chapter 9: Structure–Function Relations of
    Heterotrimetric Complexes of Sodium Channel α- and
    β-Subunits

Abhishek Deshmukh, MD
Senior Associate Consultant, Department of Cardiovascular
    Diseases, Mayo Clinic College of Medicine, Rochester, MN,
    United States
Chapter 61: Electroanatomical Mapping for Arrhythmias

Luigi Di Biase, MD, PhD, FACC, FHRS
Section Head, Electrophysiology, Director of Arrhythmia
    Services, Associate Professor of Medicine, Albert Einstein
    College of Medicine at Montefiore Hospital, New York,
    NY; Senior Researcher, Electrophysiology, Texas Cardiac
    Arrhythmia Institute at St. David's Medical Center;
    Associate Professor, Biomedical Engineering, University of
    Texas, Austin, TX, United States; Assistant Professor,
    Cardiology, University of Foggia, Foggia, Italy
Chapter 124: Catheter Ablation: Clinical Aspects

Timm M. Dickfeld, MD, PhD
Professor of Medicine, Maryland Arrhythmia and Cardiology
    Imaging Group (MACIG), Division of Cardiology, Univer-
    sity of Maryland School of Medicine, Baltimore, MD, United
    States
Chapter 62: Computed Tomography for Electrophysiology

Hans Dierckx, PhD
Department of Physics and Astronomy, Ghent University,
    Belgium
Chapter 34: Theory of Rotors and Arrhythmias

Borislav Dinov, MD
Department of Electrophysiology, Heart Centre, University of
    Leipzig, Leipzig, Germany
Chapter 85: Ventricular Tachycardia in Patients With
    Dilated Cardiomyopathy

Sanjay Dixit, MD
Associate Professor, Medicine, Cardiovascular Division, Hos-
    pital of The University of Pennsylvania; Director, Cardiac
    Electrophysiology, Cardiology-Medicine, Philadelphia
    Veterans Affairs Medical Center, Philadelphia, PA, United
    States
Chapter 134: Surgery for Ventricular Arrhythmias

Dobromir Dobrev, MD
Director, Institute of Pharmacology, Faculty of Medicine,
    University Duisburg-Essen, Essen, Germany
Chapter 42: The Molecular Pathophysiology of Atrial
    Fibrillation

Remi Dubois, PhD
Associate Professor, Ecole Superieure de Physique et de Chimie
    Industrielles – ParisTech; Team Manager, Signal Processing,
    Electrophysiology and Heart Modeling Institute, Bordeaux,
    France
Chapter 47: Panoramic Mapping of Atrial Fibrillation
    From the Body Surface

Lars Eckardt, MD, PhD
Professor, Department of Cardiology and Angiology, Division
    of Electrophysiology, Münster, Germany
Chapter 101: Drug-Induced Ventricular Tachycardia

Andrew G. Edwards, PhD
Senior Research Scientist, Simula Research Laboratory; Senior
    Research Scientist, Institute for Experimental Medical
    Research, Oslo University Hospital Ullevål, Oslo, Norway
Chapter 33: Calcium Signaling in Cardiomyocyte Models
    With Realistic Geometries

Kenneth A. Ellenbogen, MD
Kontos Professor of Medicine, Division of Cardiology, Virginia
Commonwealth University School of Medicine, Richmond,
VA, United States
Chapter 73: Atrial Tachycardia

Patrick T. Ellinor, MD, PhD
Associate Professor of Medicine, Harvard Medical School;
Cardiac Arrhythmia Service, Cardiovascular Research
Center, Massachusetts General Hospital, Boston, MA,
United States
Chapter 49: Genetics of Atrial Fibrillation

N.A. Mark Estes III, MD
Professor of Medicine, Tufts University School of Medicine;
Director, Cardiac Arrhythmia Center, The CardioVascular
Center, Tufts Medical Center, Boston, MA, United States
*Chapter 108: Sudden Cardiac Deaths in Athletes,
Including Commotio Cordis*

Larissa Fabritz, MD
Reader in Cardiovascular Sciences, Institute of Cardiovascular
Sciences, University of Birmingham; Consultant, Department
of Cardiology, University Hospitals Birmingham, Birmingham,
United Kingdom
Chapter 113: Innovations in Antiarrhythmic Drug Therapy

Vadim V. Fedorov, PhD
Associate Professor, Department of Physiology & Cell Biology
and Davis Heart & Lung Research Institute, The Ohio State
University Wexner Medical Center, Columbus, OH, United
States
*Chapter 28: Mechanisms of Normal and Dysfunctional
Sinoatrial Nodal Excitability and Propagation*

Antonio B. Fernandez, MD
Assistant Professor of Medicine, Department of Medicine,
University of Connecticut, Farmington, CT, United States;
Director, Cardiac Intensive Care Unit, Division of Cardiol-
ogy, Hartford Hospital, Hartford, CT, United States
Chapter 65: Exercise-Induced Arrhythmias

Elvis Teijeira Fernández, MD
Fellow in Electrophysiology, Bordeaux Hospital University
Center, Bordeaux, France
*Chapter 111: Ventricular Assist Devices and Cardiac
Transplantation Recipients*

David Filgueiras-Rama, MD, PhD
Assistant Health Scientist. Group Leader, Myocardial
Pathophysiology Area, Fundación Centro Nacional de
Investigaciones Cardiovasculares, Carlos III (CNIC); Cardiac
Electrophysiologist, Cardiology, Hospital Clínico San
Carlos; Centro de Investigación Biomédica en Red de Enfer-
medades Cardiovasculares (CIBERCV), Madrid, Spain
*Chapter 41: Sympathetic Innervation and Cardiac
Arrhythmias*

Michael C. Fishbein, MD
Piansky Professor of Pathology and Medicine, Department of
Pathology and Laboratory Medicine, David Geffen School of
Medicine at UCLA, Los Angeles, CA, United States
Chapter 40: Neural Activity and Atrial Tachyarrhythmias

Glenn I. Fishman, MD
William Goldring Professor of Medicine, Director, Leon H.
Charney Division of Cardiology, New York University
School of Medicine, New York, NY, United States
*Chapter 29: Cell Biology of the Specialized Cardiac
Conduction System*

David S. Frankel, MD
Assistant Professor Medicine, Fellowship Program Director, Cardiovascular Division, Electrophysiology Section, Hospital of
the University of Pennsylvania, Philadelphia, PA, United States
Chapter 84: Ischemic Heart Disease

Paul Friedman, MD
Director, Cardiac Implantable Device Lab, Division of Cardiovas-
cular Medicine, Mayo Clinic, Rochester, MN, United States
*Chapter 117: Implantable Cardioverter Defibrillator:
Clinical Aspects*

Antonio Frontera, MD
Centre Hospitalier Universitaire de Bordeaux, Hôpital
Cardiologique du Haut Lévêque, Bordeaux, France
Chapter 125: Ablation for Atrial Fibrillation

Apoor S. Gami, MD
Cardiac Electrophysiologist, Advocate Medical Group,
Elmhurst, IL, United States
*Chapter 110: Sleep-Disordered Breathing and
Arrhythmias*

Paul Garabelli, MD
Assistant Professor of Medicine, Heart Rhythm Institute,
University of Oklahoma Health Sciences Center, Oklahoma
City, OK, United States
*Chapter 44: Role of the Autonomic Nervous System in
Atrial Fibrillation*

Alfred L. George, Jr., MD
Professor and Chairman, Department of Pharmacology,
Northwestern University Feinberg School of Medicine,
Chicago, IL, United States
*Chapter 50: Mechanisms in Heritable Sodium Channel
Diseases*

Edward P. Gerstenfeld, MD
Professor of Medicine, Division of Cardiology, Department
of Medicine, University of California San Francisco, San
Francisco, CA, United States
*Chapter 81: Outflow Tract Ventricular Tachyarrhythmias:
Mechanisms, Clinical Features, and Management*

Sigfus Gizurarson, MD, PhD
Consultant, Department of Cardiology, Landspitali University
Hospital, Reykjavik, Iceland; Consultant, Department of
Cardiology, Sahlgrenska University Hospital, Gothenburg,
Sweden
*Chapter 48: Mechanisms of Human Ventricular
Tachycardia and Human Ventricular Fibrillation*

Michael R. Gold, MD, PhD
Michael E. Assey Professor of Medicine, Division of Cardiology;
Medical University of South Carolina, Charleston, SC,
United States
*Chapter 121: Newer Applications of Cardiac Pacemakers
and Extracardiac Stimulation*

Jeffrey J. Goldberger, MD
Chief, Cardiovascular Division; Professor of Medicine, Department of Medicine, University of Miami Miller School of Medicine, Miami, FL, United States
Chapter 99: Sudden Cardiac Death in Adults
Chapter 114: Impact of Nontraditional Antiarrhythmic Drugs on Sudden Cardiac Death

Andrew Grace, MB, PhD
Cambridge University Health Partners, Cambridge, United Kingdom
Chapter 118: Subcutaneous Implantable Cardioverter Defibrillators

Full Prof. Guido Grassi
Medical Clinic, San Gerardo Hospital, Milano-Bicocca University, Monza, Italy
Chapter 136: Baroreceptor Stimulation

Ruth Ann Greenfield, MD
Clinical Cardiac Electrophysiologist, Division of Cardiology, Durham VA Medical Center, Durham, NC, United States
Chapter 122: Remote Monitoring of Cardiac Implantable Electronic Devices

Wendy L. Gross, MD, MHCM
Assistant Professor of Anesthesiology, Harvard Medical School; Vice Chair, Planning and Analytics Director of Non OR Services, Department of Anesthesiology, Perioperative and Pain Medicine, Brigham and Women's Hospital, Boston, MA, United States
Chapter 132: Anesthesiology Considerations for the Electrophysiology Laboratory

Blair P. Grubb, MD
Professor of Medicine and Pediatrics, Division of Cardiovascular Medicine, The University of Toledo, Toledo, OH, United States
Chapter 104: Postural Orthostatic Tachycardia Syndrome

María S. Guillem, PhD
ITACA UPV, ITACA Institute, Universitat Politècnica de València, Valencia, Spain
Chapter 46: Body Surface Frequency–Phase Mapping of Atrial Fibrillation

Sándor Györke, PhD
Professor, Physiology and Cell Biology, The Ohio State University, Columbus, OH, United States
Chapter 6: Structural and Molecular Bases of Sarcoplasmic Reticulum Ion Channel Function

Michel Haïssaguerre, MD
Professor of Medicine, CHU Bordeaux, University of Bordeaux, LIRYC, Bordeaux, France
Chapter 47: Panoramic Mapping of Atrial Fibrillation From the Body Surface
Chapter 125: Ablation for Atrial Fibrillation
Chapter 128: Epicardial Approach in Electrophysiology
Chapter 129: Ventricular Fibrillation

Johan Hake, PhD
Department of Bioengineering, University of California San Diego, La Jolla, CA, United States; Simula Research Laboratory, Oslo, Norway
Chapter 33: Calcium Signaling in Cardiomyocyte Models With Realistic Geometries

Henry R. Halperin, MD, MA
David J. Carver Professor of Medicine, Professor of Radiology and Biomedical Engineering, Johns Hopkins University, Baltimore, MD, United States
Chapter 63: Computed Tomography and Magnetic Resonance Imaging for Electrophysiology

Brian J. Hansen, BSc
Department of Physiology & Cell Biology and Davis Heart & Lung Research Institute, The Ohio State University Wexner Medical Center, Columbus, OH, United States
Chapter 28: Mechanisms of Normal and Dysfunctional Sinoatrial Nodal Excitability and Propagation

Stéphane Hatem, MD, PhD
UPMC Univ Paris 6, INSERM UMR1166, Sorbonne University; Faculty of Medicine Pitié-Salpêtrière, Department of Cardiology, Assistance Publique - Hopitaux de Paris, Pitié-Salpêtrière Hospital, Paris, France
Chapter 20: Macromolecular Complexes and Cardiac Potassium Channels

David L. Hayes, MD
Mayo Clinic; Rochester, MN, United States
Chapter 119: Implantable Pacemakers

Jordi Heijman, PhD
Assistant Professor, Department of Cardiology, CARIM School for Cardiovascular Diseases, Maastricht University, Maastricht, The Netherlands
Chapter 42: The Molecular Pathophysiology of Atrial Fibrillation

Todd J. Herron, PhD
Associate Research Scientist, Department of Internal Medicine, Cardiovascular Medicine and Molecular & Integrative Physiology, Ann Arbor, MI, United States
Chapter 57: Highly Mature Human iPSC–Derived Cardiomyocytes as Models for Cardiac Electrophysiology and Drug Testing

Gerhard Hindricks, MD
Professor and Head, Department of Electrophysiology, Heart Centre, University of Leipzig, Leipzig, Germany
Chapter 85: Ventricular Tachycardia in Patients With Dilated Cardiomyopathy

Mélèze Hocini, MD
Associate Professor, CHU Bordeaux, University of Bordeaux, LIRYC, Bordeaux France
Chapter 47: Panoramic Mapping of Atrial Fibrillation From the Body Surface
Chapter 125: Ablation for Atrial Fibrillation
Chapter 129: Ventricular Fibrillation

Stefan H. Hohnloser, MD
Professor of Cardiology, Department of Cardiology, J.W. Goethe University, Frankfurt, Germany
Chapter 69: T-Wave Alternans

David R. Holmes, Jr., MD
Professor of Medicine, Division of Cardiovascular Diseases, Mayo Clinic College of Medicine, Rochester, MN, United States
Chapter 139: Left Atrial Appendage Closure

Masahiko Hoshijima, MD, PhD
Associate Adjunct Professor, Center for Research in Biological
    Systems and Department of Medicine, University of
    California San Diego, La Jolla, CA, United States
*Chapter 33: Calcium Signaling in Cardiomyocyte Models
    With Realistic Geometries*

Thomas J. Hund, PhD
Associate Professor, Department of Biomedical Engineering,
    The Ohio State University College of Engineering, Colum-
    bus, OH, United States
*Chapter 23: Function and Dysfunction of Ion Channel
    Membrane Trafficking and Posttranslational
    Modification*

Mathew D. Hutchinson, MD
Professor of Medicine, Sarver Heart Center, University of Arizona;
    Banner University Medical Center, Tucson, AZ, United States
*Chapter 64: Intracardiac Echocardiography for
    Electrophysiology*

Leonard Ilkhanoff, MD
Inova Medical Group, Mannassus, VA, United States
*Chapter 114: Impact of Nontraditional Antiarrhythmic
    Drugs on Sudden Cardiac Death*

Jodie Ingles, GradDipGenCouns, MPH, PhD
Conjoint Senior Lecturer, Centenary Institute of Cancer Medi-
    cine and Cell Biology, Central Clinical School, Sydney Medi-
    cal School, University of Sydney, Sydney, NSW, Australia
Chapter 71: Genetic Testing

James E. Ip, MD
Assistant Professor, Department of Medicine, Weill Cornell
    Medicine, New York, NY, United States
Chapter 79: Junctional Tachycardia

Warren M. Jackman, MD
George Lynn Cross Research Professor, Heart Rhythm
    Institute, University of Oklahoma Health Sciences Center,
    Oklahoma City, OK, United States
*Chapter 78: Electrophysiological Characteristics of
    Atrioventricular Nodal Reentrant Tachycardia:
    Implications for the Reentrant Circuits*

Nicholas Jackson, BMedSc, MB BS, FRACP
Staff Specialist, Department of Cardiology, John Hunter
    Hospital; Conjoint Lecturer, School of Medicine and Public
    Health, University of Newcastle, Newcastle, New South
    Wales, Australia
*Chapter 48: Mechanisms of Human Ventricular
    Tachycardia and Human Ventricular Fibrillation*

Pierre Jaïs, MD
Professor of Medicine, CHU Bordeaux, University of Bordeaux,
    LIRYC, Bordeaux, France
*Chapter 47: Panoramic Mapping of Atrial Fibrillation
    From the Body Surface*
*Chapter 111: Ventricular Assist Devices and Cardiac
    Transplantation Recipients*
Chapter 125: Ablation for Atrial Fibrillation
Chapter 128: Epicardial Approach in Electrophysiology

José Jalife, MD
Cyrus and Jane Farrehi Professor of Cardiovascular Research,
    Department of Internal Medicine; Professor, Department of
    Molecular and Integrative Physiology; Co-Director, Center for
    Arrhythmia Research, University of Michigan, Ann Arbor, MI,
    United States; Senior Investigator, Fundación Centro Nacional
    de Investigaciones Cardiovasculares (CNIC), Madrid, Spain
*Chapter 21: Reciprocity of Cardiac Sodium and
    Potassium Channels in the Control of Excitability and
    Arrhythmias*
*Chapter 43: Myofibroblasts, Cytokines, and Persistent
    Atrial Fibrillation*

Bong Sook Jhun, PhD
Instructor, Cardiovascular Research Center, Rhode Island Hos-
    pital; Department of Medicine, The Warren Alpert Medical
    School of Brown University, Providence RI, United States
Chapter 7: Organellar Ion Channels and Transporters

Roy M. John, MD, PhD
Director, Cardiac Arrhythmia Research; Associate Director,
    Electrophysiology Laboratory, Department of Medicine,
    Brigham and Women's Hospital, Boston, MA, United States
Chapter 89: Ventricular Arrhythmias in Heart Failure
Chapter 106: Atrioventricular Block

Monique Jongbloed, MD, PhD
Clinical Anatomist and Cardiologist, Leiden University Medical
    Center, Leiden, The Netherlands
*Chapter 102: Ventricular Arrhythmias in Congenital Heart
    Disease*

Luc Jordaens, MD, Dsc, PhD
Prof. Dr. Cardiology, University Ghent, Ghent, Belgium;
    Prof. Dr. Clinical Electrophysiology, Erasmus MC,
    Rotterdam, The Netherlands
*Chapter 90: Arrhythmias and Conduction Disturbances in
    Noncompaction Cardiomyopathy*

Jonathan M. Kalman, MBBS, PhD
Director of Cardiac Electrophysiology, Department of
    Cardiology, Royal Melbourne Hospital; Professor
    of Medicine, Department of Medicine, University of
    Melbourne, Melbourne, VIC, Australia
Chapter 72: Sinus Node Abnormalities
*Chapter 75: Typical and Atypical Atrial Flutter: Mapping
    and Ablation*

Timothy J. Kamp, MD, PhD
Professor of Medicine, Cell and Regenerative Biology,
    Tuchman Chair in Cardiology, Co-Director Stem Cell and
    Regenerative Medicine Center, University of Wisconsin–
    Madison, Madison, WI, United States
*Chapter 58: Cardiac Repair With Human Pluripotent Stem
    Cell–Derived Cardiovascular Cells and Arrhythmia Risk*

Mohamed H. Kanj, MD
Associate Director, Electrophysiology Laboratories, Robert and
    Suzanne Tomsich Department of Cardiovascular Medicine,
    Cleveland Clinic, Cleveland, OH, United States
*Chapter 116: Implantable Cardioverter Defibrillators:
    Technical Aspects*

Suraj Kapa, MD
Consultant, Department of Cardiovascular Diseases, Mayo
    Clinic College of Medicine, Rochester, MN, United States
Chapter 61: Electroanatomical Mapping for Arrhythmias

Beverly Karabin, RN, PhD, CNP
Certified Nurse Practitioner, Division of Cardiovascular Medicine, The University of Toledo, Toledo, OH, United States
Chapter 104: Postural Orthostatic Tachycardia Syndrome

Ioannis Karakikes, PhD
Stanford Cardiovascular Institute and Department of Cardiothoracic Surgery, School of Medicine, Stanford University, Stanford, CA, United States
Chapter 30: Cardiac Remodeling and Regeneration

Demosthenes G. Katritsis, MD, PhD
Director, Cardiology, Athens Euroclinic, Athens, Greece; Hon. Consultant Cardiologist, Cardiology, Guy's and St Thomas' Hospitals, London, United Kingdom
Chapter 105: Progressive Conduction System Disease

Kuljeet Kaur, PhD
Department of Internal Medicine, Center for Arrhythmia Research, University of Michigan, Ann Arbor, MI, United States
Chapter 43: Myofibroblasts, Cytokines, and Persistent Atrial Fibrillation

Paulus Kirchhof, MD, FESC, FHRS
Professor of Cardiovascular Medicine, Institute of Cardiovascular Sciences, University of Birmingham and SWBH and UHB NHS Trusts, Birmingham, United Kingdom; Chairman, AFNET, Münster, Germany
Chapter 113: Innovations in Antiarrhythmic Drug Therapy

André G. Kléber, MD
Visiting Professor, Department of Pathology, Beth Israel Deaconess Medical Center, Harvard Medical School, Boston, MA, United States
Chapter 27: Cell-to-Cell Communication and Impulse Propagation

George J. Klein, MD, FRCG(C)
Professor of Medicine, Department of Medicine, Western University, London, ON, Canada
Chapter 66: Cardiac Monitoring: Short- and Long-Term Recording

Peter Kohl, MD, PhD, FHRS, FAHA
Scientific Director, University Heart Centre Freiburg/Bad Krozingen; Director, Institute for Experimental Cardiovascular Medicine, Medical School of the University of Freiburg, Freiburg, Germany, Chair in Cardiac Biophysics and Systems Biology, National Heart and Lung Institute, Imperial College London, London, England, United Kingdom
Chapter 14: Cardiac Stretch-Activated Channels and Mechano-Electric Coupling

Jayanthi N. Koneru, MBBS
Assistant Professor, Division of Cardiology, Department of Internal Medicine, Virginia Commonwealth University, Richmond, VA, United States
Chapter 73: Atrial Tachycardia

Jacob S. Koruth, MD
Assistant Professor, Helmsley Electrophysiology Center, Mount Sinai Medical Center, New York, NY, United States
Chapter 138: Renal Sympathetic Denervation

Andrew D. Krahn, MD
Professor and Head, Division of Cardiology, University of British Columbia, Vancouver, BC, Canada
Chapter 66: Cardiac Monitoring: Short- and Long-Term Recording
Chapter 97: Idiopathic Ventricular Fibrillation

Trine Krogh-Madsen, PhD
Assistant Research Professor, Department of Medicine, Division of Cardiology, Weill Cornell Medicine, New York, NY, United States
Chapter 32: Global Optimization Approaches to Generate Dynamically Robust Electrophysiological Models

Karl Heinz Kuck, MD
Professor and Chief, Department of Cardiology, Asklepios Klinik St. Georg, Hamburg, Germany
Chapter 126: Ablation of Supraventricular Tachyarrhythmias

Saurabh Kumar, MBBS, PhD
Cardiovascular Division, Brigham and Women's Hospital, Boston, MA, United States
Chapter 75: Typical and Atypical Atrial Flutter: Mapping and Ablation
Chapter 76: Atrial Fibrillation: Mechanisms, Clinical Features, and Management

Alexander Kushnir, MD, PhD
Fellow, Division of Cardiology, New York–Presbyterian Hospital/Columbia University College of Physicians and Surgeons, New York, NY, United States
Chapter 2: Voltage-Gated Calcium Channels

Neal K. Lakdawala, MD, MSc
Instructor of Medicine, Harvard Medical School; Associate Physician, Division of Cardiovascular Medicine, Brigham and Women's Hospital, Boston, MA, United States
Chapter 89: Ventricular Arrhythmias in Heart Failure

Zachary W.M. Laksman, MD
Clinical Assistant Professor; The University of British Columbia, Vancouver, British Columbia, Canada
Chapter 97: Idiopathic Ventricular Fibrillation

Rakesh Latchamsetty, MD
Assistant Professor of Internal Medicine, University of Michigan Medical School, Ann Arbor, MI, United States
Chapter 80: Premature Ventricular Complexes

Dennis H. Lau, MBBS, PhD
Robert J. Craig Research Fellow and Staff Specialist, Centre for Heart Rhythm Disorders, South Australian Health and Medical Research Institute, University of Adelaide, Royal Adelaide Hospital, Adelaide, SA, Australia
Chapter 72: Sinus Node Abnormalities

Bruce B. Lerman, MD
H. Altschul Master Professor of Medicine, Chief, Division of Cardiology, Director, Cardiac Electrophysiology Laboratory, Department of Medicine, Division of Cardiology, Cornell University Medical Center, New York–Presbyterian Hospital, New York, NY, United States
Chapter 79: Junctional Tachycardia

Richard Z. Lin, MD
Professor, Department of Physiology and Biophysics, Stony Brook University Medical Center, Stony Brook, NY, United States
Chapter 11: Inhibition of Phosphoinositide 3-Kinase and Acquired Long QT Syndrome

Shien-Fong Lin, PhD, MBA
Professor and Director, Institute of Biomedical Engineering, National Chiao-Tung University, Hsinchu, Taiwan; Professor, Department of Medicine, Indiana University School of Medicine, Indianapolis, IN, United States
Chapter 40: Neural Activity and Atrial Tachyarrhythmias

Mark S. Link, MD
Professor of Medicine, Internal Medicine, University of Texas Southwestern Medical Center, Dallas, TX, United States
Chapter 108: Sudden Cardiac Deaths in Athletes, Including Commotio Cordis

Bin Liu, PhD
Research Scientist, The Ohio State University, Columbus, OH, United States
Chapter 6: Structural and Molecular Bases of Sarcoplasmic Reticulum Ion Channel Function

Christopher F. Liu, MD
Assistant Professor of Medicine, Division of Cardiology, Weill Cornell Medicine, Cornell University, New York, NY, United States
Chapter 79: Junctional Tachycardia

Deborah J. Lockwood, MB, BCh
Associate Professor of Medicine, Medicine/Cardiovascular, Heart Rhythm Institute, University of Oklahoma Health Sciences Center, Oklahoma City, OK, United States
Chapter 78: Electrophysiological Characteristics of Atrioventricular Nodal Reentrant Tachycardia: Implications for the Reentrant Circuits

Anatoli N. Lopatin, PhD
Associate Professor, Department of Physiology, University of Michigan, Ann Arbor, MI, United States
Chapter 4: Structural and Molecular Bases of Cardiac Inward Rectifier Potassium Channel Function

Steven A. Lubitz, MD, MPH
Assistant Professor of Medicine, Harvard Medical School; Cardiac Arrhythmia Service, Cardiovascular Research Center, Massachusetts General Hospital, Boston, MA, United States
Chapter 49: Genetics of Atrial Fibrillation

Rajiv Mahajan, MD, PhD
Leo J. Mahar Lecturer and Clinical Associate, Centre for Heart Rhythm Disorders, South Australian Health and Medical Research Institute, University of Adelaide, Royal Adelaide Hospital, Adelaide, SA, Australia
Chapter 72: Sinus Node Abnormalities

Jonathan C. Makielski, MD
Professor, Department of Medicine, University of Wisconsin, Madison, WI, United States
Chapter 98: Sudden Infant Death Syndrome

Marek Malik, PhD, MD, DSc
Professor and Senior Clinical Investigator, National Heart and Lung Institute, Imperial College London, London, England, United Kingdom
Chapter 68: Autonomic Regulation and Cardiac Risk

Francis E. Marchlinski, MD, FACC, FHRS
Professor of Medicine, Director of Cardiac Electrophysiology Program, Cardiovascular Division, Electrophysiology Section, Hospital of the University of Pennsylvania, Philadelphia, PA, United States
Chapter 84: Ischemic Heart Disease

Steven M. Markowitz, MD
Professor of Medicine, Weill Cornell Medicine, New York, NY, United States
Chapter 79: Junctional Tachycardia

Barry J. Maron, MD
Hypertrophic Cardiomyopathy Institute, Tufts Medical Center, Professor of Medicine, Tufts University School of Medicine, Boston, MA, United States
Chapter 86: Ventricular Arrhythmias in Hypertrophic Cardiomyopathy: Sudden Death, Risk Stratification, and Prevention With Implantable Defibrillators

Martin S. Maron, MD
Director of the Hypertrophic Cardiomyopathy Center, Tufts Medical Center; Assistant Professor, Tufts University School of Medicine, Boston, MA, United States
Chapter 86: Ventricular Arrhythmias in Hypertrophic Cardiomyopathy: Sudden Death, Risk Stratification, and Prevention With Implantable Defibrillators

Steven O. Marx, MD
Professor of Medicine, Columbia University College of Physicians and Surgeons, New York, NY, United States
Chapter 2: Voltage-Gated Calcium Channels

Stéphane Massé, MASc
Biomedical Engineer, Cardiology, University Health Network, Toronto, Ontario, Canada
Chapter 48: Mechanisms of Human Ventricular Tachycardia and Human Ventricular Fibrillation

Andrew D. McCulloch, PhD
Professor and Jacobs School Distinguished Scholar, Director, Cardiac Biomedical Science and Engineering Center, Departments of Bioengineering and Medicine, University of California San Diego, La Jolla, California
Chapter 33: Calcium Signaling in Cardiomyocyte Models With Realistic Geometries

Pippa McKelvie-Sebileau, PhD
Centre Hospitalier Universitaire de Bordeaux, Hopital Cardiologique du Haut Leveque, L'institut de Rythmologie et Modélisation Cardiaque, Bordeaux, France
Chapter 129: Ventricular Fibrillation

Spencer J. Melby, MD
Associate Professor of Surgery, Division of Cardiothoracic Surgery, Washington University School of Medicine, St. Louis, MO, United States
Chapter 133: Surgery for Atrial Fibrillation and Other Supraventricular Tachycardias

Andreas Metzner, MD
Department of Cardiology, Asklepios Klinik St. Georg,
Hamburg, Germany
*Chapter 126: Ablation of Supraventricular
Tachyarrhythmias*

Anushka P. Michailova, PhD†
Associate Research Scientist, Department of Bioengineering,
University of California San Diego, La Jolla, CA, United
States
*Chapter 33: Calcium Signaling in Cardiomyocyte Models
With Realistic Geometries*

Gregory F. Michaud, MD
Associate Professor of Medicine, Division of Cardiology,
Harvard Medical School, Brigham and Women's Hospital,
Boston, MA, United States
*Chapter 76: Atrial Fibrillation: Mechanisms, Clinical
Features, and Management*

John M. Miller, MD
Professor of Medicine, Department of Medicine, Indiana
University School of Medicine; Director, Cardiac
Electrophysiology Services, Indiana University Health,
Indianapolis, IN, United States
*Chapter 60: Differential Diagnosis of Narrow and Wide
Complex Tachycardias*

Jyotsna Mishra, PhD
Postdoctoral Fellow, Center for Translational Medicine,
Department of Medicine, Jefferson Medical College,
Thomas Jefferson University, Philadelphia, PA, United
States
Chapter 7: Organellar Ion Channels and Transporters

Raul D. Mitrani, MD
Division of Cardiology, University of Miami Miller School of
Medicine, Miami, FL, United States
*Chapter 114: Impact of Nontraditional Antiarrhythmic
Drugs on Sudden Cardiac Death*

Peter J. Mohler, PhD
Professor and Director, Dorothy M. Davis Heart and Lung
Research Institute, Departments of Physiology & Cell
Biology and Internal Medicine, The Ohio State University
Medical Center, Columbus, OH, United States
*Chapter 23: Function and Dysfunction of Ion Channel
Membrane Trafficking and Posttranslational
Modification*

Fred Morady, MD
McKay Professor of Cardiovascular Disease and Professor of
Internal Medicine, University of Michigan Medical School,
Ann Arbor, MI, United States
*Chapter 77: Preexcitation, Atrioventricular Reentry, and
Variants*

Robert J. Myerburg, MD
Professor of Medicine and Physiology, American Heart
Association Chair in Cardiovascular Research, Department
of Medicine, University of Miami Miller School of Medicine,
Miami, FL, United States
Chapter 99: Sudden Cardiac Death in Adults

Hiroshi Nakagawa, MD, PhD
Professor of Medicine, Heart Rhythm Institute, University of
Oklahoma Health Sciences Center, Oklahoma City, OK,
United States
*Chapter 78: Electrophysiological Characteristics of
Atrioventricular Nodal Reentrant Tachycardia:
Implications for the Reentrant Circuits*

Chrishan Joseph Nalliah, MBBS, BSc
Department of Cardiology and Department of Medicine, Royal
Melbourne Hospital, University of Melbourne, Melbourne,
VIC, Australia
*Chapter 75: Typical and Atypical Atrial Flutter: Mapping
and Ablation*

Kumaraswamy Nanthakumar, MD
Electrophysiologist, Cardiology, University Health Network;
Professor of Medicine, Department of Medicine, University
of Toronto, Toronto, Ontario, Canada
*Chapter 48: Mechanisms of Human Ventricular
Tachycardia and Human Ventricular Fibrillation*

Carlo Napolitano, MD, PhD, FHRS
Senior Scientist, Molecular Cardiology Laboratories, ICS
Maugeri IRCCS, Pavia, Italy
Chapter 56: Gene Therapy to Treat Cardiac Arrhythmias
Chapter 95: Timothy Syndrome

Sanjiv M. Narayan, MD, PhD
Professor of Medicine, Division of Cardiovascular Medicine,
Stanford University School of Medicine, Stanford, CA,
United States
Chapter 45: Rotors in Human Atrial Fibrillation

Andrea Natale, MD, FACC, FHRS, FESC
Executive Medical Director, Texas Cardiac Arrhythmia Institute
at St. David's Medical Center, Austin, TX, United States
Chapter 124: Catheter Ablation: Clinical Aspects

Stanley Nattel, MD
Professor of Medicine and Paul-David Chair in Cardiovascular
Electrophysiology, Medicine, Montreal Heart Institute and
University of Montreal, Montreal, Quebec, Canada
*Chapter 42: The Molecular Pathophysiology of Atrial
Fibrillation*

Saman Nazarian, MD, PhD
Associate Professor of Medicine, Section for Cardiac Electro-
physiology, The University of Pennsylvania Perelman School
of Medicine, Philadelphia, PA, United States
*Chapter 63: Computed Tomography and Magnetic
Resonance Imaging for Electrophysiology*
Chapter 100: Arrhythmia in Neurological Disease

Thao P. Nguyen, MD, PhD
UCLA Cardiovascular Research Laboratory, Division of
Cardiology, Department of Medicine, David Geffen School
of Medicine, University of California Los Angeles, Los
Angeles, United States
*Chapter 50: Mechanisms in Heritable Sodium Channel
Diseases*

---

† Deceased.

Akihiko Nogami, MD, PhD
Professor, Cardiovascular Division, University of Tsukuba, Tsukuba, Ibaraki, Japan
Chapter 83: Bundle Branch Reentry Tachycardia

Sami F. Noujaim, PhD
Assistant Professor, Director of Cardiac Electrophysiology Research, Department of Molecular Pharmacology and Physiology, University of South Florida Morsani College of Medicine, Tampa, FL, United States
Chapter 13: Molecular Regulation of Cardiac Inward Rectifier Potassium Channels by Pharmacological Agents
Chapter 39: Pulmonary Vein Ganglia and the Neural Regulation of the Heart Rate

Karine Nubret Le Coniat, MD
Anesthesiology Department, Centre Hospitalier Universitaire de Bordeaux, Bordeaux, France
Chapter 111: Ventricular Assist Devices and Cardiac Transplantation Recipients

Brian Olshansky, MD
Professor Emeritus, Department of Internal Medicine, University of Iowa Hospitals and Clinics, Iowa City, IA, United States
Chapter 83: Bundle Branch Reentry Tachycardia

Jin O-Uchi, MD, PhD
Assistant Professor of Medicine, Cardiovascular Research Center, Rhode Island Hospital; Department of Medicine, The Warren Alpert Medical School of Brown University, Providence, RI, United States
Chapter 7: Organellar Ion Channels and Transporters

Gavin Y. Oudit, MD, PhD, FRCPC
Division of Cardiology, University of Alberta, Edmonton, AB, Canada
Chapter 3: Voltage-Gated Potassium Channels

Feifan Ouyang, MD
Department of Cardiology, Asklepios Klinik St. Georg, Hamburg, Germany
Chapter 126: Ablation of Supraventricular Tachyarrhythmias

Cevher Ozcan, MD
Assistant Professor of Medicine, Department of Medicine, Section of Cardiology, University of Chicago, Chicago, IL, United States
Chapter 107: Sex Differences in Arrhythmias

Douglas L. Packer, MD
Division of Cardiology, Mayo Clinic College of Medicine, Rochester, MN, United States
Chapter 139: Left Atrial Appendage Closure

Sandeep V. Pandit, PhD
Adjunct Associate Research Scientist, Internal Medicine-Cardiology, University of Michigan, Ann Arbor, MI, United States
Chapter 31: Ionic Mechanisms of Atrial Action Potentials

Alexander V. Panfilov, PhD
Professor, Department of Physics and Astronomy, Ghent University, Ghent, Belgium
Chapter 34: Theory of Rotors and Arrhythmias

David S. Park, MD, PhD
Assistant Professor of Medicine, Cardiac Electrophysiology, New York University School of Medicine, New York, NY, United States
Chapter 29: Cell Biology of the Specialized Cardiac Conduction System

Bence Patocskai, MD, PhD
Intern, Universitätsmedizin Mannheim, Heidelberg University, Heidelberg, Germany
Chapter 51: Genetic, Ionic, and Cellular Mechanisms Underlying the J Wave Syndromes

Dainius H. Pauza, PhD
Professor, Institute of Anatomy, Lithuanian University of Health Sciences, Kaunas, Lithuania
Chapter 37: Innervation of the Sinoatrial Node

Neringa Pauziene, PhD
Professor, Institute of Anatomy, Lithuanian University of Health Sciences, Kaunas, Lithuania
Chapter 37: Innervation of the Sinoatrial Node

Jonathan P. Piccini, MD, MHS
Associate Professor of Medicine, Division of Cardiology Duke University Hospital; Duke Clinical Research Institute, Durham, NC, United States
Chapter 122: Remote Monitoring of Cardiac Implantable Electronic Devices

Geoffrey S. Pitt, MD, PhD
Ida and Theo Rossi Distinguished Professor of Medicine, Director, Cardiovascular Research Institute, Weill Cornell Medicine, New York, NY, United States
Chapter 19: Fibroblast Growth Factor Homologous Factors Modulate Cardiac Sodium and Calcium Channels

Sunny S. Po, MD, PhD
Professor of Medicine, Heart Rhythm Institute, University of Oklahoma Health Sciences Center, Oklahoma City, OK, United States
Chapter 44: Role of the Autonomic Nervous System in Atrial Fibrillation

Abhiram Prasad, MD, FRCP, FACC
Professor of Medicine, Department of Cardiovascular Diseases, Mayo Clinic, Rochester, MN, United States
Chapter 91: Ventricular Arrhythmias in Takotsubo Cardiomyopathy

Silvia G. Priori, MD, PhD
Professor of Cardiology, ICS Maugeri, IRCCS and Department of Molecular Medicine, University of Pavia, Pavia, Italy
Chapter 56: Gene Therapy to Treat Cardiac Arrhythmias
Chapter 95: Timothy Syndrome

Przemysław B. Radwański, PharmD, PhD
Research Assistant Professor, Pharmacy Practice and Science, The Ohio State University College of Pharmacy, Columbus, OH, United States
Chapter 6: Structural and Molecular Bases of Sarcoplasmic Reticulum Ion Channel Function

Wouter-Jan Rappel, PhD
Principal Investigator, Rappel Laboratory at the Department of Physics, UC San Diego, La Jolla, CA, United States
Chapter 45: Rotors in Human Atrial Fibrillation

Michelle Reiser, MS
Research Specialist, Department of Molecular Pharmacology and Physiology, Morsani College of Medicine, University of South Florida, Tampa, FL, United States
Chapter 13: Molecular Regulation of Cardiac Inward Rectifier Potassium Channels by Pharmacological Agents

Alejandro Jimenez Restrepo, MD
Clinical Assistant Professor of Medicine, Case Western Reserve University, Cleveland, OH, United States; Consultant Electrophysiologist, Cleveland Clinic Abu Dhabi, United Arab Emirates
Chapter 62: Computed Tomography for Electrophysiology

Richard B. Robinson, PhD
Professor of Pharmacology in the Center for Molecular Therapeutics, Professor, Department of Pharmacology, Columbia University Medical Center, New York, NY, United States
Chapter 25: Stem Cell–Derived Sinoatrial-Like Cardiomyocytes as a Novel Pharmacological Tool
Chapter 26: Gene Therapy and Biological Pacing

Dan M. Roden, MD
Professor, Departments of Medicine, Pharmacology, and Biomedical Informatics; Senior Vice President for Personalized Medicine, Vanderbilt University Medical Center, Nashville, TN, United States
Chapter 55: Pharmacogenomics of Cardiac Arrhythmias

Michael R. Rosen, MD
Gustavus A. Pfeiffer Professor of Pharmacology and Professor of Pediatrics, Columbia University, New York; Adjunct Professor, Department of Physiology and Biophysics, Stony Brook University, Stony Brook, NY, United States
Chapter 26: Gene Therapy and Biological Pacing

Raphael Rosso, MD
Head of the Atrial Fibrillation Service, Cardiology, Tel Aviv Sourasky Medical Center; Sackler School of Medicine, Tel Aviv University, Tel Aviv, Israel
Chapter 96: J-Wave Syndromes

Yoram Rudy, PhD
Fred Saigh Distinguished Professor, Professor of Biomedical Engineering, Cell Biology and Physiology, Medicine, Radiology, and Pediatrics; Director, Cardiac Bioelectricity and Arrhythmia Center (CBAC); Washington University in St. Louis, St. Louis, MO, United States
Chapter 70: Noninvasive Electrocardiographic Imaging of Arrhythmogenic Substrates and Ventricular Arrhythmias in Patients

Kristina Rysevaite-Kyguoliene, PhD
Assistant Professor, Institute of Anatomy, Lithuanian University of Health Sciences, Kaunas, Lithuania
Chapter 37: Innervation of the Sinoatrial Node

Hani N. Sabbah, PhD, FACC, FCCP, FHRS
Professor of Medicine, Wayne State University; Director of Cardiovascular Research, Henry Ford Health System, Detroit, MI, United States
Chapter 135: Vagus Nerve Stimulation for the Treatment of Heart Failure

Frederic Sacher, MD, PhD
Arrhythmia Department, Centre Hospitalier Universitaire de Bordeaux, L'institut de Rythmologie et Modélisation Cardiaque, Bordeaux, France
Chapter 111: Ventricular Assist Devices and Cardiac Transplantation Recipients
Chapter 128: Epicardial Approach in Electrophysiology

Frank B. Sachse, PhD
Associate Professor, Department of Bioengineering, Nora Eccles Harrison Cardiovascular Research and Training Institute, University of Utah, Salt Lake City, UT, United States
Chapter 12: Structural Determinants and Biophysical Properties of hERG1 Channel Gating

Ardan M. Saguner, MD
Department of Cardiology, University Hospital Zürich, Zürich, Switzerland
Chapter 126: Ablation of Supraventricular Tachyarrhythmias

Prashanthan Sanders, MBBS, PhD
Knapman Chair of Cardiology Research and Director of Cardiac Electrophysiology, Centre for Heart Rhythm Disorders, South Australian Health and Medical Research Institute, University of Adelaide, Royal Adelaide Hospital, Adelaide, SA, Australia
Chapter 72: Sinus Node Abnormalities
Chapter 75: Typical and Atypical Atrial Flutter: Mapping and Ablation

Michael C. Sanguinetti, PhD
Professor, Department of Medicine, Nora Eccles Harrison Cardiovascular Research and Training Institute, University of Utah, Salt Lake City, UT, United States
Chapter 12: Structural Determinants and Biophysical Properties of hERG1 Channel Gating

Pasquale Santangeli, MD, PhD
Assistant Professor of Medicine, Hospital of the University of Pennsylvania, Philadelphia, PA, United States
Chapter 124: Catheter Ablation: Clinical Aspects

Mohammad Sarraf, MD
Director of Structural Heart Disease, Assistant Professor, University of Alabama, Birmingham, AL, United States
Chapter 139: Left Atrial Appendage Closure

Jonathan Satin, PhD
Professor, Department of Physiology, University of Kentucky College of Medicine, Lexington, KY, United States
Chapter 10: Regulation of Cardiac Calcium Channels

Martin Jan Schalij, MD, PhD
Professor of Cardiology, Chief of Cardiology, Leiden University Medical Center, Leiden, The Netherlands
Chapter 102: Ventricular Arrhythmias in Congenital Heart Disease

Benjamin J. Scherlag, MA, PhD
Heart Rhythm Institute, University of Oklahoma Health Sciences Center, Oklahoma City, OK, United States
Chapter 44: Role of the Autonomic Nervous System in Atrial Fibrillation

Matthew R. Schill, MD
Research Fellow, Department of Surgery, Washington University in St. Louis, St. Louis, MO, United States
Chapter 133: Surgery for Atrial Fibrillation and Other Supraventricular Tachycardias

J. William Schleifer, MD
Division of Cardiovascular Diseases, Mayo Clinic Arizona, Scottsdale, AZ, United States
Chapter 103: Syncope

Richard B. Schuessler, PhD
Professor of Surgery and Biomedical Engineering, Washington University School of Medicine, St. Louis, MO, United States
Chapter 133: Surgery for Atrial Fibrillation and Other Supraventricular Tachycardias

Peter J. Schwartz, MD
Director, Center for Cardiac Arrhythmias of Genetic Origin, IRCCS Istituto Auxologico Italiano, Milano, Italy
Chapter 93: Long and Short QT Syndromes

Timon Seeger, MD
Stanford Cardiovascular Institute, School of Medicine, Stanford University, Stanford, CA, United States
Chapter 30: Cardiac Remodeling and Regeneration

Christopher Semsarian, MBBS, PhD, MPH
Head, Molecular Cardiology Program, Centenary Institute; Professor of Medicine, University of Sydney; Cardiologist, Royal Prince Alfred Hospital; NHMRC Practitioner Fellow; Sydney, NSW, Australia
Chapter 71: Genetic Testing

Prof. Gino Seravalle
Cardiology, S. Luca Hospital, Istituto Auxologico Italiano, Milan, Italy
Chapter 136: Baroreceptor Stimulation

Ashok J. Shah, MBBS, MD, DM, CCDS
CHU Bordeaux, University of Bordeaux, LIRYC, Bordeaux, France
Chapter 47: Panoramic Mapping of Atrial Fibrillation From the Body Surface
Chapter 129: Ventricular Fibrillation

Robin M. Shaw, MD, PhD
Wasserman Endowed Chair in Cardiology, Heart Institute and Department of Medicine, Cedars-Sinai Medical Center and UCLA, Los Angeles, CA, United States
Chapter 17: Ion Channel Trafficking in the Heart

Mark J. Shen, MD
Cardiology Fellow, Department of Medicine, Krannert Institute of Cardiology, Indiana University, Indianapolis, IN, United States
Chapter 40: Neural Activity and Atrial Tachyarrhythmias
Chapter 137: Spinal Cord Stimulation for Heart Failure and Arrhythmias

Win–Kuang Shen, MD
Professor and Chair, Cardiovascular Diseases, Mayo Clinic Arizona, Phoenix, AZ, United States
Chapter 103: Syncope

Shey-Shing Sheu, PhD
Professor and Associate Director, Center for Translational Medicine, Department of Medicine, Jefferson Medical College, Thomas Jefferson University, Philadelphia, PA, United States
Chapter 7: Organellar Ion Channels and Transporters

Kalyanam Shivkumar, MD, PhD, FHRS
UCLA Cardiac Arrhythmia Center, David Geffen School of Medicine, UCLA Health System, Los Angeles, CA, United States
Chapter 123: Catheter Ablation: Technical Aspects

Jennifer N.A. Silva, MD
Director, Pediatric Electrophysiology, Division of Pediatric Cardiology, Washington University School of Medicine, St. Louis, MO, United States
Chapter 130: Ablation in Pediatrics

Allan C. Skanes, MD
Professor, Arrhythmia Service, Western University; Director of Electrophysiology Laboratory, London Heart Rhythm Program, London, ON, Canada
Chapter 66: Cardiac Monitoring: Short- and Long-Term Recording

Kyoko Soejima, MD
Professor, Department of Cardiology, Kyorin University School of Medicine, Tokyo, Japan
Chapter 82: Fascicular Ventricular Arrhythmias

Virend K. Somers, MD, PhD
Department of Internal Medicine, Divisions of Hypertension and Cardiovascular Diseases, Rochester, MN, United States
Chapter 110: Sleep-Disordered Breathing and Arrhythmias

Dan Sorajja, MD
Assistant Professor of Medicine, Cardiovascular Diseases/Electrophysiology, Mayo Clinic Arizona, Phoenix, AZ, United States
Chapter 103: Syncope

Stavros Stavrakis, MD, PhD
Heart Rhythm Institute, University of Oklahoma Health Sciences Center, Oklahoma City, OK, United States
Chapter 44: Role of the Autonomic Nervous System in Atrial Fibrillation

Christian Steinberg, MD
Division of Cardiology, Quebec Heart and Lung Institute, Quebec, Quebec, Canada
Chapter 97: Idiopathic Ventricular Fibrillation

Lynne Warner Stevenson, MD
Professor of Medicine, Harvard Medical School; Director of Cardiomyopathy and Heart Failure, Cardiovascular Division, Brigham and Women's Hospital, Boston, MA, United States
Chapter 89: Ventricular Arrhythmias in Heart Failure

William G. Stevenson, MD
Director, Cardiac Arrhythmia Program, Cardiovascular Division, Brigham and Women's Hospital; Professor of Medicine, Harvard Medical School, Boston, MA, United States
Chapter 127: Catheter Ablation for Ventricular Tachycardia With or Without Structural Heart Disease
Chapter 132: Anesthesiology Considerations for the Electrophysiology Laboratory

Michael O. Sweeney, MD
Associate Professor of Medicine, Cardiovascular Division, Harvard Medical School; Cardiac Pacing and Heart Failure Device Therapy, Brigham and Women's Hospital, Boston, MA, United States
Chapter 120: Use of QRS Fusion Complex Analysis in Cardiac Resynchronization Therapy

Charles Swerdlow, MD
Cedars Sinai Heart Institute, Clinical Professor of Medicine, University of California Los Angeles and Cedars Sinai Medical Center, Los Angeles, CA, United States
Chapter 117: Implantable Cardioverter Defibrillator: Clinical Aspects

Masateru Takigawa, MD
Department of Cardiovascular Medicine, Tokyo Medical and Dental University; Cardiovascular Center, Yokosuka Kyosai Hospital, Tokyo, Japan
Chapter 125: Ablation for Atrial Fibrillation

Juan Tamargo, MD, PhD, FESC
Professor of Pharmacology, Department of Pharmacology, School of Medicine, Universidad Complutense, CIBERCV, Madrid, Spain
Chapter 54: Pharmacological Bases of Antiarrhythmic Therapy

Harikrishna Tandri, MBBS, MD
Department of Medicine, Division of Cardiology, Johns Hopkins University School of Medicine, Baltimore, MD, United States
Chapter 87: Ventricular Tachycardias in Arrhythmogenic Right Ventricular Dysplasia/Cardiomyopathy

Usha B. Tedrow, MD, MSH
Director, Clinical Cardiac Electrophysiology Program, Department of Medicine, Cardiovascular Division, Brigham and Women's Hospital; Assistant Professor of Medicine, Harvard Medical School, Boston, MA, United States
Chapter 127: Catheter Ablation for Ventricular Tachycardia With or Without Structural Heart Disease

Nathaniel Thompson, MD
Centre Hospitalier Universitaire de Bordeaux, Hôpital Cardiologique du Haut Lévêque, Bordeaux, France
Chapter 125: Ablation for Atrial Fibrillation

Paul D. Thompson, MD
Chief of Cardiology, Division of Cardiology, Hartford Hospital, Hartford, CT, United States
Chapter 65: Exercise-Induced Arrhythmias

Gordon F. Tomaselli, MD
Michel Mirowski MD Professor of Cardiology, Department of Medicine, Johns Hopkins University School of Medicine, Baltimore, MD, United States
Chapter 38: Mechanisms for Altered Autonomic and Oxidant Regulation of Cardiac Sodium Currents

Jeffrey A. Towbin, MD, MS
Executive Co-Director and Chief, Pediatric Cardiology, Heart Institute, Le Bonheur Children's Hospital; Professor, Pediatric Cardiology, University of Tennessee Health Science Center; Chief, Pediatric Cardiology, Pediatrics, St. Jude Children's Research Hospital; Vice Chair of Pediatrics for Strategy Advancement, Pediatrics, University of Tennessee Health Science Center, Memphis, TN, United States
Chapter 90: Arrhythmias and Conduction Disturbances in Noncompaction Cardiomyopathy

Natalia A. Trayanova, PhD
Murray B. Sachs Endowed Chair, Professor of Biomedical Engineering and Medicine, Johns Hopkins University, Baltimore, MD, United States
Chapter 36: Modeling the Aging Heart

Martin Tristani-Firouzi, MD
Professor, Division of Pediatric Cardiology, University of Utah School of Medicine; Associate Director, Nora Eccles Harrison Cardiovascular Research and Training Institute, Salt Lake City, UT, United States
Chapter 94: Andersen-Tawil Syndrome

Zian H. Tseng, MD, MAS
Associate Professor of Medicine in Residence, Section of Cardiac Electrophysiology, Division of Cardiology, Department of Medicine, University of California San Francisco, San Francisco, CA, United States
Chapter 81: Outflow Tract Ventricular Tachyarrhythmias: Mechanisms, Clinical Features, and Management

Akiko Ueda, MD
Assistant Professor, Department of Cardiology, Kyorin University School of Medicine, Tokyo, Japan
Chapter 82: Fascicular Ventricular Arrhythmias

Héctor H. Valdivia, MD, PhD
Frank N. Wilson Professor of Cardiovascular Medicine, Department of Internal Medicine, University of Michigan, Ann Arbor, MI, United States
Chapter 53: Inheritable Phenotypes Associated With Altered Intracellular Calcium Regulation

Virginijus Valiunas, PhD
Research Associate Professor, Department of Physiology and Biophysics, Stony Brook University, Stony Brook, NY, United States
Chapter 15: Biophysical Properties of Gap Junctions

Christian van der Werf, MD, PhD
Department of Clinical and Experimental Cardiology, AMC Heart Center, Academic Medical Center, Amsterdam, The Netherlands
Chapter 88: Ventricular Tachycardias in Catecholaminergic Cardiomyopathy (Catecholaminergic Polymorphic Ventricular Tachycardia)

George F. Van Hare, MD
Professor, Department of Pediatrics, Washington University
    School of Medicine; Director, Pediatric Cardiology, St.
    Louis Children's Hospital, St. Louis, MO, United States
Chapter 130: Ablation in Pediatrics

David Vidmar, MSc
Graduate Student, Rappel Laboratory at the Department of
    Physics, UC San Diego, La Jolla, CA, United States
Chapter 45: Rotors in Human Atrial Fibrillation

Sami Viskin, MD
Director, Cardiac Hospitalization, Tel Aviv Medical Center; Sack-
    ler School of Medicine, Tel Aviv University, Tel Aviv, Israel
Chapter 96: J-Wave Syndromes

Niels Voigt, MD
Professor of Molecular Pharmacology, Institute of Pharmacol-
    ogy and Toxicology, University Medical Center Göttingen,
    Georg-August University, Göttingen, Germany
*Chapter 42: The Molecular Pathophysiology of Atrial
    Fibrillation*

Edward P. Walsh, MD
Chief, Cardiac Electrophysiology Division, Department of
    Cardiology, Boston Children's Hospital, Boston, MA,
    United States
Chapter 109: Arrhythmias in the Pediatric Population
Chapter 131: Catheter Ablation in Congenital Heart Disease

Paul J. Wang, MD
Professor of Medicine and Bioengineering (by courtesy), Direc-
    tor, Arrhythmia Service, Department of Medicine, Stanford
    University, Stanford, CA, United States
Chapter 119: Implantable Pacemakers

Xander H.T. Wehrens, MD, PhD
Director, Cardiovascular Research Institute, Baylor College of
    Medicine, Houston, TX, United States
*Chapter 42: The Molecular Pathophysiology of Atrial
    Fibrillation*

Mark S. Weiss, MD
Assistant Professor, Department of Anesthesiology and Criti-
    cal Care, Perelman School of Medicine at the University of
    Pennsylvania, Philadelphia, PA, United States
*Chapter 132: Anesthesiology Considerations for the
    Electrophysiology Laboratory*

Arthur A.M. Wilde, MD, PhD
Professor of Cardiology, Department of Clinical and Experi-
    mental Cardiology, AMC Heart Center, Academic Medi-
    cal Center, University of Amsterdam, Amsterdam, The
    Netherlands
Chapter 52: Inheritable Potassium Channel Diseases
*Chapter 88: Ventricular Tachycardias in Catecholaminergic
    Cardiomyopathy (Catecholaminergic Polymorphic
    Ventricular Tachycardia)*

Bruce L. Wilkoff, MD
Professor of Medicine, Cleveland Clinic Lerner College of
    Medicine at Case Western Reserve University; Director,
    Cardiac Pacing and Tachyarrhythmia Devices, Associate
    Section Head, Pacing and Electrophysiology Section, Robert
    and Suzanne Tomsich Department of Cardiovascular Medi-
    cine, Cleveland Clinic, Cleveland, OH, United States
*Chapter 116: Implantable Cardioverter Defibrillators:
    Technical Aspects*

Y. Joseph Woo, MD
Norman E. Shumway Professor and Chair, Department of
    Cardiothoracic Surgery, Professor of Bioengineering (by
    courtesy), Stanford University, Stanford, CA, United States
Chapter 134: Surgery for Ventricular Arrhythmias

Joseph C. Wu, MD, PhD
Stanford Cardiovascular Institute and Department of Medicine,
    Division of Cardiology, School of Medicine, Stanford
    University, Stanford, CA, United States
Chapter 30: Cardiac Remodeling and Regeneration

Raymond Yee, B.MD.Sc, MD
Professor of Medicine, Department of Medicine, Western
    University; Director, London Heart Rhythm Program,
    University Hospital, London, ON, Canada
*Chapter 66: Cardiac Monitoring: Short- and Long-Term
    Recording*

Junaid A.B. Zaman, MA, BMBCh, MRCP
Division of Cardiovascular Medicine, Stanford University
    School of Medicine, Stanford, CA, United States
Chapter 45: Rotors in Human Atrial Fibrillation

Manuel Zarzoso, PhD
Assistant Professor, Department of Physiotherapy, University of
    Valencia, Valencia, Spain
*Chapter 13: Molecular Regulation of Cardiac Inward Rectifier
    Potassium Channels by Pharmacological Agents*
*Chapter 39: Pulmonary Vein Ganglia and the Neural
    Regulation of the Heart Rate*

Emily P. Zeitler, MD, MHS
Fellow in Clinical Cardiac Electrophysiology, Division of Car-
    diology, Duke University School of Medicine, Durham, NC,
    United States
*Chapter 122: Remote Monitoring of Cardiac Implantable
    Electronic Devices*

Katja Zeppenfeld, MD, PhD
Professor of Cardiology, Director of Clinical Electrophysiology,
    Leiden University Medical Center, Leiden, The Netherlands
*Chapter 102: Ventricular Arrhythmias in Congenital Heart
    Disease*

Tarek Zghaib, MD
Post-Doctoral Research Fellow, Johns Hopkins University
    School of Medicine, Baltimore, MD, United States
Chapter 100: Arrhythmia in Neurological Disease

Xiao-Dong Zhang, MS, PhD
Assistant Researcher, Department of Internal Medicine,
    University of California Davis, Davis, CA, United States
*Chapter 24: Feedback Mechanisms for Cardiac-Specific
    MicroRNAs and cAMP Signaling in Electrical
    Remodeling*

Douglas P. Zipes, MD
Distinguished Professor, Emeritus Professor of Medicine, Phar-
    macology, and Toxicology, Emeritus Director, Division of
    Cardiology and the Krannert Institute of Cardiology, Indiana
    University School of Medicine; Editor-in-Chief, Practice-
    Update/Cardiology, Editor-in-Chief, Trends in Cardiovas-
    cular Medicine, Indianapolis, IN, United States
*Chapter 59: Assessment of the Patient With a Cardiac
    Arrhythmia*
*Chapter 137: Spinal Cord Stimulation for Heart Failure
    and Arrhythmias*

PREFACE

Cardiac electrophysiology, both basic and clinical, continues to advance rapidly with new observations almost daily. Multiple electrophysiologic journals now publish so many articles, it is hard to stay abreast of new information vitally useful at the bench and bedside. While the sixth edition of *Cardiac Electrophysiology: From Cell to Bedside* was published in 2014, this rapid pace of new discovery compelled us to create the seventh edition in record time.

Not only have we advanced the publishing date, we have also added to the total number of chapters—from 132 to 139. In addition to all chapters being totally revised by international authorities who are experts in their fields, we have provided 19 totally new chapters in basic and clinical arenas. We have continued the full color display and the electronic version inaugurated with the sixth edition. Each chapter is crammed full with the latest information in that particular area, while the website provides space for overflow information, figures, tables, and videos.

We hope *Cardiac Electrophysiology: From Cell to Bedside* continues to be the go-to reference source for all levels of learners, from basic scientists to clinicians, for those early in their careers to those well advanced. We—the editors—have strived in our careers to blend basic with clinical in a bidirectional effort and have patterned this book with that in mind.

As before, the first half provides the foundation of basic electrophysiology, including sections on Structural and Molecular Bases of Ion Channel Function, Biophysics of Cardiac Ion Channel Function, Intermolecular Interactions and Cardiomyocyte Electrical Function, Cell Biology of Cardiac Impulse Initiation and Propagation, Models of Cardiac Excitation, Neural Control of Cardiac Electrical Activity, Arrhythmia Mechanisms, Molecular Genetics and Pharmacogenomics, and Pharmacologic, Genetic, and Cell Therapy of Ion Channel Dysfunction.

The second half is devoted to clinical cardiac electrophysiology, including sections on Diagnostic Evaluation, Supraventricular Tachyarrhythmias, Ventricular Tachyarrhythmias, Syncope and Bradyarrhythmias, Arrhythmias in Special Populations, Pharmacologic Therapy, Cardiac Implantable Electronic Devices, Catheter Ablation, Surgery for Arrhythmias, and New Approaches.

New for this edition is the addition of William G. Stevenson as an editor. Bill is well known to the electrophysiology community and joined us in preparation to take over the role of Doug Zipes for the eighth edition.

We would like to thank our spouses, Joan Zipes, Paloma Jalife, and Lynne Stevenson, for their love and support, and for putting up with the countless hours demanded of such a project.

We would also like to thank all of our colleagues who generously contributed their time, talents, and efforts to this book, and Lucia Gunzel, Dolores Meloni, and Kristine Feeherty at Elsevier for help with the publication.

Finally, we thank the readers who use our book as their learning manual and source for fact checking. We hope this edition continues the tradition of the past and meets your standards.

Douglas P. Zipes
José Jalife
William G. Stevenson

CONTENTS

VIDEO CONTENTS

1

Voltage-Gated Sodium Channels and Electrical Excitability of the Heart

William A. Catterall

Voltage-gated sodium channels initiate action potentials in nerves, cardiac myocytes, and other excitable cells.[1,2] They are responsible for the propagation of action potentials through the atria, the conduction system, and the ventricles of the heart. As shown in Fig. 1.1, action potentials in atrial and ventricular muscle fibers rise rapidly from a resting potential of about –80 mV and reach their peak within 1 ms. During this brief interval, cardiac sodium channels respond to the change in pacemaker potential as it reaches a threshold and open to allow the rapid entry of sodium ions (Na^+). Sodium channels begin to inactivate as soon as they open and are inactivated to 98% or 99% completion within a few milliseconds. The plateau phase of the cardiac action potential is generated by the opening of voltage-gated calcium channels (see Chapter 2), and the cell is finally repolarized by slower opening of voltage-gated potassium channels (see Chapter 3). The rate of conduction of the action potential through the cardiac tissue depends directly on the rate of rise of the cardiac action potential and therefore on the density of active sodium channels and their rate of activation.

Much is now known about the molecular mechanisms of activation, inactivation, and ion conduction by the sodium channel protein, as is summarized in this chapter. Multiple genes encode sodium channel subunits, and the distinct sodium channel subtypes exhibit subtle differences in functional properties and differential distribution in subcellular compartments of cardiac myocytes. These differences in the function and localization of sodium channels may contribute to their specialized functional roles in cardiac physiology and pharmacology.

Subunit Structure of Sodium Channels

Sodium channel proteins purified from excitable cells are complexes composed of an ~260-kDa α-subunit in association with one or two auxiliary β-subunits of ~33 to ~39 kDa in size.[3] Purified sodium channel complexes of α- and β-subunits are sufficient for voltage-dependent gating and ion conduction in artificial lipid membranes, and expression of the α-subunit alone is sufficient for physiological function in recipient nonexcitable cells; this indicates that the α-subunit has all of the structural elements required for voltage-dependent gating and ion conduction.[4–6] The primary sequence predicts that the sodium channel α-subunit folds into four internally repeated domains (I to IV), each of which contains six α-helical transmembrane segments (S1 to S6; Fig. 1.2).[3,6–8] In each domain, segments S1 through S4 serve as the voltage-sensing module, and segments S5 and S6 and the reentrant P-loop between them serve as the pore-forming module. One large extracellular loop connects either the S5 or S6 transmembrane segment to the P-loop in each domain, whereas the other extracellular loops are small. Large intracellular loops link the four homologous domains, and the large N-terminal and C-terminal domains also contribute substantially to the mass of the intracellular face of the sodium channels. This view of sodium channel architecture, originally derived from hydrophobicity analysis of the amino acid sequence,[7] has largely been confirmed by biochemical, electrophysiological, and structural experiments.[3,9]

Initial purification studies of sodium channels identified auxiliary β1- and β2-subunits.[4] These subunits have a single transmembrane segment, a large N-terminal extracellular domain, and a short C-terminal intracellular segment (see Fig. 1.2).[10,11] The β-subunits interact with α-subunit extracellular domains, modulating α-subunit function and enhancing their cell surface expression.[10–13] They also serve as cell adhesion molecules by interacting with extracellular matrix proteins, other cell adhesion molecules, signaling proteins, and cytoskeletal linker proteins.[14–20] These interactions are thought to localize and stabilize sodium channels in specific subcellular compartments and to bring crucial signaling molecules to the sodium channel to regulate it. Deletion of the genes encoding β-subunits causes alterations in sodium channel function; reduced action potential conduction and abnormal development of myelin folds in axons; hyperexcitability and epilepsy in the brain; and arrhythmias in the heart.[21–23]

Three-Dimensional Structure of Sodium Channels

Sodium channel architecture has been revealed in three-dimensions through determination of the crystal structure of the bacterial sodium channels at high resolution (2.7 Å) (Fig. 1.3).[9,24] This ancient sodium channel has a simple structure: four identical subunits, each similar to one homologous domain of a mammalian sodium channel but without the large intracellular and extracellular loops of the mammalian protein.[9] Knowledge of the structure has revealed a wealth of new information about the structural basis for sodium selectivity and conductance, the mechanism for blockage of the channel by therapeutically important drugs, and the mechanism of voltage-dependent gating. As viewed from the top, NavAb has a central pore surrounded by four pore-forming modules composed of S5 and S6 segments and the intervening

LEFT VENTRICLE   LEFT ATRIUM

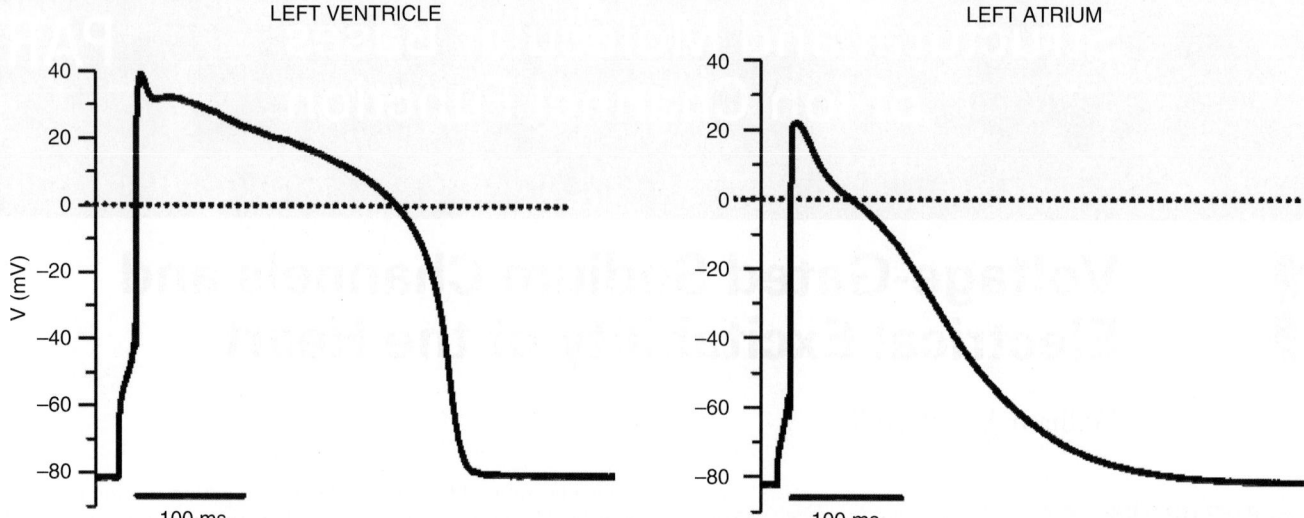

FIGURE 1.1 Cardiac action potential in sheep heart. Cardiac myocytes in the left ventricle or left atrium were impaled with a microelectrode, and the cardiac action potential was recorded. *ms,* Millisecond; *mV,* millivolt; *V,* voltage. (Courtesy J. Jalife.)

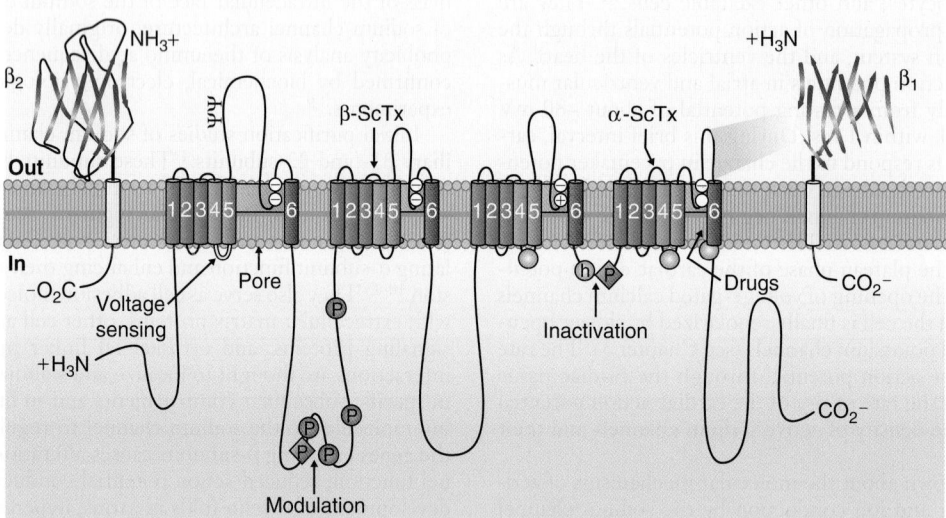

FIGURE 1.2 Transmembrane organization of sodium channel subunits. The primary structures of the subunits of the voltage-gated ion channels are illustrated as transmembrane folding diagrams. Cylinders represent probable alpha helical segments: S1 to S3, *blue*; S4, *green*; S5, *yellow*; and S6, *red*. The outer pore loop is the *shaded orange area,* and the intracellular S4–S5 helix is shown in *purple. Bold lines* represent the polypeptide chains of each subunit, with lengths approximately proportional to the number of amino acid residues in the brain sodium channel subtypes. The extracellular domains of the β1- and β2-subunits are shown as immunoglobulin-like folds. Ψ, sites of probable N-linked glycosylation. P, sites of demonstrated protein phosphorylation by protein kinase A *(circles)* and protein kinase C *(diamonds).* White circles, the outer (EEDD) and inner (DEKA) rings of amino residues that form the ion selectivity filter and the tetrodotoxin binding site. ++, S4 voltage sensors. h (in the *shaded circle),* inactivation particle in the inactivation gate loop. *Open shaded circles,* sites implicated in forming the inactivation gate receptor. The structure of the extracellular domain of the β-subunits is illustrated as an immunoglobulin-like fold based on amino acid sequence homology to the myelin P0 protein. Also shown are binding sites of α- and β-scorpion toxins and a site of interaction between α- and β1-subunits. (Modified from Catterall WA. From ionic currents to molecular mechanisms: the structure and function of voltage-gated sodium channels. *Neuron.* 2000;26:13-25.)

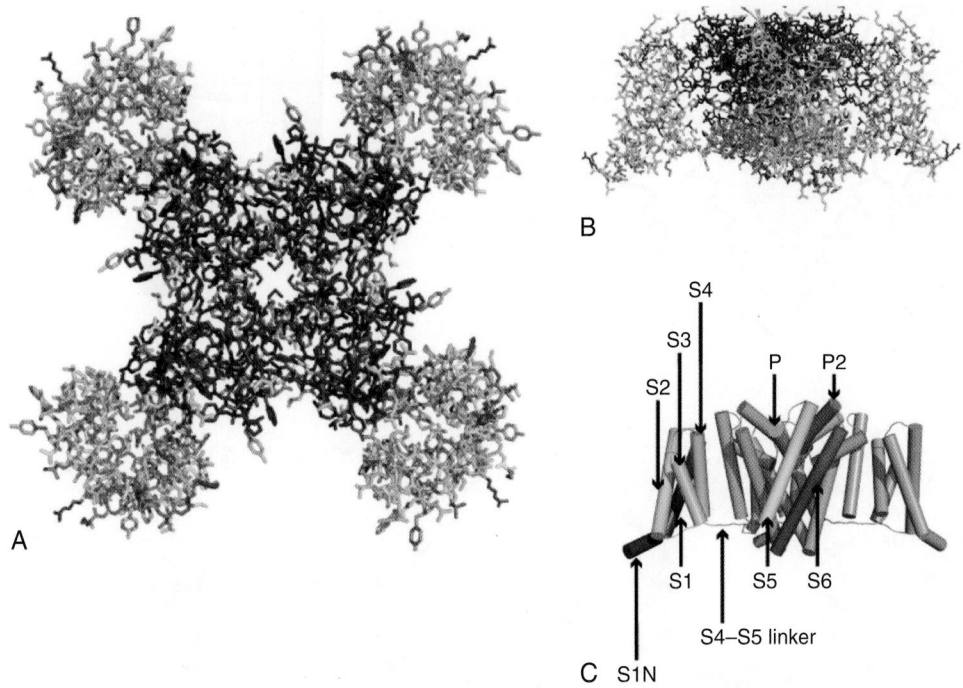

FIGURE 1.3 Three-dimensional structure of sodium channels. (A) Top view of NavAb channels colored according to crystallographic temperature factors of the main chain (blue < 50 Å² to red > 150 Å²). (B) Side view of NavAb. (C) Structural elements in NavAb. The structural components of one subunit are highlighted (1 to 6, transmembrane segments S1 to S6). (Modified from Payandeh J, Scheuer T, Zheng N, Catterall WA. The crystal structure of a voltage-gated sodium channel. *Nature.* 2011;475:353-358.)

P-loop (see Fig. 1.3A, *blue*). Four voltage-sensing modules composed of segments S1 to S4 are symmetrically located around the outer rim of the pore module (see Fig. 1.3A and B, *red* and *green*). The transmembrane architecture of NavAb shows that the adjacent subunits have swapped their functional domains such that each voltage-sensing module is most closely associated with the pore-forming module of its neighbor (see Fig. 1.3C). It is likely that this arrangement enforces concerted gating of the four subunits or domains of the sodium channels.

A comparison of the primary structures of the isoforms of auxiliary β-subunits to those of other proteins has revealed a close structural relationship to the family of proteins that contain immunoglobulin-like folds, which includes many cell adhesion molecules.[10,11,25,26] The extracellular domains of these type-I single-membrane-spanning proteins have been predicted to fold in a similar manner to that of myelin protein P0, whose immunoglobulin-like fold is formed by a sandwich of two beta sheets held together by hydrophobic interactions (see Fig. 1.2).[27] Three-dimensional structures of the extracellular domains of the β3- and β4-subunits confirm these expectations.[28,29] As would be expected from having structures that resemble cell adhesion molecules, Na_Vβ-subunits interact with extracellular matrix molecules, other cell adhesion molecules, and intracellular cytoskeletal and signaling proteins.[14–18] In addition, homophilic and heterophilic interactions of β-subunits have been demonstrated at both cellular and structural levels.[20,30]

Sodium Channel Structure and Function

The three key functions of sodium channels were defined in a classic study[1] as (1) voltage-dependent activation, (2) fast inactivation, and (3) selective ion conductance. Building on this foundation, detailed biophysical studies have revealed the ion selectivity of the channel pore, detected the movement of the voltage sensors as a capacitive gating current, and developed mechanistic models for these essential channel functions.[2,31] Recent structure-function studies that employed molecular, biochemical, structural, and electrophysiological techniques have resulted in a clear understanding of the molecular and structural basis for these sodium channel functions.

Outer Pore and Selectivity Filter

Voltage clamp studies showed that sodium channels are highly selective for sodium versus potassium and other monovalent cations.[2,32] Because of the high energy of hydration of Na⁺, theoretical considerations predicted there would be an outer, high-field-strength site that would partially dehydrate the permeating ion, and two inner sites that would conduct and rehydrate the permeant Na⁺ ion.[33] Analysis of ion selectivity and blocking by tetrodotoxin and saxitoxin led to a model in which these toxins can plug the selectivity filter in the outer pore of sodium channels.[34] Mutational analysis identified a key glutamate residue in the membrane-reentrant loop in domain I as a crucial residue for tetrodotoxin and saxitoxin binding.[35] Further studies revealed a pair of important amino acid residues, mostly negatively charged, in analogous positions in all four domains (see Fig. 1.2, *small white circles*).[36–38] The mutation to glutamates of a set of four residues in analogous positions in each domain (aspartate in domain I, glutamate in domain II, lysine in domain III, and alanine in domain IV, DEKA) confers calcium selectivity[39]; this indicates that the side chains of these amino acid residues are likely to interact with sodium ions as they are conducted through the ion selectivity filter of the pore, thus conferring sodium selectivity. Mutations in this ring of four amino acid residues have strong effects on selectivity for organic and inorganic monovalent cations, which is in agreement with the idea that they form the selectivity filter, and structure-function studies suggest specific

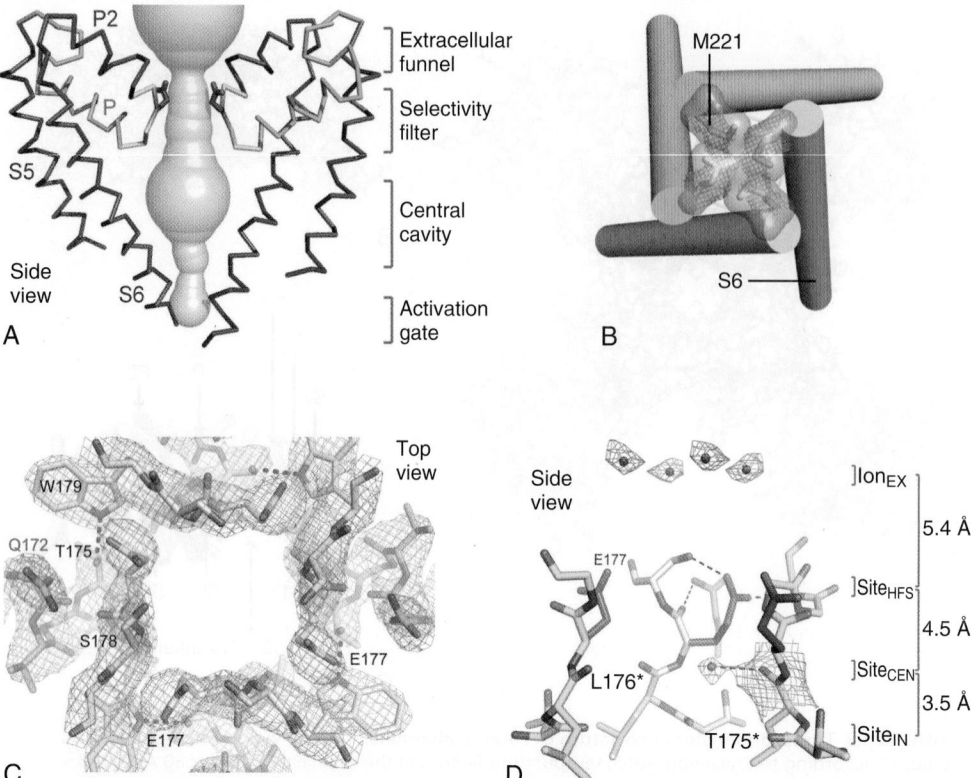

FIGURE 1.4 NavAb pore and selectivity filter. (A) Architecture of the NavAb pore. Glu177 side-chains, *purple*; pore volume, *gray*. (B) The closed activation gate at the intracellular end of the pore illustrating the close interaction of Met221 residues in closing the pore. (C) Top view of the ion selectivity filter. Symmetry-related molecules are colored *white* and *yellow*; P-helix residues are colored *green*. Hydrogen bonds between Thr175 and Trp179 are indicated by *gray dashes*. Electron-densities from F_o-F_c omit maps are contoured at 4.0 σ (*blue* and *gray*), and subtle differences can be appreciated (*small arrows*). (D) Side view of the selectivity filter. Glu177 *(purple)* interactions with Gln172, Ser178 and the backbone of Ser180 are shown in the far subunit. F_o-F_c omit map, 4.75 σ (*blue*); putative cations or water molecules *(red spheres,* Ion_{EX}). Electron-density around Leu176 *(gray;* F_o-F_c omit map at 1.75 σ) and a putative water molecule is shown *(gray sphere)*. Na^+-coordination sites: $Site_{HFS}$, $Site_{CEN}$, and $Site_{IN}$. (Modified from Payandeh J, Scheuer T, Zheng N, Catterall WA. The crystal structure of a voltage-gated sodium channel. *Nature.* 2011;475:353-358.)

structural interactions and functional roles for the P-loops from the four domains.[40–43]

The overall pore architecture in the bacterial sodium channel NavAb includes the following component structures: a large external vestibule; a narrow ion selectivity filter that contains the amino acid residues shown to determine ion selectivity in vertebrate sodium and calcium channels; a large central cavity filled with water and lined by the S6 segments; and an intracellular activation gate formed at the crossing of the S6 segments at the intracellular surface of the membrane (Fig. 1.4A).[9,24] The activation gate in the NavAb structure is tightly closed (Fig. 1.4B), and there is no space for ions or water to move through it. This general architecture resembles voltage-gated potassium channels (see Chapter 3). However, although the overall pore architecture of sodium and potassium channels is similar, the structures of their ion selectivity filters and their mechanisms of ion selectivity and conductance are completely different. Potassium channels select the potassium ion (K^+) through interacting directly with a series of four ion coordination sites formed by the backbone carbonyls of the amino acid residues that comprise the ion selectivity filter (see Chapter 3). No charged amino acid residues are involved, and no water molecules intervene between K^+ ions and the interacting backbone carbonyls in the ion selectivity filter of the potassium channels. In contrast, the NavAb ion selectivity filter has a high field strength site at its extracellular end (Fig. 1.4C), which is formed by amino acid residues that are highly conserved and are

key determinants of ion selectivity in vertebrate sodium and calcium channels (see Fig. 1.2). This high field strength site's dimensions of approximately 4.6 Å square would allow Na^+ with two to four planar waters of hydration to fit within it. This outer site is followed by two ion coordination sites formed by backbone carbonyls (Fig. 1.4D). These two carbonyl sites are perfectly designed to bind Na^+ with four planar waters of hydration but would be much too large to bind Na^+ directly. Thus the chemistry of Na^+ selectivity and conductance is opposite to that of K^+: negatively charged residues interact with Na^+ to remove most (but not all) of its waters of hydration, and Na^+ is conducted as a hydrated ion, interacting with the pore through its inner shell of bound waters.

Molecular dynamics simulations have revealed additional details of the mechanism of the ion conduction process. Remarkably, the negatively charged glutamate side chains at the high field strength site coordinate an approaching Na^+ ion and move with it into the selectivity filter in a "dunking" motion that involves rotation at a single torsion angle in the glutamate side chain.[24,44] Different numbers of glutamate side chains move with the individual Na^+ ions, and the displacement of waters of hydration is proportional to these interactions with the glutamate side chains. Thus, in contrast to classical views of a static selectivity filter, molecular dynamics simulations of sodium conduction in the structure of the NavAb selectivity filter reveal the direct catalytic participation of glutamate side chain motions in each ion-conducting event.

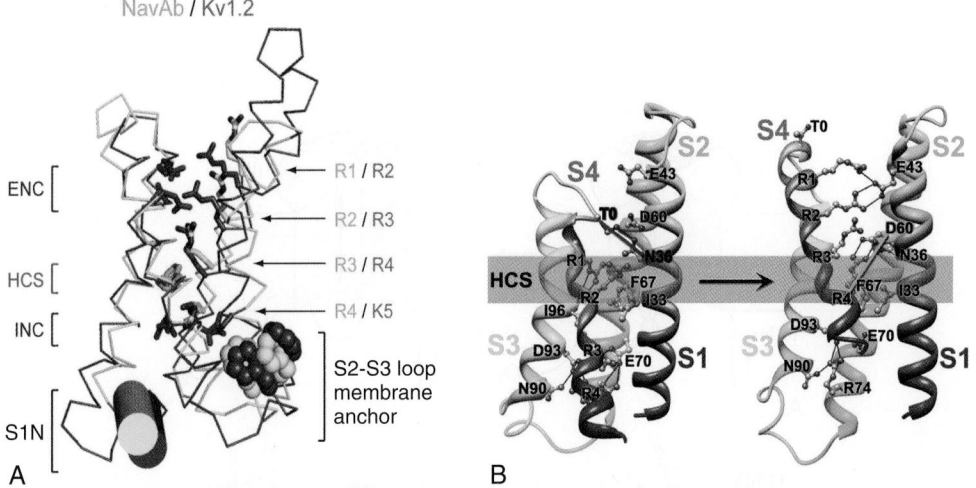

FIGURE 1.5 The voltage sensing domain (VSD). (A) Side view of the VSD illustrating the extracellular negative charge-cluster (*red,* ENC), the intracellular negative charge-cluster (*red,* INC), hydrophobic constriction site (*green,* HCS), residues of the S1N helix *(cyan)* and phenylalanines of the S2-S3 loop *(purple).* S4 segment and gating charges (R1-R4) are in *yellow.* (B) Transmembrane view of the lowest-energy Rosetta models of the VSD of NaChBac in Resting State 1 *(left)* and Activated State 3 *(right).* Side chains of the gating-charge-carrying arginines in S4 and key residues in S1, S2, and S3 segments are shown in stick representation and labeled. *Gray, blue,* and *red* atoms C, N, and O. The HCS is highlighted by *orange bars.* The majority of the lowest-energy models of Resting State 1 predict that R1 forms hydrogen bonds with the backbone carbonyl of I96 (in S3) at the extracellular edge of the HCS. On the intracellular side of the HCS, R3 makes ionic interactions with the amino acid residues of the intracellular negatively charged cluster, including E70 (in S2) and D93 (in S3), and R4 forms an ion pair with D93 (in S3). The lowest energy models for Activated State 3 predict that R1 forms an ion pair with E43 (in S1), R2 forms an ion pair with E43 (in S1), R3 forms hydrogen bond with Y156 (in S5) and makes ionic interactions with D60 (in S2) and E43 (in S1), and R4 forms an ion pair with D60 (in S2). (Modified from Payandeh J, Scheuer T, Zheng N, Catterall WA. The crystal structure of a voltage-gated sodium channel. *Nature.* 2011;475:353-358; and Yarov-Yarovoy V, De-Caen PG, Westenbroek RE, et al. Structural basis for gating charge movement in the voltage sensor of a sodium channel. *Proc Natl Acad Sci U S A.* 2012;109:E93-102.)

Voltage-Dependent Activation

The voltage dependence of the activation of sodium channels derives from outward movement of approximately 12 gating charges as a consequence of depolarization of the membrane and reduction of the membrane electrical field.[31,45] The S4 segments of each homologous domain serve as the primary voltage sensors for activation.[7,8] These contain repeated motifs of a positively charged amino acid residue followed by two hydrophobic residues, which creates a transmembrane spiral of positive charges. Upon depolarization, outward movement and rotation of S4 are thought to initiate a conformational change that opens the sodium channel pore.[7,8] This "sliding helix" or "helical screw" model is supported by strong evidence. For example, neutralization of the positively charged residues in S4 reduces the voltage-dependence of the gating.[46] The outward and rotational gating movement of the S4 segment has been detected directly by the reaction of substituted cysteine residues in S4 segments with extracellular sulfhydryl reagents following channel activation, and by analysis of the movement of fluorescent probes incorporated into these substituted cysteine residues.[47,48] Further support for this mechanism derives from a wide range of structure-function studies,[49] including extensive disulfide crosslinking studies of substituted cysteine residues that have charted the exchange of ion pair partners during activation.[50–53] In four-domain mammalian sodium channels, there is a hierarchy of activation of the four voltage sensors. Studies of fluorescently labeled S4 segments show that the voltage sensors of domains I to III activate rapidly, whereas the S4 segment of domain IV activates much more slowly.[54]

In the structure of the bacterial sodium channel NaVAb, the S4 segment is in a transmembrane position in its activated state

and its positive charges are neutralized by negative charges in the nearby S1, S2, and S3 segments[9] (Fig. 1.5A). This conformation is nearly identical to that of the voltage sensor of potassium channels (see Fig. 1.5A). In this snapshot of an activated voltage sensor, three gating charges (R1 to R3 in NaVAb) interact with the extracellular negative cluster and are located on the extracellular side of the hydrophobic constriction site, which seals the structure to prevent leak of water and ions. At the resting membrane potential, the force of the electrical field (which is negative inside the cell) would pull the positive charges inward such that gating charges R2 to R4 interact with the intracellular negative cluster.[53] Depolarization would abolish this force and allow an outward movement of the S4 helix and its gating charges, catalyzed by the exchange of ion pair partners (see Fig. 1.5B; Video 1.1).[53] After conformational changes have occurred in all four domains, the transmembrane pore can open and conduct ions (see Video 1.1).[53] This structural model shows that the S4 segment and its gating charges move through a gating pore that narrows the transmembrane electrical field to a distance of N5Å allowing a short transit through the channel protein (see Video 1.1).[53]

Pore Opening

These structural models allow the steps in the gating of a voltage-gated ion channel to be visualized.[24,53] In the closed state, the negative internal membrane potential of –70 mV to –90 mV pulls the S4 gating charges inward by electrostatic force. The inward position of the S4 segment exerts a force on the S4–S5 linker, straightens the S6 segment, and closes the pore at its inner mouth. Depolarization of the cell relieves the electrostatic force

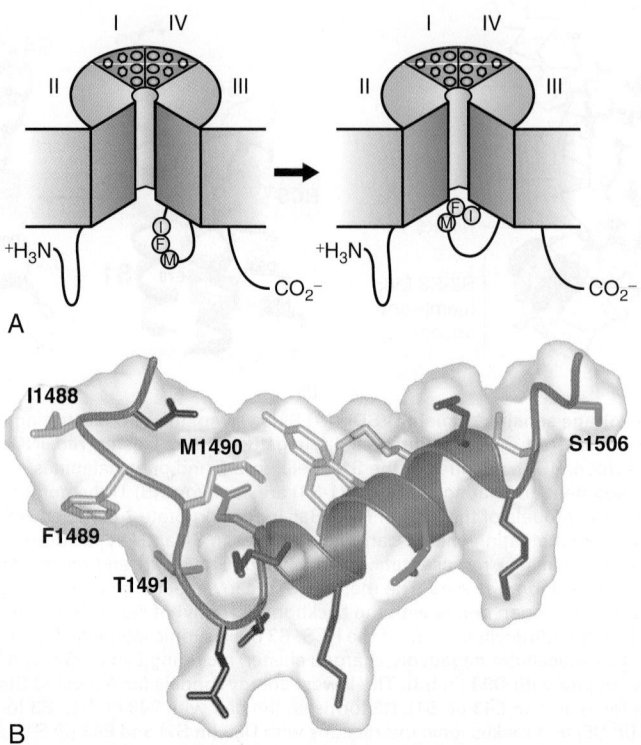

FIGURE 1.6 The molecular mechanism of fast sodium channel inactivation. (A) The hinged-lid mechanism. The intracellular loop connecting domains III and IV of the sodium channel is depicted as forming a hinged lid with the critical phenylalanine (Phe1489) within the isoleucine, phenylalanine, and methionine (IFM) motif shown occluding the mouth of the pore during the inactivation process. The *circles* represent the transmembrane helices. (B) Three-dimensional structure of the central segment of the inactivation gate as determined by multidimensional nuclear magnetic resonance. Isoleucine 1488, phenylalanine 1489, and methionine 1490 (IFM) are illustrated in *yellow*. Threonine 1491, which is important for inactivation, and serine 1506, which is a site of phosphorylation and modulation by protein kinase C, are also indicated. (Modified from Catterall WA. From ionic currents to molecular mechanisms: the structure and function of voltage-gated sodium channels. *Neuron.* 2000;26:13-25.)

pulling the S4 segment inward. In response to the change in electrostatic force, the S4 segment moves outward, with each positive gating charge interacting with the charged amino acid side chains in turn to ease their movement through the voltage-sensing module. When the R3 and R4 gating charges pass the hydrophobic constriction site in the center of the voltage sensor module, the outward force on the S4–S5 linker is sufficient to exert a torque on the pore-forming module and bend the S6 segment, resulting in the pore opening at its intracellular end. During activation of the voltage sensors of the sodium channels, the S4–S5 intracellular linkers in each domain (see Fig. 1.2) exert a force on the adjacent S6 segments, and the pore opens by bending and twisting the S6 segment (see Fig. 1.2). In bacterial voltage-gated potassium channels and sodium channels, bending of the S6 segment occurs at a critical hinge glycine residue about one-third down the length of the S6 segment[55–57]; this bending motion allows the inner mouth of the pore to open (Videos 1.1 and 1.2)[53] and allow rapid movement of the ions across the membrane.

Fast Inactivation

Fast inactivation of the sodium channel is a critical process that occurs within milliseconds of the channel opening. The generally accepted model of this process involves a conserved inactivation gate formed by the intracellular loop connecting domains III and IV (see Fig. 1.2), which serves as a hinged lid that binds to the intracellular end of the pore and blocks it (Fig. 1.6).[3] The intracellular perfusion of proteases prevents fast inactivation.[31] Site-directed antipeptide antibodies against the short, highly conserved intracellular loop that connects domains III and IV of the sodium channel α-subunit (see Fig. 1.2) were found to prevent fast sodium channel inactivation, but this was not the case for antibodies directed to other intracellular domains.[58,59] Furthermore, the accessibility of this site for antibody binding was reduced when the membrane was depolarized to induce inactivation, which suggests that the loop connecting domains III and IV forms an inactivation gate that folds into the channel structure during inactivation.[58,59] Cutting the loop between domains III and IV by expression of the sodium channel in two pieces greatly slows inactivation.[46] Mutagenesis studies of this region revealed a hydrophobic triad of isoleucine, phenylalanine, and methionine (IFM) that is critical for fast inactivation (see Fig. 1.2, *blue circle with "h"*),[60] and peptides containing this motif can serve as pore blockers and can restore inactivation to sodium channels that have a mutated inactivation gate.[61] The latch of this fast inactivation gate is formed by the three key hydrophobic residues, IFM, and adjacent threonine (T). These results support a model in which the IFM motif serves as a tethered pore blocker that binds to a receptor in the intracellular mouth of the pore. Inactivation is impaired in proportion to the hydrophilicity of the amino acid substituted for the key phenylalanine residue (F1489), suggesting that it forms a hydrophobic interaction with an inactivation gate receptor during inactivation.[62] Voltage-dependent movement of the inactivation gate has been detected by measuring the accessibility of a cysteine residue substituted for F1489.[63] This substituted cysteine residue becomes inaccessible to reaction with sulfhydryl reagents as the inactivation gate closes. Glycine and proline residues that flank the IFM motif may serve as molecular hinges that allow the inactivation gate to close like a hinged lid (see Fig. 1.6A).[64]

The three-dimensional structure of the central portion of the inactivation gate has been determined by its expression as a separate peptide and analysis of this by multidimensional nuclear magnetic resonance methods.[65] These experiments reveal a rigid alpha helix flanked on its N-terminal side by two turns, the second of which contains the IFM motif (see Fig. 1.6B). The fold of the inactivation gate peptide projects F1489 into the solvent away from the core of the peptide, an unusual position for a hydrophobic residue in a short peptide. In this position, F1489 is poised to serve as a tethered ligand that occludes the pore. The nearby threonine (T1491), which is an important residue for inactivation,[62] also is in position to interact with the inactivation gate receptor in the pore. In contrast, the methionine of the IFM motif (M1490) is buried in the core of the peptide, interacting with two tyrosine residues in the alpha helix. This hydrophobic interaction stabilizes the fold of the peptide and forces F1489 into its exposed position. The structure of the inactivation gate peptide in solution suggests that the rigid alpha helix serves as a scaffold to present the IFM motif and T1491 to a receptor in the mouth of the pore as the gate closes.

Scanning mutagenesis experiments have revealed multiple amino acid residues that may form the inactivation gate receptor within and near the intracellular mouth of the pore (see Fig. 1.2, *blue circles*); these include hydrophobic residues at the intracellular end of transmembrane segment IVS6[66] and amino acid residues in intracellular loops IIIS4–S5[67] and IVS4–S5.[68–71] Mutations of residues in each of these positions impair inactivation by destabilizing the inactivated state, as would be expected for disruption of the inactivation gate receptor. In addition, mutations in intracellular loop IVS4–S5 impair closed channel block by IFM-containing peptides, consistent with its function as the inactivation gate receptor,[69] and paired insertions of charged residues in the IIIS4–S5 loop and the IFM motif indicate that these peptide segments interact during inactivation.[67] Evidently, multiple peptide segments form a complex inactivation gate receptor into which the inactivation gate closes to occlude the inner pore.

Coupling of Activation to Fast Inactivation

Sodium channel inactivation derives most of its voltage dependence from coupling to the activation process driven by transmembrane movements of the S4 voltage sensors.[31] Increasingly strong evidence implicates the S4 segment in domain IV in this process. Mutations of charged amino acid residues at the extracellular end of the IVS4 segment have strong and selective effects on inactivation.[72] α-Scorpion toxins and sea anemone toxins uncouple activation from inactivation by binding to a receptor site at the extracellular end of the IVS4 segment and preventing its normal gating movement[73,74]; evidently, this traps it in a position that permits activation but not fast inactivation. The IIIS4 and IVS4 segments are specifically immobilized in the outward position by fast inactivation, as has been detected by covalently incorporated fluorescent probes, arguing that their movement is coupled to the inactivation process.[75] Furthermore, the S4 segments in domain IV move more slowly than those in domains I to III, which is consistent with a role in coupling activation to inactivation.[54,76] Together, these results provide strong evidence that outward movement of the S4 segment in domain IV is the signal to initiate fast inactivation of the sodium channel by closure of the intracellular inactivation gate. The molecular mechanism for coupling of this movement of IVS4 to inactivation gate closure is an interesting subject for further investigation.

Slow Inactivation

In addition to the fast inactivation process discovered by Hodgkin and Huxley in their classic work,[1] a separate slow inactivation process operating on the time scale of 100 ms to seconds also terminates the Na+ influx through Na+ channels.[77] This process is engaged during the repetitive generation of action potentials in nerve and muscle cells and limits the length of high-frequency trains of repetitive action potentials. A slow inactivation process has been detected in bacterial Na+ channels whose structures have been determined,[78] even though their homotetrameric structure means these channels do not have a structural component analogous to the intracellular loop connecting domains III and IV of vertebrate channels, which mediates fast inactivation. The structure of the slow-inactivated bacterial Na+ channel reveals that the pore has partially collapsed as a result of the movement of two opposing S6 segments toward the central axis of the pore and corresponding movement of the two adjacent pairs of S6 segments away from the axis (Fig. 1.7).[79,80] This movement is observed at the selectivity filter at the extracellular end of the pore, in the central cavity, and at the activation gate at the intracellular end of the pore (see Fig. 1.7). This asymmetrical collapse of the pore is accompanied by a subtle rotation of the voltage-sensing domain around the cylindrical exterior surface of the pore domain (see Fig. 1.7). It is likely that this pore collapse is important for stabilization of the sodium channel in the inactivated state, which requires strong, long-duration hyperpolarization for recovery to the resting state.

Inner Pore and Local Anesthetic/ Antiarrhythmic Drug Receptor Site

Sodium channels are the molecular targets for drugs used in the control of cardiac arrhythmias as well as those used in local anesthesia, the prevention of acute pain, and the treatment of epilepsy and bipolar disorder. Sodium channel–blocking drugs are also in development for the treatment of chronic pain. These drugs bind to a specific receptor site within the pore of sodium channels formed by the S6 segments in domains I, III, and IV (Fig. 1.8).[9,81–85] This binding blocks ion movement through the pore and stabilizes the inactivated state of the sodium channels. Antiarrhythmic drugs and antiepileptic drugs share similar, overlapping receptor sites.[86,87] A complete block of sodium channels would be lethal. However, these drugs selectively block sodium channels in depolarized and/or rapidly firing cells, such as axons that carry high-intensity pain information and the rapidly firing nerve and cardiac muscle cells that drive epileptic seizures or cardiac arrhythmias.[86,88,89] This selective block arises because the drugs can reach their binding site in the pore of the sodium channel more rapidly when the pore is repetitively opened, and they bind with high affinity to inactivated sodium channels that are generated in rapidly firing or depolarized cells. The conformational change observed in the central cavity during slow inactivation may be responsible for the increased affinity for drug block of the inactivated state (see Fig. 1.7). This use-dependent action of the blocking drugs is essential for their therapeutic efficacy.

High affinity binding of local anesthetics to the inactivated state of sodium channels requires two critical amino acid residues that are located on the same side of the IVS6 transmembrane segment two alpha helical turns apart (see Fig. 1.8A, Phe1764 and Tyr1771 in *blue*; etidocaine in *red*).[81–85] It is likely that the tertiary amino group of local anesthetics interacts with Phe1764, which

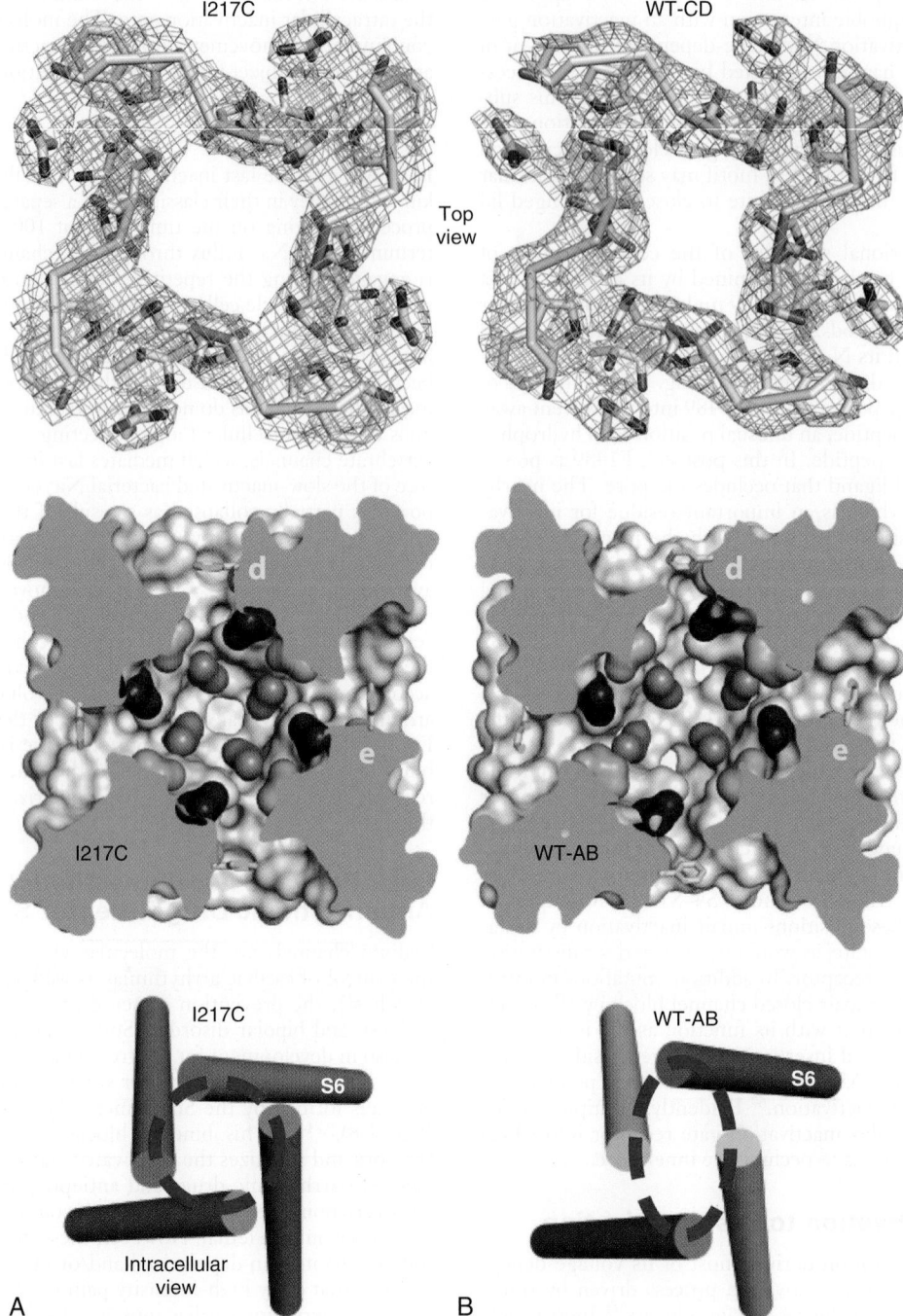

FIGURE 1.7 Structural basis for slow inactivation. (A) Structure of the functional elements of the pore in the pre-open state. *Top,* selectivity filter. *Middle,* central cavity with amino acid residues of the drug binding site shown in color. *Bottom,* activation gate. (B) Structure of the functional elements of the pore in the slow-inactivated state shown as in A. (Modified from Payandeh J, Gamal El-Din TM, Scheuer T, Zheng N, Catterall WA. Crystal structure of a voltage-gated sodium channel in two potentially inactivated states. *Nature.* 2012;486:135-139.)

is located more deeply in the pore, and that the aromatic moiety of the local anesthetics interacts with Tyr1771, which is located nearer to the intracellular end of the pore (see Fig. 1.8, *blue residues*). Subsequent work has shown that sodium channel blocking drugs of diverse structures that are used as antiarrhythmics or anticonvulsants interact with the same site as the local anesthetics but also undergo additional interactions with other nearby amino acid residues.[87,90–93]

In the structure of NavAb,[9] the amino acid residues that form the receptor sites for Na[+] channel blockers line the inner surface of the S6 segments and create a three-dimensional drug receptor site whose occupancy would block the pore (see Fig. 1.8B and C). Remarkably, fenestrations lead from the lipid phase of the membrane sideways into the drug receptor site, providing a hydrophobic access pathway for drug binding (see Fig. 1.8B and C). This form of drug binding from the membrane phase was

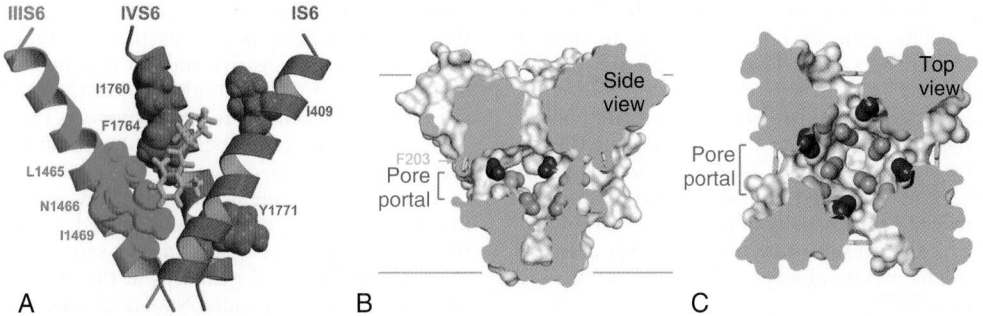

FIGURE 1.8 Drug binding in the central cavity. (A) Three-dimensional model of proposed orientation of amino acid residues within the Na+ channel pore with respect to the local anesthetic etidocaine. Only transmembrane segments IS6 *(red)*, IIIS6 *(green)*, and IVS6 *(blue)* are shown. Residues important for etidocaine binding are shown in space-filling representation. (B) Side-view through the pore module illustrating fenestrations (portals) and hydrophobic access to central cavity. Phe203 side-chains, *yellow sticks*. Surface representations of NavAb residues aligning with those implicated in drug binding and block, Thr206, *blue*; Met209, *green*; Val213, *orange*. Membrane boundaries, *gray lines*. Electron-density from an F_o-F_c omit map is contoured at 2.0 σ. (C) Top-view sectioned below the selectivity filter, colored as in (B). (Modified from Payandeh J, Scheuer T, Zheng N, Catterall WA. The crystal structure of a voltage-gated sodium channel. *Nature.* 2011;475:353-358.)

predicted in early studies of the mechanism of Na+ channel blocking by different local anesthetics.[2,88] Access to the drug-binding site in NavAb channels from the membrane phospholipid bilayer is limited by the side chain of a single amino acid residue (see Fig. 1.8B), which may control drug access and egress from the drug receptor site and possibly the entry and egress of physiological lipid modulators.

As well as being the target for these important pharmaceutical agents, sodium channels are also the molecular target for a large number of neurotoxins that paralyze prey by preventing neuromuscular function.[94,95] These toxins act at five or more distinct receptor sites and either block the pore of the channel or alter the kinetics or the voltage-dependence of gating. The pore blockers tetrodotoxin and saxitoxin bind to neurotoxin receptor site 1, which is formed by the P-loops in the four domains (see Fig. 1.2).

Sodium Channel Genes

Sodium channels are the founding members of the superfamily that includes the following ion channels: voltage-gated calcium channels; transient receptor potential channels; voltage-gated, inward rectifying, and two-pore-domain potassium channels; and the CNG (cyclic nucleotide-gated) and HCN (hyperpolarization-activated cyclic nucleotide-gated) channels.[96] In evolution, the four-domain sodium channel was last among the voltage-gated ion channels to appear, and it is only found in multicellular organisms. It is thought that sodium channels evolved via two rounds of gene duplication from ancestral single-domain bacterial sodium channels. Voltage-gated sodium channel genes are present in a variety of metazoan species including fly, leech, squid, and jellyfish. The biophysical properties, pharmacology, gene organization, and even intron-splice sites of these invertebrate sodium channels are largely similar to those of mammals.

Ten related sodium channel genes are found in vertebrates, of which nine encode voltage-gated sodium channels (Fig. 1.9).[96,97] More than 20 exons comprise each of the sodium channel α-subunit genes in mammals. Genes encoding sodium channels $Na_V1.1$, $Na_V1.2$, $Na_V1.3$, and $Na_V1.7$ are localized on chromosome 2 in humans, and these channels share similarities in sequence, biophysical characteristics, blocking by nanomolar concentrations of tetrodotoxin, and broad expression in neurons. A second cluster of genes encoding $Na_V1.5$, $Na_V1.8$, and $Na_V1.9$ channels is localized on human chromosome 3p21-24.

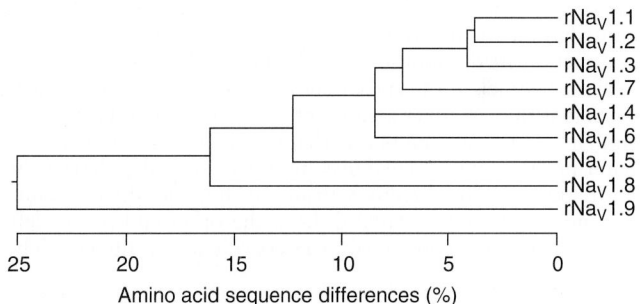

FIGURE 1.9 Amino acid sequence similarity of voltage-gated sodium channel α-subunits. A comparison of amino acid identity for rat sodium channels Nav1.1 to Nav1.9. The comparison was performed with Megalign in the program DNAStar (utilizing the Clustal method) for the four domains and the cytoplasmic linker connecting domains III and IV. (Modified from Catterall WA. From ionic currents to molecular mechanisms: the structure and function of voltage-gated sodium channels. *Neuron.* 2000;26:13-25.)

Although these sodium channels have amino acid sequences that are more than 75% identical to those of the group of channels on chromosome 2, they all contain amino acid substitutions that confer varying degrees of resistance to the pore blocker tetrodotoxin. In $Na_V1.5$, the principal cardiac isoform,[98] a single amino acid change from phenylalanine to cysteine in the pore region of domain I is responsible for a 200-fold reduction in tetrodotoxin sensitivity compared to that of the channels on chromosome 2.[99] At an identical position in $Na_V1.8$ and $Na_V1.9$, the amino acid residue is serine, and this difference results in even greater resistance to tetrodotoxin.[100] These two channels are primarily expressed in peripheral sensory neurons. In comparison to the sodium channel on chromosomes 2 and 3, $Na_V1.4$, which is expressed in skeletal muscle, and $Na_V1.6$, which is highly abundant in the central nervous system, have more than 85% sequence identity and similar functional properties, including sensitivity to tetrodotoxin in the nanomolar concentration range. A tenth sodium channel, Na_x, whose gene is located near those of the sodium channels on chromosome 2, is evolutionarily more distant.[97] It has key differences in functionally important regions of the voltage sensor and inactivation gate. It is likely that this unusual sodium channel responds to the extracellular sodium concentration and is involved in the regulation of plasma salt levels.[101]

In mammals, the Na$_V$β-subunits are encoded by four distinct genes.[10,11,25,26] The gene encoding β1 maps to human chromosome 19q13, whereas those for β2 and β4 are located on chromosome 11q22-23 and that for β3 is located nearby on chromosome 11q24. The β1- and β3-subunits associate noncovalently with the α-subunits, whereas those for β2 and β4 are covalently linked by a disulfide bond. These distinct modes of association and the corresponding similarities in amino acid sequence suggest that the similar pairs of β-subunits (β1 and β3 vs. β2 and β4) may be able to substitute for each other in interactions with sodium channel α-subunits. All four β-subunits are expressed in the heart.[102,103]

Although Na$_V$1.5 channels are primarily expressed in the heart and are often termed the *cardiac* sodium channel,[98] several of the *brain* sodium channel subtypes are also expressed at lower levels in the heart, where they are differentially localized in subcellular compartments in cell-specific and species-specific patterns. In rodents, the Na$_V$1.5 channel is highly concentrated at intercalated disks.[104–106] Small but significant levels of Na$_V$1.1 channels are present in the transverse tubules, and Na$_V$1.4 and Na$_V$1.6 channels have been detected in the cell surface membrane of ventricular myocytes.[102,105,106] The densities of these tetrodotoxin-sensitive sodium channel isoforms are in the range of 3% to 8% of Na$_V$1.5,[106] but they make a significant contribution to the coupling of cell-surface depolarization to contraction in the mouse heart.[105] The high concentration of sodium channels at the ends of mouse ventricular myocytes suggests that they conduct action potentials in a saltatory manner, similar to a myelinated nerve; that is, the large sodium current entering at the intercalated disk instantaneously depolarizes the entire myocyte and directly activates the high density of sodium channels at the intercalated disks at the other end of the cell, rather than being conducted progressively across the cell. The instantaneous depolarization of the entire cell surface would then initiate action potentials in the t-tubules conducted by the tetrodotoxin-sensitive sodium channels there. This altered mode of initiation and conduction of the cardiac action potential may be a specialization that supports the rapid beating rate of the mouse heart (600 beats/min) without loss of synchrony or force of contraction.

In contrast to rodent ventricular myocytes, Na$_V$1.5 channels in human atrial myocytes are localized in a striated pattern on the cell surface at the z-lines in each sarcomere, whereas Na$_V$1.2 channels are localized primarily at the intercalated disks, but at a lower concentration, and Na$_V$1.1 channels are localized at low density in a scattered punctate pattern over the cell surface.[107] As all of the *brain* and *skeletal muscle* sodium channel subtypes are inhibited by nanomolar concentrations of tetrodotoxin, whereas Na$_V$1.5 channels require micromolar concentrations of tetrodotoxin for inhibition, the contribution of the tetrodotoxin-sensitive sodium channels to cardiac contractility can be tested in careful dose-response experiments. Such experiments have indicated that 12% to 27% of the sodium current is conducted by the tetrodotoxin-sensitive sodium channels and that blocking of these channels reduces the amplitude and velocity of contraction of atrial muscle strips by approximately 15%.[107] The differential localization of these subtypes suggests specific functions for the Na$_V$1.2 channels in the initiation of the action potential at intercalated disks in atrial myocytes and for the Na$_V$1.5 channels in depolarizing the atrial membrane near the voltage-gated calcium channels at the z-lines in order to efficiently initiate excitation–contraction coupling. It is important to determine the distribution of sodium channel subtypes in human ventricular myocytes, but the low availability of fresh human ventricular tissue from healthy individuals presents difficulties for these experiments.

REFERENCES

1. Hodgkin AL, Huxley AF. A quantitative description of membrane current and its application to conduction and excitation in nerve. *J Physiol*. 1952;117:500–544.
2. Hille B. *Ionic Channels of Excitable Membranes*. 3rd ed. Sunderland, MA: Sinauer Associates Inc.; 2001.
3. Catterall WA. From ionic currents to molecular mechanisms: the structure and function of voltage-gated sodium channels. *Neuron*. 2000;26:13–25.
4. Catterall WA. The molecular basis of neuronal excitability. *Science*. 1984;223:653–661.
5. Hartshorne RP, Keller BU, Talvenheimo JA, Catterall WA, Montal M. Functional reconstitution of the purified brain sodium channel in planar lipid bilayers. *Proc Natl Acad Sci U S A*. 1985;82:240–244.
6. Numa S, Noda M. Molecular structure of sodium channels. *Ann N Y Acad Sci*. 1986;479:338–355.
7. Guy HR, Seetharamulu P. Molecular model of the action potential sodium channel. *Proc Natl Acad Sci U S A*. 1986;83:508–512.
8. Catterall WA. Molecular properties of voltage-sensitive sodium channels. *Annu Rev Biochem*. 1986;55:953–985.
9. Payandeh J, Scheuer T, Zheng N, Catterall WA. The crystal structure of a voltage-gated sodium channel. *Nature*. 2011;475:353–358.
10. Isom LL, De Jongh KS, Patton DE, et al. Primary structure and functional expression of the β1 subunit of the rat brain sodium channel. *Science*. 1992;256:839–842.
11. Isom LL, Ragsdale DS, De Jongh KS, et al. Structure and function of the β2 subunit of brain sodium channels, a transmembrane glycoprotein with a CAM motif. *Cell*. 1995;83:433–442.
12. McCormick KA, Isom LL, Ragsdale D, Smith D, Scheuer T, Catterall WA. Molecular determinants of Na$^+$ channel function in the extracellular domain of the beta1 subunit. *J Biol Chem*. 1998;273:3954–3962.
13. McCormick KA, Srinivasan J, White K, Scheuer T, Catterall WA. The extracellular domain of the β1 subunit is both necessary and sufficient for β1-like modulation of sodium channel gating. *J Biol Chem*. 1999;274:32638–32646.
14. Srinivasan J, Schachner M, Catterall WA. Interaction of voltage-gated sodium channels with the extracellular matrix molecules tenascin-C and tenascin-R. *Proc Natl Acad Sci U S A*. 1998;95:15753–15757.
15. Xiao ZC, Ragsdale DS, Malhotra JD, et al. Tenascin-R is a functional modulator of sodium channel β subunits. *J Biol Chem*. 1999;274:26511–26517.
16. Ratcliffe CF, Qu Y, McCormick KA, et al. A sodium channel signaling complex: modulation by associated receptor protein tyrosine phosphatase β. *Nat Neurosci*. 2000;3:437–444.
17. Ratcliffe CF, Westenbroek RE, Curtis R, Catterall WA. Sodium channel β1 and β3 subunits associate with neurofascin through their extracellular immunoglobulin-like domain. *J Cell Biol*. 2001;154:427–434.
18. Kazarinova-Noyes K, Malhotra JD, McEwen DP, et al. Contactin associates with sodium channels and increases their functional expression. *J Neurosci*. 2001;21:7517–7525.
19. Malhotra JD, Koopmann MC, Kazen-Gillespie KA, Fettman N, Hortsch M, Isom LL. Structural requirements for interaction of sodium channel β1 subunits with ankyrin. *J Biol Chem*. 2002;277:26681–26688.
20. Malhotra JD, Kazen-Gillespie K, Hortsch M, Isom LL. Sodium channel β subunits mediate homophilic cell adhesion and recruit ankyrin to points of cell-cell contact. *J Biol Chem*. 2000;275:11383–11388.
21. Chen C, Bharucha V, Chen Y, et al. Reduced sodium channel density, altered voltage dependence of inactivation, and increased susceptibility to seizures in mice lacking sodium channel β2-subunits. *Proc Natl Acad Sci U S A*. 2002;99:17072–17077.
22. Chen C, Westenbroek RE, Xu X, et al. Mice lacking sodium channel β1 subunits display defects in neuronal excitability, sodium channel expression, and nodal architecture. *J Neurosci*. 2004;24:4030–4042.
23. Lopez-Santiago LF, Meadows LS, Ernst SJ, et al. Sodium channel Scn1b null mice exhibit prolonged QT and RR intervals. *J Mol Cell Cardiol*. 2007;43:636–647.
24. Catterall WA, Zheng N. Deciphering voltage-gated Na$^+$ and Ca^{2+} channels by studying prokaryotic ancestors. *Trends Biochem Sci*. 2015;40:526–534.
25. Morgan K, Stevens EB, Shah B, et al. β3: An additional auxiliary subunit of the voltage-sensitive sodium channel that modulates channel gating with distinct kinetics. *Proc Natl Acad Sci U S A*. 2000;97:2308–2313.
26. Yu FH, Westenbroek RE, Silos-Santiago I, et al. Sodium channel β4, a new disulfide-linked auxiliary subunit with similarity to β2. *J Neurosci*. 2003;23:7577–7585.
27. Shapiro L, Doyle JP, Hensley P, Colman DR, Hendrickson WA. Crystal structure of the extracellular domain from Po, the major structural protein of peripheral nerve myelin. *Neuron*. 1996;17:435–449.
28. Gilchrist J, Das S, Van Petegem F, Bosmans F. Crystallographic insights into sodium-channel modulation by the β4 subunit. *Proc Natl Acad Sci U S A*. 2013;110:E5016–5024.
29. Namadurai S, Balasuriya D, Rajappa R, et al. Crystal structure and molecular imaging of the Nav channel β3 subunit indicates a trimeric assembly. *J Biol Chem*. 2014;289:10797–10811.
30. Brackenbury WJ, Isom LL. Na channel β subunits: overachievers of the ion channel family. *Front Pharmacol*. 2011;2:53.
31. Armstrong CM. Sodium channels and gating currents. *Physiol Rev*. 1981;61:644–683.
32. Hille B. The permeability of the sodium channel to metal cations in myelinated nerve. *J Gen Physiol*. 1972;59:637–658.
33. Hille B. Ionic selectivity, saturation, and block in sodium channels. A four-barrier model. *J Gen Physiol*. 1975;66:535–560.
34. Hille B. The receptor for tetrodotoxin and saxitoxin. A structural hypothesis. *Biophys J*. 1975;15:615–619.
35. Noda M, Suzuki H, Numa S, Stuhmer W. A single point mutation confers tetrodotoxin and saxitoxin insensitivity on the sodium channel II. *FEBS Lett*. 1989;259:213–216.
36. Terlau H, Heinemann SH, Stuhmer W, et al. Mapping the site of block by tetrodotoxin and saxitoxin of sodium channel II. *FEBS Lett*. 1991;293:93–96.

37. Lipkind GM, Fozzard HA. A structural model of the tetrodotoxin and saxitoxin binding site of the Na+ channel. *Biophys J.* 1994;66:1–13.
38. Penzotti JL, Fozzard HA, Lipkind GM, Dudley Jr SC. Differences in saxitoxin and tetrodotoxin binding revealed by mutagenesis of the Na+ channel outer vestibule. *Biophys J.* 1998;75:2647–2657.
39. Heinemann SH, Terlau H, Stuhmer W, Imoto K, Numa S. Calcium channel characteristics conferred on the sodium channel by single mutations. *Nature.* 1992;356:441–443.
40. Chiamvimonvat N, O'Rourke B, Kamp TJ, et al. Functional consequences of sulfhydryl modification in the pore-forming subunits of cardiovascular Ca2+ and Na+ channels. *Circ Res.* 1995;76:325–334.
41. Perez-Garcia MT, Chiamvimonvat N, Marban E, Tomaselli GF. Structure of the sodium channel pore revealed by serial cysteine mutagenesis. *Proc Natl Acad Sci U S A.* 1996;93:300–304.
42. Schlief T, Schonherr R, Imoto K, Heinemann SH. Pore properties of rat brain II sodium channels mutated in the selectivity filter domain. *Eur Biophys J.* 1996;25:75–91.
43. Sun YM, Favre I, Schild L, Moczydlowski E. On the structural basis for size-selective permeation of organic cations through the voltage-gated sodium channel. Effect of alanine mutations at the DEKA locus on selectivity, inhibition by Ca2+ and H+, and molecular sieving. *J Gen Physiol.* 1997;110:693–715.
44. Chakrabarti N, Ing C, Payandeh J, Zheng N, Catterall WA, Pomes R. Catalysis of Na+ permeation in the bacterial sodium channel Na$_V$Ab. *Proc Natl Acad Sci U S A.* 2013;110:11331–11336.
45. Hirschberg B, Rovner A, Lieberman M, Patlak J. Transfer of twelve charges is needed to open skeletal muscle Na+ channels. *J Gen Physiol.* 1995;106:1053–1068.
46. Stuhmer W, Conti F, Suzuki H, et al. Structural parts involved in activation and inactivation of the sodium channel. *Nature.* 1989;339:597–603.
47. Yang N, George Jr AL, Horn R. Molecular basis of charge movement in voltage-gated sodium channels. *Neuron.* 1996;16:113–122.
48. Yang N, Horn R. Evidence for voltage-dependent S4 movement in sodium channel. *Neuron.* 1995;15:213–218.
49. Catterall WA. Ion channel voltage sensors: structure, function, and pathophysiology. *Neuron.* 2010;67:915–928.
50. DeCaen PG, Yarov-Yarovoy V, Zhao Y, Scheuer T, Catterall WA. Disulfide locking a sodium channel voltage sensor reveals ion pair formation during activation. *Proc Natl Acad Sci U S A.* 2008;105:15142–15147.
51. DeCaen PG, Yarov-Yarovoy V, Sharp EM, Scheuer T, Catterall WA. Sequential formation of ion pairs during activation of a sodium channel voltage sensor. *Proc Natl Acad Sci U S A.* 2009;106:22498–22503.
52. DeCaen PG, Yarov-Yarovoy V, Scheuer T, Catterall WA. Gating charge interactions with the S1 segment during activation of a Na+ channel voltage sensor. *Proc Natl Acad Sci U S A.* 2011;108:18825–18830.
53. Yarov-Yarovoy V, DeCaen PG, Westenbroek RE, et al. Structural basis for gating charge movement in the voltage sensor of a sodium channel. *Proc Natl Acad Sci U S A.* 2012;109:E93–102.
54. Chanda B, Bezanilla F. Tracking voltage-dependent conformational changes in skeletal muscle sodium channel during activation. *J Gen Physiol.* 2002;120:629–645.
55. Jiang Y, Lee A, Chen J, Cadene M, Chait BT, MacKinnon R. Crystal structure and mechanism of a calcium-gated potassium channel. *Nature.* 2002;417:515–522.
56. Jiang Y, Lee A, Chen J, Cadene M, Chait BT, MacKinnon R. The open pore conformation of potassium channels. *Nature.* 2002;417:523–526.
57. Zhao Y, Yarov-Yarovoy V, Scheuer T, Catterall WA. A gating hinge in Na+ channels; a molecular switch for electrical signaling. *Neuron.* 2004;41:859–865.
58. Vassilev P, Scheuer T, Catterall WA. Inhibition of inactivation of single sodium channels by a site-directed antibody. *Proc Natl Acad Sci U S A.* 1989;86:8147–8151.
59. Vassilev PM, Scheuer T, Catterall WA. Identification of an intracellular peptide segment involved in sodium channel inactivation. *Science.* 1998;241:1658–1661.
60. West JW, Patton DE, Scheuer T, Wang Y, Goldin AL, Catterall WA. A cluster of hydrophobic amino acid residues required for fast Na+-channel inactivation. *Proc Natl Acad Sci U S A.* 1992;89:10910–10914.

61. Eaholtz G, Scheuer T, Catterall WA. Restoration of inactivation and block of open sodium channels by an inactivation gate peptide. *Neuron.* 1994;12:1041–1048.
62. Kellenberger S, West JW, Scheuer T, Catterall WA. Molecular analysis of the putative inactivation particle in the inactivation gate of brain type IIA Na+ channels. *J Gen Physiol.* 1997;109:589–605.
63. Kellenberger S, Scheuer T, Catterall WA. Movement of the Na+ channel inactivation gate during inactivation. *J Biol Chem.* 1996;271:30971–30979.
64. Kellenberger S, West JW, Catterall WA, Scheuer T. Molecular analysis of potential hinge residues in the inactivation gate of brain type IIA Na+ channels. *J Gen Physiol.* 1997;109:607–617.
65. Rohl CA, Boeckman FA, Baker C, Scheuer T, Catterall WA, Klevit RE. Solution structure of the sodium channel inactivation gate. *Biochemistry.* 1999;38:855–861.
66. McPhee JC, Ragsdale DS, Scheuer T, Catterall WA. A critical role for transmembrane segment IVS6 of the sodium channel α subunit in fast inactivation. *J Biol Chem.* 1995;270:12025–12034.
67. Smith MR, Goldin AL. Interaction between the sodium channel inactivation linker and domain III S4-S5. *Biophys J.* 1997;73:1885–1895.
68. Lerche H, Peter W, Fleischhauer R, et al. Role in fast inactivation of the IV/S4-S5 loop of the human muscle Na+ channel probed by cysteine mutagenesis. *J Physiol.* 1997;505(pt 2):345–352.
69. McPhee JC, Ragsdale DS, Scheuer T, Catterall WA. A critical role for the S4-S5 intracellular loop in domain IV of the sodium channel α-subunit in fast inactivation. *J Biol Chem.* 1998;273:1121–1129.
70. Tang LH, Chehab N, Wieland SJ, Kallen RG. Glutamine substitution at Alanine1649 in the S4-S5 cytoplasmic loop of domain 4 removes the voltage sensitivity of fast inactivation in the human heart sodium channel. *J Gen Physiol.* 1998;111:639–652.
71. Filatov GN, Nguyen TP, Kraner SD, Barchi RL. Inactivation and secondary structure in the D4/S4-5 region of the SkM1 sodium channel. *J Gen Physiol.* 1998;111:703–715.
72. Chen LQ, Santarelli V, Horn R, Kallen RG. A unique role for the S4 segment of domain 4 in the inactivation of sodium channels. *J Gen Physiol.* 1996;108:549–556.
73. Rogers JC, Qu Y, Tanada TN, Scheuer T, Catterall WA. Molecular determinants of high affinity binding of α scorpion toxin and sea anemone toxin in the S3-S4 extracellular loop in domain IV of the Na+ channel α subunit. *J Biol Chem.* 1996;271:15950–15962.
74. Sheets MF, Kyle JW, Kallen RG, Hanck DA. The Na channel voltage sensor associated with inactivation is localized to the external charged residues of domain IV, S4. *Biophys J.* 1999;77:747–757.
75. Cha A, Ruben PC, George AL, Fujimoto E, Bezanilla F. Voltage sensors in domains III and IV, but not I and II, are immobilized by Na+ channel fast inactivation. *Neuron.* 1999;22:73–87.
76. Capes DL, Goldschen-Ohm MP, Arcisio-Miranda M, Bezanilla F, Chanda B. Domain IV voltage-sensor movement is both sufficient and rate limiting for fast inactivation in sodium channels. *J Gen Physiol.* 2013;142:101–112.
77. Rudy B. Slow inactivation of the sodium conductance in squid giant axons. Pronase resistance. *J Physiol.* 1978;283:1–21.
78. Pavlov E, Bladen C, Winkfein R, Diao C, Dhaliwal P, French RJ. The pore, not cytoplasmic domains, underlies inactivation in a prokaryotic sodium channel. *Biophys J.* 2005;89:232–242.
79. Payandeh J, Gamal El-Din TM, Scheuer T, Zheng N, Catterall WA. Crystal structure of a voltage-gated sodium channel in two potentially inactivated states. *Nature.* 2012;486:135–139.
80. Zhang X, Ren W, DeCaen P, et al. Crystal structure of an orthologue of the NaChBac voltage-gated sodium channel. *Nature.* 2012;486:130–134.
81. Ragsdale DS, McPhee JC, Scheuer T, Catterall WA. Molecular determinants of state-dependent block of sodium channels by local anesthetics. *Science.* 1994;265:1724–1728.
82. Liu G, Yarov-Yarovoy V, Nobbs M, Clare JJ, Scheuer T, Catterall WA. Differential interactions of lamotrigine and related drugs with transmembrane segment IVS6 of voltage-gated sodium channels. *Neuropharmacology.* 2003;44:413–422.
83. Yarov-Yarovoy V, Brown J, Sharp EM, Clare JJ, Scheuer T, Catterall WA. Molecular determinants of voltage-dependent gating and binding of pore-blocking drugs in transmembrane segment IIIS6 of the Na+ channel α subunit. *J Biol Chem.* 2001;276:20–27.

84. Yarov-Yarovoy V, McPhee JC, Idsvoog D, Pate C, Scheuer T, Catterall WA. Role of amino acid residues in transmembrane segments IS6 and IIS6 of the Na+ channel α subunit in voltage-dependent gating and drug block. *J Biol Chem.* 2002;277:35393–35401.
85. Catterall WA, Swanson TM. Structural basis for pharmacology of voltage-gated sodium and calcium channels. *Mol Pharmacol.* 2015;88:141–150.
86. Catterall WA. Common-modes of drug-action on Na+ channels - local-anesthetics, antiarrhythmics and anticonvulsants. *Trends Pharmacol Sci.* 1987;8:57–65.
87. Ragsdale DS, McPhee JC, Scheuer T, Catterall WA. Common molecular determinants of local anesthetic, antiarrhythmic, and anticonvulsant block of voltage-gated Na+ channels. *Proc Natl Acad Sci U S A.* 1996;93:9270–9275.
88. Hille B. Local anesthetics: hydrophilic and hydrophobic pathways for the drug-receptor reaction. *J Gen Physiol.* 1977;69:497–515.
89. Hondeghem LM, Katzung BG. Time- and voltage-dependent interactions of antiarrhythmic drugs with cardiac sodium channels. *Biochim et Biophys Acta.* 1977;472:373–398.
90. Wright SN, Wang SY, Wang GK. Lysine point mutations in Na+ channel D4-S6 reduce inactivated channel block by local anesthetics. *Mol Pharmacol.* 1998;54:733–739.
91. Nau C, Wang SY, Wang GK. Point mutations at L1280 in Na$_V$1.4 channel D3-S6 modulate binding affinity and stereoselectivity of bupivacaine enantiomers. *Mol Pharmacol.* 2003;63:1398–1406.
92. Weiser T, Qu Y, Catterall WA, Scheuer T. Differential interaction of R-mexiletine with the local anesthetic receptor site on brain and heart sodium channel α-subunits. *Mol Pharmacol.* 1999;56:1238–1244.
93. Lipkind GM, Fozzard HA. Molecular modeling of local anesthetic drug binding by voltage-gated sodium channels. *Mol Pharmacol.* 2005;68:1611–1622.
94. Cestele S, Catterall WA. Molecular mechanisms of neurotoxin action on voltage-gated sodium channels. *Biochimie.* 2000;82:883–892.
95. Catterall WA, Cestele S, Yarov-Yarovoy V, Yu FH, Konoki K, Scheuer T. Voltage-gated ion channels and gating modifier toxins. *Toxicon.* 2007;49:124–141.
96. Yu FH, Catterall WA. The VGL-chanome: a protein superfamily specialized for electrical signaling and ionic homeostasis. *Sci STKE.* 2004:2004. re15.
97. Goldin AL, Barchi RL, Caldwell JH, et al. Nomenclature of voltage-gated sodium channels. *Neuron.* 2000;28:365–368.
98. Rogart RB, Cribbs LL, Muglia LK, Kephart DD, Kaiser MW. Molecular cloning of a putative tetrodotoxin-resistant rat heart Na+ channel isoform. *Proc Natl Acad Sci U S A.* 1989;86:8170–8174.
99. Satin J, Kyle JW, Chen M, et al. A mutant of TTX-resistant cardiac sodium channels with TTX-sensitive properties. *Science.* 1992;256:1202–1205.
100. Sivilotti L, Okuse K, Akopian AN, Moss S, Wood JN. A single serine residue confers tetrodotoxin insensitivity on the rat sensory-neuron-specific sodium channel SNS. *FEBS Lett.* 1997;409:49–52.
101. Noda M, Hiyama TY. The Na$_X$ channel: what it is and what it does. *Neuroscientist.* 2015;21:399–412.
102. Maier SK, Westenbroek RE, McCormick KA, Curtis R, Scheuer T, Catterall WA. Distinct subcellular localization of different sodium channel α and β subunits in single ventricular myocytes from mouse heart. *Circulation.* 2004;109:1421–1427.
103. Malhotra JD, Chen C, Rivolta I, et al. Characterization of sodium channel α and β subunits in rat and mouse cardiac myocytes. *Circulation.* 2001;103:1303–1310.
104. Cohen SA. Immunocytochemical localization of rH1 sodium channel in adult rat heart atria and ventricle. Presence in terminal intercalated disks. *Circulation.* 1996;94:3083–3086.
105. Maier SK, Westenbroek RE, Schenkman KA, Feigl EO, Scheuer T, Catterall WA. An unexpected role for brain-type sodium channels in coupling of cell surface depolarization to contraction in the heart. *Proc Natl Acad Sci U S A.* 2001;99:4073–4078.
106. Westenbroek RE, Bischoff S, Fu Y, Maier SK, Catterall WA, Scheuer T. Localization of sodium channel subtypes in mouse ventricular myocytes using quantitative immunocytochemistry. *J Mol Cell Cardiol.* 2013;64:69–78.
107. Kaufmann SG, Westenbroek RE, Maass AH, et al. Distribution and function of sodium channel subtypes in human atrial myocardium. *J Mol Cell Cardiol.* 2013;61:133–141.

2 Voltage-Gated Calcium Channels

Alexander Kushnir and Steven O. Marx

In the heart, the influx of Ca^{2+}, acting as a multidimensional signaling molecule, is essential for the activation of excitation–contraction coupling (E–C coupling), and also contributes to the plateau phase of the cardiac action potential, pacemaker activity in nodal cells, and the modulation of cellular processes (gene expression). The major pathway for the entry of Ca^{2+} ion into excitable cells is through voltage-gated Ca^{2+} channels. Thus voltage-gated Ca^{2+} channels are empowered to transduce membrane depolarization into cellular functions. Dysfunctions of Ca^{2+} channels have been associated with cardiac diseases.

Electrophysiological and pharmacological studies have defined six classes of voltage-gated Ca^{2+} channels: T-, L-, N-, P-, Q-, and R-type. These channel classes can be grouped by low membrane voltage activation (LVA) versus high membrane voltage activation (HVA), susceptibility to pharmacological antagonists, and rate of inactivation (Table 2.1[1-14]). Of these six classes of Ca^{2+} channels, only the long-lasting (L)-type and transient (T)-type Ca^{2+} channels are expressed in cardiomyocyte cells. Additionally, several nonvoltage-gated Ca^{2+} permeable transient receptor potential (TRP) channels are expressed in the heart.[198] In this chapter, we will review the roles of these ion channels in the function of the heart in health and disease.

Molecular Composition of Voltage-Gated Ca²⁺ Channels

Voltage-gated Ca^{2+} channels are multimers comprised of a core α_1 pore-forming subunit and several auxiliary subunits including β, $\alpha_{2\delta}$, and γ (Fig. 2.1A[17-25]). The α_1-subunit contains binding sites for most regulators and drugs, whereas the β-, $\alpha_{2\delta}$-, and γ-subunits contribute to trafficking, anchorage, and regulatory functions.[26] To date, ten α_1-subunit isoforms exhibiting diverse electrophysiological properties and response to drugs have been identified. In Ca^{2+} channel nomenclature, the chemical symbol of calcium, Ca, is followed by the subscript "V," which denotes voltage as the primary regulator and two numerical identifiers corresponding to the α_1-subunit gene subfamily and the order of discovery within that subfamily, respectively.[27,28] Sequence alignment suggests that gene duplication and divergence of an ancestral Ca^{2+} channel gene gave rise to the LVA and HVA subfamilies (see Fig. 2.1B). The Ca_V1 and Ca_V2 subfamilies arose more than 500 million years ago through duplication of the HVA gene. Four Ca_V1 genes, three Ca_V2 genes, and three Ca_V3 genes arose within these subfamilies. The amino acid sequences of these α_1-subunits are more than 70% identical within a family, but less than 40% identical among families.

$Ca_V1.1$, $Ca_V1.2$, $Ca_V1.3$, and $Ca_V1.4$ exhibit relatively long-lasting currents and are referred to as L-type Ca^{2+} channels. Relative to the L-type Ca^{2+} channels, $Ca_V3.1$, $Ca_V3.2$, and $Ca_V3.3$ exhibit transient Ca^{2+} currents and are activated at more negative potentials (see Table 2.1). These channels, known as T-type Ca^{2+} channels, contribute to automaticity and are predominantly expressed in the sinoatrial node, atrioventricular node, and in the Purkinje fiber network.[29] $Ca_V2.1$, $Ca_V2.2$, and $Ca_V2.3$, also known as P/Q-type, N-type, and R-type Ca^{2+} channels, respectively, are predominantly expressed in nerve terminals, dendrites, and neuronal cell bodies and are characterized by their response to specific pharmacological antagonists, including snake and spider toxins.[27,30]

The α_1-subunit, which contains approximately 2000 amino acid residues, is organized into four repeated domains (I to IV), each of which contains six transmembrane segments (S1 to S6) with a pore between S5 and S6 (Fig. 2.1A), similar to the Na^+ channel α-subunit.[31] The alternating positively charged arginine or lysine residues at every third or fourth position in S4 of each domain regulate voltage sensitivity. Four negatively charged glutamate residues on the pore loop located between S5 and S6 are responsible for the Ca^{2+} selectivity of the channels. Remarkably, the selectivity for Ca^{2+} can be changed to Na^+ by the mutation of only three amino acids in the pore loops of domains I, III, and IV. The pore region also contains overlapping binding sites for all major L-type Ca^{2+} channel blocking agents including dihydropyridines, phenylalkylamines, and benzothiazepines.[32] The α_{1C} C-terminus contains several protein-protein interaction motifs (see Fig. 2.1A), and their roles in regulating $Ca_V1.2$ trafficking and function in cardiomyocytes will be reviewed. The human α_{1C}-gene contains 50 exons with extensive alternative splicing.[33-35] This contributes to both gene regulation and protein diversity. For instance, $Ca_V1.2b$, the smooth muscle splice variant, is more sensitive to inhibition by dihydropyridines than $Ca_V1.2a$, the heart variant, since it contains the dihydropyridine-sensitive exon 8B.[36]

In the heart, α_{1C} exists as a 240- or 210-kDa protein depending on the extent of C-terminus truncation by posttranslational proteolytic processing. In cardiomyocytes, proteolytic cleavage of the α_{1C} C-terminus occurs in >80% of cardiac channels.[22,24,37,38] The cleaved fragment is believed to noncovalently reassemble with the truncated α_{1C} and to regulate the $Ca_V1.2$ channel function by acting as an inhibitor of channel functions.[21,39,40] Proteolytic processing has been proposed to occur via an unidentified protease at α_{1C} Ala^{1800} (see Fig. 2.1A),[24] although this is not recapitulated in heterologous expression systems.[41] In heterologous expression studies, the truncation of the α_{1C} C-terminus at residue 1821 exhibited a 2.9-fold increase in current at +10 mV compared to full-length (see Fig. 2.1C),[39,42,43] and the truncation at residue 1905 moderately reduced the $Ca_V1.2$ surface expression by ~30%, but significantly enhanced single-channel open probability (P_o).[43,44] By contrast, knock-in mice that were truncated either at Gly^{1796} or Asp^{1904} displayed a dramatic reduction in $Ca_V1.2$ surface expression and current in cardiomyocytes, and displayed cardiac failure and perinatal death.[40,45] Surprisingly, the $Ca_V1.2$ expression and function in the vascular smooth muscle were relatively unaffected in the knock-in mice, suggesting a cardiomyocyte-specific role for the α_{1C} distal C-terminus in the trafficking and regulation of $Ca_V1.2$.

The amino acid sequences of the $Ca_V\beta$ subunits, which are encoded by four β-subunit genes (Ca_V β 1-4), differ considerably. Among the β-subunits, the guanylate kinase (GK) domain, and Src-homology 3 (SH3) domain are very similar, whereas the N-termini (variable region 1), the linker between SH3 and GK

TABLE 2.1 Voltage-gated Ca²⁺ channel properties

ISOFORM	TYPE	GENE	LOCALIZATION	ANTAGONISTS	ACTIVATION THRESHOLD IN mV	V$_{50}$ ACTIVATION IN mV	V$_{50}$ INACTIVATION IN mV	τ ACTIVATION IN ms	τ INACTIVATION IN ms	PEAK OF I–V IN mV	CONDUCTANCE Ba²⁺ IN pS	REFERENCES
Ca$_v$1.1	L	*CACNA1S*	Skeletal muscle	DHP, PLK, BNZ	~20 (M)	8 to 14 (M)	−8 (M)	60 to 67 (M)	—	~30 (M)	14 (M)	1–4
Ca$_v$1.2	L	*CACNA1C*	Heart, CNS, smooth muscle, adrenal gland, pancreas, kidney, cochlea	DHP, PLK, BNZ	~20 (H)	−6 to −0.1 (H)	−28.5 to −18.4 (H)	5.2 to 7.1 (H)	9.1 to 21.1 (τ$_{fast}$), 60.9 to 133 (τ$_{slow}$) (H)	~10 (M)	25 (GP)	1,2,5,246–250
Ca$_v$1.3	L	*CACNA1D*	Heart, CNS, kidney, adrenal gland, pancreas, lung, testis, cochlea	DHP, PLK, BNZ	~40 (R)	−20.2 to −2.2 (H)	−42.7 (H)	0.5 to 2.5 (H)	3.8 to 74 (H)	~10 (R)	15 (H)	1,2,6,248,250–253
Ca$_v$1.4	L	*CACNA1F*	Retina	Unknown	~40 (H)	−11.6 to 0.6 (H)	−9.3 (H)	0.4 (τ$_{fast}$) to 6.6 (τ$_{slow}$) (H)	9.8 (H)	~10 (H)	4 (H)	1,2,7,8
Ca$_v$2.1	P/Q	*CACNA1A*	CNS, smooth muscle, pancreas, cochlea	ω-agatoxin IVA	~40 (H)	9.5 (H)	−17 (H)	0.6 to 2.2 (H)	148 to 690 (H)	~10 (H)	16.3 to 19.6 (H)	1,2,9,248,250,254
Ca$_v$2.2	N	*CACNA1B*	CNS, pancreas	ω-conotoxin-GVIA	~35 (H)	9 to 18.1 (H)	−59.4 to −53 (H)	0.93 (R)	46 to 105 (τ$_{fast}$), 291 to 453 (τ$_{slow}$) (H)	~10 (H)	19 (H)	1,2,10,248
Ca$_v$2.3	R	*CACNA1E*	CNS, heart, cochlea, pancreas, lung	SNX-482, Pb²⁺	~30 (R)	−14 to −13.3 (M)	−73 to −31 (H)	2 to 3.6 (H)	16 to 655 (H)	~10 (R)	14 to 21 (R)	1,2,11,248,250,253,255
Ca$_v$3.1	T	*CACNA1G*	Heart, CNS, pancreas, smooth muscle, kidney	Mibefradil, Kurtoxin, Ni²⁺	~60 (H)	−56 to −46 (H)	−78 to −62 (H)	1 to 7 (H)	15 to 40 (H)	~30 (H)	7.3 (H)	1,2,12,248,249
Ca$_v$3.2	T	*CACNA1H*	Heart, CNS, smooth muscle, kidney	Mibefradil, Kurtoxin, Ni²⁺	~60 (H)	−59.9 to −51.8 (H)	−86.5 to −81.7 (H)	1.6 to 8.4 (H)	12.9 to 32.6 (H)	~30 (H)	9.1 (H)	1,2,13,249
Ca$_v$3.3	T	*CACNA1I*	CNS	Mibefradil, Kurtoxin, Ni²⁺	~70 (H)	−44.9 to −41.8 (H)	−72 to −71.5 (H)	5.9 to 53 (H)	68 to 127 (H)	~30 (H)	11 (H)	1,2,14

Factors that affect range in values include prepulse duration, voltage-step dependence, charge carrier, differences between associated β subunits, and alternative splice variants of a given channel type. The fast and slow components of biexponential curves are indicated in parentheses.
CNS, Central nervous system; *GP*, guinea pig; *H*, human; *M*, mouse.

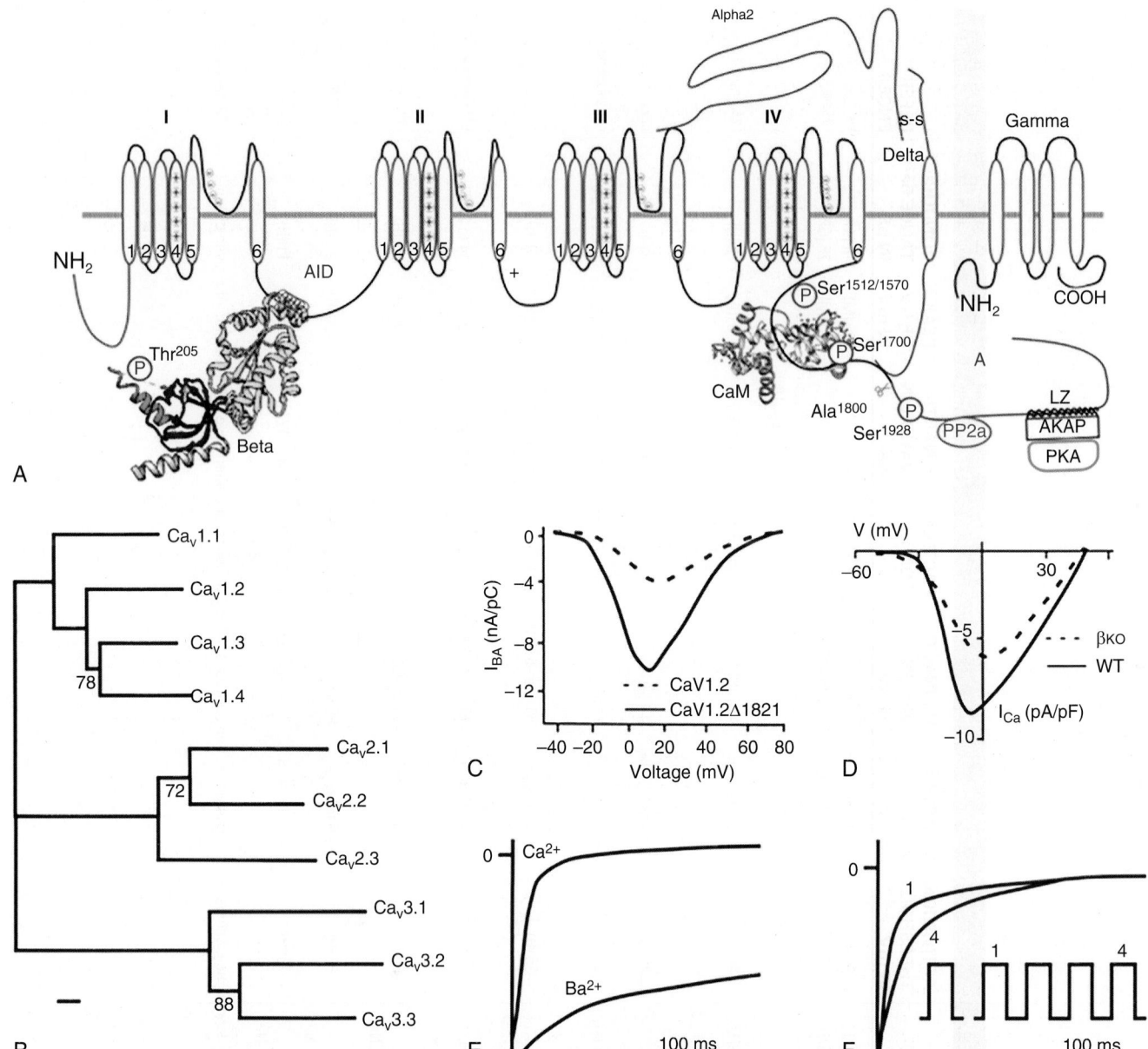

FIGURE 2.1 Voltage-gated Ca^{2+} channels. (A) Schematic representation of the cardiac α_{1C}-subunit topology and selected proteins within the Ca$_V$1.2 macromolecular complex. Positively charged residues in S4 are responsible for voltage-dependent activation, and negatively charged residues in S5-S6 mediate Ca^{2+} selectivity. The β_2-subunit (PDB accession code: 1VYT) binds to the AID domain of α_{1C}. Highlighted β_2 domains: SH3 (*blue*, residues 60–120 and 170–175), HOOK region (*green*, residues 121–169), and GK (*yellow*, residues 176–360). CaMKII phosphorylates β_2 at Thr[498] [17] and Ca$_V$1.2 at Ser[1512] and Ser[1570].[18] Calmodulin (CaM) (PDB accession code 2BE6) binds to α_{1C} at residues 1659-1692.[19,20] PKA phosphorylates Ca$_V$1.2 at Ser[1700] [21] and Ser[1928] [22] although other unidentified sites in the Ca$_V$1.2 complex are required for adrenergic regulation of Ca$_V$1.2.[23] In the heart, α_{1C} is proteo-lytically cleaved near Ala[1800] [24] although deletion of this residue does not prevent cleavage.[23] The C-terminus also includes binding sites for PP2A and AKAP-PKA. (B) Phylogenetic analysis of all 10 full human Ca$_V$ α_1 isoforms. Confidence intervals of nodes as determined by bootstrap analysis are 100% unless otherwise indicated. Scale bar = 100 amino acids. (C) Current–voltage relationship of Ca$_V$1.2 in the presence and absence of the autoinhibitory C-terminus. (D) Current–voltage curve of Ca$_V$1.2 in the presence and absence of the β_2-subunit. (E) Inactivation of L-type Ca^{2+} current in Ba^{2+} and Ca^{2+}. (F) Ca^{2+}-dependent facilitation with repeated depolarization. [B] Modified from Hulme JT, Konoki K, Lin TW, et al. Sites of proteolytic processing and noncovalent association of the distal C-terminal domain of CaV1.1 channels in skeletal muscle. *Proc Natl Acad Sci U S A.* 2005;102:5274-5279. [C] Modified from Hulme JT, Yarov-Yarovoy V, Lin TW, Scheuer T, Catterall WA. Autoinhibitory control of the CaV1.2 channel by its proteolytically processed distal C-terminal domain. *J Physiol.* 2006;576[pt 1]:87-102. [D] Modified from Meissner M, Weissgerber P, Londono JE, et al. Moderate calcium channel dysfunction in adult mice with inducible cardiomyocyte-specific excision of the cacnb2 gene. *J Biol Chem.* 2011;286:15875-15882. [E] Modified from Benitah JP, Alvarez JL, Gomez AM. L-type Ca[2+] current in ventricular cardiomyocytes. *J Mol Cell Cardiol.* 2010;48:26-36.)

(variable region 2), and the C-termini (variable region 3) are different.[46–48] All β-subunits, however, increase α_{1C} trafficking to the plasma membrane, regulate the voltage-dependence of activation, and impart the unique kinetics of inactivation. β_2 is the predominantly expressed isoform in the adult murine heart, with β_1, β_3, and β_4 not detectable by immunoblot.[49,50] In contrast, all four βs are detected in canine myocytes, suggesting species-dependence in the complement of β-isoforms expressed in cardiomyocytes. $Ca_V\beta$s primarily interact with an 18-residue sequence in the I-II intracellular linker, termed the α-interacting domain (AID), conserved among all high-voltage activated Ca^{2+} channel α_1-subunits (see Fig. 2.1A). Crystal structures show that the AID forms an α-helix that binds to the hydrophobic groove present in the $Ca_V\beta$ subunit GK domain through 10 AID side chain interactions.[51–53] Alanine-substitution of the three residues within $Ca_V1.2$ AID (Y437, W440, I441) ablates the β-binding.[54] In heterologous expression experiments, β-binding to α_{1C} is obligatory for $Ca_V1.2$ to traffic to the cell surface — deletion of the AID domain prevents α_{1C} surface expression, and α_{1C} expressed without β fails to traffic to the cell surface.[55] In mice, the global or cardiac-specific deletion of *Cacnb2* gene[56] leads to abnormal heart development and embryonic death. However, cardiomyocyte-specific, conditional deletion of the *Cacnb2* gene in adult mice causes a ~96% reduction in β_2 protein expression in cardiomyocytes, but surprisingly only a 29% reduction in Ca^{2+} current (Fig. 2.1D), with no obvious cardiac impairment.[57] β1-, β3-, and β4-deficient mice do not demonstrate significant cardiac phenotypes.[56]

The $\alpha_{2\delta}$-subunit is a 175-kDa single transmembrane protein encoded by four genes (*Cacna2d1*, *Cacna2d2*, *Cacna2d3*, *Cacna2d4*) with multiple splice variants. While the mRNAs of $\alpha_{2\delta}$1-3[58] have been identified in human myocardium, only $\alpha_{2\delta}$-1 is known to bind $Ca_V1.2$. The δ-subunit is encoded by the 3′ end of the coding sequence of the same gene as the α_2-subunit and is produced by posttranslational proteolytic processing.[31] The α_2-subunit has numerous glycosylation sites, is extracellular, and is attached to the membrane through a disulfide linkage to the δ-subunit (see Fig. 2.1A). The $\alpha_{2\delta}$ associates with multiple regions of the carboxyl-terminal half of α_1 including the S5-S6 linker in the third repeat domain. The δ component is required for this interaction.[59] The α_1-subunit is sufficient to produce functional channels, albeit with low expression levels and an abnormal kinetics/voltage dependence. Coexpression of the $\alpha_{2\delta}$-subunit and especially the β-subunit enhances expression and produces normal gating properties.[60]

Eight γ-subunit isoforms, encoded by the *CACNG1-8* genes, have been identified, although only the γ4, γ6, γ7, and γ8 cDNA have been expressed in the human heart. The γ-subunits are composed of four transmembrane domains with intracellular N- and C-terminal ends (see Fig. 2.1A). Studies on the γ1-isoform in skeletal muscle have localized the interaction site with α_1 to the first half of the γ-subunit while studies on γ6, which has an inhibitory effect on $Ca_V3.1$ current in rat atrial myocytes, have localized it to the first transmembrane domain (TM1).[61] The γ-subunits have variable effects on $Ca_V1.2$ function. γ4, γ6, and γ7 cause a leftward shift in the V_{50} for channel activation while γ8 inhibits the effects of the $\alpha_{2\delta1}$-subunit on channel function. Furthermore, these effects are different depending on what β-subunit isoform is coexpressed (β_{1b} vs β_{2b}).[62]

L-Type Ca²⁺ Channels

Electrophysiological Properties of L-Type Ca²⁺ Channels

$Ca_V1.2$-mediated Ca^{2+} current peaks at 0 to +10 mV, has a bell-shaped current–voltage relationship, and is activated at voltages positive to −40 mV (see Fig. 2.1C). Single channel Ca^{2+} conductance is 5 pS[63] and is driven by an ~10,000-fold difference in the transmembrane Ca^{2+} concentration (1.5 mM vs. 0.1 μM). The

activity of single Ca^{2+} channels alternate between different gating modes: mode 0, where the channel is unavailable for opening; mode 1, which is normal activity with brief openings occurring in rapid bursts; and mode 2 with a high open probability with long openings interrupted by brief closings.[64] The $V_{1/2}$ of activation is typically between −10 and −15 mV. Compared to $Ca_V1.2$, $Ca_V1.3$ exhibits greater negative activation thresholds, slower current inactivation rates, and stronger voltage-dependent facilitation; these are properties that enable these channels to mediate long lasting Ca^{2+} influx upon weak depolarization and contribute to pacemaking and stabilization of the plateau potentials in sinoatrial node cells and neurons.[65–67]

Following activation the channel undergoes Ca^{2+}-dependent inactivation (CDI) and voltage-dependent inactivation (VDI) (see Fig. 2.1E), which determine the duration of the action potential.[68] The molecular determinants of VDI are the cytosolic ends of the S6 transmembrane segments, the I-II linker, which is the inactivation gate, and the N- and C-termini of α_{1C}.[69] VDI is further affected by the β-subunit with protein kinase A (PKA) phosphorylation of Thr^{205} in the hook domain of the β2-subunit increasing CDI.[70] CDI occurs via Ca^{2+} binding to calmodulin (CaM),[20] which binds to the IQ domain in the α_{1C}-terminus (see Fig. 2.1A).[19,71,72] Cardiomyocytes isolated from mice expressing an α_{1C} with reduced CaM-binding affinity have reduced total α_{1C} protein and decreased $Ca_V1.2$ current.[73] CDI is believed to protect cardiomyocytes from intracellular Ca^{2+} overload at lower membrane voltages when the VDI is at its minimum. The same domain is required for Ca^{2+}-dependent facilitation in which the LTCC current increases as a function of pacing frequency (see Fig. 2.1F).[19,72]

Pharmacology of L-Type Ca²⁺ Channels

There are three main chemical classes of organic Ca^{2+} channel drugs: dihydropyridine (prototype: nifedipine), phenylalkylamines (prototype: verapamil), and benzothiazepines (prototype: (+)-cis-diltiazem), which all bind within a single overlapping region close to the pore and the proposed activation gate.[74,75] These drugs interfere with the voltage-dependent cycling of the channel.[76–78] The uncharged dihydropyridines stabilize and induce inactivated channel states and possess a higher affinity for the inactivated channel conformation, implying that their IC_{50} to block the L-type Ca^{2+} channels is much lower at depolarized voltages (voltage-dependent block).[76–79] The preferential affinity of dihydropyridines for inactivated channels explain their differential effects on the heart and the vasculature: inactivated channel states are favored in arterial smooth muscle cells due to the depolarized membrane potential.[77,80] (As discussed above, the smooth muscle $Ca_V1.2$ splice variant is also more sensitive to inhibition by dihydropyridines than the cardiac $Ca_V1.2$ splice variant due to alternative splicing.[36]) $Ca_V1.3$ is less sensitive to DHP than $Ca_V1.2$. Phenylalkylamines and benzothiazepines bind to the open and inactivated states with high affinity and stabilize the inactivated channel states, slowing recovery from inactivation, leading to use-dependent inhibition.[81,82] Therefore inhibition increases with the higher heart rates, rationalizing the use of verapamil for tachyarrhythmias. Whereas verapamil and diltiazem always reduce the inward Ca^{2+} currents, some dihydropyridines, such as (−)-BayK8644 and (+)-SDS202-791, are gating modifiers that increase current amplitudes, tail currents, and single-channel open probability.[79]

Role of L-Type Ca²⁺ Channels in the Heart

In early development, $Ca_V1.3$ is the predominant L-type Ca^{2+} channel in the heart where it contributes to automaticity. Later during embryogenesis, the expression pattern changes, and $Ca_V1.2$ becomes the dominant L-type Ca^{2+} channel in ventricular myocytes.[83] Postnatally, the expression of $Ca_V1.3$ is limited to the sinoatrial node and atrioventricular node. $Ca_V1.2$ is situated on the T-tubules in close proximity to ryanodine receptors (RyR2), which are intracellular Ca^{2+} release channels located on the sarcoplasmic reticulum (SR) (Fig. 2.2). In a process known as Ca^{2+}-induced Ca^{2+} release,[84] Ca^{2+} entry through the L-type Ca^{2+} channels triggers RyR2 to release Ca^{2+} from the SR into the cytoplasm where Ca^{2+} then binds troponin C, enabling actin–myosin cross-linking and cellular contraction.[85] L-type Ca^{2+} channels are also functional within caveolae, where Ca^{2+} influx can control signal transduction pathways (see Fig. 2.2). In healthy hearts, bridging integrator 1 (BIN1) is a membrane scaffolding protein that causes $Ca_V1.2$ to traffic to T-tubules.[86] In failing hearts, the expression of BIN1 is decreased and this reduction impairs $Ca_V1.2$ trafficking, Ca^{2+} transients, and contractility.[87]

The critical contribution of $Ca_V1.2$ to myocardial function is highlighted by the observation that $Ca_V1.2$ knockout mice are embryonically lethal by 14 days.[88] Survival in early development is likely due to the presence of $Ca_V1.3$.[83] Mice lacking $Ca_V1.3$ exhibit a reduced rate of sinoatrial node diastolic depolarization[89] and bradycardia[66] as well as atrioventricular node dysfunction.[90] Colocalization of $Ca_V1.3$ and RyR2 in the sinoatrial node likely contributes to the large increase in intracellular Ca^{2+} levels that drives diastolic depolarization.[91]

Increased Ca^{2+} influx via L-type Ca^{2+} channels can lead to arrhythmias. When the action potential duration is prolonged, recovery of the L-type Ca^{2+} channel inactivation occurs during the plateau phase, which can cause early after-depolarizations (EADs).[92] An increased L-type Ca^{2+} current also contributes to delayed after-depolarizations (DADs) and Ca^{2+}-evoked arrhythmias. Mutations in L-type Ca^{2+} channels have been associated with inherited arrhythmia syndromes including Timothy syndrome, a multisystem disorder characterized by invariant prolonged QT intervals and syndactyly, and several variably penetrant phenotypes for autism spectrum disorders, craniofacial abnormalities, and hypoglycemia.[93] The biophysical mechanism underlying the cardiac manifestations of Timothy syndrome is the prominent loss of VDI, leading to the failure of L-type Ca^{2+} channels to close during the plateau phase of the ventricular action potential.[93] Loss-of-function mutants of the pore-forming α_{1C}-, β_{2b}-, and $\alpha_{2\delta1}$-subunits have also been linked to Brugada, early repolarization, and short QT syndromes.[94–97]

Dysfunctional Ca^{2+} regulation has also been implicated in the mechanisms of cardiac hypertrophy. Transgenic cardiac overexpression of either the β_{2a}-subunit or the α_{1C}-subunit is sufficient to activate pathological hypertrophy signaling.[98] After a myocardial infarction, transgenic overexpression of β_{2a} caused greater ventricular dilation, myocyte hypertrophy and death, and depressed cardiac function.[99] The hypertrophic signaling was blocked by a caveolae-targeted L-type Ca^{2+} channel antagonist, implicating the Ca^{2+} influx via L-type Ca^{2+} channels within the caveolae as a required source for pathological cardiac hypertrophy.[100] Conversely, in $Ca_V1.2$-heterozygous null mice modest reduction in L-type Ca^{2+} current caused greater ventricular dilation, cardiac hypertrophy, and reductions in ventricular performance after pressure overload stimulation, isoproterenol infusion, and swimming. The reduction in L-type Ca^{2+} current led to the activation of the neurohormonal stress pathways and the activation of calcineurin/NFAT signaling.[101] Thus both increased and decreased L-type Ca^{2+} current is implicated in the development of hypertrophy and pathological remodeling with stress stimuli.

Regulation of L-Type Ca^{2+} Channels by Posttranslational Modifications

The association of $Ca_V1.2$ with a supramolecular complex affects its trafficking, localization, turnover, and most importantly function.[31,102,103] In addition to the $Ca_V1.2$ subunits, α_{1c}, β, $\alpha_{2\delta1}$, and γ subunits, the complex includes calmodulin,[19,71,72] kinases,[104,105] phosphatases,[106,107] scaffold proteins,[108,109] caveolin-3,[110] β_2-AR,[104] junctophilin,[111,112] and BIN1[86] (see Figs. 2.1A and 2.2).

The activation of $\beta1$- and $\beta2$-adrenergic receptors leads to an increase in L-type Ca^{2+} current[113] by redistributing the relative proportions of the gating modes such that the two most active (mode 1 and mode 2) are favored instead of the mode with sparse brief openings (mode 0).[114] Despite decades of investigative work, however, the molecular mechanisms of the β-adrenergic regulation of $Ca_V1.2$ in cardiomyocytes are incompletely known. A key obstacle for decades has been the failure to reproducibly reconstitute adrenergic regulation of heterologously expressed $Ca_V1.2$. Ser^{1928}, in the α_{1C}-subunit, was originally identified as the sole α_{1C} PKA phosphorylation site.[22,104,115–121] Phosphorylation of this residue, however, is not required for β-adrenergic agonist stimulation

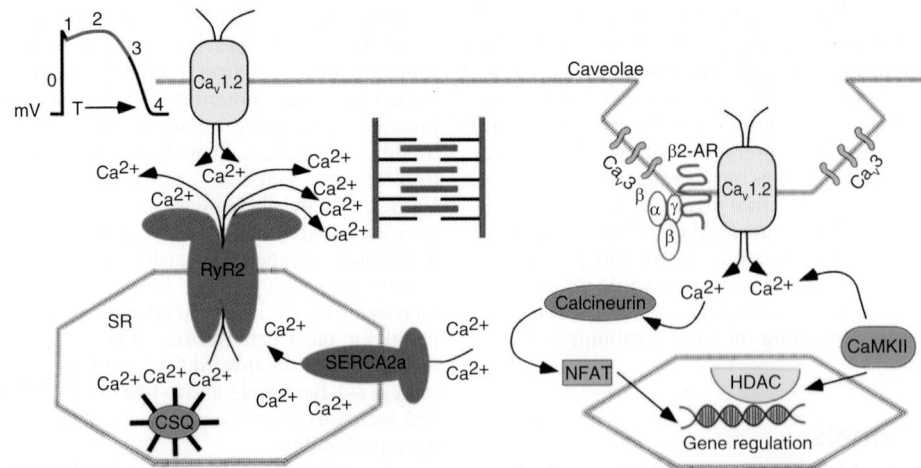

FIGURE 2.2 Localization and signaling of $Ca_V1.2$ in cardiomyocytes. Ca^{2+} influx via $Ca_V1.2$ during phase 2 of the cardiac action potential *(top left corner)* triggers ryanodine receptor (*RyR2*)-mediated Ca^{2+} release from the intracellular Ca^{2+} stores of the sarcoplasmic reticulum (*SR*). Ca^{2+} binds to troponin C, resulting in actin/myosin cross-bridging and myocardial contraction. Ca^{2+} is pumped back into the SR through SERCA2a, where it is buffered by binding to calsequestrin (*CSQ*). Regulation of $Ca_V1.2$ by $\beta2$-adrenergic receptor (*$\beta2$-AR*) occurs in localized regions called caveolae, which are formed by caveolin (*Cav3*). Ca^{2+} regulates gene transcription via multiple downstream pathways including calcineurin/NFAT and CaMKII.

of $Ca_V1.2$, as shown in guinea pig cardiomyocytes infected with an adenovirus expressing a relatively dihydropyridine-resistant S1928A-α_{1C},[122] and in α_{1C} S1928A knock-in mice.[123] Similarly, although β_{2a} Ser[459], Ser[478], and Ser[479] are PKA phosphorylated,[124] these sites are not required for β-adrenergic stimulation of $Ca_V1.2$ in cardiomyocytes.[125–127] Based upon heterologous expression studies, Ser[1700] was proposed to be a functionally relevant PKA phosphorylation site,[21,128] but this site is also not required for adrenergic-regulation of $Ca_V1.2$ in cardiomyocytes.[23]

$Ca_V1.2$ also associates with proteins containing PDZ-binding domains, although deletion of the PDZ ligand motif of α_{1C} did not affect trafficking, basal function, or adrenergic-regulation of $Ca_V1.2$ in heart.[129] The effect of $\beta2$-adrenergic receptors is dependent on its colocalization with $Ca_V1.2$ in specialized microdomains called caveolae (see Fig. 2.2).[110] Specialized microdomains have not been identified for $\beta1$-adrenergic receptors. β-adrenergic modulation of the Ca^{2+} currents in cardiomyocytes is markedly blunted by the intracellular dialysis, via a patch pipette, of peptides designed to competitively disrupt the binding of PKA to an A-kinase anchoring protein (AKAP).[109,117,130] Considerable evidence initially pointed to important roles for AKAP5 and AKAP7.[21,109,117,118] The AKAP5-null mouse, the AKAP7-null mouse, and the combined AKAP5/AKAP7-null mouse demonstrated, however, that these AKAPs are not essential for this process.[131,132] Thus PKA binding to $Ca_V1.2$ must be via an alternative AKAP, possibly containing a leucine zipper motif (see Fig. 2.1A).[109,133]

CaMKII phosphorylation of $Ca_V1.2$ causes Ca^{2+}-dependent facilitation (CDF) of the $Ca_V1.2$ current (see Fig. 2.1F), observed as a positive "staircase" of Ca^{2+} current in which the current amplitude increases and inactivation slows over a series of repetitive pulses. The significance of putative CaMKII phosphorylation sites was recently examined using two approaches: (i) a S1512A, S1570A α_{1C} knock-in mouse model, which showed reduced CaMKII-dependent potentiation of $Ca_V1.2$[18] and (ii) a viral overexpression of mutant T498A β_2-subunits in isolated rabbit cardiomyocytes, which increased the action potential duration (APD) (similar to WT β_2 expression), reduced the early afterdepolarization frequency (compared to WT β_2), and reduced the $Ca_V1.2$ current potentiation.[17] Based upon these experiments, it is likely that phosphorylation of both the α_{1C}- and β_2-subunits are required for CaMKII potentiation of $Ca_V1.2$ current.[134]

T-Type Ca^{2+} Channels

Expression and Molecular Composition of T-Type Ca^{2+} Channels

T-type Ca^{2+} channels were first discovered in invertebrates and then identified in mammalian neurons and hearts. T-type Ca^{2+} channel currents result from the function of three distinct α-subunits encoded by three genes, α_{1G} ($Ca_V3.1$), α_{1H} ($Ca_V3.2$), and α_{1I} ($Ca_V3.3$). Similar to the Ca_V1 and Ca_V2 isoforms, the poreforming α-subunit of the Ca_V3 channels has four domains, each with six transmembrane segments. In contrast to the Ca_V1 and Ca_V2 channels, however, the Ca_V3 channels do not have AID or IQ motifs. Ca_V3 channels do not require β-subunits or calmodulin, as do the Ca_V1 and Ca_V2 channels, for appropriate function. Antisense depletion of $Ca_V\beta$ subunits had no effect on T-type Ca^{2+} current in neurons,[135,136] and coexpression of the β-subunits had no major effect on the heterologously expressed T-type Ca^{2+} channels.[137] Coexpression of $\alpha_{2\delta}$ with $Ca_V3.1$ doubled T-type Ca^{2+} currents in COS-7 cells and in Xenopus oocytes, however, possibly by increasing trafficking of the channels to the membrane,[137,138] although the functional effects of this interaction in the heart is not known. In the atria, functional targeting and expression of the T-type Ca^{2+} channels requires the endosomal protein, Eps15 homology domain-containing (EDH) protein 3.[139]

The expression of the T-type Ca^{2+} channel parallels the development of pacemaker activity in the embryonic heart, such that it is expressed throughout the embryonic heart and is later restricted to the differentiating conduction system. Expression of T-type Ca^{2+} channels decreases ~80% from the embryo to the adult.[140] During fetal development, $Ca_V3.2$ (α_{1H}) is the predominant T-type isoform expressed throughout the heart.[141] In the perinatal period, the expression of $Ca_V3.2$ decreases, whereas the expression of $Ca_V3.1$ (α_{1G}) increases, becoming the predominant T-type isoform in adulthood.[142] In humans, $Ca_V3.1$ is predominantly localized to the conduction system. Some species-specific variations also exist. The $Ca_V3.3$ isoform is not expressed in the myocardium, sinoatrial node, or atrioventricular node.[12,14,143]

Electrophysiology

All three Ca_V3 clones form LVA channels. A hallmark of T-type currents is that they are transient; T-type channels generate transient macroscopic currents within milliseconds (ms) and quickly decay (in tens of ms) because of inactivation.[30] The steepest increase in conductance is at the foot of the action potential, with a depolarizing contribution limited by the degree of channel inactivation. All three recombinant Ca_V3 channels have small single-channel currents, corresponding to slope conductances in the 7–11 pS range (see Table 2.1). In contrast, $Ca_V1.2$ channels have slope conductances of 20–30 pS, and Ca_V2 channels have slope conductances in the range of 14–21 pS. Depolarization of the membrane to –70 mV is sufficient to trigger channel opening, and the current–voltage curves for all three Ca_V3 channels peak at approximately –30 mV (see Table 2.1 and Fig. 2.3A). The kinetics of the current are voltage-dependent between –70 and –20 mV. $Ca_V3.1$ and $Ca_V3.2$ both activate relatively quickly at –10 mV (1–2 ms) and inactivate 10-fold slower (11–16 ms). $Ca_V3.3$ currents activate and inactivate much slower (Fig. 2.3B).[30] All Ca_V3 channels show slow tail currents: the tail currents of $Ca_V3.1$ are the slowest (τ = 3 ms at –90 mV), whereas the tail currents of $Ca_V3.3$ are the fastest (τ = 1 ms at –90 mV). The HVA channels close 10-fold faster. The slow deactivation of T-type Ca^{2+} channels ensures T-type currents during action potential repolarization, prolonging their contribution as the membrane potential tries to repolarize.[144] Since the midpoint of the voltage-dependent steady-state inactivation of the Ca_V3 channels is –72 mV (Fig. 2.3C), T-type channels can reach inactivated states without passing through open states.[145,146] Since T-type channels can open at similar potentials at which they inactivate, they may generate window currents under steady-state conditions (see Fig. 2.3C), an optimal property for contributing to diastolic depolarization of the sinoatrial node and chronotropy. Taken together, T-type Ca^{2+} current is optimized to generate rhythmic firing patterns with rapid kinetics to drive membrane depolarization to the action potential threshold.

The T-type Ca^{2+} current is readily distinguished from the L-type Ca^{2+} current by its more depolarized (lower) activation potential (–70 mV vs. –40 mV), highly transient activation and inactivation kinetics, small single-channel conductance, and relatively low sensitivity to classical blockers of L-type Ca^{2+} channels.[30,147–149] Additionally, in contrast to high-voltage activated Ca^{2+} channels, the T-type channels do not inactivate in a Ca^{2+}-dependent manner. The "gating brake" of the channel encompasses the proximal 62 amino acids of the I-II linker, which is within the homologous position of the AID motif of Ca_V1 and Ca_V2 channels.[144,150,151]

Pharmacology

Nickel has been described as a selective blocker of R- and T-type Ca^{2+} channels over other voltage-gated Ca^{2+} channels.[30,148,152] Only $Ca_V3.2$ channels are highly nickel sensitive (IC_{50} ~10 µM),

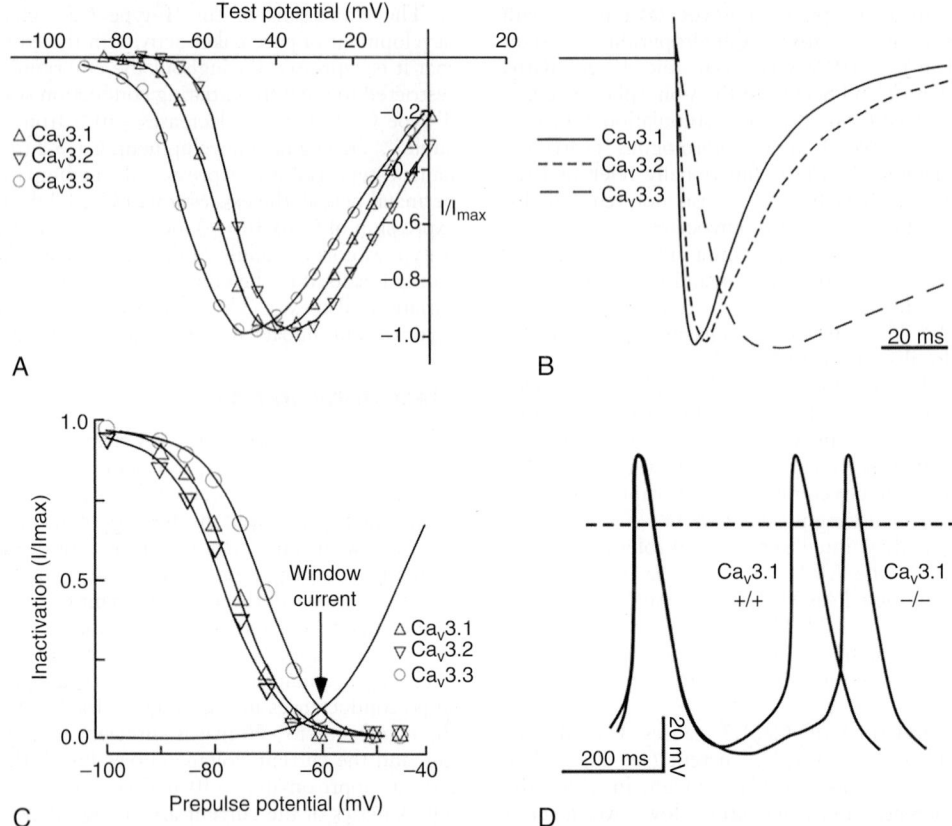

FIGURE 2.3 T-type Ca²⁺ channels in the heart. [A] Current–voltage relationship for Ca$_V$3.1, Ca$_V$3.2, and Ca$_V$3.3 heterologously expressed in HEK cells, normalized to the peak current. [B] Normalized peak current for Ca$_V$3.1, Ca$_V$3.2, and Ca$_V$3.3, demonstrating differences in kinetics of activation and inactivation for the three isoforms of T-type Ca²⁺ channels. [C] Inactivation plotted as a function of the prepulse voltage fitted with the Boltzmann equation. The superimposed activation curve demonstrates an overlap region consistent with a theoretical window current. [D] Spontaneous action potentials from sinoatrial node cells from wild-type (+/+) and Ca$_V$3.1 null (–/–) mice. ([A] and [B] Modified from McRory JE, Santi CM, Hamming KS, et al. Molecular and functional characterization of a family of rat brain T-type calcium channels. *J Biol Chem.* 2001;276:3999-4011. [C] Modified from Perez-Reyes E. Molecular physiology of low-voltage-activated t-type calcium channels. *Physiol Rev.* 2003;83:117-161. [D] Modified from Mangoni ME, Traboulsie A Leoni AL, et al. Bradycardia and slowing of the atrioventricular conduction in mice lacking CaV3.1/alpha1G T-type calcium channels. *Circ Res.* 2006;98:1422-1430.)

whereas the Ca$_V$3.1 and Ca$_V$3.2 channels are 20-fold less sensitive.[153] The nickel-mediated block is greatest at potentials that are near threshold, making nickel appear more selective than it is for LVA over HVA channels. Cav3.1 and Cav3.2 have similar activation and inactivation kinetics, but can be differentiated by their recovery from inactivation and sensitivity to blockage by nickel.[153–155]

In contrast to the highly selective Ca$_V$1 blockers, there are no highly selective drugs or peptide toxins that selectively block Ca$_V$3 channels. Low dose mibefradil (formerly called Ro-40–5967) was initially reported to preferentially block T-type Ca²⁺ current,[156] with a 10- to 30-fold selectivity for T- over L-type Ca²⁺ channels.[157,158] Mibefradil (Posicor, Roche) was FDA-approved in 1997 as a specific blocker of T-type Ca²⁺ channels, and had an indication for the treatment of essential hypertension and stable angina pectoris. It was withdrawn 1 year later due to high mortality secondary to extensive interactions with other commonly used cardiovascular drugs.[159] A mibefradil block of both HVA and LVA channels is state-dependent, having a higher affinity for inactivated states.[160,161] Subsequently, micromolar concentrations of mibefradil were found capable of blocking several types of ion channels, including Na⁺,[162] K⁺,[163] and Cl⁻[164] channels, which complicated the interpretation of mibefradil effects.[30]

T-type Ca²⁺ channels have variable sensitivities to dihydropyridine Ca²⁺ channel blockers.[165] Felodipine has an apparent affinity for the inactivated T-type channels in atrial myocytes of 13 nM,[166] implying that the blockage of T-type channels may contribute to felodipine's antihypertensive properties. Amlodipine is approximately 12-fold more selective for cardiac L-type over T-type channels and blocks the T-type channels with an apparent IC$_{50}$ of 5.7 μM.[158] The structure-activity relationships of dihydropyridines for T- and L-type channels are different. T-type channels are weakly blocked by the stereoisomers of Bay K8644,[167] whereas for L-type channels the (–) isomer is an agonist.[168] In conclusion, dihydropyridines are selective for L-type channels, but some analogs are capable of blocking T-type channels in the range of 1–10 μM.

Antiepileptics have been shown to block T-type Ca²⁺ currents. Ethosuximide, a drug used in the treatment of absence epilepsy, can block T-type channels with little effect on HVA channels in thalamic neurons in vitro.[169] With one exception,[170] however, most other studies have not confirmed the ethosuximide-induced block of T-type currents at therapeutically relevant concentrations.[171] T-type channels are also inhibited by drugs that block Na⁺ channels, such as phenytoin, although phenytoin appears to be selective for LVA channels over HVA channels.[172] T-type currents are also blocked at therapeutically relevant concentrations of some anesthetics, such as isoflurane, halothane, and nitrous oxide, and this block may contribute to their anesthetic and analgesic properties.[171,173,174] The diphenylbutylpiperidine class of antipsychotics can block the T-type channels, of which penfluridol is the most effective at blocking T-type currents in the human medullary thyroid cancer cells.[175] Thioridazine, clozapine, and haloperidol, which have comparable activity in blocking T-type channels in the human medullary thyroid carcinoma TT cell line, are much less active than fluspirilene or penfluridol.[175]

Role of T-Type Ca^{2+} Channels in the Heart

T-type Ca^{2+} current has little effect on cardiomyocyte excitation–contraction coupling[176] in the heart, but the high density of T-type Ca^{2+} current in nodal cells[177] and embryonic cardiomyocytes[178] is consistent with a role in pacemaker function. Mice deficient in CaV3.2 exhibit recurrent coronary vasospasm but normal sinoatrial rhythms,[179] whereas disruption of the gene coding CaV3.1 abolished the T-type Ca^{2+} currents in cells isolated from the sinoatrial and atrioventricular nodes, causing bradycardia and delaying atrioventricular conduction without affecting the excitability of the right atrium (Fig. 2.3D).[143] T-type Ca^{2+} channels, specifically CaV3.1, also play a role in infranodal escape automaticity as the CaV3.1 null mice had slower escape rhythms post radiofrequency atrioventricular node ablation, and higher mortality and frequency of torsades de pointes.[180] Thus the major T-type Ca^{2+} channel that contributes to the generation of the cardiac rhythm in mouse heart is CaV3.1.

The expression of the T-type Ca^{2+} channels in the heart may also be associated with cardiomyocyte proliferation and growth. T-type Ca^{2+} channels are re-expressed in hypertrophied or failing hearts, and during stimulation with certain hormones.[181–188] Re-expression of T-type Ca^{2+} channels may increase the Ca^{2+} influx during the action potential, which can contribute to the cardiac hypertrophic response. Mice with a genetic deletion of Ca$_V$3.2 are protected from both pressure overload– and angiotensin II–induced cardiac hypertrophy.[189] Unexpectedly, cardiac-specific transgenic mice with an inducible expression of Ca$_V$3.1 were partially resistant to pressure overload-, isoproterenol-, and exercise-induced cardiac hypertrophy, whereas Ca$_V$3.1 null mice displayed enhanced hypertrophic responses following pressure overload or isoproterenol.[190] These apparently conflicting findings, since Ca$_V$3.1 and Ca$_V$3.2 have similar electrophysiological characteristics, may be due to differences in structural or kinetic properties, posttranslational modifications, protein-protein interactions, or downstream signaling pathways of the T-type Ca^{2+} channels in heart.[190]

Posttranslational Regulation of T-Type Ca^{2+} Channels

The concept of whether the regulation of T-type Ca^{2+} channels by the β-adrenergic system plays a role in cardiac physiology has been controversial, perhaps due to the differences in the experimental conditions.[191] Initial reports have suggested that T-type Ca^{2+} channels in heart and brain were relatively insensitive to PKA.[1,192,193] The PKA phosphorylation of Ser^{1107} in the II–III loop of the channel α-subunit was shown to be a molecular switch that allows the Gβγ dimers to cause voltage-independent inhibition of the CaV3.2 channels.[194] The T-type Ca^{2+} currents in sinoatrial node cells from wild-type and CaV3.2 knockout mice were significantly increased by isoproterenol, suggesting that the CaV3.1 channels could be upregulated by the β-adrenergic system in vivo.[195] This regulation could play a role in heart rate regulation or arrhythmogenesis. CaMKII regulates CaV3.2 via the phosphorylation of Ser^{1198}, which is a site that is not present on CaV3.1.[196]

Transient Receptor Potential Channels

Expression and Molecular Composition of TRP Channels

The transient receptor potential (TRP) family conducts cations, and includes 28 mammalian channels divided into six subgroups [canonical TRP (TRPC), ankyrin TRP (TRPA), melastatin TRP (TRPM), polycystic TRP (TRPP), mucolipin TRP (TRPML), and vanilloid TRP (TRPV)] that are related by their cation nonselectivity and absence of voltage regulation.[197] The TRP channel primary sequence predicts six transmembrane domains (S1-S6), a pore region located between S5 and S6, and intracellular amino- and carboxy-termini (Fig. 2.4AB). Within a subfamily, the TRP channels can form homo- or heterotetramers. The composition and function of the termini differ between the TRP families. For example, amino-termini ankyrin repeats vary from ~4 in TRPC to ~29 in TRPN,[198] and the TRPC and TRPV channels contain amino-terminal NO-sensing (nitrosylation) cysteines.[199] Carboxy-terminal functional domains include an ADP-ribose (ADPR) pyrophosphatase domain on TRPM2[200] and atypical α-kinase domains on TRPM6 and TRPM7.[201] The structures of TRPA1 and TRPV1 have been solved to ~ 4 Å resolution (Fig. 2.4C).[202–204]

The mRNA from at least 13 TRP channels has been detected in the cardiovascular systems of different species. All TRPCs except TRPC5 have been expressed in the sinoatrial node[205] whereas other isoforms have been expressed in atrial and ventricular cardiomyocytes, fibroblasts, and vascular smooth muscle cells in the aorta, pulmonary arteries, coronary arteries, and mesenteric arteries.

Electrophysiology

All TRP channels are nonselective cation channels exhibiting a <10-fold selectivity for Ca^{2+} over Na$^+$, with the exceptions of the monovalent cation-selective TRPM4 and TRPM5 and the Ca^{2+}-selective TRPV5 and TRPV6.[206] TRP channels are insensitive to membrane voltage, and instead open in response to a variety of other stimuli including pressure, shear stress, mechanical stretch, oxidative stress, phospholipids, and the metabolites of phospholipids (Fig. 2.4D).[207] For example, TRPV1–4 and TRPM3 conduct Ca^{2+} in response to high temperatures[208] while TRPC5, TRPM8, and TRPA1 respond to low temperatures.[209] A decrease in intracellular free Mg^{2+} activates TRPM6 and TRPM7 while increased intracellular Ca^{2+} activates TRPM4, TRPM5, TRPM2, and TRPA1.[207] Oxidative stress activates TRPM2,[210] TRPC3/4,[211] TRPC5,[212] and TRPC6[213] while it inhibits TRPP2.[207] The TRPCs,[214] TRPVs, and TRPMs are also activated by phospholipase C and its metabolic products DAG and PIP2 via interactions between their amino- and carboxy-termini.[207] Mechanical stretch activates TRPC5,[215] TRPC6,[216] TRPP1-2,[217] and possibly TRPM7[218] while TRPV4, TRPV2, and TRPM3-4 are activated by osmotic cell swelling.[219] TRP crosstalk has also been reported. For example, TRPC6 is normally activated by angiotensin II; however this is inhibited by increased levels of intracellular Ca^{2+} due to the activation of TRPC1/C5.[205]

Pharmacology

A common problem in the study of TRP channels is the lack of specific pharmacological tools. There are several nonspecific blockers such as ruthenium red, 2-aminoethoxydiphenyl borate (2-APB), flufenamate, niflumic acid, SKF96365, clotrimazole, and pyrazole-3.[206] HC-030031 is a relatively specific antagonist of TRPA1.[220] Capsaicin is a fairly specific agonist of TRPV1,[221] and La^{3+} can be used to identify TRPC4 or TRPC5 because it potentiates these channels and blocks most other TRP- and Ca^{2+}-permeant channels.[222]

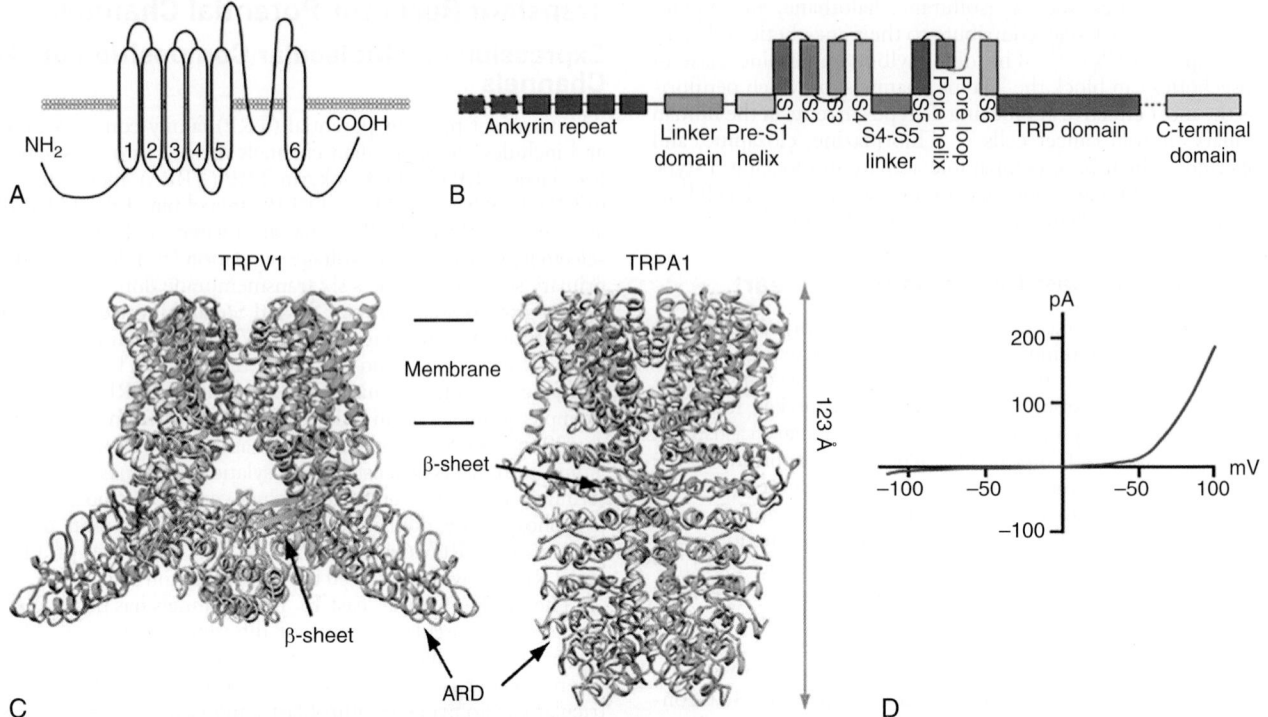

FIGURE 2.4 Transient receptor potential (TRP) channels. [A] Schematic representation of a TRP channel demonstrating six transmembrane segments with large, variable amino- and carboxy-termini. [B] Schematic linear diagram of TRPV1. [C] Side-by-side structural comparison of TRPV1 and TRPA1 as determined by electron cryomicroscopy. *ARD*, Ankyrin repeat domain. [D] TRPM7 current–voltage relationship demonstrating a near linear relationship between current and voltage. ([A] and [B] From Liao M, Cao E, Julius D, Cheng Y. Structure of the TRPV1 ion channel determined by electron cryo-microscopy. *Nature.* 2013;504:107-112. [C] From Paulsen CE, Armache JP, Gao Y, Cheng Y, Julius D. Structure of the TRPA1 ion channel suggests regulatory mechanisms. *Nature.* 2015;520:511-517. [D] Modified from Du J, Xie J, Zhang Z, et al. TRPM7-mediated Ca2+ signals confer fibrogenesis in human atrial fibrillation. *Circ Res.* 2010;106:992-1003.)

TRP Channels in Cardiac Development

TRP channels play an essential role in cardiac development. Deletion of Trpp2 (also known as Polycystin-2 [PC2]) causes defects in cardiac septation, and the embryos die before parturition; this implies that TRPP channels have a critical role in cardiac development.[223] TRPM7 is also essential for early, but not for late, development of the heart. Cardiomyocyte-specific deletion of Trpm7 before E9 caused impaired compact myocardium development with heart failure and death by E11.5.[224,225]

TRP Channels and Cardiac Conduction

TRP channels also play an essential role in cardiac action potential and arrhythmogenesis. Progressive familial heart block type I (PFHBI), a progressive cardiac bundle branch disease in the His–Purkinje system, is caused by a gain-of-function missense mutation in TRPM4, which forms a Ca^{2+}-activated nonselective cation channel.[226] The E7K mutation in the amino-terminus causes constitutive SUMOylation of the mutant TRPM4 channel and impaired endocytosis. Several other mutations of TRPM4 have been identified in autosomal dominant isolated cardiac conduction block conditions.[227,228] The mechanism by which a gain-of-function TRPM4 mutation causes conduction block is unknown.[207] TRPM4 mutations have also been linked to approximately 2.7%-6% of Brugada syndrome cases,[229] although the mechanisms by which the functional changes in TRPM4 cause the ECG changes of Brugada syndrome are not known.

Left atrial enlargement, a risk factor for atrial fibrillation, activates stretch-sensitive TRPC6 channels. Inhibition of TRPC6 by GxMTx4, a nonselective cation channel blocker, inhibits dilation-induced atrial fibrillation potentiation in rabbit hearts.[216] This suggests that TRP channels may contribute to the progression of atrial fibrillation.

TRP Channels in Cardiac Fibroblasts

Ca^{2+} signals mediated by TRPC3, TRPC6, TRPV4, and TRPM7 contribute to TGFβ1-induced fibroblast differentiation.[207] Since TRPM7-mediated Ca^{2+} signaling is required for TGFβ1-induced fibrogenesis,[230,231] it may serve as a therapeutic target for cardiac fibrosis.[207] TRPC3 enhances fibroblast proliferation and differentiation, a process that contributes to the development of atrial fibrillation. TRPC3 levels are increased in canine models of atrial fibrillation, and blocking TRPC3 with pyrazole-3 reduces fibroblast proliferation and the mean duration of atrial fibrillation.[232] In cardiac fibroblasts, TRPC6-mediated Ca^{2+} entry activates NFAT, which acts as negative regulator against endothelin-induced fibroblast differentiation.[233] Although TRPC6, TRPV4, and TRPM7 are sensitive to mechanical stimulation, only TRPV4 is required for the fibroblast differentiation induced by mechanical stimulation, based upon studies using a TRPV4 antagonist, AB159908, and TRPV4 shRNA knockdown.[234,235] To summarize, TRPC3, TRPC6, TRPV4, and TRPM7 may each play a role in cardiac fibroblast differentiation by different stimuli and under different conditions.[207]

TRP Channels and Cardiac Hypertrophy

The function of TRPC channels under normal physiological conditions is not clear but their activity has been associated with disease states. TRP channels have been localized to intracellular organelles including the sarcoplasmic reticulum and lysosomes and have contributed to diverse functions including myocardial contraction and cell death.[207] Increased expression of TRPC contributes to hypertrophy in rodent models of LV pressure overload,[236] possibly via the activation of calcineurin/NFAT signaling pathways.[237] In support of this, TRPC-deficient mice are protected from developing cardiac hypertrophy.[238] TRPC function can be inhibited by protein kinase G–dependent phosphorylation resulting in the attenuation of pathological hypertrophy; this mechanism has been linked to the antihypertrophic effects of atrial natriuretic peptide.[239] TRPC has also been linked to the cellular response to angiotensin II.[240] In humans, TRPC5[236] and TRPC6[241] expression is induced in heart failure. TRPV1 may be cardioprotective in the setting of ischemic stress, possibly by augmenting substance P release from the sensory nerves that innervate the heart.[242] Increased TRPV1 activity has also been linked to the development of pressure overload-induced cardiac hypertrophy. Thus targeting TRPCs and TRPV1 may have therapeutic potential for treating heart disease.[243] The role of TRPM2 in ischemic cardiomyopathy is controversial with some study groups demonstrating a protective role[244] and others a detrimental one.[245]

In summary, in cardiac cells, several ion channels contribute to Ca^{2+} influx, principally the L-type and T-type voltage-gated Ca^{2+} channels and TRP channels. Ca^{2+} influx is essential for many functions throughout the various regions of the heart, and altered expression and/or activity of these Ca^{2+} channels can cause Ca^{2+} overload, leading to arrhythmogenic events and adverse gene expression. Identifying mechanisms to regulate dysfunctional Ca^{2+} influx remains an important goal in designing therapeutic cardiovascular interventions.

Acknowledgments

This work was supported by National Institutes of Health grants R01 HL113136 and HL121253 to SOM.

REFERENCES

1. Alexander SP, Benson HE, Faccenda E, et al. The Concise Guide to PHARMACOLOGY 2013/14: ion channels. *Br J Pharmacol*. 2013;170:1607–1651.
2. Catterall WA, Perez-Reyes E, Snutch TP, Striessnig J. Voltage-gated calcium channels. <http://www.guidetopharmacology.org/GRAC/FamilyDisplayForward?familyId=80>; 2015 Accessed 12.04.15.
3. Dirksen RT, Beam KG. Single calcium channel behavior in native skeletal muscle. *J Gen Physiol*. 1995;105:227–247.
4. Freise D, Held B, Wissenbach U, et al. Absence of the gamma subunit of the skeletal muscle dihydropyridine receptor increases L-type Ca2+ currents and alters channel inactivation properties. *J Biol Chem*. 2000;275:14476–14481.
5. Magyar J, Iost N, Kortvely A, et al. Effects of endothelin-1 on calcium and potassium currents in undiseased human ventricular myocytes. *Pflugers Arch*. 2000;441:144–149.
6. Singh A, Gebhart M, Fritsch R, et al. Modulation of voltage- and Ca2+-dependent gating of CaV1.3 L-type calcium channels by alternative splicing of a C-terminal regulatory domain. *J Biol Chem*. 2008;283:20733–20744.
7. McRory JE, Hamid J, Doering CJ, et al. The CACNA1F gene encodes an L-type calcium channel with unique biophysical properties and tissue distribution. *J Neurosci*. 2004;24:1707–1718.
8. Koschak A, Reimer D, Walter D, et al. Cav1.4alpha1 subunits can form slowly inactivating dihydropyridine-sensitive L-type Ca2+ channels lacking Ca2+-dependent inactivation. *J Neurosci*. 2003;23:6041–6049.
9. Hans M, Urrutia A, Deal C, et al. Structural elements in domain IV that influence biophysical and pharmacological properties of human alpha1A-containing high-voltage-activated calcium channels. *Biophys J*. 1999;76:1384–1400.
10. Bleakman D, Bowman D, Bath CP, et al. Characteristics of a human N-type calcium channel expressed in HEK293 cells. *Neuropharmacology*. 1995;34:753–765.
11. Li L, Bischofberger J, Jonas P. Differential gating and recruitment of P/Q-, N-, and R-type Ca2+ channels in hippocampal mossy fiber boutons. *J Neurosci*. 2007;27:13420–13429.
12. Monteil A, Chemin J, Bourinet E, Mennessier G, Lory P, Nargeot J. Molecular and functional properties of the human alpha(1G) subunit that forms T-type calcium channels. *J Biol Chem*. 2000;275:6090–6100.
13. Williams ME, Washburn MS, Hans M, et al. Structure and functional characterization of a novel human low-voltage activated calcium channel. *J Neurochem*. 1999;72:791–799.
14. Gomora JC, Murbartian J, Arias JM, Lee JH, Perez-Reyes E. Cloning and expression of the human T-type channel Ca(v)3.3: insights into prepulse facilitation. *Biophys J*. 2002;83:229–241.
15. Bean BP. Two kinds of calcium channels in canine atrial cells. Differences in kinetics, selectivity, and pharmacology. *J Gen Physiol*. 1985;86:1–30.
16. Nilius B, Hess P, Lansman JB, Tsien RW. A novel type of cardiac calcium channel in ventricular cells. *Nature*. 1985;316:443–446.
17. Koval OM, Guan X, Wu Y, et al. CaV1.2 beta-subunit coordinates CaMKII-triggered cardiomyocyte death and afterdepolarizations. *Proc Natl Acad Sci U S A*. 2010;107:4996–5000.

18. Blaich A, Welling A, Fischer S, et al. Facilitation of murine cardiac L-type Cav1.2 channel is modulated by calmodulin kinase II-dependent phosphorylation of S1512 and S1570. *Proc Natl Acad Sci U S A*. 2010;107:10285–10299.
19. Zuhlke RD, Pitt GS, Deisseroth K, Tsien RW, Reuter H. Calmodulin supports both inactivation and facilitation of L-type calcium channels. *Nature*. 1999;399:159–162.
20. Pitt GS, Zuhlke RD, Hudmon A, Schulman H, Reuter H, Tsien RW. Molecular basis of calmodulin tethering and Ca2+-dependent inactivation of L-type Ca2+ channels. *J Biol Chem*. 2001;276:30794–30802.
21. Fuller MD, Emrick MA, Sadilek M, Scheuer T, Catterall WA. Molecular mechanism of calcium channel regulation in the fight-or-flight response. *Sci Signal*. 2010;3: ra70.
22. De Jongh KS, Murphy BJ, Colvin AA, Hell JW, Takahashi M, Catterall WA. Specific phosphorylation of a site in the full-length form of the alpha 1 subunit of the cardiac L-type calcium channel by adenosine 3′,5′-cyclic monophosphate-dependent protein kinase. *Biochemistry*. 1996;35:10392–10402.
23. Yang L, Katchman A, Samad T, Morrow JP, Weinberg RL, Marx SO. beta-adrenergic regulation of the L-type Ca2+ channel does not require phosphorylation of alpha1C Ser1700. *Circ Res*. 2013;113:871–880.
24. Hulme JT, Konoki K, Lin TW, et al. Sites of proteolytic processing and noncovalent association of the distal C-terminal domain of CaV1.1 channels in skeletal muscle. *Proc Natl Acad Sci U S A*. 2005;102:5274–5279.
25. Lipscombe D, Helton TD, Xu W. L-type calcium channels: the low down. *J Neurophysiol*. 2004;92:2633–2641.
26. Benitah JP, Alvarez JL, Gomez AM. L-type Ca(2+) current in ventricular cardiomyocytes. *J Mol Cell Cardiol*. 2010;48:26–36.
27. Catterall WA, Striessnig J, Snutch TP, Perez-Reyes E. International Union of. International Union of Pharmacology. XL. Compendium of voltage-gated ion channels: calcium channels. *Pharmacol Rev*. 2003;55:579–581.
28. Ertel EA, Campbell KP, Harpold MM, et al. Nomenclature of voltage-gated calcium channels. *Neuron*. 2000;25:533–535.
29. Mesirca P, Torrente AG, Mangoni ME. T-type channels in the sino-atrial and atrioventricular pacemaker mechanism. *Pflugers Arch*. 2014;466:791–799.
30. Perez-Reyes E. Molecular physiology of low-voltage-activated t-type calcium channels. *Physiol Rev*. 2003;83: 117–161.
31. Catterall WA. Structure and regulation of voltage-gated Ca2+ channels. *Annu Rev Cell Dev Biol*. 2000;16:521–555.
32. Striessnig J. Pharmacology, structure and function of cardiac L-type Ca(2+) channels. *Cell Physiol Biochem*. 1999;9:242–269.
33. Soldatov NM. Genomic structure of human L-type Ca2+ channel. *Genomics*. 1994;22:77–87.
34. Cheng X, Liu J, Asuncion-Chin M, et al. A novel Ca(V)1.2 N terminus expressed in smooth muscle cells of resistance size arteries modifies channel regulation by auxiliary subunits. *J Biol Chem*. 2007;282:29211–29221.
35. Abernethy DR, Soldatov NM. Structure-functional diversity of human L-type Ca2+ channel: perspectives

for new pharmacological targets. *J Pharmacol Exp Ther*. 2002;300:724–728.
36. Welling A, Ludwig A, Zimmer S, Klugbauer N, Flockerzi V, Hofmann F. Alternatively spliced IS6 segments of the alpha 1C gene determine the tissue-specific dihydropyridine sensitivity of cardiac and vascular smooth muscle L-type Ca2+ channels. *Circ Res*. 1997;81:526–532.
37. De Jongh KS, Warner C, Colvin AA, Catterall WA. Characterization of the two size forms of the alpha 1 subunit of skeletal muscle L-type calcium channels. *Proc Natl Acad Sci U S A*. 1991;88:10778–10782.
38. De Jongh KS, Merrick DK, Catterall WA. Subunits of purified calcium channels: a 212-kDa form of alpha 1 and partial amino acid sequence of a phosphorylation site on an independent beta subunit. *Proc Natl Acad Sci U S A*. 1989;86:8585–8589.
39. Hulme JT, Yarov-Yarovoy V, Lin TW, Scheuer T, Catterall WA. Autoinhibitory control of the CaV1.2 channel by its proteolytically processed distal C-terminal domain. *J Physiol*. 2006;576(pt 1):87–102.
40. Fu Y, Westenbroek RE, Yu FH, et al. Deletion of the distal C terminus of CaV1.2 channels leads to loss of beta-adrenergic regulation and heart failure in vivo. *J Biol Chem*. 2011;286:12617–12626.
41. Gerhardstein BL, Gao T, Bunemann M, et al. Proteolytic processing of the C terminus of the alpha(1C) subunit of L-type calcium channels and the role of a proline-rich domain in membrane tethering of proteolytic fragments. *J Biol Chem*. 2000;275:8556–8563.
42. Wei X, Neely A, Lacerda AE, et al. Modification of Ca2+ channel activity by deletions at the carboxyl terminus of the cardiac alpha 1 subunit. *J Biol Chem*. 1994;269:1635–1640.
43. Gao T, Cuadra AE, Ma H, et al. C-terminal fragments of the alpha 1C (CaV1.2) subunit associate with and regulate L-type calcium channels containing C-terminal-truncated alpha 1C subunits. *J Biol Chem*. 2001;276:21089–21097.
44. Gao T, Bunemann M, Gerhardstein BL, Ma H, Hosey MM. Role of the C terminus of the alpha 1C (CaV1.2) subunit in membrane targeting of cardiac L-type calcium channels. *J Biol Chem*. 2000;275:25436–25444.
45. Domes K, Ding J, Lemke T, et al. Truncation of murine CaV1.2 results in heart failure after birth. *J Biol Chem*. 2011;286:33863–33871.
46. De Waard M, Pragnell M, Campbell KP. Ca2+ channel regulation by a conserved beta subunit domain. *Neuron*. 1994;13:495–503.
47. Birnbaumer L, Qin N, Olcese R, et al. Structures and functions of calcium channel beta subunits. *J Bioenerg Biomembr*. 1998;30:357–375.
48. Buraei Z, Yang J. The ss subunit of voltage-gated Ca2+ channels. *Physiol Rev*. 2010;90:1461–1506.
49. Link S, Meissner M, Held B, et al. Diversity and developmental expression of L-type calcium channel beta2 proteins and their influence on calcium current in murine heart. *J Biol Chem*. 2009;284:30129–30137.
50. Marionneau C, Couette B, Liu J, et al. Specific pattern of ionic channel gene expression associated with pacemaker activity in the mouse heart. *J Physiol*. 2005;562(pt 1):223–234.
51. Chen YH, Li MH, Zhang Y, et al. Structural basis of the alpha1-beta subunit interaction of voltage-gated Ca2+ channels. *Nature*. 2004;429:675–680.

52. Opatowsky Y, Chen CC, Campbell KP, Hirsch JA. Structural analysis of the voltage-dependent calcium channel beta subunit functional core and its complex with the alpha 1 interaction domain. *Neuron*. 2004;42:387–399.
53. Van Petegem F, Clark KA, Chatelain FC, Minor Jr DL. Structure of a complex between a voltage-gated calcium channel beta-subunit and an alpha-subunit domain. *Nature*. 2004;429:671–675.
54. Van Petegem F, Duderstadt KE, Clark KA, Wang M, Minor Jr DL. Alanine-scanning mutagenesis defines a conserved energetic hotspot in the CaValpha1 AID-CaVbeta interaction site that is critical for channel modulation. *Structure*. 2008;16:280–294.
55. Fang K, Colecraft HM. Mechanism of auxiliary beta-subunit-mediated membrane targeting of L-type (Ca(V)1.2) channels. *J Physiol*. 2011;589(pt 18):4437–4455.
56. Weissgerber P, Held B, Bloch W, et al. Reduced cardiac L-type Ca2+ current in Ca(V)beta2-/- embryos impairs cardiac development and contraction with secondary defects in vascular maturation. *Circ Res*. 2006;99:749–757.
57. Meissner M, Weissgerber P, Londono JE, et al. Moderate calcium channel dysfunction in adult mice with inducible cardiomyocyte-specific excision of the cacnb2 gene. *J Biol Chem*. 2011;286:15875–15882.
58. Gong HC, Hang J, Kohler W, Li L, Su TZ. Tissue-specific expression and gabapentin-binding properties of calcium channel alpha2delta subunit subtypes. *J Membr Biol*. 2001;184:35–43.
59. Gurnett CA, Felix R, Campbell KP. Extracellular interaction of the voltage-dependent Ca2+ channel alpha2delta and alpha1 subunits. *J Biol Chem*. 1997;272:18508–18512.
60. Davies A, Hendrich J, Van Minh AT, Wratten J, Douglas L, Dolphin AC. Functional biology of the alpha(2)delta subunits of voltage-gated calcium channels. *Trends Pharmacol Sci*. 2007;28:220–228.
61. Lin Z, Witschas K, Garcia T, et al. A critical GxxxA motif in the gamma6 calcium channel subunit mediates its inhibitory effect on Cav3.1 calcium current. *J Physiol*. 2008;586(pt 22):5349–5366.
62. Yang L, Katchman A, Morrow JP, Doshi D, Marx SO. Cardiac L-type calcium channel (Cav1.2) associates with gamma subunits. *FASEB J*. 2011;25:928–936.
63. Guia A, Stern MD, Lakatta EG, Josephson IR. Ion concentration-dependence of rat cardiac unitary L-type calcium channel conductance. *Biophys J*. 2001;80:2742–2750.
64. McDonald TF, Pelzer S, Trautwein W, Pelzer DJ. Regulation and modulation of calcium channels in cardiac, skeletal, and smooth muscle cells. *Physiol Rev*. 1994;74:365–507.
65. Mesirca P, Torrente AG, Mangoni ME. Functional role of voltage gated Ca(2+) channels in heart automaticity. *Front Physiol*. 2015;6:19.
66. Platzer J, Engel J, Schrott-Fischer A, et al. Congenital deafness and sinoatrial node dysfunction in mice lacking class D L-type Ca2+ channels. *Cell*. 2000;102:89–97.
67. Koschak A, Reimer D, Huber I, et al. alpha 1D (Cav1.3) subunits can form l-type Ca2+ channels activating at negative voltages. *J Biol Chem*. 2001;276:22100–22106.
68. Haack JA, Rosenberg RL. Calcium-dependent inactivation of L-type calcium channels in planar lipid bilayers. *Biophys J*. 1994;66:1051–1060.
69. Hering S, Berjukow S, Sokolov S, et al. Molecular determinants of inactivation in voltage-gated Ca2+ channels. *J Physiol*. 2000;528(pt 2):237–249.
70. Brunet S, Emrick MA, Sadilek M, Scheuer T, Catterall WA. Phosphorylation sites in the Hook domain of Cabeta subunits differentially modulate Ca1.2 channel function. *J Mol Cell Cardiol*. 2015;87:248–256.
71. Peterson BZ, DeMaria CD, Adelman JP, Yue DT. Calmodulin is the Ca2+ sensor for Ca2+ -dependent inactivation of L-type calcium channels. *Neuron*. 1999;22:549–558.
72. Zuhlke RD, Pitt GS, Tsien RW, Reuter H. Ca2+-sensitive inactivation and facilitation of L-type Ca2+ channels both depend on specific amino acid residues in a consensus calmodulin-binding motif in the(alpha)1C subunit. *J Biol Chem*. 2000;275:21121–21129.
73. Poomvanicha M, Wegener JW, Blaich A, et al. Facilitation and Ca2+-dependent inactivation are modified by mutation of the Ca(v)1.2 channel IQ motif. *J Biol Chem*. 2011;286:26702–26707.
74. Cheng RC, Tikhonov DB, Zhorov BS. Structural model for phenylalkylamine binding to L-type calcium channels. *J Biol Chem*. 2009;284:28332–28342.
75. Tikhonov DB, Zhorov BS. Structural model for dihydropyridine binding to L-type calcium channels. *J Biol Chem*. 2009;284:19006–19017.
76. Striessnig J, Ortner NJ, Pinggera A. Pharmacology of L-type calcium channels: novel drugs for old targets? *Curr Mol Pharmacol*. 2015;8:110–122.
77. Bean BP, Sturek M, Puga A, Hermsmeyer K. Calcium channels in muscle cells isolated from rat mesenteric arteries: modulation by dihydropyridine drugs. *Circ Res*. 1986;59:229–235.
78. Berjukow S, Hering S. Voltage-dependent acceleration of Ca(v)1.2 channel current decay by (+)- and (-)-isradipine. *Br J Pharmacol*. 2001;133:959–966.
79. Hamilton SL, Yatani A, Brush K, Schwartz A, Brown AM. A comparison between the binding and electrophysiological effects of dihydropyridines on cardiac membranes. *Mol Pharmacol*. 1987;31:221–231.
80. Fleischmann BK, Murray RK, Kotlikoff MI. Voltage window for sustained elevation of cytosolic calcium in smooth muscle cells. *Proc Natl Acad Sci U S A*. 1994;91:11914–11918.
81. Beyl S, Timin EN, Hohaus A, Stary A, Kudrnac M, Guy Hering S. Probing the architecture of an L-type calcium channel with a charged phenylalkylamine: evidence for a widely open pore and drug trapping. *J Biol Chem*. 2007;282:3864–3870.
82. Hering S, Aczel S, Kraus RL, Berjukow S, Striessnig J, Timin EN. Molecular mechanism of use-dependent calcium channel block by phenylalkylamines: role of inactivation. *Proc Natl Acad Sci U S A*. 1997;94:13323–13328.
83. Takemura H, Yasui K, Opthof T, et al. Subtype switching of L-Type Ca 2+ channel from Cav1.3 to Cav1.2 in embryonic murine ventricle. *Circ J*. 2005;69:1405–1411.
84. Fabiato A, Fabiato F. Contractions induced by a calcium-triggered release of calcium from the sarcoplasmic reticulum of single skinned cardiac cells. *J Physiol*. 1975;249:469–495.
85. Bers DM. Cardiac excitation-contraction coupling. *Nature*. 2002;415:198–205.
86. Hong TT, Smyth JW, Gao D, et al. BIN1 localizes the L-type calcium channel to cardiac T-tubules. *PLoS Biol*. 2010;8:e1000312.
87. Hong TT, Cogswell R, James CA, et al. Plasma BIN1 correlates with heart failure and predicts arrhythmia in patients with arrhythmogenic right ventricular cardiomyopathy. *Heart Rhythm*. 2012;9:961–967.
88. Seisenberger C, Specht V, Welling A, et al. Functional embryonic cardiomyocytes after disruption of the L-type alpha1C (Cav1.2) calcium channel gene in the mouse. *J Biol Chem*. 2000;275:39193–39199.
89. Zhang Z, Xu Y, Song H, et al. Functional Roles of Ca(v)1.3 (alpha(1D)) calcium channel in sinoatrial nodes: insight gained using gene-targeted null mutant mice. *Circ Res*. 2002;90:981–987.
90. Marger L, Mesirca P, Alig J, et al. Functional roles of Ca(v)1.3, Ca(v)3.1 and HCN channels in automaticity of mouse atrioventricular cells: insights into the atrioventricular pacemaker mechanism. *Channels (Austin)*. 2011;5:251–261.
91. Christel CJ, Cardona N, Mesirca P, et al. Distinct localization and modulation of Cav1.2 and Cav1.3 L-type Ca2+ channels in mouse sinoatrial node. *J Physiol*. 2012;590(pt 24):6327–6342.
92. January CT, Riddle JM. Early afterdepolarizations: mechanism of induction and block. A role for L-type Ca2+ current. *Circ Res*. 1989;64:977–990.
93. Splawski I, Timothy KW, Decher N, et al. Severe arrhythmia disorder caused by cardiac L-type calcium channel mutations. *Proc Natl Acad Sci U S A*. 2005;102:8089–8096. discussion 8086–8088.
94. Betzenhauser MJ, Pitt GS, Antzelevitch C. Calcium channel mutations in cardiac arrhythmia syndromes. *Curr Mol Pharmacol*. 2015;8:133–142.
95. Antzelevitch C, Pollevick GD, Cordeiro JM, et al. Loss-of-function mutations in the cardiac calcium channel underlie a new clinical entity characterized by ST-segment elevation, short QT intervals, and sudden cardiac death. *Circulation*. 2007;115:442–449.
96. Burashnikov E, Pfeiffer R, Barajas-Martinez H, et al. Mutations in the cardiac L-type calcium channel associated with inherited J-wave syndromes and sudden cardiac death. *Heart Rhythm*. 2010;7:1872–1882.
97. Cordeiro JM, Marieb M, Pfeiffer R, Calloe K, Burashnikov E, Antzelevitch C. Accelerated inactivation of the L-type calcium current due to a mutation in CACNB2b underlies Brugada syndrome. *J Mol Cell Cardiol*. 2009;46:695–703.
98. Gao H, Wang F, Wang W, et al. Ca(2+) influx through L-type Ca(2+) channels and transient receptor potential channels activates pathological hypertrophy signaling. *J Mol Cell Cardiol*. 2012;53:657–667.
99. Zhang H, Chen X, Gao E, et al. Increasing cardiac contractility after myocardial infarction exacerbates cardiac injury and pump dysfunction. *Circ Res*. 2010;107:800–809.
100. Makarewich CA, Correll RN, Gao H, et al. A caveolae-targeted L-type Ca(2)+ channel antagonist inhibits hypertrophic signaling without reducing cardiac contractility. *Circ Res*. 2012;110:669–674.
101. Goonasekera SA, Hammer K, Auger-Messier M, et al. Decreased cardiac L-type Ca(2)(+) channel activity induces hypertrophy and heart failure in mice. *J Clin Invest*. 2012;122:280–290.
102. Bodi I, Mikala G, Koch SE, Akhter SA, Schwartz A. The L-type calcium channel in the heart: the beat goes on. *J Clin Invest*. 2005;115:3306–3317.
103. Dai S, Hall DD, Hell JW. Supramolecular assemblies and localized regulation of voltage-gated ion channels. *Physiol Rev*. 2009;89:411–452.
104. Davare MA, Avdonin V, Hall DD, et al. A beta2 adrenergic receptor signaling complex assembled with the Ca2+ channel Cav1.2. *Science*. 2001;293:98–101.
105. Yang L, Liu G, Zakharov SI, et al. Ser1928 is a common site for Cav1.2 phosphorylation by protein kinase C isoforms. *J Biol Chem*. 2005;280:207–214.
106. Davare MA, Horne MC, Hell JW. Protein phosphatase 2A is associated with class C L-type calcium channels (Cav1.2) and antagonizes channel phosphorylation by cAMP-dependent protein kinase. *J Biol Chem*. 2000;275:39710–39717.
107. Tandan S, Wang Y, Wang TT, et al. Physical and functional interaction between calcineurin and the cardiac L-type Ca2+ channel. *Circ Res*. 2009;105:51–60.
108. Hulme JT, Ahn M, Hauschka SD, Scheuer T, Catterall WA. A novel leucine zipper targets AKAP15 and cyclic AMP-dependent protein kinase to the C terminus of the skeletal muscle Ca2+ channel and modulates its function. *J Biol Chem*. 2002;277:4079–4087.
109. Hulme JT, Lin TW, Westenbroek RE, Scheuer T, Catterall WA. Beta-adrenergic regulation requires direct anchoring of PKA to cardiac CaV1.2 channels via a leucine zipper interaction with A kinase-anchoring protein 15. *Proc Natl Acad Sci U S A*. 2003;100:13093–13098.
110. Balijepalli RC, Foell JD, Hall DD, Hell JW, Kamp TJ. Localization of cardiac L-type Ca(2+) channels to a caveolar macromolecular signaling complex is required for beta(2)-adrenergic regulation. *Proc Natl Acad Sci U S A*. 2006;103:7500–7505.
111. Hennessey JA, Wei EQ, Pitt GS. Fibroblast growth factor homologous factors modulate cardiac calcium channels. *Circ Res*. 2013;113:381–388.
112. Jiang M, Zhang M, Howren M, et al. JPH-2 interacts with Ca-handling proteins and ion channels in dyads: contribution to premature ventricular contraction-induced cardiomyopathy. *Heart Rhythm*. 2016;13:743–752.
113. Reuter H, Scholz H. The regulation of the calcium conductance of cardiac muscle by adrenaline. *J Physiol*. 1977;264:49–62.
114. Yue DT, Herzig S, Marban E. Beta-adrenergic stimulation of calcium channels occurs by potentiation of high-activity gating modes. *Proc Natl Acad Sci U S A*. 1990;87:753–757.
115. Mitterdorfer J, Froschmayr M, Grabner M, Moebius FF, Glossmann H, Striessnig J. Identification of PK-A phosphorylation sites in the carboxyl terminus of L-type calcium channel alpha 1 subunits. *Biochemistry*. 1996;35:9400–9406.
116. Perets T, Blumenstein Y, Shistik E, Lotan I, Dascal N. A potential site of functional modulation by protein kinase A in the cardiac Ca2+ channel alpha 1C subunit. *FEBS Lett*. 1996;384:189–192.
117. Gao T, Yatani A, Dell'Acqua ML, et al. cAMP-dependent regulation of cardiac L-type Ca2+ channels requires membrane targeting of PKA and phosphorylation of channel subunits. *Neuron*. 1997;19:185–196.
118. Hall DD, Davare MA, Shi M, et al. Critical role of cAMP-dependent protein kinase anchoring to the L-type calcium channel Cav1.2 via A-kinase anchor protein 150 in neurons. *Biochemistry*. 2007;46:1635–1646.
119. Hall DD, Feekes JA, Arachchige Don AS, et al. Binding of protein phosphatase 2A to the L-type calcium channel Cav1.2 next to Ser1928, its main PKA site, is critical for Ser1928 dephosphorylation. *Biochemistry*. 2006;45:3448–3459.
120. Hell JW, Yokoyama CT, Breeze LJ, Chavkin C, Catterall WA. Phosphorylation of presynaptic and postsynaptic calcium channels by cAMP-dependent protein kinase in hippocampal neurons. *EMBO J*. 1995;14:3036–3044.
121. Hulme JT, Westenbroek RE, Scheuer T, Catterall WA. Phosphorylation of serine 1928 in the distal C-terminal domain of cardiac CaV1.2 channels during beta1-adrenergic regulation. *Proc Natl Acad Sci U S A*. 2006;103:16574–16579.
122. Ganesan AN, O'Rourke B, Maack C, Colecraft H, Sidor A, Johns DC. Reverse engineering the L-type Ca2+ channel alpha1c subunit in adult cardiac myocytes using novel adenoviral vectors. *Biochem Biophys Res Commun*. 2005;329:749–754.
123. Lemke T, Welling A, Christel CJ, et al. Unchanged beta-adrenergic stimulation of cardiac L-type calcium channels in Ca v 1.2 phosphorylation site S1928A mutant mice. *J Biol Chem*. 2008;283:34738–34744.

124. Gerhardstein BL, Puri TS, Chien AJ, Hosey MM. Identification of the sites phosphorylated by cyclic AMP-dependent protein kinase on the beta 2 subunit of L-type voltage-dependent calcium channels. *Biochemistry*. 1999;38:10361–10370.

125. Ganesan AN, Maack C, Johns DC, Sidor A, O'Rourke B. Beta-adrenergic stimulation of L-type Ca2+ channels in cardiac myocytes requires the distal carboxyl terminus of alpha1C but not serine 1928. *Circ Res*. 2006;98:e11–e18.

126. Miriyala J, Nguyen T, Yue DT, Colecraft HM. Role of CaVbeta subunits, and lack of functional reserve, in protein kinase A modulation of cardiac CaV1.2 channels. *Circ Res*. 2008;102:e54–e64.

127. Brandmayr J, Poomvanicha M, Domes K, et al. Deletion of the C-terminal phosphorylation sites in the cardiac beta-subunit does not affect the basic beta-adrenergic response of the heart and the Ca(v)1.2 channel. *J Biol Chem*. 2012;287(27):22584–22592.

128. Emrick MA, Sadilek M, Konoki K, Catterall WA. Beta-adrenergic-regulated phosphorylation of the skeletal muscle Ca(V)1.1 channel in the fight-or-flight response. *Proc Natl Acad Sci U S A*. 2010;107:18712–18717.

129. Yang L, Katchman A, Weinberg RL, et al. The PDZ motif of the alpha1C subunit is not required for surface trafficking and adrenergic modulation of CaV1.2 channel in the heart. *J Biol Chem*. 2015;290:2166–2174.

130. Hundsrucker C, Rosenthal W, Klussmann E. Peptides for disruption of PKA anchoring. *Biochem Soc Trans*. 2006;34(pt 4):472–473.

131. Nichols CB, Rossow CF, Navedo MF, et al. Sympathetic stimulation of adult cardiomyocytes requires association of AKAP5 with a subpopulation of L-type calcium channels. *Circ Res*. 2010;107:747–756.

132. Hell JW. Beta-adrenergic regulation of the L-type Ca2+ channel Ca(V)1.2 by PKA rekindles excitement. *Sci Signal*. 2010;3:pe33.

133. Jones BW, Brunet S, Gilbert ML, et al. Cardiomyocytes from AKAP7 knockout mice respond normally to adrenergic stimulation. *Proc Natl Acad Sci U S A*. 2012;109:17099–17104.

134. Sun AY, Pitt GS. Pinning down the CaMKII targets in the L-type Ca(2+) channel: an essential step in defining CaMKII regulation. *Heart Rhythm*. 2011;8:631–633.

135. Lambert RC, Maulet Y, Mouton J, et al. T-type Ca2+ current properties are not modified by Ca2+ channel beta subunit depletion in nodosus ganglion neurons. *J Neurosci*. 1997;17:6621–6628.

136. Leuranguer V, Bourinet E, Lory P, Nargeot J. Antisense depletion of beta-subunits fails to affect T-type calcium channels properties in a neuroblastoma cell line. *Neuropharmacology*. 1998;37:701–708.

137. Dolphin AC, Wyatt CN, Richards J, et al. The effect of alpha2-delta and other accessory subunits on expression and properties of the calcium channel alpha1G. *J Physiol*. 1999; 519 Pt. 1:35–45.

138. Gao B, Sekido Y, Maximov A, et al. Functional properties of a new voltage-dependent calcium channel alpha(2)delta auxiliary subunit gene (CACNA2D2). *J Biol Chem*. 2000;275:12237–12242.

139. Curran J, Musa H, Kline CF, et al. Eps15 homology domain-containing protein 3 regulates cardiac T-type Ca2+ channel targeting and function in the atria. *J Biol Chem*. 2015;290:12210–12221.

140. Senatore A, Spafford JD. Gene transcription and splicing of T-type channels are evolutionarily-conserved strategies for regulating channel expression and gating. *PLoS One*. 2012;7:e37409.

141. Ferron L, Capuano V, Deroubaix E, Coulombe A, Renaud JF. Functional and molecular characterization of a T-type Ca(2+) channel during fetal and postnatal rat heart development. *J Mol Cell Cardiol*. 2002;34: 533–546.

142. Niwa N, Yasui K, Opthof T, et al. Cav3.2 subunit underlies the functional T-type Ca2+ channel in murine hearts during the embryonic period. *Am J Physiol Heart Circ Physiol*. 2004;286:H2257–H2263.

143. Mangoni ME, Traboulsie A, Leoni AL, et al. Bradycardia and slowing of the atrioventricular conduction in mice lacking CaV3.1/alpha1G T-type calcium channels. *Circ Res*. 2006;98:1422–1430.

144. Senatore A, Guan W, Spafford JD. Cav3 T-type channels: regulators for gating, membrane expression, and cation selectivity. *Pflugers Arch*. 2014;466:645–660.

145. Serrano JR, Perez-Reyes E, Jones SW. State-dependent inactivation of the alpha1G T-type calcium channel. *J Gen Physiol*. 1999;114:185–201.

146. McRory JE, Santi CM, Hamming KS, et al. Molecular and functional characterization of a family of rat brain T-type calcium channels. *J Biol Chem*. 2001;276:3999–4011.

147. Vassort G, Alvarez J. Cardiac T-type calcium current: pharmacology and roles in cardiac tissues. *J Cardiovasc Electrophysiol*. 1994;5:376–393.

148. Huguenard JR. Low-threshold calcium currents in central nervous system neurons. *Annu Rev Physiol*. 1996;58:329–348.

149. Talavera K, Nilius B. Biophysics and structure-function relationship of T-type Ca2+ channels. *Cell Calcium*. 2006;40:97–114.

150. Arias-Olguín II, Vitko I, Fortuna M, et al. Characterization of the gating brake in the I-II loop of Ca(v)3.2 T-type Ca(2+) channels. *J Biol Chem*. 2008;283: 8136–8144.

151. Baumgart JP, Vitko I, Bidaud I, Kondratskyi A, Lory P, Perez-Reyes E. I-II loop structural determinants in the gating and surface expression of low voltage-activated calcium channels. *PLoS One*. 2008;3:e2976.

152. Randall A, Tsien RW. Pharmacological dissection of multiple types of Ca2+ channel currents in rat cerebellar granule neurons. *J Neurosci*. 1995;15:2995–3012.

153. Lee JH, Gomora JC, Cribbs LL, Perez-Reyes E. Nickel block of three cloned T-type calcium channels: low concentrations selectively block alpha1H. *Biophys J*. 1999;77:3034–3042.

154. Klockner U, Lee JH, Cribbs LL, et al. Comparison of the Ca2 + currents induced by expression of three cloned alpha1 subunits, alpha1G, alpha1H and alpha1I, of low-voltage-activated T-type Ca2 + channels. *Eur J Neurosci*. 1999;11: 4171–4178.

155. Satin J, Cribbs LL. Identification of a T-type Ca(2+) channel isoform in murine atrial myocytes (AT-1 cells). *Circ Res*. 2000;86:636–642.

156. Mishra SK, Hermsmeyer K. Selective inhibition of T-type Ca2+ channels by Ro 40-5967. *Circ Res*. 1994;75:144–148.

157. Martin RL, Lee JH, Cribbs LL, Perez-Reyes E, Hanck DA. Mibefradil block of cloned T-type calcium channels. *J Pharmacol Exp Ther*. 2000;295:302–308.

158. Perchenet L, Benardeau A, Ertel EA. Pharmacological properties of Ca(V)3.2, a low voltage-activated Ca2+ channel cloned from human heart. *Naunyn Schmiedebergs Arch Pharmacol*. 2000;361:590–599.

159. Krayenbuhl JC, Vozeh S, Kondo-Oestreicher M, Dayer P. Drug-drug interactions of new active substances: mibefradil example. *Eur J Clin Pharmacol*. 1999;55:559–565.

160. Bezprozvanny I, Tsien RW. Voltage-dependent blockade of diverse types of voltage-gated Ca2+ channels expressed in Xenopus oocytes by the Ca2+ channel antagonist mibefradil (Ro 40-5967). *Mol Pharmacol*. 1995;48:540–549.

161. McDonough SI, Bean BP. Mibefradil inhibition of T-type calcium channels in cerebellar purkinje neurons. *Mol Pharmacol*. 1998;54:1080–1087.

162. Eller P, Berjukov S, Wanner S, et al. High affinity interaction of mibefradil with voltage-gated calcium and sodium channels. *Br J Pharmacol*. 2000;130:669–677.

163. Gomora JC, Enyeart JA, Enyeart JJ. Mibefradil potently blocks ATP-activated K(+) channels in adrenal cells. *Mol Pharmacol*. 1999;56:1192–1197.

164. Nilius B, Prenen J, Kamouchi M, Viana F, Voets T, Droogmans G. Inhibition by mibefradil, a novel calcium channel antagonist, of Ca(2+)- and volume-activated Cl- channels in macrovascular endothelial cells. *Br J Pharmacol*. 1997;121:547–555.

165. Akaike N, Kanaide H, Kuga T, Nakamura M, Sadoshima J, Tomoike H. Low-voltage-activated calcium current in rat aorta smooth muscle cells in primary culture. *J Physiol*. 1989;416:141–160.

166. Cohen CJ, Spires S, Van Skiver D. Block of T-type Ca channels in guinea pig atrial cells by antiarrhythmic agents and Ca channel antagonists. *J Gen Physiol*. 1992;100:703–728.

167. Lievano A, Bolden A, Horn R. Calcium channels in excitable cells: divergent genotypic and phenotypic expression of alpha 1-subunits. *Am J Physiol*. 1994;267(2 pt 1):C411–C424.

168. Kass RS. Voltage-dependent modulation of cardiac calcium channel current by optical isomers of Bay K 8644: implications for channel gating. *Circ Res*. 1987;61(4 pt 2):I1–I15.

169. Coulter DA, Huguenard JR, Prince DA. Characterization of ethosuximide reduction of low-threshold calcium current in thalamic neurons. *Ann Neurol*. 1989;25:582–593.

170. Kostyuk PG, Molokanova EA, Pronchuk NF, Savchenko AN, Verkhratsky AN. Different action of ethosuximide on low- and high-threshold calcium currents in rat sensory neurons. *Neuroscience*. 1992;51:755–758.

171. Todorovic SM, Lingle CJ. Pharmacological properties of T-type Ca2+ current in adult rat sensory neurons: effects of anticonvulsant and anesthetic agents. *J Neurophysiol*. 1998;79:240–252.

172. Twombly DA, Yoshii M, Narahashi T. Mechanisms of calcium channel block by phenytoin. *J Pharmacol Exp Ther*. 1988;246:189–195.

173. Todorovic SM, Jevtovic-Todorovic V, Mennerick S, Perez-Reyes E, Zorumski CF. Ca(v)3.2 channel is a molecular substrate for inhibition of T-type calcium currents in rat sensory neurons by nitrous oxide. *Mol Pharmacol*. 2001;60:603–610.

174. Todorovic SM, Perez-Reyes E, Lingle CJ. Anticonvulsants but not general anesthetics have differential blocking effects on different T-type current variants. *Mol Pharmacol*. 2000;58:98–108.

175. Enyeart JJ, Biagi BA, Mlinar B. Preferential block of T-type calcium channels by neuroleptics in neural crest-derived rat and human C cell lines. *Mol Pharmacol*. 1992;42:364–372.

176. Sipido KR, Carmeliet E, Van de Werf F. T-type Ca2+ current as a trigger for Ca2+ release from the sarcoplasmic reticulum in guinea-pig ventricular myocytes. *J Physiol*. 1998;508(pt 2):439–451.

177. Hagiwara N, Irisawa H, Kameyama M. Contribution of two types of calcium currents to the pacemaker potentials of rabbit sino-atrial node cells. *J Physiol*. 1988;395:233–253.

178. Wetzel GT, Chen F, Klitzner TS. Ca2+ channel kinetics in acutely isolated fetal, neonatal, and adult rabbit cardiac myocytes. *Circ Res*. 1993;72:1065–1074.

179. Chen CC, Lamping KG, Nuno DW, et al. Abnormal coronary function in mice deficient in alpha1H T-type Ca2+ channels. *Science*. 2003;302:1416–1418.

180. Le Quang K, Benito B, Naud P, et al. T-type calcium current contributes to escape automaticity and governs the occurrence of lethal arrhythmias after atrioventricular block in mice. *Circ Arrhythm Electrophysiol*. 2013;6:799–808.

181. Xu XP, Best PM. Increase in T-type calcium current in atrial myocytes from adult rats with growth hormone-secreting tumors. *Proc Natl Acad Sci U S A*. 1990;87:4655–4659.

182. Nuss HB, Houser SR. T-type Ca2+ current is expressed in hypertrophied adult feline left ventricular myocytes. *Circ Res*. 1993;73:777–782.

183. Sen L, Smith TW. T-type Ca2+ channels are abnormal in genetically determined cardiomyopathic hamster hearts. *Circ Res*. 1994;75:149–155.

184. Martinez ML, Heredia MP, Delgado C. Expression of T-type Ca(2+) channels in ventricular cells from hypertrophied rat hearts. *J Mol Cell Cardiol*. 1999;31:1617–1625.

185. Ferron L, Capuano V, Ruchon Y, Deroubaix E, Coulombe A, Renaud JF. Angiotensin II signaling pathways mediate expression of cardiac T-type calcium channels. *Circ Res*. 2003;93:1241–1248.

186. Huang B, Qin D, Deng L, Boutjdir M, El-Sherif N. Reexpression of T-type Ca2+ channel gene and current in post-infarction remodeled rat left ventricle. *Cardiovasc Res*. 2000;46:442–449.

187. Izumi T, Kihara Y, Sarai N, et al. Reinduction of T-type calcium channels by endothelin-1 in failing hearts in vivo and in adult rat ventricular myocytes in vitro. *Circulation*. 2003;108:2530–2535.

188. Kuwahara K, Saito Y, Takano M, et al. NRSF regulates the fetal cardiac gene program and maintains normal cardiac structure and function. *EMBO J*. 2003;22:6310–6321.

189. Chiang CS, Huang CH, Chieng H, et al. The Ca(v)3.2 T-type Ca(2+) channel is required for pressure overload-induced cardiac hypertrophy in mice. *Circ Res*. 2009;104:522–530.

190. Nakayama H, Bodi I, Correll RN, et al. alpha1G-dependent T-type Ca2+ current antagonizes cardiac hypertrophy through a NOS3-dependent mechanism in mice. *J Clin Invest*. 2009;119:3787–3796.

191. Chemin J, Traboulsie A, Lory P. Molecular pathways underlying the modulation of T-type calcium channels by neurotransmitters and hormones. *Cell Calcium*. 2006;40:121–134.

192. Fisher R, Johnston D. Differential modulation of single voltage-gated calcium channels by cholinergic and adrenergic agonists in adult hippocampal neurons. *J Neurophysiol*. 1990;64:1291–1302.

193. Benham CD, Tsien RW. Noradrenaline modulation of calcium channels in single smooth muscle cells from rabbit ear artery. *J Physiol*. 1988;404:767–784.

194. Hu C, Depuy SD, Yao J, W.E. McIntire WE, Barrett PQ. Protein kinase A activity controls the regulation of T-type CaV3.2 channels by Gbetagamma dimers. *J Biol Chem*. 2009;284:7465–7473.

195. Li Y, Wang F, Zhang X, et al. beta-Adrenergic stimulation increases Cav3.1 activity in cardiac myocytes through protein kinase A. *PLoS One*. 2012;7:e39965.

196. Welsby PJ, Wang H, Wolfe JT, Colbran RJ, Johnson ML, Barrett PQ. A mechanism for the direct regulation of T-type calcium channels by Ca2+/calmodulin-dependent kinase II. *J Neurosci*. 2003;23:10116–10121.

197. Clapham DE, Julius D, Montell C, Schultz G. International Union of Pharmacology. XLIX. Nomenclature and structure-function relationships of transient receptor potential channels. *Pharmacol Rev*. 2005;57:427–450.

198. Nilius B, Owsianik G. The transient receptor potential family of ion channels. *Genome Biol.* 2011;12:218.

199. Yoshida T, Inoue R, Morii T, et al. Nitric oxide activates TRP channels by cysteine S-nitrosylation. *Nat Chem Biol.* 2006;2:596–607.

200. Perraud AL, Fleig A, Dunn CA, et al. ADP-ribose gating of the calcium-permeable LTRPC2 channel revealed by Nudix motif homology. *Nature.* 2001;411:595–599.

201. Nadler MJ, Hermosura MC, Inabe K, et al. LTRPC7 is a Mg.ATP-regulated divalent cation channel required for cell viability. *Nature.* 2001;411:590–595.

202. Paulsen CE, Armache JP, Gao Y, Cheng Y, Julius D. Structure of the TRPA1 ion channel suggests regulatory mechanisms. *Nature.* 2015;520:511–517.

203. Liao M, Cao E, Julius D, Cheng Y. Structure of the TRPV1 ion channel determined by electron cryo-microscopy. *Nature.* 2013;504:107–112.

204. Cao E, Liao M, Cheng Y, Julius D. TRPV1 structures in distinct conformations reveal activation mechanisms. *Nature.* 2013;504:113–118.

205. Ju YK, Chu Y, Chaulet H, Lai D, et al. Store-operated Ca2+ influx and expression of TRPC genes in mouse sinoatrial node. *Circ Res.* 2007;100:1605–1614.

206. Wu LJ, Sweet TB, Clapham DE. International Union of Basic and Clinical Pharmacology. LXXVI. Current progress in the mammalian TRP ion channel family. *Pharmacol Rev.* 2010;62:381–404.

207. Yue Z, Xie J, Yu AS, Stock J, Du J, Yue L. Role of TRP channels in the cardiovascular system. *Am J Physiol Heart Circ Physiol.* 2015;308:H157–H182.

208. Vriens J, Owsianik G, Hofmann T, et al. TRPM3 is a nociceptor channel involved in the detection of noxious heat. *Neuron.* 2011;70:482–494.

209. Zimmermann K, Lennerz JK, Hein A, et al. Transient receptor potential cation channel, subfamily C, member 5 (TRPC5) is a cold-transducer in the peripheral nervous system. *Proc Natl Acad Sci U S A.* 2011;108:18114–18119.

210. Hara Y, Wakamori M, Ishii M, et al. LTRPC2 Ca2+-permeable channel activated by changes in redox status confers susceptibility to cell death. *Mol Cell.* 2002;9:163–173.

211. Poteser M, Graziani A, Rosker C, et al. TRPC3 and TRPC4 associate to form a redox-sensitive cation channel. Evidence for expression of native TRPC3-TRPC4 heteromeric channels in endothelial cells. *J Biol Chem.* 2006;281:13588–13595.

212. Xu SZ, Sukumar P, Zeng F, et al. TRPC channel activation by extracellular thioredoxin. *Nature.* 2008;451:69–72.

213. Ding Y, Winters A, Ding M, et al. Reactive oxygen species-mediated TRPC6 protein activation in vascular myocytes, a mechanism for vasoconstrictor-regulated vascular tone. *J Biol Chem.* 2011;286:31799–31809.

214. Clapham DE. TRP channels as cellular sensors. *Nature.* 2003;426:517–524.

215. Gomis A, Soriano S, Belmonte C, Viana F. Hypoosmotic- and pressure-induced membrane stretch activate TRPC5 channels. *J Physiol.* 2008;586(pt 23):5633–5649.

216. Spassova MA, Hewavitharana T, Xu W, Soboloff J, Gill DL. A common mechanism underlies stretch activation and receptor activation of TRPC6 channels. *Proc Natl Acad Sci U S A.* 2006;103:16586–16591.

217. Nauli SM, Alenghat FJ, Luo Y, et al. Polycystins 1 and 2 mediate mechanosensation in the primary cilium of kidney cells. *Nat Genet.* 2003;33:129–137.

218. Numata T, Shimizu T, Okada Y. Direct mechano-stress sensitivity of TRPM7 channel. *Cell Physiol Biochem.* 2007;19:1–8.

219. Strotmann R, Harteneck C, Nunnenmacher K, Schultz G, Plant TD. OTRPC4, a nonselective cation channel that confers sensitivity to extracellular osmolarity. *Nat Cell Biol.* 2000;2:695–702.

220. McNamara CR, Mandel-Brehm J, Bautista DM, et al. TRPA1 mediates formalin-induced pain. *Proc Natl Acad Sci U S A.* 2007;104:13525–13530.

221. Caterina MJ, Schumacher MA, Tominaga M, Rosen TA, Levine JD, Julius D. The capsaicin receptor: a heat-activated ion channel in the pain pathway. *Nature.* 1997;389:816–824.

222. Strubing C, Krapivinsky G, Krapivinsky L, Clapham DE. TRPC1 and TRPC5 form a novel cation channel in mammalian brain. *Neuron.* 2001;29:645–655.

223. Wu G, Markowitz GS, Li L, et al. Cardiac defects and renal failure in mice with targeted mutations in. *Pkd2. Nat Genet.* 2000;24:75–78.

224. Sah R, Mesirca P, Mason X, et al. Timing of myo-cardial trpm7 deletion during cardiogenesis variably disrupts adult ventricular function, conduction, and repolarization. *Circulation.* 2013;128:101–114.

225. Sah R, Mesirca P, Van den Boogert M, et al. Ion channel-kinase TRPM7 is required for maintaining cardiac automaticity. *Proc Natl Acad Sci U S A.* 2013;110:E3037–E3046.

226. Kruse M, Schulze-Bahr E, Corfield V, et al. Impaired endocytosis of the ion channel TRPM4 is associated with human progressive familial heart block type I. *J Clin Invest.* 2009;119:2737–2744.

227. Stallmeyer B, Zumhagen S, Denjoy I, et al. Mutational spectrum in the Ca(2+)-activated cation channel gene TRPM4 in patients with cardiac conductance disturbances. *Hum Mutat.* 2012;33:109–117.

228. Liu H, El Zein L, Kruse M, et al. Gain-of-function mutations in TRPM4 cause autosomal dominant iso-lated cardiac conduction disease. *Circ Cardiovasc Genet.* 2010;3:374–385.

229. Liu H, Chatel S, Simard C, et al. Molecular genetics and functional anomalies in a series of 248 Brugada cases with 11 mutations in the TRPM4 channel. *PLoS One.* 2013; 8:e54131.

230. Du J, Xie J, Zhang Z, et al. TRPM7-mediated Ca2+ signals confer fibrogenesis in human atrial fibrillation. *Circ Res.* 2010;106:992–1003.

231. Yue Z, Zhang Y, Xie J, Jiang J, Yue L. Transient receptor potential (TRP) channels and cardiac fibrosis. *Curr Top Med Chem.* 2013;13:270–282.

232. Harada M, Luo X, Qi XY, et al. Transient receptor potential canonical-3 channel-dependent fibroblast regulation in atrial fibrillation. *Circulation.* 2012;126:2051–2064.

233. Davis J, Burr AR, Davis GF, Birnbaumer L, Molkentin JD. A TRPC6-dependent pathway for myofibroblast transdifferentiation and wound healing in vivo. *Dev Cell.* 2012;23:705–715.

234. Adapala RK, Thoppil RJ, Luther DJ, et al. TRPV4 channels mediate cardiac fibroblast differentiation by integrating mechanical and soluble signals. *J Mol Cell Cardiol.* 2013;54:45–52.

235. Thodeti CK, Paruchuri S, Meszaros JG. A TRP to cardiac fibroblast differentiation. *Channels (Austin).* 2013;7:211–214.

236. Bush EW, Hood DB, Papst PJ, et al. Canonical transient receptor potential channels promote cardio-myocyte hypertrophy through activation of calcineurin signaling. *J Biol Chem.* 2006;281:33487–33496.

237. Ohba T, Watanabe H, Murakami M, et al. Upregula-tion of TRPC1 in the development of cardiac hypertro-phy. *J Mol Cell Cardiol.* 2007;42:498–507.

238. Wu X, Eder P, Chang B, Molkentin JD. TRPC channels are necessary mediators of pathologic cardiac hypertrophy. *Proc Natl Acad Sci U S A.* 2010;107:7000–7005.

239. Klaiber M, Kruse M, Volker K, et al. Novel insights into the mechanisms mediating the local antihypertro-phic effects of cardiac atrial natriuretic peptide: role of cGMP-dependent protein kinase and RGS2. *Basic Res Cardiol.* 2010;105:583–595.

240. Onohara N, Nishida M, Inoue R, et al. TRPC3 and TRPC6 are essential for angiotensin II-induced cardiac hypertrophy. *EMBO J.* 2006;25:5305–5316.

241. Kuwahara K, Wang Y, McAnally J, et al. TRPC6 fulfills a calcineurin signaling circuit during pathologic cardiac remodeling. *J Clin Invest.* 2006;116:3114–3126.

242. Wang L, Wang DH. TRPV1 gene knockout impairs postischemic recovery in isolated perfused heart in mice. *Circulation.* 2005;112:3617–3623.

243. Horton JS, Buckley CL, Stokes AJ. Successful TRPV1 antagonist treatment for cardiac hypertrophy and heart failure in mice. *Channels (Austin).* 2013;7:17–22.

244. Miller BA, Wang J, Hirschler-Laszkiewicz I, et al. The second member of transient receptor potential-melas-tatin channel family protects hearts from ischemia-reperfusion injury. *Am J Physiol Heart Circ Physiol.* 2013;304:H1010–H1022.

245. Hiroi T, Wajima T, Negoro T, et al. Neutrophil TRPM2 channels are implicated in the exacerbation of myocardial ischaemia/reperfusion injury. *Cardiovasc Res.* 2013;97:271–281.

246. Saada N, Dai B, Echetebu C, Sarna SK, Palade P. Smooth muscle uses another promoter to express pri-marily a form of human Cav1.2 L-type calcium channel different from the principal heart form. *Biochem Biophys Res Commun.* 2003;302:23–28.

247. García-Palomero E, Cuchillo-Ibáñez I, García AG, Renart J, Albillos A, Montiel C. Greater diversity than previously thought of chromaffin cell Ca2+ channels, derived from mRNA identification studies. *FEBS Lett.* 2000;481:235–239.

248. Yang SN, Berggren PO. The role of voltage-gated calcium channels in pancreatic beta-cell physiology and pathophysiology. *Endocr Rev.* 2006;27:621–676.

249. Hansen PB. Functional importance of T-type voltage-gated calcium channels in the cardiovascular and renal system: news from the world of knockout mice. *Am J Physiol Regul Integr Comp Physiol.* 2015;308:R227–R237.

250. Layton MG, Robertson D, Everett AW, Mulders WH, Yates GK. Cellular localization of voltage-gated calcium channels and synaptic vesicle-associated proteins in the guinea pig cochlea. *J Mol Neurosci.* 2005;27:225–244.

251. Kang HW, Park JY, Lee JH. Molecular cloning and characterization of a hamster Cav1.3 Ca2+ channel variant with a long carboxyl terminus. *Biochim Biophys Acta.* 2011;1808:1629–1638.

252. Xie CB, Shaikh LH, Garg S, et al. Regulation of aldosterone secretion by Cav1.3. *Sci Rep.* 2016;6:24697.

253. Brennan SC, Finney BA, Lazarou M, et al. Fetal calcium regulates branching morphogenesis in the developing human and mouse lung: involve-ment of voltage-gated calcium channels. *PLoS One.* 2013;8:e80294.

254. Hansen PB, Jensen BL, Andreasen D, Friis UG, Skøtt O. Vascular smooth muscle cells express the alpha(1A) subunit of a P-/Q-type voltage-dependent Ca(2+) chan-nel, and it is functionally important in renal afferent arterioles. *Circ Res.* 2000;87:896–902.

255. Galetin T, Tevoufouet EE, Sandmeyer J, et al. Phar-macoresistant Cav 2.3 (E-type/R-type) voltage-gated calcium channels influence heart rate dynamics and may contribute to cardiac impulse conduction. *Cell Biochem Funct.* 2013;31:434–449.

3

Voltage-Gated Potassium Channels

Gavin Y. Oudit and Peter H. Backx

The cardiac action potential (AP) profile is governed by the complex interplay between depolarizing inward currents and repolarizing outward currents. Cellular patch-clamp studies have identified and classified the major currents underlying the AP profile in cardiomyocytes (CMs); most of the inward currents are generated by voltage-gated Na$^+$ channels (Na$_V$) and Ca^{2+} channels (Ca$_V$), while a large assortment of different types of K$^+$ channels provide the bulk of the outward currents (Fig. 3.1). Additional currents, generated by the Na$^+$/Ca^{2+} exchanger (inward and outward) and Na$^+$/K$^+$ ATPase (outward only) can also make contributions to the AP profile. AP profiles as well as the rate of spread of APs vary greatly between different regions of the heart as a result of tightly controlled variations in gene expression and regulation (Fig. 3.2). An example of AP diversity is provided by the regional differences in the upstroke rate of APs between the working cardiomyocytes (CMs) found in the atria and ventricles compared to the CMs in the sinoatrial (SA) and atrioventricular (AV) nodes; in the atria and ventricles, the AP upstroke is rapid and dependent on high densities of voltage-gated Na$^+$ channels (Nav) whereas in nodal tissues the AP upstroke is slow and relies primarily on inward currents generated by voltage-gated Ca^{2+} channels (Cav) due to the near absence of Na$_V$ expression.

Large numbers of distinct K$^+$ currents have been identified in CMs and the underlying K$^+$ channels are typically dynamic macromolecular complexes consisting of pore-forming α-subunits assembled with accessory subunits often in association with the cytoskeleton and various signaling complexes (Fig. 3.3, Table 3.1, and Table 3.2). K$^+$ channels can be divided into three main structural or topological classes, based on whether the genes encoding for the α-subunits have two, four, or six transmembrane segments (see Fig. 3.1). Cardiac K$^+$ channels containing α-subunits with six transmembrane segments can be either voltage-gated (K$_v$) or Ca^{2+}-activated (K$_{Ca}$) channels, while those with two transmembrane segments are inward rectifier (K$_{IR}$) channels and those with four transmembrane segments are background K$^+$ (K2P) channels (see Fig. 3.3 and Table 3.1). Quantitative and qualitative variation in the expression, biophysical properties, and the regulation of K$^+$ channels are largely responsible for the differences in the AP shapes observed between different regions of the heart (i.e., between atria versus ventricles versus His–Purkinje fibers [see Fig. 3.2] as well as within regions), during heart development, and as consequence of alterations in cardiac demands and stress (e.g., disease, exercise, inactivity, metabolic disorders). K$^+$ channel activity can change via a number of mechanisms leading to modulation of the electrical and contractile properties of the heart. Accordingly, K$^+$ channels are the molecular targets of pharmacological agents including class III antiarrhythmic drugs.

In acquired heart disease, there is reduced I$_{to}$[1,2] and I$_{Kr}$,[3,4] and the downregulation of voltage-gated K$^+$ channels can lead to AP prolongation, which can promote triggered arrhythmias via the generation of early (EADs) and delayed after-depolarizations (DADs).[5,6] In addition, regional changes in dispersion of refractoriness can lead to the unidirectional block of a wave of electrical excitation thereby creating a substrate for an arrhythmia leading to reentrant arrhythmias.[5,7] Mutations in K$^+$ channels account for long-QT, J-wave, and short-QT syndromes, familial atrial fibrillation, and altered rhythmicity. Many gaps continue to exist in our understanding of how the expression and function of K$^+$ channels are regulated and thereby influence cardiac function in normal and diseased hearts. In this chapter, we review the molecular determinants, electrophysiological properties, and the functional role of the main voltage-gated K$^+$ channels (K$_V$ channels), the Ca^{2+}-activated K$^+$ channels, and the K2P background K$^+$ channels in the heart.

General Molecular Properties of Voltage-Gated K$^+$ Channels

Alpha Pore-Forming Subunits

K$_V$ α-subunits (K$_V$α subunits) are pore-forming proteins that contain six transmembrane segments (S1–S6) with intracellular amino- and carboxy-termini. Four K$_V$α subunits assemble as tetramers along with the accessory subunits to form functional K$_V$ channels (see Fig. 3.3). Based on the sequence homology of the hydrophobic transmembrane cores, 12 classes of α-subunits exist (K$_V$1-12). The K$_v$5, K$_v$6, K$_v$8, and K$_v$9 classes are silent channels and do not produce functional channels as homotetramers.[8] Most classes of channels contain many individual channel members, and the majority of channel genes can be alternatively spliced. For example, the K$_V$1 class has eight channel members, identified as K$_V$1.1 to K$_V$1.8 with gene designations (*KCNA1* to *KCNA8*). Typically, members of a given K$_V$α class (K$_v$1.x, etc.) coassemble primarily with other members of their own class to form functional channels. The silent classes of channels are more promiscuous and coassemble with the K$_V$2 channels thus modifying their biophysical properties. The ability for K$_V$ channels to coassemble is governed largely by the specific N-terminal sequences called T1- or Nab-domains (see Fig. 3.3).[2,8] This coassembly of the different K$_V$ channel proteins allows a vast array of different heterotetrameric channels to be created, which, along with the alternative splicing, posttranslational modification, and coassembly with the auxiliary subunits, creates extensive biophysical diversity in the K$_V$ channels. A list of the major K$_V$α channels underlying the major cardiac voltage-gated currents is shown in Table 3.1.

Accessory (Auxiliary) Subunits

The expression levels and biophysical properties of the K$_V$α subunit channels are modulated by an array of accessory subunits classified as K$_V$β, KChAP, KChIP, KCNE, NCS, and DPPX (see Table 3.2). There are four classes of K$_V$β-subunits (K$_V$β11-4) that have multiple alternatively spliced variants.[9,10] Each beta-subunit contains a conserved core region with a variable N-terminal peptide and functions as a complete oxidoreductase enzyme with its active site positioned to potentially interact with the K$_V$ channel voltage-sensor domain (VSD).[10,11] K$_V$β also assembles with

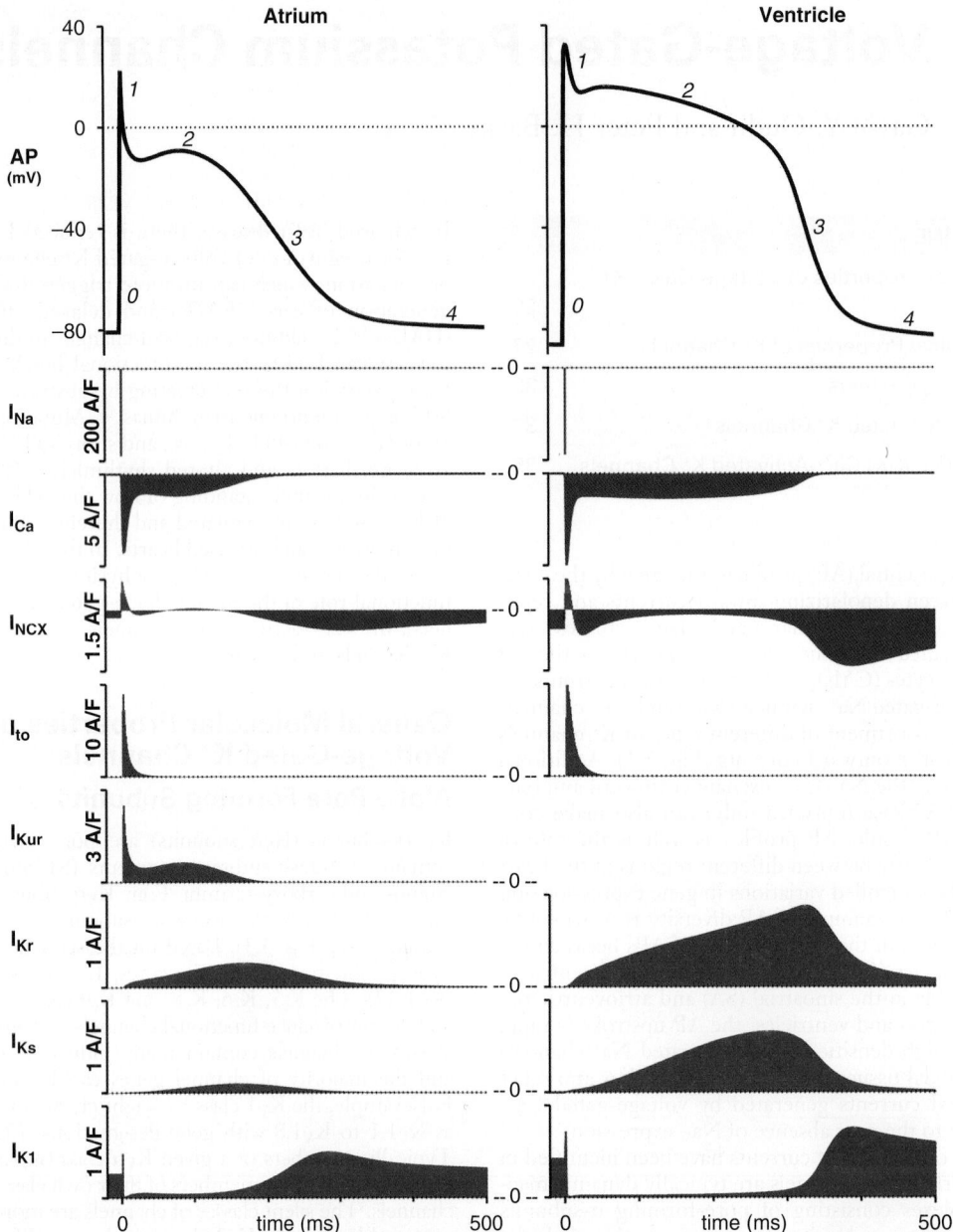

FIGURE 3.1 Representative cardiac action potential (AP) waveforms. The top panel from atrial (*left*) and ventricular (*right*) myocytes. The five phases of the action potential (AP) are labeled: *0*, upstroke of the AP represents depolarization of the membrane; *1*, initial repolarization; *2*, plateau phase; *3*, late repolarization phase; and *4*, the resting (diastolic) phase. The rate of change of the AP is directly proportional to the sum of the underlying transmembrane ion currents (lower panels). Inward currents (*blue*) depolarize the membrane, while outward currents (*red*) contribute to repolarization. Compared to an atrial AP, the ventricular AP typically has a longer duration, higher plateau potential (phase 2), and a more negative resting membrane potential (phase 4). The presence of an ultra-rapid delayed rectifier K+ current (IKur) in atrial myocytes contributes to the lower plateau phase in the atrial AP. Greater inward rectifier K+ current (IK1) in ventricular cells provides a faster phase 3 repolarization and a more negative resting membrane potential (phase 4).

a four-fold symmetry via interactions with the N-terminal T1 domain of the $K_V\alpha$-subunits $(T1_4\beta_4)$ (see Fig. 3.3).[11] $K_V\beta1.2$, $K_V\beta1.3$, and $K_V\beta3$ have been reported to be expressed in the human heart with a two-fold higher expression of $K_V\beta3$ in the ventricle than in the atrium; however, no chamber-specific difference in expression was seen for $K_V\beta1.2$ in rat hearts.[9,12] K_V channels can also be regulated by KChAP (K_V channel-associated protein), a member of the transcription factor binding protein family, by increasing the functional cell-surface expression of

specific K_v channels without affecting other channel properties (see Table 3.2).[2] KChAP is a K+ channel modulatory protein that exhibits "chaperone-like" behavior toward a subset of K+ channels. KChAP is a soluble protein that binds transiently to the cytoplasmic N-termini of its target channels and increased the channel expression in a transcription-independent manner.[2,13] K_v channel-interacting proteins (KChIPs) are Ca^{2+} binding proteins that interact with the cytoplasmic amino termini of the K_v4 α-subunits (see Fig. 3.3) and reconstitute several features of the

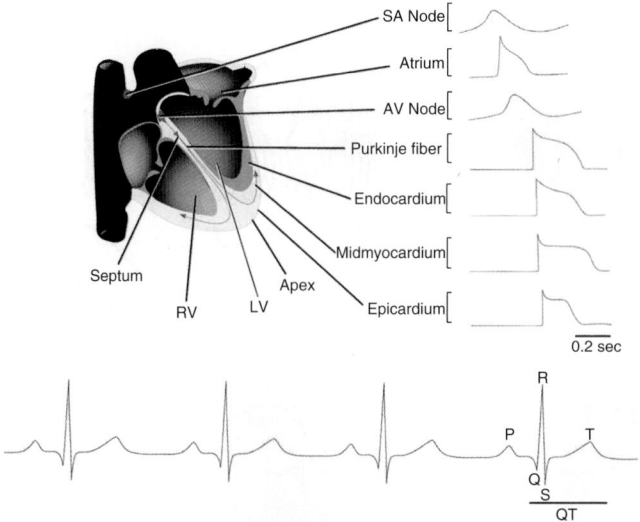

FIGURE 3.2 Illustration of the electrical events occurring in each cardiac cycle and the relationship with the electrocardiogram as well as regional differences in the action potential (AP) profile Each contraction of the heart is initiated by the generation of APs in the sinoatrial (*SA*) node, which then propagates in an orderly fashion to the atria, cardiac conduction system, and ventricles. The figure labels the type of AP profiles that is recorded in different regions of the heart. The orderly sequence of depolarizations give rise to the surface electrocardiogram that is recorded during each cardiac cycle. *AV,* Atrioventricular; *LV,* left ventricle; *RV,* right ventricle. (Modified from Nerbonne JM. Voltage-regulated potassium channels. In: Zipes D, Jalife J, eds. *Cardiac Electrophysiology.* 6th ed. Elsevier; 2014.)

native cardiac currents generated by these channels by modulating their density and inactivation kinetics.[2,14] KChIP2 is the main isoform expressed in the heart which is colocalized and coimmunoprecipitated with native K_V channels (see Table 3.2).[14] In CMs, KChIP2 has two spliced variants and is expressed predominantly in the T-tubules and nuclei.[15] Coexpression of $K_V4.2$ and KChIP2 increased the density of the $K_V4.2$ currents, indicating that KChIP2 may promote and/or stabilize expression of $K_V4.2$ at the cell surface in addition to modulating the biophysical properties so that they closely correspond to $I_{to,f}$ in cardiac myocytes.[7,14] Two other KChIP-related Ca^{2+}-binding proteins, frequenin and neuronal calcium sensor-1, are also expressed in the heart. These β-subunits increase I_{to} density and alter inactivation characteristics.[2,16,17] Another class of auxiliary subunits include MinK and MinK-related peptides called MiRP1-3, which are encoded by the *KCNE1-4* genes. MinK, MiRP1, and MiRP2 are expressed in the heart (see Table 3.2).[4,5,18,19] These proteins are single-domain transmembrane proteins with extracellular N-termini (see Fig. 3.3). They are intimately associated with the α-subunit and appear to interact with the voltage-sensor domain of the K_V channels.[4,18,20] Initial functional expression experiments suggested that MiRP1 associated wither only to modulate the channel function. However, MiRP1 can also associate with K_VLQT1.[18] Similarly, MinK also associates with both hERG and K_VLQT1 subunits and modulates their functions.[4,18,21] As such, these subunits engage in promiscuous interactions with α-subunits from different K_V gene families.

General Biophysical Properties of K_V Channels

K_V channels catalyze the rapid selective movement of K^+ ions across cell membranes by forming passageways through the lipid bilayers called pores. The pores of the K_V channels possess highly specialized structures, called selectivity filters, which allow K^+ to

move across cell membranes at near diffusion-limited rates while excluding other physiological cations. The direction of movement for K^+ is governed by its electrochemical gradients (dictated by the voltage and K^+ concentration gradients across the membrane). The activity of the K_V pore is highly regulated by voltage across the cell membrane, thus the name voltage-gated channels (see Fig. 3.3). The S1–S4 segments are collectively called the VSD. The VSD confers voltage-sensing/gating properties to the K_V channels, while the S5–S6 segments are critical for forming the channel pore and are called the pore domain (PD) (see Fig. 3.3). The K_V channel can reside in many conformations (called states): open, closed, and inactivated (Fig. 3.4). The open state conducts ions while the closed and inactivated states are nonconducting. In general, the complex interchange of different conformations of the K_V channels can be understood by applying chemical kinetic theory, which predicts that the channels can be accurately represented by a ("gating") scheme wherein there is one open state, four to five closed states, and several (or no) inactivated states. At resting membrane potentials, K_V channels are closed (i.e., deactivated). In response to increases in the membrane potential (i.e., depolarization), as occurs during an AP, K_V channels "activate" leading to a channel opening. Consistent with chemical kinetic theory, activation involves multiple stochastic transitions amongst the closed states leading ultimately to channel opening. The kinetics of the stochastic transitions depend critically on the cell membrane voltage (see Fig. 3.4). Following depolarization (and channel opening), some K_V channels subsequently transition to the inactivated state(s), for which several overlapping molecular mechanisms exist. Reentry to the closed state occurs following membrane repolarization. The voltage- and time-dependent transitions between these different functional states are referred to as gating. The molecular mechanisms and regulation of channel gating varies widely among the different K_v channels and are discussed below.

Selectivity Filter and Permeation Pore

K_V pores catalyze the selective transport of K ions across lipid bilayers at near diffusion-limited rates. This pore is formed by the pseudosymmetric arrangement of four PDs consisting of the S5 and S6 transmembrane segments linked via an external segment called the P-loop (see Fig. 3.3).[22] The overall length of the pore is about 45 Å and consists of four parts (from inside to outside): a cytoplasmic tunnel that splays open during activation, a large water-filled central cavity (10 Å in diameter), a narrow selectivity filter, and a wide shallow extracellular vestibule (see Fig. 3.3B). The selectivity filter is formed by the backbone carbonyl oxygens contributed by the residues glycine-tyrosine-glycine plus the side-chain oxygens from threonine in the sequence TXGYG (i.e., "signature sequence" for K^+ selective channels) where X represents a variable residue (see Fig. 3.3).[22] The carbonyl oxygens are symmetrically and rigidly arranged to allow optimal interaction with K^+ ions although other channel domains can modulate the structural rigidity of this region thereby altering channel selectivity.

Activation Gating Mechanisms

K_V channel activation, as for voltage-dependent Na^+ and Ca^{2+} channels, involves conformation changes in the VSD within each of the four monomers in response to membrane depolarization, which ultimately leads to a channel opening. Specifically, the fourth transmembrane segment (S4) in each monomer is studded with positively charged residues (3-6 arginines or lysines) at every third position. The precise structure of the S4 within the VSD has been the subject of considerable discussion with several structural models being proposed. Current consensus suggests that the S4 forms an extended helix embedded within the

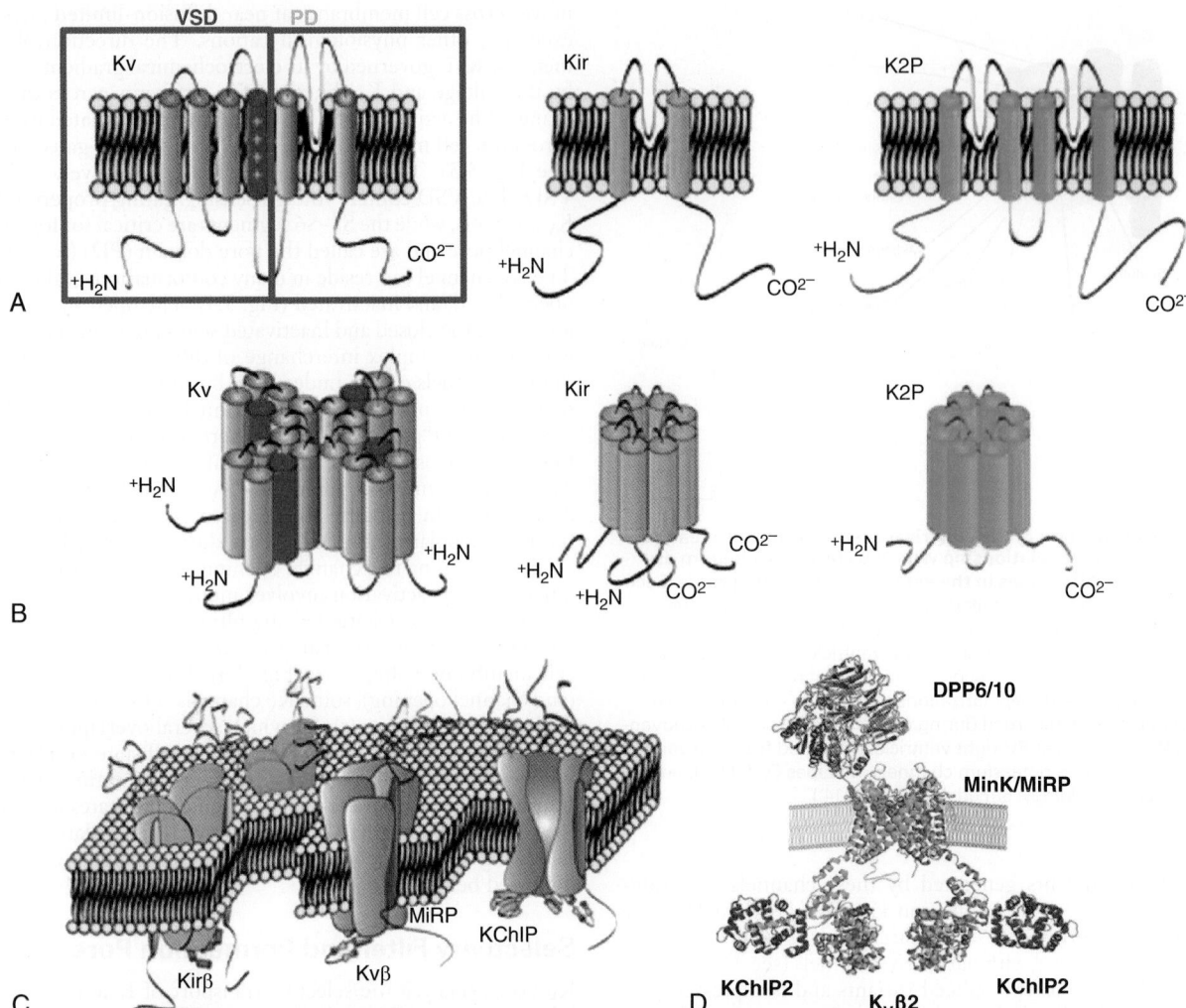

FIGURE 3.3 Molecular composition of cardiac K+ channels (A) The K_V, Kir, and two-pore (K-2-P) α-subunits are integral membrane proteins with six, two, or four membrane-spanning segments, respectively. As highlighted in the panel, channels with six transmembrane segments, such as K_V channels, possess a voltage-sensor domain (*VSD*), which is comprised of transmembrane segments S1–S4 as well as a pore-domain (*PD*) comprised of S5–S6. The VSD and PD are linked by the S4–S5 linker which couples conformational changes in the VSD to the opening (activation) and closing (deactivation and inactivation) of the PD. (B) The α-subunits assemble as tetramers for KV and Kir channels or as dimers for K-2-P channels to form K+ selective pores. (C) Functional channels are comprised of the α-subunits along with accessory subunits, some of which are cytosolic (i.e., Kvβ subunit and KChIP2) and some of which are contain transmembrane segments (see Table 3.2). (D) Predicted molecular architecture of the voltage-gated K+ channel using the Kv4.3-based $It_{o,f}$ channel. Predicted cross section of two Kv4.3 α-subunits (*blue*) based on the x-ray crystal structure of the Kv1.2 channel[135] along with various accessory subunits: KChIP2 (*red*), a cytosolic Kvβ (*green*), DPP6/10 (*brown*),[136] and MinK/MiRPs (*yellow*). KChIP2 subunits and β-subunits interact 1:1 with the α-subunits while the stoichiometry of DPP6/10 and MinK/MiRPs appear to be 1:2. (Modified from Nerbonne JM. Voltage-regulated potassium channels. In: Zipes D and Jalife J. eds. *Cardiac Electrophysiology.* 6th ed. Elsevier; 2014.)

other transmembrane segments of the channel thereby creating an energetically favorable environment provided by pairwise interactions between the S4's positive charges and the negative charges in S1–S3 as well as S5.[23,24] While important dynamic nonionic contact interactions between S4 and the other transmembrane segments also occur, S4 interactions with localized negative charges allow S4 to be energetically stable at several positions within the VSD as it moves outwardly in response to changes in membrane potential.[20] The outward movements of S4 associated with activation (depolarization) generate "ON" gating currents, while the inward movements associated with deactivation (repolarization) generate "OFF" gating currents. S4 movement is coupled directly to a short α-helical S4–S5 segment, lying

on the inner membrane-water interface, which makes multiple dynamic contacts with the S6 segment (in the same monomer), as well as with S6 and the S4–S5 linker in an adjacent monomer during the process of channel activation. These complex dynamic interactions between S4–S5 and S6 are critical for the inactivation of many K_V channels.[24] Regardless, outward movement of S4 pulls on S6 (via the S4–S5 linker) causing a rotation of the bundle crossings (formed by the Proline-Valine-Proline kinks) in the S6 helix thereby removing a hydrophobic barrier that prevents ion entry into the selectivity filter (i.e., "activation gate" or "S6-gate" opens).[20,25] Interestingly, in hyperpolarization cyclic nucleotide (HCN)-gated channels, which only open and generate inward pacemaker currents (I_f/I_h) at relatively negative membrane

TABLE 3.1 Alpha (pore-forming) subunits of cardiac potassium channels

CURRENT	DESCRIPTION	GENE	EXPRESSION	AP PHASE	ACTIVATION MECHANISM	CLONE	MOLECULAR STRUCTURE AND ASSEMBLY
$I_{to,f}$	Transient outward current (fast)	KCND2 KCND3	Atria, ventricles, Purkinje	Phase 1	Voltage (depolarization)	K_v4.2/4.3	Single pore; 6 TM domains; tetramer
$I_{to,s}$	Transient outward current (slow)	KCNA4 KCNA7 KCNC4	Ventricles	Phase 1	Voltage (depolarization)	K_v1.4/1.7/ 3.4	Single pore; 6 TM domains; tetramer
I_{Kur}	Ultra rapid delayed rectifier	KCNA5 KCNC1	Atria	Phase 2	Voltage (depolarization)	K_v1.5/3.1	Single pore; 6 TM domains; tetramer
I_{Kr}	Rapid delayed rectifier	KCNH2	Ventricles	Phase 3	Voltage (depolarization)	HERG	Single pore; 6 TM domains; tetramer
I_{Ks}	Slow delayed rectifier	KCNQ1	Ventricles	Phase 3	Voltage (depolarization)	K_vLQT1	Single pore; 6 TM domains; tetramer
I_{K1}	Inward rectifier (strong)	KCNJ2 KCNJ12	Atria, ventricles	Phase 3 and 4	Voltage (depolarization)	Kir 2.1/2.2	Single pore 2 TM domains; tetramer
I_{KATP}	ADP activated K^+ channel[a]	KCNJ11	Atria, ventricles	Phase 1 and 2	↑ADP/ATP ratio (ATP depletion)	Kir 6.2 (+SUR2A)	Single pore; 2 TM domains; tetramer
I_{KACh}	M2 receptor gated K^+ channel[a,b]	KCNJ3 KCNJ5	Atria	Phase 4	Acetylcholine (vagal tone)	Kir 3.1/3.4	Single pore; 2 TM domains tetramer
I_{Kp}	Background K^+ channels[c]	KCNK1/6 KCNK3 KCNK4	Ventricles	All phases	Metabolic parameters; membrane stretch	TWIK-1/2[a] TASK-1 TRAAK	Two pore; 4 TM domains; dimer

[a]Weak inward rectifiers.
[b]Muscarinic receptor (type 2) in atrial and nodal cells.
[c]Nonselective (permeates both Na^+ and K^+ ions).
ADP, Adenosine diphosphate; *AP,* action potential; *ATP,* adenosine triphosphate; *SUR2A,* sulphonylurea receptor isoform 2A (forms octameric complex with Kir6.2 subunits); TM, transmembrane.

TABLE 3.2 Auxiliary (accessory) subunits of voltage-gated potassium channels

SUBUNIT	GENE	MOLECULAR STRUCTURE	CBD	CURRENT	SURFACE EXPRESSION	ACTIVATION AND INACTIVATION
KChAP	KChAP	Intracellular (85 kDa)	No	I_{to} (K_v4.3)[a] ↑	↑	↔ROA, ↔ROI, ↔RFI
KChIP2[bc]	KCNIP2	Intracellular	Yes	I_{to} (K_v4.3) ↑	↑	↓ROI[d], ↑RFI; DVA
Frequenin		Intracellular (22 kDa)	Yes	I_{to} (K_v4.2)[d] ↑	↑	↓ROI[d], ↑RFI
Neuronal Ca^{2+} Sensor-1		Intracellular (25 kDa)	Yes	I_{to} (K_v4.3) ↑	↑	↓ROI, ↔RFI; DVA
DPP6, DPP10	DPP6, DPP10	Single TM domain with large EC domain (115–120 kDa)	No	I_{to} (K_v4.3) ↑	↑	↑RFI; ↔DVA
Beta-subunit1 ($K_v\beta$1.2)[c]	KCNAB1	Intracellular	No	I_{to} (K_v1.4) ↓	NR	↑ROI, ↓RFI
				I_{Kur} ↓[e]	NR	NR
Beta-subunit1 ($K_v\beta$1.3)[c]	KCNAB1	Intracellular (419 AA)	No	I_{Kur} ↔	NR	↑ROI; HVA
Beta-subunit3 ($K_v\beta$3)	KCNAB2	Intracellular (408 AA)	No	I_{to} (K_v1.4)	NR	↑ROI
				I_{to} (K_v4.3) ↑	↑	↑ROI, ↓RFI
				I_{Kur} ↔	NR	↑ROI, HVA
MiRP1	KCNE2	Single TM domain (123 AA) (N-terminal is EC)	No	I_{Kr} ↓		DVA
				I_{Ks} ↓	NR	↓ROA
				I_{to} (K_v4.3) ↑	NR	↓ROI
MinK	KCNE1	Single TM domain (129-130 AA) (N-terminal is EC)	No	I_{Kr} ↑	↔	HVA
				I_{Ks} ↑	↔	↓ROA

[a]Effect inhibited by $K_v\beta$1.2.
[b]Spliced variants.
[c]Single-nucleotide polymorphisms exist in humans.
[d]Dependent on Ca^{2+}.
[e]Antagonized by KChAP expression.
↑, Increase; ↔, no change; ↓, decrease; *AA,* amino acid; *CBD,* calcium binding domain; *DPP6,* dipeptidyl-aminopeptidase-like protein 6; *DPP10,* dipeptidyl-aminopeptidase-like protein 10; *DVA,* depolarizing shift in voltage activation; *EC,* extracellular; *HVA,* hyperpolarizing shift in voltage activation; *NR,* not reported; *RFI,* recovery from inactivation; *ROA,* rate of activation; *ROI,* rate of inactivation.

potential (i.e., <60mV), the activation gate is held open at negative potentials via interactions between S4–S5 and S6 but these interactions are broken at depolarized potentials leading to pore closure.[26] Moreover, the strength of the interactions between S4–S5 and S6 are modulated by interactions with the cyclic nucleotide binding domain located in the C-terminus of these channels.[27]

Inactivation Gating Mechanisms

Inactivation of K_V channels occurs at the functional and structural levels, and we have realized that there are multiple types of inactivation involving distinct and complex molecular mechanisms. Upon changes in membrane potential (e.g., a depolarization), K_V channels may essentially inactivate from the preopen closed states (closed-state inactivation, CSI) or from the open state(s) (open-state inactivation, OSI). Most K_V channels use both CSI and OSI. However, some K_V channels undergo more inactivation from the open state, and others undergo more inactivation from preopen closed states. We refer to these distinct behaviors as preferential OSI and preferential CSI, respectively. In either case, recovery from inactivation usually occurs when the membrane potential is returned to its initial value (e.g., repolarized). Kv4 channels, a subclass of voltage-gated K^+ (Kv) channels, undergo unstable, seemingly vestigial, OSI but prominent and physiologically relevant CSI.[27a] OSI mechanisms are relatively well known at the biophysical and structural levels (reviewed by Rasmusson and colleagues,[28] Yellen and colleagues,[28a] Aldrich,[28b] and Kurata and Fedida[29]). By contrast, the molecular basis of CSI is not fully understood. CSI may involve mechanisms related to those invoked for OSI or novel mechanisms that need further investigation. Here, we review CSI in the K_V channels, and discuss advances made in recent years towards understanding the mechanisms of CSI. Particularly, we entertain novel working hypotheses that may explain the molecular basis of CSI in the Kv4 channels. We also discuss the general applicability of the proposed CSI mechanism and present a perspective of the structural and biological implications.

Inactivation is a hallmark feature of K_V channels and refers to the process whereby channel activation/opening allows transitions to relatively stable nonconducting conformations (inactivated states) that are distinct from the closed state. When the channels are inactivated, they are often, but not necessarily (e.g., hERG channels), incapable of (re)opening unless the membrane potential is repolarized, which allows channels to "recover" back to the closed state (see Fig. 3.4). For a given K_V channel, inactivation can occur from open state(s) (OSI) or from (preopen also called "preactivated"; see Fig. 3.4) closed-states (CSI), or both. The inactivated conformations can involve structural changes in several distinct regions of the channel leading to occlusion of the pore (i.e., nonconducting conformations). Several distinct inactivation mechanisms (i.e., different conformations) have been identified in K_V channels. The two that have been best described are the N-type and C/P-type inactivations. It is now clear that inactivation in some channels (like Kv4 channels) arises from the reclosure (or recoil) of the activation gate (i.e., S6) as a result of molecular slippage between S6 and the S4–S5 linker; we will refer to this as activation gate (AG)-inactivation. The different types of inactivation can (and do) overlap in some K_V channels. Indeed, the various inactivation mechanisms often show an interdependence, suggesting that K_V channel inactivation is governed by a universal molecular gating mechanism which can manifest distinct inactivation features via modest structural and energetic adjustments. This universal model provides the molecular underpinning of the "inactivation gate" originally proposed by Hodgkin and Huxley with remarkable clarity.[30]

N-Type Inactivation

The most readily understood, and the first to be described, type of inactivation is called N-type inactivation, which was initially

Scheme 1

$$C_1 \leftrightarrow C_2 \leftrightarrow C_3 \leftrightarrow C_4 \leftrightarrow C_5 \leftrightarrow O$$

Scheme 1

$$C_1 \leftrightarrow C_2 \leftrightarrow C_3 \leftrightarrow C_4 \leftrightarrow C_5 \leftrightarrow O$$
$$\updownarrow$$
$$IO$$

Scheme 2

$$C_1 \leftrightarrow C_2 \leftrightarrow C_3 \leftrightarrow C_4 \leftrightarrow \boxed{C_5} \leftrightarrow O$$
$$\updownarrow \quad \updownarrow \quad \updownarrow \quad \updownarrow \quad \updownarrow \quad \updownarrow$$
$$IC_1 \leftrightarrow IC_2 \leftrightarrow IC_3 \leftrightarrow IC_4 \leftrightarrow \boxed{IC_5} \leftrightarrow IO$$

FIGURE 3.4 Gating schemes that describe the voltage-dependent properties of cardiac K_V channels The time- and voltage-dependent properties of K_V channels can be accurately represented using chemical kinetic theory/analysis, which assumes that channel proteins can be represented as a finite number of (energetically, structurally, and temporally) distinct conformations. Channel proteins undergo voltage-dependent transitions between these states, which are well represented by Markov dynamics. Most cardiac K_V channels can be accurately described by assuming the existence of 4–5 closed conformations (labeled C_1 to C_5) and 1 open conformation. When the voltage changes, the energy of the electrical field alters the stability of the various states. When the membranes (containing K_V channels) are highly hyperpolarized (i.e., at the resting membrane potential), C_1 is the most stable closed state. With progressive depolarization, the stability of the closed states shifts from C_1 towards C_5. C_2 to C_5 are called "preactivated" states on the channel. The open and closed conformations can be coupled (or not) to "inactivated" conformations of the channel. Some channels, like I_{Ks}, do not undergo inactivation (Scheme 1), while channels like I_{Kr} can only inactivate from the open state via C-type inactivation. Channels like $K_V1.5$, K_V4, $K_V2.1$, and $K_V1.4$ can all undergo inactivation directly from the closed states and therefore the dependence of inactivation on voltage will display a U-shaped dependence. To illustrate U-type properties, K_V4 channels undergo AG-type inactivation, which involves transitions from the C5 state to CI_5 (box in Scheme 2).

described in *Shaker* K_V channels. N-type inactivation nicely satisfies the major tenets of the "ball-and-chain" mechanism originally described in squid axon Na^+ currents by Clay Armstrong.[31] N-type inactivation occurs when the most N-terminal cytoplasmic segment (i.e., the inactivation "ball" or "particle") binds strongly to its receptor on the cytoplasmic face of the open (or preactivated channels; see Fig. 3.4) channel, leading to a physical block of the pore. Inactivation particles can also be contributed by some auxiliary β-subunits.[20,28] In addition to occluding the inner vestibule of the pore, the energetically strong binding of the "ball" with its receptor can also slow (i.e., immobilize) the "OFF" gating charge movements, which represents the slowing of the conformational changes required for channel deactivation following repolarization.

C/P-Type Inactivation (Molecular Transitions in the Selectivity Region)

This type of inactivation involves a localized collapse of the selectivity filter at the outer mouth of the pore following channel activation.[20,28] C/P-type inactivation is a prominent feature of many K_V channels and is strongly accelerated by N-type inactivation $K_v1.x$ channels. The molecular events leading to pore closure involve multiple, interdependent conformation changes identified in S5, S6, and the VSD (i.e., S4 and S4–S5 linker),[29,32] which readily explains the links between C/P-inactivation and both N-type inactivation and the profound "OFF" gating charge immobilization seen in many K_V channels. Specifically, S4 movements are linked with motion in S5 and the outer pore, which themselves interact strongly. Regardless, unlike N-type, C/P-type inactivation is prevented by K^+ and other ions (such as Cs^+ and TEA^+) binding to the extracellular face of the pore as well as the selectivity filter itself, and is promoted by extracellular H^+. The effects

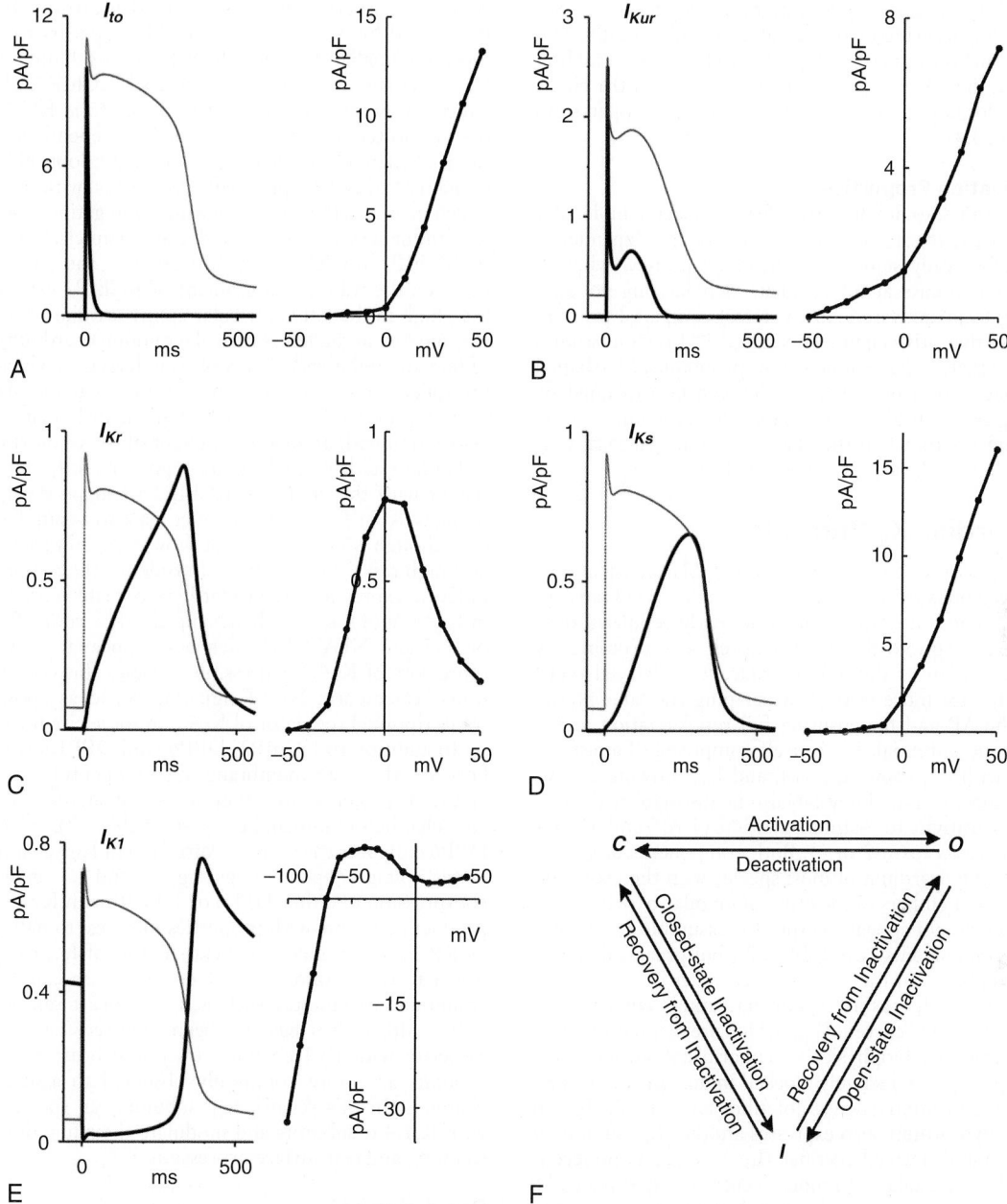

FIGURE 3.5 Current–voltage relationships in voltage-regulated K⁺ channels Panels (A) through (E) show the time courses of the major potassium currents during an action potential (superimposed dotted red line) as well as the steady-state current–voltage relationships. (A) Ventricular transient outward K⁺ current (I_{to}); (B) atrial ultra-rapid delayed rectifier K⁺ current (I_{Kur}); (C) ventricular rapid delayed rectifier K⁺ current (I_{Kr}); (D) ventricular slow delayed rectifier K⁺ current (I_{Ks}); (E) ventricular inward rectifier K⁺ current (I_{K1}). (F) Ion channel activity can be described by transitions of the protein between the different conformational states. Activation of the channel from a nonconducting closed state (C) to an open (O) conformation allows ion permeation. Both open and closed channels may enter a nonconducting inactive conformation (I). Transition of a channel from an open to closed conformation is referred to as channel deactivation.

of external K⁺ and H⁺ on C/P-type inactivation explains several electrophysiological responses observed in response to altered extracellular K⁺ and suggest a potential important role in physiological conditions.[20,28]

AG-Type Inactivation (Molecular Transitions Involving the Recoil of the Activation Gate [S6])

Channels undergoing AG-type inactivation can inactivate readily from "preactivated" closed conformations (Fig. 3.5), where

"preactivated" closed states refers to conformations in which S4 has partially moved in the outward direction in response to membrane depolarization. Although the ability to inactivate from the closed state can occur in channels undergoing N- and C/P-type inactivation as well, the molecular mechanism for AG inactivation is very distinct. An example of channels undergoing AG-type inactivation is the K_V4 channel in which the strength (i.e., energetic stability) of the physical link between the S4–S5 linker and S6 varies with position of the S4 in the VSD. Consequently, as S4 moves outward during channel activation, the S4–S5 linker can uncouple from S6, allowing elastic recoil of the S6-gate (thereby preventing channel opening). For K_V4 channels, the physical link between S6 and the S4–S5 linker is the weakest when the channels are in the closed state immediately preceding the open state (i.e., C_5; see Fig. 3.4).

U-Type Inactivation Properties

U-type inactivation does not actually refer to a specific molecular mechanism. Rather, this term refers to the voltage-dependence of the channel's steady-state inactivation properties, wherein more inactivation occurs at intermediate depolarizing voltages (corresponding to preactivated closed states) compared to more positive voltages that drive channel opening.[33,34] Previous studies have established that $K_V2.1$ channels show pronounced U-shaped steady-state inactivation properties, which can be explained by the uncoupling between S6 and the S4–S5 linker leading to the recoil of S6 and occurs when the channels are in partially activated closed states (such as C_2–C_4; see Fig. 3.4).[29,32]

Specific Cardiac K_V Currents

Two general types of K_V currents are seen in CMs: transient outward and delayed outwardly rectifying (see Table 3.1). Transient K^+ currents (I_{to1}) activate rapidly, underlie early repolarization, and contribute strongly to the phase 1 notch seen prominently in the epimyocardium of the left ventricle. The delayed rectifier currents (I_K) are more critical for shaping the later phases (2 and 3) of the AP and for ensuring full repolarization to the resting membrane potential. I_{to1} is itself comprised of a fast $I_{to,f}$ and slow $I_{to,s}$, with $I_{to,f}$ showing a fast, and $I_{to,s}$ showing a slow, recovery from inactivation. They can also be distinguished based on differential sensitivity to 4-amino-pyridine (4-AP) and the spider toxins, *Heteropoda* toxin-2 or -3. Both components of I_{to1} are expressed in the myocardium of most species with the exception of guinea pigs and members of the order of ungulates (ovine, porcine, etc.), which do not appear to express measurable $I_{to,f}$. I_K also consists of several currents (see Table 3.2), but greater diversity exists between species. In the atria and ventricles of species like humans and canines, I_K has a "rapidly activating" current (I_{ker}) and a "slowly activating" current (I_{Ks}), which are distinguished on the basis of their unique biophysical and pharmacological properties. For example, I_{Kr} is selectively blocked in humans by class III antiarrhythmic medications such as dofetilide and sotalol. Human and dog atrial myocardium also expresses another I_K component called the ultrarapid delayed rectifier (I_{Kur}), which is preferentially blocked by vernakalant. In mouse ventricles, I_K can also be separated using biophysical and pharmacological approaches into components which are called I_{Kslow1}, I_{Kslow2}, and I_{ss}, and these currents are generated by different K_V α-subunits.[35]

Transient Outward Currents (I_{to1})

Molecular Basis and Biophysical Properties of I_{to1}

Two major types of transient outward currents have been characterized in human myocardium: I_{to1} generated by K_V channels and I_{to2} generated by Ca^{2+} activated Cl^- channels whose molecular identities have only recently been identified.[36] I_{to1} has two components: $I_{to,f}$ and $I_{to,s}$. The Kv channel genes underlying $I_{to,f}$ in the heart are Kv4.2 and Kv4.3 while Kv1.4 underlies $I_{to,s}$ (see Table 3.1).[2,8,37] In humans as in other species such as the rabbit, dog, and ferret, $I_{to,f}$ appears to be encoded primarily by the Kv4.3 α-subunit, which can be alternatively spliced in the C-terminus,[38] although a recent study has linked J-wave electrocardiogram (ECG) abnormalities to a gain-of-function mutation in Kcnd2 (i.e., Kv4.2).[39] Indeed, the gain-of-function mutation in *KCND2* ($K_V4.2$) increased the peak I_{to} resulting in a loss of the epicardial AP dome and forms a molecular basis for one of the J-wave

syndrome associated with sudden cardiac arrest.[39] In rodents, $I_{to,f}$ is encoded by Kv4.2 and Kv4.3.[2,8] $I_{to,s}$ appears to be present in most mammalian species. The primary β-subunit associated with $I_{to,f}$ in humans and most other species is KChIP2, which has three alternatively spliced isoforms (see Table 3.2).[7] KChIP2 is a member of a protein family identified as Ca^{2+} dependent modulators of the K_V4 channels which contain four helix-loop-helix (EF-hands) domains[14] KChIP2 physically associates with Kv4 α-subunits which increases the current densities and gating kinetics; KChIP2 also influences the Kv1.5 and Cav channels.[40,41] These effects of KChIP2 on KV4.3 readily explains the strong correlation between the transmural gradient of KChIP2 expression and $I_{to,f}$ (i.e., high in the left ventricular epimyocardium and right ventricle, and low in the left ventricular endomyocardium) in the hearts of humans and dogs[42–48] as well as in ferrets in which KChIP2b is the splice variant linked to the ventricular $I_{to,f}$ gradients.[49] Interestingly, the KChIP2 mRNA gradient in humans was found in association with an inverse gradient of the transcriptional factors (TFs) *Irx3* and *Irx5*, which are repressors of $I_{to,f}$ in mice.[50] Consistent with the ability of KChIP2 to shape the $I_{to,f}$ pattern in humans, KChIP2 ablation in mice leads to a complete loss of $I_{to,f}$,[7] even though KChIP2 does not show regional variations in mice,[51] although this is not certain.[52] In rodents, the regional differences in Kv4.2 expression are primarily responsible regional differences in $I_{to,f}$[53,54]and these gradients appear to be controlled by the TFs of Irx5 and NFAT,[50,55]which both appear to be transcriptional repressors of $K_V4.2$ expression. Despite this correlation, activation of calcineurin/NFAT signaling can act as a powerful positive transcriptional regulator of $K_V4.2$ in some circumstances.[56]

In addition to KChIP2, DPP6, and DPP10, which are members of the transmembrane diaminopeptidyl transferase-like family of proteins, are other accessory subunits associated with K_V4 channels in human hearts (see Table 3.2).[57,58] Like KChIP2, DPP6 enhances the surface expression of K_V4 channels and modulates voltage-dependent gating[57,59] and $I_{to,f}$ generated by the coexpression of either DPP6 or DPP10 with Kv4.3 and KChIP2 produces currents with properties identical to native cardiac $I_{to,f}$. MiRP-1, the endogenous beta-subunit of I_{Kr}, can also increase the density of human $K_V4.3$ currents[60] as can KChAP which coimmunoprecipitates with $K_V4.3$ in heart samples (see Table 3.2).[13] Although it has also been reported that Kvβ1 and Kvβ2 associate with Kv4 channels in mouse hearts,[61] these auxiliary subunits are more commonly observed to associate with K_V1 channels. In this regard, $K_Vβ$ subunits can specifically associate with $K_V1.4$ α-subunits and modulate their functional properties, stability, and cell surface expression.[2,9,60]

Regulation of I_{to1}

I_{to1} is regulated by many factors involving transcriptional, translational, and posttranslational mechanisms. The molecular constituents of both $I_{to,f}$ and $I_{to,s}$ have many potential phosphorylation sites for cAMP-dependent protein kinase (PKA), protein kinase C (PKC), extracellular signal regulated kinase (ERK), and CaMKII allowing for posttranslational regulation.[62] Consistent with posttranslational, acute application of α-adrenergic agonists causes I_{to1} reductions in adult atrial, ventricular, and Purkinje fibers from various species via PKC-dependent and PKC-independent pathways.[2,63] In rabbit atrial myocytes, PKC reduces $I_{to,s}$,[64] while in heterologous expression systems, PKC causes reductions in $I_{to,f}$ currents generated by the long isoform of $K_V4.3$ only.[38] Acute α-adrenergic stimulation can reduce $I_{to,f}$ in rat ventricular CMs by an AKAP-PKA-mediated mechanism, which apparently targets K_V4 channels located in caveolae,[65] although other studies found minimal effects of acute cAMP/PKA activation in I_{to1}.[62] On the other hand, chronic exposure of ventricular myocytes to α-adrenergic receptor agonists and angiotensin II reduced the $K_V4.2$ and $K_V4.3$ expression, but increased $K_V1.4$ expression.[2,66–68] Moreover, chronic α-adrenergic receptor stimulation has been linked to reduced $K_V4.3$ transcription while chronic Ang-II appears to destabilize $K_V4.3$ mRNA.[67] These observations can help explain the downregulation of $I_{to,f}$ and K_V4 channel expression commonly observed in many types of heart disease in many species, which are associated with chronic activation of the renin-angiotensin and sympathetic nervous systems.[2] However, many signaling pathways are altered in heart disease. In this respect, CaMKII also regulates both cardiac $I_{to,f}$ (Kv4.2/4.3) and $I_{to,s}$ (Kv1.4).[69]

Heart disease is also associated with altered thyroid and aldosterone signaling. Accordingly, hypothyroidism prolongs AP durations in conjunction with reduced $I_{to,f}$ and $K_v4.2$ expression as well as increased $K_v1.4$ levels while hyperthyroidism has the opposite actions.[63,70–72] Regulation of I_{to1} by thyroid hormone explains the AP changes as well as the altered expression of $K_v1.4$, $K_v4.2$, and $K_v4.3$ seen in perinatal period, when a surge of thyroid hormone occurs.[2,70] In contrast to thyroid hormone, aldosterone mediates a receptor-specific downregulation of I_{to1} in ventricular myocytes.[73] $I_{to,f}$ also appears to be regulated by estrogens, which helps to explain gender-based differences in repolarizations in rodents, and may possibly be relevant in humans as well.[74] Other factors involved in regulating I_{to1} levels include an assortment of cytoskeletal proteins that influence channel stability, trafficking, localization, and biophysical properties, often supporting coassembly of other regulatory proteins to the channels. Some examples of cytoskeletal and structural proteins include actin, filamin, α-actinin-2, the PDZ domain–containing membrane-associated guanylate kinases (MAGUKs), the postsynaptic density protein, PSD-95, the synapse-associated protein, SAP97, and syntaxin 1A.[62] Consistent with the observation that alterations in I_{to1} are invariably associated with altered transcription of the underlying genes, *Irx5* and *NFAT* are two transcription factors that reduce $I_{to,f}$ by repressing $K_v4.2$ transcription, and this regulation is central for creating the normal regional variations of I_{to1}, which underlie the heterogeneity of repolarization between different regions of the heart.[50] Interestingly, the RNA binding protein, CIRBP, which regulates RNA splicing as well as the initiation of translation, assembly, and transport of proteins, alters the stability of $K_v4.2$ and $K_v4.3$, but not KChIP2, which might be relevant since CIRP expression is upregulated in cold, hypoxia, and several diseases.[75]

Physiological Role of I_{to1}

$I_{to,f}$ and $I_{to,s}$ have similar rates of activation ($\tau_{act} \approx 2–10$ ms) but different rates of both inactivation ($\tau_{inact} \approx 25–80$ ms for $I_{to,f}$ and $80–200$ ms for $I_{to,s}$) and recovery from inactivation ($\tau_{rec} \approx 25–80$ ms for $I_{to,f}$ and $1–2$ s for $I_{to,f}$).[2,76] When both $I_{to,f}$ and $I_{to,s}$ are present in the (ventricular) myocardium, the recovery from inactivation curves are biphasic,[2,8,37,76,77] and this can be used to separate the two currents.[35,68] These differences in inactivation are related to the distinct mechanisms underlying inactivation in K_V4 channels, which involves S6 recoil (see Fig. 3.4 and 3.5) versus in $K_V1.4$ channels, which undergo a combination of N-type and C/P-type. Because of its rapid activation kinetics, I_{to1} contributes markedly to early repolarization (phase 1) in atrial and ventricular APs (see Figs. 3.1 and 3.2) for all species. However, due to the relatively slow recovery kinetics arising C-type inactivation, $I_{to,s}$ is expected to play a limited role in repolarization compared to the fast recovering $I_{to,f}$, especially at high heart rates as seen in rodents. Consistent with this expectation, regional differences in AP profiles and durations correlate strongly with the levels of $I_{to,f}$ and its molecular constituents, not with $I_{to,s}$.[2,54,76,78,79] For example, in the left ventricular epimyocardium and in the right ventricle, APs are relatively short in all species with more prominent early notches (in species like humans and dogs). These short APs are associated with low levels of $K_{V1.4}$ and $I_{to,s}$ but high K_V4 and $I_{to,f}$ levels. By contrast, in the left ventricular endomyocardium and septum, longer APs, which lack an early notch, are associated

with lower $I_{to,f}$ and higher $I_{to,s}$. Moreover, in heart disease, AP prolongation and the loss of the AP notch occurs in conjunction with elevations in $K_V1.4$ expression and reductions in K_V4 expression along with corresponding changes in recovery kinetics,[1,80,81] a pattern that reverses the changes seen in early postnatal development.[70] The regional differences in I_{to1} as well as the changes in diseased hearts are typically seen without notable changes in KChIP2 expression.[46,82]

Importantly, regional differences in I_{to1} and its changes in both heart disease and development have important functional consequences. For example, regional variations in $I_{to,f}$-mediated AP profiles have been correlated with regional differences in contractility and Ca^{2+} transients that have been traced to the strong influence $I_{to,f}$ on L-type Ca^{2+} current profiles and NCX activity during early repolarization when excitation–contraction coupling reaches its prominence.[83,84] In large species, such as humans and dogs, rapid early repolarization may be physiologically necessary for adequate recruitment and synchronization of Ca^{2+} release events that contribute to the whole-cell Ca^{2+} transient.[83] On the other hand, slowing the rate of phase 1 repolarization (due to decreased I_{to}) can reduce trigger $I_{Ca,L}$ (via the voltage-gated Ca^{2+} channels), which increases the dispersion of sarcoplasmic reticulum (SR) Ca^{2+} release thus exacerbating impaired Ca^{2+} cycling in heart disease.[83] Also consistent with the important role of $I_{to,f}$ in myocardial electrophysiology is the observation that an increased $I_{to,f}$ level is associated with early-onset lone atrial fibrillation,[85] Brugada syndrome,[79,86] and idiopathic ventricular fibrillation.[59] However, it should be noted that $K_V1.4$-based $I_{to,s}$ may be relevant in several circumstances. For example, C-type inactivation in $I_{to,s}$ is strongly modulated by external K^+ levels and pH, making it conceivable that $I_{to,s}$ may play a larger role in repolarization in ischemia-related disease states. Another example of a possible role for $I_{to,s}$ is provided by the heart rate dependence of the J-wave, an ECG feature associated with arrhythmias. Specifically, the J-wave appears to arise as a result of prominent AP notches in the epimyocardium, and these tend to disappear at elevated heart rates within the range that is expected to affect $I_{to,s}$ but not the $I_{to,f}$ recovery from inactivation.[87]

Voltage-Gated Delayed Rectifiers Channels (I_K)

Molecular and Biophysical Properties of IK

The cardiac delayed rectifier K^+ current (I_K) has three components in human myocardium: I_{Kur}, I_{Kr}, and I_{Ks}, each having distinct voltage and time-dependent properties (see Figs. 3.1 and 3.5). I_{Kr} is generated by hERG (KCNH2) α-subunits coassembled primarily with a MinK-related peptide 1 called MiRP1 (*KCNE2*), which undergoes alternative splicing.[88] hERG also complexes with minK (the primary ancillary subunit for KvLQT1), suggesting that cardiac I_{Ks} and I_{Kr} channel expression may be interdependent.[89] hERG-based channels are characterized by their unique gating, conductance, regulation, and pharmacology. For example, hERG currents activate very slowly and show prominent inward rectifications that are linked to fast voltage-dependent inactivation and are nonabsorbing at voltages between −40 mV and +40 mV).[90,91] The slow rate of I_{Kr} activation and deactivation has been linked to the PAS domain in the N-terminus, which appears to interact with cyclic nucleotide binding domain in the C-terminus of hERG.[5,92] hERG undergoes C-type inactivation,[93] which (unlike in most other channels) depends on obligatory channel opening, thereby forcing the channel to reopen in the process of deactivation (see Fig. 3.5). These gating properties are critical for I_{Kr} to contribute prominently to late repolarization (phase 3), an essential property to prevent arrhythmias, as well as to the pacemaking in the SA node.[94] Inherited defects in I_{Kr} cause congenital long QT (LQT); hERG mutations give rise to LQT2 syndromes, and MiRP1 mutations cause LQT6 syndrome.[4,5,18,95] I_{Kr} also shows a high propensity for drug-induced block and acquired long QT syndrome, which are both associated with hERG's unique pore structure and function.[4]

Cardiac I_{Ks} is generated by the coassembly of KvLTQ1 (*KCNQ1*) plus MinK (*KCNE1*) (see Tables 3.1 and 3.2).[18,19] In the absence of MinK, KvLTQ1 displays rapidly-activating, noninactivating currents, while coexpression with minK leads to currents with very slow activation rates without inactivation, like native cardiac I_{Ks} (see Figs. 3.1 and 3.2).[5] MinK also alters the regulation of KvLQT1-based currents by pH, blockers, and temperature.[18] KvLQT1 can also coassemble with MiRP1 and MiRP2, which are both expressed in the human atrium and ventricle (see Table 3.2).[18,19] Inherited mutations interfering with I_{Ks} function cause congenital long QT, KvLQT1 mutations cause LQT1 syndrome, and MinK mutations cause LQT5 syndrome.[5,18] MinK localizes to the T-tubules surrounding the Z-line in ventricular myocytes where it is linked to the myofibrillar components via an adaptor protein; this may form a mechanoelectrical feedback system via stretch-dependent regulation of I_{Ks}.[96] Gain-of-function channelopathy leading to increased I_{Ks} and AP shortening and reentry is associated with familial atrial fibrillation (AF).[19]

I_{Kur} in human atrial myocytes is encoded by Kv1.5 (*KCNA5*), while in canines, it appears to be related to Kv3.1 channels.[77,97] These currents have also been referred to as Iss or Isus. In mouse, Kv1.5 is a prominent current in both atrial and ventricular myocytes and is referred to as $I_{K,slow1}$.[8] As the name I_{Kur} implies, these currents activate very quickly, and they undergo slow inactivation consistent with C/P-type inactivation.[29] The major ancillary subunits associated with I_{Kur} are Kvβ1.2, Kvβ1.3, Kvβ2.1, and Kvβ3.[98] In the heart, Kvβ1.2 coimmunoprecipitates with the Kv1.5 subunits, while KChAP attenuates the depression of the Kv1.5 currents produced by Kvβ1.2.[12] The N-terminal peptide in Kvb1.2, Kvβ1.3, and Kvβ3 subunits can confer additional rapid inactivation properties to Kv1.5 subunits via a proposed N-type inactivation.[9,99] In addition, both Kvβ1.3 and Kvβ3 subunits cause a hyperpolarizing shift in the voltage activation curve of human Kv1.5 current suggesting that these channels can open at more negative membrane potentials.[9] The association of Kv1.5 subunits with accessory Kvβ subunits also confers a significant degree of sensitivity of I_{Kur} to the intracellular redox state.[10]

In adult mouse CMs, neither I_{Kr} nor I_{Ks} are expressed to any measureable extent, although I_{Kr} currents are observed and important in the developing mouse heart.[100] These currents are "replaced" by $I_{K,Slow1}$ and $I_{K,slow2}$ which is linked to Kv 2.1; $I_{K,slow2}$ activates more slowly than $I_{K,slow1}$ and shows limited inactivation.

Regulation of I_K

hERG channels are regulated by PKA via phosphorylation sites located in the N- and C-terminus as well as by cAMP via a cyclic nucleotide-binding domain (CNBD) in the C-terminus.[4] PKA activation reduces hERG current, while a direct binding of cAMP to the hERG channel increases current. The summation of these effects result in a net decrease in the current.[101] These opposing effects of PKA and cAMP are also observed as voltage-shifts in the activation curves. However, when HERG is coexpressed with MiRP1 or minK, cAMP produces a net increase in the current consistent with the observation that loss-of-function mutations in the CNBD of hERG channels are associated with LQT2 syndrome.[4,101,102] In contrast, alpha-adrenergic stimulation reduces hERG currents, which is prevented by excess PIP2. This suggests that the mechanism is due to G-protein–coupled receptor stimulation of phospholipase C resulting in the consumption of endogenous PIP2. PIP2-dependent effects are primarily due to altered channel gating with no significant change in single channel conductance.[103] The physiological relevance of PIP2-hERG interactions is supported by the observations that endothelin-1 decreases I_{Kr} (and prolongs APs) in human ventricular myocytes, possibly by the local depletion of PIP2.[103,104]

Beta-adrenergic stimulation increases I_{Ks} via PKA-dependent phosphorylation of KvLQT1 channels, which involves a macromolecular complex that includes protein kinase A, protein phosphatase 1, and the targeting protein yotiao.[105] In LQT11 syndrome, there is reduced interaction between KCNQ1 and yotiao, and attenuated cAMP-induced phosphorylation of the channel, thereby eliminating the functional response of the I_{Ks} channel to cAMP.[106] Beta-adrenergic upregulation of I_{Kr} and I_{Ks} provides a key mechanistic link between the shortening of the AP duration required to maintain the diastolic period when heart rates following sympathetic activation. At elevated heart rates, the increased repolarizing currents generated by I_{Ks}, as a result of phosphorylation, are reinforced by intrinsic enhancements of I_{Ks} (as well as I_{Kr}), which occur at elevated heart rates due to their intrinsically slow deactivation properties. I_{Ks} can also be modulated by PKC activation.[18] Altered thyroid hormone status results in changes in IKs-encoding subunits with hypothyroidism resulting in increased and hyperthyroidism resulting in decreased expression of KvLQT1 and MinK.[72]

Beta- and alpha-adrenergic stimulation increases I_{Kur} via protein kinase A and C effects, respectively,[107] while the activation of the Src-family of protein tyrosine kinases reduces I_{Kur} by the phosphorylation of Src homology 3 (SH3) domains in the N-terminus of Kv1.5 channels.[108] Kv1.5 channels are also regulated by nitric oxide via a cGMP/PKG-dependent pathway.[109] The steroid hormone superfamily, including glucocorticoids, thyroid hormone, and androgens, can alter the transcription of Kv1.5 subunit. Hyperthyroidism can lead to transcriptional upregulation while hypothyroidism leads to decreased expression of Kv1.5 channel genes, although it remains to be shown whether these changes occur in atrial myocytes.[72,110] Lack of androgen leads to a reduction in the density of I_{Kur} and Kv1.5 expression, while the female sex is associated with reduced Kv1.5 expression, which may play an important role in gender-specific differences in ventricular repolarization.[111,112] Kv1.5 also interacts with membrane-associated guanylate kinase (MAGUK) proteins such as synapse-associated protein 97 (SAP97), which increases channel insertion into the membrane to the intercalated disks.[113]

Physiological Role of I_K

The delayed rectifiers play key roles in the late phase 2 and phase 3 repolarization of cardiac myocytes and Purkinje fibers (conducting tissues).[4,18] In particular, slow activation and deactivation of I_{Kr} and I_{Ks} allow K+ conductance to contribute to the late phase of phase 3 repolarization as well as providing an additional K+ conductance that contributes to the effective refractoriness of the myocardium and reinforcing the background conductance to minimize after-depolarization. These properties are also important for AP shortening at high heart rates in the atrial and ventricular myocardium.[4,114] The very rapid but incomplete voltage-dependent inactivation, ensures that I_{Kr} contribute relatively little outward current during the AP plateau (phase 2) but critically during late (phase 3) repolarization (see Figs. 3.1 and 3.5). In contrast, outward current provided by I_{Ks} increases progressively during the AP plateau and sustained during phase 3 repolarization as a result of slow deactivation (see Figs. 3.1 and 3.4D).[18] The important role of delayed rectifiers in cardiac repolarization is illustrated by the various congenital and acquired long QT syndromes that are associated with loss of function in these channels (see below).

Regional ventricular, chamber-specific and species differences in AP configuration have been linked to the differential expression of I_{Kur}, I_{Kr}, and I_{Ks} channels.[77] The short APs typical of atrial myocytes are associated with relatively high levels of I_{Kur} compared to ventricular myocytes (see Figs. 3.1 and 3.4A)[34,77] while I_{Kr} and I_{Ks} are larger in the left atrium than the right.[77] In the rabbit ventricle, I_{Kr} is more abundantly expressed in the epicardial and apical CMs consistent with relatively shorter APs in these regions, while the

I_{Ks} is more abundant at the ventricular base.[115] Moreover, in dogs and cats, I_{Kr} and I_{Ks} also show transmural differences between the feline and canine ventricle,[96,114] while hERG is more abundantly expressed in the epimyocardium but not at the base in ferrets[116]; this is consistent with the results in the guinea pig left ventricle showing higher hERG, I_{Kr}, and I_{Ks} levels in subepicardial tissue compared to other regions[117] as well as in humans.[77]

Myocardial Ca²⁺-Activated K⁺ Channels

General Molecular and Biophysical Properties

Ca²⁺-activated K⁺ channels are described in this chapter because the overall structure of these channels is equivalent to K_V channels, in that they are formed by tetrameric assembly of four genes each with six transmembrane segments. Ca²⁺-activated K⁺ channels have traditionally been divided into three classes based on their single-channel conductance: big-conductance (BK), intermediate-conductance (IK), and small-conductance (SK) channels. The corresponding protein/gene names for BK are KCa1.1/*KCNMA1* and KCa3.1/*KCNN4* for IK. SK channels have three members and are called SK1, SK2, and SK3, with protein/gene names being KCa2.1/*KCNN1*, KCa2.2/*KCNN2*, and KCa2.3/*KCNN3*.[118] Only SK channels are expressed in the myocardium with IK channels being expressed in blood vessels where they play a key role in blood pressure regulation. BK channels are found primarily in the mitochondria where they are involved in ischemia–reperfusion injuries. Since only SK channels are involved directly in cardiac electrophysiology, this review will not discuss the I_K and BK channels.

Small Conductance (SK) Ca²⁺-Activated K⁺ Channels

Molecular and Biophysical Properties of SK Channels

Although SK channels are present in the atria and ventricles, these channels selectively affect the electrophysiological properties of atria.[119] As with K_V channels, SK channels have six transmembrane segments with the N- and C-termini being located intracellularly. However, the S4 in each subunit is uncharged, and these channels do not coassemble with β-subunits. However, they do constitutively bind calmodulin in the C-terminus, and it is the Ca²⁺ binding to calmodulin (EC$_{50}$ ~ 300nM, Hill coefficient = 4–5), not voltage, that activates the SK channels.[120,121] The SK channels have small single-channel conductances of ~10 pS (in symmetric K⁺).[121]

Regulatory Properties of SK Channels

The SK2 channels have been shown to associate with protein kinase, casein kinase II, and protein phosphatase 2A (PP2A).[122] The phosphorylation of calmodulin increases the Ca²⁺ sensitivity of SK channels in neurons, and the SK2 channels also physically associate with α-actinin2, filamin A, and myosin light chain-2 (MLC2).[123] These interactions are required for channel trafficking as well as proper channel localization and are Ca²⁺ dependent, which can explain the increased SK2 channel expression and AP shortening seen in the atrial CMs isolated from hearts with atrial fibrillation.[123,124] SK2 channels also colocalize with L-type Ca²⁺ channels (Cav1.3 and Cav1.2) but this association is indirect and mediated via α-actinin2. Despite this association, SK channel activation appears to require Ca²⁺ release from the sarcoplasmic reticulum.[123]

Physiological Role of SK Channels

AP profiles are prolonged by the selective SK blocker, apamin, in human, dog, and mouse atrial CMs, with limited effects in ventricular CMs.[125,126] Apamin has also been shown to decrease the spontaneous firing rate in rabbit CMs from the SA node and the sleeves of the pulmonary veins.[127] Mice lacking the SK2 channels have prolonged AP durations in the atria only in association with AF[128] as well as reduced spontaneous firing rates and AP prolongation in AV nodal CMs.[123] Thus SK channels selectively influence atrial and pacemaker tissues, including pulmonary vein CMs while sparing the ventricular working myocardium; this suggests that these channels could be potential targets for treating AF and arrhythmias associated with the SA and AV nodes. This possibility is bolstered by genome-wide association studies of lone AF patients that have identified links with a single nucleotide polymorphism in an intron and an exon of the *KCNN3* gene.[129,130] Moreover, apamin could prevent atrial arrhythmias and electrical changes induced by periodic pacing of the coronary sinus and pulmonary veins in rabbits[131] as well as AF in paced dogs.[132] Targeting the SK channel in the treatment of AF may however be complex since SK2 ablation also increased AF vulnerability, and early after-depolarizations while treating dogs with apamin also promoted AF along with increased AP dispersion.[123] Moreover, SK1–3 levels are reduced in atria that have been isolated from chronic AF patients,[123,133] while SK currents are increased in ventricles of heart failure patients.[134]

Acknowledgments

We apologize for not being able to cite many of the original publications in this field due to space limitations. Our research is supported by operating grants from the Canadian Institutes for Health Research and Heart & Stroke Foundation.

REFERENCES

1. Kaab S, Dixon J, Duc J, et al. Molecular basis of transient outward potassium current downregulation in human heart failure: a decrease in Kv4.3 mRNA correlates with a reduction in current density. *Circulation.* 1998;98:1383–1393.

2. Oudit GY, Kassiri Z, Sah R, Ramirez RJ, Zobel C, Backx PH. The molecular physiology of the cardiac transient outward potassium current (I(to)) in normal and diseased myocardium. *J Mol Cell Cardiol.* 2001;33:851–872.

3. Tsuji Y, Opthof T, Kamiya K, et al. Pacing-induced heart failure causes a reduction of delayed rectifier potassium currents along with decreases in calcium and transient outward currents in rabbit ventricle. *Cardiovasc Res.* 2000;48:300–309.

4. Tseng GN. I(Kr): the hERG channel. *J Mol Cell Cardiol.* 2001;33:835–849.

5. Keating MT, Sanguinetti MC. Molecular and cellular mechanisms of cardiac arrhythmias. *Cell.* 2001;104:569–580.

6. Pogwizd SM, Bers DM. Na/Ca exchange in heart failure: contractile dysfunction and arrhythmogenesis. *Ann N Y Acad Sci.* 2002;976:454–465.

7. Kuo HC, Cheng CF, Clark RB, et al. A defect in the Kv channel-interacting protein 2 (KChIP2) gene leads to a complete loss of I(to) and confers susceptibility to ventricular tachycardia. *Cell.* 2001;107:801–813.

8. Nerbonne JM, Nichols CG, Schwarz TL, Escande D. Genetic manipulation of cardiac K(+) channel function in mice: what have we learned, and where do we go from here? *Circ Res.* 2001;89:944–956.

9. Deal KK, England SK, Tamkun MM. Molecular physiology of cardiac potassium channels. *Physiol Rev.* 1996;76:49–67.

10. Pongs O, Leicher T, Berger M, et al. Functional and molecular aspects of voltage-gated K+ channel beta subunits. *Ann N Y Acad Sci.* 1999;868:344–355.

11. Gulbis JM, Zhou M, Mann S, MacKinnon R. Structure of the cytoplasmic beta subunit-T1 assembly of voltage-dependent K+ channels. *Science.* 2000;289:123–127.

12. Kuryshev YA, Wible BA, Gudz TI, Ramirez AN, Brown AM. KChAP/Kvbeta1.2 interactions and their effects on cardiac Kv channel expression. *Am J Physiol Cell Physiol.* 2001;281:C290–C299.

13. Kuryshev YA, Gudz TI, Brown AM, Wible BA. KChAP as a chaperone for specific K(+) channels. *Am J Physiol Cell Physiol.* 2000;278:C931–C941.

14. An WF, Bowlby MR, Betty M, et al. Modulation of A-type potassium channels by a family of calcium sensors. *Nature.* 2000;403:553–556.

15. Deschenes I, DiSilvestre D, Juang GJ, Wu RC, An WF, Tomaselli GF. Regulation of Kv4.3 current by KChIP2 splice variants: a component of native cardiac I(to)? *Circulation.* 2002;106:423–429.

16. Guo W, Malin SA, Johns DC, Jeromin A, Nerbonne JM. Modulation of Kv4-encoded K(+) currents in the mammalian myocardium by neuronal calcium sensor-1. *J Biol Chem.* 2002;277:26436–26443.

17. Nakamura TY, Pountney DJ, Ozaita A, et al. A role for frequenin, a Ca2+-binding protein, as a regulator of Kv4 K+-currents. *Proc Natl Acad Sci U S A.* 2001;98:12808–12813.

18. Kurokawa J, Abriel H, Kass RS. Molecular basis of the delayed rectifier current I(ks)in heart. *J Mol Cell Cardiol.* 2001;33:873–882.

19. Chen YH, Xu SJ, Bendahhou S, et al. KCNQ1 gain-of-function mutation in familial atrial fibrillation. *Science*. 2003;299:251–254.

20. Yellen G. The voltage-gated potassium channels and their relatives. *Nature*. 2002;419:35–42.

21. Tinel N, Diochot S, Borsotto M, Lazdunski M, Barhanin J. KCNE2 confers background current characteristics to the cardiac KCNQ1 potassium channel. *EMBO J*. 2000;19:6326–6330.

22. Doyle DA, Morais Cabral J, Pfuetzner RA, et al. The structure of the potassium channel: molecular basis of K+ conduction and selectivity. *Science*. 1998;280:69–77.

23. Stock L, Souza C, Treptow W. Structural basis for activation of voltage-gated cation channels. *Biochemistry*. 2013;52:1501–1513.

24. Blunck R, Batulan Z. Mechanism of electromechanical coupling in voltage-gated potassium channels. *Front Pharm*. 2012;3:166.

25. Jiang Y, Lee A, Chen J, Cadene M, Chait BT, MacKinnon R. The open pore conformation of potassium channels. *Nature*. 2002;417:523–526.

26. Shin KS, Maertens C, Proenza C, Rothberg BS, Yellen G. Inactivation in HCN channels results from reclosure of the activation gate: desensitization to voltage. *Neuron*. 2004;41:737–744.

27. Decher N, Chen J, Sanguinetti MC. Voltage-dependent gating of hyperpolarization-activated, cyclic nucleotide-gated pacemaker channels: molecular coupling between the S4-S5 and C-linkers. *Journal Biol Chem*. 2004;279:13859–13865.

27a. Jerng HH, Pfaffinger PJ, Covarrubias M. Molecular physiology and modulation of somatodendritic A-type potassium channels. *Mol Cell Neurosci*. 2004;27:343–369.

28. Rasmusson RL, Morales MJ, Wang S, et al. Inactivation of voltage-gated cardiac K+ channels. *Circ Res*. 1998;82:739–750.

28a. Holmgren M, Shin KS, Yellan G. The activation gate of a voltage-gated K+ channel can be trapped in the open state by an intersubunit metal bridge. *Neuron*. 1998;21:617–621.

28b. Aldrich RW. Fifty years of inactivation. *Nature*. 2001;411:643–644.

29. Kurata HT, Fedida D. A structural interpretation of voltage-gated potassium channel inactivation. *Prog Biophys Mol Biol*. 2006;92:185–208.

30. Bahring R, Boland LM, Varghese A, Gebauer M, Pongs O. Kinetic analysis of open- and closed-state inactivation transitions in human Kv4.2 A-type potassium channels. *J Physiol*. 2001;535:65–81.

31. Bezanilla F, Armstrong CM. Inactivation of the sodium channel. I. Sodium current experiments. *J Gen Physiol*. 1977;70:549–566.

32. Bahring R, Covarrubias M. Mechanisms of closed-state inactivation in voltage-gated ion channels. *J Physiol*. 2011;589:461–479.

33. Klemic KG, Kirsch GE, Jones SW. U-type inactivation of Kv3.1 and Shaker potassium channels. *Biophys J*. 2001;81:814–826.

34. Kurata HT, Soon GS, Eldstrom JR, Lu GW, Steele DF, Fedida D. Amino-terminal determinants of U-type inactivation of voltage-gated K+ channels. *J Biol Chem*. 2002;277:29045–29053.

35. Liu J, Kim KH, London B, Morales MJ, Backx PH. Dissection of the voltage-activated potassium outward currents in adult mouse ventricular myocytes: I(to,f), I(to,s), I(K,slow1), I(K,slow2), and I(ss). *Basic Res Cardiol*. 2011;106:189–204.

36. Huang F, Wong X, Jan LY. International Union of Basic and Clinical Pharmacology. LXXXV: calcium-activated chloride channels. *Pharmacol Rev*. 2012;64:1–15.

37. Han W, Bao W, Wang Z, Nattel S. Comparison of ion-channel subunit expression in canine cardiac Purkinje fibers and ventricular muscle. *Circ Res*. 2002;91:790–797.

38. Po SS, Wu RC, Juang GJ, Kong W, Tomaselli GF. Mechanism of alpha-adrenergic regulation of expressed hKv4.3 currents. *Am J Physiol Heart Circ Physiol*. 2001;281:H2518–H2527.

39. Perrin MJ, Adler A, Green S, et al. Evaluation of genes encoding for the transient outward current (I$_{to}$) identifies the KCND2 gene as a cause of J-wave syndrome associated with sudden cardiac death. *Circ Cardiovasc Genet*. 2014;7:782–789.

40. Li H, Guo W, Mellor RL, Nerbonne JM. KChIP2 modulates the cell surface expression of Kv 1.5-encoded K(+) channels. *J Mol Cell Cardiol*. 2005;39:121–132.

41. Thomsen MB, Wang C, Ozgen N, Wang HG, Rosen MR, Pitt GS. Accessory subunit KChIP2 modulates the cardiac L-type calcium current. *Circ Res*. 2009;104:1382–1389.

42. Rosati B, Pan Z, Lypen S, et al. Regulation of KChIP2 potassium channel beta subunit gene expression underlies the gradient of transient outward current in canine and human ventricle. *J Physiol*. 2001;533:119–125.

43. Rosati B, Grau F, Rodriguez S, Li H, Nerbonne JM, McKinnon D. Concordant expression of KChIP2 mRNA, protein and transient outward current throughout the canine ventricle. *J Physiol*. 2003;548:815–822.

44. Calloe K, Cordeiro JM, Di Diego JM, et al. A transient outward potassium current activator recapitulates the electrocardiographic manifestations of Brugada syndrome. *Cardiovasc Res*. 2009;81:686–694.

45. Gaborit N, Varro A, Le Bouter S, et al. Gender-related differences in ion-channel and transporter subunit expression in non-diseased human hearts. *J Mol Cell Cardiol*. 2010;49:639–646.

46. Soltysinska E, Olesen SP, Christ T, et al. Transmural expression of ion channels and transporters in human nondiseased and end-stage failing hearts. *Pflugers Arch*. 2009;459:11–23.

47. Ambrosi CM, Yamada KA, Nerbonne JM, Efimov IR. Gender differences in electrophysiological gene expression in failing and non-failing human hearts. *PloS One*. 2013;8:e54635.

48. Antzelevitch C, Fish J. Electrical heterogeneity within the ventricular wall. *Basic Res Cardiol*. 2001;96:517–527.

49. Patel SP, Campbell DL, Strauss HC. Elucidating KChIP effects on Kv4.3 inactivation and recovery kinetics with a minimal KChIP2 isoform. *J Physiol*. 2002;545:5–11.

50. Costantini DL, Arruda EP, Agarwal P, et al. The homeodomain transcription factor Irx5 establishes the mouse cardiac ventricular repolarization gradient. *Cell*. 2005;123:347–358.

51. Guo W, Jung WE, Marionneau C, et al. Targeted deletion of Kv4.2 eliminates I(to,f) and results in electrical and molecular remodeling, with no evidence of ventricular hypertrophy or myocardial dysfunction. *Circ Res*. 2005;97:1342–1350.

52. Teutsch C, Kondo RP, Dederko DA, Chrast J, Chien KR, Giles WR. Spatial distributions of Kv4 channels and KChip2 isoforms in the murine heart based on laser capture microdissection. *Cardiovasc Res*. 2007;73:739–749.

53. Dixon JE, McKinnon D. Quantitative analysis of potassium channel mRNA expression in atrial and ventricular muscle of rats. *Circ Res*. 1994;75:252–260.

54. Wickenden AD, Jegla TJ, Kaprielian R, Backx PH. Regional contributions of Kv1.4, Kv4.2, and Kv4.3 to transient outward K+ current in rat ventricle. *J Physiol*. 1999;276:H1599–H1607.

55. Rossow CF, Dilly KW, Santana LF. Differential calcineurin/NFATc3 activity contributes to the Ito transmural gradient in the mouse heart. *Circ Res*. 2006;98:1306–1313.

56. Gong N, Bodi I, Zobel C, Schwartz A, Molkentin JD, Backx PH. Calcineurin increases cardiac transient outward K+ currents via transcriptional up-regulation of Kv4.2 channel subunits. *J Biol Chem*. 2006;281:38498–38506.

57. Radicke S, Cotella D, Graf EM, Ravens U, Wettwer E. Expression and function of dipeptidyl-aminopeptidase-like protein 6 as a putative beta-subunit of human cardiac transient outward current encoded by Kv4.3. *J Physiol*. 2005;565:751–756.

58. Cotella D, Radicke S, Bortoluzzi A, et al. Impaired glycosylation blocks DPP10 cell surface expression and alters the electrophysiology of Ito channel complex. *Pflugers Arch*. 2010;460:87–97.

59. Xiao L, Koopmann TT, Ordog B, et al. Unique cardiac Purkinje fiber transient outward current beta-subunit composition: a potential molecular link to idiopathic ventricular fibrillation. *Circ Res*. 2013;112:1310–1322.

60. Deschenes I, Tomaselli GF. Modulation of Kv4.3 current by accessory subunits. *FEBS Lett*. 2002;528:183–188.

61. Nerbonne JM. Molecular basis of functional voltage-gated K+ channel diversity in the mammalian myocardium. *J Physiol*. 2000;525 Pt(2):285–298.

62. Niwa N, Nerbonne JM. Molecular determinants of cardiac transient outward potassium current (I(to)) expression and regulation. *J Mol Cell Cardiol*. 2010;48:12–25.

63. Shimoni Y. Hormonal control of cardiac ion channels and transporters. *Prog Biophys Mol Biol*. 1999;72:67–108.

64. Murray KT, Fahrig SA, Deal KK, et al. Modulation of an inactivating human cardiac K+ channel by protein kinase C. *Circ Res*. 1994;75:999–1005.

65. Gallego M, Alday A, Alonso H, Casis O. Adrenergic regulation of cardiac ionic channels: role of membrane microdomains in the regulation of kv4 channels. *Biochim Biophys Acta*. 2014;1838:692–699.

66. Zobel C, Kassiri Z, Nguyen TT, Meng Y, Backx PH. Prevention of hypertrophy by overexpression of Kv4.2 in cultured neonatal cardiomyocytes. *Circulation*. 2002;106:2385–2391.

67. Zhang TT, Takimoto K, Stewart AF, Zhu C, Levitan ES. Independent regulation of cardiac Kv4.3 potassium channel expression by angiotensin II and phenylephrine. *Circ Res*. 2001;88:476–482.

68. Kassiri Z, Zobel C, Nguyen TT, Molkentin JD, Backx PH. Reduction of I(to) causes hypertrophy in neonatal rat ventricular myocytes. *Circ Res*. 2002;90:578–585.

69. Gray CB, Heller Brown J. CaMKIIdelta subtypes: localization and function. *Front Pharmacol*. 2014;5:15.

70. Wickenden AD, Kaprielian R, Parker TG, Jones OT, Backx PH. Effects of development and thyroid hormone on K+ currents and K+ channel gene expression in rat ventricle. *J Physiol*. 1997;504(pt 2):271–286.

71. Wickenden AD, Kaprielian R, You XM, Backx PH. The thyroid hormone analog DITPA restores I(to) in rats after myocardial infarction. *Am J Physiol Heart Circ Physiol*. 2000;278:H1105–H1116.

72. Le Bouter S, Demolombe S, Chambellan A, et al. Microarray analysis reveals complex remodeling of cardiac ion channel expression with altered thyroid status: relation to cellular and integrated electrophysiology. *Circ Res*. 2003;92:234–242.

73. Benitah JP, Perrier E, Gomez AM, Vassort G. Effects of aldosterone on transient outward K+ current density in rat ventricular myocytes. *J Physiol*. 2001;537:151–160.

74. El Gebeily G, El Khoury N, Mathieu S, Brouillette J, Fiset C. Estrogen regulation of the transient outward K(+) current involves estrogen receptor alpha in mouse heart. *J Mol Cell Cardiol*. 2015;86:85–94.

75. Lopez M, Meier D, Muller A, Franken P, Fujita J, Fontana A. Tumor necrosis factor and transforming growth factor beta regulate clock genes by controlling the expression of the cold inducible RNA-binding protein (CIRBP). *J Biol Chem*. 2014;289:2736–2744.

76. Nabauer M, Beuckelmann DJ, Uberfuhr P, Steinbeck G. Regional differences in current density and rate-dependent properties of the transient outward current in subepicardial and subendocardial myocytes of human left ventricle. *Circulation*. 1996;93:168–177.

77. Schram G, Pourrier M, Melnyk P, Nattel S. Differential distribution of cardiac ion channel expression as a basis for regional specialization in electrical function. *Circ Res*. 2002;90:939–950.

78. Di Diego JM, Sun ZQ, Antzelevitch C. I(to) and action potential notch are smaller in left vs. right canine ventricular epicardium. *J Physiol*. 1996;271:H548–H561.

79. Giudicessi JR, Ye D, Tester DJ, et al. Transient outward current (I(to)) gain-of-function mutations in the KCND3-encoded Kv4.3 potassium channel and Brugada syndrome. *Heart Rhythm*. 2011;8:1024–1032.

80. Kaprielian R, Wickenden AD, Kassiri Z, Parker TG, Liu PP, Backx PH. Relationship between K+ channel down-regulation and [Ca2+]i in rat ventricular myocytes following myocardial infarction. *J Physiol*. 1999;517(pt 1):229–245.

81. Nattel S, Maguy A, Le Bouter S, Yeh YH. Arrhythmogenic ion-channel remodeling in the heart: heart failure, myocardial infarction, and atrial fibrillation. *Physiol Rev*. 2007;87:425–456.

82. Zicha S, Xiao L, Stafford S, et al. Transmural expression of transient outward potassium current subunits in normal and failing canine and human hearts. *J Physiol*. 2004;561:735–748.

83. Sah R, Ramirez RJ, Oudit GY, et al. Regulation of cardiac excitation-contraction coupling by action potential repolarization: role of the transient outward potassium current (I(to)). *J Physiol*. 2003;546:5–18.

84. Ramirez RJ, Sah R, Liu J, Rose RA, Backx PH. Intracellular [Na(+)] modulates synergy between Na(+)/Ca (2+) exchanger and L-type Ca (2+) current in cardiac excitation-contraction coupling during action potentials. *Basic Res Cardiol*. 2011;106:967–977.

85. Olesen MS, Refsgaard L, Holst AG, et al. A novel KCND3 gain-of-function mutation associated with early-onset of persistent lone atrial fibrillation. *Cardiovasc Res*. 2013;98:488–495.

86. Delpon E, Cordeiro JM, Nunez L, et al. Functional effects of KCNE3 mutation and its role in the development of Brugada syndrome. *Circ Arrhythm Electrophysiol*. 2008;1:209–218.

87. Yan GX, Antzelevitch C. Cellular basis for the electrocardiographic J wave. *Circulation*. 1996;93:372–379.

88. Nerbonne JM, Kass RS. Molecular physiology of cardiac repolarization. *Physiol Rev*. 2005;85:1205–1253.

89. Ehrlich JR, Pourrier M, Weerapura M, et al. KvLQT1 modulates the distribution and biophysical properties of HERG. A novel alpha-subunit interaction between delayed rectifier currents. *J Biol Chem*. 2004;279:1233–1241.

90. Schonherr R, Heinemann SH. Molecular determinants for activation and inactivation of HERG, a human inward rectifier potassium channel. *J Physiol*. 1996;493(pt 3):635–642.

91. Wang S, Liu S, Morales MJ, Strauss HC, Rasmusson RL. A quantitative analysis of the activation and inactivation kinetics of HERG expressed in Xenopus oocytes. *J Physiol*. 1997;502(pt 1):45–60.

92. Gustina AS, Trudeau MC. hERG potassium channel gating is mediated by N- and C-terminal region interactions. *The Journal of general physiology.* 2011;137:315–325.

93. Kopfer DA, Hahn U, Ohmert I, et al. A molecular switch driving inactivation in the cardiac K+ channel HERG. *PloS One.* 2012;7:e41023.

94. Clark RB, Mangoni ME, Lueger A, Couette B, Nargeot J, Giles WR. A rapidly activating delayed rectifier K+ current regulates pacemaker activity in adult mouse sinoatrial node cells. *Am J Physiol Heart Circ Physiol.* 2004;286:H1757–H1766.

95. Abbott GW, Sesti F, Splawski I, et al. MiRP1 forms IKr potassium channels with HERG and is associated with cardiac arrhythmia. *Cell.* 1999;97:175–187.

96. Furukawa T, Ono Y, Tsuchiya H, et al. Specific interaction of the potassium channel beta-subunit minK with the sarcomeric protein T-cap suggests a T-tubule-myofibril linking system. *J Mol Biol.* 2001;313:775–784.

97. Nitabach MN, Llamas DA, Araneda RC, et al. A mechanism for combinatorial regulation of electrical activity: potassium channel subunits capable of functioning as Src homology 3-dependent adaptors. *Proc Natl Acad Sci U S A.* 2001;98:705–710.

98. Gaborit N, Le Bouter S, Szuts V, et al. Regional and tissue specific transcript signatures of ion channel genes in the non-diseased human heart. *J Physiol.* 2007;582:675–693.

99. Ravens U, Wettwer E. Ultra-rapid delayed rectifier channels: molecular basis and therapeutic implications. *Cardiovasc Res.* 2011;89:776–785.

100. Teng GQ, Zhao X, Lees-Miller JP, et al. Homozygous missense N629D hERG (KCNH2) potassium channel mutation causes developmental defects in the right ventricle and its outflow tract and embryonic lethality. *Circ Res.* 2008;103:1483–1491.

101. Cui J, Melman Y, Palma E, Fishman GI, McDonald TV. Cyclic AMP regulates the HERG K(+) channel by dual pathways. *Curr Biol.* 2000;10:671–674.

102. Satler CA, Walsh EP, Vesely MR, Plummer MH, Ginsburg GS, Jacob HJ. Novel missense mutation in the cyclic nucleotide-binding domain of HERG causes long QT syndrome. *Am J Med Genet.* 1996;65:27–35.

103. Bian J, Cui J, McDonald TV. HERG K(+) channel activity is regulated by changes in phosphatidyl inositol 4,5-bisphosphate. *Circ Res.* 2001;89:1168–1176.

104. Magyar J, Iost N, Kortvely A, et al. Effects of endothelin-1 on calcium and potassium currents in undiseased human ventricular myocytes. *Pflugers Arch.* 2000;441:144–149.

105. Marx SO, Kurokawa J, Reiken S, et al. Requirement of a macromolecular signaling complex for beta adrenergic receptor modulation of the KCNQ1-KCNE1 potassium channel. *Science.* 2002;295:496–499.

106. Chen L, Marquardt ML, Tester DJ, Sampson KJ, Ackerman MJ, Kass RS. Mutation of an A-kinase-anchoring protein causes long-QT syndrome. *Proc Natl Acad Sci U S A.* 2007;104:20990–20995.

107. Yue L, Feng J, Wang Z, Nattel S. Adrenergic control of the ultrarapid delayed rectifier current in canine atrial myocytes. *J Physiol.* 1999;516(pt 2):385–398.

108. Nitabach MN, Llamas DA, Thompson IJ, Collins KA, Holmes TC. Phosphorylation-dependent and phosphorylation-independent modes of modulation of shaker family voltage-gated potassium channels by SRC family protein tyrosine kinases. *J Neurosci.* 2002;22:7913–7922.

109. Nunez L, Vaquero M, Gomez R, et al. Nitric oxide blocks hKv1.5 channels by S-nitrosylation and by a cyclic GMP-dependent mechanism. *Cardiovasc Res.* 2006;72:80–89.

110. Takimoto K, Levitan ES. Glucocorticoid induction of Kv1.5 K+ channel gene expression in ventricle of rat heart. *Circ Res.* 1994;75:1006–1013.

111. Brouillette J, Trepanier-Boulay V, Fiset C. Effect of androgen deficiency on mouse ventricular repolarization. *J Physiol.* 2003;546:403–413.

112. Trepanier-Boulay V, St-Michel C, Tremblay A, Fiset C. Gender-based differences in cardiac repolarization in mouse ventricle. *Circ Res.* 2001;89:437–444.

113. Godreau D, Vranckx R, Maguy A, et al. Expression, regulation and role of the MAGUK protein SAP-97 in human atrial myocardium. *Cardiovasc Res.* 2002;56:433–442.

114. Gintant GA. Two components of delayed rectifier current in canine atrium and ventricle. Does IKs play a role in the reverse rate dependence of class III agents? *Circ Res.* 1996;78:26–37.

115. Cheng J, Kamiya K, Liu W, Tsuji Y, Toyama J, Kodama I. Heterogeneous distribution of the two components of delayed rectifier K+ current: a potential mechanism of the proarrhythmic effects of methanesulfonanilideclass III agents. *Cardiovasc Res.* 1999;43:135–147.

116. Brahmajothi MV, Morales MJ, Reimer KA, Strauss HC. Regional localization of ERG, the channel protein responsible for the rapid component of the delayed rectifier, K+ current in the ferret heart. *Circ Res.* 1997;81:128–135.

117. Bryant SM, Wan X, Shipsey SJ, Hart G. Regional differences in the delayed rectifier current (IKr and IKs) contribute to the differences in action potential duration in basal left ventricular myocytes in guinea-pig. *Cardiovasc Res.* 1998;40:322–331.

118. Berkefeld H, Fakler B, Schulte U. Ca2+-activated K+ channels: from protein complexes to function. *Physiol Rev.* 2010;90:1437–1459.

119. Nattel S. Calcium-activated potassium current: a novel ion channel candidate in atrial fibrillation. *J Physiol.* 2009;587:1385–1386.

120. Xia XM, Fakler B, Rivard A, et al. Mechanism of calcium gating in small-conductance calcium-activated potassium channels. *Nature.* 1998;395:503–507.

121. Schumacher MA, Rivard AF, Bachinger HP, Adelman JP. Structure of the gating domain of a Ca2+-activated K+ channel complexed with Ca2+/calmodulin. *Nature.* 2001;410:1120–1124.

122. Allen D, Fakler B, Maylie J, Adelman JP. Organization and regulation of small conductance Ca2+-activated K+ channel multiprotein complexes. *J Neurosci.* 2007;27:2369–2376.

123. Zhang XD, Lieu DK, Chiamvimonvat N. Small-conductance Ca2+ -activated K+ channels and cardiac arrhythmias. *Heart Rhythm.* 2015;12:1845–1851.

124. Ozgen N, Dun W, Sosunov EA, et al. Early electrical remodeling in rabbit pulmonary vein results from trafficking of intracellular SK2 channels to membrane sites. *Cardiovasc Res.* 2007;75:758–769.

125. Tuteja D, Xu D, Timofeyev V, et al. Differential expression of small-conductance Ca2+-activated K+ channels SK1, SK2, and SK3 in mouse atrial and ventricular myocytes. *Am J Physiol Heart Circ Physiol.* 2005;289:H2714–H2723.

126. Nattel S, Qi XY. Calcium-dependent potassium channels in the heart: clarity and confusion. *Cardiovasc Res.* 2014;101:185–186.

127. Chen WT, Chen YC, Lu YY, et al. Apamin modulates electrophysiological characteristics of the pulmonary vein and the sinoatrial node. *Eur J Clin Invest.* 2013;43:957–963.

128. Li N, Timofeyev V, Tuteja D, et al. Ablation of a Ca2+-activated K+ channel (SK2 channel) results in action potential prolongation in atrial myocytes and atrial fibrillation. *J Physiol.* 2009;587:1087–1100.

129. Mahida S, Mills RW, Tucker NR, et al. Overexpression of KCNN3 results in sudden cardiac death. *Cardiovasc Res.* 2014;101:326–334.

130. Olesen MS, Jabbari J, Holst AG, et al. Screening of KCNN3 in patients with early-onset lone atrial fibrillation. *Europace.* 2011;13:963–967.

131. Sosunov EA, Anyukhovsky EP, Hefer D, et al. Region-specific, pacing-induced changes in repolarization in rabbit atrium: an example of sensitivity to the rare. *Cardiovasc Res.* 2005;67:274–282.

132. Qi XY, Diness JG, Brundel BJ, et al. Role of small-conductance calcium-activated potassium channels in atrial electrophysiology and fibrillation in the dog. *Circulation.* 2014;129:430–440.

133. Yu T, Deng C, Wu R, et al. Decreased expression of small-conductance Ca2+-activated K+ channels SK1 and SK2 in human chronic atrial fibrillation. *Life Sci.* 2012;90:219–227.

134. Chang PC, Turker I, Lopshire JC, et al. Heterogeneous upregulation of apamin-sensitive potassium currents in failing human ventricles. *J Am Heart Assoc.* 2013;2:e004713.

135. Long SB, Tao X, Campbell EB, MacKinnon R. Atomic structure of a voltage-dependent K+ channel in a lipid membrane-like environment. *Nature.* 2007;450:376–382.

136. Strop P, Bankovich AJ, Hansen KC, Garcia KC, Brunger AT. Structure of a human A-type potassium channel interacting protein DPPX, a member of the dipeptidyl aminopeptidase family. *J Mol Biol.* 2004;343:1055–1065.

Structural and Molecular Bases of Cardiac Inward Rectifier Potassium Channel Function

Anatoli N. Lopatin and Justus M.B. Anumonwo

Background

Inwardly rectifying potassium (Kir) channels are important for stabilizing the resting membrane potential, establishing the threshold of excitation, and modulating the repolarization phase of the cardiac action potential.[1] Inward rectification is a process in which the conductance of the Kir channel increases with membrane hyperpolarization, but decreases with depolarization to potentials positive to the K^+ equilibrium potential. In essence, Kir channels behave as "biodiodes," preferentially passing current in one direction. The molecular basis of rectification in Kir channels is a physical occlusion of the ion permeation pathway by depolarization-induced movement of intracellular cations, such as magnesium and polyamines.[1] Only few Kir channels, however, display strong rectification.[2] Strong inward rectification not only enables the Kir channels to stabilize the resting membrane potential but also allows for the protection of the cell against an excessive loss of K^+ ions during the plateau phase of an action potential.[1] The molecular correlates of these channels are primary subunits encoded by the $KCNJ$ family of genes.[3] Mutations in $KCNJ$ genes have been associated with various channelopathies,[2] demonstrating the importance of Kir channels in normal cardiac excitation. This chapter will focus on three well-studied Kir channels in the myocardial cells: the classical inward rectifier K^+ channels (I_{K1}), the acetylcholine-activated K^+ channels (K_{ACh}), and the adenosine triphosphate (ATP)-sensitive K^+ channels (K_{ATP}). Additional information on the topics covered in this chapter can be obtained from recent review articles.[2,4,5]

A Family of Genes Encodes Inward Rectifier Potassium Channels

Channels belonging to the Kir family are structurally and functionally different from voltage-gated K^+ channels.[2,4] The genes that encode Kir channels are ascribed the $KCNJ$ nomenclature and are categorized into seven subfamilies based on the gene products (Kir1-7; Table 4.1; Fig. 4.1). In general, Kir channels consist of homomeric or heteromeric complexes of the respective Kir subunits, but as will be discussed, functionality of the

resulting channels depends partially or solely on the interactions with additional (accessory) proteins.[2] From a functional perspective, there are three distinct classes of cardiac Kir channels (I_{K1}, I_{KACh}, and I_{KATP}). As will be discussed later in this chapter, based on the degree of inward rectification, the underlying channels can be considered as strong (I_{K1}; K_{ACh}) or weak (K_{ATP}) inward rectifiers.[2]

There is ample molecular and electrophysiological evidence for the expression of Kir2, Kir3, and Kir6 subfamily members in myocardial tissue, subunits representing the molecular correlates of I_{K1}, I_{KACh}, and I_{KATP}, respectively. Given that the other members of Kir family (Kir1, Kir4, Kir5, and Kir7) are thought to be primarily important for K^+ transport in other tissues, they will not be discussed further in this chapter.

Classical Cardiac Inward Rectifier Potassium Channels

Structure and Function

Kir2 Subfamily Underlies Cardiac I_{K1}

The Kir2 subfamily consists of six members (Kir2.1-Kir2.6), of which only Kir2.1-Kir2.4 are expressed in the mammalian heart. As shown in Table 4.1, the following genes encode the mammalian Kir channels: $KCNJ2$, $KCNJ12$, $KCNJ4$, $KCNJ14$, $KCNJ17(KCNJN1)$, and $KCNJ18$ for Kir2.1 through Kir2.6, respectively. There is evidence that in the mammalian heart Kir2.1-Kir2.3 isoforms are expressed in cardiac myocytes and that Kir2.4 is probably only expressed in neuronal cells. It is now well established that members of the Kir2 subfamily underlie I_{K1}, although the subunit composition varies among species and cell types and that channel complexes are likely formed as heterotetrameric structures.

Crystal Structure of Kir2 Channels

In recent years, x-ray crystallographic structures of both bacterial and mammalian homologs of several Kir channels have been obtained.[7] Fig. 4.2 highlights some important and common features of Kir channel structure based on the results of work with Kir2.1 and Kir2.2 mammalian channels.[8] It is now firmly established that Kir channels are tetramers of distinct subunits, each having two transmembrane domains (M1 and M2), relatively small N-terminal, and large C-terminal cytoplasmic domains, and a pore-forming structure between M1 and M2 (see Fig. 4.2). The pore structure contains a pore helix directed toward the conduction pathway and the characteristic GYG (or GFG) motif, also known as the K^+ channel signature sequence, which contributes to the selectivity filter in all potassium channels. The M1 and M2 transmembrane domains in each subunit are arranged as an antiparallel coiled-coil and make contact with each other. Kir2 channels have a negatively charged amino acid (D172 in Kir2.1) located in approximately the middle of the pore, which plays a critical role in the phenomenon of inward rectification discussed later.

TABLE 4.1 Diversity of α-subunit proteins in the family of inward rectifier potassium channels

SUBFAMILY	PROTEIN	GENE	HUMAN	MOUSE	CURRENT
Kir1	Kir1.1	*KCNJ1*	11q24	9 A4	?
Kir2	Kir2.1	*KCNJ2*	17q24.3	11 E2	I_{K1}
	Kir2.2	*KCNJ12*	17p11.2	11 B2	I_{K1}
	Kir2.3	*KCNJ4*	22q13.1	15 E1	I_{K1}
	Kir2.4	*KCNJ14*	19q13.4	7 B4	?
	Kir2.5	*KCNJ17**	17p11.1		
	Kir2.6	*KCNJ18*	17p11.2		
Kir3	Kir3.1	*KCNJ3*	2q24.1	2 C1.1	I_{KACh}
	Kir3.2	*KCNJ6*	21q22.1	16 C4	
	Kir3.3	*KCNJ9*	1q23.2	1 H3	
	Kir3.4	*KCNJ5*	11q24	9 A4	I_{KACh}
Kir4	Kir4.1	*KCNJ10*	1q23.2	1 H3	
	Kir4.2	*KCNJ15*	21q22.2	16 C4	
Kir5	Kir5.1	*KCNJ16*	17q24.3	11 E2	
Kir6	Kir6.1	*KCNJ8*	12p11.23	6 G2	I_{KATP}
	Kir6.2	*KCNJ11*	11p15.1	7 B4	I_{KATP}
Kir7	Kir7.1	*KCNJ13*	2q37	1 D	?

*Also known as *KCNJN1*.[6]

Modified and updated from Nerbonne JM, Nichols CG, Schwarz TL, et al. Genetic manipulation of cardiac K⁺ channel function in mice: what have we learned, and where do we go from here? *Circ Res.* 2001;89:944-956.

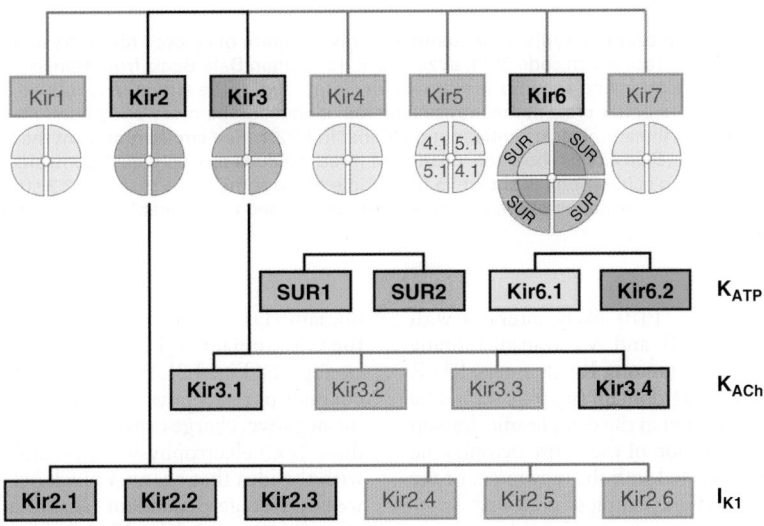

FIGURE 4.1 The family of inward rectifier potassium channels. All members of the Kir family share significant structural similarity, but only the Kir2 and Kir3 subfamilies represent channels carrying classical strongly rectifying currents. Six members of the Kir2 and four members of the Kir3 subfamilies were cloned in mammals. Heteromeric assemblies of the Kir2.1, Kir2.2, and Kir2.3 subunits underlie the I_{K1} current, and heteromeric assembly of the Kir3.1 and Kir3.4 subunits underlies the I_{KACh} current. Weakly rectifying K_{ATP} channels are composed of pore-forming Kir6.1 and Kir6.2 subunits as well as auxiliary SUR1 and SUR2 subunits. (Modified from Anumonwo JM, Lopatin AN. Cardiac strong inward rectifier potassium channels. *J Mol Cell Cardiol.* 2010;48:45-54.)

There are at least three distinct regions of the intramembrane part of the pore: the selectivity filter, a centrally located water filled cavity of approximately 10 Å in diameter, and the narrowing of the pore at the cytoplasmic side as the pore-lining M2 helixes come closer to each other (known as *bundle-crossing*). M2 helixes also possess a highly conserved glycine residue (a "hinge"; G168 in Kir2.1) that likely contributes to the channel gating by allowing the helixes to bend and change the size of the pore at the bundle crossing.

The so-called slide helix formed by the N-terminus region just preceding the M1 helix is another unique and important regulatory feature of both bacterial and mammalian Kir channels.[9] This helix intercalates between the inner leaflet of the plasma membrane and cytosol likely because of its amphiphilic nature. The important functional role of the slide helix is highlighted by the fact that many loss-of-function mutations associated with Andersen-Tawil syndrome (LQT7) are located in the slide helix.

A large C-terminal domain provided by four Kir2.x subunits consists primarily of β-strands and potentially strongly interacts with a smaller N-terminal domain. As shown in Fig. 4.2, C-terminal domain forms a large intracellular vestibule, approximately 30 Å in length, for easy ion passage and likely provides binding sites for various intracellular agents. The cytoplasmic domain harbors a number of residues (e.g., E224 and E299 in Fig. 4.2) known to contribute to inward rectification.

A membrane phospholipid phosphatidylinositol 4,5-bisphosphate (PIP_2) is an important structural and regulatory component

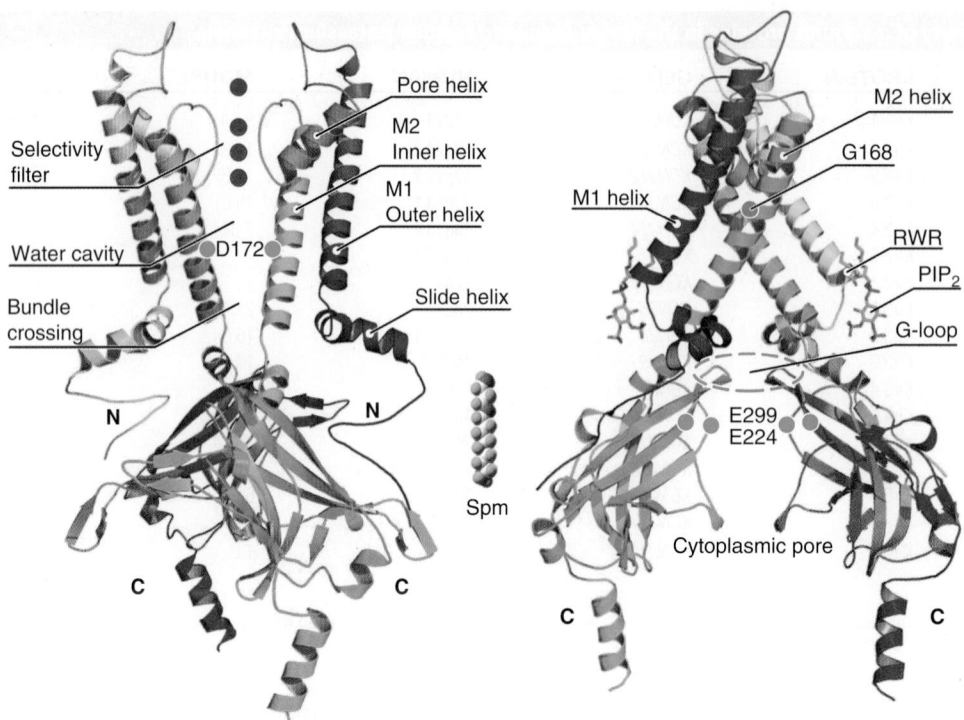

FIGURE 4.2 Architecture of a typical Kir channel. X-ray structure of chicken Kir2.2 crystallized in the presence of PIP$_2$ (accession code 3SPI, available in the Protein Data Bank; from Hansen and colleagues[8]). Only two opposing subunits are shown for clarity. *Right,* The structure is rotated approximately 90 degrees to better present the intracellular ion conduction pathway and bound molecules of PIP$_2$. Numbering of the amino acids corresponds to that in Kir2.1. *Red circles* represent the K$^+$ ions in the selectivity filter. *Blue circles* show the location of three residues most critical for inward rectification. Spermine molecule (*Spm*) is shown in the middle at the same scale as the Kir2.2 structure. Analysis and visual presentation of the structures were performed using DeepView Swiss-PdbViewer and PyMol software.

of Kir channels.[10] In the membrane, PIP$_2$ likely interacts with hydrophobic amino acids on both M1 and M2 transmembrane helices as well as with a well-conserved (among Kir channels) RWR motif located just at the end of the M1 domain (see Fig. 4.2). The interaction of PIP$_2$ with a specific region in the cytoplasmic domain leads to an approximately 6 Å translation of the entire cytoplasmic domain toward the membrane associated with the movement of the M1 helix, which ultimately leads to the opening of the gate.[8]

Mechanism of Polyamine-Induced Rectification

The key experiments conducted in mid-1990s with the first cloned members of the Kir2 subfamily have clearly demonstrated that almost all essential properties of classical strong inward rectification could be explained by a voltage-dependent block of the channel by the ubiquitous intracellular organic cations, the polyamines.[11] The micromolar concentrations of free polyamines (primarily spermine and spermidine) are sufficient to reproduce the degree of rectification observed in native cells. The strength of rectification varies among the different members of the Kir subfamily, and although every Kir channel shows some degree of inward rectification, they can be broadly grouped as either strongly rectifying (Kir2 and Kir3) or weakly rectifying (Kir1 and Kir6) channels. It is well established that the time-dependent activation of strong, inward rectifiers during membrane hyperpolarization reflects the exit of polyamines (primarily sperimine) from the pore.

Rectification Properties Are Related to Electrostatic Interactions in the Cytoplasmic Pore of a Kir Channel

Early work with cloned Kir channels established that strong inward rectification by intracellular polyamines depends on three negatively charged residues located in the second transmembrane domain (D172; the rectification controller; see Fig. 4.2) and in the C-terminal tail [E224 and E299; Kir2.1 amino acid (aa) numbering; see Fig. 4.2]. Positively charged polyamines enter the Kir channel pore to physically occlude it, which is a process aided by negative charges provided by aspartate and glutamate residues. Both electrophysiological and structural data are consistent with the idea that channel block occurs in two sequential steps. A weakly voltage-dependent (shallow) blocking step involves entry of polyamine into the Kir2.1 pore at a site provided by a ring of negative charges (E224 and E299) in the C-terminus. A more strongly voltage-dependent blocking step reflects the movement of polyamine to its deep binding site near the D172 residue. It is also believed that the strong voltage dependence of the polyamine block arises not only from the high valency (z) of polyamines (z≈4 for spermine) but also from a displacement (push) of K$^+$ ions through the pore.[12] Among the polyamines, spermine is the most voltage-dependent blocker and also has the highest potency for blocking the channel.

A characteristic feature of Kir2.1 and Kir3 channels is a flexible cytoplasmic pore-facing G-loop (see Fig. 4.2) that forms a girdle around the central axis of the Kir channel.[13] It was estimated that this girdle constricts the ion permeation pathway to approximately 3 Å. Mutations in the G-loop were shown to disrupt inward rectification. In addition to the previously described E224 and E299 residues, it was shown that A255 and A259 located farther away from the pore axis are also involved in channel rectification. Electrophysiological experiments using cysteine modifications in the pore region of a mutant Kir6.2 channel (N160D; equivalent to D172 in Kir2.1) showed that spermine binds at a deep site beyond the rectification controller residue D172, a site that is close to the extracellular mouth of the pore.

In another study, refinement of the crystal structures of bacterial KirBac1.1 and KirBac3.1 allowed identification of the shallow polyamine binding sites at the cytoplasmic interface between the two subunits.[14] These observations notwithstanding, the precise mechanism involved in rectification is still being worked out, and the exact location of polyamine binding sites in Kir channels is still a controversial issue.

Differential Properties of Kir2.x Subfamily

Consistent with their overall significant sequence homology, all Kir2 channels have the three mentioned residues (D172, E224, and E299) important for rectification at the equivalent positions. Recent studies, however, unexpectedly showed that rectification properties are rather different in the three Kir2 isoforms.[15] Specifically, the data show that Kir2.2 channels display significantly stronger voltage dependence of rectification than that observed in Kir2.1 and Kir2.3 channels. The voltage dependence of steady-state rectification is different between the Kir2.x channels, as are the single-channel conductance and kinetics properties of the currents. In particular, a polyamine unblock (activation) at negative membrane potentials in the Kir2.3 channels is several-fold slower than in Kir2.1 and Kir2.2 channels. Single-channel conductance is the smallest in Kir2.3 (approximately 10 pS), medium in Kir.2.1 (approximately 25 pS), and the largest in Kir2.2 (approximately 35 pS).

Cellular and Membrane Localization

I_{K1} currents, and thus the underlying Kir2.x subunits, display a distinct regional distribution in the heart. It has been shown that inward I_{K1} is generally more prominent in ventricular myocytes and Purkinje fibers and is significantly smaller in atrial myocytes (with one known exception of the mouse heart). The density of inward I_{K1} currents (i.e., currents normalized to membrane capacitance) is small in the pacemaker cells of the sinoatrial node in mice and rats and essentially undetectable in the rabbit sinoatrial nodes. I_{K1} cannot be detected in atrioventricular node of the rabbit but relatively large I_{K1} currents can be recorded in the guinea-pig atrioventricular node. Moreover, the density of inward I_{K1} varies across the ventricular myocardium. For example, in the mouse heart inward, I_{K1} is larger in the apical myocytes compared with the epicardial cells, and I_{K1} is larger in the right ventricular than in the left ventricular myocytes.

Molecular biological studies are also consistent with the location-dependent expression of specific Kir2 isoforms. In particular, real-time reverse-transcriptase polymerase chain reaction analysis of Kir2 transcripts in the human heart showed the following relative expression levels: in Purkinje fibers, Kir2.1 > Kir2.3 > Kir2.2, and in the right ventricle, Kir2.1 > Kir2.2 > Kir2.3; the sequence was reversed in the right atrium: Kir2.3 > Kir2.2 > Kir2.1.[16] Information on the expression patterns of the Kir2 subunits can also be gleaned from functional data using the unique properties of corresponding channels. For example, in cardiac atrial and ventricular myocytes, unitary conductance values display a wide spectrum ranging from 10 to 15 pS (as in the Kir2.3 channels) to as high as 40 to 45 pS (as in the Kir2.2 channels).

Evidence shows that I_{K1} channels are located not only in the non–T-tubular component of the sarcolemma of ventricular myocytes, but also in the intercalated discs and in the T-tubules. For example, accumulation and depletion of K^+ in T-tubules lead to changes in whole-cell I_{K1}.[17] I_{K1} accumulation/depletion phenomena are not observed in atrial cells, which essentially lack T-tubules, and in ventricular myocytes, in which T-tubules are removed by osmotic shock.[17]

Alternatively, Kir2.1, Kir2.2, and Kir2.3 subunits were localized to the T-tubular membrane using immunolabeling with specific antibodies. Intercalated discs were not studied electrophysiologically in regard to the presence of I_{K1} channels, although labeling with various Kir2 antibodies can clearly be observed at this location. Moreover, there is evidence that in canine ventricular and atrial myocytes, Kir2.3 subunits are expressed at higher levels in intercalated disc membranes relative to T-tubules.

Kir2.x Macromolecular Complexes and Channel Biogenesis

Understanding the composition, as well as assembly mechanisms of ion channel complexes in cellular microenvironments, such as the sarcolemma, intercalated discs, T-tubular membranes, and lipid rafts, has gained significant attention in recent years.[4,18] Compelling experimental evidence demonstrates that Kir2.x protein-protein and protein-lipid interactions in these microenvironments have important implications for normal channel functional properties.[8,19-22] Standard biochemical techniques, cell electrophysiology, and proteomic analyses have shown that Kir2.x channels, in macromolecular complexes, interact with the membrane-associated guanylate kinase (MAGUK) scaffolding protein family (i.e., SAP97, PSD95, and CASK, Mint and Veli) and with members of the dystrophin-associated protein complex.[18,23,24] Kir2.x proteins interact with the MAGUK proteins through the type 1 PDZ binding motif at the channel C-terminal residues. The PDZ binding motif (S/T-X-Φ; X: any amino acid, Φ: a hydrophobic amino acid) is a set of the last three (with the exception of Kir2.4) residues on the channel peptide. In one heterologous expression study of Kir2.3 isoform, it was shown that coexpression with SAP97 caused significant cellular redistribution of the Kir2.3 channel protein, with a modest increase in the cell surface expression of the channels.[23] It was also shown that the coexpression led to a wide distribution of single channel conductances, with three distinct peaks centered at 16, 29, and 42 pS. The coexpression, however, did not alter the channel open probability. In another study in rat ventricular myocytes,[24] silencing of SAP97 using adenoviral short hairpin RNA reduced I_{K1} whole-cell current density without affecting channel unitary conductance properties. In the study, silencing of the MAGUK protein blunted the sensitivity of I_{K1} to isoproterenol. Thus these results clearly demonstrate that Kir2.x channel assembly in such macromolecular platforms is critical for normal channel function. Therefore an understanding of the details of the architecture of such macromolecular scaffolds/platforms, especially the essential molecular components, is important for a better insight into channel biophysics and regulatory properties. These studies are significant, given that abnormalities in proper assembly of the platforms may play a role in arrhythmogenesis.[23-25]

Pharmacology and Regulation

Kir2.x and I_{K1} channels can be regulated in a number of ways.[2] Most studies on adrenergic stimulation show that inward I_{K1} currents are suppressed by the activation of both α- and β-receptors, although opposite effects have also been described. In addition, adrenergic regulation is clearly dependent on the type of receptors and subunit composition of the channel.

Both isoproterenol and forskolin inhibit I_{K1} in human ventricular myocytes, suggesting involvement of protein kinase A (PKA)-mediated phosphorylation of underlying Kir2.x subunits. Molecular details of the phenomenon, however, are contradictory. For example, it has been shown that the application of a catalytic subunit of cyclic adenosine monophosphate (cAMP)-dependent PKA leads to activation of Kir2.1 channels expressed in *Xenopus* oocytes, but to Kir2.1 inhibition when the channels are expressed in a mammalian cell line (COS-7). The data on PKA regulation of native I_{K1} channels is limited and somewhat controversial; however, most of the studies show that I_{K1} channels are inhibited by the exposure of the cytosolic side of the membrane to the purified catalytic subunit of PKA. Studies in exogenous-expressing systems also showed the involvement of protein kinase C in the negative regulation of Kir2.1 channels. Consistent with the latter, experiments using human atrial myocytes show that α_1-adrenergic stimulation likely reduces I_{K1} via a protein kinase C–dependent mechanism. Kir channels are also targets for phosphorylation by tyrosine kinases. In Kir2.1 channels, the site of downregulation was targeted to a single Y242 residue in the C-terminus.[26]

PIP$_2$ is an important component in membrane-delimited second messenger signaling system and a powerful activator of Kir channels.[27] There is significant evidence that PIP$_2$ regulates the channel gating primarily through specific electrostatic interactions with the cytosolic part of the channel (see Fig. 4.2).[8] It is also clear that various properties of Kir2 channels are modulated by PIP$_2$. For example, the pH sensitivity of Kir2.3 channels is strongly dependent on the strength of the channel-PIP$_2$ interaction. Cholesterol is another prominent lipid involved in the regulation of Kir2 channels. In particular, it has been shown that increased levels of cholesterol in the membrane lead to the suppression of Kir2 currents.[28]

Various common cations, such as Ca^{2+} and H^+, contribute to the regulation of Kir2 channels as well.[2] Intracellular Ca^{2+} blocks I_{K1} channels in a voltage-dependent manner. There is evidence that a transient increase in intracellular Ca^{2+} during an action potential can lead to significant blockage of I_{K1}.[29] Regulation of I_{K1} by intracellular pH (pH$_i$) is dependent on the species and the type of tissue. For example, rat and guinea pig ventricular I_{K1} is not sensitive to physiologically relevant changes in pH$_i$. In contrast, I_{K1} in sheep ventricular myocytes is inhibited by intracellular H^+ with a pKa of approximately 7.4. The difference in pH sensitivity is likely due to differences in the subunit composition of I_{K1}. For example, channels composed of Kir2.3 subunits exhibit strong sensitivity to pH$_i$ within a physiologically relevant range, whereas Kir2.1 and Kir2.2 channels are relatively insensitive to H^+.

Pharmacological tools for the modulation of Kir2.x and I_{K1} channels are limited. The most useful research tool for studying Kir2 channels is Ba^{2+} [inhibitory concentration of 50% (IC$_{50}$) for inward currents, 0.5 to 10 μM]. Ba^{2+} action is subunit dependent. For example, Ba^{2+} blocks Kir2.2 channels fivefold to sevenfold more efficiently than Kir2.1 channels. In the early 1990s, a compound RP 58866 and its active enantiomer, terikalant, were shown to be selective blockers of I_{K1} (IC$_{50}$, 5 to 20 μM). However, later studies revealed that terikalant also inhibits many other K^+ channels, some with even higher potency (IC$_{50}$ in submicromolar range for I_{Kr} channels). Similarly, it was found that a LY97119 compound (LY, a tertiary homolog of clofilium) blocks I_{K1} in the low micromolar range, but it also blocked Ito (transient outward current) at submicromolar concentrations. Perhaps chloroquine (an antimalarial drug) is the most potent blocker of I_{K1} with an IC$_{50}$ of approximately 0.5 μM. However, chloroquine does not discriminate among I_{K1}, I_{KACh}, and I_{KATP}, and it has been shown to affect other currents (e.g., I_{Na}) in the low micromolar range. Activators of Kir2 and I_{K1} channels were also described. In particular, flecainide, a widely used antiarrhythmic drug, increases Kir2.1 currents by approximately 50% at a concentration of 1 μM, but has no effect on current carried through the Kir2.2 and Kir2.3 channels.[30] Arachidonic acid and the antiinflammatory agent tenidap were shown to specifically activate Kir2.3 channels, with a greater than twofold maximum increase in inward current with an IC$_{50}$ of approximately 0.5 and 1.3 μM, respectively. Zacopride, a gastrointestinal prokinetic drug, was recently found to be a selective I_{K1} channel agonist. The activating effect, however, is modest, with a maximum increase in I_{K1} of approximately 34% at a concentration of 1 μM.

Channelopathies

There are at least four known channelopathies associated with I_{K1} channels, all originating from mutations in *KCNJ2*: ATS1, short QT (SQT) syndrome, familial atrial fibrillation (FAF), and catecholaminergic polymorphic ventricular tachycardia (CPVT) (Fig. 4.3).[2]

ATS is characterized by a triad of pathological clinical phenotypes including the morphogenesis and functioning of skeletal and cardiac muscle. One of the prominent features of ATS is cardiac electrical abnormalities, including brief episodes of ventricular tachycardia, multifocal ventricular ectopy induced by adrenergic stimulation, and prolongation of the QT interval. ATS1 is used to differentiate ATS patients carrying mutations in *KCNJ2*. Many ATS1 patients display clear QT prolongation and have been referred to, perhaps questionably in some cases, as LQT7.

LQT7/ATS1 mutations are numerous (see Fig. 4.3)[5] and result in nonfunctional channels when exogenously expressed in a heterologous system.[31,32] Because affected patients are heterozygous for the mutant and wild type (WT) alleles, and the channel is composed of four subunits, a dominant-negative effect of the mutated subunit can lead to reduced I_{K1} current in cardiac myocytes (and other cells). The dominant-negative effect of LQT7/ATS1 mutations has been demonstrated using cloned channels, although the magnitude of current inhibition is variable in different mutants.

SQT syndrome is characterized by an abnormally short QT interval (less than 300 ms) and an increased risk of developing fibrillation and sudden death. Currently, three forms of SQT syndrome have been described. SQT1 and SQT2 syndromes result from mutations in genes underlying two voltage-gated K^+ channels, hERG (*KCNH2*) and I_{Ks} (*KCNQ1*). A third variant of SQT syndrome (SQT3) originating from a mutation in *KCNJ2* has been first described by Priori and colleagues in 2005.[33] Genetic analysis revealed a charge-neutralizing substitution (D172N) in the critical place of the channel responsible for the strong inward rectification (see Fig. 4.2). Accordingly, coexpression of WT and D172N mutant subunits showed decreased rectification of the heteromeric channel. Computer simulations showed that reduced rectification of I_{K1} can explain some of the characteristic features of an electrocardiograph, such as tall and asymmetric T waves, observed in affected patients. Recently, three other mutations in the *KCNJ2* gene associated with SQT syndrome have been identified: M301K[34] and E299V[35] (see Fig. 4.2), both of which are located in the region of the channel responsible for the "shallow" polyamine binding site, and K346T[36] which is located on the outer side of C-terminal domain.

One study described the association of a single V93I mutation in *KCNJ2* with familial atrial fibrillation.[37] Electrophysiological experiments with cloned channels showed, in particular, that V93I mutation leads to a relative increase in the magnitude of the outward current, or a decrease in the strength of inward rectification. Regarding the inward rectification, the effect of the V91I mutation on Kir2.1 current resembles the mutation found in the D172N mutant channels. However, patients carrying the V93I mutation display a normal QT interval in contrast to patients affected by the D172N mutation.

Mutations in *KCNJ2* were also linked to another type of excitability disorder—catecholaminergic polymorphic ventricular tachycardia (CPVT).[38] CPVT is a heritable disorder characterized by frequent ventricular arrhythmias and sudden cardiac death associated with physical activity or adrenergic stimulation. Nine *KCNJ2* mutations associated with CPVT have been identified so far (see Fig. 4.3). These mutations can be found in both N- and C-termini as well as in the extracellular loop of the Kir2.1 channel. The electrical phenotype of these mutations included, in particular, prominent U waves, ventricular ectopy, and polymorphic ventricular tachycardia. It can be seen from Fig. 4.3 that there is a significant phenotypic overlap between ATS and CPVT.

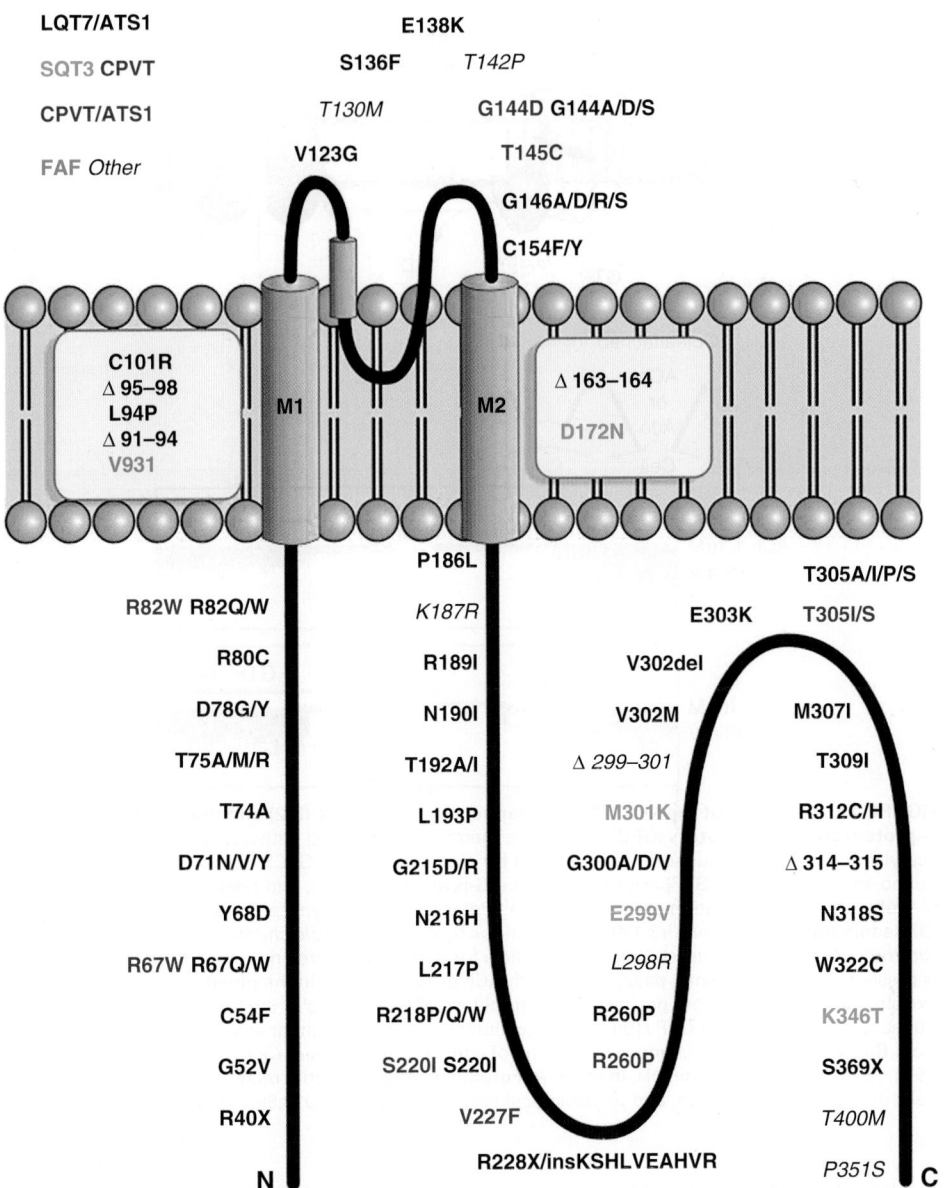

FIGURE 4.3 Channelopathies of the classical inward rectifier channel, I$_{K1}$, associated with mutations in the Kir2.1 subunit. Mutant residues are color coded to represent the long QT (LQT7/ATS1; *black*), catecholaminergic polymorphic ventricular tachycardia (CPVT; *red*), familial atrial fibrillation (FAF; *green*), short QT3 (SQT3; *blue*), and *Other* are mutations with less defined cardiovascular associations. (Modified from Anumonwo JM, Lopatin AN. Cardiac strong inward rectifier potassium channels. *J Mol Cell Cardiol*. 2010;48:45-54.)

Finally, some mutations in *KCNJ2* could not be easily classified into the four categories mentioned previously, and for this reason they are referred to as *other* in Fig. 4.3.

Acetylcholine-Activated Potassium Channels

Structure and Function

In the heart, Kir3.1/Kir3.4 channels are responsible for the effects of acetylcholine and adenosine, and they act through a coupling mechanism involving a receptor, a G protein (G$_o$/G$_i$ family), and the K$^+$ channel.[2,39] Because channel gating requires a G protein, Kir3.1/Kir3.4 channels are considered a type of K$_G$ channel.[4] For channel activation, the G-protein–coupled receptor (Fig. 4.4) can be a muscarinic (M2) or a purinergic (P1) receptor, which are activated by acetylcholine or adenosine, respectively. The ultimate result of channel activation is the opening of the Kir3.1/Kir3.4 channels, which permits K$^+$ efflux and consequently hyperpolarizes the cell membrane.

As in a typical K$^+$ channel, the ion selectivity in Kir3.x channels is conferred by the presence of the signature sequence (T-X-G-Y/F-G),[4,40] and the mechanism of rectification involves an asparagine or an aspartate residue for interactions with the polyamines (details of rectification have been discussed previously). Thus the mechanism of rectification is similar to that described for Kir2 channels, and the Kir3.x channels belong to the class of strong inward rectifier channels.[2] Membrane topology of Kir3 channels is similar to that described for Kir2 channels (see Fig. 4.2).

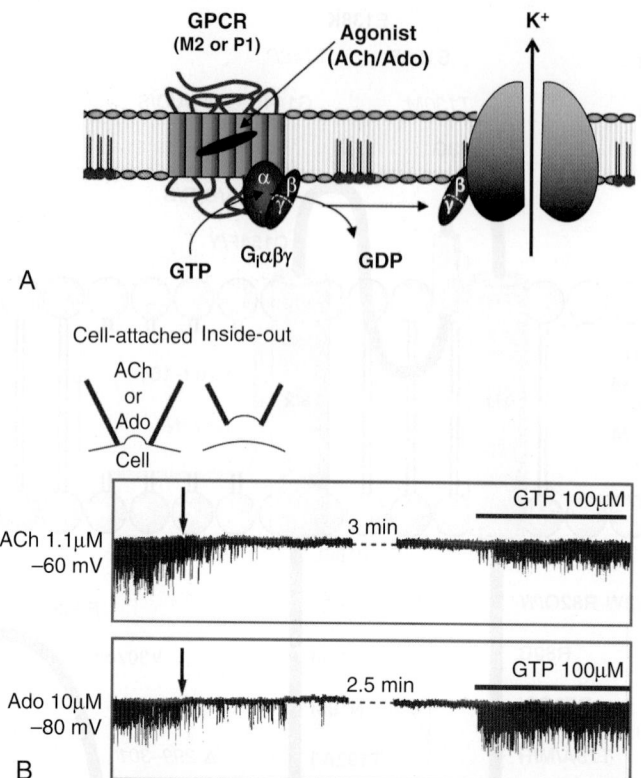

FIGURE 4.4 Activation of the Kir3.1/Kir3.4 channels by muscarinic (M2) and purinergic (P1) G-protein coupled receptors (GPCRs). (A) The membrane-delimited pathway for activation of acetylcholine (*Ach*) and adenosine (*Ado*) gated Kir channels. Ligand-GPCR interaction enhances the guanosine triphosphate (GTP) association with a G-protein α-subunit, and results in the release of the β/γ-subunits for the activation of the Kir channel. Potassium efflux hyperpolarizes the cell membrane. (B) Requirement of GTP for Kir3.1/Kir3.4 activations by ACh (*top single channel traces*) and Ado (*bottom single channel traces*). Holding potentials for experiments are annotated. Channel activity is present in the cell-attached patch mode, with ACh or Ado present in the pipette (*top inset*). Patch excision (at *arrow*; inside-out patch configuration) loss of GTP results in the loss of channel activity. Subsequent application of GTP (100 μM; intracellular side) restored channel activity. ([A] Modified from Breitwieser GE. GIRK channels: hierarchy of control. *Am J Physiol Cell Physiol.* 2005;289:C509-C511. [B] Modified from Hibino H, Inanobe A, Furutani K, et al. Inwardly rectifying potassium channels: their structure, function, and physiological roles. *Physiol Rev.* 2010;90:291-366.)

Exactly how do Kir3.1/Kir3.4 channels and G proteins interact to cause channel opening? First, a brief discussion of G proteins is necessary. G proteins are complexes consisting of an α- [molecular weight (MW), ~40,000], a β- (MW, ~35,000), and a γ- (MW, ~8000) subunit, which all transduce signals from membrane receptors [e.g., muscarinic (M2)] to an effector, such as a K_G channel.[4,39] Four subfamily members of the guanosine diphosphate (GDP) Gα subunit dictate selectivity of signaling [activation of adenylate cyclase (Gα$_s$), inhibition of adenylate cyclase (Gα$_i$), and activation of phospholipase (G$_q$)].[39] Normally, Gα is bound to GDP in the absence of an agonist, and the Gα/GDP complex is coupled to the receptor and has low guanosine triphosphatase (GTPase) activity. With vagal stimulation and ligand-receptor interaction, GDP is exchanged for guanosine triphosphate (GTP) and results in the uncoupling of Gβγ from Gα (see Fig. 4.4A). The released Gβγ-subunits in turn activate the Kir3.1/Kir3.4 channels. There is a critical requirement for GTP for channel activation (see Fig. 4.4B). A variety of experiments have determined the precise molecular interactions involved in the Gβγ-induced Kir3.1/Kir3.4 channel gating, and have shown that the cytoplasmic region of the channel is intimately involved with gating. For example, crystal structure analyses of the cytoplasmic region of Kir3.1 suggest that the C-terminus of two neighboring Kir3 channels subunits bind to each other and that an

N-terminus is positioned between the two C-terminal domains.[41] The study also showed that for Kir3.1 channels, the cytoplasmic residues L262, L333, and E336 are important in gating, and the equivalent residues are H64 and L262 in Kir3.4 channels.

Cellular and Membrane Localization

There are tissue-dependent differences in the expression of I_{KACh} in the myocardium, with a very high density of expression in nodal tissues.[2,4] Following the cloning of genes underlying Kir3 channels in the early to middle 1990s, investigators have probed myocardial tissues to examine the localization of the gene products. Overall, these studies reported an abundance of Kir3.1 and Kir3.4 mRNA in the nodal and atrial, but not ventricular, tissues, which would be consistent with tissue distribution of I_{KACh}. In one such study,[42] a comprehensive analysis was performed using Western blot and immunofluorescence to examine channel distribution in sinus-nodal, atrial, and ventricular tissues, and showed similar results for the expression patterns across species (rat, ferret, and guinea pig hearts). It was reported that, whereas there was minimal expression of Kir3.1 in the ventricles of all species tested, Kir3.1 and Kir 3.4 were highly expressed in the atrial tissue of all the species. It was noted that although there were relatively high levels of expression in the atria, significant quantitative differences in Kir3.1 and Kir3.4 protein levels were found in the different species. Furthermore, it was demonstrated that Kir3.1 and M2 receptor colocalized in the sinoatrial node. In nodal and atrial tissue, immunofluorescence showed localization of Kir3.x/M2 receptors more on the outer (lateral) membranes than in T-tubular membranes.[42] Similar quantitative differences in expression have been reported for atrial versus ventricular tissues in the human myocardium.[42,43]

Kir3.x Macromolecular Complexes and Channel Biogenesis

Similar to Kir2.x channels, multiple signaling molecules and cytoskeletal proteins directly or indirectly interact with cardiac Kir3.x channels in multiprotein scaffolds.[4] Thus scaffolds containing Kir3.x channels include a variety of clustering proteins, actin and protein kinases, and some phosphatases.[20,44] Although experimental data shows that assembly of Kir3.x channels in the multiprotein complexes is essential for normal channel function, the details of Kir3.x protein-protein/lipid interactions remain unknown.[4,20,45] Caveolae, a group of specialized sarcolemmal membrane domains of ~50–100 nm, are a subset of cholesterol and sphingolipids-enriched lipid rafts that play a role in Kir3.x channel function. Named after the clustering protein caveolin, these lipid rafts sequester Kir3.x channel complexes, a process thought to exemplify the importance of channel clustering into specific microdomains. G-protein coupled receptors (adrenergic and muscarinic) release $G\beta\gamma$ subunits following ligand biding; however, it is only the $G\beta$-subunits of the $G_{i/o}$, and not the G_s, protein that are capable of activating the Kir3.x (I_{KACh}) channels. Therefore it has been hypothesized that lipid rafts may differentially cluster G_s and G_i proteins into distinct microdomains.

Pharmacology and Regulation

It is well established that Kir3.1/Kir3.4 are generally insensitive to classical K+ channel blockers such as or 4-AP or tetraethylammonium.[4] However, experiments in cardiac myocytes isolated from rabbit hearts show that the toxin, tertiapin, is a selective blocker of I_{KACh}.[46] A channel block is highly potent, with an affinity in the nanomolar range. Cardiac Kir3.1/Kir3.4 channels are also inhibited by quinine, quinidine, and verapamil; however, affinities of the these drugs are in the micromolar range.[4] Based on the results of experiments in heterologous (oocyte) expression systems, current through Kir3.x channels is enhanced by "intoxicating" concentrations of ethanol, and an approximately 43-aa stretch on the C-terminus has been identified as important for the ethanol effect.[47] Similarly, in a heterologous expression system, Kir3.x channels displayed sensitivity to intracellular acidification, an inhibitory effect that was dependent on histidine residues in the N- and C-terminal regions of the channels.[4] A variety of other agents have also been shown to modulate Kir3.x channels. For example, similar to all Kir channels, Kir3.1/Kir3.4 require PIP_2 for channel activity.[4] Curiously, however, the PIP_2 effect is enhanced by other factors, such as the G-protein–$G\beta\gamma$ complex, as well as by intracellular cations. In general, Kir3.x channel activity is also sensitive to mechanical stretch, can be modified by phosphorylating agents, and is sensitive (negatively) to regulators of G-protein signaling.[4]

Channelopathies

Over four decades ago, a mouse with a striking locomotor deficiency (weaving) was described, and the defect has subsequently been traced to a naturally occurring gain-in-function mutation in the Kir3.2 channel.[48] Additional neurological defects attendant to this mutation earned the weaver mouse the title of the "most cantankerous rodent."[49] There is relatively little information available

on inherited cardiac channelopathies associated with the Kir3.1/Kir3.4 channels. However, alterations in Kir3.1/Kir3.4 channel activity have been reported in certain cardiac rhythm abnormalities.[50] Electrical remodeling in atrial fibrillation patients has been shown to increase the constitutively active component of I_{KACh}, which could cause an abbreviation of the action potential duration. More recently, a study was performed in a large Chinese family (49 individuals) with autosomal-dominant long QT syndrome (LQTS).[51] The locus of the LQTS-associated gene was mapped to chromosome 11q23.3-24.3. A combination of biochemistry and cell electrophysiology in heterologous expression systems was used to demonstrate that a heterozygous G387R mutation on the Kir3.4 (*KCNJ5*) gene that was identified in all affected family members was responsible for the reduced channel expression on the sarcolemma.

ATP-Sensitive Potassium Channels

Structure and Function

Among all inward rectifiers, K_{ATP} channels are the most unique in their molecular architecture.[52] As in other Kir channels, the ion conduction pathway is provided by a tetrameric arrangement of pore-forming subunits, but additional auxiliary regulatory subunits are necessary for the channel to be fully functional (Fig. 4.5B). The two known isoforms of the pore-forming subunits are encoded by Kir6.1 (*KCNJ8*) and Kir6.2 (*KCNJ11*) genes. The two isoforms of auxiliary subunits are encoded by SUR1 (*ABCC8*) and SUR2 (*ABCC9*) genes (the SUR name originates from "sulfonylureas," a class of drugs known to inhibit K_{ATP} channels by acting on the auxiliary subunit). SUR2 gene can be alternatively spliced at the very C-terminus (last 42 aa) leading to the SUR2A and SUR2B isoforms. The genomic arrangements of SUR and Kir6 genes are unique as well. Specifically, SUR1 is followed by Kir6.2 in close proximity on chromosome 11pp15.1, whereas while SUR2 is followed by Kir6.1 on chromosome 12p12.1. The consequences of this arrangement regarding the regulation at a genomic level are not clear at this time. Although the heteromeric assembly of Kir6.x subunits produces functional channels in vitro, it remains unclear whether heteromeric Kir6.x complexes exist in native tissues. In contrast, both SUR1/Kir6.2 and SUR2/Kir6.2 channels likely exist in native tissues. Membrane topology and general organization of Kir6.x subunits is highly similar to that in well-characterized Kir2.x channels (see Fig. 4.2).

K_{ATP} channels display weak rectification; however, it has been shown that just a single amino acid substitution in the so-called rectification controller region of inward rectifiers (see Fig. 4.2, Kir2.1; N160D in Kir6.2) converts Kir6.2 into a strongly rectifying channel.[53] A defining property of K_{ATP} channels is their characteristic sensitivity to intracellular ATP (hence the name ATP-dependent K+ channels). Under normal conditions, both exogenously expressed Kir6.2/SUR2 channels and native channels in cardiac myocytes are inhibited by ATP in the micromolar range (10 to 100 µM) by direct binding to the channel rather than through phosphorylation mechanisms. In the absence of intracellular Mg^{2+} ions, adenosine diphosphate (ADP) and other nucleotides also inhibit the channel. Modeling studies suggests that the ATP binding pocket is located at the interface of the N and C terminus of each Kir6.x subunit; therefore the K_{ATP} channel possesses four ATP binding sites.

The overall structure of auxiliary SUR subunit is presented in Fig. 4.5B. It is believed that SUR interacts with Kir6.x subunits to modulate channel gating through the TMD0 domain and L0 linker region. Experimental data are consistent with the idea that intracellular ATP induces dimerization of nucleotide-binding domains NBD1 and NBD2, converting them into a catalytically active site for the Mg^{2+}-dependent hydrolysis of ATP (leading to MgATP). Hydrolysis of ATP is followed by a conformational

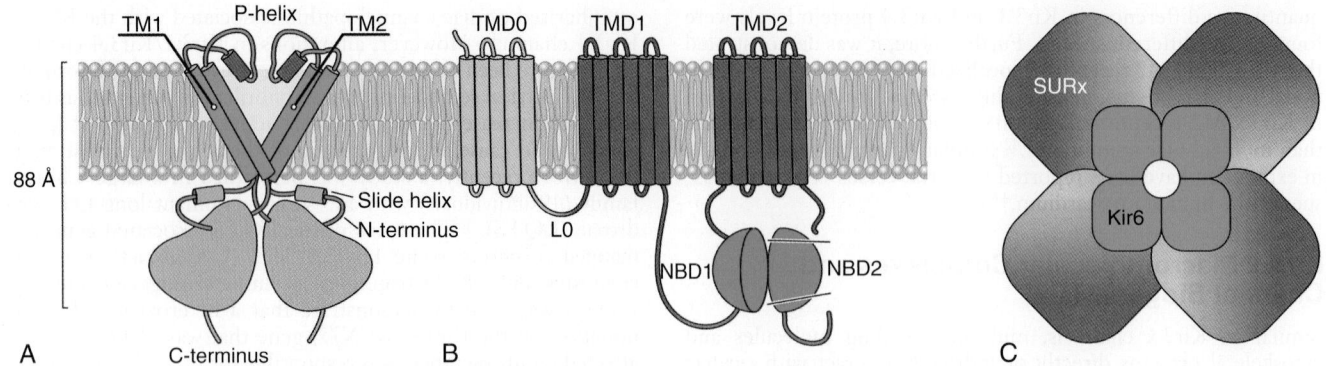

FIGURE 4.5 Molecular structure of K$_{ATP}$ channel. (A) A pore-forming subunit of K$_{ATP}$ channel is encoded by the Kir6.x genes and contains two transmembrane helical domains, TM1 and TM2; a pore-forming region (P-helix); a large C-terminal domain; and characteristic N-terminal domain (slide helix) interfacing the inner leaflet of the membrane and cytoplasmic C-terminus. (B) An auxiliary subunit to the channel is encoded by SUR1 and SUR 2A/B genes and consists of the seventeen transmembrane helices organized in several distinct domains and several important cytoplasmic regions. The TMD0 domain and L0 region are responsible for the interaction with Kir6.x subunits and regulation of gating of the channel. TMD1 and TMD2 domains are followed by nucleotide binding domains, NBD1 and NBD2, which form two nucleotide binding sites at their interface. (C) The arrangement of Kir6.x and SURx subunits in an octameric K$_{ATP}$ channel complex. Modeling studies predict one adenosine triphosphate binding site at each of the Kir6 interfaces and Mg^{2+}-nucleotide binding sites in the NBD domains of SUR subunit. (Modified from Flagg TP, Enkvetchakul D, Koster JC, et al. Muscle K$_{ATP}$ channels: recent insights to energy sensing and myoprotection. *Physiol Rev.* 2010;90:799-829.)

change that is then transduced to the Kir6.x subunit; however, MgADP is an even more potent activator of the K$_{ATP}$ channel. The latter puts the hydrolysis hypothesis into question. Accordingly, it has been suggested that NBDs can be locked in a posthydrolytic state by MgADP and other nucleotides to sustain the active state of the channel.

Cellular and Membrane Localization

K$_{ATP}$ channels are found in virtually every kind of cardiac tissues, but they are most prominent in cardiac myocytes and smooth muscle cells. Detailed experimental analysis reveals significant differences in various properties of native K$_{ATP}$ channels, suggesting a different subunit organization in every case.[54] A significant amount of evidence suggests that ventricular sarcolemmal K$_{ATP}$ channels are likely composed of Kir6.2 and SUR2A subunits. In particular, functional sarcolemmal K$_{ATP}$ channels are absent in Kir6.2 knockout mice, and various channel properties (including large single channel conductance, high sensitivity to pinacidil and cromakalim, and low sensitivity to diazoxide) are similar to those obtained from ventricular myocytes. The latter is also supported by a relatively low level of SUR1 (a pancreatic isoform) in the ventricles, and the finding that the activity of K$_{ATP}$ channels is essentially unaffected in ventricular myocytes from SUR1 knockout mice. Recent experiments with mice showed, however, that SUR1 subunit of the K$_{ATP}$ channel may be a dominant isoform in atrial tissue. In particular, the activity of the K$_{ATP}$ channels could not be detected in atrial myocytes isolated from SUR1 knockout mice, and the pharmacological profile of atrial K$_{ATP}$ channels is reminiscent of that conferred by SUR1 (higher sensitivity to diazoxide, lower to pinacidil) rather than SUR2 subunits. It remains unresolved whether this subunit composition exists in atrial tissue of other animals and humans.

K$_{ATP}$ channels in smooth muscle display a number of properties distinct from those in cardiac myocytes, suggesting unique subunit composition.[52] Significantly smaller channel densities (up to 100-fold per cell), generally low single channel conductance (~30 pS), and a lack of channel activity upon excision of the membrane patch are some of the common features of smooth muscle

K$_{ATP}$ channels. Studies with exogenously expressing systems showed that cloned K$_{ATP}$ channels originating from coexpression of Kir6.1 and SUR2B subunits resemble native K$_{ATP}$ channels in smooth muscle, for the most part. A strongest support for the Kir6.1/SUR2B composition of smooth muscle K$_{ATP}$ channels comes from experiments with genetically modified mice. Specifically, K$_{ATP}$ currents cannot be recorded in aortic smooth muscle cells isolated from either Kir6.1 or SUR2 knockout mice, whereas the activity of the K$_{ATP}$ channels is preserved in these cells in Kir6.2 knockout mice.

Mitochondrial K$_{ATP}$ channels received a lot of attention since they were first described at this location in early 1990s. In contrast to sarcolemmal K$_{ATP}$ channels, however, their molecular identity remains highly controversial.[52] Although exogenously coexpressed Kir6.1 and SUR1 subunits produce K$_{ATP}$ channels with many properties resembling those found in mitochondria, the activity of the mitochondrial K$_{ATP}$ channels in Kir6.1 knockout mice was not affected. Recent promising developments in this area include the identification of mitochondria-specific short-form of SUR2 subunits generated by a nonconventional intraexonic splicing, which can underlie the mitochondrial K$_{ATP}$ channels.[55] There is also strong evidence that the pore-forming subunit of the mitochondrial K$_{ATP}$ channels is encoded by *KCNJ1* (Kir1.1).[56]

Kir6.x/SURx Macromolecular Complexes and Channel Biogenesis

There is evidence that Kir6.x/SURx channels are assembled in multiprotein scaffolds that are necessary for normal channel function. The Kir6.x/SURx macromolecular complexes are thought to contain metabolically active protein subunits, including Na/K ATPases, as well as kinases.[57,58] In one study,[59] a number of glycolytic enzymes (glyceraldehyde-3-phosphate dehydrogenase, triose-phosphate isomerase, and pyruvate kinase), were described as protein subunits of the Kir6.x/SURx protein complex, which are obligatory for the normal function of the channel. Consequently, it has been hypothesized that this clustering of channel proteins/enzymes complexes may be needed to modulate the ATP levels in the microenvironment of the channels. Furthermore, experiments conducted in isolated cardiac myocytes as well as in heterologous expression systems, demonstrate that currents mediated by Kir6.x/SURx channels are modulated by lipid raft environment.[21,59,60]

Pharmacology and Regulation

The pharmacology of K_{ATP} channels is extensive, and the regulation is complex relative to other members of Kir family, which is in part due to the structural complexity of the channel.[4] Cardiac K_{ATP} channels are regulated by a variety of mechanisms, and important quantitative details of their modulation surely depend on the specific subunit composition. The most prominent and characteristic mechanism involves regulation by intracellular nucleotides such as ATP and ADP. Intracellular ATP is a potent blocker of the channel while ADP (in the presence of Mg^{2+} ions) has an activating effect. An overwhelming level of ATP under normal conditions keeps the channel essentially shut (native channels in cardiac myocytes are half blocked by 50 to 100 μM ATP), whereas metabolic disturbances leading to both a drop in ATP levels and a consequent rise in ADP levels result in channel opening (in the presence of intracellular Mg^{2+} ions). Experiments with isolated membrane patches show that phospholipids, especially PIP_2, are potent activators of native (and cloned) K_{ATP} channels while their hydrolysis reduces channel activity. Regulation of K_{ATP} channels by PKA-dependent phosphorylation is well documented in smooth muscles, but the data are limited in cardiac myocytes. It has been shown that the activity of atrial K_{ATP} channels can be increased by stretch suggesting the involvement of channel-cytoskeleton interactions. Intracellular pH is another potent regulator of native K_{ATP} channels with acidification leading to an increase in channel activity.

K_{ATP} channels can be inhibited or activated by a variety of drugs, all acting on the SUR subunit. Sulfonylureas such as acetohexamide, glipizide, glibenclamide, tolbutamide, and HMR 1098 are prominent inhibitors. Clinically, sulfonylureas are used exclusively for the treatment of type 2 diabetes, but they are also a useful research tool in work with cardiac preparations.

K_{ATP} channel openers (KCO) include pinacidil, cromakalim, rimakalim, nicorandil, diazoxide, and minoxidil sulfate. In contrast to sulfonylureas, KCOs are useful in treating cardiovascular disorders such as myocardial ischemia and congestive heart failure. KCOs display strong selectivity to subunit composition of K_{ATP} channels. In particular, K_{ATP} channels in pancreatic β-cells (SUR1 based) are strongly activated by diazoxide, but not affected by cromakalim or nicorandil while ventricular K_{ATP} channels (SUR2A based) are strongly activated by cromakalim or nicorandil but not by diazoxide. Smooth muscle K_{ATP} channels (SUR2B based) are activated by all these drugs. Mitochondrial K_{ATP} channels are known to be potently activated by diazoxide and inhibited by 5-hydroxydecanoate (5-HD).

Channelopathies

Mutations in genes underlying the K_{ATP} channels have been associated with cardiovascular disorders. Specifically, the F1524S and A1513T substitutions in the SUR2A gene (missense and frameshift, respectively) were linked to dilated cardiomyopathy. Both mutations were mapped to the locus of SUR2A, which is responsible for the catalytic activity of the NBD2 domains, and likely exert their actions through reduced activation of the K_{ATP} channel. The other reported mutation in the SUR2A gene was associated with adrenergic atrial fibrillation originating in the vein of Marshall, a well-known location for this type of fibrillation. As in the previous case, the underlying missense mutation in the SUR2A gene (T1547I substitution) likely affects the functioning of the NBD2 leading to a compromised channel regulation by adenine nucleotides.

Recent studies have identified multiple mutations in SUR2 gene. These mutations are associated with Cantu syndrome, which is a rare multiorgan disease that is characterized, in particular, by various abnormalities of cardiovascular system, including cardiomegaly, concentric ventricular hypertrophy, and other cardiovascular malfunctions. The mechanistic link between Cantu syndrome mutations and various cardiovascular conditions, however, remains to be established.

Recently, the gain-of-function mutation (S422L substitution) in the pore-forming Kir6.1 subunit (*KCNJ8* gene) was associated with ventricular fibrillation and linked to J-wave syndrome susceptibility,[61] and an inframe deletion (E332del) and a missense mutation (V346I) were liked to sudden infant death syndrome.[62]

Mutations in the *KCNJ11* gene encoding pore-forming Kir6.2 subunit of K_{ATP} channels were linked to diabetes mellitus and congenital hyperinsulinism although no associated cardiac abnormalities were reported.

Conclusion

The biophysical and regulatory properties of Kir channels are crucial for cardiac electrical activity. Significant experimental evidence clearly implicates several members of the Kir subfamily as molecular determinants underlying the three major inward rectifier potassium currents in native cardiac cells: I_{K1}, I_{KACh}, and I_{KATP}. The general architecture of Kir channels has been well established, and fine details of their structure and function have been revealed with the aid of several available crystal structures of the cloned channels. Nevertheless, many important questions remain unanswered. For example, how do the differences in the biophysical and regulatory properties of Kir2 isoforms affect the heteromeric channel complexes that underlie the native I_{K1} in different species and in different parts of the heart? What is the subunit composition of the mitochondrial K_{ATP} channel? How are Kir channels sorted into microdomains in the sarcolemma, such as T-tubules or intercalated discs, and how do they interact with other proteins within these microdomains? These questions undoubtedly will be the focus of much investigation in the near future.

REFERENCES

1. Lopatin AN, Nichols CG. Inward rectifiers in the heart: an update on I(K1). *J Mol Cell Cardiol.* 2001;33: 625–638.
2. Anumonwo JM, Lopatin AN. Cardiac strong inward rectifier potassium channels. *J Mol Cell Cardiol.* 2010;48:45–54.
3. Nerbonne JM, Nichols CG, Schwarz TL, Escande D. Genetic manipulation of cardiac K(+) channel function in mice: what have we learned, and where do we go from here? *Circ Res.* 2001;89:944–956.
4. Hibino H, Inanobe A, Furutani K, Murakami S, Findlay I, Kurachi Y. Inwardly rectifying potassium channels: their structure, function, and physiological roles. *Physiol Rev.* 2010;90:291–366.

5. Nguyen HL, Pieper GH, Wilders R. Andersen-Tawil syndrome: clinical and molecular aspects. *Int J Cardiol.* 2013;170:1–16.
6. Ryan DP, da Silva MR, Soong TW, et al. Mutations in potassium channel Kir2.6 cause susceptibility to thyrotoxic hypokalemic periodic paralysis. *Cell.* 2010;140:88–98.
7. Doyle DA, Morais Cabral J, Pfuetzner RA, et al. The structure of the potassium channel: molecular basis of K+ conduction and selectivity. *Science.* 1998;280: 69–77.
8. Hansen SB, Tao X, MacKinnon R. Structural basis of PIP2 activation of the classical inward rectifier K+ channel Kir2.2. *Nature.* 2011;477:495–498.

9. Enkvetchakul D, Jeliazkova I, Bhattacharyya J, Nichols CG. Control of inward rectifier K channel activity by lipid tethering of cytoplasmic domains. *J Gen Physiol.* 2007;130:329–334.
10. Logothetis DE, Jin T, Lupyan D, Rosenhouse-Dantsker A. Phosphoinositide-mediated gating of inwardly rectifying K(+) channels. *Pflugers Arch.* 2007;455:83–95.
11. Lopatin AN, Makhina EN, Nichols CG. The mechanism of inward rectification of potassium channels: "long-pore plugging" by cytoplasmic polyamines. *J Gen Physiol.* 1995;106:923–955.
12. Xu Y, Shin HG, Szep S, Lu Z. Physical determinants of strong voltage sensitivity of K(+) channel block. *Nat Struct Mol Biol.* 2009;16:1252–1258.

13. Pegan S, Arrabit C, Zhou W, et al. Cytoplasmic domain structures of Kir2.1 and Kir3.1 show sites for modulating gating and rectification. *Nat Neurosci.* 2005;8:279–287.

14. Clarke OB, Caputo AT, Hill AP, Vandenberg JI, Smith BJ, Gulbis JM. Domain reorientation and rotation of an intracellular assembly regulate conduction in Kir potassium channels. *Cell.* 2010;141:1018–1029.

15. Panama BK, Lopatin AN. Differential polyamine sensitivity in inwardly rectifying Kir2 potassium channels. *J Physiol.* 2006;571:287–302.

16. Gaborit N, Le Bouter S, Szuts V, et al. Regional and tissue specific transcript signatures of ion channel genes in the non-diseased human heart. *J Physiol.* 2007;582:675–693.

17. Cheng L, Wang F, Lopatin AN. Metabolic stress in isolated mouse ventricular myocytes leads to remodeling of t-tubules. *Am J Physiol Heart Circ Physiol.* 2011;301:H1984–H1995.

18. Leonoudakis D, Conti LR, Radeke CM, McGuire LM, Vandenberg CA. A multi-protein trafficking complex composed of SAP97, CASK, Veli and Mint1 is associated with inward rectifier Kir2 potassium channels. *J Biol Chem.* 2004;279(18):19051–19063.

19. Nattel S, Maguy A, Le Bouter S, Yeh YH. Arrhythmogenic ion-channel remodeling in the heart: heart failure, myocardial infarction, and atrial fibrillation. *Physiol Rev.* 2007;87:425–456.

20. Doupnik CA. GPCR-Kir channel signaling complexes: defining rules of engagement. *J Recept Signal Transduct Res.* 2008;28:83–91.

21. Dart C. Lipid microdomains and the regulation of ion channel function. *J Physiol.* 2010;588:3169–3178.

22. Hansen SB. Lipid agonism: the PIP2 paradigm of ligand-gated ion channels. *Biochim Biophys Acta.* 2015;1851:620–628.

23. Vikstrom KL, Vaidyanathan R, Levinsohn S, et al. SAP97 regulates Kir2.3 channels by multiple mechanisms. *Am J Physiol Heart Circ Physiol.* 2009;297:H1387–H1397.

24. Vaidyanathan R, Taffet SM, Vikstrom KL, Anumonwo JM. Regulation of cardiac inward rectifier potassium current (I(K1)) by synapse-associated protein-97. *J Biol Chem.* 2010;285:28000–28009.

25. Milstein ML, Musa H, Balbuena DP, et al. Dynamic reciprocity of sodium and potassium channel expression in a macromolecular complex controls cardiac excitability and arrhythmia. *Proc Natl Acad Sci U S A.* 2012;109:E2134–E2143.

26. Wischmeyer E, Doring F, Karschin A. Acute suppression of inwardly rectifying Kir2.1 channels by direct tyrosine kinase phosphorylation. *J Biol Chem.* 1998;273:34063–34068.

27. Huang CL, Feng S, Hilgemann DW. Direct activation of inward rectifier potassium channels by PIP2 and its stabilization by Gbetagamma. *Nature.* 1998;391:803–806.

28. Romanenko V, Fang Y, Byfield F, et al. Cholesterol sensitivity and lipid raft targeting of Kir 2.1 channels. *Biophys J.* 2004;87(6):3850–3861.

29. Zaza A, Rocchetti M, Brioschi A, Cantadori A, Ferroni A. Dynamic Ca2+-induced inward rectification of K+ current during the ventricular action potential. *Circ Res.* 1998;82:947–956.

30. Caballero R, Dolz-Gaiton P, Gomez R, et al. Flecainide increases Kir2.1 currents by interacting with cysteine 311, decreasing the polyamine-induced rectification. *Proc Natl Acad Sci U S A.* 2010;107:15631–15636.

31. Bendahhou S, Donaldson MR, Plaster NM, Tristani-Firouzi M, Fu YH, Ptacek LJ. Defective potassium channel Kir2.1 trafficking underlies Andersen-Tawil syndrome. *J Biol Chem.* 2003;278:51779–51785.

32. Plaster NM, Tawil R, Tristani-Firouzi M, et al. Mutations in Kir2.1 cause the developmental and episodic electrical phenotypes of Andersen's syndrome. *Cell.* 2001;105:511–519.

33. Priori SG, Pandit SV, Rivolta I, et al. A novel form of short QT syndrome (SQT3) is caused by a mutation in the KCNJ2 gene. *Circ Res.* 2005;96:800–807.

34. Hattori T, Makiyama T, Akao M, et al. A novel gain-of-function KCNJ2 mutation associated with short-QT syndrome impairs inward rectification of Kir2.1 currents. *Cardiovasc Res.* 2012;93:666–673.

35. Deo M, Ruan Y, Pandit SV, et al. KCNJ2 mutation in short QT syndrome 3 results in atrial fibrillation and ventricular proarrhythmia. *Proc Natl Acad Sci U S A.* 2013;110:4291–4296.

36. Ambrosini E, Sicca F, Brignone MS, et al. Genetically induced dysfunctions of Kir2.1 channels: implications for short QT3 syndrome and autism-epilepsy phenotype. *Hum Mol Genet.* 2014;23:4875–4886.

37. Xia M, Jin Q, Bendahhou S, et al. A Kir2.1 gain-of-function mutation underlies familial atrial fibrillation. *Biochem Biophys Res Commun.* 2005;332:1012–1019.

38. Watanabe H, Knollmann BC. Mechanism underlying catecholaminergic polymorphic ventricular tachycardia and approaches to therapy. *J Electrocardiol.* 2011;44:650–655.

39. Wettschureck N, Offermanns S. Mammalian G proteins and their cell type specific functions. *Physiol Rev.* 2005;85:1159–1204.

40. Bichet D, Haass FA, Jan LY. Merging functional studies with structures of inward-rectifier K(+) channels. *Nat Rev Neurosci.* 2003;4:957–967.

41. Nishida M, MacKinnon R. Structural basis of inward rectification. Cytoplasmic pore of the G protein–gated inward rectifier GIRK1 at 1.8 A resolution. *Cell.* 2002;111:957–965.

42. Dobrzynski H, Marples DD, Musa H, et al. Distribution of the muscarinic K+ channel proteins Kir3.1 and Kir3.4 in the ventricle, atrium, and sinoatrial node of heart. *J Histochem Cytochem.* 2001;49:1221–1234.

43. Koumi S, Wasserstrom JA. Acetylcholine-sensitive muscarinic K+ channels in mammalian ventricular myocytes. *Am J Physiol.* 1994;266:H1812–H1821.

44. Nikolov EN, Ivanova-Nikolova TT. Coordination of membrane excitability through a GIRK1 signaling complex in the atria. *J Biol Chem.* 2004;279:23630–23636.

45. Lober RM, Pereira MA, Lambert NA. Rapid activation of inwardly rectifying potassium channels by immobile G-protein-coupled receptors. *J Neurosci.* 2006;26:12602–12608.

46. Kitamura H, Yokoyama M, Akita H, Matsushita K, Kurachi Y, Yamada M. Tertiapin potently and selectively blocks muscarinic K(+) channels in rabbit cardiac myocytes. *J Pharmacol Exp Ther.* 2000;293:196–205.

47. Aryal P, Dvir H, Choe S, Slesinger PA. A discrete alcohol pocket involved in GIRK channel activation. *Nat Neurosci.* 2009;12:988–995.

48. Patil N, Cox DR, Bhat D, Faham M, Myers RM, Peterson AS. A potassium channel mutation in weaver mice implicates membrane excitability in granule cell differentiation. *Nat Genet.* 1995;11:126–129.

49. Herrup K. The weaver mouse: a most cantankerous rodent. *Proc Natl Acad Sci U S A.* 1996;93:10541–10542.

50. Voigt N, Trausch A, Knaut M, et al. Left-to-right atrial inward rectifier potassium current gradients in patients with paroxysmal versus chronic atrial fibrillation. *Circ Arrhythm Electrophysiol.* 2010;3:472–480.

51. Yang Y, Yang Y, Liang B, et al. Identification of a Kir3.4 mutation in congenital long QT syndrome. *Am J Hum Genet.* 2010;86:872–880.

52. Flagg TP, Enkvetchakul D, Koster JC, Nichols CG. Muscle K_{ATP} channels: recent insights to energy sensing and myoprotection. *Physiol Rev.* 2010;90:799–829.

53. Shyng S, Ferrigni T, Nichols CG. Control of rectification and gating of cloned K_{ATP} channels by the Kir6.2 subunit. *J Gen Physiol.* 1997;110:141–153.

54. Bao L, Kefaloyianni E, Lader J, et al. Unique properties of the ATP-sensitive K(+) channel in the mouse ventricular cardiac conduction system. *Circ Arrhythm Electrophysiol.* 2011;4:926–935.

55. Ye B, Kroboth SL, Pu JL, et al. Molecular identification and functional characterization of a mitochondrial sulfonylurea receptor 2 splice variant generated by intraexonic splicing. *Circ Res.* 2009;105:1083–1093.

56. Foster DB, Ho AS, Rucker J, et al. The mitochondrial ROMK channel is a molecular component of Mito-KATP. *Circ Res.* 2012;111:446–454.

57. Carrasco AJ, Dzeja PP, Alekseev AE, et al. Adenylate kinase phosphotransfer communicates cellular energetic signals to ATP-sensitive potassium channels. *Proc Natl Acad Sci U S A.* 2001;98:7623–7628.

58. Crawford RM, Ranki HJ, Botting CH, Budas GR, Jovanovic A. Creatine kinase is physically associated with the cardiac ATP-sensitive K+ channel in vivo. *FASEB J.* 2002;16:102–104.

59. Dhar-Chowdhury P, Harrell MD, Han SY, et al. The glycolytic enzymes, glyceraldehyde-3-phosphate dehydrogenase, triose-phosphate isomerase, and pyruvate kinase are components of the K(ATP) channel macromolecular complex and regulate its function. *J Biol Chem.* 2005;280:38464–38470.

60. Garg V, Sun W, Hu K. Caveolin-3 negatively regulates recombinant cardiac K(ATP) channels. *Biochem Biophys Res Commun.* 2009;385:472–477.

61. Medeiros-Domingo A, Tan BH, Crotti L, et al. Gain-of-function mutation S422L in the KCNJ8-encoded cardiac K(ATP) channel Kir6.1 as a pathogenic substrate for J-wave syndromes. *Heart Rhythm.* 2010;7:1466–1471.

62. Tester DJ, Tan BH, Medeiros-Domingo A, Song C, Makielski JC, Ackerman MJ. Loss-of-function mutations in the KCNJ8-encoded Kir6.1 K(ATP) channel and sudden infant death syndrome. *Circ Cardiovasc Genet.* 2011;4:510–515.

5 Mammalian Calcium Pumps in Health and Disease

Marisa Brini and Ernesto Carafoli

Ca^{2+}-transporting adenosine triphosphatases (ATPases) (Ca^{2+} pumps) have been described in animal and plant cells and in the cells of lower eukaryotes. This chapter will focus on those of animal cells and on the disease processes linked to their dysfunction. The three animal Ca^{2+} pumps belong to the large superfamily of P-type ATPases, which have been so defined[1] because their reaction cycle is characterized by the formation of an acid-stable phosphorylated Asp residue (the P intermediate) in a highly conserved sequence (SDKTGT[L/IV/M][T/I/S]). The family now contains hundreds of members and eight subfamilies.[2] The subfamilies have been identified based essentially on the transported substrate specificity, the evolutionary appearance of which having been accompanied by abrupt changes in sequence. The changes, however, do not involve eight conserved structurally and mechanistically important regions that define the core of the superfamily. Five branches have been identified in the phylogenetic tree of the superfamily; two animal Ca^{2+} pumps belong to subgroup II A (the sarco/endoplasmic reticulum [SR/ER] Ca^{2+} [SERCA] and secretory pathway Ca^{2+} [SPCA] pumps), and one to subgroup II B (the plasma membrane Ca^{2+} ATPase [PMCA] pump). All P-type ATPases, including the three that transport Ca^{2+} in animal cells, are multidomain proteins that share the essential properties of the reaction mechanism, have molecular masses varying between 70 and 150 kDa, and share the presence of 10 hydrophobic membrane-spanning domains (TMs) (some, however, only have six or eight). With the number of TMs being even, the N- and C-termini of all P-type pumps are on the same membrane side, i.e., the cytosol; one exception is a splice variant of the SERCA pump that has 11 TMs (see the following text). The P-type ATPases also share the sensitivity to the transition state analogue orthovanadate and, with some specific differences (see the following text), to La^{3+}. Other inhibitors only affect selected members of the superfamily. The three-dimensional (3D) structures of four P-type ATPases have become available following the landmark solution of that of the SERCA pump 16 years ago[3]; molecular modeling on templates of the SERCA pump structure has indicated that all P-type ATPases share the general principles of 3D structures. The reaction cycle of P-type ATPases originally envisaged only the E1 and E2 steps, characterized by distinct conformations and affinities for ATP and the transported ion; in Ca^{2+} pumps, for instance, in the E1 state the pump engages Ca^{2+} with high affinity at one side of the membrane, and in the E2 state its lowered affinity for Ca^{2+} releases it to the opposite membrane side.[4] Additional intermediate states were described to make the reaction cycle much more complex.[5] Importantly, each step of the reaction cycle is reversible, so that ATP can be produced by reversing the direction of the ion transport process; reversal of the SERCA pump, with production of ATP, had in fact already been demonstrated in one of the first experiments on the transport of Ca^{2+} by vesicular preparations of the sarcoplasmic reticulum.[6] A simplified version of the cycle, but adapted to the Ca^{2+} pumps, is shown in Fig. 5.1.

Several Ca^{2+} pump isoforms have been described in animal cells, differing essentially in tissue distribution, regulatory properties, and some mechanistic peculiarities. The isoform diversity reflects the existence of separate basic gene products, but also the occurrence of complex patterns of alternative splicing that very significantly increase the number of variants of each of the three pumps. The analysis of the differential properties of the Ca^{2+} pump isoforms is a major focus of investigation since it has important linkages to the general process of cellular Ca^{2+} homeostasis, which in animal cells is regulated by a number of nonmembrane Ca^{2+}-binding proteins as well as membrane-intrinsic Ca^{2+} channels and transporters. The transporters interact with Ca^{2+} with high or low affinity, and thus function either as fine tuners of cytosolic Ca^{2+} or come into play whenever the concentration of Ca^{2+} increases to levels adequate for their low affinity. The Na/Ca exchanger of the plasma membrane and the mitochondrial Ca^{2+} uptake and release systems are the low affinity regulators of cytosolic Ca^{2+}. The three pumps, by contrast, control Ca^{2+} efficiently even in the low concentrations of the cytosol at rest. Their activity is fundamental to the correct functioning of the machinery of animal cells; dysfunctions, genetic or otherwise, of their operation, may not necessarily induce cell death, but invariably generate disease phenotypes: they now define a topic that has recently undergone tremendous growth.[7]

Sarco/Endoplasmic Reticulum Ca^{2+} ATPase

The SERCA pump is a key mechanism to adjust the Ca^{2+} homeostasis in the ER lumen. Considering that the ER Ca^{2+} is involved in a multitude of signaling events and in "housekeeping" functions that control cell growth, differentiation, and apoptosis, the activity of the SERCA pump is a key element in cell wellness.

SERCA pump is inhibited by La^{3+} and orthovanadate, and the discovery of specific inhibitors like thaspigargin,[8] cyclopiazonic acid,[9] and 2.5-di(t-butyl)hydroquinone[10] represented a big advantage in the biochemical and structural characterization of the pump.

The SERCA protein is organized in the membrane with 10 TMs: numerous mutagenesis studies and the solution of its 3D structure have clarified essential molecular details of its function. They will be only briefly summarized here, and the full details are available in a number of more comprehensive reviews.[11–13] Analysis of the 3D structure of the SERCA1 pump isoform has revealed that the single polypeptide chain folds in three cytosolic domains and in one transmembrane domain (M) composed of the ten formerly predicted TMs (Fig. 5.2). The three cytosolic domains have been named according to their role in the reaction cycle: the nucleotide binding domain (N) binds ATP, the phosphorylation domain (P) drives ATP hydrolysis leading the

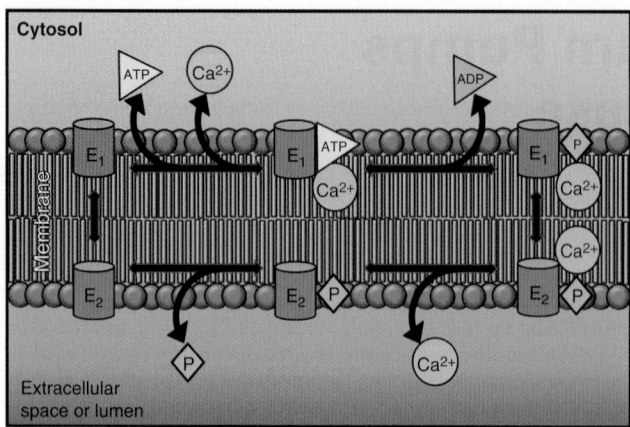

FIGURE 5.1 A simplified reaction cycle of the P-type adenosine triphosphatases (pumps) adapted to the Ca²⁺ pumps. The two original conformational states of the pumps are envisaged. The E1 pumps bind Ca²⁺ with a high affinity at one membrane side (the cytosol); the E2 pumps have much lower Ca²⁺ affinity and release Ca²⁺ to the opposite membrane side. Adenosine triphosphate (*ATP*) phosphorylates a conserved Asp in the active site.

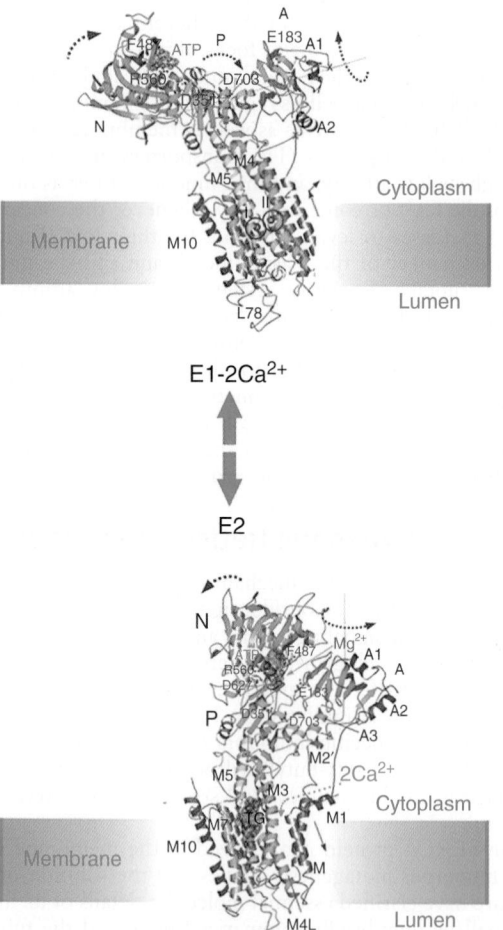

FIGURE 5.2 The three-dimensional structure of the sarco/endoplasmic reticulum Ca²⁺ pump, showing the open configuration of the three cytoplasmic domains A, N, and P in the presence of Ca²⁺ and the more compact configuration of the cytosolic sector in its absence. The two purple spheres in the upper panel represent the two bound Ca²⁺. This figure is a modified version of the original structure published by C. Toyoshima.[84] The E2 structure shown contains the inhibitor thapsigargin. The TMs are the transmembrane domains. Several residue of importance, not discussed in the text, are also shown.

phosphorylation of the catalytic Asp, and the actuator domain (A) catalyzes the dephosphorylation of the P-domain. The A and P domains are connected to the transmembrane M domain that contains the two Ca²⁺ binding sites, and the SERCA pump transports two Ca²⁺ per ATP hydrolyzed. The N domain is instead connected to the P domain. During the cycle, phosphorylation and de-phosphorylation events promote conformational changes that control the access of Ca²⁺ to the two binding sites (site 1 and site 2), which exist in high and low affinity states (Fig. 5.3). The two sites are located near the cytoplasmic surface of the membrane, but site 1 faces the cytoplasmic side and site 2 is closer to the luminal side. Once Ca²⁺ becomes bound to site 1, a conformational change increases the affinity of site 2, and permits the phosphorylation of the catalytic Asp by ATP, leading to the transition E2→E1→E1•2Ca²⁺ E1P. The binding of ATP crosslinks the P and N domains, permitting the interaction of the P domain with the A domain, which rotates, inducing the opening of the luminal gate that releases Ca²⁺ to the lumen, and permits the E1P-E2P transition. The closure of the luminal gate, and thus the E2P→E2 Pᵢ transition, then occurs, since a second rotation of the A domain locks it to the P domain. A highly conserved TGES motif (corresponding to the Thr-Gly-Glu-Ser amino acids sequence) in the A domain fills the gap between the N and P domains after the second rotation of the A domain, eventually permitting the release of Ca²⁺ into the lumen. The rearrangements of the transmembrane helices M1–M6 induced by the rotation of the A domain allow protons and water molecules to enter and stabilize the empty Ca²⁺ binding sites, and induce the retraction of the TGES from the phosphorylation site and the entrance of one water molecule to the phosphorylation site; this induces the release of phosphate (and Mg²⁺) and the complete closure of the luminal gate.

Three SERCA genes generate three isoforms. Their number is increased by alternative splicing processes. SERCA1 is almost exclusively expressed in muscle tissues, specifically in fast-twitch skeletal muscles. Interestingly, the generation of truncated, less active SERCA1 variants has been described, which contribute to reduce the Ca²⁺ concentration in the ER lumen and causes apoptotic cell death. SERCA2b and SERCA2a are the two major SERCA protein isoforms, the former having housekeeping and the latter a more specialized function. SERCA2a is found in slow skeletal and cardiac muscles (it is also expressed in low amounts in smooth muscles and in neurons). The splice variants SERCA2c and SERCA2d have also been found in low amounts in the heart. The expression of the SERCA3 pump, which has a limited cell-type distribution, is variable. In several cell types, this is induced by differentiation and is decreased during tumorigenesis and blastic transformation. In cells of hematopoietic origin and in various epithelial cells, the SERCA2 pump gene is coexpressed with that of the SERCA3 pump. All SERCA3 splice variants (SERCA3a–f) have lower Ca²⁺ affinity than the SERCA2 pump, which raises doubts on their role in the presence of higher affinity SERCA pump variants. Differences in their spatial cellular distribution could justify their copresence: the SERCA3 pump is confined to environments with high Ca²⁺ concentration, such as those close to the plasma membrane of cardiomyocytes, at basal regions in epithelial cells, and in the membrane of acidic Ca²⁺ stores in platelets. While the SERCA1a pump is the best characterized isoform in terms of structure–function relationship, the regulatory aspects of SERCA pumps have instead been better defined on the SERCA2 isoform.

The SERCA2a pump is the major isoform of developing and adult mammalian heart (SERCA2b is also expressed there, its level being unchanged during the development).[14] SERCA2a is the most abundant protein in the heart SR membrane, and its increased expression during the development paralleled the increasing rate of Ca²⁺ uptake by the SR lumen and the shortening of the relaxation time in adult compared with neonatal heart. SERCA2a pump levels are higher in atria than in ventricles, partially accounting for the shorter duration of contraction in atrial than in ventricular tissues.

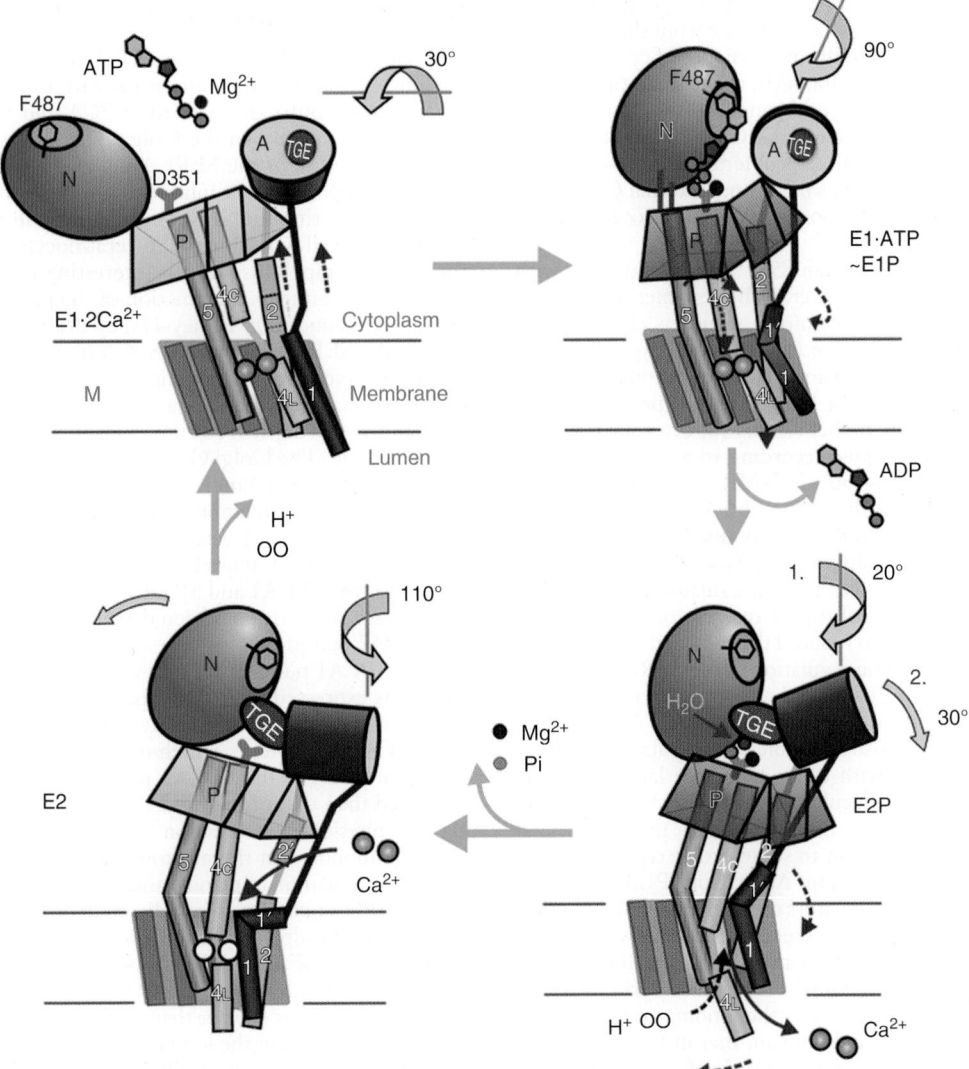

FIGURE 5.3 A cartoon describing the conformational changes of the cytosolic and membrane domains of the sarco/endoplasmic reticulum Ca²⁺ pump during the transport of Ca²⁺ across the molecule. The cartoon is taken from a review by C. Toyoshima[84] and contains details that have been discussed in the text. (From Toyoshima C. Structural aspects of ion pumping by Ca²⁺-ATPase of sarcoplasmic reticulum. *Arch Biochem Biophys*. 2008;476:3-11.)

The expression and the activity of the SERCA2a pump have been studied extensively. The primary mechanism of the regulation of the pump is mediated by phospholamban (PLB).[15] PLB is a 52 residue protein composed of a hydrophobic helical C-terminal portion inserted into the SR membrane and a hydrophilic N-terminal region that protrudes into the cytosol and contains phosphorylation sites (Ser16 and Thr17) for protein kinase A (PKA) and, possibly, Ca²⁺/calmodulin-dependent protein kinase II (CAMKII). Dephosphorylated PLB binds to the pump, decreasing its Ca²⁺ affinity; phosphorylation by PKA (and, possibly, CaMKII) releases the inhibition and increases the affinity of the pump for Ca²⁺ and thus Ca²⁺ transport. The hydrophilic N-terminal portion of PLB interacts with a domain close to the active site of the pump and, within the membrane, with transmembrane helices 2, 4, 6, and 9. It is generally believed that PLB exists both as a pentamer and as a monomer. It is not clear how the conversion between the two forms occurs, but several lines of evidence indicate that monomeric PLB is the active form. However, structural observations indicate that pentamers may also interact with the pump.[16]

Another small (31 residues) transmembrane protein, sarcolipin (SLN), originally identified as it copurified with the SERCA1a pump, has recently also received attention. SLN is predominantly expressed in the atrial compartment of the heart, and its sequence is similar to that of the transmembrane sector of PLB; modeling studies have revealed that the SLN and PLB interactions with the SERCA pump may be similar (i.e., SLN would bind to the pump in transmembrane sites of PLB).[16] Studies on SLN suggest that it is an uncoupler of the SERCA pump activity and can increase ATP hydrolysis, resulting in heat production.[17] SLN overexpression in the ventricle cells of animal models (where SLN is essentially absent) caused a decrease in the Ca²⁺ affinity of SERCA2a and slowed relaxation, suggesting that SLN may be as effective an inhibitor of SERCA pump activity as PLB. Interestingly, the overexpression of SLN in the heart of PLB null mice caused a decrease in the affinity of the SERCA2a pump for Ca²⁺ and impaired contractility. The finding that isoproterenol, a β-adrenergic agonist, relieved the inhibition suggests that SLN could mediate the β-adrenergic response in the heart. Ablation of the SLN gene increases the affinity of the SERCA pump for Ca²⁺, resulting in enhanced rates of SR Ca²⁺ uptake.[18]

The SERCA2b pump is the acknowledged housekeeping isoform. It has a dual role. By transporting Ca^{2+} from the cytosol to the ER lumen, it contributes to the maintenance of cytosolic Ca^{2+} at the low resting levels (about 100 nM), at the same time ensuring the high Ca^{2+} levels (in the mM range) in the lumen of ER that make the ER the main intracellular Ca^{2+} store that controls cellular activities (e.g., contraction, proliferation, differentiation, and cell death), and it also ensures the proper internal Ca^{2+} ambient for the ER enzymes (e.g., those involved in protein folding and lipid synthesis).

The SERCA2b pump shares an 85% sequence identity with the SERCA1a counterpart; however, it differs functionally from it and also from the SERCA2a isoform, which is characterized by a unique C-terminal extension (the so-called 2b-tail), which forms a luminal sequence extension and an additional TM segment (TM11).[19] The extension has regulatory properties: the longer pump has a two-fold higher affinity for cytosolic Ca^{2+} and a lower maximal turnover rate. According to a model based on the SERCA1a structure and on the NMR structure of TM11, the interaction of TM11 with TM7 and TM 10 has been proposed to stabilize the pump in the Ca^{2+}-bound E1 conformation, with the high-affinity Ca^{2+}-binding sites facing the cytosol. The TM11 has also been proposed as a novel regulator of the SERCA pump: the co-reconstitution of the 18-residue-long TM11 with the SERCA1a protein in vitro reduced the V_{max} and increased the Ca^{2+} affinity of the latter. The regulation of the SERCA pump by PLB and SLN, and by the 2b-tail in the 2b variant, resembles the interaction of the β- and γ-subunits of the Na^+/K^+ ATPase with the catalytic subunit α. It also resembles the regulatory interaction of the PMCA pump with calmodulin (see later), suggesting operationally similar molecular mechanisms of P-type pump regulation.[20] It could also be mentioned that the C-terminal portion of the PMCA pump can to some extent replace PLB as an inhibitor of the SERCA pump. Apart from PLB and SLN, which are the best-studied regulators of the SERCA pump, other proteins interact with it. Those interacting at the luminal side have an important role. The two chaperons calreticulin and calnexin contain a globular N-domain that binds carbohydrates, an extended P-domain that mediates the binding of ERp57 (see later), and an acidic C-terminal domain, that in the case of calreticulin binds 25 mol of Ca^{2+} per molecule of protein with low affinity (Kd, 2 mM). Luminal Ca^{2+} buffering by calnexin is less significant, and the acidic C-terminus of the protein protrudes into the cytosol. Calreticulin and calnexin have been suggested to interact through their N-domains with a putative glycosylated residue present in the C-terminal tail of the SERCA2b pump, but absent in SERCA2a. Glycosylation-independent interaction with the SERCA2b pump has been shown to occur, and molecular modeling of the SERCA2b molecule has suggested that its 2b-tail is located in luminal loops, thus making it inaccessible to interacting proteins. ERp57, a member of the protein disulfide isomerase (PDI) family of proteins with thio-oxidoreductase activity, is recruited by the SERCA2b pump/chaperone complex and to catalyze the formation of an inhibitory disulfide bridge between Cys875 and Cys887 in the luminal loop L7-8 of the SERCA2b pump.[21] It could be a regulatory mechanism, but the proposal is controversial, since mutations of either or both Cys residues resulted in loss of Ca^{2+} transport but not of the activity in SERCA1.[22]

Two other luminal Ca^{2+}-binding proteins have been shown to interact with the SERCA2 pump: the ubiquitously expressed calumenin (CALU) and the histidine-rich Ca^{2+}-binding protein (HRC). Both decrease the apparent Ca^{2+} affinity of the pump. HRC binds Ca^{2+} with high capacity and low affinity and could mediate both SR Ca^{2+} uptake and release through its interaction with SERCA, when the SR Ca^{2+} is low, and with triadin, which is part of the ryanodine receptor (RyR) Ca^{2+} release complex, when it is saturated by Ca^{2+}.[23]

Secretory Pathway Ca^{2+} ATPase

The Golgi Ca^{2+} ATPase (the SPCA pump) shares the role of loading Ca^{2+} in the Golgi apparatus with the SERCA pump.[24,25] The relative contribution of the SPCA and SERCA pumps to the total Ca^{2+} uptake in the Golgi apparatus is cell-type dependent, and the use of the SERCA pump selective inhibitor thapsigargin, which does not inhibit the SPCA pump, has permitted determination that the SERCA pump contribution is significant in numerous cell types, but not in keratinocytes, which mainly use the SPCA pump. This point is interesting because SPCA pump mutations that impair the function of the pump lead to a specific human skin condition, Hailey-Hailey disease (see later). In contrast to the SERCA pump, the SPCA pump also transports Mn^{2+} and thus serves the dual function of supplying this metal to the Golgi lumen, where it acts as a cofactor for the glycosyl-transferases, and removing it from the cytosol, where its accumulation could be toxic. The Golgi Ca^{2+} ATPase was originally discovered in yeast and named Pmr1 (plasma membrane ATPase-related) and PMA1 (plasma membrane H^+-ATPase) by two independent groups. Later, it was detected in mammals and higher vertebrates.

Two basic SPCA genes have been found in higher vertebrates coding for the SPCA1 and SPCA2 pumps. Alternative splicing of the primary transcript has been described for SPCA1, but not for the SPCA2 pump.

The SPCA1 pump is the housekeeping Ca^{2+} and Mn^{2+} pump, since it is expressed in all cell types, even if at different levels in various tissues. The alternatively spliced SPCA1 mRNA generates SPCA1a-d proteins, which differ in the C-terminal portion. The expression of the SPCA2 pump in human tissues is more restricted than that of the SPCA1 pump, suggesting a more specialized physiological function for it: the SPCA2 pump is particularly abundant in the gastrointestinal tract, trachea, thyroid, salivary and mammary glands, and prostate.

The SPCA pump is also predicted to be organized in ten TMs, with a large headpiece portion protruding into the cytosol. On the basis of the SERCA pump 3D structure, the cytosolic portion is divided in the three canonical A, P and N portions (Fig. 5.4). The SPCA pump is shorter than the SERCA and PMCA pumps, since it does not have the long cytoplasmic C-terminal tail of the PMCA pump, and its intracellular loops are shorter. The SPCA pump differs from the SERCA pump in having only one Ca^{2+} binding site, corresponding to site 2 in the SERCA1 pump. The suggested TM packing and possibly some distant residues would define the structure of the site, making it adequate to bind Mn^{2+} with high affinity and to transport it; this structural aspect is a peculiarity of the SPCA pump. Gln783 in TM6 and Val335 in TM4 appear to be essential for Mn^{2+} transport, since their mutation (in the Pmr1 yeast pump) abolished Mn^{2+} transport. Another distinction of the SPCA pump with respect to the SERCA and PMCA pumps, which function as obligatory H^+ exchangers, is the finding that it does not appear to countertransport H^+. No specific SPCA pump inhibitors have so far been described, and no endogenous activators are known. Mutagenesis studies on the Pmr1 yeast pump have generated phenotypes that are important tools that could provide information on the role of the SPCA pump in higher eukaryotic organisms. The expression levels and activity of SPCAs changed in response to altered physiological needs; the SPCA1 pump expression and activity changed in the brain after an ischemic event,[26] and the SPCA1 pump levels increased in the mammary glands during lactation. This last finding is shared by the PMCA2 pump (see the following text). The role of the SPCA pump in the maintenance of Golgi Ca^{2+} homeostasis deserves a comment, as recent evidence has indicated that the Golgi apparatus is a heterogeneous and highly dynamic Ca^{2+} store.[27] The apparatus has been shown to be an InsP3 sensitive Ca^{2+} store, implying a role for it in the generation of local cytosolic Ca^{2+} signals. The specific distribution of the SPCA pump

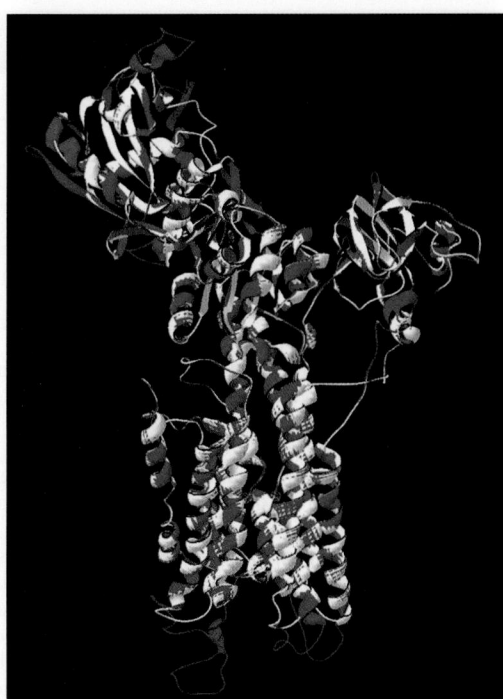

FIGURE 5.4 A molecular modeling representation of the structure of the secretory pathway Ca^{2+} pump (*white*) superimposed on a template of the sarco/endoplasmic reticulum Ca^{2+} pump (*red*). (Courtesy L. Raeymakers, Leuven, Belgium.)

in the Golgi membranes appears important because it may vary with the cell type; that is, in some cases it colocalizes with Golgi markers and in others with those of the trans-Golgi; however, general consensus has now been reached that the SPCA1 pump-containing Golgi subcompartment is insensitive (or mildly sensitive) to InsP3 and thus appears not to be involved in generating cytosolic Ca^{2+} signals. The kinetics of Ca^{2+} release from the Golgi apparatus differed from those of the ER; in particular, while the latency following agonist application and the initial rate of Ca^{2+} release were similar for the two organelles, the release of Ca^{2+} from the Golgi apparatus terminated faster than that from the ER. These findings would be compatible with distinct Ca^{2+} subcompartments in the Golgi apparatus endowed with different Ca^{2+}-regulating molecular components.

Plasma Membrane Ca^{2+} ATPase

The PMCA pump is a high-affinity, low-capacity Ca^{2+}-exporting system. Most of the initial work on the pump dealt with erythrocytes, but it gradually became clear that the pump is present and active in all animal cells, including those of excitable tissues (e.g., heart),[28] where it is generally assumed that the export of Ca^{2+} is performed solely by the Na^+/Ca^{2+} exchanger. The discovery of a PMCA pump in heart sarcolemma came as a surprise, and a role for it in the regulation of the bulk Ca^{2+} homeostasis in the cardiomyocyte was never considered realistic: according to solid and abundant evidence, and thus to general consensus, the beat-to-beat export of bulk Ca^{2+} from heart cells is indeed performed by the Na/Ca exchanger. However, it has been shown that the PMCA pump of heart sarcolemma has a specific role in Ca^{2+} signaling that is still related to the regulation of the excitation/relaxation cycle, but that is not linked to the general regulation of the homeostasis of Ca^{2+} (see the following text).

A number of comprehensive reviews (e.g., see Brini and Carafoli[11] and Brini and colleagues[29]) describe the properties of the PMCA pump; due to space limitations, this contribution will in

most cases refer to them, rather than to specific reports. The general aspects of the reaction mechanism of the PMCA pump are those of all P-type pumps (see Fig. 5.1). However, the reaction cycle of the PMCA pump differs in two important aspects from that of the SERCA pump, which is normally taken as a reference, as it is now known in atomic detail. One concerns the effect of La^{3+} on the phosphorylated Asp intermediate: in all P-type pumps, including the SERCA and SPCA pumps (see earlier), La^{3+} is supposed to replace Ca^{2+} as the metal ion that activates the phosphorylation of the catalytic Asp, thus inhibiting the formation of the phosphoenzyme. In the PMCA pump, instead, La^{3+} greatly increases the steady state level of the phosphoenzyme (a convenient observation, as it permits the detection of the PMCA in phosphate gels of membrane preparations containing much larger amounts of other P-type pumps). The other significant difference with respect to the SERCA pump, which is shared by the SPCA pump (see earlier), is the presence of only one Ca^{2+}-binding site. The single site of the PMCA pump corresponds to site 2 of the SERCA pump and coordinates Ca^{2+} to six residues (essentially the same as for the SERCA pump) in TM 4 and 6. The site that would correspond to site 1 of the SERCA pump is not operational in the PMCA pump, most likely because of the absence of an essential acidic residue in transmembrane domain 5. Interestingly, the insertion by mutagenesis of the missing acidic residue (or even of a Gln) in transmembrane 5 confers to the PMCA pump properties (high cooperativity of Ca^{2+} binding, Hill coefficient approaching 2, and negative effect of La^{3+} on the phosphorylated Asp) that resemble those of the SERCA pump, i.e., the second Ca^{2+} binding appears to have been made operational.[30] All PMCA pumps are sensitive to the classical inhibitor of P-type pumps orthovanadate and are insensitive to the specific inhibitors of the SERCA pump. Some supposedly specific inhibitors have been described (e.g., eosin or caloxin), but their specificity, and thus their usefulness, does not match that of the SERCA pump inhibitors.

In mammals, the plasma membrane Ca^{2+} ATPase is the product of four separate genes, which encode four basic pumps (PMCA1–PMCA4) differing in tissue distribution, functional properties, and interaction with protein partners.[31,32] PMCA 1 and PMCA 4 have wide tissue distribution and have traditionally been considered as the housekeeping enzymes[33,34]; this concept is still valid for the PMCA 1 pump but has recently been challenged for the PMCA 4 pump, which has now been shown to have critical Ca^{2+}-signaling roles in a number of cell types. For instance, in the spermatozoon, where it is the predominant PMCA pump form and where it is required for hyperactivated sperm motility,[35] ablation of its gene greatly limits sperm motility and generates male infertility.[36] In the heart (see previous text), where it has a role in the contractility process, which is unrelated to the beat-to-beat regulation of bulk cytosolic Ca^{2+}, it modulates the activity of the Ca^{2+}-dependent neuronal nitric oxide synthase (nNOS), which is important to the control of the excitation/contraction coupling of the cardiomyocyte.[37]

At variance with PMCA1 and PMCA4, PMCA2 and PMCA3 instead have restricted tissue distribution; they are particularly represented in neurons and have much higher affinity for calmodulin, which is the natural regulator of the PMCA pump, than the two ubiquitous isoforms (Table 5.1).

The PMCA pumps are organized in the membrane with the canonical ten TMs of the Ca^{2+} pumps. The 3D structure of the PMCA pump has not yet been solved, but molecular modeling work on SERCA pump templates has predictably indicated the same structural organization, with the cytoplasmic A, N, and P domains (Fig. 5.5). Differences, however, are also evident, beginning with the long, unstructured C-terminal tail that contains the most important regulatory sites of the pump and a phospholipid binding stretch (see the following text) in the cytosolic loop that connects TMs 2 and 3.

TABLE 5.1 Tissue distribution, calmodulin (CaM) affinity, and calpain sensitivity of the four basic plasma membrane Ca²⁺ ATPase (PMCA) pump isoforms

	PMCA1b[a]	PMCA2b	PMCA3b	PMCA4b
Tissue distribution	Ubiquitous	Restricted (Brain)	Restricted (Brain)	Ubiquitous
K_d CaM	40–50 nM	2–4 nM	8 nM	30–40 nM
Calpain sensitivity	High	Low	Low	Low

[a]The notation 1–4b refers to the full length pump, without splicing inserts (see text). The information given in the table (e.g., CaM affinities) has been extracted from several of the articles quoted in the text.

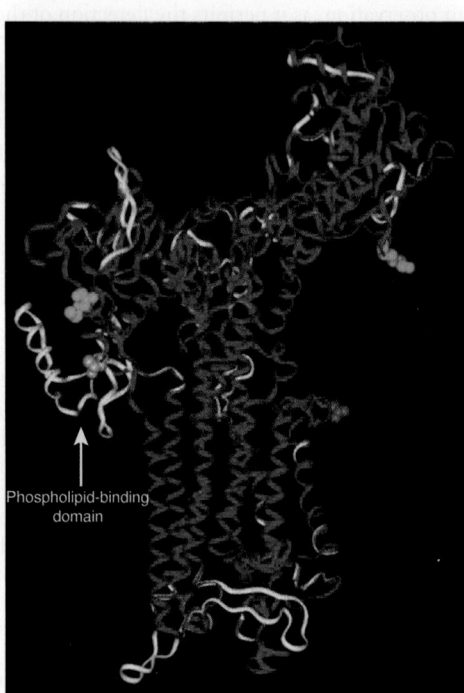

Phospholipid-binding domain

FIGURE 5.5 A molecular modeling of the structure of the plasma membrane Ca²⁺ ATPase (PMCA) pump (*yellow*) superimposed on that of the sarco/endoplasmic reticulum Ca²⁺ pump (*red*). The long, unstructured C-terminal tail of the PMCA pump is not represented. The binding region in the cytosolic loop connection TM2 and 3 of the PMCA pump is the most evident difference between the two pump structures.

As mentioned, calmodulin is the (most important) natural regulator of the PMCA pump and has been exploited to purify the enzyme using calmodulin columns.[38] Calmodulin interacts with a domain in the C-terminal tail of the pump that has the amphipathic helix configuration of canonical calmodulin binding domains. The affinity of the domain for calmodulin is very high (Kd in the nM range), and the interaction with the PMCA pump has characteristics that distinguish it from that of other targets of calmodulin regulation. The PMCA pump apparently only interacts with the C-terminal portion of calmodulin,[39] which does not collapse hairpin-like around its binding PMCA domain. The matter of the interaction of the PMCA pump with calmodulin has recently seen some unexpected developments; for example, a second calmodulin binding domain with much lower affinity for calmodulin (Kd in the μM range) has been identified downstream of the canonical one.[40] This second domain, which appears to be present only in some splice isoforms of the pump, would permit the regulation of the pump in both the nM and μM range of Ca²⁺ concentration. However, irrespective of the problem of the existence of one or two calmodulin binding domains, it is generally accepted that the mechanism of calmodulin activation depends on its ability to release the PMCA pump from the state of autoinhibition that prevails in its absence. The C-terminal tail of the pump, including the canonical calmodulin binding domain, folds over to bind to two sites next to the active site of the pump, locking it in an autoinhibited state.[41,42] The calmodulin would swing its binding domain, and presumably the entire C-terminal tail, away from the sites of autoinhibition, restoring full activity to the pump.

One of the distinctive properties of the PMCA pumps is the multiplicity of activating mechanisms. Next to calmodulin, the most important probably are acidic phospholipids, the most effective among them being the doubly phosphorylated derivative of phosphatidyl-inositol (PIP2). Acidic phospholipids bind to two sites: one is the basic C-terminal calmodulin binding domain, and the other is a stretch of about 40 predominantly basic amino acids in the cytosolic loop connecting transmembrane domains 2 and 3. The activation by acidic phospholipids could be important in vivo, and it has been calculated that the concentration of phosphatidyl-serine in the surroundings of the pump would in principle be adequate for about 50% stimulation of its activity.[43] The concentration of phosphatidyl-serine in the membrane is not known to be modulated, and it thus appears unrealistic to propose a role for it in the reversible activation of the pump. PIP2, which is the most effective activator, does instead become modulated in the membrane during Ca²⁺-mediated signaling processes; a PIP2-mediated reversible process of pump activation could thus appear be a realistic possibility. Kinases have also been found to activate the pump by phosphorylating residues in its C-terminal tail: protein kinase C acts on all pump variants, and PKA acts only on one of the isoforms. An intriguing mechanism of pump activation is that generated by a dimerization (oligomerization) process that occurs through the C-terminal calmodulin binding domain, and its physiological significance is obscure. The concentration of the PMCA pump in the plasma membrane of all animal cells is very low (probably less than 0.1% of the total membrane protein); thus the possibility of the random association of two or more pump monomers in situ to generate dimers or oligomers appears unrealistic. All mechanisms of activation act by increasing the Ca²⁺ affinity of the pump; in their absence, the Km (Ca²⁺) of the pump is as high as 20 μM but drops to 0.5 μM or less in the presence, for instance, of calmodulin or acidic phospholipids. The pump can be also activated irreversibly, and that occurs when its C-terminal tail, which includes the calmodulin binding domain, is shaved off by the Ca²⁺-dependent protease calpain. In this case, the activation is linked to the removal of the autoinhibitory C-terminal tail of the pump. The irreversible activation by calpain could become significant in conditions of pathological Ca²⁺ overload that would demand the uninterrupted maximal ability of the pump to extrude Ca²⁺ from the cytosol.

In addition to these activating mechanisms, a number of protein partners have recently been shown to become reversibly associated with the PMCA pumps, sometimes even specifically with some isoforms.[44] Interestingly, these interactions could either be activating or inhibitory; among those of special interest are those with numerous proteins that contain the PDZ binding domain, which is recognized by the extreme C-terminal portion of most

PMCA pump variants. The protein partners that are recognized by the PMCA pump via their PDZ domain include, among others, the MAGUK guanylate kinases and Ania-3, a member of the Homer family of scaffolding proteins. In addition to the C-terminal region, other portions of the PMCA molecule also interact with regulatory partners; for instance, the main intracellular loop interacts with calcineurin and the N-terminal cytosolic region with protein 14.3.3. Of particular interest is the interplay of PMCA4 with the nitric oxide synthase in the heart.[37] It has been shown that the pump tethers nNOS to a compartmentalized domain in which its activity would reduce the concentration of Ca^{2+} and thus the production of cGMP. The consequent increase of cAMP would then exert its well-known positive inotropic effects while the interaction of the pump with nNOS has a defined physiological effect; in other cases, the effects are less well understood in a physiological perspective. They vary from the modulation of activity, to the targeting to membrane domains, to the recruiting of PMCA pump variants to cell components (e.g., the cytoskeleton).

As mentioned, alternative splicing processes affect all four basic primary transcripts of the pump, greatly increasing the number of isoforms. Most of the splice variants described in the literature have also been documented at the protein level. The splicing operation occurs at two transcript sites: site A corresponds to the cytosolic loop of the pump molecule that connects transmembrane domains 2 and 3, and site C corresponds to the C-terminal calmodulin binding domain. The A site inserts are always in frame, and they affect the properties of the pumps but do not substantially alter their structure. The C site inserts, instead, may not maintain an open protein reading frame and may thus result in the truncation of the pump molecule downstream of its regular C-terminus. The full details of the splicing operations and its complexities are discussed elsewhere[11,45]: only the aspects that are especially significant to the themes of this contribution will thus be considered here. At site A one exon of 39 bp is apparently invariably inserted in the mature mRNA of pump 1, whereas an exon of 42 or 36 bp can be optionally inserted or excluded in the transcripts of pumps 3 and 4, respectively. The pump variants without the inserts are termed z and those with the extra exon x. The A splice for PMCA2 is more complex, and three exons of 33, 60, and 42 bp can be inserted or excluded; however, only some of the possible combinations have so far been detected in the mRNAs of various tissues. For example, in humans, only variant w (all exons included), variant x (only the 42 bp exon included), and variant z (no extra exon included) have been detected. Only scarce information is available on the functional consequences of the splicing operation at site A. Importantly, however, the splicing at site A has been found to alter the membrane targeting of the PMCA2 pump.[46] The insertion of all three extra exons (45 residues, the w form) determined its apical targeting in polarized MDCK epithelial cells, whereas the insertion of only one exon (14 residues, the x form), or the absence of inserts (the z form), determined the sorting of the pump to the basolateral plasma membrane.

The splicing at site C is more complex, and a large exon (154 bp in PMCA1 and PMCA3, 175 bp in PMCA4) can be optionally included in a site corresponding to the middle of the calmodulin binding domain, leading to the loss of the open reading frame and to the premature truncation of the pump. The truncated pump is termed a, and the form without insertions is termed b (an additional smaller 68-bp exon can also be optionally included in PMCA3). However, the large extra exon contains multiple internal donor sites and can thus be inserted piecemeal. The inserts of 87 and 114 bp are in frame and generate the c and d forms, whereas those of 152 and 154 bp are not in frame and generate the truncated a form. Again, the splicing operation at site C is peculiarly complex for PMCA2. A large exon of 172 bp can be inserted into its mRNA, again piecemeal, generating variants c and d (in frame) and, presumably, e (out of frame). The insertion

TABLE 5.2 Ca^{2+}-dependent ATPase activity of PMCA2 and PMCA4

	nmolATP/mg PROTEIN/min	
	− CALMODULIN	+ CALMODULIN
PMCA2	4.21	5.87
PMCA4	1.45	6.15

ATPase, Adenosine triphosphatase; *PMCA*, plasma membrane Ca^{2+} ATPase. Data from Hilfiker H, Guerini D, Carafoli E. Cloning and expression of isoform 2 of the human plasma membrane Ca^{2+} ATPase. Functional properties of the enzyme and its splicing products. *J Biol Chem.* 1994;269:26178-26183; and Elwess NL, Filoteo AG, Enyedi A, Penniston JT. Plasma membrane Ca^{2+} pump isoforms 2a and 2b are unusually responsive to calmodulin and Ca^{2+}. *J Biol Chem.* 1997;272:17981-17986.

of the full 172-bp exon generates the prematurely truncated form a, and the mRNA without inserts generates form b (an additional smaller 55-bp exon can also be optionally inserted in the case of PMCA2). Information on the consequences of the slicing operation at site C on the activity of the pump is more abundant, and recent findings may lead to important functional developments. The insertion of the novel sequence roughly in the middle of the calmodulin binding domain leads, as expected, to the lowering of the calmodulin affinity for the pump.[47,48] The consequence of this decrease in affinity should lower the ability of calmodulin to remove its binding domain from the autoinhibitory sites in the main body of the pump, decreasing pump activity. However, predictions on the effects to be expected from the insertion of the novel sequence in the calmodulin binding domain are complicated by the unexpected observation that the insert tends to reconstitute the original entire calmodulin binding domain. Eight of the first 10 residues of the insert are indeed either identical, or conservative, with respect to those of the original C-terminal half of the calmodulin binding domain they replace.

The discussion of the splicing operation has shown that the PMCA2 pump differs from the other three basic pump isoforms. Other properties of the PMCA2 pump underline the differences and set the PMCA2 pump apart from the other three basic isoforms—for instance, the very high affinity for calmodulin (see Table 5.1) and, especially, the finding that the PMCA2 pump has a peculiarly high level of activity in its absence[49,50] (Table 5.2). The anomaly is not due to the presence of tightly bound calmodulin in "purified" PMCA2 pump preparations. It could thus be reasonably related to the reduced ability of the C-terminal tail of the PMCA2 pump to autoinhibit the pump. Irrespective of the mechanism, however, the anomaly generates a pump variant that would function nearly optimally in the absence of activation by calmodulin. This would satisfy the demands particular cell types may have for a continuous and vigorous Ca^{2+}-exporting function not dependent on pump activation. One last important point on the PMCA2 pump is its high concentration in the mammary gland, where its levels increase during lactation (see earlier for the similar finding on the SPCA pump).

Ca^{2+} Pumps in the Disease Process

One of the distinctive properties of the Ca^{2+} signal is ambivalence; as must be expected, the central role of Ca^{2+} in the regulation of the most important cell activities demands its precise spatial and temporal control, and the vast array of Ca^{2+}-binding proteins and Ca^{2+} transporters expressed in all animal cells underlies the concept. Defects in the control of Ca^{2+} unavoidably generate states of cell suffering that could culminate, in cases of massive and protracted Ca^{2+} overload, in the death of the cell. This is the meaning of the ambivalence concept: having chosen Ca^{2+} as a determinant for function, cells undoubtedly benefit from its unlimited availability in their surroundings. But the coin also has a flip side; that is, the choice forces cells to live in a permanent condition of controlled risk. Increases in Ca^{2+} much above the normal level can be coped with by cells if it lasts for a limited time, thanks also to the existence of the mitochondrial uptake system that can efficiently sequester for a while large amounts of Ca^{2+}.[51] However, if the overload situation persists, the fate of the cell becomes sealed. However, apart from these extreme, and obvious, cases of Ca^{2+} catastrophe, the cellular homeostasis of Ca^{2+} can also become deregulated in less dramatic ways by defects in the individual participants in the Ca^{2+}-controlling operation. These defects are compatible with the continuation of cell life but generate cell discomfort phenotypes with diverse degrees of severity. Among them, those generated by defects of the Ca^{2+} pumps are recently receiving increasing attention. Several disease phenotypes caused by genetic and nongenetic defects of the Ca^{2+} pumps have been described. The problem with the nongenetic alterations is the frequent difficulty to decide whether the detected defects are really the sole cause of the disease phenotype and/or whether they are primitive or secondary. By contrast, the pathological genetic phenotypes are certainly causative and are mechanistically well defined. The discussion will thus focus essentially on them, limiting that of the nongenetic conditions to some special cases.

Sarco/Endoplasmic Reticulum Ca²⁺ Pump

Two human diseases associated with genetic mutations in the SERCA pump have been described, but numerous nongenetic pathological conditions (e.g., heart failure, cancer development, or diabetes) have been associated with its malfunction or decreased level of expression. Humans and some large animals develop a similar muscular disease, termed *Brody disease* in humans and *congenital pseudomyotonia* in Chianina cattle, as consequences of mutations in the gene of the SERCA1 pump. Brody disease is a rare recessive myopathy characterized by impaired relaxation, painless muscular cramps, and muscle stiffness following exercise. The clinical diagnosis is rather difficult since the symptoms are quite heterogeneous, but sometimes muscle biopsies show reduced SERCA1 pump expression. Six different mutations in the SERCA1 pump have been identified so far, four of them introducing a premature stop codon that truncates the pump, creating variants with higher instability.[52,53]

In the deficiency of SERCA1 pump function in skeletal muscles observed in Chianina cattle affected by pseudomyotonia, the SERCA1 pump activity was decreased by about 70%. Linkage analysis has shown that a mutation in the SERCA1 pump was associated with the phenotype, and subsequent mutation analysis has revealed its association with a missense Arg164His mutation in exon 6 of the gene.[54] Arg164 is a strongly conserved residue in the SERCA1 pumps, but its role in the function of the pump has not been defined. Another mutation (Arg559Cys) in the SERCA1 pump has been described in Belgian blue cattle affected by congenital muscular dystonia 1[55] and in a Dutch improved red and white cross-breed calf.[56] The disease phenotype is the same, suggesting that the loss of the SERCA pump activity could be a common element in these different myopathies.

Another disease associated with SERCA pump mutations is Darier disease, a rare human autosomal dominant skin disorder characterized by the loss of adhesion between epidermal cells and by abnormal keratinization. More than 130 mutations in the SERCA2 pump gene have been reported in human patients, distributed along all the pump sequence without evidence of clustering in specific regions.[57] An impaired ability to transport Ca^{2+} and an increased protein instability are considered the main consequence of the mutations; however, the fact that the symptoms are confined to the skin suggests that specific elements of Ca^{2+} homeostasis in keratinocytes are important to the pathogenesis

of the disorder. Alternatively, compensatory mechanisms for the SPCA pump defect could act in other tissues. No cardiac phenotypes have been described in patients carrying the SERCA2 pump mutations, even if the large majority of patients carry mutations in the region common to SERCA2a and 2b pump isoforms. Darier disease shares properties with Hailey-Hailey disease, a genetic skin disorder caused by SPCA pump mutations (see the following text), indicating that the maintaining of a proper Ca^{2+}-pumping activity is of particular relevance to the epidermis.

Nongenetic disease phenotypes linked to altered SERCA expression or activity has also been described; those associated with heart failure[58] and cancer[59] are the best documented. A general consensus has been reached on the reduction in SERCA2a pump level or activity in failing hearts of both animal models and patients. However, the mutations have been mostly ascribed to PLB rather than to the SERCA pump. A single report has described mutations in the SERCA2 gene that may predispose to heart failure.[60] The relationship between cancer and the SERCA2 and SERCA3 pumps has attracted increasing interest since 2000. Numerous alterations in the SERCA2 gene have been found in patients with colon or lung cancer. However, as is frequently the case with nongenetic alterations of Ca^{2+} pumps, whether they are primitive and directly involved in the early events of the carcinogenesis is not clear.

As for SERCA3, its expression becomes progressively lost during the multistep process of colon tumorigenesis, and its expression levels are inversely proportional to the loss of differentiation of the lesions. Finally, studies on human liver tumors have shown that the hepatitis B virus DNA could be integrated in the SERCA1 pump gene, causing the expression of a truncated mutant protein with a consequent decrease in ER Ca^{2+} content and increase in apoptosis.[61]

Secretory Pathway Ca²⁺ Pump

A skin disorder, Hailey-Hailey disease, is so far the only known genetic disease associated with an SPCA1 pump mutation. It has a dominant autosomal inheritance, and it is phenotypically characterized by the increased propensity to the formation of skin lesions, mainly at sites of sweating and friction. The lesions are due to the loss of adhesion of keratinocytes and to the abnormal keratinization of the skin. At least 87 different mutations have been described, located all along the SPCA pump sequence.[62] Some are responsible for reduced Ca^{2+} transport activity, but the large majority lead to protein instability. When the mutant SPCA pump is overexpressed in model cells, its level of protein expression is very low, despite normal levels of mRNA and correct localization to the Golgi compartment.[63-65] As mentioned, Hailey-Hailey disease shares phenotypic properties with Darier disease (see earlier). However, at variance with the keratinocytes of Darier patients, those of Hailey-Hailey patients show an abnormal response to extracellular Ca^{2+}, possibly because the upregulation of the SPCA1 pump in Darier keratinocytes could compensate for the SERCA dysfunction. Hailey-Hailey disease is essentially benign, but squamous cell carcinoma may develop from the skin lesions. Interestingly, in mice the loss of SPCA pump function causes skin cancer but not the acantholytic skin disorder that it causes in humans. This suggests that elements that favor the survival or the apoptotic death depending on the keratinocyte type may have a role in the development of the disease.

Recently, linkage analysis on chromosome 16q has revealed an association between the SPCA2 gene and specific language impairment, a common developmental disorder characterized by difficulties in language acquisition in individuals with otherwise normal development.[66] The linkage suggests a possible role of the SPCA pump in the context of language impairment.

Plasma Membrane Ca²⁺ ATPase Pump

Several genetic pathologies linked to the dysfunction of the PMCA pumps have now been described.[29,67] They affect animals (mice) and humans and are either spontaneous (e.g., those in humans) or induced by the ablation, partial disruption, or mutations of PMCA genes. The first-described disease phenotype related to a PMCA pump defect is a form of hereditary deafness that involves the PMCA2 isoform of the pump, which is abundantly expressed in the stereocilia of the hair cells of the Corti organ in the inner ear. As previously mentioned, PMCA2 has a peculiar characteristic (i.e., it has high activity even in the absence of calmodulin). This property evidently satisfies the necessity of maintaining a constant flow of Ca^{2+} from the stereocilia to the endolymph that bathes them. The tight control of the homeostasis of Ca^{2+} in the endolymph is essential for the functioning of the stereocilia bundle that gates mechanoelectrical channels through which K^+ (and Ca^{2+}) flows into the hair cell to generate (or modulate) the acoustic signals. The PMCA2 pump isoform of the stereocilia is the *wa* variant,[68] which has the site A insert that targets it to the stereocilia, and is C-terminally truncated to even further depress the calmodulin response with respect to the wild-type PMCA2 pump. The first indication of the role of the PMCA2 pump in the inner ear came from the deafness phenotype caused by the ablation of its gene.[69] Several spontaneous and induced mutations of the mouse gene were then described (see Brini and Carafoli[11] for a review) that confirmed the role of the PMCA2 *wa* variant in the function of the outer hair cells. Two human families with a hereditary deafness phenotype caused by two different point mutations in the PMCA2 gene were then also described.[70,71] The defect of the PMCA2 pump was analyzed molecularly and was characterized as a specific impairment of the long-term ability of the mutant pump to export Ca^{2+} from the cell.[71,72]

The inhibition of sperm motility and the male infertility phenotype caused by the ablation of the PMCA4 gene in mice have already been mentioned. The ablation of the PMCA4 gene, however, also has important effects on the heart function; the contractility and the amplitude of the Ca^{2+} transient linked to the L-channel activity were increased in the cardiomyocytes of the PMCA4 null mice,[37] supporting the suggestions (see earlier) for a role of the PMCA4 in the regulation of heart contractility. It may also be mentioned that the ablation of the PMCA4 gene also impaired phasic contraction and caused apoptosis in the smooth muscle of the portal vein, but only in mice that carried a null mutation in one copy of the PMCA1 pump gene.[35] Recently direct evidence has emerged on the involvement of a PMCA4 pump defect in a human disease: a missense mutation (R268Q) cosegregated in a family with autosomal dominant familial spastic paraplegia.[73] The mutation significantly decreased the efficiency of the suppression of depolarization-induced Ca^{2+} overload.[74]

A Korean genome-wide association study aimed at identifying genetic factors that influence blood pressure and hypertension risk has located the most significant single nucleotide polymorphism in the gene for the PMCA1 pump.[75,76] Based on the above-mentioned observation suggesting that the PMCA1 pump gene can function as a modifier locus for the phasic vein contraction linked to the PMCA4 pump gene, the Korean authors looked for a gene–gene interaction between variants of the PMCA1 and PMCA4 pump genes in the genome-wide association dataset and found only modest evidence for it. This pioneer study was confirmed by others[77,78] and followed by the finding that a link between PMCA1 defects and coronary artery disease existed,[79] suggesting a major role of isoform 1 in the control of Ca^{2+} handling in smooth muscles and in the regulation of blood pressure. Finally, a disease phenotype has also been identified very recently for a defect in the PMCA3 pump gene in humans. The PMCA3 pump is the least well known of the PMCA isoforms. As mentioned, it is essentially restricted to the brain (however, in rats it is also found in skeletal muscles), where it is particularly abundant in the choroid plexus. A study using X-exome sequencing has recently identified a missense G1107D mutation in the calmodulin-binding domain of the PMCA3 pump in a family with X-linked congenital cerebellar ataxia. A molecular study of the mutant PMCA3 pump expressed in model cells has revealed its impaired ability to extrude Ca^{2+}.[80] Interestingly, the in vitro characterization of PMCA3 defect has revealed that the G1107D replacement not only reduces the stability of calmodulin binding to the pump but also impairs the autoinhibition mechanism of the PMCA3 pump (Calì et al., manuscript in preparation, 2016). Recently, a few additional mutations in PMCA3 gene have been found. The first mutation (an arginine to histidine substitution [R482H]) was found in a patient with developmental delay, hypotonia, and cerebellar ataxia; in analogy with what was observed for the other PMCA3 mutation, the Ca^{2+} extrusion ability of the mutated pumps was found to be decreased.[81] Interestingly, in this case, the patient also carried compound heterozygous mutations in the *LAMA1* gene encoding laminin subunit 1α (a maternally inherited T2025M substitution and a paternally inherited R2381C substitution) that appeared to be necessary for the development of the disease. The other mutations in human PMCA3 have been reported in nonneuronal disease phenotypes; for example, a missense Y543M substitution between the catalytic Asp and the ATP-binding site has been linked to pancreatic cancer cells,[82] and an in-frame deletion of two amino acids at positions 425 and 426 in the M4 transmembrane helix has been described in aldosterone-producing adenomas.[83]

Final Comments

The pumps that transport Ca^{2+} across membranes control the homeostasis of Ca^{2+} in all animal cells. In those of nonexcitable tissues, which are not exposed to the periodical increases of cytosolic Ca^{2+} to levels that may reach the micromolar range, they are the most important or even the sole systems that maintain cytosolic Ca^{2+} at the physiological nM level. They can do so because they interact with Ca^{2+} with the appropriate high affinity. In excitable tissues, the ejection of Ca^{2+} from the cytosol is instead mostly performed by a larger, lower affinity system, the Na/Ca exchanger. Ca^{2+} pumps still exist in the internal membranes of excitable cells, and even in their plasma membrane, but their role in the control of Ca^{2+} homeostasis, at least at the peak of the Ca^{2+} transients that are essential for the physiology of these cells, is overshadowed by the activity of the exchanger. The case of heart is special because PMCA pumps have been conclusively documented in heart sarcolemma, but their role in the ejection of bulk Ca^{2+} from the sarcoplasm, especially in phase with the contraction–relaxation cycle, has always been considered unrealistic. Consistent evidence, however, now indicates that the sarcolemmal Ca^{2+} pump (isoform 4) has a Ca^{2+}-signaling role that is quantitatively unimportant, as expected, in the control of bulk sarcoplasmic Ca^{2+}, but which is still critical to the contraction-relaxation cycle in more subtle ways, linked to the modulation of the cyclic nucleotide balance. Perhaps a role of the PMCA pumps in Ca^{2+} signaling not immediately linked to the bulk ejection of Ca^{2+} will in the future be extended to other excitable cells as well.

Acknowledgment

The authors are grateful to Dr. C. Toyoshima (Tokyo, Japan) for providing the image of the SERCA pump structure in Fig. 5.2 and the cartoon in Fig. 5.3, Dr. L. Raeymaekers (Leuven, Belgium) for providing the structural model of the SPCA pump in Fig. 5.4, and Dr. S. Pantano (Montevideo, Uruguay) for providing the model of PMCA in Fig. 5.5.

The original work by the authors has been supported over the years by grants from the Italian Ministry of University and Research (FIRB2001 to E.C., PRIN 2003, 2005, 2008 to M.B), the Telethon Foundation (Project GGP04169), the Italian National Research Council (CNR), and the University of Padova (Progetto di Ateneo 2008, CPDA082825) to M.B. and the FP6 program of the European Union (FP6 Network of Excellence NeuroNe, LSH-2003-2.1.3-3, Integrated Project Eurohear), the Human Frontier Science Program Organization, and the Fondazione Cariparo (Progetti di Eccellenza 2008-2009), ERA-Net Neuron (grant nEUROsyn 2008) to E.C.

REFERENCES

1. Pedersen P, Carafoli E. Ion motive ATPases. I. Ubiquity, properties, and significance to cell function. *Trends Biochem Sci*. 1987;12:146–150.
2. Axelsen KB, Palmgren MG. Evolution of substrate specificities in the P-type ATPase Superfamily. *J Mol Evol*. 1998;46:84–101.
3. Toyoshima C, Nakasako M, Nomura H, Ogawa H. Crystal structure of the calcium pump of sarcoplasmic reticulum at 2.6 A resolution. *Nature*. 2000;405: 647–655.
4. de Meis L, Vianna AL. Energy interconversion by the Ca2+-dependent ATPase of the sarcoplasmic reticulum. *Ann RevBiochem*. 1979;48:275–292.
5. Toyoshima C, Cornelius F. New crystal structures of PII-type ATPases: excitement continues. *Curr Opin Struct Biol*. 2013;23:507–514.
6. Hasselbach W, Makinose M. The calcium pump of the "relaxing granules" of muscle and its dependence on ATP-splitting. *Biochem Z*. 1961;333:518–528.
7. Dang D, Rao R. Calcium-ATPases: gene disorders and dysregulation in cancer. *Biochim Biophys Acta*. 2016;1863:1344–1350.
8. Thastrup O, Cullen PJ, Drobak BK, Hanley MR, Dawson AP. Thapsigargin, a tumor promoter, discharges intracellular Ca2+ stores by specific inhibition of the endoplasmic reticulum Ca2(+)-ATPase. *Proc Natl Acad Sci U S A*. 1990;87:2466–2470.
9. Seidler NW, Jona I, Vegh M, Martonosi A. Cyclopiazonic acid is a specific inhibitor of the Ca2+-ATPase of sarcoplasmic reticulum. *J Biol Chem*. 1989;264:17816–17823.
10. Oldershaw KA, Taylor CW. 2,5-Di-(tert-butyl)-1,4-benzohydroquinone mobilizes inositol 1,4,5-trisphosphate-sensitive and -insensitive Ca2+ stores. *FEBS Lett*. 1990;274:214–216.
11. Brini M, Carafoli E. Calcium pumps in health and disease. *Physiol Rev*. 2009;89:1341–1378.
12. Moller JV, Nissen P, Sorensen TL, le Maire M. Transport mechanism of the sarcoplasmic reticulum Ca2+ -ATPase pump. *Curr Opin Struct Biol*. 2005;15:387–393.
13. Toyoshima C. How Ca2+-ATPase pumps ions across the sarcoplasmic reticulum membrane. *Biochim Biophys Acta*. 2009;1793:941–946.
14. Periasamy M, Bhupathy P, Babu GJ. Regulation of sarcoplasmic reticulum Ca2+ ATPase pump expression and its relevance to cardiac muscle physiology and pathology. *Cardiovasc Res*. 2008;77:265–273.
15. Kranias EG, Hajjar RJ. Modulation of cardiac contractility by the phopholamban/SERCA2a regulatome. *Circ Res*. 2012;110:1646–1660.
16. Traaseth NJ, Ha KN, Verardi R, et al. Structural and dynamic basis of phospholamban and sarcolipin inhibition of Ca(2+)-ATPase. *Biochemistry*. 2008;47:3–13.
17 Shaikh SA, Sahoo SK, Periasamy M. Phospholamban and sarcolipin: are they functionally redundant or distinct regulators of the sarco(endo)plasmic reticulum calcium ATPase? *J Mol Cell Cardiol*. 2016;91:81–91.
18. Gramolini AO, Trivieri MG, Oudit GY, et al. Cardiac-specific overexpression of sarcolipin in phospholamban null mice impairs myocyte function that is restored by phosphorylation. *Proc Natl Acad Sci U S A*. 2006;103:2446–2451.
19. Vandecaetsbeek I, Trekels M, De Maeyer M, et al. Structural basis for the high Ca2+ affinity of the ubiquitous SERCA2b Ca2+ pump. *Proc Natl Acad Sci U S A*. 2009;106:18533–18538.
20. Gorski PA, Trieber CA, Lariviere E, et al. Transmembrane helix 11 is a genuine regulator of the endoplasmic reticulum Ca2+ pump and acts as a functional parallel of beta-subunit on alpha-Na+,K+-ATPase. *J Biol Chem*. 2012;287:19876–19885.
21. Li Y, Camacho P. Ca2+-dependent redox modulation of SERCA 2b by ERp57. *J Cell Biol*. 2004;164:35–46.
22. Daiho T, Yamasaki K, Saino T, et al. Mutations of either or both Cys876 and Cys888 residues of sarcoplasmic reticulum Ca2+-ATPase result in a complete loss of Ca2+ transport activity without a loss of Ca2+-dependent ATPase activity. Role of the CYS876-CYS888 disulfide bond. *J Biol Chem*. 2001;276:32771–32778.
23. Arvanitis DA, Vafiadaki E, Fan GC, et al. Histidine-rich Ca-binding protein interacts with sarcoplasmic reticulum Ca-ATPase. *Am J Physiol Heart Circ Physiol*. 2007;293:H1581-1589.
24. Vandecaetsbeek I, Vangheluwe P, Raeymaekers L, Wuytack F, Vanoevelen J. The Ca2+ pumps of the endoplasmic reticulum and Golgi apparatus. *Cold Spring Harb Perspect Biol*. 2011;3:a004184.
25. Missiaen L, Van Acker K, Van Baelen K, et al. Calcium release from the Golgi apparatus and the endoplasmic reticulum in HeLa cells stably expressing targeted aequorin to these compartments. *Cell Calcium*. 2004;36:479–487.
26. Pavlikova M, Tatarkova Z, Sivonova M, Kaplan P, KrizanovaO, LehotskyJ. Alterations induced by ischemic preconditioning on secretory pathways Ca2+-ATPase (SPCA) gene expression and oxidative damage after global cerebral ischemia/reperfusion in rats. *Cell Mol Neurobiol*. 2009;29:909–916.
27. Pizzo P, Lissandron V, Capitanio P, Pozzan T. Ca(2+) signaling in the Golgi apparatus. *Cell Calcium*. 2011;50:184–192.
28. Caroni P, Carafoli E. An ATP-dependent Ca2+-pumping system in dog heart sarcolemma. *Nature*. 1980;283:765–767.
29. Brini M, Calì T, Ottolini D, Carafoli E. The plasma membrane calcium pump in health and disease. *FEBS J*. 2013;280:5385–5397.
30. Guerini D, Zecca-Mazza A, Carafoli E. Single amino acid mutations in transmembrane domain 5 confer to the plasma membrane Ca2+ pump properties typical of the Ca2+ pump of endo(sarco)plasmic reticulum. *J Biol Chem*. 2000;275:31361–31368.
31. Brini M, CalÃ T, Ottolini D, Carafoli E. Calcium pumps: why so many? *Compr Physiol*. 2012;2:1045–1060.
32. Krebs J. The plethora of PMCA isoforms: alternative splicing and differential expression. *Biochim Biophys Acta*. 2015;1853:2018–2024.
33. Lopreiato R, Giacomello M, Carafoli E. The plasma membrane calcium pump: new ways to look at an old enzyme. *J Biol Chem*. 2014;289:10261–10268.
34. Strehler EE. Plasma membrane calcium ATPases: from generic Ca(2+) sump pumps to versatile systems for fine-tuning cellular Ca(2.). *Biochem Biophys Res Commun*. 2015;460:26–33.
35. Okunade GW, Miller ML, Pyne GJ, et al. Targeted ablation of plasma membrane Ca2+-ATPase (PMCA) 1 and 4 indicates a major housekeeping function for PMCA1 and a critical role in hyperactivated sperm motility and male fertility for PMCA4. *J Biol Chem*. 2004;279:33742–33750.
36. Schuh K, Cartwright EJ, Jankevics E, et al. Plasma membrane Ca2+ ATPase 4 is required for sperm motility and male fertility. *J Biol Chem*. 2004;279:28220–28226.
37. Mohamed TM, Oceandy D, Zi M, et al. Plasma membrane calcium pump (PMCA4)-neuronal nitric-oxide synthase complex regulates cardiac contractility through modulation of a compartmentalized cyclic nucleotide microdomain. *J Biol Chem*. 2011;286:41520–41529.
38. Niggli V, Penniston JT, Carafoli E. Purification of the (Ca2+-Mg2+)-ATPase from human erythrocyte membranes using a calmodulin affinity column. *J Biol Chem*. 1979;254:9955–9958.
39. Elshorst B, Hennig M, Forsterling H, et al. NMR solution structure of a complex of calmodulin with a binding peptide of the Ca2+ pump. *Biochemistry*. 1999;38:12320–12332.
40. Tidow H, Poulsen LR, Andreeva A, et al. A bimodular mechanism of calcium control in eukaryotes. *Nature*. 2012;491:468–472.
41. Falchetto R, Vorherr T, Brunner J, Carafoli E. The plasma membrane Ca2+ pump contains a site that interacts with its calmodulin-binding domain. *J Biol Chem*. 1991;266:2930–2936.
42. Falchetto R, Vorherr T, Carafoli E. The calmodulin-binding site of the plasma membrane Ca2+ pump interacts with the transduction domain of the enzyme. *Protein Sci*. 1992;1:1613–1621.
43. Niggli V, Adunyah ES, Carafoli E. Acidic phospholipids, unsaturated fatty acids, and limited proteolysis mimic the effect of calmodulin on the purified erythrocyte Ca2+ -ATPase. *J Biol Chem*. 1982;256:8588–8592.
44. Ortega C, Ortolano S, Carafoli E. The plasma membrane calcium pump. In: Krebs J, Michalak M, eds. *Calcium: A Matter of Life or Death*. Vol. 41. Paris: Elsevier; 2007:179–197.
45. Strehler EE, Zacharias DA. Role of alternative splicing in generating isoform diversity among plasma membrane calcium pumps. *Physiol Rev*. 2001;81:21–50.
46. Chicka MC, Strehler EE. Alternative splicing of the first intracellular loop of plasma membrane Ca2+-ATPase isoform 2 alters its membrane targeting. *J Biol Chem*. 2003;278:18464–18470.
47. Brini M, Coletto L, Pierobon N, Kraev N, Guerini D, Carafoli E. A comparative functional analysis of plasma membrane Ca2+ pump isoforms in intact cells. *J Biol Chem*. 2003;278:24500–24508.
48. Preiano BS, Guerini D, Carafoli E. Expression and functional characterization of isoforms 4 of the plasma membrane calcium pump. *Biochemistry*. 1996;35:7946–7953.
49. Elwess NL, Filoteo AG, Enyedi A, Penniston JT. Plasma membrane Ca2+ pump isoforms 2a and 2b are unusually responsive to calmodulin and Ca2+. *J Biol Chem*. 1997;272:17981–17986.
50. Hilfiker H, Guerini D, Carafoli E. Cloning and expression of isoform 2 of the human plasma membrane Ca2+ ATPase. Functional properties of the enzyme and its splicing products. *J Biol Chem*. 1994;269:26178–26183.
51. Carafoli E. The interplay of mitochondria with calcium: an historical appraisal. *Cell Calcium*. 2012;52:1–8.
52. Odermatt A, Barton K, Khanna VK, et al. The mutation of Pro789 to Leu reduces the activity of the fast-twitch skeletal muscle sarco(endo)plasmic reticulum Ca2+ ATPase (SERCA1) and is associated with Brody disease. *Hum Genet*. 2000;106:482–491.
53. Odermatt A, Taschner PE, Khanna VK, et al. Mutations in the gene-encoding SERCA1, the fast-twitch skeletal muscle sarcoplasmic reticulum Ca2+ ATPase, are associated with Brody disease. *Nat Genet*. 1996;14:191–194.
54. Drogemuller C, Drogemuller M, Leeb T, et al. Identification of a missense mutation in the bovine ATP2A1 gene in congenital pseudomyotonia of Chianina cattle: an animal model of human Brody disease. *Genomics*. 2008;92:474–477.
55. Charlier C, Coppieters W, Rollin F, et al. Highly effective SNP-based association mapping and management of recessive defects in livestock. *Nat Genet*. 2008;40:449–454.
56. Grunberg W, Sacchetto R, Wijnberg I, et al. Pseudo-myotonia, a muscle function disorder associated with an inherited ATP2A1 (SERCA1) defect in a Dutch improved red and white cross-breed calf, Neuromuscular disorders. *NMD*. 2010;20:467–470.
57. Dhitavat J, Macfarlane S, Dode L, et al. Acrokeratosis verruciformis of Hopf is caused by mutation in ATP2A2: evidence that it is allelic to Darier's disease. *J Invest Dermatol*. 2003;120:229–232.
58. Eisner D, Caldwell J, Trafford A. Sarcoplasmic reticulum Ca-ATPase and heart failure 20 years later. *Circ Res*. 2013;113:958–961.
59. Arbabian A, Brouland JP, Gélébart P, et al. Endoplasmic reticulum calcium pumps and cancer. *Biofactors*. 2011;37: 139–149.
60. Schmidt AG, Haghighi K, Frank B, et al. Polymorphic SERCA2a variants do not account for inter-individual differences in phospholamban-SERCA2a interactions in human heart failure. *J Mol Cell Cardio*. 2003;35:867–870.
61. Chami M, Gozuacik D, Saigo K, et al. Hepatitis B virus-related insertional mutagenesis implicates SERCA1 gene in the control of apoptosis. *Oncogene*. 2000;19:2877–2886.
62. Ikeda S, Shigihara T, Mayuzumi N, Yu X, Ogawa H. Mutations of ATP2C1 in Japanese patients with Hailey-Hailey disease: intrafamilial and interfamilial phenotype variations and lack of correlation with mutation patterns. *J Invest Dermatol*. 2001;117:1654–1656.
63. Dode L, Andersen JP, Leslie N, Dhitavat J, Vilsen B, HovnanianA. Dissection of the functional differences between sarco(endo)plasmic reticulum Ca2+-ATPase (SERCA) 1 and 2 isoforms and characterization of Darier disease (SERCA2) mutants by steady-state and transient kinetic analyses. *J Biol Chem*. 2003;278:47877–47889.
64. Fairclough RJ, Lonie L, Van Baelen K, et al. Hailey-Hailey disease: identification of novel mutations in ATP2C1 and effect of missense mutation A528P on protein expression levels. *J Invest Dermatol*. 2004;123:67–71.
65. Micaroni M, Giacchetti G, Plebani R, Xiao GG, Federici L. ATP2C1 gene mutations in Hailey-Hailey disease and possible roles of SPCA1 isoforms in membrane trafficking. *Cell Death Dis*. 2016;7:e2259.

66. Newbury DF, Winchester L, Addis L, et al. CMIP and ATP2C2 modulate phonological short-term memory in language impairment. *Am J Hum Genet*. 2009;85:264–272.

67. Brini M, Carafoli E, Calì T. The plasma membrane calcium pumps: focus on the role in (neuro)pathology. *Biochem Biophys Res Commun*. 2016 Jul 29. [Epub ahead of print].

68. Grati M, Aggarwal N, Strehler EE, Wenthold RJ. Molecular determinants for differential membrane trafficking of PMCA1 and PMCA2 in mammalian hair cells. *J Cell Sci*. 2006;119:2995–3007.

69. Street VA, McKee-Johnson JW, Fonseca RC, Tempel BL, Noben-Trauth K. Mutations in a plasma membrane Ca2+-ATPase gene cause deafness in deafwaddler mice. *Nat Genet*. 1998;19:390–394.

70. Schultz JM, YangY Caride AJ, Filoteo AG, et al. Modification of human hearing loss by plasma-membrane calcium pump PMCA2. *N Engl J Med*. 2005;352:1557–1564.

71. Ficarella R, Di Leva F, Bortolozzi M, et al. A functional study of plasma-membrane calcium-pump isoform 2 mutants causing digenic deafness. *Proc Natl Acad Sci U S A*. 2007;104:1516–1521.

72. Giacomello M, De Mario A, Lopreiato R, et al. Mutations in PMCA2 and hereditary deafness: a molecular analysis of the pump defect. *Cell Calcium*. 2011;50:569–576.

73. Li M, Ho PW, Pang SY, et al. PMCA4 (ATP2B4) mutation in familial spastic paraplegia. *PLoS One*. 2014;9:e104790.

74. Ho PW, Pang SY, Li M, et al. PMCA4 (ATP2B4) mutation in familial spastic paraplegia causes delay in intracellular calcium extrusion. *Brain Behav*. 2015;5:e00321.

75. Cho YS, Go MJ, Kim YJ, et al. A large-scale genome-wide association study of Asian populations uncovers genetic factors influencing eight quantitative traits. *Nat Genet*. 2009;41:527–534.

76. Hong KW, Go MJ, Jin HS, et al. Genetic variations in ATP2B1, CSK, ARSG and CSMD1 loci are related to blood pressure and/or hypertension in two Korean cohorts. *J Hum Hypertens*. 2010;24:367–372.

77. Tabara Y, Kohara K, Kita Y. Global Blood Pressure Genetics Consortium. Common variants in the ATP2B1 gene are associated with susceptibility to hypertension: the Japanese Millennium Genome Project. *Hypertension*. 2010;56:973–980.

78. Xi B, Shen Y, Zhao X, et al. Association of common variants in/near six genes (ATP2B1, CSK, MTHFR, CYP17A1, STK39 and FGF5) with blood pressure/hypertension risk in Chinese children. *J Hum Hypertens*. 2014;28:32–36.

79. Lu X, Wang L, Chen S, et al. Genome-wide association study in Han Chinese identifies four new susceptibility loci for coronary artery disease. *Nat Genet*. 2012;44:890–894.

80. Zanni G, Calì T, Kalscheuer VM, et al. Mutation of plasma membrane Ca2+ ATPase isoform 3 in a family with X-linked congenital cerebellar ataxia impairs Ca2+ homeostasis. *Proc Natl Acad Sci U S A*. 2012;109:14514–14519.

81. Calì T, Lopreiato R, Shimony J, et al. A novel mutation in isoform 3 of the plasma membrane Ca2+ pump impairs cellular Ca2+ homeostasis in a patient with cerebellar ataxia and laminin subunit 1alpha mutations. *J Biol Chem*. 2015;290:16132–16141.

82. Jones S, Zhang X, Parsons DW, et al. Core signaling pathways in human pancreatic cancers revealed by global genomic analyses. *Science*. 2008;321:1801–1806.

83. Beuschlein F, Boulkroun S, Osswald A, et al. 2013. Somatic mutations in ATP1A1 and ATP2B3 lead to aldosterone-producing adenomas and secondary hypertension. *Nat Genet*. 2013;45:440–444. 444e1-2.

84. Toyoshima C. Structural aspects of ion pumping by Ca2+-ATPase of sarcoplasmic reticulum. *Arch Biochem Biophys*. 2008;476:3–11.

6 Structural and Molecular Bases of Sarcoplasmic Reticulum Ion Channel Function

Bin Liu, Sándor Györke, and Przemysław B. Radwański

The Sarcoplasmic Reticulum

Structural Arrangement of the Sarcoplasmic Reticulum

The sarcoplasmic reticulum (SR) is a membrane-delimited intracellular organelle that spans the sarcomere and wraps up the contractile myofilaments in striated muscle of almost all species.[1] The SR is not continuous with the external membrane, but recent data indicate that it is continuous with the nuclear envelope.[2] In striated muscle, the main function of the SR is to provide the majority of Ca^{2+} ions required to activate the myofilaments and to resequester Ca^{2+} from the myoplasm to allow for relaxation. The compartmentalization of muscle fibers into small (~2 μm) structural–functional units (sarcomeres) and the enveloping of sarcomeres by SR both ensure that Ca^{2+} diffusion from and reuptake into the SR is not a limiting step for the muscle contractile cycle.

The SR is composed of two regions: junctional SR (jSR), which directly faces invaginations of the surface membrane, called *transverse tubules* (T-tubules), and extrajunctional free SR (fSR), which is situated near the myofibrils. jSR forms extended, flattened cisternae with an average diameter of around 0.6 μm.[3] Each cisterna carries sets of closely grouped structures ("feet") that represent the cardiac SR Ca^{2+} release channels, also known as *ryanodine receptors* (RyR2s), and contains dense material, which is formed by the Ca^{2+}-binding protein, calsequestrin-2 (CASQ2).[4] On the other hand, the fSR is devoid of CASQ2, and its external surface exhibits densely distributed particles corresponding to Ca^{2+} adenosine triphosphatase (ATPase).

Molecular Players of Excitation–Contraction Coupling

During the systolic action potential, the opening of L-type Ca^{2+} channels (LCC) or dihydropyridine receptors on the invaginations of sarcolemmal membrane, dubbed the T-tubules, allow Ca^{2+} influx into the cell that in turn activates RyR2s on the SR membrane, thus triggering Ca^{2+}-induced Ca^{2+} release (CICR) from the SR.[5,6] The SR-derived Ca^{2+} thereby contributes to the Ca^{2+} transient responsible for the excitation–contraction coupling (ECC) process. Cardiac ECC is structurally organized into discrete units called *couplons*. A couplon consists of a group of LCCs within a T-tubule that juxtapose a larger cluster of RyR2s on the surface of the jSR. Within a couplon the LCCs and the RyR2s are separated by a narrow gap (~12 nm).[7] This gap forms a restricted domain ("fuzzy" space) such that local elevation of Ca^{2+} derived from LCCs results in opening of RyR2s. The resulting local Ca^{2+} signals ("sparks") then sum to form a global Ca^{2+} transient. In addition to the jSR, LCCs and RyR2s interact at peripheral couplings, the points of contact between the SR and the sarcolemmal surface.[8] The portion of peripheral couplons is substantially smaller than those localized in the interior of the myocyte owing to the smaller surface area.

In addition to LCCs, the Na^+/Ca^{2+} exchanger (NCX), distributed throughout the surface membrane,[9] plays a major role modulating CICR in the jSR of the cardiac muscle. Outside of being the dominant Ca^{2+} efflux mechanism, NCX affects Ca^{2+} concentration near jSR couplons. Specifically, in response to Na^+ influx during the systolic action potential, NCX primes the jSR couplon cleft with Ca^{2+}, thereby increasing the ECC gain.[10]

Molecular Structure of the Cardiac Ryanodine Receptor

Three isoforms of RyR have been identified in mammals, including RyR1 and RyR2, which are expressed mainly in skeletal and cardiac muscle respectively, and RyR3, which is found in several cell types but remains the least understood. All the isoforms are highly homologous with up to 70% amino acid sequence identity.[11–13] The homotetrameric RyR complex of more than 2.2 million Da is one of the largest known ion channels. Deciphering the molecular structure of this channel has long been a challenge, given the enormous size of the protein complex. Previous studies have revealed the overall RyR structure as a four-fold symmetric mushroom-like shape, with the cap of the mushroom (80% of the mass) residing in the cytosol and the stalk embedded in the SR membranes. However, several important details of the structure were missing. Recent advances in single-particle cryo-electron microscopy (EM) lead to significant progress in determining the molecular structure of the RyR protein complex, reaching an unprecedented resolution of 3.8 Å.[14] Three independent groups have pioneered this endeavor and they all agreed that the four RyR protomers are arranged in four-fold symmetry, surrounding a central transmembrane pore.[14–16] All three studies reported the structure of the skeletal isoform of RyR1, which is in general similar to that of the cardiac isoform, RyR2. Their work defined the locations of several important domains, such as the phosphorylation domains (also known as *repeat 3–4 of RyR*), Ca^{2+}-binding EF hand, and the three SPRY domains, which probably serve as a structural scaffold for the repeat domain (Fig. 6.1). Notably, the cytosolic part of the RyR protomer is built around an extended α-solenoid scaffold, which interacts with regulatory proteins and transmits conformational changes to the pore.

The existence of six transmembrane segments in each subunit of the channel tetramer was also confirmed by the three groups independently. For instance, Marks' group[15] determined that the transmembrane region is divided into two parts: the ion conducting

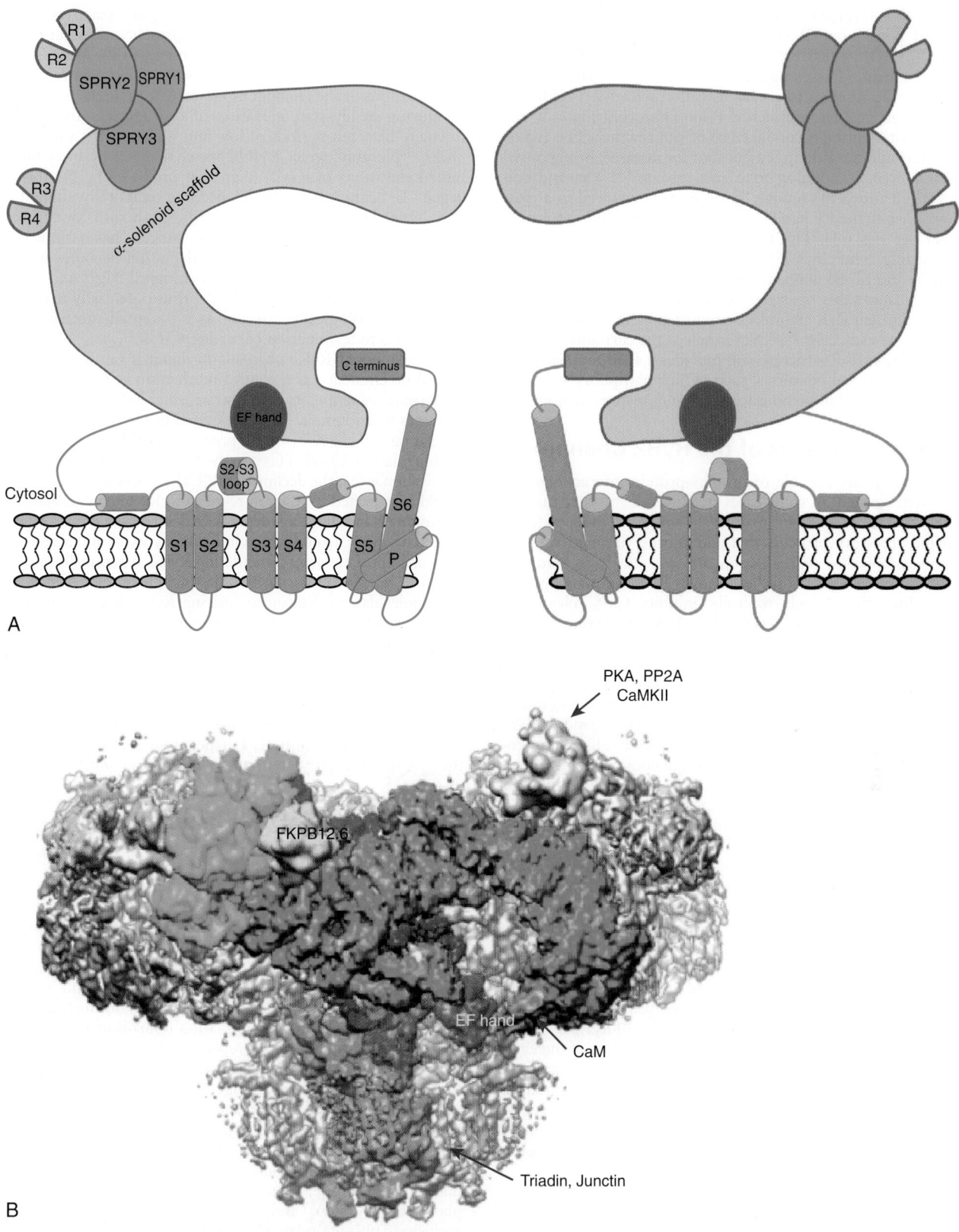

FIGURE 6.1 Representations of the ryanodine receptor (RyR) channel. (A) Color-coded scheme of RyR structure, with the α-solenoid scaffold shown in *blue*, SPRY domains in *cyan*, RyR repeats in *purple*, EF hand Ca^{2+}-binding domain in *darker purple* and transmembrane segments in *orange*. Two subunits are shown for clarity. (B) Three-dimensional surface representations of the RyR structure, with the EF hand Ca^{2+}-binding site, putative protein binding sites, and phosphorylation domain labeled. (Modified from Zalk R, Clarke OB, des Georges A, et al. Structure of a mammalian ryanodine receptor. *Nature*. 2015;517:44-49.)

pore, which is formed by S5, S6, the pore helix (p-helix), and the canonical pore loop (P-loop); and the pseudo voltage–sensor domain (pVSD), which comprises S1–S4 and interacts with the cytosolic domain. The elongated pore-forming S6 helix contains multiple acidic residues to confer its cation selectivity. Additionally, the negative charge–enriched P-loop also contributes to the ion selectivity and high conductance of the channel. The region between S5 and the P-loop is a hot spot for disease-causing mutations. Of note, in addition to Marks' group,[14,15] Yan and colleagues[14] identified the unique S2–S3 loop as involved in a close interaction with the EF hand Ca^{2+}-binding motif in the α-solenoid scaffold (see Fig. 6.1). This then suggests a novel mechanism for RyR opening, whereby Ca^{2+} binding to the EF hand is directly sensed by the S2–S3 loop, thereby eliciting subsequent conformational changes that open the ion conducting pore. Despite the largely congruent RyR architecture reported by these studies, several differences still exist.[14–16] Nevertheless, the currently available high-resolution RyR structure still provides a solid foundation to answer some critical questions, such as how phosphorylation and disease-causing mutations alter RyR structure to exert their effects.

Accessory Proteins of the RyR2 Channel

RyR2 channels are capable of protein–protein interactions that allow them to bind, in some cases steadily and in other cases in a time- and Ca^{2+}-dependent manner, to small and independently regulated accessory proteins that add another layer of versatility (and complexity) to regulation of Ca^{2+} release in vivo (see Fig. 6.1). Following are the best-known RyR2-interacting proteins: calmodulin, which tonically inhibits Ca^{2+} release[17,18]; FK506 binding protein 12.6 (FKBP12.6), which presumably stabilizes RyR2 closures[19–21]; sorcin, which inhibits Ca^{2+} release in a Ca^{2+}-dependent manner[22–24]; and the ternary complex triadin-junctin-CASQ2, along with histidine-rich Ca^{2+}-binding protein (HRC),[25] which "senses" luminal Ca^{2+} content and modulates RyR2 activity by acting either as a direct channel ligand or as an immediate source of releasable Ca^{2+}.[26,27] S100A1,[28] like calmodulin and sorcin, inhibits RyR2 more conspicuously when $[Ca^{2+}]$ is high; therefore these three proteins along with the intraluminal "sensors" might play a role in Ca^{2+}-mediated CICR termination. More recently, RyR2 has been found to hold anchoring sites for cyclic adenosine monophosphate (cAMP)-dependent protein kinase A (PKA), protein phosphatase 2 (PP2A), cAMP-specific phosphodiesterase (PDE4D3), and Ca^{2+}/calmodulin-dependent protein kinase II (CaMKII),[29] underscoring the importance of RyR2 regulation by phosphorylation. It is still unclear how this complex of proteins interplays in situ to regulate Ca^{2+} release. Deciphering the binding sites of these proteins on the RyR2 multimolecular machinery could shed light on the functional mechanisms of these proteins. For instance, previous studies have determined that the calmodulin-binding region of RyR2 resides in the cleft between the "handle" and "clamp" domains of the cytosolic part of RyR2.[30] Recent findings have further delineated the calmodulin-binding region to a solvent-exposed protrusion in the α-solenoid scaffold.[16] Additionally, the FKBP12.6 binding region has been identified at the interface between the SPRY domain and a region of the α-solenoid scaffold that does not directly interact with the SPRY domain, thus bridging the two regions.[16]

Ca^{2+} Regulation of RyR2 Channels

Ca^{2+} binds to the cytosolic and luminal domains of RyR2s and regulates the activity of the channel in a concentration- and time-dependent manner. Under stationary (nonfluctuating) $[Ca^{2+}]$, the activity of single RyR2 channels is a bell-shaped function of cytosolic $[Ca^{2+}]$ because of the presence of Ca^{2+}-activating and -inactivating sites.[31–33] Ca^{2+} in the range of 0.1 to 10 μM binds to at least one Ca^{2+}-binding domain that activates RyR2s. Higher $[Ca^{2+}]$ (100 μM–3 mM) then inactivates the channel.[33] The

affinity and cooperativity of the activating and inactivating Ca^{2+}-binding sites vary greatly under the presence of other relevant modulators (e.g., adenosine triphosphate [ATP], Mg^{2+}, and H^+) and constitute powerful mechanisms by which posttranslational modifications of the channel modulate Ca^{2+} release.

During steady-state elevation of Ca^{2+}, RyR2s are known to fluctuate between periods of low and high activity, called *gating modes*.[34] Notably, when RyR2s are challenged by brief but sustained elevations of $[Ca^{2+}]$ (e.g., that produced by photolysis of caged Ca^{2+}), the gating modes become temporally aligned such that initial bursts of high activity diminish to a lower level of steady-state open probability. This process has a time course of ~1 s and is called *adaptation*.[34] Adaptation becomes markedly accelerated in the presence of physiological Mg^{2+} and ATP, as well as upon reducing luminal Ca^{2+}, thus potentially making this process physiologically relevant as a potential mechanism that contributes to termination of cardiac CICR.[35]

Regulation of RyR2 channels by luminal (intra-SR) Ca^{2+} has gained preeminence as a control mechanism of Ca^{2+} release. Single channel experiments demonstrated that RyR2 open probability increases when luminal Ca^{2+} is elevated in the micromolar to millimolar range. The AC_{50} of this process (~1 mM) corresponds to the resting (diastolic) level of Ca^{2+} in the SR. An important physiological implication is that the decline of SR $[Ca^{2+}]$ following SR Ca^{2+} release would be expected to result in reduced RyR2 activity (deactivation). A temporary luminal Ca^{2+}-dependent deactivation of Ca^{2+} signaling indeed has been demonstrated in cardiomyocytes and is considered to be an important factor in rendering RyR2s functionally unresponsive (i.e., refractory) during the diastolic phase (discussed further). The molecular mechanism underlying RyR2 deactivation remains uncertain and is likely due to a combination of several factors including the following: (1) direct interaction of Ca^{2+} with the RyR2 domains available only from luminal side of the SR,[36] (2) indirect interaction of Ca^{2+} with the RyR2 through CASQ2- and HRC-triadin-junctin complex, and (3) reduced activation of the cytosolic sites of the RyR2 by the Ca^{2+} ions that permeate through the channel (feed-through mechanism).[37] Further studies are needed to define the specific molecular determinants of luminal regulation.

Modulation of RyR2 Channel Function

Phosphorylation

Sympathetic stimulation of the heart improves cardiac output by accelerating heart rate and increasing the force of contractions. Activation of the β-adrenergic receptor pathway by catecholamines triggers a cascade of events that increases cAMP, which in turn activates PKA and CaMKII. RyR2 channels are structural scaffolds for important kinases and phosphatases[19,29] and are one of the first proteins to undergo phosphorylation during β-adrenergic stimulation.[38–40] The phosphorylation domain of RyR2 has been located in the so-called RyR2 repeats embedded within the central regions of the protein complex.[41] More specifically, the α-helical RyR2 repeat 3 and 4 are arranged in two-fold symmetry and are connected by a flexible loop that contains up to five potential phosphorylation sites in addition to the well-studied PKA and CaMKII sites.[42] To date, three phosphorylation sites on RyR2 have been recognized: Ser2809, which was initially identified as a CaMKII phosphorylation site,[43] but was later determined to undergo phosphorylation by PKA[19] and Ser2815 and Ser2030, which seem to be exclusively phosphorylated by CaMKII[44] and PKA,[45] respectively.

Initially the effect of β-adrenergic stimulation on RyR2 had been attributed to PKA-dependent phosphorylation of Ser2809.[19] Phosphorylation of this residue reportedly resulted in increased open probability of RyR2 secondary to dissociation of FKBP12.6.[19] The resultant Ca^{2+} leak precipitated a reduction in Ca^{2+} transient amplitude and the resultant decreased systolic contractility in the failing heart. However, subsequent studies have failed to demonstrate increased RyR2 activity or facilitated

FKBP12.6 dissociation during phosphorylation of Ser2809.[46–48] On the other hand, a vast body of evidence has accumulated to suggest that RyR2 phosphorylation by CaMKII at Ser2815 stimulates RyR2 activity during both physiological modulation and in cardiac disease (discussed later). Nevertheless some controversies remain. For instance, dephosphorylation of RyR2 by PP1 and PP2a has been shown to increase rather than decrease RyR2 function.[35,49,50] Thus more work is needed to resolve the role of RyR2 phosphorylation in cardiac performance in general and in SR Ca^{2+} leak and heart failure (HF) in particular.

Oxidation and Nitrosylation

RyR2 channels (as well as RyR1 channels) can be powerfully modulated in vitro by oxidative modifications of thiol residues in free cysteines, such as S-nitrosylation, S-glutathionylation, and disulfide oxidation.[47,51–55] Both RyR2 and RyR1 channels contain approximately 100 cysteine residues per monomer, but only a few appear to be highly reactive to oxidants.[56] Furthermore, the functional response of each RyR isoform varies depending on the particular cysteine residue being modified and on the type of oxidative species that targets it, as well as on accessory protein interaction.[51,53,57] For instance, even though RyR2 and RyR1 activity depends on partial pressure of oxygen (pO_2), RyR2 does not appear to be activated through S-nitrosylation directly by nitric oxide (NO) but requires S-nitrosoglutathione for increased activity.[51] Despite the fact that functional effects of oxidation and nitrosylation are well understood, there is a gap in knowledge regarding the precise molecular reactions underlying such functional consequences.

Cytosolic Modulators

Outside of the intrinsic modulators of RyR2, such as the posttranslational modifications outlined above, extrinsic factors such as Na^+ flux have important roles in regulating Ca^{2+} release, especially in pathological states. The RyR2s of junctional and peripheral couplings are likely to face different local cytosolic Na^+ and Ca^{2+} due to differences in domain-specific ion transport systems, including LCC, neuronal Na^+ channels (Na_v1.1, 1.3, 1.6), and NCX.[58,58a] Specifically, Na^+ influx through neuronal Na^+ channels, which colocalize with junctional RyR2, can stimulate Ca^{2+} influx via the NCX, in turn facilitating RyR2 openings[58,58a] (Fig. 6.2). Outside of their unique compartmentation, what is unique about neuronal Na^+ channels is that they inactivate at relatively high potentials

and carry a substantial residual Na^+ current during depolarization.[59,60] Neuronal Na^+ channels have also been shown to exhibit substantial activity at negative membrane potentials, where they are prone to activation and do not completely inactivate.[60] Thus Na^+ flux through neuronal Na^+ channels during diastole may facilitate aberrant proarrhythmic Ca^{2+} release, particularly in a setting of "leaky" RyR2, which is often evidenced in HF or other inherited or acquired RyR2-associated disorders.[58,58a,61]

In addition to Ca^{2+}, other cytosolic factors, such as Mg^{2+}, H^+, and ATP, have important roles in regulating Ca^{2+} release, especially in pathological states (e.g., diabetes or ischemia). Most assays of RyR2 channel activity indicate that free Mg^{2+} (and H^+) inhibits RyR2 channels, whereas ATP increases their activity. Mg^{2+} inhibits RyR2 by at least two mechanisms, one being an ineffective occupation of Ca^{2+}-activation sites and the other being an effective occupation of Ca^{2+}-inactivation sites.[62] ATP, however, binds to nucleotide-binding sites on the channel protein and promotes Ca^{2+} release by acting as a ligand (i.e., without undergoing energy yielding hydrolysis).[63] The fall in pH and ATP levels (plus the concomitant rise in free Mg^{2+}) that is characteristic of prolonged ischemia is therefore expected to depress RyR2 activity and decrease Ca^{2+} release. This could intuitively deteriorate cellular contractility further but could potentially protect the heart by reducing energy consumption. The effect of other cytosolic RyR2 modulators, such as protamines, fatty acids, cyclic adenosine diphosphate (cADP) ribose, and nicotinic acid adenine nucleotide phosphate, on E-C coupling is less understood and is reviewed elsewhere.[64,65]

RyR2 Channels in Disease

RyR channels and their auxiliary proteins are involved in several cardiac diseases. This section discusses only catecholaminergic polymorphic ventricular tachycardia (CPVT) and HF as inherited and acquired, respectively, syndromes linked to the RyR2 channel complex.

Catecholaminergic Polymorphic Ventricular Tachycardia

More than 160 different mutations (and increasing) in *RYR2*, the gene encoding the RyR2 channel protein, have been associated with CPVT, an autosomal-dominant inherited cardiac syndrome characterized by exercise- or stress-induced tachyarrhythmia episodes in the absence of apparent structural heart disease.[66,67]

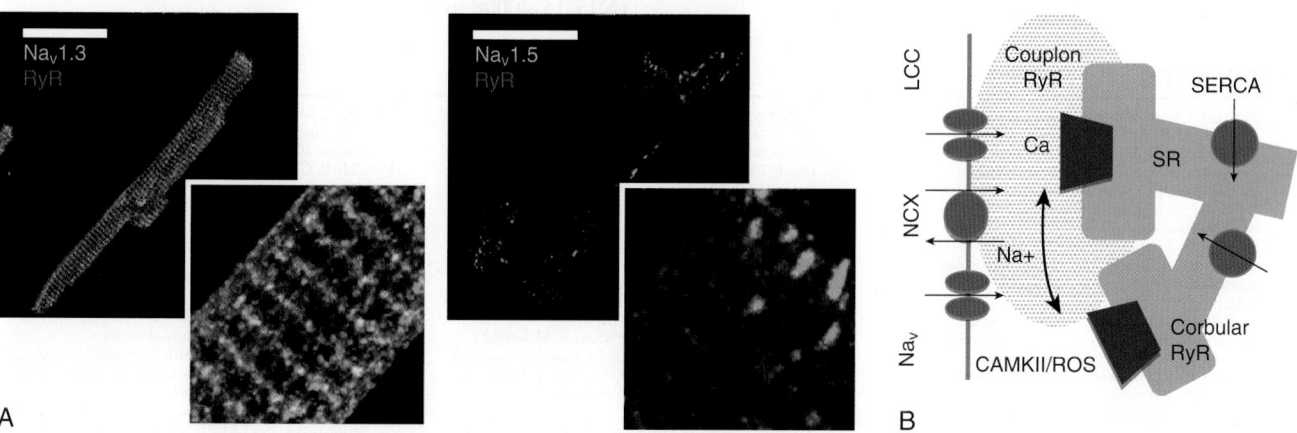

FIGURE 6.2 Subcellular organization of cardiac excitation–contraction coupling (ECC). (A) Representative confocal micrographs of isolated cardiac ventricular myocytes labeled for ryanodine receptors (RyR2) (*red*) and a representative neuronal Na^+ channel isoform (Na_v1.3; *green*). (B) Schematic representing organization of the components of ECC and Na^+/Ca^{2+} signaling. (A, Modified from Radwański PB, Brunello L, Veeraraghavan R, et al. Neuronal Na^+ channel blockade suppresses arrhythmogenic diastolic Ca^{2+} release. *Cardiovasc Res.* 2015;106:143-152.)

Additionally, mutations in genes encoding CASQ2, triadin, and calmodulin[68,69] have been linked to CPVT, suggesting that different molecular defects converge onto a common mechanism of altered Ca^{2+} cycling associated with CPVT. The majority of the RyR2 disease mutations cluster at three "hot spots" that are located in the N terminal of the protein (amino acids 1–600), in a central region (amino acids ~2100–2500), and in the C terminal domain (amino acids ~3900–end).[70] Interestingly, structural studies show that most of the mutations are located at domain-domain interfaces and thus could lead to impaired interdomain interactions.[41] The mechanism of RyR2-linked CVPT has been variably attributed to increased luminal Ca^{2+} sensitivity of RyR2, altered interdomain interactions, or loss of FKBP12.6.[66,71] On the other hand, CASQ2 and triadin mutations have been shown to be mediated by reduced ability of the mutant proteins to convey luminal deactivation to the RyR2.[72,73] At the same time, the ability of calmodulin mutations to cause CPVT[74] supports the potential importance of the cytosolic-dependent inactivation mechanism.[75] Whether and how these different molecular defects converge on RyR2 function to increase arrhythmia vulnerability in CPVT remains to be elucidated.

Aberrant Ca^{2+} release from the SR, during diastole, is accepted as the underlying mechanism that gives rise to ventricular tachyarrhythmias in CPVT.[66,72] The particular mechanism of generation of proarrhythmic aberrant SR Ca^{2+} release was examined using myocytes expressing CPVT-linked CASQ2 mutants. It was demonstrated that premature recovery of RyR2 from a state of refractoriness predisposes the SR Ca^{2+} release channels to spontaneous activation.[73] The resultant aberrant diastolic Ca^{2+} release can activate the Na^+/Ca^{2+} exchanger, which generates an inward current as it extrudes the released Ca^{2+}. The inward current, in turn, depolarizes the cell to a threshold, favoring delayed after-depolarizations and triggered arrythmia.[66] Abbreviated RyR2 refractoriness has been also shown to contribute to synchronization of aberrant Ca^{2+} release in multicellular preparations within arrhythmogenic regions of the ventricular myocardium.[73] Such release synchronization is considered to be essential for the generation of triggered activity in a conglomeration of cells because membrane depolarization occurring randomly in any isolated cell within the myocardium would be dampened by electrically connected neighboring cells acting as current sink. Temporal uniformity of systolic release and of the subsequent SR Ca^{2+} uptake provides a substrate for synchronous generation of aberrant diastolic release in multiple neighboring myocardial cells in which RyR2 refractoriness is uniformly abbreviated.[73] However, it remains to be determined to what extent aberrant Ca^{2+} release and its synchronization in different cardiac tissue types (i.e., ventricular vs. Purkinje fibers) contributes to the generation of CPVT.

Role of RyR2 Channels in Heart Failure

A broad array of primary insults to the cardiovascular system can ultimately lead to the syndrome of HF. Although the pathogenesis of contractile dysfunction at the cardiomyocyte level is extremely complex, a reduction in Ca^{2+} transient amplitude and its prolongation are hallmark features of HF. There is growing consensus that Ca^{2+} mishandling, particularly through the RyR2, leads to reduced systolic contractility and impaired diastolic relaxation. This along with altered gene transcription, resulting in maladaptive structural transformations (cardiac hypertrophy), eventually hampers basic cardiac function (congestive HF). In fact, HF is an inexorable evolving stage in transgenic mice with constitutively activated PKA[76] or CaMKII overexpression.[77] Hyperphosphorylation of Ca^{2+} cycling proteins in these animals, and of RyR2 in particular, eventually results in abnormal Ca^{2+} homeostasis, including increased diastolic leak. Growing evidence links elevated SR Ca^{2+} leak in HF to increased RyR2 phosphorylation by CaMKII on Ser 2815.[47,78,79] In support of the role of increased Ca^{2+} leak via RyR2s as a causal factor in HF, mice deficient in CASQ2 and overexpressing SERCA (to maintain sufficient substrate for SR Ca^{2+} leak) developed cardiomyopathy and died prematurely.[80]

Aside from abnormal phosphorylation, increased oxidation of reactive thiols has been shown to contribute to elevated RyR2-mediated SR Ca^{2+} leak and altered Ca^{2+} transients in failing ventricular myocytes.[47,55] Of note, during natural progression of HF, RyR2 thiol oxidation is preceded by CaMKII-mediated phosphorylation.[47,81] Both of these posttranslational modifications seem to enhance RyR2 activity and increase SR Ca^{2+} leak in similar manner as observed with genetic defects within the RyR2 complex.[81] Thus abbreviated SR Ca^{2+} refractoriness and unchecked diastolic Ca^{2+} release appear to present a common mechanism of genetic and acquired cardiac diseases associated with altered RyR2 function. An important question that awaits elucidation is why apparently mechanistically similar alterations in RyR2-mediated SR Ca^{2+} release lead to such divergent disease states as arrhythmia and HF. Some recent studies suggest that these disease states are manifestations of various stages of the same underlying process (i.e., RyR2 dysfunction)[81]; however, this remains to be confirmed.

Acknowledgment

The authors would like to acknowledge support provided by American Heart Association (15POST25460007 to BL), National Institutes of Health (grants R01-HL074045 and R01-HL063043 to SG; K99-HL127299 to PR); and Russian Science Foundation (N15-15-20008 to SG).

REFERENCES

1. Bers DM. *Excitation-contraction coupling and cardiac contractile force.* 2nd ed. Dordrecht, The Netherlands: Kluwer Academic Press; 2001:427.
2. Wu X, Bers DM. Sarcoplasmic reticulum and nuclear envelope are one highly interconnected Ca^{2+} store throughout cardiac myocyte. *Circ Res.* 2006;99:283–291.
3. Brochet DX, Yang D, Di Maio A, Lederer WJ, Franzini-Armstrong C, Cheng H. Ca^{2+} blinks: rapid nanoscopic store calcium signaling. *Proc Natl Acad Sci U S A.* 2005;102:3099–3104.
4. Tijskens P, Jones LR, Franzini-Armstrong C. Junctin and calsequestrin overexpression in cardiac muscle: the role of junctin and the synthetic and delivery pathways for the two proteins. *J Mol Cell Cardiol.* 2003;35:961–974.
5. Bers DM. Cardiac excitation-contraction coupling. *Nature.* 2002;415:198–205.
6. Fabiato A. Time and calcium dependence of activation and inactivation of calcium-induced release of calcium from the sarcoplasmic reticulum of a skinned canine cardiac Purkinje cell. *J Gen Physiol.* 1985;85:247–289.
7. Hayashi T, Martone ME, Yu Z, et al. Three-dimensional electron microscopy reveals new details of membrane systems for Ca^{2+} signaling in the heart. *J Cell Sci.* 2009;122:1005–1013.

8. Franzini-Armstrong C, Protasi F, Ramesh V. Comparative ultrastructure of Ca^{2+} release units in skeletal and cardiac muscle. *Ann N Y Acad Sci.* 1998;853:20–30.
9. Dan P, Lin E, Huang J, Biln P, Tibbits GF. Three-dimensional distribution of cardiac Na^+-Ca^{2+} exchanger and ryanodine receptor during development. *Biophys J.* 2007;93:2504–2518.
10. Torres NS, Larbig R, Rock A, Goldhaber JI, Bridge JH. Na^+ currents are required for efficient excitation-contraction coupling in rabbit ventricular myocytes: a possible contribution of neuronal Na^+ channels. *J Physiol.* 2010;588:4249–4260.
11. Marks AR, Tempst P, Hwang KS, et al. Molecular cloning and characterization of the ryanodine receptor/junctional channel complex cDNA from skeletal muscle sarcoplasmic reticulum. *Proc Natl Acad Sci U S A.* 1989;86:8683–8687.
12. Marziali G, Rossi D, Giannini G, Charlesworth A, Sorrentino V. cDNA cloning reveals a tissue specific expression of alternatively spliced transcripts of the ryanodine receptor type 3 (RyR3) calcium release channel. *FEBS Lett.* 1996;394:76–82.
13. Nakai J, Imagawa T, Hakamat Y, Shigekawa M, Takeshima H, Numa S. Primary structure and functional expression from cDNA of the cardiac ryanodine receptor/calcium release channel. *FEBS Lett.* 1990;271:169–177.

14. Yan Z, Bai XC, Yan C, et al. Structure of the rabbit ryanodine receptor RyR1 at near-atomic resolution. *Nature.* 2015;517:50–55.
15. Zalk R, Clarke OB, des Georges A, et al. Structure of a mammalian ryanodine receptor. *Nature.* 2015;517:44–49.
16. Efremov RG, Leitner A, Aebersold R, Raunser S. Architecture and conformational switch mechanism of the ryanodine receptor. *Nature.* 2015;517:39–43.
17. Yamaguchi N, Takahashi N, Xu L, Smithies O, Meissner G. Early cardiac hypertrophy in mice with impaired calmodulin regulation of cardiac muscle Ca release channel. *J Clin Invest.* 2007;117:1344–1353.
18. Gangopadhyay JP, Ikemoto N. Aberrant interaction of calmodulin with the ryanodine receptor develops hypertrophy in the neonatal cardiomyocyte. *Biochem J.* 2011;438:379–387.
19. Marx SO, Reiken S, Hisamatsu Y, et al. PKA phosphorylation dissociates FKBP12.6 from the calcium release channel (ryanodine receptor): defective regulation in failing hearts. *Cell.* 2000;101:365–376.
20. Marks AR. Ryanodine receptors, FKBP12, and heart failure. *Front Biosci.* 2002;7:d970–d977.
21. Xiao J, Tian X, Jones PP, et al. Removal of FKBP12.6 does not alter the conductance and activation of the cardiac ryanodine receptor or the susceptibility to stress-induced ventricular arrhythmias. *J Biol Chem.* 2007;282:34828–34838.

22. Meyers MB, Fischer A, Sun YJ, et al. Sorcin regulates excitation-contraction coupling in the heart. *J Biol Chem*. 2003;278:28865–28871.

23. Farrell EF, Antaramian A, Rueda A, Gomez AM, Valdivia HH. Sorcin inhibits calcium release and modulates excitation-contraction coupling in the heart. *J Biol Chem*. 2003;278:34660–34666.

24. Rueda A, Song M, Toro L, Stefani E, Valdivia HH. Sorcin modulation of Ca²⁺ sparks in rat vascular smooth muscle cells. *J Physiol*. 2006;576:887–901.

25. Liu B, Ho HT, Brunello L, et al. Ablation of HRC alleviates cardiac arrhythmia and improves abnormal Ca handling in CASQ2 knockout mice prone to CPVT. *Cardiovasc Res*. 2015;108:299–311.

26. Gyorke I, Hester N, Jones LR, Gyorke S. The role of calsequestrin, triadin, and junctin in conferring cardiac ryanodine receptor responsiveness to luminal calcium. *Biophys J*. 2004;86:2121–2128.

27. Knollmann BC. New roles of calsequestrin and triadin in cardiac muscle. *J Physiol*. 2009;587:3081–3087.

28. Prosser BL, Hernandez-Ochoa EO, Schneider MF. S100A1 and calmodulin regulation of ryanodine receptor in striated muscle. *Cell Calcium*. 2011;50:323–331.

29. Lehnart SE, Wehrens XH, Reiken S, et al. Phospho-diesterase 4D deficiency in the ryanodine-receptor complex promotes heart failure and arrhythmias. *Cell*. 2005;123:25–35.

30. Huang X, Fruen B, Farrington DT, Wagenknecht T, Liu Z. Calmodulin-binding locations on the skeletal and cardiac ryanodine receptors. *J Biol Chem*. 2012;287:30328–30335.

31. Fill M, Copello JA. Ryanodine receptor calcium release channels. *Physiol Rev*. 2002;82:893–922.

32. Capes EM, Loaiza R, Valdivia HH. Ryanodine receptors. *Skelet Muscle*. 2011;1:18.

33. Meissner G, Rios E, Tripathy A, Pasek DA. Regulation of skeletal muscle Ca²⁺ release channel (ryanodine receptor) by Ca²⁺ and monovalent cations and anions. *J Biol Chem*. 1997;272:1628–1638.

34. Fill M, Zahradnikova A, Villalba-Galea CA, Zahradnik I, Escobar AL, Gyorke S. Ryanodine receptor adaptation. *J Gen Physiol*. 2000;116:873–882.

35. Valdivia HH, Kaplan JH, Ellis-Davies GC, Lederer WJ. Rapid adaptation of cardiac ryanodine receptors: modulation by Mg²⁺ and phosphorylation. *Science*. 1995;267:1997–2000.

36. Chen W, Wang R, Chen B, et al. The ryanodine receptor store-sensing gate controls Ca²⁺ waves and Ca²⁺-triggered arrhythmias. *Nat Med*. 2014;20:184–192.

37. Laver DR, O'Neill ER, Lamb GD. Luminal Ca²⁺-regulated Mg²⁺ inhibition of skeletal RyRs reconstituted as isolated channels or coupled clusters. *J Gen Physiol*. 2004;124:741–758.

38. Takasago T, Imagawa T, Furukawa K, Ogurusu T, Shigekawa M. Regulation of the cardiac ryanodine receptor by protein kinase-dependent phosphorylation. *J Biochem*. 1991;109:163–170.

39. Benkusky NA, Weber CS, Scherman JA, et al. Intact beta-adrenergic response and unmodified progression toward heart failure in mice with genetic ablation of a major protein kinase A phosphorylation site in the cardiac ryanodine receptor. *Circ Res*. 2007;101:819–829.

40. MacDonnell SM, Garcia-Rivas G, Scherman JA, et al. Adrenergic regulation of cardiac contractility does not involve phosphorylation of the cardiac ryanodine receptor at serine 2808. *Circ Res*. 2008;102:e65–e72.

41. Yuchi Z, Lau K, Van Petegem F. Disease mutations in the ryanodine receptor central region: crystal structures of a phosphorylation hot spot domain. *Structure*. 2012;20:1201–1211.

42. Van Petegem F. Ryanodine receptors: structure and function. *J Biol Chem*. 2012;287:31624–31632.

43. Witcher DR, Kovacs RJ, Schulman H, Cefali DC, Jones LR. Unique phosphorylation site on the cardiac ryanodine receptor regulates calcium channel activity. *J Biol Chem*. 1991;266:11144–11152.

44. Wehrens XH, Lehnart SE, Reiken SR, Marks AR. Ca²⁺/calmodulin-dependent protein kinase II phosphorylation regulates the cardiac ryanodine receptor. *Circ Res*. 2004;94:e61–e70.

45. Xiao B, Zhong G, Obayashi M, et al. Ser-2030, but not Ser-2808, is the major phosphorylation site in cardiac ryanodine receptors responding to protein kinase A activation upon beta-adrenergic stimulation in normal and failing hearts. *Biochem J*. 2006;396:7–16.

46. Ai X, Curran JW, Shannon TR, Bers DM, Pogwizd SM. Ca²⁺/calmodulin-dependent protein kinase modulates cardiac ryanodine receptor phosphorylation and sarcoplasmic reticulum Ca2+ leak in heart failure. *Circ Res*. 2005;97:1314–1322.

47. Belevych AE, Terentyev D, Terentyeva R, et al. The relationship between arrhythmogenesis and impaired contractility in heart failure: role of altered ryanodine receptor function. *Cardiovasc Res*. 2011;90:493–502.

48. Xiao B, Sutherland C, Walsh MP, Chen SR. Protein kinase A phosphorylation at serine-2808 of the cardiac Ca²⁺-release channel (ryanodine receptor) does not dissociate 12.6-kDa FK506-binding protein (FKBP12.6). *Circ Res*. 2004;94:487–495.

49. Lokuta AJ, Rogers TB, Lederer WJ, Valdivia HH. Modulation of cardiac ryanodine receptors of swine and rabbit by a phosphorylation-dephosphorylation mechanism. *J Physiol*. 1995;487:609–622.

50. Terentyev D, Viatchenko-Karpinski S, Gyorke I, Terentyeva R, Gyorke S. Protein phosphatases decrease sarcoplasmic reticulum calcium content by stimulating calcium release in cardiac myocytes. *J Physiol*. 2003;552:109–118.

51. Sun J, Yamaguchi N, Xu L, Eu JP, Stamler JS, Meissner G. Regulation of the cardiac muscle ryanodine receptor by O(2) tension and S-nitrosoglutathione. *Biochemistry*. 2008;47:13985–13990.

52. Xu L, Eu JP, Meissner G, Stamler JS. Activation of the cardiac calcium release channel (ryanodine receptor) by poly-S-nitrosylation. *Science*. 1998;279:234–237.

53. Aracena P, Sanchez G, Donoso P, Hamilton SL, Hidalgo C. S-glutathionylation and S-nitrosylation inhibition and S-nitrosylation enhances Ca²⁺ activation of RyR1 channels. *J Biol Chem*. 2003;278:42927–42935.

54. Belevych AE, Terentyev D, Viatchenko-Karpinski S, et al. Redox modification of ryanodine receptors underlies calcium alternans in a canine model of sudden cardiac death. *Cardiovasc Res*. 2009;84:387–395.

55. Terentyev D, Gyorke I, Belevych AE, et al. Redox modification of ryanodine receptors contributes to sarcoplasmic reticulum Ca²⁺ leak in chronic heart failure. *Circ Res*. 2008;103:1466–1472.

56. Voss AA, Lango J, Ernst-Russell M, Morin D, Pessah IN. Identification of hyperreactive cysteines within ryanodine receptor type 1 by mass spectrometry. *J Biol Chem*. 2004;279:34514–34520.

57. Aracena-Parks P, Goonasekera SA, Gilman CP, Dirksen RT, Hidalgo C, Hamilton SL. Identification of cysteines involved in S-nitrosylation, S-glutathionylation, and oxidation to disulfides in ryanodine receptor type 1. *J Biol Chem*. 2006;281:40354–40368.

58. Radwanski PB, Brunello L, Veeraraghavan R, et al. Neuronal Na⁺ channel blockade suppresses arrhythmogenic diastolic Ca²⁺ release. *Cardiovasc Res*. 2015;106:143–152.

58a. Radwański PB, Ho HT, Veeraraghavan R, et al. Neuronal Na⁺ channels are integral components of pro-arrhythmic Na⁺/Ca²⁺ signaling nanodomain that promotes cardiac arrhythmias during β-adrenergic stimulation. *J Am Coll Cardiol Basic Trans Sci*. 2016;1:261–276.

59. Conforti L, Tohse N, Sperelakis N. Tetrodotoxin-sensitive sodium current in rat fetal ventricular myocytes–contribution to the plateau phase of action potential. *J Mol Cell Cardiol*. 1993;25:159–173.

60. Ulbricht W. Sodium channel inactivation: molecular determinants and modulation. *Physiol Rev*. 2005;85:1271–1301.

61. Radwanski PB, Greer-Short A, Poelzing S. Inhibition of Na⁺ channels ameliorates arrhythmias in a drug-induced model of Andersen-Tawil syndrome. *Heart Rhythm*. 2013;10:255–263.

62. Laver DR, Honen BN. Luminal Mg²⁺, a key factor controlling RYR2-mediated Ca²⁺ release: cytoplasmic and luminal regulation modeled in a tetrameric channel. *J Gen Physiol*. 2008;132:429–446.

63. Xu L, Mann G, Meissner G. Regulation of cardiac Ca²⁺ release channel (ryanodine receptor) by Ca²⁺, H⁺, Mg²⁺, and adenine nucleotides under normal and simulated ischemic conditions. *Circ Res*. 1996;79:1100–1109.

64. Lanner JT, Georgiou DK, Joshi AD, Hamilton SL. Ryanodine receptors: structure, expression, molecular details, and function in calcium release. *Cold Spring Harb Perspect Biol*. 2010;2: a003996.

65. Meissner G. Molecular regulation of cardiac ryanodine receptor ion channel. *Cell calcium*. 2004;35:621–628.

66. Priori SG, Chen SR. Inherited dysfunction of sarcoplasmic reticulum Ca²⁺ handling and arrhythmogenesis. *Circ Res*. 2011;108:871–883.

67. Laitinen PJ, Swan H, Piippo K, Viitasalo M, Toivonen L, Kontula K. Genes, exercise and sudden death: molecular basis of familial catecholaminergic polymorphic ventricular tachycardia. *Ann Med*. 2004;36(suppl 1):81–86.

68. Roux-Buisson N, Cacheux M, et al. Absence of triadin, a protein of the calcium release complex, is responsible for cardiac arrhythmia with sudden death in human. *Hum Mol Genet*. 2012;21:2759–2767.

69. Hwang HS, Nitu FR, Yang Y, et al. Divergent regulation of ryanodine receptor 2 calcium release channels by arrhythmogenic human calmodulin missense mutants. *Circ Res*. 2014;114:1114–1124.

70. Van Petegem F. Ryanodine receptors: allosteric ion channel giants. *J Mol Biol*. 2015;427:31–53.

71. Gyorke S. Molecular basis of catecholaminergic polymorphic ventricular tachycardia. *Heart Rhythm*. 2009;6:123–129.

72. Gyorke S, Terentyev D. Modulation of ryanodine receptor by luminal calcium and accessory proteins in health and cardiac disease. *Cardiovasc Res*. 2008;77:245–255.

73. Brunello L, Slabaugh JL, Radwanski PB, et al. Decreased RyR2 refractoriness determines myocardial synchronization of aberrant Ca²⁺ release in a genetic model of arrhythmia. *Proc Natl Acad Sci U S A*. 2013;110:10312–10317.

74. Nyegaard M, Overgaard MT, Sondergaard MT, et al. Mutations in calmodulin cause ventricular tachycardia and sudden cardiac death. *Am J Hum Genet*. 2012;91:703–712.

75. Yang Y, Guo T, Oda T, et al. Cardiac myocyte Z-line calmodulin is mainly RyR2-bound, and reduction is arrhythmogenic and occurs in heart failure. *Circ Res*. 2014;114:295–306.

76. Antos CL, Frey N, Marx SO, et al. Dilated cardiomyopathy and sudden death resulting from constitutive activation of protein kinase a. *Circ Res*. 2001;89:997–1004.

77. Zhang T, Maier LS, Dalton ND, et al. The deltaC isoform of CaMKII is activated in cardiac hypertrophy and induces dilated cardiomyopathy and heart failure. *Circ Res*. 2003;92:912–919.

78. Respress JL, van Oort RJ, Li N, et al. Role of RyR2 phosphorylation at S2814 during heart failure progression. *Circ Res*. 2012;110:1474–1483.

79. Belevych AE, Sansom SE, Terentyeva R, et al. MicroRNA-1 and -133 increase arrhythmogenesis in heart failure by dissociating phosphatase activity from RyR2 complex. *PloS One*. 2011;6: e28324.

80. Liu B, Ho HT, Velez-Cortes F, et al. Genetic ablation of ryanodine receptor 2 phosphorylation at Ser-2808 aggravates Ca²⁺-dependent cardiomyopathy by exacerbating diastolic Ca2+ release. *J Physiol*. 2014;592:1957–1973.

81. Belevych AE, Radwanski PB, Carnes CA, Gyorke S. 'Ryanopathy': causes and manifestations of RyR2 dysfunction in heart failure. *Cardiovasc Res*. 2013;98:240–247.

7

Organellar Ion Channels and Transporters

Jin O-Uchi, Bong Sook Jhun, Jyotsna Mishra, and Shey-Shing Sheu

Introduction

Historical Overview of Mitochondrial Ion Channel/Transporter Research

Mitochondria are the power plants of all kinds of tissues/cells. In heart/cardiomyocytes, mitochondria use glucose and fatty acids to produce adenosine triphosphate (ATP) that drives muscle contraction and relaxation for pumping blood that circulates through the entire body during each heartbeat unceasingly, up to a centenary human life. Indeed, mitochondria were originally found and studied mostly as a cellular "powerhouse" in the first half of the 20th century. Soon it was also recognized that Ca^{2+} stimulates oxidative phosphorylation (OXPHOS) and electron transport chain (ETC) activity, which results in the stimulation of ATP synthesis[1] (Fig. 7.1A and B). Early studies in the 1960s to 1970s revealed that isolated mitochondria can take up a large quantity of Ca^{2+}. Surprisingly, superphysiologically high Ca^{2+} concentrations ($[Ca^{2+}]$) (10–100 μM) were required to activate Ca^{2+} uptake into isolated mitochondria (see reviews[2,3]). However, in intact cells, Ca^{2+} was taken up by mitochondria during a global increase of cytosolic $[Ca^{2+}]$ ($[Ca^{2+}]_c$) (≤10 μM). This discrepancy between isolated mitochondria and intact cells was partially resolved by the finding that high $[Ca^{2+}]_c$ exists at microdomains between the mitochondria and endoplasmic reticulum (ER)/sarcoplasmic reticulum (SR) during ER/SR Ca^{2+} release via the inositol trisphosphate (IP_3) receptor and/or the ryanodine receptor (RyR), due to the juxtaposition of these two organelles. These seminal discoveries have finally positioned mitochondria as one of the key players in the dynamic regulation of physiological Ca^{2+} signaling and have promoted research in the fields of mitochondrial Ca^{2+} channels/transporters. Shortly thereafter it was also discovered that a Ca^{2+} efflux mechanism exists to dump the accumulated matrix Ca^{2+} into the cytosol. Although the functional characteristics of mitochondrial Ca^{2+} influx/efflux mechanisms had been functionally discovered over 50 years ago, the molecular identities responsible for these mechanisms have remained a mystery until very recently. The mitochondrial Ca^{2+} influx was dogmatically considered to result from a single transport mechanism mediated by a mitochondrial Ca^{2+} uniporter (MCU) principally due to nearly complete inhibition by ruthenium red (RuR) and lanthanides, and its channel nature was originally proposed over 30 years ago.[2,3] Finally, recent groundbreaking studies have made

progress, unveiling that MCU is encoded by CCDC109A.[4,5] These findings have opened up an exciting opportunity for investigating mitochondrial Ca^{2+} handling by utilizing genetic approaches. For instance, the molecular identification of MCU set a foundation for the discovery of several auxiliary subunits that associate with this pore-forming protein (e.g., EMRE and MICU1–3).[6,7] From these discoveries, a new concept in the field was uncovered with the idea that uniporter activity is not solely regulated by one single protein (MCU), but possibly by macromolecular protein complexes (called "mitochondrial Ca^{2+} uniporter protein complexes" or mtCUC).[6,7] Furthermore, several groups have shown that kinases in the cytosol can translocate into the mitochondria, interact with mtCUC, and directly modulate mtCUC function through posttranslational modifications of MCU in cardiomyocytes.[8–10] These reports also support the idea that the MCU and its regulatory proteins form macromolecular local signaling complexes at the inner mitochondrial membrane (IMM), which may significantly impact mitochondrial Ca^{2+} handling, as well as numerous mitochondrial and cellular functions. Moreover, subsequent studies have identified additional Ca^{2+} uptake pathways, which exhibit different Ca^{2+} affinity, uptake kinetics, and pharmacological characteristics from the original MCU theory (see review[3,11]) (see Fig. 7.1C). These distinct properties enable mitochondria to carry out multiple Ca^{2+}-mediated functions with optimal spatial and temporal effectiveness. Especially, in cardiomyocytes, ryanodine receptor type 1 (RyR1) was found as the first mitochondrial Ca^{2+} influx mechanism with a known molecular identity reported by our group (see "Mitochondrial Ryanodine Receptor"). Through RNA interference studies, several groups have recently proposed novel candidate proteins that are involved in mitochondrial Ca^{2+} uptake mechanisms, such as Letm1,[12] in addition to the RyR1 discovery (see "Mitochondrial Ca2+ Uniporter Protein Complex," "Mitochondrial Ryanodine Receptor," and "Letm1 (Ca^{2+}/H^+ Antiporter)").

In addition to Ca^{2+}, the movements of various electrolytes and metabolites across the IMM as well as across the outer mitochondrial membrane (OMM) are important for the regulation of major mitochondrial functions, including ATP synthesis, Ca^{2+} homeostasis, and the generation of reactive oxygen species (ROS) and reactive nitrogen species (RNS). Unlike other organelles, mitochondria possess unique double-membrane structures with distinctive phospholipids and protein compositions that allow mitochondrial membranes to maintain a mitochondrial membrane potential ($\Delta\Psi_m$) and unique architecture, including cristae (see "Overview of Mitochondrial Bioenergetics and Mitochondrial Membrane Potential"). Interestingly, IMM and OMM have different sets of ion channels/transporters as summarized in Fig. 7.1A. These include (1) proton (H^+) movement related to ETC activity and uncoupling proteins (UCPs) for the maintenance of $\Delta\Psi_m$ and ΔpH across IMM (see "Proton Fluxes and Uncoupling Proteins"); (2) K^+-selective (see "Mitochondrial K^+ Channels") and anion-selective pathways at IMM (see "Anion Channels and Mitochondrial Volume Control") and across the two membranes, such as the mitochondrial permeability transition pore (mPTP) (see "Mitochondrial Permeability Transition Pores"), which are important for the maintenance of mitochondrial volume; (3) the movement of metabolites including ATP, ADP, and phosphate

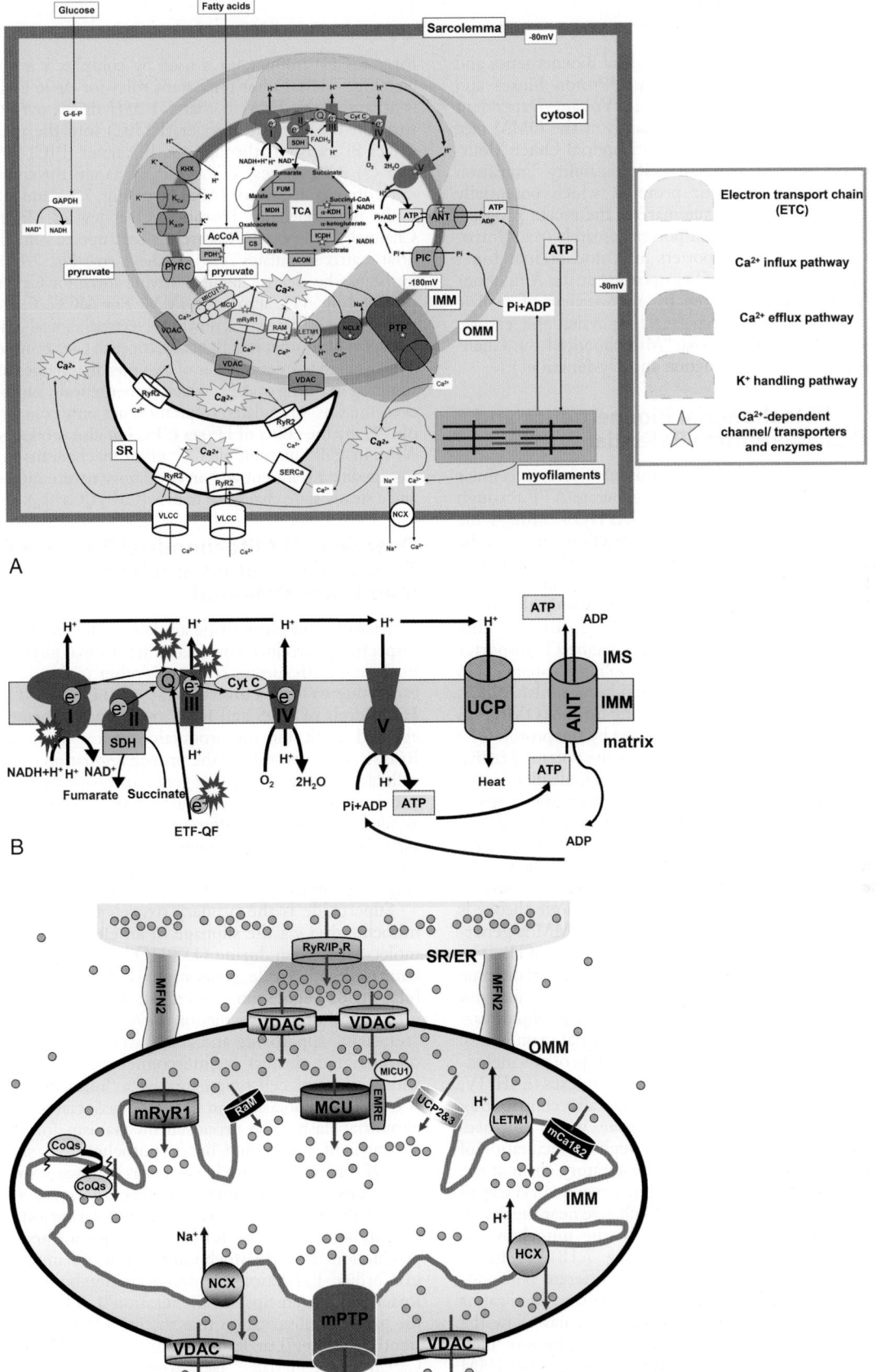

FIGURE 7.1 Overview of mitochondrial ion channels/transporters. (A) Major ion movements in mitochondria. Ca^{2+}-dependent ion channels/transporters and enzymes are indicated with *stars*. (B) Mitochondrial electron transport chain (*ETC*) and possible sites of superoxide production. *Red "explosion" symbols* indicate places where superoxide production occurs. (C) Ca^{2+} influx and efflux mechanisms: the channels/transporters whose molecular identities are still unknown are shown as *black*. *Red arrows* show Ca^{2+} movements, and *blue arrows* show other ion movements. (C, Modified from O-Uchi J, Pan S, Sheu SS. Perspectives on: SGP symposium on mitochondrial physiology and medicine: molecular identities of mitochondrial Ca^{2+} influx mechanism: updated passwords for accessing mitochondrial Ca^{2+}-linked health and disease. *J Gen Physiol.* 2012;139:435-443.)

(Pi) at IMM (see "Overview of Mitochondrial Bioenergetics and Mitochondrial Membrane Potential" and "Proton Fluxes and Uncoupling Proteins") and OMM (see "Voltage-Dependent Anion Channel"); and (4) large pores mainly at the OMM (see "Ion Channels/Transporters at the Mitochondrial Outer Membrane") or mPTP (see "Mitochondrial Permeability Transition Pores") that release proapoptotic proteins, which potentially lead to cell death. This chapter summarizes the recent progress in mitochondrial ion channel/transporter research (see "Introduction," "Ion Channels/Transporters at Mitochondrial Inner Membrane," and "Ion Channels/Transporters at the Mitochondrial Outer Membrane"), followed by an overview of cardiac mitochondrial ion channel/transporter biophysics and cardiac physiology and pathophysiology (see "Mitochondrial Ion Channels/Transporters in Cardiac Function and Dysfunction").

Overview of Mitochondrial Bioenergetics and Mitochondrial Membrane Potential

The most prominent contribution of mitochondria to cellular metabolism is based on their capacity to generate ATP through the tricarboxylic acid (TCA) cycle and OXPHOS through the ETC, which is a concerted series of redox reactions catalyzed by four multisubunit enzymes embedded in the IMM (complex I–IV) and two soluble factors, cytochrome c (cyt c) and coenzyme Q_{10} (CoQ_{10}) that function as electron shuttles within the mitochondrial intermembrane space (IMS) (see Fig. 7.1B) (see "Historical Overview of Mitochondrial Ion Channel/Transporter Research" and "Proton Fluxes and Uncoupling Proteins"). In eukaryotic cells, more than 90% of the total intracellular ATP is generated by mitochondria. The main driving force of OXPHOS is known as "chemiosmosis" and is generated by the proton (H+) movement across IMM that creates a membrane potential ($\Delta\Psi_m$, negative in the matrix) and a pH gradient (ΔpH, alkaline in the matrix). Chemiosmosis is the movement of ions across a selectively permeable membrane, down their electrochemical gradient (proton motive force: Δp), which is determined by both $\Delta\Psi_m$ and ΔpH components across the IMM ($\Delta p = \Delta\Psi_m + \Delta pH$). The chemiosmotic hypothesis was first proposed by Peter D. Mitchell in 1961.[13] The basic assumption of the chemiosmotic theory is derived from the important observation that the IMM is generally impermeable to ions, but it keeps the permeability of H+. The composition of the OMM is similar to those of the sarcolemma (SL) and ER/SR in eukaryotic cells, whereas the IMM does not possess cholesterol but has a unique dimeric phospholipid, cardiolipin, which is a typical composition for bacterial membranes. Cardiolipin has a unique ability to interact with proteins including several mitochondrial respiratory chain complexes (I, III, IV, and V) and to support their activities[14] while also contributing to the maintenance of the structure of cristae, which enhances the efficiency of ETC activity, possibly through the facilitation of the formation of super complexes of the respiratory chain at the IMM.[15] The unique structure of cardiolipin serves as a H+ trap at the IMS near the IMM, maintains the pH change near the IMM, and efficiently pools H+ or releases H+ to the mitochondrial ATP-synthase (complex V) at IMM (see Fig. 7.1B).[13,14] Interestingly, the IMM and OMM not only have different phospholipid compositions but also show different protein-to-lipid ratios (about 1 for OMM and about 4 for IMM). This may allow the proteins at the IMM to possess enzymatic and/or transport functions compared to those at the OMM, thereby making the IMM much less permeable to ions and small molecules than the OMM, which also provides the cellular compartmentalization between the mitochondrial matrix and cytosol. As shown in Fig. 7.1B, complexes I, III, and IV are engaging with the translocation of H+ from the matrix to the IMS, which establishes $\Delta\Psi_m$ and ΔpH (i.e., Δp). Therefore $\Delta\Psi_m$ is usually highly negative (around −180 mV) compared with the resting potential at plasma membranes. Finally, according to the above mechanisms, this large driving force for H+ influx (Δp) is used by complex V to produce ATP (see Fig. 7.1B). Other important roles for Δp in addition to ATP synthase at the IMM is that (1) ΔpH drives pyruvate transport through the pyruvate carrier (PYRC) into the matrix, (2) ΔpH drives Pi transport through the Pi carrier (PIC) into the matrix, and (3) $\Delta\Psi_m$ drives ATP/ADP exchange through the adenine nucleotide translocator (ANT) (see Fig. 7.1A and B).

As mentioned in "Historical Overview of Mitochondrial Ion Channel/Transporter Research," Ca2+ uptake into the mitochondrial matrix stimulates ATP synthesis (see Fig. 7.1A). At the resting state, the electrochemical driving force for Ca2+ uptake is also provided by $\Delta\Psi_m$ across the IMM. For MCU, Ca2+ is taken into the mitochondrial matrix down its electrochemical gradient without transport of another ion. Basically, for each Ca2+ transported through MCU, there is a net transfer of two positive charges into the matrix resulting in a drop of $\Delta\Psi_m$, which is energetically unfavorable. However, the Ca2+-stimulated respiration not only compensates the loss of $\Delta\Psi_m$ by the efflux of H+ via ETC but also produces a net gain of ATP. In addition, multiple Ca2+ efflux mechanisms work in concert to expedite a transient and an oscillatory nature rather than a tonic and a steady state change of matrix [Ca2+] ([Ca2+]$_m$).

Overview of Mitochondrial Reactive Oxygen Species Generation and Mitochondrial Membrane Potential

Superoxide and nitric oxide are key elements of ROS and RNS, respectively, produced in cells under normal physiological conditions, and both species react with other molecules and also with each other to form a diverse array of additional ROS and RNS.[16] High levels of ROS and RNS are known to promote cell damage and death, but the production of low to moderate levels of ROS/RNS is critical for the proper regulation of many essential cellular processes, including gene expression, signal transduction, and cardiac excitation–contraction (E–C) coupling.[17] ROS are generated by several different cellular sources: (1) membrane-associated reduced nicotinamide adenine dinucleotide phosphate (NADPH) oxidase, (2) cytosolic xanthine and xanthine oxidase, and (3) the mitochondrial ETCs at IMMs.

Superoxide is the primary oxygen free radical produced in mitochondria via the slippage of an electron from the ETC to molecular oxygen during OXPHOS (see Fig. 7.1B). This "constitutive" superoxide generation is central to the proper cellular redox regulation. Recent studies from our collaborating groups and other investigators have detected a "stochastic" and "transient" superoxide and alkalization burst from either single or restricted clusters of interconnected mitochondria across a wide variety of cell types, termed a "mitochondrial flash."[18,19] A transient depolarization of $\Delta\Psi_m$ is associated with each mitochondrial flash. The proposed mechanism for the component of transient superoxide burst, mitochondrial superoxide flash (mSOF) in cardiac muscle cells is as follows: a small increase in constitutive ROS production transiently opens a large channel named the mPTP to cause $\Delta\Psi_m$ depolarization, which subsequently stimulates the ETC to produce a burst in superoxide production (see "Mitochondrial Ion Channels/Transporters in Cardiac Excitation–Contraction/Metabolism Coupling and Reactive Oxygen Species Generation"). This idea is similar to the previous observation that the mPTP opens and closes transiently ("flicker") at its low conductance state and can release Ca2+ from the matrix[2,20] (see "Mitochondrial Permeability Transition Pores"). The frequency of mitochondrial flashes varies widely across different cell types and experimental conditions (disease models), suggesting that these flashes act as biomarkers of cellular metabolic activity and oxidative condition in physiological and pathophysiological conditions.[18,19] Future studies will clarify the contribution of altered mSOF activity to ROS overproduction and metabolic dysfunction in a wide range of mitochondrial diseases and oxidative stress related disorders.

Finally, it should be noted that mitochondrial flashes are composed of a superoxide signal with an alkalization signal within the mitochondrial matrix.[18,19] Based on chemiosmotic theory, one can envision that whenever there is a significant drop in $\Delta\Psi_m$, there should be an alkalization in ΔpH (see "Overview of Mitochondrial Bioenergetics and Mitochondrial Membrane Potential"). The functional role of this concurrent digitized superoxide and pH signal requires further investigation.

Overview of Mitochondria-Induced Apoptosis

Programmed cell death is genetically designed for self-killing of individual cells and is one of the critical mechanisms for maintaining homeostasis of multicellular organs/tissues including the heart.[21] Apoptosis is a well-established mechanism of programmed cell death activated by a variety of cellular stresses and signals.[22] In mammalian cells, the activation of caspases (a family of cysteine proteases) is the central mechanism for apoptosis. Under the resting condition, caspases are tightly kept inactive as a "proenzyme" form and/or by binding to inhibitory proteins (named inhibitors of apoptosis) in the cytosol. During apoptosis, caspases are activated by cleavage that changes the "proenzyme" form to the enzyme form and by dissociation of the inhibitors of apoptosis.[23] One of the major apoptotic pathways is derived from mitochondria, which contributes to the activation of caspases in the cytosol. This mechanism is initiated by the release of proapoptotic factors from mitochondria, including cyt c, Smac/Diablo, and HtrA2/Omi. Cyt c released to the cytosol activates caspases through its binding to apoptotic protease activating factor-1 (Apaf-1). Smac/Diablo and HtrA2/Omi bind to the inhibitory proteins to remove their inhibitory effect from caspases. Apoptotic DNases, including apoptosis inducing factor (AIF) and endonuclease G (Endo G), are also released from mitochondria in addition to the above mentioned proapoptotic factors. The release of these proapoptotic factors is regulated under the tight control of mitochondrial membrane permeability.[24] This mitochondrial membrane permeabilization is mediated via at least three distinct mechanisms: (1) physical rupture of the OMM as a result of mitochondrial swelling (usually linked to mPTP opening) (see "Mitochondrial Permeability Transition Pores"), (2) a modification of the structure of the voltage-dependent anion channel (VDAC) through its interaction with proapoptotic proteins, such as the Bcl-2 protein family (see "Voltage-Dependent Anion Channel"), and (3) formation of a new pore as a consequence of oligomerization and membrane insertion of proapoptotic proteins, including the Bcl-2 family of proteins (see "Apoptosis-Induced Channels"). The first pathway involves $\Delta\Psi_m$ depolarization and swelling of the matrix space, followed by loss of OMM integrity and rupture, thereby spilling proapoptotic proteins into the cytosol. In contrast, the other two pathways occur without $\Delta\Psi_m$ depolarization.

Ion Channels/Transporters at the Mitochondrial Inner Membrane

Mitochondrial Ca²⁺ Channels/Transporters Regulating Mitochondrial Ca²⁺ Influx

Mitochondrial Ca²⁺ Uniporter Protein Complex

Pore-Forming Subunits

MCU (CCDC109A). The MCU gene (known as CCDC109A) encodes a 40-kDa protein containing a mitochondrial target sequence (MTS) at the N-terminus.[4,5] The characteristics of MCU are summarized as follows: (1) the MCU proteins form an RuR-sensitive Ca²⁺ channel pore by oligomerization; (2) knockdown of MCU dramatically reduces mitochondrial Ca²⁺ uptake; and (3) changes in MCU expression levels do not affect basal $\Delta\Psi_m$, oxygen consumption, ATP synthesis, or mitochondrial morphology. Significant roles of MCU on mitochondrial Ca²⁺ accumulations were confirmed in various cell lines as well as

in primary cells, including cardiomyocytes.[8,25] The MCU topology was investigated by several groups, and it seems that both the N- and C-termini of MCU face the mitochondrial matrix and a short motif of amino acids for the pore-forming region is exposed to the intermembrane space. The crystal structure of the whole MCU protein has not yet been solved, but the computational analysis predicts that the MCU channel pore is formed by an MCU tetramer.[26]

MCUb (CCDC109B). Rizzuto's group reported a novel protein MCUb, which serves as an endogenous dominant-negative pore forming subunit of mtCUC.[26] MCUb, encoded by a related gene of CCDC109A named CCDC109B, is a 33-kDa protein that has two predicted transmembrane domains (TMDs), shares 50% similarity to the MCU with the key amino acid substitutions being located in the pore forming region,[26] and shows different expression profiles from the MCU in various tissues. The function of the MCUb was characterized by several groups and can be summarized as follows: (1) MCU and MCUb bind each other and form hetero-oligomers and (2) MCUb inhibits mtCUC activity. Interestingly, the ratio of MCU and MCUb mRNA expression varies in different tissues,[26] which might correlate to the size of mitochondrial Ca²⁺-selective currents recorded from mitoplasts isolated from a variety of mouse tissues.[27] For instance, heart and skeletal muscle are examples of organs that possess a high copy number of MCU mRNA,[4,5,26] but the MCUb expression in the heart is much higher compared with that in skeletal muscle.[26] Accordingly, the MCU current measured in whole mitoplast from hearts was 30 times smaller than that from skeletal muscle.[27] These observations suggest that the ratio of MCU and MCUb expression may be one of the mechanisms that characterize different mitochondrial Ca²⁺ uptake profiles in different tissue types, including heart.

Auxiliary Subunits. Rizzuto's group showed that recombinant MCU alone produces Ca²⁺ conductance in planar lipid bilayers[5,26,28] without the addition of any other auxiliary subunits (see also "Pore-Forming Subunits"). These reports strongly support the initial idea that indeed the MCU is a pore subunit and a sufficient minimal structure for the uniporter. However, in the lipid bilayers (in vitro setting) under symmetrical 100-mM Ca²⁺ conditions, the channel conductance from reconstituted channels by purified MCU proteins shows only 6–7 pS, whereas endogenous uniporter under mitoplast patch-clamp exhibits 14.3 pS. Therefore it is a reasonable speculation that, in the natural IMM environment (in situ or in vivo) and/or under asymmetrical Ca²⁺ conditions, the mtCUC conductance is different, possibly due to the coexistence of auxiliary subunits with MCU pore subunits.

EMRE. Essential MCU regulator, EMRE (known as C22ORF32) is the first identified auxiliary subunit reported that has a TMD.[29] EMRE is a 10-kDa protein with an MTS at its N-terminus and a highly conserved aspartate-rich C-terminal region.[29] It contains a predicted single TMD and is located at IMM[29] (see Fig. 7.1C). Since EMRE knockdown in mammalian cells resulted in almost complete loss-of-function of uniporter activity in situ under the condition of MCU overexpression, this protein seems likely to be an essential auxiliary subunit in the production of the mtCUC current in situ. Since the number of reports regarding EMRE is limited at this moment, there are still several important questions remaining, which need to be solved by additional experiments.

MICU1, 2, and 3. Historically, MICU1 (encoded by CBARA1/EFHA3) was the first regulatory element for the MCU pore discovered just before MCU.[30] MICU1 is a 54-kDa protein with two highly conserved EF-hand Ca²⁺-binding domains. Subsequent analysis after the discovery of MICU1[30] revealed that MICU1 shares approximately 25% sequence identity with two other human genes, *EFHA1* and *EFHA2*, which were renamed as MICU2 and MICU3.[31] These two proteins also have an N-terminal MTS and two EF-hand domains, which is similar to the structure of MICU1. Interestingly, a difference in tissue distribution patterns is observed among the three isoforms.[32,33] As shown in early studies (see "Historical Overview of Mitochondrial Ion Channel/Transporter Research"), surprisingly, high $[Ca^{2+}]$ (e.g., ≥10 μM) was required to efficiently activate Ca^{2+} uptake into isolated mitochondria. It is therefore acceptable that the transient increases in $[Ca^{2+}]_m$, in response to $[Ca^{2+}]_c$ elevation after cell-signaling activations (e.g., G_q protein-coupled receptor stimulation), are important for triggering the activation of Ca^{2+}-sensitive dehydrogenases and the acceleration of ATP production. However, scenarios where Ca^{2+} could accumulate chronically and continuously in the mitochondria even in resting $[Ca^{2+}]_c$ conditions are unfavorable situations for cells to maintain their cellular functions because mitochondrial Ca^{2+} overload causes $\Delta\Psi_m$ depolarization, ROS overproduction, and apoptotic cell death. Indeed, mitochondrial Ca^{2+} uptake rates are very slow near the resting $[Ca^{2+}]_c$, but rapidly increase if the $[Ca^{2+}]_c$ in the proximity of mitochondria reaches around 10–20 μM.[34–37] To maintain this sigmoidal response to $[Ca^{2+}]_c$, mtCUC needs to be equipped with some sort of machinery system serving as its "gatekeeper" in order to keep the channel closed at resting $[Ca^{2+}]_c$ and also to facilitate mitochondrial Ca^{2+} uptake upon high $[Ca^{2+}]_c$ stimulation. Indeed, MICU family proteins are currently the most likely candidates, but the detailed mechanisms are still under debate.

Other Proposed Auxiliary Subunits. Mitochondrial calcium uniporter regulator 1 (MCUR1) encoded by CCDC90A was proposed as a possible Class 1 auxiliary subunit for MCU by Foskett's and Madesh's groups.[38] They proposed that MCUR1 is a component of mtCUC and the direct interaction of MCU and MCUR1 are required for efficient Ca^{2+} uptake. In addition to MCUR1, Madesh's group also proposed another protein named SLC25A23 as a Class 1 auxiliary subunit.[39] This protein was originally known as a phosphate transporter across the IMM, and they reported that SLC25A23 participates in mitochondrial Ca^{2+} uptake probably via its interaction with MCU and MICU1. Since the reports regarding the protein functions of MCUR1 and SLC25A23 are limited at this time, further investigations by multiple groups will be required.

Mitochondrial Ryanodine Receptor

One of the candidates for the mitochondrial Ca^{2+} uptake mechanism with a known molecular identity is the mitochondrial RyR in cardiac cells reported by our group.[40] There are three different RyR isoforms (RyR1, RyR2, and RyR3) with different physiological and pharmacological properties. In cardiac cells, intracellular Ca^{2+} release during E–C coupling was mainly controlled by RyR2 located in the SR (see "Overview of Mitochondrial Structure and Function in the Heart"). Although RyR1 is also detectable at both mRNA and protein levels in cardiac tissue, its functional and physiological roles in the heart were not fully understood for a long time. We first showed that a low level of functional RyR is also expressed at the heart IMM and acts as a fast Ca^{2+} uptake pathway[41] (see Figs. 7.1B and 7.2). Furthermore, RyR in cardiac mitochondria exhibits remarkably similar biochemical, pharmacological, and functional properties to those of RyR1 in skeletal muscle SR, but not to those of RyR2 in cardiac SR; therefore it is called mRyR1 (mitochondrial RyR).[3] The molecular identity of mRyR1 was carefully analyzed and confirmed by a variety of functional and biochemical experiments using not only native heart, but also using the RyR1 knockout mouse heart. Recent studies from our lab using electrophysiological techniques directly demonstrated the existence of mRyR1, which clearly showed the predicted channel nature of skeletal RyR1. In a conventional lipid bilayer of mRyRs purified from a heart IMM, the activity of RyR1 but not RyR2 was observed.[42] The biophysical and pharmacological properties of native single mRyR1 channels were further characterized in heart mitoplasts using patch-clamp techniques.[43] A novel 225-pS cation-selective channel in heart mitoplasts was observed that exhibited multiple subconductance

states, which was blocked by high concentrations of ryanodine and RuR, the known inhibitors of RyRs. Ryanodine exhibited a concentration-dependent modulation of this channel, with low concentrations stabilizing a subconductance state and with high concentrations abolishing activity. The channel properties of Ca^{2+}-dependent [^{3}H]ryanodine binding and the channel modulation by caffeine in isolated cardiac mitochondria[41] implicate that the topology of mRyR1 is the same as RyR1 at the SR because of these agonist-binding sites; C- and N-terminals face toward the IMS (corresponding to cytoplasmic side of RyR1 at SR) and S1–S2, S3–S4, and S5–S6 linkers face toward mitochondrial matrix side (corresponding to the SR luminal side of RyR1 at SR). However, further studies will be needed to confirm the topology of mRyR1 using other modulators from both the matrix side and the cytosolic side.

Unlike MCU, RyR is a poorly Ca^{2+}-selective, large cation channel.[43] Therefore opening of mRyR1 might collapse $\Delta\Psi_m$, which is energetically unfavorable. This dichotomy would be explained as follows: (1) the expression number of RyR1 in a single mitochondrion is very small and the changes in $\Delta\Psi_m$ might be minimized locally assuring maintenance of a Ca^{2+}-driving force, (2) the rapid Ca^{2+}-activation and -inactivation profile of this channel (see Fig. 7.2) would minimize the $\Delta\Psi_m$ change instantly, and (3) any small decrease in $\Delta\Psi_m$ can be readily compensated by the Ca^{2+}-dependent activation of dehydrogenase during the TCA cycle and ATP synthesis. Taken together, the mRyR may be uniquely poised to sequester Ca^{2+} during transient and rapid E–C coupling processes in cardiac muscle cells (see "Mitochondrial Ion Channels/Transporters in Cardiac Excitation–Contraction/Metabolism Coupling and Reactive Oxygen Species Generation").

Letm1 (Ca^{2+}/H^+ Antiporter)

Letm1 was first found as a K^+/H^+ exchanger (KHX). Using siRNA genome-wide screening in *Drosophila*, it was proposed also as a H^+/Ca^{2+} exchanger (HCX) at the IMM[12] (see Figs. 7.1 and 7.2). Knockdown of Letm1 abolished only the initial fast mitochondrial Ca^{2+} uptake, but still showed sustained Ca^{2+} increase, suggesting that Letm1 works at low $[Ca^{2+}]_c$ for Ca^{2+} uptake (see Fig. 7.2). In addition, the detailed profile of Letm1-mediated mitochondrial Ca^{2+} handling was assessed using the liposomes containing highly purified recombinant Letm1. Letm1-mediated Ca^{2+} influx was insensitive to electroneutral (1 Ca^{2+}/2 H^+ antiport), stimulated by a pH gradient, and was insensitive both to RuR, an inhibitor of MCU, and to CGP37157, an inhibitor of the NCX.[44] However, there still remains the possibility that impaired Ca^{2+} uptake after Letm1 knockdown might be an indirect consequence of mitochondrial dysfunction and deenergization.

Mitochondrial Ca^{2+} Channels/Transporters Regulating Mitochondrial Ca^{2+} Efflux

Mitochondrial Na^+/Ca^{2+} Exchanger (NCLX)

The main mitochondrial Ca^{2+} efflux pathways are Na^+/Ca^{2+} exchanger (NCX) and/or HCX (see Figs. 7.1 and 7.2). Na^+- or Li^+-dependent Ca^{2+} transport (NCLX) was first cloned as a sixth member of the K^+-dependent NCXs suggested to be located at the ER or plasma membrane. Recently, NCLX was shown as a candidate for the mitochondrial NCX.[45] NCLX expression is particularly robust in excitable cells, whereas the activity of the HCX is primarily found in nonexcitable cells, suggesting the existence of tissue-specific mitochondrial Ca^{2+} efflux mechanisms. Indeed, the primary mitochondrial Ca^{2+} efflux mechanism is Na^{2+} dependent in cardiac mitochondria.[46]

Mitochondrial Permeability Transition Pores

The mPTP is a large, nonspecific channel that opens at the IMM and is known to form under mitochondrial stress conditions, such as mitochondrial Ca^{2+} overload and elevated oxidative stress,

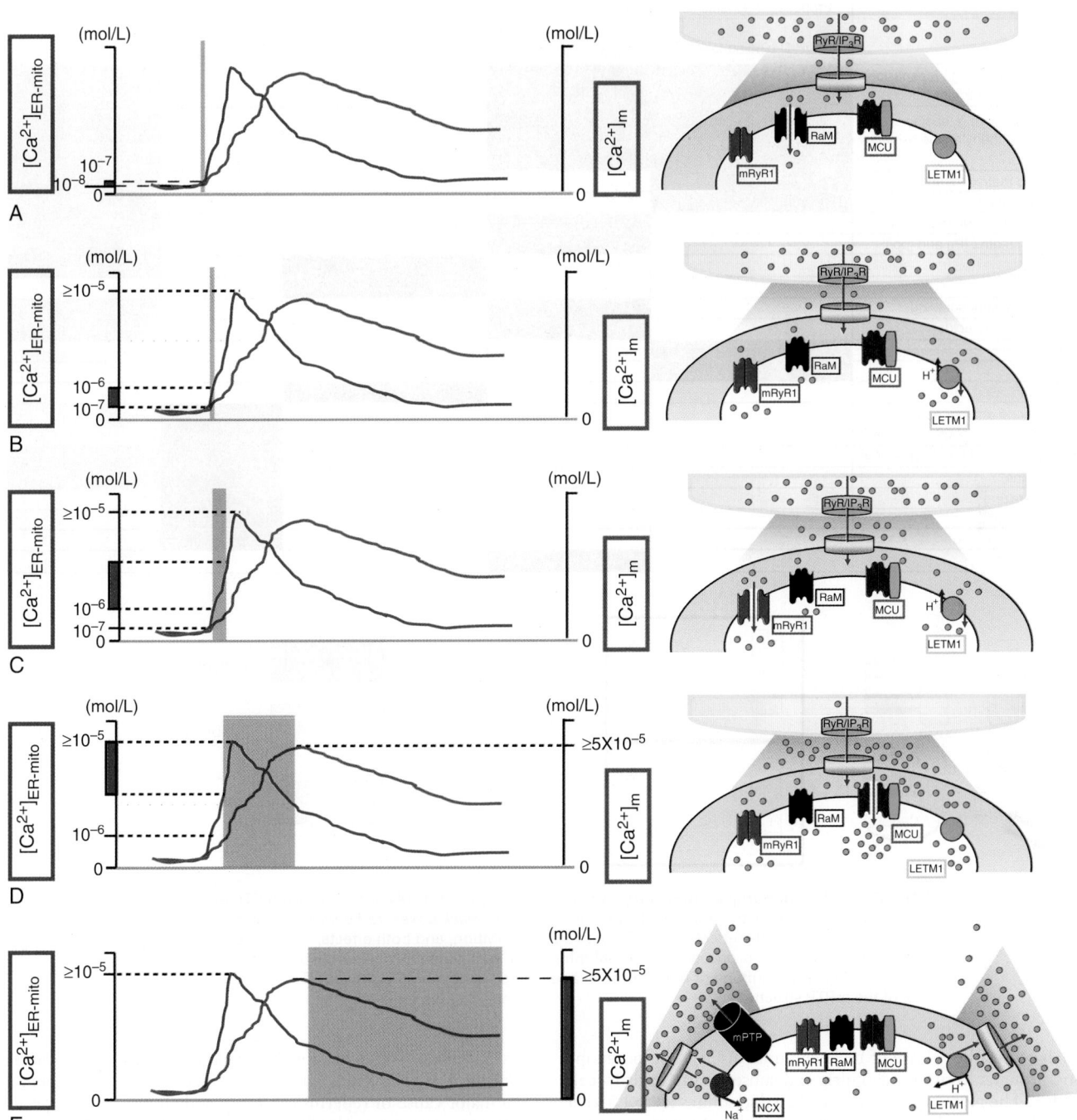

FIGURE 7.2 Activation/deactivation patterns of Ca²⁺ influx/efflux mechanisms. (A) At first, rapid mode of uptake (RaM) (*black*) is activated at very initial phase of $[Ca^{2+}]_{ER\text{-}mito}$ transient (<200 nM) with faster Ca²⁺ uptake kinetics (ms time scale). (B) Letm1 (*orange*) starts to uptake Ca²⁺ at ≥200 nM $[Ca^{2+}]_{ER\text{-}mito}$. (C) Mitochondrial ryanodine receptor 1 (*mRyR1*) (*red*) starts open at ≅1-µM $[Ca^{2+}]_{ER\text{-}mito}$ with a five-fold faster Ca²⁺ transport compared with the mitochondrial Ca²⁺ uniporter (*MCU*) and deactivates before $[Ca^{2+}]_{ER\text{-}mito}$ reaches the peak. (D) Finally, MCU (*blue*) starts to activate at >1 µM $[Ca^{2+}]_{ER\text{-}mito}$, and the activity increases in a $[Ca^{2+}]_{ER\text{-}mito}$-dependent manner. At this point, Letm1 (*orange*) shifts from Ca²⁺-uptake mode to Ca²⁺-efflux mode. (E) Mitochondrial permeability transition pore (*mPTP*) (*black*) and Na⁺/Ca²⁺ exchanger (*NCX*) (*purple*) contribute to Ca²⁺ efflux in mammalian cells and form the decay phase of the $[Ca^{2+}]_m$ transient. Letm1 also works as a Ca²⁺ efflux pathway at this phase. (Modified from O-Uchi J, Pan S, Sheu SS: Perspectives on: SGP symposium on mitochondrial physiology and medicine: molecular identities of mitochondrial Ca²⁺ influx mechanism: updated passwords for accessing mitochondrial Ca²⁺-linked health and disease. *J Gen Physiol.* 2012;139:435-443.)

Effectors	Proposed mechanisms				Effects to mPTP
	via CyP-D binding to mPTP	via change in nucleotide binding to the ANT	via Ca²⁺ binding to the mPTP	other mechanism	
Oxidative stress (e.g., reperfusion, t-butylhydroperoxide or diamide)	■	■			Activation
Thiol reagents (e.g. eosine maleimide, phenylarsine oxide, arsenite)	■	■			Activation
Increased matrix volume	■				Activation
Chaotropic agents	■				Activation
Adenine nucleotide depletion		■			Activation
Increse in matrix [Pi] and [ppi]		■			Activation
Alkalosis			■		Activation
Acidosis			■		Inhibition
Depolarization/uncoupling		■			Activation
Long chain fatty acids		■			Activation
CsA	■				Inhibition
SfA	■				Inhibition
Mg²⁺, Mn²⁺, Sr²⁺, Ba²⁺			■		Inhibition
Subiquinone analogues (e.g., decyl-ubiquinone, ubiquinone 10)				■	Activation / inhibition
Peroxynitrite and hydroxynonenal				■	Activation
Lonidamine				■	Inhibition
Trifluoperazine				■	Inhibition
Phenylglyoxal				■	Inhibition
Monobromobimane				■	Inhibition
Bongkrekic acid		■			Inhibition

A

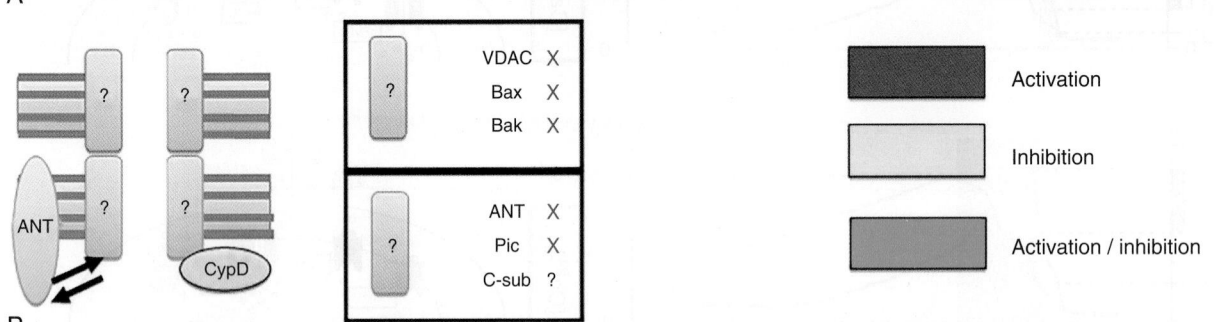

B

FIGURE 7.3 **Mitochondrial permeability transition pores (*mPTPs*).** (A) List of known mPTP effectors. Probable sites of action for the effectors are shown as *black boxes, red boxes, yellow boxes,* and a *blue box,* indicating the effects to mPTP (activation, inhibition, and both effects, respectively). (B) Scheme illustrating the proposed role of cyclophilin-D (*CypD*), adenine nucleotide translocator (*ANT*), Pi carrier (*PIC*), and c-subunit of mitochondrial adenosine triphosphate synthase (*C-sub*) in the formation of the mPTP structure.

which causes the release of huge amounts of Ca²⁺ and proapoptotic proteins from mitochondria and subsequently leads to cell death.[29] The pioneering studies showed that solutes up to 1.5 kDa can pass through this channel, suggesting that the pore diameter is approximately 3 nm. One of the important consequences of the mPTP opening is that the IMM no longer maintains a barrier to H⁺, which leads to Δp dissipation and thus inhibits ATP production (see "Overview of Mitochondrial Bioenergetics and Mitochondrial Membrane Potential"). Due to its pore size, mPTP opening also results in equilibration of cofactors and ions across the IMM including the release of accumulated Ca²⁺. This will not only lead to the disruption of metabolic gradients between the mitochondria and cytosol but also to the influx of water, which occurs concomitantly and results in swelling of the mitochondria until the OMM eventually ruptures. The OMM rupture releases cyt c and other proapoptotic proteins that potentially lead to apoptotic cell death (see "Overview of Mitochondria-Induced Apoptosis"). The mPTP opening plays a significant role in the generation of not only apoptotic cell death but also necrotic cell

death, both of which are involved in the etiology of myocardial infarction. It is also now widely recognized that mPTP opening is a major cause of reperfusion injury and an effective target for cardioprotection (see also "Role of Mitochondrial Ion Channels/Transporters in Cardioprotection Against Ischemia-Reperfusion Injury").

The properties of the mPTP are well defined, as summarized in Fig. 7.3A. However, despite extensive research by many laboratories, its exact molecular identity remains controversial (see Fig. 7.3B). Initially, the mPTP was proposed to consist of (1) the VDAC in OMM, (2) ANT and PIC in IMM, and (3) cyclophilin-D (CypD) in the matrix (see Fig. 7.3B). Indeed, pharmacological inhibitors of ANT or CypD also inhibit mPTP opening (see Fig. 7.3A). However, recent genetic studies using knockout cells or mouse models reveal that mPTP opening can still occur in the absence of VDAC, ANT, and PIC.[47–49] Therefore these proteins may be regulatory components of the mPTP rather than the channel subunits. As of now, only CypD remains potentially an essential component of mPTP. In addition to CypD, several groups reported that mitochondrial ATP synthase is a critical component of the mPTP and/or the c-subunit of mitochondrial ATP synthase serves a pore forming subunit.[50,51] Further studies, especially those using electrophysiological approaches, are required to confirm this discovery. Taken together, recent studies using the genetic approaches will provide us with further information related to the molecular identities of the mPTP, as well as to its physiological and pathophysiological properties in cardiomyocytes (see also "Role of Mitochondrial Ion Channels/Transporters in Cardioprotection Against Ischemia-Reperfusion Injury"). Interestingly, the mPTP has been also shown to open and close transiently ("flicker") at its low conductance state, which may also play a physiological role in the Ca^{2+} efflux mechanism[2] (see "Overview of Mitochondrial Reactive Oxygen Species Generation and Mitochondrial Membrane Potential"). Therefore the mPTP is also considered as one of the important Ca^{2+} efflux mechanism in both physiological and pathophysiological conditions (see Figs. 7.1 and 7.2). However, Pinton's group showed by genetically modulating the expression level of the c subunit that mPTP does not participate in mitochondrial Ca^{2+} homeostasis in HeLa cells.[52] Further studies should verify this observation in excitable cells such as cardiomyocytes.

Mitochondrial K+ Channels

Mitochondrial K_ATP Channel

Over 20 years ago, one of the K+ channel openers, nicorandil, was demonstrated to protect hearts against ischemia-reperfusion (I/R) injury (see review[53]). At first, earlier studies using pharmacological and genetic approaches in small animals indicated that the K+ channel openers, including nicorandil, were targeting K_{ATP} channels at SL (sarcK_{ATP}). Later, it became clear that in larger species, including humans, sarcK_{ATP} channels have a minor role in protecting the heart during ischemia, suggesting that other targets of these drugs such as mitochondria have essential roles in the protection of the heart from metabolic stress. Indeed, using the direct mitoplast patch-clamp technique, the presence of K_{ATP} activity was reported at the IMM, and the channels mediating this activity were named mitochondrial K_{ATP} channels (mitoK_{ATP}s) (see Fig. 7.1A) and exhibit channel properties similar to sarcK_{ATP}.[54] Currently, mitoK_{ATP} is thought to be essential for cardioprotection induced by ischemic preconditioning (IPC)[55] (see "Role of Mitochondrial Ion Channels/Transporters in Cardioprotection Against Ischemia-Reperfusion Injury"). Using a mitochondrial proteomic approach, O'Rourke's group has recently reported that one of the splice variants of the renal outer medullary K+ channel (ROMK) (Kir1.1) is a suitable candidate for the pore-forming subunit of mitoK_{ATP}.[56] This novel finding will need to be followed up using in vivo cardiac disease models. Since human ROMK mutations are well known as one of the responsible genes for the salt-wasting nephropathies (such as Bartter syndrome), further observations will be required to understand the mechanism for the sudden cardiac arrest and ventricular arrhythmias occasionally reported in these patients.

Mitochondrial K_Ca Channel

The mitochondrial K_{Ca} channel (mitoK_{Ca}) was functionally identified using the direct patch-clamp of mitoplasts obtained from cardiacmyocytes[57] (see Fig. 7.1A). This channel shows ~300-pS conductance and is inhibited by the K+ channel toxin charybdotoxin, which exhibits channel properties similar to K_{Ca} found in SL. Similar to mitoK_{ATP}, mitoK_{Ca} is thought to be essential for IPC and cardioprotection (see "Role of Mitochondrial Ion Channels/Transporters in Cardioprotection Against Ischemia-Reperfusion Injury"), but the molecular identity of this channel remains unclear.[55] Generally, big conductance Ca^{2+}-sensitive K+ (BK) channels are ubiquitously expressed in various cell types, but these channels are not functionally expressed in cardiac SL. Interestingly, a recent study showed that BK channel subunits are expressed in the IMM of neurons and cardiomyocytes and

that activation of this channel protects normoxic infant rabbit hearts.[58] Further studies, including genetic approaches, will be needed to confirm whether the protein of mitoK_{Ca} is identical or similar to the BK channels at SL.

Proton Fluxes and Uncoupling Proteins

Electron flow through the ETC is carried out by four enzyme complexes at the IMM, cyt c, and the mobile carrier CoQ_{10} (see "Overview of Mitochondrial Bioenergetics and Mitochondrial Membrane Potential"). Electron transfer processes through complexes I, III, and IV produce Δp that in turn are used to drive ATP synthase (complex V) (see Fig. 7.1B). When Δp increases, electron transport in complex III is partially inhibited; this results in the increased backup of electrons to CoQ_{10} for binding to molecular oxygen, leading to the generation of superoxide. The main route for the proton flow, driven by the electrochemical gradient, is through complex V and "proton leak." The proton leak is attributed to UCPs, which can modulate the ATP/ADP ratio.[59] Indeed, proton leak is known to contribute significantly to the control of respiration in mitochondria in state 4 and to some extent in state 3. Therefore UCPs are crucial to sustaining proton leak, preventing an excessively high H+ gradient, and ultimately avoiding excessive ROS production. There are three isoforms of UCPs (UCP1, 2, and 3) with ~60% homologies, but the isoform-specific roles of UCPs are still not clear.[60] UCP2 is ubiquitously expressed, including in the heart, whereas UCP3 is highly expressed in skeletal muscle, adipose tissue, and, to a lesser extent, the heart. The proton leak pathway via UCPs might be one of the mechanisms responsible for the cardioprotective effect of IPC, but very little is known about either the function or the regulation of UCPs in the adult heart. Further investigations with sophisticated approaches, such as genetic ablation of these proteins in cardiomyocytes, will be required to advance this important field of research.

Anion Channels and Mitochondrial Volume Control

Mitochondrial volume has been proposed to modulate the rate of substrate oxidation; thus mitochondrial swelling is a key issue in cellular pathophysiology, such as during mitophagy[61] and I/R injury.[62] As shown in "Mitochondrial Permeability Transition Pores," mPTP opening is involved in the mechanism of mitochondrial swelling. Since 1970s, the mitochondrial K+ cycle, especially counterbalancing MCU activity with the KHX, has been identified as an important component in mitochondrial volume homeostasis.[61] Not only cation movements, but also anion movements into the matrix induce mitochondrial swelling. Mitochondrial swelling experiments show that an anion-selective channel is present in the IMM. This channel is activated by matrix Mg^{2+} depletion and alkalization and is named the IMM anion channel (IMAC).[63] The physiological role of IMAC is still unknown because IMAC only appears to conduct ions under alkaline matrix conditions. However, this anion efflux through IMAC may be well designed to enable mitochondria to restore their normal volume following pathological swelling. We reported that single channel recordings of the heart IMM show a variety of anion-selective conductances, the most prominent of which is mediated by the centum picosiemen conductance channel, which matches the channel properties of IMAC.[43] Currently, the molecular identity of IMAC is still unknown.

Ion Channels/Transporters at the Mitochondrial Outer Membrane

Voltage-Dependent Anion Channel

VDAC is the most abundant protein in the OMM[64] and serves as the main pathway for the metabolite/ion transport between the cytosol and the IMS of mitochondria (see Fig. 7.1A and C). Currently, three distinct VDAC isoforms are known with high sequence homology (65%–70% identity) and similar structure.[65] The recombinant VDAC1 and two isoforms are able to form pores in lipid bilayers, but recombinant VDAC3 has no evident pore-forming ability. Usually, VDAC is seven times more permeable to Cl^- than to K^+. VDAC channels can also exist in a variety of functional states that differ in their ability to pass nonelectrolytes and conduct ions.[66] VDAC exhibits ~3 nS in 1-M NaCl in full conductance open state (Fig. 7.4B). In the open state, it shows a significant preference for anions and especially favors metabolic anions. The closed state favors cations. The permeability of VDAC to small anions by free diffusion includes K^+, Na^+, and the double positive charge ion Ca^{2+}. Ca^{2+} permeates through both the open and closed states of VDAC due to its double positive charge, which allows it to enter during the open state because the anion selectivity is not very high in VDAC. Small nonelectrolytes can also pass through the open channel, allowing the passage of metabolites (ATP, ADP, and Pi). VDAC gating has a bell-shaped voltage-dependent profile, with peak currents around 10 mV.[64] There are a variety of factors reported to modulate VDAC function, including colloidal osmotic pressure, protein(s) at the IMS, polyanions including charged proteins and nucleic acids, reduced nicotinamide adenine dinucleotide (NADH) and MgNADPH, tBid, actin, tubulin, and phosphorylation by intracellular signaling[66,67]; further, VDAC was identified as a target of various protein kinases and specific phosphorylation sites have been identified (see Fig. 7.4A). It has been reported that the phosphorylated state enhances tubulin binding to VDAC, followed by blockage of channel activity.[68]

As shown in "Overview of Mitochondria-Induced Apoptosis," recent studies have focused on the regulation of OMM permeability by a physiological or pathophysiological mechanism. While, VDAC is excluded as a component of the mPTP, VDAC is indeed one of the major factors for the regulation of cell death signaling (see "Mitochondrial Permeability Transition Pores" and Fig. 7.3B). VDAC has an interaction with the apoptosis regulators, Bcl2-family members, hexokinases, and the cytoskeleton system including tubulin, which changes the VDAC channel activity.[69] For instance, Bax forms hetero-oligomers with VDAC and activates VDAC, followed by cyt c release from IMS. Hexokinase-I has been shown to directly interact

with VDAC1, which induces antiapoptotic effects. The contribution of VDAC to cell death can be isoform- and stimulus-dependent: VDAC1 serves as a proapoptotic protein, whereas VDAC2 protects from apoptosis.[70] Recently, De Stefani and colleagues showed that the proapoptotic effect of VDAC1 is due to its physical interaction with the IP_3 receptor and its formation of the molecular route for transferring Ca^{2+} signals to mitochondria in apoptosis.[71]

Apoptosis-Induced Channels

As shown in "Overview of Mitochondria-Induced Apoptosis," the release of these proapoptotic factors including cyt c is regulated by OMM permeability and at least three distinct mechanisms. The first pathway is mediated through mPTP opening (see "Mitochondrial Permeability Transition Pores"), and the second pathway is via modification of VDAC through the interaction of Bcl-2 families (see "Voltage-Dependent Anion Channel"). The third pathway is the mitochondrial apoptosis–induced channel (MAC), which forms in the OMM during an early stage of apoptosis and directly provides a route for cyt c to release from the IMS to the cytosol (see review[72]). Unlike VDAC, MAC is partially cation-selective and has voltage-independent gating (see Fig. 7.4B). The pore size of MAC is sufficient to be permeable to 10–17-kDa proteins, which allows the passage of the 12-kDa cyt c. MAC is regulated by the Bcl-2 family. Studies using reconstituted proteins and knockout cell lines have shown that MAC activity is tightly connected to Bax/Bak expression and to their insertion and oligomerization in the OMM, suggesting that at least these two proapoptotic proteins are crucial structural components (pore) of MAC (see Fig. 7.4B). Since the molecular mass of oligomerized Bax obtained from mitochondrial membranes show very large size, MAC might associate with other mitochondrial proteins at the OMM.[73]

Mitochondrial Ion Channels/Transporters in Cardiac Function and Dysfunction

Overview of Mitochondrial Structure and Function in the Heart

In adult cardiomyocytes, mitochondria are the dominant intracellular organelle, numbering in the range of ~7000 per cell, with

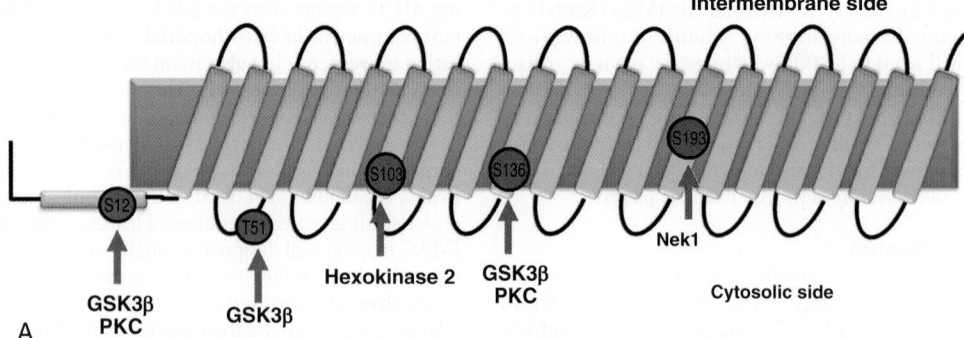

	VDAC	MAC	Bax	mPTP	TOM
Peak conductance (nS)	0.5-4	1-5	1.0-5.4	1.1±0.1	0.7±0.1
Ion selectivity	Anion	Sl. Cation	Sl. Cation	Sl. Cation	Sl. Cation
Voltage dependent	Yes	No	No	Yes	No

FIGURE 7.4 Voltage-dependent anion channel (VDAC). (A) Schematic diagram of predicted phosphorylation sites in VDAC1 structure. (B) Comparison of biophysical properties between VDAC, other outer mitochondrial membrane channels (mitochondrial anion channel [MAC] and translocase of the outer membrane of mitochondria [TOM]), mitochondrial permeability transition pores (mPTPs) and a reconstituted "Bax channel." Bax channel function was observed in the reconstituted channel using purified human Bax protein.

their mass occupying up to 35% of the cell volume.[74] There are three different subpopulations of mitochondria in the adult heart with unique sizes and shapes: interfibrillar, subsarcolemmal, and perinuclear mitochondria.[75] Interfibrillar mitochondria are aligned in longitudinal rows between myofibrils in close proximity to SR Ca^{2+} release sites. They often span a single sarcomere from Z-band to Z-band and are relatively uniform in size and shape (Fig. 7.5A and B). This unique spatial localization of interfibrillar mitochondria enables a privileged Ca^{2+}-mediated crosstalk between SR and mitochondria (see also "Mitochondrial Ion Channels/Transporters in Cardiac Excitation–Contraction/ Metabolism Coupling and Reactive Oxygen Species Generation") (see Fig. 7.5C). In contrast, subsarcolemmal and perinuclear mitochondria appear less organized and more variable in shape and size. Generally, mitochondrial morphology and dynamics, including mitochondrial fission, fusion, and movement, are well correlated with their metabolic activity.[75] In cardiomyocytes, the regulatory proteins responsible for mitochondrial dynamics, including dynamin-like protein (DLP1), mitofusin (Mfn)1, and Mfn2, are highly expressed. Recently, Maack and Dorn's group show that Mfn2 is important for the maintenance of bioenergetic responses via interorganelle Ca^{2+} crosstalk using cardiac-specific Mfn knockout mice, suggesting that Mfn2 serves as a tether of SR to mitochondria in cardiomyocytes.[76] However, there is still no data directly showing the subcellular localization of Mfn2 in native cardiomyocytes. Using cardiac-specific Mfn knockout mice, Walsh's group showed that Mfn1 and Mfn2 have important roles in the structural and metabolic development of cardiac mitochondria during the postnatal state.[77] Further studies are required to clarify the specific role of the regulatory proteins for mitochondrial form and dynamics including Mfn in adult cardiomyocytes.

Mitochondrial Ion Channels/Transporters in Cardiac Excitation–Contraction/Metabolism Coupling and Reactive Oxygen Species Generation

Ca^{2+} plays a central role in E–C coupling of cardiac muscle[78] (see Fig. 7.5C). Ca^{2+} entry via the voltage-gated L-type Ca^{2+} channel (VLCC) triggers the opening of SR-RyR2 faced toward the transverse tubules (T-tubules) and induces a release of Ca^{2+} from the SR (Ca^{2+}-induced Ca^{2+} release [CICR]). The concomitant rise of $[Ca^{2+}]_c$ activates cardiac contraction by binding to troponin C. $[Ca^{2+}]_c$ is then removed through the SR Ca^{2+} pump (SR Ca^{2+}-ATPase [SERCA]) or extruded from the cell via the sarcolemmal NCX. Usually, when the amplitude and/or frequency of the $[Ca^{2+}]_c$ transient become higher, the cardiac work increases except for the Frank-Starling mechanism. Therefore increased Ca^{2+} cycling is correlated with more ATP consumption. Accumulating evidence indicates that cardiac mitochondria take up $[Ca^{2+}]_c$ during E–C coupling and $[Ca^{2+}]_m$ accumulation serves as a signal to ensure the balance of energy supply and demand (excitation–metabolism coupling).[79] However, the kinetics of $[Ca^{2+}]_m$ uptake are still a matter of debate.

The composition and structure of Ca^{2+} microdomains located between SR and mitochondria in cardiomyocytes are still not clear. It is widely established that ER Ca^{2+} release channel IP_3 receptor is involved in Ca^{2+}-mediated crosstalk between ER and mitochondria in noncardiac cells (see Fig. 7.1C). However, Ca^{2+} release from SR in ventricular myocytes occurs exclusively via RyR2 and not from the IP_3 receptor. The majority of RyR2 were found along the T-tubule side of the SR and beneath VLCCs (see Fig. 7.5C). This unique localization tightly controls CICR in cardiomyocytes.[78] Therefore in cardiomyocytes it is a reasonable scenario that high local concentrations of Ca^{2+} after CICR in the subspace between the T-tubule membrane and SR can subsequently diffuse to nearby mitochondria to create microdomains of high Ca^{2+} around the cardiac mitochondria. Another scenario is that a smaller number of RyR2 are located in the distal end of the SR-facing mitochondria and release Ca^{2+} at the microdomain between SR and mitochondria, allowing mitochondrial Ca^{2+} channels such as MCU and RyR1 to take up Ca^{2+} into the matrix efficiently (see Fig. 7.5C). Kim's group has recently showed the possibility of functional coupling of RyR2 and VDAC2 at the SR–mitochondrial contact site in HL-1 cardiac cells,[80] but it is still unclear whether adult ventricular myocytes also possess this molecular architecture. Further studies will be required using adult cardiomyocytes with genetic manipulation to resolve the detailed localization of the channel transporters at the microdomains involved in this coupling process, including RyR2, VDAC, MCU, and mRyR1.

A second controversy related to the kinetics of $[Ca^{2+}]_m$ is whether mitochondria can take up and release Ca^{2+} in each heartbeat (an oscillator) (see Fig. 7.5D, Model I) or they act as an integrator by taking up Ca^{2+} gradually, resulting in steady state $[Ca^{2+}]_m$ increase (see Fig. 7.5D, Model II).[81] Interestingly, rabbit and guinea pig adult cardiomyocytes respond to $[Ca^{2+}]_c$ transients on a beat-to-beat basis (Model I), but rat cardiomyocyte mitochondria respond to $[Ca^{2+}]_c$ transients with a gradual $[Ca^{2+}]_m$ increase without obvious beat-to-beat $[Ca^{2+}]_m$ transients (Model II). This incapability of mitochondria to respond to $[Ca^{2+}]_c$ transients might be partly due to the slow kinetics of the mitochondrial Ca^{2+} efflux mechanism, but the mechanisms underlying these species differences in the kinetics of $[Ca^{2+}]_m$ are still unknown. Though mitochondria occupy 35% of the cytosolic space and are well-known to uptake Ca^{2+}, it is still controversial whether mitochondrial Ca^{2+} uptake contributes to the kinetics of beat-to-beat $[Ca^{2+}]_c$ transient formation in ventricular myocytes.[82] Several groups estimated that the mitochondria do not serve as a significant dynamic buffer of $[Ca^{2+}]_c$ under physiological conditions in ventricular myocytes.[83,84]

As discussed in "Historical Overview of Mitochondrial Ion Channel/Transporter Research," MCU has been widely recognized as the main mechanism for mitochondrial Ca^{2+} uptake in various cell types/tissues.[85] Indeed recent studies using adult cardiomyocytes from conditional and cardiomyocyte-specific MCU knockout mice clearly confirmed that MCU is the main mechanism for transducing the changes of $[Ca^{2+}]_c$ into changes of $[Ca^{2+}]_m$ in adult cardiomyocytes.[86,87] In addition, the possibility of additional Ca^{2+} uptake pathways, such as mRyR1 and Letm1, has been gaining recognition. Moreover, cardiac mitochondria contain two modes of Ru360-sensitive Ca^{2+} uptakes, a high Ca^{2+} affinity rapid uptake mode and a low Ca^{2+} affinity slow uptake mode, which are responsible for modulating OXPHOS and Ca^{2+} buffering, respectively.[88] Surprisingly, half maximal activation ($K_{0.5}$) of the MCU current (I_{MiCa}) observed in mitoplast patch clamp is $\cong 20$ mM, where single channel activities of MCU were specifically dissected by recognizing its unique biophysical and pharmacological characteristics.[89] This $K_{0.5}$ for purified MCU current is quite different from that determined in isolated cardiac mitochondria, which ranges from 1 to 189 µM. This discrepancy might be in part due to the differences in experimental conditions. However, the combination of multiple Ca^{2+} influx mechanisms with different $K_{0.5}$ in isolated mitochondria could also lead to this variation. Interestingly, I_{MiCa} density in the heart appears to be much smaller than in other tissues and mRNA for MICU1 is also particularly low in the heart, raising an important question about the relative contribution of MCU and other Ca^{2+} influx mechanisms especially in cardiac mitochondria (see review[3]). Indeed, the recent molecular identification of MCU studies, which employed nonexcitable cells, showed a 100-times slower and longer time course of mitochondrial Ca^{2+} transients than those recorded from cardiomyocytes,[8,9] strongly suggesting that cardiac mitochondria contain not only MCU but also other Ca^{2+} influx mechanisms, such as mRyR1 and the rapid mode of uptake (RaM), which have higher Ca^{2+} sensitivity and faster Ca^{2+}

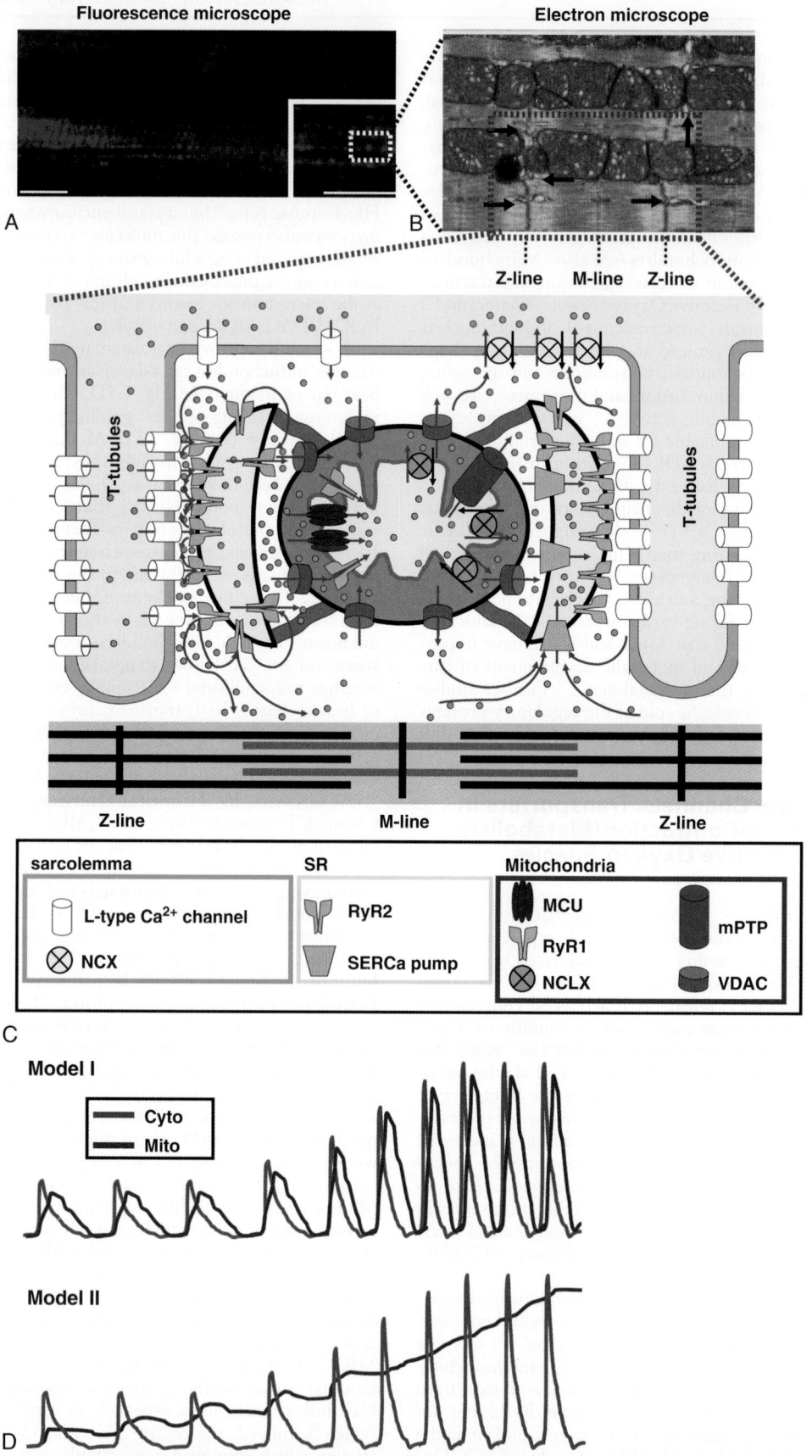

Fluorescence microscope

A

Electron microscope

B

Z-line   M-line   Z-line

T-tubules

T-tubules

Z-line   M-line   Z-line

sarcolemma	SR	Mitochondria	
⬛ L-type Ca²⁺ channel	RyR2	MCU	mPTP
⊗ NCX	SERCa pump	RyR1	VDAC
		⊗ NCLX	

C

Model I

—— Cyto
—— Mito

Model II

D

FIGURE 7.5 Overview of mitochondrial structure and function in the heart. (A) Cardiac mitochondrial structure observed in fluorescence microscope. Mouse ventricular tissue was stained by cyclophilin-D antibodies. (B) Cardiac mitochondrial ultrastructure observed in electron microscope. Mouse papillary muscle obtained from left ventricle was observed by transmission electron microscope. (C) Schematic diagram of cardiac excitation–contraction coupling including mitochondrial structure and ion channels. Left panel shows mitochondrial Ca²⁺ influx mechanisms at systole and right panel shows mitochondrial Ca²⁺ efflux mechanisms at diastole. (D) [Ca²⁺]$_m$ oscillation models in cardiomyocytes.

uptake kinetics during heartbeats. We previously showed that this Ca^{2+} uptake mode exhibits a much greater magnitude and rate of $[Ca^{2+}]_m$ than those observed in response to slow $[Ca^{2+}]_c$ pulses and is more sensitive to ryanodine (see review[3]). Moreover the $[Ca^{2+}]_c$-mRyR1 activity relationship is bimodal (see also "Mitochondrial Permeability Transition Pores"). These unique properties lead us to hypothesize that mRyR1 is an ideal candidate for sequestering Ca^{2+} quickly and transiently during the heartbeat, whereas MCU would be an ideal candidate for sequestering Ca^{2+} slowly and steadily in the higher and plateau phase of Ca^{2+} pulses, such as sustained increases in the resting $[Ca^{2+}]_c$.

In cardiomyocytes, mitochondria are the main source of ROS production and have crucial roles for the ROS signaling in physiological and pathophysiological conditions. As shown in "Overview of Mitochondrial Reactive Oxygen Species Generation and Mitochondrial Membrane Potential," recent studies discovered mSOFs in adult cardiomyocytes, which is mediated through the transient openings of the mPTP triggered by a small increase in constitutive ROS production at the ETC. Therefore, in cardiomyocytes, it seems that there is a "ROS-induced ROS release" mechanism.[90] To understand this functional coupling and cross-talk between mPTP "flickering" activity and ETC-dependent superoxide production in cardiomyocytes, the question moves to which superoxide production sites (complexes I and/or III) are important for the ignition of transient mPTP opening in intact cardiomyocytes (see Fig. 7.1B). O'Rourke's group, using intact cardiomyocytes, reported that the majority of mitochondrial ROS is from complex III,[62] whereas Dirksen's group proposed that complex I may trigger mPTP opening followed by mSOF.[91] It also remains to be determined which sites of ROS production in cardiac mitochondria are activated under pathophysiological conditions, such as during hypoxia. The next question is how the spatial and temporal organization of the mitochondrial network in cardiomyocytes can regulate mSOF size and frequency (see Fig. 7.5). It is known that the molecular architecture of the T-tubules and SR network regulates Ca^{2+} sparks from SR-RyR2 and that the alteration of these structures under heart failure can modulate the spark frequency.[92] Since mitochondrial structure and alignments are altered under the pathological heart, the state of the mitochondrial three-dimensional network and local ROS diffusion might modulate mSOF size and frequency as in the case of Ca^{2+} sparks. These questions will be resolved in the future by updating three-dimensional fluorescence image systems and by developing the computational cardiomyocyte model to include mitochondrial network.[93]

Mitochondrial Ion Channels/Transporters in Cardiac Dysfunction: Novel Therapeutic Targets

Role of Mitochondrial Ion Channels/Transporters in Cardioprotection Against Ischemia-Reperfusion Injury

Transient episodes of nonlethal myocardial I/R provide a protective effect against myocardial injuries in response to prolonged lethal ischemia. This phenomenon is known as IPC. In cardiomyocytes, both $mitoK_{ATP}$ and $mitoK_{Ca}$ channels play key roles in cardioprotection (see "Mitochondrial K^+ Channels"). Interestingly, activation of the $mitoK_{ATP}$ channel is augmented by PKC or tyrosine kinases, whereas the $mitoK_{Ca}$ channel is activated by PKA, suggesting that these two channels are regulated by independent mechanisms to protect the heart from I/R injury.[55] Opening of $mitoK_{ATP}$ and $mitoK_{Ca}$ depolarizes $\Delta\Psi_m$, which reduces the driving force for Ca^{2+} influx, thereby attenuating mitochondrial Ca^{2+} overload (see Fig. 7.1). Consequently, prevention of matrix Ca^{2+} overload inhibits mPTP opening and protects against heart cell death (see "Mitochondrial Permeability Transition Pores"). A recent clinical study has demonstrated a significant improvement in patient outcome due to a reduction in

major coronary events by antianginal therapy with a $mitoK_{ATP}$-channel opener (nicorandil, see "Mitochondrial K_{ATP} Channel") in patients with stable angina.[94] These evidences suggest that the activators of these K^+ channels and/or the activators of the upstream signaling for the regulation of these channels may provide new therapeutic strategies for ischemic heart disease.

As shown in "Overview of Mitochondria-Induced Apoptosis," OMM permeability also regulates the release of proapoptotic factors from mitochondria. Therefore it is a reasonable assumption that controlling the OMM permeability is also one of the potential therapeutic strategies for protection from I/R injury. Growing evidence shows that inhibiting VDAC interaction with Bcl-2 families and/or enhancing the hexokinases-VDAC interaction might have cardioprotective effects[95] (see "Voltage-Dependent Anion Channel").

The mPTP retained much attention from researchers as a strong candidate for a potential therapeutic target against I/R injury and myocardial infarction (see "Mitochondrial Permeability Transition Pores"). Many studies using cells or animal models clearly showed that mPTP inhibition, including CsA treatment, exhibits a cardioprotective effect, such as reducing the infarct size. Finally, recent clinical trials showed that CsA can reduce infarct size and improve recovery of contractile function during reperfusion in human patients.[96] In addition, two groups recently showed that genetic deletion of MCU inhibits mPTP opening upon acute $[Ca^{2+}]_c$ elevation during I/R and protects the heart from I/R injury,[86,87] suggesting that mitochondrial Ca^{2+} overload via MCU is a key modulator of mPTP activity in vivo. These observations indicate that delaying or preventing irreversible mPTP opening by directly (e.g., using CsA) or indirectly (e.g., preventing mitochondrial Ca^{2+} overload via MCU) inhibiting mPTP channel activity can be potential therapeutic strategies in treating ischemic heart disease. It is clear that understanding the identification of the molecular components, detailed structure, and regulation of the mPTP is crucial for designing novel and potent therapeutic drugs that are more specifically targeted to the pore (see Fig. 7.3).

Role of Mitochondrial Ion Channels/Transporters in Cardiac Arrhythmias

Cardiac arrhythmias can cause sudden cardiac death, especially during heart failure. The principal pathological processes underlying arrhythmias are heterogeneity of the cardiac action potential at the cellular level, which is commonly linked to ventricular arrhythmias.[97] Ion channels in SL have received much attention for their ability to influence action potential duration. Sarcolemmal ion channel mutations can cause alterations in the action potential duration (long and short QT syndrome) and the appearance of early or delayed after-depolarizations. Recently, increasing evidence suggests that altered cardiac ion homeostasis and structural remodeling are highly associated with elevated ROS and metabolic stress, implying the cardiac mitochondria play a key role in arrhythmia generation (see also review[98]).

Mitochondrial oxidative stress contributes to a wide range of perturbations in cardiac ion channel functions. ROS induce functional and structural alteration of Nav1.5 by both transcriptional and posttranslational mechanisms. Elevated ROS mediates SERCA inhibition, enhances SR Ca^{2+} release from RyR2, enhances VLCC current, and increases sarcolemmal NCX activity to increase the intracellular Ca^{2+} level. ROS-mediated CaMKII activation stimulates hyperphosphorylation of RyR2, resulting SR Ca^{2+} leak. These ROS-mediated network changes in the activities of ion channels/pumps are likely to contribute to the pathogenesis of arrhythmias. The conventional design of antiarrhythmic drugs target ion channels at SL to decrease ion currents. The above-mentioned observations suggest new potential therapeutic strategies to prevent arrhythmias by targeting ROS. However, general antioxidant strategies have not always been successful in antiarrhythmic therapies, in part due to the physiological levels of ROS that are essential for cell signaling and that the dominant source of ROS is from mitochondria (see "Overview of Mitochondrial Reactive Oxygen Species Generation and Mitochondrial Membrane Potential"). Therefore further improvements, such as directly targeting the sites of ROS production in mitochondria and using dosages that are within the therapeutic window, will be required.

Closing Remarks

Mitochondrial ion channels/transporters have historically been kept as an important topic in cell biology, despite the relatively slow progress in the elucidation of their molecular identities. Using multiple research tools, such as gene screening analysis, genetic manipulation, and updated biochemical, pharmacological, cell-biological, and electrophysiological techniques, has led to recent groundbreaking discoveries in the molecular identities of mtCUC, NCLX, and mPTP. The advances in cloning of mitochondrial Ca^{2+} channels/transporters will provide essential information for studying (1) the regulation of mitochondrial Ca^{2+} influx and efflux mechanisms such as posttranslational modifications of these channels/transporters, (2) the design or discovery of more specific inhibitors/activators to each channel/transporter for the potential development of therapeutic drugs, and furthermore (3) the molecular mechanisms underlying mitochondrial Ca^{2+}-mediated human diseases. However, we need to keep in mind the molecular identities of numerous mitochondrial ion channels/transporters including some K^+ channels.

In conclusion, cardiac mitochondrial ion channels/transporters are crucial in governing energy production, Ca^{2+} homeostasis, ROS generation, and cell survival and death in the heart. Revealing the molecular identities and biophysical characteristics of cardiac mitochondrial ion channels/ transporters will provide us with new therapeutic strategies for treating human cardiac diseases.

REFERENCES

1. Glancy B, Balaban RS. Role of mitochondrial Ca^{2+} in the regulation of cellular energetics. *Biochemistry.* 2012;51:2959–2973.
2. Gunter TE, Sheu SS. Characteristics and possible functions of mitochondrial Ca^{2+} transport mechanisms. *Biochim Biophys Acta.* 2009;1787:1291–1308.
3. O-Uchi J, Pan S, Sheu SS. Perspectives on: SGP symposium on mitochondrial physiology and medicine: molecular identities of mitochondrial Ca^{2+} influx mechanism: updated passwords for accessing mitochondrial Ca^{2+}-linked health and disease. *J Gen Physiol.* 2012;139:435–443.
4. Baughman JM, Perocchi F, Girgis HS, et al. Integrative genomics identifies MCU as an essential component of the mitochondrial calcium uniporter. *Nature.* 2011;476:341–345.
5. De Stefani D, Raffaello A, Teardo E, Szabo I, Rizzuto R. A forty-kilodalton protein of the inner membrane is the mitochondrial calcium uniporter. *Nature.* 2011;476:336–340.
6. De Stefani D, Patron M, Rizzuto R. Structure and function of the mitochondrial calcium uniporter complex. *Biochim Biophys Acta.* 2015;1853:2006–2011.
7. Kamer KJ, Mootha VK. The molecular era of the mitochondrial calcium uniporter. *Nat Rev Mol Cell Biol.* 2015;16:545–553.
8. O-Uchi J, Jhun BS, Xu S, et al. Adrenergic signaling regulates mitochondrial Ca^{2+} uptake through Pyk2-dependent tyrosine phosphorylation of the mitochondrial Ca^{2+} uniporter. *Antioxid Redox Signal.* 2014;21:863–879.
9. Joiner ML, Koval OM, Li J, et al. CaMKII determines mitochondrial stress responses in heart. *Nature.* 2012;491:269–273.
10. Lee Y, Min CK, Kim TG, et al. Structure and function of the N-terminal domain of the human mitochondrial calcium uniporter. *EMBO Rep.* 2015;16:1318–1333.
11. Dedkova EN, Blatter LA. Calcium signaling in cardiac mitochondria. *J Mol Cell Cardiol.* 2013;58:125–133.
12. Jiang D, Zhao L, Clapham DE. Genome-wide RNAi screen identifies Letm1 as a mitochondrial Ca^{2+}/H^+ antiporter. *Science.* 2009;326:144–147.
13. Kocherginsky N. Acidic lipids, H^+-ATPases, and mechanism of oxidative phosphorylation. physico-chemical ideas 30 years after P. Mitchell's nobel prize award. *Prog Biophys Mol Biol.* 2009;99:20–41.
14. Chicco AJ, Sparagna GC. Role of cardiolipin alterations in mitochondrial dysfunction and disease. *Am J Physiol Cell Physiol.* 2007;292:C33–C44.
15. Soubannier V, McBride HM. Positioning mitochondrial plasticity within cellular signaling cascades. *Biochim Biophys Acta.* 2009;1793:154–170.
16. Trachootham D, Lu W, Ogasawara MA, Nilsa RD, Huang P. Redox regulation of cell survival. *Antioxid Redox Signal.* 2008;10:1343–1374.
17. Santos CX, Anilkumar N, Zhang M, Brewer AC, Shah AM. Redox signaling in cardiac myocytes. *Free Radic Biol Med.* 2011;50:777–793.
18. Gong G, Liu X, Zhang H, Sheu SS, Wang W. Mitochondrial flash as a novel biomarker of mitochondrial respiration in the heart. *Am J Physiol Heart Circ Physiol.* 2015;309:H1166–H1177.
19. Wang W, Fang H, Groom L, et al. Superoxide flashes in single mitochondria. *Cell.* 2008;134:279–290.
20. Bernardi P, von Stockum S. The permeability transition pore as a Ca^{2+} release channel: new answers to an old question. *Cell Calcium.* 2012;52:22–27.

21. Mughal W, Kirshenbaum LA. Cell death signalling mechanisms in heart failure. *Exp Clin Cardiol.* 2011;16:102–108.
22. Estaquier J, Vallette F, Vayssiere JL, Mignotte B. The mitochondrial pathways of apoptosis. *Adv Exp Med Biol.* 2012;942:157–183.
23. Wang C, Youle RJ. The role of mitochondria in apoptosis*. *Annu Rev Genet.* 2009;43:95–118.
24. Kroemer G, Galluzzi L, Brenner C. Mitochondrial membrane permeabilization in cell death. *Physiol Rev.* 2007;87:99–163.
25. Drago I, De Stefani D, Rizzuto R, Pozzan T. Mitochondrial Ca^{2+} uptake contributes to buffering cytoplasmic Ca^{2+} peaks in cardiomyocytes. *Proc Natl Acad Sci U S A.* 2012;109:12986–12991.
26. Raffaello A, De Stefani D, Sabbadin D, et al. The mitochondrial calcium uniporter is a multimer that can include a dominant-negative pore-forming subunit. *EMBO J.* 2013;32:2362–2376.
27. Fieni F, Kirichok Y. Patch-clamp analysis of mitochondrial Ca^{2+} uniporter in different tissues. *J Gen Physiol.* 2011;56A.
28. Patron M, Checchetto V, Raffaello A, et al. MICU1 and MICU2 finely tune the mitochondrial Ca^{2+} uniporter by exerting opposite effects on MCU activity. *Mol Cell.* 2014;53:726–737.
29. Sancak Y, Markhard AL, Kitami T, et al. EMRE is an essential component of the mitochondrial calcium uniporter complex. *Science.* 2013;342:1379–1382.
30. Perocchi F, Gohil VM, Girgis HS, et al. MICU1 encodes a mitochondrial EF hand protein required for Ca^{2+} uptake. *Nature.* 2010;467:291–296.
31. Plovanich M, Bogorad RL, Sancak Y, et al. MICU2, a paralog of MICU1, resides within the mitochondrial uniporter complex to regulate calcium handling. *PLoS One.* 2013;8: e55785.
32. Hajnoczky G, Booth D, Csordas G, et al. Reliance of ER-mitochondrial calcium signaling on mitochondrial EF-hand Ca^{2+} binding proteins: miros, MICUs, LETM1 and solute carriers. *Curr Opin Cell Biol.* 2014;29:133–141.
33. Murgia M, Rizzuto R. Molecular diversity and pleiotropic role of the mitochondrial calcium uniporter. *Cell Calcium.* 2015;58:11–17.
34. Csordas G, Thomas AP, Hajnoczky G. Quasi-synaptic calcium signal transmission between endoplasmic reticulum and mitochondria. *EMBO J.* 1999;18:96–108.
35. Csordas G, Varnai P, Golenar T, et al. Imaging interorganelle contacts and local calcium dynamics at the ER-mitochondrial interface. *Mol Cell.* 2010;39:121–132.
36. Rizzuto R, Pinton P, Carrington W, et al. Close contacts with the endoplasmic reticulum as determinants of mitochondrial Ca^{2+} responses. *Science.* 1998;280:1763–1766.
37. Giacomello M, Drago I, Bortolozzi M, et al. Ca^{2+} hot spots on the mitochondrial surface are generated by Ca^{2+} mobilization from stores, but not by activation of store-operated Ca^{2+} channels. *Mol Cell.* 2010;38:280–290.
38. Mallilankaraman K, Cardenas C, Doonan PJ, et al. MCUR1 is an essential component of mitochondrial Ca^{2+} uptake that regulates cellular metabolism. *Nat Cell Biol.* 2012;14:1336–1343.
39. Hoffman NE, Chandramoorthy HC, Shanmughapriya S, et al. SLC25A23 augments mitochondrial Ca^{2+} uptake, interacts with MCU, and induces oxidative stress-mediated cell death. *Mol Biol Cell.* 2014;25:936–947.
40. Ryu SY, Beutner G, Dirksen RT, Kinnally KW, Sheu SS. Mitochondrial ryanodine receptors and other mitochondrial Ca^{2+} permeable channels. *FEBS Lett.* 2010;584:1948–1955.

41. Beutner G, Sharma VK, Giovannucci DR, Yule DI, Sheu SS. Identification of a ryanodine receptor in rat heart mitochondria. *J Biol Chem.* 2001;276:21482–21488.
42. Altschafl BA, Beutner G, Sharma VK, Sheu SS, Valdivia HH. The mitochondrial ryanodine receptor in rat heart: a pharmaco-kinetic profile. *Biochim Biophys Acta.* 2007;1768:1784–1795.
43. Ryu SY, Beutner G, Kinnally KW, Dirksen RT, Sheu SS. Single channel characterization of the mitochondrial ryanodine receptor in heart mitoplasts. *J Biol Chem.* 2011;286:21324–21329.
44. Tsai MF, Jiang D, Zhao L, Clapham D, Miller C. Functional reconstitution of the mitochondrial Ca^{2+}/H^+ antiporter Letm1. *J Gen Physiol.* 2014;143:67–73.
45. Palty R, Silverman WF, Hershfinkel M, et al. NCLX is an essential component of mitochondrial Na^+/Ca^{2+} exchange. *Proc Natl Acad Sci U S A.* 2010;107:436–441.
46. Takeuchi A, Kim B, Matsuoka S. The mitochondrial Na^+-Ca^{2+} exchanger, NCLX, regulates automaticity of HL-1 cardiomyocytes. *Sci Rep.* 2013;3:2766.
47. Baines CP. The mitochondrial permeability transition pore and ischemia-reperfusion injury. *Basic Res Cardiol.* 2009;104:181–188.
48. Halestrap AP. What is the mitochondrial permeability transition pore? *J Mol Cell Cardiol.* 2009;46:821–831.
49. Varanyuwatana P, Halestrap AP. The roles of phosphate and the phosphate carrier in the mitochondrial permeability transition pore. *Mitochondrion.* 2012;12:120–125.
50. Halestrap AP, Richardson AP. The mitochondrial permeability transition: a current perspective on its identity and role in ischaemia/reperfusion injury. *J Mol Cell Cardiol.* 2015;78:129–141.
51. Morciano G, Giorgi C, Bonora M, et al. Molecular identity of the mitochondrial permeability transition pore and its role in ischemia-reperfusion injury. *J Mol Cell Cardiol.* 2015;78:142–153.
52. De Marchi E, Bonora M, Giorgi C, Pinton P. The mitochondrial permeability transition pore is a dispensable element for mitochondrial calcium efflux. *Cell Calcium.* 2014;56:1–13.
53. O'Rourke B. Mitochondrial ion channels. *Annu Rev Physiol.* 2007;69:19–49.
54. Flagg TP, Enkvetchakul D, Koster JC, Nichols CG. Muscle KATP channels: recent insights to energy sensing and myoprotection. *Physiol Rev.* 2010;90:799–829.
55. Nishida H, Sato T, Ogura T, Nakaya H. New aspects for the treatment of cardiac diseases based on the diversity of functional controls on cardiac muscles: mitochondrial ion channels and cardioprotection. *J Pharmacol Sci.* 2009;109:341–347.
56. Foster DB, Ho AS, Rucker J, et al. Mitochondrial ROMK channel is a molecular component of MitoKATP. *Circ Res.* 2012;111:446–454.
57. Xu W, Liu Y, Wang S, et al. Cytoprotective role of Ca^{2+}-activated K^+ channels in the cardiac inner mitochondrial membrane. *Science.* 2002;298:1029–1033.
58. Shi Y, Jiang MT, Su J, Hutchins W, Konorev E, Baker JE. Mitochondrial big conductance KCa channel and cardioprotection in infant rabbit heart. *J Cardiovasc Pharmacol.* 2007;50:497–502.
59. Sluse FE. Uncoupling proteins: molecular, functional, regulatory, physiological and pathological aspects. *Adv Exp Med Biol.* 2012;942:137–156.
60. Mailloux RJ, Harper ME. Uncoupling proteins and the control of mitochondrial reactive oxygen species production. *Free Radic Biol Med.* 2011;51:1106–1115.

61. Nowikovsky K, Schweyen RJ, Bernardi P. Pathophysiology of mitochondrial volume homeostasis: potassium transport and permeability transition. *Biochim Biophys Acta.* 2009;1787:345–350.

62. O'Rourke B, Cortassa S, Aon MA. Mitochondrial ion channels: gatekeepers of life and death. *Physiology (Bethesda).* 2005;20:303–315.

63. Aon MA, Cortassa S, Akar FG, Brown DA, Zhou L, O'Rourke B. From mitochondrial dynamics to arrhythmias. *Int J Biochem Cell Biol.* 2009;41:1940–1948.

64. Shoshan-Barmatz V, De Pinto V, Zweckstetter M, Raviv Z, Keinan N, Arbel N.VDAC, a multi-functional mitochondrial protein regulating cell life and death. *Mol Aspects Med.* 2010;31:227–285.

65. Messina A, Reina S, Guarino F, De Pinto V. VDAC isoforms in mammals. *Biochim Biophys Acta.* 2012;1818:1466–1476.

66. Rostovtseva TK, Bezrukov SM. VDAC regulation: role of cytosolic proteins and mitochondrial lipids. *J Bioenerg Biomembr.* 2008;40:163–170.

67. Tepp K, Mado K, Varikmaa M, et al. The role of tubulin in the mitochondrial metabolism and arrangement in muscle cells. *J Bioenerg Biomembr.* 2014;46:421–434.

68. Rostovtseva TK, Bezrukov SM. VDAC inhibition by tubulin and its physiological implications. *Biochim Biophys Acta.* 2012;1818:1526–1535.

69. Shoshan-Barmatz V, Ben-Hail D.VDAC, a multifunctional mitochondrial protein as a pharmacological target. *Mitochondrion.* 2012;12:24–34.

70. Rostovtseva TK, Tan W, Colombini M. On the role of VDAC in apoptosis: fact and fiction. *J Bioenerg Biomembr.* 2005;37:129–142.

71. De Stefani D, Bononi A, Romagnoli A, et al. VDAC1 selectively transfers apoptotic Ca2+ signals to mitochondria. *Cell Death Differ.* 2012;19:267–273.

72. Dejean LM, Ryu SY, Martinez-Caballero S, Teijido O, Peixoto PM, Kinnally KW. MAC and bcl-2 family proteins conspire in a deadly plot. *Biochim Biophys Acta.* 2010;1797:1231–1238.

73. Antonsson B, Montessuit S, Sanchez B, Martinou JC. Bax is present as a high molecular weight oligomer/complex in the mitochondrial membrane of apoptotic cells. *J Biol Chem.* 2001;276:11615–11623.

74. Dedkova EN, Blatter LA. Measuring mitochondrial function in intact cardiac myocytes. *J Mol Cell Cardiol.* 2012;52:48–61.

75. Hom J, Sheu SS. Morphological dynamics of mitochondria–a special emphasis on cardiac muscle cells. *J Mol Cell Cardiol.* 2009;46:811–820.

76. Chen Y, Csordas G, Jowdy C, et al. Mitofusin 2-containing mitochondrial-reticular microdomains direct rapid cardiomyocyte bioenergetic responses via interorganelle Ca²⁺ crosstalk. *Circ Res.* 2012;111:863–875.

77. Papanicolaou KN, Kikuchi R, Ngoh GA, et al. Mitofusins 1 and 2 are essential for postnatal metabolic remodeling in heart. *Circ Res.* 2012;111:1012–1026.

78. Bers DM. Calcium cycling and signaling in cardiac myocytes. *Annu Rev Physiol.* 2008;70:23–49.

79. Liu T, O'Rourke B. Regulation of mitochondrial Ca²⁺ and its effects on energetics and redox balance in normal and failing heart. *J Bioenerg Biomembr.* 2009;41:127–132.

80. Min CK, Yeom DR, Lee KE, et al. Coupling of ryanodine receptor 2 and voltage-dependent anion channel 2 is essential for Ca2+ transfer from the sarcoplasmic reticulum to the mitochondria in the heart. *Biochem J.* 2012;447:371–379.

81. Dedkova EN, Blatter LA. Mitochondrial Ca²⁺ and the heart. *Cell Calcium.* 2008;44:77–91.

82. Boyman L, Chikando AC, Williams GS, et al. Calcium movement in cardiac mitochondria. *Biophys J.* 2014;107:1289–1301.

83. Shannon TR, Wang F, Puglisi J, Weber C, Bers DM. A mathematical treatment of integrated Ca dynamics within the ventricular myocyte. *Biophys J.* 2004;87:3351–3371.

84. Williams GS, Boyman L, Chikando AC, Khairallah RJ, Lederer WJ. Mitochondrial calcium uptake. *Proc Natl Acad Sci U S A.* 2013;110:10479–10486.

85. Gunter TE, Pfeiffer DR. Mechanisms by which mitochondria transport calcium. *Am J Physiol.* 1990;258:C755–C786.

86. Kwong JQ, Lu X, Correll RN, et al. The mitochondrial calcium uniporter selectively matches metabolic output to acute contractile stress in the heart. *Cell Rep.* 2015;12:15–22.

87. Luongo TS, Lambert JP, Yuan A, et al. The mitochondrial calcium uniporter matches energetic supply with cardiac workload during stress and modulates permeability transition. *Cell Rep.* 2015;12:23–34.

88. Wei AC, Liu T, Winslow RL, O'Rourke B. Dynamics of matrix-free Ca²⁺ in cardiac mitochondria: two components of Ca²⁺ uptake and role of phosphate buffering. *J Gen Physiol.* 2012;139:465–478.

89. Kirichok Y, Krapivinsky G, Clapham DE. The mitochondrial calcium uniporter is a highly selective ion channel. *Nature.* 2004;427:360–364.

90. Zorov DB, Juhaszova M, Sollott SJ. Mitochondrial ROS-induced ROS release: an update and review. *Biochim Biophys Acta.* 2006;1757:509–517.

91. Wei L, Dirksen RT. Perspectives on: SGP symposium on mitochondrial physiology and medicine: mitochondrial superoxide flashes: from discovery to new controversies. *J Gen Physiol.* 2012;139:425–434.

92. Prosser BL, Ward CW, Lederer WJ. Subcellular Ca²⁺ signaling in the heart: the role of ryanodine receptor sensitivity. *J Gen Physiol.* 2010;136:135–142.

93. Zhou L, Aon MA, Almas T, Cortassa S, Winslow RL, O'Rourke B. A reaction-diffusion model of ROS-induced ROS release in a mitochondrial network. *PLoS Comput Biol.* 2010;6. e1000657.

94. IONA Study Group. Effect of nicorandil on coronary events in patients with stable angina: the impact of nicorandil in angina (IONA) randomised trial. *Lancet.* 2002;359:1269–1275.

95. Camara AK, Bienengraeber M, Stowe DF. Mitochondrial approaches to protect against cardiac ischemia and reperfusion injury. *Front Physiol.* 2011;2:13.

96. Gomez L, Li B, Mewton N, et al. Inhibition of mitochondrial permeability transition pore opening: translation to patients. *Cardiovasc Res.* 2009;83:226–233.

97. Goldenberg I, Zareba W, Moss AJ. Long QT syndrome. *Curr Probl Cardiol.* 2008;33:629–694.

98. Jeong EM, Liu M, Sturdy M, et al. Metabolic stress, reactive oxygen species, and arrhythmia. *J Mol Cell Cardiol.* 2012;52:454–463.

8 Molecular Organization, Gating, and Function of Connexin-Based Gap Junction Channels and Hemichannels

Feliksas F. Bukauskas

Connexins Expression and Oligomerization

Connexins (Cxs), a large family of homologous membrane proteins, form gap junction (GJ) channels that provide a direct pathway for electrical and metabolic signaling between cells. Gap junctional communication is critically important in the spread of excitation in the heart, the communication between neurons and glia, the metabolic exchange between cells in the lens and other tissues lacking blood circulation, the organ formation during development, and the regulation of cell proliferation.[1] Each GJ channel is composed of two hemichannels (connexons). Oligomerization of six Cxs into hemichannels starts in the endoplasmic reticulum and is completed in the Golgi, from where vesicles ~100 to 150 nm in diameter containing hemichannels travel to fuse with the plasma membrane. Cxs are predicted to have four alpha-helical transmembrane domains (M1 to M4), intracellular N- and C-termini (NT and CT), two extracellular loops (E1 and E2), and a cytoplasmic loop (CL).[2] The density map of the crystal structure of human Cx26 at 3.5 Å resolution revealed that M1 and EI line the channel pore, which is narrowed by six NT domains residing in the channel vestibule. These structural data were supported by functional studies using a cysteine scanning approach[3] demonstrating that NT, M1, and E1 domains are directly involved in defining the GJ channel unitary conductance, gating properties, and permselectivity.[4] Thus far, at least 21 Cx genes have been identified in humans.

De Novo Formation of Gap Junction Channels

GJ channel *de novo* formation was examined by manipulating two separate cells into contact while monitoring electrical cell–cell coupling. This approach has been used to study the formation of GJs between the cells of *Xenopus* blastulae and myoballs, rat cardiomyocytes, insect cells, and HeLa cells transfected with Cx40.[5] Most likely, the initial step in this process is the formation of hemichannel plaques (hemiplaques) in the plasma membrane,[6,7] which should stabilize the hemichannels' lateral motion in the plasma membrane and create an outward-directed curvature that should reduce the distance between the hemichannels in apposing cells.[8] Theoretical studies show that when five or more proteins aggregate, the cluster then becomes stable despite their pairwise repulsions.[8] Subsequent steps likely include a close apposition between cells, possibly mediated by adhesion molecules and overlapping of hemiplaques that could lead to the formation of precursors of GJ channels termed "formation plaques" (FPs), which gradually transform into junctional plaques (JPs).[9] Alignment and docking of apposed hemichannels comes thereafter, followed by the formation of a high-resistance seal to isolate the nascent channel pore from the extracellular space ending with the channel pore opening. Docking of individual hemichannels furthermore stabilizes FPs and reduces the distance between the still undocked hemichannels, which may explain an acceleration of the *de novo* formation kinetics after the functional appearance of the first channels.[10] *De novo* formation of GJ channels, their clustering into JPs, GJ channels turnover, and their gating was shown to be regulated by different intracellular pathways that involve cyclic adenosine monophosphate (cAMP), G proteins, and phosphorylation.[11]

Significant progress has been made in understanding Cx trafficking, JP formation, and internalization using cells expressing Cxs fused with color variants of green fluorescent protein (GFP) or containing a tetracysteine tag.[12,13] JPs serve as "crystallization centers," attracting laterally moving hemichannels and catalyzing their docking due to the close apposition of hemichannels in the area of the JPs. By combining the fluorescence imaging of Cx-GFPs with dual whole-cell voltage clamp recording, it was shown that only cell pairs that exhibit a JP are electrically coupled.[14] Furthermore, it was shown that only a small fraction of channels assembled in a JP are functional at a given time, and this ratio varies from ~0.01 for Cx36, Cx45, and Cx57 to 0.1 for Cx43.[14–17] This fraction can be modulated reversibly in the time scale of few minutes by pH, long chain alkanols, $[Mg^{2+}]_i$, and many other chemical factors.[15,18] This indicates that this type of modulation does not involve an assembly of new GJs or their turnover.

Cell–cell communication can be organized through homotypic (same Cx isotype in both hemichannels), heterotypic (two Cx isotypes form GJ channels, but each hemichannel is assembled from one isotype), and heteromeric (different Cx isotypes at least in one of hemichannels) channels that vary in conductance, permselectivity, and gating properties. Formation of heterotypic and heteromeric GJ channels can occur in the heart, particularly in the conduction system, where cardiomyocytes coexpress several Cx isoforms. Most heterotypic junctions that can be formed in the heart exhibit asymmetric voltage gating and rectification of the current–voltage (I–V) relation.[19,20] Asymmetric junctional conductance (g_j) dependence on transjunctional voltage (V_j) can result in impeded signal transfer in one direction and facilitated transfer in the opposite direction, as it was demonstrated for Cx43/Cx45, Cx31/Cx45, and Cx40/Cx45.[5,21] Thus heterotypic GJs resemble functionally chemical synapses. An asymmetry of g_j-V_j dependence can also cause highly efficient modulation of metabolic cell–cell communication by V_j.[15,22] Both an asymmetry in g_j-V_j gating and I–V rectification tend to facilitate an initiation of a one-directional block of excitation spread, which is critical for the initiation of reentry formation.

Voltage and Chemical Gating of Connexin-Based Channels

The existence of multiple Cxs raises the questions of how they differ and how they interact. Unitary conductances of GJs formed of Cx isoforms range from ~10 pS (e.g., mCx30.2 and Cx36) to 300 pS (e.g., Cx37), and the channels vary in permselectivity from being nonselective to preferentially selective for cations or anions.[1,23] A property that appears to be common to GJs formed by any Cx isoform is the sensitivity of g_j to V_j. Fig. 8.1A[24] shows a decay of g_j until a steady-state level ($g_{j,ss}$) is reached as indicated by the arrow in response to the V_j step voltage. The symmetric reduction in $g_{j,ss}$ with positive or negative V_j has been explained by having identical V_j-sensitive gate(s) in each apposed/junctional hemichannel (aHC) of the GJ channel.[25] Normalized $g_{j,ss}$-V_j dependencies show big differences in sensitivity to V_j among the four principal Cxs of cardiomyocytes (see Fig. 8.1B). A common feature of the V_j-gating is that $g_{j,ss}$ does not decline to zero with increasing V_j, but instead reaches a residual conductance termed "g_{min}." Single channel studies have shown that g_{min} is due, at least in part, to the incomplete closure of the GJ channel by V_j, which causes channels to close to a subconductance (residual) state with fast gating transitions (~1 ms or less).[26] It was shown that V_j as

well as chemical uncouplers can also induce gating transitions to the fully closed state and that these transitions are slow at ~10 ms. Gating to different levels via fast and slow gating transitions led to the suggestion that there are two distinct V_j-sensitive gates, termed "fast and slow" or "loop" (as reviewed in Bukauskas and Verselis[5]). The fast gate closes channels to the residual state, and the slow gate closes them fully (see Fig. 8.1C). Fig. 8.1D shows an example of fast and slow gate operation during acidification with CO_2, which gradually reduces the number of operating channels. When only one channel was left to operate, the *fast* gate was governing fast transitions between the open and residual states, finally being closed by the slow gate with transitions lasting ~10 ms. The opposite sequence of events was observed during a washout from CO_2. Two distinct gating mechanisms were also demonstrated in Cx-based unapposed/nonjunctional hemichannels (uHC).[27]

Mutational studies revealed that the gating polarity of the fast gating mechanism is governed by charged residues in the N-terminal domain and that this polarity could be reversed independently from the slow gating mechanism. Modifications of Cx43, including deletion of the CT domain[28] or attachment of aequorin or enhanced green fluorescent protein (EGFP) to CT, selectively abolishes fast gating to the residual state.[5] These data demonstrate that in each hemichannel there are two molecularly distinct gating mechanisms, which require further study in determining Cx domain functioning: the *gating* and *sensorial* elements for each

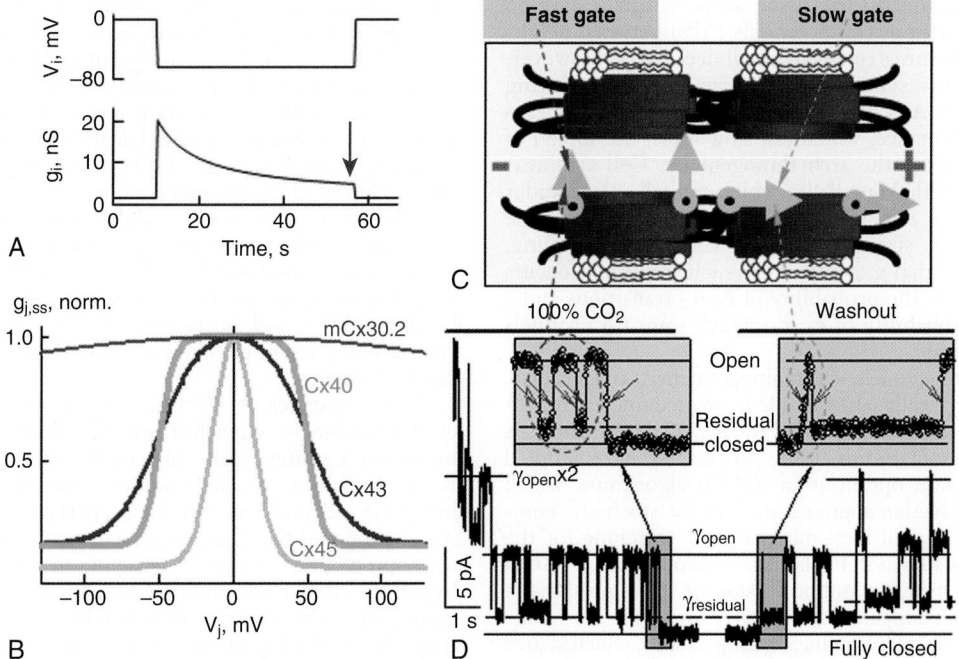

FIGURE 8.1 Gating of gap junction (GJ) channels. (A) Typically, junctional conductance (g_j) measured between cell pairs decays in response to transjunctional (V_j) voltage, reaching some steady-state level ($g_{j,ss}$) (*arrow*). (B) Normalized $g_{j,ss}$ dependencies on V_j show differences in sensitivity to V_j among four principal cardiac connexins. (C) A schematic presentation of the GJ channel containing fast and slow gating mechanisms. The fast gate (*orange*) closes the channel partially, while the slow gate (*blue*) closes the channel fully. (D) Effect of carbon dioxide (*CO_2*) on voltage gating at the single channel level in a cell pair of fibroblasts expressing connexin (*Cx*) 43. Exposure to CO_2 caused full uncoupling. I_j was monitored at $V_j = 55$ mV just before full uncoupling and at the beginning of CO_2 washout. Channels exhibited two types of I_j transition: (1) between the open and residual state (~90 pS), with a transition time of ~1 ms (*red arrows*) and (2) between the open and fully closed states (~120 pS), with a transition time of ~10 ms or more (*blue arrows*). The signals in the insets (sampled at 1-ms intervals) illustrate that the last channel closes with a transition time of ~10 ms, and the first channel opens with transition time of ~19 ms. The slow opening of the first channel during washout was followed by fast flickering between open and residual states. When two operating channels were in the residual state, g_j equals the sum of two γ_{res} (*dashed lines*). (Modified from Bukauskas FF, Peracchia C. Two distinct gating mechanisms in gap junction channels: CO_2-sensitive and voltage-sensitive. *Biophys J.* 1997;72:2137-2142.)

gate. This hypothesis has received a support from studies performed in channels formed of Cx30, Cx31, Cx32, Cx37, Cx40 Cx43, Cx45, and Cx57,[1,5] suggesting that the fast and slow gates are likely to be common to all Cx isoforms.

The gating properties of the GJ channels can be described using the Boltzmann function[25] assuming that GJ channels have two states, open and fully closed, like most ionic channels, and that each hemichannel gates independently. The accumulation of data demonstrating gating to the substate(s) and two distinct gating mechanisms stimulated the development of gating models that more intimately describes GJ channel gating.[29,30] In 2012, we developed a stochastic 16-state model (S16SM) of V_j gating, in which each aHC contains both fast and slow gating mechanisms.[26] An S16SM allows for the simulation of g_j dynamics as well as the $g_{j,ss}$-V_j plot of homotypic and heterotypic GJs depending on the individual gating parameters of the four gates. Most recent data allowed us to predict that the *fast* gate operates between open (**o**) and closed (**c**) states with transitions, **o↔c**, while the slow gate contains not one but two closed states, an *initial-closed* state (**c$_1$**) and *deep-closed* state (**c$_2$**), and operates according to a linear reaction scheme, **o↔c$_1$↔c$_2$**. Based on this concept, we developed a stochastic 36-state model (S36SM) of GJ channel gating. This model provides a mechanistic background for well-established experimental data, such as delayed g_j recovery after V_j gating, hysteresis of g_j-V_j dependence, and a low ratio of functional channels to the total number of GJ channels, which cannot be reflected using an S16SM. Also, this model demonstrates that during the spread of excitation in the neuronal networks and cardiac tissue short V_j spikes develop due to a phase shift in action potentials (APs) between neighboring cells, which causes relatively small decay of g_j. However, during an arrhythmia, such decays of g_j can accumulate during frequently repeated APs resulting in more substantial decays of junctional conductance, which can slow down the spread of excitation and increase the arrhythmogenicity. Cell acidification and overload with Mg^{2+},[18,31,32] which can take place under various pathological conditions causing depletion adenosine triphosphate (ATP), strongly facilitate cell–cell uncoupling, and we hypothesize that g_j decay under such conditions occurs due to an increase in the probability of **c$_1$→c$_2$** transitions and a decrease in the probability of **c$_2$→c$_1$**, which traps GJ channels into a *deep-closed* state.

However, gating models are multiparametric, and evaluating the values of typically >10 variable gating parameters manually from the experimental g_j-time of the $g_{j,ss}$-V_j dependencies is impractical. To automate this fitting process, we have adopted the global coordinate optimization (GCO) algorithms, which are based on the Bayesian approach to filter the stochastic component and smooth small local minima while searching for the global minimum as shown in Paulauskas and colleagues.[26] (GCO can be performed using an online version of the algorithms at http://connexons.aecom.yu.edu.)

All GJ channels display chemical gating as well, which shares several features with the slow voltage-sensitive gate (i.e., it reduces g_j to zero and closes the channels fully).[1,5] We assume that an asynchrony of conformational changes in each of the six Cx "subgates" of the slow gate lead to multistep gating transitions lasting ~10 ms or more. This may be due to the low level of cooperativity between these "slow subgates." Similar slow transitions were observed at the initial stages of channel pore opening during *de novo* channel formation, during gating induced by transmembrane voltage (V_m) or chemical uncouplers as illustrated in Fig. 8.1D. While fast gating to the residual state is induced exclusively by V_j, the slow gating mechanism can be triggered by V_j, V_m, and chemical factors. Interestingly, uncoupling induced by alkanols, Ca^{2+}, and H$^+$ was shown to be partially reversible by changes in V_m or V_j.[5] These data suggest that chemical- and voltage-sensitive gating mechanisms interact and may share the common *gating* element of the slow gate, which is triggered by sensorial elements specific for the voltage and chemical reagents.

Hemichannels: Function and Physiological Relevance

Surface expression of uHCs has been demonstrated in several cell lines and primary cultures by electron microscopic, biochemical, and electrophysiological methods.[33,34] Typically, at the single-channel level, the I–V relation of the uHCs rectifies and their unitary conductances are approximately twice the conductances of the GJ channel formed of the same Cxs.[35] It was long thought that hemichannels remained closed until docking with hemichannels from an apposed cell, since ions and metabolites can leak in the cell through open hemichannels. Furthermore, it was shown that the Cx43 uHCs have been implicated in diverse roles in cell physiology and pathology, including volume regulation, the efflux of glutamate, NAD$^+$, cAMP, IP$_3$ and ATP, acceleration of astrocytes, and cardiomyocyte death during metabolic inhibition and transduction of extracellular signals regulating apoptosis development.[36,37] The opening of hemichannels can be enhanced by cell polarization to positive potentials and the reduction of Mg^{2+} and Ca^{2+} in the extracellular milieu.[38] Conversely, the closure of hemichannels can be induced by low intracellular pH, 18-α-glycyrrhetinic acid, trivalent cations (La^{3+} or Gd^{3+}), and some chloride channel blockers.[36,39] Blocking of uHCs by chemical reagents can serve as a therapeutic approach to prevent cell death during pathological conditions. However, all above mentioned reagents are not selective, and there were multiple attempts to develop Cx-mimetic peptides that selectively blocked uHCs. It was shown that Gap19 peptide (derived from the cytoplasmic loop of Cx43) prevented the opening of Cx43 uHCs during the metabolic inhibition and protected cardiomyocytes against volume overload and cell death following ischemia/reperfusion.[40] At the same time, Cx43 GJ channels that preserved a normal spread of excitation were not affected. Gap26 and Gap27 peptides (derived from extracellular loops E1 and E2 of Cx43) prevented an increase in open probability for Cx43 uHCs that occurs under pathological conditions, when [Ca^{2+}]$_i$ is elevated.[41] Thus the development of Cx-mimetic peptides and selectively blocking uHCs, will aid to protect cells from ionic imbalance, cell swelling, loss of metabolites, and cell death under variety of diseased states.

Lately, researchers identified the presence of Cx43 hexamers/hemichannels in purified mitochondrial preparations of the mouse myocardium, which may contribute to the mitochondrial K$^+$ uptake.[42] More detailed studies revealed that Cx43 is expressed in subsarcolemmal but not in interfibrillar mitochondria, and it was proposed that Cx43 plays a critical role in mediating the cardioprotective function of ischemic preconditioning.[43,44] It is hypothesized that preconditioning leads to the opening of Cx43 hemichannels in the inner mitochondrial membrane, with subsequent loss of ATP from the mitochondrial matrix. This activates ATP-dependent K$^+$ channels that appear to be central in the protective effect.[45]

It has been shown that among cardiac Cxs, mCx30.2,[33] Cx43,[35] and Cx45[46] form functional uHCs, while Cx40 does not.[47] Typically, uHCs tend to open at a higher positivity on the cytoplasmic side. Presumably, open probability of uHCs increases during APs and to a greater extent during tachycardia when cells are depolarized for longer time. Opening of hemichannels in nodal cells would depolarize them, and locally increase the extracellular concentration of K$^+$ ions. Depolarization could inactivate inward currents driving excitability and contribute to a reduction in conduction velocity. This hypothesis raises a new mechanism that explains a long atrioventricular (AV) delay due to the mCx30.2 hemichannel function.[48] This corroborates a reduction in the PQ-interval in mCx30.2 KO mouse.[49]

Another class of membrane proteins, pannexins (Panx's) that also forms uHCs but not GJ channels, are involved in paracrine signaling and mechanosensitivity.[50] It was shown that Panx1 constitutes 300 pS uHCs in cardiomyocytes leading to the suggestion that their opening can depolarize the plasma membrane and trigger premature APs that may lead to arrhythmogenic activities.[51]

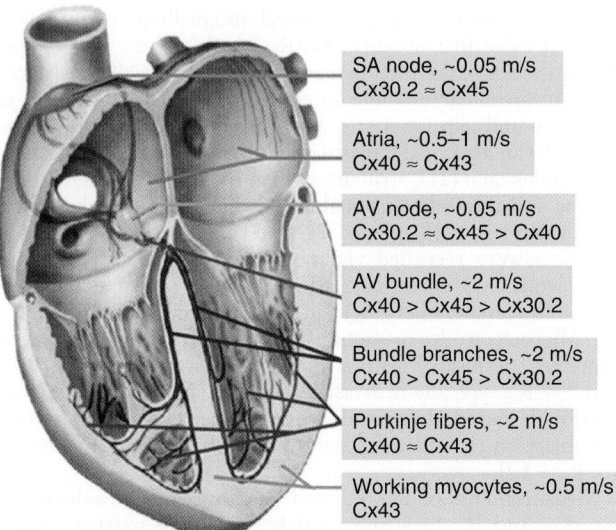

FIGURE 8.2 Schematic presentation of the heart with indications showing connexin expression patterns and conduction velocities in different regions of the heart. AV, atrioventricular; SA, sinoatrial. (Modified from Netter F, ed. *Atlas der Anatomie des Menschen*. 4th ed. New York, NY: Ciba Geigy Corp; 1993.)

Connexins Expression Pattern and Propagation of Excitation in the Heart

Until now, it was reported that four Cxs, mCx30.2, Cx40, Cx43, and Cx45, are expressed by cardiomyocytes and form GJ channels mediating the spread of excitation in the heart as well as direct intercellular metabolic communication[48]; the human ortholog of mCx30.2 is Cx31.9.[20] Expression patterns of all four cardiac Cxs are shown in Fig. 8.2. In the mammalian heart, the cardiac impulse is initiated in the spontaneously active pacemaker cells of the sinoatrial (SA) node in which the mCx30.2 and Cx45 GJs integrate thousands of pacemaker cells with various intrinsic frequencies of excitation into one functional unit. These Cxs form homotypic GJ channels with a conductance of 9 and 32 pS, respectively, as well as mCx30.2/Cx45 heterotypic GJs with a single channel conductance of ~17 pS[5,20] or even heteromeric GJs, which can exhibit a variety of single channel conductances in a range from ~9 to 32 pS.[52] Electrical coupling in the transitional region between the SA node and the atrium should not be too high, thus preserving the functional identity of pacemaker cells, but at the same time allowing for signal transfer. Fig. 8.3 shows images of cell pairs formed of HeLaCx30.2-EGFP (*red*) with HeLa cells expressing Cx40 tagged with cyan florescent protein (CFP) (*green*, part A) and Cx43-CFP (part B). Both heterotypic junctions exhibited extensive formation of JPs (*arrows*) and V$_j$-gating asymmetry typical for most of heterotypic junctions.[20] The insets in Fig. 8.3A show internalized GJ channels in the form of small vesicles. It is broadly accepted that GJ channels cannot separate into hemichannels. Most likely, an external layer of the vesicle on the left-hand side is formed of mCx30.2-EGFP while an internal layer is formed of Cx40-CFP. On the contrary, in the vesicle on the right, the external and internal layers are formed of Cx40-CFP and mCx30.2-EGFP, respectively.

Excitation transferred to the crista terminalis spreads with the velocity of 0.5–1 m/s (in the human heart) through the

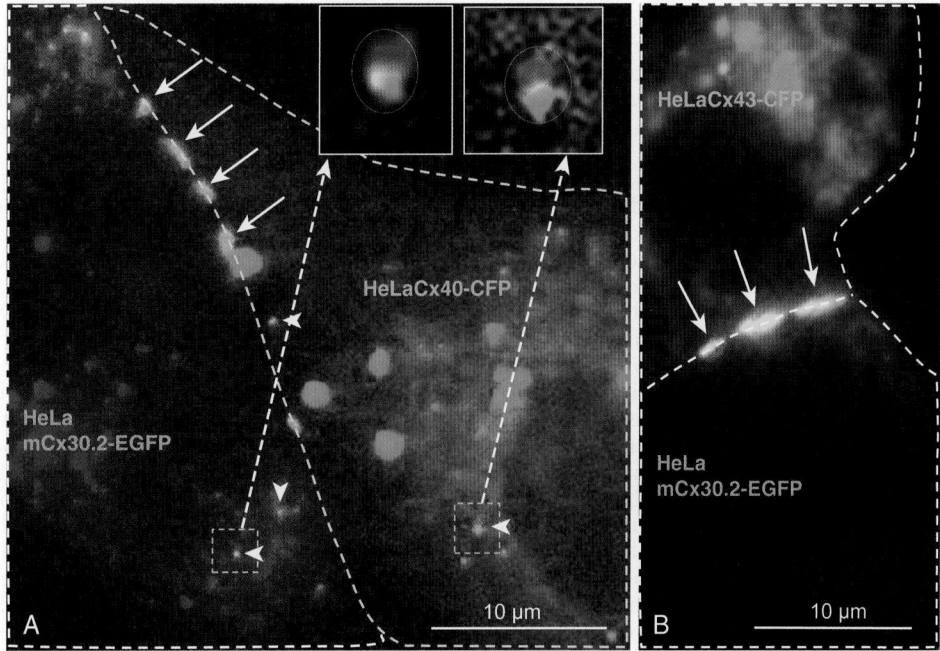

FIGURE 8.3 Formation of heterotypic gap junctions visible as multiple junctional plaques (*yellow*) indicated by *arrows* and located in between cells expressing mCx30.2-enhanced green fluorescent protein (*EGFP*) (*red*) and those expressing Cx40-cyan florescent protein (*CFP*) (A) or Cx43-CFP (B) (*both green*). The insets in A show internalized junctional plaques in the form of small vesicles (pointed by *arrowheads*) formed of two color layers. Red and green colors overlap only partially due to chromatic aberration of the different wavelengths.

right and left atria. In the atrium, Cx40 and Cx43 are most abundantly expressed,[53] and both exhibit high single channel conductances (180 pS and 115 pS, respectively),[5,54] which corroborates the fast spread of excitation and almost synchronous contraction of both atria. Presumably, cell–cell coupling in the atria is maintained by homotypic Cx40 and Cx43 GJ channels because Cx40 and Cx43 are highly incompatible to form heterotypic GJs.[21]

The excitation wave enters the AV node by passing the transitional A-N zone, and its velocity of propagation gradually decreases to ~0.05 m/s in the central region called the compact node or N region. In the normal heart, the AV node is the sole connection between the atria and ventricles, and the delay of AV conduction is necessary for the sequential contraction of atria and ventricles, which is important for optimal hemodynamics. The relatively long refractory period of the AV-nodal cells and the dependence of the conduction velocity on the frequency of excitation limit the number of impulses within a given time period, termed the Wenckebach, that can be transmitted to the ventricles. Thus the AV node protects the ventricular myocardium by reducing the frequency of APs transmitted to the His bundle during atrial fibrillation. Slow AV-nodal conduction under pathophysiological conditions can also lead to the generation of life-threatening tachycardia enclosing at least part of the *reentry* loops. In the AV-nodal cells, mainly mCx30.2 and Cx45 are expressed, and both exhibit relatively low single channel conductances. Furthermore, Cx40 is expressed in the N region, but at lesser extent.[48]

Slow conduction in the AV node may be due to the mCx30.2 uHCs that tend to depolarize the resting membrane potential[48] and may also be due to reduced excitability by lower numbers of Na+-channels, cytoarchitecture of fibers,[55] and the expression of mCx30.2 and Cx45, which both exhibit low single channel conductance that leads to relatively high resistivity of the intracellular milieu.[56,57] It was shown that only ~1% of Cx45 GJ channels are open at a given time under normal conditions.[15] Furthermore, mCx30.2 exhibits the lowest single channel conductance among all members of the Cx family and forms heterotypic as well as heteromeric channels with all other cardiac Cxs. Resulting channels also exhibit low unitary conductance (~17–18 pS), which raises a possibility that mCx30.2 demonstrates a dominant negative effect upon junctional conductance between nodal cells. This effect may also contribute to the low conduction velocity in wild-type mice and enhanced AV conduction in mCx30.2-deficient mice.[49]

After passing the transitional N-H region and entering the His bundle, the propagation of excitation quickly accelerates to ~2 m/s and remains at this level in the subendocardial network of Purkinje fibers, resulting in coordinated contraction of both ventricles. Expression of Cx40 increases in the His bundle and bundle branches where it is coexpressed with Cx43. There is also an expression of mCx30.2 and Cx45 at low levels, which becomes undetectable at the terminals of the ventricular conductive system. The His bundle and bundle branches are isolated electrically from surrounding working myocardium preserving the high speed of propagation. Cx40, due to its incapability to form heterotypic GJs with Cx43, the principal Cx of ventricular cardiomyocytes, may provide this isolation during development. Excitation from bundle branches propagates through false tendons and the endocardial layer of Purkinje cells where mainly Cx40 and Cx43 are expressed.[53] Excitation to working cardiomyocytes, preferentially expressing Cx43 is transmitted through discrete Purkinje fiber–muscle (P–M) junctions[58] distributed discretely on the endocardium surface with ~1 mm distance between them.[59] This pattern allows for Purkinje fibers to maintain their electrical identity and therefore high conduction velocity. Multiple P–M junctions preserve a satisfactorily high safety factor for signal transfer to working myocardium, and the only price

"paid" for this structural organization is a P–M delay of ~4 to 7 ms, which slightly prolongs PQ-interval.

Cell–Cell Coupling and Electrical Anisotropy in the Heart

Typically, the input resistance (R_{in}) and the length constant of electrotonic potential decay (λ; the distance at which the amplitude of electrotonic potential evoked by intracellularly injected current is reduced *e* fold) are measured in isolated heart tissue preparations to determine electrical intercellular communication. For cable-like systems, $\lambda = (R_m \cdot b/\varrho_i)^{1/2}$, where R_m is a specific resistance of the plasma membrane, ϱ_i is a specific resistance of the intracellular medium integrating averaged resistances of cytoplasm and gap junctions, and b is a ratio of the volume of the cell to an area of the plasma membrane. This applies also to two-dimensional (2D) structures when the source of excitation is the line and three-dimensional (3D) structures when the source of excitation is a 2D plane. To determine λ, the electrotonic responses were recorded via microelectrodes at different distances from intracellular current sources along the general directions of the cardiac fibers (λ_X) and in their perpendicular direction (λ_Y). Microelectrodes or suction-electrodes (~200- to 300-μm tip diameter), perfusable with a depolarizing KCl solution, were used.[60,61] R_{in} typically is measured using a single microelectrode or a double-barreled electrode when one barrel was used for current injection (I) and the second records electrotonic potential (V); $R_{in} = V/I$.

Measurements of R_{in}, λ_X, and λ_Y allow one to evaluate the $\varrho_{i,X}$, $\varrho_{i,Y}$, and R_m by using models describing passive electrical properties of syncytial structures,[62–64] where $\varrho_{i,X}$ and $\varrho_{i,Y}$ are specific resistances of the intracellular medium along and across fibers. Depending on the complexity, used models can be differentiated based on a dimension (cable, 2D sheet, or 3D volume) or structure of the syncytium (continuous with averaged electrical parameters, compartmental, or a combination of the two). In general, continuous models are more applicable to structures with well-coupled cells (e.g., heart, liver, etc.), whereas discrete models are more applicable to poorly coupled cells exemplified by neuronal networks. We formulated a continuous 2D model[62] resembling the flat-cell model,[65] a 3D model of infinite size,[63] and 3D model of finite thickness,[66] which most closely describes isolated tissue preparations and are created using methods known as "mirror reflection" or "virtual images."[64,67]

Many organs and organ systems, including the heart, exhibit an electrical anisotropy determined as a ratio, λ_X/λ_Y, which is greater than 1. Furthermore, $\lambda_X/\lambda_Y = (\varrho_{i,Y}/\varrho_{i,X})^{1/2}$, that is, an anisotropy of intracellular resistivity is higher than that estimated from λs as a square degree. By measuring the X-Y distributions of electrotonic potentials on endocardial surface of the atrium while current was injected from epicardial surface, it was shown that $\lambda_X > \lambda_Y = \lambda_Z$, where λ_Z is perpendicular to endocardial/epicardial surfaces (i.e., electrically the myocardium exhibits a cylindrical anisotropy).[66] Generally, every local myocardium domain in which the direction of cardiomyocytes remain similarly aligned exhibits a cylindrical electrical anisotropy. The magnitude of the anisotropy is determined by the ellipsoid/cylinder-like shape of the cardiomyocytes and the ratio between end-to-end and lateral gap junctions. Most proposed *reentry* mechanisms are related mainly to heterogeneities of repolarization, which break the wave of premature excitation necessary to initiate *reentry*. However, electrical anisotropy can explain *reentry* initiation by excitation during the vulnerable period of the heart, which is homogeneous with all other parameters.[68,69] Interestingly, electrical anisotropy is a property of all myocardial structural domains under normal conditions, suggesting that the heart is intended to be arrhythmogenic, whereas realization of reentry through electrical anisotropy requires premature excitations, which is acquired from pathology.

Passive Electrical Properties of the Sinoatrial Node

The first attempt to measure λ in the rabbit SA node was performed by Bonke[70] assuming that the SA node constitutes an isotropic medium. More systemic studies of intercellular communication of different SA node regions and surrounding areas were performed by measuring of λ_X, λ_Y, and R_{in}.[66,71] Intracellular recordings of APs from the different regions of the SA node allowed the determination of the region of "true" pacemakers or the central region where excitation starts earliest. Fig. 8.4B shows the averaged values of R_{in} measured along the blue dashed line crossing the central region of the SA node. R_{in} in the atrial trabeculae and crista terminalis was ~350 kOhm, which increased approaching the central region of the SA node, reaching the maximum of 1050 kOhm, and was lower in the intracellular septum at ~450 kOhm. Fig. 8.4A shows a summary of averaged data of λ_X and λ_Y in the form of crosses. Thus all regions exhibit electrical anisotropy, which is highest in the crista terminalis and atrial trabeculae. Electrical anisotropy gradually reduces, approaching the central region of the SA node, but the orientation of anisotropy remained the same as in the crista terminalis. Anisotropy of λ_X and λ_Y (529 versus 306 μm) was also reported in another study[61] in which measurements of λs were averaged for entire SA node. These data correlate with ultrastructural studies of the SA node[72] showing that "the leading (true) pacemaker cells are roughly spindle shaped with a maximum length of 20 to 30 μm and a diameter of less than 8 μm, with the long axis of the cells roughly parallel to the crista terminalis." The findings that *"the gap junctions are less developed in size and number than in atrial cells"*[72] correlate with the significantly higher R_{in} and smaller λ in the central region of SA node than in crista terminalis and trabeculae. The values of λ_X and λ_Y increased approaching the intercellular septum while the anisotropy decreased, which assumingly is due to the more dispersed orientation of the cardiomyocytes. In summary, based on λ_X, λ_Y, and R_{in} measurements and using a 3D model, it was shown that in the central region of the SA node, $\varrho_X \approx 600$ and $\varrho_Y \approx 3000$ Ohm·cm.[66] Thus the ϱ_X in SA node is ~3.5-fold bigger than the ϱ_X in the trabeculae and the crista terminalis, which is ~150 to 200 Ohm·cm and close to a specific resistance of the cytoplasm (~120 Ohm·cm[73]).

Passive Electrical Properties of the Atrioventricular Node

Division of the AV-nodal region into functionally distinct domains is based on the anatomy, AP shape, and delays in the spread of excitation.[74] Mapping of the AV node by using intracellular microelectrode recordings from different AV-nodal regions allowed us to differentiate the A-N, N, and N-H regions of the AV node based on the shape of APs and delays from the stimulus applied to the crista terminalis (Fig. 8.5A).[56] Fig. 8.5B shows that, on average, the R_{in} in all three AV-nodal domains is higher than in the crista terminalis and His bundle.

The average values of λ measured in the different domains of the AV node are shown as crosses where half of their axes are proportional to the values of λ in corresponding directions (see Fig. 8.5C). The maximal anisotropy is recorded in the crista terminalis and the His bundles, and it is significantly less expressed in the AV node mainly due to the reduction in λ_X. Data analysis revealed that in the central regions of the AV node, $R_m = 1300$ Ohm·cm^2, $\varrho_{i,X} = $ ~600, and $\varrho_{i,Y} = $ ~1200 Ohm·cm; the AV nodal cells were assumed to be 8 × 12-μm ellipsoids.[75] Thus the $\varrho_{i,X}$ in the central region of the AV node is similar to that of the SA node, while the $\varrho_{i,Y}$ is ~two-fold smaller. In both structures, the anisotropy

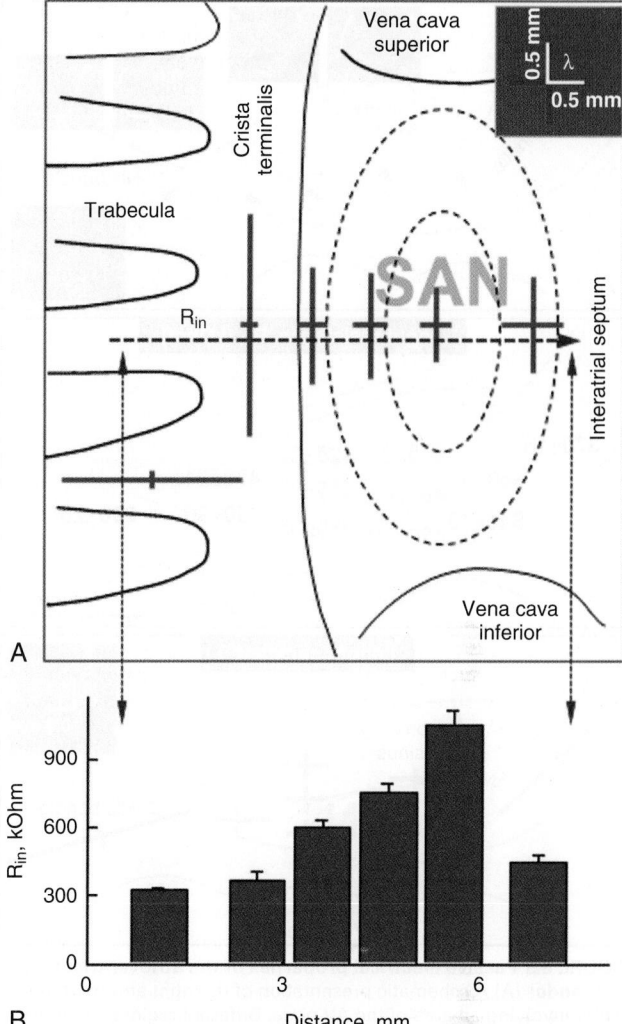

FIGURE 8.4 Passive electrical properties of the sinoatrial (SA) node. (A) A schematic presentation of the right atrium of the rabbit. The averaged data of λs measured along and across the crista terminalis are shown in the form of crosses. Values of λ were evaluated from experimental measurements (λ_{exp}) using a three-dimensional model of passive electrical properties with finite thickness. All regions exhibited electrical anisotropy, which was highest in the crista terminalis and atrial trabeculae. Electrical anisotropy is reduced in the central region of the SA node. The calibration is at the *top-right*, where lengths of white lines correspond to $\lambda = 0.5$ mm. (B) Averaged values of R_{in} measured along the *blue dashed line* starting from trabeculae and crossing the central region of the SA node. R_{in} reached maxima in the central region of the SA node (1050 kOhm) at the value that is ~two-fold higher that the R_{in} measured in trabecular structure, crista terminalis and interatrial septum.

of axial resistances is smaller than that in all other structural domains of the heart. In another study,[57] it was reported that in the AV node, the $\lambda = 430$ μm (not specifying an anisotropy) and $R_{in} = 880$ kOhm, which are comparable to our data.

Passive Electrical Properties of Conductive and Working Systems of Ventricles and Signal Transfer in P–M Contacts

After passing the AV node, excitation spreads at high speed (~2 m/s) through the His bundle, left and right bundle branches, multiple false tendons, and finally almost instantaneously excites the

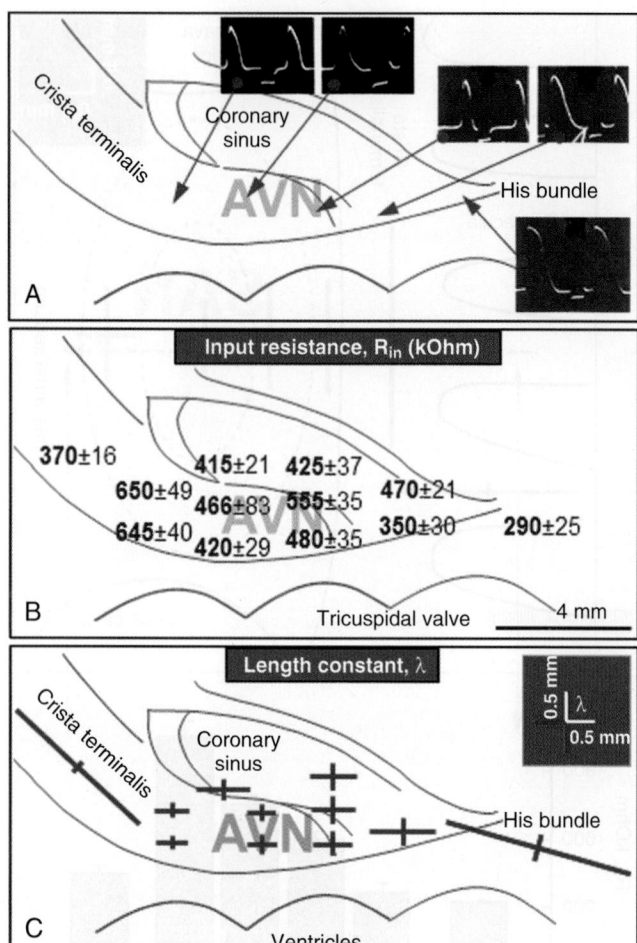

FIGURE 8.5 Passive electrical properties of the atrioventricular (AV) node. (A) A schematic presentation of the right atrium of the rabbit involving an area of the AV node. Different regions of the AV node demonstrate differences in action potential shape and stepwise responses to intracellular current steps of 50 nA applied through the recording electrode. (B) Averaged R_{in} values (in kOhm) attached to different functional regions surrounding the AV node are shown. (C) Averaged data of λs are shown in the form of crosses. All regions exhibited electrical anisotropy, which was highest in the crista terminalis and His bundle, but was smallest in the central region of the AV node. The *inset* in the *right-top corner* shows the calibration cross where the lengths of white lines correspond to λ = 0.5 mm.

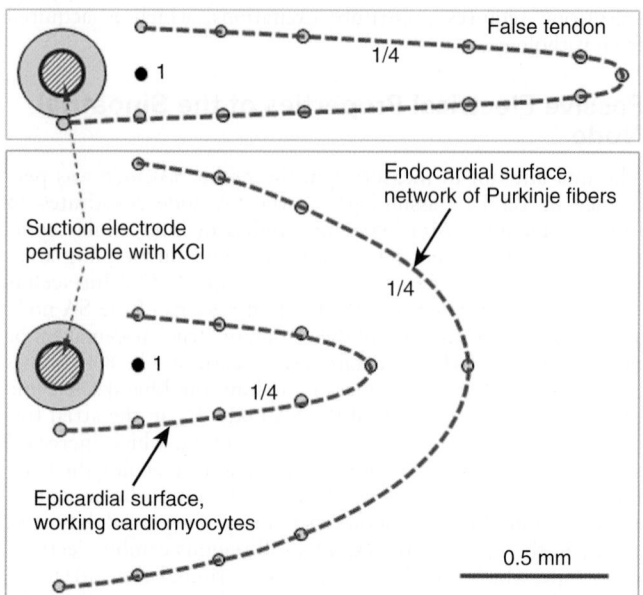

FIGURE 8.6 Isopotential lines of electrotonic potential in the false tendon, endocardial surface of Purkinje network, and working myocardium recorded from the epicardial surface in response to the intracellular current applied through the suction electrode (*dashed circle*) perfusable with potassium chloride. Isopotential lines are at the level of ¼ from that measured in the position indicated by the *filled dot*.

endocardial conductive system exhibits a relatively high λs, but smaller anisotropy that is presumably due to the mesh-like cytoarchitecture of the Purkinje terminals.

Values of $λ_{X,exp}$ in working myocardium are smaller than that in the false tendon mainly due to differences in the dimensionality of systems, such as the 3D syncytium versus a cable-like structure. In both systems, $ϱ_{iX}$ is in the range of 150–200 Ohm·cm, i.e., close to the resistivity of the cytoplasm (~120 Ohm·cm[73]); however, $ϱ_Y$ in the working myocardium is few-fold smaller than that in the false tendon, where $ϱ_{i,Y} ≈ 2$–4 kOhm·cm.

Purkinje–muscle (P–M) junctions, which were first described in Purkinje–papillary muscle preparations from ventricles of the dog heart, mediate a ~5 ms P–M delay[58] and characteristic prepotentials (notch) on the upstroke of AP of the transitional cell (Tr) located in between the P- and M-cells. Furthermore, stepwise penetrations of the microelectrode from the endocardial side in the ventricular preparations of the dog heart revealed two scenarios: (1) the AP of the P-cell was followed by the AP of the M-cell ~4–10 ms thereafter, and there were no signs of prepotential during this delay period, indicating that there is no direct electronic coupling, and (2) the AP of the P-cell was followed by the AP of the Tr cell exhibiting the prepotential and finally, the AP of the M-cell was recorded (Fig. 8.7A).[59] Interestingly, the P–M junctions were discretely distributed on the endocardium surface with distances between them of approximately 0.8 to 2 mm (see Fig. 8.7A). Consequently, excitation from the Purkinje cells is transmitted to working myocardium only at P–M junctions (*black dots*). Excitation spreads from these loci in all directions; *dashed lines* show isochrones of the spread of excitation in working myocardium. Fig. 8.7B shows that an area in which prepotentials are recorded has an elliptic shape of ~300 × 150 μm on average; the longer axis always is in parallel with the direction of the M fibers.[59] The total area of the P–M junctions constituted ~5% of the endocardial surface of the dog heart. A P–M delay is less within the zone of the P–M connection and greater outside the zone. This discrete organization of the P–M junctions in the ventricles creates conditions of electrical "independence" of the virtually 2D system of Purkinje fibers from 3D syncytium of the M-fibers. Otherwise, a strong link between P- and M-fibers would

thin layer of Purkinje fibers covering the endocardial surface of ventricles. Fig. 8.6 shows isopotential lines of electrotonic potential in false tendon, endocardial surface of Purkinje network, and working myocardium from the epicardial surface measured in response to an intracellular current applied through the suction electrode (dashed circle). Isopotential lines are ¼ from that measured in the position indicated by the filled dots.

Values of experimentally measured $λ_{X,exp}$ and $λ_{Y,exp}$ depend on the size of the current sources and dimensionality of the tissue; for example, a false tendon can be approximated as a cable, while the endocardial conductive system and working myocardium surface can be considered as 2D and 3D structures, respectively. Consequently, different models of passive electrical properties should be used to evaluate the true values of $λ_X$ and $λ_Y$, which typically are bigger than $λ_{X,exp}$ and $λ_{Y,exp}$; at the smaller diameter of the current source electrode, the values of $λ_{X,exp}$ and $λ_{Y,exp}$ are smaller. Furthermore, experimentally measured anisotropy of electronic potentials is smaller than the "true" one, i.e., $λ_X/λ_Y > λ_{X,exp}/λ_{Y,exp}$. Fig. 8.6 shows that a false tendon exhibits the highest electrical anisotropy (on average, $λ_X/λ_Y = 20$), and therefore is adapted for the high speed of excitation propagation. The

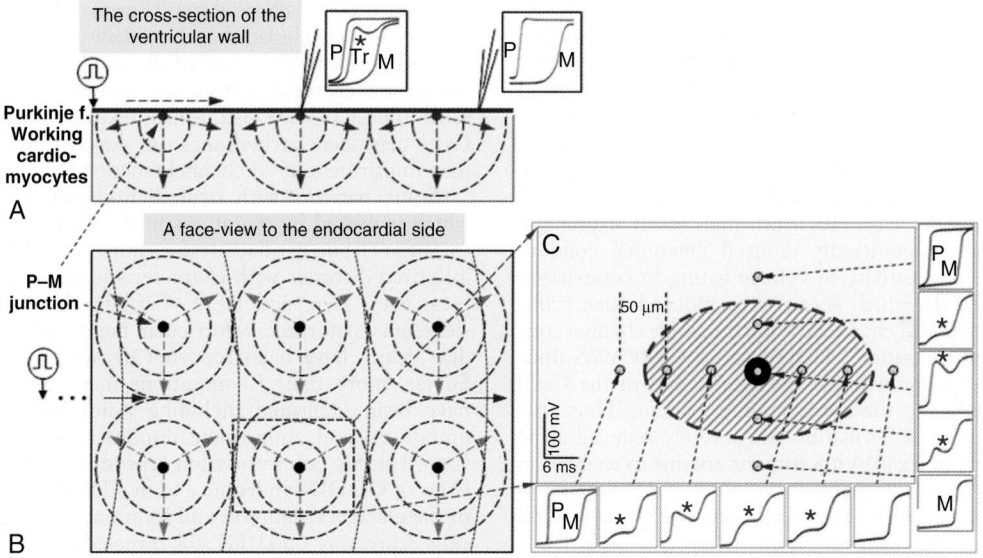

FIGURE 8.7 Schematics of discrete Purkinje fiber–muscle (P–M) junctions (*black spots*) between a subendocardial network of Purkinje fibers (*purple*) and working myocardium (*gray*). (A) A cross-section of ventricular wall. The spread of excitation in Purkinje fibers and working myocardium are shown by *purple arrows* and *black arrows*, respectively. Stepwise penetration of the microelectrode into P–M junction revealed action potentials (APs) with prepotentials (Tr) while in majority of places only APs typical for P- and M-fibers were recorded. (B) A face-view of the ventricle from the endocardial side showing the spread of excitation in the network of Purkinje fibers (*purple dashed lines*) and working myocardium (*black dashed circles*). (C) Inset from B showing that in the P–M junction an area in which APs with prepotentials are recorded has an elliptic form (*encircled with elliptic red dashed line*). (Modified from Bukauskas FF, Sakson ME, Kukushkin NI. Discrete zones of electrical connection between Purkinje terminals and muscle fibers in dog ventricles [in Russian]. *Biofizika.* 1976;21:887-892.)

reduce the speed of propagation in the thin layer of Purkinje network to that of the working myocardium, which would compromise a synchrony in activation of ventricles. The size of the P–M junctions where prepotentials are recorded allows one to speculate, using a 3D model that only few P- and M-fibers in the P–M junction form direct gap junctional contact (i.e., much smaller than the number of cells located in the area with prepotentials).

In Purkinje terminals, Cx40 and Cx43 are coexpressed with a prevalence of Cx43. Working ventricular cardiomyocytes preferentially express Cx43. It has been demonstrated that Cx40 does not form, or does so with very low efficiency, heterotypic junctions with Cx43.[21] Therefore electrical cell–cell coupling at P–M connections are organized predominately through homotypic Cx43 GJ channels.

Alterations of Cell–Cell Coupling in Connexin-Deficient Animals and Disease-Related Mutations

In order to understand the role of Cxs in cardiac impulse propagation, unrestricted and cardiomyocyte-specific null mutant mice with different cardiac Cx genes were generated. Cx43 gene deletion resulted in postnatal death due to malformation of the right ventricular outflow tract.[76] The postnatal lethality of the Cx43-deficient mice can be circumvented by cardiomyocyte-directed deletion. The resulting mice exhibit a reduced conduction velocity in the ventricles, thus demonstrating the importance of Cx43 in the maintenance of ventricular conduction.[77]

Cx40-deficient mice exhibit impaired function of automaticity,[78] slower conduction velocity in the atria and the AV-nodal region, and development of the first-degree AV block associated with bundle branch block[79,80] that correlates with the Cx40 expression pattern (see Fig. 8.2). Impaired AV-nodal conduction is reflected by a prolonged Wenckebach period and AV-nodal refractory period in these mice.[81] Moreover, the replacement of

Cx43 by Cx40, or Cx40 by Cx45 showed that some cardiac Cxs can be substituted for others.[82,83] Cx40 is critical for normal morphogenesis as a severe incidence of cardiac malformations occur in Cx40-deficient mice.[84] Cx40 is also expressed in the kidney and can influence the blood pressure through the renin–angiotensin system.[85] Cx40-null–mutated mice are hypertensive, possibly due to an increase in the number of renin-secreting cells[86] and a loss of the Cx40-mediated calcium-dependent inhibitory effect of angiotensin II.[85] The increase of blood pressure due to alterations in Cx40 expression or function of its mutations can increase arrhythmogenicity of the heart.

The impact of Cx45 on cardiac impulse propagation remains elusive, since unrestricted and cardiac-actin promoter-Cre–mediated deletion of Cx45 resulted in embryonic lethality due to endocardial cushion defects and impaired vascularization.[87]

Deletion of mCx30.2 leads to the acceleration of AV-nodal conduction without obvious morphological heart abnormalities.[49] Additionally, the Wenckebach period is shortened in these mice, which result in faster ventricular response rates during induced episodes of atrial fibrillation. Thus mCx30.2 contributes to slow AV-nodal conduction and the protection of ventricles from atrial tachyarrhythmias. No alterations of excitation propagation were found in atria, bundle branches and ventricles, where mCx30.2 expressions are absent (see Fig. 8.2).

So far, no congenital heart diseases have been linked to the mutation of mCx30.2 (hCx31.9) and Cx45, although Cx45-deficient mice show severe heart abnormalities and embryonic death. Alterations in distribution and expression levels of cardiac Cxs have been described in several noncongenital and some congestive heart failures not related with Cxs mutations.[88]

Some forms of arrhythmias appear to be genetically determined by associated mutations that lead to a decreased expression of Cx40 and modification (D1275N) of the sodium channel (*SCN5A*).[89] In addition, it was shown a predisposition to atrial standstill in patients carrying polymorphisms in the promoter region, which decreased the Cx40 expression. Furthermore, sporadic cases of atrial fibrillation not related with family history have been identified as being caused by somatic or tissue-specific genetic mutations of Cx40 and Cx43. The somatic mutation of Cx40 (Cx40*A96S) was described in patients with atrial fibrillation,[90] and it was shown that this mutation slows down the spread of excitation in the atrium due to impaired junctional conductance of Cx40*A96S GJs. Also, Cx40*A96S transgenic mice exhibited strongly reduced atrial conduction velocity and enhanced arrhythmogenicity. HeLa cell lines stably expressing Cx40*A96S revealed significantly reduced junctional conductance and enhanced sensitivity of voltage gating in comparison to Cx40 wild-type GJs, which is caused by reduced open probabilities of Cx40*A96S GJ channels, while the single channel conductance remained the same.[91] Heterozygous Cx40*A96S mice revealed normal expression levels and localization of the Cx40 protein that is similar to the corresponding patient. Thus prolonged episodes of atrial fibrillation and severely reduced atrial conduction velocity in Cx40*A96S patients are due to changes in the gating properties of GJ channels but not to the reduction of single channel conductance or the expression level of Cx40*A96S GJs, which remained unchanged.

The Cx43 somatic mutation was identified in the atrium of the patient with a long history of atrial fibrillation. It was caused by the frame shift rising from a single cytosine nucleotide deletion (c.932delC), leading to deletion of the last 72 amino acids of the putative Cx43 protein.[92] HeLa transfectants expressing c.932delC-Cx43 mutant showed a marked reduction in the ability of cell pairs to electrically couple. Cells cotransfected with c.932delC-Cx43 and Cx40 or Cx43 demonstrated a dominant negative effect of mutant on function of Cx40 and Cx43, which can explain the arrhythmogenic nature of c.932delC-Cx43 mutant.

The cardiac intercalated disc harbors mechanical and electrical junctions as well as ion channel complexes mediating propagation of electrical impulses. Cx43 colocalizes and interacts with several of the proteins located at intercalated discs in the ventricular myocardium. We have generated conditional Cx43*D378stop mice that lack the last five C-terminal amino acid residues, representing a binding motif for zonula occludens protein-1 (ZO-1), and investigated the functional consequences of this mutation on cardiac physiology and morphology.[93] Newborn and adult homozygous Cx43*D378stop mice displayed markedly impaired and heterogeneous cardiac conduction properties and died from severe ventricular arrhythmias. Cx43 and ZO-1 were colocalized at the intercalated discs in Cx43*D378stop hearts and the Cx43*D378stop GJ channels showed normal coupling properties. Patch clamp studies of isolated adult Cx43*D378stop cardiomyocytes revealed a significant decrease in sodium and potassium current densities as well as a significant loss of NaV1.5 proteins. The phenotypic lethality of the Cx43*D378stop mutation is very similar to the one previously reported for adult Cx43 KO mice. In contrast to Cx43 KO

mice, the Cx43 GJ channel is still functional in the Cx43*D378stop mutant. We concluded that the lethality of Cx43*D378stop mice was independent of the loss of the gap junctional communication but most likely resulted from impaired sodium and potassium currents. The Cx43*D378stop mice revealed for the first time that Cx43 dependent arrhythmias can develop by mechanisms other than impairment of GJ channel function.[93]

Some patients with oculodentodigital dysplasia (ODDD), which is caused by mutations in the Cx43 gene, were reported to suffer from cardiac dysfunction.[94] ODDD is a dominant inherited disorder with characteristic anomalies of the fingers, toes, eyes, face, and teeth. Cardiac abnormalities, including sick sinus syndrome, ventricular tachycardia, and sudden cardiac death, have been reported in two families with ODDD. So far, more than 50 mutations in Cx43 related to ODDD have been identified including point mutations, frame shift mutations, and amino acid duplications.[95] Mice carrying the Cx43*G138R point mutation reproduced the typical characteristics of ODDD syndrome and in addition exhibited alterations in the electrocardiogram and spontaneous arrhythmias.[96] HeLa cells expressing Cx43*G138R revealed a loss of junctional communication, while they formed functional channels with cells expressing wild-type Cx43. Cx43G138R/Cx43 heterotypic GJs were clustered in large and multiple JPs but cell–cell coupling was low and exhibited asymmetric voltage gating. Single channel conductance was similar to wild-type Cx43 but most of the GJ channels were closed due to modifications in voltage gating. Therefore we assumed that Cx43*G138R GJ channels can oligomerize into hemichannels, which can dock and form GJs channels that are preferentially closed due to changes in their gating properties.[96]

Recently, three novel point mutations of Cx43 were reported in 418 Chinese patients with congenital heart diseases.[97] The first mutation R153Q was located in the third transmembrane region of Cx43; the other two mutations, G261W and A323V, were found in the C-terminal region. All affected amino acids are highly conserved in Cx43. Most of these patients suffered from atrial and ventricular septal defects, tetralogy of Fallot, pulmonal atresia or stenosis, and other forms of cardiac malformations. The authors assume that those malformations are related with changes in function including the gating of Cx43 GJ channels, which need to be supported by more detailed studies of unitary conductances and permselectivity of those mutants.

Acknowledgments

We thank Dr. Romualdas Veteikis for helpful comments. This work was supported by a grant MIP-76/2015 from the Research Council of Lithuania and National Institutes of Health grant R01NS072238 to FFB.

REFERENCES

1. González D, Gómez-Hernández JM, Barrio LC. Molecular basis of voltage dependence of connexin channels: an integrative appraisal. *Prog. Biophys. Mol. Biol.* 2007;94:66–106.

2. Sosinsky GE, Nicholson BJ. Structural organization of gap junction channels. *Biochim Biophys Acta.* 2005;1711:99–125.

3. Kronengold J, Trexler EB, Bukauskas FF, et al. Pore-lining residues identified by single channel SCAM studies in Cx46 hemichannels. *Cell Commun Adhes.* 2003;10:193–199.

4. Trexler EB, Bukauskas FF, Kronengold J, et al. The first extracellular loop domain is a major determinant of charge selectivity in connexin46 channels. *Biophys. J.* 2000;79:3036–3051.

5. Bukauskas FF, Verselis VK. Gap junction channel gating. *Biochim. Biophys. Acta.* 2004;1662:42–60.

6. Lal R, John SA, Laird DW, et al. Heart gap junction preparations reveal hemiplaques by atomic force microscopy. *Am J Physiol.* 1995;268:C968–C977.

7. Zampighi GA, Loo DD, Kreman M, et al. Functional and morphological correlates of connexin50 expressed in Xenopus laevis oocytes. *J Gen Physiol.* 1999;113:507–524.

8. Kim KS, Neu J, Oster G. Curvature-mediated interactions between membrane proteins. *Biophysical J.* 1998;75:2274–2291.

9. Johnson RG, Reynhout JK, TenBroek EM, et al. Gap junction assembly: roles for the formation plaque and regulation by the C-terminus of connexin43. *Mol Biol Cell.* 2012;23:71–86.

10. Bukauskas FF, Weingart R. Voltage-dependent gating of single gap junction channels in an insect cell line. *Biophys J.* 1994;67:613–625.

11. Márquez-Rosado L, Solan JL, Dunn CA, et al. Connexin43 phosphorylation in brain, cardiac, endothelial and epithelial tissues. *Biochim Biophys Acta.* 2012;1818:1985–1992.

12. Gaietta G, Deerinck TJ, Adams SR, et al. Multicolor and electron microscopic imaging of connexin trafficking. *Science.* 2002;296:503–507.

13. Falk MM, Baker SM, Gumpert AM, et al. Gap junction turnover is achieved by the internalization of small endocytic double-membrane vesicles. *Mol. Biol. Cell.* 2009;20:3342–3352.

14. Bukauskas FF, Jordan K, Bukauskiene A, et al. Clustering of connexin 43-enhanced green fluorescent protein gap junction channels and functional coupling in living cells. *Proc Natl Acad Sci U S A.* 2000;97:2556–2561.

15. Palacios-Prado N, Briggs SW, Skeberdis VA, et al. pH-dependent modulation of voltage gating in connexin45 homotypic and connexin45/connexin43 heterotypic gap junctions. *Proc Natl Acad Sci U S A.* 2010;107:9897–9902.

16. Palacios-Prado N, Sonntag S, Skeberdis VA, et al. Gating, permselectivity and pH-dependent modulation of channels formed by connexin57, a major connexin of horizontal cells in the mouse retina. *J Physiol.* 2009;587:3251–3269.

17. Marandykina A, Palacios-Prado N, Rimkutė L, et al. Regulation of connexin-36 gap junction channels by n-alkanols and arachidonic acid. *J. Physiol.* 2013;591:2087–2101.

18. Skeberdis VA, Rimkute L, Skeberdyte A, et al. pH-dependent modulation of connexin-based gap junctional uncouplers. *J Physiol.* 2011;589:3495–3506.
19. Moreno AP. Biophysical properties of homomeric and heteromultimeric channels formed by cardiac connexins. *Cardiovasc Res.* 2004;62:276–286.
20. Kreuzberg MM, Sohl G, Kim J, et al. Functional properties of mouse connexin30.2 expressed in the conduction system of the heart. *Circ. Res.* 2005;96:1169–1177.
21. Rackauskas M, Kreuzberg MM, Pranevicius M, et al. Gating properties of heterotypic gap junction channels formed of connexins 40, 43 and 45. *Biophys. J.* 2007;92:1952–1965.
22. Palacios-Prado N, Bukauskas FF. Modulation of metabolic communication through gap junction channels by transjunctional voltage; synergistic and antagonistic effects of gating and ionophoresis. *Biochim Biophys Acta*. 2012:1818.
23. Harris AL. Connexin channel permeability to cytoplasmic molecules. *Prog Biophys Mol Biol.* 2007;94:120–143.
24. Bukauskas FF, Peracchia C. Two distinct gating mechanisms in gap junction channels: CO_2-sensitive and voltage-sensitive. *Biophys J.* 1997;72:2137–2142.
25. Harris AL, Spray DC, Bennett MVL. Kinetic properties of a voltage-dependent junctional conductance. *J. Gen. Physiol.* 1981;77:95–117.
26. Paulauskas N, Pranevicius H, Mockus J, et al. A stochastic 16-state model of voltage-gating of gap junction channels enclosing fast and slow gates. *Biophys. J.* 2012;102:2471–2480.
27. Trexler EB, Bennett MV, Bargiello TA, et al. Voltage gating and permeation in a gap junction hemichannel. *Proc Natl Acad Sci U S A.* 1996;93:5836–5841.
28. Elenes S, Martinez AD, Delmar M, et al. Heterotypic docking of Cx43 and Cx45 connexons blocks fast voltage gating of Cx43. *Biophys. J.* 2001;81:1406–1418.
29. Chen-Izu Y, Moreno AP, Spangler RA. Opposing gates model for voltage gating of gap junction channels. *Am. J. Physiol. Cell Physiol.* 2001;281:C1604–C1613.
30. Ramanan SV, Brink PR, Varadaraj K, et al. A three-state model for connexin37 gating kinetics. *Biophys. J.* 1999;76:2520–2529.
31. Palacios-Prado N, Chapuis S, Panjkovich A, et al. Molecular determinants of magnesium-dependent synaptic plasticity at electrical synapses formed by connexin36. *Nature Communic.* 2014;5:4667.
32. Palacios-Prado N, Hoge G, Marandykina A, et al. Intracellular magnesium-dependent modulation of gap junction channels formed by neuronal connexin36. *J Neurosci.* 2013;33:4741–4753.
33. Bukauskas FF, Kreuzberg M, Rackauskas M, et al. Properties of mouse connexin 30.2 and human connexin 31.9 hemichannels; implications for atrioventricular conduction in the heart. *Proc Natl Acad Sci U S A.* 2006;103:9726–9731.
34. De Vuyst E, Boengler K, Antoons G, et al. Pharmacological modulation of connexin-formed channels in cardiac pathophysiology. *Br J Pharmacol.* 2011;163:469–483.
35. Contreras JE, Saez JC, Bukauskas FF, et al. Gating and regulation of connexin 43 (Cx43) hemichannels. *Proc Natl Acad Sci U S A.* 2003;100:11388–11393.
36. Sáez JC, Schalper KA, Retamal MA, et al. Cell membrane permeabilization via connexin hemichannels in living and dying cells. *Exp Cell Res.* 2010;316:2377–2389.
37. Scheckenbach KE, Crespin S, Kwak BR, et al. Connexin channel-dependent signaling pathways in inflammation. *J Vasc Res.* 2011;48:91–103.
38. Paul DL, Ebihara L, Takemoto LJ, et al. Connexin46, a novel lens gap junction protein, induces voltage-gated currents in nonjunctional plasma membrane of Xenopus oocytes. *J Cell Biol.* 1991;115:1077–1089.
39. Eugenin EA, Basilio D, Sáez JC, et al. The role of gap junction channels during physiologic and pathologic conditions of the human central nervous system. *J Neuroimmune Pharmacol.* 2012;7:499–518.
40. Wang N, De Vuyst E, Ponsaerts R, et al. Selective inhibition of Cx43 hemichannels by Gap19 and its impact on myocardial ischemia/reperfusion injury. *Basic Res. Cardiol.* 2013;108:1–16.
41. Wang N, De Bock M, Antoons G, et al. Connexin mimetic peptides inhibit Cx43 hemichannel opening triggered by voltage and intracellular Ca2+ elevation. *Basic Res Cardiol.* 2012;107:1–17.
42. Miro-Casas E, Ruiz-Meana M, Agullo E, et al. Connexin43 in cardiomyocyte mitochondria contributes to mitochondrial potassium uptake. *Cardiovasc Res.* 2009;83:747–756.
43. Boengler K, Stahlhofen S, van de Sand A, et al. Presence of connexin 43 in subsarcolemmal, but not in interfibrillar cardiomyocyte mitochondria. *Basic Res Cardiol.* 2009;104:141–147.
44. Rodríguez-Sinovas A, Sánchez JA, González-Loyola A, et al. Effects of substitution of Cx43 by Cx32 on myocardial energy metabolism, tolerance to ischaemia and preconditioning protection. *J Physiol.* 2010;588:1139–1151.
45. Rottlaender D, Boengler K, Wolny M, et al. Glycogen synthase kinase 3β transfers cytoprotective signaling through connexin 43 onto mitochondrial ATP-sensitive K+ channels. *Proc Natl Acad Sci U S A.* 2012;109:E242–E251.
46. Valiunas V. Biophysical properties of connexin-45 gap junction hemichannels studied in vertebrate cells. *J. Gen. Physiol.* 2002;119:147–164.
47. Beahm DL, Hall JE. Opening hemichannels in nonjunctional membrane stimulates gap junction formation. *Biophys J.* 2004;86:781–796.
48. Kreuzberg MM, Willecke K, Bukauskas F. Connexin-mediated cardiac impulse propagation: connexin 30.2 slows atrioventricular conduction in mouse heart. *Trends in Cardiovasc. Med.* 2006;16:266–272.
49. Kreuzberg M, Schrickel J, Ghanem A, et al. Connexin30.2 containing gap junction channels decelerate impulse propagation through the atrioventricular node. *Proc. Natl. Acad. Sci. U S A.* 2006;108:5959–5964.
50. Bao L, Locovei S, Dahl G. Pannexin membrane channels are mechanosensitive conduits for ATP. *FEBS Lett.* 2004;572:65–68.
51. Kienitz MC, Bender K, Dermietzel R, et al. Pannexin 1 constitutes the large conductance cation channel of cardiac myocytes. *J Biol Chem.* 2011;286:290–298.
52. Gemel J, Lin X, Collins R, et al. Cx30.2 can form heteromeric gap junction channels with other cardiac connexins. *Biochem Biophys Res Commun.* 2008;369: 388–394.
53. Pfenniger A,AW, Kwak BR. Mutations in connexin genes and disease. *Eur J Clin Invest.* 2011;41:103–116.
54. Bukauskas FF, Elfgang C, Willecke K, et al. Biophysical properties of gap junction channels formed by mouse connexin40 in induced pairs of transfected human HeLa cells. *Biophys. J.* 1995;68:2289–2298.
55. Kleber AG, Rudy Y. Basic mechanisms of cardiac impulse propagation and associated arrhythmias. *Physiol Rev.* 2004;84:431–488.
56. Bukauskas FF, Veteikis RP. Passive electrical properties of the atrioventricular region of the rabbit heart. *Biofizika (Russian; translated in English by Pergamon press).* 1977;22:499–504.
57. De Mello WC. Passive electrical properties of the atrioventricular node. *Pflugers Arch.* 1977;37:135–139.
58. Mendez C, Mueller WJ, Merideth J, et al. Interaction of transmembrane potentials in canine Purkinje fibers and at Purkinje fiber-muscle junctions. *Circ. Res.* 1969;24:361–372.
59. Bukauskas FF, Sakson ME, Kukushkin NI. Dicrete zones of electrical connection between Purkinje terminals and muscle fibers in dog ventricles. *Biofizika (Russian; translated in English by Pergamon press).* 1976;21:887–892.
60. Adomonis VM, Bredikis II , Bukauskas FF. Suction electrode with internal perfusion. *Fiziol. Zh. SSSR Im. I M Sechenova.* 1983;69:272–275.
61. Bouman LN, Duivenvoorden JJ, Bukauskas FF, et al. Anisotropy of electrotonus in the sinoatrial node of the rabbit heart. *J Mol Cell Cardiol.* 1989;21:407–418.
62. Bukauskas FF, Kukushkin NI, Sakson ME. Model of a 2-dimensional anisotropic syncytium. *Biofizika (Russian; translated in English by Pergamon press).* 1974;19:712–716.
63. Bukauskas FF, Veteikis RP, Gutman AM. Model of a passive 3-dimensional anisotropic syncytium as a continuous medium. *Biofizika (In Russian).* 1975;20:1083–1086.
64. Bukauskas F, Bytautas A, Gutman A, et al. Simulation of passive electrical properties in two- and three-dimensional anisotropic syncytial media. In: Bukauskas F, ed. *Intercellular Communication.* Manchester/New York: Manchester University Press; 1991:203–217.
65. Woodbury JW, Crill WE. On the problem of impulse conduction in the atrium. *Nervous Inhibition.* 1961:124–135.
66. Bukauskas FF, Gutman AM, Kisunas KJ, et al. Electrical cell coupling in rabbit sino atrial node and atrium. Experimental and theoretical evaluation. In: Bouman LN, Jongsma HJ, eds. *Cardiac Rate and Rhythm. Physiological, Morphological and Developmental Aspects.* Hague/Boston/London: Martinus Nijhoff Publishers; 1982:195–216.
67. Deakin MA, Neild TO, Turner RG. The extension of two-dimensional cable theory to arteries and arterioles. *Bull Math Biol.* 1985;47:409–424.
68. Kukushkin NI, Bukauskas FF, Sakson MY, et al. Anisotropy of steady speedes and delays of the extrasystolic waves in the heart of the dog. *Biofizika.* 1975;20:687–692.
69. Spach MS, Josephson ME. Initiating reentry: the role of nonuniform anisotropy in small circuits. *J Cardiovasc Electrophysiol.* 1994;5:182–209.
70. Bonke FI. Electronic spread in the sinoatrial node of the rabbit heart. *Pflugers Arch.* 1973;339:17–23.
71. Bukauskas FF, Veteikis RP, Gutman AM, et al. Intercellular coupling in the sinus node of the rabbit heart. *Biofizika (Russian; translated in English by Pergamon press).* 1977;22:108–112.
72. Masson-Pévet M, Bleeker WK, Mackaay AJ, et al. Sinus node and atrium cells from the rabbit heart: a quantitative electron microscopic description after electrophysiological localization. *J Mol Cell Cardiol.* 1979;11:555–568.
73. Schanne OF. Measurement of cytoplasmic resistivity by means of the glass microelectrode. In: Lavellee OFS M, Herbert NC, eds. *Glass Microelectrodes.* New York: Wiley; 1969:299–321.
74. Van Capelle FJ, Janse MJ, Varghese PJ, et al. Spread of excitation in the atrioventricular node of isolated rabbit hearts studied by multiple microelectrode recording. *Circ Res.* 1972;31:602–616.
75. Torii H. Electron microscope observation of the S-A and A-V nodes and Purkinje fibers of the rabbit. *Jap. Circ. J.* 1962;26:39–77.
76. Reaume AG, De Sousa PA, Kulkarni S, et al. Cardiac malformation in neonatal mice lacking connexin43. *Science.* 1995;267:1831–1834.
77. van Rijen HV, Eckardt D, Degen J, et al. Slow conduction and enhanced anisotropy increase the propensity for ventricular tachyarrhythmias in adult mice with induced deletion of connexin43. *Circulation.* 2004;109:1048–1055.
78. Bagwe S, Berenfeld O, Vaidya D, et al. Altered right atrial excitation and propagation in connexin40 knockout mice. *Circulation.* 2005;112:2245–2253.
79. Simon AM, Goodenough DA, Paul DL. Mice lacking connexin40 have cardiac conduction abnormalities characteristic of atrioventricular block and bundle branch block. *Current biology : CB.* 1998;8:295–298.
80. van Rijen HV, van Veen TA, van Kempen MJ, et al. Impaired conduction in the bundle branches of mouse hearts lacking the gap junction protein connexin40. *Circulation.* 2001;103:1591–1598.
81. VanderBrink BA, Sellitto C, Saba S, et al. Connexin40-deficient mice exhibit atrioventricular nodal and infra-Hisian conduction abnormalities. *J Cardiovasc Electrophysiol.* 2000;11:1270–1276.
82. Alcolea S, Jarry-Guichard T, de Bakker J, et al. Replacement of connexin40 by connexin45 in the mouse: impact on cardiac electrical conduction. *Circ. Res.* 2004;94:4–6.
83. Taffet SM, Jalife J. Swapping connexin genes: how big is the gap? *Circ. Res.* 2004;94:4–6.
84. Gu H, Smith FC, Taffet SM, et al. High incidence of cardiac malformations in connexin40-deficient mice. *Circ. Res.* 2003;93:201–206.
85. Wagner C, de Wit C, Kurtz L, et al. Connexin40 is essential for the pressure control of renin synthesis and secretion. *Circ Res.* 2007;100:556–563.
86. Krattinger N, Capponi A, Mazzolai L, et al. Connexin40 regulates renin production and blood pressure. *Kidney Int.* 2007;72:814–822.
87. Kruger O, Plum A, Kim JS, et al. Defective vascular development in connexin 45-deficient mice. *Development (Cambridge, England).* 2000;127:4179–4193.
88. Dupont E, Matsushita T, Kaba RA, et al. Altered connexin expression in human congestive heart failure. *Journal of Molecular & Cellular Cardiology.* 2001;33:359–371.
89. Groenewegen WA, Firouzi M, Bezzina CR, et al. A cardiac sodium channel mutation cosegregates with a rare connexin40 genotype in familial atrial standstill. *Circ. Res.* 2003;92:14–22.
90. Gollob MH, Jones DL, Krahn AD, et al. Somatic mutations in the connexin 40 gene (GJA5) in atrial fibrillation. *N Engl J Med.* 2006;354:2677–2688.
91. Lübkemeier I, Andrié R, Lickfett L, et al. The Connexin40A96S mutation from a patient with atrial fibrillation causes decreased atrial conduction velocities and sustained episodes of induced atrial fibrillation in mice. *J Mol Cell Cardiol.* 2013;65:19–32.
92. Thibodeau IL, Xu J, Li Q, et al. Paradigm of genetic mosaicism and lone atrial fibrillation: physiological characterization of a connexin 43-deletion mutant identified from atrial tissue. *Circulation Research.* 2010;122:236–244.
93. Lübkemeier I, Requardt RP, Lin X, et al. Deletion of the last five C-terminal amino acid residues of connexin43 leads to lethal ventricular arrhythmias in mice without affecting coupling via gap junction channels. *Basic Res Cardiol.* 2013;108:1–16.
94. Paznekas WA, Boyadjiev SA, Shapiro RE, et al. Connexin 43 (GJA1) mutations cause the pleiotropic phenotype of oculodentodigital dysplasia. *Am. J. Hum. Genet.* 2003;72:408–418.
95. Zoidl G, Dermietzel R. Gap junctions in inherited human disease. *Pflugers Arch - Eur J Physiol.* 2010;460:451–466.
96. Dobrowolski R, Sasse P, Schrickel JW, et al. The conditional connexin43G138R mouse mutant represents a new model of hereditary oculodentodigital dysplasia in humans. *Hum. Mol. Genet.* 2008;17:539–554.
97. Wang B, Wen Q, Xie X, et al. Mutation analysis of Connexon43 gene in Chinese patients with congenital heart defects. *Int J Cardiol.* 2010;145:487–489.

9

Structure–Function Relations of Heterotrimetric Complexes of Sodium Channel α- and β-Subunits

Isabelle Deschênes

The cardiac voltage-gated Na$^+$ channel α-subunit (Na$_v$1.5) is a large (~220 kDa, 2016 aa) protein encoded by *SCN5A* located on chromosome 3p21 (Fig. 9.1A). *SCN5A* is composed of 28 exons spanning more than 80 Kb (see Fig. 9.1A). The *SCN5A* mRNA undergoes alternative splicing leading to different Na$_v$1.5 protein-spliced variants.[2,4–8] Overall, Na$_v$1.5 consists of four repeating transmembrane domains called DI-IV (see Fig. 9.1B). Each domain in turn consists of six transmembrane helices denoted S1–S6 (see Fig. 9.1B). It has been proposed that these repeating domains are a result of successive gene duplication of K$^+$ channels, which are analogous to a single repeat.[9] A phylogenetic study corroborated the hypothesis that Na$_v$ channels would then have evolved from voltage-gated Ca^{2+} channels with which they share structural similarities.[10] In addition to the conducting pore formed by the α-subunit, the voltage-gated Na$^+$ channel complex is also composed of several auxiliary β-subunits (β1–β4) that modulate channel gating and/or trafficking (Fig. 9.2). Attesting to the importance of both α- and β-subunits in contributing to cardiac sodium currents, mutations in both α- and β-subunits have been linked to arrhythmias.[11,12] In addition to the α- and β-subunits, the cardiac Na$^+$ channel complex also interacts with adaptor, accessory, cytoskeletal, and regulatory proteins along with other ion channels to form a large macromolecular complex.[1,2,13–20] This is the focus of Chapters 18, 21, and 22 of this book.

Upon activation, the cardiac Na$^+$ channel rapidly opens (~2 ms) and inactivates (~10 ms). Different structures in the channel contribute to this process (see Fig. 9.1B). While no crystal structure is available for the eukaryotic Na$^+$ channels, the bacterial *Arcobacter* Na$^+$ channel has been crystallized.[21] The bacterial channel has a structure akin to eukaryotic K$^+$ channels: a tetrameric arrangement of monomers. This is in contrast to the eukaryotic Na$^+$ channel, which is a single monomer with large intracellular loops connecting each transmembrane domain (see Fig. 9.1B). While the core transmembrane domains have good conservation with other channels, the large intracellular loops have been shown to mediate many of the functions of the sodium channel.[1] The four repeating domains I–IV of the Na$^+$ channel are thought to arrange in a circular fashion, forming a hydrophilic pore in the center through which sodium ions are able to pass. The links between the S5 and S6 in each domain (pore loop) form the outer pore and contain highly conserved aspartate, glutamate, lysine, and alanine residues (the "DEKA" sodium-selective motif). This sequence forms the ion selectivity and permeation pathway that primarily permits Na$^+$ ions to pass with high selectivity (see Fig. 9.1B).[22] The S4 segment of each domain consists of repeats of positively charged and hydrophobic residues thereby forming a voltage sensor that undergoes conformational changes upon depolarization and allows the channel to activate (see Fig. 9.1B).[23–26] Within milliseconds, the amplitude of the inward I_{Na} current is dramatically decreased to less than 1% of the transient amplitude (known as the late sodium current) because of the fast inactivation process.[27,28] This process is very important since it contributes to the refractoriness of cardiomyocytes by preventing premature reexcitation due to the unavailability of voltage-gated Na$^+$ channels. The structural motif in the Na$_v$ channels that underlies fast inactivation is the cytoplasmic linker between DIII and DIV containing a hydrophobic isoleucine-phenylalanine-methionine (IFM) particle that functions as a "lid" that rapidly occludes the inner mouth of the pore.[24,29–31] It is believed that these residues interact transiently with a receptor within the channel pore; while the exact identification of the residues/regions acting as the receptor is still pending, studies have suggested interactions of the inactivation particle with the S4–S5 linkers of domains III and IV and the cytoplasmic end of S6 in domain IV.[32–35] A more detailed and complete description of sodium channel structure–function and gating is provided in Chapter 1.

In the heart, Na$_v$ are crucial for the amplitude and upstroke velocity of the cardiac action potential. Therefore mutations in any of the structures involved in the gating described above can result in Na$^+$ channel gating defects, which could have substantial implications on the cardiac action potential. Considering the importance of intact voltage-gated Na$^+$ channels for proper cardiac function, substantial efforts have been undertaken in screening for mutations in *SCN5A* to detect possible factors that confer a predisposition to arrhythmogenic events. Mutations in the *SCN5A* gene are now regarded as the underlying cause of a group of arrhythmias, including long QT syndrome type 3 (LQT3), Brugada syndrome, cardiac conduction disease, sick sinus syndrome, and familial atrial fibrillation.[1–3] Functional studies using heterologous expression models have shown three major consequences leading to these different types of arrhythmias: (1) a gain-of-function in Na$^+$ currents, (2) a loss-of-function of Na$^+$ currents, and (3) both

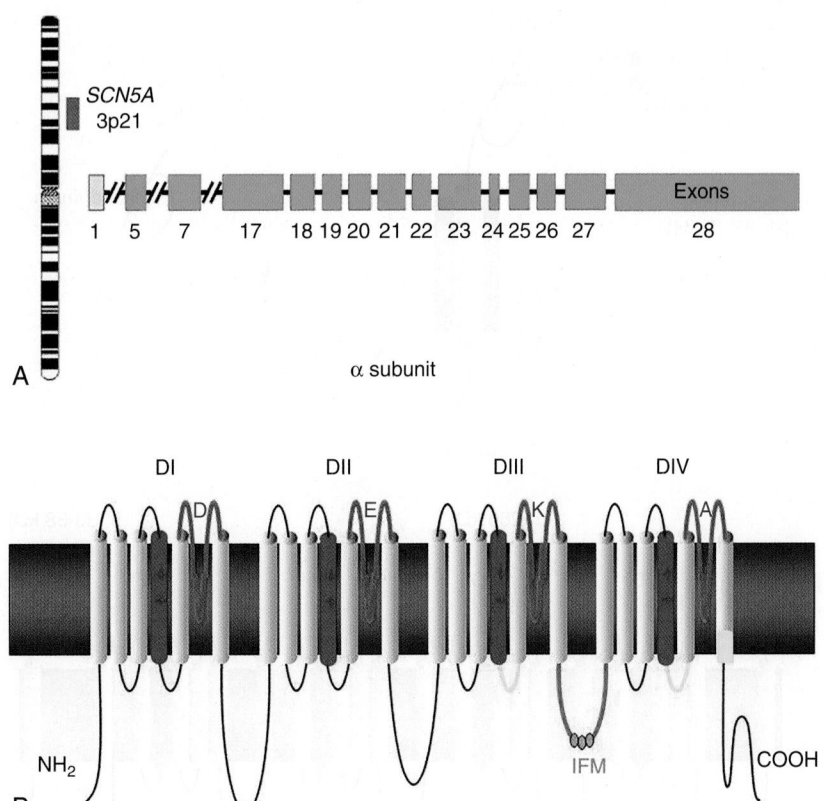

FIGURE 9.1 (A) *SCN5A* located on chromosome 3p21 is composed of 28 exons spanning more than 80 Kb. (B) Topology of cardiac Na$_v$1.5 channel (*SCN5A*). Charged S4 segments (*red*) in each domain function as voltage sensors. The links between the S5 and S6 in each domain (*pink*) form the outer pore and contain highly conserved aspartate, glutamate, lysine, and alanine residues (the "DEKA" sodium selective motif, *pink*). Isoleucine-phenylalanine-methionine (IFM) motif in DIII–DIV linker (*blue*) acts as inactivation particle to facilitate rapid voltage-dependent inactivation. The inactivation particle suggested receptor regions include the S4–S5 linkers of domains III and IV and the cytoplasmic end of S6 in domain IV (*yellow*).

gain- and loss-of-function (overlapping phenotypes). While the mechanisms involved in cardiac Na$^+$ channelopathies are covered in detail in Chapter 50, LQT3 and Brugada syndrome will be briefly described here as they relate to the current chapter.

Long QT syndrome (LQTS) is characterized by a prolonged QT interval on the surface electrocardiogram and is associated with an increased risk of sudden cardiac death due to malignant ventricular tachyarrhythmias, in particular torsade de pointes.[11] Prolongation of the QT interval may arise because of a decrease in outward currents or an increase in inward currents. However, for LQT3, most of the mutations are missense mutations and are found to cause Na$^+$ channel gain-of-function by disrupting fast inactivation and causing an abnormal persistent sodium current. Although the amplitude of the persistent Na$^+$ current is small, because it persists for hundreds of milliseconds, the influx of sodium through this mechanism is substantial enough to shift the balance toward an inward direction leading to a prolongation of the action potential. In LQT3, an increase in the current through the Na$^+$ channels causes an action potential prolongation that leads to delayed after depolarizations. The increase in currents can be caused by mutations that produce a persistent current, disrupt rapid inactivation, shift the voltage dependence of activation or inactivation, or alter recovery from inactivation. While an increase of peak Na$^+$ current can prolong the action potential, the most profound effect on the action potential is seen with the increase in the persistent current. Normally, Na$^+$ currents peak and inactivate early on during the action potential and have negligible current

that persists beyond the 5 to 10 ms peak. However, most LQT3 mutations demonstrate an increase of the persistent current, which has a profound effect on the action potential.[36,37]

Brugada syndrome is a primary electrical disorder associated with a typical electrocardiogram signature of ST-segment elevation in the right precordial leads (V1–V3) and a high risk of sudden cardiac death from ventricular tachyarrhythmias in the absence of ischemia, structural heart disease, or electrolyte abnormalities.[38,39] It is estimated that a mutation is identified in only 15% to 30% of all Brugada syndrome cases,[40] but the single largest identified contributor to Brugada syndrome is I$_{Na}$ (~25% of identified mutations in *SCN5A*). Most commonly, mutations in *SCN5A* cause loss-of-function of the sodium channel leading to the apparent accentuation of unopposed I$_{to}$ in the epicardium of the right ventricle. This leads to a loss of the "dome" of the ventricular action potential, causing heterogeneity of repolarization and reentrant arrhythmias.[17,41,42] Importantly, some of the *SCN5A* mutants identified in Brugada syndrome lead to dominant-negative effects.[43–45] Similarly, mutations in the *SCN10A* isoform, a neuronal Na$^+$ channel that has been reported in the heart, have also been linked to Brugada syndrome through a mechanism implicating the dominant cardiac isoform *SCN5A*.[46] The presence of these dominant-negative effects suggests some type of interaction/cooperation between the Na$^+$ channel α-subunits and questions the nature of the Na$^+$ channel complex. This is further discussed later.

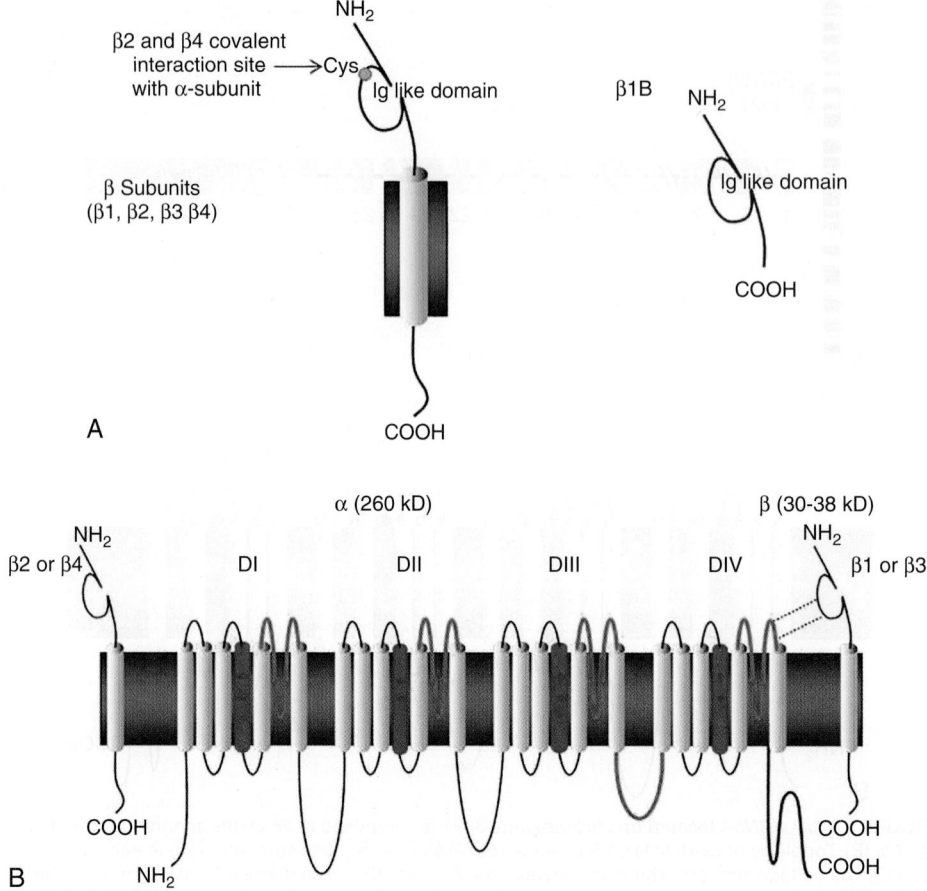

FIGURE 9.2 (A) Structures of β-subunits β1, 2, 3, 4, and β1B. (B) $Na_v1.5$ is believed to reside in a heterotrimeric complex composed of one α-subunit and two β-subunits (β1 or β3 interacting noncovalently and β2 or β4 interacting covalently).

While Brugada syndrome and LQTS are often inherited in an autosomal dominant pattern, simply carrying a dominant allele does not ensure a disease phenotype. This is known as genotype-phenotype discordance. The probability that disease-carriers actually have the disease phenotype is defined as penetrance and is not generally high for cardiac channelopathies[47]; the penetrance of LQTS has been estimated at ~40%[48] and Brugada syndrome at ~15%.[49] A major contributor to variable penetrance in cardiac arrhythmias is disease-modifying genes. Several studies have focused on the role of *SCN5A* polymorphisms as potential modifier genes. It was first demonstrated that the *SCN5A*-H558R polymorphism can rescue the cell surface expression of the Brugada syndrome *SCN5A*-R282H mutation, which could contribute to variable penetrance.[50] The ability of H558R to modulate other *SCN5A* mutations was also demonstrated in LQT3 where it was shown to restore defects in the P2006A and V1951L mutations.[51] These modulations of mutations by a polymorphism were among the first evidence questioning the nature and stoichiometry of the Na_v complex and will be further discussed later.

Sodium Channel β-Subunits

Five different β-subunits encoded by four different genes exist: β1 and β1B (a splice variant of β1) encoded by the *SCN1B* gene, and β2, β3, and β4 encoded by *SCN2B*, *SCN3B*, and *SCN4B*, respectively. These β-subunits of 30 to 38 kDa are single transmembrane spanning proteins with an extracellular N-terminus containing an immunoglobulin-like domain with homology to domains found in cell adhesion molecules and a cytoplasmic

C-terminal sequence (see Fig. 9.2A).[52] The presence of this extracellular immunoglobulin domain makes the β-subunits members of the cell adhesion molecule family.[53] In the brain, β-subunits have actually been shown to act as cell adhesion molecules.[54] Due to the splicing site found in the N-terminus region of the *SCN1B* gene, β1B does not contain a transmembrane segment; however, its N-terminus is conserved with β1 while its C-terminus differs (see Fig. 9.2A). This absence of a transmembrane segment makes it a secreted protein.[55]

Several studies in heterologous expression systems or in native cells have investigated the effect of β-subunits on Na_v. Canonically, β-subunits function in concert with α-subunits to promote channel trafficking to the plasma membrane and to modulate the Na_v biophysical properties. While there are some discrepancies in some of the observations, one consensus is with the increase in current density seen when expressing β1 with the different Na_v isoforms including $Na_v1.5$. Coexpression of β1 subunits with $Na_v1.5$ in vitro leads to increased α-subunit expression at the plasma membrane resulting in an augmentation in current density.[56–58] Interestingly though, in an *SCN1B* null mice model, increases in both tetrodotoxin (TTX)-resistant ($Na_v1.5$) and TTX-sensitive ($Na_v1.3$) currents have been observed leading to a prolonged QT interval.[59,60] For β2 and β4, little to no effect is seen on the current density when coexpressed with $Na_v1.5$.[61,62] For β3, experiments in expression systems are not clear in regard to its effect on $Na_v1.5$ current density. However, a decrease in current density is seen in ventricular myocytes isolated from an $SCN3B^{-/-}$ KO,[63] which would agree with the increase in current density seen when coexpressing β3 with $Na_v1.5$ in COS cells.[64]

β-subunits have also been shown to modulate the gating properties of Na_v, although the effects seem to be dependent on the β-subunits and the Na_v isoform studied. For β1 when coexpressed with Na_v1.5, a shift in steady-state inactivation toward hyperpolarized voltages has been observed,[61,62] while some have also observed a shift toward depolarized potentials.[65] For activation, the results are inconclusive since some studies have not seen any effect,[65,66] some have shown shifts toward hyperpolarized voltages,[67] and some have reported shifts toward depolarized voltages.[65] Silencing of β1 in canine ventricular myocytes resulted in an increase in late sodium current.[68] Finally, β1 has been reported to reduce the persistent sodium current both from expression system work[65] and based on the data obtained from the $SCN1B^{-/-}$ KO mouse.[60]

When looking at how the β2-subunit regulates the biophysical properties of Na_v1.5, no effect was seen in heterologous expression systems.[66] However, the silencing of β2 in canine ventricular myocytes resulted in an increase in late sodium current leading to action potential prolongation.[68] As it relates to β3, the most significant effect on Na_v1.5 is a shift in steady-state inactivation toward either hyperpolarized[64] or depolarized voltages[69] depending on the expression system used. However, recordings from myocytes isolated from the $SCN3B^{-/-}$ KO mouse were consistent with β3 producing a shift toward depolarized voltages.[63] Finally, β4 was shown to regulate Na_v1.5 by producing a shift in activation toward hyperpolarized voltages.[61,62,70]

Na_v Channel α- and β-Subunit Complex

The Na_v1.5 α-subunit associates with one or more β-subunits (β1–β4) (see Fig. 9.2B). The interactions between α- and β-subunits occur through two distinct mechanisms: covalently and noncovalently. β1 and β3, which share 57% sequence homology,[71] interact noncovalently with the α-subunit via their N- and C-termini.[72,73] For β1B, while it is a secreted protein, it has been shown to selectively associate with Na_v1.5 in heterologous systems.[55] β2 and β4 share 35% sequence homology[70] and engage in covalent interactions with α-subunits via a single N-terminal cysteine in the extracellular immunoglobulin loop.[70,74,75] Purification from brain tissues suggest that the Na_v α- and β-subunits assemble as an heterotrimeric complex.[75] These heterotrimeric complexes are proposed to be composed of a single pore-forming α-subunit, a noncovalently associated β-subunit (β1 or β3), and a covalently associated β-subunit (β2 or β4). While this heterotrimeric complex is well established for neuronal tissues, the stoichiometry of the Na^+ channel complex has yet to be confirmed. Interestingly, recent crystal structure for β3 shows it associates with Na_v1.5 in a trimeric complex capable of forming oligomers, rather than the canonical heterotrimeric complex of two nonidentical β-subunits with a single α-subunit.[76] In this study, the authors also showed that β3-subunits can bind to more than one site on the Na_v1.5 α-subunit and induce the formation of α-subunit oligomers, including trimers. The residues mediating this trimeric assembly are unique to β3 and are not predicted to occur in β1,[76] supporting the distinct expression patterns and postulated functional roles of these proteins. Thus the established heterotrimeric Na_v structure, predicted from the biochemical analysis of channels purified from brain, may not hold in the heart.

β-subunits are expressed throughout the heart as well as in the conduction system. Differential localization of β-subunits has been reported. In the human heart, $SCN1B$ expression is higher in the atria and endocardium than in the ventricles and epicardium, whereas $SCN2B$ and $SCN3B$ expression is found in all heart regions.[77] At the intercalated disc of ventricular myocytes, Na_v1.5 has been shown to be expressed with β1, β2, and β4.[78–81] At the t-tubules of the ventricular myocytes, the TTX-sensitive channels Na_v1.1, Na_v1.3, and Na_v1.6 are coexpressed with nonphosphorylated β1, β2, and β3.[66,78–81] The presence of β-subunits in

different regions of the heart and their associations with different channels in myocytes where they are known to regulate both expression and function of the channels predispose their involvement in cardiac channelopathies. Expectedly, human mutations in Na_v β-subunits have been linked to diseases and conditions, including Brugada syndrome ($SCN1B$ and $SCN3B$), LQTS ($SCN4B$), cardiac conduction disease ($SCN1B$), and atrial fibrillation ($SCN1B$, $SCN2B$, and $SCN3B$).[2,52,61,64,82,83]

Na_v Channel α-α Subunit Interactions and Macromolecular Complex

Unlike voltage-gated K^+ channel genes, which encode for one domain of the pore that forms a homo-tetramer, the voltage-gated Na^+ channel genes encode for an entire functional channel that has always been thought to be functional on its own, as a monomer. However, a growing body of literature has started to cast doubts on this concept. Indeed, different studies have shown that the common polymorphism Na_v1.5-H558R could partially restore I_{Na} impaired by mutations when expressed on different constructs.[50,51] Additionally, several studies have also demonstrated the presence of dominant-negative mutations found in Brugada syndrome.[43–45] In fact, recent studies demonstrated that two cardiac Na^+ channel α-subunits can actually physically interact, hence providing a mechanism explaining the presence of a dominant-negative effect of a mutant on the wild-type channel.[43,84] This α-α subunit interaction in the heart also opposes the believed heterotrimeric structure of Na_v channels composed of one α- and two β-subunits (discussed earlier). While the physical interaction between the cardiac Na_v subunits has now been established, the actual site of interaction and whether this interaction is direct or mediated through an accessory protein of the cardiac sodium channel remains to be elucidated. As described above, β3-subunits have been shown to form a trimer,[76] and as suggested by the authors, considering several sites of interaction are found on Na_v1.5, it is possible that β3 could mediate oligomerization of Na_v. The answer for this α-subunit oligomerization may be also found in the growing family of adapter, accessory, cytoskeletal, and regulatory proteins—including α1-syntrophin, ankyrin-G, βIV-spectrin, glycerol-3-phosphate dehydrogenase 1–like protein, 14-3-3, MOG1, Nedd4-2, SAP97, and calmodulin—that reside in macromolecular complexes with Na_v channels.[4,5,16–23] Recent studies demonstrate that interactions between Na_v and these related proteins: (1) regulate channel function, (2) differ depending on local membrane domain, and (3) are altered in disease. Therefore it is also possible that some of these proteins could mediate the interaction between Na_v1.5 subunits.

Interestingly, Park and colleagues[85] described in a pig transgenic model a Brugada syndrome mutant that led to a reduction in currents reflective of a dominant-negative effect. This mutant led to a truncated channel where only the first 555 amino acids were present. Assuming as with K^+ channels that a dominant-negative effect is the result of the interaction of the deficient channel with the wild-type channel leading to its loss of function, the presence of a dominant-negative effect with the truncated channel E555X suggests that the major interaction site is located within the first 555 amino acids of the channel.[85] However, recent work from Gabelli and colleagues presented a crystal structure of partial Na_v1.5 C-terminus fragments, which demonstrated the interaction with each other.[86] This suggests there might be more than one interaction site or that it could also be dependent on the partners present in the system used for the studies. Evidently, the future identification of the partner or the site mediating this interaction between Na_v1.5 α-subunits will have great implications due to the link it has with channelopathies. Removing this interaction could, for example, impair the dominant-negative effect seen with Brugada syndrome mutations.

The next obvious question relating to this interaction between $Na_v1.5$ α-subunits is whether this has implications at the biophysical level. Interestingly, multiple studies have shown that the defects of several LQT3 *SCN5A* mutations could be rescued by different SCN5A polymorphisms expressed on a separate construct not only supporting the idea of an α-α subunit interaction but also suggesting that they can biophysically interact.[51,87,88] Importantly, multiple historical evidences exist also at the single channel level that support the coupled gating of voltage-gated Na^+ channels. Aldrich and colleagues in single channel recordings noted a tendency for an even number of channels to occur within a patch.[89] A study by Iwasa and colleagues also demonstrated that the opening rate of one of two-sodium channels in a single patch in the absence of $\beta1$-subunits is greater when one channel is closed, suggesting α-α subunit interaction.[90] Furthermore, a study by Undrovinas and colleagues also demonstrated, under conditions of lysophosphatidylcholine (an ischemic metabolite) administration, two to three synchronized Na^+ channel openings from isolated patch clamp experiments. Notably, no single opening peak was present in an amplitude distribution histogram.[91] Therefore it appears that not only do $Na_v1.5$ α-subunits physically interact but they also appear to interact biophysically.

Interaction between $Na_v1.5$ α-subunits has been demonstrated, with apparent implications in arrhythmic syndromes where a mutation in one channel can affect the channel encoded by the other allele. Interestingly, *SCN5A* mRNA undergoes alternative splicing leading to different $Na_v1.5$ protein-spliced variants.[2,4–8] Up to now at least nine different splicing variants have been identified for *SCN5A*.[4] The regions where those splicing events can occur are within S3–S4 of DI, the intracellular loop linking DII and DIII, and the C-terminal region after S3 of DIV. Some of these variants lead to functional channels albeit with modified gating, while some lead to truncated channels that do not produce any currents.[4] In fact, some of these truncated splice variants could almost be compared to some of the mutations reported in Brugada syndrome. We could speculate that similarly to dominant-negative truncated channels found in Brugada syndrome,[85] these truncated splice variants could also interact with the wild-type α-subunit and lead to a reduction in sodium current. While this has not been directly demonstrated yet, the level of expression of some of these splice variants have interestingly been demonstrated to be increased in heart failure,[6] where coincidently sodium currents are decreased. Therefore the presence of these splice variants could affect the Na^+ channel α-subunit complex and modulate the level of Na^+ current in health and disease based on the level of expression of the different splice variants.

When thinking of a Na_v α-subunit complex, we also need to consider that in addition to the cardiac isoform $Na_v1.5$ and its different splice variants, other Na^+ channel isoforms are also present in the heart. The neuronal channels $Na_v1.1$-$Na_v1.3$, and $Na_v1.8$ and the skeletal muscle isoform $Na_v1.4$ have also been reported in the heart, granted with a lower expression level.[78,92–95] Importantly, their presence could likely contribute to cardiac electrophysiology, although it is still not clear exactly how. One thing that transpires, though, is that there appears to be differential targeting in the myocytes of the different isoforms. Computational work suggests that concentration of Na_v channels at the intercalated disc ($Na_v1.5$), where cells are electrically and mechanically coupled, would support electrical impulse propagation.[96,97] As for the neuronal isoforms, they do not appear to be as concentrated at the intercalated disc and do not seem to play a major role under normal conditions; however, they may play modulatory roles in excitation–contraction coupling and ventricular function.[78,93] Interestingly, mutations in the *SCN10A* isoform, a neuronal Na^+ channel expressed at low levels in myocytes, have been linked to Brugada syndrome through a mechanism implicating the dominant cardiac isoform *SCN5A*.[46] It was demonstrated that the mutations in *SCN10A* reduced the $Na_v1.5$ currents suggesting some type of interaction/cooperation between Na^+ channel α-subunits. With the data demonstrating $\beta3$-subunits can trimerize and mediate oligomerization of $Na_v1.5$, one can only speculate that with the presence of these other neuronal isoforms in the heart, we could also see heterocomplexes containing α-subunits from different isoforms along with β-subunits. Overall, this questions the nature of the Na_v complex and demonstrates that more research will be necessary.

Summary and Future Directions

Traditionally, when thinking of the cardiac Na_v responsible for the sharp upstroke of the action potential and the rapid depolarization of the heart, we assumed a heterotrimeric complex formed by the $Na_v1.5$ α-subunit and two β-subunits based on what has been reported in the brain. Interestingly though, over recent years, several studies question this traditional cardiac heterotrimeric complex. It appears that not only could there be more than one $Na_v1.5$ α-subunit in this complex but there could also be α-subunits from neuronal isoforms present. As we learn more about the constituency, localization, and function of specific Na_v macromolecular complexes within the cardiomyocyte, we anticipate the discovery of new therapeutic targets and strategies for preventing arrhythmias.

Acknowledgment

This work was supported by the National Institutes of Health grant HL094450 (to I.D.).

REFERENCES

1. Abriel H. Cardiac sodium channel Na(v)1.5 and interacting proteins: physiology and pathophysiology. *J Mol Cell Cardiol*. 2010;48:2–11.
2. Rook MB, Evers MM, Vos MA, Bierhuizen MF. Biology of cardiac sodium channel Nav1.5 expression. *Cardiovasc Res*. 2012;93:12–23.
3. Wilde AA, Brugada R. Phenotypical manifestations of mutations in the genes encoding subunits of the cardiac sodium channel. *Circ Res*. 2011;108:884–897.
4. Schroeter A, Walzik S, Blechschmidt S, Haufe V, Benndorf K, Zimmer T. Structure and function of splice variants of the cardiac voltage-gated sodium channel Na(v)1.5. *J Mol Cell Cardiol*. 2010;49:16–24.
5. Shang LL, Dudley Jr SC. Tandem promoters and developmentally regulated 5'- and 3'-mRNA untranslated regions of the mouse Scn5a cardiac sodium channel. *J Biol Chem*. 2005;280:933–940.
6. Shang LL, Pfahnl AE, Sanyal S, et al. Human heart failure is associated with abnormal C-terminal splicing variants in the cardiac sodium channel. *Circ Res*. 2007;101:1146–1154.
7. Walzik S, Schroeter A, Benndorf K, Zimmer T. Alternative splicing of the cardiac sodium channel creates multiple variants of mutant T1620K channels. *PloS One*. 2011;6:e19188.

8. Wang Q, Li Z, Shen J, Keating MT. Genomic organization of the human SCN5A gene encoding the cardiac sodium channel. *Genomics*. 1996;34:9–16.
9. Zakon HH. Adaptive evolution of voltage-gated sodium channels: the first 800 million years. *Proc Natl Acad Sci U S A*. 2012;109:10619–10625.
10. Liebeskind BJ, Hillis DM, Zakon HH. Evolution of sodium channels predates the origin of nervous systems in animals. *Proc Natl Acad Sci U S A*. 2011;108:9154–9159.
11. Moss AJ, Kass RS. Long QT syndrome: from channels to cardiac arrhythmias. *J Clin Invest*. 2005;115:2018–2024.
12. Napolitano C, Bloise R, Monteforte N, Priori SG. Sudden cardiac death and genetic ion channelopathies: long QT, Brugada, short QT, catecholaminergic polymorphic ventricular tachycardia, and idiopathic ventricular fibrillation. *Circulation*. 2012;125:2027–2034.
13. Abriel H, Kamynina E, Horisberger JD, Staub O. Regulation of the cardiac voltage-gated Na+ channel (H1) by the ubiquitin-protein ligase Nedd4. *FEBS Lett*. 2000;466:377–380.
14. Abriel H, Kass RS. Regulation of the voltage-gated cardiac sodium channel Nav1.5 by interacting proteins. *Trends Cardiovasc Med*. 2005;15:35–40.

15. Lemaillet G, Walker B, Lambert S. Identification of a conserved ankyrin-binding motif in the family of sodium channel alpha subunits. *J Biol Chem*. 2003;278:27333–27339.
16. Lowe JS, Palygin O, Bhasin N, et al. Voltage-gated Nav channel targeting in the heart requires an ankyrin-G dependent cellular pathway. *J Cell Biol*. 2008;180:173–186.
17. Mohler PJ, Rivolta I, Napolitano C, et al. Nav1.5 E1053K mutation causing Brugada syndrome blocks binding to ankyrin-G and expression of Nav1.5 on the surface of cardiomyocytes. *Proc Natl Acad Sci U S A*. 2004;101:17533–17538.
18. van Bemmelen MX, Rougier JS, Gavillet B, et al. Cardiac voltage-gated sodium channel Nav1.5 is regulated by Nedd4-2 mediated ubiquitination. *Circ Res*. 2004;95:284–291.
19. Wu L, Yong SL, Fan C, et al. Identification of a new co-factor, MOG1, required for the full function of cardiac sodium channel Nav 1.5. *J Biol Chem*. 2008;283:6968–6978.
20. Allouis M, Le Bouffant F, Wilders R, et al. 14-3-3 is a regulator of the cardiac voltage-gated sodium channel Nav1.5. *Circ Res*. 2006;98:1538–1546.

21. Payandeh J, Scheuer T, Zheng N, Catterall WA. The crystal structure of a voltage-gated sodium channel. *Nature*. 2011;475:353–358.
22. Heinemann SH, Terlau H, Stuhmer W, Imoto K, Numa S. Calcium channel characteristics conferred on the sodium channel by single mutations. *Nature*. 1992;356:441–443.
23. Catterall WA. Voltage-gated sodium channels at 60: structure, function and pathophysiology. *J Physiol*. 2012;590:2577–2589.
24. Stuhmer W, Conti F, Suzuki H, et al. Structural parts involved in activation and inactivation of the sodium channel. *Nature*. 1989;339:597–603.
25. Yang N, George Jr AL, Horn R. Molecular basis of charge movement in voltage-gated sodium channels. *Neuron*. 1996;16:113–122.
26. Yang N, Horn R. Evidence for voltage-dependent S4 movement in sodium channels. *Neuron*. 1995;15:213–218.
27. Dumaine R, Wang Q, Keating MT, et al. Multiple mechanisms of Na^+ channel–linked long-QT syndrome. *Circ Res*. 1996;78:916–924.
28. Wang DW, Yazawa K, George Jr AL, Bennett PB. Characterization of human cardiac Na^+ channel mutations in the congenital long QT syndrome. *Proc Natl Acad Sci U S A*. 1996;93:13200–13205.
29. Cha A, Ruben PC, George Jr AL, Fujimoto E, Bezanilla F. Voltage sensors in domains III and IV, but not I and II, are immobilized by Na^+ channel fast inactivation. *Neuron*. 1999;22:73–87.
30. Vassilev PM, Scheuer T, Catterall WA. Identification of an intracellular peptide segment involved in sodium channel inactivation. *Science*. 1988;241:1658–1661.
31. West JW, Patton DE, Scheuer T, Wang Y, Goldin AL, Catterall WA. A cluster of hydrophobic amino acid residues required for fast Na^+-channel inactivation. *Proc Natl Acad Sci U S A*. 1992;89:10910–10914.
32. McPhee JC, Ragsdale DS, Scheuer T, Catterall WA. A mutation in segment IVS6 disrupts fast inactivation of sodium channels. *Proc Natl Acad Sci U S A*. 1994;91:12346–12350.
33. McPhee JC, Ragsdale DS, Scheuer T, Catterall WA. A critical role for the S4-S5 intracellular loop in domain IV of the sodium channel alpha-subunit in fast inactivation. *J Biol Chem*. 1998;273:1121–1129.
34. Smith M,R, Goldin AL. Interaction between the sodium channel inactivation linker and domain III S4-S5. *Biophys J*. 1997;73:1885–1895.
35. Glaaser IW, Bankston JR, Liu H, Tateyama M, Kass RS. A carboxyl-terminal hydrophobic interface is critical to sodium channel function. Relevance to inherited disorders. *J Biol Chem*. 2006;281:24015–24023.
36. Wang Q, Shen J, Splawski I, et al. SCN5A mutations associated with an inherited cardiac arrhythmia, long QT syndrome. *Cell*. 1995;80:805–811.
37. Clancy CE, Rudy Y. Linking a genetic defect to its cellular phenotype in a cardiac arrhythmia. *Nature*. 1999;400:566–569.
38. Antzelevitch C, Brugada P, Brugada J, et al. Brugada syndrome: a decade of progress. *Circ Res*. 2002;91:1114–1118.
39. Brugada P, Brugada J. Right bundle branch block, persistent ST segment elevation and sudden cardiac death: a distinct clinical and electrocardiographic syndrome. A multicenter report. *J Am Coll Cardiol*. 1992;20:1391–1396.
40. Nielsen MW, Holst AG, Olesen S-P, Olesen MS. The genetic component of Brugada syndrome. *Front Physiol*. 2013;4:179.
41. Chen Q, Kirsch GE, Zhang D, et al. Genetic basis and molecular mechanism for idiopathic ventricular fibrillation. *Nature*. 1998;392:293–296.
42. Dumaine R, Towbin JA, Brugada P, et al. Ionic mechanisms responsible for the electrocardiographic phenotype of the Brugada syndrome are temperature dependent. *Circ Res*. 1999;85:803–809.
43. Clatot J, Ziyadeh-Isleem A, Maugenre S, et al. Dominant-negative effect of SCN5A N-terminal mutations through the interaction of Na(v)1.5 alpha-subunits. *Cardiovasc Res*. 2012;96:53–63.
44. Keller DI, Rougier JS, Kucera JP, et al. Brugada syndrome and fever: genetic and molecular characterization of patients carrying SCN5A mutations. *Cardiovasc Res*. 2005;67:510–519.
45. Mercier A, Clement R, Harnois T, et al. The beta1-subunit of Na(v)1.5 cardiac sodium channel is required for a dominant negative effect through alpha-alpha interaction. *PloS One*. 2012;7:e48690.
46. Hu D, Barajas-Martinez H, Pfeiffer R, et al. Mutations in SCN10A are responsible for a large fraction of cases of Brugada syndrome. *J Am Coll Cardiol*. 2014;64:66–79.
47. Giudicessi JR, Ackerman MJ. Determinants of incomplete penetrance and variable expressivity in heritable cardiac arrhythmia syndromes. *Transl Res*. 2013;161:1–14.
48. Berge KE, Haugaa KH, Früh A, et al. Molecular genetic analysis of long QT syndrome in Norway indicating a high prevalence of heterozygous mutation carriers. *Scand J Clin Lab Invest*. 2008;68:362–368.
49. Priori SG, Napolitano C, Gasparini M, et al. Clinical and Genetic Heterogeneity of Right Bundle Branch Block and ST-Segment Elevation Syndrome: a Prospective Evaluation of 52 Families. *Circulation*. 2000;102:2509–2515.
50. Poelzing S, Forleo C, Samodell M, et al. SCN5A polymorphism restores trafficking of a Brugada syndrome mutation on a separate gene. *Circulation*. 2006;114:368–376.
51. Shinlapawittayatorn K, Du XX, Liu H, Ficker E, Kaufman ES, Deschenes I. A common SCN5A polymorphism modulates the biophysical defects of SCN5A mutations. *Heart Rhythm*. 2011;8:455–462.
52. Meadows LS, Isom LL. Sodium channels as macromolecular complexes: implications for inherited arrhythmia syndromes. *Cardiovasc Res*. 2005;67:448–458.
53. Isom LL, Catterall WA. Na^+ channel subunits and Ig domains. *Nature*. 1996;383:307–308.
54. Brackenbury WJ, Isom LL. Na Channel beta subunits: overachievers of the ion channel family. *Front Pharmacol*. 2011;2:53.
55. Patino GA, Brackenbury WJ, Bao Y, et al. Voltage-gated Na^+ channel beta1B: a secreted cell adhesion molecule involved in human epilepsy. *J Neurosci*. 2011;31:14577–14591.
56. Nuss HB, Chiamvimonvat N, Perez-Garcia MT, Tomaselli GF, Marban E. Functional association of the beta 1 subunit with human cardiac (hH1) and rat skeletal muscle (mu 1) sodium channel alpha subunits expressed in Xenopus oocytes. *J Gen Physiol*. 1995;106:1171–1191.
57. Qu Y, Isom LL, Westenbroek RE, et al. Modulation of cardiac Na^+ channel expression in Xenopus oocytes by beta 1 subunits. *J Biol Chem*. 1995;270:25696–25701.
58. Isom LL, Scheuer T, Brownstein AB, Ragsdale DS, Murphy BJ, Catterall WA. Functional co-expression of the beta 1 and type IIA alpha subunits of sodium channels in a mammalian cell line. *J Biol Chem*. 1995;270:3306–3312.
59. Lin X, O'Malley H, Chen C, et al. Scn1b deletion leads to increased tetrodotoxin-sensitive sodium current, altered intracellular calcium homeostasis and arrhythmias in murine hearts. *The J Physiol*. 2015;593:1389–1407.
60. Lopez-Santiago LF, Meadows LS, Ernst SJ, et al. Sodium channel Scn1b null mice exhibit prolonged QT and RR intervals. *J Mol Cell Cardiol*. 2007;43:636–647.
61. Medeiros-Domingo A, Kaku T, Tester DJ, et al. SCN4B-encoded sodium channel beta4 subunit in congenital long-QT syndrome. *Circulation*. 2007;116:134–142.
62. Tan BH, Pundi KN, Van Norstrand DW, et al. Sudden infant death syndrome-associated mutations in the sodium channel beta subunits. *Heart Rhythm*. 2010;7:771–778.
63. Hakim P, Gurung IS, Pedersen TH, et al. Scn3b knockout mice exhibit abnormal ventricular electrophysiological properties. *Prog Biophys Mol Biol*. 2008;98:251–266.
64. Valdivia CR, Medeiros-Domingo A, Ye B, et al. Loss-of-function mutation of the SCN3B-encoded sodium channel β3 subunit associated with a case of idiopathic ventricular fibrillation. *Cardiovasc Res*. 2010;86:392–400.
65. Valdivia CR, Nagatomo T, Makielski JC. Late Na currents affected by alpha subunit isoform and beta1 subunit co-expression in HEK293 cells. *J Mol Cell Cardiol*. 2002;34:1029–1039.
66. Dhar Malhotra J, Chen C, Rivolta I, et al. Characterization of sodium channel alpha- and beta-subunits in rat and mouse cardiac myocytes. *Circulation*. 2001;103:1303–1310.
67. Bezzina CR, Rook MB, Groenewegen WA, et al. Compound heterozygosity for mutations (W156X and R225W) in SCN5A associated with severe cardiac conduction disturbances and degenerative changes in the conduction system. *Circ Res*. 2003;92:159–168.
68. Mishra S, Undrovinas NA, Maltsev VA, Reznikov V, Sabbah HN, Undrovinas A. Post-transcriptional silencing of SCN1B and SCN2B genes modulates late sodium current in cardiac myocytes from normal dogs and dogs with chronic heart failure. *Am J Physiol Heart Circ Physiol*. 301:H1596–H1605.
69. Fahmi AI, Patel M, Stevens EB, et al. The sodium channel beta-subunit SCN3b modulates the kinetics of SCN5a and is expressed heterogeneously in sheep heart. *J Physiol*. 2001;537:693–700.
70. Yu FH, Westenbroek RE, Silos-Santiago I, et al. Sodium channel beta4, a new disulfide-linked auxiliary subunit with similarity to beta2. *J Neurosci*. 2003;23:7577–7585.
71. Morgan K, Stevens EB, Shah B, et al. beta 3: an additional auxiliary subunit of the voltage-sensitive sodium channel that modulates channel gating with distinct kinetics. *Proc Natl Acad Sci U S A*. 2000;97:2308–2313.
72. McCormick KA, Isom LL, Ragsdale D, Smith D, Scheuer T, Catterall WA. Molecular determinants of Na^+ channel function in the extracellular domain of the beta1 subunit. *J Biol Chem*. 1998;273:3954–3962.
73. Meadows L, Malhotra JD, Stetzer A, Isom LL, Ragsdale DS. The intracellular segment of the sodium channel beta 1 subunit is required for its efficient association with the channel alpha subunit. *J Neurochem*. 2001;76:1871–1878.
74. Buffington SA, Rasband MN. Na^+ channel-dependent recruitment of Navbeta4 to axon initial segments and nodes of Ranvier. *J Neurosci*. 2013;33:6191–6202.
75. Messner DJ, Catterall WA. The sodium channel from rat brain. Separation and characterization of subunits. *J Biol Chem*. 1985;260:10597–10604.
76. Namadurai S, Balasuriya D, Rajappa R, et al. Crystal structure and molecular imaging of the Nav channel beta3 subunit indicates a trimeric assembly. *J Biol Chem*. 2014;289:10797–10811.
77. Gaborit N, Le Bouter S, Szuts V, et al. Regional and tissue specific transcript signatures of ion channel genes in the non-diseased human heart. *J Physiol*. 2007;582:675–693.
78. Maier SK, Westenbroek RE, McCormick KA, Curtis R, Scheuer T, Catterall WA. Distinct subcellular localization of different sodium channel alpha and beta subunits in single ventricular myocytes from mouse heart. *Circulation*. 2004;109:1421–1427.
79. Malhotra JD, Thyagarajan V, Chen C, Isom LL. Tyrosine-phosphorylated and nonphosphorylated sodium channel beta1 subunits are differentially localized in cardiac myocytes. *J Biol Chem*. 2004;279:40748–40754.
80. Kaufmann SG, Westenbroek RE, Maass AH, et al. Distribution and function of sodium channel subtypes in human atrial myocardium. *J Mol Cell Cardiol*. 2013;61:133–141.
81. Kaufmann SG, Westenbroek RE, Zechner C, et al. Functional protein expression of multiple sodium channel alpha- and beta-subunit isoforms in neonatal cardiomyocytes. *J Mol Cell Cardiol*. 2010;48:261–269.
82. Watanabe H, Darbar D, Kaiser DW, et al. Mutations in sodium channel beta1- and beta2-subunits associated with atrial fibrillation. *Circ Arrhythm Electrophysiol*. 2009;2:268–275.
83. Watanabe H, Koopmann TT, Le Scouarnec S, et al. Sodium channel beta1 subunit mutations associated with Brugada syndrome and cardiac conduction disease in humans. *J Clin Invest*. 2008;118:2260–2268.
84. Hoshi M, Du XX, Shinlapawittayatorn K, et al. Brugada syndrome disease phenotype explained in apparently benign sodium channel mutations. *Circ Cardiovasc Genet*. 2014;7:123–131.
85. Park DS, Cerrone M, Morley G, et al. Genetically engineered SCN5A mutant pig hearts exhibit conduction defects and arrhythmias. *J Clin Invest*. 2015;125:403–412.
86. Gabelli SB, Boto A, Kuhns VH, et al. Regulation of the Nav1.5 cytoplasmic domain by calmodulin. *Nat Commun*. 2014;5:5126.
87. Viswanathan PC, Benson DW, Balser JR. A common SCN5A polymorphism modulates the biophysical effects of an SCN5A mutation. *J Clin Invest*. 2003;111:341–346.
88. Ye B, Valdivia CR, Ackerman MJ, Makielski JC. A common human SCN5A polymorphism modifies expression of an arrhythmia causing mutation. *Physiol Genomics*. 2003;12:187–193.
89. Aldrich RW, Corey DP, Stevens CF. A reinterpretation of mammalian sodium channel gating based on single channel recording. *Nature*. 1983;306:436–441.
90. Iwasa K, Ehrenstein G, Moran N, Jia M. Evidence for interactions between batrachotoxin-modified channels in hybrid neuroblastoma cells. *Biophys J*. 1986;50:531–537.
91. Undrovinas AI, Fleidervish IA, Makielski JC. Inward sodium current at resting potentials in single cardiac myocytes induced by the ischemic metabolite lysophosphatidylcholine. *Circ Res*. 1992;71:1231–1241.
92. Lin X, Liu N, Lu J, et al. Subcellular heterogeneity of sodium current properties in adult cardiac ventricular myocytes. *Heart Rhythm*. 2011;8:1923–1930.
93. Maier SK, Westenbroek RE, Schenkman KA, Feigl EO, Scheuer T, Catterall WA. An unexpected role for brain-type sodium channels in coupling of cell surface depolarization to contraction in the heart. *Proc Natl Acad Sci U S A*. 2002;99:4073–4078.
94. Savio-Galimberti E, Gollob MH, Darbar D. Voltage-gated sodium channels: biophysics, pharmacology, and related channelopathies. *Front Pharmacol*. 2012;3:124.
95. Yang T, Atack TC, Stroud DM, Zhang W, Hall L, Roden DM. Blocking Scn10a channels in heart reduces late sodium current and is antiarrhythmic. *Circ Res*. 2012;111:322–332.
96. Kucera JP, Rohr S, Rudy Y. Localization of sodium channels in intercalated disks modulates cardiac conduction. *Circ Res*. 2002;91:1176–1182.
97. Mori Y, Fishman GI, Peskin CS. Ephaptic conduction in a cardiac strand model with 3D electrodiffusion. *Proc Natl Acad Sci U S A*. 2008;105:6463–6468.

10 Regulation of Cardiac Calcium Channels

Jonathan Satin

Overview

The super-family of voltage-gated ion channels is defined by the common ability of the protein to sense transmembrane potentials. Voltage-gated ion channels, specifically voltage-gated cation channels, share a general structural plan that consists of six α-helical transmembrane segments and a region of amino acids between transmembrane segments five and six (S5 and S6) that folds from the extracellular space in toward the cytosol to form the outer permeation pathway. The fundamental common property of voltage-sensing is conferred by a transmembrane α-helical stretch of amino acids in the fourth transmembrane segment, S4. The purpose of this chapter is to describe the regulation of cardiac Ca^{2+} channel gating. Additional detail on Ca^{2+} channels and cardiac myocyte physiology can be gleaned from several excellent reviews.[1–3] For an outstanding resource for the fundamentals of ion channel biophysics, the reader is directed to books by B. Hille[4] and L. Defelice.[5]

Voltage-gated Ca^{2+} channels tend to open in response to depolarization, and they tend to close following repolarization. A channel transiting from an open to a closed state is summarized as activation gating. Channel gating can be envisioned as a mechanical contraption that allows ionic flow across a barrier (Fig. 10.1). It requires some imagination to picture a complex molecule undergoing gating. Consider a starting gate for the Kentucky Derby horse race. In this picture, the motionless horse represents the potential energy of a calcium ion impacted by its electrochemical gradient. Once the gate opens, the calcium ion flows down its electrochemical gradient. Although the ion may interact with the gate and influence the gate, the gate is operated independently. Moreover, there are a series of sequential complex steps between the starter pushing the button for the gates to open and the actual gating event. Similarly, the initial movement of the S4 in response to voltage is transmitted in a complex, incompletely understood fashion to other domains of the channel that alter the permeation pathway allowing ionic flux.

Cardiac L-type Ca^{2+} channel gating is influenced by voltage, Ca^{2+}-ion, posttranslational modifications, and protein–protein interactions. Voltage is a major determinant of gating, and one must also consider the superimposed effects of permeating cations and the modulation of gating primarily by channel phosphorylation status. Finally, the cardiac calcium channel is a heteromultimeric protein complex. Accessory proteins and interacting proteins, either directly or via scaffolding proteins, modify cardiac Ca^{2+} channel gating. Additional details on L-type Ca^{2+} channels in the heart are found in Chapter 2, the focus on excitation-contraction coupling is covered in Chapter 16, and a more in-depth focus on Timothy syndrome is in Chapter 95.

Calcium Channel Expression in the Myocardium

L-Type Versus T-Type Channel Expression and Gating

The myocardium expresses L-type and T-type voltage-gated Ca^{2+} channels. Myocardial L-type calcium channels include Ca$_V$1.2 and Ca$_V$1.3. Mature ventricular myocardium almost exclusively expresses the Ca$_V$1.2 channel. Ca$_V$1.2 and Ca$_V$1.3 are expressed in atrial cardiomyocytes, and Ca$_V$1.3 is also expressed by sinoatrial[6] and atrioventricular nodal cells.[7] Commensurate with these tissue localizations, Ca$_V$1.2 is critically important for providing trigger calcium for excitation-contraction coupling, and Ca$_V$1.3 contributes to heart rate and cardiac conduction.[8,9] In the ventricular myocardium, there is an age- and gender-dependent gradient of I$_{Ca,L}$. Prepubertal males have elevated I$_{Ca,L}$ at the base, but developing females do not. In adulthood, the gradients are somewhat reversed in rabbits with females displaying higher I$_{Ca,L}$ at the base compared to males,[10] and this may be related to an estrogen regulation of L-type Ca^{2+} gene transcription.[11]

T-type Ca^{2+} channels in the heart are encoded by Ca$_V$3.1 and Ca$_V$3.2 pore-forming subunits.[12,13] T-type Ca^{2+} current, I$_{Ca,T}$, is not normally observed in the mature mammalian ventricular myocardium. I$_{Ca,T}$ is present in pacemaker cells,[14] atrial cells, and Purkinje fibers.[15] I$_{Ca,T}$ is also expressed in developing cardiomyocytes.[13,16,17] Consistent with the adage that pathological cardiac hypertrophy is accompanied by reexpression of the fetal gene program, I$_{Ca,T}$ is reexpressed in ventricular hypertrophy of the cat[18] and rat.[19]

The gating properties of I$_{Ca,T}$ versus I$_{Ca,L}$ are fundamentally distinct. The T-type versus L-type channels are also classified as low voltage-activated versus high-voltage activated, respectively. The activation of range of I$_{Ca,T}$ is positive to about –60 mV, whereas I$_{Ca,L}$ activates positive to about –20 mV. Closed state inactivation also follows a similar general pattern. T-type Ca^{2+} channel steady state availability is maximal for voltages less than –90 mV, whereas substantial closed state L-type channel inactivation is not observed for potentials as positive as about –40 mV. The positive shift of I$_{Ca,L}$ availability (also known as steady-state inactivation) has a practical benefit for measuring ionic current in ventricular cardiomyocytes as well. Voltage-gated Na$^+$ channels are largely inactivated at –40 mV; therefore a prepulse to –40 mV is frequently used to isolate I$_{Ca,L}$ from prominent overlapping I$_{Na}$. An alternative method used to measure I$_{Ca,L}$ in ventricular cardiomyocytes is to replace external Na$^+$ with an impermeant cation. I$_{Ca,L}$ can then be measured using the more negative holding potentials. In juvenile ventricular cardiomyocytes, hyperpolarizing the holding potential from –40 to –80 mV has only minor effects on peak I$_{Ca,L}$ (Fig. 10.2A). By contrast, embryonic ventricular cardiomyocytes exhibit I$_{Ca,T}$ and I$_{Ca,L}$. I$_{Ca,T}$ manifests itself as a current activating positive to –60 mV when a –80 mV holding

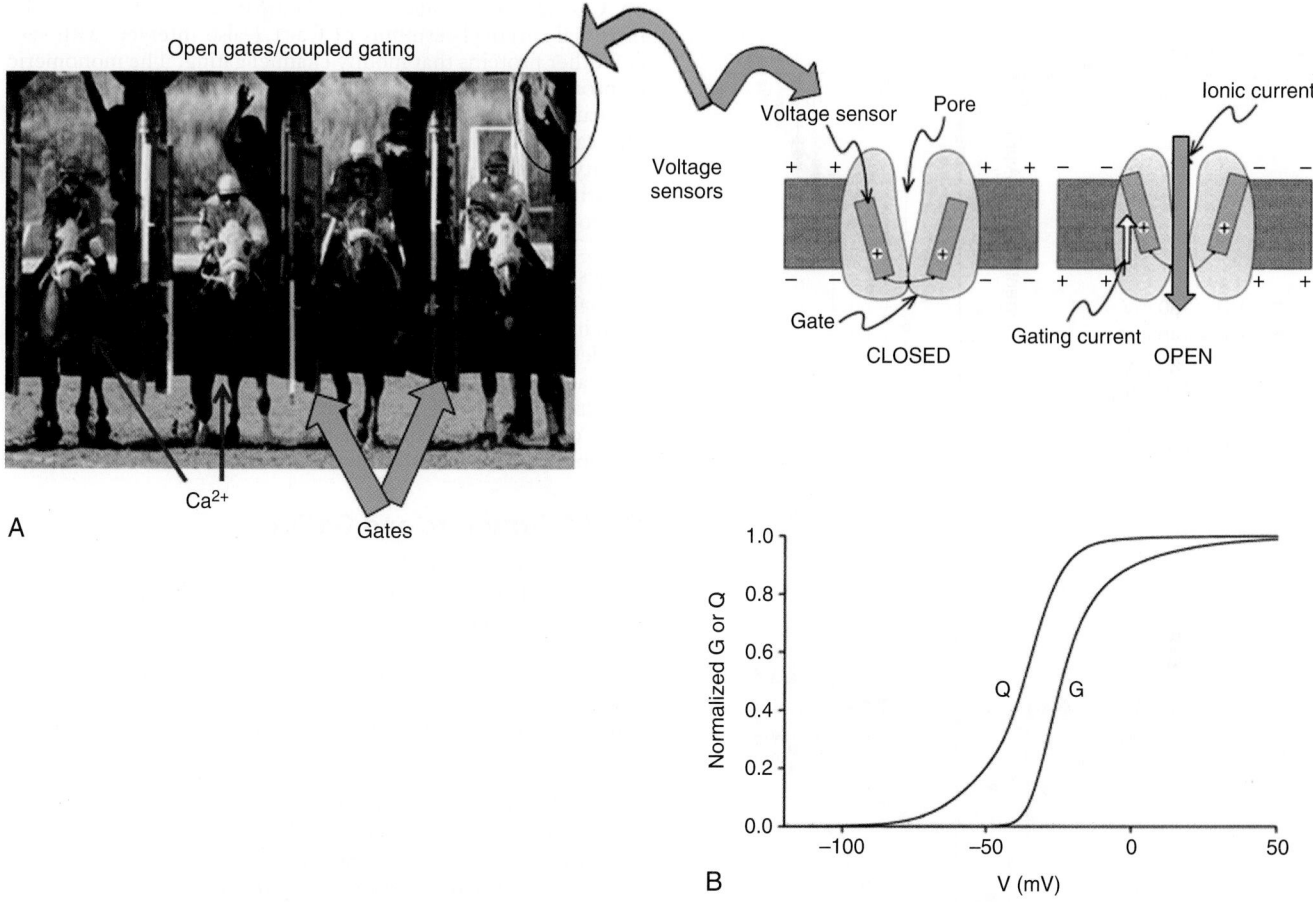

FIGURE 10.1 The relationship between voltage sensing, ion channel gating, and conductance.
(A) The schematic shows the principle features of a generalized voltage-gated ion channel and the metaphorical electrical-gated thoroughbred race horse starting gate. The α-helical transmembrane segments (S4) sense the electrical gradient. The motion of the S4 segments is transmitted allosterically through the channel protein to open the gate. Ions flow based on their electrochemical gradient.
(B) Conductance (G) and gating charge movement (Q) depend on voltage for a voltage-dependent ion channel. (B, Modified from Bezanilla F. The voltage sensor in voltage-dependent ion channels. *Physiol Rev.* 2000;80:555-592.)

potential is used, and this low-voltage activated Ca^{2+} current ($I_{Ca,T}$) is closed state inactivated by holding the potential at –40 mV (Fig. 10.2B). Heterologous expression systems transfected with pore-forming $Ca_V3.x$ subunits alone reconstitute most of the native $I_{Ca,T}$ properties.[13] In sharp contrast, native $I_{Ca,L}$ gating requires auxiliary proteins and, in some cases, is rather difficult to completely recreate in heterologous expression systems. The remainder of this chapter will focus on $Ca_V1.2$, the predominant L-type Ca^{2+} channel.

The Cardiac L-Type Calcium Channel Is a Multiprotein Complex

The pore-forming $Ca_V1.2$ Ca^{2+} channel does not gate in isolation in cardiac myocytes, and studies of ionic current in heterologous expression systems show that a functional ion channel complex requires auxiliary proteins. Although the total number of $Ca_V1.2$-interacting proteins is unknown, several important interacting partners have been identified and studied (Fig. 10.3). Early electrophysiological studies in nonexcitable cells heterologously expressing $Ca_V1.2$ alone, showed little, if any, discernable ionic current. Coexpression of $Ca_V\beta$-subunits is a requirement to study L-type Ca^{2+} current from channels generated by plasmids introduced into nonexcitable cells.[20] $Ca_V\beta$–$Ca_V1.2$ interactions

occur via a deep hydrophobic pocket of $Ca_V\beta$ complexed with the L_{I-II} domain of $Ca_V1.2$.[21] $Ca_V\beta$–$Ca_V1.2$ interactions have gating and nongating consequences. Early studies showed that $Ca_V\beta$ masks an endoplasmic reticulum retention signal on $Ca_V1.2$, thus allowing $Ca_V1.2$ to traffic to the surface membrane.[22] More recent studies show that $Ca_V\beta$–$Ca_V1.2$ binding influences a $Ca_V1.2$ carboxyl-terminal rearrangement to promote surface expression.[23] Despite the relatively high affinity $Ca_V1.2$–$Ca_V\beta$ interaction (2–54 nM), a dynamic $Ca_V\beta$–$Ca_V1.2$ interaction may also occur with respect to L-type Ca^{2+} channel gating[24] consistent with the idea that $Ca_V\beta$ modifies $Ca_V1.2$ gating in a regulated fashion.

The $Ca_V1.2$ carboxyl-terminus contains approximately 300 amino acids (size differing among splice variants) and stretches from the cytosolic border of the homologous repeat IV transmembrane S6 until the termination of the protein. The distal carboxyl terminus is proteolytically cleaved yielding an approximate 37 kDa protein that covalently reassociates with the proximal carboxyl-terminus to regulate function (see Hulme and associates[25] and also see later). The distal carboxyl terminus also can localize to the nucleus,[26] where it regulates gene transcription, including that for $Ca_V1.2$.[27] The proximal carboxyl-terminus remains contiguous with the pore-forming $Ca_V1.2$. Calmodulin (CaM) is prebound to $Ca_V1.2$ on the proximal

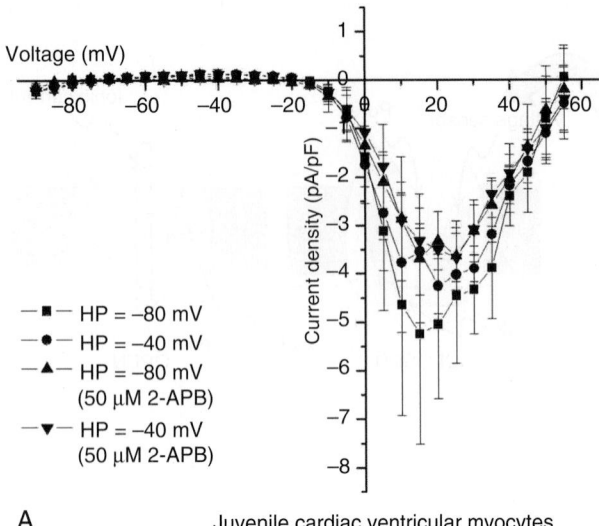

A   Juvenile cardiac ventricular myocytes

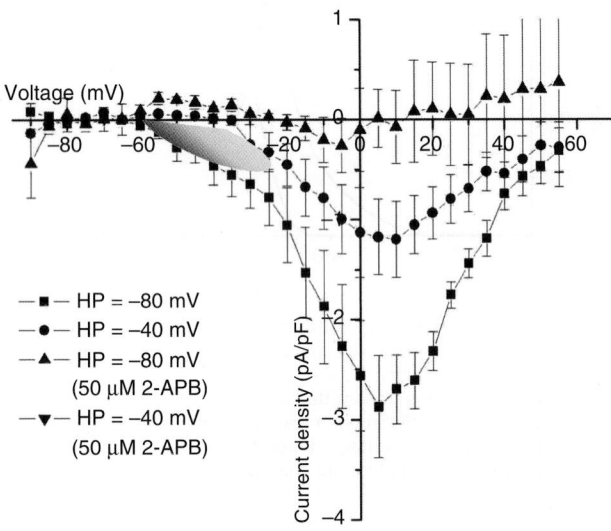

B   Embryonic cardiac ventricular myocytes

FIGURE 10.2 L-type current ($I_{Ca,L}$) is the only discernible I_{Ca} in mature cardiac myocytes. $I_{Ca,L}$ and T-type current are simultaneously functional in the developing ventricular myocardium. Current-voltage curve for juvenile (1- to 2-month-old mouse [A]) and embryonic (B) ventricular myocytes. (A) $I_{Ca,L}$ without detectable $I_{Ca,T}$ manifested as equivalent peak current for holding potentials (V_{hold}) of –80 and –40 mV. (B) $I_{Ca,T}$ is elicited from V_{hold} –80 mV and is steady-state inactivated at V_{hold} –40 resulting in no low-voltage-activated current detected on depolarization. The shaded area between –60 and –20 mV indicates the $I_{Ca,T}$ component. 2-APB does not block $Ca_V1.2$ but does inhibit non-$Ca_V1.2$ Ca^{2+} current. The 2-APB sensitivity thus illustrates the complex mixture of T- and multiple L-type currents in the developing myocardium, in contrast to the $I_{Ca,L}$ dominated by $Ca_V1.2$ in mature ventricular cardiomyocytes. (Modified from Schroder E, Wei Y, Satin J. The developing cardiac myocyte: maturation of excitability and excitation-contraction coupling. *Ann N Y Acad Sci.* 2006;1080:63-75.)

carboxyl-terminus in the IQ motif[28,29] and is a critical determinant of Ca^{2+}-dependent inactivation gating (see later). IQ is the single letter abbreviation for isoleucine and glutamine. The "I" of the IQ motif is essential for CaM binding,[30,31] and mutation of isoleucine of the IQ motif induces dilated cardiomyopathy and premature death.[32] Two CaM molecules interact with the proximal carboxyl-terminus of $Ca_V1.2$, and the CaM molecules

on $Ca_V1.2$ are arranged in an antiparallel fashion.[31,33] The proximal carboxyl-terminus of $Ca_V1.2$ also interacts with several other proteins that modify channel gating. The monomeric G-protein Rem functionally competes with CaM for channel regulation at this domain as well.[34] CaMKII tethers to the proximal carboxyl terminus and is an important modulator of $Ca_V1.2$ activity.[35] At present it is unclear how many proteins combine to form the native L-type Ca^{2+} channel complex. An unbiased proteomics screen of the closely related N-type calcium channel $Ca_V2.2$ revealed channel interactions with 207 proteins.[36] This suggests that multiple protein–protein interactions sum yielding native $I_{Ca,L}$ properties. In fact, the number of interacting proteins for the $Ca_V1.2$ carboxyl-terminal domain exceeds the restricted space suggesting that weak protein–protein interactions among multiple proteins creates the possibility of diverse mixtures of proteins for any given L-type Ca^{2+} channel complex. Some of the known $Ca_V1.2$ interacting proteins are summarized in Table 10.1.

$Ca_V1.2$ Structure and Gating

The defining functional feature of the super-family of voltage-gated ion channels is the conserved property that depolarization tends to open channels. The process of opening can be summarized by the term *activation*. According to classical ion channel biophysics, Ca_V activation is a smooth curvilinear function of voltage described by one or more Boltzmann distributions. Conversely, repolarization closes (deactivates) channels. Deactivation gating is distinguished from inactivation gating. Deactivation relates a rapid, reversible transition between an ion-conducting channel conformation and a nonconducting conformation. Inactivation is a longer-lasting nonconducting conformation that may be influenced by the position of the voltage sensors. As with the closely related Na_V channel family, Ca_V channels contain four S4 segments that presumably displace toward the extracellular space on depolarization. This S4 displacement then drives allosteric rearrangements resulting in an increase of the channel conductance. Collectively, the depolarization-dependent increase of channel conductance is referred to as activation gating.

$Ca_V1.2$ S4 segments each contain four to eight positive-charged amino acid residues (lysine, Lys; or arginine, Arg) in the register. Thus when the transmembrane potential (Vm) is negative, the S4 positive charges are electrostatically drawn toward the cytosol. Conversely, depolarization results in the relative motion of the S4 charges toward the extracellular space. The movement of charge across an electrical field creates a current. If no ionic flux occurs, and a depolarization is applied, S4 segments will move, generating what is commonly called a gating current. To measure the $Ca_V1.2$ gating currents, channel blockade is applied, or voltage is clamped to the reversal potential of the channel resulting in no net ionic flux. It should be noted that gating current yields information on the number of active channels, and the movement of the S4 segments, but gives incomplete information for activation gating. To reiterate, activation gating begins with voltage sensing (measured as gating current). Subsequent allosteric channel rearrangements result in activation gating. Gating current normalized to ionic current in a given cell is a measure of coupling between voltage sensing and allosteric rearrangements resulting in channel opening.

Inactivation gating is not simply the reverse of activation gating. There is no complete molecular structure data available for voltage-gated Ca^{2+} channels; however, voltage-gated Na^+ channels have recently been crystallized in two potentially inactivated states.[49] These crystal structure studies support the biophysical studies that suggest that inactivation gating consists of a series of complex molecular motions, whereby the voltage sensing domains (S4) shift around the pore, and two of the S6

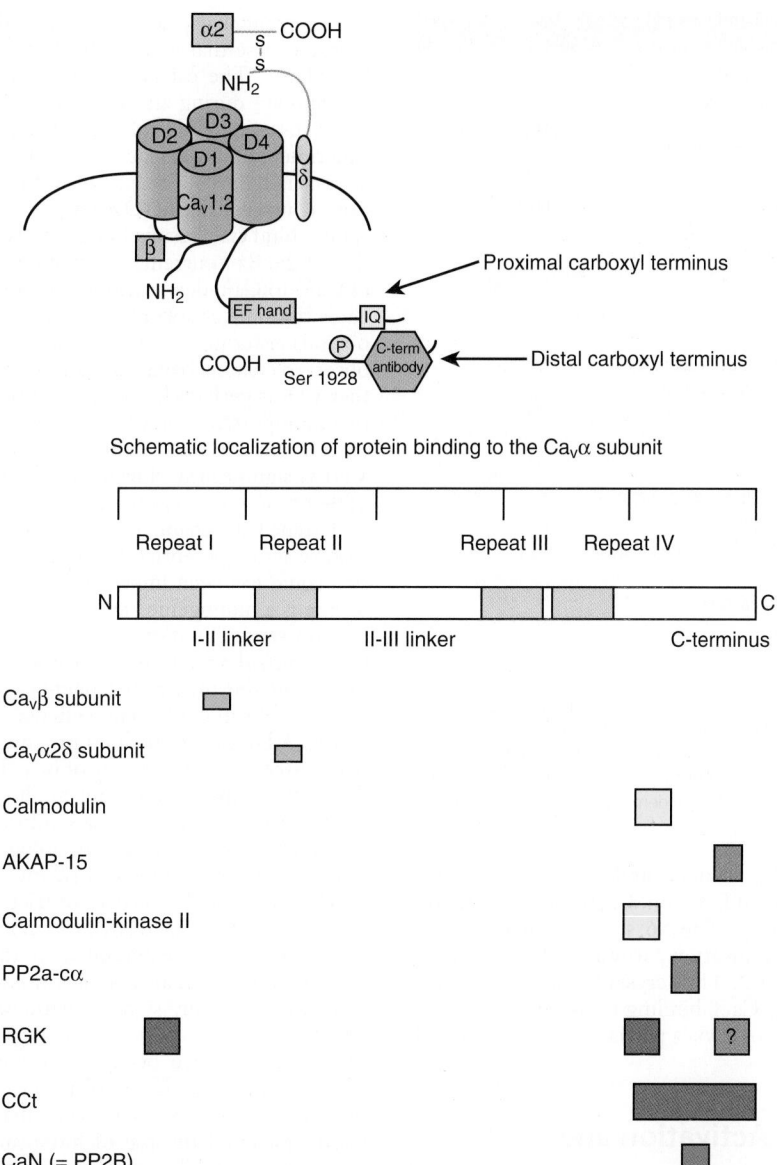

Schematic localization of protein binding to the $Ca_V\alpha$ subunit

FIGURE 10.3 Subunit structure of L-type Ca²⁺ channel complex. The upper cartoon depicts four homologous repeats of a pore-forming $Ca_V1.2$ subunit, $Ca_V\beta$ bound to L_{I-II} (linker joining repeats I and II), along with the proximal carboxyl-terminus. The IQ motif is required for calmodulin binding. The distal carboxyl-terminus is shown as a proteolytically cleaved protein. Antibodies raised against this segment show it migrating as an independent protein from the pore-forming region. The lower panel summarizes critical interacting proteins along with the approximate $Ca_V1.2$ interaction domains. *Green boxes* indicate regulators that tend to increase $I_{Ca,L}$, *yellow boxes* denote more complex effects, and *red boxes* inhibit $I_{Ca,L}$. Calcineurin (*CaN*) is denoted with a *blue box* owing to the controversial effects of CaN on $I_{Ca,L}$.

segments are transposed extracellularly while the other two S6 segments collapse on the pore. Consequentially, the permeation pathway is reshaped. Drawing on the conservation of such broad structure-function models, we can infer that similarly complex motions impart voltage-dependent inactivation (VDI) to mammalian voltage-gated Ca^{2+} channels.

The generalized structure of L-type Ca^{2+} channels ($Ca_V1.x$) shares the voltage-gated ion channel super-family plan of six α-helical transmembrane domains, arranged as four contiguous homologous repeats. There are, of course, critically important distinctions in the structure-function detail between $Ca_V1.x$ and other voltage-gated ion channels. The $Ca_V1.x$ processed transcript encodes on the order of >2100 amino acids; the precise number depends on the splice variant expression. In contrast

to T-type Ca^{2+} channels and closely related Na_V channels, Ca_V channels require various subunits to generate basal function. Perhaps the single most critical class of subunits are the $Ca_V\beta$—mainly $Ca_V\beta2$ in the myocardium.[50] $Ca_V1.x$ and $Ca_V\beta$ form tight interactions. Cytosolic $Ca_V\beta$ increases cell surface expression and increases channel gating (reviewed by Buraei and Yang[51]).

Early crystallographic studies identified a hydrophobic groove on $Ca_V\beta$ that confers Ca_V1 interactions.[21,33,52] More recent work sheds light on the α–β interactions with respect to Ca_V1 structures, and in doing so yields insight into L-type Ca^{2+} channel gating. In the 1990s, the cytoplasmic I-II linker (L_{I-II}) of $Ca_V1.2$ was identified as essential for $Ca_V\beta$ interaction.[53] Sub-domains of the cytoplasmic I-II linker (L_{I-II}) are highly

Table 10.1 Ca$_V$1.2 Interacting Proteins

PROTEIN	ASSOCIATION SITE/ INTERACTION DOMAIN ON CA$_V$1.2	REFERENCE
Ca$_V$1.2	DCT; N-terminus	37–39
Ca$_V$β2	L$_{I-II}$; PCT	Reviewed by[40]
Ca$_V$1.2–DCT	PCT	25
α2δ	uncertain	
Calmodulin (CaM)	IQ motif of PCT	See text
Calmodulin kinase II (CaMKII)	PCT	35
Rem	via Ca$_V$β2; DCT; N-terminus	34,41
Rad	via Ca$_V$β2; N-terminus	41
Calcineurin (CaN = PP2B)	DCT	42,43
PP2A	DCT	43
PDE4B	Ca$_V$1.2 by ip, no sub-domain determined	44
Akap150/79	PC–DCT scaffolds with other proteins	45
PKA	PCT-DCT via akap	46
α-actinin	PCT/DCT	47
sorcin	PCT	48

Ca$_V$1.2 by ip, indicates association demonstrating by coimmunoprecipitation with Ca$_V$1.2; *DCT*, CaV1.2 distal carboxyl-terminus; *LI-II*, cytosolic linker between homologous repeats I and II; *PCT*, Ca$_V$1.2 proximal carboxyl-terminus (defined as the cytosolic region from the termination of α-helical transmembrane segment IVS6 until the proteolytic cleavage site demarcating PCT and DCT).

conserved among the Ca$_V$1.x channels and across species consistent with the conservation of function. Ca$_V$β–L$_{I-II}$ interaction may also contribute to gating. The S6 segment of Ca$_V$1.2 is thought to form the inner permeation pathway and lies adjacent to the proximal L$_{I-II}$ of Ca$_V$1.2. Thus crystallography data supports the revised model that Ca$_V$β binding transmits changes to the inactivation gating of Ca$_V$1.2 via a partial α-helical proximal L$_{I-II}$ segment.[54]

Voltage Effects on Activation and Inactivation

Activation

Classical ion channel biophysical descriptions utilize a Boltzmann distribution to describe ion channel activation and inactivation gating.[5] Voltage determines Ca$_V$1.2 gating; therefore to study Ca$_V$1.2 gating, the voltage is experimentally controlled. To measure steady-state activation gating, cells are voltage-clamped at a relatively negative potential often approximating the diastolic potential of cardiomyocytes. Depolarizing pulses are then typically used to determine the activation range for the macroscopic current, known as the whole-cell ionic current. Typically, cardiac I$_{Ca,L}$ activates positive to about –40 mV under the conditions of physiological concentrations of external Ca^{2+}. The steady-state activation voltage range will vary with species of permeant cation; for example, Ca^{2+} versus Ba^{2+}, permeant cation concentration, phosphorylation status of the channel complex, and perhaps even dynamic protein–protein interactions with the heteromultimeric channel complex.

Inactivation

L-type Ca^{2+} channel inactivation gating is regulated by Ca^{2+} and voltage. Macroscopic (whole-cell) I$_{Ca,L}$ evoked by a step depolarization to a constant depolarized potential evokes an inward Ca^{2+} current that peaks relatively quickly, and then decays with a time course that is influenced by calcium, and to some extent by voltage. The calcium-dependent component of inactivation is dominant during a step depolarization and is discussed in the next subsection. The voltage-dependent component is uncovered experimentally by replacing Ca^{2+} with an alternative charge carrier, usually Ba^{2+}.[55] The resulting I$_{Ba,L}$ has a significantly slower time course of decay. Overexpression of the mutant CaM that cannot bind Ca^{2+} results in Ca^{2+} current decay kinetics that match that of the Ba^{2+} current,[28,56] thus supporting the key contribution of CaM to Ca^{2+}-dependent inactivation (CDI).[57] When one evaluates the time course of Ca^{2+} channel current decay, there is an obvious faster decay for I$_{Ca,L}$ than I$_{Ba,L}$ (Fig. 10.4A). This widely observed channel behavior leads to the common sense conclusion that VDI is perhaps less important than CDI. However, the relative unimportance of VDI has been challenged. On first glance, current records such as those displayed in Fig. 10.4 suggest that VDI is significantly slower than CDI. However, in the absence of β-adrenergic receptor stimulation, VDI is relatively fast.[58–60]

L-type Ca^{2+} channel inactivation limits Ca^{2+} entry during the cardiac action potential. Persistent activation such as in Timothy syndrome has been linked to inappropriate VDI. Timothy syndrome is a monogenic autosomal dominant disease likely caused by a missense mutation in Ca$_V$1.2.[61] Timothy syndrome patients have a broad spectrum of disorders, including cardiac arrhythmias, and the myocardial phenotypic changes are captured in induced pluripotent stem cell–derived cardiomyocytes.[62] The slowed VDI gating in the Timothy syndrome Ca^{2+} channels is manifested as a slower decay of I$_{Ba,L}$. In addition to explaining the fundamental disease mechanism, discovery of L-type Ca^{2+} channel involvement in Timothy syndrome revealed the importance of VDI to cardiac electrophysiology. Most recently a cardiac-only Timothy syndrome Ca$_V$1.2 mutant channel was described.[63] Mechanisms for the cardiac-restricted phenotype are unknown, although the Ca$_V$1.2–RGK protein interactions are speculated to localize the defective phenotype to the heart only.[63]

Inactivation can also be measured by evaluating channel conformation at steady-state. Regardless, it is imperative to eliminate Ca^{2+}-flux to experimentally separate CDI from VDI. Several manipulations have been performed, and each confounds the data interpretation. Equimolar replacement of Ca^{2+} with Ba^{2+} has been widely used. Some concern that Ba^{2+} weakly interacts with CaM motivated the use of monovalent cation flux to measure the channel availability. Monovalent flux measured by removal and chelation of divalent cations yields nonselective current with inactivation that is independent of current flux amplitude.[64] However, the inactivation of L-type Ca^{2+} channel in the absence of divalent cations is significantly different from that measured in the presence of divalent cations.[55] Divalent cations interacting with the permeation pathway likely alter gating behavior[65] even before the barium ions go through the channel.[66,67] Thus VDI is not purely voltage-dependent in the sense that permeating Ca^{2+} interacting with the selectivity filters may influence gating. The distinction between VDI and CDI is that in VDI ionic *flux* does not contribute to inactivation, whereas in CDI, the Ca^{2+} flux necessarily interacts with prebound cytosolic CaM and thus influences inactivation in concert with voltage.

Calcium–Calmodulin Regulates Activation and Inactivation Gating

Calcium is an important modifier of cardiac L-type Ca^{2+} channel gating.[57] CaM bound to the proximal carboxyl-terminus of the calcium channel[30,68] senses calcium ion fluxed through the channel[56,69] and the Ca^{2+} ion in the cytosol. In turn, Ca^{2+}-CaM-Ca$_V$1.2-complex imparts a relatively rapid CDI (Fig. 10.5; reviewed in Liang and colleagues[70]). CaM-modulation of I$_{Ca,L}$ targets the plateau phase of the action potential. This

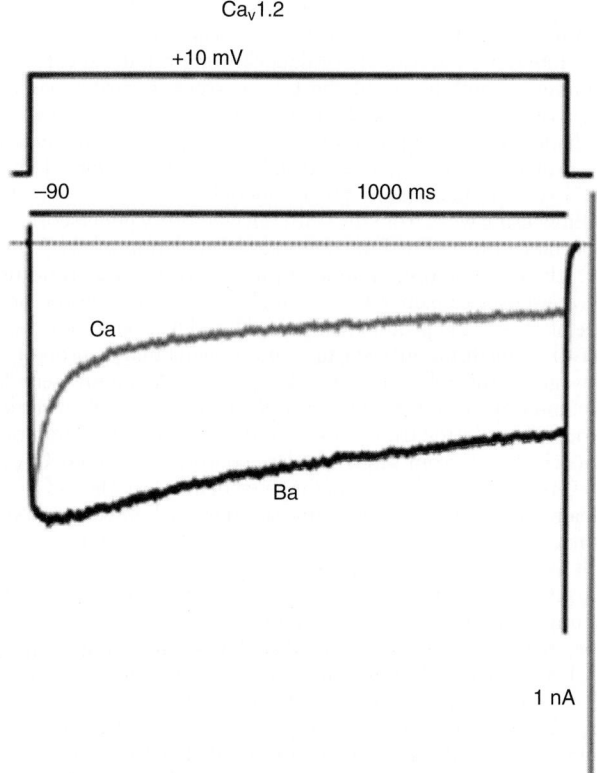

FIGURE 10.4 Voltage-dependent and calcium-dependent inactivation. HEK 293 cells expressing $Ca_V1.2$ + $Ca_V\beta2a$ +$\alpha2\delta$ recorded in the whole-cell configuration of the patch-clamp technique. Voltage stepped from V_{hold} −90 to +10 mV elicits macroscopic currents that peak within 20 ms and then decay. Currents with an external solution containing 5-mM Ba^{2+} or 5-mM Ca^{2+} are superimposed, and the peaks are normalized. Note that conductance for $I_{Ba,L} > I_{Ca,L}$. $I_{Ba,L}$ decay is a readout of voltage-dependent inactivation (VDI). $Ca_V\beta2a$ slows VDI, emphasizing the difference in decay kinetics to those for Ca^{2+}-dependent inactivation (CDI). Relatively rapid $I_{Ca,L}$ decay is dominated by CDI, albeit with VDI superimposed. (Data from Liang H, DeMaria CD, Erickson MG, et al. Unified mechanisms of Ca^{2+} regulation across the Ca^{2+} channel family. *Neuron.* 2003;39:951-960.)

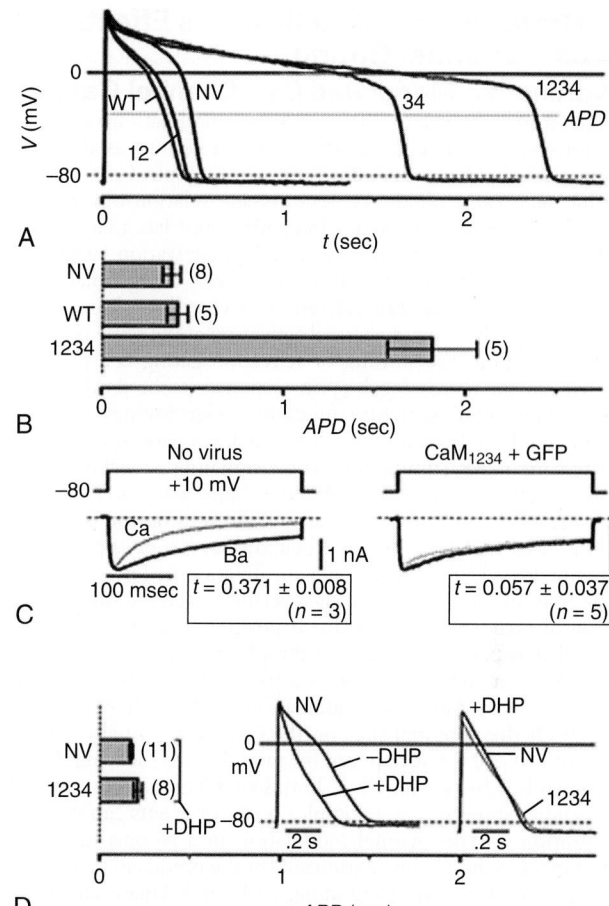

FIGURE 10.5 Ventricular cardiomyocyte action potential duration (*APD*) is regulated by Ca^{2+}-dependent inactivation (CDI) via $I_{Ca,L}$-calmodulin (*CaM*) modulation. (A) Action potentials superimposed for representative cardiomyocytes expressing exogenous CaM (wt), no virus, or CaM mutants. The numbers 12 and 34 denote CaM mutants that are unable to bind Ca^{2+} at the N- and C-termini of CaM. "1234" represents apoCaM. CaM_{1234} and CaM_{34} cause ultra-long APD consistent with the Ca^{2+} fluxing through the channel that regulates APD via a Ca^{2+}-CaM-dependent inactivation. (B) Summary data showing APD prolonged by apoCaM. (C) $I_{Ca,L}$ and $I_{Ba,L}$ superimposed in the absence of virus and in the presence of adenoviral-mediated CaM_{1234} expression. CaM_{1234} completely eliminates CDI. (D) Demonstration that the CaM_{1234} ultra-long APD is dependent on $I_{Ca,L}$. Dihydropyridine and L-type Ca^{2+} channel blockade shorten the APD in the no virus (*NV*) control, and reduces the ultra-long APD in CaM_{1234}-infected cardiomyocytes. (Modified from Alseikhan BA, DeMaria CD, Colecraft HM, Yue DT. Engineered calmodulins reveal the unexpected eminence of Ca^{2+} channel inactivation in controlling heart excitation. *PNAS.* 2002;99:17185-17190.)

was shown in an elegant series of experiments exemplified by the results shown in Fig. 10.5.[71] Engineered CaM with mutated divalent cation sites was introduced into the cardiomyocytes. The resulting $I_{Ca,L}$ showed significantly slowed decay, and the action potential duration became ultra-long (see Fig. 10.5). Moreover, prolongation of the action potential duration by divalent-cation-free CaM is reversed by the L-type Ca^{2+} channel blockade with dihydropyridine.[71]

At the single ion channel level Ca^{2+}-CaM dependent inactivation is caused by a decreased frequency of channel reopenings and a decrease of the mean open time.[72] The reopening rate is governed by an absorbing state from which the channel cannot open, whereas the decrease of the mean open time reflects a faster Ca^{2+}-driven closure of the open channels. These single channel studies showed that CDI contributes to slow macroscopic decay, despite earlier findings separating VDI from CDI based on slow versus fast macroscopic decay.

L-type Ca^{2+} channels are organized in junctional membranes in close opposition to the ryanodine receptors (RyR2). Colocalized RyR2 is present in a 4- to 10-fold excess to the number of L-type Ca^{2+} channels.[73] Therefore Ca^{2+}-induced-Ca^{2+}-release results in an amplified local elevation of subdomain Ca^{2+} with physiologically relevant gating consequences for L-type Ca^{2+} channels. L-type Ca^{2+} channels initiate sarcoplasmic reticulum (SR) Ca^{2+}-release; in

turn, this SR Ca^{2+}-release promotes L-type Ca^{2+} channel Ca^{2+}–CaM graded inactivation and creates a classical physiological negative feedback loop. Experimentally, the ability of the SR Ca^{2+} release to inactivate $I_{Ca,L}$ allows the use of $I_{Ca,L}$ as a reporter for SR Ca^{2+}-release.[74] In this way, L-type channel gating is also a sensitive caliper for subdomain cardiomyocyte cytosolic Ca^{2+}.

The physiological importance of Ca^{2+}–CaM dependent $I_{Ca,L}$ inactivation is highlighted by clinical cases of de novo CaM mutations causing cardiac arrest in infants.[75] CaM mutants associated with these arrhythmias suppress inactivation of the L-type Ca^{2+} channels[76] and prolong action potentials.[76] Despite some parallels of CaM modulation of Ca^{2+} and late Na^+ channel current, arrhythmogenic the CaM mutants only affected the L-type Ca^{2+} channel function.[77]

Posttranslational Modifications Effects on Ca^{2+} Channel Gating

β-Adrenergic-Modulated Ca^{2+} Channel Gating

β-adrenergic receptor (β-AR) stimulated modulation of $I_{Ca,L}$ is a major contributor to the cardiac response to increased sympathetic tone. β-AR agonists increase macroscopic Ca^{2+} channel conductance and shift the current voltage relationship to more negative potentials. The activation gating shift has a large effect on Ca^{2+} flux. Consider a steady-state $I_{Ca,L}$ activation curve with a 50% maximal conductance at 0 mV. All else being equal, a –10 mV shift of the steady-state activation curve will result in a >90% of maximal probability of channel activation at the same potential (Fig. 10.6). Thus the shifting of activation gating is a powerful mechanism for increasing $I_{Ca,L}$ in response to the β-AR stimulation. The detail structure–function underpinnings of β-AR modulation have been intensively studied, yet gaps in knowledge still remain. β-AR stimulation via Gs signaling activates protein kinase A (PKA). Several unambiguous substrates for PKA have been identified on $Ca_V1.2$. These include sites on the proximal- and distal-carboxyl termini.[78–80] In addition, $Ca_Vβ2$ is phosphorylated by PKA.[81,82] However, genetically modified mice carrying a knock-in of $Ca_V1.2$ containing a serine to alanine mutation in the distal carboxyl-terminus site at position 1928 rendering the channel phospho-deficient,[83] or the phospho-deficient $Ca_V1.2$-Ser1928Ala in combination with a truncated phospho-deficient $Ca_Vβ2$ retained the β-AR modulation of $I_{Ca,L}$ in cardiomyocytes.[84] Of the potential sites on the $Ca_V1.2$ proximal carboxyl-terminus, S1700 is not required for modulation,[85] leaving T1704 as a possible substrate for PKA. In this vein, heterologous expression studies showed that a complex series of events can result in recapturing L-type channel modulation in a reconstituted system. First, $Ca_V1.2$ channels truncated at the predicted proteolytic cleavage site were expressed along with an A-kinase anchoring protein 15 (akap15), and distal carboxyl-terminus.[80] The idea is that the distal carboxyl-terminus is autoinhibitory for channel gating.[25] The akap15 scaffolds the distal carboxyl-terminus to the proximal carboxyl-terminus,[25] and when expressed in optimal ratios confers PKA modulation on channels via phosphorylation of the $Ca_V1.2$ proximal carboxyl-terminus at positions S1700 and T1704.[80] In cardiomyocytes, akap150/79 is required for the β-AR

modulation of $I_{Ca,L}$.[45] This is a provocative model—namely, that PKA modulates $Ca_V1.2$ gating via the disruption of an autoinhibitory function. The paucity of data showing the distal carboxyl-terminus autoinhibition of the Ca^{2+}-current in cardiomyocytes at native stoichiometry and an incomplete understanding of the mechanisms of gating modification of L-type Ca^{2+} channels by the proteolytically separated distal carboxyl-terminus domain (DCT) creates uncertainty for this model.

Pioneering work from the Catterall laboratory underscores the importance of the DCT in the precise regulation of the L-type Ca^{2+} channel function. The identification of $Ca_V1.2$ truncation at a consensus calpain substrate site,[86–88] coupled with the presence of an ~37-kD protein recognized by a DCT-antibody[27] suggests that the distal carboxyl-terminus is generated by proteolytic cleavage of the full-length $Ca_V1.2$ protein. A requirement for Ca^{2+} and calpain activity for carboxyl terminal cleavage in cardiomyocytes is inferred from studies on the skeletal muscle homolog ($Ca_V1.1$),[86] and from sequence data conserved between $Ca_V1.1$ and $Ca_V1.2$; as yet, there is no direct evidence for either a Ca^{2+} or calpain requirement for DCT liberation in cardiomyocytes. Nevertheless, the majority of studies showing Western blots probed with anti-$Ca_V1.2$ antibodies reveal a protein migrating to ~190 kD, rather than the ~240 kD expected for the full-length that is the unproteolyzed $Ca_V1.2$. It should be noted that heterologously expressed $Ca_V1.2$ is not processed, and, interestingly, adenoviral-$Ca_V1.2$ constructs introduced into cardiomyocytes also express full-length channels. This suggests that in cardiomyocytes, native $Ca_V1.2$ mRNA and/or protein is processed relatively early during synthesis. Regardless, reassociation of DCT with $Ca_V1.2$ results in gating modifications. Coexpression of DCT with $Ca_V1.2$ truncated at the position corresponding to proteolytic cleavage results in modification of activation gating. The truncated $Ca_V1.2$ steady-state activation requires a two additive Boltzmann distributions to describe the data. DCT shifts steady-state activation by +15 mV.[25] It was also noted that the shift was greater when DCT and truncated-$Ca_V1.2$ was coexpressed, as opposed to conditions whereby DCT is retained as part of the full-length channel construct.[25] Mechanistically, DCT might restrict coupling between gating current (movement of S4 segments) and allosteric rearrangements that result in ionic flux.[25]

Facilitation

Excessive activation of CaM-kinase II (CaMKII) signaling causes arrhythmias and heart failure.[89] $Ca_Vβ2$ is a target for CaMKII-induced phosphorylation, and $Ca_Vβ2$ mediates CaMKII-triggered cardiomyocyte afterdepolarization and death.[90] The implication is that altered L-type Ca^{2+} channel gating links CaMKII activity to arrhythmias and cardiomyocyte survival. A 1-Hz train of depolarizations elicits a progressive increase in $I_{Ca,L}$ that accumulates over about 10 pulses.[91–93] This positive $I_{Ca,L}$ staircase is mediated by CaMKII-dependent phosphorylation.[94–96] In addition to the preeminent CaMKII phosphorylation targets on $Ca_Vβ2$, sites on $Ca_V1.2$ have been also identified.[35,97] Activated CaMKII promotes "Mode 2" L-type Ca^{2+} channel gating.[96] Mode 2 is the classical description of L-type channels gating with frequent relatively long-duration openings.[98] Interestingly, CaMKII tethers to multiple sites on the $Ca_V1.2$ proximal carboxyl-terminus adjacent to the CaM-binding IQ motif.[35]

Other Protein Interactions Effecting L-Type Ca^{2+} Channel Gating

RGK Proteins

L-type Ca^{2+} channel ionic current is potently inhibited by RGK GTPases including Rem, Rad, and Kir/Gem.[99,100] RGK blockade of L-type Ca^{2+} channel current does not necessarily require interference with the trafficking of $Ca_V1.2$ to the surface

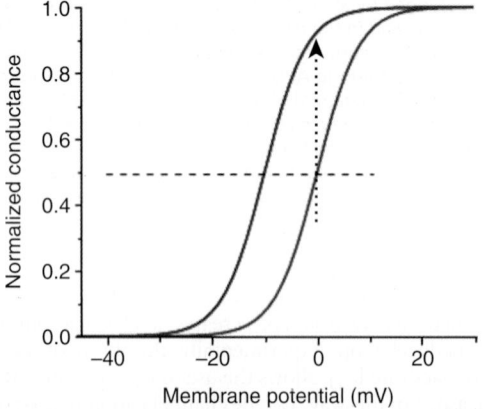

FIGURE 10.6 Steady-state activation gating shift of the voltage dependence is a potent mechanism for an increase of $I_{Ca,L}$. Single Boltzmann distributions are drawn depicting basal (*red*) and β-adrenergic stimulated (*blue*) L-type Ca^{2+} channels. For the basal state, the midpoint of activation is 0, and a –10 mV shift is simulated β-adrenergic stimulation. All else being equal, the shift of the steady-state activation curve increases channel conductance at 0 mV from 50% to >90% (*vertical arrow*). Boltzmann distribution of the form: $G_{max}/[1+\exp(V_{1/2}-V)/k]$, where G_{max} is maximal conductance, E_{rev} is reversal potential, $V_{1/2}$ is activation midpoint potential, and k is the slope factor.

membrane.[101] Rather, RGK proteins interfere with L-type Ca^{2+} channel gating. In mice carrying a deletion of Rem expression, the cardiomyocyte $I_{Ca,L}$ density is elevated at voltages corresponding to maximal activation gating, and steady-state activation is positive-shifted on the voltage axis.[102] The positive shift of steady-state activation might be a homeostatic mechanism to counteract increased current density. Moreover, Rem knockout sheds light on the contribution of Rem to L-type Ca^{2+} channel activation gating. Although all RGK family proteins, when overexpressed, profoundly block $I_{Ca,L}$ in heterologous expression systems or cardiomyocytes,[103,104] the RGK abrogation of $I_{Ca,L}$ is modified by the coexpression of CaM.[34] The overexpression of both Rem and CaM not only blunted the ability of Rem to completely block $I_{Ca,L}$, but slowed CDI (Fig. 10.7). These findings are consistent with a mechanism that includes Rem interference with CaM modulation. Initial biochemical studies showed $Ca_V\beta$–RGK interactions.[99,100] However, RGK overexpression does not necessarily inhibit the surface expression of $Ca_V1.2$.[101,105] Moreover, Rem and Rad that were engineered to prevent RGK–$Ca_V\beta$ interactions retained the ability to block L-type currents.[41] Recent studies demonstrated direct RGK–$Ca_V1.2$ interactions. Rem interacts with the $Ca_V1.2$ N-terminus[41] and the $Ca_V1.2$-PCT on a domain overlapping with the CaM interaction site.[34] RGK modulation of the L-type Ca^{2+} channel function underscores two key themes: (1) the carboxyl-terminus of $Ca_V1.2$ is a hot-spot for multiple protein interactions and (2) gating may be modified depending on the precise composition of proteins in the hetero-multimeric L-type Ca^{2+} channel complex.

Rad is highly abundant in the heart and Rad-knockout mice (Rad$^{-/-}$) show novel cardiac remodeling that provides improved systolic function that is preserved with aging.[106] Deletion of Rad in ventricular cardiomyocytes causes a β-AR-like modulated $I_{Ca,L}$, in which the maximal conductance is increased and the activation

midpoint shifts to more negative potentials.[104,107] The increased conductance speeds the L-type channel CDI. Taken together, these results suggest that Rad may tonically govern $I_{Ca,L}$, and rearrangement of Rad in the L-type channel complex contributes to current modulation.

Calcineurin

Calcineurin controls VDI of L-type Ca^{2+} channels.[108] In Timothy syndrome mutant channels, calcineurin restores aberrant VDI.[108] Calcineurin binds to both the N-terminus and the $Ca_V1.2$-DCT.[42] In neurons, the calcineurin–$Ca_V1.2$ interactions requires an akap79/150 scaffold protein.[109] In distinction, the myocardial calcineurin–$Ca_V1.2$ interaction is via direct protein-protein association.[42] Interest in calcineurin extends far beyond the L-type Ca^{2+} channel gating. Calcineurin links cytosolic Ca^{2+} to the transcription signaling that is responsible for cardiac hypertrophy.[110] The parallels of the bifunctionality for calcineurin and for $Ca_V1.2$-DCT are striking. Both proteins regulate L-type Ca^{2+} channel gating, and both proteins are involved in transcriptional regulation, calcineurin via dephosphorylation of NFAT[110] and $Ca_V1.2$-DCT via transcription regulation when translocated to the nucleus.[26,27]

$Ca_V1.2$ Coupled Gating

Early studies of single L-type Ca^{2+} channels showed that ensemble averages of single channel events do not necessarily scale to macroscopic $I_{Ca,L}$.[111] This suggested the notion that $Ca_V1.2$ may cluster and that clustering behavior may alter channel gating. Oligomerization of $Ca_V1.2$ via graded Ca^{2+}–CaM interactions amplify Ca^{2+} signaling.[112] In some Timothy syndrome mutant $Ca_V1.2$ channels, the slower VDI kinetics require akap150.[113] In

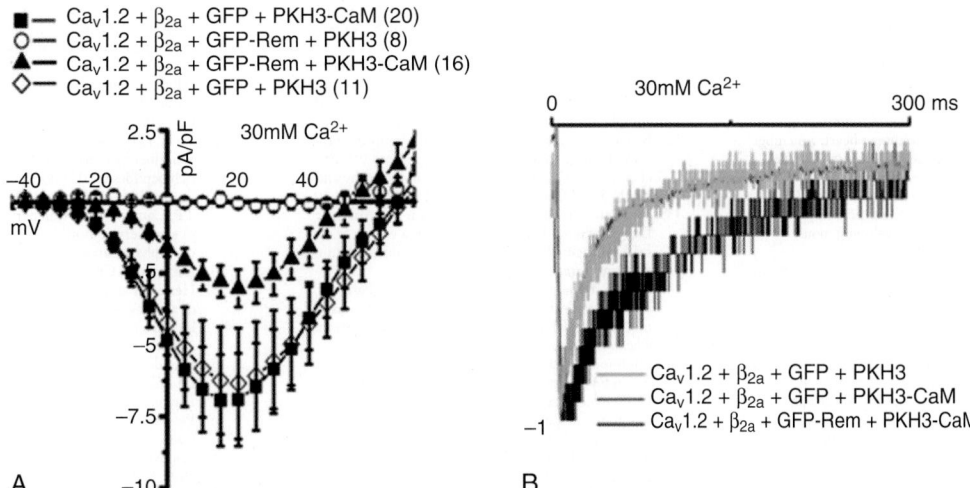

FIGURE 10.7 Ca^{2+}–calmodulin (*CaM*)-dependent inactivation is regulated by L-type Ca^{2+} channel complex interacting proteins. (A) Current voltage curves obtained from whole-cell $I_{Ca,L}$ from HEK 293 cells heterologously expressing $Ca_V1.2$ + $Ca_V\beta2a$ and either: empty vector (PKH3); CaM; Rem; or Rem + CaM. Rem expressed alone results in no detectable $I_{Ca,L}$ (*open circles*). Rem coexpressed with CaM results in about a 50% reduction of peak $I_{Ca,L}$ (*closed triangles*). CaM (*closed squares*) had no detectable effect on $I_{Ca,L}$ compared to the empty vector (*closed squares*). Thus CaM in more closely matched stoichiometries to overexpressed Rem can abrogate profound Rem blockade of current. (B) Rem may slow Ca^{2+}-CaM-dependent inactivation. $I_{Ca,L}$ elicited by a test potential step to +20 mV for empty vector (*green*); CaM (*red*) or Rem + CaM (*black*). Currents are normalized to peak value. The Rem + CaM $I_{Ca,L}$ decay kinetics are significantly slower than the empty vector or CaM alone expression. These data suggest the general notion that the native stoichiometries of the various channel complex proteins are important determinants for channel gating. (Modified from Pang C, Crump SM, Jin L, et al. Rem GTPase interacts with the proximal $Ca_V1.2$ C-terminus and modulates calcium-dependent channel inactivation. *Channels (Austin).* 2010;4:192-202.)

the absence of akap150, the Timothy syndrome slow VDI reverts to normal kinetics. Thus $Ca_V1.2$–$Ca_V1.2$ interactions bridged by akap contribute to the L-type Ca^{2+} channel inactivation gating.

N-Terminal–C-Terminal Interaction

The cardiac $Ca_V1.2$ isoform contains a relatively long N-terminus that inhibits $I_{Ba,L}$, and this long cardiac N-terminal domain is crucial for the $Ca_V\beta2$ increase of open probability.[39] The $Ca_V1.2$ N-terminal also interacts with its proximal carboxyl-terminus via Ca^{2+}–CaM.[38]

In conclusion, L-type Ca^{2+} channels provide the main route of entry into cardiomyocytes and are essential for providing the trigger Ca^{2+} for excitation-contraction coupling. The mature cardiomyocyte L-type Ca^{2+} channel is a complex of many proteins. The sum of the interactions yields distinct channel gating properties. A large number of proteins can interact with the $Ca_V1.2$ carboxyl terminus raising the notion that heterogeneous channel complexes exist, even within a given cell. Finally, the modulation of $I_{Ca,L}$ is dependent on multiple protein interactions that dictate channel gating and, in turn, cardiomyocyte function.

REFERENCES

1. Bers DM. Calcium cycling and signaling in cardiac myocytes. *Annu Rev Physiol.* 2008;70:23–49.
2. Catterall WA. Ion channel voltage sensors: structure, function, and pathophysiology. *Neuron.* 2010;67:915–928.
3. Benitah JP, Alvarez JL, Gomez AM. L-type Ca^{2+} current in ventricular cardiomyocytes. *J Mol Cell Cardiol.* 2010;48:26–36.
4. Hille B. *Ion Channels of Excitable Membranes.* 3rd ed. Sunderland, MA: Sinauer Associates, Inc.; 2001.
5. DeFelice LJ. *Electrical Properties of Cells: Patch Clamp for Biologists.* New York and London: Plenum Press; 1997.
6. Zhang Q, Timofeyev V, Qiu H, et al. Expression and roles of Cav1.3 (alpha1D) L-type Ca^{2+} channel in atrioventricular node automaticity. *J Mol Cell Cardiol.* 2011;50:194–202.
7. Zhang Z, He Y, Tuteja D, et al. Functional roles of Cav1.3(alpha1D) calcium channels in atria: insights gained from gene-targeted null mutant mice. *Circulation.* 2005;27(112): 1936-1944.
8. Mangoni ME, Couette B, Bourinet E, et al. Functional role of L-type Cav1.3 Ca^{2+} channels in cardiac pacemaker activity. *Proc Natl Acad Sci U S A.* 2003;100:5543–5548.
9. Platzer J, Engel J, Schrott-Fischer A, et al. Congenital deafness and sinoatrial node dysfunction in mice lacking class D L-type Ca^{2+} channels. *Cell.* 2000;102:89–97.
10. Sims C, Reisenweber S, Viswanathan PC, Choi BR, Walker WH, Salama G. Sex, age, and regional differences in L-type calcium current are important determinants of arrhythmia phenotype in rabbit hearts with drug-induced long QT type 2. *Circ Res.* 2008;102:e86–e100.
11. Yang X, Chen G, Papp R, Defranco DB, Zeng F, Salama G. Oestrogen upregulates L-type Ca^{2+} channels via oestrogen-receptor- by a regional genomic mechanism in female rabbit hearts. *J Physiol.* 2012;590:493–508.
12. Cribbs LL, Lee J-H, Yang J, et al. Cloning and characterization of α1H from human heart, a member of the T-type calcium channel gene family. *Circ Res.* 1998;83:103–109.
13. Cribbs LL, Martin BL, Schroder EA, Keller BB, Delisle BP, Satin J. Identification of the T-Type calcium channel (CaV3.1d) in developing mouse heart. *Circ Res.* 2001;88:403–407.
14. Hagiwara N, Irisawa H, Kameyama M. Contribution of two types of calcium currents to the pacemaker potentials of rabbit sino-atrial node cells. *J Physiol.* 1988;395:233–253.
15. Rosati B, Dun W, Hirose M, Boyden PA, McKinnon D. Molecular basis of the T- and L-type Ca^{2+} currents in canine Purkinje fibres. *J Physiol.* 2007;579:465–471.
16. Gaughan JP, Hefner CA, Houser SR. Electrophysiological properties of neonatal rat ventricular myocytes with alpha1-adrenergic-induced hypertrophy. *Am J Physiol.* 1998;275:H577–H590.
17. Wetzel GT, Chen F, Friedman WF, Klitzner TS. Calcium current measurements in acutely isolated neonatal cardiac myocytes. *Pediatr Res.* 1991;30:83–88.
18. Nuss HB, Houser SR. T-type Ca^{2+} current is expressed in hypertrophied adult feline left ventricular myocytes. *Circ Res.* 1993;73(4): 777–782.
19. Martinez ML, Heredia MP, Delgado C. Expression of T-type Ca^{2+} channels in ventricular cells from hypertrophied rat hearts. *J Mol Cell Cardiol.* Sep 1999;31:1617–1625.
20. Gao T, Chien AJ, Hosey MM. Complexes of the alpha 1C and beta subunits generate the necessary signal for membrane targeting of class C L-type calcium channels. *J. Biol. Chem.* 1999;274:2137–2144.
21. Opatowsky Y, Chen CC, Campbell KP, Hirsch JA. Structural analysis of the voltage-dependent calcium channel beta subunit functional core and its complex with the alpha 1 interaction domain. *Neuron.* 2004;42:387–399.
22. Bichet D, Cornet V, Geib S, et al. The I-II loop of the Ca^{2+} channel alpha1 subunit contains an endoplasmic reticulum retention signal antagonized by the beta subunit. *Neuron.* 2000;25:177–190.
23. Fang K, Colecraft HM. Mechanism of auxiliary beta-subunit-mediated membrane targeting of L-type (Ca(V)1.2) channels. *J Physiol.* 2011;589: 4437–4455.
24. Jangsangthong W, Kuzmenkina E, Bohnke AK, Herzig S. Single-channel monitoring of reversible L-type Ca^{2+} channel Ca(V)alpha(1)-Ca(V)beta subunit interaction. *Biophys J.* 2012;101:2661–2670.
25. Hulme JT, Yarov-Yarovoy V, Lin TW, Scheuer T, Catterall WA. Autoinhibitory control of the CaV1.2 channel by its proteolytically processed distal C-terminal domain. *J Physiol.* 2006;576:87–102.
26. Gomez-Ospina N, Tsuruta F, Barreto-Chang O, Hu L, Dolmetsch R. The C terminus of the L-type voltage-gated calcium channel ca(v)1.2 encodes a transcription factor. *Cell.* 2006;127:591–606.
27. Schroder E, Byse M, Satin J. L-type calcium channel C terminus autoregulates transcription. *Circ Res.* 2009;104:1373–1381.
28. Erickson MG, Alseikhan BA, Peterson BZ, Yue DT. Preassociation of calmodulin with voltage-gated Ca^{2+} channels revealed by FRET in single living cells. *Neuron.* 2001;27(31):973–985.
29. Pitt GS, Zuhlke RD, Hudmon A, Schulman H, Reuter H, Tsien RW. Molecular basis of CaM tethering and Ca^{2+}-dependent inactivation of L-type Ca^{2+} channels. *J. Biol. Chem.* 2001;276:30794–30802.
30. Zuhlke RD, Pitt GS, Deisseroth K, Tsien RW, Reuter H. Calmodulin supports both inactivation and facilitation of L-type calcium channels. *Nature.* 1999;399:159–162.
31. Van Petegem F, Chatelain FC, Minor Jr DL. Insights into voltage-gated calcium channel regulation from the structure of the CaV1.2 IQ domain-Ca2+/calmodulin complex. *Nat Struct Mol Biol.* 2005;12:1108–1115.
32. Blaich A, Pahlavan S, Tian Q, et al. Mutation of the CaM-binding motif IQ of the L-type Cav1.2 Ca^{2+} channel to EQ induces dilated cardiomyopathy and death. *J Biol Chem.* 2012;l287:22616–22625.
33. Van Petegem F, Clark KA, Chatelain FC, Minor Jr DL. Structure of a complex between a voltage-gated calcium channel beta-subunit and an alpha-subunit domain. *Nature.* 2004;429:671–675.
34. Pang C, Crump SM, Jin L, et al. Rem GTPase interacts with the proximal Ca(V)1.2 C-terminus and modulates calcium-dependent channel inactivation. *Channels (Austin).* May 23 2010;4:192–202.
35. Hudmon A, Schulman H, Kim J, Maltez JM, Tsien RW, Pitt GS. CaMKII tethers to L-type Ca^{2+} channels, establishing a local and dedicated integrator of Ca^{2+} signals for facilitation. *J Cell Biol.* 2005;171:537–547.
36. Muller CS, Haupt A, Bildl W, et al. Quantitative proteomics of the Cav2 channel nano-environments in the mammalian brain. *Proc Natl Acad Sci U S A.* 2010;107:14950–14957.
37. Dixon RE, Yuan C, Cheng EP, Navedo MF, Santana LF. Ca^{2+} signaling amplification by oligomerization of L-type Cav1.2 channels. *Proc Natl Acad Sci U S A.* 2012;109:1749–1754.
38. Dick IE, Tadross MR, Liang H, Tay LH, Yang W, Yue DT. A modular switch for spatial Ca^{2+} selectivity in the calmodulin regulation of CaV channels. *Nature.* 2008;451:830–834.
39. Kanevsky N, Dascal N. Regulation of maximal open probability is a separable function of Ca-v beta subunit in L-type Ca^{2+} channel, dependent on NH2 terminus of alpha(1C) (Ca(v)1.2 alpha). *J Gen Physiol.* 2006;128:15–36.
40. Minor Jr DL, Findeisen F. Progress in the structural understanding of voltage-gated calcium channel (CaV) function and modulation. *Channels (Austin).* 2010;4:459–474.
41. Yang T, Puckerin A, Colecraft HM. Distinct RGK GTPases differentially use alpha1- and auxiliary beta-binding-dependent mechanisms to inhibit CaV1.2/CaV2.2 channels. *PLoS One.* 2012;7:e37079.
42. Tandan S, Wang Y, Wang TT, et al. Physical and functional interaction between calcineurin and the cardiac L-type Ca^{2+} channel. *Circ Res.* 2009;105:51–60.
43. Xu H, Ginsburg KS, Hall DD, et al. Targeting of protein phosphatases PP2A and PP2B to the C-terminus of the L-type calcium channel Ca v1.2. *Biochemistry.* 2010;49:10298–10307.
44. Leroy J, Richter W, Mika D, et al. Phosphodiesterase 4B in the cardiac L-type Ca^{2+} channel complex regulates Ca^{2+} current and protects against ventricular arrhythmias in mice. *J Clin Invest.* 2011;121:2651–2661.
45. Nichols CB, Rossow CF, Navedo MF, et al. Sympathetic stimulation of adult cardiomyocytes requires association of AKAP5 with a subpopulation of L-type calcium channels. *Circ Res.* 2010;107:747–756.
46. Dai S, Hall DD, Hell JW. Supramolecular assemblies and localized regulation of voltage-gated ion channels. *Physiol Rev.* 2009;89:411–452.
47. Lu L, Zhang Q, Timofeyev V, et al. Molecular Coupling of a Ca2+-activated K^+ channel to L-type Ca^{2+} channels via α-actinin2. *Circ Res.* 2007;100:112–120.
48. Meyers MB, Puri TS, Chien AJ, et al. Sorcin Associates with the pore-forming subunit of voltage-dependent L-type Ca^{2+} channels. *J. Biol. Chem.* 1998;273:18930–18935.
49. Payandeh J, Gamal El-Din TM, Scheuer T, Zheng N, Catterall WA. Crystal structure of a voltage-gated sodium channel in two potentially inactivated states. *Nature.* 2012;486:135–139.
50. Foell JD, Balijepalli RC, Delisle BP, et al. Molecular heterogeneity of calcium channel beta-subunits in canine and human heart: evidence for differential subcellular localization. *Physiol Genomics.* 2004;17:183–200.
51. Buraei Z, Yang JA. The beta subunit of voltage-gated Ca^{2+} channels. *Physiol. Rev.* Oct 2010;90:1461–1506.
52. Yu H, Chen JK, Feng S, Dalgarno DC, Brauer AW, Schreiber SL. Structural basis for the binding of proline-rich peptides to SH3 domains. *Cell.* 1994;76:933–945.
53. Pragnell M, De Waard M, Mori Y, Tanabe T, Snutch TP, Campbell KP. Calcium channel beta-subunit binds to a conserved motif in the I-II cytoplasmic linker of the alpha 1-subunit. *Nature.* 1994;368:67–70.
54. Almagor L, Chomsky-Hecht O, Ben-Mocha A, Hendin-Barak D, Dascal N, Hirsch JA. The role of a voltage-dependent Ca^{2+} channel intracellular linker: a structure-function analysis. *J Neurosci.* 2012;32:7602–7613.
55. Grandi E, Morotti S, Ginsburg KS, Severi S, Bers DM. Interplay of voltage and Ca-dependent inactivation of L-type Ca current. *Prog Biophys Mol Biol.* 2010;103:44–50.
56. Peterson BZ, DeMaria CD, Adelman JP, Yue DT. Calmodulin is the Ca^{2+} sensor for Ca2+-dependent inactivation of L-type calcium channels. *Neuron.* 1999;22:549–558.
57. Ben-Johny M, Yue DT. Calmodulin regulation (calmodulation) of voltage-gated calcium channels. *J Gen Physiol.* 2014;143:679–692.
58. Mitarai S, Kaibara M, Yano K, Taniyama K. Two distinct inactivation processes related to phosphorylation in cardiac L-type Ca^{2+} channel currents. *Am J Physiol Cell Physiol.* 2000;279:C603–C610.
59. Findlay I. Beta-adrenergic and muscarinic agonists modulate inactivation of L-type Ca^{2+} channel currents in guinea-pig ventricular myocytes. *J Physiol.* 2002;545:375–388.
60. Findlay I. beta-Adrenergic stimulation modulates Ca^{2+}- and voltage-dependent inactivation of L-type Ca^{2+} channel currents in guinea-pig ventricular myocytes. *J Physiol.* 2002;541:741–751.
61. Splawski I, Timothy KW, Sharpe LM, et al. Ca(v)1.2 calcium channel dysfunction causes a multisystem disorder including arrhythmia and autism. *Cell.* 2004;119:19–31.

62. Yazawa M, Hsueh B, Jia XL, et al. Using induced pluripotent stem cells to investigate cardiac phenotypes in Timothy syndrome. *Nature.* 2011;471. 230–U120.

63. Boczek NJ, Ye D, Jin F, et al. Identification and functional characterization of a novel CACNA1C-mediated cardiac disorder characterized by prolonged QT intervals with hypertrophic cardiomyopathy, congenital heart defects, and sudden cardiac death. *Circ Arrhythm Electrophysiol.* 2015;8:1122–1132.

64. Brunet S, Scheuer T, Catterall WA. Cooperative regulation of Ca(v)1.2 channels by intracellular Mg^{2+}, the proximal C-terminal EF-hand, and the distal C-terminal domain. *J Gen Physiol.* 2009;134:81–94.

65. Josephson IR, Guia A, Lakatta EG, Stern MD. Modulation of the gating of unitary cardiac L-type Ca^{2+} channels by conditioning voltage and divalent ions. *Biophys J.* 2002;83:2575–2586.

66. Josephson IR, Guia A, Lakatta EG, Stern MD. Modulation of the gating of unitary cardiac L-type Ca^{2+} channels by conditioning voltage and divalent ions. *Biophys. J.* 2002;83:2575–2586.

67. Ferreira G, Yi J, Rios E, Shirokov R. Ion-dependent inactivation of barium current through L-type calcium channels. *J Gen Physiol.* 1997;109:449–461.

68. Erickson MG, Alseikhan BA, Peterson BZ, Yue DT. Preassociation of calmodulin with voltage-gated Ca^{2+} channels revealed by FRET in single living cells. *Neuron.* 2001;31:973–985.

69. Tadross MR, Dick IE, Yue DT. Mechanism of local and global Ca^{2+} sensing by calmodulin in complex with a Ca^{2+} channel. *Cell. Jun.* 27 2008; 133:1228–1240.

70. Liang H, DeMaria CD, Erickson MG, Mori MX, Alseikhan BA, Yue DT. Unified mechanisms of Ca^{2+} regulation across the Ca^{2+} channel family. *Neuron.* 2003;39:951–960.

71. Alseikhan BA, DeMaria CD, Colecraft HM, Yue DT. Engineered calmodulins reveal the unexpected eminence of Ca^{2+} channel inactivation in controlling heart excitation. *PNAS.* 2002;99:17185–17190.

72. Josephson IR, Guia A, Lakatta EG, Lederer WJ, Stern MD. Ca2+-dependent components of inactivation of unitary cardiac L-type Ca^{2+} channels. *J Physiol.* 2010;588:213–223.

73. Bers DM, Stiffel VM. Ratio of ryanodine to dihydropyridine receptors in cardiac and skeletal muscle and implications for E-C coupling. *Am J Physiol.* 1993;264:C1587–C1593.

74. Acsai K, Antoons G, Livshitz L, Rudy Y, Sipido KR. Microdomain [Ca$^+$] near ryanodine receptors as reported by L-type Ca^{2+} and Na$^+$/Ca^{2+} exchange currents. *J Physiol.* 2011;589:2569–2583.

75. Crotti L, Johnson CN, Graf E, et al. Calmodulin mutations associated with recurrent cardiac arrest in infants. *Circulation.* 2013;127:1009–1017.

76. Limpitikul W, Joshi-Mukherjee R, Dick IE, George AL, Yue DT. Calmodulin mutants associated with long QT syndrome suppress inactivation of cardiac L-type Ca^{2+} currents and prolong action potentials in guinea-pig ventricular myocytes. *Circulation.* 2013;128: A17783.

77. Yin G, Hassan F, Haroun AR, et al. Arrhythmogenic calmodulin mutations disrupt intracellular cardiomyocyte Ca^{2+} regulation by distinct mechanisms. *J Am Heart Assoc.* 2014;3:e000996.

78. Kamp TJ, Hell JW. Regulation of cardiac L-type calcium channels by protein kinase A and protein kinase C. *Circ Res.* 2000;87:1095–1102.

79. Hulme JT, Westenbroek RE, Scheuer T, Catterall WA. Phosphorylation of serine 1928 in the distal C-terminal domain of cardiac CaV1.2 channels during β1-adrenergic regulation. *Proc Natl Acad Sci U S A.* 2006;103:16574–165749.

80. Fuller MD, Emrick MA, Sadilek M, Scheuer T, Catterall WA. Molecular mechanism of calcium channel regulation in the fight-or-flight response. *Sci Signal.* 2010;3:ra70.

81. Perez-Reyes E, Castellano A, Kim HS, et al. Cloning and expression of a cardiac/brain beta subunit of the L-type calcium channel. PG - 1792-7. *J Biol Chem.* 1992;267:1792–1797.

82. Bunemann M, Gerhardstein BL, Gao T, Hosey MM. Functional Regulation of L-type calcium channels via protein kinase A-mediated phosphorylation of the beta 2 subunit. *J. Biol. Chem.* 1999;274: 33851–33854.

83. Lemke T, Welling A, Christel CJ, et al. Unchanged beta-adrenergic stimulation of cardiac L-type calcium channels in Ca v 1.2 phosphorylation site S1928A mutant mice. *J Biol Chem.* 2008;283:34738–34744.

84. Brandmayr J, Poomvanicha M, Domes K, et al. Deletion of the C-terminal phosphorylation sites in the cardiac beta subunit does not affect the basic beta-adrenergic response of the heart and the Cav1.2 channel. *J Biol Chem.* 2012;287:22584–22592.

85. Yang L, Katchman AN, Samad T, Morrow JP, Weinberg R, Marx SO. Beta-adrenergic regulation of the L-type Ca^{2+} channel does not require phosphorylation of alpha1C Ser1700. *Circ Res.* 2013;113:871–880.

86. Hulme JT, Konoki K, Lin TW, et al. Sites of proteolytic processing and noncovalent association of the distal C-terminal domain of CaV1.1 channels in skeletal muscle. *Proc Natl Acad Sci U S A.* 2005;102:5274–5279.

87. De Jongh KS, Colvin AA, Wang KK, Catterall WA. Differential proteolysis of the full-length form of the L-type calcium channel alpha 1 subunit by calpain. *J Neurochem.* 1994;63:1558–1564.

88. Gerhardstein BL, Gao T, Bunemann M, et al. Proteolytic processing of the C terminus of the alpha 1C subunit of L-type calcium channels and the role of a proline-rich domain in membrane tethering of proteolytic fragments. *J. Biol. Chem.* 2000;275:8556–8563.

89. Swaminathan PD, Purohit A, Hund TJ, Anderson ME. Calmodulin-dependent protein kinase II: linking heart failure and arrhythmias. *Circ Res.* 2012;110: 1661–1677.

90. Koval OM, Guan X, Wu Y, et al. CaV1.2 beta-subunit coordinates CaMKII-triggered cardiomyocyte death and afterdepolarizations. *Proc Natl Acad Sci U S A.* 2010;107:4996–5000.

91. Hryshko LV, Bers DM. Ca current facilitation during postrest recovery depends on Ca entry. *Am J Physiol.* 1990;259:H951–H961.

92. Picht E, DeSantiago J, Huke S, Kaetzel MA, Dedman JR, Bers DM. CaMKII inhibition targeted to the sarcoplasmic reticulum inhibits frequency-dependent acceleration of relaxation and Ca^{2+} current facilitation. *J Mol Cell Cardiol.* 2007;42:196–205.

93. Zygmunt AC, Maylie J. Stimulation-dependent facilitation of the high threshold calcium current in guinea-pig ventricular myocytes. *J. Physiol.* 1990;102:653–671.

94. Yuan W, Bers DM. Ca-dependent facilitation of cardiac Ca current is due to Ca-calmodulin-dependent protein kinase. *Am J Physiol.* 1994;267:H982–H993.

95. Anderson ME, Braun AP, Schulman H, Premack BA. Multifunctional Ca^{2+}/calmodulin-dependent protein kinase mediates Ca^{2+}-induced enhancement of the L-type Ca^{2+} current in rabbit ventricular myocytes. *Circ Res.* 1994;75:854–861.

96. Dzhura I, Wu Y, Colbran RJ, Balser JR, Anderson ME. Calmodulin kinase determines calcium-dependent facilitation of L-type calcium channels. *Nat Cell Biol.* 2000;2:173–177.

97. Lee TS, Karl R, Moosmang S, et al. Calmodulin kinase II is involved in voltage-dependent facilitation of the L-type Cav1.2 calcium channel: Identification of the phosphorylation sites. *J Biol Chem.* 2006;281:25560–25567.

98. Hess P, Lansman JB, Tsien RW. Different modes of Ca channel gating behaviour favoured by dihydropyridine Ca agonists and antagonists. *Nature.* 1984;311:538–544.

99. Finlin BS, Crump SM, Satin J, Andres DA. Regulation of voltage-gated calcium channel activity by the Rem and Rad GTPases. *PNAS.* 2003;100:14469–14474.

100. Beguin P, Nagashima K, Gonoi T, et al. Regulation of Ca^{2+} channel expression at the cell surface by the small G-protein kir/Gem. *Nature.* 2001;411:701–706.

101. Correll RN, Pang C, Finlin BS, Dailey AM, Satin J, Andres DA. Plasma membrane targeting is essential for Rem-mediated Ca^{2+} channel inhibition. *J Biol Chem.* 2007;282:28431–28440.

102. Magyar J, Kiper CE, Sievert G, et al. Rem-GTPase regulates cardiac myocyte L-type calcium current. *Channels (Austin).* 2012;6:1–8.

103. Crump SM, Correll RN, Schroder EA, et al. L-type calcium channel alpha-subunit and protein kinase inhibitors modulate Rem-mediated regulation of current. *Am J Physiol Heart Circ Physiol.* 2006;291:H1959–H1971.

104. Wang G, Zhu X, Xie W, et al. Rad as a novel regulator of excitation-contraction coupling and beta-adrenergic signaling in heart. *Circ Res.* 2010;106:317–327.

105. Yang T, Xu X, Kernan T, Wu V, Colecraft HM. Rem, a member of the RGK GTPases, inhibits recombinant CaV1.2 channels using multiple mechanisms that require distinct conformations of the GTPase. *J Physiol.* 2010;588:1665–1681.

106. Manning JR, Withers CN, Levitan B, Smith JD, Andres DA, Satin J. Loss of Rad-GTPase produces a novel adaptive cardiac phenotype resistant to systolic decline with aging. *Am J Physiol Heart Circ Physiol.* 2015;309:H1336–H1345.

107. Manning JR, Yin G, Kaminski CN, et al. Rad GTPase deletion increases L-type calcium channel current leading to increased cardiac contraction. *J Am Heart Assoc.* 2013;2:e000459.

108. Cohen-Kutner M, Yahalom Y, Trus M, Atlas D. Calcineurin controls voltage-dependent-inactivation (VDI) of the normal and Timothy cardiac channels. *Sci Rep.* 2012;2:366.

109. Oliveria SF, Dell'Acqua ML, Sather WA. AKAP79/150 anchoring of calcineurin controls neuronal L-type Ca^{2+} channel activity and nuclear signaling. *Neuron.* 2007;55:261–275.

110. Molkentin JD. Dichotomy of Ca^{2+} in the heart: contraction versus intracellular signaling. *J Clin Invest.* 2006;116:623–626.

111. Mazzanti M, DeFelice LJ, Liu YM. Gating of L-type Ca^{2+} channels in embryonic chick ventricle cells: dependence on voltage, current and channel density. *J Physiol.* 1991;443:307–334.

112. Dixon RE, Moreno CM, Yuan C, et al. Graded Ca^{2+}/calmodulin-dependent coupling of voltage-gated CaV1.2 channels. *eLife.* 2015;4: e05608.

113. Cheng EP, Yuan C, Navedo MF, et al. Restoration of normal L-type Ca^{2+} channel function during Timothy syndrome by ablation of an anchoring protein. *Circ Res.* 2011;109:255–261.

11

Inhibition of Phosphoinositide 3-Kinase and Acquired Long QT Syndrome

Lisa M. Ballou, Richard Z. Lin, and Ira S. Cohen

Acquired Long QT Syndrome and hERG

The first report of torsades de pointes (TdP) in a patient taking the antihistamine terfenadine at normal dosages was described in a 39-year-old woman also taking ketoconazole, cefaclor, and medroxyprogesterone. The serum concentration of terfenadine, normally low due to first pass metabolism in the liver, was excessively high, and the high levels were thought to result from an interaction between terfenadine and ketoconazole.[1] Additional reports continued to appear over the next few years linking terfenadine alone or in concert with other drugs to TdP.[2-5] Concurrent with the initial report of TdP with terfenadine in 1990 came the first accurate description of I_{Kr} and I_{Ks} as components of the plateau-delayed rectifier currents.[6] However, their potential role in terfenadine toxicity awaited the cloning of the α-subunit of the I_{Kr} channel, named hERG,[7] and its expression in oocytes.[8] In 1996, Roy and colleagues[9] were the first to report on the direct interaction of terfenadine with the I_{Kr} channel. These and other observations gave rise to the I_{Kr} hypothesis, in which blockade of this ion channel is the cause of drug-induced acquired long QT syndrome (aLQTS). (A more complete history of the development of the I_{Kr} hypothesis is reviewed in Roy and colleagues[9] and Rosen.[10])

From 1996 to the present, hundreds of compounds have been shown to reduce I_{Kr},[11] and the US Food and Drug Administration has required testing of the effects of all new drug candidates on this current.[12] Over this same time period, the I_{Kr} hypothesis has been widely accepted as the basis of the majority of cases of drug-induced aLQTS and its associated lethal arrhythmia TdP (Fig. 11.1). Complicating the picture was that, in 2012, Lu and colleagues[13] demonstrated that terfenadine inhibits phosphoinositide 3-kinase (PI3K), leading to effects on cardiac plateau currents that contribute to action potential duration (APD). In fact, a significant component of APD lengthening is not due to terfenadine's block of I_{Kr}, but instead to its inhibition of PI3K (Fig. 11.2). A comparable outcome was later described for dofetilide.[14] The importance of PI3K in regulating cardiac repolarization is underscored by evidence that aLQTS in diabetes may be due to decreased PI3K activity in the heart. These findings have led us and others to rethink the mechanistic basis for aLQTS, and for that reason we will review the role of PI3K inhibition in aLQTS and TdP.

PI3K Signal Transduction

Phosphatidylinositol is the precursor of a class of signaling lipids known as phosphoinositides that regulate multiple aspects of cell physiology. Combinatorial phosphorylation of the 3-, 4-, and 5-hydroxyl groups of the inositol moiety of phosphatidylinositol produces seven different phosphoinositides that accumulate in distinct membrane compartments. Phosphoinositides can signal directly by binding to effector proteins to modulate their localization or activity.[16]

Class IA PI3Ks preferentially phosphorylate the 3-hydroxyl of phosphatidylinositol 4,5-bisphosphate $(PI[4,5]P_2)$ to produce the second messenger $PI(3,4,5)P_3$[17,18] (Fig. 11.3). These enzymes consist of a catalytic subunit (p110α, p110β, or p110δ) tightly associated with one of several regulatory subunits (collectively referred to as p85). The p85 regulatory subunits contain Src homology 2 (SH2) domains that allow class IA PI3Ks to dock to phosphorylated tyrosyl residues in other proteins. Class IA PI3K complexes containing particular catalytic subunits are referred to as PI3Kα, PI3Kβ, and so on. Since most of the current knowledge regarding the PI3K regulation of ion channels that control the cardiac action potential comes from studies of PI3Kα, this chapter will focus on PI3Kα.

The concentration of $PI(3,4,5)P_3$ in the plasma membrane increases rapidly and transiently in response to extracellular or intracellular signals that activate class IA PI3Ks. One way in which class IA PI3Ks are activated is by binding to tyrosine-phosphorylated receptors or their adaptor proteins. It has been shown that PI3Kα is the major PI3K isoform activated by insulin or insulin-like growth factor 1 (IGF-1) in mouse ventricular myocytes.[19,20] The activation pathway includes hormone activation of the insulin or IGF-1 receptor, phosphorylation of insulin receptor substrate (IRS) proteins on tyrosyl residues, and the recruitment of PI3Kα to the receptor–IRS complex (see Fig. 11.3). The recruitment step is mediated by binding of the SH2 domains in the p85 regulatory subunit to specific phosphotyrosyl residues on the IRS proteins. The interaction of PI3Kα with phosphotyrosyl peptides increases its binding affinity to membranes containing $PI(4,5)P_2$ and relieves inhibitory contacts between the catalytic and regulatory subunits to cause an increase in $PI(3,4,5)P_3$ production.[21,22]

$PI(3,4,5)P_3$ produced by PI3Ks targets downstream effectors such as 3-phosphoinositide-dependent protein kinase 1 (PDK1) and the protein kinase Akt (also known as PKB). Pleckstrin homology (PH) domains in PDK1 and Akt bind to $PI(3,4,5)P_3$, which colocalizes the two kinases at the plasma membrane so that PDK1 can phosphorylate and partially activate Akt. Full activation of Akt occurs after phosphorylation of a second site by mTORC2, which is also controlled by $PI(3,4,5)P_3$.[23] Atypical protein kinase C (PKC) isoforms are also activated by PDK1 and mTORC2, and some isoforms contain 3-phosphoinositide–binding domains that contribute to their regulation. Akt and other protein kinases activated downstream of PI3K phosphorylate

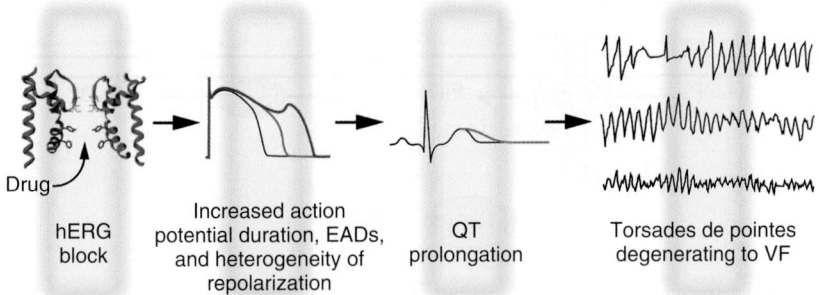

FIGURE 11.1 The original hypothesis for the genesis of acquired long QT syndrome. The product of the human ether-a-go-go related gene (*hERG*) is the α-subunit of the I_{Kr} channel. It has a large internal vestibule that can be blocked by drugs, thereby reducing I_{Kr} and prolonging action potential duration (APD). When APD is sufficiently prolonged to allow for recovery of the L-type calcium channel from inactivation, the outcome is an early afterdepolarization (*EAD*). The APD prolongation results in a prolonged QT interval while the EADs can give rise to triggered action potentials, leading to torsades de pointes, which can degenerate into ventricular fibrillation (*VF*). (From Roden DM, Viswanathan PC. Genetics of acquired long QT syndrome. *J Clin Invest.* 2005;115:2025-2032.)

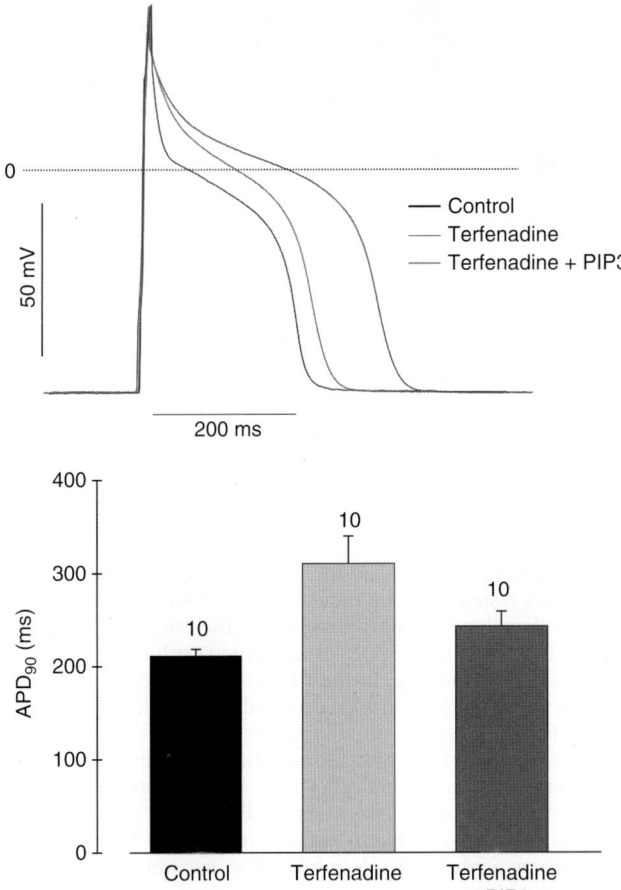

FIGURE 11.2 Terfenadine increases action potential duration (*APD*) both by blocking I_{kr} and by inhibiting phosphoinositide 3-kinase (PI3K). *Upper panel,* The control APD is shortest. A 2-hour exposure to terfenadine lengthened APD the most. After phosphatidylinositol 3,4,5-trisphosphate (*PIP3*, the second messenger produced by PI3K) is added to the pipette solution, the APD is shortened but not to control levels. The remaining increase in duration is presumed to be due to the direct block of I_{Kr}. *Lower panel,* The summary graph of APD at 90% repolarization for each group. The numbers above the bars indicate the numbers of cells studied. (Modified from Lu Z, Wu CY, Jiang YP, et al. Suppression of phosphoinositide 3-kinase signaling and alteration of multiple ion currents in drug-induced long QT syndrome. *Sci Transl Med.* 2012;4:131ra50.)

numerous targets that regulate diverse cellular processes. In addition to kinases, other PI3K effectors that contain 3-phosphoinositide–binding domains include some adaptor proteins and regulators of small GTPases.

Dephosphorylation of the 3-hydroxyl group of PI(3,4,5)P$_3$ by the lipid phosphatase PTEN terminates class IA PI3K signaling (see Fig. 11.3).

Effects of PI3kα Inhibition on Cardiac Plateau Currents

Action potential prolongation can occur via a reduction in outward currents, as in congenital LQT1 (mutations affecting I_{Ks}) and LQT2 (mutations affecting I_{Kr}), or via an increase in inward currents, as in LQT3 (mutations affecting the persistent sodium current [I_{NaP}]). All three of these currents are very small; the net current flowing during the plateau (phase 2) generates a repolarization rate of roughly 0.1 V/s, which is between 0.1% and 0.01% of the maximum upstroke velocity of the typical ventricular or Purkinje fiber action potential (300 V/s and 800 V/s, respectively). A surprising aspect of PI3Kα inhibition is that it increases I_{NaP}, which, in concert with reductions in I_{Kr} and I_{Ks}, induces APD prolongation.[13] In addition, reductions in the peak sodium current (I_{Na}) and the L-type calcium current (I_{CaL}) have been observed following PI3Kα inhibition.[13,19]

I_{NaP}

Cardiac sodium currents are generated by the α-subunit Na$_V$1.5 (SCN5a) and one or more of a number of β-subunits. The sodium channel generates the fast upstroke of the cardiac action potential (<1 ms to peak) and rapidly inactivates almost completely, leaving far fewer than 1% of the channels open in physiological conditions. This remaining current is due to two components: a very slow inactivation[24,25] over the entire range of plateau potentials, and a component that contributes steady state current over a more restricted voltage range in which the product of m^3_∞ (the probability that the three activation gates are in the open position) and h_∞ (the probability that the inactivation gate is in the open position) is nonzero.[26] It is currently unknown whether one or both of these components of I_{NaP} is increased by PI3Kα inhibition. Although very small, I_{NaP} flows several orders of magnitude longer than the peak current and thus loads a significant portion of the Na$^+$ that enters the cardiac myocyte during the action potential. Fig. 11.4A and B shows the roughly three-fold increase

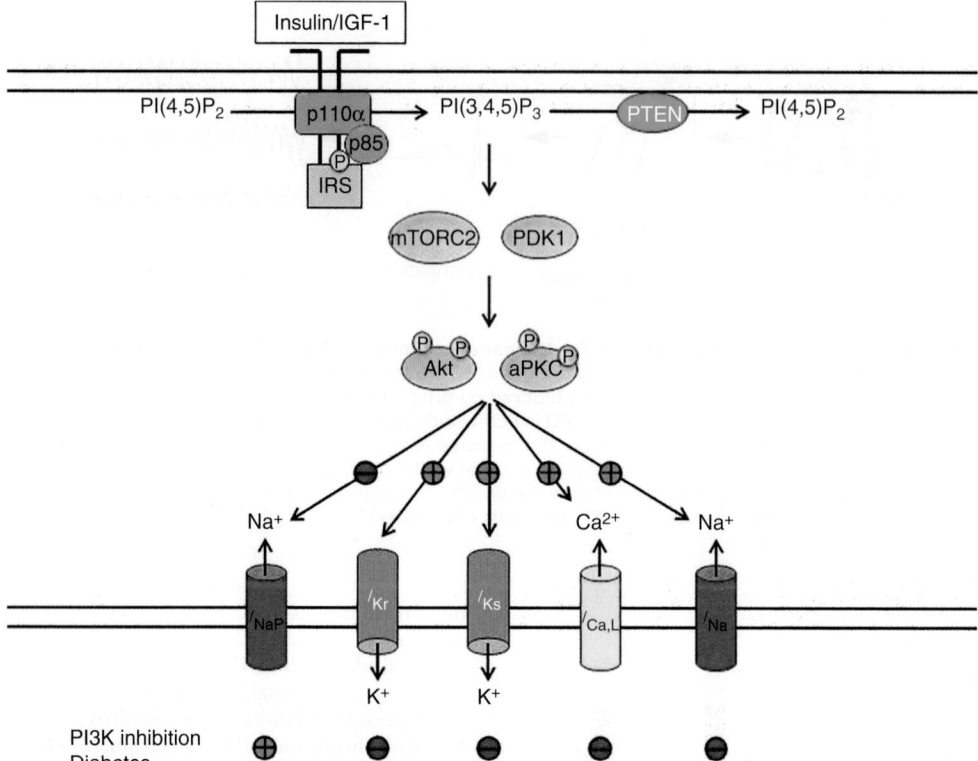

FIGURE 11.3 Activation of phosphoinositide 3-kinase α (PI3Kα) by insulin and a model of PI3Kα regulation of ion channels. Binding of insulin or insulin-like growth factor-1 (*IGF-1*) to their receptors causes tyrosine phosphorylation of insulin receptor substrate (*IRS*) proteins, which forms docking sites for the p85 regulatory subunit of the PI3Kα complex. Activated PI3Kα converts phosphatidylinositol 4,5-bisphosphate (*PI[4,5]P$_2$*) to phosphatidylinositol 3,4,5-trisphosphate (*PI[3,4,5]P$_3$*), which leads to the activation and phosphorylation of downstream effectors such as mechanistic target of rapamycin complex 2 (*mTORC2*), phosphoinositide-dependent protein kinase 1 (*PDK1*), Akt, and atypical PKC (*aPKC*) isoforms. Other effectors of PI(3,4,5)P$_3$ that are not shown might also be involved in ion channel regulation. PI3Kα signaling suppresses persistent sodium current (I_{NaP}) and enhances the rapid and slow delayed rectifiers (I_{Kr} and I_{Ks}, respectively), the L-type calcium current (I_{CaL}), and the peak sodium current (I_{Na}). PI3K inhibition and diabetes have the opposite effects on these currents. Dephosphorylation of PI(3,4,5)P$_3$ by the lipid phosphatase PTEN turns off PI3Kα signaling.

in I_{NaP} produced by a 2-hour incubation of canine ventricular myocytes with a PI3K inhibitor (PI-103) or a tyrosine kinase inhibitor (nilotinib) that leads to inhibition of PI3K signaling. The increase in I_{NaP} was reversed by long-term washout (30 minutes to 2 hours) or by using a patch pipette filled with PI(3,4,5)P$_3$, but not PI(4,5)P$_2$ or PI(3,5)P$_2$. This increase in I_{NaP} was thought to be due to PI3Kα inhibition, which was confirmed by measuring the current in myocytes from mice with the genetic deletion of p110α or p110β in the heart. I_{NaP} was larger in the PI3Kα-null myocytes than in myocytes from wild-type mice, while the loss of PI3Kβ did not affect current density. Bypassing the loss of PI3Kα by infusing knockout myocytes with PI(3,4,5)P$_3$ restored I_{NaP} to wild-type levels.[13] Thus there is clear evidence that PI3Kα regulates the cardiac sodium channel, but the specific molecular mechanism for the increase in I_{NaP} remains undetermined.

I_{Kr}

The molecular determinant of the rapid delayed rectifier, I_{Kr}, is a heteromultimer of the α-subunit hERG and the β-subunit KCNE2. Since I_{Kr} activation overlaps with that of I_{CaL} and I_{Ks}, it is identified as a difference current by using a specific I_{Kr} blocker such as E-4031 or dofetilide (but see difficulties with selectivity for both below). The difference current after short-term exposure to the blocker is I_{Kr}. Fig. 11.4C and D shows the effects of

a 2-hour incubation with nilotinib or PI-103. I_{Kr} was smaller at all voltages tested, and the reduction in current was reversed by prolonged washout of nilotinib or by the inclusion of PI(3,4,5)P$_3$, but not PI(4,5)P$_2$ or PI(3,5)P$_2$, in the pipette solution.[13]

We also examined I_{Kr} in the PI3Kα-null myocytes. The current was very small in wild-type cells and even smaller in myocytes lacking PI3Kα (Lu et al., unpublished observations). Most studies of the regulation of I_{Kr} by PI3K have been done in heterologous expression systems. In HEK293 cells stably expressing hERG, transfection of constitutively active PI3Kα or Akt enhanced function, whereas dominant negative mutants of PI3Kα or Akt or treatment with the PI3K inhibitor wortmannin reduced the current.[27]

I_{Ks}

The molecular basis of the slow delayed rectifier, I_{Ks}, is a heteromultimer of the α-subunit KCNQ1 and the β-subunit KCNE1. Like I_{Kr}, I_{Ks} is measured as a difference current after the application of a specific blocker, chromanol 293B. Also like I_{Kr}, the magnitude of I_{Ks} at all voltages is reduced after the treatment of myocytes with PI-103 or nilotinib and is restored if PI(3,4,5)P$_3$ is included in the pipette solution (see Fig. 11.4C and D). Downstream of PI3K, Akt has been shown to increase the KCNQ1/KCNE1 current in *Xenopus* oocytes.[28]

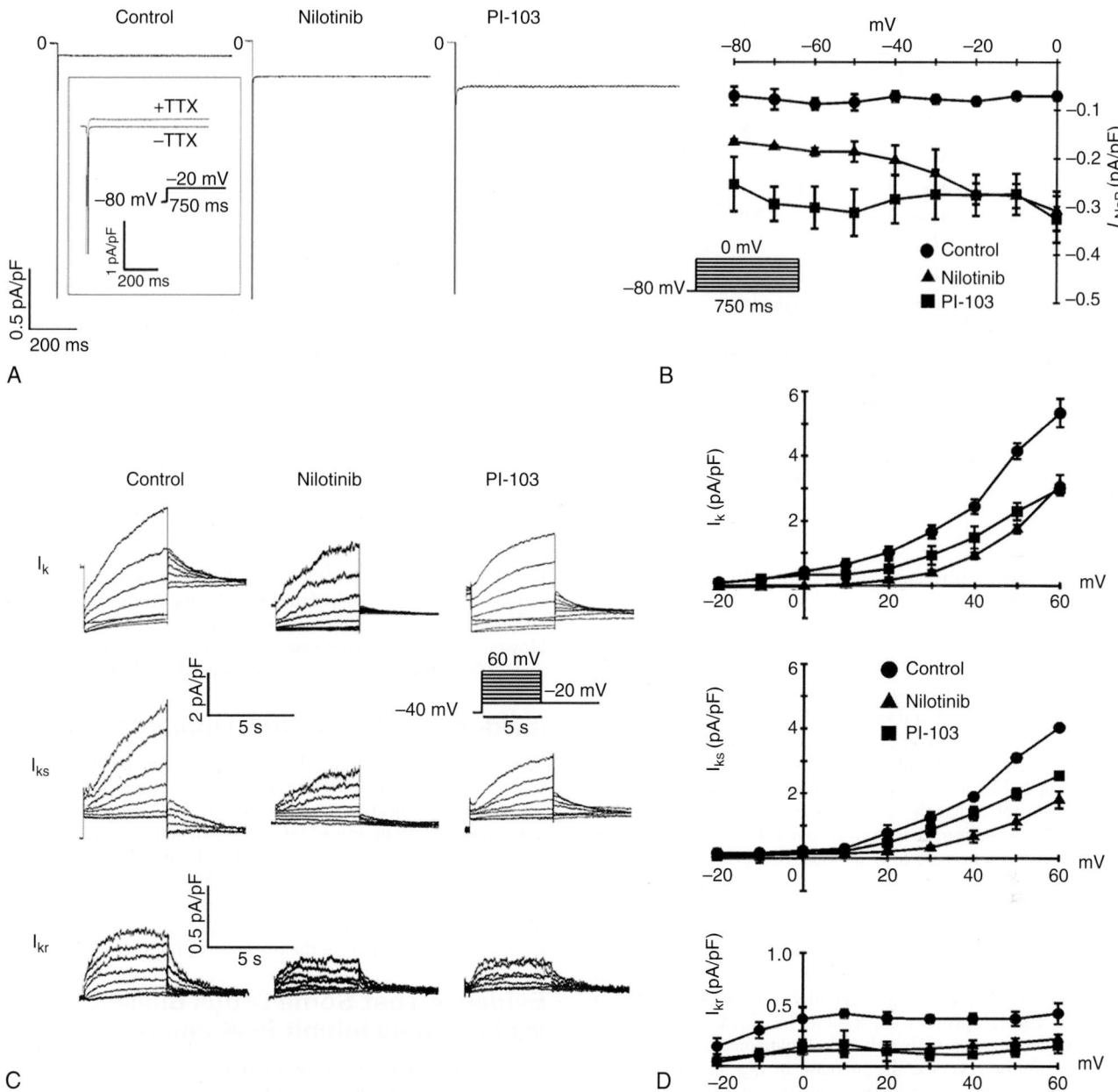

FIGURE 11.4 Effects of nilotinib, a tyrosine kinase inhibitor that decreases phosphoinositide 3-kinase (PI3K) signaling, and PI-103 (a PI3K inhibitor) on cardiac ion currents. Canine cardiac myocytes were treated with nilotinib or PI-103 for 2 hours. (A) and (B), Sample traces and current–voltage relationships of tetrodotoxin (*TTX*)-sensitive I_{NaP}. (C) and (D), Sample traces and leak-subtracted time-dependent current–voltage relationships of total outward rectifier current (I_K), I_{Kr} and I_{Ks}. (Modified from Lu Z, Wu CY, Jiang YP, et al. Suppression of phosphoinositide 3-kinase signaling and alteration of multiple ion currents in drug-induced long QT syndrome. *Sci Transl Med*. 2012;4:131ra50.)

I_{Na}

While the persistent current is increased by PI3K inhibition, the peak sodium current is reduced by roughly 50% after incubation with PI-103.[13] This reduction in I_{Na} is eliminated if $PI(3,4,5)P_3$ is added to the pipette solution, again indicating a role for the PI3K second messenger in controlling this ion channel. A reduction in I_{Na} should reduce the maximum rate of the rise in the upstroke of the cardiac action potential while having relatively little effect on the APD. Since the I–V relationship is unaltered by PI-103 or nilotinib,[13] the reduction in current is due either to a decrease in the number of channels or to a

negative shift in the inactivation curve. If the number of channels is reduced, then the actual increase in the ratio of G_{NaP}/peak G_{Na} is six-fold after PI3K inhibition. Increased PI3Kα signaling upregulated the mRNA for both SCN5a and SCN1B (the α- and β-subunits of the cardiac sodium channel, respectively) in adult mice.[29] Treatment with an Akt inhibitor did not block this effect, suggesting that the transcriptional upregulation is independent of Akt in the mouse heart.[29] On the other hand, transforming growth factor β1 increased transcription of SCN5a in the rat heart via activation of PI3K and phosphorylation of the transcription factor Foxo1 by Akt.[30] Thus there may

	I_{kr}	I_{ks}	I_{NaP}	I_{Na}	I_{CaL}	APD_{90}
Control	–	–	–	–	–	216
Nilo	.40	.45	2.0	.33	.27	343
PI-103	.40	.65	2.8	.53	.73	323
ΔI_{kr}	.40	–	–	–	–	256
ΔI_{ks}	–	.45	–	–	–	227
ΔI_{NaP}	–	–	2.0	–	–	227
ΔI_{Na}	–	–	–	.33	–	237
ΔI_{CaL}	–	–	–	–	.27	211

–, unchanged in the model

A

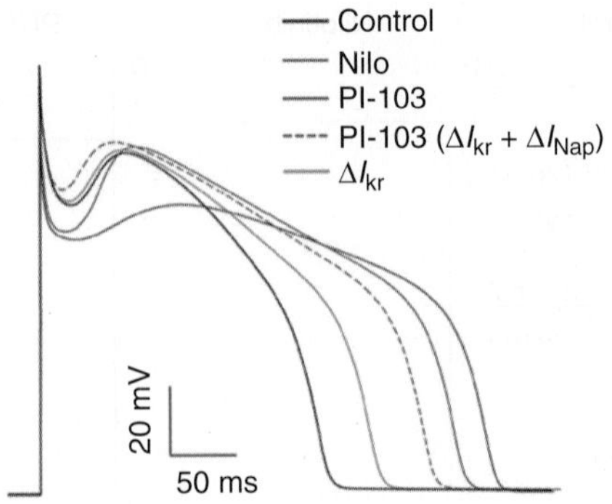

B

FIGURE 11.5 **Computer simulation of the effects of nilotinib and PI-103 on the action potential duration (APD).** (A) Table providing the fractional change in I_{Kr}, I_{Ks}, I_{NaP}, I_{Na}, and I_{CaL} caused by each drug found experimentally as well as the simulated APD at 90% repolarization (APD_{90}). The table also shows the simulated APD_{90} for isolated effects of each of the ion currents affected by nilotinib. (B) Simulated action potentials for the control, nilotinib (*Nilo*), and PI-103, with PI-103 only including the effects on I_{Kr} (ΔI_{Kr}), and PI-103 only including the effects on I_{Kr} and I_{NaP} [PI-103 ($\Delta I_{Kr} + \Delta I_{NaP}$)]. (Modified from Lu Z, Wu CY, Jiang YP, et al. Suppression of phosphoinositide 3-kinase signaling and alteration of multiple ion currents in drug-induced long QT syndrome. *Sci Transl Med.* 2012;4:131ra50.)

be species-specific differences in the downstream effectors of PI3Kα that regulate I_{Na}.

I_{CaL}

The channel that mediates I_{CaL} is a heteromultimer comprised of the α-subunit $Ca_V1.2$ and multiple distinct accessory subunits (β, γ, and δ). I_{CaL} activates positive to –40 mV and inactivates over tens to hundreds of milliseconds. Thus it provides an inward current that helps sustain the action potential plateau. Multiple studies have shown that this current is regulated at different levels by PI3Kα signaling. It is known that IGF-1 signals through PI3Kα and Akt to increase I_{CaL} in mouse myocytes.[20] Transgenic expression of constitutively active PI3Kα caused an increase in expression of $Ca_V1.2$ and some of the accessory subunits (β2 and α2δ1)[31,32] via a pathway that was not blocked by inhibition of Akt.[29] Myocytes with increased $PI(3,4,5)P_3$ levels due to deletion of the lipid phosphatase PTEN exhibited increased I_{CaL} with a negative shift in the voltage dependence of activation but no change in $Ca_V1.2$ protein expression.[20,33] Treatment of these PTEN-null myocytes with either dominant-negative PI3Kα or a PI3K inhibitor reversed the increase in I_{CaL} density and the shift in the voltage dependence of activation. Treatment with an Akt inhibitor reversed the increase in I_{CaL} density only.[20] In our experiments, we found that insulin treatment or intracellular $PI(3,4,5)P_3$ infusion of wild-type mouse myocytes did not increase the current, whereas deletion of p110α reduced I_{CaL} density by almost 25%.[19] The reduction in I_{CaL} was accompanied by a decrease in the fraction of $Ca_V1.2$ on the cell surface.[19] Intracellular delivery of PTEN or the PH domain of GRP1 to sequester $PI(3,4,5)P_3$ caused a similar reduction in I_{CaL} in wild-type myocytes.[34] Incubation of canine ventricular myocytes with PI-103, nilotinib, or an Akt inhibitor caused a reduction in I_{CaL} density, and PI-103 had the additional effect of causing a positive voltage shift in inactivation. Intracellular $PI(3,4,5)P_3$ infusion reversed current inhibition caused by PI-103.[13,19]

How Changes in Plateau Currents Caused by PI3K Inhibition Affect the Cardiac Action Potential Duration

To see how much each change in plateau membrane currents contributes to APD prolongation caused by inhibition of PI3K,

Fig. 11.5 employs a modified Hund-Rudy model of the canine action potential.[13,35] Each of the ion currents affected by PI3K inhibition induces prolongation of less than 50% of the total change. However, the combined changes in I_{NaP} and I_{Kr} account for more than 70% of the total prolongation induced by PI3K inhibition.

Incidence of Early Afterdepolarizations

Early afterdepolarizations (EADs) are a major trigger for TdP, and their occurrence in the setting of action potential prolongation is indicative of recovery of I_{CaL} from inactivation. Sympathetic stimulation of canine ventricular myocytes with isoproterenol induced EADs in 8 of 10 cells and 10 of 10 cells following their incubation with PI-103 at 50 or 500 nM, respectively (vs. EADs in 0 of 10 control myocytes).[13] These data indicate that PI3K inhibition might increase the risk of EAD-triggered ventricular arrhythmias in the presence of high sympathetic tone.

Evidence That Some Drugs Block I_{Kr} Alone, While Others Inhibit PI3K and Block I_{Kr}

PI3K inhibition by PI-103 or nilotinib caused APD prolongation only after long-term exposure to the drugs.[13] Recovery of I_{Kr} and I_{NaP} after drug washout was also a slow process. These results suggest that $PI(3,4,5)P_3$ is slowly depleted by drug treatment and gradually replenished after washout. The slow time course for the effects of PI3K inhibition is in contrast to the acute action described for classical I_{Kr} blockers. Therefore the absence of an acute effect of a drug on APD or I_{NaP} followed by an increase that develops over time is suggestive of PI3Kα inhibition. This mode of action would be supported if further electrophysiological testing shows that the increase is eliminated by adding $PI(3,4,5)P_3$, but not $PI(3,5)P_2$ or $PI(4,5)P_2$, to the pipette solution. Biochemical evidence of reduced PI3K signaling would ultimately confirm the suggested cause.

The distinct time dependence of I_{NaP} on PI3K inhibition was exploited by Yang and colleagues,[14] who asked whether some drugs that are known to acutely block I_{Kr} and are associated with variable degrees of aLQTS risk also inhibit PI3K. They used a slow rise in I_{NaP} and reversal by $PI(3,4,5)P_3$ in the pipette as evidence of PI3K inhibition. Their results demonstrated that dofetilide, E-4031, thioridazine, and erythromycin enhanced I_{NaP} (presumably by blocking PI3Kα), while haloperidol, moxifloxacin, and verapamil did not. With dofetilide, there was a substantial increase in I_{NaP} between 5 and 48 hours of treatment, and the magnitude of the effect was not saturated at 1-μM drug. Dofetilide also caused a decrease in Akt phosphorylation that is consistent with inhibition of PI3K signaling. Since an increase in I_{NaP} is known to be arrhythmogenic,[36,37] the authors concluded that the drugs that inhibit PI3K are more likely to increase the risk of TdP than agents that only reduce I_{Kr}.

Diabetes and Acquired Long QT Syndrome

Diabetic patients have a higher incidence of life-threatening cardiac arrhythmias and sudden cardiac death than nondiabetic people. Several factors including repolarization abnormalities that manifest as prolonged QTc probably increase the vulnerability of the diabetic population to these cardiac complications. QTc prolongation is a well-established risk factor for lethal ventricular arrhythmias, and its prevalence has been reported to be as high as 16% in patients with type 1 diabetes[38] and 26% in type 2 diabetic patients.[39] Prolonged QTc is an independent risk factor for mortality in people with diabetes[40–43] and is a highly significant predictor of cardiac death even in newly diagnosed diabetic subjects.[44,45]

Experiments using animal models of type 1 and type 2 diabetes have shed some light on the origins of diabetic aLQTS. QTc prolongation or APD lengthening in ventricular myocytes has been shown in diabetic rats, mice, dogs, and rabbits.[46–49] Several studies suggest that reduced cardiac insulin/PI3Kα signaling plays a role in QT interval prolongation in diabetes. First, insulin treatment reversed the repolarization defects of type 1 diabetic hearts.[50,51] Second, APD prolongation in ventricular myocytes of type 1 or type 2 diabetic mice was reversed by intracellular delivery of PI(3,4,5)P$_3$ or by adenoviral expression of constitutively active p110α.[51] Third, euglycemic mice that lack the insulin receptor only in cardiac myocytes also exhibited APD prolongation.[52] Although it is generally accepted that insulin-stimulated myocardial glucose utilization is defective in type 2 diabetes, whether or not cardiac PI3K signaling is reduced is less clear. Some human and animal studies showed an increase in insulin/PI3K/Akt signaling in diabetic versus control subjects,[53] whereas others have shown the opposite.[51,54]

Assuming that a common mechanism of suppressed PI3K signaling is responsible for aLQTS caused by diabetes and some drugs (see Fig. 11.3), one would expect to see overlap in the affected ion currents. Indeed, electrophysiological studies in myocytes from diabetic animals described reductions in a number of potassium currents including the transient outward current I_{to}, I_{Kr}, and I_{Ks},[47,48,49,50] a decrease in I_{CaL} density,[49,55] and an increase in I_{NaP}.[51] Reduced protein levels of the affected potassium or calcium ion channels were observed in some cases. The increase in I_{NaP} in cardiomyocytes of type 1 and type 2 diabetic mice was reversed by intracellular delivery of PI(3,4,5)P$_3$ or by adenoviral expression of constitutively active p110α.[51] Treatment of wild-type myocytes with an Akt inhibitor also increased I_{NaP}, but not to the extent seen in diabetic or p110α-null myocytes. Perfusion of diabetic hearts with the I_{NaP} blocker mexiletine largely reversed QTc prolongation. These results suggest that the repolarization defect in diabetes is due in large part to an increase in I_{NaP}, which is caused by suppression of PI3Kα signaling to Akt and other effectors.[51]

Although a decrease in I_{CaL} is expected to shorten QTc, examination of this current has provided insight into how defective PI3K signaling in diabetes might affect other ion channels in the heart. In a mouse model of type 1 diabetes, the amount of Ca$_V$1.2 on the surface of myocytes was reduced but the total amount of protein was the same as in nondiabetic cells.[56] Intracellular delivery of PI(3,4,5)P$_3$ or perfusion with insulin increased I_{CaL} density to the level seen in nondiabetic myocytes, but these increases were blocked by incubation with taxol to block microtubule-dependent trafficking. These results suggest that a major factor underlying the suppression of I_{CaL} in this model is reduced trafficking of the

channel to the cell surface due to reduced insulin/PI3Kα signaling.[56] The trafficking mechanism might involve Akt-dependent phosphorylation of an accessory β-subunit.[57] In a mouse model of type 2 diabetes, total expression of the Ca$_V$1.2 protein was reduced, I_{CaL} density was decreased, and steady-state activation was shifted toward more positive potentials as compared to nondiabetic controls.[58] Infusion of the diabetic myocytes with PI(3,4,5)P$_3$ or Akt caused a substantial increase in current density, and infusion of PI(3,4,5)P$_3$ or PKC-ι corrected the alteration in voltage dependence of activation.[59] Thus PI3K signaling to Akt and PKC-ι appears to regulate different aspects of Ca$_V$1.2 function.

Therapeutic Approaches

Because the I_{NaP} blocker mexiletine largely eliminated QTc prolongation in the diabetic mouse, it is worth considering whether a block of I_{NaP} might be a therapeutic approach to PI3K inhibition. To explore this possibility, Qiu and colleagues[60] looked at the action potential of canine ventricular slabs and found that moxifloxacin caused APD prolongation that reached a steady state within 30 minutes to 1 hour, while dofetilide produced a similarly rapid course of prolongation followed by a slow, continuous increase over the next 6 hours. If inhibition of PI3K causes a continuous increase in I_{NaP}, then block of this current might be beneficial at the later time point. When the authors exposed the dofetilide-treated preparations to lidocaine at low concentrations to selectively block I_{NaP}, they observed greater shortening of the APD at 6 hours than at 30 minutes. The effect of the same concentration of lidocaine on preparations exposed to moxifloxicin was small at both time points. These results support the idea that the block of I_{NaP} might be therapeutic in cases of excessive prolongation due to PI3K inhibition. They also performed an in vivo experiment with dofetilide. The QTc in the canine heart was continuously prolonged during a 6.5-hour exposure to dofetilide. Lidocaine was washed in briefly at 30 minutes and at 6.5 hours of exposure. The I_{NaP} blocker decreased the QTc to a much greater degree at 6.5 hours than at 30 minutes, suggesting that block of I_{NaP} in vivo may be a mechanism to reduce the toxicity of drugs that inhibit PI3K.

The search for selective blockers of I_{NaP} has lasted more than a decade, as I_{NaP} is increased in heart failure. However, this increase is thought to occur via a different mechanism that involves phosphorylation of the sodium channel on specific amino acid residues by calmodulin-dependent protein kinase.[61,62] Ranolazine has a high specificity for I_{NaP} over I_{Na} and is already approved for use in angina,[63] but it also blocks I_{Kr}. Thus newer and more selective agents are needed.[64]

Conclusions

aLQTS can arise from the direct block of I_{Kr}, inhibition of PI3Kα signaling, or a combination of the two. In the latter two cases, multiple ion currents are affected including I_{NaP} and I_{Kr}. It is now clear that some drugs previously thought to be pure I_{Kr} blockers, including terfenadine and dofetilide, also inhibit PI3Kα signaling. It is possible that drugs with both activities may predispose to TdP to a greater extent than pure I_{Kr} blockers. In addition, the increased incidence of aLQTS and susceptibility to arrhythmias in type 1 and type 2 diabetes may arise from the same mechanism of reduced PI3Kα signaling. Because substantial increases in I_{NaP} occur when PI3Kα is inhibited, block of this current is a promising avenue for therapy. Finally, in the interest of safety, we suggest that new drug candidates be tested for PI3Kα inhibition prior to reaching clinical trials.

Acknowledgment

We thank Michael R. Rosen for his helpful suggestions on the manuscript.

REFERENCES

1. Monahan BP, Ferguson CL, Killeavy ES, Lloyd BK, Troy J, Cantilena Jr LR. Torsades de pointes occurring in association with terfenadine use. *JAMA*. 1990;264:2788–2790.
2. Zimmermann M, Duruz H, Guinand O, et al. Torsades de pointes after treatment with terfenadine and ketoconazole. *Eur Heart J*. 1992;13:1002–1003.
3. Woosley RL, Chen Y, Freiman JP, Gillis RA. Mechanism of the cardiotoxic actions of terfenadine. *JAMA*. 1993;269:1532–1536.
4. Zechnich AD, Hedges JR, Eiselt-Proteau D, Haxby D. Possible interactions with terfenadine or astemizole. *West J Med*. 1994;160:321–325.
5. Honig PK, Woosley RL, Zamani K, Conner DP, Cantilena Jr LR. Changes in the pharmacokinetics and electrocardiographic pharmacodynamics of terfenadine with concomitant administration of erythromycin. *Clin Pharmacol Ther*. 1992;52:231–238.
6. Sanguinetti MC, Jurkiewicz NK. Two components of cardiac delayed rectifier K⁺ current. Differential sensitivity to block by class III antiarrhythmic agents. *J Gen Physiol*. 1990;96:195–215.
7. Warmke JW, Ganetzky B. A family of potassium channel genes related to eag in *Drosophila* and mammals. *Proc Natl Acad Sci U S A*. 1994;91:3438–3442.
8. Sanguinetti MC, Jiang C, Curran ME, Keating MT. A mechanistic link between an inherited and an acquired cardiac arrhythmia: hERG encodes the IKr potassium channel. *Cell*. 1995;81:299–307.
9. Roy M, Dumaine R, Brown AM. hERG, a primary human ventricular target of the nonsedating antihistamine terfenadine. *Circulation*. 1996;94:817–823.
10. Rosen MR. Of oocytes and runny noses. *Circulation*. 1996;944:607–609.
11. Redfern WS, Carlsson L, Davis AS, et al. Relationships between preclinical cardiac electrophysiology, clinical QT interval prolongation and torsade de pointes for a broad range of drugs: evidence for a provisional safety margin in drug development. *Cardiovasc Res*. 2003;58:32–45.
12. U.S. Department of Health and Human Services Food and Drug Administration Center for Drug Evaluation and Research (CDER) Center for Biologics Evaluation and Research (CBER). ICH; October 2005.
13. Lu Z, Wu CY, Jiang YP, et al. Suppression of phosphoinositide 3-kinase signaling and alteration of multiple ion currents in drug-induced long QT syndrome. *Sci Transl Med*. 2012;4:131ra150.
14. Yang T, Chun YW, Stroud DM, et al. Screening for acute IKr block is insufficient to detect torsades de pointes liability: role of late sodium current. *Circulation*. 2014;130:224–234.
15. Deleted in review.
16. Balla T. Phosphoinositides: tiny lipids with giant impact on cell regulation. *Physiol Rev*. 2013;93:1019–1137.
17. Vanhaesebroeck B, Leevers SJ, Ahmadi K, et al. Synthesis and function of 3-phosphorylated inositol lipids. *Annu Rev Biochem*. 2001;70:535–602.
18. Vanhaesebroeck B, Guillermet-Guibert J, Graupera M, Bilanges B. The emerging mechanisms of isoform-specific PI3K signalling. *Nat Rev Mol Cell Biol*. 2010;11:329–341.
19. Lu Z, Jiang YP, Wang W, et al. Loss of cardiac phosphoinositide 3-kinase p110 alpha results in contractile dysfunction. *Circulation*. 2009;120:318–325.
20. Sun H, Kerfant BG, Zhao D, et al. Insulin-like growth factor-1 and PTEN deletion enhance cardiac L-type Ca²⁺ currents via increased PI3Kalpha/PKB signaling. *Circ. Res*. 2006;98:1390–1397.
21. Hon WC, Berndt A, Williams RL. Regulation of lipid binding underlies the activation mechanism of class IA PI3-kinases. *Oncogene*. 2012;31:3655–3666.
22. Burke JE, Williams RL. Dynamic steps in receptor tyrosine kinase mediated activation of class IA phosphoinositide 3-kinases (PI3K) captured by H/D exchange (HDX-MS). *Adv Bio Regul*. 2013;53:97–110.
23. Liu P, Gan W, Chin YR, et al. PtdIns(3,4,5)P3-dependent activation of the mTORC2 kinase complex. *Cancer Discov*. 2015;5:1194–1209.

24. Gintant GA, Datyner NB, Cohen IS. Slow inactivation of a tetrodotoxin-sensitive current in canine cardiac Purkinje fibers. *Biophys J*. 1984;45:509–512.
25. Carmeliet E. Slow inactivation of the sodium current in rabbit cardiac Purkinje fibres. *Pflugers Arch*. 1987;408:18–26.
26. Attwell D, Cohen I, Eisner D, Ohba M, Ojeda C. The steady state TTX-sensitive ("window") sodium current in cardiac Purkinje fibres. *Pflugers Arch*. 1979;379:137–142.
27. Zhang Y, Wang H, Wang J, Han H, Nattel S, Wang Z. Normal function of hERG K⁺ channels expressed in HEK293 cells requires basal protein kinase B activity. *FEBS Lett*. 2003;534:125–132.
28. Embark HM, Bohmer C, Vallon V, Luft F, Lang F. Regulation of KCNE1-dependent K⁺ current by the serum and glucocorticoid-inducible kinase (SGK) isoforms. *Pflugers Arch*. 2003;445:601–606.
29. Yang KC, Tseng YT, Nerbonne JM. Exercise training and PI3Kalpha-induced electrical remodeling is independent of cellular hypertrophy and Akt signaling. *J. Mol. Cell. Cardiol*. 2012;53:532–541.
30. Kaur K, Zarzoso M, Ponce-Balbuena D, et al. TGF-beta1, released by myofibroblasts, differentially regulates transcription and function of sodium and potassium channels in adult rat ventricular myocytes. *PLoS One*. 2013;8:e55391.
31. Yang KC, Foeger NC, Marionneau C, Jay PY, McMullen JR, Nerbonne JM. Homeostatic regulation of electrical excitability in physiological cardiac hypertrophy. *J Physiol*. 2010;588:5015–5032.
32. Yano N, Tseng A, Zhao TC, Robbins J, Padbury JF, Tseng YT. Temporally controlled overexpression of cardiac-specific PI3Kalpha induces enhanced myocardial contractility—a new transgenic model. *Am J Physiol Heart Circ Physiol*. 2008;295:H1690–H1694.
33. Crackower MA, Oudit GY, Kozieradzki I, et al. Regulation of myocardial contractility and cell size by distinct PI3K- PTEN signaling pathways. *Cell*. 2002;110:737–749.
34. Lu Z, Jiang YP, Ballou LM, Cohen IS, Lin RZ. Galpha q inhibits cardiac L-type Ca²⁺ channels through phosphatidylinositol 3-kinase. *J Biol Chem*. 2005;280:40347–40354.
35. Hund TJ, Rudy Y. Rate dependence and regulation of action potential and calcium transient in a canine cardiac ventricular cell model. *Circulation*. 2004;110:3168–3174.
36. Lowe JS, Stroud DM, Yang T, Hall L, Atack TC, Roden DM. Increased late sodium current contributes to long QT-related arrhythmia susceptibility in female mice. *Cardiovasc Res*. 2012;95:300–307.
37. Shryock JC, Song Y, Rajamani S, Antzelevitch C, Belardinelli L. The arrhythmogenic consequences of increasing late INa in the cardiomyocyte. *Cardiovasc Res*. 2013;99:600–611.
38. Veglio M, Borra M, Stevens LK, Fuller JH, Perin PC. The relation between QTc interval prolongation and diabetic complications. The EURODIAB IDDM Complication Study Group. *Diabetologia*. 1999;42:68–75.
39. Veglio M, Bruno G, Borra M, et al. Prevalence of increased QT interval duration and dispersion in type 2 diabetic patients and its relationship with coronary heart disease: a population-based cohort. *J Intern Med*. 2002;251:317–324.
40. Okin PM, Devereux RB, Lee ET, Galloway JM, Howard BV. Electrocardiographic repolarization complexity and abnormality predict all-cause and cardiovascular mortality in diabetes: the strong heart study. *Diabetes*. 2004;53:434–440.
41. Rossing P, Breum L, Major-Pedersen A, et al. Prolonged QTc interval predicts mortality in patients with type 1 diabetes mellitus. *Diabet Med*. 2001;18:199–205.
42. Salles GF, Bloch KV, Cardoso CR. Mortality and predictors of mortality in a cohort of Brazilian type 2 diabetic patients. *Diabetes Care*. 2004;27:1299–1305.
43. Veglio M, Sivieri R, Chinaglia A, Scaglione L, Cavallo-Perin P. QT interval prolongation and mortality in type 1 diabetic patients: a 5-year cohort prospective study. Neuropathy Study Group of the Italian Society of the Study of Diabetes, Piemonte Affiliate. *Diabetes Care*. 2000;23:1381–1383.

44. Naas AA, Davidson NC, Thompson C, et al. QT and QTc dispersion are accurate predictors of cardiac death in newly diagnosed non-insulin dependent diabetes: cohort study. *BMJ*. 1998;316:745–746.
45. Rana BS, Lim PO, Naas AA, et al. QT interval abnormalities are often present at diagnosis in diabetes and are better predictors of cardiac death than ankle brachial pressure index and autonomic function tests. *Heart*. 2005;91:44–50.
46. Magyar J, Rusznak Z, Szentesi P, Szucs G, Kovacs L. Action potentials and potassium currents in rat ventricular muscle during experimental diabetes. *J Mol Cell Cardiol*. 1992;24:841–853.
47. Shimoni Y. Inhibition of the formation or action of angiotensin II reverses attenuated K⁺ currents in type 1 and type 2 diabetes. *J Physiol*. 2001;537:83–92.
48. Lengyel C, Virag L, Biro T, et al. Diabetes mellitus attenuates the repolarization reserve in mammalian heart. *Cardiovasc Res*. 2007;73:512–520.
49. Zhang Y, Xiao J, Lin H, et al. Ionic mechanisms underlying abnormal QT prolongation and the associated arrhythmias in diabetic rabbits: a role of rapid delayed rectifier K⁺ current. *Cell Physiol Biochem*. 2007;19:225–238.
50. Zhang Y, Xiao J, Wang H, et al. Restoring depressed hERG K⁺ channel function as a mechanism for insulin treatment of abnormal QT prolongation and associated arrhythmias in diabetic rabbits. *Am J Physiol Heart Circ Physiol*. 2006;291:H1446–H1455.
51. Lu Z, Jiang YP, Wu CY, et al. Increased persistent sodium current due to decreased PI3K signaling contributes to QT prolongation in the diabetic heart. *Diabetes*. 2013;62:4257–4265.
52. Shimoni Y, Chuang M, Abel ED, Severson DL. Gender-dependent attenuation of cardiac potassium currents in type 2 diabetic db/db mice. *J Physiol*. 2004;555:345–354.
53. Cook SA, Varela-Carver A, Mongillo M, et al. Abnormal myocardial insulin signalling in type 2 diabetes and left-ventricular dysfunction. *Eur Heart J*. 2010;31:100–111.
54. Wang B, Raedschelders K, Shravah J, et al. Differences in myocardial PTEN expression and Akt signalling in type 2 diabetic and nondiabetic patients undergoing coronary bypass surgery. *Clin Endocrinol (Oxf)*. 2011;74:705–713.
55. Wang DW, Kiyosue T, Shigematsu S, Arita M. Abnormalities of K⁺ and Ca²⁺ currents in ventricular myocytes from rats with chronic diabetes. *Am J Physiol*. 1995;269:H1288–H1296.
56. Lu Z, Jiang YP, Xu XH, Ballou LM, Cohen IS, Lin RZ. Decreased L-type Ca²⁺ current in cardiac myocytes of type 1 diabetic Akita mice due to reduced phosphatidylinositol 3-kinase signaling. *Diabetes*. 2007;56:2780–2789.
57. Viard P, Butcher AJ, Halet G, et al. PI3K promotes voltage-dependent calcium channel trafficking to the plasma membrane. *Nat Neurosci*. 2004;7:939–946.
58. Pereira L, Matthes J, Schuster I, et al. Mechanisms of [Ca²⁺]i transient decrease in cardiomyopathy of db/db type 2 diabetic mice. *Diabetes*. 2006;55:608–615.
59. Lu Z, Ballou LM, Jiang YP, Cohen IS, Lin RZ. Restoration of defective L-type Ca²⁺ current in cardiac myocytes of type 2 diabetic db/db mice by Akt and PKC-iota. *J Cardiovasc Pharmacol*. 2011;58:439–445.
60. Qiu X, Chauveau S, Evgeny AP, et al. Abstract 11490: increased late sodium current contributes to excess prolongation of canine ventricular repolarization induced by dofetilide. *Circulation*. 2015;132:A11490.
61. Wagner S, Dybkova N, Rasenack EC, et al. Ca²⁺/calmodulin-dependent protein kinase II regulates cardiac Na⁺ channels. *J Clin Invest*. 2006;116:3127–3138.
62. Maier LS. A novel mechanism for the treatment of angina, arrhythmias, and diastolic dysfunction: inhibition of late I(Na) using ranolazine. *J Cardiovasc Pharmacol*. 2009;54:279–286.
63. Kloner RA, Hines ME, Geunes-Boyer S. Efficacy and safety of ranolazine in patients with chronic stable angina. *Postgrad Med*. 2013;125:43–52.
64. Belardinelli L, Liu G, Smith-Maxwell C, et al. A novel, potent, and selective inhibitor of cardiac late sodium current suppresses experimental arrhythmias. *J Pharmacol Exp Ther*. 2013;344:23–32.

12 Structural Determinants and Biophysical Properties of hERG1 Channel Gating

Michael C. Sanguinetti and Frank B. Sachse

Physiological Role and Clinical Importance of Cardiac hERG1 Channels

The plateau phase of a ventricular action potential is terminated when outward currents conducted by several types of K^+ channels begin to dominate the inward currents conducted primarily by the L-type Ca^{2+} channels. Phase 3 repolarization of an action potential is initiated when the net current is dominated by the combined effects of the rapid and slow delayed rectifier outward K^+ currents (I_{Kr} and I_{Ks}, respectively). In the human heart, I_{Kr} is also an important determinant of the repolarization of atrial myocytes and nodal pacemaker cells. I_{Kr} is conducted by Kv11.1 channels that are more commonly known as human *ether-à-go-go* related type 1 (hERG1) K^+ channels. hERG1 protein subunits are encoded by the *KCNH2* gene (located on chromosome 7q36.1) and coassemble to form a homotetrameric channel complex. Unlike most other voltage-gated K^+ (Kv) channels, hERG1 channels activate relatively slowly in response to membrane depolarization compared with their very fast rate of inactivation. The designation of the current (I_{Kr}) as rapid is in reference to the extremely slow kinetics of the other delayed rectifier K^+ current (I_{Ks}) that is important for ventricular repolarization in humans and other large mammals.[1] hERG1 inactivation greatly reduces the contribution of these channels to net current during the plateau phase, an adaptation that is largely responsible for the prolonged action potential duration that typifies ventricular cardiomyocytes. As the transmembrane potential transitions from the plateau phase to the resting potential during phase 3 repolarization, the hERG1 channel current rapidly rebounds (channels recover from inactivation and reopen), further hastening the rate of repolarization. These features of hERG1 channel gating developed early during evolution, predating the divergence of cnidarians (sea anemones and jellyfish) and bilaterians over 550 million years ago.[2] In addition to the heart, hERG1 channels are expressed in the nervous system (e.g., hippocampus, carotid body, and astrocytes), smooth muscles throughout the gastrointestinal tract, kidney, pituitary gland, and pancreatic β-cells[3] and are overexpressed in many human primary cancers.[4] For a more in-depth description of hERG1 channel biology and biophysics, readers are directed to the outstanding review by Vandenberg and colleagues.[3]

The biophysical and pharmacological properties of hERG1 channels have been extensively studied because of their association with congenital or acquired cardiac arrhythmia.[5] In the human heart, loss of function mutations in *KCNH2* delay ventricular repolarization and cause type 2 long QT syndrome.[6] To date, over 500 mutations in *KCNH2* have been described. Delayed ventricular repolarization increases the incidence of torsades de pointes arrhythmia that can lead to syncope and sudden death. The majority of congenital *KCNH2* mutations disrupt folding or trafficking of channels to the plasma membrane,[7] while mutations that alter channel gating are relatively rare. In addition, a few congenital gain-of-function missense mutations in *KCNH2* cause short QT syndrome by suppressing channel inactivation and thus greatly increasing outward I_{Kr} during the plateau phase of ventricular action potentials. The loss of the hERG1 channel function can also result from the blocking of channels by many commonly used medications.[5] Drug-induced QT prolongation increases the risk for ventricular arrhythmia and has prompted the testing of all compounds for this unwanted side effect early in the drug discovery and development process.

hERG1 Channel Currents

Ionic Currents

The biophysical properties of I_{Kr} are difficult to study in cardiomyocytes because it is a relatively small current and it must be isolated from many other ionic currents by a combination of voltage clamp protocols and a judicious use of a cocktail of pharmacological agents. Moreover, normal healthy human cardiomyocytes are difficult to obtain by biopsy, and unused donor hearts are rare. Thus the biophysical and pharmacological properties of I_{Kr} are now most routinely studied by heterologous expression of hERG1 channels in mammalian cells (e.g., HEK293 or COS cells) transfected with plasmids that contain cDNA or *Xenopus* oocytes injected with cRNA that encodes the hERG1 protein. Using different approaches, two types of ionic channel currents (whole cell or single channel) can be measured in these cells. Most commonly, whole cell ionic currents carried by the transmembrane flux of K^+ ions via the channel pore are measured using single mammalian cells and the whole cell mode of the patch clamp technique or single *Xenopus* frog oocytes and the two-electrode voltage clamp (TEVC) technique. An example of whole cell ionic currents recorded by TEVC from an oocyte that heterologously expresses hERG1 channels is illustrated in Fig. 12.1A. The cell was voltage clamped to a holding potential of –70 mV, and the channels were activated in response to 4-s test depolarizing pulses that were applied in 10-mV increments to test potentials (Vt) that ranged between –70 and +50 mV. The rate of current onset is clearly voltage dependent, becoming faster at more depolarized potentials. Outward currents were increased in magnitude for pulses to a Vt ranging from –60 to –10 mV; however, as Vt was increased from 0 to +50 mV, the magnitude of outward currents became progressively smaller. Following each test pulse, the membrane potential was returned to the holding potential of –70 mV to elicit channel deactivation that is observed as a "tail current" that decayed with a slow time course independent of the preceding Vt and an initial magnitude that was larger in response to a more depolarized Vt. The peak outward current measured at the end of each test pulse (I_{end}) is plotted as a function of Vt in Fig. 12.1B. Most Kv channels have a nearly linear current–voltage (*I*–Vt) relationship, whereas the I_{end}–Vt relationship for hERG1 is bell-shaped and is a hallmark feature of I_{Kr}. The sigmoidal I_{tail}–Vt relationship for hERG1 (see Fig. 12.1B) is a measure of relative channel activation and indicates that channels were half-activated

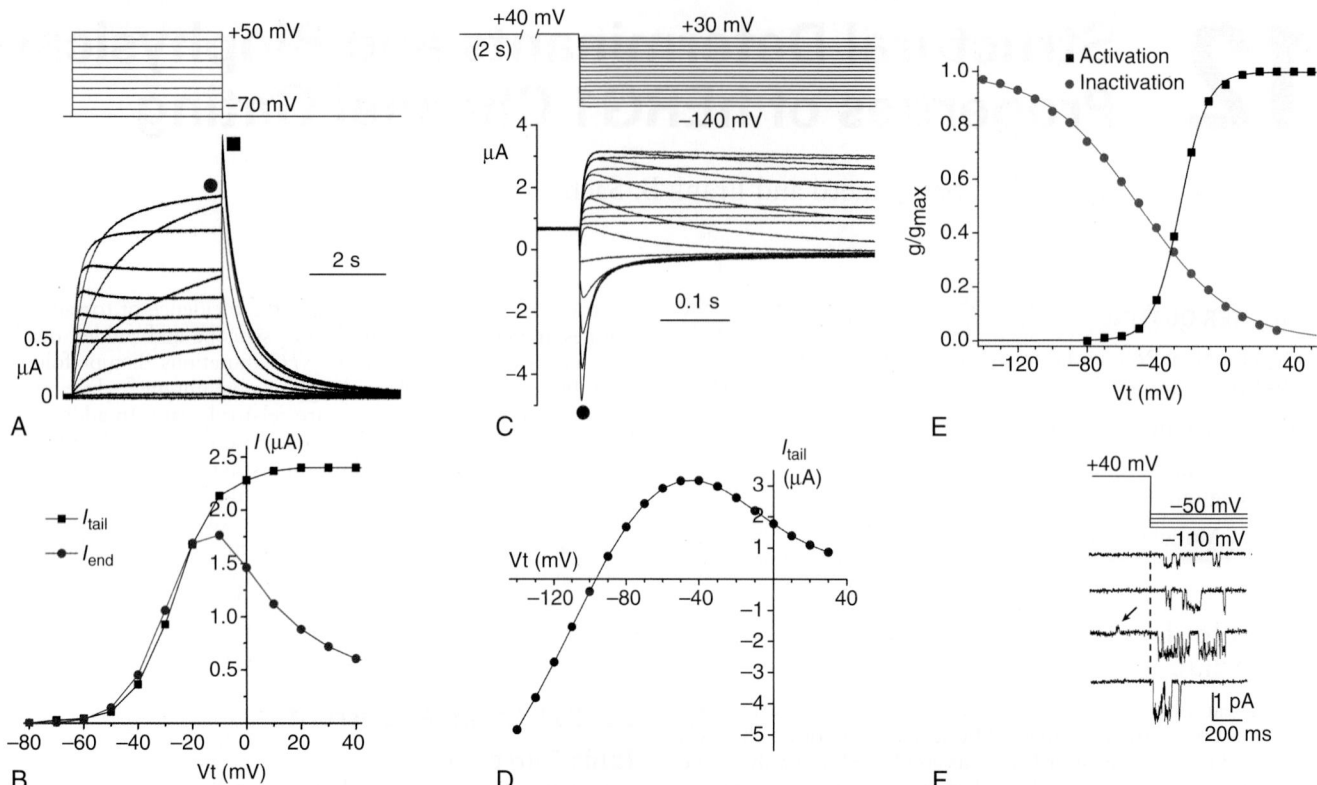

FIGURE 12.1 Ionic currents conducted by human *ether-à-go-go* related type 1 (hERG1) channels. (A) Voltage clamp protocol (*top panel*) used to elicit whole cell currents (*bottom panel*) measured using the two-electrode voltage clamp technique in a *Xenopus* oocyte, heterologously expressing hERG1 channels. (B) Current–voltage relationships for currents measured at the end of each 4-s pulse (I_{end}) and peak tail currents (I_{tail}) as illustrated by corresponding symbols in (A). (C) Voltage clamp protocol (*top panel*) used to elicit tail currents (*bottom panel*) in a *Xenopus* oocyte, heterologously expressing hERG1 channels. (D) Peak currents from (C) plotted as a function of return voltage. (E) Voltage dependence of hERG1 channel activation ($V_{0.5} = -26$ mV, z = 3.2) and inactivation ($V_{0.5} = -50$ mV, z = 0.9). For activation, g = $I_{tail}/I_{tail-max}$ (from [B]). For inactivation, g = $I_{tail}/(G_{max} \times (V_t - E_{rev})$, where E_{rev} is the reversal potential and G_{max} is the maximum slope conductance from [D]). (F) Single hERG1 channel currents recorded from a cell-attached patch of a *Xenopus* oocyte. The slope conductance calculated from these currents was 12 pS. The *arrow* points to a short opening of the channel at +40 mV. The *dotted line* indicates the onset on repolarization to the test potential indicated in the *upper panel*. ([F] Modified from Zou A, Curran ME, Keating MT, et al. Single HERG delayed rectifier K+ channels in *Xenopus* oocytes. *Am J Physiol.* 1997;272:H1309-H1314.)

at about –25 mV and maximally activated at about +20 mV when using a 4-s test pulse. Note that the peak I_{tail} measured at –70 mV is larger than the outward current elicited by its preceding test pulse despite the fact that the electrical driving force for the outward flux of K+ is smaller at –70 mV than it is for the more depolarized test pulses. This seemingly paradoxical observation can be explained by the kinetics of channel inactivation, activation, and deactivation. In response to cell depolarization, channels activate very slowly compared with the rate of inactivation (e.g., $\tau_{act} \approx 130$ ms, $\tau_{inact} \approx 5$ ms at 0 mV and room temperature). Immediately after the cell is repolarized to –70 mV, channels rapidly recover from inactivation ($\tau_{recov} \approx 10$ ms) to an open state before slowly deactivating ($\tau_{deact-fast} \approx 150$ ms, $\tau_{deact-slow} \approx 700$ ms).[3] Most importantly, because channels are far less inactivated at –70 mV compared with more depolarized test potentials, tail currents are actually larger than test currents despite the considerably smaller electrical driving force.

Another two-step voltage clamp protocol is used to characterize the voltage dependence of hERG1 channel inactivation (Fig. 12.1C). A 2-s prepulse to +40 mV is sufficient to fully activate all hERG1 channels that then rapidly enter the inactivated state. Repolarization to a variable Vt elicits a tail current that varies in amplitude and kinetics. The initial increase in tail current magnitude represents channels that recover from the inactivated state into an open state; the current then declines in magnitude as the channels deactivate

(transition from an open to a closed state) with a time course that becomes faster at more negative return potentials. A plot of peak I_{tail} as a function of Vt (Fig. 12.1D) defines the fully activated I–V relationship for hERG1, and its deviation from a linear relationship can be used to define the voltage dependence of inactivation (Fig. 12.1E). Note that the conductance–voltage (G–V) relationship for channel activation is steeper and has a voltage half-point ($V_{0.5}$) that is more positive than the G–V curve for inactivation.

Only a few studies have characterized the properties of single hERG1 channels in membrane patches, usually in the presence of high $[K^+]_e$ (e.g., 120 mM), to increase single channel current amplitudes. In cell-attached patches, single hERG1 channel activity is mostly absent at positive voltages (e.g., +40 mV in Fig. 12.1F) because the probability of channel inactivation is very high. On repolarization to a negative potential, the channel reopens after a variable delay (the period between the dotted line and initial channel openings shown in Fig. 12.1F). The delay reflects the time required for the channel to recover from inactivation and is shorter at more negative potentials. Once opened, channels briefly close and reopen repetitively until finally entering a stable closed state. Analysis of these brief open and closed times indicates that single channels have at least two open and two closed states. At –90 mV, the mean open times of single channels are about 3 and 12 ms, and the mean closed times are about 0.5 and 15 ms.[8]

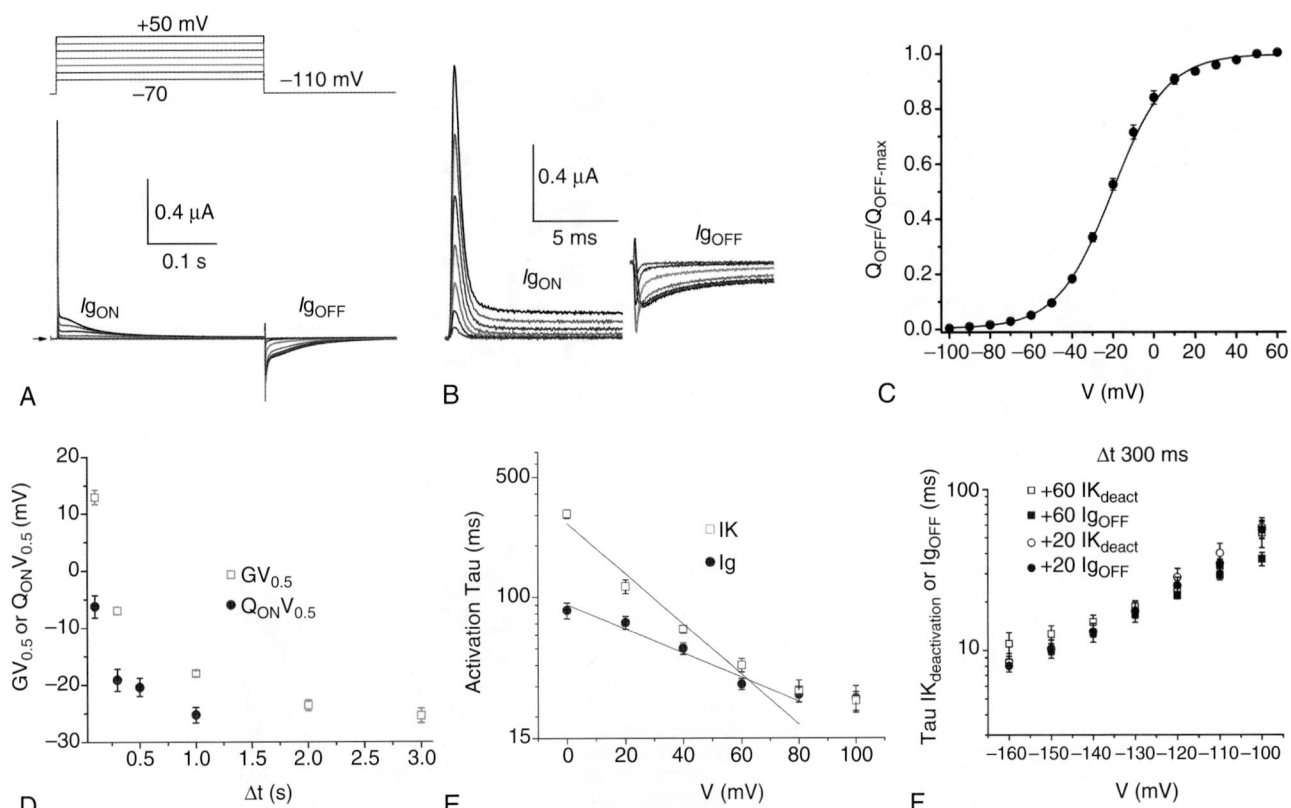

FIGURE 12.2 Human *ether-à-go-go* related type 1 (hERG1) channel gating currents. (A) hERG1 channel gating currents (*lower panel*) recorded from a *Xenopus* oocyte in response to voltage pulses applied in 10-mV increments as shown in the *upper panel*. Currents were measured using the cut-open Vaseline gap technique after a complete block of ionic currents. (B) Expanded time scale for ON gating currents (Ig_{ON}) and OFF gating currents (Ig_{OFF}). (C) Plot of normalized OFF gating charge (Q_{OFF}) for hERG1 channels as a function of test potential ($V_{0.5} = -20$ mV, z = 1.9). (D) Plot of $V_{0.5}$ from G–V and Q–V relationships as a function of pulse duration. (E) Time constants for the onset of activation of hERG1 channels measured from gating currents (Ig) or from ionic currents (IK) as a function of Vt. (F) Time constants for the onset of deactivation of hERG1 channels measured from gating currents (Ig_{OFF}) or from ionic currents ($IK_{deactivation}$) as a function of Vt. ([D–F] From Goodchild SJ, Macdonald LC, Fedida D. Sequence of gating charge movement and pore gating in hERG activation and deactivation pathways. *Biophys J.* 2015;108:1435-1447.)

Gating Currents

In response to a change in membrane potential, intramembrane displacement of the fixed charged residues (Lys and Arg) in the S4 segment of the channel protein gives rise to gating currents. Gating currents are small in magnitude compared with ionic currents and can only be measured reliably after the suppression of ionic currents with pore-blocking agents such as tetraethylammonium. In response to membrane depolarization, outward movement of the S4 segments produces an outward ON gating current (Ig_{ON}) that is comprised of an initial very fast component carrying about 10% of the total charge displacement, followed by a 100-times slower component that carries ~90% of the total charge.[9–12] In response to membrane repolarization (e.g., to –110 mV), the S4 segments move back to their resting position, generating an inward OFF gating current (Ig_{OFF}) with fast and slow components (Fig. 12.2A and B). The total charge displaced in response to depolarization (Q_{ON}) or repolarization (Q_{OFF}) is equivalent and estimated by calculating the integral of Ig_{ON} and Ig_{OFF}. The Q_{ON}–V and Q_{OFF}–V relationships for hERG1 channels are a sigmoidal function of voltage and are well described by a Boltzmann function (Fig. 12.2C), with a slope that is similar to the G–V relationship for ionic current activation (see Fig. 12.1E). However, the Q_{ON}–V relationship occurs over a more negative voltage range than the G–V relationship (Fig. 12.2D), indicating that channel opening occurs at more positive potentials than that required for the displacement of S4

voltage sensors. In addition, outward charge displacement occurs faster than the onset of ionic current activation for Vt <60 mV (Fig. 12.2E). In contrast, the rate of ionic current deactivation (channel closure) is well matched to the rate of return of Q_{OFF} over a wide range of return voltages (Fig. 12.2F). The gating charge movement is asymmetric. After a 300-ms prepulse to a potential that fully activates channels, the Q_{OFF}–V relationship is shifted by about –70 mV (a charge mode shift) compared with the Q_{ON}–V relationship in oocytes.[11] A similar shift has been observed with hERG1 channels expressed in mammalian cells.[13] The mechanisms for the stabilization of the gating charge in an activated position is uncertain, but N-terminal mutations, such as R4A+R5A, that accelerate deactivation also attenuate the mode shift,[11] suggesting that the open state of the pore is a key determinant in this phenomenon.

Structural Basis of hERG1 Channel Gating and Permeation

Similar to other Kv channels, functional hERG1 channels are formed by the coassembly of four α-subunits. Each hERG1 α-subunit (1159 amino acids, mass of 127 kDa) has six transmembrane α-helical segments (S1–S6) and very large cytoplasmic N- and C-termini. The S1–S4 segments from each subunit form independent voltage-sensor domains (VSDs). The ion-conducting pore domain includes the S5 and S6 segments, turret, and pore helices contributed by all four subunits. The S6 segments from

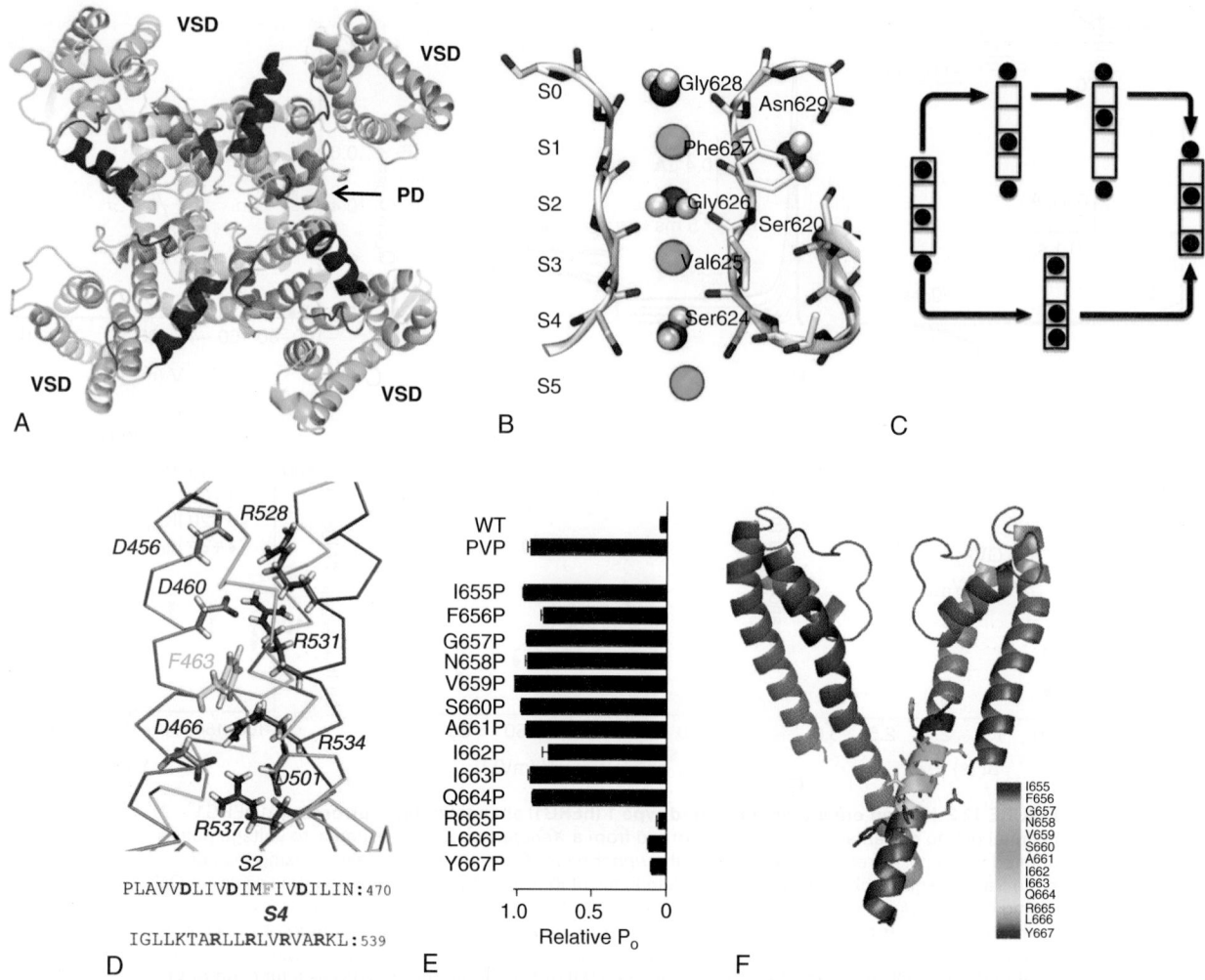

FIGURE 12.3 Structural basis of human *ether-à-go-go* related type 1 (hERG1) channel selectivity and activation gating. (A) Homology model of the hERG1 channel viewed from the outside of the membrane. The four voltage-sensor domains (*VSDs*), each containing identical S1–S4 α-helical transmembrane segments, are located on the periphery of the channel complex and surround the pore domain (*PD*) that is formed by the S5 and S6 α-helical transmembrane segments from all four subunits. The cytoplasmic N- and C-termini are not included in this model. (B) Homology model of the hERG1 channel selectivity filter. For clarity, only two of the four selectivity filter regions are shown. K+ ions (*green spheres*) and water molecules (shown as red/white van der Waals spheres) are located in every other occupancy site (designated *S0–S5*). (C) Model of K+ ion (*black spheres*) permeation through the S1–S4 occupancy sites in selectivity filter for the knock-on mechanism (*lower pathway*) and the vacancy diffusion mechanism (*upper pathway*). (D) Structural model of a hERG1 VSD, highlighting positions of the four Arg (R) residues in the S4 segment (*blue*) and three Asp (D) residues and Phe463 in the S2 segment (*pink*). The amino acid sequences of the hERG1 S2 and S4 segments include residues color coded to match the structural model. (E) The relative open probability (P$_o$) of mutant channels containing a single proline (P) substitution in the S6 segment as indicated. (F) S5–S6 region of two hERG1 subunits showing the location of mutated residues in one of the S6 segments. On the basis of the proline-scanning mutagenesis assay (E), Q664 marks the position of the intracellular activation gate. ([A] Modified from Subbotina J, Yarov-Yarovoy V, Lees-Miller J, et al. Structural refinement of the hERG1 pore and voltage-sensing domains with ROSETTA-membrane and molecular dynamics simulations. *Proteins.* 2010;78:2922-2934. ([B and C] From Ceccarini L, Masetti M, Cavalli A, Recanatini M. Ion conduction through the hERG potassium channel. *PLoS One.* 2012;7:e49017. [D] Modified from Colenso CK, Cao Y, Sessions RB, et al. Voltage sensor gating charge transfer in a hERG potassium channel model. *Biophys J.* 2014;107:L25-L28. [E and F] From Thouta S, Sokolov S, Abe Y, et al. Proline scan of the hERG channel S6 helix reveals the location of the intracellular pore gate. *Biophys J.* 2014;106:1057-1069.)

each of the four subunits line the water-filled central cavity of the pore domain. Fig. 12.3A presents a structural homology model of the hERG1 channel, viewed from the extracellular side and illustrates the peripheral arrangement of the four VSDs around the central ion-conducting pore domain. The extracellular region that links each S5 to its pore helix is called the turret, and this structure is especially large (~25 amino acids) in hERG1 channels.

Selectivity Filter and Ion Permeation

The C-terminal ends of the pore helices from each of the four subunits are tilted inward, and each is connected to a short and highly conserved "K+ signature sequence" (in hERG1:SVGFG). The selectivity filter (SF) is formed by the backbone carbonyl oxygen atoms of the VGFG residues together with the hydroxyl oxygens of the Ser residues. These oxygen atoms, contributed by all four subunits, are oriented toward each other and coordinate the short-lived binding of dehydrated K^+ ions as they passively move through the SF in accordance with the transmembrane electrochemical gradient when the channel is in an open state.[14,15] The interior of the SF contains four K^+-binding sites, designated as S1–S4, that on an average are occupied by two K^+ ions separated by water molecules (Fig. 12.3B). A fully atomistic molecular dynamics-based modeling approach[14] suggests that K^+ translocation through SF of hERG1 is mediated by both a knock-on mechanism, where an approaching K^+ ion forces a switch to the next occupancy state, and a vacancy diffusion mechanism, where ions move through the SF via the formation of transient vacancies in an adjacent binding site (Fig. 12.3C).

Voltage Sensing and Channel Activation

The amino acid sequence of the α-helical S4 segment in hERG1 subunits (GLL**K**TA**R**LL**R**LV**R**VA**RK**) contains four basic Arg residues (R528, R531, R534, and R537) and two Lys residues (K525 and K538). Only the three outermost charged residues (K525, R528, and R531) contribute to the activation gating charge.[16] The neutralization of R531 most markedly increases the energy required for channel opening.[16–18] Mutations of other basic residues in S4 of hERG1 suggest that K525 stabilizes the closed state, R531 stabilizes the open state, and R534 participates in interactions that stabilize preopen closed states.[19] As the S4 segments are moved through the cell membrane in response to changes in transmembrane potential, basic residues form transient salt bridges with acidic (Asp) residues located within the adjacent and largely immobile S1 (D411), S2 (D456 and D460), and S3 (D501) segments of the VSD. Specific salt bridges that have been suggested by experimentation are K525/K538-D411 in the closed state and R531-D460/D509 in the open state.[17,18,20,21] In the open state, basic residues on the intra- and extracellular sections of the S4 helix are separated by Phe463, which acts as a hydrophobic gating charge–transfer center that excludes water incursion across the VSD and focuses the transmembrane electric field across a region narrower than the lipid bilayer (Fig. 12.3D). Based on double mutant cycle analyses, F463 can form functional interactions with K525 and K538 at either end of the S4 segment and catalyze movement of S4 across the narrowed electrical field.[22]

In Kv channels, including hERG1, the activation gate is formed by the C-terminal ends of the S6 helices (the so-called bundle crossing). In the closed state, the crisscrossing of the S6 bundle crossing creates a narrow aperture and a barrier to K^+ flux between the cytosol and central cavity. Outward displacement of the S4 segment in response to membrane depolarization is coupled to an outward splaying of the S6 helices, thereby widening the bundle crossing aperture sufficiently to allow ions to flow into or out of the central cavity. In many Kv channels, the S6 segment contains a highly conserved Gly that acts as a hinge point for the splaying of the bundle crossing and a Pro-Val-Pro motif that kinks S6 and allows it to make contact with the S4-S5 linker (S45L) that together forms the link that enables electromechanical coupling between the movement of the S4 segment and the opening of the activation gate. However, amino acid substitution of the Gly hinge in hERG1 (Gly657) does not prevent channel opening or alter the voltage dependence of activation.[23] Moreover, introduction of the Pro-Val-Pro motif into the hERG1 channel renders it constitutively open and unable to close in response to membrane hyperpolarization. The location of the intracellular activation gate in hERG1 was determined by Pro-scanning of the S6 segment. Single Pro substitutions of S6 residues from Ile665 to Gln664 trapped channels in an open state, whereas single Pro substitutions of residues Arg665–Tyr667 did not (Fig. 12.3D to F). I663P channels trapped in an open state exhibited normal VSD movement (monitored by voltage clamp fluorimetry and gating currents), suggesting that the Pro-induced kink in S6 (above Gln664) physically disrupts the physical link between the VSD and the S6 segment and that the location of the activation gate is at Gln664.[24]

In Kv channels, S45L is an amphipathic α-helix (Asp540–Leu550 in hERG1) located near the C-terminal portion of S6 that acts as a lever to electromechanically couple VSD movement to the opening of the activation gate (the S6 bundle crossing). The mutational analysis of S45L[25] as well as crosslinking between D540C in S45L and L666C in the C-terminal portion of the S6 segment[26] suggests that S45L is also a structural link that couples voltage sensing to hERG1 channel opening and closing. However, this previously consensus view of the structural basis of electromechanical coupling may not be applicable to hERG1 and related channels. hERG1 proteins interrupted at or lacking S45L can produce channels with voltage-sensing and permeation properties that are surprisingly similar to channels formed from intact full-length subunits.[27] Split channels have normal activation properties, but deactivation is 10-fold faster, as expected for a channel with a disrupted S45L.[27] Thus the transduction of S4 voltage sensing to the intracellular activation gate does not require physical continuity between VSD and the pore domains. In hERG1, S45L can interact with the lower end of S5[28] and/or S6,[29] cyclic nucleotide-binding homology domain (CNBHD),[30] and N-terminal structures.[31–33]

Role of Intracellular Domains in Channel Gating

The cytoplasmic N- and C-termini of hERG1 channels are unusually large structures that interact to modulate channel gating. The N-terminal structure contains 376 residues. The initial 135 residues form the "eag" domain (named because it is found in all members of the eag K^+ channel family) that is composed of two structural domains: the Per-Arnt-Sim (PAS) and a PAS-cap. The N-terminal PAS-cap structure is composed of an unstructured region of nine amino acids plus an 11-amino acid amphipathic α–helix that packs its apolar face against the hydrophobic patch on the surface of the PAS β-sheet.[34] The PAS-cap connects to a PAS domain (residues 26–135), a highly ordered structure that is found in many other proteins involved with sensing environmental cues. Some PAS domains act as receptors for ligands (e.g., flavin mononucleotide, malonate), and although the hERG1 PAS domain also contains a hollow space (≈ 110 Å^3) that could accommodate binding of a ligand, none have yet been discovered.[34] Deletion of, or mutations in, the eag domain (e.g., R4A, R5A, R56Q) accelerates the rate of hERG1 channel deactivation by 10-fold, most likely because it disrupts the normal interaction between the eag domain and C-terminus of an adjacent subunit. Coexpression of eag domains together with N-terminal truncated channels can restore normal slow deactivation.[35] Based on NMR structures and the functional analysis of mutant channels, it was proposed that slow deactivation of hERG1 required an interaction between the eag domain and S45L.[31,36,37] More recent work suggests instead that the main interaction is between the eag domain and intracellular C-terminus.

The C-terminus of hERG1 is composed of a C-linker and CNBHD. The C-terminus structure has not yet been determined for hERG1; however, the C-linker/CNBHD of a mosquito erg channel was recently determined.[38] In this structure, a short β-strand (an "intrinsic ligand") occupies the pocket where a cyclic nucleotide is bound in bona fide cyclic nucleotide–gated channels (i.e., HCN and CNG channels) and explains why CNBHD of hERG1 channels are not directly modulated by cyclic nucleotides. A crystal structure of the eag domain and CNBHD complex in mouse EAG1 channels indicates that these two structures have a very large interface with a buried solvent accessible surface area of about 1400 Å.[2,39] Based on this structure, it is predicted

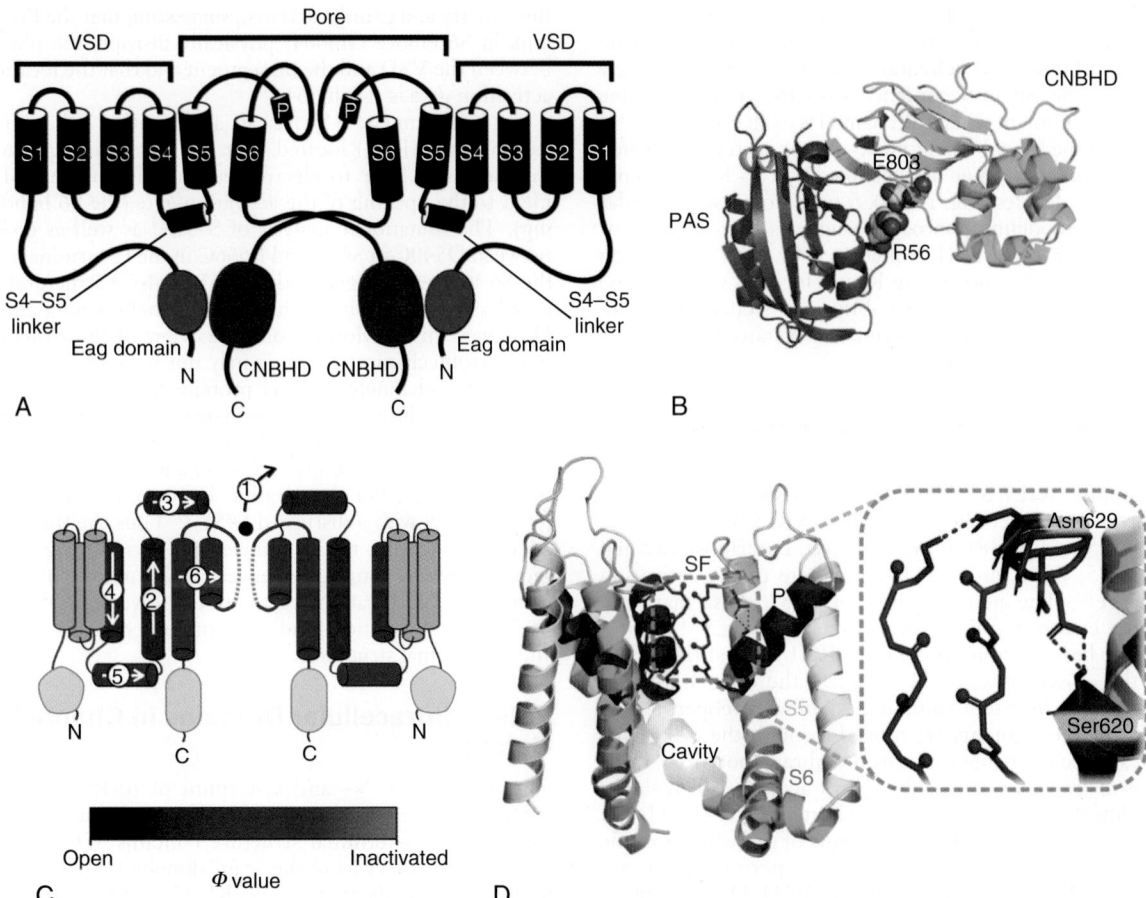

FIGURE 12.4 Structural basis of human *ether-à-go-go* related type 1 (hERG1) channel deactivation and inactivation. (A) Schematic of two hERG1 subunits indicating the α-helical transmembrane segments that form the voltage sensor domains (*S1–S4*) and the pore domain (*S5 and S6*). Also shown are the pore (*P*) helix. The N-terminal eag domain of one subunit interacts with the C-terminal cyclic nucleotide-binding homology domain (*CNBHD*) of an adjacent subunit. (B) Ribbon representation of the structures of a single Per-Arnt-Sim (*PAS*) region of the eag domain interacting with a single CNBHD, highlighting the putative salt bridge formed between Arg56 of the PAS domain with Glu803 of CNBHD. Mutation of Arg56 (R56Q) accelerates channel deactivation and causes long QT syndrome. (C) Proposed sequence of conformational changes in hERG1 subunits that underlie selectivity filter (*SF*) gating of K+ conductance based on Φ-value analysis. Sequential conformational changes associated with channel inactivation are indicated by numbering, starting with 1: the exit of K+ ions from the external side of the SF, and ending with 6: the movement of S6, the pore helix-SF linker, and the pore-S6 linker. The final step is believed to be a subtle rearrangement of SF that prevents K+ ion conductance. (D) Side view of the hERG1 channel pore domain (S5/S6 segments from three of the four subunits shown) highlighting a putative H-bonding interaction between Asn629 located at the outer end of SF and Ser620 located within the pore helix (P) that may mediate inactivation of the channel. ([A] From Gianulis EC, Liu Q, Trudeau MC. Direct interaction of eag domains and cyclic nucleotide-binding homology domains regulate deactivation gating in hERG channels. *J Gen Physiol.* 2013;142:351-366. [B] From Goodchild SJ, Macdonald LC, Fedida D. Sequence of gating charge movement and pore gating in hERG activation and deactivation pathways. *Biophys J.* 2015;108:1435-1447.[C] From Wang DT, Hill AP, Mann SA, Tan PS, Vandenberg JI. Mapping the sequence of conformational changes underlying SF gating in the K(v)11.1 potassium channel. *Nat Struct Mol Biol.* 2011;18:35-41. [D] From Kopfer DA, Hahn U, Ohmert I, et al. A molecular switch driving inactivation in the cardiac K+ channel hERG. *PLoS One.* 2012;7:e41023.)

that the C-linker/CNBHD of hERG1 channels forms a concentrically arranged tetramer with the eag domains located at the periphery,[39] with the PAS-cap of one subunit interacting with CNBHD of an adjacent subunit.[35] Experimental evidence exists for specific interactions between residues in the PAS-cap (Arg4, Arg5, and His7) and residues in the C-helix of CNBHD (Asp843, Glu847, and Asp850)[40] as well as Arg56 in the PAS-cap and Glu803 in CNBHD (Fig. 12.4B).[11] These interactions may be required for the eag domain–CNBHD complex to exert its slowing effect on channel closure. A single subunit, containing a mutation that accelerates deactivation (e.g., R56Q or R4A/R5A), induced the same rapid deactivation of a concatenated channel as

that observed for homotetrameric mutant channels. This finding indicates that the unusually slow deactivation gating of hERG1 channels requires a concerted, fully cooperative interaction between all four wild-type channel subunits.[41] The hERG1 activator RPR-260243 dramatically slows the rate of channel deactivation by binding to a hydrophobic pocket located between two adjacent hERG1 subunits. Each channel has four identical binding sites for this compound. The characterization of concatenated tetramers indicates that deactivation is slowed in proportion to the number (1–4) of RPR-26043 molecules bound.[42]

Alternative splicing of hERG1 RNA produces hERG1b, a protein with a much shorter and unique N-terminus than the full-length hERG1 (hERG1a). The N-terminus of hERG1b lacks a PAS domain and is only 36 amino acids in length. Channels formed from hERG1b alone deactivate very rapidly but can be retained in the endoplasmic reticulum because of an "RXR" endoplasmic reticulum retention signal present on the N-terminus.[43] Heteromultimeric hERG1a/1b channels are expressed in the human ventricle[44] and traffic efficiently to the plasma membrane and deactivate with kinetics that resemble native I_{Kr} measured in isolated myocytes. It has been estimated that hERG1b represents about 10%–25% of the total hERG1 mRNA in the human heart.[45] ShRNA-mediated knockdown of hERG1b subunits in cardiomyocytes derived from human-induced pluripotent stem cells reduced the I_{Kr} magnitude by 50%, lengthened action potential duration, and induced cellular correlates of arrhythmia.[46]

Structural Basis of hERG1 Channel Inactivation

The properties of hERG1 channel inactivation are still being explored, but the characterization of mutant channels and molecular dynamics simulation studies have provided remarkable insights into the mechanisms and structural basis of this gating process. Cysteine accessibility experiments suggested that conformational rearrangements in the outer mouth of the pore mediate C-type channel inactivation in Shaker channels.[47] Recently, it was proposed that C-type inactivation can occur in the absence of pore constriction[48] and might instead result from a subtle dilation of the pore at the outermost K^+-binding site within the SF.[49]

hERG1 channel inactivation is slowed by external tetraethylammonium and elevated $[K^+]_e$, similar to C-type inactivation in Shaker.[50] Elevated $[K^+]_e$ is likely to increase ion occupancy of the outermost K^+ binding site, thereby restricting the rearrangement of the SF. Mutagenesis of hERG1 identified specific residues located in the turret, SF, or pore helix that greatly attenuate or eliminate inactivation, similar to other channels that inactivate through a (usually slow) "C-type" mechanism caused by subtle rearrangement of the SF. Most notably, the combined mutation of two residues within and just outside the SF (G628C and S631C)[51] or a single point mutation in the pore helix (S620T)[52] abolishes inactivation and makes the hERG1 I–V relationship linear. The S631A mutation causes a +100-mV shift in the voltage dependence of inactivation without a significant change in the voltage dependence of activation.[53] Despite these findings, Markov modeling and the finding that S631A does not alter the kinetics of gating currents[9] argue that hERG1 inactivation is coupled to activation, similar to that proposed for other Kv channels. The potential protein rearrangements that mediate transition of hERG1 channels from an open state to an inactivated state have been probed using a technique called Φ-value analysis that examines how point mutations alter the kinetic and thermodynamic relationships between the open and inactivated states of the hERG1 channel.[54] The results of this analysis suggest a rather complex sequence of structural rearrangements that involve multiple regions of the hERG1 channel that has been compared with the opening and closing of a Japanese puzzle box (Fig. 12.4C).

The potential role of subunit interactions during hERG1 inactivation was investigated using concatenated tetramers, containing wild-type and/or mutant subunits, with defined subunit composition and stoichiometry. For mutations located within the inactivation gate proper (S620T or G628C/S631C), the presence of a single subunit in a concatenated hERG1 tetramer disrupted gating to the same extent as that observed for mutant homotetramers, indicating that the final step of hERG1 inactivation involves a concerted, all-or-none cooperative interaction among all four subunits.[55] Molecular dynamics simulations have provided potential mechanisms for how mutations disrupt fast inactivation in hERG1. The nonconductive state of the SF was most likely when the distance between the side chains of Ser620 and Asn629 (Fig. 12.4D) was reduced to favor the formation of a bidentate H-bond.[56] In the S620T mutant, the additional

methyl group adds steric bulk that may alter a potential H-bond network, whereas steric hindrance introduced by the disulfide bond formed between Cys628 and Cys631 prevents the H-bond between Ser620 and Asn629.

Pharmacology of Inactivation Gating

Most small molecule blockers of hERG1 preferentially bind to the inner pore of channels when they are in the inactivated state. The best evidence for inactivation-dependent block is the finding that mutations, such as S620T, that eliminate inactivation also greatly reduce drug potency. However, although a single S620T subunit within a concatenated tetramer is sufficient to fully disrupt inactivation gating, the potency of cisapride, dofetilide, and MK-499 is positively correlated to the number of S620T subunits contained within a tetramer, indicating that S620T substitutions allosterically disrupt drug binding independent of their effects on inactivation gating.[57] The hERG1 activator ICA-105574 (a substituted benzamide) binds to hydrophobic cavities in the pore domain. Each channel contains four identical binding sites, located between two adjacent hERG1 subunits, and occupancy of all four sites is required for maximal drug effects.[58]

Markov Models of hERG1 Channel Gating

A variety of mathematical models have been developed to gain insights into the function of hERG1 channels and its modulation in disease and by drugs. The gating of hERG1 channels has been described using Markov models or Hodgkin-Huxley type formulations, with the former approach more prevalent than the latter. Markov models describe systems, such as hERG1 channels, by a finite number of states and the transitions between them. Typical states of the hERG1 channel models are the closed (C), open (O), and inactivated (I) states. Transitions are commonly described with voltage-dependent or constant rate coefficients.

Markov models of hERG1 channels originate from the descriptions of voltage-gated K^+ channels, particularly the Markov models of I_{Kr} of ferret atrial myocytes[59] and rabbit ventricular myocytes.[60] Studies by Wang and associates[61] and Kiehn and colleagues[62] aimed at the reconstruction of ion currents through hERG1 channels with Markov models. In these studies, voltage clamp protocols were applied to characterize hERG1 channels that were expressed in *Xenopus* oocytes. Elicited current traces were described with parameters from fitting to exponential functions. Measured current traces were compared with current traces simulated with Markov models of different topologies, namely sets of states and transitions. Based on this comparison, appropriate model topologies were identified, and transition rates were defined. Analyses of the degree of sigmoidicity of current traces after channel activation suggested that models with three ($C \rightleftharpoons C \rightleftharpoons C \rightleftharpoons O$) or four closed states ($C \rightleftharpoons C \rightleftharpoons C \rightleftharpoons C \rightleftharpoons O$) are more appropriate than models with one ($C \rightleftharpoons O$) or two closed states ($C \rightleftharpoons C \rightleftharpoons O$) to reconstruct measured data.[61] Further analyses led to the development of a five-state model that accounts for inactivation from the open state only (Fig. 12.5A). In this model, all transition rates were voltage dependent with the exception of α_2 and β_2. The voltage-dependent forward (α) and backward (β) rates were defined as:

$$\alpha = \alpha_0 e^{z_\alpha V_m F/RT}$$

$$\beta = \beta_0 e^{-z_\beta V_m F/RT}$$

with the rates α_0 and β_0 at 0 mV, the charges as z_α and z_β, the temperature as T, Faraday constant as F, and the gas constant as R.

The comparison of measured versus simulated current traces in a subsequent study reinforced that a model with two closed states is inferior versus models with three closed states.[62] Furthermore, different variants of integration of the inactivated state into a model with three closed states ($C \rightleftharpoons C \rightleftharpoons C \rightleftharpoons O$) were investigated. In this study, some single channel recordings exhibited an absence

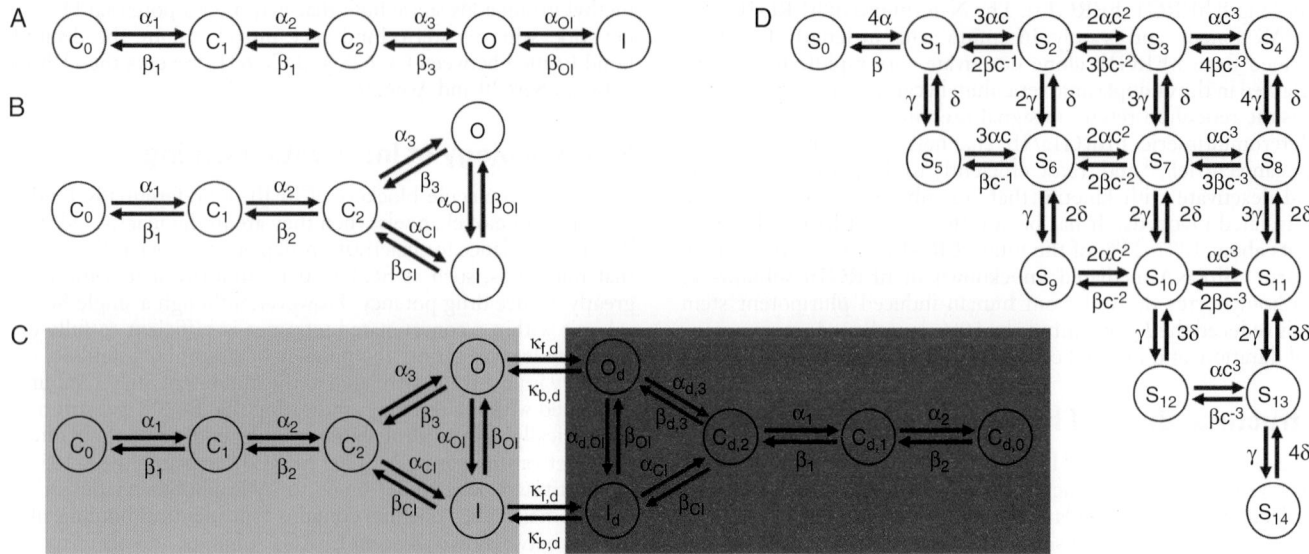

FIGURE 12.5 Schematics of Markov models for hERG1 channel gating. (A) Five-state model with inactivation through open state. (B) Five-state model with inactivation through open and closed states. (C) Two-compartment model comprising models for normal gating (*green*) and gating in the presence of a hERG1 channel activator (*red*). (D) Model for reconstruction of gating currents. ([C] Modified from Perry M, Sachse FB, Sanguinetti MC. Structural basis of action for a human *ether-à-go-go*-related gene 1 potassium channel activator. *Proc Natl Acad Sci U S A.* 2007;104:13827-13832. [D] From Abbruzzese J, Sachse FB, Tristani-Firouzi M, et al. Modification of hERG1 channel gating by Cd²⁺. *J Gen Physiol.* 2010;136:203-224.)

of channel openings during depolarization, which were nevertheless followed by openings during repolarization. Models with inactivation from the final closed state, for instance, the model presented in Fig. 12.5B, appeared more adequate to reconstruct these recordings. However, a recent study suggested an alternative interpretation of these recordings and introduced a model without direct inactivation from the final closed states that can explain the experimental data.[63] This study compared models of different topologies. The only model that effectively reproduced experimental data was based on the topology presented in Fig. 12.5A.

Several studies applied the model topologies presented in Fig. 12.5A and B to derive hERG1 channel models by the parameterization of transition rates.[64–66] Transition rates were commonly defined as voltage dependent with the exception of α_2 and β_2. Models of the topology presented in Fig. 12.5B have been implemented for several studies of hERG1 mutations. Clancy and Rudy derived hERG1 channel models of mutations linked to long QT syndrome (T474I and R56Q) and a mutation (N629D) causing reduced C-type inactivation and rendering the channel nonselective for cations.[67] These models of hERG1 channels with mutations were integrated into computational models of guinea pig ventricular myocytes. Simulations with the cell models suggested prolonged action potential duration for T474I and R56Q, as well as increased probability of early afterdepolarizations for R56Q and N629D. Loewe and associates[68] used similar computational models of human atrial myocytes to study arrhythmogenesis in several gain-of-function mutations. Simulations of single cells and two-dimensional tissues suggested that N588K and L532P shortened action potential duration and facilitated reentry.

Markov models of hERG1 channels play an important role in studies of drug effects. The first Markov model of hERG1 channels was developed for studies of dofetilide,[69] a hERG1 open–channel blocker. The model comprised four closed states, an open, an inactivated, and a nonconducting state with drug concentration-dependent transitions from the open state that accounted for the reconstruction of the drug effects. The model suggested that the apparent rate of block by the drug was modulated by the rate of inactivation. Recently, a family of Markov models was developed

to investigate the effects of dofetilide and other hERG1 channel blockers.[70,71] Similar as described above for the studies of genetic mutations, the Markov models were integrated into a cardiac myocyte model to investigate drug effects on action potentials. Comparison of simulated with measured action potentials suggested reliability of the computational approach to predict drug effects on cardiomyocyte electrophysiology.

The first Markov model for studies of effects of activators on hERG1 channels was based on a two-compartmental description (Fig. 12.5C).[72] One compartment described normal hERG1 channel gating and the other gating in the presence of the activator RPR260243. Drug-dependent transitions were defined between the open and inactivated states of the two models. Three rate constants were reduced versus the model of normal gating, which suggested that the drug affects both activation and inactivation. Wu and colleagues applied a 7-state Markov model (C⇌C⇌C⇌C⇌C⇌O⇌I) to reconstruct hERG1 channel currents in the presence of the activators ICA-105574 and PD-118057.[58] The study indicated that both activators abated transition between the open and inactivated states (O⇌I). Recently, the Markov model was applied to gain insights into mechanisms of action of the hERG1 channel activator NS1643.[73] The study suggested that the activator affected early gating transitions.

Two Markov models have been developed for the reconstruction of gating currents of hERG1 channels.[9,12] Previous studies established Markov models for gating currents of tetrameric Shaker Kv channels.[74] In these models, the gating current Ig_{ij} associated with transitions between the i-th state S_i and j-th state S_j is calculated by:

$$Ig_{ij} = \left(z_{ij,\alpha} + z_{ij,\beta} \right) \left(S_i \alpha_{ij} - S_j \beta_{ij} \right)$$

with the forward transition rate α_{ij}, backward transition rate β_{ij}, and the charges $z_{ij,\alpha}$ and $z_{ij,\beta}$. In both hERG1 models, the gating current of each channel subunit was described as a process having three states and two transitions (S0⇌S1⇌S2) with differing time constants for each transition. A schematic of the resulting Markov model is presented in Fig. 12.5D. Piper and associates[9] extended this description with two closed, two open, and three inactivated states, which allowed the reconstruction of K^+ currents through hERG1 channels. Abbruzzese and colleagues[12] split the description of gating currents (see Fig. 12.5D) from the description of K^+ currents through the channel. The two models were coupled by the definition of a transition rate of the K^+ current model that is dependent on the states of the gating current model. Interestingly, the gating current model alone was able to reproduce the major features of measured gating currents.

REFERENCES

1. Sanguinetti MC, Jurkiewicz NK. Two components of cardiac delayed rectifier K+ current. Differential sensitivity to block by class III antiarrhythmic agents. *J Gen Physiol.* 1990;96:195–215.
2. Martinson AS, van Rossum DB, Diatta FH, et al. Functional evolution of Erg potassium channel gating reveals an ancient origin for IKr. *Proc Natl Acad Sci U S A.* 2014;111:5712–5717.
3. Vandenberg JI, Perry MD, Perrin MJ, et al. hERG K+ channels: structure, function, and clinical significance. *Physiol Rev.* 2012;92:1393–1478.
4. Lastraioli E, Iorio J, Arcangeli A. Ion channel expression as promising cancer biomarker. *Biochim Biophys Acta.* 2015;1848:2685–2702.
5. Sanguinetti MC, Tristani-Firouzi M. hERG potassium channels and cardiac arrhythmia. *Nature.* 2006;440:463–469.
6. Curran ME, Splawski I, Timothy KW, et al. A molecular basis for cardiac arrhythmia: HERG mutations cause long QT syndrome. *Cell.* 1995;80:795–803.
7. Anderson CL, Delisle BP, Anson BD, et al. Most LQT2 mutations reduce Kv11.1 (hERG) current by a class 2 (trafficking-deficient) mechanism. *Circulation.* 2006;113:365–373.
8. Zou A, Curran ME, Keating MT, et al. Single HERG delayed rectifier K+ channels expressed in *Xenopus* oocytes. *Am J Physiol.* 1997;272:H1309–H1314.
9. Piper DR, Varghese A, Sanguinetti MC, et al. Gating currents associated with intramembrane charge displacement in HERG potassium channels. *Proc Natl Acad Sci U S A.* 2003;100:10534–10539.
10. Goodchild SJ, Fedida D. Gating charge movement precedes ionic current activation in hERG channels. *Channels (Austin).* 2014;8:84–89.
11. Goodchild SJ, Macdonald LC, Fedida D. Sequence of gating charge movement and pore gating in HERG activation and deactivation pathways. *Biophys J.* 2015;108:1435–1447.
12. Abbruzzese J, Sachse FB, Tristani-Firouzi M, et al. Modification of hERG1 channel gating by Cd^{2+}. *J Gen Physiol.* 2010;136:203–224.
13. Wang Z, Dou Y, Goodchild SJ, et al. Components of gating charge movement and S4 voltage-sensor exposure during activation of hERG channels. *J Gen Physiol.* 2013;141:431–443.
14. Ceccarini L, Masetti M, Cavalli A, et al. Ion conduction through the hERG potassium channel. *PLoS One.* 2012;7:e49017.
15. Zhou Y, Morais-Cabral JH, Kaufman A, et al. Chemistry of ion coordination and hydration revealed by a K+ channel-Fab complex at 2.0 A resolution. *Nature.* 2001;414:43–48.
16. Zhang M, Liu J, Tseng GN. Gating charges in the activation and inactivation processes of the HERG channel. *J Gen Physiol.* 2004;124:703–718.
17. Piper DR, Hinz WA, Tallurri CK, et al. Regional specificity of human *ether-à-go-go*-related gene channel activation and inactivation gating. *J Biol Chem.* 2005;280:7206–7217.
18. Subbiah RN, Kondo M, Campbell TJ, et al. Tryptophan scanning mutagenesis of the HERG K+ channel: the S4 domain is loosely packed and likely to be lipid exposed. *J Physiol.* 2005;569:367–379.
19. Subbiah RN, Clarke CE, Smith DJ, et al. Molecular basis of slow activation of the human *ether-à-go-go* related gene potassium channel. *J Physiol.* 2004;558:417–431.
20. Piper DR, Rupp J, Sachse FB, et al. Cooperative interactions between R531 and acidic residues in the voltage sensing module of hERG1 channels. *Cell Physiol Biochem.* 2008;21:37–46.
21. Zhang M, Liu J, Jiang M, et al. Interactions between charged residues in the transmembrane segments of the voltage-sensing domain in the hERG channel. *J Membr Biol.* 2005;207:169–181.
22. Cheng YM, Hull CM, Niven CM, et al. Functional interactions of voltage sensor charges with an S2 hydrophobic plug in hERG channels. *J Gen Physiol.* 2013;142:289–303.
23. Hardman RM, Stansfeld PJ, Dalibalta S, et al. Activation gating of hERG potassium channels: S6 glycines are not required as gating hinges. *J Biol Chem.* 2007;282:31972–31981.
24. Thouta S, Sokolov S, Abe Y, et al. Proline scan of the HERG channel S6 helix reveals the location of the intracellular pore gate. *Biophys J.* 2014;106:1057–1069.
25. Ng CA, Perry MD, Tan PS, et al. The S4-S5 linker acts as a signal integrator for HERG K+ channel activation and deactivation gating. *PLoS One.* 2012;7:e31640.
26. Ferrer T, Rupp J, Piper DR, et al. The S4-S5 linker directly couples voltage sensor movement to the activation gate in the human *ether-à-go-go*-related gene (hERG) K+ channel. *J Biol Chem.* 2006;281:12858–12864.
27. Lorinczi E, Gomez-Posada JC, de la Pena P, et al. Voltage-dependent gating of KCNH potassium channels lacking a covalent link between voltage-sensing and pore domains. *Nat Commun.* 2015;6:6672.
28. Ju P, Pages G, Riek RP, et al. The pore domain outer helix contributes to both activation and inactivation of the HERG K+ channel. *J Biol Chem.* 2009;284:1000–1008.
29. Wynia-Smith SL, Gillian-Daniel AL, Satyshur KA, et al. hERG gating microdomains defined by S6 mutagenesis and molecular modeling. *J Gen Physiol.* 2008;132:507–520.
30. Al-Owais M, Bracey K, Wray D. Role of intracellular domains in the function of the herg potassium channel. *Eur Biophys J.* 2009;38:569–576.
31. de la Pena P, Alonso-Ron C, Machin A, et al. Demonstration of physical proximity between the N terminus and the S4-S5 linker of the human *ether-à-go-go*-related gene (hERG) potassium channel. *J Biol Chem.* 2011;286:19065–19075.
32. de la Pena P, Machin A, Fernandez-Trillo J, et al. Interactions between the N-terminal tail and the gating machinery of hERG K+ channels both in closed and open/inactive states. *Pflugers Arch.* 2015;467:1747–1756.
33. Ng CA, Hunter MJ, Perry MD, et al. The N-terminal tail of hERG contains an amphipathic alpha-helix that regulates channel deactivation. *PLoS One.* 2011;6:e16191.
34. Adaixo R, Harley CA, Castro-Rodrigues AF, et al. Structural properties of PAS domains from the KCNH potassium channels. *PLoS One.* 2013;8:e59265.
35. Gustina AS, Trudeau MC. The eag domain regulates hERG channel inactivation gating via a direct interaction. *J Gen Physiol.* 2013;141:229–241.
36. Li Q, Raida M, Kang C. 1H, 13C and 15N chemical shift assignments for the N-terminal domain of the voltage-gated potassium channel-hERG. *Biomol NMR Assign.* 2010;4:211–213.
37. Wang J, Trudeau MC, Zappia AM, et al. Regulation of deactivation by an amino terminal domain in human *ether-à-go-go*-related gene potassium channels. *J Gen Physiol.* 1998;112:637–647.
38. Brelidze TI, Gianulis EC, DiMaio F, et al. Structure of the C-terminal region of an ERG channel and functional implications. *Proc Natl Acad Sci U S A.* 2013;110:11648–11653.
39. Haitin Y, Carlson AE, Zagotta WN. The structural mechanism of KCNH-channel regulation by the eag domain. *Nature.* 2013;501:444–448.
40. Muskett FW, Mitcheson JS. Resonance assignment and secondary structure prediction of the N-terminal domain of hERG (Kv11.1). *Biomol NMR Assign.* 2011;5:15–17.
41. Thomson SJ, Hansen A, Sanguinetti MC. Concerted all-or-none subunit interactions mediate slow deactivation of human *ether-à-go-go*-related gene K+ channels. *J Biol Chem.* 2014;289:23428–23436.
42. Wu W, Gardner A, Sanguinetti MC. Concatenated hERG1 tetramers reveal stoichiometry of altered channel gating by RPR-260243. *Mol Pharmacol.* 2015;87:401–409.
43. Phartiyal P, Sale H, Jones EM, et al. Endoplasmic reticulum retention and rescue by heteromeric assembly regulate human ERG 1a/1b surface channel composition. *J Biol Chem.* 2008;283:3702–3707.
44. Jones EM, Roti Roti EC, Wang J, et al. Cardiac IKr channels minimally comprise hERG 1a and 1b subunits. *J Biol Chem.* 2004;279:44690–44694.
45. Larsen AP, Olesen SP, Grunnet M, et al. Characterization of hERG1a and hERG1b potassium channels—a possible role for hERG1b in the I_{Kr} current. *Pflugers Arch.* 2008;456:1137–1148.
46. Jones DK, Liu F, Vaidyanathan R, et al. hERG 1b is critical for human cardiac repolarization. *Proc Natl Acad Sci U S A.* 2014;111:18073–18077.
47. Yellen G. The moving parts of voltage-gated ion channels. *Q Rev Biophys.* 1998;31:239–295.
48. Devaraneni PK, Komarov AG, Costantino CA, et al. Semisynthetic K+ channels show that the constricted conformation of the selectivity filter is not the C-type inactivated state. *Proc Natl Acad Sci U S A.* 2013;110:15698–15703.
49. Hoshi T, Armstrong CM. C-type inactivation of voltage-gated K+ channels: pore constriction or dilation? *J Gen Physiol.* 2013;141:151160.
50. Rasmusson RL, Morales MJ, Wang S, et al. Inactivation of voltage-gated cardiac K+ channels. *Circ Res.* 1998;82:739–750.
51. Smith PL, Baukrowitz T, Yellen G. The inward rectification mechanism of the HERG cardiac potassium channel. *Nature.* 1996;379:833–836.
52. Ficker E, Jarolimek W, Kiehn J, et al. Molecular determinants of dofetilide block of HERG K+ channels. *Circ Res.* 1998;82:386–395.
53. Zou A, Xu QP, Sanguinetti MC. A mutation in the pore region of HERG K+ channels reduces rectification by shifting the voltage dependence of inactivation. *J Physiol.* 1998;509:129–138.
54. Wang DT, Hill AP, Mann SA, et al. Mapping the sequence of conformational changes underlying selectivity filter gating in the $K_V11.1$ potassium channel. *Nat Struct Mol Biol.* 2011;18:35–41.
55. Wu W, Gardner A, Sanguinetti MC. Cooperative subunit interactions mediate fast C-type inactivation of hERG1 K+ channels. *J Physiol.* 2014;592:4465–4480.
56. Kopfer DA, Hahn U, Ohmert I, et al. A molecular switch driving inactivation in the cardiac K+ channel HERG. *PLoS One.* 2012;7:e41023.
57. Wu W, Gardner A, Sanguinetti MC. The link between inactivation and high-affinity block of hERG1 channels. *Mol Pharmacol.* 2015;87:1042–1050.
58. Wu W, Sachse FB, Gardner A, et al. Stoichiometry of altered hERG1 channel gating by small molecule activators. *J Gen Physiol.* 2014;143:499–512.
59. Liu S, Rasmusson RL, Campbell DL, et al. Activation and inactivation kinetics of an E-4031-sensitive current from single ferret atrial myocytes. *Biophys J.* 1996;70:2704–2715.
60. Clay JR, Ogbaghebriel A, Paquette T, et al. A quantitative description of the E-4031-sensitive repolarization current in rabbit ventricular myocytes. *Biophys J.* 1995;69:1830–1837.
61. Wang S, Liu S, Morales MJ, et al. A quantitative analysis of the activation and inactivation kinetics of HERG expressed in *Xenopus* oocytes. *J Physiol.* 1997;502:45–60.
62. Kiehn J, Lacerda AE, Brown AM. Pathways of HERG inactivation. *Am J Physiol.* 1999;277:H199–H210.
63. Bett GC, Zhou Q, Rasmusson RL. Models of HERG gating. *Biophys J.* 2011;101:631–642.
64. Fink M, Noble D, Virag L, et al. Contributions of HERG K+ current to repolarization of the human ventricular action potential. *Prog Biophys Mol Biol.* 2008;96:357–376.
65. Lu Y, Mahaut-Smith MP, Varghese A, et al. Effects of premature stimulation on HERG K+ channels. *J Physiol.* 2001;537:843–851.
66. Mazhari R, Greenstein JL, Winslow RL, et al. Molecular interactions between two long-QT syndrome gene products, HERG and KCNE2, rationalized by in vitro and in silico analysis. *Circ Res.* 2001;89:33–38.
67. Clancy CE, Rudy Y. Cellular consequences of HERG mutations in the long QT syndrome: precursors to sudden cardiac death. *Cardiovasc Res.* 2001;50:301–313.
68. Loewe A, Wilhelms M, Fischer F, et al. Arrhythmic potency of human *ether-à-go-go*-related gene mutations L532P and N588K in a computational model of human atrial myocytes. *Europace.* 2014;16:435–443.
69. Snyders DJ, Chaudhary A. High affinity open channel block by dofetilide of *HERG* expressed in a human cell line. *Mol Pharmacol.* 1996;49:949–955.
70. Di Veroli GY, Davies MR, Zhang H, et al. High-throughput screening of drug-binding dynamics to HERG improves early drug safety assessment. *Am J Physiol Heart Circ Physiol.* 2013;304:H104–H117.
71. DiVeroli GY, Davies MR, Zhang H, et al. hERG inhibitors with similar potency but different binding kinetics do not pose the same proarrhythmic risk: implications for drug safety assessment. *J Cardiovasc Electrophysiol.* 2014;25:197–207.
72. Perry M, Sachse FB, Sanguinetti MC. Structural basis of action for a human *ether-à-go-go*-related gene 1 potassium channel activator. *Proc Natl Acad Sci U S A.* 2007;104:13827–13832.
73. Perissinotti LL, Guo J, De Biase PM, et al. Kinetic model for NS1643 drug activation of WT and L529I variants of Kv11.1 (hERG1) potassium channel. *Biophys J.* 2015;108:1414–1424.
74. Zagotta WN, Hoshi T, Aldrich RW. Shaker potassium channel gating. III: evaluation of kinetic models for activation. *J Gen Physiol.* 1994;103:321–362.

13 Molecular Regulation of Cardiac Inward Rectifier Potassium Channels by Pharmacological Agents

Manuel Zarzoso, Michelle Reiser, and Sami F. Noujaim

The currents that flow through Kir channels include the inward rectifier (I_{K1}) and the acetylcholine-activated (I_{KACh}) and adenosine triphosphate (ATP)–sensitive (I_{KATP}) currents. Kir-like nonselective channels have recently been reported in prokaryotic cells, but their presence and relevance in eukaryotic cells and cardiomyocytes are unclear.[1] The Kir α-subunit is composed of two transmembrane domains (M1 and M2), flanking a pore-forming motif that contains the GYG sequence of the K⁺ selectivity filter and the intracellular N- and C-termini.[2] The channels can homotetramerize or heterotetramerize.[3] Kir channels lack the voltage-gating behavior that depends on the presence of an "S4" transmembrane domain, which is typically present in Kv channels. The pore forming α-subunits are composed of Kir1.x–Kir7.x proteins, which are encoded by the *KCNJ1* through *KCNJ16* genes.[3] In the heart, Kir2.x, Kir3.x, and Kir6.x are expressed (Table 13.1); however, their expression is variable among animal species and among different cardiac chambers.[4] Kir channels are characterized by inward rectification, where the currents are better conducted in the inward direction. Rectification depends on the block of the outward K⁺ flow by cytoplasmic divalent cations and positively charged polyamines. I_{K1} and I_{KACh} are considered strong rectifiers, whereas I_{KATP} is a weak rectifier.[3] Table 13.2 lists pharmacological blockers of inward rectifiers.

Inward Rectifier Potassium Current

Molecular Basis

In cardiomyocytes, Kir channels are encoded by a diverse subfamily of α-subunit genes (see Table 13.1). Several members of the Kir2.x subfamily (Kir2.1–Kir2.3) are expressed in the myocardium,[5] and it has been shown that Kir2.1 can homotetramerize or heterotetramerize with Kir2.2 and Kir2.3 to conduct cardiac I_{K1}, depending on the species and cardiac chamber.[4,6]

Crystallographic data has shown that the selectivity filter of Kir channels and their bacterial homolog contain a GYG potassium selectivity filter signature motif in the P-loop region of the channel, which is located close to the extracellular side of the membrane, followed by a water cavity, after which the pore narrows toward the intracellular side of the membrane.[2,7–9] In the cytoplasmic domain, Kir channels progressively widen, forming an intracellular ion permeation pathway.[8–11] Several studies have pinpointed residues that are critical for regulating rectification. Residue D172 was identified as a transmembrane "rectification controller" responsible for the "steep" (highly voltage-dependent) rectification. On the other hand, acidic residues in the cytoplasmic region of Kir2.1, such as E224 and E299, are involved in the "shallow" (less voltage dependent) rectification.[3,8–11] There is strong evidence that polyamines (e.g., spermine) bind with robust affinity in the vicinity of D172 and the selectivity filter, whereas E224, D259, and E299 provide low-affinity binding sites.[11,12] The proximal C-terminus and the M2 domain control the ability of Kir2.1 to interact with other Kir subunits,[13] and several sites have been identified as crucial for interaction with modulators, such as phosphatidylinositol biphosphate (PIP2), with ions, including Na⁺, and with kinases such as protein kinase C (PKC) and protein kinase A (PKA).[14,15]

Physiology

In cardiomyocytes, I_{K1} contributes to phase 3 repolarization and plays a role in establishing the resting membrane potential. There are, however, marked regional differences in the I_{K1} expression in the atria, ventricles, and specialized conduction system and also among species. For instance, I_{K1} density is higher in ventricular myocytes, including Purkinje myocytes, compared with that in the atria.[4,16] Furthermore, the I_{K1} density is small in the sinoatrial node pacemaker cells of mice and rats[17] and almost undetectable in the sinoatrial node and atrioventricular node of larger animals.[18] There are also ventricular chamber specific differences in the I_{K1} density,[19] but the density seems to be similar in epicardial, M, and endocardial cells in canine and guinea pig hearts.[20] Kir2.1 channels are considered to be abundantly expressed in the t-tubular membrane.[21,22] Detubulation of ventricular myocytes during short-term culture is accompanied by the reduction of I_{K1}.[22]

Pathophysiology

Because Kir channels are involved in the maintenance of the resting membrane potential and K⁺ transport across the membrane, they are associated with many vital physiological functions, where their aberrant malfunctioning can cause several systemic diseases, ranging from cardiovascular and neurological disorders to renal dysfunction and neonatal diabetes. Loss- or gain-of-function mutations in Kir2.1 have been identified in long QT syndrome 7, also known as Andersen-Tawil syndrome, an inherited channelopathy that leads to QT prolongation, U wave prominence, and ventricular arrhythmias, including bidirectional ventricular tachycardia.[23] Some LQT7-causing mutations affect PIP2 binding to Kir2.1, while other mutations result in a trafficking defective Kir2.1, as well as a channel loss-of-function.[24] Congenital atrial fibrillation (AF), short QT syndrome, and catecholaminergic polymorphic ventricular tachycardia have been also identified as a result of gain-of-function mutations in Kir2.1.[25] Furthermore, changes in the density and biophysical properties of I_{K1} have been observed in pathophysiology. For instance, I_{K1} is downregulated in spontaneously hypertensive rats, cardiac hypertrophy, and patients with severe heart failure and cardiomyopathies.[26,27] Reduced I_{K1} density was also observed in subendocardial Purkinje myocytes from infarcted dog hearts[28] and is also downregulated in endocardial, epicardial, and M cells from failing canine

TABLE 13.1   Inward rectifiers expressed in the mammalian heart

SUBFAMILY	PROTEIN	GENE	CURRENT
Kir2	Kir2.1	*KCNJ2*	I_{K1}
	Kir2.2	*KCNJ12*	I_{K1}
	Kir2.3	*KCNJ4*	I_{K1}
Kir3	Kir3.1	*KCNJ3*	I_{KACh}
	Kir3.4	*KCNJ5*	I_{KACh}
Kir6	Kir6.1	*KCNJ8*	I_{KATP}
	Kir6.2	*KCNJ11*	I_{KATP}

hearts.[29] The loss of I_{K1} is thought to produce membrane depolarization, action potential duration (APD) prolongation, and both early and delayed afterdepolarizations.[26,27] On the other hand, in experimental models of chronic AF and in patients, an increase in I_{K1} density is observed.[30,31] Data from experimental models have shown that Kir2.1 overexpression increases I_{K1} density, shortens APD, hyperpolarizes the resting membrane potential, and accelerates and stabilizes fibrillatory activity.[32,33]

Pharmacology

In general, blocking I_{K1} prolongs atrial node, ventricular node, and atrioventricular node action potential (AP) and refractoriness.[25,34] I_{K1} blockade could also produce a prolongation of the QT interval, membrane depolarization, and, consequently, a slowing down of conduction velocity because of increased refractoriness and a possible voltage-dependent inactivation of Na^+ channels. Barium chloride, at low micromolar concentrations, blocks I_{K1}, and at slightly higher concentrations, it blocks I_{KACh} and I_{KATP}[35] and causes devastating cardiovascular effects.[34] Compounds of the 4-aminoquinoline family, such as chloroquine (Fig. 13.1A to C) and quinidine, and pentamidine homologs can inhibit I_{K1} by directly obstructing the intracellular permeation pathway through interaction via hydrogen and Van der Waals bonding with several amino acids (E224, E259, and F259) in the water-filled cavity, with an involvement of E300 residue, which is important for intrasubunit hydrogen bonding.[36–40] Those residues have been shown to be the receptor for polyamines and divalent cationic-mediated rectification of Kir channels.[11,12] Additionally, agents such as tamoxifen that interfere with PIP2 binding to Kir 2.1 can inhibit I_{K1}.[41] Yet, quinacrine seems to inhibit I_{K1} via a direct block of the intracellular ion permeation pathway and via interfering with PIP2 regulation of the channel.[36] However, most of these drugs have direct and indirect inhibitory effects on other channels and their trafficking processes.[42,43] Thus attempts have been made to develop I_{K1}-specific blockers related to pentamidine because this compound binds residues E224, 259, and 229 and adopts a U-shaped conformation, thus blocking the channel. However, it also affects Kir2.1 membrane trafficking, decreasing Kir2.1 surface protein expression and affecting the maturation of Kv11.1 (α-subunit of I_{Kr}).[42,43] A new pentamidine analog (PA-6) was developed recently, and it has been shown to be an effective I_{K1}-specific blocker in heterologous systems and isolated canine ventricular myocytes.[40] In pathophysiological conditions associated with increased I_{K1}, blockade of this current in animal models has been shown to be antiarrhythmic and to restore normal sinus rhythm.[37,38,44]

Acetylcholine-Activated K+ Channels

Molecular Basis

The G protein–coupled inward rectifier potassium channels mediate the acetylcholine-activated inward rectifier K^+ current (I_{KACh}). Cardiac I_{KACh} flows mainly through heterotetramers of Kir3.1 and Kir3.4, which share the same membrane-spanning topology as the bacterial KcsA and Kir2.X channels.[8–11] Crystallographic studies suggested that the structure of the intracellular domain of Kir3 channels is somewhat similar to that of Kir2 channels.[11] Binding of acetylcholine (or muscarinic agonists) to the G protein–coupled muscarinic receptor (M_2) results in the dissociation of the αi- and βγ-subunits of the G protein. The βγ-subunit subsequently binds to Kir3 intracellular domains, ultimately leading to the activation of I_{KACh}.[3] It has been suggested that the Kir3.1 residues 236–244 and 320–350 form the pocket for βγ binding,[45] and Kir3.4 residues 209–2455 form a critical pocket for both βγ binding and multimeric channel assembly.[46]

Physiology

The activation of I_{KACh} channels in sinoatrial, atrioventricular, and atrial pacemaker cells leads to the hyperpolarization of the membrane potential, a slowdown of the spontaneous firing rate of pacemaker cells, and a delay in atrioventricular conduction. Vagal stimulation produces heterogeneous shortening of atrial APD and refractoriness, which may contribute to the perpetuation of AF.[47] In ventricles, I_{KACh} is considered to exert antiarrhythmic effects through direct and indirect mechanisms, including, but not limited to, the antagonism of sympathetic activity.[48] The density of I_{KACh} is much larger in the atria (approximately six times) than in the ventricles,[20] which has been proposed to be classically underestimated as a result of the presence of a large I_{K1}.[49] Kir3 channels are also expressed in sinoatrial nodes, atrioventricular nodes, and atrial cells, and the I_{KACh} density varies throughout the atrial myocardium.[25,50]

Pathophysiology

A mutation in Kir3.4, leading to loss-of-function in I_{KACh}, has been found in a family with congenital long QT syndrome. The precise mechanism by which the prolongation of the QT interval occurs is not completely understood.[51] Additionally, it has been shown in humans with chronic AF and in animal models of chronic AF that the inward rectifier potassium current (I_{KACh}) has been remodeled.[52,53] In baseline physiology, the I_{KACh} activity is minimal.[3] As discussed earlier, following parasympathetic stimulation, the channel activates. Because I_{KACh} is important in heart rate modulation, the on/off switching of the current is a tightly regulated process. In chronic AF, although the canonical acetylcholine-activated current is downregulated,[30] I_{KACh} is constitutively active, irrespective of parasympathetic stimulation, because of the possible involvement of PKC.[53] This leads to a net increase in the baseline background inward rectifier current. We have provided evidence showing that increasing the inward rectifier current leads to shortening of APD and the subsequent formation of stable electrical rotors, which activate the myocardium at high frequencies, and thus lead to fibrillation.[32,50] Consequently, it is thought that blocking I_{KACh} offers an anti-AF pharmacotherapy.[54]

Pharmacology

Stimulation of I_{KACh} activity can be performed by intracellular ATP and PIP2 as well as with μ-opioid, α2-adrenergic, and A1-adenosine receptor agonists, whereas its inhibition can be achieved by intracellular acidification, myocardial stretch, modulation of the Gi machinery and its regulators, and several antiarrhythmic drugs.[3] Chloroquine blocks I_{KACh} and has been shown to stop AF in animal models and patients.[37,55,56] We have shown that chloroquine blocks I_{KACh} in a similar mechanism to I_{K1} block (Fig. 13.1D–F), where the drug binds residues important for polyamine binding in the intracellular vestibule.[37] Currently used antiarrhythmic drugs, such as flecainide, propafenone, amiodarone, and dronedarone, block I_{KACh} with varying potency, while drugs such as disopyramide, procainamide, and

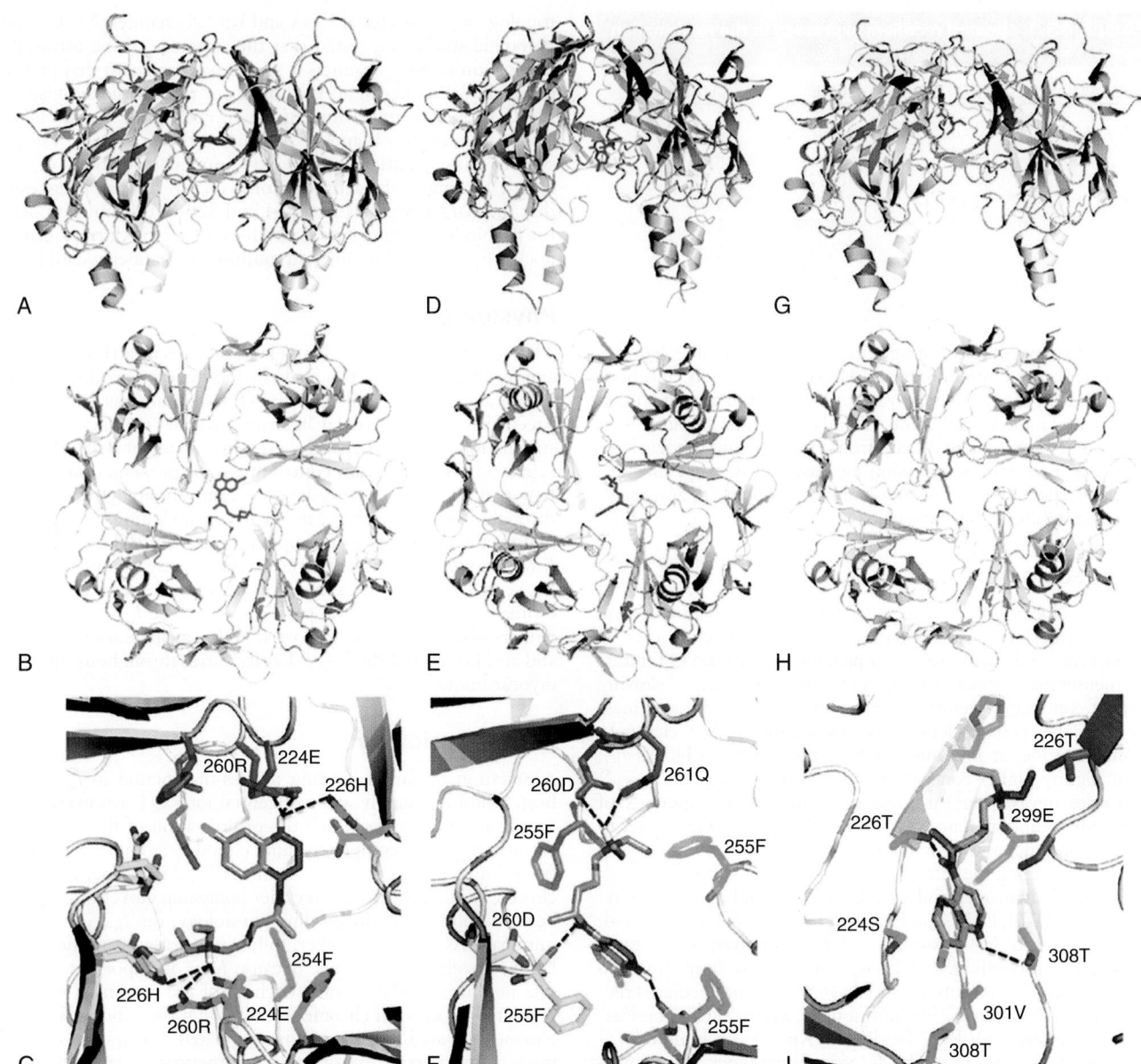

FIGURE 13.1 Molecular docking of chloroquine in the intracellular domains of Kir2.1, Kir3.1, and Kir6.1. The drug blocks the permeation pathways in Kir2.1, 3.1, and 6.1. The *ribbon structure* for the Kir proteins is in *gray*. Chloroquine is represented as *pink sticks*. The images show the lowest energy binding of chloroquine to Kir2.1 (A–C), Kir3.1 (D–F), and Kir6.2 (G–I). (A), (D), and (G) are the longitudinal view. (B), (E), and (H) are a bird's eye view from the cytoplasm. (C), (F), and (I) show the zoomed-in view on the bound chloroquine, where amino acids residues within 4 Å of the chloroquine are depicted as *sticks*. Hydrogen bonds are represented by *black dashed lines*. (From Noujaim SF, Stuckey JA, Ponce-Balbuena D, et al. Specific residues of the cytoplasmic domains of cardiac inward rectifier potassium channels are effective antifibrillatory targets. *FASEB J.* 2010;24:4302-4312.)

pilsicainide block muscarinic receptors, albeit in a nonselective manner. High-throughput screening for the identification of new and relatively specific I_{KACh} blockers of the amiloride and propafenone families[57] and of the compounds related to Kir1.1 inhibitors[58] have been undertaken. The compound VU573 was found to preferentially inhibit cardiac and neuronal I_{KACh},[58] but its use as a pharmacotherapy for AF has not been documented. The bee venom toxin tertiapin-Q has been successfully used to terminate experimental AF.[59] Likewise, it has been reported that NTC-801,[60] a benzopyrene derivative, and AZD2927,[61] a benzamide-related compound, which selectively inhibit I_{KACh} at submicromolar concentrations, exerted antiarrhythmic effects mediated by atrial-selective effective refractory period prolongation in animal models of tachypacing-induced AF.[62,63] The drugs failed to revert paroxysmal AF and atrial flutter, respectively, in patients.[60,61] This could be because of differences in the ionic bases of AF in animal models versus humans. However, it should be noted that there is no evidence that I_{KACh} is constitutively active in the atrial myocytes of patients with paroxysmal AF, let alone in atrial flutter. Therefore future efforts aimed at finding novel I_{KACh} blockers should focus on agents that are capable of inhibiting constitutively active I_{KACh} and should be used in the subset of AF patients where the current has been established to be constitutively active.

TABLE 13.2 Pharmacological blockers of inward rectifier currents

COMPOUND	I_{K1}	I_{KACh}	I_{KATP}
5-Hydroxydecanoate			81 µM
AF-DX 116		10 µM	
Ajmaline			145 µM
Amiodarone	>20 µM	1 µM	
Atropine	>0.5 µM		
AVE0118		6 µM	
Azimilide	100 µM		
Barium	0.5–10.3 µM	10–100 µM	10–100 µM
Bepridil			6.3 µM
Bretilium			>2 mM
Chloroquine	0.7 µM	0.4 µM	0.5 µM
Cibenzoline			6.6 µM
Clofilium			3.3 µM
Diltiazem			135 µM
Disopyramide		1.7 µM	17.8 µM
Dronedarone		10 nM	
Flecainide		19 µM	17.3 µM
Glibenclamide			3–6 µM
HMR1098			1.5 µM
HMR1556	>10 µM		
HMR1883			10 µM
LY97241	1–10 µM		
Nicotine	4 µM		
NTC-801		10–100 nM	
PA-6	200 nM		
Pentamidine	170 nM		
Pentobarbital	0.26–0.54 µM		
Pilsicainide		25 µM	
Pirmenol		68 µM	
Prenylamine		38 µM	
Propafenone	7.1 µM	0.7 µM	63.1 µM
Propranolol			131 µM
Quinacrine	100 µM		
Quinidine	1.2 µM	60 µM	10 µM
Risperidone	>30 µM		
RP58866	3.4–8 µM	2 µM	
Terikalant		>5 µM	
Tertiapin		30 nM	
Verapamil			85 µM
VU573		2–10 µM	

Adenosine Triphosphate–Sensitive K+ Channels

Molecular Basis

The canonical sarcolemmal ATP-sensitive potassium current flows through the heterooctameric complexes of four pore-forming Kir6 channel subunits associated with four regulatory sulfonylurea receptors (SURs). The pore-forming subunit has two membrane-spanning regions (Kir6.1 or Kir6.2), similar to Kir3 and Kir2. KCNJ8 (Kir6.1) and KCNJ11 (Kir6.2) and mainly two SUR genes, *ABCC8* (SUR1) and *ABCC9* (SUR2), encode the mammalian I_{KATP}. Although several alternatively spliced SUR protein variants are found in the heart, these regulatory subunits confer distinct physiological and pharmacological properties on the channel complex.[3,64] The closure of I_{KATP} is metabolically controlled by ATP at the Kir6 level. SUR2A has three transmembrane domains (TMD0, TMD1, and TMD2), each consisting of five, five, and six membrane-spanning regions and two nucleotide-binding folds (NBF1 and NBF2), located in the loop between TMD1 and TMD2 and in the C-terminus, respectively.[65] The SUR2A subunit is sensitive to sulfonylureas

and K+ channel openers such as pinacidil.[65] In addition, the PIP2 interaction at a site near the ATP inhibitory site provides an energetic pull to open channels, and sulfonylureas or glibenclamide interact with SUR to cause channel closure or opening, respectively.[3,64] Additionally, when the adenosine diphosphate–to–ATP ratio increases in the cell, I_{KATP} is activated. K_{ATP} channels were initially identified in the sarcolemmal membrane. It was later demonstrated that diazoxide, a mitochondrial I_{KATP} opener, can provide cardioprotection against ischemia at concentrations that did not activate the sarcolemmal I_{KATP}. Cromakalim, a sarcolemmal I_{KATP} opener, also provided cardioprotection.[66] The molecular identity of mitochondrial I_{KATP} remains elusive, given the inability to detect SUR or Kir6.1/2 subunits in the mitochondria. This led to the alternative hypotheses that renal outer medullary potassium channel (ROMK; Kir1.1) could be the pore-forming subunit of mitochondrial I_{KATP}.[67] Nevertheless, the exact molecular nature and relevance of sarcolemmal versus mitochondrial I_{KATP} remain an active field of investigation. Kir6.1 and predominantly Kir6.2, as well as SUR2A, SUR2B, and SUR1, are all expressed in the heart, and in the ventricular myocytes, sarcolemmal I_{KATP} channels are composed primarily of SUR2A and Kir6.2; however, in the atria, the regulatory SUR1 is predominantly expressed. In Purkinje cells, it seems that the current is conducted through Kir6.1 and SUR2B.[68]

Physiology

Under normal metabolic conditions, cardiac sarcolemmal I_{KATP} channels are thought to be mainly closed and do not significantly contribute to cell excitability.[64] On the other hand, it has been suggested that the sarcolemmal I_{KATP} activity is necessary for optimal adaptation to physiological or pathophysiological stress; when the heart is exposed to hemodynamic stress, sarcolemmal I_{KATP} channels might be activated and might regulate AP, thereby preventing intracellular Ca^{2+} overload because of increased Ca^{2+} influx during the plateau phase.[69] Furthermore, sarcolemmal I_{KATP} channels in the heart may be activated even under physiological conditions with increased metabolic demand. For instance, it has been reported that intracellular lactate can directly modulate I_{KATP} in the presence of moderate ATP levels in rabbit ventricular cells.[70]

Pathophysiology

It is accepted that I_{KATP} is activated when the heart is exposed to severe metabolic stress such as in anoxia, metabolic inhibition, or ischemia.[64] The activation of sarcolemmal I_{KATP} channels during myocardial ischemia shortens AP and decreases Ca^{2+} influx through L-type channels, preventing cardiac Ca^{2+} overload, preserving ATP levels, and increasing cell survival. I_{KATP} also results in APD shortening, accumulation of extracellular K+, depolarization of the resting membrane potential, and reduction in the conduction velocity, which are all proarrhythmic electrophysiological effects that leave the ischemic heart vulnerable to arrhythmias.[71] It has been shown that the activation of I_{KATP} by means of single or multiple brief periods of ischemia (ischemic preconditioning) preceding prolonged ischemia can be beneficial and can confer cardioprotection, reducing myocardial infarct size and the severity of stunning. It has been reported that the shortening of the atrial refractory period after hours of rapid atrial pacing was reversed by MR1098, suggesting that the atrial sarcolemmal I_{KATP} might be activated several hours after the induction of AF.[72] Conversely, the I_{KATP} density and mRNA level of Kir6.2 were reduced in atrial cells from patients with persistent AF.[73] While mechanistically unclear, gain-of-function mutations in I_{KATP} associated with the Kir6.1 pore subunit have been suggested as causes of J wave syndrome and idiopathic ventricular fibrillation, while loss-of-function mutations could cause sudden infant death syndrome.[64,74]

Pharmacology

I_{KATP} openers, such as pinacidil, diazoxide, bimakalim, cromakalim, rimakalim, and nicorandil, bind at distinct zones spread throughout the SUR subunits and include the regions of TMD1, NBD1, TMD2, intracellular loop joining TM13 and TM14, and TM16 and TM17 (residues K1249 and T1253).[65] Diazoxide is an effective activator of SUR1 and SUR2B but not of SUR2A, whereas pinacidil and cromakalim are activators of SUR2A and SUR2B but not of SUR1.[75] The cardioprotective effects of most of these drugs are shadowed by the hypotensive actions, resulting from the activation of vascular I_{KATP}. Moreover, because I_{KATP} density is larger in the epicardium and has been shown to be present in a left-to-right ventricular gradient, I_{KATP} openers produce an increased dispersion of AP duration and arrhythmogenesis.[76] I_{KATP} is blocked by sulfonylureas (i.e., glibenclamide, glipizide, glimepiride, tolbutamide), glinides (repaglinide, nateglinide), and various antiarrhythmic drugs. Additionally, tamoxifen inhibits the channel, partly by interfering with PIP2 binding.[77] All SUR isoforms are inhibited by glibenclamide, with SUR1 being more sensitive than SUR2.[75] Cardiac I_{KATP} blockers could be beneficial from an electrophysiological rather than a metabolic point of view, preventing APD shortening and ventricular fibrillation during myocardial ischemia and reperfusion.[76,78] However, because K_{ATP} channels are expressed in pancreatic cells and smooth muscles, I_{KATP} blockers that activate Kir6.1 and Kir6.2 channels can produce hypoglycemia and coronary vasoconstriction. Additionally, chloroquine, which blocks I_{KATP} (Fig. 13.1G to I), was shown to stop ventricular fibrillation in the presence of pinacidil.[37] It has been argued that the chronic block of I_{KATP} in the compromised myocardium may aggravate myocardial damage by intracellular Ca^{2+} overload.[74] It was further proposed that mitochondrial rather than sarcolemmal I_{KATP} is responsible for ischemic preconditioning. Diazoxide, a mitochondrial I_{KATP} agonist, mimicked preconditioning, while 5-hydroxydecanoate, considered to be a mitochondrial I_{KATP} blocker, suppressed cardioprotection, resulting from preconditioning and diazoxide.[79] However, evidence has shown that diazoxide also activates sarcolemmal I_{KATP}.[80] Therefore the selectivity of such pharmacological agents in regulating cardiac mitochondrial I_{KATP} has been questioned.[81] BMS-191095 is yet another mitochondrial I_{KATP} opener that was shown to exert cardioprotective effects by reducing infarct size without affecting AP.[82,83]

REFERENCES

1. Zubcevic L, Wang S, Bavro VN, et al. Modular design of the selectivity filter pore loop in a novel family of prokaryotic 'inward rectifier' (nirbac) channels. *Sci Rep.* 2015;5:15305.
2. Doyle DA, Morais Cabral J, Pfuetzner RA, et al. The structure of the potassium channel: molecular basis of K+ conduction and selectivity. *Science.* 1998;280:69–77.
3. Hibino H, Inanobe A, Furutani K, et al. Inwardly rectifying potassium channels: their structure, function, and physiological roles. *Physiol Rev.* 2010;90:291–366.
4. Dhamoon AS, Pandit SV, Sarmast F, et al. Unique kir2.X properties determine regional and species differences in the cardiac inward rectifier K+ current. *Circ Res.* 2004;94:1332–1339.
5. Liu GX, Derst C, Schlichthorl G, et al. Comparison of cloned Kir2 channels with native inward rectifier K+ channels from guinea-pig cardiomyocytes. *J Physiol.* 2001;532:115–126.
6. Zaritsky JJ, Redell JB, Tempel BL, et al. The consequences of disrupting cardiac inwardly rectifying K+ current (I(K1)) as revealed by the targeted deletion of the murine Kir2.1 and Kir2.2 genes. *J Physiol.* 2001;533:697–710.
7. Jiang Y, Lee A, Chen J, et al. The open pore conformation of potassium channels. *Nature.* 2002;417:523–526.
8. Nishida M, Cadene M, Chait BT, et al. Crystal structure of a Kir3.1-prokaryotic Kir channel chimera. *EMBO J.* 2007;26:4005–4015.
9. Tao X, Avalos JL, Chen J, et al. Crystal structure of the eukaryotic strong inward-rectifier K+ channel Kir2.2 at 3.1 A resolution. *Science.* 2009;326:1668–1674.
10. Nishida M, MacKinnon R. Structural basis of inward rectification: cytoplasmic pore of the G protein-gated inward rectifier GIRK1 at 1.8 A resolution. *Cell.* 2002;111:957–965.
11. Pegan S, Arrabit C, Zhou W, et al. Cytoplasmic domain structures of Kir2.1 and Kir3.1 show sites for modulating gating and rectification. *Nat Neurosci.* 2005;8:279–287.
12. Osawa M, Yokogawa M, Muramatsu T, et al. Evidence for the direct interaction of spermine with the inwardly rectifying potassium channel. *J Biol Chem.* 2009;284:26117–26126.
13. Lopatin AN, Nichols CG. Inward rectifiers in the heart: an update on I(K1). *J Mol Cell Cardiol.* 2001;33:625–638.
14. Logothetis DE, Lupyan D, Rosenhouse-Dantsker A. Diverse kir modulators act in close proximity to residues implicated in phosphoinositide binding. *J Physiol.* 2007;582:953–965.
15. Bichet D, Haass FA, Jan LY. Merging functional studies with structures of inward-rectifier K(+) channels. *Nat Rev Neurosci.* 2003;4:957–967.
16. Vaidyanathan R, O'Connell RP, Deo M, et al. The ionic bases of the action potential in isolated mouse cardiac purkinje cell. *Heart Rhythm.* 2013;10:80–87.
17. Shinagawa Y, Satoh H, Noma A. The sustained inward current and inward rectifier K+ current in pacemaker cells dissociated from rat sinoatrial node. *J Physiol.* 2000;523(pt 3):593–605.
18. Munk AA, Adjemian RA, Zhao J, et al. Electrophysiological properties of morphologically distinct cells isolated from the rabbit atrioventricular node. *J Physiol.* 1996;493(pt 3):801–818.
19. Samie FH, Berenfeld O, Anumonwo J, et al. Rectification of the background potassium current: a determinant of rotor dynamics in ventricular fibrillation. *Circ Res.* 2001;89:1216–1223.
20. Schram G, Pourrier M, Melnyk P, et al. Differential distribution of cardiac ion channel expression as a basis for regional specialization in electrical function. *Circ Res.* 2002;90:939–950.
21. Milstein ML, Musa H, Balbuena DP, et al. Dynamic reciprocity of sodium and potassium channel expression in a macromolecular complex controls cardiac excitability and arrhythmia. *Proc Natl Acad Sci U S A.* 2012;109:E2134–E2143.
22. Christe G. Localization of K(+) channels in the tubules of cardiomyocytes as suggested by the parallel decay of membrane capacitance, IK(1) and IK(ATP) during culture and by delayed IK(1) response to barium. *J Mol Cell Cardiol.* 1999;31:2207–2213.
23. Tristani-Firouzi M, Jensen JL, Donaldson MR, et al. Functional and clinical characterization of KCNJ2 mutations associated with LQT7 (Andersen syndrome). *J Clin Invest.* 2002;110:381–388.
24. Tadros R, Cadrin-Tourigny J, Abadir S, et al. Pharmacotherapy for inherited arrhythmia syndromes: mechanistic basis, clinical trial evidence and practical application. *Expert Rev Cardiovasc Ther.* 2015;13:769–782.
25. Anumonwo JM, Lopatin AN. Cardiac strong inward rectifier potassium channels. *J Mol and Cell Cardiol.* 2010;48:45–54.
26. Nabauer M, Kaab S. Potassium channel down-regulation in heart failure. *Cardiovasc Res.* 1998;37:324–334.
27. Tomaselli GF, Marban E. Electrophysiological remodeling in hypertrophy and heart failure. *Cardiovasc Res.* 1999;42:270–283.
28. Pinto JM, Boyden PA. Electrical remodeling in ischemia and infarction. *Cardiovasc Res.* 1999;42:284–297.
29. Li GR, Lau CP, Ducharme A, et al. Transmural action potential and ionic current remodeling in ventricles of failing canine hearts. *Am J Physiol Heart Circ Physiol.* 2002;283:H1031–1041.
30. Dobrev D, Graf E, Wettwer E, et al. Molecular basis of downregulation of G-protein-coupled inward rectifying K(+) current (I(KACh)) in chronic human atrial fibrillation: decrease in GIRK4 mrna correlates with reduced I(KAch) and muscarinic receptor-mediated shortening of action potentials. *Circulation.* 2001;104:2551–2557.
31. Martins RP, Kaur K, Hwang E, et al. Dominant frequency increase rate predicts transition from paroxysmal to long-term persistent atrial fibrillation. *Circulation.* 2014;129:1472–1482.
32. Noujaim SF, Pandit SV, Berenfeld O, et al. Up-regulation of the inward rectifier K+ current (I K1) in the mouse heart accelerates and stabilizes rotors. *J Physiol.* 2007;578:315–326.
33. Miake J, Marban E, Nuss HB. Functional role of inward rectifier current in heart probed by KIR2.1 overexpression and dominant-negative suppression. *J Clin Invest.* 2003;111:1529–1536.
34. de Boer TP, Houtman MJ, Compier M, et al. The mammalian K(IR).x inward rectifier ion channel family: expression pattern and pathophysiology. *Acta Physiol.* 2010;199:243–256.
35. Azam R. The pharmacology of three inwardly rectifying potassium channels in neonatal rat cardiac myocytes. *Department of Pharmacology;* 1999. PhD thesis.
36. Lopez-Izquierdo A, Arechiga-Figueroa IA, Moreno-Galindo EG, et al. Mechanisms for Kir channel inhibition by quinacrine: acute pore block of Kir2.x channels and interference in PIP2 interaction with Kir2.x and Kir6.2 channels. *Pflugers Arch.* 2011;462:505–517.
37. Noujaim SF, Stuckey JA, Ponce-Balbuena D, et al. Specific residues of the cytoplasmic domains of cardiac inward rectifier potassium channels are effective antifibrillatory targets. *FASEB J.* 2010;24:4302–4312.
38. Noujaim SF, Stuckey JA, Ponce-Balbuena D, et al. Structural bases for the different anti-fibrillatory effects of chloroquine and quinidine. *Cardiovasc Res.* 2011;89:862–869.
39. Rodriguez-Menchaca AA, Navarro-Polanco RA, Ferrer-Villada T, et al. The molecular basis of chloroquine block of the inward rectifier Kir2.1 channel. *Proc Natl Acad Sci U S A.* 2008;105:1364–1368.
40. Takanari H, Nalos L, Stary-Weinzinger A, et al. Efficient and specific cardiac IK(1) inhibition by a new pentamidine analogue. *Cardiovasc Res.* 2013;99:203–214.
41. Ponce-Balbuena D, Lopez-Izquierdo A, Ferrer T, et al. Tamoxifen inhibits inward rectifier K+ 2.X family of inward rectifier channels by interfering with phosphatidylinositol 4,5-bisphosphate-channel interactions. *J Pharmacol Exp Ther.* 2009;331:563–573.
42. Varkevisser R, Houtman MJ, Waasdorp M, et al. Inhibiting the clathrin-mediated endocytosis pathway rescues K(IR)2.1 downregulation by pentamidine. *Pflugers Arch.* 2013;465:247–259.
43. de Git KC, de Boer TP, Vos MA, et al. Cardiac ion channel trafficking defects and drugs. *Pharmacol Ther.* 2013;139:24–31.
44. Warren M, Guha PK, Berenfeld O, et al. Blockade of the inward rectifying potassium current terminates ventricular fibrillation in the guinea pig heart. *J Cardiovasc Electrophysiol.* 2003;14:621–631.
45. Yokogawa M, Osawa M, Takeuchi K, et al. NMR analyses of the gbetagamma binding and conformational rearrangements of the cytoplasmic pore of G protein-activated inwardly rectifying potassium channel 1 (GIRK1). *J Biol Chem.* 2011;286:2215–2223.
46. Wickman K, Krapivinsky G, Corey S, et al. Structure, G protein activation, and functional relevance of the cardiac G protein-gated K+ channel, IKACh. *Ann N Y Acad Sci.* 1999;868:386–398.
47. Liu L, Nattel S. Differing sympathetic and vagal effects on atrial fibrillation in dogs: role of refractoriness heterogeneity. *Am J Physiol.* 1997;273:H805–H816.
48. Brack KE, Winter J, Ng GA. Mechanisms underlying the autonomic modulation of ventricular fibrillation initiation–tentative prophylactic properties of vagus nerve stimulation on malignant arrhythmias in heart failure. *Heart Fail Rev.* 2013;18:389–408.

49. Beckmann C, Rinne A, Littwitz C, et al. G protein-activated (GIRK) current in rat ventricular myocytes is masked by constitutive inward rectifier current (I(K1)). *Cell Physiol Biochem*. 2008;21:259–268.

50. Sarmast F, Kolli A, Zaitsev A, et al. Cholinergic atrial fibrillation: I(K,Ach) gradients determine unequal left/right atrial frequencies and rotor dynamics. *Cardiovasc Res*. 2003;59:863–873.

51. Yang Y, Yang Y, Liang B, et al. Identification of a Kir3.4 mutation in congenital long QT syndrome. *Am J Hum Genet*. 2010;86:872–880.

52. Dobrev D, Friedrich A, Voigt N, et al. The G protein-gated potassium current I(K,Ach) is constitutively active in patients with chronic atrial fibrillation. *Circulation*. 2005;112:3697–3706.

53. Makary S, Voigt N, Maguy A, et al. Differential protein kinase c isoform regulation and increased constitutive activity of acetylcholine-regulated potassium channels in atrial remodeling. *Circ Res*. 2011;109:1031–1043.

54. Ferrari R, Bertini M, Blomstrom-Lundqvist C, et al. An update on atrial fibrillation in 2014: from pathophysiology to treatment. *Int J Cardiol*. 2016;203:22–29.

55. Filgueiras-Rama D, Martins RP, Mironov S, et al. Chloroquine terminates stretch-induced atrial fibrillation more effectively than flecainide in the sheep heart. *Circ Arrhythm Electrophysiol*. 2012;5:561–570.

56. Burrell Jr ZL, Martinez AC. Chloroquine and hydroxychloroquine in the treatment of cardiac arrhythmias. *N Engl J Med*. 1958;258:798–800.

57. Walsh KB. A real-time screening assay for GIRK1/4 channel blockers. *J Biomol Screen*. 2010;15:1229–1237.

58. Raphemot R, Lonergan DF, Nguyen TT, et al. Discovery, characterization, and structure-activity relationships of an inhibitor of inward rectifier potassium (Kir) channels with preference for kir2.3, kir3.X, and kir7.1. *Front Pharmacol*. 2011;2:75.

59. Hashimoto N, Yamashita T, Tsuruzoe N. Tertiapin, a selective ikach blocker, terminates atrial fibrillation with selective atrial effective refractory period prolongation. *Pharmacol Res*. 2006;54:136–141.

60. Podd SJ, Freemantle N, Furniss SS, et al. First clinical trial of specific IKAch blocker shows no reduction in atrial fibrillation burden in patients with paroxysmal atrial fibrillation: pacemaker assessment of BMS 914392 in patients with paroxysmal atrial fibrillation. *Europace*. 2016;18:340–346.

61. Walfridsson H, Anfinsen OG, Berggren A, et al. Is the acetylcholine-regulated inwardly rectifying potassium current a viable antiarrhythmic target? Translational discrepancies of AZD2927 and A7071 in dogs and humans. *Europace*. 2015;17:473–482.

62. Machida T, Hashimoto N, Kuwahara I, et al. Effects of a highly selective acetylcholine-activated K+ channel blocker on experimental atrial fibrillation. *Circ Arrhythm Electrophysiol*. 2011;4:94–102.

63. Yamamoto W, Hashimoto N, Matsuura J, et al. Effects of the selective KACh channel blocker NTC-801 on atrial fibrillation in a canine model of atrial tachypacing: comparison with class Ic and III drugs. *J Cardiovasc Pharmacol*. 2014;63:421–427.

64. Nichols CG, Singh GK, Grange DK. Katp channels and cardiovascular disease: suddenly a syndrome. *Circ Res*. 2013;112:1059–1072.

65. Seino S, Miki T. Physiological and pathophysiological roles of ATP-sensitive K+ channels. *Prog Biophys Mol Biol*. 2003;81:133–176.

66. Garlid KD, Paucek P, Yarov-Yarovoy V, et al. Cardioprotective effect of diazoxide and its interaction with mitochondrial ATP-sensitive K+ channels. Possible mechanism of cardioprotection. *Circ Res*. 1997;81:1072–1082.

67. Foster DB, Ho AS, Rucker J, et al. Mitochondrial ROMK channel is a molecular component of mitoK(ATP). *Circ Res*. 2012;111:446–454.

68. Bao L, Kefaloyianni E, Lader J, et al. Unique properties of the ATP-sensitive K(+) channel in the mouse ventricular cardiac conduction system. *Circ Arrhythm Electrophysiol*. 2011;4:926–935.

69. Zingman LV, Hodgson DM, Bast PH, Kane GC, et al. Kir6.2 is required for adaptation to stress. *Proc Natl Acad Sci U S A*. 2002;99:13278–13283.

70. Han J, So I, Kim EY, et al. ATP-sensitive potassium channels are modulated by intracellular lactate in rabbit ventricular myocytes. *Pflugers Arch*. 1993;425:546–548.

71. Nerbonne JM, Kass RS. Molecular physiology of cardiac repolarization. *Physiol Rev*. 2005;85:1205–1253.

72. Vereckei A, Gogelein H, Wirth KJ, et al. Effect of the cardioselective, sarcolemmal K(ATP) channel blocker HMR 1098 on atrial electrical remodeling during pacing-induced atrial fibrillation in dogs. *Cardiovasc Drugs*. 2004;18:23–30.

73. Balana B, Dobrev D, Wettwer E, et al. Decreased ATP-sensitive K(+) current density during chronic human atrial fibrillation. *J Mol Cell Cardiol*. 2003;35:1399–1405.

74. Nakaya H. Role of ATP-sensitive K+ channels in cardiac arrhythmias. *J Cardiovasc Pharmacol Ther*. 2014;19:237–243.

75. Glukhov AV, Flagg TP, Fedorov VV et al. Differential K(ATP) channel pharmacology in intact mouse heart. *J Mol Cell Cardiol*. 2010;48:152–160.

76. Pandit SV, Kaur K, Zlochiver S, et al. Left-to-right ventricular differences in I(KATP) underlie epicardial repolarization gradient during global ischemia. *Heart*. 2011;8:1732–1739.

77. Ponce-Balbuena D, Moreno-Galindo EG, Lopez-Izquierdo A, et al. Tamoxifen inhibits cardiac ATP-sensitive and acetylcholine-activated K+ current in part by interfering with phosphatidylinositol 4,5-bisphosphate-channel interaction. *J Pharmacol Sci*. 2010;113:66–75.

78. Vajda S, Baczko I, Lepran I. Selective cardiac plasma-membrane K(ATP) channel inhibition is defibrillatory and improves survival during acute myocardial ischemia and reperfusion. *Eur J Pharmacol*. 2007;577:115–123.

79. Sato T, Sasaki N, Seharaseyon J, et al. Selective pharmacological agents implicate mitochondrial but not sarcolemmal K(ATP) channels in ischemic cardioprotection. *Circulation*. 2000;101:2418–2423.

80. Matsuoka T, Matsushita K, Katayama Y, et al. C-terminal tails of sulfonylurea receptors control ADP-induced activation and diazoxide modulation of ATP-sensitive K(+) channels. *Circ Res*. 2000;87:873–880.

81. Das M, Parker JE, Halestrap AP. Matrix volume measurements challenge the existence of diazoxide/glibencamide-sensitive katp channels in rat mitochondria. *J Physiol*. 2003;547:893–902.

82. Gross ER, Hsu AK, Gross GJ. Gsk3beta inhibition and K(ATP) channel opening mediate acute opioid-induced cardioprotection at reperfusion. *Basic Res Cardiol*. 2007;102:341–349.

83. Grover GJ, D'Alonzo AJ, Garlid KD, et al. Pharmacologic characterization of BMS-191095, a mitochondrial K(ATP) opener with no peripheral vasodilator or cardiac action potential shortening activity. *J Pharmacol Exp Ther*. 2001;297:1184–1192.

14 Cardiac Stretch-Activated Channels and Mechano-Electric Coupling

Peter Kohl

Cardiac electrical and mechanical activities are linked not only by excitation–contraction coupling (ECC)—the processes that govern the generation of action potentials (APs) and their calcium-mediated translation into mechanical activity (see Chapter 16)—but also by mechano-electric coupling (MEC), whereby passive and active mechanical properties affect cardiac electrophysiology. In conceptual terms, cardiac MEC complements ECC, integrating cardiac electrical and mechanical activities into a regulatory loop (Fig. 14.1).

The myocardium is a truly exquisite mechano-electric transducer. A tangible example is the classic coronary-perfused heart preparation, established by Oskar Langendorff in the 19th century, which can be stopped or restarted at the flick of a finger. MEC is not restricted to isolated heart models, of course. In patients, the approach of cardiac catheters can be judged by the appearance of premature beats. Mechanically induced ectopic excitation by finger-tapping the exposed ventricular wall is used for reinstatement of sinoatrial node (SAN) rhythm in patients who are being weaned from cardiac bypass, if prior electrical defibrillation has caused asystole.

In fact, manifestations of cardiac MEC are present at all levels of structural and functional integration, from in situ and ex vivo whole heart, over in vitro tissue and cells, to subcellular domains such as membrane patches. Indeed, patch-clamp identification of cardiac stretch-activated ion channels (SACs) by Fred Sachs and coworkers[1] was pivotal not only for the development of the quantitative insight into mechanisms that underlie MEC but also for the advancement of the topic beyond the perception of a scientifically ill-founded clinical curiosity.

This chapter will discuss acute electrophysiological responses of the heart to mechanical stimulation and the involvement of SAC.

Functional Relevance of Cardiac Mechano-Electric Coupling

Effects of cardiac mechanical stimulation on heart rate and rhythm have been reported in the medical literature for well over a century. To name but a few key contributions: pioneering work by Felice Meola and Ferdinand Riedinger identified in the late 19th century *commotio cordis* (also known as *commotio thoracica*) as an independent pathological entity where cardiac rhythm disturbances of varying severity are initiated by nonpenetrating mechanical stimulation of the precordium *in the absence* of visible structural damage to the heart. In the early 20th century, Eduard Schott and Luigi Condorelli reported independently that precordial fist-thumps can be used to pace otherwise asystolic ventricles, such as in Adams-Stokes syndrome patients. At the same time, Francis Bainbridge famously identified the positive chronotropic response of the heart to increased venous return.

Thus from the very beginning of published reports in the modern medical literature, mechanical stimulation of the heart has been found to have the potential of inducing and of terminating heart rhythm disturbances, as well as of modulating cardiac pacemaker rate.

Mechanical Induction of Nonphysiological Rhythms

The fact that mechanical stimuli of sufficient amplitude can be used to pace otherwise quiescent hearts has been elegantly illustrated by Michael Franz and colleagues, using Langendorff-perfused rabbit heart preparations where the ventricles (rendered asystolic by ablation of the atrioventricular node) were stimulated by periodic inflation of an intraventricular balloon (Fig. 14.2A).

Similar behavior is believed to underlie "fist pacing" in asystolic patients. The energy levels required for mechanical induction of premature ventricular beats (PVBs) by precordial impact have been established by defibrillation pioneer Paul Zoll and colleagues in human volunteers as 0.04 to 1.5 J.[2] For comparison, the lower end of this energy range is equivalent to dropping a golf ball (46 g) from a height of 9 cm (3.5 in).

Zoll and colleagues furthermore found in anesthetized dogs that impacts with energies 10 times the PVB-induction threshold do not induce repetitive responses, such as ventricular tachycardia (VT), or ventricular fibrillation (VF), even if applied during the relative refractory period.[2] Overall, this is in keeping with the notion that arrhythmogenesis requires the combination of *trigger* and *sustaining mechanisms*, so that the consequences of isolated ectopic beats, whether mechanically induced or not, are usually benign.

While the above examples illustrate the effects of the external mechanical environment on cardiac MEC (see Fig. 14.1, *bottom box*), mechanical PVB induction may also arise as a result of the heart's own contractile activity (see Fig. 14.1, *middle box*). This is illustrated in Fig. 14.2B, which shows monophasic AP (MAP) recordings from a patient undergoing pulmonary balloon valvuloplasty. In this procedure, the stenosed right ventricular outflow valve is widened by the insertion and inflation of a balloon. During balloon inflation, right ventricular contractions are isovolumic (no ejection) and give rise to significantly increased right ventricular peak pressures. This is generally associated with AP shortening, diastolic depolarization, and the occurrence of early afterdepolarization-like events. If suprathreshold, these can trigger PVB.[3] In a pig model of balloon inflation in the descending aorta, PVB origin has been mapped to basal and apical segments of the left ventricle, indicating a role for nonhomogeneous distribution of end-systolic wall stress in PVB induction.[4] As before, against an otherwise inconspicuous myocardial background, self-sustained repetitive activity is not normally induced.

In contrast, in the presence of an arrhythmogenic structural substrate, increased intraventricular pressure favors reentrant excitation in animal models[5,6] and patients.[7] Even acutely induced nonstructural pathologies may allow mechanically induced PVB to give rise to sustained arrhythmias, as shown in whole-animal studies of pathologically prolonged QT intervals as conducted by Paul Volders and colleagues.[8] In their model, QT prolongation was induced by pharmacological block of the slowly activating delayed rectifier potassium current. On this background, additional β-adrenergic stimulation by a bolus injection of isoproterenol gives rise to ventricular after-contractions of increasing amplitude (up to 25 mm Hg). Originating from near-endocardial locations, their onset precedes (by tens of milliseconds) afterdepolarization-like epicardial

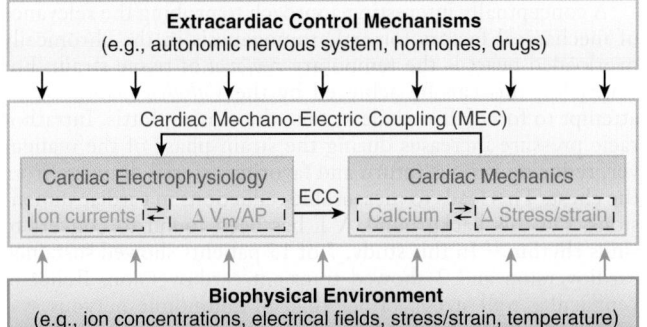

Extracardiac Control Mechanisms
(e.g., autonomic nervous system, hormones, drugs)

Cardiac Mechano-Electric Coupling (MEC)

Cardiac Electrophysiology   Cardiac Mechanics

Ion currents ⇄ Δ V$_m$/AP   ECC   Calcium ⇄ Δ Stress/strain

Biophysical Environment
(e.g., ion concentrations, electrical fields, stress/strain, temperature)

FIGURE 14.1 Schematic view of cardiac electromechanical integration. In the heart (*center box*), electrical behavior steers mechanical activity via excitation–contraction coupling (*ECC*), but in turn, it is affected by mechano-electric coupling (*MEC*). This involves a multitude of interdependent feed-forward and feedback pathways that alter transsarcolemmal and intracellular ion transport, membrane and action potential configuration (ΔV_m/AP), calcium handling, and stress/strain dynamics. Intracardiac electromechanical interactions are modulated by the biophysical environment of the heart (*bottom box*) and form a target of extracardiac control (*top box*).

potentials and alterations in descending T-wave morphology. With increasing amplitude, these apparently regional contraction-induced afterdepolarizations eventually reach the threshold for PVB induction, followed by torsades de pointes–sustained arrhythmia.[8]

Under certain conditions, acute mechanical stimulation alone can be sufficient to both trigger *and* sustain mechanisms for maintained arrhythmias, even in an otherwise healthy myocardium. A prominent example of this is commotio cordis. A number of risk factors for the mechanical induction of such rhythm disturbances have been identified on the basis of experimental observations from the pioneering work of Georg Schlomka[9] to modern-day studies by Mark Link and colleagues.[10] Key risk factors include (1) type of impact (impulse-like stimulation, whose arrhythmogenic risk is inversely related to projectile compliance and contact area); (2) impact energy (large subcontusional forces, reaching over 100 J in competitive sports); (3) impact location (precordial, or in humans also spinal, areas that offer efficient energy transmission from the body surface to the myocardium); and (4) impact timing. Factors 1 to 3 can be regarded as permissive: only if they are all present does timing become decisive.[11] This presumably explains why the vast majority of precordial (or spinal) impacts result in relatively benign heart rhythm changes, if any.

The critical time window for the worst possible outcome of commotio cordis, the induction of VF, overlaps with the T wave. The T wave, during which myocardial electrophysiological heterogeneity is maximal, has long been associated with a period of increased susceptibility to arrhythmogenesis by electrical stimulation—the so-called vulnerable (time) window. Compared with electrical stimulation (with vulnerability lasting for 100 ms or more in large animals), the vulnerable window for mechanical VF induction is surprisingly narrow (~15 ms, prior to the peak of the T wave in anesthetized pigs).[12]

Quantitative computational modeling has suggested that mechanically induced VF is favored during a short period of time only, when the mechanically stimulated tissue volume overlaps with the trailing wave of excitation.[13,14] In this setting, sustained

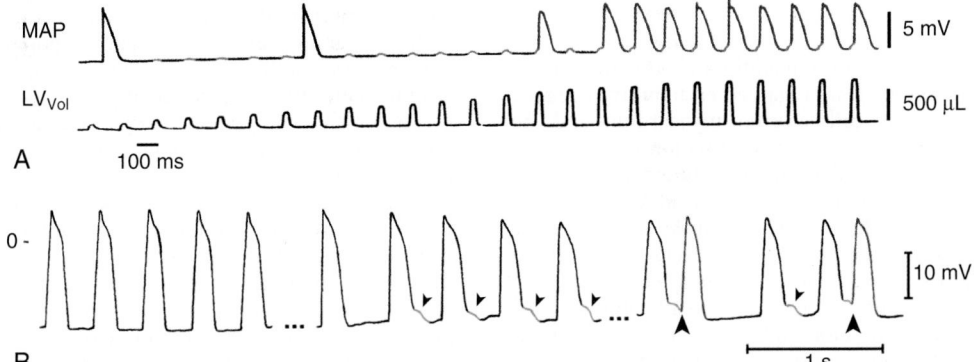

FIGURE 14.2 Mechanically induced premature ventricular beats (PVBs). (A) Mechanical pacing of the Langendorff-perfused asystolic rabbit heart. Pulsatile left ventricular (*LV*) distension (*bottom trace,* showing increasing LV balloon inflation) causes diastolic membrane depolarization (*top trace, blue highlights*). The amplitude of depolarization increases with the mechanical stimulus and, on reaching threshold levels, gives rise to the generation of action potentials (*AP; top trace, red*) with each volume pulse. Note: the first two APs are spontaneous escape beats, unrelated to the mechanical stimuli. LV$_{Vol}$, left ventricular volume increase; *MAP*, monophasic AP. (B) Cardiac contraction-induced tissue depolarization and PVB induction in patients. MAP recording before (*left*) and during (*middle and right*) inflation of a balloon in the right ventricular outflow tract, which gives rise to early afterdepolarization-like events (*blue*) and PVB induction (*red*). ([A] From Franz MR, Cima R, Wang D, et al. Electrophysiological effects of myocardial stretch and mechanical determinants of stretch-activated arrhythmias. *Circulation.* 1992;86:968-978. [B] From Levine JH, Guarnieri T, Kadish AH, et al. Changes in myocardial repolarization in patients undergoing balloon valvuloplasty for congenital pulmonary stenosis: evidence for contraction-excitation feedback in humans. *Circulation.* 1988;77:70-77.)

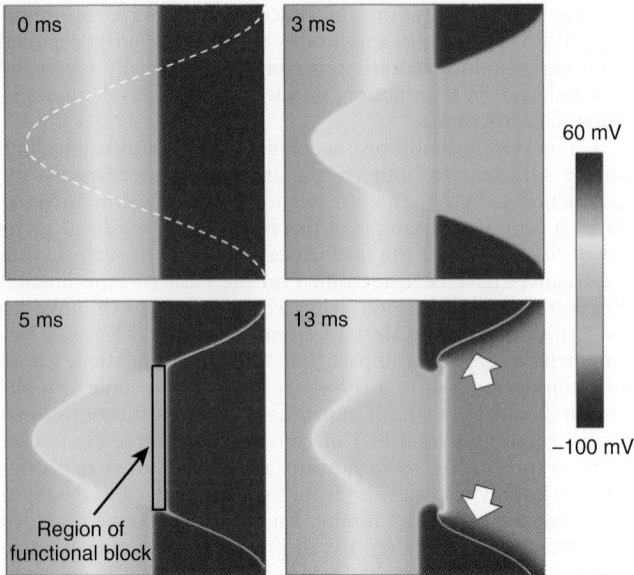

FIGURE 14.3 Effect of local mechanical stimulation during the critical window of the T wave in a two-dimensional model of ventricular free wall consisting of 256 × 256 electrotonically coupled guinea pig ventricular cell models. A local impact to the epicardium (*right-hand side of the grid*), timed to occur at 40% tissue repolarization (see trailing wave-end of the previous activation, which travels from right to left; for color-coding see scale bar), stimulates cation nonselective stretch-activated channels in the mechanically affected tissue (*white outline, top left panel*). This gives rise to depolarization in tissue that has regained excitability and early repolarization of tissue with positive membrane potentials (*top right panel*). If suprathreshold, stretch-induced depolarization causes ectopic excitation (*bottom left panel*). The intersection of the trailing wave and the mechanically induced new excitation forms a functional block zone. This causes the formation of two wavefronts that progress across the tissue almost perpendicularly to the normal direction of electrical wave propagation (*bottom right; see white arrows*) and give rise to the formation of two stable reentrant rotors of excitation. (Data from Garny A, Kohl P. Mechanical induction of arrhythmias during ventricular repolarisation: modelling cellular mechanisms and their interaction in 2D. *Ann N Y Acad Sci.* 2004;1015:133-143.)

arrhythmogenesis occurs because in addition to the mechanical PVB induction in tissue that has regained excitability (trigger), the intersection of mechanically affected myocardium and the trailing repolarization wave gives rise to a region of functional block around which reentry develops (sustaining mechanism; Fig. 14.3). The critical window for mechanical VF induction will differ therefore depending on where on the surface of the heart a mechanical stimulus is applied. However, only a limited part of myocardial tissue is in close proximity to the precordium and hence is susceptible to extracorporeally applied local mechanical stimulation. Therefore only a subset of the (location specific) critical time-windows present throughout the entire heart forms an extracorporeally accessible target for mechanical stimulation in vivo. In other words, the critical window for mechanical VF induction exists in time *and* space. This is qualitatively different from extracorporeally applied electrical stimulation, which is less focused, less application site–dependent, and therefore arrhythmogenic over a longer part of the T-wave duration.

This theoretical prediction has since been validated experimentally in a Langendorff-perfused rabbit heart, where mechanical impact-induced VF was seen only if the site of mechanical contact overlapped with a well-delineated repolarization wave edge (preparations with near-simultaneous ventricular repolarization showed no VF).[15] If the critical nature of individual repolarization dynamics were confirmed in larger species, it would imply that preparticipation risk prediction in athletes is possible on the basis of individually varying electrical repolarization patterns.

In contrast to acute effects, MEC contributions to arrhythmogenesis in *chronic* cardiac overload are more difficult to elucidate. Usually, pathologies that involve cardiac pressure and/or volume overload develop slowly, and they are associated with pronounced structural and functional remodeling. Moreover, the causes of overload and the associated tissue remodeling may both be proarrhythmogenic in their own right. Nonetheless, mechanical factors have been implicated in the domestication of atrial fibrillation,[16] whose inducibility,[17] dominant frequency,[18] and complexity[19] in patients correlate with atrial stretch. Similarly, ventricular arrhythmogenesis has been linked to pressure and volume overload.[20,21]

A conceptually interesting approach to probing the relevance of mechanical factors for arrhythmogenesis in the chronically overloaded heart is the temporary *removal* of tissue strain. For ventricles, this can be achieved by the *Valsalva maneuver*, an attempt to forcefully exhale against the closed glottis. Intrathoracic pressure increases during the strain-phase of the maneuver, reducing venous return and favoring arterial drainage from the chest. This leads to measurable reductions in cardiac dimensions. On this background, VT has been found to convert to sinus rhythm.[22] In this study, 7 of 15 patients showed sustained cardioversion and 2 showed transient cardioversion. Relief of ventricular wall stress, rather than of autonomic nervous system–mediated responses, appears to be a causal contributor to this antiarrhythmic effect, as successful cardioversion can also be observed in the presence of pharmacological[22] and/or surgical denervation of the heart, such as in transplant recipients.[23] More recently, a conceptually similar approach has been applied to patients with long-standing persistent atrial fibrillation undergoing cardiopulmonary bypass surgery. Their pathologically dilated atria were reduced in size by varying the amount of blood provided by the extracorporeal circulation, while multielectrode electrograms were recorded from both the right and left atrial surfaces. Reduction in atrial dimensions decreased atrial fibrillation cycle duration and the number of conduction block zones, illustrating that the removal of tissue stretch may be antiarrhythmogenic (spontaneous conversion to sinus rhythm was not observed in this patient population with significant structural and functional tissue remodeling).[24]

Thus acute stretch (if sufficiently large) causes diastolic depolarization. This can trigger ectopic excitation. Systolic and/or sustained stretch may contribute to arrhythmia sustenance by enhancing heterogeneities in excitability, refractoriness, and electrical load. This has implications for preventive measures (e.g., chest protector design for sports involving fast-moving projectiles), as well as for interventions such as hemodynamic unloading, cardiac assist, or biventricular pacing. In addition, defibrillation threshold increases with ventricular preload,[25] apparently not only because of geometric factors[26] but also because of regionally differing MEC-mediated strain effects that increase background electrophysiological heterogeneity.[27] This adds an interesting dimension to the discussion about whether or not a period of chest compressions (which may reduce ventricular volume and, hence, cardiac dimension) should precede defibrillation attempts in cardiac arrest victims.

Mechanical Termination of Nonphysiological Rhythms

Acute mechanical stimulation, usually by precordial thump (PT), can be used as a means of cardiopulmonary resuscitation. PT has been reported to terminate arrhythmias, including asystole, occasionally VT, and very rarely VF (Fig. 14.4).

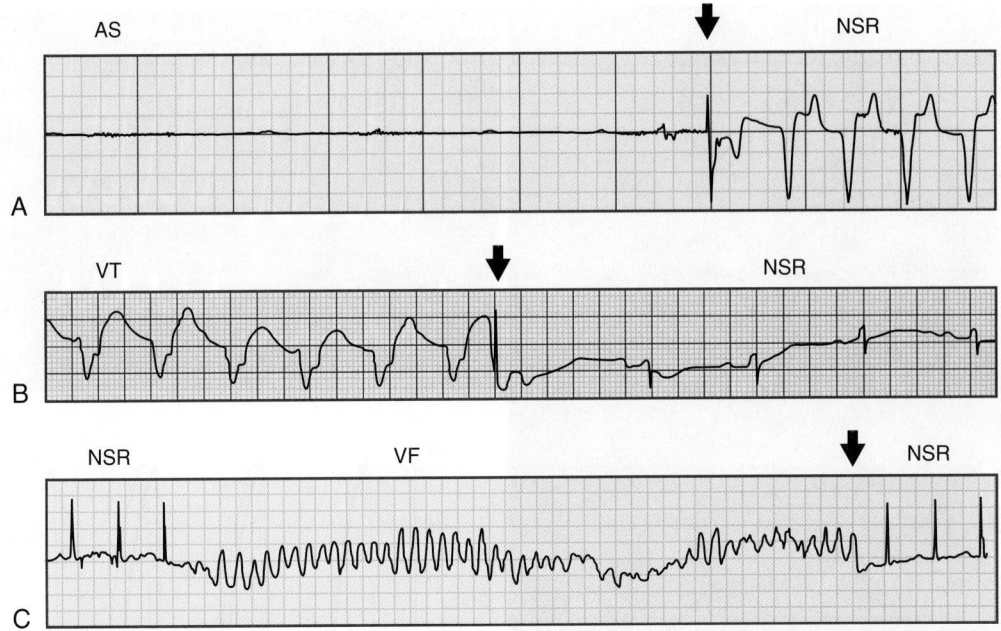

FIGURE 14.4 Electrocardiographic recordings of precordial thump (PT)-induced cardioversion in patients. (A) Conversion of ventricular asystole (*AS*) to normal sinus rhythm (*NSR*) by PT. (B) PT conversion of ventricular tachycardia (*VT*). (C) PT-induced termination of early ventricular fibrillation (*VF*). *Arrows* indicate PT application. ([A] From Pellis T, Kette F, Lovisa D, et al. Utility of precordial thump for treatment of out of hospital cardiac arrest: a prospective study. *Resuscitation.* 2009;80:17-23. [B] From Pennington JE, Taylor J, Lown B. Chest thump for reverting ventricular tachycardia. *N Engl J Med.* 1970;283:1192-1195. [C] From Barrett JS. Chest thumps and the heart beat. *N Engl J Med.* 1971;284:392-393.)

In the emergency resuscitation setting, PT is one of the fastest resuscitative procedures "at hand." PT is delivered with the ulnar side of the clenched fist, from a height of about 20 cm (~8 in), followed by active fist retraction to generate an impulse-like stimulus. The energy levels of PT applied for termination of VT and VF are one to two orders of magnitude higher than those involved in mechanical pacing of the acutely asystolic ventricle (4–10 J vs. about 0.04–1.5 J in the adult).[28] These more powerful thumps are applied preferentially to the lower sternum rather than the left sternal edge, which is targeted for fist pacing/precordial percussion.[29]

Efficacy of PT in real-life settings is difficult to calibrate and compare because patient backgrounds vary, mechanical impact properties are not normally monitored, controlled study designs are not usually possible, and published case reports suffer from "positive data" publication bias. The available information from case series that involved 10[30] to 100 patients[31] suggests that fist pacing of the bradycardic heart has higher success rates (up to 90%)[31] than PT-version of tachyarrhythmias (between 1% and 60% have been reported).[30,32] Few prospective studies have investigated the clinical utility of PT.[32–34] They show that PT is ineffective for most tachyarrhythmias, that acutely asystolic arrest (for which PT was initially described in 1920)[35] may be the most amenable target for mechanical cardioversion, and that negative side effects are rare.[32–34]

In cases where PT causes successful termination of tachyarrhythmias, it is believed to act primarily via the depolarization of tissue in the excitable gap(s).[36] However, as these gaps may be in the myocardium at sites distant from the tissue underneath the precordium, relatively high energy levels (compared to pacing in asystole) are necessary, and if there is a multitude of them (such as in VF), positive outcomes are exceedingly rare.

In an asystolic heart, fist pacing can trigger cardiac excitation and active contraction. The hemodynamic efficacy of such mechanically triggered cardiac contractions is not different from electrically stimulated beats,[37] and both are about twice as productive (in terms of volume output) as chest compressions, even if optimally performed.[38] This confers a resuscitatory value to fist pacing even in cases where normal sinus rhythm is not immediately reinstated. Of course, PT should not delay the implementation of other established resuscitation measures.

The most common manifestation of PT effects in electrocardiographic recordings, particularly of the asystolic heart, is an impact-induced electrical artifact with an electrical axis that tends to resemble the direction of normal QRS complexes. This suggests that mechanically induced excitation in the quiescent heart proceeds along a pathway that has an overall trajectory similar to that of normal activation. It is possible that the earliest excitation is triggered preferentially either in cells of the secondary/tertiary pacemaker/conduction tissue of the heart (such as Purkinje fibers, which have long been known to be mechanosensitive)[39] or in subendocardial locations, which appear to be more mechanosensitive than subepicardial tissues.[8] This may be related to transmural differences in SAC expression levels,[40,41] an area of investigation that deserves further attention across species.

Overall, the range of cardiac electrophysiological responses to mechanical stimulation is not principally different from that caused by electrical energy delivery. Both can be used to pace, cardiovert, or arrest the heart. Concepts such as the vulnerable window for VF induction apply to both electrical and mechanical stimuli. Even the effective energy ranges required for pacing, cardioversion, and defibrillation are not entirely dissimilar (external electrical defibrillation, for example, is usually achieved by extracorporeal energy application of 150–250 J; of this, only about 4% traverses the heart,[42] yielding a cardiac energy delivery of 6–10 J, similar to that for the PT-version of tachyarrhythmias). These similarities should not be surprising because mechanical energy can be converted into a transmembrane current by ion fluxes through SAC at the intervention's target site: the cardiac cell.

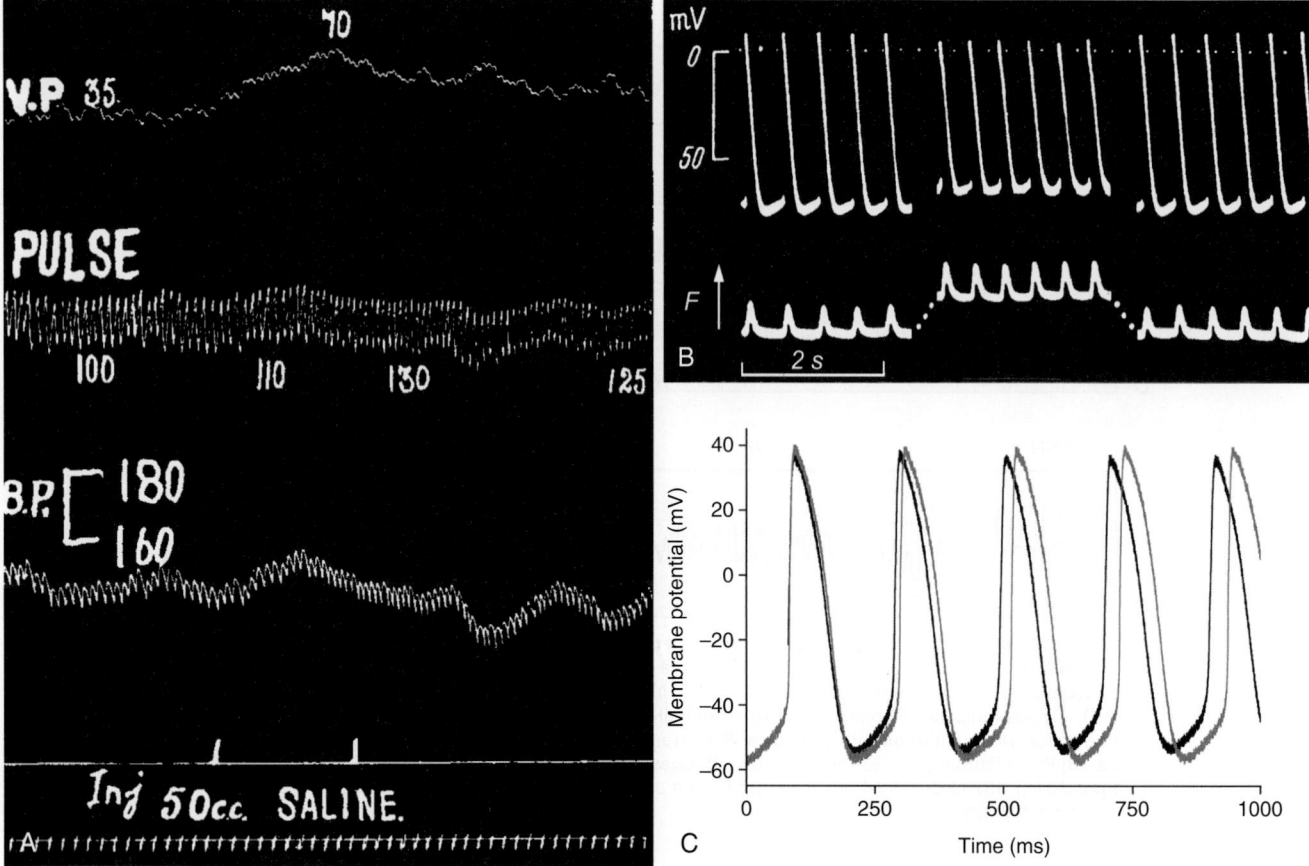

FIGURE 14.5 Positive chronotropic response to stretch in whole animal, isolated tissue, and single pacemaker cell. (A) Classic observation by Francis Bainbridge, showing that intravenous injection of saline (*bottom*) raises venous pressure (*V.P.*) (*top*) and pulse rate (*second from top*) without a coinciding change in arterial blood pressure (*B.P.*) in the anesthetized dog. (B) Sharp electrode recording of sinoatrial node (SAN) pacemaker cell potential (*top*) and tissue tension (*bottom*, contraction pointing upward) during the application of a 30% area increase to isolated right atrial tissue, containing the SAN (stretch indicated by the increase in resting tension). Telltale signs of mechano-electric coupling effects are reduction of maximum diastolic and maximum systolic potentials, and increased beating rate. (C) Axial stretch by 7% (*black curve*) of rabbit single SAN cell gives rise to electrophysiological changes that match those seen at tissue level. ([A] From Bainbridge FA. The influence of venous filling upon the rate of the heart. *J Physiol.* 1915;50:65-84. [B] From Deck KA. Dehnungseffekte am spontanschlagenden, isolierten Sinusknoten. *Pflug Arch.* 1964;280:120-130. [C] From Cooper PJ, Lei M, Cheng LX, et al. Axial stretch increases spontaneous pacemaker activity in rabbit isolated sinoatrial node cells. *J Appl Physiol.* 2000;89:2099-2104.)

Mechanical Modulation of Pacemaking

Diastolic stretch of cardiac tissues, if large enough to have any electrophysiological effect, causes membrane depolarization, whether in working myocardium (where such depolarization may trigger PVB; see Fig. 14.2) or in conduction[39] and pacemaker tissues[43] (where in many species an increase in spontaneous beating rate is seen) (Fig. 14.5). A positive chronotropic response to stretch is observed predominantly in mammals with low resting heart rates, such as guinea pig, rabbit, cat, dog, and human. In contrast, fast-beating murine hearts show a reduction in beating rate during sustained stretch, although apparently via the same underlying mechanism: the activation of SAC_{NS} (for cation nonselective SAC).[44]

From a system's point of view, early induction of the next heartbeat in response to increased venous return is advantageous (unless volume throughput is inflow limited, such as in species with already very high heart rates). In species with an upright body posture, however, a chief and overriding requirement for survival is the control of cardiac output *pressure* to ensure brain perfusion. Therefore heart rate responses to hemodynamic stimuli that affect both venous return and arterial pressure (such as most changes in body posture, for example in standard tilt table experiments) will be determined primarily by arterial pressure control patterns. This obscured the identification of the positive chronotropic response to stretch in humans until David Donald and John Shepherd dissociated the increase in venous return from arterial pressure changes by passively elevating the legs of healthy volunteers in supine position, confirming the positive chronotropic response in humans.[45]

A similar mechanosensitive behavior is believed to underlie the nonnervous component of respiratory sinus arrhythmia (RSA). Here, dynamic changes in thoraco-abdominal pressure gradients favor venous blood return to the heart during inspiration, causing a relative increase in right atrial filling and an associated increase in heart rate. While this mechanical component contributes little to RSA at rest (when modulation of vagal innervation is a dominant driver of heart rate variability), it is a major cause of RSA during peak exercise in healthy subjects (when vagal tone is reduced and respiratory effort and associated pressure gradients are enhanced)[46,47] and explains the presence of RSA in heart transplant recipients.[47]

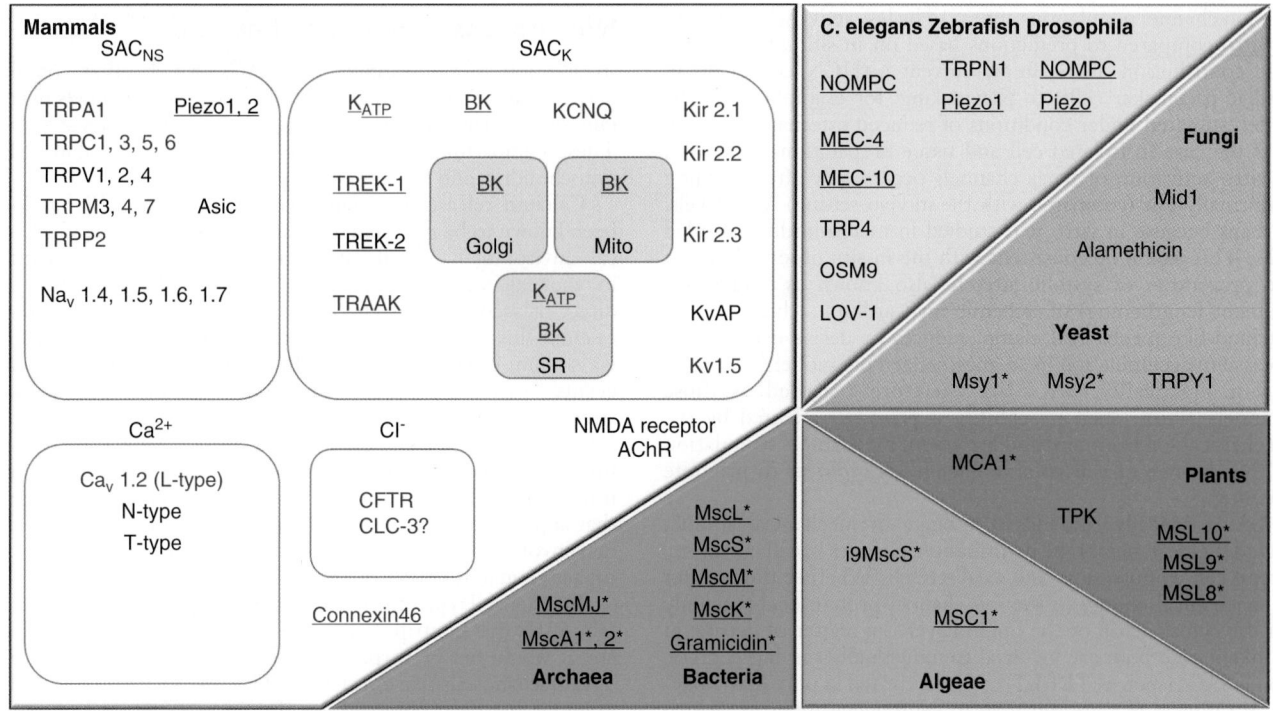

FIGURE 14.6 Mechanosensitive channel candidates throughout living organisms (selection). Several mammalian channels have homologs in other organisms. For example, NOMPC, OSM9, TRP4, TRPY1, and LOV-1 are TRP (transient receptor potential channel) homologs; MEC channels are members of the DEG/ENaC (degenerin/epithelial Na$^+$ channel) superfamily whose mammalian representative is ASIC (acid-sensing ion channel); TPK is a homolog of K_{2P} channels; and Mid1 (mating induced death) is homologous to voltage-gated calcium channels. *In red,* channels expressed in the heart; *underlined,* channels that have been identified clearly as mechano-gated; channels with no known mammalian homologs are marked by an *asterisk*. *Mito,* Mitochondria; SAC_K, stretch-activated channel, potassium selective; SAC_{NS}, stretch-activated channel, cation nonselective; *SR,* sarcoplasmic reticulum. (From Peyronnet R, Nerbonne JM, Kohl P. Cardiac mechano-gated ion channels and arrhythmias. *Circ Res.* 2016;118:311-329.)

If mechanical modulation of heart rate was the only physiologically relevant effect, one might be tempted to wonder why cardiac MEC has been preserved during evolution against its proarrhythmic potential that could have exerted a negative selection bias. This question is somewhat misleading, of course, because we do not know the evolutionary cost of removing any trait (in particular if it does not per se conflict with reproductive probability). It is possible, however, that the deleterious electrophysiological manifestations of cardiac MEC are side effects, rather than main targets, of underlying mechanisms (akin to the arrhythmogenic potential of the sodium-calcium exchanger, which—as a consequence of its electrogenicity—may give rise to depolarizing inward currents in calcium-overloaded cells, while its critical physiological function is to maintain ion concentration gradients). Thus it is conceivable that MEC is a side effect of "mechano-mechanical coupling," as perhaps required for the adjustment of individual cells' calcium concentration to external mechanical demand (see "Summary and Outlook").

Cardiac Stretch-Activated Ion Channels

Transsarcolemmal Channels

Mechanosensitive ion channels can be found in the sarcolemma of most pro- and eukaryotic cell types (Fig. 14.6). The open probability of these channels is primarily modulated by mechanical stimuli, such as stretch (e.g., SAC) or cell volume changes (volume-activated channels [VACs]). VACs in particular are believed to be a phylogenetically ancient theme, required to allow single cell organisms to adapt to potentially drastic changes in osmotic pressure in their external environment.

The mammalian heart contains both SAC and VAC.[48] SACs respond instantaneously to mechanical stimuli, whereas VACs tend to show significant lag times (up to minutes) between the onset of cell volume changes and ion channel response. VACs are understood to be important contributors to cardiac electrophysiology in chronic disease settings, such as (post-)ischemic cell swelling and hypertrophy (where VACs are constitutively activated).[49] In the context of electrophysiological responses to beat-by-beat changes in the mechanical environment, however, it is SACs that are implied as a key mechanism underlying MEC.

SACs were discovered in the 1980s, initially in cultured avian skeletal muscle by the lab of Fred Sachs[1] and were confirmed in mammalian cardiomyocytes by William Craelius and colleagues.[50] SACs show either little selectivity for (predominantly monovalent) cations (SAC_{NS}, for nonselective), or they preferentially conduct potassium ions (SAC_K). These selectivity profiles determine their transmembrane current reversal potentials, which are halfway between AP plateau and resting potentials for SAC_{NS} (usually between 0 and –25 mV), and close to the potassium equilibrium potential for SAC_K (about –95 mV in cardiomyocytes).

Like other phenomenological classifications, mechanosensitive ion channel categories are not absolute, and there is overlap with other ion channel nomenclatures. Several mechanosensitive channels are also voltage and/or ligand sensitive and vice versa. Thus the hyperpolarization-activated cyclic nucleotide–sensitive channel (HCN) is mechanically modulated,[51] as is the adenosine triphosphate (ATP)–inactivated potassium channel (K_{ATP}), whose open probability is increased by stretch in atrial[52] and ventricular myocytes.[53] Mechanosensitivity may explain why these two ion channel populations appear to be less active when studied in vitro compared to predictions based on in situ observations. The contribution of the funny current i_f (HCN equivalent in cardiac pacemaker cells) to pacemaking, for example, could be underestimated under conditions of reduced external load, such as is the case in isolated cell and tissue preparations. Likewise, in vitro activation of K_{ATP} channels occurs only after reaching abnormally low (compared with the in vivo setting) ATP levels, perhaps because in vitro it is studied in mechanically unloaded cells. This would be consistent with the in situ observation that the prevention of systolic stretch (also known as paradoxical segment lengthening) of ischemic myocardium, achieved using a tripod-like mechanical clamp, reduces or delays extracellular potassium accumulation in an anesthetized pig model.[21]

For practicality, SACs are therefore regarded as those channels whose open probability is *primarily* affected by the mechanical environment and for whom mechanical stimulation in the absence of cell volume changes is *sufficient* to promote opening.

SACs typically respond to a range of mechanical stimuli, including local membrane deformation, changes in cell curvature, lateral cell compression, and axial stretch. Whether the transfer of mechanical energy to the ion channel protein occurs mainly via the cytoskeleton or the lipid bilayer is a matter of debate; in all likelihood, both are involved to individually varying degrees. Some SACs (such as TREK1) can be activated in pure lipid bilayers.[54] Other SACs are sensitive to cytoskeletal integrity, which may either promote or prevent their opening.[55,56]

The actual mechanisms of cardiac SAC activation are not well established. Open- and closed-state data from large conductance prokaryotic mechanosensitive channels (MscL) have identified one mode of action. This involves an iris-like increase in pore dimensions during channel opening, leading to an increase in the outer circumference of the protein in the plane of the sarcolemma, combined with a reduction in transsarcolemmal size.[57] These configurational changes would be favored by increased lipid bilayer tension and by membrane thinning, both of which could underlie the mechanosensitive gating of the channel. In this context, any channel whose area projection in the plane of the cell membrane increases during opening *should* be sensitive to lipid bilayer tension. The question "why are some channels stretch-activated?" could be replaced therefore by asking "shouldn't more channels be at least modulated by their mechanical environment?" Recent reports indicate that the range of mechanically modulated ion channels is indeed significantly larger than generally assumed.[58]

At the same time, no sequence or structure homologs of MscL have been identified in mammalian myocardium (see Fig. 14.6). Recent evidence suggests, though, that transient receptor potential channels (TRPCs) such as TRPC1[59] or TRPC6[60] may underlie cardiac sarcolemmal SAC_{NS}, while cardiac SAC_K appear to include two pore-domain channels (such as TREK-1),[61] inwardly rectifying channels (such as K_{ir})[62] and ligand-activated ones (such as K_{ATP}).[52] Another promising candidate are Piezo proteins, which have been shown to assemble into very large mechanosensitive channels (protein tetramers containing over 100 transmembrane domains) in a range of species, from flies to mammals.[63] While not prominently present in myocardial tissue homogenates, first reports have identified Piezo proteins in human cardiac valve tissue.

Detailed functional characterization of SAC has been complicated by the fact that some of them (in particular SAC_{NS}) appear to be located in membrane areas that are not easily accessible to patch-clamp investigations in adult mammalian ventricular cardiomyocytes. These areas include T-tubules[64] and caveolae, which themselves form a mechanosensitive compartment that can be incorporated into the surface sarcolemma by stretch.[65,66] Single SAC_{NS} ion channel data have therefore been obtained mainly on neonatal or atrial cells.

Non-Transsarcolemmal Channels

In addition to transsarcolemmal SACs, which allow ion flux between cell interior and extracellular space, ion channels in certain subcellular compartments appear to be mechanosensitive. These compartments include the sarcoplasmic reticulum (SR), mitochondria, and nuclear envelope.

Calcium release from (and reuptake into) the SR has long been known to be modulated in cardiomyocytes by the mechanical environment, chiefly invoking length-dependent changes in the calcium buffer capacity of contractile filaments and direct or secondary effects of transsarcolemmal ion fluxes (e.g., calcium-fluxes, or sodium-fluxes that affect the calcium balance via sodium-calcium exchange). In addition, SR calcium release events ("sparks") become more frequent during acute axial cell stretch, even in resting cardiomyocytes, and also in the absence of extracellular sodium and calcium (Fig. 14.7).[67] Similarly, stimulation of cultured atrial and ventricular cardiomyocytes by application of small fluid jets can increase calcium spark rate in a way that appears to draw on mitochondrial calcium.[68] Whether this may involve mitochondrial K_{ATP} channels[69] in a mechanosensory capacity remains unknown.

In other cell types, the nuclear envelope has been found to contain SACs that contribute to calcium signaling in this domain,[70] and it would not be surprising if the same applied to the heart. The mechanosensitive ion channel TRPV4 (TRP vanilloid 4), for example, has been observed in cultured neonatal rat ventricular myocytes in the nucleus only,[71] although it is not clear whether it functions as a mechanosensor there.

Finally, connexin channels can be mechanosensitive. Connexins are best known for linking cytosols of two contacting cells (so while certainly sarcolemmal, they do not connect a cell's inside to the outside in this configuration). Noncardiac connexin46 has been shown to be mechanosensitive.[72] It will be interesting to see whether the same applies to cardiac isoforms, such as connexin43, whether located in sarcolemmal or in internal membranes, for example of cardiac mitochondria.[73] In fact, mitochondria may be more important players in cardiac MEC than customarily assumed, as they are able to generate significant intracellular forces during mitochondrial swelling[74] and hence possibly link metabolic disturbances to mechanisms involved in MEC.

Pharmacological Probes

In the absence of direct access to several relevant ion channel populations by patch-clamp approaches, SAC contributions to cardiac electrophysiology have been studied by pharmacological block. There are three main types of SAC blockers commonly used in experiments: the ionic form of gadolinium (Gd^{3+}; typically 10–100 μM), aminoglycosidic antibiotics (e.g., streptomycin; 30–50 μM), and a tarantula venom peptide (*Grammostola spatulata* mechano-toxin No. 4 [GsMTx-4]; effective at concentrations from 100 nM using the native peptide, but usually increasing to 1–5 μM with at least some of the commercially available synthetic forms).

All of these substances have drawbacks. Gadolinium suffers from a lack in specificity (overlapping concentration range for block of L-type calcium, sodium, and rapid delayed rectifier potassium channels, as well as of the sodium-calcium exchanger) and from precipitation in bicarbonate/phosphate-buffered solutions (although both Gd^{3+} and gadolinium salts may affect SAC).[75] Aminoglycosidic antibiotics are neither strictly selective (e.g., L-type calcium channel block with a half-maximal inhibition at 1–2 mM)[76] nor are they necessarily reliable tools for acute SAC block in situ (if they were, we would be unlikely to prescribe them as antibiotics).[77] Finally, high-purity GsMTx-4,[78] while selective and effective in both D- and L-configurations, still suffers from limited availability (and high cost).

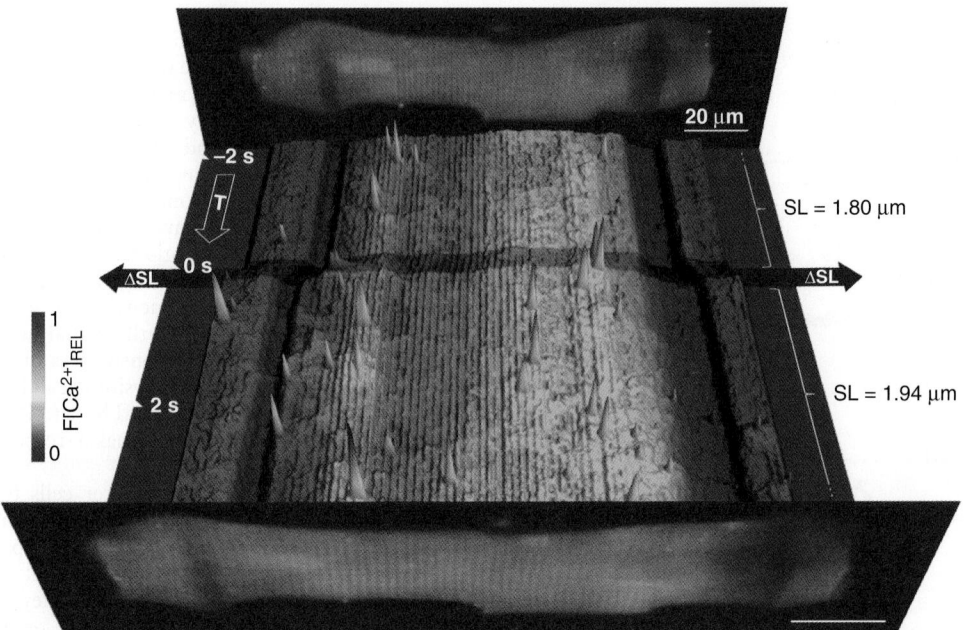

FIGURE 14.7 Time-course of relative Fluo-4 signal intensity in a rat ventricular resting cardio-myocyte, illustrating dynamic changes in spatially resolved Ca²⁺ concentration before and during axial cell stretch. *Upright panels* show cell images, averaged from 10 confocal XY scans, before (*back*) and after (*front*) stretch application. Low signal intensity areas, overlapping the cell, reveal carbon fiber positions (scale bars, 20 μm). *In between,* fluorescence intensity in each confocal XY scan was added along the Y-axis and plotted as a pseudo three dimensional–XT sequence of relative Ca²⁺ fluorescence (note corrugated appearance of background, indicative of sarcomere length [*SL*]). Axial stretch was applied by lateral movement of both carbon fibers (shading across the XT plot indicates period of carbon fiber movement), increasing SL in the affected area by ~8%. This is associated with an increase in spark rate. (Data from Iribe G, Ward CW, Camelliti P, et al. Axial stretch of rat single ventricular cardiomyocytes causes an acute and transient increase in Ca²⁺ spark rate. *Circ Res.* 2009;104:787-795. Figure design courtesy Dr. Alan Garny, University of Oxford.)

Given the above limitations, streptomycin has emerged as a popular pharmacological probe to study SAC in vitro, where it efficiently and with reasonable specificity (at micromolar concentrations) blocks whole-cell currents activated by axial cell stretch (Fig. 14.8). In this context, caution is advised when using cultured cells to study mechanosensitive behavior, as many culture media contain aminoglycosidic antibiotics. In addition, efficacy in vitro cannot simply be extrapolated to an in situ setting as it would appear that cardiac SAC, accessible to GsMTx-4, can be "protected" from acute and efficient block by streptomycin.[77]

The mechanisms of action of SAC block have not been resolved but may include screening of negative charges (popular blockers are cations with net charges ranging from 2+ for streptomycin to 5+ for GsMTx-4), interactions with the lipid bilayer, and open channel block (for details on SACs as pharmacological targets, see reviews by Ed White[79] and Remi Peyronnet and colleagues[48]).

Manifestations of Cardiac Stretch-Activated Ion Channel Activation

Cell Level Responses

Whole-cell SAC currents have been recorded from most cardiomyocyte types, including SAN pacemaker cells, Purkinje fibers, and atrial and ventricular myocytes. Their effects on cellular electrophysiology depend on the effective stretch *target* (SAC$_{NS}$ and/or SAC$_K$), stretch *timing* (relative to the cardiac cycle), and stretch *characteristics* (such as rate-of-rise and amplitude). At integrated levels (e.g., isolated organ or higher), this list further includes stimulus *location* (as even normal cardiac activity is associated with high spatial variability in electrophysiologically relevant parameters).

As a rule, diastolic stretch, if of sufficient amplitude to cause any change in membrane potential (V_m), gives rise to depolarization (Fig. 14.9). This can best be explained by the activation of SAC, whose reversal potential is positive to the resting cell membrane (i.e., SAC$_{NS}$).

The effects of stretch *during* the AP are less clear-cut because AP shortening, crossover of repolarization, and delayed repolarization have all been reported. Some of this discrepancy may be explained by differences in recording techniques, which can affect stretch targets. Thus sharp electrodes and perforated or ruptured patch can give rise to opposite AP duration changes, hinging on differential effects of these techniques on the interaction between SAC and calcium handling.[80] Stretch configuration also matters as moderate stretch initially affects only AP duration (the AP plateau is electrophysiologically more "labile" than the resting potential), while more severe distension also alters diastolic behavior, potentially causing crossover of late AP repolarization, and emergence of early afterdepolarization-like behavior (see Fig. 14.9). Another confounding aspect is related to the repolarization level at which AP duration is measured. Because early AP shortening may coincide with late AP prolongation, this may result in (apparently) contradictory changes in the reported AP duration.

While stretch of normal myocardium appears to preferentially target SAC$_{NS}$ (whose block fully eradicates whole-cell current responses in isolated cells; see Fig. 14.8), this may be different under conditions of metabolic impairment. Thus K$_{ATP}$ channels that are normally quiescent in atrial and ventricular cardiomyocytes respond to pipette suction[52] and axial cell stretch[53] when preactivated by a reduction in ATP concentration. Coactivation of a potassium-selective channel by ATP reduction and stretch will give rise to a less-positive reversal potential of the

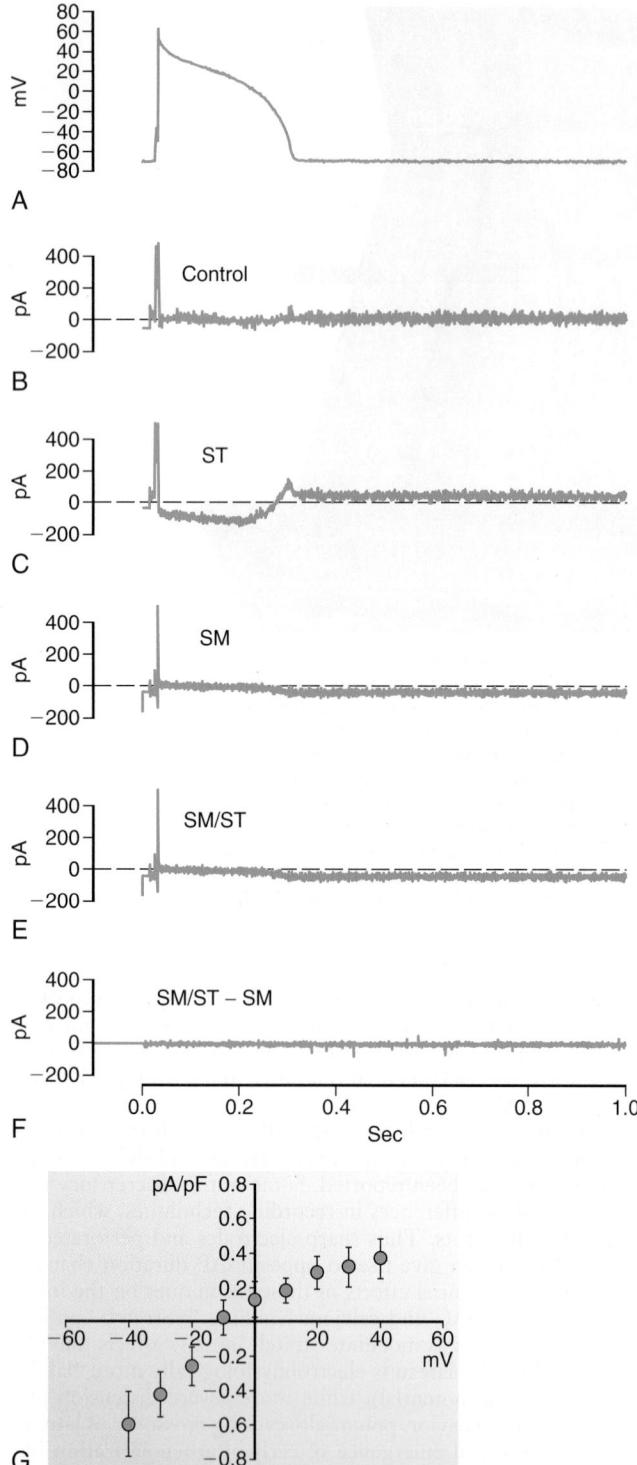

FIGURE 14.8 Action potential (AP) clamp recording of whole-cell current, induced by an axial stretch of guinea pig ventricular myocyte, in the absence and presence of 40 μM streptomycin. (A) AP recorded in control conditions and reapplied to the same cell as a voltage command (AP clamp). *Compensation* currents (B–E) illustrate the cell's response to interventions (note: *compensation* currents have the opposite polarity to native *transmembrane* currents): (B) control; (C) after application of 5% stretch (*ST*); (D) after return to control length and application of streptomycin (*SM*); (E) during 5% stretch in the presence of streptomycin (*SM/ST*). (F) Difference current (E minus D), illustrating that any streptomycin-resistant stretch-induced currents are negligible. (G) Current-voltage relation of the stretch-induced whole-cell current, measured during AP clamp repolarization from +40 to –40 mV. This current appears commensurate with SAC$_{NS}$, and is completely abolished by 40 μM streptomycin. (Unpublished data from M. Lei, P.J. Cooper, and P. Kohl.)

"net whole-cell current" induced by stretch in the ATP-starved heart. This might explain the reduced efficacy of PT (less efficient eradication of excitable gaps by reduced net inward current) in myocardium with severe metabolic impairment.[53]

Stretch effects may vary not only with disease but also with species, age, cell type, and location. Subendocardial ventricular cardiomyocytes, for example, appear to be more likely than subepicardial cells to respond to mechanical stimulation with afterdepolarization-like behavior.[8] Differences in mechanosensitivity can be caused by (1) regionally/transmurally varying levels of relevant mechanical stimuli; (2) different mechanical properties of cell and tissue components involved in transmission of external mechanical stimuli to the actual mechano-transducers; (3) variable expression or responsiveness of mechano-transducers; and (4) distinct electrophysiological background properties of affected cells and tissues. The latter appears to underlie species differences in SAN pacemaker responses to mechanical stimulation.

The response of SAN pacemaker cells to stretch seems to involve chiefly SAC$_{NS}$ activation, as shown in rabbit SAN isolated cells during axial stretch.[81] The principal effects of stretch on SAN cell AP morphology are qualitatively equivalent to those observed in SAN tissue (see Fig. 14.5). They include (in addition to truncation of diastolic and systolic V$_m$ maxima) acceleration of spontaneous diastolic depolarization and early AP repolarization (which both act to increase pacemaker rate), combined with a slowing of late AP repolarization when V$_m$ is below the SAC$_{NS}$ reversal potential (which would prolong the pacemaker cycle and reduce beating rate if it dominated the response). In other words, SAN pacemaker potential changes that move *toward* the reversal potential of SAC$_{NS}$ (–11 mV in rabbit SAN cells)[81] are accelerated by stretch, while those that move *away* from the reversal potential are slowed.

If one compares SAN pacemaker potential waveforms of slow- and fast-beating mammals (e.g., guinea pig or rabbit vs. mouse or rat), it is apparent that murine SAN pacemaker potentials have a very different AP morphology: both upstroke and initial repolarization are very fast, followed by an extended late repolarization and early depolarization phase. The percentage of the pacemaker cycle during which V$_m$ moves away from the SAC$_{NS}$ reversal potential dominates murine SAN pacemaking (71% in mouse compared with 46% in rabbit).[77] This may underlie the negative chronotropic response to sustained stretch observed in murine heart. Importantly, both negative and positive chronotropic responses to sustained stretch can be abolished by the application of GsMTx-4,[77] confirming the pivotal contribution of SAC$_{NS}$. Thus identical mechanisms may give rise to opposite responses, depending on the electrophysiological background of the affected cells. This reemphasizes the need for caution when extrapolating observations between species, such as from mouse to human.

Of course, SAN tissue in situ will not normally be stretched throughout the entire cycle, and more refined experimental study designs are needed to apply mechanical stimulation in a cycle-dependent manner. In addition, it will be interesting to explore whether individual components of the "voltage and calcium clocks" that drive pacemaking are directly mechanosensitive in native SAN cells (such as HCN or SR calcium–release channels) and whether effects secondary to other MEC actions (such as changes in intracellular calcium concentration) determine pacemaker responses to stretch.[82]

Tissue and Organ Level Effects

Cardiac arrhythmias are inherently multicellular phenomena, and it is therefore necessary to understand mechanisms, modulators, and outcomes of cardiac MEC at tissue and organ levels. However, linking macroscopic behavior to microscopic mechanisms is not without challenges in multicellular biological systems.

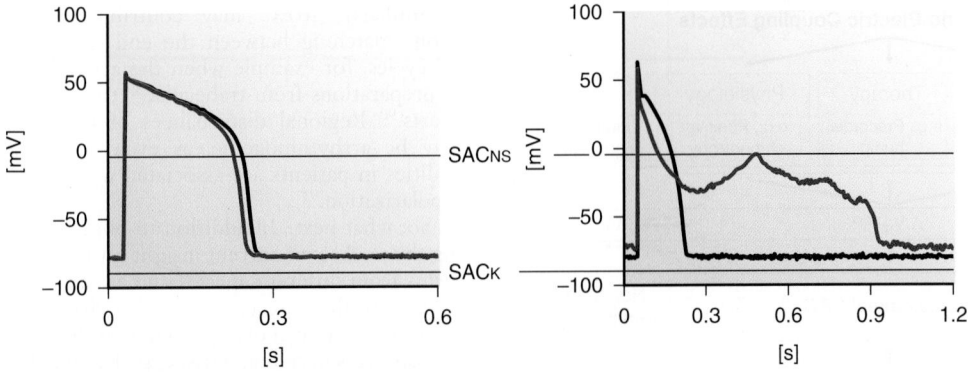

FIGURE 14.9 Effects of sustained moderate (≤5%) and severe (≥10%) axial stretch on guinea pig–isolated ventricular myocyte action potential (AP) morphology. Perforated patch-clamp recordings show AP shortening in the absence of diastolic membrane potential changes during moderate stretch, applied using a pair of carbon fibers (*left*), while more severe distension gives rise to diastolic depolarization, early AP shortening, and crossover of AP repolarization, yielding early afterpolarization-like behavior (*right*). *Black,* control; *red,* during stretch; SAC_{NS}, SAC_K: indication of differences in reversal potential of SAC populations with different ion selectivity. Note the different time scales. (Data from Kohl P, Nesbitt AD, Cooper PJ, et al. Sudden cardiac death by commotio cordis: role of mechano-electric feedback. *Cardiovasc Res.* 2001;50:280-289.)

On the "input side," quantification of mechanical interventions is even more difficult in tissue than in cells, where sarcomere length can be used as a useful indicator of axial strain, or in membrane patches, where deformation may be optically monitored (in principle at least). In most tissue preparations, except for trabeculae, thin papillary muscles, superficial muscle layers in whole heart, and live tissue slices, mechanical deformation cannot usually be quantified or graded with respect to (sub-) cellular strains. In the absence of cell deformation data, characterization of externally applied mechanical stimuli is helpful. However, because of the complex viscoelastic tissue properties that confer a strong time-varying component to the translation of external interventions to stimuli effective for MEC, this is a restricted surrogate measure only.

On the "output side," many of the standard techniques used to record electrophysiological consequences of mechanical stimulation in tissue and organ preparations report "ensemble properties" (including electrocardiogram, MAP, and optical mapping). In this context, it is important to recall that the heart contains a large number of different cell types, the majority of which are noncardiomyocytes. These include endothelial cells, fibroblasts, resident macrophages, fat, smooth muscle, and intracardiac neurons, all of which are mechanosensitive and may affect cardiac electrophysiological responses to mechanical stimulation. In addition, stretch influences conduction velocity, which is important for the interpretation of electrophysiological ensemble data and for their pathophysiological relevance. Reports in the literature on stretch-induced changes in conduction velocity include increases, reductions, and lack of change. In part at least, this will be because of the differences in the method of observation and data analysis, as metric distances (measured path length between two points) and biological distances (number of cells between two points) are differentially affected by tissue distension.

Given this complexity, the confirmation of SAC contributions to cardiac MEC in multicellular preparations has largely relied on pharmacological probes. For most SAC types, specific and efficient openers are not available (although a synthetic small molecule opener of Piezo channels has recently been identified),[83] while available blockers lack cardiomyocyte specificity (as well as the limitations discussed above). In addition, it is not sufficient for a blocker to be SAC-specific in vitro, but it must also be effective upon acute application to native tissue. This is not necessarily the case, for example, for streptomycin[77] and thus requires careful interpretation of apparently "negative" observations at the tissue level.

Despite these notes of caution, the available evidence overwhelmingly demonstrates that block of SAC_{NS} abolishes stretch-induced changes in SAN pacemaker rate. It can also prevent the mechanical induction of arrhythmogenic triggers (such as single PVB)[84] and the mechanical promotion of sustained arrhythmias (such as the preload-dependent amplification of burst pacing–induced atrial fibrillation).[85] In contrast, block of SAC_K can increase PVB inducibility.[86] Interestingly, however, SAC_K block may still prevent mechanically induced development of VF.[87] Whether this is caused by the removal of an arrhythmia-sustaining effect (ectopic excitation is still observed), a shift in the space/time–sensitive narrow vulnerable window for mechanical VF induction (as block of potassium channels alters repolarization), or another mechanism remains to be confirmed.

Summary and Outlook

The currently available data suggest that mechanical stimulation, acting via sarcolemmal SAC, gives rise to changes in cardiomyocyte V_m and AP morphology. SAC_{NS}-mediated effects in particular appear to be sufficient to quantitatively explain a majority of acute functional consequences of cardiac MEC in physiological conditions (Fig. 14.10). Sufficiency should not, however, be confused with validity, necessity, or exclusivity. Thus there are complex interactions of SAC effects with other mediators of mechano-electric integration, in particular those affecting calcium.[88] SAC may contribute to altered calcium handling either directly (such as via changes in SR calcium release or possibly via transsarcolemmal calcium flux through SAC_{NS}) or indirectly (via changes in V_m/AP morphology that alter voltage-sensitive calcium fluxes or through SAC_{NS}-mediated sodium influx with knock-on effects on the balance of transsarcolemmal ion exchange).

This could, in fact, hold the key to a better understanding of the physiological relevance of cardiac SAC. If, for example, an individual cardiomyocyte in situ was "less contractile" than its neighbors, then it would be stretched (or prevented from shortening) during systole. If this contributed to a gain of intracellular calcium (whether by additional uptake or reduced loss of calcium from the cell), then this could enable affected cells to adapt their contractility to external demand on a beat-by-beat basis. Such *matching of local contractility to dynamically varying external loads* has been shown experimentally in mechanically linked cardiac

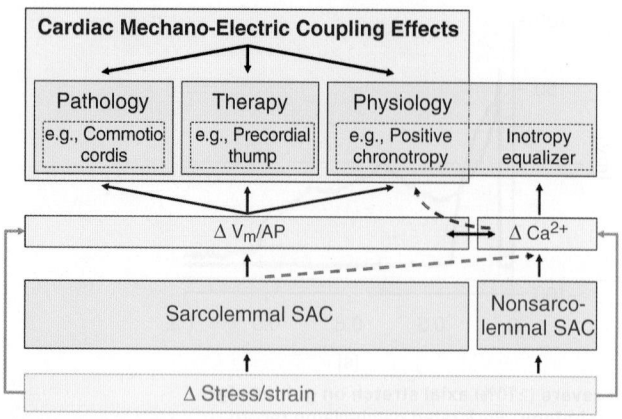

FIGURE 14.10 Schematic representation of functional relevance (*blue*) and key mechanisms (*red*) of acute cardiac mechano-electric coupling (MEC). Effects of MEC are particularly "striking" in the context of induction and termination of arrhythmias (*top left and middle*), and can be explained by the effects of stretch-activated ion channels (*SAC*) on cardiomyocyte electrophysiology. Less well documented is the physiological relevance of cardiac SAC (*top right*), which, in addition to the preload-dependent modulation of pacemaking rate, is likely to include an additional role: the matching of individual cell contractility to external demand. The latter is linked to mechanical modulation of cellular calcium handling (ΔCa^{2+}). *Dashed lines* indicate some of the possible links between classic MEC components and cell calcium, such as from SAC effects on calcium handling to the modulation of sinoatrial node pacemaking (see text for detail). *AP*, Action potential; *V_m*, membrane potential.

muscle preparations[89] and could act as an "equalizer" of the inotropic state of individual cardiomyocytes in the heart (see Fig. 14.10). This mechanism might underlie the efficient function of cells across regionally and temporally varying myocardial stress/strain dynamics in the healthy heart (in particular as, in contrast to skeletal muscle, the activity of individual cells is not controlled by neuromuscular junctions).

Similarly, MEC may contribute to a more homogeneous matching between the end of electrical and mechanical cycles, for example when the activation sequence is varied in preparations from trabeculae[89] to Langendorff-perfused pig hearts.[90] Regional disturbances of this balance, if sustained, may be arrhythmogenic, as even small wall-motion abnormalities in patients are associated with increased dispersion of repolarization.[91]

So, what next? In addition to populating and interconnecting the pockets of current insight into MEC effects and mechanisms from different species and at varying levels of structural complexity, there are a number of key challenges. These include:

- the development of improved tools to assess not only strain but also stress in cells and tissue, such as heralded by the advent of fluorescent reporters for SAC pore size[92] or cytoskeletal force for live-cell studies,[93] and by stretchable electronics for whole-heart research[94];
- the identification of mechanisms that underlie SAC activation, including the characterization of open/closed state SAC structures; assessment of differential contributions of stress, strain, or bending; and quantitative characterization of the interrelations between externally applied and internally sensed mechanical cues, including transmission to nonsarcolemmal ion channels[67];
- the integration of MEC research with mechano-mechanical and mechano-chemical transduction studies, such as involving reactive oxygen species and nitric oxide[95-97]; and
- the exploration of cross-talk between MEC and pharmacological interventions, including the identification of MEC components as drug targets and modulators.[48,98]

Acknowledgments

I am thankful to Drs. T. Alexander Quinn and Rémi Peyronnet for their helpful comments on the manuscript. Supported by the British Heart Foundation, the European Research Council Advanced Grant *CardioNECT*, the BBSRC, and the Magdi Yacoub Institute.

REFERENCES

1. Guharay F, Sachs F. Stretch-activated single ion channel currents in tissue-cultured embryonic chick skeletal muscle. *J Physiol*. 1984;352:685–701.
2. Zoll PM, Belgard AH, Weintraub MJ, et al. External mechanical cardiac stimulation. *N Engl J Med*. 1976;294:1274–1275.
3. Levine JH, Guarnieri T, Kadish AH, et al. Changes in myocardial repolarization in patients undergoing balloon valvuloplasty for congenital pulmonary stenosis: evidence for contraction-excitation feedback in humans. *Circulation*. 1988;77:70–77.
4. Haemers P, Sutherland G, Cikes M, et al. Further insights into blood pressure induced premature beats: transient depolarizations are associated with fast myocardial deformation upon pressure decline. *Nutr Metab Cardiovasc Dis*. 2015;12:2305–2315.
5. Quintanilla JG, Moreno J, Archondo T, et al. Increased intraventricular pressures are as harmful as the electrophysiological substrate of heart failure in favoring sustained reentry in the swine heart. *Heart Rhythm*. 2015;12:2172–2183.
6. Coronel R, Wilms-Schopman FJ, deGroot JR. Origin of ischemia-induced phase 1b ventricular arrhythmias in pig hearts. *J Am Coll Cardiol*. 2002;39:166–176.
7. Reiter MJ, Stromberg KD, Whitman TA, et al. Influence of intracardiac pressure on spontaneous ventricular arrhythmias in patients with systolic heart failure: insights from the REDUCEhf trial. *Circ Arrhythm Electrophysiol*. 2013;6:272–278.
8. Gallacher DJ, Van de Water A, van der Linde H, et al. In vivo mechanisms precipitating torsades de pointes in a canine model of drug-induced long-QT1 syndrome. *Cardiovasc Res*. 2007;76:247–256.
9. Schlomka G. Commotio cordis und ihre Folgen. Die Einwirkung stumpfer Brustwandtraumen auf das Herz. *Ergeb inn Med Kinderhkd*. 1934;47:1–91.
10. Link MS. Commotio cordis: sudden death from blows to the chest wall. In: Kohl P, Sachs F, Franz MR, eds. *Cardiac Mechano-Electric Coupling and Arrhythmias*. Oxford: Oxford University Press; 2011:325–239.
11. Kohl P, Nesbitt AD, Cooper PJ, et al. Sudden cardiac death by commotio cordis: role of mechano-electric feedback. *Cardiovasc Res*. 2001;50:280–289.
12. Link MS, Wang PJ, Pandian NG, et al. An experimental model of sudden cardiac death due to low-energy chest-wall impact (commotio cordis). *N Engl J Med*. 1998;338:1805–1811.
13. Garny A, Kohl P. Mechanical induction of arrhythmias during ventricular repolarisation: modelling cellular mechanisms and their interaction in 2D. *Ann N Y Acad Sci*. 2004;1015:133–143.
14. Li W, Kohl P, Trayanova N. Induction of ventricular arrhythmias following a mechanical impact: a simulation study in 3D. *J Mol Histo*. 2004;35:679–686.
15. Quinn TA, Kohl P. Critical window for mechanically-induced arrhythmias exists in time and in space. *Circulation*. 2012;126:A11162.
16. Allessie MA, Ausma J, Schotten U. Electrical, contractile and structural remodeling during atrial fibrillation. *Cardiovasc Res*. 2002;54:230–246.
17. Ravelli F, Mase M, del Greco M, et al. Acute atrial dilatation slows conduction and increases AF vulnerability in the human atrium. *J Cardiovasc Electrophysiol*. 2011;22:394–401.
18. Yoshida K, Ulfarsson M, Oral H, et al. Left atrial pressure and dominant frequency of atrial fibrillation in humans. *Heart Rhythm*. 2011;8:181–187.
19. Walters TE, Lee G, Spence S, et al. Acute atrial stretch results in conduction slowing and complex signals at the pulmonary vein to left atrial junction: insights into the mechanism of pulmonary vein arrhythmogenesis. *Circ Arrhythm Electrophysiol*. 2014;7:1189–1197.
20. Moreno J, Zaitsev AV, Warren M, et al. Effect of remodelling, stretch and ischaemia on ventricular fibrillation frequency and dynamics in a heart failure model. *Cardiovasc Res*. 2005;65:158.
21. Bollensdorff C, Lab MJ. Stretch effects on potassium accumulation and alternans in pathological myocardium. In: Kohl P, Sachs F, Franz MR, eds. *Cardiac Mechano-Electric Coupling and Arrhythmias*. 2nd ed. Oxford: Oxford University Press; 2011:173–179.
22. Waxman MB, Wald RW, Finley JP, et al. Valsalva termination of ventricular tachycardia. *Circulation*. 1980;62:843–851.
23. Ambrosi P, Habib G, Kreitmann B, et al. Valsalva manoeuvre for supraventricular tachycardia in transplanted heart recipient. *Lancet*. 1995;346:713.
24. Elvan A, Adiyaman A, Beukema RJ, et al. Electrophysiological effects of acute atrial stretch on persistent atrial fibrillation in patients undergoing open heart surgery. *Heart Rhythm*. 2013;10:322–330.
25. Dosdall DJ, Doppalapudi H, Ideker RE. Mechanical modulation of defibrillation and resuscitation efficacy. In: Kohl P, Sachs F, Franz MR, eds. *Cardiac Mechano-Electric Coupling and Arrhythmias*. Oxford: Oxford University Press; 2011:374–380.
26. Trayanova N, Li WH, Eason J, et al. Effect of stretch-activated channels on defibrillation efficacy. *Heart Rhythm*. 2004;1:67–77.
27. Li W, Gurev V, McCulloch AD, et al. The role of mechanoelectric feedback in vulnerability to electric shock. *Prog Biophys Mol Biol*. 2008;97:461–478.
28. Pellis T, Kohl P. Anti-arrhythmic effects of acute mechanical stimulation. In: Kohl P, Sachs F, Franz M, eds. *Cardiac Mechano-Electric Coupling and Arrhythmias*. Oxford: Oxford University Press; 2011:361–368.
29. Eich C, Bleckmann A, Schwarz SKW. Percussion pacing—an almost forgotten procedure for haemodynamically unstable bradycardias? A report of three case studies and review of the literature. *Brit J Anaest*. 2007;98:429–433.
30. Befeler B. Mechanical stimulation of the heart: its therapeutic value in tachyarrhythmias. *Chest*. 1978;73:832–838.

31. Klumbies A, Paliege R, Volkmann H. Mechanische Not-fallstimulation bei Asystolie und extremer Bradykardie. *Zeitschr ges Inn Med.* 1988;43:348–352.

32. Amir O, Schliamser JE, Nemer S, et al. Ineffectiveness of precordial thump for cardioversion of malignant ventricular tachyarrhythmias. *PACE.* 2007;30:153–156.

33. Haman L, Parizek P, Vojacek J. Precordial thump efficacy in termination of induced ventricular arrhythmias. *Resuscitation.* 2009;80:14–16.

34. Pellis T, Kette F, Lovisa D, et al. Utility of pre-cordial thump for treatment of out of hospital cardiac arrest: a prospective study. *Resuscitation.* 2009;80:17–23.

35. Schott E. Über Ventrikelstillstand (Adam-Stokes'sche Anfälle) nebst Bemerkungen über andersartige Arrhythmien passagerer Natur. *Dt Arch klin Med.* 1920;131:211–229.

36. Pennington JE, Taylor J, Lown B. Chest thump for reverting ventricular tachycardia. *N Engl J Med.* 1970;283:1192–1195.

37. Chan L, Reid C, Taylor B. Effect of three emergency pacing modalities on cardiac output in cardiac arrest due to ventricular asystole. *Resuscitation.* 2002;52:117–119.

38. Iseri LT, Allen BJ, Baron K, et al. Fist pacing, a forgotten procedure in bradysystolic cardiac arrest. *Am Heart J.* 1987;113:1545–1550.

39. Kaufmann R, Theophile U. Automatie-fördernde Dehnungseffekte an Purkinje-Fäden, Papillarmuskeln und Vorhoftrabekeln von Rhesus-Affen. *Pflüg Arch.* 1967;297:174–189.

40. Tan JH, Liu W, Saint DA. Differential expression of the mechanosensitive potassium channel TREK-1 in epicardial and endocardial myocytes in rat ventricle. *Exp Physiol.* 2004;89:237–242.

41. Stones R, Calaghan SC, Billeter R, et al. Transmural variations in gene expression of stretch-modulated proteins in the rat left ventricle. *Pflüg Arch.* 2007;454:545–549.

42. Lerman BB, Deale OC. Relation between transcardiac and transthoracic current during defibrillation in humans. *Circ Res.* 1990;67:1420–1426.

43. Deck KA. Dehnungseffekte am spontanschlagenden, isolierten Sinusknoten. *Pflüg Arch.* 1964;280:120–130.

44. Cooper PJ, Ravens U. Mechanical modulation of pacemaker electrophysiology. In: Kohl P, Sachs F, Franz MR, eds. *Cardiac Mechano-Electric Coupling and Arrhythmias.* 2nd ed. Oxford: Oxford University Press; 2011:95–102.

45. Donald DE, Shepherd JT. Reflexes from the heart and lungs: physiological curiosities or important regulatory mechanisms. *Cardiovasc Res.* 1978;12:449–469.

46. Casadei B, Moon J, Johnston J, et al. Is respiratory sinus arrhythmia a good index of cardiac vagal tone in exercise? *J Appl Physiol.* 1996;81:556–564.

47. Bernardi L, Salvucci F, Suardi R, et al. Evidence for an intrinsic mechanism regulating heart rate variability in the transplanted and the intact heart during submaximal dynamic exercise? *Cardiovasc Res.* 1990;24:969–981.

48. Peyronnet R, Nerbonne JM, Kohl P. Cardiac mechano-gated ion channels and arrhythmias. *Circ Res.* 2016;118:311–329.

49. Baumgarten CM, Clemo HF. Swelling-activated chloride channels in cardiac physiology and pathophysiology. *Prog Biophys Mol Biol.* 2003;82:25–42.

50. Craelius W, Chen V, El-Sherif N. Stretch activated ion channels in ventricular myocytes. *BioSci Rep.* 1988;8:407–414.

51. Lin W, Laitko U, Juranka PF, et al. Dual stretch responses of mHCN2 pacemaker channels: accelerated activation, accelerated deactivation. *Biophys J.* 2007;92:1559–1572.

52. Van Wagoner DR, Lamorgese M. Ischemia potentiates the mechanosensitive modulation of atrial ATP-sensitive potassium channels. *Ann N Y Acad Sci.* 1994;723:392–395.

53. Kohl P, Bollensdorff C, Garny A. Effects of mechanosensitive ion channels on ventricular electrophysiology: experimental and theoretical models. *Exp Physiol.* 2006;91:307–321.

54. Brohawn SG, Su ZW, Mackinnon R. Mechanosensitivity is mediated directly by the lipid membrane in TRAAK and TREK1 K⁺ channels. *Proc Natl Acad Sci U S A.* 2014;111:3614–3619.

55. Janmey PA. The cytoskeleton and cell signalling: component localization and mechanical coupling. *Physiol Rev.* 1998;78:763–781.

56. Kerr JP, Robison P, Shi GL, et al. Detyrosinated microtubules modulate mechanotransduction in heart and skeletal muscle. *Nat Comm.* 2015;6:8526.

57. Perozo E, Kloda A, Cortes DM, et al. Physical principles underlying the transduction of bilayer deformation forces during mechanosensitive channel gating. *Nat Struct Biol.* 2002;9:696–703.

58. Morris CE. Pacemaker, potassium, calcium, sodium: stretch modulation of the voltage-gated channels. In: Kohl P, Sachs F, Franz MR, eds. *Cardiac Mechano-Electric Coupling and Arrhythmias.* Oxford: Oxford University Press; 2011:42–49.

59. Maroto R, Raso A, Wood TG, et al. TRPC1 forms the stretch-activated cation channel in vertebrate cells. *Nat Cell Biol.* 2005;7:179–185.

60. Dyachenko V, Christ A, Gubanov R, et al. Misalignment of sarcomeres by mechanical stimuli: an input signal for integrin dependent modulation of ion channels? *Prog Biophys Mol Biol.* 2008;97:196–216.

61. Terrenoire C, Lauritzen I, Lesage F, et al. TREK-1-like potassium channel in atrial cells inhibited by β-adrenergic stimulation and activated by volatile anesthetics. *Circ Res.* 2001;89:336–342.

62. Tamargo J, Caballero R, Gomez R, et al. Pharmacology of cardiac potassium channels. *Cardiovasc Res.* 2004;62:9–33.

63. Coste B, Xiao B, Santos JS, et al. Piezo proteins are pore-forming subunits of mechanically activated channels. *Nature.* 2012;483:176–181.

64. Zeng T, Bett GCL, Sachs F. Stretch-activated whole cell currents in adult rat cardiac myocytes. *Am J Physiol.* 2000;278:H548–H557.

65. Kohl P, Cooper PJ, Holloway H. Effects of acute ventricular volume manipulation on in situ cardiomyocyte cell membrane configuration. *Prog Biophys Mol Biol.* 2003;82:221–227.

66. Pfeiffer ER, Wright AT, Edwards AG, et al. Caveolae in ventricular myocytes are required for stretch-dependent conduction slowing. *J Mol Cell Cardiol.* 2014;76:265–274.

67. Iribe G, Ward CW, Camelliti P, et al. Axial stretch of rat single ventricular cardiomyocytes causes an acute and transient increase in Ca²⁺ spark rate. *Circ Res.* 2009;104:787–795.

68. Belmonte S, Morad M. 'Pressure-flow'-triggered intracellular Ca²⁺ transients in rat cardiac myocytes: possible mechanisms and role of mitochondria. *J Physiol.* 2008;586:1379–1397.

69. Murata M, Akao M, O'Rourke B, et al. Mitochondrial ATP-sensitive potassium channels attenuate matrix Ca²⁺ overload during simulated ischemia and reperfusion: possible mechanism of cardioprotection. *Circ Res.* 2001;89:891–898.

70. Itano N, Okamoto S, Zhang D, et al. Cell spreading controls endoplasmic and nuclear calcium: a physical gene regulation pathway from the cell surface to the nucleus. *Proc Natl Acad Sci U S A.* 2003;100:5181–5186.

71. Zhao Y, Huang H, Jiang Y, et al. Unusual localization and translocation of TRPV4 protein in cultured ventricular myocytes of the neonatal rat. *Eur J Histochem.* 2012;56:e32.

72. Bao L, Sachs F, Dahl G. Connexins are mechanosensitive. *Am J Physiol.* 2004;278:C1389–C1395.

73. Miro-Casas E, Ruiz-Meana M, Agullo E, et al. Connexin43 in cardiomyocyte mitochondria contributes to mitochondrial potassium uptake. *Cardiovasc Res.* 2009;83:747–756.

74. Kaasik A, Kuum M, Joubert F, et al. Mitochondria as a source of mechanical signals in cardiomyocytes. *Cardiovasc Res.* 2010;87:83–91.

75. Caldwell RA, Clemo HF, Baumgarten CM. Using gadolinium to identify stretch-activated channels: technical considerations. *Am J Physiol.* 1998;275:C619–C621.

76. Belus A, White E. Effects of streptomycin sulphate on I_{CaL}, I_{Kr} and I_{Ks} in guinea-pig ventricular myocytes. *Eur J Pharmacol.* 2002;445:171–178.

77. Cooper PJ, Kohl P. Species- and preparation-dependence of stretch effects on sino-atrial node pacemaking. *Ann N Y Acad Sci.* 2005;1047:324–335.

78. Bowman CL, Gottlieb PA, Suchyna TM, et al. Mechanosensitive ion channels and the peptide inhibitor GsMTx-4: history, properties, mechanisms and pharmacology. *Toxicon.* 2007;49:249–270.

79. White E. Mechanosensitive channels: therapeutic targets in the myocardium? *Curr Pharm Des.* 2006;12:3645–3663.

80. Calaghan SC, Belus A, White E. Do stretch-induced changes in intracellular calcium modify the electrical activity of cardiac muscle? *Prog Biophys Mol Biol.* 2003;82:81–95.

81. Cooper PJ, Lei M, Cheng L-X, et al. Axial stretch increases spontaneous pacemaker activity in rabbit isolated sinoatrial node cells. *J Appl Physiol.* 2000;89:2099–2104.

82. Quinn TA, Kohl P. Mechano-sensitivity of cardiac pacemaker function: pathophysiological relevance, experimental implications, and conceptual integration with other mechanisms of rhythmicity. *Prog Biophys Mol Biol.* 2012;110:257–268.

83. Syeda R, Xu J, Dubin AE, et al. Chemical activation of the mechanotransduction channel Piezo1. *Elife.* 2015:4.

84. Hansen DE, Borganelli M, Stacy GPJ, et al. Dose-dependent inhibition of stretch-induced arrhythmias by gadolinium in isolated canine ventricles. Evidence for a unique mode of antiarrhythmic action. *Circ Res.* 1991;69:820–831.

85. Bode F, Sachs F, Franz MR. Tarantula peptide inhibits atrial fibrillation. *Nature.* 2001;409:35–36.

86. Iribe G, Jin H, Naruse K. Role of sarcolemmal BK$_{Ca}$ channels in stretch-induced extrasystoles in isolated chick hearts. *Circ J.* 2011;75:2552–2558.

87. Link MS, Wang PJ, VanderBrink BA, et al. Selective activation of the K⁺$_{ATP}$ channel is a mechanism by which sudden death is produced by low-energy chest-wall impact (commotio cordis). *Circulation.* 1999;100:413–418.

88. ter Keurs HE, Wakayama Y, Sugai Y, et al. Role of sarcomere mechanics and Ca²⁺ overload in Ca²⁺ waves and arrhythmias in rat cardiac muscle. *Ann N Y Acad Sci.* 2006;1080:248–267.

89. Solovyova O, Katsnelson L, Konovalov P, et al. Activation sequence as a key factor in spatio-temporal optimization of myocardial function. *Phil Trans Roy Soc.* 2006;364:1367–1383.

90. Opthof T, Meijborg VMF, Belterman CNW, et al. Synchronization of repolarization by mechano-electrical coupling in the porcine heart. *Cardiovasc Res.* 2015;108:181–187.

91. Opthof T, Sutton P, Coronel R, et al. The association of abnormal ventricular wall motion and increased dispersion of repolarization in humans is independent of the presence of myocardial infarction. *Front Physiol.* 2012;3:235.

92. Wang Y, Liu YX, DeBerg HA, et al. Single molecule FRET reveals pore size and opening mechanism of a mechano-sensitive ion channel. *Elife.* 2014;3:e01834.

93. Meng F, Suchyna TM, Sachs F. A fluorescence energy transfer-based mechanical stress sensor for specific proteins in situ. *FEBS J.* 2008;275:3072–3087.

94. Kim DH, Ghaffari R, Lu N, Rogers JA. Flexible and stretchable electronics for biointegrated devices. *Annu Rev Biomed Eng.* 2012;14:113–128.

95. Dyachenko V, Rueckschloss U, Isenberg G. Modulation of cardiac mechanosensitive ion channels involves superoxide, nitric oxide and peroxynitrite. *Cell Calcium.* 2009;45:55–64.

96. Prosser BL, Ward CW, Lederer WJ. X-ROS signaling: rapid mechano-chemo transduction in heart. *Science.* 2011;333:1440–1445.

97. Jian Z, Han HL, Zhang TQ, et al. Mechano-chemotransduction during cardiomyocyte contraction is mediated by localized nitric oxide signaling. *Sci Signal.* 2014;7:ra27.

98. Beyder A, Strege PR, Reyes S, et al. Ranolazine decreases mechanosensitivity of the voltage-gated sodium ion channel Nav1.5: a novel mechanism of drug action. *Circulation.* 2012;125:2698–2706.

15 Biophysical Properties of Gap Junctions

Virginijus Valiunas and Peter R. Brink

Background

The propagation of the cardiac action potential throughout the working myocardium is made possible by voltage-dependent Na^+, Ca^{2+}, and K^+ currents and by gap junction channels. One of the roles of gap junction channels is to permit the passage, from cell to cell, of currents that are essential for action potential propagation throughout the working myocardium. When considering action potential propagation, gap junctions can be best understood as components of the longitudinal resistance within the functional syncytium of the myocardium. Gap junction channels are in series with the cytoplasmic resistance. The intercellular resistance of gap junctions is in series with the intracellular resistance of the cytoplasm, and together they represent longitudinal resistance. Both resistances can affect conduction velocity within the heart, but it is the gap junction channels, composed of connexins, that dominate longitudinal resistance. Dual whole-cell patch clamp studies of cardiac myocytes have been used to quantify gap junction membrane resistance or junctional conductance in vitro. The estimates of junctional resistance for ventricular myocyte cell pairs reveal that it is often an order of magnitude less than the input resistance of an isolated myocyte, somewhere in the range of 2 to 10 MΩ or 1000 to 100 nS.[1] These values must be considered under estimates because of the series resistance of the pipettes that have similar resistance values to the junctions themselves.[1] In addition to creating an electrical syncytium for the heart, gap junctions also allow the passage of small solutes such as cyclic adenosine monophosphate (cAMP) that are able to affect the function of multiple systems within cardiac myocytes. To better understand how gap junction channels contribute to the normal functions of the heart and how they participate in cardiac arrhythmias and ischemia, it is necessary to first describe their structure and biophysical properties.

Structure of Gap Junction Channels

Structural analysis has revealed that gap junction channels are composed of two hemichannels or connexons linked together that provide an intercellular pathway between two adjacent cell interiors (Fig. 15.1A).[2] Each hemichannel is composed of six connexins. Each connexin contains four membrane-spanning domains (M1–M4; Fig. 15.1B). The N-terminus protrudes from M1 into the cytosol. M1 and M2 are connected by an extracellular loop, E1, whereas M2 and M3 are connected by a cytoplasmic loop. M3 and M4 are connected by another extracellular loop (E2), and the cytoplasmic extension of M4 is the C-terminus (see Fig. 15.1B). This general model is true for all cardiac connexins and other human connexins. Individual gap junction channels within the atrial and ventricular myocardium are found in abundance at the intercalated discs in the form of membrane complexes or plaques containing a large number of channels, ranging from hundreds to thousands. A small portion of such a plaque is depicted in Fig. 15.1A. These plaques can also form along the lateral surfaces of myocytes in normal myocardium and can become even larger structures in stressed or diseased myocardium.[3]

Only a few studies have been successful in elucidating the molecular structure of gap junction channels using electron crystallography. The first analysis was performed on a noncardiac connexin, Cx26, and more recently has been revisited, revealing structural detail to a resolution of approximately 0.35 nm.[4] Cx43 has also been analyzed using crystallographic methods with a resolution of approximately 1.0 nm.[5] Fig. 15.1C depicts a representation of the helical membrane domains and the extracellular loops of a hemichannel as viewed from within the plasma membrane of a cell. Fig. 15.1D illustrates the structure of Cx26 from the perspective of looking down its long axis directly into the channel from the cytoplasm where the four transmembrane domains of each connexin can be visualized. The structural analysis has not been sufficiently detailed to demonstrate clearly which membrane-spanning domains are forming the channel wall. However, the structure shown in Fig. 15.1D depicting the four transmembrane helices suggests that M1, M2, M3, and even M4 are potential contributors to the lining of the pore or to the cytoplasmic vestibule.

The substituted cysteine accessibility method (SCAM) is one approach that has been used to define the pore-lining regions of connexins. Substituting cysteine for other amino acids thought to be contributing to the pore wall is the first step to successful use of SCAM. This step is followed by a demonstration that the substitution does not affect normal channel activity. To establish whether the substituted group is part of the pore wall, a thiol reactive agent such as maleimide or a derivative is then perfused into the preparation while monitoring channel activity. One possible outcome is altered unitary conductance consistent, with the substituted group being a component of the pore wall. In fact, the application of SCAM to connexins has provided varied results when assessing pore-lining regions of the four membrane-spanning domains and extracellular loops and intracellular regions. The use of SCAM to elucidate the pore wall structure on Cx46 has generated data most consistent with pore-lining domains or pore-access regions in M1 and in the E1 loop,[6] but Cx32 SCAM data are more consistent with M3 as a major pore-lining helix.[6] No SCAM analysis has been performed on Cx43, Cx40, Cx45, or Cx37. Site-directed mutagenesis has also been used for Cx43 and Cx37 with various substitution strategies. In Cx43, mutations were introduced in M3 that resulted in silent channels.[6] This is not conclusive evidence that M3 participates as a functional

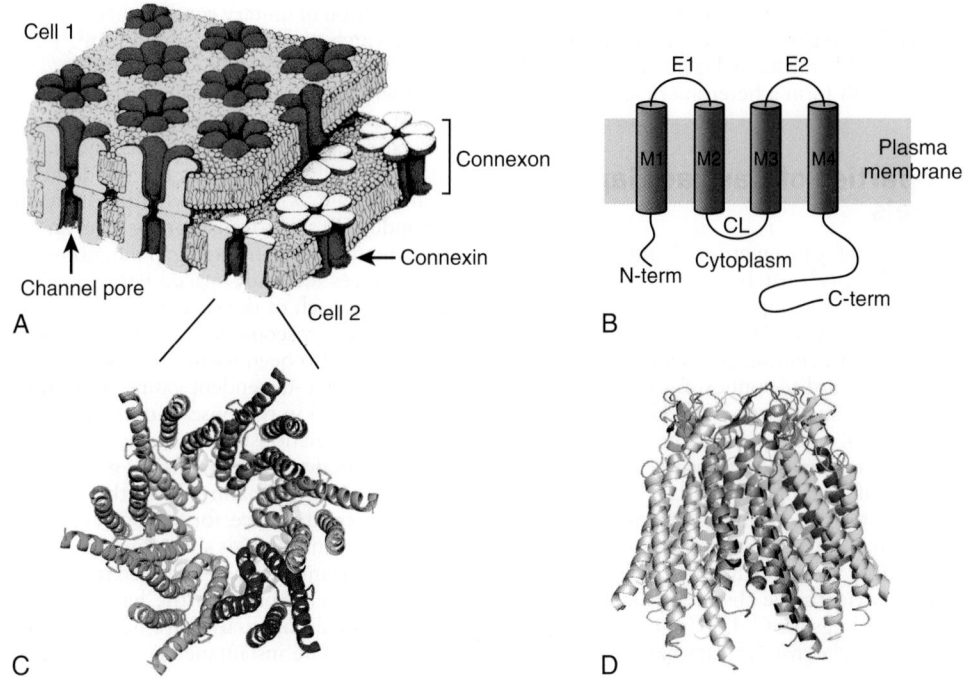

FIGURE 15.1 (A) A portion of a junctional plaque. *Yellow* bilayers are the plasma membranes of two adjacent cells. Each gap junction channel is composed of two hemichannels or connexons that are themselves composed of connexins. (B) Schematic representation of a connexin with four membrane domains, M1–M4; two extracellular loops, E1 and E2; and three cytoplasmic domains, N-terminus, cytoplasmic loop, and the C-terminus. (C) En face view of the hemichannel from the cytoplasm of a cell. (D) Molecular rendition of connexin26 (Cx26) viewed from within the plasma membrane of a cell. Each connexin is colored differently. ([A] Modified from Makowski L, Caspar DL, Phillips WC, Baker TS, Goodenough DA. Gap junction structures. VI. Variation and conservation in connexon conformation and packing. *Biophys J.* 1984;45:208-218.)

member of the pore wall, but it does not exclude the possibility. For Cx37, site-directed mutations in M3 resulted in altered conductive states, which is consistent with M3 participation in forming the pore wall, but does not exclusively demonstrate that either.[7] The crystallographic and mutagenic data lead to one possible explanation: different connexins do not use the identical structural motifs in the formation of an intercellular pore despite functional similarities. The crystallographic structure shown in Fig. 15.1C indicates that there are potential surfaces for all four domains contributing to the channel or pore and to the cytoplasmic vestibule.

Cardiac Gap Junctions: Homomeric, Heterotypic, and Heteromeric Forms

Hemichannels composed of six connexins from two closely aligned cells form a linkage via the extracellular domains E1 and E2 to create a complete gap junction channel. The heart does not express all 21 identified connexins[8] that are able to assemble into functional gap junction channels (see Fig. 15.1A and B). Instead, a select number of connexins are expressed within the human heart; they are Cx43, Cx40, Cx45, Cx46, and Cx37.[9] Their distribution within the heart is not uniform. For example, Cx43 is abundantly expressed within the ventricles but is only sparingly expressed within the atrioventricular (AV) and sinoatrial (SA) nodes.[9,10] Table 15.1 illustrates the relative connexin expression levels within the ventricles, atrium, SA node, AV node, and bundle branch/conducting system (BB/CS). Connexin 31.9, the ortholog of mouse Cx30.2 found in the mouse AV node, has thus far not been detected in the human heart. Cx30.2 has been shown to be in part responsible for conduction delay at the AV node in mice.[10] The absence of Cx31.9 in the human AV node suggests

TABLE 15.1   Connexins of the Human Heart

Ventricles	Cx43 > Cx45 >> Cx40 >> Cx46~Cx37
Atrium	Cx40 > Cx43 ~ Cx45
BB/CS	Cx40 ~ Cx43 ~ Cx45
AV node	Cx45 > Cx40 ~ Cx43
SA node	Cx45 > Cx40 > > > > Cx43

AV, Atrioventricular; *BB/CS,* bundle branch/conducting system; *SA,* sinoatrial. From Severs NJ, Bruce AF, Dupont E, et al. Remodelling of gap junctions and connexin expression in diseased myocardium. *Cardiovasc Res.* 2008;80:9-19; and Jansen JA, van Veen TA, de Bakker JM, et al. Cardiac connexins and impulse propagation. *J Mol Cell Cardiol.* 2010;48:76-82.

that the delay in humans might be the result of reduced channel numbers or the presence of heteromeric or heterotypic forms of Cx45, Cx40, and Cx43 or possibly of the existence of another unidentified connexin within the AV node whose properties mimic those of mouse Cx30.2.

As implied in Table 15.1, myocytes within the different regions of the heart are able to coexpress connexins. For example, individual atrial myocytes express Cx40, Cx43, and Cx45 simultaneously but in differing amounts, with Cx40 being the most abundantly expressed connexin. The expression of a single connexin within myocytes has the potential to generate functional gap junction channels composed of two identical hemichannels, both composed of the same connexin and referred to as a *homomeric* (i.e., homotypic) channel. Another type of gap junction channel is also possible, where each hemichannel of two opposing cells is homomeric but each cell expresses a different connexin. This type of channel is heterotypic.[8] Finally, because most myocytes express at least two and often three connexins, a hemichannel can potentially contain two or possibly three different connexins.[8,11] This type of hemichannel is heteromeric. Two heteromeric hemichannels will form a heteromeric gap junction channel.

Biophysical Properties of Cardiac Gap Junction Channels

The biophysical properties of gap junction channels are best illustrated using a dual whole-cell patch clamp on isolated cell pairs. Fig. 15.2A depicts a cell pair coupled by gap junctions with the equivalent circuit for the cell pair. All the cardiac gap junction channels have been studied in connexin-deficient cells that are then transfected with specific cardiac connexins to better understand how homotypic gap channel forms of Cx43, Cx40, Cx45, Cx46, and Cx37 behave. In all cases, each can be shown to gate closed with the application of increased transjunctional voltage (V_j). A macroscopic record of junctional currents is shown in Fig. 15.2B for Cx45 and illustrates the decline of junctional current with sustained V_j. $I_{j,inst}$ is the junctional current recorded at the onset of a voltage step, and $I_{j,ss}$ is the steady state current. In some cases, individual channel activity can be observed as shown in Fig. 15.2C. Single-channel recordings for Cx43, Cx40, and Cx45 are shown. Multichannel and single-channel data have allowed the

determination of unitary conductance ($\gamma_{j,main}$) for the cardiac connexins, which are listed in Table 15.2.[12-22] The ability to monitor unitary events has also allowed a better understanding of voltage-dependent gating in connexins, which has been shown to have at least two distinct mechanisms: fast gating and slow gating. Fast gating is characterized by a rapid transition from an open state to a residual state ($\gamma_{j,residual}$; see dashed lines in Fig. 15.2C) or closed state, whereas slow gating is manifested as a series of subconductive states transitioning from an open or closed state.[11] A systematic study on Cx30 gap junctions reported five substrate conductances unevenly spaced between $\gamma_{j,main}$ and $\gamma_{j,residual}$, suggesting that each of the six connexins of a hemichannel acts as a subgate.[23] Macroscopic recordings of junctional currents (see Fig. 15.2B) have also been useful in dissecting the molecular mechanisms of voltage-dependent gating. Plotting the steady state currents generated in response to different V_j steps (see Fig. 15.2B) reveals the relationship between junctional conductance (g_j) and transjunctional potential (V_j). g_j is derived from the ratio of $g_{j,ss}/g_{j,inst}$. A Boltzmann fit of the normalized, steady-state junctional conductance for various amplitude voltage steps for Cx43, Cx40, and Cx45 is shown in Fig. 15.2D.

An important parameter derived from the Boltzmann fit is $V_{j,o}$. This parameter represents the half-inactivation voltage or that transjunctional potential where half the channels can be considered closed. The instantaneous junctional conductance remains

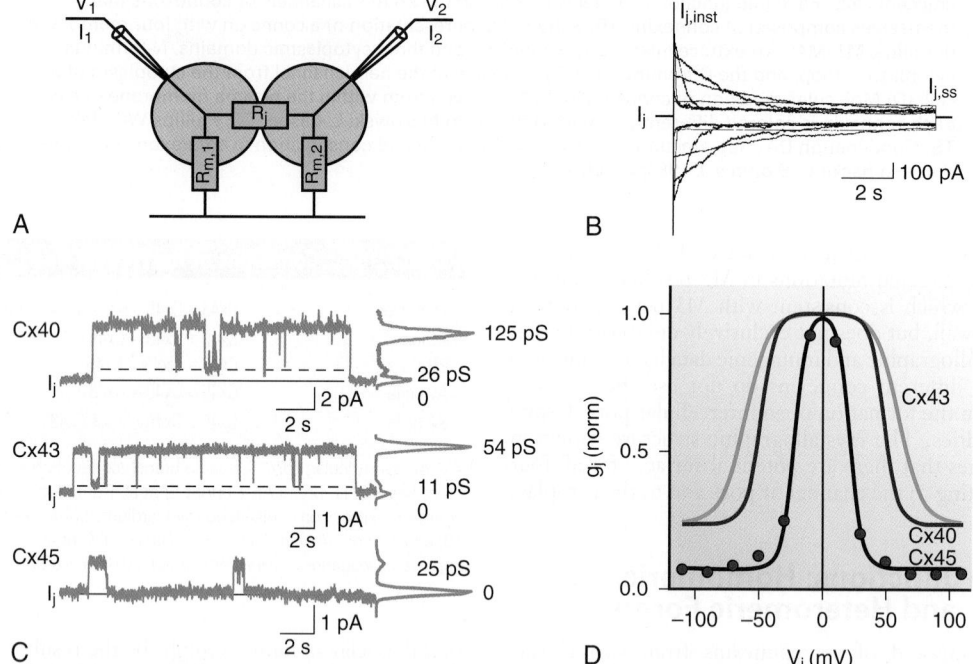

FIGURE 15.2 (A) Dual, whole-cell patch clamp equivalent circuit and superimposed cell pair. The patch electrodes ideally are significantly lower resistance than the junctional (R_j) and nonjunctional resistances (R_m). The circuit allows for the computation of junctional conductance (g_j) with the following relationships: $V_j = V_2 - V_1$, $I_1 = I_{m,1} + I_j$, $I_2 = -I_j$, and $g_j = I_j/V_j$. (B) Macroscopic record of homotypic Cx45 using V_j steps of ± 10, ± 30, ± 50, ± 70, ± 90, and ± 110 mV of 10 seconds in duration, which illustrates the voltage dependence of Cx45 and the varied time constants of inactivation with V_j. $I_{j,inst}$ is the instantaneous junctional current, and $I_{j,ss}$ is the steady-state current. (C) Single-channel properties of Cx43, Cx40, and Cx45 channels. Records of single-channel currents observed in pairs of HeLa cells transfected with Cx40, Cx43, and Cx45. *Solid line,* Zero current level; *dashed line,* residual current level. The current histograms (*right*) revealed $\gamma_{j,main}$ = 125 pS and $\gamma_{j,residual}$ = 26 pS for Cx40, $\gamma_{j,main}$ = 54 pS and $\gamma_{j,residual}$ = 11 pS for Cx43, and $\gamma_{j,main}$ = 25 pS for Cx45 cell pairs; pipette was filled with 120 mM K$^+$aspartate$^-$. (D) Normalized g_j plotted against V_j for Cx43, Cx40, and Cx45. The *red dots* represent the record shown in (B). Normalized junctional conductance (g_j) is steady state conductance $g_{j,ss}$ normalized against the instantaneous conductance $g_{j,inst}$. (Data modified from Valiunas V, Beyer EC, Brink PR. Cardiac gap junction channels show quantitative differences in selectivity. *Circ Res.* 2002;91:104-111; and Valiunas V, Gemel J, Brink PR, et al. Gap junction channels formed by coexpressed connexin40 and connexin43. *Am J Physiol Heart Circ Physiol.* 2001;281:H1675-H1689.)

relatively constant regardless of the voltage, implying that many if not all the gap junctions are patent when V_j is zero. Analysis of single and multichannel records of Cx43 (see Fig. 15.2C) have been used to determine open probability under chronic application of V_j between 20 and 40 mV, yielding values ranging from 0.5 to 0.95, consistent with the idea that gap junction channels are in the open state when there is no applied transjunctional potential. The application of V_j greater than 50 mV reduces the mean open time, whereas mean closed time remains relatively constant, which translates into reduced open probability (Po) with increased V_j amplitude.[24] This is consistent with the behavior manifest in macroscopic recordings for Cx43. Nonstationary analyses of Cx43 and Cx37 have also revealed similar results with open probabilities less than 0.95 for Cx43 and 0.7 for Cx37.[25]

Table 15.2 lists $V_{j,o}$ and unitary conductance for cardiac connexins, which includes homotypic, heterotypic, and heteromeric forms. The values of $V_{j,o}$ for homotypic channels vary from 20 mV for Cx45 to 60 mV for Cx43. Also listed are all the $V_{j,o}$ values for heterotypic forms that have thus far been determined. In addition, values for cells coexpressing Cx43/Cx40 and Cx43/Cx37 are given. Unitary conductance for the cardiac connexins varies greatly, as seen in Table 15.2. For heterotypic forms, the observed unitary conductance can be polarity-dependent.[12] Observation of cell pairs coexpressing connexins reveals a range of conductances consistent with channels of different connexin content.

The macroscopic junctional currents shown in Fig. 15.2B illustrate that the currents decline (deactivation) with a prescribed time course on the order of 0.1 to 1 second for Cx43.[26] The time constant for voltage-dependent inactivation is itself voltage-dependent and becomes shorter with larger transjunctional voltage steps. The time courses of voltage-dependent inactivation in junctional currents for Cx45, as shown in Fig. 15.2B are similar to the behavior of the other cardiac connexins, although it should be noted that Cx45 has the largest inactivation time constants of the cardiac connexins, approximately 0.1 second for large transjunctional potentials and 3 seconds for smaller transjunctional steps.[26]

Heterotypic forms that have been studied often generate asymmetric voltage-dependent current–voltage (I–V) curves; an example of heterotypic Cx43-Cx45 is shown in Fig. 15.3B, along with

TABLE 15.2 Multichannel and Single-Channel Data of Different Types of Gap Junction Channels

CHANNEL TYPE	$V_{j,o}$ (mV)	$\gamma_{j,main}$ (pS)	REFERENCES
Homotypic			
Cx43	±60	55	[12–15]
Cx40	±48	125	[2,13,14,16]
Cx45	±20	25	[17,18]
Cx46	±42	128	[19]
Cx37	±25	350	[20]
Cx40G38D	±25	220	[21]
Heterotypic			
Cx40-Cx43	−80/>100	60/100[a]	[12,14,15]
Cx40-Cx45	n.d./14	40	[12,22]
Cx43-Cx45	−100/12	40	[12,15,18]
Cx37-Cx43	−70/>100	50/175[a]	[20]
Coexpressed			
Cx40/Cx43	±70	31–130[b]	[14,22]
Cx37/Cx43	±30/>100	35–280[b]	[20]

Values represent averages derived from representative studies. Experimental conditions: room temperature; pipette solution: K+aspartate− if available.
[a]Conductance polarity dependent.
[b]Conductances from homotypic, heterotypic, and heteromeric channels are possible.

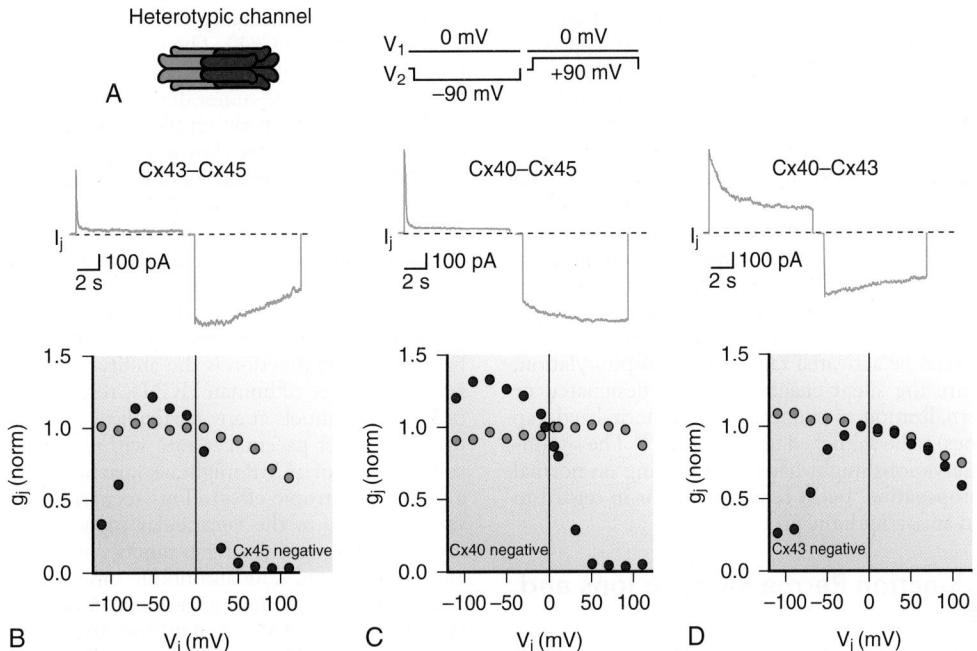

FIGURE 15.3 (A) Rendition of the heterotypic channel where each hemichannel is homomeric, but the connexins for each are different. A voltage step profile for the records shown in B–D are illustrated to the right. (B) Macroscopic current record of Cx43-Cx45 heterotypic gap junction channels. The *lower panel* shows the normalized g_j versus V_j showing both steady state $g_{j,ss}$ (*purple circles*) and instantaneous $g_{j,inst}$ (*green circles*). Cx45 gates close when the potential in the opposing cell of a pair is more positive; therefore it gates closed with a negative potential relative to its neighbor (Cx45 negative). (C) The same paradigm for a Cx40-Cx45 heterotypic junction. (D) The same paradigm for a Cx43-Cx45 heterotypic junction.

heterotypic Cx40-Cx45 (see Fig. 15.3C) and Cx40-Cx43 (see Fig. 15.3D). Note that for one voltage polarity, a voltage-dependent deactivation or decline in junctional current is present, much like the homotypic forms. For the other polarity there is, in effect, little or no voltage-dependent closure. In the case of Cx40-Cx45 and to a lesser degree Cx43-Cx45, there is an increase in junctional current, which is best illustrated by the plots of g_j versus V_j. This observation suggests that heterotypic gap junction channels have altered voltage sensing and gating relative to their homotypic parents and that Po for these forms might be significantly less than unity, or the asymmetric unitary conductance observed in heterotypic channels is itself voltage-dependent.

The Number of Functional Channels Within the Intercalated Disc

The formation of large plaques or aggregates of channels that are closely packed together is an interesting synapse-like feature of gap junctions (see Fig. 15.1), and it raises a number of questions, such as are all the channels simultaneously active or are there active and inactive or silent populations? Furthermore, is each channel functioning as an identical but independent channel, or is there evidence for nonindependent, interdependent, or cooperative behavior? Or can channels shift between states that in the case of gap junctions would be moving from mostly patent to mostly closed? Recall that active gap junction channels possess high open probabilities approaching unity. Thus accurate measurement of total junctional conductance and knowing the unitary conductance for a particular connexin allows an estimate of the total number of functioning channels operating between a cell pair. To determine whether all the channels within a plaque are functional first requires a determination of the number of channels within any one plaque; second, it requires the determination of the number of functional channels within that particular plaque. By tagging Cx43 with a fluorescent reporter such as GFP, it is possible to image plaques within cell pairs and further to directly assess the junctional conductance using a dual whole-cell patch clamp. An analysis of experiments using this dual approach of imaging and electrophysiological assessment of junctional conductance has revealed that approximately 10% of the channels are functioning within junctional membrane plaques[27]; furthermore, it appears that Cx43 channels displayed nonindependent behaviors associated with phenomena such as transitioning between an active patent state and a silent state on the order of many seconds to minutes, which represents an example of mode shifting.[24] These surprising results beg the question: why are there so many apparently silent channels (Po = 0) in presumed dynamic equilibrium with a lesser population of almost continually open (Po $\approx$ 1) channels? Are there conditions or circumstances in which the silent channels can be activated rapidly via phosphorylation, for example? Or are the silent channels already designated or identified for internalization as connexosomes (internalized gap junction membranes) to be trafficked to lysosomes?[28] The significance of these observations might have little bearing on normal action potential propagation, but it remains unclear in regard to proarrhythmic and antiarrhythmic processes.

Cardiac Gap Junction Permeability to Ions and Other Solutes

The major intracellular ion involved in intercellular current flow via gap junctions is K^+. Estimates of the number of K^+ flowing through a single gap junction channel per second in response to a voltage step of approximately 23.4 mV or the equivalent of a 10× concentration gradient ranging from approximately 18.3×10^6 ions per channel per second for Cx40 to 8.1×10^6 ions per channel per second for Cx43 and 3.7×10^6 ions per channel per second for Cx45.[13,29] A number of studies have also determined the permeability of the major cardiac connexins to a variety of exogenous fluorescent probes and endogenous second messengers such as cAMP.[30]

The permeability of gap junction channels has been defined qualitatively and quantitatively. A common qualitative approach for such studies is the use of an exogenous fluorescent probe that is introduced in one cell and is then detected in the other cell of a pair (Fig. 15.4A). For quantification of any specific probe's permeability, it is necessary to simultaneously measure the junctional conductance and the fluorescence distribution and intensity of the probe via imaging.[13]

Fig. 15.4A shows the cell-to-cell transfer of the fluorescent dye Lucifer yellow (LY). Comparison of LY permeability for Cx43, Cx40, and Cx45 is a notable example of selectivity, as illustrated in Fig. 15.4B. Lucifer yellow with a minor diameter of 0.95 nm and a net negative charge is greater than tenfold more permeable to Cx43 than to Cx40 and threefold more permeable to Cx45.[13,29] In Fig. 15.4B, the relative fluorescence intensity in a target cell of a pair is plotted at the 12-minute mark versus the simultaneously measured junctional conductance.[13]

Fig. 15.4C illustrates the differences between cAMP permeability for Cx43 and Cx40, where the *y*-axis is the ratio of a reporter channel current density relative to a control versus junctional conductance measured simultaneously.[30] cAMP permeability to Cx43 is much more permissive than that of Cx40.

For a number of the exogenous probes and select messengers, it has been possible to determine their flux relative to K^+ for specific homotypic connexins, namely Cx43 and Cx40. Fig. 15.4D is a semilog plot of flux of either an ion, a probe, or a solute relative to K^+. The monovalent cations are Li^+, Na^+, TMA, and TEA. Lucifer yellow, cAMP, and two oligonucleotides (short interfering RNA [siRNA] mimics) represent solutes of various sizes and charges. The graph illustrates what is considered a general rule for connexin channels: monovalent cations have permeabilities relative to K^+ that are similar to an Eisenmann series I or II, which is much like their mobility in free solution. As solute diameter increases, differences in permeability for the same solute begin to appear between Cx43 and Cx40. The permeabilities of two synthetic oligonucleotides are also plotted; they are long, rod-shaped molecules (morpholinos) whose minor diameters are 1.0 to 1.1 nm.[31]

The differences between the permeabilities of LY and cAMP for Cx43 and Cx40 are shown in Fig. 15.4D. It should be noted that TMA, a larger probe but of lesser charge density than cAMP, is more permeable than cAMP with a smaller minor diameter for both Cx43 and Cx40. This strongly suggests that selectivity is based on not only size but also charge.

An important aspect of gap junction–mediated transfer of second messengers is best illustrated when considering cAMP permeability. It has the potential to affect a multitude of cellular functions. One function is the ability to positively shift the voltage dependence of human HCN4, resulting in an increase in Po of HCN4 channels at any particular membrane potential that in turn can affect pacemaker rate within the heart.[32] The cell-to-cell diffusion of cAMP might also participate in the generation of a positive inotropic effect. This scenario implies a sparse innervation density in the ventricular myocardium, where only one myocyte of a number of gap junction–coupled myocytes receive autonomic input. The autonomic input to the innervated myocyte results in the rapid generation of elevated cAMP within its cytoplasm. The cAMP then diffuses to surrounding cells that are not innervated. The time to reach half concentration in adjacent cells coupled along their lateral borders would be on the order of 1 to 5 seconds, assuming the junctional permeability illustrated in Fig. 15.4 for cAMP and a cytoplasmic diffusion coefficient of approximately 1×10^{-6} cm^2/s.[33] Such a time course is consistent with the time course for sympathetically induced inotropy of the heart. The notion of sympathetic and parasympathetic innervation density being less than one-to-one for nerve to myocyte, while never having been quantitatively assessed, is consistent with observations describing low innervation density in the ventricular myocardium.[34]

Another possible role for connexins in the heart and other syncytial tissues is the passage of microRNAs and siRNAs able to affect gene expression and ultimately cellular phenotype.[35] As a general rule, cardiac connexins can be considered to be poorly selective toward monovalent cations, as an Eisenmann series 1 implies, and are only moderately more selective toward the monovalent halide anions. With increased size and charge, Cx40 and Cx45 appear to be less permissive or more selective than Cx43.

Action Potential Propagation in the Myocardium: The Role of Connexins

Two questions arise when considering the role of gap junction channels in the propagation of the cardiac action potential. First, what is the relationship between gap junction number and conduction velocity? Second, does gap junction channel voltage dependence matter? The first question has been best addressed using a combination of experimental data and computational analysis. In vitro studies of cell pairs and isolated tissues have shown that a pharmacologically induced reduction in gap junctional conductance slows conduction and ultimately can block conduction, whereas increased expression enhances conduction.[36] Similarly, many arrhythmias have been associated with reduced gap junction channel numbers, redistribution of junctional plaques on the lateral surfaces, or mutations within connexins.[3] Using both experimental and computationally derived data, it has been shown that there is a nonlinear relationship between conduction and longitudinal resistance dominated by gap junctions. Simulation of the experimental data predicts that conduction velocity is roughly proportional to the $\log_{10}$ of gap junction channel number over a range of 10 to 1000 nS (Fig. 15.5).

The second question as to whether gap junction channel voltage dependence can have a role in conduction velocity requires defining current flow longitudinally within myocytes in response to a propagating action potential. This definition then allows the determination of the transjunctional voltage experienced at the

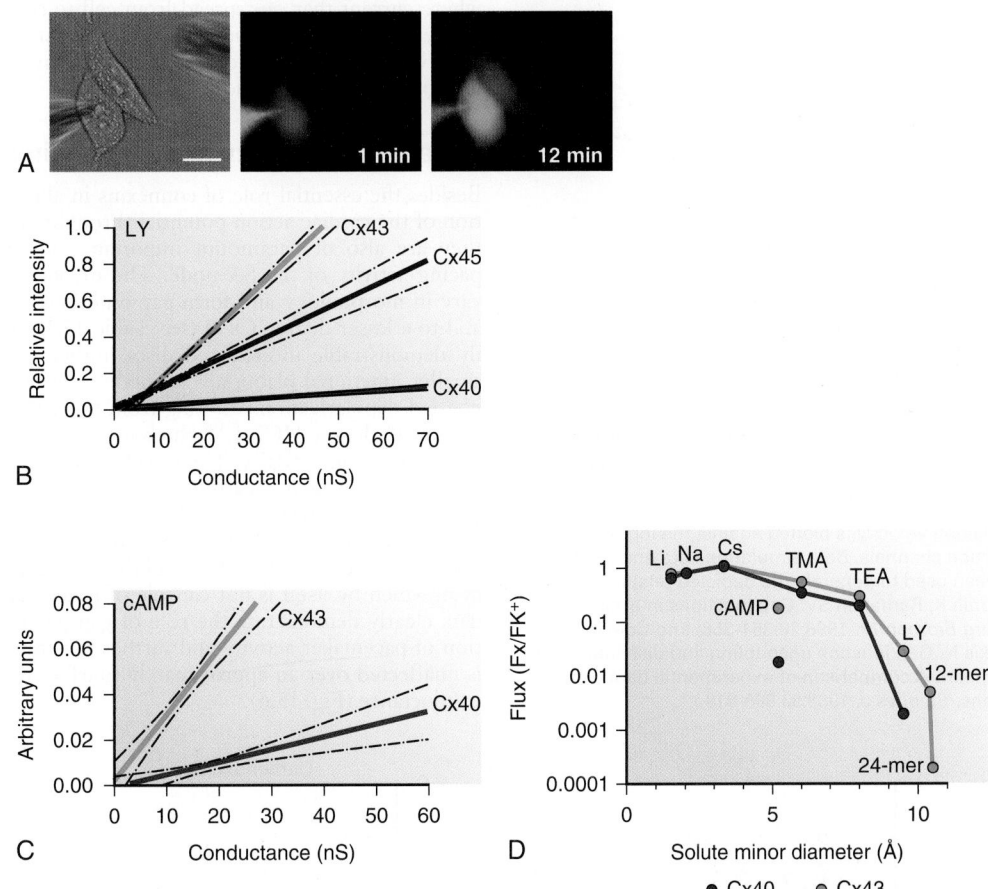

FIGURE 15.4 (A) Three images of a cell pair where the electrode on the left contains a known concentration of the fluorescent dye Lucifer yellow (*LY*). Once in whole-cell patch mode, fluorescence emission is monitored over time (1- and 12-minute records shown). Scale bar, 20 μm. (B) Relative fluorescence intensity of LY in the target cell compared with that in the source cell, plotted versus junctional conductance for Cx43, Cx40, and Cx45. All fluorescence measurements are made at the same time interval. (C) Cyclic adenosine monophosphate (*cAMP*) permeability to Cx43 and Cx40 versus conductance. cAMP is approximately 10-fold more permeable to Cx43 than to Cx40. Arbitrary units are the ratio of current density for a cAMP-activated channel before and during exposure to elevated intracellular cAMP levels. (D) Semilog plot of Li^+, Na^+, Cs^+, cAMP, TMA, TEA, and LY flux relative to K^+ ion flux for Cx43 and Cx40. Permeability of two oligonucleotides (12 and 24 nucleotides long) to Cx43 is also plotted. (Data from Valiunas V, Beyer EC, Brink PR. Cardiac gap junction channels show quantitative differences in selectivity. *Circ Res.* 2002; 91:104-111; Kanaporis G, Mese G, Valiuniene L, et al. Gap junction channels exhibit connexin-specific permeability to cyclic nucleotides. *J Gen Physiol.* 2008;131:293-305; Valiunas V, Polosina YY, Miller H, et al. Connexin-specific cell-to-cell transfer of short interfering RNA by gap junctions, *J Physiol.* 2005;568:459-468; and Brink PR. Gap junctions in vascular smooth muscle. *Acta Physiol Scand.* 1998;164:349-356.)

intercalated disc. It is assumed that a myocyte is approximately 100 μm long (L) and has a diameter of approximately 15 μm and that myoplasmic resistance is approximately 400 Ω cm. Thus the longitudinal resistance of a myocyte is approximately 2 MΩ. Assuming that conduction velocity (θ) is 50 cm/s and that the maximum rate of rise for the action potential is 100 V/s, the longitudinal voltage drop along the long axis of the cell can be determined by $V_{cell} = [(V/s)/\theta] \times L$, or 20 mV. The longitudinal current flow is then 20 mV/2 MΩ = 10 nA. For an intercalated disc with 1.8×10^5 functioning channels or a junctional conductance of approximately 1000 nS, the amount of current flowing through each patent channel is 0.05 pA. The former assumes a channel population of homotypic Cx43 channels, each with a unitary conductance of approximately 55 pS.[13] Therefore the transjunctional voltage is 1 mV per channel. For 20,000 channels the value is approximately 10 mV per channel, and for 2000 channels it is approximately 100 mV per channel. Homotypic Cx43 unitary conductances of 55 pS are observed when using K^+aspartate$^-$ pipette solutions (see Table 15.2) that best mimic the myoplasmic electrolytes. The other factor to consider is the time course of the voltage dependence. It is possible for a transjunctional voltage of 10 to 20 mV or larger, as might occur with only 1000 channels or fewer, to result in voltage-dependent channel closure. To assess this possibility, it is necessary to determine how long a transjunctional voltage will persist during the passage of an action potential. What is the duration of the transjunctional voltage for an action potential conducting at 50 cm/s? For θ = 50 cm/s, the cardiac action potential will traverse a 100-μm length in 0.2 ms or 2 ms for θ = 5 cm/s. The time course of voltage-dependent closure varies from connexin to connexin, but for the cardiac connexins a 2-ms duration would result in a small reduction in junctional conductance.

It is easy to see that only with reduced numbers of functional channels would their number or voltage dependence begin to have an effect on the propagation or conduction of the cardiac action potential. In fact, the normal AV[13] node delay of 0.12 second is thought to be in part a result of sparse gap junction density.[37] Conditions such as AV block might be manifested by reduced gap junction channel number and voltage-dependent closure, effectively elevating longitudinal resistance to a point where current that can spread from cell to cell is insufficient to trigger continued conduction. Results from animal model systems where connexin knockouts of Cx40 have been constructed are consistent with this notion.[10]

Pacemaker Activity and Connexins

Besides the essential role of connexins in allowing the propagation of the cardiac action potential throughout the myocardium, they are also of paramount importance in the generation of pacing activity of the SA node. The myocytes of the SA node vary in morphology and form gap junctions composed of Cx45 and to a lesser degree Cx40 (see Table 15.1). There are no easily demonstrable intercalated discs, rather the myocytes form smaller junctional plaques.[10] SA node cells are characterized by phase 4 depolarization resulting from the activity of HCN4 and to a lesser degree HCN1,[38] which is sufficient to elicit an action potential in the nodal cells and subsequent propagation to the surrounding atrial myocardium.

Artificial pacemaker units consisting of two coupled cells have been shown to pace at 1 Hz, where one cell of the pair is a non-myocyte cell expressing HCN and the other is a ventricular myocyte, which by itself is not capable of pacemaker activity.[39] The data clearly demonstrate the role of gap junctions in the initiation of pacemaker activity and further illustrate that pacing rate is unaffected over an approximately fourfold range of junctional conductance (Fig. 15.6).

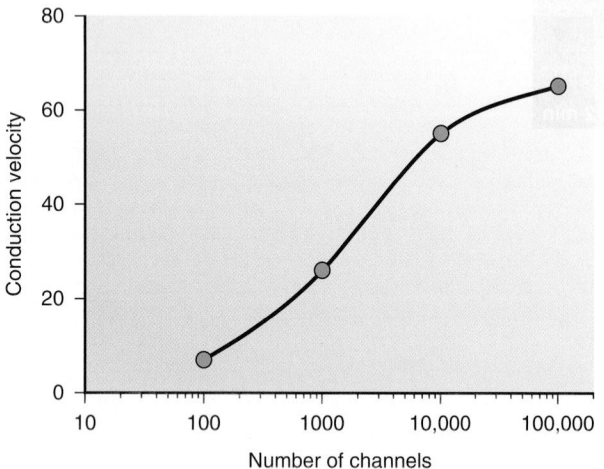

FIGURE 15.5 Conduction velocity is plotted against the log of the number of gap junction channels. Both simulation data and experimental data have been used to generate the depicted relationship. (From Brink PR, Cronin K, Ramanan SV. Gap junctions in excitable cells. *J Bioenerg Biomembr.* 1996;28:351-358; and Cole WC, Picone JB, Sperelakis N. Gap junction uncoupling and discontinuous propagation in the heart. A comparison of experimental data with computer simulations. *Biophys J.* 1988;53:809-818.)

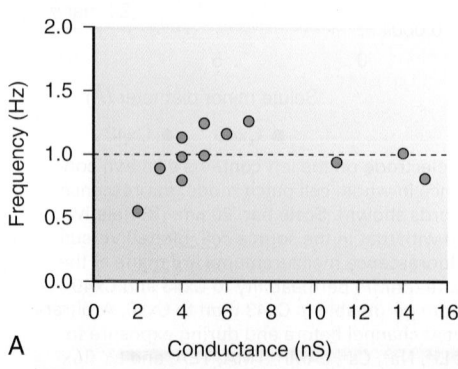
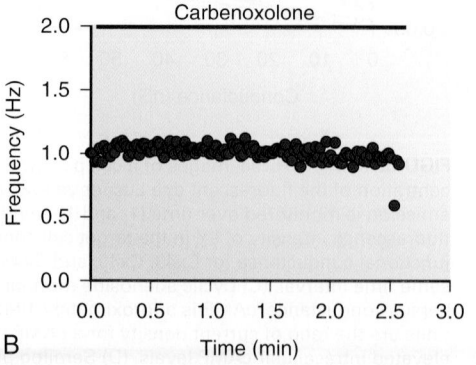

FIGURE 15.6 (A) Pacing frequency generated by a cell transfected with HCN2 coupled to a ventricular myocyte. Frequency is plotted against the measured junctional conductance. The *dashed line* corresponds to an average frequency of 1 Hz. (B) Carbenoxolone exposure results in a cessation of pacing. Pacing remains constant for more than 2 minutes and then abruptly stops. This is consistent with the notion that junctional conductance only affects propagation once a critically low level of coupling is attained. (Modified from Valiunas V, Kanaporis G, Valiuniene L, et al. Coupling an HCN2-expressing cell to a myocyte creates a two-cell pacing unit. *J Physiol.* 2009;587:5211-5226.)

Non–Voltage-Dependent Regulators of Channel Patency

There are two intrinsic intracellular elements that are able to affect junctional conductance: intracellular pH and intracellular calcium. Lowered intracellular pH, as occurs in ischemia,[40] is known to affect many cardiac membrane channels and transporters and can effectively reduce gap junction conductance.[41] Fig. 15.7 shows the effect of perfusion with 100% CO_2 on junctional conductance measured between a pair of cells expressing Cx43. A pH-sensitive fluorescent probe was used to determine intracellular pH (see Fig. 15.7B). Many investigators have observed that short exposures to elevated H^+ result in reduced coupling with subsequent recovery, as illustrated in Fig. 15.7. What is not shown in Fig. 15.7 is the result of prolonged exposure for many minutes, which results in an irreversible reaction culminating in permanent channel closure, implying both rapid and slow processes triggered by H^+. The majority of connexins are similarly affected by acidification, responding to elevated intracellular H^+ with reduced junctional conductance that is presumed to be the result of increased closed times and reduced open times. However, the mechanisms of H^+-induced closure are apparently not universal. The mechanism of pH-induced alteration of Cx43 gap junction channel open probability has been shown to be manifested by a ball-and-chain configuration between the C-terminus and the cytoplasmic loop between membrane-spanning domains M2 and M3. In contrast, Cx40 is also pH sensitive, but the mechanism of channel closure is not mediated by a ball-and-chain–like mechanism. The mechanism by which H^+ affects Cx40 channel patency has not been elucidated, but the pKa for Cx40 is essentially the same as that for Cx43 (6.7).[42] The formation of heteromeric or heterotypic forms of Cx43 and Cx40 shifts the pKa to a more alkaline value of 7.0.[42] Other cardiac connexins have not been studied as extensively as Cx43 and Cx40, with the exception of Cx46, for which the data are most consistent with a direct effect on the cytoplasmic surface. Rapid delivery of H^+ to the cytoplasmic side of Cx46 hemichannels was accomplished using an inside-out patch clamp in combination with two Cx46 constructs: a wild type with an intact C-terminus, and a deletion mutant of Cx46 missing a significant portion of the C-terminus. Both forms had the same pH sensitivity with a pKa of 6.5, clearly suggesting a site or sites for Cx46 other than the ball-and-chain mechanism of Cx43.[11]

Another intracellular ion able to affect Cx43 junctional conductance is Ca^{2+}. Elevated intracellular calcium (500 nM–1 μM) reduces the number of functioning Cx43 gap junction channels and eventually results in complete uncoupling. The mechanism of calcium-mediated channel closure has been the center of some controversy, but recently it has been demonstrated that calcium acts to reduce Cx43 gap junctional conductance via calmodulin.[43] It is possible that calcium–pH synergy is mediated through calmodulin, but there are currently no data to support such a hypothesis. Interestingly, gap junction channels composed of Cx40 are not affected by elevated intracellular calcium and do not possess the putative calmodulin binding sites found on Cx43. In addition to affecting the gating of connexins, calcium is also able to permeate connexins and has been associated with cell death within the myocardium and other syncytial tissues.[44] These findings suggest that it is Cx40 that allows the spread of elevated intracellular calcium in infarcts, whereas Cx43 is the connexin working to preserve cellular integrity by isolating healthy myocytes from those that are damaged in an ischemic episode. Calcium and calmodulin sensitivities of Cx46, Cx45, and Cx37 have not been studied as completely as they have been for Cx43 and Cx40.

Extrinsic Uncoupling Agents of Cardiac Gap Junction Channels

Anesthetics such as halothane have been shown to reduce mean open time and increase mean closed time for Cx43 and Cx40 homotypic and heteromeric channels in a dose-dependent manner. The mechanism by which halothane reduces channel open time remains unknown, but it has been suggested that interactions at the protein-lipid interface are the most likely sites of action. Another class of agents, long-chained alcohols such as octanol and heptanol, are also effective in reducing junctional conductance and are thought to act via protein-lipid interactions. Other agents that are able to reduce functional gap junction numbers are carbenoxolone, glycyrrhetinic acid, quinine derivatives, retinoic acid, arachidonic acid, and spermine.[45] All the aforementioned agents lack specificity and inhibit other systems within cells.[45] Another approach has been the use of mimetic peptides. A recent study has shown that GAP26, a polypeptide, is able to block hemichannels of Cx43 on a time scale of seconds to minutes, and longer exposure is able to effectively reduce Cx43 gap junction–mediated coupling.[46] The mimetic peptides appear to function by binding to the extracellular loops, and when the hemichannel is subsequently incorporated into a plaque or attempts to link via E1 or E2 with its counterpart in the adjacent cell, the peptide prevents formation of a functioning channel. The apparent turnover rate of approximately 30 minutes is faster than the turnover rate determined via Western blot analysis,[47] but might be related connexon docking and gap junction channel assembly or disassembly associated with the scaffolding complex protein zonula occludens, ZO-1.[48] Despite a lack of mechanistic understanding, these data demonstrate a potentially useful clinical tool if GAP26 is clearly shown to be gap junction specific. Direct proof of binding to the extracellular loops is a first necessary step, and tagged peptides must be used to assess whether

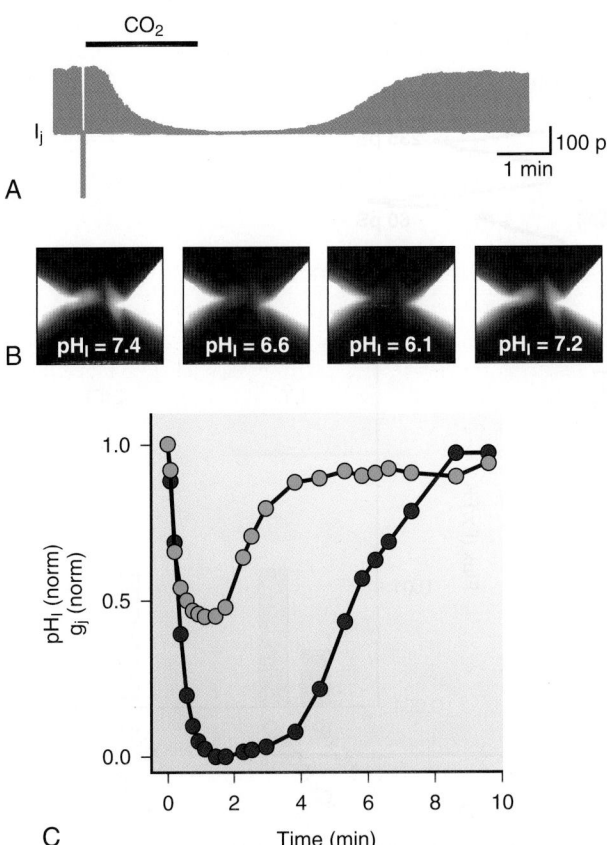

FIGURE 15.7 (A) Junctional current is reduced when 100% CO_2 is bubbled into the perfusate. The bar represents the exposure time, which is approximately 2 minutes. The time course to reduction in junctional current and subsequent recovery are not the same, but both represent examples of diffusion time within the bath and buffering capacity of the cells. (B) Intracellular pH can be monitored via pH-sensitive fluorescent dyes. A HeLa cell pair expressing Cx43 is shown. (C) Intracellular pH (pH_i) normalized to the initial pH_i (7.4) and junctional conductance (g_j) normalized to the initial g_j are plotted against time during 100% CO_2.

the peptide might affect function intracellularly, possibly via endosomal entry.

A potentially clinically relevant feature of mimetic peptides is manifest in Gap26, a mimetic peptide for Cx43 that has been shown to protect against induced myocardial ischemia in vivo.[49] Its potential to slow conduction and create proarrhythmic activity has not been tested. Overall, extrinsic uncoupling agents have proved useful in attempting to understand how gap junction channels affect cardiac action potential propagation but, as might be expected, a reduction in the number of functioning gap junction channels results in slowed conduction and, consequently, in the possibility of generating arrhythmogenic activity.[36]

Ischemia, Mutations, Arrhythmia, and Gap Junctions

Ischemia reduces or completely occludes blood flow to the myocardium, resulting in hypoxia that subsequently triggers the release of intracellular calcium and acidosis, which can result in cellular remodeling or cell death. A number of studies have demonstrated that ischemia triggers an anatomic remodeling of gap junctions within myocytes, such that fewer junctions are found in the intercalated disc and more appear on the lateral surfaces of the myocytes.[50] Such redistribution or remodeling is predicted to directly affect longitudinal resistance and reduce conduction velocity along the long axis of the myocyte. To further complicate matters, the insertion of more gap junctions laterally has the potential to create arrhythmias.[50] Studies using a canine heart failure model found

a strong correlation between reduced Cx43 expression in vivo and reentrant ventricular arrhythmias.[50] A number of studies have also found the phosphorylation state of Cx43 to be altered in ischemia and in nonischemic heart failure.[51] Phosphorylation state might also trigger anatomic remodeling in response to ischemia or other pathophysiologic challenges to the heart. Clearly, gap junction channels along with many other membrane channels participate in electrical and anatomical remodeling in response to ischemic conditions. Which one dominates in response to ischemia is most likely disease-dependent.

Atrial arrhythmias are also associated with electrical remodeling and presumed changes in connexin distribution. Of particular interest is Cx40, in which abnormal expression results in an increased tendency toward atrial fibrillation.[52–54] Three recent studies have illustrated a number of mutations of human Cx40 that are suspect. In vitro studies of the N-terminus mutation, Cx40 E9, 13K[55] have shown that it reduces the rectifying voltage dependence of the Cx43-Cx40 heterotypic channel, suggesting a possible involvement in altered longitudinal resistance. Three other mutants (L229M, V85I, and G38D) have been shown to undergo significantly faster degradation rates than wild type Cx40.[56] Degradation can be slowed to near normal by inhibition of the proteasomal degradation pathway, suggesting that junctional conductance in vivo might be reduced enough to significantly reduce longitudinal resistance. Yet another study[21] has shown that Cx40 mutants M163V, A96S, and G38D have altered permeability to anions and cations relative to wild type Cx40. Of particular interest is G38D, which has a significantly higher unitary conductance (Fig. 15.8A and B, Table 15.2).

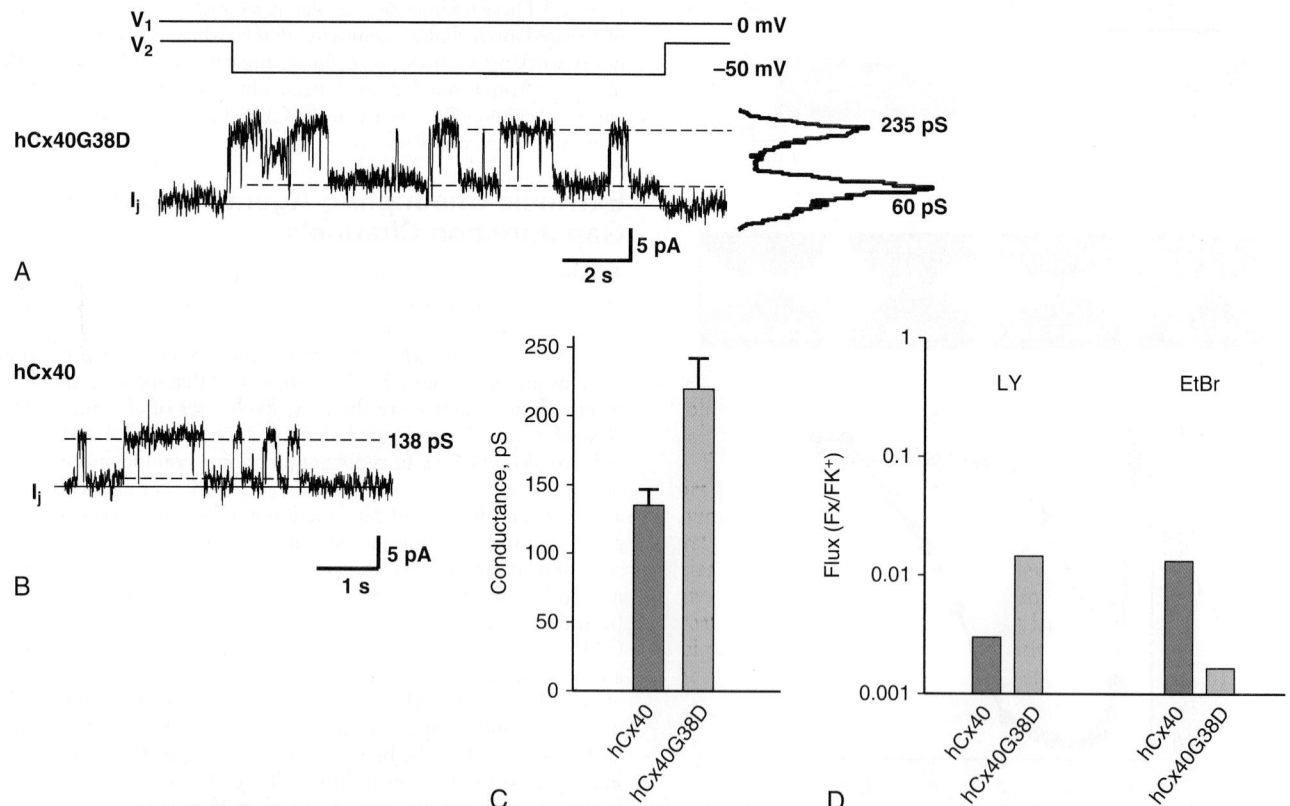

FIGURE 15.8 (A) Voltage pulse protocol (V_1 and V_2) and associated single-channel current (I_j) recorded from an N2ACx40G38 mutant cell pair. The all-points current histogram revealed $\gamma_{j,main}$ = 235 pS and $\gamma_{j,residual}$ = 60 pS, respectively; (B) Single-channel current recorded at the maintained V_j of 50 mV from a wild-type hCx40 N2A cell pair. The *dashed lines* correspond to $\gamma_{j,main}$ = 138 pS and $\gamma_{j,residual}$ = 31 pS conductance levels; pipette filled with 120 mM K$^+$aspartate$^-$. (C) Average of unitary conductances measured from hCx40 (135 ± 1.4 pS, n = 72) and hCx40G38D (220 ± 3 pS, n = 67) cell pairs. *Error bars* represent means ± SD. (D) Permeability of anionic (*LY*) and cationic (*EtBr*) fluorescent probes relative to K$^+$ ions for the G38D mutant and the wild type of Cx40. The *bars* represent LY and EtBr flux relative to K$^+$ ion plotted on a log scale. (Modified from Santa Cruz A, Meşe G, Valiuniene L, Brink PR, White TW, Valiunas V. Altered conductance and permeability of Cx40 mutations associated with atrial fibrillation. *J Gen Physiol.* 2015;146:387-398.)

The histogram in Fig. 15.8C is a summary of the unitary conductance measurements of G38D and wild-type hCx40 gap junction channels. The permeability of G38D is also significantly different than that of wild-type Cx40 as shown in Fig. 15.8D. The anion and cation fluxes relative to K^+ are inverted relative to those in wild type. The latter suggests altered second messenger permeability for solutes such as cAMP, which might in part cause aberrant pacemaker activity within the atrium.

The voltage dependence and unitary conductance of M163V are similar to that of the wild type, while both anionic and cationic permeability are significantly higher than those in wild type.[21] A96S also exhibits an elevated cation permeability.[21]

For those mutants with altered permeability, the ability to affect the distribution/diffusion of second messengers from cell to cell may be a potential source of arrhythmogenic activity.

Another study using a mouse model for A96S revealed reduced atrial conduction within the mouse heart along with a significant increase in the frequency of atrial fibrillation.[57]

For all the mutants of Cx40, altered distribution to the intercalated disc and lateral surfaces of atrial myocytes in vivo is another, as yet, untested mechanism that might result in proarrhythmic activity.

A number of studies have found strong correlations between mutations in Cx43 and disease states, with the most clearly understood being oculodentodigital dysplasia (ODDD), in which a number of mutations in Cx43 have been identified.[53,58] Interestingly, patients with ODDD do not display any cardiac anomalies. Mutations in adhesion molecules are another way to affect connexin distribution within the intercalated disc. Naxos disease arises because of a mutation within the adhesion molecule plakoglobin. This mutant form does not traffic to the intercalated disc properly.[59] As a result, Cx43 remodeling occurs with lesser junctional complexes being formed, culminating in an arrhythmogenic cardiomyopathy.

Summary

Gap junction channels are poorly selective intercellular channels that allow the movement of ions, solutes, second messengers, and even microRNAs and siRNAs from cell to cell exclusive of the extracellular milieu. Gap junctions participate in the propagation of the cardiac action potential and are expressed differentially to affect pacing rate, AV node delay, and rapid conduction in Purkinje fibers and in ventricular and atrial myocardium. The evidence is overwhelmingly clear that the cardiac connexins are essential to normal cardiac rhythm and are involved in responses to disease processes, such as the phenomenon of lateralization. Mutations in cardiac connexins resulting in or causing cardiac dysfunction must still be considered correlative rather than causative; they have not yet been unequivocally demonstrated to cause heart disease,[60] unlike Cx26, where the mutations have been shown to cause deafness.[58] For ischemic disease states, it appears that cardiac connexins are best considered as part of the effect rather than the cause. Again, the best example is remodeling associated with ischemia. In one sense, remodeling in the form of increased abundance of connexin along the lateral surfaces is most logically considered to be an attempt to circumvent a damaged intercalated disc rather than a precipitating causal event. There is a risk of creating a reentrant arrhythmia with lateralization, but it is a better alternative than significant or complete loss of longitudinal conductivity because of a dysfunctional gap junction–mediated communication at the intercalated disc.

Acknowledgments

The authors thank Dr. Robert Weingart for his guidance and mentorship. This work was supported by National Institutes of Health grants RO1 GM 088181.

REFERENCES

1. Yao JA, Gutstein DE, Liu F, et al. Cell coupling between ventricular myocyte pairs from connexin43-deficient murine hearts. *Circ Res.* 2003;93:736–743.
2. Beblo DA, Wang HZ, Beyer EC, et al. Unique conductance, gating, and selective permeability properties of gap junction channels formed by connexin40. *Circ Res.* 1995;77:813–822.
3. Severs NJ, Bruce AF, Dupont E, et al. Remodelling of gap junctions and connexin expression in diseased myocardium. *Cardiovasc Res.* 2008;80:9–19.
4. Maeda S, Nakagawa S, Suga M, et al. Structure of the connexin 26 gap junction channel at 3.5 A resolution. *Nature.* 2009;458:597–602.
5. Cheng A, Yeager M. Bootstrap resampling for voxel-wise variance analysis of three-dimensional density maps derived by image analysis of two-dimensional crystals. *J Struct Biol.* 2007;158:19–32.
6. Kovacs JA, Baker KA, Altenberg GA, et al. Molecular modeling and mutagenesis of gap junction channels. *Prog Biophys Mol Biol.* 2007;94:15–28.
7. Prochnow N, Hoffmann S, Dermietzel R, et al. Replacement of a single cysteine in the fourth transmembrane region of zebrafish pannexin 1 alters hemichannel gating behavior. *Exp Brain Res.* 2009;199:255–264.
8. Rackauskas M, Neverauskas V, Skeberdis VA. Diversity and properties of connexin gap junction channels. *Medicina (Kaunas).* 2010;46:1–12.
9. Duffy HS, Fort AG, Spray DC. Cardiac connexins: genes to nexus. *Adv Cardiol.* 2006;42:1–17.
10. Jansen JA, van Veen TA, de Bakker JM, et al. Cardiac connexins and impulse propagation. *J Mol Cell Cardiol.* 2010;48:76–82.
11. Bukauskas FF, Verselis VK. Gap junction channel gating. *Biochim Biophys Acta.* 2004;1662:42–60.
12. Valiunas V, Weingart R, Brink PR. Formation of heterotypic gap junction channels by connexins 40 and 43. *Circ Res.* 2000;86:E42–E49.
13. Valiunas V, Beyer EC, Brink PR. Cardiac gap junction channels show quantitative differences in selectivity. *Circ Res.* 2002;91:104–111.
14. Valiunas V, Gemel J, Brink PR, et al. Gap junction channels formed by coexpressed connexin40 and connexin43. *Am J Physiol Heart Circ Physiol.* 2001;281:H1675–H1689.
15. Desplantez T, Dupont E, Severs NJ, et al. Gap junction channels and cardiac impulse propagation. *J Membr Biol.* 2007;218:13–28.

16. Bukauskas FF, Elfgang C, Willecke K, et al. Biophysical properties of gap junction channels formed by mouse connexin40 in induced pairs of transfected human HeLa cells. *Biophys J.* 1995;68:2289–2298.
17. Valiunas V. Biophysical properties of connexin-45 gap junction hemichannels studied in vertebrate cells. *J Gen Physiol.* 2002;119:147–164.
18. Elenes S, Martinez AD, Delmar M, et al. Heterotypic docking of Cx43 and Cx45 connexons blocks fast voltage gating of Cx43. *Biophys J.* 2001;81:1406–1418.
19. Sakai R, Elfgang C, Vogel R, et al. The electrical behaviour of rat connexin46 gap junction channels expressed in transfected HeLa cells. *Pflugers Arch.* 2003;446:714–727.
20. Brink PR, Cronin K, Banach K, et al. Evidence for heteromeric gap junction channels formed from rat connexin43 and human connexin37. *Am J Physiol.* 1997;273:C1386–C1396.
21. Santa Cruz A, Mese G, Valiuniene L, et al. Altered conductance and permeability of Cx40 mutations associated with atrial fibrillation. *J Gen Physiol.* 2015;146:387–398.
22. Rackauskas M, Kreuzberg MM, Pranevicius M, et al. Gating properties of heterotypic gap junction channels formed of connexins 40, 43, and 45. *Biophys J.* 2007;92:1952–1965.
23. Vogel R, Valiunas V, Weingart R. Subconductance states of Cx30 gap junction channels: data from transfected HeLa cells versus data from a mathematical model. *Biophys J.* 2006;91:2337–2348.
24. Brink PR, Ramanan SV, Christ GJ. Human connexin 43 gap junction channel gating: evidence for mode shifts and/or heterogeneity. *Am J Physiol.* 1996;271:C321–C331.
25. Ramanan SV, Valiunas V, Brink PR. Non-stationary fluctuation analysis of macroscopic gap junction channel records. *J Physiol.* 2005;205:81–88.
26. Desplantez T, Halliday D, Dupont E, et al. Cardiac connexins Cx43 and Cx45: formation of diverse gap junction channels with diverse electrical properties. *Pflugers Arch.* 2004;448:363–375.
27. Bukauskas FF, Jordan K, Bukauskiene A, et al. Clustering of connexin 43-enhanced green fluorescent protein gap junction channels and functional coupling in living cells. *Proc Natl Acad Sci U S A.* 2000;97:2556–2561.
28. Kjenseth A, Fykerud T, Rivedal E, et al. Regulation of gap junction intercellular communication by the ubiquitin system. *Cell Signal.* 2010;22:1267–1273.

29. Kanaporis G, Brink PR, Valiunas V. Gap junction permeability: selectivity for anionic and cationic probes. *Am J Physiol Cell Physiol.* 2011;300:C600–C609.
30. Kanaporis G, Mese G, Valiuniene L, et al. Gap junction channels exhibit connexin-specific permeability to cyclic nucleotides. *J Gen Physiol.* 2008;2600:293–305.
31. Valiunas V, Polosina YY, Miller H, et al. Connexin-specific cell-to-cell transfer of short interfering RNA by gap junctions. *J Physiol.* 2005;568:459–468.
32. Alig J, Marger L, Mesirca P, et al. Control of heart rate by cAMP sensitivity of HCN channels. *Proc Natl Acad Sci U S A.* 2009;106:12189–12194.
33. Chen C, Nakamura T, Koutalos Y. Cyclic AMP diffusion coefficient in frog olfactory cilia. *Biophys J.* 1999;76:2861–2867.
34. Hasan W, Jama A, Donohue T, et al. Sympathetic hyperinnervation and inflammatory cell NGF synthesis following myocardial infarction in rats. *Brain Res.* 2006;1124:142–154.
35. Gommans WM, Berezikov E. Controlling miRNA regulation in disease. *Methods Mol Biol.* 2012;822: 1–18.
36. Jia Z, Bien H, Shiferaw Y, et al. Cardiac cellular coupling and the spread of early instabilities in intracellular Ca2+. *Biophys J.* 2012;102:1294–1302.
37. Greener ID, Monfredi O, Inada S, et al. Molecular architecture of the human specialised atrioventricular conduction axis. *J Mol Cell Cardiol.* 2011;50:642–651.
38. Nof E, Antzelevitch C, Glikson M. The contribution of HCN4 to normal sinus node function in humans and animal models. *Pacing Clin Electrophysiol.* 2010;33:100–106.
39. Valiunas V, Kanaporis G, Valiuniene L, et al. Coupling an HCN2-expressing cell to a myocyte creates a two-cell pacing unit. *J Physiol.* 2009;587:5211–5226.
40. Monastyrskaya K, Tschumi F, Babiychuk EB, et al. Annexins sense changes in intracellular pH during hypoxia. *Biochem J.* 2008;409:65–75.
41. Vaughan-Jones RD, Spitzer KW, Swietach P. Intracellular pH regulation in heart. *J Mol Cell Cardiol.* 2009;46:318–331.
42. Gu H, Ek-Vitorin JF, Taffet SM, et al. Coexpression of connexins 40 and 43 enhances the pH sensitivity of gap junctions: a model for synergistic interactions among connexins. *Circ Res.* 2000;86:E98–E103.

43. Xu Q, Kopp RF, Chen Y, et al. Gating of connexin 43 gap junctions by a cytoplasmic loop calmodulin binding domain. *Am J Physiol Cell Physiol.* 2012;302:C1548–C1556.

44. Decrock E, Vinken M, Bol M, et al. Calcium and connexin-based intercellular communication, a deadly catch? *Cell Calcium.* 2011;50:310–321.

45. Bodendiek SB, Raman G. Connexin modulators and their potential targets under the magnifying glass. *Curr Med Chem.* 2010;17:4191–4230.

46. Desplantez T, Verma V, Leybaert L, et al. Gap26, a connexin mimetic peptide, inhibits currents carried by connexin43 hemichannels and gap junction channels. *Pharmacol Res.* 2012;65:546–552.

47. Falk MM, Baker SM, Gumpert AM, et al. Gap junction turnover is achieved by the internalization of small endocytic double-membrane vesicles. *Mol Biol Cell.* 2009;20:3342–3352.

48. Rhett JM, Jourdan J, Gourdie RG. Connexin 43 connexon to gap junction transition is regulated by zonula occludens-1. *Mol Biol Cell.* 2011;22:1516–1528.

49. Hawat G, Benderdour M, Rousseau G, et al. Connexin 43 mimetic peptide Gap26 confers protection to intact heart against myocardial ischemia injury. *Pflugers Arch.* 2010;460:583–592.

50. Wit AL, Peters NS. The role of gap junctions in the arrhythmias of ischemia and infarction. *Heart Rhythm.* 2012;9:308–311.

51. Schulz R, Heusch G. Connexin43 and ischemic preconditioning. *Adv Cardiol.* 2006;42:213–227.

52. Chaldoupi SM, Loh P, Hauer RN, et al. The role of connexin40 in atrial fibrillation. *Cardiovasc Res.* 2009;84:15–23.

53. Molica F, Meens MJ, Morel S, et al. Mutations in cardiovascular connexin genes. *Biol Cell.* 2014;106:269–293.

54. Gollob MH, Jones DL, Krahn AD, et al. Somatic mutations in the connexin 40 gene (GJA5) in atrial fibrillation. *N Engl J Med.* 2006;354:2677–2688.

55. Lin X, Xu Q, Veenstra RD. Functional formation of heterotypic gap junction channels by connexins-40 and -43. *Channels (Austin).* 2014;8:433–443.

56. Gemel J, Simon AR, Patel D, et al. Degradation of a connexin40 mutant linked to atrial fibrillation is accelerated. *J Mol Cell Cardiol.* 2014;74:330–339.

57. Lubkemeier I, Andrie R, Lickfett L, et al. The Connexin40A96S mutation from a patient with atrial fibrillation causes decreased atrial conduction velocities and sustained episodes of induced atrial fibrillation in mice. *J Mol Cell Cardiol.* 2013;65:19–32.

58. Pfenniger A, Wohlwend A, Kwak BR. Mutations in connexin genes and disease. *Eur J Clin Invest.* 2011;41:103–116.

59. Saffitz JE. Arrhythmogenic cardiomyopathy: advances in diagnosis and disease pathogenesis. *Circulation.* 2011;124:e390–e392.

60. Makita N, Seki A, Sumitomo N, et al. A connexin40 mutation associated with a malignant variant of progressive familial heart block type I. *Circ Arrhythm Electrophysiol.* 2012;5:163–172.

16

Excitation–Contraction Coupling

Donald M. Bers

Excitation–Contraction Coupling and Relationship to Action Potentials

Cardiac excitation–contraction coupling (ECC) is the process by which the electrical activation of cardiac myocytes leads to the activation of contraction.[1-3] In its broadest use, ECC refers to everything from the initial membrane depolarization through the action potential (AP) to the activation of the Ca²⁺ transient, including how the myofilaments respond to the Ca²⁺ transient to produce contraction. Fig. 16.1 shows the temporal superposition of contraction and changes in membrane potential (E_m) and intracellular Ca²⁺ ($[Ca^{2+}]_i$), as measured in a rabbit ventricular myocyte at 37°C during 1-Hz stimulation. This chapter will focus on the initiation of normal and abnormal Ca²⁺ transients in myocytes, Ca²⁺ transport and buffering mechanisms, and the interaction of Ca²⁺ signaling with the AP and arrhythmias. In recent years it has increasingly become clear that Ca²⁺ signaling and cardiac electrophysiology are inextricably interrelated; thus understanding myocyte Ca²⁺ regulation is essential to understanding cardiac arrhythmogenesis.

Fig. 16.2 shows the structure and key mediators of ECC in myocytes. Ca²⁺ influx via Ca²⁺ current (I_{Ca}) and Ca²⁺ release from the ryanodine receptor (RyR) in the sarcoplasmic reticulum (SR) are central to myofilament activation. Ventricular myocytes have a network of transverse tubules (T-tubules) that dive into the cell center, perpendicular to the long axis of the myocyte. This T-tubular system also exhibits longitudinal extension in most myocytes. The role of the T-tubular system is to synchronize the sarcolemmal electrical signal (an AP) at junctions throughout the cell where the plasma membrane and SR are in close proximity to each other, and thereby mediate Ca²⁺-induced Ca²⁺ release. During heart failure there is evidence that the T-tubule network is less extensive and organized than in a healthy heart,[4,5] which could reduce efficacy of the ECC process.

Atrial myocytes have fewer T-tubules than ventricular myocytes,[5] and the specialized conduction fibers (sinoatrial and atrioventricular node and Purkinje fibers) have almost no T-tubules.

In cells or regions that lack T-tubules, I_{Ca} initiates SR Ca²⁺ release only at the surface membrane junctions. Then, depending on conditions discussed below, activation can more slowly propagate to the center of the myocyte (via a chain of RyR clusters) as a wave of Ca²⁺-induced Ca²⁺ release or it can fail to propagate such that the surface release produces only a small and slow $[Ca^{2+}]$ elevation near the center of the cell.

The rise in $[Ca^{2+}]_i$ activates contraction in the myofilaments. Ca²⁺ binds to troponin C on the thin filaments, thereby inducing a conformational change that allows the heads of the myosin molecules located along the thick filament to bind to the actin molecules that form the body of the thin filament (see Fig. 16.2). Myosin then uses energy stored as adenosine triphosphate (ATP) to tilt the myosin head, pulling on the actin filament to create either force or sarcomere shortening, which are responsible for isovolumic contraction and ejection of blood from the heart, respectively. Synchronization of local Ca²⁺ transients throughout the myocyte and the heart is thus essential for synchronous ventricular contraction. The strength of contraction is directly related to the $[Ca^{2+}]$ surrounding the myofilaments. Thus a myocyte (or region thereof) that has a small Ca²⁺ transient will be weaker than an adjacent area. Furthermore, this weaker myocyte can interfere with the strength of stronger neighboring regions, which can expend their strength stretching their weak neighbor and thus be unable to contribute to cardiac output. Readily appreciable consequences of this mechanical dyssynchrony include ischemia, spatially discordant cardiac alternans, and ventricular fibrillation.

Another point worth mentioning here is that Ca²⁺ signaling is highly localized, acting only within 1 to 3 μm and contrasting with electrical signals, which can spread over millimeter distances. The localized nature of Ca²⁺ signaling means that the distribution of Ca²⁺ entry into the cell and SR Ca²⁺ release must be quite uniform, even regionally within a single myocyte, to ensure proper function. In contrast, because of the electrical space constant in the heart, one could have potassium channels in every other myocyte only, and electrical signaling could be satisfactory.

For cardiac relaxation and ventricular refilling to occur, $[Ca^{2+}]_i$ must decline, allowing Ca²⁺ to dissociate from troponin C and terminating myofilament crossbridge cycling. This reduction in $[Ca^{2+}]_i$ is driven by Ca²⁺ transport, mainly via the SR Ca²⁺–adenosine triphosphatase (ATPase) and the sarcolemmal Na⁺/Ca²⁺ exchanger (NCX; discussed later). Ca²⁺ movement across the sarcolemma via Ca²⁺ channels and the 3Na⁺:1Ca²⁺ electrogenic NCX carries charge; thus it impacts the AP and excitability. Further, there are other Ca²⁺-sensitive channels whose electrophysiological impact is regulated by their local $[Ca^{2+}]_i$. Thus it is important to integrate our understanding of Ca handling into our electrophysiological framework.

Sources and Sinks of Ca²⁺ in Myocytes: Sarcolemma, Sarcoplasmic Reticulum, and Mitochondria

With reference to the cytosolic compartment, where the myofilaments reside and with which the sarcolemma, SR, mitochondria, and nucleus interface, we can consider the sources of Ca²⁺ that cause cytosolic $[Ca^{2+}]$ to rise, and sinks that cause cytosolic $[Ca^{2+}]_i$ to decline. Ca²⁺ channels (L-type and T-type) and the NCX are the main pathways of Ca²⁺ entry. However, the electrochemical driving force for Ca²⁺ influx is quite large due to a 20,000-fold concentration gradient (external = 2 mM; diastolic [Ca]ᵢ = 100 nM) and a resting Eₘ of –80 mV; thus even a slight additional Ca²⁺ permeability through a means other than these known transporters would constitute an additional nonnegligible "leak" pathway. During diastole, the Ca²⁺ channels are tightly closed and NCX (which is reversible) functions predominantly in the Ca²⁺ extrusion mode (as a small inward current).

During the AP, voltage-dependent Ca²⁺ channels open and allow Ca²⁺ to enter the cytosol flowing down its electrochemical gradient, causing an inward depolarizing current (see Chapter 2 for Ca²⁺ channel gating details). In ventricular myocytes, I_{Ca} is mediated nearly entirely by L-type Ca²⁺ channels (LTCC) and in particular by the Cav1.2 isoform. However, atrial, and especially pacemaker cells, also express the Cav1.3 LTCC isoform, which activates at a more negative Eₘ than does the Cav1.2 isoform and so can more effectively contribute to late phase 4 depolarization in pacemaker cells and thus recruit additional Cav1.2 channels.

T-type Ca²⁺ channels are also seen in atrial, pacemaker, and conduction fibers, but not in ventricular myocytes (except in neonatal myocytes and in some pathophysiological settings). These channels activate at an even more negative Eₘ than LTCCs, but also inactivate much more rapidly. T-type channels can contribute to triggered or pacemaker activity, but they produce a smaller peak I_{Ca} and integrated Ca²⁺ influx than LTCCs. Additionally, these channels cannot effectively substitute for LTCC in triggering SR Ca²⁺ release, likely due to the fact that they do not target to the sarcolemmal–SR junctions where Ca²⁺-induced Ca²⁺ release occurs during ECC. Thus the remainder of the chapter will relate mainly to Cav1.2 LTCCs.

I_{Ca} is activated by depolarization and exhibits both Eₘ- and Ca²⁺-dependent inactivation (voltage-dependent inactivation and CDI, respectively), and CDI is by far the dominant physiological mode of I_{Ca} inactivation.[6] Indeed, when CDI is abrogated experimentally, AP duration (APD) becomes extremely long and cells tend to overload with Ca²⁺. Calmodulin (CaM) is constitutively bound to the Cav1.2 in myocytes, and it senses local [Ca²⁺]ᵢ elevation and induces inactivation.[7] While Ca²⁺ entry via the channel itself can contribute to CDI, most LTCCs in cardiac myocytes are localized to junctional clefts with the SR and RyR, and the Ca²⁺-induced SR Ca²⁺ release is even more powerful in causing CDI. The integrated amount of Ca²⁺ influx via I_{Ca} in ventricular myocytes during a normal AP is 5 to 10 μmol/L cytosol, but it is about twice that concentration if SR Ca²⁺ release is blocked. To

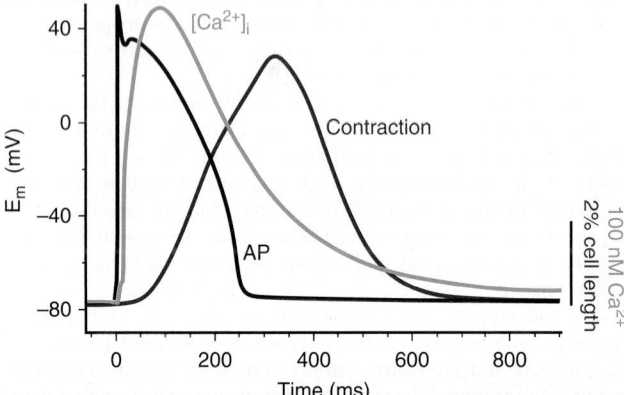

FIGURE 16.1 Example of simultaneously recorded action potential (AP), Ca²⁺ transient, and contraction. Traces from a normal rabbit ventricular myocyte under current-clamp conditions at 1-Hz stimulation and 37°C. (Membrane potential (Eₘ), [Ca]ᵢ, and contraction (shortening) were measured by Dr. Klaus Schlotthauer.)

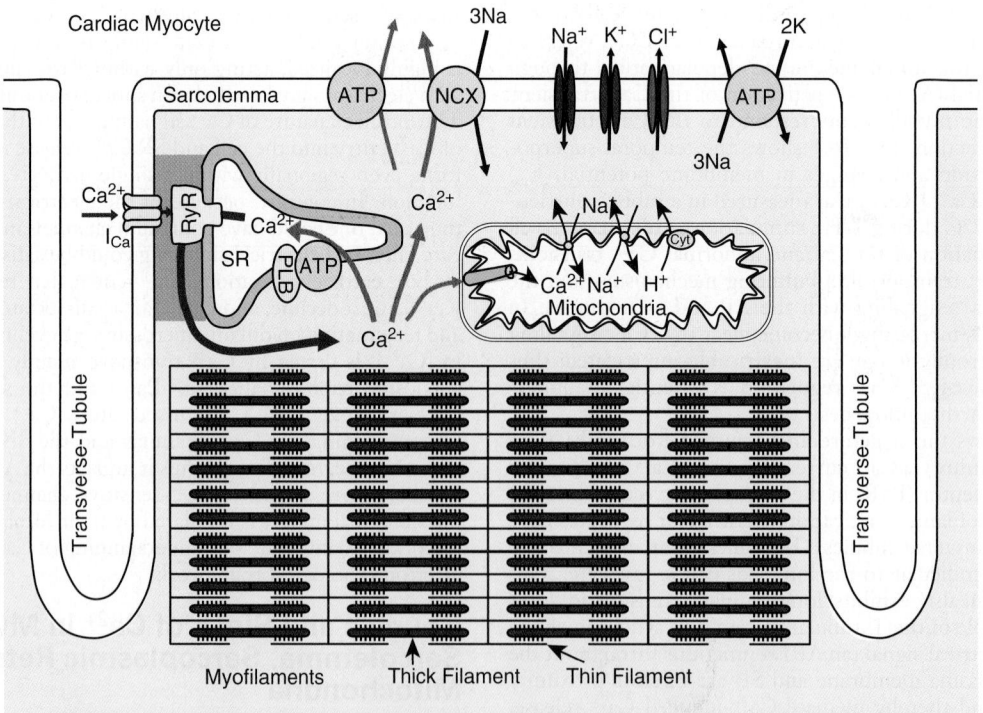

FIGURE 16.2 Schematic of Ca²⁺ handling systems in cardiac myocytes. Ca²⁺, Na⁺, K⁺, and Cl⁻ channels are shown, as are sarcolemmal and sarcoplasmic reticulum (*SR*) adenosine triphosphatase pumps (*ATP*). The SR Ca²⁺–adenosine triphosphatase is inhibited by phospholamban (*PLB*), whose inhibitory effect is reversed by phosphorylation via protein kinase A or Ca²⁺/calmodulin-dependent protein kinase. The mitochondrial cytochrome system (*Cyt*) responsible for pumping protons (*H⁺*) out of mitochondria is indicated. *NCX*, Na⁺/Ca²⁺ exchanger; *RyR*, ryanodine receptor.

place this Ca^{2+} flux in context, the amount of SR Ca^{2+} release in mammalian ventricular myocytes is normally three to ten times larger than this, depending on species and conditions. The regulation of SR Ca^{2+} release will be discussed in more detail below.

NCX can also contribute to the rise in $[Ca^{2+}]_i$, but Ca^{2+} entry via NCX is normally quite small (<1 μmol/L cytosol) and is constrained largely to the early part of the AP. NCX can bring Ca^{2+} in or out (outward or inward current) during the AP, depending on the transsarcolemmal $[Na^+]$ and $[Ca^{2+}]$ gradients and on E_m. During diastole, the E_m is negative to the electrophysiological reversal potential for NCX ($E_{NCX} = 3E_{Na} - 2E_{Ca}$), so Ca^{2+} efflux and inward I_{NCX} are thermodynamically favored (Fig. 16.3[8,9]). However, the low diastolic $[Ca^{2+}]_i$ kinetically limits the amount of transport due to low substrate concentration. The peak of the AP exceeds E_{NCX} and briefly favors Ca^{2+} influx (an outward current). However, as soon as I_{Ca} and SR Ca^{2+} release begins, the local $[Ca^{2+}]_i$ in the cleft and submembrane space ($[Ca^{2+}]_{sm}$) is much higher than the average $[Ca^{2+}]_i$ and drives Ca^{2+} extrusion via NCX (see Fig. 16.3C). The declining E_m during repolarization also more strongly favors Ca^{2+} efflux, and that situation persists throughout $[Ca^{2+}]_i$ decline

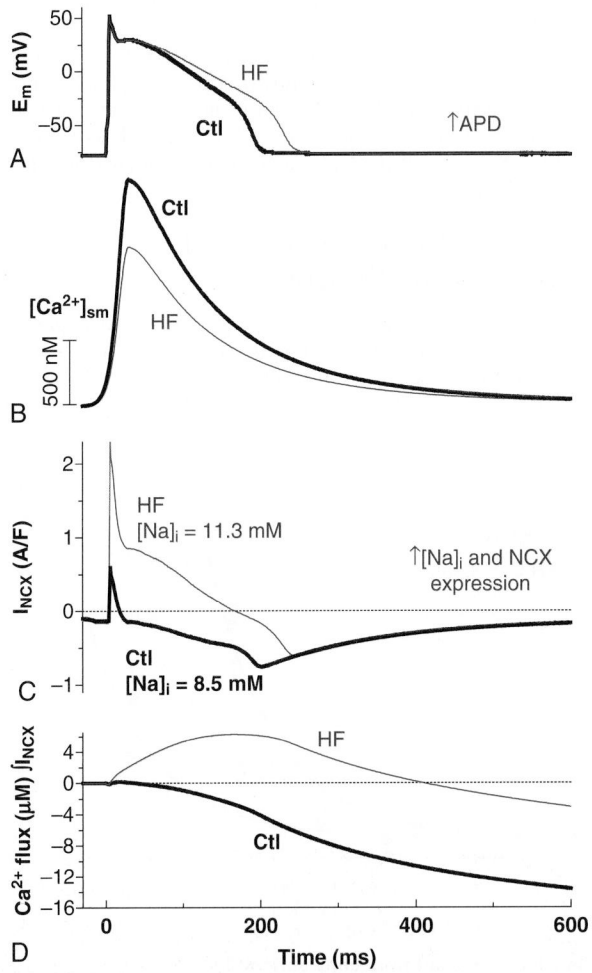

FIGURE 16.3 Na⁺/Ca²⁺ exchange (*NCX*) function in control (*Ctl*) and heart failure (*HF*) cardiac myocytes. (A) Action potentials typical of normal and HF rabbit ventricular myocytes at 37°C. (B) Submembrane $[Ca^{2+}]_i$ sensed by NCX, measured via protocols described in Weber and colleagues.[8] (C) NCX current (I_{NCX}) flowing during the action potential for normal $[Na^+]_i$ (8.5 mM) and for the higher $[Na^+]_i$ and NCX expression levels in HF. (D) Integrated Ca^{2+} flux via NCX during the action potential for the cases in (C). *APD,* Action potential duration. (Modified and redrawn from Despa S, Islam M, Weber CR, et al. Intracellular Na⁺ concentration is elevated in heart failure, but Na/K pump function is unchanged. *Circulation.* 2002;105:2543-2548.)

and diastole. Thus NCX is mainly functioning as a Ca^{2+} efflux mechanism, except in certain pathophysiological conditions. For example, in heart failure where $[Na^+]_i$ is elevated, NCX expression is elevated, Ca^{2+} transients are small, and APD is prolonged (see Fig. 16.3).[9] All of these factors shift NCX more in favor of Ca^{2+} influx, and so in heart failure Ca^{2+} entry via NCX can persist for most of the AP plateau and can significantly contribute to the Ca^{2+} transient. In a sense, this greater Ca^{2+} influx limits the extent of cardiac dysfunction in heart failure by bringing Ca^{2+} in and by indirectly helping load the SR with Ca^{2+}; however, it also means that this Ca^{2+} must be extruded during diastole, and any inability to do so could favor diastolic dysfunction.

So how much Ca^{2+} enters the cytosol during the AP, and where does it go? The total Ca^{2+} from I_{Ca}, NCX, and SR Ca^{2+} release is between 50 and 100 μmol/L cytosol. Notably, this is also the total Ca^{2+} entering the myoplasm, which contains many Ca^{2+} buffers (e.g., troponin C, the SR Ca^{2+}-ATPase, CaM, membrane lipids, ATP, etc.). The most quantitatively dominant Ca^{2+} buffers are troponin C and the SR Ca^{2+}-ATPase, which are present at ~70 and 50 μmol/L cytosol, respectively, and have affinities in the 0.5 μM-range. Overall, the cytosolic buffering is ~100:1, such that 50 to 100 μmol/L cytosol of added Ca^{2+} only raises the free $[Ca^{2+}]_i$ to ~500 to 1000 nM. However, that concentration suffices to partially saturate troponin C and activate contraction. Notably, Ca^{2+} buffering does not directly remove Ca^{2+} from the cytosol, and energy-dependent Ca^{2+} transport is required to return $[Ca^{2+}]_i$ and cytosolic buffers back to their diastolic levels.

Four transporters work in parallel to bring $[Ca^{2+}]_i$ down and drive relaxation: (1) the SR Ca^{2+}-ATPase, (2) NCX, (3) the plasma membrane Ca^{2+}-ATPase, and (4) mitochondrial Ca^{2+} uptake.[1,2] We have analyzed quantitatively how these processes compete in myocytes from different mammalian species. In rabbits (and similar in humans, canines, felines, ferrets, and guinea pigs), the percent contribution to $[Ca^{2+}]_i$ decline is roughly 70%, 28%, 1%, and 1%, respectively. Thus the SR Ca^{2+}-ATPase is the dominant transporter, by a factor of 3 over the NCX. In rat and mouse ventricular myocytes, these numbers are 92%, 7%, 0.5%, and 0.5%, and so is much more SR-dominated (14-fold over NCX). In heart failure, there is generally a downregulation of SR Ca^{2+}-ATPase and an upregulation of NCX, such that in rabbit and human heart failure, the SR and sarcolemmal removal fluxes equalize. While fewer data are available regarding atrial myocytes, the estimate for human atrial myocytes is that 66% and 25% of Ca^{2+} removal occurs via the SR Ca^{2+}-ATPase and NCX, respectively. In chronic atrial fibrillation, as in heart failure, this predominance of SR Ca^{2+}-ATPase over NCX changes to more equal contributions of sarco/endoplasmic reticulum calcium transport ATPase and NCX (46% vs. 44%).[10,11]

Mitochondria take up Ca^{2+} during normal heartbeats via the mitochondrial Ca^{2+} uniporter,[12] but as stated above, this is only ~0.5 μmol/L cytosol (~1 μmol/L mitochondria). Significant Ca^{2+} buffering occurs in this compartment packed with proteins (as in the cytosol), so the rise in free $[Ca^{2+}]$ in the mitochondria at each beat is small (~20 nM).[13] The extrusion of Ca^{2+} from mitochondria is mediated primarily by the mitochondrial Na⁺/Ca²⁺ exchanger (NCLX),[14] which differs molecularly from the sarcolemmal NCX. This Ca^{2+} extrusion occurs quite slowly, such that at higher heart rates diastolic mitochondrial $[Ca^{2+}]$ gradually accumulates to a higher steady state level.

One important effect of increased mitochondrial $[Ca^{2+}]$ is that it binds to and stimulates several dehydrogenase enzymes in the mitochondria to increase the rate of nicotinamide adenine dinucleotide (NADH) production and, consequently, the rate of ATP production.[3] This is an important feedback pathway by which the mitochondria ramp up their ATP production under conditions when the myocyte is using more ATP (i.e., when Ca^{2+} transients are more frequent and/or of higher amplitude).[15] When heart rate is reduced, the diastolic Ca^{2+} efflux is more able to keep up with the less frequent influx pulses, and mitochondrial $[Ca^{2+}]$ gradually falls.

Under severe cellular stress, mitochondria can store large amounts of Ca^{2+}, in part by progressively increasing their buffering capacity,[16] which is thought to provide temporary protection for the myocyte against the dangers of Ca^{2+} overload. However, too much Ca^{2+} in the mitochondria can lead to opening of the permeability transition pore and loss of proteins, which can cause mitochondrial death.

Balance of Fluxes, E–C Coupling Gain, and Fractional Ca²⁺ Release

By definition, the amount of Ca^{2+} that enters the cell during a steady state heartbeat must exactly equal the amount that leaves, otherwise the cell would progressively gain or lose Ca^{2+}. The same is true for the Ca^{2+} fluxes across the SR and the mitochondria at each beat, implying that the sum of the sarcolemmal Ca^{2+} entry via I_{Ca}, NCX, and leak current must equal that removed by the NCX and plasma membrane Ca^{2+}-ATPase. Likewise, the SR Ca^{2+}-ATPase must reaccumulate the amount of Ca^{2+} released by the SR. This fundamental principle helps in quantitative estimation of overall Ca^{2+} fluxes, because different measurements have different limitations.

ECC gain is often used as an index of ECC efficacy and is ideally defined as the ratio of the amount of SR Ca^{2+} release to the amount of Ca^{2+} influx that triggers this release. Using the flux balance principle and analysis of Ca^{2+} removal, the expected ECC gain should be species-dependent (~3 in rabbits or humans and ~15 in rats or mice). The method by which gain is calculated can vary, as the numerator can be peak $[Ca^{2+}]_i$ or it can be $\Delta[Ca^{2+}]_i$, and the denominator can be peak I_{Ca} or it can be the integral over the first 20 ms; for example. ECC gain is highest at negative E_m and gets progressively smaller at positive E_m. The high gain at negative E_m is because only a few LTCCs are opened (meaning that they are mostly at different individual junctions) and those that do open have very high flux (due to high driving force).[17] These LTCC openings are highly efficacious in triggering SR Ca^{2+} release. At a somewhat more positive E_m, more LTCCs are recruited, so some

junctions will have multiple open LTCCs, which will increase the denominator due to redundant I_{Ca} at some junctions, thereby reducing the calculated gain. At positive E_m, the single channel conductance gets progressively smaller as the E_m gets more positive, and successful RyR activation may require more than one LTCC to open at a given junction. Thus gain plateaus at positive E_m and does not decline as rapidly as it does at negative E_m.

Fractional SR Ca^{2+} release, which equals the amount of SR Ca^{2+} released divided by the SR Ca^{2+} content (typically assessed by rapid application of caffeine), is also a powerful measure of ECC efficacy, and it can be assessed independently of I_{Ca} or SR Ca^{2+} load, both of which are major influences on ECC efficacy. This approach has demonstrated that fractional SR Ca^{2+} release increases steeply as a function of total intra-SR $[Ca^{2+}]$ ($[Ca^{2+}]_{SRT}$; Fig. 16.4A), such that fractional release is ~50% at a normal $[Ca^{2+}]_{SRT}$ of 90 to 100 µmol Ca^{2+}/L cytosol, but at ~40% of that normal load a normal I_{Ca} trigger cannot induce any SR Ca^{2+} release.[18] This steep relationship is thought to reflect the ability of high $[Ca^{2+}]_{SR}$ to sensitize the RyR to local $[Ca^{2+}]_i$ triggers and agrees with single channel RyR recordings in lipid bilayers. The failure of ECC at moderate $[Ca^{2+}]_{SR}$ levels is also consistent with this and emphasizes the critical importance of $[Ca^{2+}]_{SR}$ in regulating the ECC process.

Regarding terminology and units for SR Ca^{2+}, a $[Ca^{2+}]_{SRT}$ of 100 µmol/L cytosol corresponds to a $[Ca^{2+}]_{SRT}$ of 1.8 mM in SR volume units (mmol/L SR), and roughly half of that Ca^{2+} is bound to low affinity intra-SR Ca^{2+} buffers, such as calsequestrin. Thus the free SR $[Ca^{2+}]$ ($[Ca^{2+}]_{SR}$) in this normal situation is roughly 900 µM.

Structure of the Couplon and Submembrane Spaces

The initiation of SR Ca^{2+} release during ECC is a local phenomenon. The close physical proximity of the L-type Ca^{2+} channel to the RyR at the junctional cleft or couplon (see Fig. 16.2) is critical for the efficacy of Ca^{2+}-induced Ca^{2+} release. Skeletal muscle expresses different isoforms of these two channels (Cav1.1 and RyR1) than those expressed in cardiac myocytes (Cav1.2 and

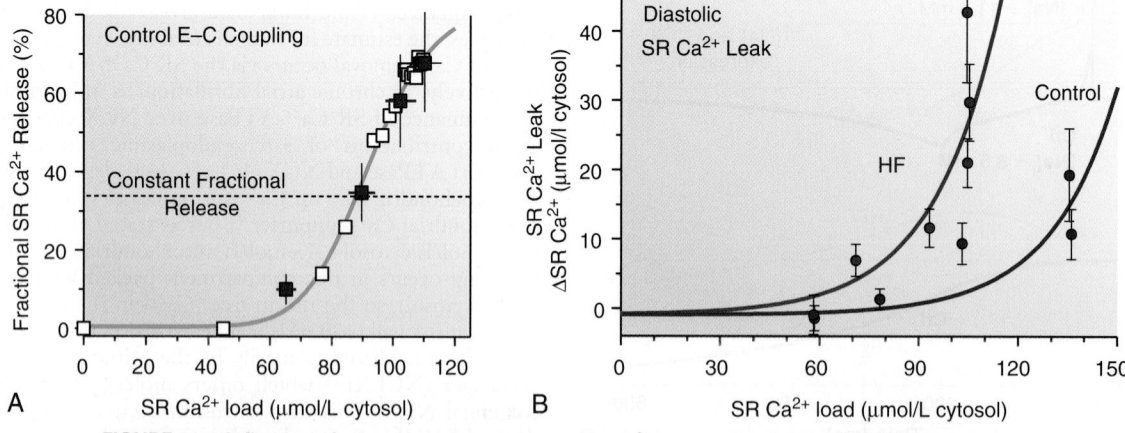

FIGURE 16.4 Influence of sarcoplasmic reticulum (*SR*) Ca²⁺ load on excitation–contraction (*E–C*) coupling efficacy and diastolic SR Ca²⁺ leak current. (A) Voltage-clamp in rabbit ventricular myocyte where SR Ca²⁺ load was varied by prepulse protocols and caffeine-induced SR Ca²⁺ depletion. Ca²⁺ current (I_Ca) amplitude at each test pulse shown was the same for each cell included, regardless of SR Ca²⁺ load. *Dashed line* shows expectation if fractional SR Ca²⁺ release was not regulated by [Ca²⁺]_SR. (B) SR Ca²⁺ load was similarly manipulated and 1 mM-tetracaine was applied to block ryanodine receptor–mediated leak current (in Na⁺-free, Ca²⁺-free solution). At a given SR Ca²⁺ load, the leak current is higher in heart failure (*HF*) myocytes. ([A] Data from Shannon TR, Ginsburg KS, Bers DM. Potentiation of fractional sarcoplasmic reticulum calcium release by total and free intra-sarcoplasmic reticulum calcium concentration. *Biophys J.* 2000;78:334-343. [B] Data from Shannon TR, Pogwizd SM, Bers DM. Elevated sarcoplasmic reticulum Ca²⁺ leak in intact ventricular myocytes from rabbits in heart failure. *Circ Res.* 2003;93:592-594.)

RyR2), and the ECC process is more highly evolved in skeletal muscle. That is, in skeletal muscle, Cav1.1 physically communicates with RyR1 such that the depolarization-induced change in Ca^{2+} channel structure is sufficient to activate RyR1, even without any Ca^{2+} influx through the channel. The structure of these skeletal muscle junctions is relatively rigid, in that every other RyR1 tetrameric channel in a corner-to-corner array has four L-type Ca^{2+} channels directly above it and communicating with it.[19] In the heart, there are similarly structured arrays of RyR2 tetramers (~100 RyR per junction), and Cav1.2 channels are clustered in these junctional clefts. However, these LTCCs appear to be distributed randomly within the cluster with one Cav1.2 per 4 to 10 RyR tetramers. The majority of these couplons (short cylinders ~200 nm in diameter and ~15 nm deep located between SR and sarcolemmal membranes) are in the T-tubule, but ~25% exist along the external sarcolemma, and both function similarly with respect to ECC.[1]

In a rabbit ventricular myocyte, these junctions occupy ~21% of the T-tubule membrane but only 5% of the surface sarcolemma. Both of these values are a bit higher in the rat, but the couplons occupy 11% to 20% of the total sarcolemma. NCX and the Na^+/K^+-ATPase are more concentrated in T-tubules than in the surface membrane, but most of the NCX are not located in junctions.[20] It is unclear what protein or signal dictates the localization of RyR2 and Cav1.2 to the junction, but junctophilin is a candidate protein that interacts with both membranes and RyR2.[21] Notably, in atrial myocytes there are clusters of RyR2 organized in transverse arrays much like in ventricles, even where T-tubules are lacking in atria.

Compelling electrophysiological data show that the local submembrane $[Ca^{2+}]$ sensed by sarcolemmal ion channels and transporters, even those outside the junctional cleft, differs significantly from that sensed in the general cytoplasm by myofilaments and cytosolic fluorescent indicators,[8] meaning that Ca^{2+}-sensitive ionic currents will sense Ca^{2+} transients to be larger and faster rising than those sensed by globally situated Ca^{2+} indicators (see Fig. 16.3 and below).

E–C Coupling: Ca^{2+}-Induced Ca^{2+} Release, Ca^{2+} Sparks, and Ca^{2+} Waves

ECC requires Ca^{2+} influx via the Cav1.2 channel or a surrogate pathway, which raises cleft $[Ca^{2+}]_i$ to activate RyR opening and SR Ca^{2+} release. Indeed, if extracellular Ca^{2+} is removed or I_{Ca} is inhibited there is an immediate (<1 s) abolition of cardiac Ca^{2+} transients (an effect not seen in skeletal muscle). Under physiological conditions, there are enough L-type Ca^{2+} channels in each junction[12–17] to assure that at least one will open during each AP, and that suffices to raise local $[Ca^{2+}]_i$ enough to activate at least one of the ~100 RyRs in the cleft. Once a single RyR channel opens, it can recruit more RyRs within the cleft, and we think that about 6 to 15 individual RyR openings may constitute a normal local release event. Within the tiny cleft space, local $[Ca^{2+}]$ likely rises to a peak higher than 100 µM. However, as Ca^{2+} diffuses away, the local $[Ca^{2+}]_i$ at sites outside the cleft are much lower and decline as one gets further away due to a three-dimensional diffusion (peak $[Ca^{2+}]_i$ ~500 to 1000 nM). Throughout the myocyte and the heart, these local release events are synchronized by the AP and almost simultaneous activation of I_{Ca} at each junction. This synchronization is critical for functionally effective ECC.

Spontaneous SR Ca^{2+} release events (Ca^{2+} sparks) can also occur in the absence of Ca^{2+} current (Fig. 16.5) because RyR

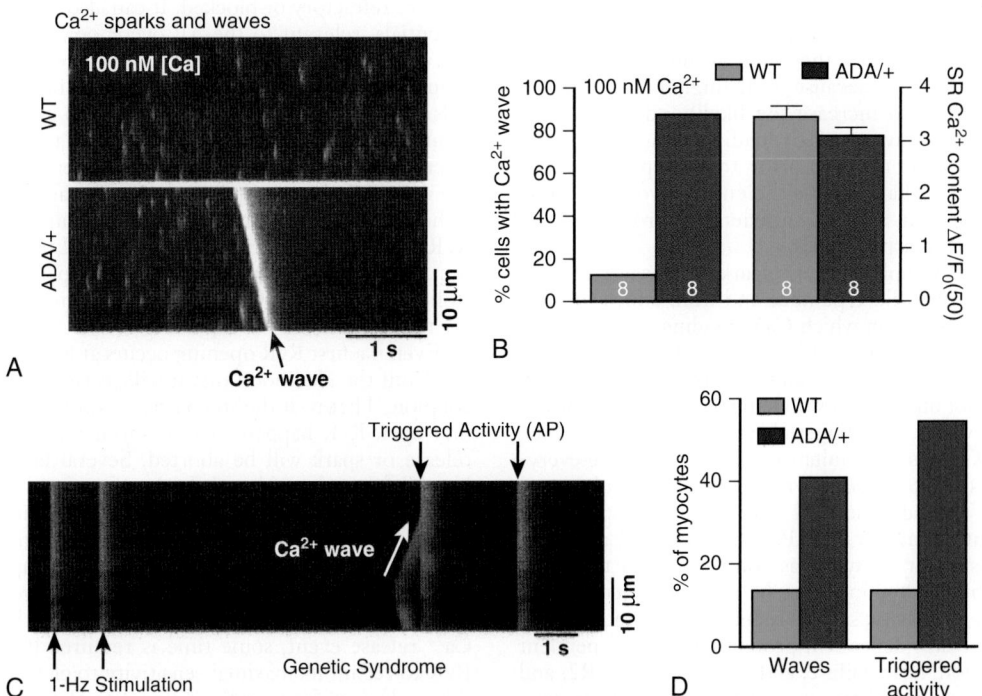

FIGURE 16.5 Ca^{2+} sparks and waves in cardiac myocytes. (A) Linescan confocal images showing numerous Ca^{2+} sparks in mouse ventricular myocytes (wild-type [*WT*] and knock-in mice [*ADA/+*]), in which 50% of the ryanodine receptors have a mutation that prevents calmodulin binding to the ryanodine receptor.[22] (B) Percent of myocytes that demonstrate Ca^{2+} waves and sarcoplasmic reticulum (*SR*) Ca^{2+} content measured by rapid caffeine-induced Ca^{2+} transient. (C) Ca^{2+} waves and triggered action potentials (*APs*) in an ADA/+ mouse myocyte after field stimulation was stopped. (D) Percent of myocytes that demonstrated Ca^{2+} waves and triggered APs (triggered activity). (Data from Wang L, Myles RC, De Jesus NM, et al. Optical mapping of sarcoplasmic reticulum Ca^{2+} in the intact heart: ryanodine receptor refractoriness during alternans and fibrillation. *Circ Res.* 2014;114:1410-1421.)

opening is stochastic and is influenced by $[Ca^{2+}]_i$, $[Ca^{2+}]_{SR}$, and RyR modulation (e.g., by phosphorylation, oxidation, or disease-related mutations, as seen in RyR2 or calsequestrin with catecholaminergic polymorphic ventricular tachycardia). Even if the normal open probability is 10^{-4} per second and there are 1 million RyR per cell, one could expect ~100 RyR openings per second in each cell. Each one of these can participate in the same local positive feedback of Ca^{2+}-induced Ca^{2+} release and cause the firing of a single junction, similar to that initiated by the I_{Ca} trigger. These stochastic Ca^{2+} sparks are considered to be the fundamental unit of SR Ca^{2+} release, and the normal ECC Ca^{2+} transient is the spatiotemporal summation of ~15,000 of these local Ca^{2+} release events with one happening at each junction.

Under normal conditions, the SR Ca^{2+} release at one junction does not trigger the release of Ca^{2+} from a neighboring junction, which would be either 2 μm away longitudinally (at the next Z-line) or ~0.5 μm away transversely. That is, we normally see spatially discrete Ca^{2+} sparks because the $[Ca^{2+}]_i$ is too low at that distance to activate the next junction, which requires a higher local $[Ca^{2+}]_i$ near the mouth of a Ca^{2+} channel. However, there are conditions where this tight local control is lost and Ca^{2+} waves can propagate and, importantly, become arrhythmogenic.

What conditions favor Ca^{2+} waves? The same conditions that increase RyR excitability and the frequency of Ca^{2+} sparks tend to increase the ability of Ca^{2+} sparks to propagate as Ca^{2+} waves.[1] The simplest and best-known case of such a condition is that of cellular and SR Ca^{2+} overload. Since RyR opening is favored by both high local cleft $[Ca^{2+}]$ and elevated $[Ca^{2+}]_{SR}$, Ca^{2+} spark frequency increases when Ca^{2+} loading is favored (e.g., Na^+/K^+-ATPase inhibition, AP prolongation, β-adrenergic activation, or increased heart rate). In these cases there is also greater SR Ca^{2+} release during each Ca^{2+} spark due to a higher $[Ca^{2+}]_{SR}$ and driving force, and this can superimpose on an elevated $[Ca^{2+}]_i$ background. These factors will increase the rise in $[Ca^{2+}]_i$ that a Ca^{2+} spark causes at a neighboring junction. Furthermore, the neighboring junction has a higher sensitivity to $[Ca^{2+}]_i$ because of the higher $[Ca^{2+}]_{SR}$, and these effects synergize to increase the likelihood that a Ca^{2+} spark becomes a Ca^{2+} wave. As Ca^{2+} loading progresses, small abortive mini-waves often occur prior to the appearance of full-blown Ca^{2+} waves that traverse the entire myocyte. These cell-wide Ca^{2+} waves can activate sufficient inward NCX current to cause triggered arrhythmias.

Fig. 16.5 shows examples of Ca^{2+} sparks and waves in ventricular myocytes from wild-type mice and from knock-in mice harboring one RyR allele, in which CaM binding to the RyR is prevented (ADA/+; see Yang et al.[22]). Normal CaM binding to the RyR tends to quiet RyR gating, and the ADA/+ cells in which half the RyRs cannot bind CaM exhibit an increased frequency of Ca^{2+} sparks, Ca^{2+} waves, and triggered activity. Indeed, the Ca^{2+} wave in Fig. 16.5C leads to simultaneous SR Ca^{2+} release everywhere in the cell (*downward black arrows*), which can only occur if the Ca^{2+} wave caused a delayed afterdepolarization (DAD) that was sufficient to trigger an AP. These mice also exhibit increased propensity for arrhythmias compared with the wild-type animal.[22] Thus arrhythmias can be induced by conditions that enhance RyR sensitivity, such as reduced CaM binding, oxidative stress, Ca^{2+}-CaM dependent protein kinase II–dependent RyR phosphorylation, heart failure, and mutations in RyR2, and calsequestrin that are linked to catecholaminergic polymorphic ventricular tachycardia in patients.

SR Ca^{2+} leak during diastole is composed of leak that is detectable as Ca^{2+} sparks plus Ca^{2+} leak that is not detectable as Ca^{2+} sparks.[23,24] Thus while Ca^{2+} sparks can provide a convenient readout concerning SR Ca^{2+} leak, the Shannon-Bers tetracaine block protocol assesses all RyR-dependent leak and was the first to demonstrate that SR Ca^{2+} leak was increased in heart failure[25,26] (Fig. 16.6). Notably, a small but significant component of

the SR Ca^{2+} leak is not mediated by either the RyR or the related inositol trisphosphate receptor.[23]

Atrial myocytes that lack T-tubules cannot use I_{Ca} to synchronize release at internal RyR clusters that exist along the Z-lines. Instead the normal mode of ECC in these cells includes propagated Ca^{2+}-induced Ca^{2+} release (Ca^{2+} waves) to activate the center of the cell.[27] The cause of this difference is unknown: it may be due to atrial myocytes having a higher Ca^{2+} load under baseline conditions compared with ventricular myocytes, or it may be due to a structural or regulatory difference in RyRs in these cells compared with that in other cells. Regardless of the cause, this tendency might predispose atrial myocytes to the production of potentially arrhythmogenic Ca^{2+} waves.

How does SR Ca^{2+} release terminate? Since Ca^{2+}-induced Ca^{2+} release is an inherently positive feedback system, it is important to consider how SR Ca^{2+} release terminates. Since Ca^{2+} release normally terminates when $[Ca^{2+}]_{SR}$ levels are only ~50% depleted (during either global ECC events or Ca^{2+} sparks), a mechanism that breaks the positive feedback must exist. Compelling evidence indicates that luminal $[Ca^{2+}]_{SR}$ strongly influences cardiac RyR gating, such that RyR opening is favored at high $[Ca^{2+}]_{SR}$ and Ca^{2+} spark initiation is enhanced; conversely, RyR closing is favored at lower $[Ca^{2+}]_{SR}$. Experiments show that Ca^{2+} release terminates at ~400 μM $[Ca^{2+}]_{SR}$ during Ca^{2+} sparks, ECC, and when there is little spatial gradient of $[Ca^{2+}]_{SR}$.[28] Thus an internal brake seems to prevent this positive feedback from continuing to completion. As $[Ca^{2+}]_{SR}$ decreases, this internal brake seems to occur at a similar $[Ca^{2+}]_{SR}$ to that at which ECC and Ca^{2+} sparks fail (see Fig. 16.4), and these are probably functionally related effects.

Why does a specific junction fail to activate? Several factors could be responsible. First, the depolarization could fail to activate sufficient entry via I_{Ca}, which could happen if the Ca^{2+} channels are refractory or blocked. It can also happen at very positive potentials, relevant to the AP overshoot. At positive potentials, the unitary current through Ca^{2+} channels is reduced due to a reduced driving force, and thus the opening of more Ca^{2+} channels in the junction may be necessary to raise cleft $[Ca^{2+}]$ sufficiently to assure RyR activation. Notably, the early repolarization often seen (phase 1) of the cardiac AP serves to rapidly increase the driving force for Ca^{2+} entry via activated LTCCs.[29] Second, if the $[Ca^{2+}]_{SR}$ is low, the cleft $[Ca^{2+}]$ required to activate the first RyR is higher, so the same I_{Ca} might fail to initiate RyR activation.[30] Indeed, the dependence of Ca^{2+} spark frequency and diastolic Ca^{2+} leak on $[Ca^{2+}]_{SR}$ is similar to that for fractional SR Ca^{2+} release during ECC (see Fig. 16.4).

Even if a first RyR opening occurs at low $[Ca^{2+}]_{SR}$, several factors limit the likelihood that it will recruit the other RyRs in the couplon. That is, if the stochastic closure of both the I_{Ca} and the first open RyR happens before another RyR is recruited, a full release or spark will be aborted. Several factors contribute. At low $[Ca^{2+}]_{SR}$, the reduced driving force and shorter open time create both a lower cleft $[Ca^{2+}]$ that lasts a shorter time, and the neighboring RyRs are also less sensitive (meaning that more than the normal trigger is required to attain amplification). Third, the RyR can also be refractory. While RyR refractoriness is not exactly like Na^+ channel refractoriness, it is clear that after a SR Ca^{2+} release event, some time is required (0.5 to 10 s) for the RyR to regain its maximal sensitivity to cleft $[Ca^{2+}]$.[31] Note that this is distinct from and additional to the time that it takes for the SR Ca^{2+}-ATPase to refill the SR between beats. This RyR refractoriness may be an important intrinsic protection against arrhythmogenic Ca^{2+} waves, although it may also be involved in the development of alternans. Notably, this RyR refractoriness is not absolute, and increased Ca^{2+} loads can hasten recovery, allowing an abrupt appearance of Ca^{2+} waves at a certain threshold of SR Ca^{2+} load. Fourth, physical disruption of the couplon can reduce the efficacy of I_{Ca} to activate the RyR, which may occur

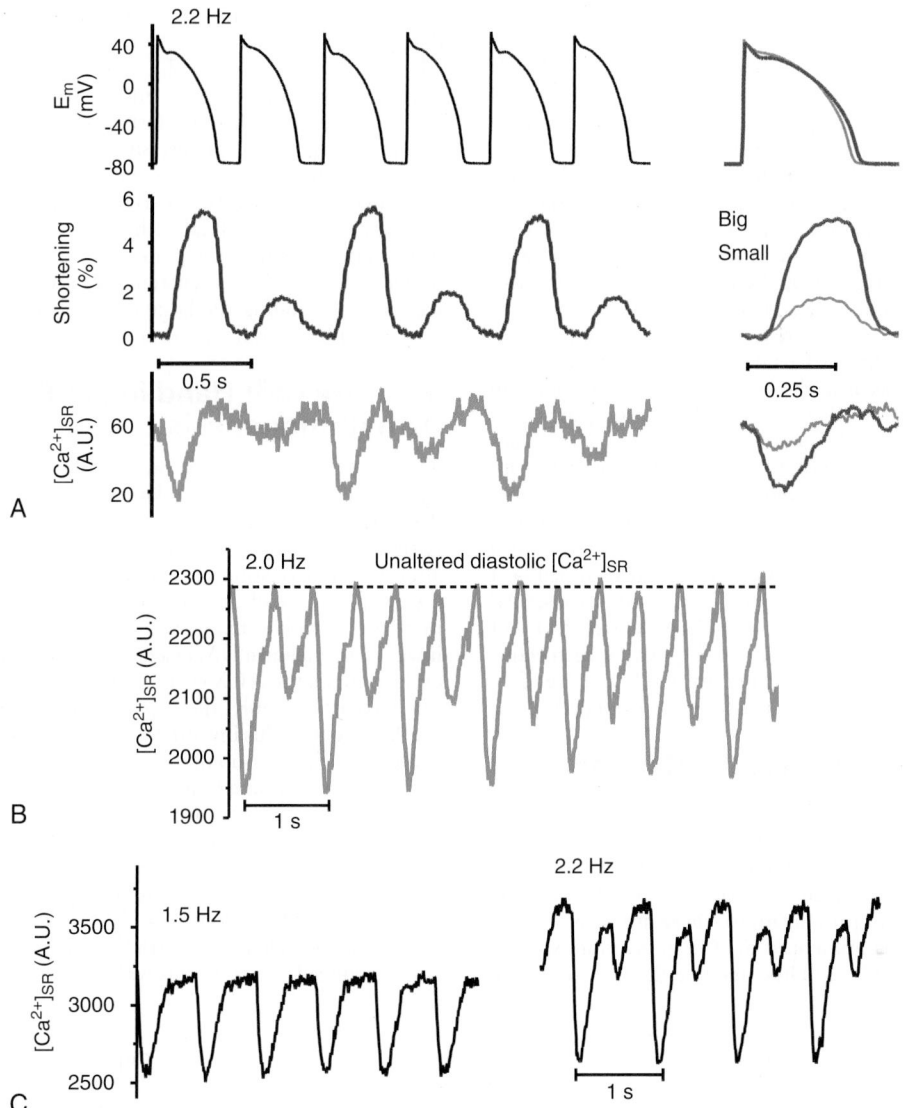

FIGURE 16.6 Cardiac alternans in rabbit ventricular myocytes. (A) E_m, myocyte shortening, and intra-sarcoplasmic reticulum (*SR*) free [Ca²⁺] ($[Ca^{2+}]_{SR}$) assessed using fluo-5N trapped inside the SR. The large and small beats are superimposed at right. (B) Frequently, alternans are observed without any change in diastolic $[Ca^{2+}]_{SR}$ between large and small beats. (C) At a stimulus frequency of 1.5 Hz, this cell did not demonstrate alternans, but as $[Ca^{2+}]_{SR}$ rose further at 2.2 Hz, the cell exhibited stable alternans. (Data redrawn from Picht E, DeSantiago J, Blatter LA, et al. Cardiac alternans do not rely on diastolic sarcoplasmic reticulum calcium content fluctuations. *Circ Res.* 2006;99:740-748.)

when junctophilin 2 is knocked down[32] and also in heart failure when T-tubular organization is lost[33]; in these cases, the efficacy of local ECC could be compromised. In the most extreme locations, it would become rather like the situation in non–T-tubular regions of atrial myocytes where the local I_{Ca} cannot trigger Ca²⁺ release and release is instead triggered mainly by propagated Ca²⁺-induced Ca²⁺ release.

Cardiac Alternans

Alternans was first observed in pulse pressure, but Ca²⁺ transient amplitude and APD alternans also occur, and T-wave alternans has been recognized as a precursor for ventricular tachycardia and ventricular fibrillation. As heart rate increases, it reaches a threshold above which Ca²⁺, contractile, and APD alternans begin to appear, more or less hand-in-hand (see Fig. 16.6). Because Ca²⁺ alternans persists under voltage clamp (where no E_m change occurs) and because several cardiac ion currents are

$[Ca^{2+}]_i$-dependent in ways that explain APD alternans, it is generally accepted that Ca²⁺ alternans causes APD alternans.[34] In alternans, larger Ca²⁺ transients are generally associated with longer APDs (concordant Ca²⁺-E_m alternans; see Fig. 16.6), but the opposite can be true as well (discordant Ca²⁺-E_m alternans). While there are several Ca²⁺-dependent ionic currents (see later), APD alternans can be adequately explained by effects on I_{Ca} and NCX. During the large beat there is faster I_{Ca} inactivation because of more robust CDI, which should shorten APD. However, the larger Ca²⁺ transient will also drive greater inward NCX current, which prolongs APD. So, in concordant Ca²⁺-E_m alternans, the NCX effect is predominant. Conversely, the I_{Ca} effect can predominate for the more rare discordant alternans. Ca²⁺ alternans can also exist out of phase within a single myocyte, reemphasizing the idea that Ca²⁺ signals are highly localized compared with E_m signals. At the level of the whole heart, alternans can also be spatially concordant (all regions in phase with each other) or discordant, and the latter is more likely to degenerate into ventricular tachycardia or ventricular fibrillation.

So why do Ca^{2+} transients alternate during alternans? Possibilities include refractoriness of I_{Ca}, changes in SR Ca^{2+} load, and refractoriness of SR Ca^{2+} release. As heart rate increases and alternans occur, I_{Ca} is not different between the large and small beats.[31] Alternans also occurs even when diastolic $[Ca^{2+}]_{SR}$ and SR Ca^{2+} load are the same at the beginning of the large and small beats (see Fig. 16.6); in this case, the initial event is due to refractoriness of the RyR at the small beat,[31] which creates a small beat where some RyR junctions fail to fire and can recover by the next and thus larger beat. However, the large–small Ca^{2+} transients can also influence SR Ca^{2+} load. At the small beat, because there is less I_{Ca} inactivation and less Ca^{2+} extrusion via NCX, there will tend to be net gain of cell and SR Ca^{2+}; the opposite will occur at the large beat. This phenomenon may be why alternations in SR Ca^{2+} load often accompany alternans (see Fig. 16.6). Indeed, the direction is such that such changes will tend to amplify the extent of Ca^{2+} alternans. Recent work with direct $[Ca^{2+}]_{SR}$ measurements in whole heart[35] has suggested that heart rate–induced alternans starts when RyR refractoriness is limited but diastolic $[Ca^{2+}]_{SR}$ is unaltered (release alternans, as seen in Fig. 16.6B), which progresses to $[Ca^{2+}]_{SRT}$ alternans (small beat enhances Ca^{2+} uptake, as seen in Fig. 16.6C), which then causes AP duration alternans due to changes in Ca^{2+}-dependent currents. At even higher heart rates, the refractoriness of I_{Ca} may be encroached upon, depending on both the diastolic interval and $[Ca^{2+}]_i$ (i.e., E_m- and $[Ca^{2+}]_i$-dependent recovery from inactivation, respectively).

Ca²⁺ Fluxes Can Influence the Cardiac Action Potential

In addition to the manner by which Ca^{2+} carries ionic current (I_{Ca}, NCX) and the predictable consequences of this Ca^{2+} current on the AP configuration (reduced I_{Ca} inactivation as in Timothy syndrome can cause APD prolongation), there are several other channels whose gating is influenced by $[Ca^{2+}]_i$ or, more specifically, by submembrane $[Ca^{2+}]$. These include the Ca^{2+}-activated

Cl^- current ($I_{Cl(Ca)}$), the Ca^{2+}-activated K^+ current ($I_{K(Ca)}$), and the delayed rectifier current (I_{Ks}), and these currents can all influence AP configuration as well. $I_{Cl(Ca)}$ is more prominent at positive E_m than the other currents and contributes to the early repolarization phase of the AP, during which submembrane $[Ca^{2+}]$ is especially high. $I_{K(Ca)}$ is very small or nonexistent in ventricular myocytes but is more prominent in atrial myocytes and, again, most likely participates in early repolarization. I_{Ks} is known to increase with higher $[Ca^{2+}]_i$, but the kinetics of this effect and how it interfaces with the β-adrenergic effects on I_{Ks} are not well understood. All of these currents are sensitive to changes in Ca^{2+} transients, including the large increases in Ca^{2+} transient associated with physiological β-adrenergic activation.

Myocyte Ca²⁺ Handling in Rhythmicity and Arrhythmogenesis

The focus in this section is on the role of Ca^{2+} in triggered activity, especially early afterdepolarizations (EADs) and delayed afterdepolarizations (DADs) (Fig. 16.7). The mechanism for DADs is fairly simple and is an extension of properties described above. If after AP repolarization the conditions favor Ca^{2+} sparks and waves (i.e., Ca^{2+} overload and/or enhanced RyR sensitivity), more of these events will occur and will generate a Ca^{2+}-activated transient inward current and a DAD (see Fig. 16.7A), which is carried almost exclusively via the NCX current (not the $I_{Cl(Ca)}$ or nonselective cation current). Notably, the negative diastolic E_m favors an inward NCX current. If this inward NCX current is sufficient to bring the myocyte to the threshold, then an AP can be triggered.

EADs that initiate before repolarization is complete are a bit more complicated because they occur via at least two possible mechanisms. One mechanism is fundamentally the same as that for DADs (i.e., spontaneous SR Ca^{2+} release and inward NCX current; Fig. 16.7B). EADs are typically observed under conditions where APD is long (e.g., I_{Kr} block or long QT syndromes), and this tends to load cells with Ca^{2+} due to prolonged Ca^{2+} entry and a reduced diastolic interval for Ca^{2+} efflux. However, the

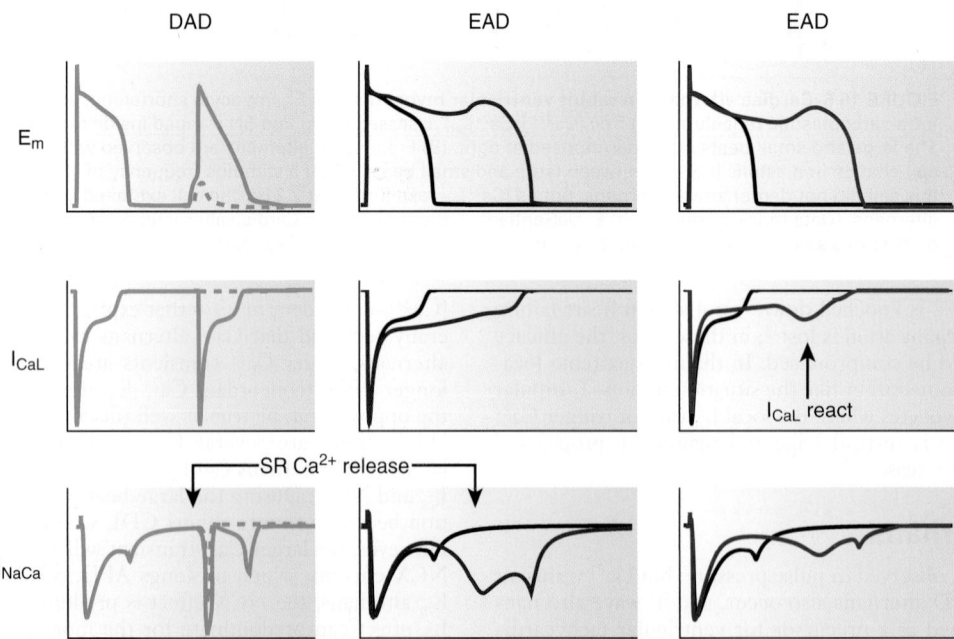

FIGURE 16.7 Delayed afterdepolarization (*DAD*) and early afterdepolarization (*EAD*) and related Ca²⁺ current (I$_{Ca}$) and Na⁺/Ca²⁺ exchange current (I$_{NCX}$). During the DAD, sarcoplasmic reticulum (*SR*) Ca²⁺ release activates I$_{NCX}$ that in one case (*solid trace*) is sufficient to trigger an action potential and in the other case (*dashed trace*) is not. The purple EAD shows a situation where the EAD is initiated by SR Ca²⁺ release and I$_{NCX}$, while the red EAD is initiated by reactivation of L-type Ca²⁺ current.

depolarized E_m reduces inward I_{NCX} at any given $[Ca^{2+}]_i$, making this current more impactful as repolarization proceeds than it is at positive plateau potentials. The second, and historically precedent, mechanism is that some LTCCs become available again during long APD and reactivate, creating an inward current surge and a net depolarization (see Fig. 16.7C). A third EAD mechanism was recently described,[36,37] involving reactivation of Na⁺ channels. This novel mechanism is relevant to rodent ventricular and human atrial APs in which early repolarization is fast and the plateau occurs at a quite negative E_m (below that at which Ca^{2+} channels are activated). That plateau is promoted by a larger SR Ca^{2+} release and a late inward I_{NCX}, which allows the reactivation of a tiny fraction of normal Na⁺ channels to drive net depolarization and EADs. Good experimental and theoretical evidence exists for all three of these mechanisms, and they are not mutually exclusive. For example, an SR Ca^{2+} release event may produce only a very small plateau I_{NCX} and a depolarization that may then be amplified by recruiting I_{Ca} (or I_{Na}, depending on E_m) to cause a larger EAD.

Sinoatrial and atrioventricular node myocytes show spontaneous Ca^{2+} transients and APs. Notably, the SR Ca^{2+} release and I_{NCX} mechanism described above for triggered DAD activity in atrial and ventricular myocytes is an important part of normal pacemaker activity in the sinoatrial node. These cells most likely have a relatively Ca^{2+}-loaded physiological state, ancillary I_{Ca} that activates at more negative E_m (via T-type and Cav1.3 channels), lower stabilizing I_{K1} current, and a more favorable source–sink relationship compared to ventricular myocytes.

In conclusion, cardiac electrophysiology and Ca^{2+} handling are inextricably linked functionally, and whereas E_m influences $[Ca^{2+}]_i$ and contraction, changes in $[Ca^{2+}]_i$ and Ca^{2+} transporters feedback and alter E_m in fundamentally important ways. These can alter AP morphology and excitability and can be important in pacemaking activity and arrhythmias. The Ca^{2+} regulation discussed in this chapter is also under intense regulatory control by numerous signaling pathways in normal and diseased hearts. This includes but is not limited to sympathetic α- and β-adrenergic pathways and regulation by CaM and Ca^{2+}/CaM-dependent protein kinase II.

REFERENCES

1. Bers DM. *Excitation-Contraction Coupling and Cardiac Contractile Force*. 2nd ed. The Netherlands: Kluwer Academic Press Dordrecht; 2001:427.
2. Bers DM. Cardiac excitation-contraction coupling. *Nature*. 2002;415:198–205.
3. Bers DM. Calcium cycling and signaling in cardiac myocytes. *Annu Rev Physiol*. 2008;70:23–49.
4. Lyon AR, MacLeod KT, Zhang Y, et al. Loss of T-tubules and other changes to surface topography in ventricular myocytes from failing human and rat heart. *Proc Natl Acad Sci U S A*. 2009;106:6854–6859.
5. Dibb KM, Clarke JD, Horn MA, et al. Characterization of an extensive transverse tubular network in sheep atrial myocytes and its depletion in heart failure. *Circ Heart Fail*. 2009;2:482–489.
6. Morotti S, Grandi E, Summa A, et al. Theoretical study of L-type Ca^{2+} current inactivation kinetics during action potential repolarization and early afterdepolarizations. *J Physiol*. 2012;590:4465–4481.
7. Zuhlke RD, Pitt GS, Deisseroth K, et al. Calmodulin supports both inactivation and facilitation of L-type calcium channels. *Nature*. 1999;399:159–162.
8. Weber CR, Piacentino 3rd V, Ginsburg KS, et al. Na^+-Ca^{2+} exchange current and submembrane $[Ca(2+)]$ during the cardiac action potential. *Circ Res*. 2002;90:182–189.
9. Despa S, Islam MA, Weber CR, et al. Intracellular Na^+ concentration is elevated in heart failure but Na/K pump function is unchanged. *Circulation*. 2002;105:2543–2548.
10. Grandi E, Pandit SV, Voigt N, et al. Human atrial action potential and Ca^{2+} model: sinus rhythm and chronic atrial fibrillation. *Circ Res*. 2011;109:1055–1066.
11. Voigt N, Li N, Wang Q, et al. Enhanced sarcoplasmic reticulum Ca^{2+} leak and increased Na^+-Ca^{2+} exchanger function underlie delayed afterdepolarizations in patients with chronic atrial fibrillation. *Circulation*. 2012;125:2059–2070.
12. De Stefani D, Raffaello A, Teardo E, et al. A forty-kilodalton protein of the inner membrane is the mitochondrial calcium uniporter. *Nature*. 2011;476:336–340.
13. Lu X, Ginsburg KS, Kettlewell S, et al. Measuring local gradients of intramitochondrial $[Ca^{2+}]$ in cardiac myocytes during sarcoplasmic reticulum Ca^{2+} release. *Circ Res*. 2013;112:424–431.
14. Palty R, Sekler I. The mitochondrial Na^+/Ca^{2+} exchanger. *Cell Calcium*. 2012;52:9–15.
15. Kwong JQ, Lu X, Correll RN, et al. The mitochondrial calcium uniporter selectively matches metabolic output to acute contractile stress in the heart. *Cell Rep*. 2015;12:15–22.
16. Wei AC, Liu T, Winslow RL, et al. Dynamics of matrix-free Ca^{2+} in cardiac mitochondria: two components of Ca^{2+} uptake and role of phosphate buffering. *J Gen Physiol*. 2012;139:465–478.
17. Altamirano J, Bers DM. Voltage dependence of cardiac excitation-contraction coupling: unitary Ca^{2+} current amplitude and open channel probability. *Circ Res*. 2007;101:590–597.
18. Shannon TR, Ginsburg KS, Bers DM. Potentiation of fractional sarcoplasmic reticulum calcium release by total and free intra-sarcoplasmic reticulum calcium concentration. *Biophys J*. 2000;78:334–343.
19. Block BA, Imagawa T, Campbell KP, et al. Structural evidence for direct interaction between the molecular components of the transverse tubule/sarcoplasmic reticulum junction in skeletal muscle. *J Cell Biol*. 1988;107:2587–2600.
20. Scriven DR, Dan P, Moore ED. Distribution of proteins implicated in excitation-contraction coupling in rat ventricular myocytes. *Biophys J*. 2000;79:2682–2691.
21. Ziman AP, Gomez-Viquez NL, Bloch RJ, et al. Excitation-contraction coupling changes during postnatal cardiac development. *J Mol Cell Cardiol*. 2010;48:379–386.
22. Yang Y, Guo T, Oda T, et al. Cardiac myocyte Z-line calmodulin is mainly RyR2-bound, and reduction is arrhythmogenic and occurs in heart failure. *Circ Res*. 2014;114:295–306.
23. Zima AV, Bovo E, Bers DM, et al. Ca^{2+} spark-dependent and -independent sarcoplasmic reticulum Ca^{2+} leak in normal and failing rabbit ventricular myocytes. *J Physiol*. 2010;588:4743–4757.
24. Bers DM. Cardiac sarcoplasmic reticulum calcium leak: basis and roles in cardiac dysfunction. *Annu Rev Physiol*. 2014;76:107–127.
25. Shannon TR, Pogwizd SM, Bers DM. Elevated sarcoplasmic reticulum Ca^{2+} leak in intact ventricular myocytes from rabbits in heart failure. *Circ Res*. 2003;93:592–594.
26. Shannon TR, Ginsburg KS, Bers DM. Quantitative assessment of the SR Ca^{2+} leak-load relationship. *Circ Res*. 2002;91:594–600.
27. Huser J, Lipsius SL, Blatter LA. Calcium gradients during excitation-contraction coupling in cat atrial myocytes. *J Physiol*. 1996;494:641–651.
28. Picht E, Zima AV, Shannon TR, et al. Dynamic calcium movement inside cardiac sarcoplasmic reticulum during release. *Circ Res*. 2011;108:847–856.
29. Sah R, Ramirez RJ, Oudit GY, et al. Regulation of cardiac excitation-contraction coupling by action potential repolarization: role of the transient outward potassium current (I(to)). *J Physiol*. 2003;546:5–18.
30. Sato D, Bers DM. How does stochastic ryanodine receptor-mediated Ca leak fail to initiate a Ca spark? *Biophys J*. 2011;101:2370–2379.
31. Picht E, DeSantiago J, Blatter LA, et al. Cardiac alternans do not rely on diastolic sarcoplasmic reticulum calcium content fluctuations. *Circ Res*. 2006;99:740–748.
32. van Oort RJ, Garbino A, Wang W, et al. Disrupted junctional membrane complexes and hyperactive ryanodine receptors after acute junctophilin knockdown in mice. *Circulation*. 2011;123:979–988.
33. Song LS, Sobie EA, McCulle S, et al. Orphaned ryanodine receptors in the failing heart. *Proc Natl Acad Sci U S A*. 2006;103:4305–4310.
34. Weiss JN, Nivala M, Garfinkel A, et al. Alternans and arrhythmias: from cell to heart. *Circ Res*. 2011;108:98–112.
35. Wang L, Myles RC, De Jesus NM, et al. Optical mapping of sarcoplasmic reticulum Ca^{2+} in the intact heart: ryanodine receptor refractoriness during alternans and fibrillation. *Circ Res*. 2014;114:1410–1421.
36. Morotti S, McCulloch AD, Bers DM, et al. Atrial-selective targeting of arrhythmogenic phase-3 early afterdepolarizations in human myocytes. *J Mol Cell Cardiol*. 2016;96:63–71.
37. Edwards AG, Grandi E, Hake JE, et al. Nonequilibrium reactivation of Na^+ current drives early afterdepolarizations in mouse ventricle. *Circ Arrhythm Electrophysiol*. 2014;7:1205–1213.

17 Ion Channel Trafficking in the Heart

Robin M. Shaw

Overview of Ion Channel Trafficking in the Heart

A remarkable aspect of cardiac ion channel biology is that individual ion channels have half-lives of the order of hours. For example, Cx43 gap junction proteins have a half-life of 1 to 3 hours,[1,2] while calcium channels have half-lives that are reported to be 2 to 8 hours.[3,4] The short life span of ion channels suggests that there needs to be efficiency in their life cycle and movements, which is in the order of formation, delivery to the correct subdomain on the plasma membrane, behavior once in the membrane, and internalization back into the cell.

Cardiomyocytes (CMs) use common intracellular organelles and machinery to produce and shuttle ion channel proteins to their specific organelles and functional subdomains at the cell membrane. After gene transcription in the nuclei, proteins are translated and subjected to posttranslational modification in the endoplasmic reticulum (ER) and then further modified in the Golgi apparatus. For ion channels, sorting and delivery to their subcellular destination begins in the Golgi complex, which is usually found adjacent to the lateral side of each nucleus in mammalian ventricular CMs. Colocalized with each Golgi is the centrosome at which microtubules are nucleated and extend throughout the cell.[5] The sorting of proteins mainly occurs at the trans-Golgi network (TGN).[6] Cargo proteins are sorted into post-Golgi carriers, which are docked onto molecular motors and delivered to the cell periphery along microtubules.[7] These extending microtubules form an intricate and dynamic outgoing network capable of shuttling ion channel–containing vesicles to their destinations. In the context of trafficking, one can consider the Golgi to be the "loading dock" and the microtubules to be the "highways" along which packets of channels are delivered to the plasma membrane.

The mechanisms by which microtubules exert their specificity in interacting with membrane subdomains are now being elucidated. Our report in 2007[8] and subsequent studies[9–11] have led to the targeted delivery model of ion channel delivery. The targeted delivery model has since been supported by multiple other reports.[12–15]

Targeted Delivery

Targeted delivery is the understanding that channels, once formed and after exiting the Golgi, can be rapidly directed across the cytoplasm to their respective specific membrane subdomains. The highways for transport are microtubules whose negative ends originate at Golgi-oriented microtubule–organizing centers and whose positive ends are growing outward and can be captured at the plasma membrane by membrane anchor proteins and complexes. The specificity of delivery is a combination of individual channels, which are plus end–tracking proteins (+TIPs) at the positive ends of microtubules that guide microtubule growth and capture, and the membrane-bound anchor complexes that capture the microtubule, thus completing the highway for channel delivery (Fig. 17.1). The actin cytoskeleton serves as en route rest stop stations to redirect microtubules,[16] providing additional sorting sites. Targeted delivery is explained in this review with two different types of channels: Cx43 hemichannels to intercalated disks and Ca$_V$1.2 channels to T-tubules, followed by an exploration of critical components in the machinery.

Cx43 Trafficking in the Heart

Connexins are ubiquitous transmembrane proteins that are encoded by over 20 different genes in humans, with Cx43 being the most commonly expressed in all organ systems, particularly the heart.[17,18] An extensively studied and well-appreciated function of connexins is their ability to form gap junctions. To form a gap junction, six connexin monomers from one cell oligomerize to form a transmembrane channel referred to as a connexon or hemichannel. The connexons from one cell then dock and couple with apposing connexons on neighboring cells and coalesce into dense gap junction plaques.[19–21] Gap junctions are specialized channels that aid in the intercellular exchange of small metabolites, secondary messengers, and ions carrying electrical signals between neighboring cells, thereby allowing cells to cooperate both electrically and metabolically.[19,20,22]

In the heart, the localization of Cx43 gap junctions at the intercalated disks is crucial to provide the intercellular coupling necessary for rapid action potential propagation through the myocardium and synchronized cardiac contraction.[23–25] Altered Cx43 localization and losses in cell–cell gap junction coupling occur during cardiac disease[26] and contribute to abnormal impulse propagation and arrhythmogenic substrates, leading to sudden cardiac death.[27–33] In addition, a large number of studies in recent years have demonstrated a decrease in expression and/or lateralization and heterogeneous distribution of Cx43 in the myocardium of patients with hypertrophic cardiomyopathies,[34–36] dilated cardiomyopathies,[37,38] ischemic cardiomyopathies,[35–37] and clinical congestive heart failure.[39] In general, altered Cx43 localization is a result of a diseased myocardium, with consequences that include lethal arrhythmias. The mislocalization of Cx43 during disease reflects impaired trafficking to the intercalated disks. Thus to preserve rapid and organized

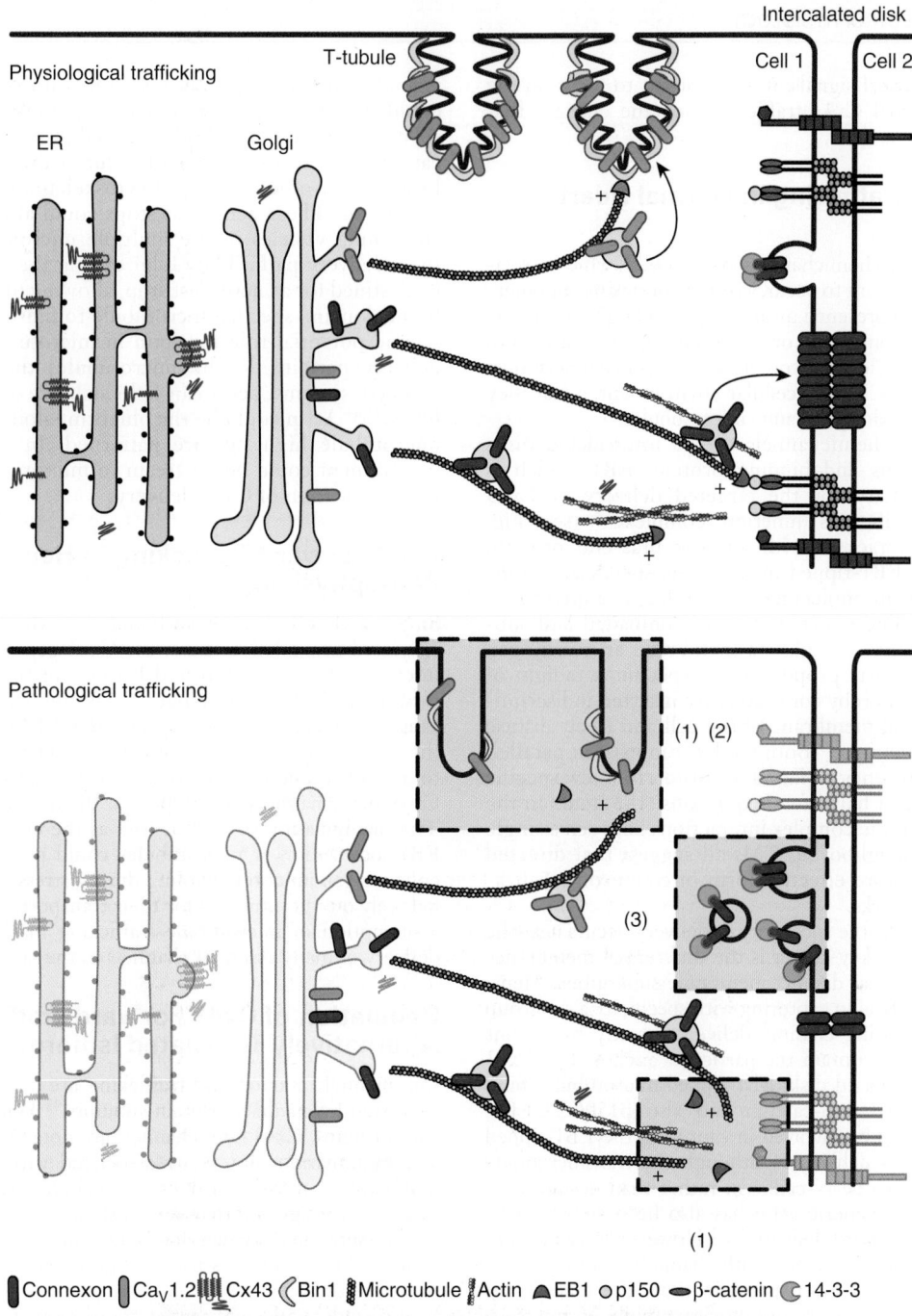

Connexon | Ca$_V$1.2 | Cx43 | Bin1 | Microtubule | Actin | EB1 | p150 | β-catenin | 14-3-3

N-cadherin | MT plus-end binding protein | Desmosome | Desmoplakin

FIGURE 17.1 Channel trafficking in healthy and failing hearts. *Top panel,* Ion channel proteins are synthesized by ribosomes, and in the case of Cx43, multiple isoforms are produced as a result of alternative translation. Ion channel proteins are translocated to the rough endoplasmic reticulum (*ER*), transported through the Golgi apparatus, and then to the trans-Golgi network. Channel proteins are then sorted into vesicular carriers and docked onto microtubules at the trans-Golgi network and subsequently delivered to their subcellular destinations in cooperation with actin "rest stops" along the route. Microtubule plus end–binding proteins interact with anchor proteins of specific membrane subdomains, allowing the targeted delivery of cargo proteins. The interaction between EB1, a microtubule plus end–binding protein, and the adherens junction complex ensures the targeted delivery of Cx43 hemichannels to the intercalated disks, whereas the association of microtubules and bridging integrator 1 (*BIN1*), a membrane scaffolding protein, warrants the delivery of Ca$_V$1.2, a voltage-gated L-type calcium channel protein, to T-tubules. Channel proteins on the plasma membrane undergo internalization for degradation. *Bottom panel,* In failing cardiomyocytes, the expression of ion channels on the cell surface and the morphology of T-tubules are altered. As highlighted in *light green,* possible mechanisms underlying these changes include (*1*) dissociation of microtubule plus end–binding proteins from microtubules, (*2*) reduced expression of membrane scaffolding proteins, and (*3*) increased internalization. Under oxidative stress, EB1 dissociates from the tip of microtubules, impairing the attachment of microtubules to the adherens junction and the Cx43 delivery to intercalated disks. During acute cardiac ischemia, the 14-3-3–mediated internalization of Cx43 is increased, diminishing the amount of Cx43 channels on the plasma membrane. In failing hearts, the expression of BIN1 is significantly reduced, resulting in the detachment of microtubules from the sarcolemma and reduction in Ca$_V$1.2 delivery to T-tubules. The dense membrane folds in T-tubules are also lost as a result of the low expression of BIN1.

propagation of electrical signals, it is important to focus on the mechanisms of normal Cx43 trafficking and the changes that occur with disease.

Cx43 Forward Trafficking in Normal Heart Physiology

Cx43 oligomerizes into hemichannels at the TGN, which is relatively late for such an event to occur, as other connexins oligomerize in ER. This may represent a means of controlling heteromeric hemichannel formations with other connexin isoforms.[25] On exiting the TGN, vesicles that contain Cx43 hemichannels must navigate the complex CM intracellular environment, a feat they achieve by trafficking along dynamic microtubules.

Trafficking Cx43 hemichannels to the intercalated disks involves a major plus end–binding protein, EB1, which is known to be necessary for the targeted delivery of Cx43 hemichannels to adherens junction complexes[8] (see Fig. 17.1). Through interaction with another plus-end protein, p150GLUED, the EB1-tipped microtubule specifically complexes with β-catenin molecules at the fascia adherens of intercalated disks. The vesicular cargo is unloaded and subsequently inserted into the plasma membrane at nearby gap junctions. Other reports propose a less specific paradigm of connexin delivery, whereby connexons are inserted indiscriminately into the lateral membrane of the cell and freely diffuse to gap junction structures.[19] Both models can exist in parallel. However, the inefficiency of lateral diffusion to a few specific subdomains, the short half-life of connexins (1–3 hours in the myocardium),[1,2] and the complex interactions between a single cell with multiple neighboring CMs all suggest that directed targeting can be a more effective form of connexon localization to intercalated disks.

In targeted delivery, the specificity of delivery occurs near the membrane, in which a key aspect is the differential membrane-bound anchor proteins at distinct membrane subregions. Membrane anchors are critical in capturing with specificity a subgroup of microtubules, allowing channel delivery directly to regions of the membrane that contain the particular anchor. For Cx43 delivery to the intercalated disk, EB1-tipped microtubules bind to N-cadherin–associated β-catenin and also p150GLUED.[8] Desmoplakin may also be involved in capturing the EB1-tipped microtubule for Cx43 delivery,[40] although the transmembrane domain still appears to be N-cadherin rather than desmosomal desmoglein.[41] Nonsarcomeric actin has also been shown to be necessary for Cx43 forward delivery.[16,42] However, it remains to be determined how actin interacts with channels and the microtubule apparatus. At any given point in time, the majority of intracellular Cx43 channels are not moving rapidly on microtubules but rather are stationary and associated with nonsarcomeric actin.[16,42]

Other than microtubules, there is an increasing appreciation for the involvement of the nonsarcomeric actin cytoskeleton in the targeted delivery of Cx43. The fundamental question remains with regard to why actin is involved in Cx43 trafficking. If vesicles that contain Cx43 can depart the Golgi and ride a microtubule highway straight to its proper subdomain, is there a need for actin filaments that appear to slow down vesicle transport? Actin can have at least two important roles in Cx43 forward delivery. The first is to help contribute specificity to delivery. Vesicles transported along microtubules on kinesin motors move rapidly at a rate of about 1 micron per second.[8] Thus delivery to most locations in a cell membrane can occur within a minute. Association with important accessory proteins and posttranslational modification of channels, both of which can affect delivery destination, probably also happen en route between the Golgi and membrane. Hopping off the microtubule highway on an actin "way station," which

is analogous to a highway rest stop with convenience stores, could allow Cx43 and the vesicle containing it to pick up accessory proteins and enable the needed posttranslational modification. Such rest stops would occur at the Z-disk, subcortical locations, or other important cytoskeleton intersections in the cytoplasm. These actin rest stops could also allow the Cx43-containing vesicles to use multiple microtubule highways in their delivery path. The Golgi exiting the microtubule could be destined for an actin rest stop, allowing for a different membrane domain–specific microtubule to finish the delivery. The second potential role for actin in microtubule-based forward delivery pertains to the microtubules themselves. In non-myocyte systems, actin can help stabilize and guide microtubules.[43,44] Actin could be the blueprint along and across which microtubule highways are patterned. In this respect, actin involvement could be upstream to microtubules in determining the location of Cx43 delivery.

Cx43 Forward Trafficking in Heart Pathophysiology

Smyth and colleagues have found that when isolated CMs are subjected to oxidative stress, the Cx43 gap junction delivery to intercalated disks is impaired because of the disruption of the forward trafficking machinery.[10] Specifically, oxidative stresses cause the microtubule plus-end protein EB1 to disassociate from the tips of microtubules, impairing microtubule attachment to adherens junction structures and the subsequent delivery of Cx43 hemichannels to the plasma membrane[10] (see Fig. 17.1). The manipulation of EB1 as well as the upstream regulators of EB1 localization at microtubules could potentially preserve or enhance gap junction coupling during stress. As many ion channels rely on microtubules for their transport, it is likely that such a disruption of microtubule trafficking machinery inhibits the delivery of many essential channels to the sarcolemma.

Regulation of Cx43 Forward Trafficking by Its Alternatively Translated Isoforms

Ion channel function and trafficking are usually dependent and regulated by auxiliary protein subunits.[45] With regard to accessory proteins, Cx43 hemichannels are notable for, despite extensive examination, not being associated with their own unique β-subunits that assist in their trafficking. It turns out that *Cx43* mRNA, through alternative translation, encodes its own trafficking subunits,[46] which are N-terminal truncations of the full protein. These isoforms also have potential roles in noncanonical functions of Cx43.

To understand alternative translation, it should be recognized that traditional translation of mRNA begins with the first coding triplet, which is always an AUG (methionine). Most transcribed genes (mRNA strands) have other AUG sites downstream of the first one. The Cx43 protein has six methionines, corresponding to the different AUG triplet translation start sites beyond the first one (Fig. 17.2). Alternative translation occurs when ribosomal translation is initiated not at the first triplet but at a downstream triplet. By initiating translation at downstream sites, alternative translation creates truncated proteins that lack the respective nontranslated upstream (N-terminal) portions of the proteins.

Cx43 is a product of the *GJA1* gene, and we have recently reported that the coding region of the *GJA1* mRNA occurs as a polycistronic molecule with different N-terminal truncated isoforms of the Cx43 protein, arising from the internal translation of the same mRNA molecule.[46] Smyth and Shaw have found that the *GJA1* mRNA produces the expected full-length 43-kDa proteins and proteins that are approximately 32, 29, 26, 20, 11, and 7 kDa in size (see Fig. 17.2), with the 20-kDa isoform (GJA1-20k)

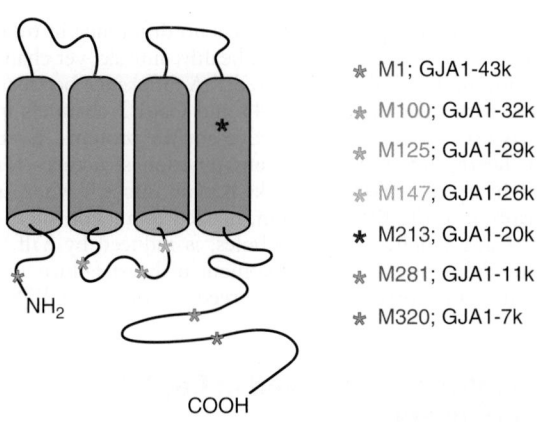

M1; GJA1-43k

M100; GJA1-32k

M125; GJA1-29k

M147; GJA1-26k

M213; GJA1-20k

M281; GJA1-11k

M320; GJA1-7k

Transmembrane domain · Methionine location corresponding to the AUG start site for the indicated Cx43 isoform

FIGURE 17.2 Alternatively translated isoforms of Cx43. Schematic presentation of the protein structure of full length Cx43 (*GJA1-43k*) with methionine locations corresponding to the respective AUG start sites of the various Cx43 isoforms marked by *asterisks* and *color coded*. Cx43 alternative translation creates N-terminal truncated proteins, lacking the respective nontranslated upstream (N-terminal) portions of the Cx43 protein. The six different Cx43 isoforms that result from the alternative translation are GJA1-32k, GJA1-29k, GJA1-26k, GJA1-20k, GJA1-11k, and GJA1-7k.

being the predominant isoform in human heart tissues and several other cell lines.[46] This is the first evidence that alternative translation is possible for human ion channels and in the human heart. These results have since been supported by a separate report that shows that the GJA1-20k isoform is expressed in many cell lines that express high levels of full-length Cx43.[47] In addition, it has been reported that this 20-kDa isoform is induced by hypoxic stimuli in the mouse brain and is the result of internal translation from an IRES element.[48]

Smyth and Shaw have found that at least one of the alternatively translated isoforms, GJA1-20k, is important for increasing Cx43 trafficking to the plasma membrane.[46] Loss of all four Cx43 isoforms, namely GJA1-32k, GJA1-29k, GJA1-26k, and GJA1-20k, severely abrogated the formation of Cx43 gap junctions at the membrane.[46] Interestingly, the reintroduction of the GJA1-20k isoform was sufficient to rescue the transport of Cx43 to the cell surface. The majority of ectopically expressed GJA1-20k remained localized primarily at the cytoplasmic reticular structures, which were confirmed to be the ER/Golgi network. The interaction between full-length GJA1-43k and GJA1-20k isoforms in ER was confirmed using coimmunoprecipitation assays where Brefeldin A (an inhibitor of the protein transport from ER to the Golgi) resulted in increased interactions between these two peptides. These data suggest a role of the GJA1-20k isoform early in the Cx43 vesicular transport pathway and also suggest that this isoform functions as a cytoplasmic chaperone auxiliary protein for trafficking of de novo GJA1-43k molecules through the ER/Golgi complex to the membrane.[46] We also found that the mammalian target of rapamycin (mTOR) signaling pathway increases the expression of the GJA1-20k isoform and Cx43 trafficking.[46] It remains to be determined how GJA1-20k contributes to the specificity of trafficking delivery. We expect that GJA1-20k is involved in cytoskeleton organization.

Cx43 Internalization in Healthy Cardiomyocytes

Endocytosis of Cx43 can occur either through the internalization of uncoupled hemichannels or entire gap junctions, which require

the engulfment of gap junctions from the opposing neighboring cell plasma membrane as well. The internalized double-membrane intracellular structures are known as nonfunctional annular gap junctions. Both the lysosome and proteasome have been implicated in the degradation of Cx43,[49] and interestingly, autophagy is now known to be involved in the degradation of annular gap junctions in failing hearts.[50] Studies have shown that the recycling of gap junctions occurs during cell cycle progression in cell lines,[51] but whether gap junctions are recycled in CMs remains a controversial issue. It is exciting to consider that a delicate balance and competition exists between the various posttranslational modifications of Cx43, including phosphorylation[2,52,53] and ubiquitination[54–57] that may act as checkpoints within the same connexin molecule, or connexon hemichannel. This would then allow a specific series of events to permit the internalization and degradation of the hemichannel or annular gap junction.

In the case of Cx43, phosphorylation is the most well studied, and its importance has been highlighted by recent findings that casein kinase–dependent phosphorylation alters the gap junction remodeling and decreases arrhythmic susceptibility.[52] Many residues on the C-terminus of Cx43, specifically 22 serines, 5 tyrosines, and 4 threonines, are potentially subjected to phosphorylation. To make matters even more complex, Cx43 exists as a hexamer on the plasma membrane, and it is currently not known how phosphorylation differs between individual connexins of the same connexon. It is likely that a cascade of phosphorylation events occurs preceding the ubiquitination of Cx43, which then leads to channel internalization and degradation.[53,58]

Cx43 Internalization in Diseased Cardiomyocytes

Our experience with Cx43 protein is that posttranslational modification preferentially affects ion channel internalization. Pathological gap junction remodeling is strongly associated with altered phosphorylation of Cx43.[25,59,60] Rather than individual independent phosphorylation events of singular residues at the C-terminus, it is likely that internalization results from a sophisticated cascade of posttranslational modifications. The Cx43 C-terminus contains a phosphorylation-dependent 14-3-3–binding motif at serine 373 (within 10 amino acids of the protein end). The 14-3-3 proteins are known to regulate protein transport and have been implicated in facilitating de novo Cx43 transport from ER to the Golgi apparatus.[61,62] The phosphorylation of Ser373 and the subsequent 14-3-3 binding provide a gateway to a signaling cascade of downstream phosphorylation of Ser368, leading to gap junction ubiquitination, internalization, and degradation during acute cardiac ischemia.[2]

The C-terminus of Cx43 is the main protein–protein interaction domain responsible for Cx43 binding to its partners within cells.[63] In close proximity to the Cx43 14-3-3–binding motif is a PDZ domain at the distal end of the C-terminus. It is through this PDZ domain that Cx43 interacts with ZO-1,[64] and this interaction has been demonstrated to regulate Cx43 gap junction plaque size and assembly.[65,66] Disruption of Cx43/ZO-1 complexing has been reported to increase gap junction plaque size in cultured cells.[67,68] Phosphorylation of Cx43 Ser373 can disrupt interaction with ZO-1,[69] and indeed, it would be sterically unlikely for both 14-3-3 and ZO-1 to bind the same Cx43 protomer simultaneously. However, increased Cx43/ZO-1 interaction has also been associated with gap junction remodeling, highlighting the complex nature of these dynamic posttranslational and protein complexing events.[70,71]

Ca$_V$1.2 Channel Trafficking in the Heart

The calcium-handling proteins that are important in cardiac excitation–contraction coupling, in particular the voltage-gated

L-type calcium channels (LTCCs), are mostly enriched in T-tubules. Enrichment of LTCCs (with pore forming subunit $Ca_V1.2$) at the T-tubules helps bring these channels in close proximity (~15 nm) to the intracellular sarcoplasmic reticulum (SR)-based calcium sensing and releasing channel ryanodine receptors (RyR). This is important for an efficient calcium-induced calcium release (CICR) process during each heartbeat. On membrane depolarization, initial calcium influx occurs through $Ca_V1.2$ channels, and the close association between $Ca_V1.2$ and RyR permits efficient CICR and subsequent sarcomeric contraction.[72]

T-tubules, which are continuously extended from the surface sarcolemma, are lipid bilayers that are embedded with transmembrane or lipid-associated proteins.[73] Cardiac T-tubules occur at regular intervals along the lateral sides of the cell, closely coincident with the sarcomeric Z-disks. The physiological function of cardiac T-tubules depends on the proteins that are localized at and within the vicinity of T-tubules, including transmembrane ion channels and ion handling proteins. Specific membrane scaffolding proteins and cytoskeletal structural proteins are required to localize to T-tubules for the organization and regulation of the T-tubule network and structure. By differentially compartmentalizing proteins involved in ion handling and signaling, T-tubules serve as a signaling hub-like organelle to regulate the myocyte function. The expression of transmembrane ion channels, ion transporters, and pumps have been well characterized in cardiac T-tubules.[74]

$Ca_V1.2$ Forward Trafficking in Normal Heart Physiology

Enrichment of $Ca_V1.2$ channels in the T-tubules is essential for the efficient contractile function of the myocardium. We found that the trafficking of $Ca_V1.2$ vesicles from the TGN to T-tubules also occurs in a microtubule-dependent manner[9] (see Fig. 17.1). Moreover, consistent with the targeted delivery model just as with Cx43 connexons, dynamic microtubules preferentially interact with a specific membrane anchor protein, BIN1, to insure targeted delivery of $Ca_V1.2$ to T-tubules[9] (see Fig. 17.1). BIN1 contains a membrane curvature BAR domain (which confers the ability to form membrane curvatures), a coiled-coil domain, and an SH3 protein–protein interaction domain. Perhaps the most compelling evidence for BIN1 utilizing the cytoskeleton is the finding that the deletion of the coiled-coil and SH3 domains does not affect membrane invagination but abrogates $Ca_V1.2$ colocalization with these structures. Therefore it is through specific interactions with the BIN1 membrane scaffolding protein and not with the T-tubule structures that the targeting of $Ca_V1.2$ delivery is achieved.[9] The specificity of targeted delivery is also contributed by +TIPs at the plus ends of the growing microtubules. For example, EB1 works in concert with p150GLUED to target Cx43 channels to adherens junctions at intercalated disks,[8] while the other +TIP CIIP170 has been reported to interact with BIN1,[75] possibly facilitating BIN1-directed delivery of LTCCs to T-tubules.

A subpopulation of $Ca_V1.2$ channels, on the other hand, can be delivered to caveolae through the interaction between the subunits of LTCC complex and the caveolae structural protein caveolin 3.[76] In addition, the fibroblast growth factor homologous factors have been shown to be potent regulators of $Ca_V1.2$ localization to the sarcolemmal membrane[77] by interacting with the C-terminal domains of ion channels.

$Ca_V1.2$ Forward Trafficking in Heart Pathophysiology

In failing hearts, the forward trafficking of $Ca_V1.2$ channels to T-tubules is also impaired.[11] Biochemical assessment of $Ca_V1.2$

channel content in failing hearts indicates no difference in total channel content compared with that in healthy muscle, yet channel localization to T-tubules is impaired.[11] A difference between the impaired forward delivery of Cx43 and $Ca_V1.2$ channels in failing hearts exists with their respective anchor proteins. Even in diseased heart muscle, the adherens junction structures for the Cx43 delivery to intercalated disks remain intact,[10] whereas the transcription of the BIN1 protein, needed to anchor microtubules for $Ca_V1.2$ delivery to T-tubules, is reduced by half.[11] In animal models, the successful treatment of heart failure and recovery of function correlates with the recovery of muscle BIN1 levels.[78,79]

Accessory Proteins Involved in $Ca_V1.2$ Targeted Delivery

As mentioned earlier, ion channel function and trafficking are usually dependent and regulated by auxiliary protein subunits,[45] including their own unique β-subunits that assist in their trafficking. In the case of LTCC, accessory β-subunits exist with the expression of four different isoforms (β1–β4) at the myocardium, varying across species. In mouse hearts, only the β2-subunit (with five splice variants β2a–2e)[80] has been detected, whereas all four isoforms have been detected in canine myocardium.[81] By masking the ER retention signal at the intracellular I-II loop of $Ca_V1.2$ protein, β-subunits are critical in facilitating the ER exiting of the $Ca_V1.2$ channel. However, the role of β-subunits in the targeted delivery of LTCCs remains unclear. We speculate that the β-subunit may be the one directly binding to membrane anchor proteins to facilitate the delivery of LTCCs to membrane subdomains. We also speculate that the specificity of the LTCC delivery can be determined by the binding of BIN1 or caveolin 3–like membrane anchor proteins with different β-subunit isoforms and splice variants.

T-Tubules and $Ca_V1.2$ Regulation in Normal Heart Physiology

A recent development in cardiac membrane biology is the finding that T-tubule invaginations are not simply straight and planar but instead contain complex folds that are tight and narrow enough to limit the free flow of extracellular ions.[82] Hong and colleagues found that BIN1 is responsible for these microfolds within T-tubules, thus affecting extracellular ion diffusion and controlling the driving force of $Ca_V1.2$ channel activity.[82] BIN1-folded subdomains within T-tubules may also limit LTCC lateral diffusion once the channels are inserted into the T-tubule membrane to maintain functional LTCC-RyR dyads. Therefore BIN1-like membrane scaffold proteins may help localize particular pools of ion channel proteins to membrane subdomains for the compartmentalized regulation of the ion channel activity and function.

T-Tubules and $Ca_V1.2$ Regulation in Heart Pathophysiology

In failing hearts, LTCCs also have diminished forward trafficking, resulting in intracellular accumulation of the channels.[11] There already exists significant evidence that gross T-tubule network remodeling occurs in failing hearts.[83–85] The mechanisms of T-tubule remodeling in failing hearts is being actively researched. Junctophilin-2 trafficked by microtubules has been implicated in impaired T-tubule maintenance during heart failure.[86] However, the role of junctophilin-2 in T-tubule remodeling during heart failure has been questioned because of a lack of decrease with heart failure as T-tubule structures are diminished[78,79] or return with the recovery of T-tubule structures in treated heart failure.[78] In these same studies, BIN1 decreased with the decrease in T-tubule density in heart failure,[78,79] and then BIN1 recovered along with T-tubule density during functional recovery of the myocardium.[78]

During extended in vitro culture, isolated mature ventricular myocytes lose T-tubules in 3 days. Interestingly, actin stabilization by cytochalasin D can preserve T-tubules in cultured myocytes.[82,87,88] To that end, the cardiac isoform of BIN1 recently described by Hong and associates was found to promote N-WASP-dependent actin polymerization.[82] Exogenous BIN1 introduced by an adenovirus not only rescued the T-tubule membrane intensity[82] but also the surface $Ca_V1.2$ channels[11] in isolated CMs cultured in vitro. Altogether, these data support the concept that actin is important for T-tubule maintenance, and the mechanism can be mediated by cardiac BIN1.[82] It is worth noting that the loss of BIN1 to levels that occur in end-stage heart failure[11] results in impaired actin-associated T-tubule microfolds.[82] Furthermore, BIN1-deficient mice exhibit T-tubule remodeling similar to that observed in mice with failing hearts.[82]

$Ca_V1.2$ Internalization

General internalization of LTCCs is poorly understood, with a particular lack of studies in CMs. In oocytes, the LTCC β-subunit can enhance dynamin-dependent internalization,[89] and in neurons, $Ca_V1.2$ channels may undergo depolarization and calcium-dependent internalization.[90] We found in CMs that a dynamin GTPase inhibitor dynasore can increase surface LTCC expression, indicating dynamin-dependent endocytosis of cardiac $Ca_V1.2$ channels.[9] Furthermore, a small GTPase Rab11 is implicated in the endosomal transport of LTCCs, thereby limiting the surface expression of LTCCs.[91]

Conclusions

An individual CM is a highly complex and dynamic system with an internal organization designed to maintain an efficient cell–cell communication and excitation–contraction coupling. To maintain intracellular homeostasis and overall synchrony across the myocardium, CMs regulate the ion channel intracellular movement and localization through highly sophisticated and highly efficient protein trafficking machineries. In diseased hearts, the CM structures and organizations are negatively affected by environmental conditions of stress, impacting the channel trafficking and function. As the physiological movements of cardiac channels are elucidated and then disease-related changes of these movements are understood, interventions can be designed to promote positive intracellular remodeling. Therefore new therapies for the failing heart should focus on specific organelles and pathways that regulate CM channel trafficking.

REFERENCES

1. Beardslee MA, Laing JG, Beyer EC, et al. Rapid turnover of connexin43 in the adult rat heart. *Circ Res.* 1998;83:629–635.
2. Smyth JW, Zhang SS, Sanchez JM, et al. A 14-3-3 mode-1 binding motif initiates gap junction internalization during acute cardiac ischemia. *Traffic.* 2014;15:684–699.
3. Chien AJ, Zhao X, Shirokov RE, et al. Roles of a membrane-localized beta subunit in the formation and targeting of functional L-type Ca2+ channels. *J Biol Chem.* 1995;270:30036–30044.
4. Di Biase V, Tuluc P, Campiglio M, et al. Surface traffic of dendritic CaV1.2 calcium channels in hippocampal neurons. *J Neurosci.* 2011;31:13682–13694.
5. de Forges H, Bouissou A, Perez F. Interplay between microtubule dynamics and intracellular organization. *Int J Biochem Cell Biol.* 2012;44:266–274.
6. Gu F, Crump CM, Thomas G. Trans-Golgi network sorting. *Cell Mol Life Sci.* 2001;58:1067–1084.
7. Luini A, Mironov AA, Polishchuk EV, et al. Morphogenesis of post-Golgi transport carriers. *Histochem Cell Biol.* 2008;129:153–161.
8. Shaw RM, Fay AJ, Puthenveedu MA, et al. Microtubule plus-end-tracking proteins target gap junctions directly from the cell interior to adherens junctions. *Cell.* 2007;128:547–560.
9. Hong TT, Smyth JW, Gao D, et al. BIN1 localizes the L-type calcium channel to cardiac T-tubules. *PLoS Biol.* 2010;8:e1000312.
10. Smyth JW, Hong TT, Gao D, et al. Limited forward trafficking of connexin 43 reduces cell-cell coupling in stressed human and mouse myocardium. *J Clin Invest.* 2010;120:266–279.
11. Hong TT, Smyth JW, Chu KY, et al. BIN1 is reduced and Cav1.2 trafficking is impaired in human failing cardiomyocytes. *Heart Rhythm.* 2012;9:812–820.
12. Ligon LA, Holzbaur EL. Microtubules tethered at epithelial cell junctions by dynein facilitate efficient junction assembly. *Traffic.* 2007;8:808–819.
13. Levy JR, Holzbaur EL. Special delivery: dynamic targeting via cortical capture of microtubules. *Dev Cell.* 2007;12:320–322.
14. Hendricks AG, Lazarus JE, Perlson E, et al. Dynein tethers and stabilizes dynamic microtubule plus ends. *Curr Biol.* 2012;22:632–637.
15. Chkourko HS, Guerrero-Serna G, Lin X, et al. Remodeling of mechanical junctions and of microtubule-associated proteins accompany cardiac connexin43 lateralization. *Heart Rhythm.* 2012;9:1133–1140. e6.
16. Smyth JW, Vogan JM, Buch PJ, et al. Actin cytoskeleton rest stops regulate anterograde traffic of connexin 43 vesicles to the plasma membrane. *Circ Res.* 2012;110:978–989.
17. Willecke K, Eiberger J, Degen J, et al. Structural and functional diversity of connexin genes in the mouse and human genome. *Biol Chem.* 2002;383:725–737.
18. Beyer EC. Gap junctions. *Int Rev Cytol.* 1993;137C:1–37.
19. Laird DW. Life cycle of connexins in health and disease. *Biochem J.* 2006;394:527–543.
20. Noorman M, van der Heyden MA, van Veen TA, et al. Cardiac cell-cell junctions in health and disease: electrical versus mechanical coupling. *J Mol Cell Cardiol.* 2009;47:23–31.
21. Unwin PN, Zampighi G. Structure of the junction between communicating cells. *Nature.* 1980;283:545–549.
22. Saez JC, Berthoud VM, Branes MC, et al. Plasma membrane channels formed by connexins: their regulation and functions. *Physiol Rev.* 2003;83:1359–1400.
23. Rohr S. Role of gap junctions in the propagation of the cardiac action potential. *Cardiovasc Res.* 2004;62:309–322.
24. Shaw RM, Rudy Y. Ionic mechanisms of propagation in cardiac tissue. Roles of the sodium and L-type calcium currents during reduced excitability and decreased gap junction coupling. *Circ Res.* 1997;81:727–741.
25. Hesketh GG, Van Eyk JE, Tomaselli GF. Mechanisms of gap junction traffic in health and disease. *J Cardiovasc Pharmacol.* 2009;54:263–272.
26. Saffitz JE, Hames KY, Kanno S. Remodeling of gap junctions in ischemic and nonischemic forms of heart disease. *J Membr Biol.* 2007;218:65–71.
27. Gutstein DE, Morley GE, Vaidya D, et al. Heterogeneous expression of Gap junction channels in the heart leads to conduction defects and ventricular dysfunction. *Circulation.* 2001;104:1194–1199.
28. van Rijen HV, van Veen TA, Gros D, et al. Connexins and cardiac arrhythmias. *Adv Cardiol.* 2006;42:150–160.
29. Danik SB, Liu F, Zhang J, et al. Modulation of cardiac gap junction expression and arrhythmic susceptibility. *Circ Res.* 2004;95:1035–1041.
30. Lerner DL, Yamada KA, Schuessler RB, et al. Accelerated onset and increased incidence of ventricular arrhythmias induced by ischemia in Cx43-deficient mice. *Circulation.* 2000;101:547–552.
31. Poelzing S, Rosenbaum DS. Altered connexin43 expression produces arrhythmia substrate in heart failure. *Am J Physiol Heart Cir Physiol.* 2004;287:H1762–H1770.
32. Lo CW. Role of gap junctions in cardiac conduction and development: insights from the connexin knockout mice. *Circ Res.* 2000;87:346–348.
33. Saffitz JE. Arrhythmogenic cardiomyopathy and abnormalities of cell-to-cell coupling. *Heart Rhythm.* 2009;6:S62–S65.
34. Sepp R, Severs NJ, Gourdie RG. Altered patterns of cardiac intercellular junction distribution in hypertrophic cardiomyopathy. *Heart.* 1996;76:412–417.
35. Peters NS. New insights into myocardial arrhythmogenesis: distribution of gap-junctional coupling in normal, ischaemic and hypertrophied human hearts. *Clin Sci (Lond).* 1996;90:447–452.
36. Jongsma HJ, Wilders R. Gap junctions in cardiovascular disease. *Circ Res.* 2000;86:1193–1197.
37. Kostin S, Rieger M, Dammer S, et al. Gap junction remodeling and altered connexin43 expression in the failing human heart. *Mol Cell Biochem.* 2003;242:135–144.
38. Kitamura H, Ohnishi Y, Yoshida A, et al. Heterogeneous loss of connexin43 protein in nonischemic dilated cardiomyopathy with ventricular tachycardia. *J Cardiovasc Electrophysiol.* 2002;13:865–870.
39. Dupont E, Matsushita T, Kaba RA, et al. Altered connexin expression in human congestive heart failure. *J Mol Cell Cardiol.* 2001;33:359–371.
40. Patel DM, Dubash AD, Kreitzer G, et al. Disease mutations in desmoplakin inhibit Cx43 membrane targeting mediated by desmoplakin-EB1 interactions. *J Cell Biol.* 2014;206:779–797.
41. Shaw RM. Desmosomal hotspots, microtubule delivery, and cardiac arrhythmogenesis. *Dev Cell.* 2014;31:139–140.
42. Zhang SS, Hong S, Kleber AG, et al. A micropatterning approach for imaging dynamic Cx43 trafficking to cell-cell borders. *FEBS Lett.* 2014;588:1439–1445.
43. Bartolini F, Ramalingam N, Gundersen GG. Actin-capping protein promotes microtubule stability by antagonizing the actin activity of mDia1. *Mol Biol Cell.* 2012;23:4032–4040.
44. Wittmann T, Bokoch GM, Waterman-Storer CM. Regulation of leading edge microtubule and actin dynamics downstream of Rac1. *J Cell Biol.* 2003;161:845–851.
45. Smyth JW, Shaw RM. Forward trafficking of ion channels: what the clinician needs to know. *Heart Rhythm.* 2010;7:1135–1140.
46. Smyth JW, Shaw RM. Autoregulation of connexin43 gap junction formation by internally translated isoforms. *Cell Rep.* 2013;5:611–618.
47. Salat-Canela C, Sese M, Peula C, et al. Internal translation of the connexin 43 transcript. *Cell Commun Signal.* 2014;12:31.
48. Ul-Hussain M, Olk S, Schoenebeck B, et al. Internal ribosomal entry site (IRES) activity generates endogenous carboxyl-terminal domains of Cx43 and is responsive to hypoxic conditions. *J Biol Chem.* 2014;289:20979–20990.
49. Laing JG, Tadros PN, Westphale EM, et al. Degradation of connexin43 gap junctions involves both the proteasome and the lysosome. *Exp Cell Res.* 1997;236:482–492.
50. Hesketh GG, Shah MH, Halperin VL, et al. Ultrastructure and regulation of lateralized connexin43 in the failing heart. *Circ Res.* 2010;106:1153–1163.
51. Boassa D, Solan JL, Papas A, et al. Trafficking and recycling of the connexin43 gap junction protein during mitosis. *Traffic.* 2010;11:1471–1486.
52. Remo BF, Qu J, Volpicelli FM, et al. Phosphatase-resistant gap junctions inhibit pathological remodeling and prevent arrhythmias. *Circ Res.* 2011;108:1459–1466.
53. Leithe E, Rivedal E. Ubiquitination and down-regulation of gap junction protein connexin-43 in response to 12-O-tetradecanoylphorbol 13-acetate treatment. *J Biol Chem.* 2004;279:50089–50096.
54. Martins-Marques T, Catarino S, Marques C, et al. Heart ischemia results in connexin43 ubiquitination localized at the intercalated discs. *Biochimie.* 2015;112:196–201.
55. Martins-Marques T, Catarino S, Zuzarte M, et al. Ischaemia-induced autophagy leads to degradation of gap junction protein connexin43 in cardiomyocytes. *Biochem J.* 2015;467:231–245.

56. Basheer WA, Harris BS, Mentrup HL, et al. Cardiomyocyte-specific overexpression of the ubiquitin ligase Wwp1 contributes to reduction in Connexin 43 and arrhythmogenesis. *J Mol Cell Cardiol*. 2015;88:1–13.

57. Girao H, Catarino S, Pereira P. Eps15 interacts with ubiquitinated Cx43 and mediates its internalization. *Exp Cell Res*. 2009;315:3587–3597.

58. Leithe E, Rivedal E. Epidermal growth factor regulates ubiquitination, internalization and proteasome-dependent degradation of connexin43. *J Cell Sci*. 2004;117:1211–1220.

59. Beardslee MA, Lerner DL, Tadros PN, et al. Dephosphorylation and intracellular redistribution of ventricular connexin43 during electrical uncoupling induced by ischemia. *Circ Res*. 2000;87:656–662.

60. Marquez-Rosado L, Solan JL, Dunn CA, et al. Connexin43 phosphorylation in brain, cardiac, endothelial and epithelial tissues. *Biochim Biophys Acta*. 2012;1818:1985–1992.

61. Majoul IV, Onichtchouk D, Butkevich E, et al. Limiting transport steps and novel interactions of Connexin-43 along the secretory pathway. *Histochem Cell Biol*. 2009;132:263–280.

62. Batra N, Riquelme MA, Burra S, et al. 14-3-3theta facilitates plasma membrane delivery and function of mechanosensitive connexin 43 hemichannels. *J Cell Sci*. 2014;127:137–146.

63. Giepmans BN. Gap junctions and connexin-interacting proteins. *Cardiovasc Res*. 2004;62:233–245.

64. Giepmans BN, Moolenaar WH. The gap junction protein connexin43 interacts with the second PDZ domain of the zona occludens-1 protein. *Curr Biol*. 1998;8:931–934.

65. Laing JG, Chou BC, Steinberg TH. ZO-1 alters the plasma membrane localization and function of Cx43 in osteoblastic cells. *J Cell Sci*. 2005;118:2167–2176.

66. Rhett JM, Jourdan J, Gourdie RG. Connexin 43 connexon to gap junction transition is regulated by zonula occludens-1. *Mol Biol Cell*. 2011;22:1516–1528.

67. Hunter AW, Barker RJ, Zhu C, et al. Zonula occludens-1 alters connexin43 gap junction size and organization by influencing channel accretion. *Mol Biol Cell*. 2005;16:5686–5698.

68. Hunter AW, Jourdan J, Gourdie RG. Fusion of GFP to the carboxyl terminus of connexin43 increases gap junction size in HeLa cells. *Cell Commun Adhes*. 2003;10:211–214.

69. Chen J, Pan L, Wei Z, et al. Domain-swapped dimerization of ZO-1 PDZ2 generates specific and regulatory connexin43-binding sites. *EMBO J*. 2008;27:2113–2123.

70. Bruce AF, Rothery S, Dupont E, et al. Gap junction remodeling in human heart failure is associated with increased interaction of connexin43 with ZO-1. *Cardiovasc Res*. 2008;77:757–765.

71. Kieken F, Mutsaers N, Dolmatova E, et al. Structural and molecular mechanisms of gap junction remodeling in epicardial border zone myocytes following myocardial infarction. *Circ Res*. 2009;104:1103–1112.

72. Orchard C, Brette F. T-Tubules and sarcoplasmic reticulum function in cardiac ventricular myocytes. *Cardiovasc Res*. 2008;77:237–244.

73. Lindner E. Submicroscopic morphology of the cardiac muscle. *Z Zellforsch Mikrosk Anat*. 1957;45:702–746.

74. Brette F, Orchard C. Resurgence of cardiac t-tubule research. *Physiology (Bethesda)*. 2007;22:167–173.

75. Meunier B, Quaranta M, Daviet L, et al. The membrane-tubulating potential of amphiphysin 2/BIN1 is dependent on the microtubule-binding cytoplasmic linker protein 170 (CLIP-170). *Eur J Cell Biol*. 2009;88:91–102.

76. Balijepalli RC, Foell JD, Hall DD, et al. Localization of cardiac L-type Ca(2+) channels to a caveolar macromolecular signaling complex is required for beta(2)-adrenergic regulation. *Proc Natl Acad Sci U S A*. 2006;103:7500–7505.

77. Hennessey JA, Wei EQ, Pitt GS. Fibroblast growth factor homologous factors modulate cardiac calcium channels. *Circ Res*. 2013;113:381–388.

78. Lyon AR, Nikolaev VO, Miragoli M, et al. Plasticity of surface structures and beta2-adrenergic receptor localization in failing ventricular cardiomyocytes during recovery from heart failure. *Circ Heart Fail*. 2012;5:357–365.

79. Caldwell JL, Smith CE, Taylor RF, et al. Dependence of cardiac transverse tubules on the BAR domain protein amphiphysin ii (BIN-1). *Circ Res*. 2014;115:986–996.

80. Meissner M, Weissgerber P, Londono JE, et al. Moderate calcium channel dysfunction in adult mice with inducible cardiomyocyte-specific excision of the cacnb2 gene. *J Biol Chem*. 2011;286:15875–15882.

81. Foell JD, Balijepalli RC, Delisle BP, et al. Molecular heterogeneity of calcium channel beta-subunits in canine and human heart: evidence for differential subcellular localization. *Physiol Genomics*. 2004;17:183–200.

82. Hong T, Yang H, Zhang SS, et al. Cardiac BIN1 folds T-tubule membrane, controlling ion flux and limiting arrhythmia. *Nat Med*. 2014;20:624–632.

83. Heinzel FR, Bito V, Biesmans L, et al. Remodeling of T-tubules and reduced synchrony of Ca2+ release in myocytes from chronically ischemic myocardium. *Circ Res*. 2008;102:338–346.

84. Wei S, Guo A, Chen B, et al. T-tubule remodeling during transition from hypertrophy to heart failure. *Circ Res*. 2010;107:520–531.

85. Wagner E, Lauterbach MA, Kohl T, et al. Stimulated emission depletion live-cell super-resolution imaging shows proliferative remodeling of T-tubule membrane structures after myocardial infarction. *Circ Res*. 2012;111:402–414.

86. Zhang C, Chen B, Guo A, et al. Microtubule-mediated defects in junctophilin-2 trafficking contribute to myocyte transverse-tubule remodeling and Ca2+ handling dysfunction in heart failure. *Circulation*. 2014;129:1742–1750.

87. Leach RN, Desai JC, Orchard CH. Effect of cytoskeleton disruptors on L-type Ca channel distribution in rat ventricular myocytes. *Cell Calcium*. 2005;38:515–526.

88. Tian Q, Pahlavan S, Oleinikow K, et al. Functional and morphological preservation of adult ventricular myocytes in culture by sub-micromolar cytochalasin D supplement. *J Mol Cell Cardiol*. 2012;52:113–124.

89. Gonzalez-Gutierrez G, Miranda-Laferte E, Neely A, et al. The Src homology 3 domain of the beta-subunit of voltage-gated calcium channels promotes endocytosis via dynamin interaction. *J Biol Chem*. 2007;282:2156–2162.

90. Green EM, Barrett CF, Bultynck G, et al. The tumor suppressor eIF3e mediates calcium-dependent internalization of the L-type calcium channel CaV1.2. *Neuron*. 2007;55:615–632.

91. Best JM, Foell JD, Buss CR, et al. Small GTPase Rab11b regulates degradation of surface membrane L-type Cav1.2 channels. *Am J Physiol Cell Physiol*. 2011;300:C1023–C1033.

18 Microdomain Interactions of Macromolecular Complexes and Regulation of the Sodium Channel Na$_v$1.5

Hugues Abriel

Na$_v$1.5 and Interacting Proteins

Among the many ionic currents known to be involved in the genesis of the cardiac action potential, the Na$^+$ current (I$_{Na}$) has been studied for more than 60 years[1] and remains a major focus of research. The basic structure and function of the cardiac Na$^+$ channel Na$_v$1.5 and its central role in cardiac pathologies are covered in other chapters of this book. This chapter summarizes published data on the proteins interacting with Na$_v$1.5 that form distinct macromolecular and multiprotein complexes. The roles of the four β-subunits are not reviewed since this topic is covered in other chapters of this book. Over the past several years, Na$_v$1.5 has been shown to interact with a growing list of regulatory proteins (Fig. 18.1A and B, Table 18.1[2–44]). The genes coding for several of these interacting proteins have been found in patients with inherited arrhythmias, such as congenital long QT syndrome (LQTS)[45] and Brugada syndrome (BrS).[46] The proteins interacting with Na$_v$1.5 have been classified as (1) anchoring/adaptor proteins involved in trafficking, targeting, and anchoring the channel protein to specific membrane compartments; (2) enzymes, such as protein kinases or ubiquitin ligases, interacting with and modifying the channel structure via posttranslational modifications[47]; and (3) proteins modulating the biophysical properties of Na$_v$1.5 upon binding (see Table 18.1). These classifications are not mutually exclusive. It has been recently shown[48] that Na$_v$1.5 channels may also interact with each other (i.e., multimerize). However, the stoichiometry and molecular determinants of these interactions remain unknown.

Localization of Na$_v$1.5 in Cardiac Cells: Evidence for Distinct Pools

Immunofluorescence staining experiments have shown that Na$_v$1.5 is expressed in distinct membrane compartments—that is, the intercalated disks and the "lateral membrane" of cardiac cells[2,15,49–53] (Fig. 18.2). Our group proposed a model of Na$_v$1.5 localization at two distinct pools based on strong molecular and in vivo evidence showing that Na$_v$1.5 belongs to the dystrophin multiprotein complex,[5] reviewed in Gillet and colleagues.[54] Dystrophin and syntrophin proteins are not expressed at the intercalated disks of human,[55] rat,[56] or mouse cardiomyocytes[15] (Fig. 18.3A). Recent studies have presented evidence supporting this multiple-pool model of Na$_v$1.5. The group of Roden investigated a knock-in mouse model harboring the p.D1275N mutation in the gene SCN5A, which codes for Na$_v$1.5 and is found in patients with dilated cardiomyopathy. They observed a marked reduction in the expression of Na$_v$1.5 exclusively at the lateral membrane.[57] More recently, Makara and coworkers[2] reported that ankyrin-G specifically permitted the targeting of Na$_v$1.5 to the intercalated disks. It is, however, likely that this "two pool" expression model of Na$_v$1.5 is an oversimplification, as there is both functional[58] and morphological evidence[3,50] for a T-tubular population of Na$_v$1.5 (see Fig. 18.3). In a recent paper, Na$_v$1.5 was found to be colocalized with SAP97 at the T-tubules.[59] Findings[60] suggest that this "third" pool does not depend on the syntrophin/dystrophin complex since it does not depend on the syntrophin interaction domain found in the C-terminus of Na$_v$1.5.

The relationship between the expression of Na$_v$1.5 at the intercalated disks and other "disk" proteins has been studied. It was observed that the intercalated disk pool of Na$_v$1.5 is dependent on the expression of key proteins known to be well expressed at the disks, such as connexin-43,[61,62] plakophilin 2,[17–19] and desmoglein-2.[11] Super-resolution microscopy techniques also demonstrated that Na$_v$1.5 proteins form distinct clusters approximately 100 nm in size and overlapping with N-cadherin at the disks.[63] Similar clusters are also observed in other membrane compartments of cardiac cells.[63]

Thus not only does Na$_v$1.5 interact with many different partner proteins, but its localization in different cellular and membrane compartments is also diverse and shows an unexpected complexity. One of the obvious conclusions of these observations is that there is not just one cardiac Na$^+$ channel Na$_v$1.5, but rather a multiplicity of them with variable functions and regulatory mechanisms.

Proteins Interacting With Na$_v$1.5 Without Demonstrated Roles in Arrhythmias

This section lists the proteins that interact with Na$_v$1.5 that currently have no demonstrable pathological roles. The past has shown that proteins from this list may then be found to be involved in pathological phenotypes. These interacting proteins were discovered either by performing protein–protein interaction screens, such as yeast two-hybrid assays, or by using proteomic-based protein identification assays. The sites of interaction, often protein–protein interaction domains, were mapped on the sequence of Na$_v$1.5, as described in Fig. 18.1A. This list does not follow any specific logic related to importance but is mainly dictated by the chronological order of the published studies.

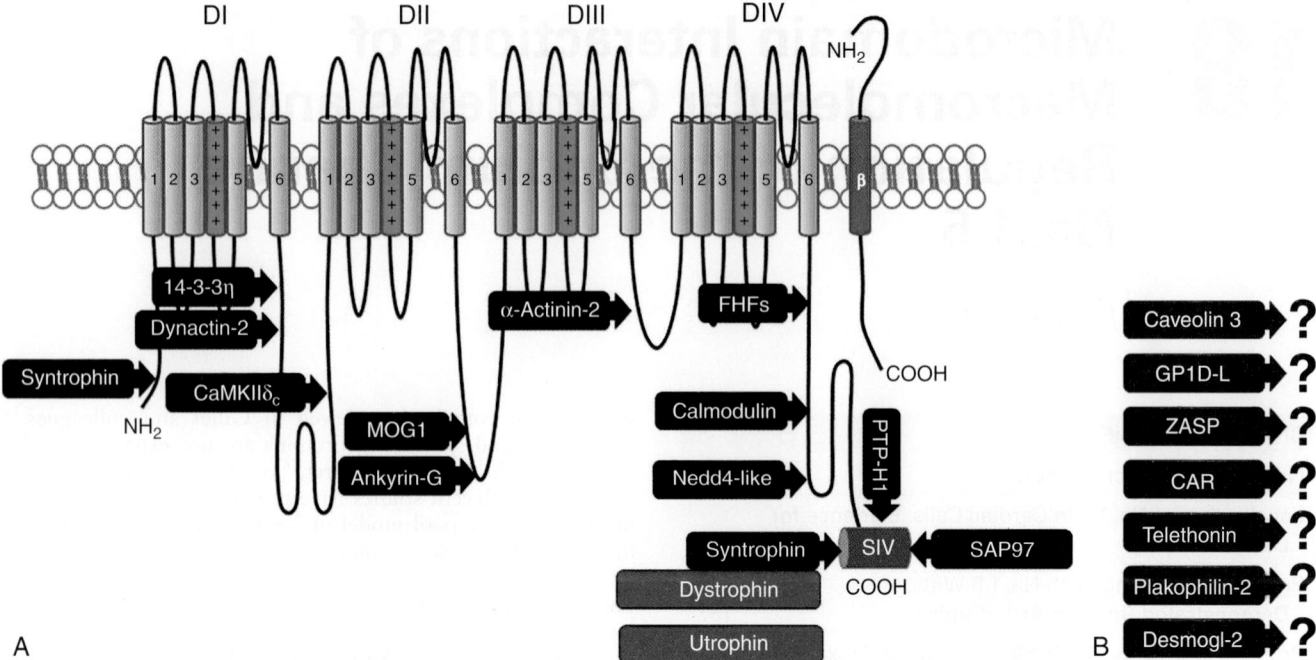

FIGURE 18.1 Schematic representation of the α- and β-subunits of Na$_V$1.5 and interacting proteins. (A) The predicted membrane topology of the α-subunit of Na$_V$1.5 is illustrated. DI-DIV indicates the four homologous domains of the α-subunit; segments S5 and S6 are the pore-lining segments, and the S4 helices (*green*) serve as voltage sensors. The two first intracellular loops display many sites for phosphorylation, whereas the C-terminal domain bears several protein–protein interaction motifs. Only one β-subunit, out of the four known to be able to interact with sodium channels, is shown (*red* one-transmembrane domain protein on right side). The proteins, beside the β-subunits, are reported to interact with Na$_V$1.5, for which a binding site to one of the intracellular domains is represented schematically. (B) For these seven proteins, the interaction with Na$_V$1.5 has been only shown by coimmunoprecipitation experiments, but the binding sites within Na$_V$1.5 are still unknown (*question marks*). These interactions may be indirect (i.e., requiring adaptor proteins). *FHFs,* Fibroblast growth factor homologous factors.

Table 18.1   Summary of proteins (or families of proteins) that have been reported to interact with and regulate Na$_V$1.5

PROTEIN	TYPE OF PROTEIN	MAIN EFFECTS ON Na$_V$1.5	MUTATED IN CARDIAC DISORDER	INTERACTION DOMAIN ON Na$_V$1.5	UniProt REFERENCE	REFERENCES
Ankyrin-G	Anchoring-adaptor	Trafficking and anchoring to the cell membrane, in particular the intercalated disks	Na$_V$1.5-binding site mutated in one BrS patient	VPIAxxSD motif in intracellular loop DII-III	Q12955 (ANK3_ HUMAN)	2–4
Syntrophin proteins	Anchoring-adaptor	Adapt to dystrophin and utrophin complex and stabilization at the lateral membrane of the myocytes	Gene of α1-syntrophin mutated in LQTS and SIDS	PDZ domain–binding motif in C-terminus and internal PDZ-binding domain in N-terminus	Q13424 (SNTA1_ HUMAN)	5–8
MOG1	Anchoring-adaptor	Involved in trafficking of Na$_V$1.5 by unknown mechanisms	Gene mutated in BrS	Intracellular loop between DII-III	Q9HD47 (MOG1_ HUMAN)	9,10
Desmoglein-2	Anchoring-adaptor	Overexpression of ARVC mutants in mice reduces I$_{Na}$	Gene mutated in ARVC	Not determined	Q14126 (DSG2_ HUMAN)	11
α-Actinin-2	Anchoring-adaptor	Involved in trafficking of Na$_V$1.5 by unknown mechanisms	n/a	Intracellular loop between DIII-IV	P35609 (ACTN2_ HUMAN)	12
Dynactin-2	Anchoring-adaptor	Involved in trafficking of Na$_V$1.5 by unknown mechanisms	n/a	Intracellular loop between DI-II	Q13561 (DCTN2_ HUMAN)	13
CAR	Anchoring-adaptor	Involved in trafficking of Na$_V$1.5 by unknown mechanisms	n/a	Not determined	P78310 (CXAR_ HUMAN)	14

Table 18.1 Summary of proteins (or families of proteins) that have been reported to interact with and regulate Na$_V$1.5—cont'd

PROTEIN	TYPE OF PROTEIN	MAIN EFFECTS ON Na$_V$1.5	MUTATED IN CARDIAC DISORDER	INTERACTION DOMAIN ON Na$_V$1.5	UniProt REFERENCE	REFERENCES
SAP97	Anchoring adaptor	Not yet determined	n/a	PDZ domain–binding motif in C-terminus	Q12959 (DLG1_ HUMAN)	15,16
Plakophilin-2	Anchoring and alteration of biophysical properties	Silencing reduces I$_{Na}$, shifts negatively steady-state inactivation, and slows recovery from inactivation	Gene mutated in ARVC and BrS	Not determined	Q99959 (PKP2_ HUMAN)	17–20
14-3-3η (eta)	Alteration of biophysical properties	Modulation of steady-state inactivation	n/a	Intracellular loop between DI-II	Q04917 (1433F_ HUMAN)	21
Caveolin-3	Alteration of biophysical properties	Mutant of caveolin-3 induces persistent current	Gene mutated in LQTS and SIDS	Not determined	P56539 (CAV3_ HUMAN)	22,23
Calmodulin	Alteration of biophysical properties	Many discrepant effects but may confer intracellular calcium sensitivity to Na$_V$1.5. May permit multimerization of Na$_V$1.5 proteins.	n/a	IQ-motif (1900-1920) in C-terminus and loop between DIII-IV	P62158 (CALM_ HUMAN)	24–29
FHF proteins	Alteration of biophysical properties	Modulation of steady-state inactivation, recovery from inactivation, and also density at cell membrane	Gene mutated in BrS	Residues 1773-1832 in C-terminus	P61328 (FGF12_ HUMAN)	30–33
Telethonin	Alteration of biophysical properties	Modulation of voltage dependence of activation	Gene mutated in patient with GI disorder	Not determined	O15273 (TELT_ HUMAN)	34
GPD1-L	Alteration of biophysical properties	Loss-of-function variants reduce I$_{Na}$ by modulating PKC-dependent phosphorylation of Na$_V$1.5	Gene mutated in BrS	Not determined	Q8N335 (GPD1L_ HUMAN)	35–37
ZASP	Alteration of biophysical properties	Loss-of-function variant of ZASP reduces I$_{Na}$ and modulates the voltage dependence of activation and inactivation	Gene mutated in dilated cardiomyopathy and cardiac noncompaction	Not determined	O75112 (LDB3_ HUMAN)	38
Nedd4-like E3 ubiquitin ligases	Enzyme	Ubiquitylation and internalization	n/a	PY-motif in C-terminus	Q96PU5 (NED4L_ HUMAN)	39,40
Calmodulin kinase II δc	Enzyme	Phosphorylation of residues in intracellular loop I and modulation of biophysical activity	n/a	Intracellular loop between DI-II and via betaIV-spectrin	Q13557 (KCC2D_ HUMAN)	41–43
Protein-tyrosine-phosphatase-H1	Enzyme	Dephosphorylation (site unknown) and modulation of biophysical activity	n/a	PDZ-domain binding motif in C-terminus	P26045 (PTN3_ HUMAN)	44

This table does not take into account the four beta sodium channel subunits.
ARVC, Arrhythmogenic right ventricular cardiomyopathy; *BrS*, Brugada syndrome; *FHF*, fibroblast growth factor homologous factor; *GI*, gastrointestinal; *LQTS*, long QT syndrome; *PKC*, protein kinase C; *SIDS*, sudden infant death syndrome.

Ubiquitin-Protein Ligases of the Nedd4/Nedd4-Like Family

Ubiquitylation of target proteins tags them for proteasome-dependent degradation[64] but also serves multiple "nondegradative" functions, in particular the trafficking of membrane proteins.[65] Ubiquitin is a small protein of 76 amino acids found in all animal cells.[66] It covalently binds to lysine residues of target proteins. This protein ubiquitylation is performed by E3 ubiquitin-protein ligases.[66] Ubiquitylated membrane proteins are subsequently internalized and can be targeted for lysosomal or proteasomal degradation. Alternatively, they can also be deubiquitylated by specific proteases and recycled back to the membrane.[67,68] Many different ion channels have been recently reported to be regulated by the Nedd4-like family of E3 ubiquitin-protein ligases. Nedd4-like enzymes specifically bind to target proteins that have consensus domains known as PY motifs with the sequence [L/P]PxY.[39,68–72] Nedd4/Nedd4-like enzymes harbor several WW domains[73] that can interact with these PY motifs. When expressed in *Xenopus* oocytes, Na$_V$1.5-mediated I$_{Na}$ is decreased by Nedd4-2–mediated ubiquitylation.[74] My group investigated the molecular determinants of this regulation[40] and found that the ubiquitin-protein ligase Nedd4-2 directly binds to the PY motif of Na$_V$1.5 and ubiquitylates

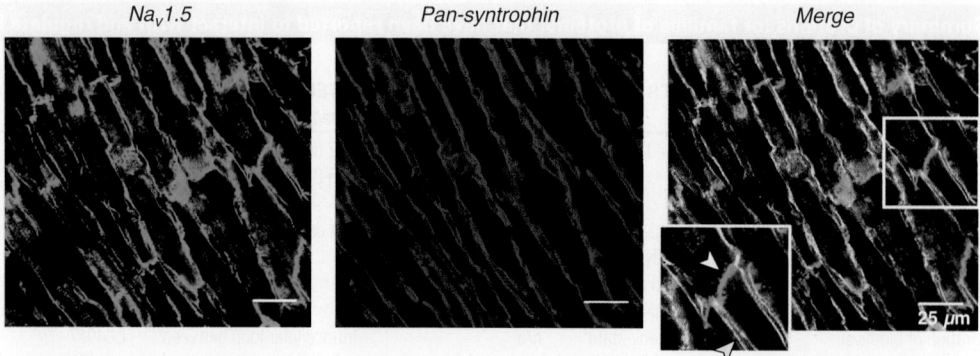

FIGURE 18.2 Stainings of cardiac sections leading to the concept of multiple pools of Na$_v$1.5 channels in cardiac cells. Sections of mouse ventricular myocardium with anti-Na$_v$1.5 staining (*left panel*), anti–pan-syntrophin staining (*middle panel*), and overlay (*right panel, merge*). From these stainings, it is clear that syntrophin proteins are not expressed at the intercalated disks (*white arrowhead*) where Na$_v$1.5 is present. This defines the intercalated disk pool of Na$_v$1.5 that has been proposed to interact with SAP97 (see Fig. 18.1A). *Yellow arrowhead* shows the lateral membrane pool of Na$_v$1.5 colocalized with syntrophin proteins.

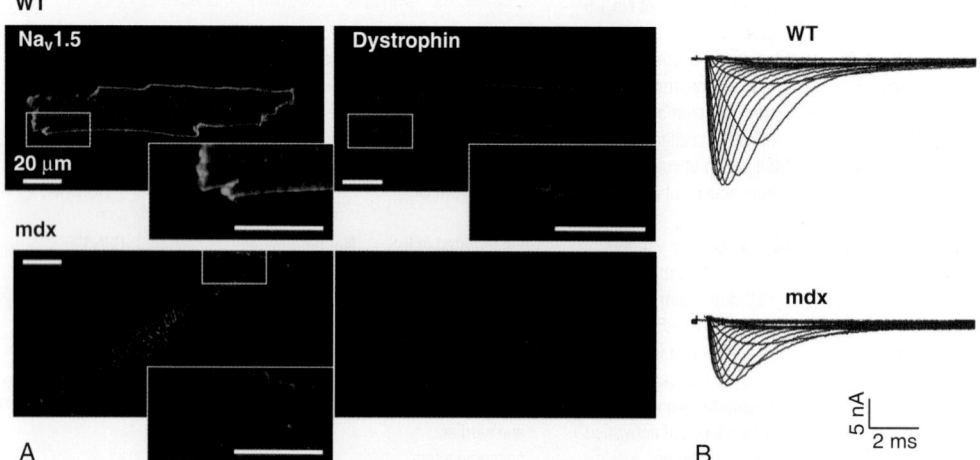

FIGURE 18.3 Reduction of Na$_v$1.5 and sodium current in dystrophin-deficient mouse cardiomyocytes. (A) Isolated mouse cardiomyocytes from wild-type (*WT*) and mdx (dystrophin-deficient) mice with Na$_v$1.5 staining (*green*) and dystrophin staining (*red*). Whereas Na$_v$1.5 channels are found at the intercalated disks and at the lateral membrane compartment, it is apparent that dystrophin is excluded from the intercalated disks. The Na$_v$1.5 pool at the disks has been shown to colocalize with SAP97. (B) Sodium current recordings from whole-cell patch-clamp experiments of freshly isolated WT and mdx mouse cardiomyocytes. It can be inferred that the reduction in current is caused by the specific loss of Na$_v$1.5 channels from the lateral membrane pool. ([A] Modified from Petitprez S, Zmoos AF, Ogrodnik J, et al. SAP97 and dystrophin macromolecular complexes determine two pools of cardiac sodium channels Nav1.5 in cardiomyocytes. *Circ Res.* 2011;108:294-304; with permission from Wolters Kluwer Health. [B] Modified from Gavillet B, Rougier JS, Domenighetti AA, et al. Cardiac sodium channel Nav1.5 is regulated by a multiprotein complex composed of syntrophins and dystrophin. *Circ Res.* 2006;99:407-414; with permission from Wolters Kluwer Health.)

the channel. Since there was no reduction in the total level of Na$_v$1.5 protein upon coexpression with Nedd4-2, we concluded that this was most likely caused by an increased internalization rate rather than by Na$_v$1.5 degradation.[39] Inhibition of the proteasome has been linked to an increase in I$_{Na}$ and Na$_v$1.5 expression in neonatal rat cardiomyocytes.[75] Ubiquitylated Na$_v$1.5 was found to be present in mouse cardiac tissue,[40] further suggesting that membrane turnover or the stability of Na$_v$ channels can be regulated in vivo via ubiquitylation.[71,76] It has been recently proposed[77] that the observed increase in Na$_v$1.5 expression at the cell membrane following phosphoinositide 3-kinase inhibition may be caused by increased phosphorylation and subsequent inhibition of Nedd4-2. Altogether these results suggest that the ubiquitin-proteasome system is involved in several

aspects of Na$_v$1.5 regulation, the intricacies of which remain to be elucidated.

14-3-3η (eta) Protein

The 14-3-3 protein family is composed of dimeric cytosolic adaptor ubiquitous proteins.[78] The members of this family are involved in many cellular functions, such as the binding and regulation of trafficking of various membrane proteins.[79] Allouis and colleagues performed yeast two-hybrid and coimmunoprecipitation experiments[21] showing that the isoform 14-3-3η interacts with the N-terminal part of the intracellular loop linking domains I to II (see Fig. 18.1A and Table 18.1). Furthermore, it was observed that 14-3-3 and Na$_v$1.5 are colocalized at the intercalated disks of myocytes. No influence on the Na$_v$1.5-mediated peak current was observed when Na$_v$1.5 and 14-3-3η were coexpressed in COS cells, suggesting that this protein does not influence Na$_v$1.5 trafficking. In this expression system, 14-3-3 shifted the inactivation curve toward negative potentials and delayed recovery from inactivation, illustrating that 14-3-3 proteins are able to modify the biophysical properties of ion channels. Since different isoforms of 14-3-3 proteins are expressed in cardiac cells,[21] their exact roles in normal cardiac function and their implications in disease states require further investigation.

Calmodulin

Intracellular Ca^{2+} has been shown to modulate the function of many ion channels, including voltage-gated Na$^+$ channels.[80,81] Many cardiac ion channels use calmodulin (CaM), a ubiquitous intracellular Ca^{2+}-binding protein involved in many different cellular processes,[82] as a Ca^{2+}-sensing partner. The Na$_v$1.5 C-terminal domain has an "IQ motif" with a consensus sequence of IQxxxRxxxxR (see Table 18.1), which is very similar to that found in voltage-gated Ca^{2+} channels.[83] The IQ motif is also found in all isoforms of the Na$_v$ family.[84] Several studies[24 26,30] have shown a direct interaction between CaM and the IQ motif of Na$_v$1.5. Recent work by Wang and associates described a crystal structure with an IQ motif ternary complex of Na$_v$1.5, FGF13, and CaM. The functional consequences of this CaM–Na$_v$1.5 interaction are controversial. Several studies[27,84,85] have published inconsistent results that have been difficult to reconcile. A few groups[24,26,27,85] reported that the voltage dependence and stability of the inactivated state were dependent on CaM and the IQ motif. In addition, it has been proposed that CaM may not be the only sensor for the Ca^{2+}-dependent regulation of Na$_v$1.5, as the proximal part of the Na$_v$1.5 C-terminal domain is similar to an EF-hand motif, which is known to bind Ca^{2+}.[86,87] Whether this domain binds intracellular calcium is still under debate.[28,30,88–90] Recently, it has been reported that CaM may serve as an adapter protein promoting Na$_v$1.5–Na$_v$1.5 interaction, thus allowing multimerization of the channel.[29]

Ca^{2+}/Calmodulin-Dependent Protein Kinase II

Ca^{2+}/calmodulin-dependent protein kinase II (CaMKII) is a serine/threonine protein kinase expressed in many cell types, where it transduces intracellular Ca^{2+} increases into the phosphorylation of target proteins, including cardiac ion channels.[91] CaMKIIδc is the predominant cardiac isoform upregulated in human and animal heart failure models.[92,93] Na$_v$1.5 has been found to colocalize and coimmunoprecipitate with CaMKIIδc.[41,42,94] Ashpole and colleagues[42] have shown that CaMKIIδc interacts with the first intracellular loop of Na$_v$1.5 (see Fig. 18.1) and that the residues Ser-516 and Thr-594 may be phosphorylated by this kinase. Hund and associates[43] found that Ser-571 was also a target of CaMKII within the same intracellular loop of Na$_v$1.5 and that this regulation was dependent on the correct expression of betaIV-spectrin, which interacts with ankyrin-G at the intercalated disks. Overexpression of the CaMKIIδc enzyme in rabbit myocytes and transgenic mice induced a Ca^{2+}-dependent hyperpolarizing shift of the steady-state inactivation curve, slowed the recovery from inactivation, and increased the persistent I$_{Na}$. These biophysical property alterations of I$_{Na}$ are similar to some congenital LQTS type 3 mutation–dependent modifications.[95] In mice, transgenic overexpression of CaMKIIδc leads to chronic heart failure and episodes of ventricular tachycardia. Using dog ventricular myocytes, it has also been shown that CaMKII activity increases the persistent/late I$_{Na}$.[96] It is unclear whether these arrhythmias are the direct consequence of the Na$_v$1.5 biophysical alterations or related to other heart failure mechanisms. Nevertheless, CaMKII is an important component in the pathogenesis of arrhythmias and potentially a new drug target.[91]

Protein Tyrosine Phosphatase PTPH1

Ion channels are also regulated by phosphorylation of tyrosine residues, a process that depends both on the phosphorylation activity of tyrosine protein kinases and the dephosphorylation by phosphatases.[97] It was demonstrated that the overexpression of the protein tyrosine kinase Fyn in HEK293 cells altered several of the biophysical properties of Na$_v$1.5 via the phosphorylation of Tyr-1495.[98] This residue is close to the Ile-Phe-Met cluster (IFM) in the intracellular loop linking domains III–IV (see Fig. 18.1A), which is known to mediate the rapid inactivation process of voltage-gated Na$^+$ channels.[99] Fyn coexpression in HEK293 cells shifted the steady-state inactivation curve toward depolarized potentials and accelerated the recovery from Na$_v$1.5 inactivation.[98] The site of interaction of Fyn with Na$_v$1.5 remains to be investigated. My colleagues and I reported[44] that the protein tyrosine phosphatase PTPH1 interacts with the PDZ domain–binding motif of Na$_v$1.5.[100] PTPH1 coexpression in HEK293 cells shifted the availability curve of wild-type Na$_v$1.5 toward hyperpolarized potentials. This effect was abolished when the PDZ domain–binding motif of the Na$_v$1.5 C-terminus was removed by an early stop mutation. These results suggest that tyrosine phosphorylation of Na$_v$1.5 modulates the stability of the inactivated state. The fact that several proteins (e.g., PTPH1, syntrophin proteins, and SAP97) interact with the same binding domain supports the coexistence of different multiprotein complexes with Na$_v$1.5 in cardiac cells.[101]

Telethonin

Telethonin is a small 19-kDa protein expressed in striated muscle cells, including cardiac cells. Mutations in the gene coding for telethonin, TCAP, lead to hypertrophic and dilated cardiomyopathy and limb-girdle muscular dystrophy.[102,103] This protein has been shown to interact with the sarcomeric protein titin,[104] as well as with the β-subunit of the KCNQ1 channel (KCNE1), which mediates the cardiac IKs current.[105] Telethonin can be coprecipitated with Na$_v$1.5 from mouse cardiac tissue, and the two proteins colocalize in cardiomyocytes.[34] The site of interaction on Na$_v$1.5 has not yet been mapped. When the endogenous expression of telethonin in HEK293 cells was reduced, the voltage-dependent activation of the Na$_v$1.5-mediated current shifted toward positive potential values. In addition, coexpression experiments of telethonin and Na$_v$1.5 in HEK293 cells altered several of the kinetic properties of the channel.[34] Furthermore, a point mutation in TCAP was found in a patient with abnormal gut motility,[34] consistent with the fact that Na$_v$1.5 and telethonin are expressed in the neurons of the intestinal mucosa.[106] The precise role of telethonin in the regulation of Na$_v$1.5 in the heart (and other tissues) remains to be clarified.

α-Actinin-2

α-Actinin-2 is a protein of the F actin–crosslinking protein family (similar to spectrin and dystrophin) that interacts with and regulates the trafficking of several potassium channels,[107] in particular Kv1.5. A recent study[12] used pull-down experiments to show that α-actinin-2 interacts with the intracellular III–IV loop of Na$_v$1.5. Coexpression of α-actinin-2 in tsA201 cells increased the measured I$_{Na}$ densities as well as the Na$_v$1.5 protein at the cell surface. Colocalization of Na$_v$1.5 and α-actinin-2 was mainly found at the lateral membrane at the level of the Z-lines; α-actinin-2 seems to be an alternative to the dystrophin/syntrophin complex and ankyrin-G for the connection of Na$_v$1.5 to the cytoskeletal network. Whether these anchoring proteins have overlapping or clearly distinct functions remains to be investigated.

Synapse-Associated Protein 97

Proteins of the membrane-associated guanylate kinase (MAGUK) family are mainly expressed at the cell–cell junctions and are characterized by numerous protein–protein interaction domains, including PDZ domains.[108] The MAGUK proteins regulate the function and localization of many membrane proteins (including ion channels) in neurons, epithelial cells, and cardiomyocytes. Synapse-associated protein 97 (SAP97) and zonula occludens 1 (ZO-1) are the predominant MAGUK proteins expressed in cardiac cells.[109] SAP97 regulates the targeting, localization, and function of cardiac K+ channels, such as Kir2.x,[110] K_v1.5,[111] and Kv4.x,[112] via their PDZ domain–binding motifs located in the C-termini. My colleagues and I recently obtained evidence for the coexistence of at least two pools of Na_v1.5 channels in cardiomyocytes: one located at the lateral membrane with the dystrophin multiprotein complex and the other with SAP97 at the intercalated disks.[15] We demonstrated that the interaction of Na_v1.5 and SAP97 was dependent on the PDZ domain–binding motif that most likely interacts with one of the PDZ domains of SAP97. In a recent study[16] we generated a cardiac-specific SAP97-deficient mouse line. Unexpectedly, neither the I_{Na} nor the Na_v1.5 expression at the intercalated disks were modified. This finding suggests that the localization and stabilization of Na_v1.5 at the intercalated disk depends on other proteins such as ankyrin-G.[2] The functional role of this likely SAP97-Na_v1.5 interaction thus remains to be further explored. SAP97 expression has been found at the intercalated disks[15,111] and in the T-tubule compartment of cardiac cells.[59] Milstein and colleagues[59] demonstrated that Na_v1.5 expression is coregulated with the potassium channel K_{ir}2.1, both of which interact with SAP97. However, a recent work by Matamoros and coworkers[6] presented evidence suggesting the SAP97 is not a sufficient condition for this coregulation and demonstrating a key role for α1-syntrophin. Note that while no modification of I_{Na} and Na_v1.5 expression was observed in cardiac-specific SAP97-deficient mice,[16] we observed a reduction of the K_{ir}2.1-mediated current I_{K1}.

Dynactin-2

Dynactin-2 (also called dynamitin/p50) is a 50-kDa subunit protein of the large multiprotein complex–forming dynein, one of the ubiquitous cytoskeletal motors of cells.[113] Dynein uses microtubules as tracks to transport cargo organelles across different cellular compartments. As recently observed from a yeast two-hybrid screen,[13] dynactin-2 binds to the N-terminal domain of the first intracellular loop of Na_v1.5 (see Fig. 18.1A). Both proteins colocalize mainly at the intercalated disks of mouse adult cardiomyocytes. While no change in the intrinsic Na_v1.5 biophysical properties was observed upon coexpression of dynactin-2 and the channel in HEK293 cells, the peak I_{Na} was reduced. Biotinylation assays also demonstrated a reduction of Na_v1.5 channels at the cell surface of dynactin-2–overexpressing cells. This reduction of Na_v1.5 channels at the plasma membrane may be caused by disruption of the dynein machinery when dynactin-2 is overexpressed.[13] These findings suggest a model involving the dynein complex participating in the trafficking of Na_v1.5 vesicles along microtubules to the plasma membrane, similar to a model proposed for connexin-43.[114]

Coxsackievirus and Adenovirus Receptor

Among the myriad proteins expressed at the intercalated disks, the coxsackievirus and adenovirus receptor (CAR) protein has recently been shown to be colocalized and coprecipitated with Na_v1.5.[14] Motivated by a genome-wide association study suggesting that CAR may be a genetic determinant of ischemia-induced ventricular fibrillation,[115] Marsman and coworkers[14] observed

that the hearts of CAR-deficient mice (at the heterozygote state) showed reduced ventricular conduction. Myocytes of these hearts displayed reduced I_{Na} specifically at the intercalated disks, but the molecular determinants of this CAR-dependent regulation of Na_v1.5 are not yet understood. It is, however, intriguing that there are a large number of Na_v1.5 regulatory partners at the intercalated disks, suggesting that this regulation is complex and leads to a fine-tuned expression and function of Na_v1.5 in this membrane compartment.

Proteins Interacting With Na_v1.5 That Are Linked to Cardiac Arrhythmias

This section summarizes the proteins interacting with Na_v1.5 for which genes have been found to be mutated in patients with cardiac arrhythmias.

Caveolin-3

Caveolae are plasma membrane invaginations with an enrichment of signaling molecules and ion channels.[116] Caveolin proteins are important constituents of these caveolae. Caveolin-3, encoded by the gene CAV3, is the predominant isoform expressed in striated muscle cells, including cardiomyocytes. Mutations in CAV3 have been linked to limb-girdle muscular dystrophy, rippling muscle disease, and familial hypertrophic cardiomyopathy.[117] CAV3 has also recently been shown to be mutated in patients with congenital LQTS[22] (LQTS type 9) and sudden infant death syndrome (SIDS).[23] Caveolin-3 was coimmunoprecipitated with Na_v1.5 in rat cardiac tissue[118] and HEK293 cells.[22] The site of interaction between caveolin-3 and Na_v1.5 has not yet been determined (see Fig. 18.1B). Immunohistostainings of cardiac cells demonstrated that these two proteins are mainly colocalized at the lateral membrane.[22,118,119] Dystrophin is also a component of caveolae,[120] suggesting that the interaction between caveolin-3 and Na_v1.5 could be indirect via proteins of the dystrophin multiprotein complex.[5] The precise role of the Na_v1.5/caveolin-3 interaction in normal physiology remains to be clarified. The coexpression of Na_v1.5 and the mutants of caveolin-3 found in patients with LQTS and SIDS in HEK293 cells was shown to increase the inward Na+ persistent current.[22,23] In an earlier study, it was reported that β-adrenergic stimulation by isoproterenol led to a rapid increase of peak I_{Na} in rat cardiac myocytes.[118] This phenomenon is most likely independent of protein kinase A (PKA), since a PKA inhibitor did not reduce this effect. The increase was, however, completely abolished by antibodies against caveolin-3. The precise molecular and cellular mechanisms underlying these observations require further investigation.

α-1 Syntrophin and the Dystrophin/Utrophin Complex[7]

In 2006, Gavillet and coworkers demonstrated that Na_v1.5 interacts with the important muscle protein dystrophin via adaptor syntrophin proteins.[5] Similar to its binding with SAP97 and PTP-H1, this interaction is dependent on the C-terminal PDZ domain–binding motif of Na_v1.5 (see Fig. 18.1A), which is composed of the last three residues (Ser-Ile-Val) of the protein. In the hearts of dystrophin-deficient mice (mdx), the best-studied animal model of Duchenne muscular dystrophy, the protein level of Na_v1.5 was decreased.[5] The decreased expression of the Na+ channel resulted in reduced cellular I_{Na} and conduction defects[15] (see Fig. 18.3). The reduced expression of the Na_v1.5 protein could not be explained by a decrease in SCN5A mRNA levels,[5] suggesting that a defect in the translational process or a lack of dystrophin may reduce the stability of the Na_v1.5 protein. It seems that the ubiquitin proteasome system plays a crucial role in this destabilization of Na_v1.5 at the lateral membrane since a 1-week-long treatment with the proteasome inhibitor MG132 almost completely rescued the Na$_v$1.5 expression and I$_{Na}$ in mdx hearts.[121] Albesa and associates[8] showed that utrophin, a homolog protein of dystrophin, was upregulated in mdx hearts and interacted with Na$_v$1.5 similarly to dystrophin. Cardiac cells deficient in both dystrophin and utrophin displayed a larger decrease in Na$_v$1.5 expression and in I$_{Na}$.[8] Two missense mutations in *SNTA1*, which encodes α1-syntrophin, have been described in patients with congenital LQTS,[122,123] further supporting the important role of this multiprotein complex in the regulation of Na$_v$1.5. The *SNTA1* mutation, p.A390V,[122] was reported to disrupt a previously undescribed macromolecular complex comprising neuronal nitric oxide synthase (nNOS), plasma membrane Ca-ATPase type 4b with syntrophin, and Na$_v$1.5. The overexpression of the mutant syntrophin protein in cardiac myocytes increased the persistent Na$^+$ current, a finding that is consistent with the LQTS phenotype in affected individuals. Since syntrophin is excluded from the intercalated disks,[15] syntrophin-dependent regulation of the persistent current is most likely exclusively related to the lateral pool of Na$_v$1.5. This suggests that Na$_v$1.5-dependent late current at the lateral membrane may be different than those at the intercalated disks. Recently, α1-syntrophin has been shown to not only interact with the canonical C-terminal PDZ-binding motif of Na$_v$1.5[51] but also with an internal PDZ motif located in the proximal part of the N-terminus of the channel[6] (see Fig. 18.1A). The authors presented convincing evidence supporting the central role of this Na$_v$1.5–N-terminal interaction with α1-syntrophin in the observed Na$_v$1.5-Kir2.1 and Kir2.2 coregulation of expression. This finding provides a molecular understanding for this channel–channel interaction that may play a role in pathophysiology.[59]

Glycerol-3-Phosphate Dehydrogenase–Like Protein

Mutations in the gene coding for Na$_v$1.5, *SCN5A*, are found in ~20% of patients with BrS. Other possible causative genes are still being investigated. London and colleagues described a locus on chromosome 3[124] in a large family with BrS, but simultaneously excluded *SCN5A*. A missense mutation of the gene coding for the glycerol-3-phosphate dehydrogenase–like protein (GPD1-L) was later found.[35] GPD1-L is expressed in cardiac tissue, and coexpression experiments using HEK293 cells showed that mutant GPD1-L reduced I$_{Na}$. Three more mutations of the *GPD1L* gene have been found in individuals that died of SIDS.[36] Expression of these variants in neonatal mouse cardiomyocytes decreased I$_{Na}$, suggesting that a proportion of SIDS patients may have decreased I$_{Na}$, as is observed in BrS patients. Valdivia and associates[37] observed an interaction between Na$_v$1.5 and GPD1-L by performing pull-down experiments. The site of interaction has not yet been investigated. The mechanisms by which the genetic variants of GPD1-L reduce the Na$^+$ current have been studied in expression systems.[37] A pathway has been proposed whereby Ser-1503 can be phosphorylated by PKC and leads to reduced I$_{Na}$. It has been shown that the activity of PKC depends on GPD1-L function and that the mutant GPD1-L variants lead to a further decrease of the I$_{Na}$. These observations linking the redox state of the cells with the activity of Na$_v$1.5 are very interesting and should be investigated using native cardiac cells and tissues.

MOG1

Multicopy suppressor of *gsp1* (MOG1) is a small 29-kDa protein, which is encoded by the *RANGRF* gene. MOG1 binds to the GTP-binding nuclear protein Ran and is involved in regulating nuclear protein trafficking.[125] MOG1 is found in the nucleus and the cytosol of cardiac cells, and its mRNA is well expressed in cardiac tissue.[125] Wu and colleagues[9] demonstrated that MOG1

interacts with the intracellular loop between domains II and III of Na$_v$1.5 (see Fig. 18.1A). This interaction was first determined through a yeast two-hybrid screen, followed by pull-down and coimmunoprecipitation experiments.[9] The two proteins were also shown to colocalize in mouse ventricular cells, mostly at the intercalated disks. MOG1 coexpression in HEK293 cells increased the Na$_v$1.5-mediated current without altering its biophysical properties, suggesting that MOG1 is a cofactor for optimal channel expression at the cell membrane. The role of MOG1 in regulating the surface expression of Na$_v$1.5 was confirmed in a more recent study.[10] This study described two genetic variants of MOG1 found in patients with BrS, which led to reduced expression of Na$_v$1.5 at the cell membrane of rat atrial cardiomyocytes and a decreased current. This work puts *MOG1* on the increasingly long list of susceptibility genes for BrS and illustrates the heterogeneity of mechanisms found in this syndrome.

Plakophilin-2

Plakophilin-2 is a desmosomal protein found in the intercalated disks of cardiac cells. Its human gene (*PKP2*) is mutated in patients with arrhythmogenic right ventricular cardiomyopathy (ARVC).[126] By performing pull-down and coimmunoprecipitation experiments, Delmar's group[17,18] demonstrated that Na$_v$1.5 interacts with not only plakophilin-2 but also ankyrin-G and connexin-43.[18] Whether the interactions between these different proteins of the intercalated disks are direct or indirect, as well as the site of interaction with Na$_v$1.5, remains to be determined. It was, however, convincingly shown that these proteins are colocalized at the intercalated disks, and that silencing of plakophilin-2 in cardiomyocytes reduces I$_{Na}$ and alters some of its biophysical properties. The influence of plakophilin-2 integrity on Na$_v$1.5 was demonstrated in vivo by studying a mouse model expressing only one allele of plakophilin-2.[19] Reduced expression of plakophilin-2 decreased I$_{Na}$ without changing the localization or the total expression of Na$_v$1.5 in the mouse heart. Recent clinical findings have demonstrated that *PKP2* loss-of-function variants found in BrS also reduce Na$_v$1.5 expression at the site of cell contact and I$_{Na}$.[20] These findings clearly support the notion of the coregulation of desmosomal proteins and the Na$_v$1.5 complex at the intercalated disks.

Desmoglein-2

The most recently described protein interacting with Na$_v$1.5 is desmoglein-2, another protein of the desmosomal complex of cardiac cells found to be mutated in patients with ARVC.[127] Desmoglein-2 was shown[11] to coimmunoprecipitate with Na$_v$1.5 in mouse cardiac tissue. The study of a transgenic mouse model overexpressing one mutant of desmoglein-2 (p.N271S) revealed a reduction of I$_{Na}$ and electrical impulse propagation. There was, however, no reduction in Na$_v$1.5 total expression. These results are very similar to those seen with the plakophilin-2 mutants (see earlier) and further support a cross-talk mechanism between the desmosomal proteins and Na$_v$1.5, whose molecular details remain to be investigated.

Ankyrin-G

The ankyrin proteins organize, transport, and anchor membrane proteins to the actin and spectrin cytoskeletons of cells.[128] In the human genome, *ANK1–3* are the three genes encoding ankyrins. The expression of ankyrin-B (*ANK2*) and ankyrin-G (*ANK3*) has been demonstrated in the heart.[128] Mutations of *ANK2* have been linked to congenital LQTS type 4,[129] sinoatrial node dysfunction, atrial fibrillation, conduction slowing, and sudden cardiac death. This collection of diseases defines "ankyrin-B cardiac syndrome."[130] There is currently no evidence that Na$_v$1.5 is directly regulated by ankyrin-B, even though in ankyrin-B–deficient mouse cardiac cells, Na+ channels display late openings similar to those seen in Na$_v$1.5 congenital LQTS type 3 mutant channels.[131] On the other hand, ankyrin-G was shown to directly interact with the ankyrin-binding motif of the linker loop between domains II and III of Na$_v$1.5[4] (see Fig. 18.1A and Table 18.1). Ankyrin-G is predominantly located at the intercalated disks, where it not only interacts with Na$_v$1.5 but also with the actin-associated protein betaIV-spectrin and CaMKII.[43] In ankyrin-G–deficient mouse cardiomyocytes, the Na$_v$1.5 intercalated disk pool was markedly reduced, but not the lateral pool. This illustrates further the distinct molecular mechanisms of regulation of Na$_v$1.5 expression in the different cardiac cell compartments.[2] A clear T-tubular localization of ankyrin G has also been observed.[43] An SCN5A mutation, p.E1053K, in the ankyrin-binding motif was found in a BrS patient and was shown to disrupt the interaction between Na$_v$1.5 and ankyrin-G.[3] Expression of wild-type and mutant Na$_v$1.5 channels in adult rat myocytes[3] was achieved using viral vectors, and while wild-type Na$_v$1.5 channels were correctly transported to the intercalated disks and lateral membranes, the E1053K channels remained in the cytoplasm.[3,132]

Fibroblast Growth Factor Homologous Factors

Fibroblast growth factor homologous factors (FHFs) are cytosolic proteins that are homologous to fibroblast growth factors but are not secreted. Several recent studies have shown that FHFs modulate both cardiac Na+ and Ca2+ channels.[133] The murine homolog FGF13[31] and human homolog FGF12[32] bind to the conserved proximal part of the C-terminal domain of Na$_v$1.5 [31](see Fig. 18.1A). Reduced expression of FGF13 in murine ventricular myocytes decreased I$_{Na}$ and channel availability.[31] Related to arrhythmias, the genetic variant (p.Q7R) of the gene coding for human FGF12 was recently identified in one BrS patient.[32] When expressed in rat myocytes, this variant reduced I$_{Na}$ and channel availability, hence leading to a loss of function, which is consistent with the BrS phenotype. Whether this gene and FHF-dependent regulatory mechanisms are involved in other types of arrhythmias remains to be investigated.

Z-Band Alternatively Spliced PDZ Motif Protein

The human gene LDB3Z4 encodes the Z-band alternatively spliced PDZ motif protein (ZASP protein) that is expressed in the human heart. Mutations in LDB3Z4 cause inherited cardiomyopathies, such as dilated cardiomyopathy and left ventricular noncompaction.[134] Based on the fact that conduction alterations are often observed in such cardiomyopathies, the role of the ZASP variant p.D117N on Na$_v$1.5 and I$_{Na}$ has been recently investigated.[38] Coexpression of this mutant ZASP variant with Na$_v$1.5 reduced I$_{Na}$ and rightward-shifted the voltage dependence of activation and inactivation in cellular expression systems. Interaction of ZASP with Na$_v$1.5 was demonstrated with pull-down experiments. The molecular details of this interaction are not yet known. ZASP is therefore a candidate protein for Na$_v$1.5-dependent disorders.[30,31,33,100,135–137]

Conclusions and Perspectives

This chapter summarizes the most recent findings related to the rapidly growing list of Na$_v$1.5-associated proteins. More and more of these proteins are found to be mutated in patients with genetic forms of arrhythmias, clearly illustrating their important roles in the pathophysiology of disease. Most of the detailed molecular and cellular mechanisms involved in the regulation of Na$_v$1.5 are, however, still poorly understood, thus providing many challenges for future studies in this field. It is clear that an important concept is emerging from the reviewed findings. The cardiac Na+ channel Na$_v$1.5 is most likely part of several multiprotein macromolecular complexes defining multiple populations of Na$_v$1.5 channels in cardiac cells. These associated proteins may interact at different life cycle stages of the Na$_v$1.5 subunit and in many different intracellular compartments. Na$_v$1.5 may encounter hundreds of proteins during its lifespan, from biosynthesis until degradation. Among the most intriguing questions that remain to be answered are the following: Where are the other pools of Na$_v$1.5 located in cardiac cells, and what are their molecular determinants? What are the specific roles and cross-talk mechanisms between the proteins of the intercalated disks and Na$_v$1.5? And what are the specific functions of the different populations of Na$_v$1.5 in cardiac cells? Finally, it is intriguing to speculate about possible noncanonical roles of Na$_v$1.5, such as its involvement in intercellular adhesion[63] or mechanosensation.[138]

Acknowledgment

This work has been supported by a grant of the Swiss National Science Foundation to H. A. (310030_165741).

REFERENCES

1. Fozzard HA. Cardiac sodium and calcium channels: a history of excitatory currents. *Cardiovasc Res.* 2002;55:1–8.
2. Makara MA, Curran J, Little SC, et al. Ankyrin-G coordinates intercalated disc signaling platform to regulate cardiac excitability in vivo. *Circ Res.* 2014;115:929–938.
3. Mohler PJ, Rivolta I, Napolitano C, et al. Nav1.5 E1053K mutation causing Brugada syndrome blocks binding to ankyrin-G and expression of Nav1.5 on the surface of cardiomyocytes. *Proc Natl Acad Sci U S A.* 2004;101:17533–17538.
4. Lemaillet G, Walker B, Lambert S. Identification of a conserved ankyrin-binding motif in the family of sodium channel alpha subunits. *J Biol Chem.* 2003;278:27333–27339.
5. Gavillet B, Rougier JS, Domenighetti AA, et al. Cardiac sodium channel Nav1.5 is regulated by a multiprotein complex composed of syntrophins and dystrophin. *Circ Res.* 2006;99:407–414.
6. Matamoros M, Perez-Hernandez M, Guerrero-Serna G, et al. Nav1.5 N-terminal domain binding to alpha1-syntrophin increases membrane density of human Kir2.1, Kir2.2 and Nav1.5 channels. *Cardiovasc Res.* 2016;110:279–290.
7. Gee SH, Madhavan R, Levinson SR, Caldwell JH, Sealock R, Froehner SC. Interaction of muscle and brain sodium channels with multiple members of the syntrophin family of dystrophin-associated proteins. *J Neurosci.* 1998;18:128–137.

8. Albesa M, Ogrodnik J, Rougier J-S, Abriel H. Regulation of the cardiac sodium channel Nav1.5 by utrophin in dystrophin-deficient mice. *Cardiovasc Res.* 2011;89:320–328.
9. Wu L, Yong SL, Fan C, et al. Identification of a new co-factor, MOG1, required for the function of cardiac sodium channel Nav1.5. *J Biol Chem.* 2008;283:6968–6978.
10. Kattygnarath D, Maugenre S, Neyroud N, et al. MOG1: a new susceptibility gene for Brugada syndrome. *Circ Cardiovasc Genet.* 2011;4:261–248.
11. Rizzo S, Lodder EM, Verkerk AO, et al. Intercalated disc abnormalities, reduced Na+ current density and conduction slowing in desmoglein-2 mutant mice prior to cardiomyopathic changes. *Cardiovasc Res.* 2012;95:409–418.
12. Ziane R, Huang H, Moghadaszadeh B, Beggs AH, Levesque G, Chahine M. Cell membrane expression of cardiac sodium channel Na(v)1.5 is modulated by alpha-actinin-2 interaction. *Biochemistry.* 2010;49:166–178.
13. Chatin B, Colombier P, Gamblin AL, Allouis M, Le BF. Dynamitin impacts cell surface expression of voltage-gated sodium channel Nav1.5. *Biochem J.* 2014;463:339–349.
14. Marsman RF, Bezzina CR, Freiberg F, et al. Coxsackie and adenovirus receptor is a modifier of cardiac conduction and arrhythmia vulnerability in the setting of myocardial ischemia. *J Am Coll Cardiol.* 2014;63:549–559.
15. Petitprez S, Zmoos AF, Ogrodnik J, et al. SAP97 and dystrophin macromolecular complexes determine two pools of cardiac sodium channels Nav1.5 in cardiomyocytes. *Circ Res.* 2011;108:294–304.

16. Gillet L, Rougier J-S, Shy D, et al. Cardiac-specific ablation of synapse-associated protein SAP97 in mice decreases potassium currents but not sodium current. *Heart Rhythm.* 2015;12:181–192.
17. Sato PY, Musa H, Coombs W, et al. Loss of plakophilin-2 expression leads to decreased sodium current and slower conduction velocity in cultured cardiac myocytes. *Circ Res.* 2009;105:523–526.
18. Sato PY, Coombs W, Lin X, et al. Interactions between ankyrin-g, plakophilin-2, and connexin43 at the cardiac intercalated disc. *Circ Res.* 2011;109:193–201.
19. Cerrone M, Noorman M, Lin X, et al. Sodium current deficit and arrhythmogenesis in a murine model of plakophilin-2 haploinsufficiency. *Cardiovasc Res.* 2012;95:460–468.
20. Cerrone M, Lin X, Zhang M, et al. Missense mutations in plakophilin-2 cause sodium current deficit and associate with a Brugada syndrome phenotype. *Circulation.* 2014;129:1092–1103.
21. Allouis M, Le Bouffant F, Wilders R, et al. 14-3-3 is a regulator of the cardiac voltage-gated sodium channel Nav1.5. *Circ Res.* 2006;98:1538–1546.
22. Vatta M, Ackerman MJ, Ye B, et al. Mutant caveolin-3 induces persistent late sodium current and is associated with long-QT syndrome. *Circulation.* 2006;114:2104–2112.
23. Cronk LB, Ye B, Kaku T, et al. Novel mechanism for sudden infant death syndrome: persistent late sodium current secondary to mutations in caveolin-3. *Heart Rhythm.* 2007;4:161–166.

24. Tan HL, Kupershmidt S, Zhang R, et al. A calcium sensor in the sodium channel modulates cardiac excitability. *Nature*. 2002;415:442–447.
25. Deschenes I, Neyroud N, DiSilvestre D, Marban E, Yue DT, Tomaselli GF. Isoform-specific modulation of voltage-gated Na^+ channels by calmodulin. *Circ Res*. 2002;90:E49–E57.
26. Kim J, Ghosh S, Liu H, Tateyama M, Kass RS, Pitt GS. Calmodulin mediates Ca^{2+} sensitivity of sodium channels. *J Biol Chem*. 2004;279:45004–45012.
27. Young KA, Caldwell JH. Modulation of skeletal and cardiac voltage-gated sodium channels by calmodulin. *J Physiol*. 2005;565:349–370.
28. Potet F, Chagot B, Anghelescu M, et al. Functional interactions between distinct sodium channel cytoplasmic domains through the action of calmodulin. *J Biol Chem*. 2009;284:8846–8854.
29. Gabelli SB, Boto A, Kuhns VH, et al. Regulation of the NaV1.5 cytoplasmic domain by calmodulin. *Nat Commun*. 2014;5:5126.
30. Wang C, Chung BC, Yan H, Lee SY, Pitt GS. Crystal structure of the ternary complex of a NaV C-terminal domain, a fibroblast growth factor homologous factor, and calmodulin. *Structure*. 2012;20:1167–1176.
31. Wang C, Hennessey JA, Kirkton RD, et al. Fibroblast growth factor homologous factor 13 regulates Na^+ channels and conduction velocity in murine hearts. *Circ Res*. 2011;109:775–782.
32. Hennessey JA, Marcou CA, Wang C, et al. FGF12 is a candidate Brugada syndrome locus. *Heart Rhythm*. 2013;10:1886–1894.
33. Liu CJ, Dib-Hajj SD, Renganathan M, Cummins TR, Waxman SG. Modulation of the cardiac sodium channel Nav1.5 by fibroblast growth factor homologous factor 1B. *J Biol Chem*. 2003;278:1029–1036.
34. Mazzone A, Strege PR, Tester DJ, et al. A mutation in telethonin alters Nav1.5 function. *J Biol Chem*. 2008;283:16537–16544.
35. London B, Michalec M, Mehdi H, et al. Mutation in glycerol-3-phosphate dehydrogenase 1 like gene (GPD1-L) decreases cardiac Na^+ current and causes inherited arrhythmias. *Circulation*. 2007;116:2260–2268.
36. Van Norstrand DW, Valdivia CR, Tester DJ, et al. Molecular and functional characterization of novel glycerol-3-phosphate dehydrogenase 1 like gene (GPD1-L) mutations in sudden infant death syndrome. *Circulation*. 2007;116:2253–2259.
37. Valdivia CR, Ueda K, Ackerman MJ, Makielski JC. GPD1L links redox state to cardiac excitability by PKC-dependent phosphorylation of the sodium channel SCN5A. *Am J Physiol Heart Circ Physiol*. 2009;297:H1446–H1452.
38. Xi Y, Ai T, De Lange E, et al. Loss of function of hNav1.5 by a ZASP1 mutation associated with intraventricular conduction disturbances in left ventricular noncompaction. *Circ Arrhythm Electrophysiol*. 2012;5:1017–1026.
39. Rougier J-S, van Bemmelen MX, Bruce MC, et al. Molecular determinants of voltage-gated sodium channel regulation by the Nedd4/Nedd4-like proteins. *Am J Cell Physiol*. 2005;288:C692–C701.
40. van Bemmelen MX, Rougier J-S, Gavillet B, et al. Cardiac voltage-gated sodium channel Nav1.5 is regulated by Nedd4-2 mediated ubiquitination. *Circ Res*. 2004;95:284–291.
41. Wagner S, Dybkova N, Rasenack EC, et al. Ca/calmodulin-dependent protein kinase II regulates cardiac Na channels. *J Clin Invest*. 2006;116:3127–3128.
42. Ashpole NM, Herren AW, Ginsburg KS, et al. Ca^{2+}/calmodulin-dependent protein kinase II (CaMKII) regulates cardiac sodium channel NaV1.5 gating by multiple phosphorylation sites. *J Biol Chem*. 2012;287:19856–19869.
43. Hund TJ, Koval OM, Li J, et al. A bIV-spectrin/CaMKII signaling complex is essential for membrane excitability in mice. *J Clin Invest*. 2010;120:3508–3519.
44. Jespersen T, Gavillet B, van Bemmelen MX, et al. Cardiac sodium channel Nav1.5 interacts with and is regulated by the protein tyrosine phosphatase PTPH1. *Biochem Biophys Res Commun*. 2006;348:1456–1463.
45. Cerrone M, Priori SG. Genetics of sudden death: focus on inherited channelopathies. *Eur Heart J*. 2011;32:2109–2118.
46. Mizusawa Y, Wilde AA. Brugada syndrome. *Circ Arrhythm Electrophysiol*. 2012;5:606–616.
47. Marionneau C, Abriel H. Regulation of the cardiac Na^+ channel NaV1.5 by post-translational modifications. *J Mol Cell Cardiol*. 2015;82:36–47.
48. Clatot J, Ziyadeh-Isleem A, Maugenre S, et al. Dominant-negative effect of SCN5A N-terminal mutations through the interaction of Nav1.5 alpha-subunits. *Cardiovasc Res*. 2012;96:53–63.
49. Haufe V, Camacho JA, Dumaine R, et al. Expression pattern of neuronal and skeletal muscle voltage-gated Na+ channels in the developing mouse heart. *J Physiol*. 2005;564:683–696.
50. Leoni AL, Gavillet B, Rougier JS, et al. Variable Na(v)1.5 protein expression from the wild-type allele correlates with the penetrance of cardiac conduction disease in the Scn5a mouse model. *PLoS ONE*. 2010;5:e9298.
51. Shy D, Gillet L, Ogrodnik J, et al. PDZ-domain-binding motif regulates cardiomyocyte compartment-specific $Na_v1.5$ channel expression and function. *Circulation*. 2014;130:147–160.
52. Maier SKG, Westenbroek RE, McCormick KA, Curtis R, Scheuer T, Catterall WA. Distinct subcellular localization of different sodium channel α and β subunits in single ventricular myocytes from mouse heart. *Circulation*. 2004;109:1421–1427.
53. Kucera JP, Rohr S, Rudy Y. Localization of sodium channels in intercalated disks modulates cardiac conduction. *Circ Res*. 2002;91:1176–1182.
54. Gillet L, Shy D, Abriel H. NaV1.5 and interacting proteins in human arrhythmogenic cardiomyopathy. *Future Cardiol*. 2013;9:467–470.
55. Kaprielian RR, Stevenson S, Rothery SM, Cullen MJ, Severs NJ. Distinct patterns of dystrophin organization in myocyte sarcolemma and transverse tubules of normal and diseased human myocardium. *Circulation*. 2000;101:2586–2594.
56. Stevenson SA, Cullen MJ, Rothery S, Coppen SR, Severs NJ. High-resolution en-face visualization of the cardiomyocyte plasma membrane reveals distinctive distributions of spectrin and dystrophin. *Eur J Cell Biol*. 2005;84:961–971.
57. Watanabe H, Yang T, Stroud DM, et al. Striking in vivo phenotype of a disease-associated human SCN5A mutation producing minimal changes in vitro. *Circulation*. 2011;124:1001–1011.
58. Brette F, Orchard CH. Density and sub-cellular distribution of cardiac and neuronal sodium channel isoforms in rat ventricular myocytes. *Biochem Biophys Res Comm*. 2006;348:1163–1166.
59. Milstein ML, Musa H, Balbuena DP, et al. Dynamic reciprocity of sodium and potassium channel expression in a macromolecular complex controls cardiac excitability and arrhythmia. *Proc Natl Acad Sci U S A*. 2012;109:E2134–E2143.
60. Shy D, Gillet L, Abriel H. Targeting the sodium channel NaV1.5 to specific membrane compartments of cardiac cells: not a simple task! *Circ Res*. 2014;115:901–903.
61. Jansen JA, Noorman M, Musa H, et al. Reduced heterogeneous expression of Cx43 results in decreased Nav1.5 expression and reduced sodium current which accounts for arrhythmia vulnerability in conditional Cx43 knockout mice. *Heart Rhythm*. 2011;9:600–607.
62. Desplantez T, McCain M, Beauchamp P, et al. Connexin 43 ablation in fetal atrial myocytes decreases electrical coupling, partner connexins and sodium current. *Cardiovasc Res*. 2012;94:58–65.
63. Leo-Macias A, Agullo-Pascual E, Sanchez-Alonso JL, et al. Nanoscale visualization of functional adhesion/excitability nodes at the intercalated disc. *Nat Commun*. 2016;7:10342.
64. Glickman MH, Ciechanover A. The ubiquitin-proteasome proteolytic pathway: destruction for the sake of construction. *Physiol Rev*. 2002;82:373–428.
65. Staub O, Rotin D. Role of ubiquitylation in cellular membrane transport. *Physiol Rev*. 2006;86:669–707.
66. Hershko A, Ciechanover A. The ubiquitin system. *Annu Rev Biochem*. 1998;67:425–479.
67. Hicke L, Dunn R. Regulation of membrane protein transport by ubiquitin and ubiquitin-binding proteins. *Annu Rev Cell Dev Biol*. 2003;19:141–172.
68. Abriel H, Staub O. Ubiquitylation of ion channels. *Physiology*. 2005;20:398–407.
69. Rotin D, Kumar S. Physiological functions of the HECT family of ubiquitin ligases. *Nat Rev Mol Cell Biol*. 2009;10:398–409.
70. Fotia AB, Ekberg J, Adams DJ, Cook DI, Poronnik P, Kumar S. Regulation of neuronal voltage-gated sodium channels by the ubiquitin-protein ligases Nedd4 and Nedd4-2. *J Biol Chem*. 2004;279:28930–28935.
71. Jespersen T, Membrez M, Nicolas CS, et al. The KCNQ1 potassium channel is down-regulated by ubiquitylating enzymes of the Nedd4/Nedd4like family. *Cardiovasc Res*. 2007;74:64–74.
72. Albesa M, Grilo LS, Gavillet B, Abriel H. Nedd4-2-dependent ubiquitylation and regulation of the cardiac potassium channel hERG1. *J Mol Cell Cardiol*. 2011;51:90–98.
73. Staub O, Rotin D. WW domains. *Structure*. 1996;4:495–499.
74. Abriel H, Kamynina E, Horisberger JD, Staub O. Regulation of the cardiac voltage-gated Na^+ channel (H1) by the ubiquitin-protein ligase Nedd4. *FEBS Lett*. 2000;466:377–380.
75. Kang L, Zheng M, Morishima M, Wang Y, Kaku T, Ono K. Bepridil up-regulates cardiac Na^+ channels as a long-term effect by blunting proteasome signals through inhibition of calmodulin activity. *Br J Pharmacol*. 2009;157:404–414.
76. Ingham RJ, Gish G, Pawson T. The Nedd4 family of E3 ubiquitin ligases: functional diversity within a common modular architecture. *Oncogene*. 2004;23:1972–1984.
77. Ballou LM, Lin RZ, Cohen IS. Control of cardiac repolarization by phosphoinositide 3-kinase signaling to ion channels. *Circ Res*. 2015;116:127–137.
78. Morrison DK. The 14-3-3 proteins: integrators of diverse signaling cues that impact cell fate and cancer development. *Trends Cell Biol*. 2009;19:16–23.
79. Mrowiec T, Schwappach B. 14-3-3 proteins in membrane protein transport. *Biol Chem*. 2006;387:1227–1236.
80. Saimi Y, Kung C. Calmodulin as an ion channel subunit. *Annu Rev Physiol*. 2002;64:289–311.
81. Pitt GS. Calmodulin and CaMKII as molecular switches for cardiac ion channels. *Cardiovasc Res*. 2007;73:641–647.
82. Chin D, Means AR. Calmodulin: a prototypical calcium sensor. *Trends Cell Biol*. 2000;10:322–328.
83. Pitt GS, Zuhlke RD, Hudmon A, Schulman H, Reuter H, Tsien RW. Molecular basis of calmodulin tethering and Ca^{2+}-dependent inactivation of L-type Ca^{2+} channels. *J Biol Chem*. 2001;276:30794–30802.
84. Herzog RI, Liu C, Waxman SG, Cummins TR. Calmodulin binds to the C terminus of sodium channels Nav1.4 and Nav1.6 and differentially modulates their functional properties. *J Neurosci*. 2003;23:8261–8270.
85. Motoike HK, Liu H, Glaaser IW, Yang AS, Tateyama M, Kass RS. The Na+ channel inactivation gate is a molecular complex: a novel role of the COOH-terminal domain. *J Gen Physiol*. 2004;123:155–165.
86. Shah VN, Wingo TL, Weiss KL, Williams CK, Balser JR, Chazin WJ. Calcium-dependent regulation of the voltage-gated sodium channel hH1: intrinsic and extrinsic sensors use a common molecular switch. *Proc Natl Acad Sci U S A*. 2006;103:3592–3597.
87. Wingo TL, Shah VN, Anderson ME, Lybrand TP, Chazin WJ, Balser JR. An EF-hand in the sodium channel couples intracellular calcium to cardiac excitability. *Nat Struct Mol Biol*. 2004;11:219–225.
88. Chagot B, Potet F, Balser JR, Chazin WJ. Solution NMR structure of the C-terminal EF-hand domain of human cardiac sodium channel NaV1.5. *J Biol Chem*. 2008;284:6436–6445.
89. Miloushev VZ, Levine JA, Arbing MA, Hunt JF, Pitt GS, Palmer AG 3rd . Solution structure of the NaV1.2 C-terminal EF-hand domain. *J Biol Chem*. 2009;284:6446–6454.
90. Casini S, Verkerk AO, van Borren MM, et al. Intracellular calcium modulation of voltage-gated sodium channels in ventricular myocytes. *Cardiovasc Res*. 2009;81:72–81.
91. Couchonnal LF, Anderson ME. The role of calmodulin kinase II in myocardial physiology and disease. *Physiology*. 2008;23:151–159.
92. Maier LS. Role of CaMKII for signaling and regulation in the heart. *Front Biosci*. 2009;14:486–496.
93. Maier LS, Bers DM. Calcium, calmodulin, and calcium-calmodulin kinase II: heartbeat to heartbeat and beyond. *J Mol Cell Cardiol*. 2002;34:919–939.
94. Yoon JY, Ho WK, Kim ST, Cho H. Constitutive CaMKII activity regulates Na+ channel in rat ventricular myocytes. *J Mol Cell Cardiol*. 2009;47:475–484.
95. Kass RS. The channelopathies: novel insights into molecular and genetic mechanisms of human disease. *J Clin Invest*. 2005;115:1986–1989.
96. Maltsev VA, Reznikov V, Undrovinas NA, Sabbah HN, Undrovinas A. Modulation of the late sodium current by Ca^{2+}, calmodulin, and CaMKI I in normal and failing dog cardiomyocytes: similarities and differences. *Am J Heart Circ Physiol*. 2008;294:1597–1608.
97. Davis MJ, Wu X, Nurkiewicz TR, et al. Regulation of ion channels by protein tyrosine phosphorylation. *Am J Physiol Heart Circ Physiol*. 2001;281:H1835–H1862.
98. Ahern CA, Zhang JF, Wookalis MJ, Horn R. Modulation of the cardiac sodium channel NaV1.5 by Fyn, a Src family tyrosine kinase. *Circ Res*. 2005;96:991–998.
99. Hartmann HA, Tiedeman AA, Chen SF, Brown AM, Kirsch GE. Effects of III-IV linker mutations on human heart Na^+ channel inactivation gating. *Circ Res*. 1994;75:114–122.
100. Wehrens XHT, Abriel H, Cabo C, Benhorin J, Kass RS. Arrhythmogenic mechanism of an LQT-3 mutation of the human heart Na^+ channel alpha-subunit: a computational analysis. *Circulation*. 2000;102:584–590.
101. Shy D, Gillet L, Abriel H. Cardiac sodium channel Nav1.5 distribution in myocytes via interacting proteins: the multiple pool model. *Biochim Biophys Acta*. 2013;1833:886–894.
102. Faulkner G, Lanfranchi G, Valle G. Telethonin and other new proteins of the Z-disc of skeletal muscle. *IUBMB Life*. 2001;51:275–282.
103. Hayashi T, Arimura T, Itoh-Satoh M, et al. Tcap gene mutations in hypertrophic cardiomyopathy and dilated cardiomyopathy. *J Am Coll Cardiol*. 2004;44:2192–2201.
104. Mues A, van der Ven PFM, Young P, Furst DO, Gautel M. Two immunoglobulin-like domains of the Z-disc portion of titin interact in a conformation-dependent way with telethonin. *FEBS Letters*. 1998;428:111–114.
105. Furukawa T, Ono Y, Tsuchiya H, et al. Specific interaction of the potassium channel beta-subunit minK with the sarcomeric protein T-cap suggests a T-tubule-myofibril linking system. *J Mol Biol*. 2001;313:775–784.
106. Ou Y, Gibbons SJ, Miller SM, et al. SCN5A is expressed in human jejunal circular smooth muscle cells. *Neurogastroenterol Motil*. 2002;14:477–486.

107. Steele DF, Eldstrom J, Fedida D. Mechanisms of cardiac potassium channel trafficking. *J Physiol.* 2007;582:17–26.

108. Funke L, Dakoji S, Bredt DS. Membrane-associated guanylate kinases regulate adhesion and plasticity at cell junctions. *Ann Rev Biochem.* 2000;74:219–245.

109. Godreau D, Vranckx R, Maguy A, et al. Expression, regulation and role of the MAGUK protein SAP-97 in human atrial myocardium. *Cardiovasc Res.* 2002;56:433–442.

110. Leonoudakis D, Conti LR, Anderson S, et al. Protein trafficking and anchoring complexes revealed by proteomic analysis of inward rectifier potassium channel (Kir2.x) associated proteins. *J Biol Chem.* 2004;279:22331–22346.

111. Godreau D, Vranckx R, Maguy A, Goyenvalle C, Hatem SN. Different isoforms of synapse-associated protein, SAP97, are expressed in the heart and have distinct effects on the voltage-gated K⁺ channel Kv1.5. *J Biol Chem.* 2003;278:47046–47052.

112. El-Haou S, Balse E, Neyroud N, et al. Kv4 potassium channels form a tripartite complex with the anchoring protein SAP97 and CaMKII in cardiac myocytes. *Circ Res.* 2009;104:758–769.

113. Cianfrocco MA, DeSantis ME, Leschziner AE, Reck-Peterson SL. Mechanism and regulation of cytoplasmic dynein. *Annu Rev Cell Dev Biol.* 2015;31:83–108.

114. Shaw RM, Fay AJ, Puthenveedu MA, von ZM, Jan YN, Jan LY. Microtubule plus-end-tracking proteins target gap junctions directly from the cell interior to adherens junctions. *Cell.* 2007;128:547–560.

115. Bezzina CR, Pazoki R, Bardai A, et al. Genome-wide association study identifies a susceptibility locus at 21q21 for ventricular fibrillation in acute myocardial infarction. *Nat Genet.* 2010;42:688–691.

116. Williams TM, Lisanti MP. The caveolin genes: from cell biology to medicine. *Ann Med.* 2004;36:584–595.

117. Cohen AW, Hnasko R, Schubert W, Lisanti MP. Role of caveolae and caveolins in health and disease. *Physiol Rev.* 2004;84:1341–1379.

118. Yarbrough TL, Lu T, Lee HC, Shibata EF. Localization of cardiac sodium channels in caveolin-rich membrane domains: regulation of sodium current amplitude. *Circ Res.* 2002;90:443–449.

119. Shibata EF, Brown TL, Washburn ZW, Bai J, Revak TJ, Butters CA. Autonomic regulation of voltage-gated cardiac ion channels. *J Cardiovasc Electrophysiol.* 2006;17:S34–S42.

120. Doyle DD, Goings G, Upshaw-Earley J, et al. Dystrophin associates with caveolae of rat cardiac myocytes: relationship to dystroglycan. *Circ Res.* 2000;87:480–488.

121. Rougier J-S, Gavillet B, Abriel H. Proteasome inhibitor (MG132) rescues Nav1.5 protein content and the cardiac sodium current in dystrophin-deficient mdx5cv mice. *Front Physiol.* 2013;4:51.

122. Ueda K, Valdivia C, Medeiros-Domingo A, et al. Syntrophin mutation associated with long QT syndrome through activation of the nNOS-SCN5A macromolecular complex. *Proc Natl Acad Sci U S A.* 2008;105:9355–9360.

123. Wu G, Ai T, Kim JJ, et al. Alpha-1-syntrophin mutation and the long QT syndrome: a disease of sodium channel disruption. *Circ Arrhythm Electrophysiol.* 2008;1:193–201.

124. Weiss R, Barmada MM, Nguyen T, et al. Clinical and molecular heterogeneity in the Brugada syndrome: a novel gene locus on chromosome 3. *Circulation.* 2002;105:707–713.

125. Marfatia KA, Harreman MT, Fanara P, Vertino PM, Corbett AH. Identification and characterization of the human MOG1 gene. *Gene.* 2001;266:45–56.

126. Gerull B, Heuser A, Wichter T, et al. Mutations in the desmosomal protein plakophilin-2 are common in arrhythmogenic right ventricular cardiomyopathy. *Nat Genet.* 2004;36:1162–1164.

127. Pilichou K, Nava A, Basso C, et al. Mutations in desmoglein-2 gene are associated with arrhythmogenic right ventricular cardiomyopathy. *Circulation.* 2006;113:1171–1179.

128. Cunha SR, Mohler PJ. Cardiac ankyrins: essential components for development and maintenance of excitable membrane domains in heart. *Cardiovasc Res.* 2006;71:22–29.

129. Mohler PJ, Schott JJ, Gramolini AO, et al. Ankyrin-B mutation causes type 4 long-QT cardiac arrhythmia and sudden cardiac death. *Nature.* 2003;421:634–639.

130. Mohler PJ, Le Scouarnec S, Denjoy I, et al. Defining the cellular phenotype of "ankyrin-B syndrome" variants. Human ANK2 variants associated with clinical phenotypes display a spectrum of activities in cardiomyocytes. *Circulation.* 2007;115:432–441.

131. Chauhan VS, Tuvia S, Buhusi M, Bennett V, Grant AO. Abnormal cardiac Na⁺ channel properties and QT heart rate adaptation in neonatal ankyrin(B) knockout mice. *Circ Res.* 2000;86:441–447.

132. Lowe JS, Palygin O, Bhasin N, et al. Voltage-gated Nav channel targeting in the heart requires an ankyrin-G dependent cellular pathway. *J Cell Biol.* 2008;180:173–186.

133. Pablo JL, Pitt GS. Fibroblast growth factor homologous factors: new roles in neuronal health and disease. *Neuroscientist.* 2016;22:19–25.

134. Vatta M, Mohapatra B, Jimenez S, et al. Mutations in Cypher/ZASP in patients with dilated cardiomyopathy and left ventricular non-compaction. *J Am Coll Cardiol.* 2003;42:2014–2027.

135. Olsen SK, Garbi M, Zampieri N, et al. Fibroblast growth factor (FGF) homologous factors share structural but not functional homology with FGFs. *J Biol Chem.* 2003;278:34226–34236.

136. Goetz R, Dover K, Laezza F, et al. Crystal structure of a fibroblast growth factor homologous factor (FHF) defines a conserved surface on FHFS for binding and modulation of voltage-gated sodium channels. *J Biol Chem.* 2009;284:17883–17896.

137. Lou JY, Laezza F, Gerber BR, et al. Fibroblast growth factor 14 is an intracellular modulator of voltage-gated sodium channels. *J Physiol.* 2005;569:179–193.

138. Beyder A, Strege PR, Reyes S, et al. Ranolazine decreases mechanosensitivity of the voltage-gated sodium ion channel NaV1.5: a novel mechanism of drug action. *Circulation.* 2012;125:2698–2706.

19 Fibroblast Growth Factor Homologous Factors Modulate Cardiac Sodium and Calcium Channels

Geoffrey S. Pitt

The discovery and early investigations of fibroblast growth factor homologous factors (FHFs) have been previously reviewed.[1] In brief, FHFs were discovered during a search for novel retinal-specific genes that initially identified a complementary DNA (cDNA) encoding a predicted protein with limited homology to members of the fibroblast growth factor (FGF) superfamily and subsequently to the identification of three related cDNAs.[2] Originally named *FHF-1*, *FHF-2*, *FHF-3*, and *FHF-4*, the FHF genes are now known as *FGF12*, *FGF13*, *FGF11*, and *FGF14*, respectively. In the mouse, the FHFs are variably expressed in the brain and retina. *Fgf13* is also present in the mouse heart. Although the FHFs contain an FGF-like core domain, the FHFs each lack the signal sequence found in canonical FGFs, are not known to be secreted, and do not appear to function as extracellular growth factors. Moreover, specific structural differences between the FGF-like core and canonical FHFs have been suggested to prevent FHFs from being able to activate FGF receptors.[3] Nevertheless, induced misexpression of FHF orthologs present during chick limb development was shown to affect limb morphogenesis in a growth factor–like manner.[4]

A yeast two-hybrid screen that uncovered FHFs as binding partners for the intracellular C-termini of voltage-gated Na+ channels focused attention on the regulation of Na$_V$ channels.[5] In heterologous systems and in neurons, various FHFs affect the current density and/or inactivation kinetics of specific Na$_V$ channels in a pairwise manner.[6–11] The binary logic of the specific regulatory effects of the FHF–Na$_V$ channel pairs has been difficult to decipher. Depending on the individual FHF, its specific splice variant, the specific Na$_V$1 channel, and the cell type in which channel function is assessed, the regulatory effects can vary greatly. For example, FGF14 decreased the Na$_V$1.5 current density when the two were coexpressed in HEK293 cells, but it moderately increases the current density of Na$_V$1.1 in the same cell system.[10]

Contemporaneously with the identification of Na$_V$ C-terminal domains as FHF-binding partners, the independent identification of *FGF14* as the locus for spinocerebellar ataxia 27[12] and the development of an ataxia phenotype in *Fgf14* knockout mice[7,13] implied that regulation of neuronal Na$_V$ channels by FHFs and consequent neuronal excitability is essential for normal physiology.

While most studies of Na$_V$ channel regulation by FHFs have focused on the central nervous system, the presence of *Fgf13* expression in developing mouse heart prompted an investigation into homologous roles for FHF regulation of cardiac Na$_V$ channels. Knockdown experiments in ventricular cardiomyocytes of adult mice and rats demonstrated that FHFs do, indeed, regulate cardiac Na+ channel function.[14] This will be discussed in more detail in the following text.

The Structure of Fibroblast Growth Factor Homologous Factors

FHFs have a core FGF-like domain surrounded by an extended N-terminus and C-terminus. The N-terminus for each FHF derives from alternative splicing of the respective first exon, producing two distinct isoforms with the exception of *FGF13*, which utilizes alternative splicing of four exons to generate a total of five isoforms.[15] In heterologous expression systems, one of the alternatively spliced isoforms for *FGF12* and *FGF13* shows nuclear localization,[2,15] but roles for FHFs within the nucleus have not yet been determined.

Crystal structures for the FGF-like core domains of FGF12 and FGF13 have been determined both in the presence and absence of their channel Na$_V$ C-terminal domain binding partners. Like FGFs, FHFs contain 12 antiparallel β-strands arranged in a structure with pseudo threefold-symmetry called a β-trefoil.[3,16,17] As previously noted, nonhomologous substitutions of several amino acids known to be critical for FGF interaction with FGF receptors may introduce steric clashes or remove hydrogen bonds, thus providing a basis for the inability of FHFs to bind to or activate FGF receptors.[3] When FHFs are bound to a Na$_V$ channel C-terminal domain, there are minimal structural changes.[18,19]

The crystal structures of FHFs bound to a Na$_V$ channel C-terminal domain, within ternary complexes that also contain calmodulin,[18,19] identify the components necessary for interaction between FHFs and Na$_V$ channel C-termini. Specific amino acids conserved among all four FHFs form protrusions that fit into Na$_V$ C-terminal domain crevices that comprised amino acids conserved across the Na$_V$ channel family.[18–20] Critical among these protrusions on the FHF are the side chains of Leu[56] and Arg[57] (numbered according to the FGF13U isoform), which interact with Na$_V$1.5 His[1849] and Asp[1852]. Mutation of Arg[57] is sufficient to completely abrogate interaction with the Na$_V$ channel.[20] Likewise, mutation of His[1849] in Na$_V$1.5 markedly reduces the interaction with FHFs and provides a basis for understanding an inherited arrhythmia syndrome,[21] as discussed in more detail later. Another residue in FHFs that has been found to be important for interaction includes a glutamine

(Gln[7] in FGF12B) that, when mutated to an Arg, reduces interaction with $Na_V1.5$ and has been associated with Brugada syndrome.[22]

Fibroblast Growth Factor Homologous Factors Regulate Voltage-Gated Sodium Channels

FHFs regulate multiple aspects of Na_V channel function. These processes are mediated through the direct contacts between FHFs and Na_V channel C-terminal domains as previously described. Defining the specific ways in which FHFs affect Na_V channel function, however, has been challenging because, although FHFs have profound effects on Na_Vs in heterologous expression systems and in native cells, the specific effects depend upon the individual FHF and Na_V pair studied, and the observed effects do not always faithfully recapitulate the consequences in a native cell environment. For the cardiac $Na_V1.5$ channel, knockdown and expression experiments in ventricular cardiomyocytes of adult rats show that FHFs increase $Na_V1.5$ current density and increase channel availability (i.e., inducing a depolarizing shift steady-state inactivation).[14,22] Recent analyses of an inducible, cardiac-specific *Fgf13* knockout mouse revealed similar consequences on cardiac Na_V currents recorded from isolated ventricular cardiomyocytes.[23] In contrast, the analysis of recordings from HEK293 cells in which FGF13 and $Na_V1.5$ are coexpressed show a reduction in Na_V channel current density compared to recordings from cells in which only $Na_V1.5$ is expressed,[24] emphasizing the utility of analyzing the consequences in a native environment. The reasons for these discrepancies between native cells and heterologous expression systems are not clear but may indicate influences of the Na_V channel macromolecular complex that are not present in the heterologous expression system.

FHFs also regulate the neuronal $Na_V1.6$ channel,[8,25–27] which is found in ventricular cardiomyocytes and where $Na_V1.6$ appears to participate in the depolarization necessary for excitation within T-tubules.[28] Thus the consequences of FHF knockdown or knockout on ventricular Na_V currents may include effects upon regulation of $Na_V1.6$ as well as the loss of regulation of the dominant $Na_V1.5$.

Arrhythmia Mutations Result From Aberrant Fibroblast Growth Factor Homologous Factor–Voltage-Gated Sodium Channels Interaction

The direct interactions between FHFs and Na_V channels and the potent regulatory effects of FHFs on Na_V channels through these direct interactions prompted queries into whether mutations in FHFs were associated with arrhythmia syndromes. Further rationale for such queries arose from the consequences of Na_V channel mutations on Na_V channel function and arrhythmogenesis as well as previously discovered disease-associated mutations in other Na_V channel auxiliary subunits. Perhaps a mutation in an FHF would similarly be detrimental.

Querying a database of previously genotype-negative Brugada syndrome patients uncovered a p.K7R mutation in FGF12B, the most prominent FHF in the human heart.[22] Support for causality of this mutation in the arrhythmia can be derived from two main lines of evidence. First, the p.K7R mutant FGF12 bound the $Na_V1.5$ C-terminal domain with decreased affinity. Second, in contrast to wild-type FGF12, expression of the p.K7R mutant FGF12 failed to rescue the reduced Na_V current in ventricular cardiomyocytes of adult rats after the knockdown of FGF13, the endogenous FHF in rat hearts.

More recently, a disruption of the interaction between FGF12 and $Na_V1.5$ by a mutation within the FHF surface on $Na_V1.5$ was found in a five-generation kindred with a history of atrial and ventricular arrhythmias and sudden cardiac death.[21] The mutation, p.H1849R, sits at the base of the binding pocket into which the critical Arg residue (Arg[52] in FGF12 or Arg[57] in FGF13, as previously discussed) protrudes. Binding assays demonstrated that the p.H1849R mutation in the $Na_V1.5$ C-terminal domain markedly reduced the affinity to interact with the FHF. Functional studies showed that this reduced interaction correlated with striking changes in the kinetics of $Na_V1.5$ channel inactivation in a heterologous expression system. Further, expression of the p.H1849R mutant $Na_V1.5$ in neonatal cardiomyocytes, in which the endogenous $Na_V1.5$ was knocked out, prolonged the action potential and induced spontaneous activity. Thus, disruption of the interaction between FGF12 and $Na_V1.5$ channel, whether by mutation in the FHF or in the $Na_V1.5$ channel, can alter channel function and cause arrhythmias.

Fibroblast Growth Factor Homologous Factors Regulate Voltage-Gated Calcium Channels

A proteomic screen for FHF interactors in ventricular cardiomyocytes identified junctophilin-2 (JPH2), a protein that organizes the close apposition of the L-type Ca^{2+} channel $Ca_V1.2$ and the ryanodine receptor type 2 (RyR2) in the dyad.[29] This prompted an investigation into whether FHFs, through interactions with JPH2, affected $Ca_V1.2$ function. Indeed, knockdown of FGF13 in cultured adult ventricular cardiomyocytes altered $Ca_V1.2$ channel subcellular localization, at least in part by affecting normal trafficking of $Ca_V1.2$ to the sarcolemma, and reduced the number of functional $Ca_V1.2$ channels at the sarcolemma. As a result, induced Ca^{2+} transients were reduced but excitation–contraction coupling gain was unaffected. Thus, in this cultured ventricular cardiomyocyte system, FHFs appear to affect $Ca_V1.2$ channel function through a mechanism different from how FHFs affect $Na_V1.5$ channels. For $Ca_V1.2$ channels, FHF-dependent regulation appears to be mediated through the JPH2 interaction and the $Ca_V1.2$ macromolecular complex rather than through a direct interaction with the channel. The arrhythmogenic p.K7R mutation in FGF12 did not affect $Ca_V1.2$ function in the same assays that demonstrated altered $Na_V1.5$ channel function.[22] These data thus suggest that the FGF12 domain(s) responsible for $Na_V1.5$ channel regulation are separate from the domains that affect $Ca_V1.2$ channel function. Analogous to these results, knockdown of *Fgf14* in cerebellar neurons of rats reduces the number of presynaptic voltage-gated $Ca_V2.1$ and $Ca_V2.2$ channels and decreases the amount of presynaptic Ca^{2+} entry.[30] As for $Ca_V1.2$ in cardiomyocytes, there is no apparent direct interaction between FGF14 and presynaptic voltage-gated Ca^{2+} channels.

Despite the profound effects of FGF13 knockdown on $Ca_V1.2$ channel function in cultured adult ventricular cardiomyocytes, no human mutations in FHFs or $Ca_V1.2$ channels have yet been reported that alter the FHF modulation of $Ca_V1.2$ channels and thereby contribute to arrhythmogenesis or cardiomyopathy. One possibility is that the defects noted after FHF knockdown in culture may be alleviated by compensatory mechanisms in vivo that are not present in culture. Indeed, action potential morphology and duration are differentially affected after cardiac-specific *Fgf13* knockout in mouse compared to *Fgf13* knockdown in cultured ventricular cardiomyocytes of adult rats. While species-specific differences could explain this difference, other measures of channel function have been consistent between rat and mouse.[29] A detailed analysis of the *Fgf13* knockout model will likely be helpful in addressing this discrepancy.

Novel Fibroblast Growth Factor Homologous Factor Roles and Future Directions

While the targeted investigations into the effects of FHF on cardiac Na_V channels followed directly from the known effects of FHFs on neuronal Na_V channels, the initial research demonstrating a connection between these noncanonical members of the FGF superfamily and Na_V channels followed a circuitous route. As is frequent in such cases, the appreciated influences of a specific regulatory factor increase as the investigations proceed. This has certainly held true for FHFs, as demonstrated by their recently discovered regulation of voltage-gated Ca^{2+} channels, as previously discussed. Moreover, an analysis of the action potential morphologies in the FHF knockdown and knockout models offers hints at additional effects. The changes in the action potential duration and morphology cannot readily be explained by the documented effects on Na_V and/or voltage-gated Ca^{2+} channels.

Rather, these specific effects suggest an involvement of K^+ channels. Further, there is little rationale to limit the regulatory focus of FHFs on ion channels. Other potential FHF interactors, such as microtubules in neurons[31] and kinase scaffolds,[32] have previously been reported. The specific roles for these interactions are not yet clear, but the availability of new inducible cardiac-specific knockout mice provides an opportunity to determine the various ways in which FHFs contribute to cardiac physiology. Finally, the ability of FHFs to function in a growth factor–like manner as well as to regulate chick limb development and, separately, the nuclear localization of certain FHF isoforms may suggest additional functions of FHFs in the heart.

Acknowledgment

This work was supported by the National Institutes of Health [R01 HL112918, R01 HL122967, R01 HL071165].

REFERENCES

1. Goldfarb M.. Fibroblast growth factor homologous factors: evolution, structure, and function. *Cytokine Growth Factor Rev.* 2005;16:215–220.
2. Smallwood PM, Munoz-Sanjuan I, Tong P, et al. Fibroblast growth factor (FGF) homologous factors: new members of the FGF family implicated in nervous system development. *Proc Natl Acad Sci U S A.* 1996;93:9850–9857.
3. Olsen SK, Garbi M, Zampieri N, et al. Fibroblast growth factor (FGF) homologous factors share structural but not functional homology with FGFs. *J Biol Chem.* 2003;278:34226–34236.
4. Munoz-Sanjuan I, Simandl BK, Fallon JF, Nathans J. Expression of chicken fibroblast growth factor homologous factor (FHF)-1 and of differentially spliced isoforms of FHF-2 during development and involvement of FHF-2 in chicken limb development. *Development.* 1999;126:409–421.
5. Liu C, Dib-Hajj SD, Waxman SG. Fibroblast growth factor homologous factor 1B binds to the C terminus of the tetrodotoxin-resistant sodium channel rNav1.9a (NaN). *J Biol Chem.* 2001;276:18925–18933.
6. Dover K, Solinas S, D'Angelo E, Goldfarb M. Long-term inactivation particle for voltage-gated sodium channels. *J Physiol.* 2010;588:3695–3711.
7. Goldfarb M, Schoorlemmer J, Williams A, et al. Fibroblast growth factor homologous factors control neuronal excitability through modulation of voltage-gated sodium channels. *Neuron.* 2007;55:449–463.
8. Laezza F, Lampert A, Kozel MA, et al. FGF14 N-terminal splice variants differentially modulate Nav1.2 and Nav1.6-encoded sodium channels. *Mol Cell Neurosci.* 2009;42:90–101.
9. Liu CJ, Dib-Hajj SD, Renganathan M, Cummins TR, Waxman SG. Modulation of the cardiac sodium channel Nav1.5 by fibroblast growth factor homologous factor 1B. *J Biol Chem.* 2003;278:1029–1036.
10. Lou JY, Laezza F, Gerber BR, et al. Fibroblast growth factor 14 is an intracellular modulator of voltage-gated sodium channels. *J Physiol.* 2005;569:179–193.
11. Rush AM, Wittmack EK, Tyrrell L, Black JA, Dib-Hajj SD, Waxman SG. Differential modulation of sodium

channel Na(v)1.6 by two members of the fibroblast growth factor homologous factor 2 subfamily. *Eur J Neurosci.* 2006;23:2551–2562.
12. van Swieten JC, Brusse E, de Graaf BM, et al. A mutation in the fibroblast growth factor 14 gene is associated with autosomal dominant cerebral ataxia. *Am J Hum Genet.* 2003;72:191–199.
13. Wang Q, Bardgett ME, Wong M, et al. Ataxia and paroxysmal dyskinesia in mice lacking axonally transported FGF14. *Neuron.* 2002;35:25–38.
14. Wang C, Hennessey JA, Kirkton RD, et al. Fibroblast growth factor homologous factor 13 regulates Na⁺ channels and conduction velocity in murine hearts. *Circ Res.* 2011;109:775–782.
15. Munoz-Sanjuan I, Smallwood PM, Nathans J. Isoform diversity among fibroblast growth factor homologous factors is generated by alternative promoter usage and differential splicing. *J Biol Chem.* 2000;275:2589–2597.
16. Goetz R, Dover K, Laezza F, et al. Crystal structure of a fibroblast growth factor homologous factor (FHF) defines a conserved surface on FHFs for binding and modulation of voltage-gated sodium channels. *J Biol Chem.* 2009;284:17883–17896.
17. Zhu X, Komiya H, Chirino A, et al. Three-dimensional structures of acidic and basic fibroblast growth factors. *Science.* 1991;251:90–93.
18. Wang C, Chung BC, Yan H, Lee SY, Pitt GS. Crystal structure of the ternary complex of a NaV C-terminal domain, a fibroblast growth factor homologous factor, and calmodulin. *Structure.* 2012;20:1167–1176.
19. Wang C, Chung BC, Yan H, Wang HG, Lee SY, Pitt GS. Structural analyses of Ca²⁺/CaM interaction with NaV channel C-termini reveal mechanisms of calcium-dependent regulation. *Nat Commun.* 2014;5:4896.
20. Yan H, Pablo JL, Wang C, Pitt GS. FGF14 modulates resurgent sodium current in mouse cerebellar Purkinje neurons. *Elife.* 2014;3:e04193.
21. Musa H, Kline CF, Sturm AC, et al. SCN5A variant that blocks fibroblast growth factor homologous factor regulation causes human arrhythmia. *Proc Natl Acad Sci U S A.* 2015;112:12528–12533.

22. Hennessey JA, Marcou CA, Wang C, et al. FGF12 is a candidate Brugada syndrome locus. *Heart Rhythm.* 2013a;10:1886–1894.
23. Wang X, Tang H, Wei EQ, et al. Conditional knockout of Fgf13 in murine hearts increases arrhythmia susceptibility and reveals novel ion channel modulatory roles. *J Mol Cell Cardiol.* 2017;104:63–74.
24. Yang J, Wang Z, Sinden DS, et al. FGF13 modulates the gating properties of the cardiac sodium channel Nav1.5 in an isoform-specific manner. *Channels (Austin).* 2016;10:410–420.
25. Shakkottai VG, Xiao Y, Xu L, et al. FGF14 regulates the intrinsic excitability of cerebellar Purkinje neurons. *Neurobiol Dis.* 2009;33:81–88.
26. Venkatesan K, Liu Y, Goldfarb M. Fast-onset long-term open-state block of sodium channels by A-type FHFs mediates classical spike accommodation in hippocampal pyramidal neurons. *J Neurosci.* 2014;34:16126–16139.
27. Wittmack EK, Rush AM, Craner MJ, Goldfarb M, Waxman SG, Dib-Hajj SD. Fibroblast growth factor homologous factor 2B: association with Nav1.6 and selective colocalization at nodes of Ranvier of dorsal root axons. *J Neurosci.* 2004;24:6765–6775.
28. Noujaim SF, Kaur K, Milstein M, et al. A null mutation of the neuronal sodium channel NaV1.6 disrupts action potential propagation and excitation-contraction coupling in the mouse heart. *FASEB J.* 2012;26:63–72.
29. Hennessey JA, Wei EQ, Pitt GS. Fibroblast growth factor homologous factors modulate cardiac calcium channels. *Circ Res.* 2013b;113:381–388.
30. Yan H, Pablo JL, Pitt GS. FGF14 regulates presynaptic Ca²⁺ channels and synaptic transmission. *Cell Rep.* 2013;4:66–75.
31. Wu QF, Yang L, Li S, et al. Fibroblast growth factor 13 is a microtubule-stabilizing protein regulating neuronal polarization and migration. *Cell.* 2012;149:1549–1564.
32. Schoorlemmer J, Goldfarb M. Fibroblast growth factor homologous factors and the islet brain-2 scaffold protein regulate activation of a stress-activated protein kinase. *J Biol Chem.* 2002;277:49111–49119.

20 Macromolecular Complexes and Cardiac Potassium Channels

Stéphane Hatem and Elise Balse

In the heart, the main repolarizing currents are carried by potassium ions. Several of the potassium currents shape and control the action potential (AP). The inward rectifier K+ current is crucial for maintaining the membrane potential near the equilibrium potential for potassium, namely –90 mV during diastole. Voltage-dependent outward currents regulate the duration and termination of the plateau phase of the AP, whereas delayed rectifier and inward rectifier currents control the final repolarization phase of the AP. The molecular basis of potassium currents is diverse, with more than 40 genes encoding potassium channels expressed in the heart. In addition, a number of auxiliary units and protein partners contribute to the trafficking and anchoring of potassium channels at the plasma membrane and to their organization in macromolecular complexes. These partners confer important properties to potassium currents, contributing to the plasticity of cardiac electrical properties both in normal conditions and during cardiac diseases. Not only proteins but also lipids of the plasma membrane appear to be major partners for potassium channels. This chapter will focus on the description of partners involved in the formation of macromolecular potassium channel complexes and their role in cardiac excitability.

The Four General Classes of Accessory Subunits

Kvβ Family

The first identified auxiliary subunits of potassium channels are Kvβ-subunits that associate with Kv channels (referred to as α-subunits). Initially purified from bovine brain,[1,2] nine β-subunits encoded by four genes have been identified. In mammals, three genes, namely Kβ1.1, Kvβ1.2, and Kvβ1.3, are expressed in the heart, and variants from alternative splicing are also found.[3] Kvβ subunits are localized in the cytosol with a conserved C-terminal and a variable N-terminal.

Two main roles have been described for Kvβ subunits. Trimmer and coworkers reported that Kvβ1 and Kvβ3 associate with α-subunits early during their biosynthesis in the endoplasmic reticulum (ER) and exert a chaperone-like effect, facilitating their stable expression in the plasma membrane.[4,5] The C-terminal domain of Kvβ interacts with the α-subunit (stoichiometry of 1α-1β) to regulate channel trafficking. However, this chaperone property of the Kvβ-subunit has not been found for all Kv channels[6,7] (Fig. 20.1).

The most drastic effect of Kvβ on the voltage-dependent outward current is to accelerate its rate of inactivation. Kv channels inactivate through two main mechanisms: the rapid N-type inactivation called the "ball and chain" model and the slow C-type inactivation.[8] For instance, Kv channels such as Kv1.5, which do not have an N-terminus acting as an open channel blocker, are inactivated through a mechanism that involves slow conformational changes of the outer mouth of the pore, referred to as C-type inactivation. The coexpression of Kvβ1 with Kvα-subunits with a C-type inactivation results in a fast inactivating current with increased membrane depolarization. For instance, the Kv1.5-encoded current, which is a main component of I_{Kur} in atrial myocytes, is transformed by Kvβ1.3 subunits into a transient outward I_{to}-type current.[9] This effect on current kinetics is associated with a shift of the voltage-dependent activation and inactivation toward more negative potentials. The effect of Kvβ1 on channel inactivation is mediated by its N-terminal domain, which blocks the inner cavity of the α-subunit pore, resembling the "ball and chain" process.[8,10] In addition, by binding to the C-terminus of the channel, Kvβ can accelerate C-type inactivation.[11] In heterologous expression systems, the coexpression of Kvβ1.3 with Kv1.5 is necessary for a protein kinase A (PKA) (cyclic adenosine monophosphate [cAMP]-dependent protein kinase)-mediated increase in K+ current. In addition, protein kinase C (PKC) has little effect on Kv1.5 channels alone, whereas when coexpressed with Kvβ1.2, the protein kinase reduces the K+ current.[12] These observations are consistent with the presence of multiple phosphorylation sites on the β- and α-subunits[13] and may provide an explanation for the effects of β-adrenergic or PKC stimulation on I_{Kur} in human atrial myocytes.[14] The duration and frequency of membrane depolarization can persistently modify the rate of inactivation of I_{kur} in human atrial myocytes. This effect is modulated by the activation of calcium-calmodulin–dependent protein kinase-II (CaMKII) and may also involve the interaction between Kvβ and Kvα1.5 subunits.[15]

Another illustration of the important role of Kvβ in regulating Kv channels has been provided by the study on pharmacological properties of the Kv1.5 channel. The contribution of I_{kur} to AP shortening during atrial fibrillation[16–19] and the fact that the Kv1.5 channel is more abundantly expressed in the atrial than in the ventricular myocardium explain the efforts to develop selective I_{Kur} blockers as potential atrial-specific antiarrhythmic agents. Some of these molecules compete with β-subunits to bind in the inner cavity of the Kv1.5 channel pore and are responsible for an apparent open-channel block of I_{kur}. For instance, Kvβ1.3 decreases the drug affinity of Kv1.5 for local anesthetic and antiarrhythmic drugs (e.g., bupivacaine[20,21]; AVE0118[22]; vernakalant[23]). In atrial myocytes, the analog of tedisamil, bertosamil, accelerates the rate of inactivation of the outward current with membrane depolarization, which is consistent with a competition between the drug and endogenous Kvβ at the inner face of the pore.[24]

Finally, an oxidoreductase activity has been reported for the Kvβ subunit as indicated by the observation that Kvβ2.1 confers oxygen sensitivity to Kv4.2.[25] This enzymatic activity is likely because of the presence of a binding site for the cofactor nicotinamide adenine dinucleotide phosphate (NADP+) and catalytic domains. However, in vivo data are lacking.

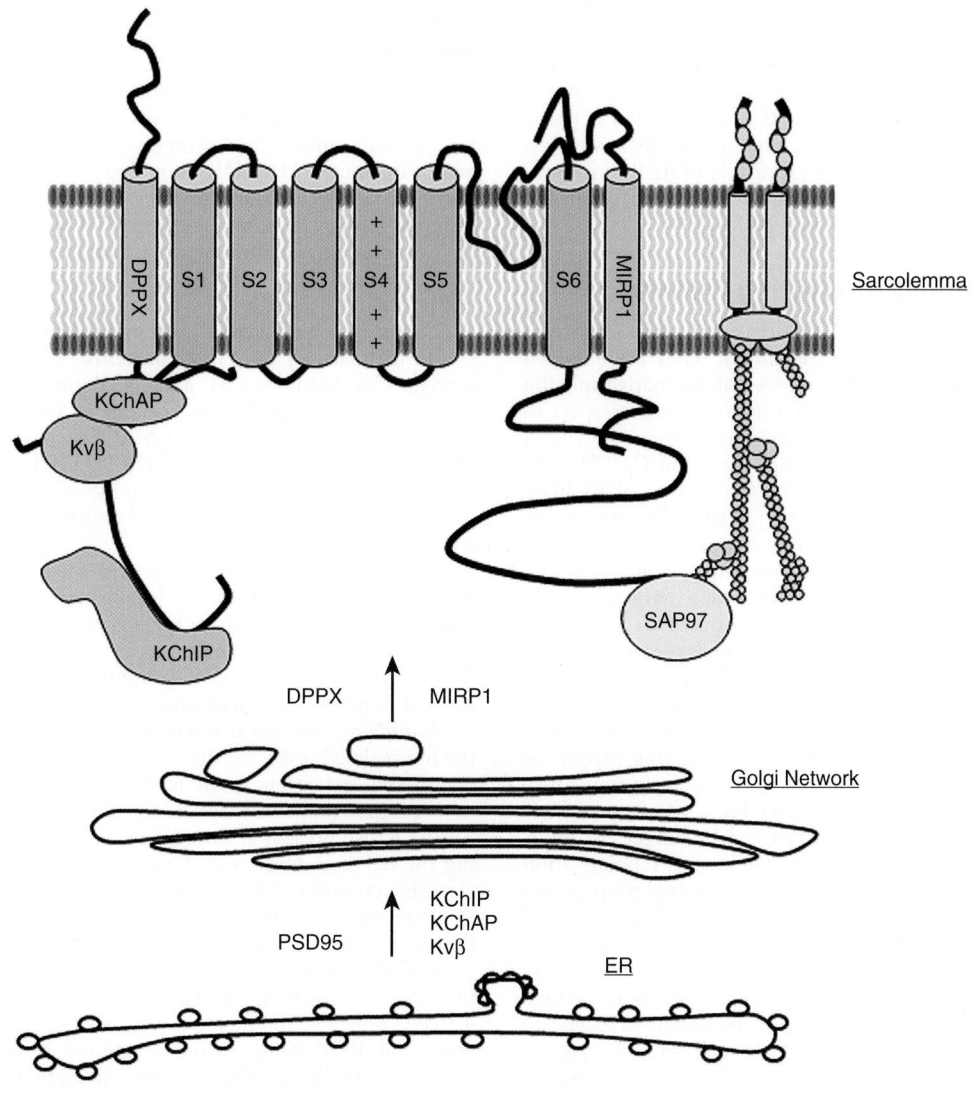

FIGURE 20.1 Main partners of Kv4 channels from their synthesis and assembly to their organization in macromolecular complexes at the plasma membrane of cardiomyocytes. *DPP,* Dipeptidyl aminopeptidase protein; *ER,* endoplasmic reticulum; *KChAP,* K+ channel–associated protein; *KChIP,* K+ channel–interacting protein; *MIRP1,* minK-related peptide.

minK and minK-Related Proteins

Originally considered to be the α-subunit of the delayed rectifier potassium current Iks, minimal K+ channel protein (minK)[26] is a small transmembrane protein (14–20 kDa) encoded by KCNE1. The first interaction described for minK is with the Kv7.1 channel (KvLQT1). Expressed alone, Kv7.1 underlies a voltage-dependent outward current of very small amplitude. In contrast, when coexpressed with minK, this channel is responsible for a large slow delayed-type current, Iks.[27,28] minK can interact with other channels such as *human ether-à-go-go–related* gene (hERG; or Kv11.1), which are responsible for the activation of the rapid delayed rectifier I_{kr}. However, this observation was only reported in heterologous expression systems. In mice, the deletion of KCNE1 is associated with an impaired QT-RR adaptability in the electrocardiogram (ECG), a prolongation of the epicardial AP duration, and the frequent episodes of atrial tachycardia,[29,30] pointing to the physiological importance of this ancillary subunit for cardiac electrophysiology.

Four other peptides that belong to the minK family have been identified and called minK-related peptide (MiRP; KCNE2-5).[7]

In the heart, MiRP1 (KCNE2) is expressed mainly in nodal tissue and Purkinje cells. In vitro MiRP1 can interact with several potassium channels, including Kv7.1,[31] Kv4,[32] and hERG.[33] The hERG channel is regulated by PKA, which increases the current amplitude through the shift of the voltage-dependent activation of the channels. This regulation is an important target for the sympathetic regulation and the subsequent adaptation of cardiac repolarization to an increased heart rate. It has been reported that KCNE2 facilitates the PKA regulation of I_{kr} by stabilizing the hERG channel in its phosphorylated form.[34] Transgenic models had contributed to the establishment of the physiological role of MiRP1 in the heart. Mice with the specific deletion of KCNE2 have a prolonged ventricular AP duration and reduced density of fast and slow components of the outward potassium current, which is consistent with the ability of KCNE2 to interact with various potassium channels.[7,35]

Genetic studies in patients suffering from inherited or drug-induced long QT syndrome have also provided important information regarding the physiological role of this family of potassium partners. Mutations of genes that encode minK and MiRP1 have been found in the familial forms of long QT syndrome, LQT5 and LQT6, respectively.[33] Some mutations of KCNE2 are responsible for the decrease in I_{kr} because of the acceleration of hERG inactivation. This results in a less repolarizing current during the termination of AP, causing the prolongation of phase 3 and risk for triggered activity.[36] Other mutations have been shown to modify the pharmacological profile of hERG, providing a molecular explanation for iatrogenic long QT syndrome and torsades de pointes[33,37,38] (see Fig. 20.1).

Potassium Channel–Interacting Protein

K+ channel–interacting protein (KChIP) is another important family of ancillary subunits of K+ channels. They are encoded by four genes, KChIP1–4, with a number of alternative splicing variants. KChIP isoforms differ from each other with respect to their N-terminus, while they share 70% homology notably with four conserved "EF hand-like" domains that bind Ca^{2+}.[39] Only KChIP2 is expressed in the heart. The C-terminus of KChIP2 interacts directly with the N-terminus of Kv4 channels at the cytosol face of the membrane, which is characterized by a rapid N-terminal inactivation. In expression systems, the interaction of KChIP with Kv4 α-subunits is associated with a marked increase in the amplitude of $I_{to,f}$,[39,40] an effect attributed to the capacity of KChIP in preventing the retention of Kv4 α-subunits in ER.[40] The other effect of KChIP on Kv4 channels is to regulate their rate of inactivation and recovery from inactivation.[39,40] Of note, the three cardiac isoforms of KChIP2 differ with respect to their effects on the functional expression and gating properties of potassium channels and might not have the same regulatory effects on cardiac electrophysiology[7] (see Fig. 20.1).

Endocardial myocytes are characterized by longer AP durations than epicardial myocytes. Such a gradient of repolarization from endo- to epicardium is essential for the oriented propagation of the depolarization wave, prevention of retrograde activation of the myocardium, and risk for arrhythmogenic reentry. In mammals, the gradient is because of regional differences in the density of the fast component of the transient outward current $I_{to,f}$, which is the highest density of $I_{to,f}$ to have been observed in myocytes of the epicardial layer.[41,42] In large mammals such as humans, $K_v4.3$ is the predominant molecular basis of $I_{to,f}$. This channel is homogeneously distributed in the ventricular wall and cannot explain the gradient of $I_{to,f}$.[41,42] In contrast, at both the transcript and protein levels, the concentration of KChIP2 increases from endo- to epicardium. This gradient is likely to contribute to the gradual expression of $I_{to,f}$ in human and dog ventricles.[43,44] In rodents, the gradient of repolarization is not because of KChIP but because of the gradual increase in the expression of Kv4.2 from endo- to epicardium. However, despite such species specificities, mouse models have helped establish the importance of KChIP2 in the normal activation of voltage-dependent outward current I_{to}, which is suppressed in KChIP2 knockout mice.[45]

A third partner contributes to the formation of the Kv4 macromolecular complex, the transmembrane dipeptidyl aminopeptidase-protein (DPP). This integral transmembrane protein that interacts with the extracellular matrix may separately or jointly with KChIP associate with Kv4 subunits at the N-terminus to modulate the trafficking and targeting of the channel[46] (see Fig. 20.1).

Potassium Channel–Associated Protein

Only a few studies have been conducted on the K+ channel–associated protein (KChAP). This small protein of 574 amino acids, expressed in the heart, is a cytoplasmic subunit that interacts transiently with several voltage-dependent Kv channels, including Kv1.x, Kv2.1, and Kv4.3.[47,48] In vitro, KChAP upregulates the Kv channel's surface expression through a chaperone effect[47,48] (see Fig. 20.1).

The Membrane-Associated Guanylate Kinase Proteins

In 1995, Kim and colleagues reported that neuronal *Shaker* channels are clustered by PSD95, a protein belonging to a family of multidomain membrane proteins called membrane-associated guanylate kinase (MAGUK) homologs.[49] Since then a number of channels have been found to interact with MAGUK proteins in different tissues, including the heart.[50] These anchoring proteins are now viewed as central organizers of specialized plasma membrane domains such as the intercalated disks of cardiomyocytes (CMs).

The presence of several protein–protein interacting domains is the hallmark of MAGUK proteins. This includes an SH3 domain (Src homology 3), a GUK domain with homology to the enzyme guanylate kinase, and one or several PDZ domain(s) (PSD-95 Dlg and ZO-1). Most MAGUK proteins contain three PDZ domains. The PDZ domain of MAGUK proteins expressed in the heart recognizes a C-terminal-Ser/thr-X-ψ-Val sequence (where X refers to any amino acid and ψ refers to hydrophobic amino acid)[51,52] (Fig. 20.2).

Several MAGUK proteins are expressed in the heart: SAP97, ZO-1, CASK, and MAGI3. For instance, the gap junction channel connexin43 interacts with ZO-1, which regulates its localization at the intercalated disks and probably also its internalization.[53–55] The other cardiac MAGUK protein that has been extensively studied is SAP97. In atrial and ventricular myocytes, SAP97 is predominantly located at the extremities of myocytes, notably at the intercalated disks.[56–61] In vitro, it has been shown that SAP97 is targeted exclusively at the level of myocyte–myocyte contacts in membrane domains that contain adherens and gap junctions.[62] SAP97 is also present at the adrenergic synapse in myocytes, facing the nerve endings, and therefore is part of the β-adrenergic signaling complex.[63] These results help explain the role of SAP97 in targeting potassium channels in specialized cell–cell contact domains of the sarcolemma.

SAP97 interacts with several cardiac ion channels, including Nav1.5, Kir2.x, Kv4.x, Kv1.5, HCN-2, and HCN-4.[49,56,57,60,61,64,65] In most cases, SAP97 interacts with the consensus PDZ-binding domain located at the C-terminus of ion channels. Beside this classical interaction, indirect interactions involving the N-terminus of channel SAP97 and α-actinin have been reported and can also contribute to the role of SAP97 in the organization of potassium channels in macromolecular complexes.[66,67]

In native myocytes and heterologous expression systems, SAP97 enhances the functional expression of ion channels, resulting in the upregulation of corresponding currents. Using single channel recordings, it has been possible to measure the increased activity of single Kv1.5 channels in cells that overexpress SAP97.[62] In keeping with the accumulation of α-subunits in the membrane protein fraction of CMs that overexpress SAP97, these data indicate that SAP97 enhances the density of channels at the plasma membrane.[68] Cardiac-specific ablation of SAP97 is associated with a drastic reduction in the density of the transient outward potassium current I_{to}, together with the prolongation of both AP duration and QT interval of ECG in mouse, suggesting that, in situ also, SAP97 is an important partner of Kv channels.[69]

SAP97 can enhance the functional expression of ion channels through various mechanisms, including increased forward trafficking, membrane stabilization, and aggregation of channels and formation of signalosomes. For instance, in CMs that overexpress SAP97, potassium channels are immobilized and concentrated at the level of myocyte–myocyte contacts (see Fig. 20.2). Along the same line, it has been reported that the increased expression of SAP97 by heat shock protein indirectly enhances the functional expression of Kv1.5 by inhibiting

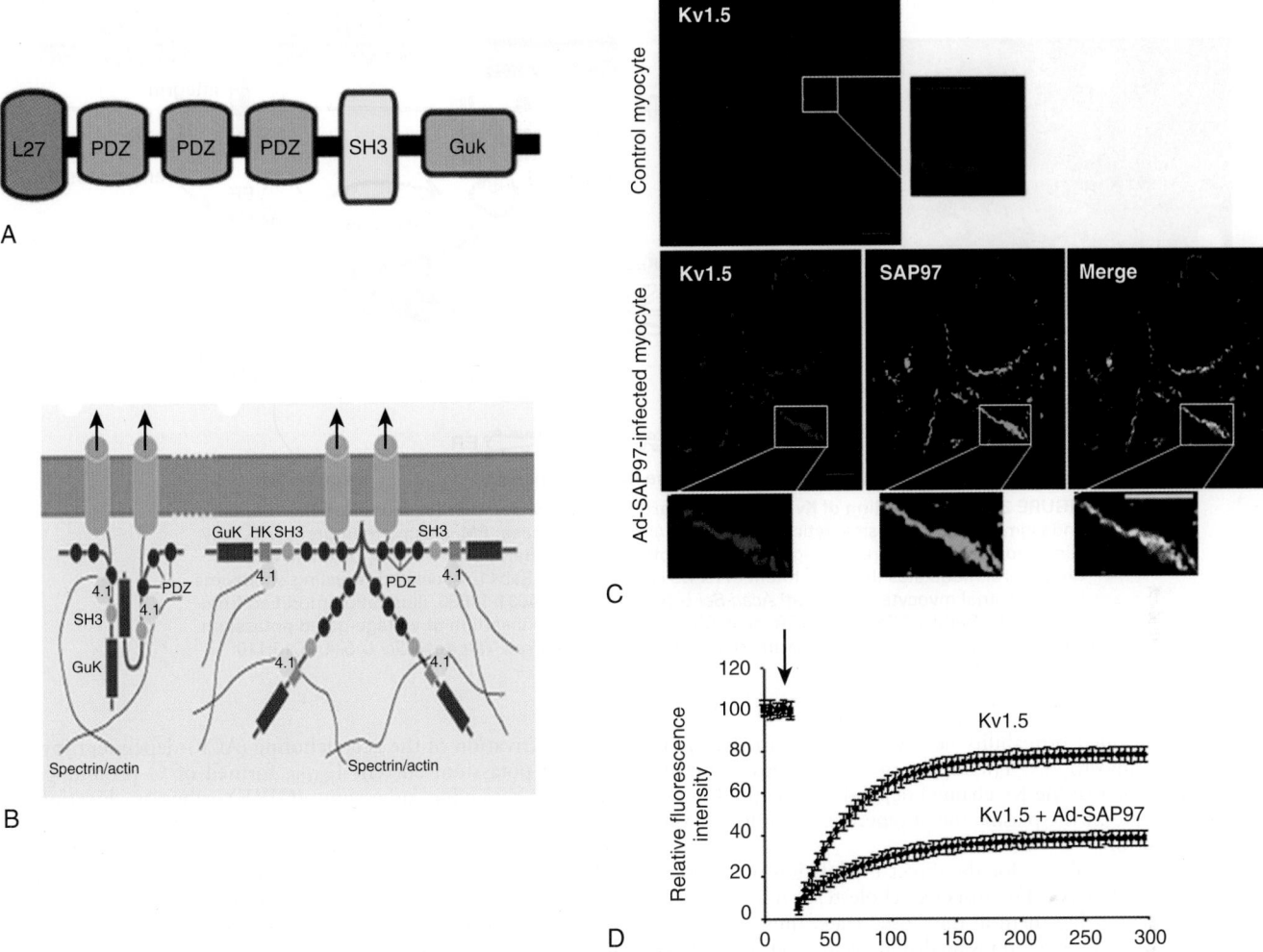

FIGURE 20.2 The anchoring protein SAP97 of the membrane-associated guanylate kinase (MAGUK) family. (A) Molecular organization of MAGUK proteins. (B) Scheme of possible interactions of MAGUK protein and with potassium channels. (C) The overexpression of SAP97 (*Ad-SAP97*) is associated with the accumulation of green fluorescent protein–tagged Kv1.5 channels at the plasma membrane level, and (D) the immobilization of Kv1.5 channel in cardiomyocytes. (From Abi-Char J, El-Haou S, Balse E, et al. The anchoring protein SAP97 retains Kv1.5 channels in the plasma membrane of cardiac myocytes. *Am J Physiol Heart Circ Physiol.* 2008;294:H1851-H1861.)

channel endocytosis, thereby promoting their accumulation in the plasma membrane.[70]

By its capacity to oligomerize, SAP97 contributes to the formation of channel networks that may gather different ion channel families, as suggested by the observations that SAP97 regulates the formation of Nav1.5/Kir2.1 complexes.[65,71,72] The macromolecular complex composed of Kir2.1/Nav1.5 and SAP97 allows a reciprocal modulation of the two channels: the increase in the functional expression of one channel modulates in return the activity of the other and contributes to normal cardiac excitability.[65] Another example of the role played by SAP97 in the functional interactions among channels is provided by the observation of its involvement in the organization of the plakoglobin, connexin43, and Nav1.5 macromolecular complex at the intercalated disks.[73]

Finally, the ability to interact with multiple proteins and form networks confers to SAP97 a role of linker between ion channels or receptors and signaling pathways[74–76] Concerning potassium channels, such a role has been described for the G-protein regulation of the inward rectifier K$^+$ channel[77] and the regulation of Kv4 channels by CaMKII.[56]

Membrane Lipids and Potassium Channel Complexes

Potassium channels are embedded in a lipid environment that can constitute an important modulator for channel activity. Lipids can regulate potassium channels through several mechanisms, including conformational changes of the protein, modulations of the delivery of channels to the plasma membrane, and clustering into macromolecular complexes.

Lipids and the Biophysical Properties of Potassium Channels

There is an interrelation among membrane stiffness, bilayer deformation energy, and changes in channel conformation.[78] For instance, the effects of cholesterol on the open probability of Kir or Ca^{2+} channels are due to an increase in the bilayer stiffness and energy necessary for the transition of channels from the closed to the open state.[78–80] Using the paddle chimera voltage-dependent (Kv) channel, it has been shown that the rate of channel opening, voltage dependence of open probability,

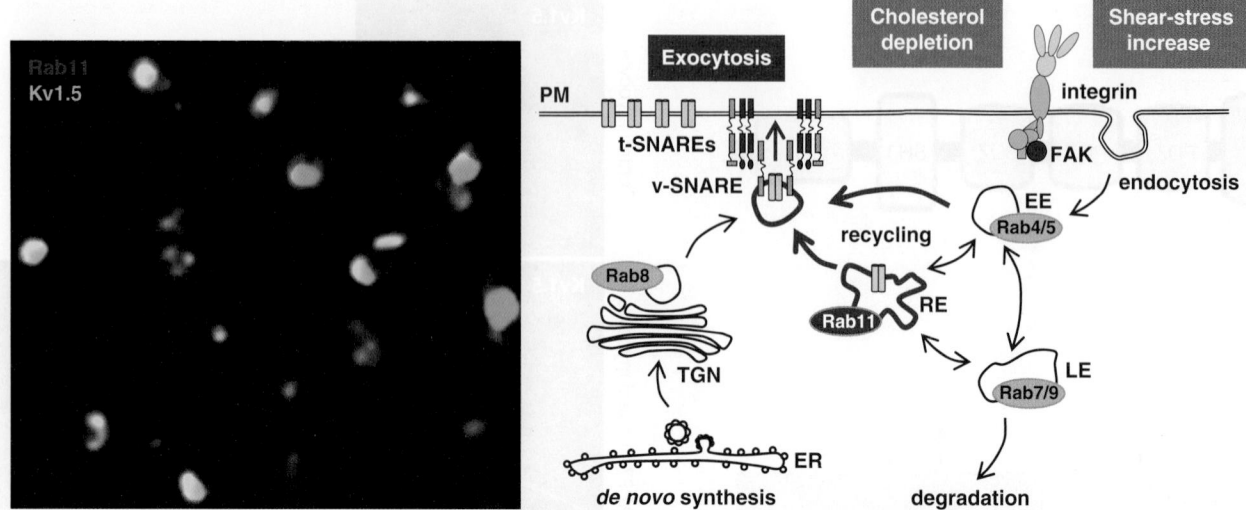

FIGURE 20.3 The recycling of Kv channels in cardiomyocytes (see text for more details). *EE,* Early endosome; *ER,* endoplasmic reticulum; *FAK,* focal adhesion kinase; *PM,* plasma membrane; *RE,* recycling endosome; *TGN,* trans-Golgi network. (Photograph from Balse E, El-Haou S, Dillanian G, et al. Cholesterol modulates the recruitment of Kv1.5 channels from Rab11-associated recycling endosome in native atrial myocytes. *Proc Natl Acad Sci U S A.* 2009;106:14681-14686. Illustration modified from Boycott HE, Barbier CSM, Eichel CA, et al. Shear stress triggers insertion of voltage-gated potassium channels from intracellular compartments in atrial myocytes. *Proc Natl Acad Sci U S A.* 2013;110: E3955-E3964.)

and maximum open probability achievable vary with the lipid membrane composition.[81] The explanation is that movement of the voltage sensor of the Kv channel depends on the fluidity or mechanical state of the plasma membrane, hence indirectly on lipid composition.[82,83]

There is also evidence for the direct modulation of channel function by cholesterol. For instance, cholesterol inhibits Kir2 channels by stabilizing them in the closed state, thus rendering them silent. Such a regulation is mediated via interaction of cholesterol with a specific region of the cytosolic C-terminal domain of the channel. The optical isomer of cholesterol, epicholesterol, which displays similar effects on membrane biophysical properties as cholesterol, fails to modulate Kir2 channels, indicating specificity in cholesterol–channel interactions.[83] Cholesterol may bind to two hydrophobic regions in the transmembrane domain of Kir2.1 located between adjacent subunits of the channel, and thus modulate the hinging motion at the center of the pore-lining transmembrane helix that underlies the channel gating, either directly or through the interface between the N- and C-termini of the channel.[84] This finding is reminiscent of observations that other membrane lipids, such as arachidonic acid, can induce rapid inactivation in otherwise noninactivating Kv channels by binding to a specific site near the selectivity filter.[85]

Lipid Rafts and Clustering of Potassium Channels

Cholesterol and sphingolipid, two structural lipids of the plasma membrane, pack together to form cholesterol-enriched domains referred to as lipid rafts. A subset of lipid rafts that form small invaginations of the plasma membrane, named caveolae, contain the scaffolding protein caveolin. Caveolae are particularly abundant in CMs.[86] Lipid rafts are considered to be platforms where proteins are delivered and clustered together with signaling pathways to form dynamic macromolecular complexes. Several potassium channels are localized in lipid rafts, notably in caveolae.[87–89] The importance of lipid-raft integrity for the normal functional expression of potassium channels is illustrated

by the activation of the acetylcholine (ACh)-dependent inward rectifier potassium current I_{KACh}, formed of G protein–gated inwardly rectifying potassium (GIRK) subunits. Fixation of ACh to its inhibitory G protein (G$_i$)–coupled muscarinic 2 (M2) receptor leads to the release of G$_{\beta\gamma}$ subunits and the activation of GIRK channels.[90] Other receptors coupled to the stimulatory G protein (G$_s$), such as the β-adrenergic receptor, fail to activate GIRK channels. In contrast to G$_s$, which is exclusively localized in raft fractions, the M2 signaling pathway is localized in both the lipid raft and nonlipid raft fractions. Thus one explanation for the specific effect of G$_i$ on GIRK is that a distinct localization in lipid rafts of signaling cascades may act as a mechanism of selectivity, such that free G$_{\beta\gamma}$ released from lipid rafts is much less efficient in activating GIRK. However, there is a disagreement between studies conducted in heterologous expression systems and those conducted in native myocytes on the localization of potassium channels in lipid rafts and notably caveolae. Contrary to CHO cells, in the atrial and ventricular myocardium, the Kv1.5 channel does not target caveolae. This channel is present predominantly at the level of the intercalated disks where caveolin 3 is poorly expressed.[68,91,92] Moreover, the two proteins cannot be coprecipitated from cardiac protein samples.[93] However, it is possible that in native CMs, Kv1.5 channels are only transiently localized in lipid rafts during their trafficking from delivery sites in the plasma membrane to their final targeting into specialized domains.[91,94]

Caveolae are an important route of endocytosis for many proteins in the myocardium. As already described, cholesterol content regulates the shape and size of lipid rafts such that depletion of cholesterol causes the flattening of caveolae.[95–98] This explains why drugs that sequester cholesterol, such as filipin, nystatin, and cyclodextrins, block endocytosis mediated by caveolae. More recently, cholesterol has also been reported to play a role in internalization through the clathrin-mediated endocytosis pathways.[99,100] Given that the endocytosis rate would control the number of potassium channels in the sarcolemma, any alteration of the endocytosis step could affect the properties of potassium currents in CMs (Fig. 20.3).

Macromolecular Complex Involved in the Delivery of Potassium Channels

Ion channels and receptors are delivered to the plasma membrane from intracellular compartments exiting the Golgi network (de novo synthesis) or from recycling pathways. Ion channels traffic via endosomes associated to specific Rab GTPases that regulate their fate, notably their recycling or degradation.[101,102] Each step of trafficking, from the Golgi exit to the insertion in the plasma membrane, is dependent on the fusion of an endosome vesicle to an acceptor membrane and requires the formation of soluble N-ethyl-maleimide-sensitive factor attachment protein receptor (SNARE) complexes. In atrial myocytes, the reduction of membrane cholesterol content using methyl-β-cyclodextrin (MβCD) is associated with a time-dependent increase in I_{Kur} that can be completely prevented by the SNARE complex inhibitor N-ethylmaleimide (NEM) and the inhibition of Rab11. These observations suggested that lipids can play a role in the ion channel delivery and recycling.[68,103,104]

Rab11-mediated recycling has been described for other potassium channels, such as KCNQ1/KCNE1 potassium channel,[105] as well as for cardiac pacemaker channels HCN2 and HCN4[106] and the glucose transporter GluT4.[107] Recently, the Rab11-dependent recycling of Kv1.5 has been shown to be stimulated by changes in mechanical forces experienced by atrial myocytes. Increasing shear stress activated a large K^+ current with a parallel increase of single channel activity and Kv1.5 channel surface expression. As the response was prevented by both NEM and the Ca^{2+} chelator BAPTA, the current increase was primarily attributable to Kv1.5 exocytosis from intracellular compartments. Interestingly, the Kv1.5 channel delivery was triggered by the activation of the integrin/focal adhesion kinase signaling, suggesting that mechanical constraints are translated from the extracellular environment to the cytoplasm of CMs, defining signaling macromolecular complexes involved in the regulation of ion channel turnover.[108]

Conclusion

The classical view of well-individualized potassium currents being the functional expression of distinct potassium channels constitutively expressed at the cell surface is challenged by the molecular dissection of potassium channel macromolecular complexes. The emerging picture is that the activity of the potassium channel is the result of continuing and dynamic processes of protein and lipid interactions, from the synthesis of the α-subunit to its specific targeting into submembrane domains of the sarcolemma for interactions with macromolecular complexes and correct functions. Such a complex regulation over time (turnover) and space (tethering) suggests an important plasticity for these protein complexes that could be a major determinant of the physiological adaptation of cardiac excitability and the pathogenesis of electrical disorders. For instance, it is possible that potassium channels are recruited or recycled in response to various physiological stimuli or during pathological conditions as in other excitable tissues. For example, during chronic hemodynamic atrial overload, the Kv1.5 protein level is reduced, whereas the atrial-specific current I_{Kur} is increased.[108] This basal increase in I_{Kur} is accompanied by an increased integrin expression and focal adhesion kinase activation, leading to more functional channels at the cell surface during conditions of excessive mechanical stress. Internalization can also be involved in disease conditions. Indeed, Guo and colleagues reported that the external potassium concentration can modulate the availability of hERG channels in such a way that the low external potassium concentration increases the channel internalization, resulting in the suppression of I_{Kr}.[109] This phenomenon could contribute to the prolongation of the QT interval during hypokalemia. Interestingly, antiarrhythmic agents, such as quinidine, specifically accelerate the internalization of Kv1.5 channels but not of other K_V channels, which can also be blocked by quinidine.[101] Altogether, the foregoing highlights the importance of alterations in the macromolecular environment of ion channels in the development of arrhythmias.

Another emerging concept is the heterogeneity of macromolecular channel complexes, which can be composed of α-subunits of different types, depending on their membrane localization and their role in the activation and propagation of the electrical activity. This is suggested by the recent discovery of Nav1.5/Kir complexes at the lateral membrane and Cx43/Nav1.5 complexes at the level of the intercalated disks.[65,110] Many more studies conducted on CMs or using experimental models are needed to establish new schemes of cardiac electrophysiology that integrate a large diversity of molecular actors involved in the formation of potassium channels. Progress also will occur with the development of new tools to study protein processing, assembly, and interactions in native myocytes.

REFERENCES

1. Parcej DN, Scott VE, Dolly JO. Oligomeric properties of alpha-dendrotoxin-sensitive potassium ion channels purified from bovine brain. *Biochemistry (Mosc).* 1992;31:11084–11088.
2. Scott VE, Rettig J, Parcej DN, et al. Primary structure of a beta subunit of alpha-dendrotoxin-sensitive K+ channels from bovine brain. *Proc Natl Acad Sci U S A.* 1994;91:1637–1641.
3. England SK, Uebele VN, Kodali J, et al. A novel K+ channel beta-subunit (hKv beta 1.3) is produced via alternative mRNA splicing. *J Biol Chem.* 1995;270:28531–28534.
4. Shi G, Nakahira K, Hammond S, et al. Beta subunits promote K+ channel surface expression through effects early in biosynthesis. *Neuron.* 1996;16:843–852.
5. Nagaya N, Papazian DM. Potassium channel alpha and beta subunits assemble in the endoplasmic reticulum. *J Biol Chem.* 1997;272:3022–3027.
6. Leicher T, Roeper J, Weber K, et al. Structural and functional characterization of human potassium channel subunit beta 1 (KCNA1B). *Neuropharmacology.* 1996;35:787–795.
7. Pongs O, Schwarz JR. Ancillary subunits associated with voltage-dependent K+ channels. *Physiol Rev.* 2010;90:755–796.
8. Rasmusson RL, Morales MJ, Wang S, et al. Inactivation of voltage-gated cardiac K+ channels. *Circ Res.* 1998;82:739–750.
9. Uebele VN, England SK, Gallagher DJ, et al. Distinct domains of the voltage-gated K+ channel Kv beta 1.3 beta-subunit affect voltage-dependent gating. *Am J Physiol.* 1998;274:C1485–C1495.
10. Rettig J, Heinemann SH, Wunder F, et al. Inactivation properties of voltage-gated K+ channels altered by presence of beta-subunit. *Nature.* 1994;369:289–294.

11. Morales MJ, Wee JO, Wang S, et al. The N-terminal domain of a K+ channel beta subunit increases the rate of C-type inactivation from the cytoplasmic side of the channel. *Proc Natl Acad Sci U S A.* 1996;93:15119–15123.
12. Williams CP, Hu N, Shen W, et al. Modulation of the human Kv1.5 channel by protein kinase C activation: role of the Kvbeta1.2 subunit. *J Pharmacol Exp Ther.* 2002;302:545–550.
13. Kwak YG, Hu N, Wei J, et al. Protein kinase A phosphorylation alters Kvbeta1.3 subunit-mediated inactivation of the Kv1.5 potassium channel. *J Biol Chem.* 1999;274:13928–13932.
14. Li GR, Yang B, Feng J, et al. Transmembrane ICa contributes to rate-dependent changes of action potentials in human ventricular myocytes. *Am J Physiol.* 1999;276:H98–H106.
15. Tessier S, Godreau D, Vranckx R, et al. Cumulative inactivation of the outward potassium current: a likely mechanism underlying electrical memory in human atrial myocytes. *J Mol Cell Cardiol.* 2001;33:755–767.
16. Dobrev D, Carlsson L, Nattel S. Novel molecular targets for atrial fibrillation therapy. *Nat Rev Drug Discov.* 2012;11:275–291.
17. Hatem SN, Coulombe A, Balse E. Specificities of atrial electrophysiology: clues to a better understanding of cardiac function and the mechanisms of arrhythmias. *J Mol Cell Cardiol.* 2010;48:90–95.
18. Le Grand BL, Hatem S, Deroubaix E, et al. Depressed transient outward and calcium currents in dilated human atria. *Cardiovasc Res.* 1994;28:548–556.
19. Ravens U, Wettwer E. Ultra-rapid delayed rectifier channels: molecular basis and therapeutic implications. *Cardiovasc Res.* 2011;89:776–785.

20. Arias C, Guizy M, David M, et al. Kvbeta1.3 reduces the degree of stereoselective bupivacaine block of Kv1.5 channels. *Anesthesiology.* 2007;107:641–651.
21. Gonzalez T, Arias C, Caballero R, et al. Effects of levobupivacaine, ropivacaine and bupivacaine on HERG channels: stereoselective bupivacaine block. *Br J Pharmacol.* 2002;137:1269–1279.
22. Decher N, Kumar P, Gonzalez T, et al. Binding site of a novel Kv1.5 blocker as a 'foot in the door' against atrial fibrillation. *Mol Pharmacol.* 2006;70:1204–1211.
23. Eldstrom J, Wang Z, Xu H, et al. The molecular basis of high-affinity binding of the antiarrhythmic compound vernakalant (RSD1235) to Kv1.5 channels. *Mol Pharmacol.* 2007;72:1522–1534.
24. Tessier S, Rucker-Martin C, Mace L, et al. The antiarrhythmic agent bertosamil induces inactivation of the sustained outward K+ current in human atrial myocytes. *Br J Pharmacol.* 1997;122:291–301.
25. Perez-Garcia MT, Lopez-Lopez JR, Gonzalez C. Kvbeta1.2 subunit coexpression in HEK293 cells confers O2 sensitivity to kv4.2 but not to Shaker channels. *J Gen Physiol.* 1999;113:897–907.
26. Takumi T, Ohkubo H, Nakanishi S. Cloning of a membrane protein that induces a slow voltage-gated potassium current. *Science.* 1988;242:1042–1045.
27. Barhanin J, Lesage F, Guillemare E, et al. K(V)LQT1 and lsK (minK) proteins associate to form the I(Ks) cardiac potassium current. *Nature.* 1996;384:78–80.
28. Sanguinetti MC, Curran ME, Zou A, et al. Coassembly of K(V)LQT1 and minK (IsK) proteins to form cardiac I(Ks) potassium channel. *Nature.* 1996;384:80–83.

29. Drici MD, Arrighi I, Chouabe C, et al. Involvement of IsK-associated K+ channel in heart rate control of repolarization in a murine engineered model of Jervell and Lange-Nielsen syndrome. *Circ Res.* 1998;83:95–102.

30. Temple J, Frias P, Rottman J, et al. Atrial fibrillation in KCNE1-null mice. *Circ Res.* 2005;97:62–69.

31. Tinel N, Diochot S, Borsotto M, et al. KCNE2 confers background current characteristics to the cardiac KCNQ1 potassium channel. *EMBO J.* 2000;19:6326–6330.

32. Zhang M, Jiang M, Tseng GN. minK-related peptide 1 associates with Kv4.2 and modulates its gating function: potential role as beta subunit of cardiac transient outward channel? *Circ Res.* 2001;88:1012–1019.

33. Abbott GW, Sesti F, Splawski I, et al. MiRP1 forms IKr potassium channels with HERG and is associated with cardiac arrhythmia. *Cell.* 1999;97:175–187.

34. Cui J, Kagan A, Qin D, et al. Analysis of the cyclic nucleotide binding domain of the HERG potassium channel and interactions with KCNE2. *J Biol Chem.* 2001;276:17244–17251.

35. Roepke TK, Kontogeorgis A, Ovanez C, et al. Targeted deletion of kcne2 impairs ventricular repolarization via disruption of IK(slow1) and I(to,f). *FASEB J.* 2008;22:3648–3660.

36. Isbrandt D, Friederich P, Solth A, et al. Identification and functional characterization of a novel KCNE2 (MiRP1) mutation that alters HERG channel kinetics. *J Mol Med Berl.* 2002;80:524–532.

37. Lu Y, Mahaut-Smith MP, Huang CL, et al. Mutant MiRP1 subunits modulate HERG K+ channel gating: a mechanism for pro-arrhythmia in long QT syndrome type 6. *J Physiol.* 2003;551:253–262.

38. Sesti F, Abbott GW, Wei J, et al. A common polymorphism associated with antibiotic-induced cardiac arrhythmia. *Proc Natl Acad Sci U S A.* 2000;97:10613–10618.

39. An WF, Bowlby MR, Betty M, et al. Modulation of A-type potassium channels by a family of calcium sensors. *Nature.* 2000;403:553–556.

40. Bähring R, Dannenberg J, Peters HC, et al. Conserved Kv4 N-terminal domain critical for effects of Kv channel-interacting protein 2.2 on channel expression and gating. *J Biol Chem.* 2001;276:23888–23894.

41. Nerbonne JM, Guo W. Heterogeneous expression of voltage-gated potassium channels in the heart: roles in normal excitation and arrhythmias. *J Cardiovasc Electrophysiol.* 2002;13:406–409.

42. Oudit GY, Kassiri Z, Sah R, et al. The molecular physiology of the cardiac transient outward potassium current (I(to)) in normal and diseased myocardium. *J Mol Cell Cardiol.* 2001;33:851–872.

43. Deschênes I, DiSilvestre D, Juang GJ, et al. Regulation of Kv4.3 current by KChIP2 splice variants: a component of native cardiac I(to)? *Circulation.* 2002;106:423–429.

44. Rosati B, Grau F, Rodriguez S, et al. Concordant expression of KChIP2 mRNA, protein and transient outward current throughout the canine ventricle. *J Physiol.* 2003;548:815–822.

45. Kuo HC, Cheng CF, Clark RB, et al. A defect in the Kv channel-interacting protein 2 (KChIP2) gene leads to a complete loss of I(to) and confers susceptibility to ventricular tachycardia. *Cell.* 2001;107:801–813.

46. Nadal MS, Ozaita A, Amarillo Y, et al. The CD26-related dipeptidyl aminopeptidase-like protein DPPX is a critical component of neuronal A-type K+ channels. *Neuron.* 2003;37:449–461.

47. Kuryshev YA, Gudz TI, Brown AM, et al. KChAP as a chaperone for specific K(+) channels. *Am J Physiol Cell Physiol.* 2000;278:C931–C941.

48. Wible BA, Yang Q, Kuryshev YA, et al. Cloning and expression of a novel K+ channel regulatory protein, KChAP. *J Biol Chem.* 1998;273:11745–11751.

49. Kim E, Niethammer M, Rothschild A, et al. Clustering of Shaker-type K+ channels by interaction with a family of membrane-associated guanylate kinases. *Nature.* 1995;378:85–88.

50. Balse E, Steele DF, Abriel H, et al. Dynamic of ion channel expression at the plasma membrane of cardiomyocytes. *Physiol Rev.* 2012;92:1317–1358.

51. Nourry C, Grant SGN, Borg JP. PDZ domain proteins: plug and play!. *Sci STKE Signal Transduct Knowl Environ.* 2003 RE7:2003.

52. Songyang Z, Fanning AS, Fu C, et al. Recognition of unique carboxyl-terminal motifs by distinct PDZ domains. *Science.* 1997;275:73–77.

53. Barker RJ, Price RL, Gourdie RG. Increased association of ZO-1 with connexin43 during remodeling of cardiac gap junctions. *Circ Res.* 2002;90:317–324.

54. Itoh M, Morita K, Tsukita S. Characterization of ZO-2 as a MAGUK family member associated with tight as well as adherens junctions with a binding affinity to occludin and alpha catenin. *J Biol Chem.* 1999;274:5981–5986.

55. Jesaitis LA, Goodenough DA. Molecular characterization and tissue distribution of ZO-2, a tight junction protein homologous to ZO-1 and the Drosophila discs-large tumor suppressor protein. *J Cell Biol.* 1994;124:949–961.

56. El-Haou S, Balse E, Neyroud N, et al. Kv4 potassium channels form a tripartite complex with the anchoring protein SAP97 and CaMKII in cardiac myocytes. *Circ Res.* 2009;104:758–769.

57. Godreau D, Vranckx R, Maguy A, et al. Expression, regulation and role of the MAGUK protein SAP-97 in human atrial myocardium. *Cardiovasc Res.* 2002;56:433–442.

58. Leonoudakis D, Conti LR, Radeke CM, et al. A multi-protein trafficking complex composed of SAP97, CASK, Veli, and Mint1 is associated with inward rectifier Kir2 potassium channels. *J Biol Chem.* 2004;279:19051–19063.

59. Murata M, Buckett PD, Zhou J, et al. SAP97 interacts with Kv1.5 in heterologous expression systems. *Am J Physiol Heart Circ Physiol.* 2001;281:H2575–H2584.

60. Peters CJ, Chow SS, Angoli D, et al. In situ co-distribution and functional interactions of SAP97 with sinoatrial isoforms of HCN channels. *J Mol Cell Cardiol.* 2009;46:636–643.

61. Petitprez S, Zmoos AF, Ogrodnik J, et al. SAP97 and dystrophin macromolecular complexes determine two pools of cardiac sodium channels Nav1.5 in cardiomyocytes. *Circ Res.* 2011;108:294–304.

62. Abi-Char J, El-Haou S, Balse E, et al. The anchoring protein SAP97 retains Kv1.5 channels in the plasma membrane of cardiac myocytes. *Am J Physiol Heart Circ Physiol.* 2008;294:H1851–H1861.

63. Shcherbakova OG, Hurt CM, Xiang Y, et al. Organization of beta-adrenoceptor signaling compartments by sympathetic innervation of cardiac myocytes. *J Cell Biol.* 2007;176:521–533.

64. Leonoudakis D, Mailliard W, Wingerd K, et al. Inward rectifier potassium channel Kir2.2 is associated with synapse-associated protein SAP97. *J Cell Sci.* 2001;114:987–998.

65. Milstein ML, Musa H, Balbuena DP, et al. Dynamic reciprocity of sodium and potassium channel expression in a macromolecular complex controls cardiac excitability and arrhythmia. *Proc Natl Acad Sci U S A.* 2012;109:E2134–E2143.

66. Eldstrom J, Choi WS, Steele DF, et al. SAP97 increases Kv1.5 currents through an indirect N-terminal mechanism. *FEBS Lett.* 2003;547:205–211.

67. Mathur R, Choi WS, Eldstrom J, et al. A specific N-terminal residue in Kv1.5 is required for upregulation of the channel by SAP97. *Biochem Biophys Res Commun.* 2006;342:1–8.

68. Abi-Char J, Maguy A, Coulombe A, et al. Membrane cholesterol modulates Kv1.5 potassium channel distribution and function in rat cardiomyocytes. *J Physiol.* 2007;582:1205–1217.

69. Gillet L, Rougier J-S, Shy D, et al. Cardiac-specific ablation of synapse-associated protein SAP97 in mice decreases potassium currents but not sodium current. *Heart Rhythm Off J Heart Rhythm Soc.* 2015;12:181–192.

70. Ting YK, Morikawa K, Kurata Y, et al. Transcriptional activation of the anchoring protein SAP97 by heat shock factor (HSF)-1 stabilizes K(v) 1.5 channels in HL-1 cells. *Br J Pharmacol.* 2011;162:1832–1842.

71. Kim E, Sheng M. Differential K+ channel clustering activity of PSD-95 and SAP97, two related membrane-associated putative guanylate kinases. *Neuropharmacology.* 1996;35:993–1000.

72. Godreau D, Vranckx R, Maguy A, et al. Different isoforms of synapse-associated protein, SAP97, are expressed in the heart and have distinct effects on the voltage-gated K+ channel Kv1.5. *J Biol Chem.* 2003;278:47046–47052.

73. Asimaki A, Kapoor S, Plovie E, et al. Identification of a new modulator of the intercalated disc in a zebrafish model of arrhythmogenic cardiomyopathy. *Sci Transl Med.* 2014;6:240ra74.

74. Bassand P, Bernard A, Rafiki A, et al. Differential interaction of the tSXV motifs of the NR1 and NR2A NMDA receptor subunits with PSD-95 and SAP97. *Eur J Neurosci.* 1999;11:2031–2043.

75. Mauceri D, Gardoni F, Marcello E, et al. Dual role of CaMKII-dependent SAP97 phosphorylation in mediating trafficking and insertion of NMDA receptor subunit NR2A. *J Neurochem.* 2007;100:1032–1046.

76. Gardoni F, Schrama LH, Dalen JJ van, et al. AlphaCaM-KII binding to the C-terminal tail of NMDA receptor subunit NR2A and its modulation by autophosphorylation. *FEBS Lett.* 1999;456:394–398.

77. Vaidyanathan R, Taffet SM, Vikstrom KL, et al. Regulation of cardiac inward rectifier potassium current (I(K1)) by synapse-associated protein-97. *J Biol Chem.* 2010;285:28000–28009.

78. Lundbaek JA, Birn P, Girshman J, et al. Membrane stiffness and channel function. *Biochemistry (Mosc).* 1996;35:3825–3830.

79. Andersen OS, Koeppe 2nd RE. Bilayer thickness and membrane protein function: an energetic perspective. *Annu Rev Biophys Biomol Struct.* 2007;36:107–130.

80. Elinder F, Madeja M, Arhem P. Surface charges of K channels. Effects of strontium on five cloned channels expressed in Xenopus oocytes. *J Gen Physiol.* 1996;108:325–332.

81. Long SB, Tao X, Campbell EB, et al. Atomic structure of a voltage-dependent K+ channel in a lipid membrane-like environment. *Nature.* 2007;450:376–382.

82. Schmidt D, MacKinnon R. Voltage-dependent K+ channel gating and voltage sensor toxin sensitivity depend on the mechanical state of the lipid membrane. *Proc Natl Acad Sci U S A.* 2008;105:19276–19281.

83. Epshtein Y, Chopra AP, Rosenhouse-Dantsker A, et al. Identification of a C-terminus domain critical for the sensitivity of Kir2.1 to cholesterol. *Proc Natl Acad Sci U S A.* 2009;106:8055–8060.

84. Rosenhouse-Dantsker A, Noskov S, Durdagi S, et al. Identification of novel cholesterol-binding regions in Kir2 channels. *J Biol Chem.* 2013;288:31154–31164.

85. Oliver D, Lien CC, Soom M, et al. Functional conversion between A-type and delayed rectifier K+ channels by membrane lipids. *Science.* 2004;304:265–270.

86. Palade GE. An electron microscope study of the mitochondrial structure. *J Histochem Cytochem.* 1953;1:188–211.

87. Balijepalli RC, Kamp TJ. Caveolae, ion channels and cardiac arrhythmias. *Prog Biophys Mol Biol.* 2008;98:149–160.

88. Dart C. Lipid microdomains and the regulation of ion channel function. *J Physiol.* 2010;588:3169–3178.

89. Maguy A, Hebert TE, Nattel S. Involvement of lipid rafts and caveolae in cardiac ion channel function. *Cardiovasc Res.* 2006;69:798–807.

90. Schwarzer S, Nobles M, Tinker A. Do caveolae have a role in the fidelity and dynamics of receptor activation of G-protein-gated inwardly rectifying potassium channels? *J Biol Chem.* 2010;285:27817–27826.

91. Locke D, Liu J, Harris AL. Lipid rafts prepared by different methods contain different connexin channels, but gap junctions are not lipid rafts. *Biochemistry (Mosc).* 2005;44:13027–13042.

92. Yarbrough TL, Lu T, Lee HC, et al. Localization of cardiac sodium channels in caveolin-rich membrane domains: regulation of sodium current amplitude. *Circ Res.* 2002;90:443–449.

93. Eldstrom J, Van Wagoner DR, Moore ED, et al. Localization of Kv1.5 channels in rat and canine myocyte sarcolemma. *FEBS Lett.* 2006;580:6039–6046.

94. Schubert AL, Schubert W, Spray DC, et al. Connexin family members target to lipid raft domains and interact with caveolin-1. *Biochemistry (Mosc).* 2002;41:5754–5764.

95. Hailstones D, Sleer LS, Parton RG, et al. Regulation of caveolin and caveolae by cholesterol in MDCK cells. *J Lipid Res.* 1998;39:369–379.

96. Rothberg KG, Ying YS, Kamen BA, et al. Cholesterol controls the clustering of the glycophospholipid-anchored membrane receptor for 5-methyltetrahydrofolate. *J Cell Biol.* 1990;111:2931–2938.

97. Rubinstein Jr RA, Shelbourne KD, McCarroll JR, et al. The accuracy of the clinical examination in the setting of posterior cruciate ligament injuries. *Am J Sports Med.* 1994;22:550–557.

98. Schnitzer JE, Oh P, Pinney E, et al. Filipin-sensitive caveolae-mediated transport in endothelium: reduced transcytosis, scavenger endocytosis, and capillary permeability of select macromolecules. *J Cell Biol.* 1994;127:1217–1232.

99. Rodal SK, Skretting G, Garred O, et al. Extraction of cholesterol with methyl-beta-cyclodextrin perturbs formation of clathrin-coated endocytic vesicles. *Mol Biol Cell.* 1999;10:961–974.

100. Subtil A, Gaidarov I, Kobylarz K, et al. Acute cholesterol depletion inhibits clathrin-coated pit budding. *Proc Natl Acad Sci U S A.* 1999;96:6775–6780.

101. McEwen DP, Schumacher SM, Li Q, et al. Rab-GTPase-dependent endocytic recycling of Kv1.5 in atrial myocytes. *J Biol Chem.* 2007;282:29612–29620.

102. Steele DF, Eldstrom J, Fedida D. Mechanisms of cardiac potassium channel trafficking. *J Physiol.* 2007;582:17–26.

103. Balse E, El-Haou S, Dillanian G, et al. Cholesterol modulates the recruitment of Kv1.5 channels from Rab11-associated recycling endosome in native atrial myocytes. *Proc Natl Acad Sci U S A.* 2009;106:14681–14686.

104. O'Connell KM, Rolig AS, Whitesell JD, et al. Kv2.1 potassium channels are retained within dynamic cell surface microdomains that are defined by a perimeter fence. *J Neurosci.* 2006;26:9609–9618.

105. Seebohm G, Strutz-Seebohm N, Birkin R, et al. Regulation of endocytic recycling of KCNQ1/KCNE1 potassium channels. *Circ Res.* 2007;100:686–692.

106. Hardel N, Harmel N, Zolles G, et al. Recycling endosomes supply cardiac pacemaker channels for regulated surface expression. *Cardiovasc Res.* 2008;79:52–60.

107. Uhlig M, Passlack W, Eckel J. Functional role of Rab11 in GLUT4 trafficking in cardiomyocytes. *Mol Cell Endocrinol.* 2005;235:1–9.

108. Boycott HE, Barbier CSM, Eichel CA, et al. Shear stress triggers insertion of voltage-gated potassium channels from intracellular compartments in atrial myocytes. *Proc Natl Acad Sci U S A.* 2013;110:E3955–E3964.

109. Guo J, Massaeli H, Xu J, et al. Extracellular K+ concentration controls cell surface density of IKr in rabbit hearts and of the HERG channel in human cell lines. *J Clin Invest.* 2009;119:2745–2757.

110. Delmar M. Connexin43 regulates sodium current; ankyrin-G modulates gap junctions: the intercalated disc exchanger. *Cardiovasc Res.* 2012;93:220–222.

21

Reciprocity of Cardiac Sodium and Potassium Channels in the Control of Excitability and Arrhythmias

Eva Delpón and José Jalife

The current understanding of the relationship between the sodium current (I_{Na}) and inward rectifier potassium current (I_{K1}), the two most important ionic currents that control ventricular excitability, began in 1955 with the seminal work by Dr. Weidmann.[1] It also derives from the basic and clinical studies on arrhythmogenesis in ion channel diseases and heart failure, which have demonstrated that the modification in the peak density of either I_{Na} or I_{K1} changes cell excitability and conduction velocity (CV). However, until recently, the pathophysiological consequences of a molecular interplay between the individual channels at the center of such diseases had not been investigated.[2] In the heart, I_{K1} is the major current responsible for the maintenance of the resting membrane potential (RMP), whereas I_{Na} provides the largest fraction of the inward depolarizing current that flows during an action potential (AP).[3] It is well known that by controlling RMP and AP duration (APD) at the end of repolarization, I_{K1} modifies the Na^+ channel availability and therefore cell excitability.[4] In addition, I_{K1}–I_{Na} interactions are important for stabilizing and controlling the frequency of the electrical rotors that are responsible for the most dangerous cardiac arrhythmias, including ventricular tachycardia (VT) and ventricular fibrillation (VF).[5,6]

Recent data obtained from adult transgenic mice, single adult rat ventricular myocytes (ARVMs), neonatal rat ventricular myocyte (NRVM) monolayers, and heterologous expression systems (HEK 293 and CHO cells) have demonstrated that the I_{Na}–I_{K1} interplay is much more complex than previously considered. It comprises model independent, reciprocal modulation of the expression of their respective channel proteins ($Na_V1.5$ and Kir2.1) within a macromolecular complex that involves the membrane-associated guanylate kinase (MAGUK)-type protein synapse-associated protein 97 (SAP97),[2] α1-syntrophin, and possibly additional scaffolding proteins. In adult transgenic mice overexpressing Kir2.1 (Kir2.1 OE), peak I_{Na} density is twice as large as that measured in cells from control hearts. In heterozygous Kir2.1 knockout (KO) mice (Kir2.1$^{-/+}$), $Na_V1.5$ protein and I_{Na} are significantly reduced. Similarly, in single ARVMs, I_{K1} increased significantly on the adenoviral transfer of $Na_V1.5$. In NRVM monolayers, the co-overexpression of $Na_V1.5$ with Kir2.1 increased CV, abbreviated APD, and increased rotor frequency beyond those produced by Kir2.1 OE alone.[2] Furthermore, recent data in the literature suggest that conditions that result in $Na_V1.5$ protein reduction, such as those occurring in dystrophin-deficient mdx^{5cv} mice, are accompanied by a concomitant reduction in Kir2.1 protein levels.[7] Importantly, the finding that coexpression of $Na_V1.5$ can reduce internalization of Kir2.1 is a central mechanistic observation.[2] The purpose of this chapter is to discuss those results in the context of cardiac excitability and the mechanisms of reentrant arrhythmias. It will be shown that sodium and potassium channel interactions depend on more than membrane voltage alone. Altogether, the evidence that will be discussed suggests that cardiac cells undergo model-independent coregulation that involves the posttranslational mechanisms of Kir2.1 and $Na_V1.5$, with important functional consequences for myocardial excitation, impulse velocity, and arrhythmogenesis. Moreover, the evidence suggests that similar interactions are applicable to other sarcolemmal ion channels, which could themselves have unique effects on myocardial function.

Sodium Channels and Cardiac Excitation

In the heart, I_{Na} is the major current that excites working atrial and ventricular myocytes and the Purkinje fibers. Normally closed at the resting potential (approximately –85 mV in the adult ventricular myocardium), sodium channels open upon depolarization beyond the threshold, allowing an influx of Na^+ ions down their electrochemical gradients. This inward current causes "all-or-none" membrane depolarization at a rapid rate (~500 V/s in the Purkinje fibers) in a process that moves the membrane potential to positive values. The rapid voltage-dependent activation of the sodium channel is immediately followed by an inactivation process that is also triggered by an initial depolarization. The inactivation process causes I_{Na} to be brief and results in the termination of the current. These properties are important for the rapid (~50 cm/s) conduction of the electrical impulse in the myocardium.

From the clinical standpoint, multiple mutations in the *SCN5A* gene that codes for $Na_V1.5$ have been identified in association with the long QT syndrome (LQTS), Brugada syndrome, idiopathic VF, cardiac conduction defects, sick sinus syndrome, and dilated cardiomyopathy associated with atrial fibrillation.[8] Such mutations illustrate the pathophysiological importance of these channels.

Homozygous KO *SCN5A*$^{-/-}$ mouse embryos die during midgestation, most likely because of severe defects in ventricular morphogenesis,[9] which provides evidence for an essential role of $Na_V1.5$ in cardiac development.[8] However, heterozygous KO mice (*SCN5A*$^{+/-}$) show normal survival but exhibit slow atrial, atrioventricular (AV), and intraventricular conductions; prolonged ventricular refractoriness; and enhanced ventricular arrhythmia inducibility.[8,9] Ventricular myocytes isolated from adult $SCN5A^{+/-}$ mice demonstrate an approximately 50% reduction in sodium conductance.[9] However, an important question that has recently begun to be addressed is whether, as has been demonstrated in other model systems, changes in $Na_V1.5$ expression alter the level of functional expression of other membrane ion channels, particularly Kir2.1.[2] Based on recent results,[2] it would be reasonable to expect a significant reduction in Kir2.1 (and its respective ionic current I_{K1}) and RMP depolarization of adult ventricular myocytes as a consequence of one $SCN5A$ allele being absent. Should that be the case, one would predict that I_{K1}, RMP, and excitability would be rescued to normal levels by the virally mediated gene transfer of $Na_V1.5$ into adult ventricular myocytes isolated from these mice.

Cardiac-specific overexpression of the $SCN5A$ gene in mice resulted in a shorter P-wave duration and PR interval.[10,11] In a recent study using a transgenic mouse line overexpressing the human $SCN5A$ gene, levels for the cardiac sodium channel mRNA transcript ($Scn5a$) and protein ($Na_V1.5$) were each increased by approximately ten-fold in ventricular tissues from transgenic mice.[11] The immunohistochemical analysis revealed that in transgenic mouse hearts, the $Na_V1.5$ signal intensity was greatly enhanced compared with that in the wild-type (WT) mouse hearts throughout both the atrial and ventricular working myocardium.[11] Moreover, peak I_{Na} in transgenic ventricular myocytes was double that in WT ventricular myocytes, while surprisingly, it was not modified in transgenic atrial myocytes.[11] Unfortunately, I_{K1} density and Kir2.1 expression were not analyzed.

The Inward Rectifier Potassium Current

Kir channels are responsible for I_{K1}, and they are involved in the depolarization, repolarization, and resting phases of the cardiac AP.[12,13] Among the three strong inward rectifier potassium channels (Kir2.1, 2.2, and 2.3) that are expressed in the heart, Kir2.1 (encoded by the $KCNJ2$ gene) is the most abundant in the ventricles. It is usually accepted that, near the resting potential, the ventricular I_{K1} conductance is much larger than that of any other current, with the exception of the adenosine triphosphate (ATP)-sensitive potassium current (I_{KATP}), which, however, is generally not active because KATP channels are not open under normal conditions. It is thus likely that the physiological and/or pathophysiological modulation of I_{K1} will have a significant effect on excitability. Kir channels show strong rectification between −50 and 0 mV, which means they remain closed during the AP plateau; they open only when the membrane potential repolarizes to levels between −30 and −80 mV, which occurs during the late phases of AP.[14] Rectification is achieved by a voltage-dependent blockade by intracellular polyamines (spermine, spermidine, putrescine) and magnesium,[14] which are known to interact with at least three amino acid residues located inside the pore of the channel complex.[15] Investigators have used several strategies to modify and study Kir2.1, including a KO mouse,[16] a Kir2.1-OE mouse model,[17] antisense oligonucleotide targeting,[18] and a DNA transfection of a dominant-negative construct.[19] These studies have helped to define the role of I_{K1} in cardiac excitability.[20,21] As shown by Zaritzky and colleagues, ventricular myocytes from Kir2.1 KO ($KCNJ2^{-/-}$) mice lack I_{K1} in whole-cell recordings under physiological conditions, which demonstrated that Kir2.1 is the major determinant of I_{K1}.[16] In that model, sustained outward K^+ and Ba^{2+} currents through the L- and T-type channels were not significantly altered by the mutation. However, the direct consequences of Kir2.1 disruption on $Na_V1.5$ function were never studied in homozygous Kir2.1 KO mice. Recently, the authors took advantage of the availability of the

heterozygous Kir2.1 KO ($KCNJ2^{-/+}$) mouse model to study the functional consequences of reducing Kir2.1, and therefore I_{K1}, at both the cellular and organism levels. In particular, as discussed in detail later, the $KCNJ2^{-/+}$ mouse was used to address the question of whether the reduced Kir2.1 protein is associated with the reduced expression of $Na_V1.5$ and I_{Na}.[2]

Loss-of-function mutations in the $KCNJ2$ gene have been identified in patients affected by Andersen-Tawil syndrome (ATS), also known as LQTS type 7, which is characterized by prolonged repolarization.[22] In addition to being expressed in the heart, Kir2.1 is expressed in other organs, such as skeletal muscle. As a result, ATS is associated with hypokalemic periodic paralysis and skeletal developmental abnormalities, including clinodactyly, low-set ears, mandibular hypoplasia, short stature, and scoliosis.[22] In the heart, I_{K1} reduction leads to QT prolongation and predisposes to arrhythmias; however, QT prolongation is less prominent in patients with ATS than in those with other LQTS types.[23] Moreover, although patients with ATS develop ventricular tachyarrhythmias, including torsades de pointes, sudden cardiac death is rare.[23]

In patients with short QT syndrome type 3, a gain-of-function mutation (D172N) in the $KCNJ2$ gene was demonstrated.[24] The D172N mutation causes a significant increase in the outward component of the current–voltage (I–V) relationship of I_{K1} and is associated with an accelerated repolarization, which can be arrhythmogenic. However, the direct involvement of I_{K1} in arrhythmia mechanisms was not demonstrated in affected patients; therefore the Kir2.1 OE mouse model[25] was used to study the effect of I_{K1} increase on VF at the molecular level.[26] An increase of I_{K1} was shown to shorten repolarization and the QT interval and to exert a proarrhythmic effect in both atria and ventricles of this transgenic mouse model.[25,26] Optical mapping and numerical studies in these mice demonstrated that by hyperpolarizing RMP, I_{K1} overexpression enhanced the availability of sodium channels during sustained reentry, which contributed to the observed increase in the frequency and stability of rotors and VF.[26] Recent experiments with the same Kir2.1-OE mouse model have shown that Kir2.1, and therefore I_{K1}, upregulation leads to a significant increase in the I_{Na} density. These results strongly support the hypothesis that a change in the functional expression of $Na_V1.5$ could be the result of protein-protein–type interactions with Kir2.1. Such interactions can be mediated through common partners in a macromolecular protein complex.[2]

Intermolecular Interactions Involving PDZ Domains

PDZ domain–mediated interactions are among the most frequently encountered protein–protein interactions in cell biology.[27] PDZ stands for *postsynaptic density protein* (PSD-95), *disks*-large (the *Drosophila* septate junction protein), and *zona occludens*-1 (the epithelial tight junction protein).[28] The primary function of PDZ domains is to mediate protein–protein interactions by recognizing the very last three C-terminal amino acids of their target proteins.[29–31] PDZs can combine with other interaction modules (such as WW, SH3, and PTB domains) and help to direct the specificity of receptor tyrosine kinases and protein trafficking, establish and maintain cell polarity, and coordinate synaptic signaling.[32–35] Their pathophysiological importance is highlighted by significant neuronal and developmental defects observed in PDZ KO mice[36–40] and by their implication in human inherited diseases.[41–43]

More than 70 PDZ domain–containing proteins (hereafter referred to as PDZ domain proteins) have been identified that interact with different ion channels, receptors, and signaling molecules.[32] PDZ domain proteins are multidomain proteins that serve to link different proteins to form macromolecular complexes via interactions with their various domains. For example, the protein structure of SAP97 contains three PDZ domains, an SH3 domain, a HOOK domain, and an inactive guanylate kinase (GK) domain. The oligomerization site of SAP97 is contained within its unique amino terminal domain, which mediates the multimerization of SAP97 into dimeric and tetrameric species in solution.[44] Interactions via its HOOK domain enable SAP97 to bind protein 4.1; therefore SAP97 is able to link proteins bound to its PDZ domains to the actin–spectrin membrane cytoskeleton or to protein components of the actin–spectrin membrane cytoskeleton, such as protein 4.1.[44] On the other hand, the most abundant cardiac isoform of syntrophin (α1-syntrophin) exhibits two pleckstrin homology domains (PH1 and PH2) in the N-terminal region of the protein that allow the binding of α1-syntrophin to phosphatidylinositol lipids. PH1 is split in two PH domains (PH1a and PH1b) between which is located a type I PDZ domain. The C-terminal region of syntrophin is unique to this class of proteins and is called the syntrophin-unique (SU) domain.[45]

The complement of interacting proteins varies among the different PDZ domain proteins and provides a mechanism to recruit ion channel proteins into distinct macromolecular complexes, depending on which scaffolding proteins they bind (e.g., see Tiffany and coworkers[46]). The cellular localization of PDZ domain proteins can also vary, and it has been suggested that ion channel–PDZ domain protein interactions might be an important mechanism for plasma membrane expression and distribution of ion channels.[46–48] For example, ZO-1 and SAP97 are found in overlapping but distinct subcellular locations in the heart. ZO-1 is located exclusively in the intercalated disk, whereas SAP97 is found at the intercalated disk, lateral membranes,[46,48,49] and the T-tubules.[2]

Na$_V$1.5-Interacting Proteins

Almost 15 proteins have been shown to interact and form a multiprotein complex with Na$_V$1.5, making up the Na$_V$1.5 "channelosome," which is comprehensively described in Chapter 18.[8,50] Some of the interacting proteins modify Na$_V$1.5 gating properties when binding to the channel (such is the case of telethonin). Others are anchoring proteins (ankyrin-G, SAP97, and α1-syntrophin among others) or enzymes (Nedd4-like E3 ubiquitin ligases) that produce posttranslational modifications. Interestingly, most of these proteins interact with the C-terminal domain of Na$_V$1.5 (244 amino acid residues), which in addition to the C-terminal PDZ–binding domain, bears both PY and IQ motifs. The C-terminus of Na$_V$1.5 has been shown to interact with the fibroblast growth factor–homologous factor 1B, calmodulin, Nedd4-like ubiquitin-protein ligase, dystrophin and syntrophin, SAP97, Fyn, and protein–tyrosine phosphatase (PTPH1).[51–54] Na$_V$1.5 cytoplasmic loops I and II also exhibit interacting domains for proteins such as 14-3-3 and ankyrin-G, respectively. Ankyrin-G, similar to SAP97 and α1-syntrophin, helps to promote the localization of sodium channels to the cell membrane in ventricular myocytes.[50] In 2004, Mohler and associates[50] identified a point mutation (E1053K) in the ankyrin-binding motif of Na$_V$1.5 that was associated with Brugada syndrome. The E1053K mutation abolishes the binding of Na$_V$1.5 to ankyrin-G and prevents the accumulation of Na$_V$1.5 at cell surface sites in ventricular myocytes.[50] The data suggested that the association of Na$_V$1.5 with ankyrin-G is required for Na$_V$1.5 localization, and therefore its function at excitable membranes in ventricular myocytes. Concerted ankyrin-G interaction with potassium (K$_V$7) and Na$_V$ channels has also been demonstrated in neurons,[55] but Kir2.1 has not been shown to interact with ankyrin-G. There is a possibility that a defect in ankyrin-mediated Na$_V$1.5 trafficking and localization on the membrane could alter the Kir2.1 functional expression. This idea has not yet been explored in any detail.

To date, at least four anchoring proteins have been shown to interact with both Na$_V$1.5 and Kir2.1 channels (caveolin 3, plakoglobin, SAP97, and α1-syntrophin),[2,56] but only two of them are PDZ domain proteins: SAP97 and α1-syntrophin.

Na$_V$1.5 Interacts With SAP97

The three last amino acids (Ser-Ile-Val, SIV) of the Na$_V$1.5 C-terminus constitute a PDZ-binding motif that is known to interact with type I PDZ domains found in the proteins of the MAGUK family.[57] MAGUK proteins act as scaffolding proteins involved in intermolecular interactions and protein trafficking to the cell membrane. Petitprez and colleagues[58] and Milstein and associates[2] independently reported that SAP97, one of the cardiac MAGUK proteins, is involved in the turnover and regulation of the biophysical properties of Na$_V$1.5. Using Na$_V$1.5 C-terminal fusion proteins in pull-down experiments with human and mouse heart protein extracts, Petitprez and coworkers demonstrated that the association between SAP97 and Na$_V$1.5 depended on the PDZ domain–binding motif of Na$_V$1.5. Na$_V$1.5 constructs did not pull down either PSD95 or ZO-1, two other MAGUK proteins that are expressed in the human heart; thus the interaction appeared to be specific for SAP97.[59] In patch-clamp experiments, Petitprez and associates[58] further demonstrated that silencing the SAP97 expression reduced the whole-cell I$_{Na}$ without decreasing the total protein content in HEK293 cells that stably express Na$_V$1.5 channels. Similar results were obtained by Milstein and colleagues.[2] Taken together with the demonstrated colocalization of Na$_V$1.5 and SAP97 at both intercalated disks[58] and T-tubules,[2] these findings supported the existence of an interaction between Na$_V$1.5 and SAP97 in cardiac tissue. This interaction could have a role in determining the channel density at the plasma membrane.

Na$_V$1.5 Interacts With Syntrophins

Like other ion channels, Na$_V$1.5 has been reported to be part of the dystrophin multiprotein complex.[60] Gavillet and associates[7] demonstrated that Na$_V$1.5 interacts with dystrophin via syntrophin adaptor proteins through the PDZ domain–binding motif at the Na$_V$1.5 C-terminus.[52] Dystrophin-deficient mice (*mdx*^{5cv}) have reduced protein levels of Na$_V$1.5 in ventricular lysates; this is directly associated with reduced I$_{Na}$ in isolated ventricular myocytes and with conduction defects documented on an electrocardiogram. Immunostaining of frozen mouse heart slices demonstrated the colocalization of Na$_V$1.5 and dystrophin specifically at lateral membranes but not at intercalated disks.[7] Furthermore, as mentioned, ΔPDZ mice displayed reduced Na$_V$1.5 expression and decreased I$_{Na}$ specifically at the lateral myocyte membrane. The authors demonstrated that in vivo truncation of the PDZ-binding domain abolished the interaction between Na$_V$1.5 and syntrophin specifically localized to the lateral membrane.[61] Consistently, ventricular CV was preferentially decreased in the transversal direction to the myocardial fiber orientation. Biochemical analysis suggested that the deletion of the PDZ-binding motif affected the Na$_V$1.5 proteasomal degradation rather than internalization.[61] Recently, it has been described that in addition to the C-terminal canonical PDZ–binding domain, Na$_V$1.5 channels exhibit another internal PDZ-binding domain located at the N-terminal region. Site-directed mutagenesis analysis revealed that the internal PDZ-binding domain (20-SLA-22) allows binding to α1-syntrophin. Therefore these results suggested that Na$_V$1.5 channels bind to α1-syntrophin by means of two different PDZ-binding motifs.[62]

A study by Ueda and coworkers[63] demonstrated that α1-syntrophin (encoded by the *SNTA1* gene), connects Na$_V$1.5 to the neuronal nitric oxide synthase (nNOS)–plasma membrane Ca-ATPase (PMCA) complex in the heart. These results implicated *SNTA1* as a susceptibility gene for inherited LQTS. The cardiac isoform of PMCA, PMCA4b, participates in the nNOS complex to inhibit nitric oxide synthesis.[64] Furthermore, the study by Ueda and associates[63] identified a rare missense mutation (p.A390V) in α1-syntrophin that was found in an LQTS patient. The A390V mutation selectively disrupted the association of α1-syntrophin with PMCA4b, increased $Na_V1.5$ nitrosylation, and increased late sodium current, all suggesting that the *SNTA1* mutation was pathogenic.

Two Pools of $Na_V1.5$ Channels

Petitprez and colleagues[58] have suggested that there are at least two pools of $Na_V1.5$ channels in ventricular myocytes: one targeted to lateral membranes by the syntrophin–dystrophin complex, and another targeted to intercalated disks by SAP97. Thereafter, Abriel and associates developed a knock-in mouse model that expressed $Na_V1.5$ that lacked the PDZ-binding domain (ΔPDZ).[61] In that in vivo model, the authors reported a significant decrease in I_{Na} in ventricular myocytes from the ΔPDZ mice compared with that from the WT mice, coupled with a loss of $Na_V1.5$ at the lateral membrane. Conversely, $Na_V1.5$ at the intercalated disk was unaffected in ΔPDZ myocytes.[61] Consistent with these findings, the cardiac-specific ablation of SAP97 in mice decreased cardiac I_{K1} as well as transient outward (I_{to}) and ultrarapid delayed rectifier (I_{Kur}) currents but not I_{Na}.[65] Altogether, the above in vivo findings suggested that $Na_V1.5$ channels are targeted to intercalated disks that are independent of the PDZ domain protein association. Therefore although the experimental evidence supporting a direct $Na_V1.5$-SAP97 interaction via the $Na_V1.5$-SIV motif and a SAP97 PDZ domain is strong, the exact role of SAP97 in regulating $Na_V1.5$ function remains incompletely understood.

Kir2.1 Interacts With Both SAP97 and α-Syntrophin

Members of the Kir2.x subfamily (Kir2.1, Kir2.2, and Kir2.3) each have a C-terminal motif that enables an interaction with PDZ domain proteins. However, the C-terminal motifs are not identical among the isoforms. *RRESEI* is found in Kir2.1 and Kir2.2, whereas *RRESAI* is found in Kir2.3.[66] It is noteworthy that the PDZ-binding motif sequence on Kir2.x overlaps a consensus sequence (RRxS) for protein kinase A–dependent phosphorylation. Consistent with this finding, Kir2.3 binding to PDZ domain proteins is modulated in vitro by the phosphorylation of Kir2.3 proteins.[67]

A number of PDZ domain–containing proteins have already been shown to bind Kir2.x channels. In two studies,[68,69] affinity purification was used to isolate PDZ domain proteins from cardiac and brain tissue extracts. Cardiac SAP97, CASK, Veli3, and Mint1 were found in a complex with Kir2.2 channels. For the most part, the consequences (e.g., channel expression and biophysics of interactions between Kir2.x channels and PDZ domain proteins) are unknown. An association of PDZ domain proteins with many other ion channels or receptors has been shown to affect various aspects of protein trafficking in the secretory and endocytic pathways. In general, PDZ domain–mediated protein-protein interactions can alter the rate of channel/receptor trafficking to the plasma membrane or alter the rate at which a given cell surface channel and/or receptor is endocytosed.[70–72] It has also been suggested that binding to PDZ domain proteins is important for anchoring Kir2.x channels at the plasma membrane[49]; however, until recently, this hypothesis had not been directly tested, with the exception of the interaction of PSD-95 (a neuronal scaffolding protein) and Kir2.1 (discussed later).[73]

In 2004, Leonoudakis and coworkers[69] used a proteomics approach to identify proteins associated with Kir2 channels via the channel's C-terminal PDZ–binding motif. On the basis of the immunoaffinity purification and affinity chromatography from skeletal and cardiac muscle and the brain, they demonstrated that

in addition to MAGUK-type proteins, Kir2.x channels interact with various components of the dystrophin-associated protein complex, including α1-, β1-, and β2-syntrophin; dystrophin; and dystrobrevin. Their affinity pull-down experiments revealed that Kir2.1, Kir2.2, Kir2.3, and Kir4.1 all bind to scaffolding proteins but with different affinities for the dystrophin-associated protein complex, including dystrophin, syntrophin, and dystrobrevin,[69] as well as MAGUK proteins such as SAP97, CASK, and Veli. Indeed, recent experiments in human atrial myocytes revealed that Kir2.3 channels bind to SAP97 but not to α1-syntrophin. Furthermore, site-directed mutagenesis experiments in heterologous expression systems demonstrated that the lack of affinity for α1-syntrophin of Kir2.3 channels is a consequence of the sequence of their PDZ-binding domain.[62,74] Moreover, immunofluorescence localization studies demonstrated that Kir2.2 colocalizes with syntrophin, dystrophin, and dystrobrevin at skeletal muscle neuromuscular junctions[68,69] and that Kir2.1 colocalizes with α1-syntrophin in ventricular myocytes.[62] Overall, these results suggested that Kir2.x channels associate with protein complexes that are important to traffic and target channels to specific subcellular locales, as well as to anchor and stabilize channels in the plasma membrane.

Reciprocal Regulation of $Na_V1.5$ and Kir2.1

Voltage-clamp experiments presented in Fig. 21.1 show a reciprocal regulation of $Na_V1.5$ and Kir2.1 in ARVMs. $Na_V1.5$ was overexpressed using the adenoviral (Ad) construct (Ad-$Na_V1.5$)[2]; a control group of myocytes was infected with an adenovirus encoding green fluorescent protein (Ad-GFP). Average I_{Na}-density–voltage (I–V) plots are shown in Fig. 21.1A. There was a significant increase ($p < .005$) in I_{Na} density compared with that in control cells. There was no significant difference for $V_{1/2}$ values between control and Ad-$Na_V1.5$–treated cells.[2] $Na_V1.5$ overexpression also resulted in a significant increase in I_{K1} density in both the inward ($p < .01$) and outward ($p < .05$) directions (see Fig. 21.1B). Next, the possibility that Kir2.1 overexpression would increase $Na_V1.5$ functional expression was considered.[2] Infection with Ad-Kir2.1 resulted in an increase of I_{K1} in ARVMs (Fig. 21.1C). Peak inward (–100 mV) and outward (–60 mV) currents were significantly larger ($p < .01$) than those in control (Ad-GFP) cells. As hypothesized, peak I_{Na} density was also increased ($p < .005$; see Fig. 21.1D) with no changes in the voltage dependence of activation or inactivation.[2] These results suggest that common molecular mechanisms are involved in the regulation of Kir2.1 and $Na_V1.5$ functional expressions.[2] Neither the stoichiometry of the $Na_V1.5$-Kir2.1 interaction nor the relationship between current densities and the amount of DNA used for cell infection has been elucidated to date. As suggested by Abriel,[8] there may be intrinsic mechanisms that avoid "overloading" of the cardiac cell membrane with $Na_V1.5$. Assuming that there is a limited number of docking sites or complexes to which the $Na_V1.5$ and/or Kir2.1 channel bind in the adult heart, these complexes (i.e., including its localization, stoichiometry, available components) could then provide an upper limit as to how many functional $Na_V1.5$ and/or Kir2.1 channels can be brought to the membrane in adult mouse myocytes.[8]

SAP97 and Syntrophin Are Involved in $Na_V1.5$-Kir2.1 Interactions

Both $Na_V1.5$ and Kir2.1 have PDZ-binding domains at their respective C-terminus; therefore the potential role of SAP97 in the reciprocal I_{Na}–I_{K1} interactions discussed in the previous sections was examined. As described elsewhere in detail,[2] adenoviral transfer was used to knock down SAP97 expression (Ad-shSAP97) in ARVMs, and the properties of I_{K1} and I_{Na} were then studied under these conditions. As illustrated in Fig. 21.2,

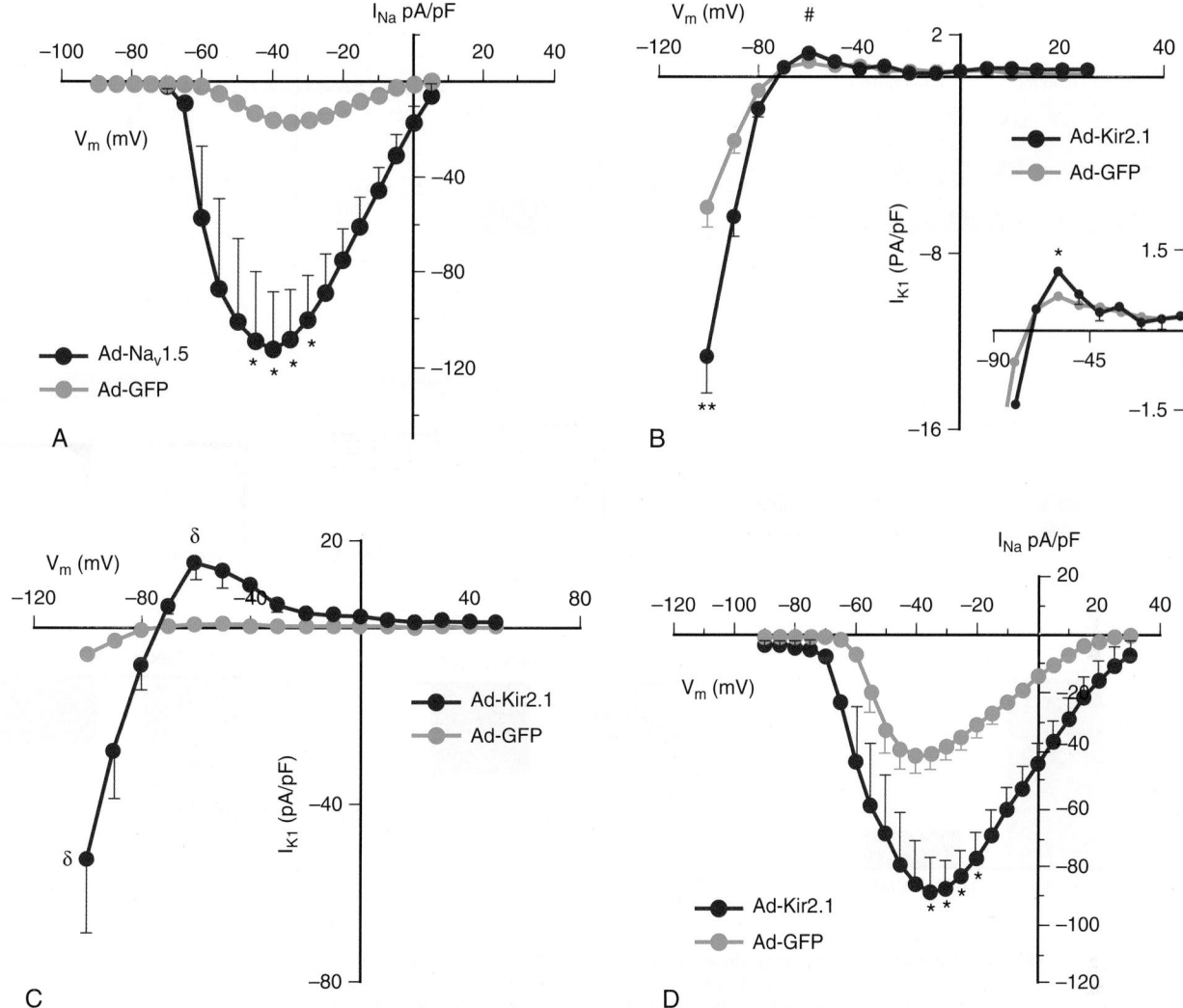

FIGURE 21.1 Reciprocal regulation of Na$_V$1.5 and Kir2.1 in adult rat ventricular myocytes. (A) and (B) Na$_V$1.5 overexpression increases both sodium current (I_{Na}) and inward rectifier potassium current (I_{K1}) densities. (A) Superimposed I_{Na} density–voltage relationships (5 mmol/L [Na$^+$]$_o$) for adenovirus encoding green fluorescent protein (*Ad-GFP; green; N = 1, n = 7*) and Ad-Na$_V$1.5 (*purple; N = 2, n = 6*)-infected cells. (B) Superimposed I_{K1} density–voltage relationship for Ad-GFP (*green; N = 3, n = 8*) and Ad-Na$_V$1.5 (*purple; N = 3, n = 8*)-infected cells. The *inset* shows the magnification of the outward component of the I_{K1} I–V relationship. (C) and (D) Kir2.1 overexpression increases both I_{K1} and I_{Na} densities. (C) Superimposed I_{K1} density–voltage relationships for Ad-GFP (*green; N = 3, n = 8*) and Ad-Kir2.1 (*purple; N = 2, n = 5*). (D) Superimposed I_{Na} density–voltage relationships (20 mmol/L [Na$^+$]$_o$) for Ad-GFP (*green; N = 2, n = 6*) and Ad-Kir2.1 (*purple; N = 4, n = 7*). #$p < .05$; $\delta p < .01$; *$p < .005$ unpaired t test with Welch's correction. (Modified from Milstein ML, Musa H, Balbuena DP, et al. Dynamic reciprocity of sodium and potassium channel expression in a macromolecular complex controls cardiac excitability and arrhythmia. *Proc Natl Acad Sci U S A.* 2012;109:E2134-E2143.)

an approximately 56% reduction in the relative levels of SAP97 (day 3 postinfection) (see Fig. 21.2B) was accompanied by an approximately 50% reduction in the I_{K1} density compared with that in control cells (see Fig. 21.2C). Similarly, silencing SAP97 expression also reduced whole-cell I_{Na} density at several tested voltages (see Fig. 21.2D). Peak inward I_{Na} density was reduced by approximately 60% compared with that in control cells ($p < .005$).

Kir2.1 and Na$_V$1.5 also associate with syntrophin as demonstrated in Fig. 21.2. Syntrophin was detected in ventricular membrane fractions after immunoprecipitation with antibodies raised to Kir2.1 (see Fig. 21.2E) or to Na$_V$1.5 (see Fig. 21.2F). Lentiviral transfer was used to knock down α1-syntrophin (shRNA SNTA1) in ARVMs, which led to an 80% reduction in α1-syntrophin expression (see Fig. 21.2I). Examples of I_{K1} and I_{Na} traces recorded in ARVMs infected with either a scrambled

shRNA (scrambled) or shRNA SNTA1 demonstrated that both I_{K1} and I_{Na} were significantly decreased in myocytes in which α1-syntrophin expression was decreased (see Fig. 21.2G and H). Quantification of these effects demonstrated that I_{K1} and I_{Na} densities significantly diminished by 44% and 60%, respectively (see Fig. 21.2J and K).

Na$_V$1.5-Kir2.1 Interactions Are Posttranslational and Model-Independent

The availability of a transgenic mouse model overexpressing Kir2.1[26] gave us the opportunity to ensure that the interactions were not an artifact of adenoviral infection and to discard any species-related differences in the interactions. Therefore additional patch-clamp experiments were conducted in ventricular

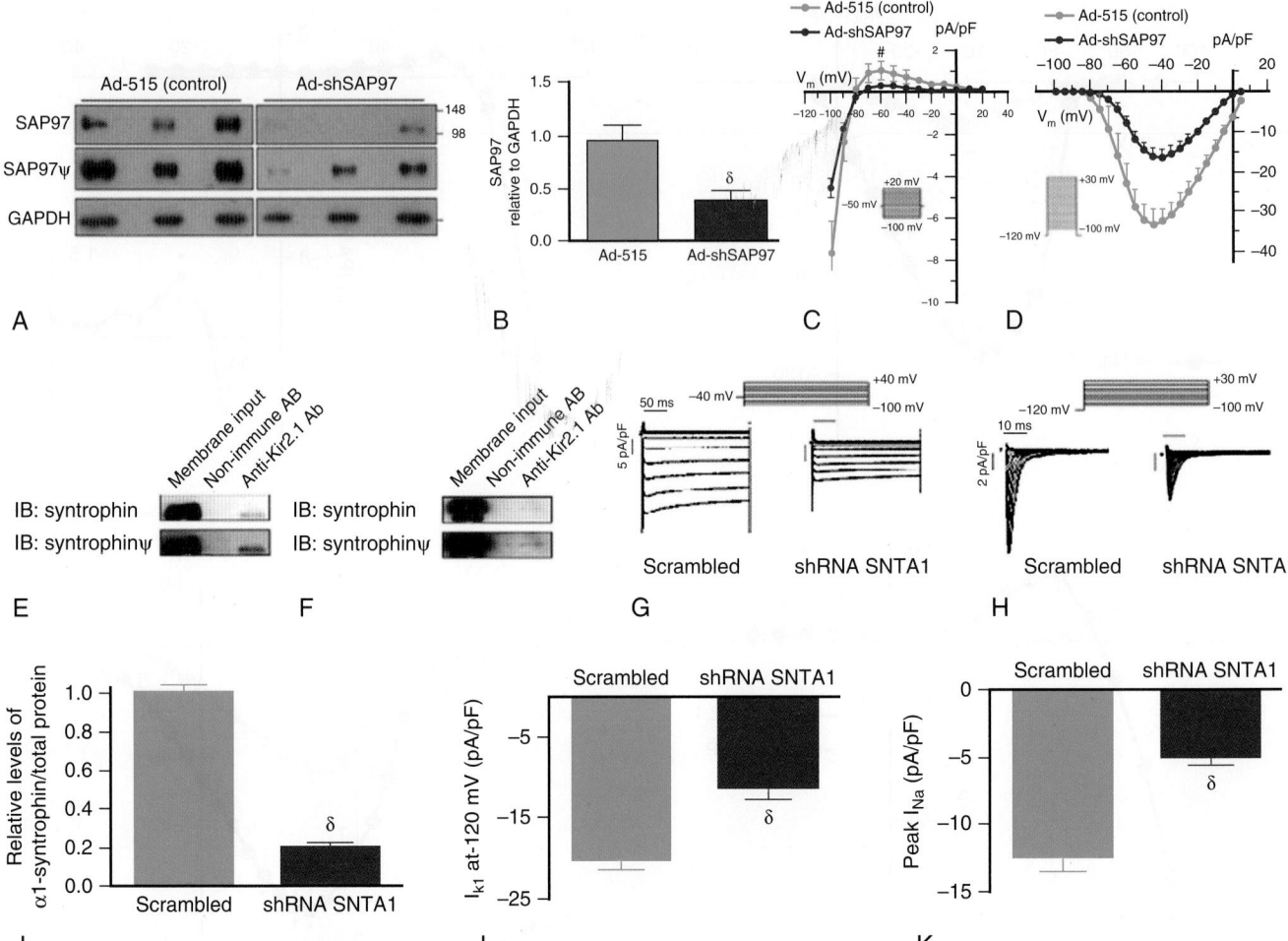

FIGURE 21.2 SAP97 and syntrophin are involved in Na$_V$1.5-Kir2.1 interactions. (A) Immunoblot showing the immunodetection of SAP97 expression (*top* and *middle*) and glyceraldehyde-3-phosphate dehydrogenase (*GAPDH*) (loading control; *bottom*) from cells infected with either a control (Ad-515) or shSAP97 (Ad-shSAP97) adenovirus. *Middle* (SAP97), the longer exposure of the same immunoblot (denoted by ψ). (B) Densitometric analysis of SAP97 expression normalized to GAPDH levels in the control (*green*) and SAP97-silenced (*purple*) cells. Values represent data (mean ± SEM) from two different preparations harvested 3 days after infection. The SAP97 expression was effectively knocked down by approximately 56% on day 3. (C) Inward rectifier potassium current (I_{K1}) density is reduced after SAP97 silencing in adult rat ventricular myocytes (ARVMs). The peak inward current density at −100 mV and peak outward current density at −60 were significantly different ($p = .02$ and $p = .04$, respectively) between myocytes infected with shSAP97 ($N = 4$, $n = 11$) and those infected with Ad-515 (control; $N = 2$, $n = 6$). *Inset*, The protocol used to measure the current. (D) Effects of SAP97 knockdown on the sodium current (I_{Na}) density in ARVMs. I_{Na} density–voltage relationships of the control (Ad-515) and SAP97-silenced (Ad-shSAP97) cells are superimposed. For both the control and silenced conditions, $N = 2$ and $n = 11$. *Inset*, The voltage clamp step protocol. $^{\#}p < .05$; $^{\delta}p < .01$; $^{*}p < .005$ unpaired t test with Welch's correction. (E) and (F) Kir2.1 and Na$_V$1.5 each associate with syntrophin in the rat heart ventricle. Syntrophin is detected following immunoprecipitation with specific antibodies raised to Kir2.1 (E) or Na$_V$1.5 (F). Coimmunoprecipitation reactions used membrane-enriched preparations generated from rat heart ventricles (ψ images were digitally enhanced for clarity). *IB*, Antibody used for immunoblotting; *IP*, antibody used for immunoprecipitation. (G–K) Effects on I_{K1} and I_{Na} densities produced by SNTA1 silencing in an ARVM. (G) and (H) I_{K1} traces recorded in two ARVMs from the same heart that were cultured and infected with a lentiviral construction, encoding either scrambled shRNA+GFP (scrambled; *left*) or shRNA for α1-syntrophin shRNA+GFP (shRNA SNTA1; *right*). (H) I_{Na} traces recorded in two ARVMs from the same heart that were cultured with scrambled (*left*) or shRNA for α1-syntrophin (*right*). (I) Densitometric analysis of α1-syntrophin expression normalized to total protein in control (*green*) and shRNA SNTA1 (*purple*)-infected cells ($^{\delta}p < .01$ unpaired t test followed by Newman-Keuls test). (J) and (K) Peak I_{K1} at −120 mV (J) and peak I_{Na} (K) densities recorded in myocytes infected with either scrambled or ShRNA-SNTA1 lentiviral constructions. Both I_{K1} and I_{Na} densities significantly decreased ($^{\delta}p < .01$ unpaired t test followed by Newman-Keuls test) in ShRNA SNTA1 myocytes compared with those infected with scrambled shRNA. Each bar represents the mean ± SEM of eight cells from two rats. ([A–F] Modified from Milstein ML, Musa H, Balbuena DP, et al. Dynamic reciprocity of sodium and potassium channel expression in a macromolecular complex controls cardiac excitability and arrhythmia. *Proc Natl Acad Sci U S A.* 2012;109:E2134-E2143. [G-K] Modified from Matamoros M, Pérez-Hernández M, Guerrero-Serna G, et al. Na$_V$1.5 N-terminal domain binding to α1-syntrophin increases membrane density of human Kir2.1, Kir2.2 and Na$_V$1.5 channels. *Cardiovasc Res.* 2016;110:279-290.)

myocytes isolated from these adult transgenic mice, which are known to have approximately 12-fold greater I_{K1} density than littermate WT mice.[75] A comparison of I_{Na} density in WT and Kir2.1-OE mice is shown in Fig. 21.3. Representative I_{Na} tracings from each genotype are presented in the *left inset* (see Fig. 21.3A). Compared with WT, the I-V relationship for I_{Na} in myocytes from Kir2.1-OE mice shows significantly larger I_{Na} density at several tested voltages (see Fig. 21.3A, *right inset; p <* .005). Consistent with functional consequences observed with Kir2.1 overexpression (see Fig. 21.3A), increased Kir2.1 expression in the mouse heart leads to altered membrane protein expression of SAP97, syntrophin, and $Na_V1.5$ in the transgenic Kir2.1-OE mouse heart (see Fig. 21.3B and C). The relative levels of SAP97, syntrophin, and $Na_V1.5$ were significantly increased by factors of 1.6, 1.9, and 2.2, respectively, compared with the levels in WT littermates ($p <$ .01; see Fig. 21.3B and C). These data demonstrate that the reciprocal regulation between Kir2.1 and $Na_V1.5$ (and their respective currents) also occurs in the mouse heart and thus is not model-specific or unique to ARVMs. It also provides assurance that the observed reciprocal regulation in rat myocytes was not a virally mediated artifact of overexpression. However, real-time polymerase chain reaction (RT-PCR) analyses showed that although the *Kcnj2* mRNA transcript was significantly elevated in the transgenic Kir2.1-OE mice, mRNA levels encoding for SAP97, $Na_V1.5$, and syntrophin were unchanged in the hearts of these mice compared with those of WT littermates (Fig. 21.4A).

Additional RT-PCR experiments (Fig. 21.4B) demonstrated that the expression levels of *SCN5A*, *DLG1* (encoding SAP97), and *SNTA1* mRNA transcripts were unchanged in ventricles of heterozygous *Kcnj2* KO mice[16] compared with those in WT littermates. Yet, as shown in Fig. 21.5, a 50% allelic reduction of *KCNJ2* gene expression by homologous recombination resulted in a significant decrease in the relative membrane protein levels of $Na_V1.5$, SAP97, and syntrophin ($p <$ .05). The results suggest that regardless of whether these reciprocal changes lead to the downregulation or upregulation of channel proteins, they appear to involve posttranscriptional or posttranslational mechanisms.

$Na_V1.5$-Kir2.1 Interactions Involve Membrane Trafficking

The results discussed in the previous section demonstrate that the synergistic and reciprocal effects of Kir2.1 and $Na_V1.5$ expressions on channel current density occur at posttranslational levels. Recently, it was suggested that these channel proteins share a common trafficking pathway where the synergistic effects act to modulate the surface levels of Kir2.1 and $Na_V1.5$ channels.[2] However, the mechanisms that control Kir2.1 or $Na_V1.5$ plasma membrane targeting or localization remain poorly explored. The balance between anterograde and retrograde trafficking pathways determines the steady-state cell surface expression of channel proteins. Disease-associated mutations in both Kir2.1 and $Na_V1.5$ have been shown to affect anterograde trafficking by inhibiting steps early in the secretory pathway to cause intracellular retention. Yet, it is unknown whether the retention of Kir2.1 results in the retention of $Na_V1.5$ or vice versa. In contrast, once at the plasma membrane, endocytosis is the initial step in retrograde movement, after which internalized proteins can follow multiple routes to different intracellular fates.[76] One well-recognized outcome is the targeting of internalized proteins to lysosomes followed by degradation. Alternatively, trafficking through recycling endosomes allows proteins to return to the plasma membrane, thereby protecting them from degradation.[77] Data presented recently in collaboration with Dr. Jeffrey Martens show that Kir2.1 undergoes constitutive internalization in HL-1 myocytes, which contributes to the control of Kir2.1

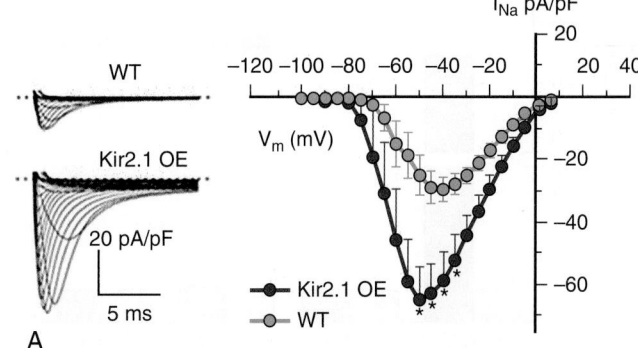

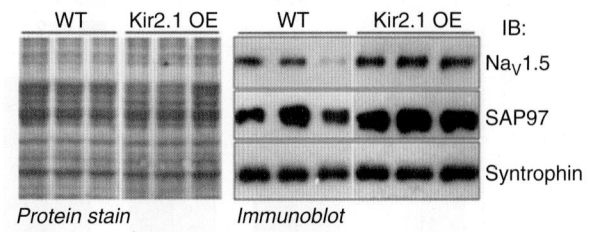

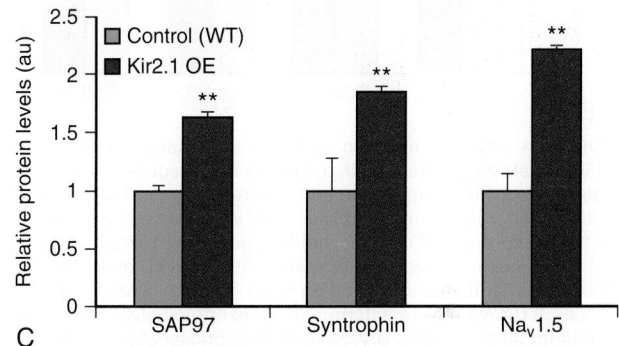

FIGURE 21.3 Reciprocal regulation of sodium current (I_{Na}) and $Na_V1.5$ in Kir2.1-overexpressing (OE) mice. (A) Superimposed I_{Na} density–voltage relationships in wild-type (WT; *green*) and Kir2.1 OE (*purple*) mice. The *left inset* shows representative examples of I_{Na} traces in each group. The *dotted line* denotes 0 pA. (WT N = 4, n = 10; Kir2.1 OE N = 2, n = 6. *p < .005, unpaired t test with Welch's correction. (B) Relative levels of syntrophin, SAP97, and $Na_V1.5$ are significantly increased in hearts of transgenic mice overexpressing Kir2.1. Crude membrane vesicles were prepared from the ventricles of control (WT) and Kir2.1 OE mice. Samples (16 μg/lane) were analyzed with sodium dodecyl sulfate polyacrylamide gel electrophoresis and immunoblotted using specific antibodies for syntrophin, SAP97, or $Na_V1.5$, as indicated. Representative immunoblots following the detection of protein immunoreactivity with horseradish peroxidase–conjugated secondary antibodies and chemiluminescence (*right*). The corresponding Amido black nitrocellulose (protein stain) is shown on the *left* to demonstrate the analysis of equal total protein. Protein concentrations were also verified by Lowry assay. (C) Densitometric analysis of data shown in (B) (*top*) comparing the relative protein levels between WT and Kir2.1 OE mice. Results are expressed as mean signal intensities and represent data from three animals for each genotype (N = 3 per genotype; $^\delta p$ < .01, mean ± SEM). (Modified from Milstein ML, Musa H, Balbuena DP, et al. Dynamic reciprocity of sodium and potassium channel expression in a macromolecular complex controls cardiac excitability and arrhythmia. *Proc Natl Acad Sci U S A.* 2012;109:E2134-E2143.)

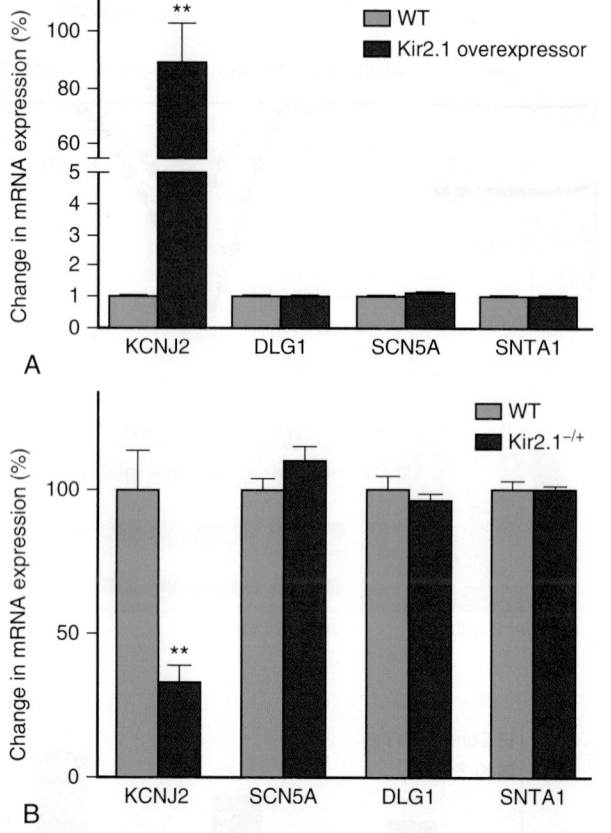

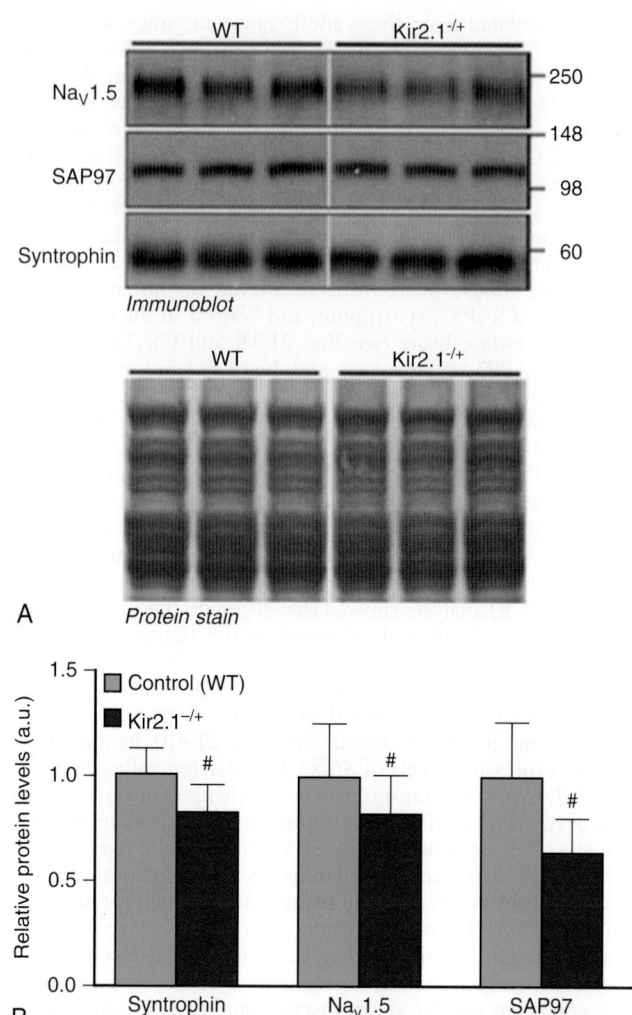

FIGURE 21.4 SAP97, syntrophin, and Na$_V$1.5 messenger RNA (*mRNA*) levels are unchanged in the hearts of transgenic mouse models of Kir2.1 overexpression and underexpression. Total RNA was extracted from ventricular tissues that were harvested from Kir2.1-overexpressing (OE) mice, heterozygous Kir2.1 knockout (*Kir2.1$^{-/+}$*) mice, or respective littermate wild-type (*WT*) mice. The mRNA levels for the genes encoding Kir2.1 (*KCNJ2*), SAP97 (*DLG1*), and Na$_V$1.5 (*SCN5A*) were determined by real-time polymerase chain reaction for all genotypes. Glyceraldehyde-3-phosphate dehydrogenase was used as an endogenous control for data normalization in each sample. Relative quantification of mRNA expression was calculated using the $2^{\Delta\Delta-Ct}$ method. (A) The bar graph compares mRNA expression for all genes between control and transgenic Kir2.1 OE ventricles. (B) Na$_V$1.5, SAP97, and syntrophin mRNA levels are unchanged in the hearts of heterozygous Kir2.1 knockout (Kir2.1$^{-/+}$) mice. $N = 4$ for all genotypes. **$p < .005$. (Modified from Milstein ML, Musa H, Balbuena DP, et al. Dynamic reciprocity of sodium and potassium channel expression in a macromolecular complex controls cardiac excitability and arrhythmia. *Proc Natl Acad Sci U S A*. 2012;109:E2134-E2143.)

FIGURE 21.5 Transgenic reduction of Kir2.1 gene expression leads to a significant decrease in relative protein levels of Na$_V$1.5 and SAP97 as well as syntrophin. Crude membrane vesicles were prepared from the ventricles of control (wild-type [*WT*]) and Kir2.1$^{-/+}$ mice. See Fig. 21.3 for methods that describe the sodium dodecyl sulfate polyacrylamide gel electrophoresis and immunoblotting. (A) Representative immunoblots following the detection of protein immunoreactivity with horseradish peroxidase–conjugated secondary antibodies and chemiluminescence (*top*). The corresponding Amido black nitrocellulose (protein stain) is shown at the *bottom* to demonstrate the analysis of equal total protein. Protein concentrations were also verified by Lowry assay. (B) Densitometric analysis comparing relative protein levels between WT and Kir2.1$^{-/+}$ mice. Results are expressed as mean signal intensity ($N = 7$ per genotype. #$p < .05$, mean ± SEM. (Modified from Milstein ML, Musa H, Balbuena DP, et al. Dynamic reciprocity of sodium and potassium channel expression in a macromolecular complex controls cardiac excitability and arrhythmia. *Proc Natl Acad Sci U S A*. 2012;109:E2134-E2143.)

steady-state surface density.[2] In addition, it was demonstrated that Na$_V$1.5 promotes cell surface expression of Kir2.1 in ventricular myocytes, at least in part, by reducing its internalization.[2] However, it remains unclear how Na$_V$1.5 or the macromolecular complex formation with SAP97 and/or α1-syntrophin affects this process. Elucidation of the mechanisms that control the surface expression of Kir2.1 and Na$_V$1.5 will contribute significantly to the currently limited understanding of protein transport in the heart and to channelopathies that involve altered trafficking.

Reciprocal Na$_V$1.5-Kir2.1 Interactions Control Reentry Frequency

The electrophysiological interplay between I$_{Na}$ and I$_{K1}$ is essential for controlling cardiac excitability and determining the stability and frequency of reentry and VT/VF.[5,26] In fact, I$_{K1}$ upregulation is a substrate for very fast electrical rotors in the

structurally normal ventricles.[26] I$_{K1}$ upregulation hyperpolarizes RMP and thus increases sodium channel availability during reentry in a voltage-dependent manner. Recently, Milstein and associates[2] demonstrated that in NRVM monolayers, voltage dependency is not the only mechanism by which Na$_V$1.5-Kir2.1 interactions control reentry dynamics and lead to faster rotors. Fig. 21.6 shows reproduced phase maps and rotation frequency plots obtained from optical mapping experiments that investigated the electrophysiological consequences of the Na$_V$1.5-Kir2.1 molecular interplay when one or both protein channels were overexpressed.[2] A single stationary rotor maintained the

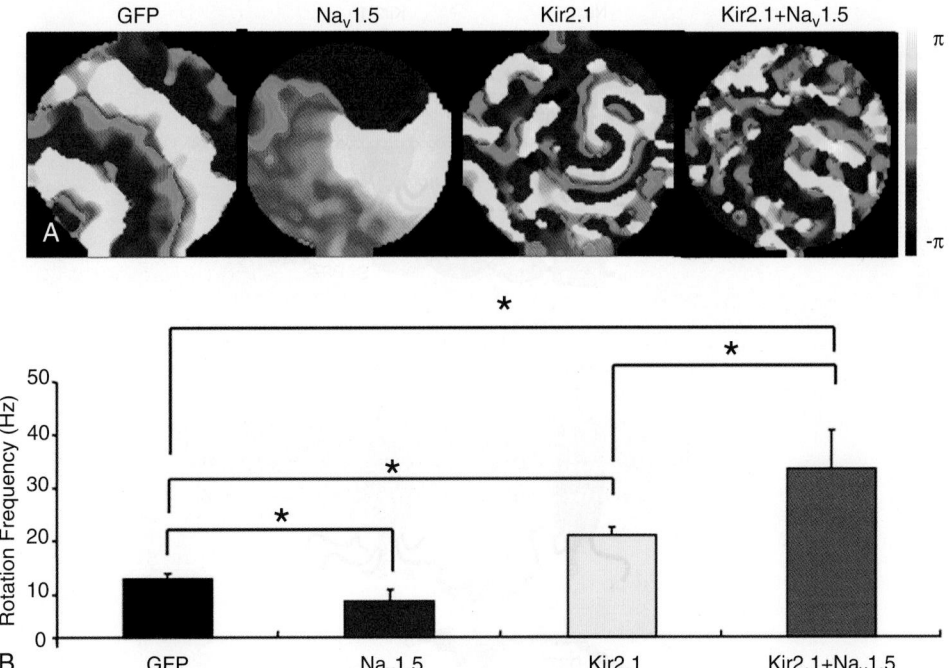

FIGURE 21.6 Molecular Na$_V$1.5-Kir2.1 interactions modulate reentry frequency in neonatal rat ventricular myocyte monolayers. (A) Phase maps for single rotations obtained from representative optical mapping movies of monolayers infected with adenovirus encoding green fluorescent protein (Ad-*GFP*), Ad-Na$_V$1.5, Ad-Kir2.1, or Ad-Kir2.1+Ad-Na$_V$1.5. The color bar indicates the phase in the excitation–recovery cycle. (B) Reentry frequencies in monolayers infected with Ad-GFP (*black; n* = 11), Ad-Na$_V$1.5 (*blue; n* = 13), Ad-Kir2.1 (*yellow; n* = 11), or Ad-Kir2.1+Ad-Na$_V$1.5 (*red; n* = 13). $^\delta p < .01$, analysis of variance. (Modified from Milstein ML, Musa H, Balbuena DP, et al. Dynamic reciprocity of sodium and potassium channel expression in a macromolecular complex controls cardiac excitability and arrhythmia. *Proc Natl Acad Sci U S A.* 2012;109:E2134-E2143.)

electrical activity in each monolayer. It was previously shown in single NRVMs that Na$_V$1.5 overexpression alone prolonged APD, whereas Kir2.1 overexpression had the opposite effect.[2] In Fig. 21.6A, APD prolongation induced by Na$_V$1.5 overexpression in the monolayer was manifested as a lengthening of the wavelength and slowing of the reentry frequency. However, the shortened APD of the Kir2.1 OE monolayers significantly decreased the wavelength and increased the rotation frequency (see Fig. 21.6B). Most remarkable was the fact that the combined overexpression of Na$_V$1.5+Kir2.1 hyperpolarized RMP, resulting in a shortened APD and a faster CV.[2] Consequently, the frequency of reentry was even higher than that produced by Ad-Kir2.1 infection alone. These results suggest that the reciprocal intermolecular interplay of Kir2.1 and Na$_V$1.5 could have profound consequences on the frequency and stability of reentry in the heart.

Concluding Remarks

The results discussed in this chapter provided the first evidence that two major ion channel proteins, Na$_V$1.5 and Kir2.1, that control cardiac electrical function are part of a common macromolecular complex that involves at least two distinct scaffolding proteins, SAP97 and syntrophin (Fig. 21.7). Most likely, their interactions offer a means for their reciprocal regulation, with vital functional consequences for myocardial excitation, CV, and arrhythmogenesis.[2] It is tempting to speculate that the complex formed by these two major ion channels, along with their protein partners, represents a molecular sensing system in the cell that might enable it to monitor and accordingly adjust the expression levels of proteins involved in generating and maintaining the cardiac impulse as well as adjusting to pathophysiological conditions. Most exciting, the demonstrated intermolecular interaction between these two essential channels, controlling cardiac excitability, opens a new pathway in the study of molecular mechanisms that underlie sudden cardiac death in highly prevalent heart diseases, including heart failure, and in inherited cardiac arrhythmias wherein defects in the functional expression of Kir2.1 have been clearly demonstrated.[78,79] Moreover, a mechanistic link among Kir2.1-Na$_V$1.5 interactions, arrhythmogenesis, and heart failures is further underscored by demonstrating that the I$_{Na}$ density decreases in chronic heart failure.[80] The regulation of expressions and mechanisms of interactions between Kir2.1 and Na$_V$1.5 discussed here could contribute to the development of more efficacious treatments for arrhythmia in heart diseases, particularly heart failures and inherited arrhythmogenic diseases in which a defect in the membrane expression of Na$_V$1.5 channel might affect the functional expression of Kir2.1 and vice versa.

Acknowledgments

The authors thank Ricardo Caballero for comments on the manuscript. This work was supported by R01 Grant HL122352 from the US National Heart Lung and Blood Institute (JJ) and the Leducq Foundation (JJ), as well as Ministerio de Economía (SAF2014-58769-P) and Red de Investigación Cardiovascular (RD12/0042/0011) (ED).

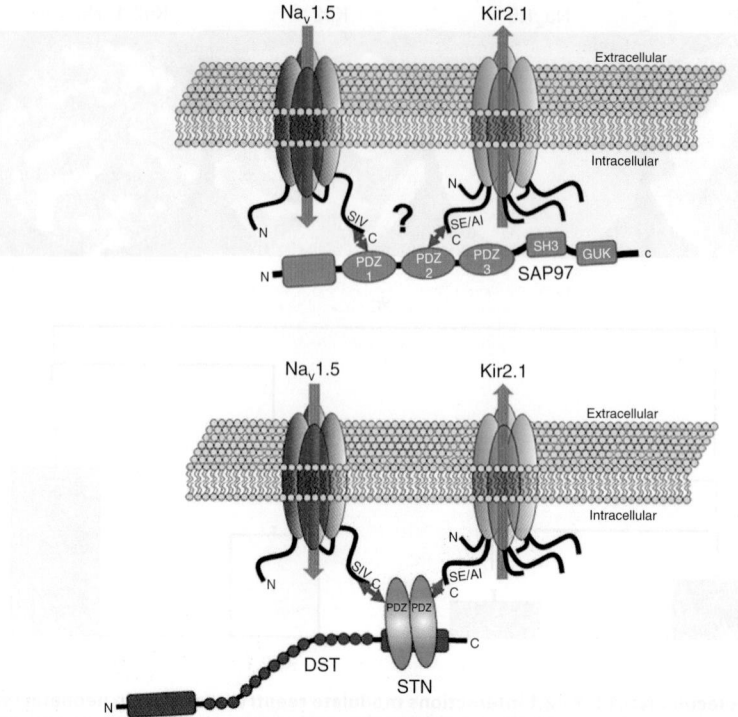

FIGURE 21.7 Schematic diagrams of possible interactions between Kir2.1, Na$_V$1.5, SAP97 (*top*) and α1-syntrophin, as well as their possible connection with the dystrophin-associated protein complex (*bottom*). The subcellular localization and channel activity of both Na$_V$1.5 and Kir2.1 are regulated by protein–protein interactions via their respective C-terminal PDZ–binding motifs with such PDZ domain–containing proteins as SAP97 and syntrophin. As shown here, the C-terminus of individual Na$_V$1.5 and Kir2.1 channels may each bind to the same SAP97 (*top*) or syntrophin (*bottom*) molecule but at different PDZ domains. It is possible that these interactions occur as part of a macromolecular complex (a "channelosome") in different cellular microdomains and result in changes in the expression of Na$_V$1.5 or Kir2.1, thereby influencing their functions in the cell membrane. *GUK*, Guanylate kinase-like domain of SAP97; *SH3*, src kinase homology domain of SAP97; *SNT,* syntrophin.

REFERENCES

1. Weidmann S. The effect of the cardiac membrane potential on the rapid availability of the sodium-carrying system. *J Physiol.* 1955;127:213–224.
2. Milstein ML, Musa H, Balbuena DP, et al. Dynamic reciprocity of sodium and potassium channel expression in a macromolecular complex controls cardiac excitability and arrhythmia. *Proc Natl Acad Sci U S A.* 2012;109:E2134–E2143.
3. Fozzard HA, Hanck DA. Structure and function of voltage-dependent sodium channels. Comparison of brain II and cardiac isoforms. *Physiol Rev.* 1996;76:887–926.
4. Lopatin AN, Nichols CG. Inward rectifiers in the heart. An update on I$_{K1}$. *J Mol Cell Cardiol.* 2001;33:625–638.
5. Noujaim SF, Berenfeld O, Kalifa J, et al. Universal scaling law of electrical turbulence in the mammalian heart. *Proc Natl Acad Sci U S A.* 2007;104:20985–20989.
6. Noujaim SF, Kaur K, Milstein M, et al. A null mutation of the neuronal sodium channel Nav1.6 disrupts action potential propagation and excitation-contraction coupling in the mouse heart. *FASEB J.* 2012;26:63–72.
7. Gavillet B, Rougier JS, Domenighetti AA, et al. Cardiac sodium channel Nav1.5 is regulated by a multiprotein complex composed of syntrophins and dystrophin. *Circ Res.* 2006;99:407–414.
8. Abriel H. Roles and regulation of the cardiac sodium channel Na v 1.5: recent insights from experimental studies. *Cardiovasc Res.* 2007;76:381–389.
9. Papadatos GA, Wallerstein PM, Head CE, et al. Slowed conduction and ventricular tachycardia after targeted disruption of the cardiac sodium channel gene SCN5A. *Proc Natl Acad Sci U S A.* 2002;99:6210–6215.
10. Zhang T, Yong SL, Tian XL, et al. Cardiac-specific overexpression of SCN5A gene leads to shorter P wave duration and PR interval in transgenic mice. *Biochem Biophys Res Commun.* 2007;355:444–450.
11. Liu GX, Remme CA, Boukens BJ, et al. Overexpression of SCN5A in mouse heart mimics human syndrome of enhanced atrioventricular nodal conduction. *Heart Rhythm.* 2015;12:1036–1045.

12. Nichols CG, Makhina EN, Pearson WL, et al. Inward rectification and implications for cardiac excitability. *Circ Res.* 1996;78:1–7.
13. Shimoni Y, Clark RB, Giles WR. Role of an inwardly rectifying potassium current in rabbit ventricular action potential. *J Physiol.* 1992;448:709–727.
14. Nichols CG, Lopatin AN. Inward rectifier potassium channels. *Annu Rev Physiol.* 1997;59:171–191.
15. Yang J, Jan YN, Jan LY. Control of rectification and permeation by residues in two distinct domains in an inward rectifier K$^+$ channel. *Neuron.* 1995;14:1047–1054.
16. Zaritsky JJ, Redell JB, Tempel BL, et al. The consequences of disrupting cardiac inwardly rectifying K$^+$ current I$_{K1}$ as revealed by the targeted deletion of the murine Kir2.1 and Kir2.2 genes. *J Physiol.* 2001;533:697–710.
17. Li J, McLerie M, Lopatin AN. Transgenic upregulation of I$_{K1}$ in the mouse heart leads to multiple abnormalities of cardiac excitability. *Am J Physiol Heart Circ Physiol.* 2004;287:H2790–H2802.
18. Nakamura TY, Artman M, Rudy B, et al. Inhibition of rat ventricular I$_{K1}$ with antisense oligonucleotides targeted to Kir2.1 mRNA. *Am J Physiol.* 1998;274:H892–H900.
19. Preisig-Muller R, Schlichthorl G, Goerge T, et al. Heteromerization of Kir2.X potassium channels contributes to the phenotype of Andersen's syndrome. *Proc Natl Acad Sci U S A.* 2002;99:7774–7779.
20. Miake J, Marban E, Nuss HB. Functional role of inward rectifier current in heart probed by Kir2.1 overexpression and dominant-negative suppression. *J Clin Invest.* 2003;111:1529–1536.
21. McLerie M, Lopatin A. Dominant-negative suppression of I$_{K1}$ in the mouse heart leads to altered cardiac excitability. *J Mol Cell Cardiol.* 2003;35:367–378.
22. Plaster NM, Tawil R, Tristani-Firouzi M, et al. Mutations in Kir2.1 cause the developmental and episodic electrical phenotypes of Andersen's syndrome. *Cell.* 2001;105:511–519.

23. Anderson CL, Delisle BP, Anson BD, et al. Most LQT2 mutations reduce Kv11.1 (hERG) current by a class 2 (trafficking-deficient) mechanism. *Circulation.* 2006;113:365–373.
24. Priori SG, Pandit SV, Rivolta I, et al. A novel form of short QT syndrome (SQT3) is caused by a mutation in the KCNJ2 gene. *Circ Res.* 2005;96:800–807.
25. Li J, McLerie M, Lopatin AN. Transgenic upregulation of I$_{K1}$ in the mouse heart leads to multiple abnormalities of cardiac excitability. *Am J Physiol Heart Circ Physiol.* 2004;287:H2790–H2802.
26. Noujaim SF, Pandit SV, Berenfeld O, et al. Upregulation of the inward rectifier K$^+$ current (I$_{K1}$) in the mouse heart accelerates and stabilizes rotors. *J Physiol.* 2007;578:315–326.
27. Stiffler MA, Grantcharova VP, Sevecka M, et al. Uncovering quantitative protein interaction networks for mouse PDZ domains using protein microarrays. *J Am Chem Soc.* 2006;128:5913–5922.
28. Stanfield PR, Nakajima S, Nakajima Y. Constitutively active and g-protein coupled inward rectifier K$^+$ channels: Kir2.0 and Kir3.0. *Rev Physiol Biochem Pharmacol.* 2002;145:47–179.
29. Kim E, Niethammer M, Rothschild A, et al. Clustering of shaker-type K$^+$ channels by interaction with a family of membrane-associated guanylate kinases. *Nature.* 1995;378:85–88.
30. Kornau HC, Schenker LT, Kennedy MB, et al. Domain interaction between NMDA receptor subunits and the postsynaptic density protein PSD-95. *Science.* 1995;269:1737–1740.
31. Sato T, Irie S, Kitada S, et al. Fap-1: a protein tyrosine phosphatase that associates with Fas. *Science.* 1995;268:411–415.
32. Garner CC, Nash J, Huganir RL. PDZ domains in synapse assembly and signaling. *Trends Cell Biol.* 2000;10:274–280.
33. Bilder D. PDZ proteins and polarity: functions from the fly. *Trends Genet.* 2001;17:511–519.

34. Sheng M, Sala C. PDZ domains and the organization of supramolecular complexes. *Annu Rev Neurosci.* 2001;24:1–29.

35. Nourry C, Grant SG, Borg JP. PDZ domain proteins: plug and play! *Sci STKE.* 2003;179:re7.

36. Hildebrand JD, Soriano P. Shroom, a PDZ domain-containing actin-binding protein, is required for neural tube morphogenesis in mice. *Cell.* 1999;99:485–497.

37. Zhadanov AB, Provance Jr DW, Speer CA, et al. Absence of the tight junctional protein af-6 disrupts epithelial cell-cell junctions and cell polarity during mouse development. *Curr Biol.* 1999;9:880–888.

38. Bladt F, Tafuri A, Gelkop S, et al. Epidermolysis bullosa and embryonic lethality in mice lacking the multi-PDZ domain protein grip1. *Proc Natl Acad Sci U S A.* 2002;99:6816–6821.

39. Laverty HG, Wilson JB. Murine cask is disrupted in a sex-linked cleft palate mouse mutant. *Genomics.* 1998;53:29–41.

40. Caruana G, Bernstein A. Craniofacial dysmorphogenesis including cleft palate in mice with an insertional mutation in the discs large gene. *Mol Cell Biol.* 2001;21:1475–1483.

41. Boeda B, El-Amraoui A, Bahloul A, et al. Myosin VIIa, harmonin and cadherin 23, three Usher I gene products that cooperate to shape the sensory hair cell bundle. *EMBO J.* 2002;21:6689–6699.

42. Verpy E, Leibovici M, Zwaenepoel I, et al. A defect in harmonin, a PDZ domain-containing protein expressed in the inner ear sensory hair cells, underlies Usher syndrome type 1c. *Nat Genet.* 2000;26:51–55.

43. Boerkoel CF, Takashima H, Stankiewicz P, et al. Periaxin mutations cause recessive Dejerine-Sottas neuropathy. *Am J Hum Genet.* 2001;68:325–333.

44. Marfatia SM, Byron O, Campbell G, et al. Human homologue of the *Drosophila* discs large tumor suppressor protein forms an oligomer in solution. Identification of the self-association site. *J Biol Chem.* 2000;275:13759–13770.

45. Bhat HF, Adams ME, Khanday FA. Syntrophin proteins as Santa Claus: role(s) in cell signal transduction. *Cell Mol Life Sci.* 2013;70:2533–2554.

46. Tiffany AM, Manganas LN, Kim E, et al. Psd-95 and sap97 exhibit distinct mechanisms for regulating K+ channel surface expression and clustering. *J Cell Biol.* 2000;148:147–158.

47. Melnyk P, Zhang L, Shrier A, et al. Differential distribution of Kir2.1 and Kir2.3 subunits in canine atrium and ventricle. *Am J Physiol Heart Circ Physiol.* 2002;283:H1123–H1133.

48. Murata M, Buckett PD, Zhou J, et al. SAP97 interacts with Kv1.5 in heterologous expression systems. *Am J Physiol Heart Circ Physiol.* 2001;281:H2575–H2584.

49. Leonoudakis D, Mailliard W, Wingerd K, et al. Inward rectifier potassium channel Kir2.2 is associated with synapse-associated protein SAP97. *J Cell Sci.* 2001;114:987–998.

50. Mohler PJ, Rivolta I, Napolitano C, et al. Nav1.5 E1053K mutation causing Brugada syndrome blocks binding to ankyrin-G and expression of Nav1.5 on the surface of cardiomyocytes. *Proc Natl Acad Sci U S A.* 2004;101:17533–17538.

51. Wu L, Yong SL, Fan C, et al. Identification of a new co-factor, MOG1, required for the full function of cardiac sodium channel Nav1.5. *J Biol Chem.* 2008;283:6968–6978.

52. Abriel H, Kass RS. Regulation of the voltage-gated cardiac sodium channel Nav1.5 by interacting proteins. *Trends Cardiovasc Med.* 2005;15:35–40.

53. Jespersen T, Gavillet B, van Bemmelen MX, et al. Cardiac sodium channel Nav1.5 interacts with and is regulated by the protein tyrosine phosphatase PTPH1. *Biochem Biophys Res Commun.* 2006;348:1455–1462.

54. Chauhan-Patel R, Spruce AE. Differential regulation of potassium currents by FGF-1 and FGF-2 in embryonic *Xenopus laevis* myocytes. *J Physiol.* 1998;512:109–118.

55. Pan Z, Kao T, Horvath Z, et al. A common ankyrin-G-based mechanism retains KCNQ and Nav channels at electrically active domains of the axon. *J Neurosci.* 2006;26:2599–2613.

56. Asimaki A, Kapoor S, Plovie E, et al. Identification of a new modulator of the intercalated disc in a zebrafish model of arrhythmogenic cardiomyopathy. *Sci Transl Med.* 2014;6:240ra74.

57. Gardoni F, Marcello E, Di Luca M. Postsynaptic density-membrane associated guanylate kinase proteins (PSD-MAGUKS) and their role in CNS disorders. *Neuroscience.* 2009;158:324–333.

58. Petitprez S, Zmoos AF, Ogrodnik J, et al. SAP97 and dystrophin macromolecular complexes determine two pools of cardiac sodium channels Nav1.5 in cardiomyocytes. *Circ Res.* 2011;108:294–304.

59. Godreau D, Vranckx R, Maguy A, et al. Expression, regulation and role of the MAGUK protein SAP-97 in human atrial myocardium. *Cardiovasc Res.* 2002;56:433–442.

60. Gee SH, Madhavan R, Levinson SR, et al. Interaction of muscle and brain sodium channels with multiple members of the syntrophin family of dystrophin-associated proteins. *J Neurosci.* 1998;18:128–137.

61. Shy D, Gillet L, Ogrodnik J, et al. PDZ domain-binding motif regulates cardiomyocyte compartment-specific NaV1.5 channel expression and function. *Circulation.* 2014;130:147–160.

62. Matamoros M, Pérez-Hernández M, Guerrero-Serna G, et al. Nav1.5 N-terminal domain binding to α1-syntrophin increases membrane density of human Kir2.1, Kir2.2 and Nav1.5 channels. *Cardiovasc Res.* 2016;110:279–290.

63. Ueda K, Valdivia C, Medeiros-Domingo A, et al. Syntrophin mutation associated with long QT syndrome through activation of the nNOS-SCN5A macromolecular complex. *Proc Natl Acad Sci U S A.* 2008;105:9355–9360.

64. Oceandy D, Cartwright EJ, Emerson M, et al. Neuronal nitric oxide synthase signaling in the heart is regulated by the sarcolemmal calcium pump 4b. *Circulation.* 2007;115:483–492.

65. Gillet L, Rougier JS, Shy D, et al. Cardiac-specific ablation of synapse-associated protein SAP97 in mice decreases potassium currents but not sodium current. *Heart Rhythm.* 2015;12:181–192.

66. Wang L, Piserchio A, Mierke DF. Structural characterization of the intermolecular interactions of synapse-associated protein-97 with the Nr2b subunit of N-methyl-d-aspartate receptors. *J Biol Chem.* 2005;280:26992–26996.

67. Cohen NA, Sha Q, Makhina EN, et al. Inhibition of an inward rectifier potassium channel (Kir2.3) by G-protein betagamma subunits. *J Biol Chem.* 1996;271:32301–32305.

68. Leonoudakis D, Conti LR, Radeke CM, et al. A multiprotein trafficking complex composed of SAP97, CASK, Veli, and Mint1 is associated with inward rectifier Kir2 potassium channels. *J Biol Chem.* 2004;279:19051–19063.

69. Leonoudakis D, Conti LR, Anderson S, et al. Protein trafficking and anchoring complexes revealed by proteomic analysis of inward rectifier potassium channel (Kir2.x)-associated proteins. *J Biol Chem.* 2004;279:22331–22346.

70. Hruska-Hageman AM, Benson CJ, Leonard AS, et al. Psd-95 and Lin-7b interact with acid-sensing ion channel-3 and have opposite effects on H+- gated current. *J Biol Chem.* 2004;279:46962–46968.

71. Lin Y, Skeberdis VA, Francesconi A, et al. Postsynaptic density protein-95 regulates NMDA channel gating and surface expression. *J Neurosci.* 2004;24:10138–10148.

72. Jugloff DG, Khanna R, Schlichter LC, et al. Internalization of the Kv1.4 potassium channel is suppressed by clustering interactions with PSD-95. *J Biol Chem.* 2000;275:1357–1364.

73. Leyland ML, Dart C. An alternatively spliced isoform of PSD-93/chapsyn 110 binds to the inwardly rectifying potassium channel, Kir2.1. *J Biol Chem.* 2004;279(42):43427–43436.

74. Caballero R, Pérez-Hernández M, Matamoros M, et al. Nav1.5 differentially regulates expression of Kir2.1 and Kir2.3 channels. *Heart Rhythm.* 2013;10:S394–S395.

75. Piao L, Li J, McLerie M, et al. Transgenic upregulation of IK1 in the mouse heart is proarrhythmic. *Basic Res Cardiol.* 2007;102:416–428.

76. Jordens I, Marsman M, Kuijl C, et al. Rab proteins, connecting transport and vesicle fusion. *Traffic.* 2005;6:1070–1077.

77. Mellman I. Endocytosis and molecular sorting. *Annu Rev Cell Dev Biol.* 1996;12:575–625.

78. Bendahhou S, Donaldson MR, Plaster NM, et al. Defective potassium channel Kir2.1 trafficking underlies Andersen-Tawil syndrome. *J Biol Chem.* 2003;278:51779–51785.

79. Li GR, Lau CP, Leung TK, et al. Ionic current abnormalities associated with prolonged action potentials in cardiomyocytes from diseased human right ventricles. *Heart Rhythm.* 2004;1:460–468.

80. Maltsev VA, Sabbab HN, Undrovinas AI. Down-regulation of sodium current in chronic heart failure: effect of long-term therapy with carvedilol. *Cell Mol Life Sci.* 2002;59:1561–1568.

22

The Intercalated Disc: A Molecular Network That Integrates Electrical Coupling, Intercellular Adhesion, and Cell Excitability

Marina Cerrone, Esperanza Agullo-Pascual, and Mario Delmar

Introduction and Historical Perspective

A heartbeat results from the added output of millions of cells that contract in synchrony. To achieve this function, complex molecular networks work in concert, with exquisite temporal precision. The accurate timing of the molecular events demands a comparable precision on the location of each molecule within the cell. Indeed, molecular networks organize within well-confined microdomains, where physical proximity allows for prompt and efficient interaction. In turn, the loss of molecular organization at a nanoscale can be a core component in the pathophysiology of a disease.

This chapter focuses on the intercalated disc, a region of specialization formed at the end–end site of contact between cardiomyocytes (CMs). When first observed using light microscopy (in 1866), the intercalated disc was considered "a cementing material" at cardiac cell boundaries. The 1893 article by Przewoski "Du mode de reunion des cellules myocardiques de l'homme adulte" supported the idea that the intercalated disc was necessary for cell–cell adhesion. However, the scientific community at the time was divided on whether cardiac cells were separate from each other or fused into a single syncytium. The latter hypothesis was in fact favored by most during the early twentieth century. The advent of electron microscopy tilted and eventually settled this debate. The studies of Sjostrand and Andersson[1] and others showed that the intercalated disc consisted of a double membrane, flanked by the termination of myofibrils in the dense material. Their observations led Muir[2] to conclude that "the discs represent the junctions between neighboring cardiac muscle cells." He also wrote "... there is no valid

evidence to contest the statement that the intercalated discs are specialized regions of cellular adhesion." Since then and as a result of the pioneering electrophysiological experiments of Weidmann[3] and other ultrastructural observations,[4] the intercalated disc has been recognized as an area of specialization that provides a physical continuum between cardiac cells through mechanical junctions (desmosomes, adherens junctions, and area composita) and intercellular channels (gap junctions).

The availability of immunofluorescence microscopy demonstrated that other molecular complexes, not detectable by electron microscopy, are also present in the intercalated disc. Of particular relevance to this chapter is the fact that channel protein complexes involved in both depolarization and repolarization localize preferentially to the intercalated disc. This physical proximity allows for a key functional consequence: molecules traditionally defined as junctional, such as connexin43 (Cx43) and plakophilin-2 (PKP2), actually regulate the function of ion channels responsible for the action potential. In turn, molecules accessory to ion channels are also relevant for cell adhesion and for gap junction function.[5–7] When taken together, the data support the notion that the intercalated disc is not just the site of residence of independent "junctional" and "nonjunctional" complexes that are oblivious to the presence and function of others. It is, rather, the home of a protein-interacting network (a "connexome"[8]) where molecules multitask to achieve jointly, intimately related functions—that is, the entry and exit of charges into cells, transfer of charges between cells, and anchoring of cells to each other; this provides a mechanically stable environment critical for ion channel functions.

In the following sections, we will update the current knowledge on the composition of selected molecular complexes of the intercalated disc, their interactions, and the possible mechanisms by which the dysfunction of intercalated disc molecules may lead to arrhythmia. In the end, we converge with other investigators to challenge the notions that (1) connexins are only involved in the formation of gap junctions, (2) sodium channels are only important for single cell excitability, (3) desmosomal molecules are only relevant to cell adhesion, and (4) it is only through modifications of those functions that these proteins participate in the genesis of lethal cardiac arrhythmias or are potentially valuable as targets for antiarrhythmic therapy.

Intercalated Disc Proteins in Inherited and Acquired Diseases

The function of intercalated disc components is relevant not only to normal physiology but also to the understanding of disease. It is not the purpose of this chapter to review clinical aspects of arrhythmias. But it seems worth mentioning at the outset selected examples where novel findings regarding intercalated disc biology may provide insight into arrhythmia mechanisms.

Initial studies on the relationship between desmosome integrity and cardiac electrophysiology were propelled by the finding that most familial cases of arrhythmogenic right ventricular

THE INTER

interacting with
interact with ior
disc.

Desmosom
Sodium Cha

The observation
whether Cx43 i
ogy that interac
tion of the VGS
its possible cros
CMs were treate
trol cells were t

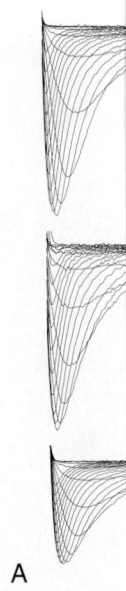

A

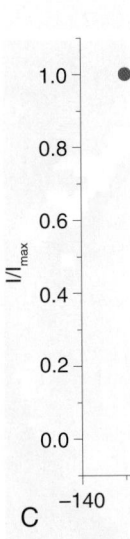

C

cardiomyopathy (ARVC), where a genetic link has been found, associate with mutations in genes that code for desmosomal molecules (reviewed in Corrado and Thiene[9]). The latter brought forth the question of how a molecule, considered purely relevant to cell adhesion, altered the electrical behavior of the heart. The associations between desmosomal proteins and ion channel function (particularly the sodium current [I_{Na}]) are extensively reviewed in this chapter. (Of note, a recent publication refers to this disease as "arrhythmogenic cardiomyopathy" [AC] to denote the occurrence of left ventricular involvement.[9])

A number of studies have demonstrated the remodeling of gap junction proteins (in particular Cx43) in a number of inherited and acquired arrhythmia-related diseases (e.g., see references[10–14]). The Fishman laboratory provided evidence that aberrant posttranslational phosphorylation of Cx43 could be the common pathway that leads to pathological gap junction remodeling and arrhythmias.[11,15] While the relationship between Cx43 remodeling and arrhythmia exists, it is unclear whether these arrhythmias are exclusively consequential to changes in the gap junction formation.[16] Recent data show that reduced Cx43 expression alters sodium and potassium current function, and these changes could become part of the arrhythmogenic substrate.[17–19]

Disruption of the voltage-gated sodium channel (VGSC) complex is considered an important molecular substrate for arrhythmogenesis. Extensive reviews on the relationship between mutations in proteins of the VGSC complex and arrhythmias are available (e.g., see Wilde and Brugada[20]). Of particular interest in the context of this review is the observation that the haploinsufficiency of a desmosomal protein or the overexpression of a mutant desmosomal protein lead to I_{Na} deficit and increased arrhythmia susceptibility.[21,22]

The latter brings back the previously formulated concept that ARVC and Brugada syndrome (a channelopathy caused by mutations on genes of the VGSC complex) share common features.[23]

Structural Features of the Intercalated Disc

In its classical definition, the intercalated disc is composed of three electron-dense structures: adherens junctions, desmosomes, and gap junctions (Fig. 22.1). Additional reviews on the characteristics of these structures can be found elsewhere (e.g., see references[24,25]). These structures are described briefly later, and the structural/molecular definition of the intercalated disc is expanded to include the area composita, intercellular space, and "nonjunctional" ion channel complexes.

Adherens Junctions

Adherens junctions are specialized structures essential for the mechanical coupling between neighboring cells. The three morphologically different forms of adherens junctions are puncta adherentia, zonula adherens, and fascia adherens, the last name corresponding to the morphology found in the cardiac intercalated disc.[26] Cell–cell mechanical anchoring occurs at two crucial points: the extracellular space, within which cadherins tightly bind to each other, and the intracellular space, within which the cytoplasmic end of the cadherin is indirectly attached to the actin cytoskeleton. The association between cadherins and the cytoskeleton involves at least two molecular "hinges." Cadherin binds to β-catenin and plakoglobin, and both molecules in turn bind to α-catenin (among others), the latter being in direct contact with actin. However, this is only a simplified

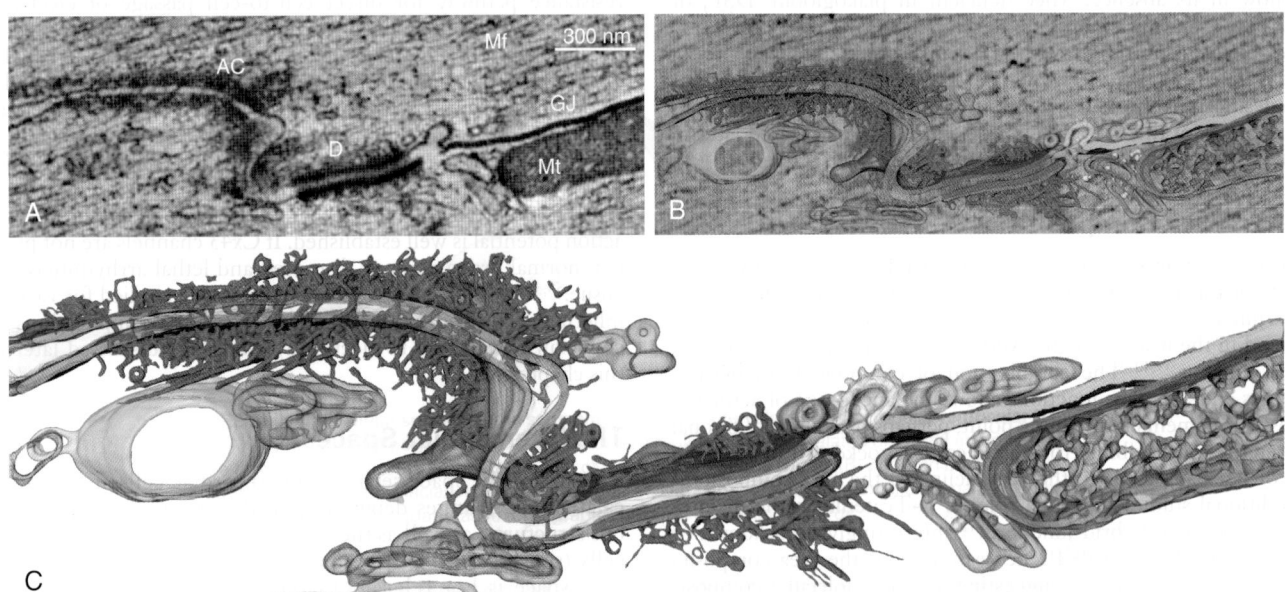

FIGURE 22.1 Electron microscopy tomography section and three-dimensional (3D)-rendered representation of a portion of an intercalated disc from mouse ventricular tissues. (A) An XY virtual section of a tomogram is shown. Different typical intercalated disc structures (desmosome [*D*], gap junction [*GJ*], and area composita [*AC*]) as well as other structures typically present in myocytes (myofibrils [*Mf*] and mitochondria [*Mt*]) are visible. (B) Overlay of the tomographic slice and 3D-rendered models, resulting from the segmentation of different structures of interest: cellular membranes forming the intercalated disc (*red*); a gap junction (*light pink*); a budding vesicle (*white*) with a rough surface (possibly clatherin coating) between a desmosome and gap junction; a complex network of filaments adjacent to the desmosome and area composita (*dark blue*); tubular and cisternae structures that form an intricate connected network in close proximity to the intercalated disc (*light blue*), often decorated with electron-dense particles, of dimensions compatible with ribosomes (*yellow*); a multivesicular body (*green*); and a mitochondrion (*magenta*) in close contact with the gap junction. (C) 3D-rendered model of all structures of interest segmented in the tomogram, where all spatial interrelations are observed. (Modified from Leo-Macias A, Liang FX, Delmar M. Ultrastructure of the intercellular space in adult murine ventricle revealed by quantitative tomographic electron microscopy. *Cardiovasc Res.* 2015;107:442-452.)

associated w
cause a redu
diseases, suc
duction defe
atrial fibrilla
spectrum tha
and may ma
same family.
linked to a
dence of atri

β-Subunits
The Na$_V$ β-s
are coded by
gle-span trar
minus facing
presents a co
the one in
associates wi
gether, β-sul
VGSC mult
those relevar
cells.[75] Furtl
that null mic
SCN5A mRI
did not affec
disc; on the
the T-tubule
observed. Tl
homeostasis.
of β-subunits
the data sho
β-subunits ca
the regulatio
function and

**Subcellular
Channel**
Recent studi
surface of th
tion and func
on whether
the midsectio
two separate
two subpopu
cytes, where
the second su
disc, where N
and ZO1, as
the Abriel lab
sion or the d
not affect the
SAP97 expre
for Na$_V$1.5 i
colleagues[79])
Lin and a
bution of Na
Using cell-a
showed that
disc than at
resistant char
tive shift in t
these channe
resting poter
channels at t
strated that tl
paired, stron
sodium chan

of intercellular junctions (PKP2) and another complex primarily involved in supporting cell excitability (the VGSC complex). The results supported the hypothesis that arrhythmias that occur in patients with ARVC may have as a substrate not only changes in the macroscopic architecture of the tissue (as would be expected once the fibrofatty infiltrations populate the heart) or in the integrity of intercellular coupling but also changes in the electrical properties of CMs. Of relevance, these results revealed that a property "of the single cell" (excitability; I_{Na}) is in fact subject to modulation by proteins classically defined as belonging to the "group" of intercellular junction molecules.

PKP2 mutations associated with ARVC have all been found in only one allele. We therefore characterized the relationship between PKP2 abundance and sodium current function in mice haploinsufficient for the pkp2 gene (PKP2-Hz).[21] Of note, one of the most common mutations in PKP2 is the presence of a stop codon at amino acid position 79 (R79x).[100] This early truncation is functionally equivalent to haploinsufficiency.[101] Patch clamp experiments showed decreased amplitude (Fig. 22.5A) and a shift in gating and kinetics of I_{Na} in PKP2-Hz myocytes compared with those in control myocytes. To further unmask I_{Na} deficiency, we exposed myocytes, Langendorff-perfused hearts, and anesthetized animals to a pharmacological challenge (flecainide). The extent of the flecainide-induced I_{Na} block, impaired ventricular conduction, and altered electrocardiographic parameters were larger in PKP2-Hz hearts than in control hearts. As shown in Fig. 22.5B and C and described by Cerrone and associates,[21] flecainide provoked ventricular arrhythmias and death in PKP2-Hz

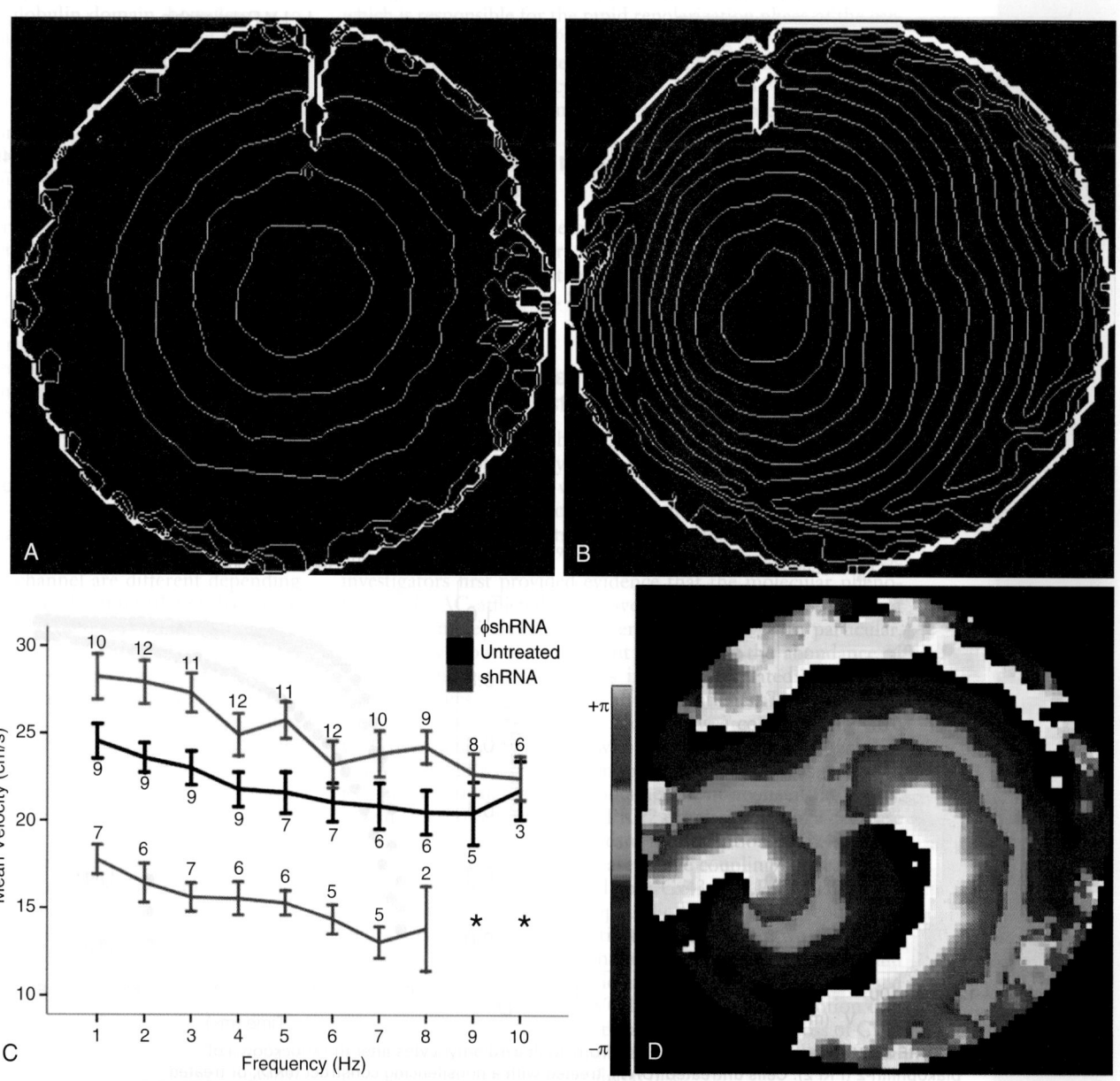

FIGURE 22.4 Optical mapping of action potential propagation in monolayers of neonatal rat ventricular myocytes. Isochrone maps from monolayers treated with a nonsilencing construct (A) or silenced for plakophilin-2 (PKP2) (B). Conduction velocity as a function of pacing frequency illustrated in (C). A phase map of spontaneous reentrant activity in a PKP2-deficient monolayer is illustrated in (D). (From Sato PY, Musa H, Coombs W, et al. Loss of plakophilin-2 expression leads to decreased sodium current and slower conduction velocity in cultured cardiac myocytes. *Circ Res.* 2009;105:523-526.)

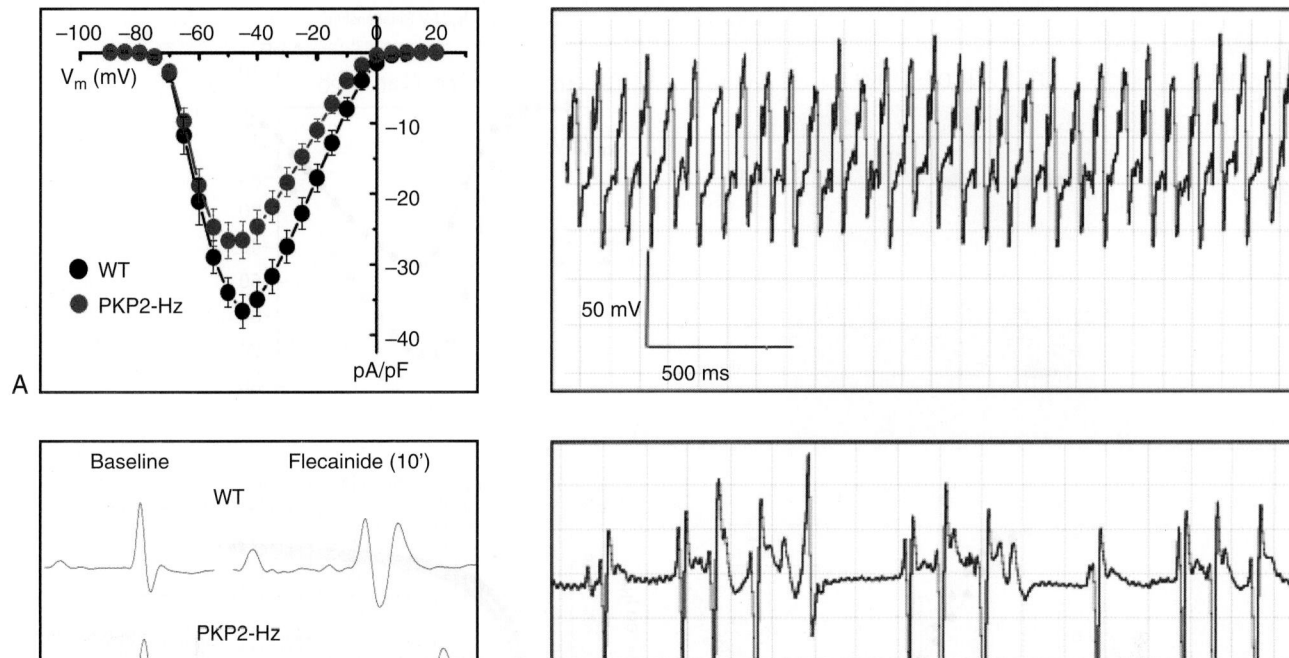

FIGURE 22.5 Electrocardiographic features of plakophilin-2 (*PKP2*)-Hz mice at baseline and in response to flecainide. (A) Average peak sodium current density as a function of voltage command in wild-type (*WT*) (*black*) and PKP2-Hz (*red*) myocytes. (B) Examples of electrocardiogram traces from WT (*top*) and PKP2-Hz (*bottom*) mice. Recordings obtained at baseline (*left*) and 10 minutes after flecainide administration (40 mg/Kg i.p., *right*). (C) Ventricular tachycardia in PKP2-Hz mice. Overall, the flecainide caused a prolongation of the P and QRS durations and of the PR and QTc intervals that were significantly more pronounced in the PKP2-Hz mice than in the control mice. Six out of 12 PKP2-Hz mice showed ventricular arrhythmias. None of the tested 11 WT mice showed ventricular arrhythmias. Arrhythmic death occurred in three PKP2-Hz mice and none in the control mice. (From Cerrone M, Noorman M, Lin X, et al. Sodium current deficit and arrhythmogenesis in a murine model of plakophilin-2 haploinsufficiency. *Cardiovasc Res.* 2012;95:460-468.)

mice but not in the wild-type mice. These results showed that PKP2 haploinsufficiency led to an I_{Na} deficit in murine hearts, thus documenting for the first time the relationship between the "desmosomal molecule" PKP2 and the VGSC complex in a living heart. Our results supported the contention that I_{Na} dysfunction may contribute to the generation and/or maintenance of arrhythmias in patients with desmosomal deficiencies.

The relationship between desmosomal molecules and VGSC has also been demonstrated in mice that overexpress a desmoglein-2 (DSG-2) mutation.[22] This is a very interesting model, given that severe arrhythmias and sudden death in these mice often occur prior to structural damage; the latter mimics a phenomenon often observed in humans affected with AC, where arrhythmias and/or electrocardiographic changes have been described early in the history of the disease before any overt structural changes in the myocardium.[24,58,102] Electrophysiological analysis of these DSG-2 transgenic mutant mice revealed prolonged ventricular activation time, decreased conduction velocity in both longitudinal and transverse directions, and increased arrhythmia susceptibility, prior to signs of fibrosis or necrosis in the myocardium. The authors also observed a decrease in maximal upstroke velocity and decreased I_{Na} amplitude. Altogether, the data demonstrate that a decrease in PKP2 abundance,[21] as well as the overexpression of a DSG-2 mutation,[22] lead to impaired I_{Na} function in hearts with no histological features of ARVC. These data demonstrate the interaction between desmosomal molecules and VGSC in vivo and suggest

that as originally proposed by our laboratory,[78] impaired sodium current may be a substrate for lethal arrhythmias in the concealed phase of ARVC. More recent studies have confirmed these observations.[103]

The question remains as to whether other desmosomal proteins also interact with $Na_V1.5$ and whether these interactions occur in the human heart. Gomes and coworkers[104] reported that mice haploinsufficient for DSP present an average peak I_{Na} density similar to that in control mice; yet, careful analysis of their results suggests the possibility of technical limitations in their voltage clamp recordings, which could have masked small differences between the groups (discussed in Cerrone and colleagues[21]). On the other hand, in the same study, the authors showed that patients with heterozygous mutations in DSP and without overt structural disease had significant regional conduction delays and heterogeneous $Na_V1.5$ distribution.

Connexin43 Regulates Sodium and Potassium Currents

The loss of Cx43 expression leads to propagation block and arrhythmias. Interpretation of this result has centered mostly on the role of Cx43 as the pore-forming subunit of gap junctions. However, the latter does not exclude the possibility that Cx43 could also interact with other channel complexes and affect their function. In fact, there is no reason to confine Cx43 to a single task in a single structure.

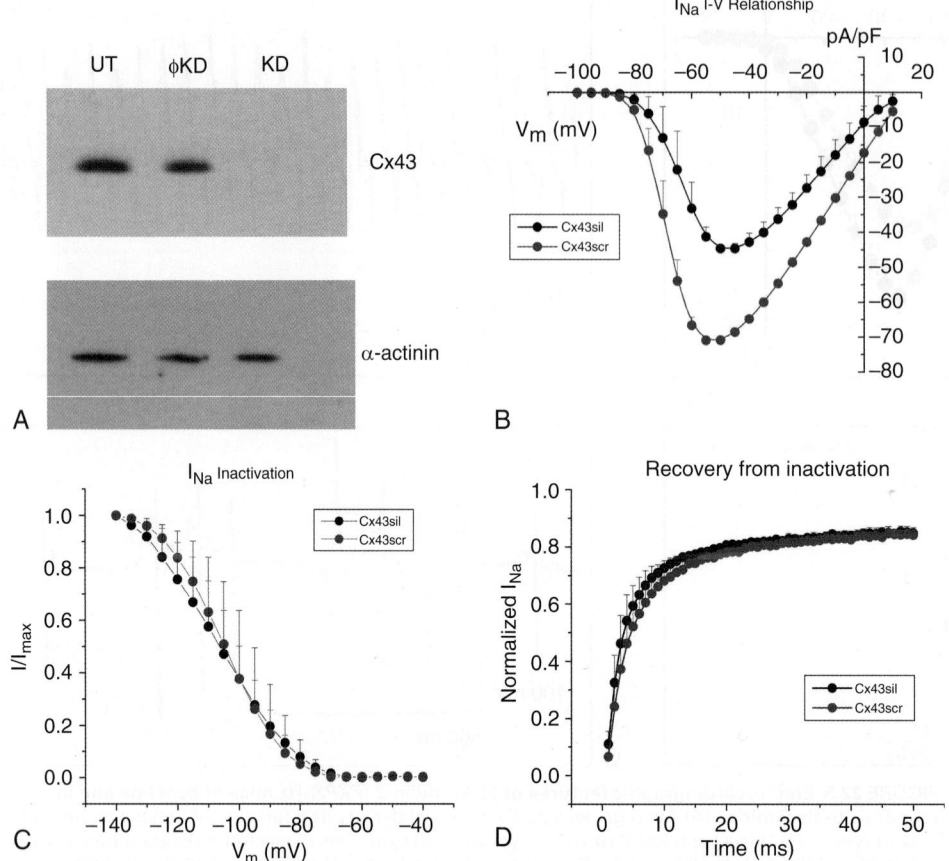

FIGURE 22.6 Decreased Cx43 expression leads to reduced sodium current (I_{Na}) in isolated adult rat ventricular myocytes. (A) Western blot for Cx43 in cells untreated (*UT*), treated with an oligonucleotide that prevented Cx43 expression (*KD*), or a nontargeting construct (*φKD*). (B) Peak sodium current density was lower in cells that lack Cx43. (C) and (D) Loss of Cx43 expression did not affect steady-state inactivation or recovery from inactivation kinetics. (From Jansen JA, Noorman M, Musa H, et al. Reduced heterogeneous expression of Cx43 results in decreased Na$_V$1.5 expression and reduced sodium current that accounts for arrhythmia vulnerability in conditional Cx43 knockout mice. *Heart Rhythm*. 2012;9:600-607.)

The first indication of an interaction between Cx43 and other ion channel complexes came from the work of Malhotra and associates, which showed the coprecipitation of Na$_V$1.5 with Cx43.[105] The physical proximity of these molecules was observed by Rhett and colleagues,[106] although their association occurs outside the domain of the gap junction plaque (see "The Connexome, Visual Proteomics, and the Existence of 'Mini-Nodes of Ranvier' at the Intercalated Disc"). Not only are Cx43 and Na$_V$1.5 in close proximity, but also these two molecules are functionally intertwined. Indeed, as shown in Fig. 22.6, Jansen and associates reported that the siRNA-mediated loss of Cx43 expression in adult ventricular myocytes led to a decrease in the amplitude of I_{Na}.[18] The functional effect coincided with decreased colocalization of Cx43 and Na$_V$1.5 at the intercalated disc. A similar decrease in I_{Na} was later reported by Desplantez and colleagues in fetal atrial myocytes of Cx43-deficient mice.[19] Overall, the data demonstrate that Cx43 expression is necessary for proper sodium current function and for the accumulation of Na$_V$1.5 at the cardiac intercalated disc.[107]

VGSC is not the only electrically functional complex of the intercalated disc that is disrupted subsequent to the loss of Cx43 expression. In fact, the first report that correlated Cx43 expression to nonjunctional currents was by Danik and associates.[17] These authors noted that the action potential duration recorded from the ventricles of Cx43 conditional knockout animals were

significantly shorter than that from control animals. This shortening was associated with higher levels of sustained repolarizing current and higher levels of inward rectifier current in myocytes from RV. Overall, the data show that Cx43 is not only a gap junction–forming molecule in the heart but also a component of a molecular network that regulates excitability and repolarization.

Cx43 as a Microtubule Anchoring Point and the Control of Sodium Current Amplitude

The observations described later related to the complete loss of Cx43 expression. More recently, Lübkemeier and coworkers reported that a cardiac-specific, tamoxifen-activated knock-in murine model of a Cx43 mutation caused sudden death in the absence of a structural disease.[108] The mutation in question was a loss of the last five amino acids of the Cx43 sequence (i.e., truncation Cx43D378stop). The original thought was to create a murine model where Cx43 could not bind to the PDZ domain–containing protein (particularly, ZO-1). The results were surprising in two fronts. First, the association between Cx43 and ZO-1 was unaffected by the mutation. Second, the mice died because of ventricular fibrillation within 3 weeks of tamoxifen administration. A detailed analysis showed that the Cx43D378stop mutation did not affect the formation or function of gap junctions. On the other hand, there was a significant reduction in both sodium and potassium currents. Subsequent studies that utilized superresolution microscopy showed that the Cx43D378stop mutation altered the anchoring of the microtubule plus end to the N-cadherin-rich region of the cell end, thus impairing the microtubule-mediated delivery of $Na_V1.5$ and consequently caused a reduction in the sodium current amplitude (Fig. 22.7).[43] Immunoelectron microscopy imaging demonstrated that Cx43 was not only located at the interplicate region (forming gap junctions) but also in the plicate region of the intercalated disc in the area heavily populated by adhesion molecules, where it likely contributed to the targeted delivery of Nav1.5 by microtubules (Fig. 22.8). Targeted delivery has been demonstrated previously both for the intercalated disc[109] and T-tubular domain of CMs.[110]

AnkG and Cx43 Are Necessary to Maintain Intercellular Adhesion

In the earlier sections, we described that desmosome molecules, relevant to intercellular adhesion (namely PKP2 and DSG-2), are actually important to preserve I_{Na} amplitude and electrical coupling between cardiac cells. If the system works as a unit, decreased protein levels of either Cx43 or a component of VGSC would in turn affect the intercellular adhesion strength. Consistent with this hypothesis, we showed that the intercellular adhesion strength is decreased in the monolayers of neonatal rat ventricular myocytes treated with siRNA to prevent AnkG expression.[107] Similarly, the loss of Cx43 expression in cultured cells significantly impaired the

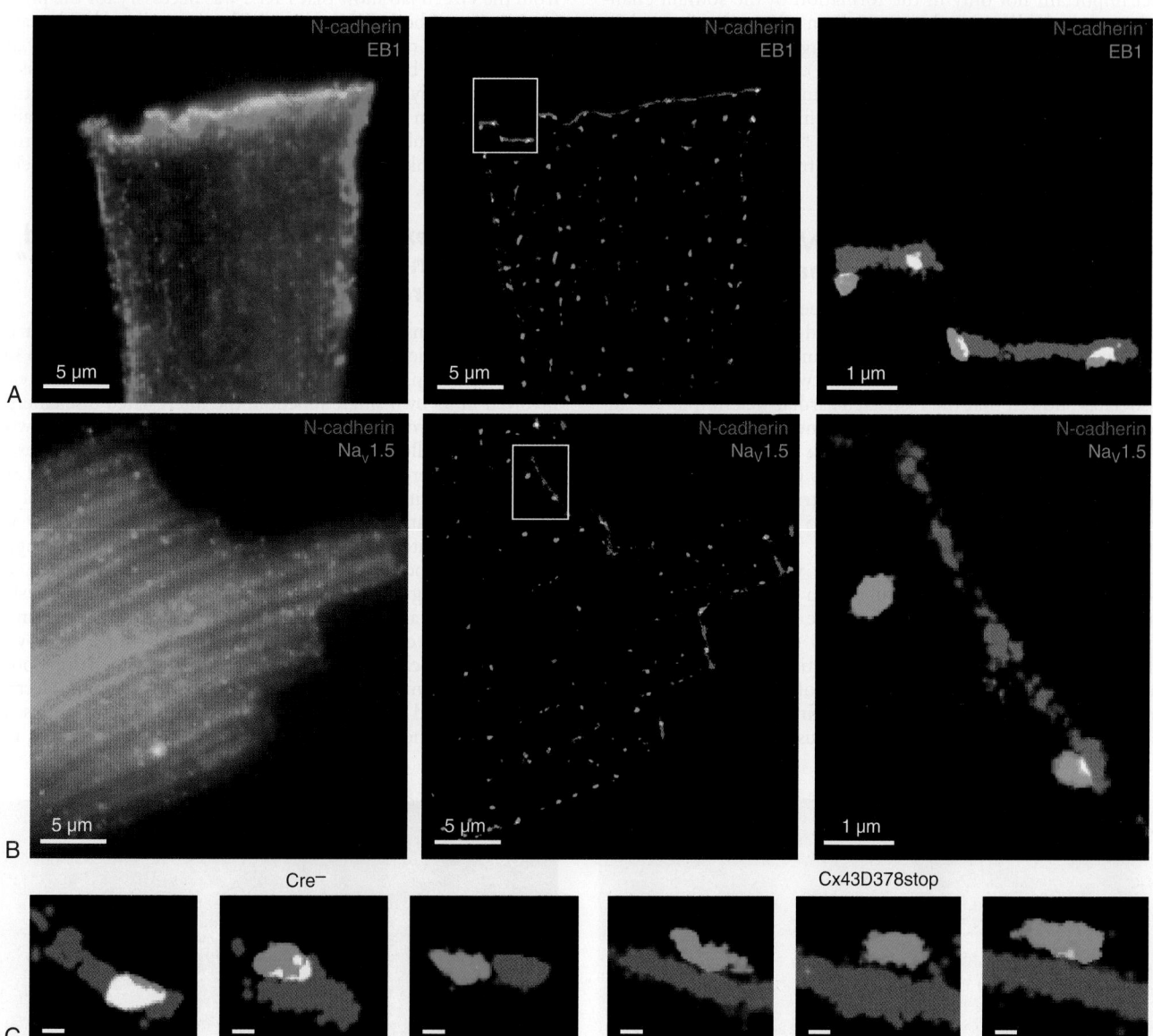

FIGURE 22.7 Localization of N-cadherin, EB1, and Na$_V$1.5 in adult mouse ventricular myocytes.
(A) N-cadherin (*magenta*) and EB1 (*green*) labeling. *Left panel* shows total internal reflection fluorescence (TIRF) image generated by the projection of 2000 frames collected to generate the superresolution fluorescence microscopy (SRFM) image. *Central panel* shows same region by SRFM. *White box* is enlarged in the *right panel*. (B) TIRF (*left*) and SRFM (*middle*) images of N-cadherin (*magenta*) and Na$_V$1.5 (*green*). Inset is enlarged in the *right panel*. (C) Enlargement shows proximity between N-cadherin and Na$_V$1.5 clusters at the intercalated disc in Cre⁻ myocytes compared with Cx43D378stop. Scale bar: 200 nm. (Modified from Agullo-Pascual E, Lin X, Leo-Macias A, et al. Super-resolution imaging reveals that loss of the C-terminus of connexin43 limits microtubule plus-end capture and Na$_V$1.5 localization at the intercalated disc. *Cardiovasc Res.* 2014;104:371-381.)

intercellular adhesion strength,[7] a result consistent with previous observations.[111]

The "α Personality" of the β-Subunit: Intercellular Adhesion Strength

The finding that mutations in desmosomal molecules associate with familial cases of ARVC has brought to light the important link between cell adhesion and sodium channel function. Yet, in retrospect, the link between these two seemingly unrelated functions was first established several years ago by the Isom lab, after they isolated and discovered the β-1-subunit of the sodium channel.[112,113] They subsequently demonstrated that "sodium channel β-subunits" also mediate cell adhesion,[114] a fact important not only in the formation of the sodium channel complex[114,115] but also in sodium channel-independent functions such as cell migration, cell aggregation, and interaction with the cytoskeleton (see Isom[116]). Studies that followed demonstrated their critical role in cancer (see Brackenbury and Isom[117] for review). Overall, these findings emphasize that cataloging molecules as "adhesion" or "sodium channel complex" is artificial and in fact, incorrect from a functional point of view.

Other Intercellular Adhesion Molecules That Crosstalk With Cardiac Ion Channels

Two other adhesion molecules have been associated with cardiac electrical function: N-cadherin, and the coxsackievirus and adenovirus receptor (CAR). N-cadherin is well recognized as critical to the mechanical coupling between cells. Yet, Li and associates showed that the restricted cardiac deletion of N-cadherin also led to severe arrhythmias and a loss of Cx43 from the intercalated disc.[118] The Radice lab reported that in addition to the effects on coupling, the loss of N-cadherin led to a decreased density of the repolarizing current $I_{K,slow}$, concurrent with the decreased expressions of $K_V1.5$ and its accessory protein Kcne2.[84]

CAR is another case of a molecule whose identity is burdened by its birth name. Undoubtedly a receptor for both coxsackievirus and adenovirus, studies have demonstrated that the immunoglobulin extracellular domains of CAR were capable of homophilic binding and could participate in intercellular adhesion in epithelial cells. The role of this molecule in cell adhesion in the heart is less well defined. Interestingly, the cardiac-restricted deletion of CAR causes significant slowing

of the atrioventricular (AV) propagation and disruption of gap junctions at the intercalated disc.[119,120] Separate studies show that a loss of CAR expression causes a significant reduction in the sodium current amplitude, specifically at the intercalated disc.[121]

The Intercalated Disc and the Intracellular Signaling Platforms

A function-beyond-adhesion well known to mechanical junctions is that of supporting intracellular signaling platforms. While this has been extensively described for the cadherin-catenin axis,[122] it has not been until recently that the role of PKP2 in intracellular signaling has been brought to light. In particular, studies from the Green lab show that PKP2 was necessary for the proper functioning of both PKCα[123] and RhoA signaling.[124] The latter may play a key role in the activation of the Hippo pathway and Wnt signaling, both potentially involved in the pathogenesis of AC.[54] Separately, work from the Mohler lab has shown that the ankyrin/spectrin core at the intercalated disc scaffolds a signaling platform to regulate cardiac excitability.[125] Interestingly, a crosstalk between AnkG and PKP2-supported platforms was unveiled by these studies.

The Connexome, Visual Proteomics, and the Existence of "Mini-Nodes of Ranvier" at the Intercalated Disc

The observations described throughout this chapter disrupt the notion that molecules can be classified as only belonging to one functional group. Rather than silos of molecular complexes each involved in its own single function, the intercalated disc emerges as a complex protein-interacting network where molecules work together to collectively achieve electrical coupling, cell excitability, and intercellular adhesion strength. We have named this protein-interacting network the "connexome" (Fig. 22.9). Its physical localization is a matter of active investigation.[106,126] We have implemented a combination of superresolution imaging techniques to localize clusters of $Na_V1.5$ in the intercalated disc domain (see Agullo-Pascual and colleagues[43] and unpublished results). Using a "visual proteomics" approach, implementing a combination of correlative light-electron microscopy, angle-view scanning patch clamp, three-dimensional direct stochastic optical reconstruction microscopy, focused ion beam–scanning electron microscopy, and Monte-Carlo and random-walk simulations, we reached the conclusion that $Na_V1.5$ organizes into clusters that

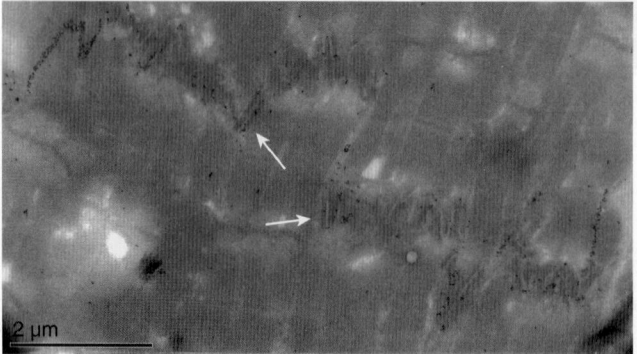

FIGURE 22.8 Immunoelectron microscopy of mouse adult ventricular intercalated disc decorated with gold particles targeting Cx43. Notice the abundant clustering along gap junctions but also at areas with clear intercellular space (*arrows*). (From Agullo-Pascual E, Lin X, Leo-Macias A, et al. Super-resolution imaging reveals that loss of the C-terminus of connexin43 limits microtubule plus-end capture and Na$_V$1.5 localization at the intercalated disc. *Cardiovasc Res.* 2014;104:371-381.)

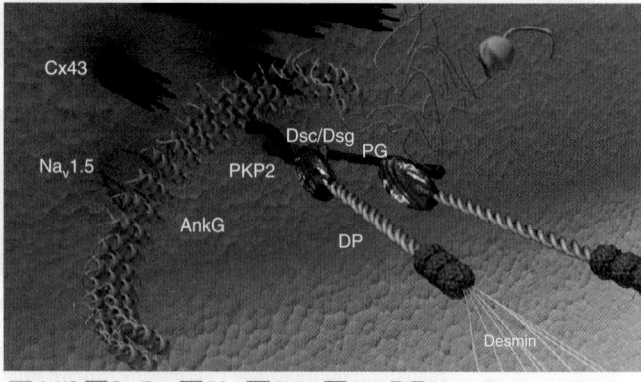

FIGURE 22.9 Diagrammatic representation of the potential interactions between the voltage-gated sodium channel, gap junctions, and desmosomes. (From Sato PY, Coombs W, Lin X, Nekrasova O, et al. Interactions between ankyrin-G, plakophilin-2, and connexin43 at the cardiac intercalated disc. *Circ Res.* 2011;109:193-201.)

gather adjacent to N-cadherin-rich domains, likely at the area composita. These nodes that contain both adhesion and excitability molecules are reminiscent of the nodes of Ranvier, as well as the axon initial segment, where Nav channels are packed into clusters in close association with adhesion molecules.[127] As in the case of neurons,[128] AnkG may be critical for the organization of the structure and retention of channels within the tightly packed node. Additional preliminary studies from our lab suggest that the interaction between sodium channels and adhesion molecules is also present in cardiac costameres, forming nodes that contain $Na_V1.5$ and dystroglycan (unpublished) and are likely supported by the syntrophin/dystrophin complex, which is well known to be involved in the regulation of the sodium channel.[77,80] Previous studies have shown that sodium channels are mechanosensitive.[129] Our observations are consistent with this notion and suggest that the association of the points of mechanical anchoring is important for mechanical stability and therefore electrical function.

The Mini-Node of Ranvier and the Possibility of Ephaptic Transmission

Several mathematical models of cardiac action potential propagation assume that gap junctions are the only path for the transfer of charge between cells. Accordingly, they predict that decreases in junctional conductance result in decreases in conduction velocity. This notion contrasts sharply with actual data that show that only extreme reductions in Cx43 abundance (and electrical coupling) lead to significant changes in conduction velocity.[55,97,130] These results have given new impetus to the notion that under poor gap junction–mediated coupling, propagation can be maintained via a separate "electric field mechanism,"[60,61,63,131] also referred to as "ephaptic transmission."[63,67] This alternative postulates that the large I_{Na} in the proximal side of an intercellular cleft generates a negative extracellular potential within the cleft, which depolarizes the distal membrane and activates its sodium channels. Thus propagation can continue downstream in the absence of gap junctions provided there is a large I_{Na} at the intercalated disc and a narrow intercellular cleft that separates the two apposing cells.

The success or failure of propagation under the model described earlier depends heavily on the dimensions of the intercellular cleft at the site where the sodium channel clusters are located and on the dimensions of the sodium channel cluster itself (and hence the current density that it can generate). It was not until recently that a three-dimensional reconstruction of the intercellular space at the intercalated disc was generated[66] (see Fig. 22.2). The results of Leo-Macias and colleagues show that the intercellular cleft in the vicinity of adhesion complexes was approximately 90 nm. Unpublished observations from our laboratory indicate that this is also the position of the mini-node of Ranvier, described earlier. A quick analysis of published literature suggests that 90 nm is too large a cleft to enable ephaptic transmission. On the other hand, Gourdie and Poelzing used a different experimental approach to explore sodium channel localization; these authors reached the conclusion that sodium channels organized in the periphery of gap junction plaques, separated by gaps of 30 nm or less and therefore within distances permissive of electric field–mediated charge transmission.[67] These seemingly discrepant results demonstrate the need for further studies. Most importantly, they highlight the fact that solving the molecular organization of the intercalated disc is crucial for the advancement of our understanding of cell–cell communication and action potential propagation in the heart.

Brugada Syndrome and Arrhythmogenic Cardiomyopathy: Bookends of a Common Spectrum

The evidence provided by different studies,[78,107] showing that PKP2 not only participates in intercellular coupling but also interacts with the VGSC complex, brought us to postulate that some mutations in PKP2 could cause decreased sodium current availability and enhanced propensity for arrhythmias even in the absence of structural cardiomyopathic changes typical of AC. Loss-of-function of the sodium channel has been associated with Brugada syndrome, an inherited condition characterized by a grossly normal structured heart and an increased risk for ventricular fibrillation.[132] Mutations on the *SCN5a* gene, coding for $Na_V1.5$, account for the majority of genotype-positive cases of Brugada syndrome. Our group speculated that some mutations in PKP2 could cause decreased sodium current and yield a Brugada syndrome phenotype in the absence of overt cardiomyopathic changes. Indeed, by sequencing the DNA of 200 patients affected by Brugada syndrome and having a negative genotype, Cerrone and associates detected novel missense mutations on the PKP2 gene in five patients. They showed that when these mutants were transiently expressed in HL-1 cells deficient in native PKP2, they caused a decrease in the sodium current amplitude, while transfection with the wild-type PKP2 rescued the current to normal values.[133] These findings were further supported by experiments in induced pluripotent stem (iPS) cell–derived human CMs from a patient carrying a complete loss-of-function in PKP2 and affected by AC. Human CMs (that did not have PKP2) showed a decreased sodium current. The current was rescued by the transfection of wild-type PKP2, whereas transfection with one PKP2 mutant linked to Brugada syndrome was unable to restore it. For the first time, these experiments provided evidence that not only the complete loss of PKP2 but also specific single amino acid mutations could affect the sodium channel function, resulting in an arrhythmic phenotype. Interestingly, when Brugada syndrome was initially described, it was suggested that this condition shared features with AC. Additionally, although structural cardiomyopathy is not part of the typical Brugada syndrome spectrum, it has been shown that some patients may have minor structural anomalies and localized RV fibrosis. On the other end of the spectrum, there have been several reports of patients affected by AC, with an occurrence of fatal or nearly fatal ventricular fibrillation before any fibrofatty infiltration was detected. The evidence of a possible common genetic substrate supports the concept that the two phenotypes could be at the boundaries of a shared common condition, whose aspects range from an increased arrhythmic propensity to structural fibrotic damage. This concept is further supported by the evidence that specific *SCN5a* mutations could yield a dilated cardiomyopathy phenotype in the absence of electrocardiogram (ECG) changes that are known for Brugada syndrome. It remains unclear how mutations in the sodium channel could lead to structural damages in the myocardium. Based on the crosstalk between intercalated disc structures described in this chapter, we are tempted to speculate that the integrity of the sodium channel complex is also relevant to the intercellular adhesion strength (e.g., see references[21,22,107]).

Conclusions

Through the previous sections, we have summarized evidence that shows that molecules classically defined as belonging to mechanical junctions, VGSC and gap junctions, interact with each other. We have also described how through these interactions, the function of one complex is altered by changes in the expression of molecules of a different group. The evidence suggests that intercalated disc molecules are not necessarily constrained to a single function (e.g., Cx43 is not only limited to making gap junctions). Rather, we propose that the molecules of the intercalated disc multitask within a protein-interacting network (the connexome), working in concert toward one common function: the propagation of excitatory current from one cell to the next. From this perspective, Cx43 is a molecule that is relevant to cell excitability (by modulating I_{Na}),[18,19] sodium channels can support cell–cell electrical coupling and intercellular adhesion strength,[60,61] and "adhesion molecules" are actually required for the proper functioning of electrical complexes.[21] The results have important consequences in translational medicine. We questioned whether the anatomy of the intercalated disc is compatible with the notion of ephaptic transmission. Furthermore, we demonstrated that Brugada syndrome and AC are not completely separate diseases but rather are bookends of a common spectrum. We also propose that cardiomyopathies consequent to mutations in the gene that codes for Na$_V$1.5 may result, at least in part, from a deficiency in intercellular adhesion strength. Noncanonical functions of intercalated disc molecules and the concept of a connexome can help in our understanding of the molecular bases of disease. Overall, the implication of these interactions to the understanding of arrhythmia mechanisms and treatments emerges as an exciting area of future investigation.

Acknowledgments

Supported by grants RO1-HL106632 and RO1-GM67691 from the National Institutes of Health (MD), a Foundation Leducq Transatlantic Network (MD). A Scientist Development Grant (14SDG18580014) from the American Heart Association (MC) and a Postdoctoral Fellowship from the American Heart Association (EA-P).

REFERENCES

1. Sjostrand FS, Andersson E. Electron microscopy of the intercalated discs of cardiac muscle tissue. *Experientia*. 1954;10:369–370.
2. Muir AR. An electron microscope study of the embryology of the intercalated disc in the heart of the rabbit. *J Biophys Biochem Cytol*. 1957;3:193–202.
3. Weidmann S. The electrical constants of Purkinje fibres. *J Physiol*. 1952;118:348–360.
4. Sjostrand FS, Andersson-Cedergren E, Dewey MM. The ultrastructure of the intercalated discs of frog, mouse and guinea pig cardiac muscle. *J Ultrastruct Res*. 1958;1:271–287.
5. Delmar M. Connexin43 regulates sodium current; ankyrin-G modulates gap junctions: the intercalated disc exchanger. *Cardiovasc Res*. 2012;93:220–222.
6. Delmar M, Liang FX. Connexin43 and the regulation of intercalated disc function. *Heart Rhythm*. 2012;9:835–838.
7. Agullo-Pascual E, Delmar M. The noncanonical functions of Cx43 in the heart. *J Membr Biol*. 2012;245:477–482.
8. Agullo-Pascual E, Cerrone M, Delmar M. Arrhythmogenic cardiomyopathy and Brugada syndrome: diseases of the connexome. *FEBS Lett*. 2014;588:1322–1330.
9. Corrado D, Thiene G. *Arrhythmogenic Cardiomyopathy*. Philadelphia: Saunders; 2011.
10. Fontes MS, van Veen TA, de Bakker JM, et al. Functional consequences of abnormal Cx43 expression in the heart. *Biochim Biophys Acta*. 2012;1818:2020–2029.
11. Qu J, Volpicelli FM, Garcia LI, et al. Gap junction remodeling and spironolactone-dependent reverse remodeling in the hypertrophied heart. *Circ Res*. 2009;104:365–371.
12. Akar FG, Nass RD, Hahn S, et al. Dynamic changes in conduction velocity and gap junction properties during development of pacing-induced heart failure. *Am J Physiol Heart Circ Physiol*. 2007;293:H1223–1230.
13. Zhang Y, Wang H, Kovacs A, et al. Reduced expression of Cx43 attenuates ventricular remodeling after myocardial infarction via impaired TGF-beta signaling. *Am J Physiol Heart Circ Physiol*. 2010;298:H477–487.
14. Smyth JW, Hong TT, Gao D, et al. Limited forward trafficking of connexin 43 reduces cell-cell coupling in stressed human and mouse myocardium. *J Clin Invest*. 2010;120:266–279.
15. Remo BF, Qu J, Volpicelli FM, et al. Phosphatase-resistant gap junctions inhibit pathological remodeling and prevent arrhythmias. *Circ Res*. 2011;108:1459–1466.
16. Chkourko HS, Guerrero-Serna G, Lin X, et al. Remodeling of mechanical junctions and of microtubule-associated proteins accompany cardiac connexin43 lateralization. *Heart Rhythm*. 2012;9:1133–1140. e1136.
17. Danik SB, Rosner G, Lader J, et al. Electrical remodeling contributes to complex tachyarrhythmias in connexin43-deficient mouse hearts. *FASEB J*. 2008;22:1204–1212.
18. Jansen JA, Noorman M, Musa H, et al. Reduced heterogeneous expression of Cx43 results in decreased Nav1.5 expression and reduced sodium current that accounts for arrhythmia vulnerability in conditional Cx43 knockout mice. *Heart Rhythm*. 2012;9:600–607.
19. Desplantez T, McCain ML, Beauchamp P, et al. Connexin43 ablation in fetal atrial myocytes decreases electrical coupling, partner connexins, and sodium current. *Cardiovasc Res*. 2012;94:58–65.
20. Wilde AA, Brugada R. Phenotypical manifestations of mutations in the genes encoding subunits of the cardiac sodium channel. *Circ Res*. 2011;108:884–897.
21. Cerrone M, Noorman M, Lin X, et al. Sodium current deficit and arrhythmogenesis in a murine model of plakophilin-2 haploinsufficiency. *Cardiovasc Res*. 2012;95:460–468.

22. Rizzo S, Lodder EM, Verkerk AO, et al. Intercalated disc abnormalities, reduced Na+ current density and conduction slowing in desmoglein-2 mutant mice prior to cardiomyopathic changes. *Cardiovasc Res*. 2012;95:409–418.
23. Corrado D, Buja G, Basso C, et al. What is the Brugada syndrome? *Cardiol Rev*. 1999;7:191–195.
24. Delmar M, McKenna WJ. The cardiac desmosome and arrhythmogenic cardiomyopathies: from gene to disease. *Circ Res*. 2010;107:700–714.
25. Bass-Zubek AE, Godsel LM, Delmar M, et al. Plakophilins: multifunctional scaffolds for adhesion and signaling. *Curr Opin Cell Biol*. 2009;21:708–716.
26. Gottardi CJ, Niessen CM, Gumbiner BM. The adherens junction. In: Beckerle MC, ed. *Cell Adhesion*. Oxford: Oxford University Press; 2001:259–287.
27. Gates J, Peifer M. Can 1000 reviews be wrong? Actin, alpha-catenin, and adherens junctions. *Cell*. 2005;123:769–772.
28. Bannon LJ, Goldfinger LE, Jones JCR, et al. Desmosomes and hemidesmosomes. In: Beckerle MC, ed. *Cell Adhesion*. Oxford: Oxford University Press; 2001:324–368.
29. Hatsell S, Cowin P. Deconstructing desmoplakin. *Nat Cell Biol*. 2001;3:E270–272.
30. North AJ, Bardsley WG, Hyam J, et al. Molecular map of the desmosomal plaque. *J Cell Sci*. 1999;112(Pt 23):4325–4336.
31. Al-Amoudi A, Castano-Diez D, Devos DP, et al. The three-dimensional molecular structure of the desmosomal plaque. *Proc Natl Acad Sci U S A*. 2011;108:6480–6485.
32. Chen X, Bonne S, Hatzfeld M, et al. Protein binding and functional characterization of plakophilin 2. Evidence for its diverse roles in desmosomes and beta-catenin signaling. *J Biol Chem*. 2002;277:10512–10522.
33. Gallicano GI, Kouklis P, Bauer C, et al. Desmoplakin is required early in development for assembly of desmosomes and cytoskeletal linkage. *J Cell Biol*. 1998;143:2009–2022.
34. Grossmann KS, Grund C, Huelsken J, et al. Requirement of plakophilin 2 for heart morphogenesis and cardiac junction formation. *J Cell Biol*. 2004;167:149–160.
35. Ruiz P, Brinkmann V, Ledermann B, et al. Targeted mutation of plakoglobin in mice reveals essential functions of desmosomes in the embryonic heart. *J Cell Biol*. 1996;135:215–225.
36. Sen-Chowdhry S, Syrris P, McKenna WJ. Genetics of right ventricular cardiomyopathy. *J Cardiovasc Electrophysiol*. 2005;16:927–935.
37. Delmar M. Desmosome-ion channel interactions and their possible role in arrhythmogenic cardiomyopathy. *Pediatr Cardiol*. 2012;33:975–979.
38. Franke WW, Borrmann CM, Grund C, et al. The area composita of adhering junctions connecting heart muscle cells of vertebrates. I. Molecular definition in intercalated disks of cardiomyocytes by immunoelectron microscopy of desmosomal proteins. *Eur J Cell Biol*. 2006;85:69–82.
39. Borrmann CM, Grund C, Kuhn C, et al. The area composita of adhering junctions connecting heart muscle cells of vertebrates. II. Colocalizations of desmosomal and fascia adhaerens molecules in the intercalated disk. *Eur J Cell Biol*. 2006;85:469–485.
40. Pieperhoff S, Franke WW. The area composita of adhering junctions connecting heart muscle cells of vertebrates. VI. Different precursor structures in non-mammalian species. *Eur J Cell Biol*. 2008;87:413–430.
41. Pieperhoff S, Schumacher H, Franke WW. The area composita of adhering junctions connecting heart muscle cells of vertebrates. V. The importance of plakophilin-2 demonstrated by small interference RNA-mediated knockdown in cultured rat cardiomyocytes. *Eur J Cell Biol*. 2008;87:399–411.

42. Li J, Goossens S, van Hengel J, et al. Loss of alphaT-catenin alters the hybrid adhering junctions in the heart and leads to dilated cardiomyopathy and ventricular arrhythmia following acute ischemia. *J Cell Sci*. 2012;125:1058–1067.
43. Agullo-Pascual E, Lin X, Leo-Macias A, et al. Super-resolution imaging reveals that loss of the C-terminus of connexin43 limits microtubule plus-end capture and NaV1.5 localization at the intercalated disc. *Cardiovasc Res*. 2014;104:371–381.
44. Agullo-Pascual E, Reid DA, Keegan S, et al. Super-resolution fluorescence microscopy of the cardiac connexome reveals plakophilin-2 inside the connexin43 plaque. *Cardiovasc Res*. 2013;100:231–240.
45. Cerrone M, Delmar M. Desmosomes and the sodium channel complex: implications for arrhythmogenic cardiomyopathy and Brugada syndrome. *Trends Cardiovasc Med*. 2014;24:184–190.
46. Clevers H. Wnt/beta-catenin signaling in development and disease. *Cell*. 2006;127:469–480.
47. Chen X, Shevtsov SP, Hsich E, et al. The beta-catenin/T-cell factor/lymphocyte enhancer factor signaling pathway is required for normal and stress-induced cardiac hypertrophy. *Mol Cell Biol*. 2006;26:4462–4473.
48. Chen S, Guttridge DC, You Z, et al. Wnt-1 signaling inhibits apoptosis by activating beta-catenin/T cell factor-mediated transcription. *J Cell Biol*. 2001;152:87–96.
49. Longo KA, Kennell JA, Ochocinska MJ, et al. Wnt signaling protects 3T3-L1 preadipocytes from apoptosis through induction of insulin-like growth factors. *J Biol Chem*. 2002;277:38239–38244.
50. Ross SE, Hemati N, Longo KA, et al. Inhibition of adipogenesis by Wnt signaling. *Science*. 2000;289:950–953.
51. Garcia-Gras E, Lombardi R, Giocondo MJ, et al. Suppression of canonical Wnt/beta-catenin signaling by nuclear plakoglobin recapitulates phenotype of arrhythmogenic right ventricular cardiomyopathy. *J Clin Invest*. 2006;116:2012–2021.
52. Lombardi R, Dong J, Rodriguez G, et al. Genetic fate mapping identifies second heart field progenitor cells as a source of adipocytes in arrhythmogenic right ventricular cardiomyopathy. *Circ Res*. 2009;104:1076–1084.
53. Lombardi R, da Graca Cabreira-Hansen M, Bell A, et al. Nuclear plakoglobin is essential for differentiation of cardiac progenitor cells to adipocytes in arrhythmogenic right ventricular cardiomyopathy. *Circ Res*. 2011;109:1342–1353.
54. Chen SN, Gurha P, Lombardi R, et al. The hippo pathway is activated and is a causal mechanism for adipogenesis in arrhythmogenic cardiomyopathy. *Circ Res*. 2014;114:454–468.
55. Danik SB, Liu F, Zhang J, et al. Modulation of cardiac gap junction expression and arrhythmic susceptibility. *Circ Res*. 2004;95:1035–1041.
56. Yao JA, Gutstein DE, Liu F, et al. Cell coupling between ventricular myocyte pairs from connexin43-deficient murine hearts. *Circ Res*. 2003;93:736–743.
57. Kaplan SR, Gard JJ, Carvajal-Huerta L, et al. Structural and molecular pathology of the heart in Carvajal syndrome. *Cardiovasc Pathol*. 2004;13:26–32.
58. Kaplan SR, Gard JJ, Protonotarios N, et al. Remodeling of myocyte gap junctions in arrhythmogenic right ventricular cardiomyopathy due to a deletion in plakoglobin (Naxos disease). *Heart Rhythm*. 2004;1:3–11.
59. Oxford EM, Everitt M, Coombs W, et al. Molecular composition of the intercalated disc in a spontaneous canine animal model of arrhythmogenic right ventricular dysplasia/cardiomyopathy. *Heart Rhythm*. 2007;4:1196–1205.
60. Mori Y, Fishman GI, Peskin CS. Ephaptic conduction in a cardiac strand model with 3D electrodiffusion. *Proc Natl Acad Sci U S A*. 2008;105:6463–6468.

61. Tsumoto K, Ashihara T, Haraguchi R, et al. Roles of subcellular Na+ channel distributions in the mechanism of cardiac conduction. *Biophys J*. 2011;100:554–563.
62. Veeraraghavan R, Salama ME, Poelzing S. Interstitial volume modulates the conduction velocity-gap junction relationship. *Am J Physiol Heart Circ Physiol*. 2012;302:H278–286.
63. Sperelakis N. An electric field mechanism for transmission of excitation between myocardial cells. *Circ Res*. 2002;91:985–987.
64. Kant S, Krull P, Eisner S, et al. Histological and ultrastructural abnormalities in murine desmoglein 2-mutant hearts. *Cell Tissue Res*. 2012;348:249–259.
65. Kostetskii I, Li J, Xiong Y, et al. Induced deletion of the N-cadherin gene in the heart leads to dissolution of the intercalated disc structure. *Circ Res*. 2005;96:346–354.
66. Leo-Macias A, Liang FX, Delmar M. Ultrastructure of the intercellular space in adult murine ventricle revealed by quantitative tomographic electron microscopy. *Cardiovasc Res*. 2015;107:442–452.
67. Veeraraghavan R, Lin J, Hoeker GS, et al. Sodium channels in the Cx43 gap junction perinexus may constitute a cardiac ephapse: an experimental and modeling study. *Pflugers Arch*. 2015;467:2093–2105.
68. Cohen SA. Immunocytochemical localization of rH1 sodium channel in adult rat heart atria and ventricle. Presence in terminal intercalated disks. *Circulation*. 1996;94:3083–3086.
69. Maier SK, Westenbroek RE, Schenkman KA, et al. An unexpected role for brain-type sodium channels in coupling of cell surface depolarization to contraction in the heart. *Proc Natl Acad Sci U S A*. 2002;99:4073–4078.
70. Motoike HK, Liu H, Glaaser IW, et al. The Na+ channel inactivation gate is a molecular complex: a novel role of the COOH-terminal domain. *J Gen Physiol*. 2004;123:155–165.
71. Lin X, Liu N, Lu J, et al. Subcellular heterogeneity of sodium current properties in adult cardiac ventricular myocytes. *Heart Rhythm*. 2011;8:1923–1930.
72. Lin X, O'Malley H, Chen C, et al. Scn1b deletion leads to increased tetrodotoxin-sensitive sodium current, altered intracellular calcium homeostasis and arrhythmias in murine hearts. *J Physiol*. 2015;593:1389–1407.
73. McNair WP, Sinagra G, Taylor MR, et al. SCN5A mutations associate with arrhythmic dilated cardiomyopathy and commonly localize to the voltage-sensing mechanism. *J Am Coll Cardiol*. 2011;57:2160–2168.
74. Patino GA, Isom LL. Electrophysiology and beyond: multiple roles of Na+ channel beta subunits in development and disease. *Neurosci Lett*. 2010;486:53–59.
75. Meadows LS, Isom LL. Sodium channels as macromolecular complexes: implications for inherited arrhythmia syndromes. *Cardiovasc Res*. 2005;67:448–458.
76. Lopez-Santiago LF, Meadows LS, Ernst SJ, et al. Sodium channel Scn1b null mice exhibit prolonged QT and RR intervals. *J Mol Cell Cardiol*. 2007;43:636–647.
77. Petitprez S, Zmoos AF, Ogrodnik J, et al. SAP97 and dystrophin macromolecular complexes determine two pools of cardiac sodium channels Nav1.5 in cardiomyocytes. *Circ Res*. 2011;108:294–304.
78. Sato PY, Musa H, Coombs W, et al. Loss of plakophilin-2 expression leads to decreased sodium current and slower conduction velocity in cultured cardiac myocytes. *Circ Res*. 2009;105:523–526.
79. Gillet L, Rougier JS, Shy D, et al. Cardiac-specific ablation of synapse-associated protein SAP97 in mice decreases potassium currents but not sodium current. *Heart Rhythm*. 2015;12:181–192.
80. Shy D, Gillet L, Ogrodnik J, et al. PDZ domain-binding motif regulates cardiomyocyte compartment-specific NaV1.5 channel expression and function. *Circulation*. 2014;130:147–160.
81. Mays DJ, Foose JM, Philipson LH, et al. Localization of the Kv1.5 K+ channel protein in explanted cardiac tissue. *J Clin Invest*. 1995;96:282–292.
82. Murata M, Buckett PD, Zhou J, et al. SAP97 interacts with Kv1.5 in heterologous expression systems. *Am J Physiol Heart Circ Physiol*. 2001;281:H2575–2584.
83. Milstein ML, Musa H, Balbuena DP, et al. Dynamic reciprocity of sodium and potassium channel expression in a macromolecular complex controls cardiac excitability and arrhythmia. *Proc Natl Acad Sci U S A*. 2012;109:E2134–2143.
84. Cheng L, Yung A, Covarrubias M, et al. Cortactin is required for N-cadherin regulation of Kv1.5 channel function. *J Biol Chem*. 2011;286:20478–20489.
85. Barry DM, Trimmer JS, Merlie JP, et al. Differential expression of voltage-gated K+ channel subunits in adult rat heart. Relation to functional K+ channels? *Circ Res*. 1995;77:361–369.
86. Takeuchi S, Takagishi Y, Yasui K, et al. Voltage-gated K(+)channel, Kv4.2, localizes predominantly to the transverse-axial tubular system of the rat myocyte. *J Mol Cell Cardiol*. 2000;32:1361–1369.
87. Melnyk P, Zhang L, Shrier A, et al. Differential distribution of Kir2.1 and Kir2.3 subunits in canine atrium and ventricle. *Am J Physiol Heart Circ Physiol*. 2002;283:H1123–1133.
88. Hong M, Bao L, Kefaloyianni E, et al. Heterogeneity of ATP-sensitive K+ channels in cardiac myocytes: enrichment at the intercalated disk. *J Biol. Chem*. 2012;287:41258–41267.
89. Saffitz JE. Dependence of electrical coupling on mechanical coupling in cardiac myocytes: insights gained from cardiomyopathies caused by defects in cell-cell connections. *Ann N Y Acad Sci*. 2005;1047:336–344.
90. Oxford EM, Musa H, Maass K, et al. Connexin43 remodeling caused by inhibition of plakophilin-2 expression in cardiac cells. *Circ Res*. 2007;101:703–711.
91. Fidler LM, Wilson GJ, Liu F, et al. Abnormal connexin43 in arrhythmogenic right ventricular cardiomyopathy caused by plakophilin-2 mutations. *J Cell Mol Med*. 2009;13:4219–4228.
92. Li MW, Mruk DD, Lee WM, et al. Connexin 43 and plakophilin-2 as a protein complex that regulates blood-testis barrier dynamics. *Proc Natl Acad Sci U S A*. 2009;106:10213–10218.
93. Asimaki A, Tandri H, Huang H, et al. A new diagnostic test for arrhythmogenic right ventricular cardiomyopathy. *N Engl J Med*. 2009;360:1075–1084.
94. Asimaki A, Tandri H, Duffy ER, et al. Altered desmosomal proteins in granulomatous myocarditis and potential pathogenic links to arrhythmogenic right ventricular cardiomyopathy. *Circ Arrhythm Electrophysiol*. 2011;4:743–752.
95. Noorman M, Hakim S, Kessler E, et al. Remodeling of the cardiac sodium channel, connexin43, and plakoglobin at the intercalated disk in patients with arrhythmogenic cardiomyopathy. *Heart Rhythm*. 2013;10:412–419.
96. Eckardt D, Theis M, Degen J, et al. Functional role of connexin43 gap junction channels in adult mouse heart assessed by inducible gene deletion. *J Mol Cell Cardiol*. 2004;36:101–110.
97. Morley GE, Vaidya D, Jalife J. Characterization of conduction in the ventricles of normal and heterozygous Cx43 knockout mice using optical mapping. *J Cardiovasc Electrophysiol*. 2000;11:375–377.
98. Thomas SP, Kucera JP, Bircher-Lehmann L, et al. Impulse propagation in synthetic strands of neonatal cardiac myocytes with genetically reduced levels of connexin43. *Circ Res*. 2003;92:1209–1216.
99. Deo M, Sato PY, Musa H, et al. Relative contribution of changes in sodium current versus intercellular coupling on reentry initiation in 2-dimensional preparations of plakophilin-2-deficient cardiac cells. *Heart Rhythm*. 2011;8:1740–1748.
100. van der Zwaag PA, Cox MG, van der Werf C, et al. Recurrent and founder mutations in the Netherlands: plakophilin-2 p.Arg79X mutation causing arrhythmogenic right ventricular cardiomyopathy/dysplasia. *Neth Heart J*. 2010;18:583–591.
101. Joshi-Mukherjee R, Coombs W, Musa H, et al. Characterization of the molecular phenotype of two arrhythmogenic right ventricular cardiomyopathy (ARVC)-related plakophilin-2 (PKP2) mutations. *Heart Rhythm*. 2008;5:1715–1723.
102. Bauce B, Basso C, Rampazzo A, et al. Clinical profile of four families with arrhythmogenic right ventricular cardiomyopathy caused by dominant desmoplakin mutations. *Eur Heart J*. 2005;26:1666–1675.
103. Asimaki A, Kapoor S, Plovie E, et al. Identification of a new modulator of the intercalated disc in a zebrafish model of arrhythmogenic cardiomyopathy. *Sci Transl Med*. 2014;6: 240ra274.
104. Gomes J, Finlay M, Ahmed AK, et al. Electrophysiological abnormalities precede overt structural changes in arrhythmogenic right ventricular cardiomyopathy due to mutations in desmoplakin-A combined murine and human study. *Eur Heart J*. 2012;33:1942–1953.
105. Malhotra JD, Thyagarajan V, Chen C, et al. Tyrosine-phosphorylated and nonphosphorylated sodium channel beta1 subunits are differentially localized in cardiac myocytes. *J Biol Chem*. 2004;279:40748–40754.
106. Rhett JM, Ongstad EL, Jourdan J, et al. Cx43 associates with Na(v)1.5 in the cardiomyocyte perinexus. *J Membr Biol*. 2012;245:411–422.
107. Sato PY, Coombs W, Lin X, et al. Interactions between ankyrin-G, plakophilin-2, and connexin43 at the cardiac intercalated disc. *Circ Res*. 2011;109:193–201.
108. Lübkemeier I, Requardt RP, Lin X, et al. Deletion of the last five C-terminal amino acid residues of connexin43 leads to lethal ventricular arrhythmias in mice without affecting coupling via gap junction channels. *Basic Res Cardiol*. 2013;108:348–364.
109. Shaw RM, Fay AJ, Puthenveedu MA, et al. Microtubule plus-end-tracking proteins target gap junctions directly from the cell interior to adherens junctions. *Cell*. 2007;128:547–560.
110. Hong T, Yang H, Zhang SS, et al. Cardiac BIN1 folds T-tubule membrane, controlling ion flux and limiting arrhythmia. *Nat Med*. 2014;20:624–632.
111. Meyer RA, Laird DW, Revel JP, et al. Inhibition of gap junction and adherens junction assembly by connexin and A-CAM antibodies. *J Cell Biol*. 1992;119:179–189.
112. Hartshorne RP, Catterall WA. Purification of the saxitoxin receptor of the sodium channel from rat brain. *Proc Natl Acad Sci U S A*. 1981;78:4620–4624.
113. Isom LL, De Jongh KS, Patton DE, et al. Primary structure and functional expression of the beta 1 subunit of the rat brain sodium channel. *Science*. 1992;256:839–842.
114. Malhotra JD, Kazen-Gillespie K, Hortsch M, et al. Sodium channel beta subunits mediate homophilic cell adhesion and recruit ankyrin to points of cell-cell contact. *J Biol Chem*. 2000;275:11383–11388.
115. Dhar Malhotra J, Chen C, Rivolta I, et al. Characterization of sodium channel alpha- and beta-subunits in rat and mouse cardiac myocytes. *Circulation*. 2001;103:1303–1310.
116. Isom LL. Sodium channel beta subunits: anything but auxiliary. *Neuroscientist*. 2001;7:42–54.
117. Brackenbury WJ, Isom LL. Na channel beta subunits: overachievers of the ion channel family. *Front Pharmacol*. 2011;2:53.
118. Li J, Patel VV, Kostetskii I, et al. Cardiac-specific loss of N-cadherin leads to alteration in connexins with conduction slowing and arrhythmogenesis. *Circ Res*. 2005;97:474–481.
119. Lim BK, Xiong D, Dorner A, et al. Coxsackievirus and adenovirus receptor (CAR) mediates atrioventricular-node function and connexin 45 localization in the murine heart. *J Clin Invest*. 2008;118:2758–2770.
120. Lisewski U, Shi Y, Wrackmeyer U, et al. The tight junction protein CAR regulates cardiac conduction and cell-cell communication. *J Exp Med*. 2008;205:2369–2379.
121. Marsman RF, Bezzina CR, Freiberg F, et al. Coxsackie and adenovirus receptor is a modifier of cardiac conduction and arrhythmia vulnerability in the setting of myocardial ischemia. *J Am Coll Cardiol*. 2014;63:549–559.
122. Swope D, Li J, Radice GL. Beyond cell adhesion: the role of armadillo proteins in the heart. *Cell Signal*. 2013;25:93–100.
123. Bass-Zubek AE, Hobbs RP, Amargo EV, et al. Plakophilin 2: a critical scaffold for PKC alpha that regulates intercellular junction assembly. *J Cell Biol*. 2008;181:605–613.
124. Godsel LM, Dubash AD, Bass-Zubek AE, et al. Plakophilin 2 couples actomyosin remodeling to desmosomal plaque assembly via RhoA. *Mol Biol Cell*. 2010;21:2844–2859.
125. Makara MA, Curran J, Little SC, et al. Ankyrin-G coordinates intercalated disc signaling platform to regulate cardiac excitability in vivo. *Circ Res*. 2014;115:929–938.
126. Rhett JM, Jourdan J, Gourdie RG. Connexin 43 connexon to gap junction transition is regulated by zonula occludens-1. *Mol Biol Cell*. 2011;22:1516–1528.
127. Salzer JL. Clustering sodium channels at the node of Ranvier: close encounters of the axon-glia kind. *Neuron*. 1997;18:843–846.
128. Leterrier C, Dargent B. No Pasaran! Role of the axon initial segment in the regulation of protein transport and the maintenance of axonal identity. *Semin Cell Dev Biol*. 2014;27:44–51.
129. Beyder A, Rae JL, Bernard C, et al. Mechanosensitivity of Nav1.5, a voltage-sensitive sodium channel. *J Physiol*. 2010;588:4969–4985.
130. Kirchhoff S, Kim JS, Hagendorff A, et al. Abnormal cardiac conduction and morphogenesis in connexin40 and connexin43 double-deficient mice. *Circ Res*. 2000;87:399–405.
131. Kucera JP, Rohr S, Rudy Y. Localization of sodium channels in intercalated disks modulates cardiac conduction. *Circ Res*. 2002;91:1176–1182.
132. Chen Q, Kirsch GE, Zhang D, et al. Genetic basis and molecular mechanism for idiopathic ventricular fibrillation. *Nature*. 1998;392:293–296.
133. Cerrone M, Lin X, Zhang M, et al. Missense mutations in plakophilin-2 cause sodium current deficit and associate with a Brugada syndrome phenotype. *Circulation*. 2014;129:1092–1103.

23 Function and Dysfunction of Ion Channel Membrane Trafficking and Posttranslational Modification

Thomas J. Hund and Peter J. Mohler

Over the course of a human lifetime, the heart will beat more than 2 billion times. Furthermore, the cardiovascular system must be essentially fail-proof across the decades of human life as any loss of function even for only minutes may be fatal. To ensure robust cardiac excitation–contraction coupling, the heart has evolved elaborate pathways to regulate excitability across diverse cardiac cell types (sinus node myocytes, atrial myocytes, cardiac Purkinje fibers, ventricular myocytes) with the ability to fine-tune the cellular response to acute and chronic physiological or pathological stimuli. Human cell excitability is centrally governed by the activity of ion channels and transporters that control the movement of charged ions across membrane networks to tune electrochemical gradients (Fig. 23.1). Moreover, congenital or acquired defects that alter ion channel biophysics (activation, inactivation) have been directly linked with a host of human arrhythmia syndromes, including sinus node disease, atrial fibrillation, conduction disorders, and potentially fatal ventricular arrhythmias. While these diseases comprise the majority of cardiac "channelopathies," two new and related classes of alternative pathways for cardiac channelopathies have emerged because of the defects in ion channel or transporter trafficking or ion channel posttranslational modification (PTM). This chapter will highlight how dysfunction in these two alternative pathways has been linked to arrhythmia phenotypes.[1]

Defects in Ion Channel Trafficking and Cardiac Arrhythmia

Steady-state ion channel/transporter function is regulated by membrane protein synthesis, trafficking, membrane stabilization, internalization/recycling, and degradation. Ultimately, these pathways control the ensemble of ion channels and transporters that regulate the cardiac action potential (AP) (see Fig. 23.1). As noted earlier, each excitable cardiomyocyte harbors unique combinations of membrane ion channels and transporters that control membrane depolarization and repolarization. In this way, the sinus node myocyte is able to maintain a more depolarized resting membrane potential than an atrial or ventricular myocyte to support automaticity. As reviewed in Chapter 17, ion channels and transporters are synthesized in the endoplasmic reticulum and, following modification in the Golgi and trans-Golgi network, move through the endosome pathway to their final destination at the plasma membrane or sarcoplasmic reticulum (SR) membrane. In response to external and cellular cues, membrane proteins are internalized for degradation or recycling. Defects in all of these cellular pathways have been implicated in human disease but may involve diversity in mechanisms of dysfunction.[2]

Defects in Ion Channel Processing/Folding Result in Cardiac Arrhythmia

As previously noted, membrane protein trafficking first requires a newly synthesized protein to travel from the endoplasmic reticulum through the multiple layers of the Golgi apparatus. These organelles not only serve to modify membrane proteins with appropriate carbohydrate moieties but also serve as "quality control" pathways to ensure that immature or misfolded proteins are removed from the biosynthetic pathway and ultimately targeted for degradation. Directly related to this chapter, the human ether-à-go-go (hERG1) protein ($K_v11.1$, encoded by *KCNH2*) serves as the α-subunit for I_{Kr}, a voltage-dependent K$^+$ current critical for cardiac repolarization (see Fig. 23.1).[3,4] Human loss-of-function mutations in hERG1 lead to aberrant repolarization, resulting in AP prolongation, and the second most common form of human long QT syndrome, LQT2.[3,4] Notably, a large fraction of the more than 200 hERG1 loss-of-function variants linked with LQT2 are associated with misfolding and ultimately altered trafficking and rapid degradation of the immature polypeptide.[5] Defects in membrane protein folding are certainly not limited to cardiac voltage-gated K$^+$ channels. For example, there are numerous examples of voltage-gated Na$_v$ channel defects linked to altered protein folding, again resulting in reduced membrane expression because of premature degradation.[6]

Defects in Ion Channel Anterograde Trafficking Result in Cardiac Arrhythmia

Beyond defects in folding, defects in properly folded ion channel trafficking have been linked with defects in ion channel and membrane excitability. In a normal myocyte, forward (anterograde) trafficking of hERG1 requires the Golgi and trans-Golgi chaperone activity of two heat shock proteins, Hsp70 and Hsp90. Interestingly, human hERG1 LQT2 mutations R752W and G601S *increase* the binding activity of the K$^+$ channel α-subunit for these chaperones such that they are unable to disassemble from the chaperones, thereby reducing their exit from the Golgi and trans-Golgi network and limiting their delivery to the myocyte membrane.[7–9] K$_v$LQT1 (encoded by *KCNQ1*) serves as the α-subunit for the voltage-dependent K$^+$ current I_{Ks} (see Fig. 23.1; mutations cause LQT1). Proper delivery of K$_v$LQT1 to the myocyte membrane (as well as membrane regulation) requires the chaperone activity of its β-subunit minK (encoded by *KCNE1*). Notably, while select human minK arrhythmia mutations do not affect I_{Ks} function while at the membrane, these variants (e.g., minK L51H) alter anterograde trafficking.[10] Conversely, K$_v$LQT1 human arrhythmia mutations (e.g., *KCNQ1* T587M) also limit forward protein trafficking through the biosynthetic pathway.[11] Finally, it is important to note that human channel mutations may ultimately alter membrane current through multiple mechanisms. For example, *KCNQ1* H258R results in reduced forward trafficking to the plasma membrane.[12] However, this same variant alters K+ channel biophysical properties to increase K+ conductance.[12] Thus a single human channel variant may affect two

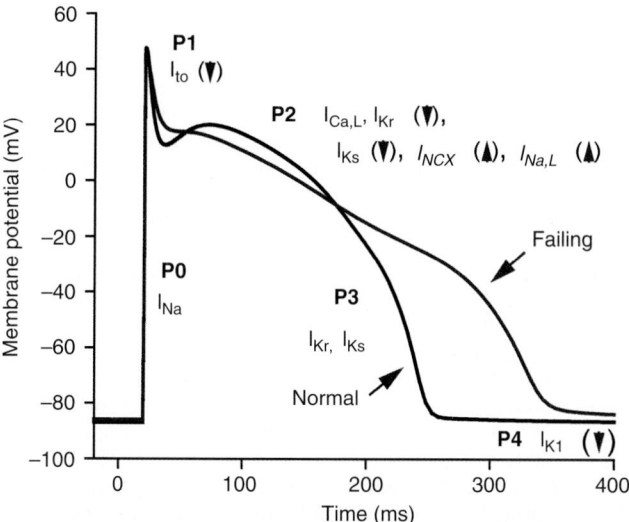

FIG. 23.1 Ion channels regulate cardiac action potential (AP) duration in health and disease. The cycle of events that underlie the normal AP (*black line*) involves rapid membrane depolarization (phase 0, P0) dictated primarily by the activation of voltage-gated Na+ current (I_{Na}). Rapid inactivation of I_{Na} combined with the activation of voltage-gated transient outward K+ current (I_{to}) causes early repolarization (phase 1, P1). A delicate balance of depolarizing currents (primarily L-type Ca2+ [$I_{Ca,L}$], Na+/Ca2+ exchanger [I_{NCX}], and late Na+ [$I_{Na,L}$]) and repolarizing currents [fast and slow delayed rectifier K+ (I_{Kr}, I_{Ks})] shapes the AP plateau (phase 2, P2). The inactivation of $I_{Ca,L}$ together with further increases in I_{Kr} and I_{Ks} eventually enable late repolarization (phase 3, P3) and the activation of the inward rectifier K+ current (I_{K1}), which returns the membrane to its resting state (phase 4, P4). Defects in the ion channel expression and posttranslational modification disrupt the normal AP cycle in diseases, such as heart failure, increasing the risk for life-threatening arrhythmias and contractile dysfunctions (representative AP shown in *red*). AP waveforms were simulated using a mathematical model of the canine AP paced to steady state at a cycle length of 2000 ms.[1] The failing AP was produced by decreasing maximal conductances for I_{to} (73% decrease), I_{Kr} (45% decrease), I_{Ks} (57% decrease), and I_{K1} (32% decrease) and by increasing I_{NCX} (75% increase) and $I_{Na,L}$ (300% increase) (changes indicated by *red arrows*).

disparate channel functions, resulting in potentially counteracting phenotypes to regulate cellular excitability.

Finally, the importance of proper ion channel membrane trafficking is further illustrated by the link between defects in the endosomal transport protein Eps15 homology domain–containing protein 3 (EHD3) and abnormal atrial and ventricular cell membrane excitability. In the ventricles, EHD3 function is requisite for normal membrane expression and distribution of the Na+/Ca2+ exchanger (NCX) and Ca$_v$1.2.[13] Furthermore, in the atria, an unbiased screen confirmed by functional studies revealed a requirement of EHD3 for the localization of T-type Ca2+ channel membrane expression and function.[14]

Defects in Ion Channel/Transporter Membrane Targeting/Scaffolding Cause Arrhythmia

As noted earlier, defects in ion channel/transporter navigation of the early biosynthetic pathway may result in altered membrane protein expression and ultimately defects in membrane excitability. However, as reviewed later, equally important to early protein folding and endoplasmic reticulum and Golgi transitions are the retention and regulation of ion channels and transporters at the plasma membrane. Since 2000, we have learned of multiple examples of dysfunction in membrane protein targeting and scaffolding that cause human arrhythmia. Notably, these mutations may occur within the ion channel or transporter. Alternatively, mutations in proteins that target or scaffold ion channels/transporters may also result in electrical phenotypes.

Na$_v$1.5 (encoded by *SCN5A*; reviewed in Chapter 1) is a large 24 transmembrane–spanning ion channel critical for the rapid upstroke of the cardiac AP (Fig. 23.2). Defects in Na$_v$1.5 have been linked with multiple forms of cardiac dysfunction, including sinus node dysfunction, atrial fibrillation, conduction disorders, and ventricular arrhythmia.[15] Similar to cardiac K+ channels, Na$_v$1.5 channels do not simply exist as single polypeptides but instead are regulated by a host of accessory proteins (see Fig. 23.2). The first and best characterized Na$_v$1.5-interacting protein is a family of Na$_v$ channel β-subunits (four genes, multiple isoforms). Relevant to this chapter, Na$_v$ channel β-subunits are tightly linked with Na$_v$1.5 channel trafficking in the heart, and Na$_v$ channel β-subunit mutations are now linked with multiple forms of inherited arrhythmias. Beyond Na$_v$ channel β-subunits, Na$_v$1.5 is now known to associate with a host of cytosolic proteins that have clear roles in Na+ current (I_{Na}) regulation. For example, ankyrin-G is a member of a family of membrane adapter proteins (ankyrins-R, -B, and -G, encoded by *ANK1*, *ANK2*, and *ANK3*, respectively) first identified in the erythrocyte plasma membrane. In the nervous system, ankyrin-G targets Na$_v$ channels to

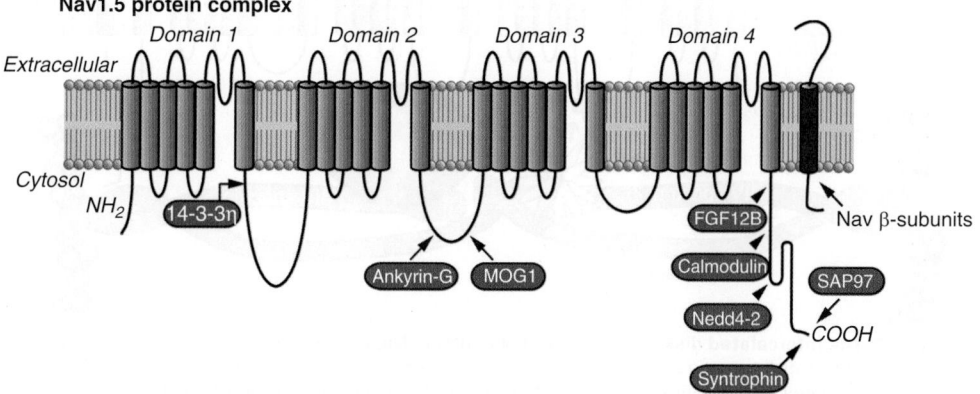

FIG. 23.2 Na$_v$1.5 interacting proteins. The figure depicts proteins defined to directly associate with Na$_v$1.5 in either in vitro or in vivo systems. Additional proteins have been linked with Na$_v$1.5; however, the mechanism for interaction is currently unknown (e.g., caveolin 3).

axon initial segments and nodes of Ranvier, and mice that lack ankyrin-G in the cerebellum display severe ataxia.[16] Notably, ankyrin-G is also highly expressed in the heart and in ventricular cardiomyocytes and is highly enriched at the myocyte intercalated disk, where it directly associates with a nine–amino acid motif in the DII-DIII loop of $Na_v1.5$ (Fig. 23.3).[17,18] Reduction of ankyrin-G in neonatal and adult cardiomyocytes results in reduced $Na_v1.5$ and I_{Na} at the intercalated disk, and a recently generated mouse model that selectively lacks ankyrin-G in the heart results in altered $Na_v1.5$ membrane expression, as well as rate, conduction, and arrhythmia disorders.[17,19] Consistent with these findings, a human Brugada syndrome mutation in *SCN5A* located in the ankyrin-G–binding motif that reduces ankyrin-G/$Na_v1.5$ interaction results in reduced $Na_v1.5$ membrane expression.[18] However, since 2010, additional members of the ankyrin-G/$Na_v1.5$ intercalated disk complex have been identified that demonstrate additional nontrafficking roles for ankyrin-G. For example, ankyrin-G directly associates with the actin-binding molecule β_{IV} spectrin (see Fig. 23.3).[20] Ankyrin-G is required for β_{IV} spectrin expression and localization at the intercalated disk, and β_{IV} spectrin recruits the Ca^+/calmodulin-dependent protein kinase II (CaMKIIδ) to the disk.[20] As discussed later in this chapter, this interaction is critical for the posttranslational regulation of $Na_v1.5$ and has major consequences for the arrhythmogenic $I_{Na,late}$ (I_{Na} persistent current).[20,21] Ankyrin-G has also been linked with plakophilin-2 at the intercalated disk membrane[19,22] and thus may play an additional role in myocyte membrane excitability and structure.

While ankyrin-G is central for $Na_v1.5$ targeting to the intercalated disk, $Na_v1.5$ targeting to the lateral myocyte membrane is controlled by interaction with α1-syntrophin (encoded by *SNTA1*). Specifically, α1-syntrophin (via its PDZ domain) interacts with the C-terminal residues of $Na_v1.5$ (see Fig. 23.2). Notably, mice that lack α1-syntrophin or its binding partner dystrophin display defects in lateral membrane $Na_v1.5$ expression/localization and a significant decrease in I_{Na}.[23,24] As further proof of the importance of this interaction for cardiac I_{Na}, human α1-syntrophin mutations are linked to human arrhythmia.[25] Mechanistically, this arrhythmia disorder likely results from defects in $Na_v1.5$ trafficking as well as $Na_v1.5$ posttranslational regulation (discussed later in this chapter).[25]

Finally, new $Na_v1.5$ partners are emerging rapidly with significant roles in channel trafficking and membrane regulation. As discussed in Chapter 19, the family of fibroblast growth factor homologous factors (FHFs) has an important modulatory role for Na_v channels in the brain and heart (see Fig. 23.2).[26,27] In the heart, FHFs play dual roles in $Na_v1.5$ channel trafficking and membrane regulation. Moreover, human FGF12 variants are now identified in patients with Brugada syndrome.[28] Furthermore, in 2015, human $Na_v1.5$ mutations that directly alter the interaction of FHFs and $Na_v1.5$ were linked with atrial fibrillation and ventricular fibrillation.[29] Functionally, channels that lack FHF-binding activity display delayed inactivation, resulting in increased I_{Na} late in AP and afterdepolarizations.[29] In summary, these three $Na_v1.5$-interacting proteins illustrate the complexity of the mechanisms that underlie $Na_v1.5$ regulation in the heart and further confirm the impact of dysfunction in these pathways for human disease pathogenesis. Additional important $Na_v1.5$-associated proteins include caveolin 3, calmodulin, MOG-1, 14-3-3, Nedd4, and SAP97 (see Fig. 23.2).[30]

Since 2003, we have learned that defects in membrane scaffolding proteins may impact multiple ion channels and transporters, as well as cytoskeletal and signaling proteins, resulting in complex cardiac phenotypes. The best example is ankyrin-B (encoded by *ANK2*). Structurally similar to ankyrin-G, ankyrin-B is localized to cardiac transverse-tubule/SR membranes with β_{II} spectrin.[31,32] Ankyrin-B directly associates with multiple cardiac ion channels and transporters, including NCX, Na/K ATPase, Kir6.2, $Ca_v1.3$, and the SR inositol 1,4,5 trisphosphate receptor (IP3 receptor).[33-36] Moreover, ankyrin-B directly associates with the large Rho-GEF obscurin, the molecular chaperone Hsp40,[37] dynactin,[38] EHD3,[13,39] and the regulatory subunit of protein phosphatase 2A (PP2A, B56α).[40,41] Mice that lack global ankyrin-B expression are postembryonic lethal, whereas mice heterozygous for an ankyrin-B mutation are viable but display reduced heart rate, atrial fibrillation, conduction defects, and polymorphic ventricular arrhythmia in response to catecholamines.[36,42-44] At the cellular level, the loss of ankyrin-B alters trafficking and membrane expression of its key binding partners, ultimately resulting in defects in intracellular Ca^+ regulation, altered adrenergic balance, and extrasystoles.[36] More notably, human mutations in *ANK2* are now linked with a complex cardiac phenotype that includes bradycardia, AF, and catecholaminergic ventricular arrhythmia.[36,42,43] To date, nearly 10 different *ANK2* loss of function variants have been identified[45,46] that alter association with protein partners[31] or impact ankyrin-B stability.[47]

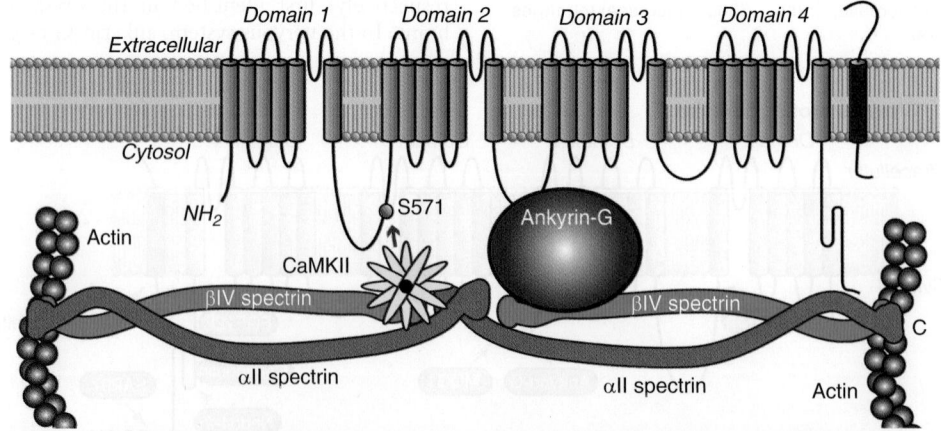

FIG. 23.3 The intercalated disk protein complex controls $Na_v1.5$ targeting and regulation. Ankyrin-G controls disk targeting of $Na_v1.5$ via interaction with β_{IV}/αII-spectrin and actin. β_{IV} spectrin directly associates with calcium/calmodulin-dependent protein kinase II (*CaMKII*) to target the molecule within angstroms of its target $Na_v1.5$. CaMKII directly phosphorylates $Na_v1.5$ at residue Ser571 to regulate the arrhythmogenic $I_{Na,late}$. CaMKII also directly phosphorylates other sites on $Na_v1.5$ (not shown).

Channel Dysfunction Induced by Altered Posttranslational Modifications

As previously discussed, proper ion channel function depends on the proper folding and trafficking of the protein to the membrane. Once at the membrane, ion channel function may be rapidly tuned via a large number of PTMs, including phosphorylation, nitrosylation, acetylation, oxidation, and glycosylation. While channelopathies caused by genetic mutations affecting channel gating and/or membrane trafficking are a major health problem, a more common cause of channel dysfunction is because of abnormal PTM. Dysregulation of cell signaling pathways occurs in many forms of acquired disease, including heart failure (HF), myocardial infarction, and diabetes. Furthermore, primary defects in ion channels or associated proteins induced by mutations or pharmacological agents may cause downstream changes in cell signaling that exacerbate the substrate for disease and arrhythmias (e.g., catecholaminergic polymorphic ventricular tachycardia [CPVT], ankyrin-B syndrome, or cardiac glycoside cytotoxicity). Ultimately, alterations in cellular signaling may actively promote aberrant ion channel function, resulting in cell and organ phenotypes and disease.

Dysregulation of Cell Signaling in Heart Failure

Altered ion channel PTM downstream of aberrant cell signaling has been linked to arrhythmias in a wide range of cardiac diseases, including myocardial infarction, ischemia, diabetes, hypertrophy, and HF.[1,48] HF remains a major health burden worldwide and stands as perhaps the best characterized example of the link between altered cell signaling, channel dysfunction, and disease/arrhythmias. HF presents with a range of etiologies, but common clinical characteristics include decreased myocardial contractility, an enlarged and/or dilated heart, and a high incidence of cardiac arrhythmia.[49] At the cellular level, myocytes from failing hearts display a prolonged AP duration and defects in Ca^{2+} cycling that serve as potential triggers for arrhythmias (see Fig. 23.1). Dysregulation of Ca^{2+} homeostasis also promotes contractile dysfunction and disease progression.[50–52] While the precise mechanisms that underlie electrical and mechanical dysfunction in HF remain to be determined, it is clear that altered ion channel PTM is an important determinant of the pathology. Excessive activity of the sympathetic nervous and renin–angiotensin systems in the setting of HF perturbs intracellular signaling networks that involve protein kinase A (PKA) and CaMKII among others. In turn, an altered PTM of multiple ion channel complexes (described later) have been linked to arrhythmias and disease progression.[53]

Sodium Channel Dysfunction Induced by Altered Posttranslational Modifications in Heart Failure

Voltage-gated Na^+ channels (Na_v) generate a large depolarizing current necessary for the rapid AP upstroke (see Fig. 23.1). Central to normal cell membrane excitability, Na_v rapidly activates in response to an extracellular stimulus followed by an almost instantaneous inactivation, which allows the membrane potential to return to rest prior to the next cycle. Even under normal conditions, a small percentage (<1%) of channels fails to inactivate, resulting in a miniscule persistent (late) Na^+ current throughout the AP duration. Phosphorylation of the voltage-gated Na^+ channel by CaMKII has been shown to have complex effects on channel function, including a decrease in steady-state channel availability, slower recovery from inactivation, and an increase in late current.[21,54–57] A consistent finding in failing myocytes is

an increase in late Na^+ current.[21,58,59] Multiple potential CaMKII phosphorylation sites have been identified on $Na_v1.5$ that may be causative targets for altered channel function in HF (Fig. 23.4).[20,21,56,57,60,61] Studies using an antibody specific for $Na_v1.5$, phosphorylated at Ser571 in the $Na_v1.5$ DI-DII linker, revealed increased phosphorylation of this site in failing human and mouse hearts (see Fig. 23.4).[21,57,58] Furthermore, knock-in mice with an ablation of Ser571 (Ser571Ala mice) are resistant to increased late Na^+ current, AP prolongation, and maladaptive remodeling after transaortic constriction, thereby supporting an important role for CaMKII-dependent PTM of $Na_v1.5$ at this site in HF. Interestingly, recent phosphor-proteomic studies have revealed decreased phosphorylation in human HF at a different site (Ser516), suggesting a more complex profile of altered $Na_v1.5$ PTM in HF (see Fig. 23.4).[60] At the same time, it is possible that the altered PTM of Na_v aside from phosphorylation may be involved in the aberrant channel activity in the disease. For example, S-nitrosylation of $Na_v1.5$ has been shown to increase late current with likely relevance for HF, where increased nitric oxide may occur downstream of the β-adrenergic signaling pathway (see Fig. 23.4).[62,63]

The preponderance of data support the notion that altered PTM of $Na_v1.5$ contributes to an increased late current in HF, but how does increased late I_{Na} help shape the pathological substrate? Stated differently, does late I_{Na} serve a dual role in both creating the arrhythmia substrate and promoting disease progression? There is now ample evidence to support the notion that increased late I_{Na} promotes AP prolongation and susceptibility to arrhythmogenic afterdepolarizations by subtly perturbing the very delicate balance between depolarizing (primarily L-type Ca^{2+} current) and repolarizing currents during the AP plateau phase (see Fig. 23.1).[21,58,64] At the same time, late I_{Na}, integrated over the AP duration, may also contribute to accumulation of intracellular Na^+, which in turn leads to elevation of intracellular Ca^{2+} via a forward-mode NCX.[65] Not only does this Ca^{2+} accumulation further exacerbate the arrhythmia substrate but it also may provide a feed-forward mechanism for further activation of Ca^{2+}-dependent signaling that ultimately sets the heart down an irrevocable maladaptive remodeling pathway.

Calcium Cycling Dysfunction Induced by Altered Posttranslational Modifications in Heart Failure

Similar to $Na_v1.5$, RyR2 is phosphorylated by multiple kinases, including CaMKII and PKA. Phosphorylation of RyR2 at specific residues (e.g., Ser2808, Ser2814, and Ser2030)[66–68] has been shown to alter Ca^{2+} sensitivity. Although the relative importance of specific RyR2 phosphorylation events in HF remains controversial,[69,70] it is clear that increased phosphorylation of RyR2 promotes diastolic leak of Ca^{2+} from SR in failing myocytes.[71–73] Enhanced Ca^{2+} leak, in turn, serves a dual role as both a potential trigger for arrhythmia and a source of contractile dysfunction.[74–76]

SR Ca^{2+} uptake is also altered in failing myocytes through PTM of phospholamban (PLB), an SR-associated phosphoprotein that reversibly regulates activity of SR Ca^{2+}-ATPase (SERCA2a). PLB is phosphorylated by PKA, CaMKII, and protein kinase C (PKC) to relieve its inhibition of SERCA2a and increase SR Ca^{2+} uptake. Interestingly, phosphorylation of PLB at PKA and CaMKII sites has been reported to decrease in failing myocytes perhaps because of the increased phosphatase activity.[77] This decrease in phosphorylated PLB together with changes in SERCA2a/PLB stoichiometry actually suppress Ca^{2+} uptake and promote contractile dysfunction. PLB is also subject to S-nitrosylation with β-adrenergic stimulation, although a role for this pathway in disease is unknown.[78]

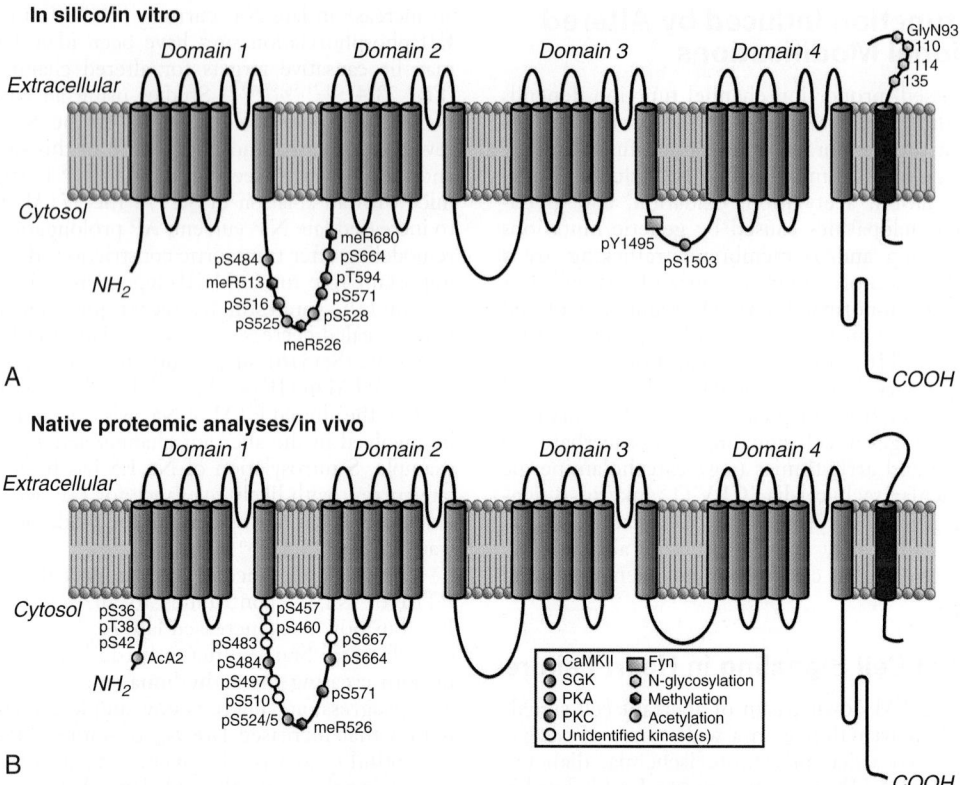

FIG. 23.4 Na$_v$1.5 is regulated by posttranslational modifications. Both the Na$_v$1.5 α- and β-subunits are highly regulated by posttranslational modifications. Noted in (A) are sites/modifications identified through in silico or in vitro studies. (B) Sites detected in proteomic screens or defined in vivo are depicted. A legend for these sites is shown in (B). *PKA*, Protein kinase A; *PKC*, protein kinase C; *SGK*, serum/glucocorticoid regulated kinase.

Altered Posttranslational Modifications Downstream of Defects in Ion Channel Complex

The altered PTM of ion channel and transporter complexes downstream of the neurohumoral imbalance promotes arrhythmias and contractile dysfunction in disease. However, primary inherited or acquired defects in ion channels or associated proteins may also disrupt cell signaling pathways, leading to altered PTM and arrhythmias. A clear example of this mechanism is found in ankyrin-B syndrome (see earlier), an inherited disease characterized by stress-induced arrhythmias and caused by mutations in the *ANK2* gene.[36] As discussed earlier, ankyrin-B is an adapter protein involved in the membrane targeting of several ion channels and transporters that are important for normal Ca^{2+} cycling as well as PP2A via a direct interaction with the B56alpha isoform of the PP2A regulatory subunit.[79] The loss of ankyrin-B function has been shown to alter PTM of select ion channels, including RyR2, to promote arrhythmia.[80] In fact, the genetic inhibition of CaMKII was shown to suppress arrhythmias in a mouse model of ankyrin-B syndrome.[80] Likewise, CPVT is an inherited disease characterized by stress-induced arrhythmias in the absence of structural defects or overt electrocardiographic abnormalities. CPVT is primarily caused by gene mutations in RyR2 with an autosomal recessive variant linked to mutations in calsequestrin (*CASQ2*).[81] A hallmark of CPVT is increased Ca^{2+} sensitivity of RyR2 either because of a lower

threshold for store overload Ca^{2+}-induced release or impaired SR Ca^{2+} buffering capacity. Similar to ankyrin-B syndrome, CaMKII inhibition was shown to suppress stress-induced arrhythmias in a mouse model of CPVT (RyR2-R4496C).[82] In a similar vein, the cardiotoxic effects of cardiac glycosides have been partially ascribed to defects in cell signaling and altered PTM of RyR2.[83]

Summary

As illustrated in this chapter, cardiac excitability is regulated by the synchronized activities of a large group of ion channels and transporters. These molecules are critical for regulating charge movement, and since the mid-1990s we have acquired considerable knowledge regarding their mechanisms of action as well as the pathways that underlie their regulation. Clearly ion channels are not simply isolated molecules that float in the lipid bilayer but instead are members of highly ordered membrane complexes that are controlled through both transcriptional and posttranslational mechanisms, including protein trafficking and PTMs. While we have uncovered a number of these regulatory pathways to date, we are clearly just beginning to understand how these pathways control cardiac excitability in health and disease. It will be critical in the future to better define these pathways to discover potential new therapeutic modalities to tune automaticity in disease.

REFERENCES

1. Christensen MD, Dun W, Boyden PA, et al. Oxidized calmodulin kinase II regulates conduction following myocardial infarction: a computational analysis. *PLoS Comput Biol.* 2009;5:e1000583.
2. Curran J, Mohler PJ. Alternative paradigms for ion channelopathies: disorders of ion channel membrane trafficking and posttranslational modification. *Annu Rev Physiol.* 2015;77:505–524.
3. Curran ME, Splawski I, Timothy KW, et al. A molecular basis for cardiac arrhythmia: HERG mutations cause long QT syndrome. *Cell.* 1995;80:795–803.
4. Sanguinetti MC, Jiang C, Curran ME, et al. A mechanistic link between an inherited and an acquired cardiac arrhythmia: HERG encodes the IKr potassium channel. *Cell.* 1995;81:299–307.
5. Anderson CL, Delisle BP, Anson BD, et al. Most LQT2 mutations reduce Kv11.1 (hERG) current by a class 2 (trafficking-deficient) mechanism. *Circulation.* 2006;113:365–373.
6. Gui J, Wang T, Jones RP, et al. Multiple loss-of-function mechanisms contribute to SCN5A-related familial sick sinus syndrome. *PLoS ONE.* 2010;5:e10985.
7. Ficker E, Dennis A, Kuryshev Y, et al. HERG channel trafficking. *Novartis Found Symp.* 2005;266:57–69.
8. Bukau B, Horwich AL. The Hsp70 and Hsp60 chaperone machines. *Cell.* 1998;92:351–366.
9. Ficker E, Dennis AT, Wang L, et al. Role of the cytosolic chaperones Hsp70 and Hsp90 in maturation of the cardiac potassium channel HERG. *Circ Res.* 2003;92:e87–e100.
10. Bianchi L, Shen Z, Dennis AT, et al. Cellular dysfunction of LQT5-minK mutants: abnormalities of IKs, IKr and trafficking in long QT syndrome. *Hum Mol Genet.* 1999;8:1499–1507.
11. Yamashita F, Horie M, Kubota T, et al. Characterization and subcellular localization of KCNQ1 with a heterozygous mutation in the C terminus. *J Mol Cell Cardiol.* 2001;33:197–207.
12. Labro AJ, Boulet IR, Timmermans JP, et al. The rate-dependent biophysical properties of the LQT1 H258R mutant are counteracted by a dominant negative effect on channel trafficking. *J Mol Cell Cardiol.* 2010;48:1096–1104.
13. Curran J, Makara MA, Little SC, et al. EHD3-dependent endosome pathway regulates cardiac membrane excitability and physiology. *Circ Res.* 2014;115:68–78.
14. Curran J, Musa H, Kline CF, et al. Eps15 Homology domain-containing protein 3 regulates cardiac T-type Ca2+ channel targeting and function in the atria. *J Biol Chem.* 2015;290:12210–12221.
15. Hund TJ, Mohler PJ. Nav channel complex heterogeneity: new targets for the treatment of arrhythmia? *Circulation.* 2014;130:132–134.
16. Zhou D, Lambert S, Malen PL, et al. AnkyrinG is required for clustering of voltage-gated Na channels at axon initial segments and for normal action potential firing. *J Cell Biol.* 1998;143:1295–1304.
17. Lowe JS, Palygin O, Bhasin N, et al. Voltage-gated Nav channel targeting in the heart requires an ankyrin-G dependent cellular pathway. *J Cell Biol.* 2008;180:173–186.
18. Mohler PJ, Rivolta I, Napolitano C, et al. Nav1.5 E1053K mutation causing Brugada syndrome blocks binding to ankyrin-G and expression of Nav1.5 on the surface of cardiomyocytes. *Proc Natl Acad Sci U S A.* 2004;101:17533–17538.
19. Makara MA, Curran J, Little SC, et al. Ankyrin-G coordinates intercalated disc signaling platform to regulate cardiac excitability in vivo. *Circ Res.* 2014;115:929–938.
20. Hund TJ, Koval OM, Li J, et al. A beta(IV)-spectrin/CaMKII signaling complex is essential for membrane excitability in mice. *J Clin Invest.* 2010;120:3508–3519.
21. Glynn P, Musa H, Wu X, et al. Voltage-gated sodium channel phosphorylation at Ser571 regulates late current, arrhythmia, and cardiac function in vivo. *Circulation.* 2015;132:567–577.
22. Sato PY, Coombs W, Lin X, et al. Interactions between ankyrin-G, Plakophilin-2, and Connexin43 at the cardiac intercalated disc. *Circ Res.* 2011;109:193–201.
23. Gavillet B, Rougier JS, Domenighetti AA, et al. Cardiac sodium channel Nav1.5 is regulated by a multiprotein complex composed of syntrophins and dystrophin. *Circ Res.* 2006;99:407–414.
24. Shy D, Gillet L, Ogrodnik J, et al. PDZ-domain-binding motif regulates cardiomyocyte compartment-specific Nav1.5 channel expression and function. *Circulation.* 2014;130:147–160.
25. Ueda K, Valdivia C, Medeiros-Domingo A, et al. Syntrophin mutation associated with long QT syndrome through activation of the nNOS-SCN5A macromolecular complex. *Proc Natl Acad Sci U S A.* 2008;105:9355–9360.
26. Wei EQ, Barnett AS, Pitt GS, et al. Fibroblast growth factor homologous factors in the heart: a potential locus for cardiac arrhythmias. *Trends Cardiovasc Med.* 2011;21:199–203.
27. Wang C, Hennessey JA, Kirkton RD, et al. Fibroblast growth factor homologous factor 13 regulates Na+ channels and conduction velocity in murine hearts. *Circ Res.* 2011;109:775–782.
28. Hennessey JA, Marcou CA, Wang C, et al. FGF12 is a candidate Brugada syndrome locus. *Heart Rhythm.* 2013;10:1886–1894.
29. Musa H, Kline CF, Sturm AC, et al. SCN5A variant that blocks fibroblast growth factor homologous factor regulation causes human arrhythmia. *Proc Natl Acad Sci U S A.* 2015;112:12528–12533.
30. Abriel H, Rougier JS, Jalife J. Ion channel macromolecular complexes in cardiomyocytes: roles in sudden cardiac death. *Circ Res.* 2015;116:1971–1988.
31. Smith SA, Sturm AC, Curran J, et al. Dysfunction in the betaII spectrin-dependent cytoskeleton underlies human arrhythmia. *Circulation.* 2015;131:695–708.
32. Mohler PJ, Yoon W, Bennett V. Ankyrin-B targets beta2-spectrin to an intracellular compartment in neonatal cardiomyocytes. *J Biol Chem.* 2004;279:40185–40193.
33. Li J, Kline CF, Hund TJ, et al. Ankyrin-B regulates Kir6.2 membrane expression and function in heart. *J Biol Chem.* 2010;285:28723–28730.
34. Kline CF, Kurata HT, Hund TJ, et al. Dual role of K ATP channel C-terminal motif in membrane targeting and metabolic regulation. *Proc Natl Acad Sci U S A.* 2009;106:16669–16674.
35. Kline CF, Cunha SR, Lowe JS, et al. Revisiting ankyrin-InsP3 receptor interactions: ankyrin-B associates with the cytoplasmic N-terminus of the InsP3 receptor. *J Cell Biochem.* 2008;104:1244–1253.
36. Mohler PJ, Schott JJ, Gramolini AO, et al. Ankyrin-B mutation causes type 4 long-QT cardiac arrhythmia and sudden cardiac death. *Nature.* 2003;421:634–639.
37. Mohler PJ, Hoffman JA, Davis JQ, et al. Isoform specificity among ankyrins. An amphipathic alpha-helix in the divergent regulatory domain of ankyrin-b interacts with the molecular co-chaperone Hdj1/Hsp40. *J Biol Chem.* 2004;279:25798–25804.
38. Ayalon G, Davis JQ, Scotland PB, et al. An ankyrin-based mechanism for functional organization of dystrophin and dystroglycan. *Cell.* 2008;135:1189–1200.
39. Gudmundsson H, Hund TJ, Wright PJ, et al. EH domain proteins regulate cardiac membrane protein targeting. *Circ Res.* 2010;107:84–95.
40. DeGrande ST, Little SC, Nixon DJ, et al. Molecular mechanisms underlying cardiac protein phosphatase 2A regulation in heart. *J Biol Chem.* 2013;288:1032–1046.
41. Little SC, Curran J, Makara MA, et al. Protein phosphatase 2A regulatory subunit B56alpha limits phosphatase activity in the heart. *Sci Signal.* 2015;8:ra72.
42. Cunha SR, Hund TJ, Hashemi S, et al. Defects in ankyrin-based membrane protein targeting pathways underlie atrial fibrillation. *Circulation.* 2011;124:1212–1222.
43. Le Scouarnec S, Bhasin N, Vieyres C, et al. Dysfunction in ankyrin-B-dependent ion channel and transporter targeting causes human sinus node disease. *Proc Natl Acad Sci U S A.* 2008;105:15617–15622.
44. Mohler PJ, Splawski I, Napolitano C, et al. A cardiac arrhythmia syndrome caused by loss of ankyrin-B function. *Proc Natl Acad Sci U S A.* 2004;101:9137–9142.
45. Mohler PJ, Le Scouarnec S, Denjoy I, et al. Defining the cellular phenotype of "ankyrin-B syndrome" variants: human ANK2 variants associated with clinical phenotypes display a spectrum of activities in cardiomyocytes. *Circulation.* 2007;115:432–441.
46. Cunha SR, Mohler PJ. Cardiac ankyrins: essential components for development and maintenance of excitable membrane domains in heart. *Cardiovasc Res.* 2006;71:22–29.
47. Lorenzo DN, Healy JA, Hostettler J, et al. Ankyrin-B metabolic syndrome combines age-dependent adiposity with pancreatic beta cell insufficiency. *J Clin Invest.* 2015;125:3087–3102.
48. Anderson ME. Oxidant stress promotes disease by activating CaMKII. *J Mol Cell Cardiol.* 2015;89:160–167.
49. Marban E. Heart failure: the electrophysiologic connection. *J Cardiovasc Electrophysiol.* 1999;10:1425–1428.
50. Kaab S, Nuss HB, Chiamvimonvat N, et al. Ionic mechanism of action potential prolongation in ventricular myocytes from dogs with pacing-induced heart failure. *Circ Res.* 1996;78:262–273.
51. Kaab S, Dixon J, Duc J, et al. Molecular basis of transient outward potassium current downregulation in human heart failure: a decrease in Kv4.3 mRNA correlates with a reduction in current density. *Circulation.* 1998;98:1383–1393.
52. Narayan SM, Bayer JD, Lalani G, et al. Action potential dynamics explain arrhythmic vulnerability in human heart failure: a clinical and modeling study implicating abnormal calcium handling. *J Am Coll Cardiol.* 2008;52:1782–1792.
53. Anderson ME, Brown JH, Bers DM. CaMKII in myocardial hypertrophy and heart failure. *J Mol Cell Cardiol.* 2011;51:468–473.
54. Aiba T, Hesketh GG, Liu T, et al. Na+ channel regulation by Ca2+/calmodulin and Ca2+/calmodulin-dependent protein kinase II in guinea-pig ventricular myocytes. *Cardiovasc Res.* 2010;85:454–463.
55. Wagner S, Dybkova N, Rasenack EC, et al. Ca2+/calmodulin-dependent protein kinase II regulates cardiac Na+ channels. *J Clin Invest.* 2006;116:3127–3138.
56. Ashpole NM, Herren AW, Ginsburg KS, et al. Ca2+/calmodulin-dependent protein kinase II (CaMKII) regulates cardiac sodium channel NaV1.5 gating by multiple phosphorylation sites. *J Biol Chem.* 2012;287:19856–19869.
57. Koval OM, Snyder JS, Wolf RM, et al. Ca2+/calmodulin-dependent protein kinase II-based regulation of voltage-gated Na+ channel in cardiac disease. *Circulation.* 2012;126:2084–2094.
58. Toischer K, Hartmann N, Wagner S, et al. Role of late sodium current as a potential arrhythmogenic mechanism in the progression of pressure-induced heart disease. *J Mol Cell Cardiol.* 2013;61:111–122.
59. Undrovinas NA, Maltsev VA, Belardinelli L, et al. Late sodium current contributes to diastolic cell Ca2+ accumulation in chronic heart failure. *J Physiol Sci.* 2010;60:245–257.
60. Herren AW, Weber DM, Rigor RR, et al. CaMKII phosphorylation of Na(V)1.5: novel in vitro sites identified by mass spectrometry and reduced S516 phosphorylation in human heart failure. *J Proteome Res.* 2015;14:2298–2311.
61. Marionneau C, Lichti CF, Lindenbaum P, et al. Mass spectrometry-based identification of native cardiac Nav1.5 channel alpha subunit phosphorylation sites. *J Proteome Res.* 2012;11:5994–6007.
62. Bers DM. Adrenergic fight-or-flight: S-NO falls on PKA targets. *Circ Res.* 2015;117:747–749.
63. Cheng J, Valdivia CR, Vaidyanathan R, et al. Caveolin-3 suppresses late sodium current by inhibiting nNOS-dependent S-nitrosylation of SCN5A. *J Mol Cell Cardiol.* 2013;61:102–110.
64. Maltsev VA, Undrovinas A. Late sodium current in failing heart: friend or foe? *Prog Biophys Mol Biol.* 2008;96:421–451.
65. Morotti S, Edwards AG, McCulloch AD, et al. A novel computational model of mouse myocyte electrophysiology to assess the synergy between Na+ loading and CaMKII. *J Physiol.* 2014;592:1181–1197.
66. Reiken S, Gaburjakova M, Guatimosim S, et al. Protein kinase A phosphorylation of the cardiac calcium release channel (ryanodine receptor) in normal and failing hearts. Role of phosphatases and response to isoproterenol. *J Biol Chem.* 2003;278:444–453.
67. Wehrens XH, Lehnart SE, Reiken SR, et al. Ca2+/calmodulin-dependent protein kinase II phosphorylation regulates the cardiac ryanodine receptor. *Circ Res.* 2004;94:e61–e70.
68. Xiao B, Zhong G, Obayashi M, et al. Ser-2030, but not Ser-2808, is the major phosphorylation site in cardiac ryanodine receptors responding to protein kinase A activation upon beta-adrenergic stimulation in normal and failing hearts. *Biochem J.* 2006;396:7–16.
69. Dobrev D, Wehrens XH. Role of RyR2 phosphorylation in heart failure and arrhythmias: controversies around ryanodine receptor phosphorylation in cardiac disease. *Circ Res.* 2014;114:1311–1319.
70. Houser SR. Role of RyR2 phosphorylation in heart failure and arrhythmias: protein kinase A-mediated hyperphosphorylation of the ryanodine receptor at serine 2808 does not alter cardiac contractility or cause heart failure and arrhythmias. *Circ Res.* 2014;114:1320–1327.
71. Ai X, Curran JW, Shannon TR, et al. Ca2+/calmodulin-dependent protein kinase modulates cardiac ryanodine receptor phosphorylation and sarcoplasmic reticulum Ca2+ leak in heart failure. *Circ Res.* 2005;97:1314–1322.
72. Curran J, Hinton MJ, Rios E, et al. Beta-adrenergic enhancement of sarcoplasmic reticulum calcium leak in cardiac myocytes is mediated by calcium/calmodulin-dependent protein kinase. *Circ Res.* 2007;100:391–398.
73. Shannon TR, Pogwizd SM, Bers DM. Elevated sarcoplasmic reticulum Ca2+ leak in intact ventricular myocytes from rabbits in heart failure. *Circ Res.* 2003;93:592–594.
74. Pogwizd SM, Bers DM. Na/Ca exchange in heart failure: contractile dysfunction and arrhythmogenesis. *Ann N Y Acad Sci.* 2002;976:454–465.
75. Pogwizd SM, Hoyt RH, Saffitz JE, et al. Reentrant and focal mechanisms underlying ventricular tachycardia in the human heart. *Circulation.* 1992;86:1872–1887.
76. Pogwizd SM, McKenzie JP, Cain ME. Mechanisms underlying spontaneous and induced ventricular arrhythmias in patients with idiopathic dilated cardiomyopathy. *Circulation.* 1998;98:2404–2414.

77. Mattiazzi A, Kranias EG. The role of CaMKII regulation of phospholamban activity in heart disease. *Front Pharmacol.* 2014;5:5.

78. Irie T, Sips PY, Kai S, et al. S-nitrosylation of calcium-handling proteins in cardiac adrenergic signaling and hypertrophy. *Circ Res.* 2015;117:793–803.

79. Bhasin N, Cunha SR, Mudannayake M, et al. Molecular basis for PP2A regulatory subunit B56alpha targeting in cardiomyocytes. *Am J Physiol Heart Circ Physiol.* 2007;293:H109–H119.

80. DeGrande S, Nixon D, Koval O, et al. CaMKII inhibition rescues proarrhythmic phenotypes in the model of human ankyrin-B syndrome. *Heart Rhythm.* 2012;9:2034–2041.

81. Napolitano C, Liu N, Priori SG. Role of calmodulin kinase in catecholaminergic polymorphic ventricular tachycardia. *Heart Rhythm.* 2011;8:1601–1605.

82. Liu N, Ruan Y, Denegri M, et al. Calmodulin kinase II inhibition prevents arrhythmias in RyR2(R4496C+/-) mice with catecholaminergic polymorphic ventricular tachycardia. *J Mol Cell Cardiol.* 2011;50:214–222.

83. Ho HT, Liu B, Snyder JS, et al. Ryanodine receptor phosphorylation by oxidized CaMKII contributes to the cardiotoxic effects of cardiac glycosides. *Cardiovasc Res.* 2014;101:165–174.

24 Feedback Mechanisms for Cardiac-Specific MicroRNAs and cAMP Signaling in Electrical Remodeling

Xiao-Dong Zhang and Nipavan Chiamvimonvat

Overview of Cardiac MicroRNAs

MicroRNA Biology

MicroRNAs (miRNAs) are endogenously expressed, noncoding RNAs of ~22 nucleotides in length. The initial identification of miRNAs can be dated back to 1993, when two groups of investigators reported the posttranscriptional regulation of the *lin-14* gene by small transcripts of the *lin-4* gene in *Caenorhabditis elegans*, suggesting that *lin-4* regulates *lin-14* translation via an antisense RNA–RNA interaction.[1,2] These landmark findings opened the era of miRNAs in biological sciences. Since then, the significance and essential roles of miRNAs in biological processes have been intensely studied and miRNAs have been shown to participate in nearly all developmental and pathological processes. Importantly, recent studies suggest that miRNAs may represent potential biomarkers and therapeutic targets for human diseases.[3–8]

Genes encoding miRNAs constitute one of the most abundant gene families. They are widely distributed in animals, plants, protists, and viruses.[4,9] To date, ~2600 miRNAs have been identified in the human genome according to the recent release of the miRNA database (miRBase).[4,10] MiRNAs are encoded by introns of noncoding or coding transcripts, but some miRNAs are encoded by their own genes.[4] Further, miRNAs can be transcribed either individually or in clusters as polycistronic transcripts.

The maturation of miRNAs involves two steps of endonucleolytic cleavage following transcription in the nucleus where they are transcribed by RNA polymerase II to form primary miRNAs (pri-miRNAs), usually over 1 kb in length. Pri-miRNAs are cleaved in the nucleus by the microprocessor,[11] a protein complex primarily composed of the RNase III enzyme ribonuclease 3 (also known as RNASEN or Drosha) and its cofactor DiGeorge syndrome critical region gene 8 (DGCR8 or Pasha).[12,13] The hairpin loop is first recognized by DGCR8, which recruits RNASEN to cut the pri-miRNAs at the base of the stem structure, releasing the stem-loop portion of ~65 nucleotides termed precursor miRNAs (pre-miRNAs).[14] The pre-miRNAs then translocate out of the nucleus via the ATP-dependent Exportin-5 protein (Xpo5).[15,16] In the cytoplasm, pre-miRNAs interact with a second RNase III enzyme, Dicer, and

its cofactor, HIV-1 transactivating response (TAR) RNA-binding protein (TRBP).[17,18] Dicer cleaves off the loop structure, leaving only the stem region, referred to as the miRNA duplex,[19,20] since the two strands of the stem are no longer covalently connected and only held together by base pairing. This cleavage allows the duplex to be unwound and separated in an ATP-independent[21] fashion by Dicer, TRBP, and argonaute 2 (AGO2), which together form the RNA-induced silencing complex (RISC).[22,23] Through the interaction of the miRNA duplex and RISC, the duplex is unwound and one strand, the guide strand, is loaded onto AGO2.[24] The other strand, the passenger strand, is degraded. The guide strand is the mature and fully functional miRNA unit and can target a variety of coding messenger RNAs to promote degradation and translational repression.

A hallmark of miRNAs is their tremendous potential to target a large number of genes, often in common pathways. With an estimated 60% of human messenger RNA having conserved miRNA targets, miRNAs represent one of the key regulators and informative biomarkers of a set of genes controlling different cellular processes rather than single genes.[25,26] To comprehensively evaluate the influence of miRNAs on multiple proteins through the integration of various downstream genes, the global evaluation of miRNA in the signaling cascade becomes essential.[27]

MicroRNA in the Heart

miRNAs in the heart have been extensively studied since the mid-2000s.[28–30] Cardiac-specific miRNAs play critical roles in heart development, myocardial regeneration, and cardiac remodeling. *MiR-1* and *miR-133* are muscle-specific miRNAs representing the most abundant miRNAs expressed in the heart.[31,32] Mouse embryos lacking Dicer in the developing heart die from cardiac failure before birth and exhibit a poorly developed ventricular myocardium.[33] Dicer is necessary for cardiac outflow tract alignment and chamber septation.[34] Conditional *Dicer* gene deletion in 3-week-old mice provokes premature death and induces rapid and dramatic biventricular enlargement accompanied by cardiac hypertrophy, myofiber disarray, ventricular fibrosis, and strong induction of fetal gene transcripts in adult mice.[35] Cardiomyocyte-specific deletion of DGCR8, an essential partner of Drosha, in newborn hearts induces dilated cardiomyopathy and heart failure.[36] Several miRNAs, including *miR-1*, *miR-133*, *miR-208a*, *miR-208b*, *miR-499*, the *miR-15* family, and the *miR-17~92* cluster of miRNAs, have been reported to be important for cardiac development.[28,37]

MiRNAs are also essential in myocardial regeneration. The global loss of miRNAs in embryonic stem cells by deletion of *Dicer* and *Drosha* or *DGCR8* leads to defective differentiation and proliferation.[38,39] Muscle-specific *miR-1* and *miR-133* have been identified to influence muscle lineage commitment and regulate muscle proliferation and differentiation.[39,40] A recent study analyzing the roles of *miR-1* and *miR-133a* in the differentiation of pluripotent stem cells shows the importance of *miR-1* and *miR-133a* in controlling cardiac fate of the pluripotent cells.[41] *MiR-499* is a cardiac-specific miRNA and is essential for cardiac commitment of human embryonic stem cells.[42–44] MiR-NAs are also potent regulators of cell-fate reprograming, and several miRNAs, including *miR-1*, *-133a*, *-208a*, and *-499*, have been shown to be capable of converting cardiac fibroblasts into cardiomyocytes.[45]

Critical Roles of MicroRNAs in the Regulation of Cardiac Ion Channel Expression

Recent studies have provided strong evidence for the critical roles of miRNAs in ion channel regulation.[46,47] *MiR-1-2* deletion in mice induces abnormal cardiac electrical activity, including slow heart rate, shortened PR interval, and prolonged QRS complexes with increased incidence of sudden death.[33] Abnormality in cardiac excitability may result partially from upregulation of the iroquois homeobox domain 5 (Irx5), which is a confirmed target of *miR-1*. Irx5 is a known homeodomain transcriptional inhibitor of the *Kcnd2* gene encoding for the pore-forming $K_v4.2$ subunit of the transient outward K^+ channel. As a result, the expression of *Kcnd2* is downregulated, leading to decreased transient outward K^+ currents (I_{to}).

MiR-1 has been shown to target Kir2.1 channel, and overexpression of *miR-1* suppresses the expression of the Kir2.1 channel and connexin43.[48] Additionally, *miR-1* inhibits the expression of other ion channel genes, including *Scn5a*, *Cacna1c*, *Kcna5*, and *Kcne1*.[49] The protein phosphatase 2 (PP2A) regulatory subunit, B56alpha, is a target of *miR-1*, and *miR-1* overexpression increases phosphorylation of L-type Ca^{2+} channels and ryanodine receptor 2 (RyR2) by suppressing PP2A, which enhances RyR2 activity and cardiac excitation–contraction coupling.[50]

In contrast, *miR-133* is reported to depress PP2A activities, resulting in abnormal RyR2 function and Ca^{2+} cycling in heart failure leading to increased propensity to cardiac arrhythmias.[51] In addition, *miR-133* may also regulate pacemaker channels, hyperpolarization-activated cyclic nucleotide–gated channels (HCN2 and HCN4).[52] *MiR-208* is a cardiac-specific miRNA, and analysis of mice lacking *miR-208a* indicates that *miR-208a* is required for proper cardiac conduction and expression of the gap junction protein connexin40.[53]

One recent study examined the roles of Dicer1, a critical enzyme processor for the maturation of miRNAs in the heart.[54] Delivery of a *Cre* recombinase–expressing adenovirus (Ad-GFP-Cre) to the left ventricles of a conditional *Dicer1* knockout mouse model (*Dicer1^{tm1Bdb}/f*), which contains a floxed RNase III domain critical for Dicer1, results in cardiac-specific knockout of the Dicer1 enzyme. Similar to *miR-1-2* deletion, knockout of *Dicer1* in adult mouse cardiomyocytes results in decreased I_{to} and prolonged action potential duration (APD). In addition, an increased Ca^{2+} current (I_{Ca}) is observed. This model allows the evaluation of the roles of miRNAs on ionic currents without the interference of organ level changes, such as hypertrophy or fibrosis. Parallel experiments in neonatal *Dicer1^{tm1Bdb}/f* mouse cardiomyocytes by transduction of Ad-GFP-Cre resulted in increased *Cacna1c* transcripts encoding for the $Ca_v1.2$ (α_{1c}) pore-forming subunit of the L-type Ca^{2+} channel and decreased *Kcnd2* transcripts encoding for the $K_v4.2$ pore-forming subunit for the transient outward K^+ channel. Moreover, there is a significant increase in the expression of the known *Kcnd2* transcriptional inhibitor, Irx5, a validated target of *miR-1*.[35,55,56] Taken together, these studies support the critical role of miRNAs in the regulation of cardiac ion channel expression.

MicroRNA Signature of Cardiovascular Diseases

Apart from the critical roles of miRNAs in normal cardiac development and myocardial regeneration, the expression and function of miRNAs in the diseased heart demonstrate significant alterations

resulting from pathological remodeling, characterized by distinct miRNA signatures in cardiovascular diseases.[28,37,57] A signature pattern of cardiac miRNAs has been reported in cardiac hypertrophy and heart failure, and more than 12 miRNAs have been identified to be up- or downregulated associated with pathological processes.[58] Many miRNAs are downregulated through different stages after transverse aortic constriction in a mouse model, and muscle-specific *miR-1* is singularly downregulated as early as day one and persists through day seven postoperation.[59] The significance of miRNAs in cardiac pathogenesis highlights the potential of miRNAs as novel diagnostic markers and therapeutic targets for the treatment of cardiovascular diseases. Challenges remain regarding the roles and regulatory mechanisms of distinct miRNAs during different pathological processes and disease progression. Moreover, cardiac diseases such as hypertrophy and heart failure result in significant electrical remodeling, changes in miRNA expression, and a multitude of alterations in intracellular signaling, all of which are highly interdependent and coregulated. Readers are referred to extensive publications and reviews on the subject. This chapter will focus on the feedback mechanisms and regulation of miRNAs and 3′, 5′-cyclic adenosine monophosphate (cAMP) signaling in cardiac electrical remodeling.

Functional Roles of MicroRNAs in Cardiac cAMP Signaling and Electrical Remodeling

cAMP Signaling in the Heart

cAMP is a diffusible intracellular second messenger generated by adenylyl cyclases (ACs) in response to the binding of hormones and neurotransmitters to G protein–coupled receptors. cAMP orchestrates a network of intracellular events by activating a multitude of intracellular targets including protein kinase A (PKA), the exchange protein directly activated by cAMP (Epac), and cyclic nucleotide–gated ion channels. In cardiomyocytes, cAMP is a key regulator of cardiac function and represents the major second messenger of the β-adrenergic receptor (β-AR) pathway, producing positive chronotropic, inotropic, and lusitropic effects during sympathetic stimulation. Further, cAMP activates PKA leading to the subsequent phosphorylation of several key proteins, including L-type Ca^{2+} channel, phospholamban, ryanodine receptor (RyR2), and troponin I.[60–63] Accumulated studies provide evidence for the specificity of cAMP-signaling complexes achieved via subcellular compartmentalization to allow fast, effective, and precise integration of the signaling networks.[60,64,65] For example, subcellular compartmentalization of AC-cAMP-PKA signaling complexes allows cAMP to gain access to a subset of cAMP-dependent PKA, and PKA can only interact with a subset of relevant cellular substrates.

cAMP Signaling in Cardiac Electrical Remodeling

Chronic activation of the β-AR/cAMP signaling pathway has been shown to trigger pathological remodeling, ultimately leading to heart failure accompanied by significant downregulation of β_1-AR expression.[66–68] Electrical remodeling has been well documented in cardiac hypertrophy and failure, with APD prolongation and downregulation of K^+ currents.[69] Several ion channels, including voltage-gated Na^+, Ca^{2+}, and K^+ channels, can be modulated by the β-AR/cAMP signaling pathway,[70] and thus cAMP represents one of the key molecules mediating cardiac electrical remodeling.

MicroRNA and cAMP Signaling

A recent study tested the effects of a β-blocker, propranolol, on *miR-1* expression in a rat myocardial infarction (MI) model.[71] In ischemic myocardium, *miR-1* expression was upregulated and administration of propranolol reversed the upregulation of *miR-1* and reduced the incidence of arrhythmias. Moreover, the study identified the presence of a cAMP response element (CRE) in the *miR-1* promoter region, suggesting a potential role for β-AR/cAMP signaling in the regulation of *miR-1* expression. A subsequent study examined in detail the expression profile of miRNAs and the functional implications under conditions of β-AR activation or inhibition in rat heart.[72] Rats were treated with isoproterenol or propranolol, and the expression of 349 miRNAs was analyzed. Isoproterenol and propranolol induced differential miRNA expression profiles. In the isoproterenol-treated group, 43 miRNAs were upregulated and 9 miRNAs were downregulated; in the propranolol-treated group, only 5 miRNAs were upregulated, whereas 28 miRNAs were downregulated. Isoproterenol and propranolol exert opposite effects on the expression of 11 miRNAs that are abundantly expressed in the heart, suggesting a specific role of the β-AR/cAMP signaling pathway in the regulation of cardiac miRNAs. The effects of long-term stimulation of β-AR on the expression of the GTP-binding protein, Rem, were examined. While *miR-132* and *miR-214* expression was upregulated five-fold and nine-fold, respectively, Rem expression was reduced. Moreover, Rem was identified as a target of *miR-132*.[73] *MiR-132* has been shown to regulate both cardiac hypertrophy and cardiomyocyte autophagy,[74] and it is well established that β-AR overstimulation leads to development of hypertrophy.[75,76]

CRE-Binding, CRE-Modulator, and Inducible cAMP Early Repressor Proteins

β-AR/cAMP signaling can activate two regulatory proteins, CRE-binding protein (CREB) and CRE-modulator (CREM), which are regulators of the CREB signaling pathway and a predicted target of *miR-1*.[77,78] Recent studies have documented the beneficial effects of preserving β-adrenergic sensitivity after an MI[79,80] and the essential role of CREM in chronic β-adrenergic signaling.[81] In addition, cardiac-specific knockout of *Creb* leads to electrical remodeling in cardiomyocytes similar to that seen post-MI with a loss of I_{to} and prolonged APDs.[82] These studies highlight the critical roles of CREM and CREB in cardiac electrical remodeling.

One isoform of CREM, termed the inducible cAMP early repressor (ICER), arises from an alternative internal promoter and is induced by β-adrenergic signaling.[83] ICER contains only the CRE DNA–binding domain and acts as a powerful repressor of CREB signaling, thus constituting a negative autoregulatory loop. Under physiological conditions, ICER acts in a negative feedback fashion to prevent overactivation of CREB-dependent genes. However, under chronic pathological conditions, excessive β-adrenergic signaling drives a progressive increase in ICER expression that may contribute to inhibition of CREB-dependent gene expression and β-adrenergic desensitization.[84,85] Continuous infusion of isoproterenol increases ICER in the rat heart in vivo, and overexpression of ICER significantly attenuates isoproterenol-induced cardiac hypertrophy but also stimulates cardiac myocyte apoptosis.[84] Therefore ICER represents a critical regulator of the β-AR/cAMP signaling pathway in the heart.

Feedback Mechanisms for Cardiac MicroRNAs and cAMP Signaling in Cardiac Electrical Remodeling

Roles of MicroRNAs in Electrical Remodeling in Cardiac Hypertrophy and Failure

Electrical remodeling with action potential prolongation represents one of the hallmarks of cardiac hypertrophy and failure.[69,86–93] Prolongation of the cardiac action potential results in part from the downregulation of the underlying outward K⁺ currents.[94–99] However, the mechanistic underpinning for the downregulation of the K⁺ currents remains incompletely understood.

Recent studies have provided strong evidence for the significant roles of miRNAs in ion channel regulation and cardiac electrical remodeling in heart failure.[46,47] Further, *miR-1* and *miR-133a* have been identified to be critical players in hypertrophy-induced cardiac electrical remodeling.[58,59,71,100,101] *MiR-1* overexpression has been identified in patients with coronary artery disease, and overexpression of *miR-1* exacerbates arrhythmogenesis in normal or infarcted rat hearts. Potential underlying mechanisms include suppression of *Kcnj2* gene expression (encoding for the pore-forming Kir2.1 subunit of the inwardly rectifying K⁺ channel) and *Gja1* gene expression (encoding connexin43) by *miR-1*.[48]

Loss of miRNAs may underlie the well-documented electrical remodeling seen in pathological cardiac hypertrophy and failure.[35,36] Specifically, cardiac *miR-1* and *miR-133a* are significantly reduced in different hypertrophy models.[58,59,100] However, the mechanistic basis leading to miRNA dysregulation in diseased conditions remains incompletely understood. In a recent study, a decrease in the enzyme Dicer1 was documented in end-stage heart failure patients, and the level of Dicer1 was rescued by a left ventricular assist device implantation.[102] In the acute phase of MI, levels of *miR-1* and *miR-133a* increase and can be detected in the circulation.[103,104] However, these miRNA levels quickly decline.[105,106] Myocardia from patients with ischemic heart failure exhibit decreased levels of *miR-1* and *miR-133a*, which are restored after implantation of a left ventricular assist device.[107] In particular, *miR-1* has been shown to enhance I_{to} by repressing Irx5, and loss of *miR-1* may underlie the I_{to} remodeling seen post-MI.[35,55,56] Therefore loss of miRNAs may underlie the well-documented remodeling in cardiac hypertrophy and failure (Fig. 24.1).[35,36,55]

MiR-133 has been reported to be essential to the control of cardiac hypertrophy.[100] In this study, three murine models of cardiac hypertrophy, including transverse aortic arch–constricted (TAC) mice, transgenic mice with selective cardiac overexpression of a constitutively active mutant of the Akt kinase, and exercised rats, were thoroughly examined and assessed for expression levels of *miR-133* and *miR-1*. Cardiac hypertrophy in all three models resulted in reduced expression levels of both *miR-133* and *miR-1*, and this decrease was particularly prominent in the left ventricle and atria. The reduced expression of *miR-133* and *miR-1* was also identified in diseased human ventricles and atria. Additionally, in vivo inhibition of *miR-133* by a single infusion of an antagomir caused marked and sustained cardiac hypertrophy, and in vitro overexpression of *miR-133* or *miR-1* inhibited cardiac hypertrophy. Another study tested the effects of restoring *miR-133a* levels on the hypertrophic remodeling.[101] Cardiac α-myosin heavy chain (*MYH6*) promoter–directed expression of a *miR-133a* genomic precursor was used to induce the overexpression of *miR-133a* in normal and pressure-overloaded adult mouse heart, and it was found that increased expression of *miR-133a* had no effect on postnatal cardiac development assessed by measures of structure, function, and messenger RNA profile. However, QT duration corrected for heart rate (QTc) and APD in isolated ventricular myocytes was significantly increased in *miR-133a*–overexpressed mice. The fast component of I_{to} was also decreased. Interestingly, transgenic expression of *miR-133a* prevented TAC-associated *miR-133a* downregulation and improved myocardial fibrosis and diastolic function without affecting the extent of hypertrophy, and I_{to} downregulation normally observed post-TAC was absent in *miR-133a* transgenic mice.[101] *MiR-212* has been found to be upregulated in heart failure.[108] Bioinformatics analysis revealed a potential target in the 3′ UTR of Kir2.1 (*Kcnj2*) for *miR-212*, and overexpression of *miR-212* downregulates Kir2.1 channels.

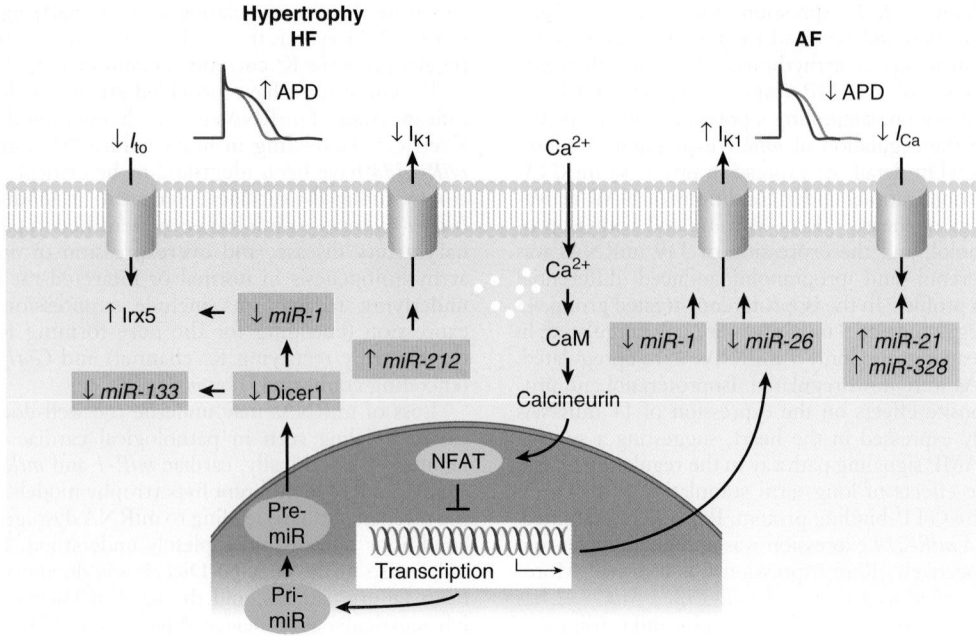

FIGURE 24.1 Roles of microRNAs in electrical remodeling in cardiac hypertrophy and failure and in atrial fibrillation. *AF,* Atrial fibrillation; *APD,* action potential duration; *HF,* heart failure; *NFAT,* nuclear factor of activated T cells.

Roles of MicroRNAs in Electrical Remodeling in Atrial Fibrillation

Atrial fibrillation (AF) represents the most common arrhythmia clinically. The inward-rectifier K+ current (I_{K1}) has been shown to be a major component of AF-related electrical remodeling. Several miRNAs have been predicted to target the gene encoding Kir2.1, *Kcnj2*, including *miR-1*, *miR-212*, and *miR-26*. Specifically, *miR-26* has been shown to be downregulated in atrial samples from animal models and in patients with AF, leading to the upregulation of I_{K1} and the Kir2.1 protein.[109] Moreover, it is demonstrated that *Kcnj2* is a target of *miR-26*. The same study further provides new mechanistic insight into the documented alterations in *miR-26*. Specifically, nuclear factor of activated T cells (NFAT), a known factor in AF-associated remodeling, negatively regulates *miR-26* transcription (see Fig. 24.1).[109]

In patients with persistent AF, *miR-1* levels are greatly reduced, contributing to the upregulation of Kir2.1 subunits and increased I_{K1}, abbreviation of the atrial refractoriness, and maintenance of AF.[110] L-type Ca2+ channels and RyR2 are also reported to be regulated by *miR-1*. Overexpression of *miR-1* inhibits protein phosphatase 2A (PP2A) and increases the phosphorylation of L-type Ca2+ channels and RyR2, resulting in the enhancement of Ca2+ release and cardiac arrhythmogenesis.[50]

In contrast to the downregulation of *miR-1* and *miR-26*, several miRNAs have been found to be upregulated in AF. *MiR-21* was recently identified to be upregulated in atrial myocytes in chronic AF patients and was associated with the reduction of the L-type Ca2+ current density and decreased expression of pore-forming subunits of Ca$_v$1.2 (α_{1c}) Ca2+ channel (*CACNA1C*). Further computational analyses and experimental study demonstrated that *CACNA1C* as well as the β2 subunit of the Ca2+ channel (*CACNB2*) are potential targets for *miR-21*.[111] An additional study also found that *miR-328* levels were elevated in a canine model of AF and in patients with AF relative to non-AF subjects. Further computational prediction and experimental studies identified *CACNA1C* and *CACNB1* as the potential targets for *miR-328*.[112]

Delivery of *miR-1/133a* Prevents Electrical Remodeling Post–Myocardial Infarction

It has previously been shown that delivery of *miR-1* and the cotranscribed *miR-133a* by in vivo tail vein injections in a clinically relevant ischemia-reperfusion mouse model can significantly improve cardiac function post-MI.[54] In both the ischemia-reperfusion model and in patients, the long-term effects of MI include hypertrophy, fibrosis, electrical remodeling, and progression toward heart failure. In this study, control MI mice received nonsilencing miRNA mimics and exhibited an increased heart weight/body weight (HW/BW) ratio with significant increases in the transcripts for atrial natriuretic peptide (*Nppa*) and angiotensinogen (*Agt*). Cardiac hypertrophy was prevented in the *miR-1/133a*–injected MI mice and the transcript levels for *Nppa* and *Agt*, as well as the skeletal α-actin (*Acta1*) levels, returned to the sham levels. *Agt* is a predicted target of *miR-133a*, and local release of angiotensinogen has been described as pathological in MI.[113] *Nppa* and *Acta1* are not predicted targets of *miR-1* or *miR-133a*, but their expression has been linked to both miRNAs through indirect mechanisms.[100,101]

In vivo or in vitro overexpression of *MiR-1* and *miR-133a* has been shown to increase the expression of *Kcnd2* or enhance the I_{to}.[55,56,101] To directly test the roles of *miR-1* and *miR-133a* on electrical remodeling, patch-clamp recordings of I_{to}, I_{Ca}, and APD were performed in cardiomyocytes isolated from mice that had received a *miR-1/133a* injection.[54] In MI mice, peak I_{to} current was significantly reduced, leading to prolonged APD. Moreover, delivery of *miR-1* and *miR-133a* resulted in the recovery of peak I_{to} density toward sham levels together with normalization of the voltage-dependent activation of I_{to} toward sham control. Indeed, after MI, there was a 35% decrease in K$_v$4.2 channel transcripts (*Kcnd2*) and a 77% increase in Irx5. *MiR-1/133a* delivery prevented the increase in *Irx5* expression and increased *Kcnd2* levels to 85% of sham levels. In addition, consistent with the findings observed after *Dicer1* knockout, peak I_{Ca} density was significantly reduced by miRNA delivery.

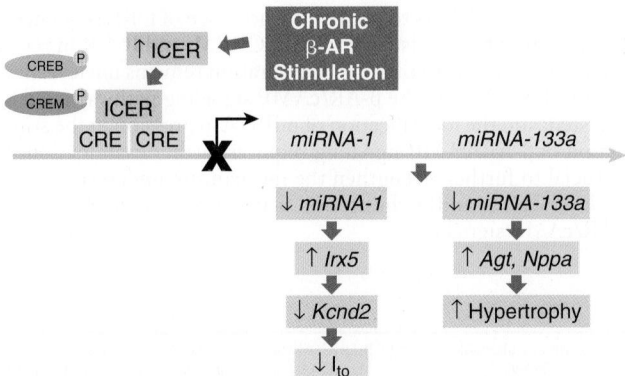

FIGURE 24.2 Feedback mechanisms for cardiac microRNAs (*miRNAs*) and cyclic adenosine monophosphate (cAMP) signaling in cardiac electrical remodeling. *β-AR*, Beta-adrenergic receptor; *CRE*, cAMP response element; *CREB*, CRE-binding protein; *CREM*, CRE-modulator; *ICER*, inducible cAMP early repressor.

CRE-Modulator and Inducible cAMP Early Repressor Are Targets of *miR-1*

The beneficial effects of overexpression of *miR-1/133a* on hypertrophy-induced cardiac electrical remodeling have been documented.[40,52,54] However, the targets of *miR-1/133a* have not been completely identified. CREM represents an important key regulator of cardiac gene expression, which is essential for normal left ventricular contractile performance and response to β-AR stimulation.[81] In cardiac hypertrophy, one isoform of CREM, ICER, is upregulated by cardiac hypertrophic stimuli, which inhibits the CRE-mediated transcription in cardiac myocytes and acts as a negative regulator of hypertrophy.[84,85] Indeed, it was recently demonstrated using a luciferase reporter system that CREM and ICER are *miR-1* targets.[54] The predicted *miR-1* binding sequence was identified in the 3′ untranslated regions of all CREM isoforms except CREM7 and 8, which correspond to τ-like isoforms not found in the heart.[114] Importantly, the *miR-1*–binding sequence is identified in the two ICER isoforms of CREM. It is further demonstrated that delivery of *miR-1/133a* reduces the elevated *Icer* expression levels in MI mouse heart and returns the level toward the sham control.

Additionally, an isoproterenol infusion mouse model was used to test the roles of β-adrenergic signaling on the expression of ICER and miRNAs in the heart. Indeed, chronic isoproterenol challenge results in a significant increase in *Icer* expression similar to that seen in the post-MI heart. In addition, the expression levels of *miR-1* and *Kcnd2* are reduced. More importantly, similar to the MI model, treatment with *miR-1/133a* by tail vein injections normalizes the levels of *Icer*.[54]

As demonstrated in Fig. 24.2, a feedback mechanism for the regulation of miRNAs was proposed for CRE, ICER, and cardiac electrical remodeling in pathological conditions of the heart subjected to chronic activation of the β-AR/cAMP signaling pathway. Both CREM and ICER are direct targets of *miR-1*, and increased expression of ICER post-MI leads to reduction of *miR-1* and *miR-133* and the consequences of electrical remodeling. Since CREM and ICER are *miR-1* targets,[54] the reduced *miR-1* expression further maintains the elevated expression of ICER forming a feedback signaling pathway.

Therapeutic Potentials of MicroRNA Delivery in Cardiac Electrical Remodeling

The intense and exciting studies of cardiac miRNAs since the mid-2000s have elucidated the critical roles of miRNAs in cardiac development, myocardial regeneration, and cardiac remodeling during hypertrophy and failure. The temporally and spatially regulated expression of miRNAs forms a dynamic network to fine-tune gene expression in physiological and pathological conditions. Importantly, the emerging miRNA signature of cardiovascular diseases provides the tantalizing possibility for the use of cardiac miRNAs as diagnostic biomarkers and as potential targets for therapeutics in cardiovascular diseases.

Electrical remodeling has been shown to occur in several cardiac pathological conditions, including hypertrophy, heart failure, and AF. During the remodeling process, miRNAs may directly target the transcripts of ion channels, transporters, and their associated regulatory proteins to modify their expression and alter the excitability of cardiomyocytes. Alternatively, miRNAs may target the signaling pathways that regulate ion channel expression and function. Moreover, miRNAs have been shown to regulate a set of genes that control different cellular processes rather than single genes.[25,26] This pattern of regulation adds to the intricacy and complexity of the gene expression as well as to the efficiency and economy of the cells in the fine-tuning process.

Significant roles of multiple miRNAs in cardiac electrical remodeling have been identified. Indeed, dysregulation of miRNAs in the heart represents a major cause of maladaptive process, leading to adverse cardiac remodeling. A single miRNA may modulate multiple target genes, leading to cardiac electrical remodeling. Therefore miRNA therapeutic strategies may include miRNA reexpression to recover reduced miRNA levels or anti-miRNA to suppress overexpressed miRNAs in diseased heart.[28,30,115] Multiple miRNAs are dysregulated in specific cardiac diseases, and a single miRNA may regulate a network of genes. Several new techniques and approaches have been developed[115]; however, challenges remain regarding the current knowledge gaps in our understanding of the intricate and intertwining miRNA regulatory mechanisms underlying cardiovascular diseases.

Summary and Future Perspectives

Extensive studies of cardiac miRNA since the mid-2000s have elucidated the distinct roles of miRNAs in cardiac physiology and pathology. With the aid of bioinformatics analyses and advanced molecular biological techniques, many target genes of miRNAs in the heart have been identified and the functions of a multitude of cardiac miRNAs have been revealed. Cardiac electrical remodeling represents an adaptive change in cardiac electrophysiological function against stress.[116] Cardiac hypertrophy, heart failure, and arrhythmia are the major causes leading to electrical remodeling involving alterations in the expression ion channels and transporters in the heart. MiRNAs represent critical players in regulating gene expression in the heart, which has been documented in cardiac development, myocardial regeneration, and cardiac remodeling. Several cardiac ion channels have been identified to be the targets of a specific miRNA, and the altered expression levels of miRNAs have been demonstrated to cause the abnormal function of cardiac ion channels in the diseased human heart as well as in animal models.

Cardiac electrical remodeling is tightly linked to abnormal β-AR/cAMP signaling. An important finding reveals the presence of a CRE sequence in the *miR-1* promoter region, suggesting β-AR/cAMP signaling in the heart may regulate the expression of miRNAs.[71] One recent study further tested the mechanistic underpinnings among *miR-1/133a*, cAMP signaling, and electrical remodeling in a clinically relevant mouse model of MI and revealed a novel feedback mechanism underlying cardiac miRNAs and the electrical remodeling in pathological conditions with heightened β-AR stimulation.[54] At the translational level, the study provides a molecular basis for the potential roles for *miR-1* and *miR-133* therapy post-MI and offers a proof-of-concept for miRNA intervention.

β-AR/cAMP signaling in the heart has been extensively studied. The altered miRNA expression by β-AR/cAMP signaling and the regulation of the signaling pathways by miRNAs provide a new and exciting mechanistic insight as well as treatment strategy for cardiac diseases. Because of the broad spectrum of the target proteins and the spatial and temporal control of β-AR/cAMP signaling, miRNA regulation may have a wide-ranging impact on the downstream effectors of the signaling. Indeed, many open questions remain. Computational analyses are necessary to analyze other cardiac miRNAs to predict the presence of CRE sequences; the molecular mechanisms of CREB, CREM, and ICER in regulating miRNA transcription and maturation remains unclear; new targets of miRNAs in the β-AR/cAMP signaling pathway need to be tested; and the identification of miRNA expression in the stimulation of β-AR/cAMP signaling requires further examination. It is crucial to further strengthen the mechanistic understanding of the interactions and orchestration between cardiac miRNAs and β-AR/cAMP signaling.

REFERENCES

1. Lee RC, Feinbaum RL, Ambros V. The *C. elegans* heterochronic gene lin-4 encodes small RNAs with antisense complementarity to lin-14. *Cell*. 1993;75:843–854.
2. Wightman B, Ha I, Ruvkun G. Posttranscriptional regulation of the heterochronic gene lin-14 by lin-4 mediates temporal pattern formation in. *C. elegans*. *Cell*. 1993;75:855–862.
3. Soifer HS, Rossi JJ, Saetrom P. MicroRNAs in disease and potential therapeutic applications. *Mol Ther*. 2007;15:2070–2079.
4. Ha M, Kim VN. Regulation of microRNA biogenesis. *Nat Rev Mol Cell Biol*. 2014;15:509–524.
5. Sayed D, Abdellatif M. MicroRNAs in development and disease. *Physiol Rev*. 2011;91:827–887.
6. Kim YK. Extracellular microRNAs as biomarkers in human disease. *Chonnam Med J*. 2015;51:51–57.
7. Wang J, Chen J, Sen S. MicroRNA as biomarkers and diagnostics. *J Cell Physiol*. 2016;231:25–30.
8. Goretti E, Wagner DR, Devaux Y. MiRNAs as biomarkers of myocardial infarction: a step forward towards personalized medicine? *Trends Mol Med*. 2014;20:716–725.
9. Griffiths-Jones S, Saini HK, van Dongen S, Enright AJ. MiRBase: tools for microRNA genomics. *Nucleic Acids Res*. 2008;36:D154–D158.
10. Kozomara A, Griffiths-Jones S. MiRBase: annotating high confidence microRNAs using deep sequencing data. *Nucleic Acids Res*. 2014;42:D68–D73.
11. Gregory RI, Yan KP, Amuthan G, et al. The Microprocessor complex mediates the genesis of microRNAs. *Nature*. 2004;432:235–240.
12. Wu H, Xu H, Miraglia LJ, Crooke ST. Human RNase III is a 160-kDa protein involved in preribosomal RNA processing. *J Biol Chem*. 2000;275:36957–36965.
13. Lee Y, Ahn C, Han J, et al. The nuclear RNase III Drosha initiates microRNA processing. *Nature*. 2003;425:415–419.
14. Han J, Lee Y, Yeom KH, et al. Molecular basis for the recognition of primary microRNAs by the Drosha-DGCR8 complex. *Cell*. 2006;125:887–901.
15. Lund E, Guttinger S, Calado A, Dahlberg JE, Kutay U. Nuclear export of microRNA precursors. *Science*. 2004;303:95–98.
16. Yi R, Qin Y, Macara IG, Cullen BR. Exportin-5 mediates the nuclear export of pre-microRNAs and short hairpin RNAs. *Genes Dev*. 2003;17:3011–3016.
17. Chendrimada TP, Gregory RI, Kumaraswamy E, et al. TRBP recruits the Dicer complex to Ago2 for microRNA processing and gene silencing. *Nature*. 2005;436:740–744.
18. Lau PW, Potter CS, Carragher B, MacRae IJ. Structure of the human Dicer-TRBP complex by electron microscopy. *Structure*. 2009;17:1326–1332.
19. Vermeulen A, Behlen L, Reynolds A, et al. The contributions of dsRNA structure to Dicer specificity and efficiency. *RNA*. 2005;11:674–682.
20. Kim VN. MicroRNA biogenesis: coordinated cropping and dicing. *Nat Rev Mol Cell Biol*. 2005;6:376–385.
21. Maniataki E, Mourelatos Z. A human, ATP-independent, RISC assembly machine fueled by pre-miRNA. *Genes Dev*. 2005;19:2979–2990.
22. Wang HW, Noland C, Siridechadilok B, et al. Structural insights into RNA processing by the human RISC-loading complex. *Nat Struct Mol Biol*. 2009;16:1148–1153.
23. Meister G, Landthaler M, Peters L, et al. Identification of novel argonaute-associated proteins. *Curr Biol*. 2005;15:2149–2155.
24. Gregory RI, Chendrimada TP, Cooch N, Shiekhattar R. Human RISC couples microRNA biogenesis and posttranscriptional gene silencing. *Cell*. 2005;123:631–640.
25. Friedman RC, Farh KK, Burge CB, Bartel DP. Most mammalian mRNAs are conserved targets of microRNAs. *Genome Res*. 2009;19:92–105.
26. Cummins JM, Velculescu VE. Implications of micro-RNA profiling for cancer diagnosis. *Oncogene*. 2006;25:6220–6227.
27. Inui M, Martello G, Piccolo S. MicroRNA control of signal transduction. *Nat Rev Mol Cell Biol*. 2010;11:252–263.
28. Hata A. Functions of microRNAs in cardiovascular biology and disease. *Annu Rev Physiol*. 2013;75:69–93.
29. Topkara VK, Mann DL. Role of MicroRNAs in cardiac remodeling and heart failure. *Cardiovasc Drug Ther*. 2011;25:171–182.
30. Orenes-Pinero E, Montoro-Garcia S, Patel JV, Valdes M, Marin F, Lip GYH. Role of microRNAs in cardiac remodelling: new insights and future perspectives. *Int J Cardiol*. 2013;167:1651–1659.
31. Lagos-Quintana M, Rauhut R, Yalcin A, Meyer J, Lendeckel W, Tuschl T. Identification of tissue-specific microRNAs from mouse. *Curr Biol*. 2002;12:735–739.
32. Rao PK, Kumar RM, Farkhondeh M, Baskerville S, Lodish HF. Myogenic factors that regulate expression of muscle-specific microRNAs. *Proc Natl Acad Sci U S A*. 2006;103:8721–8726.
33. Zhao Y, Ransom JF, Li A, et al. Dysregulation of cardiogenesis, cardiac conduction, and cell cycle in mice lacking miRNA-1-2. *Cell*. 2007;129:303–317.
34. Saxena A, Tabin CJ. MiRNA-processing enzyme Dicer is necessary for cardiac outflow tract alignment and chamber septation. *Proc Natl Acad Sci U S A*. 2010;107:87–91.
35. da Costa Martins PA, Bourajjaj M, Gladka M, et al. Conditional dicer gene deletion in the postnatal myocardium provokes spontaneous cardiac remodeling. *Circulation*. 2008;118:1567–1576.
36. Rao PK, Toyama Y, Chiang HR, et al. Loss of cardiac microRNA-mediated regulation leads to dilated cardiomyopathy and heart failure. *Circ Res*. 2009;105:585–594.
37. Notari M, Pulecio J, Raya A. Update on the pathogenic implications and clinical potential of microRNAs in cardiac disease. *Biomed Res Int*. 2015;2015:105620.
38. Martinez NJ, Gregory RI. MicroRNA gene regulatory pathways in the establishment and maintenance of ESC identity. *Cell Stem Cell*. 2010;7:31–35.
39. Ohtani K, Dimmeler S. Control of cardiovascular differentiation by microRNAs. *Basic Res Cardiol*. 2011;106:5–11.
40. Chen JF, Mandel EM, Thomson JM, et al. The role of microRNA-1 and microRNA-133 in skeletal muscle proliferation and differentiation. *Nat Genet*. 2006;38:228–233.
41. Izarra A, Moscoso I, Canon S, et al. MiRNA-1 and miRNA-133a are involved in early commitment of pluripotent stem cells and demonstrate antagonistic roles in the regulation of cardiac differentiation. *J Tissue Eng Regen Med*. 2014. [E-pub ahead of print].
42. Fu JD, Rushing SN, Lieu DK, et al. Distinct roles of microRNA-1 and -499 in ventricular specification and functional maturation of human embryonic stem cell-derived cardiomyocytes. *PLoS One*. 2011;6:e27417.
43. Wilson KD, Hu S, Venkatasubrahmanyam S, et al. Dynamic microRNA expression programs during cardiac differentiation of human embryonic stem cells: role for miR-499. *Circ Cardiovasc Genet*. 2010;3:426–435.
44. Sluijter JP, van Mil A, van Vliet P, et al. MicroRNA-1 and -499 regulate differentiation and proliferation in human-derived cardiomyocyte progenitor cells. *Arterioscler Thromb Vasc Biol*. 2010;30:859–868.
45. Jayawardena TM, Egemnazarov B, Finch EA, et al. MicroRNA-mediated in vitro and in vivo direct reprogramming of cardiac fibroblasts to cardiomyocytes. *Circ Res*. 2012;110:1465–1473.
46. Topkara VK, Mann DL. Clinical applications of miRNAs in cardiac remodeling and heart failure. *Per Med*. 2010;7:531–548.
47. Divakaran V, Mann DL. The emerging role of microRNAs in cardiac remodeling and heart failure. *Circ Res*. 2008;103:1072–1083.
48. Yang B, Lin H, Xiao J, et al. The muscle-specific microRNA miR-1 regulates cardiac arrhythmogenic potential by targeting GJA1 and KCNJ2. *Nat Med*. 2007;13:486–491.
49. Yang B, Lu Y, Wang Z. Control of cardiac excitability by microRNAs. *Cardiovasc Res*. 2008;79:571–580.
50. Terentyev D, Belevych AE, Terentyeva R, et al. MiR-1 overexpression enhances Ca^{2+} release and promotes cardiac arrhythmogenesis by targeting PP2A regulatory subunit B56alpha and causing CaMKII-dependent hyperphosphorylation of RyR2. *Circ Res*. 2009;104:514–521.
51. Belevych AE, Sansom SE, Terentyeva R, et al. MicroRNA-1 and -133 increase arrhythmogenesis in heart failure by dissociating phosphatase activity from RyR2 complex. *PLoS One*. 2011;6:e28324.
52. Luo X, Zhang H, Xiao J, Wang Z. Regulation of human cardiac ion channel genes by microRNAs: theoretical perspective and pathophysiological implications. *Cell Physiol Biochem*. 2010;25:571–586.
53. Callis TE, Pandya K, Seok HY, et al. MicroRNA-208a is a regulator of cardiac hypertrophy and conduction in mice. *J Clin Invest*. 2009;119:2772–2786.
54. Myers R, Timofeyev V, Li N, et al. Feedback mechanisms for cardiac-specific microRNAs and cAMP signaling in electrical remodeling. *Circ Arrhythm Electrophysiol*. 2015;8:942–950.
55. Costantini DL, Arruda EP, Agarwal P, et al. The homeodomain transcription factor Irx5 establishes the mouse cardiac ventricular repolarization gradient. *Cell*. 2005;123:347–358.
56. He W, Jia Y, Takimoto K. Interaction between transcription factors Iroquois proteins 4 and 5 controls cardiac potassium channel Kv4.2 gene transcription. *Cardiovasc Res*. 2009;81:64–71.
57. Romaine SP, Tomaszewski M, Condorelli G, Samani NJ. MicroRNAs in cardiovascular disease: an introduction for clinicians. *Heart*. 2015;101:921–928.
58. van Rooij E, Sutherland LB, Liu N, et al. A signature pattern of stress-responsive microRNAs that can evoke cardiac hypertrophy and heart failure. *Proc Natl Acad Sci U S A*. 2006;103:18255–18260.
59. Sayed D, Hong C, Chen IY, Lypowy J, Abdellatif M. MicroRNAs play an essential role in the development of cardiac hypertrophy. *Circ Res*. 2007;100:416–424.
60. Zaccolo M. cAMP signal transduction in the heart: understanding spatial control for the development of novel therapeutic strategies. *Brit J Pharmacol*. 2009;158:50–60.
61. Guellich A, Mehel H, Fischmeister R. Cyclic AMP synthesis and hydrolysis in the normal and failing heart. *Pflugers Arch*. 2014;466:1163–1175.
62. Bers DM. Cardiac excitation-contraction coupling. *Nature*. 2002;415:198–205.
63. Bers DM. Calcium cycling and signaling in cardiac myocytes. *Annu Rev Physiol*. 2008;70:23–49.
64. Zaccolo M. Spatial control of cAMP signalling in health and disease. *Curr Opin Pharmacol*. 2011;11:649–655.
65. Perera RK, Nikolaev VO. Compartmentation of cAMP signalling in cardiomyocytes in health and disease. *Acta Physiol*. 2013;207:650–662.
66. Michel MC, Maisel AS, Brodde OE. Mitigation of beta 1- and/or beta 2-adrenoceptor function in human heart failure. *Br J Clin Pharmacol*. 1990;30:37S–42S.
67. Engelhardt S, Hein L, Wiesmann F, Lohse MJ. Progressive hypertrophy and heart failure in beta1-adrenergic receptor transgenic mice. *Proc Natl Acad Sci U S A*. 1999;96:7059–7064.
68. Lefkowitz RJ, Rockman HA, Koch WJ. Catecholamines, cardiac beta-adrenergic receptors, and heart failure. *Circulation*. 2000;101:1634–1637.
69. Nass RD, Aiba T, Tomaselli GF, Akar FG. Mechanisms of disease: ion channel remodeling in the failing ventricle. *Nat Clin Pract Cardiovasc Med*. 2008;5:196–207.
70. Zipes DP. *Cardiac Electrophysiology From Cell to Bedside*. Philadelphia: Saunders; 2009.
71. Lu Y, Zhang Y, Shan H, et al. MicroRNA-1 downregulation by propranolol in a rat model of myocardial infarction: a new mechanism for ischaemic cardioprotection. *Cardiovasc Res*. 2009;84:434–441.
72. Hou Y, Sun Y, Shan H, et al. Beta-adrenoceptor regulates miRNA expression in rat heart. *Med Sci Monit*. 2012;18:BR309–BR314.
73. Carrillo ED, Sampieri R, Hernandez A, Garcia MC, Sanchez JA. MiR-132 regulates Rem expression in cardiomyocytes during long-term beta-adrenoceptor agonism. *Cell Physiol Biochem*. 2015;36:141–154.
74. Ucar A, Gupta SK, Fiedler J, et al. The miRNA-212/132 family regulates both cardiac hypertrophy and cardiomyocyte autophagy. *Nat Comm*. 2012;3:1078.

75. Stanton HC, Brenner G, Mayfield Jr ED. Studies on isoproterenol-induced cardiomegaly in rats. *Am Heart J*. 1969;77:72–80.

76. Zierhut W, Zimmer HG. Significance of myocardial alpha- and beta-adrenoceptors in catecholamine-induced cardiac hypertrophy. *Circ Res*. 1989;65:1417–1425.

77. Ruppert S, Cole TJ, Boshart M, Schmid E, Schutz G. Multiple mRNA isoforms of the transcription activator protein CREB: generation by alternative splicing and specific expression in primary spermatocytes. *EMBO J*. 1992;11:1503–1512.

78. Laoide BM, Foulkes NS, Schlotter F, Sassonecorsi P. The functional versatility of CREM is determined by its modular structure. *EMBO J*. 1993;12:1179–1191.

79. White DC, Hata JA, Shah AS, Glower DD, Lefkowitz RJ, Koch WJ. Preservation of myocardial beta-adrenergic receptor signaling delays the development of heart failure after myocardial infarction. *Proc Natl Acad Sci U S A*. 2000;97:5428–5433.

80. Bathgate-Siryk A, Dabul S, Pandya K, et al. Negative impact of beta-arrestin-1 on post-myocardial infarction heart failure via cardiac and adrenal-dependent neurohormonal mechanisms. *Hypertension*. 2014;63:404–412.

81. Muller FU, Lewin G, Matus M, et al. Impaired cardiac contraction and relaxation and decreased expression of sarcoplasmic Ca2+-ATPase in mice lacking the CREM gene. *FASEB J*. 2003;17:103–105.

82. Schulte JS, Seidl MD, Nunes F, et al. CREB critically regulates action potential shape and duration in the adult mouse ventricle. *Am J Physiol Heart Circ Physiol*. 2012;302:H1998–H2007.

83. Molina CA, Foulkes NS, Lalli E, Sassonecorsi P. Inducibility and negative autoregulation of CREM—an alternative promoter directs the expression of ICER, an early response repressor. *Cell*. 1993;75:875–886.

84. Tomita H, Nazmy M, Kajimoto K, Yehia G, Molina CA, Sadoshima J. Inducible cAMP early repressor (ICER) is a negative-feedback regulator of cardiac hypertrophy and an important mediator of cardiac myocyte apoptosis in response to beta-adrenergic receptor stimulation. *Circ Res*. 2003;93:12–22.

85. Ma D, Fu L, Shen J, et al. Interventional effect of valsartan on expression of inducible cAMP early repressor and phosphodiesterase 3A in rats after myocardial infarction. *Eur J Pharmacol*. 2009;602:348–354.

86. Houser S, Freeman A, Jaeger J. Resting potential changes associated with Na-K pump in failing heart muscle. *Am J Physiol*. 1981;240:H168–H176.

87. Aronson R, Nordin C. Electrophysiological properties of hypertrophied myocytes isolated from rats with renal hypertension. *Eur Heart J*. 1984;5:339–345.

88. Gelband H, Bassett A. Depressed transmembrane potentials during experimentally induced ventricular failure in cats. *Circ Res*. 1973;32:625–634.

89. Kleiman R, Houser S. Calcium currents in normal and hypertrophied isolated feline ventricular myocytes. *Am J Physiol*. 1988;255:H1434–H1442.

90. Hart G. Cellular electrophysiology in cardiac hypertrophy and failure. *Cardiovasc Res*. 1994;28:933–946.

91. Beuckelmann D, Näbauer M, Erdmann E. Alterations of K+ currents in isolated human ventricular myocytes from patients with terminal heart failure. *Circ Res*. 1993;73:379–385.

92. Nordin C, Siri P, Aronson R. Electrophysiological characteristics of single myocytes isolated from hypertrophied guinea-pig hearts. *J Mol Cell Cardiol*. 1989;21:729–739.

93. Scamps F, Mayoux E, Charlemagne D, Vassort G. Calcium current in single cells isolated from normal and hypertrophied rat heart. Effects of b-adrenergic stimulation. *Circ Res*. 1990;67:199–208.

94. Näbauer M, Beuckelmann D, Erdmann E. Characteristics of transient outward current in human ventricular myocytes from patients with terminal heart failure. *Circ Res*. 1993;73:386–394.

95. Kaab S, Dixon J, Duc J, et al. Molecular basis of transient outward potassium current downregulation in human heart failure: a decrease in Kv4.3 mRNA correlates with a reduction in current density. *Circulation*. 1998;98:1383–1393.

96. Kääb S, Nuss H, Chiamvimonvat N, et al. Ionic mechanism of action potential prolongation in ventricular myocytes from dogs with pacing-induced heart failure. *Circ Res*. 1996;78:262–273.

97. Kaprielian R, Wickenden AD, Kassiri Z, Parker TG, Liu PP, Backx PH. Relationship between K+ channel down-regulation and [Ca2+]i in rat ventricular myocytes following myocardial infarction. *J Physiol (Lond)*. 1999;517:229–245.

98. Nabauer M, Kaab S. Potassium channel down-regulation in heart failure. *Cardiovasc Res*. 1998;37:324–334.

99. Armoundas AA, Wu R, Juang G, Marban E, Tomaselli GF. Electrical and structural remodeling of the failing ventricle. *Pharmacol Ther*. 2001;92:213–230.

100. Care A, Catalucci D, Felicetti F, et al. MicroRNA-133 controls cardiac hypertrophy. *Nat Med*. 2007;13:613–618.

101. Matkovich SJ, Wang W, Tu YZ, et al. MicroRNA-133a protects against myocardial fibrosis and modulates electrical repolarization without affecting hypertrophy in pressure-overloaded adult hearts. *Circ Res*. 2010;106:166–175.

102. Chen JF, Murchison EP, Tang R, et al. Targeted deletion of Dicer in the heart leads to dilated cardiomyopathy and heart failure. *Proc Natl Acad Sci U S A*. 2008;105:2111–2116.

103. Cheng C, Wang Q, You WJ, Chen MH, Xia JH. MiRNAs as biomarkers of myocardial infarction: a metaanalysis. *PLoS One*. 2014;9:e88566.

104. Goretti E, Wagner DR, Devaux Y. MiRNAs as biomarkers of myocardial infarction: a step forward towards personalized medicine? *Trends Mol Med*. 2014;20:716–725.

105. Dimmeler S, Zeiher AM. Circulating microRNAs: novel biomarkers for cardiovascular diseases? *Eur Heart J*. 2010;31:2705–2707.

106. Zile MR, Mehurg SM, Arroyo JE, Stroud RE, DeSantis SM, Spinale FG. Relationship between the temporal profile of plasma microRNA and left ventricular remodeling in patients after myocardial infarction. *Circ Cardiovasc Genet*. 2011;4:614–619.

107. Schipper ME, van Kuik J, de Jonge N, Dullens HF, de Weger RA. Changes in regulatory microRNA expression in myocardium of heart failure patients on left ventricular assist device support. *J Heart Lung Transplant*. 2008;27:1282–1285.

108. Thum T, Galuppo P, Wolf C, et al. MicroRNAs in the human heart: a clue to fetal gene reprogramming in heart failure. *Circulation*. 2007;116:258–267.

109. Luo X, Pan Z, Shan H, et al. MicroRNA-26 governs profibrillatory inward-rectifier potassium current changes in atrial fibrillation. *J Clin Invest*. 2013;123:1939–1951.

110. Girmatsion Z, Biliczki P, Bonauer A, et al. Changes in microRNA-1 expression and IK1 up-regulation in human atrial fibrillation. *Heart Rhythm*. 2009;6:1802–1809.

111. Barana A, Matamoros M, Dolz-Gaiton P, et al. Chronic atrial fibrillation increases microRNA-21 in human atrial myocytes decreasing L-type calcium current. *Circ Arrhythm Electrophysiol*. 2014;7:861–868.

112. Lu Y, Zhang Y, Wang N, et al. MicroRNA-328 contributes to adverse electrical remodeling in atrial fibrillation. *Circulation*. 2010;122:2378–2387.

113. Schunkert H, Ingelfinger JR, Hirsch AT, et al. Evidence for tissue-specific activation of renal angiotensinogen mRNA expression in chronic stable experimental heart failure. *J Clin Invest*. 1992;90:1523–1529.

114. Foulkes NS, Mellstrom B, Benusiglio E, Sassone-Corsi P. Developmental switch of CREM function during spermatogenesis: from antagonist to activator. *Nature*. 1992;355:80–84.

115. Pan ZW, Lu YJ, Yang BF. MicroRNAs: a novel class of potential therapeutic targets for cardiovascular diseases. *Acta Pharmacologica Sinica*. 2010;31:1–9.

116. Nattel S. Electrophysiologic remodeling: are ion channels static players or dynamic movers? *J Cardiovasc Electrophysiol*. 1999;10:1553–1556.

25

Stem Cell–Derived Sinoatrial-Like Cardiomyocytes as a Novel Pharmacological Tool

Andrea Barbuti and Richard B. Robinson

Since the early 1990s, there have been numerous studies manipulating stem cells of various origins to produce cardiac-like cell preparations.[1] However, the result is generally a heterogeneous population of cells, the majority of which are reminiscent of, but quite distinct from, adult ventricular myocytes.[2,3] Further, most research studies and review articles have focused on optimizing and characterizing these ventricular-like cells, which might be suitable to repair the working myocardium following myocardial infarction or heart failure.

More recently, investigators have begun exploring whether the sinoatrial node (SAN) subtype within this heterogeneous cell population, which typically represents just a small percentage of the cells, can be preferentially generated and/or selected.[4] There could be multiple applications for a relatively pure preparation of adult SAN–like cells:

1. It would provide an ideal model system for studying the ionic basis of normal and abnormal automaticity within the SAN. Further, patient-specific induced pluripotent stem cells (iPSCs) could represent a model preparation for exploring the cellular/molecular basis of congenital bradycardic and/or tachycardic disorders, as previously demonstrated with ventricular-like cells of patients with genetic mutations that cause long QT syndrome.[5]
2. This preparation might provide an ideal source with which to create a "biological pacemaker" to replace current electronic pacemakers in treating rhythm disorders.[6]
3. The development of ivabradine[7] has demonstrated a therapeutic market for bradycardic drugs, and high-throughput screening of new molecules would benefit from spontaneously active nodal-like lines.

To realize this potential, there is a need to develop a methodology that improves on the current yield of just a few percent nodal-like cells and/or permits selection of nodal-like cells from within a mixed population. Furthermore, it is not yet known if one cell source (adult stem cells, embryonic stem cells [ESCs],

or iPSCs) is more suitable than another for each potential application. It also should be noted that thus far no approach has produced truly mature cardiac cells, at least with respect to ventricular function.[8] This issue is somewhat less clear for nodal-like cells because there is less (but nonzero) functional distinction between cells of the young and adult SAN.

In this chapter we review the current state of the art and discuss what remains to be accomplished before a preparation of stem cell–derived human nodal-like cells can be employed in therapeutic and basic science applications. A critical issue is the appropriate definition/identification of cells of nodal lineage from within the heterogeneous population that results from driving stem cells down a cardiac lineage. Therefore we first briefly review the critical molecular and functional characteristics of the adult SAN cell. We then review what is known about normal SAN development because this is relevant to devising novel approaches aimed at preferentially driving stem cells down a nodal lineage. Finally, we review the existing literature on the preparation, selection, and characterization of nodal-like cells derived from mouse and human stem cell sources and consider current limitations and potential future directions.

The Adult Sinoatrial Node

The SAN is heterogeneous with respect to cell size, density of ionic currents, connexin expression, and other molecular markers,[9] all of which may impact function. Thus in selecting molecular or cellular screening criteria to identify cells of SAN origin, one must first settle on a collection of characteristics that are most representative of the SAN as a whole and most relevant to its function. Consequently, the resulting homogeneous preparation will recapitulate only a subset of the complex functionality of the syncytial SAN.

The most obvious and relevant feature of the SAN is spontaneous activity, and there are some clear qualitative commonalities throughout the SAN that contribute to this behavior, such as a relative low abundance of the inward rectifier K current, I_{K1}. The paucity of background outward current during diastole allows a small inward current to drive the cell to the threshold for firing. In this regard, the second typical feature of SAN cells is the presence of the so-called pacemaker current, I_f, generated by the *HCN* (hyperpolarization-activated cyclic nucleotide-gated) gene family, which is highly expressed in the SAN and activates at diastolic potentials. While there is a continuing debate on the importance of this current,[10] there is no question that HCN subunits (specifically HCN4) are highly expressed throughout the SAN of different species, *HCN4* mutations result in cardiac rhythm disorders,[11] and an I_f-selective blocker slows (but does not stop) the sinus rate.[7] Thus both functionally and as a molecular marker, HCN4 expression is a minimal criterion for identifying a nodal-like cell. However, as we argue later in the chapter, HCN4 is a general marker of pacemaker cells rather than a specific sinoatrial marker. That is, not all pacemaker cells are of nodal lineage. Furthermore, in the immature heart I_f activation at physiologically relevant voltages is not restricted to the SAN.[12] Therefore both HCN4 expression and a positively activating I_f are necessary, but not sufficient, selection criteria.

Other studies have explored the role of calcium homeostasis in SAN basal and adrenergically stimulated automaticity.[13,14] Such studies suggest that potential additional identifying characteristics of the SAN cell are a high abundance of the L-type calcium channel isoform Cav1.3 and T-type isoforms Cav3.1 and Cav3.2.[15,16] More recent data suggest that the I_f and calcium homeostasis pathways may not be independent and that it is the adenylyl cyclase (AC) signaling cascade that provides the interconnection. Unlike working myocardium, SAN expresses several AC isozymes that are activated by Ca^{2+} in the ~100-nM range, specifically AC1 and AC8.[17,18] The presence of Ca^{2+}-activated AC isozymes may contribute to the observation that basal cyclic adenosine monophosphate (cAMP) is higher in SAN than elsewhere in the heart.[19,20] By considering the specific transmembrane channels and other proteins contributing to the regulation of automaticity, one can create functional criteria to assess the "nodal" characteristics of cardiomyocytes derived from stem cells, as well as a list of positive or negative molecular markers to aid in the selection or subsequent identification of cells of the nodal lineage. Besides the previously described channel isoforms and other proteins that are either highly expressed or relatively absent in the SAN, there are additional molecular markers of nodal cells such as neurofilament-M (NF-M) and the connexin isoforms Cx45 and Cx30.2,[16,21] as well as transcription factors that may also serve as molecular markers. These are summarized in Table 25.1[22–38] and described in subsequent sections.

Sinoatrial Node Development

In order to generate a fully functional sinoatrial-like cell from an undifferentiated stem cell, it is important to know how sinoatrial cells form during normal embryological development. Although in 1907 Keith and Flack anatomically identified the SAN,[39] when and from which embryological structure it developed was less clear. In 1967, Van Mierop demonstrated that at very early stages of chick development (8–9 somites), action potentials could be recorded in both the sinoatrial and bulboventricular regions, with sinoatrial action potentials always preceding the bulboventricular ones even if hearts beat faintly or not at all.[40] Later, it was shown that spontaneous activity can be measured in the cardiac primordia even before their fusion into a linear heart tube.[41] However, the fact that cardiomyocytes composing the early embryonic heart tube share some of the functional and structural properties (glycolytic metabolism or poorly organized sarcomeres) of the SAN hindered the identification of sinoatrial precursors. What is needed are unique and specific markers that allow tracking of the SAN cell fate during development. The very first marker described to discriminate sinoatrial and conduction system cells from atrial and ventricular cardiomyocytes was NF-M, and its expression could be detected in a subpopulation of cardiomyocytes already at E9.5.[37,38] The fact that NF-M was at that time recognized as a neuronal protein led to erroneously believe in a neuroectodermic origin of the cardiac conduction system.

One of the most reliable markers for identifying mature sinoatrial and conduction system cells is HCN4.[11] HCN4 is responsible for the generation of I_f, the current responsible for the initiation of slow diastolic depolarization that rhythmically drives the membrane potential at the threshold for firing an action potential. In the mouse, *HCN4* mRNA can be detected as early as E7.5 in the precardiac mesoderm (cardiac crescent) and later (E8) in the sinus venosus, the structure from which the sinus node develops. For all the subsequent phases of development, *HCN4* expression specifically delineates the formation of the SAN and

TABLE 25.1 Markers defining the sinoatrial node (SAN) and SAN-like stem cells

EMBRYONIC SAN	POSTNATAL SAN	SPECIES	REFERENCES	CD166 mESC[16]	SHOX2-NEO mESC[22]	CD166 hESC[23]	GATA6-GFP hESC[24]
Tbx18[+]		h, m	25,26	+	n.r.	n.r.	n.r.
Tbx3[+]	Tbx3[+]	m, r, h	15,27,28	+	+	n.r.	+
Shox2[+]		m	29	+	+	n.r.	n.r.
Isl-1[+]	Isl-1[+]	m	30	+	−	+	n.r.
mef2C		m	24	+	+	+	n.r.
Nkx2.5[−]		m	27,31	low	low	+	+
Pitx2c[−]		m	30	n.r.	n.r.	n.r.	n.r.
HCN4[+]	HCN4[+]	h, m, r, rb	15,32–34	+	n.r.	+	+
HCN1[+]	HCN1[+]	h, m, r, rb	35	+	n.r.	+	+
CaV1.3[+]	CaV1.3[+]	h, m	15,16,36	+	n.r.	n.r.	n.r.
	CaV3.2[+]	m	36	+	n.r.	n.r.	n.r.
CaV3.1[+]	CaV3.1[+]	h	15	+	n.r.	n.r.	+
Cx30.2[+]	Cx30.2[+]	m	28,34	+	+	n.r.	n.r.
Cx40[−]	Cx40[−]	m	28,34	n.r.	n.r.	n.r.	n.r.
CX43[−]	CX43[−]	m, h	15,28,34	n.r.	n.r.	−	n.r.
HCN2[−]	HCN2[−]	h, m, r, rb	15,35	n.r.	n.r.	n.r.	n.r.
	Kir2.1[−]	r, rb, h	15,36	n.r.	n.r.	n.r.	n.r.
	ssTnI[+]	m	36	+	n.r.	n.r.	n.r.
NF-M[+]	NF-M[+]	rb	37,38	n.r.	n.r.	n.r.	n.r.
	AC1	g	17	n.r.	n.r.	n.r.	n.r.
	AC8	g	17	n.r.	n.r.	n.r.	n.r.
CD166[+]		m, h	16	+/−	n.r.	n.r.	n.r.
Nppa[−]	Nppa[−]	m, h	15,27,34	n.r.	−	n.r.	+

g, Guinea pig; *h*, human; *hESC*; human embryonic stem cell; *m*, mouse; *mESC*, mouse embryonic stem cell; *n.r.*, not reported; *r*, rat; *rb*, rabbit.

the conduction system.[32,42] *HCN4* expression, however, also can be detected in a subset of cells of the first heart field that will contribute to ventricles[42] and will not be a part of the mature cardiac conduction system. These HCN4-expressing derivatives of the first heart field represent the spontaneously beating cells that start peristaltic contraction as soon as the heart tube is formed (E7.5–E8.5).[34] HCN4 thus seems to represent a functional marker of pacemaker cells rather than a specific marker of SAN precursors.

Since the mid-2000s, it has been possible to identify the progenitors of the SAN cells quite early during heart development and well before SAN formation. In the embryo, the sinus venosus (right and left sinus horns) develops into the sinus venarum, the SAN (in the right side), and the coronary sinus (in the left side) that form the systemic venous return of the heart.[43] In the mouse, the sinus venosus originates around E9.5 from the recruitment and proliferation of mesenchymal cells expressing the transcription factor Tbx18 that are different from both the Nkx2.5+ first heart field or from the Isl-1+ second heart field precursors.[43] Tbx18+/Nkx2.5−/Isl-1− progenitors separate quite early (around E8) from the rest of the cardiac mesoderm. Around E8.5, a

subpopulation of these precursors starts to express Isl-1 (Tbx18+/Isl-1+/Nkx2.5−), and then this population matures to form the SAN[26] (Fig. 25.1).

For the SAN to develop correctly, several conditions need to be met within the sinus venosus: (1) the genetic program for the maintenance of pacemaker properties needs to be promoted in the right sinus horn, (2) the genetic program for chamber specification needs to be inhibited in the right horn, and (3) the pacemaker genetic program needs to be inhibited in the left horn. Three transcription factors have been found to be fundamental for these processes: tbx3, shox-2, and pitx2. Starting at E9.5, the Tbx18+/Isl-1+/Nkx2.5− progenitors within the sinus venosus start to express Tbx3, which specifically inhibits the atrial genes Nppa and Cx40.[27] These atrial genes are instead promoted by Tbx5 and Nkx2.5 whose expression is indeed complementary to that of Tbx3. In fact, Tbx3 deficiency in the mouse causes the expression of Cx40, Cx43, and Nppa genes within the SAN, while ectopic expression of Tbx3 in the atria causes the repression of atrial genes and the activation of Hcn4 and Cx30.2.[28,34] The importance of Tbx3 in maintaining the pacemaker properties is further supported by the fact that its expression remains elevated in the

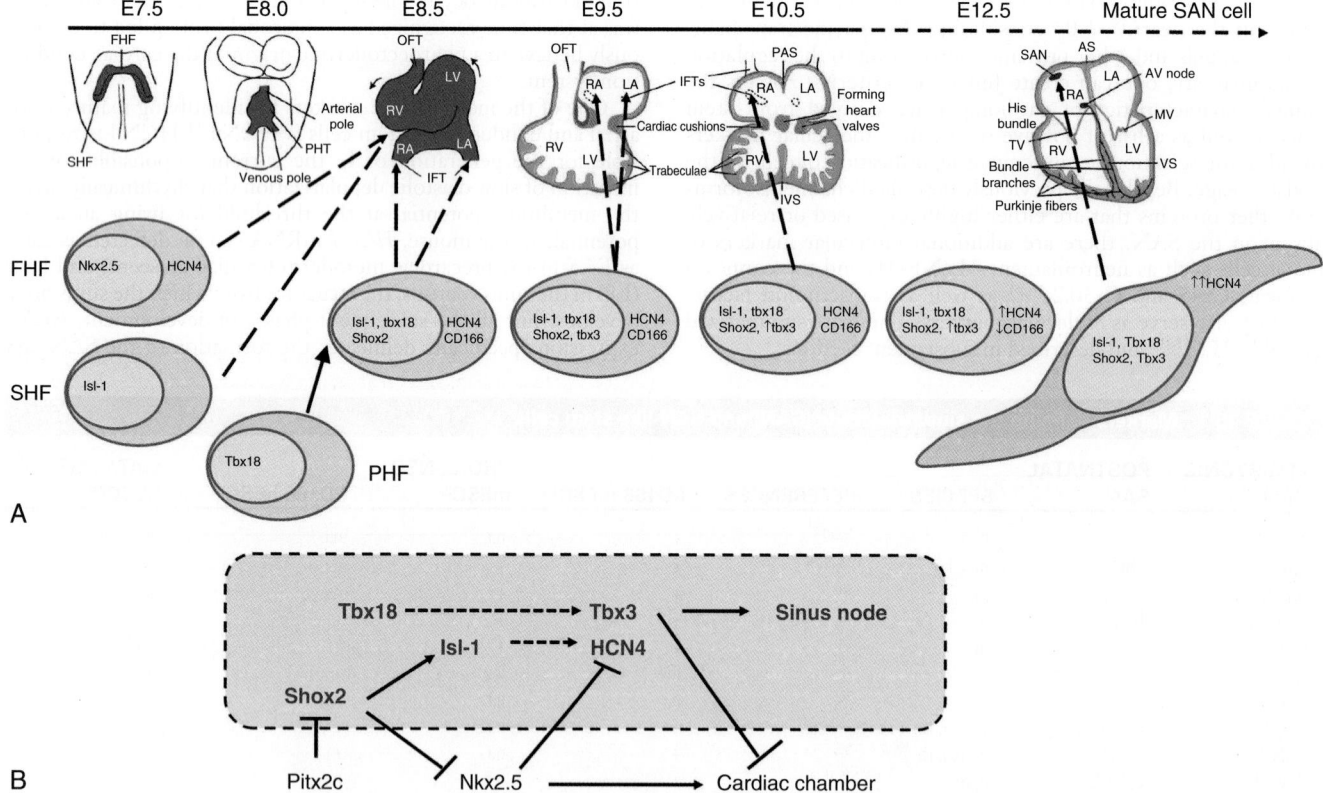

FIGURE 25.1 (A) Time course of mouse heart development (*top*) together with precursors that give rise to the mature sinoatrial node (*SAN*). At each time point, the genes involved in the generation of spontaneous electrical activity and in the development of SA node cells from spontaneously firing mesodermal precursors are shown (*bottom*). Pacemaker activity is first detected at E7.5 in mesodermal cells of the first heart field that express Nkx2.5 and HCN4. At E8, the posterior heart field (*PHF*) precursors characterized by the expression of Tbx18 proliferate, and at E8.5, they start to form the sinus venosus. The sinus venosus, expressing Tbx18, Shox2, HCN4, and CD166, becomes the leading pacemaker. From E9.5, a subgroup of sinus venosus precursors start to express Isl-1 and Tbx3, generating the SA node precursors. These cells increase the expression of bothTbx3 and HCN4, while decreasing the expression of CD166. Postnatal SAN cells are characterized by the transcription factors Isl-1, Tbx18, Shox2, and Tbx3 and high levels of HCN4. (B) Schematic representation of the relationship between factors inducing (↓) or inhibiting (⊥) SAN specifications; the *pink area* within the *dotted line* represents the sinoatrial lineage. *Dotted arrows* represent indirect associations with not yet clarified mediators. *FHF*, First heart field; *IFT*, inflow tract; *LA*, left atrium; *LV*, left ventricle; *MV*, mitral valve; *OFT*, outflow tract; *RA*, right atrium; *RV*, right ventricle; *SHF*, second heart field; *TV*, tricuspid valve; *VS*, ventricular septum.

postnatal and adult SAN while its deficiency induces the ectopic expression of atrial genes in the SAN region.[27,44]

Shox2 is an evolutionary conserved transcriptional factor whose expression is specifically restricted to the sinus venosus and later in development to the SAN and the sinus valves. Zebrafish embryos injected with an anti-Shox2 morpholino displayed both severe bradycardia and lethal sinus arrhythmias.[29,45] In the mouse, Shox2 knockdown induces a hypoplastic SAN and bradycardia compared to wild-type animals, and all Shox[−/−] embryos die at mid-gestation.[29]

Shox2, like Tbx18, has an expression pathway complementary to that of the transcription factor Nkx2.5. Interestingly, in Shox2[−/−] embryos, the compromised SAN region expressed Nkx2.5.[45] Nkx2.5 is widely expressed in the developing heart, with the exception of the portions of the conduction system.[31] Nkx2.5 activates, together with Tbx5, the genetic pathway leading to cardiac chamber formation; in particular, it can bind to Cx40 and Nppa promoters and activate their expression.[27] Indeed, the Nkx2.5-positive SAN region of the Shox2[−/−] embryos expresses Cx40 and Cx43 typical of chamber myocardium. Shox2 is thus responsible for repressing Nkx2.5 expression and "protecting" the SAN from becoming chamber myocardium. Shox2-null mice display a downregulation of the second heart field marker Isl-1 specifically in the SAN,[46] while no alterations of Isl-1 expression are detected in other cardiac regions (e.g., the outflow tract). Morpholino-mediated downregulation of either Shox2 or Isl-1 induced pronounced bradycardia in zebrafish. Interestingly, transient cardiac-specific Isl-1 expression was sufficient to rescue the bradycardic phenotype, suggesting that Shox2 controls Isl-1 expression in the SAN, and this pathway is important for the proper development of pacemaker functions.[46] Recently, it has been demonstrated that induction of Isl-1 knockdown specifically in the SAN causes bradycardia and a decrease in cell proliferation during development that consequently results in a significant reduction of the number of sinoatrial cells.

With the progression of development, the expression of both Shox2 and Isl-1 is restricted to the right side of the sinus venosus in the region coinciding with the forming SAN.[31] This asymmetry is guaranteed by the transcription factor Pitx2c (see Fig. 25.1). The inflow tract of Pitx2c knockout mice appears normal at E9.5 when the SAN is yet to develop, but at E10.5, two primordial SANs start to form, one as expected on the right side and another on the left side. The left-sided SAN has a gene expression profile indistinguishable from that of the right-sided SAN. This evidence clearly demonstrates that the physiological role of Pitx2c in the heart is to specifically repress the SAN gene program in the left sinus horn, allowing the correct asymmetric development of the conduction system.[30]

Because nodal cells and immature ventricular cardiomyocytes both have a depolarized maximum diastolic potential and a slow pacemaker depolarization that make them functionally similar, the knowledge of their distinct embryological origin may be helpful in the effort to separate and enrich a population of SAN-like cells from differentiating stem cells.

Sinoatrial Node Precursor

In order to select and isolate a population of SAN precursors from the developing heart or from differentiating stem cells in vitro, two conditions are necessary: (1) the availability of a well-defined marker of such precursors and (2) a selection approach enabling the separation. The elucidation of the genetic program leading to the development of SAN has provided novel candidate markers for identifying SAN precursors. Selection then requires either the expression of a reporter gene (e.g., fluorescent proteins) under the transcriptional control of a SAN-specific promoter or the availability of an antibody recognizing a membrane protein specific to the cell of interest.

Transgenic mice expressing the reporter genes Lac-Z or GFP in the Tbx18 locus have been developed and used to dissect GFP(Tbx18)[+] mesenchyme, fated to become the sinus venosus, from E9.5 embryos.[25,30] This Tbx18-derived mesenchyme did not show any autorhythmic activity and stained negative for Nkx2.5, HCN4, and myosin heavy chain (MHC) (MF20); curiously, day-matched explants derived from the forming ventricle were beating spontaneously. However, after 4 days in culture, GFP(Tbx18)[+] explants began to express MF20 and HCN4, but not Nkx2.5, and 50% of them started to beat spontaneously at a rate significantly higher than that of the ventricular explants.[25,30] Unfortunately, this Tbx18-based strategy requires genetic manipulation of the organism (mouse) for expressing the reporter gene, and this hampers the use of Tbx18 as a selection marker for human SAN precursors.

In 2006, Hirata and colleagues showed that the activated leukocyte cell adhesion molecule (ALCAM), also known as CD166 or DS-GRASP, is specifically expressed in the murine tubular heart and sinus venosus during early stages of cardiogenesis (around E8.5), but this specificity is lost at later stages when the expression broadens to other organs.[47] Furthermore, selection of Flk-1[−]/CD166[+] cells obtained from E8.5 yolk sac resulted in a population of cardiovascular precursors that in culture formed clusters of spontaneously beating cells.[48] More recently, it has been demonstrated that at E10.5, CD166 and HCN4 are coexpressed in the same regions of the developing mouse heart, and at E12, although they still colocalize to the SAN region, CD166 expression becomes more widespread and extends to other cardiac and noncardiac regions.[16] These data indicate that within a restricted and well-defined developmental window, CD166 can identify SAN precursors.

Mouse Stem Cells

The possibility of driving stem cell differentiation toward the cardiac lineage provides the opportunity to use them for clinically relevant applications, such as heart regeneration and cardiovascular drug screening. Spontaneously contracting cardiomyocytes were first observed in 1983 upon mouse embryonic carcinoma induction with dimethyl sulfoxide (DMSO)[49] and then later upon spontaneous differentiation of mouse ESCs (mESCs).[50] The discovery of stem/progenitor cells in postnatal/adult tissues of mesodermal origin with a certain degree of plasticity raised the possibility of generating novel cardiomyocytes from an autologous source of cells. Hematopoietic stem cells (HSCs), endothelial progenitor cells, mesenchymal stem cells (MSCs), skeletal myoblasts, and cardiac stem cells have all been reported to possess the potential of somehow differentiating into cardiomyocytes. However, most of these cells are not able to beat spontaneously.[4]

Only three types of adult mouse stem cells have so far displayed the potential to differentiate into spontaneously beating cardiomyocytes: MSCs,[51] dedifferentiated fat cells (DFATs),[52] and cardiac mesoangioblasts (MABs).[53,54] MSCs isolated from mouse bone marrow and treated with 3 μM 5-azacytidine lost the fibroblast-like morphology, acquired an elongated shape, and started to contract spontaneously. They expressed several cardiac transcription factors (GATA4, Nkx2.5, and Mef2C), structural sarcomeric proteins (β-MHC, α-MHC, and α-actin), and atrial natriuretic peptide (ANP); furthermore, most of these MSC-derived cardiomyocytes exhibited action potentials typical of sinoatrial-like pacemaker cells. With further maturation in culture, however, around 30% to 40% of cells displayed ventricular-like action potentials.[51]

Two types of adipose tissue are present in the body: white adipose tissue (WAT) and brown adipose tissue (BAT). Both WAT and BAT cells have been shown to differentiate into functional cardiomyocytes. In 2010 it was reported that 10% to 15%

of dedifferentiated WAT cells (dubbed DFAT cells) spontaneously differentiated into cardiomyocyte-like cells[52] expressing several cardiac markers. A fraction of DFAT cardiomyocytes were autorhythmic and responded to isoproterenol with an increase in beating rate, which could be prevented by propranolol, a β-adrenergic antagonist. Unfortunately, a molecular analysis for sinoatrial genes is lacking except for the evidence that DFAT-derived cardiomyocytes expressed high levels of Mef2C, a direct activator of HCN4 transcription, and only a faint signal for Nkx2.5, a known inhibitor of the sinoatrial gene program.[52] More recently, BAT-derived cells have been shown to differentiate into beating cardiomyocytes with a heterogeneous morphology after 5 to 7 days in culture in cytokine-containing medium.[55] Round and fusiform cells expressed many cardiac genes, some of which (GATA6, Tbx3, HF-1b, Cx45, and HCN channels) are typical of cells of the conduction system, while multinucleated myotube–like cells expressed the myogenic mastergenes MyoD, myogenin, and myf5 but lacked atrial natriuretic factor (ANF). Superfusion of β-adrenergic and muscarinic agonists modulated the rate of spontaneous firing by +57% and –80%, respectively. In vivo data show that injection of BAT-derived cells in the atrioventricular (AV) region of mice with stable AV-block induced partial or complete AV conduction recovery in four out of eight mice, suggesting that these cells are functional pacemaker cells. However, molecular analysis showed that these cells mainly expressed the working myocardium genes HCN2 and Cx40, with only a modest expression of the sinoatrial isoform HCN4. These data indicate that BAT-derived cells may be immature working cardiomyocytes rather than true pacemaker/sinoatrial-like cells.[55]

The third type of adult stem cell able to differentiate into spontaneously active cardiomyocytes is represented by the cardiac MABs,[54] and 50% to 80% of these cells displayed a very high spontaneous cardiogenic potential upon serum deprivation. Undifferentiated MABs have already been shown to express cardiac (Nkx2.5, GATA4, Tbx5, Cx43, and ANF) and SAN markers (GATA6, Isl-1, Tbx2, and Tbx3) together with adult stem cell markers (Sca-1, c-kit).[34,56] Upon spontaneous differentiation, MAB-derived cardiomyocytes were able to fire either triggered or spontaneous action potentials.[53,54] One-third of all differentiating MABs had several features of sinoatrial cells: (1) their firing rate was modulated by autonomic agonists; (2) they displayed an I_f similar to that of mature SAN cells, carried mostly by the HCN4 isoform; and (3) they did not express I_{K1} and expressed the low-conductance junctional protein Cx45.[53]

Generating Sinoatrial-Like Cells From Mouse Embryonic Stem Cells

In 1981 the first ESC lines were generated by Evans and Kaufman[57]; these blastocyst-derived ESC lines spontaneously differentiated in vitro to form cystic embryoid bodies (EBs), which are cell aggregates that recapitulate the initial stages of in vivo murine embryonic development and display a high capacity to form beating cardiomyocytes.[58] A large number of spontaneously beating cardiomyocytes can be obtained by culturing ESCs for 2 days in hanging drops containing between 300 and 500 undifferentiated mESCs that, by gravity, interact to form EBs. After 4 to 5 days of culture in suspension, EBs are plated. Following this protocol, 80% to 90% of the EBs display one or more spontaneously beating regions.[50] This protocol represents the gold standard for cardiac differentiation of mESCs; it works independently of the mESC line used and of the laboratory applying it, and this reproducibility is what sets mESCs apart from adult stem cells concerning the generation of pacemaker cardiomyocytes.

Within the EBs, however, cardiomyocytes are heterogeneous with respect to action potential waveform: at early differentiation

stages (9–11 days), most cardiomyocytes display pacemaker-like action potentials, whereas at later stages (16–20 days), atrial-, ventricular-, and sinoatrial-like action potentials can be distinguished.[2,59] Abi-Gerges and coworkers were the first to report that 65% of beating cardiomyocytes isolated from EBs at early stages of differentiation had an I_f, with properties resembling those of native sinoatrial cells. At later stages, the percentage of cells displaying I_f decreased to 45% but, as expected for a maturation process, current density increased.[60]

Because neonatal ventricular cardiomyocytes are also able to spontaneously fire action potentials and express I_f,[12] these features are not sufficient to catalog a cell as sinoatrial-like, and several other conditions need to be considered. The expression of HCN4 and Cx45 characterizes both sinoatrial precursors and sinoatrial cells[32,34,61]; furthermore, HCN1 has been reported in the adult SAN,[33] while HCN2 and Cx43 are mainly expressed by neonatal ventricular cardiomyocytes.[16,62] Van Kempen and colleagues showed that ESC-derived cardiomyocytes express HCN1 and HCN4 mRNA.[63] Using an mESC line expressing the GFP under the transcriptional control of the α-MHC promoter, Yanagi and colleagues[64] showed that mESC-derived beating cells express the HCN1 and HCN4 pacemaker channels as well as the T-type calcium isoforms Cav3.1 and 3.2, typical of SAN myocytes.[36] mESC-derived cardiomyocytes can be grouped, on the basis of electrophysiological analysis, into two distinct populations: one with a fast activating I_f and the other with slow-activating I_f,[65] a feature also found in native mouse SAN cells.[66]

Improvements in the Generation of Sinoatrial Node–Like Cells

Because of the heterogeneity in mESC-derived cardiomyocytes, different approaches have been pursued to obtain a specific subtype of cardiomyocyte: (1) a cell engineering approach using fluorescence molecules under the transcriptional control of specific promoters; (2) a pharmacological approach, by adding specific molecules to the culture medium; and (3) a selection approach of the desired cells on the basis of expression of endogenous markers.

Cell Engineering

In 2004, Gassanov and colleagues[67] generated a mESC line carrying the expression of enhanced green fluorescent protein (EGFP) under the ANP promoter. EGFP-positive cells had three different morphologies: triangle-shaped, spindle-shaped, and round-shaped in the proportions of approximately 20%, 60%, and 20%, respectively. Triangle-shaped cells were mostly quiescent, with a few cells firing at a relatively slow rate (around 1 Hz), and displayed atrial-like action potentials. Spindle-shaped cells were spontaneous, fired at significantly higher rates (close to 3 Hz), and had a larger I_f that activated at more positive potentials and with faster kinetics than triangle-shaped cells.[67]

A more focused approach for the isolation of sinoatrial-like cells was accomplished by engineering ESCs to express EGFP under the transcriptional control of the α-MHC promoter[68]; α-MHC is indeed highly expressed in the atria and in the forming sinus node but only faintly in the ventricles.[69] After selection, two populations of EGFP+ could be recognized: an EGFP-bright round-cell population that, based on multielectrode array analysis, constituted the leading pacemaker within the EBs and an EGFP-dim triangle-shaped cell population with electrophysiological properties similar to those of atrial-like cells. Cells with ventricular-like action potential were not present. At early stages of differentiation, both EGFP-bright and -dim cells expressed the pacemaker current I_f with gating compatible with a role in spontaneous activity ($V_{1/2} = -78$ mV); however, at later differentiation stages, the spontaneous rate of atrial-like cells declined in parallel with a decrease in I_f density.

EGFP-bright cells may represent *bona fide* sinoatrial-like cells because, despite maintaining I_f expression, a significantly lower fraction of them expressed I_{K1} compared to atrial-like cells (30% vs. >80%), and I_{K1} density was also lower.[68] Thanks to the possibility of separating EGFP-bright from EGFP-dim cells, this work represents the first approach actually able to specifically select/enrich a population of mESC-derived sinoatrial-like cardiomyocytes with the proper electrical features needed to sustain spontaneous electrical activity.

At the same time, an independent group generated an mESC line expressing both the reporter gene LacZ, under the control of the minK promoter (minK-LacZ), and the enhanced red fluorescence protein (ERFP), under the control of the chicken GATA6 enhancer (cGATA6-ERFP).[70] MinK, a β-subunit functionally interacting with hERG or KvLQT1 channels to give rise to native rapid and slow components of inward rectifying K+ currents (I_{Kr} and I_{Ks}, respectively), was used because it is expressed in the sinoatrial-conduction system regions.[71] GATA6 was used instead because it is expressed in the developing AV conduction system.[56] Using this cell line, the authors demonstrated that cells coexpressing GATA6 and minK were the pacemaker cells within the beating EBs. However, GATA6/minK cells displayed both sinoatrial- and atrial-like action potentials and indeed expressed moderate levels of the conduction system genes Tbx3, Cx45, and Cav1.3 and very low levels of the genes of the pacemaker channels HCN4 and HCN1, but they expressed moderate to high levels of the chamber myocardium genes Nkx2.5, Cx43, HCN2, and MLC-2a.[70]

Because HCN4 is a fundamental functional marker of pacemaker cells,[32] selection of mESC-derived cardiomyocytes on the basis of HCN4 expression could constitute a suitable approach. Indeed, mESCs expressing EGFP under the control of the HCN4 gene promoter have been generated.[16,72] Differentiation of these cell lines produced EBs with a strong EGFP signal in the spontaneously contracting areas; EGFP+ regions expressed HCN4 as well as other proteins, such as caveolin-3, HCN1, and CaV3.2, which are highly expressed in mature SAN cells.[16,72] Surprisingly, however, this strategy failed to yield a pure/enriched population of sinoatrial-like cells, and in fact, the majority of the selected EGFP+ cells were quiescent. Because EGFP became detectable only around day 7 of differentiation and peaked a week later, it is possible that by this time, HCN4 also was expressed by other cell types, including neuronal precursors,[32] as evidenced by the fact that HCN4-driven EGFP+ cells expressed low levels of the neuronal marker nestin.[72]

In the elucidation of the genetic program leading to the normal development of the SAN, some genes specifically delineating the SAN were identified. In 2013, Hashem and Calycomb[22] engineered mESCs with a vector containing the neomycin resistance gene under the control of the Shox2 gene promoter. Neomycin-selected cells expressed both general cardiac genes and genes specific for the sinoatrial/conduction system program, including Tbx2, Tbx3, GATA6, Cx45, Cx30.2, Cav1.3, Cav3.1, and HCN4. In addition, the ventricular and atrial genes Nkx2.5 and ANF were only modestly expressed; however, no electrophysiological data have been provided that could definitely identify these cells as sinoatrial-like[72] (see Table 25.1).

A significant enrichment in mESC-derived pacemaker-like cells was recently obtained with a forward reprogramming approach followed by antibiotic selection. mESCs were first engineered to stably express high levels of the human TBX3 cDNA; this intervention increased the number of pacemaker-like, HCN4-expressing cells within the EBs. This cell line was further manipulated to introduce a neomycin resistance cassette under the control of the Myh6 promoter. Neomycin selection induced the formation of beating aggregates expressing HCN4, Cx30.2, and Cx45, with a spontaneous rate and an I_f similar to that of native murine SAN cells. These cells were responsive to the HCN blocker ZD-7288 and to autonomic agonists and, more importantly, were able to electrically couple to and pace ventricular slices.[73]

All the selection methods described so far have a major drawback in that they require the manipulation of the cell genome. Genome manipulation can either lead to the inactivation of one of the allele pairs (in the case of homologous recombination) that causes a haploinsufficiency scenario or requires the random insertion of the construct carrying the exogenous reporter DNA in the genome, with the risk of activation of oncogenes or inactivation of other important genes. These possibilities make this methodology unsafe for therapeutic applications.

Pharmacological Approach

As an alternative or perhaps complementary approach to cell engineering, pharmacological strategies have also been pursued. Some of these approaches, although not specifically intended to push toward the pacemaker lineage, did enrich the cardiomyocyte population in sinoatrial-like cells.

Using the previously described ANP-EGFP ESC line, Gassanov and colleagues found that the incubation of differentiating ESCs with the cytokine endothelin-1 (ET-1) up to day 14 increased the proportion of EGFP+ spindle-shaped sinoatrial-like cells in a dose-dependent manner; 100 nM ET-1 induced a 30% commitment of the total EGFP+ cells toward the sinoatrial lineage and induced a parallel decrease of atrial-like cells from 60% to 40%.[67] Coincubation of the cells with both ET-1 and either BQ123 or BQ788, which are selective endothelin A and endothelin B receptor antagonists, respectively, prevented the increase of sinoatrial-like cells. Although the overall enrichment was poor, this work represents the first evidence of the possibility to pharmacologically push mESC differentiation toward the nodal phenotype.

A better yield of mESC-derived pacemaker-like cardiomyocytes was obtained using 1-ethyl-2-benzimidazolinone (EBIO), a drug able to keep Ca2+-activated potassium channels (SKCas) in the open state.[74] Following EBIO treatment, the number of cardiomyocytes displaying pacemaker-like action potentials and expressing I_f increased from 7% (in nontreated cells) to 60%. The enrichment in sinoatrial-like cells was also supported by molecular data demonstrating a robust membrane expression of HCN4; Cx30.2; and sinoatrial-specific transcription factors Tbx2, Tbx3, Shox2, and Isl-1. EBIO effects were mediated by SK4, which is the SKCa channel isoform most abundantly expressed in the atrium, the conduction system, and differentiating mESCs. Either blocking the SK4 channel with its specific inhibitor clotrimazole or its specific knockdown using small hairpin RNA completely prevented the EBIO-induced upregulation of HCN4 and of cardiac differentiation in general.[74]

Similarly, incubating EBs from day 5 to 7 with 0.5 mM suramin, a compound that was shown to induce the formation of heart structures in *Xenopus* embryos,[75] increased the proportion of sinoatrial-like cells to 50%–70% of the total cardiomyocytes, as assessed by action potential shape. Furthermore, the expression levels of HCN4 and Tbx3 doubled following suramin treatment, and at the same time, mESC differentiation toward the neuronal and skeletal muscle phenotypes was prevented.[76] Some degree of enrichment in the SAN was also obtained very recently through stimulation of the purinergic P2 receptor pathway by adenosine diphosphate (ADP) and adenosine triphosphate (ATP). Both ADP (5 μM) and ATP (10 μM) significantly increased the number and beating rate of EBs and also upregulated HCN4 and Cx45 mRNA expression. However, no direct functional quantification was provided to estimate the real degree of enrichment in sinoatrial-like cardiomyocytes.[77]

Even if these pharmacological approaches do not provide a sufficiently pure population of sinus node–like cells, they do not require manipulation of the ESC genome and thus if combined and associated with a proper selection/isolation method, may become relevant from a clinical perspective.

The ideal approach for obtaining a pure population of differentiated sinoatrial-like cells would comprise using an extracellular marker, to be used for cell sorting, in the selection of the proper cell lineages. Unfortunately, extracellular markers that can be used to specifically recognize sinoatrial-like cells are presently not available. So far, the only nongenomic approaches to select an enriched population of cardiomyocytes from pluripotent stem cells have used either tetramethylrhodamine methyl ester perchlorate (TMRM), a fluorescent molecule specifically marking mitochondria,[78] or the extracellular markers CD166 (or ALCAM or DS-GRASP)[16,23,47,79,80] and CD172a (or SIRPA).[81]

TMRM was effective in selecting cardiomyocytes from all the analyzed species (mouse, marmoset, rat, and human) but lacked specificity for sinoatrial-like cells, and, indeed, TMRM-selected α-actinin$^+$ cardiomyocytes also expressed Nkx2.5.[78] SIRPA also does not seem to be a good selection marker for sinoatrial cells because it is expressed both in human atrial and ventricular cardiomyocytes from the fetal stages to adulthood but was not detected in mouse heart, indicating that its expression is not conserved during evolution.[81] Furthermore, because functional data have not been provided for both TMRM- and SIRPA-selected cells, it remains to be established if, at a particular differentiation stage, these approaches may be effective in enriching sinoatrial-like cells.

CD166, an adhesion molecule, was shown to be enriched in cardiac progenitors from E7.75 to E9.5 embryonic hearts.[79] In 2006 Hirata and colleagues demonstrated that at E8.5, CD166 protein expression was restricted to the linear cardiac tube and inflow tract. By E9.5, its expression broadened to other organs as well and, after E12.5, expression of CD166 in the heart was completely lost. At E8.25, CD166 marked the cardiac troponin T-positive cells of the sinus venosus.[47] Based on this evidence and other data showing that CD166 was specifically coexpressed with HCN4 in the embryonic heart at E10.5, but not at later stages, it has been used to select a pure population of SAN precursors from differentiating ESCs.[16] CD166$^+$ ESC–derived cells that were sorted between days 6 and 8 of differentiation expressed high levels of genes important for SAN development and function, such as Tbx18, Shox2, Tbx3, and isl-1; the pacemaker channels, HCN4 and HCN1; the calcium channels, CaV1.3 and CaV3.2; the connexins Cx30.2 and Cx45; and the skeletal (and sinoatrial) slow isoform of troponin I, ssTnI. The atrial and ventricular genes Nkx2.5, HCN2, Cx43, Myh6, and Mlc2v were instead expressed at low levels in CD166$^+$ cells (see Table 25.1). From a functional point of view, in CD166-selected cells, the contribution of L- and T-type calcium and I$_f$ currents to the membrane electrical activity was identical to that of native mouse sinoatrial cells. CD166-selected cells also assumed the spindle-shaped morphology, typical of native sinoatrial cells after 3 weeks of culture, a feature never observed before in vitro in stem cell–derived cardiomyocytes[16] (Fig. 25.2). CD166-based selection appears at present to be the best methodology available for the specific selection of SAN precursors.

Human Stem Cells

Embryonic Stem Cells

The human counterpart of mESCs, human ESCs (hESCs), were first generated in 1998 by Thomson and colleagues from embryos produced by in vitro fertilization.[82] hESCs have been successfully differentiated into beating cardiomyocytes even though at the moment a fully reproducible differentiation protocol, similar to the hanging drop method applied to mESC differentiation, is lacking. The development of a spontaneously beating

area within differentiating hESCs was shown in 2001 by Kehat and colleagues.[83] These contracting regions were composed of small (10–30 μm in diameter) round-shaped cells resembling the murine counterpart.[67,68] Besides presenting spontaneous and repetitive calcium transients, they were modulated by autonomic neurotransmitters and expressed several cardiac markers of various lineages, such as GATA4, Nkx2.5, cTnI, cTnT, MLC-2a and -2v, α-MHC, and ANF.[83] Two years later, however, came the first evidence of the presence of ventricular-atrial and sinoatrial cells in beating hESC-derived cells.[3,84] The first work investigating the contribution of various ion channels/currents to the spontaneous activity of hESC-derived cells found a robust expression of I$_{Na}$ and I$_f$ but not of the I$_{K1}$.[85] Curiously, pharmacological data suggested that automaticity of these pacemaker cells depended more on I$_{Na}$ than on I$_f$ and I$_{CaL}$ because the application of tetrodotoxin (TTX) slowed or stopped the beating, while neither 100 nM of the L-type calcium channel blocker nifedipine nor the f-channel blocker Cs^{2+} (2 mM) had any effect on the rate. This evidence, together with the mRNA analysis showing the expression of Na$_v$1.5, Cav1.2, and HCN2 and the lack of expression of Cav1.3 and HCN4, suggests that these hESC-derived cardiomyocytes more likely represent immature ventricular cardiomyocytes than nodal-like pacemaker cells.[85] Later, Sartiani and colleagues conducted a comparative study on spontaneously beating hESC-derived cardiomyocytes at early (15–30 days) and late (55–110 days) stages of differentiation.[86] Early cardiomyocytes expressed a robust I$_f$, which, however, displayed a maturation-dependent decrease in amplitude and a slowing of activation kinetics. mRNA analysis highlighted that maturation decreased the expression levels of the sinoatrial isoforms HCN1 and HCN4, whereas HCN2 levels remained constantly high. Despite this, cells responded to the I$_f$ inhibitor zatebradine (10 μM) with a significant reduction in rate, suggesting an important role of HCN channels in their pacemaking mechanisms.[86] In another study, the same group confirmed that HCN4 mRNA expression decreased during maturation of hESC-derived cardiomyocytes, but HCN4 protein levels actually increased. After 110 days of differentiation, HCN4 is expressed at a high density in a restricted number of cells.[87] Overall, electrophysiological and expression data indicate that sinoatrial-like cells may be scarce, but present, in differentiating hESCs that are more prone to differentiation into chamber myocardium. The presence of pacemaker-like cardiomyocytes in hESC-derived cardiomyocytes at early differentiation stages was also confirmed by Weisbrod and colleagues.[88] They found that I$_f$ was expressed in most beating cells, and its inhibition by both zatebradine and ZD 7288 significantly decreased the rate; however, this decrease was present only in 58% of them. Spontaneous activity also was blocked by the inhibition of I$_{CaL}$ with nifedipine but was completely insensitive to sodium channel block by 10-μM TTX. Weisbrod and colleagues also found that all the hESC-derived pacemaker cells functionally expressed the Ca^{2+}-activated potassium channel SK4 whose inhibition by either clotrimazole or TRAM-34 completely stopped spontaneous beating. Even though at the moment it is not known if SK4 channels are expressed in native SAN cells, the fact that activation of this channel with EBIO significantly increased the differentiation of mESC-derived sinoatrial-like cells[74] and that at later stages of differentiation, only 30% of hESC-derived beating cells responded to TRAM-34[88] suggest that SK4 expression may provide a novel way to functionally distinguish sinoatrial-like cells from immature working cardiomyocytes. All these functional data together with the relatively high expression of HCN4, HCN2, Cav1.3, NCX-1, and Tbx3,[88] known to be abundant in the nodal and paranodal areas of human heart,[15] indicate that hESC-derived pacemaker cells are true sinoatrial-like cells rather than immature chamber cardiomyocytes.

It is important to mention that when the beating portions of hESC-derived EBs were coupled in vitro to neonatal ventricular

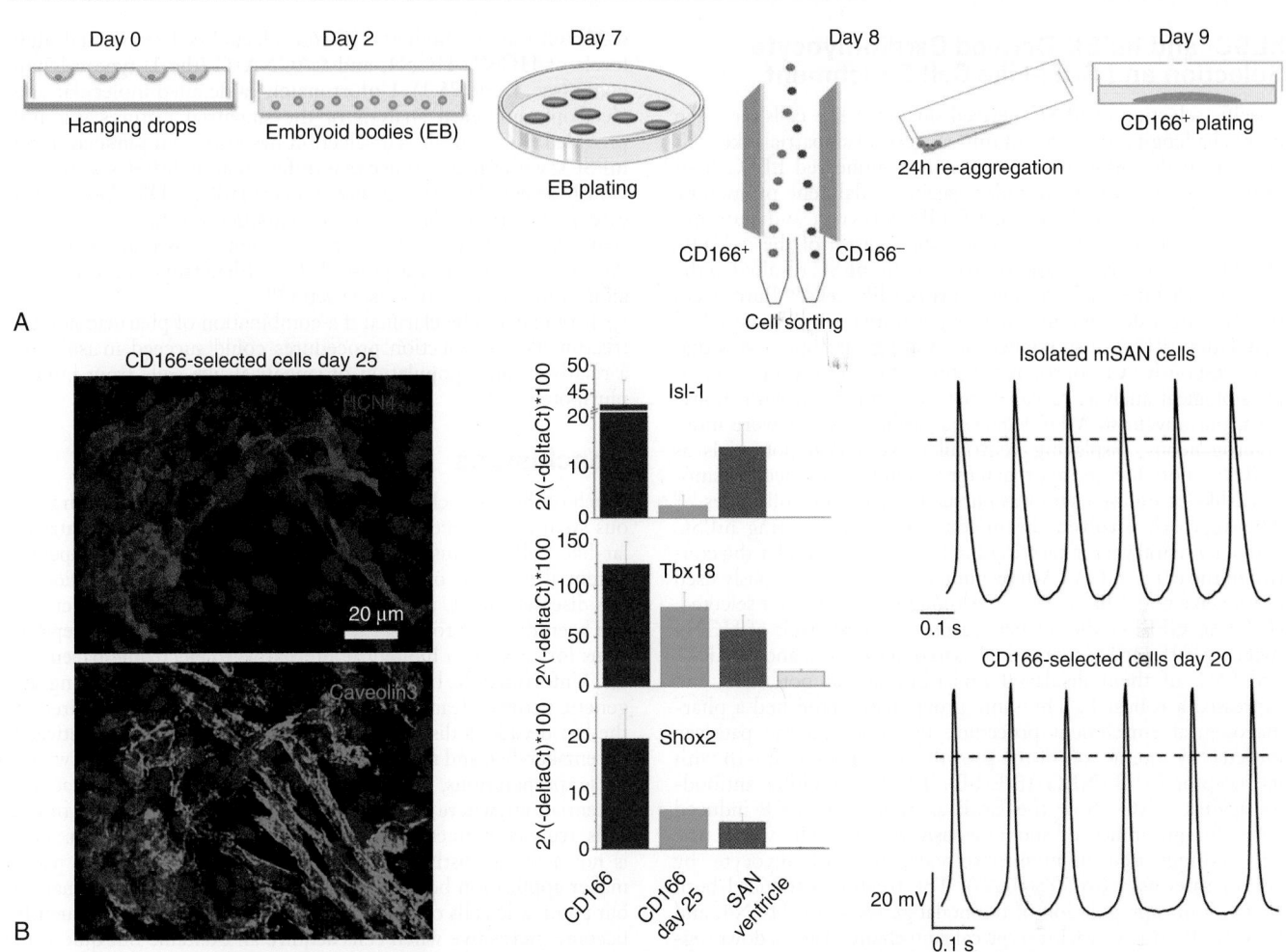

FIGURE 25.2 (A) Schematic representation of the protocol used to obtain CD166-selected sinoatrial-like cardiomyocytes from mouse embryonic stem cells (mESCs). (B) (*left*): Confocal images of a portion of an aggregate of CD166-derived cells after 25 days in culture stained with anti-HCN4 (*red*) and anticaveolin3 (*green*) antibodies; (*center*): Comparison of the expression levels of three transcription factors linked to sinoatrial node (*SAN*) development in CD166-selected cells just after sorting and after 25 days in culture, in the SAN and in the ventricle; (*right*): Representative action potential recordings from a mouse sinoatrial cell (*top*) and from mESC-derived CD166-selected cells after 20 days of culture (*bottom*).

cardiomyocytes or injected in vivo in the hearts of swine[89] and guinea pigs,[90] they were able to impose their regular rhythm. Even if the injected cell population was heterogeneous, it is, nevertheless, likely that sinoatrial-like cells contributed to the generation of the observed spontaneous rhythmic activity because perfusion of the f-channel blocker ZD7288 reduced, whereas isoproterenol increased, the rate.[89,90]

Induced Pluripotent Stem Cells

Even if hESC represents a potential human cellular model and a cell source with a great potential for therapeutics, ethical and legislative issues have slowed research on this cell type while at the same time producing a "selective pressure," in response to which a new type of human pluripotent stem cell has emerged: human induced pluripotent stem cells (hiPSCs).[91] In recent years, progress has been made in the methodology for driving hiPSCs toward the cardiac lineage.[92,93] The specific issue of electrophysiological characteristics of these cells has been covered by several reviews.[93–95] Here we will consider only those works that report data concerning cell automaticity and the presence of nodal-like cells.

In 2009 Zhang and colleagues[96] compared molecular and electrophysiological properties of cardiomyocytes obtained from hiPSCs with those of commercial hESCs lines. Ventricular-, atrial-, and nodal-like cells could be generated in similar proportions from both cell sources (hESCs and hiPSCs). Nodal-like cells represented between 13% and 20% in hiPSCs and 11% and 20% in the hESCs. Spontaneous rate as well as chronotropic responsiveness to isoproterenol also was similar in autorhythmic cells of both preparations. Similarly, Ma and colleagues[97] reported similar proportions of nodal-like cells (22%). Unfortunately, as in the prior study, nodal-like cells were defined uniquely by action potential parameters, and, curiously, individual currents (including the pacemaker current I_f) were measured solely in ventricular-like cells. Lee and colleagues[98] also compared hESC and hiPSC lines, reporting a higher percentage of nodal-like cells than those reported in earlier studies (45% and 43%, respectively).

Overall, the current knowledge concerning the nodal-like nature of cardiomyocytes derived from hiPSCs is limited, but data seem to show that they behave like hESC cells even though it remains to be determined if the spontaneously beating cells represent a true nodal lineage or simply immature "ventricular-like" cells with pacemaker activity.

hESC- and hiPSC-Derived Cardiomyocyte Selection and SAN-Like Cell Enrichment

Specific selection of hESC-derived sinoatrial-like cells has been more challenging than that of mESC-derived sinoatrial-like cells because of the difficulty of generating engineered hESC lines expressing reporter genes under specific nodal gene promoters. One of the first methods used GFP expression and puromycin resistance under the transcriptional control of the α-MHC (MYH6) promoter,[99] an approach that with mESC resulted in the specific enrichment of atrial and sinoatrial-like cells.[68] Puromycin selection of differentiating hESCs generated a highly enriched population (91%) of spontaneously beating cardiomyocytes that were responsive to isoproterenol stimulation. However, electrophysiological analysis revealed that, in comparison with mouse cells, puromycin (α-MHC)-selected cardiomyocytes were more heterogeneous, displaying ventricular-like action potentials as well.[99] A more focused approach for enriching and selecting sinoatrial-like cardiomyocytes was pursued by Zhu and colleagues.[100] The approach involved the infection of differentiating hiPSC with a lentiviral vector carrying the EGFP cDNA under the control of the chicken GATA-6 promoter, a strategy previously used to visualize nodal-like cells.[53,70] Although cells were not selected, cGATA6-GFP+ cardiomyocytes expressed high levels of HCN4 together with cardiac troponin T, sarcomeric actin, and β-MHC, and 95% of them displayed nodal-like action potentials and expressed a robust I_f. The same group also established a pharmacological enrichment procedure by inhibiting the pathway initiated by interaction of the growth factor neuregulin-1β with its receptor ErbB (NRG-1β/ErbB). The use of either antibodies against NRG-1β or the ErbB antagonist AG1478 induced an early appearance of spontaneously beating cells within the EBs and increased the number of nodal-like cardiomyocytes by almost three-fold (to 50%–60%). The treatment induced both a significant upregulation of the nodal genes Tbx3, HCN4, and CACNA1G (the Cav3.1 T-type calcium channel) and a downregulation of chamber genes CACNA1C (the Cav1.2 L-type calcium channel) and SCN5A (the Na$_v$1.5 sodium channel).[100] To date, this approach remains the most effective in generating hESC-derived sinoatrial-like cells that could be appropriate for in vitro drug screening applications.

Cell selection approaches using extracellular antigens have also been exploited with both hESC and hiPSC. The selection of CD166+ cells that works so well in mESCs[16] was actually first used on hESCs, for enriching the population of cardiomyocytes,[23] and later on hiPSCs.[80] Rust and colleagues have, for example, sorted CD166+ cells from hESCs after 12 days of differentiation, a stage at which the expression of CD166 and other cardiac markers (Nkx2.5, Gata4, Isl-1, Mef2C, Tbx5, and

α-MHC) was the highest. CD166-selected cells expressed high levels of HCN1, HCN4, and CACNA1C (the L-type calcium gene) (see Table 25.1). Unfortunately, a detailed molecular and electrophysiological analysis of the sinoatrial features was not provided.[23] CD166-based selection has also been pursued using hiPSCs, with the difference that differentiating hiPSCs were previously selected for the cardiovascular marker KDR. Also in this case, no functional data on action potential waveform or ion currents were collected, and the only evidence was that more than 90% of CD166+ cells expressed the cardiac troponin T protein along with the smooth muscle actin.[80]

It remains to be clarified if a combination of pharmacological treatments and selection procedures could succeed in isolating a relatively pure population of sinoatrial-like cells from human pluripotent cells.

Conclusions

Much of the research on derivation of cardiomyocytes from various stem cell sources has been directed at generating ventricular-like cells because such cells have tremendous therapeutic potential in terms of improving cardiac mechanical function in the diseased heart. Research on cells with pacemaking activity has been directed toward the potential use of such cell preparations for creating a biological alternative to electronic pacemakers. Unfortunately, because much of the knowledge regarding the genetic pathway leading to SAN formation has been acquired in the last decade, a distinction has not always been made between pacemaker-like and nodal-like cells; therefore the extent to which these preparations, which have reported "nodal-like" action potentials anywhere from a few percent to as high as 45% of the cells, truly contain cells of nodal lineage remains uncertain. This is not a trivial distinction with respect to the biological pacemaker application because such a pacemaker based on immature but automatic cells of the ventricular lineage might subsequently become ineffective when cells acquire an excitable but quiescent phenotype typical of mature ventricular cells.

Furthermore, because most of the research and protocols for stem cell differentiation toward nodal lineage have been developed in mouse cells, few studies have attempted to select or enrich specifically for human cells of nodal lineage on the basis of intracellular or surface markers. These results are promising, but much more progress needs to be made both on translating mouse research to humans and in determining the optimal markers to be used, as well as in developing methodologies to enrich the preparations for these markers. If successful, there would be a diverse range of applications for a purified human cell line of nodal lineage that recapitulates the key characteristics of SAN pacemaking.

REFERENCES

1. Matsa E, Sallam K, Wu JC. Cardiac stem cell biology: glimpse of the past, present, and future. *Circ Res.* 2014;114:21–27.
2. Maltsev VA, Rohwedel J, Hescheler J, et al. Embryonic stem cells differentiate in vitro into cardiomyocytes representing sinusnodal, atrial and ventricular cell types. *Mech Dev.* 1993;44:41–50.
3. Mummery C, Ward-van Oostwaard D, Doevendans P, et al. Differentiation of human embryonic stem cells to cardiomyocytes: role of coculture with visceral endoderm-like cells. *Circulation.* 2003;107:2733–2740.
4. Barbuti A, Robinson RB. Stem cell–derived nodal-like cardiomyocytes as a novel pharmacologic tool: insights from sinoatrial node development and function. *Pharmacol Rev.* 2015;67:368–388.
5. Sallam K, Li Y, Sager PT, et al. Finding the rhythm of sudden cardiac death: new opportunities using induced pluripotent stem cell–derived cardiomyocytes. *Circ Res.* 2015;116:1989–2004.
6. Rosen MR, Robinson RB, Brink PR, et al. The road to biological pacing. *Nat Rev Cardiol.* 2011;8:656–666.
7. DiFrancesco D. The role of the funny current in pacemaker activity. *Circ Res.* 2010;106:434–446.

8. Yang X, Pabon L, Murry CE. Engineering adolescence: maturation of human pluripotent stem cell–derived cardiomyocytes. *Circ Res.* 2014;114:511–523.
9. Boyett MR, Dobrzynski H, Lancaster MK, et al. Sophisticated architecture is required for the sinoatrial node to perform its normal pacemaker function. *J Cardiovasc Electrophysiol.* 2003;14:104–106.
10. Lakatta EG, DiFrancesco D. What keeps us ticking: a funny current, a calcium clock, or both? *J Mol Cell Cardiol.* 2009;47:157–170.
11. Baruscotti M, Barbuti A, Bucchi A. The cardiac pacemaker current. *J Mol Cell Cardiol.* 2010;48:55–64.
12. Robinson RB, Yu H, Chang F, et al. Developmental change in the voltage-dependence of the pacemaker current, if, in rat ventricle cells. *Pflugers Arch.* 1997;433:533–535.
13. Ju YK, Allen DG. How does beta-adrenergic stimulation increase the heart rate? The role of intracellular Ca²⁺ release in amphibian pacemaker cells. *J Physiol.* 1999;516:793–804.
14. Lakatta EG, Vinogradova TM, Maltsev VA. The missing link in the mystery of normal automaticity of cardiac pacemaker cells. *Ann N Y Acad Sci.* 2008;1123:41–57.

15. Chandler NJ, Greener ID, Tellez JO, et al. Molecular architecture of the human sinus node: insights into the function of the cardiac pacemaker. *Circulation.* 2009;119:1562–1575.
16. Scavone A, Capilupo D, Mazzocchi N, et al. Embryonic stem cell–derived CD166+ precursors develop into fully functional sinoatrial-like cells. *Circ Res.* 2013;113:389–398.
17. Mattick P, Parrington J, Odia E, et al. Ca²⁺-stimulated adenylyl cyclase isoform AC1 is preferentially expressed in guinea-pig sino-atrial node cells and modulates the If pacemaker current. *J Physiol.* 2007;582:1195–1203.
18. Younes A, Lyashkov AE, Graham D, et al. Ca²⁺-stimulated basal adenylyl cyclase activity localization in membrane lipid microdomains of cardiac sinoatrial nodal pacemaker cells. *J Biol Chem.* 2008;283:14461–14468.
19. Vinogradova TM, Lyashkov AE, Zhu W, et al. High basal protein kinase A–dependent phosphorylation drives rhythmic internal Ca²⁺ store oscillations and spontaneous beating of cardiac pacemaker cells. *Circ Res.* 2006;98:505–514.
20. Kryukova YN, Protas L, Robinson RB. Ca²⁺-activated adenylyl cyclase 1 introduces Ca²⁺-dependence to beta-adrenergic stimulation of HCN2 current. *J Mol Cell Cardiol.* 2012;52:1233–1239.

21. Boyett MR, Inada S, Yoo S, et al. Connexins in the sinoatrial and atrioventricular nodes. *Adv Cardiol.* 2006;42:175–197.

22. Hashem SI, Claycomb WC. Genetic isolation of stem cell–derived pacemaker-nodal cardiac myocytes. *Mol Cell Biochem.* 2013;383:161–171.

23. Rust W, Balakrishnan T, Zweigerdt R. Cardiomyocyte enrichment from human embryonic stem cell cultures by selection of ALCAM surface expression. *Regen Med.* 2009;4:225–237.

24. Vedantham V, Evangelista M, Huang Y, et al. Spatiotemporal regulation of an Hcn4 enhancer defines a role for Mef2c and HDACs in cardiac electrical patterning. *Dev Biol.* 2013;373:149–162.

25. Wiese C, Grieskamp T, Airik R, et al. Formation of the sinus node head and differentiation of sinus node myocardium are independently regulated by Tbx18 and Tbx3. *Circ Res.* 2009;104:388–397.

26. Mommersteeg MT, Dominguez JN, Wiese C, et al. The sinus venosus progenitors separate and diversify from the first and second heart fields early in development. *Cardiovasc Res.* 2010;87:92–101.

27. Hoogaars WM, Tessari A, Moorman AF, et al. The transcriptional repressor Tbx3 delineates the developing central conduction system of the heart. *Cardiovasc Res.* 2004;62:489–499.

28. Hoogaars WM, Engel A, Brons JF, et al. Tbx3 controls the sinoatrial node gene program and imposes pacemaker function on the atria. *Genes Dev.* 2007;21:1098–1112.

29. Espinoza-Lewis RA, Yu L, He F, et al. Shox2 is essential for the differentiation of cardiac pacemaker cells by repressing Nkx2-5. *Dev Biol.* 2009;327:376–385.

30. Mommersteeg MT, Hoogaars WM, Prall OW, et al. Molecular pathway for the localized formation of the sinoatrial node. *Circ Res.* 2007;100:354–362.

31. Liu H, Espinoza-Lewis RA, Chen C, et al. The role of Shox2 in SAN development and function. *Pediatr Cardiol.* 2012;33:882–889.

32. Garcia-Frigola C, Shi Y, Evans SM. Expression of the hyperpolarization-activated cyclic nucleotide-gated cation channel HCN4 during mouse heart development. *Gene Expr Patterns.* 2003;3:777–783.

33. Brioschi C, Micheloni S, Tellez JO, et al. Distribution of the pacemaker HCN4 channel mRNA and protein in the rabbit sinoatrial node. *J Mol Cell Cardiol.* 2009;47:221–227.

34. Christoffels VM, Smits GJ, Kispert A, et al. Development of the pacemaker tissues of the heart. *Circ Res.* 2010;106:240–254.

35. Stieber J, Herrmann S, Feil S, et al. The hyperpolarization-activated channel HCN4 is required for the generation of pacemaker action potentials in the embryonic heart. *Proc Nat Acad Sci U S A.* 2003;100:15235–15240.

36. Marionneau C, Couette B, Liu J, et al. Specific pattern of ionic channel gene expression associated with pacemaker activity in the mouse heart. *J Physiol.* 2005;562:223–234.

37. Gorza L, Schiaffino S, Vitadello M. Heart conduction system: a neural crest derivative? *Brain Res.* 1988;457:360–366.

38. Vitadello M, Vettore S, Lamar E, et al. Neurofilament M mRNA is expressed in conduction system myocytes of the developing and adult rabbit heart. *J Mol Cell Cardiol.* 1996;28:1833–1844.

39. Keith A, Flack M. The form and nature of the muscular connections between the primary divisions of the vertebrate heart. *J Anat Physiol.* 1907;41:172–189.

40. Van Mierop LH. Location of pacemaker in chick embryo heart at the time of initiation of heartbeat. *Am J Physiol.* 1967;212:407–415.

41. Kamino K. Optical approaches to ontogeny of electrical activity and related functional organization during early heart development. *Physiol Rev.* 1991;71:53–91.

42. Liang X, Wang G, Lin L, et al. HCN4 dynamically marks the first heart field and conduction system precursors. *Circ Res.* 2013;113:399–407.

43. Christoffels VM, Mommersteeg MT, Trowe MO, et al. Formation of the venous pole of the heart from an Nkx2-5-negative precursor population requires Tbx18. *Circ Res.* 2006;98:1555–1563.

44. Morris GM, D'Souza A, Dobrzynski H, et al. Characterization of a right atrial subsidiary pacemaker and acceleration of the pacing rate by HCN over-expression. *Cardiovasc Res.* 2013;100:160–169.

45. Blaschke RJ, Hahurij ND, Kuijper S, et al. Targeted mutation reveals essential functions of the homeodomain transcription factor Shox2 in sinoatrial and pacemaking development. *Circulation.* 2007;115:1830–1838.

46. Hoffmann S, Berger IM, Glaser A, et al. Islet1 is a direct transcriptional target of the homeodomain transcription factor Shox2 and rescues the Shox2-mediated bradycardia. *Basic Res Cardiol.* 2013;108:339.

47. Hirata H, Murakami Y, Miyamoto Y, et al. ALCAM (CD166) is a surface marker for early murine cardiomyocytes. *Cells Tissues Organs.* 2006;184:172–180.

48. Murakami Y, Hirata H, Miyamoto Y, et al. Isolation of cardiac cells from E8.5 yolk sac by ALCAM (CD166) expression. *Mech Dev.* 2007;124:830–839.

49. Edwards MK, Harris JF, McBurney MW. Induced muscle differentiation in an embryonal carcinoma cell line. *Mol Cell Biol.* 1983;3:2280–2286.

50. Wobus AM, Wallukat G, Hescheler J. Pluripotent mouse embryonic stem cells are able to differentiate into cardiomyocytes expressing chronotropic responses to adrenergic and cholinergic agents and Ca^{2+} channel blockers. *Differentiation.* 1991;48:173–182.

51. Makino S, Fukuda K, Miyoshi S, et al. Cardiomyocytes can be generated from marrow stromal cells in vitro. *J Clin Invest.* 1999;103:697–705.

52. Jumabay M, Zhang R, Yao Y, et al. Spontaneously beating cardiomyocytes derived from white mature adipocytes. *Cardiovasc Res.* 2010;85:17–27.

53. Barbuti A, Galvez BG, Crespi A, et al. Mesoangioblasts from ventricular vessels can differentiate in vitro into cardiac myocytes with sinoatrial-like properties. *J Mol Cell Cardiol.* 2010;48:415–423.

54. Galvez BG, Sampaolesi M, Barbuti A, et al. Cardiac mesoangioblasts are committed, self-renewable progenitors, associated with small vessels of juvenile mouse ventricle. *Cell Death Differ.* 2008;15:1417–1428.

55. Takahashi T, Nagai T, Kanda M, et al. Regeneration of the cardiac conduction system by adipose tissue-derived stem cells. *Circ J.* 2015;79:2703–2712.

56. Davis DL, Edwards AV, Juraszek AL, et al. A GATA-6 gene heart-region-specific enhancer provides a novel means to mark and probe a discrete component of the mouse cardiac conduction system. *Mech Dev.* 2001;108:105–119.

57. Evans MJ, Kaufman MH. Establishment in culture of pluripotential cells from mouse embryos. *Nature.* 1981;292:154–156.

58. Doetschman TC, Eistetter H, Katz M, et al. The in vitro development of blastocyst-derived embryonic stem cell lines: formation of visceral yolk sac, blood islands and myocardium. *J Embryol Exp Morphol.* 1985;87:27–45.

59. Hescheler J, Fleischmann BK, Lentini S, et al. Embryonic stem cells: a model to study structural and functional properties in cardiomyogenesis. *Cardiovasc Res.* 1997;36:149–162.

60. Abi-Gerges N, Ji GJ, Lu ZJ, et al. Functional expression and regulation of the hyperpolarization activated nonselective cation current in embryonic stem cell–derived cardiomyocytes. *J Physiol.* 2000;523:377–389.

61. Alcolea S, Theveniau-Ruissy M, Jarry-Guichard T, et al. Downregulation of connexin 45 gene products during mouse heart development. *Circ Res.* 1999;84:1365–1379.

62. Yasui K, Liu W, Opthof T, et al. If current and spontaneous activity in mouse embryonic ventricular myocytes. *Circ Res.* 2001;88:536–542.

63. van Kempen M, van Ginneken A, de Grijs I, et al. Expression of the electrophysiological system during murine embryonic stem cell cardiac differentiation. *Cell Physiol Biochem.* 2003;13:263–270.

64. Yanagi K, Takano M, Narazaki G, et al. Hyperpolarization-activated cyclic nucleotide-gated channels and T-type calcium channels confer automaticity of embryonic stem cell–derived cardiomyocytes. *Stem Cells.* 2007;25:2712–2719.

65. Barbuti A, Crespi A, Capilupo D, et al. Molecular composition and functional properties of f-channels in murine embryonic stem cell–derived pacemaker cells. *J Mol Cell Cardiol.* 2009;46:343–351.

66. Mangoni ME, Nargeot J. Properties of the hyperpolarization-activated current (If) in isolated mouse sino-atrial cells. *Cardiovasc Res.* 2001;52:51–64.

67. Gassanov N, Er F, Zagidullin N, et al. Endothelin induces differentiation of ANP-EGFP expressing embryonic stem cells towards a pacemaker phenotype. *FASEB J.* 2004;18:1710–1712.

68. Kolossov E, Lu Z, Drobinskaya I, et al. Identification and characterization of embryonic stem cell–derived pacemaker and atrial cardiomyocytes. *FASEB J.* 2005;19:577–579.

69. Lyons GE, Schiaffino S, Sassoon D, et al. Developmental regulation of myosin gene expression in mouse cardiac muscle. *J Cell Biol.* 1990;111:2427–2436.

70. White SM, Claycomb WC. Embryonic stem cells form an organized, functional cardiac conduction system in vitro. *Am J Physiol Heart Circ Physiol.* 2005;288:H670–H679.

71. Kupershmidt S, Yang T, Anderson ME, et al. Replacement by homologous recombination of the minK gene with lacZ reveals restriction of minK expression to the mouse cardiac conduction system. *Circ Res.* 1999;84:146–152.

72. Morikawa K, Bahrudin U, Miake J, et al. Identification, isolation and characterization of HCN4-positive pacemaking cells derived from murine embryonic stem cells during cardiac differentiation. *Pacing Clin Electrophysiol.* 2010;33:290–303.

73. Jung JJ, Husse B, Rimmbach C, et al. Programming and isolation of highly pure physiologically and pharmacologically functional sinus-nodal bodies from pluripotent stem cells. *Stem Cell Reports.* 2014;2:592–605.

74. Kleger A, Seufferlein T, Malan D, et al. Modulation of calcium-activated potassium channels induces cardiogenesis of pluripotent stem cells and enrichment of pacemaker-like cells. *Circulation.* 2010;122:1823–1836.

75. Grunz H. Suramin changes the fate of Spemann's organizer and prevents neural induction in Xenopus laevis. *Mech Dev.* 1992;38:133–141.

76. Wiese C, Nikolova T, Zahanich I, et al. Differentiation induction of mouse embryonic stem cells into sinus node–like cells by suramin. *Int J Cardiol.* 2011;147:95–111.

77. Mazrouei S, Sharifpanah F, Bekhite MM, et al. Cardiomyogenesis of embryonic stem cells upon purinergic receptor activation by ADP and ATP. *Purinergic Signal.* 2015;11:491–506.

78. Hattori F, Chen H, Yamashita H, et al. Nongenetic method for purifying stem cell–derived cardiomyocytes. *Nat Methods.* 2010;7:61–66.

79. Masino AM, Gallardo TD, Wilcox CA, et al. Transcriptional regulation of cardiac progenitor cell populations. *Circ Res.* 2004;95:389–397.

80. Lin B, Kim J, Li Y, et al. High-purity enrichment of functional cardiovascular cells from human iPS cells. *Cardiovasc Res.* 2012;95:327–335.

81. Dubois NC, Craft AM, Sharma P, et al. SIRPA is a specific cell-surface marker for isolating cardiomyocytes derived from human pluripotent stem cells. *Nat Biotechnol.* 2011;29:1011–1018.

82. Thomson JA, Itskovitz-Eldor J, Shapiro SS, et al. Embryonic stem cell lines derived from human blastocysts. *Science.* 1998;282:1145–1147.

83. Kehat I, Kenyagin-Karsenti D, Snir M, et al. Human embryonic stem cells can differentiate into myocytes with structural and functional properties of cardiomyocytes. *J Clin Invest.* 2001;108:407–414.

84. He JQ, Ma Y, Lee Y, et al. Human embryonic stem cells develop into multiple types of cardiac myocytes: action potential characterization. *Circ Res.* 2003;93:32–39.

85. Satin J, Kehat I, Caspi O, et al. Mechanism of spontaneous excitability in human embryonic stem cell derived cardiomyocytes. *J Physiol.* 2004;559:479–496.

86. Sartiani L, Bettiol E, Stillitano F, et al. Developmental changes in cardiomyocytes differentiated from human embryonic stem cells: a molecular and electrophysiological approach. *Stem Cells.* 2007;25:1136–1144.

87. Bosman A, Sartiani L, Spinelli V, et al. Molecular and functional evidence of HCN4 and caveolin-3 interaction during cardiomyocyte differentiation from human embryonic stem cells. *Stem Cells Dev.* 2013;22:1717–1727.

88. Weisbrod D, Peretz A, Ziskind A, et al. SK4 Ca^{2+} activated K^+ channel is a critical player in cardiac pacemaker derived from human embryonic stem cells. *Proc Natl Acad Sci U S A.* 2013;110:E1685–E1694.

89. Kehat I, Khimovich L, Caspi O, et al. Electromechanical integration of cardiomyocytes derived from human embryonic stem cells. *Nat Biotechnol.* 2004;22:1282–1289.

90. Xue T, Cho HC, Akar FG, et al. Functional integration of electrically active cardiac derivatives from genetically engineered human embryonic stem cells with quiescent recipient ventricular cardiomyocytes: insights into the development of cell-based pacemakers. *Circulation.* 2005;111:11–20.

91. Takahashi K, Tanabe K, Ohnuki M, et al. Induction of pluripotent stem cells from adult human fibroblasts by defined factors. *Cell.* 2007;131:861–872.

92. Yoshida Y, Yamanaka S. iPS cells: a source of cardiac regeneration. *J Mol Cell Cardiol.* 2011;50:327–332.

93. Karakikes I, Ameen M, Termglinchan V, et al. Human induced pluripotent stem cell–derived cardiomyocytes: insights into molecular, cellular, and functional phenotypes. *Circ Res.* 2015;117:80–88.

94. Poon E, Kong CW, Li RA. Human pluripotent stem cell-based approaches for myocardial repair: from the electrophysiological perspective. *Mol Pharm.* 2011;8:1495–1504.

95. Hoekstra M, Mummery CL, Wilde AA, et al. Induced pluripotent stem cell derived cardiomyocytes as models for cardiac arrhythmias. *Front Physiol.* 2012;3:346.

96. Zhang J, Wilson GF, Soerens AG, et al. Functional cardiomyocytes derived from human induced pluripotent stem cells. *Circ Res.* 2009;104:e30–e41.

97. Ma J, Guo L, Fiene SJ, et al. High purity human-induced pluripotent stem cell–derived cardiomyocytes: electrophysiological properties of action potentials and ionic currents. *Am J Physiol Heart Circ Physiol.* 2011;301:H2006–H2017.

98. Lee YK, Ng KM, Lai WH, et al. Calcium homeostasis in human induced pluripotent stem cell–derived cardiomyocytes. *Stem Cell Rev.* 2011;7:976–986.

99. Anderson D, Self T, Mellor IR, et al. Transgenic enrichment of cardiomyocytes from human embryonic stem cells. *Mol Ther.* 2007;15:2027–2036.

100. Zhu WZ, Xie Y, Moyes KW, et al. Neuregulin/ErbB signaling regulates cardiac subtype specification in differentiating human embryonic stem cells. *Circ Res.* 2010;107:776–786.

26 Gene Therapy and Biological Pacing

Michael R. Rosen, Ofer Binah, Peter R. Brink, Richard B. Robinson, and
Ira S. Cohen

Introduction

The natural pacemaker of the heart, the sinoatrial node (the true "biological pacemaker") is a complex structure whose anatomy facilitates the transmission of impulses to the rest of the heart while also protecting the heart from excitation due to impulses arising elsewhere. The unique ion channel complement of the sinoatrial node allows it to initiate impulses rhythmically throughout the life of the organism, while its autonomic neural supply and circulating hormones ensure ready adjustment to physiological demands for altering heart rate.

Like any biological system, the sinoatrial node is affected by aging and pathology in ways that can lead to dysfunction. For much of human history, this dysfunction, expressed as sinoatrial arrest or block or as atrioventricular block, was accompanied by syncope, a marginal quality of life, and—over varying time spans—death (see Adams[1] and Stokes[2]). The major therapy until the mid-20th century was a stopgap: ephedrine or sublingual isoproterenol, administered every two hours.

In the 1960s, electronic pacing became available via devices that could be implanted transvenously with little risk.[3,4] Early units were relatively massive—resembling hockey pucks—but they were lifesaving. Technology improved and the size of the pacing units diminished over the second half of the 20th century; improvement and innovation continue in the current era.

However, electronic pacing is not perfect: while it restores individuals to their lives, their families, and their society, it is not the seamlessly functioning structure exemplified by the sinoatrial node. As possible alternatives to electronic pacing, investigators have explored gene and cell therapies that would replace or mimic the function of the sinoatrial node, albeit not its structure.

Seen in this light, cardiac pacing appears to be coming full circle—from biological to electronic and back to biological—but success is not yet within our grasp. To provide a perspective and a view of the future, this chapter will first discuss the normal and pathological mechanisms underlying sinoatrial node function and dysfunction and the rationale for developing biological pacemakers. Then this chapter will consider strategies for building biological pacemakers and will review successes and failures to date. Finally, the chapter will finish with a discussion of challenges for the future.

The Normal Cardiac Pacemaker

The mammalian sinoatrial node was identified structurally in 1907 by Keith and Flack,[5] and its function to initiate the cardiac impulse was demonstrated electrophysiologically by Lewis and colleagues in 1910.[6] These investigators recognized they were dealing with a heterogeneous structure that appeared to be the dominant site of origin of the normal heartbeat. Yet, the mechanisms of sinoatrial node function remained a mystery for decades. One school of thought held that the node—and indeed the entire cardiac conducting system—consisted of specialized neural fibers, with a neural impulse initiating the heartbeat.[7] The finding that the sinus rhythm continued after cardiac denervation[8] argued against central neural origin; however, the belief in a role for local neuronal activity as the cause of the heartbeat persisted.[7]

The modern era of molecular biophysics has determined the why and wherefore of the origin of cardiac impulses. However, the origin of the sinoatrial node cells remains under active investigation (e.g., see Mommersteeg and associates[9]). As shown in Fig. 26.1A, multiple currents contribute to the sinoatrial node action potential.[10–13] A small inward rectifier K^+ current, I_{K1}, maintains the resting membrane potential of normal sinoatrial node cells at a more highly depolarized state than that of most other cardiac myocytes, which means that Ca^{2+}, rather than Na^+, is the inward charge carrier during the upstroke of action potentials initiated in sinoatrial node cells. The result is a slowly propagating impulse similar to that found in the normal atrioventricular node, the atrioventricular valves, and the coronary sinus.

As sinoatrial node cells repolarize to their maximum diastolic potentials, their hyperpolarization permits the opening of hyperpolarization-activated cyclic nucleotide-gated (HCN) channels through which an inward Na^+ current, referred to as I_f, flows and begins to depolarize the membrane (see Fig. 26.1A–B).[10–12] A major contributor to pacemaker activity is the Ca^{2+} clock mechanism, which depends on Ca^{2+} cycling between intracellular uptake and release sites, as well as Ca^{2+} entry via L- and T-type Ca^{2+} channels.[13,14] This impacts the activity of the Na^+/Ca^{2+} exchanger which directly modulates phase-4 depolarization.[13,14] All these events occur against the backdrop of an outward (repolarizing), K^+ current, such that any increase in inward current and/or decrease in outward current will increase the slope of phase-4 depolarization and pacemaker rate.

HCN channels have six transmembrane spanning domains; they are ubiquitous in heart and are found elsewhere in the body, as well (see Fig. 26.1B). There are four channel isoforms, HCN1–4, with isoforms 1 and 4 found in the sinoatrial node, 2 found in much of the conducting system and myocardium, and 3 found largely in neural tissues.[12] Each has differing activation and deactivation kinetics and differing cyclic adenosine monophosphate (AMP) sensitivity. The critical aspects of these channels with regard to pacemaker activity are their activation on hyperpolarization and their modulation by autonomic neurohumors.

The sympathetic and parasympathetic nervous systems are the principal modulators of phase-4 depolarization. Their respective neurohumors, norepinephrine and acetylcholine, act via β-adrenergic or muscarinic receptor-G protein–linked pathways to increase (β-adrenergic) or decrease (muscarinic) cyclic AMP synthesis (see Fig. 26.1B). Cyclic AMP binding to a site near the carboxy-terminus of the HCN channel shifts channel activation positively, resulting in an increase in phase-4 depolarization.[12]

Whereas all the currents described above contribute to phase-4 depolarization and to pacemaker rate, the initiator of the process appears to be I_f.[10,11] Yet, not all pacemaker activity is attributable

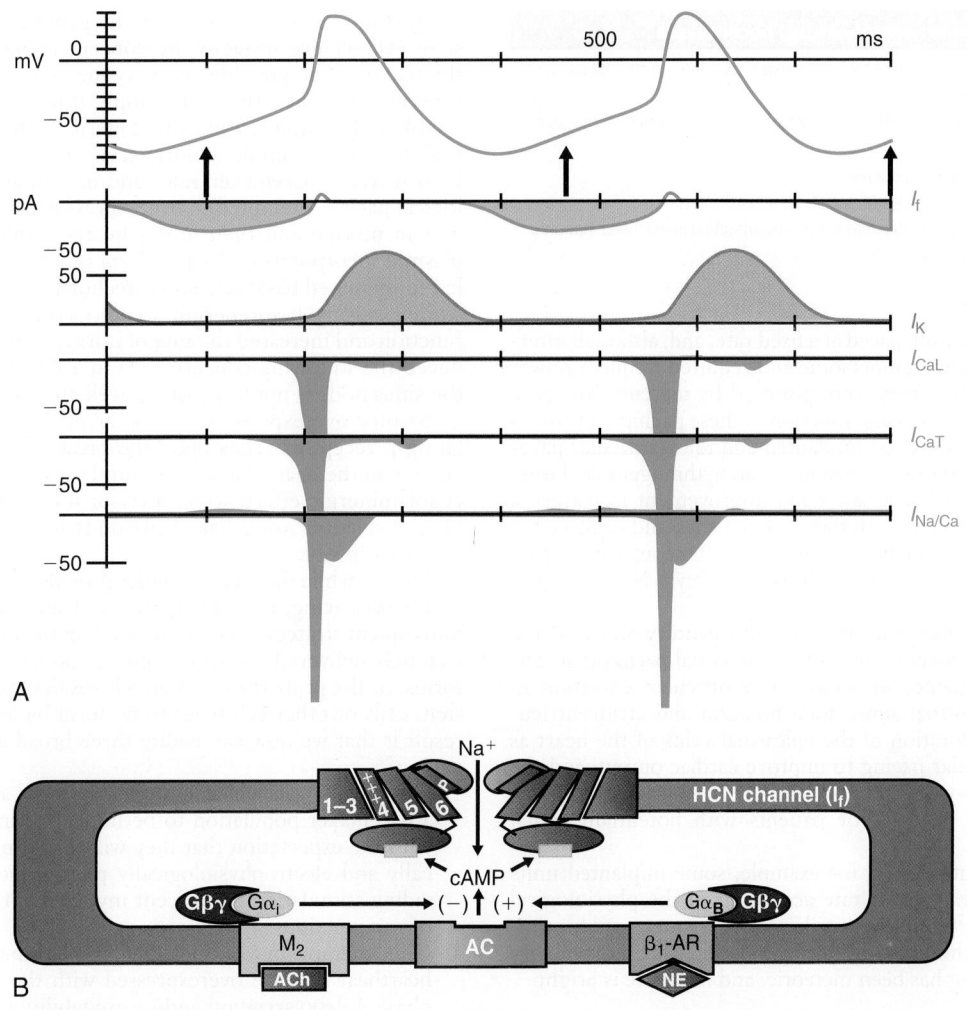

FIGURE 26.1 (A) The sinoatrial node action potential and the currents contributing to impulse generation. (B) The hyperpolarization-activated cyclic nucleotide-gated (*HCN*) channel. See text for discussion.

to I_f: administration of I_f blocking drugs in experimental models and in the clinic have resulted in significant slowing of sinus rate but not in termination of the rhythm.[15,16] The inability to suppress sinus node function using any one channel blocker highlights the redundancy within the sinoatrial pacemaker, which helps enable it to continue to function even under challenge.

To summarize, the primary biological pacemaker is structurally and functionally complex. In settings of disordered sinoatrial node impulse initiation or propagation that interferes with normal cardiac function one has the choice of attempting to remake or repair the sinoatrial node—a difficult and, as yet, impossible task—or to reproduce aspects of its function. The overall goals of such a treatment are to restore the quality of life and to prolong life itself.

Pathologies Impacting Normal Pacemaker Function and a Brief History of Therapies

Adams[1] in 1827 and Stokes[2] in 1846 noted the clinical characteristics of an event that had likely afflicted mankind for centuries: they described patients who became pale, whose pulse became slow or was absent, and who then collapsed. We now recognize that the pathology behind these events is high-degree heart block. In the 20th century, the availability of synthetic catecholamines and later of β-agonists afforded a new type of treatment: sublingual isoproterenol every 2 hours.[17]

While this therapy increased the rate of idioventricular pacemakers to more closely approximate the normal physiological range in many patients, it also caused ventricular tachycardia in some cases. Moreover, this stopgap therapy could not ensure long-term patient survival.

The answer to this dilemma faced by patients and physicians was the electronic pacemaker. The origin of electronic pacing is traceable to a report by McWilliam in 1889 of a means for delivering shocks at about 60 to 70 times per minute to a patient whose heartbeat had failed.[18] In 1928, Lidwell and Booth used an electrical power source attached to a needle plunged into the heart to revive "a stillborn infant."[19] The term *cardiac pacemaker* is attributed to Hyman, who used a hand-cranked device to generate electrical shocks in 1932.[20] However, the modern era in pacing commenced in the early 1950s when Hopps[21] in Canada and Zoll[22] in the United States reported devices that delivered transcutaneous shocks. Weirich and associates reported pacing via shocks delivered through an intramyocardial needle in the setting of a postsurgical complete heart block in 1957,[23] the same year in which Bakken fabricated the first portable external pacemaker.[24]

Initially, pacemaker implantation in the human heart required a thoracotomy for intramyocardial electrode placement.[4] The first temporary transvenous approach was reported by Furman and Schwedel in 1959.[3] The early 1960s then saw the rapid adoption of transvenous pacing with implanted units. These pacemakers

- Not fully responsive to the autonomic nervous system—to the demands of exercise and emotion
- Require monitoring and maintenance, including, at times, battery and/or electrode replacement
- Not optimal for pediatric patients
- Problems with infection, interference from other devices
- Often cannot implant at sites that optimize contraction in individual patients
- Palliate but do not cure

had no sensing function, paced at a fixed rate, and, although internally implanted, were cumbersome and required frequent power pack changes because they were powered by mercury batteries. Moreover, the lack of sensing function in these pacing units often led to competition between implanted and idioventricular pacemakers and, in far too many instances, arrhythmogenesis. However, the 1960s and 1970s saw rapid improvement in batteries, electrodes, and software, such that pacemakers could be placed in a demand mode, in which they sensed spontaneously occurring heartbeats and reset appropriately (see Jeffrey,[4] Nelson,[24] and Zivin and colleagues[25]).

Advances continued through the 20th century and into the current decade: atrioventricular (AV) sequential pacing that synchronized the sequence of atrial and ventricular activation in patients having normal sinus node function and atrioventricular block; the exploration of the epicardial veins of the heart as sites for biventricular pacing to improve cardiac output; and the evolution of cardioverter-defibrillators that could sense, shock, and then pace if needed, for patients with potentially lethal tachyarrhythmias.

Innovation continues as, for example, some implanted units are now able to vary heart rate according to the physiological needs of the body,[26] and leadless electrodes are now used to stimulate the heart without incorporating a catheter.[27] So the history of electronic pacing has been meteoric, and its future is bright.

Rationale for Developing Biological Pacemakers

Given the above description of electronic pacemakers, why bother with biological pacing—or indeed with any other approach? Simply because the electronic pacemaker, while a superior treatment, is not a cure. Box 26.1 summarizes why biological pacemakers are being investigated to normalize cardiac rhythm in a way that more nearly approximates the physiological state than do electronic pacemakers. If the development of biological pacing succeeds, then doctors would likely treat patients with the two technologies in tandem for some time to maximize patient safety. But the eventual goal would be the phasing out of electronic pacing. As such, biological pacing represents a disruptive technology.

Strategies, Successes, and Failures in Developing Biological Pacemakers

In the late 1980s, biological pacing was a pipe-dream occasionally discussed around coffee tables among investigators working on mechanisms of impulse initiation. The discussions were likely stimulated by DiFrancesco's discovery of the pacemaker current, I_f,[10,11] and usually began with statements like, "Wouldn't it be wonderful if we could put pacemaker currents into diseased sinus nodes or ventricles and create a site of normal impulse initiation." This was the stuff of science fiction, but as we have learned time and again, science fiction often explores desirable outcomes before the development of the needed technology—the works of Jules Verne being a prime example.

By the late 1990s, advances in genetic manipulation and stem cell science brought the concept of biological pacing to the realm of the possible, as everyone ventured to state in lectures and in print rather than simply at the coffee table. Several templates for exploration of biological pacing are suggested by Fig. 26.1. For example, β-adrenergic stimulation can modulate I_f to increase pacemaker rate, and an initial strategy for biological pacing attempted to overexpress $β_2$-adrenergic receptors first in murine and then in pig hearts.[28] Injection of a naked plasmid incorporating the $β_2$-adrenergic receptor into pig atria led to increased basal rate and catecholamine response.[28] While overexpressing β-adrenergic receptors augmented sinus node function and increased the rate of normal rhythms, it also introduced the following concerns: (1) in a diseased heart in which the sinus node is not functioning well and/or there is AV block, β-receptor overexpression can be arrhythmogenic; (2) upregulating β-receptors relies upon the presence of pacemaker cells already in the heart that will respond normally to increased catecholaminergic effect, which may or may not be the case; and (3) transfection using naked plasmids has marginal success in the heart in situ.

Hence, while these early studies provided proof of concept for biological pacing, the strategy was not one that could advance. Subsequent strategies have depended on the manipulation of ion channels delivered via viral vectors, the use of stem cell platforms, or the properties of channels resident in or deliverable to stem cells or other cell types to perform biological pacing. The result is that we now can codify three broad areas of biological pacing[29]:

1. Cell therapy, in which human stem cells are converted into a pacemaker population to be implanted in the myocardium with the expectation that they will function as a morphologically and electrophysiologically phenotypic pacemaker, providing stimulation to adjacent myocardium via the formation of gap junctions
2. Gene therapy, in which ion channels or other genes regulating heartbeat rate are overexpressed with the intent to increase phase-4 depolarization and/or excitability in native myocytes, thereby generating an electrophysiologically phenotypic pacemaker
3. Hybrid therapy, in which stem cells carry genes that modify phase-4 depolarization and create electrophysiologically phenotypic pacemakers by coupling to native myocytes, or in which transcription factors are delivered to native myocardial cells in situ, converting them to morphologically and electrophysiologically phenotypic pacemakers

Cell Therapy

Four different cell types have been used to create morphologically and electrophysiologically phenotypic biological pacemakers. One is the human embryonic stem cell that has been forced along a cardiogenic lineage.[30] Within this lineage a subset of cells manifest typical pacemaker characteristics, including action potentials showing prominent phase-4 depolarization.[30] The underlying populations of ion channels include a very weak I_{K1} and a robust I_f, which together would tend to generate depolarization during phase 4.[31] Unlike the sinoatrial node, however, the major contributor of the inward current is reportedly Na^+, rather than the L-type Ca^{2+} current.[31]

Clusters of these cells in culture initiate and propagate spontaneous rhythms, and when implanted into the ventricles of pigs in complete heart block, they have initiated stable spontaneous rhythms that persist for up to 3 months.[30] The major issues with this approach are the need to use immunosuppression and the questions regarding the eventual fate of the cells (whether they will persist as pacemaker cells or instead mature into nonbeating ventricular myocytes or into other inimical cell types).

Other attempts to work with cells containing full ion channel complements have included the grafting of fetal[32] or neonatal[33] pacemaker cells. These research directions have not yet been published in sufficient detail to permit the objective evaluation of the possibilities they offer. A fourth cell therapy approach has involved the generation of induced pluripotent stem cells (iPSCs), initially from dermal fibroblasts[34] and then from keratinocytes.[35] At the cellular level, good pacemaker function has been demonstrated with this approach. The advantage of iPSCs is that they permit the development of pacemaker cells that have the full complement of pacemaker genes, similar to the embryonic stem cell. An advantage of the iPSCs over embryonic stem cells is that iPSCs can be used autologously, thereby creating no immune response. Questions remain regarding the possibility of tumor development, although the oncogenes originally used to create iPSCs no longer need be used.[36,37] In addition, there are questions regarding whether autologous stem cells developed from tissues of aging populations, such as most patients requiring pacemakers, will be as robust as those from young individuals.

We have used iPSCs generated from human keratinocytes to develop a population of cardiomyocyte-like cells having pacemaker properties as well as the basic features of the excitation–contraction coupling machinery.[35] Interestingly, these cardiomyocyte-like cells show a beat rate variability that matches the heart rate variability seen in the cell donors.[39–41] The data suggest that heart rate variability, long thought to reflect autonomic input to the heart, is fundamentally determined by the ionic channels, exchangers, and pumps of the cells themselves, modified by autonomic input. Additionally, we see that cells derived from mature keratinocytes (and, by extension, any mature cells similarly treated) can be reprogrammed to develop to recapitulate the properties of a developing cardiomyocyte and to include the potential to act as a pacemaker.

With this in mind, iPSC-derived cardiomyocyte-like cells have been studied as biological pacemakers, implanted as xenografts into the hearts of immunosuppressed dogs.[42] Function of these cells has approximated that of other biological pacemakers that are based on HCN genes, and we are working to improve the pacemaker characteristics here. While having to immunosuppress confers a major clinical disadvantage, the vision for potential clinical application of iPSC-derived biological pacemakers is that they would be prepared and administered autologously, obviating the need for immunosuppression.

Gene Therapy

As a means to increase phase-4 depolarization and/or excitability and pacemaker rate, gene therapy usually employs a viral vector to deliver a gene or genes, the introduction of which results in loss of outward currents or gain of inward currents. The outcome is that working myocardial cells (with myocyte morphology) develop a pacemaker electrophysiological phenotype.

Gene Therapies Generating Loss- or Gain-of-Function Ion Channels

Referring to Fig. 26.1A, the initial ion channel–based approach reported transfection of guinea pig ventricles with an adenoviral vector incorporating a dominant negative Kir2.1 construct to reduce the repolarizing current, I_{K1}.[43] As shown on ECG in the intact heart and with microelectrode and ion current recordings, an ectopic ventricular rhythm was expressed that was associated with phase-4 depolarization and reduced I_{K1} in myocytes. A shortcoming of this approach was that reducing repolarizing current increases action potential duration, and a subsequent publication showed that this approach to biological pacing created the repolarization characteristics of Anderson syndrome.[44]

Our group has worked primarily with means to modify and magnify the pacemaker current, I_f.[10,11] We first demonstrated in neonatal rat myocytes in cell culture that using an adenoviral vector to overexpress the HCN2 channel isoform produced a robust and rapid pacemaker that far exceeded in rate and stability the rhythm normally recorded in nontransfected cultures.[45,46] For this reason, we adopted the strategy of using HCN genes to build biological pacemakers and centered the approach on HCN2.[47] An additional attraction of working with HCN channels was that their inward current flows only during diastole. With this means of increasing an inward current, there is no prolongation of action potential duration, thereby avoiding the problem inherent in I_{K1} downregulation.

Our initial in vivo study involved injecting an adenoviral construct containing the HCN2 gene and the green fluorescent protein (GFP) gene into the canine left atria and, several days later, using vagal stimulation to suppress sinus rhythm.[47] The result was escape beats originating from the implant site. Cells that were disaggregated from this site showed an I_f (actually an I_{HCN2}) about 100 times greater in magnitude than that in native atrial myocytes. Additional vagal stimulation terminated firing of this pacemaker locus, consistent with parasympathetic control.

A follow-up study used a custom designed electrode catheter to locate the left bundle branch system in dogs and to inject the same adenoviral–HCN2 complex into the bundle branch.[48] When the vagi were stimulated to terminate sinus rhythm and induce atrioventricular block, a rhythm emerged from the injection site. Microelectrode studies demonstrated spontaneous and rapid impulse initiation at these bundle branch sites. Subsequently, we found that in dogs in radiofrequency-induced complete heart block, a biological pacemaker inserted into the left bundle branch system drove the heart regularly and stably.[49] These rhythms were mapped to their bundle branch origins (Fig. 26.2).

For the 2 weeks during which stable HCN2 expression occurred, about 70% of beats originated from the injection site. Basal rates averaged 50 to 60 beats/min.[49] The remaining 30% of beats were provided by the demand electronic pacemaker set at an escape rate of 45 beats/min. A control group of saline-injected animals with electronic pacemakers also set at 45 beats/min had 90% of beats electronically stimulated, with the remainder of the beats arising from various idioventricular sites. Finally, the biological pacemaker manifested an approximate 50% rate increase in response to catecholamine injection. Taking this finding together with our earlier report,[47] we concluded that both vagal and sympathetic (or at least β-adrenergic) modulation of biological pacing is possible.

Optimizing Pacemaker Gene Constructs

Attempts are ongoing to improve on the function of HCN2 using designer-based K+ channel genes,[50] mutant or chimeric HCN channels,[49,51,52] and combinations of two channels. We first studied a mutant HCN2 (E324A) that showed enhanced catecholamine responsiveness, but found only modest improvement over wild-type HCN2.[49] We then designed a chimera, HCN212, whose transmembrane portion included the pore of HCN1 (which has a more positive activation voltage than HCN2) and the amino- and carboxy-termini of HCN2, the latter terminus incorporating the cyclic AMP binding site.[52] We hypothesized that this channel would generate faster basal pacemaker rates than HCN2 while exhibiting greater autonomic responsiveness than HCN1 alone. However, HCN212 outcomes were excessive, such that ventricular tachycardias having rates greater than 200 beats/min occurred. While this result was unfortunate with regard to construct design, it permitted us to test whether I_f blockade might be useful in suppressing arrhythmias generated by biological pacemakers. The I_f blocker, ivabradine, was highly effective here.[52]

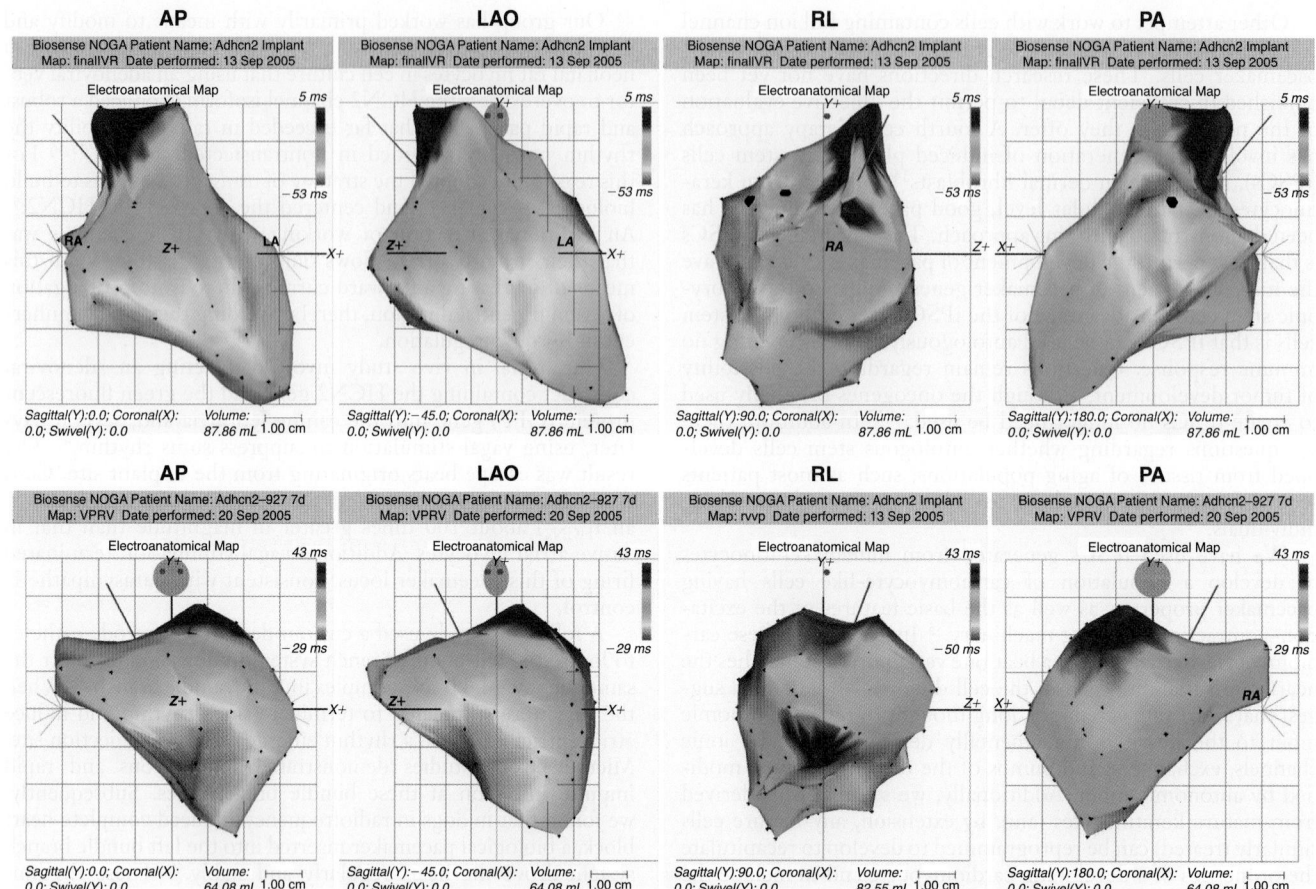

FIGURE 26.2 Noncontact mapping of the left ventricle with the Carto system in a dog with complete heart block, an electronic right ventricular apical endocardial pacemaker, and an HCN2 adenoviral construct administered into the proximal left bundle branch. Panels demonstrate four projections, showing early (*red*) through late (*blue*) activation. Upper panels show an impulse activating left ventricular endocardium at several sites simultaneously, reflecting arrival of an impulse initiated in the left bundle branch system. Lower panels show early activation of left ventricular septum via the electronic pacemaker. *AP*, Anteroposterior; *LAO*, left anterior oblique; *PA*, posteroanterior; *RL*, right lateral.

Another mutant gene was reported by Kashiwakura and colleagues.[50] They used a K+ channel engineered to carry inward Na+ current having many of the properties of I_f. The shortcoming was the absence of a cyclic AMP binding site, without which there is no autonomic modulation. Although these and other constructs so far developed have not offered an advantage over the wild-type channels, it is anticipated that continued efforts at discovery will develop robust alternatives.

Combinations of two genes have shown promising outcomes. One approach uses the dominant negative Kir2.1 construct described above.[53] This construct was tested in an adenoviral vector together with an HCN gene to increase inward current. The intent was to decrease hyperpolarizing current and increase inward current simultaneously in a small region of the ventricle, which was done successfully in pigs[53] and is proposed by the investigators as a potential treatment in settings where electronic pacemakers have become infected, necessitating hardware extraction from the heart. The concern here is that the adenoviral vector, which itself can cause inflammation, and the additional catheter manipulation necessary may contribute to the inflammatory process in the heart. Therefore this approach will likely be tested in a large animal model of endocarditis before advancing the therapy.

Another approach uses HCN2 together with the skeletal muscle Na+ channel, SkM1.[54] SkM1 not only improves propagation of the cardiac impulse at depolarized membrane potentials,[55] but moves the threshold potential to more negative voltages.[54] The net result is that impulse initiation occurs earlier in phase 4, speeding the pacemaker rate. When tested in a canine model of complete heart block, the outcome was basal rates in the range of 80 beats/min, with responses to catecholamine or exercise up to 140 to 150 beats/min. In addition, in this setting there was no need for the backup electronic pacemaker to fire.[54]

A different attempt to improve function uses the Ca2+-stimulated adenylyl cyclase (AC1) gene expressed alone or in combination with HCN2.[56] Basal beating rates were excessively high, around 140 beats/min with HCN2/AC1 and only in the 50 to 65 beats/min range with AC1 alone. Escape times in both groups were 1 to 2 seconds following overdrive pacing and the percent of electronic beats was 2% to 7%. Instantaneous and long-term heart rate variability and circadian rhythm in 24-h recordings showed a greater sensitivity to parasympathetic modulation in animals injected with AC1 than in those injected with HCN2/AC1 and showed a high degree of sympathetic modulation in those injected with HCN2/AC1.

In vitro and in vivo data suggested that enhancement of not only I_f but also other Ca2+-based pacemaker mechanisms occurs with AC1, and this is a concern.[56] However, given the robust autonomic response to this intervention, its continued exploration is warranted, although better control of basal rates will be a requisite.

Hybrid Therapy

Delivery of Transcription Factors to Modify Morphology and Phenotype of Working Myocytes

Whereas the gene therapies described above focus on adding or subtracting function but not on altering morphology of endogenous working myocardium or conducting tissue, the transcription factor approach is intended to transform working myocardial cells into pacemaker cells. Initial studies reported delivery of the transcription factor TBX3 to myocytes in culture, resulting in transformation of a subset of cells into a pacemaker phenotype.[57] However, subsequent administration of TBX3 to hearts in a small animal model reportedly conferred no pacemaker function. In contrast, TBX18 not only induced biological pacemaker function in a guinea pig model,[58] it also did so in a porcine model.[59] Here, radiofrequency ablation was used to induce complete heart block in pigs implanted with backup electronic pacemakers. Then either a vector containing the gene encoding TBX18 or one encoding a reporter gene was injected into the right ventricular upper septum of each pig. Heart rates in the TBX18 recipients were faster than those in the reporter gene recipients over a 14-day period, and the rhythms generated were autonomically responsive. Cardiomyocytes with nodal morphology and a sinus node–like electrophysiological phenotype were identified at the site of injection. The duration of the transcriptional change in this model is uncertain, but research is proceeding and the investigators have suggested that they might propose to use this approach to treat individuals with pacemaker lead infections.

Use of Cells to Carry Pacemaker Genes

This hybrid approach is a cell therapy using cell types that do not have the proper ion channel population to generate pacemaker function but have other characteristics that make them candidates for platform therapy. These cells can be loaded with a gene or genes of interest that result in delivery of a pacemaker signal to adjacent cells. While some work has been reported using fibroblasts as platforms and fusing them with ventricular myocytes,[60] the more completely reported approach to date has used adult human mesenchymal stem cells (hMSCs).[61–63] Gene chip analysis has shown that hMSCs do not have any appreciable signal for the pacemaker genes, HCN1–4, but they do have a robust signal for the cardiac connexins, Cx40 and Cx43.[62] We hypothesized that if we could load hMSCs with a pacemaker gene, they might couple adequately to myocytes such that the depolarizing signal generated by I_f would be transmitted to adjacent myocytes, causing them to depolarize (Fig. 26.3).[64–66] Both dye transfer and current injection experiments in cell pairs showed that hMSCs could indeed communicate with myocytes.[62] This prompted us to load these cells with HCN2 via electroporation (avoiding any viral vector) (Fig. 26.4A–C) and to implant them in the canine left ventricle.[61,63] An initial study used vagal stimulation to suppress sinoatrial node impulse initiation and atrioventricular conduction. Here, an escape rhythm that pace-mapped to the injection site was generated by the hMSC-based pacemakers (Fig. 26.4D). Connexins at the interstices between hMSCs and cardiac myocytes also were noted (Fig. 26.4E).

In a subsequent study of dogs in complete heart block, hMSCs generated pacemaker function for at least 6 weeks when 700,000 cells or more, approximately 50% of which were loaded with HCN2, were implanted at a single left ventricular site.[63] Longer term follow-up has revealed an issue of major concern: by 8 to 10 weeks most hMSCs had migrated from the site of administration. For this reason, attempts are now being made to encapsulate

Rationale for Stem Cell–Based Pacemaker

Natural pacemaker

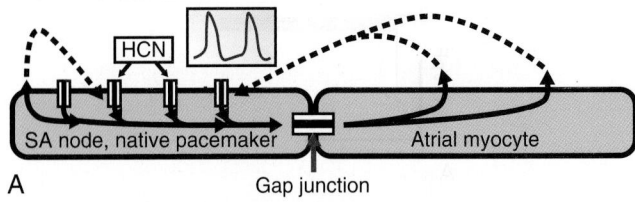

A   Gap junction

hMSC as platform for a biological pacemaker

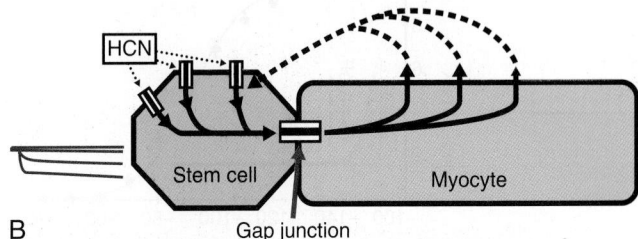

B   Gap junction

FIGURE 26.3 Initiation of spontaneous rhythms by wild-type pacemaker cells as well as by genetically engineered stem cell pacemakers. (A) In a native pacemaker cell (or in a myocyte engineered to incorporate pacemaker current via gene transfer) action potentials (*inset*) are initiated via inward current flowing through transmembrane hyperpolarization-activated cyclic nucleotide-gated (*HCN*) channels. These channels open when the membrane repolarizes to its maximum diastolic potential and close when the membrane has depolarized during the action potential. Current flowing via gap junctions to adjacent myocytes results in their excitation and the propagation of impulses through the conducting system. **(B)** A stem cell has been engineered to incorporate HCN channels in its membrane. These channels can only open, and current can only flow through them (*inset*), when the membrane is hyperpolarized; such hyperpolarization can only be delivered if an adjacent myocyte is tightly coupled to the stem cell via gap junctions. In the presence of such coupling and the opening of the HCN channels to induce local current flow, the adjacent myocyte will be excited and initiate an action potential that then propagates through the conducting system. The depolarization of the action potential will result in the closing of the HCN channels until the next repolarization restores a high negative membrane potential. In summary, wild-type and genetically engineered pacemaker cells incorporate in each cell all the machinery needed to initiate and propagate action potentials. In contrast, in the stem cell–myocyte pairing, two cells together work as a single functional unit whose operation is critically dependent on the gap junctions that form between the two disparate cell types. *hMSC,* Human mesenchymal stem cell; *SA,* sinoatrial.

them in nanofabrics to maintain them at the site of administration while still permitting gap junction formation and transmission of signals across the fabric.

Critical questions regarding these and other stem cells concern not only the possibility of evolution of these cells into inimical or ineffective cell types but also of rejection or apoptosis.[65,66] In a 6-week trial of hMSCs xenotransplanted into canine hearts there was no rejection (Fig. 26.5),[63] which is consistent with the hypothesis that hMSCs are immunoprotected, most likely by one of several humoral factors they release.[67,68] However, we have seen robust rejection of occasional lots of hMSCs by canine hearts, which is not unexpected with xenotransplantation. As for the eventual human application of hMSCs, studies of their allogeneic administration to human subjects for myocardial repair have not reported any rejection response, but there has been a high degree of cell loss (summarized in Zimmett and Hare[67]) mirroring experience in the canine. Clearly, issues remain regarding how to best bring this therapy to human subjects.

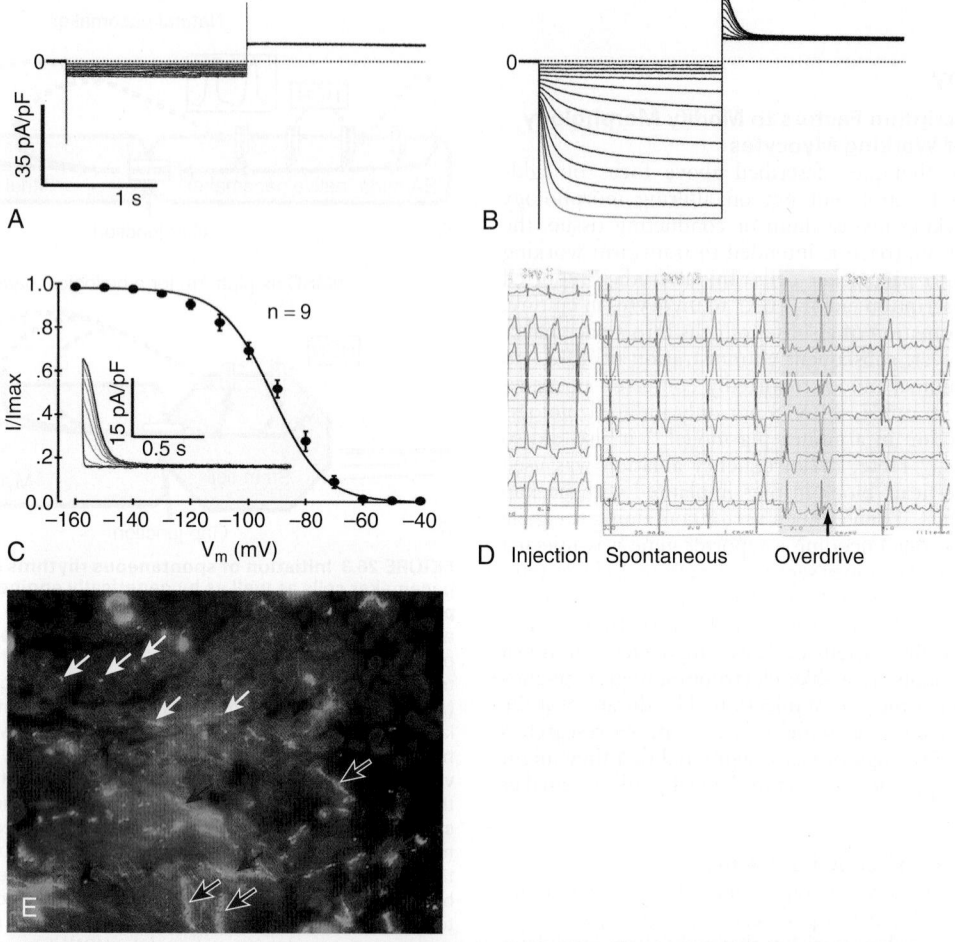

FIGURE 26.4 Example of loading human mesenchymal stem cells (hMSCs) with a gene of interest, studying it biophysically, and determining its effect on the heart. (A) Pacemaker current, I_f, is not seen in a nonelectroporated hMSC. (B) Functional expression of I_f in hMSCs transfected with the mHCN2 gene. (C) Fit by the Boltzmann equation to the normalized tail currents of I_f gives a midpoint of –91.8 +/– 0.9 mV and a slope of 8.8 +/– 0.5 mV ($n = 9$). I_f is fully activated around –140 mV, with an activation threshold of –60 mV. *Inset* shows representative tail currents used for activation curves. Voltage protocol: hold at –30 mV, hyperpolarize × 1.5 s from –40 to –160 mV in 10-mV increments followed by 1.5-s voltage step to +20 mV. (D) Pacemaker function in canine heart in situ. *Top to bottom,* electrocardiogram leads I, II, III, aVR, aVL, and aVF. (1) Pacing from hMSC injection site showing electrocardiogram configuration; (2) spontaneous rhythm pace-maps to site of injection, suggesting it is initiated at the injection site; (3) last two beats of overdrive pacing (*black arrow*) at 80 beats/min followed by escape rhythm. Escape time = 1.3 s. E, Immunostaining for connexin43 (Cx43) in a region of interface between an injection site and myocardium. 4′,6-diamidino-2-phenylindole staining reveals nuclei. *Purple arrows* are intercalated disks; *white arrows* show Cx43 staining between hMSCs; and *red arrows* show Cx43 staining between hMSCs and myocytes.

Challenges

Some of the challenges we will discuss are unique to biological pacing; other challenges hold for a variety of other approaches to gene and cell therapy. A major challenge is to identify the optimal construct, and the groups working in this area continue attempts at optimizing mutants and chimeras. HCN2 alone manifests properties that likely are adequate for first generation biological pacing. However, it might be preferable to have a construct that maintains basal rates in the 60 to 70 beats/min range and reaches peaks of 120 to 140 beats/min on catecholamine stimulation, as has been reported for the HCN2/SkM1 combination.[54]

Although vagal and β-adrenergic responsiveness are characteristics of HCN2-based biological pacemakers, further

understanding of autonomic control is required. Use of HCN2 in both viral and hMSC constructs has demonstrated that vagal control depends on the site at which the pacemaker is implanted.[69] In vagally innervated regions, Poincaré plots of heart rate variability are consistent with vago-sympathetic input. In contrast, on the lateral free wall of the left ventricle, where there is little to no vagal innervation, there is no evidence of vagal input and only sympathetic responsiveness is seen.

Preclinical and clinical testing of biological pacing also are major challenges. At the preclinical level, questions that arise relate largely to safety, efficacy, and duration of action. Another challenge is to effectively utilize the relationship between biological and electronic pacing. When and if biological pacing is ready for clinical trial, it cannot simply be administered alone to human subjects in need of support of their ventricular rate. Rather, it

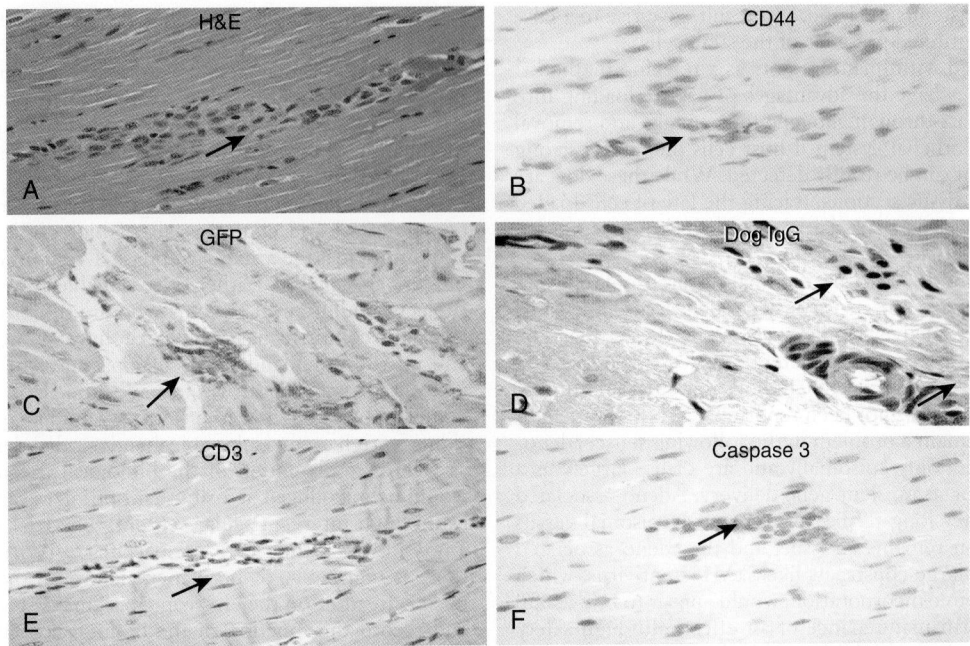

FIGURE 26.5 Human mesenchymal stem cells (hMSCs) 6 weeks after left ventricular anterior wall intramyocardial injection. Hematoxylin and eosin (*H&E*) staining identifies basophilic cells (A) that are CD44 positive (B) and green fluorescent protein (*GFP*) positive (peroxidase stain) (C). hMSCs do not display labeling/binding of dog IgG to their surface (D), evidence against humoral rejection. CD3-positive T lymphocytes are rarely noted in association with clusters of hMSCs (E), evidence against cellular rejection; staining is negative for activated caspase 3 (F), evidence against apoptosis. (Original magnification, ×400.)

will have to be used together with electronic pacemakers, as these are the current state of the art. For this reason, we have tested integration of biological and electronic pacemakers in tandem operation.[49] Tandem biological–electronic pacemaker therapy manifests (1) a seamless interface between biological and electronic components, maintaining heart rate greater than 45 beats/min; (2) conservation of total electronic beats delivered, which should prolong battery life; (3) the utility of employing the memory function of the electronic pacemaker to track the function of the biological component; and (4) a more physiological and catecholamine-responsive heart rate than is provided by electronic pacemakers alone.

The need to reclaim normal cardiac activation in the setting of normal sinus rhythm and complete heart block has also led investigators to engineer bypass tracts such that sinus impulses can gain access to the ventricles. This design would facilitate atrioventricular conduction and would potentially rival the function of atrioventricular sequential pacing. However, this work is still in its infancy relative to biological pacing. In one innovative approach, rat skeletal myoblasts were placed on an artificial matrix and inserted into the atrioventricular groove of rats whose adjacent atrium and ventricle had been denuded of epicardium. Atrioventricular conduction and survival of transplanted cells was then documented.[70] Replication of these results and information regarding long-term success of this approach are awaited.

What studies are needed if biological pacing is to move into clinical testing? Long-term trials are needed in which either viral or stem cell constructs show reliable effect and no toxicity. The hallmark for comparison is the electronic pacemaker. The trials should show that regardless of whether a viral vector, a cell platform delivery system, or a pacemaker cell is used, the therapy provides function that supports life with an adequate basal rate and response to autonomic input. This activity must emanate uniquely from the site of implantation with no evidence of wandering constructs or cells to other sites in the heart that might compete with the site of implantation.

TABLE 26.1 Methods of cell tracking	
AGENT	**LIMITATIONS**
Reporter Proteins	
LacZ/β-gal	Require secondary detection
Green fluorescent protein	Unstable, may be weaker than autofluorescence
Ex Vivo Staining	
Fluorescence in situ hybridization	Expensive, false positives
Surface markers	Lost/unexpressed over time; require secondary detection
Inorganic	
Radiometals	Toxicity, uniformity of loading
Fluorescent microspheres	Significant aggregation, unstable signal
Nanoparticles (i.e., quantum dots)	New technology, many unknowns

Satisfying these demands is no mean feat: it requires following the beat-by-beat function of the heart for 6- to 12-month periods while concurrently ensuring that viral vectors are not causing untoward effects on the heart or other tissues and that cells, whether hMSCs, ESC- or iPSC-derived, or other, are not being destroyed or transforming into forms that are malignant or, if nonmalignant, then nonfunctional.

A variety of methods are available for tracking cells (Table 26.1). Ideally tracking should use markers that stay with the cell forever, cannot pass from cell to cell, and whose signal can be read from the body surface via imaging techniques. To date, no method has been adequate. Variations on MRI to track iron or ferritin particles loaded into stem cells have been most frequently used for in vivo studies. The shortcoming is that if a cell dies, these particles can be taken up by or reside in other cells and/or reside extracellularly. On being read via MRI they may be identified as a persistent signal and, as a result, give rise to a false conclusion of a continued presence of the stem cells.

We have worked with quantum dots as a tracking method.[71] These nanoparticles have the advantages of passive loading into cells, inability to pass through gap junctions, uptake and removal by the reticuloendothelial system if host cells die, and a strong emission signal that can be readily detected. While these dots are easily identified in tissue sections, tracing the fate of cells loaded with quantum dots using standard imaging techniques in vivo remains a major challenge.

Another issue important to large animal research and to future applicability to human subjects is construct delivery. While catheters are available to deliver viral vectors in specific settings, the ideal delivery system, a flexible catheter with electrode recording capability at its tip and a large enough bore that it will not inflict damage on stem cells, has not been reported.

Viral vectors remain a problem in the following sense: adenoviral vectors express only episomally and are of use largely as a proof of concept or a transient gene delivery. Adeno-associated virus provides better long-term expression, but episomal versus genomic expression remains an issue, and the adeno-associated virus cannot carry large constructs like SkM1. Lentivirus, which does result in genomic incorporation, would appear to be a useful vector for long-term maintenance of an effect, although safety issues remain a concern. In addition, while lentivirus readily supports gene expression in cell culture, achieving consistent expression in vivo has been a challenge.

Cell systems must be optimized and their persistence documented. Autologous cells elicit no immune response when readministered to the donor. However, use of these cells would make biological pacing into a designer therapy whose expense and quality control from patient to patient would be highly challenging in comparison to electronic pacing. It has been shown that hMSCs can be administered allogeneically to human subjects with no adverse reactions, although long-term persistence is still an issue.[66] These cells may ultimately offer a readily standardized cell type, but more research is needed to test this. Human ESCs have required the use of immunosuppression in experiments to date.[30] Whether this will be the case in human experimentation remains to be seen, but a lifetime of electronic pacing appears far preferable to a lifetime of immunosuppression. If the issues surrounding iPSC-derived pacemaker cells (in many cases mirroring those with embryonic stem cells) can be overcome, these cells might be the optimal cell type to carry forward, as autologous administration obviates the need for immunosuppression, and, to date, migration of these cells has not appeared to be an issue in canine experiments.[42]

The choice of promoter and the regulation of nucleic acids are additional issues. To date, many of us have worked with a cytomegalovirus (CMV) promoter. However, there can be temporal changes in the expression of promoters,[72] such that CMV is not the best long-term choice. Moreover, because of safety concerns, a cardiac-specific (and maybe even cardiac region–specific) promoter would be of importance, especially with regard to viral delivery.

Duration of effect and robustness of expression will be influenced by processes regulating protein expression. The discovery that microRNA may reduce expression and/or that alterations in protein degradation alter expression of proteins can impact RNA/DNA expression, DNA regulatory sequences, and the modulation of expression. All of these processes will continue to be explored over the coming years.

One issue on which some progress has been made is the design of preclinical and clinical trials of biological pacemakers. One could not envisage a standard phase-1 trial in which healthy volunteers are sought. Rather, a reasonable trial design in human subjects would enroll patients who are in chronic atrial fibrillation and complete heart block or have significant bradycardia and in whom demand ventricular pacing is needed. The canine equivalent of this trial would have animals in ablation-induced complete heart block. Either setting would incorporate implantation of a right ventricular apical endocardial demand pacemaker, as well as implantation of the biological pacemaker. The latter would be introduced at a site that optimizes cardiac output, such as the high interventricular septum. The trial would proceed in a way in which the electronic pacemaker provides a safety net if there is temporary or permanent failure in the biological pacemaker. In addition the electronic pacemaker can be used to track and record the function of the biological pacemaker. The biological unit, in turn, would likely conserve battery power in the electronic unit; our work to date has shown that tandem biological–electronic operation sees the electronic unit firing only 30% of the time, which would prolong the life of the battery.[49] In addition, the biological component would be the heart's primary pacemaker, would provide autonomic responsiveness, and would provide cardiac activation and output characteristics superior to that provided by the electronic unit. As reviewed above, proof-of-concept experiments of tandem pacing have been promising and have shown no competition between biological and electronic units.[49]

Conclusions

Modern media mania expects this morning's ideas to be this afternoon's cures. But it would be irresponsible to try to make biological pacing fit this mold. Because electronic pacing provides the luxury of a competent backstop, biological pacing should be optimized and adequately tested before human experimentation begins. The advantage of this cautious approach is that the difficult questions that must be asked and the difficult experiments that must be done will not only aid in advancing our knowledge in this field, but will likely find beneficial application in a variety of areas of gene and cell therapy.

Acknowledgment

Some of the studies discussed in this chapter were supported by USPHS-NHLBI grants HL-28958 and HL111401.

REFERENCES

1. Adams R. Cases of diseases of the heart, accompanied with pathological observations. *Dublin Hospital Reports.* 1827;4:353–453.
2. Stokes W. Observations on some cases of permanently slow pulse. *Dublin Q J Med Sci.* 1846;2:73–85.
3. Furman S, Schwedel JB. An intracardiac pacemaker for Stokes-Adams seizures. *N Eng J Med.* 1959;261:943–948.
4. Jeffrey K. The invention and reinvention of cardiac pacing. *Cardiol Clin.* 1992;10:561–571.
5. Keith A, Flack MW. The form and nature of the muscular connections between the primary divisions of the vertebrate heart. *J Anat Physiol.* 1907;41:172–189.
6. Lewis T, Oppenheimer BS, Oppenheimer A. The site of origin of the mammalian heart beat; the pacemaker in the dog. *Heart.* 1910;2:147–169.

7. Fye WB. The origin of the heart beat: a tale of frogs, jellyfish, and turtles. *Circulation.* 1987;76:493–500.
8. Geison G. The Royal institution lectures of 1869. In: *Michael Foster and the Cambridge School of Physiology.* Princeton, NJ: Princeton University Press; 1978:200.
9. Mommersteeg MT, Hoogaars WM, Prall OW, et al. Molecular pathway for the localized formation of the sinoatrial node. *Circ Res.* 2007;100:354–362.
10. DiFrancesco D. A study of the ionic nature of the pacemaker current in calf Purkinje fibres. *J Physiol.* 1981;314:377–393.
11. DiFrancesco D. Block and activation of the pacemaker channel in calf Purkinje fibres effects of potassium, caesium and rubidium. *J Physiol.* 1982;222:329–347.

12. Biel M, Schneider A, Wahl C. Cardiac HCN channels structure, function, and modulation. *Trends Cardiovasc Med.* 2002;12:202–216.
13. Lakatta EG, Maltsev VA, Vinogradova TM. A coupled SYSTEM of intracellular Ca²⁺ clocks and surface membrane voltage clocks controls the timekeeping mechanism of the heart's pacemaker. *Circ Res.* 2010;106:659–673.
14. Lakatta EG, DiFrancesco D. What keeps us ticking: a funny current, a calcium clock, or both? *J Mol Cell Cardiol.* 2009;47:157–170.
15. Thollon C, Bedut S, Villeneuve N, et al. Use-dependent inhibition of hHCN4 by ivabradine and relationship with reduction in pacemaker activity. *Br J Pharmacol.* 2007;150:37–46.

16. Borer JS, Fox K, Jaillon P, et al. for the ivabradine Investigators Group. Antianginal and antiischemic effects of ivabradine, an I_f inhibitor, in stable angina. A randomized, double-blind, multicentered, placebo-controlled trial. *Circulation.* 2003;107:817–823.

17. Scherf D, Schott A. *Extrasystoles and Allied Arrhythmias.* 2nd ed. Chicago: Year Book Medical Publishers; 1973.

18. McWilliam JA. Electrical stimulation of the heart in man. *Brit Med J.* 1889;1:348–350.

19. Lidwell MC. Cardiac disease in relation to anaesthesia. In: *Transactions of the Third Session.* Sydney, Australia: Australasian Medical Congress; 1929:160. Sept. 2–7.

20. Furman S, Szarka G, Layvand D. Reconstruction of Hyman's second pacemaker. *Pacing Clin Electrophysiol.* 2005;28:446–453.

21. Bigelow WG, Callaghan JC, Hopps JA. General hypothermia for experimental intracardiac surgery; the use of electrophrenic respirations, an artificial pacemaker for cardiac standstill, and radio-frequency rewarming in general hypothermia. *Trans Meet Am Surg Assoc Am Surg Assoc.* 1950;68:211–219.

22. Zoll PM. Resuscitation of the heart in ventricular standstill by external electric stimulation. *New Engl J Med.* 1952;247:768–771.

23. Weirich W, Gott V, Lillehei C. The treatment of complete heart block by the combined use of a myocardial electrode and an artificial pacemaker. *Surg Forum.* 1957;8:360–363.

24. Nelson G. A brief history of cardiac pacing. *Tex Heart Inst J.* 1993;20:12–18.

25. Zivin A, Mehra R, Bardy GH. Cardiac pacemakers. In: Spooner PM, Rosen MR, eds. *Foundations of Cardiac Arrhythmias.* New York: Marcel Dekker Inc; 2001:571–598.

26. Gregoratos G, Cheitlin MD, Conill A. ACC/AHA Guidelines for Implantation of Cardiac Pacemakers and Antiarrhythmia Devices: Executive Summary—a Report of the American College of Cardiology/American Heart Association Task Force on Practice Guidelines (Committee on Pacemaker Implantation). *Circulation.* 1998;97:1325–1335.

27. Lee KL. In the wireless era: leadless pacing. *Expert Rev Cardiovasc Ther.* 2010;8:171–174.

28. Edelberg JM, Huang DT, Josephson ME, et al. Molecular enhancement of porcine cardiac chronotropy. *Heart.* 2001;86:559–562.

29. Rosen MR. Gene therapy and biological pacing. *New Engl J Med.* 2014;371:1158–1159.

30. Kehat I, Khimovich L, Caspi O, et al. Electromechanical integration of cardiomyocytes derived from human embryonic stem cells. *Nat Biotechnol.* 2004;22:1282–1289.

31. Satin J, Kehat I, Caspi O, et al. Mechanism of spontaneous excitability in human embryonic stem cell derived cardiomyocytes. *J Physiol.* 2004;559:479–496.

32. Lin G, Cai J, Jiang H, et al. Biological pacemaker created by fetal cardiomyocyte transplantation. *J Biomed Sci.* 2005;12:513–519.

33. Cai J, Lin G, Jiang H, et al. Transplanted neonatal cardiomyocytes as a potential biological pacemaker in pigs with complete atrioventricular block. *Transplantation.* 2006;81:1022–1026.

34. Zhang J, Wilson GF, Soerens AG, et al. Functional cardiomyocytes derived from human. *Circ Res.* 2009;104:e30–e41.

35. Novak A, Shtrichman R, Germanguz I, et al. Enhanced reprogramming and cardiac differentiation of human keratinocytes derived from plucked hair follicles, using a single excisable lentivirus. *Cell Reprogramm.* 2010;12:665–678.

36. Efe JA, Hilcove S, Kim J, et al. Conversion of mouse fibroblasts into cardiomyocytes using a direct reprogramming strategy. *Nature Cell Biology.* 2011;13:215–222.

37. Warren L, Manos PD, Ahfeldt T, et al. Highly efficient reprogramming to pluripotency and directed differentiation of human cells with synthetic modified mRNA. *Cell Stem Cell.* 2010;7:618–630.

38. Deleted in review.

39. Mandel Y, Weissman A, Schick R, et al. Human embryonic and induced pluripotent stem cells-derived cardiomyocytes exhibit beat rate variability and power-law behavior. *Circulation.* 2012;125:883–893.

40. Binah O, Weissman A, Itskovitz-Eldor J, et al. Integrating beat rate variability: from single cells to hearts. *Heart Rhythm.* 2013;10:928–932.

41. Ben-Ari M, Schick R, Barad L, et al. From beat rate variability in induced pluripotent stem cell-derived pacemaker cells to heart rate variability in human subjects. *Heart Rhythm.* 2014;11:1808–1818.

42. Chauveau S, Anyukhovsky EP, Potapova IS, et al. Keratinocyte-derived cardiomyocytes provide in vivo biological pacemaker function. *Eur Heart J.* 2016;8:257.

43. Miake J, Marbán E, Nuss HB. Gene therapy: biological pacemaker created by gene transfer. *Nature.* 2002;419:132–133.

44. Miake J, Marbán E, Nuss HB. Functional role of inward rectifier current in heart probed by Kir2.1 overexpression and dominant-negative-suppression. *J Clin Invest.* 2003;111:1529–1536.

45. Yu H, Wu J, Potapova I, et al. MinK-related peptide 1: a β subunit for the HCN ion channel subunit family enhances expression and speeds activation. *Circ Res.* 2001;88:E84–E87.

46. Qu J, Barbuti A, Protas L, et al. HNC2 overexpression in newborn and adult ventricular myocytes: distinct effects on gating and excitability. *Circ Res.* 2001;89:E8–E14.

47. Qu J, Plotnikov AN, Danilo Jr P, et al. Expression and function of a biological pacemaker in canine heart. *Circulation.* 2003;107:1106–1109.

48. Plotnikov AN, Sosunov EA, Qu J, et al. A biological pacemaker implanted in the canine left bundle branch provides ventricular escape rhythms having physiologically acceptable rates. *Circulation.* 2004;109:506–512.

49. Bucchi A, Plotnikov AN, Shlapakova I, et al. Wild-type and mutant HCN channels in a tandem biological-electronic cardiac pacemaker. *Circulation.* 2006;114:992–999.

50. Kashiwakura Y, Cho HC, Barth AS, et al. Gene transfer of a synthetic pacemaker channel into the heart: a novel strategy for biological pacing. *Circulation.* 2006;114:1682–1686.

51. Tse HF, Xue T, Lau CP, et al. Bioartificial sinus node constructed via in vivo gene transfer of an engineered pacemaker HCN channel reduces the dependence on electronic pacemaker in a sick-sinus syndrome model. *Circulation.* 2006;114:1000–1011.

52. Plotnikov AN, Bucchi A, Shlapakova I, et al. HCN212-channel biological pacemakers manifesting ventricular tachyarrhythmias are responsive to treatment with I_f blockade. *Heart Rhythm.* 2008;5:282–288.

53. Cingolani E, Yee K, Shehata M, et al. Biological pacemaker created by percutaneous gene delivery via venous catheters in a porcine model of complete heart block. *Heart Rhythm.* 2011;8:S112.

54. Boink GJ, Duan L, Nearing BD, et al. HCN2/SkM1 gene transfer into canine left bundle branch induces stable, autonomically responsive biological pacing at physiological heart rates. *J Am Coll Cardiol.* 2013;61:1192–1201.

55. Protas L, Dun W, Lu J, et al. Expression of skeletal but not cardiac Na+ channel isoform preserves normal conduction in a depolarized cardiac syncytium. *Cardiovasc Res.* 2009;81:528–535.

56. Boink GJ, Nearing BD, Shlapakova IN, et al. Ca2+-stimulated adenylyl cyclase AC1 generates efficient biological pacing as single gene therapy and in combination with HCN2. *Circulation.* 2012;126:528–536.

57. Bakker ML, Boink GJ, Boukens BJ, et al. T-box transcription factor TBX3 reprogrammes mature cardiac myocytes into pacemaker-like cells. *Cardiovasc Res.* 2012;94:439–449.

58. Kapoor N, Liang E, Marbán E, et al. Direct conversion of quiescent cardiomyocytes to pacemaker cells by expression of Tbx18. *Nat Biotechnol.* 2013;31:54–62.

59. Hu Y-F, Dawkins JF, Cho HC, et al. Biological pacemaker created by minimally invasive somatic reprogramming in pigs with complete heart block. *Sci Transl Med.* 2014;6. 245ra94.

60. Cho HC, Kashiwakura Y, Marban E. Creation of a biological pacemaker by cell fusion. *Circ Res.* 2007;100:1112–1115.

61. Potapova I, Plotnikov A, Lu Z, et al. Human mesenchymal stem cell use as a gene delivery system to create cardiac pacemakers. *Circ Res.* 2004;94:841–959.

62. Valiunas V, Doronin S, Valiuniene L, et al. Human mesenchymal stem cells make cardiac connexins and form functional gap junctions. *J Physiol.* 2004;555:617–626.

63. Plotnikov AP, Shlapakova I, Szabolcs MJ, et al. Xeno-grafted adult human mesenchymal stem cells provide a platform for sustained biological pacemaker function in canine heart. *Circulation.* 2007;116:706–713.

64. Rosen MR, Brink PR, Cohen IS, et al. Genes, stem cells and biological pacemakers. *Cardiovasc Res.* 2004;64:12–23.

65. Rosen M. Biological pacemaking: in our lifetime? *Heart Rhythm.* 2005;2:418–428.

66. Rosen MR, Robinson RB, Brink PR, et al. The road to biological pacing. *Nat Rev Cardiol.* 2011;8:656–666.

67. Zimmett JM, Hare JM. Emerging role for bone marrow derived mesenchymal stem cells in myocardial regenerative therapy. *Basic Res Cardiol.* 2005;100:471–481.

68. Tse WT, Pendleton JD, Beyer WM, et al. Suppression of allogeneic T-cell proliferation by human marrow stromal cells: implications in transplantation. *Transplantation.* 2003;75:389–397.

69. Shlapakova IN, Nearing BD, Lau DH, et al. Biological pacemakers in canines exhibit positive chronotropic response to emotional arousal. *Heart Rhythm.* 2010;7:1835–1840.

70. Choi YH, Stamm C, Hammer PE, et al. Cardiac conduction through engineered tissue. *Am J Pathol.* 2006;169:72–85.

71. Rosen AB, Kelly DJ, Schuldt AJ, et al. Finding fluorescent needles in the cardiac haystack: tracking human mesenchymal stem cells labeled with quantum dots for quantitative in vivo 3-D fluorescence analysis. *Stem Cells.* 2007;25:2128–2138.

72. Reinhard E, Nedivi E, Wegner J, et al. Neural selective activation and temporal regulation of a mammalian GAP-43 promoter in zebrafish. *Development.* 1994;120:1767–1775.

27 Cell-to-Cell Communication and Impulse Propagation

André G. Kléber

Cardiac Cell-to-Cell Communication by Gap Junctions

The existence of low-resistance pathways between cardiac cells had been postulated from experimental assessment of electrical interactions (cable analysis) between cardiac Purkinje fibers before the existence of gap junction channels was known (see Weidmann[1]). During the subsequent decades, ion channels between cardiac cells were identified, formed by two connexon hemichannels, each composed of six connexin molecules. The main connexins of the myocardium, Cx43, Cx40, and Cx45, have been defined in terms of genetic code, amino acid sequence, and molecular function. Introduction of the whole-cell dual voltage-clamp technique made it possible to directly measure intercellular electrical conductance and single-channel conductance between a pair of cells obtained from enzymatic dissociation of cardiac tissue or from neoformation in cultured cells. Later, transfection techniques were used to study the biophysical properties of specific cardiac connexins in heterologous expression systems and to define the properties of pure or mixed connexons and connexins (homomeric vs. heteromeric connexons, and homologous vs. heterologous connexin channels) in terms of biophysical and diffusive properties.[2–5]

Similar to ion channels, the electrical behavior of gap junction channels is sensitive to the electrical field across the channel and to variations of the intercellular milieu (Ca^{2+}, pH, Mg^{2+}, and ATP).[6] Gap junction channels have a high turnover rate with a half-life at the intercalated disk of only a few hours.[7,8] Connexon hemichannels are transported along microtubular highways and uploaded to the periphery of the gap junction plaques by mechanisms that are dependent on interaction between microtubular plus-end proteins and proteins of the composite junctions.[9–12]

The dynamic balance of gap junction channel expression at the intercalated disk is maintained by continuous internalization.[7,8] Proteins such as ZO-1 and CAR take part in these processes and are involved in interactions with other proteins of the intercellular junction and plaque size control (see Kleber[13] for discussion). The total of these behaviors indicates that gap junction channels form a highly dynamic, regulated system that interacts with other functional protein complexes and explains why changes in composition and function can contribute importantly to disease phenotypes.

Cx43, Cx40, and Cx45 in the Myocardium

Cx43, Cx40, and Cx45 are the three major connexins of the myocardium.[14–16] A fourth connexin, Cx32.1, has been described in murine nodal tissues.[17] Cx43 is the dominant connexin in ventricular myocardium, Cx40 is dominant in the ventricular conduction system, and Cx45 is present in the atrioventricular and sinoatrial nodes and, in lower amounts, in atrial and ventricular myocardium.

Coexpression of Cx43 and Cx45 (ventricle), Cx43, Cx40, and Cx45 (atria), and Cx40 and Cx45 (Purkinje system) raises the question of whether these connexins form mixed heteromeric connexons and/or heterotypic gap junction channels of relevance for cardiac electrical coupling and propagation. Homomeric/homotypic Cx43 and Cx40 gap junction channels have a relatively large unitary electrical conductance, γ_j (approximately 100 pS and 174 pS, respectively), whereas γ_j of Cx45 is considerably smaller (approximately 30 pS).[3]

The question of the role of mixed Cx43/Cx40/Cx45 channels is especially important for atrial tissue showing a wide spectrum of electrical propagation velocities (from 0.2 to 1.6 m/s; see Kleber and colleagues[18]). In both atria, Cx43 and Cx40 are both abundantly expressed and colocalize in intercalated disks, the ratio of Cx40:Cx43 expression being larger in the right atrium than in the left.[19] It has been shown in *human* atria that the ratio of Cx40:Cx43 expression is an important determinant of propagation velocity, with Cx40 dominance decreasing local velocity and Cx43 dominance increasing it.[20] A very similar behavior was observed in vitro in patterned atrial strands cultured from myocytes with genetic Cx43 and Cx40 ablation.[21] These findings contrast to measurements of macroscopic excitation in murine atria with Cx40 ablation in vivo, which yielded slowed or unchanged propagation (see Beauchamp and associates[21] for discussion and references). The reasons for these controversial findings are not evident, but the possibility that malformations may affect macroscopic measurements in whole atria with genetic Cx40 cannot be excluded.[22] The important question is whether colocalization of Cx43/Cx40/Cx45 immunosignals in the atria reflects the existence of separate gap junction channels or if instead mixed Cx40/Cx43/Cx45 heteromeric connexins and/or heterotypic channels exist in the atrial myocardium. An answer to this question is important because mixed Cx40/Cx43 channels may have electrical conductances different from pure homomeric/homotypic Cx43 and Cx40 channels[2,23] and thus may differently affect propagation velocity. It is well known that Cx45 can form heteromeric connexons with Cx43 and Cx40. However, the question of whether heteromeric Cx40/Cx43 connexons or heterotypic Cx40/Cx43 gap junction channels exist in the atria has remained unanswered. In heterologous expression systems, controversial results about the existence and function of mixed Cx40/Cx43 channel systems have been reported.[2,23,24]

A further, not yet fully resolved, question relates to the role of Cx45. Cx45 is expressed in the early stages of cardiac development in all cardiac regions.[25,26] In adult hearts it is detected in the sinoatrial and atrioventricular nodes and, in small amounts, in atrial and ventricular tissue from human, rat, and murine hearts.[19,21,27,28] Germline ablation of Cx43 in murine ventricular pairs with persistence of Cx45 expression produces a >90% reduction in electrical cell-to-cell coupling.[28] This finding indicates that Cx45 contributes very little to electrical coupling per se. However, a regulatory role has been attributed to Cx45 in cardiac failure, in which Cx45 is upregulated together with a decrease in Cx43 and a reduction in gap junction size.[29] This finding may indicate that Cx45 is involved in the regulation of gap junction size, as is also suggested from results following coexpression of Cx43 with Cx45 in a rat liver epithelial cell line.[30] Recently, it has been shown that genetic deletion of the coxsackie–adenovirus receptor (CAR) is associated with a marked reduction or deletion of Cx45. Conditional ablation of CAR increased cell-to-cell dye diffusion between ventricular cells, further suggesting that Cx45 may be a significant modulator of ventricular cell-to-cell communication.[31]

How Safe Is Propagation in Tissue With Reduced Cell-to-Cell Coupling?

The role of gap junction channels as one of the key elements in cardiac propagation is well acknowledged. Early experimental and theoretical studies looked at the effect of a decrease in gap junction conductance on propagation velocity in a general way by implicating or inducing a uniform change of intercellular electrical conductance in the tissue.[32] The effect of a uniform decrease in intercellular electrical conductance in best understood by considering the concept of conduction safety (SF). Several formalisms describing SF have been published (for references see Boyle and Vigmond[33]). The formalism describing SF in linear uniform tissue states that: $SF = (\int_A I_c \cdot dt + \int_A I_{out} \cdot dt)/(\int_A I_m \cdot dt); A \mid Q_m > 0$.[34] In simple terms, the numerator of this equation equals the electrical charge produced by a given cell in the propagating wavefront and consists of the sum of electrical charges needed to produce the action potential (capacitive component, $\int_A I_c \cdot dt$) and the charge flowing to excite the cells downstream (axial component, $\int_A I_{out} \cdot dt$). The denominator corresponds to the electrical charge ($\int_A I_m \cdot dt$) exciting this same cell, which is produced by the excited cells upstream of the propagating front. From this formalism it follows that propagation becomes decremental and eventually blocked, when SF decreases to <1, or, in other words, when more electrical charge is needed to excite a given cell than this same cell can produce by its machinery of excitation.[34] The theoretical dependence of propagation velocity on cell-to-cell coupling and the associated change in SF is illustrated in Fig. 27.1A. Several distinct features specifically related to cellular coupling can be derived from this figure. First, changes in cell-to-cell coupling that remain close to the normal level of coupling produce relatively small changes in propagation velocity. Second, cell-to-cell uncoupling can produce extremely slow propagation (on the order of 1 cm/s) if the conductance between cells is reduced by >100-fold. This behavior also predicts preservation of propagation, albeit very slow, even at extreme levels of uncoupling. This prediction made from theoretical studies has been verified in experimental work either using engineered strands of neonatal rat ventricular myocytes exposed to an uncoupling agent or using cells with germline ablation of Cx43, as depicted in Fig. 27.1B.[28,35] At such reduced levels, propagation becomes highly discontinuous, with fast excitation of the cytoplasm and long delays at the cell border. The explanation for this behavior, which

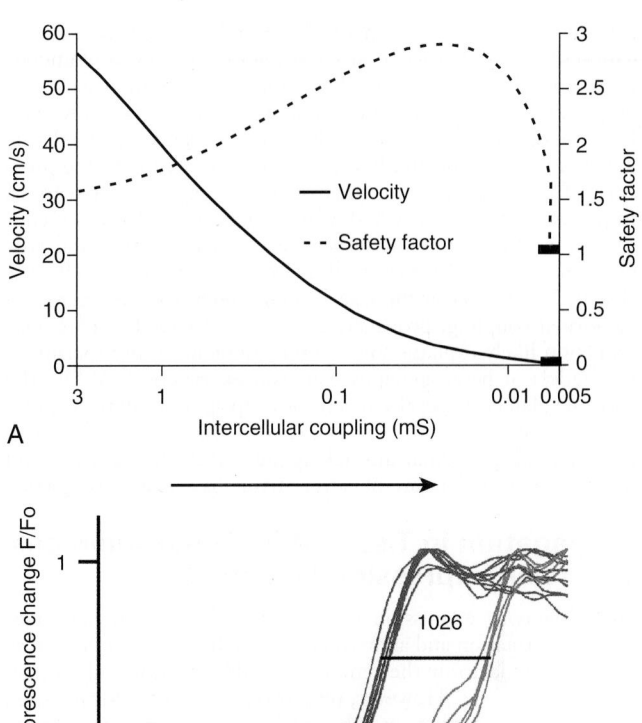

FIGURE 27.1 Dependence of safety and velocity of propagation on intercellular coupling. (A) Theoretical dependence of propagation velocity (*filled line*) and safety factor (*dotted line*) on intercellular coupling. Note log scale on the abscissa. (B) Optical measurement of action potential upstrokes in a patterned strand of neonatal rat ventricular myocytes. Signals in *red* are measured in an upstream cell and signals in *blue* in the adjacent cell downstream at a resolution of 6 μm. For each color, crowding of signal depicts the almost simultaneous excitation of a single cell. The long delay of excitation of >1 ms is confined to the cell boundary. This excitation corresponded to a propagation velocity of 2.1 cm/s and 95% uncoupling due to residual connexin45 (Cx45) in absence of genetically ablated connexin43 (Cx43). This "saltatory" type of cellular excitation is typical for uncoupled tissue and is in accordance with theoretical studies. ([A] From Shaw RM, Rudy Y. Ionic mechanisms of propagation in cardiac tissue. Roles of the sodium and l-type calcium currents during reduced excitability and decreased gap junction coupling. *Circ Res.* 1997;81:727-741. [B] From Beauchamp P, Choby C, Desplantez T, et al. Electrical propagation in synthetic ventricular myocyte strands from germline connexin43 knockout mice. *Circ Res.* 2004;95:170-178.)

is typical for cell-to-cell uncoupling and contrasts to the behavior during block of depolarizing ion currents (I_{Na} and $I_{L,Ca}$),[34,35] is given by the biphasic behavior of the margin of safety of propagation. Two processes with opposing effects determine the biphasic time course of SF. First, the axial currents flowing into a given cell from excited tissue upstream decrease due to an increase in the resistance between the cells. This "source effect" causes the membrane capacitance of a given cell to charge more slowly and to reach the excitation threshold later than normal, and therefore causes propagation to slow. At the same time, the excitatory electrical charge flowing downstream, due to the increased intercellular resistance between the downstream cells, is distributed over fewer cells and is therefore conserved at the site of excitation within the wavefront (a decrease of the so-called sink effect). In other words, cell-to-cell uncoupling protects the excitatory current from downstream dissipation and therefore makes propagation safer (an increase of SF). Only at extreme levels of uncoupling do failure and, eventually, propagation block occur. The biophysical principle of source–sink interaction is not only valid for states of cell-to-cell uncoupling; it represents a general rule independent of scale and holds also for propagation in the presence of discontinuities in tissue structure (e.g., infarct scars[32]). Importantly, however, very slow propagation is only preserved if sites of increased coupling resistance are closely spaced and produce an effective decrease in the electrical sink. If this effect is absent, for instance at the transition between tissue of decreased to normal coupling, propagation block is observed.[36] This phenomenon likely explains some observations made in experimental models of heterogeneous connexin expression.[37] While the above-explained general concept of propagation safety is useful for linear structures with homogeneous changes of cell-to-cell coupling, other formalisms taking into account the two- and three-dimensional nature of cardiac tissue have been described.[33]

Propagation in Tissue With Heterogeneous Connexin Expression Is Robust

Heterogeneous expression of connexins, leading to heterogeneous propagation and arrhythmogenesis, has been implicated as an important factor in the genesis of atrial fibrillation and ventricular arrhythmias.[38] However, only two studies have documented a direct association between the incidence of ventricular arrhythmias in heart failure patients and heterogeneous connexin expression.[39,40] Cx43 immunofluorescence measured in specimens from such patients with ventricular arrhythmias showed a heterogeneous pattern with scattered absence of Cx43 signals. Similarly, in a mouse model of conditional cardiac Cx43 ablation, the occurrence of ventricular arrhythmias and sudden cardiac death is associated with a marked heterogeneity in connexin expression and a decrease in macroscopic propagation velocity to levels ≤50% of normal (Fig. 27.2).[41] Recent work using cell engineering techniques made an attempt to quantitatively study electrical cell-to-cell coupling in tissue consisting of a defined mixture of wild-type (WT) cells and cells with genetic Cx43 (Cx43$^{-/-}$) ablation. With respect to the normal interface between WT cells, the electrical conductance between WT/Cx43$^{-/-}$ cell pairs and Cx43$^{-/-}$/Cx43$^{-/-}$ cell pairs was markedly reduced (Fig. 27.3C), and the whole-cell dual voltage-clamp experiments showed the presence of mixed Cx43/Cx45 channels in the WT/Cx43$^{-/-}$ cell pairs and homomeric/homotypic gap junction channels in the Cx43$^{-/-}$/Cx43$^{-/-}$ cell pairs.[42,43] While immunofluorescence showed the expected coexistence of Cx43 and Cx45 at the cell interface in the WT/WT pairs, no Cx43 or Cx45 signals were observed in mixed WT/CX43$^{-/-}$ pairs or in Cx43$^{-/-}$/Cx43$^{-/-}$ cell pairs (see Fig. 27.3A). These experiments demonstrated that absence of connexin immunofluorescence does not equal the absence of gap junction channels and that electrical intercellular conductance is a more sensitive indicator of residual, reduced electrical coupling than is immunofluorescence. A very similar conclusion was drawn from experiments comparing quantitative immunofluorescence with intercellular conductance in engineered cell pairs.[44]

The experimental model of engineered cell strands consisting of controlled mixtures of wild-type–green fluorescent protein (WT-GFP) and Cx43$^{-/-}$ cells was also used to measure the effect of Cx43 inhomogeneity on propagation velocity, as illustrated in Fig. 27.3B.[45] The change in macroscopic propagation velocity along engineered strands revealed a relatively preserved velocity in mixtures containing ≥50% WT-GFP cells and a marked decrease in cell mixtures with ≤50% WT-GFP cells (see Fig. 27.3D). The explanation for this preserved propagation at a relatively fast level, even in the presence of 50% of cells devoid of Cx43 expression, is illustrated in Fig. 27.4, which illustrates the pattern of cell-to-cell propagation recorded at high spatial and temporal resolution. Both the sequence of activation times and the shapes of the action potential upstrokes reveal a "mixed" type of propagation, with fast continuous conduction[32] meandering through the clusters with normal Cx43 expression and delayed activation of Cx43$^{-/-}$ cells showing a prolonged foot potential before the rapid action potential upstroke, characteristic of discontinuous conduction.[32] Very similar results were recently presented in a study comparing heterogeneous propagation in patterned strands of neonatal myocytes with theoretical simulations.[46] Although local propagation delays at cell borders can be as long as several milliseconds, they are too short to produce microentry in markedly uncoupled tissue.[28,35,45] Restriction of Cx43 ablation to small cell clusters and eventual excitation of all cells probably explain why optical recordings of macroscopic velocities in the mouse model with conditional Cx43 ablation show relatively smooth isochronal activation.[47] Furthermore, the observation that Cx43 immunosignals are absent from the interface between Cx43-expressing and Cx43-nonexpressing cells suggests that the degree of Cx43 ablation (proportion of Cx43$^{-/-}$ cells) is overestimated if calculated from the percent-loss of Cx43 immunosignal. Overall, these results demonstrate that propagation in tissue with heterogeneous connexin expression is very robust, with a small probability of local conduction block formation.

In contrast to mouse models of microscopic connexin inhomogeneity (conditional Cx43 ablation or mixed Cx43$^{+/+}$/Cx43$^{-/-}$ engineered strands[45,47]), macroscopic connexin inhomogeneity was produced by injecting Cx43$^{-/-}$ embryonic stem cells into Cx43$^{+/+}$ host blastocysts.[37] The hearts of the surviving chimeric mice, characterized by a "patchy" or mosaic-like regional ablation of Cx43 with macroscopic interfaces, were highly arrhythmogenic and showed an irregular epicardial activation pattern with decreased contractility.[37] Comparison of this model with the other mouse models suggests that both the average degree of Cx43 ablation and the scale of heterogeneity determine the effects on electrical and contractile behavior. A biophysical explanation for irregular electrical activation with macroscopic, mosaic-like Cx43 ablation was given by theoretical work, which simulated propagation at an interface between two large strand segments with different degrees of cell-to-cell coupling.[36] In such a case, propagation from a segment of low intercellular coupling to a segment of normal intracellular coupling encounters a large downstream sink at the transition. As a consequence, there is a large local decrease of safety factor and a conduction delay, which is nearly one order of magnitude larger than the delay observed with uniform cell-to-cell uncoupling. This increased delay, which most likely accounts for the highly irregular propagation patterns and the increased arrhythmogenicity in mice with mosaic–chimeric Cx43 ablation, is due to the absence of the protective effect of low-resistance coupling downstream, as explained above.

Cell-to-Cell Coupling, Tissue Architecture, and Ion Currents Form an Interacting System

The morphology of atrial and ventricular tissues is highly discontinuous at several levels. Ventricular tissue is organized in layers, which rotate with respect to their longitudinal axis of anisotropy.[48–50] Atrial and subendocardial ventricular tissue are trabeculated,[51] and age or disease may cause additional microfibrosis.[50,52–54] As recognized early on by the seminal work of M.S. Spach (see Spach and Kootsey[55] and Kleber and Rudy[32] for review), a common consequence of these structural discontinuities for impulse propagation exists, namely that propagating waves encounter sites of structural and electrical mismatch. In the context of this chapter, it is important to mention that local changes in cell-to-cell coupling can have a marked influence on propagation at such sites (Fig. 27.5). Fig. 27.5A*i* illustrates a simple engineered tissue structure, "archetypical" for source–sink

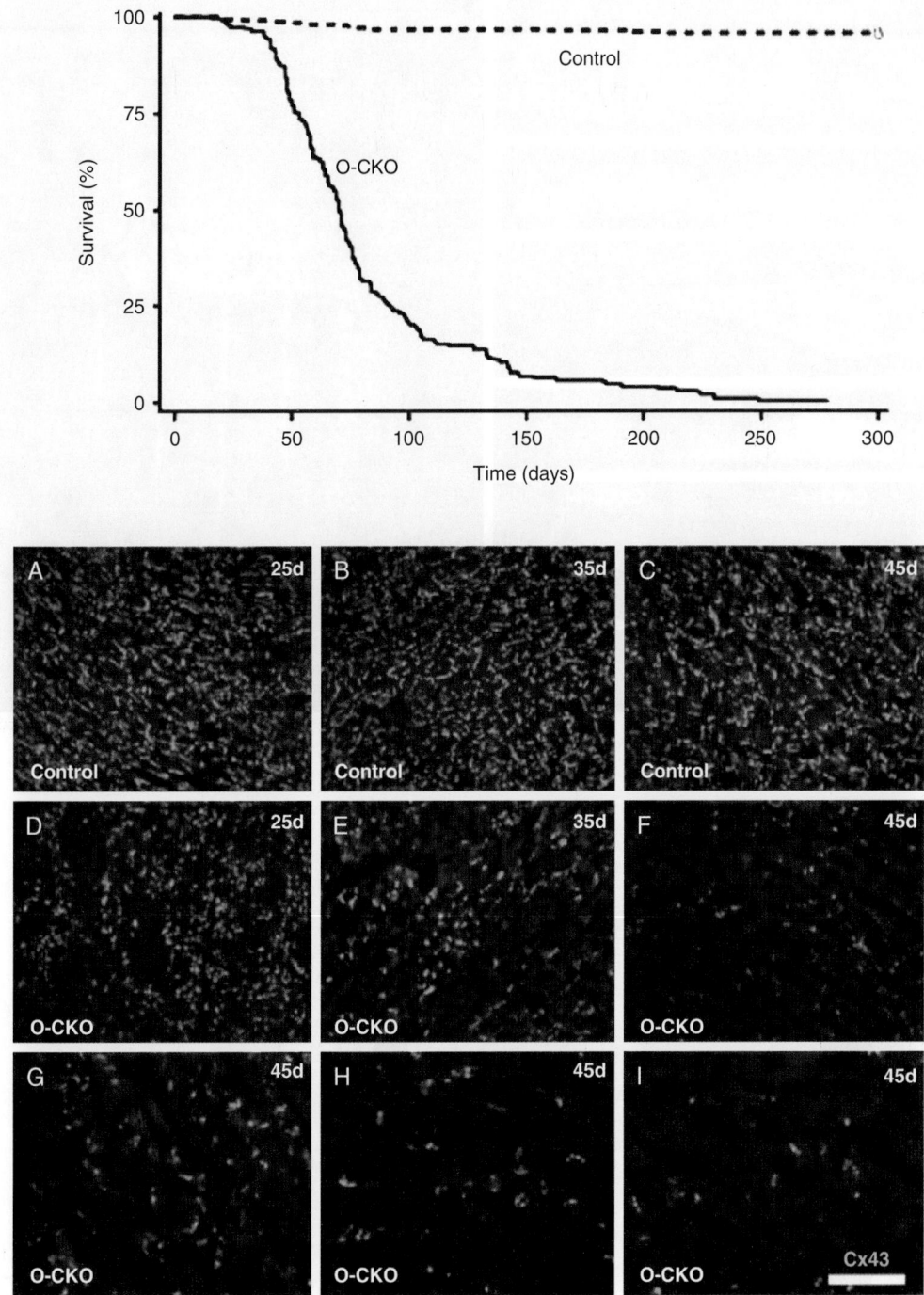

FIGURE 27.2 Mouse model of heterogeneous connexin43 (Cx43) expression with delayed conditional Cx43 knockout (*O-CKO*). *Top,* Kaplan–Meier survival curve showing onset of sudden death at approximately 30 to 40 days. *Bottom:* Cx43 immunofluorescence signals in ventricle between 25 and 45 days after birth in control (A–C) and O-CKO mice (D–F). G–H depict inhomogeneity of Cx43 expression by comparison of three different regions of interest. (From Danik SB, Liu F, Zhang J, et al. Modulation of cardiac gap junction expression and arrhythmic susceptibility. *Circ Res.* 2004;95:1035-1041.)

mismatch, consisting of a cardiac strand (50 μm in width) connected to a large area (bulk).[56] In such structures, propagation from the strand to the large area is determined by a small source (strand) emerging into a large sink (bulk). As a consequence, unidirectional block occurs at the transition in case the source is too small (narrow strand diameter, h) to excite the large sink (see Fig. 27.5A*ii*). In contrast, propagation from the bulk to the strand is safe because, in the reverse direction, a large source (bulk) will excite the small sink. In the situation of source–sink mismatch, the degree of cell-to-cell coupling acts as a modulator of propagation, and a decrease in cell-to-cell coupling can restore unidirectional block to bidirectional propagation as demonstrated in Fig. 27.5A*iii*. The exact mechanism is illustrated in Fig. 27.5B, in which the strand segment and the bulk are represented by a network of excitable cells interconnected by longitudinal (*black*) and transverse (*red*) resistors, mimicking cell-to-cell coupling.[57]

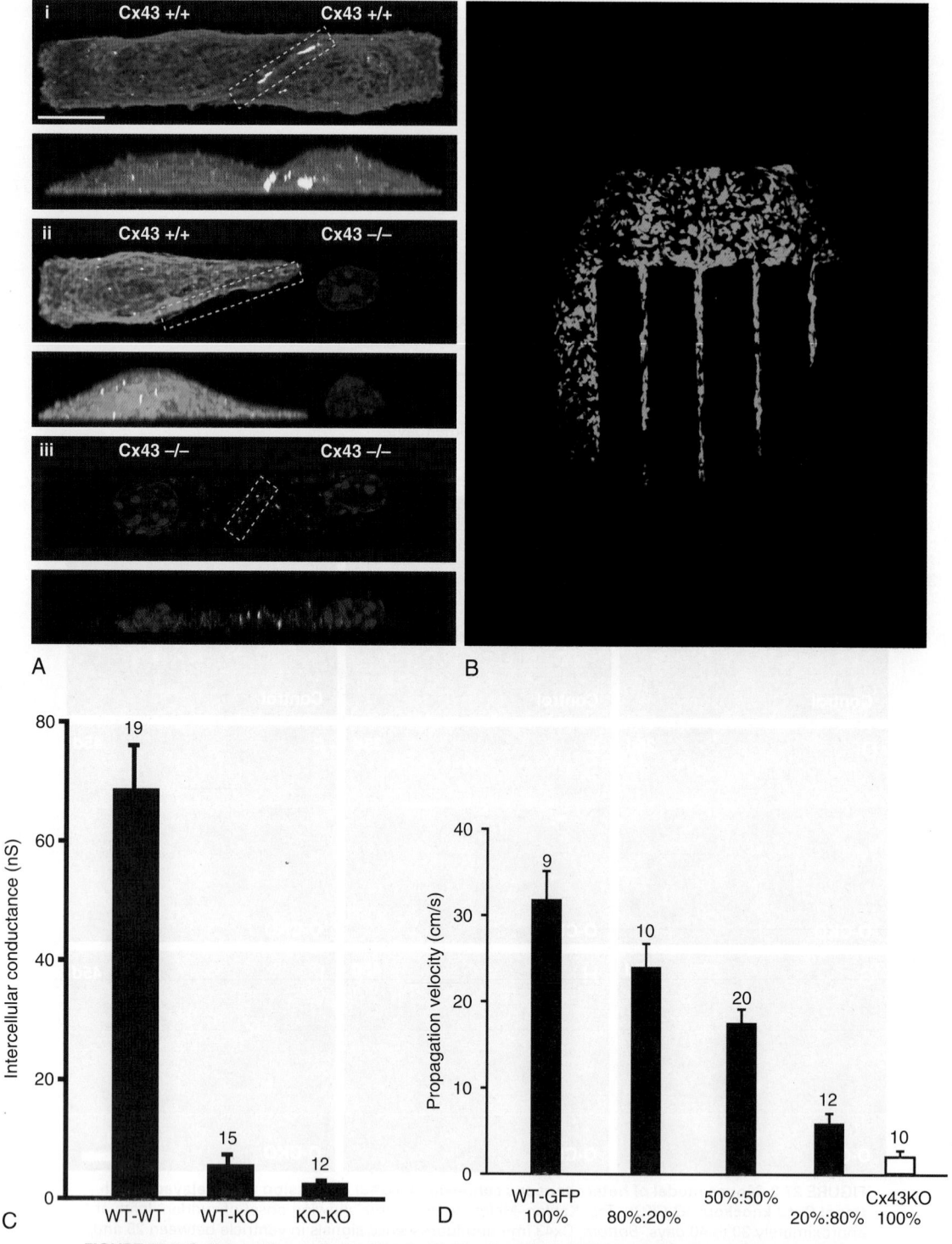

FIGURE 27.3 Cell-to-cell coupling and propagation in tissue with heterogeneous expression of connexin43 (Cx43). Wild-type cells (*WT*) are expressing green fluorescent protein (*GFP*). (A) *i:* Top and side view of WT/WT cell pair. *ii:* Top and side view of WT/knockout (*KO*) cell pair. *iii:* Top and side view of KO/KO cell pair. Cx43 immunofluorescence: *orange*; Cx45 immunofluorescence: *white*. Note superimposition of Cx43 and Cx45 immunofluorescence at the intercalated disk in the WT/WT cell pairs. Immunofluorescence signals are absent at the interface between a WT and a Cx43$^{-/-}$ myocyte, and small Cx45-positive signals can be observed between Cx43$^{-/-}$ cells. (B) Engineered strands (100 μm in width) composed of WT (*green*, 50%) and Cx43$^{-/-}$ cells (50%) used for measurement of propagation velocity. (C) Intercellular conductance between the pairs illustrated in A. Note that a small finite electrical conductance is present in WT/KO and KO/KO cells, despite the absence of Cx43 and Cx45 immunofluorescence signals. (D) Dependence of macroscopic velocity on the proportions of WT-GPF and KO cells in the engineered strands. The percentage ratios correspond to WT-GFP:Cx43 KO cells. Note the rapid decrease of velocity when the relative amount of WT-GFP cells is <50%. (Modified from Beauchamp P, Desplantes T, McCain ML, et al. Electrical coupling and propagation in engineered ventricular myocardium with heterogeneous expression of connexin43. *Circ Res.* 2012;110:1445-1453.)

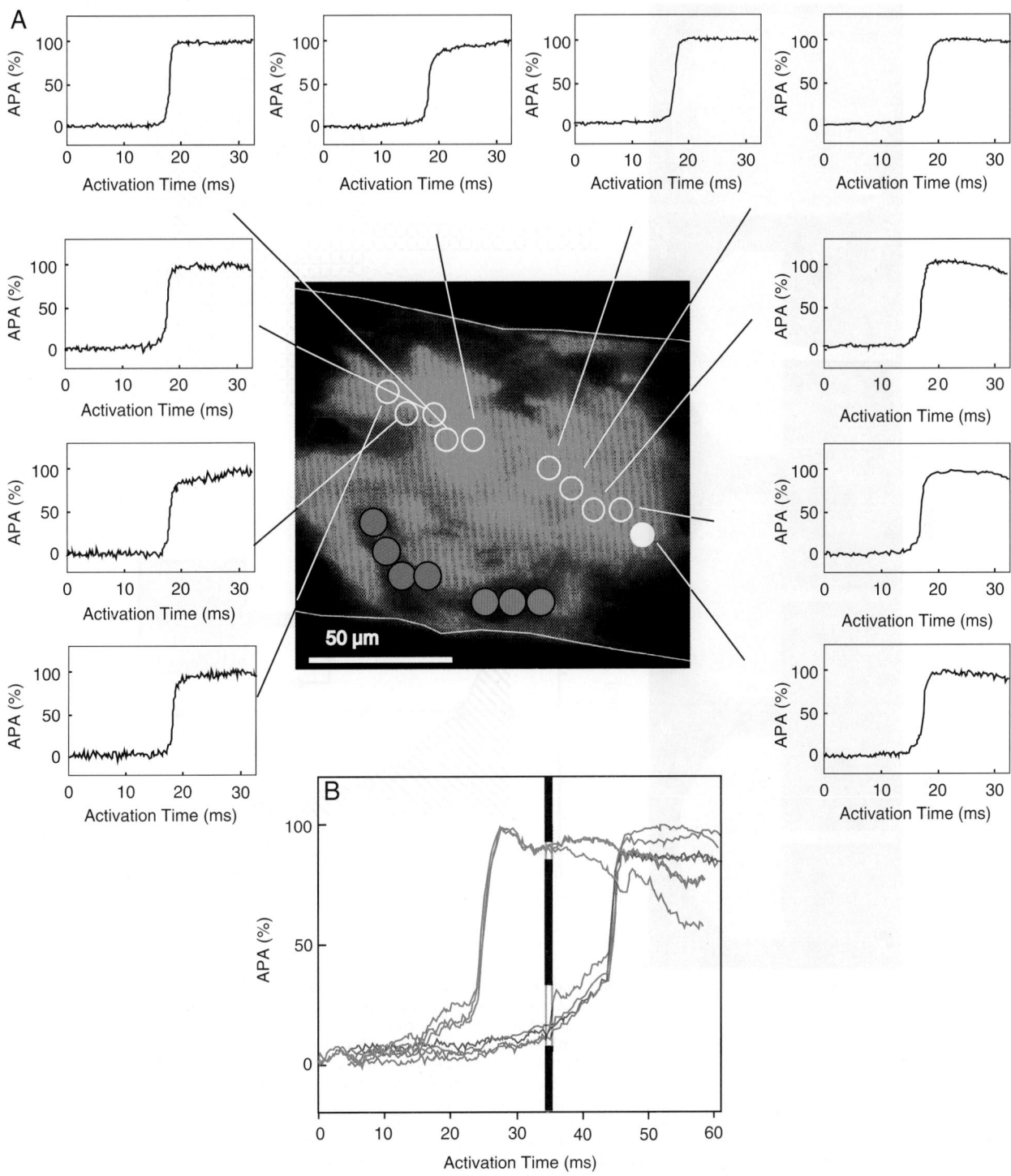

FIGURE 27.4 Multisite high-resolution optical measurement of propagation in engineered strands with mixed connexin43 (Cx43) expression. The center shows a strand segment 100 μm in width, with wild-type–green fluorescent protein (WT-GFP) cells emitting green fluorescence. (A) shows action potentials with smooth and steep upstrokes illustrating rapid sequential activation (velocity 32 cm/s) of the WT-GFP cells, starting from the *filled white circle* meandering along a path indicated by the *white circles*. (B) shows activation of two cell areas with genetic Cx43 ablation with a region (*blue*) preceding the activation of the WT-GFP cells and a region (*red*) with markedly delayed activation. The width of the bar in the middle of B corresponds to the activation window of the WT-GFP cell cluster shown in A. It illustrates the extreme degree of discontinuity. Note that the existence of a "foot" of the action potentials in the knockout (KO) cell is typical for discontinuous activation. While activation was microscopically highly irregular, no local propagation blocks were observed and all cells became electrically excited. (From Beauchamp P, Desplantez T, McCain ML, et al. Electrical coupling and propagation in engineered ventricular myocardium with heterogeneous expression of connexin43. *Circ Res.* 2012;110:1445-1453.)

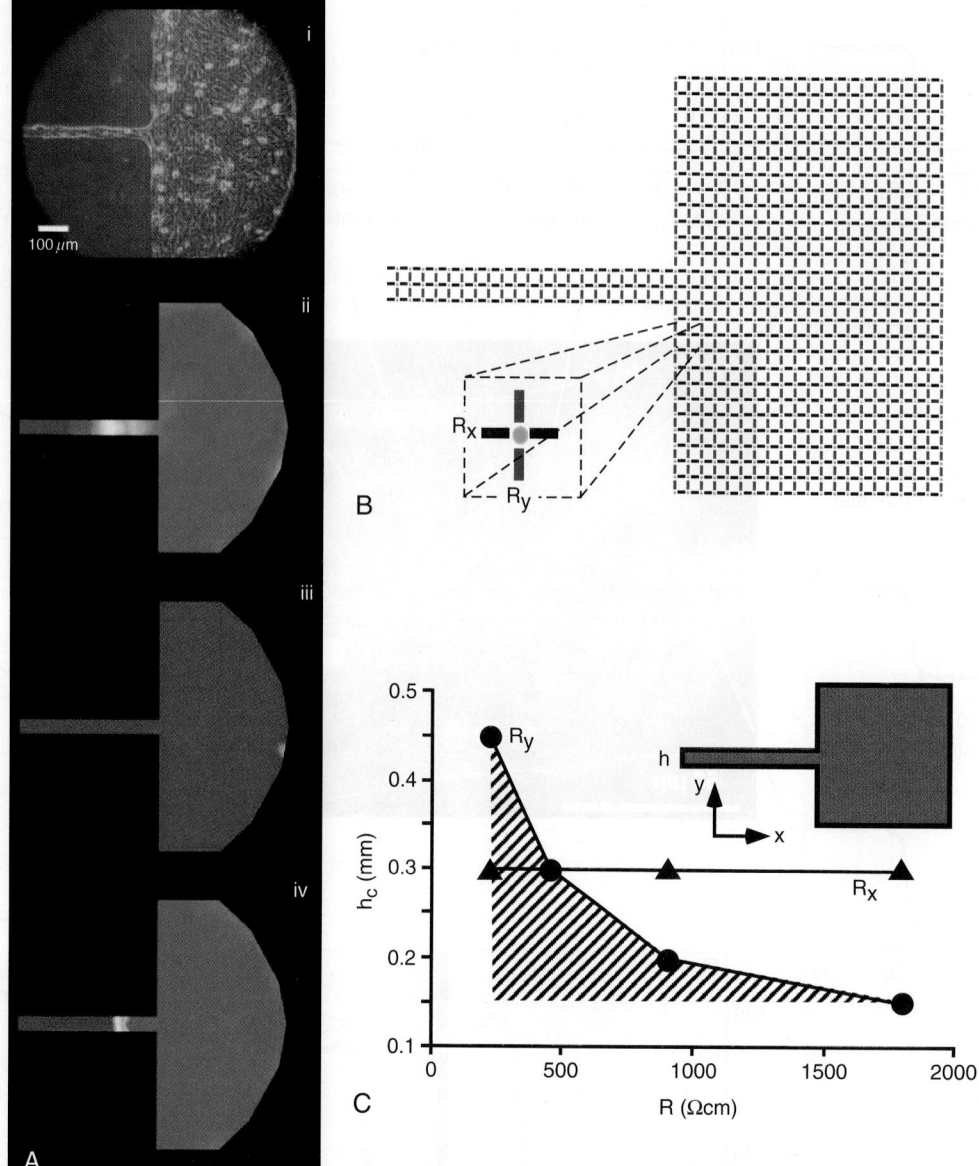

FIGURE 27.5 Interaction between cell-to-cell coupling and discontinuous propagation.
(A) Experimental demonstration of the effect of cell-to-cell uncoupling on source-sink mismatch
at a site of a tissue discontinuity. (A) *i*: Picture of an engineered culture of neonatal rat ventricular
myocytes with a narrow strand (width 50 μm) emerging into a bulk. *ii*: Propagation from the strand
into the bulk produces propagation block at the transition. Cells at action potential level are depicted
in *red* and tissue at resting potential level in *blue*. *iii*: Partial uncoupling with palmitoleic acid restores
propagation. *iv*: Total uncoupling produces propagation block. This phenomenon is occurring in reverse sequence upon washout of the uncoupling agent (not shown). (B) Sketch of simplified electrical
equivalent circuit showing excitable elements (cells) in *green*, intercellular resistors representing
gap junctions in the x-direction in *black*, and intercellular resistors representing gap junctions in the
y-direction in *red* (for explanation see text). (C) Numerical presentation of the dependence of the
critical strand width, h_c, producing propagation block on cell-to-cell coupling (expressed as intercellular resistance). *Hatched area* corresponds to propagation block. Note (i) very strong dependence of
block on cell-to-cell coupling, especially close to normal levels of coupling and (ii) block dependence
on changes in y-resistor, R_y, but not x-resistors, R_x. ([A] Modified from Rohr S, Kucera JP, Fast VG,
et al. Paradoxical improvement of impulse conduction in cardiac tissue by partial cellular uncoupling.
Science. 1997;275:841-844. [C] Modified from Fast VG, Kléber AG: Block of impulse propagation at an
abrupt tissue expansion: evaluation of the critical strand diameter in 2- and 3-dimensional computer
models. *Cardiovasc Res.* 1995;30:449-459.)

Reduction of cell-to-cell coupling reduces the loss of local electrical current into the sink at the transition site and restores propagation. This explanation becomes evident from the fact that only the increase of lateral elements of cell-to-cell coupling contributes to the decrease of the sink effect and restoration of propagation.[57] In the extreme hypothetical case, when the longitudinal resistors are left unchanged and the transverse resistors are made infinite, propagation into the lateral sink is no longer possible and propagation gets linear (i.e., the source–sink mismatch is eliminated). The numerical dependence of source–sink-related propagation block in cell-to-cell coupling is illustrated in Fig. 27.5C. The above examples make it clear that no essential difference exists between the biophysical mechanisms of source-to-sink mismatch at a transition of linear strand segments with different degrees of cell-to-cell coupling and those of a transition from a small to a large tissue structure.[36] Repetitive alternations of sink and sources due to tissue structure, such as branching tissue fibers (scars), can cause a decrease of the downstream sink, a high margin of safety for propagation, and very slow propagation in the order of 1 cm/s.[58] The propagation behavior at macroscopic alternations is very similar to the situation of uniform cell-to-cell uncoupling illustrated in Fig. 27.1 and underlines the above statement of "scale independence," stating that the biophysical rules of source-to-sink mismatch apply to both the cellular and the network scale.[32]

In normal linear propagation, Na^+ inward current, which produces the upstroke of the cardiac action potential, drives propagation by contributing a major portion to the charge flowing downstream. The L-type Ca^{2+} current, which is activated later and more slowly, does not contribute significantly to propagation (<1%–2%) in the normal condition.[34] Since a decrease of cell-to-cell coupling resistance is associated with a delay at the cell border, the action potential of the driven cells is created with delay with respect to the driver cell. This delay can become so long that the upstroke of the driven cell falls into the late upstroke or early plateau phase of the driver cell. As a consequence, the L-type Ca^{2+} current becomes a main charge carrier for propagation in uncoupled tissue.[36]

The above discussion illustrates that the three main functional elements determining cardiac propagation—the action potential, the degree of cell-to-cell coupling, and the cellular network structure—show a high degree of interdependence at sites of source-to-sink mismatch. Therefore effects of changes in these determinants (i.e., in disease) should be considered within the context of a whole complex system. Interestingly, interacting ion currents, cell-to-cell coupling, and structural determinants of heart tissue not only affect cardiac propagation via biophysical interaction, they also form a highly interactive system at the level of molecular expression in the cell, as discussed in the last paragraph in this chapter.

Ephaptic Impulse Transmission: Revival of an Old Concept to Explain Cardiac Cell-to-Cell Impulse Transfer

The observation that cardiac tissue consists of individual cells, but functions as an electrical syncytium, raised the question of how the electrical impulse would be transferred between cells. Already in the 1960s two opposite hypotheses prevailed and became a matter of friendly controversy among investigators.[59] The first hypothesis postulated low-resistance pathways between cardiac cells, based on measurements of passive electrical properties, the diffusion constant for K^+, and the observation that a full electrical resistive local circuit was necessary for propagation to occur (implicating resistive connections between cardiac cells).[60] The second hypothesis stated that electrical impulse transfer would be possible without direct electrical connections between cardiac cells.[61] These two hypotheses, which at low levels of

cell-to-cell coupling may represent complementary rather than opposite mechanisms, attracted attention initiated by the observation that propagation in cardiac ventricular tissue with conditional Cx43 ablation was maintained at approximately 50% of the normal level, despite an approximately 90% reduction of Cx43 immunofluorescence signal.[47,62] The opportunities to perform detailed theoretical modeling of the cardiac cell junction offered the possibility to selectively assess the roles of these two postulated hypotheses using settings of critical biophysical parameters within a wide range.[63,64] Impulse transmission involving ephaptic transmission at a cardiac cell border is schematically illustrated in Fig. 27.6A. In contrast to models that represent the cell junction by a simple resistor, the cleft model of a cardiac cell junction contains an excitable element, which faces the cell junction toward a high intercellular cleft resistance (R_{cleft}), and a radial resistance (R_{radial}) that connects the cleft to the "normal" extracellular space. In the model, the high cleft resistance is varied by changing the cleft width. Inward Na^+ current flowing during depolarization through the Na^+ channels in the cleft is forced to flow through the narrow intercellular cleft toward the extracellular space. Field effect or ephaptic transmission between cells implicates that the flow of inward Na^+ current during depolarization creates an electrical field across the cleft or an intracleft potential with respect to the extracellular space. This transient intracleft potential is negative with respect to the extracellular reference and thus acts to depolarize the membrane potential of the downstream cell. In turn, depolarization may lead to local activation of juxtaposed Na^+ channels located in the cleft membrane and excitation of the downstream cell. As a mechanism opposing field effect transmission, depletion of Na^+ ions in the intercalated disk or "cleft" is predicted to reduce the transmembrane Na^+ gradient and the Na^+ inward current in the Na^+ channels in the intercalated disk.[63] Depletion is inversely related to the cleft width and is caused by the high diffusion barrier between the cleft and the normal extracellular space, which prevents equilibrium of extracellular Na^+ during inward Na^+ current flow.

In essence, two variables affecting ephaptic impulse transmission are of interest: the cleft width and the fraction of total Na^+ channels expressed in the intercalated disk. Two detailed models have been used thus far (a 1D- vs a 3D-model),[63,64] both of which agree with respect to the main results. Fig. 27.7B illustrates the complex dependence of propagation velocity on cleft width at different degrees of resistive cell-to-cell coupling via gap junctions and with the assumption that *all Na^+ channels* are clustered at the cell junction. At *normal to moderate reduction of cell-to-cell coupling* by gap junctions, decreasing the cleft width *decreases* propagation velocity significantly. This effect is due to the fact that Na^+ depletion in the cleft will decrease the driving force for Na^+ ions.[64] At very high degrees of cell-to-cell uncoupling, decreasing cleft width below a certain threshold (<40 nm) maintains propagation velocity, and propagation is inversely related to the cleft width. This effect is due to the negative electrical field built up in the cleft ("field effect"), which depolarizes the membrane of the juxtaposed cell to threshold for activation of Na^+ channels. At larger cleft width, propagation is determined by residual coupling through gap junction channels. As shown in Fig. 27.7C, cell-to-cell transfer of the electrical impulse without any resistive coupling is theoretically only possible if close to 100% of Na^+ channels are clustered in the cleft. With 50% of Na^+ channels located in the intercalated disk, ephaptic impulse transmission can contribute to very slow conduction in states of marked gap junction uncoupling. However, ephaptic transmission cannot maintain propagation in the absence of conducting gap junction channels. As shown in Fig. 27.7C, the question of Na^+ channel expression in different compartments of the cell membrane becomes important. All recent experimental studies carried out in adult or neonatal cardiac tissue point to a distinct pool of Na^+ on the surface membrane (registered with Z-lines)

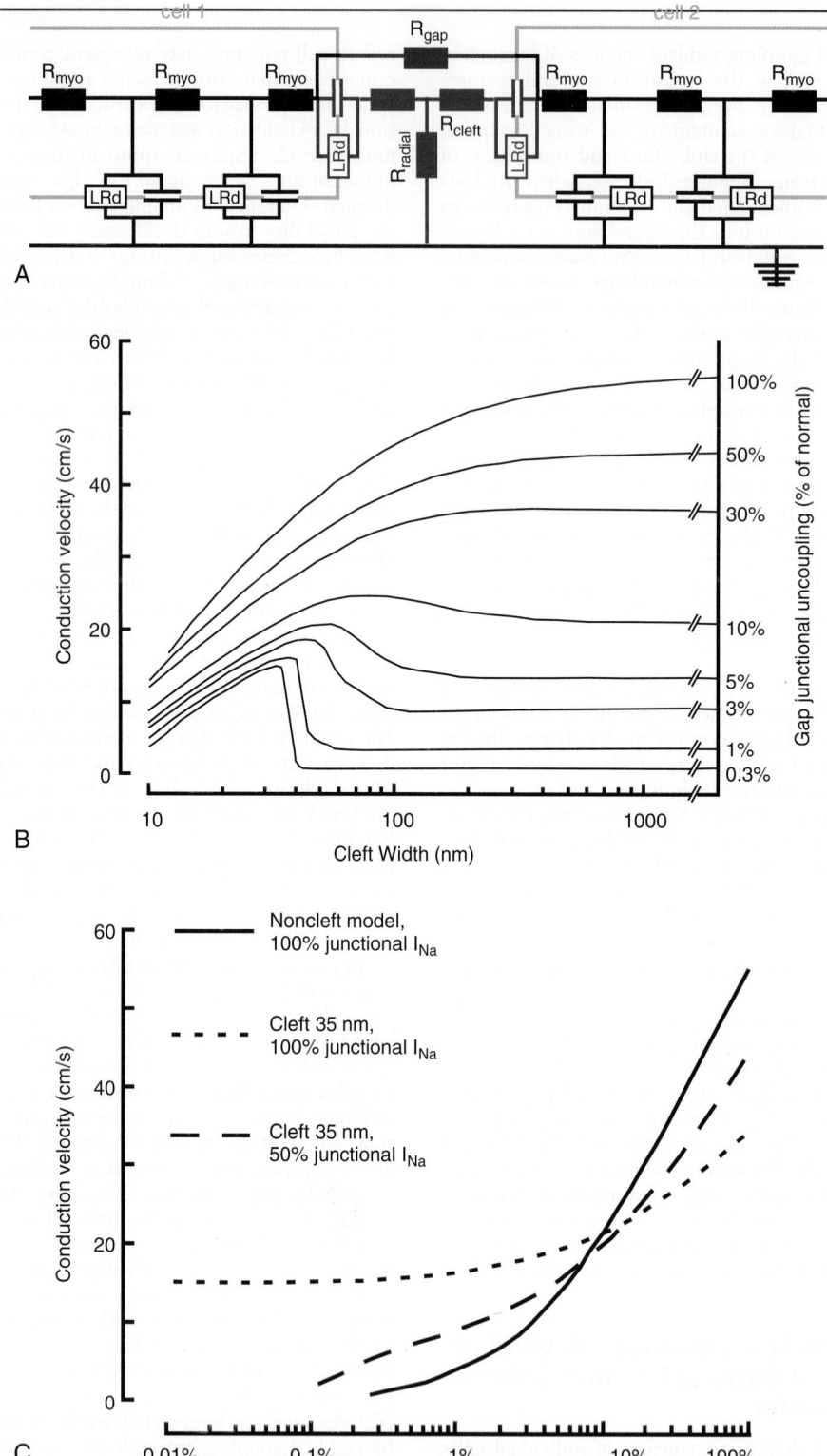

FIGURE 27.6 Modeling ephaptic impulse transmission. (A) Schematic presentation of the electrical circuitry between two cells (*green*) used in the model. The classical electrical circuitry usually used to represent a cell is drawn in *black* and consists of myoplasmic (*myo*) resistors and excitable elements (*LRd*) in parallel with a membrane capacitor. The cells are linked by a resistor (*blue*), representing electrical coupling by gap junctions. For simulation of ephaptic transmission, excitable elements are added to each cell (*red*), which face the intercellular cleft and are connected to the extracellular space by a cleft and a radial resistor (*red*). (B) Dependence of propagation velocity on cleft width at different degrees of gap junction coupling. In the presence of normal gap junction coupling, the field effect caused by current flow through the Na+ channels facing the cleft produces *propagation slowing*. At a very large degree of cell-to-cell uncoupling (0.3%–5%), propagation is markedly slowed or blocked at a cleft width >40–50 μm. At a smaller width, propagation resumes due to ephaptic transmission but is again inversely dependent on cleft width. This dependence occurs if 100% of the Na+ channels reside in the intercellular cleft. (C) Dependence of propagation velocity on gap junctional coupling in three models. *Filled line,* Classical noncleft model. *Dashed line,* Cleft model with 100% of Na+ channels residing in the intercalated disk. *Dotted line,* Cleft model with 50% of Na+ channels residing in the intercalated disk. (Modified from Kucera JP, Rohr S, Rudy Y. Localization of sodium channels in intercalated disks modulates cardiac conduction. *Circ Res.* 2002;91:1176-1182.)

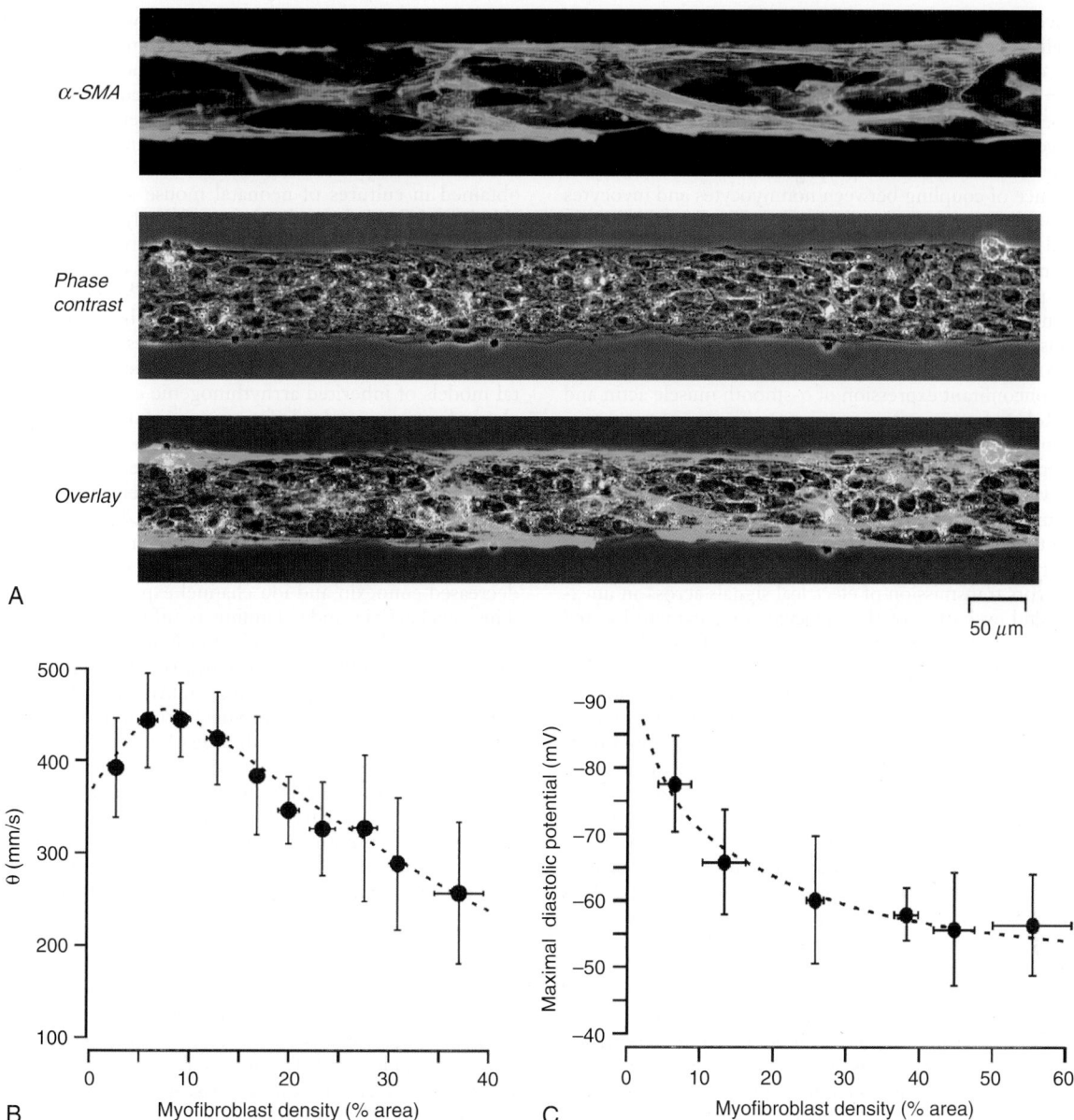

FIGURE 27.7 Effect of myofibroblast–myocyte coupling on propagation. (A) Myofibroblasts cultured on top of cardiomyocytes identified by immunosignals (*green*) for α-smooth muscle actin. (B) Conduction velocities along cell strands showing a biphasic dependence on myofibroblast density, the first phase being due to supernormal conduction.[72–74] (C) Increasing myofibroblast densities cause a reduction in maximal diastolic membrane potential of electrically coupled cardiomyocytes. (Modified from Miragoli M, Gaudesius G, Rohr S. Electrotonic modulation of cardiac impulse conduction by myofibroblasts. *Circ Res.* 2006;98:801-810.)

and make a unique clustering of Na^+ channels at the intercalated disk unlikely.[65–69] At present, the importance and contribution of ephaptic transmission to cardiac propagation is difficult to define because of lack of conclusive experimental data. While impulse transmission is maintained at very low degrees of gap junction coupling,[28,45] total inhibition of resistive coupling by means of a gap junction channel blocker produces rapid propagation block in neonatal cultured tissue.[28] Recently, the groups of Poelzing and Gourdie have strongly advocated the existence of ephaptic impulse transmission as an important mechanism contributing to *normal* impulse propagation.[70,71] However, evidence from detailed theoretical modeling of the perinexus region of the intercalated disk at a nanometer scale, including the consequences of changes in ion concentrations and corresponding experimental data, is still lacking.

Coupling Between Cardiomyocytes and Nonmyocytes and Its Effect on Propagation

It has been known for several decades that in a small percentage of transplanted hearts, the rhythm of the implant can be partially controlled by the sinus node remaining in place after explanation of the diseased heart (so-called atrial:atrial conduction).[75,76,77] Such an observation indicates that electrical impulses can cross the fibrous scar between the cardiac tissue of the original heart and the newly implanted organ, or, alternatively, it indicates formation of an "electrical anastomosis" by regenerated myocardial tissue. The fact that these electrical anastomoses are interrupted by ablation indicates that they are restricted to small defined locations and do not represent distributed electrical connections between myocardial and scar tissue. Much effort has been made to define cell-to-cell coupling and propagation between nonmyocyte and myocyte tissue in in vitro models. At a biophysical level, three major questions appear to be relevant: (1) To what extent do nonmyocytes, such as fibrocytes and myofibroblasts, couple to working myocardium? (2) What is the effect of coupling between nonmyocytes and myocytes on propagation velocity? (3) What is the relevance of coupling between nonmyocytes and myocytes in vitro? Coupling between nonmyocytes and myocytes is highly variable and depends on connexin expression by nonmyocytes. In cultures of neonatal myocytes from small rodents, nonmyocytes are mostly present as myofibroblasts, which express α-smooth muscle actin, Cx43, Cx45, and possibly Cx40.[78–80] The degree of expression is variable and depends on paracrine signaling. Transforming growth factor-β (TGF-β) is a major signal upstream leading to concomitant expression of α-smooth muscle actin and Cx43 (see Rohr[80] for review).

The nonmyocytes can bridge excitable tissue for relatively extended lengths of the nonexcitable gap. In patterned cell cultures, gap widths up to 300 μm have been reported to pass the electrical impulse from one excitable compartment to the other.[81] In addition to cell–cell coupling by gap junctions, the high input resistance (reflecting a high membrane resistance) of the nonmyocytes favors transmission of electrical signals across an unexcitable gap and excitation of the myocyte compartment located beyond. The second question relates to the role of myofibroblasts in cell cultures. In cultures of cardiac myocytes, fibroblasts are often considered a contamination and are eliminated by one or more preplating steps of different duration and by addition of mitosis inhibitors. Absence of this inhibitor leads to rapid division of nonmyocytes, which consistently leads to formation of a partial or continuous cell layer of nonmyocytes overgrowing the myocytes. The unexcitable nonmyocytes may then act as an electrotonic sink and draw current from the process of propagation in the myocyte layer via cell–cell coupling. The resulting change in propagation velocity is highly significant (see Fig. 27.7).[82] This dependence of propagation velocity on coupling to myofibroblasts is likely to be an important factor explaining the large variation of propagation velocity reported in cell cultures.

While multiple paracrine interactions between myocytes and nonmyocytes (fibroblasts and vascular endothelial cells) have been described,[83] the importance of direct electrical interaction through cell-to-cell coupling by gap junctions in vivo is based on limited and partially indirect information.[80,84] Dye transfer between fibroblasts and myocytes, mainly mediated by Cx45, has been shown in explanted sinoatrial nodes.[79] Upregulated expression of Cx43 in fibroblasts, probably related to increased TGF-β signaling, has been reported from cells isolated from murine infarcts (when compared to noninfarcted regions from the same hearts).[85]

Remodeling Proteins of the Intercalated Disk: Interactions Between Mechanical Junctions and Gap Junctions

Recent work indicates that proteins of the intercalated disk that are involved in intercellular mechanical and electrical function share common regulatory mechanisms. These mechanisms appear to be complex and have as yet only partially been elucidated.[86,87] A first indication of a close interaction between functional protein complexes at the intercalated disk was offered from experiments defining neoformation of cell junctions in cultured adult rat cardiomyocytes.[88–90] During cell–cell adherence, formation of mechanical junctions precedes integration of connexins into the intercalated disk in a spatiotemporally defined manner, which suggests that mechanical junctions play an important role in the regulation and expression of gap junction channels and ion channels. Two types of observations provide further support for

the hypothesis of mutual interaction between the expression of proteins of the composite junctions (combined fascia adherens junctions and desmosomes[91]), connexins, and ion channels at the intercalated disk. First, tamoxifen-induced ablation of Cx43 in the ventricle was associated with an absence of $Na_V1.5$ immunosignal at the intercalated disk, and silencing of Cx43 led to a marked decrease of inward Na^+ current.[39] A similar finding was obtained in cultures of neonatal mouse atrial myocytes, where ablation of Cx43 showed an approximately 50% decrease of I_{Na}. Second, silencing of plakophilin-2 or expression of mutated plakophilin-2 is associated with a significant decrease in Na^+ channel expression at the intercalated disk,[92,93] suggesting (similar to connexin expression) a close relationship between the integrated function of composite junctions and expression of ion channels at the intercalated disk. Observations in patients and in experimental models of inherited arrhythmogenic cardiomyopathy (ACM) also indicate a pivotal role for proteins of desmosomal and adherence junctions in the integration of connexins and ion channels into the intercalated disk. Although the detailed mechanisms of decreased Cx43 expression at the intercalated disk in ACM have not yet been clarified, and a detailed discussion is beyond the scope of this chapter, evidence obtained thus far suggests a defect in the trafficking machinery as the mechanism underlying decreased connexin and ion channel expression in this disorder. This mechanistic understanding is inferred from the observation that the decrease of Cx43 and $Na_V1.5$ signals at the intercalated disk occurs in the presence of unchanged total cellular Cx43 and $Na_V1.5$ levels.[94,95] Importantly, trafficking of connexin hemichannels along microtubules[96] to the periphery of the gap junction plaques[7] requires tethering of microtubules to β-catenin, a protein of the fascia adherens scaffold, via the microtubule plus-end-tracking protein EB1 and the intermediate "glue" protein p150.[10] Moreover, EB1 also binds to the desmosomal protein desmoplakin,[9] pointing to additional protein–protein interactions between the EB1-tipped microtubules (transporting ion channel cargo) and proteins of the mechanical junctions. Importantly, ion channels and connexins are further modulated by a multitude of proteins of the intercalated disk. Among those, the MAGUK proteins, SAP97 and ZO-1, are likely to play a role in regulating the stochiometry of $Na_V1.5$ and Kv2.1 channels at the intercalated disk and the size of the gap junctions via specific PDZ-binding domains.[65,67] Overall, more experimental work is needed to understand the multitude of complex protein–protein interactions at the intercalated disk, which may affect cell-to-cell coupling and propagation.

The observation that remodeling of electrical cell-to-cell coupling via gap junctions can be associated with a change in ion channel expression makes it difficult to correlate changes in connexin expression to changes in propagation velocity without information about concomitant changes in ion channels, such as $Na_V1.5$ and Kv2.1. Some studies involving marked electrical uncoupling of myocyte strands using genetic ablation or drug inhibition of gap junction channel conductance have shown that a marked decrease in gap junction coupling is necessary for significant changes in propagation velocity to occur,[28,35] in accordance with theoretical experiments.[34] However, other studies have suggested that relatively moderate changes in local Cx expression lead to a measurable decrease in propagation velocity.[97] Therefore the possibility needs to be taken into account that $Na_V5.1$ and Kv2.1 channel expression, which might vary according to experimental and pathological conditions, might accompany changes in connexin expression and affect propagation.

Summary

The recent findings of the molecular interaction between and common regulation of mechanical junction proteins, ion channels, and connexins, at the levels of trafficking to or regulation within the intercalated disk, point to the difficulty in explaining the importance of remodeling of connexins and gap junction channels for propagation as isolated, independent events within a complex molecular phenotype. In addition, another level of complexity is added by the functional interaction of electrical cell-to-cell coupling, cellular network architecture, and ion current flow in producing linear or circulating electrical propagation waves.

REFERENCES

1. Weidmann S. Heart: electrophysiology. *Annu Rev Physiol.* 1974;36:155–169.
2. Cottrell GT, Burt JM. Functional consequences of heterogeneous gap junction channel formation and its influence in health and disease. *Biochim Biophys Acta.* 2005;1711:126–141.
3. Harris AL. Emerging issues of connexin channels: biophysics fills the gap. *Q Rev Biophys.* 2001;34:325–472.
4. Moreno AP. Biophysical properties of homomeric and heteromultimeric channels formed by cardiac connexins. *Cardiovasc Res.* 2004;62:276–286.
5. Spray DC, Bennett MV. Physiology and pharmacology of gap junctions. *Annu Rev Physiol.* 1985;47:281–303.
6. Spray DC, White RL, Mazet F, Bennett MV. Regulation of gap junctional conductance. *Am J Physiol.* 1985;248:H753–H764.
7. Gaietta G, Deerinck TJ, Adams SR, et al. Multicolor and electron microscopic imaging of connexin trafficking. *Science.* 2002;296:503–507.
8. Smyth JW, Zhang SS, Sanchez JM, et al. 14-3-3 mode-1 binding motif initiates gap junction internalization during acute cardiac ischemia. *Traffic.* 2014;15:684–699.
9. Patel DM, Dubash AD, Kreitzer G, Green KJ. Disease mutations in desmoplakin inhibit Cx43 membrane targeting mediated by desmoplakin-EB1 interactions. *J Cell Biol.* 2014;206:779–797.
10. Shaw RM, Fay AJ, Puthenveedu MA, von Zastrow M, Jan YN, Jan LY. Microtubule plus-end-tracking proteins target gap junctions directly from the cell interior to adherens junctions. *Cell.* 2007;128:547–560.
11. Smyth JW, Shaw RM. Visualizing cardiac ion channel trafficking pathways. *Methods Enzymol.* 2012;505:187–202.
12. Smyth JW, Shaw RM. The gap junction life cycle. *Heart Rhythm.* 2012;9:151–153.
13. Kleber AG. Gap junctions and conduction of cardiac excitation. *Heart Rhythm.* 2011;8:1981–1984.
14. Davis LM, Rodefeld ME, Green K, Beyer EC, Saffitz JE. Gap junction protein phenotypes of the human heart and conduction system. *J Cardiovasc Electrophysiol.* 1995;6:813–822.
15. Saffitz JE, Davis LM, Darrow BJ, Kanter HL, Laing JG, Beyer EC. The molecular basis of anisotropy: role of gap junctions. *J Cardiovasc Electrophysiol.* 1995;6:498–510.
16. van Veen AA, van Rijen HV, Opthof T. Cardiac gap junction channels: modulation of expression and channel properties. *Cardiovasc Res.* 2001;51:217–229.
17. Bukauskas FF, Kreuzberg MM, Rackauskas M, et al. Properties of mouse connexin 30.2 and human connexin 31.9 hemichannels: implications for atrioventricular conduction in the heart. *Proc Natl Acad Sci U S A.* 2006;103:9726–9731.
18. Kleber AG, Janse MJ, Fast VG. Normal and abnormal conduction in the heart. In: Page E, Fozzard HA, Solaro RJ, eds. *Handbook of Physiology, Section 2: The Cardiovascular System.* vol I. The Heart. New York: Oxford University Press; 2001:455–529.
19. Vozzi C, Dupont E, Coppen SR, Yeh HI, Severs NJ. Chamber-related differences in connexin expression in the human heart. *J Mol Cell Cardiol.* 1999;31:991–1003.
20. Kanagaratnam P, Rothery S, Patel P, Severs NJ, Peters NS. Relative expression of immunolocalized connexins 40 and 43 correlates with human atrial conduction properties. *J Am Coll Cardiol.* 2002;39:116–123.
21. Beauchamp P, Yamada KA, Baertschi AJ, et al. Relative contributions of connexins 40 and 43 to atrial impulse propagation in synthetic strands of neonatal and fetal murine cardiomyocytes. *Circ Res.* 2006;99:1216–1224.
22. Gu H, Smith FC, Taffet SM, Delmar M. High incidence of cardiac malformations in connexin40-deficient mice. *Circ Res.* 2003;93:201–206.
23. Valiunas V, Gemel J, Brink PR, Beyer EC. Gap junction channels formed by coexpressed connexin40 and connexin43. *Am J Physiol Heart Circ Physiol.* 2001;281:H1675–H1689.
24. Cottrell GT, Burt JM. Heterotypic gap junction channel formation between heteromeric and homomeric Cx40 and Cx43 connexons. *Am J Physiol Cell Physiol.* 2001;281:C1559–C1567.
25. Vaidya D, Tamaddon HS, Lo CW, et al. Null mutation of connexin43 causes slow propagation of ventricular activation in the late stages of mouse embryonic development. *Circ Res.* 2001;88:1196–1202.
26. Alcolea S, Theveniau-Ruissy M, Jarry-Guichard T, et al. Downregulation of connexin 45 gene products during mouse heart development. *Circ Res.* 1999;84:1365–1379.

27. Johnson CM, Kanter EM, Green KG, et al. Redistribution of connexin45 in gap junctions of connexin43-deficient hearts. *Cardiovasc Res.* 2002;53:921–935.
28. Beauchamp P, Choby C, Desplantez T, et al. Electrical propagation in synthetic ventricular myocyte strands from germline connexin43 knockout mice. *Circ Res.* 2004;95:170–178.
29. Yamada KA, Rogers JG, Sundset R, Steinberg TH, Saffitz JE. Up-regulation of connexin45 in heart failure. *J Cardiovasc Electrophysiol.* 2003;14:1205–1212.
30. Grikscheit K, Thomas N, Bruce AF, et al. Coexpression of connexin 45 with connexin 43 decreases gap junction size. *Cell Commun Adhes.* 2008;15:185–193.
31. Lisewski U, Shi Y, Wrackmeyer U, et al. The tight junction protein CAR regulates cardiac conduction and cell-cell communication. *J Exp Med.* 2008;205:2369–2379.
32. Kleber AG, Rudy Y. Basic mechanisms of cardiac impulse propagation and associated arrhythmias. *Physiol Rev.* 2004;84:431–488.
33. Boyle PM, Vigmond EJ. An intuitive safety factor for cardiac propagation. *Biophys J.* 2010;98:L57–L59.
34. Shaw RM, Rudy Y. Ionic mechanisms of propagation in cardiac tissue. Roles of the sodium and L-type calcium currents during reduced excitability and decreased gap junction coupling. *Circ Res.* 1997;81:727–741.
35. Rohr S, Kucera JP, Kleber AG. Slow conduction in cardiac tissue, I: effects of a reduction of excitability versus a reduction of electrical coupling on microconduction. *Circ Res.* 1998;83:781–794.
36. Wang Y, Rudy Y. Action potential propagation in inhomogeneous cardiac tissue: safety factor considerations and ionic mechanism. *Am J Physiol Heart Circ Physiol.* 2000;278:H1019–H1029.
37. Gutstein DE, Morley GE, Vaidya D, et al. Heterogeneous expression of gap junction channels in the heart leads to conduction defects and ventricular dysfunction. *Circulation.* 2001;104:1194–1199.
38. Severs NJ, Bruce AF, Dupont E, Rothery S. Remodelling of gap junctions and connexin expression in diseased myocardium. *Cardiovasc Res.* 2008;80:9–19.
39. Jansen JA, Noorman M, Musa H, et al. Reduced heterogeneous expression of Cx43 results in decreased Nav1.5 expression and reduced sodium current that accounts for arrhythmia vulnerability in conditional Cx43 knockout mice. *Heart Rhythm.* 2012;9:600–607.
40. Kitamura H, Ohnishi Y, Yoshida A, et al. Heterogeneous loss of connexin43 protein in nonischemic dilated cardiomyopathy with ventricular tachycardia. *J Cardiovasc Electrophysiol.* 2002;13:865–870.
41. Danik SB, Liu F, Zhang J, et al. Modulation of cardiac gap junction expression and arrhythmic susceptibility. *Circ Res.* 2004;95:1035–1041.
42. Elenes S, Martinez AD, Delmar M, Beyer EC, Moreno AP. Heterotypic docking of Cx43 and Cx45 connexons blocks fast voltage gating of Cx43. *Biophys J.* 2001;81:1406–1418.
43. Desplantez T, Halliday D, Dupont E, Weingart R. Cardiac connexins Cx43 and Cx45: formation of diverse gap junction channels with diverse electrical properties. *Pflugers Arch.* 2004;448:363–375.
44. McCain ML, Desplantez T, Geisse NA, et al. Cell-to-cell coupling in engineered pairs of rat ventricular cardiomyocytes: relation between Cx43 immunofluorescence and intercellular electrical conductance. *Am J Physiol - Heart and Circ.* 2012;302:H443–H450.
45. Beauchamp P, Desplantez T, McCain ML, et al. Electrical coupling and propagation in engineered ventricular myocardium with heterogeneous expression of connexin43. *Circ Res.* 2012;110:1445–1453.
46. Prudat Y, Kucera JP. Nonlinear behaviour of conduction and block in cardiac tissue with heterogeneous expression of connexin 43. *J Mol Cell Cardiol.* 2014;76:46–54.
47. Gutstein DE, Morley GE, Tamaddon H, et al. Conduction slowing and sudden arrhythmic death in mice with cardiac-restricted inactivation of connexin43. *Circ Res.* 2001;88:333–339.
48. Caldwell BJ, Trew ML, Sands GB, Hooks DA, LeGrice IJ, Smaill BH. Three distinct directions of intramural activation reveal nonuniform side-to-side electrical coupling of ventricular myocytes. *Circ Arrhythm Electrophysiol.* 2009;2:433–440.
49. Gilbert SH, Benoist D, Benson AP, et al. Visualization and quantification of whole rat heart laminar structure using high-spatial resolution contrast-enhanced MRI. *Am J Physiol Heart Circ Physiol.* 2012;302:H287–H298.

50. Pope AJ, Sands GB, Smaill BH, LeGrice IJ. Three-dimensional transmural organization of perimysial collagen in the heart. *Am J Physiol Heart Circ Physiol.* 2008;295:H1243–H1252.
51. Spach MS, Miller WT 3rd, Dolber PC, Kootsey JM, Sommer JR, Mosher CE Jr. The functional role of structural complexities in the propagation of depolarization in the atrium of the dog. Cardiac conduction disturbances due to discontinuities of effective axial resistivity. *Circ Res.* 1982;50:175–191.
52. Dolber PC, Spach MS. Thin collagenous septa in cardiac muscle. *Anat Rec.* 1987;218:45–55.
53. Spach MS, Heidlage JF, Dolber PC, Barr RC. Mechanism of origin of conduction disturbances in aging human atrial bundles: experimental and model study. *Heart Rhythm.* 2007;4:175–185.
54. Rutherford SL, Trew ML, Sands GB, LeGrice IJ, Smaill BH. High-resolution 3-dimensional reconstruction of the infarct border zone: impact of structural remodeling on electrical activation. *Circ Res.* 2012;111:301–311.
55. Spach MS, Kootsey JM. The nature of electrical propagation in cardiac muscle. *Am J Physiol.* 1983;244:H3–H22.
56. Rohr S, Kucera JP, Fast VG, Kleber AG. Paradoxical improvement of impulse conduction in cardiac tissue by partial cellular uncoupling. *Science.* 1997;275:841–844.
57. Fast VG, Kleber AG. Block of impulse propagation at an abrupt tissue expansion: evaluation of the critical strand diameter in 2- and 3-dimensional computer models. *Cardiovasc Res.* 1995;30:449–459.
58. Kucera JP, Kleber AG, Rohr S. Slow conduction in cardiac tissue, II: effects of branching tissue geometry. *Circ Res.* 1998;83:795–805.
59. Weidmann S. Cardiac action potentials, membrane currents, and some personal reminiscences. *Annu Rev Physiol.* 1993;55:1–14.
60. Barr L, Dewey MM, Berger W. Propagation of action potentials and the structure of the nexus in cardiac muscle. *J Gen Physiol.* 1965;48:797–823.
61. Sperelakis N, Hoshiko T, Berne RM. Nonsyncytial nature of cardiac muscle: membrane resistance of single cells. *Am J Physiol.* 1960;198:531–536.
62. Danik SB, Rosner G, Lader J, Gutstein DE, Fishman GI, Morley GE. Electrical remodeling contributes to complex tachyarrhythmias in connexin43-deficient mouse hearts. *FASEB J.* 2008;22:1204–1212.
63. Kucera JP, Rohr S, Rudy Y. Localization of sodium channels in intercalated disks modulates cardiac conduction. *Circ Res.* 2002;91:1176–1182.
64. Mori Y, Fishman GI, Peskin CS. Ephaptic conduction in a cardiac strand model with 3D electrodiffusion. *Proc Natl Acad Sci U S A.* 2008;105:6463–6468.
65. Abriel H, Rougier JS, Jalife J. Ion channel macromolecular complexes in cardiomyocytes: roles in sudden cardiac death. *Circ Res.* 2015;116:1971–1988.
66. Gillet L, Rougier JS, Shy D, et al. Cardiac-specific ablation of synapse-associated protein SAP97 in mice decreases potassium currents but not sodium current. *Heart Rhythm.* 2015;12:181–192.
67. Milstein ML, Musa H, Balbuena DP, et al. Dynamic reciprocity of sodium and potassium channel expression in a macromolecular complex controls cardiac excitability and arrhythmia. *Proc Natl Acad Sci U S A.* 2012;109:E2134–E2143.
68. Petitprez S, Zmoos AF, Ogrodnik J, et al. SAP97 and dystrophin macromolecular complexes determine two pools of cardiac sodium channels Nav1.5 in cardiomyocytes. *Circ Res.* 2011;108:294–304.
69. Shy D, Gillet L, Ogrodnik J, et al. PDZ domain-binding motif regulates cardiomyocyte compartment-specific NaV1.5 channel expression and function. *Circulation.* 2014;130:147–160.
70. Veeraraghavan R, Lin J, Hoeker GS, Keener JP, Gourdie RG, Poelzing S. Sodium channels in the Cx43 gap junction perinexus may constitute a cardiac ephapse: an experimental and modeling study. *Pflugers Arch.* 2015;467:2093–2105.
71. Veeraraghavan R, Gourdie RG, Poelzing S. Mechanisms of cardiac conduction: a history of revisions. *Am J Physiol Heart Circ Physiol.* 2014;306:H619–H627.
72. Peon J, Ferrier GR, Moe GK. The relationship of excitability to conduction velocity in canine Purkinje tissue. *Circ Res.* 1978;43:125–135.
73. Spear JF, Moore EN. Supernormal excitability and conduction in the His-Purkinje system of the dog. *Circ Res.* 1974;35:782–792.

74. Spear JF, Moore EN. Supernormal conduction in the canine bundle of His and proximal bundle branches. *Am J Physiol*. 1980;238:H300–H306.

75. Bexton RS, Hellestrand KJ, Cory-Pearce R, Spurrell RA, English TA, Camm AJ. Unusual atrial potentials in a cardiac transplant recipient. Possible synchronization between donor and recipient atria. *J Electrocardiol*. 1983;16:313–321.

76. Lefroy DC, Fang JC, Stevenson LW, Hartley LH, Friedman PL, Stevenson WG. Recipient-to-donor atrioatrial conduction after orthotopic heart transplantation: surface electrocardiographic features and estimated prevalence. *Am J Cardiol*. 1998;82:444–450.

77. Rothman SA, Miller JM, Hsia HH, Buxton AE. Radio-frequency ablation of a supraventricular tachycardia due to interatrial conduction from the recipient to donor atria in an orthotopic heart transplant recipient. *J Cardiovasc Electrophysiol*. 1995;6:544–550.

78. Miragoli M, Gaudesius G, Rohr S. Electrotonic modulation of cardiac impulse conduction by myofibroblasts. *Circ Res*. 2006;98:801–810.

79. Camelliti P, Green CR, LeGrice I, Kohl P. Fibroblast network in rabbit sinoatrial node: structural and functional identification of homogeneous and heterogeneous cell coupling. *Circ Res*. 2004;94:828–835.

80. Rohr S. Arrhythmogenic implications of fibroblast-myocyte interactions. *Circ Arrhythm Electrophysiol*. 2012;5:442–452.

81. Gaudesius G, Miragoli M, Thomas SP, Rohr S. Coupling of cardiac electrical activity over extended distances by fibroblasts of cardiac origin. *Circ Res*. 2003;93:421–428.

82. Miragoli M, Salvarani N, Rohr S. Myofibroblasts induce ectopic activity in cardiac tissue. *Circ Res*. 2007;101:755–758.

83. Howard CM, Baudino TA. Dynamic cell-cell and cell-ECM interactions in the heart. *J Mol Cell Cardiol*. 2014;70:19–26.

84. Kohl P, Gourdie RG. Fibroblast-myocyte electrotonic coupling: does it occur in native cardiac tissue? *J Mol Cell Cardiol*. 2014;70:37–46.

85. Zhang Y, Kanter EM, Yamada KA. Remodeling of cardiac fibroblasts following myocardial infarction results in increased gap junction intercellular communication. *Cardiovasc Pathol*. 2010;19:e233–e240.

86. Delmar M. Connexin43 regulates sodium current; ankyrin-G modulates gap junctions: the intercalated disc exchanger. *Cardiovasc Res*. 2012;93:220–222.

87. Delmar M, Liang FX. Connexin43 and the regulation of intercalated disc function. *Heart Rhythm*. 2012;9:835–838.

88. Geisler SB, Green KJ, Isom LL, et al. Ordered assembly of the adhesive and electrochemical connections within newly formed intercalated disks in primary cultures of adult rat cardiomyocytes. *J Biomed Biotechnol*. 2010;2010:624719.

89. Hertig CM, Butz S, Koch S, Eppenberger-Eberhardt M, Kemler R, Eppenberger HM. N-cadherin in adult rat cardiomyocytes in culture. II. Spatio-temporal appearance of proteins involved in cell-cell contact and communication. Formation of two distinct N-cadherin/catenin complexes. *J Cell Sci*. 1996;109:11–20.

90. Kostin S, Hein S, Bauer EP, Schaper J. Spatiotemporal development and distribution of intercellular junctions in adult rat cardiomyocytes in culture. *Circ Res*. 1999;85:154–167.

91. Li J, Radice GL. A new perspective on intercalated disc organization: implications for heart disease. *Dermatol Res Pract*. 2010;2010:207835.

92. Sato PY, Musa H, Coombs W, et al. Loss of plakophilin-2 expression leads to decreased sodium current and slower conduction velocity in cultured cardiac myocytes. *Circ Res*. 2009;105:523–526.

93. Cerrone M, Noorman M, Lin X, et al. Sodium current deficit and arrhythmogenesis in a murine model of plakophilin-2 haploinsufficiency. *Cardiovasc Res*. 2012;95:460–468.

94. Asimaki A, Kapoor S, Plovie E, et al. Identification of a new modulator of the intercalated disc in a zebrafish model of arrhythmogenic cardiomyopathy. *Sci Transl Med*. 2014;6:240ra74.

95. Asimaki A, Kleber AG, MacRae CA, Saffitz JE. Arrhythmogenic cardiomyopathy—new insights into disease mechanisms and drug discovery. *Prog Pediatr Cardiol*. 2014;37:3–7.

96. Smyth JW, Vogan JM, Buch PJ, et al. Actin cytoskeleton rest stops regulate anterograde traffic of connexin 43 vesicles to the plasma membrane. *Circ Res*. 2012;110:978–989.

97. Eloff BC, Lerner DL, Yamada KA, Schuessler RB, Saffitz JE, Rosenbaum DS. High resolution optical mapping reveals conduction slowing in connexin43 deficient mice. *Cardiovasc Res*. 2001;51:681–690.

28 Mechanisms of Normal and Dysfunctional Sinoatrial Nodal Excitability and Propagation

Brian J. Hansen, Thomas A. Csepe, and Vadim V. Fedorov

The sinoatrial node (SAN) is the primary pacemaker of the heart and is responsible for regular cardiac rhythm. Since its discovery by Keith and Flack[1] in the early 20th century, many important advances have been made in terms of understanding the complex structure and function of the SAN and the role these factors have in cardiac physiology and pathophysiology. Decades of research have provided greater understanding of the anatomy,[2–4] molecular biology,[5,6] and electrophysiology[7,8] of the human SAN. Three-dimensional (3D) histological and immunofluorescence reconstructions of the SAN, as well as molecular studies regarding gene and protein expression, have helped to demonstrate the unique structural and molecular heterogeneity of the SAN pacemaker complex.[5,6,9] Furthermore, recent optical imaging of the SAN in human and animal hearts has provided important insights into the functional features of this profoundly complex structure in normal and diseased states.[10] This chapter reviews the current knowledge of SAN structure, excitability, and conduction with specific reference to these recent discoveries in the human heart.

Structural and Molecular Characteristics of the Sinoatrial Node Pacemaker Complex

Anatomy and Structure of the Human Sinoatrial Node

Anatomically located at the junction of the superior vena cava and right atrium in the mammalian heart (Fig. 28.1A), the SAN is a complex multicompartment structure characterized by small clusters of pacemaker myocytes that are arranged in parallel rows that frequently anastomose.[3,4,11] The SAN pacemaker cells are striated like normal working myocardial cells but are smaller in both length and diameter.[5] The clusters of specialized cardiomyocytes are enmeshed within strands of dense connective tissue, nerve fibers, and capillaries, creating the SAN pacemaker complex. In the normal adult human heart, the SAN is 12- to 20-mm long and 2- to 6-mm wide and has a banana-shaped 3D structure that traverses intramurally. The head (superior third) of the SAN is typically separated from the epicardium by less than 1 mm of fibrous tissue and fat[1,3,4,11] (Fig. 28.1B). The SAN is normally tilted in such a way that the SAN head lies more subepicardially and the SAN tail more subendocardially, but the 3D human SAN structure

is highly variable, making its exact location difficult to define in patients.[3,11] The human SAN is typically centered on the sinus node artery, which arises from the right coronary artery in 55% of patients and from the left circumflex artery in the other 45%. The sinus node artery marks an important anatomical landmark of the SAN complex and may help to avoid accidental injury to the SAN during surgical procedures[3,11,12] (see Fig. 28.1A and C). The normal adult SAN structure consists of 40% to 55% fibrotic connective tissue, which creates a honeycomb-like fibrotic matrix composed of a network of collagen sheaths.[13,14] This fibrotic scaffolding houses sophisticated SAN myocytes while also providing mechanical protection to the SAN. Apart from sinoatrial conduction pathways (SACPs), which provide a discrete and continuous electrical connection between the SAN and atria, fibrosis, fatty tissue, and/or discontinuous myofibers create a structural border surrounding the SAN, thus electrically insulating the SAN pacemaker cells from the hyperpolarizing effect of the surrounding myocardium and thereby efficiently regulating normal sinus rhythm (SR) (see Fig. 28.1B).[8,15]

Molecular Characteristics of the Mammalian and Human Sinoatrial Node

A unique composition of ion channels and Ca^{2+}-handling proteins are essential for SAN pacemaker automaticity and distinguishes the SAN complex from the surrounding atria. Importantly, direct molecular[5,6] and ion current studies[16] on the human SAN, rather than animal models, are limited. It is generally accepted that mammalian SAN pacemaker cells are depolarized (–60 mV) compared with the surrounding atrial myocardium (–85 mV) and lack a stable resting potential because of the absence of the background inward rectifier K^+ current I_{K1}.[2] Instead, the SAN pacemaker cells exhibit slow diastolic depolarization due to the synergistic membrane and Ca^{2+} clock mechanisms.[17] The membrane voltage clock is attributed to the hyperpolarization-activated funny current (I_f), of which the molecular α-subunits are represented by hyperpolarization-activated cyclic nucleotide-gated (HCN1, HCN2, and HCN4) channels. The Ca^{2+} clock contributes to SAN diastolic depolarization through activation of the Na^+/Ca^{2+} exchanger current by spontaneous localized Ca^{2+} release from the sarcoplasmic reticulum via type 2 ryanodine receptors. The slow diastolic depolarization leads to spontaneous generation of the SAN pacemaker action potential (AP). Importantly, central SAN pacemaker cells lack the fast Na^+ current I_{Na} responsible for the fast depolarization and conduction in atrial and ventricular cells. Instead, SAN conduction is very slow[8,18,19] as AP upstroke is generated by small, slow Ca^{2+} current $I_{Ca,L}$,[20] which is modulated by sympathetic and parasympathetic stimulation.

Slow conduction within the SAN complex is also affected by its unique expression of gap junction proteins. The SAN lacks the high conductance gap junction proteins connexin (Cx)43 and Cx40, which are the major gap junction proteins responsible for electrical coupling between cardiomyocytes in the working atrial myocardium. Instead, animal and human studies have shown the

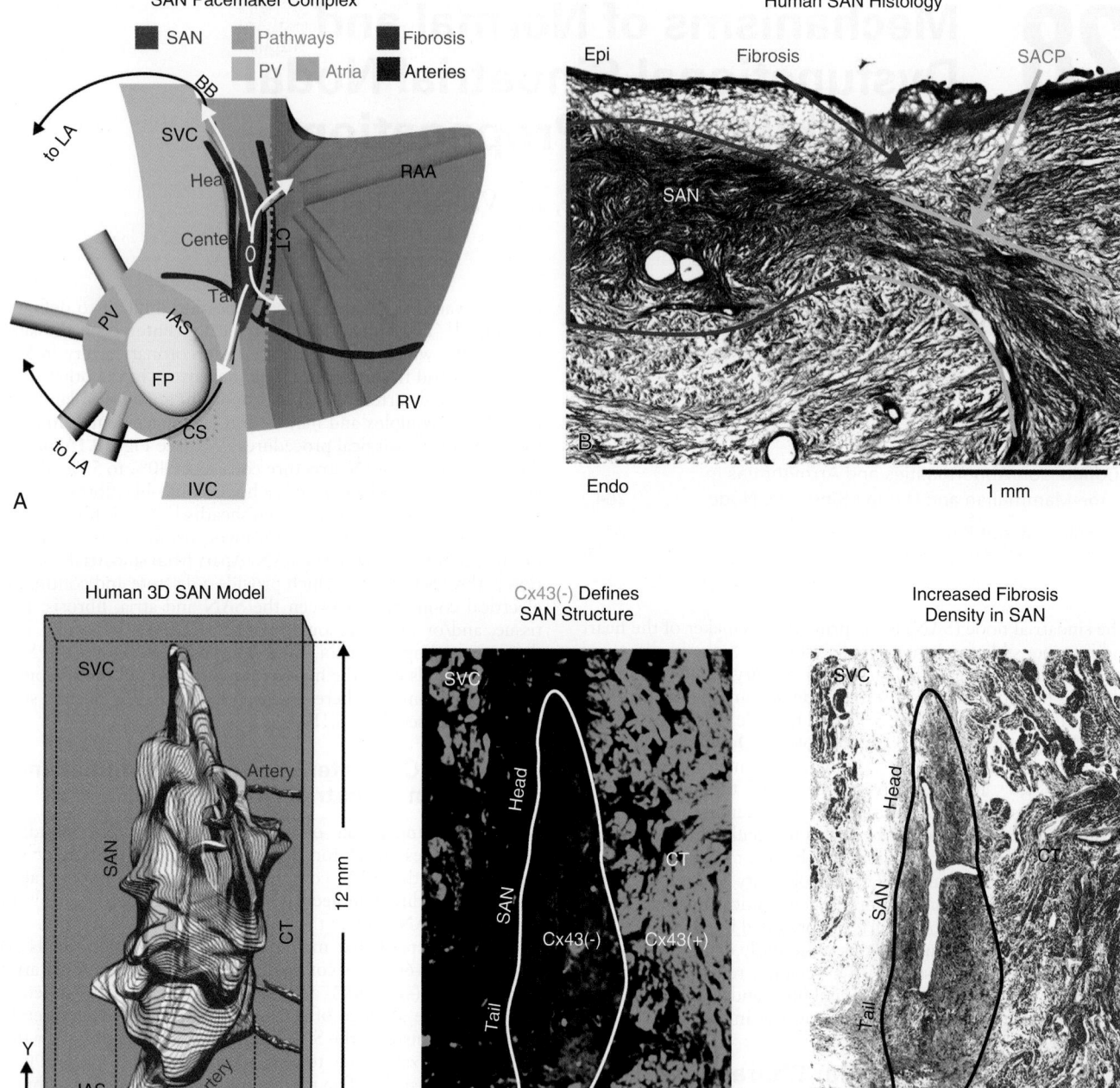

FIGURE 28.1 The three-dimensional (*3D*) structure of the human sinoatrial node (*SAN*) pacemaker complex. (A) Epicardial view of the 3D SAN model on the basis of the structural and functional data from optical mapping. SAN (*red*) is isolated from the surrounding atrium (*green*) by three bifurcating coronary arteries (*blue*) and fibrosis (*purple*). The *yellow bundles* show sinoatrial conduction pathways (*SACPs*) that electrically connect SAN to the atrium. (B) A histological cross-section of a human SAN (*red outline*) connected to the atria by SACP (*orange outline*). (C) Computational 3D human SAN from serial-sectioned histological slides shows nodal (*blue*) and arterial (*red*) tissue. (D) Immunostaining defines human SAN borders based on connexin 43 (*Cx43*) negativity in SAN and high Cx43 expression in the atrial myocardium. (E) Masson's trichrome staining used to further characterize the human SAN as a region of compact fibrosis (*blue*). *BB*, Bachmann's bundle; *CS*, coronary sinus; *CT*, crista terminalis; *Endo*, endocardium; *Epi*, epicardium; *IAS*, interatrial septum; *IVC*, inferior vena cava; *LA*, left atria; *PV*, pulmonary vein; *RAA*, right atrial appendage; *RV*, right ventricle; *SVC*, superior vena cava. ([A] Data modified from Fedorov VV, Glukhov AV, Chang R. Conduction barriers and pathways of the sinoatrial pacemaker complex: their role in normal rhythm and atrial arrhythmias. *Am J Physiol Heart Circ Physiol.* 2012;302:H1773-1783. [B] Data modified from Fedorov VV, Glukhov AV, Chang R, et al. Optical mapping of the isolated coronary-perfused human sinus node. *J Am Coll Cardiol.* 2010;56:1386-1394. [C–E] Data modified from Csepe TA, Zhao J, Hansen BJ, et al. Human sinoatrial node structure: 3D microanatomy of sinoatrial conduction pathways. *Prog Biophys Mol Biol.* 2016;120:164-178.)

28

presence of Cx45, a low conductance connexin that is expected to provide weak electrical coupling in the SAN.[5,21] Moreover, a weaker cell-to-cell electrical connection may increase the safety of conduction.[22]

The specialized SAN structure and connexin distribution, as well as the combination of ion channels responsible for SAN automaticity, present multiple molecular markers to distinguish the SAN from surrounding atrial tissue.[5,23] The high fibrosis level in the SAN (40%–50% tissue composition) compared with that in the atria (5%–20%) allows Mason trichrome or immunostaining of fibroblasts to identify the SAN (see Fig. 28.1B and E). Cx43 and potentially Cx40 negativity can also be successfully used as molecular markers of human SAN tissue[8] (Fig. 28.2). A recent molecular mapping study[6] of HCN isoform distribution in the human heart revealed that HCN1 may be exclusively expressed in the SAN pacemaker compartment, emphasizing its functional importance and potential utility as a new specific molecular marker of the human SAN (see Fig. 28.2). It is important to consider that protein expression may vary significantly between different compartments of the SAN (head vs. center vs. tail).[6,24,25]

Sinoatrial Conduction Pathways

SAN pacemaker clusters require anatomical and functional barriers for protection from the hyperpolarizing influence of the surrounding atria, yet a direct myofiber connection between the two structures must still exist for SAN cells to excite the right atrium. The idea of a discrete connection between the SAN and the atria has been proposed by multiple structural and functional studies,[3,8,19,26,27] but a lack of resolution in both the functional and structural mapping techniques has led to debates regarding the connection between the SAN and the atria. One hypothesis is that a structural border of fibrosis, fat layers, and myocyte discontinuity surround and electrically insulate the SAN and that the functional and structural connection between the SAN and atria is limited to discrete SACPs.[3,8,19,26,27] An alternative hypothesis is that SAN and atrial cells are extensively connected by diffuse interdigitations of the SAN border with the atrial myocardium and that no discrete pathways exist.[9,11]

Recently, our laboratory utilized serial high-resolution histology sections to reconstruct two optically mapped SANs, allowing us to identify and define the structural features of the functionally identified SACPs.[12] In the normal heart studied, several discrete branching myofiber tracts formed the SACP structure and made continuous, uninterrupted physical connections between the SAN and the atria. These myofiber tracts were composed of cells with transitional morphology (including shape and cell diameter) between the SAN and atrial cells. Furthermore, Cx43 immunolabeling showed a progressive transition from Cx43-negative SAN pacemaker cells to intermediate expression in the SACP region and distinct Cx43 gap junction expression in the

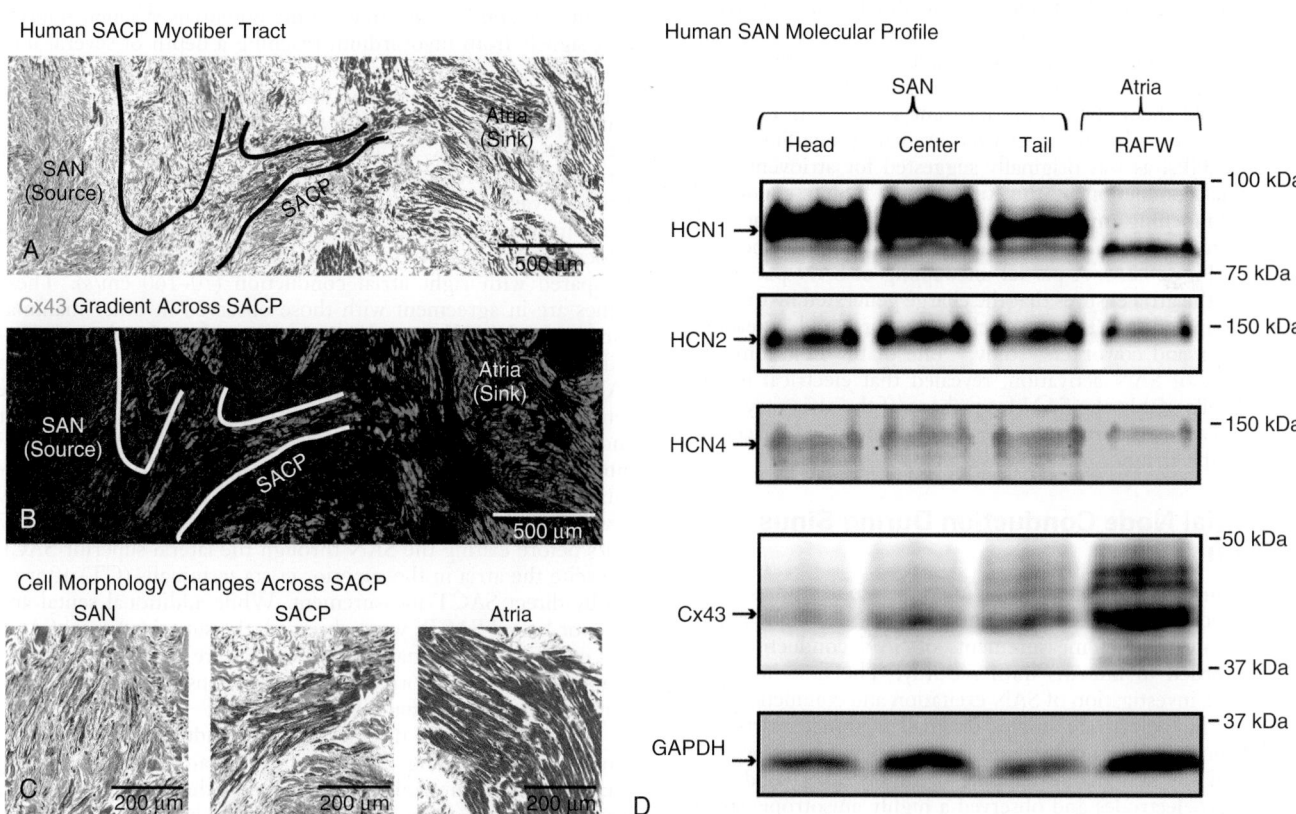

FIGURE 28.2 Structural and molecular characteristics of the human sinoatrial node (*SAN*) pacemaker complex. (A) Histological staining with lateral sinoatrial conduction pathway (*SACP*) outlined. (B) A sister section to panel (A) immunostained for connexin 43 (*Cx43; green*) and vimentin (*red*) compiled from a mosaic of high-resolution confocal images. (C) High-resolution images of histological regions show the myofiber morphology of SAN, SACP, and atrial tissue. (D) Representative immunoblot for hyperpolarization-activated cyclic nucleotide-gated (*HCN*) channels and Cx43 protein distribution in the human SAN head, center, tail, and right atrial free wall (*RAFW*). *GAPDH*, glyceraldehyde 3-phosphate dehydrogenase. ([A–C] Data modified from Csepe TA, Zhao J, Hansen BJ, et al. Human sinoatrial node structure: 3D microanatomy of sinoatrial conduction pathways. *Prog Biophys Mol Biol.* 2016;120:164-178. [D] Data modified from Li N, Csepe TA, Hansen BJ, et al. Molecular mapping of sinoatrial node HCN channel expression in the human heart. *Circ Arrhythm Electrophysiol.* 2015;8:1219-1227.)

atria. Future detailed functional, structural, and molecular studies on explanted human SANs are needed to confirm and expand these findings.

Sinoatrial Node Conduction Properties During Normal Sinus Rhythm

Source–Sink Relationships Allow the Small Sinoatrial Node to Drive the Large Atria

The specific structural and molecular features of the human SAN are extremely important for its successful function as the leading pacemaker of the heart.[15,19] As described earlier, normal SAN automaticity is dependent on a relatively depolarized state (about –60 mV). Electrotonic influence from the surrounding atrial myocardium at a resting potential of about –85 mV could hyperpolarize SAN pacemaker cells and inhibit automaticity[28]; however, this is prevented by a structural and functional insulation in the form of fibrosis and fat surrounding the SAN complex.[15] Moreover, the specialized SAN structure and its electrical coupling with the atria plays a crucial role in the synchronization of pacemaker clusters inside of the SAN (mutual entrainment), allowing for stability of SR, a relationship shown by earlier microelectrode and computer simulation studies conducted by the Jalife group.[29]

Another important consideration in the normal function of the SAN is the source–sink relationship between the SAN leading pacemaker and atria. SAN pacemaker cell clusters are small and rely on a relatively weak AP generated by the slow $I_{Ca,L}$ upstroke. This means that the SAN is a relatively weak source of current, while the atrial cells, being much larger with a more negative resting potential, pose a very large sink of current before reaching the threshold themselves. This apparent source–sink mismatch may be overcome by the specialized branching myofiber structure of SACPs, as was originally suggested for atrioventricular (AV) nodal conduction by the Rudy group.[30] Slow conduction through branching myofiber tracts of SACPs[19] gives the SAN enough time to build up a sufficient charge to excite the large atria (see Fig. 28.2A). A partial uncoupling of SAN pacemaker cells from the atria ensures that the charge generated by the SAN is not dissipated into the atria before the threshold is reached. The Joyner and coworkers' study,[31] one of the first computer simulations of SAN activation, revealed that electrical uncoupling of cells within the SAN from those of the atria may be an essential feature of normal electrical communication between the SAN and the atrium.

Sinoatrial Node Conduction During Sinus Rhythm

Despite numerous detailed direct microelectrode studies of the leading pacemaker and conduction in the SAN of many animal species, only indirect measurements of SAN conduction have been recorded in humans until recently. The first important steps in the investigation of SAN excitation and conduction were made by microelectrode studies of small mammal hearts.[32] In 1965, Sano and Yamagashi[33] and then Bleeker and associates[18] performed the systematic mapping of rabbit SAN conduction using microelectrodes and observed a highly anisotropic spread of activation (Fig. 28.3A). Bleeker and colleagues[18] estimated that intrinsic rabbit sinoatrial conduction time (SACT), or the time between the first SAN activation and the first atrial activation, was about 25 to 40 ms and calculated the conduction velocity near the leading pacemaker site to be 2 to 8 cm/s or less. However, SANs of small mammals are essentially two-dimensional structures.[18,34] This makes it easier to study using microelectrodes but raises concerns of its relevance to the 3D structure of large canine[26] or human[3,7] SANs, where it is practically impossible to utilize the same microelectrode techniques.

In 1980, Hariman and associates[35] were the first to describe a technique for recording sinus node electrograms (SNEs) using conventional electrode catheters and high amplifications. Subsequently, several investigators employed both unipolar and remote bipolar catheter electrodes to investigate automatic activity and conduction of the SAN pacemaker complex in patients with and without SAN dysfunction (SND).[36–38] The SNE recordings required strong contact to the surface near the anatomical location of the SAN to record the slow and relatively small SAN deflection that preceded the fast and large atrial upstroke[39] (see Fig. 28.3B). This slow SAN upstroke represents the cumulative signals from intramural SAN tissue, and thus SNE allows for a more direct estimate of SACT in humans. However, SNE recordings were never validated by structural confirmation of SAN location, and interpretation of the recordings was difficult and uncertain, which prevented the broad utilization of SNE recording techniques.[38] Bromberg and colleagues demonstrated that epi- and endocardial surface electrodes cannot properly determine the leading pacemaker sites and the slow propagation of SAN APs due to the 3D intramural structure of canine and human SANs.[26]

The limitations of surface electrode mapping were overcome by optical mapping with voltage-sensitive dyes,[19] particularly the new near-infrared dye di-4-ANBDQBS,[8] which was able to resolve the origin of activation and conduction inside the intramural SAN structure in canine and human hearts. Such high resolution is possible because optical APs (OAPs) represent a weighted average of transmembrane potentials through fluorescent signals from myocardium reaching a depth of several millimeters.[40] As such, SAN OAPs have specific morphological criteria: slow diastolic depolarization and upstrokes with multiple components corresponding to activation in SAN and atrial tissue layers.[19] Analytical approaches allow the separation[19] and/or extraction[41] of the slow SAN upstroke components from the fast atrial activation that resolves intramural SAN conduction separately from atrial activation. Human intranodal SAN conduction velocities, ranging from 1 to 16 cm/s,[8] are significantly slower compared with right atrial conduction (70–160 cm/s). These values are in agreement with those observed in other mammalian species.[2,18,19,33] Fig. 28.3C shows an example of near-infrared optical mapping of the explanted coronary-perused human SAN during stable SR.[12] Depicted in the figure are two separate activation patterns: SAN excitation from the leading pacemaker and atrial excitation originating from the insertion of the SACP into the atrial myocardium (see Fig. 28.3C and D). SAN activation originated in the SAN center–tail region, preferentially propagated superiorly at 14.3 ± 1.5 cm/s, and slowed to 6.8 ± 1.7 cm/s before exiting the SAN through the lateral superior SACP to excite the atria in the superior crista terminalis (CT) after 65 ms by direct SACT measurement. While additional septal and inferior lateral SACPs were observed, the superior lateral SACP and corresponding atrial breakthrough were the primary excitation patterns during normal SR, which is consistent with previous clinical and experimental observations.[8,42]

Moreover, cardiac disease and drug-induced structural and molecular remodeling can significantly alter pacemaker cell excitability and intracellular coupling in the SAN, which may lead to variations from the classical hierarchy of head–tail leading pacemakers[25,43] as well as the emergence of latent atrial pacemakers.[23,44,45]

Sinoatrial Node Pacemaker Complex Conduction Determines the Atrial Activation Pattern

Both epi-[7] and endocardial[43,46,47] surface electrode mapping studies have demonstrated anatomically widespread sites of earliest atrial activation during SR that may even excite

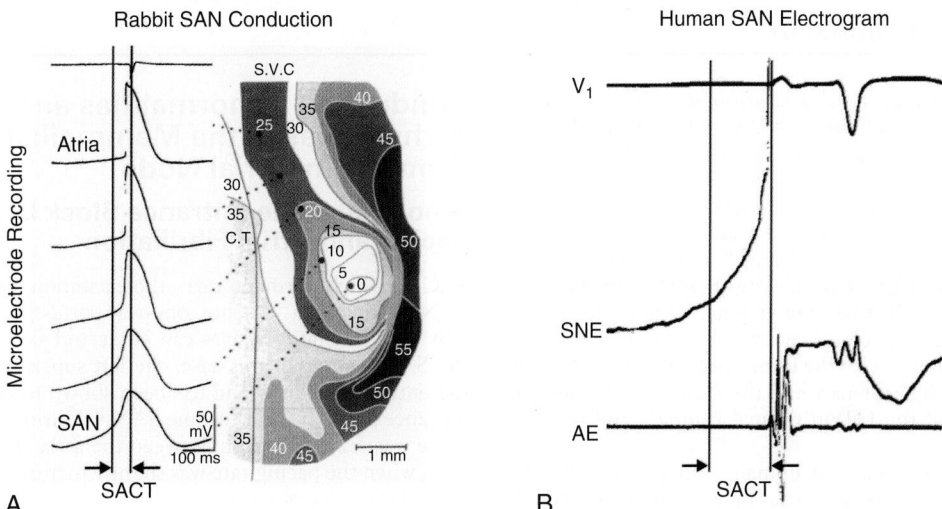

Rabbit SAN Conduction

Microelectrode Recording

Atria

SAN

50 mV

100 ms

SACT

A

Human SAN Electrogram

V₁

SNE

AE

SACT

B

Human SAN Conduction from Optical Mapping

SAN Activation

SAN Histology

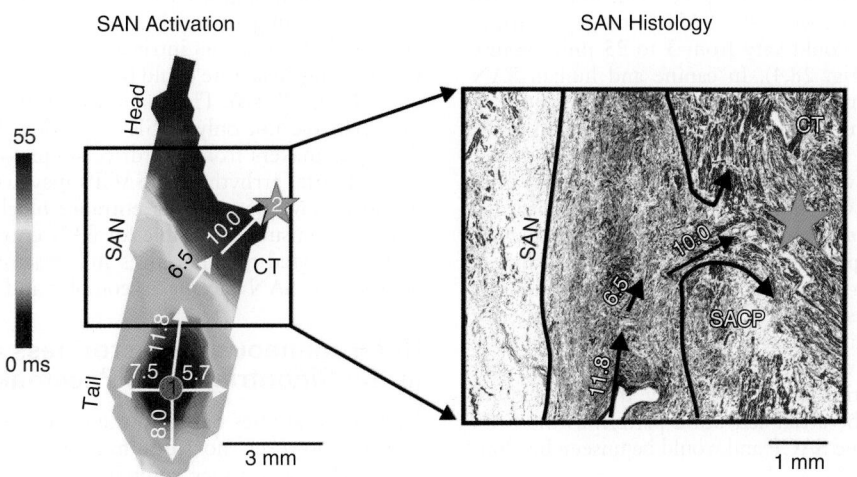

Atrial Activation

Direct SAN Conduction Time

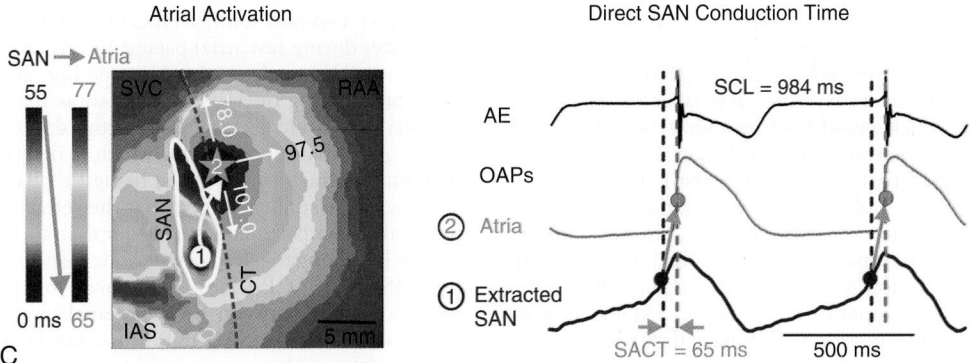

C

FIGURE 28.3 In vivo and ex vivo analyses of sinoatrial node (*SAN*) conduction. (A) Action potentials from microelectrode recordings in the route of preferential conduction in the rabbit atria. Toward the periphery, action potentials show an increase in amplitude and V_{max} and a decrease in the rate of diastolic depolarization. The numbers on the map give the activation time in milliseconds. (B) Human sinus node electrogram (*SNE*), atrial electrogram (*AE*), and V1 lead of electrocardiogram show the sinoatrial conduction time (*SACT*) in a patient. (C) *Top left,* Optical mapping of a human SAN reveals conduction within the SAN complex traveled from the leading pacemaker (1) to the lateral border of SAN. *White arrows* indicate the path of conduction, and the conduction velocity (cm/s) at that point was labeled. The *gray circle with "1"* denotes extracted SAN and location of optical action potential (*OAP*) #1, and the *green star with "2"* denotes atrial breakthrough (*exit point*) and location of OAP #2. *Top right,* Histological section shows the sinoatrial conduction pathway region with myofibers branching off from the compact nodal tissue. *Bottom left,* Optical mapping of SAN conduction and resulting atrial activation. *Bottom right,* AEs and OAPs from the atria and SAN demonstrate the direct measurement of SAN conduction time. *CT,* Crista terminalis; *IAS,* interatrial septum; *RAA,* right atrial appendage; *SCL,* sinus cycle length; *SVC,* superior vena cava. ([A] Modified from Bleeker WK, Mackaay AJ, Masson-Pevet M, et al. Functional and morphological organization of the rabbit sinus node. *Circ Res.* 1980;46:11-22. [B] Data modified from Gomes JA, Winters SL. The origins of the sinus node pacemaker complex in man: demonstration of dominant and subsidiary foci. *J Am Coll Cardiol.* 1987;9:45-52. [C] Data modified from Csepe TA, Zhao J, Hansen BJ, et al. Human sinoatrial node structure: 3D microanatomy of sinoatrial conduction pathways. *Prog Biophys Mol Biol.* 2016;120:164-178.)

simultaneously. Such multifocal activation started simultaneously during normal SR in humans in 2 to 5 foci located more than 1 cm apart. Pioneering atrial epicardial multielectrode mapping studies in canine and human hearts[7] by the Schuessler and Boineau group have led to the suggestion of a widely distributed "atrial pacemaker complex." Atrial breakthroughs were reported to arise over a region of 7.5 cm[7,46] along the CT. That region is significantly larger than the length of the human anatomical SAN body (10–20 mm).[3,4] In vivo mapping studies have also suggested the presence of a pacemaker hierarchy within the atrial pacemaker complex, with the fastest pacemakers preferentially located at the superior part and the slowest ones located at the inferior part of the CT in normal canine[48] and human hearts.[7,47]

Optical mapping of explanted human[8] and canine[19] hearts revealed that the majority of the atrial breakthroughs observed in the earlier experiments represent exit points of SAN electrical wave propagation through SACPs, rather than actual leading pacemaker sites. In Fig. 28.3C, the atrial breakthrough site is about 7.5 mm away from the leading pacemaker in the human SAN,[12] but the distance between the SAN leading pacemaker and atrial breakthroughs could vary from 3 to 25 mm because of multiple SACPs[8,19] (Fig. 28.4). In canine and human SAN studies,[8,10,15,19,25,41] intramural optical mapping revealed three to five discrete atrial breakthrough sites, which corresponded to the superior, lateral, inferior, and septal SACPs.

Fig. 28.4A and B shows two examples of superior and inferior patterns of atrial activation that were recorded by epicardial multielectrode[7] (*center panels*) and optical mapping[8] (*right panels*). The SAN activation maps demonstrated that these two different atrial activation patterns corresponded to atrial activations by the SAN excitation waves exiting through superior and inferior SACPs rather than two different leading pacemakers. Fig. 28.4C shows optical mapping examples of the leading pacemaker shift from the SAN center to the head. Importantly, this shift did not lead to any changes of the atrial activation pattern as the SAN waves exited from the same SACP and would be unseen by clinical mapping.

SAN pacemaking and conduction vary greatly due to SAN excitation dependence on the $I_{Ca,L}$ current,[2,16] which is regulated by the autonomic nervous system and its agonists.[17,49] Moreover, SAN conduction, especially in SACPs, could also be affected by different antiarrhythmic drugs that affect the membrane excitability of both SAN pacemaker cells and the surrounding atria, which could lead to a shift in preferential SACP and/or leading pacemaker. For instance, canine optical mapping[10] revealed that isoproterenol (Iso), a sympathetic agonist, accelerated SR and produced a superior shift in the leading pacemaker inside the SAN complex, whereas acetylcholine (ACh), a parasympathetic agonist, had the opposite effect. Moreover, perfusion with Iso and ACh generally results in a preferential use of superior and inferior SACPs, respectively. The inferior and superior SACPs have different conduction properties and sensitivities to autonomic stimulations by ACh and Iso[10]; this is potentially because of the heterogeneous expression of muscarinic and β-adrenergic receptors[24] and/or pacemaker ion channels[5,6,25] in the different compartments of the SAN pacemaker complex, although this has yet to be studied directly in human SACPs.

Moreover, optical mapping studies[8,10,15,19] have revealed that the presence of multiple functional SACPs could lead to beat-to-beat variations in atrial activation and that several simultaneous atrial breakthrough sites along the CT could be misinterpreted as multipacemaker activity. This issue may also explain the low efficacy of clinical ablation treatments for SAN arrhythmias, such as SAN-inappropriate tachycardia[50] due to targeting one of multiple exit points rather than the leading SAN pacemaker, that could be more than 2 cm away.

Conduction Abnormalities and Arrhythmias in the Mammalian and Human Sinoatrial Node

Sinoatrial Node Entrance Block During Atrial Pacing and Atrial Fibrillation

SACPs, which normally carry the excitation wavefront from the SAN to the atria, are not one-way roads.[10] Fig. 28.5A shows that atrial excitation waves can enter and slowly propagate into the SAN center. In this case, the left superior SACP is used as the entrance pathway and has been shown to be the preferential entrance pathway in the canine SAN.[10] During slow atrial pacing, there was 1:1 conduction between the atria and the SAN. However, when the pacing rate was slightly increased, a Wenckebach-like 2:1 entrance block into the SAN was observed. A high degree (5:1) of SAN entrance block during low potassium–induced atrial fibrillation (AF) was demonstrated in a classical microelectrode study of the rabbit SAN by Kirchhof and Allessie.[51] Furthermore, our optical mapping studies[10,41] showed that the SAN center, the common leading pacemaker site, cannot be paced faster than 10% to 50% above its intrinsic spontaneous rate, although the surrounding atrial rate could be 5 to 10 times faster than the normal SR (Fig. 28.5B). These studies revealed that SACPs may play a crucial role not only in SR regulation, but also in protecting SAN pacemakers from overdrive suppression during atrial pacing and atrial arrhythmias. SACPs may act like a low-pass filter for atrial waves by creating entrance block during atrial pacing. The mechanism responsible for SAN entrance block during AF is likely related to differences in refractoriness and excitability between the SAN pacemaker complex and surrounding atria.

Heterogeneous Refractoriness and Excitability in the Sinoatrial Node Pacemaker Complex

Only a few studies have reported SAN refractoriness measurements[52]; however, no study has been reported that paced the intact SAN pacemaker complex independent of the surrounding atria, keeping direct measurements of the SAN complex refractoriness elusive. To evaluate the activation of the SAN pacemaker complex and specifically SACP conduction filtering properties during fast atrial pacing and AF, we utilized dominant frequency (DF) analysis of OAPs (see Fig. 28.5B).[10,53,54] During atrial tachypacing or AF, DF maps show the minimal activation interval that could be captured by the different SAN compartments and atrial myocardium, which is determined by the local functional refractoriness of the tissue.[15,24] Based on detailed DF analysis, these studies suggest that the refractory periods of SAN pacemaker compartments are longer than those in SACPs, which in turn have longer refractory periods than the surrounding atrial tissue (SAN > SACP > atria). Moreover, functional refractoriness may also differ between SAN pacemaker compartments (SAN center > SAN head > SAN tail). Importantly, AP duration (APD) does not always determine the refractoriness of pacemaker cells because of the presence of postrepolarization refractoriness that is dependent on the excitability of the slow upstroke $I_{Ca,L}$ current.[52] As such, conditions that affect $I_{Ca,L}$ current excitability and pacemaker cell refractoriness can directly affect the entrance block ratio during tachypacing or AF and can be exaggerated by autonomic stimulation[52] and in patients with SNDs. Furthermore, some conditions, such as autonomic stimulation[10] or adenosine perfusion,[41] could have a heterogeneous effect on different compartments of the SAN complex.

Insight into how changes in refractoriness and excitability may affect SAN function can be gained by considering the experimental effects of ACh and adenosine, a natural metabolite of the heart.[25] ACh and adenosine activate a potassium-outward current ($I_{KACh,Ado}$) and suppress both the inward-calcium current ($I_{Ca,L}$)

Human Atrial Activation Defined by Superior SACP

Exit Through
Superior SACP

In Vivo
Epi Electrode Mapping

Ex Vivo
Optical Mapping

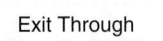
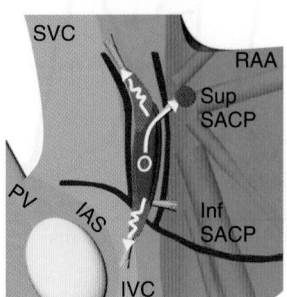
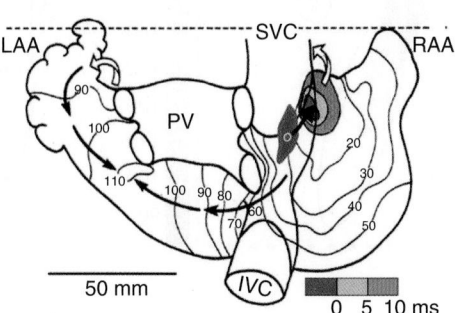
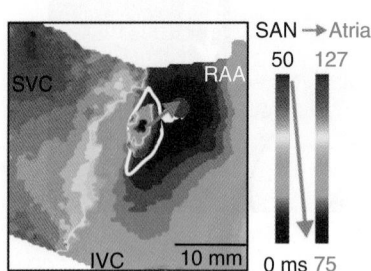

Human Atrial Activation Defined by Inferior SACP

Exit Through
Inferior SACP

In Vivo
Epi Electrode Mapping

Ex Vivo
Optical Mapping

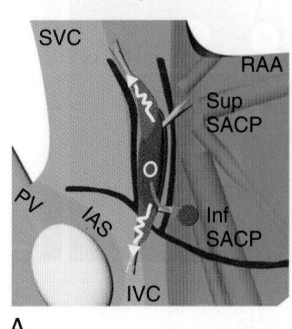
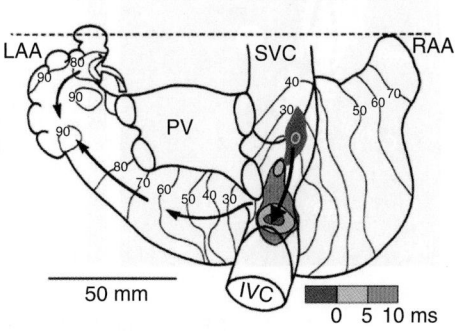
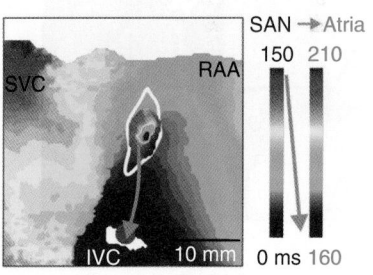

A

SAN Leading Pacemaker Shift Masked by Atrial Activation

Pacemaker Shift

SAN Center Pacemaker

SAN Head Pacemaker

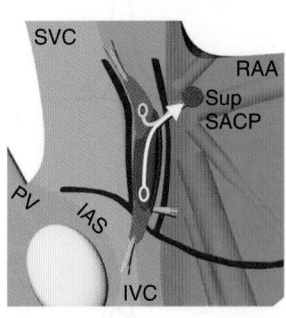
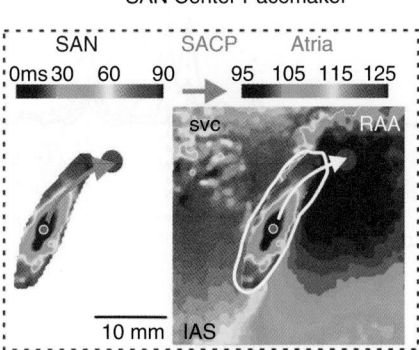
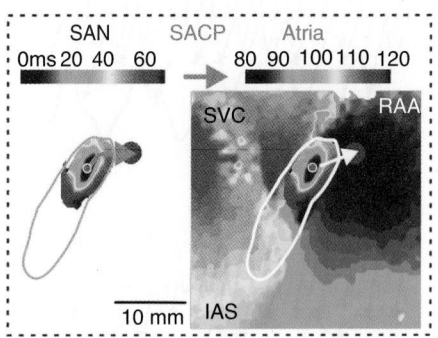

B

FIGURE 28.4 The sinoatrial conduction pathway (*SACP*) determines the atrial activation pattern during sinus rhythm. (A) *Left,* Sinoatrial node (*SAN*) models showing a single dominant pacemaker using the superior (*top*) and inferior (*bottom*) SACPs. The existence of several SAN pathways explains why, even during the presence of one leading pacemaker inside of SAN, the earliest atrial activation could arise in different sites (*exit points, magenta circles*). *Middle,* Multielectrode epicardial mapping of the human heart showing a change in the location of the earliest atrial activation (*exit point*) activated by SAN through the superior (*top*) and inferior (*bottom*) SACPs. *Right,* Optical mapping of the canine SAN revealed activation through superior and inferior pathways without a shift in the leading pacemaker location altered the atrial activation pattern. (B) The SAN model showing that a shift of the leading pacemaker from the SAN tail to the SAN head may not change the atrial activation pattern when the preferential SACP is maintained. *IAS,* Interatrial septum; *IVC,* inferior vena cava; *LAA,* left atrial appendage; *PV,* pulmonary vein; *RAA,* right atrial appendage; *SVC,* superior vena cava. ([A] Data modified from Fedorov VV, Glukhov AV, Chang R. Conduction barriers and pathways of the sinoatrial pacemaker complex: their role in normal rhythm and atrial arrhythmias. *Am J Physiol Heart Circ Physiol.* 2012;302:H1773-1783; and Boineau JP, Canavan TE, Schuessler RB, et al. Demonstration of a widely distributed atrial pacemaker complex in the human heart. *Circulation.* 1988;77:1221-1237. [B] Data modified from Glukhov AV, Hage LT, Hansen BJ, et al. Sinoatrial node reentry in a canine chronic left ventricular infarct model: role of intranodal fibrosis and heterogeneity of refractoriness. *Circ Arrhythm Electrophysiol.* 2013;6:984-994.)

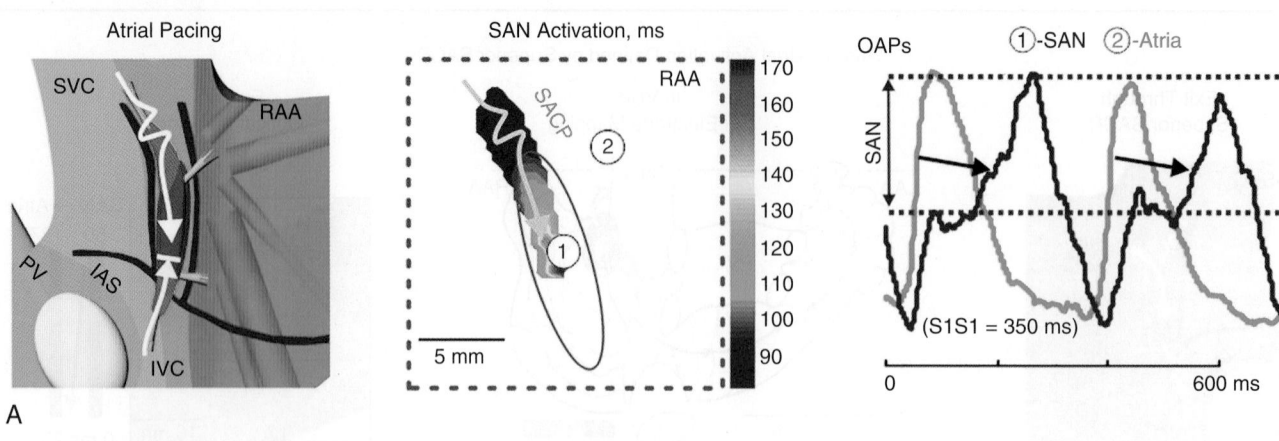

Atrial Pacing

SAN Activation, ms

OAPs ①-SAN ②-Atria

(S1S1 = 350 ms)

A

Protective Entrance Block During Tachypacing

SACP Entrance Block Protects the SAN

Dominant Frequency (DF), Hz

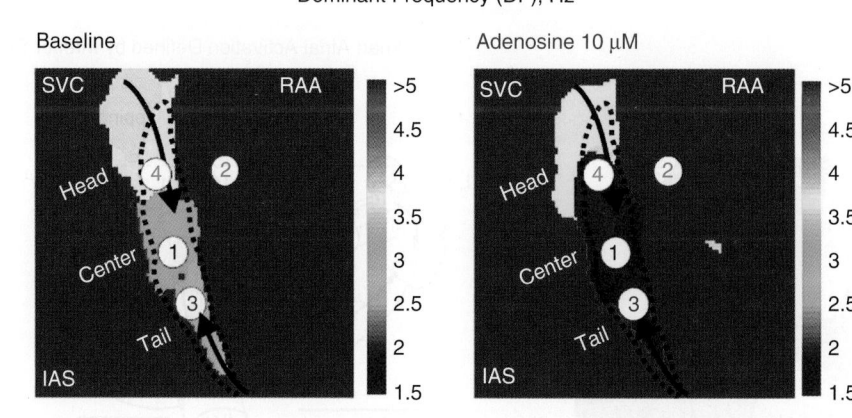

Baseline

Adenosine 10 μM

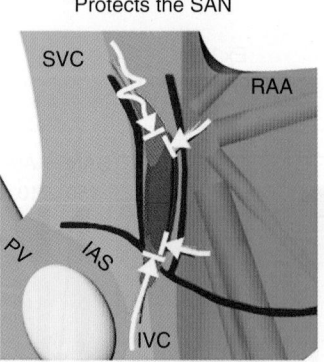

OAPs During Atrial Pacing 7.5 Hz

DF Spectrum During Atrial Pacing 7.5 Hz

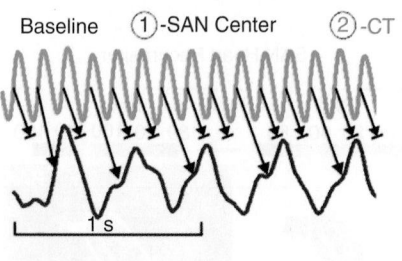

Baseline ①-SAN Center ②-CT

Adenosine 10 μM

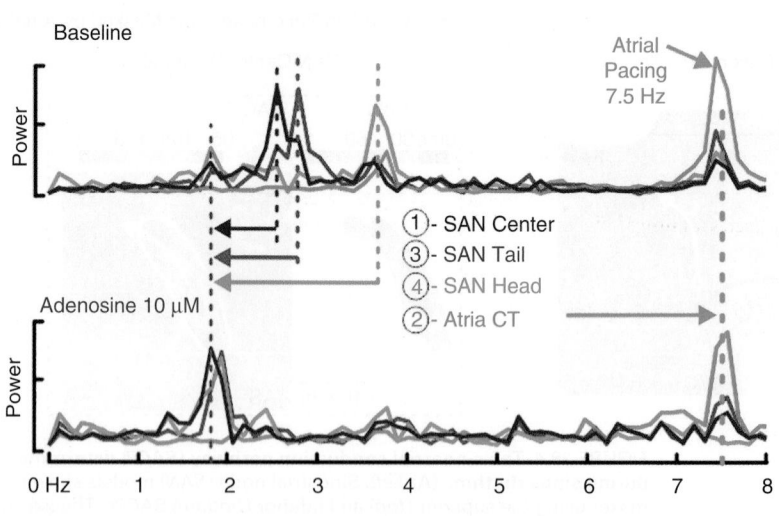

Baseline

Atrial Pacing 7.5 Hz

①- SAN Center
③- SAN Tail
④- SAN Head
②- Atria CT

Adenosine 10 μM

B

FIGURE 28.5 Entrance conduction properties of the sinoatrial node (*SAN*) pacemaker complex. (A) *Left to right,* The SAN model showing atrial conduction pacing of SAN through a sinoatrial conduction pathway (SACP). Optical mapping shows SAN activity during slow atrial pacing in a canine. Optical action potentials (*OAPs*) from SAN (*blue, 1*) and atrial myocardium (*green, 2*). (B) *Top left,* The SAN model showing that atrial conduction does not pace SAN because of the entrance block in SACPs. *Top right,* Dominant frequency (*DF*) maps during rapid pacing in canine SAN. SAN is outlined by a *dashed line.* At baseline, the activation frequency decreased from the SAN head and tail to the SAN center. Administration of 10 μM adenosine reduced SACP refractoriness and thus activation frequencies throughout the SAN. *Bottom left,* OAPs during rapid atrial pacing at baseline and 10 μM adenosine from the SAN center (*blue, 1*) and crista terminalis (*CT; green, 2*). *Bottom right,* Adenosine induced a decrease in the SAN activation frequency. Frequency power spectra of DF maps above from the SAN center (1), CT (2), SAN tail (3), and SAN head (4). *IAS,* Interatrial septum; *IVC,* inferior vena cava; *PV,* pulmonary vein; *RAA,* right atrial appendage; *SVC,* superior vena cava. ([A] Data modified from Fedorov VV, Chang R, Glukhov AV, et al. Complex interactions between the sinoatrial node and atrium during reentrant arrhythmias in the canine heart. *Circulation.* 2010;122:782-789. [B] Data modified from Lou Q, Glukhov AV, Hansen B, et al. Tachy-brady arrhythmias: the critical role of adenosine-induced sinoatrial conduction block in posttachycardia pauses. *Heart Rhythm.* 2013;10:110-118.)

and the hyperpolarization-activated current (I_f), all of which may decrease the excitability of SAN pacemaker cells.[49,55,56] ACh has been shown to heterogeneously affect rabbit SAN refractoriness[52] and excitability.[57] West and Belardinelli demonstrated that the response to adenosine was also heterogeneous in the rabbit SAN,[55] which echoes the heterogeneous conduction depression and pacemaker shifts observed in our canine studies.[10,41] The heterogeneous sensitivity to ACh and adenosine might be explained by the SAN pacemaker tissue near the SACPs being more susceptible to overdrive suppression by the neighboring atria (see Fig. 28.5B). Rapid stimulation is filtered more in the SACPs and thus prevents overdrive suppression of the leading pacemaker in the SAN center (see Fig. 28.5B). Moreover, higher ACh and adenosine concentrations or vagal stimulation could even lead to transient unexcitability of SAN pacemaker cells.[34,57] This temporal unexcitability could lead to a pacemaker shift outside of the SAN, intranodal conduction blocks, and reentrant arrhythmias, including atrial flutter, AF, and SAN reentry.[10,58]

Sinoatrial Node Exit Block

While conduction from rapid atrial pacing and AF may get filtered by the entrance block previously described, the effects of overdrive suppression still impact the SAN pacemaker complex. Atrial tachycardia can directly depress excitability of the SAN complex by inactivation of the $I_{Ca,L}$ current. Watanabe and associates[59] showed that overdrive suppression of the single rabbit SAN pacemaker cell by fast pacing transiently reduced the $I_{Ca,L}$ current to 15% of baseline, which led to temporal depression of excitability and rhythm slowing. In the intact SAN pacemaker complex, the entrance block and filtering properties of SACPs would cause the pacemaker tissue near the SACPs to experience more overdrive suppression than the central SAN compartment. The leading pacemaker located in the SAN center may recover before cells in other compartments or the SACPs and may manifest as an exit block after the cessation of tachycardia (Fig. 28.6). Importantly, ACh and adenosine may potentiate a pacing-induced depression of excitability in pacemaker cells near the SACPs (see earlier paragraph), leading to a high probability of postpacing-induced exit block and, consequently, tachy–brady syndrome.[41]

Sinoatrial Node Recovery Time

Postpacing recovery time of SR (SAN recovery time or SNRT) is widely used in clinical electrophysiology laboratories to evaluate the SAN pacemaker and diagnose SND. However, clinical atrial electrograms can only measure the time between the last paced atrial beat and the first spontaneous atrial beat, which provides only an indirect measurement of SNRT (or SNRTi) (see Fig. 28.6A). Moreover, the results can be normal despite the patient having SND symptoms or vice versa as it significantly depends on the autonomic tone. The presence of an entrance block can also significantly affect the SNRTi results and may even lead to a falsely short SNRTi if the last paced atrial beat measured does not pace the SAN.[41] Importantly, when presented with an extended pause after pacing is stopped, SNRTi does not differentiate between the exit block and automaticity failure as the cause. These long postpacing pauses are frequent in diseased hearts, especially during high vagal tone and adenosine, and clinical studies with SNE (see Fig. 28.6A) and optical mapping (see Fig. 28.6B) are necessary to elucidate the mechanism because these methods allow for the measurement of direct SNRT (SNRTd), which is the time from the last paced atrial beat to the first spontaneous SAN upstroke.

Our optical canine and human mapping studies[12,25,41,58] showed that pacing-induced atrial pauses (>1.5 s) are attributable to an exit block (see Fig. 28.6), which is consistent with the majority of clinical studies with SNE.[60] Fig. 28.6B shows

a representative example of intramural optical mapping of a canine chronic heart failure (HF) model with SND.[25] Cessation of atrial pacing was followed by a long atrial pause of 6252 ms. However, the SAN optical recording indicated that the SAN had recovered long before the first recovered atrial beat and was active during the atrial pause, indicating that SAN automaticity was not the main reason for the long pause (see Fig. 28.6B). These findings support the fact that entrance block within the SACPs can prevent overdrive suppression of the SAN central pacemaker but can also lead to temporal exit block and long atrial pauses.

Tachy–Brady Syndrome: Pacemaker Arrest or Sinoatrial Exit Block?

Tachy–brady syndrome or tachy–brady arrhythmia has been explained to be the heart rate alternation between too fast and too slow, where the termination of paroxysmal tachycardia may be followed by long atrial pauses lasting several seconds, which can provoke another tachyarrhythmia paroxysm.[14,61] These post-tachycardia atrial pauses could theoretically result from either sinus arrest and/or SAN exit block. Several clinical studies have demonstrated the presence of a SAN exit block using SNE (see Fig. 28.6A).[37,62] SNE typically shows regular SAN activity during atrial pauses in patients with tachy–brady syndrome[62] and SND.[37,60] Moreover, because of the technical limitations of SNE, it is not always clear whether the absence of SAN activity during long pauses is a result of sinus arrest or a pacemaker shift.[37] These clinical observations and the optical mapping of canine and human SANs strongly suggest an important role for a SAN exit block, rather than a sinus pacemaker arrest, in tachy–brady syndrome.

Sinoatrial Node Reentry

SAN reentrant tachycardia, also called SAN macroreentry, is a reentrant tachyarrhythmia involving the SAN and surrounding atrial tissue and may account for 2% to 17% of all atrial arrhythmias.[63,64] SAN reentrant tachycardia is one of the most intriguing cardiac arrhythmias because of the electrocardiographic similarity of the P wave to the normal SR that may lead to an underdiagnosis of these arrhythmias in clinics.[63] The electrocardiographic similarity of atrial activation during SAN macroreentry and normal SR is due to the reentrant excitation that still exits SAN through the preferential SACP, just as in a normal SR.

Recently, we were able to unmask the detailed activation patterns during SAN reentrant arrhythmias in canine models of chronic postmyocardial infarction and HF[58] using intramural optical mapping (Fig. 28.7). Depending on the excitable state of multiple SACPs, as well as intranodal compartments, two scenarios of SAN reentry maintenance could be observed. First, in SAN macroreentry, described in the preceding paragraph, the reentrant wave could normally propagate through an active SACP and then activate the atrial myocardium. After about 50 ms, the wave could reexcite a SAN compartment via another SACP and thus form a macroreentry circuit with two main pathways: a slow path (6–8 mm) located inside the SAN (~300–350 ms) and another fast atrial pathway (10–20 mm) located outside of the SAN between two SACPs (~50 ms). SAN macroreentry describes the classical clinical electrocardiographic view of SAN reentrant tachycardia.[58] Second, in SAN microreentry, SAN reentrant waves can circulate inside of the SAN around an intranodal longitudinal functional block such as fibrosis (1–3 mm). Interestingly, SAN macroreentry will always lead to heart rate accelerations or tachycardia, but SAN microreentry can present with symptoms of tachycardia or, more importantly, bradycardia because of an exit block in the SACP[58] (see Fig. 28.7A). Thus SAN reentry should be strongly considered when clinicians attempt to diagnose a variety of arrhythmias.

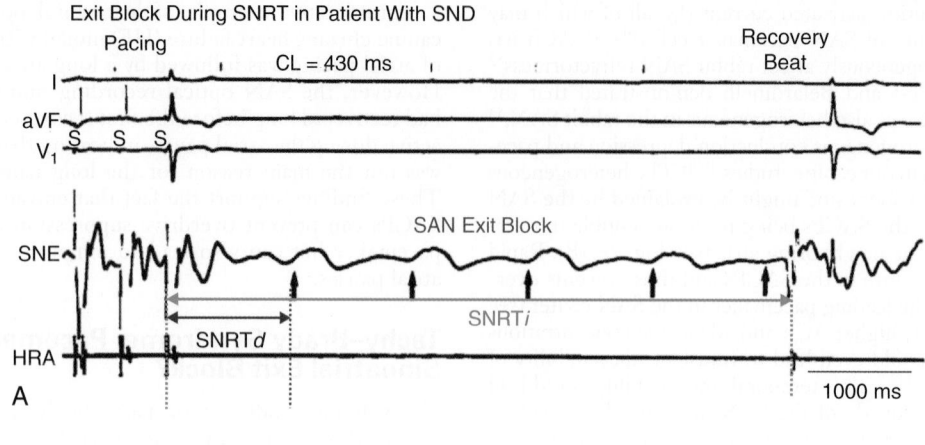

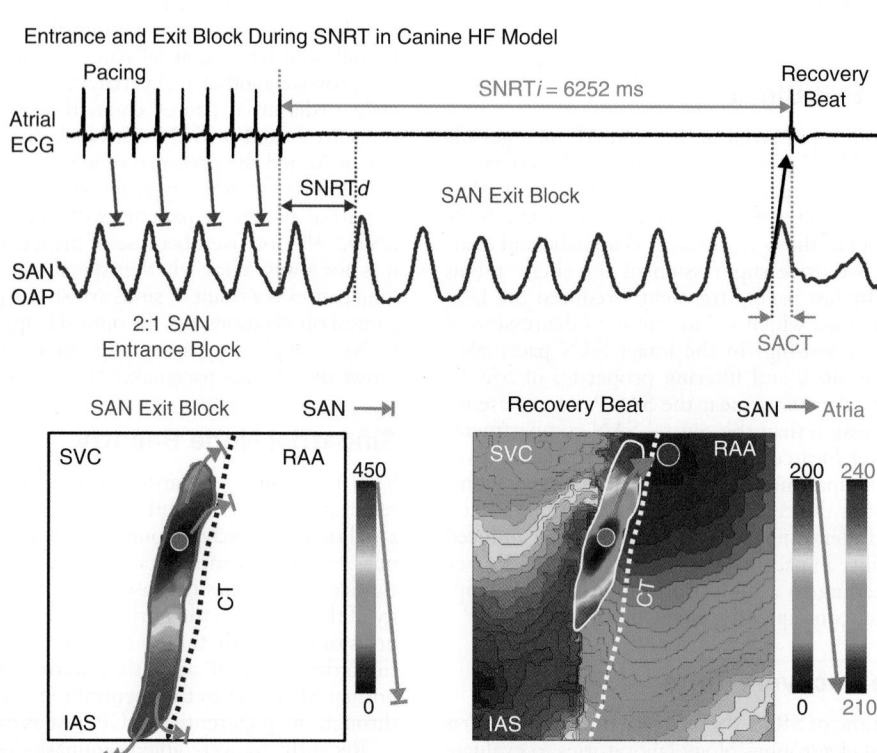

FIGURE 28.6 Sinoatrial node (*SAN*) exit block during long atrial pauses. (A) A sinus node electrogram (*SNE*) shows four isolated sinus node signals (*black arrows*) during a pacing-induced atrial pause in a SAN dysfunction (*SND*) patient. (B) *Top*, SAN optical action potential (*OAP*) and atrial electrocardiogram (*ECG*) recordings during and after pacing (2:1 SAN entrance block) during the administration of 10 μM adenosine in a canine heart failure (*HF*) model. Direct (*SNRTd*) and indirect (*SNRTi*) measurements of sinoatrial recovery time and sinoatrial conduction time (*SACT*) are shown. *Bottom*, The optical activation maps of pacing-induced SAN exit block (*left*) and a recovery beat (*right*), the first beat with recovered sinoatrial conduction. Two *color bars* indicate the activation times in SAN and atria when applicable. *CT*, crista terminalis; *IAS*, interatrial septum; *RAA*, right atrial appendage; *SVC*, superior vena cava. ([A] Data modified from Wu D, Yeh S, Lin F, et al. Sinus automaticity and sinoatrial conduction in severe symptomatic sick sinus syndrome. *J Am Coll Cardiol*. 1992;19:355-364. [B] Data modified from Lou Q, Hansen BJ, Fedorenko O, et al. Upregulation of adenosine A1 receptors facilitates sinoatrial node dysfunction in chronic canine heart failure by exacerbating nodal conduction abnormalities revealed by novel dual-sided intramural optical mapping. *Circulation*. 2014;130:315-324.)

Because of the intramural 3D SAN structure and transmural differences in activation between the subepicardial and subendocardial layers, SAN intranodal block and reentry cannot always be resolved through the optical mapping of a single surface (see Fig. 28.7B). Using dual-sided intramural mapping,[25] we were able to identify regions of conduction block not only at the SAN conduction pathways (entrance and exit block) but also within the SAN (intranodal block), which led to incidences of intranodal microreentry. Importantly, the phenomenon of SAN reentry was not observed in control dogs. Histological analysis revealed that these arrhythmias required intranodal fibrotic strands, which were not present in healthy hearts, indicating a critical role of a structural substrate for SAN macro- and microreentry.[25,58]

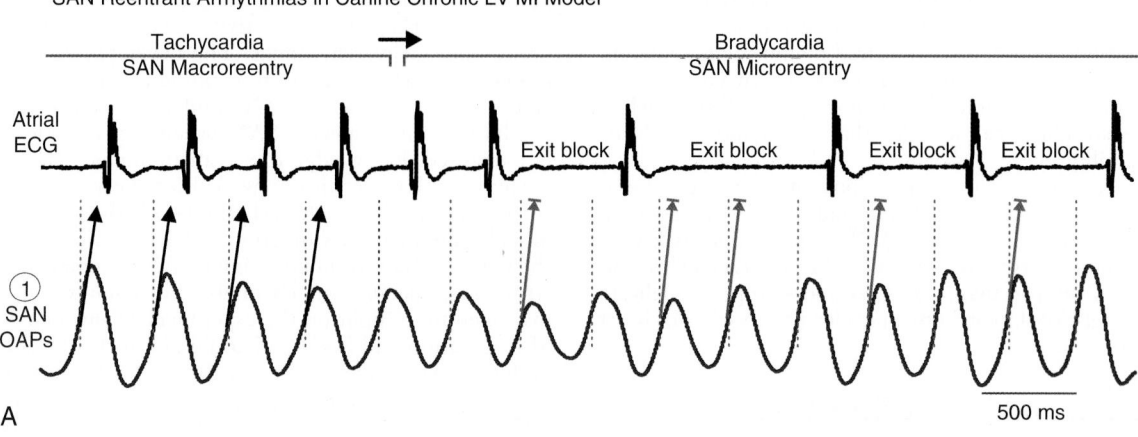

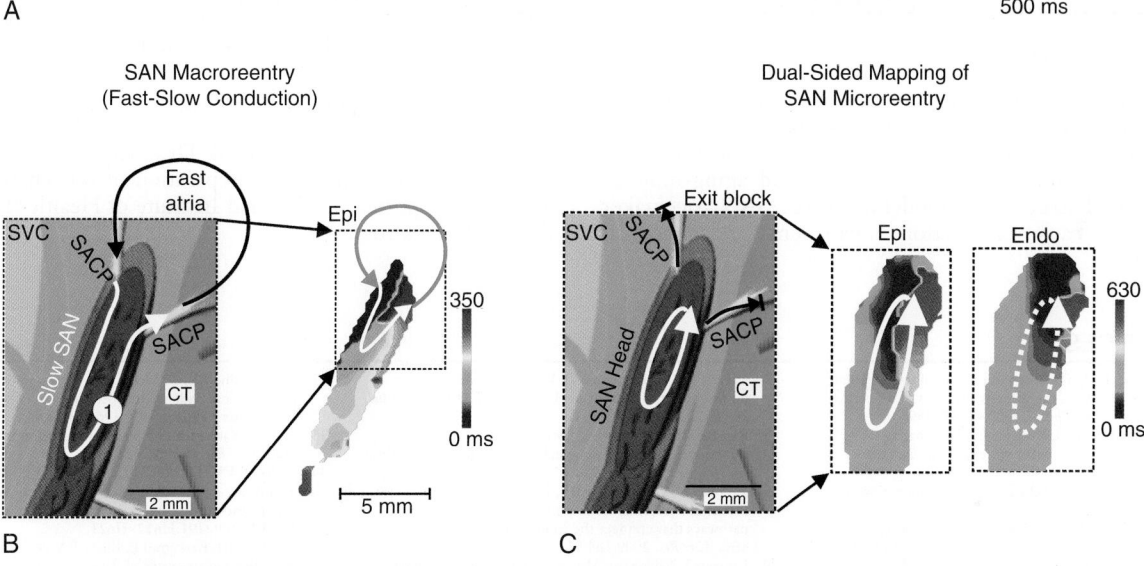

FIGURE 28.7 Sinoatrial node (*SAN*) reentry unmasked by optical mapping. (A) Atrial electrocardiogram (*ECG*) and SAN optical action potentials (*OAPs*) show tachycardia and bradycardia because of SAN macro- and microreentry, respectively. (B) The SAN model (*left*) and epicardial optical activation map (*right*) of fast-slow SAN macroreentry in a canine model of chronic left ventricular myocardial infarction (*LV MI*). (C) The SAN model (*left*) and dual-sided optical activation maps (*right*) of SAN microreentry within SAN and exit block in sinoatrial conduction pathways (SACPs). Microreentry in this case was only visualized from the epicardium due to the three-dimensional intramural structure of SAN. *CT*, Crista terminalis; *Endo*, endocardium; *Epi*, epicardium; *SVC*, superior vena cava. ([A] and [B] Data modified from Glukhov AV, Hage LT, Hansen BJ, et al. Sinoatrial node reentry in a canine chronic left ventricular infarct model: role of intranodal fibrosis and heterogeneity of refractoriness. *Circ Arrhythm Electrophysiol.* 2013;6:984-994. [C] Data modified from Lou Q, Hansen BJ, Fedorenko O, et al. Upregulation of adenosine A1 receptors facilitates sinoatrial node dysfunction in chronic canine heart failure by exacerbating nodal conduction abnormalities revealed by novel dual-sided intramural optical mapping. *Circulation.* 2014;130:315-324.)

Sinoatrial Node Conduction Impairments and Sinoatrial Node Dysfunction

Conduction impairments in the different compartments of the SAN pacemaker complex could lead to a variety of heart rhythm disturbances and SND. SND is conceptualized as a spectrum of arrhythmias, including bradycardia, sinus pauses/arrest, exit block, tachy–brady syndrome, and SAN reentrant arrhythmias.[43,65,66] Importantly, patients with SND usually exhibit combined abnormalities in SAN automaticity and conduction.[60] Repetitive SAN exit block seems to play a major role in causing long atrial pauses after the termination of atrial tachyarrhythmia in patients with preserved anterograde SAN conduction during spontaneous SR (see Fig. 28.6A). Overdrive suppression of sinus node automaticity may also contribute to the long pause. However, current diagnostic methods cannot always distinguish between depressions of SAN automaticity and conduction and

thus fail to identify the functional–structural cause of the dysfunction unless there are postmortem anatomical evaluations.[66,67]

SND is largely a disease of the elderly, and its incidence increases in an exponential manner with age.[65] SND can be induced by a number of different pathophysiological conditions such as autonomic and hormone imbalances, genetic mutations, drug side effects, SAN ischemia, inflammatory conditions, HF, and AF.[25,43,68,69] The degenerative loss of SAN pacemaker cells and their replacement with fibrosis tissue is frequently evident upon pathological examination of specimens from aged patients with SND.[67] Moreover, recent SND animal models[25,44,70,71] found upregulated fibrosis in the dysfunctional SAN pacemaker complex.

Upregulated interstitial fibrosis may lead to disruption of the continuity of electrically coupled myocytes, which alters the delicate balance between depolarized cells and the resting tissue ahead, thereby disrupting SAN automaticity and slowing conduction, particularly in SACPs, and ultimately leading to exit block (see Fig. 28.6) and/or reentrant arrhythmias (Fig. 28.7). Importantly, SAN impaired by fibrotic remodeling may still generate physiologically adequate pacemaker rhythm, but it would be vulnerable to exit block in the SACPs when exposed to an additional stimulus that may depress SAN or atrial excitability.[25,58]

Moreover, many genetic mutations and disease-induced remodeling of ion channels (HCN4[72] and SCN5A[73]), structural proteins (ankyrin-B[74]), receptors (A1[25]), gap junctions (Cx40[54]), and Ca^{2+} handling proteins[23] may also alter the excitability and conduction of the pacemaker complex and disrupt the delicate source–sink relationship and ultimately lead to a variety of heart rhythm disorders.

Conclusion and Future Directions

The human SAN pacemaker complex has a unique molecular profile and 3D structure that consists of several discrete compartments responsible for the spontaneous generation of electrical impulses (pacemaker clusters) and the delivery of these electrical impulses to the atria (SACP), which allow for robust physiological regulation of SR. Disease- and aging-induced molecular and structural remodeling in the SAN pacemaker complex may cause conduction impairments and abnormal impulse propagation (intranodal conduction block, exit and entrance block, reentrant activity) and thus various types of brady- and tachyarrhythmias. The development of new integrated 3D electroanatomical mapping methodologies that are able to directly measure SAN conduction and link functional results to patient-specific SAN pacemaker complex structure is warranted. Knowledge of a realistic human 3D SAN pacemaker complex is critically needed for the successful targeted treatment of SAN tachyarrhythmias.[50] Moreover, computer models of human SAN function and dysfunction incorporating the realistic 3D intramural human SAN pacemaker and SACP structures, specific ion channels, and connexin distribution may shed more light on the exact mechanisms behind normal SR regulation and SND and could aid in the development of biological pacemakers.[75] Eventually the field may move toward the development of new therapies where diseased areas of the SAN complex (e.g., SACPs impaired by fibrosis) can be defined and selectively treated by gene/cell interventions.

Acknowledgment

We would like to sincerely thank Dr. Avirup Guha for many useful discussions during the preparation of this chapter. This work was supported by National Institute of Health HL115580 (Vadim V. Fedorov).

REFERENCES

1. Keith A, Flack M. The form and nature of the muscular connections between the primary divisions of the vertebrate heart. *J Anat Physiol.* 1907;41:172–189.
2. Boyett MR, Honjo H, Kodama I. The sinoatrial node, a heterogeneous pacemaker structure. *Cardiovasc Res.* 2000;47:658–687.
3. James TN. Anatomy of the human sinus node. *Anat Rec.* 1961;141:109–139.
4. Truex RC, Smythe MQ, Taylor MJ. Reconstruction of the human sinoatrial node. *Anat Rec.* 1967;159:371–378.
5. Chandler NJ, Greener ID, Tellez JO, et al. Molecular architecture of the human sinus node: insights into the function of the cardiac pacemaker. *Circulation.* 2009;119:1562–1575.
6. Li N, Csepe TA, Hansen BJ, et al. Molecular mapping of sinoatrial node HCN channel expression in the human heart. *Circ Arrhythm Electrophysiol.* 2015;8:1219–1227.
7. Boineau JP, Canavan TE, Schuessler RB, et al. Demonstration of a widely distributed atrial pacemaker complex in the human heart. *Circulation.* 1988;77:1221–1237.
8. Fedorov VV, Glukhov AV, Chang R, et al. Optical mapping of the isolated coronary-perfused human sinus node. *J Am Coll Cardiol.* 2010;56:1386–1394.
9. Chandler N, Aslanidi O, Buckley D, et al. Computer three-dimensional anatomical reconstruction of the human sinus node and a novel paranodal area. *Anat Rec (Hoboken).* 2011;294:970–979.
10. Fedorov VV, Chang R, Glukhov AV, et al. Complex interactions between the sinoatrial node and atrium during reentrant arrhythmias in the canine heart. *Circulation.* 2010;122:782–789.
11. Sanchez-Quintana D, Cabrera JA, Farre J, et al. Sinus node revisited in the era of electroanatomical mapping and catheter ablation. *Heart.* 2005;91:189–194.
12. Csepe TA, Zhao J, Hansen BJ, et al. Human sinoatrial node structure: 3D microanatomy of sinoatrial conduction pathways. *Prog Biophys Mol Biol.* 2016;120:164–178.
13. Shiraishi I, Takamatsu T, Minamikawa T, et al. Quantitative histological analysis of the human sinoatrial node during growth and aging. *Circulation.* 1992;85:2176–2184.
14. Csepe TA, Kalyanasundaram A, Hansen BJ, et al. Fibrosis: a structural modulator of sinoatrial node physiology and dysfunction. *Front Physiol.* 2015;6:37.
15. Fedorov VV, Glukhov AV, Chang R. Conduction barriers and pathways of the sinoatrial pacemaker complex: their role in normal rhythm and atrial arrhythmias. *Am J Physiol Heart Circ Physiol.* 2012;302:H1773–H1783.
16. Verkerk AO, Wilders R, van Borren MM, et al. Pacemaker current (I(f)) in the human sinoatrial node. *Eur Heart J.* 2007;28:2472–2478.

17. Lakatta EG, DiFrancesco D. What keeps us ticking: a funny current, a calcium clock, or both? *J Mol Cell Cardiol.* 2009;47:157–170.
18. Bleeker WK, Mackaay AJ, Masson-Pevet M, et al. Functional and morphological organization of the rabbit sinus node. *Circ Res.* 1980;46:11–22.
19. Fedorov VV, Schuessler RB, Hemphill M, et al. Structural and functional evidence for discrete exit pathways that connect the canine sinoatrial node and atria. *Circ Res.* 2009;104:915–923.
20. Kodama I, Nikmaram MR, Boyett MR, et al. Regional differences in the role of the Ca2+ and Na+ currents in pacemaker activity in the sinoatrial node. *Am J Physiol.* 1997;272:H2793–H2806.
21. Boyett MR, Inada S, Yoo S, et al. Connexins in the sinoatrial and atrioventricular nodes. *Adv Cardiol.* 2006;42:175–197.
22. Rohr S, Kucera JP, Fast VG, et al. Paradoxical improvement of impulse conduction in cardiac tissue by partial cellular uncoupling. *Science.* 1997;275:841–844.
23. Dobrzynski H, Anderson RH, Atkinson A, et al. Structure, function and clinical relevance of the cardiac conduction system, including the atrioventricular ring and outflow tract tissues. *Pharmacol Ther.* 2013;139:260–288.
24. Beau SL, Hand DE, Schuessler RB, et al. Relative densities of muscarinic cholinergic and beta-adrenergic receptors in the canine sinoatrial node and their relation to sites of pacemaker activity. *Circ Res.* 1995;77:957–963.
25. Lou Q, Hansen BJ, Fedorenko O, et al. Upregulation of adenosine A1 receptors facilitates sinoatrial node dysfunction in chronic canine heart failure by exacerbating nodal conduction abnormalities revealed by novel dual-sided intramural optical mapping. *Circulation.* 2014;130:315–324.
26. Bromberg BI, Hand DE, Schuessler RB, et al. Primary negativity does not predict dominant pacemaker location: implications for sinoatrial conduction. *Am J Physiol.* 1995;269:H877–H887.
27. Schuessler RB. Abnormal sinus node function in clinical arrhythmias. *J Cardiovasc Electrophysiol.* 2003;14:215–217.
28. Kirchhof CJ, Bonke FI, Allessie MA, et al. The influence of the atrial myocardium on impulse formation in the rabbit sinus node. *Pflugers Arch.* 1987;410:198–203.
29. Jalife J. Mutual entrainment and electrical coupling as mechanisms for synchronous firing of rabbit sino-atrial pace-maker cells. *J Physiol.* 1984;356:221–243.
30. Kucera JP, Rudy Y. Mechanistic insights into very slow conduction in branching cardiac tissue: a model study. *Circ Res.* 2001;89:799–806.
31. Joyner RW, van Capelle FJ. Propagation through electrically coupled cells. How a small SA node drives a large atrium. *Biophys J.* 1986;50:1157–1164.

32. De Carvalho AP, de Mello WC, Hoffman BF. Electrophysiological evidence for specialized fiber types in rabbit atrium. *Am J Physiol.* 1959;196:483–488.
33. Sano T, Yamagishi S. Spread of excitation from the sinus node. *Circ Res.* 1965;16:423–430.
34. Fedorov VV, Hucker WJ, Dobrzynski H, et al. Postganglionic nerve stimulation induces temporal inhibition of excitability in the rabbit sinoatrial node. *Am J Physiol.* 2006;291:H612–H623.
35. Hariman RJ, Krongrad E, Boxer RA, et al. Methods for recording electrograms of the sinoatrial node during cardiac surgery in man. *Circulation.* 1980;61:1024–1029.
36. Gomes JA, Kang PS, El Sherif N. The sinus node electrogram in patients with and without sick sinus syndrome: techniques and correlation between directly measured and indirectly estimated sinoatrial conduction time. *Circulation.* 1982;66:864–873.
37. Asseman P, Berzin B, Desry D, et al. Persistent sinus nodal electrograms during abnormally prolonged postpacing atrial pauses in sick sinus syndrome in humans: sinoatrial block vs overdrive suppression. *Circulation.* 1983;68:33–41.
38. Reiffel JA, Kuehnert MJ. Electrophysiological testing of sinus node function: diagnostic and prognostic application-including updated information from sinus node electrograms. *Pacing Clin Electrophysiol.* 1994;17:349–365.
39. Gomes JA, Winters SL. The origins of the sinus node pacemaker complex in man: demonstration of dominant and subsidiary foci. *J Am Coll Cardiol.* 1987;9:45–52.
40. Macianskiene R, Martisiene I, Navalinskas A, et al. Evaluation of excitation propagation in the rabbit heart: optical mapping and transmural microelectrode recordings. *PLoS One.* 2015;10:e0123050.
41. Lou Q, Glukhov AV, Hansen B, et al. Tachy-brady arrhythmias: the critical role of adenosine-induced sinoatrial conduction block in post-tachycardia pauses. *Heart Rhythm.* 2013;10:110–118.
42. Stiles MK, Brooks AG, Roberts-Thomson KC, et al. High-density mapping of the sinus node in humans: role of preferential pathways and the effect of remodeling. *J Cardiovasc Electrophysiol.* 2010;21:532–539.
43. Sanders P, Morton JB, Kistler PM, et al. Electrophysiological and electroanatomic characterization of the atria in sinus node disease: evidence of diffuse atrial remodeling. *Circulation.* 2004;109:1514–1522.
44. Glukhov AV, Kalyanasundaram A, Lou Q, et al. Calsequestrin 2 deletion causes sinoatrial node dysfunction and atrial arrhythmias associated with altered sarcoplasmic reticulum calcium cycling and degenerative fibrosis within the mouse atrial pacemaker complex. *Eur Heart J.* 2015;36:686–697.
45. Fedorov VV, Ambrosi CM, Kostecki G, et al. Anatomic localization and autonomic modulation of AV junctional rhythm in failing human hearts. *Circ Arrhythm Electrophysiol.* 2011;4:515–525.

46. Cosio FG, Martin-Penato A, Pastor A, et al. Atrial activation mapping in sinus rhythm in the clinical electrophysiology laboratory: observations during Bachmann's bundle block. *J Cardiovasc Electrophysiol.* 2004;15:524–531.

47. Joung B, Hwang HJ, Pak HN, et al. Abnormal response of superior sinoatrial node to sympathetic stimulation is a characteristic finding in patients with atrial fibrillation and symptomatic bradycardia. *Circ Arrhythm Electrophysiol.* 2011;4:799–807.

48. Schuessler RB, Boineau JP, Wylds AC, et al. Effect of canine cardiac nerves on heart rate, rhythm, and pacemaker location. *Am J Physiol.* 1986;250:H630–H644.

49. Belardinelli L, Giles WR, West A. Ionic mechanisms of adenosine actions in pacemaker cells from rabbit heart. *J Physiol.* 1988;405:615–633.

50. Jacobson JT, Kraus A, Lee R, et al. Epicardial/endocardial sinus node ablation after failed endocardial ablation for the treatment of inappropriate sinus tachycardia. *J Cardiovasc Electrophysiol.* 2014;25:236–241.

51. Kirchhof CJ, Allessie MA. Sinus node automaticity during atrial fibrillation in isolated rabbit hearts [see comments]. *Circulation.* 1992;86:263–271.

52. Prystowsky EN, Grant AO, Wallace AG, et al. An analysis of the effects of acetylcholine on conduction and refractoriness in the rabbit sinus node. *Circ Res.* 1979;44:112–120.

53. Mandapati R, Skanes A, Chen J, et al. Stable microreentrant sources as a mechanism of atrial fibrillation in the isolated sheep heart. *Circulation.* 2000;101:194–199.

54. Bagwe S, Berenfeld O, Vaidya D, et al. Altered right atrial excitation and propagation in connexin40 knockout mice. *Circulation.* 2005;112:2245–2253.

55. West GA, Belardinelli L. Sinus slowing and pacemaker shift caused by adenosine in rabbit SA node. *Pflugers Arch.* 1985;403:66–74.

56. Zaza A, Rocchetti M, DiFrancesco D. Modulation of the hyperpolarization-activated current (I(f)) by adenosine in rabbit sinoatrial myocytes. *Circulation.* 1996;94:734–741.

57. Vinogradova TM, Fedorov VV, Yuzyuk TN, et al. Local cholinergic suppression of pacemaker activity in the rabbit sinoatrial node. *J Cardiovasc Pharmacol.* 1998;32:413–424.

58. Glukhov AV, Hage LT, Hansen BJ, et al. Sinoatrial node reentry in a canine chronic left ventricular infarct model: role of intranodal fibrosis and heterogeneity of refractoriness. *Circ Arrhythm Electrophysiol.* 2013;6:984–994.

59. Watanabe EI, Honjo H, Boyett MR, et al. Inactivation of the calcium current is involved in overdrive suppression of rabbit sinoatrial node cells. *Am J Physiol.* 1996;271:H2097–H2107.

60. Wu DL, Yeh SJ, Lin FC, et al. Sinus automaticity and sinoatrial conduction in severe symptomatic sick sinus syndrome. *J Am Coll Cardiol.* 1992;19:355–364.

61. Moss AJ, Davis RJ. Brady-Tachy syndrome. *Prog Cardiovasc Dis.* 1974;16:439–454.

62. Yeh SJ, Lin FC, Wu D. Complete sinoatrial block in two patients with bradycardia-tachycardia syndrome. *J Am Coll Cardiol.* 1987;9:1184–1188.

63. Goya M, Iesaka Y, Takahashi A, et al. Radiofrequency catheter ablation for sinoatrial node reentrant tachycardia: electrophysiologic features of ablation sites. *Jpn Circ J.* 1999;63:177–183.

64. Gomes JA, Hariman RJ, Kang PS, et al. Sustained symptomatic sinus node reentrant tachycardia: incidence, clinical significance, electrophysiologic observations and the effects of antiarrhythmic agents. *J Am Coll Cardiol.* 1985;5:45–57.

65. Jensen PN, Gronroos NN, Chen LY, et al. Incidence of and risk factors for sick sinus syndrome in the general population. *J Am Coll Cardiol.* 2014;64:531–538.

66. Mandel WJ, Jordan JL, Karagueuzian HS. Disorders of sinus function. *Curr Treat Options Cardiovasc Med.* 1999;1:179–186.

67. Thery C, Gosselin B, Lekieffre J, et al. Pathology of sinoatrial node. Correlations with electrocardiographic findings in 111 patients. *Am Heart J.* 1977;93:735–740.

68. Zicha S, Fernandez-Velasco M, Lonardo G, et al. Sinus node dysfunction and hyperpolarization-activated (HCN) channel subunit remodeling in a canine heart failure model. *Cardiovasc Res.* 2005;66:472–481.

69. Yeh YH, Burstein B, Qi XY, et al. Funny current downregulation and sinus node dysfunction associated with atrial tachyarrhythmia: a molecular basis for tachycardia-bradycardia syndrome. *Circulation.* 2009;119:1576–1585.

70. Hao X, Zhang Y, Zhang X, et al. TGF-beta1-mediated fibrosis and ion channel remodeling are key mechanisms in producing the sinus node dysfunction associated with SCN5A deficiency and aging. *Circ Arrhythm Electrophysiol.* 2011;4:397–406.

71. Swaminathan PD, Purohit A, Soni S, et al. Oxidized CaMKII causes cardiac sinus node dysfunction in mice. *J Clin Invest.* 2011;121:3277–3288.

72. Schweizer PA, Schroter J, Greiner S, et al. The symptom complex of familial sinus node dysfunction and myocardial noncompaction is associated with mutations in the HCN4 channel. *J Am Coll Cardiol.* 2014;64:757–767.

73. Benson DW, Wang DW, Dyment M, et al. Congenital sick sinus syndrome caused by recessive mutations in the cardiac sodium channel gene (SCN5A). *J Clin Invest.* 2003;112:1019–1028.

74. Le SS, Bhasin N, Vieyres C, et al. Dysfunction in ankyrin-B-dependent ion channel and transporter targeting causes human sinus node disease. *Proc Natl Acad Sci U S A.* 2008;105:15617–15622.

75. Rosen MR. Gene therapy and biological pacing. *N Engl J Med.* 2014 September 18;371:1158–1159.

29 Cell Biology of the Specialized Cardiac Conduction System

David S. Park and Glenn I. Fishman

The cardiac conduction system (CCS) consists of the impulse generating but slowly conducting sinoatrial and atrioventricular nodes (SAN and AVN, respectively) and the rapidly conducting ventricular conduction system (VCS). The SAN is the dominant pacemaker and is located at the junction between the superior vena cava (SVC) and the right atrium (RA). Cardiac impulses originating from the SAN rapidly propagate throughout the pectinated atrial myocardium (PAM) resulting in synchronous contraction of the atrial chambers. Upon reaching the AVN, which is located within the triangle of Koch in the low RA, the cardiac impulse slows, giving the ventricles adequate time to fill. As the cardiac impulse enters the VCS, which consists of the His bundle, bundle branches, and the Purkinje fiber network (PFN), conduction accelerates and enables synchronized ventricular chamber contraction. The His bundle and bundle branches are ensheathed in fibrous insulation; therefore only the PFN is coupled to the ventricular myocardium in a more apical location. This configuration allows for apex-to-base ventricular activation that optimizes blood propulsion toward the aorta and pulmonary artery. Therefore the CCS initiates each heartbeat, synchronizes atrial and ventricular chamber contraction, and optimizes the vector of myocardial contraction to maximize cardiac output.

The framework of the CCS is laid down early during heart development. Paff and associates[1] noted that the chick electrocardiogram (ECG) converts from a sinusoidal waveform to the mature configuration before identifiable components of the CCS are formed (Fig. 29.1).[1] They also noted that atrioventricular (AV) block was achievable with digitalis at the 18-somite stage before a discernible PR interval is evident, suggesting that the AVN primordium develops with the early heart tube (see Fig. 29.1B).[1] After the 18-somite stage, cardiac chamber formation initiates, and the ECG begins to manifest evidence of fast conduction, as demonstrated by the presence of high-frequency P-waves and QRS complexes (see Fig. 29.1C). The evolution of the chick ECG suggests that the slowly conducting nodal elements are present in the early-looped heart and that the fast conducting elements are incorporated during chamber formation. It is therefore the interposition of the slowly conducting AV canal (AVC) myocardium between the rapidly conducting atrial and ventricular chamber myocardium that generates the mature ECG configuration. The rapidly conducting components are enriched in high-conductance gap junction proteins, Connexin40 (Cx40, encoded by *Gja5*) and Cx43 (encoded by *Gja1*), and in the α-subunit of the cardiac sodium channel, $Na_V1.5$ (encoded by *Scn5a*); the slowly conducting SAN and AVN express low-conductance gap junction proteins, Cx30.2 (encoded by *Gjd3*)

and Cx45 (encoded by *Gja7*), express little to no $Na_V1.5$.[2] How these electrophysiologically distinct regions are specified and what defines the boundaries between slow and fast conduction have been the focus of intense research over the past 50 years. In this chapter, we will discuss the developmental origins of the CCS and the transcriptional networks that govern its formation.

Histological Analysis of the Developing Mammalian Cardiac Conduction System

Viragh and Challice performed histological analysis of the developing CCS in mouse embryos ranging from 8 to 12 days postcoitum (E8–E12). Conduction cells were distinguished from working cardiomyocytes by the following characteristics: (1) periodic acid–Schiff (PAS)–positive staining, (2) poorly organized contractile apparatus, (3) enriched glycogen content, and (4) reduced number of T-tubules. Using these features, the temporospatial distribution of conduction cells was then tracked during cardiac development.[3–5]

At E9 the origin of contraction was noted to be in the right sinus horn well before the appearance of the SAN primordium.[5] Within the dorsolateral wall of the sinus horns, loose mesenchymal cells were noted to transform into the early sinus musculature, which covers the sinus side of the sinoatrial venous valves. This aggregation of early sinus muscle tissue was the presumed site of SAN development. The SAN primordium was recognizable at E11 in the medioanterior wall of the right SVC within the early sinus muscle. A left-sided SAN developed simultaneously in the medioanterior region of the left common cardinal vein, but ultimately resorbed and incorporated into the wall of the left atrium.[5]

The SAN and AV conduction systems develop simultaneously. At E9–10, the AVC is a well-defined constriction, with the inner cell layer making numerous interconnections with the trabecular compartment, which is the source of the VCS.[3,4] At E11, the primordium of the AVN was identified as a PAS+ cell cluster in the inner dorsal AVC. These PAS+ AVC cells were contiguous with the crest of the developing interventricular (IV) septum, positioning the AV nodal anlage in direct communication with the primordial His bundle and bundle branches. During this time, the outer cell layer of the AVC was undergoing apoptosis. In the trabecular region, glycogen-rich, PAS+ cells were seen immediately subjacent to the endocardium; these nascent Purkinje cells formed extensive connections with the developing bundle branches.[3,4] Consequently, all components of the AV conduction system were in contact with each other throughout cardiogenesis.

The work of Viragh and Challice demonstrated that conduction system development is inextricably linked to cardiogenesis. Yet, significant questions remained regarding the cellular origins of the conduction system, the mechanism by which the pool of conduction cells expands, and the factors that dictate CCS specification and patterning.

Cellular Origins of the Cardiac Conduction System

The neuronal qualities of the CCS led many to believe that its cellular origins were from neural crest derivatives. However, lineage-tracing studies in the chick and mouse have demonstrated that all conductive components of the CCS are myocardial in origin.[6–11]

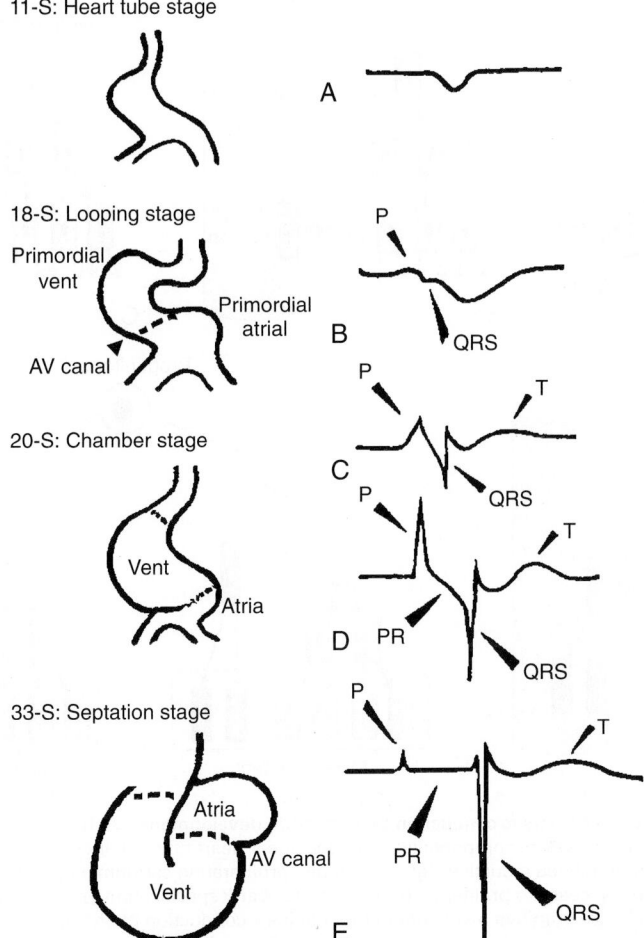

FIGURE 29.1 Schematic of chick heart development *(left panels)* with corresponding electrocardiograms at different somite stages: (A) 11. (B) 18. (C and D) 20. (E) 33. *AV,* Atrioventricular. (From Paff GH, Boucek RJ, Harrell TC. Observations on the development of the electrocardiogram. *Anat Rec.* 1968;160:575-582.)

Models of Cardiac Conduction System Development

The prevailing models of conduction system development are: (1) the ring model,[12] (2) the inductive recruitment or ingrowth model,[6] (3) the early specification or outgrowth model,[13] and (4) the biphasic model[8] (Fig. 29.2). The ring model was based on early observations that the specialized conduction system formed within four constriction points in the D-looped heart (see Fig. 29.2A).[12] Four rings were noted to form from the venous pole to the arterial pole: sinoatrial (SA) ring, atrioventricular (AV) ring, primary (P) ring, and ventriculoarterial (VA) ring.[14,15] The ring hypothesis, which proposed a preexisting template for ring formation in the linear heart tube, has largely been discredited. It is now known that the linear heart tube is composed of clonally related myocardial cells from the first heart field.[16]

Cheng and associates[6] proposed the recruitment model or "ingrowth model" based on several observations noted during chick VCS development (see Fig. 29.2B). First, the proliferative capacity of developing VCS components was found to be significantly lower than that of working myocytes. Second, lineage-tracing studies showed that individually labeled myocyte clones gave rise to both conduction cells and working myocytes. Third, cell birth dating experiments demonstrated that new conductive cells were added to the developing His bundle in lamellar fashion. These observations led the authors to conclude that the specialized conduction system expands

through a process of inductive recruitment of neighboring myocytes.[6] However, what constituted the early framework upon which new conduction cells were added or the nature of the molecular signal used for inductive recruitment was not speculated upon.

The early specification model, or outgrowth model, states that conduction cells expand from a progenitor pool that retains its specialized conduction phenotype (see Fig. 29.2C).[13,18] The conduction gene programming is retained by the expression of transcriptional repressors that suppress a working myocardial phenotype, which is the default pathway. In support of this hypothesis, persistent expression of repressive transcription factors, such as *Tbx2*, *Tbx3*, muscle segment homeobox 2 (*Msx2*), and inhibitor of differentiation 2 (*Id2*), has been identified within primordial conduction regions.[13,18,19] *Tbx3* is expressed as a continuous band linking the SAN and AVN, and the proximal VCS.[13] Heterologous expression of *Tbx2* or *Tbx3* is able to suppress chamber-type myocardial genes (*Nppa*, encoding ANF) and high-conductance gap junction proteins (Cx43 and Cx40) and in the case of TBX3, to elicit ectopic pacemaker formation.[13,18–20] Consistent with these findings, *Tbx3* and Cx43 exhibit complementary expression patterns in the developing heart.[13]

Lastly, a biphasic model of conduction system development has been proposed (see Fig. 29.2D).[8] In this model, once conduction cells are specified from myocardial precursors, they retain the capacity to undergo limited rounds of cell division. Analysis of labeled myocyte clones revealed two classes of conduction

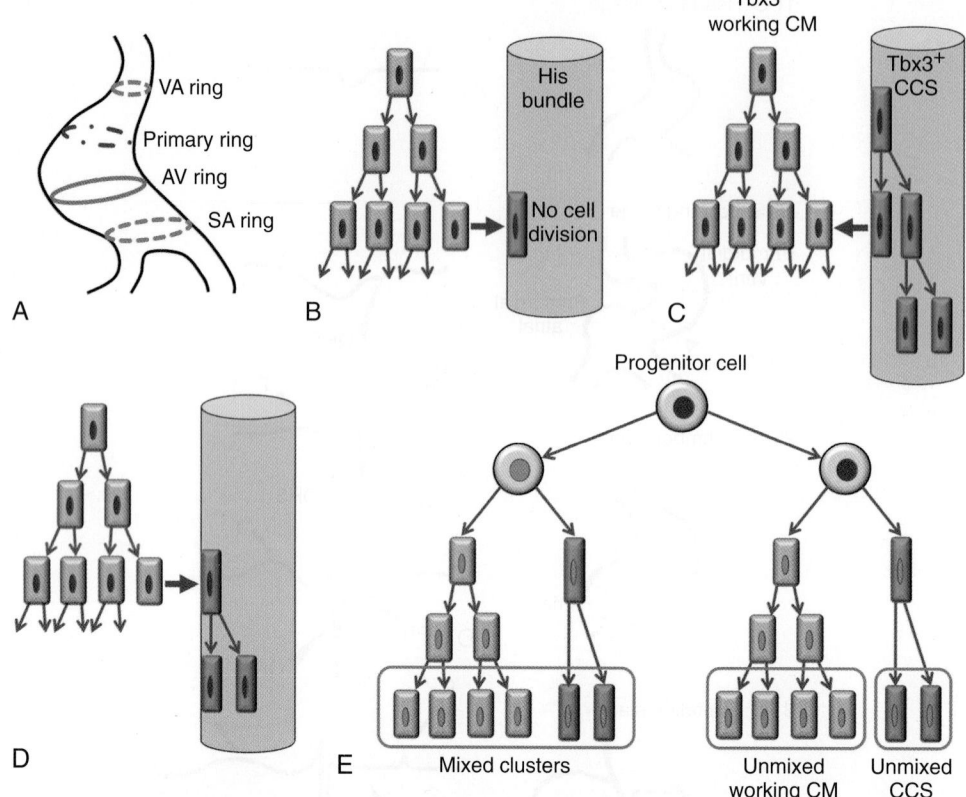

FIGURE 29.2 Models of cardiac conduction system (CCS) development. (A) Ring model. Prespecification of conduction system components within the linear heart tube. (B) Inductive recruitment or ingrowth model. Undefined inductive signals "recruit" proliferating cardiomyocytes (CM) to a conduction lineage and then cease to proliferate (*red arrow*). (C) Early specification or outgrowth model. Tbx3+ CCS cells expand from primitive myocardium that retains a conduction phenotype. Loss of Tbx3 (or Tbx2) expression results in a phenotypic change from a CCS cell to a working cardiomyocyte, the default pathway (*red arrow*). (D) The biphasic model incorporates both the ingrowth and outgrowth models. (E) Retrospective clonal analysis of LacZ-labeled, cardiomyocyte clones (*blue nuclei*). Mixed clusters of conduction and working cardiomyocytes are consistent with a common myocardial progenitor. Unmixed clusters of CCS-only cells demonstrate the potential for limited rounds of cell proliferation. *AV*, Atrioventricular; *SA*, sinoatrial; *VA*, ventriculoarterial. (Modified from Miquerol L, Beyer S, Kelly RG. Establishment of the mouse ventricular conduction system. *Cardiovasc Res.* 2011;91:232-242.)

clusters, mixed and unmixed (see Fig. 29.2E). The mixed clusters represented single myocyte clones that gave rise to both conductive and working myocytes. The unmixed clones were composed exclusively of either working myocytes or conduction myocytes, but not both. Conduction-only, unmixed clones were identified throughout the central and peripheral VCS, indicating that once specified, all components of the conduction system are capable of approximately four to five rounds of cell division. Based on these findings, the authors concluded that mammalian VCS development appears to utilize both ingrowth and outgrowth modes of expansion.[8] However, these findings are not incompatible with the early specification/outgrowth model, as mixed clusters may represent conduction cells that have lost Tbx2/Tbx3 expression and have now defaulted to the chamber pathway.

Molecular Markers of the Cardiac Conduction System

Visualization of the developing CCS has been greatly enhanced by the development of conduction system reporter mice (Table 29.1[21-45]). Each reporter mouse delineates different components of the CCS at various developmental time points using LacZ, green fluorescent protein (GFP), or Cre transgenes. The CCS-LacZ,[46] Contactin-2-EGFP (Cntn2-EGFP),[47] and Cx40-eGFP[48] mouse lines are representative examples of well-established markers of the specialized conduction system. (Fig. 29.3A–C). Using the CCS-LacZ and Cntn2-EGFP reporter lines, novel regulators of Purkinje cell specification and function have been identified, such as the transcription factor ETV1.[49] The *Etv1* nuclear-LacZ (*Etv1*[nlz])[49a] reporter gene is expressed throughout the CCS but has the highest levels of expression in regions of rapid conduction, namely the pectinated atrial myocardium and the trabeculated ventricular myocardium, which matures into the VCS[49] (Fig. 29.3D). Etv1-nlz reporter demonstrates overlapping expression with Cntn2-EGFP in Purkinje cells throughout the VCS[49] (Fig. 29.3E). While some CCS reporters delineate the entire conduction system, others are more restricted in their expression pattern. All CCS reporter lines have some degree of expression outside of the specialized conduction system, such as in the atria, coronary arteries, cardiac nerves, valves, or extracardiac sites.

Transcription Factor Regulatory Networks

A rich hierarchy of gene networks dictates the specification and patterning of CCS components (Fig. 29.4). Unifying all of these networks is the balance struck between prochamber myocardial programming versus antichamber programming. As mentioned previously, the T-box transcription factors dictate much of this

TABLE 29.1 Mouse models of the cardiac conduction system

MOUSE	GENETIC MANIPULATION	DEVELOPMENTAL STAGES	CARDIAC CONDUCTION SYSTEM					OTHER CARDIAC EXPRESSION
			SAN	AVN	HB	BB	PFN	
minK-CreERT2[21,22]	Transgenic	E9.5-adult	−	+	+	+	+	A, V, and IVS
Cx40-CreERT2[23]	Knockin	E9.5-adult	−	±	+	+	+	A, EC, and CA
HCN4-CreERT2[24–26]	Knockin	E6.5-adult	+	+	+	+	+	LV and EC
Hcn4-CreERT2[27]	Transgenic	E7.5-adult	+	+	+	+	+	LV and EC
Tbx2-Cre[28]	Knockin	E9.5-adult	−	+	−	−	−	AVC
cGATA6-Cre[29]	Transgenic	E8.5-neonates	−	+	+	−	−	A and LV
Tbx3-Cre[30]	Knockin	E11.5-adult	+	+	+	−	−	No
Tbx18-Cre[26,28]	Knockin	E10.5-adult	+	−	−	−	−	EPI, EPDCs, and SH
Isl1-Cre[26,31]	Knockin	E8.5-adult	+	−	−	RBB	RPF	OFT, RV, and A
Shox2-Cre[32]	Knockin	E9.0-adult	+	−	−	−	−	No
Shox2-LacZ[32]	Knockin	E9.5-12.5	+	−	−	−	−	IVS
HCN4-nEGFP[26,31]	Knockin	E7.5-adult	+	+	+	+	+	LV (~E12.5) and EC
HCN4-nLacZ[26]	Knockin	E7.5-adult	+	+	+	+	+	LV (~E12.5), EC
cGATA6-lacZ[29]	Transgenic	E7.5-neonates	−	+	+	−	−	A and LV
Troponin I-lacZ[33]	Transgenic	E9.5-adult	−	+	−	−	−	A and ring
Des1-nLacZ[34]	Transgenic	E8-E18	−	−	−	+	+	No
HF-1b-LacZ[35]	Knockin	E8.5-adult	−	+	+	+	+	RA
CCS-lacZ[46]	Transgenic	All stages	±	+	+	+	+	RA and VV
mink-lacZ[21,22]	Knockin	E8.5-adult	−	+	+	+	+	OFT, IVS, AS, and VV
HOP-lacZ[36]	Knockin	E16.5-adult	−	+	+	+	+	A and V
Cntn2-lacZ[47]	Knockin	Adult	+	+	+	+	+	No
Cntn2-GFP[47]	Transgenic	Adult	+	+	+	+	+	No
Popdc1-LacZ[37]	Knockin	Adult	+	?	+	+	−	CMC
Popdc2-LacZ[37]	Knockin	Adult	+	+	+	+	−	CMC
Cx40-EGFP[48]	Knockin	E9.5-adult	−	±	+	+	+	EC and A
Cx45-LacZ[38,39]	Knockin	E9.5-adult	+	+	+	+	−	A and V
Cx30-LacZ[40]	Knockin	Adult	+	+	+	+	−	No
Cx30.2-LacZ[41,38]	Knockin	E10.5-adult	+	+	+	+	+?	No
Tbx3-AVC-GFP[42]	Transgenic	E9.5-adult	−	+	−	−	−	AVC
Tbx18-GFP[43]	Knockin	E10.5-?	+	−	−	−	−	EPI, EPDCs, and SH
ISL1-nLacZ[31]	Knockin	E9.5-adult	+	−	−	−	−	OFT, RV, and A
Irx3-tauLacZ[44]	Knockin	E10-adult	−	−	+	+	+	No
mlrx3-EGFP[44]	Transgenic	E14.5-P3	−	−	+	+	+	No
Id2-LacZ[45]	Transgenic	Transient E14.5	−	−	+	+	−	No
Etv1-nlz[49,49a]	Knockin	E9-adult	−	+	+	+	+	A, VV, Val

A, Atria; *AS*, atrial septum; *AVC*, atrioventricular canal; *AVN*, atrioventricular node; *BB*, bundle branch; *CA*, coronary artery; *CMC*, cardiomyocyte; *EC*, endothelial cell; *EPDCs*, epicardial-derived cells; *EPI*, epicardium; *HB*, His bundle; *IVS*, interventricular septum; *LV*, left ventricle; *OFT*, outflow tract; *PF*, Purkinje fiber; *RA*, right atria; *RBB*, right bundle branch; *RPF*, right Purkinje fiber; *RV*, right ventricle; *SAN*, sinoatrial node; *SH*, sinus horn; *Val*, valves; *V*, ventricle; *VV*, venous valve.
Modified from Liang X, Evans SM, Sun Y. Insights into cardiac conduction system formation provided by HCN4 expression. *Trends Cardiovasc Med.* 2015;25:1-9.

equilibrium, tilting the scales toward or away from a conduction lineage. The T-box factors can function as transcriptional activators or repressors and are known to be critical regulators of cardiac specification and differentiation.[50] Seven *TBX* family members are expressed in the developing heart, four of which (*TBX1, TBX5, TBX20,* and *TBX3*) have been linked to human congenital heart disease.[51–53] The major cardiac transcriptional activators, TBX5 and TBX20, act in concert with NKX2-5 and GATA4 to drive prochamber myocardial gene expression, such as *Scn5a*/Na$_V$1.5, *Nppa,* and *Gja5*/Cx40.[54–56a] The transcriptional repressors, TBX2, TBX3, and TBX18, compete with TBX5 for NKX2-5 binding to suppress chamber-specific gene expression, thus maintaining a nodal gene expression profile.[13,18,19,30,57]

The delicate balance between TBX activators and repressors and the expression of cofactors, such as NKX2-5, dictates the rich conduction phenotypes seen in the mature CCS. Both *TBX5* and *NKX2-5* have been implicated in inherited disorders of the CCS and are critical determinants of many elements of the slow and fast conduction systems.[45,58–60] Mutations in *TBX5* result in Holt-Oram Syndrome (HOS), an autosomal dominant condition characterized by preaxial radial ray limb deformities and cardiac septation defects.[50] HOS patients manifest variable degrees of CCS dysfunction, including sinus bradycardia and AV block, even in the absence of overt structural heart disease.[50] *NKX2-5* mutations cause nonsyndromic congenital heart disease associated with AV block.[60] Proper CCS development is highly dependent on appropriate gene dosage of both of these factors.[45,59,61,62]

NKX2-5 and TBX5 are broadly expressed beyond the borders of the CCS, and both have a role in specifying working myocyte as well as specialized conduction cell gene programming, suggesting that they function with CCS-restricted cofactors to elicit conduction specification.[54,56] Numerous regulatory feedback and feedforward loops have now been identified in CCS compartments that enhance the specialized conduction phenotype while simultaneously repressing the working myocyte gene profile (see Fig. 29.4). These CCS-restricted cofactors will be discussed in their regional context.

The Sinoatrial Node

The mammalian SAN is a large comma-shaped structure with its head region located at the junction between the right SVC and the atrium and the tail region situated along the crista terminalis.

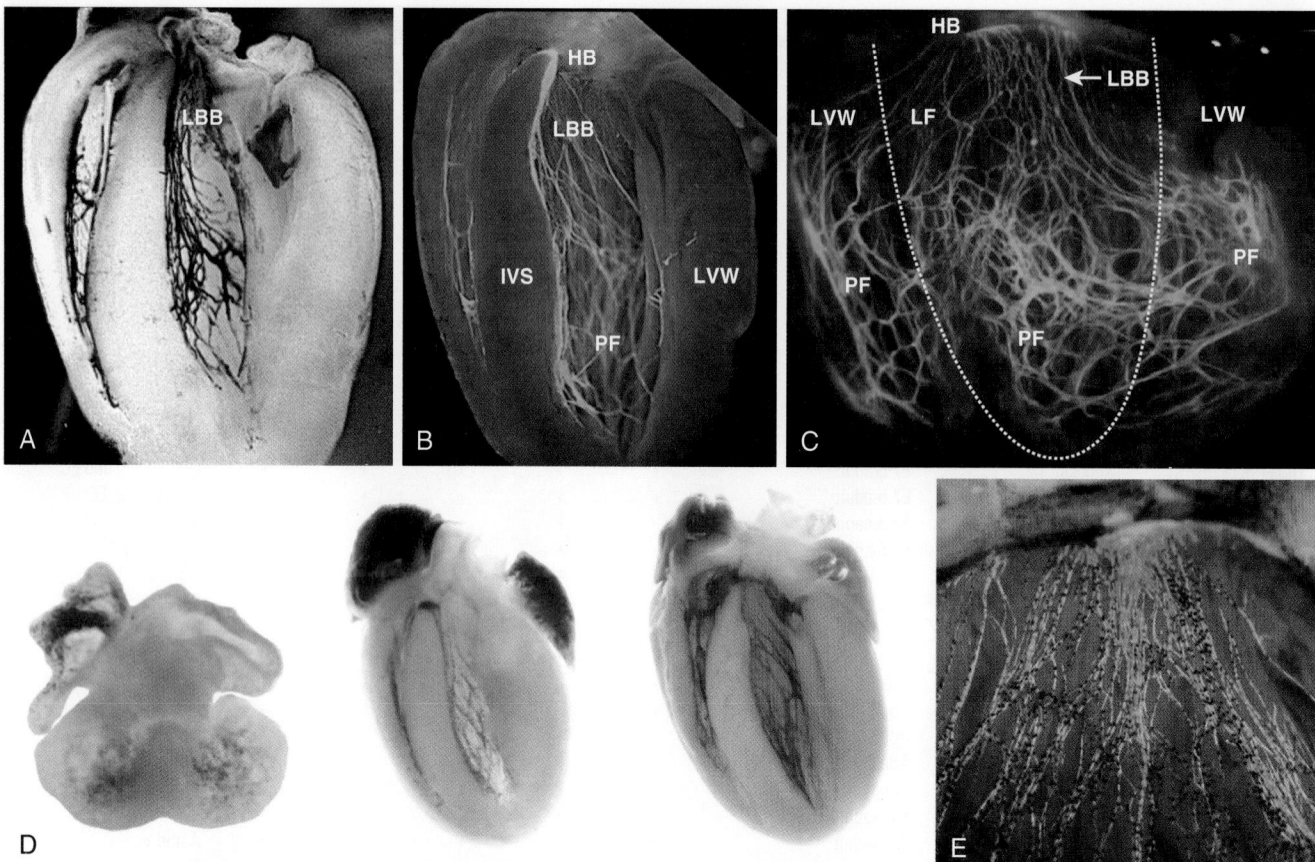

FIGURE 29.3 Cardiac conduction system reporter mice. (A) CCS-LacZ. (B) Contactin2-eGFP (Cntn2-eGFP). (C) Connexin-40-eGFP. (D) *Etv1* nuclear LacZ (*Etv1$^{nlz/+}$*) reporter mice at various stages of development (*left to right*): Embryonic day 12.5, postnatal day 1, and postnatal day 21.[49] (E) Dual conduction system reporter mice: *Etv1$^{nlz/+}$*; Cntn2-eGFP demonstrating overlapping expression in the left bundle branch fascicles.[49] *HB,* His bundle; *IVS,* interventricular septum; *LBB,* left bundle branch; *LF,* left flank of the IVS; *LVW,* left ventricular free wall; *PF,* Purkinje fiber. ([C] From Miquerol L, Meysen S, Mangoni M, et al. Architectural and functional asymmetry of the His-Purkinje system of the murine heart. *Cardiovasc Res.* 2004;63:77-86. [D] From Shekhar A, Lin X, Liu FY, et al. Transcription factor ETV1 is essential for rapid conduction in the heart. *J Clin Invest.* 2016;126:4444-4459. [E] From *J Clin Invest.* 2016;126 [cover image].)

As mentioned previously, the inflow tract and then sinus venosus (SV) serve as the dominant pacemaking regions from E8–E10.5. The SAN becomes morphologically identifiable by E11.5 and assumes the role of primary pacemaker. Automaticity of the SAN is dependent on two interdependent clock mechanisms: the membrane voltage and calcium clocks.[63] A key pacemaker channel of the membrane voltage clock is the hyperpolarization-activated cyclic nucleotide–gated potassium channel HCN4, which generates the funny current (I_f). Components of the calcium clock include the ryanodine receptor (*Ryr2*), the sodium-calcium exchanger (*Ncx*), and the voltage-dependent calcium channel, T-type, alpha-1G subunit (*Cacna1g*). Expression of pacemaker-enriched channels is determined by the unique transcription factor profile of the SAN.

Proper SAN development is dependent on the appropriate temporospatial expression of T-box proteins (*Tbx5, Tbx3,* and *Tbx18*) and homedomain factors (*Shox2* and *Isl1*) (see Fig. 29.4B). The SAN originates from myocardium of the sinus horns, which possesses a unique SV signature (*Shox2$^+$;Tbx3$^+$;Tbx18$^+$; Isl1$^+$; Nkx2-5$^-$*).[64] The head region maintains this SV signature while the tail region loses *Tbx18* expression and weakly upregulates *Nkx2-5.*[43,65] NKX2-5 positively regulates chamber myocardial gene programming, such as *Gja5*/Cx40 and *Nppa*, while negatively regulating the expression of pacemaker genes *Hcn4* and *Tbx3.*[66]

TBX5 expression in the inflow tract is a critical regulator of the SAN signature through its actions on TBX3 and SHOX2.[61,67] Homozygous *Tbx5$^{del/del}$* mice die embryonically at E10.5 due to severe hypoplasia of the sinoatrial region and primitive LV.[55] Mice haploinsufficient for *Tbx5* exhibit significant sinus node dysfunction (SND).[55,59] Gene profiling of *Tbx5* heterozygous hearts has identified *Tbx3* and *Shox2* as significantly downregulated targets, and both factors are reduced in the inflow tract region.[61,67]

Tbx3 is expressed throughout the developing and mature CCS (except in the PFN) and represses chamber-specific programming. Like *Tbx5*, *Tbx3* displays critical dose dependency for proper differentiation and homeostatic maintenance of the conduction system.[68] Analysis of *Tbx3* mutant mice revealed a dose-dependent SAN phenotype with variable degrees of SND and inappropriate expression of chamber-specific genes (*Gja1*/Cx43, *Gja5*/Cx40, *Nppa*, and *Scn5a*) within the SAN region.[30,68] While the overall structure of the SAN was normal, SAN volume was reduced by approximately 45%–60%, although this phenotype was not consistently seen in all *Tbx3* mutants when adjusted for weight.[20,30,43,68] Ectopic overexpression of *Tbx3* in atrial myocardium suppressed chamber-specific genes and upregulated the SAN gene profile (*Hcn4, Gjd3*/Cx30.2, and *Cacna1g*).[30] Taken together, these data suggest that *Tbx3* is not essential for SAN structural formation but is important for establishing and maintaining proper pacemaker gene programming.

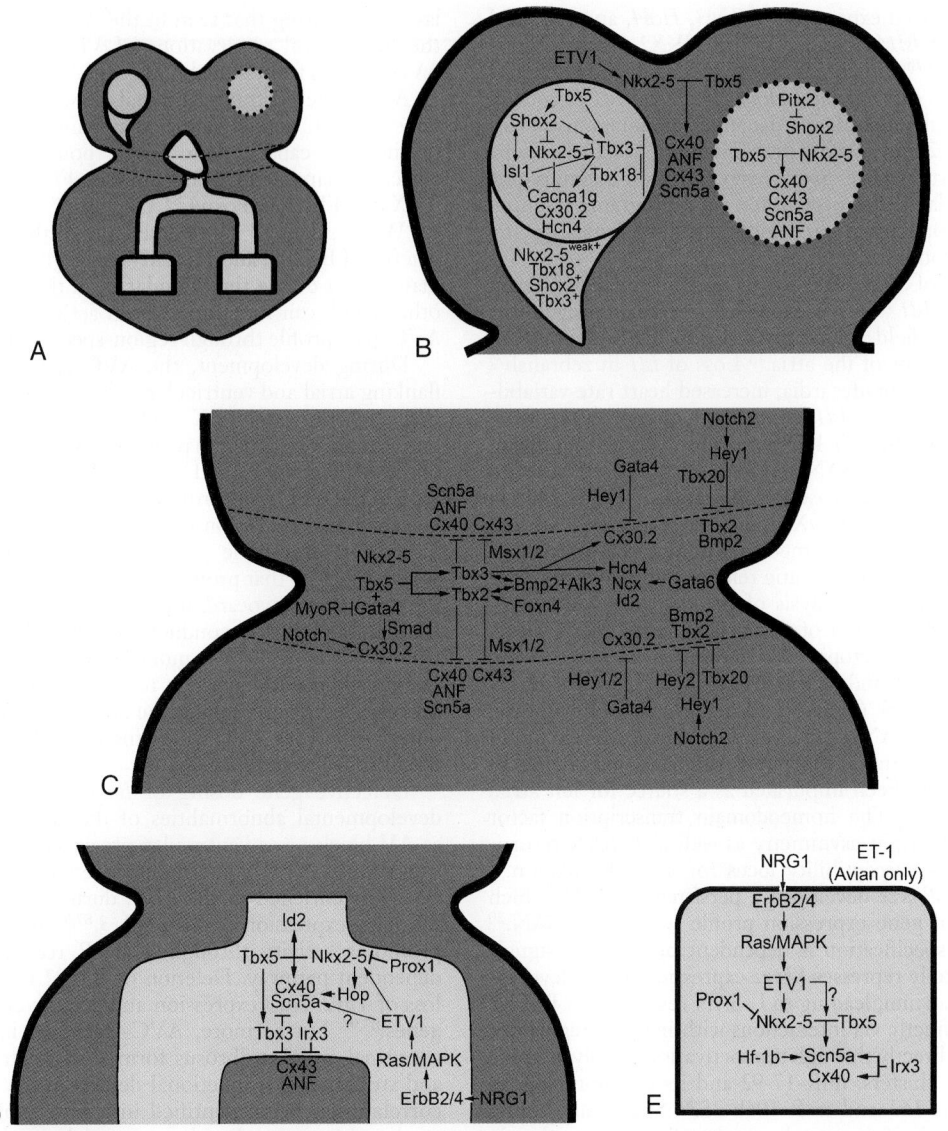

FIGURE 29.4 Transcription factor regulatory networks. (A) Schematic of the cardiac conduction system. (B) Right sinoatrial node (head and tail domains), atrial myocardium, and left sinoatrial node (*stippled circle*). (C) Atrioventricular canal/node region flanked by atrial and ventricular myocardium. (D) His bundle and bundle branches and ventricular myocardium. (E) Purkinje fiber.

Tbx3 expression and transcriptional repressor activity in the SAN is coordinated by Baf250a, a key component of the chromatin-remodeling complex SWI/SNF.[69] SAN-specific knockout of *Arid1a* (encodes Baf250a) under tamoxifen induction resulted in SND.[69] Transcriptome analysis and chromatin immunoprecipitation (ChIP) studies of Baf250a identified *Tbx3* as a direct transcriptional target.[69] Importantly, Baf250a acted coordinately with TBX3 and histone deacetylase 3 (HDAC3) to repress *Nkx2-5* expression within the SAN.[69]

Tbx18 is expressed in the sinus horn myocardium during development and is important for SAN formation. Loss of *Tbx18* resulted in marked reduction in the volume of the SAN head, either due to failure to expand the mesenchymal precursor pool or failure to differentiate into SAN cells.[43] The tail region, on the other hand, was unaffected.[43] Despite this reduction in SAN volume, sinus node function was normal due to residual SAN tail tissue.[43] *Tbx3* and *Tbx18* double heterozygous embryos demonstrated normal SAN development, indicating a lack of interaction on a genetic level. Similar to *Tbx3*, heterologous expression of *Tbx18* led to transcriptional repression of Cx43.[70] Transduced

Tbx18 expression in vivo converted working ventricular myocytes into SAN-like cells based on morphology, automaticity, and epigenetic features.[71]

Shox2 is essential for development of the SAN.[72] Mice deficient in *Shox2* were embryonic lethal due to severe bradycardia in the setting of SAN hypoplasia.[72,73] Evaluation of the *Shox2*[−/−] SAN revealed reduced levels of *Tbx3* and *Hcn4*, indicating a failure of differentiation.[73] Downregulation of *Tbx3* results in ectopic expression of Nkx2-5 and chamber myocardial genes (*Nppa*, *Gja1*/Cx43, and *Gja5*/Cx40) within the SAN head region.[72] Luciferase reporter assays revealed that SHOX2 negatively regulates expression of *Nkx2-5*, a known inhibitor of *Tbx3* and *Hcn4* expression.[20] Thus SHOX2 promotes SAN head development by repressing *Nkx2-5* expression, thereby preventing atrial myocardialization of the SAN head.[73]

The SAN tail represents a distinct region as it expresses both *Shox2* and *Nkx2-5*. Selective deletion of *Shox2* driven by *Nkx2-5*[IRESCre/+] in the tail region was associated with SND and lack of SAN tail structures.[65] At E12.5, the SAN tail in *Nkx2-5*[IRESCre/+]; *Shox*[flox/flox] mice began to exhibit hypoplasia and reduced expression of *Tbx3*, *Hcn4*, and the LIM homeodomain factor *Isl1*.[65] Graded loss of NKX2-5 using *Nkx2-5*[Cre/IRESCre/+];*Shox*[flox/flox] mice was able to rescue the SAN phenotype and reestablish expression of *Hcn4*, *Tbx3*, and *Isl1* to control levels.[65] These results identified a dynamic and antagonistic balance between *Shox2* and *Nkx2-5* in maintaining pacemaker gene programming. Furthermore, *Shox2* overexpression in embryonic stem cells upregulated the pacemaker gene program, resulting in enhanced automaticity in vitro and induced biological pacing under transplant conditions.[74]

Gene profiling of *Shox2* KO RA tissue confirmed significant downregulation of *Isl1*.[75] *Isl1* is expressed in cardiac progenitors of the second heart field, which gives rise to the SAN, outflow tract, RV, and portions of the atria.[76] Loss of *Isl1* in zebrafish[75] and mice[77] resulted in bradycardia, increased heart rate variability, and frequent pauses. An *Isl1* compound hypomorph (*Isl1*[nLacZ/fl:Neo]) and *Hcn4*-restricted *Isl1* KO both demonstrated significant reduction in the size of the SAN and SV, which was attributed to increased apoptosis and decreased proliferation.[77] *Isl1* is a direct transcriptional target of SHOX2, and overexpression of *Isl1* functionally rescued the *Shox2*-mediated bradycardia phenotype in zebrafish, confirming an epistatic relationship between *Shox2* and *Isl1*.[75] Transcriptome analysis of *Isl1*-deficient SAN demonstrated reduced expression of pacemaker genes (*Tbx3*, *Hcn4*, *Hcn1*, and *Cacna1g*) and ectopic expression of atrial genes (*Nppa*, *Gja1*/Cx43, *Gja5*/Cx40, and *Scn5a*).[78]

The left-sided SAN (L-SAN) forms in parallel with the right-sided SAN (R-SAN), but regresses during development and incorporates into the left atrium.[5] Abnormal persistence of L-SAN remnants has been implicated as a source for left atrial arrhythmic triggers.[79] The homeodomain transcription factor *Pitx2c* regulates left-right asymmetry as well as L-SAN resorption[80] and is a key susceptibility locus for atrial fibrillation.[81] Mice deficient in *Pitx2c* developed a persistent L-SAN, which shares an identical gene expression profile with the R-SAN.[20] As such, L-SAN specification is dependent on SHOX2 signaling. PITX2C directly represses *Shox2* expression in the developing left SVC and atrium, leading to L-SAN regression.[79] PITX2 regulates *Shox2* directly via interactions with intronic regulatory elements[79] and indirectly through transactivation of polycistronic microRNA (miR) clusters, miR-17-92 and its two homologous clusters, miR-106a-363 and miR-106b-25.[82] Specifically, miR-17-92 and miR-106b-25 negatively regulate *Shox2* expression in the left superior caval vein and *Tbx3* expression in the left AVC.[82]

Atrioventricular Canal and Atrioventricular Node

The mammalian AVN is a complex, heterogeneous structure that serves as the only conduction pathway between the atria and ventricles. Histological and electrophysiological (EP) evaluation of the AVN revealed three distinct layers termed: (*i*) atrionodal (AN), (*ii*) compact nodal (N), and (*iii*) nodo-His (NH, also known as lower nodal cells).[83] The compact or true nodal region had characteristic nodal action potentials, such as slow upstroke of phase 0, lower peak amplitudes, and diastolic depolarization of phase 4.[83,84] The AN and NH transition regions exhibited hybrid action potential morphologies intermediate to nodal cells and atrial or His bundle myocytes, respectively.[83,84] The AN and NH regions were enriched in $Na_V1.5$, Cx43, and/or Cx40, whereas the N region had little to no $Na_V1.5$ and high levels of Cx45 and Cx30.2, resulting in the different action potential morphologies and conduction velocities.[28,41,83,85]

Lineage tracing studies and differential gene expression analysis indicate that the compact AVN (N) derives from AVC myocardium, while the lower nodal cells (NH) are ventricular in origin.[42,86] In the adult heart, remnants of the AVC persist as rings of myocardial tissue that possess distinct electrophysiological

layers, mirroring that seen in the AVN.[28] These results validate the histological observations of Viragh and Challice that the AVN derives from dorsal AVC cells.[3,4]

A multitiered transcriptional network establishes and maintains the AVC gene signature that maintains slow conduction, low proliferative capacity, and proper boundary formation with the adjacent chamber myocardium (see Fig. 29.4C). BMP2/TBX2/TBX3,[87] TBX5,[88] Foxn4,[88] GATA6,[89] NKX2-5,[62] and canonical Wnt signaling[90,91] are activators of the AVC gene signature, whereas TBX20[92] and Notch2/Hey signaling[93] are negative regulators that define the boundaries of the AVC. GATA4, on the other hand, can function as both activator and repressor of the AVC gene profile through region-specific histone modification.[94]

During development, the AVC can be distinguished from flanking atrial and ventricular myocardium by the enrichment of BMP2, TBX2, and TBX3. This transcriptional signature maintains the slow conduction properties and low proliferative capacity of the AVC.[95] BMP2 and TBX2/TBX3 function in a feedforward loop in the AVC myocardium directing endocardial epithelial-to-mesenchymal transition (EMT) and AV cushion formation.[87,96] Expansion of cardiac jelly displaces the endocardium (which secretes factors that promote Cx40 expression in myocytes) from the underlying myocardium, establishing a secondary mechanism for maintaining slow conduction in the AVC.[97] Paracrine signals from AVC myocytes also induce epicardial cells to undergo EMT and invade the AV junction to create the annulus fibrosus. This process electrically isolates the atria and ventricles, except at the dorsal wall of the AVC where the lower AV nodal cells penetrate the fibrous insulation.

Defective gene dosing of *Bmp2*, *Tbx2*, and *Tbx3* leads to developmental abnormalities of the AVC, which can manifest as AV block or as ventricular preexcitation (i.e., Wolff-Parkinson-White, WPW) due to defective annulus fibrosus formation. BMP2 is enriched in the AVC during development and drives the local expression of *Tbx2*/*Tbx3*.[87,96] BMP2 upregulates *Tbx2* promoter activity through a BMP receptor (ALK3)/SMAD–dependent pathway. Deletion of BMP2 in the AVC resulted in loss of *Tbx2*/*Tbx3* expression and ectopic expression of chamber genes.[87,96] Furthermore, AVC-restricted loss of ALK3 led to abnormal annulus fibrosus formation, ventricular preexcitation, and structural and functional defects in the AVN.[98,99] A human correlate has been identified in a rare familial form of WPW syndrome associated with a microdeletion involving the BMP2 gene.[100]

TBX2 and TBX3 are essential for maintaining the slow conduction phenotype of the AVC/AVN.[13,18,19] *Tbx2* and *Tbx3* are differentially expressed in the AVC, with *Tbx2* more dominant in the left AVC and *Tbx3* more dominant in the right AVC.[101] Evaluation of a *Tbx3* allelic series demonstrated an exquisite dose:phenotype correlation, with diminishing *Tbx3* levels directly correlating with the severity of AV conduction disease and fetal demise.[68] AV block was exclusively seen in the embryos with the lowest *Tbx3* gene dosage. Consistent with its known repressive function, *Tbx3*-deficient embryos showed ectopic expression of chamber genes within the SAN, AVC, AV bundle, and bundle branches.[68,102] Regional deletion of *Tbx3* within the AV bundle primordium or the AVC caused AV block. Therefore *Tbx3* expression is required throughout the multi-tiered AV conduction axis to maintain slow conduction properties in the AVC. Furthermore, conditional deletion of *Tbx3* at an adult time point resulted in AV block, indicating that TBX3 is critical for proper maintenance of the AV conduction axis.[68]

Tbx2 deficiency resulted in embryonic lethality due to defects in AVC differentiation and outflow tract septation.[103] Ectopic expression of chamber-type genes was noted in the AVC of *Tbx2*-deficient hearts, with the left AVC more affected than the right.[101,103] Accordingly, *Tbx2* deficiency had minimal impact on AV node formation, which is predominantly a right-sided structure. However, loss of myocardial *Tbx2* resulted in structural defects in the left annulus fibrosus, resulting in accessory pathway formation and ventricular preexcitation.[101]

Mice lacking both *Tbx2* and *Tbx3* exhibited failure of AVC formation.[96] *Tbx2−/−;Tbx3−/−* hearts showed a lack of AV constriction and cushion formation with a reduction in *Bmp2* levels.[96] Chamber myocardial genes, *Nppa* and *Gja5*/Cx40, were ectopically expressed in the AVC of double KO hearts.[96] In contrast, forced expression of *Tbx2* or *Tbx3* in the chamber myocardium activated myocardial BMP2 signaling and endocardial Notch1 signaling, resulting in ectopic subendocardial cushion formation and EMT.[96] *Tbx3* overexpression also activated *Gja7*/Cx45 and suppressed *Gja5*/Cx40 and *Bmp10* (a major activator of chamber myocardial cell cycling).[96] *Tbx2* overexpression suppressed *Nppa* and *Gja5*/Cx40. Both TBX2 and TBX3 were shown to interact with AVC-enriched MSX1 and MSX2 to negatively regulate Cx43 expression.[19] Therefore the BMP2 and TBX2/TBX3 feed-forward loop ensures proper localization of slow conduction and AV cushion formation within the AVC.

TBX5 is enriched in the AVC during development and is essential for normal development of the AVC/AVN.[61] Mice haploinsufficient for *Tbx5* had significant maturation defects in the AVC and AVN and exhibited first- and second-degree AV block.[55,59] The immature configuration of the AVC/AVN resulted in significant slowing of AV nodal conduction time, as measured by prolonged Atrio-His (A-H) intervals during invasive EP testing.[59]

TBX5 regulates the expression of GATA4 and partners with it to drive the expression Cx30.2 in the AVC by directly interacting with a highly conserved region within the *Gjd3*/Cx30.2 promoter.[58,61] Unlike *Tbx5+/−* mice, which have maturation defects of the AVN, the AVN of *Gata4+/−* mice were structurally normal but had reduced expression of Cx30.2, resulting in PR interval shortening, indicative of loss of slow conduction.[58] The inhibitory beta helix-loop-helix transcription factor MyoR directly repressed the action of GATA4 on the Cx30.2 minimal AVC enhancer.[104] Consistent with these findings, MyoR-null mice had increased expression of Cx30.2 and prolonged AV conduction.[104]

GATA6 has also been shown to be important for proper development of the AVN.[89] Mice with myocardial-specific ablation of the carboxyl zinc-finger domain of GATA6 displayed prolonged conduction through the AVN.[89] Evaluation of *Gata6* mutant mice revealed smaller AV nodes and aberrant cell cycling in AV bundle cells.[89] Furthermore, *Gata6* mutant hearts had reduced expression of genes involved in normal pacemaker function (*Hcn4* and *Ncx*) or conduction system specification (*Id2*).[89]

Foxn4, an upstream regulator of *tbx2b*, was recently identified from a zebra fish mutagenesis screen.[88] *Foxn4* mutants displayed structural and functional defects in the AVC. Several AVC-restricted genes were mislocated, such as *bmp4* and endocardial *notch1b*, whereas *tbx2b* was completely absent from the AVC.[88] Highly conserved Foxn4- and Tbx5-binding sites were identified in the *tbx2b* promoter, and *tbx2b* expression in the AVC proved highly sensitive to mutagenesis of the Foxn4- or Tbx5-binding sites.[88]

NKX2-5, a member of the homeodomain family, plays a central role in cardiac development. Loss of the *Nkx2-5* homolog, *tinman*, in the fruit fly resulted in failure of cardiogenesis.[105] Mice deficient in *Nkx2-5* died *in utero* at E9–10 due to arrested cardiac development in the linear heart tube stage. The hearts of these mice underwent partial looping morphogenesis, lacked endocardial cushions and trabeculae, and had underdeveloped AV canals.[106] *Nkx2-5*-null embryos lacked minK-LacZ reporter staining in the region of AVN primordium.[62] *Nkx2-5+/neo* mice exhibited an overall reduction in the size of the AVN and VCS. Histological evaluation of the *Nkx2-5+/neo* AVN revealed that compact nodal cells (Cx40−/Cx45+) were markedly reduced while the lower nodal cells (Cx40+/Cx45+) remained intact.[62] Consistent

with these findings, *Nkx2-5+/neo* mice had prolonged PR intervals on surface ECG and displayed abnormal AVN physiology on electrophysiology (EP) testing.[62] In humans, *NKX2-5* mutations cause nonsyndromic congenital heart disease associated with AV nodal conduction disease that in some progresses to complete heart block.[60] Some of these individuals die of sudden cardiac death, and histological evaluation of the AVN has revealed significant myocyte dropout and fatty replacement.[107]

In the chick heart, NOTCH2, HEY1, and HEY2 signaling delimit the AVC myocardium. *Hey1* (expressed in atrium and ventricle) and *Hey2* (expressed in ventricle only) are expressed in complementary fashion to *Bmp2* in the looped heart.[93] NOTCH2 acts directly through HEY1 to suppress BMP2, while HEY2 suppresses BMP2 in a NOTCH-independent manner.[93] Mouse and zebra fish hearts deficient in *Hey2* displayed abnormally expanded AVC regions that were enriched in *Bmp2* or *bmp4*, respectively.[93] *Tbx2* expression in the AVC is also delimited by atrial and ventricular chamber expression of TBX20.[92] Observations of *Tbx20* KO embryos showed precocious upregulation and ectopic expression of *Tbx2* throughout the cardiac crescent and early heart tube. In vitro reporter assays demonstrated that TBX20 inhibits *Tbx2* promoter activity through its actions on the ALK3/SMAD signaling pathway.[92]

Recently, GATA-dependent regulatory switches have been identified that delimit AVC enriched gene expression.[94] GATA binding sites were present within AVC enhancer regions, and mutation of these sites caused de-repression of these enhancers in the chamber myocardium. Analysis of AVC-enriched genes, such as *Tbx2*, *Tbx3*, *Bmp2*, *Msx2*, *Id2*, *Gjd3*/Cx30.2, and *Cacna1g*, showed significant enrichment in histone H3 lysine 27 (H3K27) acetylation marks, a modification associated with active enhancers.[94] GATA4 was shown to act in conjunction with BMP2/SMAD signaling on AVC enhancers, leading to recruitment of histone acetyl transferase (HAT) to activate gene transcription.[94] In the chamber myocardium, GATA4 recruited pancardiac HDACs and chamber-specific HEY1 and HEY2, leading to H3K27 deacetylation and repression.[94]

The endocardium plays a crucial role in establishing the conduction properties of the AVC. Zebra fish lacking endocardial cells (cloche) showed no AV conduction delay.[108] Knockdown of endocardial factors, neuregulin or notch1b, resulted in loss of slow conduction in the AVC.[108] In contrast, knockdown of endothelin-1 in fish[108] or knockout of endothelin receptors in mice[109] had no effect on AVC conduction properties. The role of Notch signaling in AVC/AVN development in the mammalian heart was studied in loss-of-function and gain-of-function Notch mutants.[110] The dominant negative Notch mutant, DNMAML, driven by Mlc2v^Cre/+, displayed reduced AV nodal volumes due to loss of Cx30.2 expressing cells. Mlc2v^Cre/+/DNMAML had shortened PR and AH intervals on EP testing, consistent with loss of slow AV nodal conduction.[110] Constitutive Notch activation, on the other hand, resulted in enlarged AV nodes and accessory pathway formation due to abnormal boundary formation between the AVC and ventricular myocardium.[110] Gain-of-function Notch mutants demonstrated a robust upregulation of conduction system markers, such as *Cntn2*, *Tbx5*, and *Nkx2-5*. Notch activation also upregulated nodal genes (*Gjd3*/Cx30.2 and HCN1) and Purkinje-enriched genes (*Scn5a*/Na$_V$1.5). In addition, Notch activation reprogrammed ventricular myocytes in vivo and newborn ventricular myocytes in vitro into a Purkinje-type lineage. These results suggest that Notch signaling may fate restrict cardiomyocytes toward a conduction lineage.[111]

Notch gain-of-function mice showed reduced levels of canonical Wnt signaling in the AVC.[91] In fish, canonical Wnt signaling was shown to establish the expression domain of BMP4 and Tbx2b in the AVC.[90] Loss of Wnt signaling in mouse cardiomyocytes resulted in tricuspid atresia, hypoplastic right ventricle, and loss of AVC myocardium.[91] Conversely, ectopic Wnt signaling expanded the boundaries of the AVC and forced a slow conduction fate by inhibiting chamber myocardial genes in both fish[90] and mice.[91]

Proximal Ventricular Conduction System

The proximal VCS consists of the His bundle and bundle branches. These fast-conducting components of the CCS derive from ventricular myocardial precursors. Formation of the proximal VCS is critically dependent on the coexpression of NKX2-5 and TBX5, as combined haploinsufficiency of these two factors results in a specification defect of the His bundle and bundle branches, although AV conduction remained intact up to the early postnatal period.[45] During development, overlapping expression of NKX2-5 and TBX5 in addition to tissue-specific regulators, such as the transcription factor ETV1,[70] drives the expression of genes required for fast conduction properties ($Gja5$/Cx40$^+$, $Scn5a$/Na$_V$1.5$^+$) while also maintaining phenotypic distinctiveness (TBX3$^+$; Id2$^+$; Cx43$^-$) from working myocytes (see Fig. 29.4D). Both NKX2-5 and TBX5 have cell-autonomous roles in VCS development and perturbation of either factor leads to significant CCS structural and functional abnormalities.

$Nkx2$-5 haploinsufficient mice exhibited marked hypoplasia of the AVN and VCS, resulting in PR and QRS interval prolongation.[62,107,112] Ventricular-restricted, $Nkx2$-5 KO mice displayed progressive AV conduction disease, advancing to complete heart block by 6 months to 1 year of age. Histological analysis revealed a diminutive AVN and an atrophic VCS that worsened with age.[62,107,113,114] These mice accurately phenocopied the progressive postnatal AV conduction disease seen in patients with $NKX2$-5 mutations.[107] The phenotypic manifestations of $NKX2$-5 haploinsufficiency are highly pleotropic in man and mouse models, which suggests that $NKX2$-5 is subject to upstream regulatory control by genetic modifiers. One such modifier is Prospero-Related Homeobox Protein 1 (Prox1), which functions in concert with HDAC3 to regulate $Nkx2$-5 expression.[115] Combined haploinsufficiency of $Nkx2$-$5^{cre/+}$;$Prox1^{loxP/+}$ rescued the $Nkx2$-$5^{cre/+}$ conduction phenotype on a structural and functional level. Compound heterozygotes rescued the hypoplastic phenotype of the AVN and significantly restored cellularity of the VCS, resulting in normalization of ECG parameters.[115] In light of these findings, PROX1 appears to function as an upstream regulator of $Nkx2$-5 gene dosage, which ensures accurate gene expression within the AVN and VCS.

ETV1 is a member of the PEA3 group of transcription factors and was found to be highly expressed in the pectinated atrial myocardium (PAM) and His-Purkinje system where it regulates the expression of NKX2-5, Na$_V$1.5, and Cx40.[49] $Etv1$-deficient mice exhibited conduction defects in the atria and His-Purkinje system with a third of animals displaying bundle branch blocks. Similar to $Nkx2$-5 haploinsufficient mice, $Etv1$ KO mice displayed VCS hypoplasia, and some animals exhibited discontinuity between the His bundle and proximal right bundle branch. A phenome-wide association study (PheWAS) identified an association between an $ETV1$ sequence variant and bundle branch block and AV block in humans.[49]

Mice haploinsufficient for $Tbx5$ exhibited patterning and maturation defects of the VCS. The His bundle and left bundle branch remained immature in all $Tbx5^{del/+}$ mice, and many of the mice had absent right bundle branches. The expression of TBX5-responsive genes, $Nppa$ and $Gja5$/Cx40, were significantly downregulated.[59] NKX2-5 and TBX5 coordinately drive the expression of $Nppa$, $Gja5$/Cx40, and $Id2$ within the proximal VCS.[45] Id2 is believed to function as an inhibitor of muscle differentiation allowing specification toward a conduction lineage.[45] $Id2$-null mice displayed structural and functional VCS abnormalities similar to those seen in $Tbx5^{+/-}$ mice, suggesting they

function within the same transcriptional regulatory network. Indeed, combined haploinsufficiency of $Tbx5^{+/-}$; $Id2^{+/-}$ resulted in a specification defect of the His bundle and bundle branches.[107] Therefore NKX2-5, TBX5, and Id2 function as a VCS transcriptional unit that together with tissue-specific regulators imparts fast conduction properties, while also inhibiting myocardial gene programming.

TBX5 is essential for maintaining the fast conduction properties of the VCS. Using a VCS-specific, tamoxifen-inducible Cre driver (minKCreERT2), $Tbx5$ was knocked out of the adult mouse AVN and VCS, resulting in sudden death as early as 5 weeks after Cre induction.[116] $Tbx5^{minKCreERT2}$ VCS conduction was severely impaired, leading to spontaneous arrhythmias, including Mobitz type II AV block and ventricular tachycardia. Selective ablation of $Tbx5$ in the VCS resulted in a corresponding loss of $Gja5$/Cx40 and $Scn5a$ expression.[116,117]

GWAS focused on CCS parameters have identified several loci ($TBX5$, $TBX3$, $NKX2$-5, $SCN10A$, and $SCN5A$) that modulate PR and QRS duration in the general population.[118–122] Given the importance of TBX5 and TBX3 in CCS specification and function, the $Scn5a$ locus was screened for TBX-responsive elements. A TBX-responsive enhancer was identified approximately 15-kb downstream of $Scn5a$, and the expression pattern of this enhancer mirrored $Scn5a$ expression in the AV bundle and bundle branches.[117] Using a complementary approach, the genome-wide occupancy profile of TBX3 was carried out using ChIP-massive parallel sequencing (ChIP-Seq) analysis.[123] Two TBX3/TBX5–responsive enhancers were located within the $Scn5a$/$Scn10a$ locus. The orthologous human fragments had similar expression patterns to their mouse counterparts within the developing VCS, providing evidence that these enhancers were functionally conserved in humans.[123] The GWAS single nucleotide polymorphism (SNP), rs6801957, was located in a conserved enhancer site in the $SCN10A$ locus. Interestingly, rs6801957 alters a highly conserved residue in the consensus T-box binding site, altering its ability to respond to TBX5 activation and TBX3 repression.[123] Using high-resolution chromatin conformation capture-sequencing (4C-seq), direct associations between the $Scn10a$ intronic enhancer and the promoters of $Scn5a$ and $Scn10a$ were established.[124] The $SCN10A$ variant rs6801957 modulated $Scn5a$ expression in transgenic mouse models and in humans harboring the SNP variant.[124] These data reaffirm the fidelity of GWAS in identifying gene regulatory networks that underlie phenotypic variations in humans on a population scale.

The maintenance of Cx40 in the proximal VCS is vital for proper function of the His bundle and bundle branches. Mice deficient in Cx40 exhibited slowed conduction through the VCS and displayed bundle branch block.[125,126] During development, Cx40 is expressed in the ventricular trabeculae, which makes extensive interconnections with the primary interventricular ring and the AVC myocardium.[3,4,127] Cx40 expression in the ventricular trabeculae dictates the switch in ventricular activation from the primary interventricular ring pattern to the mature apical-to-basal sequence.[127] The regional localization of Cx40 and the enriched expression of $Scn5a$ within the trabecular myocardium that ultimately gives rise to the VCS is dependent on endocardially secreted factors, such as Neuregulin-1 (NRG1), and on several transcription factors, which function downstream of NKX2-5, TBX5, and ETV1: HF-1b, HOP, and IRX3.

HF-1b is a zinc-finger transcription factor with enriched expression within the compact myocardial layers and the VCS.[35] Mice deficient in Hf-$1b$ manifested SND, intermittent AV block, and sudden cardiac death due to spontaneous ventricular arrhythmias. Hf-$1b^{-/-}$ hearts displayed both a reduced number of Cx40$^+$ distal Purkinje fibers, as well as an abnormal intracellular distribution of Cx40, suggesting a defect in trafficking. This phenotype was predominantly seen in the ventricular apex; apical working myocytes were also smaller in size and had significantly reduced levels of Cx43.[128] In addition, the coronary arterial structure and function were also perturbed within the apical region.[128] Therefore the defects in Cx40 and Cx43 expression within the ventricular apex may be multifactorial and will need further investigation.

Homeodomain-only protein (HOP) is a unique member of the homeobox transcription factors that does not directly bind DNA.[36] It is known to function downstream of NKX2-5 and inhibits serum response factor (SRF)-dependent transcription.[107] *Hop* is expressed in the CCS, with significant enrichment beyond the neonatal time period. *Hop*$^{-/-}$ mice have structurally normal hearts and CCS anatomy but manifest slowed conduction in the VCS on EP testing. Expression of Cx40 was significantly reduced in the atria and the VCS, while levels of Cx43 remained normal.[36] Therefore HOP is not required for CCS specification and patterning, but plays an important role in optimizing fast conduction in the VCS through its action on Cx40 expression.

The Iroquois homeobox 3 (IRX3) transcription factor is expressed in the VCS and regulates its fast conduction properties.[44] *Irx3* KO mice exhibited prolonged QRS duration on EKG and right bundle branch block due to VCS hypoplasia and defects in the right bundle branch formation.[128a] Cx40 levels were also reduced in *Irx3* KO Purkinje cells with ectopic expression of Cx43. IRX3 directly represses the expression of Cx43 and activates Cx40 expression through an indirect mechanism.[44] IRX3 directly interacts with NKX2-5 and TBX5 and is believed to act cooperatively with these factors to drive Purkinje-specific gene expression. Ambulatory cardiac monitoring of *Irx3*-deficient mice revealed an increased propensity for spontaneous ventricular arrhythmias.[129] *Irx3* mutant mice also demonstrated intermittent AV block.[129] Screening of patients with documented ventricular fibrillation identified two missense mutations in *IRX3* (*IRX3*^{R421P} and *IRX3*^{P485T}).[94] Both *IRX3* mutants had reduced ability to increase *Gja5*/Cx40 and *Scn5a* levels in heterologous expression systems. Taken together, ETV1, HF-1b, HOP, and IRX3 function cooperatively with NKX2-5 and TBX5 to upregulate expression of *Gja5*/Cx40 and *Scn5a* in the VCS to optimize fast conduction.

The Purkinje Fiber Network

The PFN represents the most distal aspect of the VCS. In mammals, the PFN derives from the trabecular myocardium, likely through a process of recruitment, and so, the complex patterning of the PFN directly mirrors the complexity of the trabecular network.[7] Paracrine signals from the overlying endocardium, such as Endothelin-1 (ET-1) in chickens and Neuregulin-1 (NRG1) in mammals, direct underlying trabecular myocytes toward a Purkinje lineage (see Fig. 29.4E).[130]

In mammals, NRG1 is essential for Purkinje fiber specification, whereas ET-1 signaling was found to be dispensable for CCS development.[109] Using CCS-LacZ hearts in an in vitro culture system, NRG1 but not ET-1 was sufficient to expand the pool of LacZ+ Purkinje cells in a time window between E8.5–E10.5. The increase in LacZ+ cells could not be explained by changes in proliferation or apoptosis and suggested that NRG1 was able to direct embryonic cardiomyocytes toward a conduction phenotype.[131] The marked upregulation of CCS-LacZ+ cells in NRG1-treated hearts was associated with changes in the ventricular activation pattern by optical mapping.[131] NRG1 also induced a Purkinje gene profile in dissociated mouse embryonic ventricular myocytes and in intact embryonic hearts.[132] There was no cumulative effect of coadministration of NRG1 and ET-1

on Purkinje gene programming.[132] Therefore NRG1 is sufficient to activate a potent gene regulatory network for Purkinje fiber specification.

Using the in vitro CCS-LacZ heart culture assay, a dual screen that employed signal transduction and transcriptional profiling screens identified that NRG1 acts through the Ras-MAPK pathway to regulate the transcription factor ETV1.[49] Loss of *Etv1* reduced the levels of NKX2-5, Cx40, and Na$_V$1.5 in the PAM and VCS to ventricular levels, resulting in conduction defects in these tissues and VCS hypoplasia due to a loss of terminal Purkinje fibers. *Etv1*-deficient hearts also exhibited loss of the unique biophysical features of the sodium current normally present in atrial and Purkinje myocytes, resulting in a "ventricularized" sodium current.[49]

Nkx2-5 gene dosage is critical for proper maturation of the PFN.[133] Inappropriately high or low levels of *Nkx2-5* can negatively impact proper Purkinje development.[133] Consistent with other models of *Nkx2-5* deficiency, adult *Nkx2-5*$^{+/-}$/*Cx40*$^{eGFP/+}$ mice showed marked reduction in PFN cellularity, despite the trabecular region appearing qualitatively normal during development.[112] The reduction of Purkinje fibers in *Nkx2-5*$^{+/-}$ hearts occurred mainly after birth and was due to either reduced PF recruitment or loss of PF in the postnatal period.[112] Evaluation of the remaining Purkinje fibers revealed that they were of normal size and had normal electrophysiological properties.[112] Therefore the conduction defects seen in *Nkx2-5*$^{+/-}$/*Cx40*$^{eGFP/+}$ hearts appeared to be due to a reduction in the number of Purkinje cells rather than electrophysiological defects at the cellular level.[112] Based on chimeric analysis, postnatal development of the PFN was critically dependent on the dose of *Nkx2-5*, which behaved in a cell-autonomous manner.[112]

In summary, the genetic programs that dictate the CCS are fundamentally based on the intricate balance between activating and repressing T-box transcription factors, *Nkx2-5* gene dosage, and expression of tissue-specific modifiers that enhance slow or fast conduction properties. These transcriptional networks are further controlled by regulatory feedback and feedforward loops established by paracrine signaling cues originating from the endocardium.

Conclusion

Since the first anatomical descriptions of the CCS in the early 20th century, our knowledge of the developmental origins of the CCS has grown dramatically. Every fundamental discovery, from the cellular origins of the CCS to the transcriptional networks that govern the properties of slow and fast conduction, has created a broader and richer understanding of how each heartbeat is initiated and propagated. Incorporating newer modalities, such as GWAS, PheWAS, RNA-Seq, ChIP-Seq, and 4/5/Hi-C-seq, will further enhance our understanding of how these transcription factor networks regulate CCS specification on a genome-wide scale. Additionally, advances in genome-editing tools, such as CRISPR/CAS9, allow for rapid generation of knockout mouse models and validation of genetic variations in vivo. Ultimately, new insights will shape the future therapy of heart rhythm disorders.

Acknowledgments

This work was supported by National Institutes of Health Grants R01HL82727, R01HL105983, New York State N08G-132 to GIF, and the American Heart Association Scientist Development Grant (#17SDG33411201) to DSP.

REFERENCES

1. Paff GH, Boucek RJ, Harrell TC. Observations on the development of the electrocardiogram. *Anat Rec.* 1968;160:575–582.
2. Kreuzberg MM, Willecke K, Bukauskas FF. Connexin-mediated cardiac impulse propagation: connexin 30.2 slows atrioventricular conduction in mouse heart. *Trends Cardiovasc Med.* 2006;16:266–272.
3. Viragh S, Challice CE. The development of the conduction system in the mouse embryo heart. II. Histogenesis of the atrioventricular node and bundle. *Dev Biol.* 1977;56:397–411.
4. Viragh S, Challice CE. The development of the conduction system in the mouse embryo heart. I. The first embryonic A-V conduction pathway. *Dev Biol.* 1977;56:382–396.
5. Viragh S, Challice CE. The development of the conduction system in the mouse embryo heart. *Dev Biol.* 1980;80:28–45.
6. Cheng G, Litchenberg WH, Cole GJ, Mikawa T, Thompson RP, Gourdie RG. Development of the cardiac conduction system involves recruitment within a multipotent cardiomyogenic lineage. *Development.* 1999;126:5041–5049.
7. Gourdie RG, Mima T, Thompson RP, Mikawa T. Terminal diversification of the myocyte lineage generates Purkinje fibers of the cardiac conduction system. *Development.* 1995;121:1423–1431.
8. Miquerol L, Moreno-Rascon N, Beyer S, et al. Biphasic development of the mammalian ventricular conduction system. *Circ Res.* 2010;107:153–161.
9. Kitajima S, Miyagawa-Tomita S, Inoue T, Kanno J, Saga Y. Mesp1-nonexpressing cells contribute to the ventricular cardiac conduction system. *Dev Dyn.* 2006;235:395–402.
10. Poelmann RE, Jongbloed MR, Molin DG, et al. The neural crest is contiguous with the cardiac conduction system in the mouse embryo: a role in induction? *Anat Embryol (Berl).* 2004;208:389–393.
11. Miquerol L, Bellon A, Moreno N, et al. Resolving cell lineage contributions to the ventricular conduction system with a Cx40-GFP allele: a dual contribution of the first and second heart fields. *Dev Dyn.* 2013;242:665–677.
12. Wenink AC. Development of the human cardiac conducting system. *J Anat.* 1976;121:617–631.
13. Hoogaars WM, Tessari A, Moorman AF, et al. The transcriptional repressor Tbx3 delineates the developing central conduction system of the heart. *Cardiovasc Res.* 2004;62:489–499.
14. Jongbloed MR, Mahtab EA, Blom NA, Schalij MJ, Gittenberger-de Groot AC. Development of the cardiac conduction system and the possible relation to predilection sites of arrhythmogenesis. *ScientificWorldJournal.* 2008;8:239–269.
15. Wessels A, Vermeulen JL, Verbeek FJ, et al. Spatial distribution of "tissue-specific" antigens in the developing human heart and skeletal muscle. III. An immunohistochemical analysis of the distribution of the neural tissue antigen G1N2 in the embryonic heart; implications for the development of the atrioventricular conduction system. *Anat Rec.* 1992;232:97–111.
16. Meilhac SM, Kelly RG, Rocancourt D, Eloy-Trinquet S, Nicolas JF, Buckingham ME. A retrospective clonal analysis of the myocardium reveals two phases of clonal growth in the developing mouse heart. *Development.* 2003;130:3877–3889.
17. Deleted in review.
18. Christoffels VM, Hoogaars WM, Tessari A, Clout DE, Moorman AF, Campione M. T-box transcription factor Tbx2 represses differentiation and formation of the cardiac chambers. *Dev Dyn.* 2004;229:763–770.
19. Boogerd KJ, Wong LY, Christoffels VM, et al. Msx1 and Msx2 are functional interacting partners of T-box factors in the regulation of Connexin43. *Cardiovasc Res.* 2008;78:485–493.
20. Mommersteeg MT, Hoogaars WM, Prall OW, et al. Molecular pathway for the localized formation of the sinoatrial node. *Circ Res.* 2007;100:354–362.
21. Kondo RP, Anderson RH, Kupershmidt S, Roden DM, Evans SM. Development of the cardiac conduction system as delineated by minK-lacZ. *J Cardiovasc Electrophysiol.* 2003;14:383–391.
22. Kupershmidt S, Yang T, Anderson ME, et al. Replacement by homologous recombination of the minK gene with lacZ reveals restriction of minK expression to the mouse cardiac conduction system. *Circ Res.* 1999;84:146–152.
23. Beyer S, Kelly RG, Miquerol L. Inducible Cx40-Cre expression in the cardiac conduction system and arterial endothelial cells. *Genesis.* 2011;49:83–91.
24. Hoesl E, Stieber J, Herrmann S, et al. Tamoxifen-inducible gene deletion in the cardiac conduction system. *J Mol Cell Cardiol.* 2008;45:62–69.
25. Spater D, Abramczuk MK, Buac K, et al. A HCN4+ cardiomyogenic progenitor derived from the first heart field and human pluripotent stem cells. *Nat Cell Biol.* 2013;15:1098–1106.

26. Liang X, Wang G, Lin L, et al. HCN4 dynamically marks the first heart field and conduction system precursors. *Circ Res.* 2013;113:399–407.
27. Wu M, Peng S, Zhao Y. Inducible gene deletion in the entire cardiac conduction system using Hcn4-CreERT2 BAC transgenic mice. *Genesis.* 2014;52:134–140.
28. Aanhaanen WT, Mommersteeg MT, Norden J, et al. Developmental origin, growth, and three-dimensional architecture of the atrioventricular conduction axis of the mouse heart. *Circ Res.* 2010;107:728–736.
29. Davis DL, Edwards AV, Juraszek AL, Phelps A, Wessels A, Burch JB. A GATA-6 gene heart-region-specific enhancer provides a novel means to mark and probe a discrete component of the mouse cardiac conduction system. *Mech Dev.* 2001;108:105–119.
30. Hoogaars WM, Engel A, Brons JF, et al. Tbx3 controls the sinoatrial node gene program and imposes pacemaker function on the atria. *Genes Dev.* 2007;21:1098–1112.
31. Sun Y, Liang X, Najafi N, et al. Islet 1 is expressed in distinct cardiovascular lineages, including pacemaker and coronary vascular cells. *Dev Biol.* 2007;304:286–296.
32. Sun C, Zhang T, Liu C, Gu S, Chen Y. Generation of Shox2-Cre allele for tissue specific manipulation of genes in the developing heart, palate, and limb. *Genesis.* 2013;51:515–522.
33. Di Lisi R, Sandri C, Franco D, Ausoni S, Moorman AF, Schiaffino S. An atrioventricular canal domain defined by cardiac troponin I transgene expression in the embryonic myocardium. *Anat Embryol (Berl).* 2000;202:95–101.
34. Li Z, Marchand P, Humbert J, Babinet C, Paulin D. Desmin sequence elements regulating skeletal muscle-specific expression in transgenic mice. *Development.* 1993;117:947–959.
35. Nguyen-Tran VT, Kubalak SW, Minamisawa S, et al. A novel genetic pathway for sudden cardiac death via defects in the transition between ventricular and conduction system cell lineages. *Cell.* 2000;102:671–682.
36. Ismat FA, Zhang M, Kook H, et al. Homeobox protein Hop functions in the adult cardiac conduction system. *Circ Res.* 2005;96:898–903.
37. Froese A, Breher SS, Waldeyer C, et al. Popeye domain containing proteins are essential for stress-mediated modulation of cardiac pacemaking in mice. *J Clin Invest.* 2012;122:1119–1130.
38. Kreuzberg MM, Sohl G, Kim JS, Verselis VK, Willecke K, Bukauskas FF. Functional properties of mouse connexin30.2 expressed in the conduction system of the heart. *Circ Res.* 2005;96:1169–1177.
39. Kruger O, Plum A, Kim JS, et al. Defective vascular development in connexin 45-deficient mice. *Development.* 2000;127:4179–4193.
40. Gros D, Theveniau-Ruissy M, Bernard M, et al. Connexin 30 is expressed in the mouse sino-atrial node and modulates heart rate. *Cardiovasc Res.* 2010;85:45–55.
41. Kreuzberg MM, Schrickel JW, Ghanem A, et al. Connexin30.2 containing gap junction channels decelerate impulse propagation through the atrioventricular node. *Proc Natl Acad Sci U S A.* 2006;103:5959–5964.
42. Horsthuis T, Buermans HP, Brons JF, et al. Gene expression profiling of the forming atrioventricular node using a novel tbx3-based node-specific transgenic reporter. *Circ Res.* 2009;105:61–69.
43. Wiese C, Grieskamp T, Airik R, et al. Formation of the sinus node head and differentiation of sinus node myocardium are independently regulated by Tbx18 and Tbx3. *Circ Res.* 2009;104:388–397.
44. Zhang SS, Kim KH, Rosen A, et al. Iroquois homeobox gene 3 establishes fast conduction in the cardiac His-Purkinje network. *Proc Natl Acad Sci U S A.* 2011;108:13576–13581.
45. Moskowitz IP, Kim JB, Moore ML, et al. A molecular pathway including Id2, Tbx5, and Nkx2-5 required for cardiac conduction system development. *Cell.* 2007;129:1365–1376.
46. Rentschler S, Vaidya DM, Tamaddon H, et al. Visualization and functional characterization of the developing murine cardiac conduction system. *Development.* 2001;128:1785–1792.
47. Pallante BA, Giovannone S, Fang-Yu L, et al. Contactin-2 expression in the cardiac Purkinje fiber network. *Circ Arrhythm Electrophysiol.* 2010;3:186–194.
48. Miquerol L, Meysen S, Mangoni M, et al. Architectural and functional asymmetry of the His-Purkinje system of the murine heart. *Cardiovasc Res.* 2004;63:77–86.
49. Shekhar A, Lin X, Liu FY, et al. Transcription factor ETV1 is essential for rapid conduction in the heart. *J Clin Invest.* 2016;126:4444–4459.
49a. Arber S, Ladle DR, Lin JH, Frank E, Jessell TM. ETS gene Er81 controls the formation of functional connections between group Ia sensory afferents and motor neurons. *Cell.* 2000;101:485–498.

50. Basson CT, Bachinsky DR, Lin RC, et al. Mutations in human TBX5 [corrected] cause limb and cardiac malformation in Holt-Oram syndrome. *Nat Genet.* 1997;15:30–35.
51. Stennard FA, Harvey RP. T-box transcription factors and their roles in regulatory hierarchies in the developing heart. *Development.* 2005;132:4897–4910.
52. Linden H, Williams R, King J, Blair E, Kini U. Ulnar Mammary syndrome and TBX3: expanding the phenotype. *Am J Med Genet A.* 2009;149A:2809–2812.
53. Meneghini V, Odent S, Platonova N, Egeo A, Merlo GR. Novel TBX3 mutation data in families with ulnar-mammary syndrome indicate a genotype-phenotype relationship: mutations that do not disrupt the T-domain are associated with less severe limb defects. *Eur J Med Genet.* 2006;49:151–158.
54. Hiroi Y, Kudoh S, Monzen K, et al. Tbx5 associates with Nkx2-5 and synergistically promotes cardiomyocyte differentiation. *Nat Genet.* 2001;28:276–280.
55. Bruneau BG, Nemer G, Schmitt JP, et al. A murine model of Holt-Oram syndrome defines roles of the T-box transcription factor Tbx5 in cardiogenesis and disease. *Cell.* 2001;106:709–721.
56. Garg V, Kathiriya IS, Barnes R, et al. GATA4 mutations cause human congenital heart defects and reveal an interaction with TBX5. *Nature.* 2003;424:443–447.
56a. Luna-Zurita L, Stirnimann CU, Glatt S, et al. Complex interdependence regulates heterotypic transcription factor distribution and coordinates cardiogenesis. *Cell.* 2016;164:999–1014.
57. Habets PE, Moorman AF, Clout DE, et al. Cooperative action of Tbx2 and Nkx2.5 inhibits ANF expression in the atrioventricular canal: implications for cardiac chamber formation. *Genes Dev.* 2002;16:1234–1246.
58. Munshi NV, McAnally J, Bezprozvannaya S, et al. Cx30.2 enhancer analysis identifies Gata4 as a novel regulator of atrioventricular delay. *Development.* 2009;136:2665–2674.
59. Moskowitz IP, Pizard A, Patel VV, et al. The T-Box transcription factor Tbx5 is required for the patterning and maturation of the murine cardiac conduction system. *Development.* 2004;131:4107–4116.
60. Schott JJ, Benson DW, Basson CT, et al. Congenital heart disease caused by mutations in the transcription factor NKX2-5. *Science.* 1998;281:108–111.
61. Mori AD, Zhu Y, Vahora I, et al. Tbx5-dependent rheostatic control of cardiac gene expression and morphogenesis. *Dev Biol.* 2006;297:566–586.
62. Jay PY, Harris BS, Maguire CT, et al. Nkx2-5 mutation causes anatomic hypoplasia of the cardiac conduction system. *J Clin Invest.* 2004;113:1130–1137.
63. Lakatta EG, Maltsev VA, Vinogradova TM. A coupled SYSTEM of intracellular Ca²⁺ clocks and surface membrane voltage clocks controls the timekeeping mechanism of the heart's pacemaker. *Circ Res.* 2010;106:659–673.
64. Mommersteeg MT, Dominguez JN, Wiese C, et al. The sinus venosus progenitors separate and diversify from the first and second heart fields early in development. *Cardiovasc Res.* 2010;87:92–101.
65. Ye W, Wang J, Song Y, et al. A common Shox2-Nkx2-5 antagonistic mechanism primes the pacemaker cell fate in the pulmonary vein myocardium and sinoatrial node. *Development.* 2015;142:2521–2532.
66. Espinoza-Lewis RA, Liu H, Sun C, Chen C, Jiao K, Chen Y. Ectopic expression of Nkx2.5 suppresses the formation of the sinoatrial node in mice. *Dev Biol.* 2011;356:359–369.
67. Puskaric S, Schmitteckert S, Mori AD, et al. Shox2 mediates Tbx5 activity by regulating Bmp4 in the pacemaker region of the developing heart. *Hum Mol Genet.* 2010;19:4625–4633.
68. Frank DU, Carter KL, Thomas KR, et al. Lethal arrhythmias in Tbx3-deficient mice reveal extreme dosage sensitivity of cardiac conduction system function and homeostasis. *Proc Natl Acad Sci U S A.* 2012;109:E154–E163.
69. Wu M, Peng S, Yang J, et al. Baf250a orchestrates an epigenetic pathway to repress the Nkx2.5-directed contractile cardiomyocyte program in the sinoatrial node. *Cell Res.* 2014;24:1201–1213.
70. Kapoor N, Galang G, Marban E, Cho HC. Transcriptional suppression of connexin43 by TBX18 undermines cell-cell electrical coupling in postnatal cardiomyocytes. *J Biol Chem.* 2011;286:14073–14079.
71. Kapoor N, Liang W, Marban E, Cho HC. Direct conversion of quiescent cardiomyocytes to pacemaker cells by expression of Tbx18. *Nat Biotechnol.* 2013;31:54–62.
72. Blaschke RJ, Hahurij ND, Kuijper S, et al. Targeted mutation reveals essential functions of the homeodomain transcription factor Shox2 in sinoatrial and pacemaking development. *Circulation.* 2007;115:1830–1838.
73. Espinoza-Lewis RA, Yu L, He F, et al. Shox2 is essential for the differentiation of cardiac pacemaker cells by repressing Nkx2-5. *Dev Biol.* 2009;327:376–385.

74. Ionta V, Liang W, Kim EH, et al. SHOX2 overexpression favors differentiation of embryonic stem cells into cardiac pacemaker cells, improving biological pacing ability. *Stem Cell Reports*. 2015;4:129–142.

75. Hoffmann S, Berger IM, Glaser A, et al. Islet1 is a direct transcriptional target of the homeodomain transcription factor Shox2 and rescues the Shox2-mediated bradycardia. *Basic Res Cardiol*. 2013;108:339.

76. Cai CL, Liang X, Shi Y, et al. Isl1 identifies a cardiac progenitor population that proliferates prior to differentiation and contributes a majority of cells to the heart. *Dev Cell*. 2003;5:877–889.

77. Liang X, Zhang Q, Cattaneo P, et al. Transcription factor ISL1 is essential for pacemaker development and function. *J Clin Invest*. 2015;125:3256–3268.

78. Vedantham V, Galang G, Evangelista M, Deo RC, Srivastava D. RNA sequencing of mouse sinoatrial node reveals an upstream regulatory role for Islet-1 in cardiac pacemaker cells. *Circ Res*. 2015;116:797–803.

79. Wang J, Klysik E, Sood S, Johnson RL, Wehrens XH, Martin JF. Pitx2 prevents susceptibility to atrial arrhythmias by inhibiting left-sided pacemaker specification. *Proc Natl Acad Sci U S A*. 2010;107:9753–9758.

80. Ammirabile G, Tessari A, Pignataro V, et al. Pitx2 confers left morphological, molecular, and functional identity to the sinus venosus myocardium. *Cardiovasc Res*. 2012;93:291–301.

81. Gudbjartsson DF, Arnar DO, Helgadottir A, et al. Variants conferring risk of atrial fibrillation on chromosome 4q25. *Nature*. 2007;448:353–357.

82. Wang J, Bai Y, Li N, et al. Pitx2-microRNA pathway that delimits sinoatrial node development and inhibits predisposition to atrial fibrillation. *Proc Natl Acad Sci U S A*. 2014;111:9181–9186.

83. de Carvalho A, de Almeida D. Spread of activity through the atrioventricular node. *Circ Res*. 1960;8:801–809.

84. Efimov IR, Mazgalev TN. High-resolution, three-dimensional fluorescent imaging reveals multilayer conduction pattern in the atrioventricular node. *Circulation*. 1998;98:54–57.

85. Ko YS, Yeh HI, Ko YL, et al. Three-dimensional reconstruction of the rabbit atrioventricular conduction axis by combining histological, desmin, and connexin mapping data. *Circulation*. 2004;109:1172–1179.

86. Aanhaanen WT, Brons JF, Dominguez JN, et al. The Tbx2+ primary myocardium of the atrioventricular canal forms the atrioventricular node and the base of the left ventricle. *Circ Res*. 2009;104:1267–1274.

87. Ma L, Lu MF, Schwartz RJ, Martin JF. Bmp2 is essential for cardiac cushion epithelial-mesenchymal transition and myocardial patterning. *Development*. 2005;132:5601–5611.

88. Chi NC, Shaw RM, De Val S, et al. Foxn4 directly regulates tbx2b expression and atrioventricular canal formation. *Genes Dev*. 2008;22:734–739.

89. Liu F, Lu MM, Patel NN, Schillinger KJ, Wang T, Patel VV. GATA-binding factor 6 contributes to atrioventricular node development and function. *Circ Cardiovasc Genet*. 2015;8:284–293.

90. Verhoeven MC, Haase C, Christoffels VM, Weidinger G, Bakkers J. Wnt signaling regulates atrioventricular canal formation upstream of BMP and Tbx2. *Birth Defects Res A Clin Mol Teratol*. 2011;91:435–440.

91. Gillers BS, Chiplunkar A, Aly H, et al. Canonical wnt signaling regulates atrioventricular junction programming and electrophysiological properties. *Circ Res*. 2015;116:398–406.

92. Singh R, Horsthuis T, Farin HF, et al. Tbx20 interacts with smads to confine tbx2 expression to the atrioventricular canal. *Circ Res*. 2009;105:442–452.

93. Rutenberg JB, Fischer A, Jia H, Gessler M, Zhong TP, Mercola M. Developmental patterning of the cardiac atrioventricular canal by Notch and Hairy-related transcription factors. *Development*. 2006;133:4381–4390.

94. Stefanovic S, Barnett P, van Duijvenboden K, Weber D, Gessler M, Christoffels VM. GATA-dependent regulatory switches establish atrioventricular canal specificity during heart development. *Nat Commun*. 2014;5:3680.

95. Park DS, Tompkins RO, Liu F, et al. Pocket proteins critically regulate cell cycle exit of the trabecular myocardium and the ventricular conduction system. *Biol Open*. 2013;2:968–978.

96. Singh R, Hoogaars WM, Barnett P, et al. Tbx2 and Tbx3 induce atrioventricular myocardial development and endocardial cushion formation. *Cell Mol Life Sci*. 2012;69:1377–1389.

97. Bressan M, Yang PB, Louie JD, Navetta AM, Garriock RJ, Mikawa T. Reciprocal myocardial-endocardial interactions pattern the delay in atrioventricular junction conduction. *Development*. 2014;141:4149–4157.

98. Gaussin V, Morley GE, Cox L, et al. Alk3/Bmpr1a receptor is required for development of the atrioventricular canal into valves and annulus fibrosus. *Circ Res*. 2005;97:219–226.

99. Stroud DM, Gaussin V, Burch JB, et al. Abnormal conduction and morphology in the atrioventricular node of mice with atrioventricular canal targeted deletion of Alk3/Bmpr1a receptor. *Circulation*. 2007;116:2535–2543.

100. Lalani SR, Thakuria JV, Cox GF, et al. 20p12.3 microdeletion predisposes to Wolff-Parkinson-White syndrome with variable neurocognitive deficits. *J Med Genet*. 2009;46:168–175.

101. Aanhaanen WT, Boukens BJ, Sizarov A, et al. Defective Tbx2-dependent patterning of the atrioventricular canal myocardium causes accessory pathway formation in mice. *J Clin Invest*. 2011;121:534–544.

102. Bakker ML, Boukens BJ, Mommersteeg MT, et al. Transcription factor Tbx3 is required for the specification of the atrioventricular conduction system. *Circ Res*. 2008;102:1340–1349.

103. Harrelson Z, Kelly RG, Goldin SN, et al. Tbx2 is essential for patterning the atrioventricular canal and for morphogenesis of the outflow tract during heart development. *Development*. 2004;131:5041–5052.

104. Harris JP, Bhakta M, Bezprozvannaya S, et al. MyoR modulates cardiac conduction by repressing Gata4. *Mol Cell Biol*. 2015;35:649–661.

105. Ranganayakulu G, Elliott DA, Harvey RP, Olson EN. Divergent roles for NK-2 class homeobox genes in cardiogenesis in flies and mice. *Development*. 1998;125:3037–3048.

106. Tanaka M, Chen Z, Bartunkova S, Yamasaki N, Izumo S. The cardiac homeobox gene Csx/Nkx2.5 lies genetically upstream of multiple genes essential for heart development. *Development*. 1999;126:1269–1280.

107. Pashmforoush M, Lu JT, Chen H, et al. Nkx2-5 pathways and congenital heart disease; loss of ventricular myocyte lineage specification leads to progressive cardiomyopathy and complete heart block. *Cell*. 2004;117:373–386.

108. Milan DJ, Giokas AC, Serluca FC, Peterson RT, MacRae CA. Notch1b and neuregulin are required for specification of central cardiac conduction tissue. *Development*. 2006;133:1125–1132.

109. Hua LL, Vedantham V, Barnes RM, et al. Specification of the mouse cardiac conduction system in the absence of Endothelin signaling. *Dev Biol*. 2014;393:245–254.

110. Rentschler S, Harris BS, Kuznekoff L, et al. Notch signaling regulates murine atrioventricular conduction and the formation of accessory pathways. *J Clin Invest*. 2011;121:525–533.

111. Rentschler S, Yen AH, Lu J, et al. Myocardial Notch signaling reprograms cardiomyocytes to a conduction-like phenotype. *Circulation*. 2012;126:1058–1066.

112. Meysen S, Marger L, Hewett KW, et al. Nkx2.5 cell-autonomous gene function is required for the postnatal formation of the peripheral ventricular conduction system. *Dev Biol*. 2007;303:740–753.

113. Wakimoto H, Kasahara H, Maguire CT, Izumo S, Berul CI. Developmentally modulated cardiac conduction failure in transgenic mice with fetal or postnatal overexpression of DNA nonbinding mutant Nkx2.5. *J Cardiovasc Electrophysiol*. 2002;13:682–688.

114. Kasahara H, Wakimoto H, Liu M, et al. Progressive atrioventricular conduction defects and heart failure in mice expressing a mutant Csx/Nkx2.5 homeoprotein. *J Clin Invest*. 2001;108:189–201.

115. Risebro CA, Petchey LK, Smart N, et al. Epistatic rescue of Nkx2.5 adult cardiac conduction disease phenotypes by Prospero-related homeobox protein 1 and HDAC3. *Circ Res*. 2012;111:e19–e31.

116. Arnolds DE, Moskowitz IP. Inducible recombination in the cardiac conduction system of minK: CreERT(2) BAC transgenic mice. *Genesis*. 2011;49:878–884.

117. Arnolds DE, Liu F, Fahrenbach JP, et al. TBX5 drives Scn5a expression to regulate cardiac conduction system function. *J Clin Invest*. 2012;122:2509–2518.

118. Sotoodehnia N, Isaacs A, de Bakker PI, et al. Common variants in 22 loci are associated with QRS duration and cardiac ventricular conduction. *Nat Genet*. 2010;42:1068–1076.

119. Chambers JC, Zhao J, Terracciano CM, et al. Genetic variation in SCN10A influences cardiac conduction. *Nat Genet*. 2010;42:149–152.

120. Holm H, Gudbjartsson DF, Arnar DO, et al. Several common variants modulate heart rate, PR interval and QRS duration. *Nat Genet*. 2010;42:117–122.

121. Pfeufer A, van Noord C, Marciante KD, et al. Genome-wide association study of PR interval. *Nat Genet*. 2010;42:153–159.

122. Smith JG, Magnani JW, Palmer C, et al. Genome-wide association studies of the PR interval in African Americans. *PLoS Genet*. 2011;7: e1001304.

123. van den Boogaard M, Wong LY, Tessadori F, et al. Genetic variation in T-box binding element functionally affects SCN5A/SCN10A enhancer. *J Clin Invest*. 2012;122:2519–2530.

124. van den Boogaard M, Smemo S, Burnicka-Turek O, et al. A common genetic variant within SCN10A modulates cardiac SCN5A expression. *J Clin Invest*. 2014;124:1844–1852.

125. van Rijen HV, van Veen TA, van Kempen MJ, et al. Impaired conduction in the bundle branches of mouse hearts lacking the gap junction protein connexin40. *Circulation*. 2001;103:1591–1598.

126. Tamaddon HS, Vaidya D, Simon AM, Paul DL, Jalife J, Morley GE. High-resolution optical mapping of the right bundle branch in connexin40 knockout mice reveals slow conduction in the specialized conduction system. *Circ Res*. 2000;87:929–936.

127. Sankova B, Benes Jr J, Krejci E, et al. The effect of connexin40 deficiency on ventricular conduction system function during development. *Cardiovasc Res*. 2012;95:469–479.

128. Hewett KW, Norman LW, Sedmera D, et al. Knockout of the neural and heart expressed gene HF-1b results in apical deficits of ventricular structure and activation. *Cardiovasc Res*. 2005;67:548–560.

128a. Kim KH, Rosen A, Hussein SM, et al. Irx3 is required for postnatal maturation of the mouse ventricular conduction system. *Sci Rep*. 2016;6:19197.

129. Koizumi A, Sasano T, Kimura W, et al. Genetic defects in a His-Purkinje system transcription factor, IRX3, cause lethal cardiac arrhythmias. *Eur Heart J*. 2016;37:1469–1475.

130. Gourdie RG, Wei Y, Kim D, Klatt SC, Mikawa T. Endothelin-induced conversion of embryonic heart muscle cells into impulse-conducting Purkinje fibers. *Proc Natl Acad Sci U S A*. 1998;95:6815–6818.

131. Rentschler S, Zander J, Meyers K, et al. Neuregulin-1 promotes formation of the murine cardiac conduction system. *Proc Natl Acad Sci U S A*. 2002;99:10464–10469.

132. Patel R, Kos L. Endothelin-1 and Neuregulin-1 convert embryonic cardiomyocytes into cells of the conduction system in the mouse. *Dev Dyn*. 2005;233:20–28.

133. Harris BS, Spruill L, Edmonson AM, et al. Differentiation of cardiac Purkinje fibers requires precise spatiotemporal regulation of Nkx2-5 expression. *Dev Dyn*. 2006;235:38–49.

30 Cardiac Remodeling and Regeneration

Timon Seeger, Caressa Chen, Ioannis Karakikes, and Joseph C. Wu

Abbreviations

AF: Atrial fibrillation
AHA: American Heart Association
AMI: Acute myocardial infarction
BMC: Bone marrow–derived cells
CAD: Coronary artery disease
CDC: Cardiosphere-derived cells
CHF: Chronic heart failure
CPC: Cardiac progenitor cells
DCM: Dilated cardiomyopathy
EHM: Engineered heart muscle
ESC: Embryonic stem cell
ESC-CM: Embryonic stem cell–derived cardiomyocyte
ET-1: Endothelin-1
HCM: Hypertrophic cardiomyopathy
HF: Heart failure
ICAM-1: Intercellular adhesion molecule-1
IL: Interleukin
iPSC: Induced pluripotent stem cell
iPSC-CM: Induced pluripotent stem cell–derived cardiomyocyte
HFpEF: Heart failure with preserved ejection fraction
HFrEF: Heart failure with reduced ejection fraction
IRI: Ischemia-reperfusion injury
LVAD: Left ventricular assist device
LV: Left ventricle
LVEF: Left ventricular ejection fraction
MSC: Mesenchymal stem cells
SA: Sinoatrial
VCAM-1: Vascular cell adhesion molecule-1

Heart failure (HF) remains the leading cause of death in the United States.[1] However, the molecular and pathophysiological mechanisms leading to failing cardiac function are still poorly understood. Available therapies are limited to relieving symptoms and slowing disease progression. None of the treatments leads to regeneration of cardiac tissue, and the only treatment option for end-stage HF is heart transplantation. This chapter provides an overview of the pathophysiological processes of cardiac remodeling that lead to chronic HF (CHF) and the progressive impairment of heart function. Approaches to enhance or stimulate regeneration and associated benefits and risks are discussed.

Pathophysiology of Cardiac Remodeling

Cardiac remodeling is the pathophysiological process after cardiac injury on the molecular, cellular, and interstitial levels that alters the size, shape, and function of the heart.[2] Several disease entities and pathophysiological conditions lead to cardiac remodeling.

Chronic Heart Failure

CHF is a common clinical presentation defined by symptoms such as dyspnea, fatigue, exertional intolerance, and signs (e.g., edema, gallop rhythm, and pulmonary rales) that are caused by a variety of cardiovascular diseases.[3] In most cases, the underlying cardiovascular abnormalities do not originate from the myocardium itself in the beginning, but lead to CHF caused by pathological cardiac remodeling and dysfunction. Of particular importance are atherosclerotic coronary artery disease (CAD), arterial hypertension with pathological cardiac hypertrophy, and valvular diseases, which result in pressure or volume overload and HF.

In addition, a heterogeneous group of diseases of the myocardium has been classified by the American Heart Association (AHA) as cardiomyopathies (Fig. 30.1) that can cause HF.[4] These cardiomyopathies can present with ventricular hypertrophy (hypertrophic cardiomyopathy; HCM) and dilation (dilated cardiomyopathy; DCM) or disorganization of the myocardium (left ventricular [LV] noncompaction, arrhythmogenic right ventricular dysplasia, or restrictive cardiomyopathy) that are associated with mechanical and/or electrical dysfunctions leading to HF. With diverse underlying causes, cardiomyopathies are classified as *primary* cardiomyopathies (genetic, nongenetic, or acquired), *secondary* cardiomyopathies, or cardiomyopathies as a part of a generalized systemic (multiorgan) disorder (see Fig. 30.1).[4]

Historically, HF was attributed to a decline in systolic function with an LV ejection fraction (LVEF) of ≤40% (HF with reduced ejection fraction; HFrEF). However, it is estimated that around 50% of patients presenting with symptoms of HF actually have a preserved LV systolic function with an LVEF of ≥50% (HF with preserved ejection fraction; HFpEF), whereas an LVEF of 41% to 49% is known as HFpEF borderline.[5,6] Although the systolic function of the LV is not significantly reduced in HFpEF, cardiac relaxation is impaired and reduced diastolic function affects the filling of the ventricles.

Depending on the underlying disease, the most prominent mechanisms in cardiac remodeling are cardiomyocyte loss (i.e., in the setting of myocardial ischemia), cardiomyocyte hypertrophy, invasion and activation of immune cells, and activation of cardiac fibroblasts that lead to fibrosis and inflammation.[7]

Heart Failure With Preserved Ejection Fraction

Initially, HFpEF was defined as decreased ventricular filling originating from the pathological dysfunction of ventricular cardiomyocytes.[8] However, the impaired diastolic function and symptoms of HF involve a complex interplay of volume overload, insufficiency of perfusion, and inadequate filling times.[9] The most powerful risk factors for HFpEF are arterial hypertension, age, gender (female), and atrial fibrillation (AF).[10,11] The majority of patients with arterial hypertension–associated HFpEF have concentric LV remodeling (either concentric hypertrophy or increased mass/volume ratio and accordingly relative wall thickness in the absence of LV hypertrophy).[12] However, HFpEF is strongly associated with more than pathological cardiac hypertrophy. Autopsies in the hearts of HFpEF patients revealed epicardial CAD, coronary microvascular rarefaction, and myocardial fibrosis accompanied by cardiac hypertrophy.[13] These findings further highlight the complexity of cardiac remodeling in HFpEF. A new paradigm suggests that a chronic systemic inflammatory response to high-prevalence comorbidities, such as obesity, diabetes

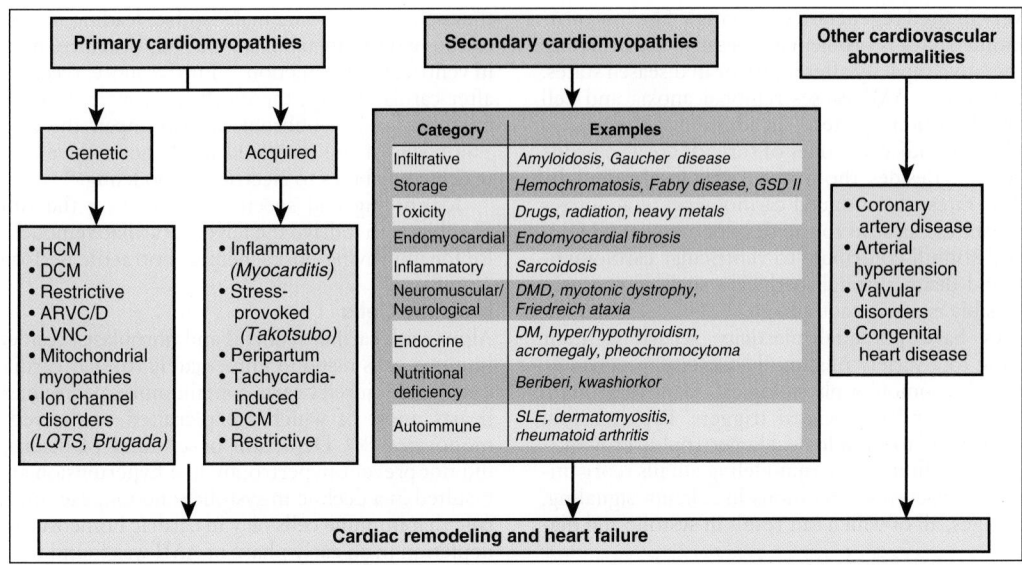

FIGURE 30.1 American Heart Association classification of cardiomyopathies organized by cause and initial involvement of the myocardium as well as other cardiovascular disorders directly leading to cardiac remodeling and heart failure. *ARVC/D,* Arrhythmogenic right ventricular cardiomyopathy/dysplasia; *DCM,* dilated cardiomyopathy; *DM,* diabetes mellitus; *DMD,* Duchenne muscular dystrophy; *GSD,* glycogen storage disease; *HCM,* hypertrophic cardiomyopathy; *LQTS,* long QT syndrome; *LVNC,* left ventricular noncompaction cardiomyopathy; *SLE,* systemic lupus erythematosus. (Modified from Maron BJ. Contemporary definitions and classification of the cardiomyopathies: an American Heart Association scientific statement from the Council on Clinical Cardiology, Heart Failure and Transplantation Committee; Quality of Care and Outcomes Research and Function. *Circulation.* 2006;113:1807-1816.)

mellitus, chronic obstructive pulmonary disease, and salt-sensitive hypertension, is associated with cardiac mesenchymal alterations that promote contractile dysfunction in HFpEF.[14]

In HFpEF, increasing the passive stiffness of cardiomyocytes and extracellular matrix as well as altering cellular levels during LV remodeling may promote the transition from LVH to HFrEF.[15] In addition to concentric hypertrophy, eccentric hypertrophy is also observed, suggesting that a distinct subgroup of patients may develop HFrEF.[16] A recently published meta-analysis reported a 5-year overall mortality rate of 32% in HFpEF patients compared to 40% in HFrEF patients.[17] However, no specific treatment has been shown to be effective in HFpEF, and treatment is based on HFrEF-tested guidelines. Given our aging population, the overall absolute number of deaths attributable to HFpEF is likely to increase in the coming years.[18]

Heart Failure in Ischemic Heart Disease

CAD and subsequent ischemia of the cardiac muscle is the leading cause of HFrEF.[6] Acute or subacute ischemia, as well as chronic hypoxia due to pathological occluding of the microcirculation, results in a multistep remodeling of the heart and ultimately HFrEF.[19] After the occlusion of a coronary artery, a lack of oxygen and nutritional supply downstream leads to apoptosis and necrosis of cardiomyocytes.[20] Within the first day following an acute myocardial infarction (AMI), cardiomyocyte death triggers an inflammatory reaction, attracting immune cells and stimulating invasion of inflammatory cells.[21] In this highly changeable environment, collagenases and other neutral proteinases contribute to the removal of necrotic tissue and alter the structure of connective tissue. Within the first week post-MI, the normal collagen structure virtually disappears[22] and myofibroblasts reconstitute a new collagen network, which is essential for scar formation.[21] After several weeks, a stable collagen structure forms a solid scar with little cellularity.[23] To preserve cardiac output, the infarcted area induces an adaptive hypertrophic growth response in the remote zones of the ventricle.[24] Subsequently, the hemodynamic burden

drives dilation of the ventricle, leading to the decline of systolic as well as diastolic functions.[24] The overall post-MI remodeling is a strong prognostic determinant and is closely related to the incidence of arrhythmias and sudden cardiac death.[25]

Early reperfusion of the occluded vessel is crucial for minimizing the infarct size and reducing mortality.[26] Although reperfusion—either spontaneous or consequent to reperfusion therapy—halts ischemic injury, it can cause additional injury, contributing to up to 50% of the final infarct size.[27,28] Ischemia-reperfusion injury (IRI) leads to myocardial damage that can be compounded by arrhythmias, myocardial stunning (reversible postischemic contractile dysfunction), endothelial dysfunction, microvascular obstruction (inability to reperfuse an ischemic region due to capillary damage), and lethal myocardial injury.[29] The molecular mechanisms underlying IRI are complex and involve the overproduction of reactive oxygen species, calcium overload, damage due to rapid restoration of pH, and inflammation.[28] Despite numerous clinical trials testing approaches to lower or block IRI, no effective therapies to minimize these adverse effects of revascularization have been established.[30]

Cardiac Remodeling

Remodeling of the heart due to pathological stimuli affects and involves all cell types. In particular, cardiomyocytes and cardiac fibroblasts transitioning into myofibroblasts play a major role. However, recent evidence indicates that immune cells significantly contribute to cardiac remodeling because immunoreactive inflammation affects the cardiac vasculature and microcirculation. In the following section, we provide an overview of the processes within each cell type throughout the course of cardiac remodeling.

Cardiomyocytes

Cardiomyocytes carry out the contractile function of the heart. The majority of them are terminally differentiated postmitotic cells exhibiting very limited regenerative potential. The low turnover rate of cardiomyocytes is problematic because the heart has insufficient regenerative capacity after injury or in diseased states. As previously mentioned, AMI causes regional anoxia and cell death, particularly of cardiomyocytes.[31] In addition to the acutely affected area, cells in the adjacent zones of survival are also prone to death after AMI.[32] Besides the massive cell loss caused by AMI, even the low rates of continued cardiomyocyte apoptosis in chronic disease states can lead to the development of CHF.[33] Pathophysiological stimuli contribute to ventricular cardiomyocyte remodeling and death through pathways such as necrosis, apoptosis, and possibly excessive autophagy.[34]

Cardiomyocytes have potential plasticity regarding their cell size in response to a variety of stimuli. Exercise, pregnancy, and postnatal growth promote a physiological adaptive growth, whereas neurohumoral and mechanical triggers, hypertension, and myocardial injury lead to pathological hypertrophic growth.[35] On the cellular level, cardiomyocyte remodeling entails reorganization of sarcomeric structures, alterations in calcium signaling, and metabolic changes, all of which can result in systolic and diastolic dysfunction.[34]

Pathological stimuli also lead to alterations in electrophysiological processes (excitation–contraction coupling, rearrangement of ion-channels) within cardiomyocytes, resulting in electrical remodeling.[36] A central feature of electrical remodeling is alterations in transmembrane calcium fluxes, which have been shown to contribute to the pathogenesis of hypertrophy and HF. Additional aspects of electrical remodeling are discussed in the following section.

Cardiac Fibroblasts and Fibrosis

Cardiac fibroblasts are the most abundant cell type in the adult heart, with cardiomyocytes estimated to constitute 30% of cardiac cells and fibroblasts representing the majority of the remaining 70%.[37,38] Cardiac fibroblasts maintain the composition of the extracellular matrix, an acellular scaffold, and the organizational network that distributes the mechanical force throughout the myocardium and is essential for cardiac function.[39] The peripheral positioning of cardiac fibroblasts allows them to act as sources and sensors of mechanical, chemical, and electrical stimuli, enabling contractile coordination and electrical coupling between cardiomyocytes. In addition, recent studies provided evidence that fibroblasts are also protective for cardiomyocytes in IRI.[40] Taken together, cardiac fibroblasts are crucial for cardiac homeostasis,[41] and in the developing heart, fibroblasts are essential for cardiomyocyte proliferation.[42] Modulation of cardiac fibroblasts to a more embryonic state could trigger cardiomyocyte regeneration in heart disease.

Despite their critical role in homeostasis, fibroblasts are also major mediators in maladaptive cardiac remodeling and HF. Stimuli including chronic pressure or volume overload, autocrine and/or paracrine release of growth factors, and cytokines activate the profibrotic signaling pathways, leading to secretion of collagens and proteases and remodeling of extracellular matrix. Fibrotic remodeling is classified as reparative/replacement fibrosis or scarring that accompanies cardiomyocyte death and reactive fibrosis that appears as "interstitial" or "perivascular" and is not directly associated with cardiomyocyte death.[43,44] Fibrosis can also be initiated indirectly by the secretion of fibrogenic mediators (such as tumor necrosis factor [TNF]-α, transforming growth factor-β, and endothelin [ET]-1) by immune cells, cardiomyocytes, and vascular cells.[41] The increased cytokine and growth factor release causes fibroblasts to transform into myofibroblasts, which proliferate, migrate, and remodel the cardiac interstitium through increased secretion of proteases and collagen.[45] In addition, myofibroblasts secrete growth factors and cytokines (i.e., interleukin 1-β [IL-1β], IL-6, and TNF), which can further activate inflammation and drive cardiac remodeling.[46] Initially, all of these changes are critical to the reparative wound healing response. However, over time,

these changes become maladaptive, leading to fibrosis that affects cardiomyocyte metabolism and performance, ultimately resulting in ventricular dysfunction.[47] Furthermore, recent data suggest that after cardiac injury, the mechanical interactions between cardiomyocytes and myofibroblasts also impair the cardiac conduction as a result of the increased mechanosensitive channel activation, which contributes to electrical remodeling.[48]

Identifying and specifically targeting the subsets of cardiac fibroblasts that drive the adverse cardiac remodeling holds promise for improving postischemic contractile performance.

Immune Cells

Along with cardiomyocytes and fibroblasts, resident and invading immune cells respond immediately to early cardiac injury.[49] Diseased and injured hearts contain more macrophages than healthy hearts, most of which are recruited or derived from invading monocytes.[50,51] Depletion of a subset of macrophages in mice did not prevent hypertrophy in a hypertension animal model but resulted in a decline in systolic function, exemplifying the crucial role that immune cells play in cardiac homeostasis.[52] Macrophage depletion in an early phase of AMI was found to lead to increased necrotic debris and neutrophils, resulting in an impaired repair mechanism. Meanwhile, depletion of macrophages at a later stage prevented collagen deposition and diminished remodeling, suggesting heterogeneity in cardiac macrophage composition and function.[53,50] The rapid response of neutrophils to an acute injury was shown to be protective in AMI animal models, but their precise role in hypertrophy remains poorly understood.[51]

In addition, T-cells are recruited during the inflammatory stage of postinfarction remodeling. Depletion of T-cells in cardiac pressure overload models reduced cardiac fibrosis, decreased the number of infiltrating macrophages, and attenuated cardiac dysfunction.[54] However, T-cells are a very heterogeneous cell population, and some subpopulations of T-cells have beneficial effects in postinfarction remodeling. For example, increasing T-regulatory cells attenuated fibrosis and improved cardiac function after AMI.[55] Targeting deleterious, inflammatory subpopulations of immune cells or manipulating immune cell phenotypes may be a novel therapeutic approach to blunt remodeling or even increase regeneration after cardiac injury.

Vascular Remodeling: Endothelial and Smooth Muscle Cells

Vascular endothelial cells are strategically positioned between the vascular wall and the bloodstream, playing a critical role in the pathogenesis of cardiac hypertrophy, remodeling, and failure. Through secretion of growth factors such as ET-1 (a potent vasoconstrictor with inotropic properties) and the expression of adhesion molecules, endothelial cells modulate vascular tone, thrombogenicity, and inflammation. When expressed, proteins such as the intercellular adhesion molecule-1 (ICAM-1) and the vascular cell adhesion molecule-1 (VCAM-1) promote inflammation by recruiting immune cells. The correlation between ET-1 expression levels and the degree of CHF has been well established.[56] ET-1 contributes to essential hypertension, CAD, and chronic renal failure progression and promotes cardiac fibrosis.[57] Furthermore, endothelial cells release proangiogenic growth factors that affect both heart size and cardiac function. Disruption of coordinated tissue growth and angiogenesis in the heart contributes to the progression from adaptive cardiac hypertrophy to CHF.[58] In response to pressure overload, complete blockade promotes the transition from compensatory cardiac hypertrophy to failure.[59]

Lastly, vascular smooth muscle cells can move from the tunica media to the intima, where they contribute to vascular remodeling by synthesis of extracellular matrix components, specifically proteoglycans.[60] When activated by proinflammatory cytokines, the smooth muscle cells produce more collagen, leading to arterial fibrosis and the release of matrix-remodeling proteinases.[61]

Cardiac Remodeling and Arrhythmias

Disease-related electrical remodeling is a fundamental mechanism underlying the often life-threatening arrhythmias associated with HF. Electrical remodeling leads to pathophysiological changes at various stages and in cell types within the cardiac conduction system.

The sinoatrial (SA) node undergoes significant remodeling characterized by anatomical and structural changes in CHF patients.[62] Fibrosis during cardiac remodeling may lead to SA node reentry and exit block, thereby causing AF, ventricular arrhythmias, and cardiac arrest.[63] Even transient episodes of atrial tachyarrhythmias, which occur commonly in HF, can induce significant electrical remodeling in the SA node and consequent nodal dysfunction.[64]

Cardiac Purkinje cells play an important role in the generation of ventricular arrhythmias, particularly those related to triggered activity.[65] In addition, CHF causes remodeling of important potassium and calcium currents, which, with HF-induced ion channel changes, may promote arrhythmogenic afterdepolarizations.[36]

Atrial Fibrillation

AF is the most common type of arrhythmia after MI, occurring in up to 39% of patients, and is associated with high morbidity and mortality.[66,67] The mechanisms of AF are complex and involve structural and electrical remodeling in both the atrial and ventricular myocardia.[68] The relationship between ventricular remodeling, especially ventricular fibrosis, and the onset of AF is not well understood.[69] However, the remodeling of atrial myocytes during HF is a major contributor to the pathogenesis of AF.[39] Atrial structural and functional changes may develop as a result of pathological systemic processes in cardiac conditions, including hypertension, valvular disease, and HF, or AF itself.[62] Certain aspects of the structural remodeling in AF, such as interstitial fibrosis, cellular hypertrophy, and degeneration, are irreversible and develop concurrently with electrical alterations.[39] These changes may reduce the efficacy of medical therapy for chronic AF in CHF patients.

Ventricular Arrhythmia

A prolonged ventricular action potential is a common feature of HF and is responsible for triggering abnormal impulses by increasing the risk of intracellular calcium overload. The changes in the ion channels, which contribute to prolonged action potential duration, are thoroughly reviewed elsewhere.[37,39] Lengthening of ventricular action potential duration is also common in hypertrophy, a phenotype that contrasts with the shortened action potential in the stressed (fibrillating) atrium.[34]

In recent years, a large body of evidence has defined the association between LV hypertrophy, ventricular arrhythmia, and sudden cardiac death.[70] The risk of arrhythmia increases with the extent of LV hypertrophy, and hypertrophy also serves as a predictive risk factor for mortality.[71,72] Patients with LV hypertrophy have a 3.4-fold increased risk of developing supraventricular tachycardias and 2.8-fold increased risk of developing ventricular tachycardia or fibrillation.[73] Myocardial electric remodeling is manifested as abnormalities of repolarization (prolonged QTc and $T_{peak}-T_{end}$ intervals) and depolarization (prolonged QRS interval), both of which facilitate the phenomenon of reentry. Lastly, the amount of fibrotic scar in the myocardium correlates strongly with the increased incidence of arrhythmias and sudden cardiac death.

Approaches to Enhance Cardiac Regeneration

Cardiomyocytes were considered to be postmitotic, but recent reports have shown a cardiomyocyte turnover rate of around 1% per year, a number which declines with age.[74,75] However, this turnover does not contribute to significant regeneration, and the loss of cardiomyocytes therefore leads to irreversible HF. Given the poor cardiac regenerative capacity of adult mammals, considerable efforts have been made to create new muscle in the setting of an injured heart. Regenerative therapy approaches can be divided into two major categories that are discussed here: stimulation of intrinsic cardiac regenerative potential and extrinsic cell-based therapies (Fig. 30.2).

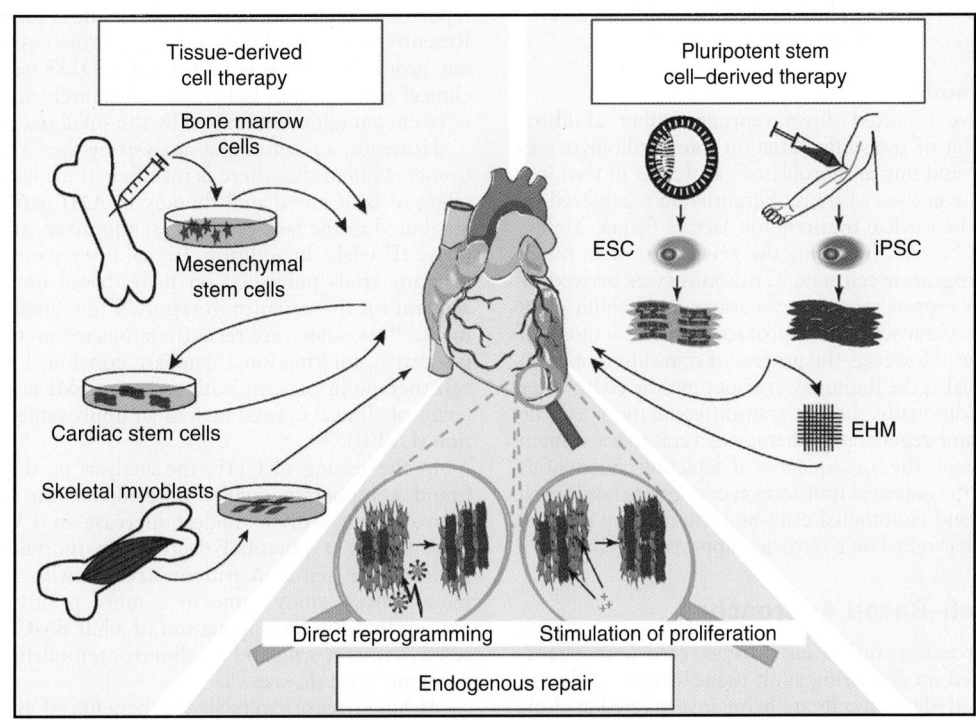

FIGURE 30.2 Major approaches for cardiac regeneration. *EHM,* Engineered heart muscle; *ESC,* embryonic stem cells; *iPSC,* induced pluripotent stem cells.

Enhancement of Intrinsic Regeneration

Lower vertebrates such as zebra fish and amphibians demonstrate an intrinsic cardiac regenerative potential. Their cardiomyocytes are mainly mononucleated and retain the ability to proliferate throughout adulthood.[76] In the adult mammalian heart, most cardiomyocytes are binucleated and polyploid, and the vast majority of them have exited the cell cycle. Interestingly, mammals are born with mononucleated cardiomyocytes that have the ability to divide, and mammalian hearts can fully regenerate myocardium without scar formation after apex dissection or induced AMI in the early postnatal period.[77,78] This regenerative potential is present during the first days after birth and requires both cardiomyocyte proliferation and angiogenesis. However, the mechanisms underlying neonatal mammalian cardiac regeneration are poorly understood. A recent study demonstrated that immune cells, especially macrophages, play a role in the regenerative processes.[79] In addition, molecular studies have implicated specific signaling pathways in cardiomyocyte proliferation, particularly the Hippo-YAP pathway and the transcription factor Meis1.[80] A better understanding of the pathways regulating mammalian cardiomyocyte proliferation will allow us to augment and exploit intrinsic regeneration as a potential therapeutic approach in HF.

Reports from patients with nonischemic dilated cardiomyopathy treated with LV assist devices (LVADs) suggest an intrinsic regenerative potential of the adult heart. Following LVAD therapy, some patients displayed myocardial recovery,[81] but the mechanisms underlying the recovery remained unclear. However, ventricular unloading in combination with pharmacological therapy was thought to support intrinsic regenerative capacities.[82] Based on these findings, in a recent prospective study, myocardial biopsies from implantation as well as explantation of LVADs in DCM patients were compared.[83] Patients with more than 6 months of LVAD therapy had the most profound changes in their cardiomyocyte population, showing a reversal of a hypertrophic state to a more hyperplastic state. These data fall in line with changes in the regenerating heart observed in early postnatal mammals, as previously mentioned. A deeper understanding of the underlying mechanisms for these findings could be combined with a defined temporary unloading of the diseased heart to create a promising regenerative therapy for systolic HF.

Direct Reprogramming

Recent studies have reported direct reprogramming of fibroblasts with induction of transdifferentiation into cardiomyocytes in vitro in mouse[84] and human fibroblasts[85] as well as in vivo in a mouse model.[86] The process of transdifferentiation is achieved by overexpression of the cardiac transcription factors Gata4, Mef2c, Tbx5, Hand2, and Nkx2.5, bypassing the generation of an intermediate stem or progenitor cell state. Cardiomyocytes derived by transdifferentiation express sarcomeric markers and exhibit electrophysiological and transcriptional profiles similar to those of fetal cardiomyocytes. However, the process of transdifferentiation remains controversial as the findings were not reproduced by other investigators.[87] Additionally, before transdifferentiation can be established as a major regenerative therapy, several issues remain to be addressed, namely the consequences of depleting endogenous cardiac fibroblasts, the potential transfection of nontarget cells such as smooth muscle and endothelial cells, and the delivery method itself, which so far has relied on a retroviral approach in vivo.[88]

Exogenous Cell–Based Approaches

In contrast to approaches stimulating intrinsic cardiac regeneration, therapies based on delivering adult tissue–derived cells and pluripotent stem cell–derived cells are being investigated in clinical trials. The following section provides an overview of the cell sources currently being investigated and discusses associated benefits, risks, and possible adverse reactions.

Adult Tissue–Derived Progenitor Cell Therapy

Transplantation of exogenous cells began in the mid-1990s, when myoblasts injected into an infarcted area were reported to improve myocardial function.[89,90] Since then, progenitor cells from adult primary tissues such as skeletal muscle, bone marrow, and the adult heart have been transplanted in patients either via endomyocardial or intracoronary application.

Skeletal Myoblasts. Myoblasts were a promising cell source for cell therapy and were shown to benefit myocardial performance in numerous preclinical trials. A pilot clinical study in which myoblasts were injected to treat ischemic HF reported positive findings after a 6-month follow-up.[91,92] Although ensuing clinical trials involving skeletal myoblast therapy were encouraging, the first prospective randomized, placebo-controlled phase II skeletal myoblast trial (MAGIC trial) exhibited a lack of efficacy and was discontinued prematurely.[93] The disappointing results were due to several reasons: low initial cell retention, a high rate of subsequent cell death, and the inability of engrafted myoblasts to establish functional electromechanical connections with the host cardiomyocytes. In addition, a trend toward excess arrhythmias was observed in myoblast-treated patients despite the use of the prophylactic antiarrhythmic drug amiodarone. This confirmed early safety concerns that were raised in phase I trials.

By contrast, the SEISMIC trial argued that injection of autologous skeletal myoblasts in HF patients was safe and provided symptomatic relief, as demonstrated by increased exercise tolerance.[94] Nevertheless, no significant effect on global LVEF was observed. The negative results of MAGIC+SEISMIC trials and the arrhythmogenic potential associated with skeletal myoblasts have caused a shift to other sources for cell therapy in HF.

Bone Marrow Cells. Autologous bone marrow–derived cells (BMCs) are the most prevalent cell type studied in clinical trials thus far. In 2001 it was reported that BMCs selected on the basis of c-kit expression could regenerate the heart by engrafting and differentiating into cardiomyocytes in vivo.[95] However, subsequent studies using parabiotic systems and lineage tracing could not demonstrate any differentiation of the transplanted BMCs into cardiomyocytes.[96,97] In addition, in initial studies, the injection of BMCs directly into the myocardium or coronary vasculature was reported to induce modest improvement in cardiac function.[98–100] Recently, fractions of bone marrow purified using the hematopoietic progenitor markers CD34 and CD133 have been studied in clinical trials in both ischemic and nonischemic HF. The results were encouraging but limited by the small size of the trials.[101,102]

However, a recent meta-analysis by the Cochrane Collaboration concluded that there is insufficient evidence for a beneficial effect of BMC-mediated therapy in AMI patients,[103] which was attributed to the lack of larger, randomized, adequately powered phase III trials. In addition, factual discrepancies were identified in many trials published on BMC-based therapies, which may account for the variance in reported functional cardiac improvement.[104] Another very recently published meta-analysis of a collaborative, multinational database concluded that intracoronary cell therapy in patients with a recent AMI was not beneficial in terms of clinical events, such as an improvement in systolic function (LVEF).[105]

In the setting of CHF, the analysis by the Cochrane group found a moderate quality of evidence for functional cardiac improvement with a modest increase in LVEF, with limited evidence for a potential decrease in mortality and long-term performance status in patients treated with BMCs.[106] Another meta-analysis study came to a more positive conclusion suggesting that the transplantation of adult BMCs improves LVEF, reduces infarct size, and ameliorates remodeling in patients with ischemic heart disease.[107]

Although controversial, the benefits of BMC-based cardiac cell therapy could be predominantly paracrine mediated, with cells releasing factors that lead to neovascularization, cardiac repair, and cytoprotection.[108]

The debate regarding whether BMCs serve as an evidence-based therapy in the setting of AMI or HF is ongoing. To this end, the BAMI trial (The Effect of Intracoronary Reinfusion of Bone Marrow-derived Mononuclear Cells on All-Cause Mortality in Acute Myocardial Infarction), a multicenter, interventional, randomized, open-label trial was started in September 2013 (clinical trial identifier NCT01569178). The primary endpoint of this study is the 3-year all-cause mortality, with results expected in 2018.

Beside the ongoing discussion about the effectiveness of BMC therapy in cardiac diseases, the administration of cells has been proven to be safe, with a low procedural complication rate (around 2%). Importantly, there is no evidence that intracoronary administration of BMCs induces life-threatening arrhythmias in patients with CHF.[109]

Mesenchymal Stem Cells. About 0.01% of the cells in bone marrow are multipotent mesenchymal stem cells (MSCs).[110] After bone marrow aspiration, MSCs are purified and expanded ex vivo before being transplanted into the heart. Compared to BMCs, using MSCs as a source of cell therapy showed improved cardiac function in initial trials[111]; however, a direct comparison of BMCs and MSCs injected transendocardially in CHF patients showed only insignificant functional changes.[112]

Aside from modest beneficial effects similar to BMCs, a major limitation of autologous MSC transplantation is the obligatory 4- to 6-week in vitro cell expansion. In the POSEIDON trial, autologous and allogenic MSCs were applied transendocardially in postinfarction HF patients. Both MSC sources appeared to be safe, with comparable, modest effects on ventricular remodeling.[113] To potentially increase the effectiveness of cell therapy on cardiac regeneration, the C-CURE trial exposed autologous MSCs to a cocktail of cardiogenic cytokines prior to endomyocardial injections in postinfarction HF patients.[114] The trial confirmed feasibility and safety and reported a slightly higher increase in LVEF (7%) than that reported by studies using unconditioned MSCs.

Similar to BMCs, the complication rate associated with MSC treatment is very low. Furthermore, there are hints that MSCs may protect against arrhythmias after MI by positively affecting potassium channel remodeling.[115]

Endogenous Cardiac Stem Cells. In 2003, endogenous cardiac progenitor cells (CPCs) were first proposed as cells expressing the tyrosine protein kinase (CD117 or c-kit), with the potential to self-renew; to differentiate into myocytes, smooth muscle, and endothelial cells; and to regenerate the heart after injury.[116] Since then, other markers such as Sca-1[117] and the transcription factor *Islet-1*[118] have been used to characterize subsets of CPCs. Other candidate CPCs were isolated on the basis of their unique behavior. Side population cells were named after their ability to efflux a DNA-binding dye with an adenosine triphosphate (ATP)–binding cassette,[119] whereas cardiosphere-derived cells (CDCs) came from self-assembling multicellular clusters formed in culture.[120] However, two independent lineage-tracing studies in transgenic mice have shown that CPCs, in particular those expressing c-kit, marginally contribute to cardiomyocytes in the heart,[121] with the vast majority displaying an endothelial phenotype.[122] Hence their potential therapeutic value in cardiac muscle regeneration therapies remains controversial.[123]

Beside these controversies, recent clinical trials have studied ex vivo expanded autologous CPCs for cell therapy. A clinical phase I trial (SCIPIO trial) utilizing c-kit+ was initiated. C-*kit*+ cells were isolated from the atrial appendage during bypass surgery, tested and expanded ex vivo, and, finally, injected intracoronary around 120 days after surgery.[124] While the study was still in progress, early results were published with marked improvement of cardiac function 4 months after cell therapy[124] and also after 1 year of follow-up.[125] Recently, concerns were raised regarding the integrity of the trial,[126] and the final results of the study are still outstanding after completion of the study in September 2013.

Another source of cardiac-derived cell therapy tested in clinical trials are CDCs. These are derived by ex vivo expansion after explant culture of endomyocardial biopsies.[120] However, recent reports highlighted the very limited potential of CDCs to differentiate into cardiomyocytes.[127] Their therapeutic benefit in vivo has been proposed to be secondary to stimulating endogenous unknown repair mechanisms, which might involve myogenesis.[128,129] In the first clinical phase I trial using CDCs in HF patients (CADUCEUS Trial), there was no significant difference in the LVEF, end-systolic, or end-diastolic volumes between the treatment and the control groups. Although the CDC-treated patients were reported to have increased viable myocardium and contractility as well as reduced scar mass at 6-month posttreatment, they also exhibited high levels of nonsustained ventricular tachycardia, and serious events at the 1-year follow-up were observed.[130] Ongoing studies are currently evaluating allogenic CDCs in DCM and postinfarction HF patients (DYNAMIC and ALLSTAR).

A novel approach of combining CDCs and growth factors with a controlled release of the basic fibroblast growth factor (bFGF) has been shown to be effective in a porcine model.[131] A subsequent clinical phase I trial (ALCADIA) demonstrated the safety of the combined administration in CHF patients. Larger, randomized, and placebo-controlled trials are needed to also prove effectiveness.

Pluripotent Stem Cell Therapy

Pluripotent stem cells hold great potential for regenerative therapies due to their ability to differentiate into every cell type of the human body. Human embryonic stem cells (ESCs) are the most studied, but the process involves the destruction of human embryos that raises ethical concerns and thus greatly restricts their use. Induced pluripotent stem cells (iPSCs) overcome this problem as they can be derived from any terminally differentiated cell of any individual. The transcription factors OCT4, SOX2, KLF4, and c-MYC are highly expressed in ESCs, and the forced expression of these four factors can reprogram terminally differentiated cells into a stem cell–like cell state.[132,133] Since the first description of iPSCs in 2006, intensive efforts have been made to improve the reprogramming techniques and to eliminate random integration of the exogenous genes, which is an important prerequisite for potential clinical applications.[134] Human iPSCs and ESCs possess comparable differentiation potential, allowing for the directed differentiation into numerous tissue cell types, including cardiomyocytes. In recent years, progress has been made in optimizing the efficiency of differentiation protocols, making it possible to reproducibly generate large-scale numbers of iPSC- and ESC-derived cardiomyocytes (iPSC-CMs and ESC-CMs)[135-137] Cardiomyocytes derived from human ESCs and iPSCs, particularly the autologous iPSC-CMs, are extremely valuable for disease modeling and drug screening.[138] The ability to derive iPSCs from any individual has great implications in precision medicine.

Beside these preclinical applications, ESC-CMs or iPSC-CMs may serve as the optimal source for regenerative therapies in cardiac injury and HF. Preclinical trials using ESC-CMs in HF models showed promising results in mice, rats,[100] pigs,[139] and nonhuman primates.[140,141] After optimizing generation of ESC-CMs to ensure quality and safety of the graft as well as cell delivery systems, the first clinical trial in postinfarction HF patients was initiated in May 2013. This French study tested ESC-derived mesoderm/cardiomyocyte progenitor cells surgically delivered using a fibrin patch (ESCORT; clinical accession number NCT02057900).[142] In the first 3-month follow-up, investigators reported no major complications (e.g., arrhythmias, tumor formation, or adverse effects from immunosuppression therapy).[143]

Discussion of Pluripotent Cell–Based Therapies

Although significant progress has been made toward the use of pluripotent stem cell–derived cardiomyocytes for regenerative therapy, several concerns remain to be addressed as discussed in the following sections.

Route of Delivery: Injection Based Versus Engineered Patch Based. Injection-based delivery allows for better integration into host myocardium, whereas patch-based delivery is superior in cell retention, survival, and preservation of heart function.[143-145] Even during long-term observations, cells delivered via patch remain in situ.[146] However, the patch does not integrate with existing tissue or generate new tissue, but rather harnesses endogenous repair pathways through a paracrine effect. In a recent study using ESC-CMs in nonhuman primates, intramyocardial delivery resulted in long-term graft survival, although epicardially applied patches did not remain adherent.[147]

Electrical Coupling and Arrhythmias. In a recent study, ESC-CMs were injected into the infarcted hearts of monkeys, and successful cardiomyocyte engraftment with vascularization of the graft by the host was observed.[147] While engraftment allowed constructs to electrically couple with the host myocardium, nonfatal ventricular arrhythmias were observed in the first weeks after transplantation. In contrast, in an earlier study by the same group, ESC-CMs injected in guinea pigs also showed electrical coupling but were protective against arrhythmias.[139] One possible explanation is the different beat rates across species (macaques: 100–130 beats/min, guinea pigs: 230 beats/min, rats: 400 beats/min, and mice: 600 beats/min).[139] Hence grafts could cause arrhythmias through inherent automaticity and triggered activity, or the graft itself could promote reentry due to interference with the electrical excitation of the host myocardium.

Immunogenicity and Tumorigenicity. ESC lines are well established and characterized, with the advantage of avoiding the risk of genetic alterations associated with reprogramming. However, because ESCs are an allogenic cell source, they might require life-long immunosuppression if administered to HF patients. Furthermore, autologous, syngenic transplantation of undifferentiated iPSCs was shown to induce an immune response.[148] By comparison, differentiated cells derived from iPSCs or ESCs were shown to induce very limited or no immune response.[149] Preclinical studies in small animals have shown no significant immune response following transplantation of ESC- or iPSC-CMs.[139,140] However, because ESC- and iPSC-CMs exhibit a relatively immature phenotype, this by itself could lead to an activation of the immune system when applied to humans. The initiation of pilot preclinical studies in large animals such as nonhuman primates could provide valuable insights into possible adverse immune responses of pluripotent stem cell–derived cardiomyocytes, especially autologous iPSC-CMs.

Another risk for using iPSC-CMs is that despite well-established, nonintegrative reprogramming methods, genetic alterations may still arise due to the reprogramming and/or extensive cell culture. Furthermore, incomplete or partial reprogramming of a very small proportion may increase the risk of tumorigenicity. Pluripotent stem cell–derived cells carry the inherent risk of residual pluripotent cells and thus the potential to form teratomas.[144] Long-term follow-ups in large animal studies or human trials are not yet available, so the exact risk remains uncertain, but preclinical trials thus far suggest a minimal risk. In nonhuman primates, transplanted ESCs after AMI led to teratoma formation in the scar, but no teratomas were found after the transplantation of differentiated cardiomyocytes.[140] Additionally, engineered heart muscle (EHM) derived from human ESC-CMs were implanted into immunocompromised rats after AMI with no evidence of tumor or teratoma formation.[150] Research to eliminate potential premature cells from the transplants is ongoing and could eliminate this potential tumorigenic risk.[151]

Human pluripotent stem cell–derived cardiomyocytes have a tremendous potential to create a truly regenerative approach in HF, although challenges in safety and regenerative efficacy remain. Nonetheless, the first clinical trial using ESC-derived cells has been initiated, and the results are expected to drive future research and optimization of cell therapy.

Outlook

Recent years have seen extensive efforts to create new cardiac regeneration therapies, and several innovative approaches have now advanced from preclinical testing into clinical trials.[152] Transplantation of adult tissue–derived cells after AMI or in CHF is under active investigation. However, true cardiomyocyte regeneration and therapeutic outcomes remain elusive, and some of the modest observed benefits are attributed to paracrine signaling of the transplanted cells. Recent advances in generating pluripotent cell–derived cardiomyocytes from ESCs or iPSCs, as well as extensive preclinical research, have brought this approach closer to the clinic. The tremendous regenerative potential of these pluripotent cell–derived cardiomyocytes may be realized once current concerns such as tumorigenicity, immunogenicity, immaturity of the transplanted cardiomyocytes, and arrhythmogenicity are resolved.[153] Beside cell-based regenerative therapies, cardiac regeneration based on restoring or stimulating intrinsic cardiac regenerative potential is equally promising but needs to advance from the preclinical phase.

In the future, cardiac regeneration may be achieved by combining different approaches, including the use of extrinsic cell therapy and reactivation/stimulation of a silenced intrinsic cardiac regeneration program.

Acknowledgments

We thank Blake Wu for the critical reading, and we received funding support from the American Heart Association (AHA) 13 EIA 14420025, Innovation in Regulatory Science Award (Burroughs Wellcome Fund), National Institutes of Health (NIH) R01 HL130020, NIH R01 HL128170, NIH R01 HL123968, (JCW), the Sarnoff Cardiovascular Research Foundation (CS), the German Research Foundation (TS), and NIH K99 HL104002, AHA 15BGIA22730027 (I.K.).

REFERENCES

1. Mozaffarian D, Benjamin EJ, Go AS, et al. Heart disease and stroke statistics—2015 update: a report from the American Heart Association. *Circulation.* 2014;131:e29–e322.
2. Cohn JN, Ferrari R, Sharpe N. Cardiac remodeling—concepts and clinical implications: a consensus paper from an international forum on cardiac remodeling. *J Am Coll Cardiol.* 2000;35:569–582.
3. Borlaug BA, Redfield MM. Diastolic and systolic heart failure are distinct phenotypes within the heart failure spectrum. *Circulation.* 2011;123:2006–2013.
4. Maron BJ. Contemporary definitions and classification of the cardiomyopathies: an American Heart Association scientific statement from the Council on Clinical Cardiology, Heart Failure and Transplantation Committee; Quality of Care and Outcomes Research and Function. *Circulation.* 2006;113:1807–1816.
5. Yancy CW, Jessup M, Bozkurt B, et al. 2013 ACCF/AHA guideline for the management of heart failure: a report of the American College of Cardiology Foundation/American Heart Association Task Force on practice guidelines. *Circulation.* 2013;128:e240–e327.
6. Borlaug BA, Paulus WJ. Heart failure with preserved ejection fraction: pathophysiology, diagnosis, and treatment. *Eur Heart J.* 2011;32:670–679.
7. Shimizu I, Minamino T. Physiological and pathological cardiac hypertrophy. *J Mol Cell Cardiol.* 2016;97:245–262.
8. Soufer R, Wohlgelernter D, Vita NA, et al. Intact systolic left ventricular function in clinical congestive heart failure. *Am J Cardiol.* 1985;55:1032–1036.
9. Packer M. Can brain natriuretic peptide be used to guide the management of patients with heart failure and a preserved ejection fraction? The wrong way to identify new treatments for a nonexistent disease. *Circ Heart Fail.* 2011;4:538–540.
10. Brouwers FP, de Boer RA, van der Harst P, et al. Incidence and epidemiology of new onset heart failure with preserved vs. reduced ejection fraction in a community-based cohort: 11-year follow-up of PREVEND. *Eur Heart J.* 2013;34:1424–1431.
11. Lee DS, Gona P, Vasan RS, Larson MG, et al. Relation of disease pathogenesis and risk factors to heart failure with preserved or reduced ejection fraction: insights from the Framingham Heart Study of the National Heart, Lung, and Blood Institute. *Circulation.* 2009;119:3070–3077.
12. Lam CSP, Roger VL, Rodeheffer RJ, et al. Cardiac structure and ventricular-vascular function in persons with heart failure and preserved ejection fraction from Olmsted County, Minnesota. *Circulation.* 2007;115:1982–1990.
13. Mohammed SF, Hussain S, Mirzoyev SA, Edwards WD, Maleszewski JJ, Redfield MM. Coronary microvascular rarefaction and myocardial fibrosis in heart failure with preserved ejection fraction. *Circulation.* 2015;131:550–559.

14. Paulus WJ, Tschöpe C. A novel paradigm for heart failure with preserved ejection fraction: Comorbidities drive myocardial dysfunction and remodeling through coronary microvascular endothelial inflammation. *J Am Coll Cardiol*. 2013;62:263–271.
15. Heinzel FR, Hohendanner F, Jin G, Sedej S, Edelmann F. Myocardial hypertrophy and its role in heart failure with preserved ejection fraction. *J Appl Physiol*. 2015;119:1233–1242.
16. Katz DH, Beussink L, Sauer AJ, Freed BH, Burke MA, Shah SJ. Prevalence, clinical characteristics, and outcomes associated with eccentric versus concentric left ventricular hypertrophy in heart failure with preserved ejection fraction. *Am J Cardiol*. 2013;112:1158–1164.
17. Somaratne JB, Berry C, McMurray JJ, Poppe KK, Doughty RN, Whalley GA. The prognostic significance of heart failure with preserved left ventricular ejection fraction: a literature-based meta-analysis. *Eur J Heart Fail*. 2009;11:855–862.
18. Gottdiener JS, McClelland RL, Marshall R, et al. Outcome of congestive heart failure in elderly persons: influence of left ventricular systolic function. The Cardiovascular Health Study. *Ann Intern Med*. 2002;137:631–639.
19. Fraccarollo D, Galuppo P, Bauersachs J. Novel therapeutic approaches to post-infarction remodelling. *Cardiovasc Res*. 2012;94:293–303.
20. Oerlemans MIFJ, Koudstaal S, Chamuleau SA, de Kleijn DP, Doevendans PA, Sluijter JPG. Targeting cell death in the reperfused heart: pharmacological approaches for cardioprotection. *Int J Cardiol*. 2013;165:410–422.
21. Ertl G, Frantz S. Healing after myocardial infarction. *Cardiovasc Res*. 2005;66:22–32.
22. Whittaker P, Boughner DR, Kloner RA. Role of collagen in acute myocardial infarct expansion. *Circulation*. 1991;84:2123–2134.
23. Willems IE, Havenith MG, De Mey JG, Daemen MJ. The alpha-smooth muscle actin-positive cells in healing human myocardial scars. *Am J Pathol*. 1994;145:868–875.
24. Dorn GW. Novel pharmacotherapies to abrogate postinfarction ventricular remodeling. *Nat Rev Cardiol*. 2009;6:283–291.
25. Gaudron P, Kugler I, Hu K, Bauer W, Eilles C, Ertl G. Time course of cardiac structural, functional and electrical changes in asymptomatic patients after myocardial infarction: their inter-relation and prognostic impact. *J Am Coll Cardiol*. 2001;38:33–40.
26. O'Gara PT, Kushner FG, Ascheim DD, et al. 2013 ACCF/AHA guideline for the management of ST-elevation myocardial infarction: a report of the American College of Cardiology Foundation/American Heart Association Task Force on Practice Guidelines. *Circulation*. 2013;127:e362–e425.
27. Matsumura K, Jeremy RW, Schaper J, Becker LC. Progression of myocardial necrosis during reperfusion of ischemic myocardium. *Circulation*. 1998;97:795–804.
28. Yellon DM, Hausenloy DJ. Myocardial reperfusion injury. *N Engl J Med*. 2007;357:1121–1135.
29. Altamirano F, Wang ZV, Hill JA. Cardioprotection in ischaemia-reperfusion injury: novel mechanisms and clinical translation. *J Physiol*. 2015;593:3773–3788.
30. Hausenloy DJ, Erik Bøtker H, Condorelli G, et al. Translating cardioprotection for patient benefit: position paper from the Working Group of Cellular Biology of the Heart of the European Society of Cardiology. *Cardiovasc Res*. 2013;98:7–27.
31. Pfeffer MA, Braunwald E. Ventricular remodeling after myocardial infarction. Experimental observations and clinical implications. *Circulation*. 1990;81:1161–1172.
32. Olivetti G, Quaini F, Sala R, et al. Acute myocardial infarction in humans is associated with activation of programmed myocyte cell death in the surviving portion of the heart. *J Mol Cell Cardiol*. 1996;28:2005–2016.
33. Wencker D, Chandra M, Nguyen K, et al. A mechanistic role for cardiac myocyte apoptosis in heart failure. *J Clin Invest*. 2003;111:1497–1504.
34. Burchfield JS, Xie M, Hill JA. Pathological ventricular remodeling: mechanisms: part 1 of 2. *Circulation*. 2013;128:388–400.
35. Hill JA, Olson EN. Cardiac plasticity. *N Engl J Med*. 2008;358:1370–1380.
36. Wang Y, Hill JA. Electrophysiological remodeling in heart failure. *J Mol Cell Cardiol*. 2010;48:619–632.
37. Kakkar R, Lee RT. Intramyocardial fibroblast myocyte communication. *Circ Res*. 2010;106:47–57.
38. Chen W, Frangogiannis NG. Fibroblasts in post-infarction inflammation and cardiac repair. *Biochim Biophys Acta*. 2013;1833:945–953.
39. Baum J, Duffy HS. Fibroblasts and myofibroblasts: what are we talking about? *J Cardiovasc Pharmacol*. 2011;57:376–379.
40. Abrial M, Da Silva CC, Pillot B, et al. Cardiac fibroblasts protect cardiomyocytes against lethal ischemia-reperfusion injury. *J Mol Cell Cardiol*. 2014;68:56–65.
41. Souders CA, Bowers SLK, Baudino TA. Cardiac fibroblast: the renaissance cell. *Circ Res*. 2009;105:1164–1176.
42. Ieda M, Tsuchihashi T, Ivey KN, et al. Cardiac fibroblasts regulate myocardial proliferation through beta1 integrin signaling. *Dev Cell*. 2009;16:233–244.
43. Weber KT. Cardiac interstitium in health and disease: the fibrillar collagen network. *J Am Coll Cardiol*. 1989;13:1637–1652.
44. Anderson KR, Sutton MG, Lie JT. Histopathological types of cardiac fibrosis in myocardial disease. *J Pathol*. 1979;128:79–85.
45. Brown RD, Ambler SK, Mitchell MD, Long CS. The cardiac fibroblast: therapeutic target in myocardial remodeling and failure. *Annu Rev Pharmacol Toxicol*. 2005;45:657–687.
46. Corda S, Samuel JL, Rappaport L. Extracellular matrix and growth factors during heart growth. *Heart Fail Rev*. 2000;5:119–130.
47. Porter KE, Turner NA. Cardiac fibroblasts: at the heart of myocardial remodeling. *Pharmacol Ther*. 2009;123:255–278.
48. Thompson SA, Copeland CR, Reich DH, Tung L. Mechanical coupling between myofibroblasts and cardiomyocytes slows electric conduction in fibrotic cell monolayers. *Circulation*. 2011;123:2083–2093.
49. Heidt T, Courties G, Dutta P, et al. Differential contribution of monocytes to heart macrophages in steady-state and after myocardial infarction. *Circ Res*. 2014;115:284–295.
50. Nahrendorf M, Swirski FK, Aikawa E, et al. The healing myocardium sequentially mobilizes two monocyte subsets with divergent and complementary functions. *J Exp Med*. 2007;204:3037–3047.
51. Litt MR, Jeremy RW, Weisman HF, Winkelstein JA, Becker LC. Neutrophil depletion limited to reperfusion reduces myocardial infarct size after 90 minutes of ischemia. Evidence for neutrophil-mediated reperfusion injury. *Circulation*. 1989;80:1816–1827.
52. Zandbergen HR, Sharma UC, Gupta S, et al. Macrophage depletion in hypertensive rats accelerates development of cardiomyopathy. *J Cardiovasc Pharmacol Ther*. 2009;14:68–75.
53. Frantz S, Hofmann U, Fraccarollo D, et al. Monocytes/macrophages prevent healing defects and left ventricular thrombus formation after myocardial infarction. *FASEB J*. 2013;27:871–881.
54. Laroumanie F, Douin-Echinard V, Pozzo J, et al. CD4+ T cells promote the transition from hypertrophy to heart failure during chronic pressure overload. *Circulation*. 2014;129:2111–2124.
55. Tang T-T, Yuan J, Zhu Z-F, et al. Regulatory T cells ameliorate cardiac remodeling after myocardial infarction. *Basic Res Cardiol*. 2012;107:232.
56. Agapitov AV, Haynes WG. Role of endothelin in cardiovascular disease. *J Renin Angiotensin Aldosterone Sys*. 2002;3:1–15.
57. Widyantoro B, Emoto N, Nakayama K, et al. Endothelial cell-derived endothelin-1 promotes cardiac fibrosis in diabetic hearts through stimulation of endothelial-to-mesenchymal transition. *Circulation*. 2010;121:2407–2418.
58. Shiojima I, Sato K, Izumiya Y, et al. Disruption of coordinated cardiac hypertrophy and angiogenesis contributes to the transition to heart failure. *J Clin Invest*. 2005;115:2108–2118.
59. Izumiya Y, Shiojima I, Sato K, Sawyer DB, Colucci WS, Walsh K. Vascular endothelial growth factor blockade promotes the transition from compensatory cardiac hypertrophy to failure in response to pressure overload. *Hypertension*. 2006;47:887–893.
60. Lee RT, Yamamoto C, Feng Y, et al. Mechanical strain induces specific changes in the synthesis and organization of proteoglycans by vascular smooth muscle cells. *J Biol Chem*. 2001;276:13847–13851.
61. Heusch G, Libby P, Gersh B, Yellon D, Böhm M, Lopaschuk G, et al. Cardiovascular remodelling in coronary artery disease and heart failure. *Lancet*. 2014;383:1933–1943.
62. Sanders P, Morton JB, Davidson NC, et al. Electrical remodeling of the atria in congestive heart failure: electrophysiological and electroanatomic mapping in humans. *Circulation*. 2003;108:1461–1468.
63. Csepe TA, Kalyanasundaram A, Hansen BJ, Zhao J, Fedorov VV. Fibrosis: a structural modulator of sinoatrial node physiology and dysfunction. *Front Physiol*. 2015;6:37.
64. Hadian D, Zipes DP, Olgin JE, Miller JM. Short-term rapid atrial pacing produces electrical remodeling of sinus node function in humans. *J Cardiovasc Electrophysiol*. 2002;13:584–586.
65. Berenfeld O, Jalife J. Purkinje-muscle reentry as a mechanism of polymorphic ventricular arrhythmias in a 3-dimensional model of the ventricles. *Circ Res*. 1998;82:1063–1077.
66. Jabre P, Jouven X, Adnet F, et al. Atrial fibrillation and death after myocardial infarction: a community study. *Circulation*. 2011;123:2094–2100.
67. Zareba W, Steinberg JS, McNitt S, Daubert JP, Piotrowicz K, Moss AJ. Implantable cardioverter-defibrillator therapy and risk of congestive heart failure or death in MADIT II patients with atrial fibrillation. *Heart Rhythm*. 2006;3:631–637.
68. Dzeshka MS, Lip GYH, Snezhitskiy V, Shantsila E. Cardiac fibrosis in patients with atrial fibrillation: mechanisms and clinical implications. *J Am Coll Cardiol*. 2015;66:943–959.
69. Dzeshka MS, Lip GYH, Snezhitskiy V, Shantsila E. Cardiac fibrosis in patients with atrial fibrillation: mechanisms and clinical implications. *J Am Coll Cardiol*. 2015;66:943–959.
70. Stecker EC, Vickers C, Waltz J, et al. Population-based analysis of sudden cardiac death with and without left ventricular systolic dysfunction: two-year findings from the Oregon Sudden Unexpected Death Study. *J Am Coll Cardiol*. 2006;47:1161–1166.
71. Liao Y, Cooper RS, McGee DL, Mensah GA, Ghali JK. The relative effects of left ventricular hypertrophy, coronary artery disease, and ventricular dysfunction on survival among black adults. *JAMA*. 1995;273:1592–1597.
72. Turakhia MP, Schiller NB, Whooley MA. Prognostic significance of increased left ventricular mass index to mortality and sudden death in patients with stable coronary heart disease (from the Heart and Soul Study). *Am J Cardiol*. 2008;102:1131–1135.
73. Chatterjee S, Bavishi C, Sardar P, et al. Meta-analysis of left ventricular hypertrophy and sustained arrhythmias. *Am J Cardiol*. 2014;114:1049–1052.
74. Bergmann O, Bhardwaj RD, Bernard S, et al. Evidence for cardiomyocyte renewal in humans. *Science*. 2009;324:98–102.
75. Mollova M, Bersell K, Walsh S, et al. Cardiomyocyte proliferation contributes to heart growth in young humans. *Proc Natl Acad Sci U S A*. 2013;110:1446–1451.
76. Mahmoud AI, Porrello ER. Turning back the cardiac regenerative clock: lessons from the neonate. *Trends Cardiovasc Med*. 2012;22:128–133.
77. Porrello ER, Mahmoud AI, Simpson E, et al. Transient regenerative potential of the neonatal mouse heart. *Science*. 2011;331:1078–1080.
78. Porrello ER, Mahmoud AI, Simpson E, et al. Regulation of neonatal and adult mammalian heart regeneration by the miR-15 family. *Proc Natl Acad Sci U S A*. 2013;110:187–192.
79. Aurora AB, Porrello ER, Tan W, et al. Macrophages are required for neonatal heart regeneration. *J Clin Invest*. 2014;124:1382–1392.
80. Porrello ER, Olson EN. A neonatal blueprint for cardiac regeneration. *Stem Cell Res*. 2014;13:556–570.
81. Ambardekar AV, Buttrick PM. Reverse remodeling with left ventricular assist devices: a review of clinical, cellular, and molecular effects. *Circ Heart Fail*. 2011;4:224–233.
82. Birks EJ, George RS, Hedger M, et al. Reversal of severe heart failure with a continuous-flow left ventricular assist device and pharmacological therapy: a prospective study. *Circulation*. 2011;123:381–390.
83. Canseco DC, Kimura W, Garg S, et al. Human ventricular unloading induces cardiomyocyte proliferation. *J Am Coll Cardiol*. 2015;65:892–900.
84. Ieda M, Fu J-D, Delgado-Olguin P, et al. Direct reprogramming of fibroblasts into functional cardiomyocytes by defined factors. *Cell*. 2010;142:375–386.
85. Fu J-D, Stone NR, Liu L, et al. Direct reprogramming of human fibroblasts toward a cardiomyocyte-like state. *Stem Cell Reports*. 2013;1:235–247.
86. Qian L, Huang Y, Spencer CI, et al. In vivo reprogramming of murine cardiac fibroblasts into induced cardiomyocytes. *Nature*. 2012;485:593–598.
87. Chen JX, Krane M, Deutsch M-A, et al. Inefficient reprogramming of fibroblasts into cardiomyocytes using Gata4, Mef2c, and Tbx5. *Circ Res*. 2012;111:50–55.
88. Matsa E, Sallam K, Wu JC. Cardiac stem cell biology. *Circ Res*. 2014;114:21–27.
89. Taylor DA, Atkins BZ, Hungspreugs P, et al. Regenerating functional myocardium: improved performance after skeletal myoblast transplantation. *Nat Med*. 1998;4:929–933.
90. Murry CE, Wiseman RW, Schwartz SM, Hauschka SD. Skeletal myoblast transplantation for repair of myocardial necrosis. *J Clin Invest*. 1996;98:2512–2523.
91. Smits PC, van Geuns R-JM, Poldermans D, et al. Catheter-based intramyocardial injection of autologous skeletal myoblasts as a primary treatment of ischemic heart failure: clinical experience with six-month follow-up. *J Am Coll Cardiol*. 2003;42:2063–2069.
92. Siminiak T, Kalawski R, Fiszer D, et al. Autologous skeletal myoblast transplantation for the treatment of postinfarction myocardial injury: phase I clinical study with 12 months of follow-up. *Am Heart J*. 2004;148:531–537.
93. Menasché P, Alfieri O, Janssens S, et al. The Myoblast Autologous Grafting in Ischemic Cardiomyopathy (MAGIC) trial: first randomized placebo-controlled study of myoblast transplantation. *Circulation*. 2008;117:1189–1200.
94. Duckers HJ, Houtgraaf J, Hehrlein C, et al. Final results of a phase IIa, randomised, open-label trial to evaluate the percutaneous intramyocardial transplantation of autologous skeletal myoblasts in congestive heart failure patients: the SEISMIC trial. *EuroIntervention*. 2011;6:805–812.
95. Orlic D, Kajstura J, Chimenti S, et al. Bone marrow cells regenerate infarcted myocardium. *Nature*. 2001;410:701–705.

96. Murry CE, Soonpaa MH, Reinecke H, et al. Haemato-poietic stem cells do not transdifferentiate into cardiac myocytes in myocardial infarcts. *Nature*. 2008;428:664–668.

97. Balsam LB, Wagers AJ, Christensen JL, Kofidis T, Weissman IL, Robbins RC. Haematopoietic stem cells adopt mature haematopoietic fates in ischaemic myocardium. *Nature*. 2004;428:668–673.

98. Assmus B, Schächinger V, Teupe C, et al. Transplantation of progenitor cells and regeneration enhancement in acute myocardial infarction (TOPCARE-AMI). *Circulation*. 2002;106:3009–3017.

99. Strauer BE, Brehm M, Zeus T, et al. Repair of infarcted myocardium by autologous intracoronary mononuclear bone marrow cell transplantation in humans. *Circulation*. 2002;106:1913–1918.

100. Fernández-Avilés F, San Román JA, García-Frade J, et al. Experimental and clinical regenerative capability of human bone marrow cells after myocardial infarction. *Circ Res*. 2004;95:742–748.

101. Vrtovec B, Poglajen G, Lezaic L, et al. Effects of intracoronary CD34+ stem cell transplantation in nonischemic dilated cardiomyopathy patients: 5-year follow-up. *Circ Res*. 2013;112:165–173.

102. Patel AN, Geffner L, Vina RF, et al. Surgical treatment for congestive heart failure with autologous adult stem cell transplantation: a prospective randomized study. *J Thorac Cardiovasc Surg*. 2005;130:1631–1638.

103. Fisher SA, Zhang H, Doree C, Mathur A, Martin-Rendon E. Stem cell treatment for acute myocardial infarction. *Cochrane Database Syst Rev*. 2015;9:CD006536.

104. Nowbar AN, Mielewczik M, Karavassilis M, et al. Discrepancies in autologous bone marrow stem cell trials and enhancement of ejection fraction (DAMASCENE): weighted regression and meta-analysis. *BMJ*. 2014;348. g2688–g2688.

105. Gyöngyösi M, Wojakowski W, Lemarchand P, et al. Meta-Analysis of Cell-based CaRdiac stUdiEs (ACCRUE) in patients with acute myocardial infarction based on individual patient data. *Circ Res*. 2015;116:1346–1360.

106. Fisher SA, Brunskill SJ, Doree C, Mathur A, Taggart DP, Martin-Rendon E. Stem cell therapy for chronic ischaemic heart disease and congestive heart failure. *Cochrane Database Syst Rev*. 2014;4:CD007888.

107. Afzal MR, Samanta A, Shah ZI, et al. Adult bone marrow cell therapy for ischemic heart disease: evidence and insights from randomized controlled trials. *Circ Res*. 2015;117:558–575.

108. Tang X-L, Rokosh G, Sanganalmath SK, et al. Intracoronary administration of cardiac progenitor cells alleviates left ventricular dysfunction in rats with a 30-day-old infarction. *Circulation*. 2010;121:293–305.

109. Leistner DM, Schmitt J, Palm S, et al. Intracoronary administration of bone marrow-derived mononuclear cells and arrhythmic events in patients with chronic heart failure. *Eur Heart J*. 2011;32:485–491.

110. Dimmeler S, Burchfield J, Zeiher AM. Cell-based therapy of myocardial infarction. *Arterioscler Thromb Vasc Biol*. 2008;28:208–216.

111. Chen S, Fang W, Ye F, et al. Effect on left ventricular function of intracoronary transplantation of autologous bone marrow mesenchymal stem cell in patients with acute myocardial infarction. *Am J Cardiol*. 2004;94:92–95.

112. Heldman AW, DiFede DL, Fishman JE, et al. Transendocardial mesenchymal stem cells and mononuclear bone marrow cells for ischemic cardiomyopathy: the TAC-HFT randomized trial. *JAMA*. 2014;311:62–73.

113. Hare JM, Fishman JE, Gerstenblith G, et al. Comparison of allogeneic vs autologous bone marrow–derived mesenchymal stem cells delivered by transendocardial injection in patients with ischemic cardiomyopathy: the POSEIDON randomized trial. *JAMA*. 2012;308:2369–2379.

114. Bartunek J, Behfar A, Dolatabadi D, et al. Cardiopoietic stem cell therapy in heart failure: the C-CURE (Cardiopoietic stem Cell therapy in heart failURE) multicenter randomized trial with lineage-specified biologics. *J Am Coll Cardiol*. 2013;61:2329–2338.

115. Cai B, Wang G, Chen N, et al. Bone marrow mesenchymal stem cells protected post-infarcted myocardium against arrhythmias via reversing potassium channels remodelling. *J Cell Mol Med*. 2014;18:1407–1416.

116. Beltrami AP, Barlucchi L, Torella D, et al. Adult cardiac stem cells are multipotent and support myocardial regeneration. *Cell*. 2003;114:763–776.

117. Oh H, Chi X, Bradfute SB, et al. Cardiac muscle plasticity in adult and embryo by heart-derived progenitor cells. *Ann N Y Acad Sci*. 2004;1015:182–189.

118. Laugwitz K-L, Moretti A, Lam J, et al. Postnatal isl1+ cardioblasts enter fully differentiated cardiomyocyte lineages. *Nature*. 2005;433:647–653.

119. Hierlihy AM, Seale P, Lobe CG, Rudnicki MA, Megeney LA. The post-natal heart contains a myocardial stem cell population. *FEBS Lett*. 2002;530:239–243.

120. Smith RR, Barile L, Cho HC, et al. Regenerative potential of cardiosphere-derived cells expanded from percutaneous endomyocardial biopsy specimens. *Circulation*. 2007;115:896–908.

121. van Berlo JH, Kanisicak O, Maillet M, et al. c-kit+ cells minimally contribute cardiomyocytes to the heart. *Nature*. 2014;509:337–341.

122. Sultana N, Zhang L, Yan J, et al. Resident c-kit(+) cells in the heart are not cardiac stem cells. *Nat Commun*. 2015;6:8701.

123. Koudstaal S, Jansen OF, Lorkeers SJ, Gaetani R, et al. Concise review: heart regeneration and the role of cardiac stem cells. *Stem Cells Transl Med*. 2013;2:434–443.

124. Bolli R, Chugh AR, D'Amario D, et al. Cardiac stem cells in patients with ischaemic cardiomyopathy (SCIPIO): initial results of a randomised phase 1 trial. *Lancet*. 2011;378:1847–1857.

125. Chugh AR, Beache GM, Loughran JH, et al. Administration of cardiac stem cells in patients with ischemic cardiomyopathy: the SCIPIO trial: surgical aspects and interim analysis of myocardial function and viability by magnetic resonance. *Circulation*. 2012;126:S54–S64.

126. The Lancet Editors, Expression of concern: the SCIPIO trial. *Lancet*. 2014;383:1279.

127. Gago-Lopez N, Awaji O, Zhang Y, et al. THY-1 receptor expression differentiates cardiosphere-derived cells with divergent cardiogenic differentiation potential. *Stem Cell Reports*. 2014;2:576–591.

128. Li T-S, Cheng K, Malliaras K, et al. Direct comparison of different stem cell types and subpopulations reveals superior paracrine potency and myocardial repair efficacy with cardiosphere-derived cells. *J Am Coll Cardiol*. 2012;59:942–953.

129. Malliaras K, Ibrahim A, Tseliou E, et al. Stimulation of endogenous cardioblasts by exogenous cell therapy after myocardial infarction. *EMBO Mol Med*. 2014;6:760–777.

130. Makkar RR, Smith RR, Cheng K, et al. Intracoronary cardiosphere-derived cells for heart regeneration after myocardial infarction (CADUCEUS): a prospective, randomised phase 1 trial. *Lancet*. 2012;379:895–904.

131. Takehara N, Tsutsumi Y, Tateishi K, et al. Controlled delivery of basic fibroblast growth factor promotes human cardiosphere-derived cell engraftment to enhance cardiac repair for chronic myocardial infarction. *J Am Coll Cardiol*. 2008;52:1858–1865.

132. Takahashi K, Yamanaka S. Induction of pluripotent stem cells from mouse embryonic and adult fibroblast cultures by defined factors. *Cell*. 2006;126:663–676.

133. Takahashi K, Tanabe K, Ohnuki M, et al. Induction of pluripotent stem cells from adult human fibroblasts by defined factors. *Cell*. 2007;131:861–872.

134. Malik N, Rao MS. A review of the methods for human iPSC derivation. *Methods Mol Biol*. 2013;997:23–33.

135. Burridge PW, Matsa E, Shukla P, et al. Chemically defined generation of human cardiomyocytes. *Nat Methods*. 2014;11:855–860.

136. Karakikes I, Ameen M, Termglinchan V, Wu JC. Human induced pluripotent stem cell-derived cardiomyocytes: insights into molecular, cellular, and functional phenotypes. *Circ Res*. 2015;117:80–88.

137. Karakikes I, Senyei GD, Hansen J, et al. Small molecule-mediated directed differentiation of human embryonic stem cells toward ventricular cardiomyocytes. *Stem Cells Transl Med*. 2014;3:18–31.

138. Karakikes I, Termglinchan V, Wu JC. Human-induced pluripotent stem cell models of inherited cardiomyopathies. *Curr Opin Cardiol*. 2014;29:214–219.

139. Shiba Y, Fernandes S, Zhu W-Z, et al. Human ES-cell-derived cardiomyocytes electrically couple and suppress arrhythmias in injured hearts. *Nature*. 2012;489:322–325.

140. Blin G, Nury D, Stefanovic S, et al. A purified population of multipotent cardiovascular progenitors derived from primate pluripotent stem cells engrafts in post-myocardial infarcted nonhuman primates. *J Clin Invest*. 2010;120:1125–1139.

141. Chong JJH, Murry CE. Cardiac regeneration using pluripotent stem cells–progression to large animal models. *Stem Cell Res*. 2014;13:654–665.

142. Menasché P, Vanneaux V, Fabreguettes J-R, et al. Towards a clinical use of human embryonic stem cell-derived cardiac progenitors: a translational experience. *Eur Heart J*. 2015;36:743–750.

143. Menasché P, Vanneaux V, Hagège A, et al. Human embryonic stem cell-derived cardiac progenitors for severe heart failure treatment: first clinical case report. *Eur Heart J*. 2015;36:2011–2017.

144. Gerbin KA, Murry CE. The winding road to regenerating the human heart. *Cardiovasc Pathol*. 2015;24:133–140.

145. Hamdi H, Furuta A, Bellamy V, et al. Cell delivery: intramyocardial injections or epicardial deposition? A head-to-head comparison. *Ann Thorac Surg*. 2009;87:1196–1203.

146. Hamdi H, Planat-Benard V, Bel A, et al. Long-term functional benefits of epicardial patches as cell carriers. *Cell Transplant*. 2014;23:87–96.

147. Chong JJH, Yang X, Don CW, et al. Human embryonic-stem-cell-derived cardiomyocytes regenerate non-human primate hearts. *Nature*. 2014;510:273–277.

148. Zhao T, Zhang Z-N, Rong Z, Xu Y. Immunogenicity of induced pluripotent stem cells. *Nature*. 2011;474:212–215.

149. Araki R, Uda M, Hoki Y, et al. Negligible immunogenicity of terminally differentiated cells derived from induced pluripotent or embryonic stem cells. *Nature*. 2013;494:100–104.

150. Riegler J, Tiburcy M, Ebert A, et al. Human Engineered Heart Muscles Engraft and Survive Long Term in a Rodent Myocardial Infarction Model. *Circ Res*. 2015;117:720–730.

151. Zhang L, Pan Y, Qin G, et al. Inhibition of stearoyl-coA desaturase selectively eliminates tumorigenic Nanog-positive cells: improving the safety of iPS cell transplantation to myocardium. *Cell Cycle*. 2014;13:762–771.

152. Nguyen PK, Rhee JW, Wu JC. Adult stem cell therapy and heart failure, 2000 to 2016: a systematic review. *JAMA Cardiol*. 2016;1:831–841.

153. Nguyen PK, Neofytou E, Rhee JW, Wu JC. Potential strategies to address the major clinical barriers facing stem cell regenerative therapy for cardiovascular disease: a review. *JAMA Cardiol*. 2016;1:935–962.

31

Ionic Mechanisms of Atrial Action Potentials

Sandeep V. Pandit

Our knowledge regarding the ionic bases of the atrial action potential has evolved continuously since the early transmembrane recordings made in isolated human atrial tissue almost 50 years ago.[1] The advent of the patch-clamp technique in the early 1980s[2] and the subsequent detailed characterization of the biophysical properties of various ionic currents in the human atrial cells[3–6] led to the development of the first detailed quantitative mathematical models of the human atrial action potential in 1998.[7,8] This was subsequently followed by increased recognition that intracellular Ca^{2+} ($[Ca^{2+}]_i$) homeostasis plays a major role in influencing the atrial repolarization in both normal and pathophysiological conditions, particularly in atrial fibrillation (AF).[9–14] It resulted in formulations of newer quantitative models that encapsulate the nonlinear interactions between ionic currents and $[Ca^{2+}]_i$ to simulate the human atrial excitation–contraction (E–C) coupling.[15,16] Studies have also documented regional variations in atrial electrophysiology,[17] influences of age-related changes,[18] and ionic bases of atrial remodeling occurring due to AF[14] and/or ventricular dysfunction.[19] This chapter provides an overview of the principal ionic determinants of the atrial action potentials at the cellular level in health and disease (mainly humans and sometimes from experimental animal models), their regional heterogeneities and age-related changes, and their behavior during functional reentry due to one or more spiral waves (rotors), which are either stable or meandering and have now been shown to sustain AF in both animal models[20] and, more recently, in humans.[21,22]

Ionic Bases of Atrial Action Potentials in the Healthy Myocardium

We recently developed a mathematical model of the human atrial cell electrophysiology[15] on the basis of the available experimental data. The atrial formulation was derived from a computational model of the human ventricular cell.[23] Updated versions of this cellular model have been published,[24,25] and the use of computational modeling in investigating atrial electrophysiology and AF was addressed in a recent review.[26] By incorporating the experimentally known ionic differences between atrial and ventricular myocytes, the Grandi-Pandit-Voigt model[15] reconstructs essential aspects of atrial E–C coupling in humans. It allows for a

systematic comparison of the main ionic currents underlying the human atrial action potential (Fig. 31.1, in *red*) and for highlighting key differences with those underlying the ventricular action potential (see Fig. 31.1. in *black*).

Action Potential Characteristics

The human atrial action potential typically exhibits a triangular morphology (compared to a spike-and-dome shape with a prominent plateau phase of the ventricular counterpart).[1,27] The human atrial action potential duration at 90% repolarization (APD_{90}) at 1 Hz is highly variable, ranging between 150 and 500 ms, possibly influenced by recording conditions and ionic concentrations.[27–30] The atrial resting membrane potential (V_{rest}) has been found to vary between –65 and –80 mV and is more depolarized than that in the human ventricle[27–30] (see Fig. 31.1). The depolarized V_{rest} in atrial cells compared to ventricular cells is mainly attributed to differences in the density of the inward rectifier K^+ current, I_{K1}[15] (also see the subsequent text). The maximum upstroke velocities (V_{max}) for atrial action potentials have been experimentally reported to vary between ~150 and 300 V/s in contrast to higher values of 300–400 V/s for human ventricular cells.[27–30] The characteristic human atrioventricular action potential property/shape differences are replicated in most mammalian species, except for the murine myocardium (rat/mouse), where both atrial and ventricular cells display short, triangular action potentials.[31]

The Inward, Depolarizing Currents (Na^+, Ca^{2+})

The initiation of the atrial action potential is due to the rapid activation of the inward Na^+ current, I_{Na}, which is also the principal determinant of V_{max}. The functional differences in human ventricular and atrial I_{Na} biophysical properties were reported to be minimal,[32] but recent studies have shown that the molecular correlates of I_{Na} in the human atrial and ventricular myocardium are different. Although $Na_V1.5$ was found to be the main α-subunit encoding atrial/ventricular I_{Na}, the transcript for the β-subunit, $Na_Vβ1$, was more prominently expressed in the human atrium.[33] In addition, recent reports in canine atrial cells suggest that atrial I_{Na} has a higher current density and a more negative steady-state, half-inactivation voltage value compared to ventricular cells.[34] Similar differences were reported in guinea pig atrial and ventricular cells.[35] Furthermore, due to the more depolarized V_{rest}, the availability of atrial I_{Na} is less and results in a smaller I_{Na} underlying the atrial action potential compared to the ventricular counterpart as seen in Fig. 31.1. Recent reports also suggest that although the tetrodotoxin (TTX)-sensitive late Na^+ current (I_{NaL}) is detectable in cells isolated from the right atrial tissue of patients in sinus rhythm, this is mainly observed at room temperature, and the I_{NaL} density is negligible at more physiological temperatures (37°C).[36] The L-type Ca^{2+} current (I_{CaL}) is mainly responsible for the plateau phase of the atrial action potential and the Ca^{2+}-induced Ca^{2+} release in human

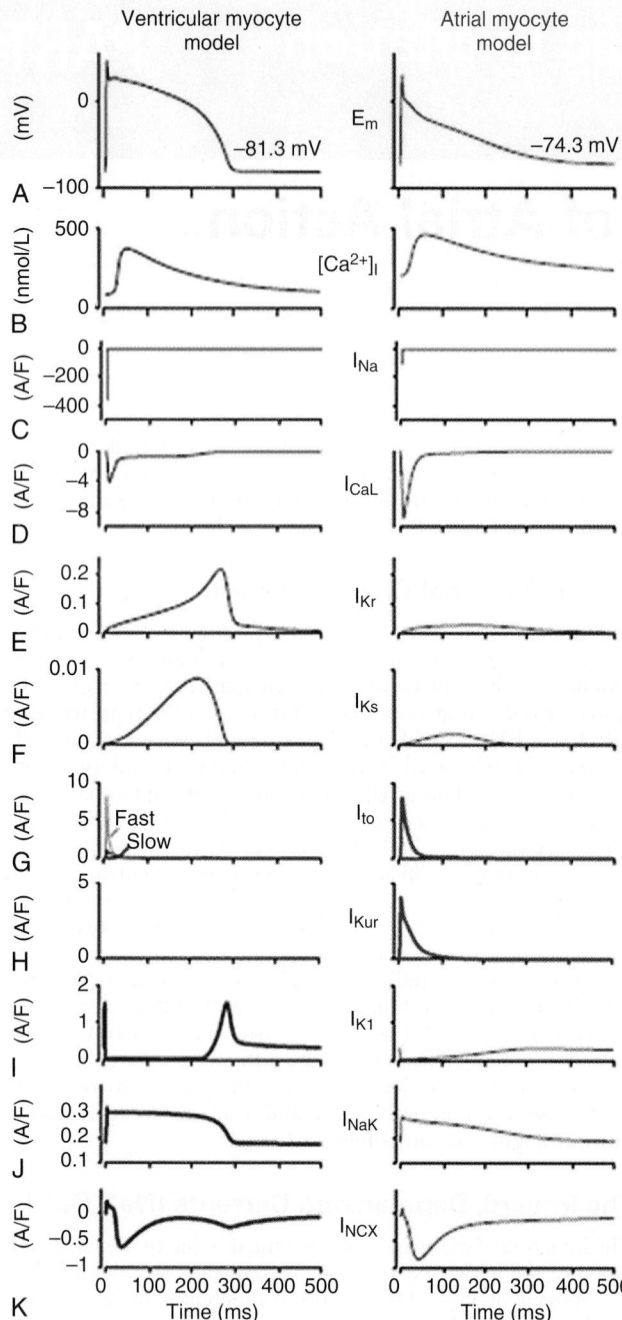

FIGURE 31.1 Key ionic currents underlying ventricular (*black*) and atrial (*red*) action potentials. Depicted in this figure are (A) action potentials; (B) Ca²⁺ transients ([Ca²⁺]ᵢ); (C) sodium current, I_{Na}; (D) calcium current, I_{CaL}; (E) rapid delayed rectifier current, I_{Kr}; (F) slow delayed rectifier current, I_{Ks}; (G) transient outward current, I_{to}; (H) ultra-rapid delayed rectifier current, I_{Kur}; (I) inward rectifier current, I_{K1}; (J) Na⁺-K⁺ pump current, I_{NaK}; and (K) Na⁺-Ca²⁺ exchanger current, I_{NCX}. (Modified from Grandi E, Pandit SV, Voigt N, et al. Human atrial action potential and Ca²⁺ model sinus rhythm and chronic atrial fibrillation. *Circ Res.* 2011;109:1055-1066.)

represents membrane voltage and E_{Ca} represents reversal potential for I_{CaL}) and results in an I_{CaL} with a larger magnitude underlying the human atrial cell action potential (compared to its ventricular counterpart), as seen in Fig. 31.1.[15] Differences in regulation of human atrial (but not ventricular) I_{CaL} by second messengers such as serotonin[39] and phosphodiesterases[40] (PDE) have also been reported and may further influence action potential morphology.

The Outward, Repolarizing K⁺ Currents (K⁺)

The key current that sets the V_{rest}, i.e., I_{K1}, has a much smaller density (approximately five- to six-fold less) in human atrial cells, compared to its ventricular counterpart,[15] and partially explains the depolarized V_{rest} in atrial as opposed to the ventricular cells (see Fig. 31.1). The smaller density of I_{K1} is also responsible, in part, for the slower late phase of repolarization in the atrium. The main molecular correlate of I_{K1}, Kir2.1, is more robustly expressed in the human ventricle compared to the atrium.[33] The human atrium also expresses the fast, depolarization-activated, 4-aminopyridine (4-AP)–sensitive, Ca²⁺-independent transient outward K⁺ current, I_{to1}.[3,27,41] This current is responsible for the initial repolarization phase of the atrial action potential[15,27] (see Fig. 31.1). Interestingly, despite having almost a two-fold higher density in the atrium than in the ventricle,[15] the magnitude of I_{to1} underlying the atrial and ventricular action potentials is similar, likely due to action potential morphologies (see Fig. 31.1). The main molecular correlates of human atrial I_{to1} are Kv4.3/KChiP2 (α/β-subunits, respectively).[33] The slow component of $I_{to1,slow}$ (mainly encoded by Kv1.4) is absent in the human atrium but present in the ventricle.[15,33] More recently, a late sustained component of I_{to1} has been identified in human atrial cells and is hypothesized to be due to the interaction of dipeptidyl peptidase–like protein (DPP) 10 (DPP10a) with Kv4.3 channels.[42] DPP10a and Kv4.3 proteins have also been shown to be colocalized in human atrial cells.[42] However, the precise role of this late component of I_{to1} in influencing atrial repolarization remains unknown. A Ca²⁺-dependent transient outward K⁺ current, I_{to2}, has been reported in human atrial cells, but its molecular correlate as well as contribution to the action potential remain unclear.[41] Human atrial cells also express three functional delayed rectifier K⁺ currents, which contribute to repolarization: the ultra-rapid delayed rectifier K⁺ current, I_{Kur} (molecular correlate Kv1.5),[4,5,43] and the rapid and slow delayed rectifier K⁺ currents, I_{Kr} and I_{Ks} (molecular correlates hERG and KvLQT1, respectively).[6,44,45] I_{Kur} is present only in the atrium (not ventricle), is active during the plateau phase (see Fig. 31.1.), and is blocked by low concentrations of 4-AP (100 μM)[4,5]; its atrial-selective nature has made it an attractive target for many antiarrhythmic drugs in development for terminating and/or preventing recurrence of AF.[14] Compared to I_{Kur}, the contribution of I_{Kr} and I_{Ks} to the human atrial action potential is small (see Fig. 31.1),[15] in part, due to their small density and, in part, due to the triangular shape and plateau phase at relatively negative membrane voltages, which preclude both I_{Kr} and I_{Ks} from activating fully. However, there is considerable variability in the shape of the human atrial action potentials, and I_{Kr}/I_{Ks} are likely to contribute more in cells showing a prominent plateau phase and dome (the so-called type-1 action potentials).[6]

Besides the traditional transient outward and delayed rectifier currents, recent experiments have shed more light on other K⁺ channels that may potentially contribute to atrial repolarization in humans. Studies from the Chiamvimonvat laboratory first suggested that the Ca²⁺-activated K⁺ current I_{KCa} (putative molecular correlate SK2) may modulate the human atrial action potential.[46] However, this finding is controversial as other investigators did not find a role for this current in other species (canine/rat).[47] A recent study in human atrial trabeculae/cells suggested that SK2 channels were widely expressed in undiseased cells and that blocking these currents prolonged the APD and effective refractory period (ERP) in a frequency-dependent manner (more block at low frequencies) and also depolarized the V_{rest} by about 2 to 4 mV.[48] A putative

atrial cells.[37] Patch-clamp experiments suggested that the T-type Ca²⁺ current (I_{CaT}) was not present in human atrial cells.[37] Experimental studies conducted in the Lederer lab reported differences in the biophysical properties of I_{CaL} between human atrial and ventricular cells in the current density and the steady-state inactivation properties.[38] At the transcript level, a higher expression of the α-subunits Cav1.3 and Cav3.1 has been reported in the atrium than in the ventricle.[33] Moreover, a more "negative voltage" of the triangular plateau phase causes a larger driving force ($V_m - E_{Ca}$; where V_m

role for the neural voltage-gated K⁺ channel Kv1.1 (encoded by the *KCNA1* gene) has been suggested recently; patch-clamp studies revealed the presence of a dendrotoxin-K (DTX-K)–sensitive outward current in human atrial cells.[49] However, its precise contribution to atrial repolarization was not explored.

$[Ca^{2+}]_i$, $[Na^+]_i$, Electrogenic Pumps and Exchangers

The human atrial action potential is also modulated by $[Ca^{2+}]_i$, which directly influences the inactivation of I_{CaL},[50] and the magnitude and temporal profile of the electrogenic Na⁺-Ca²⁺ exchanger current, I_{NCX}[9,51] (molecular transcript NCX1[33]), and has an indirect influence on the Na⁺-K⁺ pump current, I_{NaK}, by influencing intracellular Na⁺ ion ($[Na^+]_i$) accumulation[15] (molecular transcripts Na/K ATPase α1,α3, β1[33]). I_{NCX} is the main Ca²⁺ extrusion and Na⁺ influx pathway in cardiomyocytes. It extrudes one Ca²⁺ in exchange for three Na⁺, thus generating an inward current that influences cardiac repolarization and arrhythmogenesis.[15] The Na⁺/K⁺ pump (NKA) is the main route of Na⁺ efflux in cardiac cells, thus regulating $[Na^+]_i$. By extruding three Na⁺ in exchange for two K⁺, it generates an outward current that is known to influence both V_{rest} and repolarization.[15] $[Na^+]_i$ has also been recently shown to inhibit the outward component of I_{K1} in human atrial cells.[52] We recently simulated the $[Ca^{2+}]_i$ homeostasis in human atrial cells, and our results showed that whereas I_{NaK} is primarily a repolarizing outward current, I_{NCX} can be both outward and inward; it contributes to repolarization in the early phase of the action potential and is a negative current (depolarizing influence) during the later phase of the action potential, when it extrudes Ca²⁺ ions from the atrial cells (see Fig. 31.1).[15] I_{NaK} and I_{NCX} also influence the frequency dependence of the human atrial APD.[15]

Other Ion Channels

Besides the previously discussed currents, other ion channels are activated under specific conditions and can influence the human atrial action potential. These include the acetylcholine-activated K⁺ current, I_{KACh}[28,53,54] (molecular correlates Kir3.1/3.4[33]); the ATP-sensitive K⁺ current, I_{KATP}[55,56] (molecular correlate Kir6.1/6.2/SuR2[33]); the Ca²⁺-dependent nonselective cation current,[57,58] which may be encoded by the transient receptor potential channel (TRPC1)[59]; and the hyperpolarization-activated funny current, I_f[60] (molecular correlates HCN1/HCN4[33]). Stretch-activated ion channels (I_{SAC}) have been reported in human atrial cells[61] and influence both V_{rest} and APD; however, their molecular correlates remain unknown. Swelling-induced, outwardly rectifying chloride channels, I_{Cl^-},[62] (putative molecular correlates Cl3,Cl6,Cl7[33]) have been reported in human atrial cells. However, no information is available on the contribution of I_{Cl^-} to the APD. The transcripts of two-pore channels (TWIK1, TASK1) have also been reported to be present in the human atrium.[33] Different groups have recently reported the presence of either TASK-1 or TASK-3 in the human atria.[63–65] TASK-1 current was recorded in human atrial cells,[63,64] and TASK-3 expression was reported in the human right atrium (RA) and shown to be localized to the plasma membrane.[65] Schmidt and colleagues found the presence of TASK-1 (K2P3.1) transcripts and proteins in human atrial tissue and showed that the functional block of this current via the pharmacological inhibitor A293 prolonged the APD_{90} significantly in cells derived from patients in sinus rhythm at room temperature; this finding was also supported by concomitant computer simulations.[65] Whether the TWIK current can also contribute to the APD remains to be determined.

Ionic Bases of Regional Heterogeneity in Atrial Action Potentials

The atrium is a complicated three-dimensional (3D) structure, and the heterogeneities in the electrical properties between different regions such as the left atrium (LA), the RA, and the pulmonary veins (PVs) and their ionic basis have been extensively studied in many species, including mouse,[66,67] rabbit,[68] dogs,[69] and sheep.[70] Information regarding such heterogeneity in humans is more limited, but recent studies have begun to address the putative ionic/molecular basis of these differences. The frequencies of excitation in AF have been reported to show regional gradients during paroxysmal AF with the LA-PV regions displaying the highest frequencies.[71] This is highly indicative of underlying differences in biophysical properties of some ionic currents, and these variations, which are more prominent in disease conditions, are discussed later. In patients in normal sinus rhythm, Caballero and colleagues reported a higher density of I_{Kur} in the right than in the left atrial cardiomyocytes.[45] Incorporating such data in human atrial mathematical models did not result in appreciable differences between the LA/RA action potentials in normal sinus rhythm.[15] However, large variations in human atrial action potential shapes (mainly triangular, with some dome shaped) have been reported in cells isolated from the right atrial appendage, and this has been attributed to differences in current density ratios of I_{to1}/I_{Kr} in these cells.[6] The carbachol-activated K⁺ current (I_{KACh}) was reported to be 70% larger in the RA than in the LA in sinus rhythm patients, with correspondingly higher protein expressions of its molecular correlates (Kir3.1/Kir3.4) in the RA versus the LA.[72] To the best of my knowledge, there is no report on ionic mechanisms underlying human PV cells. Thus available data regarding the regional variations in human atrial electrophysiology/underlying ionic mechanisms under healthy conditions are very limited, and further studies are needed in this regard. We briefly review the atrial action potential heterogeneity/ionic mechanisms from other animal species in the next paragraph.

In healthy hearts of dogs and mice, the APD is shorter in LA than in RA, primarily on account of the differences in current densities of the delayed rectifier K⁺ currents: I_{Kr} in dogs and I_{Kur} and the steady-state K⁺ current, I_{ss}, in mice display higher current densities in LA than in RA.[67,73,74] In sheep atrial cells, the I_{KACh} was shown to have a higher density in LA than in RA, whereas the density of I_{K1} was similar.[70,75] In contrast, the I_{KACh} current density was higher in RA than in LA in mice,[76] similar to humans in sinus rhythm.[72] The density of I_{Na} has been reported to be higher in LA than in RA in dogs.[77] However, our recent studies in sheep did not find any differences in the densities of I_{Na} and I_{CaL} between LA and RA.[70] Besides those between LA and RA, differences within the RA have also been reported. For example, the action potential properties of the pectinate muscles and crista terminalis in the rabbit RA are different[78]; such differences have been attributed to differences in various ion channels (Na⁺, Ca²⁺, and K⁺) and have been integrated in a mathematical model.[79] Furthermore, differences in the electrophysiological properties of cells isolated from the LA and the PV regions have been extensively studied by the Nattel group in dogs[69] and the Chen group in rabbits.[68] Canine PV cells exhibit a depolarized V_{rest}, smaller V_{max}, and shorter APD than that exhibited by LA cells.[69] This has been attributed to a higher density of I_{Kr}, I_{Ks}, and I_{KCa} and a lower density of I_{CaL} and I_{to1} in PV cells than in LA cells, whereas the densities of I_{NCX} and I_{CaT} were found to be similar between PV and LA cells.[69] Interestingly, the Ca²⁺-handling properties were not different between the canine PV and LA cells.[80] Computational models have been recently developed to account for these ionic heterogeneities and their effects on reentry (see the subsequent text).[81] As reported in the ventricle, epi-endocardial differences also exist in the atrium. A recent study in pigs reported a shorter refractory period in the atrial epicardium than in the endocardium.[82] This is in line with a shorter atrial epicardial APD recorded in the canine right atrial free wall than in the endocardium.[83] The canine atrial endocardium was also more sensitive to APD shortening following the addition of acetylcholine.[83]

However, the ionic mechanisms underlying the atrial epicardium-endocardium differences remain unexplored.

Ionic Bases of Atrial Action Potential Variations With Age

Age-related changes in atrial action potential differences in humans have been most systematically investigated between infants (neonatal) and adults.[29,30] Adult cells displayed a more prominent initial notch than that displayed by neonatal atrial cells.[29,30] The properties of I_{to1} were significantly different as well; I_{to1} displayed a significantly higher density, faster inactivation, and a slower recovery from inactivation in neonatal than in adult human atrial cells.[29] Correspondingly, the protein density of Kv4.3 was higher and KChiP2 was lower in neonatal than in adult cells.[29] The properties of I_{CaL} were also different: the basal density was smaller and the protein density of Giα3 was larger in neonatal than in adult cells, resulting in a different response to lower dosage of β-adrenergic stimulation.[84] In addition, Ca^{2+} transients, which influence both adult and neonatal human atrial action potentials,[15,85] may display inherently different biophysical properties but remain unexplored. It is well known that the propensity for AF increases with age,[18] but very few studies have been conducted to explore potential differences between adult and aged human atrial electrophysiology, and most of the knowledge in this area has been derived from animal models (rat, rabbit, or dog). This topic was reviewed comprehensively in a recent article, and we briefly describe the salient points therein.[18] V_{rest} was found to be more depolarized in rats/dogs,[86,87] whereas APD_{90} was more prolonged in rats/rabbits/dogs in aged atria compared to that in adult atria.[18,88–90] The density of I_{Na} was not different,[77] but the density of I_{CaL} was reported to be smaller in canine atrial cells.[90,91] Furthermore, the density of I_{to1} was higher, its steady-state half-inactivation value showed more positive values, and recovery from inactivation was slower in canine aged atrial cells than in their adult counterparts.[91] The density of the sustained outward K^+ current, I_{sus}, was also reported to be larger in aged canine atrial cells.[91] In addition to the changes in ionic currents and action potentials, an increased level of interstitial fibrosis and modifications in intercellular coupling have also been reported in aged tissue compared to those in adult tissue[92] and may further enhance the susceptibility to AF with age. Ca^{2+} handling is also different between the aged and adult atrial tissue, and recent studies in human right atrial myocytes show that aging is associated with a reduction in the sarcoplasmic reticulum (SR) calcium content, calcium transient amplitude, I_{CaL} density, and protein expression of sarco-endoplasmic reticulum Ca^{2+} ATPase (SERCA)-2 and calsequestrin-2.[93]

Action Potential and Ionic Remodeling in Chronic Atrial Fibrillation

AF is the most common cardiac arrhythmia seen in the clinic, and it affects an estimated 33 million people worldwide.[94] It is one of the main causes of embolic stroke.[14] AF is characterized by a rapid and irregular activation of the atria, at a rate of 5 to 10 Hz.[14] Several studies have investigated the ionic mechanisms involved in the remodeling that occurs in the atria of patients with long-standing chronic AF (cAF), and they have shown that electrophysiological remodeling contributes to the development of a substrate that facilitates the tendency for persistence of AF.[14] Electrical remodeling induces changes in the biophysical properties of the Na^+, Ca^{2+}, and K^+ currents, which lead to a shortening of the APD.[14,15] Abnormal $[Ca^{2+}]_i$ homeostasis also plays an important role in AF-induced electrical remodeling.[13–15] The changes in E–C coupling have been comprehensively reviewed elsewhere,[14] and the important underlying ionic mechanisms are discussed in the following text.

Effect of Atrial Fibrillation on Action Potential and $[Ca^{2+}]_i$

Atrial cells from patients in cAF display shorter APD than those from healthy individuals in normal sinus rhythm (Fig. 31.2A).[14,15,95–99] Furthermore, the normal human atrial APD_{90} shortens when paced at progressively faster frequencies, but in cAF, this shortening is severely attenuated.[14,15,95,96] The peak amplitude of $[Ca^{2+}]_i$ is reduced in atrial myocytes from cAF patients compared to those from healthy individuals (see Fig. 31.2B), although the SR Ca^{2+} content is unaltered.[12–15] $[Ca^{2+}]_i$ decays more slowly in cAF compared to that in sinus rhythm.[12,15] Our recently published mathematical model of the human atrial cell provided novel insights into the ionic mechanisms underlying the altered APD/$[Ca^{2+}]_i$ in cAF (see Fig. 31.2A and B; *black*: sinus rhythm, *red*: cAF), and the salient points are discussed in the following text.

Ionic Remodeling in Chronic Atrial Fibrillation

Sarcolemmal Ion Channels

I_{Na}. Bosch and associates reported that the density of I_{Na} and the voltage dependence of steady-state activation were not altered in cAF in humans, whereas the steady-state inactivation was shifted to the right by ~10 mV,[98] and no changes were detected in the mRNA levels of the Na^+ channel gene SCN5A.[100] In contrast, data from Sossalla and coworkers showed that the expression of $Na_V1.5$ and the peak I_{Na} density were both decreased (slightly) in the atrial myocardium of patients with cAF.[101] Additionally, the late Na^+ current component, I_{NaL} (see *inset*, Fig. 31.2), was reported to be significantly increased in cAF patients.[101] Sossalla and colleagues proposed that this increase could be due to the increase in neuronal Na^+ channel isoforms ($Na_V1.1$ expression is increased)[101]; mediated by Ca^{2+}/calmodulin-dependent protein kinase II (CaMKII), which is increased in AF[102] and known to regulate I_{NaL}[103]; or due to increased oxidative stress in AF, which can also augment I_{NaL}.[104,105] Simulations suggest that an increased I_{NaL} does not contribute significantly to repolarization in cAF, where the overall APD_{90} is still shorter than that in normal healthy cells.[15] A recent report from the Ravens laboratory showed that although I_{NaL} was detected at room temperature in right atrial myocytes from patients in both sinus rhythm and AF (and larger in the latter), its contribution and the purported increase in AF was not significant at more physiological temperatures.[36] In an atrial-tachypaced sheep model of AF, the density of I_{Na} was significantly reduced in cAF patients compared to that in controls, but changes in I_{NaL} were not explored.[70]

I_{CaL}. A reduction in I_{CaL} density by ~50% in cAF compared to that in sinus rhythm (see Fig. 31.2A, *third row*) is one of the most consistent experimentally observed electrophysiological findings in both humans and animal models of AF.[14,15,70,95,96,106] Christ and associates[106] demonstrated that decreased I_{CaL} density in cAF was not accompanied by altered expression of the corresponding α_{1c}- and β_{2a}-channel subunits (although other studies found different results[70,107]) and proposed that lower basal I_{CaL} was due to decreased channel phosphorylation in cAF, which results from an altered ratio of protein kinase/phosphatase activity in favor of increased phosphatase activity. It has been shown that blocking I_{CaL} with nifedipine in normal human atrial cells results in an action potential characteristic that is typically seen in AF[95] with respect to morphology, duration, and impaired rate-dependent adaptation. In other words, a reduction in I_{CaL} seems to be a critical component of the remodeled atrial action potential in cAF.[14,15]

I_f. A recent report provided the first evidence that the conductance of I_f was significantly increased around the threshold for activation (–60 to –80 mV) during cAF in humans, and it was suggested that this could mediate atrial ectopy.[60] However, this

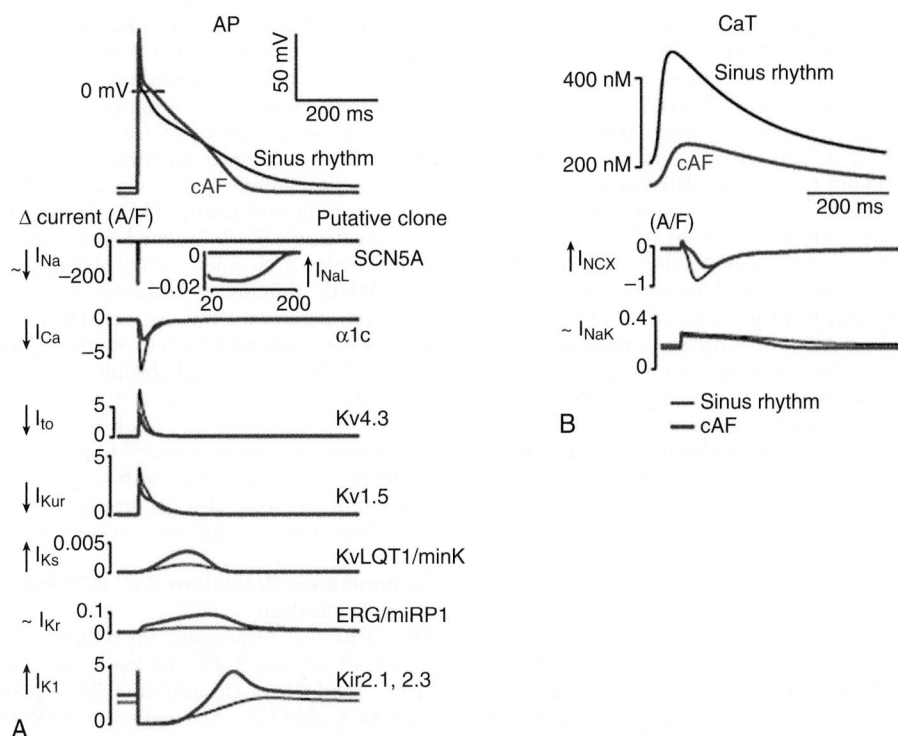

FIGURE 31.2 (A) Comparison between ionic currents and action potentials as well as (B) Ca^{2+} transients (*CaT*), pumps (I_{NaK}), and exchangers (I_{NCX}) in atrial cells from normal sinus rhythm patients *(black)* versus chronic AF (*cAF*) patients *(red)*. AP, Action potential, I_{Ca}, inward calcium current; I_{K1}, inward rectifier K^+ current; I_{Ks}, slow delayed rectifier K^+ current; I_{Kur}, ultra-rapid delayed rectifier K^+ current; I_{Na}, inward Na^+ current. (Modified from Grandi E, Pandit SV, Voigt N, et al. Human atrial action potential and Ca^{2+} model sinus rhythm and chronic atrial fibrillation. *Circ Res.* 2011;109:1055-1066.)

conclusion must be interpreted with caution, given the increase in other K^+ currents, such as I_{K1}[14,15] (see the subsequent text).

I_{to1} and I_{Kur}. Human cAF is associated with strong reduction of I_{to1} (see Fig. 31.2A, *fourth row*) density[45,96,98,108-110] and downregulation of its α-subunit Kv4.3.[111] I_{to1} is also reduced in the sheep model of AF.[70] The role of DPP10a, which has been recently postulated to encode a late component of I_{to1},[42] however, has not been explored in cAF. I_{Kur} (see Fig. 31.2A, *fifth row*) was reported to be reduced in cAF,[45,108,110,112] along with a diminished expression of Kv1.5 in some studies.[100,108] However, others have reported no changes in I_{Kur} density.[96,98,109] Inconsistent results regarding I_{Kur} function have been commented on previously by Christ and colleagues and attributed to different strategies for identification of I_{Kur} (e.g., pharmacological or with I_{to1}-inactivating prepulse) and to a fraction of I_{Kur} that is not accounted for by Kv1.5.[112] The reduction in I_{to1} and I_{Kur} explains the slight prolongation in earlier phases of the action potential (see Fig. 31.2A, *first row*).[15] Caballero and coworkers have recently looked at differences in current density and AF-induced alterations in the right versus left human atrium.[45] They demonstrated that cAF reduced the I_{to1} amplitude and density more markedly in the LA than in the RA, thus creating a right-to-left gradient, whereas I_{Kur} was more markedly reduced in the RA than in the LA, thus dissipating the left-to-right gradient detected in sinus rhythm.[45] Recent experimental work using relatively selective inhibitors of I_{Kur} in human atrial tissue (XEND0103) has shed further light on their role in cAF; at low frequencies, the APD_{90} was prolonged in cAF, but not in sinus rhythm.[113]

I_{Ks} and I_{Kr}. Until now, no direct experimental evidence has been provided regarding the involvement of I_{Kr} in AF-induced electrical remodeling. However, E-4031, a relatively selective blocker of I_{Kr}, has been shown to prolong APD_{90} in atrial

trabeculae from patients in cAF,[114] and this data provides strong indirect evidence indicating that I_{Kr} contributes functionally to repolarization in the diseased human atrium. Recently, Caballero and associates provided the first demonstration that cAF significantly increased the amplitude of I_{Ks} in both atria.[45] They suggested that I_{Ks} increase could contribute to cAF-induced shortening of APD and could further promote fibrillatory conduction, especially with its accumulation at higher pacing frequencies, as shown in neonatal rat ventricular myocytes, where I_{Ks} was overexpressed.[115]

I_{K1} and I_{KACh}. In human cAF, increases in both current density[28,72,95] and mRNA levels of I_{K1}[28] have been reported (see Fig. 31.2A, *eighth row*). Our recent study in a sheep experimental model also showed that the I_{K1} density and the underlying encoding protein expression (Kir2.3) were increased in cAF compared to those in controls.[70] Increased I_{K1} causes a more negative V_{rest} in cAF versus sinus rhythm human atrial myocytes.[15,28] Patients with cAF also exhibit agonist-independent constitutive I_{KACh} activity that contributes to the enhanced basal inward rectifier current and may result from abnormal channel phosphorylation by protein kinase C (PKC).[28,72,116] Constitutively active I_{KACh} is considered to support the maintenance of AF, together with increased I_{K1}, by stabilizing reentrant activity sustained by rotors (faster activation, less meander[117]; also see the subsequent text). Recently, Voigt and colleagues found significant left-to-right gradients in I_{K1} and constitutively active I_{KACh} in patients with paroxysmal AF, which had dissipated in cAF; this possibly contributes to the left-to-right dominant frequency gradients that are often more evident in paroxysmal AF.[72]

Other K^+ Currents. Gene expression and electrophysiological studies in patients with AF demonstrated reduced mRNA levels of Kir6.2[111] and current activation,[55] but increased current was also reported.[56] The density of the Ca^{2+}-activated K^+ current and its underlying transcripts (SK2, SK3) were reduced in the atria from patients in cAF compared to those in sinus rhythm, and the contribution of this current to APD in cAF when assessed pharmacologically was not significant.[48] The current encoded by neural voltage-gated K^+ channel Kv1.1 and the underlying protein expression was found to be upregulated in human atrial cells isolated from AF patients compared to those from controls, but its role in modulating APD remains to be investigated.[49] There are contradictory reports regarding the contribution of TASK-1 current in cAF; one group could not detect the TASK-1 current in myocytes isolated from patients in AF or in canine atrial tachypaced models of AF.[63] In contrast, others found that TASK-1 current was upregulated and contributed significantly to the APD in myocytes isolated from cAF patients, and the mRNA and protein levels of the underlying molecular correlates ($K_{2p}3.1$) were also increased in cAF.[65] The reasons for the discrepant findings regarding the TASK current remain unclear. The remodeling of many other ion channels that were present in the human atrium due to cAF (such as TRP, stretch, chloride, and TWIK) has not been investigated to date.

Ca^{2+} and Na^+ Handling

I_{NCX}. Increased expression[11,12] and abnormal function of I_{NCX} protein[11-15] have been reported in human cAF and in a sheep model of cAF.[70] An increase in I_{NCX} may be an adaptive response to cellular Ca^{2+} loading and contributes to diminish the Ca^{2+} overload induced by rapid atrial pacing. The decay rate of caffeine-evoked $[Ca^{2+}]_i$ (attributable to Ca^{2+} removal by I_{NCX}) is faster in human cAF than in sinus rhythm myocytes.[14] Note that simulated I_{NCX} during an action potential is smaller in AF than in sinus rhythm (see Fig. 31.2B, *second row*) due to the reduced amplitude of $[Ca^{2+}]_i$ (see Fig. 31.2B, *first row*). Na^+ overload-induced Ca^{2+} influx via reverse-mode NCX has been implicated in Ca^{2+} overload and related arrhythmogenesis, whereas increased Ca^{2+} extrusion via forward mode has been linked to delayed-afterdepolarizations (DADs).[13,14] Indeed, Na^+ and Ca^{2+} loading is more favored at increased atrial rates (with AF). Although DADs may be important in initiating arrhythmias in paroxysmal AF via I_{NCX},[24] their role in mediating DADs in cAF is unclear because an increased I_{K1} in cAF[14,15] will tend to oppose the occurrence of such DADs. Indirect support for this hypothesis was provided by recent studies in the atrial trabeculae isolated from cAF patients, which showed that arrhythmic events in response to catecholamines were in fact reduced.[118]

I_{NaK}. Workman and associates found no difference in I_{NaK} in myocytes from cAF patients compared to those from sinus rhythm and concluded that I_{NaK} was not involved in AF-induced electrophysiological remodeling in patients.[119] Our simulations show different I_{NaK} currents underlying the action potential in cAF versus sinus rhythm (see Fig. 31.2B, *third row*) because of altered Na^+ loading.

Our simulations also indicate that the APD rate adaptation in sinus rhythm atrial cells involves the accumulation of $[Na^+]_i$ at high frequencies, which causes outward shifts in Na^+/Ca^{2+} exchanges and I_{NaK}. The model also predicts that E–C coupling remodeling in cAF would reduce Na^+ accumulation, thus causing a blunted APD rate–dependent response.[15] Interestingly, a recent report indicates that the concentration of $[Na^+]_i$ is significantly reduced in an atrial-tachypaced rabbit experimental model of AF.[120] However, the precise mechanisms and significance of this important finding, and whether it is also true for human cAF, remains unclear.

Ryanodine Receptors

Spontaneous Ca^{2+}-release events (Ca^{2+} sparks) and Ca^{2+} waves through leaky ryanodine receptor (RyR) channels have been reported in myocytes from hearts in AF[12-14,99,120,121] despite

unaltered SR Ca^{2+} content. One potential contributor to RyR hyperactivity may be oxidative stress, which is known to play a critical role in AF pathophysiology[104] and increase RyR open probability. Neef and colleagues suggested that the CaMKII-dependent increase in the SR Ca^{2+} leak caused by RyR hyperphosphorylation in AF is a potential arrhythmogenic mechanism[99] because elimination of Ca^{2+} via inward I_{NCX} could lead to cell depolarization and cause DADs. Voigt and associates directly measured single RyRs isolated from cAF patients and demonstrated a higher channel open probability in cAF that responded to CaMKII inhibition.[12] However, in contrast, norepinephrine-induced I_{CaL} response was decreased by the inhibition of CaMKII in myocytes from patients with sinus rhythm but not from those in cAF.[118] Agonist-evoked phosphorylation by CaMKII at phospholamban (PLN), but not at ryanodine, was reduced in cAF, and this was suggested to underlie a decrease in agonist-evoked arrhythmias in cAF patients.[118] Our recent studies in the sheep model of cAF showed that both total RyR2 and phosphorylated RyR2 proteins were also decreased.[70] Thus the role of RyR in mediating DADs in cAF remains controversial.

Sarcoplasmic Reticulum Ca^{2+} ATPase and Phospholamban

The SERCA is responsible for pumping Ca^{2+} back into the SR after Ca^{2+} release.[14] The endogenous inhibitor PLN regulates SERCA and releases its inhibition when phosphorylated by either PKA or CaMKII.[14] A decrease in SERCA activity, associated with smaller SERCA protein expression, is evident in human cAF and explains the slower $[Ca^{2+}]_i$ decay than in sinus rhythm.[14,15] On the other hand, reduced inhibition of SERCA by hyperphosphorylated PLN[12] in cAF could help maintain a normal SR Ca^{2+} load despite increased RyR activity. In the sheep model of cAF, the protein levels of SERCA and PLN were reduced, whereas CaMKII levels remained unchanged.[70]

To summarize, the findings of APD shortening as well as changes in Na^+, Ca^{2+}, and K^+ currents and electrogenic pumps and exchangers due to cAF in humans have been largely reproducible in canine/goat/rabbit/sheep models of tachypaced-induced AF and suggest that electrical remodeling, including changes in APD and ionic mechanisms, occurs over a period of 1 to 2 weeks.[14] In contrast, structural remodeling occurs over longer periods of atrial tachypacing (months) and is mostly irreversible.[14] Finally, the role of Ca^{2+} handling in inducing arrhythmogenesis in cAF remains controversial, with conflicting results in both patients and animal models, and needs further systematic investigation.

Alterations in Atrial Electrophysiology During Ventricular Dysfunction

Atrial remodeling that increases the propensity for AF also occurs with cardiac disorders, such as coronary artery disease, congestive heart failure, and left ventricular (LV) systolic dysfunction.[122] In atrial cells isolated from patients with LV dysfunction, the APD was either unaltered[123] or prolonged.[124] In sinus rhythm patients with reduced LV ejection fraction (<45%), the APD_{90} was shorter than that in patients with higher ejection fractions,[19] and there was a significant correlation between cellular ERP shortening and decreasing of the LV ejection fraction.[19] Furthermore, multivariate analysis adjusting for 10 relevant clinical covariates confirmed that LV dysfunction was independently associated with atrial cellular ERP shortening, which may therefore be expected to contribute to a predisposition to AF in these patients. The ionic remodeling due to heart failure/LV dysfunction in the human atrium remains poorly understood. I_{CaL} was either decreased in patients with coronary artery disease, aortic valve disease, or mitral valve disease[125] or unchanged in LV dysfunction/heart failure patients.[19,126] Schreieck and colleagues found an increased I_{to1} density in the human atrial myocytes of patients with reduced LV function, with no change in its voltage dependence or decay, but with faster recovery from activation.[123] However, this I_{to1} increase may have been confounded by the lower proportion of patients treated with β-blockers in the reduced LV function group because such treatment is associated with decreased I_{to1} in human atrium.[127] In contrast, Workman and associates found that LV dysfunction was associated with decreased I_{to1}, a positive shift in its activation voltage, and no change in its decay kinetics.[19] Koumi and colleagues reported depolarized V_{rest} in atrial myocytes from heart failure patients, possibly due to reduced density of I_{K1} and I_{KACh}.[124] Workman and associates reported unchanged I_{K1} in LV dysfunction,[19] although Ba^{2+}-sensitive I_{K1} or I_{KACh} were not measured. Unchanged atrial I_{Kur} has also been reported in human LV dysfunction.[19] Cardiac dilatation is known to develop frequently during the course of cardiac failure.[128] In trabeculae and myocytes taken from dilated atria, the APD was shorter and the plateau was markedly depressed compared to trabeculae and myocytes from nondilated atria.[128] However, it must be noted that the ventricular dysfunction was not quantified in these patients. AP changes were explained with more severely depressed I_{CaL} compared to the reduction in total outward current.[128] Overall, the ionic bases of altered atrial APD in patients with ventricular dysfunction, and how it predisposes to more frequent AF episodes culminating in cAF, remains poorly understood.

The changes in atrial electrical remodeling due to ventricular dysfunction (mainly tachypaced-induced or myocardial infarction–induced heart failure) have also been studied in animal models, and the most systematic studies have been conducted in dogs by the Nattel group.[129,130] In the atria of dogs with short-term (2–5 weeks) tachypaced-induced heart failure, the APD did not change at slower pacing frequencies but increased in duration at rapid pacing frequencies.[130] The densities of I_{CaL}, I_{to1}, and I_{Ks} were reduced, but there was no change in their voltage dependencies or kinetics. The densities of the K^+ currents, I_{K1}, I_{Kur}, I_{Kr}, and I_{CaT}, were not altered but that of I_{NCX} was increased.[130] Further, substantial dysregulation in $[Ca^{2+}]_i$ and its regulatory proteins was reported, which led to an increased diastolic $[Ca^{2+}]_i$ level, $[Ca^{2+}]_i$ amplitude, SR load, and spontaneous release events.[131] In contrast, for a long-term tachypaced canine model of ventricular heart failure (4 months), the APD was significantly shortened.[132] The ionic changes reported included an increased I_{to1} and decreased I_{K1}, I_{Kur}, and I_{Ks}.[132] Upon studying the I_{CaL} under action potential clamp conditions, the heart failure atrial action potential reduced the integral of I_{CaL} in control, healthy cells, with a larger reduction in myocytes from heart failure dogs.[132] These data point toward a complex electrical phenotype and underlying ionic mechanism changes in the atrium in the presence of heart failure, depending upon the severity of the condition (short-term versus long-term ventricular pacing), and in part mirrors the complex and varied phenotype seen in patients with ventricular dysfunction.[122]

Ventricular dysfunction is also known to increase atrial fibrosis[133] (and in some cases, cAF-enhanced fibrosis can also occur independently of heart failure, such as in our recent study in sheep[70]). Recent studies (mostly computational) have investigated the putative bases of fibroblast effects on atrial electrophysiology, mainly occurring as a result of coupling between myocytes and atrial fibroblasts.[134,135] Simulations indicate that such coupling can modulate V_{rest} and repolarization, predisposing the atrium to arrhythmogenesis.[134,135] However, direct experimental evidence of such coupling in the atrium (or the heart) is still not available.[136] Besides coupling, fibroblasts/myofibroblasts can influence atrial ion channels and excitability through secretion of factors such as transforming growth factor (TGF)-β1 and platelet-derived growth factor (PDGF) and also by direct physical contact that can lead to dedifferentiation.[133]

Ionic Basis of Reentry (Spiral Waves) in the Atrium

We conclude the chapter with a very brief summary about the ionic basis of spiral waves and rotors, focusing on studies mostly from our laboratory (for more detailed information, see recent reviews[20,26]). These rotors have now been shown to sustain AF in many experimental and recent clinical studies.[20–22]

The initiation of atrial arrhythmias can occur at the cellular level in the form of afterdepolarizations, either early or late (EADs and DADs), or automaticity.[14] The ionic mechanisms underlying these arrhythmogenic action potentials are somewhat similar to their ventricular counterpart. For example, our computer simulations showed that in the presence of a Kv1.5 mutation that renders I_{Kur} inactive, β-adrenergic stress can give rise to EADs, primarily on account of the reactivation of I_{CaL}.[15] Similarly, abnormal Ca^{2+} homeostasis leading to enhanced Ca^{2+} leaks, in combination with an increased density of I_{NCX}, was shown to underlie an increased propensity for DADs in cells isolated from cAF patients compared to normal healthy ones.[14] These arrhythmogenic action potentials can lead to vortex shedding and wavebreaks in cardiac tissue, which can then generate rotors.[20,137]

We[70,117,138] and others[139–142] have studied the ionic and/or structural basis of these rotors. In a simple two-dimensional (2D) homogeneous and isotropic sheet (size: 5 cm × 5 cm) that incorporated mathematical models of human atrial cells (500 × 500 cells), rotors were simulated by cross-field stimulation.[117] The ionic conditions seen experimentally in cAF were mimicked in two cases using the Courtemanche atrial model[8]: (1) in which a downregulation in I_{CaL}, I_{to1}, and I_{Kur} was implemented (CAF1)[143] and (2) where in addition to reducing the densities of I_{CaL}, I_{to1}, and I_{Kur}, the density of I_{K1} was increased two-fold (CAF2), as was found in experiments.[108] The resulting APD shortening and restitution are shown for CAF1 and CAF2 (Fig. 31.3A and B, respectively; the *DI* in Fig. 31.3B represents diastolic interval for an S1–S2 stimulus protocol). The increase in I_{K1}, in addition to shortening the APD further, also caused a hyperpolarization of V_{rest} (see Fig. 31.3A). Both conditions allowed for the maintenance of stable rotors in 2D sheets, as illustrated in Fig. 31.3C. However, the rotors had different properties: the rotor in the CAF2 condition had a higher frequency of rotation (8.4 Hz) compared to that in CAF1 (5.7 Hz).[117] Furthermore, the meander of the spiral wave tip was also smaller in the CAF2 condition (see Fig. 31.3C). Thus an increase in I_{K1} caused the rotors to become more stable (faster frequency, less meander). Further analyses (not shown) revealed that the key mechanism underlying the rotor acceleration was the removal of the I_{Na} inactivation (increased availability) on account of the faster repolarization and hyperpolarized V_{rest}.[117] Since I_{Na} is the key determinant of excitation, this allowed for a faster rotor activity. Interestingly, when I_{CaL} in CAF1 condition was further reduced, it shortened APD, but did not hyperpolarize V_{rest}, and the rotor was able to accelerate only a little (6.3 Hz), thus providing further support to the key role of I_{K1} in accelerating reentry. These simulations have been supported by experimental results in mice and dogs. Transgenic mice overexpressing I_{K1} were able to sustain much faster and sustained rotors (frequency ~44 Hz) compared to those sustained by wild-type mice (~26 Hz).[144] Furthermore, the Nattel lab compared AF frequencies in dogs with matched ERPs in two models of AF, one in which APD was shortened due to cholinergic activation of I_{KACh}, an I_{K1}, and one in which the APD was shortened due to atrial tachypacing (thus the ionic mechanism of shortening was both a reduction in I_{CaL} and an increase in I_{K1}).[145] It was found that the frequency of AF was higher in the case where the APD was shortened due to I_{KACh} alone than in the case where shortening was induced by remodeling of both I_{CaL} and I_{K1} in tachypaced hearts.[145] These experiments provide support to the notion that inward rectifier currents are critical determinants of reentry and its activation frequency.[20]

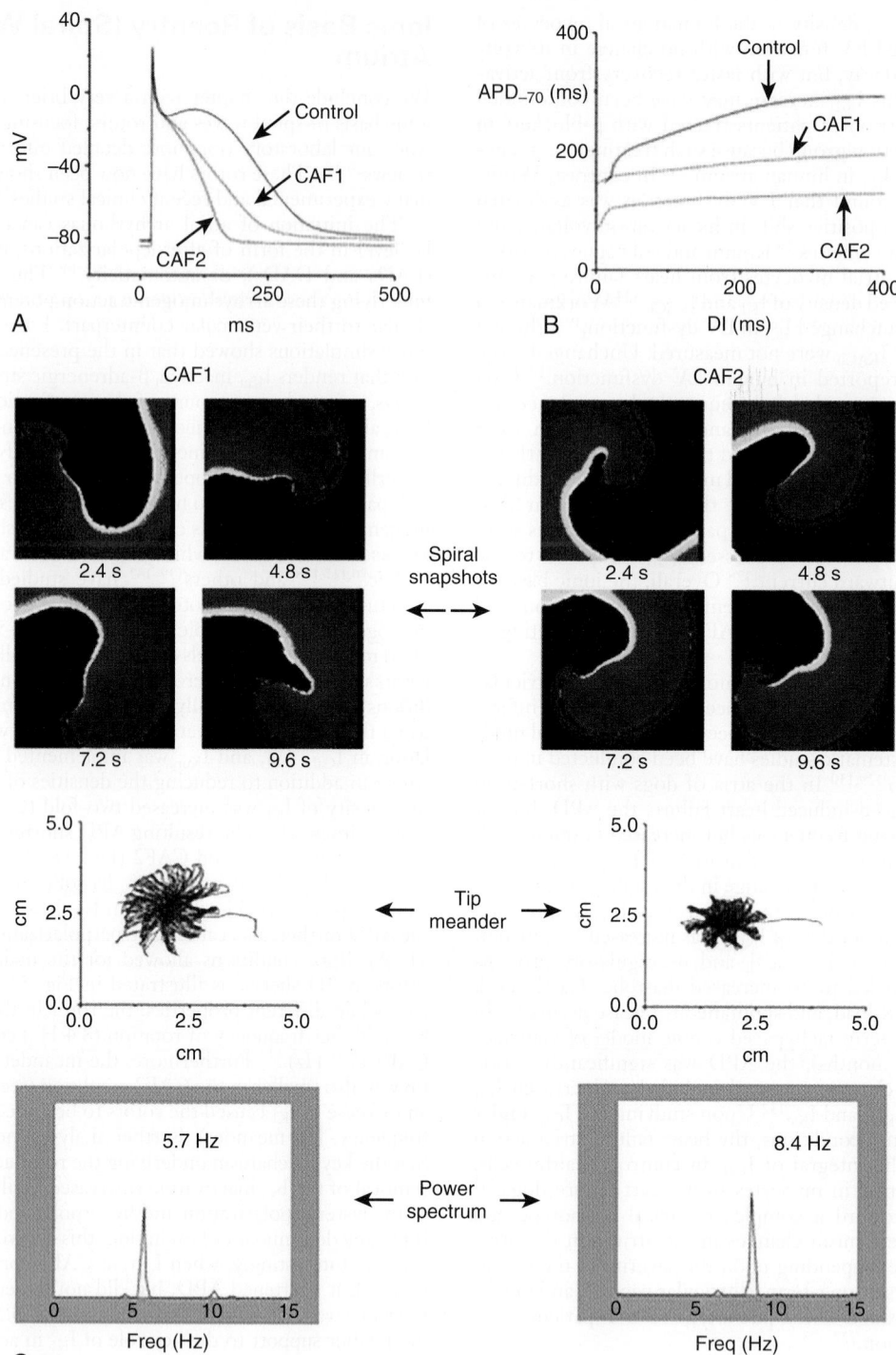

FIGURE 31.3 (A) Action potentials in control and chronic atrial fibrillation (*CAF1, CAF2*). (B) Electrical restitution plotted as *APD₋₇₀* versus the diastolic interval (*DI*) in control and chronic atrial fibrillation. (C) Spiral waves (phase movie), tip meander, and power spectral densities in chronic atrial fibrillation conditions CAF1 and CAF2. Phase movies are shown at separate times (2.4, 4.8, 7.2, and 9.6 s). The tip meander is plotted in a 5 × 5 cm², two-dimensional atrial sheet. *APD*, Action potential duration. (Modified from Pandit SV, Berenfeld O, Anumonwo JM, et al. Ionic determinants of functional reentry in a 2-D model of human atrial cells during simulated chronic atrial fibrillation. *Biophys J.* 2005;88:3806-3821.)

This effect has been verified in the human atria by the infusion of adenosine, which was shown to increase the AF frequency of excitation.[146] The role of other K^+ currents in sustaining rotors in AF is less clear. When the maximum conductance of I_{to1} and I_{Kur} were reduced by 90%, the rotor was terminated, but when

the same was done for I_{Kr} and I_{Ks}, the rotor activity remained sustained.[117] Our simulations were devoid of any ionic and structural heterogeneities, which play an important role in sustaining AF; thus more work is needed to be able to define the ionic bases of reentry in detailed 3D structural models of the atria[147] that incorporate ionic heterogeneities[17] as well as interstitial fibrosis.[148] A recent simulation study using 2D and pseudo-3D funnel-shaped models partially addressed these questions, wherein the effect of ionic heterogeneities between the PVs and the LA were explored.[81] The main finding from this study was that the rotors were attracted to the PV, and this was mainly attributable to the differences in the density of I_{K1} compared to other currents.[81] Furthermore, simulations in a 3D human biatrial finite element model based on patient-derived computed tomography showed that areas of fibrosis anchored the rotors.[141] Computer simulations have also been conducted to investigate the role of the so-called epicardial-endocardial dissociation in maintaining AF.[149] However, these do not account for possible ionic heterogeneities in the epicardial-endocardial layers, partly because of lack of quantitative experimental data for the same at this stage. Lastly, simulations that incorporate more recent ionic models with detailed Ca^{2+} formulations,[15] in combination with further experiments, are needed to obtain more detailed quantitative insights into whether Ca^{2+} homeostasis is important in maintaining rotors in AF. Although important in initiating arrhythmias in paroxysmal AF (not cAF), $[Ca^{2+}]_i$ is unlikely to play a critical role in sustaining rotors, likely because of the refractoriness of RyR at high activation rates (8–10 Hz). Although this has been shown to be true in experimental models of ventricular fibrillation in rabbits,[150] additional experiments and simulations will be necessary to confirm this hypothesis in AF.

REFERENCES

1. Trautwein W, Kassebaum DG, Nelson RM, Hecht HH. Electrophysiological study of human heart muscle. *Circ Res.* 1962;10:306–312.
2. Hamill OP, Marty A, Neher E, Sakmann B, Sigworth FJ. Improved patch-clamp techniques for high-resolution current recording from cells and cell-free membrane patches. *Pflugers Arch.* 1981;391:85–100.
3. Shibata EF, Drury T, Refsum H, Aldrete V, Giles W. Contributions of a transient outward current to repolarization in human atrium. *Am J Physiol.* 1989;257:H1773–H1781.
4. Firek L, Giles WR. Outward currents underlying repolarization in human atrial myocytes. *Cardiovasc Res.* 1995;30:31–38.
5. Fedida D, Wible B, Wang Z, et al. Identity of a novel delayed rectifier current from human heart with a cloned K+ channel current. *Circ Res.* 1993;73:210–216.
6. Wang Z, Fermini B, Nattel S. Delayed rectifier outward current and repolarization in human atrial myocytes. *Circ Res.* 1993;73:276–285.
7. Nygren A, Fiset C, Firek L, et al. Mathematical model of an adult human atrial cell: the role of K+ currents in repolarization. *Circ Res.* 1998;82:63–81.
8. Courtemanche M, Ramirez RJ, Nattel S. Ionic mechanisms underlying human atrial action potential properties: insights from a mathematical model. *Am J Physiol.* 1998;275:H301–H321.
9. Bénardeau A, Hatem SN, Rücker-Martin C, et al. Contribution of Na+/Ca2+ exchange to action potential of human atrial myocytes. *Am J Physiol.* 1996;271:H1151–H1161.
10. Hatem SN, Bénardeau A, Rücker-Martin C, et al. Different compartments of sarcoplasmic reticulum participate in the excitation-contraction coupling process in human atrial myocytes. *Circ Res.* 1997;80:345–353.
11. El-Armouche A, Boknik P, Eschenhagen T, et al. Molecular determinants of altered Ca2+ handling in human chronic atrial fibrillation. *Circulation.* 2006;114:670–680.
12. Voigt N, Li N, Wang Q, et al. Enhanced sarcoplasmic reticulum Ca2+ leak and increased Na+-Ca2+ exchanger function underlie delayed afterdepolarizations in patients with chronic atrial fibrillation. *Circulation.* 2012;125:2059–2070.
13. Nattel S, Dobrev D. The multidimensional role of calcium in atrial fibrillation pathophysiology: mechanistic insights and therapeutic opportunities. *Eur Heart J.* 2012;33:1870–1877.
14. Heijman J, Voigt N, Nattel S, Dobrev D. Cellular and molecular electrophysiology of atrial fibrillation initiation, maintenance, and progression. *Circ Res.* 2014;114:1483–1499.
15. Grandi E, Pandit SV, Voigt N, et al. Human atrial action potential and Ca2+ model: sinus rhythm and chronic atrial fibrillation. *Circ Res.* 2011;109:1055–1066.
16. Koivumäki JT, Korhonen T, Tavi P. Impact of sarcoplasmic reticulum calcium release on calcium dynamics and action potential morphology in human atrial myocytes: a computational study. *PLoS Comput Biol.* 2011;7:e1001067.
17. Schram G, Pourrier M, Melnyk P, Nattel S. Differential distribution of cardiac ion channel expression as a basis for regional specialization in electrical function. *Circ Res.* 2002;90:939–950. Review.
18. Dun W, Boyden PA. Aged atria: electrical remodeling conducive to atrial fibrillation. *J Interv Card Electrophysiol.* 2009;25:9–18.
19. Workman AJ, Pau D, Redpath CJ, et al. Atrial cellular electrophysiological changes in patients with ventricular dysfunction may predispose to AF. *Heart Rhythm.* 2009;6:445–451.
20. Pandit SV, Jalife J. Rotors and the dynamics of cardiac fibrillation. *Circ Res.* 2013;112:849–862.

21. Narayan SM, Krummen DE, Rappel WJ. Clinical mapping approach to diagnose electrical rotors and focal impulse sources for human atrial fibrillation. *J Cardiovasc Electrophysiol.* 2012;23:447–454.
22. Haissaguerre M, Hocini M, Denis A, et al. Driver domains in persistent atrial fibrillation. *Circulation.* 2014;130:530–538.
23. Grandi E, Pasqualini FS, Bers DM. A novel computational model of the human ventricular action potential and Ca transient. *J Mol Cell Cardiol.* 2010;48:112–121.
24. Voigt N, Heijman J, Wang Q, et al. Cellular and molecular mechanisms of atrial arrhythmogenesis in patients with paroxysmal atrial fibrillation. *Circulation.* 2014;129:145–156.
25. Chang KC, Bayer JD, Trayanova NA. Disrupted calcium release as a mechanism for atrial alternans associated with human atrial fibrillation. *PLoS Comput Biol.* 2014;10:e1004011.
26. Trayanova NA. Mathematical approaches to understanding and imaging atrial fibrillation: significance for mechanisms and management. *Circ Res.* 2014;114:1516–1531.
27. Amos GJ, Wettwer E, Metzger F, Li Q, Himmel HM, Ravens U. Differences between outward currents of human atrial and subepicardial ventricular myocytes. *J Physiol.* 1996;491:31–50.
28. Dobrev D, Graf E, Wettwer E, et al. Molecular basis of downregulation of G-protein-coupled inward rectifying K+ current (I(K,ACh)) in chronic human atrial fibrillation: decrease in GIRK4 mRNA correlates with reduced I(K,ACh) and muscarinic receptor-mediated shortening of action potentials. *Circulation.* 2001;104:2551–2557.
29. Wang Y, Xu H, Kumar R, Tipparaju SM, Wagner MB, Joyner RW. Differences in transient outward current properties between neonatal and adult human atrial myocytes. *J Mol Cell Cardiol.* 2003;35:1083–1092.
30. Escande D, Loisance D, Planche C, Coraboeuf E. Age-related changes of action potential plateau shape in isolated human atrial fibers. *Am J Physiol.* 1985;249:H843–H850.
31. Xu H, Li H, Nerbonne JM. Elimination of the transient outward current and action potential prolongation in mouse atrial myocytes expressing a dominant negative Kv4 alpha subunit. *J Physiol.* 1999;519:11–21.
32. Sakakibara Y, Wasserstrom JA, Furukawa T, et al. Characterization of the sodium current in single human atrial myocytes. *Circ Res.* 1992;71:535–546.
33. Gaborit N, Le Bouter S, Szuts V, et al. Regional and tissue specific transcript signatures of ion channel genes in the non-diseased human heart. *J Physiol.* 2007;582:675–693.
34. Burashnikov A, Di Diego JM, Zygmunt AC, Belardinelli L, Antzelevitch C. Atrium-selective sodium channel block as a strategy for suppression of atrial fibrillation: differences in sodium channel inactivation between atria and ventricles and the role of ranolazine. *Circulation.* 2007;116:1449–1457.
35. Li GR, Lau CP, Shrier A. Heterogeneity of sodium current in atrial vs epicardial ventricular myocytes of adult guinea pig hearts. *J Mol Cell Cardiol.* 2002;34:1185–1194.
36. Poulet C, Wettwer E, Grunnet M, et al. Late sodium current in human atrial cardiomyocytes from patients in sinus rhythm and atrial fibrillation. *PLoS One.* 2015;10:e0131432.
37. Li GR, Nattel S. Properties of human atrial ICa at physiological temperatures and relevance to action potential. *Am J Physiol.* 1997;272:H227–H235.
38. Cohen NM, Lederer WJ. Calcium current in single human cardiac myocytes. *J Cardiovasc Electrophysiol.* 1993;4:422–437.
39. Ouadid H, Seguin J, Dumuis A, Bockaert J, Nargeot J. Serotonin increases calcium current in human atrial myocytes via the newly described 5-hydroxytryptamine4 receptors. *Mol Pharmacol.* 1992;41:346–351.

40. Rivet-Bastide M, Vandecasteele G, Hatem S, et al. cGMP-stimulated cyclic nucleotide phosphodiesterase regulates the basal calcium current in human atrial myocytes. *J Clin Invest.* 1997;99:2710–2718.
41. Escande D, Coulombe A, Faivre JF, Deroubaix E, Coraboeuf E. Two types of transient outward currents in adult human atrial cells. *Am J Physiol.* 1987;252:H142–H148.
42. Turnow K, Metzner K, Cotella D, et al. Interaction of DPP10a with Kv4.3 channel complex results in a sustained current component of human transient outward current Ito. *Basic Res Cardiol.* 2015;110:5.
43. Wang Z, Fermini B, Nattel S. Sustained depolarization-induced outward current in human atrial myocytes. Evidence for a novel delayed rectifier K+ current similar to Kv1.5 cloned channel currents. *Circ Res.* 1993;73:1061–1076.
44. Wang Z, Fermini B, Nattel S. Rapid and slow components of delayed rectifier current in human atrial myocytes. *Cardiovasc Res.* 1994;28:1540–1546.
45. Caballero R, de la Fuente MG, Gómez R, et al. In humans, chronic atrial fibrillation decreases the transient outward current and ultrarapid component of the delayed rectifier current differentially on each atria and increases the slow component of the delayed rectifier current in both. *J Am Coll Cardiol.* 2010;55:2346–2354.
46. Xu Y, Tuteja D, Zhang Z, et al. Molecular identification and functional roles of a Ca2+-activated K+ channel in human and mouse hearts. *J Biol Chem.* 2003;278:49085–49094.
47. Nagy N, Szuts V, Horváth Z, et al. Does small-conductance calcium-activated potassium channel contribute to cardiac repolarization? *J Mol Cell Cardiol.* 2009;47:656–663.
48. Skibsbye L, Poulet C, Diness JG, et al. Small-conductance calcium-activated potassium (SK) channels contribute to action potential repolarization in human atria. *Cardiovasc Res.* 2014;103:156–167.
49. Glasscock E, Voigt N, McCauley MD, et al. Expression and function of Kv1.1 potassium channels in human atria from patients with atrial fibrillation. *Basic Res Cardiol.* 2015;110:505.
50. Sun H, Leblanc N, Nattel S. Mechanisms of inactivation of L-type calcium channels in human atrial myocytes. *Am J Physiol.* 1997;272:H1625–H1635.
51. Li GR, Nattel S. Demonstration of an inward Na+-Ca2+ exchange current in adult human atrial myocytes. *Ann N Y Acad Sci.* 1996;779:525–528.
52. Voigt N, Heijman J, Trausch A, et al. Impaired Na+-dependent regulation of acetylcholine-activated inward-rectifier K+ current modulates action potential rate dependence in patients with chronic atrial fibrillation. *J Mol Cell Cardiol.* 2013;61:142–152.
53. Koumi S, Arentzen CE, Backer CL, Wasserstrom JA. Alterations in muscarinic K+ channel response to acetylcholine and to G protein-mediated activation in atrial myocytes isolated from failing human hearts. *Circulation.* 1994;90:2213–2224.
54. Heidbüchel H, Vereecke J, Carmeliet E. Three different potassium channels in human atrium. Contribution to the basal potassium conductance. *Circ Res.* 1990;66:1277–1286.
55. Balana B, Dobrev D, Wettwer E, Christ T, Knaut M, Ravens U. Decreased ATP-sensitive K+ current density during chronic human atrial fibrillation. *J Mol Cell Cardiol.* 2003;35:1399–1405.
56. Wu G, Huang CX, Tang YH, et al. Changes of $I_{K,ATP}$ current density and allosteric modulation during chronic atrial fibrillation. *Chin Med J (Engl).* 2005;118:1161–1166.
57. Guinamard R, Chatelier A, Demion M, et al. Functional characterization of a Ca2+-activated non-selective cation channel in human atrial cardiomyocytes. *J Physiol.* 2004;558:75–83.

58. Koster OF, Szigeti GP, Beuckelmann DJ. Characterization of a $[Ca^{2+}]_i$-dependent current in human atrial and ventricular cardiomyocytes in the absence of Na^+ and K^+. *Cardiovasc Res*. 1999;41:175–187.
59. Zhang YH, Wu HJ, Che H, et al. Functional transient receptor potential canonical type 1 channels in human atrial myocytes. *Pflugers Arch*. 2013;465:1439–1449.
60. Stillitano F, Lonardo G, Giunti G, et al. Chronic atrial fibrillation alters the functional properties of If in the human atrium. *J Cardiovasc Electrophysiol*. 2013;24:1391–1400.
61. Kamkin A, Kiseleva I, Wagner KD, et al. Characterization of stretch-activated ion currents in isolated atrial myocytes from human hearts. *Pflugers Arch*. 2003;446:339–346.
62. Demion M, Guinamard R, El Chemaly A, Rahmati M, Bois P. An outwardly rectifying chloride channel in human atrial cardiomyocytes. *J Cardiovasc Electrophysiol*. 2006;17:60–68.
63. Harleton E, Besana A, Chandra P, et al. TASK-1 current is inhibited by phosphorylation during human and canine chronic atrial fibrillation. *Am J Physiol Heart Circ Physiol*. 2015;308:H126–H134.
64. Rinné S, Kiper AK, Schlichthörl G, et al. TASK-1 and TASK-3 may form heterodimers in human atrial cardiomyocytes. *J Mol Cell Cardiol*. 2015;81:71–80.
65. Schmidt C, Wiedmann F, Voigt N, et al. Upregulation of K(2P)3.1 K^+ current causes action potential shortening in patients with chronic atrial fibrillation. *Circulation*. 2015;132:82–92.
66. Lomax AE, Rose RA, Giles WR. Electrophysiological evidence for a gradient of G protein-gated K^+ current in adult mouse atria. *Br J Pharmacol*. 2003;140:576–584.
67. Lomax AE, Kondo CS, Giles WR. Comparison of time- and voltage-dependent K+ currents in myocytes from left and right atria of adult mice. *Am J Physiol Heart Circ Physiol*. 2003;285:H1837–H1848.
68. Tsai WC, Chen YC, Lin YK, Chen SA, Chen YJ. Sex differences in the electrophysiological characteristics of pulmonary veins and left atrium and their clinical implication in atrial fibrillation. *Circ Arrhythm Electrophysiol*. 2011;4:550–559.
69. Ehrlich JR, Cha TJ, Zhang L, et al. Cellular electrophysiology of canine pulmonary vein cardiomyocytes: action potential and ionic current properties. *J Physiol*. 2003;551:801–813.
70. Martins RP, Kaur K, Hwang E, et al. Dominant frequency increase rate predicts transition from paroxysmal to long-term persistent atrial fibrillation. *Circulation*. 2014;129:1472–1482.
71. Atienza F, Almendral J, Jalife J, et al. Real-time dominant frequency mapping and ablation of dominant frequency sites in atrial fibrillation with left-to-right frequency gradients predicts long-term maintenance of sinus rhythm. *Heart Rhythm*. 2009;6:33–40.
72. Voigt N, Trausch A, Knaut M, et al. Left-to-right atrial inward rectifier potassium current gradients in patients with paroxysmal versus chronic atrial fibrillation. *Circ Arrhythm Electrophysiol*. 2010;3:472–480.
73. Li D, Zhang L, Kneller J, Nattel S. Potential ionic mechanism for repolarization differences between canine right and left atrium. *Circ Res*. 2001;88:1168–1175.
74. Hu Y, Jones SV, Dillmann WH. Effects of hyperthyroidism on delayed rectifier K+ currents in left and right murine atria. *Am J Physiol Heart Circ Physiol*. 2005;289. H1448–H1455. Erratum in: *Am J Physiol Heart Circ Physiol*. 2006;290:H489.
75. Sarmast F, Kolli A, Zaitsev A, et al. Cholinergic atrial fibrillation: I(K,ACh) gradients determine unequal left/right atrial frequencies and rotor dynamics. *Cardiovasc Res*. 2003;59:863–873.
76. Lomax AE, Rose RA, Giles WR. Electrophysiological evidence for a gradient of G protein-gated K+ current in adult mouse atria. *Br J Pharmacol*. 2003;140:576–584.
77. Baba S, Dun W, Hirose M, Boyden PA. Sodium current function in adult and aged canine atrial cells. *Am J Physiol Heart Circ Physiol*. 2006;291:H756–H761.
78. Yamashita T, Nakajima T, Hazama H, Hamada E, Murakawa Y, et al. Regional differences in transient outward current density and inhomogeneities of repolarization in rabbit right atrium. *Circulation*. 1995;92:3061–3069.
79. Aslanidi OV, Boyett MR, Dobrzynski H, Li J, Zhang H. Mechanisms of transition from normal to reentrant electrical activity in a model of rabbit atrial tissue: interaction of tissue heterogeneity and anisotropy. *Biophys J*. 2009;96:798–817.
80. Coutu P, Chartier D, Nattel S. Comparison of Ca2+-handling properties of canine pulmonary vein and left atrial cardiomyocytes. *Am J Physiol Heart Circ Physiol*. 2006;291:H2290–H300.
81. Calvo CJ, Deo M, Zlochiver S, Millet J, Berenfeld O. Attraction of rotors to the pulmonary veins in paroxysmal atrial fibrillation: a modeling study. *Biophys J*. 2014;106:1811–1821.
82. Michowitz Y, Nakahara S, Bourke T, et al. Electrophysiological differences between the epicardium and the endocardium of the left atrium. *Pacing Clin Electrophysiol*. 2011;34:37–46.
83. Anyukhovsky EP, Rosenshtraukh LV. Electrophysiological responses of canine atrial endocardium and epicardium to acetylcholine and 4-aminopyridine. *Cardiovasc Res*. 1999;43:364–370.
84. Tipparaju SM, Kumar R, Wang Y, Joyner RW, Wagner MB. Developmental differences in L-type calcium current of human atrial myocytes. *Am J Physiol Heart Circ Physiol*. 2004;286:H1963–H1969.
85. Wagner MB, Wang Y, Kumar R, Tipparaju SM, Joyner RW. Calcium transients in infant human atrial myocytes. *Pediatr Res*. 2005;57:28–34.
86. Su N, Duan J, Moffat MP, Narayanan N. Age-related changes in electrophysiological responses to muscarinic receptor stimulation in rat myocardium. *Can J Physiol Pharmacol*. 1995;73:1430–1436.
87. Anyukhovsky EP, Sosunov EA, Chandra P, et al. Age-associated changes in electrophysiologic remodeling: a potential contributor to initiation of atrial fibrillation. *Cardiovasc Res*. 2005;66:353–363.
88. Toda N. Age-related changes in the transmembrane potential of isolated rabbit sino-atrial nodes and atria. *Cardiovasc Res*. 1980;14:58–63.
89. Huang C, Ding W, Li L, Zhao D. Differences in the aging-associated trends of the monophasic action potential duration and effective refractory period of the right and left atria of the rat. *Circ J*. 2006;70:352–357.
90. Xu GJ, Gan TY, Tang BP, et al. Age-related changes in cellular electrophysiology and calcium handling for atrial fibrillation. *J Cell Mol Med*. 2013;17:1109–1118.
91. Dun W, Yagi T, Rosen MR, Boyden PA. Calcium and potassium currents in cells from adult and aged canine right atria. *Cardiovasc Res*. 2003;58:526–534.
92. Spach MS, Heidlage JF, Dolber PC, Barr RC. Mechanism of origin of conduction disturbances in aging human atrial bundles: experimental and model study. *Heart Rhythm*. 2007;4:175–185.
93. Herraiz-Martínez A, Álvarez-García J, Llach A, et al. Ageing is associated with deterioration of calcium homeostasis in isolated human right atrial myocytes. *Cardiovasc Res*. 2015;106:76–86.
94. Rahman F, Kwan GF, Benjamin EJ. Global epidemiology of atrial fibrillation. *Nat Rev Cardiol*. 2014;11:639–654.
95. Van Wagoner DR, Pond AL, Lamorgese M, Rossie SS, McCarthy PM, Nerbonne JM. Atrial L-type Ca^{2+} currents and human atrial fibrillation. *Circ Res*. 1999;85:428–436.
96. Workman AJ, Kane KA, Rankin AC. The contribution of ionic currents to changes in refractoriness of human atrial myocytes associated with chronic atrial fibrillation. *Cardiovasc Res*. 2001;52:226–235.
97. Boutjdir M, Le Heuzey J, Lavergne T, et al. Inhomogeneity of cellular refractoriness in human atrium: factor of arrhythmia? *Pacing Clin Electrophysiol*. 1986;9:1095–1100.
98. Bosch RF, Zeng X, Grammer JB, Popovic K, Mewis C, Kuhlkamp V. Ionic mechanisms of electrical remodeling in human atrial fibrillation. *Cardiovasc Res*. 1999;44:121–131.
99. Neef S, Dybkova N, Sossalla S, et al. CaMKII-dependent diastolic SR Ca^{2+} leak and elevated diastolic Ca^{2+} levels in right atrial myocardium of patients with atrial fibrillation. *Circ Res*. 2010;106:1134–1144.
100. Brundel BJ, Van Gelder IC, Henning RH, et al. Ion channel remodeling is related to intraoperative atrial effective refractory periods in patients with paroxysmal and persistent atrial fibrillation. *Circulation*. 2001;103:684–690.
101. Sossalla S, Kallmeyer B, Wagner S, et al. Altered Na^+ currents in atrial fibrillation effects of ranolazine on arrhythmias and contractility in human atrial myocardium. *J Am Coll Cardiol*. 2010;55:2330–2342.
102. Tessier S, Karczewski P, Krause EG, et al. Regulation of the transient outward K^+ current by Ca^{2+}/calmodulin-dependent protein kinases II in human atrial myocytes. *Circ Res*. 1999;85:810–819.
103. Wagner S, Dybkova N, Rasenack EC, et al. Ca^{2+}/calmodulin-dependent protein kinase II regulates cardiac Na^+ channels. *J Clin Invest*. 2006;116:3127–3138.
104. Mihm MJ, Yu F, Carnes CA, et al. Impaired myofibrillar energetics and oxidative injury during human atrial fibrillation. *Circulation*. 2001;104:174–180.
105. Wagner S, Ruff HM, Weber SL, et al. Reactive oxygen species-activated Ca/calmodulin kinase II{delta} is required for late I_{Na} augmentation leading to cellular Na and Ca overload. *Circ Res*. 2011;108:555–565.
106. Christ T, Boknik P, Wohrl S, et al. L-type Ca^{2+} current downregulation in chronic human atrial fibrillation is associated with increased activity of protein phosphatases. *Circulation*. 2004;110:2651–2657.
107. Brundel BJ, van Gelder IC, Henning RH, et al. Gene expression of proteins influencing the calcium homeostasis in patients with persistent and paroxysmal atrial fibrillation. *Cardiovasc Res*. 1999;42:443–454.
108. Van Wagoner DR, Pond AL, McCarthy PM, Trimmer JS, Nerbonne JM. Outward K^+ current densities and Kv1.5 expression are reduced in chronic human atrial fibrillation. *Circ Res*. 1997;80:772–781.
109. Grammer JB, Bosch RF, Kuhlkamp V, Seipel L. Molecular remodeling of Kv4.3 potassium channels in human atrial fibrillation. *J Cardiovasc Electrophysiol*. 2000;11:626–633.
110. Brandt MC, Priebe L, Bohle T, Sudkamp M, Beuckelmann DJ. The ultrarapid and the transient outward K^+ current in human atrial fibrillation. Their possible role in postoperative atrial fibrillation. *J Mol Cell Cardiol*. 2000;32:1885–1896.
111. Brundel BJ, Van Gelder IC, Henning RH, et al. Alterations in potassium channel gene expression in atria of patients with persistent and paroxysmal atrial fibrillation: differential regulation of protein and mRNA levels for K^+ channels. *J Am Coll Cardiol*. 2001;37:926–932.
112. Christ T, Wettwer E, Voigt N, et al. Pathology-specific effects of the $I_{Kur}/I_{to}/I_{K,ACh}$ blocker AVE0118 on ion channels in human chronic atrial fibrillation. *Br J Pharmacol*. 2008;154:1619–1630.
113. Ford J, Milnes J, El Haou S, et al. The positive frequency-dependent electrophysiological effects of the I(kur) inhibitor Xen-D0103 are desirable for the treatment of atrial fibrillation. *Heart Rhythm*. 2016;13:555–564.
114. Wettwer E, Christ T, Endig S, et al. The new antiarrhythmic drug vernakalant: ex vivo study of human atrial tissue from sinus rhythm and chronic atrial fibrillation. *Cardiovasc Res*. 2013;98:145–154.
115. Muñoz V, Grzeda KR, Desplantez T, et al. Adenoviral expression of IKs contributes to wavebreak and fibrillatory conduction in neonatal rat ventricular cardiomyocyte monolayers. *Circ Res*. 2007;101:475–483.
116. Dobrev D, Friedrich A, Voigt N, et al. The G protein-gated potassium current $I_{K,ACh}$ is constitutively active in patients with chronic atrial fibrillation. *Circulation*. 2005;112:3697–3706.
117. Pandit SV, Berenfeld O, Anumonwo JM, et al. Ionic determinants of functional reentry in a 2-D model of human atrial cells during simulated chronic atrial fibrillation. *Biophys J*. 2005;88:3806–3821.
118. Christ T, Rozmaritsa N, Engel A, et al. Arrhythmias, elicited by catecholamines and serotonin, vanish in human chronic atrial fibrillation. *Proc Natl Acad Sci U S A*. 2014;111:11193–11198.
119. Workman AJ, Kane KA, Rankin AC. Characterisation of the Na, K pump current in atrial cells from patients with and without chronic atrial fibrillation. *Cardiovasc Res*. 2003;59:593–602.
120. Greiser M, Kerfant BG, Williams GS, et al. Tachycardia-induced silencing of subcellular Ca^{2+} signaling in atrial myocytes. *J Clin Invest*. 2014;124:4759–4772.
121. Chelu MG, Sarma S, Sood S, et al. Calmodulin kinase II-mediated sarcoplasmic reticulum Ca^{2+} leak promotes atrial fibrillation in mice. *J Clin Invest*. 2009;119:1940–1951.
122. Neuberger HR, Mewis C, van Veldhuisen DJ, et al. Management of atrial fibrillation in patients with heart failure. *Eur Heart J*. 2007;28:2568–2577.
123. Schreieck J, Wang Y, Overbeck M, Schomig A, Schmitt C. Altered transient outward current in human atrial myocytes of patients with reduced left ventricular function. *J Cardiovasc Electrophysiol*. 2000;11:180–192.
124. Koumi S, Arentzen CE, Backer CL, Wasserstrom JA. Alterations in muscarinic K^+ channel response to acetylcholine and to G protein-mediated activation in atrial myocytes isolated from failing human hearts. *Circulation*. 1994;90:2213–2224.
125. Dinanian S, Boixel C, Juin C, et al. Downregulation of the calcium current in human right atrial myocytes from patients in sinus rhythm but with a high risk of atrial fibrillation. *Eur Heart J*. 2008;29:1190–1197.
126. Cheng TH, Lee FY, Wei J, Lin CI. Comparison of calcium-current in isolated atrial myocytes from failing and nonfailing human hearts. *Mol Cell Biochem*. 1996;157:157–162.
127. Marshall GE, Russell JA, Tellez JO, et al. Remodelling of human atrial K^+ currents but not ion channel expression by chronic β-blockade. *Pflugers Arch*. 2012;463:537–548.
128. Le Grand BL, Hatem S, Deroubaix E, Couetil JP, Coraboeuf E. Depressed transient outward and calcium currents in dilated human atria. *Cardiovasc Res*. 1994;28:548–556.
129. Li D, Fareh S, Leung TK, Nattel S. Promotion of atrial fibrillation by heart failure in dogs: atrial remodeling of a different sort. *Circulation*. 1999;100:87–95.
130. Li D, Melnyk P, Feng J, et al. Effects of experimental heart failure on atrial cellular and ionic electrophysiology. *Circulation*. 2000;101:2631–2638.
131. Yeh YH, Wakili R, Qi XY, et al. Calcium-handling abnormalities underlying atrial arrhythmogenesis and contractile dysfunction in dogs with congestive heart failure. *Circ Arrhythm Electrophysiol*. 2008;1:93–102.
132. Sridhar A, Nishijima Y, Terentyev D, et al. Chronic heart failure and the substrate for atrial fibrillation. *Cardiovasc Res*. 2009;84:227–236.
133. Jalife J, Kaur K. Atrial remodeling, fibrosis, and atrial fibrillation. *Trends Cardiovasc Med*. 2015;25:475–484.

134. Maleckar MM, Greenstein JL, Giles WR, Trayanova NA. Electrotonic coupling between human atrial myocytes and fibroblasts alters myocyte excitability and repolarization. *Biophys J.* 2009;97:2179–2190.

135. Aguilar M, Qi XY, Huang H, Comtois P, Nattel S. Fibroblast electrical remodeling in heart failure and potential effects on atrial fibrillation. *Biophys J.* 2014;107:2444–2455.

136. Rohr S. Arrhythmogenic implications of fibroblast-myocyte interactions. *Circ Arrhythm Electrophysiol.* 2012;5:442–452.

137. Cabo C, Pertsov AM, Davidenko JM, Baxter WT, Gray RA, Jalife J. Vortex shedding as a precursor of turbulent electrical activity in cardiac muscle. *Biophys J.* 1996;70:1105–1111.

138. Deo M, Ruan Y, Pandit SV, et al. KCNJ2 mutation in short QT syndrome 3 results in atrial fibrillation and ventricular proarrhythmia. *Proc Natl Acad Sci U S A.* 2013;110:4291–4296.

139. Kneller J, Zou R, Vigmond EJ, Wang Z, Leon LJ, Nattel S. Cholinergic atrial fibrillation in a computer model of a two-dimensional sheet of canine atrial cells with realistic ionic properties. *Circ Res.* 2002;90:E73–E87.

140. Krogh-Madsen T, Abbott GW, Christini DJ. Effects of electrical and structural remodeling on atrial fibrillation maintenance: a simulation study. *PLoS Comput Biol.* 2012;8:e1002390.

141. Gonzales MJ, Vincent KP, Rappel WJ, Narayan SM, McCulloch AD. Structural contributions to fibrillatory rotors in a patient-derived computational model of the atria. *Europace.* 2014;16. suppl 4:iv3–iv10.

142. McDowell KS, Vadakkumpadan F, Blake R, et al. Mechanistic inquiry into the role of tissue remodeling in fibrotic lesions in human atrial fibrillation. *Biophys J.* 2013;104:2764–2773.

143. Courtemanche M, Ramirez RJ, Nattel S. Ionic targets for drug therapy and atrial fibrillation-induced electrical remodeling: insights from a mathematical model. *Cardiovasc Res.* 1999;42:477–489.

144. Noujaim SF, Pandit SV, Berenfeld O, et al. Up-regulation of the inward rectifier K^+ current (I K1) in the mouse heart accelerates and stabilizes rotors. *J Physiol.* 2007;578:315–326.

145. Katsouras G, Sakabe M, Comtois P, et al. Differences in atrial fibrillation properties under vagal nerve stimulation versus atrial tachycardia remodeling. *Heart Rhythm.* 2009;6:1465–1472.

146. Atienza F, Almendral J, Moreno J, et al. Activation of inward rectifier potassium channels accelerates atrial fibrillation in humans: evidence for a reentrant mechanism. *Circulation.* 2006;114:2434–2442.

147. Harrild D, Henriquez C. A computer model of normal conduction in the human atria. *Circ Res.* 2000;87:E25–E36.

148. Tanaka K, Zlochiver S, Vikstrom KL, et al. Spatial distribution of fibrosis governs fibrillation wave dynamics in the posterior left atrium during heart failure. *Circ Res.* 2007;101:839–847.

149. Gharaviri A, Verheule S, Eckstein J, Potse M, Kuijpers NH, Schotten U. A computer model of endo-epicardial electrical dissociation and transmural conduction during atrial fibrillation. *Europace.* 2012;14(suppl 5):v10–v16.

150. Wang L, Myles RC, De Jesus NM, Ohlendorf AK, Bers DM, Ripplinger CM. Optical mapping of sarcoplasmic reticulum Ca^{2+} in the intact heart: ryanodine receptor refractoriness during alternans and fibrillation. *Circ Res.* 2014;114:1410–1421.

32 Global Optimization Approaches to Generate Dynamically Robust Electrophysiological Models

Trine Krogh-Madsen and David J. Christini

Mathematical models of cardiomyocyte electrophysiology are widely used tools in cardiac arrhythmia research. Applications span an impressive range, including predicting antiarrhythmic effects of pharmacological agents, illuminating ionic mechanisms underlying arrhythmogenesis, and linking genetic variations to cellular- and tissue-level phenotypes. Computational models have been formulated and developed for a broad array of species, cell types (e.g., sinoatrial node, atrial, Purkinje fiber, and ventricular), and cell locations (e.g., endo-, mid-, and epicardium).

Unfortunately, many of the scores of mathematical models used to investigate cardiac physiology and arrhythmia mechanisms suffer from important limitations. Most models have been developed through a suboptimal process involving manual tuning of conductance parameters to subjectively match a simple target objective such as a single action potential. Consequently, models often fail to accurately simulate behavior that is dynamically dissimilar (i.e., with the complexity that is typical in vivo) to the simple target objective to which the model was fit.

These simple-objective/manual-tuning shortcomings are compounded by inconsistency that comes from using data collected over multiple experiments, often from different labs using varying conditions. Furthermore, model development typically ignores the biological variability present at both the intersubject and intercell levels, even though such population heterogeneity can be critical to arrhythmogenesis and drug response. In short, hand-tuned models are based on limited data and attempt to create representative behavior for a cardiac myocyte, although individual cells are anything but standardized.

In this chapter, we discuss recent advances aimed at overcoming these limitations in model development. In particular, we will focus on (1) the use of a genetic algorithm, which is an automated, global search heuristic to replace manual tuning in determining model parameters and (2) the use of complex target data sets to generate models capable of reproducing arrhythmia-relevant dynamics.

Introduction

The electrical activity underlying the cardiac action potential emerges from a complicated process. This activity involves a large number of proteins, including ion channels and transporters that often have nonlinear dependencies on components such as the transmembrane potential and the concentration of ion species. As an additional level of complexity, different components influence one another through feedback loops. Complex systems such as this often exhibit emergent properties that are not easily predicted from the characteristics of the individual parts.[1] Consider, as an example, triggering of early afterdepolarizations in a cell due to block of the rapid delayed rectifier potassium current (I_{Kr}). Whether this proarrhythmic event is triggered or not depends not only on the extent of I_{Kr}-block in a particular cell, but also on the availability of compensating current (such as the slow delayed rectifier potassium current, I_{Ks}), as well as on the exact activities of the inward currents that actually generate the afterdepolarization (i.e., the L-type calcium current, I_{CaL}, and/or the sodium–calcium exchange current, I_{NCX}), which in turn have additional dependencies on the dynamic intracellular calcium concentration.

Because of this complexity, mathematical models of cardiomyocyte electrophysiology are valuable tools for illumination of both normal and pathophysiological electrical activity, as a model allows access to all variables at all time points during specific interventions. A large number of cardiac cell models have been developed, generally incorporating an increasing level of detail and specificity.[2,3] Model applications have a wide span, including predicting antiarrhythmic or proarrhythmic effects of pharmacological agents, illuminating ionic mechanisms underlying arrhythmias, and studying consequences of genetic variations.[4-6]

Limitations to the Cardiac Ionic Model Development Process

Unfortunately, the reality of mathematical modeling does not always live up to the potential just described. Models have in many cases been applied successfully, but often fail to accurately simulate complex dynamics. Two examples are that (1) the rate dependence of the action potential is inaccurate for several human atrial and ventricular cell models and (2) models may not exhibit expected arrhythmia-relevant dynamics, such as early afterdepolarizations and repolarization alternans.[7,8] We believe that several limitations inherent to the traditional model-development process contribute to these deficiencies[9,10]:

1. *Interlaboratory variations and data inconsistency*: Models are typically constructed based on voltage-clamp data of individual currents. For several reasons, including specialization in biological interests and experimental techniques, these data usually come from multiple laboratories. Therefore the data have often been obtained under different experimental protocols (with varying conditions such as temperature and solution composition) and from animals with divergent characteristics (including sex, age, and breed), factors that all impact cellular electrophysiology.[11]

2. *Intercell variability:* In addition to such externally imposed variations, individual cardiac myocytes exhibit intrinsic cell-to-cell variability in electrical activity. Even cells originating

from the same region of a given heart form a heterogeneous population.[10,12] Both local cell-to-cell and interheart biological variability in electrophysiological properties are typically disregarded when formulating mathematical cardiomyocyte models, which instead rely on population-averaged data to generate a "representative" model. However, the extent to which such a model actually represents a heterogeneous population is unknown; moreover, the fidelity of an average model in predicting the effects of perturbations to a particular cell (e.g., the response to a pharmacological agent) is limited.[13,14]

3. *Manual parameter tuning:* Average voltage-clamp data are combined with equations for the individual currents to build a composite model, a step that often requires adjustment of model parameters for the model to reproduce desired whole-cell behavior. This tuning is typically done manually by tweaking parameters in a cumbersome process until the model generates output that is deemed to sufficiently reproduce the desired target behavior (e.g., an action potential). However, an automated search heuristic, which can test many more parameter combinations in a directed manner, is much more likely to find the best fit to the data.

4. *Dynamically simple data:* The data to which models are tuned is typically relatively simple, such as a single action potential. However, a host of different parameter combinations may in fact result in simple outputs that appear equivalent; dynamically simple data are therefore insufficient at uniquely identifying model parameters.[10,15–17] Consequently, a model tuned to simple data would not be expected to accurately predict the more complex dynamics associated with cardiac arrhythmias, as different channel compositions change many properties of electrical activity.[17] This limitation is severe, as one of the fundamental ambitions of cardiac modeling is to illuminate mechanisms underlying arrhythmias.

Using Complex Electrophysiological Protocols and Optimization to Generate Models

Two central strategies have been applied in efforts to overcome these inherent limitations to model development: use of automated, global search methods and use of target data beyond a single action potential. The two strategies work best when combined, in which case they generate a powerful parameter estimation methodology.

To see in more detail why more complex data are advantageous for model development, consider the following. The action potential is generated from the algebraic sum of many inward and outward currents, and its duration is largely controlled by the relatively small net outward current during the slow repolarization associated with phase 2 of the cardiac action potential. This net current can come about by a near-balance of a range of levels of the individual inward and outward currents, with different amounts of cancellation between opposite going currents and compensation among similar currents. This idea is exemplified in Fig. 32.1, which schematically shows hypothetical ranges of combinations of conductances of I_{CaL}, I_{Ks}, and I_{Kr} that may generate action potentials of very similar duration.

However, other variables and electrophysiological features will not be equivalent among cells or models with different current combinations. For example, the membrane resistance will generally vary among cells with diverse current balances, as will the response to current block or different pacing rates.[17,18] Therefore use of such data as additional targets during model development effectively reduces the range of parameter combinations that produce acceptable outputs (see Fig. 32.1).

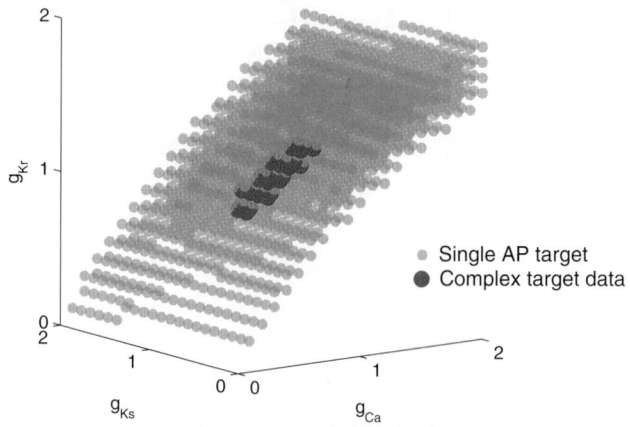

FIGURE 32.1 Nonuniqueness schematic. A range of combinations of conductance parameters (here exemplified as normalized values of the maximal conductances of the L-type calcium current [g_{CaL}], slow delayed rectifier potassium current [g_{Ks}], and rapid delayed rectifier potassium current [g_{Kr}]) may generate very similar action potentials, for example by compensation between I_{Ks} and I_{Kr} or cancellation between I_{CaL} and I_{Ks}/I_{Kr} (*gray*). A smaller range of parameters matches a more complex data sequence, e.g., an action potential and concurrent membrane resistance, seen as the reduction of the region of parameter space for which similar outputs are found (*red*).

Genetic Algorithm Optimization

For the purpose of estimating parameter values in models, solving an optimization problem means determining the set of parameters that minimizes the differences between model output and target data. As discussed in this section, the genetic algorithm is a search method that is highly suitable for finding such solutions.

The genetic algorithm is one of several optimization strategies inspired by evolutionary dynamics. The premise behind the genetic algorithm is that an initial pool of random parameter sets evolve toward a best parameter set by means of computational correlates of (i) survival of the fittest (i.e., selection of parameter sets resulting in model output closest to the target objective), (ii) reproduction and generations (pairing of parent models to create new offspring models), (iii) crossover (parameter exchange), and (iv) mutation (parameter modification).

How these operations guide the evolution of parameter sets is shown in Fig. 32.2 for an application of a genetic algorithm to estimate parameters in a cardiac electrophysiology model. In this representation, the genes of the genetic algorithm are the parameters to be estimated, which in this case are the maximal conductances or fluxes of the ion channels and transporters (see Fig. 32.2A). Different model instantiations, or individuals in the context of biological evolution, will have different combinations of these gene values. For each individual, an output can be obtained by simulating the model with its particular set of parameter values. This output can then be compared against the desired target objective, resulting in an error measure (see Fig. 32.2A). Note that the progression of the genetic algorithm to minimize this error correlates with the notion of maximizing an opposite fitness measure in Darwinian evolution.

The genetic algorithm starts out with a population of models with randomized parameter values (see Fig. 32.2B). A selection process then eliminates individuals based on their error values, such that poorly matching solutions are discarded. The surviving models form a mating pool and are recombined to generate new offspring models in the process of crossover. One way to implement this process is by a so-called uniform crossover (illustrated in Fig. 32.2B), in which parameters from two parents are

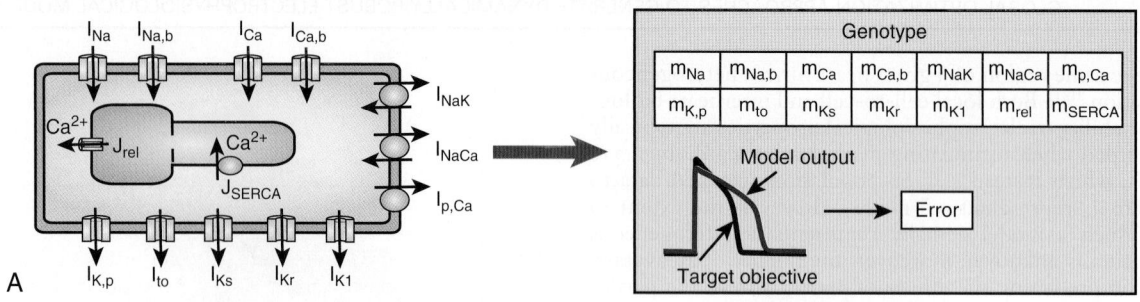

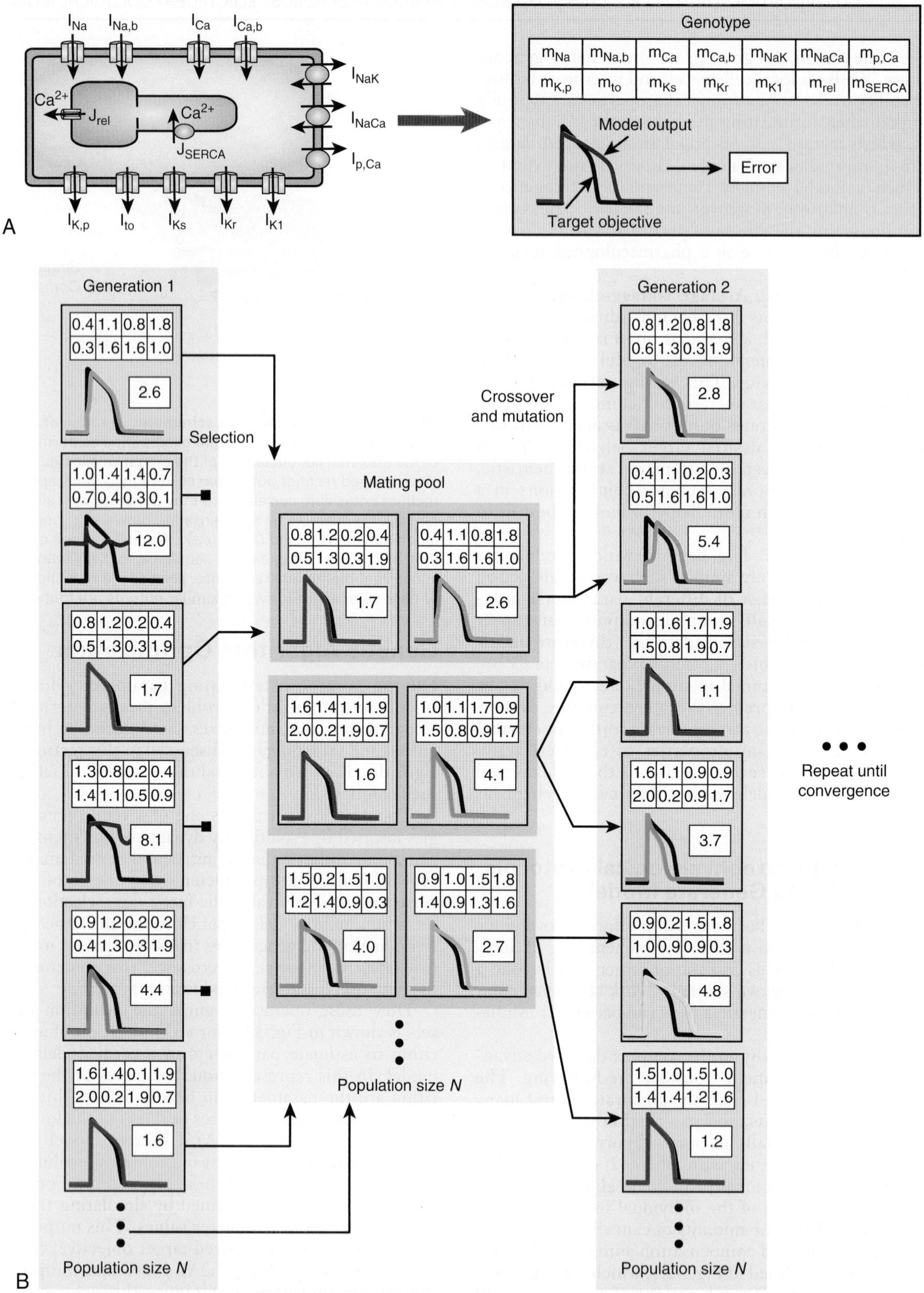

FIGURE 32.2 Schematic of genetic algorithm principles. (A) A mathematical model of a cardiac myocyte containing equations for ion transport across the sarcolemmal membrane and between intracellular compartments is characterized by its *genotype,* which are values of the parameters to be estimated (here multiplicative factors for the maximal conductances and fluxes of the ion channels and transporters). Each model instantiation, with its own particular parameter values, produces a simulated *output* (here, a single action potential), which can be used to calculate an associated *error* between model output and desired target objective. (B) The genetic algorithm progresses in generations, mimicking biological evolution. The first generation consists of *N* individual model instantiations with randomized parameter values (for purposes of clarification and simplicity only a subset is shown). Models that match the target poorly tend to be discarded in a *selection* process that favors models with closer fits (i.e., lower errors). Selected models are then combined in the *mating pool* and swap parameter values in a *crossover* process, forming new offspring. The genes inherited by the offspring may undergo *mutation,* where parameter values are perturbed. The actions of selection, crossover, and mutation are repeated through generations until a set convergence limit or another stopping criterion is reached.

swapped on a gene-by-gene basis with equal probability between two children. Following crossover, the genes of the offspring may undergo mutation to generate new values (see Fig. 32.2B).

The processes of selection, crossover, and mutation are repeated through generations of model pools, until a convergence or stop criterion is reached (e.g., that the reduction in error between consecutive generations is less than a set value or that the error of the best individual is below a certain threshold).

In addition to the randomization of the parameters of the individuals in the first generation, genetic algorithms rely on stochastic processes during the simulated evolution to maintain population diversity and prevent the search from converging on a suboptimal solution (i.e., a local, rather than the global, minimum of the error in the parameter search space). Elements of randomness can be incorporated into all the key operations of the algorithm. For example, for the selection process, we use a so-called pairwise tournament selection; this method randomly pairs two individuals and chooses the one with the lower error to continue to the mating pool while discarding the other. How mating pool members are combined, how genes are interchanged when generating offspring, and how genes are mutated, also readily succumb to randomization.

Example: Genetic Algorithm Optimization to Single Action Potential

A specific example of parameter estimation by a genetic algorithm in an ionic cardiomyocyte model is shown in Fig. 32.3. In this case, we illustrate the performance of the genetic algorithm by fitting the model to its own output, such that the optimization should return the known parameters. The particular model is the guinea pig ventricular myocyte model presented by Faber and Rudy.[19]

In this setup, each generation consists of 500 individuals. As their parameters are randomized, most individuals generate output that is very different from the single action potential target (see Fig. 32.3A and C). However, some model instantiations fit the target well by chance (see Fig. 32.3B). As the optimization progresses, errors decrease as fits get closer to the target (see Fig. 32.3F and G). For example, in the 10th generation, the model with the lowest error produces an action potential that is almost identical to the objective (see Fig. 32.3D), and in the 100th generation, the best fit is essentially indistinguishable from the target (see Fig. 32.3E).

Importantly, the closest reproduction of the target found by the genetic algorithm is not obtained through a complete recovery of the known parameters (i.e., in Fig. 32.3, a parameter scaling of 1). In particular, the conductance of the plateau potassium current (parameter 7) is overestimated, while I_{Kr} conductance and maximal SERCA flux (parameters 5 and 9) are underestimated. This exactly exemplifies the situation in Fig. 32.1, where different combinations of parameter values can produce nearly identical action potentials. While continuing the progression of the genetic algorithm could possibly eventually lead to more accurate recovery of these parameters, it is more likely that using a single action potential as the target simply provides insufficient information to constrain parameters better.

Setting up a Genetic Algorithm Optimization

Before turning to a discussion on selecting objectives to better constrain parameters in cardiac cell models, a few more words are needed on how to set up a genetic algorithm optimization, as several choices are available,[20] including both model- and physiology-based choices, such as which parameters to include and how to determine their allowed ranges. Wider bounds and, in particular, more parameters translate into much harder optimization problems, as the addition of each parameter expands the parameter search space by one dimension. A larger parameter space requires more target data to constrain the parameters and increases the computational costs. Therefore estimating all the 100+ parameters that modern cardiac electrophysiology models typically include would require both an immense amount of target data and prohibitively long computational time. Practical approaches therefore include optimizing only conductance parameters, as shown in Fig. 32.3 and elsewhere,[21,22] and not including parameters controlling the time- and voltage-dependence of channel gating. This simplification builds on the assumption that "a channel is a channel" and that variation among cells and subjects is primarily due to differences in channel density. A limitation to this reduction is that any baseline mismatch in gating between model and target will not be rectified. Other strategies for achieving a manageable optimization problem (using genetic algorithm or other optimization methods) include using simplified cell models[23–26] or focusing on a single current only.[27,28]

Designing a genetic algorithm optimization also involves determining settings for the genetic algorithm itself, such as the number of individuals per generation; the details of the selection, crossover, and mutation operators; the potential use of elitism strategies in which a certain number of individuals with the lowest errors are guaranteed to continue in the evolution; the stop or convergence criteria; and the number of individual runs of the algorithm, as each randomized run-through will produce a different result. The choices are interconnected (e.g., more parameters and larger search ranges require more individuals). Variations of the search methods may also include dynamic changes in the settings during the optimization (e.g., by allowing generous parameter perturbations early in the evolution with later restrictions to fine, local, parameter modifications).[29,30] As the best settings for a genetic algorithm tend to depend on both model and objective, the settings may need to be chosen specifically for a given optimization problem (e.g., by testing the ability of the algorithm to recover known parameters).

The main computational cost of running a genetic algorithm for cardiac cell model parameterization is the numerical integration of the many individual models. As these are independent within each generation, the genetic algorithm is readily parallelizable and can be implemented to run on many cores, including those of a graphics processing unit (GPU), thus dramatically reducing execution times.[31] In our hands, relatively simple optimizations such as that in Fig. 32.3 can be run in less than an hour using central processing units (CPUs) on a 3.2 GHz, 6-core, 6 GB memory machine. Using the more complex objectives described in the next section increases CPU time to around 8 hours per run. Hence, although optimization can be computationally costly, the approaches described here are not unattainable.

Use of Complex Objectives in Optimization

While it is clear that a single action potential provides insufficient information to accurately estimate the main conductances in cardiac cell models, questions remain as to precisely what types of data sets comprise more desirable objectives and how a protocol is designed to best generate complex target data. Several different categories of objectives have been adopted previously, including the use of membrane potential recordings obtained at multiple pacing frequencies, as well as currents and membrane resistance data recorded with different voltage-clamp protocols. To enable application to isolated cardiac myocytes, an additional consideration is that protocols

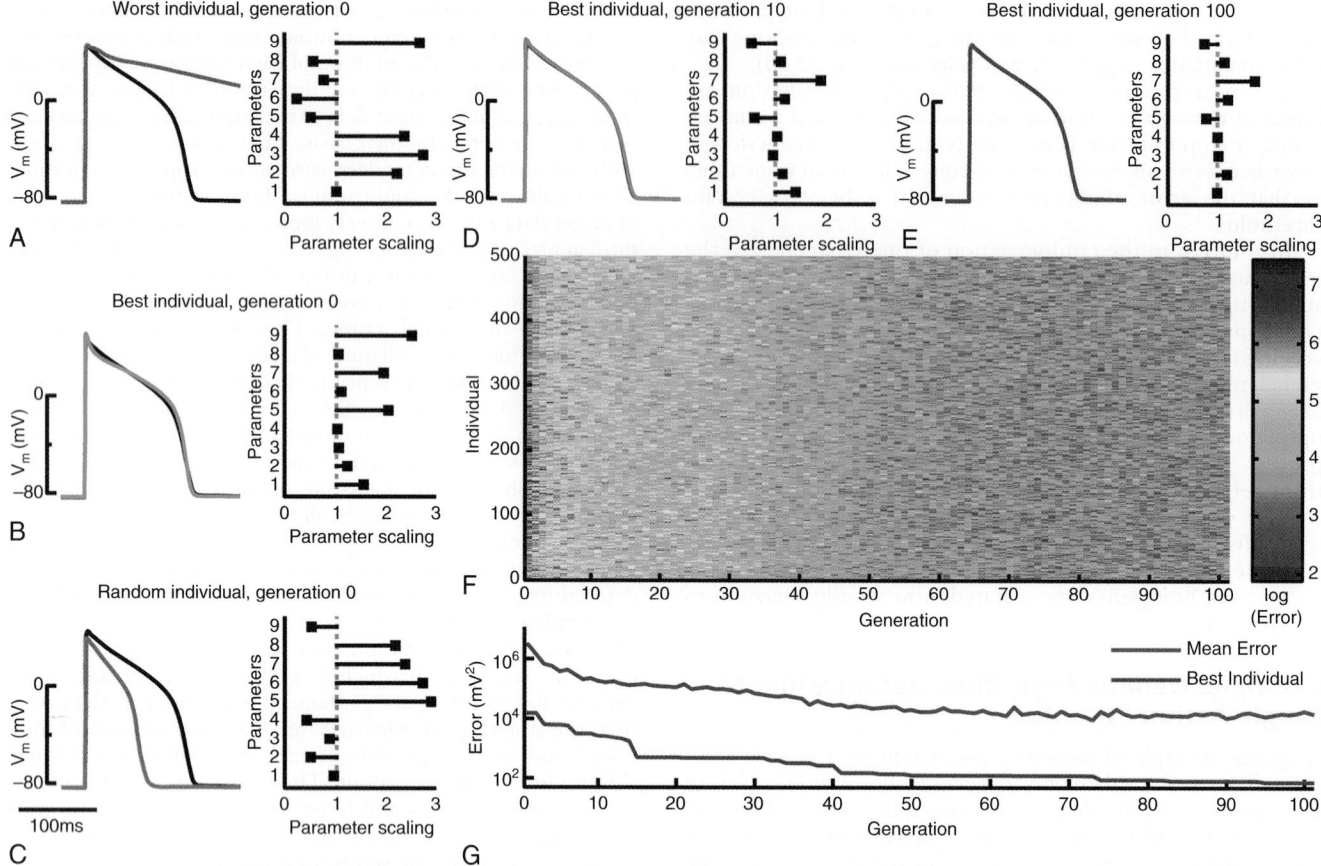

FIGURE 32.3 Genetic algorithm optimization to single action potential objective. (A–C) The randomized individuals in the initial generation of the genetic algorithm run produce a wide range of outputs, including repolarization failure as well as action potentials close to the desired target (*black trace*). Model output is color coded according to the error value (*color bar in* [F]), which is calculated as the sum of squared differences between model output and target objective. Bar graphs indicate scaled parameter values for each individual, with a value of 1 representing the original model value to be recovered by the genetic algorithm search. Parameters 1 through 9 correspond to: the sodium current (I_{Na}), L-type calcium current (I_{CaL}), T-type calcium current (I_{CaT}), inwardly rectifying potassium current (I_{K1}), rapid delayed rectifier potassium current (I_{Kr}), slow delayed rectifier potassium current (I_{Ks}), plateau potassium current (I_{Kp}), sarcolemmal calcium pump current (I_{pCa}), and maximal flux of the sarco/endoplasmic reticulum calcium ATPase (J_{SERCA}), respectively. These nine parameters are represented by normalized scaling factors, which we allow to change between 0.01% and 300% in the optimization process. (D–E) With progression of the genetic algorithm, the best individual in each generation, which represents the best solution so far, becomes very similar to the optimization objective. Note, however, that the parameter values of even the best solutions are different from those of the baseline model, demonstrating how different parameter combinations can generate equivalent action potentials. (F–G) The advancement of the reduction in error is seen across the population of 500 individuals. (From Groenendaal W, Ortega FA, Kherlopian AR, et al. Cell-specific cardiac electrophysiology models. *PLoS Comput Biol.* 2015;11:e1004242.)

must be sufficiently short to avoid significant current rundown while being long enough to allow for the dynamic richness needed.

Voltage-Based Optimization

One way to increase the complexity of the optimization objective is to perturb the action potential waveform. Indeed, addition of a voltage waveform perturbed by nonconstant current injection to a single action potential objective can lead to improvements in parameter estimation.[15]

Because of the rate dependence of the cardiac action potential, additional data that can help constrain model parameters in an optimization can readily be obtained by recording at different pacing rates. As the rate dependence is of clear importance

to arrhythmogenesis, such data are essential for models to reproduce accurately. Indeed, the inclusion of such additional data can have the dual goal of better constraining parameters and better reproducing rate-dependent dynamics. In early work, Syed et al. found that when optimizing a model to a series of experimental action potentials recorded when pacing at a single fixed rate (2 Hz), the resulting model did not reproduce well the dynamics recorded at a different pacing rate (1 Hz, Fig. 32.4A).[21] Optimizing the model to multiple data sets obtained at different pacing rates (1, 2, 3, and 4 Hz) resulted in much better fits (Fig. 32.4B). In contrast, when the target data instead consisted of action potentials obtained by simulating a second computational model, no such improvement was found by adding data from multiple pacing rates,[21] suggesting that the gain is model/system dependent.

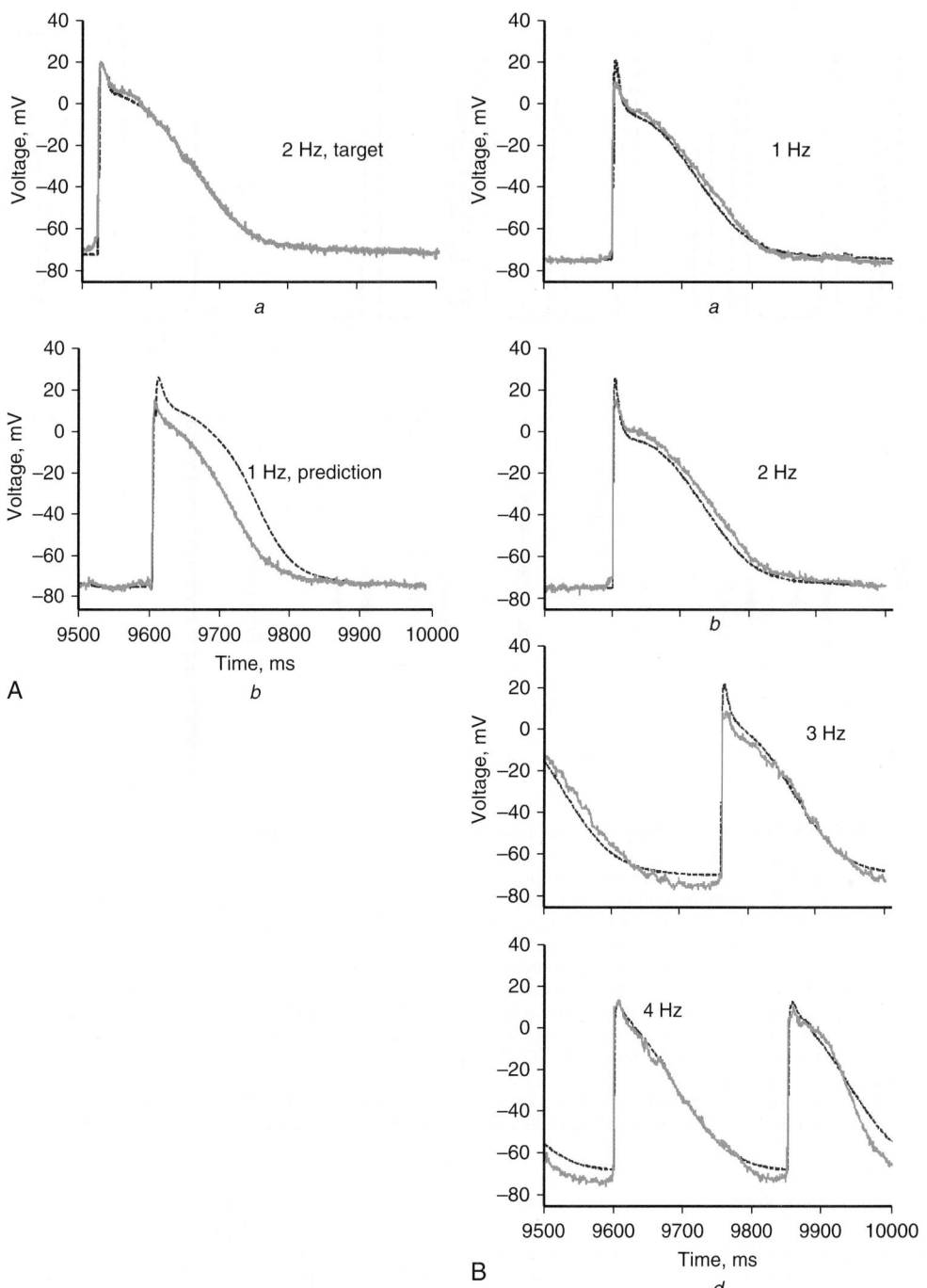

FIGURE 32.4 Addition of action potentials recorded at different rates improves optimization. (A) Optimizing an atrial cell model to canine atrial tissue action potentials recorded at 2 Hz (*a*) results in a poor model prediction of the action potential at 1 Hz (*b*). Note, however, that part of this mismatch may be due to what seems like an unusual shortening of the action potential recorded at 1 Hz. (B) The fits can be much better when data recorded at 1, 2, 3, and 4 Hz are included in the objective. (Modified from Syed Z, Vigmond E, Nattel S, et al. Atrial cell action potential parameter fitting using genetic algorithms. *Med Biol Eng Comput.* 2005;43:561-571.)

Rather than matching the action potential waveform at a few different rates, another strategy is to match the full action potential duration restitution curve. Determining this relationship at many pacing rates requires long stimulation and simulation times, and this approach may therefore not (yet) be amenable for optimizing biophysically detailed models, but it has been applied to simpler models.[23,26] An important caveat is that a model may reproduce the action potential duration restitution curve and still

have action potentials whose morphologies do not actually match those of the target.[21]

As a way to both sample the rate dependence more quickly and to maintain waveform data, the use of stochastically paced action potentials can be useful. This approach has the added advantage that it somewhat mimics arrhythmic dynamics and is thus of greater relevance to arrhythmia simulation. Adopting again the process of optimizing a model to itself and measuring the

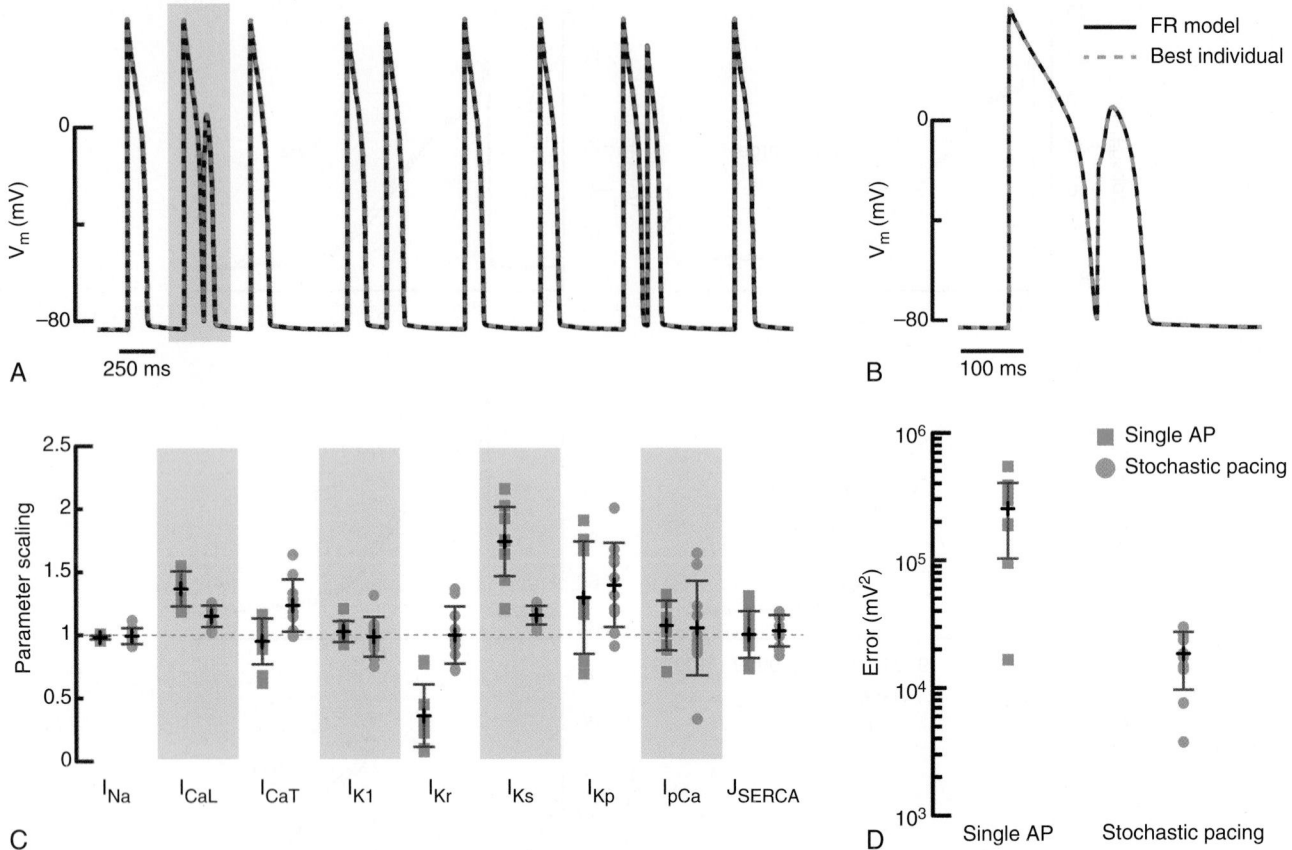

FIGURE 32.5 Stochastic pacing objective improves parameter estimation and predictability. (A) The stochastic stimulation optimization target (Faber-Rudy model[19] *black trace*) is closely matched by the best fit obtained from a genetic algorithm search using that sequence as the objective (*light blue dashed line*). (B) Close-up of the shaded region in (A). (C) The stochastic pacing objective leads to some improvement in parameter recovery (*light blue circles*) compared to the single action potential objective (*green squares*), most notably for the rapid delayed rectifier potassium current (I_{Kr}), L-type calcium current (I_{CaL}), and slow delayed rectifier potassium current (I_{Ks}) conductances. Because of the inherent randomness of the genetic algorithm, each optimization was run ten times. Symbols indicate the best individual from each of the ten runs, plus signs (*black*) give their mean, error bars (*gray*) show standard deviation, and the dashed line at parameter scaling 1 indicates the original model parameter values to be recovered. (D) When presented with a novel stimulation sequence to test predictive power, models optimized to the stochastic stimulation sequence perform significantly better than models optimized using only a single action potential. (Modified from Groenendaal W, Ortega FA, Kherlopian AR, et al. Cell-specific cardiac electrophysiology models. *PLoS Comput Biol.* 2015;11:e1004242.)

ability of the optimization method to recover parameter values, we compared the use of a single action potential objective versus using a 6-second series of randomly timed action potentials as the objective (Fig. 32.5).[10] As was the case for the single action potential, the stochastic pacing objective was fit very closely by the best model (see Fig. 32.5A). Several parameters were more accurately recovered when using the dynamically richer stochastic pacing protocol (see Fig. 32.5C). This improvement was especially marked for the maximal conductances of I_{Kr}, I_{Ks}, and I_{CaL}. During a single action potential, these currents are correlated with compensatory (I_{Kr} and I_{Ks}) or antagonistic (I_{Ks} and I_{CaL}) effects,[10] which makes uniquely determining parameters difficult for the genetic algorithm. However, during the stochastic stimulation sequence, the currents replace or oppose each other less well due to their distinct kinetics, which helps the genetic algorithm identify their conductances, as depicted generally in Fig. 32.1.

In addition to fitting error and parameter accuracy, an important means to assess the outcome of an optimization is to measure the ability of optimized models to predict new dynamics. We subjected models to a novel sequence of randomly timed stimuli and assessed their predictive power based on the differences

in response between the optimized and the target models. This predictive error was significantly reduced for models trained to the more complex stochastic pacing sequence compared with the single action potential optimization (see Fig. 32.5D). Thus the use of the stochastic pacing protocol improves this optimization as measured both at the level of the parameter estimation and as a manifestation of better predictive power.

Current-Based Optimization

Parameter identification typically gains precision when including a new variable in the objective. This suggests that adding recordings of a different variable, for example current recorded during voltage-clamp, may yield much better optimization results than using longer trains of the same data variable. Using this motivation, we added membrane current to the objective. Specifically, we aimed to design a voltage-clamp protocol for which individual steps were meant to induce a different ion current in isolation (Fig. 32.6A).[10] For example, the protocol starts with a hyperpolarizing step to activate primarily I_{K1}. In this way, only a model with accurate conductance values for each isolated

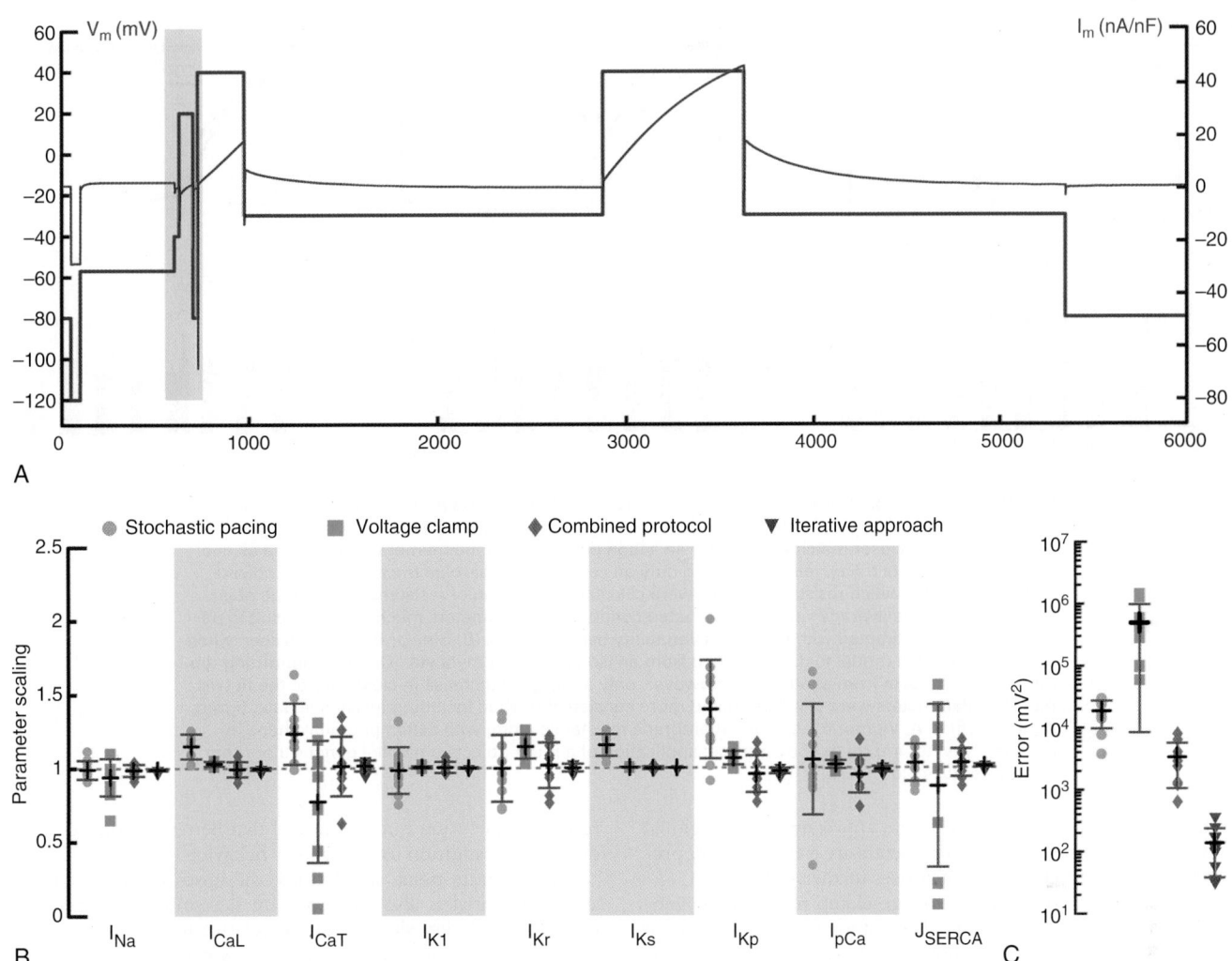

FIGURE 32.6 Addition of voltage-clamp data enhances parameter estimation and boosts predictive power. (A) Voltage-clamp protocol (*blue*) and total current response (*red*). (B) Increased accuracy in the parameter estimation from using stochastic stimulation (*light blue circles*) or voltage-clamping (*green squares*) alone, to using the combined stochastic pacing and voltage-clamp protocol (*orange diamonds*). Further improvement is obtained when using the iterative optimization of running the genetic algorithm twice, with the second run being restricted to a local region in parameter space defined by the first runs (*magenta triangles*). Symbols indicate results from the individual runs; error bars give the mean (*black*) ± standard deviation (*gray*). (C) The error in predicting the response to a novel stochastic pacing sequence is large for the voltage-clamp objective alone, which does not train models according to membrane potential. Adding the voltage-clamp protocol to the stochastic pacing protocol results in predictions better than those obtained from models optimized to stochastic stimulation alone. The prediction error is further reduced when using the iterative optimization approach (*magenta triangles*). (Modified from Groenendaal W, Ortega FA, Kherlopian AR, et al. Cell-specific cardiac electrophysiology models. *PLoS Comput Biol.* 2015;11:e1004242.)

current will match the target well and will propagate in the optimization evolution.

The protocol effectively isolated I_{K1}, I_{Ks}, and I_{CaL}, and these currents were accurately estimated in an optimization using the total current during the voltage-clamp as the objective (Fig. 32.6B). Combining the stochastic pacing and the voltage-clamp protocol into one objective resulted in more accurate parameter recovery for most of the conductances (see Fig. 32.6B). Along with the variations in the ability to pinpoint parameters, the different objectives also lead to models with different predictive abilities (Fig. 32.6C). Not surprisingly, models generated by optimizing to the voltage-clamp protocol only are less capable of predicting the response to a stochastic pacing sequence, as they have not been trained to match voltage waveforms. Interestingly, models optimized using the combined stochastic pacing

and voltage-clamp protocol predict the novel stochastic pacing dynamics better than models optimized using only the stochastic pacing objective. This result may be counter-intuitive, as one might hypothesize that fitting to another variable and another type of dynamics would compromise the ability of the model to accurately simulate the response to stochastic pacing. Instead the more complex protocol leads to more faithful parameter estimation and thus results in increased predictive power.

Fig. 32.6 also demonstrates how methodological advancements to the genetic algorithm itself can improve optimization. We added a second genetic algorithm iteration after each initial run, with the parameter search range restricted to the span of the best solutions found in the first iteration.[10,30] This approach allows for a finer search in the local region of parameter space determined by the first evolution and therefore relies on the

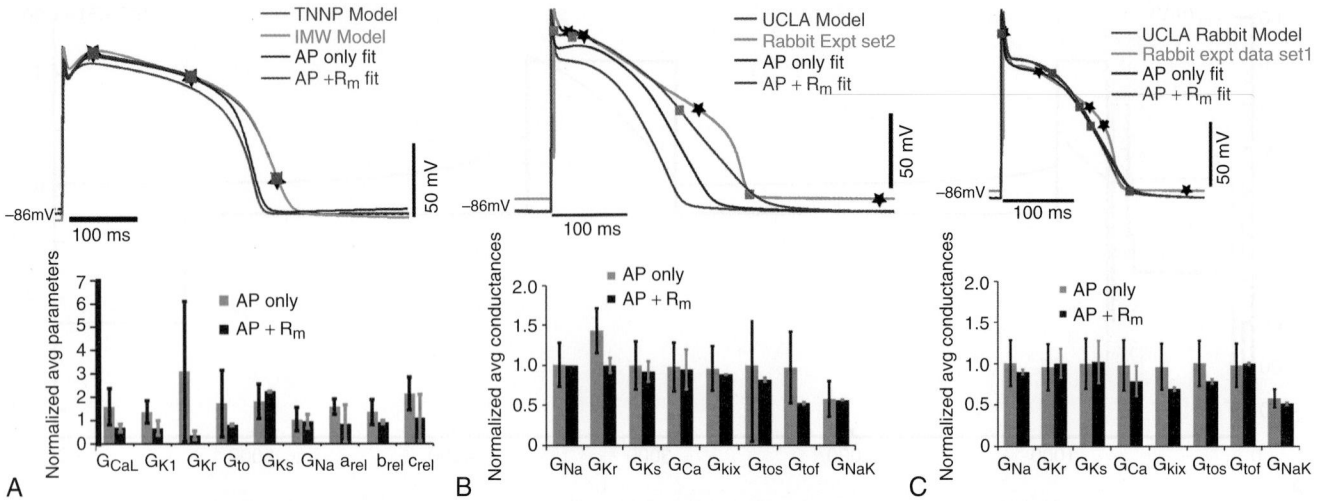

FIGURE 32.7 Addition of membrane resistance data to single action potential objective. (A) Optimizing one human cell model (*red trace*) to fit target data generated by another model (*green trace*) results in a closer match when using an action potential and the membrane resistance as dual objectives (*magenta trace*), relative to using only an action potential (*blue trace*). Symbols indicate voltage points for which resistance values were calculated. Addition of resistance data to the objective did not change average values of estimated conductance parameters much, but did result in parameters being estimated with much less variability between runs. (B) Similar benefit was seen when optimizing a rabbit model to data recorded from an isolated rabbit myocyte. (C) When optimizing the rabbit model to data from another cell, however, only a marginal increase in closeness of the fit was reported. Parameters were still determined more consistently when including resistance data. (From Kaur J, Nygren A, Vigmond EJ. Fitting membrane resistance along with action potential shape in cardiac myocytes improves convergence: application of a multi-objective parallel genetic algorithm. *PLoS One.* 2014;9:e107984.)

ability of the initial iteration to locate approximately the global minimum. With this addition, parameters are estimated very precisely and the predictive error decreases further.

The utilization of complex voltage-clamp protocols to generate current objectives has also been studied in the context of parameterization of Markov models of ion currents.[27,28] These models typically contain many more parameters than Hodgkin–Huxley–type models and thus require more data for parameter identification. It therefore becomes imperative for protocols to generate objectives that disentangle key features efficiently. Using parameter sensitivities as a measure of whether a certain objective can uniquely identify parameters, it is indeed feasible to design relatively short protocols with the same ability to identify parameters as classic voltage-clamp protocols that systematically parse through voltage and time dependencies.[27] This approach of using sensitivity measures should be applicable to other optimization problems, including that of determining conductance parameters.

Membrane Resistance, Upstroke Velocity, and Tissue Considerations

As mentioned in the Introduction, identical-looking action potentials with different ion current balances may have different membrane resistance profiles. Therefore membrane resistance may help restrain parameters in an optimization. Indeed, Kaur et al. demonstrated that adding resistance values, calculated at several different voltage values during the action potential, to a single action potential objective can improve fits and reduce variability in estimated parameters (Fig. 32.7).[18] The extent to which fits are improved by the inclusion of resistance values can depend on the particular model used and on how different its action potential and resistance are to the objective data (see Fig. 32.7). As membrane resistance controls source–sink dynamics between coupled cells, accurate resistance capture is important when simulating cardiac tissue.[18] Therefore a significant gain obtained by

resistance inclusion can be a model that better reproduces tissue dynamics in addition to the cellular behavior.

For accurate tissue simulations, the upstroke velocity of the action potential is also an important determinant. Because the upstroke is of very short duration relative to the action potential, optimizing only to action potentials may not yield accurate matching of the upstroke velocity. This deficiency can be alleviated by including in the objective the rate of change of the membrane potential.[26]

If the explicit goal of the parameter estimation is to generate accurate tissue models, one can also take the approach of optimizing a tissue model directly to data from tissue recordings,[25] which may also include optimizing to conduction velocity and even to the conduction velocity restitution curve. This approach has been applied when optimizing simple models only,[23,24] as it is highly expensive computationally.

Thus several individual objectives, both at the cellular level and at the tissue level, may be useful for tissue model development, but as tissue-level optimization is computationally demanding, we have previously called for more rigorous ways to parameterize cellular models so that they exhibit appropriate behavior in tissue.[9]

Conclusions and Outlook

We have discussed in this chapter different approaches for improving model generation. The overall strategy is to use a combination of automated global search techniques and complex target objectives to estimate model parameters. Rich target data may be generated by diverse pacing or clamping protocols, by perturbations such as drug block,[26,28] and by using different types of variables (e.g., membrane potential, resistance, and current). We have previously suggested that intracellular calcium concentration also presents an important variable to include in ionic model optimization.[10] However, which types of data are best for a particular model remains practically unexplored. The question of how data variables are optimally explored and sampled for use as target objectives is also undetermined. Using sensitivity measures to determine what parameters are identifiable with a given protocol may be one approach to tackle this issue.[10,27]

Optimization Methods

The genetic algorithm is only one of several methods that can be applied to solve the kind of parameter estimation problems discussed here. Other techniques include particle swarm, gradient descent methods, and simulated annealing.[15,24,26,32–35] Comparative testing of these methodologies has been carried out for applications to neuronal model optimization,[35] but not for cardiac cell applications. Outside a specific comparative study, to compare the accuracy and efficiency of different methods becomes almost impossible, as these methods have been applied to different types of models (including sophisticated ionic and simple phenomenological models) and have used different metrics of success (e.g., error of best fit, accuracy of parameter values, and predictive ability) and different objectives. The genetic algorithm may be particularly appealing to physiologists as it is effective for application to a range of optimization problems, is easy to implement (toolboxes exist) and parallelize, and builds on biologically intuitive concepts.

Cell- and Patient-Specific Modeling

When the target data sequences can be acquired from protocols in individual cells, the parameter estimation can generate cell-specific models, thus solving the problems of cell-to-cell variability and data inconsistency outlined in the Introduction. This method requires the protocols to be sufficiently short to be run in single cells before significant rundown of currents or other damage occurs. Such cell-specific models may allow modelers to generate accurate predictions of dynamics (e.g., early afterdepolarizations) in a given cell with its specific mix of cellular components.

Cell-specific models can be utilized to study population heterogeneity, both at the level of intraheart spatial variations and interheart variability.[9,10,14] Ultimately, studies of subject-level population heterogeneity can provide insights into why some patients are more prone than others to experience arrhythmias with particular interventions and hence can guide precision medicine.

Model Validation

No existing framework currently exists for validation of such optimized cell-specific models; the traditional approach of comparing model output to average or perceived representative experimental data is insufficient. A proper process should validate both estimated parameters and model output on a cell-by-cell basis. Validation of model output could include quantification of the ability of the models to predict novel dynamics, as done previously.[10] Testing the accuracy of optimized parameters is less straightforward, but could conceivably be tested through drug-induced perturbations to individual currents. Importantly, development of these validation steps needs to proceed in parallel with further development of the model parameter optimization methodologies in order for the model development enterprise to progress properly.[36,37]

REFERENCES

1. Krogh-Madsen T, Christini DJ. Nonlinear dynamics in cardiology. *Annu Rev Biomed Eng.* 2012;14:179–203.
2. Fink M, et al. Cardiac cell modelling: observations from the heart of the cardiac physiome project. *Prog Biophys Mol Biol.* 2011;104:2–21.
3. Noble D, Garny A, Noble PJ. How the Hodgkin-Huxley equations inspired the cardiac Physiome Project. *J Physiol.* 2012;590:2613–2628.
4. Rudy Y, Silva JR. Computational biology in the study of cardiac ion channels and cell electrophysiology. *Quart Rev Biophys.* 2006;39:57–116.
5. Trayanova NA. Whole-heart modeling: applications to cardiac electrophysiology and electromechanics. *Circ Res.* 2011;108:113–128.
6. Roberts BN, Yang PC, Behrens SB, Moreno JD, Clancy CE. Computational approaches to understand cardiac electrophysiology and arrhythmias. *Am J Physiol Heart Circ Physiol.* 2012;303:H766–H783.
7. O'Hara T, Virág L, Varró A, Rudy Y. Simulation of the undiseased human cardiac ventricular action potential: model formulation and experimental validation. *PLoS Comput Biol.* 2011;7:e1002061.
8. Gonzales MJ, Vincent KP, Rappel WJ, Narayan SM, McCulloch AD. Structural contributions to fibrillatory rotors in a patient-derived computational model of the atria. *Europace.* 2014;16:iv3–iv10.
9. Krogh-Madsen T, Sobie EA, Christini DJ. Improving cardiomyocyte model fidelity and utility via dynamic electrophysiology protocols and optimization algorithms. *J Physiol.* 2016;594:2525–2536.
10. Groenendaal W, et al. Cell-specific cardiac electrophysiology models. *PLoS Comput Biol.* 2015;11:e1004242.
11. Niederer SA, Fink M, Noble D, Smith NP. A meta-analysis of cardiac electrophysiology computational models. *Exp Physiol.* 2009;94:486–495.
12. Bénardeau A, et al. Contribution of Na⁺/Ca²⁺ exchange to action potential of human atrial myocytes. *Am J Physiol.* 1996;271:H1151–H1161.
13. Marder E. Variability, compensation, and modulation in neurons and circuits. *Proc Natl Acad Sci U S A.* 2011;108:15542–15548.

14. Sarkar AX, Christini DJ, Sobie EA. Exploiting mathematical models to illuminate electrophysiological variability between individuals. *J Physiol.* 2012;590:2555–2567.
15. Dokos S, Lovell NH. Parameter estimation in cardiac ionic models. *Prog Biophys Mol Biol.* 2004;85:407–431.
16. Sarkar AX, Sobie EA. Regression analysis for constraining free parameters in electrophysiological models of cardiac cells. *PLoS Comput Biol.* 2010;6:e1000914.
17. Zaniboni M, Riva I, Cacciani F, Groppi M. How different two almost identical action potentials can be: A model study on cardiac repolarization. *Math Biosci.* 2010;228:56–70.
18. Kaur J, Nygren A, Vigmond EJ. Fitting membrane resistance along with action potential shape in cardiac myocytes improves convergence: application of a multi-objective parallel genetic algorithm. *PLoS One.* 2014;9:e107984.
19. Faber GM, Rudy Y. Action potential and contractility changes in [Na⁺]ᵢ overloaded cardiac myocytes: a simulation study. *Biophys J.* 2000;78:2392–2404.
20. de Jong KA. *Evolutionary Computation: A Unified Approach.* Cambridge, MA: MIT Press; 2006.
21. Syed Z, Vigmond E, Nattel S, Leon LJ. Atrial cell action potential parameter fitting using genetic algorithms. *Med Biol Eng Comput.* 2005;43:561–571.
22. Bot CT, Kherlopian AR, Ortega FA, Christini DJ, Krogh-Madsen T. Rapid genetic algorithm optimization of a mouse computational model: Benefits for anthropomorphization of neonatal mouse cardiomyocytes. *Front Physio.* 2012;3:1–14.
23. Bueno-Orovio A, Cherry EM, Fenton FH. Minimal model for human ventricular action potentials in tissue. *J Theor Biol.* 2008;253:544–560.
24. Weber FM, et al. Adaptation of a minimal four-state cell model for reproducing atrial excitation properties. *Comp Cardiol Proc.* 2008;35:61–64.
25. Al Abed A, Guo T, Lovell NH, Dokos S. Optimisation of ionic models to fit tissue action potentials: application to 3D atrial modelling. *Comput Math Methods Med.* 2013;2013:951234.

26. Guo T, Al Abed A, Lovell NH, Dokos S. Optimisation of a generic ionic model of cardiac myocyte electrical activity. *Comput Math Methods Med.* 2013;2013:706195.
27. Fink M, Noble D. Markov models for ion channels: versatility versus identifiability and speed. *Philos Transact A Math Phys Eng Sci.* 2009;367:2161–2179.
28. Zhou Q, et al. Identification of Iₖᵣ kinetics and drug binding in native myocytes. *Ann Biomed Eng.* 2009;37:1294–1309.
29. Druckmann S, et al. A novel multiple objective optimization framework for constraining conductance-based neuron models by experimental data. *Front Neurosci.* 2007;1:7–18.
30. Hobbs KH, Hooper SL. Using complicated, wide dynamic range driving to develop models of single neurons in single recording sessions. *J Neurophysiol.* 2008;99:1871–1883.
31. Tomaiuolo M, Bertram R, Leng G, Tabak J. Models of electrical activity: calibration and prediction testing on the same cell. *Biophys J.* 2012;103:2021–2032.
32. Chen F, Chu A, Yang X, Lei Y, Chu J. Identification of the parameters of the Beeler-Reuter ionic equation with a partially perturbed particle swarm optimization. *IEEE Trans Biomed Eng.* 2012;59:3412–3421.
33. Wang W, et al. Optimal estimation of ion-channel kinetics from macroscopic currents. *PLoS One.* 2012;7:e35208.
34. Guo TT, Al Abed A, Lovell NH, Dokos SS. A generic ionic model of cardiac action potentials. *Conf Proc IEEE Eng Med Biol Soc.* 2010;2010:1465–1468.
35. Vanier MC, Bower JM. A comparative survey of automated parameter-search methods for compartmental neural models. *J Comput Neurosci.* 1999;7:149–171.
36. Carusi A, Burrage K, Rodriguez B. Bridging experiments, models and simulations: an integrative approach to validation in computational cardiac electrophysiology. *Am J Physiol Heart Circ Physiol.* 2012;303:H144–H155.
37. Pathmanathan P, Gray RA. Ensuring reliability of safety-critical clinical applications of computational cardiac models. *Front Physio.* 2013;4:358.

33 Calcium Signaling in Cardiomyocyte Models With Realistic Geometries

Andrew G. Edwards, Johan Hake, Anushka P. Michailova,
Masahiko Hoshijima, and Andrew D. McCulloch

The microarchitecture of cellular substructures involved in calcium signaling is highly organized in all forms of mammalian striated muscle, and the cardiac ventricular myocyte (VM) is no exception. The ultrastructural characteristics of the T-tubular system and sarcoplasmic reticulum (SR) play an important role in normal cardiac electrophysiology, and their degradation has dire consequences in a number of pathological contexts. Below we discuss several electrophysiologically important aspects of VM ultrastructure and place emphasis on structure–function relationships in the healthy and diseased myocardium. Because interaction within and between these structures often occurs at or below the limit of resolution for traditional live-imaging techniques, quantitative computational modeling has made an essential contribution to the understanding of how structure determines function. As such, we highlight ongoing computational efforts that make use of reconstructed subcellular geometries to describe VM physiology at the optical diffraction limit and below.

Electrophysiological Structure of the Ventricular Myocyte

Anatomy of the Myocyte Sarcolemma

The plasma membrane of ventricular myocytes, and of most mammalian striated muscle, exhibits regular invaginations that project into the cell perpendicular to its surface (Fig. 33.1). These structures align with the sarcomeric Z-disk and were originally termed transverse tubules (T-tubules) for their dominant orientation with respect to the long axis of the cell. However, in most species a large number of longitudinal branches have also been observed,[1,2] causing different authors to describe the lattice architecture variously as the transverse-axial-tubular system (TATS),[3] sarcolemmal tubule system,[4] T-system,[5] and sarcolemmal Z-rete.[6] At a macroscopic level, the T-tubular lattice impacts myocyte function by at least two important mechanisms. First, it expands the VM surface area and thereby increases the density (per unit cell volume) of all sarcolemmal transport mechanisms. Second, it provides a platform for regionalization of specialized signaling structures. Here we focus on structures that are directly involved in cardiac Ca²⁺ signaling, the best described of which are the calcium release unit (CRU; see Fig. 33.1, *right panel*) and the cardiac couplon.

A Brief Ultrastructural History of Cardiac Excitation–Contraction Coupling

Initial impressions of the shape and structure of the CRU first appeared roughly half a century ago, and well before the function of the couplon was understood or the term itself had been coined.[7] At that time, transmission electron microscopy (EM) had shown junctions between the SR and T-tubular membranes, which in cardiac muscle were termed dyads for their characteristic two-component appearance in longitudinal tissue sections. A few years later, Constantin and associates[8] identified these SR structures as the site of intracellular calcium storage, and Winegrad's landmark study[9] followed shortly after to show that these structures were also the site of intracellular Ca²⁺ release. Fawcett and McNutt[5] accordingly refined Porter and Palade's well-known sketch of the cardiac sarcomere,[10] and their rendition remains popular today (see Fig. 33.1, *left panel*). In this schematic, Ca²⁺ is released from specialized projections of the SR, which closely juxtapose the T-tubular membrane. These projections were also originally named for their anatomical appearance in transmission EM (i.e., junctional SR [jSR] and terminal cisternal SR) or for their characteristics of physical separation (i.e., heavy SR). Over the next several decades, classic studies were published by a number of groups to define Ca²⁺-induced Ca²⁺ release (CICR) as the essential mechanism of EC coupling occurring at cardiac dyads and as being responsible for activating contraction of the heart.[11,12] Key aspects of CICR are detailed in Chapters 2 and 6, but to review briefly, voltage-dependent opening of local L-type Ca²⁺ channels (LCC) permits influx of Ca²⁺, which binds to and activates nearby ryanodine receptors (RyR) in the jSR membrane. This RyR activation results in release, from the jSR, of the bulk of the Ca²⁺ that goes on to participate in contraction.[12]

Since the early 1990s, it has become clear that a number of important properties of cardiac EC coupling are critically dependent upon the biophysical characteristics of Ca²⁺-mediated interaction between the LCC and RyR. These processes and phenomena will be discussed in detail below, but at this point it behooves us to introduce several terms that have been adopted to reflect fundamental structure–function relationships in the current paradigm of EC coupling, known as "local control."[13] First, the term CRU refers to a grouping of jSR terminals and RyR clusters, which together constitute a discrete functional ensemble.[14] The RyR clusters that comprise a CRU are activated together in an all-or-nothing fashion, but are otherwise functionally isolated from others by a sufficiently large diffusion distance. CRU structure is usually drawn schematically, as in Fig. 33.1, with a single jSR terminal with a densely packed array of RyR. However, as we shall see, it is likely that real CRUs exhibit heterogeneous morphologies incorporating multiple RyR clusters and probably also multiple functionally coupled jSR terminals.[15] The term "couplon" was introduced to explicitly define the combination of an LCC cluster and an associated CRU, which together are capable of functionally interacting to contribute to EC coupling.[7] For this reason the couplon is, by definition, the elementary site of EC

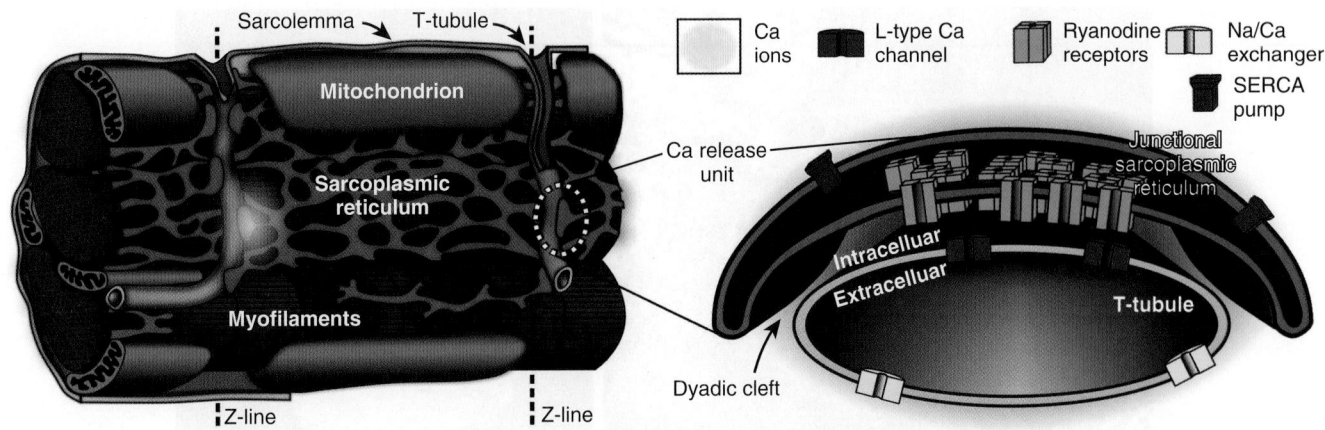

FIGURE 33.1 Overview of structures involved in cardiac Ca²⁺ handling and excitation–contraction coupling. T-tubules are invaginations of the sarcolemma that facilitate spatiotemporal synchronization of intracellular Ca²⁺ release by bringing L-type Ca²⁺ channels (LCCs) into close proximity with the majority of the cell's volume. Ca²⁺ release units (CRUs) juxtapose the T-tubules along their length, and the narrow space separating the junctional sarcoplasmic reticulum and T-tubules is named the dyadic cleft. LCCs reside in the sarcolemma, predominantly at dyadic clefts, and the surface of the release unit that faces the T-tubule (the dyadic surface) contains ryanodine receptors (RyRs). A ventricular myocyte typically has around 20,000 CRUs, and these are synchronously activated during an action potential (AP). Upon arrival of the AP, LCCs open and permit Ca²⁺ influx, which then triggers further Ca²⁺ release from the sarcoplasmic reticulum via binding to local RyRs. Ca²⁺ release from a single CRU is called a Ca²⁺ spark. After a spark, the sarco-endoplasmic reticulum Ca²⁺ ATPase (*SERCA*) pump and Na⁺/Ca²⁺ exchanger either resequester the released Ca²⁺ into the sarcoplasmic reticulum or extrude it from the cell, respectively. (*Left panel* is retouched from Fawcett DW, McNutt NS. The ultrastructure of the cat myocardium. I. Ventricular papillary muscle. *J Cell Biol.* 1969;42:1-45.)

coupling in the heart (see Fig. 33.1) and, along with the CRU, will be a feature of much further discussion in this chapter.

Role of Imaging in Defining Cardiac Ultrastructure and Subcellular Modeling

Much of our knowledge of cardiac ultrastructure has been permitted by steadily improving approaches to both EM and light microscopy (LM). In combination with tomographic reconstruction algorithms, high voltage EM (HVEM) has both enhanced resolution and improved penetration of thick section preparations, which has now permitted three-dimensional (3D) reconstruction of the T-tubule system and associated EC coupling structures.[15,16] Improvements in acquisition and analysis of LM images have also now permitted imaging at or below the optical diffraction limit. This progress has brought the living T-tubule,[6,17] and even the detailed morphology of individual RyR clusters,[18,19] into view. Together, these techniques have been central to defining the structural characteristics of VM microdomains, describing protein localization in and around those domains, and permitting the geometrically detailed quantitative approaches described here.

Structure–Function Relationships at the Nanometer Scale (Calcium Release Unit and Couplon)

Couplon and Calcium Release Unit Microarchitecture

The small space between the jSR and T-tubular membranes provides a confined volume (the "dyadic cleft," "junctional cleft," or "fuzzy space") in which large and rapid changes in local [Ca²⁺] can be generated by the local transporters, particularly LCCs and RyRs. This constrained architecture is fundamental to high-fidelity coupling between those transporters

and is maintained by the specialized anchoring protein, junctophilin, which tethers the jSR to the T-tubular membrane.[19–21] In healthy myocytes, junctophilin keeps the distance between the jSR and the T-tubule to within 12 to 15 nm and appears to be interspersed among the RyR molecules within the dyadic surface of the jSR membrane.[19]

The exact number of LCCs and RyRs inside the couplon is still debated. Early studies employed transmission EM to measure the cross-sectional diameter of individual CRU terminals, and to show that, in mammalian cardiac muscle, RyRs form dense clusters at these terminals.[22] Assuming that the CRU terminals are circular (i.e., that the size corresponds to the diameter) and densely packed with receptors, these authors were able to approximate the number of RyRs per couplon. This estimate suggested that 130–150 receptors are present in mouse ventricular couplons.[22] Given that the RyR tetramer is 30 nm at each side, a dyad containing 100 RyRs would have to be 440 nm in diameter and 1.8×10^{-12} μl in volume. Recent studies have challenged these initial estimates.[15,18,23] Using 3D EM tomography, Hayashi and colleagues[15] reported that the size of each dyad is almost an order of magnitude smaller than previously reported (mean of 0.44×10^{-12} μl), with a large fraction of tiny dyads (median 0.28×10^{-12} μl). They also showed that the density of RyRs within each CRU was sparse. By segmenting the T-tubule (*green*), the jSR (*yellow*), the dyadic space (*white*), and the RyR occupancy (*blue*), they observed spaces within the dyad that did not contain any RyRs (Fig. 33.2E). Interestingly, Hayashi and associates also found that 80% of all dyads have a neighboring dyad within 25 nm, which is dramatically closer than previously thought. Using super resolution LM, Baddeley and coworkers[18] found support for most of these surprising results. They similarly observed RyR clusters to be much smaller, more closely arranged, and irregularly shaped than had been reported or assumed in earlier work. It is not completely clear why Franzini-Armstrong and associates[22] retrieved such different estimates of couplon size compared with those of more recent studies, although it is at least clear that the early assumption of a circular dyadic geometry is

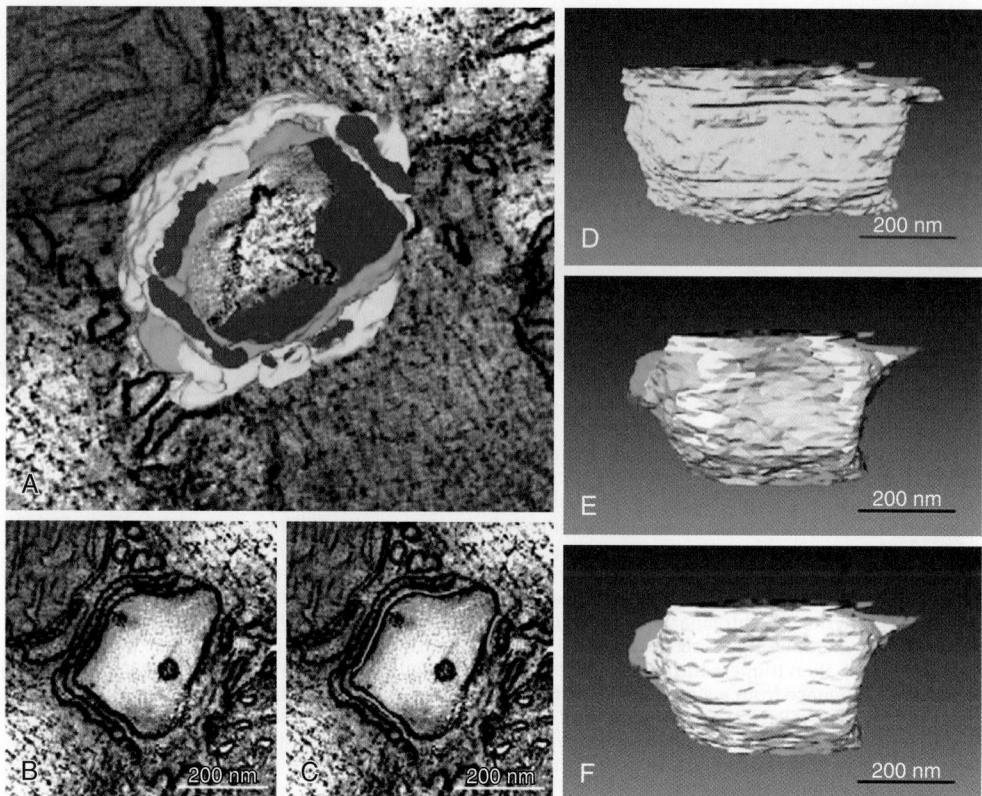

FIGURE 33.2 Fine anatomy of dyadic clefts in the mouse myocardium. (A) High-resolution mesh models of a T-tubule (*green*) and junctional sarcoplasmic reticulum (jSRs) (*yellow*) shown with a slice image, which were constructed by dual-axis electron microscopic tomography. (B and C) The ultra-thin serial slice images of this structure revealed inhomogeneous distribution of ryanodine receptor (RyR) feet in dyadic cleft spaces (B) and their RyR foot–rich subdomains were segmented (*light blue lines* in [C]). (D) through (F) The intraanatomy of three closely assembled dyadic clefts. From the complete mesh model (D), jSR membranes are removed to expose eight RyR foot–rich subdomains (the surface meshes of these subdomains are shown in *light blue* in [E]) that partially occupy dyadic cleft spaces (the whole dyadic cleft spaces are indicated as the junctional regions of T-tubule membranes, in *white*). Both jSR meshes and meshes that identify the RyR-rich subdomains are removed in (F). Scale bars: 200 nm. (From Hayashi T, Martone ME, Yu Z, et al. Three-dimensional electron microscopy reveals new details of membrane systems for Ca^{2+} signaling in the heart. *J Cell Sci.* 2009;122:1005-1013.)

oversimplified, which may contribute to this discrepancy. Based on agreement among recent structural studies, and even earlier functional work,[24] it is probably safe to conclude that the number of RyRs in *the average* CRU is on the order of tens rather than being greater than 100. Perhaps most importantly, it has come to be appreciated that anchoring our understanding of cardiac EC coupling on the notion of an average dyadic structure is probably profoundly oversimplified.

Localization of Ca^{2+}-Handling Proteins in Cardiac Microdomains

Immunofluorescence-based colocalization studies have definitively shown that the LCCs present in ventricular myocytes exhibit a punctate pattern of distribution and that ~90% of these puncta are coincident with RyR.[25,26] Thus the vast majority of LCCs are probably components of couplon structures. The number of LCCs within each couplon is less certain, as is the number of active LCCs required to trigger local Ca^{2+} release during physiological EC coupling. One range of estimates suggests that 17 to 53 LCCs are likely to be involved in couplon activation[27–29]; however, others have observed higher coupling fidelities, and therefore suggested that fewer LCCs are required to trigger local SR Ca^{2+} release.[30] Part of the uncertainty here is due to discrepancy in the estimates of

RyR cluster size, which are necessary to extrapolate the LCC number in some studies (e.g., see Polakova and colleagues[28]). Otherwise differences in the details of approach across studies, such as the potential ranges for LCC activation and partial pharmacological inhibition of the LCC pool, have made it difficult to determine truly physiologically representative constraints for EC coupling. Localization of the myocardial Na^+/Ca^{2+} exchanger (NCX) is also worth mentioning at this point, as its potential involvement in EC coupling is a long-debated topic that has recently been revisited.[31] While NCX does exhibit a punctate distribution in the T-tubules, precise colocalization of NCX with RyR occurs for only ~10% of the total NCX signal.[26,32] With this in mind, the latter authors also noted that ~40% of the NCX puncta reside within 150 nm of the nearest RyR cluster. Thus while NCX is probably not selectively concentrated within the dyadic portion of the T-tubular membrane, it is likely to be nearby.

The protein exhibiting the strongest colocalization with RyR is calsequestrin (CSQN), for which 95% of all labeling is coincident with RyR, and, further, only ~10% of RyR occur in the absence of CSQN. These observations are consistent with our understanding of CSQN function, which through its ability to rapidly buffer Ca^{2+}, acts both to limit the thermodynamic gradient that opposes SR Ca^{2+} reuptake and to provide a large local supply of Ca^{2+} for RyR-mediated Ca^{2+} release. Finally, localization of the sarco-endoplasmic

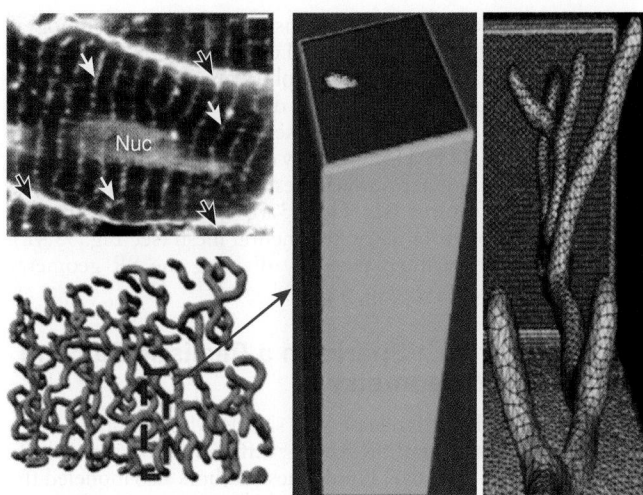

FIGURE 33.3 The rodent ventricular T-tubular network and single-tubule geometric model. *Upper left panel*: Cardiac sarcolemma including T-tubules is visualized by 2-photon microscopy: external membrane (*blue arrows*); T-tubules (*white arrows*); nucleus (*Nuc*); scale bar: 2 µm. *Lower left panel*: Geometric model of the T-tubule subsystem extracted from the 2-photon image. *Middle and right panels*: Expanded view of single T-tubule geometry and its surrounding half-sarcomeres. (Modified from Cheng Y, Yu Z, Hoshijima M, et al. Numerical analysis of Ca²⁺ signaling in rat ventricular myocytes with realistic transverse-axial tubular geometry and inhibited sarcoplasmic reticulum. *PLoS Comput Biol*. 2010;6:e1000972.)

reticulum Ca^{2+} ATPase (SERCA2) is less clear than that of either RyR or CSQN. It is generally agreed that both the major (SERCA2a) and the minor (SERCA2b) cardiac splice variants are present at the Z-disk and therefore in the vicinity of the jSR.[33–35] However, fluorescent labeling also appears to decorate the M-line SR,[33] and no investigation to date has definitively demonstrated that SERCA2 exists within the same functional domain as RyR and CSQN. As mentioned in Section 2.3, our quantitative approaches suggest that uncertainty in SERCA2 localization at this level may be functionally important, particularly with respect to Ca^{2+} spark dynamics.

Three-Dimensional Imaging and Generation of Model Geometries

The realistic model geometries described in this chapter are reconstructed from either LM or EM data, depending on the spatial scale being modeled. With important structural characteristics at ~10 to 20 nm, detailed geometries of the cardiac CRU are beyond the resolution of LM, whereas the T-system is amenable to LM imaging of dyes that associate with the sarcolemmal membrane, as are the geometries of certain intracellular structures, such as RyR clusters. For both EM and LM data, the gap between imaging and simulation involves two major steps: (1) extracting features (boundary or skeleton) from imaging data and (2) constructing geometric models (represented by meshes) from the detected features. Thus the simple requirement of this approach is that the imaging modality provides sufficient resolution and dimension to both (1) capture the volume of the desired microarchitectural feature and (2) permit sufficiently accurate segmentation of that feature. To this end, image preprocessing is usually necessary for better feature extraction, particularly when the original image is noisy or the contrast between features and background is low. With 3D two-photon microscopy (T-PM) images, Yu and collaborators developed a set of image processing and analysis tools, which, combined with the mesh generator, GAMer, have been used to generate high-quality meshes for 3D T-tubular systems in mice (Fig. 33.3, *lower left*),[16,36] and the murine cardiac CRU (Fig. 33.4[15]).

Subcellular Modeling at the Nanometer Scale

Few biological processes have required mathematical approaches to the extent that they have been required for understanding cardiac EC coupling. Iterative development of local control models has been instrumental in forming our concept of the cardiac dyad and RyR regulation, and this will remain the case while techniques for live Ca^{2+} imaging are fluorophore-based. In this way, interaction between biophysically formulated models and functional data gained from LM and patch-clamp electrophysiology have formed the basis for studying whole-cell EC coupling and single Ca^{2+} sparks for 20 years.[36,37] While these efforts have provided tremendous insight to fundamental processes in EC coupling, the vast majority have been conducted in idealized geometries based on structural averages. This section describes the key principles gleaned from these models and looks forward to how models built upon realistic dyadic geometries can be expected to extend these principles.

Reconstructing Ca²⁺ Sparks in Idealized Geometries

A set of four specific properties of macroscopic EC coupling and isolated RyR function have been used to drive and constrain the development of SR Ca^{2+} release models: (1) RyR activation should exhibit a steep and nonlinear dependence upon submembrane cytosolic [Ca^{2+}], (2) reliable termination of release should be achieved by experimentally defined RyR gating properties, (3) the total Ca^{2+} released from the SR should be about an order of magnitude larger than that entering through activated LCCs (i.e., EC-coupling gain should be high), and (4) the total Ca^{2+} released from the SR should be proportional to the macroscopic LCC current (i.e., SR Ca^{2+} release should be graded by I_{CaL}).

The multiscale aspects of modeling EC coupling became obvious quite early, as (3) and (4) are whole-cell measures, while EC coupling is controlled locally within each of the ~20,000 couplons in a myocyte. The first attempts to model EC coupling used the mean cytosolic [Ca^{2+}] as a trigger for RyR release. None of these early models, however, were able to reconcile (1)–(3) with (4).[13] The remedy was to let local [Ca^{2+}] within each CRU control the gating of the local RyRs,[13,38,39] and thus "local control" models were born. These models kept a steep all-or-none control of RyR release within each couplon, and graded release was accomplished by a probabilistic recruitment of the CRUs in proportion with I_{CaL}.

While modelers made quick progress with these approaches, a number of experimental uncertainties posed repeated challenges. The inability to directly measure local SR Ca^{2+} release current for a single CRU (due to the inability to patch-clamp intracellular structures) has forced modelers to (1) estimate these quantities from indirect measures, such as Ca^{2+} spark fluorescence,[40] or (2) reconstruct the release current from lipid bilayer recordings of RyRs extracted from their native environment.[41] Complicating the latter approach, isolated RyRs often exhibit marked variability[42] and surprisingly large species differences for reconstituted proteins.[43,44] Together, these factors have often discouraged modelers from rigorously constraining Ca^{2+} release models to bilayer RyR recordings.[45,46] Indeed, most existing integrative models abandon this level of constraint in favor of functionalistic approaches.[47] As a result, understanding of how models based on bilayer experiments should be incorporated into integrative models is still incomplete, and whether these models are capable of fulfilling all four EC coupling properties above is unknown.

Functionally, these uncertainties have manifested as challenges in replicating certain measurable spark characteristics. In particular, faithful spark termination (property (2) above) has been surprisingly difficult to achieve while satisfying constraints based on data for reconstituted RyR and fluorescence-based Ca^{2+}

measures. One major unresolved issue is the unknown strong means of RyR inactivation or deactivation that is required to terminate sparks before the jSR is almost completely depleted of Ca^{2+}. Functionalistic and integrated whole-cell models have generally implemented RyR inactivation due to cytosolic $[Ca^{2+}]$, which is a convenient means of enforcing RyR closure but only occurs at supraphysiological (mM) $[Ca^{2+}]$.[47] Similarly, luminal SR $[Ca^{2+}]$ has long been known to activate RyR at physiological concentrations,[48,49] but simulations indicate that this mechanism needs to be much stronger than observed in experiments to terminate sparks at significant residual jSR $[Ca^{2+}]$ content.[50] Recent models have argued that the more important role of luminal Ca^{2+} is to support flow-through cytosolic activation of RyR, where depleted luminal SR is less able to maintain a critical dyadic $[Ca^{2+}]$ for regenerative RyR opening;[50] different authors have variously termed this process "inductance decay"[43,44] or "pernicious attrition."[51]

While the use of idealized geometries has permitted these focused studies of RyR gating, all have necessarily made assumptions about the geometries themselves, flux distributions within those geometries, and their relationships to optical recording volumes and conditions. Many of these assumptions are likely to impact comparisons between models and comparisons with fluorescence-based measures of CRU function. For example, two possible explanations for the discrepancy between near complete SR depletion during simulated sparks and less severe depletion observed experimentally as Ca^{2+} "blinks" are that (1) the experimental recording volume may cause averaging over both active and inactive jSR terminals and (2) the dynamics of the low-affinity fluorophore (Fluo5) used to measure SR $[Ca^{2+}]$ combines with intra-SR Ca^{2+} diffusion rates to prevent the fluorescent signal from reflecting true depletion. To constrain these aspects as much as possible and to move toward fully realistic simulation frameworks, researchers have begun designing models on the

basis of subcellular geometries reconstructed from EM tomography. Specific to the CRU, Hake and colleagues combined recent developments in 3D EM tomography with new techniques in computational mesh generation to develop a 3D model of the Ca^{2+} spark.[52] The CRU geometry (see Fig. 33.4A) was manually segmented from 3D EM tomography data for a mouse ventricular myocyte.[15] An annotated surface mesh was then generated from the segmented features (see Fig. 33.4B–E) and was eventually transformed into a volumetric tetrahedral mesh (see Fig. 33.4F). The SR was compartmentalized by dividing the SR geometry into individual parts (see Fig. 33.4G).

Modeling of Ca^{2+} Sparks in a Realistic Calcium Release Unit Geometry

In Hake's model, Ca^{2+} release was simulated by coupling Ca^{2+} diffusion within the local SR to Ca^{2+} diffusion in the cytosol. By including the SR Ca^{2+} dye, Fluo5, these authors also modeled the impact of dye dynamics on experimental measurements of luminal $[Ca^{2+}]$. Specific RyR dynamics were not used to define release termination in this model. Instead release was terminated such that the modeled Fluo5 signal decayed to a level corresponding with experimentally measured values.[53] In this way, Hake and associates applied a functionalistic termination criterion to directly relate experimentally measured Fluo5 fluorescence with jSR $[Ca^{2+}]$ at the end of a spark. Importantly, these dynamics included local competition between Fluo5 and CSQN, and a maximal RyR release flux that was within the range of the best available experimental estimates. Interestingly, these analyses suggest that the jSR $[Ca^{2+}]$ at spark termination is indeed low (~10% of resting value, Fig. 33.5C), even though Fluo5 fluorescence decays to only 60% of the resting value.[52] The available Ca^{2+} reserve within the neighboring SR compartments (44%) was also comparable with experimentally measured values.[54]

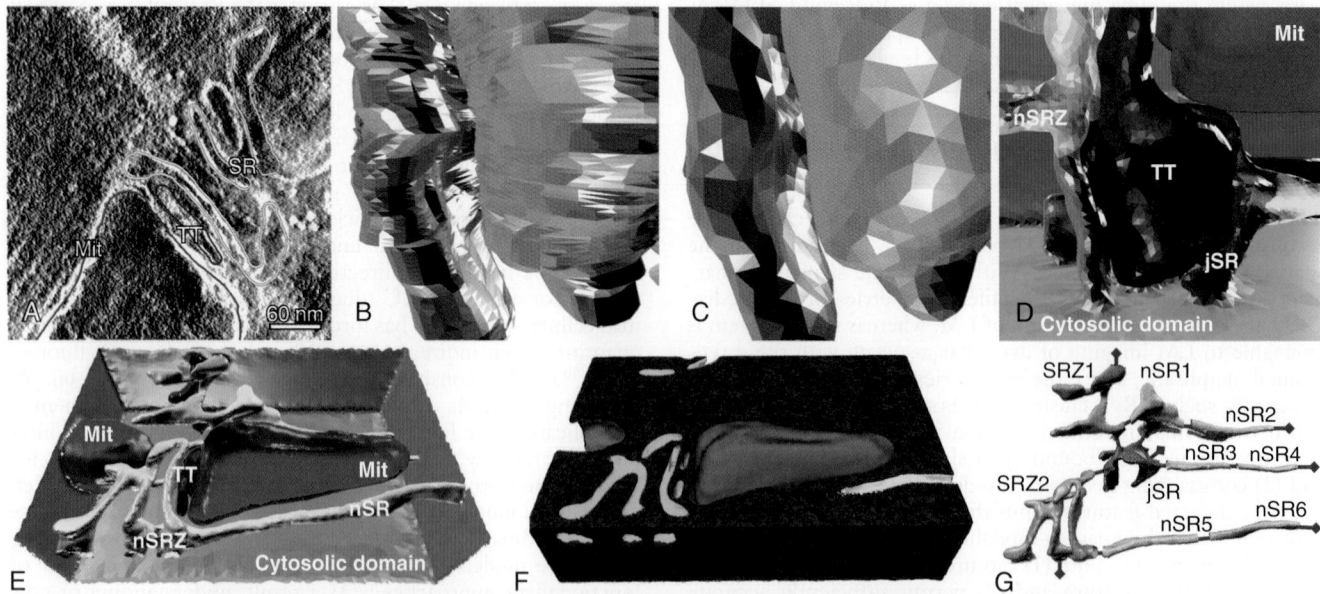

FIGURE 33.4 Generation of reconstructed geometries is a multistage process. (A) Features are first segmented from electron tomography data. (B) From the segmented data, an initial low-quality surface mesh is generated. (C) The quality of the surface mesh is improved. (D) The surface mesh is annotated, for easy application of boundary fluxes. The *blue* is the T-tubule (*TT*), the *red, orange,* and *yellow* is the sarcoplasmic reticulum and the *purple* is a mitochondrion (*Mit*). (E) The full, annotated surface mesh. The dimensions of the mesh are 1430 × 940 × 406 nm. (F) The surface mesh is converted to an annotated volumetric mesh using TetGen. (G) The geometry included a full representation of the local sarcoplasmic reticulum. *jSR,* Junctional sarcoplasmic reticulum; *nSR,* network sarcoplasmic reticulum. ([A], [D], [E], and [G] from Hake J, Edwards AG, Yu Z, et al. Modeling cardiac calcium sparks in a three-dimensional reconstruction of a calcium release unit. *J Physiol.* 2012;590:4403-4422.)

Another advantage of the realistic geometry used in this model is that it inherently provides the correct surface area to volume relationship for the local structures, which is crucial to finding correct quantitative relationships between the local surface fluxes represented in the model by the RyRs, SERCA, and NCX. SERCA localized close to the CRU will experience a much larger cytosolic $[Ca^{2+}]$ during the spark than peripherally located pumps, as illustrated by the cytosolic $[Ca^{2+}]$ gradients

shown in Fig. 33.5B. Interestingly, Hake and colleagues identified a new potential role for the SERCA pump during the Ca^{2+} spark. By pumping Ca^{2+} back into the SR during the spark, local SERCA activity was able to slow down depletion of luminal Ca^{2+} and hence increase spark duration. This phenomenon was possible because, at the late phase of a Ca^{2+} spark when luminal Ca^{2+} in the jSR is low and cytosolic Ca^{2+} close to the CRU is high, the SERCA pump operates under thermodynamically optimal

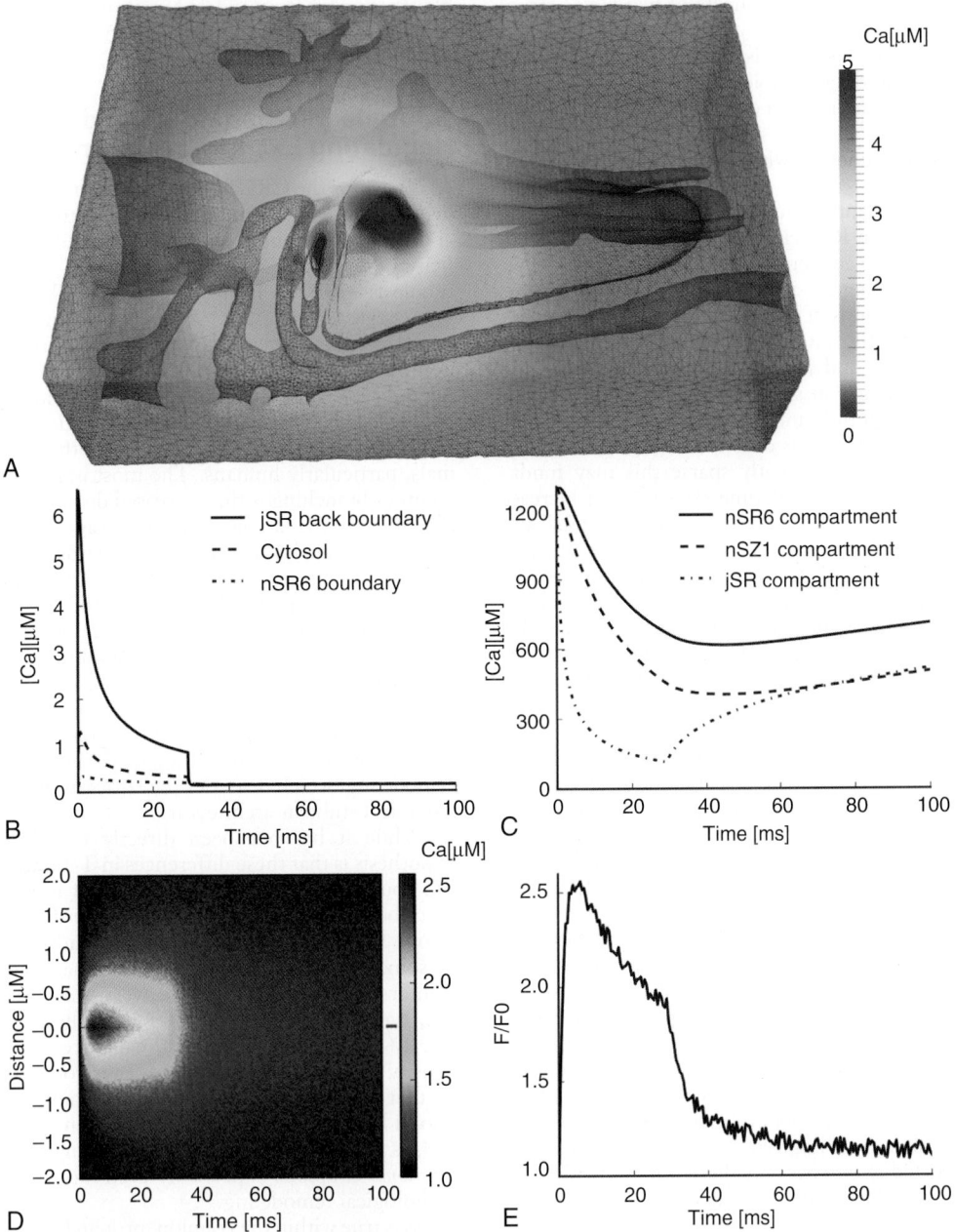

FIGURE 33.5 Large Ca²⁺ gradients within a single calcium release unit (CRU). (A) A volumetric representation of the $[Ca^{2+}]$ in the cytosolic domain after 5 ms. (B) The average $[Ca^{2+}]$ at three different positions in the CRU: backside boundary of junctional sarcoplasmic reticulum (*jSR*) (*continuous line*), the whole cytosolic domain (*dashed line*), and at the boundary of the sixth network sarcoplasmic reticulum compartment (*dash-dotted line*). (C) The free Ca^{2+} content in three SR domains during a spark: the sixth nSR compartment (*continuous line*), the first Z-line SR compartment (*dashed line*), and the jSR compartment (*dash-dotted line*). (D) A generated line-scan image from the Cytosolic Fluo4 signal with added noise. The full-width half-maximum is 1.0 μm, and the full-duration half-maximum is 28.5 ms. (E) A Fluo4 trace from the *red marker* at the right of the line-scan image. (From Hake J, Edwards AG, Yu Z, et al. Modeling cardiac calcium sparks in a three-dimensional reconstruction of a calcium release unit. *J Physiol.* 2012;590:4403-4422.)

conditions. This modulatory role needs to be investigated further, but it is a clear prediction of the model, which was made possible by the correct surface area:volume relationship for the local SR components.

Future Work

As mentioned above, models employing realistic geometries may help to constrain certain aspects of RyR gating and average CRU function, but the most important questions for CRU physiology are in understanding the effects of two major structural characteristics:

1. Irregular or heterogeneous RyR distributions, with particular emphasis on understanding the role of RyR cluster geometry and spacing in CRU function and definition,
2. The effects of normal and disease-induced changes to protein localization and function within and around the dyadic microdomain.

Super resolution LM approaches are already being used to define the heterogeneity in RyR cluster geometry that has heretofore been inaccessible via conventional confocal LM. However, relatively few data describing the associated membrane structures are available under conditions of disease-induced CRU remodeling. Both rat models of HF[55] and human failing tissue samples[56] exhibit reduced T-tubule and jSR areas and volume densities. The effects of these changes in size would be expected to have little impact on spark amplitude and duration so long as the ratio of RyR number and jSR volume is constant.[57] However, if RyR density in CRUs becomes sufficiently sparse this may fundamentally alter the spark and CICR time course[58] and increase the propensity for subspark release events, such as "quarks" and "sparklets." At this time, no study has assessed these characteristics in detailed reconstructed geometries from healthy or diseased tissue. One hypothetical characteristic of HF that has been quantitatively interrogated is the effect of increased dyadic width (T-tubule to jSR release surface) on CICR coupling. This alteration has not been observed but is expected to accompany the loss or redistribution of the tethering protein junctophilin.[59] While there appears to be little effect of dyadic volume on the amplitude or kinetics of the spark, it does appear to potently modulate the ability of a trigger flux to initiate a spark, and therefore the fidelity (single couplon), gain (whole cell), and synchrony of EC coupling.[60] This again would be expected to promote subspark release events and contribute to the "silent" or "invisible" SR Ca^{2+} leak that conspires with altered expression of SERCA and NCX to reduce SR Ca^{2+} load in HF.

As described above, similar super resolution approaches have already been used to good effect for defining gross spatial colocalization of sarcolemmal proteins (particularly LCC and NCX). Combining super resolution LM with EM through correlative LM/EM will be critical to creating and constraining these models within realistic membrane geometries, and this effort has already begun for dyadic structures.[61] To date, only several studies have looked at the effect of altered phosphorylation of RyR, LCC, and SERCA/phospholamban in failing cells[62–64]; however, meaningful use of reconstructed geometries for these questions will first require new experimental data and better constraints.

Structure–Function Relationships at the Micron Scale (T-Tubule and T-System)

The problem of extending local control to whole cell Ca^{2+} signaling is an inherently multiscale problem and has been addressed by a number of approaches of varying complexity.[65] Virtually all of these efforts have employed idealized and repetitive geometries. In part this is due to the technical constraints in imaging large enough volumes at the necessary resolution, but even given sufficiently large reconstructed geometries, major computational challenges also exist for solving detailed electrodiffusive models in 3D and at sufficient spatial resolution. The two related structure–function relationships that most require detailed geometric modeling at this spatial scale are (1) the impact of heterogeneous CRU structure on the ensemble behaviors that underlie triggered and spontaneous SR Ca^{2+} release and (2) the roles that T-tubule and T-system structure and the corresponding molecular localization play in modulating these ensemble effects and whole-cell ionic homeostasis. Because both the T-system and CRU ensemble structures are remodeled in chronic cardiac disease, this type of model may provide key insight to fundamental mechanisms of pathological dysfunction.

T-Tubule Microanatomy and Its Role in Regulating Excitation–Contraction Coupling

As is true for the CRU, advancements in imaging modalities have driven progress in defining the architecture of cardiac T-tubules, and these studies have consistently found a strong-species specificity of T-tubular structure. In the rat, the average ventricular tubule is ~250 nm in diameter and exhibits longitudinal (axial) branches every 6.87 μm.[6] Rabbit and human myocytes generally have larger T-tubular diameters (~450 nm) and exhibit less pronounced branching.[1,17,66,67] This frequency of T-tubular branching indicates a key aspect of species differences in the relationship between T-tubular structure and function: the T-tubular rete of rodents is generally more intricate than that of larger mammals, particularly humans. The most important outcome of this complex branching is the decreased distance from any part of the cytoplasm to the sarcolemmal membrane in the rodent cell. Two-dimensional analyses of transverse sections indicate that ~64% of the cytoplasm resides within 250 nm of a T-tubular membrane in the human compared with ~94% in the rat.[1] It is generally held that this intricate lattice-like structure facilitates more synchronous Ca^{2+} release in the rodent, and thereby reduces intracellular heterogeneity of ECC, which may be necessary to support efficient contraction at the very high heart rates of these animals. As described at the end of this chapter, this principle probably also applies in the converse under circumstances of pathological remodeling, which degrades the lattice architecture and results in a sparse T-tubular architecture.

While it has not been directly tested, a commonly held hypothesis is that these differences in T-tubular density influence EC coupling by altering the density of functional couplons. As described above, CRU nearest-neighbor distances (from the edge of one CRU to the edge of its closest adjacent CRU) appear to be somewhere on the order of tens of nanometers in the rat.[15,18] Center to center distances between CRU are larger on average, typically 300 to 800 nm.[18,22,25] These distances are ~15% to 50% greater in the human, which results in an RyR cluster density (per unit cell volume) that is roughly halved compared to that in the rat.[68] Remodeling accompanying heart failure, also in humans, reduces RyR cluster density by a further 20%,[67] and, as is described below, recent data suggest that the density of *functional* couplons is probably even more severely degraded by pathological remodeling.

As is true within the couplon, protein localization is a key component of T-tubular structure–function relationships, and a number of sarcolemmal transporters are selectively enriched within the T-tubules. Functionalistic approaches involving experimental detubulation or rapid changes in permeant ion concentration indicate that currents carried by the LCC,[69,70] the NCX,[71] and the Na^+-K^+ ATPase[71,72] exhibit a dominant T-tubular distribution. The fold-enrichment ($I_{CaL}:I_{NaCa}:I_{NaK}$) of each of these currents, *with respect to the surface sarcolemm*a and after accounting for differences in corresponding membrane areas, is approximately 6:3:3.[69] Interestingly, the neuronal Na^+ current (I_{NaN}), which has recently been proposed to be a driver of reverse mode I_{NaCa},[31] exhibits strong T-tubular localization (~ninefold), as does the steady-state K^+ current (I_{SS}).[66] Other K^+ currents appear to be homogeneously distributed. Many of these current carriers are sensitive to local ionic concentrations, particularly Na^+ and Ca^{2+}, which is just one reason that spatially realistic quantitative models will be fundamental to developing a complete understanding of the function of these current carriers.

Subcellular Modeling in Idealized Geometries at the Micron Scale

Whole-cell computational models have proven to be powerful tools for predicting and analyzing interactions among sarcolemmal ion fluxes, the action potential (AP), and intracellular Ca^{2+}-handling under normal and pathological conditions. Excellent reviews from Noble and associates offer a complete view of successes and failures in modeling pursuits of this type.[73,74] Using whole-cell modeling approaches, Orchard and collaborators also investigated how changes in T-system volume and distribution of ion fluxes between the surface and the T-tubular membrane affect whole-cell electrophysiology.[75,76] However, as was the case for modeling of the couplon, an important limitation of these whole-cell models is that they treat subcellular spaces as lumped compartments and are thus unable to dissect the impact of structural changes in the T-system and other organelles. To overcome this limitation, recent modeling approaches have introduced simplified representations of T-system geometry to enable introduction of spatial control of Ca^{2+} handling. In rodents, Lu and coworkers[77] and Yao and Yu[78] assumed a cylindrical T-tubule geometry. These studies suggested that the Ca^{2+} transient is tightly regulated by the localization of sarcolemmal Ca^{2+} transporters and is strongly reliant upon the presence of Ca^{2+} buffers, when SR Ca^{2+} fluxes are pharmacologically inhibited. Hatano and collaborators[79,80] extended the approach of Lu and associates by developing a detailed 3D geometric model of a guinea pig cardiomyocyte in which the subcellular structures (T-tubules, myofibrils, SR, and mitochondria) were modeled using simplified geometries. Their analyses of sarcomere dynamics revealed that the dyssynchronous contraction caused by detubulation led to impairment of contractile efficiency.

The use of idealistic shapes, however, may alter the diffusion distances in the longitudinal and axial directions and, consequently, the predicted Ca^{2+} dynamics. Using published images of T-system ultrastructure from rodents and rabbits, recent investigations have examined Ca^{2+} dynamics in 3D reconstructions of single and multitubule geometric domains.[81–83] Before discussing work that has made use of this relatively new paradigm in subcellular modeling, it is best to briefly describe the process by which these geometries are generated.

Modeling the Effects of Normal T-Tubule Ultrastructure on Subcellular Ca^{2+} Signals

Cheng and collaborators[81] used the Yu and colleagues[16] geometry to investigate the role of individual T-tubular architecture and Ca^{2+} buffer activity in determining the characteristics of Ca^{2+} signaling in rat ventricular myocytes. A small compartment containing a single T-tubule and its surrounding half-sarcomeres were considered because the entire T-tubular system in ventricular myocytes is roughly periodic.[15,84] The surrounding half-sarcomeres were modeled as a rectangular box of 2 μm × 2 μm in the plane of the external sarcolemma and 5.96 μm in depth (see Fig. 33.3, *middle*). As Yu's T-tubule model did not include a realistic cell surface, one of the box faces (*top red surfaces* in Fig. 33.3) was assumed to be the external sarcolemma. The T-tubule inside this compartment was extracted from the T-PM data corresponding to the region indicated in Fig. 33.3 (*lower left*). The T-tubule

diameter varied from 0.19 μm to 0.469 μm and the T-tubule depth was 5.645 μm. The volume of the model compartment was ~23.31 μm³. The compartment membrane area was ~9.00 μm² where the percentage of cell membrane within the T-tubule was 64% (~5.75 μm²) and that within the external membrane was 36% (~3.25 μm²). Four exogenous and endogenous Ca^{2+} buffers (Fluo-3, ATP, calmodulin, and troponin C) were modeled within the cytosolic domain (Fig. 33.6, *left panel*). When 100-μM Fluo-3 was included, along with ~1.7-fold enrichment of the LCC and threefold enrichment of NCX in the T-tubular membrane, the model-predicted [Ca^{2+}] dynamics closely resembled experimental data collected in rat VMs with blocked SR Ca^{2+} fluxes[85] (see Fig. 33.6, *right panels*). Counterintuitively, when LCC density was heterogeneously distributed within the T-tubule model, the spatial heterogeneity of cytosolic [Ca^{2+}] was reduced relative to a homogeneous sarcolemmal LCC distribution. Strongly nonuniform spatial Ca^{2+} gradients, not observed during experiments, were found when the LCC and NCX fluxes were uniformly distributed along the sarcolemma. This unexpected result may be due to the high curvature of the membrane near the mouth of the T-tubule, which increases the LCC flux per unit cytosolic volume in that region. When the LCC distribution is homogeneous this effect is exaggerated at these points of high curvature. A second important finding of this study, which may also contribute to the effects regarding LCC distribution, is that including the mobile Ca^{2+} buffering effect of 100-μM Fluo-3 was able to mask spatial nonuniformities in cytosolic [Ca^{2+}] that occurred in the absence of dye, even when Ca^{2+} transporters were heterogeneously distributed (see Fig. 33.6). Thus during physiological Ca^{2+} influx (i.e., no Fluo-3), large and steep Ca^{2+} gradients might be expected in the narrow subsarcolemmal space (~40–50 nm in depth). Interestingly, in rabbit cells, Kekenes-Huskey and associates revealed qualitatively similar results to Cheng and colleagues. When SR Ca^{2+} fluxes were blocked, local [Ca^{2+}] gradients within the cytosol and subsarcolemmal regions were highly sensitive to details of T-tubule ultrastructure and membrane Ca^{2+} flux distribution.[82] For this reason, it seems likely that several of the key effects of single T-tubule microarchitecture on local Ca^{2+} dynamics are conserved across species.

These two models are the first to have combined sophisticated computational methods and detailed structural information to understand the role of T-tubular microarchitecture in defining cardiac Ca^{2+} microdomains. Important limitations of these studies are (1) the relatively small size of the modeled compartments, which contained only a single realistic T-tubule, and (2), as described above, significant branching of the rat T-tubular lattice suggests that our assumption that the modeled compartment is a repeating unit inside the cell is, to some extent, unrealistic.

In attempting to reach beyond these limitations, Yu and associates recently extended the approach of Cheng and coworkers by reconstructing a 3D geometry of several T-tubules in the mouse.[83] Briefly, this study affirmed that local Ca^{2+} dynamics are sharply impacted by T-system ultra-structure and Ca^{2+} fluxes at the surface membrane. Finally, Soeller and associates constructed a model of stochastic Ca^{2+} dynamics in rat myocytes using measured 3D distributions of RyR clusters, which are adjacent to the T-system.[86] These authors found that the spatial irregularities of RyR cluster distribution may significantly impact Ca^{2+} dynamics, although the role of T-tubular microanatomy was not directly assessed in that study.

Modeling Calcium Release Unit Ensemble Behavior in Realistic Geometries

Only one study to date has attempted to assess CRU ensemble behavior based on reconstruction of a half-sarcomere myocyte geometry.[87] These authors created a hybrid model in which RyR cluster distributions and their spatial relationships to myofibrillar

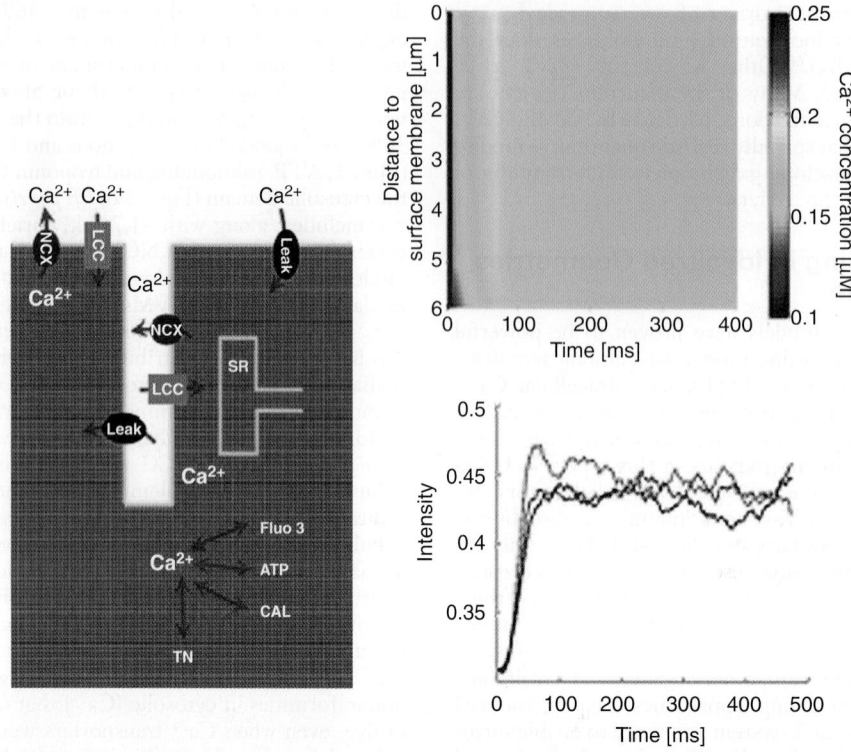

FIGURE 33.6 *Left panel*: Diagram illustrating Ca²⁺ entry and extrusion via the sarcolemma, and Ca²⁺ buffering and diffusion inside the cytosol with sarcoplasmic reticulum (*SR*) Ca²⁺ fluxes pharmacologically blocked: L-type Ca²⁺ channel (*LCC*); Na⁺/Ca²⁺ exchanger (*NCX*); membrane Ca²⁺ leak (*Leak*); troponin C (*TN*), adenosine triphosphate (*ATP*); calmodulin (*CAL*); Ca²⁺ fluorophore (*Fluo-3*). *Upper right panel*: Calcium concentrations visualized as line-scan images in the transverse cell direction. LCC current density is heterogeneously distributed along the length of the T-tubule. Na⁺/Ca²⁺ flux density was three times higher in the T-tubule, and the Ca²⁺ leak current was homogeneously distributed. Line-scan was positioned 200 nm from the T-tubule membrane at an angle of 120 degrees. *Lower right panel*: Local Ca²⁺ time-courses with replot from experimental data.[85] The replots are taken along the scan line at 0 μm (*blue*), 3.96 μm (*green*), and 5.65 μm (*red*) from the near-surface location. The scan line in the Cheng and colleagues experiments was located 200 nm from the surface of the T-tubule. (Modified from Cheng Y, Yu Z, Hoshijima M, et al. Numerical analysis of Ca²⁺ signaling in rat ventricular myocytes with realistic transverse-axial tubular geometry and inhibited sarcoplasmic reticulum. *PLoS Comput Biol*. 2010;6:e1000972.)

proteins were described statistically. These statistical descriptions were then mapped onto an EM tomogram of a myocyte cross-section (240 nm thick), which was segmented to separate the mitochondrial and myofibrillar volumes included within the sarcolemmal boundary. To extend the geometry beyond the 240 nm section thickness that could be imaged at required resolution, the authors assumed that most RyR clusters are localized at the Z-disk and that myofibrillar geometry is relatively constant over the length of a sarcomere, thus allowing them to extend the geometry symmetrically to the depth of a full half-sarcomere (0.9 μm). This yielded a final geometry of a 94.8 μm² myocyte cross section with a 0.9 μm longitudinal depth, containing 123 RyR Ca²⁺ release sites. Some structural details present in the images were not segmented for inclusion in the model, for example T-tubules and SR structures, because the authors constrained their investigation to the impact of RyR cluster localization on Ca²⁺ dynamics during the very early phase of Ca²⁺ release. These simulations helped to define the relative number of clusters that are required to remain silent in order to be observed as a point of delayed Ca²⁺ release in confocal linescans, a measure that is used to infer changes to the synchrony of Ca²⁺ release during disease. Another potentially important finding of the model was the suggestion that mitochondria, which were presumed not to act as Ca²⁺ sinks, provide a meaningful structural barrier to Ca²⁺ diffusion, and thereby contribute to subcellular Ca²⁺ heterogeneity.

While these and other findings will be subject to further scrutiny in coming years, this model serves as a first step toward simulating ensemble effects in cardiomyocyte ECC with realistic geometries and protein distributions.

Toward a Quantitative Understanding of Pathological T-tubule Remodeling

Over the last 5 to 15 years, remodeling of the T-tubular lattice has emerged as a consistent characteristic of a number of cardiac pathologies[88] across a range of species, including humans.[67,89] The characteristics and pathology-specificity of these processes are not yet firmly established. However, various investigations have observed a reduction in the number or density of T-tubules,[89] expansion of T-tubular diameter,[67] and/or an increase in the prevalence of axial/longitudinal tubule elements.[90] A consistent functional outcome associated with these remodeling processes is reduced synchrony of CICR,[88,91] which is generally thought to contribute to contractile dysfunction.

The precise mechanisms by which remodeling leads to CICR dyssynchrony is not completely clear, although decoupling of RyR clusters appears to be the dominant endpoint.[92,93] This decoupling may occur through orphaning of entire T-tubules from the surface membrane, such that they can no longer conduct the AP to their associated CRUs, or through local changes in couplon geometry that orphan individual receptor clusters. As mentioned above, it is also possible that reduced overall CRU density causes heterogeneity in Ca^{2+} release accompanying T-tubule loss.[67] The approach presented by Heinzel and colleagues[91] offers some promise for describing these structure–function relationships experimentally. These authors measured regional CICR kinetics and T-tubular density in the same patch-clamped myocytes. While they did not quantitatively correlate delayed CICR to distance from the local T-tubule, they were able to characterize spark kinetics at sites that were designated as decoupled based on the latency of their activation.

To date, no modeling study has attempted to explicitly simulate the effects of T-tubular remodeling with realistic geometries. As mentioned above, some efforts have taken idealized approaches to understanding how increases in junctional cleft width promote heterogeneity in CICR latency[94] or EC coupling gain,[21] but more complex structural changes have not been investigated. These questions remain an obvious target of the approaches described in this chapter.

Continued advancement in ultrastructural imaging will be critical to pursuing these goals, particularly for defining intracellular membrane structures at high resolution in larger dimensions

than is currently possible and in associating those structures with correct localization of ECC proteins. To this end, the ability of destructive techniques, such as focused ion beam (FIB) and block-phase milling of tissue samples for SEM, have the potential to markedly extend the imaging volumes used to construct the simulation geometries and is a very exciting advancement. Correlative LM/EM is also likely to provide important information at specific ultrastructures and cardiac microdomains. As these imaging techniques improve, procedures for efficiently and accurately solving computationally intensive simulations will need to keep pace with the available geometries and molecular localization data, which will be aided in part by continued increases in available computational power; however, pipelines and open source tools for generating meshes and solving multiphysics problems will require continuous and evolutionary refinement.

Acknowledgment

The authors dedicate this chapter to the memory of Dr. Anushka Michailova who was a pioneer in the field of computational modeling of cardiac myocyte calcium signaling for three decades and a cherished colleague.

REFERENCES

1. Jayasinghe I, Crossman Dj, Soeller C, Cannell M. Comparison of the organization of T-tubules, sarcoplasmic reticulum and ryanodine receptors in rat and human ventricular myocardium. *Clin Exp Pharmacol Physiol.* 2012;39:469–476.

2. Sommer JR, Waugh RA. The ultrastructure of the mammalian cardiac muscle cell—with special emphasis on the tubular membrane systems. A review. *Am J Pathol.* 1976;82:192–232.

3. Forbes MS, Hawkey LA, Sperelakis N. The transverse-axial tubular system (TATS) of mouse myocardium: its morphology in the developing and adult animal. *Am J Anat.* 1984;170:143–162.

4. Bers D. *Excitation Contraction Coupling and Cardiac Contractile Force.* Dortrecht/Boston/London: Kluwer Academic Publishers; 2001.

5. Fawcett DW, McNutt NS. The ultrastructure of the cat myocardium. I. Ventricular papillary muscle. *J Cell Biol.* 1969;42:1–45.

6. Soeller C, Cannell MB. Examination of the transverse tubular system in living cardiac rat myocytes by 2-photon microscopy and digital image-processing techniques. *Circ Res.* 1999;84:266–275.

7. Stern MD, Pizarro G, Rios E. Local control model of excitation-contraction coupling in skeletal muscle. *J Gen Physiol.* 1997;110:415–440.

8. Constantin LL, Franzini-Armstrong C, Podolsky RJ. Localization of calcium-accumulating structures in striated muscle fibers. *Science.* 1965;147:158–160.

9. Winegrad S. Autoradiographic studies of intracellular calcium in frog skeletal muscle. *J Gen Physiol.* 1965;48:455–479.

10. Porter KR, Palade GE. Studies on the endoplasmic reticulum. III. Its form and distribution in striated muscle cells. *J Biophys Biochem Cytol.* 1957;3:269–300.

11. Endo M, Tanaka M, Ogawa Y. Calcium induced release of calcium from the sarcoplasmic reticulum of skinned skeletal muscle fibres. *Nature.* 1970;228:34–36.

12. Fabiato A, Fabiato F. Contractions induced by a calcium-triggered release of calcium from the sarcoplasmic reticulum of single skinned cardiac cells. *J Physiol.* 1975;249:469–495.

13. Stern MD. Theory of excitation-contraction coupling in cardiac muscle. *Biophys J.* 1992;63:497–517.

14. Isenberg G, Han S. Gradation of Ca(2+)-induced Ca^{2+} release by voltage-clamp pulse duration in potentiated guinea-pig ventricular myocytes. *J Physiol.* 1994;480(Pt 3):423–438.

15. Hayashi T, Martone ME, Yu Z, et al. Three-dimensional electron microscopy reveals new details of membrane systems for Ca^{2+} signaling in the heart. *J Cell Sci.* 2009;122(Pt 7):1005–1013.

16. Yu Z, Holst MJ, Hayashi T, et al. Three-dimensional geometric modeling of membrane-bound organelles in ventricular myocytes: bridging the gap between microscopic imaging and mathematical simulation. *J Struct Biol.* 2008;164:304–313.

17. Savio-Galimberti E, Frank J, Inoue M, et al. Novel features of the rabbit transverse tubular system revealed by quantitative analysis of three-dimensional reconstructions from confocal images. *Biophys J.* 2008;95:2053–2062.

18. Baddeley D, Jayasinghe ID, Lam L, Rossberger S, Cannell MB, Soeller C. Optical single-channel resolution imaging of the ryanodine receptor distribution in rat cardiac myocytes. *Proc Natl Acad Sci U S A.* 2009;106:22275–22280.

19. Jayasinghe ID, Baddeley D, Kong CH, Wehrens XH, Cannell MB, Soeller C, et al. Nanoscale organization of junctophilin-2 and ryanodine receptors within peripheral couplings of rat ventricular cardiomyocytes. *Biophys J.* 2012;102:L19–L21.

20. Takeshima H, Komazaki S, Nishi M, Iino M, Kangawa K. Junctophilins: a novel family of junctional membrane complex proteins. *Mol Cell.* 2000;6:11–22.

21. van Oort RJ, Garbino A, Wang W, et al. Disrupted junctional membrane complexes and hyperactive ryanodine receptors after acute junctophilin knockdown in mice. *Circulation.* 2011;123:979–988.

22. Franzini-Armstrong C, Protasi F. Ramesh V. Shape, size, and distribution of Ca^{2+} release units and couplons in skeletal and cardiac muscles. *Biophys J.* 1999;77:1528–1539.

23. Asghari P, Scriven DR, Hoskins J, Fameli N, van Breemen C, Moore ED. The structure and functioning of the couplon in the mammalian cardiomyocyte. *Protoplasma.* 2012;249(suppl 1):S31–S38.

24. Bridge JH, Ershler PR, Cannell MB. Properties of Ca^{2+} sparks evoked by action potentials in mouse ventricular myocytes. *J Physiol.* 1999;518:469–478.

25. Scriven DR, Asghari P, Schulson MN, Moore ED. Analysis of Cav1.2 and ryanodine receptor clusters in rat ventricular myocytes. *Biophys J.* 2010;99:3923–3929.

26. Scriven DR, Dan P, Moore ED. Distribution of proteins implicated in excitation-contraction coupling in rat ventricular myocytes. *Biophys J.* 2000;79:2682–2691.

27. Louch WE, Hake J, Jolle GF, et al. Control of Ca^{2+} release by action potential configuration in normal and failing murine cardiomyocytes. *Biophys J.* 2010;99:1377–1386.

28. Polakova E, Zahradníková Jr A, Pavelková J, Zahradník I, Zahradníková A. Local calcium release activation by DHPR calcium channel openings in rat cardiac myocytes. *J Physiol.* 2008;586:3839–3854.

29. Sobie EA, Ramay HR. Excitation-contraction coupling gain in ventricular myocytes: insights from a parsimonious model. *J Physiol.* 2009;587:1293–1299.

30. Altamirano J, Bers DM. Voltage dependence of cardiac excitation-contraction coupling: unitary Ca^{2+} current amplitude and open channel probability. *Circ Res.* 2007;101:590–597.

31. Torres NS, Larbig R, Rock A, Goldhaber JI, Bridge JH. Na$^+$ currents are required for efficient excitation-contraction coupling in rabbit ventricular myocytes: a possible contribution of neuronal Na$^+$ channels. *J Physiol.* 2010;588:4249–4260.

32. Jayasinghe ID, Cannell MB, Soeller C. Organization of ryanodine receptors, transverse tubules, and sodium-calcium exchanger in rat myocytes. *Biophys J.* 2009;97:2664–2673.

33. Dally S, Corvazier E, Bredoux R, Bobe R, Enouf J. Multiple and diverse coexpression, location, and regulation of additional SERCA2 and SERCA3 isoforms in nonfailing and failing human heart. *J Mol Cell Cardiol.* 2010;48:633–644.

34. Greene AL, Lalli MJ, Ji Y, et al. Overexpression of SERCA2b in the heart leads to an increase in sarcoplasmic reticulum calcium transport function and increased cardiac contractility. *J Biol Chem.* 2000;275:24722–24727.

35. Vangheluwe P, Louch WE, Ver Heyen M, Sipido K, Raeymaekers L, Wuytack F. Ca^{2+} transport ATPase isoforms SERCA2a and SERCA2b are targeted to the same sites in the murine heart. *Cell Calcium.* 2003;34:457–464.

36. Soeller C, Cannell MB. Analysing cardiac excitation-contraction coupling with mathematical models of local control. *Prog Biophys Mol Biol.* 2004;85:141–162.

37. Williams GS, Smith GD, Sobie EA, Jafri MS. Models of cardiac excitation-contraction coupling in ventricular myocytes. *Math Biosci.* 2010;226:1–15.

38. Greenstein JL, Winslow RL. An integrative model of the cardiac ventricular myocyte incorporating local control of Ca^{2+} release. *Biophys J.* 2002;83:2918–2945.

39. Hinch R, Greenstein JL, Tanskanen AJ, Xu L, Winslow RL. A simplified local control model of calcium-induced calcium release in cardiac ventricular myocytes. *Biophys J.* 2004;87:3723–3736.

40. Cheng H, Lederer WJ, Cannell MB. Calcium sparks: elementary events underlying excitation-contraction coupling in heart muscle. *Science.* 1993;262:740–744.

41. Zahradnik I, Gyorke S, Zahradnikova A. Calcium activation of ryanodine receptor channels–reconciling RyR gating models with tetrameric channel structure. *J Gen Physiol.* 2005;126:515–527.

42. Laver DR, van Helden F. Three independent mechanisms contribute to tetracaine inhibition of cardiac calcium release channels. *J Mol Cell Cardiol.* 2011;51:357–369.

43. Cannell MB, Kong CHT, Intiaz MS, Laver DR. Control of sarcoplasmic reticulum Ca^{2+} release by stochastic RyR gating within a 3D model of the cardiac dyad and importance of induction decay for CICR termination. *Biophys J.* 2013;104:2149–2159.

44. Laver DR, Kong CH, Imtiaz MS, Cannell MB. Termination of calcium-induced calcium release by induction decay: an emergent property of stochastic channel gating and molecular scale architecture. *J Mol Cell Cardiol.* 2013;54:98–100.

45. Tanskanen AJ, Greenstein JL, Chen A, Sun SX, Winslow RL. Protein geometry and placement in the cardiac dyad influence macroscopic properties of calcium-induced calcium release. *Biophys.* 2007;92:3379–3396.

46. Winslow RL, Cortassa S, O'Rourke B, Hashambhoy YL, Rice JJ, Greenstein JL. Integrative modeling of the cardiac ventricular myocyte. *Wiley Interdiscip Rev Syst Biol Med.* 2011;3:392–413.

47. Laver DR, Honen BN. Luminal Mg^{2+}, a key factor controlling RYR2-mediated Ca^{2+} release: cytoplasmic and luminal regulation modeled in a tetrameric channel. *J Gen Physiol.* 2008;132:429–446.

48. Chen W, Wang R, Chen B, et al. The ryanodine receptor store-sensing gate controls Ca^{2+} waves and Ca^{2+}-triggered arrhythmias. *Nat Med.* 2014;20:184–192.

49. Gyorke S, Gyorke I, Lukyanenko V, Terentyev D, Viatchenko-Karpinski S, Wiesner TF. Regulation of sarcoplasmic reticulum calcium release by luminal calcium in cardiac muscle. *Front Biosci.* 2002;7:d1454–d1463.

50. Stern MD, Rios E, Maltsev VA. Life and death of a cardiac calcium spark. *J Gen Physiol.* 2013;142:257–274.

51. Gillespie D, Fill M. Pernicious attrition and inter-RyR2 CICR current control in cardiac muscle. *J Mol Cell Cardiol.* 2013;58:53–58.

52. Hake J, Edwards AG, Yu Z, et al. Modeling cardiac calcium sparks in a three-dimensional reconstruction of a calcium release unit. *J Physiol.* 2012;590:4403–4422.

53. Zima AV, Picht E, Bers DM, Blatter LA. Termination of cardiac Ca²⁺ sparks: role of intra-SR [Ca²⁺], release flux, and intra-SR Ca²⁺ diffusion. *Circ Res.* 2008;103:e105–e115.

54. Antoons G, Mubagwa K, Nevelsteen I, Sipido KR. Mechanisms underlying the frequency dependence of contraction and [Ca²⁺](i) transients in mouse ventricular myocytes. *J Physiol.* 2002;543(Pt 3):889–898.

55. Wu HD, Xu M, Li RC, et al. Ultrastructural remodelling of Ca²⁺ signalling apparatus in failing heart cells. *Cardiovasc Res.* 2012;95:430–438.

56. Zhang HB, Li RC, Xu M, et al. Ultrastructural uncoupling between T-tubules and sarcoplasmic reticulum in human heart failure. *Cardiovasc Res.* 2013;98:269–276.

57. Polakova E, Sobie AE. Alterations in T-tubule and dyad structure in heart disease: challenges and opportunities for computational analyses. *Cardiovasc Res.* 2013;98:233–239.

58. Louch WE, Hake J, Mørk HK, et al. Slow Ca²⁺ sparks de-synchronize Ca²⁺ release in failing cardiomyocytes: evidence for altered configuration of Ca²⁺ release units? *J Mol Cell Cardiol.* 2013;58:41–52.

59. Wei S, Guo A, Chen B, et al. T-tubule remodeling during transition from hypertrophy to heart failure. *Circ Res.* 2010;107:520–531.

60. Koh X, Srinivasan B, Ching HS, Levchenko A. A 3D Monte Carlo analysis of the role of dyadic space geometry in spark generation. *Biophys J.* 2006;90:1999–2014.

61. Das T, Hoshijima M. Adding a new dimension to cardiac nano-architecture using electron microscopy: coupling membrane excitation to calcium signaling. *J Mol Cell Cardiol.* 2013;58:5–12.

62. Hashambhoy YL, Greenstein JL, Winslow RL. Role of CaMKII in RyR leak, EC coupling and action potential duration: a computational model. *J Mol Cell Cardiol.* 2010;49:617–624.

63. Saucerman JJ, Bers DM. Calmodulin binding proteins provide domains of local Ca²⁺ signaling in cardiac myocytes. *J Mol Cell Cardiol.* 2008;52:312–316.

64. Stokke MK, Briston SJ, Jølle GF, et al. Ca²⁺ wave probability is determined by the balance between SERCA2-dependent Ca²⁺ reuptake and threshold SR Ca²⁺ content. *Cardiovasc Res.* 2011;90:503–512.

65. Williams GS, Smith GD, Sobie EA, Jafri MS, et al. Models of cardiac excitation-contraction coupling in ventricular myocytes. *Math Biosci.* 2010;226:1–15.

66. Brette F, Orchard C. T-tubule function in mammalian cardiac myocytes. *Circ Res.* 2003;92:1182–1192.

67. Crossman DJ, Ruygrok PR, Soeller C, Cannell MB. Changes in the organization of excitation-contraction coupling structures in failing human heart. *PLoS One.* 2011;6:e17901.

68. Soeller C, Crossman D, Gilbert R, Cannell MB. Analysis of ryanodine receptor clusters in rat and human cardiac myocytes. *Proc Natl Acad Sci U S A.* 2007;104:14958–14963.

69. Brette F, Orchard C. Resurgence of cardiac T-tubule research. *Physiology (Bethesda).* 2007;22:167–173.

70. Pasek M, Brette F, Nelson A, et al. Quantification of T-tubule area and protein distribution in rat cardiac ventricular myocytes. *Prog Biophys Mol Biol.* 2008;96:244–257.

71. Despa S, Brette F, Orchard CH, Bers DM. Na/Ca exchange and Na/K-ATPase function are equally concentrated in transverse tubules of rat ventricular myocytes. *Biophys J.* 2003;85:3388–3396.

72. Despa S, Bers DM. Functional analysis of Na⁺/K⁺-ATPase isoform distribution in rat ventricular myocytes. *Am J Physiol Cell Physiol.* 2007;293:C321–C327.

73. Noble D. Successes and failures in modeling heart cell electrophysiology. *Heart Rhythm.* 2011;8:1798–1803.

74. Noble D, Garny A, Noble PJ. How the Hodgkin-Huxley equations inspired the cardiac Physiome Project. *J Physiol.* 2012;590:2613–2628.

75. Pasek M, Simurda J, Christe G. The functional role of cardiac T-tubules explored in a model of rat ventricular myocytes. *Philos Trans A Math Phys Eng Sci.* 2006;364:1187–1206.

76. Pasek M, Simurda J, Orchard CH. Role of T-tubules in the control of trans-sarcolemmal ion flux and intracellular Ca²⁺ in a model of the rat cardiac ventricular myocyte. *Eur Biophys J.* 2012;41:491–503.

77. Lu S, Michailova AP, Saucerman JJ, et al. Multiscale modeling in rodent ventricular myocytes. *IEEE Eng Med Biol Mag.* 2009;28:46–57.

78. Yao G, Yu Z. A localized meshless approach for modeling spatial-temporal calcium dynamics in ventricular myocytes. *Int J Numer Method Biomed Eng.* 2012;28:187–204.

79. Hatano A, Okada JI, Hisada T, et al. Critical role of cardiac T-tubule system for the maintenance of contractile function revealed by a 3D integrated model of cardiomyocytes. *J Biomech.* 2012;45:815–823.

80. Hatano A, Okada JI, Washio T, Hisada T, Sugiura S. A three-dimensional simulation model of cardiomyocyte integrating excitation-contraction coupling and metabolism. *Biophys J.* 2011;101:2601–2610.

81. Cheng Y, Yu Z, Hoshijima M, et al. Numerical analysis of Ca²⁺ signaling in rat ventricular myocytes with realistic transverse-axial tubular geometry and inhibited sarcoplasmic reticulum. *PLoS Comput Biol.* 2010;6:e1000972.

82. Kekenes-Huskey PM, Cheng Y, Hake J, et al. Contributions of structural T-tubule heterogeneities and membrane Ca²⁺ flux localization to local Ca²⁺ signaling in rabbit ventricular myocytes. *Biophys J.* (Annual Meeting Abstract). 2011;100:557.

83. Yu Z, Yao G, Hoshijima M, Michailova A, Holst M. Multiscale modeling of calcium dynamics in ventricular myocytes with realistic transverse tubules. *IEEE Trans Biomed Eng.* 2011;58:2947–2951.

84. Bers DM, Despa S. Na⁺ transport in cardiac myocytes: implications for excitation-contraction coupling. *IUBMB Life.* 2009;61:215–221.

85. Cheng H, Cannell MB, Lederer WJ. Propagation of excitation-contraction coupling into ventricular myocytes. *Pflugers Arch.* 1994;428:415–417.

86. Soeller C, Jayasinghe ID, Li P, Holden AV, Cannell MB. Three-dimensional high-resolution imaging of cardiac proteins to construct models of intracellular Ca²⁺ signalling in rat ventricular myocytes. *Exp Physiol.* 2009;94:496–508.

87. Rajagopal V, Bass G, Walker CG, et al. Examination of the effects of heterogeneous organization of RyR clusters, myofibrils and mitochondria on Ca²⁺ release patterns in cardiomyocytes. *PLoS Comput Biol.* 2015;11:e1004417.

88. Louch WE, Sejersted OM, Swift F. There goes the neighborhood: pathological alterations in T-tubule morphology and consequences for cardiomyocyte Ca²⁺ handling. *J Biomed Biotechnol.* 2010;2010:503906.

89. Lyon AR, MacLeod KT, Zhang Y, et al. Loss of T-tubules and other changes to surface topography in ventricular myocytes from failing human and rat heart. *Proc Natl Acad Sci U S A.* 2009;106:6854–6859.

90. Louch WE, Mørk HK, Sexton J, et al. T-tubule disorganization and reduced synchrony of Ca²⁺ release in murine cardiomyocytes following myocardial infarction. *J Physiol.* 2006;574:519–533.

91. Heinzel FR, Bito V, Biesmans L, et al. Remodeling of T-tubules and reduced synchrony of Ca²⁺ release in myocytes from chronically ischemic myocardium. *Circ Res.* 2008;102:338–346.

92. Biesmans L, Macquaide N, Heinzel FR, Bito V, Smith GL, Sipido KR. Subcellular heterogeneity of ryanodine receptor properties in ventricular myocytes with low T-tubule density. *PLoS One.* 2011;6:e25100.

93. Song LS, Sobie EA, McCulle S, Lederer WJ, Balke CW, Cheng H. Orphaned ryanodine receptors in the failing heart. *Proc Natl Acad Sci U S A.* 2006;103:4305–4310.

94. Cannell MB, Crossman DJ, Soeller C. Effect of changes in action potential spike configuration, junctional sarcoplasmic reticulum micro-architecture and altered T-tubule structure in human heart failure. *J Muscle Res Cell Motil.* 2006;27:297–306.

34 Theory of Rotors and Arrhythmias

Alexander V. Panfilov and Hans Dierckx

Each heartbeat is controlled by an electrical wave of excitation that propagates through the heart and initiates cardiac contraction. Abnormal regimes of wave propagation may result in cardiac arrhythmias. Death from cardiac arrhythmias remains one of the largest causes of death in the industrialized world. Understanding the conditions leading to abnormal wave propagation in the heart is of great interest for theoretical and practical cardiology.

In most cases, cardiac arrhythmias result from formation of so-called reentrant sources of excitation. To introduce them, we need two important properties of cardiac tissue: the ability to conduct pulses of excitation and the existence of a refractory period (R) during which the tissue cannot be excited. After a time, R, the tissue recovers and can be excited again. As a result, two colliding waves of excitation cannot continue to propagate due to the existence of the refractory state. Therefore colliding waves will extinguish or annihilate each other (Fig. 34.1A). A consequence of the annihilation phenomenon is illustrated in Fig. 34.1B and C. Consider the interaction of two excitation sources (e.g., pacemakers) with different frequency. The faster source will extend its influence to a larger spatial domain at each excitation because the wave from the faster source (the upper source in Fig. 34.1B and C) will arrive to the point of previous wave collision at an earlier time than the wave from the slower source, and hence the next collision point will shift toward the slower source (see Fig. 34.1C). As a result, the faster source will eventually organize the cardiac excitation.

The same properties enable the existence of circus movement and reentry. Fig. 34.2A illustrates such circular movement in a ring of cardiac tissue. If the rotation period of a wave along this circle is longer than the refractory period, one obtains a sustained rotation or a reentrant source. The period of rotation (T) can be estimated from the length of circle (L) and the velocity of propagation (v) as T = L/v, and sustained rotation is possible only if T > R. Similarly, the rotation around a circular obstacle in a two-dimensional (2D) sheet of cardiac cells will produce a spiral-shaped wave (Fig. 34.2B and C).[1,2] The period of such a spiral wave will still be determined by the size of the obstacle and will again be given by T = L/v. An important finding for 2D tissue was the understanding that such rotation is also possible in tissue without any obstacles.[3] In this case, the excitation from a wave break (Fig. 34.2D) will propagate along the refractory tail of the wave until the end of the refractory period (Fig. 34.2E), then it will make a half-turn and will further follow the refractory tail (Fig. 34.2F). In this situation the wave rotates around its own refractory tail, which serves as a functional obstacle for wave propagation. Such spiral waves rotating in tissue without obstacles

are often called rotors. An essential difference between rotors and spiral waves rotating around obstacles (anatomical reentry) is that the rotation period of a rotor is close to the refractory period of the tissue. This property can be understood from Fig. 34.2F where it is seen that the wave front closely follows the refractory tail of the wave. Therefore rotors are believed to be responsible for the most dangerous arrhythmias (i.e., various types of tachycardia and fibrillation where the heart rate is very high).

Rotors do not uniquely exist in the heart; they were first found in the Belousov-Zhabotinsky chemical reaction[4] and many other physical and biological systems.[5] The group of J. Jalife has extensively studied properties of rotors in cardiac tissue and their relation to cardiac arrhythmias using a range of experimental setups, from simple 2D preparations[6] up to the whole heart level.[7] The importance of rotors for cardiac arrhythmias is widely recognized and can be found in most medical textbooks on cardiology.[8] This chapter will describe and explain some basic properties of rotors. It will also discuss some recent developments in the theoretical studies of rotors and their possible application in practical research.

Basic Rotor Dynamics

Details of the schematic process of rotor formation depicted in Fig. 34.2D–I reveal that after the break formation, the wave tip does not rotate instantly, but along a circle of some radius. This phenomenon is a consequence of so-called curvature effects. The simplest manifestation of curvature effects is the dependency of the wave's propagation velocity on the curvature of its front. Indeed, an expanding circular front increases the circumference of the wave, and thus its local electrical currents are spread onto a larger area. Consequently, propagation velocity decreases and waves with extremely high curvature may even be blocked. When the wave tip tries to make a rotation to form a rotor (see Fig. 34.2D), it also increases the length of the wave front, which increases the wave front curvature. As a result, the wave rotates along a circle of some radius that highly depends on the excitability of the wave front. In highly excitable tissue, the rotation is almost instantaneous, as shown in Fig. 34.2D–E. In this case, the small excitable gap between the wave front and wave back brings the period of the rotor close to the refractory period. However, if the tissue is less excitable, the radius of such rotation and the excitable gap are larger (see Fig. 34.2F and H–I), and therefore the period of a rotor can be substantially longer than the refractory period. Also, if the rotation along such a circle takes sufficient time for tissue to recover, a circular tip trajectory is expected. If, however, the tissue is not yet recovered, the curling wave front will face the refractory wave back, leading to strong front–tail interactions, which disturb the rotation of the tip. The main conclusion from this simple analysis is that we have two main determinants of the period of the rotor: the refractory period, which mainly depends on the recovery dynamics of the action potential, and curvature effects, which mainly depend on the excitability of the wave front and determine the excitable gap. In addition, if the rotation of the tip cannot be completed due to the refractory tail of the wave, we expect a noncircular, complex rotation of the wave tip, which is normally called meandering. From the above analysis, we expect meander to happen either if the radius of rotation is small or if the refractory period is long.

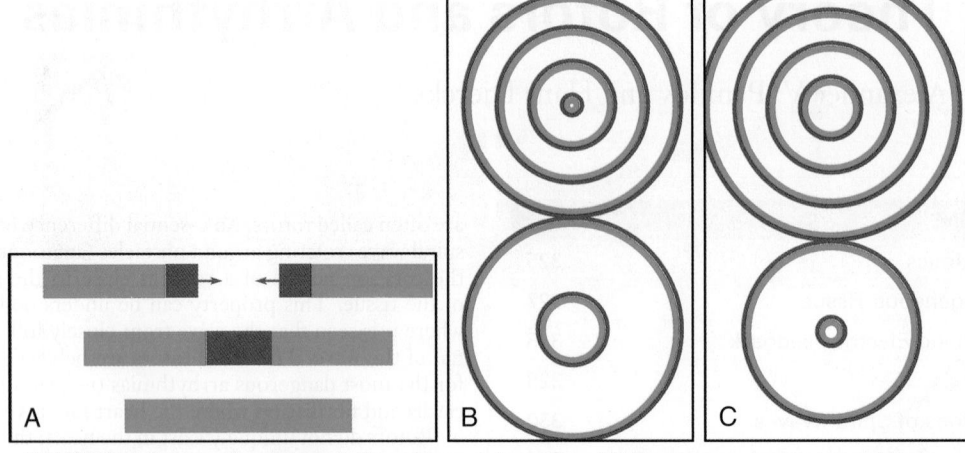

FIGURE 34.1 Schematic representation of wave interaction. (A) Two waves moving toward each other collide and annihilate. (B) and (C) Interaction of two ectopic sources of excitation with different frequencies.

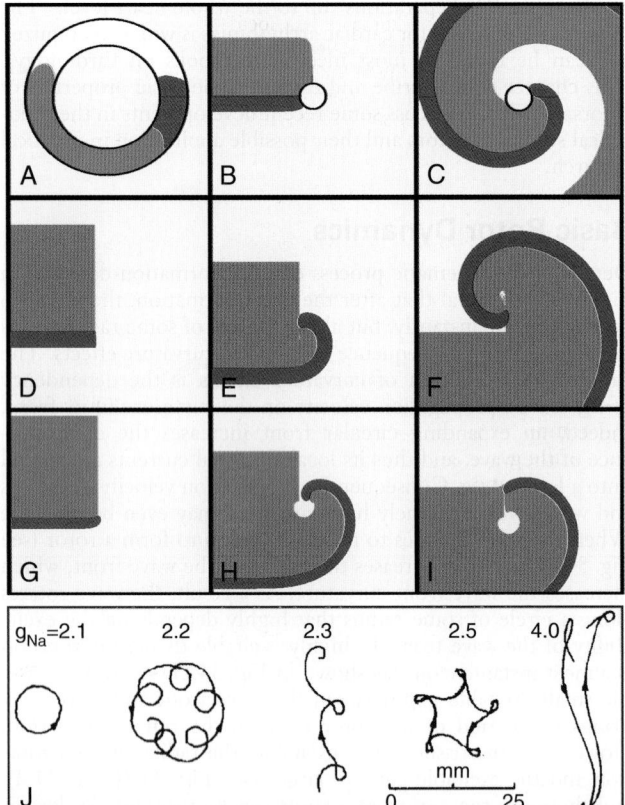

FIGURE 34.2 Schematic representation of source of excitation in the heart. (A) One-dimensional anatomical reentry. (B) and (C), Formation of a spiral wave rotating around an obstacle. (D–F) Formation of a rotor in the case of high excitability of the tissue. (G–I) Formation of a rotor in the case of low excitability of the tissue. (J) Meandering of rotors in the Beeler-Reuter model for different sodium conductances (g_{Na}). ([J] From Efimov V, Krinsky I, Jalife J. Dynamics of rotating vortices in the Beeler-Reuter model of cardiac tissue. *Chaos, Solitons & Fractals.* 1995;5:513-526.)

The meandering of rotors was first described by Zykov[9] in low-dimensional models of excitable media, where he showed that meandering patterns can exhibit epicycloidal rotation (inward petals) or hypocycloidal rotation (outward petals) with few intermediate regimes. These types of dynamics turned out

to be very general and further research confirmed such meandering in many detailed models of cardiac tissue.[10–12] Fig. 34.2J shows meandering patterns obtained in the Beeler-Reuter model of cardiac tissue at various values for the conductance of the sodium current. The meandering pattern changes from circular core to inward petals, then to outward petals, and finally to a so-called linear core. Such dynamics of rotors can be clinically important: the stable rotation along a circular trajectory has been implicated in monomorphic tachycardia, while meandering has been related to both polymorphic ventricular tachycardia and torsades de pointes.[13–15] Unfortunately it is still not understood how meandering of a rotor can be predicted from cardiac cell properties, such as the action potential shape or action potential duration (APD) and conduction velocity (CV) restitution. However, some insights can be obtained from the simple schematic description that was given in Fig. 34.2. Experimental data from a series of papers from Kodama's group,[16,17] in which the dynamics of rotors in rabbit hearts was investigated using a high-resolution optical mapping system, illustrate its value. A quasi-2D preparation was created in a subepicardial layer of the left ventricle by endocardial cryoablation, and how rotor dynamics are affected was studied by blocking different ion channels.

The information depicted in Fig. 34.2 leads to the conclusion that decreasing the curling radius of the rotor tip or increasing the refractory period leads to increased front–tail interaction and therefore meandering. One must then consider how blocking of the major ionic currents will affect these processes.

It is known that I_{Na} blockade reduces the excitability and does not substantially affect the APD. In accordance with Fig. 34.2, blocking I_{Na} should mainly increase the radius of rotation and therefore increase the period of the rotor through an increase of the excitable gap. It should also reduce front–tail interactions and thus stabilize the rotor by reducing its possible meandering. Kodama and colleagues[16] studied the effects of the sodium channel blockers, pilsicainide, disopyramide, and cibenzoline, and found that blocking sodium channels indeed increased the period of the rotor, widened the excitable gap, and made rotation more stable, confirming our predictions.

Blocking potassium current, I_{Kr} or I_{Ks}, should increase the APD, but not the excitable gap, thus increasing the rotor period and meandering. In Kodama and associates,[16] the application of the I_{Kr} blocker nifekalant increased the period of the rotor due to longer APD and not due to an increase of the excitable gap. Also, in accordance with expectations, nifekalant increased rotor meandering.

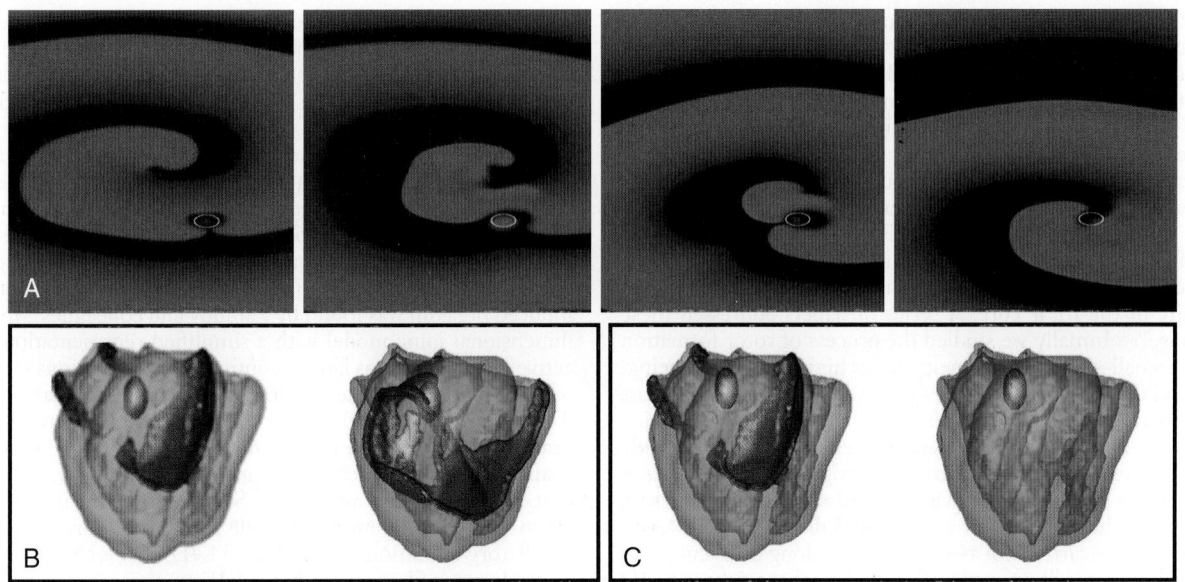

FIGURE 34.3 Attraction of rotors by an ionic heterogeneity. (A) Positions of a rotor after 7 s, 7.42 s, 8.45 s, and 9.29 s after spiral initiation in two-dimensional cardiac tissue. The rotor is initially located at 4.1 cm from the heterogeneity. (B) Attraction of the rotor in an anatomical model of ventricles of the human heart. (C) Removal of rotor by a heterogeneity located in the proximity of the basal region of the heart. (Modified from Defauw A, Vandersickel N, Dawyndt P, et al. Small size ionic heterogeneities in the human heart can attract rotors. *Am J Physiol Heart Circ Physiol.* 2014;307:H1456-H1468.)

Finally, blocking the calcium current I_{CaL} should decrease the APD, but since in healthy conditions front propagation is mainly controlled by the sodium current, it should not affect the radius of rotation. Thus one would expect block of I_{CaL} to decrease the period, and reduce meandering, but not to change the excitable gap. However, the results obtained in the experiments with block of I_{CaL} are controversial. In a study by Ishiguro and colleagues,[17] application of the I_{CaL} blocker verapamil decreased the rotor period and increased its stability. However, in a recent study performed on an atrial murine cell culture by Climent and associates,[18] verapamil was shown to increase the average meandering of rotors, as well as the rotor period. In both cases, administration of verapamil decreased APD. The different actions of verapamil may be due to different excitability of the tissues used in these experiments, as suggested by the different effects of verapamil on the rotor period. In Climent and coworkers,[18] the rotor period increased despite APD shortening, implying that the excitable gap increased, which increased the size of the rotor core. Such a phenomenon is well known from modeling studies of rotors in cardiac tissues under conditions of low excitability. In Ishiguro and associates,[17] verapamil decreased the period mainly due to a decreased APD; however, the application of verapamil combined with the sodium channel blocker pilsicainide resulted in a longer period together with a destabilization of rotors and large drift, similar to the results obtained by Climent and colleagues.[18] Therefore the effect of I_{CaL} blockade depends on the excitability of the tissue and can be monitored by the excitable gap. However, based on our simple theory, it still should result in reduction of front–tail interactions and not increase the meandering. The increased meandering observed experimentally may indicate either the limitation of such a simplified theoretical approach or may result from an increased rotor core size. The resulting drift may also arise from other mechanisms not related to meandering, such as anisotropy or heterogeneity of the tissue, which are discussed later in this chapter. Note that the research of the Kodama group also provides additional examples of drug action and hypothermia on rotor dynamics.[18a] Most of these examples can also be interpreted via the same approach, by weighting the effects of the refractory period and excitability.

Rotors in Heterogeneous Tissue

Heterogeneity of the heart is well documented. Even in normal ventricles there are substantial differences in APD between the basal and apical regions, between left and right ventricles,[7] and across the myocardial wall.[19–22] Heterogeneities can directly impact rotor dynamics in several ways. A gradient of heterogeneity induces a drift of rotors.[23–25] This drift is generally directed at some angle to the gradient, and thus can be decomposed into two components: the longitudinal component, along the direction of the gradient, and the transverse component, orthogonal to the gradient direction. The transverse component depends on the direction of rotation of the rotor; thus changing the rotation direction would also alter the sign of the transverse drift component. This is an obvious consequence of symmetry. Indeed, observing drift in a mirror positioned along the gradient of heterogeneity would change the direction of the rotation, as well as the direction of the transverse drift. Multiple numerical studies showed that the longitudinal component is always directed toward the region of the longer period of rotor rotation.[23–25] The mechanism of this phenomenon is still unknown. For cardiac arrhythmias, this means that, due to drift, the cycle length of an arrhythmia will increase, which should present some antiarrhythmic effect. Drift in the opposite direction, however, may result in a very natural mechanism for the "mother rotor"-type of fibrillation.[7] Indeed, in this case the rotor will fasten its rotation and the cycle length of the arrhythmia will decrease, which would lead to secondary wave breaks at the heterogeneities. Extensive analysis of drift direction in low-dimensional models of cardiac tissue shows a possibility of existence of drift to the direction of lower period.[26] However, this retrograde drift occurs only in a very narrow range of parameters and so far has not been reproduced in ionic models.

Localized heterogeneities, a different type of heterogeneity, were also found to affect rotor dynamics. Recent experimental studies of wedge preparations from explanted human hearts performed in the laboratory of I. Efimov showed the existence of large APD heterogeneities of small spatial size.[25] For example, the data showed that APD could change about 60 ms on a space scale of only 3 mm. Several important issues are related to the existence of such heterogeneities. It is well established that large APD heterogeneities are smoothened due to electrotonic effects, whose typical spatial length is estimated at approximately 0.3 to 1 cm,[27,28] meaning that observed differences in APD at the tissue level actually indicate much larger differences in APD at the single cell level. To reconstruct the underlying heterogeneity is important, and the extent of heterogeneity can be estimated (e.g., using a Green function approach).[27] Furthermore, a small spatial scale of heterogeneity may indicate that the effect of such heterogeneities on rotor dynamics is small and can occur only in the proximity of the rotor core. A series of papers addressed these questions.[29,30] Initially we studied the process of rotor formation around a small-sized heterogeneity under high-frequency pacing. We found that despite the small size of the heterogeneity, rotors may form around it. In most cases a single rotor occurred, which was always anchored at the heterogeneity.[29] The next study addressed the effects of localized heterogeneities on existing rotors. It was shown that even very small-sized heterogeneities could attract the rotors from a substantial distance.[30] However, this attraction occurred, not as a drift, but as a long transient process. This process is illustrated in Fig. 34.3A, where a rotor in 2D tissue is located at a distance of 4 cm from a small heterogeneity. The rotor initially generates wave breaks close to the heterogeneity. The breakup region extends in space, approaches the rotor core and subsequently gives rise to a new rotor. As a result of such interaction the rotor distant from the heterogeneity vanishes, and the newly formed rotor anchors to the heterogeneity (see Fig. 34.3A, right frame). A similar situation was observed in an anatomical model of the heart (Fig. 34.3B): a rotor initially located at a distance from a heterogeneity (see Fig. 34.3B) shifts and anchors to it. As in the 2D example above, the pinning process occurs as a result of wave break formation at the heterogeneity and subsequent interaction of the wave breaks with the initial rotor. Interestingly enough, if such heterogeneity was located close to the base of the heart, it also attracted the rotors. However, after attraction the rotor disappeared via collision with the upper boundary of the ventricular wall (Fig. 34.3C). Attraction was observed for distances of at least 5 cm from the heterogeneity over a time interval of 10 sec. In most cases, rotors at larger distances were also attracted, but required more time.

Rotors and Mechano-Electric Feedback

Another phenomenon that can affect rotor dynamics is the mechanical contraction of the heart. Cardiac contraction affects excitation via several mechanisms, one of the most important being via special ion channels that are activated by stretch.[31,32] There are several groups of such stretch-activated channels (SAC): cation nonselective, potassium-selective, and chloride-selective channels. In most cases, stretch contributes to the depolarization of cardiac tissue. Such depolarization may affect rotor dynamics in several ways. First, a strong external mechanical stimulus can produce additional local excitation of the heart. If this excitation occurs during a vulnerable phase, it may result in the onset of new rotors via the S1–S2 mechanism. It has been suggested that such a mechanism may explain the mechanical induction of heart rhythm disturbances that occur in the absence of structural damage to the chest, a phenomenon known as *commotio cordis*.[33,34] The impact induces a secondary (S2) beat during the vulnerable period, which initiates a rotor(s) and thereby triggers a cardiac arrhythmia. More recently, it was also demonstrated that external mechanical stretch can induce another form of vulnerability where a figure-of-eight reentry with opposite rotation direction is formed.[35] This mechanism occurred in a very narrow range of parameters. However, it was common when the mechanical S2 stimulus was not external, and was instead formed by the stretch generated by the propagating wave itself.[35]

Effects of depolarization induced by the propagating waves were also presented in a study performed with an advanced electromechanical, anatomically accurate model[36] showing that stretch-induced depolarization in ischemic regions can initiate rotors at the whole organ level.

Another effect of mechanical stretch is associated with the accommodation phenomenon,[37,38] which means that depolarization of a cell reduces the availability of sodium channels. As stretch causes local depolarization, it may locally inhibit sodium current, which may block wave propagation in the stretched area and generate new rotors. Such a phenomenon of mechanically induced breakup was found by Panfilov and colleagues[39] in a low-dimensional ionic model with a simplified representation of the active tension and was later reconfirmed in simulations in an anatomical model of the left ventricle of the human heart with the TP06 human ventricular cell model and the Niederer-Hunter-Smith model for active tension development.[40] Fig. 34.4A shows a single rotor (indicated by a single rotor filament in Fig. 34.4B) that is stable in the absence of SACs. However, if SACs were taken into consideration, the same rotor would break down in a fibrillatory excitation pattern (Fig. 34.4D) that is characterized by multiple rotor filaments in Fig. 34.4E.

The possible effects of SACs on rotor dynamics in a regime of spiral breakup have also been investigated.[41] The opening of SACs with a reversal potential of –60 mV diminished scroll wave breakup, as it resulted in flattening of the APD restitution curve. Opening of SACs with a reversal potential of –10 mV also inhibited the breakup for low SAC conductance, whereas new wave breaks were created at high SAC conductance, via the same mechanism of decreased availability of I_{Na} due to depolarization caused by stretch.

Mechanical stretch can induce rotor drift.[39] Fig. 34.4C shows a rotor that is stable in the absence of mechanical contraction. However, if SACs are taken into account a drift toward the center of the tissue is seen. The drift can be explained by the so-called resonance phenomenon, where rotor drift is induced by periodic temporal modulation of the tissue properties.[42] Particularly, it has been shown that modulating the properties of cardiac tissue with a frequency close to the frequency of the rotor causes rotor drift.[43,44] Mechanical contraction obviously generates a periodic change of stretch, which is transformed via SACs into a periodic modulation of the electrical tissue properties. Since the frequency of such modulation coincides with the rotor frequency, it results in rotor drift via the resonance mechanism. The drift induced by stretch was demonstrated in low-dimensional models[39] and was later confirmed in the TP06 ionic model for human ventricular tissue.[45] Also theoretical studies of such drift were performed using the response function approach, and it was confirmed that the net spiral wave drift is proportional to the first Fourier component of the induced stretch in the neighborhood of the rotor's rotation center.[46] In Dierckx and associates[46] a theoretical approach for predicting the direction of rotor drift based on the excitation pattern of the tissue was also proposed. However, all studies of drift have been so far performed in 2D models only. These studies are very difficult to project to anatomically accurate situations, as in that case stretch will be determined by shape, anisotropy of cardiac tissue, and mechanical boundary conditions. All these factors will obviously affect rotor drift and, together, will determine its final destination.

Rotors and Fibrosis

Fibrosis of cardiac tissue is one of the main components of structural remodeling of cardiac tissue that occurs during aging, disease, or injury.[47,48] As fibroblasts are unexcitable cells, their increased numbers, together with collagen deposition during fibrosis, affects the processes of wave propagation, rotor initiation, and rotor dynamics. The impact of fibrosis on these

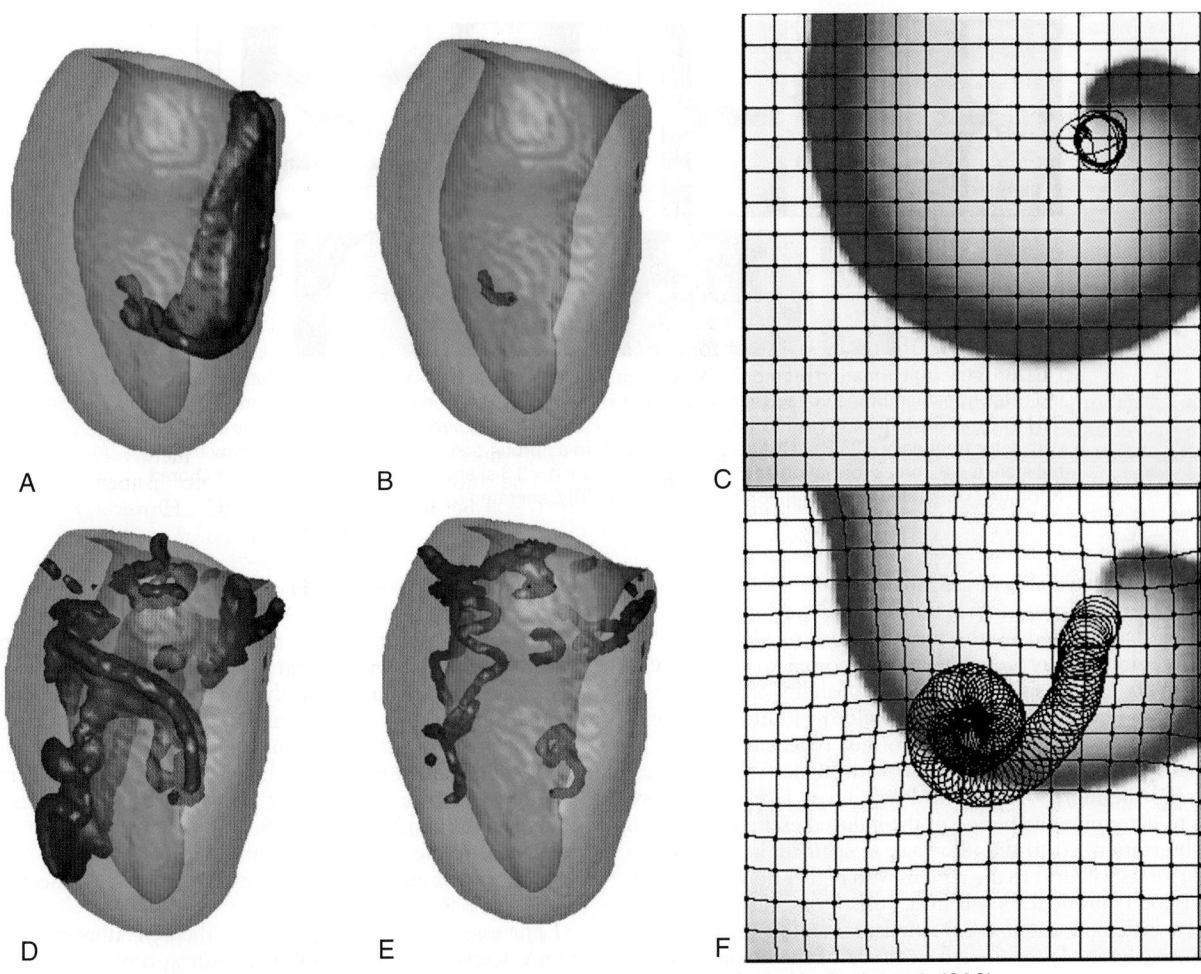

FIGURE 34.4 Breakup and drift of rotors induced by stretch-activated ionic channels (SAC).
(A) and (B) The rotor in an anatomical model of the human heart remains stable in the absence of
SAC ([A] shows the wave front and [B] the filament). In presence of SAC with high conductance, the
spiral wave breaks into the fibrillatory pattern with multiple filaments. (D) and (E) Simulations in the
TP06 model for human cardiac tissue.[40] If SAC conductivity is not sufficient to induce a breakup, it
causes a drift of a rotor: (C) dynamics without contraction; (F) with contraction. Simulations in a low
dimensional model of cardiac tissue.[39]

processes depends on its spatial organization. The main textures
of fibrosis are compact, patchy, interstitial, and diffuse, which differ by degree of spatial organization of fibroblasts and collagen.[47]
Most numerical studies of rotor dynamics have focused on the
two extreme cases of compact and diffuse fibrosis.

Compact fibrosis is characterized by large, dense, nonconducting areas that can be considered in modeling studies as
unexcitable obstacles to a propagating wave. Rotors can anchor
to such obstacles.[6] In addition, several papers have investigated
the possibility of rotor formation around those obstacles under
high-frequency stimulation and have shown that rotor formation is possible, however, only when the frequency of the external forcing is high enough and exceeds some critical value.[49,50]
Interestingly, the critical frequency to generate new rotors
turned out to lie very close to the frequency of the rotor itself.
This property was initially shown in a low-dimensional model of
cardiac tissue[49,50] and later in the TP06 ionic model for human
ventricular cells.[51] In a wide range of parameters accounting for
modified conductivities of I_{Na}, I_{CaL}, I_{Ks}, I_{Kr}, and I_{K1}, the critical
frequency of rotor induction coincided almost identically with
the frequency of a rotor spinning in the same tissue. Fig. 34.5
shows wave dynamics around an obstacle representing an infarction scar. For frequencies below the rotor frequency (3.83 Hz)

(see Fig. 34.5A, 1–2) no rotors are formed, but for a frequency of
3.85 Hz, breaks form separated from the scar (see Fig. 34.5A, 3),
which evolve into several rotors after termination of stimulation
(see Fig. 34.5A, 4).

Rotor dynamics were also widely studied for the case of diffuse fibrosis. Diffuse fibrosis was found to increase the rotor
period.[52–55] A direct consequence of this period increase is a
reduced probability for restitution-induced breakup. The longer
rotation period results in a wider excitable gap, which lowers the
slope of the restitution curve at the rotor frequency, and finally
decreases the probability of onset of the breakup.[52,53] However,
fibrosis by itself promoted onset of new rotors due to source–sink
mismatch.[53,54] Several attempts have been made to characterize
the conditions for the onset of rotors. Alonso and coworkers[56]
studied rotor initiation in a conducting network with a fraction
of nonconducting links. Such texture can be considered to be a
generic model of diffuse fibrosis. Rotor generation is determined
by the proximity of the fraction of nonconducting links to the
percolation threshold (within 5%–10%). Here, the percolation
threshold equals the degree of nonconducting elements at which
the network becomes disconnected, thereby inhibiting wave
propagation. Furthermore, rotor formation depends on the excitability and size of the heterogeneous region.

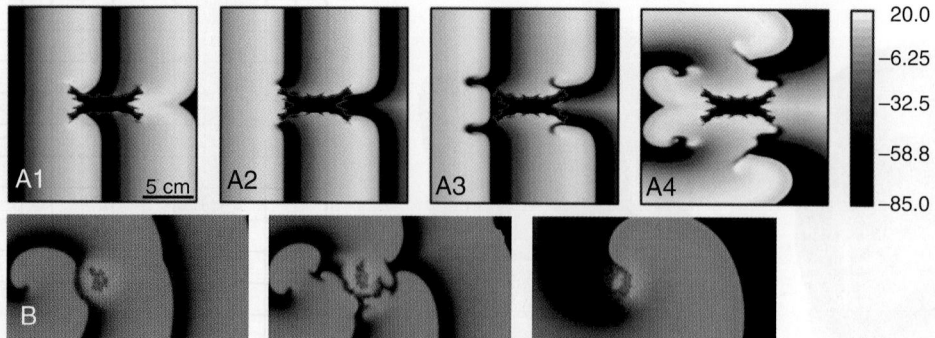

FIGURE 34.5 (A) Formation of rotors around an unexcitable scar at high-frequency stimulation. Color indicates transmembrane voltage in mV. *Panels 1 and 2,* No breaks, frequency of stimulation 3.2 Hz and 3.8 Hz. *Panel 3,* Multiple break formation at 3.85 Hz. *Panel 4,* Rotors persist after stimulation is stopped with rotor frequency 3.83 Hz. (B) Attraction of a rotor to a fibrotic scar. Subsequent frames show the initial state (t = 0), break formation and spreading of rotors (t = 3.3 s) and ultimate survival of an anchored rotor. ([A] Generated by Dr. Rupamanjari Majumder. [B] Generated by Dr. Ivan Kazbanov.)

Recently we have also investigated the effects of fibrosis heterogeneity on the onset of arrhythmias. Study of various textures of fibrosis that differed by the mean amount of fibrosis and by the degree and size of heterogeneity[57] showed that the spatial heterogeneity of fibrosis increases the probability of the onset of arrhythmias. This effect is more pronounced with the increase of both the spatial size and the degree of heterogeneity and can be explained by the presence of regions with higher values of local fibrosis. Furthermore, the maximal local fibrosis level was demonstrated to determine the period of the induced excitation pattern. This observation led to the idea that, in spatially heterogeneous fibrosis, rotors will drift to the regions with higher fibrotic content, and thus local fibrotic scars will attract the rotors. This anticipated process was demonstrated in 2D simulation and in an anatomical patient-specific model of the left ventricle of the human heart.[58] Fig. 34.5B shows the process of attraction in a 2D setup. A rotor was initially located 4 cm from a fibrotic region. During rotation, the rotor induced additional wave breaks in the fibrotic region. These breaks spread toward the rotor and, after interaction, the initial rotor disappeared by collision with the boundary. However the rotor close to the scarred region anchors to the fibrotic region and rotates around it. This process appears to be very similar to the attraction to a small size ionic heterogeneity illustrated in Fig. 34.3 and probably has the same mechanism.

Rotor dynamics have also been studied in more complex fibrotic textures, such as the effects of fibrosis in atrial tissue in an anatomically accurate ionic model.[59,60] Inducibility of rotors by high frequency pacing depends on the distance between a given pacing location and the closest fibrotic region, with only midrange distances resulting in arrhythmia. Also, persistent rotors were moving within restricted regions of tissue that were determined by the distribution of the fibrosis. Similar results were obtained by Gonzales and associates[60] in a patient-specific model of human atria. Moreover, regions of fibrosis were identified that may anchor rotors.

Another significant area of research dealt with the possible effect of myocyte–fibroblast coupling on wave propagation and rotor dynamics[54,61]; however, a detailed discussion of these results falls outside the scope of this chapter. The formation of rotors at an anatomical obstacle in a slightly different setup has been demonstrated experimentally in cardiac tissue.[62,63]

Response Functions of Spiral Waves

One new approach to the study of rotor dynamics in the heart uses so-called response functions, which allows the prediction of

the reaction of a rotor on any external perturbation by testing its reaction to standard elementary perturbations. This method is a common tool in physics and engineering, called perturbation theory, and is widely used in the most advanced theoretical fields, such as quantum electrodynamics, quantum chemistry, and particle physics. For rotor dynamics, the method was introduced in 1988 by Keener,[64] who combined it with singular perturbation theory and applied it to three-dimensional (3D) rotor filaments. The term *response functions* was later coined by Biktasheva and coworkers (2003).[65] Response functions have been successfully applied to predict the dynamics of 3D rotor filaments[64,66–71] and drift of 2D spiral waves due to external fields,[72] inhomogeneities,[73–75] or anisotropy.[76]

The essence of response function theory is illustrated in Fig. 34.6A. Consider a stably rotating rotor at time t. Perturbing it for a short period of time will result in a shift of this rotor in space (i.e., the center of its rotation jumps over some distance in the x and y directions. In addition, the perturbation will also cause an extra shift of the rotation phase (ϕ). Now, suppose a localized perturbation of small amplitude (σ) and duration (Δt) is applied at any point (x_0, y_0) (e.g., by an electrode stimulus), and these shifts are determined. For small stimuli the shifts in the x and y directions and the phase shift will be proportional to Δt and σ, such that (Δx, Δy, $\Delta \phi$) = ($\sigma W^x \Delta t$, $\sigma W^y \Delta t$, $\sigma W^0 \Delta t$), where W^x, W^y, and W^0 are constants that depend only on the position (x_0, y_0) where the stimulus was delivered, relative to the spiral position and orientation. If this experiment is repeated by disturbing each state variable for every relative position (x_0, y_0), a set of functions, $\mathbf{W}^x(x_0,y_0)$, $\mathbf{W}^y(x_0,y_0)$, and $\mathbf{W}^0(x_0,y_0)$, will be obtained, which are known as response functions[65]; examples are shown in Fig. 34.1B and C. For rigidly rotating (nonmeandering) rotors, response functions are time-independent in a coordinate system that corotates with the spiral wave. Thus response functions are rotating in the same sense as the rotors and therefore explicitly depend on time. By knowing the three response functions, you can predict the spiral's reaction to any perturbation $\mathbf{h}(x,y,t)$ by decomposing $\mathbf{h}$ as a sum over elementary perturbations. By linear superposition, the drift velocity (V^x, V^y) and frequency shift $\omega-\omega_0$ are well approximated by[64,77]:

$$V^x(t) = \iint \mathbf{W}^x(x, y, t)\, \mathbf{h}(x, y, t)\, dx\, dy,$$
$$V^y(t) = \iint \mathbf{W}^y(x, y, t)\, \mathbf{h}(x, y, t)\, dx\, dy, \qquad (1)$$
$$\omega - \omega_0 + \iint \mathbf{W}^0(x, y, t)\, \mathbf{h}(x, y, t)\, dx\, dy.$$

If one knows the reaction terms from the right-hand side of a cardiac model, response functions need not be determined by application of the perturbations described above, but can be explicitly

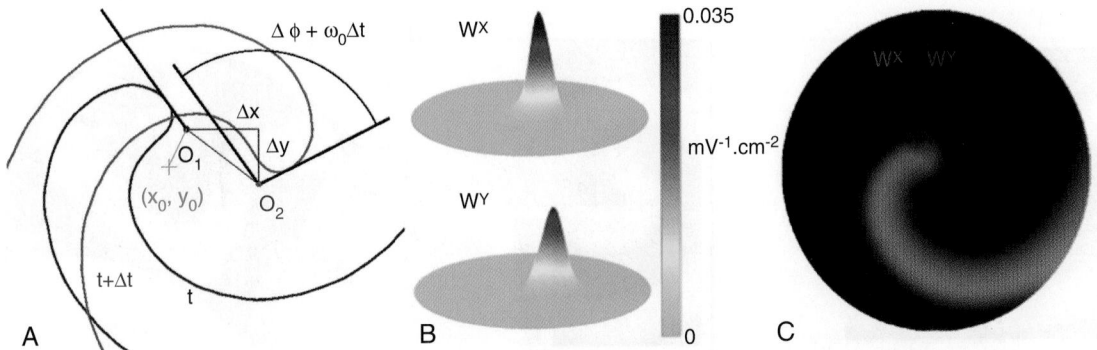

FIGURE 34.6 Rotor response functions. (A) At time t, a small stimulus is delivered at a point (x_0, y_0) relative to the rotation center O1 of the rotor (*blue*). After a small transient time (Δt), one observes the same rotor (*A, red*), whose rotation center has shifted over Δx, Δy. Recording the shifts in x and y for all possible stimulus positions (x_0, y_0) yields the response functions $W^x(x_0, y_0)$ and $W^y(x_0, y_0)$ shown in (B). In (C) the response function densities are strongly localized to the spiral wave core region, which shows that rotors are insensitive to external stimuli far from their core. (Response functions in [B] and [C] were calculated by V. Biktashev for the Beuler-Reuter model of cardiac tissue.)

computed by numerically solving an eigenvalue problem. The full derivation would be too mathematical for the scope of this chapter and can be found in specialized papers (e.g., see Biktashev and Holden[77]).

Numerical solutions of response functions have been found for simple excitation models[68,74,78] up to the Beeler-Reuter[79] cardiac model.[80] Interestingly, *all computed response functions are strongly localized near the spiral wave core*; an example is shown in Fig. 34.6, where the translational response functions for the voltage component of the Beeler-Reuter model are presented on a disk of radius 4 mm. *The response functions are nonzero only in a region of about 2 mm² at the core of the rotor, meaning that any perturbation outside this region will not affect rotor dynamics.* For example, an ablation line 4 mm away from the rotor core will not remove it and will not even change its period, core size, etc. Also, for the depicted rotation phase, W^x and W^y are both positive, indicating that a positive voltage stimulus ahead of the rotor tip will cause net shifts in the positive x and y directions. Also, if rotor rotation is disturbed by any means that change the balance of ionic currents on the membrane, such as stretch activated current or heterogeneous expression of any ion channel, the effect of such disturbance will now easily be found by using these response functions and Eq.(1). On a general note, response functions show which regions affect rotor dynamics, and thus they give an accurate estimate of the scale of heterogeneity that is essential for rotor dynamics, the characteristic obstacle sizes that will affect rotors, necessary ablation textures, and many other factors related to rotor dynamics, including their drift and meandering.

Response functions have already been used for direct calculations (Fig. 34.7). Additionally, important results can be found even without explicit knowledge of the response functions, in the sense that general expressions for drift of spiral waves, scroll waves, and wave fronts have been derived (e.g., see references[64,66,70,81]) after which the model-dependent coefficients may be fit to simulations or experiments. Current challenges in response function theory in view of applications include the extension of this theory to nonstationary (meandering) cores and the development of efficient methods to compute response functions in detailed ionic models. It would be also important to develop the methods to measure response functions directly in experiments or from clinical recordings and to apply them for a better understanding of the effect of drugs on rotor dynamics. Novel approaches to most of these problems are under development and substantial progress in this area is expected.

Curved-Space Approach to Cardiac Anisotropy

Anisotropy is an important property of cardiac tissue, since the electrical signal or action potential travels 2 to 3 times faster along the local myofiber direction than in the directions transverse to it.[82] Therefore typical excitation patterns after point stimulation on the epicardial surface appear as ellipses or more complex patterns rather than circular disks. Anisotropy of cardiac tissue has a substantial effect on wave propagation in the heart and affects rotor dynamics in various ways. For example, the idea of anisotropic reentry[83] is one of the founding hypotheses for heart rhythm disturbances. Below several manifestations of anisotropy using a novel approach, in which anisotropy can be treated as a geometrical property of cardiac tissue, are discussed.

To illustrate this viewpoint, consider a rotating spiral wave in a sheet of tissue with horizontally aligned myofibers, as shown in Fig. 34.7A. Since conduction velocity $v_x > v_y$, the rotating spiral appears to be stretched horizontally, with a factor equal to the ratio $v_x{:}v_y$ of principal conduction velocities. Mathematically, *the effect of anisotropy can be accounted for by measuring distances in terms of arrival time of electrical signals, rather than in terms of inches or centimeters.* In everyday life, an online route planner or navigation device will also report the travel time, rather than distance in miles or kilometers.

This concept of distance can be related to the anisotropic diffusion tensor ($\boldsymbol{D}$) in the cardiac monodomain equations, since the propagation velocity in a given direction is known to scale as $v = \alpha\sqrt{D}$, where D is the diffusion coefficient in that direction, and α is a tissue-dependent constant. To find an explicit expression for the distance, Fig. 34.7B introduces rescaled coordinates as $x' = x/v_x$ and $y' = y/v_y$, which is equivalent to using different yardsticks in different directions such that the propagation velocity becomes isotropic and equal to 1. Then, the squared travel time for a plane wave to propagate from (x, y) to $(x+dx, y+dy)$ equals:

$$dt^2 = dx'^2 + dy'^2 = \frac{dx^2}{v_x^2} + \frac{dx^2}{v_x^2}$$
$$= \alpha^{-2}\left(\frac{dx^2}{D^{xx}} + \frac{dy^2}{D^{yy}}\right) = (dxdy)\cdot\boldsymbol{g}\cdot\left(\frac{dx}{dy}\right) \qquad (2)$$

This result is presented in such form, as it is a standard way to measure a distance in mathematical physics, where one

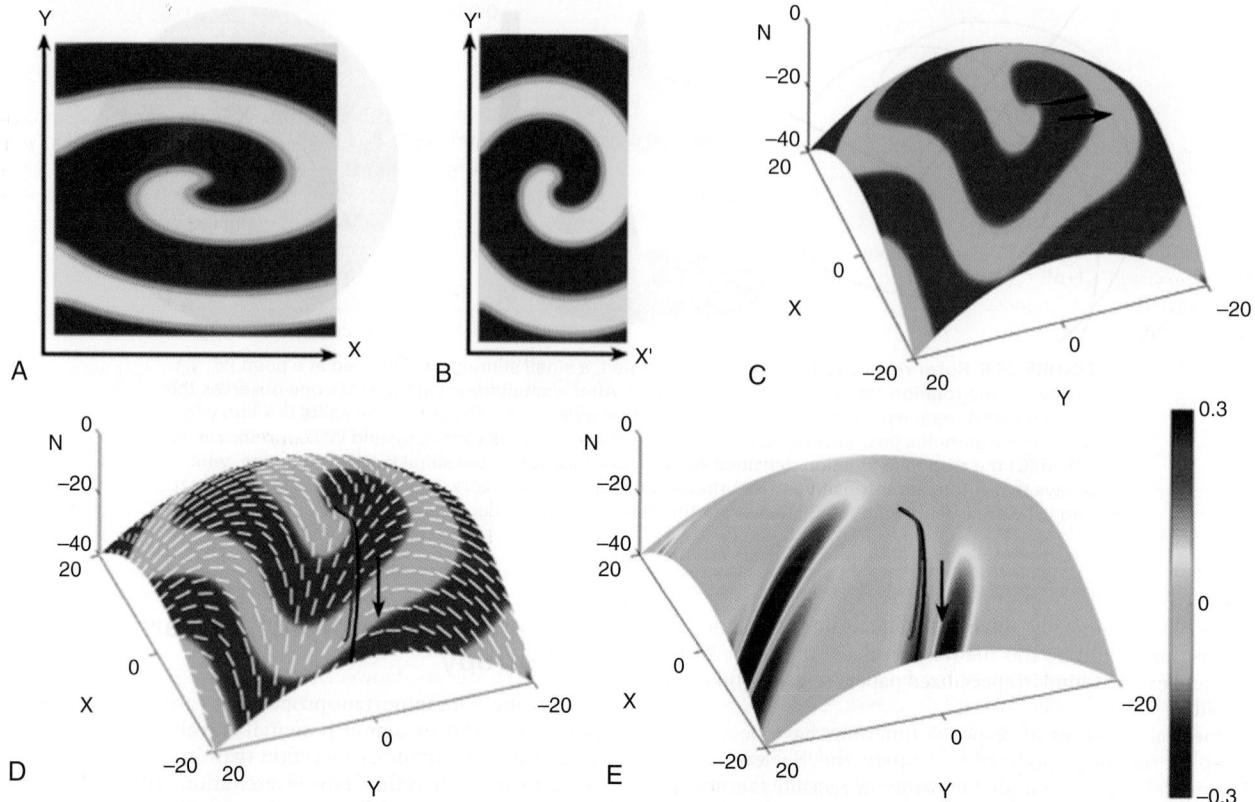

FIGURE 34.7 Curved-space approach to cardiac anisotropy. (A) A reentrant wave in a tissue region with horizontally aligned myofibers can be made isotropic by scaling of the X axis. (B) A procedure that can be mathematically extended to locally varying finer rotation in three spatial dimensions. The curved-space approach enables theoretical prediction (*red*) of rotor drift (*black*) on curved surfaces (e.g., on a paraboloid surface with isotropic diffusion). (C) By combining extrinsic or visual curvature and intrinsic or anisotropy-induced curvature, one can compute the Ricci scalar curvature (E) using Eq.(6). With this knowledge, the dynamics of rotors on an anisotropic curved surface can be predicted (D), for the rotor drifts under a fixed angle with the gradient of the Ricci curvature.

generalizes Pythagoras' theorem via the metric tensor, g. It allows the measurement of distances via coordinates not only in our usual Euclidean space, but also in more complex situations (e.g., on a sphere or on another more complex surface). In such situations, the metric tensor provides a way to compute relative distances given a set of coordinates. In cardiac modeling, one finds from Eq.(1) that:

$$g(\vec{x}) = \alpha^{-2} D^{-1}(\vec{x}). \qquad (3)$$

This relation fundamentally means that if local diffusion in a given direction is high, the points in this direction effectively lie closer to each other because depolarization waves travel faster between them. The prefactor, α^{-2}, is a constant which relates the diffusion coefficient and the propagation velocity and has units of travel time (milliseconds).

The idea of using the space defined by Eq.(3), which in mathematical physics is called a Riemannian or curved space, was first introduced by Wellner and associates (2002)[84] to describe the equilibrium shape of rotor filaments in anisotropic cardiac tissue. The physical interpretation as an arrival time space was demonstrated by Ten Tusscher,[85] and its implications were further studied.[69,86–88]

The properties of Riemannian spaces are well studied in modern physics and mathematics, allowing the application of the methods and the obtained results to cardiac modeling. For example, cardiac tissue is an example of a curved space (i.e., a space where the shortest path between two points is a curve and not a straight line). Indeed, if myofiber orientation

varies in space, the wave between two distant points propagates along some complex curve, which is almost never a straight line.

Many important results on wave propagation in anisotropic tissue have been found using a curved-space approach:

Application to Wave Fronts

Let us start with a simple example. A common anisotropy pattern in the heart is rotational anisotropy of the ventricular wall, where the fiber orientation angle rotates through the thickness of the myocardium.[89] It turns out that such fiber architecture forms a curved space with negative curvature.[86] General considerations tell us that in spaces with negative curvature, the geodesics (i.e., the lines of shortest distance) diverge, similar to the geodesics on the saddle surface displayed in Fig. 34.7C. By Huygens' principle, the activation of points ahead of the wave front occurs via geodesics. Therefore since the heart is a negatively curved space, a propagating wave front expands itself in space faster than it would without fiber rotation. As a result, the rotational anisotropy will result in more efficient wave spread, and the transmural rotation of myofibers increases the efficiency of excitation.[86]

A second insight on wave propagation in a curved space was found in the relation between the velocity, c, and wave front curvature, K, which is sometimes called the eikonal-curvature equation. This relation was first studied in isotropic media[90,91] and was later generalized to anisotropic cardiac tissue.[92] By combining the curved-space viewpoint with response function theory, it was shown that the equation for anisotropic myocardium formally looks the same as in isotropic media[81]:

$$c = c_0 - \gamma K, \tag{4}$$

where c_0 is the velocity of a plane wave and, in isotropic media, K is the mean curvature (i.e., the sum of the inverse principal radii of curvature). However, in anisotropic media, the meaning of K is very different. K here must be computed only after a local rescaling of coordinates, which takes into account different wave propagation velocities in different directions and also the local variations in anisotropy around the wave front. When that expression is further simplified, all factors affecting the wave velocity are found:

$$c = \sqrt{D_\perp} c_0 - \gamma \left(D^{ij} K_{ij} + K_{ansio} \right), \tag{5}$$

where $D_\perp = \vec{N} \cdot D \cdot \vec{N}$ with $\vec{N}$ the Euclidean unit normal vector to the wave front, K_{ij} is the curvature tensor measured in standard 3D rectangular coordinates, and $K_{ansio} = (\vec{\nabla} \cdot D) \cdot \vec{N} - \frac{1}{2} \vec{N} \cdot D \cdot \vec{\nabla} \ln D_\perp$ is another term that comes from the curvature of space itself, meaning that a wave front that appears as planar in usual Euclidean space ($K_{ij} = 0$) may still be curved due to locally varying myofiber rotation. Note that a similar expression can be obtained using singular perturbation theory.[92,93] However, application of the curved-space formalism provides a direct physical interpretation of the curvature effects. Indeed, by its definition, the curvature, K, measures the relative rate-of-change in the cross-sectional area if one progresses orthogonally to the wave front surface,[94] such that $K = \partial_n A / A$. Therefore the wave front curvature K in Eq.(4) is just an "electrotonic load" on wave propagation, and it can result in "source–sink mismatch" and possibly wave break–formation induced by anisotropy. This mechanism was studied by Zemlin and colleagues[95] in the Luo-Rudy model for cardiac cells. Later, such mechanisms were also confirmed in experiments in a cell culture with neonatal rat cardiomyocytes[96] and reproduced in a TP06 model for human ventricular tissue.[97] Kudryashova and associates[97] also suggested that block of the I_{K1} current may be an efficient way to prevent wave block–formation due to anisotropy. This result, however, requires further investigation.

Spiral Wave Drift

Both anisotropy of cardiac tissue[98,99] and curvature of a 2D medium[100] can cause spiral wave drift. Dierckx and colleagues (2013) showed that both kinds of spiral wave drift may be understood and unified from a curved-space perspective. Using response function theory, the drift of the rotor can be found from the following equations[76]:

$$\partial_t \vec{X} = -q_1 \vec{\nabla} R - q_2 \vec{n} \times \vec{\nabla} R \tag{6}$$

Here, q_1 and q_2 are scaling factors, X is the rotor core position, and R is the Ricci curvature scalar R, which is the main determinant of the drift. In general, the Ricci curvature scalar of a 2D surface is simply twice its Gaussian curvature K_G (e.g., for a sphere it is $2/(\text{radius})^2$). However, in curved space, R also depends on anisotropy and can be computed as

$$R = 2 D_1 K_G - 2 (D_1 - D_2) \vec{\nabla} (\vec{e}_f (\vec{\nabla} \vec{e}_f)). \tag{7}$$

Here, K_G is the Gaussian curvature of the surface (i.e., the product of the inverse principal radii of curvature), $\vec{e}_f$ is the local fiber direction, and D_1 and D_2 are the diffusion coefficients along and transverse to the local myofiber direction.[76] The first term in Eq. (7) accounts for the visible curvature of the surface (e.g., the atrial wall), whereas the second term arises from local myofiber divergence. Even the general forms of Eqs.(6–7) allow us to obtain some interesting results. For example, it was known that in the isotropic case, the rotor on a surface normally drifts to the regions where the Gaussian curvature of the surface is maximal.[101] This property directly follows from Eq.(6), since for $q_1 < 0$, drift is directed toward the largest Gaussian curvature. In contrast, for $q_1 > 0$, the drift will be in the opposite direction (i.e., to the most negative Gaussian curvature). However, in the presence of anisotropy, both the curvature of the surface and the anisotropy will be essential. A numerical example is given in Fig. 34.7D and E where a linearly varying fiber rotation, as in Rogers and associates,[98] was applied to a paraboloid surface. Using response functions, the coefficients $q_1 = 0.643$ and $q_2 = 0.357$ in Eq.(6) were computed for Barkley's model.[102] Without anisotropy ($D_1 = D_2$, Fig. 34.7D), the rotor drifts toward lower Gaussian curvature (i.e., moves away from the paraboloid top since q_1 is positive). The predicted trajectory (*red*) is confirmed by numerical simulations (*black*). In the presence of anisotropy, however, the drift magnitude and direction are much harder to predict. Nevertheless, with the curved-space approach, one can compute the intrinsic curvature, R, using Eq.(7) and then apply Eq.(6) to find the drift trajectory (*red curve* in Fig. 34.7E), which closely matches the numerical simulations (*black*). Note that the drift trajectories with and without anisotropy are markedly different, but both are well predicted by the theory (Eqs.[6–7]).

Acknowledgments

The authors thank I. Kazbanov, R. Majumder, and V.N. Biktashev for help in preparation of the manuscript.

REFERENCES

1. Mines GR. On dynamic equilibrium of the heart. *J Physiol.* 1913;46:349–482.
2. Wiener N, Rosenblueth A. The mathematical formulation of the problem of conduction of impulses in a network of connected excitable elements, specifically in cardiac muscle. *Arch Inst Cardiol Mex.* 1946;16:205–265.
3. Selfridge O. Studies on flutter and fibrillation. Some notes on the theory of flutter. *Arch Inst Cardiol de Mexico.* 1948;18:177–187.
4. Zaikin AN, Zhabotinsky AM. Concentration wave propagation in two-dimensional liquid-phase self-oscillating system. *Nature.* 1970;225:535–537.
5. Winfree AT, Strogatz SH. Organizing centres for three-dimensional chemical waves. *Nature.* 1984;311:611–615.
6. Davidenko JM, Pertsov AM, Salomonsz R, Baxter W, Jalife J. Stationary and drifting spiral waves of excitation in isolated cardiac muscle. *Nature.* 1991;355:349–351.
7. Samie FH, Berenfeld O, Anumonwo J, et al. Rectification of the background potassium current: a determinant of rotor dynamics in ventricular fibrillation. *Circ Res.* 2001;89:1216–1223.
8. Katz AM. *Physiology of the Heart.* 5th ed. Wolters Kluwer; 2011.

9. Zykov VS. *Simulation of Wave Processes in Excitable Media.* Manchester: Manchester University Press; 1987.
10. Efimov IR, Krinsky VI, Jalife J. Dynamics of rotating vortices in the Beeler-Reuter model of cardiac tissue. *Chaos, Solitons and Fractals.* 1995;5:513–526.
11. Qu Z, Xie F, Garfinkel A, Weiss J. Origins of spiral wave meander and breakup in a two-dimensional cardiac tissue model. *Ann Biomed Eng.* 2000;28:755–771.
12. Ten Tusscher KH, Noble D, Noble PJ, Panfilov AV. A model for human ventricular tissue. *Am J Physiol Heart Circ Physiol.* 2004;286:H1573–H1589.
13. Abildskov JA, Lux RL. The mechanism of simulated torsade de pointes in a computer model of propagated excitation. *J Cardiovasc Electrophysiol.* 1991;2:224–237.
14. Gray RA, Jalife J, Panfilov A, et al. Non-stationary vortex-like reentrant activity as a mechanism of polymorphic ventricular tachycardia in the isolated rabbit heart. *Circulation.* 1995;91:2454–2469.
15. Garfinkel A, Qu Z. Nonlinear dynamics of excitation and propagation in cardiac tissue. In: Zipes DP, Jalife J, eds. *Cardiac Electrophysiology: From Cell to Bedside.* 3rd ed. Philadelphia: Saunders; 1999:315–320.
16. Kodama I, Honjo H, Yamazaki M, et al. Optical imaging of spiral waves: pharmacological modification of

spiral-type excitations in a 2-dimensional layer of ventricular myocardium. *J Electrocardiol.* 2005;38:126–130.
17. Ishiguro YS, Honjo H, Opthof T, et al. Early termination of spiral wave reentry by combined blockade of Na⁺ and L-type Ca²⁺ currents in a perfused two-dimensional epicardial layer of rabbit ventricular myocardium. *Heart Rhythm.* 2009;6:684–692.
18. Climent AM, Guillem MS, Fuentes L, et al. The role of atrial tissue remodeling on rotor dynamics: an in-vitro study. *Am J Physiol Heart Circ Physiol.* 2015;309:H1964–H1973.
18a. Harada M, Honjo H, Yamazaki M, et al. Moderate hypothermia increases the chance of spiral wave collision in favor of self-termination of ventricular tachycardia/fibrillation. *Am J Physiol Heart Circ Physiol.* 2008;294:H1896–H1905.
19. Burton FL, Cobbe SM. Dispersion of ventricular repolarization and refractory period. *Cardiovasc Res.* 2001;50:10–23.
20. Liu DW, Antzelevitch C. Characteristics of the delayed rectifier current (IKr and IKs) in canine ventricular epicardial, midmyocardial, and endocardial myocytes. A weaker IKs contributes to the longer action potential of the M cell. *Circ Res.* 1995;76:351–365.

21. Schram G, Pourrier M, Melnyk P, Nattel S. Differential distribution of cardiac ion channel expression as a basis for regional specialization in electrical function. *Circ Res.* 2002;90:939–950.

22. Glukhov AV, Fedorov VV, Lou Q, et al. Transmural dispersion of repolarization in failing and nonfailing human ventricle. *Circ Res.* 2010;106:981–991.

23. Rudenko AN, Panfilov AV. Drift and interaction of vortices in two-dimensional heterogeneous active medium. *Studia Biophysica.* 1983;98:183–188.

24. Ivanitsky G, Krinsky V, Panfilov AV, Tsiganov M. Two regimes of the drift of reverberators in nonhomogeneous active media. *Biofizika.* 1989;34:297–299.

25. Ten Tusscher KH, Panfilov AV. Reentry in heterogeneous cardiac tissue described by the Luo-Rudy ventricular action potential model. *Am J Physiol Heart Circ Physiol.* 2003;284:H542–H548.

26. Sridhar S, Sinha S, Panfilov AV. Anomalous drift of spiral waves in heterogeneous excitable media. *Phys Rev E.* 2010;82:051908/1-051908/5.

27. Defauw A, Kazbanov IV, Dierckx H, Dawyndt P, Panfilov AV. Action potential duration heterogeneity of cardiac tissue can be evaluated from cell properties using Gaussian Green's function approach. *PLoS One.* 2013;8:e79607.

28. Sampson KJ, Henriquez CS. Electrotonic influences on action potential duration dispersion in small hearts: a simulation study. *Am J Physiol Heart Circ Physiol.* 2005;289:H350–H360.

29. Defauw A, Dawyndt P, Panfilov AV. Initiation and dynamics of a spiral wave around an ionic heterogeneity in a model for human cardiac tissue. *Phys Rev E Stat Nonlin Soft Matter Phys.* 2013;88:062703.

30. Defauw A, Vandersickel N, Dawyndt P, Panfilov AV. Small size ionic heterogeneities in the human heart can attract rotors. *Am J Physiol Heart Circ Physiol.* 2014;307:H1456–H1468.

31. Kohl P, Day K, Noble D. Cellular mechanisms of cardiac mechanoelectric feedback in a mathematical model. *Can J Cardiol.* 1998;14:111–119.

32. Kohl P, Hunter PJ, Noble D. Stretch-induced changes in heart rate and rhythm: clinical observations, experiments and mathematical models. *Prog Biophys Mol Biol.* 1999;71:91–138.

33. Garny A, Kohl P. Mechanical induction of arrhythmias during ventricular repolarization: modeling cellular mechanisms and their interaction in two dimensions. *Ann N Y Acad Sci.* 2004;1015:133–143.

34. Li W, Kohl P, Trayanova N. Induction of ventricular arrhythmias following mechanical impact: a simulation study in 3D. *J Mol Histol.* 2004;35:679–686.

35. Weise LD, Panfilov AV. New mechanism of spiral wave initiation in a reaction-diffusion mechanics system. *PLoS One.* 2011;6; e27264/1–e27264/9.

36. Jie X, Gurev V, Trayanova N. Mechanisms of mechanically induced spontaneous arrhythmias in acute regional ischemia. *Circ Res.* 2010;106:185–192.

37. Hill AV. Excitation and accommodation in nerve. *Proc R Soc London.* 1936;119:305–355.

38. Hodgkin AL, Huxley AF. A quantitative description of membrane current and its application to conduction and excitation in nerve. *J Physiol.* 1952;117:500–544.

39. Panfilov AV, Keldermann RH, Nash MP. Drift and breakup of spiral waves in reaction–diffusion–mechanics systems. *Proc Natl Acad Sci U S A.* 2007;104:7922–7926.

40. Keldermann RH, Nash MP, Gelderblom H, Wang VY, Panfilov AV. Electromechanical wavebreak in a model of the human left ventricle. *Am J Physiol Heart Circ Physiol.* 2010;299:H134–H143.

41. Hu Y, Gurev V, Constantino J, Bayer JD, Trayanova NA. Effects of mechano-electric feedback on scroll wave stability in human ventricular fibrillation. *PLoS One.* 2013;8:e60287.

42. Agladze KI, Davydov VA, Mikhailov AS. An observation of resonance of spiral waves in distributed excitable medium. *JETP Lett.* 1987;45:767–769.

43. Panfilov AV, Müller SC, Zykov VS, Keener J. Elimination of spiral waves in cardiac tissue by multiple electrical shocks. *Phys Rev E.* 2000;61:4644–4647.

44. Biktashev VN, Holden AV. Design principles of a low voltage cardiac defibrillator based on the effect of feedback resonant drift. *J Theor Biol.* 1994;169:101–112.

45. Weise LD, Panfilov AV. A discrete electromechanical model for human cardiac tissue: effects of stretch-activated currents and stretch conditions on restitution properties and spiral wave dynamics. *PLoS One.* 2013;8; e59317/1–e59317/13.

46. Dierckx H, Arens S, Li BW, Weise LD, Panfilov AV. A theory for spiral wave drift in reaction-diffusion-mechanics systems. *New J Phys.* 2015;17;043055/1-043055/20.

47. de Jong S, van Veen TA, van Rijen HV, de Bakker JM. Fibrosis and cardiac arrhythmias. *J Cardiovasc Pharmacol.* 2011;57:630–638.

48. Nguyen TP, Qu Z, Weiss JN. Cardiac fibrosis and arrhythmogenesis: the road to repair is paved with perils. *J Mol Cell Cardiol.* 2014;70:83–91.

49. Panfilov AV, Keener JP. Effects of high frequency stimulation in excitable medium with obstacle. *J Theor Biol.* 1993;163:439–448.

50. Agladze KI, Keener JP, Müller SC, Panfilov AV. Rotating spiral waves created by geometry. *Science.* 1994;264:1746–1748.

51. Majumder R, Pandit R, Panfilov AV. Turbulent electrical activity at sharp-edged inexcitable obstacles in a model for human cardiac tissue. *Am J Physiol Heart Circ Physiol.* 2014;307:H1024–H1035.

52. Panfilov AV. Spiral breakup in an array of coupled cells: the role of the intercellular conductance. *Phys Rev Lett.* 2002;88:118101.

53. Ten Tusscher KH, Panfilov AV. Influence of diffuse fibrosis on wave propagation in human ventricular tissue. *Europace.* 2007;9:v138–v145.

54. Zlochiver S, Munoz V, Vikstrom KL, Taffet SM, Berenfeld O, Jalife J. Electrotonic myofibroblast-to-myocyte coupling increases propensity to reentrant arrhythmias in two-dimensional cardiac monolayers. *Biophys J.* 2007;95:4469–4480.

55. Alonso S, Bär M, Panfilov AV. Effects of reduced discrete coupling on filament tension in excitable media. *Chaos.* 2011;21; 013118/1-013118/7.

56. Alonso S, Bär M. Reentry near the percolation threshold in a heterogeneous discrete model for cardiac tissue. *Phys Rev Lett.* 2013;110:158101.

57. Kazbanov IV, Ten Tusscher KH, Panfilov AV. Effects of heterogeneous diffuse fibrosis on arrhythmia formation. *Sci Rep.* 2016;6:20835.

58. Vandersickel N, Masaya Watanabe M, Tao Q, Fostier J, Zeppenfeld K, Panfilov AV. Attraction of arrhythmia sources by fibrotic regions via dynamical anchoring. *J Physiology.* Under revision.

59. McDowell KS, et al. Virtual electrophysiological study of atrial fibrillation in fibrotic remodeling. *PLoS One.* 2015;10(2):e0117110.

60. Gonzales MJ, Vincent KP, Rappel WJ, Narayan SM, McCulloch AD. Structural contributions to fibrillatory rotors in a patient-derived computational model of the atria. *Europace.* 2014;16(suppl 4):iv3–iv10.

61. Ashihara T, et al. The role of fibroblasts in complex fractionated electrograms during persistent/permanent atrial fibrillation: implications for electrogram-based catheter ablation. *Circ Res.* 2012;110:275–284.

62. Cabo C, Pertsov AM, Davidenko J, Jalife J. Electrical turbulence as a result of the critical curvature for propagation in cardiac tissue. *Chaos.* 1998;8:116–126.

63. Cabo C, et al. Vortex shedding as a precursor of turbulent electrical activity in cardiac muscle. *Biophys J.* 1996;70:1105–1111.

64. Keener JP. The dynamics of three-dimensional scroll waves in excitable media. *Physica D.* 1988;31:269–276.

65. Biktasheva IV, Biktashev VN. Wave-particle dualism of spiral waves dynamics. *Phys Rev E Stat Nonlin Soft Matter Phys.* 2003;67:026221.

66. Biktashev VN, Holden AV, Zhang H. Tension of organizing filaments of scroll waves. *Phil Trans R Soc Lond A.* 1994;347:611–630.

67. Mikhailov AS, Davydov VA, Zykov VS. Complex dynamics of spiral waves and motion of curves. *Physica D.* 1994;70:1–39.

68. Henry H, Hakim V. Scroll waves in isotropic excitable media: linear instabilities, bifurcations, and restabilized states. *Phys Rev E.* 2002;65:046235.

69. Verschelde H, Dierckx H, Bernus O. Covariant string-like dynamics of scroll wave filaments in anisotropic cardiac tissue. *Phys Rev Lett.* 2007;99:168104.

70. Dierckx H, Verschelde H, Selsil Ö, Biktashev VN. Buckling of scroll waves. *Phys Rev Lett.* 2012;109(17):174102.

71. Dierckx H, Verschelde H. Effective dynamics of twisted and curved scroll waves using virtual filaments. *Phys Rev E.* 2013;88:062907.

72. Henry H. Spiral wave drift in an electric field and scroll wave instabilities. *Phys Rev E.* 2004;70:026204.

73. Biktashev VN, Barkley D, Biktasheva IV. Orbital motion of spiral waves in excitable media. *Phys Rev Lett.* 2010;104:058302.

74. Biktasheva IV, Barkley D, Biktashev VN, Foulkes AJ. Computation of the drift velocity of spiral waves using response functions. *Phys Rev E.* 2010;81:066202.

75. Dierckx H, Bernus O, Verschelde H. A geometric theory for scroll wave filaments in anisotropic excitable media. *Physica D - nonlinear phenomena.* 2009;238:941–950.

76. Dierckx H, Brisard E, Verschelde H, Panfilov AV. Drift laws for scroll waves on curved anisotropic surfaces. *Phys Rev E.* 2013;88:012908.

77. Biktashev VN, Holden AV. Resonant drift of autowave vortices in 2D and the effects of boundaries and inhomogeneities. *Chaos, Solitons and Fractals.* 1995;5:575–622.

78. Biktasheva IV, Holden AV, Biktashev VN. Localization of response functions of spiral waves in the FitzHugh-Nagumo system. *Int J Bifurcation Chaos.* 2006;16:1547–1555.

79. Beeler GW, Reuter H. Reconstruction of the action potential of ventricular myocardial fibres. *J Physiol.* 1977;268:177–210.

80. Biktashev VN, Biktasheva IV, Sarvazyan NA. Evolution of spiral and scroll waves of excitation in a mathematical model of ischaemic border zone. *PLoS One.* 2011;6:e24388.

81. Dierckx H, Bernus O, Verschelde H. An accurate eikonal-curvature relation for wave fronts in locally anisotropic reaction-diffusion systems. *Phys Rev Lett.* 2011;107:108101.

82. Caldwell BJ, et al. Three distinct directions of intramural activation reveal nonuniform side-to-side electrical coupling of ventricular myocytes. *Circ Arrhythm Electrophys.* 2009;2:433–440.

83. Schalij MJ, Boersma L, Huijberts M, Allessie MA. Anisotropic reentry in a perfused 2-dimensional layer of rabbit ventricular myocardium. *Circulation.* 2000;102:2650–2658.

84. Wellner M, Berenfeld OM, Jalife J, Pertsov AM. Minimal principle for rotor filaments. *Proc Natl Acad Sci U S A.* 2002;99:8015–8018.

85. Ten Tusscher KH, Panfilov AV. Eikonal formulation of the minimal principle for scroll wave filaments. *Phys Rev Lett.* 2004;93:108106.

86. Young RJ, Panfilov AV. Anisotropy of wave propagation in the heart can be modeled by a Riemannian electrophysiological metric. *Proc Natl Acad Sci U S A.* 2010;107:15063–15068.

87. Wellner M, Zemlin C, Pertsov AM. Frustrated drift of an anchored scroll wave filament and the geodesic principle. *Phys Rev.* 2010;82:036122.

88. Dierckx H, Wellner M, Bernus O, Verschelde H. Generalized minimal principle for rotor filaments. *Phys Rev Lett.* 2015;114:178104.

89. Streeter DD, Spotnitz MM, Patel DP, Ross Jr J, Sonnenblick EH. Fiber orientation in the canine left ventricle during diastole and systole. *Circ Res.* 1969;24:339–347.

90. Kuramoto Y. Instability and turbulence of wavefronts in reaction-diffusion systems. *Prog Theor Phys.* 1980;63:1885–1903.

91. Keener JP. A geometrical theory for spiral waves in excitable media. *Siam J Appl Math.* 1986;46:1039–1056.

92. Keener JP. An eikonal equation for action potential propagation in myocardium. *J Math Biol.* 1991;29:629–651.

93. Franzone PC, Guerri L, Tentoni S. Mathematical modeling of the excitation process in myocardial tissue: influence of fiber rotation on wavefront propagation and potential field. *Math Biosci.* 1990;101:155–235.

94. Misner CW, Thorne KS, Wheeler JA. *Gravitation.* New York: W.H. Freeman and Co; 1973.

95. Zemlin CW, Pertsov AM. Bradycardic onset of spiral wave re-entry: structural substrates. *Europace.* 2007;9:59–63.

96. Kudryashova NN, Teplenin AS, Orlova YV, Selina LV, Agladze K. Arrhythmogenic role of the border between two areas of cardiac cell alignment. *J Mol Cell Cardiol.* 2014;76:227–234.

97. Kudryashova NN, Kazbanov IV, Panfilov AV, Agladze K. Conditions for waveblock due to anisotropy in a model of human ventricular tissue. *PLoS One.* 2015;10:e0141832.

98. Rogers JM, McCulloch AD. Nonuniform muscle fibre orientation causes spiral wave drift in a finite element model of cardiac action potential propagation. *J Cardiovasc Electr.* 1994;5:496–509.

99. Davydov VA, Morozov VG, Davydov NV, Yamaguchi T. Propagation of autowaves in excitable media with chiral anisotropy. *Phys Lett A.* 2004;325:334–339.

100. Davydov VA, Manz N, Steinbock O, Zykov VS, Müller SC. Excitation fronts on a periodically modulated curved surface. *Phys Rev Lett.* 2000;85:868–871.

101. Davydov VA, Zykov VS, Yamaguchi T. Drift of spiral waves on non-uniformly curved surfaces. *Macromol Symp.* 2000;160:99–106.

102. Barkley D. A model for fast computer simulation of waves in excitable media. *Physica D.* 1991;49:61–70.

35 Computational Approaches for Accurate Rotor Localization in the Human Atria

Omer Berenfeld

Experimental and clinical data from our laboratory support the hypothesis that both acute and persistent atrial fibrillation (AF) in the sheep, and in some groups of human patients, is not random. Studies analyzing the spatiotemporal organization of waves and dominant frequency (DF) in the isolated sheep heart demonstrate that AF maintenance in this model depends on localized reentrant, or "rotor," sources in the left atrium (LA) and fibrillatory conduction in their periphery.[1–6] Subsequent translational studies analyzing the organization of DFs in human AF suggested that in paroxysmal AF, reentrant AF sources were localized primarily to the LA posterior wall near the pulmonary veins (PVs), but elsewhere in persistent AF.[7–11] More direct evidence for the presence and role of rotors in driving human AF has been recently provided in numerous invasive[12–14] and noninvasive[15,16] mapping studies. Several of these studies showed that AF could be eliminated by directly ablating AF-driving sources that exhibit high-frequency periodic activity, based on either electrogram visual analysis, dominant frequency analysis, or panoramic endocardial mapping.[8–10,12–14,17–19] These results demonstrated that AF ablation based on a target-specific strategy aimed at eliminating localized sources, whether identified as rotors, focal discharges, or high frequency sites, is at least as efficacious as and safer than empirically isolating all the PVs.

Nevertheless, controversies regarding the particular role of rotors as a mechanism underlying AF maintenance persist[20,21] and may arise as a result of different mapping and processing methods.[22] Thus the focus of this chapter is to present and discuss computational methods for better understanding of the localization of rotors with optical and electrical methods. The chapter begins with a brief mechanistic description of the rotor, followed by phase- and frequency-domain approaches used to enhance the accuracy in the understanding of rotor dynamics in AF. The chapter then illustrates and discusses the application of the phase and frequency approaches in optical mapping in a sheep model of AF and in noninvasive mapping of patients with AF. Better understating and localization of rotors responsible for AF maintenance will arguably help design the most suitable ablation strategy for each individual AF patient.

The Action Potential Rotor

Cardiac muscle belongs to a class of systems called "excitable media" because each of its component cells can switch between bistable states designated as resting and excited (action potential) electrical potential states. When cells are coupled to form a two- or three-dimensional (2D or 3D, respectively) syncytium, the governing electrical, diffusion, and biochemical principles of such a system render them capable of generating action potential waves that may self-organize and swirl continuously, forming vortices, which are termed rotors.[23–25] Fig. 35.1 reproduces one of the first ever visualized rotors in cardiac tissue.[26] Fig. 35.1A, taken from an optical mapping experiment, shows selected snapshots of action potential depolarizations (*white*) forming a periodic wave front with a full-cycle phase spectrum pivoting around a phase singularity point (SP) in space that is otherwise an ordinary normal point like any other point in the medium.[23] In Fig. 35.1B, a time–space plot along a line crossing the center of the rotation in Fig. 35.1A (*red line*) together with superimposed traces at various times to illustrate the fact that the area around the SP is characterized with a low-amplitude activity that remains unexcited although it is eminently excitable.[27] Such an area is known generally as the core of the rotor as illustrated in the diagram of Fig. 35.1C, which represents a counterclockwise spinning rotor with a characteristic isopotential activation front whose velocity decreases as the wave front curvature increases with decreased distance from the core. At the point of critical curvature, the propagation of the action potential is blocked and only electrotonically mediated depolarizing currents invade the core region. The unexcited core exerts in return an electrotonic-repolarizing influence on the excited regions within its immediate surroundings, acting to reduce their action potential amplitude and duration. The closer such regions are to the center, the briefer the repolarization will be. In fact, at the point of critical curvature the action potential duration (APD)-shortening effect is such that the wave front and the wave tail merge. Thus a unique feature of rotors, one that distinguishes them from so-called "anatomical reentry" (i.e., reentry around an inexcitable center), is the fusion of the wave front with its repolarizing tail.[28] Front–tail fusion at the SP is the basis for the identification and localization of rotors in the heart.

In practice, rotor localization is difficult. As illustrated in Fig. 35.1, the voltage near the rotor SP can be very small in comparison with the action potential amplitude, and in addition the center of rotation may meander and drift. Therefore marking the activations for rotor localization might be inaccurate. Spatiotemporal characterization and localization of rotors can, however, be markedly enhanced by analyzing separately the instantaneous and stationary properties that are derived from analyses of the phase and the frequency domains, respectively, as discussed in the following sections.

Phase Representation of the Action Potential Time Course

In 1998 Gray and colleagues introduced a unique phase mapping algorithm that markedly enhanced the characterization of

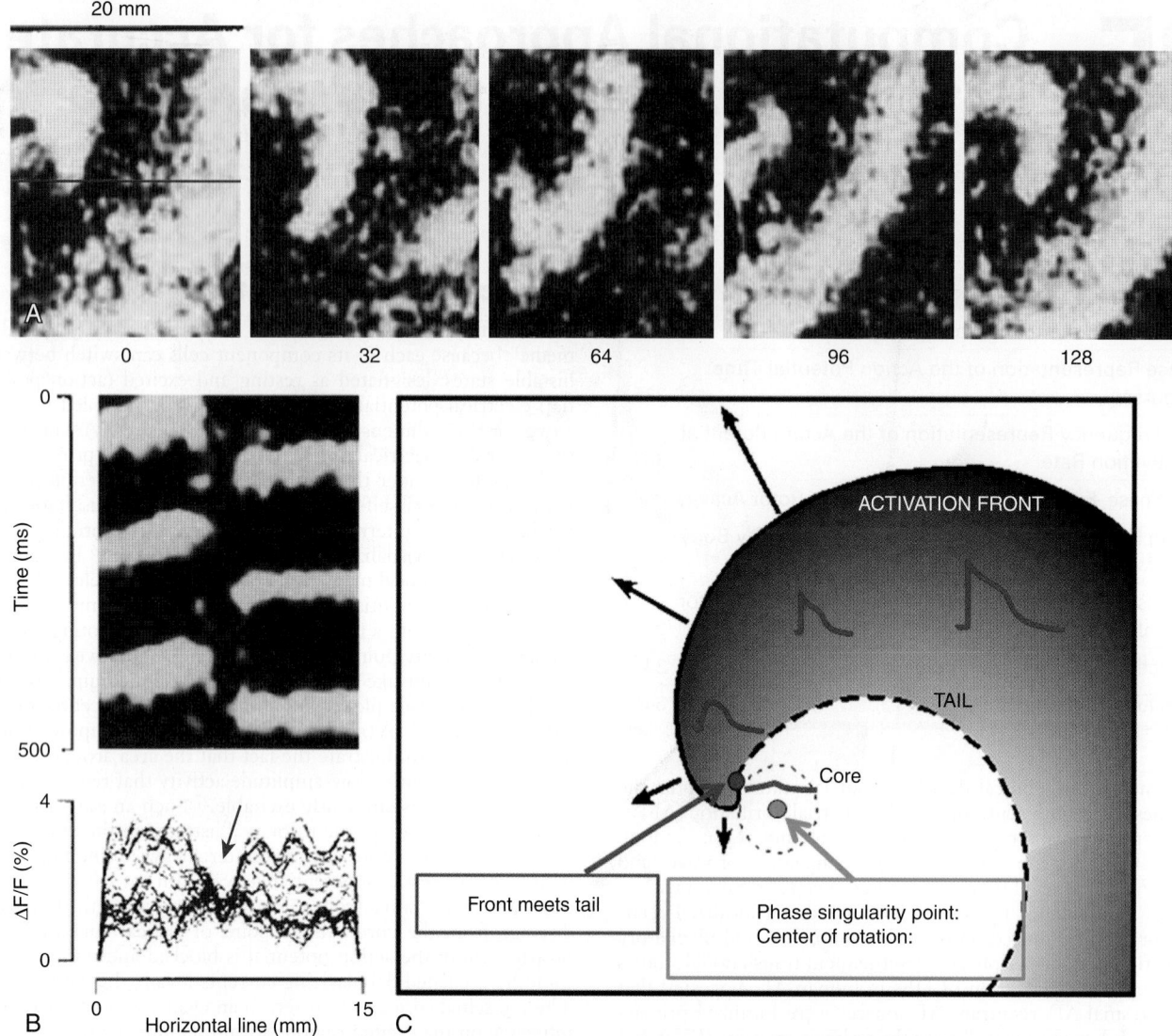

FIGURE 35.1 Rotor in optical mapping (the gold standard) and low amplitude at the core region. (A) A clockwise-rotating rotor in canine epicardial muscle shown in optical mapping of voltage-sensitive fluorescence (F). *White,* Maximal depolarization; *black,* resting potentials; numbers, time in ms. (B) *Top:* time–space plot of F along a line (*red line*) through the center of the core of a stationary rotor as shown in (A). *Bottom:* superimposed 50 traces of ΔF/F during about six rotations from top. (C) A diagram of a counterclock rotor showing an isopotential wave front and repolarization tail rotating around a functional core (*dashed circle*). The point where the wave front fuses with the repolarization (*red*) and the center of rotation (*green*) are marked. Arrows' lengths indicate conduction velocity level. Action potentials (*red traces*) illustrate reduction in duration and amplitude from the periphery of the rotor toward its core center. ([A] and [B] Modified from Davidenko JM, Pertsov AV, Salomonsz R, et al. Stationary and drifting spiral waves of excitation in isolated cardiac muscle. *Nature.* 1992;355:349-351.)

complex spatiotemporal patterns of cardiac fibrillation.[29] Transmembrane signal derived from the fluorescence of a potentiometric dye recorded by each pixel location of a high-resolution video camera focused on the ventricular epicardium exhibited repetitive action potentials, each of which was transformed into a quasi-closed trajectory in 2D phase–space that could be represented by its phase.[29] Accordingly, since the action potential recorded by a single pixel during fibrillation is a function of time, the fluorescence of each pixel at time t, $F(t)$, was plotted against the fluorescence of the same pixel offset by a time interval τ, $F(t-\tau)$. A cyclic return map of $F(t)$ vs. $F(t-\tau)$ was constructed that allowed the phase of the action potential sequence, $\theta(t)$, to be defined as the angle of the coordinate $x = F(t)$ and $y = F(t-\tau)$ in

a 2D fluorescence space around the mean fluorescence for that given pixel, with repeating values between 0 and 2π (or between 0 and 360 degrees), represented as a continuous color scheme.[29–32] The value of the time lag τ is chosen such that the phase can be uniquely specified during the course of a wave rotation. In nonlinear dynamics, an optimal choice of τ for such a task is one that minimizes the mutual dependence of the two variables.[33] Thus the value of τ can be chosen such that it is the lowest lag that significantly minimizes the correlation between $F(t)$ and $F(t-\tau)$.[32] However, the above criterion is difficult to implement, as it needs to be evaluated separately for each signal. The simple possibility for minimizing the correlation by selecting the lag time τ to be a quarter of the average interbeat interval[32] is also hampered

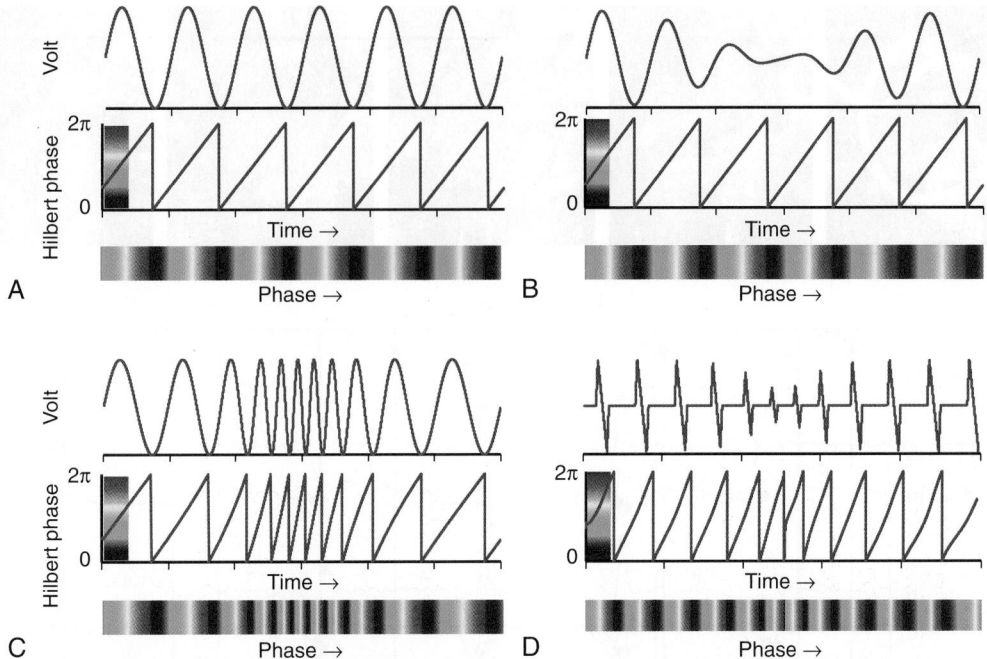

FIGURE 35.2 Phase representation of the action potential using the Hilbert transform. Top traces are simulated traces of voltage and bottom traces are the phases of the voltage time series (between 0 and 2π or between 0 and 360 degrees) calculated with the Hilbert transform. Horizontal color bars are the time course phase representation of the voltage time series. (A) Harmonic voltage wave with fixed amplitude and frequency shows a fixed periodic increase in phases from blue to red. (B) A harmonic voltage wave with a fixed frequency and a significant transient amplitude reduction shows a periodic phase time course independent of the amplitude alteration. (C) A harmonic voltage wave with fixed amplitude and a transient acceleration in frequency shows a corresponding transient acceleration in the periodicity of the phase time course. (D) A unipolar-like voltage wave with a transient reduction in amplitude and acceleration shows the corresponding phase time course that is not affected by the altered morphology and amplitude of the voltage wave.

because of the variability in the frequency content of the signals during fibrillation. Fortunately, the Hilbert transform automatically provides an optimal $F(t-\tau)$ counterpart for $F(t)$, enabling the most reliably possible phase calculation of the action potential sequences, regardless of their varying frequency content.

Fig. 35.2 presents a few examples demonstrating the performance and robustness of the Hilbert transform approach in resolving the time course phase of quasi-periodic signals. In Fig. 35.2A, a simulated harmonic wave with a constant frequency and amplitude, shown in the upper trace, is subject to Hilbert transform and phase calculation, as shown in the lower trace. The time course of the phase is seen to repeat its linear increase between 0 and 2π radians (or between 0 and 360 degrees), which can be color coded and displayed as a color bar time series (bottom). Fig. 35.2B reproduces a similar processing on a wave simulated to have a constant frequency and a transient but significant amplitude reduction, such as that expected near the pivoting point of a rotor, as shown in Fig. 35.1. As can be appreciated by the phase trace and color-coded time series at the bottom, the phase calculation based on the Hilbert transform is not affected by the transient amplitude reduction and displays the correct phase time course as in Fig. 35.2A. Fig. 35.2C demonstrates that the Hilbert transform correctly calculates the instantaneous phase even when the frequency in not constant. Fig. 35.2D shows the calculation of the Hilbert-based phase of a signal that is simulated to have not only transient alterations in amplitude and frequency, but also a nonharmonic morphology that is more comparable to surface electrical unipolar recordings. As can be appreciated, the calculated phase time course accurately follows the simulated cycles even in this case, showing the robustness of the method. Despite the examples shown in Fig. 35.2 supporting the utilization of the

Hilbert-based phase calculation, it should be noted that the interpretation of the phase as the stage of the action potential cycle in experimental and clinical cases is not always straightforward. The interpretation could benefit from additional processing and filtering justified on physiological grounds, as will be demonstrated below.

The Frequency Representation of the Action Potential Activation Rate

The local activation rate is widely used to characterize the stationary organization of the arrhythmia and as a guide to localize and terminate AF sources by ablation.[8,34] As such, reliable assessment of the activation rate is important for accurate detection and study of rotors in AF. The activation rate can be determined either as the average cycle length (CL), in the time domain, or the dominant frequency (DF), in the frequency domain, of the local time-course activation. Thus we have performed a systematic investigation into the question of whether the assessment of the activation time is more reliable in the time or the frequency domain.[35]

We mapped AF in an isolated sheep heart using our custom-built optical system simultaneously with a commercial catheter-based electrode (Reflexion Spiral, Model 402804, St. Jude Medical, St. Paul, MN) and recording system (EnSite NavX, St. Jude Medical), as shown in Fig. 35.3A. Please note that the CCD camera of the optical system cannot give simultaneous information at the exact same location where the electrical signals are recorded because the tissue is masked by the circular electrode. Therefore to increase reliability of the correlation between optical and electrical data, we performed comparisons only in five

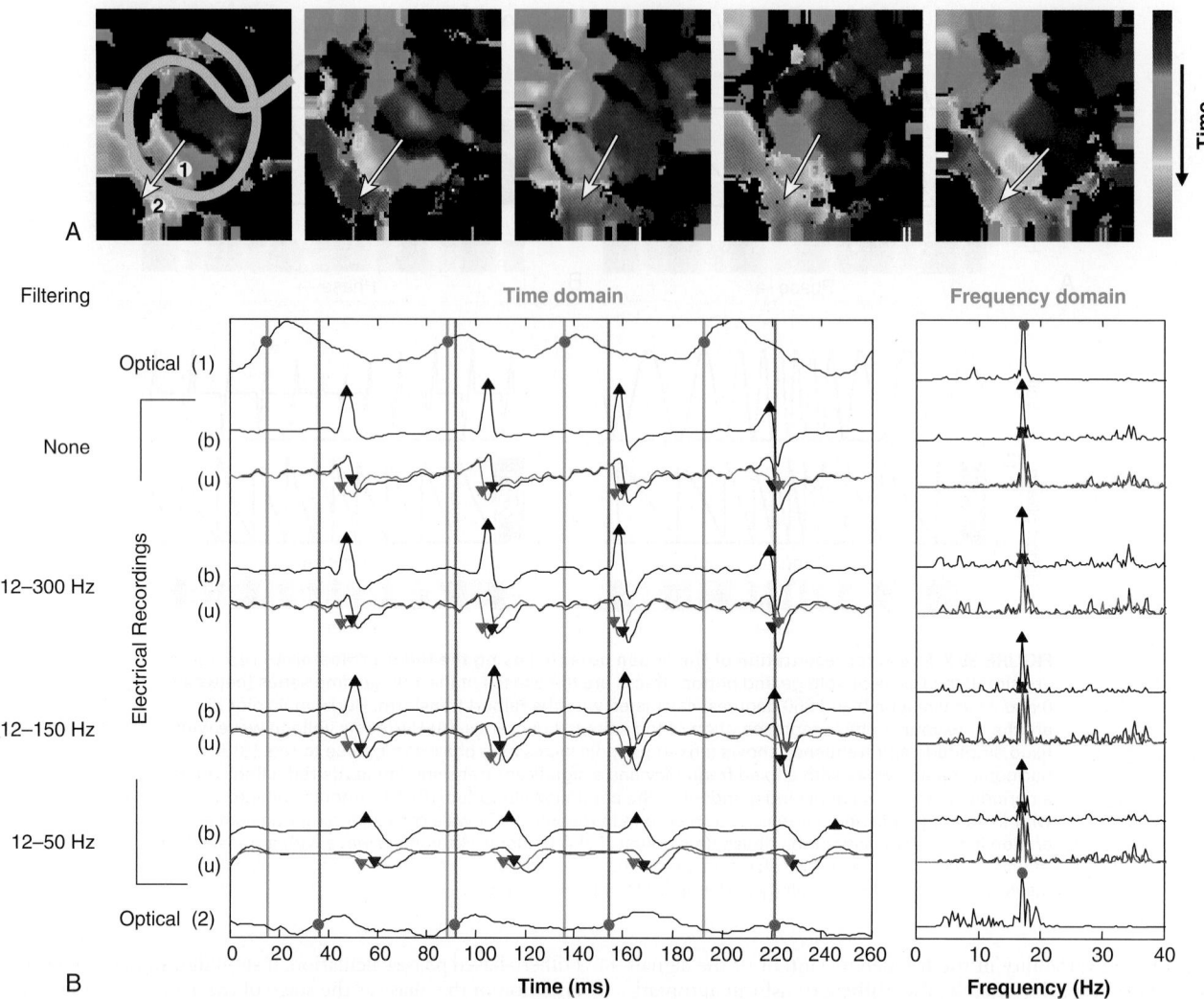

FIGURE 35.3 Comparison between optical and electrical mapping. (A) Activation maps during atrial fibrillation showing sample sequential waves propagating in the direction of the white arrow and crossing the circular catheter (*superimposed gray shade*) near electrodes 11 and 12 in this animal. Sites 1 and 2 in the left-most panel indicate pixels used for optical data analysis and correlation with electrode signals. (B) Sample comparison between simultaneous nearby optical (*top and bottom*) and electrical (*middle: u,* unipolar; *b,* bipolar) time and frequency analysis. *Left:* sample 260-ms episode showing spatiotemporal periodicity during atrial fibrillation. *Red circles* = activation times of optical signals; *red and blue triangles* = activation times of the unipolar signals; *black triangles* = activation times of the corresponding bipolar signals; *green line* = activation times of pixel 1 (*top*); *purple line* = activation time of pixel 2 (*bottom*). *Right:* corresponding power spectra of 5-second-long signals including the episodes shown on left. *Circles and triangles* = dominant-frequency peaks (*blue triangles are overlapped by red triangles*). (Modified from Berenfeld O, Ennis S, Hwang E, et al. Time- and frequency-domain analyses of atrial fibrillation activation rate: the optical mapping reference. *Heart Rhythm.* 2011;8:1758-1765.)

5-second-long episodes showing AF waves that traveled repeatedly on the two opposing sides of the catheter with a relatively fixed interbeat interval for four or more cycles (i.e., waves exhibiting spatiotemporal periodicity, STP). These waves included some that traveled uninterruptedly either across or in parallel with the catheter to allow interpolation of the optical data with the electrical signals from the catheter that masked the tissue underneath. Fig. 35.3A shows an example of such STP waves: Five (out of eight observed) sequential impulses are shown to cross (*white arrows*) the circular catheter (*gray outline*) at about 6 to 7 o'clock. Waves traveling on the two sides of the catheter, but parallel to it, were also identified but are not shown here. In most cases, the STPs during the AF episode did not last for the entire 5-second duration of the recording, but rather they altered their patterns.

Superimposed on the leftmost activation map of Fig. 35.3A are two markers indicating locations selected for pixel signals used in the comparison with the electrical recordings. Fig. 35.3B shows 260-millisecond-long samples out of 5-second-long time series and their corresponding power spectra obtained simultaneously from optical and electrical recordings in a pair of flanking pixels and a pair of electrodes between the pixels. The top and bottom traces are signals from the pixels marked in the activation map. They show the typical oscillatory feature of activation during fibrillation, as detected by fluorescence mapping. These optical traces flank electrical recordings from the catheter electrodes between the two pixels. All electrical traces correspond to the same location and timing, but were grouped for the four different processing routines employed: unprocessed

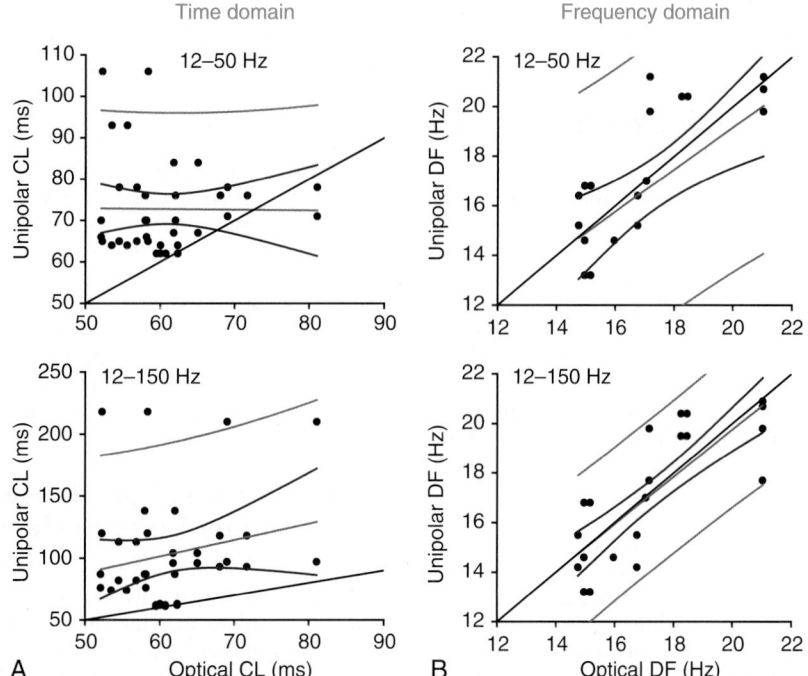

FIGURE 35.4 Correlations of activation rate assessments in the time (A) and frequency (B) domains between electrical and optical recordings during atrial fibrillation in five isolated sheep hearts. (A) Correlation of unipolar and optical cycle length (*CL*) for 12–50 Hz (*top*, n = 40) and 12–150 Hz (*bottom*, n = 38) filtering. (B) Correlation of unipolar and optical dominant frequency (*DF*) for 12–50 Hz (*top*, n = 28) and 12–150 Hz (*bottom*, n = 28) filtering. Line colors: *black*, unity; *red*, best fit; *blue*, 95% confidence; *purple*, 95% predictable scatter boundaries. (Modified from Berenfeld O, Ennis S, Hwang E, et al. Time- and frequency-domain analyses of atrial fibrillation activation rate: the optical mapping reference. *Heart Rhythm.* 2011;8:1758-1765.)

signal (None) and the 12–300, 12–150, and 12–50 Hz bandpass filtering modes.

The traces in Fig. 35.3B are marked with detected activation times. For the optical traces, the 50% amplitude level was marked down as the activation (*red circles with green and purple vertical lines*). For the electrical unipolars and bipolars, the time of activation was determined here as the minimal time-derivative (*red and blue triangles*) and maximal deflection (*black triangles*), respectively. Comparing the four main unipolar and bipolar deflections in Fig. 35.3B, one notices a general qualitative correspondence to the fluorescence deflections. However, differences become evident when considering the activation times: only the fourth electrical activation coincides with the optical activation (*green and purple vertical lines*, except 12–50 Hz filter) while the other waves appear more delayed. Note also that, as more aggressive filtering is applied (i.e., from None, to 12–300, 12–150, and finally 12–50 Hz), the activation times are progressively delayed relative to the camera pixels, suggesting that different filtering modes introduce different phase shifts into the analyzed signals. Overall, in 81% of waves analyzed in four different animals during 5-second-long episodes of AF, the 12–50 Hz filtering setting results in delayed activation time detection by the bipolars relative to the corresponding pixels. The best coincidence between maximal voltage activation times of bipolars and optical signals was obtained with the 12–300 Hz filtering setting. However, only about 35% of the bipolar waves were fully concordant with the flanking pixels. In about 37% of waves, the bipolars activated earlier and in 28% of waves, they activated later than the flanking pixels, often within the same recording.

The automatic 5-second average CLs for the signals exemplified in Fig. 35.3B ranged as follows: optical signals, 60–71 ms; unipolars, 55–65 ms; and bipolars, 60–76 ms. The corresponding power spectra shown at the right-hand side of Fig. 35.3B, in

contrast, presented an invariable DF of 17 Hz (59 ms) for all the signals. The origin of the variability in relative activation timing and rates may be related to complex spatiotemporal patterns of activation in the small area comprising the pixels, the two recording unipolars, and/or different noise handling. In any event, the same variability may underlie discrepancies between electrical versus optical and time versus frequency methods shown further below and may become important when using one type of recordings and analysis as a reference.

From the foregoing description, it is evident that the correlation between time and frequency domain measurements is different for the electrical versus the optical data analyzed. To further understand that discrepancy, the performance of the time- and frequency-domain analyses was studied separately in the electrical versus optical modalities. Fig. 35.4 presents analysis for the same areas as in Fig. 35.3. The unipolar signals included those subjected to 12–50 and 12–150 Hz filtering modes to test for the possible effect of phase shifts on the analysis. Fig. 35.4A shows the time–domain analysis comparing the CL of the activity in the unipolars and the optical signals. The identity y = x line falls mostly outside the 95% confidence interval for both filtering modes with respective adjusted R^2 values of –0.03 and 0.02, leading to the conclusion that the average CL of the unipolars does not correlate with the average CL of the optical data. Fig. 35.4B shows the frequency–domain analysis. In contrast to the CL correlations, the 95% confidence interval of the unipolar–optical DF correlation includes the identity relationship y = x for both filtering modes. The DF adjusted R^2 value of 0.68 for 12–150 Hz filtering is higher than the value of 0.31 for 12–50 Hz filtering ($p < .001$), and both DF adjusted R^2 values are higher than those of the CL ($p < .001$). Altogether, our comparisons of electrical vs. optical correlations demonstrate that the DF dispersion determined for both unipolar and bipolar signals follows the dispersion of the optical signals closer than the average CL dispersion.[35] In particular, the DF of unipolar signals is more reliable than the average CL for measuring the local activation rate during AF.

The Phase–Frequency Domain Analysis of Rotor Activity

The key requirement to be able to detect rotors is to process effectively the dynamic spatiotemporal fibrillation process in each space and time point; the space–phase processing of a quasi-periodic time series is designed to accomplish precisely that. Fig. 35.5 shows a diagram of a mapping setup with a demonstration of a combined frequency–phase domain analysis of AF waves in isolated, but intact, sheep heart experiments of AF.[36] Fig. 35.5A shows the configuration of the setup with epicardial and endocardial CCD cameras for simultaneous mapping the left atrial appendage (LAA) and posterior LA (PLA), respectively. Following the transformation of the time series of each pixel signal recorded by the cameras into the phase domain, a new phase field, θ(t), is produced over all pixels in the mapped areas, as shown in Fig. 35.5B. The snapshots in Fig. 35.5B correspond to activity at selected time points during AF and show a dynamic process of continuously changing wave patterns in which the upstroke of the action potential, and hence the activation wave front, is represented by the color *green*, while the plateau of the action potential corresponds to the colors *red* and *yellow*. The refractory tail of the action potential corresponds to the colors *blue* and *purple*. In particular, phase SPs which were defined as the points where all phases converged to[23,32] indicate the presence of reentrant activity in the PLA at 0–301 ms snapshots and then in the LAA at the 301–541 ms snapshots.

To further establish the role of the patterns of activation underlying the DF values in the PLA and the LAA, we used phase movies to compare the number of waves leaving versus entering the mapped PLA region (1-second-long segments). Data from five hearts at 10-minute intervals demonstrated that the number

of waves propagating outward consistently exceeded those propagating inward (6.6 ± 0.2 versus 2.9 ± 0.2, respectively; $p < .05$).[36] In addition, rotors and breakthroughs in the PLA were analyzed by counting the total number of rotations/cm^2 (regardless of lifespan of rotors) and breakthroughs/cm^2 in 2-second-long segments. Whether those breakthroughs are the surface expression of intramural reentrant activity is not certain but is possible.[37] As soon as the rotor enters in the LAA field of view, the patterns of activation there switch from breakthroughs to reentry and the drifting rotor becomes the main source driving the AF. Fig. 35.5C shows the DF maps at periods when the LAA rotor activates its surroundings (left), and thereafter when the rotor abandoned the LAA (right). Concomitant transition in the highest DF (HDF) values from the PLA to the LAA when the rotor appears in the LAA area (8.7 Hz) and a reduction to 7.4 Hz once the rotor disappears further confirm the essential role of LAA rotor in this AF episode.[36]

Torso Reduces Sensitivity of Rotor Detection by Body Surface Mapping

The dynamics of the body surface SPs depend dramatically on the HDF-filtering, which calls for extreme caution when interpreting body surface phase map interpretation.[15] Unfortunately, the ability to derive inferences from simultaneous recordings of AF in the atrial cavities and the body surface is limited, leading us to rely on computer simulations for assistance. To guide processing and interpretation of the recorded body surface potentials, we simulated the electric potentials behavior on a computerized model of the atria within the torso during various impulse propagation episodes with different patterns. This approach enabled derivation of testable predictions about the manifestation of atrial reentrant activity on both the internal volume and the torso surface. We constructed a generic atria-torso model consisting of a spherical shell of active tissue, representing the atria, within a passive torso modeled as a uniform volume conductor bounded by a spherical

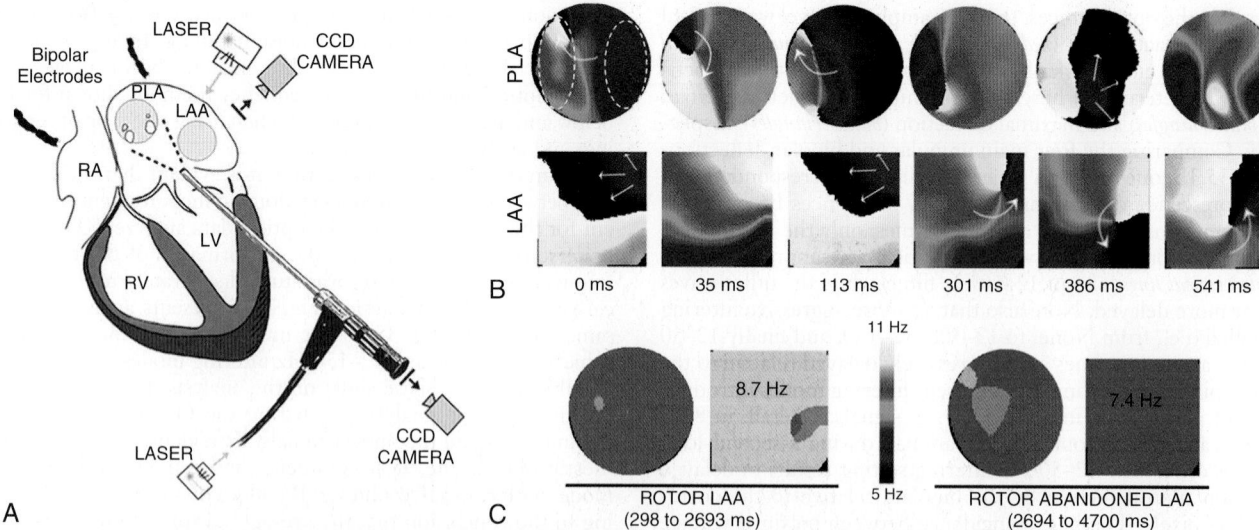

FIGURE 35.5 Patterns of activation in the posterior left atrium (*PLA*) and left atrial appendage (*LAA*) of isolated hearts during atrial fibrillation in a sheep. (A) Ex vivo epicardial and endocardial mapping setup includes synchronized dual charge-coupled device (*CCD*) cameras, as well as bipolar electrodes placed in the right atrium (*RA*) and the roof of the left atrium. Bipolar signals are also obtained from the pulmonary veins. (B) Snapshots from a phase movie show a rotor appearing in the field of view of the LAA. The patterns of activation switch from breakthroughs (0–113 ms) to a meandering rotor (301–541 ms). (C) The highest dominant frequency is in the LAA when the rotor stays in the field of view and goes back to PLA when the rotor drifts outside the LAA. *RA,* Right atrium; *RV,* right ventricle. (Modified from Filgueiras-Rama D, Price NF, Martins RP, et al. Long-term frequency gradients during persistent atrial fibrillation in sheep are associated with stable sources in the left atrium. *Circ Arrhythm Electrophysiol.* 2012;5:1160-1167.)

surface with no-flux conditions (Fig. 35.6A).[15] The electrical potential resulting from the wave propagation simulated on the atrial sphere was studied everywhere on 20 concentric spheres by using the Boundary Element Method. The potentials on the outermost sphere, defined as the torso surface, and in the internal layers were analyzed to characterize the time course of the potential distribution everywhere; in particular, the patterns and time course of the phase SPs everywhere resulting from atrial rotors were characterized. (It is important to note that the phase analysis here is performed on a time series of potentials in the volume conductor torso that result from action potentials in the atria, but not on the time series of the action potentials themselves.) To increase reliability of SP detection in 3D space, the phase values were obtained along three different circles in the three different main planes surrounding each evaluated point[31]; an evaluated point was defined as an SP only when the phase of each of at least two of these closed paths was gradually and monotonically increasing or decreasing for a total of 2π. A filament was defined as the connection between SPs across spherical layers that lasted at least one full rotation.[15]

We explored the effect of the torso on the ability to detect body surface rotors. Fig. 35.6 reproduces simulation results from a model with two regions of equal size in the LA, one representing normal tissue and the other representing fibrotic tissue. The epicardial activity (left-most row) consisted of an LA rotor with a stable SP and a much more disorganized activity with several unstable SPs in the fibrotic area. The latter appeared progressively more organized with distance from the epicardium (Fig. 35.6B). Fig. 35.6C explains why the body surface is seen as more

organized in comparison with the atrial epicardial surface; most of the filaments in the torso originate at SPs involving a small piece of fibrotic tissue and do not originate at the driving rotor. As can be seen, spatial smoothing stabilizes filaments and eliminates all but a single filament pair reaching the surface. To understand how the filaments originating on the epicardium disappear inside the torso, the filaments were color coded according to their chirality. Fig. 35.6C clearly shows that filaments are continuous and do not vanish inside the passive volume conductor; rather a filament does not reach the surface once it joins its counterrotating neighbor. Overall, mutual cancelation of filament pairs reduces the average number of SPs at increasing distances from the epicardium (Fig. 35.6D). At the outermost layer, only two SPs can be observed: one which is the "true" SP and another that we term the "mirror" SP which appears following the extinction of SPs at the fibrotic area and the extension of the stable LA rotor filament to the contralateral aspect of the torso. Mutual cancellation of filaments can indeed result in a failure to detect "true" SPs originating at small atrial areas; an effect that may be counteracted by the HDF filtering, as shown below.

Highest Dominant Frequency-Filtering Effect on Rotor Localization

Frequency analysis, and in particular the highest HDF, are reliable[35,38] and important in the mechanistic interpretation of the role of rotors in AF.[15] We therefore utilized the same computer model shown in Fig. 35.6A to study the effect of the HDF bandpass filtering on the detection of rotor activity. Fig. 35.7 shows analysis

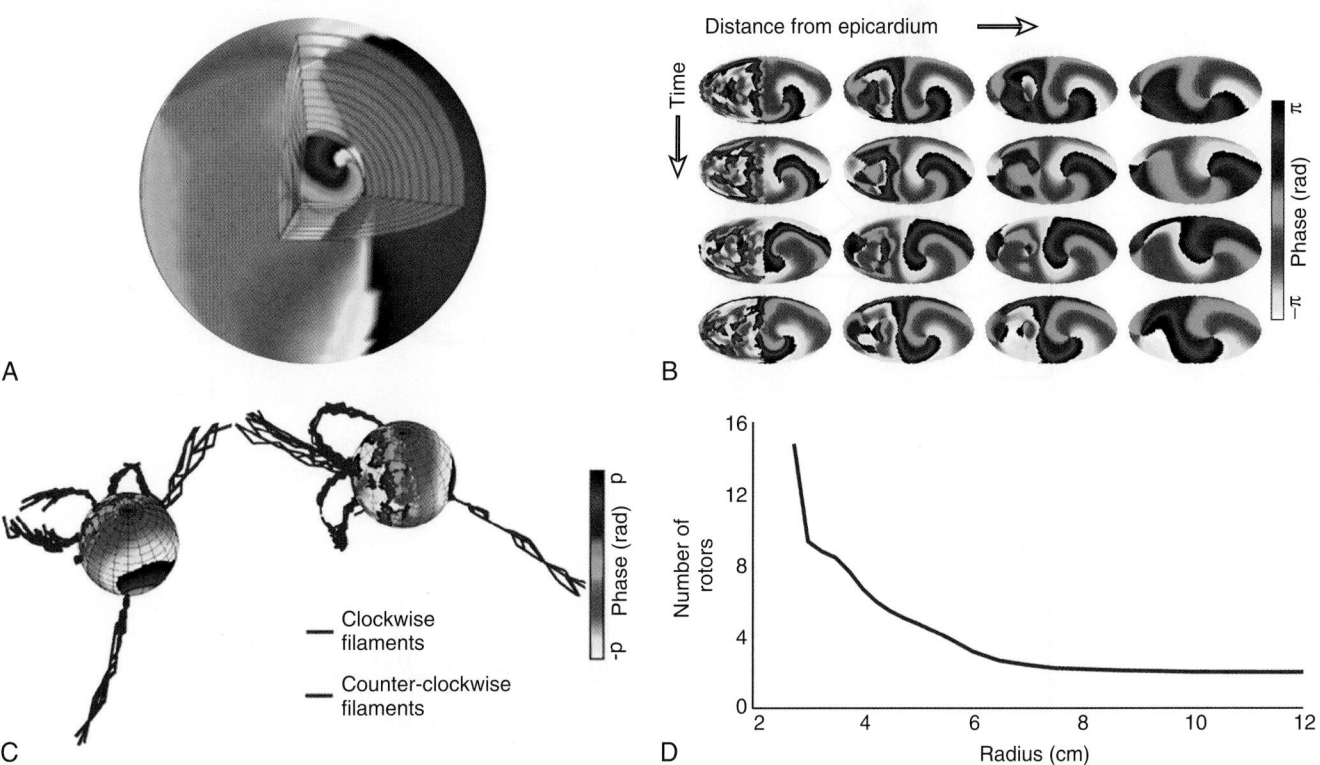

FIGURE 35.6 A simulation of the natural filtering of the rotors filaments by the torso. (A) The model combining concentric spheres of the atria and the torso. (B) Phase maps at four time instants (*top to bottom*) in four concentric layers from the atria to the torso surface (*left to right;* each ellipse is an open representation of a spherical layer) showing the phase maps of simulated epicardial and consequential layers activity. The simulated activity was of a diving rotor in a left atrium–like hemisphere and fibrotic right atrial hemisphere model. (C) Phase map of epicardial sphere and distribution of filaments (*clockwise rotations in blue; counterclockwise rotations in red*) inside the torso during 10 ms simulation. (D) Average number of rotors per distance from the epicardium. ([B] to [D] from Rodrigo M, Guillem MS, Climent AM, et al. Body surface localization of left and right atrial high-frequency rotors in atrial fibrillation patients: a clinical-computational study. *Heart Rhythm.* 2014;11:1584-1591.)

of the results of a simulation in which a single functional rotor in an LA-like hemisphere was spinning at 7.2 Hz, while the RA-like hemisphere was passively activated at a lower frequency (3.9 Hz). Fig. 35.7A shows the phase map on the epicardium, and it shows the time courses of filaments extending to the torso from the LA rotor and a wavebreak SP at the LA–RA interface for unfiltered potentials. Note that both filaments exhibit strong deflections in their trajectory to the torso. The deflection angle of the filaments before HDF filtering is not stationary over time, and instead the filaments' trajectories inscribe wide conic outlines. However, after HDF filtering (Fig. 35.7B), filaments became stable and their deflections were significantly reduced to follow straight paths

from the epicardium to the body surface. We hypothesize that the HDF-filtering stabilizing effect on the filament is via the minimization of the influence of the atrial activity that is not activated at the HDF. To corroborate such a hypothesis, all the RA dipoles were summed into a single equivalent dipole and its vector projection was plotted on the RA–LA interface (Y, Z) plane (Fig. 35.7C). In addition, the trajectory of the body surface SP that was originated by the stable LA rotor projection on the same (Y, Z) plane was plotted. Fig. 35.7E–F show the match in the time course and rotation frequency between the RA equivalent dipole rotation and the SP trajectory. Accordingly, we conclude that SPs arising at the interface between LA and RA as a consequence of abrupt changes

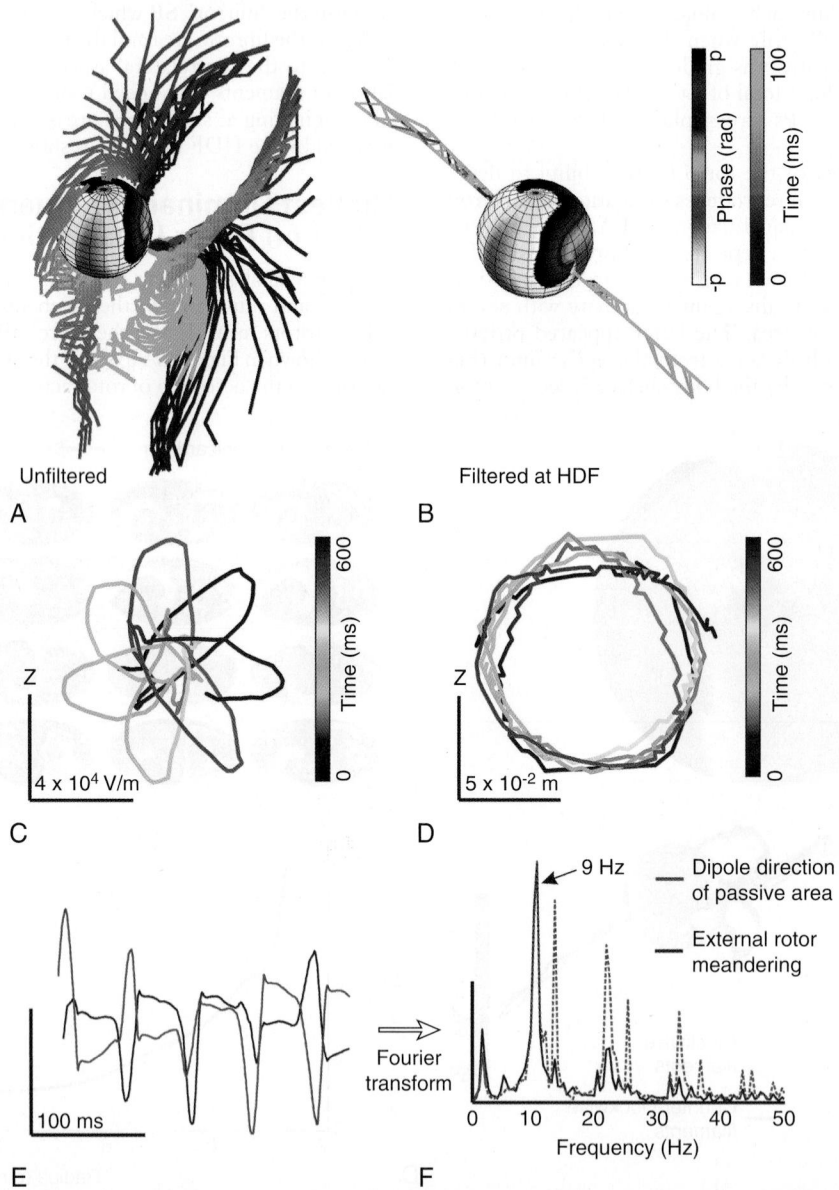

FIGURE 35.7 Highest dominant frequency (*HDF*) filtering to highlight driving rotor in a simulation of a fast and stable rotor in a left atrium–like hemisphere and unstable wavebreak at the hemispheres' interfaces. (A) and (B) Phase maps of the epicardial spheres and temporal configurations of filaments inside the torso for unfiltered potentials (A) and for HDF-filtered (B) potentials. (C) Tracking of the surface singularity point that arises from the stable rotor without HDF filtering. (D) Tracking of the direction of the far field dipole produced by the nonrotor right atrial hemisphere on the YZ plane (virtual interface plane). (E) and (F) Temporal evolution and spectral distribution of the Y coordinate for panels (C) and (D). (Modified from Rodrigo M, Guillem MS, Climent AM, et al. Body surface localization of left and right atrial high-frequency rotors in atrial fibrillation patients: a clinical-computational study. *Heart Rhythm.* 2014;11:1584-1591.)

in propagation direction that reached the outermost layer disappear after HDF filtering, since their activation frequencies did not match with the HDF. In addition, we note that, as in the case of Fig. 35.6C, a mirror filament appears with opposite direction and chirality as compared with the true rotor originating at the SP on the LA epicardium. The respective relations of the mirror and the true SPs with the driving rotor will be discussed below.

Detection of Driving Rotors in Body Surface Mapping

Mathematically, rotors, as well as reentries in general, appear always in pairs such that their summed topological charge is zero.[39] Thus either the torso natural low-pass filtering (see Fig. 35.6) or the HDF bandpass filtering (see Fig. 35.7) would result in a couple of SPs on the mapped surface if the AF is associated with either rotors or anatomical reentry. The dynamics and role of the paired rotors in driving a tachyarrhythmia is however not necessarily equal; while one of the rotors may be spinning at a fast frequency and driving the arrhythmia, its counterpart may be unstable and rotating more slowly. We termed the SP linked to the former as the "true" and to the latter as the "mirror." Fig. 35.8A illustrates the concept of true and mirror rotor filaments. The atrial activity in Fig. 35.8A consists of a stable and fast LA rotor with a fixed SP and an unstable wavebreak with unstable SP at the interface of the LA hemisphere with the slower activity at

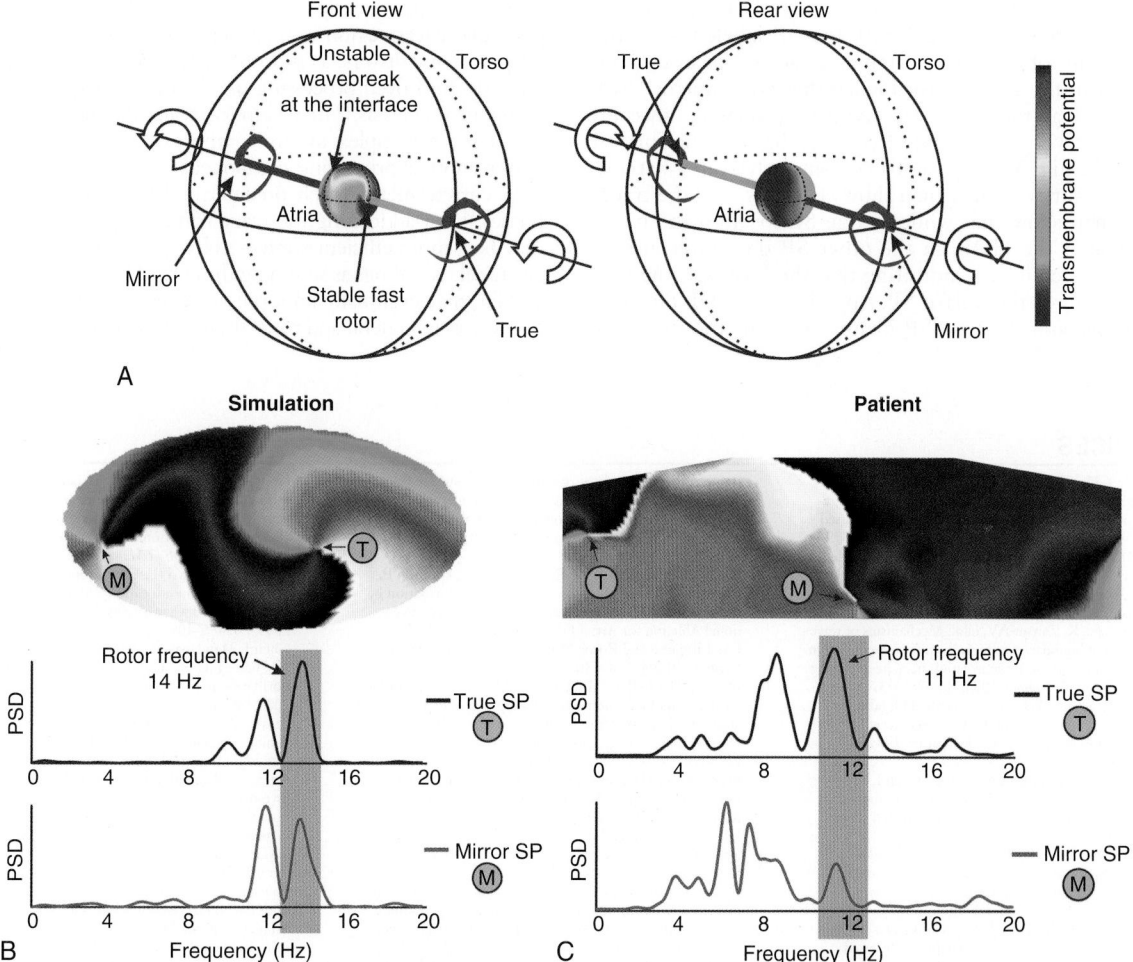

FIGURE 35.8 The role of the surface reentries is determined by their power spectra. (A) A diagram demonstrating the concept of true and mirror surface singularity points (*SP*) at surface phase maps. The figure shows two opposing viewpoints of a simulated activity in a model that includes atrial tissue, torso volume, and torso surface. Atrial voltage maps are represented according to a color scale from blue to red. The atrial activity consists of a stable and fast rotor with a fixed SP and an unstable wavebreak with unstable SP at the interface of the left atrial hemisphere, with the slower activity at the right atrial hemisphere. Upon bandpass filtering of the surface data at the frequency of the stable left atrial rotor, two stable reentries (*red* wavefont patterns on the surface of the torso are the pivoting rotors with the chirality indicated by the *circular arrows*) with two fixed SPs become visible on the torso surface; one is termed the true (*T, green filament*) SP and the other the mirror SP (*M, blue filament*) based on the trajectory of the filament connecting them with the source atrial rotor. (B) Surface phase map in a half left atrial and half fibrotic atrial model (see Fig. 35.6) and power spectra of surface potentials at the true rotor location (*blue, T*) and at the mirror rotor location (*red, M*). (C) Surface phase map after highest dominant frequency filtering from a patient during atrial fibrillation and power spectra of surface potentials before the filtering at the true rotor location (*blue, T*) and at the mirror rotor location (*red, M*). *PSD,* Power spectral density. (From Rodrigo M, Guillem MS, Climent AM, et al. Body surface localization of left and right atrial high-frequency rotors in atrial fibrillation patients: a clinical-computational study. *Heart Rhythm.* 2014;11:1584-1591.)

the RA hemisphere. Upon bandpass filtering of the surface data at the frequency of the stable LA rotor, two stable reentries with two fixed SPs become visible on the torso surface; one is termed the true SP and the other the mirror SP, based on the trajectory of the filament connecting them with the source atrial rotor. The true SP is connected to the source rotor directly (*green filament*), and the mirror SP is connected to the source rotor intersecting the contralateral atrial wall (*blue filament*), whereas no stable rotor at the frequency of the LA rotor is present (see rear view panel on the right side).

The discrimination between true and mirror rotors can be performed based on the spectral properties of surface recordings at the HDF. Fig. 35.8B shows a surface phase map with two SPs that resulted from HDF filtering of a simulation with only one stable rotor (see Fig. 35.6). The SP labeled T is the endpoint of the filament that connects directly to the epicardial SP (hence the label "true" SP); the SP labeled M is the surface endpoint of a filament originating at the epicardial wall contralateral to the stable rotor (hence the term "mirror" SP). On the phase map these SPs seem undistinguishable; however, the spectral power at the rotor frequency band is maximal at the "true" SP. Fig. 35.8C shows a similar analysis in a patient. The patient's surface phase map shows two SPs, and the traces below the map show that while in one SP location the maximal power is at the HDF, in the other SP the power at that frequency is much lower, indicating that the former is the true SP and the latter is the mirror SP. Applying the HDF filtering, phase analysis, and the true-SP identification method to body surface mapping data, we localized driving rotors in about 70% of the AF time in 14 patients to either the LA or RA.[15]

Concluding Remarks

AF ablation should aim at terminating rotor or reentrant activity, and therefore it is important to localize rotors as precisely as possible. As rotors come in pairs, the strategy should be to target both, even if one of them is faster than the other. Knowing the frequency of the rotor helps localize it, so to localize more than the fastest rotor at the HDF, it would be necessary to know the rotation frequency of all SPs, which may be a difficult task requiring reliable panoramic information with high resolution and fidelity. Despite many recent advances in AF mapping, the current electrical recording systems may not be sufficient to characterize every AF case to identify ablation targets, particularly in those cases in which AF waves are complex, the driver region is very small, or if the atrial substrate can support many drivers, as is probably the case in long-lasting persistent AF. Improved processing of AF waves, such as with principal component analysis,[40] may help to extract the meaningful information from a complex dynamic. Improved automatic detection of SPs is another processing component of the localization that may help; current methods rely on deterministic closed-path integrals of phases,[31] but addressing the fuzzy nature of the SP trajectories[41,42] may be a more efficient strategy. However, the basic nature of the electrical recordings as summing the contribution of all sources, near and far, may eventually limit our accuracy in characterizing fibrillation waves in general and rotor drivers in particular.

REFERENCES

1. Berenfeld O, Mandapati R, Dixit S, et al. Spatially distributed dominant excitation frequencies reveal hidden organization in atrial fibrillation in the Langendorff-perfused sheep heart. *J Cardiovasc Electrophysiol*. 2000;11:869–879.
2. Berenfeld O, Zaitsev AV, Mironov SF, Pertsov AM, Jalife J. Frequency-dependent breakdown of wave propagation into fibrillatory conduction across the pectinate muscle network in the isolated sheep right atrium. *Circ Res*. 2002;90:1173–1180.
3. Kalifa J, Tanaka K, Zaitsev AV, et al. Mechanisms of wave fractionation at boundaries of high-frequency excitation in the posterior left atrium of the isolated sheep heart during atrial fibrillation. *Circulation*. 2006;113:626–633.
4. Mandapati R, Skanes A, Chen J, Berenfeld O, Jalife J. Stable microreentrant sources as a mechanism of atrial fibrillation in the isolated sheep heart. *Circulation*. 2000;101:194–199.
5. Mansour M, Mandapati R, Berenfeld O, Chen J, Samie FH, Jalife J. Left-to-right gradient of atrial frequencies during acute atrial fibrillation in the isolated sheep heart. *Circulation*. 2001;103:2631–2636.
6. Skanes AC, Mandapati R, Berenfeld O, Davidenko JM, Jalife J. Spatiotemporal periodicity during atrial fibrillation in the isolated sheep heart. *Circulation*. 1998;98:1236–1248.
7. Atienza F, Martins RP, Jalife J. Translational research in atrial fibrillation: a quest for mechanistically based diagnosis and therapy. *Circ Arrhythm Electrophysiol*. 2012;5:1207–1215.
8. Atienza F, Almendral J, Jalife J, et al. Real-time dominant frequency mapping and ablation of dominant frequency sites in atrial fibrillation with left-to-right frequency gradients predicts long-term maintenance of sinus rhythm. *Heart Rhythm*. 2009;6:33–40.
9. Atienza F, Almendral J, Moreno J, et al. Activation of inward rectifier potassium channels accelerates atrial fibrillation in humans: evidence for a reentrant mechanism. *Circulation*. 2006;114:2434–2442.
10. Sanders P, Berenfeld O, Hocini M, et al. Spectral analysis identifies sites of high-frequency activity maintaining atrial fibrillation in humans. *Circulation*. 2005;112:789–797.
11. Atienza F, Calvo D, Almendral J, et al. Mechanisms of fractionated electrograms formation in the posterior left atrium during paroxysmal atrial fibrillation in humans. *J Am Coll Cardiol*. 2011;57:1081–1092.
12. Miller JM, Kowal RC, Swarup V, et al. Initial independent outcomes from focal impulse and rotor modulation ablation for atrial fibrillation: multicenter FIRM registry. *J Cardiovasc Electrophysiol*. 2014;25:921–929.
13. Narayan SM, Krummen DE, Clopton P, Shivkumar K, Miller JM. Direct or coincidental elimination of

stable rotors or focal sources may explain successful atrial fibrillation ablation: on-treatment analysis of the CONFIRM trial (conventional ablation for AF with or without focal impulse and rotor modulation). *J Am Coll Cardiol*. 2013;62:138–147.
14. Narayan SM, Krummen DE, Shivkumar K, Clopton P, Rappel WJ, Miller JM. Treatment of atrial fibrillation by the ablation of localized sources: CONFIRM (Conventional Ablation for Atrial Fibrillation With or Without Focal Impulse and Rotor Modulation) trial. *J Am Coll Cardiol*. 2012;60:628–636.
15. Rodrigo M, Guillem MS, Climent AM, et al. Body surface localization of left and right atrial high-frequency rotors in atrial fibrillation patients: a clinical-computational study. *Heart Rhythm*. 2014;11:1584–1591.
16. Haissaguerre M, Hocini M, Denis A, et al. Driver domains in persistent atrial fibrillation. *Circulation*. 2014;130:530–538.
17. Dobrev D, Nattel S. New antiarrhythmic drugs for treatment of atrial fibrillation. *Lancet*. 2010;375:1212–1223.
18. Jais P, Haissaguerre M, Shah DC, et al. A focal source of atrial fibrillation treated by discrete radiofrequency ablation. *Circulation*. 1997;95:572–576.
19. Dixit S, Gerstenfeld EP, Ratcliffe SJ, et al. Single procedure efficacy of isolating all versus arrhythmogenic pulmonary veins on long-term control of atrial fibrillation: a prospective randomized study. *Heart Rhythm*. 2008;5:174–181.
20. Narayan SM, Jalife J. Crosstalk proposal: rotors have been demonstrated to drive human atrial fibrillation. *J Physiol*. 2014;592:3163–3166.
21. Allessie MA, de Groot N. Crosstalk opposing view: rotors have not been demonstrated to be the drivers of atrial fibrillation. *J Physiol*. 2014;592:3167–3170.
22. Berenfeld O, Oral H. The quest for rotors in atrial fibrillation: different nets catch different fishes. *Heart Rhythm*. 2012;9:1440–1441.
23. Winfree AT. Electrical instability in cardiac muscle: phase singularities and rotors. *J Theor Biol*. 1989;138:353–405.
24. Winfree AT. Vortex action potentials in normal ventricular muscle. *Ann N Y Acad Sci*. 1990;591:190–207.
25. Winfree AT. Electrical turbulence in three-dimensional heart muscle. *Science*. 1994;266:1003–1006.
26. Davidenko JM, Pertsov AV, Salomonsz R, Baxter W, Jalife J. Stationary and drifting spiral waves of excitation in isolated cardiac muscle. *Nature*. 1992;355:349–351.
27. Athill CA, Ikeda T, Kim YH, et al. Transmembrane potential properties at the core of functional reentrant wave fronts in isolated canine right atria. *Circulation*. 1998;98:1556–1567.
28. Pertsov AM, Davidenko JM, Salomonsz R, Baxter WT, Jalife J. Spiral waves of excitation underlie reentrant activity in isolated cardiac muscle. *Circ Res*. 1993;72:631–650.

29. Gray RA, Pertsov AM, Jalife J. Spatial and temporal organization during cardiac fibrillation. *Nature*. 1998;392:75–78.
30. Bray MA, Wikswo JP. Considerations in phase plane analysis for nonstationary reentrant cardiac behavior. *Phys Rev E Stat Nonlin Soft Matter Phys*. 2002;65:051902.
31. Bray MA, Wikswo JP. Use of topological charge to determine filament location and dynamics in a numerical model of scroll wave activity. *IEEE Trans Biomed Eng*. 2002;49:1086–1093.
32. Chen J, Mandapati R, Berenfeld O, Skanes AC, Gray RA, Jalife J. Dynamics of wavelets and their role in atrial fibrillation in the isolated sheep heart. *Cardiovasc Res*. 2000;48:220–232.
33. Fraser AM, Swinney HL. Independent coordinates for strange attractors from mutual information. *Phys Rev A Gen Phys*. 1986;33:1134–1140.
34. Atienza F, Almendral J, Ormaetxe JM, et al. RADAR-AF investigators. Comparison of radiofrequency catheter ablation of drivers and circumferential pulmonary vein isolation in atrial fibrillation: a noninferiority randomized multicenter RADAR-AF trial. *J Am Coll Cardiol*. 2014;64:2455–2467.
35. Berenfeld O, Ennis S, Hwang E, et al. Time- and frequency-domain analyses of atrial fibrillation activation rate: the optical mapping reference. *Heart Rhythm*. 2011;8:1758–1765.
36. Filgueiras-Rama D, Price NF, Martins RP, et al. Long-term frequency gradients during persistent atrial fibrillation in sheep are associated with stable sources in the left atrium. *Circ Arrhythm Electrophysiol*. 2012;5:1160–1167.
37. Tanaka K, Zlochiver S, Vikstrom KL, et al. Spatial distribution of fibrosis governs fibrillation wave dynamics in the posterior left atrium during heart failure. *Circ Res*. 2007;101:839–847.
38. Guillem MS, Climent AM, Millet J, et al. Noninvasive localization of maximal frequency sites of atrial fibrillation by body surface potential mapping. *Circ Arrhythm Electrophysiol*. 2013;6:294–301.
39. Pertsov AM, Wellner M, Vinson M, Jalife J. Topological constraint on scroll wave pinning. *Phys Rev Lett*. 2000;84:2738–2741.
40. Rabinovitch A, Biton Y, Braunstein D, et al. Singular value decomposition of optically-mapped cardiac rotors and fibrillatory activity. *J Phys D Appl Phys*. 2015;48:095401.
41. Tomii N, Yamazaki M, Arafune T, Honjo H, Shibata N, Sakuma I. Detection algorithm of phase singularity using phase variance analysis for epicardial optical mapping data. *IEEE Trans Biomed Eng*. 2016;63:1795–1803.
42. Seitz J, Bars C, Théodore G, et al. AF Ablation guided by spatiotemporal electrogram dispersion without pulmonary vein isolation: a wholly patient-tailored approach. *J Am Coll Cardiol*. 2017;69:303–321.

36 Modeling the Aging Heart

Natalia A. Trayanova and Patrick M. Boyle

Introduction

The Aging Heart

The aging heart is characterized by a number of morphological and structural changes manifested at the different levels of biological hierarchy.[1] These changes lead to the functional decline of the aging heart and particularly to its diminished ability to meet the increases in demand. The progressive changes in cardiac anatomy and physiology occur even in apparently healthy individuals.[2] Age-dependent remodeling of the heart in healthy populations is predominantly associated with cardiomyocyte (CM) hypertrophy and fibrotic remodeling, accompanied by a decline in diastolic function, as demonstrated by the Framingham Heart Study[3] and the Baltimore Longitudinal Study on Aging.[4]

As reviewed extensively by Biernacka and colleagues,[1] animal model studies provide consistent evidence of aging-related CM hypertrophy accompanied by an increase in myocardial collagen content. Additionally, histological analysis of non-hypertensive aging hearts reveals progressive loss of CMs because of necrotic and apoptotic cell death.[5,6] Animal experiments have also revealed an increased collagen deposition in the aging heart.[7] The findings are similar in human hearts. The aging human heart exhibits a progressive increase in left ventricular (LV) mass despite a reduction in the total myocyte number.[8] Collagen content in the normal human heart increases with age[9]; studies involving human subjects have documented an age-related increase in cardiac fibrosis.[10,11] Furthermore, myocardium from senescent individuals exhibits increased collagen deposition and thicker endomysial and perimysial collagen fibers.[12] Autopsy studies of cardiac tissue from human subjects free of pathological conditions have shown that collagen content increases by almost 50% between the third and seventh decade of life.[9]

The differences between the normal and senescent heart are illustrated in Fig. 36.1. In the normal heart, thin layers of perimysium and endomysium surround myocardial bundles and individual myocytes, respectively. In the senescent heart, there is increased deposition of perimysial and endomysial collagen, referred to as interstitial fibrosis. Interstitial fibrosis initially progresses without myocyte loss and is accompanied by CM hypertrophy as part of an adaptive response aimed at preserving cardiac output while normalizing wall stress. Eventually, however, replacement fibrosis occurs as CMs undergo necrosis and apoptosis.[13] Finally, in the aging heart, there is transition of fibroblasts to myofibroblasts.[1] Fibroblasts primarily regulate collagen turnover in tissues; however, under certain conditions that remain controversial,[14] fibroblasts are activated and undergo phenotypic transition into myofibroblasts, the key effector cells in fibrotic remodeling.

Aging, Arrhythmias, and Fibrotic Remodeling

As described in the preceding section, fibrotic remodeling has been identified as the hallmark of the aging heart. There is a large body of evidence demonstrating that increased fibrotic remodeling in the heart is strongly correlated with an increased incidence of atrial and ventricular tachyarrhythmias and sudden cardiac death.[15–23] While the exact mechanisms of arrhythmogenesis are not fully understood, it is widely believed that impaired electrical conduction plays an important role. Indeed, increased amounts of fibrosis have been found to lead to partial decoupling of myocytes, reduced excitability, unidirectional block,[24,25] conduction slowing, zig-zag course of wave propagation, localized source–sink mismatch, and conduction block,[26,27] and thus in the establishment of arrhythmogenic substrate.[28–31] Furthermore, clinical studies suggest that it is not only just the amount but also the architecture of the fibrosis that is important for arrhythmogenic propensity.[26]

The molecular mechanisms associated with fibrosis are complex,[32] and the spatial patterns of fibrosis vary widely among individuals.[33,34] This has hindered the mechanistic inquiry, and the link between the substrate fibrotic remodeling and reentry dynamics in patients remains elusive. Better understanding of this relationship will increase knowledge of arrhythmia pathophysiology in the aging heart and will help pave the way toward personalized antiarrhythmia treatment planning in patients with fibrotic remodeling.

Computer Modeling as a Tool in Arrhythmia Research

Computer modeling has emerged as a powerful platform for the investigation of heart rhythm disorders. Biophysically detailed simulations can explain experimental observations and help reveal the manner in which the organ-scale arrhythmogenic phenomena (ectopic heartbeats, conduction failure, electrical turbulence, etc.) emerge from pathological effects at the tissue, cell, and protein levels. The development of this extensive "virtual heart" methodology[35–39] has been built on a strong foundation of integration between experiments and simulations. Furthermore, recent advancements in single-cell action potential (AP) modeling have produced building blocks for constructing models of the atria,[40–42] ventricles,[43–46] and cardiac conduction system,[47–51] with unprecedented levels of biophysical detail and accuracy. Such developments have helped to fuel the exciting progress made in simulating cardiac electrical behavior at the organ level.[52–61] Initial progress has also been made in using three-dimensional (3D) cardiac simulations to address problems in clinical practice via studies utilizing clinical imaging of the heart.[62–68] Since the mid-2000s, computer modeling has become an indispensable tool in arrhythmia research.

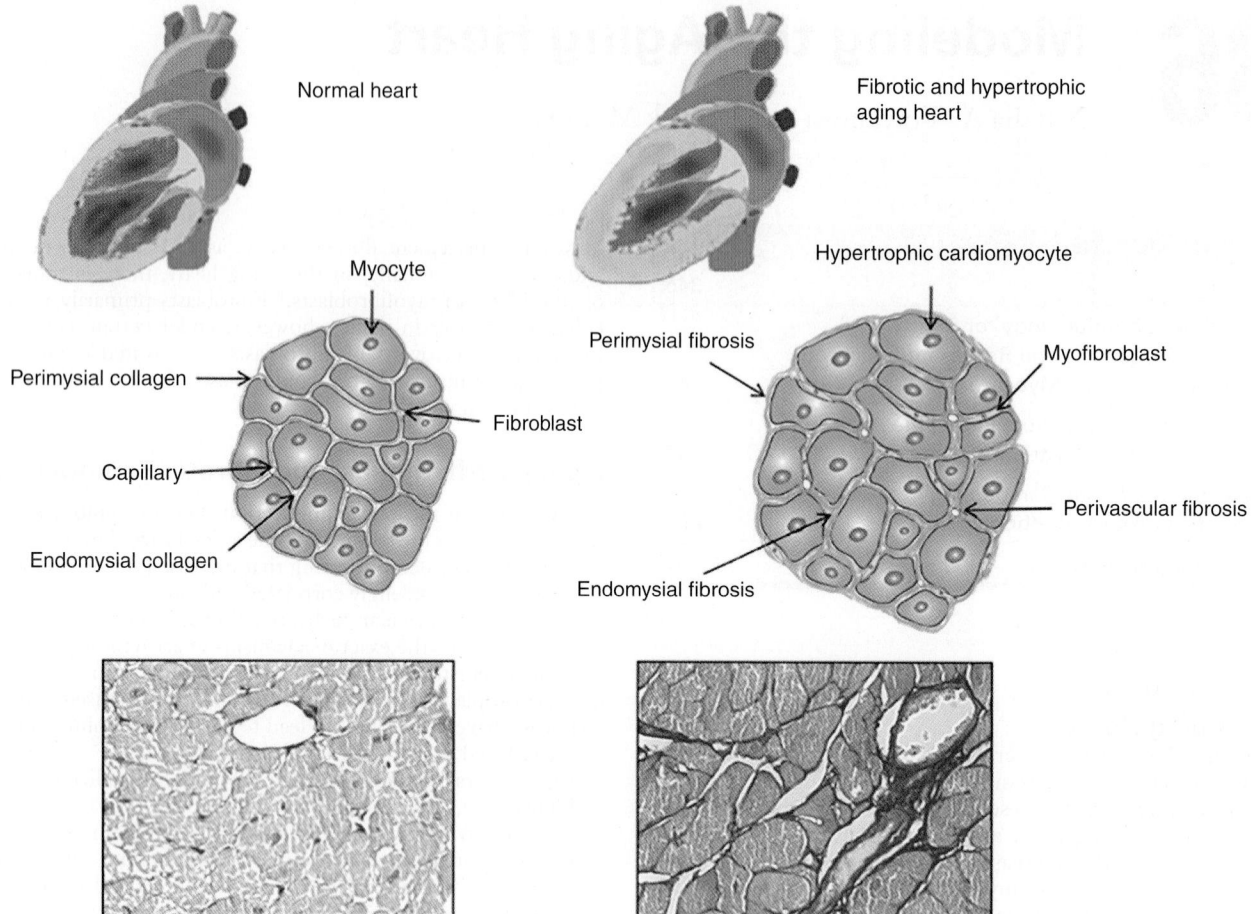

FIGURE 36.1 Age-dependent remodeling of the human heart is highlighted by schematic comparison of normal (*left*) and senescent (*right*) properties of organ size/shape (*top row*) and cardiac tissue properties (*middle row*). Histopathological images (*bottom row*) show remodeled tissue in C57BL/6 mice of different ages (*left*, 2 months old; *right*, 2 years old). Red-stained regions indicate collagenous tissue. (From Biernacka A, Frangogiannis NG. Aging and cardiac fibrosis. *Aging Dis.* 2011;2:158-173.)

Chapter Scope

In this chapter, we review the current state-of-the-art in modeling atrial and ventricular arrhythmogenesis that arises from fibrotic remodeling in the heart, as well as the contributions these modeling studies have made to our understanding of the mechanisms of arrhythmias in the aging heart. Because of the rapid advancement of structural imaging methodologies in cardiac electrophysiology, a larger emphasis is placed on studies that have used such imaging methodologies to construct geometrically realistic structural models of cardiac tissue or the organ itself, where the regional remodeling properties of the myocardium can also be represented in a realistic manner. We emphasize how the acquired knowledge can be used to pave the way for clinical applications of cardiac function modeling under the conditions of fibrotic remodeling.

Overview of Methodology for Simulating Arrhythmogenesis and Representing Fibrotic Remodeling in the Myocardium

Computer modeling of arrhythmogenesis has made enormous progress since the mid-2000s, enabling the simulation of electrical function in cardiac tissue as well as in the entire organ. A schematic of the current state-of-the-art general approach to 3D multiscale (from the molecule to the organ) arrhythmia modeling (atrial or ventricular) is shown in Fig. 36.2A. Ionic exchanges

across cell membranes via ionic channels, pumps, and exchangers, represented by an AP ionic model comprising numerous ordinary differential and algebraic equations, drive current flow in the tissue. In the multiscale atrial or ventricular model, propagation of the wave of AP is simulated by solving[69–71] a reaction-diffusion partial differential equation describing current flow through tissue composed of myocytes that are electrically connected via low-resistance gap junctions. Cardiac tissue has orthotropic passive electrical conductivities that arise from the cellular organization of the myocardium (cardiac muscle) into fibers and laminar sheets. Global conductivity values in the atrial or ventricular model are obtained by combining fiber and sheet organization with myocyte-specific local conductivity values.

Local fiber directions are typically mapped on the basis of histological sectioning information[72,73] or on diffusion tensor magnetic resonance imaging (DTMRI),[74] sometimes using an atlas heart.[75] The *left panel* of Fig. 36.2B presents fiber orientation, as reconstructed from DTMR images, in the canine ventricles shown in Fig. 36.2A. In cases where neither histological nor DTMRI information is available, rule-based approaches have been used to assign fiber orientation consistent with measurements, either manually or using a semiautomatic rule-based approach.[76–79] This particularly applies to atrial fiber orientation (see Fig. 36.2B, *right panel*) because DT imaging of the thin atrial walls has yet to provide reliable information about atrial fiber architecture.

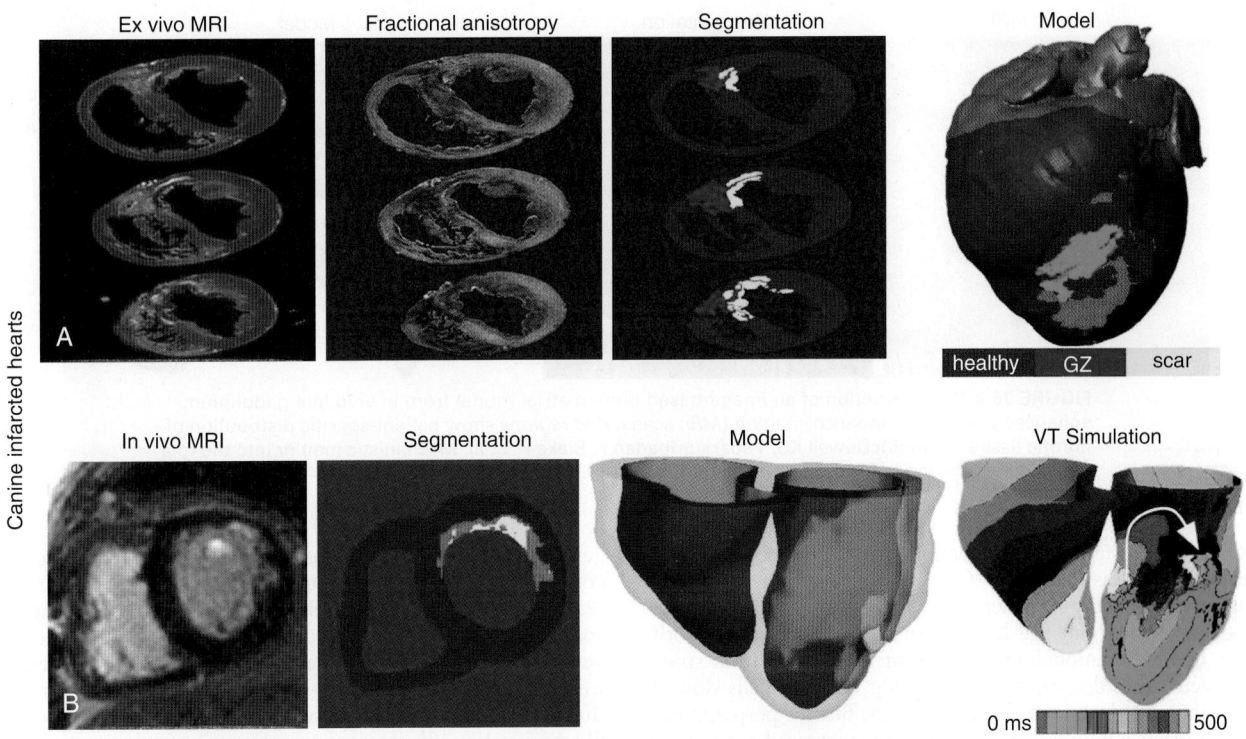

Ex vivo MRI	Fractional anisotropy	Segmentation	Model

Canine infarcted hearts

A

healthy   GZ   scar

In vivo MRI	Segmentation	Model	VT Simulation

B

0 ms   500

FIGURE 36.2 Schematic representation of the approach to image-based cardiac modeling, including (A) representation of electrophysiological features at the cell, tissue, and organ scales and (B) incorporation of myocardial fiber orientations. Bioelectric impulses initiated at the cellular level (action potentials) propagate at the tissue level because of syncytial coupling of cardiomyocytes via gap junctions. Three-dimensional models of the canine heart (*left*) and human atria (*right*) shown here were reconstructed according to the approaches described by Arevalo et al.[67] and Krueger et al.,[76] respectively. *MRI*, Magnetic resonance imaging; *VT*, ventricular tachycardia. (From Trayanova NA, Boyle PM, Arevalo HJ, et al. Exploring susceptibility to atrial and ventricular arrhythmias resulting from remodeling of the passive electrical properties in the heart: a simulation approach. *Front Physiol.* 2014;5:435; and Arevalo H, Plank G, Helm P, et al. Tachycardia in post-infarction hearts: insights from 3D image-based ventricular models. *PLoS One.* 2013;8:e68872.)

The electrical properties of the myocardium in the models (see Fig. 36.2A) can be regionally altered to represent fibrosis, with regional changes represented in various models: (1) changes in gap junction resistance between cells, resulting in changes in conductivity values; (2) deposition of collagen, forming either local resistive barriers between fibers or replacing myocytes; and (3) proliferation of myofibroblasts, which may or may not interact with CMs electrically.

Multiscale models of arrhythmias are typically modular, allowing the use of any cellular ionic models, of different species and have different levels of biophysical detail. Furthermore, solutions are executed on user-specified organ geometries, which can be two-dimensional (2D) or 3D, and are idealized or anatomically accurate, the latter representing either averaged geometries obtained from histological sectioning[72,73] or the geometry and structure of individual hearts (atria and/or ventricles).[67,80–82]

Clinical MRI scans with a contrast agent (late gadolinium enhancement [LGE]) have been used to visualize the fibrotic remodeling in atria and ventricles.[20,83–86] Fig. 36.3 presents a patient-specific atrial model generation from clinical LGE-MR images, using a model construction pipeline as described in a recent paper.[87] It has to be noted, however, that the segmentation of LGE-MRI fibrotic regions and even segmentation of the geometry of the thin atria from clinical MRI is fraught with uncertainty and is an area of intense image-processing research.

Numerical approaches for simulating the electrical behavior of the heart have been described in detail in many papers, some of which offer comprehensive reviews on the subject.[38,71,79,88–92]

Modeling Fibrotic Remodeling in the Atria and Its Contribution to Atrial Fibrillation

Atrial fibrillation (AF) is the most common cardiac arrhythmia and a major contributor to mortality and morbidity, affecting 1%–2% of the worldwide population.[93] More than 2.5 million Americans have AF according to the American Heart Association, and the incidence increases markedly with advancing age. Aging has been found to be the strongest independent risk factor for AF,[93–96] with AF having an estimated prevalence of approximately 9% in adults aged over 80 years.

Clinical research has provided ample evidence that a large number of patients with persistent AF have extensive atrial fibrotic remodeling.[33,34,97] Since the mid-2000s, catheter ablation has emerged as a potential approach to treat AF. However, the efficacy of this procedure remains limited, with a particularly low success rate (~50%) in patients with persistent AF.[98] Modeling studies of AF under the condition of fibrotic remodeling have attempted to address issues related to both the dynamics of AF and its termination by ablation.

Models of the fibrotic atria have accounted for different aspects of fibrotic remodeling in an attempt to elucidate the mechanisms leading to altered conduction and those responsible for the reentrant drivers and organization of AF. The simplest model representation of atrial structural remodeling was based on the assumption that a component of structural remodeling, gap junction remodeling (connexin-43 [Cx43] downregulation, hypophosphorylation, and lateralization), occurs throughout the atria in a uniform fashion. Two such studies have been conducted thus

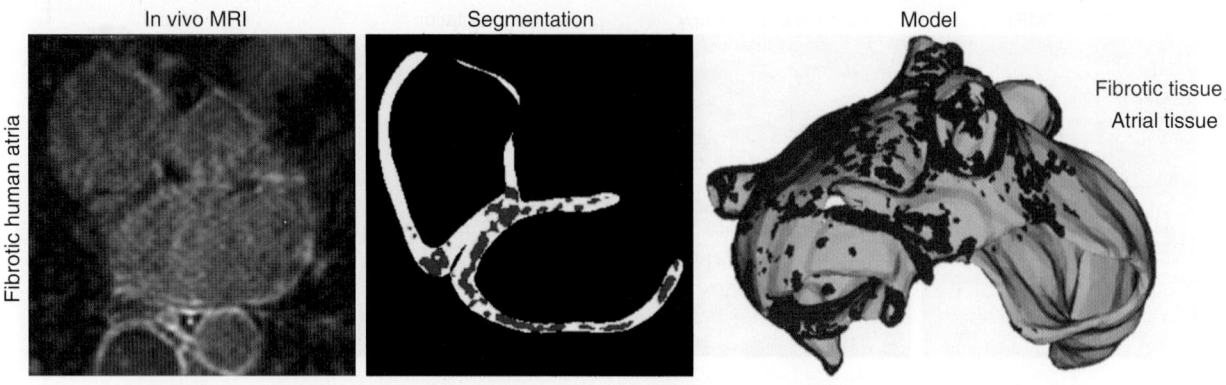

In vivo MRI   Segmentation   Model

Fibrotic human atria

Fibrotic tissue
Atrial tissue

FIGURE 36.3 Reconstruction of an image-based human atrial model from in vivo late gadolinium-enhanced magnetic resonance imaging (*MRI*) scans. *Red regions* show patient-specific distribution of fibrotic tissue. (From McDowell KS, Vadakkumpadan F, Blake R, et al. Mechanistic inquiry into the role of tissue remodeling in fibrotic lesions in human atrial fibrillation. *Biophys J.* 2013;104:2764-2773.)

far. One study assumed that the coupling strength between computational cells was decreased (Cx43 downregulation and hypophosphorylation only),[99] whereas the other modeled increased anisotropy throughout the left atrium (LA) (representing both aspects of Cx43 remodeling).[100] One of these simulation studies showed[99] that decreasing the coupling between cells slowed conduction and decreased the wavelength, further perpetuating AF. The other study[100] demonstrated that increased anisotropy throughout the fibrotic human LV was an additional mechanism for the breakup of ectopic waves emanating from the pulmonary veins (PVs) into multiple reentrant circuits; higher anisotropy ratios resulted in sustained reentrant activity, even though the ectopic focus was no longer present. Similar conclusions were obtained from a human atrial model[101] where the locations of the fibrotic (i.e., high-anisotropy ratio) regions were implemented from patient LGE-MRI scans.

The next component of fibrosis, collagen deposition, was first represented in seminal studies by Spach and associates,[102] who simulated diffuse fibrosis by removing lateral gap junctions in human atrial tissue; increased heterogeneity in intercellular coupling was found to lead to vulnerability for partial wave block and reentry. Subsequently, collagen deposition has been represented in models as insulating barriers in several ways: (1) by randomly removing the electrical connections between two 2D layers of atrial tissue, the endocardial and the epicardial, to model an increased level of dissociation between these two layers (a form of reactive interstitial fibrosis), mimicking experimental observations in goats[103]; (2) by introducing a set of random collagenous septa-disconnecting cardiac fibers in the transverse direction[104] (reactive interstitial fibrosis again); and (3) by incorporating non-conductive regions of various sizes throughout the tissue[25,29,105] (reparative fibrosis), either randomly throughout the atria or based on imaging data. Endoepicardial dissociation resulted[103] in a number of AF reentrant waves that were significantly higher than those in cases without dissociation, thereby exacerbating AF complexity. The increase in collagen content in interstitial spaces between fibers was not found to affect longitudinal conduction[29,106,107] but caused slowed propagation in the transverse direction, with the degree of slowing dependent of the length of the collagenous septa.[104]

Atrial models incorporating transverse collagen deposition[25,29,105] (as in reparative fibrosis) have highlighted the significant interruption and disarray in atrial conduction patterns caused by it. Importantly, collagen deposition rather than Cx43 remodeling was found to be the major factor in atrial conduction disturbances under heart failure conditions[29] (Fig. 36.4A). Furthermore, it was established that not only the total amount but also the specific spatial distribution of collagen deposition (e.g., as

generated by a stochastic algorithm) governed the occurrences of conduction block.[105] To evaluate the consequences of structural remodeling (on AF dynamics in the posterior LA, Tanaka and colleagues[25] used 2D models of transmural posterior LA sections generated from histological data; patchy distributions of collagen were also reconstructed from that data. Simulations demonstrated that whether the mechanism sustaining AF was reentrant or focal, fibrous patches of large size were the major factor responsible for the different dynamics of AF waves in remodeled versus control hearts; they anchored reentrant circuits and impaired wave propagation to generate delays and signal fractionation (Fig. 36.4B).

A third component of fibrotic remodeling, fibroblast proliferation and phenotype switching, has also been represented in computational models of the atria, particularly in view of the fact that fibroblasts, in addition to being part of the structural remodeling of the atria, could potentially also exert electrophysiological influences on neighboring myocytes, possibly either through electrical coupling[108] or via paracrine effects.[109] The first study to explicitly incorporate fibroblast presence as a representation of fibrotic remodeling was the 2D atrial model by Ashihara and coworkers.[110] Within the fibrotic region, coupling of fibroblasts (kinetics governed by a fibroblast ionic model) to atrial myocytes caused shorter AP duration (APD), slower conduction, and lower excitability as well as spiral wave breakups. This effect was exacerbated when fibroblast density increased (Fig. 36.5A[111,112]). Interestingly, when fibroblasts were substituted by collagen in the model, wave breakups were not observed.

All three elements of fibrotic remodeling (gap junction remodeling, collagen deposition, and myofibroblast proliferation) were combined together in the LA model generated from LGE-MRI data of a patient with permanent AF,[106,107] accurately capturing both the atrial geometry and the distribution of fibrotic lesions. Electrophysiological remodeling associated with persistent AF was also incorporated. The model was used to examine the mechanisms for AF initiation by PV ectopic stimulation. The study found that for fibrotic lesions typical of human remodeled atria under the conditions of persistent AF, gap junction remodeling in the fibrotic lesions was a necessary but not sufficient condition for the development of AF following a PV ectopic beat. The sufficient condition was myofibroblast proliferation in these lesions where myofibroblasts exerted either electrotonic or paracrine influences on myocytes within the lesions. Deposition of collagen in the lesions assisted the myofibroblasts' paracrine or electrotonic effects by additionally shortening APD (Fig. 36.5B). Recently, using the same methodology, McDowell and associates[113] provided the first proof-of-concept that patient-specific atrial models, which combine atrial structure and fibrosis distribution from clinical MRIs, and representations of remodeled

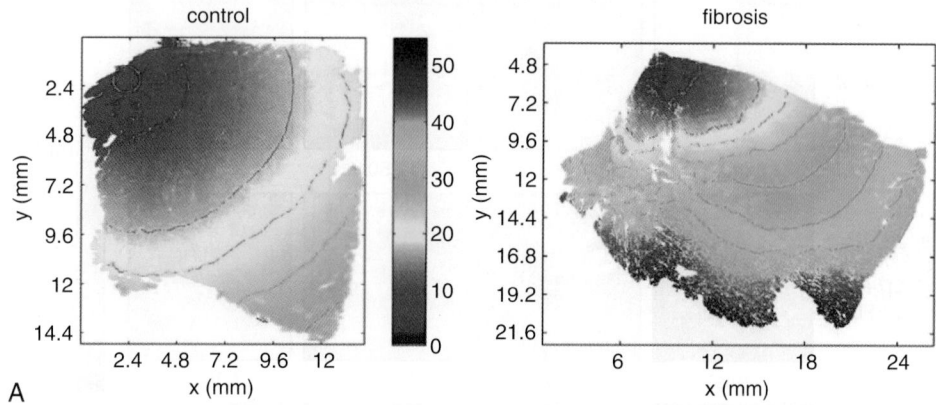

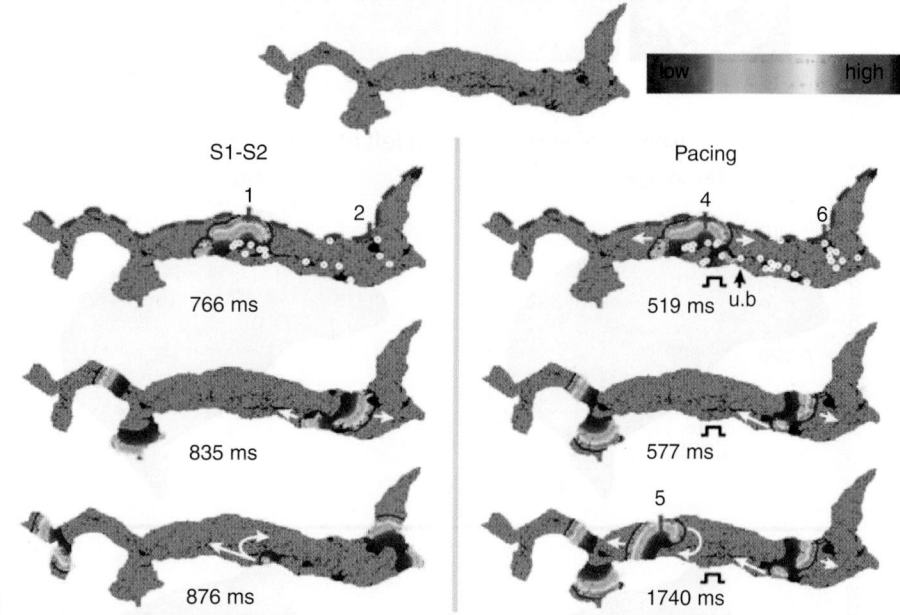

FIGURE 36.4 (A) Simulations of excitatory wavefront propagation in two-dimensional (*2D*) sections of canine atrial tissues under control (*left*) and fibrotic (*right*) conditions. Fibrosis is modeled as regions of collagen, which is represented as an electrical insulator. (B) Simulations conducted using a similar methodology to (A) but in a transmural slice from the canine posterior left atrium under heart failure conditions. *Red dashed lines* demarcate the epicardial surface. *Colors* indicate transmembrane voltage; *u.b*, unidirectional block; *white circles* indicate wavebreak sites. ([A] From Burstein B, Comtois P, Michael G, et al. Changes in connexin expression and the atrial fibrillation substrate in congestive heart failure. *Circ Res.* 2009;105:1213-1222. [B] From Tanaka K, Zlochiver S, Vikstrom KL, et al. Spatial distribution of fibrosis governs fibrillation wave dynamics in the posterior left atrium during heart failure. *Circ Res.* 2007;101:839-847.)

atrial electrophysiology could be used to predict optimal ablation targets in patients. The study reconstructed four patient-specific atrial models, two of which had persistent AF associated with fibrosis, and analyzed AF to determine the ablation targets. When the restricted regions encompassing the meander of the persistent phase singularities were modeled as ablation lesions, AF could no longer be induced. The study demonstrated that a patient-specific modeling approach to identify noninvasive AF ablation targets prior to the clinical procedure was feasible. While these studies have demonstrated the utility of patient-specific modeling of the atria, the electrophysiological representation of fibrotic remodeling, particularly the role of myofibroblasts in altering the AP dynamics (via gap-junction coupling), remains, however, very

controversial. Despite a significant research effort in recent years, there continues to be a lack of experimental data in support of this assertion.

The most recent studies[114–115b] on fibrosis and AF have focused on the relationship between the spatial pattern of fibrotic distribution and AF reentrant dynamics and, in particular, how the fibrotic distribution impacts the locations of the AF-driving reentrant sources. These studies used a large number of patient-specific atrial models (n = 20) with individualized atrial fibrosis distribution reconstructed again from LGE-MRI. In these studies, in addition to including AP changes associated with persistent AF, fibrotic regions were represented with remodeled electrophysiology, anisotropy, and conduction properties but without

Human atrial cell monolayer models
with fibroblast proliferation

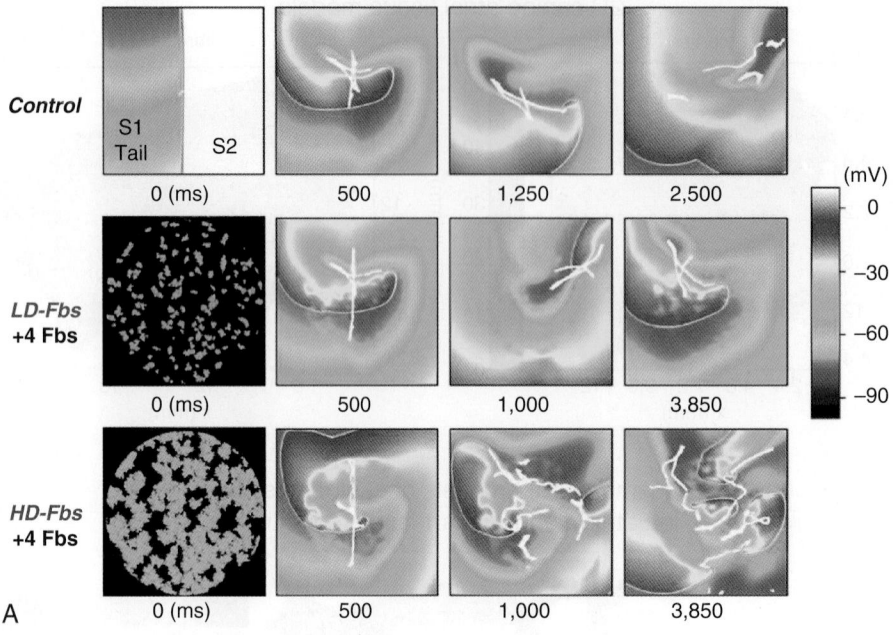

A

Models of fibrotic human left atrial tissue

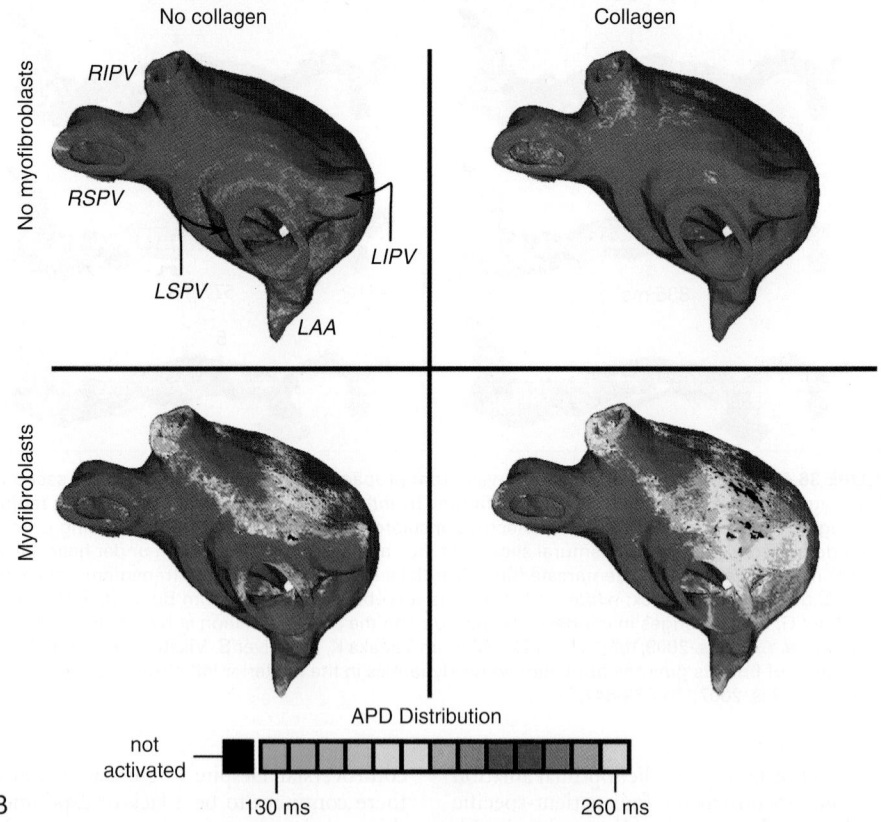

B

FIGURE 36.5 (A) Effects of fibroblast-myocyte coupling on spiral wave behavior in a two-dimensional model of human atrial tissue (width and height = 4.5 cm). *Top, middle, and bottom rows* illustrate propagation dynamics control, low fibrosis (*LD-Fbs*; 12.5%), and high fibrosis (*HD-Fbs*; 50%) conditions, respectively. In fibrotic regions (*green*), each point is modeled as an atrial myocyte (100 pF) coupled to four fibroblasts (6.3 pF), using a previously described method.[111]111 (B) Action potential duration (*APD*) distribution in a three-dimensional (3D) human atrial model under four different combinations of two parameters: (1) with (*top*) or without (*bottom*) myofibroblast infiltration (and myocyte-myofibroblast coupling, as described previously[111,112]), and (2) with (*left*) or without (*right*) diffuse collagen deposition. Anatomical landmarks: right inferior, right superior, left inferior, and left superior pulmonary veins (*RIPV, RSPV, LIPV, LSPV*, respectively); left atrial appendage (*LAA*). (From Ashihara T, Haraguchi R, Nakazawa K, et al. The role of fibroblasts in complex fractionated electrograms during persistent/permanent atrial fibrillation: implications for electrogram-based catheter ablation. *Circ Res*. 2012;110:275-284. [B] From McDowell KS, Vadakkumpadan F, Blake R, et al. Mechanistic inquiry into the role of tissue remodeling in fibrotic lesions in human atrial fibrillation. *Biophys J*. 2013;104:2764-2773.)

explicitly representing any electrophysiological effects associated with the controversial myocyte–fibroblast coupling. Instead, ionic current modifications were implemented that were consistent with changes in atrial myocyte electrophysiology when subjected to elevated transforming growth factor β1, a key component of the fibrogenic signaling pathway.[116,117] Conductivity values and anisotropy ratios in fibrotic regions reflected decreased intercellular coupling because of replacement fibrosis, collagen deposition (interstitial fibrosis), and gap junction remodeling.[28,29] In this manner, fibrotic remodeling representation not only better reflected new experimental data but also ensured computational tractability of studies involving a large number of patient atria.

Fig. 36.6A presents four patient-specific models, in which programmed electrical stimulation was conducted to determine the AF propensity of the fibrotic substrate. In each model, maps of fibrosis complexity were built by computing local spatial metrics for a surrounding volume within 1.5 mm of every point. The metrics included fibrosis density (D; proportion of LGE tissue), clustering (C; diffuse or patchy) by Moran's I, and disorganization by Shannon entropy (H). The phase singularities of the induced reentries persisted near fibrosis cluster boundaries (Fig. 36.6B). Fibrosis spatial patterns in regions that harbored the organizing centers of persistent reentries were complex, with median values higher than those in the rest of the atria for all spatial metrics (Fig. 36.6C). The locations of the organizing centers were strongly correlated (81%) with tissue regions that had a highly complex fibrosis spatial pattern ($D \geq 0.8$, $C \geq 0.8$, and $H \geq 0.8$), where there was extensive intermingling with nonfibrotic tissue; only a small subvolume (<4%) of each model had this pattern (Fig. 36.6D). This study demonstrated that in personalized models of AF under the conditions of fibrosis, the phase singularities of the persistent reentrant circuits were exclusively harbored in regions with complex fibrosis spatial patterns. The study concluded that identifying locations with such properties could help optimize AF ablation.

An important question arose from the latter simulation study—because AF reentrant sources were found to be harbored near the edges of fibrotic regions, does the prevalence of such regions correlate with AF inducibility? If so, could this metric serve as a better predictor of AF inducibility than total atrial fibrosis burden (FB)? The latter quantity (total FB) has been previously linked to higher risk of persistent AF.[118] A simulation study[115] using the same patient-specific models as above quantified the spatial distribution of fibrosis using the fibrosis density metric D, with its median (D_{50}) and upper quartile (D_{75}) values estimating the prevalence of regions with highly intermingled fibrotic and nonfibrotic tissue. Simulations demonstrated that noninducible atrial models had low FB ($\leq 11\%$) and D_{75} (≤ 0.1) values. In AF-inducible models, higher inducibility was associated with increased FB and D_{75}. Inducibility was correlated both with FB (Fig. 36.6E) and D_m, a linear combination of D_{50} and D_{75}. Statistical analysis demonstrated that D_m had a higher predictive power than FB. This simulation study demonstrated that fibrosis spatial pattern analysis could be a novel avenue for persistent AF risk stratification, a conclusion that could have important clinical implications.

Modeling of Fibrotic Remodeling in the Ventricles and the Link to Arrhythmias

Computer modeling has also been used to examine the mechanisms of ventricular arrhythmias in the aging heart, although unlike atrial simulation research, such studies are few and far between. One of the first studies that examined the effects of fibrotic remodeling on ventricular propagation was by Pertsov and colleagues[119]; they used a simplified ventricular representation to study wave propagation in tissue with inexcitable obstacles, representing collagenous septa. The study found that fibrotic

strands led to widening and fractionation of electrograms and influenced the rotation of spiral waves. Similar electrogram fractionation was documented by Turner and associates[120] in a model of human ventricular tissue with string-like fibrotic obstacles.

In a series of studies,[121–124] Panfilov and colleagues studied the effects of diffuse fibrosis on wave propagation, vulnerability to arrhythmia, spiral and scroll wave dynamics, and steep restitution-mediated spiral breakup. It was found that despite the small size of the obstacles (length, 0.25–0.5 mm) relative to the wavelength in human ventricular tissue (1–3 cm), the presence of diffuse fibrosis had significant effects on wave propagation and led to the formation of a vulnerable window, during which wave break and spiral wave formations occurred. Furthermore, fibrosis resulted in an increase in spiral wave rotation period, suggesting that the average period of ventricular arrhythmias increases with increasing amounts of diffuse fibrosis. Finally, the presence of diffuse fibrosis suppressed spiral breakup caused by steep APD restitution (Fig. 36.7), similar to model findings in atrial tissue reviewed above.[110] The latter suggests that mechanisms different from restitution-induced spiral breakup might be more likely to account for the onset of fibrillation in the presence of large amounts of diffuse fibrotic tissue.

Concluding Remarks

As this chapter demonstrates, mathematical modeling and computer simulations of atrial and ventricular electrophysiology have made significant contributions to the dissection of the mechanisms and relationships underlying atrial and ventricular arrhythmias in the aging heart. As this trend will continue in the future, modeling as a tool in arrhythmia research will necessitate continuous adaptation and integration of new elements, including model redesign and evaluation, improvements in the execution time of biophysically detailed atrial and ventricular models, implementation of consistent strategies for comparison with experimental and clinical measurements, and investing in efforts to ensure repeatability and consistency of modeling results. The advancement of modeling representation of the aging heart will continue to be strongly dependent on developments in experimental and imaging methodologies, which provide data to enrich as well as constrain and validate the models. Of particular importance will be the capability to better resolve the pathophysiological structure of the aging atria and ventricles and to fully characterize the complex pathophysiological changes, at all levels of biological complexity, of fibrotic remodeling and other components of natural aging changes in the heart. Once the molecular and structural mechanisms associated with remodeling in the aging heart are fully elucidated, this will constitute a major impetus for computational studies, as a more physiologically faithful modeling construct could be developed. This will allow the research community to fully harness the capability of computational modeling to predict emergent phenomena at the organ level, which originate from molecular and structural remodeling. Major challenges that lie ahead for computer models of the aging heart include elucidating the dynamics of persistent AF and detecting rotor locations, as well as understanding the multitude of factors that drive progression of AF in some, but not all, patients. Furthermore, arrhythmia risk stratification for sudden cardiac death in the elderly remains a challenge, and thus patient-specific models of nonischemic cardiomyopathy will need to be developed to address this need.

Acknowledgments

This work was supported by the National Institutes of Health (DP1-HL123271 and R01-HL1034280) and the National Science Foundation (CDI 1124804).

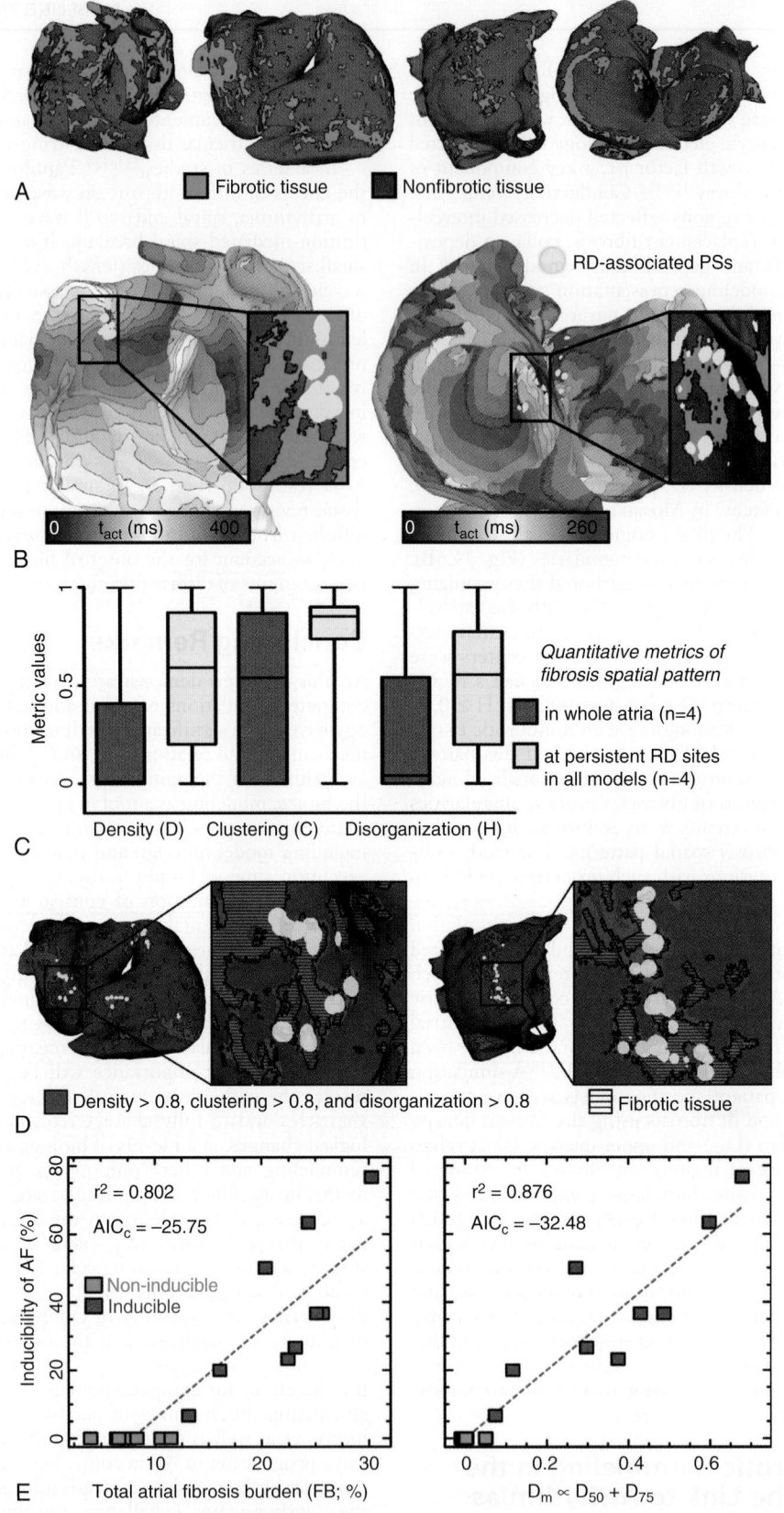

FIGURE 36.6 (A) Atrial models reconstructed using late gadolinium-enhanced magnetic resonance imaging scans for four patients with persistent atrial fibrillation (*AF*). (B) Activation maps recorded during episodes of reentrant arrhythmia induced by rapid atrial pacing. *Golden spheres* indicate organizing centers (i.e., phase singularities; PSs) of reentrant drivers (RDs; i.e., rotors). (C) Comparison of fibrosis spatial pattern metrics computed at atrial points where PSs occurred (*gold*) or did not occur (*gray*) for all arrhythmic episodes induced in all four models. In all cases, interquartile ranges (IQRs) were significantly different ($p < .05$): density (IQR_D, 0.58 vs. 0.01), clustering (IQR_C, 0.85 vs. 0.54), and disorganization (IQR_H, 0.55 vs. 0.04). (D) Three-dimensional maps for two atrial models showing that PS locations from all arrhythmic episodes superimposed were colocalized with regions that had high values (>0.8) of all three fibrosis spatial pattern metrics. (E) Inducibility of AF in 20 patient-specific atrial models (proportion of pacing sites out of 30 that initiated reentrant arrhythmia) is compared with two predictive metrics: fibrosis burden (*FB; left*) and D_m (*right*). Statistical analysis (via Akaike information criterion *[AICc]*) showed that D_m had better predictive power than FB (likelihood of FB producing better predictions than D_m was ~3%). (From Boyle PM, Zahid S, Schwarz E, et al. Local complexity of the fibrosis spatial pattern determines the locations of stable reentrant sources in persistent atrial fibrillation: analysis from patient-specific models. *Heart Rhythm.* 2015;12:S7; and Boyle PM, Zahid S, Schwarz E, et al. Prevalence of regions with highly intermingled fibrotic and non-fibrotic tissue is a better predictor of arrhythmia inducibility than total fibrosis burden: analysis of patient-specific models of persistent atrial fibrillation. *Heart Rhythm.* 2015;12:S80.)

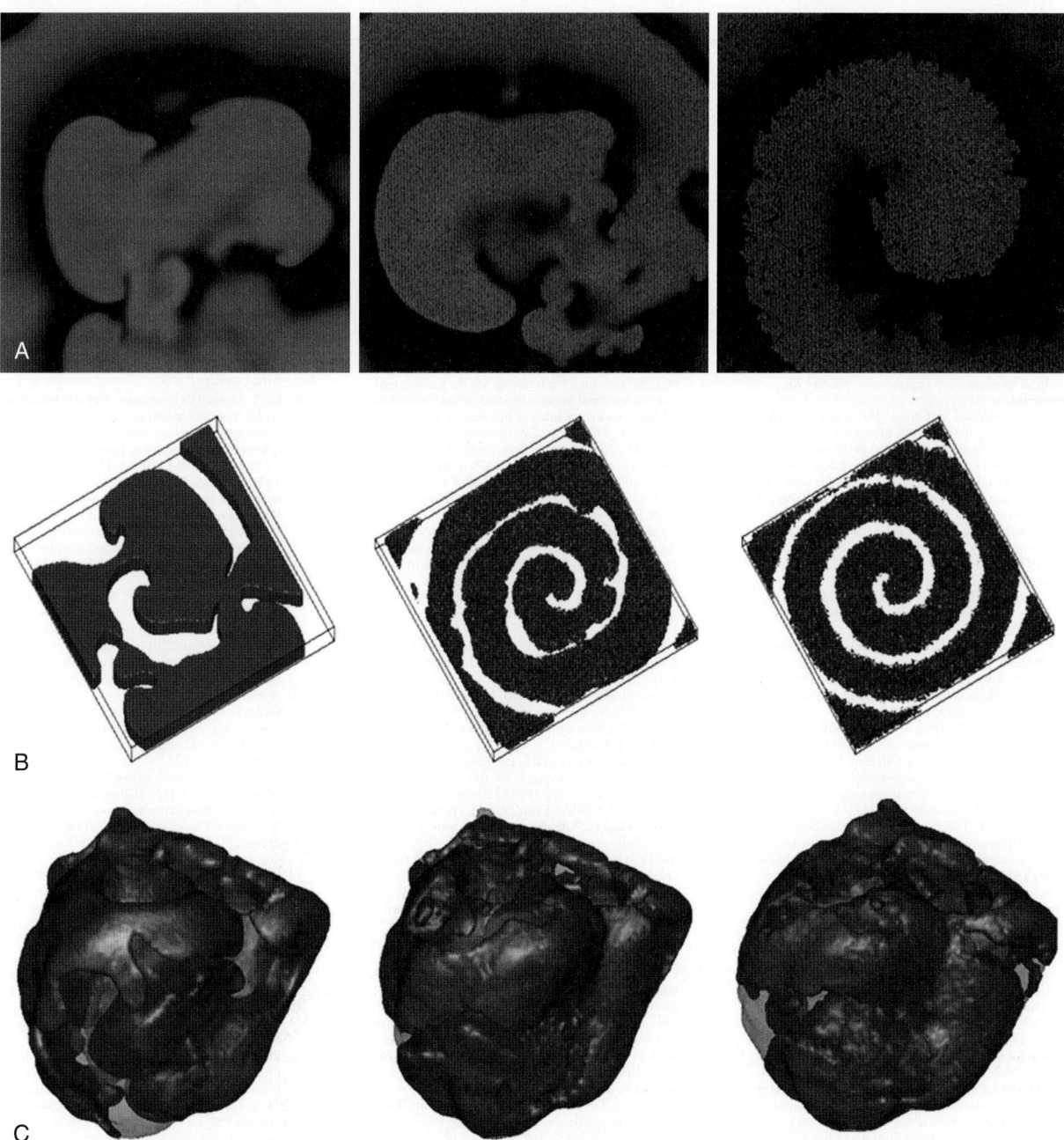

FIGURE 36.7 Simulations of fibrotic tissue in a two-dimensional sheet (A), three-dimensional slab (B), and ventricular model (C) with 0%, 10%, and 35%, respectively, of diffuse fibrosis (*left, middle,* and *right columns,* respectively). Spiral wave breakup is suppressed by diffuse fibrosis. (From Ten Tusscher KH, Panfilov AV. Influence of diffuse fibrosis on wave propagation in human ventricular tissue. *Europace.* 2007;9:vi38-vi45.)

REFERENCES

1. Biernacka A, Frangogiannis NG. Aging and cardiac fibrosis. *Aging Dis*. 2011;2:158–173.
2. Pugh KG, Wei JY. Clinical implications of physiological changes in the aging heart. *Drugs Aging*. 2001;18:263–276.
3. Dannenberg AL, Levy D, Garrison RJ. Impact of age on echocardiographic left ventricular mass in a healthy population (the Framingham Study). *Am J Cardiol*. 1989;64:1066–1068.
4. Lakatta EG. Age-associated cardiovascular changes in health: impact on cardiovascular disease in older persons. *Heart Fail Rev*. 2002;7:29–49.
5. Kajstura J, Cheng W, Sarangarajan R, et al. Necrotic and apoptotic myocyte cell death in the aging heart of Fischer 344 rats. *Am J Physiol*. 1996;271:H1215–H1228.
6. Anversa P, Palackal T, Sonnenblick EH, et al. Myocyte cell loss and myocyte cellular hyperplasia in the hypertrophied aging rat heart. *Circ Res*. 1990;67:871–885.
7. Mukherjee D, Sen S. Collagen phenotypes during development and regression of myocardial hypertrophy in spontaneously hypertensive rats. *Circ Res*. 1990;67:1474–1480.
8. Olivetti G, Melissari M, Capasso JM, et al. Cardiomyopathy of the aging human heart. Myocyte loss and reactive cellular hypertrophy. *Circ Res*. 1991;68:1560–1568.
9. Gazoti Debessa CR, Mesiano Maifrino LB, Rodrigues de Souza R. Age related changes of the collagen network of the human heart. *Mech Ageing Dev*. 2001;122:1049–1058.
10. Song Y, Yao Q, Zhu J, et al. Age-related variation in the interstitial tissues of the cardiac conduction system; and autopsy study of 230 Han Chinese. *Forensic Sci Int*. 1999;104:133–142.
11. Burkauskiene A, Mackiewicz Z, Virtanen I, et al. Age-related changes in myocardial nerve and collagen networks of the auricle of the right atrium. *Acta Cardiol*. 2006;61:513–518.
12. de Souza RR. Aging of myocardial collagen. *Biogerontology*. 2002;3:325–335.
13. Isoyama S, Nitta-Komatsubara Y. Acute and chronic adaptation to hemodynamic overload and ischemia in the aged heart. *Heart Fail Rev*. 2002;7:63–69.
14. Moore-Morris T, Tallquist MD, Evans SM. Sorting out where fibroblasts come from. *Circ Res*. 2014;115:602–604.
15. Strain JE, Grose RM, Factor SM, et al. Results of endomyocardial biopsy in patients with spontaneous ventricular tachycardia but without apparent structural heart disease. *Circulation*. 1983;68:1171–1181.
16. Segawa I, Suzuki T, Kato M, et al. Relation between myocardial histological changes and ventricular tachycardia in cardiomyopathy: a study by 24-hour ECG-monitoring and endomyocardial biopsy. *Heart Vessels Suppl*. 1990;5:37–40.
17. Varnava AM, Elliott PM, Mahon N, et al. Relation between myocyte disarray and outcome in hypertrophic cardiomyopathy. *Am J Cardiol*. 2001;88:275–279.
18. Hsia HH, Marchlinski FE. Characterization of the electroanatomic substrate for monomorphic ventricular tachycardia in patients with nonischemic cardiomyopathy. *Pacing Clin Electrophysiol*. 2002;25:1114–1127.
19. John BT, Tamarappoo BK, Titus JL, et al. Global remodeling of the ventricular interstitium in idiopathic myocardial fibrosis and sudden cardiac death. *Heart Rhythm*. 2004;1:141–149.
20. Assomull RG, Prasad SK, Lyne J, et al. Cardiovascular magnetic resonance, fibrosis, and prognosis in dilated cardiomyopathy. *J Am Coll Cardiol*. 2006;48:1977–1985.
21. Everett TH, Olgin JE. Atrial fibrosis and the mechanisms of atrial fibrillation. *Heart Rhythm*. 2007;4:S24–S27.
22. Nakai T, Chandy J, Nakai K, et al. Histologic assessment of right atrial appendage myocardium in patients with atrial fibrillation after coronary artery bypass graft surgery. *Cardiology*. 2007;108:90–96.
23. Saito T, Tamura K, Uchida D, et al. Histopathological features of the resected left atrial appendage as predictors of recurrence after surgery for atrial fibrillation in valvular heart disease. *Circ J*. 2007;71:70–78.
24. Spach MS, Dolber PC, Heidlage JF. Interaction of inhomogeneities of repolarization with anisotropic propagation in dog atria. A mechanism for both preventing and initiating reentry. *Circ Res*. 1989;65:1612–1631.
25. Tanaka K, Zlochiver S, Vikstrom KL, et al. Spatial distribution of fibrosis governs fibrillation wave dynamics in the posterior left atrium during heart failure. *Circ Res*. 2007;101:839–847.
26. Kawara T, Derksen R, de Groot JR, et al. Activation delay after premature stimulation in chronically diseased human myocardium relates to the architecture of interstitial fibrosis. *Circulation*. 2001;104:3069–3075.
27. de Bakker JM, van Rijen HM. Continuous and discontinuous propagation in heart muscle. *J Cardiovasc Electrophysiol*. 2006;17:567–573.
28. Li D, Fareh S, Leung TK, et al. Promotion of atrial fibrillation by heart failure in dogs: atrial remodeling of a different sort. *Circulation*. 1999;100:87–95.
29. Burstein B, Comtois P, Michael G, et al. Changes in connexin expression and the atrial fibrillation substrate in congestive heart failure. *Circ Res*. 2009;105:1213–1222.
30. Verheule S, Sato T, Everett T, et al. Increased vulnerability to atrial fibrillation in transgenic mice with selective atrial fibrosis caused by overexpression of TGF-beta1. *Circ Res*. 2004;94:1458–1465.
31. Hansen BJ, Zhao J, Csepe TA, et al. Atrial fibrillation driven by micro-anatomic intramural re-entry revealed by simultaneous sub-epicardial and sub-endocardial optical mapping in explanted human hearts. *Eur Heart J*. 2015;36:2390–2401.
32. Jalife J, Kaur K. Atrial remodeling, fibrosis, and atrial fibrillation. *Trends Cardiovasc Med*. 2015;25:475–484.
33. Marrouche NF, Wilber D, Hindricks G, et al. Association of atrial tissue fibrosis identified by delayed enhancement MRI and atrial fibrillation catheter ablation: the DECAAF study. *JAMA*. 2014;311:498–506.
34. Cochet H, Mouries A, Nivet H, et al. Age, atrial fibrillation, and structural heart disease are the main determinants of left atrial fibrosis detected by delayed-enhanced magnetic resonance imaging in a general cardiology population. *J Cardiovasc Electrophysiol*. 2015;26:484–492.
35. Noble D. Modeling the heart—from genes to cells to the whole organ. *Science*. 2002;295:1678–1682.
36. Vigmond E, Vadakkumpadan F, Gurev V, et al. Towards predictive modelling of the electrophysiology of the heart. *Exp Physiol*. 2009;94:563–577.
37. Gurev V, Lee T, Constantino J, et al. Models of cardiac electromechanics based on individual hearts imaging data: image-based electromechanical models of the heart. *Biomech Model Mechanobiol*. 2011;10:295–306.
38. Trayanova NA. Whole-heart modeling: applications to cardiac electrophysiology and electromechanics. *Circ Res*. 2011;108:113–128.
39. Winslow RL, Trayanova N, Geman D, et al. Computational medicine: translating models to clinical care. *Sci Transl Med*. 2012;4:158rv11.
40. Courtemanche M, Ramirez RJ, Nattel S. Ionic mechanisms underlying human atrial action potential properties: insights from a mathematical model. *Am J Physiol*. 1998;275:H301–H321.
41. Nygren A, Fiset C, Firek L, et al. Mathematical model of an adult human atrial cell: the role of K+ currents in repolarization. *Circ Res*. 1998;82:63–81.
42. Grandi E, Pandit SV, Voigt N, et al. Human atrial action potential and Ca^{2+} model: sinus rhythm and chronic atrial fibrillation. *Circ Res*. 2011;109:1055–1066.
43. ten Tusscher KH, Panfilov AV. Alternans and spiral breakup in a human ventricular tissue model. *Am J Physiol Heart Circ Physiol*. 2006;291:H1088–H1100.
44. Fink M, Noble D, Virag L, et al. Contributions of HERG K+ current to repolarization of the human ventricular action potential. *Prog Biophys Mol Biol*. 2008;96:357–376.
45. Grandi E, Pasqualini FS, Bers DM. A novel computational model of the human ventricular action potential and Ca transient. *J Mol Cell Cardiol*. 2010;48:112–121.
46. O'Hara T, Virag L, Varro A, et al. Simulation of the undiseased human cardiac ventricular action potential: model formulation and experimental validation. *PLoS Comput Biol*. 2011;7:e1002061.
47. Stewart P, Aslanidi OV, Noble D, et al. Mathematical models of the electrical action potential of Purkinje fibre cells. *Philos Trans A Math Phys Eng Sci*. 2009;367:2225–2255.
48. Aslanidi OV, Sleiman RN, Boyett MR, et al. Ionic mechanisms for electrical heterogeneity between rabbit Purkinje fiber and ventricular cells. *Biophys J*. 2010;98:2420–2431.
49. Sampson KJ, Iyer V, Marks AR, et al. A computational model of Purkinje fiber single cell electrophysiology: implications for the long QT syndrome. *J Physiol*. 2010;588:2643–2655.
50. Li P, Rudy Y. A model of canine purkinje cell electrophysiology and Ca(2+) cycling: rate dependence, triggered activity, and comparison to ventricular myocytes. *Circ Res*. 2011;109:71–79.
51. Vaidyanathan R, O'Connell RP, Deo M, et al. The ionic bases of the action potential in isolated mouse cardiac Purkinje cell. *Heart Rhythm*. 2013;10:80–87.
52. Moreno JD, Zhu ZI, Yang P-C, et al. A computational model to predict the effects of class I anti-arrhythmic drugs on ventricular rhythms. *Sci Transl Med*. 2011;3:98ra83.
53. Tandri H, Weinberg SH, Chang KC, et al. Reversible cardiac conduction block and defibrillation with high-frequency electric field. *Sci Transl Med*. 2011;3:102ra96.
54. Trayanova NA, O'Hara T, Bayer JD, et al. Computational cardiology: how computer simulations could be used to develop new therapies and advance existing ones. *Europace*. 2012;14:v82–v89.
55. Boyle PM, Williams JC, Ambrosi CM, et al. A comprehensive multiscale framework for simulating optogenetics in the heart. *Nat Commun*. 2013;4:2370.
56. Boyle PM, Masse S, Nanthakumar K, et al. Transmural IK(ATP) heterogeneity as a determinant of activation rate gradient during early ventricular fibrillation: mechanistic insights from rabbit ventricular models. *Heart Rhythm*. 2013;10:1710–1717.
57. Boyle PM, Veenhuyzen GD, Vigmond EJ. Fusion during entrainment of orthodromic reciprocating tachycardia is enhanced for basal pacing sites but diminished when pacing near Purkinje system end points. *Heart Rhythm*. 2013;10:444–451.
58. Boyle PM, Park CJ, Arevalo HJ, et al. Sodium current reduction unmasks a structure-dependent substrate for arrhythmogenesis in the normal ventricles. *PLoS ONE*. 2014;9:e86947.
59. Clayton R, Bishop M. Computational models of ventricular arrhythmia mechanisms: recent developments and future prospects. *Drug Discov Today Dis Models*. 2014;14:17–22.
60. Hu Y, Gurev V, Constantino J, et al. Optimizing cardiac resynchronization therapy to minimize ATP consumption heterogeneity throughout the left ventricle: a simulation analysis using a canine heart failure model. *Heart Rhythm*. 2014;11:1063–1069.
61. Trayanova NA, Boyle PM. Advances in modeling ventricular arrhythmias: from mechanisms to the clinic. *Wiley Interdiscip Rev Syst Biol Med*. 2014;6:209–224.
62. Ashikaga H, Arevalo H, Vadakkumpadan F, et al. Feasibility of image-based simulation to estimate ablation target in human ventricular arrhythmia. *Heart Rhythm*. 2013;10:1109–1116.
63. Relan J, Chinchapatnam P, Sermesant M, et al. Coupled personalization of cardiac electrophysiology models for prediction of ischaemic ventricular tachycardia. *Interface Focus*. 2011;1:396–407.
64. Zhu X, Wei D, Okazaki O. Computer simulation of clinical electrophysiological study. *Pacing Clin Electrophysiol*. 2012;35:718–729.
65. Wong J, Abilez OJ, Kuhl E. Computational optogenetics: a novel continuum framework for the photoelectrochemistry of living systems. *J Mech Phys Solids*. 2012;60:1158–1178.
66. Pop M, Sermesant M, Mansi T, et al. Correspondence between simple 3-D MRI-based computer models and in-vivo EP measurements in swine with chronic infarctions. *IEEE Trans Biomed Eng*. 2011;58:3483–3486.
67. Arevalo H, Plank G, Helm P, et al. Tachycardia in post-infarction hearts: insights from 3D image-based ventricular models. *PLoS One*. 2013;8:e68872.
68. Ringenberg J, Deo M, Filgueiras-Rama D, et al. Effects of fibrosis morphology on reentrant ventricular tachycardia inducibility and simulation fidelity in patient-derived models. *Clin Med Insights Cardiol*. 2014;8:1–13.
69. Vigmond EJ, Aguel F, Trayanova NA. Computational techniques for solving the bidomain equations in three dimensions. *IEEE Trans Biomed Eng*. 2002;49:1260–1269.
70. Vigmond EJ, Hughes M, Plank G, et al. Computational tools for modeling electrical activity in cardiac tissue. *J Electrocardiol*. 2003;36:69–74.
71. Plank G, Zhou L, Greenstein JL, et al. From mitochondrial ion channels to arrhythmias in the heart: computational techniques to bridge the spatio-temporal scales. *Philos Trans A Math Phys Eng Sci*. 2008;366:3381–3409.
72. Nielsen PM, Le Grice IJ, Smaill BH, et al. Mathematical model of geometry and fibrous structure of the heart. *Am J Physiol*. 1991;260:H1365–H1378.
73. Vetter FJ, McCulloch AD. Three-dimensional analysis of regional cardiac function: a model of rabbit ventricular anatomy. *Prog Biophys Mol Biol*. 1998;69:157–183.
74. Helm PA, Tseng HJ, Younes L, McVeigh ER, Winslow RL. Ex vivo 3D diffusion tensor imaging and quantification of cardiac laminar structure. *Magn Reson Med*. 2005;54:850–859.
75. Vadakkumpadan F, Arevalo H, Ceritoglu C, et al. Image-based estimation of ventricular fiber orientations for personalized modeling of cardiac electrophysiology. *IEEE Trans Med Imaging*. 2012;31:1051–1060.
76. Krueger MW, Schmidt V, Tobón C, et al. Modeling atrial fiber orientation in patient-specific geometries: a semi-automatic rule-based approach. International conference on functional imaging and modeling of the heart. *Springer*. 2011:223–232.
77. Trayanova NA, Boyle PM, Arevalo HJ, et al. Exploring susceptibility to atrial and ventricular arrhythmias resulting from remodeling of the passive electrical properties in the heart: a simulation approach. *Front Physiol*. 2014;5:435.
78. Bayer J, Blake R, Plank G, et al. A novel rule-based algorithm for assigning myocardial fiber orientation to computational heart models. *Ann Biomed Eng*. 2012;40:2243–2254.

79. Dossel O, Krueger MW, Weber FM, et al. Computational modeling of the human atrial anatomy and electrophysiology. *Med Biol Eng Comput.* 2012;50:773–799.

80. Bishop MJ, Plank G, Burton RA, et al. Development of an anatomically detailed MRI-derived rabbit ventricular model and assessment of its impact on simulations of electrophysiological function. *Am J Physiol Heart Circ Physiol.* 2010;298:H699–H718.

81. Vadakkumpadan F, Arevalo H, Prassl AJ, et al. Image-based models of cardiac structure in health and disease. *Wiley Interdiscip Rev Syst Biol Med.* 2010;2:489–506.

82. Deng D, Arevalo H, Pashakhanloo F, et al. Accuracy of prediction of infarct-related arrhythmic circuits from 2 image-based models reconstructed from low and high resolution 3 MRI. *Front Physiol.* 2015;6:282.

83. Nazarian S, Bluemke DA, Lardo AC, et al. Magnetic resonance assessment of the substrate for inducible ventricular tachycardia in nonischemic cardiomyopathy. *Circulation.* 2005;112:2821–2825.

84. Oakes RS, Badger TJ, Kholmovski EG, et al. Detection and quantification of left atrial structural remodeling with delayed-enhancement magnetic resonance imaging in patients with atrial fibrillation. *Circulation.* 2009;119:1758–1767.

85. Roes SD, Borleffs CJW, van der Geest RJ, et al. Infarct tissue heterogeneity assessed with contrast-enhanced MRI predicts spontaneous ventricular arrhythmia in patients with ischemic cardiomyopathy and implantable cardioverter-defibrillator. *Circ Cardiovasc Imaging.* 2009;2:183–190.

86. Akoum N, Daccarett M, McGann C, et al. Atrial fibrosis helps select the appropriate patient and strategy in catheter ablation of atrial fibrillation: a DE-MRI guided approach. *J Cardiovasc Electrophysiol.* 2011;22:16–22.

87. Prakosa A, Malamas P, Zhang S, et al. Methodology for image-based reconstruction of ventricular geometry for patient-specific modeling of cardiac electrophysiology. *Prog Biophys Mol Biol.* 2014;115:226–234.

88. Rodriguez B, Trayanova N. Upper limit of vulnerability in a defibrillation model of the rabbit ventricles. *J Electrocardiol.* 2003;36:51–56.

89. Vigmond EJ, Hughes M, Plank G, et al. Computational tools for modeling electrical activity in cardiac tissue. *J Electrocardiol.* 2003;36:69–74.

90. Jacquemet V, Kappenberger L, Henriquez CS. Modeling atrial arrhythmias: impact on clinical diagnosis and therapies. *IEEE Rev Biomed Eng.* 2008;1:94–114.

91. Vigmond EJ, Weber dos Santos R, Prassl AJ, et al. Solvers for the cardiac bidomain equations. *Prog Biophys Mol Biol.* 2008;96:3–18.

92. Niederer SA, Kerfoot E, Benson AP, et al. Verification of cardiac tissue electrophysiology simulators using an N-version benchmark. *Philos Trans A Math Phys Eng Sci.* 2011;369:4331–4351.

93. Andrade J, Khairy P, Dobrev D, et al. The clinical profile and pathophysiology of atrial fibrillation: relationships among clinical features, epidemiology, and mechanisms. *Circ Res.* 2014;114:1453–1468.

94. Heeringa J, van der Kuip DA, Hofman A, et al. Prevalence, incidence and lifetime risk of atrial fibrillation: the Rotterdam study. *Eur Heart J.* 2006;27:949–953.

95. Rietbrock S, Heeley E, Plumb J, et al. Chronic atrial fibrillation: Incidence, prevalence, and prediction of stroke using the Congestive heart failure, Hypertension, Age >75, Diabetes mellitus, and prior Stroke or transient ischemic attack (CHADS2) risk stratification scheme. *Am Heart J.* 2008;156:57–64.

96. Piccini JP, Hammill BG, Sinner MF, et al. Incidence and prevalence of atrial fibrillation and associated mortality among Medicare beneficiaries, 1993-2007. *Circ Cardiovasc Qual Outcomes.* 2012;5:85–93.

97. Oakes RS, Badger TJ, Kholmovski EG, et al. Detection and quantification of left atrial structural remodeling with delayed-enhancement magnetic resonance imaging in patients with atrial fibrillation. *Circulation.* 2009;119:1758–1767.

98. Verma A, Jiang CY, Betts TR, et al. Approaches to catheter ablation for persistent atrial fibrillation. *N Engl J Med.* 2015;372:1812–1822.

99. Krogh-Madsen T, Abbott GW, Christini DJ. Effects of electrical and structural remodeling on atrial fibrillation maintenance: a simulation study. *PLoS Comput Biol.* 2012;8:1002390.

100. Plank G, Prassl AJ, Wang JI, et al. Atrial fibrosis promotes the transition of pulmonary vein ectopy into reentrant arrhythmias. *Heart Rhythm.* 2008;5:S78.

101. Krueger MW, Rhode KS, O'Neill MD, et al. Patient-specific modeling of atrial fibrosis increases the accuracy of sinus rhythm simulations and may explain maintenance of atrial fibrillation. *J Electrocardiol.* 2014;47:324–328.

102. Spach MS, Heidlage JF, Dolber PC, et al. Electrophysiological effects of remodeling cardiac gap junctions and cell size: experimental and model studies of normal cardiac growth. *Circ Res.* 2000;86:302–311.

103. Eckstein J, Maesen B, Linz D, et al. Time course and mechanisms of endo-epicardial electrical dissociation during atrial fibrillation in the goat. *Cardiovasc Res.* 2011;89:816–824.

104. Jacquemet V, Henriquez CS. Genesis of complex fractionated atrial electrograms in zones of slow conduction: a computer model of microfibrosis. *Heart Rhythm.* 2009;6:803–810.

105. Comtois P, Nattel S. Interactions between cardiac fibrosis spatial pattern and ionic remodeling on electrical wave propagation. *Conf Proc IEEE Eng Med Biol Soc.* 2011;2011:4669–4672.

106. McDowell KS, Vadakkumpadan F, Blake R, et al. Mechanistic inquiry into the role of tissue remodeling in fibrotic lesions in human atrial fibrillation. *Biophys J.* 2013;104:2764–2773.

107. McDowell KS, Vadakkumpadan F, Blake R, et al. Methodology for patient-specific modeling of atrial fibrosis as a substrate for atrial fibrillation. *J Electrocardiol.* 2012;45:640–645.

108. Camelliti P, Green CR, LeGrice I, et al. Fibroblast network in rabbit sinoatrial node: structural and functional identification of homogeneous and heterogeneous cell coupling. *Circ Res.* 2004;94:8288–8235.

109. Pedrotty DM, Klinger RY, Kirkton RD, et al. Cardiac fibroblast paracrine factors alter impulse conduction and ion channel expression of neonatal rat cardiomyocytes. *Cardiovasc Res.* 2009;83:688–697.

110. Ashihara T, Haraguchi R, Nakazawa K, et al. The role of fibroblasts in complex fractionated electrograms during persistent/permanent atrial fibrillation: implications for electrogram-based catheter ablation. *Circ Res.* 2012;110:275–284.

111. Maleckar MM, Greenstein JL, Giles WR, et al. Electrotonic coupling between human atrial myocytes and fibroblasts alters myocyte excitability and repolarization. *Biophys J.* 2009;97:2179–2190.

112. Maleckar MM, Greenstein JL, Giles WR, et al. K+ current changes account for the rate dependence of the action potential in the human atrial myocyte. *Am J Physiol Heart Circ Physiol.* 2009;297:H1398–H1410.

113. McDowell KS, Zahid S, Vadakkumpadan F, et al. Virtual electrophysiological study of atrial fibrillation in fibrotic remodeling. *PLoS ONE.* 2015;10:e0117110.

114. Boyle PM, Zahid S, Schwarz E, et al. Local complexity of the fibrosis spatial pattern determines the locations of stable reentrant sources in persistent atrial fibrillation: analysis from patient-specific models. *Heart Rhythm.* 2015;12:S7.

115. Boyle PM, Zahid S, Schwarz E, et al. Prevalence of regions with highly intermingled fibrotic and non-fibrotic tissue is a better predictor of arrhythmia inducibility than total fibrosis burden: analysis of patient-specific models of persistent atrial fibrillation. *Heart Rhythm.* 2015;12:S80.

115a. Zahid S, Cochet H, Boyle PM, et al. Patient-derived models link re-entrant driver localization in atrial fibrillation to fibrosis spatial pattern. *Cardiovasc Res Physiol.* 2016;110:443–454.

115b. Zahid S, Whyte KN, Schwarz EL, et al. Feasibility of using patient-specific models and the "minimum cut" algorithm to predict optimal ablation targets for left atrial flutter. *Heart Rhythm.* 2016;13:1687–1698.

116. Avila G, Medina IM, Jimenez E, et al. Transforming growth factor-beta1 decreases cardiac muscle L-type Ca2+ current and charge movement by acting on the Cav1.2 mRNA. *Am J Physiol Heart Circ Physiol.* 2007;292:H622–H631.

117. Ramos-Mondragon R, Vega AV, Avila G. Long-term modulation of Na+ and K+ channels by TGF-beta1 in neonatal rat cardiac myocytes. *Pflugers Arch.* 2011;461:235–247.

118. Platonov PG, Mitrofanova LB, Orshanskaya V, et al. Structural abnormalities in atrial walls are associated with presence and persistency of atrial fibrillation but not with age. *J Am Coll Cardiol.* 2011;58:2225–2232.

119. Pertsov A. Scale of geometric structures responsible for discontinuous propagation in myocardial tissue. In: Spooner P, Joyner R, Jalife J, eds. *Discontinuous Conduction in the Heart.* Armonk, NY: Futura Publishing Company; 1997.

120. Turner I, L-H Huang C, Saumarez RC. Numerical simulation of paced electrogram fractionation: relating clinical observations to changes in fibrosis and action potential duration. *J Cardiovasc Electrophysiol.* 2005;16:151–161.

121. Panfilov AV. Spiral breakup in an array of coupled cells: the role of the intercellular conductance. *Phys Rev Lett.* 2002;88:118101.

122. Ten Tusscher K, Panfilov AV. Influence of nonexcitable cells on spiral breakup in two-dimensional and three-dimensional excitable media. *Phys Rev E Stat Nonlin Soft Matter Phys.* 2003;68:062902.

123. Ten Tusscher K, Panfilov AV. Wave propagation in excitable media with randomly distributed obstacles. *Multiscale Model Simul.* 2005;3:265–282.

124. Ten Tusscher KH, Panfilov AV. Influence of diffuse fibrosis on wave propagation in human ventricular tissue. *Europace.* 2007;9:vi38–vi45.

37 Innervation of the Sinoatrial Node

Dainius H. Pauza, Kristina Rysevaite-Kyguoliene, and Neringa Pauziene

The cardiac conduction system (CCS) initiates, conducts, and controls the heart rhythm. It comprises the sinoatrial node (SAN), atrioventricular node, penetrating bundle, and ventricular bundle branches.

The human SAN described in sagittal sections is a wedge-shaped structure situated at the junction of the superior vena cava (SVC) with the musculature of the terminal crest; the node is always arranged about a central SAN artery.[1–3] Nodal cells are fascicular in nature and are embedded in a prominent fibrous tissue matrix. The cells around the SAN artery are more densely packed and less eosinophilic than those at the nodal borders. Nodal cells are smaller than the adjacent atrial myocardial cells, and a distinct border is observed between the node and adjacent atrial myocardium.[3] The human SAN is located beneath the epicardium of the terminal crest with a layer of atrial muscle in between the SAN and the endocardium. The SAN has a wide body and a thin head and tail, which are located more toward the endocardial surface than toward the body.[2] The SAN measures 30 mm in length, 2 mm in height, and up to 7 mm in width.[2] The mammalian SAN is a complex three-dimensional (3D) structure that is anatomically and functionally isolated from the atrial myocardium (*crista terminalis* and interatrial septum) except for several SA exit pathways.[4] This conduction barrier is formed by the SAN arteries, connective tissue, and fat, as well as an abrupt change in connexin43 (Cx43) expression between atrial and nodal cells.[5,6] In the rat and rabbit hearts, CCS cells that are immunoreactive for hyperpolarization activated cyclic nucleotide-gated potassium channel 4 (HCN4) and Cx45 but negative for Cx43 extend downward from the SVC in the interatrial groove and are capable of independent pacemaker activity.[7] The nodal cells are positive for acetylcholinesterase (AChE) in contrast to the surrounding atrial myocytes, but this staining is much less intense than that displayed by neural AChE activity.[8]

In the mouse heart, HCN4-immunoreactive SAN cardiomyocytes (CMs) are widely distributed around the root of the SVC and form a well-defined horseshoe-shaped boundary by the side of the terminal groove and along the course of the SAN artery.[9] On electron microscope, the SAN CMs, described as P cells, contain sparse myofibrils, scanty sarcoplasmic reticulum, and numerous glycogen particles and are evidently smaller in size compared with regular atrial CMs. The mouse SAN also involves another type of CMs called transitional or T cells, which contain a slightly increased number of myofibrils.[9–14] However, frequently the structure of the SAN cells in rats and mice do not correspond with the classical description because the SAN pacemaker cells of these animals lack glycogen particles,[15] their transverse profiles vary in size and shape, and the morphological pattern of myofibrils of numerous conductive myocytes may be similar to myofibrils in regular atrial CMs.[9] Thus the structure and architecture of SAN cells in mammals appear to be more complex than previously considered.[16]

General Neuroanatomy of the Heart

Autonomic innervation of the heart involves both the extrinsic and intrinsic cardiac nervous systems. The former collectively includes the autonomic neurons in the brainstem or along the spinal cord (e.g., the vagosympathetic trunk) and their axons en route to the heart; the latter consists of the autonomic ganglia and axons located in the heart itself or along the great vessels in the thorax.[17] Studies in different animal species demonstrate significant variations in morphologic pattern of cardiac innervations.[18–27] In humans, as well as in other mammalians, extrinsic cardiac nerves access the heart via the heart hilum (HH).[28] From the arterial part of the HH (i.e., around the ascending aorta and pulmonary trunk), nerves extend predominantly into the ventricles, while from the venous part of the HH (i.e., around the pulmonary veins [PVs] and venae cavae), accessing nerves proceed on both the atria and ventricles. In the arterial part of the HH, plentiful nerves are regularly located in a fat pad between the ascending aorta and pulmonary trunk, but occasionally these nerves may be found in front of, behind, and on both sides of the aorta and pulmonary trunk.[23] Within the venous part of the human HH, neural access sites are concentrated at the following locations: the left atrial nerve fold (ligament of Marshall), between the right superior PV (RSPV) and SVC, between the RSPV and left superior PV, between the left superior PV and left inferior PV, between the RSPV and right inferior PV, and rarely, from the left and right sides of the inferior vena cava.[23] Rarely, human hearts contain thin accessing nerves in front of and dorsal to the SVC.[23] The number of nerves in any access and the thickness of the nerves on the HH level vary from heart to heart, but commonly, two to five nerves proceed through any neural access site.[23]

In the human heart, nerves from the accessing sites in the HH extend into the epicardium, in which they course by seven pathways.[23] Two nerve pathways start from the arterial part of the HH. From there, the nerves extend to the left side by the left ventral coronary groove as well as to the right side by the right ventral coronary groove. Nerves that pass onto the heart through the venous

37

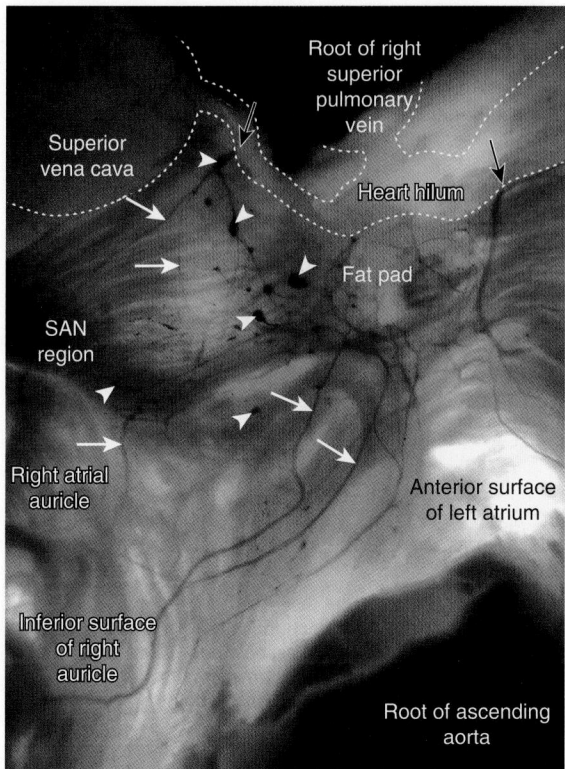

FIGURE 37.1 Macrophotograph of the ventral surface of a newborn human heart histochemically stained for acetylcholinesterase, demonstrating the right ventral nerve subplexus associated with the sinoatrial node (*SAN*) region. *White dashed lines* indicate the heart hilum. *White arrowheads* indicate some intrinsic ganglia; *black arrows* indicate preganglionated nerves, and *white arrows* point to postganglionated nerves.

part of the HH proceed by five pathways: the anterior interatrial groove and the groove situated dorsally between the roots of the SVC and RSPV nerves extending mainly to the right atrium, the left atrial nerve fold (Marshall ligament) to the lateral surface of the left atrium, and the ventral and dorsal surfaces of the left atrium epicardial nerves, which course to the left atrium and dorsal wall of the left ventricle.[23] Very close to both parts of the HH, the nerves proceeding by these pathways reach the epicardial ganglia, which as ganglionated fields (GFs) are distributed in consistent regions, interconnecting complexly among themselves via thin nerves.[23] Although sparse thin epicardial nerves also interconnect ganglia situated on different neural pathways, all GFs are clearly separated by wide regions of the heart surface, in which the epicardial neural plexus is devoid of ganglia.[23] Within the boundaries of the GFs, epicardial nerves extending from the HH branch out, become thin, and pass into the ganglia. In GFs, some epicardial nerves originate from numerous intrinsic ganglia, appear thicker, and course away from GFs to pass directly into the structures they innervate, in which they gradually disappear from view in two ways: either via penetration into myocardium or becoming gradually thinner in the epicardium (Figs. 37.1 and 37.2). Because the latter nerves are mostly devoid of ganglia, they are called postganglionated nerves (postGNs), while others that proceed from the HH into the GFs are called preganglionated nerves (preGNs). Because of characteristic disposition, appearance, and interrelations of the preGNs, GFs, and postGNs, it has been suggested that the entire epicardial neural plexus of humans may be considered as being composed of seven ganglionated subplexuses, each of which contains its own preGNs, GF, and postGNs.[23] The subplexal organization of the epicardial neural plexus has been confirmed in other mammalian species examined so far by employing the technique of histochemical staining of nerves in total heart preparations.[18,22,26,27,29–32] The largest GFs, involving

up to 84% of all cardiac ganglia, are distributed throughout the atria. The GFs of the different epicardial ganglionated subplexuses contain unequal numbers of ganglia, but their architecture is generally similar; that is, ganglia of various shapes and sizes are complexly interconnected in a network of thin epicardial nerves.

The human intrinsic cardiac ganglia range in size from those containing a few neurons to large ganglia measuring up to 0.5 × 1 mm and involving more than 2800 nerve cell bodies.[1,23] On average, the adult human heart contains about 800 epicardial ganglia that involve more than 43,000 neurons.[23] Depending on the age, the number of intrinsic ganglia per one heart may significantly fluctuate. For instance, in human adult hearts, the mean number is 700, while in human fetuses, neonates, infants, and children, the mean is larger than 900.[23] Importantly, the number of intrinsic cardiac ganglia and nerve cells strictly depends on species. The sheep heart contains 769 ± 52 epicardial ganglia in which 17,000 neurons reside.[29] The estimated total number of the intrinsic ganglia per porcine heart is 362 ± 52, comprising about 12,000 neurons.[30] The intracardiac neurons in adult guinea pigs are concentrated within 329 ± 15 ganglia that enclose approximately 2500 nerve cells.[19] The mean number of intrinsic cardiac neurons in old rats is nearly 6600, but juvenile rats contain significantly fewer such neurons, only 5000.[18] Correspondingly, rabbit and mouse hearts involve nearly 2100 and 1100 intrinsic cardiac neurons.[26,27,33]

Nerve Supply of the Sinoatrial Node Area

In the human heart as well as in the hearts of some other mammalian species, both the dorsal right atrial (DRA) and ventral right atrial (VRA) neural subplexuses supply epicardial nerves to the SAN neural network.[18,22,26,29,34,35] PreGNs of the VRA subplexus in the human heart enter the epicardium at the superior interatrial groove, where a large epicardial fat pad is consistently located near the HH (see Fig. 37.1). The epicardial ganglia of the VRA subplexus distribute on the VRA region, inferior surface of the right auricle, and in part on the ventral side of the root of the SVC.[23] The size and number of ganglia inside this GF vary from one heart to another, but the largest number and density of epicardial ganglia are usually located at the junction of the SVC with the anterior wall of the right atrium. The VRA subplexus accumulates approximately 11% of the human epicardial ganglia.[23] Although the thickest postGNs of the VRA subplexus are mainly oriented in the inferior surface of the right auricle and the ventral atrial regions, some upper postGNs of this subplexus innervate the SAN region, as well as penetrate into the lower part of the interatrial septum.[23] Noteworthy, the third part of the postGNs of this subplexus passes onto the left atrium via a remarkable crest of the ventral surface of the left atrium, located behind the root of the aorta, and reaches the root region of the left coronary artery (see Fig. 37.1).

In humans, the DRA subplexus does not extend beyond the dorsal and lateral surfaces of the right atrium. Its preGNs enter the epicardium in a narrow groove between the SVC and RSPV and join the GF distributed on the sinuses of both caval veins (see Fig. 37.2).[23] Although the extent of this GF varies from one heart to another, the largest number and density of ganglia are concentrated on the dorsal side of the root of the SVC and in part, over the interatrial septum (see Fig. 37.2).[23] In some hearts, epicardial ganglia of the DRA subplexus are more widely distributed and reach the lateral sides of the root of the SVC and even overlap with the ganglia of the VRA subplexus.[23] Overall, the ganglia of the DRA subplexus comprise about 26% of all ganglia per heart.[23] PostGNs of the DRA subplexus spread widely into the DRA and lateral right atrium, including the SAN region and superior surface of the right auricle.[23]

It is estimated that about 1000 intrinsic neurons residing within the right ganglionic cluster at the interatrial groove of the left atrium are involved in the neural regulation of the mouse SAN.[9,32] Recent physiological data definitely confirmed the significance of the DRA subplexus for the neural control of SAN function.[36,37]

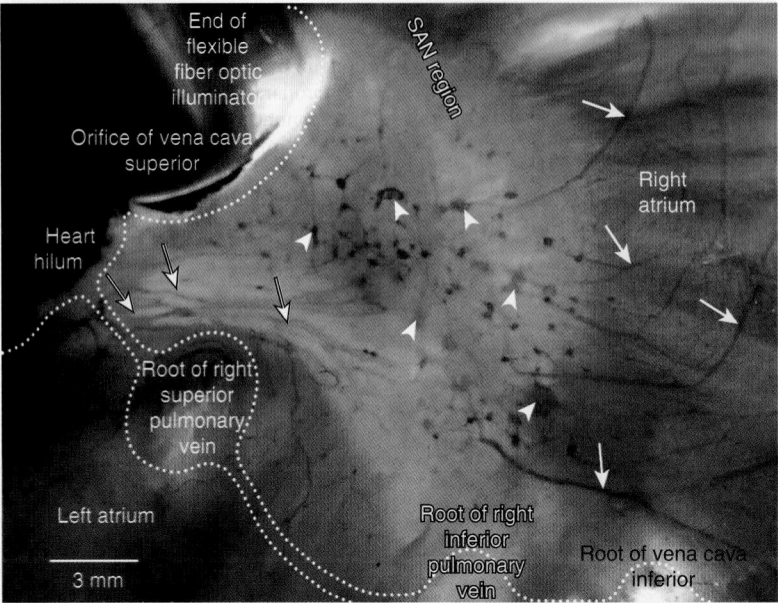

FIGURE 37.2 Macrophotograph of the dorsal surface of a newborn human heart histochemically stained for acetylcholinesterase, demonstrating the dorsal right atrial nerve subplexus associated with the sinoatrial node (*SAN*) region. *White dashed lines* indicate the heart hilum. *White arrowheads* indicate some intrinsic ganglia; *black arrows* indicate preganglionated nerves, and *white arrows* point to postganglionated nerves.

Morphology and Immunohistochemistry of the Sinoatrial Node Innervation in Humans and Other Mammals

All regions of the CCS possess a significantly higher density of nerve fibers than the adjacent working myocardium.[3,20,38,39] The SAN is defined as the most densely innervated region of the human CCS.[3] The highest density of nerve fibers immunoreactive for general neuronal marker protein gene product (PGP) 9.5 has also been observed in the guinea pig SAN compared with a significantly lower density of nerve fibers in the surrounding right atrium.[8] More than a three-fold higher density of PGP 9.5–immunoreactive innervation relative to that of the surrounding atrial myocardium is confirmed in the pig heart.[20]

Fluorescence immunohistochemistry has shown that the mouse SAN CMs positive for HCN4 are accompanied by a dense fine meshwork of nerve fibers. Slender and narrow HCN4-immunoreactive myocytes from the main mass of the SAN extend toward the right auricle, the root of the right PV, and the root of the caudal vein (Fig. 37.3). Compared with the right atrial areas adjacent to the root of the right cranial vein (the right cranial vein prevailing in many mammalian species corresponds to the SVC in humans), the density of nerve fibers amid the cardiac pacemaker cells positive for HCN4 is three- to four-fold higher.[9]

The density of nerve fibers and their phenotypes vary between the zones of the SAN, and such variability is species dependent.[8,20,21,38] Significantly more nerve fibers are distributed in the central zone of the human SAN surrounding the nodal artery compared with the nodal periphery, including the perivascular innervation of small arteries and arterioles in the atrial myocardium.[3] However, no significant difference was found in the total percentage of the stained area of nerves immunoreactive for PGP 9.5 between the central and peripheral nodal regions of the pig heart.[20]

Electron microscopic data conclusively demonstrate that all nerve fibers identified in the mouse SAN are exclusively composed of unmyelinated nerve fibers and involve axons with both cholinergic and adrenergic neurotransmitters.[9] The axons within unmyelinated nerve fibers have varicosities with abundant round, small, clear, and a few dense-cored vesicles. A number of unmyelinated nerve fibers have axons that are incompletely enveloped

by Schwann cells with a fragment of their plasma membrane in direct contact with the basal lamina surrounding the whole unmyelinated nerve fiber (Fig. 37.4). These unmyelinated nerve fibers have varicosities and are distributed regularly in the vicinity of cardiac pacemaker cells.[9] The density of nerve fibers within the distinct zones of the root of the right cranial vein (SVC, in humans) is significantly higher than that in the neighboring atrial zones, which correlates well between corresponding data of fluorescent and electron microscopy. Unmyelinated nerve fibers with numerous axonal varicosities are situated predominantly close to cardiac pacemaker cells. The closest unmyelinated nerve fibers are located 0.06 μm from cardiac pacemaker cells, but occasionally some were 2 μm or more away from such cells. In the mouse SAN, the average distance between cardiac pacemaker cells and unmyelinated nerve fibers is less than 0.5 μm,[9] whereas it is only about 80 nm in the guinea pig SAN.[40] SAN cells are closely associated with at least one unmyelinated nerve fiber or axon, but the majority of these cells usually are in close proximity to two to three unmyelinated nerve fibers.[9]

Nerve fibers immunoreactive for tyrosine hydroxylase (TH) are observed within large nerves running adjacent to AChE-positive nerves located within the nodal tissue but close to the border with the atrial musculature and also at the nodal surfaces adjacent to both the SVC and the terminal crest.[20] TH immunoreactivity is detectable in a significantly lower proportion of nerves and nerve fibers than that for AChE activity, representing approximately 30% of the total nodal innervations in pig hearts. Axonal profiles of TH immunoreactivity distribute in nerves that also possess AChE-positive fibers.[20] TH-immunoreactive nerves represented 40%–45% of the total SAN innervation as displayed by PGP 9.5 immunoreactivity in the guinea pig heart; however, unlike AChE-positive nerves, a large number of TH-immunoreactive nerves are associated with perivascular plexuses both in and around the SAN.[8] A meshwork rich in both cholinergic and adrenergic nerve fibers and possessing axons with a high amount of varicosities fills the mouse SAN region. Choline acetyltransferase (ChAT)-immunoreactive and TH-immunoreactive nerve fibers are equally abundant in the mouse SAN.[9]

Neuropeptide Y (NPY)–immunoreactive nerves are distributed similarly and occupy a similar area as TH-immunoreactive nerves. NPY-immunoreactive nerve fibers represent the

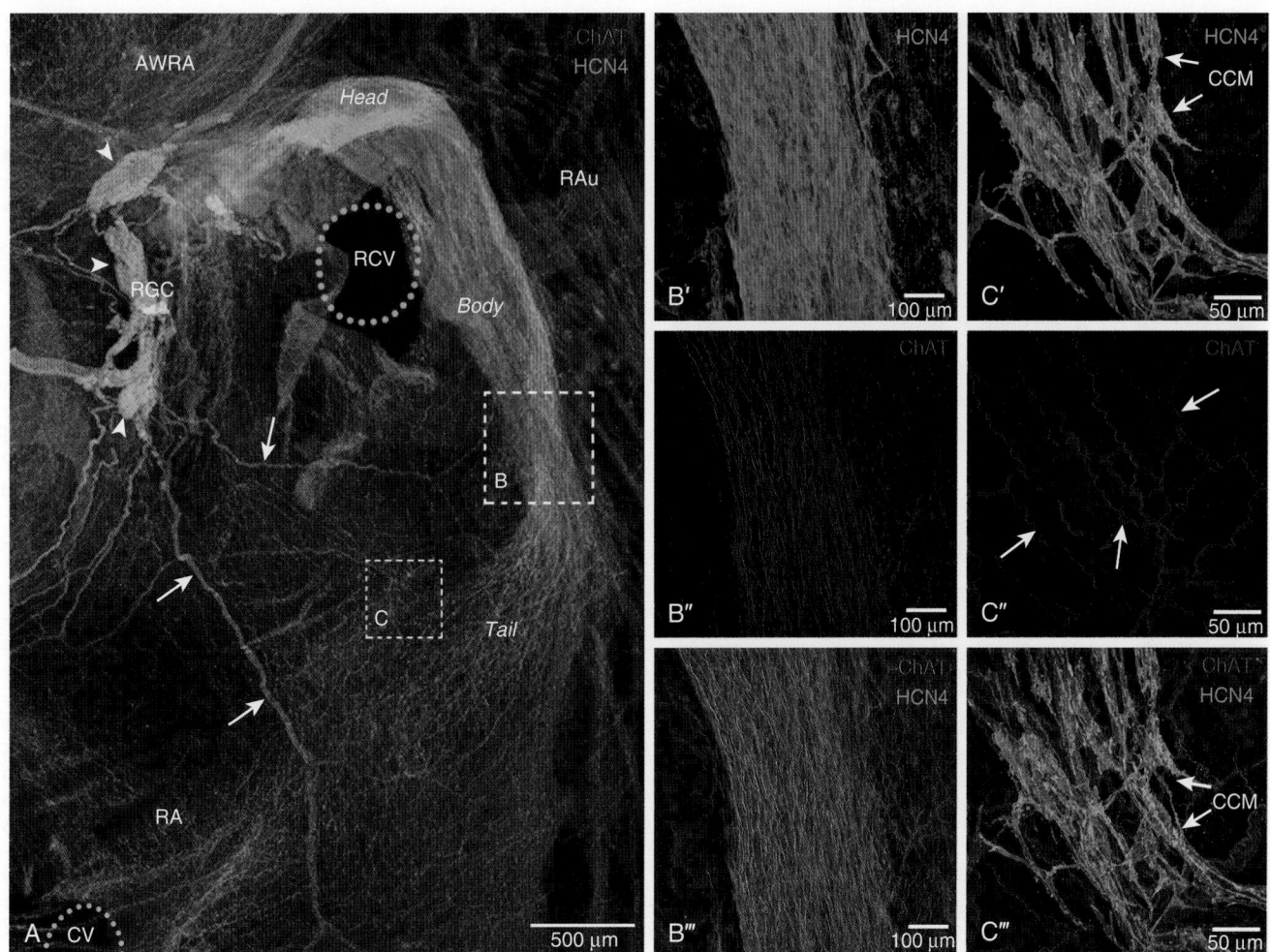

FIGURE 37.3 Whole-mount preparation of mouse atria demonstrates the distribution of conductive myocytes immunoreactive for hyperpolarization-activated cyclic nucleotide–gated channel 4 (*HCN4*) and neural structures positive for choline acetyltransferase (*ChAT*; intrinsic nerves, ganglia, and nerve fibers). Atrial appendages, left atrium, interatrial septum, and roots of pulmonary veins were dissected to flatten the right atrial wall. Cholinergic (ChAT) neural structures (nerves and ganglia) are labeled *red*, while cells positive for HCN4 are labeled *green*, and the merged immunoreactivity (ChAT + HCN4) is shown in panels (A), (B‴), and (C‴). In panel (A), *arrowheads* indicate some intrinsic cardiac ganglia in the right-sided ganglionic cluster (*RGC*), from where the epicardial postganglionated nerves (*arrows*) extend toward the sinoatrial node region and right atrium. The *boxed areas* (B and C) in panel (A) are enlarged as panels (B′–B‴) and (C′–C‴) to display the overlapped distribution of the cholinergic nerve fibers (*white arrows*) and pacemaker cells immunoreactive for HCN4. The head, body, and tail in panel (A) indicate the corresponding portions of the mouse SAN region. *AWRA*, Anterior wall of right atrium; *CCM*, conductive cardiomyocyte; *CV*, orifice of caudal vein; *RA*, right atrium; *RAu*, right auricle; *RCV*, orifice of right cranial vein.

predominant peptide-containing nerve subpopulation in the SAN and are significantly higher than NPY-containing nerves in the surrounding right atrium in the pig[20] and the guinea pig heart.[8] Examinations by Steele and Choate[41] of the guinea pig heart determined that the entire SAN was densely innervated by sympathetic axons, the majority of which were NPY immunoreactive. However, only a few axons were revealed to be immunoreactive for TH. In the human heart, the relative density of sympathetic nerve fibers immunoreactive for NPY and TH is significantly greater in the central SAN region compared with the periphery SAN region.[3]

After NPY, the other predominant peptidergic nerve subpopulations are immunoreactive for the sensory peptide substance P (SP) and calcitonin gene–related peptide (CGRP).[8,41] Somatostatin (SOM)-immunoreactive nerves are less abundant than SP- and CGRP-containing nerves and possess a distinct pattern of distribution compared with other nerve populations. Vasoactive intestinal peptide (VIP)-immunoreactive nerves are very sparse in both the SAN and the surrounding right atrium. Nerve fibers displaying immunoreactivity for VIP are rare in the pig SAN area. When found, these fibers are closely associated with small blood vessels, mainly arterioles, within the nodal tissue and also, to a lesser extent, in the atrial myocardium.[20] Altogether, these nerves appear to represent a relatively minor component of the sinus nodal innervation exhibiting a percentage of stained area 10- to 40-fold less than that of NPY- and TH-immunoreactive nerves, respectively.[3,8] Individual VIP- and SOM-immunoreactive nerve fibers scatter among SAN cells, whereas SP- and CGRP-immunoreactive nerve fibers occur mainly in epicardial nerves and are also found surrounding cell bodies in cardiac ganglia. No difference is found between the area of SP- and CGRP-stained nerves.[3] The great majority of CGRP-immunoreactive neural tissue in the canine heart exists adjacent to the SAN where varicose nerve processes course in numerous large nerve

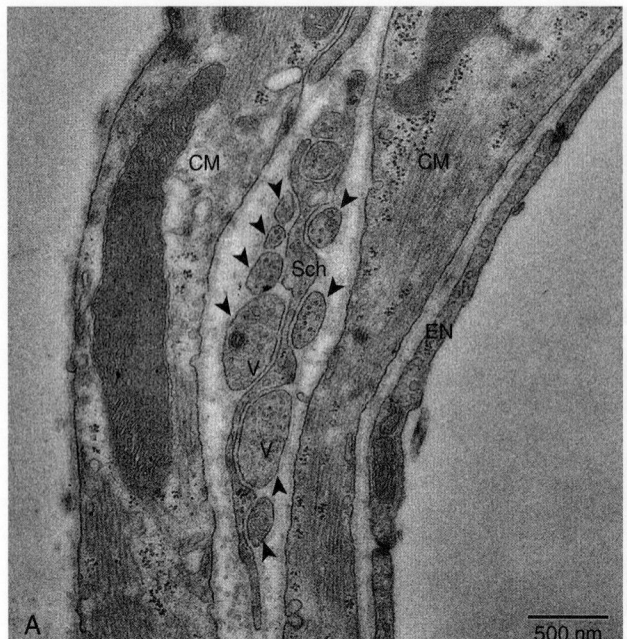

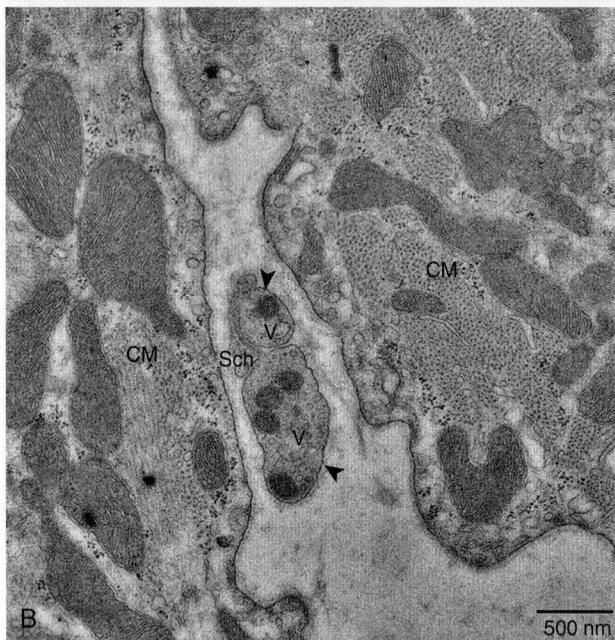

FIGURE 37.4 (A and B) Electron micrographs of unmyelinated nerve fibers closely inserted between cardiomyocytes (*CM*) of the mouse sinoatrial node. Practically all axons in both nerve fibers are incompletely enveloped by Schwann cells, and their plasma membrane is in direct contact with the basal lamina (*arrowheads*). Many axons are filled with neurotransmitter vesicles (*V*). Note irregularly arranged myofibrils in the cytoplasm of CMs. *EN,* Endothelial cell of capillary; *Sch,* Schwann cell.

by placing them in organotypic culture to allow degeneration of extrinsic axons. These experiments demonstrated several distinct populations of parasympathetic nerves innervating only a small, discrete part of the SAN. Such populations were immunoreactive for NPY, SOM, or VIP alone or for SOM combined with NPY, SOM with dynorphin B, and SOM with SP. These results highlighted a remarkable difference in the pattern of innervation of the SAN by the sympathetic and parasympathetic nervous systems.

Intrinsic Ganglia and Neuronal Somata Related With the Sinoatrial Node

Numerous ganglionic cells immunoreactive for general neuronal marker PGP 9.5 are distributed in the human epicardium overlying the SAN region, with most ganglia occurring on the root of the SVC.[3,23,35] In the guinea pig heart, the peripheral SAN regions and epicardial tissues possess several large PGP 9.5-immunoreactive ganglia. Isolated ganglionic cell bodies are also observed in the SAN itself.[8] No ganglion cell bodies displaying TH or NPY immunoreactivity were observed in the SAN region of the pig heart.[20]

Examinations of the canine and human right atrial ganglionated plexus (RAGP) located at the fat pad between the superior and inferior PVs demonstrate that this ganglionated plexus has a major role in the regulation of heart rate and may serve as an integration center for inputs from other parts of the cardiac ganglionated plexus.[36,43–46] Using the acute biopsy samples from the human RAGP, Hoover and coworkers[47] revealed that numerous cardiac ganglionic cells from this location contain neuronal nitric oxide synthase (nNOS). Staining for nNOS is also prominent in axons within these ganglia and in nerve fibers connecting to or bordering ganglia. A small population of neurons from the RAGP (about 20%) showed immunoreactivity for noradrenergic neuronal markers and for TH and vesicular monoamine transporter 2 (VMAT2). In addition, some VMAT2 immunoreactive axons in the ganglia appeared to surround neuronal somata. TH-positive nerve fibers were far less common, but they were also labeled for VMAT2.[47] The neuropeptides VIP, CGRP, and SP were localized within nerve fibers in the cardiac ganglia. SP was always colocalized with CGRP, but many CGRP-positive nerve fibers were not positive for SP.[47] The study by Hoover and coworkers[47] demonstrated that neurons of the human RAGP receive a plethora of noncholinergic inputs that include nerve fibers staining for VIP, CGRP, SP, nNOS, and noradrenergic markers.[47] Moreover, the presence of several distinct populations of autonomic cardiac neurons in the human RAGP indicates a high complexity in neuronal regulation of heart rate. The right-sided ganglionic cluster of the mouse heart consists of about 86% ChAT-immunoreactive, 14% biphenotypic, and 3% TH-immunoreactive neurons,[33] and all epicardial nerves entering the SAN region from this cluster include both the cholinergic and adrenergic nerve fibers.[32]

Concluding Remarks

The heart rhythm is regulated by both extrinsic and intrinsic cardiac nerves. While the extrinsic nerves more generally control various cardiac functions, such as chronotropy and contractility, the intrinsic cardiac nerve structures are more specific in their respective functional roles.[36,37,48–50] Stimulation of parasympathetic nerves that innervate the SAN increased atrial cycle length and shortened atrial refractoriness in humans without affecting atrioventricular nodal conduction.[44,46] Chronic neural stimulation of the DRA subplexus has been found feasible for rate control during atrial fibrillation,[51] while stimulation of the VRA subplexus may contribute to rapid SVC firing.[49] The right atrial ganglionated subplexuses have been shown to play a

bundles.[42] Immunoreactivity for CGRP is localized to isolated nerve fibers within AChE-positive nerves. CGRP-positive nerve fibers occupy a significantly lower percentage stained area than the subpopulation of nerves immunoreactive for NPY and represent approximately 8% of the total neural population. SOM-immunoreactive nerves are relatively sparse compared with either NPY- or CGRP-immunoreactive nerves, representing less than 4% of the overall innervation.

In the study by Steele and Choate,[41] intrinsic parasympathetic neurons from the guinea pig heart were extrinsically denervated

unique role in regulating the SAN activity.[37,52,53] On the basis of the results from acute ablation and stimulation experiments in anesthetized dogs, it may be concluded that the main connection between the right vagosympathetic trunk and the SAN goes through the VRA subplexus, and this subplexus serves as the integration center for both the right and left vagosympathetic trunks to modulate the sinus rate.[36] Autonomic imbalance in sympathetic and parasympathetic activities is an important feature of heart failure and is associated with increased mortality.[54] Experimental studies in dogs demonstrate that heart failure is associated with increased sympathetic nerve discharges from the stellate ganglion as well as with abnormal heart rate responses. In heart failure, denervation of the DRA subplexus and decreased nerve activity from this subplexus contribute to SAN dysfunction.[55,56]

Acknowledgments

The authors wish to express thanks to Audrys G. Pauza, MSc, for his graphical assistance in preparing this chapter. The authors are also exceptionally grateful to Prof. José Jalife from the Center for Arrhythmia Research, University of Michigan, Ann Arbor, Michigan, USA, for his careful reading of the manuscript and friendly editorial assistance. Funding for this study was partly allocated from Grants MIP-11184 and MIP-13037 provided by the Research Council of Lithuania.

REFERENCES

1. Armour JA, Murphy DA, Yuan BX, et al. Gross and microscopic anatomy of the human intrinsic cardiac nervous system. *Anat Rec.* 1997;247:289–298.
2. Chandler N, Aslanidi O, Buckley D, et al. Computer three-dimensional anatomical reconstruction of the human sinus node and a novel paranodal area. *Anat Rec.* 2011;294:970–979.
3. Crick SJ, Wharton J, Sheppard MN, et al. Innervation of the human cardiac conduction system. A quantitative immunohistochemical and histochemical study. *Circulation.* 1994;89:1697–1708.
4. Fedorov VV, Glukhov AV, Chang R, et al. Optical mapping of the isolated coronary-perfused human sinus node. *J Am Coll Cardiol.* 2010;56:1386–1394.
5. Fedorov VV, Schuessler RB, Hemphill M, et al. Structural and functional evidence for discrete exit pathways that connect the canine sinoatrial node and atria. *Circ Res.* 2009;104:915–923.
6. Chandler NJ, Greener ID, Tellez JO, et al. Molecular architecture of the human sinus node: insights into the function of the cardiac pacemaker. *Circulation.* 2009;119:1562–1575.
7. Yamamoto M, Dobrzynski H, Tellez J, et al. Extended atrial conduction system characterised by the expression of the HCN4 channel and connexin45. *Cardiovasc Res.* 2006;72:271–281.
8. Crick SJ, Sheppard MN, Anderson RH, et al. A quantitative study of nerve distribution in the conduction system of the guinea pig heart. *J Anat.* 1996;188:403–416.
9. Pauza DH, Rysevaite K, Inokaitis H, et al. Innervation of sinoatrial nodal cardiomyocytes in mouse. A combined approach using immunofluorescent and electron microscopy. *J Mol Cell Cardiol.* 2014;75:188–197.
10. Ayettey AS, Navaratnam V, Yates RD. Ultrastructure of the internodal myocardium in the rat. *J Anat.* 1988;158:77–90.
11. Bleeker WK, Mackaay AJ, Masson-Pévet M, et al. Functional and morphological organization of the rabbit sinus node. *Circ Res.* 1980;46:11–22.
12. Stoletzki S, Schmiedl A, Richter J. Intercalated clear cells or pale cells in the sinus node of canine hearts? An ultrastructural study. *Anat Rec.* 2000;260:33–41.
13. James TN, Sherf L, Fine G, et al. Comparative ultrastructure of the sinus node in man and dog. *Circulation.* 1966;34:139–163.
14. Lowe JE, Hartwich T, Takla M, et al. Ultrastructure of electrophysiologically identified human sinoatrial nodes. *Basic Res Cardiol.* 1988;83:401–409.
15. Calvet-Márquez S, Domènech-Mateu JM. Presence or absence of glycogen-beta particles in sinoatrial node cells. *Acta Anat (Basel).* 1994;150:267–273.
16. Balbi T, Ghimenton C, Pasquinelli G, et al. Advancement in the examination of the human cardiac sinus node: an unexpected architecture and a novel cell type could interest the forensic science. *Am J Forensic Med Pathol.* 2011;32:112–118.
17. Ardell JL. Intrathoracic neuronal regulation of cardiac function. In: Armour JA, Ardell JL, eds. *Basic and Clinical Neurocardiology.* Oxford, UK: Oxford University Press; 2004:118–152.
18. Batulevicius D, Pauziene N, Pauza DH. Topographic morphology and age-related analysis of the neuronal number of the rat intracardiac nerve plexus. *Ann Anat.* 2003;185:449–459.
19. Batulevicius D, Pauziene N, Pauza DH. Architecture and age-related analysis of the neuronal number of the guinea pig intrinsic cardiac nerve plexus. *Ann Anat.* 2005;187:225–243.

20. Crick SJ, Sheppard MN, Ho SY, et al. Localisation and quantitation of autonomic innervation in the porcine heart I: conduction system. *J Anat.* 1999;195:341–357.
21. Hoover DB, Ganote CE, Ferguson SM, et al. Localization of cholinergic innervation in guinea pig heart by immunohistochemistry for high-affinity choline transporters. *Cardiovasc Res.* 2004;62:112–121.
22. Pauza DH, Skripka V, Pauziene N, et al. Anatomical study of the neural ganglionated plexus in the canine right atrium: implications for selective denervation and electrophysiology of the sinoatrial node in dog. *Anat Rec.* 1999;255:271–294.
23. Pauza DH, Skripka V, Pauziene N, et al. Morphology, distribution, and variability of the epicardiac neural ganglionated subplexuses in the human heart. *Anat Rec.* 2000;259:353–382.
24. Pauza DH, Pauziene N, Pakeltyte G, et al. Comparative quantitative study of the intrinsic cardiac ganglia and neurons in the rat, guinea pig, dog and human as revealed by histochemical staining for acetylcholinesterase. *Ann Anat.* 2002;184:125–136.
25. Pauziene N, Pauza DH, Stropus R. Morphological study of the heart innervation of bats Myotis daubentoni and Eptesicus serotinus (Microchiroptera: Vespertilionidae) during hibernation. *Eur J Morphol.* 2000;38:195–205.
26. Rysevaite K, Saburkina I, Pauziene N, et al. Morphologic pattern of the intrinsic ganglionated nerve plexus in mouse heart. *Heart Rhythm.* 2011;8:448–454.
27. Saburkina I, Gukauskiene L, Rysevaite K, et al. Morphological pattern of intrinsic nerve plexus distributed on the rabbit heart and interatrial septum. *J Anat.* 2014;224:583–593.
28. Pauza DH, Pauziene N, Tamasauskas KA, et al. Hilum of the heart. *Anat Rec.* 1997;248:322–324.
29. Saburkina I, Rysevaite K, Pauziene N, et al. Epicardial neural ganglionated plexus of ovine heart: anatomic basis for experimental cardiac electrophysiology and nerve protective cardiac surgery. *Heart Rhythm.* 2010;7:942–950.
30. Batulevicius D, Skripka V, Pauziene N, et al. Topography of the porcine epicardiac nerve plexus as revealed by histochemistry for acetylcholinesterase. *Auton Neurosci.* 2008;138:64–75.
31. Batulevicius D, Pauziene N, Pauza DH. Key anatomic data for the use of rat heart in electrophysiological studies of the intracardiac nervous system. *Medicina (Kaunas).* 2004;40:253–259.
32. Pauza DH, Saburkina I, Rysevaite K, et al. Neuroanatomy of the murine cardiac conduction system: a combined stereomicroscopic and fluorescence immunohistochemical study. *Auton Neurosci.* 2013;176:32–47.
33. Rysevaite K, Saburkina I, Pauziene N, et al. Immunohistochemical characterization of the intrinsic cardiac neural plexus in whole-mount mouse heart preparations. *Heart Rhythm.* 2011;8:731–738.
34. Pauziene N, Pauza DH, Stropus R. Morphology of human intracardiac nerves: an electron microscope study. *J Anat.* 2000;197:437–459.
35. Saburkina I, Pauza DH. Location and variability of epicardiac ganglia in human fetuses. *Anat Embryol.* 2006;211:585–594.
36. Hou Y, Scherlag BJ, Lin J, et al. Ganglionated plexi modulate extrinsic cardiac autonomic nerve input: effects on sinus rate, atrioventricular conduction, refractoriness, and inducibility of atrial fibrillation. *J Am Coll Cardiol.* 2007;50:61–68.
37. Hou Y, Scherlag BJ, Lin J, et al. Interactive atrial neural network: determining the connections between ganglionated plexi. *Heart Rhythm.* 2007;4:56–63.

38. Crick SJ, Sheppard MN, Anderson RH, et al. A quantitative assessment of innervation in the conduction system of the calf heart. *Anat Rec.* 1996;245:685–698.
39. Steele PA, Gibbins IL, Morris JL. Projections of intrinsic cardiac neurons to different targets in the guinea-pig heart. *J Auton Nerv Syst.* 1996;56:191–200.
40. Choate JK, Klemm M, Hirst GD. Sympathetic and parasympathetic neuromuscular junctions in the guinea-pig sino-atrial node. *J Auton Nerv Syst.* 1993;44:1–15.
41. Steele PA, Choate JK. Innervation of the pacemaker in guinea-pig sinoatrial node. *J Auton Nerv Syst Elsevier.* 1994;47:177–187.
42. Ursell PC, Ren CL, Albala A, et al. Nonadrenergic noncholinergic innervation. Anatomic distribution of calcitonin gene-related peptide-immunoreactive tissue in the dog heart. *Circ Res.* 1991;68:131–140.
43. Cardinal R, Pagé P, Vermeulen M, et al. Spatially divergent cardiac responses to nicotinic stimulation of ganglionated plexus neurons in the canine heart. *Auton Neurosci.* 2009;145:55–62.
44. Carlson MD, Geha AS, Hsu J, et al. Selective stimulation of parasympathetic nerve fibers to the human sinoatrial node. *Circulation.* 1992;85:1311–1317.
45. Bluemel KM, Wurster RD, Randall WC, et al. Parasympathetic postganglionic pathways to the sinoatrial node. *Am J Physiol.* 1990;259:H1504–H1510.
46. Quan KJ, Lee JH, Geha AS, et al. Characterization of sinoatrial parasympathetic innervation in humans. *J Cardiovasc Electrophysiol.* 1999;10:1060–1065.
47. Hoover DB, Isaacs ER, Jacques F, et al. Localization of multiple neurotransmitters in surgically derived specimens of human atrial ganglia. *Neuroscience.* 2009;164:1170–1179.
48. Armour JA. Potential clinical relevance of the "little brain" on the mammalian heart. *Exp Physiol.* 2008;93:165–176.
49. Lu Z, Scherlag BJ, Niu G, et al. Functional properties of the superior vena cava (SVC)-aorta ganglionated plexus: evidence suggesting an autonomic basis for rapid SVC firing. *J Cardiovasc Electrophysiol.* 2010;21:1392–1399.
50. Choi E-K, Shen MJ, Han S, et al. Intrinsic cardiac nerve activity and paroxysmal atrial tachyarrhythmia in ambulatory dogs. *Circulation.* 2010;121:2615–2623.
51. Mischke K, Zarse M, Schmid M, et al. Chronic augmentation of the parasympathetic tone to the atrioventricular node: a nonthoracotomy neurostimulation technique for ventricular rate control during atrial fibrillation. *J Cardiovasc Electrophysiol.* 2010;21:193–199.
52. Nakajima K, Furukawa Y, Kurogouchi F, et al. Autonomic control of the location and rate of the cardiac pacemaker in the sinoatrial fat pad of parasympathetically denervated dog hearts. *J Cardiovasc Electrophysiol.* 2002;13:896–901.
53. Armour JA. Cardiac neuronal hierarchy in health and disease. *Am J Physiol Regul Integr Comp Physiol.* 2004;287:R262–R271.
54. Mortara A, La Rovere MT, Pinna GD, et al. Arterial baroreflex modulation of heart rate in chronic heart failure: clinical and hemodynamic correlates and prognostic implications. *Circulation.* 1997;96:3450–3458.
55. Ogawa M, Zhou S, Tan AY, et al. Left stellate ganglion and vagal nerve activity and cardiac arrhythmias in ambulatory dogs with pacing-induced congestive heart failure. *J Am Coll Cardiol.* 2007;50:335–343.
56. Shinohara T, Shen MJ, Han S, et al. Heart failure decreases nerve activity in the right atrial ganglionated plexus. *J Cardiovasc Electrophysiol.* 2012;23:404–412.

38 Mechanisms for Altered Autonomic and Oxidant Regulation of Cardiac Sodium Currents

Gordon F. Tomaselli

Sodium Channels: Structural Aspects of Oxidant and Autonomic Regulation

The voltage-dependent sodium (Na) channel (Na_V1 family) is a multisubunit transmembrane glycoprotein that is highly regulated in health and disease (see Chapters 1 and 9). Voltage-dependent ion channels, such as the Na channel, facilitate the apparently incongruous rapid ($>10^6$ ions per second) yet highly selective flux of ions across the lipid bilayer down their respective electrochemical gradients. All ion channels exhibit two essential properties: gating and selective permeation. Gating is the opening and closing of the channel pore in response to a specific biological stimulus, such as transmembrane voltage. Ion selectivity is in part determined by molecular sieving and, perhaps more importantly, by different energetic strategies for transiently binding the permeant ion in the pore. Both processes are exquisitely regulated by a number of signaling cascades that are active during normal physiological and pathological conditions associated with cardiac arrhythmias.

As has been described elsewhere in this volume, voltage-gated ion channels share common structural themes: a modular architecture, an ion-selective pore with highly conserved pore-lining residues for channels with similar selectivity, a common gating strategy using a charged-membrane voltage sensor, and auxiliary subunits that regulate trafficking and function. $Na_V1.5$ channels are among the most abundant ion channels in working cardiac muscles ($\sim10^6$ copies/myocyte) and carry the major inward current (I_{Na}) for excitation. Expression of the $Na_V1.5$ channel pore-forming α-subunit is sufficient for current generation, and it determines the ion selectivity and conductance properties. The Na_V1 channel family transmembrane domain sequences are highly conserved from the eel electroplax to humans[1,2]; however, there is significant divergence in key regulatory channel domains, such as the cytoplasmic loops and carboxyl terminus. There are long and short variants of the linker between domains I and II, and the long version of this linker contains multiple putative phosphorylation sites for several physiologically relevant kinases (Fig. 38.1).

Four genes (SCN1B-SCN4B) encode five different β-subunit proteins ($Na_V \beta1$, 1B, 2, 3, and 4), each with a single membrane-spanning domain (type 1 topology) and a large extracellular V-like immunoglobulin fold often found in cell adhesion molecules.[3] The only exception is the $Na_V \beta1B$ splice variant that is secreted and lacks the small carboxyl-terminal cytoplasmic domains characteristic of the other isoforms. β-Subunits are present in a wide range of tissues, and their general function is to promote the expression and specific subcellular localization of $Na_V\beta$ subunits.[3] The structure of $Na_V\beta$ subunits is similar to that of classes of cell adhesion molecules[4]; β-subunits promote adhesion and can do so even in the absence of Na_V1 α-subunits (thus could influence conduction). The distinct kinetic, voltage-dependent, and pharmacological properties of Na_V channels are dependent on the specific α-β–subunit combination and cell expression systems.[5]

The role of β-subunits in the function and regulation of $Na_V1.5$ channels in the heart is uncertain. However, variants in a number of β-subunits have been implicated in the production of cardiac arrhythmias, sudden infant death syndrome (SIDS), and sudden unexplained death in epilepsy (SUDEP). Mutations in SCN1B, SCN2B, and SCN3B have been described in Brugada syndrome (BrS); SCN3B in SIDS and idiopathic ventricular fibrillation (IVF); and SCN4B in long QT syndrome (LQTS) and SIDS. The presence of an arrhythmic phenotype in scn1b and scn3b null mice is consistent with a functional effect of these subunits in the heart, although the interpretation in scn1b–/– mice is complicated by the presence of a complex neurological and developmental phenotype.[3]

Myocardial Metabolism and Oxidant Stress

Under resting conditions, in excess of 95% of myocardial adenosine triphosphate (ATP) production comes from oxidative-phosphorylation in the mitochondria,[6,7] and other than the contractile apparatus, mitochondria occupy the largest volume of the ventricular myocyte ($\sim30\%$–35% in humans).[8] Normally, the rate of oxidative phosphorylation is linked to the rate of ATP hydrolysis to match energy supply and demand. Acetyl CoA generated from fatty acid β-oxidation, and reduced nicotinamide adenine dinucleotide (NADH) and flavin adenine dinucleotide ($FADH_2$) in the tricarboxylic acid (TCA) cycle in the mitochondrial matrix. NADH and $FADH_2$ provide electrons to the electron transport chain where oxidation–reduction reactions occur at complexes I, III, and IV with the generation of superoxide radicals resulting from electron leak. The proton gradient and steeply negative mitochondrial membrane potential serve to generate ATP.[6] Most of the ATP generated is used for contraction but it is estimated that up to one-third supports ion homeostasis.[9] Low levels of reactive oxygen and nitrogen species (ROS/RNS), such as superoxide and hydroxyl radicals, nitric oxide (NO), and hydrogen peroxide (H_2O_2), are important physiological signaling molecules. However, excess levels of ROS/RNS can produce deleterious effects

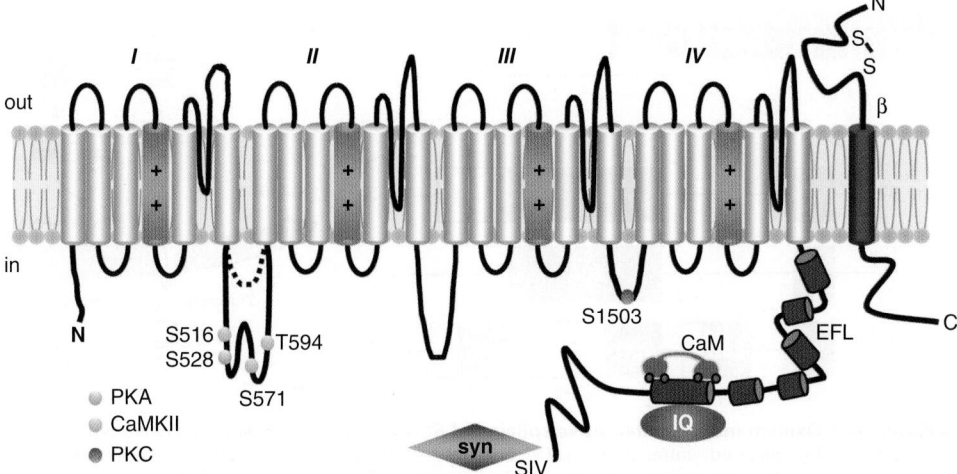

FIGURE 38.1 Schematic of the cardiac sodium (Na) channel. There is a voltage-sensing, membrane-spanning repeat (*orange cylinder*) in each of the four domains. Voltage-dependent Na channels (Na$_V$1) are associated with one or more β-subunits, each with an extracellular V-like immunoglobulin fold. Interacting proteins and sites involved in oxidant and kinase regulation of the Na$_V$1.5 channel are illustrated. Syntrophin (*syn*) binds to the C-terminal class I PDZ ligand (*SIV*) in Na$_V$1.5. Functionally important phosphorylation sites for protein kinase A (*PKA*) and Ca^{2+}/calmodulin-dependent protein kinase II (*CaMKII*) are in the I–II linker of long isoforms of the channel (*solid line*), and short isoforms (*dotted line*) contain no consensus phosphorylation sites. Protein kinase C (*PKC*) phosphorylation occurs in the III–IV linker. The proximal C-terminus contains an EF hand-like motif (*EFL*) and is richly invested with regulatory proteins including calmodulin (*CaM*) that bind to an *IQ* motif in the distal part of the structured C-terminus.

on cellular function and protein structure, which is referred to as oxidant stress. Other than mitochondria, the sources of ROS in the heart are NADPH oxidase (NOX), nitric oxide synthase (NOS), and xanthine oxidase (XO) that generate superoxide radical or NO. NO, although a weak oxidant, can generate other more potent ROS by reaction with superoxide and via guanylyl cyclase (GC)/protein kinase G (PKG) signaling and may directly or indirectly increase late Na current (I$_{Na-L}$).[10–12]

Modulation of Cardiac Voltage-Dependent Sodium Channels in Health and Disease

Na channels are responsible for the upstroke of the action potential (AP) and are the principal determinants of conduction velocity in both atrial and ventricular myocardia. The main isoform in both chambers is Na$_V$1.5, although β-subunit expression is distinct. Differences in the biophysical properties of Na currents in atrial compared to ventricular myocytes have been described, with larger current densities and a hyperpolarized availability curve in atrial compared to ventricular myocytes.[13,14] The resting potential in atrial cells is more depolarized, resulting in less Na current available to contribute to the upstroke of the atrial AP compared with its ventricular counterpart (see Chapter 1). The role of remodeled atrial Na currents in human atrial fibrillation is controversial. In one study, no change in current density or voltage dependence of activation with a modest but significant depolarizing shift in availability was observed.[15] In contrast, another group noted a decrease in peak I$_{Na}$ density and reduced expression of Na$_V$1.5 immunoreactive protein, with an increase in I$_{Na-L}$.[16] The putative mechanisms for the remodeling of atrial I$_{Na}$ in atrial fibrillation include altered expression of Na$_V$1 channel isoforms, disordered Ca^{2+},[15,17] or oxidant[18]-mediated signaling. Ca^{2+}/calmodulin-dependent protein kinase II (CaMKII) and oxidant-mediated alterations in Na channel function in atrial fibrillation may produce an increase in I$_{Na-L}$; however, other changes in ionic currents result in shorter AP durations (APDs) in control atria compared to fibrillating atria and atrial myocytes.[17–20]

In addition to their key roles in excitation and repolarization, Na channels may contribute to Ca^{2+} loading of heart cells. Functional alteration of Na$_V$1.5 currents may contribute to deleterious remodeling of cellular and tissue electrophysiological properties in the heart. Neurohumoral activation and oxidant stress are characteristic of a number of cardiac conditions associated with heightened arrhythmic risk, such as myocardial ischemia and heart failure (HF). In the setting of such acquired heart diseases, cardiac structure and cellular electrophysiology are remodeled, and the arrhythmic substrate is further complicated by changes in autonomic signaling, alterations in ROS/RNS, and changes in Ca^{2+} homeostasis. The relationship among these potentially pathogenic factors is changeable as is their impact on mechanical and electrical function of the heart. For example, myocardial ischemia may enhance oxidant burden, increase sympathetic activation, and alter autonomic balance.[21–23] Moreover, oxidant stress may indirectly influence Na channel function and arrhythmic risk via promoting coronary artery disease,[24,25] altering autonomic function,[26] and/or promoting apoptotic cell death and progressive cardiac damage.[22,27]

HF is characterized by sympathetic activation, and many salutary therapeutics target this signaling cascade, which is an initially compensatory response that ultimately becomes maladaptive. The changes in I$_{Na}$ in the failing heart described in the following text are likely multifactorial, with contributions from altered autonomic balance,[28,29] oxidant stress,[30–32] and disordered Ca^{2+} homeostasis.[33,34] A number of other heart diseases may alter Na channel function through changes in metabolism or autonomic imbalance. Hypertrophic cardiomyopathy is associated with alterations in coupling of metabolism to contraction.[35] Heritable arrhythmia syndromes have been associated with mutations in molecules that are key components of autonomic (A-kinase anchor protein 9 [AKAP9], caveolin-3 [Cav3])[11,36–38] or metabolic/oxidant signaling (glycerol-3 phosphate dehydrogenase 1-like [GPD1-L], α1-syntrophin).[39–41] Arrhythmogenic cardiomyopathy and alterations in the intercalated disk are associated with alterations in myocyte metabolism and autonomic activation,[42–46] as is diabetic cardiomyopathy,[47,48] all with possible effects on cardiac Na currents.

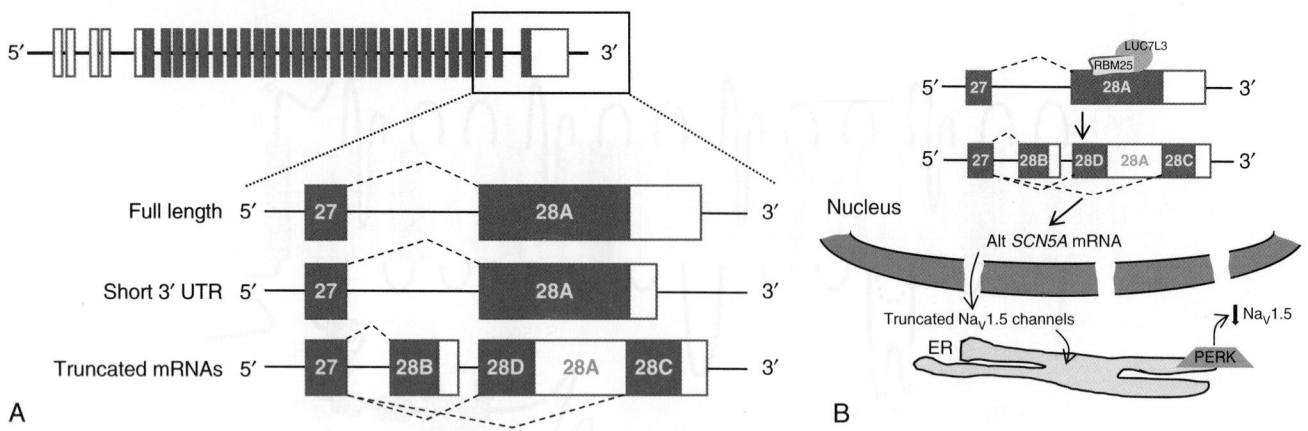

FIGURE 38.2 Oxidant induced alternative splicing of *SCN5A*. (A) 3′ Alternative splice variants of SCN5A and the translated, untranslated (*UTR*), and untranscribed sequences are represented by *filled boxes*, *open boxes*, and *lines*, respectively. (B) Oxidant stress leads to variant splicing involving exon 28 of *SCN5A* mediated by RBM25/LUC7L3. Aberrant splicing produces an increase in truncated sodium (Na) channel mRNAs and proteins, eliciting an unfolded protein response (UPR) and activation of protein kinase R–like endoplasmic reticulum kinase (*PERK*), which reduces translation of full-length Na$_V$1.5. Abnormal mRNA splicing and variant-mediated UPR activation contribute to decreased Na current in heart failure. (Modified from Gao G, Xie A, Zhang J, et al. Unfolded protein response regulates cardiac sodium current in systolic human heart failure. *Circ Arrhythm Electrophysiol.* 2013;6:1018-1024.)

The functional responses of Na$_V$1.5 currents to oxidant stress or sympathetic activation may profoundly influence cardiac electrophysiology. Downregulation of the current will potently affect conduction in the His–Purkinje system and working myocardium in a way that may promote reentry. Enhancement of I$_{Na-L}$ will primarily prolong APD and increase the possibility of arrhythmogenic early afterdepolarizations (EADs) and exaggerated dispersion of repolarization. To the extent that gain-of-function changes in Na$_V$1.5 currents promote intracellular Na$^+$ loading, this effect may perpetuate dysregulated cellular metabolism; enhanced ROS production; and maladaptive metabolic, electrical, and mechanical remodeling. Increased [Na$^+$]$_i$ will promote intracellular Ca^{2+} loading through the action of the Na$^+$-Ca^{2+} exchanger (NCX). Increased intracellular Na$^+$ and Ca^{2+} both can drive an increase in mitochondrial Ca^{2+}, impairing function, further increasing mitochondrial ROS production.[49]

Cardiac Metabolism, Oxidant Stress, and Voltage-Dependent Sodium Channels

Impaired metabolism and oxidant stress impact many signaling pathways involved in cardiac excitation and contraction and profoundly influences the risk for developing cardiac arrhythmias and sudden cardiac death (SCD). Ion transporters, connexins, ligand- and voltage-gated K channels, plasma membrane and sarcoplasmic reticulum (SR) Ca channels, and protein kinases may all be impacted by alterations in cellular metabolism and oxidant stress.[50] It is essential to understand that any changes in Na$_V$ channel function produced by oxidants and consequently the impact on cardiac electrophysiology occurs in the context of modulation of a broad array of channels, transporters, and their regulators. This section will focus on the consequences of metabolic and oxidant regulation of cardiac Na currents.

Na$_V$ channels may be regulated by metabolism and oxidants in a number of ways at several levels in the heart. The functional consequences may reduce or produce a gain-of-function of cardiac I$_{Na}$. Currents may decrease as a result of altered transcription, translation, enhanced turnover, or posttranslational modifications that impede function. In most cases of oxidant stress, gain-of-function is a result of impaired inactivation and development of an exaggerated late current (I$_{Na-L}$).

Alterations in mRNA transcripts in structural heart disease, such as HF, may be important drivers of remodeling of cardiac electrophysiology.[51,52] Functionally important changes in the transcriptional regulation of Na$_V$ channels have been described in animal models and human heart disease. The cardiac Na channel promoter contains oxidant-sensitive response elements that are involved in the regulation of transcription and RNA splicing. Oxidant stress in the form of angiotensin II (ang II) or H$_2$O$_2$ exposure in H9c2 cells and rodent ventricular myocytes has been shown to reduce Na$_V$1.5 mRNA levels, decrease peak I$_{Na}$, slow current decay, and increase I$_{Na-L}$. The transcriptional and functional effects of ang II were antagonized by pretreatment with ROS scavengers or inhibitors of NAPDH oxidase. Mutation of a nuclear factor κB (NFκB)–binding site in the mouse *scn5a* promoter eliminated ang II-dependent reduction in Na$_V$1.5 mRNA and functional changes in I$_{Na}$.[53]

Human HF is associated with an increase in intrinsically unfolded proteins[54] and the unfolded protein response (UPR). An increase in *SCN5A* alternative splicing associated with an increase in truncated mRNA variants of the channel contributing to the UPR has been demonstrated in human HF[55] and induced pluripotent stem cell–derived cardiomyocytes (hiPSC-CMs) exposed to ang II or hypoxia. Alternative splicing of *SCN5A* in human HF is associated with upregulation of a number of mRNA splicing factors, prominently RBM25 and LUC7L3.[56] These factors increase alternative, cryptic splicing of the terminal exon (exon 28) of *SCN5A* producing truncated mRNAs and proteins that elicit a UPR. Protein kinase R–like ER kinase (PERK) is an effector of the UPR that selectively destabilizes mRNAs, including Na$_V$1.5; moreover, PERK inhibition prevents oxidant-induced alternative splicing of Na$_V$1.5 transcripts.[57] Oxidant stress appears to be able to alter Na$_V$1.5 transcription via activation of NFκB and induction of a UPR, reducing peak Na current and altering channel function (Fig. 38.2).

There are a number of posttranscriptional mechanisms by which ROS can alter ion channel and specifically Na$_V$1.5 channel function. Well-recognized effects of ROS on cardiac Na current include an increase in late openings, slowing of current decay, and increasing the magnitude of noninactivating or late currents. In rodent ventricular myocytes, H$_2$O$_2$ prolonged the APD and acutely enhanced cell shortening. These effects were inhibited by

μM levels of tetrodotoxin (TTX) and mimicked by Na channel–selective toxins that inhibit inactivation.[58] These changes were caused by attenuated inactivation of cardiac Na channels reflected in late openings of single Na channels. The peroxide-induced altered Na channel gating and AP prolongation could be prevented by inhibition of protein kinase C (PKC) and reduced glutathione.[58,59] Similar changes in Na channel gating are observed in the setting of hypoxia and myocardial ischemia with an increase in I_{Na-L}, increased the mean open probability and duration of late Na channel openings.[60–62] In some cell systems, there appears to be a reciprocal relationship between peak and I_{Na-L} mediated by oxidant-induced alteration in gating modes,[63,64] suggesting that oxidant exposure may produce changes in both conduction and repolarization mediated by alterations in Na currents.

The presence of enhanced oxidant stress in a number of clinically relevant conditions such as ischemia and HF that contribute to arrhythmogenic risk suggests that I_{Na-L} may be a therapeutic target for the treatment of arrhythmic and contractile complications of these conditions.[60,65] Drugs like ranolazine have been shown to reduce the hypoxia- or oxidant-induced increase in I_{Na-L} and APD prolongation.[60,65,66] Other therapeutics may be useful in suppressing oxidant-induced I_{Na-L}; for example, milrinone reduced I_{Na-L} and APD prolongation in hypoxia and oxidant stress, an effect that was abrogated by the protein kinase A (PKA) inhibitor H-89.[67]

Oxidant stress can alter cellular metabolism in the heart. It perpetuates disturbances in cellular metabolism, producing a feed forward increase in ROS and a disturbance in levels of important regulatory nucleotides. It has been suggested that alterations in cardiac metabolism and dysregulation of pyridine nucleotides are involved in forms of BrS associated with mutations in GPD1-L. Coexpression of GPD1-L harboring a BrS mutation (A280V) decreased surface expression of $Na_V1.5$.[40] The application of NADH or transfection of mutant GPD1-L in mammalian tissue culture cells or neonatal rat ventricular myocytes (NRVMs) reduced peak Na current, without altering the $Na_V1.5$ mRNA or surface protein expression. This effect could be reversed by treatment with NAD, PKC inhibitors such as chelerythrine, or ROS scavengers such as superoxide dismutase. The effect of NAD to reverse the NADH-induced reduction of Na currents was antagonized by PKA inhibition. The NAD and NADH effects were mimicked by forskolin and phorbol esters, respectively. The regulation of $Na_V1.5$ by pyridine nucleotides is consistent with a link between metabolism and I_{Na} that appears to require PKC activation and is mediated by oxidative stress.[68]

The source of ROS involved in the signaling cascade associated with changes in NAD/NADH balance or disease-causing mutations in GPD1-L appears to be the mitochondria. The ability of increased NADH or expression of GPD1-L mutations to reduce $Na_V1.5$ currents is inhibited by scavengers of mitochondrial superoxide; inhibitors of electron transport chain complexes I, II, or III; voltage-dependent ion channels; or benzodiazepine receptors. In contrast, inhibitors of NOS, NOX, or xanthine oxidases do not inhibit the NADH-induced Na current reduction.[69] This reinforces the interplay of regulation through phosphorylation by PKA, PKC, and CaMKII as well as oxidation, suggesting that effects of metabolism and oxidants are very likely to be condition dependent.

The details of the signaling pathway associated with GPD1-L and metabolically mediated downregulation of Na currents have been debated. PKC activation may increase ROS production and inhibit I_{Na}. GPD1-L associates with $Na_V1.5$ channels, and the BrS and SIDS mutations cause a loss of enzymatic function, resulting in a glycerol-3-phosphate PKC–dependent phosphorylation of $Na_V1.5$ in the III–IV linker–reducing current. It has been suggested that since the GPD1-L reaction is NAD dependent, activation of this pathway may be relevant to modulation of Na currents in ischemia and HF.[41]

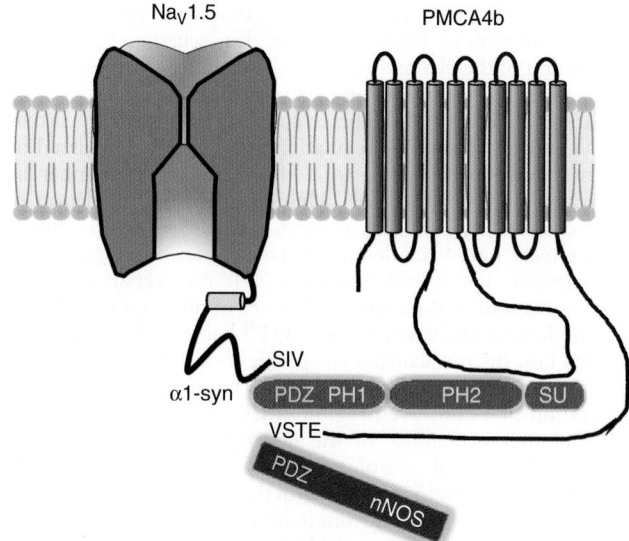

FIGURE 38.3 $Na_V1.5$ macromolecular signaling complex. $\alpha1$-syntrophin ($\alpha1$-syn) in the heart brings neuronal nitric oxide synthase (*nNOS*) and an endogenous inhibitor plasma membrane calcium-adenosine triphosphatase 4b (*PMCA4b*) in close proximity to $Na_V1.5$. $\alpha1$-syn binds to C-terminus of $Na_V1.5$ via a PDZ-binding domain. PMCA4b interacts with $\alpha1$-syn between the second pleckstrin homology domain (*PH2*) and a syntrophin unique (*SU*) motif. Nitric oxide (NO) produced by nNOS increases the persistent current. NO production is inhibited by PMCA4b, and mutations in $\alpha1$-syn that disturb the spatial relationships in the complex may lead to increases in late current. (Modified from Ueda K, Valdivia C, Medeiros-Domingo A, et al. Syntrophin mutation associated with long QT syndrome through activation of the nNOS-SCN5A macromolecular complex. *Proc Natl Acad Sci U S A.* 2008;105:9355-9360.)

Other oxidants may regulate Na_V1 currents with varying functional effects that depend on the mechanism of activation of signaling as well as the species and expression system. NO is a diffusible and labile signaling molecule derived from L-arginine by NOSs. NOSs are a family of constitutive (NOS1 or neuronal [nNOS] and NOS3 or endothelial [eNOS]) and inducible (NOS2 or inducible [iNOS]) enzymes[70] that are expressed in the heart and that regulate ion channels and cardiac function through the production of NO.[71] In the heart, the major source of NO is the coronary endothelium; it is also produced in cardiomyocytes by constitutive forms of NOS.[72] NO is a complex endogenous regulator of Na currents in the heart. Persistent Na current or I_{Na-L} can be increased by the photo release of caged NO or the application of NO donors in adult rat ventricular myocytes. The effect of NO to increase I_{Na-L} is blocked by inhibitors of NOS and N-ethylmaleimide, independent of GC activation, and it is robust in excised membrane patches.[10] This is consistent with a direct effect of the reactive nitrogen species, perhaps mediated by S-nitrosylation of thiol residues on the channel or closely related proteins.[73] Constitutive NOS isoforms (nNOS and eNOS) are Ca^{2+}/calmodulin (CaM)-dependent and linked to syntrophin,[74–76] a peripheral membrane protein that can localize NOS to PDZ-binding proteins such as $Na_V1.5$ channels. The proximity of constitutive NOS and $Na_V1.5$ channels may facilitate channel regulation by an evanescent signal such as NO (Fig. 38.3).

In a study of guinea pig and mouse ventricular myocytes, NO-containing solution and NO donors at relatively high concentrations reduced peak I_{Na} without altering the kinetics and voltage dependence of gating or single-channel current amplitude. The reduction in I_{Na} was insensitive to sulfhydryl-reducing agents, suggesting that S-nitrosylation or oxidation of the channel or regulatory protein was not involved in the regulatory cascade that reduced current amplitude. In contrast, the NO inhibition of cardiac I_{Na} could be blocked by reduction of cGMP and cAMP and by inhibition of PKA.[12] It is not clear whether PKA phosphorylation of the channel is the mediator of this form of inhibition, and there are conflicting data regarding the effects of PKA activation on native[77-79] and heterologously expressed[80,81] cardiac I_{Na}. Moreover, adrenergic regulation of I_{Na} may be mediated by channel phosphorylation or in a PKA-independent manner by the action of G-proteins.[79,82] Multiple forms of regulation of Na_V1 channels by NO and nitrogen radicals, with varied functional effects, have been demonstrated and may differ depending upon species, type of expression system (native versus heterologous expression), and manner of delivery of nitrogen radicals.

A molecular understanding of LQTS has provided important insights into the mechanisms of specific forms of NO regulation of cardiac Na channels. A form of LQTS has been associated with a mutation in a conserved region of α1-syntrophin (*SNTA1*).[39] Syntrophin is a member of the dystrophin-associated protein family and serves as a molecular scaffold for macromolecular complexes. Syntrophin interacts with the C-terminal PDZ ligand of the $Na_V1.5$ channel and binds nNOS and a cardiac plasma membrane calcium-ATPase (PMCA4b), an inhibitor of nNOS (see Fig. 38.3).[75,76] A mutation is a conserved, protein-binding region of *SNTA1* (A390V) that has been associated with LQTS and disrupts the interaction between PMCA4b and syntrophin, bringing nNOS into close proximity to $Na_V1.5$ in the absence of an endogenous inhibitor. nNOS-induced *S*-nitrosylation of $Na_V1.5$ increases the late current, leading to AP and QT prolongation, and in this study, the peak I_{Na} in the presence of the mutant *SNTA1* was increased compared to the expression of the channel alone or with the wild-type *SNTA1* in mammalian expression cells or NRVMs.[39] It is certainly possible that the mutant syntrophin exerts other effects by *S*-nitrosylation of $Na_V1.5$ or associated proteins or via activation of cGMP. Other mutations in *SNTA1* have been associated with LQTS[83] and SIDS.[84] A series of six rare variants were discovered in regions of varying conservation of *SNTA1*, and three of the mutations of highly conserved amino acids produced potentially arrhythmogenic changes in expressed $Na_V1.5$ function. When compared to the expression of $Na_V1.5$ with wild-type *SNTA1*, each of the mutant syntrophins increased both the peak I_{Na} and I_{Na-L} densities, slowed current decay, and produced a depolarizing shift in the steady-state inactivation curve, all of which could conspire to prolong the APD.[84]

Mutations in other proteins associated with LQTS and SIDS have been implicated in disrupting physiological regulation of $Na_V1.5$ by NO signaling. Caveolae are specialized membrane microdomains rich in cholesterol and specific sphingolipids. The major scaffolding protein in caveolae in heart cells is caveolin 3 (Cav3). A number of ion channels and transporters as well as regulatory proteins are concentrated in caveolae, including voltage-dependent Na and Ca channels, G protein–coupled receptors, PKA, PKC, receptor and nonreceptor tyrosine kinases, and NOS, to name a few.[37,85] Cav3 binding to nNOS inhibits synthase activity and nNOS-dependent *S*-nitrosylation of $Na_V1.5$ with the effect of decreasing I_{Na-L}. Mutations in Cav3 have been identified in patients with LQTS[36] and SIDS[86]; in general, these variants are of highly conserved residues, often in the intramembrane domain. Expression of mutant Cav3 with $Na_V1.5$ in expression systems significantly increased the density of I_{Na-L} when compared to $Na_V1.5$ expressed alone or when the channel was expressed with wild-type Cav3.[11,36,86] Cav3 is part of a macromolecular complex with $Na_V1.5$, syntrophin 1, and nNOS; the mutations in Cav3 eliminate the suppression of nNOS, increasing local NO levels and I_{Na-L}. The mechanisms by which Cav3 mutations disable their nNOS inhibitory activity are uncertain, but in some cases, mutant Cav3 can still bind to nNOS.[11] The channel-based mechanism(s) for the *S*-nitrosylation–induced increase in I_{Na-L} and other changes in gating have not been fully

elucidated. Moreover, it is possible that alterations in nNOS signaling may modulate the functional expression of a number of currents in the heart to enhance arrhythmic risk. In addition to rare, inherited arrhythmia syndromes, augmented NOS activity has been described in HF and may contribute to increased risk of arrhythmias and SCD.[87,88] It is interesting to note that common variants in other nNOS regulators, such as NOS1 adaptor protein (NOS1AP), have been associated with the QT interval[89] and SCD.[90]

Autonomic Regulation of Voltage-Dependent Sodium Channels

Sympathetic nerve stimulation (SNS) results in well-defined changes in the cellular and tissue electrophysiological properties, including enhanced conduction in working myocardium and shortening of the APD and refractory periods. β-Adrenergic receptor (AR) stimulation mediates many of the changes in cardiac electrophysiology. Activation of β-receptors regulates the function of many ion channels in the heart, including Na, K, and Ca channels.[91-93] β-AR regulation of cardiac Na channels may occur via several distinct mechanisms. Indirect, PKA-dependent and direct, PKA-independent signaling pathways impact cardiac Na channel function. The indirect pathway engages canonical signaling, including PKA phosphorylation of the Na channel α-subunit. The linker between the first and second transmembrane domains (I–II linker) is a key region for phosphorylation of the cardiac Na channel by a number of kinases, such as PKA[80,94-96] and CaMKII (see Fig. 38.1).[97-101] Divergent functional effects of protein kinases that act primarily on residues in I–II linker of the channel have been described. The differences may be the result of the chronicity of exposure to the kinase,[33] the system (native versus expressed channels) being studied, and the presence of accessory subunits.[98] In adult ventricular myocytes, the consensus is that β-AR stimulation shifts the voltage dependence of inactivation gating in the hyperpolarizing direction and hastens current decay.[77,79,102-104] There is general, but not complete, consensus on the relative importance of PKA phosphorylation sites in the I–II linker.[96] It is possible that the functional effects of a phosphorylation event is conditioned or modified by another posttranslational modification. There is also evidence that PKA-dependent phosphorylation may promote trafficking to the membrane.[96,105]

PKA-independent regulation, referred to as direct or membrane-delimited regulation, of cardiac Na channels has been described. In ventricular myocytes, ion channels, such as $Na_V1.5$, $Ca_V1.2$, and $K_V1.5$, are enriched in caveolae and colocalized with Cav3. Caveoli are a ready reservoir of select cell membrane proteins; β-AR stimulation opens caveoli through a Gαs-involved pathway and increases membrane density of resident ion channels.[93,106] It is important to remember that sympathetic stimulation will generate a number of simultaneous effects that could impact $Na_V1.5$ function. In addition to caveolin-associated augmentation of surface expression and channel phosphorylation, sympathetic activation will increase L-type Ca channel activity and intracellular Ca^{2+}, activating Ca^{2+}-dependent enzymes such as CaMKII, which will increase I_{Na-L}[33,97] (see Chapter 18). Other mechanisms whereby intracellular Ca^{2+} may directly modulate Na channel function continue to emerge.[107-109] CaM regulates Na_V1 channel gating through binding to an IQ-like motif in the C-terminus (see Fig. 38.1).[108-110] At low levels of Ca^{2+}, CaM binding consistently increases the open probability of Na_V1 channels, including $Na_V1.5$.[108] Calcium binding to CaM produces Ca^{2+}-dependent inactivation, analogous to that described in L-type Ca channels. This is a prominent effect in $Na_V1.4$ but not in $Na_V1.5$ channels.

In the neurohumorally driven failing heart, sympathetic nervous system activation is prominent, peak I_{Na} is reduced, and

I_{Na-L} is enhanced.[34,111] The features of the failing heart that might contribute to alterations in cardiac Na channel function include intracellular Na^+ overload with enhanced NCX[112,113] and increased mitochondrial ROS production.[49] The consequences of the increase in Ca^{2+} exchanged for Na^+ and in ROS burden are an increase in total immunoreactive, activated, and oxidized CaMKII[32-34] and augmented PKC activity.[114] The enhanced sympathetic drive in the failing heart is associated with uncoupling of β-AR activation from downstream signaling.[115,116] Notably, in the dyssynchronously contracting failing heart, resynchronization by biventricular or left ventricular (LV) pacing serves to decrease sympathetic drive and recouple β-AR activation to downstream signaling via a reduction in $G\alpha i$.[116,117] Moreover, resynchronization of contraction even in the context of ongoing LV dysfunction reduces I_{Na-L}, immunoreactive levels, and activation of CaMKII.[34]

PKA regulation may be relevant to the phenotypic expression of heritable Na channelopathies. For example, we identified an *SCN5A* mutation in a patient with BrS that produces both chronic reduction in I_{Na} and absence of augmentation of the current by adrenergic stimulation. The disease-causing mutation, R526H, eliminates the basic priming residue in a consensus PKA phosphorylation recognition sequence. S528A replaces the phosphorylation target residue and alters channel trafficking and regulation by PKA in a manner that is comparable to the disease-causing mutation and similar to previously described defects in PKA-mediated I_{Na} potentiation.[96] Both the R526H and S528A mutant channels produced a reduction in peak I_{Na} that was further reduced by oxidant stress. Such metabolic stressors are typically accompanied by activation of the sympathetic nervous system, which may partially offset the redox-induced reduction in peak I_{Na} and would dampen stress-induced electrocardiogram changes in BrS. Unlike the wild-type $Na_V1.5$ channels, neither the direct activation of adenylyl cyclase nor β-AR stimulation with isoproterenol had a significant effect on peak I_{Na} density of the mutant channel variants. In such circumstances, ventricular arrhythmias would not be induced by sympathetic activation but instead would be mitigated by an increase in sympathetic tone. This concept is consistent with the utility of isoproterenol in the treatment of arrhythmic storm in patients with BrS.[118-120] The elimination of a PKA site appears to be central to both the autonomic regulation and trafficking deficits in this Na channelopathy.[94]

The effect of parasympathetic activation on Na_V1 channel function is less well studied. The recognition of cholinergic regulation of excitation and contraction and its emerging therapeutic role in ischemic heart disease[121] and HF[122] has prompted searches for functional effects on ion channels. There is limited evidence for a direct regulation of cardiac Na currents by parasympathetic activity, but reversal of the effects of β-AR stimulation by acetylcholine has been described,[123] and cholinergic modulation of some forms of LQT3 may provoke arrhythmias.[124] The potential beneficial effects of parasympathetic activation, including heart rate reduction, adrenergic antagonism, and antiinflammatory and antiapoptotic effects,[125,126] mandate a more complete understanding of their impact on active membrane properties of the heart.

REFERENCES

1. Gellens ME, George Jr AL, Chen LQ, et al. Primary structure and functional expression of the human cardiac tetrodotoxin-insensitive voltage-dependent sodium channel. *Proc Natl Acad Sci U S A.* 1992;89:554–558.
2. Noda M, Shimizu S, Tanabe T, et al. Primary structure of Electrophorus electricus sodium channel deduced from cDNA sequence. *Nature.* 1984;312:121–127.
3. O'Malley HA, Isom LL. Sodium channel beta subunits: emerging targets in channelopathies. *Annu Rev Physiol.* 2015;77:481–504.
4. Isom LL, Catterall WA. Na+ channel subunits and Ig domains. *Nature.* 1996;383:307–308.
5. Calhoun JD, Isom LL. The role of non-pore-forming beta subunits in physiology and pathophysiology of voltage-gated sodium channels. *Handb Exp Pharmacol.* 2014;221:51–89.
6. Taegtmeyer H. Energy metabolism of the heart: from basic concepts to clinical applications. *Curr Probl Cardiol.* 1994;19:59–113.
7. Stanley WC, Recchia FA, Lopaschuk GD. Myocardial substrate metabolism in the normal and failing heart. *Physiol Rev.* 2005;85:1093–1129.
8. Schaper J, Meiser E, Stammler G. Ultrastructural morphometric analysis of myocardium from dogs, rats, hamsters, mice, and from human hearts. *Circ Res.* 1985;56:377–391.
9. Suga H. Ventricular energetics. *Physiol Rev.* 1990;70:247–277.
10. Ahern GP, Hsu SF, Klyachko VA, Jackson MB. Induction of persistent sodium current by exogenous and endogenous nitric oxide. *J Biol Chem.* 2000;275:28810–28815.
11. Cheng J, Valdivia CR, Vaidyanathan R, Balijepalli RC, Ackerman MJ, Makielski JC. Caveolin-3 suppresses late sodium current by inhibiting nNOS-dependent S-nitrosylation of SCN5A. *J Mol Cell Cardiol.* 2013;61:102–110.
12. Ahmmed GU, Xu Y, Hong Dong P, Zhang Z, Eiserich J, Chiamvimonvat N. Nitric oxide modulates cardiac Na+ channel via protein kinase A and protein kinase G. *Circ Res.* 2001;89:1005–1013.
13. Li GR, Lau CP, Shrier A. Heterogeneity of sodium current in atrial vs epicardial ventricular myocytes of adult guinea pig hearts. *J Mol Cell Cardiol.* 2002;34:1185–1194.
14. Burashnikov A, Di Diego JM, Zygmunt AC, Belardinelli L, Antzelevitch C. Atrium-selective sodium channel block as a strategy for suppression of atrial fibrillation: differences in sodium channel inactivation between atria and ventricles and the role of ranolazine. *Circulation.* 2007;116:1449–1457.
15. Bosch RF, Zeng X, Grammer JB, Popovic K, Mewis C, Kuhlkamp V. Ionic mechanisms of electrical remodeling in human atrial fibrillation. *Cardiovasc Res.* 1999;44:121–131.

16. Sossalla S, Kallmeyer B, Wagner S, et al. Altered Na+ currents in atrial fibrillation effects of ranolazine on arrhythmias and contractility in human atrial myocardium. *J Am Coll Cardiol.* 2010;55:2330–2342.
17. Neef S, Dybkova N, Sossalla S, et al. CaMKII-dependent diastolic SR Ca2+ leak and elevated diastolic Ca2+ levels in right atrial myocardium of patients with atrial fibrillation. *Circ Res.* 2010;106:1134–1144.
18. Mihm MJ, Yu F, Carnes CA, et al. Impaired myofibrillar energetics and oxidative injury during human atrial fibrillation. *Circulation.* 2001;104:174–180.
19. Voigt N, Li N, Wang Q, et al. Enhanced sarcoplasmic reticulum Ca2+ leak and increased Na+-Ca2+ exchanger function underlie delayed afterdepolarizations in patients with chronic atrial fibrillation. *Circulation.* 2012;125:2059–2070.
20. Tessier S, Karczewski P, Krause EG, et al. Regulation of the transient outward K+ current by Ca2+/calmodulin-dependent protein kinases II in human atrial myocytes. *Circ Res.* 1999;85:810–819.
21. Remme WJ. The sympathetic nervous system and ischaemic heart disease. *Eur Heart J.* 1998;19(suppl F):F62–F71.
22. Zweier JL, Talukder MA. The role of oxidants and free radicals in reperfusion injury. *Cardiovasc Res.* 2006;70:181–190.
23. Simpson PJ, Lucchesi BR. Free radicals and myocardial ischemia and reperfusion injury. *J Lab Clin Med.* 1987;110:13–30.
24. Stocker R, Keaney Jr JF. Role of oxidative modifications in atherosclerosis. *Physiol Rev.* 2004;84:1381–1478.
25. Bornfeldt KE, Tabas I. Insulin resistance, hyperglycemia, and atherosclerosis. *Cell Metab.* 2011;14:575–585.
26. Dhalla NS, Adameova A, Kaur M. Role of catecholamine oxidation in sudden cardiac death. *Fundam Clin Pharmacol.* 2010;24:539–546.
27. Aiba T, Noda T, Hidaka I, et al. Acetylcholine suppresses ventricular arrhythmias and improves conduction and connexin-43 properties during myocardial ischemia in isolated rabbit hearts. *J Cardiovasc Electrophysiol.* 2015;26:678–685.
28. Aiba T, Tomaselli GF. Electrical remodeling in the failing heart. *Curr Opin Cardiol.* 2010;25:29–36.
29. Nass RD, Aiba T, Tomaselli GF, Akar FG. Mechanisms of disease: ion channel remodeling in the failing ventricle. *Nat Clin Pract Cardiovasc Med.* 2008;5:196–207.
30. Roul D, Recchia FA. Metabolic alterations induce oxidative stress in diabetic and failing hearts: different pathways, same outcome. *Antioxid Redox Signal.* 2015;22:1502–1514.

31. Sag CM, Wagner S, Maier LS. Role of oxidants on calcium and sodium movement in healthy and diseased cardiac myocytes. *Free Radic Biol Med.* 2013;63:338–349.
32. Wagner S, Ruff HM, Weber SL, et al. Reactive oxygen species-activated Ca/calmodulin kinase IIdelta is required for late I(Na) augmentation leading to cellular Na and Ca overload. *Circ Res.* 2011;108:555–565.
33. Wagner S, Dybkova N, Rasenack EC, et al. Ca2+/calmodulin-dependent protein kinase II regulates cardiac Na+ channels. *J Clin Invest.* 2006;116:3127–3138.
34. Aiba T, Barth AS, Hesketh GG, et al. Cardiac resynchronization therapy improves altered Na channel gating in canine model of dyssynchronous heart failure. *Circ Arrhythm Electrophysiol.* 2013;6:546–554.
35. Song W, Vikhorev PG, Kashyap MN, et al. Mechanical and energetic properties of papillary muscle from ACTC E99K transgenic mouse models of hypertrophic cardiomyopathy. *Am J Physiol Heart Circ Physiol.* 2013;304:H1513–H1524.
36. Vatta M, Ackerman MJ, Ye B, et al. Mutant caveolin-3 induces persistent late sodium current and is associated with long-QT syndrome. *Circulation.* 2006;114:2104–2112.
37. Balijepalli RC, Kamp TJ. Caveolae, ion channels and cardiac arrhythmias. *Prog Biophys Mol Biol.* 2008;98:149–160.
38. Chen L, Marquardt ML, Tester DJ, Sampson KJ, Ackerman MJ, Kass RS. Mutation of an A-kinase-anchoring protein causes long-QT syndrome. *Proc Natl Acad Sci U S A.* 2007;104:20990–20995.
39. Ueda K, Valdivia C, Medeiros-Domingo A, et al. Syntrophin mutation associated with long QT syndrome through activation of the nNOS-SCN5A macromolecular complex. *Proc Natl Acad Sci U S A.* 2008;105:9355–9360.
40. London B, Michalec M, Mehdi H, et al. Mutation in glycerol-3-phosphate dehydrogenase 1 like gene (GPD1-L) decreases cardiac Na+ current and causes inherited arrhythmias. *Circulation.* 2007;116:2260–2268.
41. Valdivia CR, Ueda K, Ackerman MJ, Makielski JC. GPD1L links redox state to cardiac excitability by PKC-dependent phosphorylation of the sodium channel SCN5A. *Am J Physiol Heart Circ Physiol.* 2009;297:H1446–H1452.
42. Wichter T, Schafers M, Rhodes CG, et al. Abnormalities of cardiac sympathetic innervation in arrhythmogenic right ventricular cardiomyopathy: quantitative assessment of presynaptic norepinephrine reuptake and postsynaptic beta-adrenergic receptor density with positron emission tomography. *Circulation.* 2000;101:1552–1558.

43. Djouadi F, Lecarpentier Y, Hebert JL, Charron P, Bastin J, Coirault C. A potential link between peroxisome proliferator-activated receptor signalling and the pathogenesis of arrhythmogenic right ventricular cardiomyopathy. *Cardiovasc Res*. 2009;84:83–90.
44. Saffitz JE, Asimaki A, Huang H. Arrhythmogenic right ventricular cardiomyopathy: new insights into mechanisms of disease. *Cardiovasc Pathol*. 2010;19:166–170.
45. Paul M, Meyborg M, Boknik P, et al. Autonomic dysfunction in patients with arrhythmogenic right ventricular cardiomyopathy: biochemical evidence of altered signaling pathways. *Pacing Clin Electrophysiol*. 2014;37:173–178.
46. Cerrone M, Delmar M. Desmosomes and the sodium channel complex: implications for arrhythmogenic cardiomyopathy and Brugada syndrome. *Trends Cardiovasc Med*. 2014;24:184–190.
47. Casis O, Echevarria E. Diabetic cardiomyopathy: electromechanical cellular alterations. *Curr Vasc Pharmacol*. 2004;2:237–248.
48. Cesario DA, Brar R, Shivkumar K. Alterations in ion channel physiology in diabetic cardiomyopathy. *Endocrinol Metab Clin North Am*. 2006;35:601–610. ix-x.
49. Kohlhaas M, Liu T, Knopp A, et al. Elevated cytosolic Na^+ increases mitochondrial formation of reactive oxygen species in failing cardiac myocytes. *Circulation*. 2010;121:1606–1613.
50. Yang KC, Kyle JW, Makielski JC, Dudley Jr SC. Mechanisms of sudden cardiac death: oxidants and metabolism. *Circ Res*. 2015;116:1937–1955.
51. Gao Z, Barth AS, DiSilvestre D, et al. Key pathways associated with heart failure development revealed by gene networks correlated with cardiac remodeling. *Physiol Genomics*. 2008;35:222–230.
52. Barth AS, Kumordzie A, Frangakis C, Margulies KB, Cappola TP, Tomaselli GF. Reciprocal transcriptional regulation of metabolic and signaling pathways correlates with disease severity in heart failure. *Circ Cardiovasc Genet*. 2011;4:475–483.
53. Shang LL, Sanyal S, Pfahnl AE, et al. NF-kappaB-dependent transcriptional regulation of the cardiac scn5a sodium channel by angiotensin II. *Am J Physiol Cell Physiol*. 2008;294:C372–C379.
54. Barth AS, Kumordzie A, Colantuoni C, Margulies KB, Cappola TP, Tomaselli GF. Reciprocal regulation of metabolic and signaling pathways. *BMC Genomics*. 2010;11:197.
55. Shang LL, Pfahnl AE, Sanyal S, et al. Human heart failure is associated with abnormal C-terminal splicing variants in the cardiac sodium channel. *Circ Res*. 2007;101:1146–1154.
56. Gao G, Xie A, Huang SC, et al. Role of RBM25/LUC7L3 in abnormal cardiac sodium channel splicing regulation in human heart failure. *Circulation*. 2011;124:1124–1131.
57. Gao G, Xie A, Zhang J, et al. Unfolded protein response regulates cardiac sodium current in systolic human heart failure. *Circ Arrhythm Electrophysiol*. 2013;6:1018–1024.
58. Ward CA, Giles WR. Ionic mechanism of the effects of hydrogen peroxide in rat ventricular myocytes. *J Physiol*. 1997;500:631–642.
59. Ma JH, Luo AT, Zhang PH. Effect of hydrogen peroxide on persistent sodium current in guinea pig ventricular myocytes. *Acta Pharmacol Sin*. 2005;26:828–834.
60. Ma J, Song Y, Shryock JC, et al. Ranolazine attenuates hypoxia- and hydrogen peroxide-induced increases in sodium channel late openings in ventricular myocytes. *J Cardiovasc Pharmacol*. 2014;64:60–68.
61. Weiss S, Benoist D, White E, Teng W, Saint DA. Riluzole protects against cardiac ischaemia and reperfusion damage via block of the persistent sodium current. *Br J Pharmacol*. 2010;160:1072–1082.
62. Ju YK, Saint DA, Gage PW. Hypoxia increases persistent sodium current in rat ventricular myocytes. *J Physiol*. 1996;497:337–347.
63. Wang W, Ma J, Zhang P, Luo A. Redox reaction modulates transient and persistent sodium current during hypoxia in guinea pig ventricular myocytes. *Pflugers Arch*. 2007;454:461–475.
64. Luo A, Ma J, Zhang P, Zhou H, Wang W. Sodium channel gating modes during redox reaction. *Cell Physiol Biochem*. 2007;19:9–20.
65. Song Y, Shryock JC, Wagner S, Maier LS, Belardinelli L. Blocking late sodium current reduces hydrogen peroxide-induced arrhythmogenic activity and contractile dysfunction. *J Pharmacol Exp Ther*. 2006;318:214–222.
66. Song Y, Shryock JC, Belardinelli L. A slowly inactivating sodium current contributes to spontaneous diastolic depolarization of atrial myocytes. *Am J Physiol Heart Circ Physiol*. 2009;297:H1254–H1262.
67. Zheng J, Ma J, Zhang P, Hu L, Fan X, Tang Q. Milrinone inhibits hypoxia or hydrogen dioxide-induced persistent sodium current in ventricular myocytes. *Eur J Pharmacol*. 2009;616:206–212.
68. Liu M, Sanyal S, Gao G, et al. Cardiac Na+ current regulation by pyridine nucleotides. *Circ Res*. 2009;105:737–745.
69. Liu M, Liu H, Dudley Jr SC. Reactive oxygen species originating from mitochondria regulate the cardiac sodium channel. *Circ Res*. 2010;107:967–974.
70. Nathan C, Xie QW. Nitric oxide synthases: roles, tolls, and controls. *Cell*. 1994;78:915–918.
71. Barouch LA, Harrison RW, Skaf MW, et al. Nitric oxide regulates the heart by spatial confinement of nitric oxide synthase isoforms. *Nature*. 2002;416:337–339.
72. Balligand JL, Kelly RA, Marsden PA, Smith TW, Michel T. Control of cardiac muscle cell function by an endogenous nitric oxide signaling system. *Proc Natl Acad Sci U S A*. 1993;90:347–351.
73. Hammarstrom AK, Gage PW. Nitric oxide increases persistent sodium current in rat hippocampal neurons. *J Physiol*. 1999;520 Pt: 451–461.
74. Gee SH, Madhavan R, Levinson SR, Caldwell JH, Sealock R, Froehner SC. Interaction of muscle and brain sodium channels with multiple members of the syntrophin family of dystrophin-associated proteins. *J Neurosci*. 1998;18:128–137.
75. Oceandy D, Cartwright EJ, Emerson M, et al. Neuronal nitric oxide synthase signaling in the heart is regulated by the sarcolemmal calcium pump 4b. *Circulation*. 2007;115:483–492.
76. Williams JC, Armesilla AL, Mohamed TM, et al. The sarcolemmal calcium pump, alpha-1 syntrophin, and neuronal nitric-oxide synthase are parts of a macromolecular protein complex. *J Biol Chem*. 2006;281:23341–23348.
77. Sunami A, Fan Z, Nakamura F, et al. The catalytic subunit of cyclic AMP-dependent protein kinase directly inhibits sodium channel activities in guinea-pig ventricular myocytes. *Pflugers Arch*. 1991;419:415–417.
78. Ono K, Kiyosue T, Arita M. Isoproterenol, DBcAMP, and forskolin inhibit cardiac sodium current. *Am J Physiol*. 1989;256:C1131–C1137.
79. Matsuda JJ, Lee H, Shibata EF. Enhancement of rabbit cardiac sodium channels by beta-adrenergic stimulation. *Circ Res*. 1992;70:199–207.
80. Frohnwieser B, Chen LQ, Schreibmayer W, Kallen RG. Modulation of the human cardiac sodium channel alpha-subunit by cAMP-dependent protein kinase and the responsible sequence domain. *J Physiol*. 1997;498:309–318.
81. Schreibmayer W, Frohnwieser B, Dascal N, et al. Beta-adrenergic modulation of currents produced by rat cardiac Na^+ channels expressed in Xenopus laevis oocytes. *Receptors Channels*. 1994;2:339–350.
82. Lu T, Lee HC, Kabat JA, Shibata EF. Modulation of rat cardiac sodium channel by the stimulatory G protein alpha subunit. *J Physiol*. 1999;518:371–384.
83. Wu G, Ai T, Kim JJ, et al. alpha-1-syntrophin mutation and the long-QT syndrome: a disease of sodium channel disruption. *Circ Arrhythm Electrophysiol*. 2008;1:193–201.
84. Cheng J, Van Norstrand DW, Medeiros-Domingo A, et al. Alpha1-syntrophin mutations identified in sudden infant death syndrome cause an increase in late cardiac sodium current. *Circ Arrhythm Electrophysiol*. 2009;2:667–676.
85. Parton RG, Simons K. The multiple faces of caveolae. *Nat Rev Mol Cell Biol*. 2007;8:185–194.
86. Cronk LB, Ye B, Kaku T, et al. Novel mechanism for sudden infant death syndrome: persistent late sodium current secondary to mutations in caveolin-3. *Heart Rhythm*. 2007;4:161–166.
87. Damy T, Ratajczak P, Shah AM, et al. Increased neuronal nitric oxide synthase-derived NO production in the failing human heart. *Lancet*. 2004;363:1365–1367.
88. Bendall JK, Damy T, Ratajczak P, et al. Role of myocardial neuronal nitric oxide synthase-derived nitric oxide in beta-adrenergic hyporesponsiveness after myocardial infarction-induced heart failure in rat. *Circulation*. 2004;110:2368–2375.
89. Arking DE, Pfeufer A, Post W, et al. A common genetic variant in the NOS1 regulator NOS1AP modulates cardiac repolarization. *Nat Genet*. 2006;38:644–651.
90. Kao WH, Arking DE, Post W, et al. Genetic variations in nitric oxide synthase 1 adaptor protein are associated with sudden cardiac death in US white community-based populations. *Circulation*. 2009;119:940–951.
91. Buckley U, Shivkumar K, Ardell JL. Autonomic regulation therapy in heart failure. *Curr Heart Fail Rep*. 2015;12:284–293.
92. Fukuda K, Kanazawa H, Aizawa Y, Ardell JL, Shivkumar K. Cardiac innervation and sudden cardiac death. *Circ Res*. 2015;116:2005–2019.
93. Shibata EF, Brown TL, Washburn ZW, Bai J, Revak TJ, Butters CA. Autonomic regulation of voltage-gated cardiac ion channels. *J Cardiovasc Electrophysiol*. 2006;17(suppl 1):S34–S42.
94. Aiba T, Farinelli F, Kostecki G, et al. A mutation causing Brugada syndrome identifies a mechanism for altered autonomic and oxidant regulation of cardiac sodium currents. *Circ Cardiovasc Genet*. 2014;7:249–256.
95. Murphy BJ, Rogers J, Perdichizzi AP, Colvin AA, Catterall WA. cAMP-dependent phosphorylation of two sites in the alpha subunit of the cardiac sodium channel. *J Biol Chem*. 1996;271:28837–28843.
96. Zhou J, Shin HG, Yi J, Shen W, Williams CP, Murray KT. Phosphorylation and putative ER retention signals are required for protein kinase A-mediated potentiation of cardiac sodium current. *Circ Res*. 2002;91:540–546.
97. Aiba T, Hesketh GG, Liu T, et al. Na^+ channel regulation by Ca^{2+}/calmodulin and Ca^{2+}/calmodulin-dependent protein kinase II in guinea-pig ventricular myocytes. *Cardiovasc Res*. 2010;85:454–463.
98. Ashpole NM, Herren AW, Ginsburg KS, et al. Ca^{2+}/calmodulin-dependent protein kinase II (CaMKII) regulates cardiac sodium channel $Na_V1.5$ gating by multiple phosphorylation sites. *J Biol Chem*. 2012;287:19856–19869.
99. Glynn P, Musa H, Wu X, et al. Voltage-gated sodium channel phosphorylation at Ser571 regulates late current, arrhythmia, and cardiac function in vivo. *Circulation*. 2015;132:567–577.
100. Hund TJ, Koval OM, Li J, et al. A beta(IV)-spectrin/CaMKII signaling complex is essential for membrane excitability in mice. *J Clin Invest*. 2010;120:3508–3519.
101. Koval OM, Snyder JS, Wolf RM, et al. Ca^{2+}/calmodulin-dependent protein kinase II-based regulation of voltage-gated Na+ channel in cardiac disease. *Circulation*. 2012;126:2084–2094.
102. Sorbera LA, Morad M. Modulation of cardiac sodium channels by cAMP receptors on the myocyte surface. *Science*. 1991;253:1286–1289.
103. Gintant GA, Liu DW. Beta-adrenergic modulation of fast inward sodium current in canine myocardium. Syncytial preparations versus isolated myocytes. *Circ Res*. 1992;70:844–850.
104. Ono K, Fozzard HA, Hanck DA. Mechanism of cAMP-dependent modulation of cardiac sodium channel current kinetics. *Circ Res*. 1993;72:807–815.
105. Hallaq H, Yang Z, Viswanathan PC, et al. Quantitation of protein kinase A–mediated trafficking of cardiac sodium channels in living cells. *Cardiovasc Res*. 2006;72:250–261.
106. Palygin OA, Pettus JM, Shibata EF. Regulation of caveolar cardiac sodium current by a single Gsalpha histidine residue. *Am J Physiol Heart Circ Physiol*. 2008;294:H1693–H1699.
107. Adams PJ, Ben-Johny M, Dick IE, Inoue T, Yue DT. Apocalmodulin itself promotes ion channel opening and Ca^{2+} regulation. *Cell*. 2014;159:608–622.
108. Ben-Johny M, Yang PS, Niu J, Yang W, Joshi-Mukherjee R, Yue DT. Conservation of Ca^{2+}/calmodulin regulation across Na and Ca^{2+} channels. *Cell*. 2014;157:1657–1670.
109. Gabelli SB, Boto A, Kuhns VH, et al. Regulation of the $Na_V1.5$ cytoplasmic domain by calmodulin. *Nat Commun*. 2014;5:5126.
110. Deschenes I, Neyroud N, DiSilvestre D, Marban E, Yue DT, Tomaselli GF. Isoform-specific modulation of voltage-gated Na^+ channels by calmodulin. *Circ Res*. 2002;90:E49–E57.
111. Valdivia CR, Chu WW, Pu J, et al. Increased late sodium current in myocytes from a canine heart failure model and from failing human heart. *J Mol Cell Cardiol*. 2005;38:475–483.
112. Pogwizd SM, Schlotthauer K, Li L, Yuan W, Bers DM. Arrhythmogenesis and contractile dysfunction in heart failure: Roles of sodium-calcium exchange, inward rectifier potassium current, and residual beta-adrenergic responsiveness. *Circ Res*. 2001;88:1159–1167.
113. Aiba T, Hesketh GG, Barth AS, et al. Electrophysiological consequences of dyssynchronous heart failure and its restoration by resynchronization therapy. *Circulation*. 2009;119:1220–1230.
114. Ma J, Luo A, Wu L, et al. Calmodulin kinase II and protein kinase C mediate the effect of increased intracellular calcium to augment late sodium current in rabbit ventricular myocytes. *Am J Physiol Cell Physiol*. 2012;302:C1141–C1151.
115. Chakir K, Depry C, Dimaano VL, et al. Galphas-biased beta2-adrenergic receptor signaling from restoring synchronous contraction in the failing heart. *Sci Transl Med*. 2011;3:100ra88.
116. Chakir K, Daya SK, Aiba T, et al. Mechanisms of enhanced beta-adrenergic reserve from cardiac resynchronization therapy. *Circulation*. 2009;119:1231–1240.
117. Chakir K, Zhu W, Tsang S, et al. RGS2 is a primary terminator of beta(2)-adrenergic receptor-mediated G(i) signaling. *J Mol Cell Cardiol*. 2011;50:1000–1007.
118. Maury P, Couderc P, Delay M, Boveda S, Brugada J. Electrical storm in Brugada syndrome successfully treated using isoprenaline. *Europace*. 2004;6:130–133.
119. Tanaka H, Kinoshita O, Uchikawa S, et al. Successful prevention of recurrent ventricular fibrillation by intravenous isoproterenol in a patient with Brugada syndrome. *Pacing Clin Electrophysiol*. 2001;24:1293–1294.

120. Miyazaki T, Mitamura H, Miyoshi S, Soejima K, Aizawa Y, Ogawa S. Autonomic and antiarrhythmic drug modulation of ST segment elevation in patients with Brugada syndrome. *J Am Coll Cardiol*. 1996;27:1061–1070.

121. Huang WA, Shivkumar K, Vaseghi M. Device-based autonomic modulation in arrhythmia patients: the role of vagal nerve stimulation. *Curr Treat Options Cardiovasc Med*. 2015;17:379.

122. Zannad F, De Ferrari GM, Tuinenburg AE, et al. Chronic vagal stimulation for the treatment of low ejection fraction heart failure: results of the NEural Cardiac TherApy foR Heart Failure (NECTAR-HF) randomized controlled trial. *Eur Heart J*. 2015;36:425–433.

123. Matsuda JJ, Lee HC, Shibata EF. Acetylcholine reversal of isoproterenol-stimulated sodium currents in rabbit ventricular myocytes. *Circ Res*. 1993;72:517–525.

124. Fabritz L, Damke D, Emmerich M, et al. Autonomic modulation and antiarrhythmic therapy in a model of long QT syndrome type 3. *Cardiovasc Res*. 2010;87:60–72.

125. De Ferrari GM, Schwartz PJ. Vagus nerve stimulation: from pre-clinical to clinical application: challenges and future directions. *Heart Fail Rev*. 2011;16:195–203.

126. DeMazumder D, Kass DA, O'Rourke B, Tomaselli GF. Cardiac resynchronization therapy restores sympathovagal balance in the failing heart by differential remodeling of cholinergic signaling. *Circ Res*. 2015;116:1691–1699.

39 Pulmonary Vein Ganglia and the Neural Regulation of the Heart Rate

Guillaume Bassil, Manuel Zarzoso, and Sami F. Noujaim

Intrinsic Nervous System of the Heart

Initially, the intrinsic cardiac nervous system (ICNS) was thought to be composed of parasympathetic postganglionic neurons and their axonal projections, along with intramyocardial chromaffin cells, which act as a simple relay region under the control of the central nervous system. However, later studies have shown that the ICNS represents the final relay center for the coordination of regional cardiac function and is composed of sensory (afferent), interconnecting (local circuit), and motor (adrenergic and cholinergic efferent) neurons. These neurons communicate with intrathoracic extracardiac ganglia, forming a distributive network that processes both centripetal and centrifugal neuronal impulses for cardiac control, under the influence of the central nervous system, and circulating catecholamines.[1–3]

The number of cardiac ganglia is variable and species dependent.[4] Their location, shape, and size is also variable, but in many mammals, including humans, intrinsic cardiac ganglia are usually distributed at specific atrial regions: around the sinoatrial node (SAN), roots of caval and pulmonary veins (PVs), and near the atrioventricular node (AVN).[5,6] Intrinsic cardiac ganglia are also thought to be present within the ventricles, although in a smaller number compared to the atria.[7]

The ICNS regulates several aspects of cardiac function such as heart rate (HR), atrial and ventricular refractoriness, conduction, contractility, and blood flow.[8] Furthermore, the ICNS modulates intrathoracic and central cardiovascular–cardiac reflexes and coordinates parasympathetic and sympathetic efferent postganglionic neuronal input to the heart.[1]

It has been suggested that intrinsic cardiac ganglionated plexi (GPs) exert influence over adjacent myocardial regions,[9–11] where vagal deceleration of HR can be selectively mediated by neurons located at the junction of the right atrium and superior vena cava, while the effects on AVN transmission can be controlled by the neurons of a fat pad at the junction of the inferior vena cava and the inferior left atrium.[11]

On the other hand, Armour proposed that intrinsic cardiac ganglia in atrial or ventricular GPs can selectively influence the electrical and mechanical events not only in adjacent tissues but also in all cardiac chambers.[1] For instance, it has been reported that the cholinergic neurons of the right atrial ganglionated plexi (RAGPs) can decrease the rate of discharge of SAN, depress the AVN conduction, and also affect ventricular contractility[12] and that the repolarization of ventricular muscle can be influenced by atrial as well as ventricular ganglia.[13]

Pulmonary Vein Ganglia and Heart Rate Control

Neuroanatomy

The PV ganglia (PVG) are located at the roots of the PVs and form a circuit via interconnecting nerve fibers (Fig. 39.1). They have received special attention because they may play a role in promoting pathophysiological conditions such as atrial fibrillation (AF).[14]

Recent studies have focused on the macroscopic and microscopic neuroanatomy of the PVs and have provided detailed descriptions of their nerve distribution and characteristics. In human hearts, it was found that nerve fibers and ganglia have distinct distribution patterns in the PVs, with a higher nerve density at the ostia than at distal PVs, and are more abundant epicardially, rather than endocardially.[15] In addition, Tan and colleagues performed immunostaining of 192 PV-atrial segments from eight human hearts using antityrosine hydroxylase (anti-TH) and anticholine acetyltransferase (anti-ChAT) antibodies to label adrenergic and cholinergic elements, respectively.[16] They found a similar macroscopic distribution in the PV area for both nerve types and noted adrenergic and cholinergic immunofluorescence colocalization in about 90% of ganglia. A significant proportion of ganglion cells (30%) expressed both TH-positive and CHAT-positive nerves simultaneously. More recently, Vaitkevicius and associates performed a detailed investigation in 35 intact (nonsectioned) left atrial–PV complexes stained with the Karnovsky–Roots acetylcholinesterase precipitation reaction to determine the characteristics and distribution of the neural routes by which autonomic nerves supply the human PVs.[17] They found that three epicardial subplexuses located at the inferior portion of PVs are the source of nerve supply where nerves extend to the PVs from the cardiac GP only. Based on the correlation between the areas of epicardial ganglia and the number of somas they contain, it was estimated that approximately 8000 intrinsic nerve cells (2000 associated with each PV) contribute to the neural control of PVs in humans.[17]

Nerve fibers originating from PVG can extend to different regions of the heart. For instance, the long-term impact of radiofrequency ablation (RFA) of PVG on the structure of epicardial nerves located distally from the ablation sites was examined in the sheep heart.[18] Ablation of PVG resulted in the degeneration of remote epicardial nerves after 2–3 months. There was disorganization in the neural structures of the dorsal left atrium, coronary sinus, ventricle, and AVN. These experiments suggested that there could be anatomical links between the PVG and areas distal to the surrounding PVs. In mouse whole-mount atrial preparations, it was shown that PVG formed a circuit via interconnecting nerve fibers. Most importantly, nerves emerged from the PV ganglionic circuit and advanced toward the SAN area and innervated it,[19] demonstrating that there was a direct neuroanatomical communication between the PVG and the SAN.[19]

Control of Heart Rate

It is well known that the SAN can be regulated by intrinsic ganglia located in its vicinity, and this regulation has been assumed

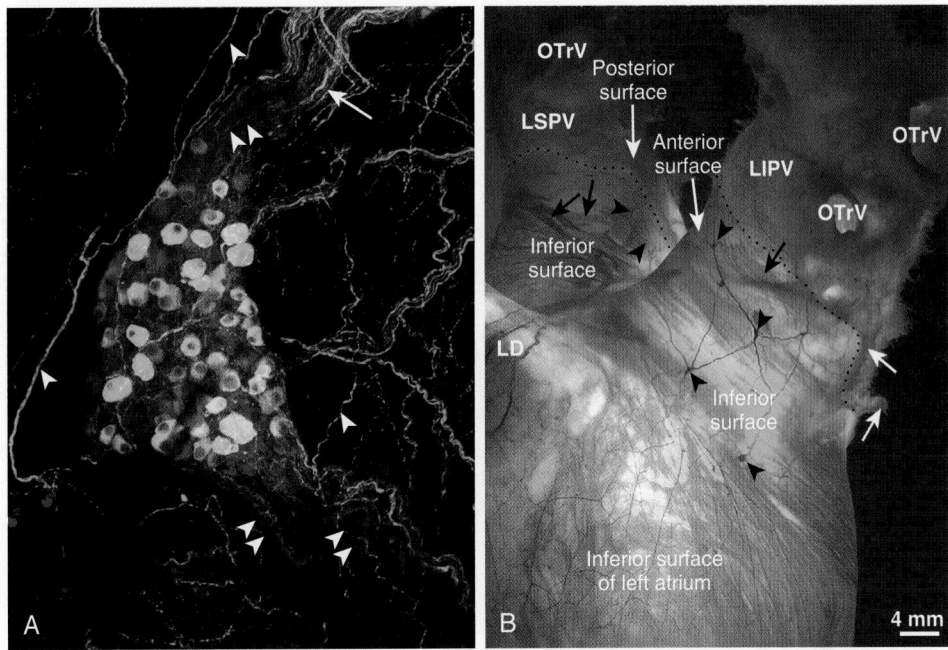

FIGURE 39.1 Neuroanatomical characterization of pulmonary vein (PV) whole-mount preparations. (A) Immunofluorescence image of whole mount mouse PV ganglion stained for tyrosine hydroxylase (sympathetic marker, *green*) and choline acetyltransferase (parasympathetic, *red*). *Single arrowheads* point to sympathetic nerve fibers, *double arrowheads* to parasympathetic fibers, and *arrow* to biphenotypic fibers. (B) A macrophotograph of inferior surface of human embryonic left PVs showing the course of epicardial ganglionated nerves (extending from the middle and left dorsal neural subplexuses to the PV roots) is shown. *Dotted line,* Limits of the cardiac hilum; *black arrowheads,* epicardial ganglia; *solid black arrows,* myocardial sleeves stained histochemically for acetylcholinesterase. *LD,* left dorsal subplexus; *LIPV,* left inferior pulmonary vein; *LSPV,* left superior pulmonary vein; *OTrV,* orifice of tributaries of pulmonary vein. ([B] Modified from Vaitkevicius R, Saburkina I, Rysevaite K, et al. Nerve supply of the human pulmonary veins: an anatomical study. *Heart Rhythm.* 2009;6:221-228.)

to be parasympathetic.[8,20–22] Indeed, experimental studies have shown that ganglia of the fat pad located near the right superior PV, at the junction of the right atrium and superior vena cava (RAGP), mediate a selective negative chronotropic effect.[23] Similarly, the posterior atrial ganglia (found in a fat pad on the right atrium), while having a modest role in producing vagal bradycardia,[22] can mediate more pronounced parasympathetic effects.[23] A third fat pad located between the medial superior vena cava and aortic root appears to be the "head station" of vagal fibers that project to both atria.[24]

In humans, radiofrequency (RF) application to PVG can produce a bradycardic response during ablation,[25,26] and PVG can be stimulated by high-frequency trains of pulses to elicit a decrease in HR.[14] The bradycardic responses have been attributed to an evoked vagal reflex, but the link between these ganglia and SAN has not been fully elucidated. Hou and colleagues[27,28] investigated the interactions between the extrinsic and intrinsic cardiac nervous system in the context of SAN modulation. They proposed a complex interaction between the RAGP and the superior left ganglionated plexus (SLGP), located adjacent to the base of the left superior PV between the left atrial appendage and the left pulmonary artery. They suggested that the main neural pathway between the left vagosympathetic trunk and the SAN traverses the SLGP and RAGP sequentially before proceeding to the SAN, and the stimulation of the right and left vagosympathetic chains produced a negative chronotropic effect (measured as the mean of 20 beats after stimulation), reflecting only a parasympathetic response.

Zarzoso and colleagues[19] studied the effects of PVG high-frequency stimulation of different train durations (200–2000 ms) on SAN activity modulation in the isolated murine heart. The immediate effect of PVG stimulation was a 24% ± 9%

increase in the mean P-P interval of the first three beats after stimulation (Fig. 39.2A), which became more pronounced with longer-stimulus trains. Autonomic blockade with 1-µM atropine and 0.5-µM propranolol abolished all PVG nerve–stimulation effects. High-frequency, low-amplitude stimulation of the right atrial appendage did not affect the cardiac cycle length (see Fig. 39.2B).

Analysis of the time course of beat-to-beat changes during the first 20 intervals following high-frequency stimulation showed that upon PVG with 200-ms trains, the initial slowing of HR was followed by a progressive return toward baseline (see Fig. 39.2C), whereas with the longest trains (1500 ms), an acceleration in HR took place after the 14th beat. Autonomic blockade with atropine and propranolol abolished all nerve stimulation effects. Therefore the experiments pointed out that the SAN can be directly modulated by the remotely located ganglia of the PVs. Hou and coworkers[28] investigated the effects of the interplay between different GPs on sinus rate and AVN conduction. Their study suggested that interconnections exist between GPs, which collectively modulate the responses of the SAN and AVN to ECNS input, and that these interconnections and their effects on SAN and AVN modulation should be considered while identifying targets for AF ablation.[28]

Modulation of Sinoatrial Node Activation Pattern

The location of the earliest site of activation in the SAN is not fixed. It can shift to different zones in response to stimuli such as sympathetic and parasympathetic stimulation, changes in temperature, pharmacological agents, and modifications in extracellular ions.

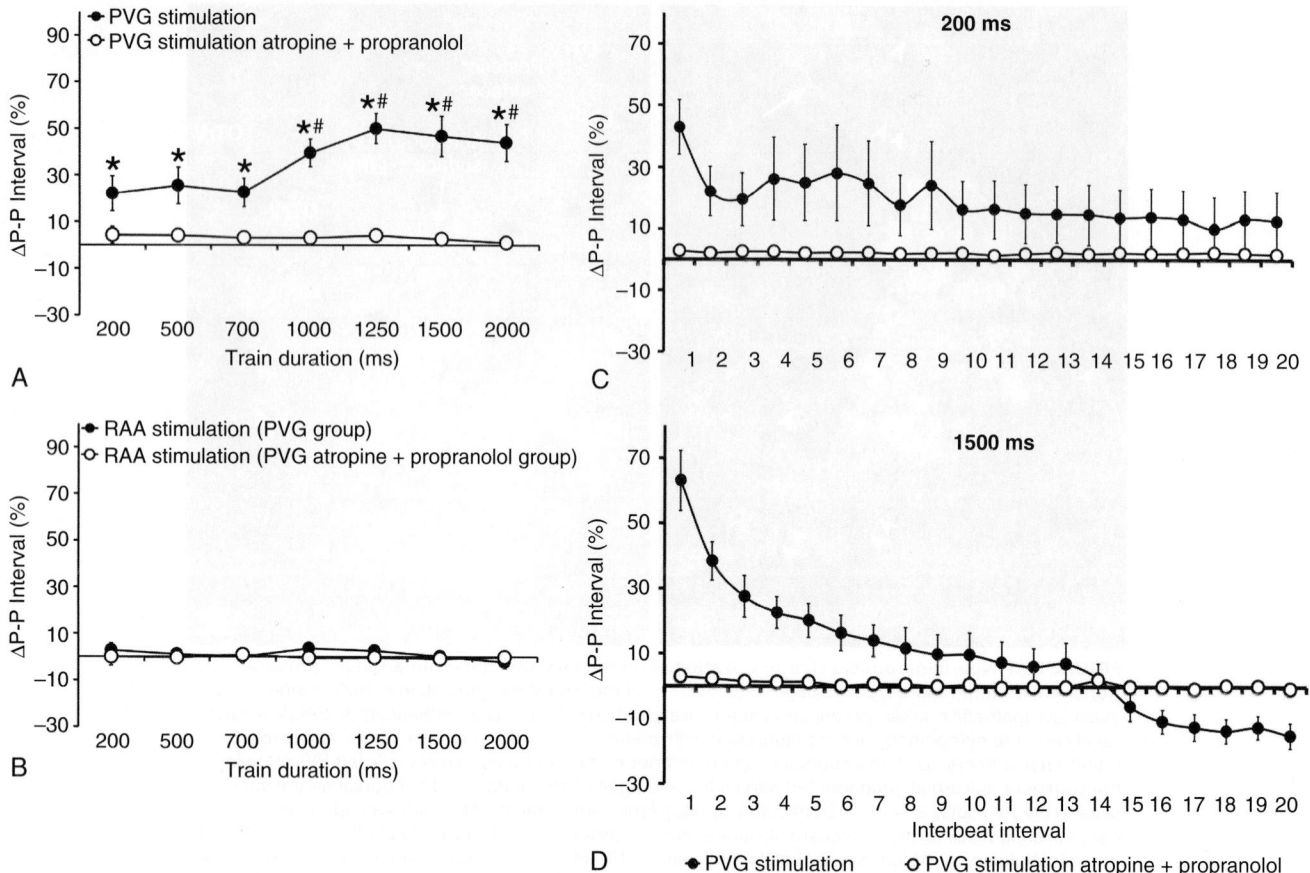

FIGURE 39.2 Pulmonary vein ganglia (*PVG*) stimulation using high-frequency, low-amplitude stimulation modulates heart rate. (A) The percentage change, with respect to baseline at pre-PVG stimulation, in the average of the first three P-P intervals post-PVG stimulation at different stimulus train durations. Atropine + propranolol abolished the PVG stimulation effects on the P-P interval. $*p < .05$ vs. PVG stimulation atropine + propranolol; $\#p < .05$ vs. 200-ms train. (B) The same stimulation parameters applied to the right atrial appendage (*RAA*) produced no effect on heart rate. (C) and (D) Time-course effects (20 beats after stimulation) of PVG stimulation with 200-ms train (C) and 1500-ms train (D). (Modified from Zarzoso M, Rysevaite K, Milstein ML, et al. Nerves projecting from the intrinsic cardiac ganglia of the pulmonary veins modulate sinoatrial node pacemaker function. *Cardiovasc Res.* 2013;99:566-575.)

For instance, in vivo studies in the dog reported that stimulation of the stellate ganglia and the vagus nerve cause, respectively, cranial and caudal shifts of the earliest activation site.[29] Schuessler and colleagues[30] reported that vagal stimulation, either from the right or left vagosympathetic trunk, caused a downward shift in the earliest activation site. In isolated rabbit and canine SAN preparations, it has been shown that the site of earliest activation shifted downward, upward, or remained the same after nerve stimulation.[30–32] This was in line with what has been recently shown in isolated rabbit and murine SAN preparations subjected to direct high-frequency stimulation or isoproterenol/acetylcholine (ACh) administration.[33–35] The role of PVG stimulation on the modulation of SAN cycle length and pattern of activation was studied in the mouse heart. PVG stimulation caused downward (70% of cases) or upward (30%) displacement of the earliest activation site,[19] consistent with the dominant parasympathetic effects of PVG. Fig. 39.3 shows a downward shift of the earliest site of activation immediately after PVG stimulation.[19]

The mechanism by which pacemaker shifts occur after parasympathetic stimulation has been studied using numerical simulations.[36] It was proposed that the SAN is comprised of electrically coupled oscillators (pacemaker cells) with different intrinsic firing rates. Through reciprocal phase-dependent interactions, the coupled oscillators mutually entrain, resulting in the emergence

of an origin of activation. Those mutually entrained oscillators, or pacemaker cells, respond to exogenous perturbations, such as ACh, through changes in maximum diastolic potential, action potential duration, and cycle length. In the simulations, ACh caused a downward shift in the dominant pacemaker region in addition to an increase in the cycle length of the array. By the 10th beat, the array returned to its control pattern and rate of activation.[36] This is similar to the experiments shown in Fig. 39.2. It has also been suggested that nerve stimulation can produce a pacemaker shift from the center to the periphery of the SAN because of electrophysiological and neuroanatomical heterogeneities inherent to the SAN.[31,37,38]

Clinical Implications

Animal data strongly suggest a possible role for ganglia in SAN and AVN functions. However, extrapolation of such findings to the clinical setting is not obvious. It is unclear whether during PV isolation, the delivered RF energy to the PVs can stimulate PVG and produce the somewhat frequently observed decrease in HR.[26,39,40] The mechanism was thought to be caused by the activation of afferent fibers in the PVG, thus evoking a vagal reflex response and resulting in the observed HR decrease.[39,41] The experiments of Zarzoso and associates[19] suggested that the

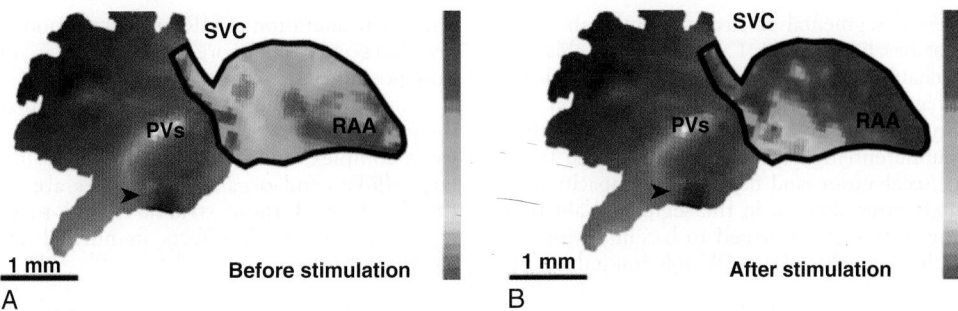

FIGURE 39.3 Modulation of the sinoatrial node activation pattern induced by pulmonary vein ganglia (PVG) stimulation in isolated mouse heart preparations. The leading pacemaker site shifted upward in 32% (7 out of 22) and downward in 68% (15 out of 22) of observations after applying 1000-ms train of stimulation to the PVG. (A) and (B) show activation maps of representative examples of a downward shift after PVG stimulation. The site of earliest activation is depicted in *red. Arrowheads* point to the tip of the stimulation electrode. Map scale, 0–6 ms. *PVs,* pulmonary veins; *RAA,* right atrial appendage; *SVC,* superior vena cava. (Modified from Zarzoso M, Rysevaite K, Milstein ML, et al. Nerves projecting from the intrinsic cardiac ganglia of the pulmonary veins modulate sinoatrial node pacemaker function. *Cardiovasc Res.* 2013;99:566-575.)

local neuronal circuitry between PVGs and the SAN are sufficient to influence HR. Moreover, it has been demonstrated in animal models, and in patients, that PVG ablation may lead to the degeneration of the ventricular innervation and may cause cardiac autonomic dysfunction for up to a year and may even predispose to ventricular arrhythmogenesis.[18,42,43]

Pulmonary Vein Ganglia and Atrial Fibrillation

The autonomic nervous system plays an important role in AF,[44] and AF triggers were shown to originate from the densely innervated PV roots.[41] Studies suggested that AF can be initiated by electrical stimulation of the GP at the roots of the PVs and that ablation of these arrhythmogenic foci can stop AF.[45–47] Nevertheless, the exact mode of action of the GP remains unclear. As previously mentioned, while some investigators show that the GPs function as local centers of integration between the heart and the ECNS, others argued that GPs can act independently of higher autonomic centers and can directly affect cardiac function.[48] To determine the relative role of the intrinsic cardiac nerve activity in triggering atrial arrhythmias and AF, Choi and colleagues[49] performed continuous in vivo nerve recordings from extrinsic cardiac nerve activity (vagus nerve and left stellate ganglion) and the ICNS (SLGP at the base of the left superior PV and ligament of Marshall) in dogs subjected to rapid atrial pacing. It was found that activity of the ICNS preceded the onset of paroxysmal atrial tachyarrhythmias, suggesting that these intrinsic ganglia are an important trigger of paroxysmal AF and atrial tachycardias. It is thought that higher autonomic centers might have inhibitory effects on GPs. Loss of this inhibitory tone could lead to possible GP hyperactivity, which might contribute to increased AF susceptibility.[50–52] Lo and coworkers tested such a hypothesis in live dogs by ablating the junction between the ICNS and ECNS and monitoring for AF development over 10 weeks. Dogs with ablated junctions had a progressive increase in AF occurrence compared to sham, which did not have AF.[53] It was also demonstrated that GP neurons remain viable and capable of increasing neurotransmitter release up to several weeks after ECNS denervation[54] and that the stimulation of GP at the roots of the right superior PV provides the substrate for progression of the focal PV firing into AF.[55]

Evidence suggests that both sympathetic and parasympathetic innervations play a role in AF initiation and maintenance. Patterson and colleagues[56] recorded action potentials from myocardial cells in an excised, superfused PV–atrial sleeve preparation. PVG activation by low-threshold stimulation caused action potential and refractory period shortenings of PV myocardial cells, along with the initiation of rapid firing reminiscent of early

afterdepolarizations. Shortening of the action potential was abrogated by atropine and afterdepolarizations were suppressed by β_1-blockade.[56] In addition, Lemola and associates[45] demonstrated that intact PVs are not needed for the maintenance of experimental cholinergic AF, and they proposed that the PVG, not the PVs themselves, are important in vagally mediated AF maintenance. Although both limbs of the autonomic nervous system play a role in AF, cholinergic stimulation is argued to be the main factor for spontaneous AF initiation.[57]

RFA of the PVG in human and experimental studies can result in successful denervation and prevention of AF inducibility.[25,58] Circumferential PV ablation, which produces a concomitant autonomic denervation by PVG destruction, seems to correlate well with a lower recurrence of AF episodes.[25] It was shown that high-frequency stimulation applied to PVG can initiate PV rapid firings and promote paroxysmal AF, and ablation of the GPs eliminated those rapid firings,[58] thus suggesting an important role of the ICNS in the genesis of AF in structurally normal hearts.

Selective ablation of intrinsic cardiac ganglia in the PVs using RFA has been proposed as either a single treatment for patients with AF[26,59] or in combination with PVs isolation.[60,61] These studies showed that RFA of selected sites, where high-frequency stimulation induces vagal reflexes, can prevent AF recurrence[26,59,62]; however, anatomical PVG ablation yields significantly lower success rates compared to combined PVG and PV ablation.[60,63]

Even though studies have demonstrated the efficacy of PVG ablation, other factors must be taken into consideration. Studies conducted in dogs showed that nerve sprouting occurred within 2 hours of RFA in the right atrium and persisted for at least 1 month after the intervention, even at remote sites with respect to the site of RFA.[64] Removal of the epicardial fat pads and GP ablation greatly reduced the effects of vagal stimulation, not only in the atrial conduction system but also in the atrial myocardium, with possible reinnervation occurring 4 weeks afterward.[65] More recently, the long-term impact of RFA at the roots of the PVs on the structure of epicardial nerves located distally from the PVs was investigated.[18] After 2–3 months, alterations in the structure and degeneration of remote atrial and ventricular nerves occurred.[18] This suggested that long-term autonomic dysfunction is a potential risk related to RFA of PVG. In humans, an upregulation of nerve growth factor (NGF) expression has been reported after RFA. Even though RFA did not increase transcardiac NGF immediately after the procedure, significant systemic increases were observed on the first day after the procedure and persisted for at least 2 days.[66] Furthermore, ablation of ganglia could lead to autonomic dysfunction. Bauer and colleagues[43] studied the short- and long-term effects of segmental and circumferential PV ablation on cardiac autonomic function in patients who received segmental or circumferential ablation. Holter monitoring at baseline and for 1 year after the ablation procedure showed changes in HR acceleration and deceleration capacity as well as HR variability. Cardiac acceleration and deceleration capacity significantly decreased immediately after ablation in the circumferential ablation group and lasted for 1 year after ablation. Acceleration and deceleration capacity also decreased immediately after ablation in the segmental ablation group. However, the parameters returned to baseline within 1 month. Thus the authors concluded that PV ablation induces an immediate alteration of HR autonomic modulation, and this suppression seems to be more long term in circumferential PV ablation, possibly due to the more extensive PVG damage.

The role played by the intrinsic cardiac nervous system, including the network of ganglia in the PVs, in atrial excitability is complex, and its understanding is incomplete. Molecular, cellular, and organ level studies are required to explore the function of these structures and to shed more mechanistic light on their effects in normal and abnormal atrial electrophysiology.

REFERENCES

1. Armour JA. Potential clinical relevance of the "little brain" on the mammalian heart. *Exp Physiol.* 2008;93:165–176.
2. Armour JA, Murphy DA, Yuan BX, et al. Gross and microscopic anatomy of the human intrinsic cardiac nervous system. *Anat Rec.* 1997;247:289–298.
3. Armour JA. Intrinsic cardiac neurons involved in cardiac regulation possess alpha 1-, alpha 2-, beta 1- and beta 2-adrenoceptors. *Can J Ccardiol.* 1997;13:277–284.
4. Pauza DH, Pauziene N, Pakeltyte G, et al. Comparative quantitative study of the intrinsic cardiac ganglia and neurons in the rat, guinea pig, dog and human as revealed by histochemical staining for acetylcholinesterase. *Ann Anat.* 2002;184:125–136.
5. Arora RC, Waldmann M, Hopkins DA, et al. Porcine intrinsic cardiac ganglia. *Anat Rec.* 2003;271:249–258.
6. Pauza DH, Skripka V, Pauziene N. Morphology of the intrinsic cardiac nervous system in the dog: a whole-mount study employing histochemical staining with acetylcholinesterase. *Cells, Tissues, Organs.* 2002;172:297–320.
7. Batulevicius D, Skripka V, Pauziene N, et al. Topography of the porcine epicardiac nerve plexus as revealed by histochemistry for acetylcholinesterase. *Auton Neurosci.* 2008;138:64–75.
8. Tsuboi M, Furukawa Y, Nakajima K, et al. Inotropic, chronotropic, and dromotropic effects mediated via parasympathetic ganglia in the dog heart. *Am J Physiol Heart Circ Physiol.* 2000;279:H1201–H1207.
9. Chen PS, Chen LS, Fishbein MC, et al. Role of the autonomic nervous system in atrial fibrillation: pathophysiology and therapy. *Circ Res.* 2014;114:1500–1515.
10. Chen J, Wasmund SL, Hamdan MH. Back to the future: the role of the autonomic nervous system in atrial fibrillation. *Pacing Clin Electrophysiol.* 2006;29:413–421.
11. Gatti PJ, Johnson TA, Phan P, et al. The physiological and anatomical demonstration of functionally selective parasympathetic ganglia located in discrete fat pads on the feline myocardium. *J Auton Nerv Syst.* 1995;51:255–259.
12. Yuan BX. Cardiac responses induced by bradykinin activation of canine ganglial plexus between aorta and pulmonary artery. *Zhongguo Yao Li Xue Bao.* 1993;14:31–34.
13. Cardinal R, Page P, Vermeulen M, et al. Spatially divergent cardiac responses to nicotinic stimulation of ganglionated plexus neurons in the canine heart. *Auton Neurosci.* 2009;145:55–62.
14. Nishida K, Maguy A, Sakabe M, et al. The role of pulmonary veins vs. autonomic ganglia in different experimental substrates of canine atrial fibrillation. *Cardiovasc Res.* 2011;89:825–833.
15. Chevalier P, Tabib A, Meyronnet D, et al. Quantitative study of nerves of the human left atrium. *Heart Rhythm.* 2005;2:518–522.
16. Tan AY, Li H, Wachsmann-Hogiu S, et al. Autonomic innervation and segmental muscular disconnections at the human pulmonary vein-atrial junction: implications for catheter ablation of atrial-pulmonary vein junction. *J Am Coll Cardiol.* 2006;48:132–143.
17. Vaitkevicius R, Saburkina I, Rysevaite K, et al. Nerve supply of the human pulmonary veins: an anatomical study. *Heart Rhythm.* 2009;6:221–228.
18. Puodziukynas A, Kazakevicius T, Vaitkevicius R, et al. Radiofrequency catheter ablation of pulmonary vein roots results in axonal degeneration of distal epicardial nerves. *Auton Neurosci.* 2012;167:61–65.
19. Zarzoso M, Rysevaite K, Milstein ML, et al. Nerves projecting from the intrinsic cardiac ganglia of the pulmonary veins modulate sinoatrial node pacemaker function. *Cardiovasc Res.* 2013;99:566–575.
20. Lazzara R, Scherlag BJ, Robinson MJ, et al. Selective in situ parasympathetic control of the canine sinoatrial and atrioventricular nodes. *Circ Res.* 1973;32:393–401.
21. Gray AL, Johnson TA, Ardell JL, et al. Parasympathetic control of the heart. II. A novel interganglionic intrinsic cardiac circuit mediates neural control of heart rate. *J Appl Physiol (1985).* 2004;96:2273–2278.
22. Mick JD, Wurster RD, Duff M, et al. Epicardial sites for vagal mediation of sinoatrial function. *Am J Physiol.* 1992;262:H1401–H1406.
23. Randall WC, Ardell JL, Wurster RD, et al. Vagal postganglionic innervation of the canine sinoatrial node. *J Auton Nerv Syst.* 1987;20:13–23.
24. Chiou CW, Eble JN, Zipes DP. Efferent vagal innervation of the canine atria and sinus and atrioventricular nodes. The third fat pad. *Circulation.* 1997;95:2573–2584.
25. Pappone C, Santinelli V, Manguso F, et al. Pulmonary vein denervation enhances long-term benefit after circumferential ablation for paroxysmal atrial fibrillation. *Circulation.* 2004;109:327–334.
26. Pokushalov E, Romanov A, Shugayev P, et al. Selective ganglionated plexi ablation for paroxysmal atrial fibrillation. *Heart Rhythm.* 2009;6:1257–1264.
27. Hou Y, Scherlag BJ, Lin J, et al. Ganglionated plexi modulate extrinsic cardiac autonomic nerve input: effects on sinus rate, atrioventricular conduction, refractoriness, and inducibility of atrial fibrillation. *J Am Coll Cardiol.* 2007;50:61–68.
28. Hou Y, Scherlag BJ, Lin J, et al. Interactive atrial neural network: determining the connections between ganglionated plexi. *Heart Rhythm.* 2007;4:56–63.
29. Goldberg JM. Intra-SA-nodal pacemaker shifts induced by autonomic nerve stimulation in the dog. *Am J Physiol.* 1975;229:1116–1123.
30. Schuessler RB, Bromberg BI, Boineau JP. Effect of neurotransmitters on the activation sequence of the isolated atrium. *Am J Physiol.* 1990;258:H1632–H1641.
31. Shibata N, Inada S, Mitsui K, et al. Pacemaker shift in the rabbit sinoatrial node in response to vagal nerve stimulation. *Exp Physiol.* 2001;86:177–184.
32. Mackaay AJ, Op't Hof T, Bleeker WK, et al. Interaction of adrenaline and acetylcholine on cardiac pacemaker function. Functional inhomogeneity of the rabbit sinus node. *J Pharmacol Exp Ther.* 1980;214:417–422.
33. Glukhov AV, Fedorov VV, Anderson ME, et al. Functional anatomy of the murine sinus node: high-resolution optical mapping of ankyrin-b heterozygous mice. *Am J Physiol Heart Circ Physiol.* 2010;299:H482–H491.
34. Fedorov VV, Chang R, Glukhov AV, et al. Complex interactions between the sinoatrial node and atrium during reentrant arrhythmias in the canine heart. *Circulation.* 2010;122:782–789.
35. Abramochkin DV, Kuzmin VS, Sukhova GS, et al. Modulation of rabbit sinoatrial node activation sequence by acetylcholine and isoproterenol investigated with optical mapping technique. *Acta Physiol.* 2009;196:385–394.
36. Michaels DC, Matyas EP, Jalife J. Mechanisms of sinoatrial pacemaker synchronization: a new hypothesis. *Circ Res.* 1987;61:704–714.
37. Mabe AM, Hoover DB. Structural and functional cardiac cholinergic deficits in adult neurturin knockout mice. *Cardiovasc Res.* 2009;82:93–99.
38. Beau SL, Hand DE, Schuessler RB, et al. Relative densities of muscarinic cholinergic and beta-adrenergic receptors in the canine sinoatrial node and their relation to sites of pacemaker activity. *Circ Res.* 1995;77:957–963.
39. Lemery R, Birnie D, Tang AS, et al. Feasibility study of endocardial mapping of ganglionated plexuses during catheter ablation of atrial fibrillation. *Heart Rhythm.* 2006;3:387–396.
40. Scherlag BJ, Nakagawa H, Jackman WM, et al. Electrical stimulation to identify neural elements on the heart: their role in atrial fibrillation. *J Interv Cardiac Electrophysiol.* 2005;13(suppl 1):37–42.
41. Haissaguerre M, Jais P, Shah DC, et al. Spontaneous initiation of atrial fibrillation by ectopic beats originating in the pulmonary veins. *N Engl J Med.* 1998;339:659–666.
42. Osman F, Kundu S, Tuan J, et al. Ganglionic plexus ablation during pulmonary vein isolation–predisposing to ventricular arrhythmias? *Indian Pacing Electrophysiol J.* 2010;10:104–107.
43. Bauer A, Deisenhofer I, Schneider R, et al. Effects of circumferential or segmental pulmonary vein ablation for paroxysmal atrial fibrillation on cardiac autonomic function. *Heart Rhythm.* 2006;3:1428–1435.
44. Coumel P, Attuel P, Lavallee J, et al. The atrial arrhythmia syndrome of vagal origin. *Arch Mal Coeur Vaiss.* 1978;71:645–656.
45. Lemola K, Chartier D, Yeh YH, et al. Pulmonary vein region ablation in experimental vagal atrial fibrillation: role of pulmonary veins versus autonomic ganglia. *Circulation.* 2008;117:470–477.
46. Lin J, Scherlag BJ, Lu Z, et al. Inducibility of atrial and ventricular arrhythmias along the ligament of Marshall: role of autonomic factors. *J Cardiovasc Electrophysiol.* 2008;19:955–962.
47. Lin J, Scherlag BJ, Zhou J, et al. Autonomic mechanism to explain complex fractionated atrial electrograms (CFAE). *J Cardiovasc Electrophysiol.* 2007;18:1197–1205.
48. Wickramasinghe SR, Patel VV. Local innervation and atrial fibrillation. *Circulation.* 2013;128:1566–1575.
49. Choi EK, Shen MJ, Han S, et al. Intrinsic cardiac nerve activity and paroxysmal atrial tachyarrhythmia in ambulatory dogs. *Circulation.* 2010;121:2615–2623.
50. Zhang Y, Scherlag BJ, Lu Z, et al. Comparison of atrial fibrillation inducibility by electrical stimulation of either the extrinsic or the intrinsic autonomic nervous systems. *J Interv Cardiac Electrophysiol.* 2009;24:5–10.
51. Scherlag BJ, Nakagawa H, Jackman WM, et al. Non-pharmacological, non-ablative approaches for the treatment of atrial fibrillation: experimental evidence and potential clinical implications. *J Cardiovasc Transl Res.* 2011;4:35–41.
52. Male S, Scherlag BJ. Role of neural modulation in the pathophysiology of atrial fibrillation. *Indian J Med Res.* 2014;139:512–522.
53. Lo LW, Scherlag BJ, Chang HY, et al. Paradoxical long-term proarrhythmic effects after ablating the "head station" ganglionated plexi of the vagal innervation to the heart. *Heart Rhythm.* 2013;10:751–757.
54. Smith FM, McGuirt AS, Hoover DB, et al. Chronic decentralization of the heart differentially remodels canine intrinsic cardiac neuron muscarinic receptors. *Am J Physiol Heart Circ Physiol.* 2001;281:H1919–H1930.
55. Scherlag BJ, Yamanashi W, Patel U, et al. Autonomically induced conversion of pulmonary vein focal firing into atrial fibrillation. *J Am Coll Cardiol.* 2005;45:1878–1886.
56. Patterson E, Po SS, Scherlag BJ, et al. Triggered firing in pulmonary veins initiated by in vitro autonomic nerve stimulation. *Heart Rhythm.* 2005;2:624–631.
57. Sharifov OF, Fedorov VV, Beloshapko GG, et al. Roles of adrenergic and cholinergic stimulation in spontaneous atrial fibrillation in dogs. *J Am Coll Cardiol.* 2004;43:483–490.
58. Lu Z, Scherlag BJ, Lin J, et al. Autonomic mechanism for initiation of rapid firing from atria and pulmonary veins: Evidence by ablation of ganglionated plexi. *Cardiovasc Res.* 2009;84:245–252.
59. Scanavacca M, Pisani CF, Hachul D, et al. Selective atrial vagal denervation guided by evoked vagal reflex to treat patients with paroxysmal atrial fibrillation. *Circulation.* 2006;114:876–885.
60. Katritsis DG, Giazitzoglou E, Zografos T, et al. Rapid pulmonary vein isolation combined with autonomic ganglia modification: a randomized study. *Heart.* 2011;8:672–678.
61. Ohkubo K, Watanabe I, Okumura Y, et al. Combined effect of pulmonary vein isolation and ablation of cardiac autonomic nerves for atrial fibrillation. *Int Heart J.* 2008;49:661–670.
62. Mikhaylov E, Kanidieva A, Sviridova N, et al. Outcome of anatomic ganglionated plexi ablation to treat paroxysmal atrial fibrillation: a 3-year follow-up study. *Europace.* 2011;13:362–370.
63. Pokushalov E, Romanov A, Artyomenko S, et al. Ganglionated plexi ablation for longstanding persistent atrial fibrillation. *Europace.* 2010;12:342–346.
64. Okuyama Y, Pak HN, Miyauchi Y, et al. Nerve sprouting induced by radiofrequency catheter ablation in dogs. *Heart Rhythm.* 2004;1:712–717.
65. Sakamoto S, Schuessler RB, Lee AM, et al. Vagal denervation and reinnervation after ablation of ganglionated plexi. *Thorac Cardiovasc Surg.* 2010;139:444–452.
66. Kangavari S, Oh YS, Zhou S, et al. Radiofrequency catheter ablation and nerve growth factor concentration in humans. *Heart Rhythm.* 2006;3:1150–1155.

40 Neural Activity and Atrial Tachyarrhythmias

Mark J. Shen, Michael C. Fishbein, Lan S. Chen, Shien-Fong Lin, and Peng-Sheng Chen

Atrial tachyarrhythmias, including atrial tachycardia (AT) and atrial fibrillation (AF), continue to burden public health, with AF being the most common sustained arrhythmia in the developed world.[1] AF is associated with dreadful complications, such as stroke and heart failure (HF). *The cardiac autonomic nervous system (ANS) plays an important role in normal cardiac electrophysiology and arrhythmogenesis.*[2] Multiple experimental studies have contributed to a better understanding of the underlying mechanisms by which the cardiac ANS induces atrial tachyarrhythmias. Work from our laboratory on this subject used direct nerve recordings in ambulatory canines to study spontaneous arrhythmias.[3–8] This chapter focuses on the role of neural activity in atrial tachyarrhythmias. It also discusses neuromodulation as a treatment strategy for patients with AF and a new discovery that allows estimation of sympathetic tone using skin sympathetic nerve activity (SKNA).

Cardiac Autonomic Nervous System

Extrinsic Cardiac Nerves

The cardiac ANS can be divided into extrinsic and intrinsic components (Fig. 40.1).[9] The extrinsic cardiac ANS has sympathetic and parasympathetic components. The sympathetic fibers are largely derived from major autonomic ganglia along the cervical and thoracic spinal cord. These autonomic ganglia include the superior cervical ganglia, which communicate with C1–3; the stellate (cervicothoracic) ganglia (Fig. 40.2A), which communicate with C7–8 to T1–2; and the thoracic ganglia (as low as the 7th thoracic ganglion).[10] Because preganglionic sympathetic efferents arising from the T1–T4 spinal cord that project to the heart transit through the stellate ganglia via the paravertebral chain, T1–T2 surgical excision is sufficient to functionally interrupt central control of peripheral sympathetic efferent activity.[11] The parasympathetic preganglionic fibers are carried almost entirely within the vagus nerve and are divided into superior, middle, and inferior branches (see Fig. 40.2A). Most of the parasympathetic nerve fibers converge at a distinct fat pad between the superior vena cava and the aorta (known as the "third fat pad") en route to the sinus and atrioventricular nodes.[12] In ambulatory dogs, the vagal and fat pad nerve activities may activate in a coordinated fashion, indicating a direct functional connection between the two nerve structures.[7] While parasympathetic nerve fibers are carried by the vagal nerve, the human and canine vagal nerves may also contain significant sympathetic nerve structures.[5,13–15] An example is shown in Fig. 40.2B. Low-output vagal stimulation may selectively activate these sympathetic nerve structures and accelerate the heart rate.[16] Therefore the terms "vagal" and "parasympathetic" should not be used interchangeably. Commonly used terms such as "vagal tone" and "vasovagal response" may be anatomically incorrect.

Intrinsic Cardiac Nerves

In addition to the extrinsic cardiac ANS, the heart is also innervated by an exquisitely complex intrinsic cardiac ANS.[17] Armour and colleagues provided a detailed map of the distribution of autonomic nerves in human hearts.[18] Throughout the heart, numerous cardiac ganglia, each of which contains 200–1000 neurons,[18,19] form synapses with the sympathetic and parasympathetic fibers that enter the pericardial space. The vast majority of these ganglia are organized into ganglionated plexi (GPs) on the surface of the atria and ventricles.[18] The intrinsic cardiac ANS thus forms a complex network composed of GPs (concentrated within epicardial fat pads) and the interconnecting ganglia and axons.[18,20,21] These GPs may function as the "integration centers" that modulate the intricate autonomic interactions between the extrinsic cardiac ANS and the intrinsic cardiac ANS.[22] In the atria, GPs are concentrated in distinct locations on the chamber walls.[18] Specifically, the sinus node is primarily innervated by the right atrial GP, whereas the atrioventricular node is innervated by the inferior vena cava–inferior atrial GP (IVC–IAGP), which is located at the junction of the inferior vena cava and the left atrium.[9,10,19,22] Another region with a high density of GPs is the PV–LA junction, and these GPs are characterized by colocalization of adrenergic and cholinergic nerves (Fig. 40.2C).[23] The importance of these GPs will be discussed later in this chapter.

Neural Activities in Atrial Electrophysiology and Arrhythmogenesis

Normal Neural Influences on Atrial Electrophysiology

Sympathetic activation of the heart serves to enhance cardiac output during "fight-or-flight" reactions by increasing calcium entry and the spontaneous release of calcium from the sarcoplasmic reticulum.[24,25] On the other hand, parasympathetic activation of the heart can reduce the atrial effective refractory period,[26] augment spatial electrophysiological heterogeneity of the atria,[27] and promote early afterdepolarizations toward the end of phase 3 in the cardiac action potential.[28]

Abnormal Neural Activities in Atrial Arrhythmogenesis

Experimental models have shown that acetylcholine infusion in the sinus node artery invariably induces AF in dogs;

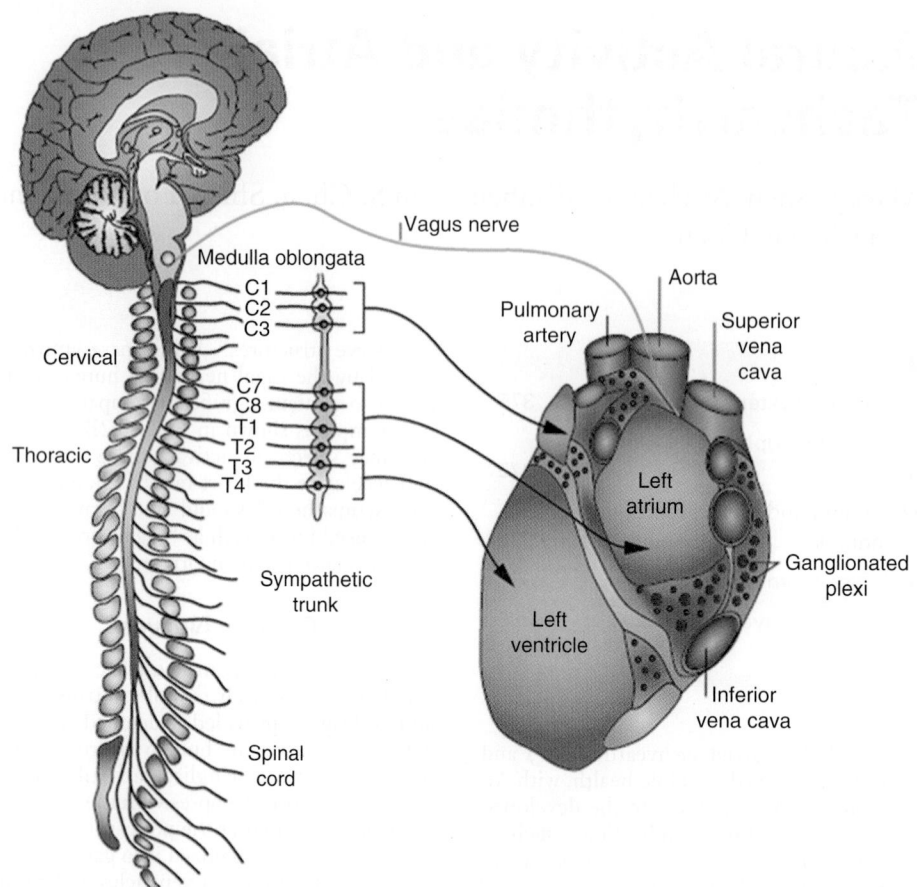

FIGURE 40.1 The scheme of autonomic innervation of the heart. The cardiac sympathetic ganglia consist of cervical ganglia, stellate (cervicothoracic) ganglia, and thoracic ganglia. Parasympathetic innervation comes from the vagus nerves. (From Shen MJ, Choi EK, Tan AY, et al. Neural mechanisms of atrial arrhythmias. *Nat Rev Cardiol.* 2011;9:30-39.)

acetylcholine-mediated AF was facilitated by the β-adrenoceptor agonist isoproterenol, which decreased the threshold concentration of acetylcholine required for the induction of AF and prolonged episodes of AF.[29] Mechanistically, if simultaneous sympathetic and vagal activations occur, then action potential duration (APD) is shortened while the Ca^{2+} transient is large and long. A short APD and a large Ca^{2+} transient create a condition for late phase 3 early after-depolarization (EAD) that can induce triggered activity and AF.[28,30] As pulmonary veins naturally have short APDs, they are particularly prone to develop these Ca^{2+} transient–triggered arrhythmias.[31–33] Electrical stimulation to the GPs around the pulmonary veins can stimulate both adrenergic and cholinergic nerves and can reliably trigger arrhythmias by this mechanism (Fig. 40.3).

Recording Stellate Ganglion and Vagal Nerve Activity From Ambulatory Canines

Ambulatory Nerve Recording

Most of the above-mentioned studies were performed either with a Langendorff-perfused heart or in anesthetized animals. These methods have limited applicability to human arrhythmias—a perfused heart lacks hemodynamic reflexes and background neurohormonal influences; acute studies are typically short-term observations without spontaneously occurring arrhythmias. At least two noninvasive methods have emerged that sought to correlate cardiac ANS with arrhythmias in an ambulatory setting over a longer monitoring period. The first one is heart rate

variability analysis. Power spectral analysis of heart rate variability in electrocardiogram (ECG) recordings taken over a period of time is used to reflect cardiac sympathetic tone or sympathovagal balance. Analysis of baroreflex sensitivity is another example. An increase in aortic pressure or volume can trigger the firing of stretch-sensitive neurons in the afferent baroreceptor, which sends impulses to the medulla and leads to decreased efferent sympathetic and increased efferent parasympathetic activity to restore pressure homeostasis.[34] These analyses provide significant prognostic value in that a depressed heart rate variability or baroreflex sensitivity following myocardial infarction is associated with higher cardiac mortality.[35] Nonetheless, these noninvasive methods have substantial limitations for at least two reasons. First, they measure only relative changes in autonomic nerve activity rather than the absolute intensity of sympathetic or parasympathetic discharges. Second, such analyses require an intact sinus node that mediates adequate cardiac responses to autonomic activities. Patients with AF often have associated sinus node dysfunction,[36,37] rendering analyses of heart rate variability or baroreflex sensitivity in patients with arrhythmias unreliable. Therefore to better translate into clinical scenarios, a technique that enables chronic direct nerve activity recordings would be highly desirable to demonstrate whether autonomic activity is a direct trigger of cardiac arrhythmias.

Such a study was carried out in 2006 when Jung and associates first continuously recorded the activity of the stellate ganglia in healthy dogs using implanted radio transmitters for an average of 41.5 days.[4] The results showed the feasibility of chronic cardiac nerve recordings and demonstrated a circadian variation

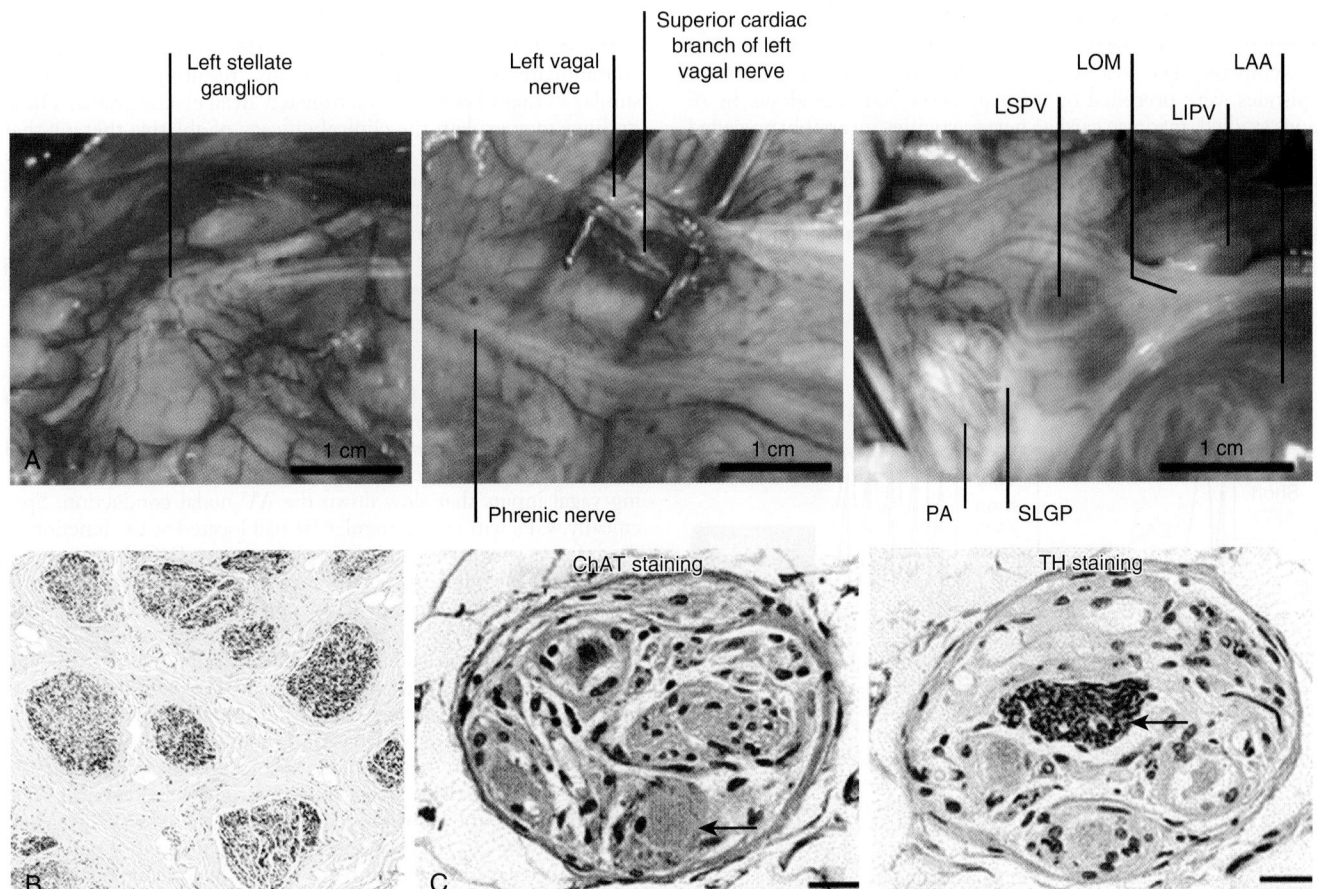

FIGURE 40.2 Anatomy and histology of cardiac autonomic nervous system. (A) Photographs of the left stellate ganglion (*left image*) and the superior cardiac branch of the left vagal nerve (*middle image*) in a dog heart. The ligament of Marshall (*LOM*) originates from the coronary sinus and connects to the left superior pulmonary vein (*LSPV*); the superior left ganglionated plexi (*SLGP*) is located between the left-atrial appendage (*LAA*) and the LSPV (*right image*). (B) Cross section of human vagal nerve stained with TH (*brown*), confirming the presence of sympathetic nerves. (C) Colocalization of adrenergic and cholinergic nerves in the intrinsic cardiac ganglia. The same ganglion contained cholinergic ganglion cells (*arrow, left image*) and adrenergic nerve fibers (*arrow, right image*). *ChAT,* Choline acetyltransferase; *LIPV,* left inferior pulmonary vein; *PA,* pulmonary artery; *TH,* tyrosine hydroxylase. ([A] Modified from Choi EK, Shen MJ, Han S, et al. Intrinsic cardiac nerve activity and paroxysmal atrial tachyarrhythmia in ambulatory dogs. *Circulation.* 2010;121:2615-2623. [B] Modified from Seki A, Green HR, Lee TD, et al. Sympathetic nerve fibers in human cervical and thoracic vagus nerves. *Heart Rhythm.* 2014;11:1411-1417. [C] Modified from Tan AY, Li H, Wachsmann-Hogiu S, et al. Autonomic innervation and segmental muscular disconnections at the human pulmonary vein–atrial junction: implications for catheter ablation of atrial-pulmonary vein junction. *J Am Coll Cardiol.* 2006;48:132-143.)

of sympathetic outflow to the heart.[4] Multiple subsequent studies[3,6,7,38–40] with direct nerve activity recordings in animal models of disease have provided insights to understanding the role of the cardiac ANS in arrhythmogenesis, and these studies will be discussed later.

Paroxysmal Atrial Tachyarrhythmias

Chronic ambulatory nerve recordings allow us to study the temporal relationships of autonomic nerve discharges and spontaneous paroxysmal AF and AT. Tan and colleagues[6] implanted a pacemaker and a radiotransmitter in dogs to simultaneously record nerve activities of the left stellate ganglion and left vagal nerve, as well as a surface ECG over a period of several weeks. Intermittent rapid atrial pacing commenced, and the nerve activity was monitored when the pacemaker was turned off. The authors found that there is a circadian variation of the frequencies of atrial tachyarrhythmias, similar to that found in human patients with symptomatic paroxysmal AF. More importantly,

they also found that simultaneous sympathovagal discharges are a common trigger for premature atrial contractions and are the most frequent trigger of paroxysmal AT (Fig. 40.4A) and AF (Fig. 40.4B).[6] Cryoablation of bilateral stellate ganglia and the superior cardiac branches of the left vagus nerve eliminated all episodes of paroxysmal atrial arrhythmias, indicating a (not necessarily causal) relationship between ANS activity and the generation of these arrhythmias. In a different canine model of pacing-induced heart failure, simultaneous sympathovagal discharge was again the most frequent trigger of atrial tachyarrhythmias.[5] These arrhythmias could be prevented by cryoablation of the stellate ganglion and the T2–4 thoracic sympathetic ganglia.[38] These findings echo the results discussed earlier by Sharifov and coworkers and Patterson and colleagues that showed that simultaneous sympathetic and parasympathetic activations are particularly proarrhythmic at the atrial level.[29,33]

Subsequently, Choi and associates[3] went a step further and recorded intrinsic nerve activity from the superior left GP, the ligament of Marshall, the left stellate ganglion, and the left thoracic vagus nerve in dogs subjected to intermittent, rapid atrial pacing. Similarly, a vast majority of paroxysmal AF and AT were preceded by sympathovagal coactivations, while a minority (10%–20%) of episodes were preceded by intrinsic nerve activities alone. In all dogs studied, intrinsic cardiac nerve activities invariably preceded atrial tachyarrhythmia episodes (Fig. 40.5A). The importance of intracardiac ganglia around the pulmonary veins in triggering paroxysmal atrial tachyarrhythmias is supported by a study that showed ablation of these ganglia reduced the inducibility of AF

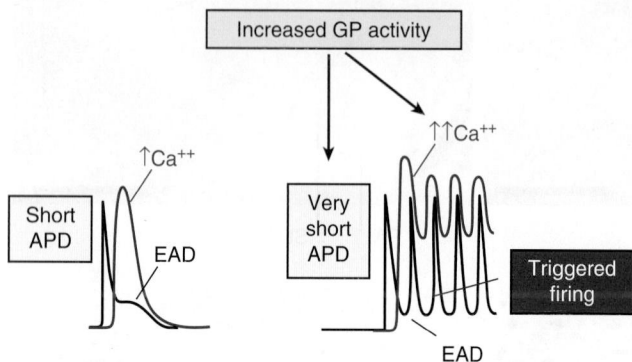

FIGURE 40.3 Pulmonary vein myocytes have an abbreviated action potential duration (*APD*) at baseline. Sympathetic activation increases calcium transient and if the duration of the calcium transient exceeds APD, forward mode of the sodium-calcium exchanger will activate, generating an early after-depolarization (*EAD*). As ganglionated plexi (*GP*) have colocalizing cholinergic and adrenergic nerves, with increased GP activity, the combination of APD shortening and calcium transient enhancement results in EAD formation and triggered firing. (Data from Patterson E, Po SS, Scherlag BJ, et al. Triggered firing in pulmonary veins initiated by in vitro autonomic nerve stimulation. *Heart Rhythm.* 2005;2:624-631.)

in dogs with atrial tachypacing.[41] Another interesting observation of this study[3] is that the activities of intrinsic cardiac nerves might contaminate local atrial electrograms, resulting in recordings similar to that of complex fractionated atrial electrograms. These findings may explain the clinical efficacy of ablative therapy that targets those intrinsic cardiac ganglia[42–44] or targets sites with complex fractionated atrial electrograms.[45] Because linear lesions from standard pulmonary vein–directed ablation run through areas with high concentrations of GPs,[46] autonomic modification or denervation might be a potential mechanism that contributes to the effectiveness of such ablation procedures.

Persistent Atrial Fibrillation

In most patients with AF, rate control is not inferior to rhythm control as a management strategy.[47] The cardiac ANS, particularly the vagal tone, is important in modulating dromotropy (AV nodal conduction). Therefore rate control can be achieved by augmenting vagal inputs that slow down the AV nodal conduction. Specifically, GPs within a triangular fat pad located at the junction of the inferior vena cava and inferior left atrium (IVC–IAGP) mediate most vagal input to the AV node.[48] Electrical stimulation of these GPs may slow the ventricular rate during AF in canines[49] and human patients.[50] An elegant study by Park and colleagues[8] that simultaneously recorded bilateral cervical vagal nerve activities and IVC–IAGP nerve activity in a canine model of persistent AF gives insight into how these nerve activities interact and contribute to ventricular rate changes during AF. Left-sided cervical vagal nerve activity was found to be associated with ventricular rate reduction during AF in five of six dogs while, for right-sided cervical vagal nerve activities, the association occurred in one of six dogs. More importantly, IVC–IAGP discharges were invariably associated with ventricular rate reduction during AF. In comparison, right or left cervical vagal nerve activities were associated with ventricular

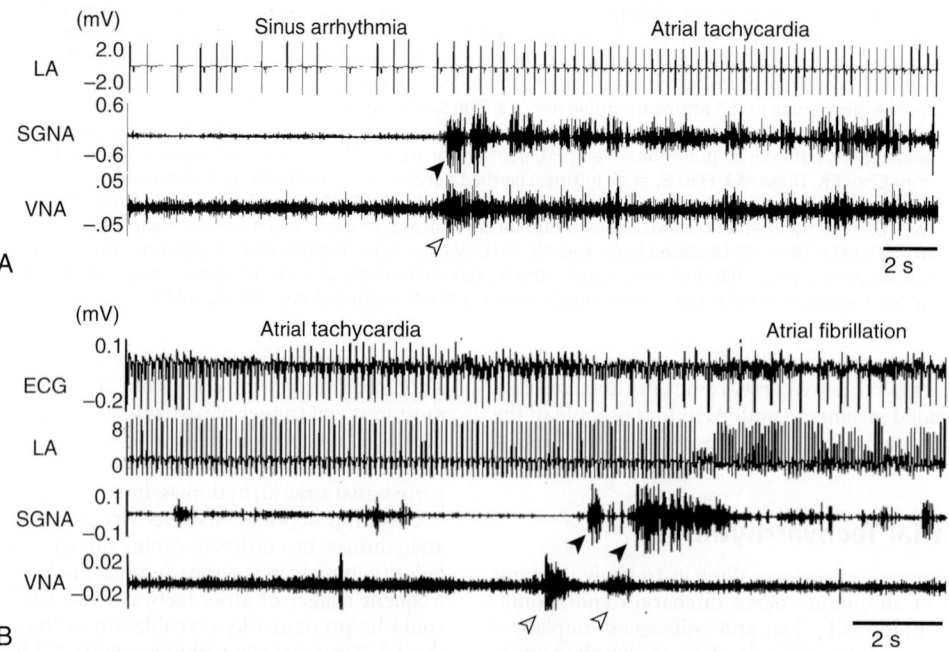

FIGURE 40.4 Paroxysmal atrial arrhythmias in dogs with intermittent rapid atrial pacing. (A) Simultaneous sympathetic (*black arrowheads*) and parasympathetic (*hollow arrowheads*) coactivation preceded the onset of paroxysmal atrial tachycardia. (B) During an episode of atrial tachycardia, simultaneous sympathetic (*black arrowheads*) and parasympathetic (*hollow arrowheads*) coactivation resulted in the conversion of atrial tachycardia to atrial fibrillation. *ECG,* Electrocardiogram; *LA,* left atrium; *SGNA,* stellate ganglion nerve activity; *VNA,* vagal nerve activity. (Modified from Tan AY, Zhou S, Ogawa M, et al. Neural mechanisms of paroxysmal atrial fibrillation and paroxysmal atrial tachycardia in ambulatory canines. *Circulation.* 2008;118:916-925.)

rate reduction only when coactivated with the IVC–IAGP nerve activity (Fig. 40.5B). IVC–IAGP discharges alone without cervical vagal input are sufficient to cause transient AV conduction delay. These studies also suggest that vagal nerves do not directly innervate the AV node. Rather, they activate IVC–IAGP to control the ventricular rate during AF.

In a population-based study that followed patients with lone, paroxysmal AF over 30 years, roughly half of the patients progressed to persistent or permanent AF.[51] The exact mechanism by which some patients progressed while others did not remains elusive. Moreover, among those who did progress to a more chronic form of AF, the time to progression varied considerably. Reasons for such interindividual disparities in the susceptibility to progression of AF are also poorly understood. In the two studies mentioned earlier, by Tan and coworkers[6] and Choi and colleagues,[3] intermittent rapid atrial pacing initially induced paroxysmal AF. However, if pacing continued, sustained AF was induced. The duration it took to reach sustained (>48 hours) AF varied among the dogs. This model thus provided a great resource to study characteristics that may predict the susceptibility of pacing-induced sustained AF. At baseline prior to the commencement of atrial pacing, two differential patterns

exist of interactions among cardiac autonomic structures (Fig. 40.6).[40] Among them, dogs with a linear sympathovagal correlation (Group 1) tended to undergo a faster development of sustained AF than those with L-shaped sympathovagal correlation (Group 2). In addition, prior to the development of sustained AF, Group 1 dogs had more paroxysmal AF and AT compared with Group 2. These data imply that different forms of sympathovagal discharge patterns might also be present in human patients and that differential ANS discharge patterns may predetermine which patients will be at greater risk of progression from paroxysmal to persistent or permanent AF.

Recording Nerve Activities From the Skin
Subcutaneous Nerve Recording

As the thoracic subcutaneous tissue contains abundant sympathetic nerves[52] that can be traced back to the ipsilateral stellate ganglion,[53] subcutaneous nerve activity (SCNA) might serve as a surrogate for stellate ganglion nerve activity (SGNA) and be more easily accessible for recording. A proof-of-concept study was first carried out by Robinson and associates from our laboratory.[54]

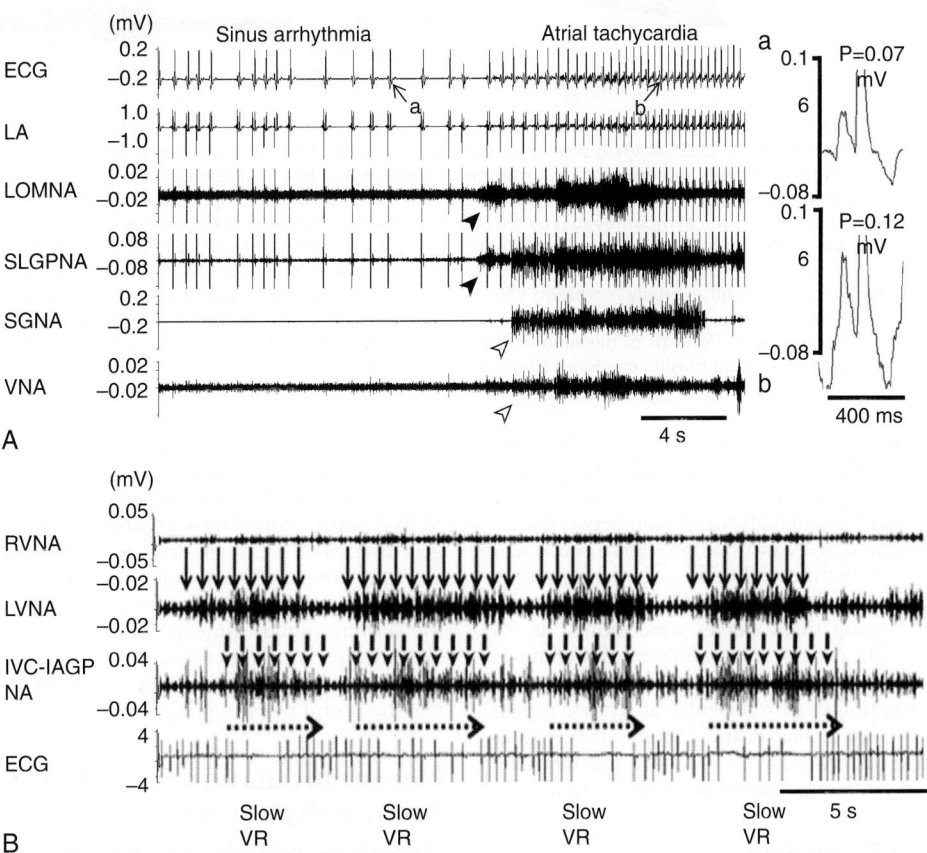

FIGURE 40.5 The effect of intrinsic cardiac nerve activity (*NA*). (A) Intrinsic cardiac nerve activities from ligament of Marshall and superior left ganglionated plexi (*black arrowheads*) occurred before extrinsic cardiac nerve activities (*hollow arrowheads*) in an episode of paroxysmal atrial tachycardia. The magnified pseudo-electrocardiogram (*ECG*) shows the different P wave morphologies during sinus rhythm (*a*) and during atrial tachycardia (*b*). (B) During persistent atrial fibrillation, inferior vena cava–inferior left atrial ganglionated plexi (*IVC–IAGP*) activity is associated with reduced ventricular rate (*VR*). In this example, IVC–IAGP mostly coactivated with left cervical vagus nerve. *LOMNA,* Ligament of Marshall nerve activity; *LVNA,* left vagal nerve activity; *RVNA,* right vagal nerve activity; *SGNA,* stellate ganglion nerve activity; *SLGPNA,* superior left ganglionated plexi nerve activity; *VNA,* vagal nerve activity. ([A] Modified from Choi EK, Shen MJ, Han S, et al. Intrinsic cardiac nerve activity and paroxysmal atrial tachyarrhythmia in ambulatory dogs. *Circulation.* 2010;121:2615-2623. [B] Modified from Park HW, Shen MJ, Han S, et al. Neural control of ventricular rate in ambulatory dogs with pacing-induced sustained atrial fibrillation. *Circ Arrhythm Electrophysiol.* 2012;5:571-580.)

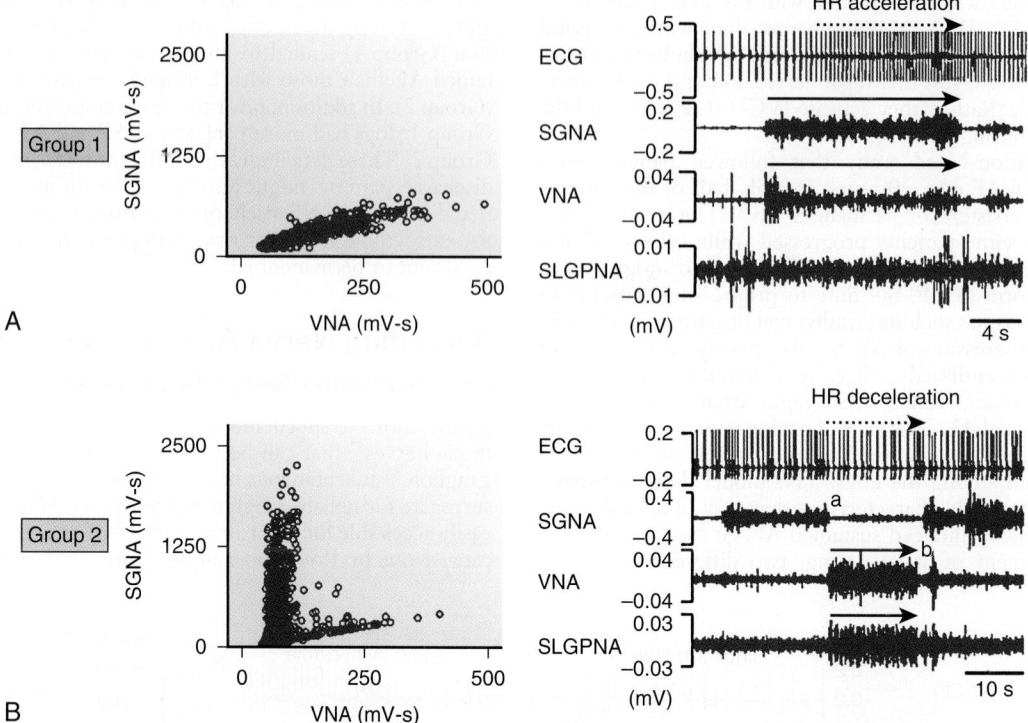

FIGURE 40.6 Patterns of autonomic interactions. (A) Representative stellate ganglion nerve activity–vagal nerve activity (*SGNA–VNA*) scatter plot of a Group 1 dog. Each dot represents an SGNA–VNA pair of nerve activity integrated over 1 minute. The entire plot has 1440 data points to cover a 24-hour period. A linear sympathovagal correlation was observed and the *right panel* shows an example of simultaneous sympathovagal coactivation (*arrows*) observed in a Group 1 dog that led to heart rate (*HR*) acceleration. (B) Representative SGNA–VNA scatter plot from a Group 2 dog that demonstrated an L-shaped correlation. *Right panel* shows an example of a recording from a Group 2 dog showing that simultaneously increased VNA and superior left ganglionated plexi nerve activity (*SLGPNA*) (*arrows*) resulted in HR deceleration. *ECG,* Electrocardiogram. (Modified from Shen MJ, Choi EK, Tan AY, et al. Patterns of baseline autonomic nerve activity and the development of pacing-induced sustained atrial fibrillation. *Heart Rhythm.* 2011;8:583-589.)

Bipolar electrodes were secured in the left thoracic subcutaneous tissue to represent SCNA. Dogs were ambulating while SCNA and SGNA (from left stellate ganglion) were continuously recorded. The investigators found high correlation between integrated SCNA and integrated SGNA with a correlation coefficient of 0.7 (Fig. 40.7A). Both activities exhibited a circadian variation. No crosstalk between channels was found. Histological analysis confirmed that rich sympathetic nerves were located at the recording site (Fig. 40.7B). A subsequent study by Doytchinova and colleagues showed that SCNA can be used as an estimate of SGNA to predict susceptibility to ventricular tachyarrhythmias in a canine model of sudden cardiac death.[55] In ambulatory dogs with healed myocardial infarction, SCNA is more accurate than heart rate variability in estimating cardiac sympathetic tone.[56]

Cutaneous Nerve Recording

Recording SCNA still requires a skin incision for implanting the subcutaneous electrodes. For clinical applications for cardiac risk stratification, it is highly desirable to develop a completely noninvasive method. The skin of the canine upper thorax is extensively innervated by sympathetic nerves from the stellate ganglion.[57] Jiang and coworkers securely taped ECG patch electrodes onto dogs' skin in multiple configurations to represent lead I, lead II, and also left- and right-sided chest wall.[58] Signals were high-passed at 100 Hz to display skin nerve activity (SKNA). Simultaneous SGNA was recorded from the left stellate ganglion. High correlation was

found between SKNA and SGNA in the ambulatory setting (Fig. 40.7C). The SKNA recorded from the left-sided chest wall (upper third of the thorax) has the highest correlation to SGNA, with a correlation coefficient of 0.743. These data suggest that SKNA can be used to estimate cardiac sympathetic activity in dogs. Subsequent clinical studies showed that SKNA can also be recorded using conventional ECG electrodes on the skin in human subjects.[59] The cold water pressor test and Valsalva maneuver increase the SKNA while stellate ganglion block suppresses SKNA. These findings suggest that SKNA may be useful in estimating sympathetic tone in humans.

Neuromodulation for Atrial Tachyarrhythmias

Ganglionated Plexi Ablation

Since the seminal work by Haïssaguerre and colleagues[60] that discovered that a rapidly firing focus in or close to the pulmonary veins can be the trigger of paroxysmal AF, pulmonary vein isolation (PVI) has been the most widely used ablation approach to treat AF. However, the long-term results of PVI remain unsatisfactory, particularly for persistent AF.[61] Two potential reasons can explain this phenomenon. First, sustained PV isolation is not achieved in those who have recurrent AF. However, in a study that systematically examined the prevalence of PV reconnection during a repeat procedure in patients with and without AF recurrence, reconnection of at least one PV was found in

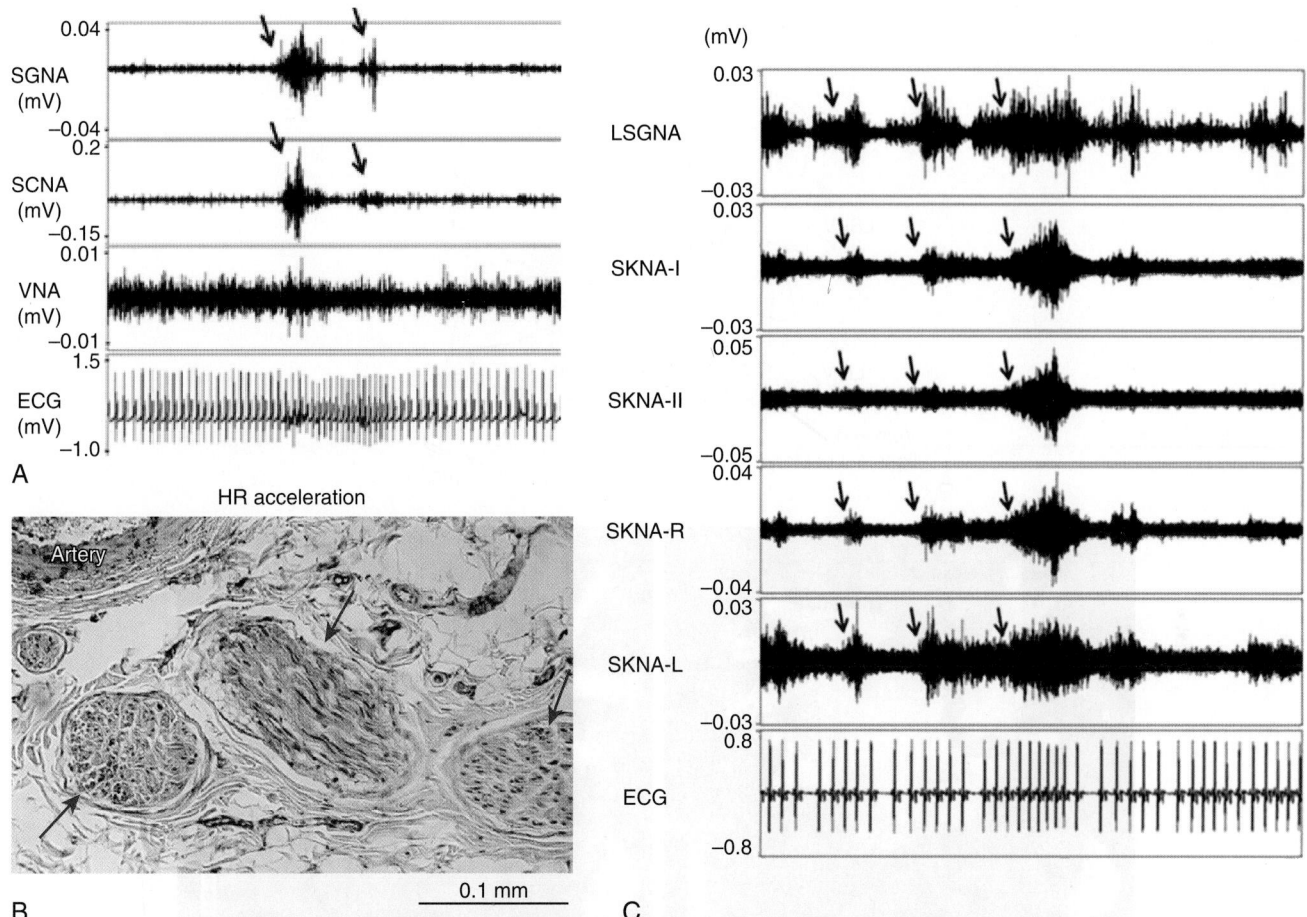

FIGURE 40.7 Subcutaneous nerve activity (*SCNA*) and skin nerve activity (*SKNA*). (A) An example of SCNA coactivated with stellate ganglion nerve activity (*SGNA*) leading to heart rate (*HR*) acceleration. A second coactivation caused HR to slow down. (B) Immunohistochemical staining of the subcutaneous tissue demonstrates tyrosine hydroxylase-positive (*brown; arrows*) nerve structures, consistent with the presence of sympathetic innervation. (C) Simultaneous recording in an ambulatory dog from SGNA and SKNA from different location such as lead I, II, right-sided chest wall (*R*), and left-sided chest wall (*L*). SKNA correlates well with SCNA and causes HR acceleration. *ECG*, Electrocardiogram. ([A and B] Modified from Robinson EA, Rhee KS, Doytchinova A, et al. Estimating sympathetic tone by recording subcutaneous nerve activity in ambulatory dogs. *J Cardiovasc Electrophysiol.* 2015;26:70-78. [C] Modified from Jiang Z, Zhao Y, Doytchinova A, et al. Using skin sympathetic nerve activity to estimate stellate ganglion nerve activity in dogs. *Heart Rhythm.* 2015;12:1324-1332.)

the vast majority of patients (>90%) in each group,[62] suggesting that, contrary to popular belief, sustained PV isolation may not be a prerequisite for freedom from AF recurrence. The second, and more plausible, explanation would be that failure of eliminating the trigger (or substrate) in standard PVI contributes to the high recurrence rate after ablation; this trigger may be the GPs surrounding the PVs. In experimental models, these GPs are more important than PVs in triggering AF.[41] A recent study found that, at a follow-up (mean follow-up time of 508 days) in patients with paroxysmal AF who underwent an extensive PVI procedure, those with positive GP responses after PVI had a significantly higher recurrence rate of atrial tachyarrhythmias (51%) than those without positive GP responses (8%).[63] The hypothesis that GP ablation, whether as an adjunctive procedure[42,64] or as a stand-alone treatment,[65,66] may yield a better clinical efficacy has been tested and yielded inconsistent results in smaller trials.[42,43,67–69] The hitherto largest randomized, multicenter trial, by Katritsis and associates,[70] enrolled 242 patients of paroxysmal AF and compared the efficacy of PVI, GP ablation alone, and PVI followed by GP ablation (Fig. 40.8); this study found that freedom from AF was achieved in 56%, 48%, and 74%, respectively, after 2 years of follow-up.

Renal Sympathetic Denervation

Catheter-based renal sympathetic denervation is now widely applied clinically as a treatment for resistant hypertension.[71] Renal denervation ablates both efferent and afferent renal sympathetic nerves as they run together. By ablating the efferent nerves, renal denervation decreases the renal norepinephrine spillover by 47%[72] and attenuates the activity of the renin–angiotensin–aldosterone system,[73] which can be important in the pathogenesis of AF.[74] Ablating the afferent nerves decreased feedback activation to the central nervous system and thereby decreased sympathetic input to the heart. In a porcine model of obstructive sleep apnea, renal denervation was shown to attenuate the shortening of the atrial effective refractory period that was presumably caused by combined sympathovagal activation.[75] Pokushalov and colleagues compared the efficacy of combined renal denervation with PVI to PVI alone in a study enrolling 27 patients with paroxysmal or persistent AF.[76] The authors found that at a 1-year follow-up, 69% of patients who received both procedures were free of AF, compared with 29% of those in the PVI-only group. A more recent study showed that renal denervation may improve the results of PVI in patients with persistent AF and/or severe

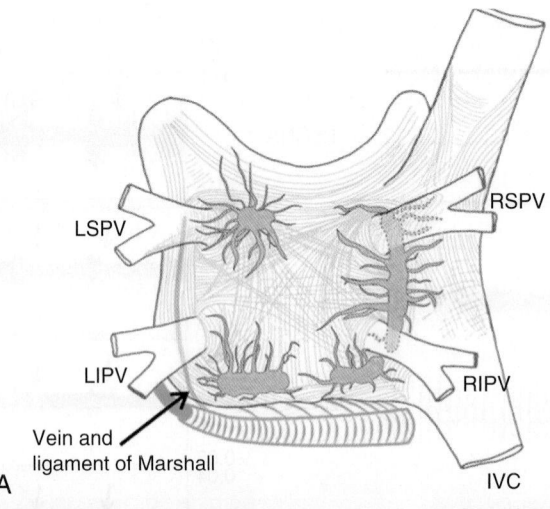

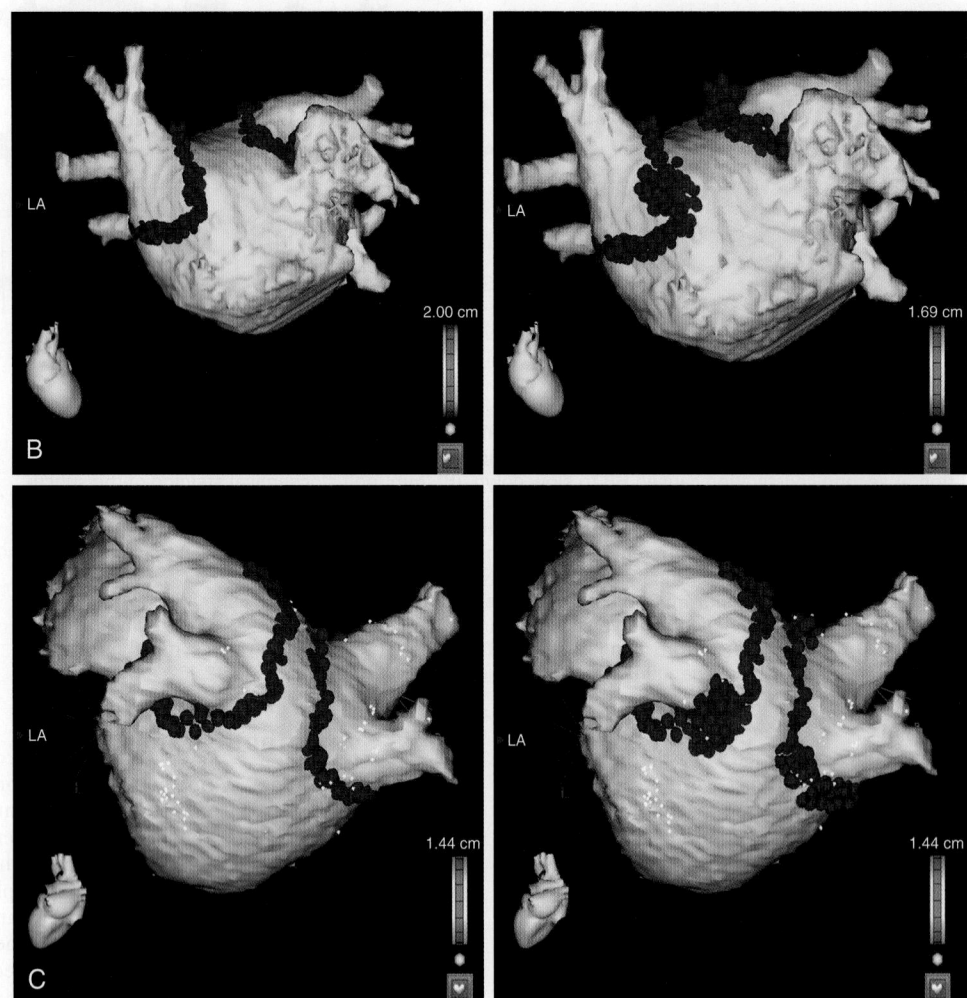

FIGURE 40.8 Major left atrial ganglionated plexi (GPs) proposed for ablation. (A) Anatomic location of the four GPs. Schematic posterior view of the left and right atria shows the five major left atrial autonomic GP and axons (superior left GP [SLGP], inferior left GP [ILGP], anterior right GP [ARGP], inferior right GP [IRGP], and ligament of Marshall) are shown in *yellow*; while in *blue* is shown the coronary sinus. (B) Anatomic ablation of the SLGP and ARGP. (C) Anatomic ablation of the ILGP and IRGP. Following pulmonary vein isolation, the ablation lesions are expanded in order to cover the anatomic site of presumed GP clusters. *IVC,* Inferior vena cava; *LA,* left atrium; *LIPV,* left inferior pulmonary vein; *LSPV,* left superior pulmonary vein; *RIPV,* right inferior pulmonary vein; *RSPV,* right superior pulmonary vein. (Modified from Katritsis DG, Pokushalov E, Romanov A, et al. Autonomic denervation added to pulmonary vein isolation for paroxysmal atrial fibrillation: a randomized clinical trial. *J Am Coll Cardiol.* 2013;62:2318-2325.)

resistant hypertension.[77] We are still at an early stage of application of renal denervation in treating AF and many questions remain to be answered. One important question is whether the antiarrhythmic property of renal denervation is beyond normalization of blood pressure. In a goat model of persistent AF, renal denervation reduced atrial sympathetic nerve sprouting and atrial fibrosis.[78] Moreover, by increasing the conduction velocity with less conduction block, renal denervation reduced AF complexity (defined as the ratio of number of waves to AF cycle length). The authors hypothesized that this is because renal denervation contributes to a lower degree of atrial remodeling characterized by better endo-epicardial electrical connections. Another interesting hypothesis would be that renal denervation directly inhibits arrhythmogenic cardiac autonomic nerve activities from the stellate ganglia or GPs. A recent study in dogs showed that renal denervation can damage the stellate ganglion and remodel the brain stem.[79]

Low-Level Vagus Nerve Stimulation

Although vagus nerve stimulation is a reliable technique used for the experimental induction of AF, low-level cervical vagus nerve stimulation (LL–VNS) at a stimulus strength of 1 V below the threshold needed to reduce heart rate can lower intrinsic cardiac nerve activity and, paradoxically, suppress electrically induced AF in open-chest, anesthetized dogs.[80] The antifibrillatory effects are still present even when the stimulus strength is 50% below the threshold. LL–VNS reverses the electrical remodeling caused by rapid atrial pacing.[80,81] To test if this is true in ambulatory animals chronically, Shen and coworkers used direct nerve recordings to demonstrate that continuous LL–VNS suppressed paroxysmal atrial tachyarrhythmias in ambulatory dogs via suppression of stellate-ganglion nerve activity.[7] This reduction was most apparent in the early morning, when the incidence of AF is the highest (Fig. 40.9A).[82] Histologically, LL–VNS caused structural remodeling in the left stellate ganglion characterized by a significant reduction of ganglion cells that stained positive for tyrosine hydroxylase, an enzyme critical in the biosynthesis of adrenalines (Fig. 40.9B). Subsequent studies by the same investigators showed that in the left stellate ganglion, LL–VNS also resulted in the upregulation of the small-conductance calcium-activated potassium channel type 2 and increased its expression in the cell membrane (Fig. 40.9C and D).[83] These changes may facilitate hyperpolarization of the ganglion cells and reduce the frequency of neuronal discharges.[84] Thus LL–VNS can functionally and structurally remodel the left stellate ganglion, reducing sympathetic outflow to the heart, hence its anti-AF property.[85]

Other Forms of Neural Stimulation

Acupuncture is widely practiced for pain control, and one effect of acupuncture is the modulation of autonomic tones. Lomuscio and colleagues[86] showed that acupuncture at Neiguan, Shenmen, and Xinshu acupoints could prevent arrhythmia recurrences in patients with persistent AF after electrical cardioversion. The efficacy was comparable to amiodarone.[86] In another study, acupuncture resulted in a significant reduction in the number and duration of symptomatic AF episodes in a small group of patients with paroxysmal AF.[87] An alternative somatic sensory stimulation is low-level tragus stimulation. Yu and associates[88] developed this noninvasive approach by delivering low-level stimulation to the auricular branch of the vagus nerve at the tragus of the ear. The authors found that low-level tragus stimulation can reverse pacing-induced atrial remodeling and suppress AF inducibility, suggesting its possible value in the treatment of AF. More recently, the same approach was shown to suppress AF in humans and was associated with a reduction in inflammatory cytokines.[89] Spinal cord stimulation (SCS) is also being investigated in the treatment of AF. Bernstein and colleagues demonstrated that acute application of SCS at the T_1–T_5 level prolonged the atrial effective refractory period without a noticeable effect on the heart rate or atrioventricular conduction, and it substantially decreased AF burden and inducibility by rapid atrial pacing.[90] SCS and the previously mentioned tragus stimulation both may possibly work through activation of vagal tones to the heart. This notion is supported by the fact that the electrophysiological and antiarrhythmic effects of both SCS and tragus stimulation are abolished after transection of bilateral cervical vagal nerves.[88,91] In addition, SCS is associated with reversion of deleterious neuronal remodeling during atrial tachypacing, such as upregulation of nerve growth factor and downregulation of the small-conductance calcium-activated potassium channel type 2 in the stellate ganglion and intrinsic cardiac ganglia.[92] These findings were similar to the effects seen in direct vagal nerve stimulation.[83] These early results are exciting, but the limitations of these studies are considerable, including small sample size. Further investigations and clinical trials enrolling larger number of patients will be needed to test the efficacy of cutaneous neuromodulation in the management of AF.

Conclusions

Cardiac ANS is important in atrial arrhythmogenesis. Ambulatory nerve recordings demonstrate that intrinsic ANS activations invariably precede the onset of paroxysmal atrial tachyarrhythmias and sympathovagal coactivations (from the left stellate ganglion and the left thoracic vagal nerve) are common triggers of these arrhythmias. Neuromodulation with various strategies is shown to be effective in treating AF. This can be done by GP ablation or by LL–VNS, SCS, renal denervation, or low-level tragus stimulation. The promising early results need to be tested in larger randomized clinical trials before widespread use can be recommended to treat patients with AF, a serious disease with ever-increasing prevalence. Subcutaneous or skin nerve recordings correlate well with nerve activity recorded invasively from the stellate ganglion. These relatively noninvasive recording methods can be easily translated to clinical practice for cardiovascular risk stratification and to provide mechanistic insights into clinical efficacy of neuromodulation in treating AF.

Acknowledgments

This study was supported in part by NIH Grants P01 HL78931, R01 HL71140, R41HL124741, R42DA043391, a Medtronic-Zipes Endowment and the Indiana University Health–Indiana University School of Medicine Strategic Research Initiative.

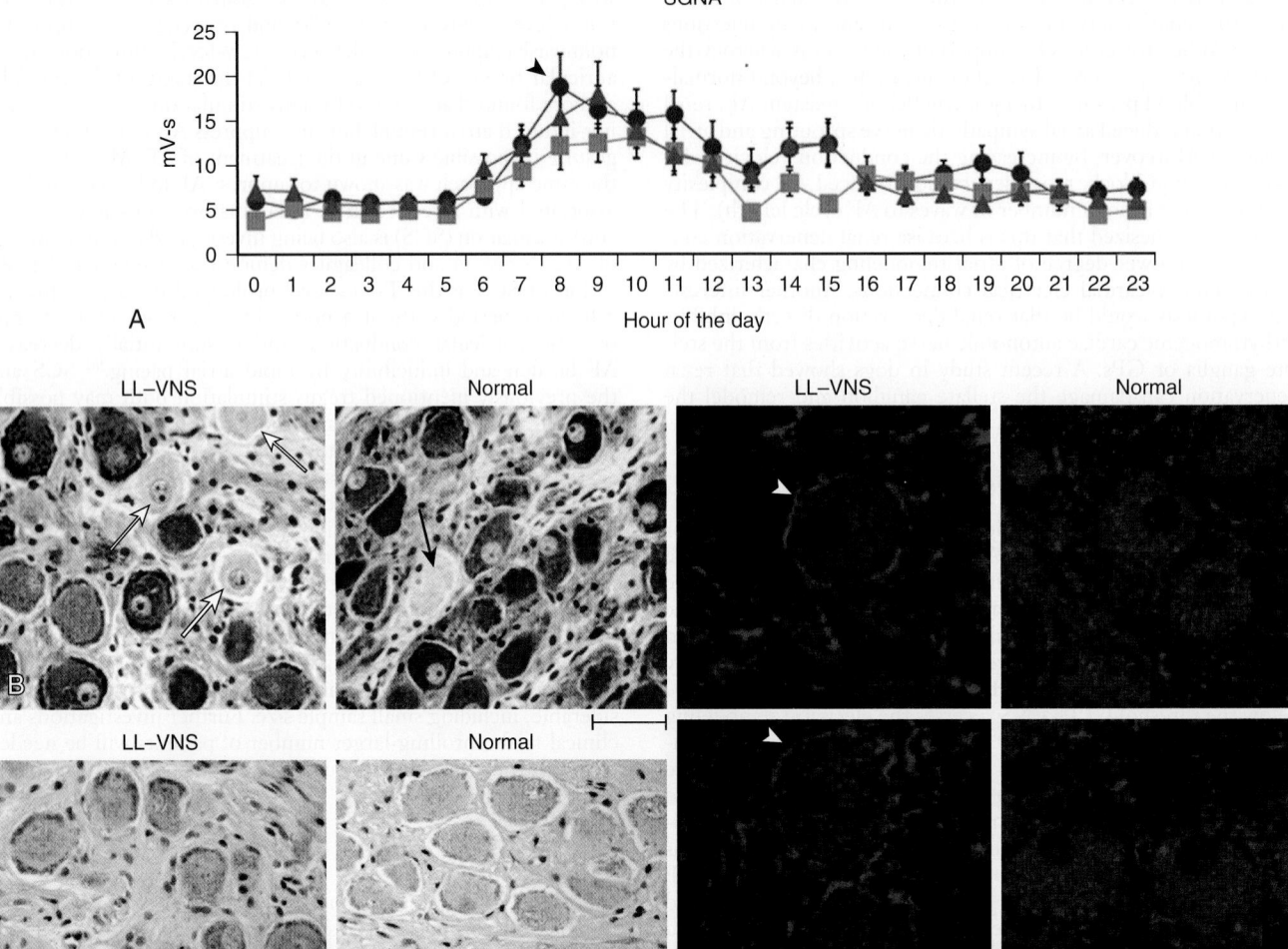

FIGURE 40.9 Effects of low-level vagus nerve stimulation (*LL–VNS*). (A) LL–VNS significantly reduced stellate ganglion nerve activity (*SGNA*) and the reduction is most pronounced at 8 a.m. (*black arrowhead*). (B) Following LL–VNS, there is a significant increase in the number of tyrosine hydroxylase–negative ganglion cells (*hollow arrows*). In control, tyrosine hydroxylase–negative cells are fewer (*black arrows*). Calibration bar = 50 μm. (C) In dogs that underwent LL–VNS, there is also an upregulation of ganglion cells that are stained more strongly positive for small-conductance calcium-activated potassium channel subtype 2 (SK2) (*black arrowhead*). Increased SK2 current may hyperpolarize the ganglion cells and reduce the frequency of neuronal discharges. Calibration bar = 50 μm. (D) Immunofluorescence confocal microscope images show an increase of expression of SK2 protein in the periphery of the cells (*white arrowheads*) while they show a decrease in the cytosol. This intracellular trafficking of SK2 protein to the cell membrane is evident after LL–VNS. ([A and B] Modified from Shen MJ, Shinohara T, Park HW, et al. Continuous low-level vagus nerve stimulation reduces stellate ganglion nerve activity and paroxysmal atrial tachyarrhythmias in ambulatory canines. *Circulation.* 2011;123:2204-2212. [C and D] Modified from Shen MJ, Hao-Che Chang X, Park HW, et al. Low-level vagus nerve stimulation upregulates small conductance calcium-activated potassium channels in the stellate ganglion. *Heart Rhythm.* 2013;10:910-915.)

REFERENCES

1. Benjamin EJ, Chen PS, Bild DE, et al. Prevention of atrial fibrillation: report from a national heart, lung, and blood institute workshop. *Circulation.* 2009;119:606–618.
2. Shen MJ, Zipes DP. Role of the autonomic nervous system in modulating cardiac arrhythmias. *Circ Res.* 2014;114:1004–1021.
3. Choi EK, Shen MJ, Han S, et al. Intrinsic cardiac nerve activity and paroxysmal atrial tachyarrhythmia in ambulatory dogs. *Circulation.* 2010;121:2615–2623.
4. Jung BC, Dave AS, Tan AY, et al. Circadian variations of stellate ganglion nerve activity in ambulatory dogs. *Heart Rhythm.* 2006;3:78–85.
5. Ogawa M, Zhou S, Tan AY, et al. Left stellate ganglion and vagal nerve activity and cardiac arrhythmias in ambulatory dogs with pacing-induced congestive heart failure. *J Am Coll Cardiol.* 2007;50:335–343.
6. Tan AY, Zhou S, Ogawa M, et al. Neural mechanisms of paroxysmal atrial fibrillation and paroxysmal atrial tachycardia in ambulatory canines. *Circulation.* 2008;118:916–925.
7. Shen MJ, Shinohara T, Park HW, et al. Continuous low-level vagus nerve stimulation reduces stellate ganglion nerve activity and paroxysmal atrial tachyarrhythmias in ambulatory canines. *Circulation.* 2011;123:2204–2212.
8. Park HW, Shen MJ, Han S, et al. Neural control of ventricular rate in ambulatory dogs with pacing-induced sustained atrial fibrillation. *Circ Arrhythm Electrophysiol.* 2012;5:571–580.
9. Armour JA. Functional anatomy of intrathoracic neurons innervating the atria and ventricles. *Heart Rhythm.* 2010;7:994–996.
10. Kawashima T. The autonomic nervous system of the human heart with special reference to its origin, course, and peripheral distribution. *Anat Embryol (Berl).* 2005;209:425–438.
11. Buckley U, Yamakawa K, Takamiya T, Andrew Armour J, Shivkumar K, Ardell JL. Targeted stellate decentralization: implications for sympathetic control of ventricular electrophysiology. *Heart Rhythm.* 2016;13:282–288.
12. Chiou CW, Eble JN, Zipes DP. Efferent vagal innervation of the canine atria and sinus and atrioventricular nodes–the third fat pad. *Circulation.* 1997;95:2573–2584.
13. Seki A, Green HR, Lee TD, et al. Sympathetic nerve fibers in human cervical and thoracic vagus nerves. *Heart Rhythm.* 2014;11:1411–1417.
14. Onkka P, Maskoun W, Rhee KS, et al. Sympathetic nerve fibers and ganglia in canine cervical vagus nerves: localization and quantitation. *Heart Rhythm.* 2013;10:585–591.
15. Kawagishi K, Fukushima N, Yokouchi K, Sumitomo N, Kakegawa A, Moriizumi T. Tyrosine hydroxylase-immunoreactive fibers in the human vagus nerve. *J Clin Neurosci.* 2008;15:1023–1026.
16. Rhee KS, Hsueh CH, Hellyer JA, et al. Cervical vagal nerve stimulation activates the stellate ganglion in ambulatory dogs. *Korean Circ J.* 2015;45:149–157.
17. Shen MJ, Choi EK, Tan AY, et al. Neural mechanisms of atrial arrhythmias. *Nat Rev Cardiol.* 2011;9:30–39.
18. Armour JA, Murphy DA, Yuan BX, Macdonald S, Hopkins DA. Gross and microscopic anatomy of the human intrinsic cardiac nervous system. *Anat Rec.* 1997;247:289–298.
19. Pauza DH, Skripka V, Pauziene N, Stropus R. Morphology, distribution, and variability of the epicardiac neural ganglionated subplexuses in the human heart. *Anat Rec.* 2000;259:353–382.
20. Yuan BX, Ardell JL, Hopkins DA, Losier AM, Armour JA. Gross and microscopic anatomy of the canine intrinsic cardiac nervous system. *Anat Rec.* 1994;239:75–87.
21. Pauza DH, Skripka V, Pauziene N. Morphology of the intrinsic cardiac nervous system in the dog: a whole-mount study employing histochemical staining with acetylcholinesterase. *Cells Tissues Organs.* 2002;172:297–320.
22. Hou Y, Scherlag BJ, Lin J, et al. Ganglionated plexi modulate extrinsic cardiac autonomic nerve input: effects on sinus rate, atrioventricular conduction, refractoriness, and inducibility of atrial fibrillation. *J Am Coll Cardiol.* 2007;50:61–68.
23. Tan AY, Li H, Wachsmann-Hogiu S, Chen LS, Chen PS, Fishbein MC. Autonomic innervation and segmental muscular disconnections at the human pulmonary vein-atrial junction: implications for catheter ablation of atrial-pulmonary vein junction. *J Am Coll Cardiol.* 2006;48:132–143.
24. ter Keurs HE, Boyden PA. Calcium and arrhythmogenesis. *Physiol Rev.* 2007;87:457–506.
25. Bers DM. Cardiac excitation-contraction coupling. *Nature.* 2002;415:198–205.
26. Wijffels MC, Kirchhof CJ, Dorland R, Allessie MA. Atrial fibrillation begets atrial fibrillation. A study in awake chronically instrumented goats. *Circulation.* 1995;92:1954–1968.
27. Fareh S, Villemaire C, Nattel S. Importance of refractoriness heterogeneity in the enhanced vulnerability to atrial fibrillation induction caused by tachycardia-induced atrial electrical remodeling. *Circulation.* 1998;98:2202–2209.

28. Burashnikov A, Antzelevitch C. Reinduction of atrial fibrillation immediately after termination of the arrhythmia is mediated by late phase 3 early afterdepolarization-induced triggered activity. *Circulation.* 2003;107:2355–2360.
29. Sharifov OF, Fedorov VV, Beloshapko GG, Glukhov AV, Yushmanova AV, Rosenshtraukh LV. Roles of adrenergic and cholinergic stimulation in spontaneous atrial fibrillation in dogs. *J Am Coll Cardiol.* 2004;43:483–490.
30. Choi EK, Chang PC, Lee YS, et al. Triggered firing and atrial fibrillation in transgenic mice with selective atrial fibrosis induced by overexpression of TGF-beta1. *Circ J.* 2012;76:1354–1362.
31. Patterson E, Jackman WM, Beckman KJ, et al. Spontaneous pulmonary vein firing in man: relationship to tachycardia-pause early afterdepolarizations and triggered arrhythmia in canine pulmonary veins in vitro. *J Cardiovasc Electrophysiol.* 2007;18:1067–1075.
32. Patterson E, Lazzara R, Szabo B, et al. Sodium-calcium exchange initiated by the Ca²⁺ transient: an arrhythmia trigger within pulmonary veins. *J Am Coll Cardiol.* 2006;47:1196–1206.
33. Patterson E, Po SS, Scherlag BJ, Lazzara R. Triggered firing in pulmonary veins initiated by in vitro autonomic nerve stimulation. *Heart Rhythm.* 2005;2:624–631.
34. La Rovere MT, Specchia G, Mortara A, Schwartz PJ. Baroreflex sensitivity, clinical correlates, and cardiovascular mortality among patients with a first myocardial infarction. A prospective study. *Circulation.* 1988;78:816–824.
35. La Rovere MT, Bigger Jr JT, Marcus FI, Mortara A, Schwartz PJ. Baroreflex sensitivity and heart-rate variability in prediction of total cardiac mortality after myocardial infarction. ATRAMI (Autonomic Tone and Reflexes After Myocardial Infarction) Investigators. *Lancet.* 1998;351:478–484.
36. Elvan A, Wylie K, Zipes DP. Pacing-induced chronic atrial fibrillation impairs sinus node function in dogs–electrophysiological remodeling. *Circulation.* 1996;94:2953–2960.
37. Gomes JA, Kang PS, Matheson M, Gough Jr WB, El Sherif N. Coexistence of sick sinus rhythm and atrial flutter-fibrillation. *Circulation.* 1981;63:80–86.
38. Ogawa M, Tan AY, Song J, et al. Cryoablation of stellate ganglia and atrial arrhythmia in ambulatory dogs with pacing-induced heart failure. *Heart Rhythm.* 2009;6:1772–1779.
39. Zhou S, Jung BC, Tan AY, et al. Spontaneous stellate ganglion nerve activity and ventricular arrhythmia in a canine model of sudden death. *Heart Rhythm.* 2008;5:131–139.
40. Shen MJ, Choi EK, Tan AY, et al. Patterns of baseline autonomic nerve activity and the development of pacing-induced sustained atrial fibrillation. *Heart Rhythm.* 2011;8:583–589.
41. Nishida K, Maguy A, Sakabe M, Comtois P, Inoue H, Nattel S. The role of pulmonary veins vs. autonomic ganglia in different experimental substrates of canine atrial fibrillation. *Cardiovasc Res.* 2011;89:825–833.
42. Nakagawa H, Scherlag BJ, Wu R, et al. Addition of selective ablation of autonomic ganglia to pulmonary vein antrum isolation for treatment of paroxysmal and persistent atrial fibrillation. *Circulation.* 2006;110:III-459.
43. Pappone C, Santinelli V, Manguso F, et al. Pulmonary vein denervation enhances long-term benefit after circumferential ablation for paroxysmal atrial fibrillation. *Circulation.* 2004;109:327–334.
44. Pokushalov E, Romanov A, Shugayev P, et al. Selective ganglionated plexi ablation for paroxysmal atrial fibrillation. *Heart Rhythm.* 2009;6:1257–1264.
45. Nademanee K, McKenzie J, Kosar E, et al. A new approach for catheter ablation of atrial fibrillation: mapping of the electrophysiologic substrate. *J Am Coll Cardiol.* 2004;43:2044–2053.
46. Bauer A, Deisenhofer I, Schneider R, et al. Effects of circumferential or segmental pulmonary vein ablation for paroxysmal atrial fibrillation on cardiac autonomic function. *Heart Rhythm.* 2006;3:1428–1435.
47. Wyse DG, Waldo AL, DiMarco JP, et al. A comparison of rate control and rhythm control in patients with atrial fibrillation. *N Engl J Med.* 2002;347:1825–1833.
48. Ardell JL, Randall WC. Selective vagal innervation of sinoatrial and atrioventricular nodes in canine heart. *Am J Physiol.* 1986;251:H764–H773.
49. Zhuang S, Zhang Y, Mowrey KA, et al. Ventricular rate control by selective vagal stimulation is superior to rhythm regularization by atrioventricular nodal ablation and pacing during atrial fibrillation. *Circulation.* 2002;106:1853–1858.
50. Rossi P, Bianchi S, Barretta A, et al. Post-operative atrial fibrillation management by selective epicardial vagal fat pad stimulation. *J Interv Card Electrophysiol.* 2009;24:37–45.
51. Jahangir A, Lee V, Friedman PA, et al. Long-term progression and outcomes with aging in patients with lone atrial fibrillation: a 30-year follow-up study. *Circulation.* 2007;115:3050–3056.

52. Donadio V, Nolano M, Provitera V, et al. Skin sympathetic adrenergic innervation: an immunofluorescence confocal study. *Ann Neurol.* 2006;59:376–381.
53. Baron R, Janig W, With H. Sympathetic and afferent neurones projecting into forelimb and trunk nerves and the anatomical organization of the thoracic sympathetic outflow of the rat. *J Auton Nerv Syst.* 1995;53:205–214.
54. Robinson EA, Rhee KS, Doytchinova A, et al. Estimating sympathetic tone by recording subcutaneous nerve activity in ambulatory dogs. *J Cardiovasc Electrophysiol.* 2015;26:70–78.
55. Doytchinova A, Patel J, Zhou S, et al. Subcutaneous nerve activity and spontaneous ventricular arrhythmias in ambulatory dogs. *Heart Rhythm.* 2015;122:612–620.
56. Chan YH, Tsai WC, Shen C, et al. Subcutaneous nerve activity is more accurate than heart rate variability in estimating cardiac sympathetic tone in ambulatory dogs with myocardial infarction. *Heart Rhythm.* 2015;12:1619–1627.
57. Taniguchi T, Morimoto M, Taniguchi Y, Takasaki M, Totoki T. Cutaneous distribution of sympathetic postganglionic fibers from stellate ganglion: a retrograde axonal tracing study using wheat germ agglutinin conjugated with horseradish peroxidase. *J Anesth.* 1994;8:441–449.
58. Jiang Z, Zhao Y, Doytchinova A, et al. Using skin sympathetic nerve activity to estimate stellate ganglion nerve activity in dogs. *Heart Rhythm.* 2015;12:1324–1332.
59. Doytchinova A, Hassel JL, Yuan Y, et al. Simultaneous non-invasive recording of skin sympathetic nerve activity and electrocardiogram. *Heart Rhythm.* 2017;14:25–33.
60. Haissaguerre M, Jais P, Shah DC, et al. Spontaneous initiation of atrial fibrillation by ectopic beats originating in the pulmonary veins. *N Engl J Med.* 1998;339:659–666.
61. Verma A, Jiang CY, Betts TR, et al. Approaches to catheter ablation for persistent atrial fibrillation. *N Engl J Med.* 2015;372:1812–1822.
62. Jiang RH, Po SS, Tung R, et al. Incidence of pulmonary vein conduction recovery in patients without clinical recurrence after ablation of paroxysmal atrial fibrillation: mechanistic implications. *Heart Rhythm.* 2014;11:969–976.
63. Kurotobi T, Shimada Y, Kino N, et al. Features of intrinsic ganglionated plexi in both atria after extensive pulmonary isolation and their clinical significance after catheter ablation in patients with atrial fibrillation. *Heart Rhythm.* 2015;12:470–476.
64. Katritsis DG, Giazitzoglou E, Zografos T, Pokushalov E, Po SS, Camm AJ. Rapid pulmonary vein isolation combined with autonomic ganglia modification: a randomized study. *Heart Rhythm.* 2010;8:672–678.
65. Katritsis D, Giazitzoglou E, Sougiannis D, Goumas N, Paxinos G, Camm AJ. Anatomic approach for ganglionic plexi ablation in patients with paroxysmal atrial fibrillation. *Am J Cardiol.* 2008;102:330–334.
66. Scanavacca M, Pisani CF, Hachul D, et al. Selective atrial vagal denervation guided by evoked vagal reflex to treat patients with paroxysmal atrial fibrillation. *Circulation.* 2006;114:876–885.
67. Lemery R, Birnie D, Tang AS, Green M, Gollob M. Feasibility study of endocardial mapping of ganglionated plexuses during catheter ablation of atrial fibrillation. *Heart Rhythm.* 2006;3:387–396.
68. Cummings JE, Gill I, Akhrass R, Dery M, Biblo LA, Quan KJ. Preservation of the anterior fat pad paradoxically decreases the incidence of postoperative atrial fibrillation in humans. *J Am Coll Cardiol.* 2004;43:994–1000.
69. Scherlag BJ, Nakagawa H, Jackman WM, et al. Electrical stimulation to identify neural elements on the heart: their role in atrial fibrillation. *J Interv Card Electrophysiol.* 2005;13(suppl 1):37–42.
70. Katritsis DG, Pokushalov E, Romanov A, et al. Autonomic denervation added to pulmonary vein isolation for paroxysmal atrial fibrillation: a randomized clinical trial. *J Am Coll Cardiol.* 2013;62:2318–2325.
71. Krum H, Schlaich M, Whitbourn R, et al. Catheter-based renal sympathetic denervation for resistant hypertension: a multicentre safety and proof-of-principle cohort study. *Lancet.* 2009;373:1275–1281.
72. Symplicity HTNI Investigators, Esler MD, Krum H, Sobotka PA, et al. Renal sympathetic denervation in patients with treatment-resistant hypertension (The Symplicity HTN-2 Trial): a randomised controlled trial. *Lancet.* 2010;376:1903–1909.
73. Zhao Z, Xie Y, Wen H, et al. Role of the transient outward potassium current in the genesis of early afterdepolarizations in cardiac cells. *Cardiovasc Res.* 2012;95:308–316.
74. Tsai CT, Lai LP, Lin JL, et al. Renin-angiotensin system gene polymorphisms and atrial fibrillation. *Circulation.* 2004;109:1640–1646.
75. Linz D, Mahfoud F, Schotten U, et al. Renal sympathetic denervation suppresses postapneic blood pressure rises and atrial fibrillation in a model for sleep apnea. *Hypertension.* 2012;60:172–178.
76. Pokushalov E, Romanov A, Corbucci G, et al. A randomized comparison of pulmonary vein isolation with versus without concomitant renal artery denervation in patients with refractory symptomatic atrial fibrillation and resistant hypertension. *J Am Coll Cardiol.* 2012;60:1163–1170.

77. Pokushalov E, Romanov A, Katritsis DG, et al. Renal denervation for improving outcomes of catheter ablation in patients with atrial fibrillation and hypertension: early experience. *Heart Rhythm*. 2014;11:1131–1138.

78. Linz D, van Hunnik A, Hohl M, et al. Catheter-based renal denervation reduces atrial nerve sprouting and complexity of atrial fibrillation in goats. *Circ Arrhythm Electrophysiol*. 2015;8:466–474.

79. Tsai W-C, Chan YH, Chinda K, et al. Effects of renal sympathetic denervation on the stellate ganglion and the brain stem in dogs. *Heart Rhythm*. 2017;14:255–226.

80. Yu L, Scherlag BJ, Li S, et al. Low-level vagosympathetic nerve stimulation inhibits atrial fibrillation inducibility: direct evidence by neural recordings from intrinsic cardiac ganglia. *J Cardiovasc Electrophysiol*. 2010;22:455–463.

81. Sheng X, Scherlag BJ, Yu L, et al. Prevention and reversal of atrial fibrillation inducibility and autonomic remodeling by low-level vagosympathetic nerve stimulation. *J Am Coll Cardiol*. 2011;57:563–571.

82. Viskin S, Golovner M, Malov N, et al. Circadian variation of symptomatic paroxysmal atrial fibrillation. Data from almost 10,000 episodes. *Eur Heart J*. 1999;20:1429–1434.

83. Shen MJ, Hao-Che Chang X, Park HW, et al. Low-level vagus nerve stimulation upregulates small conductance calcium-activated potassium channels in the stellate ganglion. *Heart Rhythm*. 2013;10:910–915.

84. Adelman JP, Maylie J, Sah P. Small-conductance Ca^{2+}-activated K^+ channels: form and function. *Annu Rev Physiol*. 2012;74:245–269.

85. Chinda K, Tsai WC, Chan YH, et al. Intermittent left cervical vagal nerve stimulation damages the stellate ganglia and reduces ventricular rate during sustained atrial fibrillation in ambulatory dogs. *Heart Rhythm*. 2016;13:771–780.

86. Lomuscio A, Belletti S, Battezzati PM, Lombardi F. Efficacy of acupuncture in preventing atrial fibrillation recurrences after electrical cardioversion. *J Cardiovasc Electrophysiol*. 2011;22:241–247.

87. Lombardi F, Belletti S, Battezzati PM, Lomuscio A. Acupuncture for paroxysmal and persistent atrial fibrillation: an effective non-pharmacological tool? *World J Cardiol*. 2012;4:60–65.

88. Yu L, Scherlag BJ, Li S, et al. Low-level transcutaneous electrical stimulation of the auricular branch of the vagus nerve: a noninvasive approach to treat the initial phase of atrial fibrillation. *Heart Rhythm*. 2013;10:428–435.

89. Stavrakis S, Humphrey MB, Scherlag BJ, et al. Low-level transcutaneous electrical vagus nerve stimulation suppresses atrial fibrillation. *J Am Coll Cardiol*. 2015;65:867–875.

90. Bernstein SA, Wong B, Vasquez C, et al. Spinal cord stimulation protects against atrial fibrillation induced by tachypacing. *Heart Rhythm*. 2012;9:1426–1433.

91. Olgin JE, Takahashi T, Wilson E, Vereckei A, Steinberg H, Zipes DP. Effects of thoracic spinal cord stimulation on cardiac autonomic regulation of the sinus and atrioventricular nodes. *J Cardiovasc Electrophysiol*. 2002;13:475–481.

92. Wang S, Zhou X, Huang B, et al. Spinal cord stimulation suppresses atrial fibrillation by inhibiting autonomic remodeling. *Heart Rhythm*. 2016;13:274–281.

41 Sympathetic Innervation and Cardiac Arrhythmias

David Filgueiras-Rama

The autonomic nervous system plays an important role in the genesis of several cardiac arrhythmias, both in the atria and in the ventricles. Adrenergic and cholinergic stimulation exert electrophysiological effects that can predispose the heart to the initiation and maintenance of complex arrhythmias.[1-4] Shortening of the atrial effective refractory period or enhanced triggered activity upon vagal nerve or adrenergic stimulation have been associated with atrial fibrillation (AF).[4-6] An adrenergic milieu may also facilitate ventricular arrhythmias in heart failure, especially in the context of electrophysiological remodeling and an increase in intraventricular pressure.[3,7]

Modulation of the autonomic response is a complex process, in which the final effect is the product of interactions among central, peripheral, and intracardiac components.[8] Moreover, the underlying substrate is also modulated by changes in parasympathetic and sympathetic innervation in the diseased heart (neural remodeling) that can promote ventricular arrhythmias and sudden death.[9] Therefore this chapter begins with the anatomy of the cardiac sympathetic nervous system and pathological changes associated with neural remodeling in different clinical and experimental settings. This is followed with an overview of currently techniques for assessing autonomic function in cardiovascular disease. The chapter goes on to describe basic electrophysiological effects of the sympathetic nervous system that can facilitate atrial or ventricular arrhythmias. Finally, different clinical and experimental strategies to modulate and/or control the autonomic imbalance will be discussed.

Anatomy of Cardiac Sympathetic Innervation

The cardiac sympathetic nervous system includes central components in cortical areas and specific regions of the brainstem, as well as peripheral extrinsic and intrinsic cardiac nerves. Sympathetic nerve activity requires complex interplay among several cortical areas that further interact with specific regions of the brainstem (Fig. 41.1).[10] Moreover, sympathetic nerve control activity seems to be heterogeneous within cortical centers, because stimulation of the motor cortex results in an increase in sympathetic activity, which can also be observed during stimulation of the right insular cortex.[11] The brainstem strongly regulates central sympathetic activity within specific regions, such as the nucleus tractus solitarius, the nucleus ambiguus, and the dorsal motor nucleus.[10] These regions interact with the peripheral components at the level of the spinal cord to establish the net sympathetic effect on the heart. Thus signals processed within the thoracic spinal cord feed information back via the paravertebral ganglia to the cervical sympathetic chain, which sends sympathetic input directly to the heart (see Fig. 41.1).

The sympathetic chain consists of several ganglia (three cervical ganglia and three to four thoracic ganglia) arising from preganglionic sympathetic fibers coming from the spinal cord. The right and left cervicothoracic ganglia (C8–T1 ganglia) are called the right stellate and left stellate ganglia, respectively. Preganglionic neurons can synapse on neurons within the ganglia at the same thoracic level, or they can travel through the sympathetic chain and synapse on neurons of ganglia at other spinal levels. Acetylcholine is the preganglionic neurotransmitter within the ganglia.

The sympathetic chain ganglia give rise to postganglionic axons that target the heart and other organs (see Fig. 41.1). The sympathetic cardiac effect can also be modulated by prevertebral ganglia, which are related to the pelvic viscera. These ganglia provide both efferent and afferent information, which in turn can influence the cervical and thoracic sympathetic chain signaling and therefore directly affect cardiac and vascular responsiveness.[12] In fact, diminishing or increasing neural responsiveness to pelvic organs could attenuate or increase sympathetic tone, which may become more relevant in certain diseases, such as hypertension.[13]

Postganglionic nerve fibers from the sympathetic chain ganglia form the left and right cardiac nerves, defined by the cardiac plexus at the base of the heart.[14,15] The cardiac plexus is divided into a superficial and a deep portion, with the superficial plexus lying beneath the aortic arch, just in front of the right pulmonary artery, and the deep plexus lying in front of the tracheal bifurcation behind the aortic arch. The superficial portion usually has a ganglion (ganglion of Wrisberg) located just below the aortic arch and to the right of the ligamentum arteriosum, which reflects a junction point prior to the division of the major branches to the back and anterior part of the heart, following the trajectory of the coronary arteries (see Fig. 41.1). The deep cardiac plexus further divides into a right and a left half, which send branches to the anterior and posterior part of the heart, running in line with the coronary arteries and connecting back to the superficial cardiac plexus. The deep plexus also provides fibers to the right and left atria and to the pulmonary plexus, which supplies the region of the pulmonary artery and the right ventricular outflow tract. Within this general architecture, the divisions of the cardiac nerve plexus are complex and can differ between patients.[16] Acetylcholinesterase staining of neural tissue in the whole heart of large mammals allows the visualization and location of the surrounding nerves and ganglia.[17] More specifically, sympathetic cardiac nerves can be identified by immunolabeling for tyrosine hydroxylase. Interestingly, staining for tyrosine hydroxylase and myelin basic protein has confirmed the presence of myelinated sympathetic nerves on all surfaces of the epicardium and endocardium.[18]

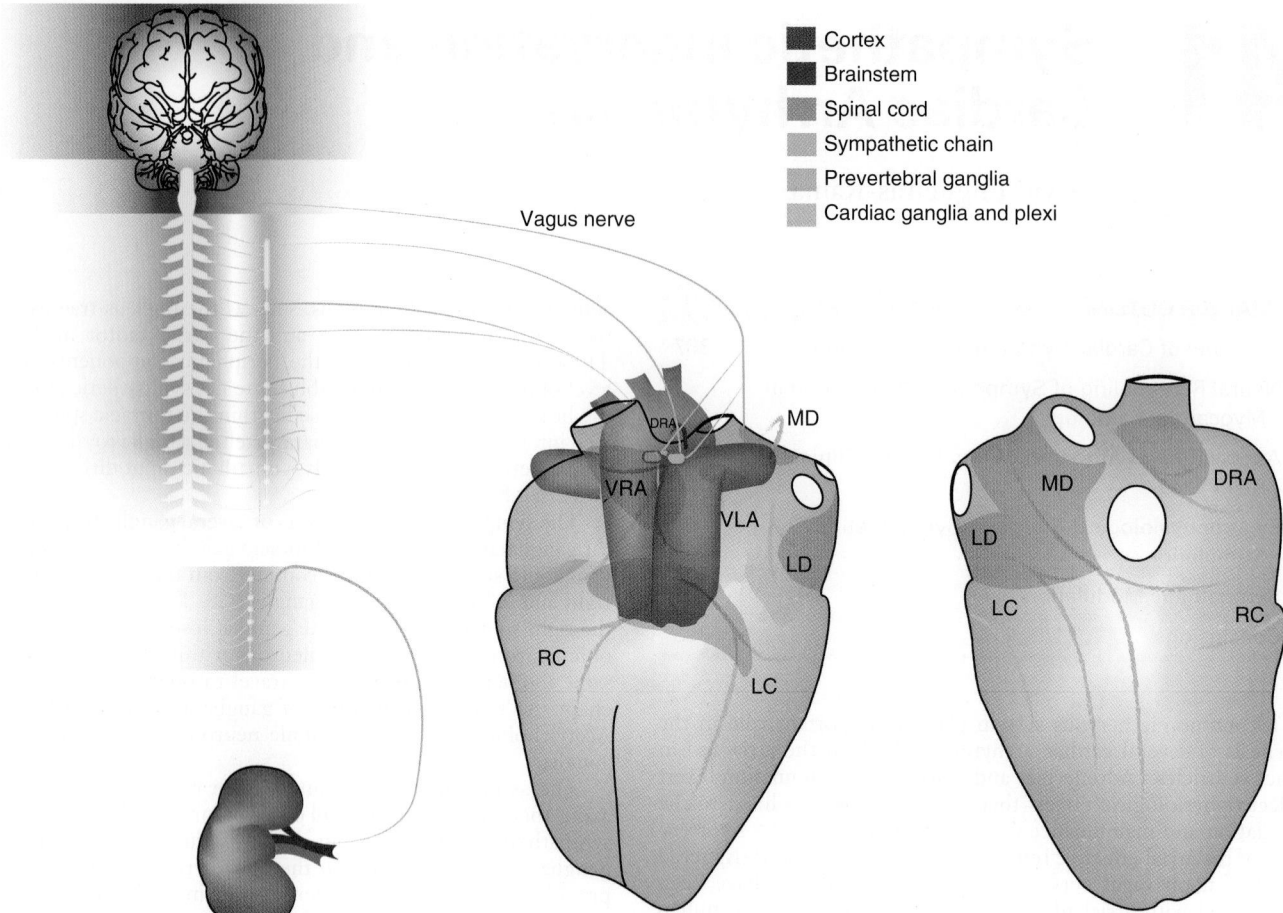

■ Cortex
■ Brainstem
■ Spinal cord
■ Sympathetic chain
■ Prevertebral ganglia
■ Cardiac ganglia and plexi

FIGURE 41.1 Anatomy of cardiac sympathetic innervation. *DRA,* Dorsal right atrial ganglionated subplexus; *LC,* left coronary ganglionated subplexus; *LD,* left dorsal ganglionated subplexus; *MD,* middle dorsal ganglionated subplexus; *RC,* right coronary ganglionated subplexus; *VLA,* ventral left atrial ganglionated subplexus; *VRA,* ventral right atrial ganglionated subplexus.

Extensive neural processing also occurs at the level of the heart through the intrinsic cardiac nervous system. Generally, both parasympathetic and sympathetic preganglionic nerve endings need to first synapse in a cardiac ganglion. These ganglia act as nerve centers that respond to parasympathetic and sympathetic signals to control net neural output and provide feedback to one another; they also generate local stimuli independent of the extrinsic cardiac nervous system.[19] Cardiac ganglia are mainly distributed around the epicardial side of the atria especially on the dorsal and dorsolateral surfaces of the left atrium. The ganglia can also be found around the junction between the atria and ventricles at the level of the mitral and tricuspid annulus and at peri-great vessel areas (right and left ventricular outflow tracts, aorta, and pulmonary roots).[20] The total number of ganglia ranges from 700 to 1500, with a population of neurons over 14,000 that can decrease by as much as 50% with age or myocardial ischemia.[21] The functional distribution of the atrial ganglia can be gauged from their preferential influence on the sinoatrial versus the atrioventricular node. However, there is extensive crosslinking among ganglia, enabling multiple levels of unidirectional and bidirectional feedback.[22] Much less is known about ventricular ganglia and their role in cardiac electrical and functional properties; however, they might play a role in nerve sprouting and ventricular arrhythmogenesis after myocardial infarction.[23]

Additional direct cardiac innervation is provided by cardiac sensory afferent fibers that mainly run along the sympathetic cardiac nerves. Sensory afferent fibers participate in cardiac pain by activating autonomic pathways and reflex feedback.[24]

Neural Remodeling of Sympathetic Innervation in Myocardial Pathology

Several cardiac diseases and pathological conditions cause autonomic nervous system remodeling, with a range of changes, including denervation, an increase in synaptic density or sympathetic activation, and nerve sprouting in specific pathological regions.

Heart Failure

Sympathetic efferent neural activity is increased in chronic heart failure, which is associated with parasympathetic withdrawal.[25,26] This imbalance contributes to myocardial hypertrophy and accelerates heart failure progression.[27] Thus chronic sympathetic stimulation induces myocyte enlargement, interstitial growth, and remodeling, which increase myocardial mass and may lead to enlargement of the left ventricular chamber.[28] Alterations in cardiac loading result in both increased release and decreased uptake of norepinephrine at adrenergic nerve endings. Decreased norepinephrine uptake results in chronically elevated stimulation of the cardiac β-adrenergic receptor system, which exerts effects on several key organs (e.g., the heart, kidney, and peripheral vasculature).

Chronic human heart failure significantly disorganizes cardiomyocyte β-adrenergic receptor signaling and function and diminishes the adrenergic reserve. Overstimulation of cardiac β-adrenergic receptors by an excess of sympathetic nervous

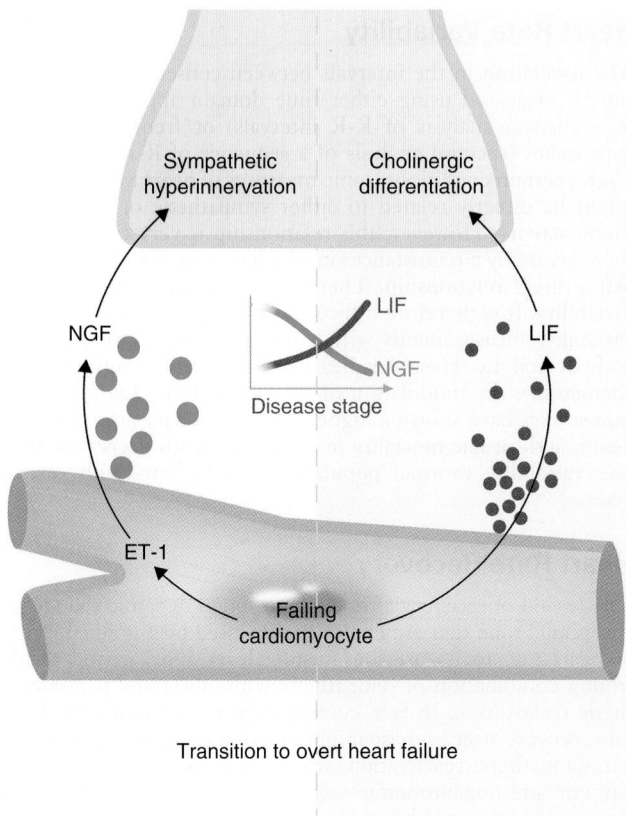

FIGURE 41.2 Neural remodeling of sympathetic innervation in heart failure. *ET-1,* Endothelin-1; *LIF,* leukemia inhibitory factor; *NGF,* nerve growth factor.

system-derived catecholamine can trigger upregulation of the G-protein-coupled receptor kinase GRK2 which leads to a reduction in cardiac β-adrenergic receptor density and responsiveness and results in cardiac inotropic reserve depletion.[29] It has been also suggested that sympathetic nerve endings are probably damaged by norepinephrine-derived free radicals.[30] In fact, Kimura et al. have shown that long-term exposure of severely decompensated heart failure rats to high norepinephrine concentration in the plasma causes a reduction in myocardial nerve growth factor (NGF) and associated sympathetic fiber loss (anatomic denervation).[31] During the transition to overt heart failure, sympathetic neural tone is upregulated and NGF expression is elevated, contributing to hyperinnervation of cardiac sympathetic nerves. Failing cardiomyocytes induce NGF via an endothelin-1 (ET-1)-mediated pathway and upregulate the leukemia inhibitory factor (LIF). NGF leads to hyperinnervation, whereas LIF induces cholinergic differentiation (Fig. 41.2). Thus the expression of catecholaminergic markers (tyrosine hydroxylase and dopamine β-hydroxylase) decreases, while cholinergic and juvenile markers (choline transporter, choline acetyltransferase, and polysialyated neural cell adhesion molecule) increase.[32] Therefore there is a paradoxical reduction in norepinephrine synthesis concomitant with downregulation of catecholaminergic markers, norepinephrine reuptake into the sympathetic nerve terminals, and depression of norepinephrine levels in the myocardium. Many neurons in the stellate ganglia and left ventricle also express parasympathetic markers, which have been related to cholinergic trans-differentiation of cardiac adrenergic neurons into cholinergic neurons by LIF.[33]

Several mechanisms have been proposed to explain sympathetic activation in heart failure: (1) abnormalities in baroreceptors, which transmit signals to the central nervous system and then transduce processed signals to the heart[34]; (2) the

chemoreceptor reflex under hypoxic and hypercapnic conditions sensed in the carotid body[35]; (3) responses mediated by the brainstem and suprabulbar regions, as in the presence of reduced nitric oxide, increased oxidative stress, and activation of angiotensin II type 1 receptor[36]; and (4) activation of efferent and afferent renal nerves, which involves signals from afferent renal sensory nerves later processed in the hypothalamus, in the nucleus of the solitary tract, and in other cortical areas.[37,38]

Myocardial Infarction

Cardiac autonomic activity can be activated within seconds after the onset of acute ischemia. This activity can affect survival, depending on whether the profibrillatory action of sympathetic activity or the protective action of vagal activation is predominant.[39] From a broader perspective, it is possible to identify three specific phases in the evolution of post–myocardial infarction neural remodeling into ventricular dysfunction and heart failure. (1) sympathetic reflex activation and acute sympathetic denervation, (2) sympathetic reinnervation and nerve sprouting, and (3) later innervation loss in advanced heart failure.

After transmural myocardial infarction sympathetic fibers within the scar area die and the surviving myocardium distal to the necrotic region undergoes sympathetic denervation.[40] Post-myocardial infarction reinnervation reflects neural, structural, and electrophysiological remodeling after the ischemic damage, and is mainly directed by NGF expressed in the ischemic heart. The increase in NGF protein in the infarct site is very fast and precedes the increase in NGF mRNA, which suggests a rapid release from storage areas.[41] It also seems that NGF specifically increases in the border zone area of the myocardial lesion, and nerve sprouting markers can also be documented when NGF is injected into the left stellate ganglion.[41] In fact, stellate ganglion activity increases within a few seconds after myocardial infarction and is associated with intramyocardial nerve sprouts and synaptic density in both the left and right stellate ganglia. From the stellate ganglia, the nerve-sprouting signal induces a generalized enhancement in cardiac nerve density throughout the heart, especially at the noninfarcted left ventricular free wall site. This nerve sprouting and sympathetic hyperinnervation within the heart can be observed beyond the first week after the infarction and might be in part sustained by an increase in systemic NGF concentration.[42] Therefore NGF levels seem to increase abruptly in the first hours after myocardial infarction, whereas experimental evidence has shown a progressive decrease in NGF expression over time after coronary occlusion, following a prolonged exposure to elevated concentrations of catecholamine due to advanced heart failure.[43] In experimental dog hearts, norepinephrine infusion for 8 weeks can reduce NGF expression, possibly via α-adrenergic receptor stimulation, which may have an inhibitory effect on NGF release.[44] Pathological evidence from explanted human hearts indicates that, in end-stage heart failure, areas deprived of neural endings are contiguous with hyperinnervated areas,[45] which also show high electrophysiological heterogeneity.

Atrial Fibrillation

Abnormal autonomic innervation has been documented both in AF animal models and in humans. In dogs with pacing-induced AF there is a heterogeneous increase in atrial sympathetic innervation.[46] Similarly, an increase in sympathetic nerve densities is sometimes observed in patients with persistent AF.[47] AF incidence and duration is also increased in response to other pathological conditions, such as myocardial infarction, associated with atrial nerve sprouting and sympathetic hyperinnervation.[48] In fact, adrenergic stimulation promotes structural remodeling via other actions mediated by calmodulin-dependent kinase type II (CaMKII) and oxidative stress, among other signaling pathways. This structural remodeling facilitates reentrant activity and AF perpetuation, especially in the presence of persistent AF, which is also associated with electrical and functional changes.[49]

Adrenergic activation can promote focal activity via enhanced automaticity, early afterdepolarizations, or delayed afterdepolarization-associated triggered activity. Automaticity is enhanced when the inward rectifier potassium current (I_{K1}) decreases,[50] which may result from α-adrenergic stimulation or increased funny current, produced by β-adrenergic activation.[51] β-Adrenergic activation can also increase the likelihood of early afterdepolarizations. Despite the association of focal activity with AF maintenance, it seems more likely to be related to reentry initiation than to maintenance of the arrhythmia.[52,53]

Other Pathological Conditions

Remodeling of the cardiac sympathetic nervous system has been also observed in other conditions, such as hypertension and cardiac hypertrophy. Elevated cardiac and renal sympathetic tones are core features of human hypertension and are associated with disease progression and mortality. Hypertensive left ventricular hypertrophy is associated with increased sympathetic activity largely confined to the heart, suggesting that disease development is related to increased cardiac norepinephrine release.[54] Approximately 50% of patients with hypertension have increased sympathetic activity in the kidneys and skeletal muscle vessels.[55] In hypertension, single-fiber sympathetic recording demonstrates increased fiber firing frequencies and multiple firings within a cardiac cycle, which are not seen in health.[56] Cardiac hypertrophy is also associated with upregulation of NGF, which leads to sympathetic hyperinnervation.[32] Increased renal sympathetic nerve activity directly affects renal physiology through vasoconstriction and an increased renin secretion rate.[57] In addition, under such conditions, afferent signals from the kidneys are transmitted to the central nervous system, which enhances the sympathetic outflow to the heart, kidneys, and other organs.[58] A higher sympathetic nervous activation was also documented in obesity-related hypertension and end-stage renal disease hypertension.[59,60]

Assessment of Autonomic Function and Clinical Relevance

Autonomic modulation plays an important role in arrhythmogenesis. However, the autonomic nervous system is highly complex, and it is not easy to establish a simple relationship between a physiological marker and autonomic activity. Among the different markers that can reflect autonomic activity, heart rate and electrocardiogram (ECG) parameters are noninvasive and easy to measure.

Heart Rate

Sympathetic and parasympathetic effects on the intrinsic heart rate predominantly determine the actual heart rate, although nonautonomic contributions (e.g., hypoxia and temperature) also affect the intrinsic heart rate. Heart rate provides a static index of the net effects of autonomic input to the sinus node, although it does not reflect direct information about individual sympathetic or parasympathetic input. However, this simple measure has prognostic value, as reflected in population-based studies, in which high resting heart rate (net predominance of sympathetic effect) was associated with increased all-cause mortality, death from cardiovascular disease, and sudden death.[61,62]

Heart Rate Variability

The oscillation in the intervals between consecutive heartbeats can be measured using either time domain approaches (based on statistical analysis of R-R intervals) or frequency domain approaches (spectral analysis of a sequence of R-R intervals).[63] Under certain conditions, some measures of heart rate variability might be directly related to either sympathetic or parasympathetic activity. However, this relationship is very complex, and there are many circumstances in which it is not possible to establish a direct relationship. There is also marked interindividual variability. It is therefore difficult to correlate specific heart rate variability measurements with either sympathetic or parasympathetic activity. However, heart rate variability can be used to characterize the modulation of autonomic tone. Large population studies have shown a higher risk of coronary artery disease, death, and cardiac mortality in individuals with decreased heart rate variability (normal population and patients with cardiac disease).[64]

Heart Rate Recovery

The period of recovery after exercise shows dynamic changes in autonomic tone that are clinically expressed by a gradual return of heart rate to its previous resting level. This period results from a combination of sympathetic withdrawal and parasympathetic reactivation. In fact, current data suggest that early heart rate recovery after exercise might be predominantly explained by parasympathetic reactivation, with less contribution from sympathetic and nonautonomic components.[65,66] Clinical data have shown that impaired heart rate recovery (slow rate recovery to the resting level) has prognostic implications under a broad range of exercise conditions.[67] However, the underlying autonomic influence associated with an increased risk of death in patients with abnormal heart rate recovery is not completely understood.

Baroreflex Sensitivity

Baroreceptor reflexes can be modulated by cardiac afferent sympathetic activity activated by mechanical and chemical stimuli.[68] Baroreflex sensitivity represents an index of autonomic input to the sinus node and is measured by the reflex changes in R-R interval in response to induced changes in blood pressure. It is usually measured by characterizing the magnitude of induced bradycardia in response to a pressor challenge (e.g., phenylephrine). A reduction in baroreflex control of heart rate has been consistently reported in hypertension, diabetes, coronary artery disease, myocardial infarction, and heart failure.[69] Rather than a risk factor, baroreflex sensitivity assessed by the phenylephrine test has been shown to be a modifiable risk factor[70]; thus an improved prognosis was observed for those patients in whom exercise training was able to induce a notable increase in baroreflex sensitivity.

Heart Rate Turbulence

Heart rate turbulence denotes the baroreflex-mediated short-term oscillation of sinus rhythm cycle length after spontaneous ventricular premature complexes.[71] Heart rate turbulence is represented by two numeric descriptors: turbulence onset, reflecting the initial acceleration of heart rate after a premature ventricular complex, and turbulence slope, describing subsequent deceleration of heart rate following a premature ventricular beat. Heart rate turbulence could be considered to be an indirect measure and surrogate of baroreflex sensitivity. High-risk patients with myocardial infarction are characterized by depressed heart rate turbulence, expressed as the lack of an immediate acceleration, or even a deceleration, of a sinus rhythm, and then a blunted rate of subsequent deceleration with lower turbulence slope values (flattened slope).[71] Abnormal turbulence slope has been also associated with a higher risk of sudden death during follow-up in apparently healthy individuals older than 65 years.[72]

T-Wave Alternans

Microvolt-level beat-to-beat variation of the amplitude of the T-wave is an independent marker of risk for sudden cardiac death.[73] At the cellular level, T-wave alternans directly probe dysregulation of repolarization.[74] There is evidence supporting the role of calcium transient alternans in the development of repolarization alternans,[75] although action potential duration restitution may also be involved. The sympathetic tone may affect both mechanisms by increasing calcium transients, enhancing triggered activity, and affecting action potential duration and restitution.[76,77] β-Adrenergic stimulation enhances virtually all processes controlling calcium entry, storage, and release in the heart. Under conditions predisposing to calcium-dependent triggered activity (e.g., heart failure),[77] the enhanced calcium-loading/release conditions produced by adrenergic stimulation strongly promote arrhythmogenesis.

Continuous Recording of Sympathetic Activity

Noninvasive methods based on ECG parameters or baroreflex sensitivity do not provide the absolute intensity of sympathetic or parasympathetic discharges and may be affected by baseline conditions, such as heart failure–related sinus node dysfunction.[78] Chronic and continuous cardiac nerve recordings have been obtained using implanted radio transmitters in animal models.[79] The data have shown that left atrial pacing–induced AF or atrial tachycardia episodes are invariably preceded by intracardiac nerve activity. Moreover, there was a significant temporal relationship between extracardiac and intracardiac nerve activities, although intracardiac nerve activity could also activate alone. Continuous recordings of both sympathetic and vagal nerve activity have shown that different baseline patterns of activation may be prone to fast atrial pacing-induced AF.[80] Continuous recordings of the left stellate ganglion activity after myocardial infarction in dogs have also demonstrated that increased left stellate ganglion and subcutaneous nerve activity preceded the episodes of premature ventricular contractions and ventricular tachycardia.[81]

Electrophysiological Effects of Sympathetic Stimulation

Sympathetic nerve stimulation has been associated with proarrhythmic effects in several studies.[82,83] β-Adrenergic stimulation activates a guanosine-5′-triphosphate (GTP)-binding protein (Gs), which stimulates adenylcyclase to produce cyclic adenosine monophosphate (cAMP), which in turn activates protein kinase A (PKA). This kinase phosphorylates several proteins related to excitation–contraction coupling (e.g., L-type Ca^{2+} [ICaL], ryanodine receptors, phospholamban, and troponin I), which greatly enhance calcium transient amplitude. These effects are amplified by Ca^{2+}/calmodulin-dependent protein kinase type II (CaMKII). Adrenergically induced phospholamban phosphorylation dissociates phospholamban from the sarcoplasmic reticulum Ca^{2+}-ATPase, which pumps Ca^{2+} into the sarcoplasmic reticulum (Fig. 41.3). This mechanism is responsible for maintaining sarcoplasmic reticulum Ca^{2+} stores and restoring low diastolic Ca^{2+} levels after the systolic Ca^{2+} transient.

Sympathetic activity also has significant effects on cardiac ion channels, besides the increase in voltage-dependent Ca^{2+} entry through the plasma membrane upon I_{CaL} phosphorylation. Thus the slow rectifier K^+ current (I_{Ks}) is strongly enhanced by β-adrenergically induced PKA phosphorylation,[84] which may

counterbalance the increased inward current resulting from adrenergic enhancement of I_{CaL}. β-Adrenergic activation also increases the funny current to enhance automaticity.[51] This automaticity is further enhanced via α-adrenergic stimulation and inhibition of the inward rectifier K^+ current (I_{K1}) (see Fig. 41.3).[85]

Under pathological conditions with enhanced Ca^{2+}-loading/release, as in heart failure, hyperphosphorylation of ryanodine receptors can cause diastolic leak of sarcoplasmic reticulum Ca^{2+},[86] which especially favors arrhythmogenesis within a coexisting pathological substrate. Experimental data from animal models have shown an increase in action potential duration dispersion upon sympathetic stimulation, both during ischemia and in normal canine and porcine hearts. Left stellate ganglion stimulation significantly increased activation recovery interval dispersion (as a surrogate of action potential duration dispersion) in pigs with normal hearts, which indeed was associated with ventricular fibrillation in two of eight pig hearts.[87] Electrical stimulation of the left ansa subclavia (nerve cord connecting the inferior cervical ganglion and middle cervical ganglia) significantly increased ventricular fibrillation incidence in open-chest dogs during acute coronary occlusion.[88] Moreover, dispersion in refractoriness has also been documented during ventricular fibrillation in dogs undergoing regional ischemia and sympathetic stimulation. Thus left stellate ganglion stimulation during ischemia produced no response, or it even further prolonged the ventricular fibrillation intervals at ischemic sites compared with regional ischemia without sympathetic stimulation. Moreover, ventricular fibrillation intervals shortened at nonischemic sites, whereas dispersion in refractoriness across the ischemic border increased by 14%–59%.[89]

Atrial sympathetic innervation can also be affected several weeks after myocardial infarction, which may prime the atria to fibrillate. Data from dogs with chronic myocardial infarction have shown both an increase in atrial sympathetic innervation and more heterogeneous innervation. The latter was associated with increased heterogeneity of monophasic action potential duration and its restitution slope. Both circumstances were significantly associated with higher incidence and longer AF duration compared with controls.[48]

Sympathetic Modulation

From the foregoing it is possible to assert that either medical or surgical strategies aimed at reducing the sympathetic tone might diminish the risk of cardiac arrhythmia in certain pathological conditions. The cardiac sympathetic nervous system can be modulated at multiple levels (e.g., the brainstem and cortical areas, the spinal cord and sympathetic chain, and the cardiac plexus); these can affect neural-mediated triggers for arrhythmia and also modify the myocardial substrate, which can make myocytes stress-resistant. Different techniques have been developed to achieve sympathetic modulation (Fig. 41.4), beyond the routine use of β-adrenergic blocking agents.

Vagus Nerve Stimulation

This technique may require a surgical intervention and implantation of a neurostimulator, which consists of a bipolar helical lead positioned around the vagus nerve in the cervical region, with the terminal end connected to the pulse generator.[90] Chronic stimulation decreases ventricular tachycardia and ventricular fibrillation in animal models at different ischemic stages.[91,92] Suppression of ventricular arrhythmia has also shown potential benefits in animal models with heart failure. However, current available data in humans with heart failure do not establish any benefit of vagus nerve stimulation in improving left ventricular remodeling and systolic function when combined with current medical therapy.[90] Moreover, during short-term follow-up, there

3 Na+
Na/K ATPase
2 K+
K+
Na+,K+
Automatic cells
AR β1
Gαs
AC
β
γ
ATP
cAMP
P
IKs
PLM
If
PKA
K+
K+
IK1
CaMKII
P
P
Ca2+
RyR2
Sarcoplasmic reticulum
P
PLB
PKC
ICaL
IP3R
SERCA
CaM
IP3 + DAG
Ca2+
PLCβ
PIP2
Regular contraction
Adrenergic stimulation
Gαq
γ
β
Contraction
AR α

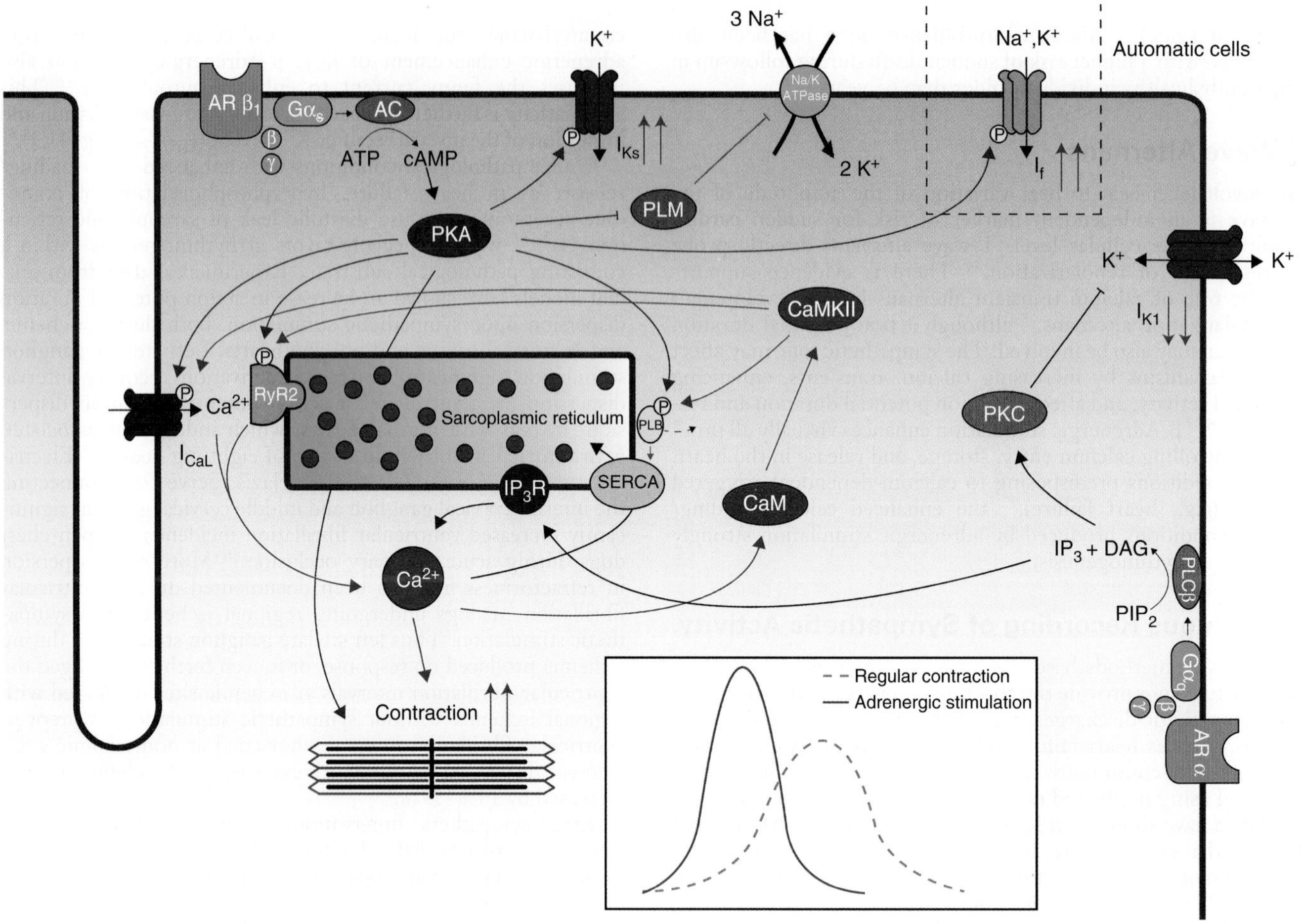

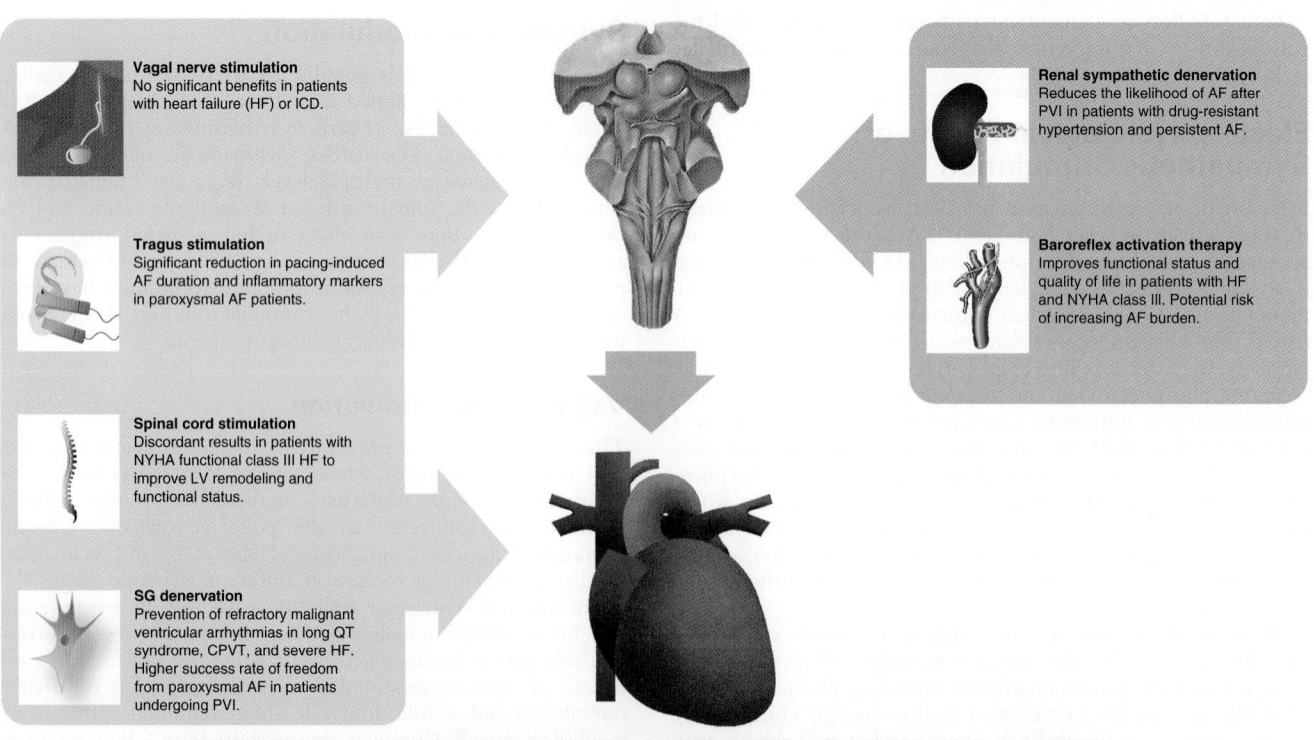

FIGURE 41.3 Effects of adrenergic stimulation in the cardiomyocyte. *AC,* Adenylcyclase; *AR β1, α1,* adrenergic receptor β1, α1; *CaM,* calmodulin; *CaMKII,* Ca^{2+}/CaM-dependent protein kinase type II; *DAG,* diacylglycerol; *IP_3,* inositol triphosphate; *IP_3R,* inositol triphosphate receptor; *PKA,* protein-kinase A; *PLB,* phospholamban; *PLC,* phospholipase C; *PLM,* phospholemman; *RYR2,* ryanodine receptor2; *SERCA,* sarcoplasmic/endoplasmic reticulum Ca^{2+}-ATPase.

Vagal nerve stimulation
No significant benefits in patients with heart failure (HF) or ICD.
Tragus stimulation
Significant reduction in pacing-induced AF duration and inflammatory markers in paroxysmal AF patients.
Spinal cord stimulation
Discordant results in patients with NYHA functional class III HF to improve LV remodeling and functional status.
SG denervation
Prevention of refractory malignant ventricular arrhythmias in long QT syndrome, CPVT, and severe HF. Higher success rate of freedom from paroxysmal AF in patients undergoing PVI.
Renal sympathetic denervation
Reduces the likelihood of AF after PVI in patients with drug-resistant hypertension and persistent AF.
Baroreflex activation therapy
Improves functional status and quality of life in patients with HF and NYHA class III. Potential risk of increasing AF burden.

FIGURE 41.4 Current techniques to achieve sympathetic modulation. *AF,* Atrial fibrillation; *CPVT,* catecholaminergic polymorphic ventricular tachycardia; *ICD,* implantable cardioverter defibrillator; *LV,* left ventricle; *PVI,* pulmonary vein isolation; *SG,* stellate ganglia.

seem to be no significant differences in the occurrence of implantable cardioverter defibrillator shock delivery and/or antitachycardia pacing between groups with and without the neurostimulator.

Unlike classic suprathreshold vagus nerve stimulation, low-level vagus nerve stimulation, rather than being proarrhythmic, has been shown to exert both anticholinergic and antiadrenergic effects,[93,94] which may prevent and even reverse electrophysiological remodeling induced by fast atrial pacing in animal models. Moreover, the incidence of AF and atrial tachyarrhythmias is significantly reduced during stimulation.[94] A noninvasive strategy to stimulate the vagus nerve has been tested in paroxysmal AF patients eligible for an ablation procedure.[95] Low-level vagus nerve stimulation was achieved by transcutaneous stimulation of the tragus (the anterior protuberance of the ear), where the auricular branch of the vagus nerve is accessible. Stimulation is accomplished by attaching a metal clip onto the tragus, which serves as the cathode, with another clip at an adjacent site for the anode. This proof-of-concept randomized clinical study showed that low-level tragus stimulation for 1 hour significantly reduced pacing-induced AF duration and decreased inflammatory markers.[95]

Baroreflex Activation Therapy and Spinal Cord Stimulation

These two therapies appear to share the dual effect of reducing sympathetic tone and enhancing vagal tone, which can lead to antiarrhythmic effects.

Stimulation of the carotid baroreceptor is a centrally mediated invasive approach to increase parasympathetic activity and decrease sympathetic outflow. An implantable device consisting of a carotid sinus lead and a pulse generator delivers electrical stimulation titrated to avoid side effects such as excessive reduction in heart rate or blood pressure. The therapy has been shown to significantly improve functional status, quality of life, and N-terminal pro–brain natriuretic peptide levels (NT-proBNP) in patients with heart failure in New York Heart Association (NYHA) functional class III.[96]

Despite findings that reduced sympathetic activity might improve heart failure and decrease ventricular arrhythmia, parallel increases in vagal tone may promote AF. Thus electrical baroreflex stimulation has been shown to shorten the atrial effective refractory period and increase AF inducibility in pigs.[97] Therefore the antiarrhythmic effects of the therapy are still unclear and need further investigation.

Spinal cord stimulation in the thoracic region has been associated with a decrease in the incidence of ischemic-related ventricular tachycardia and ventricular fibrillation episodes in a canine model of postinfarction and superimposed rapid pacing-related heart failure.[98] Current clinical data from a small randomized clinical study (DEFEAT-HF) did not show significant differences in left ventricular end-systolic volume index after 6 months of follow up in patients with heart failure in NYHA functional class III.[99] These results are discordant with previous data from a pilot study (SCS HEART), in which the authors observed significant improvement in NYHA functional class, peak maximum oxygen consumption, and left ventricular ejection fraction, among other parameters.[100] Despite fundamental differences between these two studies, the results raise concerns about appropriate patient selection, anatomic site of stimulation, and device duty cycles.

Sympathetic Denervation

Surgical cardiac sympathetic denervation has been used successfully in the past in patients with long QT syndrome, severe heart failure, and catecholaminergic ventricular tachycardia.[101–103] Left and bilateral cervicothoracic sympathectomy involves removal of the lower one-third to one-half of the left or bilateral stellate ganglia and the T2–T4 thoracic ganglia. Despite minimally invasive

approaches by video-assisted thoracoscopic sympathectomy, this procedure is not exempt from side effects, such as Horner syndrome, which makes it currently reserved for patients whose arrhythmias are refractory to medical therapy and/or who are receiving frequent implantable cardioverter defibrillator shocks.[104]

Partial sympathetic denervation can also be achieved by ganglionated plexi ablation of the intrinsic cardiac autonomic nervous system. This can potentially affect both initiation and maintenance of AF. In fact, a combination of anatomic ganglionated plexi ablation with pulmonary vein isolation yields a higher rate of freedom from AF in paroxysmal AF patients than either procedure alone.[105] Although these results may seem promising, there are concerns about the long-term consequences of glanglionated plexi damage in ventricular innervation and the risk of arrhythmia. Thus experimental data in sheep undergoing epicardial radiofrequency ablation of the left and middle pulmonary vein roots showed overt degeneration of remote atrial and ventricular epicardial nerves 2–3 months after the procedure. These nerves are likely to generate long-term autonomic dysfunction.[106] Moreover, ganglionated plexi ablation in dogs prolongs ventricular effective refractory periods and action potential duration, without significant effects on effective refractory period dispersion or the risk of ventricular arrhythmia in normal hearts. However, after ganglionated plexi ablation, the incidence of ventricular arrhythmia was significantly increased and ventricular fibrillation was significantly facilitated in dogs undergoing acute myocardial ischemia, compared with a group of dogs without ablation.[107] Interestingly, the occurrence of ventricular arrhythmia was attenuated with additional stellate ganglion ablation. These data suggest that ganglionated plexi ablation may dramatically reduce the parasympathetic control of the heart, indirectly increasing sympathetic activity, which may be particularly arrhythmogenic in pathological substrates, such as myocardial ischemia.

Renal artery sympathetic denervation can also affect whole-body sympathetic activation. Beneficial effects have been reported in patients with severe drug-resistant hypertension and persistent AF who are undergoing pulmonary vein isolation. A recent meta-analysis from two prospective double-blind, randomized studies showed that renal denervation reduces the likelihood of AF after pulmonary vein isolation in such patients.[108] This procedure has also been shown to have potential benefits in reducing the occurrence of ventricular tachycardia and ventricular fibrillation in a pig model of acute myocardial ischemia.[109]

Conclusions

The sympathetic nervous system exerts significant electrophysiological effects that favor both arrhythmogenesis within a coexisting pathological substrate and additional remodeling of the autonomic nervous system, as in heart failure or myocardial infarction. Therapies aimed at modulating the effects of the sympathetic system at different levels have shown promising potential for reducing the burden of atrial and ventricular arrhythmias. The combination of noninvasive ECG markers and newly developed imaging techniques may help to better assess autonomic activity and improve the selection of patients who will benefit the most from sympathetic modulation. Current recommendations reserve sympathetic modulation for patients with arrhythmias refractory to medical therapy and/or ablation.

Acknowledgments

The CNIC is supported by the Spanish Ministry of Economy and Competitiveness (MINECO) and the Pro-CNIC Foundation, and is a Severo Ochoa Center of Excellence (MINECO award SEV-2015-0505. Supported in part by Jesús Serra Foundation. I thank José Manuel Alfonso and Daniel Enríquez-Vázquez for their contribution in the illustration of the figures.

REFERENCES

1. Armour JA, Hageman GR, Randall WC. Arrhythmias induced by local cardiac nerve stimulation. *Am J Physiol.* 1972;223:1068–1075.

2. Hirose M, Leatmanoratn Z, Laurita KR, et al. Partial vagal denervation increases vulnerability to vagally induced atrial fibrillation. *J Cardiovasc Electrophysiol.* 2002;13:1272–1279.

3. Brunner-La Rocca HP, Esler MD, Jennings GL, et al. Effect of cardiac sympathetic nervous activity on mode of death in congestive heart failure. *Eur Heart J.* 2001;22:1136–1143.

4. Patterson E, Po SS, Scherlag BJ, et al. Triggered firing in pulmonary veins initiated by in vitro autonomic nerve stimulation. *Heart Rhythm.* 2005;2:624–631.

5. Tai CT, Chiou CW, Chen SA. Interaction between the autonomic nervous system and atrial tachyarrhythmias. *J Cardiovasc Electrophysiol.* 2002;13:83–87.

6. Coumel P, Attuel P, Lavallee J, et al. The atrial arrhythmia syndrome of vagal origin. *Arch Mal Coeur Vaiss.* 1978;71:645–656.

7. Quintanilla JG, Moreno J, Archondo T, et al. Increased intraventricular pressures are as harmful as the electrophysiological substrate of heart failure in favoring sustained reentry in the swine heart. *Heart Rhythm.* 2015;12:2172–2183.

8. Kapa S, DeSimone CV, Asirvatham SJ. Innervation of the heart: an invisible grid within a black box. *Trends Cardiovasc Med.* 2016;26:245–257.

9. Vaseghi M, Shivkumar K. The role of the autonomic nervous system in sudden cardiac death. *Prog Cardiovasc Dis.* 2008;50:404–419.

10. Sequeira H, Viltart O, Ba-M'Hamed S, et al. Cortical control of somato-cardiovascular integration: neuroanatomical studies. *Brain Res Bull.* 2000;53:87–93.

11. Oppenheimer SM, Kedem G, Martin WM. Left-insular cortex lesions perturb cardiac autonomic tone in humans. *Clin Auton Res.* 1996;6:131–140.

12. Szurszewski JH. Physiology of mammalian prevertebral ganglia. *Annu Rev Physiol.* 1981;43:53–68.

13. Oshima N, Kumagai H, Onimaru H, et al. Monosynaptic excitatory connection from the rostral ventrolateral medulla to sympathetic preganglionic neurons revealed by simultaneous recordings. *Hypertens Res.* 2008;31:1445–1454.

14. Kawashima T. Anatomy of the cardiac nervous system with clinical and comparative morphological implications. *Anat Sci Int.* 2011;86:30–49.

15. Janes RD, Brandys JC, Hopkins DA, et al. Anatomy of human extrinsic cardiac nerves and ganglia. *Am J Cardiol.* 1986;57:299–309.

16. Pauza DH, Skripka V, Pauziene N, et al. Morphology, distribution, and variability of the epicardiac neural ganglionated subplexuses in the human heart. *Anat Rec.* 2000;259:353–382.

17. Pauza DH, Rysevaite-Kyguoliene K, Vismantaite J, et al. A combined acetylcholinesterase and immunohistochemical method for precise anatomical analysis of intrinsic cardiac neural structures. *Ann Anat.* 2014;196:430–440.

18. Marron K, Wharton J, Sheppard MN, et al. Distribution, morphology, and neurochemistry of endocardial and epicardial nerve terminal arborizations in the human heart. *Circulation.* 1995;92:2343–2351.

19. Armour JA. The little brain on the heart. *Cleve Clin J Med.* 2007;74:S48–S51.

20. Lachman N, Syed FF, Habib A, et al. Correlative anatomy for the electrophysiologist, part II: cardiac ganglia, phrenic nerve, coronary venous system. *J Cardiovasc Electrophysiol.* 2011;22:104–110.

21. Armour JA, Murphy DA, Yuan BX, et al. Gross and microscopic anatomy of the human intrinsic cardiac nervous system. *Anat Rec.* 1997;247:289–298.

22. Beaumont E, Salavatian S, Southerland EM, et al. Network interactions within the canine intrinsic cardiac nervous system: implications for reflex control of regional cardiac function. *J Physiol.* 2013;591:4515–4533.

23. Chen LS, Zhou S, Fishbein MC, et al. New perspectives on the role of autonomic nervous system in the genesis of arrhythmias. *J Cardiovasc Electrophysiol.* 2007;18:123–127.

24. Longhurst JC, Tjen ALSC, Fu LW. Cardiac sympathetic afferent activation provoked by myocardial ischemia and reperfusion. Mechanisms and reflexes. *Ann N Y Acad Sci.* 2001;940:74–95.

25. Ajiki K, Murakawa Y, Yanagisawa-Miwa A, et al. Autonomic nervous system activity in idiopathic dilated cardiomyopathy and in hypertrophic cardiomyopathy. *Am J Cardiol.* 1993;71:1316–1320.

26. Porter TR, Eckberg DL, Fritsch JM, et al. Autonomic pathophysiology in heart failure patients. Sympathetic-cholinergic interrelations. *J Clin Invest.* 1990;85:1362–1371.

27. Zhang Y, Popovic ZB, Bibevski S, et al. Chronic vagus nerve stimulation improves autonomic control and attenuates systemic inflammation and heart failure progression in a canine high-rate pacing model. *Circ Heart Fail.* 2009;2:692–699.

28. Babick A, Elimban V, Zieroth S, et al. Reversal of cardiac dysfunction and subcellular alterations by metoprolol in heart failure due to myocardial infarction. *J Cell Physiol.* 2013;228:2063–2070.

29. Floras JS. The "unsympathetic" nervous system of heart failure. *Circulation.* 2002;105:1753–1755.

30. Albino Teixeira A, Azevedo I, Branco D, et al. Sympathetic denervation caused by long-term noradrenaline infusions; prevention by desipramine and superoxide dismutase. *Br J Pharmacol.* 1989;97:95–102.

31. Kimura K, Kanazawa H, Ieda M, et al. Norepinephrine-induced nerve growth factor depletion causes cardiac sympathetic denervation in severe heart failure. *Auton Neurosci.* 2010;156:27–35.

32. Kimura K, Ieda M, Kanazawa H, et al. Cardiac sympathetic rejuvenation: a link between nerve function and cardiac hypertrophy. *Circ Res.* 2007;100:1755–1764.

33. Kanazawa H, Ieda M, Kimura K, et al. Heart failure causes cholinergic transdifferentiation of cardiac sympathetic nerves via gp130-signaling cytokines in rodents. *J Clin Invest.* 2010;120:408–421.

34. La Rovere MT, Bigger Jr JT, Marcus FI, et al. Baroreflex sensitivity and heart-rate variability in prediction of total cardiac mortality after myocardial infarction. ATRAMI (Autonomic Tone and Reflexes After Myocardial Infarction) Investigators. *Lancet.* 1998;351:478–484.

35. Chua TP, Clark AL, Amadi AA, et al. Relation between chemosensitivity and the ventilatory response to exercise in chronic heart failure. *J Am Coll Cardiol.* 1996;27:650–657.

36. Yu Y, Zhang ZH, Wei SG, et al. Brain perivascular macrophages and the sympathetic response to inflammation in rats after myocardial infarction. *Hypertension.* 2010;55:652–659.

37. Calaresu FR, Ciriello J. Renal afferent nerves affect discharge rate of medullary and hypothalamic single units in the cat. *J Auton Nerv Syst.* 1981;3:311–320.

38. Cechetto DF. Cortical control of the autonomic nervous system. *Exp Physiol.* 2014;99:326–331.

39. Schwartz PJ, La Rovere MT, Vanoli E. Autonomic nervous system and sudden cardiac death. Experimental basis and clinical observations for post-myocardial infarction risk stratification. *Circulation.* 1992;85:I77–I91.

40. Inoue H, Zipes DP. Time course of denervation of efferent sympathetic and vagal nerves after occlusion of the coronary artery in the canine heart. *Circ Res.* 1988;62:1111–1120.

41. Zhou S, Chen LS, Miyauchi Y, et al. Mechanisms of cardiac nerve sprouting after myocardial infarction in dogs. *Circ Res.* 2004;95:76–83.

42. D'Elia E, Pascale A, Marchesi N, et al. Novel approaches to the post-myocardial infarction/heart failure neural remodeling. *Heart Fail Rev.* 2014;19:611–619.

43. Kaye DM, Vaddadi G, Gruskin SL, et al. Reduced myocardial nerve growth factor expression in human and experimental heart failure. *Circ Res.* 2000;86:E80–E84.

44. Qin F, Vulapalli RS, Stevens SY, et al. Loss of cardiac sympathetic neurotransmitters in heart failure and NE infusion is associated with reduced NGF. *Am J Physiol Heart Circ Physiol.* 2002;282:H363–H371.

45. Chen GP, Caldwell JH. Evaluating presynaptic and postsynaptic innervation in heart failure. *Curr Cardiol Rep.* 2009;11:141–147.

46. Chang CM, Wu TJ, Zhou S, et al. Nerve sprouting and sympathetic hyperinnervation in a canine model of atrial fibrillation produced by prolonged right atrial pacing. *Circulation.* 2001;103:22–25.

47. Nguyen BL, Fishbein MC, Chen LS, et al. Histopathological substrate for chronic atrial fibrillation in humans. *Heart Rhythm.* 2009;6:454–460.

48. Miyauchi Y, Zhou S, Okuyama Y, et al. Altered atrial electrical restitution and heterogeneous sympathetic hyperinnervation in hearts with chronic left ventricular myocardial infarction: implications for atrial fibrillation. *Circulation.* 2003;108:360–366.

49. Martins RP, Kaur K, Hwang E, et al. Dominant frequency increase rate predicts transition from paroxysmal to long-term persistent atrial fibrillation. *Circulation.* 2014;129:1472–1482.

50. Sanchez-Chapula JA, Salinas-Stefanon E, Torres-Jacome J, et al. Blockade of currents by the antimalarial drug chloroquine in feline ventricular myocytes. *J Pharmacol Exp Ther.* 2001;297:437–445.

51. DiFrancesco D. The role of the funny current in pacemaker activity. *Circ Res.* 2010;106:434–446.

52. Filgueiras-Rama D, Jalife J. Mechanisms underlying atrial fibrillation. In: Antzelevitch C, ed. *Basic Science for Clinical Electrophysiologist.* Saunders; 2011:141–156.

53. Satoh T, Zipes DP. Cesium-induced atrial tachycardia degenerating into atrial fibrillation in dogs: atrial torsades de pointes? *J Cardiovasc Electrophysiol.* 1998;9:970–975.

54. Schlaich MP, Kaye DM, Lambert E, et al. Relation between cardiac sympathetic activity and hypertensive left ventricular hypertrophy. *Circulation.* 2003;108:560–565.

55. Parati G, Esler M. The human sympathetic nervous system: its relevance in hypertension and heart failure. *Eur Heart J.* 2012;33:1058–1066.

56. Greenwood JP, Stoker JB, Mary DA. Single-unit sympathetic discharge: quantitative assessment in human hypertensive disease. *Circulation.* 1999;100:1305–1310.

57. DiBona GF. Sympathetic nervous system and the kidney in hypertension. *Curr Opin Nephrol Hypertens.* 2002;11:197–200.

58. Ciriello J, Calaresu FR. Hypothalamic projections of renal afferent nerves in the cat. *Can J Physiol Pharmacol.* 1980;58:574–576.

59. Lambert E, Straznicky N, Schlaich M, et al. Differing pattern of sympathoexcitation in normal-weight and obesity-related hypertension. *Hypertension.* 2007;50:862–868.

60. Converse Jr RL, Jacobsen TN, Toto RD, et al. Sympathetic overactivity in patients with chronic renal failure. *N Engl J Med.* 1992;327:1912–1918.

61. Kannel WB, Kannel C, Paffenbarger Jr RS, et al. Heart rate and cardiovascular mortality: the Framingham Study. *Am Heart J.* 1987;113:1489–1494.

62. Shaper AG, Wannamethee G, Macfarlane PW, et al. Heart rate, ischaemic heart disease, and sudden cardiac death in middle-aged British men. *Br Heart J.* 1993;70:49–55.

63. Heart rate variability: standards of measurement, physiological interpretation and clinical use. Task Force of the European Society of Cardiology and the North American Society of Pacing and Electrophysiology. *Circulation.* 1996;93:1043–1065.

64. Tsuji H, Larson MG, Venditti Jr FJ, et al. Impact of reduced heart rate variability on risk for cardiac events. The Framingham Heart Study. *Circulation.* 1996;94:2850–2855.

65. Kannankeril PJ, Le FK, Kadish AH, et al. Parasympathetic effects on heart rate recovery after exercise. *J Investig Med.* 2004;52:394–401.

66. Rosenwinkel ET, Bloomfield DM, Arwady MA, et al. Exercise and autonomic function in health and cardiovascular disease. *Cardiol Clin.* 2001;19:369–387.

67. Jouven X, Empana JP, Schwartz PJ, et al. Heart-rate profile during exercise as a predictor of sudden death. *N Engl J Med.* 2005;352:1951–1958.

68. Schwartz PJ, Pagani M, Lombardi F, et al. A cardiocardiac sympathovagal reflex in the cat. *Circ Res.* 1973;32:215–220.

69. La Rovere MT, Pinna GD, Raczak G. Baroreflex sensitivity: measurement and clinical implications. *Ann Noninvasive Electrocardiol.* 2008;13:191–207.

70. La Rovere MT, Bersano C, Gnemmi M, et al. Exercise-induced increase in baroreflex sensitivity predicts improved prognosis after myocardial infarction. *Circulation.* 2002;106:945–949.

71. Schmidt G, Malik M, Barthel P, et al. Heart-rate turbulence after ventricular premature beats as a predictor of mortality after acute myocardial infarction. *Lancet.* 1999;353:1390–1396.

72. Stein PK, Sanghavi D, Sotoodehnia N, et al. Association of Holter-based measures including T-wave alternans with risk of sudden cardiac death in the community-dwelling elderly: the Cardiovascular Health Study. *J Electrocardiol.* 2010;43:251–259.

73. Rosenbaum DS, Jackson LE, Smith JM, et al. Electrical alternans and vulnerability to ventricular arrhythmias. *N Engl J Med.* 1994;330:235–241.

74. Pastore JM, Girouard SD, Laurita KR, et al. Mechanism linking T-wave alternans to the genesis of cardiac fibrillation. *Circulation.* 1999;99:1385–1394.

75. Hirata Y, Kodama I, Iwamura N, et al. Effects of verapamil on canine Purkinje fibres and ventricular muscle fibres with particular reference to the alternation of action potential duration after a sudden increase in driving rate. *Cardiovasc Res.* 1979;13:1–8.

76. Taggart P, Sutton P, Chalabi Z, et al. Effect of adrenergic stimulation on action potential duration restitution in humans. *Circulation.* 2003;107:285–289.

77. Yeh YH, Wakili R, Qi XY, et al. Calcium-handling abnormalities underlying atrial arrhythmogenesis and contractile dysfunction in dogs with congestive heart failure. *Circ Arrhythm Electrophysiol.* 2008;1:93–102.

78. Piccirillo G, Ogawa M, Song J, et al. Power spectral analysis of heart rate variability and autonomic nervous system activity measured directly in healthy dogs and dogs with tachycardia-induced heart failure. *Heart Rhythm.* 2009;6:546–552.

79. Choi EK, Shen MJ, Han S, et al. Intrinsic cardiac nerve activity and paroxysmal atrial tachyarrhythmia in ambulatory dogs. *Circulation.* 2010;121:2615–2623.

80. Shen MJ, Choi EK, Tan AY, et al. Patterns of baseline autonomic nerve activity and the development of pacing-induced sustained atrial fibrillation. *Heart Rhythm.* 2011;8:583–589.

81. Doytchinova A, Patel J, Zhou S, et al. Subcutaneous nerve activity and spontaneous ventricular arrhythmias in ambulatory dogs. *Heart Rhythm.* 2015;12:612–620.

82. Meredith IT, Broughton A, Jennings GL, et al. Evidence of a selective increase in cardiac sympathetic activity in patients with sustained ventricular arrhythmias. *N Engl J Med.* 1991;325:618–624.

83. Schwartz PJ, Stone HL. Left stellectomy in the prevention of ventricular fibrillation caused by acute myocardial ischemia in conscious dogs with anterior myocardial infarction. *Circulation.* 1980;62:1256–1265.

84. Han W, Wang Z, Nattel S. Slow delayed rectifier current and repolarization in canine cardiac Purkinje cells. *Am J Physiol Heart Circ Physiol.* 2001;280:H1075–H1080.

85. Sato R, Koumi S. Modulation of the inwardly rectifying K⁺ channel in isolated human atrial myocytes by alpha 1-adrenergic stimulation. *J Membr Biol.* 1995;148:185–191.

86. Bers DM. Cardiac excitation-contraction coupling. *Nature.* 2002;415:198–205.

87. Vaseghi M, Zhou W, Shi J, et al. Sympathetic innervation of the anterior left ventricular wall by the right and left stellate ganglia. *Heart Rhythm.* 2012;9:1303–1309.

88. Euler DE, Nattel S, Spear JF, et al. Effect of sympathetic tone on ventricular arrhythmias during circumflex coronary occlusion. *Am J Physiol.* 1985;249:H1045–H1050.

89. Opthof T, Coronel R, Vermeulen JT, et al. Dispersion of refractoriness in normal and ischaemic canine ventricle: effects of sympathetic stimulation. *Cardiovasc Res.* 1993;27:1954–1960.

90. Zannad F, De Ferrari GM, Tuinenburg AE, et al. Chronic vagal stimulation for the treatment of low ejection fraction heart failure: results of the NEural Cardiac TherApy foR Heart Failure (NECTAR-HF) randomized controlled trial. *Eur Heart J.* 2015;36:425–433.

91. Vanoli E, De Ferrari GM, Stramba-Badiale M, et al. Vagal stimulation and prevention of sudden death in conscious dogs with a healed myocardial infarction. *Circ Res.* 1991;68:1471–1481.

92. Myers RW, Pearlman AS, Hyman RM, et al. Beneficial effects of vagal stimulation and bradycardia during experimental acute myocardial ischemia. *Circulation.* 1974;49:943–947.

93. Sheng X, Scherlag BJ, Yu L, et al. Prevention and reversal of atrial fibrillation inducibility and autonomic remodeling by low-level vagosympathetic nerve stimulation. *J Am Coll Cardiol.* 2011;57:563–571.

94. Shen MJ, Shinohara T, Park HW, et al. Continuous low-level vagus nerve stimulation reduces stellate ganglion nerve activity and paroxysmal atrial tachyarrhythmias in ambulatory canines. *Circulation.* 2011;123:2204–2212.

95. Stavrakis S, Humphrey MB, Scherlag BJ, et al. Low-level transcutaneous electrical vagus nerve stimulation suppresses atrial fibrillation. *J Am Coll Cardiol.* 2015;65:867–875.

96. Abraham WT, Zile MR, Weaver FA, et al. Baroreflex activation therapy for the treatment of heart failure with a reduced ejection fraction. *JACC Heart Fail.* 2015;3:487–496.

97. Linz D, Mahfoud F, Schotten U, et al. Effects of electrical stimulation of carotid baroreflex and renal denervation on atrial electrophysiology. *J Cardiovasc Electrophysiol.* 2013;24:1028–1033.

98. Issa ZF, Zhou X, Ujhelyi MR, et al. Thoracic spinal cord stimulation reduces the risk of ischemic ventricular arrhythmias in a postinfarction heart failure canine model. *Circulation.* 2005;111:3217–3220.

99. Zipes DP, Neuzil P, Theres H, et al. Determining the feasibility of spinal cord neuromodulation for the treatment of chronic systolic heart failure: The DEFEAT-HF Study. *JACC Heart Fail.* 2016;4:129–136.

100. Tse HF, Turner S, Sanders P, et al. Thoracic spinal cord stimulation for heart failure as a restorative treatment (SCS HEART study): first-in-man experience. *Heart Rhythm.* 2015;12:588–595.

101. Schwartz PJ, Priori SG, Cerrone M, et al. Left cardiac sympathetic denervation in the management of high-risk patients affected by the long-QT syndrome. *Circulation.* 2004;109:1826–1833.

102. Wilde AA, Bhuiyan ZA, Crotti L, et al. Left cardiac sympathetic denervation for catecholaminergic polymorphic ventricular tachycardia. *N Engl J Med.* 2008;358:2024–2029.

103. Schwartz PJ. Cardiac sympathetic denervation to prevent life-threatening arrhythmias. *Nat Rev Cardiol.* 2014;11:346–353.

104. Priori SG, Blomstrom-Lundqvist C, Mazzanti A, et al. 2015 ESC Guidelines for the management of patients with ventricular arrhythmias and the prevention of sudden cardiac death: the Task Force for the Management of Patients with Ventricular Arrhythmias and the Prevention of Sudden Cardiac Death of the European Society of Cardiology (ESC) Endorsed by: Association for European Paediatric and Congenital Cardiology (AEPC). *Eur Heart J.* 2015;36:2793–2867.

105. Katritsis DG, Pokushalov E, Romanov A, et al. Autonomic denervation added to pulmonary vein isolation for paroxysmal atrial fibrillation: a randomized clinical trial. *J Am Coll Cardiol.* 2013;62:2318–2325.

106. Puodziukynas A, Kazakevicius T, Vaitkevicius R, et al. Radiofrequency catheter ablation of pulmonary vein roots results in axonal degeneration of distal epicardial nerves. *Auton Neurosci.* 2012;167:61–65.

107. He B, Lu Z, He W, et al. Effects of ganglionated plexi ablation on ventricular electrophysiological properties in normal hearts and after acute myocardial ischemia. *Int J Cardiol.* 2013;168:86–93.

108. Pokushalov E, Romanov A, Katritsis DG, et al. Renal denervation for improving outcomes of catheter ablation in patients with atrial fibrillation and hypertension: early experience. *Heart Rhythm.* 2014;11:1131–1138.

109. Linz D, Wirth K, Ukena C, et al. Renal denervation suppresses ventricular arrhythmias during acute ventricular ischemia in pigs. *Heart Rhythm.* 2013;10:1525–1530.

42 The Molecular Pathophysiology of Atrial Fibrillation

Stanley Nattel, Jordi Heijman, Niels Voigt, Xander H.T. Wehrens, and Dobromir Dobrev

CHAPTER OUTLINE

Atrial fibrillation (AF) is a highly prevalent and clinically relevant arrhythmia, for which all current therapeutic approaches have important limitations. An improved understanding of the mechanistic basis of AF has evolved over decades, particularly with respect to molecular aspects. Mechanistic insights have contributed greatly to the contemporary management of AF and are expected to further improve arrhythmia therapy in the future.[1] The purpose of this chapter is to review findings in the molecular pathophysiology of AF and to discuss their potential value for improving management.

This chapter will begin with an overview of the etiological determinants of AF, then discuss briefly the principal mechanisms contributing to AF, and finally review the molecular basis of specific arrhythmia determinants.

Etiological Determinants

Heart Disease

The majority of AF cases have associated cardiac disease (Fig. 42.1). Cardiac senescence is a major predisposing factor, largely mediated by structural remodeling which causes fibrotic alterations and microconduction slowing, as well as atrial enlargement.[2] Heart failure (HF), hypertensive heart disease, valvular disease, and ischemic heart disease are major contributors to the occurrence of AF. Less common conditions leading to AF include pericarditis, myocarditis, and various cardiomyopathies. Cardiac surgery is followed by postoperative AF, with a typical presentation and therapeutic response, in about 30% of cases.

Genetic Determinants

There has been a rapid increase in knowledge of genetic determinants of AF since the mid-2000s.[3–6] A wide range of disease-causing mutations has been established (Table 42.1), and additional AF susceptibility gene loci have been identified with genome-wide association studies (GWASs; Table 42.2) (see Chapter 49).

Rare variants linked to monogenic forms of AF have high penetrance and provide important insights into AF mechanisms, whereas common genetic variants identified using GWAS provide new insights into genetics-based population determinants of AF, while raising challenging pathophysiological issues.[6]

Extracardiac Contributors

A variety of extracardiac conditions can affect AF occurrence. Heavy alcohol consumption promotes AF,[7] and hyperthyroidism is a well-recognized factor.[8] Obesity is increasingly recognized as an AF risk factor,[9] with obstructive sleep apnea, often associated with obesity, also being an important contributor. Autonomic tone may set the conditions for AF initiation and maintenance. The AF-promoting properties of vagal activation are well known, and there is increasing evidence for an important role of combined sympathovagal discharge.[10]

General Mechanisms and Atrial Fibrillation Forms

Focal ectopic firing and reentrant activity are the primary AF arrhythmia mechanisms (Fig. 42.2A). Focal activity can be transient, producing isolated atrial extrasystoles or self-limited tachycardias and can contribute to AF generation by acting as a trigger to initiate reentry in a vulnerable substrate. In addition, sustained focal ectopic activity can produce rapid "driver" activity that is conducted heterogeneously to generate fibrillatory conduction maintaining the irregular activity typical of AF.[11,12] Clinical AF can be paroxysmal (self-terminating) or persistent (terminating only with medical intervention). With increasing duration, persistent AF becomes increasingly resistant to therapy, and "long-standing persistent AF," lasting >1 year, often becomes permanent when attempts to restore sinus rhythm fail or are abandoned. Repetitively firing focal ectopic drivers are believed to produce paroxysmal forms. Reentrant activity generates more persistent AF, tending to become more fixed, therapy-resistant, and irreversible as the substrate evolves.[13,14] Besides progression of AF-associated comorbidities, the evolution of the substrate is promoted by AF-induced remodeling related to the rapid atrial rate, cardiac dysfunction, neurohumoral effects, and consequences of atrial metabolic disturbances (Fig. 42.2B). The remodeling induced by long-standing AF involves both functional and structural components that promote a transition toward complex reentrant mechanisms, as quantified in recent noninvasive mapping studies.[15,16] These analyses have shown pronounced temporal and interpatient variability in AF activity, suggesting dynamic and complex interactions between AF mechanisms.

CAUSES OF ATRIAL FIBRILLATION

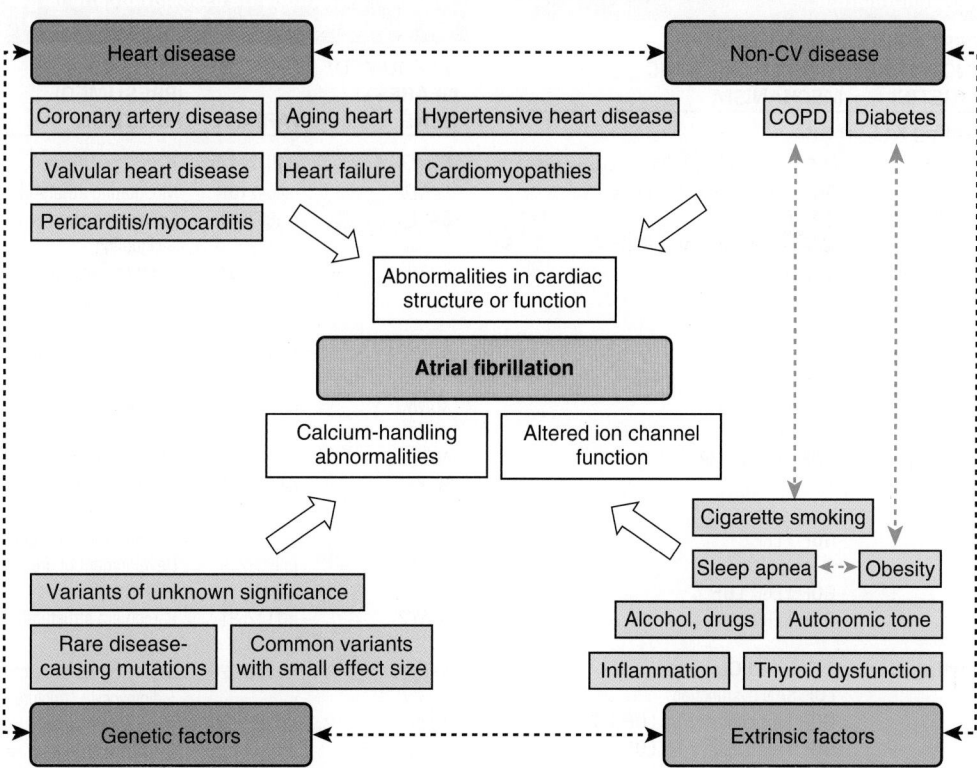

FIGURE 42.1 Etiological contributors to atrial fibrillation. *COPD,* Chronic obstructive pulmonary disease; *CV,* cardiovascular.

Focal Ectopic Activity

Several mechanisms produce abnormal impulse formation and can cause focal ectopic activity. Spontaneous automatic activity depends on the balance between inward and outward currents during phase 4 of the action potential (AP). Increased phase 4 inward currents carried by Na^+ or Ca^{2+}, particularly time-dependent hyperpolarization-activated currents like the "funny current," I_f, and/or decreased phase 4 outward currents, produce spontaneous phase 4 depolarization that can reach threshold and cause ectopic firing.

Focal ectopic activity may also result from afterdepolarizations, which are subdivided into early afterdepolarizations (EADs; arising before the end of phase 3) or delayed afterdepolarizations (DADs; occurring after full repolarization). Normal cardiomyocyte Ca^{2+} handling is crucial for cardiac contractility (Fig. 42.3A). DADs (Fig. 42.3B) are thought to be the predominant cause of focal atrial ectopic firing. DADs are caused by a diastolic Ca^{2+} leak from the sarcoplasmic reticulum (SR) via SR Ca^{2+}-release channels or "ryanodine receptors" (RyRs, RyR2 being the cardiac isoform). Systolic Ca^{2+} release through RyR2s mediates cardiac excitation–contraction coupling. Relaxation is mediated by diastolic Ca^{2+} removal from the cytosol into the SR by a Ca^{2+} uptake pump, the SR Ca^{2+}-ATPase (SERCA2a). RyR2s are sensitive to both cytosolic and intraluminal SR Ca^{2+} concentrations, and diastolic releases result from SR Ca^{2+} overload or when oversensitive RyR2s have an abnormally low Ca^{2+} threshold for Ca^{2+} release. Excess cytosolic Ca^{2+} is handled by the sarcolemmal Na^+/Ca^{2+} exchanger (NCX), which moves three Na^+ ions (charge +3) into the cell for each Ca^{2+} ion (charge +2) extruded into the extracellular space, generating net inward current (called "transient inward current," I_{ti}), which depolarizes the cell, producing a DAD. When DADs reach threshold, they induce premature AP firing (*dashed line* in Fig. 42.3B), which promotes its own perpetuation by synchronizing release events and allowing more Ca^{2+} to enter the cell.[17] Repeated DAD-triggered APs can generate focal atrial tachycardias. RyR2 function is regulated by channel phosphorylation; hyperphosphorylation enhances RyR2 Ca^{2+} sensitivity and promotes DAD formation. Calsequestrin (CSQ) is the principal Ca^{2+} storage buffer of the SR. Inadequate CSQ function/expression increases the free SR Ca^{2+} concentration and promotes diastolic RyR2 Ca^{2+} release.[18]

EADs generally occur when AP duration (APD) is excessively prolonged. With very long APs, L-type Ca^{2+} currents may have enough time to recover from inactivation and carry inward Ca^{2+} current to generate an EAD and stimulate a spontaneous extrasystole.

Reentry

The two principal competing conceptual frameworks for understanding functional reentry[19] are shown in Fig. 42.4 (top). The leading-circle model (Fig. 42.4A) posits reentry around a central zone that is continuously activated by centripetal waves emanating from a reentering activation wavefront. In this model, reentry establishes itself in a circuit with dimension equal to the distance travelled during one refractory period ("wavelength," refractory period times conduction velocity; CV). When the wavelength is small because of slow conduction or brief refractoriness, multiple circuits can be accommodated in the atria and spontaneous self-termination is unlikely. In the spiral-wave model (Fig. 42.4B), reentry is maintained by rotors established by tissue excitability properties (depending on both conduction and refractoriness), which determine rotor period, stability, and size (greater excitability generates smaller, more stable, and faster rotors). Anatomical obstacles or complexities favor reentry by anchoring reentry circuits. Fig. 42.4C illustrates the effect of structural remodeling. Progressive atrial dilation creates longer conduction pathways for reentry. Tissue fibrosis slows conduction, makes conduction more heterogeneous, and creates conduction barriers that favor

TABLE 42.1 Amino acid–coding (AAC) missense variants associated with atrial fibrillation

GENE	(PRESUMED) FUNCTIONAL TARGET(S)	(PRESUMED) ARRHYTHMOGENIC MECHANISM
AAC Variants Affecting K⁺ Currents		
ABCC9	I_{KATP}	LOF: Impaired APD adaptation during stress
KCNA5	I_{Kur}	GOF: ↓ ERP; LOF: ↑ APD, EADs, TA
KCND3	I_{to}	GOF: ↓ ERP
KCNE1	I_{Ks}	GOF: ↓ ERP; LOF: ↑ APD, EADs
KCNE2	KCNQ1/KCNE2 K⁺-current	GOF: ↓ ERP
KCNE3	I_{to}/I_{Kr}	GOF: ↓ ERP
KCNE4	I_{Ks} (?)	?
KCNE5	I_{Ks}	GOF: ↓ ERP
KCNH2	I_{Kr}	GOF: ↓ ERP; LOF: ?
KCNK3	I_{K2P}	LOF: ↑ APD, SAN dysfunction
KCNJ2	I_{K1}	GOF: ↓ ERP, ↓ RMP
KCNJ4	I_{K1}	?
KCNJ5	$I_{K,ACh}$	?
KCNJ8	I_{KATP}	GOF: ↓ ERP
KCNJ12	I_{K1}	?
KCNQ1	I_{Ks}	GOF: ↓ ERP; LOF: ?
NPPA	I_{Ks}	GOF: ↓ ERP, ?
AAC Variants Affecting Na⁺ and Related Currents		
HCN4	I_f	LOF: SAN dysfunction
SCN5A	I_{Na}	GOF: ↑ excitability / TA; LOF: ↓ CV
SCN10A	I_{Na}	GOF: ↑ excitability / TA; LOF: ↓ CV
SCN1B	I_{Na}	LOF: ↓ CV
SCN1Bb	I_{Na}/I_{to}	Mixed: ↓ I_{Na}, ↑ I_{to}, ↓ ERP
SCN2B	I_{Na}	LOF: ↓ CV
SCN3B	I_{Na}	LOF: ↓ CV
SCN4B	I_{Na}	?
AAC Variants Affecting Ca²⁺ Handling and Current		
CACNA1C	$I_{Ca,L}$	?
CACNA2D2	$I_{Ca,L}$	?
CASQ2	Ca²⁺-buffering	?
JPH2	RyR2-channel	GOF: ↑ SCaEs, TA
RYR2	RyR2-channel	GOF: ↑ SCaEs, TA, ↓ CV
AAC Variants Not Directly Affecting Sarcolemmal Ion Currents		
GATA4, GATA5, GATA6	TF	LOF: ?
GJA1	Connexin43	LOF: ↓ CV
GJA5	Connexin40	LOF: ↓ CV
GREM2	BMP antagonist	GOF: Abnormal cardiac development, ↓ CV
LMNA	Lamin A/C	Structural remodeling, ↓ CV
MYH6	Contractile proteins	?
NKX2-5, NKX2-6	TF	LOF: ?
NUP155	Nuclear pore complex	LOF: Impaired nuclear permeability, remodeling, ↓ APD
PITX2c	TF	LOF: ?
ZFHX3	TF	?

APD, Action potential duration; *↓ CV*, slow/heterogeneous conduction; *↓ ERP*, reduced effective refractory period; *GOF*, gain of function variants; *LOF*, loss of function variants; *↓ RMP*, resting membrane potential hyperpolarization; *↑ SCaEs*, spontaneous diastolic Ca²⁺-release events; *TA*, triggered activity; *TF*, transcription factor; *?*, unknown mechanism.
Based on recent overviews.[3–6]

TABLE 42.2 Genetic variants associated with atrial fibrillation in genome-wide association and large-scale genotyping studies in patients of European descent

(PRESUMED/ NEAREST) GENE	VARIANT	(PRESUMED) FUNCTION	RELATIVE RISK
C9orf3	rs10821415	?	1.13 (1.08–1.18)
CAND2	rs4642101	Modulating atrial APD	1.10 (1.06–1.14)
CAV1	rs3807989	Cellular structure and signaling	0.88 (0.84–0.91)
GJA1	rs13216675	Electrical coupling controlling conduction velocity	1.10 (1.06–1.14)
HCN4	rs7164883	Regulation of I_f and automaticity	1.16 (1.10–1.22)
KCNN3	rs6666258	Regulation of I_{SK}, modulating APD	1.18 (1.13–1.23)
NEURL	rs12415501	Modulating atrial APD	1.18 (1.13–1.23)
PITX2	rs6817105	Left/right division and pulmonary vein sleeve development	1.64 (1.54–2.21)
PRRX1	rs3903239	Development of great vessels	1.14 (1.10–1.18)
SYNE2	rs1152591	Sarcomere structural protein	1.13 (1.09–1.18)
SYNPO2L / MYOZ1	rs10824026	Regulating actin and cardiomyocyte structure	0.85 (0.81–0.9)
TBX5	rs10507248	Transcription factor controlling conduction system development	1.12 (1.08–1.16)
ZFHX3	rs2106261	?	1.24 (1.17–1.30)

Based on recent overviews.[3–6]

the development of stable rotors and/or multiple simultaneous irregular reentry circuits that can sustain AF. In addition, fibroblast proliferation can promote arrhythmogenesis via cardiomyocyte–fibroblast interactions that alter AP properties and reduce conduction speed.

Molecular Control Mechanisms
Molecular Control of Gene Expression in Atrial Fibrillation

There is extensive evidence for an important role of altered gene-control in AF pathogenesis. Fig. 42.5 presents a simplified schematic of dysregulated molecular control mechanisms of gene expression that are implicated in AF. These are recognized to occur in at least four different contexts: (1) AF-inducing mutations in transcription factors (TFs); (2) gene variants identified by GWAS that are in or related to TFs, which are the presumptive immediate mediators of AF substrate control; (3) AF-induced signaling changes that are involved in AF-induced atrial remodeling; and (4) changes in gene expression that mediate the AF-promoting effects of predisposing diseases and risk factors. Many of these are discussed in detail below, but a general overview is provided here. The tissue-specific cellular phenotype is controlled primarily by selective expression of genes in the genome. Transcription patterns from DNA to messenger RNA (mRNA) are tissue- and disease-specific, largely under the regulation of TFs that bind to specific DNA sequences and enhance or suppress transcription of associated sequences. Mutations in the TFs *GATA*, *NKX2-5*, and *TBX5* cause various forms of congenital heart disease and predispose to AF.[20] In addition, GWASs have identified a number of single nucleotide polymorphisms (SNPs) believed to control AF risk via TFs, like the 4q25 variants for which *PITX2* is the

Atrial fibrillation – triggers and substrates

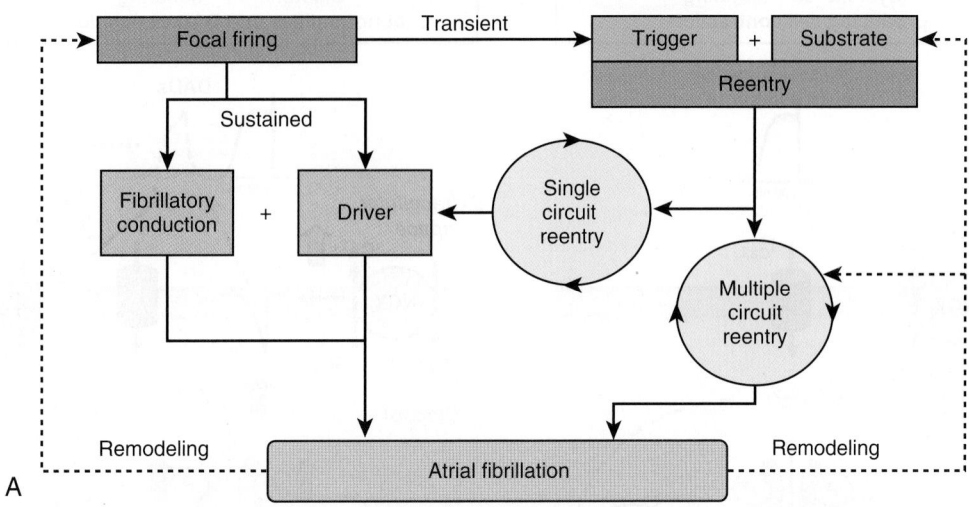

A

Atrial fibrillation – forms and progression

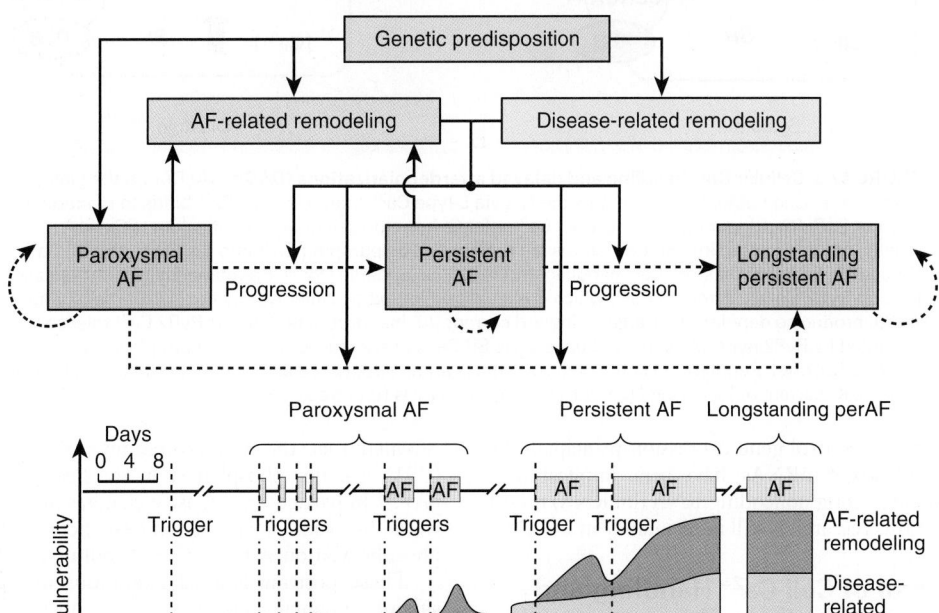

B

FIGURE 42.2 Mechanistic basis of atrial fibrillation (*AF*) and associated clinical forms. (A) Focal firing usually results from local ectopic activity. Organized discrete reentrant activity and focal firing can maintain AF by producing regularly firing drivers that are irregularly conducted (fibrillatory conduction) in the heterogeneous atrial substrate. (B) AF can progress from paroxysmal (self-terminating) forms, believed to result primarily from focal drivers, to persistent and longstanding persistent (>1 year) forms due to AF-related remodeling and/or disease progression, resulting in development of an increasingly vulnerable substrate. Substrate vulnerability, AF-related remodeling, and disease progression are further modulated by genetic predisposition. There is overlap between mechanisms and pronounced patient-to-patient heterogeneity.

closest gene, the 16q22 SNPs in an intron (noncoding segment) of *ZFHX3*, and the 1q24 variants of *PRRX1* (see Table 42.2). AF itself causes reprogramming of gene expression, in particular by increasing cellular Ca^{2+} loading and thereby activating a variety of signaling systems.[21] Prominent among these is the nuclear factor of activated T-lymphocytes (NFAT)/calcineurin system, which regulates the expression of a range of important ion channels.[21] AF-inducing conditions (in many cases along with AF itself) act

through a number of cell membrane receptors controlling signaling pathways like the renin-angiotensin-aldosterone and transforming growth factor-β systems, which induce atrial remodeling through a range of downstream TFs. Reactive oxygen species, particularly those derived from NADPH oxidase, also play a key role. Nuclear-delimited signaling likely also occurs, although we are just beginning to understand these pathways and their role in disease states.[22] Finally, a range of small noncoding RNA sequences,

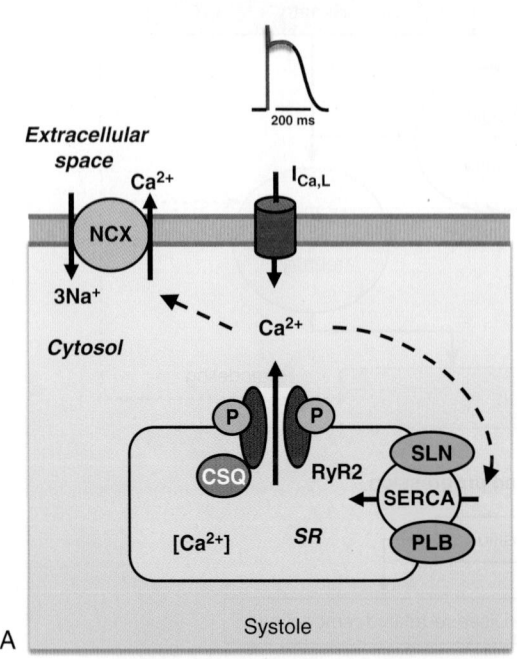
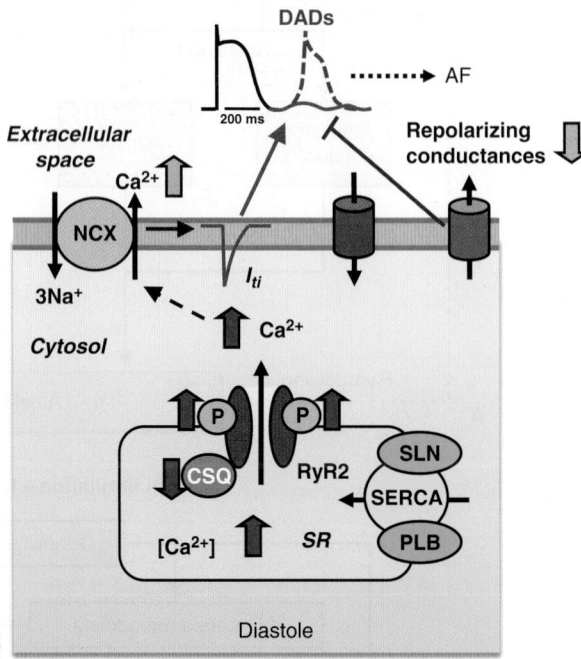

FIGURE 42.3 Cellular Ca²⁺ handling and delayed afterdepolarizations (*DADs*). (A) During the plateau phase of the action potential, Ca²⁺ enters the cell via L-type Ca²⁺ channels. This Ca²⁺ binds to ryanodine—receptor 2 (*RyR2*), triggering a much larger Ca²⁺ release from the sarcoplasmic reticulum (*SR*), which initiates cellular contraction. SR Ca²⁺ stores are maintained by pumping Ca²⁺ into the SR by the SR Ca²⁺-ATPase (*SERCA*). (B) Diastolic Ca²⁺ handling abnormalities underlie DADs. Spontaneous SR Ca²⁺ releases through RyR2 elevate cytosolic Ca²⁺, which is exchanged for extracellular Na⁺ by the Na⁺/Ca²⁺ exchanger (*NCX*), producing depolarizing transient inward current (*I_{ti}*). Inappropriate diastolic RyR2 Ca²⁺ release is promoted by RyR2 hyperphosphorylation, excess SR Ca²⁺, or decreased SR Ca²⁺ binding to calsequestrin (*CSQ; red arrows*). Repolarizing conductances oppose I_{ti} and suppress diastolic depolarization, so reduced diastolic K⁺ current or increased NCX current can favor DADs (*orange arrows*).

called microRNAs, which control gene expression principally by blocking translation of target mRNAs, have been implicated in AF-inducing remodeling. Long noncoding RNA (lncRNA) might also contribute,[23] but this research is still in its infancy in the atria.

Molecular Control of Cell Ca²⁺ Handling and Delayed Afterdepolarizations Generation

Normal cell Ca²⁺ handling is crucial for cellular contraction and relaxation (see Fig. 42.3A; also see Chapter 16). Abnormal SR Ca²⁺ handling is seen in both paroxysmal and chronic AF (pAF and cAF) patients,[24–29] promoting spontaneous RyR2-mediated diastolic SR Ca²⁺ releases. Moreover, patients with rare inherited variants in RyR2 linked to catecholaminergic polymorphic ventricular tachycardia (CPVT) also commonly exhibit AF as a result of abnormal SR Ca²⁺ release.[30]

Fig. 42.6 summarizes the detailed molecular pathobiology of DAD-inducing diastolic RyR2 Ca²⁺ release in nongenetic forms of AF. Protein kinase A (PKA) phosphorylation of RyR2 at Ser2808[26] and Ca²⁺/calmodulin-dependent protein kinase II (CaMKII) phosphorylation at Ser2814 are increased in dogs and goats with pacing-induced AF and in human cAF patients.[24,29–32] CaMKII activity is normally autoinhibited. Ca²⁺/calmodulin binding removes autoinhibition, activating CaMKII and causing autophosphorylation that activates CaMKII and makes it Ca²⁺-independent. Similar activation may result from CaMKII oxidation. Changes in the RyR2 phosphorylation state at PKA and CaMKII sites may result not only from changed kinase activity, but also from alterations in phosphatases (dephosphorylating enzymes).[31] Proteomic studies

revealed that the serine/threonine protein phosphatase type-1 (PP1), a major phosphatase in the heart, is also dysregulated in pAF.[33] In particular, extensive changes in PP1 regulatory subunits were observed, which may underlie heterogeneous changes in the phosphorylation status of Ca²⁺-handling proteins in AF patients.

These posttranslational alterations increase RyR2 Ca²⁺ sensitivity, enhancing channel open probability.[24,26] Mice deficient in the RyR2 inhibitory FK-505 binding protein 12.6, mice with gain-of-function mutations in RyR2, and mice with constitutively phosphorylated RyR2 channels at S2814 (S2814D mice) all exhibit increased susceptibility to pacing-induced AF in association with increased atrial cell SR Ca²⁺ leak and triggered activity.[24,30,34,35] AF-promoting effects of angiotensin may in part be due to oxidative stress acting via CaMKII oxidation on diastolic RyR2 Ca²⁺ release.[36] RyR2 dysfunction can be induced by Ca²⁺ overload resulting from phospholamban hyperphosphorylation, which removes phospholamban inhibition of SERCA2a and enhances SR Ca²⁺ uptake,[31] as has been reported for pAF.[29] Phospholamban hyperphosphorylation can be produced by enhanced PKA or CaMKII activity or by decreased phosphatase function. Reduced phosphatase function can be a consequence of increased activity of the inhibitory protein, I-1, typically caused by I-1 hyperphosphorylation.[31]

Increases in NCX expression and/or function are also commonly noted in persistent AF,[24,28,31,37] causing I_{ti} resulting from any specific amount of diastolic SR Ca²⁺ leak to be larger in AF, likely contributing to the increased risk of DADs and triggered ectopic activity.[24,38] Cardiac IP₃ receptors (IP₃R2) act as Ca²⁺-transporting pathways and can facilitate SR Ca²⁺ leak to promote arrhythmogenesis. IP₃R2 expression is increased by ATR

Mechanisms of Reentry

Functional Determinants

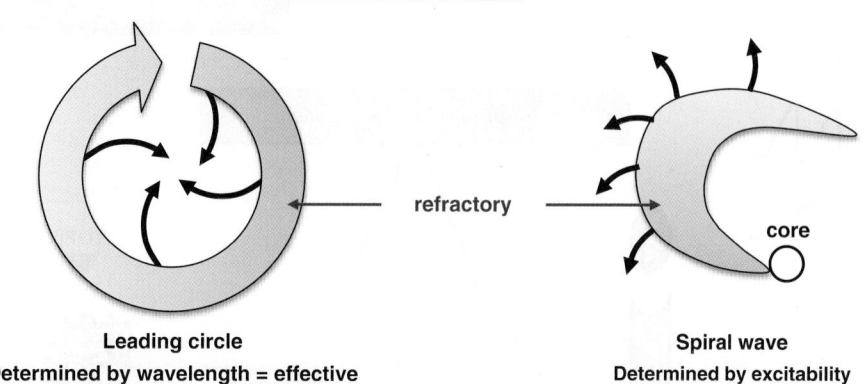

Leading circle
Determined by wavelength = effective refractory period × conduction velocity

A

Spiral wave
Determined by excitability and wave curvature

B

Structural Remodeling

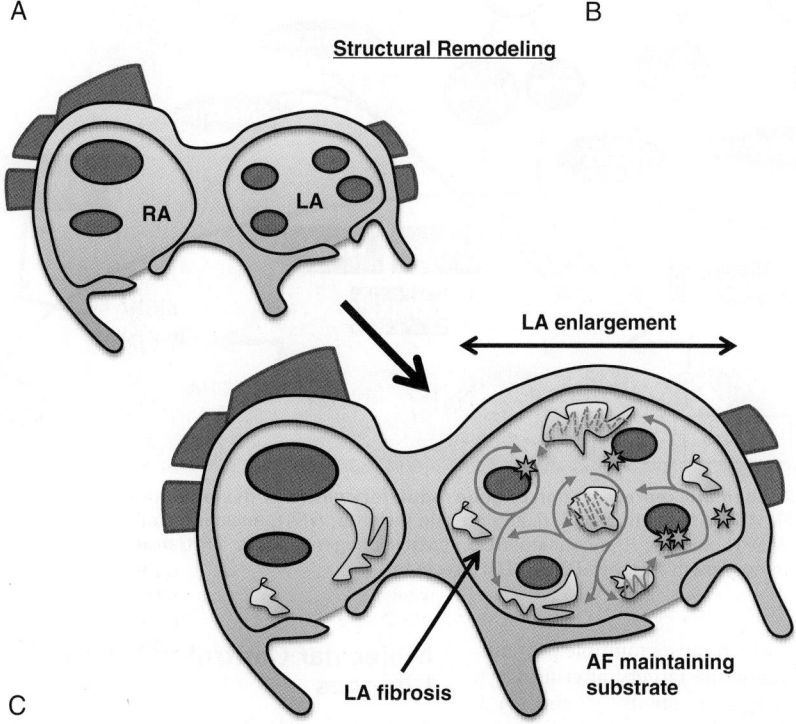

C

FIGURE 42.4 Determinants of reentry. *Top,* Basic concepts of reentry. The leading circle model (A) posits reentry around a central zone that is continuously activated by centripetal waves emanating from the reentering activation wavefront. The spiral wave model (B) describes reentry as a "rotor" established by tissue excitability properties. (C) Structural remodeling (atrial enlargement and fibrosis, most typically affecting the left atrium [*LA*]), produces relatively fixed reentry substrates that reverse poorly if at all. *AF,* Atrial fibrillation.

and is greater in the atria than in the ventricles.[39] IP$_3$R2-coupled amplification of atrial SR Ca^{2+}-release events and related arrhythmogenesis may thus contribute to AF-related ectopic activity.

Congestive heart failure (CHF) is a very important cause of AF. Focal drivers and triggered activity play a role in CHF-related AF.[40] In experimental dilated cardiomyopathy, CHF increases SR Ca^{2+} load and reduces CSQ expression, thereby promoting spontaneous SR Ca^{2+} release.[41] Increased SR Ca^{2+} load also contributes to arrhythmogenic SR Ca^{2+} releases in pAF patients.[29] Altered RyR2 activity due to an inherited mutation in the structural protein junctophilin-2 was shown to cause AF in patients with hypertrophic cardiomyopathy, and a relative lack of junctophilin-2 due to increased RyR2 protein

expression may contribute to RyR2 dysfunction in pAF.[42] The increased RyR2 protein expression in pAF is at least in part due to a reduction in the inhibitory miRNA-106b-25 complex.[43] Coronary artery disease (CAD) is also an important risk factor for AF. Atrial ischemia promotes AF maintenance.[44] In a dog model of chronic occlusive CAD affecting the atrium, frequent spontaneous atrial ectopy is associated with an increased incidence of atrial cardiomyocyte–triggered activity.[44] Triggered activity is likely due to spontaneous SR Ca^{2+}-release events and increased NCX function in cardiomyocytes from the ischemic border zone.[44]

In addition to the rare genetic variants in RyR2, two AF-promoting genetic variants have been linked to DAD mechanisms: (1) a mutation of the gene encoding the adapter protein ankyrin-B

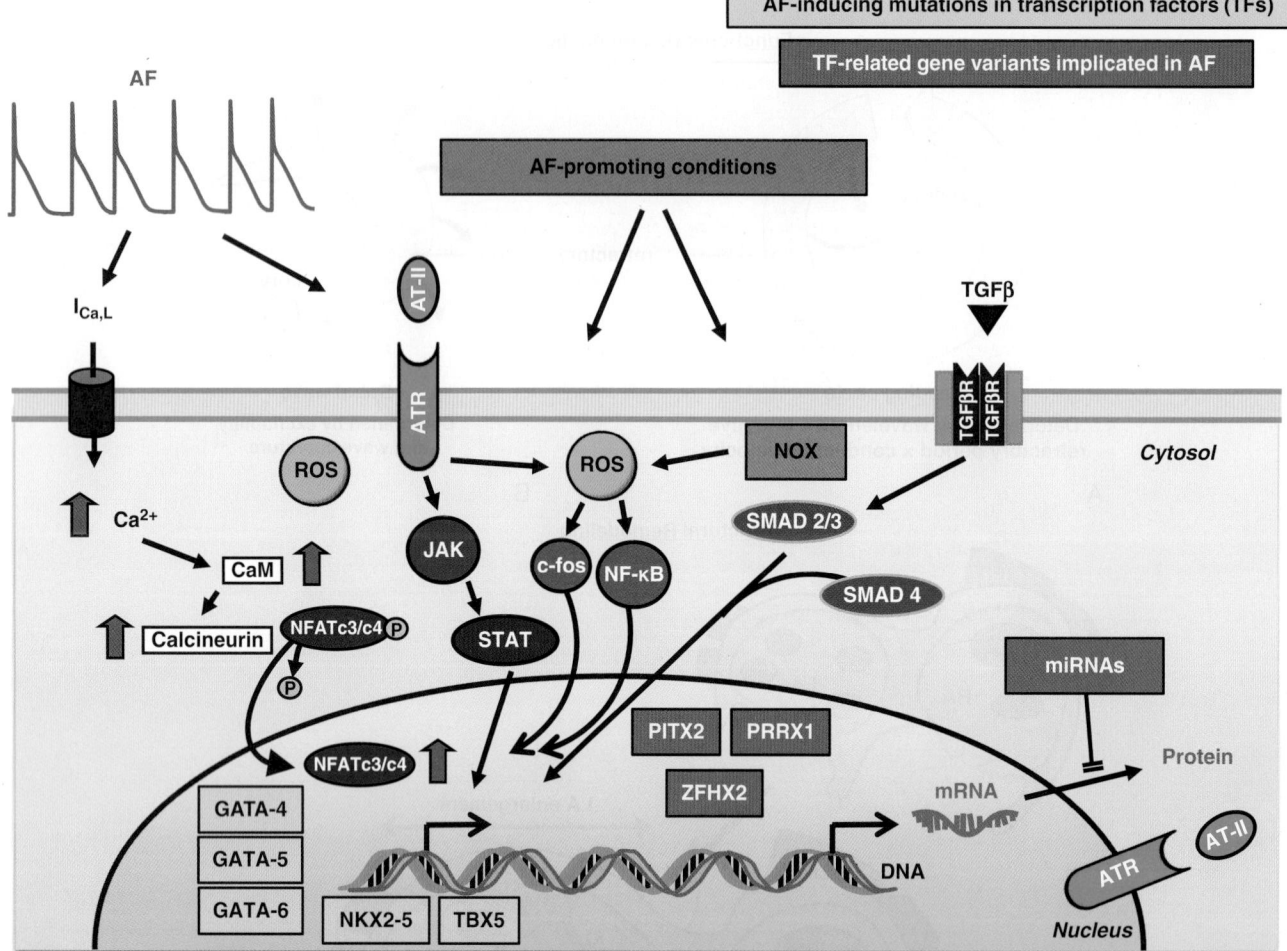

FIGURE 42.5 A schematic representation of gene regulatory pathway dysregulation in atrial fibrillation (AF). *AT-II,* Angiotensin-II; *ATR,* angiotensin receptor; *NFAT,* nuclear factor of activated T-cells; *NOX,* NADPH-oxidase; *P,* phosphate; *ROS,* reactive oxygen species; *TF,* transcription factor; *TGFβ,* transforming growth factor-β; *TGFβR,* TGFβ-receptor.

(long-QT syndrome-4 [LQTS4]), which causes multiple proteins to be poorly addressed to their membrane targets, altering Ca^{2+} handling and leading to DADs/triggered activity[45,46] and (2) a predicted loss-of-function SNP of the *SLN* gene encoding the SERCA2a inhibitory protein sarcolipin, which could increase SR Ca^{2+} load and thereby affect DAD susceptibility.[47]

β-Adrenoceptor activation phosphorylates RyR2, promoting diastolic SR Ca^{2+} release events.[47] Conditions that directly cause DAD-promoting abnormalities in Ca^{2+} handling may require adrenergic stimulation to induce Ca^{2+} sparks and triggered activity.[44] Spontaneous AF paroxysms occur in dog models of autonomic hyperinnervation,[48] with sympathovagal discharge preceding AF paroxysms.[49] Vagal activation promotes arrhythmogenesis by reducing APD, allowing afterdepolarizations induced by adrenergic stimulation to induce ectopic firing in pulmonary veins.[50–52] Finally, although Ca^{2+}-handling abnormalities and DADs occur in atrial cardiomyocytes from pAF and cAF patients, atrial aftercontractions are less frequent in multicellular atrial trabeculae from AF patients compared with sinus rhythm controls.[53] Similarly, high atrial rates alone may not produce proarrhythmic Ca^{2+}-handling abnormalities, but may even cause Ca^{2+}-handling silencing to counteract the potentially cytotoxic effects of chronically elevated intracellular Ca^{2+}.[54] Thus much more work is needed to precisely define the role of abnormal Ca^{2+} handling in AF pathophysiology.

Molecular Control of L-Type Ca^{2+} Current Changes

AF,[55] and indeed all very rapid atrial tachyarrhythmias,[56] remodel atrial electrical properties to promote AF initiation and maintenance (atrial tachycardia remodelling [ATR]). A major AF-promoting component of ATR is refractory period reduction due to APD abbreviation (see Fig. 42.4B). Reduced depolarizing L-type Ca^{2+} current ($I_{Ca,L}$), along with increased repolarizing inward-rectifier K^+ currents, underlie ATR-induced APD shortening.[57–64] The molecular basis of $I_{Ca,L}$ reduction in persistent AF is illustrated in Fig. 42.7A. Rapid atrial activation induces Ca^{2+} loading, activating Ca^{2+}/calmodulin/calcineurin/NFAT signaling, which causes downregulation of Cav1.2 α-subunit mRNA.[65–67] Other contributors to $I_{Ca,L}$ downregulation may include decreased expression of accessory $β_1$, $β_{2a}$, $β_{2b}$, $β_3$, and $α_2δ_2$ subunits[59,68,69]; Cav1.2 dephosphorylation via PP1 and type-2A (PP2A) protein phosphatases[31,59,70]; increased Cav1.2 α-subunit S-nitrosylation[71]; and metabolic stress.[72] MicroRNAs are centrally involved in cardiac remodeling,[73] and recent work implicated increased miRNA-328 and miR-21 in AF promotion due to $I_{Ca,L}$ downregulation mediated by inhibition of translation and mRNA destabilization.[74,75] In 82 patients with Brugada syndrome/short QT electrocardiogram (ECG) phenotypes,

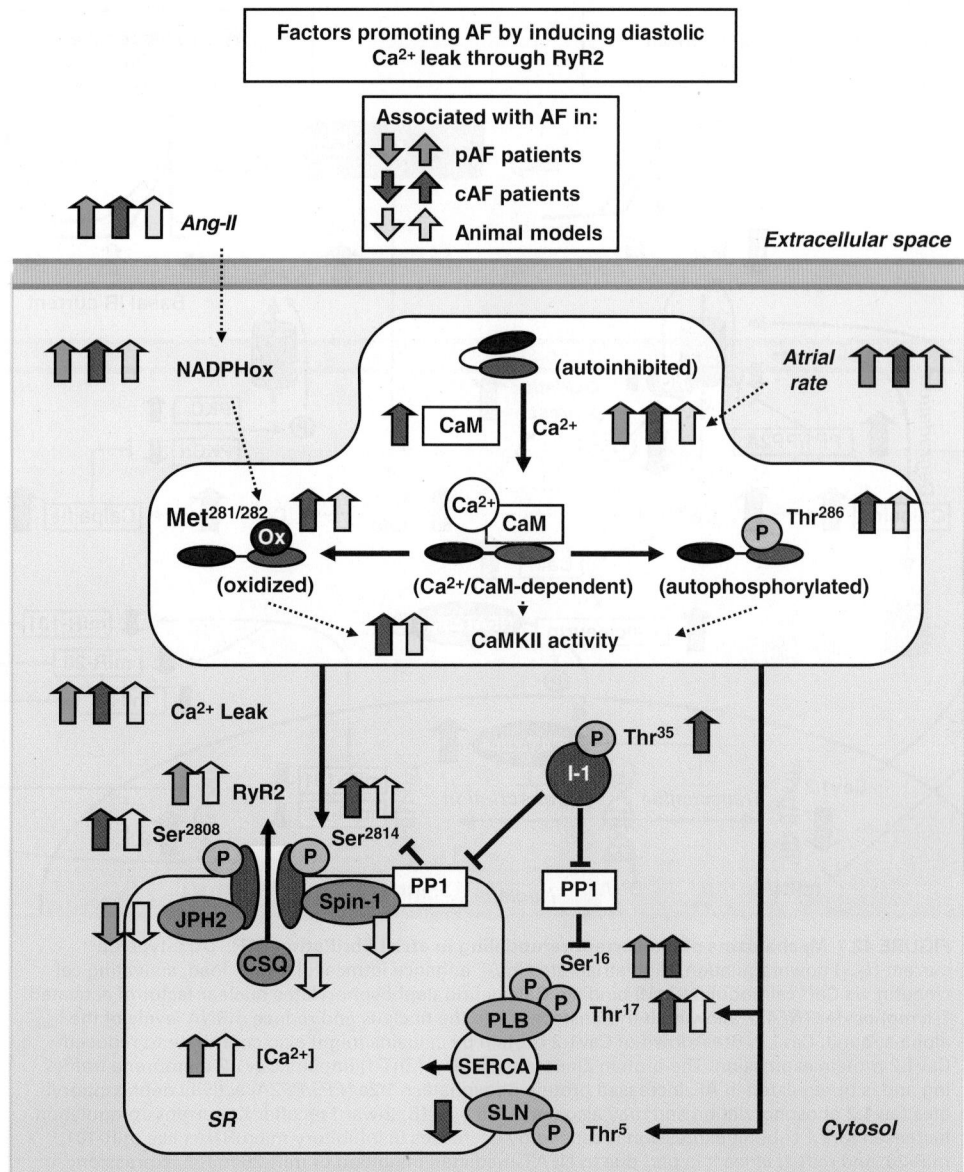

FIGURE 42.6 Molecular basis of delayed afterdepolarization–inducing diastolic Ca²⁺ releases.
Ryanodine receptor (RyR) dysfunction is caused by RyR hyperphosphorylation or excess Ca²⁺ loads.
Phospholamban (*PLB*) inhibits sarcoplasmic reticulum (*SR*) Ca²⁺-ATPase (*SERCA*). PLB hyperphosphorylation removes this inhibitory effect, enhances SERCA function, and can lead to Ca²⁺ overload. High atrial rate during atrial fibrillation (*AF*) enhances cellular Ca²⁺ entry. Increased cell Ca²⁺
promotes Ca²⁺/calmodulin (*CaM*) binding to Ca²⁺/calmodulin-dependent protein kinase-II (*CaMKII*),
disinhibiting the catalytic subunit. After CaMKII catalytic subunit activation, oxidation at Met281/282
or phosphorylation at Thr286 causes persistent CaMKII activity. Inhibitor-1 (*I-1*) suppresses protein
phosphatase-1 (*PP1*) function in the SR and contributes to PLB and RyR phosphorylation. These
factors have been associated with AF in samples from paroxysmal AF (*pAF*) patients (*blue arrows*),
chronic (*cAF*) patients (*red arrows*), or animal models (*yellow arrows*).

loss-of-function mutations of the *CACNA1C* and *CACNB2*
genes, encoding $I_{Ca,L}$ α- and β-subunits, were observed along
with AF in individual patients.[76] Patients with full-blown short
QT syndromes of various phenotypes have reduced APDs and
are also predisposed to AF.[6]

Molecular Control of K⁺ Current and Basis of Atrial Fibrillation–Promoting Alterations

Inward-rectifier K⁺ current enhancement promotes AF maintenance by reducing APD (favoring reentry) and stabilizing/accelerat-
ing arrhythmia-maintaining rotors by removing voltage-dependent

I_{Na} inactivation through membrane hyperpolarization.[11,77] Upregulation of other K⁺ currents, like two-pore K⁺ currents, small-
conductance Ca²⁺-dependent K⁺ currents, and Kv1.1-mediated
K⁺ currents, may further contribute to APD-shortening in persistent AF.[78–80] Fig. 42.7B shows how I_{K1} and agonist-independent
(constitutive) $I_{K,ACh}$ ($I_{K,AChc}$) are upregulated in persistent AF. I_{K1}
increases because of upregulation of the underlying Kir2.1 sub-
unit[60–64,69,81–83] caused by reduced Kir2.1 inhibitory microRNAs,
like miR-1, miR-26, and miR-101.[83,84] Kir2.1 dephosphorylation
(activation) via increased PP1 and PP2A function[31,59,70,85] may
also contribute. CHR upregulates fibroblast Kir2.1 expression and
related I_{K1} currents, thereby causing membrane hyperpolarization,

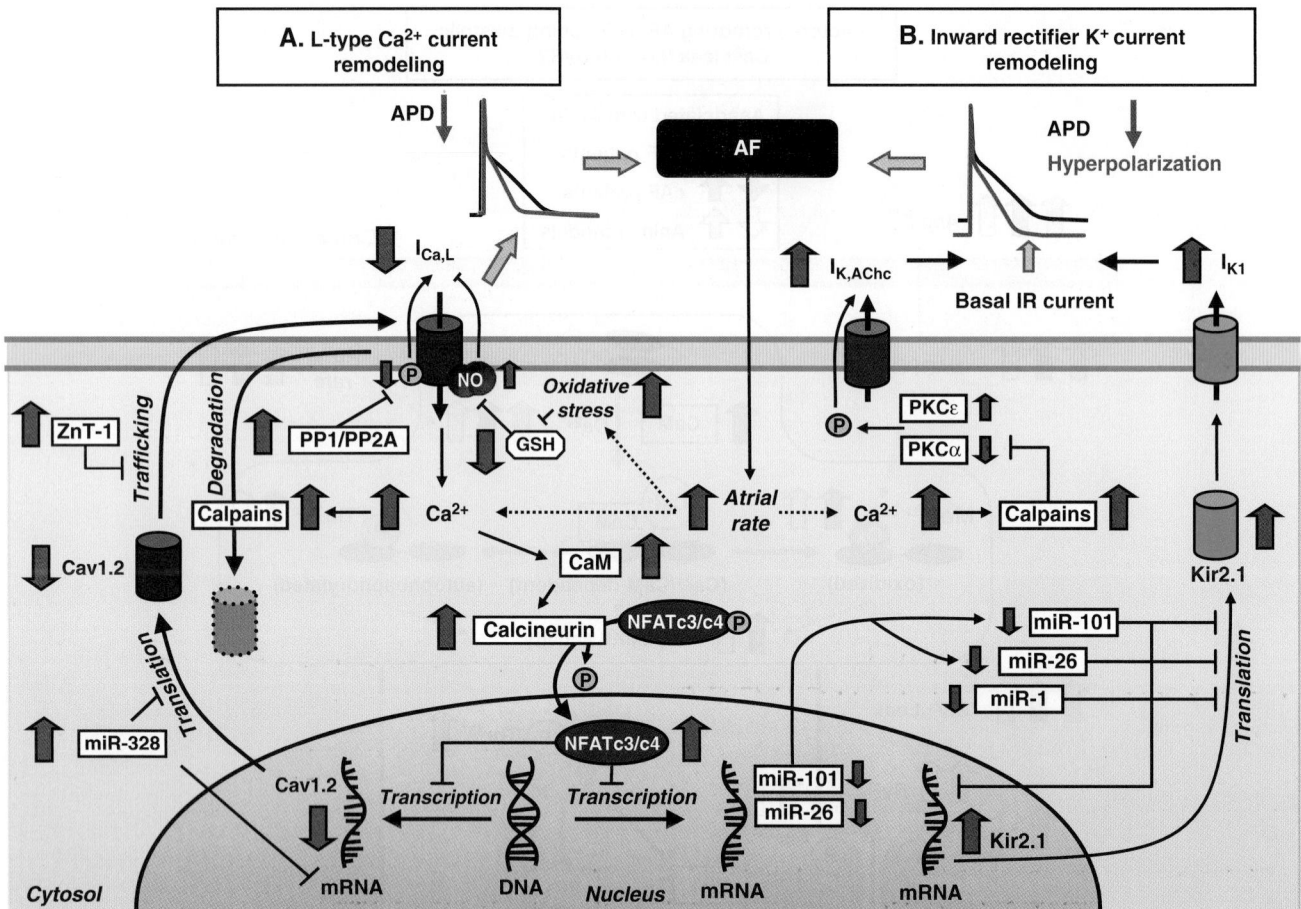

FIGURE 42.7 Mechanisms of ion current remodeling in atrial fibrillation (AF). (A) L-type Ca^{2+} current ($I_{Ca,L}$) downregulation. High atrial rates in AF enhance intracellular Ca^{2+} load, activating calcineurin via Ca^{2+}/calmodulin (*CaM*) binding. Calcineurin dephosphorylates nuclear factor of activated T-lymphocytes (*NFAT*), allowing it to translocate into the nucleus and reduce mRNA levels of the $I_{Ca,L}$ alpha-subunit, Cav1.2. Breakdown of Cav1.2 protein by calpains might also contribute to reduced Cav1.2 protein expression. The protein Zinc transporter-1 (*ZnT-1*) impairs Cav1.2 membrane trafficking and is upregulated in AF. Increased protein phosphatase 1/2a (*PP1/PP2A*) activity dephosphorylates Cav1.2 phosphorylation and may also decrease $I_{Ca,L}$. (B) Inward rectifier K^+ current upregulation. Increased Kir2.1 subunit expression is caused by decreases in inhibitory microRNAs like miR-101, miR-26, and miR-1, at least in part due to NFAT-mediated inhibition of miR-26/miR-1 expression. Constitutively active acetylcholine-activated K^+ current ($I_{K,AChc}$) is increased because of increased membrane abundance of the stimulatory protein kinase C (*PKC*) isoform, PKCε, and decreased cellular expression of the inhibitory isoform, PKCα, due to enhanced calpain-mediated breakdown.

increasing Ca^{2+} entry, and enhancing atrial fibroblast proliferation,[86] contributing to structural remodeling (see below). The changes in fibroblast I_{K1} are likely mediated by miRNA-26a downregulation, positioning miRNA-26a as a common determinant of both electrical and structural remodeling.

Agonist-induced muscarinic receptor–mediated $I_{K,ACh}$ activation is reduced in AF.[60,61] This process involves a reduction in Kir3.1 and Kir3.4 channel subunits and is associated with a loss of physiological Na^+-mediated $I_{K,ACh}$ activation.[87] However, agonist-independent (constitutive) $I_{K,AChc}$ is increased, both in dog models[60,63,82,88] and in human AF patients.[62,64,81,89] Increased $I_{K,AChc}$ is due to greater channel opening probability, with no change in single-channel conductance, kinetics, or density.[62,82] A key role is played by altered protein kinase C (PKC)-mediated $I_{K,AChc}$ phosphorylation, with increased phosphorylation by stimulatory Ca^{2+}-dependent isoforms and reduced inhibitory classical Ca^{2+}-independent isoform function.[88,89] $I_{K,AChc}$ inhibition suppresses atrial tachyarrhythmias in ATR preparations,[63] suggesting that $I_{K,AChc}$ contributes to ATR-induced arrhythmogenic remodeling.

The most common AF-promoting monogenic paradigm is accelerated atrial repolarization due to gain-of-function K^+ channel mutations (see Table 42.1). Vagal enhancement is known to promote clinical AF and is central in some cases.[90] $I_{K,ACh}$ hyperpolarizes atrial cardiomyocytes and reduces APD in a spatially heterogeneous manner. Vagal enhancement strongly favors AF initiation and persistence by facilitating the initiation and subsequent stability of reentrant rotors.[90] Kir3.4 knockout strongly suppresses $I_{K,ACh}$ and prevents cholinergic AF.[91]

Molecular Determinants of Atrial Conduction Disturbances

Conduction Abnormalities due to Ion Channel Dysfunction

Conduction abnormalities favor reentry. Gap junctions are essential for efficient cell coupling and conduction. There are discrepant results about AF-related atrial gap junctional remodeling in the literature.[69,92,93] Some of the variability may be due to differences in AF duration, underlying heart disease, and species-related factors.[94] Spatially heterogeneous connexin40 remodeling occurs in the goat model of electrically maintained AF, consistent with clinical data indicating that gene variants that affect connexin40 promoter function may predispose to AF.[95–97] Connexin43 dephosphorylation/lateralization occurs in CHF, but CHF-induced conduction slowing and AF promotion are unchanged with CHF recovery, despite disappearance of connexin abnormalities.[98] Recent evidence indicates that connexin43 gene transfer can improve conduction and suppress AF in porcine models, supporting the importance of gap junction protein remodeling in AF.[99,100]

Atrial ischemic disease causes localized conduction slowing, which allows for AF-sustaining local reentry stabilized around a line of conduction block.[44] With acute ischemia, gap junction uncoupling predominates.[101]

A number of AF-associated gene variants affect ion channels that control cardiac conduction. *GJA5* encodes connexin40, an atrial-selective gap junction ion channel. Connexin40 knockout causes conduction abnormalities and atrial arrhythmia susceptibility.[102] An AF-causing *GJA5* missense somatic mutation was identified in idiopathic AF patients.[96] *GJA5* promoter variants believed to decrease gene transcription increase AF susceptibility.[95,97,103]

I_{Na} provides the energy for conduction and governs CV. I_{Na} density decreases in canine ATR, with corresponding decreases in SCN5A subunit mRNA and protein.[57] In humans with AF, SCN5A mRNA expression appears unchanged.[69] Atrial cardiomyocytes from AF patients showed a slightly reduced I_{Na}.[104]

Cardiac Na^+ channel gene (*SCN5A*) loss-of-function mutations cause AF, presumably via reentry-promoting conduction slowing (see Table 42.1). *SCN5A* mutations were initially associated with AF in a family presenting a complex and variable phenotype including dilated cardiomyopathy, AF, sinus node dysfunction, and conduction defects.[105] *SCN5A* mutations and SNPs were subsequently found in idiopathic AF subjects.[106,107] Loss-of-function *SCN5A* mutations are the most common cause of Brugada syndrome,[108] which typically presents as VF/sudden death, but can also cause AF.[96] Recently, mutations in SCN10A, as well as in Na^+ channel β-subunits like *SCN1B*, *SCN2B*, and *SCN3B*, have been implicated in AF.[109–112]

Structural Remodeling

Atrial fibrosis plays an important role in AF in different etiologies.[13,44,113,114] The underlying signaling pathways and clinical manifestations have recently been reviewed.[115] The development of atrial fibrosis is likely determined by multiple signals acting simultaneously. Cardiomyocytes and fibroblasts interact extensively through autocrine and paracrine factors, and possibly electrically as well.[13,116] Fibroblasts produce extracellular matrix (ECM) proteins and mediators that affect cardiomyocyte phenotype, whereas cardiomyocytes generate products like reactive oxygen species (ROS), platelet-derived growth factor (PDGF), transforming growth factor-β (TGF-β), and connective tissue growth factor (CTGF) that modulate fibroblast function.

Angiotensin II (AT-II) plays an important role in AF,[117] likely in large measure via fibroblast modulation. AT-II type 1 receptors (AT1Rs) promote fibrosis via enhanced actions of TGF-β, Smad2/3, Smad4, Arkadia, and activated extracellular signal-regulated (ERK) mitogen-activated protein-kinase (MAPK).[118] Arkadia promotes ubiquitination and removal of Smad7, thereby increasing TGF-β signaling by removing Smad7 antagonism.[119] In addition, AT1Rs act through Shc/Grb2/SOS to activate Ras, which enhances MAPK phosphorylation,[120] and through phospholipase C (PLC). PLC breaks down phosphatidylinositol 4,5-bisphosphate (PIP₂), yielding diacylglycerol (DAG) and inositol 1,4,5-trisphosphate (IP3). DAG activates PKC, and IP3 mobilizes intracellular Ca^{2+}, both actions contributing to remodeling. The JAK/STAT pathway, also AT1R-sensitive, activates transcription factors such as AP-1 and NF-κB, which cause further cardiomyocyte remodeling. AT2R activation counters AT1R-mediated MAPK activation by enhancing dephosphorylation via PP2A and phosphotyrosine phosphatase (PTP).[120]

TGF-β₁ is a key player in cardiac fibrosis and is secreted by both fibroblasts and cardiomyocytes.[121] Overactivity of cardiac TGF-β₁ causes atrial-selective fibrosis, conduction abnormalities, and AF promotion.[122] TGF-β₁ mediates AT-II effects in both paracrine and autocrine fashions.[123] TGF-β₁ acts through SMADs to activate fibroblasts and enhance collagen production.[13,116,119] Rapidly firing atrial cardiomyocytes produce AT-II and ROS, acting via enhanced TGF-β production to differentiate cardiac fibroblasts into ECM-secreting myofibroblasts.[124,125] Progressive fibrosis likely contributes to conduction disturbances that make long-lasting AF very difficult to treat.[14]

PDGF stimulates fibroblast proliferation and differentiation.[13,116,122] PDGF receptors contain two transmembrane domains that dimerize upon stimulation and then activate an internal tyrosine kinase. Tyrosine kinase autophosphorylation of PDGF receptors induces Ras/MEK1/2, MAPK, JAK/STAT, and PLC signaling. PDGF overexpression induces cardiac fibrosis and dysfunction.[126] Atrial-selective PDGF expression and action may contribute to the greater fibrotic responses typically seen for atria versus ventricles.[121]

CTGF lies downstream to TGF-β₁ and AT-II in profibrotic signaling pathways. CTGF activates fibroblasts through Src kinase and MAPKs.[127] CTGF has emerged as a potential central player in atrial structural remodeling.[128–130]

MicroRNAs appear to contribute importantly to atrial structural remodeling. MiR-29 inhibits collagen gene expression,[131] and its downregulation likely contributes to atrial fibrosis in CHF.[132] MiR-30 and miR-133 are also downregulated in CHF, suppress CTGF translation,[133] and may participate in atrial fibrosis.[134] In contrast to miR-29, miR-20, and miR-133, atrial miR-21 expression increases in CHF.[134] MiR-21 targets the *Sprouty-1* (*Spry-1*) gene, which promotes fibroblast MAPK phosphorylation and enhances fibroblast survival.[135] Although the significance of this finding for ventricular remodeling has been disputed,[136] more recent work strongly suggests an important role of miR-21 upregulation in CHF-associated atrial fibrosis and AF promotion.[137]

SNPs in genes determining atrial structural integrity, inflammation, and neurohumoral control have been associated with AF by conventional approaches. Examples include genes encoding angiotensin-converting enzyme (ACE),[138,139] matrix metalloproteinase-2 (MMP2), and interleukin-10.[140] However, these results have not been replicated in hypothesis-free large-scale population studies. GWASs have implicated SNPs on chromosome 4q25, with *PITX2c* being the closest potential target gene, and a SNP in chromosome 16q22 near the zinc finger homeobox 3 transcription factor gene (*ZFHX3*).[50,51,141] *PITX2c* is involved in cardiac development, particularly sidedness and pulmonary vein aspects[142,143] implicating possible structural abnormalities as the way in which it may be involved in AF. *ZFHX3* is a tumor suppressor[144,145] that induces expression of PDGF receptors and protects against oxidant stress,[146] also suggesting structural remodeling as a potential mechanism of AF promotion.

Atrial Ca^{2+}-handling abnormalities may also contribute to reentry-promoting structural remodeling. Increased fibroblast Ca^{2+} entry through TRP channels promotes fibroblast proliferation and structural remodeling.[147] Genetic inhibition of RyR2 hyperphosphorylation prevents excessive SR Ca^{2+} leak, suppresses atrial dilatation, and reduces atrial conduction abnormalities in mice with cardiac-restricted overexpression of a repressor form of the cAMP response element modulator.[148]

Future Directions

The largest and most important challenge related to the molecular basis of AF is translating our increased knowledge into practical clinical applications. It is widely hoped that targeting the molecular mechanisms of AF will permit the development of novel, safer, and more specific treatment approaches. Recent advances suggest that biological therapies capable of specifically modifying the AF substrate may be in sight.[149] The challenges in moving from scientific discovery to practical therapeutic innovation in this area are substantial, but the history of this field suggests that conceptual advances do ultimately result in tangible improvements in patient management options.[1]

Acknowledgments

The authors thank Jennifer Bacchi for excellent secretarial help.

Funding

Supported by the Canadian Institutes of Health Research (MGP6957 and MOP44365), the Quebec Heart and Stroke Foundation, the Foundation Leducq (European-North American Atrial Fibrillation Research Alliance, ENAFRA, grant 07CVD03), the German Federal Ministry of Education and Research through Atrial Fibrillation Competence Network (grant 01Gi0204) and DZHK (German Centre for Cardiovascular Research), the Deutsche Forschungsgemeinschaft (Do 769/1-3), the European Union (European Network for Translational Research in Atrial Fibrillation, EUTRAF, grant 261057). NIH-NHLBI grants (R01-HL089598, R01-HL091947, R01-HL117641, R41-HL129570), and the American Heart Association (13EIA14560061).

REFERENCES

1. Heijman J, Algalarrondo V, Voigt N, Wehrens XHT, Nattel S. The value of basic research insights into atrial fibrillation mechanisms as a guide to therapeutic innovation: a critical analysis. *Cardiovasc Res.* 2016;109:467–479.
2. Nattel S. From guidelines to bench: implications of unresolved clinical issues for basic investigations of atrial fibrillation mechanisms. *Can J Cardiol.* 2011;27:19–26.
3. Darbar D. The role of pharmacogenetics in atrial fibrillation therapeutics—is personalized therapy in sight? *J Cardiovasc Pharmacol.* 2016;67:9–18.
4. Olesen MS, Nielsen MW, Haunso S, Svendsen JH. Atrial fibrillation: the role of common and rare genetic variants. *Eur J Hum Genet.* 2014;22:297–306.
5. Sinner MF, Tucker NR, Lunetta KL, et al. Integrating genetic, transcriptional, and functional analyses to identify five novel genes for atrial fibrillation. *Circulation.* 2014;130:1225–1235.
6. Tucker NR, Ellinor PT. Emerging directions in the genetics of atrial fibrillation. *Circ Res.* 2014;114:1469–1482.
7. Mukamal KJ, Tolstrup JS, Friberg J, Jensen G, Gronbaek M. Alcohol consumption and risk of atrial fibrillation in men and women: the Copenhagen City Heart Study. *Circulation.* 2005;112:1736–1742.
8. Auer J, Scheibner P, Mische T, Langsteger W, Eber O, Eber B. Subclinical hyperthyroidism as a risk factor for atrial fibrillation. *Am Heart J.* 2001;142:838–842.
9. Schoonderwoerd BA, Smit MD, Pen L, Van Gelder IC. New risk factors for atrial fibrillation: causes of 'not-so-lone atrial fibrillation'. *Europace.* 2008;10:668–673.
10. Chou CC, Chen PS. New concepts in atrial fibrillation: neural mechanisms and calcium dynamics. *Cardiol Clin.* 2009;27:35–43, viii.
11. Nattel S, Burstein B, Dobrev D. Atrial remodeling and atrial fibrillation: mechanisms and implications. *Circ Arrhythm Electrophysiol.* 2008;1:62–73.
12. Berenfeld O, Zaitsev AV, Mironov SF, Pertsov AM, Jalife J. Frequency-dependent breakdown of wave propagation into fibrillatory conduction across the pectinate muscle network in the isolated sheep right atrium. *Circ Res.* 2002;90:1173–1180.
13. Burstein B, Nattel S. Atrial fibrosis: mechanisms and clinical relevance in atrial fibrillation. *J Am Coll Cardiol.* 2008;51:802–809.
14. de Groot NM, Houben RP, Smeets JL, et al. Electro-pathological substrate of longstanding persistent atrial fibrillation in patients with structural heart disease: epicardial breakthrough. *Circulation.* 2010;122:1674–1682.
15. Cuculich PS, Wang Y, Lindsay BD, et al. Noninvasive characterization of epicardial activation in humans with diverse atrial fibrillation patterns. *Circulation.* 2010;122:1364–1372.
16. Haissaguerre M, Hocini M, Denis A, et al. Driver domains in persistent atrial fibrillation. *Circulation.* 2014;130:530–538.
17. Lou Q, Belevych AE, Radwanski PB, et al. Alternating membrane potential/calcium interplay underlies repetitive focal activity in a genetic model of calcium-dependent atrial arrhythmias. *J Physiol.* 2015;593:1443–1458.
18. MacLennan DH, Chen SR. Store overload-induced Ca²⁺ release as a triggering mechanism for CPVT and MH episodes caused by mutations in RYR and CASQ genes. *J Physiol.* 2009;587:3113–3115.
19. Comtois P, Kneller J, Nattel S. Of circles and spirals: bridging the gap between the leading circle and spiral wave concepts of cardiac reentry. *Europace.* 2005;7(suppl 2):10–20.
20. Mahida S. Transcription factors and atrial fibrillation. *Cardiovasc Res.* 2014;101:194–202.
21. Nattel S, Dobrev D. The multidimensional role of calcium in atrial fibrillation pathophysiology: mechanistic insights and therapeutic opportunities. *Eur Heart J.* 2012;33:1870–1877.
22. Tadevosyan A, Vaniotis G, Allen BG, Hebert TE, Nattel S. G protein-coupled receptor signalling in the cardiac nuclear membrane: evidence and possible roles in physiological and pathophysiological function. *J Physiol.* 2012;590:1313–1330.

23. Ruan Z, Sun X, Sheng H, Zhu L. Long non-coding RNA expression profile in atrial fibrillation. *Int J Clin Exp Pathol.* 2015;8:8402–8410.
24. Voigt N, Li N, Wang Q, et al. Enhanced sarcoplasmic reticulum Ca²⁺ leak and increased Na⁺-Ca²⁺ exchanger function underlie delayed afterdepolarizations in patients with chronic atrial fibrillation. *Circulation.* 2012;125:2059–2070.
25. Hove-Madsen L, Llach A, Bayes-Genis A, et al. Atrial fibrillation is associated with increased spontaneous calcium release from the sarcoplasmic reticulum in human atrial myocytes. *Circulation.* 2004;110:1358–1363.
26. Vest JA, Wehrens XH, Reiken SR, et al. Defective cardiac ryanodine receptor regulation during atrial fibrillation. *Circulation.* 2005;111:2025–2032.
27. Liang X, Xie H, Zhu PH, et al. Ryanodine receptor-mediated Ca²⁺ events in atrial myocytes of patients with atrial fibrillation. *Cardiology.* 2008;111:102–110.
28. Neef S, Dybkova N, Sossalla S, et al. CaMKII-dependent diastolic SR Ca²⁺ leak and elevated diastolic Ca²⁺ levels in right atrial myocardium of patients with atrial fibrillation. *Circ Res.* 2010;106:1134–1144.
29. Voigt N, Heijman J, Wang Q, et al. Cellular and molecular mechanisms of atrial arrhythmogenesis in patients with paroxysmal atrial fibrillation. *Circulation.* 2014;129:145–156.
30. Chelu MG, Sarma S, Sood S, et al. Calmodulin kinase II-mediated sarcoplasmic reticulum Ca2+ leak promotes atrial fibrillation in mice. *J Clin Invest.* 2009;119:1940–1951.
31. El-Armouche A, Boknik P, Eschenhagen T, et al. Molecular determinants of altered Ca²⁺ handling in human chronic atrial fibrillation. *Circulation.* 2006;114:670–680.
32. Greiser M, Neuberger HR, Harks E, et al. Distinct contractile and molecular differences between two goat models of atrial dysfunction: AV block-induced atrial dilatation and atrial fibrillation. *J Mol Cell Cardiol.* 2009;46:385–394.
33. Chiang DY, Lebesgue N, Beavers DL, et al. Alterations in the interactome of serine/threonine protein phosphatase type-1 in atrial fibrillation patients. *J Am Coll Cardiol.* 2015;65:163–173.
34. Sood S, Chelu MG, van Oort RJ, et al. Intracellular calcium leak due to FKBP12.6 deficiency in mice facilitates the inducibility of atrial fibrillation. *Heart Rhythm.* 2008;5:1047–1054.
35. Li N, Wang T, Wang W, et al. Inhibition of CaMKII phosphorylation of RyR2 prevents induction of atrial fibrillation in FKBP12.6 knockout mice. *Circ Res.* 2012;110:465–470.
36. Purohit A, Swaminathan PD, Chen B, et al. Angiotensin II promotes atrial fibrillation in mice by CaMKII oxidation. *Circulation.* 2011;124:A14037.
37. Lenaerts I, Bito V, Heinzel FR, et al. Ultrastructural and functional remodeling of the coupling between Ca²⁺ influx and sarcoplasmic reticulum Ca²⁺ release in right atrial myocytes from experimental persistent atrial fibrillation. *Circ Res.* 2009;105:876–885.
38. Dobrev D, Voigt N, Wehrens XH. The ryanodine receptor channel as a molecular motif in atrial fibrillation: pathophysiological and therapeutic implications. *Cardiovasc Res.* 2012;89:734–743.
39. Zhao ZH, Zhang HC, Xu Y, et al. Inositol-1,4,5-trisphosphate and ryanodine-dependent Ca²⁺ signaling in a chronic dog model of atrial fibrillation. *Cardiology.* 2007;107:269–276.
40. Ryu K, Shroff SC, Sahadevan J, Martovitz NL, Khrestian CM, Stambler BS. Mapping of atrial activation during sustained atrial fibrillation in dogs with rapid ventricular pacing induced heart failure: evidence for a role of driver regions. *J Cardiovasc Electrophysiol.* 2005;16:1348–1358.
41. Yeh YH, Wakili R, Qi XY, et al. Calcium-handling abnormalities underlying atrial arrhythmogenesis and contractile dysfunction in dogs with congestive heart failure. *Circ Arrhythm Electrophysiol.* 2008;1:93–102.

42. Beavers DL, Wang W, Ather S, et al. Mutation E169K in junctophilin-2 causes atrial fibrillation due to impaired RyR2 stabilization. *J Am Coll Cardiol.* 2013;62:2010–2019.
43. Chiang DY, Kongchan N, Beavers DL, et al. Loss of microRNA-106b-25 cluster promotes atrial fibrillation by enhancing ryanodine receptor type-2 expression and calcium release. *Circ Arrhythm Electrophysiol.* 2014;7:1214–1222.
44. Nishida K, Qi XY, Wakili R, et al. Mechanisms of atrial tachyarrhythmias associated with coronary occlusion in a chronic canine model. *Circulation.* 2011;123:137–146.
45. Cunha SR, Hund TJ, Hashemi S, et al. Defects in ankyrin-based membrane protein targeting pathways underlie atrial fibrillation. *Circulation.* 2011;124:1212–1222.
46. Mohler PJ, Schott JJ, Gramolini AO, Dilly KW, Guatimosim S, et al. Ankyrin-B mutation causes type 4 long-QT cardiac arrhythmia and sudden cardiac death. *Nature.* 2003;421:634–639.
47. Nyberg MT, Stoevring B, Behr ER, Ravn LS, McKenna WJ, Christiansen M. The variation of the sarcolipin gene (SLN) in atrial fibrillation, long QT syndrome and sudden arrhythmic death syndrome. *Clin Chim Acta.* 2007;375:87–91.
48. Tan AY, Zhou S, Ogawa M, et al. Neural mechanisms of paroxysmal atrial fibrillation and paroxysmal atrial tachycardia in ambulatory canines. *Circulation.* 2008;118:916–925.
49. Choi EK, Shen MJ, Han S, et al. Intrinsic cardiac nerve activity and paroxysmal atrial tachyarrhythmia in ambulatory dogs. *Circulation.* 2010;121:2615–2623.
50. Burashnikov A, Antzelevitch C. Reinduction of atrial fibrillation immediately after termination of the arrhythmia is mediated by late phase 3 early afterdepolarization-induced triggered activity. *Circulation.* 2003;107:2355–2360.
51. Patterson E, Po SS, Scherlag BJ, Lazzara R. Triggered firing in pulmonary veins initiated by in vitro autonomic nerve stimulation. *Heart Rhythm.* 2005;2:624–631.
52. Chou CC, Nguyen BL, Tan AY, et al. Intracellular calcium dynamics and acetylcholine-induced triggered activity in the pulmonary veins of dogs with pacing-induced heart failure. *Heart Rhythm.* 2008;5:1170–1177.
53. Christ T, Rozmaritsa N, Engel A, et al. Arrhythmias, elicited by catecholamines and serotonin, vanish in human chronic atrial fibrillation. *Proc Natl Acad Sci U S A.* 2014;111:11193–11198.
54. Greiser M, Kerfant BG, Williams GS, et al. Tachycardia-induced silencing of subcellular Ca²⁺ signaling in atrial myocytes. *J Clin Invest.* 2014;124:4759–4772.
55. Wijffels MC, Kirchhof CJ, Dorland R, Allessie MA. Atrial fibrillation begets atrial fibrillation. A study in awake chronically instrumented goats. *Circulation.* 1995;92:1954–1968.
56. Shiroshita-Takeshita A, Mitamura H, Ogawa S, Nattel S. Rate-dependence of atrial tachycardia effects on atrial refractoriness and atrial fibrillation maintenance. *Cardiovasc Res.* 2009;81:90–97.
57. Yue L, Feng J, Gaspo R, Li GR, Wang Z, Nattel S. Ionic remodeling underlying action potential changes in a canine model of atrial fibrillation. *Circ Res.* 1997;81:512–525.
58. Van Wagoner DR, Pond AL, Lamorgese M, Rossie SS, McCarthy PM, Nerbonne JM. Atrial L-type Ca²⁺ currents and human atrial fibrillation. *Circ Res.* 1999;85:428–436.
59. Christ T, Boknik P, Wohrl S, et al. L-type Ca²⁺ current downregulation in chronic human atrial fibrillation is associated with increased activity of protein phosphatases. *Circulation.* 2004;110:2651–2657.
60. Ehrlich JR, Cha TJ, Zhang L, et al. Characterization of a hyperpolarization-activated time-dependent potassium current in canine cardiomyocytes from pulmonary vein myocardial sleeves and left atrium. *J Physiol.* 2004;557:583–597.

61. Dobrev D, Graf E, Wettwer E, et al. Molecular basis of downregulation of G-protein-coupled inward rectifying K$^+$ current (I$_{K,ACh}$) in chronic human atrial fibrillation: decrease in GIRK4 mRNA correlates with reduced I$_{K,ACh}$ and muscarinic receptor-mediated shortening of action potentials. *Circulation.* 2001;104:2551–2557.

62. Dobrev D, Friedrich A, Voigt N, et al. The G protein-gated potassium current I$_{K,ACh}$ is constitutively active in patients with chronic atrial fibrillation. *Circulation.* 2005;112:3697–3706.

63. Cha TJ, Ehrlich JR, Chartier D, Qi XY, Xiao L, Nattel S. Kir3-based inward rectifier potassium current: potential role in atrial tachycardia remodeling effects on atrial repolarization and arrhythmias. *Circulation.* 2006;113:1730–1737.

64. Voigt N, Friedrich A, Bock M, et al. Differential phosphorylation-dependent regulation of constitutively active and muscarinic receptor-activated I$_{K,ACh}$ channels in patients with chronic atrial fibrillation. *Cardiovasc Res.* 2007;74:426–437.

65. Yue L, Melnyk P, Gaspo R, Wang Z, Nattel S. Molecular mechanisms underlying ionic remodeling in a dog model of atrial fibrillation. *Circ Res.* 1999;84: 776–784.

66. Qi XY, Yeh YH, Xiao L, et al. Cellular signaling underlying atrial tachycardia remodeling of L-type calcium current. *Circ Res.* 2008;103:845–854.

67. Sun H, Chartier D, Leblanc N, Nattel S. Intracellular calcium changes and tachycardia-induced contractile dysfunction in canine atrial myocytes. *Cardiovasc Res.* 2001;49:751–761.

68. Bosch RF, Scherer CR, Rub N, et al. Molecular mechanisms of early electrical remodeling: transcriptional downregulation of ion channel subunits reduces I$_{Ca,L}$ and I$_{to}$ in rapid atrial pacing in rabbits. *J Am Coll Cardiol.* 2003;41:858–869.

69. Gaborit N, Steenman M, Lamirault G, et al. Human atrial ion channel and transporter subunit gene-expression remodeling associated with valvular heart disease and atrial fibrillation. *Circulation.* 2005;112:471–481.

70. Greiser M, Halaszovich CR, Frechen D, et al. Pharmacological evidence for altered src kinase regulation of I$_{Ca,L}$ in patients with chronic atrial fibrillation. *Naunyn Schmiedebergs Arch Pharmacol.* 2007;375:383–392.

71. Carnes CA, Janssen PM, Ruehr ML, et al. Atrial glutathione content, calcium current, and contractility. *J Biol Chem.* 2007;282:28063–28073.

72. Harada M, Tadevosyan A, Qi X, et al. Atrial fibrillation activates AMP-dependent protein kinase and its regulation of cellular calcium handling: potential role in metabolic adaptation and prevention of progression. *J Am Coll Cardiol.* 2015;66:47–58.

73. Luo X, Yang B, Nattel S. MicroRNAs and atrial fibrillation: mechanisms and translational potential. *Nat Rev Cardiol.* 2015;12:80–90.

74. Lu Y, Zhang Y, Wang N, et al. MicroRNA-328 contributes to adverse electrical remodeling in atrial fibrillation. *Circulation.* 2010;122:2378–2387.

75. Barana A, Matamoros M, Dolz-Gaiton P, et al. Chronic atrial fibrillation increases microRNA-21 in human atrial myocytes decreasing L-type calcium current. *Circ Arrhythm Electrophysiol.* 2014;7:861–868.

76. Antzelevitch C, Pollevick GD, Cordeiro JM, et al. Loss-of-function mutations in the cardiac calcium channel underlie a new clinical entity characterized by ST-segment elevation, short QT intervals, and sudden cardiac death. *Circulation.* 2007;115:442–449.

77. Pandit SV, Berenfeld O, Anumonwo JM, et al. Ionic determinants of functional reentry in a 2-D model of human atrial cells during simulated chronic atrial fibrillation. *Biophys J.* 2005;88:3806–3821.

78. Glasscock E, Voigt N, McCauley MD, et al. Expression and function of Kv1.1 potassium channels in human atria from patients with atrial fibrillation. *Basic Res Cardiol.* 2015;110:505.

79. Qi XY, Diness JG, Brundel BJ, et al. Role of small-conductance calcium-activated potassium channels in atrial electrophysiology and fibrillation in the dog. *Circulation.* 2014;129:430–440.

80. Schmidt C, Wiedmann F, Voigt N, et al. Upregulation of K$_2$p3.1 K$^+$ current causes action potential shortening in patients with chronic atrial fibrillation. *Circulation.* 2015;132:82–92.

81. Voigt N, Trausch A, Knaut M, et al. Left-to-right atrial inward rectifier potassium current gradients in patients with paroxysmal versus chronic atrial fibrillation. *Circ Arrhythm Electrophysiol.* 2010;3:472–480.

82. Voigt N, Maguy A, Yeh YH, et al. Changes in I$_{K,ACh}$ single-channel activity with atrial tachycardia remodelling in canine atrial cardiomyocytes. *Cardiovasc Res.* 2008;77:35–43.

83. Girmatsion Z, Biliczki P, Bonauer A, et al. Changes in microRNA-1 expression and I$_{K1}$ up-regulation in human atrial fibrillation. *Heart Rhythm.* 2009;6:1802–1809.

84. Luo X, Pan Z, Shan H, et al. MicroRNA-26 governs profibrillatory inward-rectifier potassium current changes in atrial fibrillation. *J Clin Invest.* 2013;123:1939–1951.

85. Karle CA, Zitron E, Zhang W, et al. Human cardiac inwardly-rectifying K$^+$ channel Kir2.1b is inhibited by direct protein kinase C-dependent regulation in human isolated cardiomyocytes and in an expression system. *Circulation.* 2002;106:1493–1499.

86. Qi XY, Huang H, Ordog B, et al. Fibroblast inward-rectifier potassium current upregulation in profibrillatory atrial remodeling. *Circ Res.* 2015;116:836–845.

87. Voigt N, Heijman J, Trausch A, et al. Impaired Na$^+$-dependent regulation of acetylcholine-activated inward-rectifier K$^+$ current modulates action potential rate dependence in patients with chronic atrial fibrillation. *J Mol Cell Cardiol.* 2013;61:142–152.

88. Makary S, Voigt N, Maguy A, et al. Differential protein kinase C isoform regulation and increased constitutive activity of acetylcholine-regulated potassium channels in atrial remodeling. *Circ Res.* 2011;109:1031–1043.

89. Voigt N, Makary S, Nattel S, Dobrev D. Voltage-clamp-based methods for the detection of constitutively active acetylcholine-gated I$_{K,ACh}$ channels in the diseased heart. *Methods Enzymol.* 2010;484:653–675.

90. Kneller J, Zou R, Vigmond EJ, Wang Z, Leon LJ, Nattel S. Cholinergic atrial fibrillation in a computer model of a two-dimensional sheet of canine atrial cells with realistic ionic properties. *Circ Res.* 2002;90:E73–E87.

91. Kovoor P, Wickman K, Maguire CT, et al. Evaluation of the role of I$_{K,ACh}$ in atrial fibrillation using a mouse knockout model. *J Am Coll Cardiol.* 2001;37:2136–2143.

92. Nattel S, Maguy A, Le Bouter S, Yeh YH. Arrhythmogenic ion-channel remodeling in the heart: heart failure, myocardial infarction, and atrial fibrillation. *Physiol Rev.* 2007;87:425–456.

93. Dhein S, Hagen A, Jozwiak J, et al. Improving cardiac gap junction communication as a new antiarrhythmic mechanism: the action of antiarrhythmic peptides. *Naunyn Schmiedebergs Arch Pharmacol.* 2010;381:221–234.

94. Nishida K, Michael G, Dobrev D, Nattel S. Animal models for atrial fibrillation: clinical insights and scientific opportunities. *Europace.* 2010;12:160–172.

95. Firouzi M, Ramanna H, Kok B, et al. Association of human connexin40 gene polymorphisms with atrial vulnerability as a risk factor for idiopathic atrial fibrillation. *Circ Res.* 2004;95:e29–e33.

96. Gollob MH, Jones DL, Krahn AD, et al. Somatic mutations in the connexin 40 gene (GJA5) in atrial fibrillation. *N Engl J Med.* 2006;354:2677–2688.

97. Juang JM, Chern YR, Tsai CT, et al. The association of human connexin 40 genetic polymorphisms with atrial fibrillation. *Int J Cardiol.* 2007;116:107–112.

98. Burstein B, Comtois P, Michael G, et al. Changes in connexin expression and the atrial fibrillation substrate in congestive heart failure. *Circ Res.* 2009;105:1213–1222.

99. Bikou O, Thomas D, Trappe K, et al. Connexin 43 gene therapy prevents persistent atrial fibrillation in a porcine model. *Cardiovasc Res.* 2011;92:218–225.

100. Igarashi T, Finet JE, Takeuchi A, et al. Connexin gene transfer preserves conduction velocity and prevents atrial fibrillation. *Circulation.* 2012;125:216–225.

101. Dhein S. Cardiac ischemia and uncoupling: gap junctions in ischemia and infarction. *Adv Cardiol.* 2006;42:198–212.

102. Hagendorff A, Schumacher B, Kirchhoff S, Luderitz B, Willecke K. Conduction disturbances and increased atrial vulnerability in connexin40-deficient mice analyzed by transesophageal stimulation. *Circulation.* 1999;99: 1508–1515.

103. Wirka RC, Gore S, Van Wagoner DR, et al. A common connexin-40 gene promoter variant affects connexin-40 expression in human atria and is associated with atrial fibrillation. *Circ Arrhythm Electrophysiol.* 2011;4:87–93.

104. Sossalla S, Kallmeyer B, Wagner S, et al. Altered Na$^+$ currents in atrial fibrillation effects of ranolazine on arrhythmias and contractility in human atrial myocardium. *J Am Coll Cardiol.* 2010;55:2330–2342.

105. Olson TM, Michels VV, Ballew JD, et al. Sodium channel mutations and susceptibility to heart failure and atrial fibrillation. *JAMA.* 2005;293:447–454.

106. Chen LY, Ballew JD, Herron KJ, Rodeheffer RJ, Olson TM. A common polymorphism in SCN5A is associated with lone atrial fibrillation. *Clin Pharmacol Ther.* 2007;81:35–41.

107. Ellinor PT, Nam EG, Shea MA, Milan DJ, Ruskin JN, MacRae CA. Cardiac sodium channel mutation in atrial fibrillation. *Heart Rhythm.* 2008;5:99–105.

108. Hedley PL, Jorgensen P, Schlamowitz S, et al. The genetic basis of Brugada syndrome: a mutation update. *Hum Mutat.* 2009;30:1256–1266.

109. Watanabe H, Darbar D, Kaiser DW, et al. Mutations in sodium channel beta1- and beta2-subunits associated with atrial fibrillation. *Circ Arrhythm Electrophysiol.* 2009;2:268–275.

110. Olesen MS, Jespersen T, Nielsen JB, et al. Mutations in sodium channel beta-subunit SCN3B are associated with early-onset lone atrial fibrillation. *Cardiovasc Res.* 2011;89:786–793.

111. Wang P, Yang Q, Wu X, et al. Functional dominant-negative mutation of sodium channel subunit gene SCN3B associated with atrial fibrillation in a Chinese GeneID population. *Biochem Biophys Res Commun.* 2010;398:98–104.

112. Jabbari J, Olesen MS, Yuan L, et al. Common and rare variants in SCN10A modulate the risk of atrial fibrillation. *Circ Cardiovasc Genet.* 2015;8:64–73.

113. Lamirault G, Gaborit N, Le Meur N, et al. Gene expression profile associated with chronic atrial fibrillation and underlying valvular heart disease in man. *J Mol Cell Cardiol.* 2006;40:173–184.

114. Li D, Fareh S, Leung TK, Nattel S. Promotion of atrial fibrillation by heart failure in dogs: atrial remodeling of a different sort. *Circulation.* 1999;100:87–95.

115. Dzeshka MS, Lip GY, Snezhitskiy V, Shantsila E. Cardiac fibrosis in patients with atrial fibrillation: mechanisms and clinical implications. *J Am Coll Cardiol.* 2015;66:943–959.

116. Yue L, Xie J, Nattel S. Molecular determinants of cardiac fibroblast electrical function and therapeutic implications for atrial fibrillation. *Cardiovasc Res.* 2011;89: 744–753.

117. Ehrlich JR, Hohnloser SH, Nattel S. Role of angiotensin system and effects of its inhibition in atrial fibrillation: clinical and experimental evidence. *Eur Heart J.* 2006;27:512–518.

118. He X, Gao X, Peng L, et al. Atrial fibrillation induces myocardial fibrosis through angiotensin II type 1 receptor-specific Arkadia-mediated downregulation of Smad7. *Circ Res.* 2011;108:164–175.

119. Koinuma D, Shinozaki M, Komuro A, et al. Arkadia amplifies TGF-beta superfamily signalling through degradation of Smad7. *EMBO J.* 2003;22:6458–6470.

120. Hunyady L, Catt KJ. Pleiotropic AT1 receptor signaling pathways mediating physiological and pathogenic actions of angiotensin II. *Mol Endocrinol.* 2006;20:953–970.

121. Burstein B, Libby E, Calderone A, Nattel S. Differential behaviors of atrial versus ventricular fibroblasts: a potential role for platelet-derived growth factor in atrial-ventricular remodeling differences. *Circulation.* 2008;117:1630–1641.

122. Verheule S, Sato T, Everett TT, et al. Increased vulnerability to atrial fibrillation in transgenic mice with selective atrial fibrosis caused by overexpression of TGF-beta1. *Circ Res.* 2004;94:1458–1465.

123. Attisano L, Wrana JL. Signal transduction by the TGF-beta superfamily. *Science.* 2002;296:1646–1647.

124. Burstein B, Qi XY, Yeh YH, Calderone A, Nattel S. Atrial cardiomyocyte tachycardia alters cardiac fibroblast function: a novel consideration in atrial remodeling. *Cardiovasc Res.* 2007;76:442–452.

125. Tsai CT, Tseng CD, Hwang JJ, et al. Tachycardia of atrial myocytes induces collagen expression in atrial fibroblasts through transforming growth factor β1. *Cardiovasc Res.* 2011;89:805–815.

126. Ponten A, Folestad EB, Pietras K, Eriksson U. Platelet-derived growth factor D induces cardiac fibrosis and proliferation of vascular smooth muscle cells in heart-specific transgenic mice. *Circ Res.* 2005;97:1036–1045.

127. Gudbjartsson DF, Arnar DO, Helgadottir A, et al. Variants conferring risk of atrial fibrillation on chromosome 4q25. *Nature.* 2007;448:353–357.

128. Cardin S, Libby E, Pelletier P, et al. Contrasting gene expression profiles in two canine models of atrial fibrillation. *Circ Res.* 2007;100:425–433.

129. Adam O, Lavall D, Theobald K, et al. Rac1-induced connective tissue growth factor regulates connexin 43 and N-cadherin expression in atrial fibrillation. *J Am Coll Cardiol.* 2010;55:469–480.

130. Ko WC, Hong CY, Hou SM, et al. Elevated expression of connective tissue growth factor in human atrial fibrillation and angiotensin II-treated cardiomyocytes. *Circ J.* 2011;75:1592–1600.

131. van Rooij E, Sutherland LB, Thatcher JE, et al. Dysregulation of microRNAs after myocardial infarction reveals a role of miR-29 in cardiac fibrosis. *Proc Natl Acad Sci U S A.* 2008;105:13027–13032.

132. Dawson K, Wakili R, Ördög B, et al. MicroRNA29: a mechanistic contributor and potential biomarker in atrial fibrillation. *Circulation.* 2013;127:1466–1475.

133. Duisters RF, Tijsen AJ, Schroen B, et al. miR-133 and miR-30 regulate connective tissue growth factor: implications for a role of microRNAs in myocardial matrix remodeling. *Circ Res.* 2009;104:170–178.

134. Chen Y, Wakili R, Luo X, et al. Distinct atrial and ventricular microRNA expression changes in experimental dilated cardiomyopathy: cell-type specificity and time course. *J Mol Cell Cardiol.* 2014;12:113–124.

135. Thum T, Gross C, Fiedler J, et al. MicroRNA-21 contributes to myocardial disease by stimulating MAP kinase signalling in fibroblasts. *Nature.* 2008;456:980–984.

136. Patrick DM, Montgomery RL, Qi X, et al. Stress-dependent cardiac remodeling occurs in the absence of microRNA-21 in mice. *J Clin Invest.* 2010;120: 3912–3916.

137. Cardin S, Guasch E, Luo X, et al. A role for microRNA in atrial profibrillatory fibrotic remodeling associated with experimental postinfarction heart failure. *Circ Arrhythm Electrophysiol.* 2012;5:1027–1035.

138. Fatini C, Sticchi E, Gensini F, et al. Lone and secondary nonvalvular atrial fibrillation: role of a genetic susceptibility. *Int J Cardiol.* 2007;120:59–65.

139. Bedi M, McNamara D, London B, Schwartzman D. Genetic susceptibility to atrial fibrillation in patients with congestive heart failure. *Heart Rhythm.* 2006;3:808–812.

140. Kato K, Oguri M, Hibino T, et al. Genetic factors for lone atrial fibrillation. *Int J Mol Med.* 2007;19:933–939.

141. Benjamin EJ, Rice KM, Arking DE, et al. Variants in ZFHX3 are associated with atrial fibrillation in individuals of European ancestry. *Nat Genet.* 2009;41:879–881.

142. Mommersteeg MT, Brown NA, Prall OW. Pitx2c and Nkx2-5 are required for the formation and identity of the pulmonary myocardium. *Circ Res.* 2007;101:902–909.

143. Mommersteeg MT, Hoogaars WM, Prall OW, et al. Molecular pathway for the localized formation of the sinoatrial node. *Circ Res.* 2007;100:354–362.

144. Kim CJ, Song JH, Cho YG, et al. Down-regulation of ATBF1 is a major inactivating mechanism in hepatocellular carcinoma. *Histopathology.* 2008;52:552–559.

145. Sun X, Frierson HF, Chen C, et al. Frequent somatic mutations of the transcription factor ATBF1 in human prostate cancer. *Nat Genet.* 2005;37:407–412.

146. Kim TS, Kawaguchi M, Suzuki M, et al. The ZFHX3 (ATBF1) transcription factor induces PDGFRB, which activates ATM in the cytoplasm to protect cerebellar neurons from oxidative stress. *Dis Model Mech.* 2010;3:752–762.

147. Harada M, Luo X, Qi XY, et al. Transient receptor potential canonical-3 channel-dependent fibroblast regulation in atrial fibrillation. *Circulation.* 2012;126:2051–2064.

148. Li N, Chiang DY, Wang S, et al. Ryanodine receptor-mediated calcium leak drives progressive development of an atrial fibrillation substrate in a transgenic mouse model. *Circulation.* 2014;129:1276–1285.

149. Donahue JK. Biological therapies for atrial fibrillation: ready for prime time? *J Cardiovasc Pharmacol.* 2016;67:19–25.

43 Myofibroblasts, Cytokines, and Persistent Atrial Fibrillation

Kuljeet Kaur and José Jalife

Atrial fibrillation (AF) is the most common sustained cardiac arrhythmia observed in clinical practice. It is the most important cause of embolic stroke and is associated with increased morbidity and mortality.[1] Yet despite more than 100 years of basic and clinical research, we still do not fully understand its fundamental mechanisms and have not learned how to effectively treat it. When AF lasts continuously for more than 7 days, it is designated as persistent AF.[2] Spontaneous, pharmacological, or ablative resumption of sinus rhythm (SR) is infrequent in persistent AF, with prompt recurrences or commonly failed cardioversions. Episodes lasting more than 1 year are termed "long-term persistent AF." While persistent AF is usually accompanied by comorbidities like hypertension, heart failure (HF), and ischemic heart disease, fundamental mechanisms governing AF perpetuation are poorly understood, which explains in part why AF prevention and treatment remain suboptimal. Nevertheless, it is reasonable to speculate that the continuous high frequency and heterogeneous bombardment of atrial cells and tissues by electrical fibrillatory waves during long-lasting AF lead to a modification of the molecular substrate, with consequent electrical and structural remodeling, substantial enough to increase the likelihood of perpetuation of the electrical sources that maintain the arrhythmia.

Fibrosis has been implicated in initiation and maintenance of arrhythmia, affecting electrical propagation through slow, discontinuous conduction with "zigzag" propagation,[3,4] reduced regional coupling,[5] abrupt changes in fibrotic bundle size,[6] and microanatomical reentry.[7] In the past, most clinical, experimental, and numerical studies have regarded fibrosis as electrically insulating obstacles. However, heart injury promotes differentiation of fibroblasts into myofibroblasts,[8] which are hypercontractile and hypersecretory of soluble proteins termed "cytokines" that are known to affect atrial extracellular matrix (ECM) through the secretion of collagen and the generation of fibrosis. Myofibroblasts have been shown to electrotonically couple to myocytes in vitro.[9–13] However, electrical coupling between fully differentiated myocytes and fibroblasts has never been demonstrated in normal atrial or ventricular muscles. Nevertheless, it is tempting to speculate whether electrical remodeling associated with cardiac ischemia or sustained AF, in response to heterocellular electrical communication, occurs only in response to injury after fibroblasts have phenotypically switched to myofibroblasts and myocytes have undergone dedifferentiation in the embryonic stage.[8,14] On the other hand, it is

probable that cytokines released from myofibroblasts in the fibrillating atria contribute to ion channel dysfunction and electrical remodeling.[9,10] Regardless of the mechanisms involved, it is likely that both myofibroblasts and fibrosis play critical roles in atrial electroanatomical remodeling and further facilitate perpetuation of AF.

AF per se may promote cardiac fibrosis, and it is notable that although numerous studies indicate a clear association between AF and fibrosis, the underlying pathological basis of AF-induced fibrosis remains poorly understood. Arguably, early identification and prevention of molecular and cellular mechanisms of the atrial fibrotic process might halt AF progression and improve its response to both pharmacological and nonpharmacological therapies. This highlights the importance of investigating the biology of fibroblasts as "sentinel cells"[15]; their role in the fibrotic process; the impact of their interactions with myocytes; their effect on sarcolemmal ion channel behavior, cardiac excitability, and atrial impulse propagation; and their possible role in the mechanisms underlying the transition from paroxysmal to persistent or permanent AF. In this chapter, we present a brief and necessarily incomplete review of possible mechanisms underlying AF-induced fibrosis. We pay particular attention to the role played by activated fibroblasts (myofibroblasts) and the cytokines released by them during the mechanisms of electrical and structural remodeling. Our objective is two-fold: first, to examine our understanding of the molecular mechanisms of fibrosis; and second, to help predict how myofibroblasts impinge on the electrical function of atrial myocytes by means of signaling molecules and result in the electrophysiological remodeling that contributes to AF perpetuation.

Cardiac Fibroblasts and Myofibroblasts

Cardiac fibroblasts are critical players in normal cardiac function.[11] Although occupying a small portion of the myocardial tissue volume, cardiac fibroblasts account for 50%–70% of the cells in a normal adult mammalian heart[12] and even more in pathological conditions, where cardiac fibrosis ensues due to the transformation of fibroblasts to myofibroblasts, which is a key event in connective tissue remodeling (Fig. 43.1).[11,13,15] Cardiac myofibroblast proliferation and migration with concomitant collagenous matrix accumulation leading to fibrosis develop during myocardial remodeling in ischemic, hypertensive, hypertrophic, and dilated cardiomyopathies,[16] arrhythmogenic right ventricular cardiomyopathy (ARVC),[17] and HF. Similarly, myofibroblasts are active contributors to atrial fibrosis,[11] which is part of the maladaptive atrial response to AF.[18] Myofibroblasts are phenotypically transformed (active) fibroblasts, containing α-smooth muscle actin (αSMA) and expressing integrins, fibronectin, and other adhesion proteins (see Fig. 43.1). They were first identified by Gabbiani and Majno, who termed them "myofibroblasts,"[19] after demonstrating their contractility in response to chemical mediators of inflammation and strips of granulation tissue. These wound-healing fibroblast-like cells are involved in each of the fibrous tissue responses

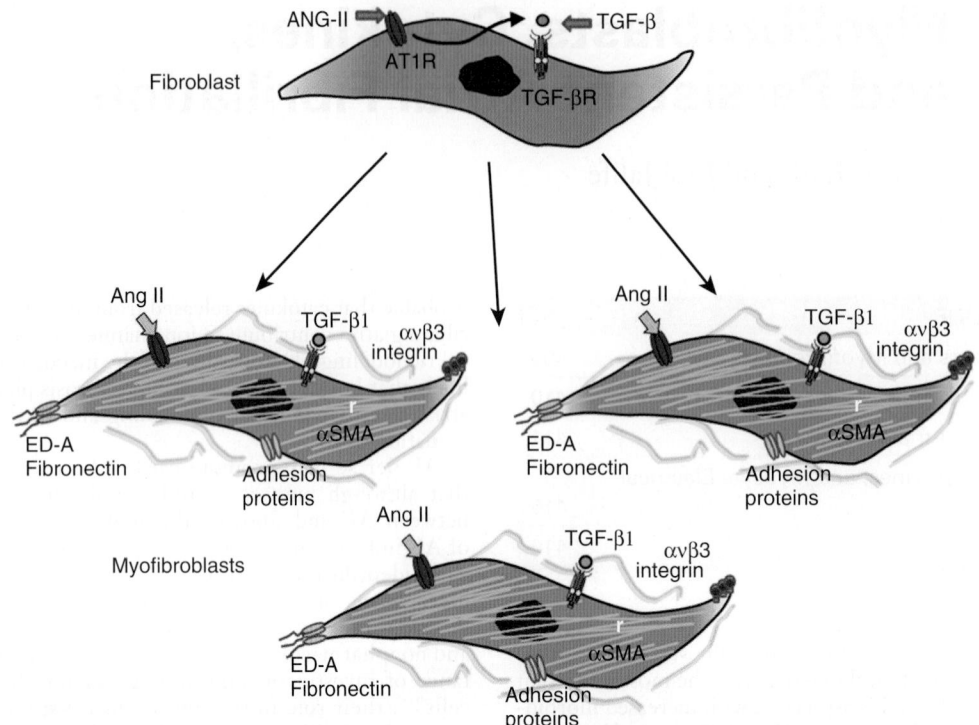

FIGURE 43.1 The phenotypic transformation (activation) of fibroblasts into myofibroblasts is highly controlled by the renin-angiotensin-aldosterone system and downstream activation of soluble proteins termed "cytokines," particularly transforming growth factor (*TGF*)-β1. Myofibroblasts proliferate and hypersecrete α-smooth muscle actin (*αSMA*), which makes them hypercontractile and promotes their expression of integrins and other adhesion proteins, as well as extracellular matrix genes, including fibronectin and fibrillar collagen types I and III. *Ang II*, Angiotensin II.

present throughout the body. Yet their role in the mechanism underlying structural and electrophysiological remodeling secondary to sustained AF has not been fully elucidated. Much of the information on the specific role played by myofibroblasts in atrial fibrosis and AF perpetuation derives from what is known about hypertensive heart disease, in which there is impaired tissue compliance and symptomatic failure linked to interstitial fibrosis and the expression of ECM genes, including fibrillar collagen types I and III and fibronectin. It has also been shown that fibroblast proliferation and collagen deposition are significantly and heterogeneously increased in all atrial regions after prolonged AF[20,21] and that atrial fibrosis development is highly controlled by the renin-angiotensin-aldosterone system and downstream activation of soluble proteins termed "cytokines," particularly transforming growth factor (TGF)-β1 and platelet-derived growth factor (PDGF).[9,10]

Molecular Regulation of Cardiac Fibroblasts

Micro RNAs (miRNAs or miRs) are naturally occurring small noncoding RNA molecules that are partially complementary to one or more messenger RNAs.[22] A number of ubiquitously distributed miRs have been shown to be involved in structural or electrical remodeling, and several have been suggested to exhibit a strong arrhythmogenic potential.[23] It is highly probable that multiple miRs contribute to controlling cardiac arrhythmogenesis and that different miRs are involved in different types of arrhythmias under different pathophysiological conditions, including AF.[24-26]

A detailed study of miRNA expression in tachypaced dog hearts revealed that miRNA changes are cell specific.[27] For example, miR-29b, which is responsible for the degradation of collagen-1A1, collagen-3A1, and fibrillin genes, is expressed in fibroblasts at five times higher levels than in atrial myocytes.[28] In tachypaced-induced HF dogs, fibroblasts from the left atrial appendage showed a greater decrease in miR-29b expressions than those from the left ventricle (LV), thereby supporting the idea that atrial fibroblasts are more profibrotic than ventricular fibroblasts.[27] In another study, miR-29b plasma levels were decreased in patients with congestive HF (CHF) or AF and were further decreased in patients with both AF and CHF. miR-29b expression was also reduced in the atria of chronic AF patients. In the same study, viral-mediated knockdown of miR-29b in mice significantly increased atrial collagen-1A1 mRNA expression and cardiac tissue collagen content. Altogether, the above data substantiated possible roles of miR-29b in atrial fibrotic remodeling and as a biomarker.[28]

Recent studies indicate that fibroblasts respond to high-frequency electrical excitation by undergoing significant electrophysiological remodeling. In one such study, atrial fibroblasts isolated from ventricular tachypacing–induced HF dogs exhibited increased Ba^{2+}-sensitive inward rectifier potassium current (I_{K1}) and increased *KCNJ2* mRNA expressions with miRNA-26a downregulation.[29] As a result of the increased I_{K1}, fibroblasts from tachypaced dogs demonstrated hyperpolarized resting membrane potentials leading to enhanced calcium entry and increased proliferation.[30]

Cardiac fibroblasts express a variety of transient receptor potential (TRP) channels,[31] some of which have been identified as important activators of myofibroblast differentiation.[32] Most TRP channels are activated by a number of ligands and by mechanical stretch and allow Ca^{2+} and Na^+ entry. One of the so-called canonical channels, TRPC3, is highly expressed in cardiac fibroblasts.[33] TRPC3 increases extracellular signal–regulated kinase (ERK) activation and contributes to increased fibrosis. Atrial samples from AF patients and from tachypacing-induced

43

AF goats showed increased TRPC3 mRNA expression compared with that in respective control samples.[34] Cultured left atrial fibroblasts from dogs maintained in AF for 1 week showed increased TRPC3 with increased ERK phosphorylation and ECM gene expression.[34] Inhibition of TRPC3 channels by pyrazole-3 in dogs suppressed AF substrate development, atrial fibroblast proliferation rate, αSMA expression, and ERK phosphorylation, suggesting a role for increased calcium influx via TRPC3 channels in AF and atrial fibrosis.[34] TRPM6 was shown to be upregulated in atrial tissue of AF patients who also had increased atrial cell size, fibrosis, collagen, and TGF-β1 expression.[35] Of interest, atrial fibroblasts from chronic AF patients exhibit increased TRPM7 current and calcium influx.[36] Silencing TRPM7 in atrial fibroblasts decreased TRPM7 current and calcium influx and reduced fibroblast-to-myofibroblast differentiation and TGF-β–mediated fibrosis. On the other hand, TGF-β treatment increased TRPM7 expression in atrial cells.[36] TGF-β has been shown to involve TRPV4 in its effect on fibrosis markers in fibroblasts. TGF-β treatment increases TRPV4 expression, leading to increased calcium influx.[37]

Inflammation and Atrial Fibrillation

A mechanistic role of inflammation in human AF remains uncertain. To fully understand the role of myofibroblasts and/or cytokines in fibrosis and AF perpetuation, it will be necessary to fully understand the role played by inflammation, which is known to be involved in the pathogenesis of fibrosis in several cardiovascular diseases.[38] Increasing evidence from animal models now suggests that inflammatory pathways are directly linked to cellular and subcellular mechanisms known to also lead to AF.[38] Activated inflammatory cells, such as neutrophils, lymphocytes, monocytes, and resident macrophages; proinflammatory cytokines; and activated platelets are important players in this picture (Fig. 43.2). Moreover, inflammatory cascades alter ion channel function in myocytes and are also strongly associated with fibrosis.[38] Inflammatory stimuli, such as nicotinamide adenine dinucleotide phosphate (NADPH) oxidase–derived reactive oxygen species (ROS), cytokines, growth factors, angiotensin II (Ang II), and other hormones, and mechanical stretch are well-known triggers of fibroblast proliferation, migration, and differentiation into myofibroblasts, which are critical players in the development of fibrosis.[38]

Absence of programmed cell death 1 (PD-1) gene in mice increased circulating levels of inflammatory cytokines interleukin (IL)-2, -4, -6, -10, and -17; interferon-γ; and tumor necrosis factor (TNF)-α. These mice exhibited increased atrial fibrosis and decreased atrial effective refractory period, thus making these animals more prone to atrial arrhythmias.[39] Furthermore, intense endurance exercise increases susceptibility to AF in mice and is associated with macrophage infiltration and fibrosis. Exercise-induced atrial remodeling was prevented by treatment with the TNF-α inhibitor (etanercept) and was not seen in mice lacking TNF-α gene. The study indicated that TNF-α–induced inflammation is a major player in exercise-induced AF.[40]

The idea that AF promotes inflammation has been derived from studies demonstrating that chronic human AF is associated with increased atrial oxidative stress and peroxynitrite formation.[41] Thereafter, long-term rapid atrial pacing experiments in dogs demonstrated a pacing-induced shortening of the atrial effective refractory period, which was associated with decreased tissue ascorbate levels and increased protein nitration. The latter is a biomarker of peroxynitrite formation.[42] Oral ascorbate supplementation attenuated all changes. In a parallel study, supplemental ascorbate was administered to 43 patients before and for 5 days after cardiac bypass graft surgery.[42] The incidence of postoperative AF was 16.3% in patients receiving ascorbate

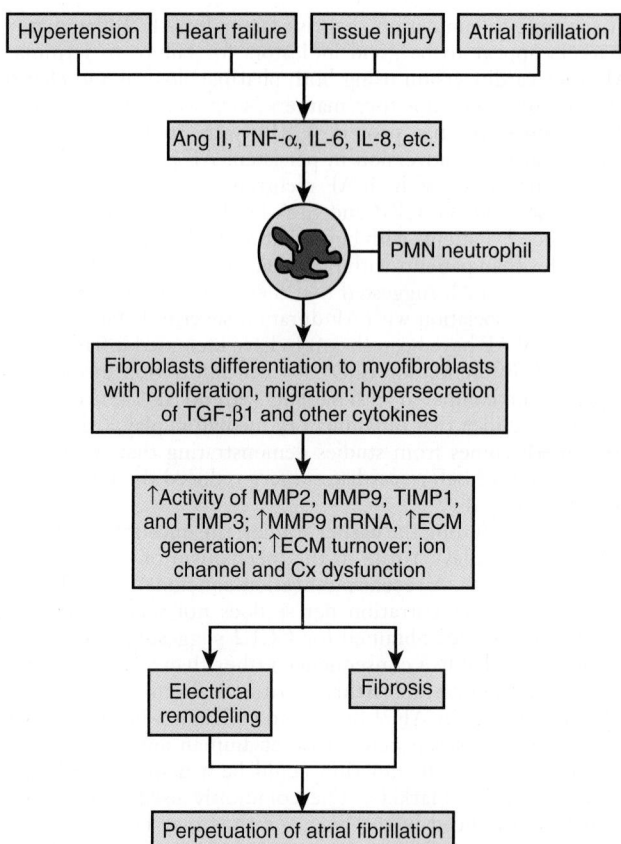

FIGURE 43.2 Possible inflammatory pathways involved in the perpetuation of atrial fibrillation. Hypertension, heart failure, tissue injury, or sustained atrial fibrillation lead to the release of proinflammatory cytokines and hormones, such as angiotensin II (*Ang II*), tumor necrosis factor (*TNF*)-α, interleukin (*IL*)-6, and IL-8, which promote activation of leukocytes with subsequent activation of fibroblasts into myofibroblasts, which proliferate and become hypersecretory of a number of cytokines. As a result, connexin and ion channel dysfunction occurs along with myocyte apoptosis and matrix generation and turnover, which lead to electrical and structural remodeling (fibrosis) that contributes to atrial fibrillation perpetuation. *ECM*, Extracellular matrix; *PMN*, polymorphonuclear; *TGF*, transforming growth factor.

compared with 34.9% in control subjects. More recently, rapid atrial pacing in a porcine model increased the activity of profibrotic enzymes matrix metalloproteinases (MMPs) 2 and 9 in the atrial interstitium, increased the MMP9 mRNA expression, and increased the activity of tissue inhibitor of matrix metalloproteinases (TIMPs) 1 and 3.[43] Fig. 43.2 illustrates a likely scenario linking sustained AF to inflammation with subsequent electrical remodeling, fibrosis, and AF perpetuation. Proinflammatory cytokines and hormones, such as Ang II, TNF-α, IL-6, and IL-8, related to cardiovascular diseases and tissue injury, promote activation of leukocytes with subsequent release of cytokines and ROS. As a result, connexin and ion channel dysfunction occurs, along with myocyte apoptosis, as well as matrix generation and turnover, which leads to electrical and structural remodeling that predisposes to AF.[38]

Clinical studies have identified inflammation as a pathogenic factor in AF and have shown a correlation between inflammatory markers and AF incidence.[44] In a 5-year follow-up of an original Framingham Heart Study cohort of about 800 patients with no history of AF, subjects' white blood cell counts were significantly associated with AF development after correction for standard risk factors for AF.[45] As a standard indicator of general inflammation, white blood cell count is also an indicator of the role of systemic inflammation as a risk factor for AF. Inflammatory markers appear to be good indicators for failure to terminate AF after cardioversion using both pharmacological and electrical methods. Inflammatory markers, such as serum amyloid A (SAA) and C-reactive protein (CRP), were studied before and 3 weeks after cardioversion in persistent AF patients[46]; 33% of patients presented with an AF recurrence at 3 weeks after cardioversion, and the CRP and SAA levels were associated with recurrence.[46] Patients with persistent AF had a higher inflammatory index than patients with proximal AF, as measured by serum CRP levels, which suggested that there was progressive inflammation in association with AF duration/severity.[47] Patients with a history of AF have been shown to have increased inflammatory cluster of differentiation (CD) 45+ cell infiltration in the atrial myocardium compared with patients with no AF.[48] Further support for the idea that inflammatory mediators play a significant role in AF comes from studies demonstrating that hydrocortisone treatment before cardiac surgery reduced the incidence of postoperative AF.[49]

Notwithstanding the earlier studies, the question of whether inflammation plays a role in the mechanism of AF remains a matter of debate. A recent publication concluded that elevated plasma CRP concentration per se does not increase the risk for AF, and values obtained for CCL2 suggested that inflammation is probably a consequence rather than a cause of AF.[50] Moreover, rheumatoid arthritis patients do not appear to be at a higher risk for AF.[51] Soeki and colleagues have suggested that the data discrepancies between human and animal studies in regard to inflammation could be a matter of selection of inflammation markers. The commonly used marker CRP is mainly produced in the liver and thus may be a poor indicator of cardiac inflammation as a risk factor for AF. On the other hand, pentraxin 3, which is a locally produced inflammation marker, was shown to be differentially upregulated in AF patients, with serum samples from the left atrial appendage being greater than the periphery. However, levels of other inflammatory markers studied were not different from control, indicating an inconsistency between animal and human studies.[52]

Cytokines and Human Atrial Fibrillation

The development of interstitial fibrosis and its impact on atrial contractile and electrical function have been found to be central for AF maintenance.[21,53,54] Fibroblast proliferation and collagen deposition are significantly and heterogeneously increased in all atrial regions after prolonged AF,[20,21] a process that is highly controlled by the renin-angiotensin-aldosterone system and the downstream activation of soluble cytokines such as TGF-β1 and PDGF. Originally termed "cytokines" by Stanley Cohen in 1974, these proteins are major players in immune reactions.[55] However, while immune cells are a major source of cytokines, a number of other cell types, including heart cells, can synthesize and release them.[56] Multiple studies have demonstrated close relationships between elevated cytokines and AF. In patients with either paroxysmal or persistent AF, serum levels of vascular endothelial growth factor (VEGF), IL-8, soluble intercellular adhesion molecule 1(sICAM-1), and TGF-β1 are upregulated at baseline,[57] and increased VEGF has been shown to associate independently with AF occurrence.[58] IL-18 levels are also higher in persistent AF patients with atrial dilatation.[59] Graded increases in TNF-α and N-terminal probrain natriuretic peptide (NTpBNP) have been shown in various AF groups, with the levels being highest in permanent AF.[60] A cross-sectional analysis of the Heart and Soul Study patients suggested a genetic link between IL-6 polymorphism 174CC and AF. Patients with this polymorphism have high IL-6 levels.[61]

Increased serum levels of cytokines and other inflammatory markers also correlate with the failure of rhythm control in AF.[62] For example, it has been shown that the expression of IL-2 associates with the outcome of cardioversion with amiodarone; serum IL-2 levels were lower in successfully cardioverted patients compared with noncardioverted patients. In addition, the baseline IL-2 level was a strong indicator of therapeutic success.[62] In patients with paroxysmal or persistent AF, elevated plasma IL-6 and CRP levels appear to be independent predictors of failure of pulmonary vein isolation.[63] In another study, baseline levels of CRP, TNF-α, sICAM-1, and oxidative stress markers were elevated in patients with AF compared with controls and were higher in patients with than those without persistent AF recurrence; however, IL-6 levels were equally elevated in the two subgroups.[64] In yet another clinical study, the serum IL-6, CRP, and CD40L levels decreased in patients with no AF recurrence after ablation, whereas the same indicators did not decrease in patients who failed ablation.[65] An AF-related release of cytokines during SR was suggested by another study in which CRP and IL-6 levels were similar in AF and SR patients. In AF patients, single episodes of AF increased these protein levels.[66]

Along with increases in the proinflammatory proteins, AF is also associated with decreases in antiinflammatory mediators. Peroxisome proliferator–activated receptor-γ (PPARγ), a multifunctional nuclear receptor protein, regulates a number of transcription factors and has been shown to be antiinflammatory.[67] mRNA and protein levels of PPARγ were shown to be decreased in hypertensive patients with AF compared with those with no AF and were further decreased in persistent AF patients compared with paroxysmal patients. In addition, there was a negative correlation between the levels of inflammatory cytokines and PPARγ.[68]

Transforming Growth Factor-β1 and Atrial Fibrillation

Members of the TGF-β family of pleiotropic cytokines are implicated in a wide variety of cell functions.[69] They regulate inflammation, ECM deposition, cell proliferation, differentiation, and growth. In mammalian species, three structurally similar isoforms of TGF-β (TGF-β1, 2, and 3), encoded by three distinct genes, have been identified.[70] The most prevalent is TGF-β1. It is widely expressed in many cell types, whereas the other isoforms are found in a more limited range of cells and tissues.[69] The binding of TGF-β family ligands induces the association between type I and II receptors in a heterodimeric complex (Fig. 43.3). The type II receptor kinase phosphorylates the type I receptor, inducing its serine/threonine kinase activity. Receptor-regulated Smads (R-Smads) are then activated by phosphorylation by the type I receptor kinase. Activated R-Smads form complexes with common-partner Smads (Co-Smad) and translocate into the nucleus.[18] Once there, these proteins bind other transcriptional factors, including both transcriptional coactivators and corepressors.

Knowledge about the effects of TGF-β1 in advancing cardiac hypertrophy and fibrosis in vivo is derived in part from studies in transgenic mice. TGF-β1–overexpressing mice demonstrated significant cardiac hypertrophy accompanied by interstitial fibrosis.[71] On the other hand, cardiac-restricted expression of a mutant TGF-β1 that enhances local TGF-β activity was associated with atrial but not ventricular fibrosis,[72] which suggested that the susceptibility of the atrial myocardium to the fibrogenic actions of TGF-β was greater than that of the ventricular myocardium. Microarray analysis of cardiac samples from such mice revealed that chamber-specific fibrosis occurred because of an increased phosphorylation of SMAD in atrial tissue compared with that in ventricular tissue. Increased atrial fibrosis in transgenic mice

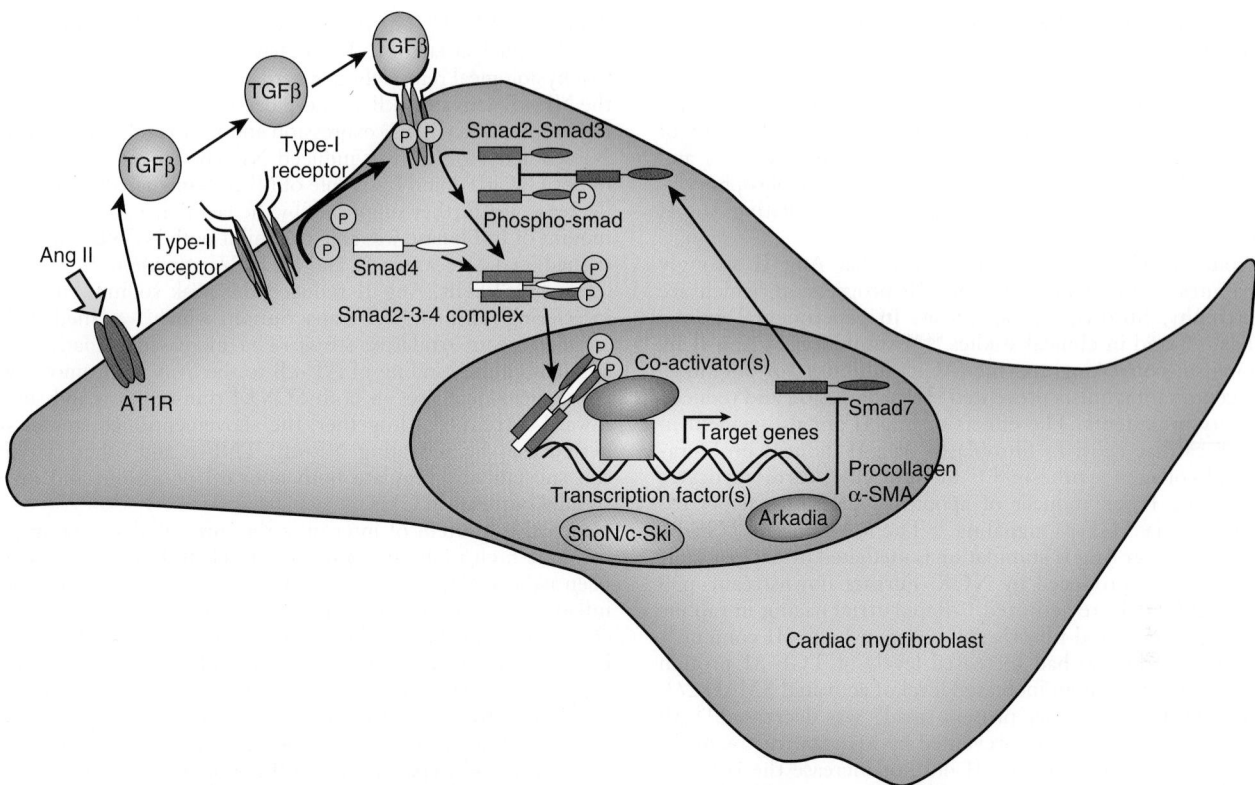

FIGURE 43.3 Angiotensin II (*Ang II*) induces fibrosis through activation of the transforming growth factor (*TGF*)-β signaling pathway in the myofibroblast. Activation of the angiotensin type 1 receptor (*AT1R*) increases the expression of TGF-β1, which leads to phosphorylation of type I and II TGF-β1 membrane receptors. This leads to the formation of a complex that activates Smad2 and Smad3 through phosphorylation, promoting the consolidation of the Smad2-3-4 complex with subsequent translocation to the nucleus, leading to increased transcription of profibrillatory genes. Ang II/AT1R–specific activation of Arkadia-mediated polyubiquitination and degradation of Smad7 is considered to decrease the inhibitory feedback regulation of TGF-β1/Smad signaling and serve as a key mechanism for atrial fibrillation–induced atrial fibrosis.[18]

was mitigated by TGF-β1 receptor 1 kinase inhibition, which provided evidence that atria have increased kinase activity and thus may be more sensitive to the effects of phosphorylated proteins.[73] Along with increased kinase activity in atria, atrial fibroblasts showed higher NADPH oxidase activity than ventricular cells. Atrial fibroblasts treated with TGF-β had greater response in terms of collagen and fibronectin production. This difference in atrial and ventricular fibroblasts was abolished when NADPH oxidase 4 (NOX4) was eliminated.[74] Fibrotic remodeling of the atrium in this transgenic model was sufficient to increase vulnerability to AF.[75]

A single nucleotide polymorphism at codon 25, 915 G>C, which is associated with myocardial infarction and atrial stiffness, is also associated with increased plasma TGF-β1 levels in patients with essential hypertension and AF.[76] Lower atrial voltage, especially in the left atrium, has been associated with AF. Plasma TGF-β1 levels have been shown to strongly correlate with left atrial voltage and volume, suggesting that TGF-β1 is an indicator of AF.[77] In an interesting study in which right atrial appendages were taken from SR and AF patients and were divided into five groups (SR; paroxysmal/chronic persistent AF of <6 months; chronic permanent AF of 7–24 months, 25–60 months, and >60 months), there was a gradual increase in fibrosis as AF progressed.[78] As with collagen, there were also progressive increases in the expression of TGF-β1 mRNA, protein, and TGF-β receptor II protein. However, the TGF-β1 effect appeared to decline with increasing AF duration, suggesting a biphasic change in TGF-β1–mediated signaling in AF.[78] TGF-β1 inhibition using

tranilast in dogs subjected to atrial tachypacing reduced AF inducibility and duration. TGF-β1 inhibition had no effect on pacing-induced decrease in $Ca_V1.2$ and $K_V4.3$ but significantly reduced fibrosis and TGF-β1 expression.[79]

In an isolated cell system, pacing of an HL-1 cell line for 24 hours increased TGF-β1 release and synthesis with increasing pacing frequency.[80] The increase in TGF-β1 expression was associated with increased oxidative stress that was measured using a fluorescent dye and was prevented at a lower pacing frequency with TGF-β1 antibody; this suggested that TGF-β1 increased the oxidative stress. The same study also indicated that increased myosin loss in paced cells was due to TGF-β1.[80]

Angiotensin II and Transforming Growth Factor-β1

Elevations in Ang II and TGF-β1 levels are often found under conditions that lead to HF progression. Ang II enhances TGF-β1 expression via the SMAD pathway activation of the transcription factor activator protein 1 (AP-1), and this pathway is involved in hypertrophic growth of the heart muscle and in the development of cardiac fibrosis (see Fig. 43.3).[81] Ang II can also lead to fibrosis via a TGF-β1–independent Smad-mediated activation of Ang II receptor type 1 receptors (AT1Rs) and mitogen-activated protein kinases (MAPKs).[82] It has been reported that Ang II–induced LV remodeling and fibrosis is dependent on both ERK and Smad activation; inhibition of either pathway is equally efficacious in restoring LV function and architecture.[83] However, it is unknown whether ERK is also involved in Smad signaling in AF-induced atrial fibrosis. Finally, angiotensin-induced increased fibrosis measured by increased collagen content was inhibited by class I histone deacetylase (HDAC) inhibitors. HDACs can alter cell cycle progression in cardiac fibroblasts and could be one of the main mechanisms of increased fibroblast proliferation and fibrosis. HDACs were suggested to increase ERK phosphorylation, which indicated that ERK is involved in mediating Ang II effects.[84]

From the previous data, it is clear that Ang II strongly contributes to the main causes of HF progression, which are hypertrophy, fibrosis, and apoptosis. In experimental animal models[85–87] and in clinical studies,[88–90] inhibition of Ang II by angiotensin-converting enzyme (ACE) inhibitors or angiotensin receptor antagonists prevented HF progression and reduced mortality in patients. The effects of Ang II are also evident in isolated cardiac cells. In fibroblasts, Ang II induces proliferation and collagen synthesis.[91,92] In ventricular cardiomyocytes (CMs), Ang II, an inducer of apoptosis, promotes hypertrophy in part via TGF-β1 signaling.[81] The induction of TGF-β1 expression under Ang II stimulation is mediated by oxygen radicals, which are produced by NOX. Further downstream, p38 MAPK and AP-1 are activated.[93] Rapid atrial pacing in rabbits for 4 weeks increased fibrosis and collagen I and III content.[18] The paced atria also had increased levels of TGF-β1 protein and mRNA as well as an increased level of activated SMAD 2/3, but the TGF-β inhibitory protein smad7 was decreased.[18] All of the above changes were prevented by losartan treatment. In addition, treatment with Ang II did not increase the collagen levels in cells overexpressing smad7,[18] suggesting that there is strong feedback between the Ang II and TGF-β1 pathways (see Fig. 43.3); this also demonstrated the significance of increased TGF-β1–mediated pathways in fibrosis associated with rapid atrial pacing.

Ang II participates in the development of AF-induced myocardial fibrosis through the activation of AT1R and AT2R.[94–96] AT1R antagonism significantly attenuated AF-related fibrosis in dogs.[97] In a rabbit model of atrial tachypacing, treatment with losartan decreased the deposition of cardiac collagens in a dose-dependent manner, suggesting that activation of AT1Rs is an important mechanism for AF-induced atrial fibrosis.[18]

Effects of Other Cytokines on Ion Channels and Atrial Fibrillation

Macrophage Migration Inhibitory Factor

Macrophage migration inhibitory factor (MIF) is another multifaceted protein that can regulate the synthesis and release of other cytokines such as TNF-α, IL-1, and interferons.[98] These cytokines are found in the sera of AF patients. In a recent study, atrial samples from AF patients showed increased MIF expression levels, and cells isolated from the right atrial appendage showed a significantly reduced peak Ca^{2+} current compared with that observed in SR patients. mRNA and protein levels of the pore-forming $α_{1C}$ subunit of L-type Ca^{2+} channel were also decreased.[99] The MIF-induced decrease in Ca^{2+} current was confirmed in HL-1 cells. Phosphorylation of Src was increased by MIF treatment in the atrial cells. Yet treatment with protein phosphatase (PP) 1 (a specific Src antagonist) antagonized the MIF-mediated effects on both the Ca^{2+} current and LCC protein expression.[99] The results supported the involvement of MIF in the electrical remodeling that accompanies AF, through impairment of L-type Ca^{2+} channel expression and function via the activation of c-Src kinases in atrial myocytes.

Effects of TNF-α on Ionic Currents

When mice are treated with TNF-α for 6 weeks, their ventricular myocytes exhibit reduced transient outward potassium currents I_{to} and I_{Kur}.[100] In addition, TNF-α increases the action potential duration (APD).[101] The main downstream signaling molecule for TNF-α, nuclear factor (NF)-κB, has also been implicated in electrophysiological remodeling in cardiac cells.[102] Overexpression of the NF-κB activator IκB kinase-β decreased K_v channel–interacting protein 2 (KChIP2) expression and I_{to}. In addition, the classic NF-κB activator TNF-α induced NF-κB–dependent reductions of both KChIP2 and I_{to}. A role of NF-κB–mediated ionic current decrease was further supported by the fact that a phosphorylation mutant of IκB kinase was able to inhibit both NF-κB– and TNF-α–mediated decrease in I_{to} and KChIP2 expression.[103]

In H9c2 cells, Ang II reduced the peak sodium current by interfering with *SCN5A* transcription, which was mediated by an increase in oxidative stress. The increased oxidative stress augmented the binding of NF-κB to the *SCN5A* promoter with consequent decreases in both *SCN5A* transcription and sodium inward current.[102] Altogether, the abovementioned studies suggested that by activating NF-κB, TNF-α and other cytokines can substantially regulate both outward potassium and inward sodium currents in CMs.

Another protein of interest is the intracellular inflammatory cytokine high mobility group box 1 (HMGB1), which has also been associated with various cardiac insults.[104] HMGB1 promotes inflammation when released via active secretion from necrotic cells or by activation of the NF-κB pathway. HMGB1 treatment in Cos cells transfected with Kv4.2 or Kv4.3 cDNA decreased the respective transmembrane currents.[105] In neonatal rat ventricular myocytes, HMGB1 treatment for 24 hours decreased I_{to}, as well as the sustained component of the transient outward current, but it increased cell capacitance and therefore cell size. This protein decreased mRNA and protein levels of both Kv4.2 and Kv4.3 without affecting KChIP2 expression. HMGB1 modestly inhibited L-type Ca^{2+} current but not I_{K1}.[105]

Leukemia Inhibitory Factor

In HEK-293 cells transfected with the α-subunit of the T-type calcium channel, 12-hour treatment with leukemia inhibitory factor (LIF) caused a significant increase in the functional expression of the channels as indicated by changes in current density.[106] LIF increased phosphorylation of STAT3 and ERK in these cells. Treatment with the ERK inhibitor U0126 inhibited LIF-induced increased calcium current.[106]

Platelet-Derived Growth Factor

Recently, we examined the effects of a 24-hour exposure to the AB isoform of platelet-derived growth factor (PDGF) (PDGF-AB) on atrial myocytes obtained from persistent AF sheep,[107] and emphasized on the expression, subcellular localization, and electromechanical function of the voltage-gated L-type calcium current ($I_{Ca,L}$) and channel ($Ca_V1.2$).[9] As reproduced in Fig. 43.4, PDGF-AB caused significant reduction in APD at both 50% (APD50) and 80% (APD80) repolarization. PDGF-neutralizing antibody (N-ab) prevented this effect (Fig. 43.4A to D). In Fig 43.4E and F, both atrial myocytes isolated from a persistent AF animal and atrial myocytes isolated from an unpaced heart but incubated with PDGF-AB could be rapidly stimulated, up to 10 Hz. In contrast, myocytes from unpaced atria and myocytes treated with PDGF in the presence of N-ab were unable to respond in a 1:1 manner to pacing frequencies of 3 Hz or higher (see Fig. 43.4D to G). In Fig. 43.5, $I_{Ca,L}$ was reduced in PDGF-AB–treated cells but retained a normal I-V profile in the presence of N-ab (Fig. 43.5A and B). Other biophysical properties of $I_{Ca,L}$ were unaffected. Finally, we examined the effects of PDGF-AB on the $Ca_V1.2$ protein expression in lysates from atrial cells cultured in the presence or absence of PDGF-AB for a period of 24 hours. As shown in Fig. 43.5D and E, PDGF-AB significantly reduced the whole-cell $Ca_V1.2$ immunoreactive protein in treated cells compared with untreated cells. Densitometry analysis revealed a 37% reduction in $Ca_V1.2$ protein in cells treated with PDGF ($p ≤ .05$). The sodium–calcium exchanger (NCX1)

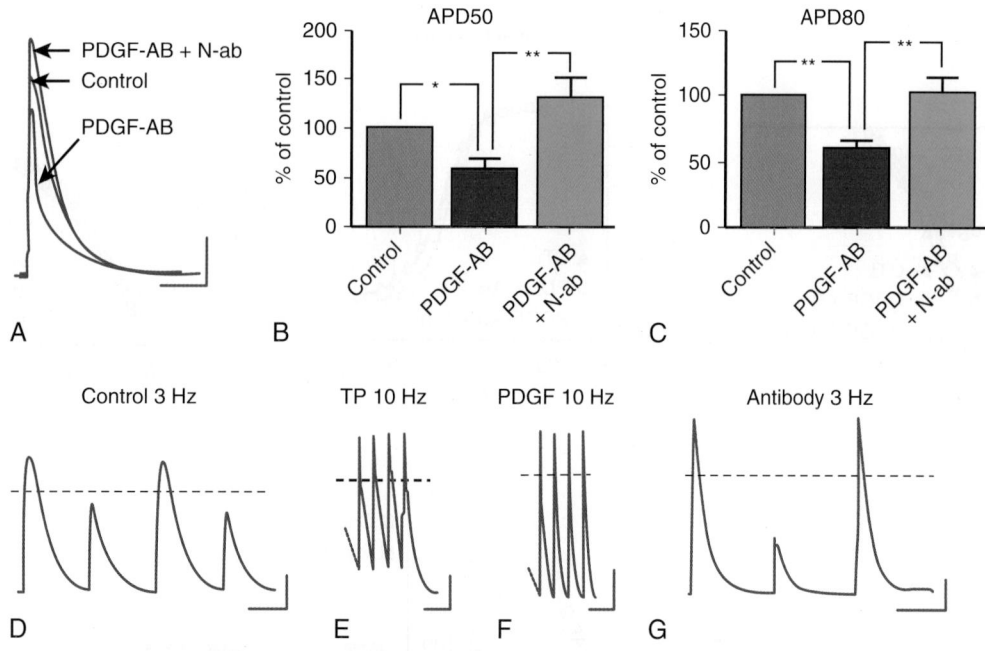

FIGURE 43.4 (A–C) Platelet-derived growth factor-AB (*PDGF-AB*; 1 ng/mL) shortens sheep atrial myocyte APD50 and APD80 by 40% and 39%, respectively (*$p < .05$; **$p < .01$). Neutralizing antibody (*N-ab*) blocks the effect (all conditions; n ≥ 9). (D–G) After a 24-hour incubation with PDGF-AB, atrial myocytes could be stimulated up to 10 Hz (F) similar to cells from a tachypaced (*TP*) animal (E). In contrast, atrial cells from an unpaced animal (D) as well as those exposed to PDGF-AB+N-ab (G) could not be paced higher than 3 Hz. Scale bars = 20 mV, 100 ms (A), and 200 ms (D–F). (From Kaur K, Zarzoso M, Ponce-Balbuena D, et al. TGF-beta1, released by myofibroblasts, differentially regulates transcription and function of sodium and potassium channels in adult rat ventricular myocytes. *PLoS One.* 2013;8:e55391.)

was used as the negative control. GAPDH was used as a loading control. Altogether, the results demonstrated the profound electrical, cellular, and mechanical remodeling that can occur in the presence of PDGF-AB. Such results offer at least a partial mechanistic explanation for the manner in which some cytokines released from myofibroblasts contribute to the electromechanical remodeling known to occur during the rapid activation of the atria and to AF perpetuation.[9]

Myofibroblasts, Cytokines, and Myocyte Electrical Remodeling

The significance of investigating the interactions between myofibroblasts and myocytes from normal and diseased hearts is highlighted by the fact that myofibroblasts are the primary mediators of wound healing in the injured heart and are the dominant cell type in the infarcted scar.[108–110] They also contribute to fibrosis in the atria and ventricles through their ability to produce fibrillar and nonfibrillar collagens,[110,111] and to ECM remodeling through their production of focal adhesion–associated proteins (see Fig. 43.1).[109,112,113] The importance of these studies is also enhanced by the knowledge that paracrine factors released from myofibroblasts lead to myocyte hypertrophy and diastolic dysfunction.[11,114] The best studied factors include TGF-β, PDGF, FGF-2, and members of the IL-6 family of proteins.[11,114,115]

Despite the importance of myofibroblasts and fibrosis in myocardial infarction, cardiomyopathies, HF, and AF, whether and how the abovementioned factors affect CM electrical function or excitation–contraction coupling has not been adequately addressed. Clearly, there is a need to examine the electrophysiological consequences of paracrine, mechanical, and electrical myocyte–myofibroblast interactions on myocyte electrophysiology, which is underscored by the recent discovery

that attachment of myofibroblasts to adult CMs in vitro results in structural remodeling of myocytes.[8,14] Whether such maladaptive behavior results in electrical remodeling has never been investigated. Finally, while dye transfer experiments have suggested that intercellular coupling exists between cocultured adult rabbit ventricular myocytes and myofibroblasts,[14,116] to our knowledge, no such evidence exists in vivo either in the atria or the ventricles of the adult heart. In addition, no dual patch clamping experiments have been conducted to rigorously quantify the conductance of junctional channels between adult myocytes and myofibroblasts.

Early reports on the consequences of culturing neonatal myocytes in cardiac fibroblast-conditioned medium (FCM) showed increased protein expression,[117] APD prolongation, and $K_V4.2$ downregulation in myocytes.[118] Pedrotty and colleagues[119] demonstrated that the exposure of neonatal rat ventricular myocyte (NRVM) monolayers to FCM produced a dose-dependent reduction in conduction velocity, a prolongation of APD, a depolarization of the resting membrane potential, and a reduction of the AP upstroke velocity. Fibroblast proliferation, myocyte apoptosis, and Cx43 expression were not affected. However, mRNA levels of $Na_V1.5$, Kir2.1, and $K_V4.3$ were all reduced by the exposure to the FCM.[119] More recently, Vazquez and associates[120] showed that in NRVM monolayers treated with FCM harvested from infarcted hearts, the conduction velocity could be higher or lower than in NRVM treated with FCM from normal hearts, depending on cell density. In addition, the optical APD_{70} was slightly shorter in the former than in the latter.[120] While these effects of neonatal fibroblasts on NRVMs are of interest, they should not be extrapolated to the adult heart, particularly those derived from the myocardial infarction scar. In fact, there is evidence in the literature suggesting that the phenotypic changes produced by paracrine factors released by cardiac fibroblasts may be different in the developing versus the adult

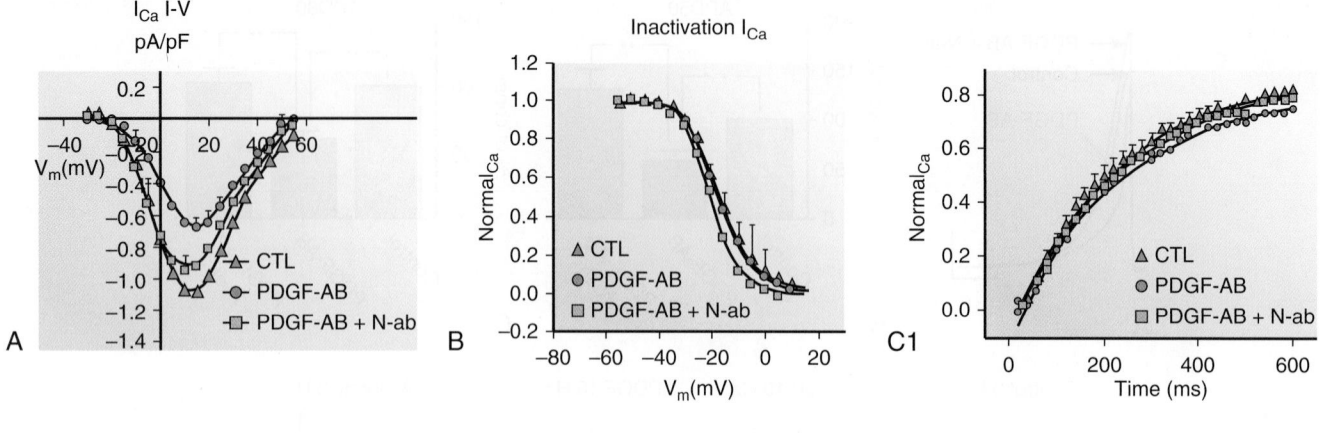

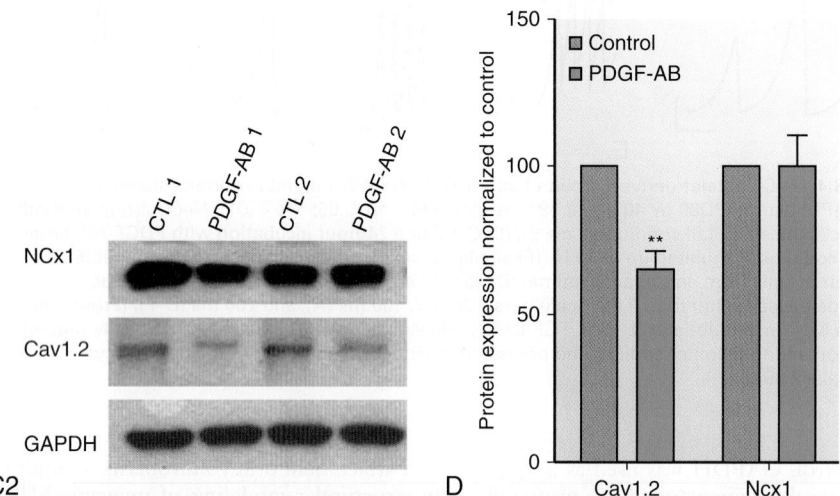

FIGURE 43.5 Recombinant platelet-derived growth factor-AB (*PDGF-AB*) decreases L-type calcium current ($I_{Ca,L}$), calcium transients in unpaced atrial myocytes. (A) Whole-cell recordings of $I_{Ca,L}$ from atrial myocytes treated with PDGF-AB for 24 hours (*circles*) demonstrated a significant ($p < .005$) reduction in peak amplitudes relative to untreated myocytes (*triangles*) at several voltages. Preincubation with a neutralizing antibody (*N-ab*) prevented these effects (*squares*). (B and C1) The voltage-dependent inactivation and time dependence of recovery remain unchanged (n = 9, 9, and 4 for control [*CTL*], PDGF-AB, and PDGF-AB+N-ab, respectively). (C2 and D) Western blot analyses demonstrate that 24-hour exposure to PDGF-AB downregulates whole-cell CaV1.2 proteins. Results from three experiments, each performed in duplicate (A), are shown in (B). CaV1.2 proteins were reduced by 35% (n = 3; **$p < .01$). Sodium–calcium exchanger (*NCX1*) remained unaffected and was used as the negative control. Glyceraldehyde 3-phosphate dehydrogenase (*GAPDH*) was used as the loading control. (From Kaur K, Zarzoso M, Ponce-Balbuena D, et al. TGF-beta1, released by myofibroblasts, differentially regulates transcription and function of sodium and potassium channels in adult rat ventricular myocytes. *PLoS One*. 2013;8:e55391.)

myocyte.[121] In addition, while the use of FCM is important, it leaves the uncertainty of which specific cytokines are the ones producing the electrophysiological changes. Finally, despite the potential importance of both electrical and structural remodeling in AF, a role for specific regulation by cytokines released from atrial fibroblasts on atrial myocyte electrical function and/or excitation–contraction coupling has not been established. Therefore in adult atria myocytes, there is a need to investigate the electrophysiological effects of specific cytokines that are known to be released by myofibroblasts and upregulated in the fibrillating atria.

Concluding Remarks

In view of the striking effects that myofibroblast paracrine factors have on atrial and ventricular function, the evidence that cytokines are significantly unregulated and may play an important role in atrial structural remodeling and the relative dearth of information about whether they are involved in electrical remodeling in the adult heart, it appears important to examine the paracrine effects of myofibroblast-derived cytokines on AP of atrial myocytes, as well as the ionic and molecular mechanisms. In vitro experiments should address questions related to the effects of conditioned media derived from atrial myofibroblasts (i.e., activated fibroblasts expressing αSMA) obtained from normal and chronically fibrillating hearts. Thereafter, research should focus on the effects of specific cytokines and their signaling pathways that have been shown to be involved in atrial remodeling (e.g., TGF-β1 and PDGF). The use of clinically relevant large animal models of persistent AF that are capable of recapitulating the features of sustained AF in patients, including TGF-β1 elevation, the presence of interstitial fibrosis, the upregulation of a major inward rectifier current, and the frequency characteristics and spatial distribution of the fibrillatory waves will be essential in this endeavor. Clearly, although both pharmacological and ablative treatments of persistent AF have shown some efficacy, the clinical needs are far from being met, and the field is facing many challenges. Two of these challenges are the expected increase in the incidence of AF in the general population and the potentially adverse long-term consequences of the extensive ablative therapy that is usually needed to terminate persistent AF. Thus novel antiarrhythmic strategies targeting not only fibrosis but also the molecular mechanisms underlying myocyte remodeling are highly desirable. As such, finding new target genes with pleiotropic effects on both myocytes and nonmyocyte cells, which are important for pathological remodeling in AF, may become an important goal in therapy.

Acknowledgments

Supported in part by National Heart, Lung and Blood Institute R01 (HL122352) NIH/NHLBI, the Leducq Foundation; and the University of Michigan Health System–Peking University Health Science Center Joint Institute for Translational and Clinical Research (UMHS-PUHSC).

REFERENCES

1. Kannel WB, Wolf PA, Benjamin EJ, et al. Prevalence, incidence, prognosis, and predisposing conditions for atrial fibrillation: population-based estimates. *Am J Cardiol.* 1998;82:2N–9N.
2. Calkins H, Kuck KH, Cappato R, et al. 2012 HRS/EHRA/ECAS expert consensus statement on catheter and surgical ablation of atrial fibrillation: recommendations for patient selection, procedural techniques, patient management and follow-up, definitions, endpoints, and research trial design. *Europace.* 2012;14:528–606.
3. de Bakker JM, van Capelle FJ, Janse MJ, et al. Slow conduction in the infarcted human heart. 'Zigzag' course of activation. *Circulation.* 1993;88:915–926.
4. Bian W, Tung L. Structure-related initiation of reentry by rapid pacing in monolayers of cardiac cells. *Circ Res.* 2006;98:e29–e38.
5. Spach MS, Boineau JP. Microfibrosis produces electrical load variations due to loss of side-to-side cell connections: a major mechanism of structural heart disease arrhythmias. *Pacing Clin Electrophysiol.* 1997;20:397–413.
6. de Bakker JM, Stein M, van Rijen HV. Three-dimensional anatomic structure as substrate for ventricular tachycardia/ventricular fibrillation. *Heart Rhythm.* 2005;2:777–779.
7. Valderrabano M, Kim YH, Yashima M, et al. Obstacle-induced transition from ventricular fibrillation to tachycardia in isolated swine right ventricles: insights into the transition dynamics and implications for the critical mass. *J Am Coll Cardiol.* 2000;36:2000–2008.
8. Driesen RBVF, Dispersyn GD, Thoné F, et al. Structural adaptation in adult rabbit ventricular myocytes: influence of dynamic physical interaction with fibroblasts. *Cell Biochem Biophys.* 2006;44:119–128.
9. Musa H, Kaur K, O'Connell R, et al. Inhibition of platelet-derived growth factor-AB signaling prevents electromechanical remodeling of adult atrial myocytes that contact myofibroblasts. *Heart Rhythm.* 2013;10:1044–1051.
10. Kaur K, Zarzoso M, Ponce-Balbuena D, et al. TGF-beta1, released by myofibroblasts, differentially regulates transcription and function of sodium and potassium channels in adult rat ventricular myocytes. *PLoS One.* 2013;8:e55391.
11. Souders CA, Bowers SL, Baudino TA. Cardiac fibroblast: the renaissance cell. *Circ Res.* 2009;105:1164–1176.
12. Baudino TA, Carver W, Giles W, et al. Cardiac fibroblasts: friend or foe? *Am J Physiol Heart Circ Physiol.* 2006;291:H1015–H1026.
13. Vasquez C, Benamer N, Morley GE. The cardiac fibroblast: functional and electrophysiological considerations in healthy and diseased hearts. *J Cardiovasc Pharmacol.* 2011;57:380–388.
14. Driesen RBDG, Verheyen FK, van den Eijnde SM, et al. Partial cell fusion: a newly recognized type of communication between cardiomyocytes and fibroblasts. *Cardiovasc Res.* 2005;68:37–46.
15. Baum J, Duffy HS. Fibroblasts and myofibroblasts: what are we talking about? *J Cardiovasc Pharmacol.* 2011;57:376–379.
16. Manabe I, Shindo T, Nagai R. Gene expression in fibroblasts and fibrosis: involvement in cardiac hypertrophy. *Circ Res.* 2002;91:1103–1113.
17. Brown RD, Ambler SK, Mitchell MD, et al. The cardiac fibroblast: therapeutic target in myocardial remodeling and failure. *Annu Rev Pharmacol Toxicol.* 2005;45:657–687.
18. He X, Gao X, Peng L, et al. Atrial fibrillation induces myocardial fibrosis through angiotensin II type 1 receptor-specific Arkadia-mediated downregulation of Smad7. *Circ Res.* 2011;108:164–175.
19. Gabbiani G, Majno G. Dupuytren's contracture: fibroblast contraction? An ultrastructural study. *Am J Pathol.* 1972;66:131–146.
20. Burstein B, Qi XY, Yeh YH, et al. Atrial cardiomyocyte tachycardia alters cardiac fibroblast function: a novel consideration in atrial remodeling. *Cardiovasc Res.* 2007;76:442–452.

21. Burstein B, Libby E, Calderone A, et al. Differential behaviors of atrial versus ventricular fibroblasts: a potential role for platelet-derived growth factor in atrial-ventricular remodeling differences. *Circulation.* 2008;117:1630–1641.
22. Ambros V. MicroRNA pathways in flies and worms: growth, death, fat, stress, and timing. *Cell.* 2003;113:673–676.
23. Lu Y, Zhang Y, Wang N, et al. MicroRNA-328 contributes to adverse electrical remodeling in atrial fibrillation. *Circulation.* 2010;122:2378–2387.
24. Chiang DY, Kongchan N, Beavers DL, et al. Loss of microRNA-106b-25 cluster promotes atrial fibrillation by enhancing ryanodine receptor type-2 expression and calcium release. *Circ Arrhythm Electrophysiol.* 2014;7:1214–1222.
25. Horie T, Baba O, Kuwabara Y, et al. MicroRNA-33 deficiency reduces the progression of atherosclerotic plaque in ApoE-/- mice. *J Am Heart Assoc.* 2012;1:e003376.
26. McManus DD, Tanriverdi K, Lin H, et al. Plasma microRNAs are associated with atrial fibrillation and change after catheter-ablation (the miRhythm study). *Heart Rhythm.* 2015;12:3–10.
27. Chen Y, Wakili R, Xiao J, et al. Detailed characterization of microRNA changes in a canine heart failure model: relationship to arrhythmogenic structural remodeling. *J Mol Cell Cardiol.* 2014;77:113–124.
28. Dawson K, Wakili R, Ordog B, et al. MicroRNA29: a mechanistic contributor and potential biomarker in atrial fibrillation. *Circulation.* 2013;127:1466–1475. 1475e1–e28.
29. Aguilar M, Qi XY, Huang H, et al. Fibroblast electrical remodeling in heart failure and potential effects on atrial fibrillation. *Biophys J.* 2014;107:2444–2455.
30. Qi XY, Huang H, Ordog B, et al. Fibroblast inward-rectifier potassium current upregulation in profibrillatory atrial remodeling. *Circ Res.* 2015;116:836–845.
31. Yue Z, Zhang Y, Xie J, et al. Transient receptor potential (TRP) channels and cardiac fibrosis. *Cur Top Med Chem.* 2013;13:270–282.
32. Yue Z, Xie J, Yu A, et al. Role of TRP channels in the cardiovascular system. *Am J Physiol Heart Circ Physiol.* 2015;308:H157–H182.
33. Yue Z, Zhang Y, Xie J, et al. Transient receptor potential (TRP) channels and cardiac fibrosis. *Curr Top Med Chem.* 2013;13:270–282
34. Harada M, Luo X, Qi XY, et al. Transient receptor potential canonical-3 channel-dependent fibroblast regulation in atrial fibrillation. *Circulation.* 2014;126:2051–2064.
35. Zhang YJ, Ma N, Su F, et al. Increased TRPM6 expression in atrial fibrillation patients contribute to atrial fibrosis. *Exp Mol Pathol.* 2015;98:486–490.
36. Du J, Xie J, Zhang Z, et al. TRPM7-mediated Ca^{2+} signals confer fibrogenesis in human atrial fibrillation. *Circ Res.* 2010;106:992–1003.
37. Adapala RK, Thoppil RJ, Luther DJ, et al. Trpv4 channels mediate cardiac fibroblast differentiation by integrating mechanical and soluble signals. *J Mol Cell Cardiol.* 2013;54:45–52.
38. Friedrichs K, Klinke A, Baldus S. Inflammatory pathways underlying atrial fibrillation. *Trends Mol Med.* 2011;17:556–563.
39. Fu G, Cao Y, Lu J, et al. Programmed cell death-1 deficiency results in atrial remodeling in C57BL/6 mice. *Int J Mol Med.* 2013;31:423–429.
40. Aschar-Sobbi R, Izaddoustdar F, Korogyi AS, et al. Increased atrial arrhythmia susceptibility induced by intense endurance exercise in mice requires TNFalpha. *Nat Commun.* 2015;6:6018.
41. Mihm MJ, Yu F, Carnes CA, et al. Impaired myofibrillar energetics and oxidative injury during human atrial fibrillation. *Circulation.* 2001;104:174–180.

42. Carnes CA, Chung MK, Nakayama T, et al. Ascorbate attenuates atrial pacing-induced peroxynitrite formation and electrical remodeling and decreases the incidence of postoperative atrial fibrillation. *Circ Res.* 2001;89:E32–E38.
43. Chen CL, Huang SK, Lin JL, et al. Upregulation of matrix metalloproteinase-9 and tissue inhibitors of metalloproteinases in rapid atrial pacing-induced atrial fibrillation. *J Mol Cell Cardiol.* 2008;45:742–753.
44. Kaski JC, Arrebola-Moreno AL. Inflammation and thrombosis in atrial fibrillation. *Rev Esp Cardiol.* 2011;64:551–553.
45. Rienstra M, Sun JX, Magnani JW, et al. White blood cell count and risk of incident atrial fibrillation (from the Framingham Heart Study). *Am J Cardiol.* 2012;109:533–537.
46. Barassi A, Pezzilli R, Morselli-Labate AM, et al. Serum amyloid A and C-reactive protein independently predict the recurrences of atrial fibrillation after cardioversion in patients with preserved left ventricular function. *Can J Cardiol.* 2012;28:537–541.
47. Yao SY, Chu JM, Chen KP, et al. Inflammation in lone atrial fibrillation. *Clin Cardiol.* 2009;32:94–98.
48. Chen MC, Chang JP, Liu WH, et al. Increased inflammatory cell infiltration in the atrial myocardium of patients with atrial fibrillation. *Am J Cardiol.* 2008;102:861–865.
49. Weis F, Beiras-Fernandez A, Schelling G, et al. Stress doses of hydrocortisone in high-risk patients undergoing cardiac surgery: effects on interleukin-6 to interleukin-10 ratio and early outcome. *Crit Care Med.* 2009;37:1685–1690.
50. Alegret JM, Aragones G, Elosua R, et al. The relevance of the association between inflammation and atrial fibrillation. *Eur J Clin Invest.* 2013;43:324–331.
51. Kim SC, Liu J, Solomon DH. The risk of atrial fibrillation in patients with rheumatoid arthritis. *Ann Rheum Dis.* 2014;73:1091–1095.
52. Soeki T, Bando S, Uematsu E, et al. Pentraxin 3 is a local inflammatory marker in atrial fibrillation. *Heart Vessels.* 2014;29:653–658.
53. Kostin S, Klein G, Szalay Z, et al. Structural correlate of atrial fibrillation in human patients. *Cardiovasc Res.* 2002;54:361–379.
54. Boldt A, Wetzel U, Lauschke J, et al. Fibrosis in left atrial tissue of patients with atrial fibrillation with and without underlying mitral valve disease. *Heart.* 2004;90:400–405.
55. Cohen S. Cytokine: More than a new word, a new concept proposed by Stanley Cohen thirty years ago. *Cytokine.* 2004;28:242–247.
56. Kaur K, Dhingra S, Slezak J, et al. Biology of TNF alpha and IL-10, and their imbalance in heart failure. *Heart Fail Rev.* 2009;14:113–123.
57. Scridon A, Morel E, Nonin-Babary E, et al. Increased intracardiac vascular endothelial growth factor levels in patients with paroxysmal, but not persistent atrial fibrillation. *Europace.* 2012;14:948–953.
58. Choudhury A, Freestone B, Patel J, et al. Relationship of soluble CD40 ligand to vascular endothelial growth factor, angiopoietins, and tissue factor in atrial fibrillation: a link among platelet activation, angiogenesis, and thrombosis? *Chest.* 2007;132:1913–1919.
59. Luan Y, Guo Y, Li S, et al. Interleukin-18 among atrial fibrillation patients in the absence of structural heart disease. *Europace.* 2010;12:1713–1718.
60. Li J, Solus J, Chen Q, et al. Role of inflammation and oxidative stress in atrial fibrillation. *Heart Rhythm.* 2010;7:438–444.
61. Marcus GM, Whooley MA, Glidden DV, et al. Interleukin-6 and atrial fibrillation in patients with coronary artery disease: data from the Heart and Soul Study. *Am Heart J.* 2008;155:303–309.

62. Rizos I, Tsiodras S, Rigopoulos AG, et al. Interleukin-2 serum levels variations in recent onset atrial fibrillation are related with cardioversion outcome. *Cytokine.* 2007;40:157–164.

63. Henningsen KM, Nilsson B, Bruunsgaard H, et al. Prognostic impact of hs-CRP and IL-6 in patients undergoing radiofrequency catheter ablation for atrial fibrillation. *Scand Cardiovasc J.* 2009;43:285–291.

64. Leftheriotis DI, Fountoulaki KT, Flevari PG, et al. The predictive value of inflammatory and oxidative markers following the successful cardioversion of persistent lone atrial fibrillation. *Int J Cardiol.* 2009;135:361–369.

65. Osmancik P, Peroutka Z, Budera P, et al. Changes in cytokine concentrations following successful ablation of atrial fibrillation. *Eur Cytokine Netw.* 2010;21:278–284.

66. Marcus GM, Smith LM, Ordovas K, et al. Intracardiac and extracardiac markers of inflammation during atrial fibrillation. *Heart Rhythm.* 2010;7:149–154.

67. Choi JM, Bothwell AL. The nuclear receptor PPARs as important regulators of T-cell functions and autoimmune diseases. *Mol Cells.* 2012;33:217–222.

68. Chen X, Bing Z, He J, et al. Downregulation of peroxisome proliferator-activated receptor-gamma expression in hypertensive atrial fibrillation. *Clin Cardiol.* 2009;32:337–345.

69. Dobaczewski M, Chen W, Frangogiannis NG. Transforming growth factor (TGF)-beta signaling in cardiac remodeling. *J Mol Cell Cardiol.* 2011;51:600–606.

70. Schiller M, Javelaud D, Mauviel A. TGF-beta-induced SMAD signaling and gene regulation: consequences for extracellular matrix remodeling and wound healing. *J Dermatol Sci.* 2004;35:83–92.

71. Rosenkranz S, Flesch M, Amann K, et al. Alterations of beta-adrenergic signaling and cardiac hypertrophy in transgenic mice overexpressing TGF-beta(1). *Am J Physiol Heart Circ Physiol.* 2002;283:H1253–H1262.

72. Nakajima H, Nakajima HO, Salcher O, et al. Atrial but not ventricular fibrosis in mice expressing a mutant transforming growth factor-beta(1) transgene in the heart. *Circ Res.* 2000;86:571–579.

73. Rahmutula D, Marcus GM, Wilson EE, et al. Molecular basis of selective atrial fibrosis due to overexpression of transforming growth factor-beta1. *Cardiovasc Res.* 2013;99(4):769–779.

74. Yeh YH, Kuo CT, Chang GJ, et al. Nicotinamide adenine dinucleotide phosphate oxidase 4 mediates the differential responsiveness of atrial versus ventricular fibroblasts to transforming growth factor-beta. *Circ Arrhythm Electrophysiol.* 2013;6:790–798.

75. Verheule S, Sato T, Everett TT, et al. Increased vulnerability to atrial fibrillation in transgenic mice with selective atrial fibrosis caused by overexpression of TGF-beta1. *Circ Res.* 2004;94:1458–1465.

76. Wang Y, Hou X, Li Y. Association between transforming growth factor beta1 polymorphisms and atrial fibrillation in essential hypertensive subjects. *J Biomed Sci.* 2010;17:23.

77. Kim SK, Park JH, Kim JY, et al. High plasma concentrations of transforming growth factor-beta and tissue inhibitor of metalloproteinase-1: potential non-invasive predictors for electroanatomical remodeling of atrium in patients with non-valvular atrial fibrillation. *Circ J.* 2011;75:557–564.

78. Gramley F, Lorenzen J, Koellensperger E, et al. Atrial fibrosis and atrial fibrillation: the role of the TGF-beta1 signaling pathway. *Int J Cardiol.* 2010;143:405–413.

79. Nakatani Y, Nishida K, Sakabe M, et al. Tranilast prevents atrial remodeling and development of atrial fibrillation in a canine model of atrial tachycardia and left ventricular dysfunction. *J Am Coll Cardiol.* 2013;61:582–588.

80. Yeh YH, Kuo CT, Chan TH, et al. Transforming growth factor-beta and oxidative stress mediate tachycardia-induced cellular remodelling in cultured atrial-derived myocytes. *Cardiovasc Res.* 2011;91:62–70.

81. Schroder D, Heger J, Piper HM, et al. Angiotensin II stimulates apoptosis via TGF-beta1 signaling in ventricular cardiomyocytes of rat. *J Mol Med (Berl).* 2006;84:975–983.

82. Rodriguez-Vita J, Sanchez-Lopez E, Esteban V, et al. Angiotensin II activates the Smad pathway in vascular smooth muscle cells by a transforming growth factor-beta-independent mechanism. *Circulation.* 2005;111:2509–2517.

83. de Boer RA, Pokharel S, Flesch M, et al. Extracellular signal regulated kinase and SMAD signaling both mediate the angiotensin II driven progression towards overt heart failure in homozygous TGR(mRen2)27. *J Mol Med (Berl).* 2004;82:678–687.

84. Williams SM, Golden-Mason L, Ferguson BS, et al. Class I HDACs regulate angiotensin II-dependent cardiac fibrosis via fibroblasts and circulating fibrocytes. *J Mol Cell Cardiol.* 2014;67:112–125.

85. Pfeffer JM, Pfeffer MA. Angiotensin converting enzyme inhibition and ventricular remodeling in heart failure. *Am J Med.* 1988;84:37–44.

86. Pinto YM, Pinto-Sietsma SJ, Philipp T, et al. Reduction in left ventricular messenger RNA for transforming growth factor beta(1) attenuates left ventricular fibrosis and improves survival without lowering blood pressure in the hypertensive TGR(mRen2)27 rat. *Hypertension.* 2000;36:747–754.

87. Kim S, Yoshiyama M, Izumi Y, et al. Effects of combination of ACE inhibitor and angiotensin receptor blocker on cardiac remodeling, cardiac function, and survival in rat heart failure. *Circulation.* 2001;103:148–154.

88. Solvd investigators. Effect of enalapril on survival in patients with reduced left ventricular ejection fractions and congestive heart failure. *N Engl J Med.* 1991;325:293–302.

89. Pfeffer MA, Braunwald E, Moye LA, et al. Effect of captopril on mortality and morbidity in patients with left ventricular dysfunction after myocardial infarction. Results of the survival and ventricular enlargement trial. The SAVE investigators. *N Engl J Med.* 1992;327:669–677.

90. Pitt B, Poole-Wilson PA, Segal R, et al. Effect of losartan compared with captopril on mortality in patients with symptomatic heart failure: randomised trial—the Losartan Heart Failure Survival Study ELITE II. *Lancet.* 2000;355:1582–1587.

91. Schorb W, Booz GW, Dostal DE, et al. Angiotensin II is mitogenic in neonatal rat cardiac fibroblasts. *Circ Res.* 1993;72:1245–1254.

92. Bouzegrhane F, Thibault G. Is angiotensin II a proliferative factor of cardiac fibroblasts? *Cardiovasc Res.* 2002;53:304–312.

93. Wenzel S, Taimor G, Piper HM, et al. Redox-sensitive intermediates mediate angiotensin II-induced p38 MAP kinase activation, AP-1 binding activity, and TGF-beta expression in adult ventricular cardiomyocytes. *FASEB J.* 2001;15:2291–2293.

94. Boldt A, Scholl A, Garbade J, et al. ACE-inhibitor treatment attenuates atrial structural remodeling in patients with lone chronic atrial fibrillation. *Basic Res Cardiol.* 2006;101:261–267.

95. Hirayama Y, Atarashi H, Kobayashi Y, et al. Angiotensin-converting enzyme inhibitors are not effective at inhibiting further changes in the atria in patients with chronic atrial fibrillation: speculation from analysis of the time course of fibrillary wave amplitudes. *Jpn Heart J.* 2004;45:93–101.

96. Chrysostomakis SI, Karalis IK, Simantirakis EN, et al. Angiotensin II type 1 receptor inhibition is associated with reduced tachyarrhythmia-induced ventricular interstitial fibrosis in a goat atrial fibrillation model. *Cardiovasc Drugs Ther.* 2007;21:357–365.

97. Nakashima H, Kumagai K. Reverse-remodeling effects of angiotensin II type 1 receptor blocker in a canine atrial fibrillation model. *Circ J.* 2007;71:1977–1982.

98. Calandra T, Bernhagen J, Metz CN, et al. MIF as a glucocorticoid-induced modulator of cytokine production. *Nature.* 1995;377:68–71.

99. Rao F, Deng CY, Wu SL, et al. Involvement of Src in L-type Ca²⁺ channel depression induced by macrophage migration inhibitory factor in atrial myocytes. *J Mol Cell Cardiol.* 2009;47:586–594.

100. Grandy SA, Fiset C. Ventricular K+ currents are reduced in mice with elevated levels of serum TNFalpha. *J Mol Cell Cardiol.* 2009;47:238–246.

101. Fernandez-Velasco M, Ruiz-Hurtado G, Hurtado O, et al. TNF-alpha downregulates transient outward potassium current in rat ventricular myocytes through iNOS overexpression and oxidant species generation. *Am J Physiol Heart Circ Physiol.* 2007;293:H238–H245.

102. Shang LL, Sanyal S, Pfahnl AE, et al. NF-kappaB-dependent transcriptional regulation of the cardiac scn5a sodium channel by angiotensin II. *Am J Physiol Cell Physiol.* 2008;294:C372–C379.

103. Panama BK, Latour-Villamil D, Farman GP, et al. Nuclear factor kappaB downregulates the transient outward potassium current I(T$_{o,f}$) through control of KChiP2 expression. *Circ Res.* 2011;108:537–543.

104. Kohno T, Anzai T, Naito K, et al. Role of high-mobility group box 1 protein in post-infarction healing process and left ventricular remodelling. *Cardiovasc Res.* 2009;81:565–573.

105. Liu W, Deng J, Xu J, et al. High-mobility group box 1 (HMGB1) downregulates cardiac transient outward potassium current (I$_{to}$) through downregulation of Kv4.2 and Kv4.3 channel transcripts and proteins. *J Mol Cell Cardiol.* 2010;49:438–448.

106. Dey D, Shepherd A, Pachuau J, et al. Leukemia inhibitory factor regulates trafficking of T-type Ca²⁺ channels. *Am J Physiol Cell Physiol.* 2011;300:C576–C587.

107. Martins RP, Kaur K, Hwang E, et al. Dominant frequency increase rate predicts transition from paroxysmal to long-term persistent atrial fibrillation. *Circulation.* 2014;129:1472–1482.

108. Dixon IM. The soluble interleukin 6 receptor takes its place in the pantheon of interleukin 6 signaling proteins: phenoconversion of cardiac fibroblasts to myofibroblasts. *Hypertension.* 2010;56:193–195.

109. Santiago JJ, Dangerfield AL, Rattan SG, et al. Cardiac fibroblast to myofibroblast differentiation in vivo and in vitro: expression of focal adhesion components in neonatal and adult rat ventricular myofibroblasts. *Dev Dyn.* 2010;239:1573–1584.

110. Dobaczewski M, Bujak M, Zymek P, et al. Extracellular matrix remodeling in canine and mouse myocardial infarcts. *Cell Tissue Res.* 2006;324:475–488.

111. Espira L, Czubryt MP. Emerging concepts in cardiac matrix biology. *Can J Physiol Pharmacol.* 2009;87:996–1008.

112. Thum T, Gross C, Fiedler J, et al. MicroRNA-21 contributes to myocardial disease by stimulating MAP kinase signalling in fibroblasts. *Nature.* 2008;456:980–984.

113. Cleutjens JP, Verluyten MJ, Smiths JF, et al. Collagen remodeling after myocardial infarction in the rat heart. *Am J Pathol.* 1995;147:325–338.

114. Kakkar R, Lee RT. Intramyocardial fibroblast myocyte communication. *Circ Res.* 2010;106:47–57.

115. Banerjee IFJ, Souders CA, Bowers SL, et al. The role of interleukin-6 in the formation of the coronary vasculature. *Microsc Microanal.* 2009;15:415–421.

116. Chilton L, Giles WR, Smith GL. Evidence of intercellular coupling between co-cultured adult rabbit ventricular myocytes and myofibroblasts. *J Physiol.* 2007;583:225–236.

117. Harada M, Itoh H, Nakagawa O, et al. Significance of ventricular myocytes and nonmyocytes interaction during cardiac hypertrophy: evidence for endothelin-1 as a paracrine hypertrophic factor from cardiac nonmyocytes. *Circulation.* 1997;96:3737–3744.

118. Guo W, Kamiya K, Yasui K, et al. Paracrine hypertrophic factors from cardiac non-myocyte cells downregulate the transient outward current density and Kv4.2 K+ channel expression in cultured rat cardiomyocytes. *Cardiovasc Res.* 1999;41:157–165.

119. Pedrotty DM, Klinger RY, Kirkton RD, et al. Cardiac fibroblast paracrine factors alter impulse conduction and ion channel expression of neonatal rat cardiomyocytes. *Cardiovasc Res.* 2009;83:688–697.

120. Vasquez C, Mohandas P, Louie KL, et al. Enhanced fibroblast-myocyte interactions in response to cardiac injury. *Circ Res.* 2010;107:1011–1020.

121. Ieda M, Tsuchihashi T, Ivey KN, et al. Cardiac fibroblasts regulate myocardial proliferation through beta1 integrin signaling. *Dev Cell.* 2009;16:233–244.

44 Role of the Autonomic Nervous System in Atrial Fibrillation

Stavros Stavrakis, Benjamin J. Scherlag, Paul Garabelli, and Sunny S. Po

The Cardiac Autonomic Nervous System

The autonomic nervous system can be viewed as the interface between the central nervous system and the viscera, glands, and blood vessels. It is divided into three main components: sympathetic, parasympathetic, and enteric.[1] Integration of the neural trafficking among the afferent and efferent autonomic nerves as well as their associated autonomic neurons maintains a delicate homeostasis of the function of the entire body. In mammalian hearts, the efferent sympathetic preganglionic neurons are located in the intermediolateral columns of the gray matter of the spinal cord; the preganglionic fibers of these neurons pass through or synapse with the paravertebral ganglia (e.g., the stellate ganglia). The stellate ganglia, receiving neural inputs mainly from spinal nerves C6–T2, are the key neural structures for cardiac sympathetic innervation.[1] The efferent parasympathetic preganglionic neurons are located in the motor nuclei of the vagus nerves (e.g., nucleus ambiguus) in the brain stem, from which the vagus nerves carry the preganglionic parasympathetic fibers to the heart. The parasympathetic postganglionic neurons are concentrated mainly in the ganglionated plexi (GP) embedded in epicardial fat pads, and the efferent postganglionic parasympathetic fibers are distributed over the entire heart. The afferent autonomic fibers, both sympathetic and parasympathetic, course along the cardiac plexus in the thorax and eventually reach the sensory neurons in the nodose ganglia at the base of the skull as well as the dorsal root ganglia of the spinal cord. These afferent nerves and ganglia mediate important cardiorespiratory reflexes (e.g., baroreflex) and pain sensation from the heart to the brain.[2,3]

The Extrinsic and Intrinsic Cardiac Autonomic Nervous System

The cardiac autonomic nervous system (CANS) regulates vascular tone, contractility, and electrophysiology by transducing and integrating the afferent and efferent autonomic trafficking.[2,3] Autonomic control of the heart is mediated by highly integrated intrinsic and extrinsic CANS.[2,3] The extrinsic CANS mainly consists of ganglia and their axons located outside the heart. The nucleus ambiguus, dorsal vagal nucleus, and vagus nerves constitute most of the parasympathetic limb of the extrinsic CANS, whereas the neurons in the intermediolateral column of the spinal cord, the stellate ganglia, and their axons en route to the heart constitute most of the sympathetic limb. The intrinsic CANS is mainly composed of sympathetic and parasympathetic nerves as well as GP on the heart itself, or along the great vessels in the thorax such as the pulmonary artery, aorta, superior vena cava (SVC), and pulmonary veins (PVs). The stellate ganglia serve as the "head stage" for the sympathetic innervation of the heart. The postganglionic sympathetic fibers, mainly from the stellate ganglia, constitute the vast majority of the sympathetic innervation to both the atrium and ventricle. The major atrial GP are embedded in the epicardial fat pads and contain up to several hundred autonomic neurons (Fig. 44.1A–C). The distribution of the major ventricular GP is limited to the proximal segments of the coronary arteries; they are in general small and not as extensive on the ventricles.[2–5]

The intrinsic CANS appears to function interdependently as well as independently from the extrinsic CANS, evidenced by its retaining of nearly full control of the cardiac physiology after autotransplantation.[2,3] Armour elegantly described the intrinsic CANS as "the little brain on the heart." A cooperative interaction between the extrinsic and intrinsic CANS maintains a homeostasis that facilitates balanced cardiac physiological functions. The major atrial GP are located adjacent to the PV–atrial junction or the junction of the right atrium and the SVC or inferior vena cava. Chiou and colleagues discovered that the efferent parasympathetic fibers in the vagus nerve converge at a GP before innervating the heart.[6] This right pulmonary artery–aortico (RPA–Ao) GP, at the junction of the right pulmonary artery, aorta, and SVC, was coined as the "head stage" GP because the bradycardia response induced by vagus nerve stimulation in canine hearts was nearly abolished if the RPA–Ao GP was ablated.[6]

The different nomenclature used by anatomists introduced a great deal of confusion for scientific communication.[2–5] In this chapter, we use the nomenclature based on clinical anatomy, e.g., GP's relation to PVs (see Fig. 44.1A–C). The superior left GP (SLGP) and inferior left GP (ILGP) are located adjacent to the PV–atrial junction of the left superior PV and left inferior PV, respectively.[7] The anterior right GP (ARGP) is situated at the caudal end of the sinoatrial node near the right superior PV–atrial junction. The inferior right GP (IRGP) extends from the inferior right PV–atrial junction to the crux of the heart near the junction of the right atrium and inferior vena cava.

It was once thought that the ARGP specifically innervates the sinus node, while the IRGP at the crux of the heart only innervates the AV node. Recent studies have indicated that the intrinsic CANS forms a complex neural network and GP serve as the "integration centers" to control the physiological functions of the heart.[2,3,8] For example, high-frequency stimulation (HFS, 20 Hz) to the SLGP also markedly slowed the sinus rate (SR), proving that the ARGP is not the only GP innervating the sinus node. Ablation of the ARGP greatly attenuated, but did not eliminate, the SR slowing response induced by SLGP stimulation, indicative of the ARGPs' role as the gateway GP for the sinus node and the presence of other neural pathways bypassing the ARGP. Ablation of the four major atrial GP and ligament of

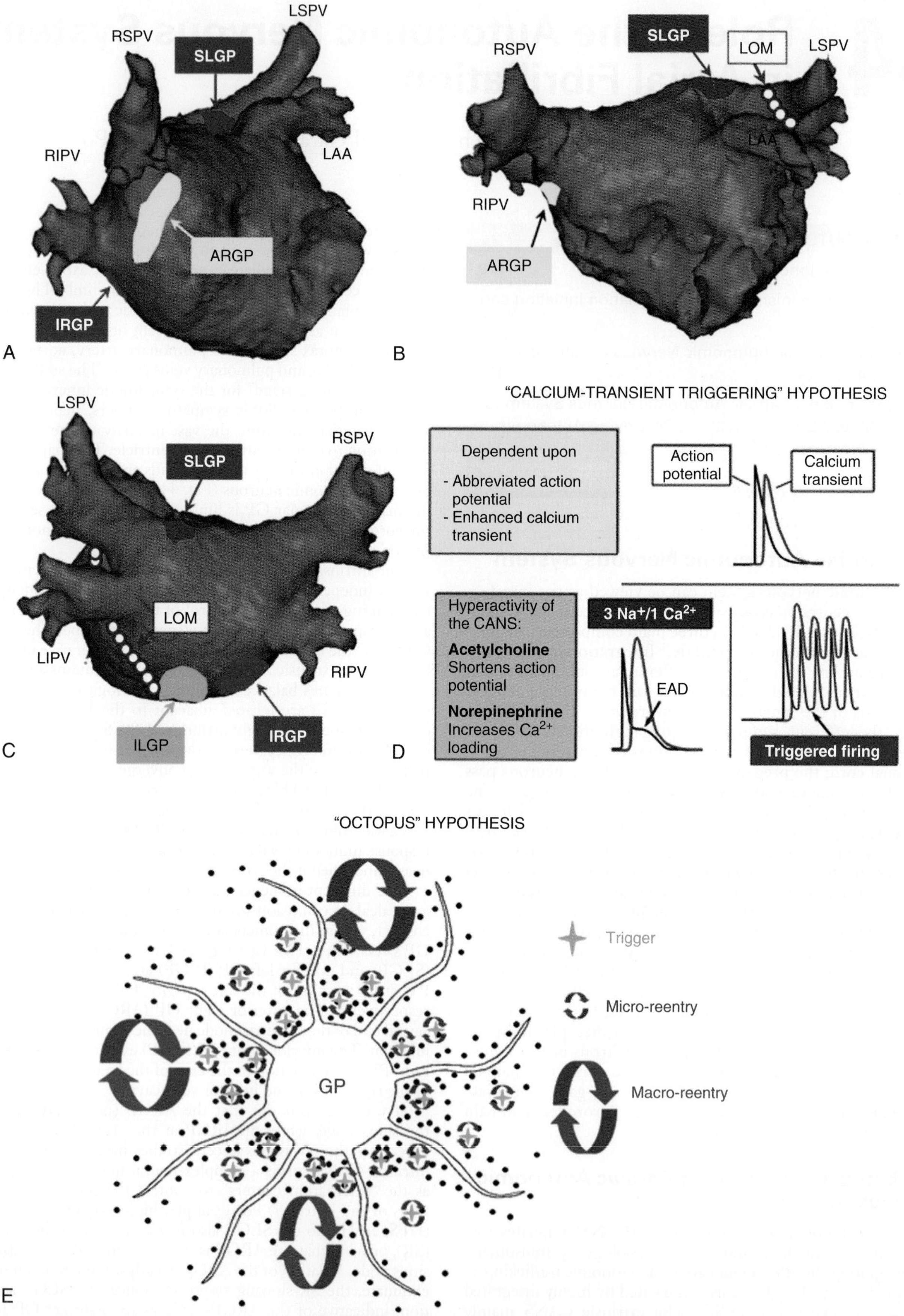

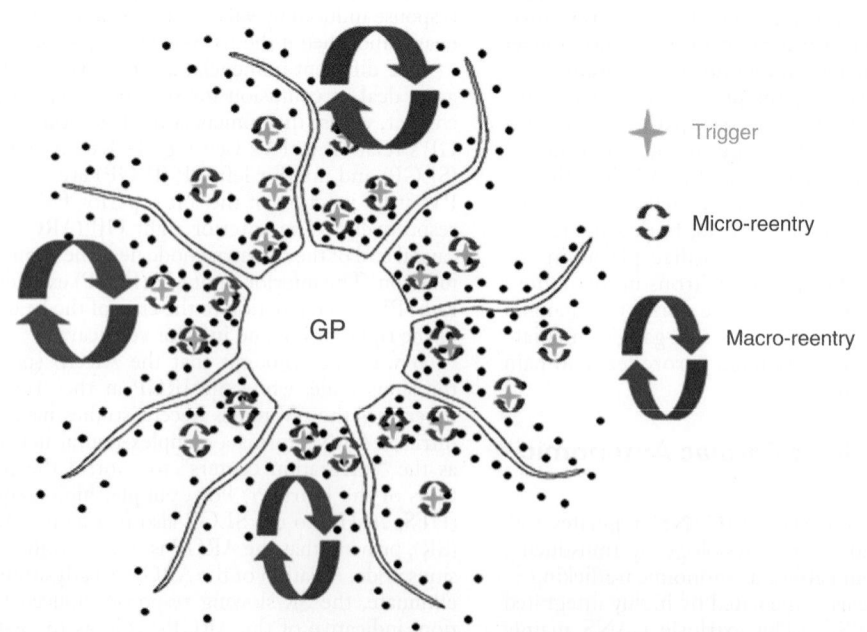

FIGURE 44.1 For legend, see opposite page.

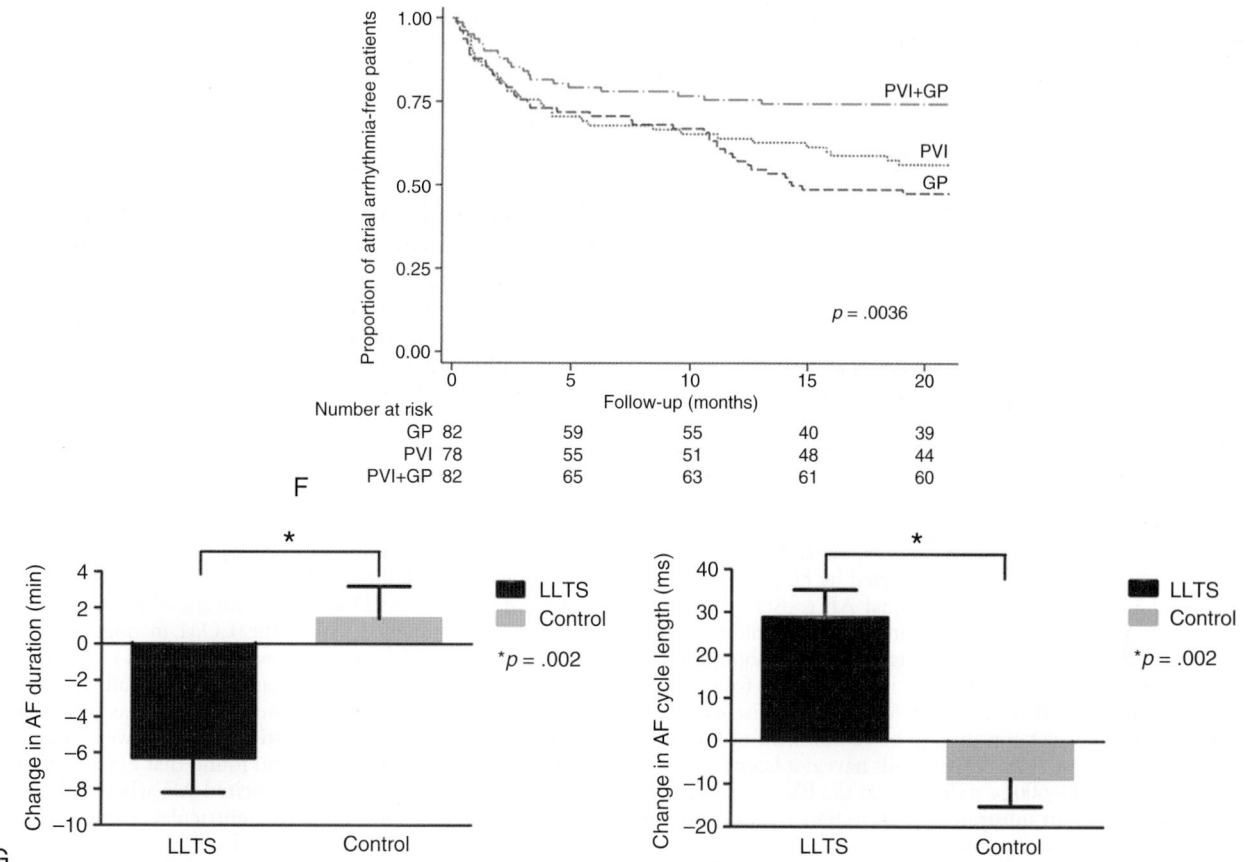

FIGURE 44.1 (A)–(C) Location of the major atrial ganglionated plexi (*GP*) and ligament of Marshall (*LOM*). (A) Right anterior oblique view. (B) Anteroposterior caudal view. (C) Posteroanterior view. (D) Ca²⁺ transient hypothesis. Simultaneous activation of the sympathetic and parasympathetic systems induces early afterdepolarization and subsequently triggered firing (see text for details). (E) Octopus hypothesis. Hyperactivity of the autonomic neurons (head of the octopus) causes excessive release of the neurotransmitters from the autonomic nerves (tentacle) at multiple sites. This leads to triggered firing and reentry at multiple sites to initiate and maintain atrial fibrillation (AF). (F) Results of a randomized clinical trial including GP ablation for paroxysmal AF. The addition of GP ablation to standard pulmonary vein isolation (*PVI*) significantly increased freedom from AF at follow-up. (G) Antiarrhythmic effects of low-level tragus stimulation (*LLTS*) in humans. Pacing-induced AF duration (*left panel*) and AF cycle length (*right panel*) were significantly decreased by LLTS compared to control. *ARGP*, Anterior right GP; *CANS*, cardiac autonomic nervous system; *EAD*, early afterdepolarization; *ILGP*, inferior left GP; *IRGP*, inferior right GP; *LIPV*, left inferior pulmonary vein; *LSPV*, left superior pulmonary vein; *RIPV*, right inferior pulmonary vein; *RSPV*, right superior pulmonary vein; *SLGP*, superior left GP. ([D] Modified from Patterson E, Lazzara R, Szabo B, et al. Sodium-calcium zexchange initiated by the Ca²⁺ transient: an arrhythmia trigger within pulmonary veins. *J Am Coll Cardiol.* 2006;47:1196-1206. [F] Modified from Katritsis DG, Pokushalov E, Romanov A, et al. Autonomic denervation added to pulmonary vein isolation for paroxysmal atrial fibrillation: a randomized clinical trial. *J Am Coll Cardiol.* 2013;62:2318-2325. [G] Modified from Stavrakis S, Humphrey MB, Scherlag BJ, et al. Low-level transcutaneous electrical vagus nerve stimulation suppresses atrial fibrillation. *J Am Coll Cardiol.* 2015;65:867-875.)

Marshall (LOM) exerts potent inhibitory effects on the activity of the CANS, supporting clinical implications targeting these GP to treat atrial fibrillation (AF).[9]

Noncholinergic, Nonadrenergic Neurotransmitters in the Intrinsic Cardiac Autonomic Nervous System

Until the 1990s, it was believed that the sympathetic component of the intrinsic CANS is composed exclusively of postganglionic sympathetic fibers, and all cardiac autonomic neurons are parasympathetic neurons expressing cholinergic markers. With the advances in immunohistochemistry, subpopulations of cardiac autonomic neurons expressing various neurotransmitter markers have been identified.[10] The presence of the peptidergic, nitrergic, and noradrenergic neurons, along with their associated neurotransmitters, such as neuropeptide-Y, vasostatin, galactin, vasoactive intestinal peptide (VIP), nitric oxide synthase, and angiotensin-II, strongly indicate that the autonomic control of cardiac physiology involves a milieu of neurotransmitters beyond acetylcholine and norepinephrine.[10–14] Neuropeptide-Y coreleased by prolonged sympathetic activation reduces acetylcholine release from the neighboring vagal nerve ending, and it is a good example of sympathovagal cross-talk.[11] These noncholinergic, nonadrenergic neurotransmitters often exert effects similar to cholinergic or adrenergic agonists or antagonists. Using cholinergic and adrenergic blockers alone to "eliminate" the CANS control is clearly an oversimplified approach.[15,16] Liu and associates demonstrated that until an antagonist of VIP ([Ac-Tyr1,D-phe2]-VIP) was administered, vagal stimulation continued to induce AF in canine hearts despite GP ablation+atropine+esmolol.[14] The release of these neurotransmitters/modulators is often highly dependent on the level of neuronal stimulation, and they tend to be slowly diffusing molecules that often function as neuromodulators rather than classical neurotransmitters. Better understanding of the arrhythmogenic potential of these noncholinergic, nonadrenergic neurotransmitters may facilitate the development of new antiarrhythmic agents to treat AF.

Autonomic Mechanisms of Atrial Fibrillation Initiation and Maintenance

In 1978, Coumel and coworkers described a group of patients with AF of vagal origin, manifesting an absence of structural heart disease and nocturnal onset of AF preceded by a slow heart rate.[17] As the vast majority of AF patients appeared not to have the typical findings described by Coumel, vagal AF was viewed as a rarity. The landmark findings reported by Haisseguerre and colleagues demonstrated that paroxysmal AF resistant to drugs and cardioversion, in most cases, originated from rapid focal firing in the PVs.[18] Subsequent studies verified the pathophysiological roles of the PV muscle sleeve as an ideal substrate for reentry, and periodic acid–Schiff (PAS)–positive cells were discovered in the PV myocardium that appeared to be reminiscent of Purkinje cells.[19] However, these PAS-positive cells have not been shown to elicit rapid firing (300–600 beats/min), and the PV sleeve, despite being an ideal reentrant substrate, cannot initiate reentry without a spontaneous, well-timed premature beat.

Since the early 2000s, AF ablation has evolved from eliminating the focal trigger(s) within the PVs (focal PV ablation) to circumferentially isolating the PV–atrial antrum (CPVI). Ironically, the mechanism(s) responsible for the following fundamental questions remain poorly understood: (1) Why do PVs elicit rapid firing? (2) How does PV firing initiate AF? and (3) How does AF maintain itself, particularly in the first few hours before structural remodeling starts? The recent, disappointing long-term outcome (<50% success, 5 years, single procedure) of the standard CPVI[20,21] clearly indicates that a better understanding of the mechanisms underlying AF initiation and maintenance is crucial for identifying more effective ablation targets, thereby providing more effective methods for treating AF.

The "Ca^{2+} Transient Triggering" Hypothesis

Clinical studies have demonstrated that activation of both the sympathetic and parasympathetic nervous systems commonly precedes the initiation of paroxysmal AF.[22,23] This finding was later corroborated by multiple basic studies.[24–26] Patterson and associates[26] proposed a "Ca^{2+} transient triggering" hypothesis to explain the initiation of rapid PV firing. This hypothesis states that norepinephrine (by sympathetic activation) augments the Ca^{2+} transient, and acetylcholine (by parasympathetic activation) shortens the PV action potential duration (APD). The abbreviated APD contrasts with the longer Ca^{2+} transient, allowing loading of the myocytes with excess Ca^{2+}. This leads to activation of the forward mode of the Na$^+$/Ca^{2+} exchanger, causing early afterdepolarizations and subsequently triggered firing from the PVs (see Fig. 44.1D). This hypothesis also helps explain the observation that PV firing often occurs at the distal segments of the PVs where the APD is the shortest.[27] Zhou and coworkers proposed an "octopus hypothesis" in which the autonomic neurons in the major atrial GP function like the head of an octopus, while their axons are analogous to the tentacles.[28] When the head of the octopus becomes hyperactive, excessive release of neurotransmitters

from its tentacles can initiate triggered firing and macro- and microreentry at multiple atrial sites to initiate and maintain AF (see Fig. 44.1E). The "octopus hypothesis" also implies that targeting the head of the octopus, i.e., the GP, is perhaps the most effective means to mitigate a hyperactive state of the CANS and subsequently the associated arrhythmias.

Rapid Firing From the Nonpulmonary Vein Sites: Ligament of Marshall and Superior Vena Cava

Although PV firing accounts for nearly 90% of the initiation of paroxysmal AF, non-PV sites such as the LOM and SVC are alternative sites for rapid firing and AF initiation.[29,30] Notably, the initiation pattern of paroxysmal AF from the LOM, SVC, and PVs is remarkably similar. LOM itself is richly innervated and had been named the "left atrial neural fold" by some anatomists, signifying the abundance of its autonomic neural elements.[5] However, there are substantial discrepancies in the relative abundance of sympathetic versus parasympathetic innervation reported by different groups.[31–34] Based on both electrophysiological and immunohistochemical findings, Ulphani and colleagues[31] found the LOM as a parasympathetic conduit in normal dogs, whereas Doshi and associates[32] demonstrated sympathetic predominance within the LOM in dogs with chronic AF. In contrast, Makino and coworkers found in human hearts that the LOM–LSPV junction was sympathetically predominant, whereas the LOM–coronary sinus junction was predominantly parasympathetic.[33] Such innervation gradients were later corroborated by Lin and colleagues, who found that HFS at the LOM–coronary sinus junction mainly elicited AF, whereas HFS at the LOM–LSPV junction induced ventricular tachycardia, atrial tachycardia, or junctional tachycardia.[34] However, it is unquestionable that the LOM provides an ideal substrate for triggered firing if the sympathetic versus parasympathetic balance is altered or if both become hyperactive.

Another common site for non-PV firing is the SVC–atrial junction, where high density of autonomic innervation has been shown.[6] In patients, the site of rapid firing and successful ablation was usually the posteroseptal aspect of the SVC–RA junction adjacent to the RPV–Ao junction, suggesting that this "head stage" GP may be the autonomic basis of SVC firing. Lu and associates delivered HFS to this GP and elicited rapid firing and AF only at the SVC, not at atrium or PV.[35] Ablation of this GP only prolonged the refractory period at SVC sites. These findings indicate that the RPA–Ao GP may provide specific autonomic innervation to the atrial sleeve investing the SVC–atrial junction, and hyperactivity of this GP may be the basis for the SVC firing. Intuitively, elimination of the RPA–Ao GP may alleviate AF because acute stimulation of the RPA–Ao GP induces rapid firing and AF from the SVC–RA junction. Paradoxically, ablation of this "head stage" GP led to progressive increases of the AF burden[33] in a chronic canine model, suggesting that the RPA–Ao GP might relay inhibitory vagal output from the extrinsic to the intrinsic CANS. The seemingly conflicting role of this "head stage" GP underscores the complex interplay between the intrinsic and extrinsic CANS in the occurrence and suppression of AF.

Perpetuation of Atrial Fibrillation: The First Few Hours and Beyond

Electrical remodeling (e.g., shortening of the refractory period) and structural remodeling (e.g., fibrosis) are indispensable factors to perpetuate AF over a period of several weeks or months.[36–38] However, how AF perpetuates itself within the first few minutes or hours after its initiation (e.g., before the occurrence of structural remodeling) is poorly understood. Any modality that provides early termination of AF will have a great impact on AF therapy. Yu and coworkers recorded the neural activity of the canine ARGP or SLGP during 6 hours of AF that was simulated by rapid atrial pacing.[39] Rapid atrial pacing not only shortened the atrial refractory period but also progressively enhanced the neural activity within the GP, providing direct evidence of autonomic remodeling during AF. Yu and colleagues proposed that electrical and autonomic remodeling formed a vicious cycle. A hyperactive state of the intrinsic CANS (e.g., GP) facilitates AF initiation. AF then shortens the refractory period further and augments the GP activity to perpetuate AF itself. This "vicious cycle" hypothesis helps answer the aforementioned fundamental questions: (1) Why do PVs elicit rapid firing? (2) How does PV firing initiate AF? and (3) How does AF maintain itself? Autonomic remodeling as a part of the answer to the third question was further corroborated by a study by Zhang and associates[40] in a rabbit model of rapid atrial pacing for 24 hours. In the first 12 hours of rapid atrial pacing, both sympathetic and vagal activity progressively increased. Then, vagal activity remained elevated, but the sympathetic activity began to attenuate. Progressive increases of neural elements that stained positive for growth-associated protein 43 (GAP43), choline acetyltransferase, and tyrosine hydroxylase were also noted during 24-hour pacing, suggesting progressive autonomic remodeling.

As previously discussed, AF begets electrical, structural, and autonomic remodeling. As AF burden increases, the increased GP activity may spread to peripheral atrial sites. The excessive neurotransmitter release locally engenders more atrial substrates (e.g., shortened and dispersed refractory period, higher intracellular Ca^{2+} load, and inflammation) to sustain AF. Importantly, higher autonomic activity, particularly sympathetic activity, is associated with inflammation that is known to facilitate atrial fibrosis and structural remodeling.[41–43] We hypothesize that the "metastasizing" activity within the intrinsic CANS may be a crucial element in facilitating the progression of AF from the paroxysmal form to more advanced forms, in which higher global CANS activity promotes electrical remodeling, inflammation, and structural remodeling, thereby facilitating AF progression.

Autonomic Basis for Complex Fractionated Atrial Electrograms

In 2004, Nademanee and coworkers described the technique for targeting complex fractionated atrial electrograms (CFAEs) to treat patients with paroxysmal AF.[44] Although CFAEs may simply be caused by the physical properties of the myocardial fibers, such as anisotropic conduction or zones of slow conduction, two other hypotheses also help account for the formation of CFAEs: the rotor and the autonomic hypotheses. The rotor hypothesis indicates that CFAEs are formed when the meandering rotor(s) encounters heterogeneous substrates (e.g., dispersion of refractoriness).[45] CFAEs are therefore the byproduct of the reentrant rotors, which break down at the boundaries of these rotors. Notably, infusion of acetylcholine into the animal heart is required to maintain a stable rotor, implying that the rotor hypothesis is also related to autonomic activity. The autonomic hypothesis stems from the locations of the CFAEs originally described by Nademanee and colleagues[44]; according to this hypothesis, the distribution of the CFAEs correlates well with the locations of the major atrial GP. Lin and associates showed in a canine model that CFAEs can be produced by the topical application of acetylcholine[46] at sites on the atria showing regular but rapid activation during AF. Furthermore, CFAEs could be eliminated by ablating the GP at a distance from those sites, indicating that activation of the intrinsic CANS is critical in the formation of CFAEs. Clinical studies later corroborated that CFAEs tend to occur at the presumed GP sites.[47] Ablation of GP greatly reduced the extent of CFAE distribution around the GP, implying a possible causal relationship between CANS activity and CFAEs.[7,46]

Several clinical studies independently reported that combined cholinergic and adrenergic blockade attenuated, but failed to eliminate, CFAEs in patients undergoing AF ablation,[15,16] casting doubt on the autonomic mechanism for CFAEs. The CFAEs recorded in patients with paroxysmal AF appeared to be more sensitive to autonomic blockers compared with CFAEs in those with persistent AF, underlying the importance of other mechanisms (e.g., fibrosis) responsible for the formation of CFAEs. Of note, a large milieu of noncholinergic, nonadrenergic neurotransmitters has been identified within the intrinsic CANS.[10–12] Failure to eliminate CFAEs by cholinergic and adrenergic blockade cannot exclude the autonomic mechanism underlying CFAEs. AF ablations targeting CFAEs as a stand-alone therapy or an adjunct therapy to CPVI have not been shown to improve outcomes compared to CPVI alone in patients with paroxysmal or persistent AF.[48,49] As previously discussed, CFAEs are probably an electrophysiological epiphenomenon of a host of underlying pathophysiological conditions such as fibrosis, inflammation, and autonomic hyperactivity. Attempts to eliminate CFAE may not have enough effects on the conditions responsible for CFAEs or the suppression of the various forms of AF.

Ablating the Cardiac Autonomic Nervous System to Treat Atrial Fibrillation

To ablate the CANS to treat AF, the most practical targets are the major atrial GP (e.g., the head of the "octopus"[28]). An accidental finding was reported by Pappone and coworkers describing a group of paroxysmal AF patients undergoing CPVI.[50] When a parasympathetic response was evoked by ablation, elimination of all evoked parasympathetic responses around the PV ostia resulted in an outstanding success rate (99%) in terms of freedom from AF. Scanavacca and colleagues showed the feasibility of selective GP ablation using an endocardial approach, and the results of some, but not all, GP ablations were disappointing.[51] With a better understanding of the anatomy and physiology of the major atrial GP, the results of GP ablation improved substantially. A major limitation of GP ablation is that despite their consistent location adjacent to the PV–atrial junction, the extent of each "hyperactive" GP that needs to be ablated to treat AF is largely unknown. Pokushalov and associates randomized 80 paroxysmal AF patients to two groups: (1) selective GP ablation guided by parasympathetic responses induced by HFS (20 Hz) and (2) ablation of GP selected by their presumed anatomical locations.[52] At 13.1 ± 1.9 months, 42.5% of patients with HFS-guided GP ablation and 77.5% of patients with anatomical GP ablation were free of symptomatic AF (p = .02). Their difference may be attributed to significantly more radiofrequency applications delivered in the latter group, covering a larger area for each GP.

While GP-only ablation appeared to produce results similar to those of the standard CPVI, the combination of CPVI and GP ablation seemed to lead to higher success rates than CPVI alone.[7,53] Recently, Katritsis and coworkers randomized 242 patients with PAF to circumferential PVI alone, anatomical GP ablation alone, and circumferential PVI plus anatomical PVI ablation.[54] After 2 years of follow-up, freedom from AF or atrial tachycardia was achieved in 56%, 48%, and 74% of patients in the PVI, GP ablation, and PVI+GP ablation groups, respectively (p = .0036), indicating additional benefits provided by GP ablation (see Fig. 44.1F). Moreover, in another randomized study comprising 264 patients with persistent AF, the addition of GP ablation to PVI conferred superior clinical results compared to the addition of linear lesions to PVI (freedom from AF at 3 years, 34% in the PVI plus linear lesions group versus 49% in the PVI plus GP group; p = .035).[55] While the debate of adding GP ablation to CPVI continues, it cannot be overemphasized that CPVI transects the LOM, almost three of four major atrial GP at the

PV–atrial junction (see Fig. 44.1A–C), and numerous autonomic nerves. Thus the contribution of autonomic denervation to the efficacy of CPVI cannot be overlooked.

The disappointing long-term results of a single AF ablation (CPVI) raises further questions: (1) Is the isolated or destroyed myocardium the real trigger or substrate for AF? and (2) What is the cause of AF recurrence after ablation? The premise of CPVI, at least for paroxysmal AF, is to ensure that rapid firing inside the CPVI line does not exit into the left atrium to initiate AF. A common but intriguing observation of CPVI is that rapid firing tends to cease after CPVI, implying that the real arrhythmogenic tissue is either along the CPVI line or in the left atrium. In a recent study of patients with paroxysmal AF, isoproterenol and adenosine triphosphate (ATP) were coadministered to provoke PV firing before and after CPVI.[56] PV firing was induced in 58.0% and 18.2% of patients before and after CPVI, respectively ($p < .01$). PV firing was induced in 2 of 88 patients after CPVI, which was eliminated by GP ablation *outside* the CPVI line. These findings strongly suggest that the real source of PV firing is located in the atrium; PV firing may be an epiphenomenon.

Although the resumption of conduction between PV and atrium is considered the main cause for recurrence, mapping of the PV–atrial junction in patients without clinical recurrence after AF ablation is rarely done. Jiang and colleagues studied 43 and 32 patients with and without recurrence of atrial tachyarrhythmia for 12 months after CPVI, respectively.[57] Repeat mapping of the PV–LA junctions revealed that 29 of 32 patients without arrhythmia recurrence (90.5%) had at least one PV that was not electrically isolated from the LA. When compared to patients with recurrence, no significant differences were seen in the proportion of patients with reconnection or the location of the reconnection. These findings suggest that sustained PV isolation may not be required for freedom from the clinical recurrence of AF and question the real cause of AF recurrence after ablation.

Modulation of the Cardiac Autonomic Nervous System to Treat Atrial Fibrillation Without Destroying Autonomic Neural Elements

The consequences of neural degeneration and regeneration after ablation are poorly understood. If autonomic denervation and regeneration are critical elements in the efficacy and failure of CPVI, respectively, suppression of the hyperactive CANS by modulating, instead of destroying, the autonomic neural elements may be a more effective approach. Inspired by a clinical report by Tai et al.[58] showing that PV firing in paroxysmal AF patients could be inhibited by increased vagal reflex caused by phenylephrine-induced hypertension, the Oklahoma group hypothesized that by taking advantage of neural plasticity, low-level vagal stimulation (LL-VS) at voltages not slowing the heart rate or AV conduction may inhibit the CANS and subsequently suppress AF inducibility. A series of acute canine studies corroborated that LL-VS markedly lengthened the atrial and PV refractory period and inhibited the AF inducibility.[59–62] Notably, LL-VS was capable of preventing AF initiation as well as terminating AF. The antiarrhythmic effects were mediated by the suppression of the recorded neural activity of the major atrial GP and the stellate ganglia.[60,61] Chronic canine studies by Shen and associates not only verified these findings but also discovered that suppression of the stellate ganglion activity is responsible for the effects of LL-VS on AF.[63] Notably, in acute canine studies, low-level transcutaneous stimulation of the tragus, where the auricular branch of the vagus nerve is located, worked as well as stimulating the cervical vagus nerve, indicating that transcutaneous LL-VS may be a clinically feasible approach to treat AF and other autonomic-based diseases without permanently injuring the myocardium or intrinsic CANS.[64] This approach was recently tested in a pilot randomized clinical trial. Stavrakis and coworkers randomized 40 patients to either low-level tragus stimulation (LLTS) for 1 hour or sham stimulation. LLTS for only 1 hour was enough to suppress effective refractory period (ERP) shortening and AF inducibility, as well as shorten the AF duration and prolong AF cycle length in paroxysmal AF patients (see Fig. 44.1G).[65] It is noteworthy that the inflammatory markers, including tumor necrosis factor (TNF)-α, were also reduced by 1 hour of LLTS, indicating that LLTS may have an antiinflammatory effect as well. Future studies are required to evaluate the chronic antiarrhythmic and antiinflammatory effects of LLTS.

Perspectives

Although the results of GP ablation to treat AF have been promising, several recent lines of evidence suggest that AF can be targeted from afar, without destroying myocardium. The use of transcutaneous vagus nerve stimulation, as previously illustrated, is an example. Another example is renal artery denervation. While it remains unclear which sympathetic pathways are modified by renal artery denervation, a more direct relationship between autonomic modulation and AF appeared in a clinical study by Pokushalov and colleagues.[66] Patients with concomitant AF and drug-resistant hypertension were randomized into two groups: CPVI versus CPVI plus renal artery denervation. After a follow-up of 12 months, 29% of patients with CPVI alone were AF free, whereas 69% of those with PVI plus renal artery denervation were AF free ($p = .03$).

Using injections of botulinum toxin in the epicardial fat pads to achieve temporary denervation of the major atrial GP, a neuromodulatory approach was also used to treat AF following cardiac surgery. In this randomized controlled trial, the injection of botulinum toxin in the epicardial fat pads ($n = 30$) compared to injection of saline alone ($n = 30$) resulted in a significantly lower incidence of AF not only at 30 days but also at 12 months of follow-up (0% vs. 27%, respectively, $p = .002$).[67] In addition, the mean AF burden assessed using implantable loop recorders was significantly lower in the botulinum toxin injection group than in the placebo group ($p < .001$). The results of neuromodulation, such as LLTS or temporary autonomic denervation using botulinum toxin injection in the GP, highlight a potential new paradigm for treating arrhythmias. Instead of solely targeting the myocardial substrates, modulation of CANS activity may alter both the neural and myocardial substrates for arrhythmias and mitigate the arrhythmias with minimal myocardial damage.

REFERENCES

1. Goetz CG. Autonomic nervous system. In: Goetz CG, ed. *Textbook of Clinical Neurology*. 3rd ed. Philadelphia: Saunders; 2007:383–404.
2. Armour JA. Functional anatomy of intrathoracic neurons innervating the atria and ventricles. *Heart Rhythm*. 2010;7:994–996.
3. Armour JA. The little brain on the heart. *Cleve Clin J Med*. 2007;74:S48–S51.
4. Saburkina I, Rysevaite K, Pauziene N, et al. Epicardial neural ganglionated plexus of ovine heart: anatomic basis for experimental cardiac electrophysiology and nerve protective cardiac surgery. *Heart Rhythm*. 2010;7:942–950.
5. Pauza DH, Skripka V, Pauziene N. Morphology of the intrinsic cardiac nervous system in the dog: a whole-mount study employing histochemical staining with acetylcholinesterase. *Cells Tissues Organs*. 2002;172:297–320.
6. Chiou CW, Eble JN, Zipes DP. Efferent vagal innervation of the canine atria and sinus and atrioventricular nodes. The third fat pad. *Circulation*. 1997;95:2573–2584.
7. Po SS, Nakagawa H, Jackman WM. Localization of left atrial ganglionated plexi in patients with atrial fibrillation. *J Cardiovasc Electrophysiol*. 2009;20:1186–1189.
8. Hou Y, Scherlag BJ, Zhou J, et al. Interactive atrial neural network: determining the connections between ganglionated plexi. *Heart Rhythm*. 2007;4:56–63.
9. Lu Z, Scherlag BJ, Lin J, et al. Autonomic mechanism for initiation of rapid firing from atria and pulmonary vein: evidence by ablation of ganglionated plexi. *Cardiovasc Res*. 2009;84:245–252.
10. Hoover DB, Isaacs ER, Jacques F, et al. Localization of multiple neurotransmitters in surgically derived specimens of human atrial ganglia. *Neuroscience*. 2009;164:1170–1179.

11. Herring N, Paterson DJ. Neuromodulators of peripheral cardiac sympatho-vagal balance. *Exp Physiol.* 2009;94:46–53.

12. Herring N, Cranley J, Lokale MN, et al. The cardiac sympathetic co-transmitter galanin reduces acetylcholine release and vagal bradycardia: implications for neural control of cardiac excitability. *J Mol Cell Cardiol.* 2012;52:667–676.

13. Brack KE, Coote JH, Ng NA. Vagus nerve stimulation protects against ventricular.fibrillation independent of muscarinic receptor activation. *Cardiovasc Res.* 2011;91:437–446.

14. Liu Y, Scherlag BJ, Fan Y, et al. Inducibility of atrial fibrillation after GP ablations and 'autonomic blockade': evidence for the pathophysiological role of the non-adrenergic and non-cholinergic neurotransmitters. *J Cardiovasc Electrophysiol.* 2013;24:188–195.

15. Knecht S, Wright M, Matsuo S, et al. Impact of pharmacological autonomic blockade on complex fractionated atrial electrograms. *J Cardiovasc Electrophysiol.* 2010;21:766–772.

16. Chaldoupi SM, Linnenbank AC, Wittkampf FH, et al. Complex fractionated electrograms in the right atrial free wall and the superior/posterior wall of the left atrium are affected by activity of the autonomic nervous system. *J Cardiovasc Electrophysiol.* 2012;23:26–33.

17. Coumel P, Attuel P, Lavallée J, et al. The atrial arrhythmia syndrome of vagal origin. *Arch Mal Coeur Vaiss.* 1978;71:645–656.

18. Haïssaguerre M, Jaïs P, Shah DC, et al. Spontaneous initiation of atrial fibrillation by ectopic beats originating in the pulmonary veins. *N Engl J Med.* 1998;339:659–666.

19. Perez-Lugones A, McMahon JT, Ratliff NB, et al. Evidence of specialized conduction cells in human pulmonary vein of patients with atrial fibrillation. *J Cardiovasc Electrophysiol.* 2003;14:803–809.

20. Ouyang F, Tilz R, Chun J, et al. Long-term results of catheter ablation in paroxysmal atrial fibrillation: lessons from a 5-year follow-up. *Circulation.* 2010;122:2368–2377.

21. Weerasooriya R, Khairy P, Litalien J, et al. Catheter ablation for atrial fibrillation: are results maintained at 5 years of follow-up? *J Am Coll Cardiol.* 2011;57:160–166.

22. Bettoni M, Zimmermann M. Autonomic tone variations before the onset of paroxysmal atrial fibrillation. *Circulation.* 2002;105:2753–2759.

23. Amar D, Zhang H, Miodownik S, Kadish A. Competing autonomic mechanisms precedes the onset of postoperative atrial fibrillation. *J Am Coll Cardiol.* 2003;42:1262–1268.

24. Ogawa M, Zhou S, Tan AY, et al. Left stellate ganglion and vagal nerve activity and cardiac arrhythmias in ambulatory dogs with pacing-induced congestive heart failure. *J Am Coll Cardiol.* 2007;50:335–343.

25. Sharifov OF, Fedorov VV, Beloshapko G, et al. Roles of adrenergic and cholinergic stimulation in spontaneous atrial fibrillation in dogs. *J Am Coll Cardiol.* 2004;43:483–490.

26. Patterson E, Lazzara R, Szabo B, et al. Sodium-calcium exchange initiated by the Ca^{2+} transient: an arrhythmia trigger within pulmonary vein. *J Am Coll Cardiol.* 2006;21(47):1196–1206.

27. Po SS, Li Y, Tang D, et al. Rapid and stable re-entry within the pulmonary vein as a mechanism initiating paroxysmal atrial fibrillation. *J Am Coll Cardiol.* 2005;45:1871–1877.

28. Zhou J, Scherlag BS, Edwards J, et al. Gradients of atrial refractoriness and inducibility of atrial fibrillation due to ganglionated plexi stimulation. *J Cardiovas Electrophysiol.* 2007;18:83–90.

29. Chang HY, Lo LW, Lin YJ, et al. Long-term outcome of catheter ablation in patients with atrial fibrillation originating from the superior vena cava. *J Cardiovasc Electrophysiol.* 2012;23:955–961.

30. Hwang C, Fishbein MC, Chen PS. How and when to ablate the ligament of Marshall. *Heart Rhythm.* 2006;3:1505–1507.

31. Ulphani JS, Arora R, Cain JH, et al. The ligament of Marshall as a parasympathetic conduit. *Am J Physiol Heart Circ Physiol.* 2007;293:H1629–H1635.

32. Doshi RN, Wu TJ, Yashima M, Kim YH, et al. Relation between ligament of Marshall and adrenergic atrial tachyarrhythmia. *Circulation.* 1999;100. 876–683.

33. Makino M, Inoue S, Matsuyama TA, et al. Diverse myocardial extension and autonomic innervation on ligament of Marshall in humans. *J Cardiovasc Electrophysiol.* 2006;17:594–599.

34. Lin J, Scherlag BJ, Lu Z, et al. Inducibility of atrial and ventricular arrhythmias along the ligament of Marshall: role of autonomic factors. *J Cardiovasc Electrophysiol.* 2008;19:955–962.

35. Lu Z, Scherlag BJ, Niu G, et al. Functional properties of the superior vena cava (SVC)-aorta ganglionated plexi: evidence suggesting an autonomic basis for rapid SVC firing. *J Cardiovasc Electrophysiol.* 2010;21:1392–1399.

36. Wijffels MC, Kirchhof CJ, Dorland R, Allessie MA. Atrial fibrillation begets atrial fibrillation. A study in awake chronically instrumented goats. *Circulation.* 1995;92:1954–1968.

37. Everett 4th TH, Olgin JE. Atrial fibrosis and the mechanisms of atrial fibrillation. *Heart Rhythm.* 2007;4:S24–S27.

38. Yue L, Xie J, Nattel S. Molecular determinants of cardiac fibroblast electrical function and therapeutic implications for atrial fibrillation. *Cardiovasc Res.* 2011;89:744–753.

39. Yu L, Scherlag BJ, Sha Y, et al. Interactions between atrial electrical remodeling and autonomic remodeling: how to break the vicious cycle. *Heart Rhythm.* 2012;9:804–809.

40. Zhang L, Po SS, Wang H, et al. Autonomic remodeling: how atrial fibrillation begets atrial fibrillation in the first 24 hours. *J Cardiovasc Pharmacol.* 2015;66:307–315.

41. Frustaci A, Chimenti C, Bellocci F, et al. Histological substrate of atrial biopsies in patients with lone atrial fibrillation. *Circulation.* 1997;96:1180–1184.

42. Gao G, Dudley Jr SC. Redox regulation, NF-kappaB, and atrial fibrillation. *Antioxid Redox Signal.* 2009;11:2265–2277.

43. Andrade J, Khairy P, Dobrev D, Nattel S. The clinical profile and pathophysiology of atrial fibrillation: relationships among clinical features, epidemiology, and mechanisms. *Circ Res.* 2014;114:1453–1468.

44. Nademanee K, Mckenzie J, Kosar E, et al. A new approach for catheter ablation of atrial fibrillation: Mapping of the electrophysiologic substrate. *J Am Coll Cardiol.* 2004;43:2044–2053.

45. Kalifa J, Tanaka K, Zaitsev AV, et al. Mechanisms of wave fractionation at boundaries of high-frequency excitation in the posterior left atrium of the isolated sheep heart during atrial fibrillation. *Circulation.* 2006;113:626–633.

46. Lin J, Scherlag BJ, Lu Z, et al. Autonomic mechanism for complex fractionated atrial electrograms. *J Cardiovasc Electrophysiol.* 2008;19:835–842.

47. Katritsis D, Sougiannis D, Batsikas K, et al. Autonomic modulation of complex fractionated atrial electrograms in patients with paroxysmal atrial fibrillation. *J Interv Card Electrophysiol.* 2011;31:217–223.

48. Verma A, Jiang CY, Betts TR, et al. Approaches to catheter ablation for persistent atrial fibrillation. *N Engl J Med.* 2015;372:1812–1822.

49. Providência R, Lambiase PD, Srinivasan N, et al. Is there still a role for CFAE ablation in addition to pulmonary vein isolation in patients with paroxysmal and persistent atrial fibrillation? a meta-analysis of 1,415 patients. *Circ Arrhythm Electrophysiol.* 2015;8:1017–1029.

50. Pappone C, Santinelli V, Manguso F, et al. Pulmonary vein denervation enhances long-term benefit after circumferential ablation for paroxysmal atrial fibrillation. *Circulation.* 2004;109:327–334.

51. Scanavacca M, Pisani CF, Hachul D, et al. Selective atrial vagal denervation guided by evoked vagal reflex to treat patients with paroxysmal atrial fibrillation. *Circulation.* 2006;29(114):876–885.

52. Pokushalov E, Romanov A, Shugayev P, et al. Selective ganglionated plexi ablation for paroxysmal atrial fibrillation. *Heart Rhythm.* 2009;6:1257–1264.

53. Katritsis DG, Giazitzoglou E, Zografos T, et al. Rapid pulmonary vein isolation combined with autonomic ganglia modification: a randomized study. *Heart Rhythm.* 2011;8:672–678.

54. Katritsis DG, Pokushalov E, Romanov A, et al. Autonomic denervation added to pulmonary vein isolation for paroxysmal atrial fibrillation: a randomized clinical trial. *J Am Coll Cardiol.* 2013;62:2318–2325.

55. Pokushalov E, Romanov A, Katritsis DG, et al. Ganglionated plexus ablation vs linear ablation in patients undergoing pulmonary vein isolation for persistent/long-standing persistent atrial fibrillation: a randomized comparison. *Heart Rhythm.* 2013;10:1280–1286.

56. Jiang RH, Jiang CY, Sheng X, et al. Marked suppression of pulmonary vein firing after circumferential pulmonary vein isolation in patients with atrial fibrillation: is pulmonary vein firing an epiphenomenon? *J Cardiovasc Electrophysiol.* 2014;25:111–118.

57. Jiang RH, Po SS, Tung R, et al. Incidence of pulmonary vein conduction recovery in patients without clinical recurrence after ablation of paroxysmal atrial fibrillation: mechanistic implications. *Heart Rhythm.* 2014;11:969–976.

58. Tai CT, Chiou CW, Wen ZC, et al. Effect of phenylephrine on focal atrial fibrillation originating in the pulmonary veins and superior vena cava. *J Am Coll Cardiol.* 2000;36:788–793.

59. Li S, Scherlag BJ, Yu L, et al. Low level vagosympathetic stimulation: a paradox and potential new modality for the treatment of focal atrial fibrillation. *Circ Arrhythm Electrophysiol.* 2009;2:645–651.

60. Sha Y, Scherlag BJ, Yu L, et al. Low-level right vagal stimulation: anticholinergic and antiadrenergic effects. *J Cardiovasc Electrophysiol.* 2011;22:1147–1153.

61. Yu L, Scherlag BJ, Li S, et al. Low-level vagosympathetic nerve stimulation inhibits atrial fibrillation inducibility: direct evidence by neural recordings from intrinsic cardiac ganglia. *J Cardiovasc Electrophysiol.* 2011;22:4554–4563.

62. Sheng X, Scherlag BJ, Yu L, et al. Prevention and reversal of atrial fibrillation inducibility and autonomic remodeling by low level vagosympathetic nerve stimulation. *J Am Coll Cardiol.* 2011;57:563–571.

63. Shen MJ, Shinohara T, Park HW, et al. Continuous low-level vagus nerve stimulation reduces stellate ganglion nerve activity and paroxysmal atrial tachyarrhythmias in ambulatory canines. *Circulation.* 2011;123:2204–2212.

64. Yu L, Scherlag BJ, Li S, et al. Low-level transcutaneous electrical stimulation of the auricular branch of the vagus nerve: a noninvasive approach to treat the initial phase of atrial fibrillation. *Heart Rhythm.* 2013;10:428–435.

65. Stavrakis S, Humphrey MB, Scherlag BJ, et al. Low-level transcutaneous electrical vagus nerve stimulation suppresses atrial fibrillation. *J Am Coll Cardiol.* 2015;65:867–875.

66. Pokushalov E, Romanov A, Corbucci G, et al. A randomized comparison of pulmonary vein isolation with versus without concomitant renal artery denervation in patients with refractory symptomatic atrial fibrillation and resistant hypertension. *J Am Coll Cardiol.* 2012;60:1163–1170.

67. Pokushalov E, Kozlov B, Romanov A, et al. Botulinum toxin injection in epicardial fat pads for prevention of atrial fibrillation after cardiac surgery: one year follow up of a randomized pilot study. *Circ Arrhythm Electrophysiol.* 2015;8:1334–1341.

45 Rotors in Human Atrial Fibrillation

Sanjiv M. Narayan, Junaid A.B. Zaman, David Vidmar, and Wouter-Jan Rappel

There is an urgent clinical need to better define the mechanisms for atrial fibrillation (AF). Pharmacological therapy is often used to maintain sinus rhythm or limit ventricular rate in AF but has modest results.[1,2] Ablation by pulmonary vein isolation (PVI) is often successful in individual cases, yet single procedure success remains 40%–60% in meta-analyses[3] and randomized trials of paroxysmal[4] and persistent[5] AF even with latest generation catheters.[6,7] These limitations motivate translational studies[8] to define precise mechanistic targets for drug discovery[9] and ablation.

Mechanistic concepts for human AF have rapidly progressed in recent years. A major mechanistic debate is whether AF is sustained by disorganized self-regenerating activity with no source(s),[10,11] which mandates widespread ablation, or whether disorganization in AF is driven by localized sources,[12] which may respond to localized ablation. The debate is fueled by clinical experience that localized ablation may on occasion eliminate persistent AF,[13,14] that extensive ablation does not in general improve outcome,[15,16] and that AF exhibits consistent gradients in rate, organization, and spatial vector[17] that are difficult to explain by disorganized mechanisms alone.

The localized source hypothesis, in which AF is sustained by rotors or focal sources, has been demonstrated through optical mapping of AF in animal models[12] and diseased human atria[18] and may explain these observations. Moreover, new mapping tools have revealed rotors and focal sources in AF patients[14] that show many similarities to human AF optical mapping studies,[18] where ablation can improve outcomes.[19–22]

One potential explanation for this mechanistic debate is that it reflects differences in the mapping methods used by each side. For instance, classical rules for interpreting electrograms (e.g., qS, rS shape) were developed for a single wavefront (e.g.. atrial flutter), activating all tissue within the recording envelope of the electrode in 1:1 fashion. However, this may need to be revisited in AF, where each electrode records an envelope containing an undefined number of spatiotemporally varying wavelets and collisions.[23,24] It is thus not surprising that maps differ for techniques that do or do not use these rules. More surprising is that nearly all studies of optical imaging that map action potentials (APs) show that AF is sustained by rotors and focal sources across a variety of model systems,[12] including human atria,[18] whereas nearly all mapping studies of AF using classical electrogram rules in many of the same species (including humans) do not.

This chapter examines the physiological determinants of AF in human atria and compares the methods to map these mechanisms in computational models, translational studies, and clinical trials. Our interpretation of the literature is that human AF, at least in patients who present for catheter ablation, is best explained by a small number of localized rotors or focal sources that drive AF via a process of "fibrillatory conduction." We will support this argument with historical AF studies and contemporary clinical trials.

Mechanisms for the Initiation of Human Atrial Fibrillation

Arrhythmias may require dynamic and fixed mechanisms.[25] In AF, triggers such as ectopic beats,[26] bursts of atrial flutter,[27] or varying autonomic balance[28,29] may or may not dynamically initiate AF despite relatively fixed atrial architecture, surface curvature, and fibrosis.[30]

The dynamics of atrial repolarization and conduction may explain how triggers initiate clinical AF. In Fig. 45.1A, a single ectopic beat produces dramatic oscillations of human left atrial AP duration (APD)[27,31,32] because of the fashion in which APD shortens with diastolic interval (DI, time from end repolarization to depolarization of the next beat) or restitution (Fig. 45.1B).[33] Classically, a restitution slope of >1 enables an early beat (with short DI) to dramatically shorten APD and lengthen DI of the next beat, producing APD alternans that can be discordant in space to precipitate a wave break. Atrial conduction velocity is also rate dependent. Fig. 45.1C shows that triggers can dramatically slow human atrial conduction immediately preceding AF onset, producing a spiral wave reentry at AF onset (Fig. 45.1D).[34] Although it is unclear how these dynamics interact with atrial anatomy[35] or fibrosis,[36] a recent study showed that each of the multiple distinct AF initiations (spiral wave reentry) arose at spatially conserved sites for diverse triggers in either atrium, suggesting that functional mechanisms are spatially determined.

Mechanisms That Sustain Human Atrial Fibrillation

Once initiated by triggers from PVs,[26] other thoracic veins,[37] or other sites,[38] disorganized wavefronts in AF can be sustained by two hypothesized mechanisms. In one mechanism, AF is caused by spatially variable mechanisms, particularly a multitude of short-lived spiral waves (wavelets) with a limited spatial extent. In the multiwavelet hypothesis,[10] disorganized activity generates new wavelets in a stochastic fashion. A related version posits that focal activity occurs randomly in time and space,[39] resulting in colliding and fragmenting wavefronts. Of note, this hypothesis does not require "special" tissue regions so that AF can occur in homogeneous or heterogeneous tissue. The second alternative mechanism is that certain "special" regions of the atria harbor sources in the form of spiral waves or focal sources. These localized sources generate wavefronts that break down and are known in this context as fibrillatory conduction.

The multiwavelet mechanism implies a finite probability that wavelets self-terminate by encountering a nonconducting tissue boundary so that AF duration is determined by rates of wavelet creation and extinction. Fig. 45.2 shows computer simulations of unstable spiral waves and multiwavelet reentry in homogeneous two-dimensional domains with nonconducting boundaries. In Fig. 45.2A, the number of spiral tips fluctuates and is approximately five for this 4.5×4.5-cm domain and parameter set. Because the number of tips is stochastic, there is a finite probability that the

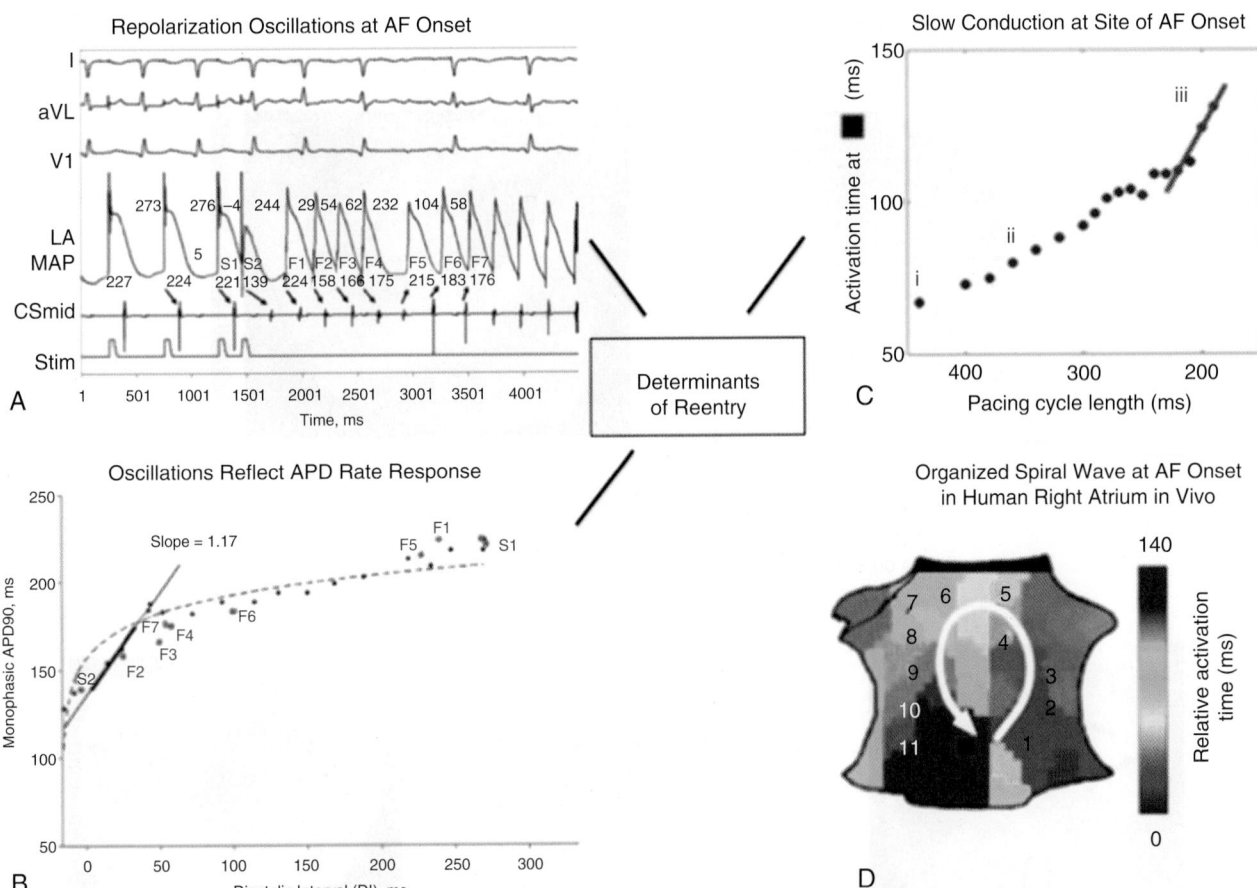

FIGURE 45.1 Dynamic initiating mechanisms for human atrial fibrillation (*AF*). (A) Clinical electrograms show ectopic beat (S2) causing AF (varying rapid cycle lengths). (B) A steep action potential duration (*APD*) restitution curve enables S2 to produce repolarization oscillations preceding AF. (C) A conduction restitution curve shows dynamic slowing at the site of AF onset imminently preceding AF onset (iii, *red slope*). (D) Critical activation delay facilitates formation of a counterclockwise spiral, initiating AF in the right atrium that was conserved across AF initiations from diverse triggers.

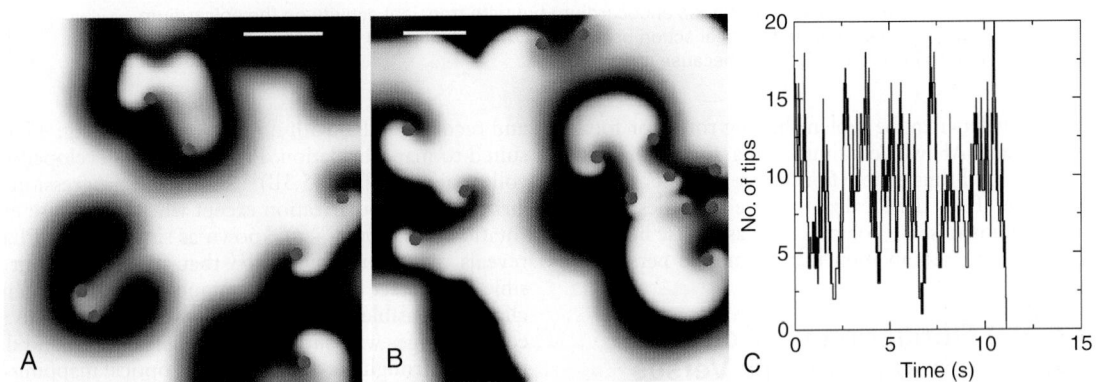

FIGURE 45.2 Multiwavelet reentry has a stochastic probability of terminating. A snapshot of simulations with multiwavelet activation color coded with white (*black*), corresponding to depolarized (repolarized) tissue. The position of the spiral tips is marked by *red dots*. The spatial domain in (A) is 4.5 × 4.5 cm, while the domain in (B) is 5.625 × 5.625 cm in size. Scale bar = 1 cm. Panel (C) shows the number of spiral tips as a function of time for one of the simulations, showing the abrupt termination of atrial fibrillation.

number of tips spontaneously reaches 0, resulting in AF termination. In 100 simulations with different random initial conditions, average spontaneous termination time was ≈3.3 seconds. Fig. 45.2B shows a simulation of identical parameters in a larger domain (5.625 × 5.625 cm), with eight spiral wave tips and a

termination time of approximately 15 seconds. The result of a typical simulation, presenting the number of spiral tips as a function of time, is shown in Fig. 45.2C. Multiwavelet reentry should thus last longer for larger domains,[40] as seen clinically, but with a finite probability of termination, unless waves are regenerated.

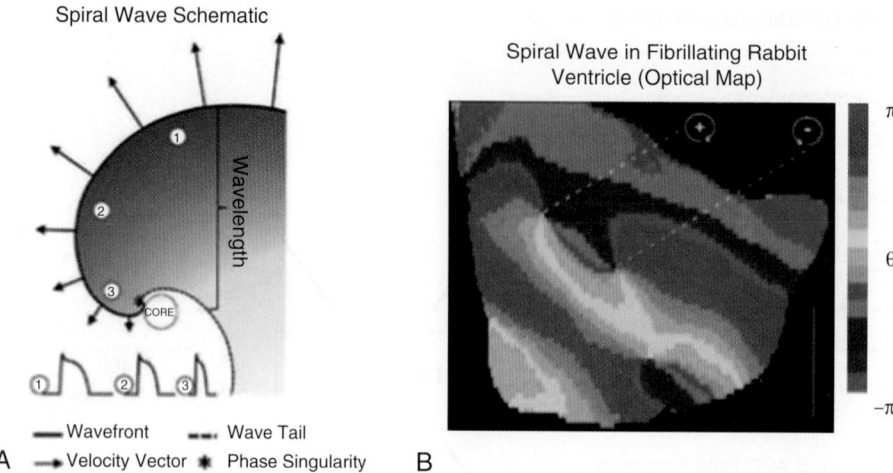

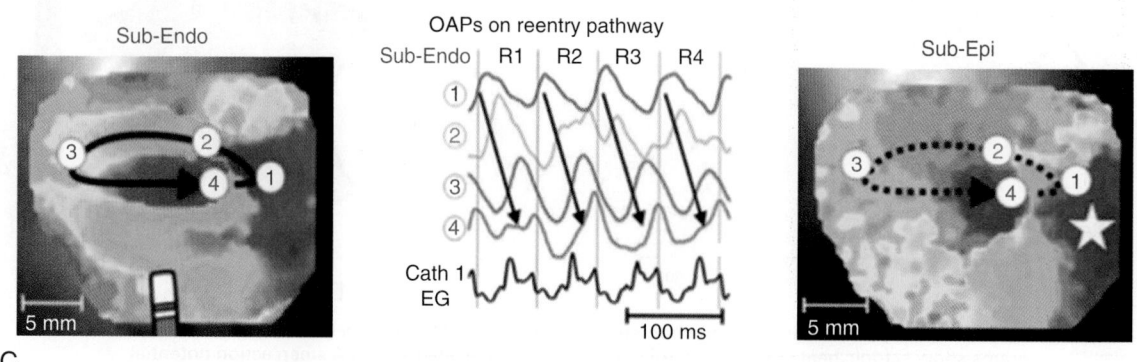

FIGURE 45.3 Spiral wave reentry as drivers of cardiac fibrillation. (A) Schematic of spiral wave, showing wavefront curvature as conduction velocity slows toward the core (*).[12] (B) First experimental demonstration of spiral waves (in rabbit ventricular fibrillation). The phase is depicted in color with chirality indicated by + (clockwise) or – (counterclockwise). Three phase singularities are seen; the bottom one has no chirality label.[43] (C) Optical mapping of human atria in atrial fibrillation shows stable microreentrant sources on the endocardium but with transient activity on the epicardium. Notably, despite consistent optical action potentials (*OAPs*) at sites 1–4 on the endocardium, the electrograms (Cath 1 EG) vary because of crosstalk.[18]

Alternatively, wavelets may be replenished by rotors or focal sources, in which case AF will continue while source(s) exist. Rotor elimination would thus enable fibrillatory wavelets to stochastically terminate. Thus the localized source hypothesis may explain how AF sustains in small volumes such as mouse hearts[41] and, clinically, how targeted ablation may terminate persistent AF.[13,14,42]

Mapping Atrial Fibrillation via Activation and Recovery: Action Potentials Versus Electrogram Surrogates

Mapping Considerations

Because AF is characterized by rapid spatiotemporally varying wavelets where successive activations may occur at the limits of recovery, AF mapping should ideally detect activation and recovery at high temporal resolution and multiple sites without crosstalk (contamination) from adjacent or remote myocardium.

Mapping Human Atrial Fibrillation Using Action Potentials

Optical mapping of voltage-sensitive dyes provides high spatial and temporal resolution for simultaneously mapping activation

and recovery (APs) with minimal crosstalk (Fig. 45.3) and is well suited to map fibrillation. Phase analysis developed by Gray and colleagues (see Fig. 45.3B)[43] shows the progression from depolarization to repolarization except where the phase exhibits a full rotation (i.e., – π to + π), known as singularities. Phase mapping reveals rotors in fibrillation[12] that are difficult but not impossible[44] to detect by other techniques. Optical mapping is not yet clinically feasible because of dye toxicity, the need to register successive images without immobilizing the heart, and difficulties of imaging through blood.[45] However, optical mapping has recently been applied to explanted diseased atria from AF patients[18] (see Fig. 45.3C).

In patients, activation and recovery can be measured in AF[27,32] with monophasic AP (MAP) catheters that are validated against intracellular recordings[46] and that can capture minimal far field.[47] However, challenges in the recording of MAPs at multiple sites in patients have limited this approach to a few centers.[27,48]

Traditionally, mapping of human AF has thus used electrograms[11] that provide high temporal resolution and can be recorded at multiple sites. However, a number of potential pitfalls must be recognized when using unipolar or bipolar electrodes to map spatiotemporal activation during AF.

Electrogram-Based Mapping of Human Atrial Fibrillation

Recordings from bipolar electrodes, as used in most clinical AF mapping studies, compare extracellular potential at two closely spaced poles. It is well appreciated that bipolar signals critically depend on the alignment of the electrode pair relative to an activation front, which, if it reaches both poles simultaneously, will not be recorded and thus will produce incorrect activation times. Fig. 45.4A shows a computer simulation of a stable spiral surrounded by fibrillatory breakdown. The activation front arriving at the bipolar electrode (*white dots* in the coherent domain)

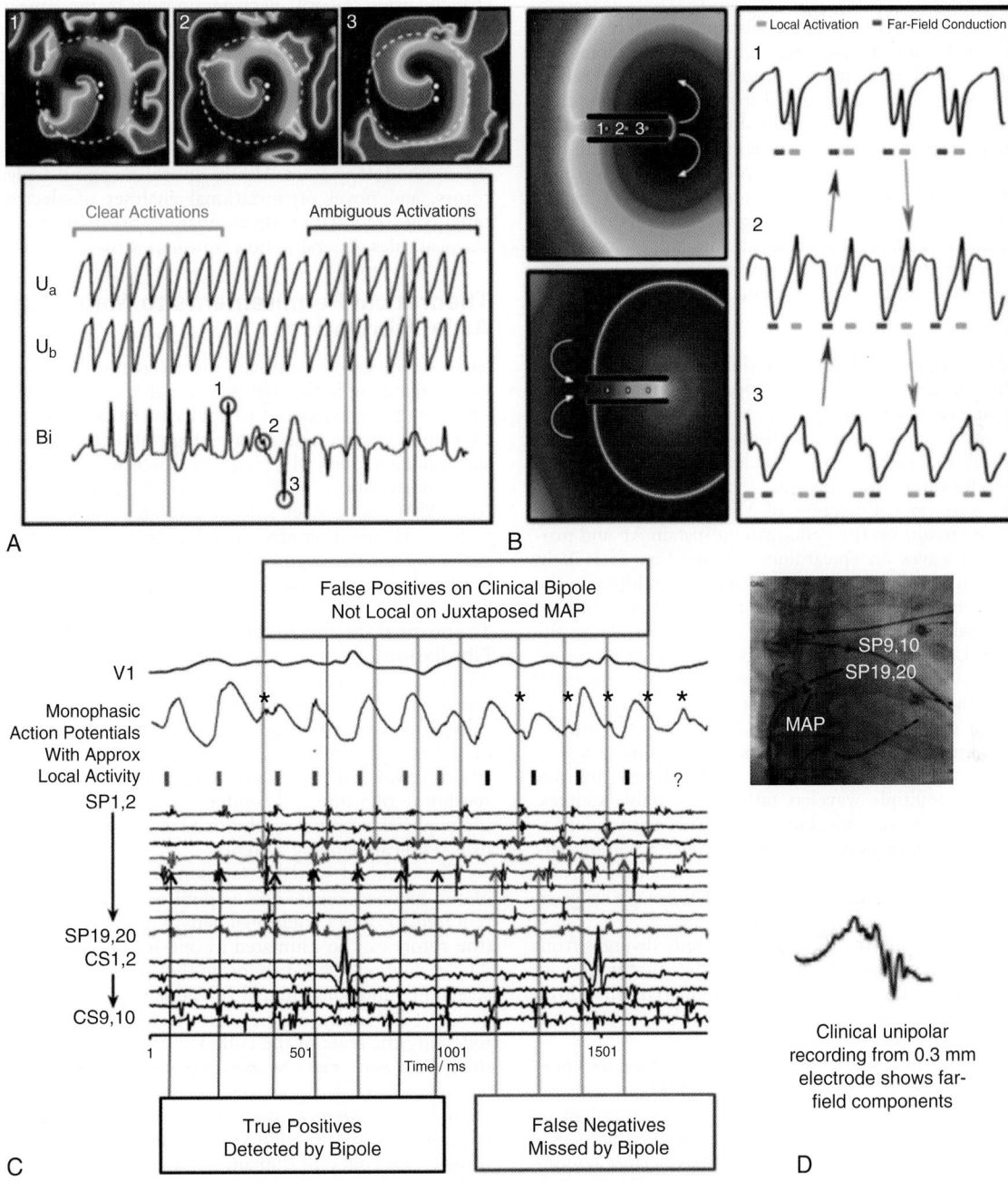

FIGURE 45.4 Potential pitfalls of classical electrogram interpretation in atrial fibrillation (AF). Computational and clinical studies. (A) *Upper panels* show snapshots of a simulation consisting of a stable spiral surrounded by fibrillatory conduction (warm/cold color corresponds to depolarized/repolarized tissue). *White dots* mark the locations of bipolar electrodes. Traces *Ua* and *Ub* represent unipolar activation, while the trace *Bi* shows the resulting bipolar electrogram. Points marked *1, 2,* and *3* correspond to snapshots in the *upper panels*. Note that the marking of activation times based on the bipolar electrogram becomes problematic as the direction of the incoming wavefront changes relative to the electrode positions, producing an incorrect marking. (B) Snapshots of a figure-of-eight reentry through a narrow isthmus, created by two nonconducting zones shown in *black*. Unipolar electrodes in the isthmus, indicated by *white dots*, show complex morphologies that represent local (*green*) and also far-field (*red*) activations. This may cause the activation times that are marked unipolar to be incorrect, as indicated by the *red arrows*. (C) Clinical AF recording showing that bipolar electrograms often miss local activity on a MAP catheter and depict far-field signals similar to local activity. Both effects will dramatically alter AF activation maps.[23] (D) Far-field components on unipolar electrodes reflect a wide recording field that integrates noncoherent waves.[11]

is missed at point no. 2 (corresponding to snapshot 2) because any slight tip movement alters the activation direction relative to the bipole. This may result in ambiguous activation markings or electrograms that miss activation times. Clinically, we have demonstrated that bipolar signals in AF may completely miss local activation and also detect unrelated far-field activations on an opposed MAP catheter[23] (see Fig. 45.4C).

Unipolar electrode recordings can also be misinterpreted in AF because, unlike optical mapping techniques, they integrate considerable far-field activation. Unipolar signals may reflect far-field components, even if recorded from small 0.3-mm electrodes[11] (see Fig. 45.4D), as shown in simulations.[49] Note that unipolar signals may be challenging even in a simple rhythm; Fig. 45.4B shows simulated macroreentry through a narrow isthmus. Unipolar electrograms at isthmus locations 1, 2, and 3 display multiple deflections representing local (*green*) and far-field (*red*) components that make local activation time difficult to assign and can easily result in incorrect maps (*red arrows*). Electrograms may be more complex in a fibrotic milieu and may further influence classical analysis.

Differing Mechanisms of Human Atrial Fibrillation Revealed by Optical/Electrogram Approaches

It is notable that optical mapping studies show that fibrillation is sustained by rotors across most animal models,[12] including studies from clinical AF patients,[18] whereas electrogram studies using classical mapping rules mostly do not.

In human atria, optical mapping of AF has shown that stable microreentrant circuits on the endocardium sustain AF and produce disordered waves on epicardium[18,50] (see Fig. 45.3C). In these studies, endocardial sources were single or multiple, in the right or left atrium, and were stable within 1-cm² areas related to microfibrosis and anatomical complexity (that was greater on the endocardium). Localized ablation at endocardial circuits terminated AF. These recent studies confirmed that localized sources may drive AF in human atria, and in preliminary studies, they correlated with novel clinical mapping tools.[51] Optical studies are subject to limitations, such as the use of uncoupling agents and pinacidil,[18,50] although by shortening refractoriness, this may actually facilitate multiple wavelets rather than stable sources. Moreover, in this context, optical mapping serves as an independent modality to examine activation waves during AF without far-field contamination and is well suited to examine classical rules to interpret electrograms in AF[51] and validate novel electrogram indices.

Electrogram mapping for AF, in fact, not only diverges from optical mapping but also differs between studies that used classical rules to create AF activation maps compared with those that used repetition, consistency, vectors, or other electrogram features.

In intraoperative mapping of subjects with longstanding persistent AF during valvular repair[52] or induced AF in controls without clinical AF,[11,53] the Maastricht group produced maps that showed disordered waves with no rotational activity that supported the Moe hypothesis, while Lee and associates demonstrated transient focal activity.[39] These studies are elegant with limitations that the Maastricht group simultaneously mapped only <10%–20% of the >100-cm² atrial areas in longstanding AF patients,[54] that these studies did not test interventions to support causality, and that rules for interpreting local activation[55,56] await comparison to optical maps. A minority of electrogram mapping studies showed rotational activity in AF, such as Schuessler and colleagues,[57] who showed stable reentry in canine right but not left atrium; Walters and coworkers,[17] who showed unstable rotations in some patients; and the mathematical inverse solution from the body surface that revealed transient rotational activity (in stable regions over time) in human AF.[58]

Studies that analyzed novel electrogram features, such as dominant frequency or electrogram morphology, do show

"organization" consistent with AF sources, such as repeating frequency gradients,[59,60] electrogram shapes,[61,62] and propagation vectors,[17,63] over time. These results appear to contradict the disordered AF hypothesis and again highlight differences in AF stability based on methodology; these studies also show more stable AF activation[19,59] than disordered activation maps constructed using classical electrogram rules by the same groups.[39,58] Atienza and colleagues showed that sites of high dominant frequency in paroxysmal AF patients were consistent with rotors[64] and that ablation at these sites alone was noninferior to wider anatomical PVI in the Radiofrequency Ablation of Drivers of Atrial Fibrillation (RADAR-AF) trial.[65]

The results of AF mapping are thus exquisitely sensitive to the methodology used. While optical mapping typically shows rotors, and novel organizational analyses of electrograms are often consistent with sources, analyses of AF electrograms using classical rules generally show transient activity and disorder.

Theoretical Requirements to Map Human Atrial Fibrillation

In 2001, we set out to clarify the mechanisms for human AF by widely mapping both atria using the dynamic physiology of activation and repolarization to approximate the strengths of optical mapping in the electrophysiology laboratory without invasive surgical techniques. Mapping was achieved by contact baskets[66,67] and repolarization,[31,32,68] conduction[34,69] dynamics were defined from MAP and basket studies, and algorithms were developed to filter AF electrograms physiologically rather than using rules based on qS, rS shape criteria. Our initial hypothesis was that localized sources do *not* exist in human AF.

Theoretical Design Requirements to Map Human Atrial Fibrillation

The minimum spatial and temporal resolution required to map human AF can be estimated from tissue characteristics.[70] Specifically, temporal resolution must be able to distinguish activation on neighboring recording sites and can be found by dividing the spatial resolution by dynamic conduction velocity. For a spatial resolution of 5 mm and conduction velocities of 150–50 cm/s,[69] the required temporal resolution (3.3–10 ms) is readily achievable using clinical mapping systems.

The required spatial resolution depends on the length scale of the mapped event. For a spiral wave, the spatial resolution required to detect rotational activity around a rigid spiral core (the rotor) can be estimated as one-fourth of wavelength ($\lambda/4$). The resolution needed to locate the spiral tip, however, is more stringent and is determined by the length scale of the reentrant path R_{locus}. Finally, a minimum electrode grid size is required, reflecting the scale of the coherent domain R_{rotor}. Grids smaller than R_{rotor} may miss the spiral tip and rotational activity. These length scales (λ, R_{locus}, and R_{rotor}) have been determined experimentally. The reentrant path R_{locus} ranges from 1 to >3 cm,[44,71,72] requiring a resolution of 0.5 cm to theoretically map the smallest rotors. The coherent domain has an area of >5 cm²,[73] so that if a plaque is directly placed over the rotor, its field of view should be >2.5 × 2.5 cm. Wavelength λ can be estimated as minimum conduction velocity × shortest refractory period.[74] In human AF, experimentally, this is $V_{min} \approx 20$ cm/s[69] × $APD_{min} \approx 110$ ms[31,32] for λ min of ≈2–3 cm, requiring a spatial resolution of ≈0.5–1 cm for the smallest rotor domains; however, a resolution of 1 cm or so may be sufficient if reentrant sources are larger (for instance in optical maps of human atria[18]).

Numerical Validation of Design Requirements for Atrial Fibrillation Mapping

We have recently validated our design requirements for human AF mapping using in silico simulations.[75] Fig. 45.5 shows a simulated stable rotor with wavelength λ = 3.2 cm and coherent

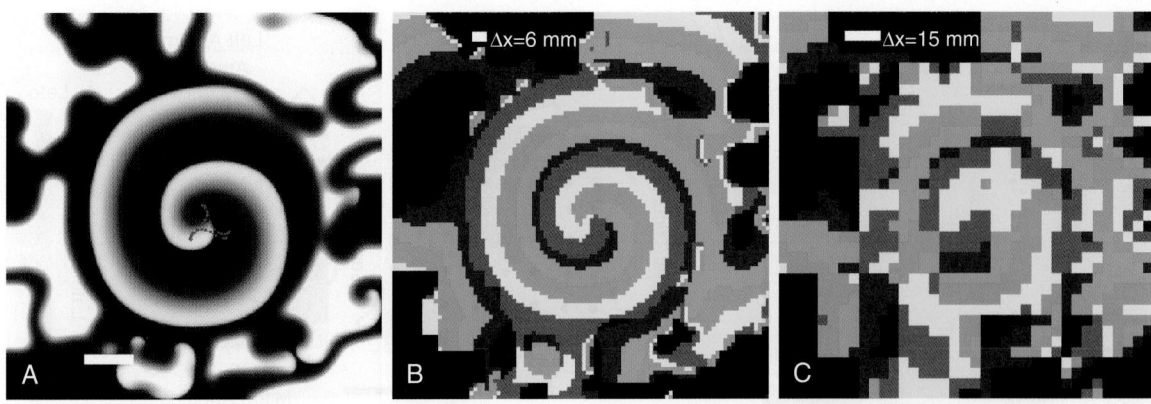

FIGURE 45.5 Required spatial resolution to map spiral wave reentry. (A) A snapshot of a simulation of a stable spiral, with a tip trajectory shown in *red*, surrounded by fibrillatory conduction. Scale bar = 1 cm. (B) The corresponding computed isochronal map, with *red* representing the most recent activation, using a resolution of 6 mm (indicated by scale bar). (C) Same as (B), but now with a spatial resolution of 15 mm. Although the rotor is difficult to see, it is still detectable on successive isochrones (movies).[70]

domain L_{rotor} = 6 cm, beyond which activity breaks down. A spatial resolution of $\Delta x \approx \lambda/4$ = 8 mm should reveal this spiral wave. Fig. 45.5B shows a color-coded isochronal map in human AF with *red/blue* indicating most/least recent activation for a spatial resolution Δx = 6 mm that detects the rotor. Further coarsening of resolution reduces the ability to identify a rotational pattern in a single snapshot (see Fig. 45.5C), although successive snapshots (i.e., movies) may still resolve the rotor.

Practical Requirements to Map Human Atrial Fibrillation

To simply detect a rotational AF source, optical mapping of human AF confirms that a resolution of ≈1 cm should resolve microreentrant AF sources (≈0.5–1.5 cm),[18,50] and larger spatial domains of AF sources in some clinical mapping studies[14,20,42] suggest that coarser resolution may also be effective in some cases. For the scientific goal of resolving rotor migration, however, finer spatial resolution is required.

A practical clinical approach to globally map atria at this resolution is to use a basket catheter (Fig. 45.6). Smaller pentarray or circular catheters may partially or completely miss a precessing rotor of the scale discussed and attempting to "piece together" sequentially mapped atrial patches during spatiotemporally varying AF is theoretically challenging. Accordingly, several basket designs are emerging, with typical electrode separations of finer than 4–6 mm along and 4–10 mm between splines. Spatial resolution is greater at the poles than at the equator, and one strategy is to place the basket poles over a region of interest identified from an initial global map.[67]

The theoretical temporal resolution to map human AF of 3.3–10 ms[70] is best achieved by dedicating one amplifier channel per electrode, which limits the practical number of recordable electrodes. Multiplexing is an alternative to recording more channels (e.g., 2 × 64 = 128, 3 × 64 = 192, or n × 64) every n-th timeslice rather than continuously. However, if sampling falls below the temporal resolution threshold, the AF map will lose accuracy.

Focal Impulse and Rotor Mapping Reveals That Rotors and Focal Sources Sustain Human Atrial Fibrillation

Using focal impulse and rotor mapping (FIRM) to map AF, based on the abovementioned physiological and technical considerations, several groups have demonstrated that localized rotors and focal sources sustain human AF. These source regions meet classical criteria as AF drivers, and, in a preliminary optical mapping study of AF in human atria, were identified simultaneously on both FIRM maps and optical maps[51]; further details are awaited. Ablation of human AF rotors has been shown to terminate AF in some studies and to improve the success of ablation. Many of these results have been verified by other groups using different methods.[19,76]

Demonstration of Rotors and Focal Sources in Human Atrial Fibrillation

For validation, Fig. 45.6B shows biatrial maps of sinus rhythm. The atria are projected onto grids that retain relative electrode locations, with the limitation that nonuniform electrode spacings appear uniform (akin to the Mercator versus Peters geographical projections of the Earth). Sinus activation is represented by *contour lines* (isochrones) from the sinoatrial node (*red*), crossing Bachmann's bundle to conclude in the inferolateral left atrium (*blue*). Fig. 45.6D shows right atrial activation in reverse typical flutter, and Fig. 45.6F shows a FIRM map of a simple focal atrial tachycardia (AT) with coherent 1:1 activation in ipsilateral and contralateral atria.

During AF, maps can reveal spatially organized regions as well as disorganized activation. *Rotors* are defined as a phase singularity (core) that yields spiral rotational waves that drive surrounding disorganization, or *focal impulses*, defined as centrifugal activation from a point of origin. Rotors and focal sources are used as ablation targets if they are stable in several recording epochs over tens of seconds to minutes and can exclude rotational and/or focal activations that do not occur in the same location over time (transient). Fig. 45.6C shows an AF rotor in the right atrium (*clockwise*) causing disorganization peripherally and in the left atrium. This is quite different than the 1:1 coherent activity from reverse typical flutter in Fig. 45.6D. Fig. 45.6E shows a focal source driving AF that differs from a simple AT (see Fig. 45.6F).

AF sources have been reported by multiple groups, first in the CONventional ablation with or without Focal Impulse and Rotor Modulation (CONFIRM) trial[14] and now extending to multicenter studies of paroxysmal, persistent, and long-standing persistent AF.[20–22,77] In the original CONFIRM trial (in 2011), a single AF map of both atria revealed 2.1 ± 1.0 concurrent AF sources in nearly all patients, with higher numbers in persistent AF,[14] sleep apnea, and obesity (particularly in the right atrium) patients.[78] Studies using contemporary software that enables AF remapping successively after ablation shows up to five biatrial rotors in longstanding persistent AF.[21]

AF sources may be conserved over time for the timescale initially reported for mapping (115 ± 57 minutes[79]), and in a

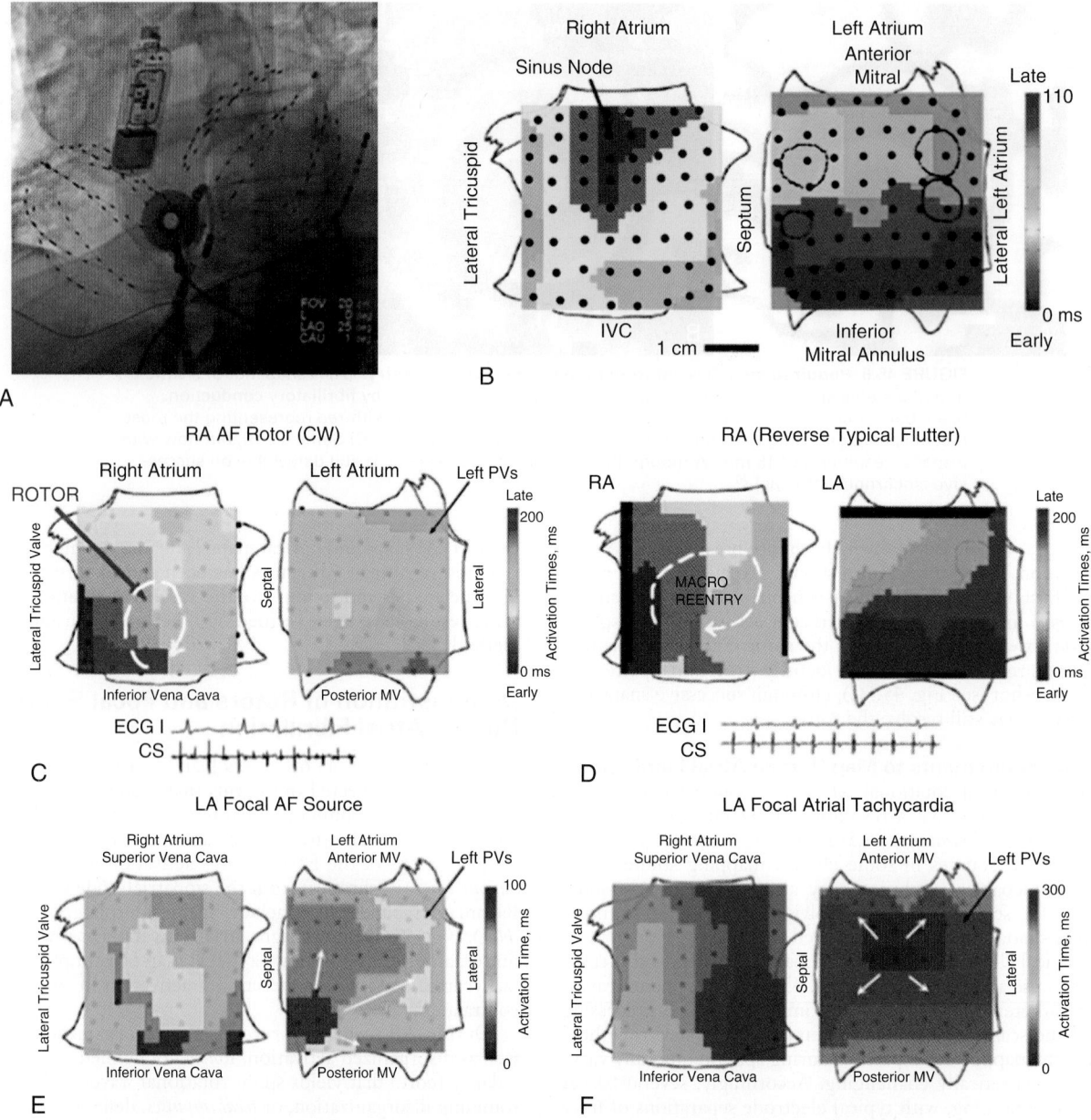

FIGURE 45.6 Contact basket mapping of sinus rhythm, atrial tachycardia, and atrial fibrillation (AF). (A) Fluoroscopy of 64-pole basket in the left atrium (*LA*). Ablation and coronary sinus (*CS*) catheters are also shown. The basket is typically placed first for right atrial (*RA*), then for LA mapping. (B) Sinus rhythm map on a biatrial schematic. The activation is color coded from the sinus node across RA and via Bachmann's bundle to the septal then the lateral inferior LA. RA is opened between its poles with the tricuspid annulus lateral and medial; LA is opened along its equator, with the mitral annulus opened superiorly and inferiorly. (C) Clockwise (*CW*) right atrial rotor in AF, showing noncoherent (non-1:1) propagation in RA and LA. In contrast, (D) CW (reverse) typical flutter with 1:1 propagation to LA. (E) Focal source for paroxysmal AF in low septal LA, with fibrillatory activation to the remaining LA and RA. In contrast, (F) Focal atrial tachycardia (nonfibrillatory) from the high posterior LA shows 1:1 activation centrifugally to the remaining LA, then across the CS to the RA (CL 300 ms). *ECG*, Electrocardiogram; *IVC*, inferior vena cava; *MV*, mitral valve; *PVs*, pulmonary veins. ([A] From Narayan S, Krummen D, Shivkumar K, et al. Treatment of atrial fibrillation by the ablation of localized sources. *J Am Coll Cardiol*. 2012;60:628-636. [B -E] Modified from Narayan S, Krummen D, Rappel WJ. Clinical mapping approach to diagnose electrical rotors and focal impulse sources for human atrial fibrillation. *J Cardiovasc Electrophysiol*. 2012;23:447-454.)

subset of subjects who failed conventional ablation and were remapped[79] over months. AF sources may also interact, particularly if there are several sources in the same atrium, so that a rotor may be temporarily obscured by fibrillatory conduction from a competing source and then reappear in the same location (spatial stability) for prolonged periods (temporal stability).[77] This may also represent a failure to detect intramural migration of an endocardial rotor as shown in human optical AF maps.[18]

AF rotors and focal sources lie in diverse locations. Right atrial sources represent approximately one-third of all sources,[20,67,77] as now echoed by other techniques.[19] This may explain the 70%–80% success ceiling of multiple left atrial ablation procedures[80] and the documented benefits of right atrial ablation in some patients.[81] In spontaneous and induced AF patients, maps of AF show similar source locations for both forms of AF per patient. There have been few complications during mapping.[14,20–22,77]

Evidence That Rotors and Focal Sources Drive Human Atrial Fibrillation

Three lines of evidence support rotors and focal sources as mechanisms that sustain human AF. First, mapping of directionality shows that activation emanates from sources to drive disordered AF in human atria.[82] Second, local ablation of rotors alone has been shown to acutely terminate AF at multiple centers.[14,22,42] Of note, termination of persistent AF by localized ablation is difficult to explain by disordered nonhierarchical models and has now been confirmed by groups using other methods to identify rotors.[19] Third, on long-term follow-up in many (nonrandomized) trials, rotor ablation improves upon the benefit of conventional ablation alone, and in early series and case reports, rotor ablation alone may be effective in paroxysmal AF patients where mapping is optimal.[83]

Activation Emanates From Human Atrial Fibrillation Sources

Rotors and focal sources exhibit 1:1 activation within their spatial domain, with peripheral disorganization (Figs. 45.6 and 45.7). We used directionality analysis to establish that activation emanates from rather than toward sustained AF sources, as used to prove the role of AF sources in animal models.[12,84] Fig. 45.7 shows (A) a left atrial AF rotor with (B) activation emanating to the remaining atria, and (C) a left atrial focal AF source with (D) activation emanating to the remaining atria. Directionality was conserved close to the center of each source but not farther away, which was consistent with the mechanism that AF sources are organized and sustain fibrillatory activity.[82]

Targeted Ablation at Atrial Fibrillation Rotors and Focal Sources Alone Can Acutely Terminate Persistent and Paroxysmal Atrial Fibrillation

Several groups have shown that source ablation alone can terminate AF[14,20,22,42,85] to sinus rhythm or AT, analogous to optical mapping studies in human atria.[18] This finding is difficult to explain by the multiwavelet hypothesis and supports localized sources. In each case, focused radiofrequency or cryoablation focused on the ≈2-cm² areas of source precession, shown by phase analysis in patients,[82] terminated AF in 30%–50% of cases across studies[14,21,22,42] (see Fig. 45.7). This is comparable with lower AF termination rates in patients treated with conventional ablation.[86,87] It is unclear why termination rates by source ablation differs among centers, which may reflect patient selection or ablation method, but long-term successes have been reported by rotor elimination without AF termination,[21] concordant with other findings that termination may not predict outcome from AF ablation.[88]

Mechanisms for AF termination by localized ablation are the subject of ongoing study[89] and are required to explain clinical reports where single[13,90] or very limited[82] interventions can terminate persistent AF to sinus rhythm without linear ablation (or PVI). We recently suggested a mechanistic framework to explain how local ablation may terminate AF to sinus rhythm[89] by interacting with structural and functional nonuniformities known to exist in the atria of AF patients[91] that anchor microreentrant AF drivers in optical maps of human atria[18,50] and that may be central to AF onset.[36]

Fig. 45.8 shows an ablation lesion that eliminates a zone of slow conduction that anchors a rotor,[12,92] that may occur near patchy fibrosis, and that results in rotor tip migration to regions of preserved conduction with boundary collision and AF termination to sinus rhythm. Fig. 45.8B shows a mechanism in which ablation increases the wave path to create an excitable gap that is invaded by fibrillatory waves to terminate AF. Several other mechanisms may operate depending on atrial properties, and so the mechanism of AF termination by rotor ablation in specific

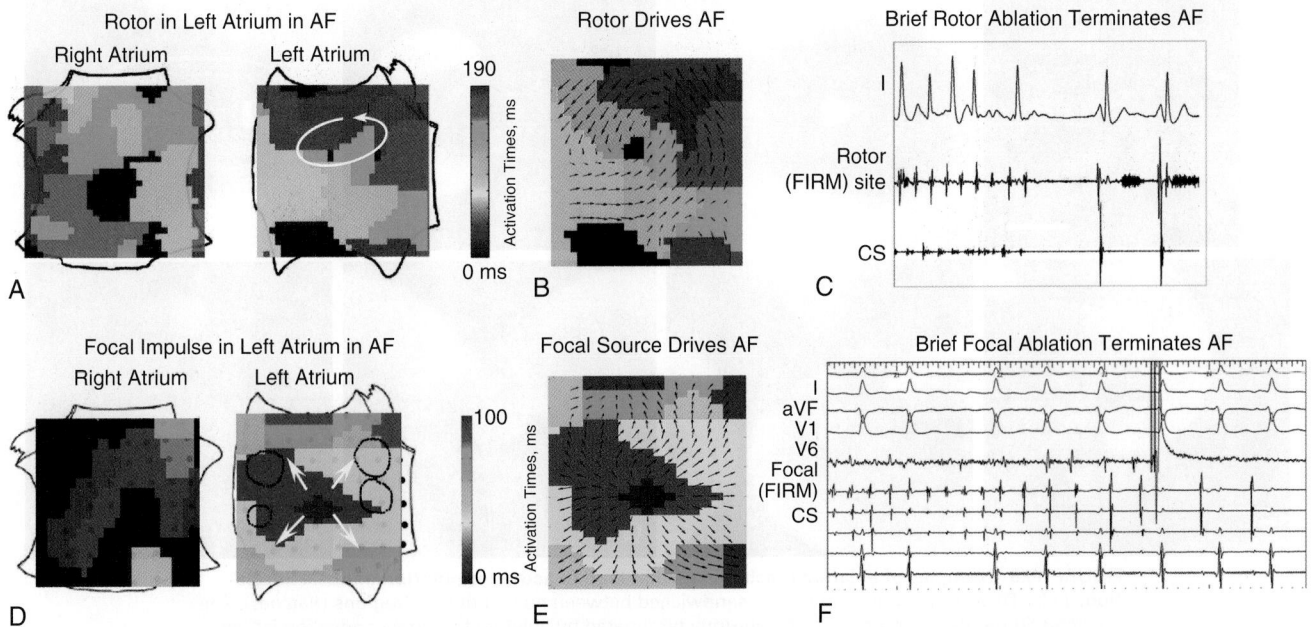

FIGURE 45.7 Activation emanates from localized atrial fibrillation (*AF*) sources to the surrounding atria, and localized ablation terminates human AF. (A) Left atrial AF rotor. (B) Directionality shows propagation from AF rotor to remaining atria. (C) AF termination to sinus rhythm by brief localized ablation at rotor. (D) Left atrial AF focal source. (E) Directionality shows propagation from AF focal source to remaining atria. The *arrows* indicate activation direction[84] between isochrones (*color bar*). (F) AF termination to sinus rhythm by brief localized ablation at focal source.

patients likely depends on the rotor location and its dynamic relationship with atrial nonuniformities.

Long-Term Follow-up After Focal Impulse and Rotor Mapping–Guided Ablation

A number of multicenter and single center studies now show that ablation of localized rotors and focal sources for human AF can improve success compared with conventional ablation, and randomized clinical trials are underway.

The CONFIRM trial was a prospective case cohort study[14] of 107 AF patients with standard ablation indications who underwent FIRM-guided ablation followed by conventional ablation or conventional ablation alone in 1:2 fashion. Overall, 72% of patients had persistent or longstanding persistent AF with a wide range of ages (20–81 years), left ventricular ejection fractions (20%–75%), and comorbidities. In the trial, source ablation used a single biatrial map because remapping after ablation was not possible using early mapping software. Conventional ablation consisted of PVI (and a roof line in persistent AF patients). Patients were carefully monitored using cardiac-implanted electronic devices during follow-up in 86% of patients. The single procedure freedom from AF was 82.4% in FIRM-guided patients compared with 44.9% in FIRM-blinded cases ($p < .001$) at up to 1 year.[14] A subsequent long-term study has shown that the benefit of FIRM-guided ablation in this cohort was maintained for a median of 2.5 years (Fig. 45.9).[93] Patients undergoing FIRM-guided ablation had more comorbidities and more AF monitoring than those in the conventional group. There was no difference in adverse events between groups, with inability to complete source ablation in a small number of patients such as to avoid esophageal heating or other factors. Some early mapping studies have recently reported disappointing results[94] for unclear reasons that may reflect small number of cases per operator, challenging patients, or other technical issues,[95] yet several groups have recently reported similar results to CONFIRM when FIRM-guided ablation (FIRM plus PVI) was used in an aggregate of over 500 patients.[20–22,96]

Other groups also have reported qualitatively similar results using other approaches to map AF sources. Using a body surface potential-based approach, Haissaguerre and associates reported rotational or focal source regions in all persistent AF patients. Ablation of these sites reduced ablation time compared with the traditional Bordeaux stepwise approach, with 1-year freedom from AF of 85% (with 16% rate of AT).[19,76]

The most significant limitation of these studies thus far is their nonrandomized design, although subjects were prospectively treated for prespecified endpoints. Strengths of these trials include the fact that success has been reported even in patients with advanced disease or after multiple failed conventional procedures.[20,21] Randomized clinical trials are underway for FIRM-guided, body surface potential mapping, and other approaches to rotor ablation, and these data are eagerly awaited.

Conclusions

Considerable evidence now supports the role of localized rotors and focal sources in sustaining human AF. Several modalities reveal that AF is typically sustained by a small number (typically 2–4) of sources, in spatially stable atrial regions over time, making them attractive ablation targets. Rotors identified by these methods meet many criteria as sustaining mechanisms for clinical AF, share many similarities with AF drivers on optical mapping of human atria, and have improved ablation success rates in studies from many centers.

These studies challenge historical data that AF is due to self-sustaining disorganization and highlight that reported AF mechanisms depend on the mapping modality used. While most optical mapping studies show that AF is sustained by rotors, most classical electrogram mapping studies do not. It remains to be determined if this is because classical electrogram rules are obfuscated by far-field signals or other factors. Notably, clinical

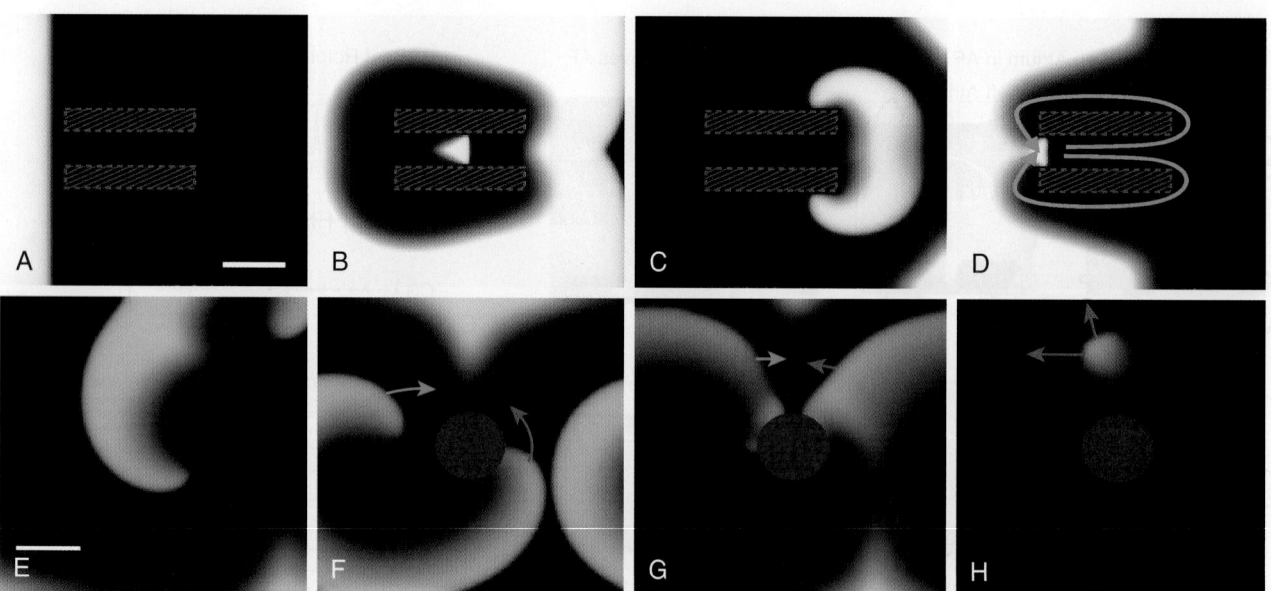

FIGURE 45.8 Examples of ablation mechanisms that lead to acute termination of atrial fibrillation. In (A–D), a slow-conducting zone is sandwiched between nonconducting regions (*hatche*s). The resulting figure-of-eight reentry can be abruptly terminated by ablating the slow-conducting isthmus. (E–H) present an example in which an excitable gap created by ablation is invaded by fibrillatory waves to rapidly terminate spiral wave reentry. Before ablation, multiple waves exist (E) and the abrupt creation of an ablation lesion (*blue disk*) leads to an activation front that rotates around the lesion (*red arrow*, F). The distance between the front and back of the wave is large enough that an incoming wave (*green arrow*) can excite the tissue. This results in a wave collision (G) and dislodgement of reentry (H). Scale bars = 1 cm.

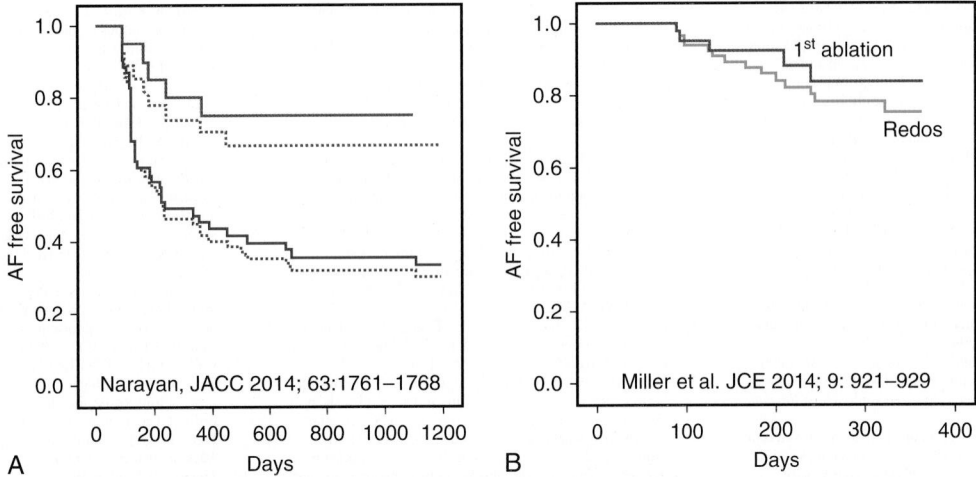

FIGURE 45.9 Cumulative freedom from atrial fibrillation (_AF_) in patients off antiarrhythmic medications. (A) Extended follow-up of CONventional ablation with or without Focal Impulse and Rotor Modulation (CONFIRM) trial for all cases (_bold lines_) and those at first ablation (_dashed lines_), for FIRM+ pulmonary vein isolation (PVI; _blue_), and PVI (_red_). Intention-to-treat analysis, and _p_ values reflect the complete follow-up period. (B) First Independent Outcomes from FIRM in n = 78 patients (2/3 persistent AF) at 10 centers. ([A] Modified from Narayan SM, Baykaner T, Clopton P, et al. Ablation of rotor and focal sources reduces late recurrence of atrial fibrillation compared to trigger ablation alone: extended follow-up of the CONFIRM [CONventional ablation with or without Focal Impulse and Rotor Modulation] trial. _J Am Coll Cardiol._ 2014;63:1761-1768. [B] Modified from Miller JM, Kowal RC, Swarup V, et al. Initial independent outcomes from focal impulse and rotor modulation ablation for atrial fibrillation: multicenter FIRM registry. _J Cardiovasc Electrophys._ 2014;25:921-929.)

studies that report AF rotors largely used mapping approaches that did not use classical rules to interpret unipolar and bipolar AF electrograms. To reconcile this debate, future studies should compare the results from simultaneous classical electrogram mapping, novel clinical mapping, and optical mapping as recently reported.[97] This may help develop and validate novel electrogram indices to analyze AF.

Future studies should also define how structural factors influence the formation and stabilization of AF rotors and the mechanisms of conduction breakdown (fibrillatory conduction). This may lead to additive benefit of imaging approaches in guiding patient management. Together, such studies may also enable more precise endophenotyping of AF patients. Mechanistic definition of AF at the cellular and genetic level may eventually enable preventive therapy for AF, as well as novel ablation, drug discovery, and potentially regenerative therapies for AF.

Acknowledgments

This work was supported by grants from the NIH to Dr. Narayan (HL83359, HL103800) and to Dr. Rappel (HL122384). Drs. Narayan and Rappel are the authors of intellectual property owned by the University of California Regents and licensed to Topera, Inc. and have held equity in Topera. Dr. Narayan reports consulting fees and honoraria from the American College of Cardiology, Medtronic, St. Jude, Abbott, and Uptodate. Dr. Zaman is funded by a Fulbright award and by a fellowship from the British Heart Foundation. Dr. Zaman and Mr. Vidmar report no other conflicts.

REFERENCES

1. Roy D, Talajic M, Nattel S, et al. Rhythm control versus rate control for atrial fibrillation and heart failure. _N Engl J Med._ 2008;358:2667–2677.
2. Van Gelder IC, Groenveld HF, Crijns HJ, et al. Lenient versus strict rate control in patients with atrial fibrillation. _N Engl J Med._ 2010;362:1363–1373.
3. Ganesan AN, Shipp NJ, Brooks AG, et al. Long-term outcomes of catheter ablation of atrial fibrillation: a systematic review and meta-analysis. _J Am Heart Assoc._ 2013;2:e004549.
4. Reddy VY, Dukkipati SR, Neuzil P, et al. Randomized, controlled trial of the safety and effectiveness of a contact force-sensing irrigated catheter for ablation of paroxysmal atrial fibrillation: results of the TactiCath Contact Force Ablation Catheter Study for Atrial Fibrillation (TOCCASTAR) study. _Circulation._ 2015;132:907–915.
5. Verma A, Narayan SM. Is human longstanding persistent atrial fibrillation more stable than assumed? _JACCCEP._ 2015;1:25–28.
6. Calkins H. Demonstrating the value of contact force sensing: more difficult than meets the eye. _Circulation._ 2015;132:901–903.
7. Dukkipati SR, Cuoco F, Kutinsky I, et al. Pulmonary vein isolation using the visually guided laser balloon: a prospective, multicenter, and randomized comparison to standard radiofrequency ablation. _J Am Coll Cardiol._ 2015;66:1350–1360.

8. Nattel S. New ideas about atrial fibrillation 50 years on. _Nature._ 2002;415:219–226.
9. Dobrev D, Nattel S. New antiarrhythmic drugs for treatment of atrial fibrillation. _Lancet._ 2010;375:1212–1223.
10. Moe GK, Rheinboldt W, Abildskov JA. A computer model of atrial fibrillation. _Am Heart J._ 1964;67:200–220.
11. de Groot NM, Houben RP, Smeets JL, et al. Electropathological substrate of longstanding persistent atrial fibrillation in patients with structural heart disease: epicardial breakthrough. _Circulation._ 2010;122:1674–1682.
12. Pandit SV, Jalife J. Rotors and the dynamics of cardiac fibrillation. _Circ Res._ 2013;112:849–862.
13. Herweg B, Kowalski M, Steinberg JS. Termination of persistent atrial fibrillation resistant to cardioversion by a single radiofrequency application. _Pacing Clin Electrophysiol._ 2003;26:1420–1423.
14. Narayan SM, Krummen DE, Shivkumar K, et al. Treatment of atrial fibrillation by the ablation of localized sources: the Conventional Ablation for Atrial Fibrillation With or Without Focal Impulse and Rotor Modulation: CONFIRM trial. _J Am Coll Cardiol._ 2012;60:628–636.
15. Verma A, Jiang CY, Betts TR, et al. Approaches to catheter ablation for persistent atrial fibrillation. _N Engl J Med._ 2015;372:1812–1822.
16. Wong KC, Paisey JR, Sopher M, et al. No Benefit of Complex Fractionated Atrial Electrogram (CFAE) Ablation in Addition to Circumferential Pulmonary Vein Ablation and Linear Ablation: BOCA Study. _Circ Arrhythm Electrophysiol._ 2015;8:1316–1324.

17. Walters TE, Lee G, Morris G, et al. Temporal stability of rotors and atrial activation patterns in persistent human atrial fibrillation: a high density epicardial mapping study of prolonged recordings (transient rotors in human persistent AF). _J Am Coll Cardiol: Clinical Electrophysiology._ 2015;1:18–25.
18. Hansen BJ, Zhao J, Csepe TA, et al. Atrial fibrillation driven by micro-anatomic intramural re-entry revealed by simultaneous sub-epicardial and sub-endocardial optical mapping in explanted human hearts. _Eur Heart J._ 2015;36:2390–2401.
19. Haissaguerre M, Hocini M, Denis A, et al. Driver domains in persistent atrial fibrillation. _Circulation._ 2014;130:530–538.
20. Miller JM, Kowal RC, Swarup V, et al. Initial independent outcomes from focal impulse and rotor modulation ablation for atrial fibrillation: multicenter FIRM registry. _J Cardiovasc Electrophys._ 2014;25:921–929.
21. Sommer P, Kircher S, Rolf S, et al. Successful repeat catheter ablation of recurrent longstanding persistent atrial fibrillation with rotor elimination as the procedural endpoint: a case series. _J Cardiovasc Electrophysiol._ 2016;27:274–280.
22. Tomassoni G, Duggal SA, Muir ME, et al. Long-term follow-up of FIRM-guided ablation of atrial fibrillation: a single-center experience. _J Innov Cardiac Rhythm Management._ 2015;2145–2151.

23. Narayan SM, Wright M, Derval N, et al. Classifying fractionated electrograms in human atrial fibrillation using monophasic action potentials and activation mapping: evidence for localized drivers, rate acceleration and non-local signal etiologies. *Heart Rhythm*. 2011a;8:244–253.
24. Narayan SM, Zaman JA. Mechanistically-based mapping of human cardiac fibrillation. *J Physiol*. 2016;594:2399–2415.
25. Weiss JN, Garfinkel A, Karagueuzian HS, et al. Perspective: a dynamics-based classification of ventricular arrhythmias. *J Mol Cell Cardiol*. 2015;82:136–152.
26. Haissaguerre M, Hsieh MH, Tai CT, et al. Spontaneous initiation of atrial fibrillation by ectopic beats originating in the pulmonary veins. *N Engl J Med*. 1998;339:659–666.
27. Narayan SM, Bode F, Karasik PL, et al. Alternans of atrial action potentials as a precursor of atrial fibrillation. *Circulation*. 2002b;106:1968–1973.
28. Patterson E, Po SS, Scherlag BJ, et al. Triggered firing in pulmonary veins initiated by in vitro autonomic nerve stimulation. *Heart Rhythm*. 2005;2:624–631.
29. Katritsis DG, Giazitzoglou E, Zografos T, et al. Rapid pulmonary vein isolation combined with autonomic ganglia modification: a randomized study. *Heart Rhythm*. 2011;8:672–678.
30. Engelman ZJ, Trew ML, Smaill BH. Structural heterogeneity alone is a sufficient substrate for dynamic instability and altered restitution. *Circ Arrhythm Electrophysiol*. 2010;3:195–203.
31. Narayan SM, Kazi D, Krummen DE, et al. Repolarization and activation restitution near human pulmonary veins and atrial fibrillation initiation: a mechanism for the initiation of atrial fibrillation by premature beats. *J Am Coll Cardiol*. 2008c;52:12221230.
32. Narayan SM, Franz MR, Clopton P, et al. Repolarization alternans reveals vulnerability to human atrial fibrillation. *Circulation*. 2011b;123:2922–2930.
33. Franz MR, Swerdlow CD, Liem LB, et al. Cycle length dependence of human action potential duration in vivo. Effects of single extrastimuli, sudden sustained rate acceleration and deceleration, and different steady-state frequencies. *J Clin Invest*. 1988a;82:972–979.
34. Schricker A, Rostamian A, Lalani G, et al. Human atrial fibrillation initiates by organized not disorganized mechanisms. *Circ Arrhythm Electrophysiol*. 2014;7:816–824.
35. Gonzales MJ, Vincent KP, Rappel WJ, et al. Structural contributions to fibrillatory rotors in a patient-derived computational model of the atria. *Europace*. 2014;16:iv3–iv10.
36. Marrouche NF, Wilber D, Hindricks G, et al. Association of atrial tissue fibrosis identified by delayed enhancement MRI and atrial fibrillation catheter ablation: the DECAAF study. *JAMA*. 2014;311:498–506.
37. Chen SA, Hsieh MH, Tai CT, et al. Initiation of atrial fibrillation by ectopic beats originating from the pulmonary veins: electrophysiological characteristics, pharmacological responses, and effects of radiofrequency ablation. *Circulation*. 1999a;100:1879–1886.
38. Dixit S, Marchlinski FE, Lin D, et al. Randomized ablation strategies for the treatment of persistent atrial fibrillation: RASTA study. *Circ Arrhythm Electrophysiol*. 2012;5:287–294.
39. Lee S, Sahadevan J, Khrestian CM, et al. Simultaneous bi-atrial high density (510-512 electrodes) epicardial mapping of persistent and long-standing persistent atrial fibrillation in patients: new insights into the mechanism of its maintenance. *Circulation*. 2015;132:2108–2117.
40. Qu Z. Critical mass hypothesis revisited: role of dynamical wave stability in spontaneous termination of cardiac fibrillation. *Am J Physiol Heart Circ Physiol*. 2006;290:H255–H263.
41. Vaidya D, Morley GE, Samie FH, et al. Reentry and fibrillation in the mouse heart. A challenge to the critical mass hypothesis. *Circ Res*. 1999;85:174–181.
42. Shivkumar K, Ellenbogen KA, Hummel JD, et al. Acute termination of human atrial fibrillation by identification and catheter ablation of localized rotors and sources: first multicenter experience of focal impulse and rotor modulation (FIRM) ablation. *J Cardiovasc Electrophysiol*. 2012;23:1277–1285.
43. Gray RA, Pertsov AM, Jalife J. Spatial and temporal organization during cardiac fibrillation. *Nature*. 1998;392:75–78.
44. Skanes AC, Mandapati R, Berenfeld O, et al. Spatiotemporal periodicity during atrial fibrillation in the isolated sheep heart. *Circulation*. 1998;98:1236–1248.
45. Lee P, Taghavi F, Yan P, et al. In situ optical mapping of voltage and calcium in the heart. *PLoS One*. 2012;7:e42562.
46. Franz MR, Chin MC, Sharkey HR, et al. A new, single-catheter technique for simultaneous measurement of action potential duration and refractory period *in vivo*. *J Am Coll Cardiol*. 1990;16:878–886.
47. Knollmann BC, Tranquillo J, Sirenko SG, et al. Microelectrode study of the genesis of the monophasic action potential by contact electrode technique. *J Cardiovasc Electrophysiol*. 2002;13:1246–1252.
48. Kim BS, Kim YH, Hwang GS, et al. Action potential duration restitution kinetics in human atrial fibrillation. *J Am Coll Cardiol*. 2002;39:1329–1336.
49. Jacquemet V, Virag N, Ihara Z, et al. Study of unipolar electrogram morphology in a computer model of atrial fibrillation. *J Cardiovasc Electrophysiol*. 2003;14:S172–S179.
50. Zhao J, Hansen BJ, Csepe TA, et al. Integration of high resolution optical mapping and 3D micro-CT imaging to resolve the structural basis of atrial conduction in the human heart. *Circ Arrhythm Electrophysiol*. 2015;8:1514–1517.
51. Hansen BJ, Briggs C, Moore BT, et al. Human atrial fibrillation drivers seen simultaneously by focal impulse and rotor mapping and high-resolution optical mapping [abstract]. *Circulation*. 2015;132:A18402.
52. Allessie MA, de Groot NM, Houben RP, et al. Electropathological substrate of long-standing persistent atrial fibrillation in patients with structural heart disease: longitudinal dissociation. *Circ Arrhythm Electrophysiol*. 2010;3:606–615.
53. Konings K, Kirchhof CJ, Smeets JR, et al. High-density mapping of electrically induced atrial fibrillation in humans. *Circulation*. 1994;89:1665–1680.
54. Jadidi AS, Cochet H, Shah AJ, et al. Inverse relationship between fractionated electrograms and atrial fibrosis in persistent atrial fibrillation—a combined MRI and high density mapping. *J Am Coll Cardiol*. 2013;62:802–812.
55. Houben R, de Groot N, Lindemans F, et al. Automatic mapping of human atrial fibrillation by template matching. *Heart Rhythm*. 2006;3:1221–1228.
56. Houben RP, Allessie MA. Processing of intracardiac electrograms in atrial fibrillation. Diagnosis of electropathological substrate of AF. *IEEE Eng Med Biol Mag*. 2006;25:40–51.
57. Schuessler RB, Grayson TM, Bromberg BI, et al. Cholinergically mediated tachyarrhythmias induced by a single extrastimulus in the isolated canine right atrium. *Circ Res*. 1992;71:1254–1267.
58. Cuculich PS, Wang Y, Lindsay BD, et al. Noninvasive characterization of epicardial activation in humans with diverse atrial fibrillation patterns. *Circulation*. 2010;122:1364–1372.
59. Sahadevan J, Ryu K, Peltz L, et al. Epicardial mapping of chronic atrial fibrillation in patients: preliminary observations. *Circulation*. 2004;110:3293–3299.
60. Wu TJ, Doshi RN, Huang HL, et al. Simultaneous biatrial computerized mapping during permanent atrial fibrillation in patients with organic heart disease. *J Cardiovasc Electrophysiol*. 2002;13:571–577.
61. Ravelli F, Faes L, Sandrini L, et al. Wave similarity mapping shows the spatiotemporal distribution of fibrillatory wave complexity in the human right atrium during paroxysmal and chronic atrial fibrillation. *J Cardiovasc Electrophysiol*. 2005;16:1071–1076.
62. Ng J, Gordon D, Passman RS, et al. Electrogram morphology recurrence patterns during atrial fibrillation. *Heart Rhythm*. 2014;11:2027–2034.
63. Gerstenfeld E, Sahakian A, Swiryn S. Evidence for transient linking of atrial excitation during atrial fibrillation in humans. *Circulation*. 1992;86:375–382.
64. Atienza F, Almendral J, Moreno J, et al. Activation of inward rectifier potassium channels accelerates atrial fibrillation in humans: evidence for a reentrant mechanism. *Circulation*. 2006;114:2434–2442.
65. Atienza F, Almendral J, Moreno J, et al. Comparison of radiofrequency catheter ablation of drivers and circumferential pulmonary vein isolation in atrial fibrillation: a noninferiority randomized multicenter RADAR-AF trial. *J Am Coll Cardiol*. 2014;64:2455–2467.
66. Krummen DE, Peng KA, Bullinga JR. Centrifugal gradients of rate and organization in human atrial fibrillation. *Pacing Clin Electrophysiol*. 2009;32:1366–1378.
67. Narayan SM, Krummen DE, Rappel WJ. Clinical mapping approach to identify rotors and focal beats in human atrial fibrillation. *J Cardiovasc Electrophysiol*. 2012;23:447–454.
68. Lalani GG, Schricker AA, Clopton P, et al. Frequency analysis of atrial action potential alternans: a sensitive clinical index of individual propensity to atrial fibrillation. *Circ Arrhythm Electrophysiol*. 2013;6:859–867.
69. Lalani G, Schricker A, Gibson M, et al. Atrial conduction slows immediately before the onset of human atrial fibrillation: a bi-atrial contact mapping study of transitions to atrial fibrillation. *J Am Coll Cardiol*. 2012;59:595–606.
70. Rappel WJ, Narayan SM. Theoretical considerations for mapping activation in human cardiac fibrillation. *Chaos*. 2013;23:023113.
71. Hill BC, Courtney KR. Design of a multi-point laser scanned optical monitor of cardiac action potential propagation: application to microreentry in guinea pig atrium. *Ann Biomed Eng*. 1987;15:567–577.
72. Kirchhof C, Chorro F, Scheffer GJ, et al. Regional entrainment of atrial fibrillation studied by high-resolution mapping in open-chest dogs. *Circulation*. 1003;88:736–749.
73. Cherry EM, Fenton FH. Visualization of spiral and scroll waves in simulated and experimental cardiac tissue. *New J Phys*. 2008;10:125016.
74. Rensma P, Allessie M, Lammers W, et al. Length of excitation wave and susceptibility to reentrant atrial arrhythmias in normal conscious dogs. *Circ Res*. 1998;62:395–410.
75. Fenton F, Karma A. Vortex dynamics in three-dimensional continuous myocardium with fiber rotation: Filament instability and fibrillation. *Chaos*. 1998;8:20–47.
76. Lin YJ, Lo MT, Lin C, et al. Prevalence, characteristics, mapping, and catheter ablation of potential rotors in nonparoxysmal atrial fibrillation. *Circ Arrhythm Electrophysiol*. 2013;6:851–858.
77. Swarup V, Baykaner T, Rostamian A, et al. Stability of rotors and focal sources for human atrial fibrillation. *J Cardiovasc Electrophysiol*. 2014;25:1284–1292.
78. Baykaner T, Clopton P, Lalani GG, et al. Targeted ablation at stable atrial fibrillation sources improves success over conventional ablation in high risk patients: a substudy of the CONFIRM trial. *Can J Cardiol*. 2013;29:1218–1226.
79. Narayan SM, Krummen DE, Enyeart MW, et al. Computational mapping approach identifies stable and long-lived electrical rotors and focal sources in human atrial fibrillation. *PLos One*. 2012;7:e46034.
80. Calkins CH. 2012 HRS/EHRA/ECAS Expert Consensus Statement on Catheter and Surgical Ablation of Atrial Fibrillation: Recommendations for Patient Selection, Procedural Techniques, Patient Management and Follow-up, Definitions, Endpoints, and Research Trial Design. *Heart Rhythm*. 2012;9:632–696.
81. Hocini M, Nault I, Wright M, et al. Disparate evolution of right and left atrial rate during ablation of long-lasting persistent atrial fibrillation. *J Am Coll Cardiol*. 2010;55:1007–1016.
82. Narayan SM, Shivkumar K, Krummen DE, et al. Panoramic electrophysiological mapping but not individual electrogram morphology identifies sustaining sites for human atrial fibrillation (AF rotors and focal sources relate poorly to fractionated electrograms). *Circ Arrhythm Electrophysiol*. 2013;6:58–67.
83. Narayan SM, Krummen DE, Donsky A, et al. Precise rotor elimination without concomitant pulmonary vein isolation for the successful elimination of paroxysmal atrial fibrillation. PRECISE-PAF. *Heart Rhythm*. 2013;10:1414-LB1401-1405.
84. Kalifa J, Tanaka K, Zaitsev AV, et al. Mechanisms of wave fractionation at boundaries of high-frequency excitation in the posterior left atrium of the isolated sheep heart during atrial fibrillation. *Circulation*. 2006;113:626–633.
85. Lin T, Kuck KH, Ouyang F, et al. First in-human robotic rotor ablation for atrial fibrillation. *Eur Heart J*. 2014;35:1432.
86. Elayi CS, Di Biase L, Barrett C, et al. Atrial fibrillation termination as a procedural endpoint during ablation in long-standing persistent atrial fibrillation. *Heart Rhythm*. 2010;7:1216–1223.
87. Latchamsetty R, Oral H. Is ablation to termination the best strategy for ablation of persistent atrial fibrillation? Ablation to termination is not the best strategy during ablation. *Circ Arrhythm Electrophysiol*. 2015;8:972–980.
88. Miller J, Kowal RC, Swarup V, et al. Similar long-term freedom from persistent or paroxysmal atrial fibrillation after ablation of patient-specific rotors and focal sources: multicenter FIRM study (abstract: featured poster). *Heart Rhythm*. 2014;11:(suppl 5):PO01–PO127.
89. Rappel WJ, Zaman JA, Narayan SM. Mechanisms for the termination of atrial fibrillation by localized ablation: computational and clinical studies. *Circ Arrhythm Electrophysiol*. 2015;8:1325–1333.
90. Tzou WS, Saghy L, Lin D. Termination of persistent atrial fibrillation during left atrial mapping. *J Cardiovasc Electrophysiol*. 2011;22:1171–1173.
91. Ho SY, Anderson RH, Sanchez-Quintana D. Atrial structure and fibers: morphologic bases of atrial conduction. *Cardiovasc Res*. 2002;54:325–336.
92. Lin JW, Garber L, Qi YR, et al. Region [corrected] of slowed conduction acts as core for spiral wave reentry in cardiac cell monolayers. *Am J Physiol Heart Circ Physiol*. 2008;294:H58–H65.
93. Narayan SM, Baykaner T, Clopton P, et al. Ablation of rotor and focal sources reduces late recurrence of atrial fibrillation compared to trigger ablation alone: extended followup of the CONFIRM (CONventional ablation with or without Focal Impulse and Rotor Modulation) trial. *J Am Coll Cardiol*. 2014;63:1761–1768.
94. Buch E, Share M, Tung R, et al. Long-term clinical outcomes of focal impulse and rotor modulation for treatment of atrial fibrillation: a multi-center experience. *Heart Rhythm*. 2016;13:636–641.
95. Jalife J, Filgueiras Rama D, Berenfeld O. Letter by Jalife et al regarding article, "quantitative analysis of localized sources identified by focal impulse and rotor modulation mapping in atrial fibrillation." *Circ Arrhythm Electrophysiol*. 2015;8:1296–1298.
96. Miller JM, Das MK, Jain R, Garlie J, Brewster J, Dandamudi G. Clinical benefit of ablating localized sources for human atrial fibrillation: The Indiana University FIRM Registry. *J Am Coll Cardiol*. 2017;69:1247–1256.
97. Alhusseini M, Vidmar D, Meckler GL, et al. Two independent mapping techniques identify rotational activity patterns at sites of local termination during persistent atrial fibrillation. *J Cardiovasc Electrophys*. 2017. In press.

46 Body Surface Frequency–Phase Mapping of Atrial Fibrillation

Felipe Atienza, Andreu M. Climent, and María S. Guillem

Studies that analyze the spatiotemporal organization of waves and dominant frequency (DF) in isolated sheep hearts have demonstrated that atrial fibrillation (AF) maintenance in this model depends on reentrant sources most often localized to the posterior wall of the left atrium (LA) with fibrillatory conduction in its periphery.[1–6] Recently, we translated the analysis on the organization of DF to human AF and found that AF reentrant sources are localized primarily to the pulmonary veins (PVs) and the LA posterior wall in the case of paroxysmal AF but elsewhere in the case of persistent AF.[7–9] Several studies suggested that instead of empirically targeting PVs,[10] AF should be eliminated by directly ablating AF-driving sources or "rotors" that exhibit a high frequency of activation.[8–16] Sanders and colleagues[14] were able to retrospectively identify localized sites of high-frequency activity with different DF distributions in paroxysmal and permanent AF patients. Ablation at these sites resulted in prolongation of the AF cycle length and termination of the majority of paroxysmal AF episodes, indicating their role in AF maintenance.[14] In a later study, we demonstrated that using advanced signal analysis systems for real-time DF mapping in humans was feasible and safe.[8] Moreover, ablation of high-frequency sites to abolish DF gradients was associated with a favorable long-term outcome.[8] In summary, these observational studies showed that AF could be eliminated by directly ablating AF-driving sources that exhibit high-frequency periodic activity, considered as surrogates of rotor location, using endocardial sequential mapping. Based on these studies, we designed the multicenter randomized Radiofrequency Ablation of Drivers of Atrial Fibrillation (RADAR-AF) clinical trial to compare the efficacy and safety of localized high-frequency source ablation versus the standard circumferential PV isolation (CPVI) strategy in drug-refractory AF patients.[17] The trial demonstrated that in paroxysmal AF patients, selective ablation of high-frequency sites responsible for AF maintenance was as effective as empirical CPVI and was associated with a lower incidence of adverse events.[18] However, in persistent AF patients, the combination of CPVI with highest DF (HDF) site ablation offered no incremental benefit and tended to increase the complication rate. Several factors might account for the results obtained in persistent AF patients, such as the sequential nature and low resolution of DF mapping in remodeled atria patients, leading to an electrogram (EGM) complexity that precluded accurate DF measurements and/or the inability of DF mapping to detect the underlying mechanisms of AF maintenance in these patients.

In recent years, other investigators have shown localized rotational activity driving AF using either spiral[19] or PentaRay catheters[20] or EGM similarity computational approaches as surrogates for human AF rotors.[21–23] However, to date, the focal impulse and rotors modulation (FIRM) ablation strategy is the most extensively validated mapping technique that has been able to localize and facilitate ablation of rotors (see Chapter 45). In the Conventional Ablation for AF With or Without FIRM (CONFIRM) multicenter trial, Narayan and colleagues performed direct rotor-guided ablation using computed endocardial recordings in a mix of paroxysmal and persistent AF patients and reported significantly higher AF freedom rates than in patients who underwent the standard CPVI approach.[24–26]

Overall, there is compelling evidence for localized AF–sustaining sources, including rotors, in all different types of AF. However, although AF-driving sources in paroxysmal AF are most commonly located in the LA junction with PVs, persistent AF patients frequently present extrapulmonary vein sources that may also shift location in time.[8,14,18,21,24,25] Therefore it would be desirable to noninvasively localize the sources responsible for AF maintenance before the procedure to identify patients who are most suitable for ablation and to design the ideal ablation strategy for each individual AF patient prior to the procedure. Here we present the results of our endeavors to develop a noninvasive mapping system that enables reliable identification of AF-driving sources.

Spectral Analysis of Body Surface Potential Mapping

Previous studies from our group and others have highlighted the major role of high-frequency sources in AF maintenance in animals and humans.[1–6,8,9,11,13–15] We conducted a correlation study as an initial step to explore the possibility of using body surface potential mapping (BSPM) to identify high-frequency intracardiac sources noninvasively together with endocardial mapping (CARTO) prior to the AF ablation procedure.[27] We used a custom-made, adjustable vest with 64 electrodes covering the entire torso surface.[27] The vest included recording electrodes on the anterior (N = 28), posterior (N = 34), and lateral (N = 2) sides of the torso (Fig. 46.1A), together with three limb leads used to generate the Wilson terminal. Surface unipolar electrocardiogram (ECG) recordings were obtained using a commercial system for biopotential measurements (Active Two, Biosemi, The Netherlands).[28] Ventricular activity was removed from the unipolar recordings prior to analysis either numerically or by applying adenosine.[9]

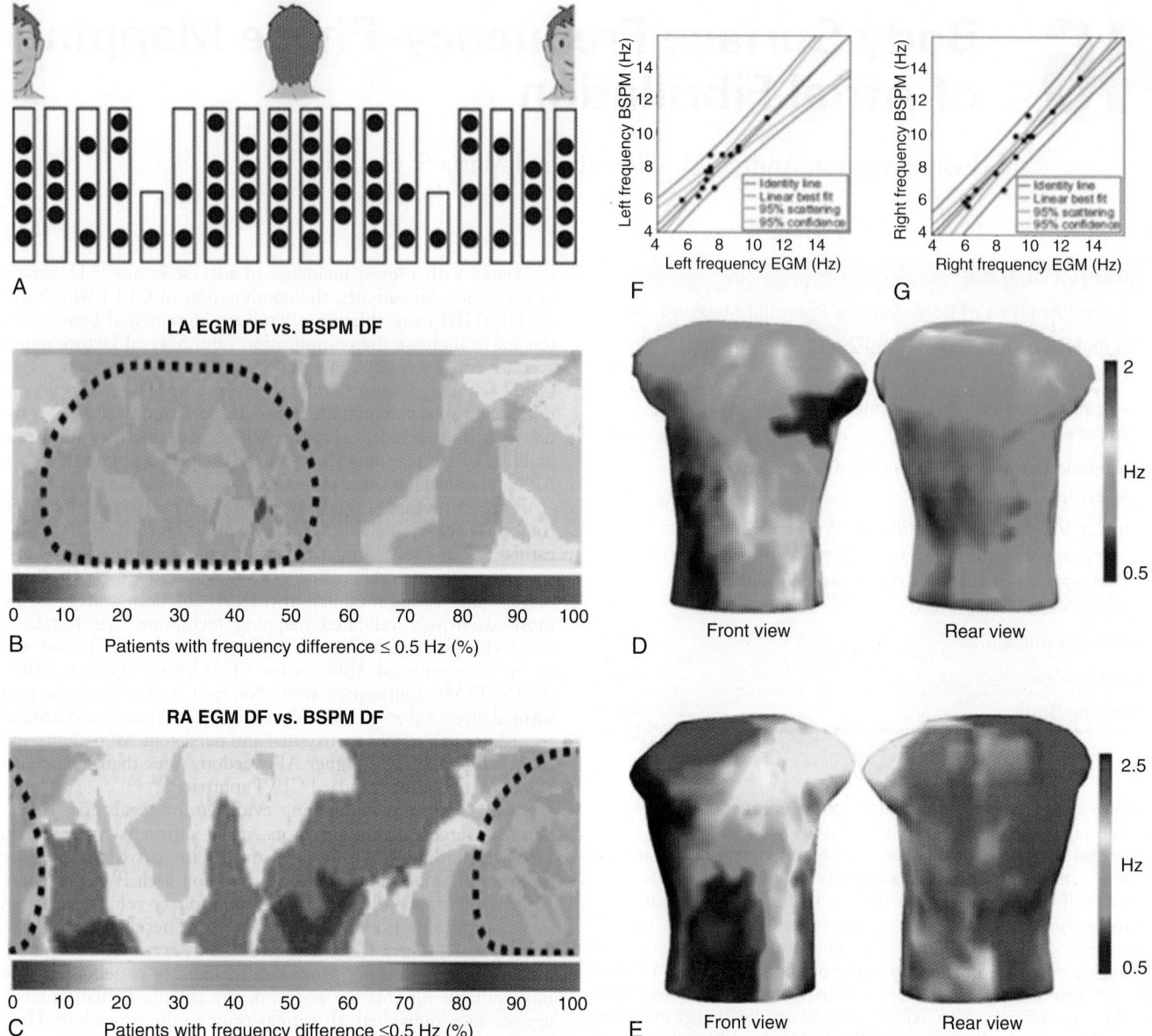

FIGURE 46.1 Correspondence between intracardiac and surface dominant frequencies (*DF*). (A) Schematic location of body surface electrodes. *Circles* represent the location of recording electrodes. (B and C) Summary maps showing the percent of patients with surface DFs <0.5 Hz different than the maximum left (B) and maximum right (C) intracardiac DFs. Areas outlined by the *dashed curves* represent the portion of the torso with the best correspondence with the left and right electrograms (EGMs). (D and E) Summary maps showing the torso projections of the matching portions (*in blue*) with a mean frequency difference between surface DFs and maximum left (D) and maximum right (E) DFs found in EGMs. (F) A correlation plot showing the highest DFs found in left EGMs versus the highest DFs found on the left portion of the torso. (G) Correlation plot showing the highest DFs found in the right EGMs versus the highest DFs found on the right portion of the torso. *BSPM*, Body surface potential maps; *CS*, coronary sinus; *DF*, dominant frequency; *LA*, left atrium; *LIPV*, left inferior pulmonary vein; *LSPV*, left superior pulmonary vein; *RA*, right atrium; *SL*, surface left; *SP*, surface posterior; *SR*, surface right; *SVC*, superior vena cava. (Modified from Guillem MS, Climent AM, Millet J, et al. Noninvasive localization of maximal frequency sites of atrial fibrillation by body surface potential mapping. *Circ Arrhythm Electrophysiol.* 2013;6:294-301.)

Surface leads and simultaneously recorded intracardiac signals presented closely related spectral components. In Fig. 46.2, we present spectral analyses of data from a representative patient with a right-to-left DF frequency pattern in which the presence of a distinct atrial site with high-frequency activity in the anterolateral RA wall could be determined noninvasively. In Fig. 46.2A, three representative EGMs illustrate the range of activation rates across the atria, with DFs ranging from 7

Hz in LA to 7.5 Hz in the coronary sinus (CS) to 12.75 Hz in RA. Simultaneously recorded surface leads also showed different DFs at nearly the same frequency range that was found in EGM recordings, as shown in Fig. 46.2B by three representative leads that corresponded to the surface left (SL), surface posterior (SP), and surface right (SR) regions. Surface DFs mostly correlated with the activation rate of the nearest atrial tissue: the highest endocardial DF point was observed at

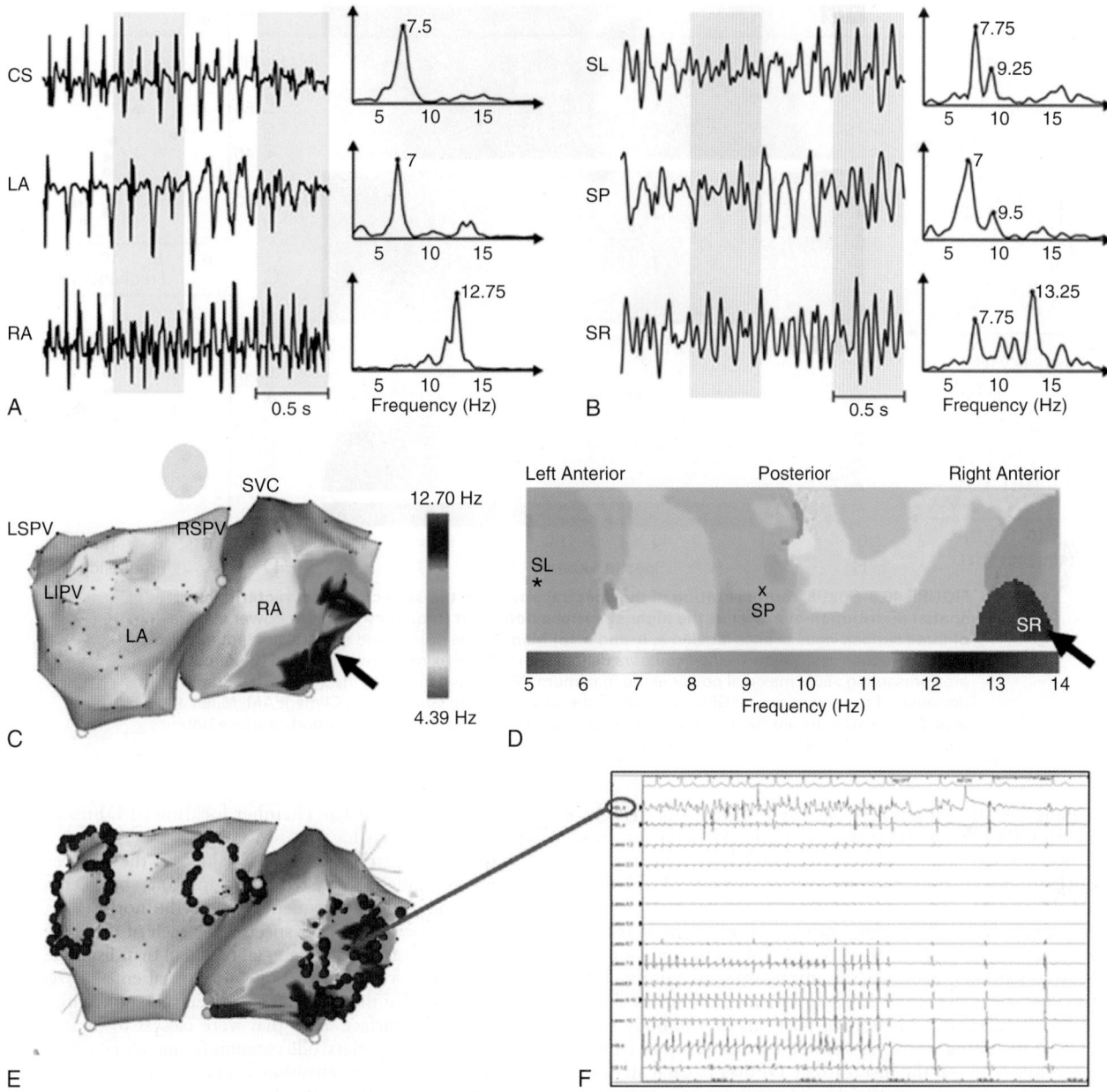

FIGURE 46.2 Recorded electrograms (*EGMs*) and electrocardiograms and their dominant frequency (*DF*) distribution in a sample patient with a right-to-left DF gradient. (A) EGMs recorded at different endocardial atrial sites and their corresponding power spectra. (B) Selected body surface potential mapping (*BSPM*) leads and their corresponding power spectra. (C) Real-time biatrial DF map. *Black arrow* indicates the right atrial (*RA*) region with the highest DF at the RA (*in purple*). (D) DF map on the torso surface with superimposed locations of electrodes from (B). *Black arrow* indicates the torso region with the highest DF at the RA (*in purple*). (E) Posterior view, biatrial DF map with superimposed *red dots* showing encircling ablation lesions around the right and left pulmonary vein (PV) antra, and a coin-like circumferential set of lesions at the RA posterolateral endocardial wall, leading to atrial fibrillation (AF) termination (F). (F) Tracings during RA maximum dominant frequency (DFmax) site ablation leading to AF termination. Electrocardiogram lead I and intracardiac EGMs recorded from ablation catheter and lasso catheter located at the RA appendage, coronary sinus catheter, and His catheter. (Modified from Guillem MS, Climent AM, Millet J, et al. Noninvasive localization of maximal frequency sites of atrial fibrillation by body surface potential mapping. *Circ Arrhythm Electrophysiol.* 2013;6:294-301.)

the nearest point on the torso surface (13.25 Hz on the right torso). Intracardiac CARTO DF maps obtained prior to adenosine infusion and surface DF distributions obtained during adenosine infusion showed good correspondence (Fig. 46.2C and D). However, direct comparison of frequencies from CARTO and surface maps was unattainable because of their sequential nature and because adenosine accelerates AF activation in humans, increasing DF values recorded using BSPM compared with baseline intracardiac recordings.[9] Nevertheless, despite these limitations, the outcome of ablation clearly supported the ability of the BSPM system to capture the intracardiac right atrial (RA)-HDF site that was responsible for AF

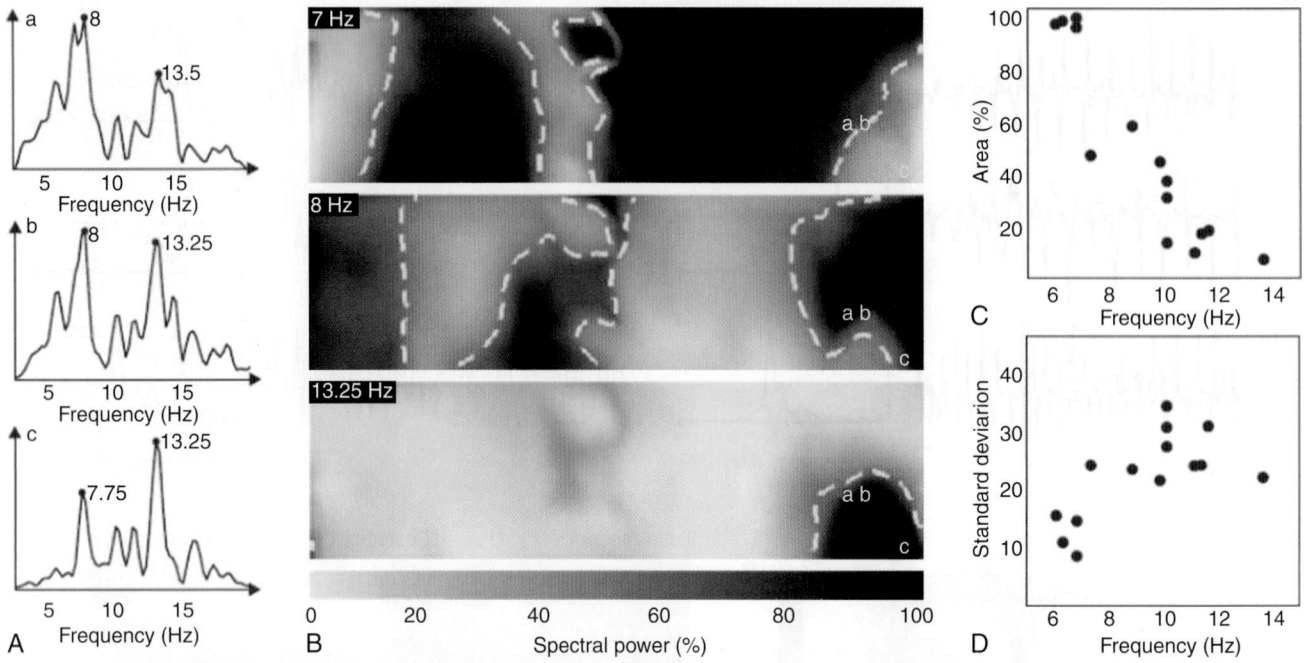

FIGURE 46.3 Spatial representation of the spectral power on the surface and characteristics of spatial distribution of power at the highest surface dominant frequency (DF). (A) Power spectra of three surface leads in sites labeled *a, b,* and *c.* (B) Maps of the normalized spectral content at three discrete frequencies. *Yellow dashed contours* delineate the 50% maximal power borders. (C) Percentage area presenting >50% maximal power at the maximum DF (DFmax) found on the surface. (D) Standard deviation of the power map at DFmax found on the surface. (From Guillem MS, Climent AM, Millet J, et al. Noninvasive localization of maximal frequency sites of atrial fibrillation by body surface potential mapping. *Circ Arrhythm Electrophysiol.* 2013;6:294-301.)

maintenance in this patient. As per the protocol, the patient underwent CPVI first with no changes in the AF behavior, followed by targeted ablation of the RA-HDF site that terminated AF to stable sinus rhythm after 4 minutes of ablation (Fig. 46.2E and F).

We then analyzed the correspondence between intracardiac and surface AF frequencies in RA and LA in a series of 14 consecutive patients, grouped the intracardiac maximum DF (DFmax) values measured in LA and RA, and correlated them with DFs of EGMs from matching portions on the body surface. These matching portions were defined as those in which the difference between the intracardiac DFmax in each atrium, and the surface DFmax was ≤0.5 Hz. Overall, there was a good correspondence between DFmax found in each atrial chamber and the right and left matching portions on the body surface. The correlation between left leads and left intracardiac EGMs was 0.92 (see Fig. 46.1B, D, and F), whereas the correlation between right surface leads and right intracardiac EGMs was 0.96 (see Fig. 46.1C, E, and G). The attempted correlation of the surface leads with EGMs of the atrial chamber on the opposite side yielded much lower correlation values (RA body surface leads vs. intracardiac LA EGMs, 0.26; $p < .0001$ vs. r = 0.96; left body surface leads vs. intracardiac RA EGMs, 0.46; $p = .0052$ vs. r = 0.92). Such a strong, side-specific correspondence of frequencies enabled a reliable determination of atrial frequency gradients noninvasively. The DF gradients on the 64 electrodes of BSPM showed a good correlation with the DF gradients obtained using simultaneous intracardiac EGMs (correlation coefficient = 0.93). On the other hand, surface frequency gradients estimated by the standard precordial ECG leads yielded poor correspondence with gradients estimated from intracardiac EGMs, with a correlation coefficient equal to 0.41 when considering all six standard leads. These results demonstrate that the surface DFmax can accurately detect the

value of the intracardiac chamber location of DFmax, regardless of whether it is localized to LA or RA.[27]

The spatial distribution of DF values on the surface was not continuous, and abrupt stepwise transitions between adjacent domains and different frequencies were the norm (Fig. 46.2D). Fig. 46.3A shows the power spectral for each of the three sample leads on the right anterior torso (a, b, and c) that displayed significant power at 7–8 Hz and 13.25 Hz for the patient analyzed in Fig. 46.2, showing that the power at any given spectral component was highest for the surface leads that were closest to its intracardiac origin. Each surface electrode contains frequency components that are also related to the activation frequency of many atrial regions and not only the closest atrial tissue. However, the highest frequency components were typically found to occupy the small DF domains on the body surface. In fact, there was a negative correlation ($\varrho = .92$) between the frequency of HDF and the area at which that frequency presented at least 50% of the power of the highest peak of the spectrum (Fig. 46.3C). The power of high spectral components also showed higher spatial variability than that of low spectral components, as depicted in Fig. 46.3D, with a correlation coefficient of 0.66.[27]

Therefore, based on correlations between simultaneous real-time endocardial DF mapping and body surface recordings, we can conclude that spatial gradients of activation frequency in human AF can be detected and quantified noninvasively, enabling the identification of the atrium-driving AF on the basis of the surface DF distribution. Although most surface leads predominantly reflect the rate of activation of the overall atrial tissue, high-frequency sources are reflected on the surface electrodes closest to the atria that harbor HDF as measured by intracardiac EGMs. These results also demonstrate that the portion of the torso at which these high-frequency components are dominant relates inversely with the frequency, and thus HDF is reflected in a small area of the body surface. Thus, during AF in humans, the DF

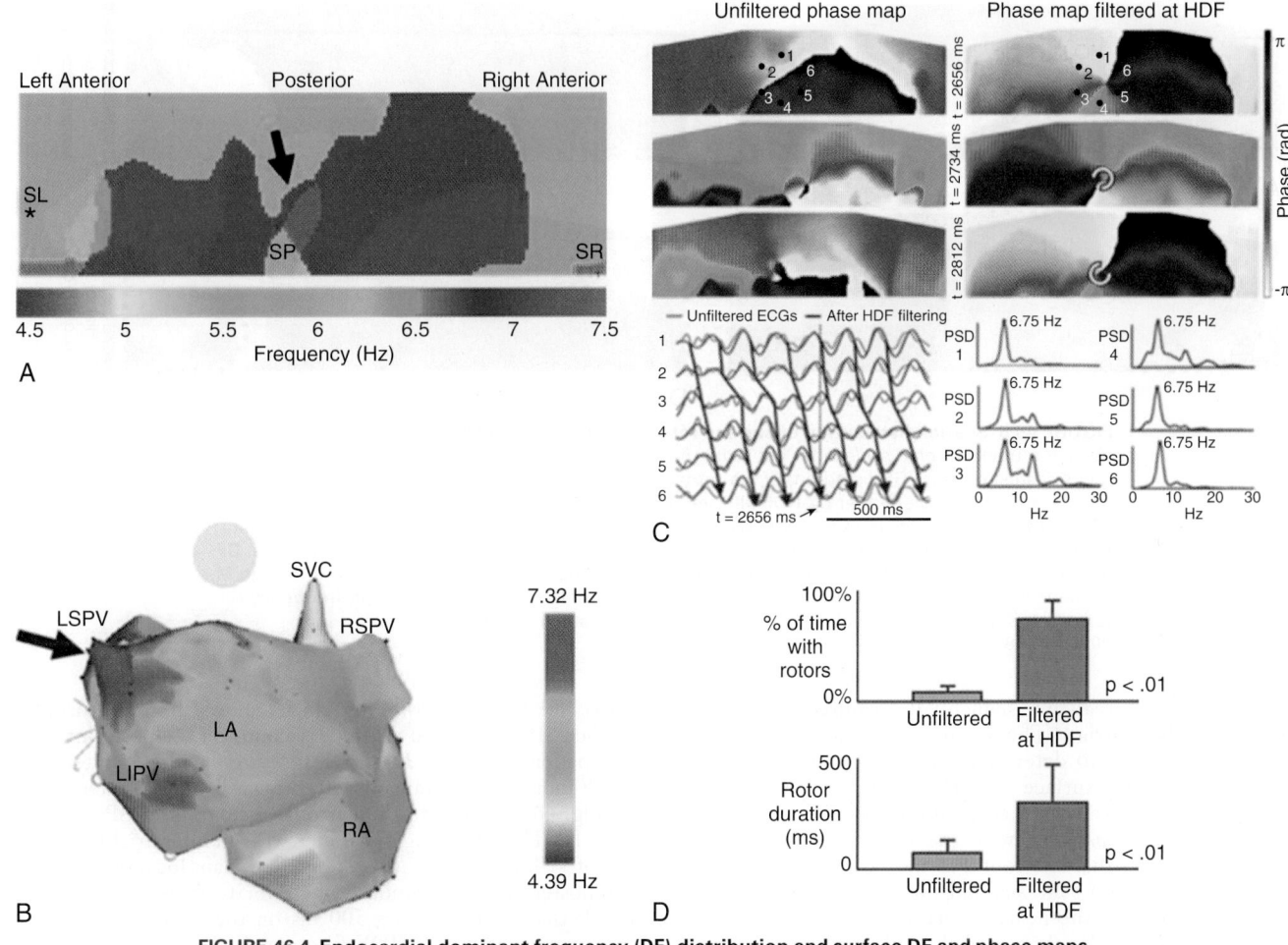

FIGURE 46.4 Endocardial dominant frequency (DF) distribution and surface DF and phase maps in patients with a left-to-right DF gradient. (A) DF map on the torso surface with selected surface body surface potential mapping leads: surface left (*SL*), surface posterior (*SP*) and surface right (*SR*). *Black arrow* points to the body surface region (SP) with highest DF. (B) Intracardiac DF map of patient in (A). *Black arrow* points to the left atrial (*LA*) region with highest DF at the left superior pulmonary vein (*LSPV*), closest to the SP body surface recording. (C) Surface phase maps at three selected times for unfiltered (*left superior panel*) and for highest dominant frequency (*HDF*)-filtered (*right superior panel*) surface potentials. Electrocardiograms (*ECGs*) at positions 1--6 marked in superior panels before and after HDF filtering and power spectral density (*PSD*) for unfiltered ECGs. Time marker at 2656 ms corresponds to the top map in the HDF-filtered data in right superior panel. (D) Percentage of time with rotors and rotor duration in surface phase maps from unfiltered and HDF-filtered surface potentials over the entire cohort. *CS*, Coronary sinus; *LIPV*, left inferior pulmonary vein; *RA*, right atrium; *RSPV*, right superior pulmonary vein; *SVC*, superior vena cava. (From Guillem MS, Climent AM, Millet J, et al. Noninvasive localization of maximal frequency sites of atrial fibrillation by body surface potential mapping. *Circ Arrhythm Electrophysiol.* 2013;6:294-301; and Rodrigo M, Guillem MS, Climent AM, et al. Body surface localization of left and right atrial high-frequency rotors in atrial fibrillation patients: a clinical-computational study. *Heart Rhythm.* 2014;11:1584-1591.)

distribution on the BSPM replicates the epicardial distribution of DFs and can identify small areas containing high-frequency sources that result in fibrillatory conduction to the reminder of the atria.

Noninvasive Mapping of Rotors in Human Atrial Fibrillation

The ability of BSPM to detect rotors and propagation patterns during AF was described by our group.[28] Phase maps computed from the TQ intervals in 64 surface potentials showed complex patterns in which reentries could be identified, but they were unstable and of very short duration. Very similar observations were reported during AF using an inverse solution electrocardiographic imaging (ECGI) system, where isochronal activation maps presented multiple wavelets, but only 15% of patients presented activation maps that could be attributed to rotors.[29] Haissaguerre used the ECGI system with additional signal processing that included filtering, wavelet transformation, and phase mapping and observed active AF sources, such as unstable rotors and PV foci.[30] A subsequent ECGI study of 103 persistent AF patients reported that up to 80.5% activations were caused by reentries, most of them unstable, with a median of 2.6 repetitive rotations (maximum of eight rotations) and a mean duration of 449 ± 89 ms, clustered in one to five discrete regions whose ablation terminated AF in a substantial proportion of patients (see Chapter 47).[31]

Using a different approach, we conducted a clinical–computational study in a sample of 14 AF patients in whom we simultaneously recorded surface ECGs using a 67-electrode

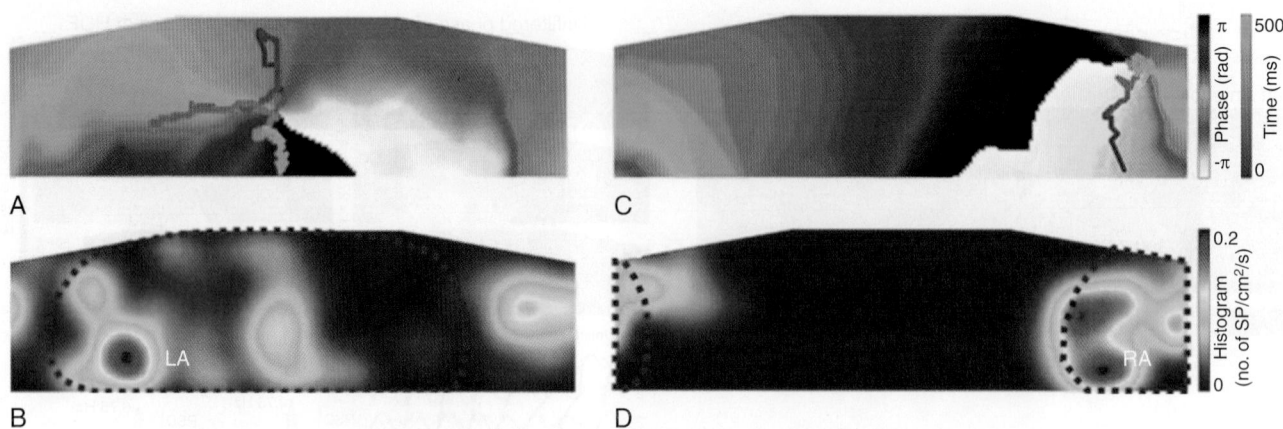

FIGURE 46.5 Spatial distribution of surface rotors in human atrial fibrillation. (A) Phase map and rotor tracking (*blue scale*) after left atrial (*LA*) highest dominant frequency (HDF) filtering in an LA-fastest patient. (B) Histogram of the rotor position for all rotors detected in patients with an interatrial DF gradient after LA-HDF filtering. LA-detected region is outlined with a *dotted line.* (C) Phase map and rotor tracking (*blue scale*) after right atrial (*RA*)-HDF filtering in an RA-fastest patient. (D) Histogram of the rotor position for all rotors detected in patients with an interatrial DF gradient after RA-HDF filtering. RA-detected region is outlined with a *dotted line.* (FromRodrigo M, Guillem MS, Climent AM, et al. Body surface localization of left and right atrial high-frequency rotors in atrial fibrillation patients: a clinical-computational study. *Heart Rhythm.* 2014;11:1584-1591.)

vest together with real-time sequentially acquired intracardiac EGMs from both atria.[32] The power spectral density of all signals was computed to determine local DFs and their distribution on the body surface.[27] As shown in Fig. 46.4, surface DFs (*panel A*) showed good correlation with the endocardial DF distribution (*panel B*), with the highest activation rate of the LA endocardial site found at the nearest point on the torso surface (*central posterior*) and the lowest activation rate of the RA found at the nearest portion of the surface ECG (*right inferior*).[27,32] We then used this information to process and interpret our noninvasive data to localize driving rotors, which as predicted by theory should coincide with HDFs in the atria. Unfiltered surface phase maps of the unipolar voltage time series recorded during AF showed unstable patterns that drifted erratically (Fig. 46.4C, *left superior panel*). However, after band-pass filtering of the potential signal around the HDF (6.8 Hz), surface phase maps showed more stable and longer lasting rotor activity for the same AF episode (Fig. 46.4C, *right superior panel*). In Fig. 46.4C *left lower panel*, the *arrows* connecting sequential activations in ECGs recorded around the SP in the *upper panels* show a clear reentrant pattern, which, after HDF filtering, transformed into long-lasting rotational patterns with stable SPs. Considering data from all patients, the HDF band-pass filtering of the body surface potentials increased the time with observed rotors from 8.3% ± 5.7% at baseline to 73.1% ± 16.8% after filtering and increased the duration of continuous visible rotation from 160 ± 43 ms to 342 ± 138 ms, respectively (Fig. 46.4D).[32] Of the average HDF of 9.2 ± 2.3 Hz for BSPM or 9.3 ± 2.0 Hz for intracardiac recordings, the latter corresponded to an average of 2.9 ± 0.7 continuous rotations per SP observed in our cohort of 14 AF patients.[32] Our BSPM phase maps, obtained after filtering the surface potentials, displayed patterns that resembled those reported by the ECGI system in their complexity.[29–31]

Regions of Body Surface Rotational Activity in Human Atrial Fibrillation

Rotors, defined as true singularity points (SPs) with at least 60% of their spectral content at the HDF band, drifted on the surface mapped area, but they tended to concentrate at certain torso

areas (see Chapter 35).[32] Fig. 46.5A shows the trajectory of a surface SP that drifted during 2 seconds on the posterior torso of a patient following LA-HDF filtering (band-pass filtering at HDF found in simultaneous left intracardiac EGM recordings). In Fig. 46.5B, the two-dimensional histogram of SP locations after LA-HDF filtering in patients with an interatrial DF gradient of >1 Hz (n = 10) shows the predominant location of SPs on the posterior torso. Similarly, Fig. 46.5C shows the trajectory of SP that drifted during 500 ms on the right anterior torso in a patient after RA-HDF filtering. In Fig. 46.5D, the two-dimensional histogram of SP locations after RA-HDF filtering in patients with an interatrial DF gradient shows a predominant localization on the right anterior torso. The locations of the maximal numbers of true LA or RA SPs (*dark red regions*) are shown in *panels B and D* and reside well within the areas demarcated by HDFs originating either at the LA or RA (see Fig. 46.1B and C), respectively, found on our previous surface atrial DF distribution correlation study.[27]

Simulations for Noninvasive Rotors Mapping Interpretation

In general, the AF activation patterns reported using various noninvasive systems (i.e., BSMP, ECGI) using different signal processing methods[29–32] appear to be simpler than epicardial maps recorded in other studies that do not report stable rotors.[28,33,34] To clarify the relationship between surface mapping recordings and the intracardiac AF activity, particularly the effect of filtering and phase processing, we reproduced our mapping processing in computer simulations.[32] Using a simplified spherical model of the excitable atria surrounded by a passive torso, we could track spatiotemporal potentials and phase singularities of rotors everywhere (Fig. 46.6A and D). Action potential rotors simulated on the atrial sphere produce rotating potentials in the torso, and their phase SPs extend into the torso to form axes of pivoting potentials termed filaments.

Two relevant outcomes emerged from our spherical simplified computer simulations that have been recently corroborated using anatomically realistic mathematical models (Fig. 46.6B and E). First, the number of SPs is reduced with the distance from the atria, and in some cases, filaments arising from the atrial SPs did

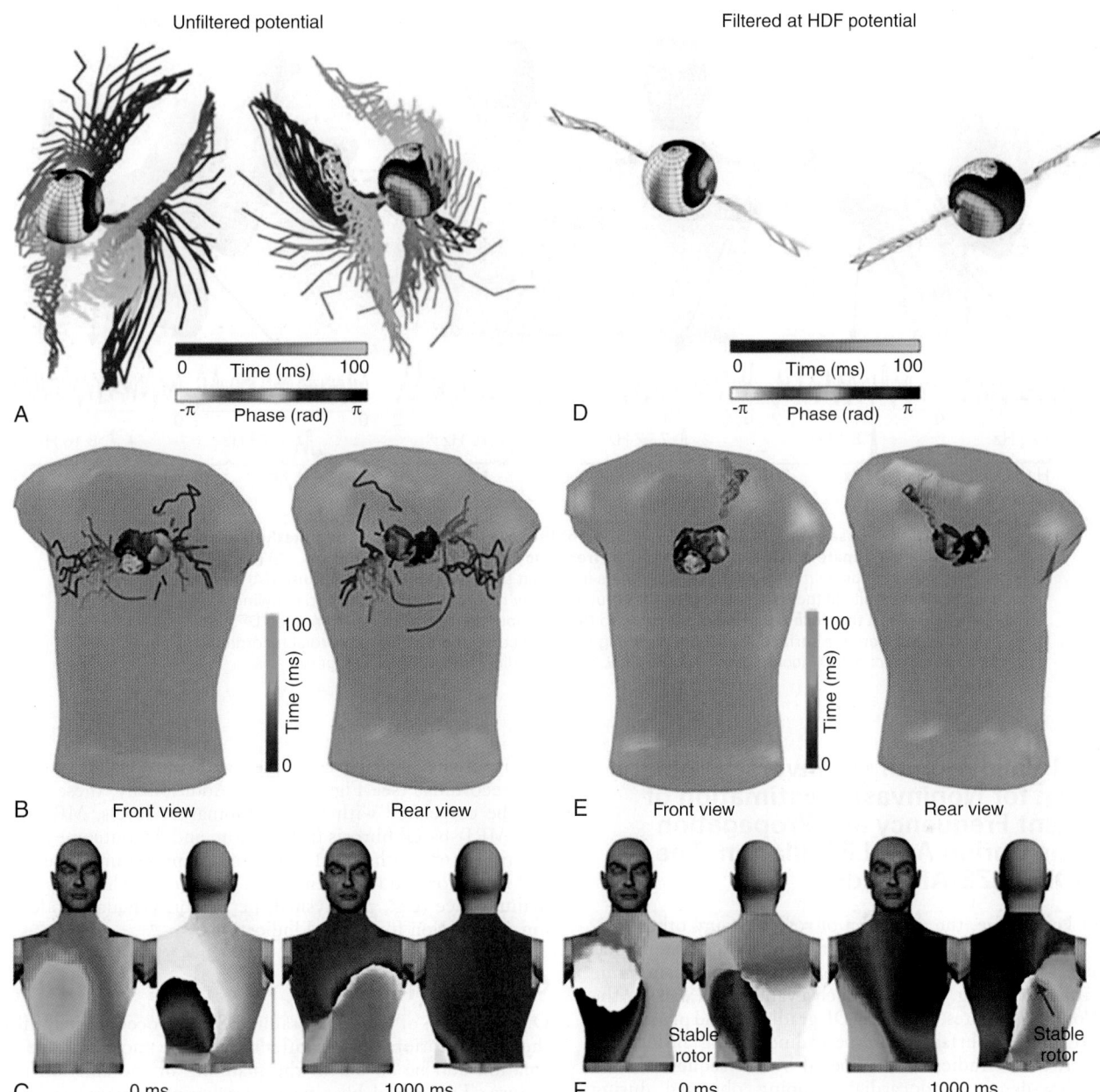

FIGURE 46.6 Effect of surface electrocardiogram recordings filtering on phase maps. (A and D) Phase map of epicardial sphere and temporal distribution of filaments for unfiltered potentials (A) and for highest dominant frequency (*HDF*)-filtered potentials (D) of a simplified spherical model of the excitable atria surrounded by a passive torso. (B and E) Temporal distribution of filaments for unfiltered potentials (B) and for left atrial (LA) HDF-filtered potentials (E) of a realistic three-dimensional (3D) mathematical model with an LA-fastest atrial fibrillation pattern. (C and F) Phase maps for unfiltered potentials (C) and for LA HDF–filtered potentials (F) of the same 3D mathematical simulation in (B and E). (From Rodrigo M, Guillem MS, Climent AM, et al. Body surface localization of left and right atrial high-frequency rotors in atrial fibrillation patients: a clinical-computational study. *Heart Rhythm.* 2014;11:1584-1591.)

not reach the outer surface due to the mutual cancelation effect of the counter-rotating filaments; this reduced the sensitivity for rotor detection from the body surface (see Chapter 35 for further details). Second, in the absence of any signal filtering, filaments originating from a relatively stable SP span and diverge, describing a cone and ultimately become unstable on the torso surface (see Fig. 46.6A and B), resulting in uninterpretable propagation patterns (Fig. 46.6C). However, as shown in Fig. 46.6D and E, HDF filtering significantly reduces the filaments' deflection and stabilizes them to follow a straight path from the epicardium to

the surface, enabling the detection of stable propagation patterns (Fig. 46.6F). These findings explain why body surface phase maps in our study[32] and those produced by the ECGI system[30,31] are simpler compared with the expected complexity of epicardial potentials during AF.

Thus our simulations indicate that all SPs and rotors detected on the torso surface are the ends of filaments originating at atrial surface rotors. Second, our HDF band-pass filtering out the effect of propagation at distal regions to the rotor allows the uncovering of the AF driver location for better physiological interpretation and treatment.

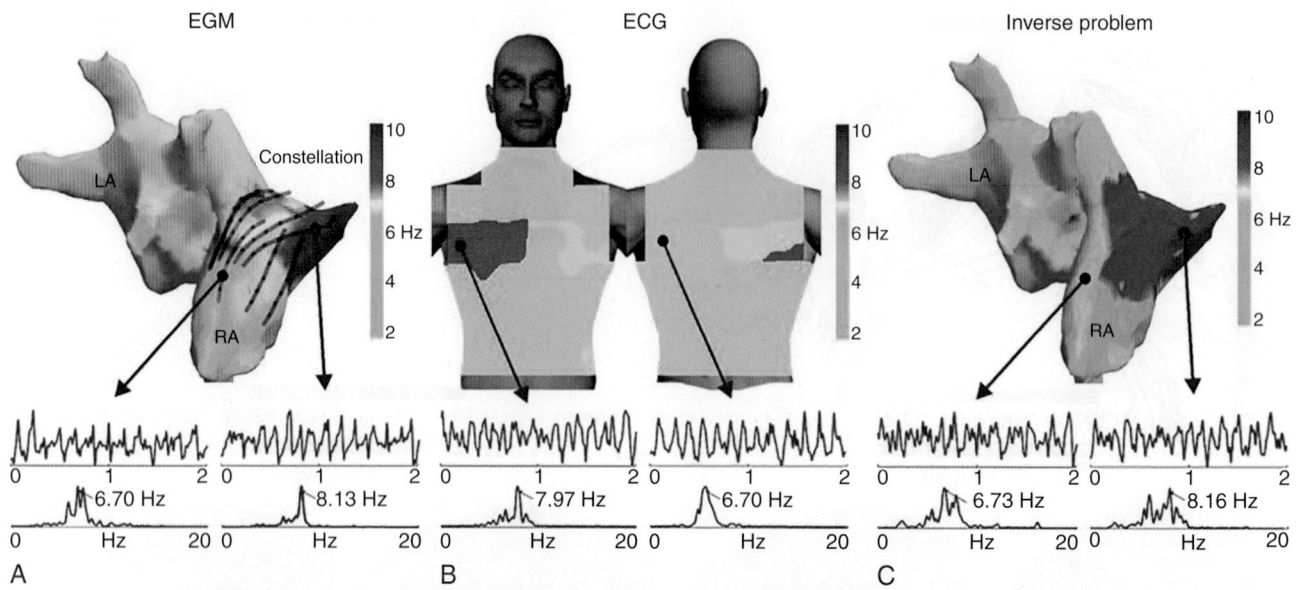

FIGURE 46.7 Case example of clinical validation of the inverse problem solution method to non-invasively estimate epicardial high dominant frequency (DF) regions distribution. (A) Biatrial DF map obtained using multipolar basket catheters in the left atrium (*LA*) and right atrium (*RA*) showing a highest DF site at the RA appendage. (B) Simultaneously recorded surface DF map showing maximal DF site at the closest portion of the torso to the RA appendage. (C) Inverse computed DF maps calculated from the surface recordings showing excellent correlation with endocardial recordings, in terms of maximal DF location and values. *ECG*, Electrocardiogram; *EGM*, electrogram.

Clinical Validation of the Inverse Problem Solution for Noninvasive Estimation of Dominant Frequency and Propagation Patterns During Atrial Fibrillation: The PERSONALIZE-AF Study

To our knowledge, the detection of rotors or any other activation patterns using different surface mapping systems has not been validated until today using simultaneous panoramic intracardiac mapping. However, such a validation exists for the detection of HDF sites, interatria DF gradients, and phase maps of HDF-filtered surface ECG recordings using BSPM.[27,32] However, these studies are hampered by the sequential, relatively low-density endocardial mapping obtained during simultaneous surface recordings. Thus, to further confirm this contention, we recently designed the PERSONALIZED-AF study (www.clinicaltrials.gov: NCT02497248) to clinically validate the technology for the noninvasive identification of mechanisms responsible for AF maintenance by body surface electrical mapping. To achieve this goal, surface ECG recordings of the atrial activity will be used to compute the DF distribution and phase maps of AF activity by means of the inverse problem solution and correlate them with simultaneously obtained high-density endocardial recordings (see Fig. 46.7).[35,36] Magnetic resonance (MR) images of the heart will be obtained prior to the procedure, enabling atrial three-dimensional (3D) model reconstruction (Fig. 46.8). The torso surface anatomy and body surface electrode position will be coregistered at the beginning of the procedure using a proprietary computerized system. During the electrophysiological study, body surface ECG recordings from 59 electrodes evenly distributed along the torso will be simultaneously obtained together with multipolar high-density endocardial recordings from basket catheters in both atria. Inverse calculated DFs and phase maps computed using BSPM recordings and the

3D atrial shell will be correlated with intracardiac endocardial recordings (see Fig. 46.8).[35,36] Additionally, these results will be correlated with fibrosis biomarker levels, MR imaging (MRI)-based fibrosis distribution, and AF outcomes of AF ablation at 6 months and 1 year after the procedure. The study will be performed in patients with different mechanisms of AF maintenance (e.g., paroxysmal, persistent, valvular) undergoing AF ablation for clinical indications.

Clinical Implications

Our approach of a full panoramic BSPM procedure may allow the identification of AF patients who are most suitable for ablation and be an aid in the planning of the ablation procedure. This could be especially relevant in paroxysmal AF patients, in whom selective ablation of high-frequency sites responsible for AF maintenance has proved to be as effective as empirical CPVI, and was associated with a lower incidence of adverse events.[18] In this subset of patients, a priori knowledge of the AF-driving chambers and DF site locations may help in planning and performing the ablation procedure, potentially decreasing the time required for the search and elimination of the HDF sites. Moreover, in persistent AF patients without a clear DF gradient, BSPM may help in patient selection because the absence of an interchamber DF gradient is associated with lower ablation success rates.[8] Nevertheless, additional mapping and ablation strategies are needed in persistent AF patients in whom the combination of CPVI with high-frequency site ablation (HFSA) did not provide incremental value and was associated with an increased complications risk.[18] In this context, the combination of DF, phase mapping, and other signal analysis techniques (causality analysis)[36] may allow the identification of AF-driving sources from the body surface. Finally, body surface potential maps could also arguably be used to test the effect of different drugs and predict the effect of noninvasive treatments and interventions.

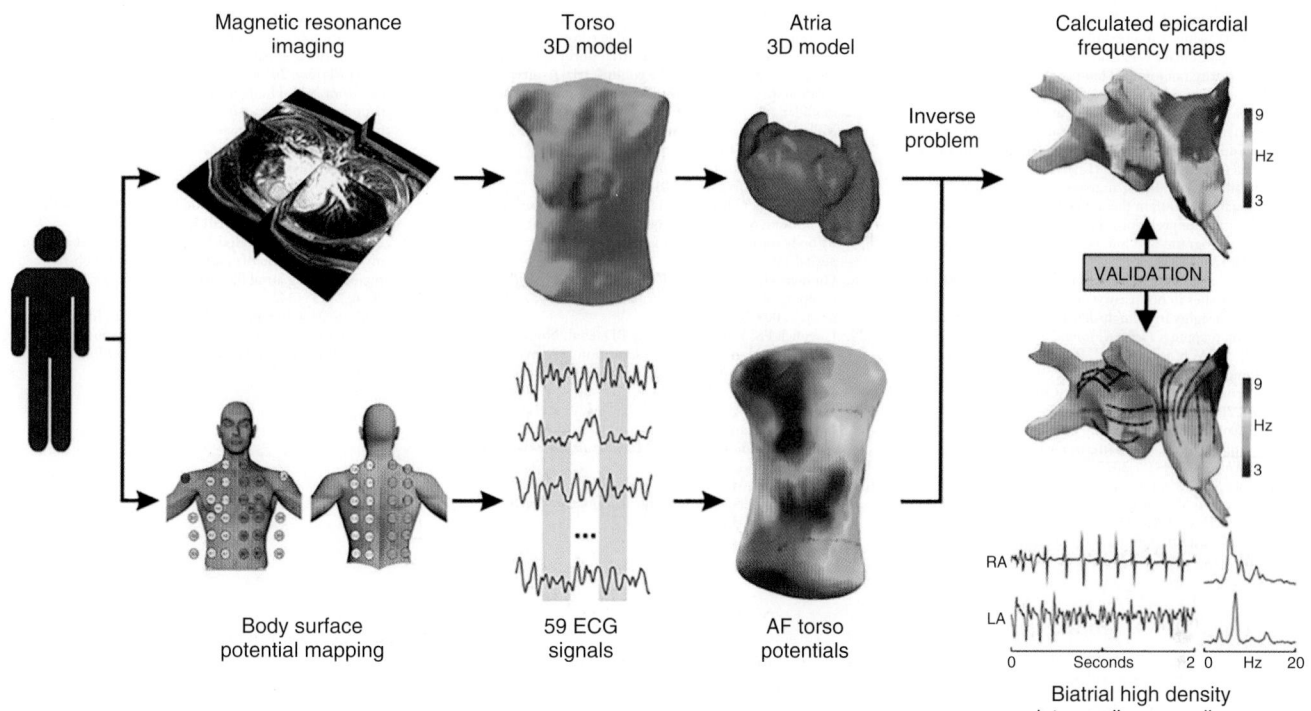

FIGURE 46.8 PERSONALIZE-AF protocol. Clinical validation of the inverse problem solution method for the noninvasive estimation of dominant high-frequency distribution and phase map reconstruction during atrial fibrillation (*AF*) (see text for details). *ECG,* Electrocardiogram; *3D,* three-dimensional.

Conclusions

Global atrial noninvasive frequency analysis is feasible and allows identification of high-frequency sources prior to the arrival to the electrophysiology laboratory for AF ablation. Importantly, our clinical–computational BSPM study on patterns of activity suggests that body surface data contains features that can be linked to reentrant drivers of AF. Narrow band-pass filtering allows selecting the electrical activity projected on the torso at the HDF, which stabilizes the projection of rotors that potentially drive AF on the surface. Phase maps of HDF-filtered surface ECG recordings allow the noninvasive localization of atrial reentries during AF. Different rotor mapping techniques have recently emerged as a mechanistic approach for AF treatment. However, notice that nowadays, noninvasive mapping is the only existent technology that allows a simultaneous recording of the entire activity from both the LA and RA. Thus the ability of BSPM to detect the site(s) driving AF may enable a noninvasive, fast, and personalized diagnosis and treatment of AF patients.

Funding Sources

Supported in part by the Instituto de Salud Carlos III (Ministry of Economy and Competitiveness, Spain: PI13-01882, PI13-00903 and PI14/00857, DTS16/00160); Spanish Society of Cardiology (Grant for Clinical Research in Cardiology 2009, 2015), and Spanish Ministry of Science and Innovation (Red RIC, PLE2009-0152).

Acknowledgment

We thank Miguel Rodrigo, MS, for critical discussions and figure designs.

REFERENCES

1. Skanes AC, Mandapati R, Berenfeld O, et al. Spatiotemporal periodicity during atrial fibrillation in the isolated sheep heart. *Circulation.* 1998;98:1236–1248.
2. Berenfeld O, Mandapati R, Dixit S, et al. Spatially distributed dominant excitation frequencies reveal hidden organization in atrial fibrillation in the Langendorff-perfused sheep heart. *J Cardiovasc Electrophysiol.* 2000;11:869–879.
3. Mandapati R, Skanes A, Chen J, et al. Stable microreentrant sources as a mechanism of atrial fibrillation in the isolated sheep heart. *Circulation.* 2000;101:194–199.
4. Mansour M, Mandapati R, Berenfeld O, et al. Left-to-right gradient of atrial frequencies during acute atrial fibrillation in the isolated sheep heart. *Circulation.* 2001;103:2631–2636.
5. Berenfeld O, Zaitsev AV, Mironov SF, et al. Frequency-dependent breakdown of wave propagation into fibrillatory conduction across the pectinate muscle network in the isolated sheep right atrium. *Circ Res.* 2002;90:1173–1180.
6. Kalifa J, Tanaka K, Zaitsev AV, et al. Mechanisms of wave fractionation at boundaries of high-frequency excitation in the posterior left atrium of the isolated sheep heart during atrial fibrillation. *Circulation.* 2006;113:626–633.

7. Atienza F, Martins RP, Jalife J. Translational research in atrial fibrillation: a quest for mechanistically based diagnosis and therapy. *Circ Arrhythm Electrophysiol.* 2012;5:1207–1215.
8. Atienza F, Almendral J, Jalife J, et al. Real-time dominant frequency mapping and ablation of dominant frequency sites in atrial fibrillation with left-to-right frequency gradients predicts long-term maintenance of sinus rhythm. *Heart Rhythm.* 2009;6:33–40.
9. Atienza F, Almendral J, Moreno J, et al. Activation of inward rectifier potassium channels accelerates atrial fibrillation in humans: evidence for a reentrant mechanism. *Circulation.* 2006;114:2434–2442.
10. Pappone C, Rosanio S, Oreto G, et al. Circumferential radiofrequency ablation of pulmonary vein ostia: a new anatomic approach for curing atrial fibrillation. *Circulation.* 2000;102(21):2619–2628.
11. Morillo CA, Klein GJ, Jones DL, et al. Chronic rapid atrial pacing. Structural, functional, and electrophysiological characteristics of a new model of sustained atrial fibrillation. *Circulation.* 1995;91:1588–1595.

12. Haissaguerre M, Jaïs P, Shah DC, et al. Spontaneous initiation of atrial fibrillation by ectopic beats originating in the pulmonary veins. *N Engl J Med.* 1998;339:659–666.
13. Nademanee K, McKenzie J, Kosar E, et al. A new approach for catheter ablation of atrial fibrillation: mapping of the electrophysiologic substrate. *J Am Coll Cardiol.* 2004;43:2044–2053.
14. Sanders P, Berenfeld O, Hocini M, et al. Spectral analysis identifies sites of high-frequency activity maintaining atrial fibrillation in humans. *Circulation.* 2005;112:789–797.
15. Lin YJ, Tai CT, Kao T, et al. Frequency analysis in different types of paroxysmal atrial fibrillation. *J Am Coll Cardiol.* 2006;47:1401–1407.
16. Dixit S, Gerstenfeld EP, Ratcliffe SJ, et al. Single procedure efficacy of isolating all versus arrhythmogenic pulmonary veins on long-term control of atrial fibrillation: a prospective randomized study. *Heart Rhythm.* 2008;5:174–181.
17. Jalife J, Atienza F, López-Salazar B, et al. Molecular, cellular and pathophysiological mechanisms of human atrial fibrillation. *Nat Clin Pract Cardiovasc Med* (CNIC Edition). 2009;6:15–21.

18. Atienza F, Almendral J, Ormaetxe JM, et al. Comparison of radiofrequency catheter ablation of drivers and circumferential pulmonary vein isolation in atrial fibrillation: a noninferiority randomized multicenter RADAR-AF trial. *J Am Coll Cardiol*. 2014;64(23):2455–2467.

19. Atienza F, Calvo D, Almendral J, et al. Mechanisms of fractionated electrograms formation in the posterior left atrium during paroxysmal atrial fibrillation in humans. *J Am Coll Cardiol*. 2011;57:1081–1092.

20. Ghoraani B, Dalvi R, Gizurarson S, et al. Localized rotational activation in the left atrium during human atrial fibrillation: relationship to complex fractionated atrial electrograms and low-voltage zones. *Heart Rhythm*. 2013;10:1830–1838.

21. Lin YJ, Tsao HM, Chang SL, et al. Role of high dominant frequency sites in nonparoxysmal atrial fibrillation patients: insights from high-density frequency and fractionation mapping. *Heart Rhythm*. 2010;7:1255–1262.

22. Lin YJ, Lo MT, Lin C, et al. Prevalence, characteristics, mapping, and catheter ablation of potential rotors in nonparoxysmal atrial fibrillation. *Circ Arrhythm Electrophysiol*. 2013;6:851–858.

23. Ng J, Gordon D, Passman RS, et al. Electrogram morphology recurrence patterns during atrial fibrillation. *Heart Rhythm*. 2014;11:2027–2034.

24. Narayan SM, Krummen DE, Shivkumar K, et al. Treatment of atrial fibrillation by the ablation of localized sources: CONFIRM (conventional ablation for atrial fibrillation with or without focal impulse and rotor modulation) trial. *J Am Coll Cardiol*. 2012;60:628–636.

25. Narayan SM, Krummen DE, Clopton P, et al. Direct or coincidental elimination of stable rotors or focal sources may explain successful atrial fibrillation ablation: On-treatment analysis of the confirm trial (conventional ablation for AF with or without focal impulse and rotor modulation). *J Am Coll Cardiol*. 2013;62:138–147.

26. Miller JM, Kowal RC, Swarup V, et al. Initial independent outcomes from focal impulse and rotor modulation ablation for atrial fibrillation: multicenter FIRM registry. *J Cardiovasc Electrophysiol*. 2014;25:921–929.

27. Guillem MS, Climent AM, Millet J, et al. Noninvasive localization of maximal frequency sites of atrial fibrillation by body surface potential mapping. *Circ Arrhythm Electrophysiol*. 2013;6:294–301.

28. Guillem MS, Climent AM, Castells F, et al. Noninvasive mapping of human atrial fibrillation. *J Cardiovasc Electrophysiol*. 2009;20:507–513.

29. Cuculich PS, Wang Y, Lindsay BD, et al. Noninvasive characterization of epicardial activation in humans with diverse atrial fibrillation patterns. *Circulation*. 2010;122:1364–1372.

30. Haissaguerre M, Hocini M, Shah AJ, et al. Noninvasive panoramic mapping of human atrial fibrillation mechanisms: a feasibility report. *J Cardiovasc Electrophysiol*. 2013;24:711–717.

31. Haissaguerre M, Hocini M, Denis A, et al. Driver domains in persistent atrial fibrillation. *Circulation*. 2014;130:530–538.

32. Rodrigo M, Guillem MS, Climent AM, et al. Body surface localization of left and right atrial high-frequency rotors in atrial fibrillation patients: a clinical-computational study. *Heart Rhythm*. 2014;11:1584–1591.

33. de Groot NM, Houben RP, Smeets JL, et al. Electropathological substrate of longstanding persistent atrial fibrillation in patients with structural heart disease: Epicardial breakthrough. *Circulation*. 2010;122:1674–1682.

34. Lee S, Sahadevan J, Khrestian CM, et al. High density mapping of atrial fibrillation during vagal nerve stimulation in the canine heart: restudying the Moe hypothesis. *J Cardiovasc Electrophysiol*. 2013;24:328–335.

35. Pedrón-Torrecilla J, Rodrigo M, Climent A, et al. Noninvasive estimation of epicardial dominant high-frequency regions during atrial fibrillation. *J Cardiovasc Electrophysiol*. 2016;27:435–442.

36. Rodrigo M, Climent AM, Liberos A, et al. Identification of dominant excitation patterns and sources of atrial fibrillation by causality analysis. *Ann Biomed Eng*. 2016;44:2364–2376.

47 Panoramic Mapping of Atrial Fibrillation From the Body Surface

Pierre Jaïs, Ashok J. Shah, Remi Dubois, Mélèze Hocini, and Michel Haïssaguerre

A twelve-lead electrocardiogram (ECG) involves measuring electrical potentials from limited sites on the torso to get an approximate recording of the electrical activity of the heart; however, this technique has not really evolved for more than 100 years. Despite the limited resolution of the ECG, some diagnoses of possible mechanisms have been made and likely sites of origin of cardiac arrhythmia have been demonstrated with this test. Several decades of research have led to the development of a 252-lead ECG–based three-dimensional (3D) mapping tool to refine noninvasive diagnosis and improve the management of heart rhythm disorders.[1] Here, we describe the clinical potential of this noninvasive mapping technique in the diagnosis of the most common cardiac electrical disorder, atrial fibrillation (AF), and its utility in guiding the catheter ablation of the most challenging form of this disorder, persistent AF.

Noninvasive Mapping Technique

The signal acquisition from the patient and subsequent computational methods used in the reconstruction of noninvasive maps using multiple surface electrocardiographic electrodes have been previously described.[1] Briefly, a 252-electrode vest is applied to the patient's torso and connected to the noninvasive imaging system, and all 252 leads are recorded. It is followed by a noncontrast thoracic computed tomography (CT) scan to obtain high-resolution images of the heart and the vest electrodes. The 3D-epicardial bicameral (atria or ventricles) geometries are reconstructed from segmental CT images, wherein the relative positions of body surface electrodes on the torso geometry are also prominently visualized. The system reconstructs epicardial potentials, unipolar electrograms, and activation maps from torso potentials during each beat/cycle using mathematical reconstruction algorithms. Details of the mathematical methods have been provided in detail elsewhere.[2–6]

Atrial Fibrillation

In the area of AF, noninvasive mapping further contributes to our understanding of AF pathophysiology and facilitates catheter ablation. Currently, pulmonary vein (PV) isolation (PVI) remains the cornerstone of catheter ablation for AF.[7,8] Recently, there has been emerging evidence that AF may be driven and maintained by localized reentrant and focal sources in the atria.[9–13]

Mapping these localized sources proves to be difficult because AF is essentially a dynamic rhythm. Previous mapping techniques utilizing single-point catheters, regional multielectrode catheters,[13] or surgical plaques[10] have been restricted by several factors, such as the inability to map both atria simultaneously, catheter contact issues, and limited surgical access.[14] With the advent of noninvasive mapping, AF may be mapped beat-to-beat in a panoramic fashion, allowing the identification of potential driving sources.[12,15]

Noninvasive Mapping Approach (Fig. 47.1)

Atrial cardiac potentials are much finer than ventricular potentials. To noninvasively map the atria accurately, several key barriers need to be overcome.[14–16] As aforementioned, individual, patient-specific 3D biatrial geometry is obtained from high-resolution, noncontrast CT scans performed with a 252-electrode vest applied to the patient's torso.[12,15] The exact locations of body surface electrodes in relation to the cardiac geometry are obtained during the same CT scan.

Consecutive windows with R-R pauses ≥1000 ms during AF are analyzed. To avoid QRST interference, only the T-Q segments are selected for analysis. In patients with rapid ventricular rates, diltiazem may be administered to slow atrioventricular (AV) conduction to create adequate recording windows.[15] Filtering processes are applied to remove artifacts in signal morphology.[12,14]

Activation maps are computed utilizing the intrinsic deflection–based method on unipolar electrograms ($-dV/dT\text{max}$).[14–16] With the global recording of cardiac signals, phase mapping algorithms may be applied to create AF maps, whereby a representation of the depolarization and repolarization wavefronts is computed from the isophase values corresponding, respectively, to $\pi/2$ and $-\pi/2$.[15] Movies of wave propagation patterns are then displayed on the individualized biatrial geometry of each patient.

With the above technique, two general types of AF drivers have been identified: (1) reentrant, when a wave is observed to fully rotate around a functional core on phase progression, and (2) focal, when a wavefront originates from a focal site with centrifugal activation. Reentrant drivers are verified by sequential activation of local unipolar electrograms around a pivot point that covers the entire local cycle length (CL), and focal drivers are confirmed by a QS pattern on unipolar electrograms. Due to the meandering nature of reentrant drivers observed in AF, the CT-based biatrial geometry is divided into regional domains for classification.[15] An aggregated driver-density map is then created in each individual patient that summates all the drivers recorded in each window and is projected on the patient's biatrial geometry.

Paroxysmal Atrial Fibrillation

In paroxysmal AF, noninvasive mapping successfully identifies focal drivers, most of which arise from the PVs.[12,14] Centrifugal spread of the wavefront is demonstrated both by activation and phase mapping.[12,14] The most remarkable finding is the observation of repetitive activation breakthroughs emanating from one or several PVs (simultaneously or sequentially), which generate reentrant drivers/rotor activity along the PV ostia. The validity of mapping is confirmed by termination of AF during isolation of the culprit PV.[12] The mutual interplay between focal discharges from the PV and ensuing reentrant activity therefore confirms

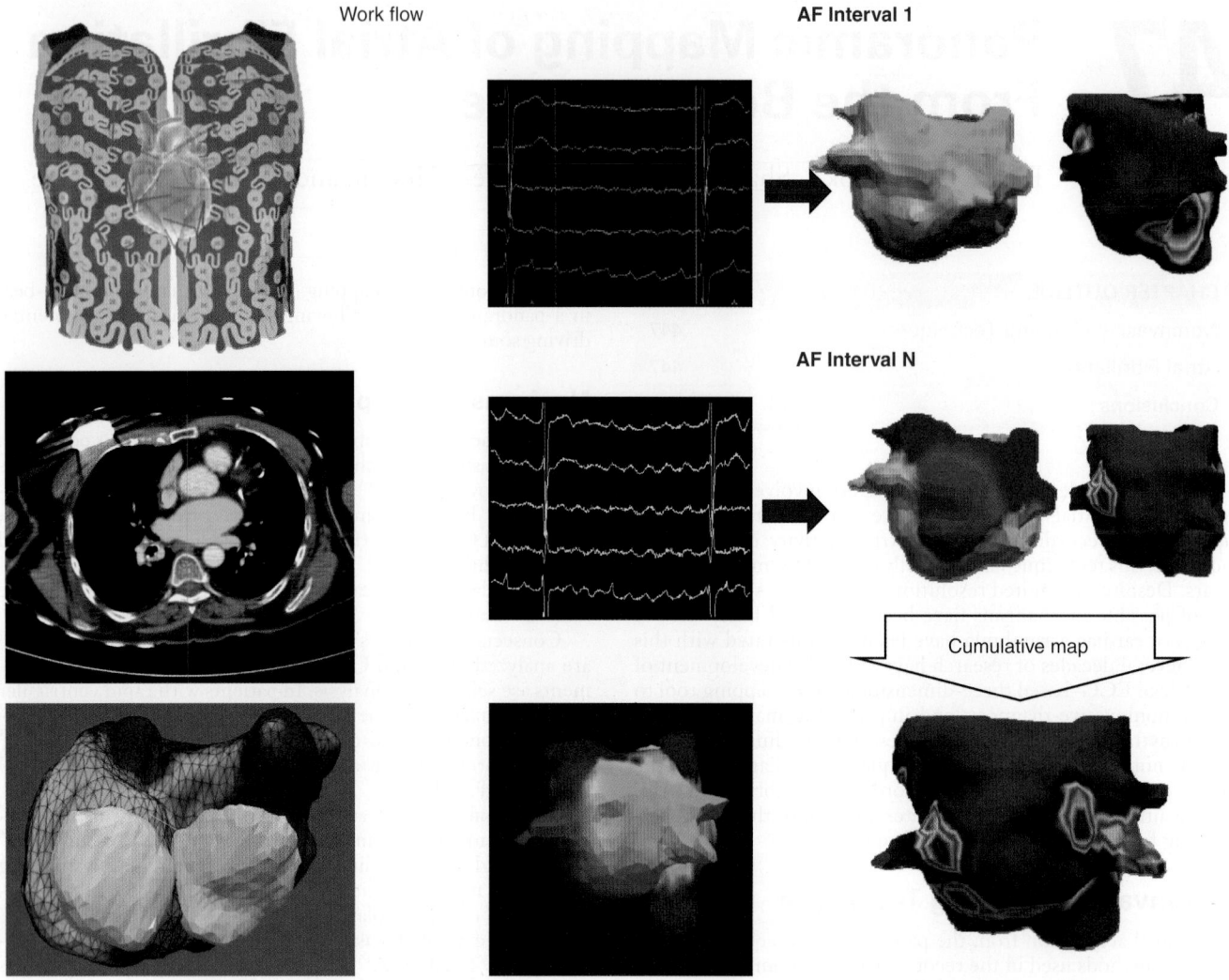

FIGURE 47.1 *Left panel:* Individual, patient-specific three-dimensional biatrial geometry is obtained from segmented high-resolution noncontrast computed tomography scans performed with a 252-electrode vest applied to the patient's torso. *Right panel:* Consecutive windows with R-R pauses ≥ 1000 ms during atrial fibrillation (*AF*) are analyzed. At least 10 pauses of 1 second were used to create a cumulative map that shows the hierarchy of regions hosting drivers and therefore determines the order for ablation.

prior experimental observations made by Jalife and associates[17] and Chen and coworkers[18] on optical maps.

To guide catheter ablation, we noninvasively mapped 20 consecutive patients with clinical paroxysmal AF.[19] The invasive procedure consisted of multispline mapping at sites of noninvasively identified sources and radiofrequency (RF) application at these sites as targets of ablation, with the endpoint of AF termination. Noninvasive maps showed single or repetitive discharges from one or several PVs, coexisting with rotor drifting along the venous ostia in the posterior wall. The PV discharges either extinguished or reset preexisting rotor. The rotor was not temporally stationary for more than mean two rotations. The anterior left as well as the right atrium was passively activated by the left atrial waves traveling over the Bachman bundle or the coronary sinus or both. In total, 344 drivers (255 rotors [74%] and 89 PV discharges/foci [26%]) were mapped in 17 of 20 patients. Among them, 95% of rotors and 81% of foci were found to be in the PV and posterior left atrial region, respectively. The first ablated PV region terminated AF in 50% of patients (and prolonged AF CL in 30%). The second targeted PV region terminated AF in an additional 40% of patients. PV

ectopics were identified after AF termination in 30% of patients. Later, circumferential PVI was undertaken and achieved in all patients.

The findings of noninvasive mapping reinforce the arrhythmogenic role of PVs in paroxysmal AF. The posterior left atrial PV regions are the most frequent (>90%) ablation target sites, leading to termination of paroxysmal AF, which is in concurrence with the key role of PVI that has been described as the cornerstone of AF ablation in contemporary guidelines.

Persistent Atrial Fibrillation

In persistent AF, the identification of AF drivers helps pinpoint the targets for substrate ablation. In a cohort of patients with paroxysmal and persistent AF, Cuculich and colleagues[14] described diverse AF activation patterns that included multiple wavelets, rotors, and focal sources with the use of noninvasive activation mapping. However, no phase mapping algorithm was used in that study, and this may explain the limited number of rotors reported by the authors. We were interested in attempting to understand why activation mapping was not showing as many reentrant activities as shown by phase mapping. Part of the answer may relate to the resolution used for activation mapping. In an experiment on isolated hearts of sheep with AF, we did run optical activation mapping and phase mapping (using an optimized algorithm designed for this purpose) and could demonstrate that similar patterns were observed with both modalities.[20] This observation, combined with the ability to record consistent atrial unipolar potentials covering the local CL on the trajectory of the reentrant activities, was considered to provide a strong validation for phase mapping.[15]

In a recent study by Haïssaguerre and colleagues,[15] 103 consecutive patients undergoing catheter ablation for persistent AF were investigated using noninvasive phase mapping. A median of four driver regions was identified in patients with persistent AF. Of the recorded driver activity, 80.5% of AF drivers were reentrant and 19.5% were focal. Reentrant AF drivers were commonly located in the right PV/septal region, left PV/left appendage region, left inferior wall/coronary sinus region, and the superior right atrium; however, the exact locations varied among individuals.[15] Reentrant activities were noted to be short-lasting, with the median number of continuous rotations being 2.6, but periodic (i.e., they would often recur at the same or adjacent site). On the other hand, an average of six events was noted from a focal site.

In a subset of patients in this study, electrogram characteristics of AF driver versus nondriver regions were compared using an invasive multielectrode catheter. Regions harboring reentrant AF drivers more often demonstrated prolonged fractionated electrograms, and the recorded electrograms spanned across a large part of the AF CL. Studies are underway to delineate the electrogram characteristics of these reentrant activities. However, fractionation alone is nonspecific as it can be influenced by contiguous anatomical structures, slow or anisotropic conduction, and the direction or overlap of multiple wavefronts.[21] A previous study, however, has indicated that these reentrant drivers tend to harbor in the patchy zones bordering dense fibrotic areas.[15,22,23]

The aggregated driver-density map derived from noninvasive mapping serves as a roadmap for ablation. Point-by-point lesions are applied at the area harboring reentrant or focal drivers, starting with the region of highest driver-density and proceeding in a decreasing order (Fig. 47.2 A–D). Local CL slowing is pursued as an endpoint of regional ablation, where initial electrograms are often rapid and fractionated. They are targeted until they become slower and less complex, usually harboring synchronous activation on distal and proximal electrodes of the ablation catheter (indicative of passive activation). Fig. 47.2 shows the example of an aggregated map to guide ablation reentrant drivers. In the ablation approach undertaken by Haïssaguerre and associates,[15] following ablation of all driver regions, linear ablation was undertaken if AF persisted. In the most recent studies performed in Bordeaux, the linear lesions were no longer used to terminate AF, but were used only in case of macroreentrant atrial tachycardia (AT). As in the index study,[15] we keep ablating all intermediate ATs upon termination of AF. Using this approach, AF was acutely terminated in 80% of patients. The number of driver regions targeted to achieve AF termination increased with the duration of persistent AF; a single dominant region was identified in only 9% of patients. Fig. 47.2 shows a typical record form of ablation procedure and demonstrates a continuity of mechanisms between AF and AT.

Among 90 patients who completed a 12-month follow-up, 64% were in stable sinus rhythm (SR), 22% were in AT, and 20% were in AF.[15] Importantly, the strategy of driver-based ablation guided by noninvasive mapping achieved 12-month clinical outcomes similar to those achieved by the conventional stepwise approach, but with half the ablation time (28 vs. 65 minutes for AF termination).[15] In this setting, persistent AF ablation guided by noninvasive mapping of localized drivers offers the ability of a direct therapy to localized AF driver regions and the potential to minimize the extent of ablation.

One of the advantages when mapping with this technology is that the vest can be left on the torso of the patient during the ablation procedure. This is demonstrated in Fig. 47.3 and offers the opportunity to assess the impact of catheter ablation on AF drivers, as depicted by noninvasive phase mapping. One of the limitations of this mapping is that some of the activities, particularly from the septal region, are not directly visible but rather project on the anterior and posterior right atrium as shown in Fig. 47.3. This phenomenon is under investigation as we have started a systematic remapping study to document the impact of PVI. Another limitation should be acknowledged here. The phase mapping algorithm has been optimized for AF mapping and for a range of frequencies and is therefore not suitable for AT mapping. This is, however, possible using the usual activation mapping that is embedded in the system. Some expertise is still required to achieve the results published on this topic.[24]

In some cases, remapping AF persistent after ablation of all driver regions has shown the emergence of a second set of drivers that may be new or possibly preexisting but were unveiled after the first set of drivers had been eliminated. The characteristics of the second set of drivers emerging after initial ablation and how this added information can help ablation will be studied in the near future.

Conclusions

Both paroxysmal and persistent AF can be mapped noninvasively to guide catheter ablation. AF-maintaining localized reentrant and focal sources are predominantly located in the PV antra and contiguous posterior left atrium in paroxysmal AF. The impact of panoramic AF mapping is modest in paroxysmal AF as PVI fits the vast majority of patients, but this mapping strategy is particularly relevant for early persistent AF. The results are best with uninterrupted AF for less than 6 months—with few biatrial regions hosting drivers—and disappointing after a year. Most of the AF drivers are unstable reentries. The pre- and periprocedural utility of the system in panoramic 3D mapping expresses its high accuracy and potential to reduce invasive procedural and ablation times. Cardiac geometry acquisition using an alternative technique is required to reduce cumulative radiation exposure.

Persistent AF 3-4 months

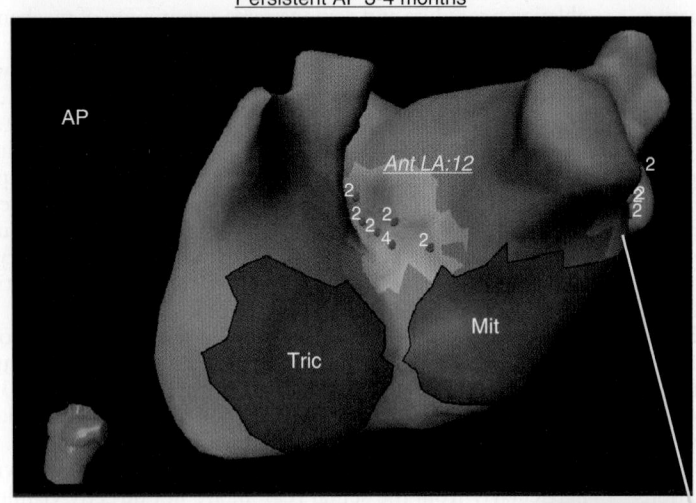

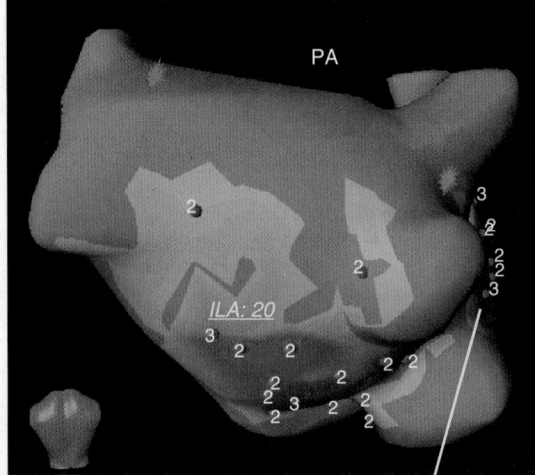

- No DC shock
- No structural heart disease
- LAA CL 145
- RAA CL 146

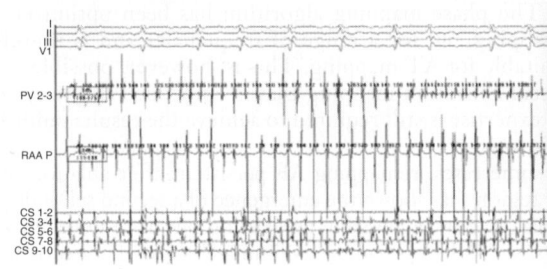

A

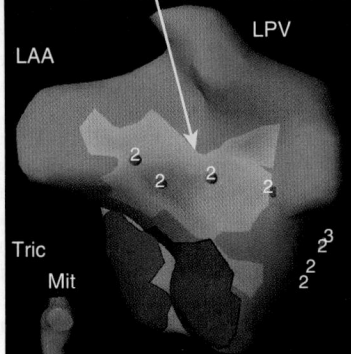

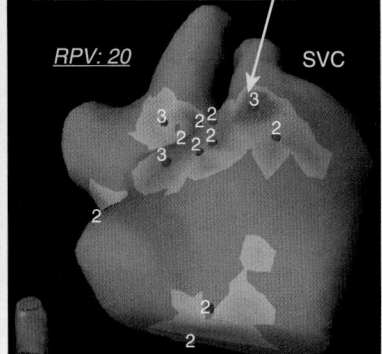

Pause during ablation site 1 (ILA, 12 min of RF)

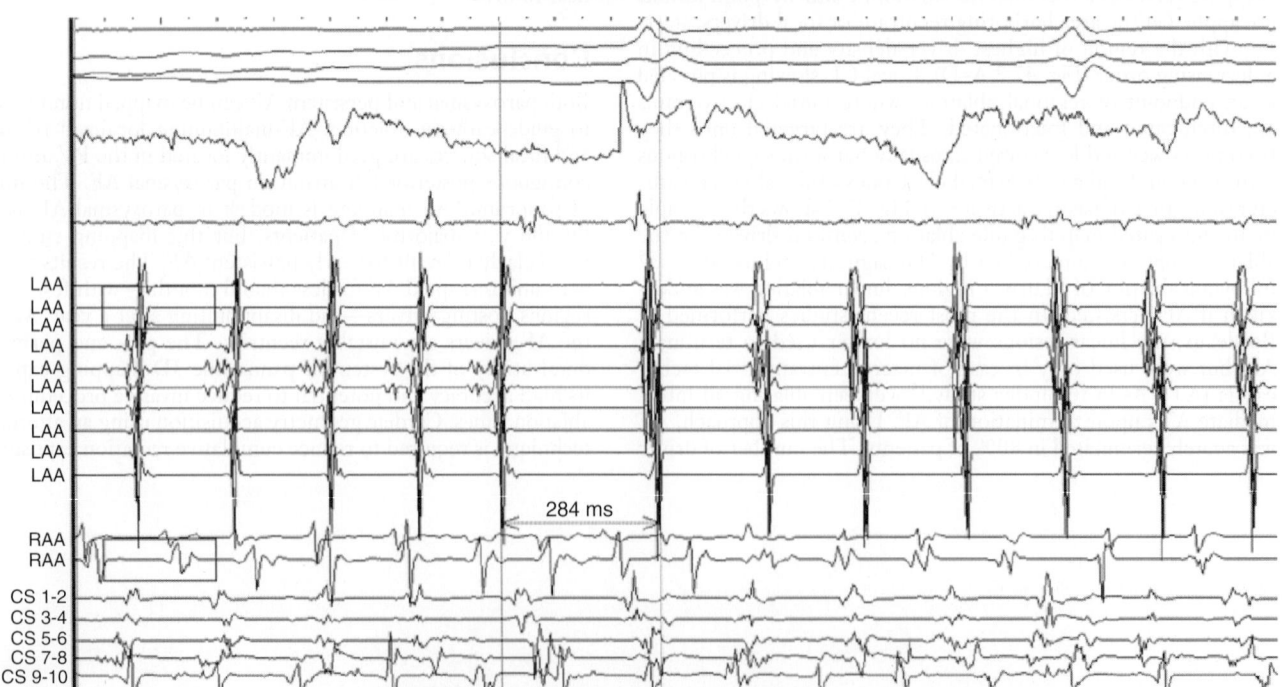

284 ms

B

FIGURE 47.2 For legend, see opposite page.

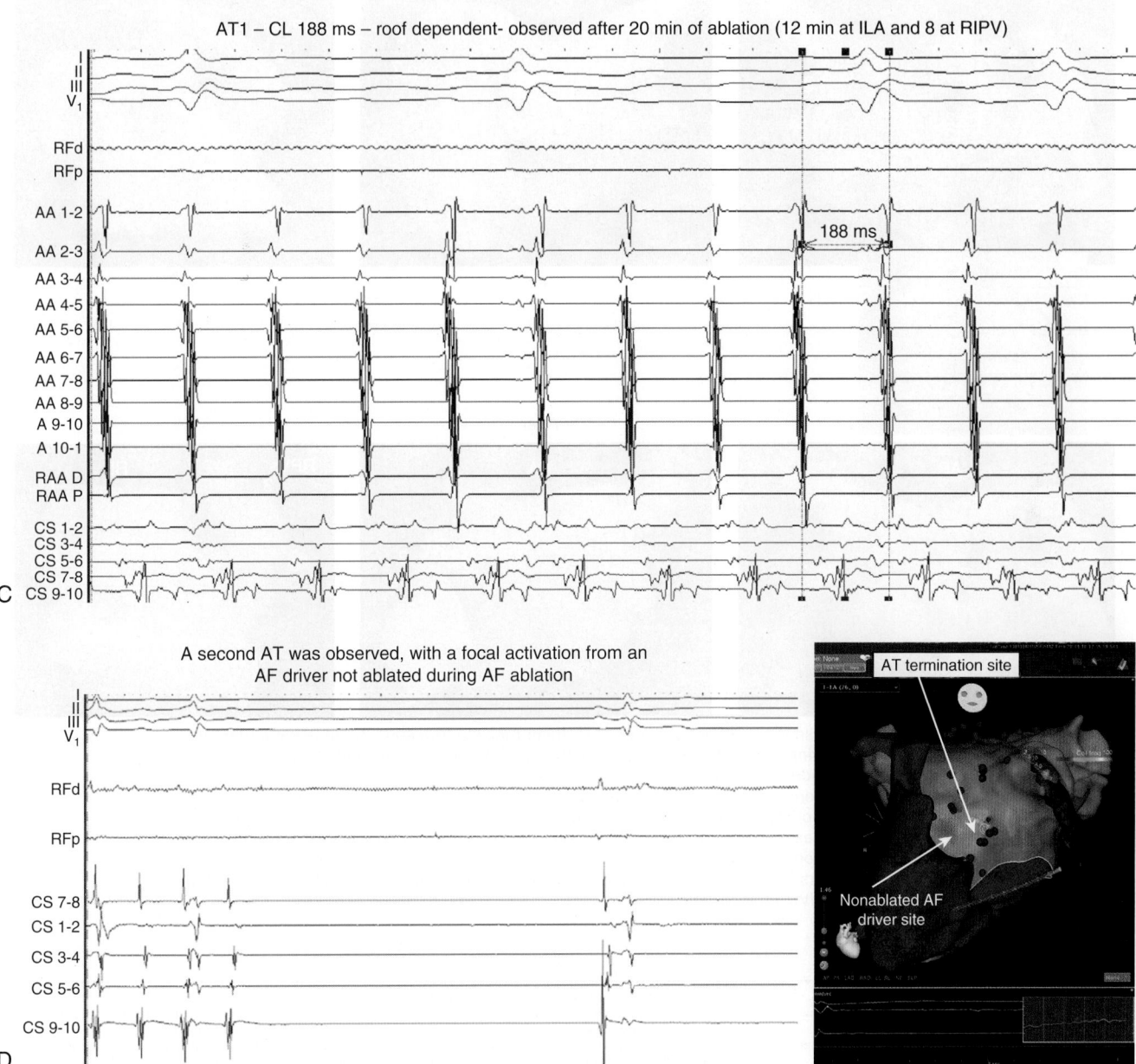

FIGURE 47.2 (A) In this patient suffering from early persistent atrial fibrillation (*AF*), the baseline AF cycle length (*CL*) is about 145 ms. The short duration of uninterrupted AF, the absence of structural heart disease (SHD) or severe left atrial dilatation (<50 mm in a parasternal echo view), and a baseline AF CL >140 ms are predictive of AF termination. The first targeted region was the inferior left atrium (*ILA*), followed by the right pulmonary veins (*RPV*), as revealed by phase mapping of 14 accumulated pauses (*not shown*), each more than 1 second. The areas with rotors (AF drivers) are depicted in *red* and the numbers represent the number of their full rotations. (B) During radiofrequency (RF) ablation of the first target site—the ILA—some degree of AF slowing and organization was observed, demonstrating the impact of targeted ablation. (C) Ablation around the next target site—the RPV—terminated AF into a roof-dependent atrial tachycardia (AT), which was terminated by linear ablation of the left atrial roof. (D) The roof-dependent AT terminated into focal AT from the anterior left atrium (*Ant LA*). Interestingly, the focal AT location was identified as the AF driver site, third in the order of ablation, but not ablated since the AF terminated into AT during ablation of the second target site. Mechanistically, focal anterior left atrial AT, while obviously not the consequence of local ablation, can be considered to have participated in AF maintenance and was found to have emerged following the elimination of more dominant AF sources by ablation. *LAA,* Left atrial appendage; *LPV,* left pulmonary veins; *RAA,* right atrial appendage; *SVC,* superior vena cava.

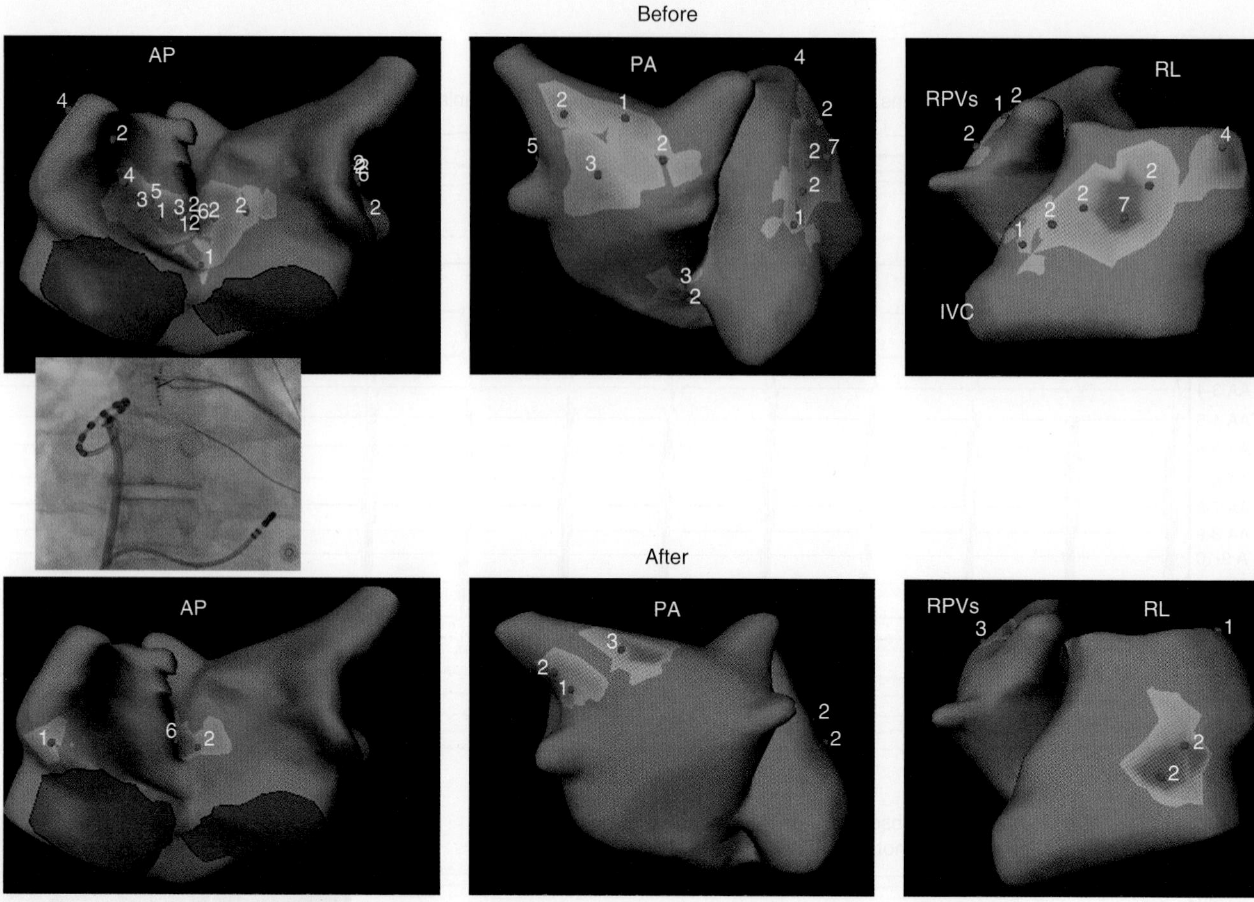

Before

After

FIGURE 47.3 Comparison of atrial fibrillation (AF) driver maps before and after ablation of the first set of drivers involving the right pulmonary veins (*RPVs*). RPV ablation was undertaken for 3 minutes using a multielectrode circular ablation catheter, nMARQ (Biosense Webster, Diamond Bar, CA). AF persisted and was remapped. The post-RPV ablation maps revealed that the number of rotors on the anterior and posterior right atrium in the anteroposterior (*AP*), posteroanterior (*PA*), and right lateral (*RL*) views had decreased. It is noteworthy that the RPV rotors project onto the adjacent right atrium. Thus the RPV ablation eliminated the majority of the rotors projecting on the adjacent right atrium. The areas with rotors (AF drivers) are depicted in *red*, and the numbers represent the number of full rotations of rotors. *IVC*, Inferior vena cava.

REFERENCES

1. Oster HS, Taccardi B, Lux RL, Ershler PR, Rudy Y. Noninvasive electrocardiographic imaging: reconstruction of epicardial potentials, electrograms, and isochrones and localization of single and multiple electrocardiac events. *Circulation.* 1997;96:1012–1024.
2. Tikhonov AN, Arsenin VY. *Solutions of Ill-Posed Problems.* New York: Wiley; 1977.
3. Calvetti D, Lewis B, Reichel L. GMRes, L-curves, and discrete ill-posed problems. *BIT Numer Math.* 2002;42:44–65.
4. Rudy Y, Oster HS. The electrocardiographic inverse problem. *Crit Rev Biomed Eng.* 1992;20:25–45.
5. Rudy Y, Burnes JE. Noninvasive electrocardiographic imaging. *Ann Noninvasive Electrocardiol.* 1999;4:340–358.
6. Ramanathan C, Jia P, Ghanem RN, Calvetti D, Rudy Y. Noninvasive electrocardiographic imaging (ECGI): application of the generalized minimal residual (GMRes) method. *Ann Biomed Eng.* 2003;31:981–994.
7. Haïssaguerre M, Jais P, Shah DC, et al. Spontaneous initiation of atrial fibrillation by ectopic beats originating in the pulmonary veins. *N Engl J Med.* 1998;339:659–666.
8. Calkins H, Kuck KH, Cappato R, et al; Heart Rhythm Society Task Force on Catheter and Surgical Ablation of Atrial Fibrillation. 2012 HRS/EHRA/ECAS expert consensus statement on catheter and surgical ablation of atrial fibrillation: recommendations for patient selection, procedural techniques, patient management and follow-up, definitions, endpoints, and research trial design: a report of the Heart Rhythm Society (HRS) Task Force on Catheter and Surgical Ablation of Atrial Fibrillation. Developed in partnership with the European Heart Rhythm Association (EHRA), a registered branch of the European Society of Cardiology (ESC) and the European Cardiac Arrhythmia Society (ECAS); and in collaboration with the American College of Cardiology (ACC), American Heart Association (AHA), the Asia Pacific Heart Rhythm Society (APHRS), and the Society

of Thoracic Surgeons (STS). Endorsed by the governing bodies of the American College of Cardiology Foundation, the American Heart Association, the European Cardiac Arrhythmia Society, the European Heart Rhythm Association, the Society of Thoracic Surgeons, the Asia Pacific Heart Rhythm Society, and the Heart Rhythm Society. *Heart Rhythm.* 2012;9:632–696 e21.
9. Schuessler RB, Grayson TM, Bromberg BI, Cox JL, Boineau JP. Cholinergically mediated tachyarrhythmias induced by a single extrastimulus in the isolated canine right atrium. *Circ Res.* 1992;71:1254–1267.
10. Sahadevan J, Ryu K, Peltz L, et al. Epicardial mapping of chronic atrial fibrillation in patients: preliminary observations. *Circulation.* 2004;110:3293–3299.
11. Narayan SM, Krummen DE, Shivkumar K, Clopton P, Rappel WJ, Miller JM. Treatment of atrial fibrillation by the ablation of localized sources: CONFIRM (Conventional Ablation for Atrial Fibrillation With or Without Focal Impulse and Rotor Modulation) trial. *J Am Coll Cardiol.* 2012;60:628–636.
12. Haïssaguerre M, Hocini M, Shah AJ, et al. Noninvasive panoramic mapping of human atrial fibrillation mechanisms: a feasibility report. *J Cardiovasc Electrophysiol.* 2013;24:711–717.
13. Haïssaguerre M, Hocini M, Sanders P, et al. Localized sources maintaining atrial fibrillation organized by prior ablation. *Circulation.* 2006;113:616–625.
14. Cuculich PS, Wang Y, Lindsay BD, et al. Noninvasive characterization of epicardial activation in humans with diverse atrial fibrillation patterns. *Circulation.* 2010;122:1364–1372.
15. Haïssaguerre M, Hocini M, Denis A, et al. Driver domains in persistent atrial fibrillation. *Circulation.* 2014;130:530–538.
16. Rudy Y. Noninvasive electrocardiographic imaging of arrhythmogenic substrates in humans. *Circ Res.* 2013;112:863–874.

17. Jalife J, Berenfeld O, Mansour M. Mother rotors and fibrillatory conduction: a mechanism of atrial fibrillation. *Cardiovasc Res.* 2002;54:204–216.
18. Chen J, Mandapati R, Berenfeld O, Skanes AC, Gray RA, Jalife J. Dynamics of wavelets and their role in atrial fibrillation in the isolated sheep heart. *Cardiovasc Res.* 2000;48:220–232.
19. Zellerhoff S, Hocini M, Dubois R, et al. Mechanisms driving paroxysmal AF displayed by noninvasive panoramic imaging (AB 35-05). *Heart Rhythm.* 2013;10:S41–S95.
20. Gutbrod SR, Walton R, Gilbert S, et al. Quantification of the transmural dynamics of atrial fibrillation by simultaneous endocardial and epicardial optical mapping in an acute sheep model. *Circ Arrhythm Electrophysiol.* 2015;8:456–465.
21. Lim HS, Haïssaguerre M. Focused review: mapping human atrial fibrillation to guide catheter ablation. In: Bonow, RO, Mann, DL, Zipes, DP, Libby, P, eds. *Braunwald's Heart Disease: A Textbook of Cardiovascular Medicine.* 9th ed; 2013(digital edition).
22. Jadidi AS, Cochet H, Shah AJ, et al. Inverse relationship between fractionated electrograms and atrial fibrosis in persistent atrial fibrillation: combined magnetic resonance imaging and high-density mapping. *J Am Coll Cardiol.* 2013;62:802–812.
23. Lim HS, Yamashita S, Cochet H, Haïssaguerre M. Delineating atrial scar by electroanatomic voltage mapping versus cardiac magnetic resonance imaging: where to draw the line? *J Cardiovasc Electrophysiol.* 2014;25:1053–1056.
24. Shah AJ, Hocini M, Xhaet O, et al. Validation of novel 3-dimensional electrocardiographic mapping of atrial tachycardias by invasive mapping and ablation: a multicenter study. *J Am Coll Cardiol.* 2013;62:889–897.

48 Mechanisms of Human Ventricular Tachycardia and Human Ventricular Fibrillation

Nicholas Jackson, Sigfus Gizurarson, Stéphane Massé, and Kumaraswamy Nanthakumar

Ventricular tachyarrhythmias are the most common cause of sudden cardiac death (SCD) in the Western world, and every year, more than 400,000 SCDs are reported in Europe and the United States.[1] Knowledge and insights into the mechanisms of both ventricular tachycardia (VT) and ventricular fibrillation (VF) have translated into key therapies to reduce morbidity and mortality from these conditions. Understanding the mechanisms that trigger VT and VF, and the substrates that sustain them, have been critical in developing these therapies. Such critical treatments range from medications and catheter ablation that reduce the burden of arrhythmias and the related symptoms to advanced device therapies that decrease mortality by rapidly detecting and treating arrhythmias with pacing and defibrillation.

Despite advances in cardiac care, the increasing number of patients with heart failure and conditions that lead to ventricular arrhythmias creates a significant burden of care for these patients with the currently established treatment paradigms. In addition, many patients are not offered effective treatment with therapies such as catheter ablation because of the perceived complexity of the procedure and concomitant risks. This underscores the need for a greater understanding and awareness of ventricular arrhythmia treatments and for the pathophysiology that underlies them. Most basic and translational research has been performed in animal models and has been extrapolated to humans. These studies have been invaluable in providing a framework for understanding ventricular arrhythmia mechanisms; however, human studies are critical to confirm their findings and determine their relevance to clinical practice. Hence this chapter mainly focuses on the insights derived from studies conducted in humans as they pertain to the mechanisms of VT and VF.

Mechanisms of Human Ventricular Tachycardia

The vast majority of ventricular arrhythmias occur in the setting of structural heart disease, although this may be subclinical at the time of presentation. In both ischemic and nonischemic cardiomyopathies (NICMs), there are varying degrees of myocardial fibrosis and myocyte disarray, reduction and redistribution of gap junctions, and ion channel dysfunction that provide the substrate for arrhythmia. Abnormal substrate may lead to ventricular arrhythmias by three fundamental mechanisms: abnormal automaticity or triggered activity (focal mechanisms), and reentry. The relative frequency by which each of these mechanisms occurs depends on the characteristics of the substrate involved. Although these three mechanisms are believed to be operative in humans, studies of human ventricular arrhythmias have primarily centered around reentry. For completeness, we have reviewed the principles of abnormal automaticity and triggered activity without human studies.

Focal Ventricular Tachycardia

The term focal ventricular arrhythmia is used to describe ventricular arrhythmias that arise from and are sustained by one localized region of cardiac tissue. In general, these arrhythmias occur because of abnormal automaticity and triggered activity; however, depending on the mapping tool used, they may occasionally include microreentrant and transmurally reentrant mechanisms. Abnormal automaticity occurs in myocytes with a reduced resting membrane potential (less negative) and results from spontaneous impulses of the cardiac action potential (AP).[2] Failure to achieve the normal diastolic resting membrane potential might result from a failure of potassium conduction to normally increase during repolarization, from a reduction in background outward potassium current, or from an increased background inward current. Impairment of the Na^{2+}/K^+ exchanger may also lead to loss of the maximum diastolic potential.[2] Abnormal automaticity has been described in both Purkinje fibers and ischemic ventricular myocytes. It differs from triggered activity in that a reduction in the resting membrane potential is present. In general, arrhythmias because of abnormal automaticity cannot be overdrive-suppressed by rapid pacing.[3]

Focal arrhythmias because of triggered activity are further divided into those caused by early afterdepolarizations (EADs) or delayed afterdepolarizations (DADs). EADs occur when a myocyte fails to completely repolarize from the previous AP. As the membrane potential is at an intermediate value, oscillatory depolarizations can reach threshold values and initiate another response.[2] Once an EAD occurs, the membrane potential may return to normal or may be followed by repetitive depolarizations at rapid rates. EADs are often associated with bradycardia or slow heart rate and have been linked to numerous ion channel disturbances, including L-type calcium, potassium rectifier current, and late sodium currents. With QT prolongation, phase 2/3 of the AP prolongs and arrhythmias due to EADs are more likely to occur. Repetitive firing from EADs has also been demonstrated in the setting of hypokalemia, exposure to myocyte toxins, and with high concentrations of catecholamines.

DADs occur following phase 3 of the AP when the resting membrane potential has returned to normal or less than normal. Because the amplitude of a DAD increases as the preceding cycle length decreases, these premature depolarizations frequently exhibit a self-sustaining nature.[2] Although the exact mechanism for DADs is uncertain, they can be reduced by agents that block the slow inward channels and are increased in amplitude by catecholamines and by increases in extracellular calcium concentration. Digitalis toxicity is a typical cause of DADs. Digitalis impairs the Na/K ATPase and decreases extrusion of Na. Increased intracellular Na then allows for increased Na/Ca exchange and results in increased intracellular Ca oscillations. Oscillatory changes in Ca cause a change in membrane conductance that allows the transient inward current to cause DADs.

Reentrant Ventricular Tachycardia After Healed Myocardial Infarction

In electrophysiology, the term reentry is used when an electrical impulse or wavefront follows a specific path that returns upon itself to form a continuous circuit of electrical activation. In order for reentry to occur in this way, two functionally or anatomically distinct pathways are required with proximal and distal connections and differing electrophysiological properties. The characteristics of these pathways must be such that an impulse can block in one pathway (the effective refractory period of that pathway is exceeded), while propagation down the other pathway is sufficiently delayed such that recovery of excitability has occurred in the blocked pathway and the wavefront can reenter the blocked pathway in the retrograde direction.[4]

Mechanisms of Maintenance of Human Ventricular Tachycardia

Reentry is the most common mechanism of VT in the presence of structural heart disease and myocardial fibrosis.[5] In the era of modern electrophysiology, Hein Wellens first studied reentry in the human heart by performing programmed stimulation in five patients with recurrent VT and known structural heart disease.[6] By delivering a drive train and single extrastimulus from the right ventricle (RV), VT could be reliably induced and then terminated with one or two (closely coupled) RV extrastimuli. A single extrastimulus delivered during VT was followed by an interval shorter than a compensatory pause. Reliable induction and termination of VT with extrastimuli and the capacity to reset VT with a single extrastimulus were most consistent with a reentrant mechanism. This concept of programmed stimulation to induce arrhythmias paved the way for the interventional phase of cardiovascular electrophysiology.

Although reentry was believed to be the predominant mechanism underlying VT in these early studies, it was not definitively demonstrated in humans until 1978 when Josephson and colleagues[7] were able to demonstrate reentry in three patients with recurrent VT by recording continuous diastolic activity on the endocardium during VT using a sequential mapping technique. A critical degree of fractionation and delay in local activation was required for VT initiation, and VT cessation was preceded by loss of continuous diastolic activity.[7] These early studies provided further evidence for reentrant mechanisms in scar-related VT but had inherent limitations from sequential mapping. Subsequent examination of ventricular arrhythmia mechanisms by programmed stimulation has shown that the hallmark of reentry is the capacity to reset or entrain the rhythm in the presence of QRS fusion.[4]

The advent of high-density multielectrode arrays for intraoperative mapping, combined with high-gain and hard-wired bipolar recordings, enabled further understanding of reentrant pathways in human VT. By simultaneously mapping the left ventricular (LV) endo- and epicardium in patients with infarct-related VT, Downar and associates[8] found that the diastolic pathways in VT were often complex with multiple paths of entry and exit. Both spontaneous and induced block occurred within these reentrant pathways, resulting in intermittent VT cycle length changes. If conduction block occurred near the exit site of a diastolic pathway, then the VT terminated or utilized a different exit pathway, often resulting in changes to the VT cycle length and morphology. Multiple different VT morphologies were observed to share common portions of diastolic pathways, and termination of VT could result from block close to the entrance or exit sites.[8]

In the current era of electroanatomical mapping, we can conceptualize the VT circuit as consisting of some or all of the following distinct parts: the isthmus (critical diastolic channel), an inner loop (a circuit constrained within scar tissue), an outer loop (working ventricular myocardium that is not constrained by scar), and bystander regions (channels adjacent to or distant from the isthmus that are not critical to the maintenance of VT).[5] Fig. 48.1 demonstrates these regions in three different theoretical reentry circuits originating from the same chronic infarct model. A combination of activation mapping with entrainment maneuvers during VT can enable identification of these regions for catheter ablation as pioneered in the electrophysiology lab by Stevenson.[5]

Further studies using electroanatomical mapping systems and activation/entrainment mapping of VT circuits have shown that isthmus and exit sites are invariably located within regions of scar and/or scar border zones.[9] This is consistent with the work of de Bakker and coworkers,[10] who examined the histology from endocardial specimens in patients undergoing endocardial resection for intractable VT. Histology showed isolated fibers of surviving myocytes interspersed between regions of dense myocardial fibrosis.[10] This leads to the concept that regions of scar form anatomical barriers around which reentry can occur and that surviving myocardial bundles within this scar provide sufficiently slow or circuitous conduction to allow for recovery of excitability of adjacent tissue and the initiation of reentry. Ventricular remodeling following myocardial infarction not only leads to fibrosis and myocyte disarray but also to a decrease and redistribution of gap junctions and ion channel dysfunction, further perpetuating the uncoupling of cardiomyocyte bundles observed in these areas.[11] Structural changes lead to zigzag conduction that is often seen in the diastolic isthmus of the VT circuit. Structural and functional factors then contribute to heterogeneity in myocardial conduction and refractoriness that is exacerbated by differing heart rates, ischemia, autonomic tone, and ectopic beats that are frequently the initiators of VT.

Though it is believed that there is slow conduction in the diastolic isthmus of VT, original studies indicated that absolute velocity was on average 70 cm/s, and it was in fact circuitous or zigzag conduction in confined anatomical regions that led to this misconception of slow conduction. Using high-density mapping of the diastolic circuit in VT, Josephson[11] recently demonstrated that there was no slow conduction at the isthmus but that the greatest slowing was observed postexit as wavefront curvature increased.

Mechanisms of Initiation of Human Ventricular Tachycardia

Ventricular scar forms the substrate and sets the stage for reentrant arrhythmias, but in humans, less is known about the exact mechanisms of VT initiation. Berger and colleagues[12] studied Holter recordings of 16 patients with ischemic VT. They found that VT was induced by 1–5 ventricular extrasystoles that often

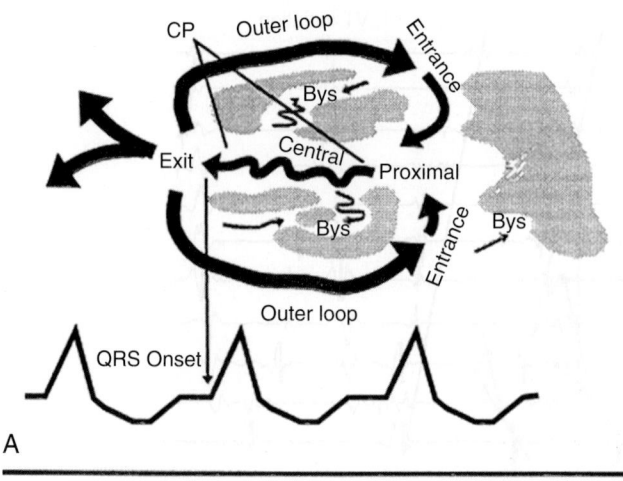

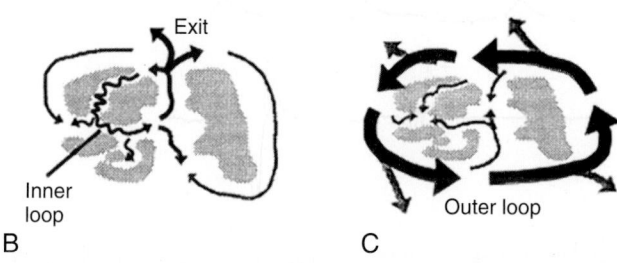

FIGURE 48.1 Three theoretical reentry circuits are shown originating from the same chronic infarct. In each panel, the reentry circuit is indicated by the *black arrows*. *Gray arrows* indicate excitation wavefronts from the circuit that depolarize tissue that is not in the circuit (bystanders *[Bys]*). *Gray stippled* areas are unexcitable regions in the chronic infarct. (A) Circuit that contains two loops and a common pathway (*CP*) through which conduction is slowed, creating a "figure-eight" configuration. The CP is a relatively small mass of tissue in the chronic infarct, depolarization of which generates low-amplitude signals that are not detectable in the standard body surface electrocardiogram. The CP has an exit as well as central and proximal regions. The QRS complex is inscribed after the excitation wavefront leaves the CP at the exit (*arrow* to the QRS onset at *bottom*) and begins propagating around the border of the scar through two outer loops. The excitation wavefronts then enter the infarct region through entrances to reach the proximal portion of the CP. Several regions that are in the chronic infarct but do not participate in the circuit are labeled as Bys. (B) Circuit that is contained entirely within the chronic infarct. This circuit consists of an exit as well as central, proximal, and inner loop regions. (C) Circuit that is a single outer loop. The reentry wavefront circulates around the margins of the chronic infarct. Excitation wavefronts collide in the paths within the chronic infarct; these paths behave as bystanders. (From Stevenson WG, Friedman PL, Sager PT, et al. Exploring postinfarction reentrant ventricular tachycardia with entrainment mapping. *J Am Coll Cardiol.* 1997;29:1180-1189).

had a resemblance to the ensuing VT morphology. It is likely that these represent true ectopy but may also include so-called transitional beats. These transitional beats are frequently seen during VT initiation at the line of functional block, and hence diastolic pathways for VT are gradually evolving. Segal and associates[13] studied the mechanisms of VT initiation in nine patients by mapping with a noncontact balloon catheter deployed in the LV. They found that in addition to areas of anatomical fixed block (dense scar), functional block was frequently observed, forming a critical part of the diastolic pathway. In most of the observed VTs in their study, lines of functional block (and hence the diastolic pathway) formed over up to six transitional beats before stable reentrant VT was established. They also observed that the initiation of VT was dependent on unidirectional block in the area that subsequently became the VT exit site.[13]

In a recent study, Jackson and coworkers[14] advanced this concept further by elucidating that areas that undergo unidirectional block reveal decremental conduction when stressed with extrastimuli prior to block. These findings were only decipherable because of high density–fixed contact mapping, and thus the same regions could be studied at stimulation, initiation, and during VT. Using this method, Jackson and colleagues studied the role of decremental conduction in scar and scar border zones during the initiation of reentrant VT. Decremental conduction is a well-recognized phenomenon in the induction of reentrant supraventricular tachycardias[15]; however, it is less well characterized in VT. The concept was developed from surgically mapped VT cases and further validated with mathematical modeling. Fig. 48.2 shows VT initiation where a pacing train and extrastimuli first lead to decremental conduction followed by unidirectional block and then initiation of VT. With the introduction of a premature extrastimulus, there is marked delay of the local electrograms across all bipoles from A to J. With S3, there is block at the VT exit site (bipole J), and this combination of delayed conduction and unidirectional block then leads to the initiation of reentrant VT. Fig. 48.2B highlights reversal in polarity of the local electrogram at bipole H with initiation of VT. This is critical for reentry initiation because following block at bipole H, wavefront collision no longer occurs in the isthmus, bipoles H–K are instead activated in the opposite direction, and a continuous reentry circuit ensues. Mathematical modeling demonstrated that the effect of decreased conduction velocity with an extrastimulus (conduction velocity restitution) was magnified by zigzag conduction within the diastolic isthmus to create the critical conduction delay required for reentry initiation.[14]

The inability to perform activation mapping of noninducible and hemodynamically unstable VTs led to new mapping techniques based on defining the scar areas and substrate to try to determine which regions of the myocardium might theoretically sustain VT without actually having to map during tachycardia or even perform induction. Although good clinical success rates have been reported, there are inherent limitations to this technique, relating to the sensitivity and specificity of the ablation strategy. In patients with VT following myocardial infarction, the scar regions may be abundant with fractionated signals, double potentials, and late potentials over a large area of the ventricle. These abnormal electrograms may be caused by a variety of conditions, including wavefront collision, functional conduction block or slowing, wave break or fusion, and structural complexities such as branching and joining muscle bundles and fiber disarray.[16] Because a number of these preceding features have been associated with reentry, the ablation of these abnormal signals has been proposed to treat patients with VT. Subsequent studies have shown, however, that these abnormal signals frequently represent passive regions of abnormal conduction in the myocardium and that such abnormal signals have a low specificity for critical regions of VT circuits.[17] Two approaches that have shown improved specificity for identifying the VT isthmus include looking for late potentials that lie within scar tissue channels[17] and looking for local potentials that delay with an extrastimulus, thus exhibiting the decremental conduction that is required for reentry initiation.[14]

Although it is convenient to employ anatomical targets such as scar channels and border zones as constructs for VT circuits, this oversimplification does not include the role of functional block and may be a key reason for the modest results of current substrate-based VT ablation techniques.

Ventricular Tachycardia Early Following Myocardial Infarction

In the previous section, we discussed reentry in the setting of healed myocardial infarction. Although other VT mechanisms in this setting are uncommon, they are, however, more prevalent in the acute phases

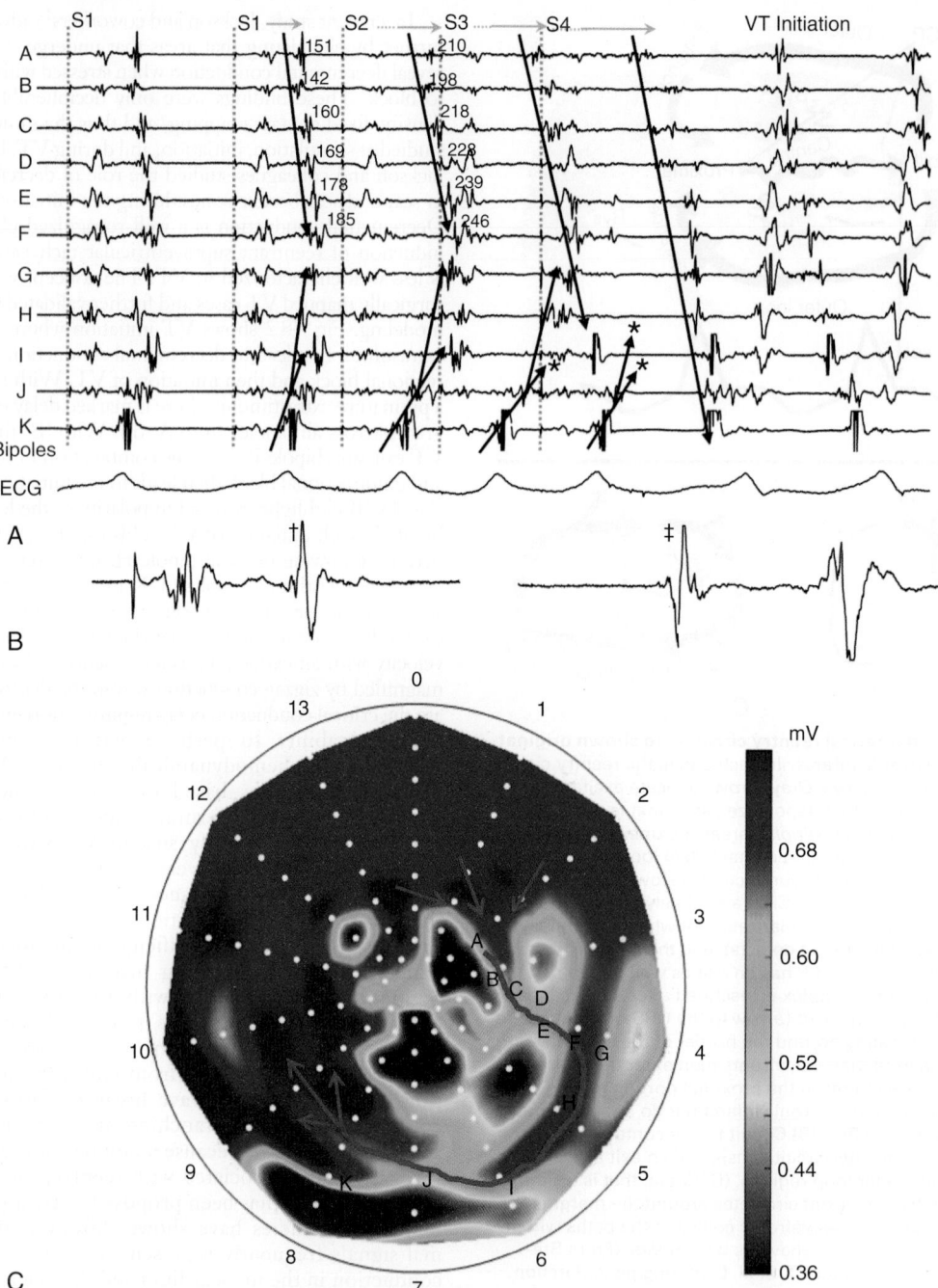

FIGURE 48.2 Pacing induced decremental conduction followed by unidirectional block leads to initiation of ventricular tachycardia (VT). (A) The bipoles A–K are located sequentially within the diastolic pathway of the VT circuit. With the introduction of a premature stimulus (S2), there is marked delay of the local activation (delayed local electrograms) across all bipoles from A to J. With S3, there is block (*) of the local potential on bipole I and subsequently with S4, there is block (*) at the VT exit site (bipole J). Block at the VT exit site and conduction delay through the entrance to the diastolic isthmus sets up the environment for the reentrant circuit to begin. Bipoles A–J then span the entire diastolic limb of the VT circuit. (B) is an enlarged image of bipole H from (A). The split potential following S1 is enlarged to clearly show the polarity of the local component (†). With S4, block to bipole H occurs through the exit site of the VT isthmus, and this bipole is subsequently activated via the VT entrance site from the opposite direction. This change in direction of activation leads to an exact polarity change in the local electrogram (‡). (C) is a corresponding scar map of the left ventricle with the voltage scale on the right. Apical electrodes are at the center, basal electrodes at the periphery, and spline 0 is oriented to the anterior interventricular groove. Heterogeneous scar is found at the apex and extends to the inferobasal region. The diastolic pathway of the VT shown in (A) is drawn (*red arrow*), and the corresponding electrodes are labeled. *ECG*, Electrocardiogram. (From Jackson N, Gizurarson S, Viswanathan K, et al. Decrement evoked potential mapping: the basis of a mechanistic strategy for ventricular tachycardia ablation. *Circ Arrhythm Electrophysiol.* 2015;8:1433-1442.)

after myocardial ischemia, whether reperfusion has occurred or not. For obvious reasons, studies in humans are difficult to perform, and most studies are observational or have an experimental animal setup.

During the early stages of coronary occlusion, ventricular arrhythmias predominantly occur because of reentry within the ischemic myocardium where depressed transmembrane potentials lead to slow conduction and block.[18] The premature ventricular contractions (PVCs) that initiate reentry may be reentrant themselves or may be due to triggered activity from Purkinje fibers[19] in ischemic regions in response to increased catecholamine levels.[20] In the subacute period following acute myocardial infarction (6 hours to 3 days), rapid VT may result from abnormal automaticity in surviving Purkinje fibers and possibly triggered activity.[18] These delayed arrhythmias may be promoted by increased cardiac sympathetic nerve activity[21] or by increased sensitivity of Purkinje fibers to catecholamines.[18] Beyond the subacute period following acute myocardial infarction, ventricular arrhythmias are more likely to result from reentry involving zigzag conducting in surviving myocardial fibers in regions of infarction,[18] similar to that observed later in the healed postmyocardial infarct state. Careful plunge needle studies of subacute infarct-related VT have confirmed reentrant rather than focal mechanisms.[22]

Ventricular Tachycardia in Nonischemic Substrates

The mechanisms of VT have not been studied as widely in NICMs. In general, monomorphic VT is less common in NICMs than in ICMs; however, as myocardial scar and functional elements of the VT circuit often lie away from the endocardium, complete mapping is more challenging.[23] In one study of 26 patients with VT and NICM, 16 (62%) had VT due to a reentrant mechanism involving scar in the myocardium, 5 (19%) had VT due to bundle branch reentry, and 7 (27%) had a focal mechanism for VT.[23] Another study of 19 patients with NICM suggested that these patients exhibit a smaller area of abnormal electrical signals on the endocardium than those with ICM and that low voltage regions were confined to the basal LV (perivalvular).[24] The majority of mapped VTs in these patients originated from the ventricular base in regions of abnormal endocardial electrograms.[24] In general, VT recurrence following ablation therapy is more common in patients with NICM than in those with ICM.[25] This may reflect a greater incidence of epicardial and midmyocardial substrates that are less amenable to catheter ablation or to a more dynamic disease progression in patients with NICM over time.

Patients with congenital heart defects having previous corrective surgery involving the ventricles also represent a small but challenging subset of patients in whom dense anatomical scar is frequently observed in the areas of patches and ventriculotomy. Typical patients are those with repaired tetralogy of Fallot, who commonly have surgical patches and scar tissue in the area of the the RV outflow tract and septum. Downar and associates[26] reported a small study of four patients who were carefully mapped in the operating room with a customized balloon. In these patients, all induced VTs were macroreentrant, with the exit sites located in the RV outflow tract. In addition, they demonstrated that VT induction was dependent on functional block to form the critical isthmus of reentry. Modern era clinical mapping studies[27] have demonstrated similar findings, and ablation strategies based on these principles have been largely successful for VT suppression in these patients.

Mechanisms of Human Ventricular Fibrillation

Mechanisms of Initiation of Human Ventricular Fibrillation

The same previously discussed triggers that may initiate VT may also initiate VF when critically timed. Detailed human

studies on such isolated triggers that initiate VF are difficult to perform; however, given the potential therapeutic target for ablation, studies from the catheterization laboratory have suggested closely coupled Purkinje fiber ectopics may play a role in VF initiation.[28,29] In two studies of idiopathic VF (VF occurring in structurally normal hearts that was not preceded by VT), ectopy from the Purkinje system initiated VF in 87%[29] and 75%[28] of cases, and ablation of these triggering beats reduced the recurrence of VF during follow-up. Purkinje fibers are capable of rapid burst activity, which may set up heterogeneous conduction block within vulnerable myocardium to initiate VF.

Mechanisms of Maintenance of Human Ventricular Fibrillation

Mechanistic studies regarding human VF maintenance pose a considerable challenge because of the catastrophic hemodynamic state. Unlike hemodynamically tolerated VT, there is no means to ethically study nonperfused VF in the human heart beyond the early phase. Therefore the Toronto VF research program innovated clinically relevant models in the catheterization laboratory, and operating room, and used human Langendorff models to understand the mechanisms of human VF as it progresses. The clinical relevance of these models was validated by comparing the characteristics of human VF at defibrillation threshold testing before cardiac transplantation to the characteristics of the very same hearts in a Langendorff model following transplant.[30]

Short-Duration Ventricular Fibrillation

Initial studies by Nanthakumar and coworkers[31] in nine patients using 20-cm[2] segments of the human LV epicardium during intraoperative mapping revealed large sweeping wavefronts with significant organization that followed repetitive pathways. This organization was not consistent with the previously conceived notion of VF maintenance by multiple reentrant wavefronts, thus challenging the disorganized nature of VF. This organization was consistent, however, with Walcott and colleagues,[32] who at DFT testing mapped VF with a multipolar catheter and found sweeping well-organized wavefronts that spanned large portions of the LV endocardium.[32]

In a first in human analysis, Nanthakumar and associates[33] established an optical mapping program to study VF in human Langendorff hearts. Transformation of the optical data to phase-based analysis demonstrated for the first time the presence of phase singularity points, wave breaks, and rotor formation in human VF. Large wavefronts (the 8-cm length of the optical field) were frequently seen, suggesting there are a limited number on the human heart during VF. Fig. 48.3 shows a sequence of phase maps from optical data that track a phase singularity point and a dominant frequency map of the area where this rotor was located. The region of the rotor demonstrates the highest activation rate with no conduction block, while regions with lower activation rates are seen where the wavefronts fragment and conduction block occurs. These studies largely involved high-density mapping of limited regions of the ventricle with extrapolation to the entire ventricle. As such, a global mapping strategy was needed to better understand organization in VF.

Masse and coworkers[34] demonstrated in an elegant simultaneous endo- and epicardial mapping study that indeed phase singularities and rotors contributed to VF organization as suspected by the limited high-density mapping studies. In addition, wavefront patterns indicated a complex and transient organizational phenomenon that suggested that scroll waves were meandering in the LV (although this study did not map the myocardium transmurally). These findings were in agreement with the data acquired by Nash and colleagues.[35]

In an attempt to improve the understanding of VF, Umapathy and associates[36] introduced the concept of phase mapping to clinical electrophysiology. Critical findings from phase mapping include the identification of phase singularities that colocalize

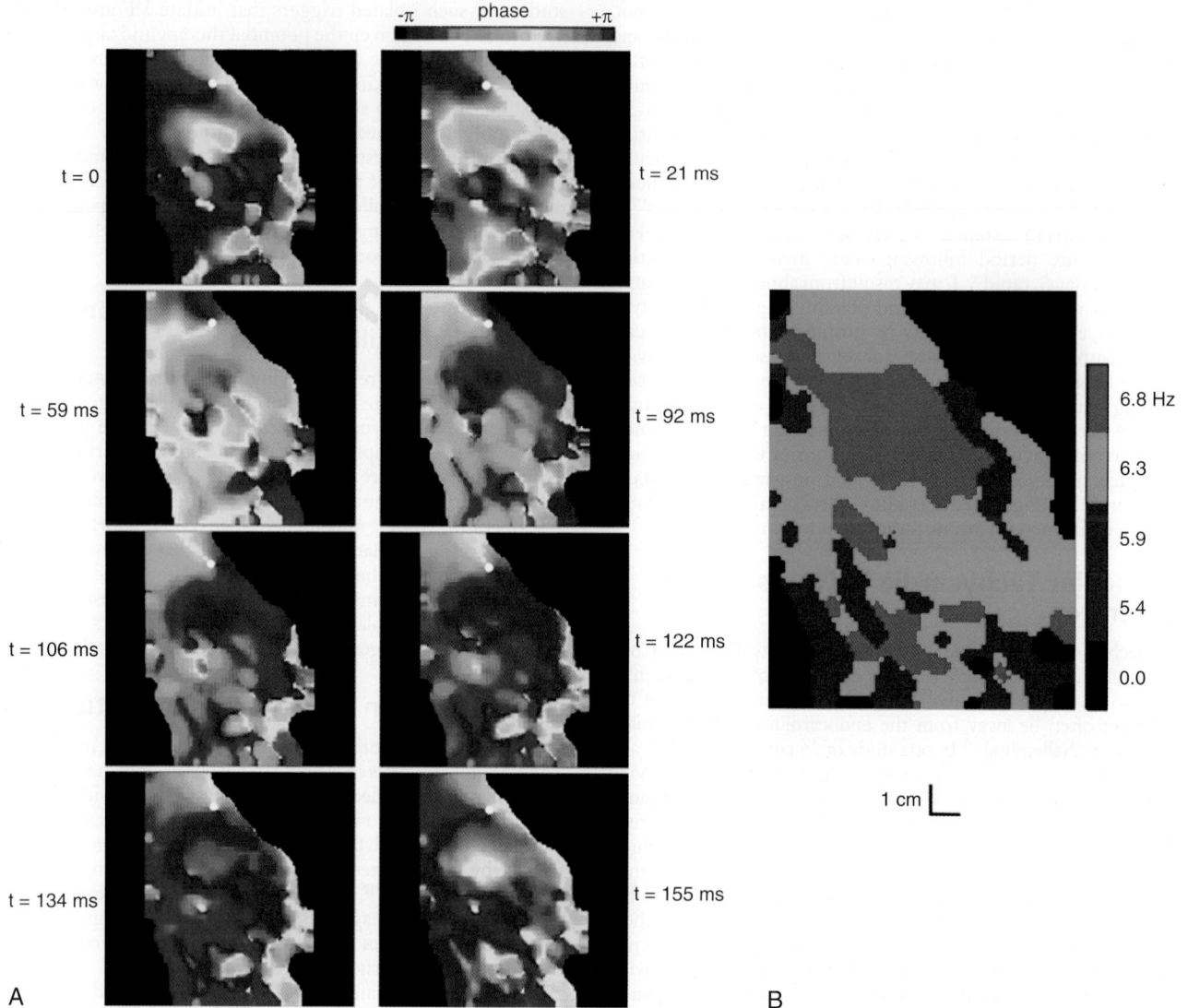

FIGURE 48.3 Optical mapping of ventricular fibrillation in a human heart. (A) shows sequential phase maps of the optical data that allow tracking of phase singularity points. A prominent phase singularity is shown at *top* as a *white dot*. Circulating wavefronts that turn 360 degrees around the dot are shown in snapshots. These snapshots reveal a cycle length of 155 ms for this rotor. (B) shows a dominant frequency map displaying the area where the rotor was located, with no conduction block to the wavefronts, having the highest activation rate, and the area where the wavefronts fragment and have conduction block with lower activation rates. (From Nanthakumar K, Jalife J, Masse S, et al. Optical mapping of Langendorff-perfused human hearts: establishing a model for the study of ventricular fibrillation in humans. *Am J Physiol Heart Circ Physiol.* 2007;293:H875-H880.)

with scar boundaries and anatomical heterogeneities and that these anatomical heterogeneities modulate their spatial meandering. Phase singularities correlate with the location of wave breaks, and the organization of electrical activity in human VF relates to wavefronts emanating from a few rotors.[36] Because VF is a nonstationary process, Umapathy and coworkers[37] went from simply analyzing phase and dominant frequency maps to instantaneous mean frequency maps to better understand its spatiotemporal evolution. In 13 isolated human hearts, there were significant spatiotemporal changes in the evolution of VF frequency, suggesting that instantaneous mean frequency better tracks frequency patterns and conduction block in VF than phase mapping.[37]

In an effort to understand the transmural mechanism of VF, Nair and colleagues[38] used transmural plunge needles to study electrical activation in 13 Langendorff perfused hearts (obtained after cardiac transplantation) immediately following

the onset of VF. Simultaneous transmural activation across these plunge needles was the most common pattern of activation seen following VF onset. Simultaneous endo- and epicardial mapping, combined with high-resolution–fixed space mapping (high-density plaque with plunge needles) and optical mapping, confirmed the presence of transmural scroll waves and not multiple wavelets as driving VF in its early stages (Fig. 48.4).[38] Subsequent histological examination showed that scroll waves were more likely to anchor to regions with greater intramural fibrosis.[38]

Human VF displays regional frequency variation, and this was quantified and related to bipolar voltage maps in human Langendorff hearts. In 35 VF episodes of eight myopathic human hearts, the LV had a larger dominant frequency span than the RV, with no significant difference between the LV free wall and septum.[39] Furthermore, regions of abnormal myocardium correlated with dominant frequencies in only 50% of cases, indicating that ion

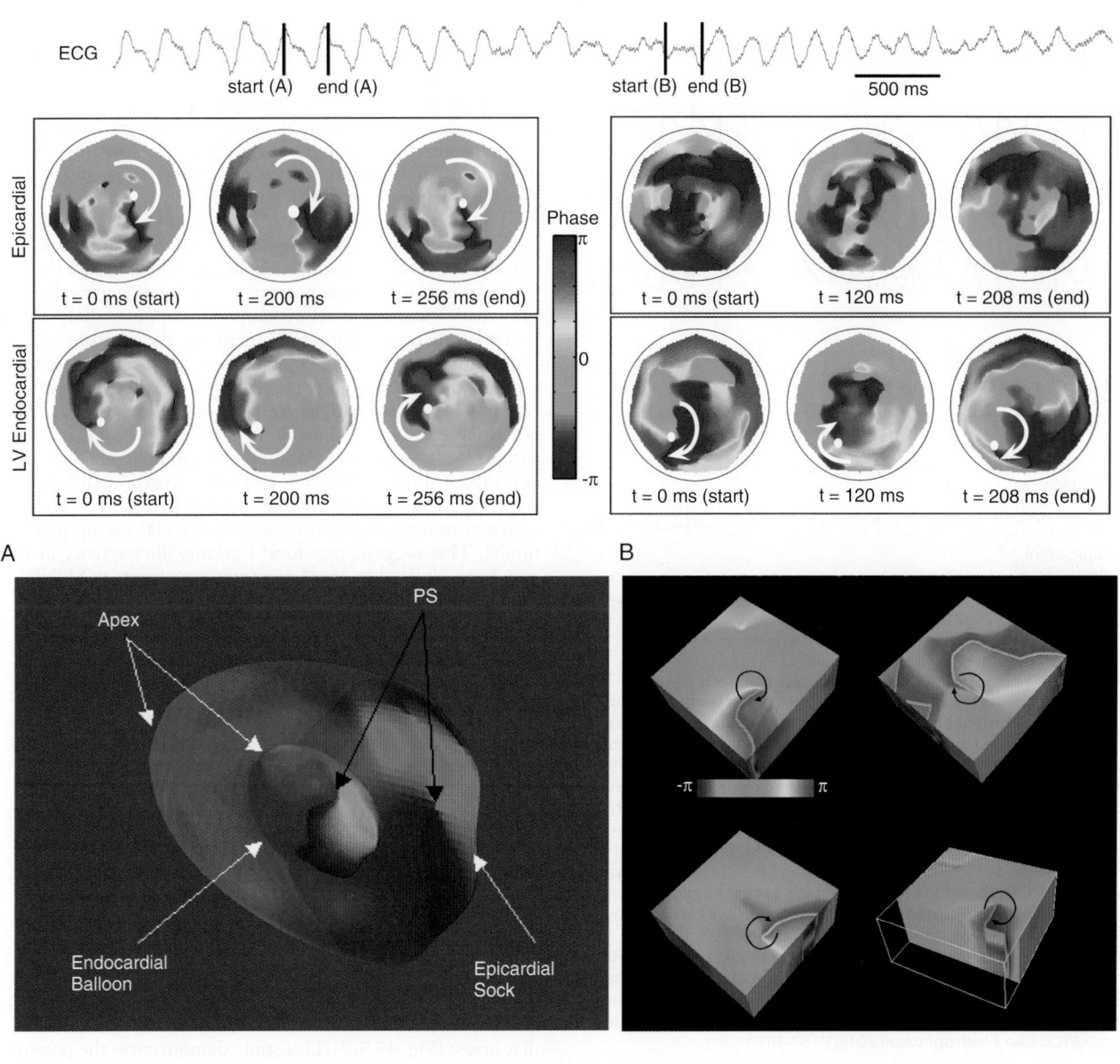

FIGURE 48.4 Three-dimensional mapping of ventricular fibrillation (VF). (A) shows a series of phase map snapshots during the organized phase of VF that reveal a rotor on the left ventricle (*LV*) endocardium and a rotor on the epicardium with a lower rotational speed than the endocardial rotor. (B) depicts the same VF episode at a later time, during a disorganized portion of VF, revealing continuing presence of the same endocardial rotor but absence of rotor on the epicardium. (C) shows a three-dimensional model of the heart superimposed with epicardial and endocardial phase maps. *Black arrows* indicate the location of phase singularities. The mean cycle length of VF shown in this figure is 200 ms. (D) shows high-resolution plunge needle mapping that illustrates a transmural rotor. Phase maps showing scroll waves at different time instances are shown. Endocardial sections are shown on the *left* and epicardial sections on the *right. ECG*, Electrocardiogram; *PS*, phase singularity. ([A and B] From Massé S, Downar E, Chauhan V, et al. Ventricular fibrillation in myopathic human hearts: mechanistic insights from in vivo global endocardial and epicardial mapping. *Am J Physiol Heart Circ Physiol.* 2007;292:H2589-H2597. [C] Modified from Nair K, Umapathy K, Farid T, et al. Intramural activation during early human ventricular fibrillation. *Circ Arrhythm Electrophysiol.* 2011;4:692-703.)

channel heterogeneity and dynamic physiological factors may play an important role in maintaining VF.[39]

Physiological determinants of VF maintenance were evaluated by Toal and associates.[40] Variation in AP duration (APD) is a key determinant in the occurrence of wave break and reentry. Oscillations in APD can increase to a point where regions of the myocardium become refractory to depolarization, and wave break

and reentry may ensue. The determinants of APD variability in VF were studied in seven myopathic human hearts by recording monophasic APs from the interventricular septum during sinus rhythm and VF.[40] Short-term memory (the influence of APD and diastolic interval from preceding beats) was the key determinant of APD variability in early human VF, followed by APD/diastolic interval restitution.[40] In a human myopathic trabecular muscle

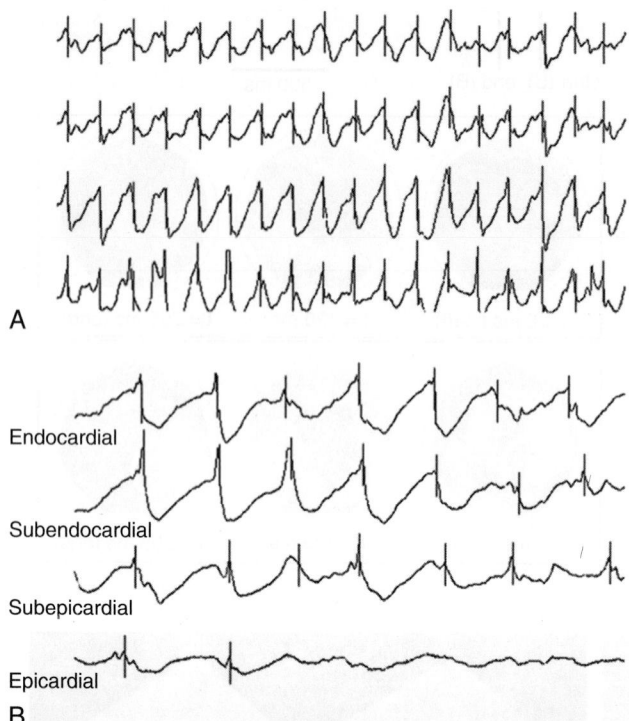

FIGURE 48.5 Examples of activation patterns in both short-duration ventricular fibrillation (SDVF; onset) and long-duration VF (LDVF; 10 minutes) on transmural plunge needles. (A) shows unipolar needle electrograms at VF onset with local activation markers included. In this SDVF needle segment, each transmural activation is entirely simultaneous. (B) shows examples of six activation sequences on unipolar needle recordings during LDVF. Transmural activation during this segment of LDVF is not simultaneous but exhibits a number of different patterns. From *left* to *right*, Epicardial to endocardial activation, endocardial to epicardial activation, endocardial to epicardial activation with wave break, simultaneous activation with wave break, endocardial to epicardial activation with wave break, nonuniform multidirectional pattern with wave break, and endocardial to epicardial activation with wave break. Local activation is marked at the maximum negative dV/dt. (From Jackson N, Massé S, Zamiri N, et al. Mechanisms of long-duration ventricular fibrillation in human hearts and experimental validation in canine Purkinje fibers. *JACC Clin Electrophysiol.* 2015;1:187-197.)

model, rate-dependent AP amplitude alternans was also seen to precede functional conduction block.[41]

Long-Duration Human Ventricular Fibrillation

In modern studies using electroanatomical mapping techniques with human and animal models, long-duration VF (LDVF) has been defined as VF that has a duration of more than 1–3 minutes.[42]

Building on the work of prior animal models, Jackson and coworkers[42] examined human VF from onset to 10 minutes in 12 cardiomyopathic human Langendorff hearts. Electrical activation was mapped with combinations of epi- and endocardial arrays and transmural plunge needles. Fig. 48.5 shows examples of activation patterns in both short-duration VF (SDVF; onset) and LDVF (10 minutes) using transmural plunge needles. Transmural activation was most frequently simultaneous during SDVF, whereas activation patterns originating at the endocardium and variably propagating toward the epicardium were most common in LDVF. Both endo- and epicardial cycle lengths increased over

time in human VF; however, an activation rate gradient developed between the endo- and epicardium in LDVF only. The incidence of reentry also decreased from SDVF to LDVF, suggesting that focal endocardial activations with midmyocardial wave break were responsible for this activation frequency gradient. Fig. 48.6 is a transmural spatiotemporal activation plot that illustrates the differences in transmural activation rates and patterns in two 3-second snapshots of SDVF and LDVF.

To determine the origin of focal endocardial activations in LDVF, Jackson and colleagues constructed bi- and unipolar isochronal maps of endocardial activation and compared them with the locations of Purkinje potentials with basal ventricular pacing prior to VF induction. With unipolar mapping, sharp Purkinje potentials become more prominent on the endocardium over time, while lower frequency signals with a slower cycle length are seen on the epicardium (Fig. 48.7). The earliest sites of activation in LDVF frequently correspond to the locations of Purkinje potentials on isochronal mapping (see Fig. 48.7). This may relate to a greater resistance of Purkinje fibers to ischemia than ventricular myocardium and to their receiving oxygen by diffusion from the LV.[43] In addition to this, we showed that focal Purkinje fiber activity can be induced with rapid ventricular pacing in a canine model. This suggests that focal Purkinje fiber activity in LDVF may be modulated by rapid reentrant wavefronts in SDVF.

Ionic Determinants of Ventricular Fibrillation Dynamics

To clarify the importance of molecular remodeling in VF dynamics, we studied ion channel remodeling in myopathic human hearts and related this to local electrical activation. Compared with normal hearts, significant differences were seen in the expression of multiple ion channels in myopathic hearts.[44] This analysis yielded potential critical candidates in VF maintenance and led to the finding that blockade of K_{ATP} channels decreased ischemia-dependent spatiotemporal heterogeneity of refractoriness and promoted spontaneous defibrillation in early VF.[45] In addition, modeling studies indicated that refractoriness in low K_{ATP} regions contributed to the development of transmural activation rate gradients in VF.[46] Most recently Zamiri and associates demonstrated that stabilization of ryanodine receptors using dantrolene facilitates defibrillation, prevents myocardial stunning, and improves survival from VF in an in vivo swine model of cardiac arrest (Fig. 48.8).[47] This study demonstrates the potential of translational research in improving human VF outcomes.

Conclusions

Despite advances in therapy, human VF and VT remain an important cause of SCD. VT may originate from focal sources but is most commonly a reentrant arrhythmia that is initiated and maintained by structural and functional elements. Conduction velocity restitution and circuitous conduction pathways lead to decremental conduction properties that precede unidirectional block and the initiation of reentrant VT. These same regions that demonstrate decremental properties due to structural and functional factors are also critical for the maintenance of reentrant VT and may provide targets for therapeutic benefit.

Human VF is initially organized as migrating transmural scroll waves that demonstrate transient patterns and show a propensity to regions of increased intramural fibrosis. Elucidating ion channel determinants of VF dynamics may form an exciting new avenue to modulate human VF maintenance. As human VF progresses over time, there is no evidence of sustained rotors or scroll wave organization but a rhythm characterized by focal, endocardial Purkinje fiber activations with midmyocardial wave break.

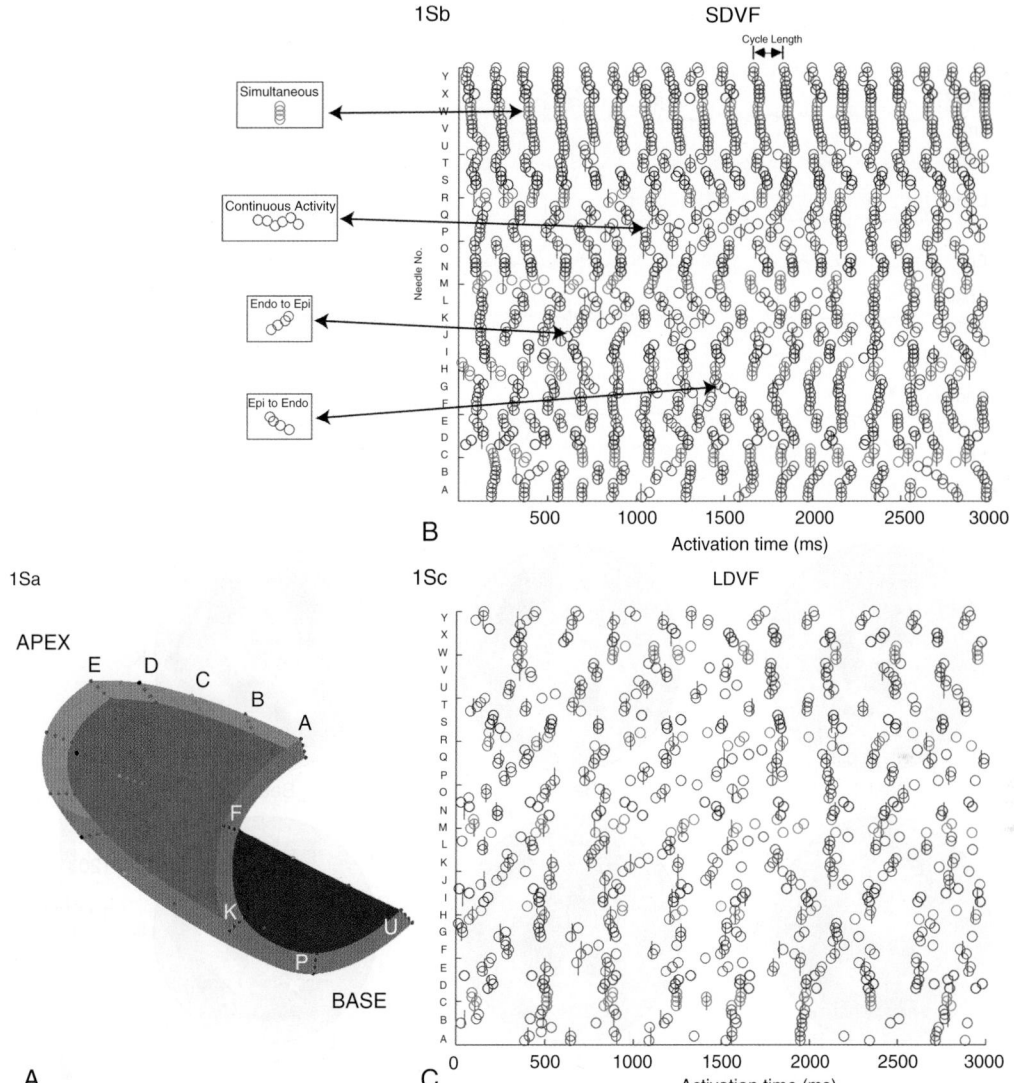

FIGURE 48.6 Transmural spatiotemporal activation plots of short-duration ventricular fibrillation (*SDVF*) and long-duration VF (*LDVF*). (A) shows the locations of 25 plunge needles (labeled *A* through *Y*) in the left ventricular myocardium with the true septum removed from the graphic. (B) SDVF and (C) LDVF are transmural spatiotemporal activation plots showing cycle length and activation patterns over a 3-second period at onset and after 10 minutes of VF, respectively. Time is indicated on the X axis with the 25 plunge needles shown on the Y axis (basal needles are in *red*, apical needles are in *purple*, and so forth). Each needle has four electrodes represented by a *colored circle*, beginning from the endocardial pole shown at the *bottom*, to the subendocardial, subepicardial, and epicardial poles. The inset shows how different activation sequences are represented on the plot in (B). Peaks of activation on the graph represent times when most local activation times (LATs) occur, and the largest peaks are assigned as "beats" (see *arrows* in [B]). The interval between beats defined the cycle length (see *arrows* in [B]). In SDVF, the peaks of LATs are relatively uniform, while in LDVF, the number of peak LATs varies from needle to needle, creating a less heterogeneous appearance of transmural activation. (From Jackson N, Massé S, Zamiri N, et al. Mechanisms of long-duration ventricular fibrillation in human hearts and experimental validation in canine Purkinje fibers. *JACC Clin Electrophysiol.* 2015;1:187-197.)

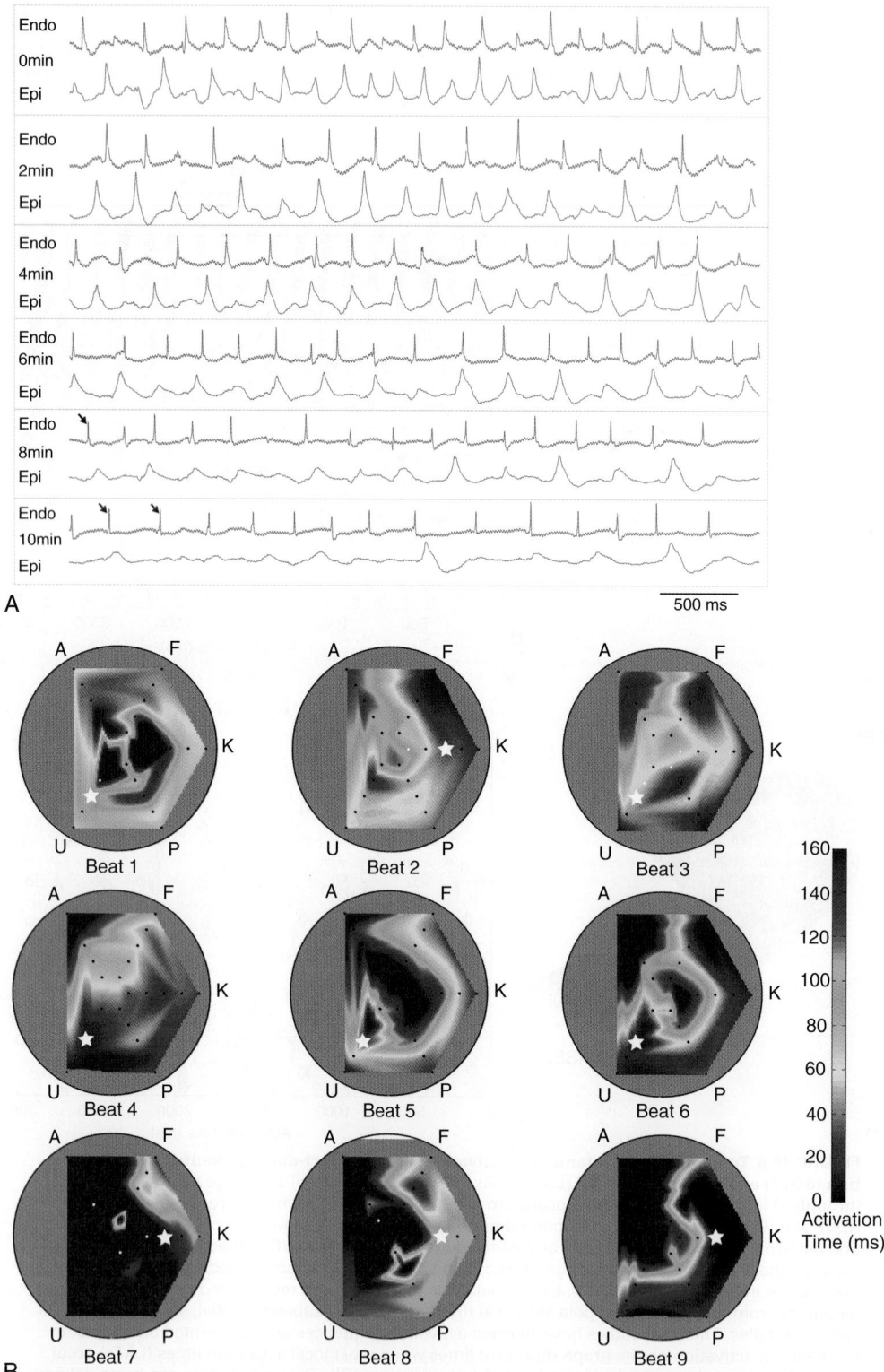

FIGURE 48.7 Purkinje potentials become more prevalent over time as ventricular fibrillation (VF) progresses. (A) shows unipolar needle recordings every 2 minutes from short-duration VF (time zero) through to long-duration VF (10 minutes), with endocardial activation shown above epicardial activation at each time point. As VF progresses, more frequent sharp Purkinje potentials can be seen on the endocardium (*arrows*). Purkinje potentials are high frequency spikes that appear to fire regularly but propagate variably to the epicardium, where lower frequency activations with significantly longer cycle lengths are seen. (B) shows isochronal maps of ventricular activation that correspond with the endocardial needle electrodes shown at 10 minutes in (A). Apical electrodes are shown at the center and basal electrodes at the periphery. On beats 3, 4, 5, 6, and 9, the earliest ventricular activation occurs in the regions of identified Purkinje potentials (*stars*) and propagates variably from there. Early activations on other beats may represent unidentified Purkinje activation or activation from working ventricular myocardium. (From Jackson N, Massé S, Zamiri N, et al. Mechanisms of long-duration ventricular fibrillation in human hearts and experimental validation in canine Purkinje fibers. *JACC Clin Electrophysiol*. 2015;1:187-197.)

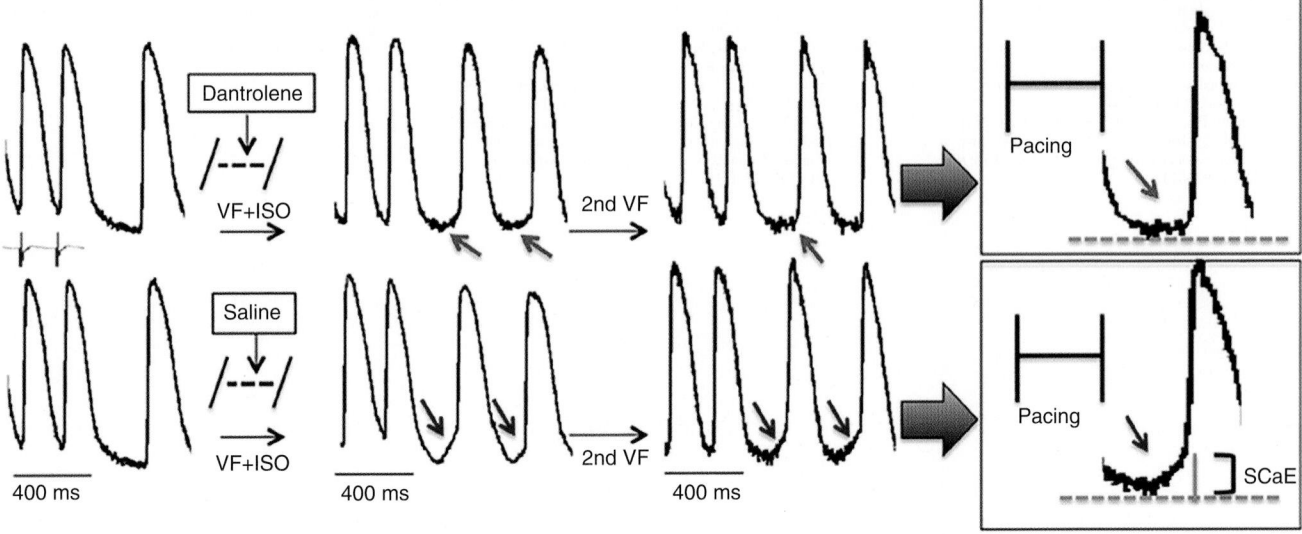

FIGURE 48.8 Dantrolene reduced diastolic spontaneous calcium elevation amplitude and increased calcium alternans threshold in rabbit hearts. (A) Representatives of calcium transients and diastolic spontaneous calcium elevations (*SCaE; blue arrows*) in dantrolene-treated (*top*) and control (*bottom*) rabbit hearts. Dantrolene infusion significantly decreased or completely abolished diastolic SCaE (*red arrow*). Amplitude of SCaE was calculated by measuring the difference between the onset of SCaE and the onset of the first spontaneous calcium transient and is normalized to the amplitude of calcium transients during pacing. One arbitrary unit equals the mean amplitude of calcium transients during pacing. *ISO,* isoproterenol; *VF,* ventricular fibrillation. (From Zamiri N, Masse S, Ramadeen A, et al. Dantrolene improves survival after ventricular fibrillation by mitigating impaired calcium handling in animal models. *Circulation.* 2014;129:875-885.)

REFERENCES

1. Kirchhof P, Breithardt G, Eckardt L. Primary prevention of sudden cardiac death. *Heart.* 2006;92:1873–1878.
2. Hoffman BF, Rosen MR. Cellular mechanisms for cardiac arrhythmias. *Circ Res.* 1981;49:1–15.
3. Dangman KH, Hoffman BF. Studies on overdrive stimulation of canine cardiac Purkinje fibers: maximal diastolic potential as a determinant of the response. *J Am Coll Cardiol.* 1983;2:1183–1190.
4. Josephson ME. *Josephson's Clinical Cardiac Electrophysiology: Techniques and Interpretations.* 4th ed. Philadelphia: Lippincott Williams & Wilkins; 2008.
5. Stevenson WG, Friedman PL, Sager PT, et al. Exploring postinfarction reentrant ventricular tachycardia with entrainment mapping. *J Am Coll Cardiol.* 1997;29:1180–1189.
6. Wellens HJ, Schuilenburg RM, Durrer D. Electrical stimulation of the heart in patients with ventricular tachycardia. *Circulation.* 1972;46:216–226.
7. Josephson ME, Horowitz LN, Farshidi A. Continuous local electrical activity. A mechanism of recurrent ventricular tachycardia. *Circulation.* 1978;57:659–665.
8. Downar E, Saito J, Doig JC, et al. Endocardial mapping of ventricular tachycardia in the intact human ventricle. III. Evidence of multiuse reentry with spontaneous and induced block in portions of reentrant path complex. *J Am Coll Cardiol.* 1995;25:1591–1600.
9. Hsia HH, Lin D, Sauer WH, et al. Anatomic characterization of endocardial substrate for hemodynamically stable reentrant ventricular tachycardia: identification of endocardial conducting channels. *Heart Rhythm.* 2006;3:503–512.
10. de Bakker JM, van Capelle FJ, Janse MJ, et al. Reentry as a cause of ventricular tachycardia in patients with chronic ischemic heart disease: electrophysiologic and anatomic correlation. *Circulation.* 1988;77:589–606.
11. Josephson ME, Anter E. Substrate mapping for ventricular tachycardia: assumptions and misconceptions. *JACC: Clin Electrophysiol.* 2015;1:341–352.
12. Berger MD, Waxman HL, Buxton AE, et al. Spontaneous compared with induced onset of sustained ventricular tachycardia. *Circulation.* 1988;78:885–892.
13. Segal OR, Chow AW, Peters NS, et al. Mechanisms that initiate ventricular tachycardia in the infarcted human heart. *Heart Rhythm.* 2010;7:57–64.
14. Jackson N, Gizurarson S, Viswanathan K, et al. Decrement evoked potential mapping: the basis of a mechanistic strategy for ventricular tachycardia ablation. *Circ Arrhythm Electrophysiol.* 2015;8:1433–1442.

15. Lai WT, Lee CS, Sheu SH, et al. Electrophysiological manifestations of the excitable gap of slow-fast AV nodal reentrant tachycardia demonstrated by single extrastimulation. *Circulation.* 1995;92:66–76.
16. de Bakker JM, Wittkampf FH. The pathophysiologic basis of fractionated and complex electrograms and the impact of recording techniques on their detection and interpretation. *Circ Arrhythm Electrophysiol.* 2010;3:204–213.
17. Mountantonakis SE, Park RE, Frankel DS, et al. Relationship between voltage map "channels" and the location of critical isthmus sites in patients with post-infarction cardiomyopathy and ventricular tachycardia. *J Am Coll Cardiol.* 2013;61:2088–2095.
18. Janse MJ, Wit AL. Electrophysiological mechanisms of ventricular arrhythmias resulting from myocardial ischemia and infarction. *Physiol Rev.* 1989;69:1049–1169.
19. Arnar DO, Bullinga JR, Martins JB. Role of the Purkinje system in spontaneous ventricular tachycardia during acute ischemia in a canine model. *Circulation.* 1997;96:2421–2429.
20. Janse MJ, Kleber AG, Capucci A, et al. Electrophysiological basis for arrhythmias caused by acute ischemia. Role of the subendocardium. *J Mol Cell Cardiol.* 1986;18:339–355.
21. Jardine DL, Charles CJ, Ashton RK, et al. Increased cardiac sympathetic nerve activity following acute myocardial infarction in a sheep model. *J Physiol.* 2005;565:325–333.
22. Downar E, Parson ID. Mechanisms underlying ventricular arrhythmias of acute myocardial ischemia and reperfusion. *Circulation.* 1981;64:216.
23. Delacretaz E, Stevenson WG, Ellison KE, et al. Mapping and radiofrequency catheter ablation of the three types of sustained monomorphic ventricular tachycardia in nonischemic heart disease. *J Cardiovasc Electrophysiol.* 2000;11:11–17.
24. Hsia HH, Callans DJ, Marchlinski FE. Characterization of endocardial electrophysiological substrate in patients with nonischemic cardiomyopathy and explanted ventricular tachycardia. *Circulation.* 2003;108:704–710.
25. Dinov B, Fiedler L, Schonbauer R, et al. Outcomes in catheter ablation of ventricular tachycardia in dilated nonischemic cardiomyopathy compared with ischemic cardiomyopathy: results from the Prospective Heart Centre of Leipzig VT (HELP-VT) Study. *Circulation.* 2014;129:728–736.
26. Downar E, Harris L, Kimber S, et al. Ventricular tachycardia after surgical repair of tetralogy of Fallot: results of intraoperative mapping studies. *J Am Coll Cardiol.* 1992;20:648–655.

27. Zeppenfeld K, Schalij MJ, Bartelings MM, et al. Catheter ablation of ventricular tachycardia after repair of congenital heart disease: electroanatomic identification of the critical right ventricular isthmus. *Circulation.* 2007;116:2241–2252.
28. Haissaguerre M, Shah DC, Jais P, et al. Role of Purkinje conducting system in triggering of idiopathic ventricular fibrillation. *Lancet.* 2002;359:677–678.
29. Knecht S, Sacher F, Wright M, et al. Long-term follow-up of idiopathic ventricular fibrillation ablation: a multicenter study. *J Am Coll Cardiol.* 2009;54:522–528.
30. Nair K, Farid T, Masse S, et al. Studying semblances of a true killer: experimental model of human ventricular fibrillation. *Am J Physiol Heart Circ Physiol.* 2012;302:H1533–H1537.
31. Nanthakumar K, Walcott GP, Melnick S, et al. Epicardial organization of human ventricular fibrillation. *Heart Rhythm.* 2004;1:14–23.
32. Walcott GP, Kay GN, Plumb VJ, et al. Endocardial wave front organization during ventricular fibrillation in humans. *J Am Coll Cardiol.* 2002;39:109–115.
33. Nanthakumar K, Jalife J, Masse S, et al. Optical mapping of Langendorff-perfused human hearts: establishing a model for the study of ventricular fibrillation in humans. *Am J Physiol Heart Circ Physiol.* 2007;293:H875–H880.
34. Masse S, Downar E, Chauhan V, et al. Ventricular fibrillation in myopathic human hearts: mechanistic insights from in vivo global endocardial and epicardial mapping. *Am J Physiol Heart Circ Physiol.* 2007;292:H2589–H2597.
35. Nash MP, Mourad A, Clayton RH, et al. Evidence for multiple mechanisms in human ventricular fibrillation. *Circulation.* 2006;114:536–542.
36. Umapathy K, Nair K, Masse S, et al. Phase mapping of cardiac fibrillation. *Circ Arrhythm Electrophysiol.* 2010;3:105–114.
37. Umapathy K, Masse S, Sevaptsidis E, et al. Spatiotemporal frequency analysis of ventricular fibrillation in explanted human hearts. *IEEE Trans Biomed Eng.* 2009;56:328–335.
38. Nair K, Umapathy K, Farid T, et al. Intramural activation during early human ventricular fibrillation. *Circ Arrhythm Electrophysiol.* 2011;4:692–703.
39. Umapathy K, Masse S, Sevaptsidis E, et al. Regional frequency variation during human ventricular fibrillation. *Med Eng Phys.* 2009;31:964–970.
40. Toal SC, Farid TA, Selvaraj R, et al. Short-term memory and restitution during ventricular fibrillation in human hearts: an in vivo study. *Circ Arrhythm Electrophysiol.* 2009;2:562–570.

41. Sivagangabalan G, Masse S, Nair K, et al. Action potential amplitude alternans and conduction block in human hearts. *Can J Cardiol*. 2011;27:263.e25.

42. Jackson N, Massé S, Zamiri N, et al. Mechanisms of long-duration ventricular fibrillation in human hearts and experimental validation in canine Purkinje fibers. *JACC Clin Electrophysiol*. 2015;1:187–197.

43. Friedman PL, Stewart JR, Fenoglio Jr JJ, et al. Survival of subendocardial Purkinje fibers after extensive myocardial infarction in dogs. *Circ Res*. 1973;33:597–611.

44. Sivagangabalan G, Nazzari H, Bignolais O, et al. Regional ion channel gene expression heterogeneity and ventricular fibrillation dynamics in human hearts. *PLoS One*. 2014;9:e82179.

45. Farid TA, Nair K, Masse S, et al. Role of KATP channels in the maintenance of ventricular fibrillation in cardiomyopathic human hearts. *Circ Res*. 2011;109:1309–1318.

46. Boyle PM, Masse S, Nanthakumar K, et al. Transmural IK(ATP) heterogeneity as a determinant of activation rate gradient during early ventricular fibrillation: mechanistic insights from rabbit ventricular models. *Heart Rhythm*. 2013;10:1710–1717.

47. Zamiri N, Masse S, Ramadeen A, et al. Dantrolene improves survival after ventricular fibrillation by mitigating impaired calcium handling in animal models. *Circulation*. 2014;129:875–885.

49 Genetics of Atrial Fibrillation

Steven A. Lubitz and Patrick T. Ellinor

The pathophysiology of atrial fibrillation (AF) remains incompletely characterized; however, epidemiological studies demonstrate a heritable basis for the arrhythmia. In recent years, the appreciation of AF heritability has stimulated the search for the genetic underpinnings of the disease. Genetic mapping studies have identified rare mutations and common variants associated with AF. In addition to validating the suspected electrophysiological mechanisms underlying AF, recent genetic discoveries have identified previously unrecognized pathways involved in the development of AF. Investigators are now searching for causal variants at many identified loci, investigating the biological mechanisms linking AF susceptibility loci to disease, and assessing the clinical implications of recent genetic discoveries.

Heritability of Atrial Fibrillation

Reports of familial clustering of AF date back to the early 1940s.[1,2] Familial AF was generally regarded as a rare condition for many years thereafter. However, since the early 2000s, a major paradigm shift occurred with the widespread recognition of the heritability underlying AF.[3-7] In the community-based Framingham Heart Study, it was found that 27% of individuals with AF had a first-degree relative with AF confirmed by electrocardiography.[7] Familial AF was associated with a 40% increased risk of AF in other family members over a subsequent 8-year period (Fig. 49.1). The risk associated with familial AF persisted even after adjusting for established clinical risk factors for AF. A study from Denmark demonstrated that AF was more common among monozygotic twins as compared to dizygotic twins, implicating a genetic predisposition for the arrhythmia even among those raised with shared environmental exposures.[6]

In numerous reports, the heritability of AF appears to be greatest among younger individuals[3,5,7] and those without structural heart disease.[3,4] Premature familial AF, or that occurring in family members aged ≤65 years, was associated with a two-fold increased risk of AF compared to individuals without familial AF in the Framingham Heart Study.[7] Nevertheless, data from this study provide evidence that the heritability of AF is present in the elderly as well.[7]

Large Families With Atrial Fibrillation Are Rare but Informative

Early attempts to identify the genetic basis of AF utilized classical linkage analysis to identify monogenic disease loci in families. Linkage analysis relies upon the fact that genetic recombination during meiosis shuffles regions of the genome. Assessing genetic markers at known locations of the genome can help determine which loci transmit along with disease.

The first genetic locus for AF was described in 1997 by Brugada and colleagues,[8] who identified an AF susceptibility region on chromosome 10 in a large family with autosomal dominant AF (Table 49.1[9-75]). Since this initial report, linkage analysis has occasionally been used to identify genetic mutations underlying AF in a number of large families with AF.

Chen and associates narrowed an AF susceptibility locus to a region on chromosome 11p15 in a family with autosomal dominant AF, spanning four generations.[11] The investigators extended their analysis by sequencing *KCNQ1*, a candidate gene in the region that encodes a potassium channel α-subunit. In the first transmembrane segment of the channel, they discovered a highly conserved serine residue that was mutated to glycine in all affected family members. Subsequent characterization revealed that the mutant protein increases the repolarizing I_{Ks} current density when expressed with the KCNE1 subunit. This gain-of-function mutation is expected to result in shortened atrial refractory periods and thereby promote reentry, a well-founded mechanism underlying AF.[76] Our group, led by Das and coworkers, used a similar approach to map a mutation in the third transmembrane domain of *KCNQ1*.[12] The S209P variant demonstrated a similar gain-of-function effect, again implicating *KCNQ1* as a disease-susceptibility gene for AF.

Linkage analysis also has identified mutations in *SCN5A* that segregate with AF, conduction abnormalities, cardiomyopathy, and possibly early-onset ischemic stroke.[77-79] *SCN5A* encodes a sodium channel α-subunit responsible for the depolarizing I_{Na} current. The D1275N mutation that results in an aspartic acid for asparagine substitution was independently identified by different investigators[77-79] and associates with atrial standstill when cosegregating with connexin 40 (*GJA5*) mutations.[80]

In another large, multigenerational family with AF, Hodgson-Zingman and colleagues mapped a frameshift mutation to *NPPA*, which encodes atrial natriuretic peptide (ANP).[70] The deletion of two base-pairs eliminates a stop codon and results in additional 12 amino acids at the carboxy terminus of the mature

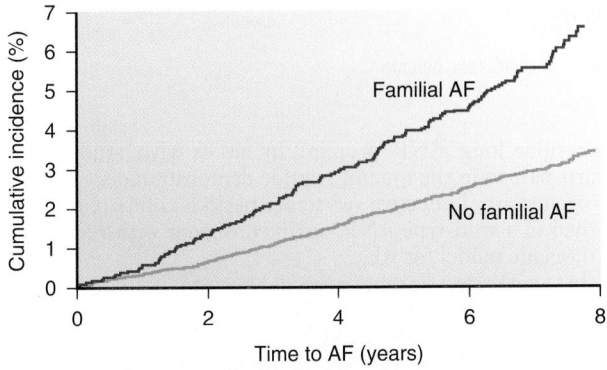

FIGURE 49.1 The risk of atrial fibrillation (*AF*) is increased in individuals with a first-degree relative with antecedent AF in the Framingham Heart Study. The estimated 8-year risk of AF is increased by 40% among individuals with a first-degree relative with AF as compared to those without familial AF. (Modified from Lubitz SA, Yin X, Fontes JD, et al. Association between familial atrial fibrillation and risk of new-onset atrial fibrillation. *JAMA*. 2010;304:2263-2269.)

TABLE 49.1 Atrial fibrillation susceptibility genes identified by linkage analysis or candidate gene association studies

GENE	GENE PRODUCT	PRESUMED MECHANISM OF ACTION	REFERENCES
Potassium Channels			
KCNH2	α-subunit of $K_v11.1$ channel (HERG)	Modulation of I_{Kr}	9,10
KCNQ1	α-subunit of $K_v7.1$ channel	Increased I_{Ks}	11–18
KCNE1	β-subunit of $K_v7.1$ channel (minK)	Increased I_{Ks}	19,20
KCNE2	β-subunit of $K_v7.1$ channel (MiRP1)	Increased I_{Ks}	21,22
KCNE5	β-subunit of $K_v7.1$ channel	Increased I_{Ks}	23
KCNJ2	β-subunit of $K_{ir}2.1$ channel	Increased I_{K1}	24–26
KCNA5	α-subunit of $K_v1.5$ channel	Modulation of I_{Kur}	21,27,28
KCNJ8	α-subunit of $K_{ir}6.1$ channel	Increased I_{KATP}	29
KCND3	α-subunit of $K_v4.3$ channel	Increased I_{to} current	30
ABCC9	SUR2A subunit of K_{ATP} channel	Decreased I_{KATP}	31
KCNN3	Ca-activated K channel KCa2.3	Modulation of SK_{Ca} current	32,33
Sodium Channels			
SCN5A	α-subunit of $Na_v1.5$	Modulation of I_{Na}	34–38
SCN10A	α-subunit of $Na_v1.5$	Potential modulation of $Na_v1.5$	39,40
SCN1B	β-subunit of $Na_v1.5$	Reduced I_{Na}	41,42
SCN2B	β-subunit of $Na_v1.5$	Reduced I_{Na}	41
SCN3B	β-subunit of $Na_v1.5$	Reduced I_{Na}	35,43
SCN4B	β-subunit of $Na_v1.5$	Not characterized	44
Other Ion Channels or Related Proteins			
HCN4	Hyperpolarization activated cyclic nucleotide gated K channel 4	Modulation of the pacemaking I_f current	45
CAV1	Caveolin 1	Altered ion channel signaling	46,47
Gap Junction Proteins			
GJA1	Connexin 43 (Cx43)	Reduced intercellular electrical coupling	48
GJA5	Connexin 40 (Cx40)	Impaired intercellular electrical coupling	49–51
Transcription Factors			
GATA4	GATA4	Decreased activity	52–54
GATA5	GATA5	Decreased activity	55–57
GATA6	GATA6	Decreased activity	58–60
NKX2-5	NKD2.5	Decreased activity	61–63
PITX2	PITX2	Decreased activity	64–67
ZFHX3	ATBF-1	Altered binding activity	64
Other Genes			
C9orf3	Aminopeptidase-O	Unclear	64,68
JPH2	Junctophilin-2: modulation of RyR activity	Decreased RyR stabilization	69
NPPA	Natriuretic peptide precursor A	Altered ANP signaling	70–72
NUP155	Nucleoporin	Reduced nuclear membrane permeability	73
RYR2	Ryanodine receptor	Increased activity	74,75
SYNE2	Neseprin-2	Unclear	64,68

ANP, Atrial natriuretic peptide.

28-residue-long ANP protein. In an ex vivo study, rabbit hearts bathed in the mutant peptide demonstrated significantly shortened atrial effective refractory periods compared to those bathed in a wild-type ANP, again consistent with reentry as a pathogenic model for AF.

In aggregate, linkage analysis has implicated potassium (KCNQ1[11,12]) and sodium (SCN5A[77–79]) channel mutations, a nuclear envelope protein (NUP155[81,82]), NPPA,[70] and loci on chromosomes 6[83] and 10[8,84] in the etiology of AF. Newer genetic techniques such as exome and whole-genome sequencing have emerged in recent years that make mapping of these families even more efficient. However, the large, multigenerational families required for linkage analysis remain rare. More often AF is observed in smaller families, and thus it is often hard to establish the causality of apparently disease-causing mutations with such limited genetic information.

Candidate Gene Association Studies

In contrast to linkage analysis, in which inferences about recombination are made on the basis of segregation of markers in a pedigree, investigators have also selected and screened individual candidate genes for mutations in cohorts of patients with and without AF. As an extrapolation of initial studies on KCNQ1, numerous additional candidate gene association studies have focused on cardiac ion channels (see Table 49.1 and Fig. 49.2).

In one report, genetic variants in KCNQ1 were identified that predisposed to AF in a stretch-sensitive fashion,[85] illustrating the potential for a concealed predisposition for AF to be elicited by an acquired exposure (e.g., valvular disease, heart failure). In another report implicating KCNQ1, a mutation was identified in a patient with long QT syndrome.[86] Diverging effects on I_{Ks} were observed depending on whether the mutant protein was expressed with

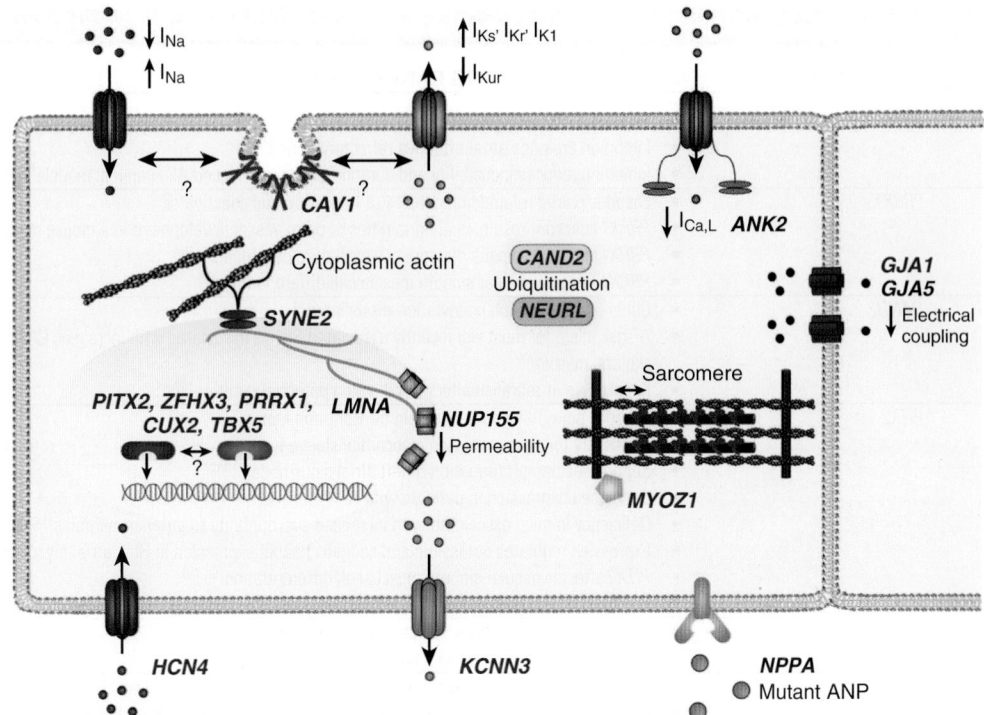

FIGURE 49.2 Genes implicated in the pathogenesis of atrial fibrillation. A depiction of a myocyte indicates the putative location and function of each implicated gene product. Genes associated with atrial fibrillation mapped via linkage or candidate gene testing are depicted in *black*. Potential candidate genes associated with atrial fibrillation mapped via genome-wide association studies are depicted in *blue*. ANP, Atrial natriuretic peptide.

KCNE1 or *KCNE2* β-subunits, each of which are differentially expressed in the atria and ventricles, leading the authors to speculate that the mutation was the cause of both long QT syndrome and AF. Gain-of-function mutations in both *KCNQ1*[87] and *KCNH2*[88] have been discovered in AF in the context of short QT syndrome.

In contrast to the enhanced atrial repolarization mechanism invoked by most potassium channel mutations, a nucleotide substitution resulting in a premature stop codon in *KCNA5* has been described; it manifested a loss-of-function of the Kv1.5 channel protein.[27] The mutation effectively abolished I_{Kur} and prolonged the action potential duration, increasing the susceptibility to early afterdepolarization–induced atrial tachycardia and fibrillation. This mechanism has been described as "atrial torsades," and the observations from this report underscore the heterogeneity of mechanisms that can lead to AF.

Candidate gene association studies in patients with AF also have identified variants in genes encoding sodium channel subunits. Both loss-of-function[34] and gain-of-function[89,90] mutations in *SCN5A* have been identified in patients with lone AF. Mutations in sodium channel β-subunits, *SCN1B* and *SCN2B*, have been described that decrease sodium current amplitude and alter channel gating kinetics when coexpressed with *SCN5A*.[91] These mutations are speculated to predispose to AF either through shortening of the atrial action potential duration or conduction slowing, both of which may facilitate reentry.

Mutations in *GJA5*, which encodes the gap junction connexin 40, have been described in 4 of 15 patients with AF who were screened in one candidate gene association study.[92] The *GJA5* mutations in three of the four patients were present in cardiac tissue but not in lymphocyte specimens, suggesting that these mutations were acquired somatic, rather than inherited, mutations. Other candidate gene association studies have linked common genetic variations in *GJA5* to AF.[93,94] Nevertheless, more recent data, generated using modern next-generation

sequencing and variant calling approaches in left atrial appendage samples from 25 patients with AF, did not support a role for somatic variation underlying AF susceptibility.[95]

Beyond the previously described variation in potassium, sodium, and gap junction proteins, there have been an ever-increasing number of candidate gene studies reporting AF-related mutations (see Table 49.1). However, the validity and generalizability of the identified variants remain unclear due to the small sample sizes, which are typically in the range of ~50–300 AF cases. Furthermore, these studies have usually examined only one or a small number of genes at a time in AF cases. Thus with limited power and sampling of a small fraction of the genome, it is hard to determine whether any AF "mutation" is plausibly related to AF. Future exome or whole-genome studies in large studies consisting of thousands of cases and controls should help define which, if any, of these genes are causally related to AF.

Genome-Wide Association Studies

Since 2000, systematic efforts to examine human genetic variation, such as the international HapMap[96] and 1000 Genomes[97] projects, have increased the appreciation of genetic diversity in different ancestral groups. The HapMap project revealed the presence of about 10 million common genetic variants occurring with a frequency of 5% or greater in the general population, and most of these variants were single nucleotide polymorphisms (SNPs). Such efforts provided a reference against which observed genetic variation could be compared in cohorts of individuals assembled for investigation. High-density chips were developed that allowed the simultaneous genotyping of hundreds of thousands of SNPs across the genome, enabling efficient genetic profiling of many individuals.

Genome-wide associations emerged in which genotypes at each of the hundreds of thousands to millions of known SNP

TABLE 49.2 **Atrial fibrillation susceptibility loci identified by genome-wide association study**

CHROMOSOME	CANDIDATE GENE(S)	FACTORS SUPPORTING CANDIDATE GENE
1q21[102,103]	KCNN3	• Encodes a calcium-activated potassium channel • Inhibition prolongs atrial effective refractory period[104,105] • Inhibition reduces inducibility and duration of pacing-induced AF in animal models[104,105]
1q24[103]	PRRX1	• Encodes paired related homeobox 1, a transcriptional coactivator • PRRX1 knockout results in abnormalities of great vessel development in a mouse model[106] • PRRX1 knockout impairs pulmonary vasculature development[107] • PRRX1 affects vascular smooth muscle cell differentiation[108]
3p25[109]	CAND2	• Cullin-associated and neddylation-dissociated 2 • AF risk allele for most significantly associated SNP is associated with increased CAND2 expression in skeletal muscle[109] • Knockdown in zebrafish alters atrial action potential duration[109]
4q25[99–103]	PITX2	• Encodes paired-like homeodomain transcription factor 2 • Necessary for pulmonary vein myocardial sleeve formation[110] • Suppresses default formation of left atrial sinus node[111,112] • Decreased expression in patients with AF[113,114] • Deficiency in mice associated with increased susceptibility to atrial arrhythmias[114] • Expression regulates potassium and sodium channel expression in HL-1 atrial myocytes[113] • PITX2 affects vascular smooth muscle cell differentiation[108,115] • PITX2 conditional postnatal knockdown causes sinus node dysfunction and alters ion channel gene expression[116]
6q22[109]	GJA1	• Encodes connexin 43, a component of gap junctions • Mutations are associated with cardiac malformations[117,118]
7q31[103]	CAV1	• Encodes caveolin 1, a cellular membrane protein involved in signal transduction[119] • Knockout associated with dilated cardiomyopathy[120] and cardiac hypertrophy[121] • Directly modulates endothelial cell KCNN3 trafficking[122] and indirectly modulates cardiac KCNH2 trafficking[123]
9q22[103]	C9orf3	• Encodes aminopeptidase-O • Unclear relation to AF
10q22[103]	SYNPO2L/MYOZ1	• MYOZ1 encodes myozenin 1, expressed in cardiomyocytes and localizes to Z-disc[124]
10q24[109]	NEURL	• Encodes neuralized E3 ubiquitin protein ligase 1 • Knockdown in zebrafish alters atrial action potential duration[109]
10q24[109]	CUX2	• Encodes cut-like homeobox 2 • Japanese-specific susceptibility locus for AF • Unclear relation to AF
12q24[109]	TBX5	• Encodes the transcription factor T-box 5 • Critically involved in cardiac conduction system formation[125,126] • Mutations in TBX5 cause Holt-Oram syndrome,[127] which may include conduction abnormalities as well as atrial and ventricular septal defects • Variants in TBX5 have been associated with PR-interval duration,[128,129] an endophenotype for AF[130]
14q23[103]	SYNE2	• Encodes spectrin repeat containing nuclear envelope 2 • Located in sarcomere and involved in maintaining nuclear structural integrity; binds lamin[131] • Mutations underlie some cases of Emery-Dreifuss muscular dystrophy which is characterized by muscle atrophy, cardiomyopathy, and cardiac conduction abnormalities
15q24[103]	HCN4	• Encodes hyperpolarization activated cyclic nucleotide gated potassium channel 4 • Highly expressed in sinoatrial node • HCN4 channel is responsible for the inward phase 4 depolarizing pacemaker current (funny current, I_f)[132] • Mutations in HCN4 are associated with sick sinus syndrome and bradycardia[133]
16q22[103]	ZFHX3	• Encodes the transcription factor zinc finger homeobox 3 • Partial deletion of 16q22 associated with congenital heart disease[134] • Variants at 16q22 associated with Kawasaki disease[135]

AF, Atrial fibrillation; *SNP,* single-nucleotide polymorphism.

positions were tested for association with human traits. Unlike linkage analysis, genome-wide association testing does not require multigenerational cohorts for assessment of variant transmission. In contrast to candidate gene association studies, the presence of genome-wide genotyping allowed investigators to efficiently test variants in genes or genetic regions that were not previously suspected of being involved in AF pathogenesis.

Unique study design and interpretation considerations are applicable to genome-wide association studies (GWASs). First, owing to the massive number of tests performed in each GWAS, stringent significance thresholds (e.g., $p < 5 \times 10^{-8}$) are used to guard against false-positive test results that occur by chance with multiple hypothesis testing. Second, common genetic variants

associated with disease are expected to confer small or modest disease risks in contrast to rare and large-effect genetic variants observed in monogenic forms of AF. Third, the stringent significance thresholds used and modest relative risks expected in GWASs necessitate extremely large sample sizes to adequately power genetic variant discovery. Diverse international collaborations have formed over the past several years and contributed to the success of GWASs. As of 2016, 2366 studies encompassing 16,755 SNP-human trait associations have been published.[98]

GWASs have identified 14 genomic regions associated with AF (Table 49.2[99–135] and Fig. 49.3). Association signals at these loci often span tens of thousands of base pairs and encompass both coding and noncoding regions of the genome. The

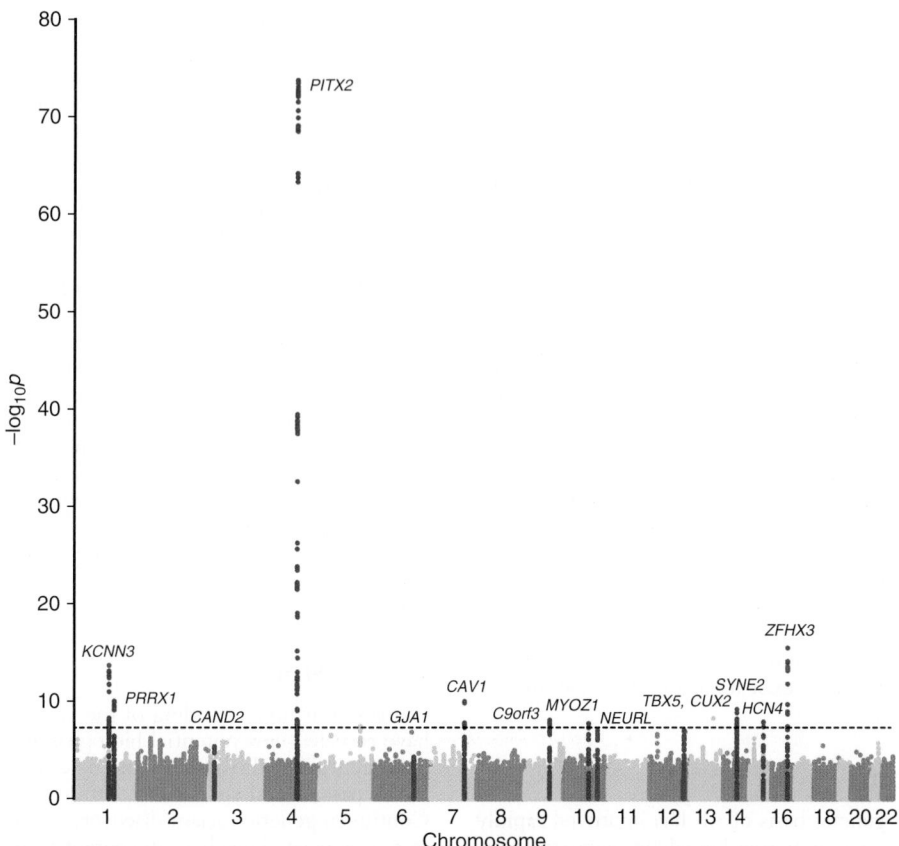

FIGURE 49.3 Fourteen genetic loci have been associated with atrial fibrillation in genome-wide association studies. The chromosome and position of each of 2.2 million tested single nucleotide polymorphisms are plotted on the *x*-axis, and the $-\log_{10}p$ (*p*-value) is plotted on the *y*-axis. The *dotted horizontal line* represents the traditional genome-wide significance threshold ($p < 5 \times 10^{-8}$). Loci represented in *red* indicate those that were significantly associated with atrial fibrillation in genome-wide association studies,[103] and those represented in *blue* indicate subthreshold loci further validated through large-scale genotyping or functional characterization.[109] The closest gene at each associated locus is indicated.

AF-associated SNPs are not usually the causal genetic variants, but rather markers that tag causal genetic elements located nearby. To date, the causal variants at the known AF GWAS loci have not been identified. Nevertheless, candidate genes at these loci frequently exist and have implicated transcription factors involved in cardiac and pulmonary development, ion channels, and other molecules in the etiology of AF (see Fig. 49.2). Ongoing studies have begun to explore the mechanisms by which these genomic regions potentially underlie AF.

The most significantly associated variants associated with AF exist at the chromosome 4q25 locus and were reported in the first GWAS for AF in 2007.[99] Review of this discovery provides an example of the power of GWASs and the follow-up work involved in identifying causal elements at a particular susceptibility locus.

Investigators first identified genetic variants at the chromosome 4q25 locus that were highly associated with AF in approximately 550 individuals with and 4500 without AF from Iceland.[99] The association between SNPs at chromosome 4q25 and AF has been widely replicated in samples of European,[99,136–139] Han Chinese,[99,140] African American,[141,142] and Japanese[103] ancestry, demonstrating the fundamental role of this locus in the pathophysiology of AF.

The top variants associated with AF lie in a region of the genome without any known genes and are approximately 150,000 base-pairs away from the nearest gene at the locus, the paired-like homeodomain 2 transcription factor (*PITX2*). Among the genes at 4q25, *PITX2* is a plausible candidate for involvement in AF. Mutations in *PITX2* are found in Axonfeld-Reiger syndrome[143] and Peter anomaly,[144] which are characterized by ocular abnormalities but not AF. *PITX2* encodes a transcription factor involved in cardiac and pulmonary development. In mice deficient in one isoform of the protein that is expressed in the heart, Pitx2c, myocardial sleeves are not formed in the pulmonary veins.[110] Given the importance of pulmonary vein ectopic foci in the pathogenesis of AF,[145] the relations between *PITX2* and pulmonary vein myocardial cell development are particularly intriguing. Additionally, Pitx2c is responsible for suppressing the default formation of a sinus node in the developing left atrial region.[111,112]

Decreased expression of Pitx2c was noted in patients with AF as compared to those with sinus rhythm,[113,114] suggesting that Pitx2c deficiency or downregulation may predispose to AF. Increased inducibility of AF was observed in heterozygous Pitx2c knockout mice subjected to programmed atrial stimulation.[114] Pitx2c expression appears to regulate expression of certain sodium and potassium channels in HL-1 atrial cardiomyocytes, demonstrating a direct role for Pitx2c in cellular electrophysiology.[113] Data from investigations in mice further suggest that loss of *PITX2* function may increase susceptibility to AF indirectly through the inhibition of micro-RNAs responsible for the posttranscriptional regulation of factors involved in sinus node development.[146] Furthermore, conditional, postnatal knockdown of *PITX2* in mice caused sinus node dysfunction and altered expression of ion channel genes and others involved in calcium handling, suggesting that *PITX2* perturbation may exert electrophysiological effects beyond the developmental stage.[116]

How genetic variants at chromosome 4q25 specifically contribute to AF risk is unknown, but it is suspected that variants exert regulatory effects on distant gene targets.[147–149] Indeed, at least four independent susceptibility signals for AF at the chromosome 4q25 locus have been identified in conserved noncoding regions of chromosome 4q25.[150,151] A risk score comprising four variants at chromosome 4q25 explained between a four- and five-fold gradient of AF risk in over 7000 cases of European ancestry and nearly 60,000 referent individuals.[151] The gradient of risk was similar in samples of about 7000 individuals with and 3000 without Japanese ancestry. These observations indicate that the 4q25 locus is critical to AF susceptibility and that genetic susceptibility to AF is shared across at least some ancestral groups.

After the discovery of AF-associated variants on chromosome 4q25, GWASs demonstrated additional associations on chromosome loci 16q22[100,101] and 1q21.[102] In 2012, the largest meta-analysis of GWASs of AF was published, which included 6707 individuals with and 52,426 individuals without AF.[103] In addition to the three previously identified AF susceptibility loci, six novel loci for AF were discovered.[103] In a subsequent multidisciplinary approach in Europeans and Japanese involving large-scale replication genotyping of SNPs associated with AF below the stringent significance threshold of $p < 5 \times 10^{-8}$, paired with functional characterization, five additional AF susceptibility loci were identified.[109] Although causal variants at these loci have not been identified, candidate genes exist at most of these loci and are summarized in Table 49.2.

Future Directions

Understanding of the genetic basis of AF has improved rapidly in the past several years, yet numerous knowledge gaps still exist. The heritability underlying AF is incompletely explained by top variants at genetic loci.[7] Despite associations between variations at some loci and AF across different ancestral groups, significant undiscovered genetic differences may underlie differences in the AF prevalence between races.[152] Importantly, causal variants at established loci remain undiscovered.

The application of technological advancements such as next-generation exome sequencing and whole-genome sequencing, as well as novel functional assays, is underway and may provide a greater understanding of the genetic architecture related to AF at associated loci. Functional characterization of genetic variation at AF loci will involve a combination of bioinformatics and experimentation in cellular and animal model systems. Such follow-up work will take time to reveal the mechanisms by which genetic variation associates with AF, but it may ultimately facilitate the development of new therapeutics for this common arrhythmia.

The potential clinical applications of genetic variants associated with AF remain largely unexplored. Investigation into the predictive utility of AF genetic variants for incident arrhythmia and AF-related morbidities, such as stroke and heart failure, are warranted. Systematic assessment of pharmacogenetic interactions between AF-related therapeutics and genetic variants is necessary to determine whether use of such information can enhance the efficacy of care and minimize adverse effects.

Conclusions

Gains in our understanding of the genetic underpinnings of AF have revealed new potential biological pathways involved in the pathogenesis of the arrhythmia. The field has advanced rapidly in the past several years and continues to evolve at a brisk pace. Continued genetic variant discovery and biological characterization of associated loci have the potential to reveal new therapeutic targets for the management of patients with AF.

REFERENCES

1. Levy RL. Paroxysmal auricular fibrillation and flutter without signs of organic cardiac disease in two brothers. *J Mt Sinai Hosp.* 1942;8:765–770.
2. Wolff L. Familial auricular fibrillation. *N Engl J Med.* 1943;229:396–398.
3. Fox CS, Parise H, D'Agostino Sr RB, et al. Parental atrial fibrillation as a risk factor for atrial fibrillation in offspring. *JAMA.* 2004;291:2851–2855.
4. Ellinor PT, Yoerger DM, Ruskin JN, MacRae CA. Familial aggregation in lone atrial fibrillation. *Hum Genet.* 2005;118:179–184.
5. Arnar DO, Thorvaldsson S, Manolio TA, et al. Familial aggregation of atrial fibrillation in Iceland. *Eur Heart J.* 2006;27:708–712.
6. Christophersen IE, Ravn LS, Budtz-Joergensen E, et al. Familial aggregation of atrial fibrillation: a study in Danish twins. *Circ Arrhythm Electrophysiol.* 2009;378–383.
7. Lubitz SA, Yin X, Fontes JD, et al. Association between familial atrial fibrillation and risk of new-onset atrial fibrillation. *JAMA.* 2010;304:2263–2269.
8. Brugada R, Tapscott T, Czernuszewicz GZ, et al. Identification of a genetic locus for familial atrial fibrillation. *N Engl J Med.* Mar 1997;336:905–911.
9. Hong K, Bjerregaard P, Gussak I, Brugada R. Short QT syndrome and atrial fibrillation caused by mutation in KCNH2. *J Cardiovasc Electrophysiol.* 2005;16:394–396.
10. Sinner MF, Pfeufer A, Akyol M, et al. The non-synonymous coding I_{Kr}-channel variant KCNH2-K897T is associated with atrial fibrillation: results from a systematic candidate gene-based analysis of KCNH2 (HERG). *Eur Heart J.* 2008;29:907–914.
11. Chen YH, Xu SJ, Bendahhou S, et al. KCNQ1 gain-of-function mutation in familial atrial fibrillation. *Science.* 2003;299:251–254.
12. Das S, Makino S, Melman YF, et al. Mutation in the S3 segment of KCNQ1 results in familial lone atrial fibrillation. *Heart Rhythm.* 2009;6:1146–1153.
13. Hong K, Piper DR, Diaz-Valdecantos A, et al. De novo KCNQ1 mutation responsible for atrial fibrillation and short QT syndrome in utero. *Cardiovasc Res.* 2005;68:433–440.
14. Christophersen IE, Budtz-Jorgensen E, Olesen MS, Haunso S, Christensen K, Svendsen JH. Familial atrial fibrillation predicts increased risk of mortality: a study in Danish twins. *Circ Arrhythm Electrophysiol.* 2013;6:10–15.
15. Hayashi K, Konno T, Tada H, et al. Functional characterization of rare variants implicated in susceptibility to lone atrial fibrillation. *Circ Arrhythm Electrophysiol.* 2015;8:1095–1104.
16. Hasegawa K, Ohno S, Ashihara T, et al. A novel KCNQ1 missense mutation identified in a patient with juvenile-onset atrial fibrillation causes constitutively open I_{Ks} channels. *Heart Rhythm.* 2014;11:67–75.
17. Ki CS, Jung CL, Kim HJ, et al. A KCNQ1 mutation causes age-dependant bradycardia and persistent atrial fibrillation. *Pflugers Arch.* 2014;466:529–540.
18. Bartos DC, Anderson JB, Bastiaenen R, et al. A KCNQ1 mutation causes a high penetrance for familial atrial fibrillation. *J Cardiovasc Electrophysiol.* 2013;24:562–569.
19. Olesen MS, Bentzen BH, Nielsen JB, et al. Mutations in the potassium channel subunit KCNE1 are associated with early-onset familial atrial fibrillation. *BMC Med Genet.* 2012;13:24.
20. Liang C, Li X, Xu Y, et al. KCNE1 rs1805127 polymorphism increases the risk of atrial fibrillation: a meta-analysis of 10 studies. *PLoS One.* 2013;8:e68690.
21. Yang Y, Xia M, Jin Q, et al. Identification of a KCNE2 gain-of-function mutation in patients with familial atrial fibrillation. *Am J Hum Genet.* 2004;75:899–905.
22. Nielsen JB, Bentzen BH, Olesen MS, et al. Gain-of-function mutations in potassium channel subunit KCNE2 associated with early-onset lone atrial fibrillation. *Biomark Med.* 2014;8:557–570.
23. Ravn LS, Aizawa Y, Pollevick GD, et al. Gain of function in I_{Ks} secondary to a mutation in KCNE5 associated with atrial fibrillation. *Heart Rhythm.* 2008;5:427–435.
24. Deo M, Ruan Y, Pandit SV, et al. KCNJ2 mutation in short QT syndrome 3 results in atrial fibrillation and ventricular proarrhythmia. *Proc Natl Acad Sci U S A.* 2013;110:4291–4296.
25. Hattori T, Makiyama T, Akao M, et al. A novel gain-of-function KCNJ2 mutation associated with short-QT syndrome impairs inward rectification of Kir2.1 currents. *Cardiovasc Res.* 2012;93:666–673.
26. Xia M, Jin Q, Bendahhou S, et al. A Kir2.1 gain-of-function mutation underlies familial atrial fibrillation. *Biochem Biophys Res Commun.* 2005;332:1012–1019.
27. Olson TM, Alekseev AE, Liu XK, et al. Kv1.5 channelopathy due to KCNA5 loss-of-function mutation causes human atrial fibrillation. *Hum Mol Genet.* 2006;15:2185–2191.
28. Christophersen IE, Olesen MS, Liang B, et al. Genetic variation in KCNA5: impact on the atrial-specific potassium current I_{Kur} in patients with lone atrial fibrillation. *Eur Heart J.* 2013;34:1517–1525.
29. Delaney JT, Muhammad R, Blair MA, et al. A KCNJ8 mutation associated with early repolarization and atrial fibrillation. *Europace.* 2012;14:1428–1432.
30. Olesen MS, Refsgaard L, Holst AG, et al. A novel KCND3 gain-of-function mutation associated with early-onset of persistent lone atrial fibrillation. *Cardiovasc Res.* 2013;98:488–495.
31. Olson TM, Alekseev AE, Moreau C, et al. KATP channel mutation confers risk for vein of Marshall adrenergic atrial fibrillation. *Nat Clin Pract Cardiovasc Med.* 2007;4:110–116.
32. Ling TY, Wang XL, Chai Q, et al. Regulation of the SK3 channel by microRNA-499–potential role in atrial fibrillation. *Heart Rhythm.* 2013;10:1001–1009.
33. Mahida S, Mills RW, Tucker NR, et al. Overexpression of KCNN3 results in sudden cardiac death. *Cardiovasc Res.* 2014;101:326–334.
34. Ellinor PT, Nam EG, Shea MA, Milan DJ, Ruskin JN, MacRae CA. Cardiac sodium channel mutation in atrial fibrillation. *Heart Rhythm.* 2008;5:99–105.
35. Olesen MS, Jespersen T, Nielsen JB, et al. Mutations in sodium channel beta-subunit SCN3B are associated with early-onset lone atrial fibrillation. *Cardiovasc Res.* 2011;89:786–793.
36. Darbar D, Kannankeril PJ, Donahue BS, et al. Cardiac sodium channel (SCN5A) variants associated with atrial fibrillation. *Circulation.* 2008;117:1927–1935.
37. Ziyadeh-Isleem A, Clatot J, Duchatelet S, et al. A truncating SCN5A mutation combined with genetic variability causes sick sinus syndrome and early atrial fibrillation. *Heart Rhythm.* 2014;11:1015–1023.
38. Olesen MS, Yuan L, Liang B, et al. High prevalence of long QT syndrome-associated SCN5A variants in patients with early-onset lone atrial fibrillation. *Circ Cardiovasc Genet.* 2012;5:450–459.

39. Jabbari J, Olesen MS, Yuan L, et al. Common and rare variants in SCN10A modulate the risk of atrial fibrillation. *Circ Cardiovasc Genet.* 2015;8:64–73.

40. Savio-Galimberti E, Weeke P, Muhammad R, et al. SCN10A/Nav1.8 modulation of peak and late sodium currents in patients with early onset atrial fibrillation. *Cardiovasc Res.* 2014;104:355–363.

41. Watanabe H, Darbar D, Kaiser DW, et al. Mutations in sodium channel beta1- and beta2-subunits associated with atrial fibrillation. *Circ Arrhythm Electrophysiol.* 2009;2:268–275.

42. Olesen MS, Holst AG, Svendsen JH, Haunso S, Tfelt-Hansen J. SCN1Bb R214Q found in 3 patients: 1 with Brugada syndrome and 2 with lone atrial fibrillation. *Heart Rhythm.* 2012;9:770–773.

43. Wang P, Yang Q, Wu X, et al. Functional dominant-negative mutation of sodium channel subunit gene SCN3B associated with atrial fibrillation in a Chinese GeneID population. *Biochem Biophys Res Commun.* 2010;398:98–104.

44. Li RG, Wang Q, Xu YJ, et al. Mutations of the SCN4B-encoded sodium channel beta4 subunit in familial atrial fibrillation. *Int J Mol Med.* 2013;32:144–150.

45. Macri V, Mahida SN, Zhang ML, et al. A novel trafficking-defective HCN4 mutation is associated with early-onset atrial fibrillation. *Heart Rhythm.* 2014;11:1055–1062.

46. Chen S, Wang C, Wang X, et al. Significant association between CAV1 Variant rs3807989 on 7p31 and atrial fibrillation in a Chinese Han population. *J Am Heart Assoc.* 2015;4(5).

47. Liu Y, Ni B, Lin Y, et al. The rs3807989 G/A polymorphism in CAV1 is associated with the risk of atrial fibrillation in Chinese Han populations. *Pacing Clin Electrophysiol.* 2015;38:164–170.

48. Thibodeau IL, Xu J, Li Q, et al. Paradigm of genetic mosaicism and lone atrial fibrillation: physiological characterization of a connexin 43-deletion mutant identified from atrial tissue. *Circulation.* 2010;122:236–244.

49. Gollob MH, Jones DL, Krahn AD, et al. Somatic mutations in the connexin 40 gene (GJA5) in atrial fibrillation. *N Engl J Med.* 2006;354:2677–2688.

50. Wirka RC, Gore S, Van Wagoner DR, et al. A common connexin-40 gene promoter variant affects connexin-40 expression in human atria and is associated with atrial fibrillation. *Circ Arrhythm Electrophysiol.* 2011;4:87–93.

51. Shi HF, Yang JF, Wang Q, et al. Prevalence and spectrum of GJA5 mutations associated with lone atrial fibrillation. *Mol Med Rep.* 2013;7:767–774.

52. Wang J, Sun YM, Yang YQ. Mutation spectrum of the GATA4 gene in patients with idiopathic atrial fibrillation. *Mol Biol Rep.* 2012;39:8127–8135.

53. Jiang JQ, Shen FF, Fang WY, Liu X, Yang YQ. Novel GATA4 mutations in lone atrial fibrillation. *Int J Mol Med.* Dec 2011;28:1025–1032.

54. Yang YQ, Wang MY, Zhang XL, et al. GATA4 loss-of-function mutations in familial atrial fibrillation. *Clin Chim Acta.* 2011;412:1825–1830.

55. Gu JY, Xu JH, Yu H, Yang YQ. Novel GATA5 loss-of-function mutations underlie familial atrial fibrillation. *Clinics (Sao Paulo).* 2012;67:1393–1399.

56. Wang XH, Huang CX, Wang Q, et al. A novel GATA5 loss-of-function mutation underlies lone atrial fibrillation. *Int J Mol Med.* 2013;31:43–50.

57. Yang YQ, Wang J, Wang XH, et al. Mutational spectrum of the GATA5 gene associated with familial atrial fibrillation. *Int J Cardiol.* 2012;157:305–307.

58. Li J, Liu WD, Yang ZL, Yang YQ. Novel GATA6 loss-of-function mutation responsible for familial atrial fibrillation. *Int J Mol Med.* 2012;30:783–790.

59. Yang YQ, Li L, Wang J, et al. GATA6 loss-of-function mutation in atrial fibrillation. *Eur J Med Genet.* 2012;55:520–526.

60. Yang YQ, Wang XH, Tan HW, Jiang WF, Fang WY, Liu X. Prevalence and spectrum of GATA6 mutations associated with familial atrial fibrillation. *Int J Cardiol.* 2012;155:494–496.

61. Yuan F, Qiu XB, Li RG, et al. A novel NKX2-5 loss-of-function mutation predisposes to familial dilated cardiomyopathy and arrhythmias. *Int J Mol Med.* 2015;35:478–486.

62. Yu H, Xu JH, Song HM, et al. Mutational spectrum of the NKX2-5 gene in patients with lone atrial fibrillation. *Int J Med Sci.* 2014;11:554–563.

63. Huang RT, Xue S, Xu YJ, Zhou M, Yang YQ. A novel NKX2.5 loss-of-function mutation responsible for familial atrial fibrillation. *Int J Mol Med.* 2013;31:1119–1126.

64. Tsai CT, Hsieh CS, Chang SN, et al. Next-generation sequencing of nine atrial fibrillation candidate genes identified novel de novo mutations in patients with extreme trait of atrial fibrillation. *J Med Genet.* 2015;52:28–36.

65. Wang J, Zhang DF, Sun YM, Yang YQ. A novel PITX2c loss-of-function mutation associated with familial atrial fibrillation. *Eur J Med Genet.* 2014;57:25–31.

66. Zhou YM, Zheng PX, Yang YQ, Ge ZM, Kang WQ. A novel PITX2c loss-of-function mutation underlies lone atrial fibrillation. *Int J Mol Med.* 2013;32:827–834.

67. Yang YQ, Xu YJ, Li RG, Qu XK, Fang WY, Liu X. Prevalence and spectrum of PITX2c mutations associated with familial atrial fibrillation. *Int J Cardiol.* 2013;168:2873–2876.

68. Martin RI, Babaei MS, Choy MK, et al. Genetic variants associated with risk of atrial fibrillation regulate expression of PITX2, CAV1, MYOZ1, C9orf3, and FANCC. *J Mol Cell Cardiol.* 2015;85:207–214.

69. Beavers DL, Wang W, Ather S, et al. Mutation E169K in junctophilin-2 causes atrial fibrillation due to impaired RyR2 stabilization. *J Am Coll Cardiol.* 2013;62:2010–2019.

70. Hodgson-Zingman DM, Karst ML, Zingman LV, et al. Atrial natriuretic peptide frameshift mutation in familial atrial fibrillation. *N Engl J Med.* 2008;359:158–165.

71. Ren X, Xu C, Zhan C, et al. Identification of NPPA variants associated with atrial fibrillation in a Chinese GeneID population. *Clin Chim Acta.* 2010;411:481–485.

72. Abraham RL, Yang T, Blair M, Roden DM, Darbar D. Augmented potassium current is a shared phenotype for two genetic defects associated with familial atrial fibrillation. *J Mol Cell Cardiol.* 2010;48:181–190.

73. Zhang X, Chen S, Yoo S, et al. Mutation in nuclear pore component NUP155 leads to atrial fibrillation and early sudden cardiac death. *Cell.* 2008;135:1017–1027.

74. Zhabyeyev P, Hiess F, Wang R, Liu Y. Wayne Chen SR, Oudit GY. S4153R is a gain-of-function mutation in the cardiac Ca²⁺ release channel ryanodine receptor associated with catecholaminergic polymorphic ventricular tachycardia and paroxysmal atrial fibrillation. *Can J Cardiol.* 2013;29:993–996.

75. Kazemian P, Gollob MH, Pantano A, Oudit GY. A novel mutation in the RYR2 gene leading to catecholaminergic polymorphic ventricular tachycardia and paroxysmal atrial fibrillation: dose-dependent arrhythmia-event suppression by beta-blocker therapy. *Can J Cardiol.* 2011;27:870. e877–e810.

76. Nattel S. New ideas about atrial fibrillation 50 years on. *Nature.* 2002;415:219–226.

77. McNair WP, Ku L, Taylor MR, et al. SCN5A mutation associated with dilated cardiomyopathy, conduction disorder, and arrhythmia. *Circulation.* 2004;110:2163–2167.

78. Olson TM, Michels VV, Ballew JD, et al. Sodium channel mutations and susceptibility to heart failure and atrial fibrillation. *JAMA.* 2005;293:447–454.

79. Laitinen-Forsblom PJ, Makynen P, Makynen H, et al. SCN5A mutation associated with cardiac conduction defect and atrial arrhythmias. *J Cardiovasc Electrophysiol.* 2006;17:480–485.

80. Groenewegen WA, Firouzi M, Bezzina CR, et al. A cardiac sodium channel mutation cosegregates with a rare connexin40 genotype in familial atrial standstill. *Circ Res.* 2003;92:14–22.

81. Oberti C, Wang L, Li L, et al. Genome-wide linkage scan identifies a novel genetic locus on chromosome 5p13 for neonatal atrial fibrillation associated with sudden death and variable cardiomyopathy. *Circulation.* 2004;110:3753–3759.

82. Zhang X, Chen S, Yoo S, et al. Mutation in nuclear pore component NUP155 leads to atrial fibrillation and early sudden cardiac death. *Cell.* 2008;135:1017–1027.

83. Ellinor PT, Shin JT, Moore RK, Yoerger DM, MacRae CA. Locus for atrial fibrillation maps to chromosome 6q14-16. *Circulation.* 2003;107:2880–2883.

84. Volders PG, Zhu Q, Timmermans C, et al. Mapping a novel locus for familial atrial fibrillation on chromosome 10p11-q21. *Heart Rhythm.* 2007;4:469–475.

85. Otway R, Vandenberg JI, Guo G, et al. Stretch-sensitive KCNQ1 mutation: a link between genetic and environmental factors in the pathogenesis of atrial fibrillation? *J Am Coll Cardiol.* 2007;49:578–586.

86. Lundby A, Ravn LS, Svendsen JH, Olesen SP, Schmitt N. KCNQ1 mutation Q147R is associated with atrial fibrillation and prolonged QT interval. *Heart Rhythm.* 2007;4:1532–1541.

87. Hong K, Piper DR, Diaz-Valdecantos A, et al. De novo KCNQ1 mutation responsible for atrial fibrillation and short QT syndrome in utero. *Cardiovasc Res.* 2005;68:433–440.

88. Hong K, Bjerregaard P, Gussak I, Brugada R. Short QT syndrome and atrial fibrillation caused by mutation in KCNH2. *J Cardiovasc Electrophysiol.* 2005;16:394–396.

89. Makiyama T, Akao M, Shizuta S, et al. A novel SCN5A gain-of-function mutation M1875T associated with familial atrial fibrillation. *J Am Coll Cardiol.* 2008;52:1326–1334.

90. Li Q, Huang H, Liu G, et al. Gain-of-function mutation of Nav1.5 in atrial fibrillation enhances cellular excitability and lowers the threshold for action potential firing. *Biochem Biophys Res Commun.* 2009;380:132–137.

91. Watanabe H, Darbar D, Kaiser DW, et al. Mutations in sodium channel beta1- and beta2-subunits associated with atrial fibrillation. *Circ Arrhythm Electrophysiol.* 2009;2:268–275.

92. Gollob MH, Jones DL, Krahn AD, et al. Somatic mutations in the connexin 40 gene (GJA5) in atrial fibrillation. *N Engl J Med.* 2006;354:2677–2688.

93. Firouzi M, Ramanna H, Kok B, et al. Association of human connexin40 gene polymorphisms with atrial vulnerability as a risk factor for idiopathic atrial fibrillation. *Circ Res.* 2004;95:e29–e33.

94. Juang JM, Chern YR, Tsai CT, et al. The association of human connexin 40 genetic polymorphisms with atrial fibrillation. *Int J Cardiol.* 2007;116:107–112.

95. Roberts JD, Longoria J, Poon A, et al. Targeted deep sequencing reveals no definitive evidence for somatic mosaicism in atrial fibrillation. *Circ Cardiovasc Genet.* 2015;8:50–57.

96. International HapMap Consortium. The International HapMap Project. *Nature.* 2003;426:789–796.

97 International Genome Sample Resource. Homepage. http://www.1000genomes.org.

98 Hindorff LA, Junkins HA, Mehta JP, Manolio TA. A catalog of published genome-wide association studies. Available at: http://www.genome.gov/gwastudies. Accessed January 25, 2016.

99. Gudbjartsson DF, Arnar DO, Helgadottir A, et al. Variants conferring risk of atrial fibrillation on chromosome 4q25. *Nature.* 2007;448:353–357.

100. Benjamin EJ, Rice KM, Arking DE, et al. Variants in ZFHX3 are associated with atrial fibrillation in individuals of European ancestry. *Nat Genet.* 2009; 41:879–881.

101. Gudbjartsson DF, Holm H, Gretarsdottir S, et al. A sequence variant in ZFHX3 on 16q22 associates with atrial fibrillation and ischemic stroke. *Nat Genet.* 2009;41:876–878.

102. Ellinor PT, Lunetta KL, Glazer NL, et al. Common variants in KCNN3 are associated with lone atrial fibrillation. *Nat Genet.* 2010;42:240–244.

103. Ellinor PT, Lunetta KL, Albert CM, et al. Meta-analysis identifies six new susceptibility loci for atrial fibrillation. *Nat Genet.* 2012;44:670–675.

104. Diness JG, Sorensen US, Nissen JD, et al. Inhibition of small-conductance Ca²⁺-activated K⁺ channels terminates and protects against atrial fibrillation. *Circ Arrhythm Electrophysiol.* 2010;3:380–390.

105. Skibsbye L, Diness JG, Sorensen US, Hansen RS, Grunnet M. The duration of pacing-induced atrial fibrillation is reduced in vivo by inhibition of small conductance Ca²⁺-activated K⁺ channels. *J Cardiovasc Pharmacol.* 2011;57:672–681.

106. Bergwerff M, Gittenberger-de Groot AC, Wisse LJ, et al. Loss of function of the Prx1 and Prx2 homeobox genes alters architecture of the great elastic arteries and ductus arteriosus. *Virchows Arch.* 2000;436:12–19.

107. Ihida-Stansbury K, McKean DM, Gebb SA, et al. Paired-related homeobox gene Prx1 is required for pulmonary vascular development. *Circ Res.* 2004;94:1507–1514.

108. Shang Y, Yoshida T, Amendt BA, Martin JF, Owens GK. Pitx2 is functionally important in the early stages of vascular smooth muscle cell differentiation. *J Cell Biol.* 2008;181:461–473.

109. Sinner MF, Tucker NR, Lunetta KL, et al. Integrating genetic, transcriptional, and functional analyses to identify five novel genes for atrial fibrillation. *Circulation.* 2014;130:1225–1235.

110. Mommersteeg MT, Brown NA, Prall OW, et al. Pitx2c and Nkx2-5 are required for the formation and identity of the pulmonary myocardium. *Circ Res.* 2007;101:902–909.

111. Wang J, Klysik E, Sood S, Johnson RL, Wehrens XH, Martin JF. Pitx2 prevents susceptibility to atrial arrhythmias by inhibiting left-sided pacemaker specification. *Proc Natl Acad Sci U S A.* 2010;107:9753–9758.

112. Mommersteeg MT, Hoogaars WM, Prall OW, et al. Molecular pathway for the localized formation of the sinoatrial node. *Circ Res.* 2007;100:354–362.

113. Chinchilla A, Daimi H, Lozano-Velasco E, et al. PITX2 insufficiency leads to atrial electrical and structural remodeling linked to arrhythmogenesis. *Circ Cardiovasc Genet.* 2011;4:269–279.

114. Kirchhof P, Kahr PC, Kaese S, et al. PITX2c is expressed in the adult left atrium, and reducing Pitx2c expression promotes atrial fibrillation inducibility and complex changes in gene expression. *Circ Cardiovasc Genet.* 2011;4:123–133.

115. Yoshida T, Hoofnagle MH, Owens GK. Myocardin and Prx1 contribute to angiotensin II-induced expression of smooth muscle alpha-actin. *Circ Res.* 2004;94:1075–1082.

116. Tao Y, Zhang M, Li L, et al. Pitx2, an atrial fibrillation predisposition gene, directly regulates ion transport and intercalated disc genes. *Circ Cardiovasc Genet.* 2014;7:23–32.

117. Britz-Cunningham SH, Shah MM, Zuppan CW, Fletcher WH. Mutations of the Connexin43 gap-junction gene in patients with heart malformations and defects of laterality. *N Engl J Med.* 1995;332:1323–1329.

118. Reaume AG, de Sousa PA, Kulkarni S, et al. Cardiac malformation in neonatal mice lacking connexin43. *Science*. 1995;267:1831–1834.

119. Gratton JP, Bernatchez P, Sessa WC. Caveolae and caveolins in the cardiovascular system. *Circ Res*. 2004;94:1408–1417.

120. Zhao YY, Liu Y, Stan RV, et al. Defects in caveolin-1 cause dilated cardiomyopathy and pulmonary hypertension in knockout mice. *Proc Natl Acad Sci U S A*. 2002;99:11375–11380.

121. Cohen AW, Park DS, Woodman SE, et al. Caveolin-1 null mice develop cardiac hypertrophy with hyperactivation of p42/44 MAP kinase in cardiac fibroblasts. *Am J Physiol Cell Physiol*. 2003;284:C457–C474.

122. Lin MT, Adelman JP, Maylie J. Modulation of endothelial SK3 channel activity by Ca^{2+}-dependent caveolar trafficking. *Am J Physiol Cell Physiol*. 2012;303: C318–C327.

123. Lin J, Lin S, Choy PC, et al. The regulation of the cardiac potassium channel (HERG) by caveolin-1. *Biochem Cell Biol*. 2008;86:405–415.

124. Frey N, Olson EN. Calsarcin-3, a novel skeletal muscle-specific member of the calsarcin family, interacts with multiple Z-disc proteins. *J Biol Chem*. 2002;277:13998–14004.

125. Moskowitz IP, Pizard A, Patel VV, et al. The T-Box transcription factor Tbx5 is required for the patterning and maturation of the murine cardiac conduction system. *Development*. 2004;131:4107–4116.

126. Moskowitz IP, Kim JB, Moore ML, et al. A molecular pathway including Id2, Tbx5, and Nkx2-5 required for cardiac conduction system development. *Cell*. 2007;129:1365–1376.

127. Postma AV, van de Meerakker JB, Mathijssen IB, et al. A gain-of-function TBX5 mutation is associated with atypical Holt-Oram syndrome and paroxysmal atrial fibrillation. *Circ Res*. 2008;102:1433–1442.

128. Pfeufer A, van Noord C, Marciante KD, et al. Genome-wide association study of PR interval. *Nat Genet*. 2010;42:153–159.

129. Holm H, Gudbjartsson DF, Arnar DO, et al. Several common variants modulate heart rate, PR interval and QRS duration. *Nat Genet*. 2010;42:117–122.

130. Schnabel RB, Sullivan LM, Levy D, et al. Development of a risk score for atrial fibrillation (Framingham Heart Study): a community-based cohort study. *Lancet*. 2009;373:739–745.

131. Zhang Q, Ragnauth CD, Skepper JN, et al. Nesprin-2 is a multi-isomeric protein that binds lamin and emerin at the nuclear envelope and forms a subcellular network in skeletal muscle. *J Cell Sci*. 2005;118:673–687.

132. DiFrancesco D. The role of the funny current in pacemaker activity. *Circ Res*. 2010;106:434–446.

133. Dobrzynski H, Boyett MR, Anderson RH. New insights into pacemaker activity: promoting understanding of sick sinus syndrome. *Circulation*. 2007;115:1921–1932.

134. Yamamoto T, Dowa Y, Ueda H, et al. Tetralogy of Fallot associated with pulmonary atresia and major aortopulmonary collateral arteries in a patient with interstitial deletion of 16q21-q22.1. *Am J Med Genet A*. 2008;146A:1575–1580.

135. Burgner D, Davila S, Breunis WB, et al. A genome-wide association study identifies novel and functionally related susceptibility loci for Kawasaki disease. *PLoS Genet*. 2009;5:e1000319.

136. Kaab S, Darbar D, van Noord C, et al. Large scale replication and meta-analysis of variants on chromosome 4q25 associated with atrial fibrillation. *Eur Heart J*. 2009;30:813–819.

137. Body SC, Collard CD, Shernan SK, et al. Variation in the 4q25 chromosomal locus predicts atrial fibrillation after coronary artery bypass graft surgery. *Circ Cardiovasc Genet*. 2009;2:499–506.

138. Kiliszek M, Franaszczyk M, Kozluk E, et al. Association between variants on chromosome 4q25, 16q22 and 1q21 and atrial fibrillation in the Polish population. *PLoS One*. 2011;6:e21790.

139. Viviani Anselmi C, Novelli V, Roncarati R, et al. Association of rs2200733 at 4q25 with atrial flutter/fibrillation diseases in an Italian population. *Heart*. 2008;94:1394–1396.

140. Shi L, Li C, Wang C, et al. Assessment of association of rs2200733 on chromosome 4q25 with atrial fibrillation and ischemic stroke in a Chinese Han population. *Hum Genet*. 2009;126:843–849.

141. Schnabel RB, Kerr KF, Lubitz SA, et al. Large-scale candidate gene analysis in whites and African Americans identifies IL6R polymorphism in relation to atrial fibrillation: the National Heart, Lung, and Blood Institute's Candidate Gene Association Resource (CARe) project. *Circ Cardiovasc Genet*. 2011;4:557–564.

142. Delaney JT, Jeff JM, Brown NJ, et al. Characterization of genome-wide association-identified variants for atrial fibrillation in African Americans. *PLoS One*. 2012;7:e32338.

143. Semina EV, Reiter R, Leysens NJ, et al. Cloning and characterization of a novel bicoid-related homeobox transcription factor gene, RIEG, involved in Rieger syndrome. *Nat Genet*. 1996;14:392–399.

144. Doward W, Perveen R, Lloyd IC, Ridgway AE, Wilson L, Black GC. A mutation in the RIEG1 gene associated with Peters' anomaly. *J Med Genet*. 1999;36:152–155.

145. Haissaguerre M, Jais P, Shah DC, et al. Spontaneous initiation of atrial fibrillation by ectopic beats originating in the pulmonary veins. *N Engl J Med*. 1998;339:659–666.

146. Wang J, Bai Y, Li N, et al. Pitx2-microRNA pathway that delimits sinoatrial node development and inhibits predisposition to atrial fibrillation. *Proc Natl Acad Sci U S A*. 2014;111:9181–9186.

147. Nobrega MA, Ovcharenko I, Afzal V, Rubin EM. Scanning human gene deserts for long-range enhancers. *Science*. 2003;302:413.

148. Lettice LA, Heaney SJ, Purdie LA, et al. A long-range Shh enhancer regulates expression in the developing limb and fin and is associated with preaxial polydactyly. *Hum Mol Genet*. 2003;12:1725–1735.

149. Kleinjan DA, van Heyningen V. Long-range control of gene expression: emerging mechanisms and disruption in disease. *Am J Hum Genet*. 2005;76:8–32.

150. Lubitz SA, Sinner MF, Lunetta KL, et al. Independent susceptibility markers for atrial fibrillation on chromosome 4q25. *Circulation*. 2010;122:976–984.

151. Lubitz SA, Lunetta KL, Lin H, et al. Novel genetic markers associate with atrial fibrillation risk in Europeans and Japanese. *J Am Coll Cardiol*. 2014;63:1200–1210.

152. Marcus GM, Alonso A, Peralta CA, et al. European ancestry as a risk factor for atrial fibrillation in African Americans. *Circulation*. 2010;122:2009–2015.

50 Mechanisms in Heritable Sodium Channel Diseases

Thao P. Nguyen and Alfred L. George, Jr.

The discovery of the first mutation in the *SCN5A* gene encoding the human cardiac voltage-gated sodium channel in 1995 launched a new era in our understanding of the molecular and genetic basis of arrhythmias. Subsequent work has revealed an unexpectedly large number of clinically and pathophysiologically diverse conditions (Box 50.1) associated with an ever-increasing number of mutations in this gene and in genes encoding important regulatory or interacting proteins. Sodium channel dysfunction or dysregulation caused by gain- or loss-of-function mutations leads to arrhythmias in either the ventricles or atria or in both with potentially life-threatening consequences. The diversity of clinical disorders (phenotypes) associated with *SCN5A* is explained partly by corresponding heterogeneity in mutant channel dysfunction and resulting cellular electrophysiological effects. Understanding the functional consequences of *SCN5A* mutations has led to tremendous progress in elucidating arrhythmia mechanisms in these genetic disorders and has inspired new therapeutic strategies.

This chapter will focus primarily on pathophysiological aspects of genetic cardiac sodium channel diseases with emphasis on the biophysical mechanisms that underlie these disorders. The goal of this review is to provide the reader with a basic mechanistic foundation for clinical diagnosis, risk stratification, and management. Such mechanistic insights will not be possible without a basic appreciation of the channel structure, function, and trafficking as provided in depth by other chapters that are cited throughout this review.

Cardiac Sodium Channel

SCN5A encodes the pore-forming subunit of the major voltage-gated sodium channel expressed in the human heart. This gene spans approximately 100 kilobases on the short arm of chromosome 3 (3p21) and consists of 28 canonical exons ranging in size from 53 (exon 24) to 3257 (exon 28) base pairs (Fig. 50.1A). The full-length product of *SCN5A* is a 2016-amino acid protein designated as $Na_V1.5$, but other nomenclature (i.e., hH1) prevalent in older literature has been used to describe recombinant forms. Native $Na_V1.5$ is localized to the intercalated disks and lateral plasma membranes of cardiomyocytes.

Alternatively spliced messenger RNAs (mRNAs) transcribed from *SCN5A* have been detected in the heart.[1] One splice variant expressed in the adult heart is generated by alternative usage of splice acceptor sequences at the junction between intron 17 and exon 18,

resulting in either inclusion or exclusion of glutamine at position 1077 in the protein.[2] Approximately half of the mature *SCN5A* mRNA in the heart encodes the 2015-amino acid alternative form of the protein that arises from this alternative splicing event, and this impacts the functional properties of certain genetic variants.[3,4] In the fetal and neonatal heart, another alternatively spliced form of $Na_V1.5$ is expressed that utilizes an alternative exon 6 (exon 6a; see Fig. 50.1A), resulting in seven amino acid differences within a voltage-sensor domain (D1/S3–S4).[1,5] This fetal-expressed $Na_V1.5$ splice variant exhibits developmental regulation in mouse and human hearts[6] and exhibits distinct biophysical properties including a more depolarized voltage dependence of activation. Other alternative splicing events have less certain physiological relevance.[1]

Transcription of human *SCN5A* is under the control of a promoter that precedes the first exon and other determinants of transcriptional activity located in the first intron.[7] Common genomic variants within the *SCN5A* promoter may influence the expression of the gene and have clinical relevance. One particular combination of variants constituting a common haplotype within the *SCN5A* promoter has been associated with longer PR interval and QRS duration as well as the extent of QRS widening during challenge with sodium channel-blocking drugs in Asians.[8] Another common variant within an adjacent gene (*SCN10A*) encoding a peripheral nerve-expressed sodium channel ($Na_V1.8$) has been associated with altered cardiac conduction and Brugada syndrome (BrS).[9,10] This variant occurs within a binding site for two related T-box transcription factors (TBX3 and TBX5) that are involved in control of *SCN5A* expression through long-range chromatin interactions.[11,12]

Structurally, the channel has a four-fold symmetry consisting of structurally homologous domains (D1–D4), each containing four transmembrane segments (S1–S4) that comprise the voltage sensor, and a separate pore domain (S5–S6) important for determining ion selectivity. The S4 segment, which functions as the main voltage-sensing element, is amphipathic with basic amino acids (arginine or lysine) at every third position surrounded by hydrophobic residues. Activation of voltage-gated channels is evoked by a membrane depolarization that acts to propel the S4 segments in an outward direction away from the negative electrostatic cell interior. Subsequent conformational changes involving the S6 segment open the ion pore and permit rapid movement of ions through a passageway created by the pore domain. Chapter 1 presents a more complete discussion of the structure and function of sodium channels.

The cardiac sodium channel resides in the myocyte plasma membrane as a multiprotein complex consisting of the pore-forming (α) subunit ($Na_V1.5$), auxiliary (β) subunits, and other interacting proteins. A family of four sodium channel β-subunits (β_1, β_2, β_3, and β_4) encoded by the genes *SCN1B*, *SCN2B*, *SCN3B*, and *SCN4B*, respectively, are expressed in heart and likely interact with $Na_V1.5$ possibly to modulate channel function or subcellular localization, but the stoichiometry of these interactions is

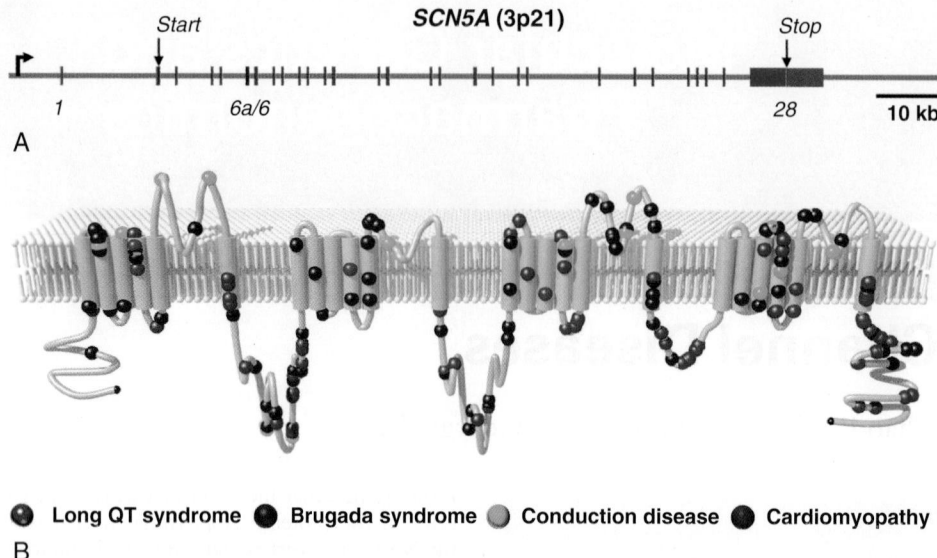

FIGURE 50.1 *SCN5A* gene structure and mutations. (A) Schematic of the *SCN5A* gene illustrating 28 canonical exons and 1 alternative exon (*vertical lines*: red for canonical coding exons, *blue* for alternative exon 6a, and *dark gray* for noncoding exons or portions of exons). A *bent arrow* indicates the approximate location of the transcription start site near the promoter. Locations of the translation start and stop codons are indicated. (B) Locations of representative mutations associated with arrhythmia syndromes are superimposed on a two-dimensional membrane topology map of the sodium channel protein. Approximately half of known Brugada syndrome mutations are displayed. (Image prepared using software supplied by Dr. André Linnenbank, University of Amsterdam.)

BOX 50.1   Disorders of the cardiac sodium channel gene, *SCN5A*

Ventricular Arrhythmia/Sudden Death
Congenital long QT syndrome (LQTS) type 3
Brugada syndrome type 1
Idiopathic ventricular fibrillation
Sudden unexplained nocturnal death syndrome
Sudden infant death syndrome

Impaired Cardiac Conduction
Progressive cardiac conduction system disease (Lenègre)
Familial atrioventricular block
Congenital sick sinus syndrome
Atrial standstill

Latent Arrhythmia Susceptibility
Drug-induced LQTS
Arrhythmia susceptibility in African-Americans (S1103Y)

Other
Mixed phenotypes/overlap syndromes
Dilated cardiomyopathy with arrhythmia
Atrial fibrillation

Cardiac voltage-gated sodium channels are critical mediators of phase 0 depolarization and control the velocity of impulse propagation through the heart. Sodium channels switch between three major functional states (*closed, open,* and *inactivated*) in response to changes in the membrane potential. Only open channels generate electrical current by allowing the selective passage of sodium ions into cells. The functional state of sodium channels can be monitored in electrophysiological recording experiments by using specific voltage-clamp protocols to elicit *activation* (closed → open), *fast inactivation* (open → inactivated), and *recovery from inactivation* (inactivated → closed), which occur on a millisecond time scale. In addition to these rapid transitions, sodium channels are also susceptible to *slow inactivation* if the membrane remains depolarized for a longer time. Slow inactivation occurs over a time course of several seconds and may contribute to determining the availability of active channels under various physiological conditions. The structural basis for sodium channel function is discussed in Chapters 1 and 9.

Consequences of Sodium Channel Dysfunction

More than 750 *SCN5A* mutations have been identified in patients with the arrhythmia predisposition syndromes presented in Box 50.1. The types of mutations include missense (e.g., amino acid substitutions), nonsense (e.g., premature stop codon), insertions or deletions, and splice-site mutations. Some mutation types, particularly those predicted to truncate the encoded protein (nonsense, insertions, or deletions affecting the reading frame), destroy the functionality of the channel (*loss-of-function*) by deleting critical domains or preventing protein translation through nonsense-mediated decay of the mRNA. Splice-site mutations may also severely disrupt channel function if exons are skipped or intron sequences are retained in the final mRNA. However, a large number of *SCN5A* mutations result in single amino acid substitutions for which functional predictions are difficult. Several missense mutations and a few in-frame insertion/deletion

unknown.[13] Several other proteins expressed in the heart, including ankyrins, caveolin-3, calmodulin, α_1-syntrophin, glycerol-3-phosphate dehydrogenase 1-like protein (GPD1L), fibroblast growth factor homologous factors, Nedd4-like ubiquitin-protein ligase, multicopy suppressor of *gsp1* (MOG1), and 14-3-3η, also interact directly or indirectly with sodium channels.[14] Some of these proteins have been implicated in rare cases of inherited arrhythmia susceptibility, suggesting that they mediate important functional interactions.[15] Further information about the regulation of sodium channels in the context of multiprotein complexes is provided in Chapters 18 and 21.

TABLE 50.1 Pathophysiology of sodium channel dysfunction in heritable arrhythmia syndromes

DISORDER	FUNCTIONAL MECHANISMS	CELLULAR CONSEQUENCES
Long QT syndrome	Enhanced persistent current (gain of function)	Impaired repolarization
Brugada syndrome	Reduced sodium current density (loss of function)	Impaired conduction, especially in right ventricular outflow tract
Conduction system disease	Reduced sodium current density (loss of function)	Impaired conduction
Cardiomyopathy-arrhythmia	Altered activation gating Aberrant gating pore current (gain of function)	Enhanced diastolic sodium current Altered intracellular ion homeostasis

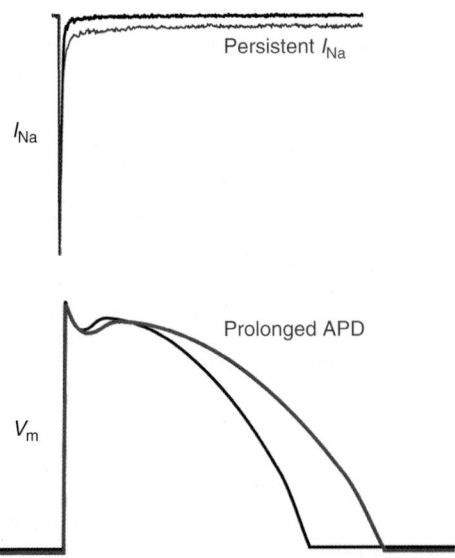

FIGURE 50.2 Enhanced persistent sodium current (I_{Na}) in LQT3. *Upper panel* is a representative current recording from a cell expressing either wildtype cardiac sodium channels (*black trace*) or an *SCN5A* mutation associated with LQT3 (*red trace*), illustrating enhanced persistent I_{Na}. Lower panel illustrates a normal ventricular action potential waveform (*black line*) and an illustration of prolonged action potential duration (*APD; red line*) as occurs in long QT syndrome.

alleles have been studied in vitro to determine the molecular basis for arrhythmia predisposition in these syndromes, and common patterns of sodium channel dysfunction have emerged.

At the cellular and tissue levels, abnormal sodium channel function can be predicted to cause delayed repolarization, impaired impulse propagation, altered intracellular ion homeostasis, or combinations of these pathophysiological effects (Table 50.1). These pathogenic outcomes will be used as the framework for discussing mechanisms of sodium channel dysfunction in specific disorders.

Delayed Repolarization

Congenital Long QT Syndrome

Congenital long QT syndrome (LQTS) is an inherited condition of abnormal myocardial repolarization. It is characterized clinically by an increased risk of potentially fatal ventricular arrhythmias, especially torsades de pointes, manifesting as syncope, cardiac arrest, and sudden unexplained death in otherwise healthy young adults and children. The disease is typically recognized in late childhood or early adolescence, but extreme cases may present during early infancy or in the perinatal period.[16] The syndrome is most often transmitted in families as an autosomal dominant trait (Romano-Ward syndrome; see also Chapter 93).

Approximately 10% of autosomal dominant LQTS cases are explained by *SCN5A* mutations,[17] and this form of the disease is referred to as LQT3. The proportion of sodium channel mutations in LQTS cases presenting during the perinatal and neonatal time periods may be higher.[18] The first *SCN5A* mutation described was an in-frame deletion of three highly conserved amino acid residues (delKPQ 1505–1507) located within the cytoplasmic loop connecting domains 3 and 4 of $Na_V1.5$,[19] a structural domain required for fast inactivation.

Since the discovery of the first *SCN5A* mutation in 1995, more than 200 mostly missense *SCN5A* mutations have been reported in association with LQT3 (see Fig. 50.1B). Although mutations are found throughout the channel sequence, there are a small number of structural regions where multiple mutations are clustered. One of these regions is the S4 segment of domain 4 (D4), a critical structural determinant of voltage sensing. Another mutation cluster can be found in the aforementioned cytoplasmic inactivation gate. Finally, several mutations are found in the proximal carboxyl terminus, which includes binding sites for several interacting proteins that can modulate sodium channel function[14] and has been implicated as part of a Ca^{2+} and calmodulin regulatory apparatus.[20]

Persons with *SCN5A* mutations associated with LQTS often present with distinct clinical features including sinus bradycardia and a tendency for cardiac events to occur during sleep or rest.[21]

In addition to bradycardia, certain features of the surface electrocardiogram (ECG), such as narrow and late-onset peaked or biphasic T-waves, may offer additional clues to the presence of an *SCN5A* mutation in the setting of LQTS.[22] Cardiac events are less frequent in the setting of *SCN5A* mutations as compared to the two major forms of LQTS caused by potassium channel mutations (LQT1 and LQT2).[23,24] However, in children and adults, the risk of dying after a cardiac event is greater among those with LQT3 than among those with either LQT1 or LQT2.

In LQT3, most *SCN5A* mutations exhibit a dominant *gain-of-function* phenotype at the molecular level characterized by defective inactivation, leading to enhanced persistent sodium current (Fig. 50.2).[25] Some mutant channels may also exhibit accelerated recovery from inactivation, a phenomenon consistent with an unstable inactivated state. At the level of single sodium channels, enhanced persistent sodium current has been correlated with a greater tendency for channel reopening, which may occur in bursts.[25] A more severe slowing of inactivation may be present in mutations associated with unusually severe LQTS,[16,26] while a small number of mutations alter the voltage dependence of activation and/or inactivation with less dramatic effects on the level of persistent current.[27,28]

Enhanced persistent sodium current has also been observed when wildtype $Na_V1.5$ channels were coexpressed with LQTS-associated mutations in certain auxiliary subunits and interacting proteins. Specifically, mutations in *SCN4B* encoding the β_4 auxiliary subunit,[29] *CAV3* encoding the vesicular trafficking protein caveolin-3,[30] and *SNTA1* encoding the adapter protein α_1-syntrophin[31,32] exert their pathological effects by disturbing sodium channel inactivation, leading to enhanced persistent current. The mechanism responsible for enhanced persistent current associated with *SNTA1* mutations involves activation of neuronal nitric oxide synthase (nNOS) complexed with $Na_V1.5$, leading to increased cell levels of nitric oxide and nitrosylation of the sodium channel. Activation of nNOS is the result of disrupted scaffolding of a plasma membrane Ca^{2+}-adenosine triphosphatase (ATPase) (PMCA4b) that normally inhibits the enzyme in a multiprotein complex with $Na_V1.5$ and α_1-syntrophin.[32]

Enhanced persistent sodium current provides an explanation for delayed repolarization in LQTS.[33] Cardiac action potentials last several hundred milliseconds due to a prolonged depolarization phase (plateau), a result of opposing inward (mainly Na^+ and Ca^{2+}) and outward (K^+) ionic currents. Repolarization occurs when the net outward current exceeds the net inward current. Enhanced persistent sodium current will shift this balance toward inward current and delay the onset of repolarization, thus lengthening the action potential duration and the corresponding QT interval. Delayed repolarization predisposes to ventricular arrhythmias mainly by increasing the probability of early afterdepolarization (EAD) and through increased dispersion of action potential duration.[34] These phenomena promote conditions that allow electrical signals from depolarized regions of the heart to prematurely reexcite adjacent myocardium that has already repolarized, the basis for a reentrant arrhythmia. Purkinje cells may have a greater sensitivity to the effects of LQT3 mutations and might contribute uniquely to arrhythmia susceptibility.[35]

The pathogenic effects of enhanced persistent sodium current in LQTS have also been strongly supported by computer simulations of cardiac action potentials[33,36] in electrophysiological investigations of cardiomyocytes from genetically engineered mice and human cardiomyocytes differentiated from induced pluripotent stem cells (iPSCs). Mice engineered to carry the delKPQ mutation have spontaneous life-threatening ventricular arrhythmias.[37,38] At the cellular level, cardiomyocytes from these mice with LQT3 exhibit prolonged action potential duration and frequent EADs, findings that were exaggerated by slow pacing rates. These cells have enhanced persistent sodium currents, and there is faster recovery from inactivation, features that were predicted from studies performed in noncardiac cells.[37] There is further evidence from the delKPQ mouse that delayed afterdepolarization (DAD) caused by a Ca^{2+}-dependent diastolic transient inward current, possibly evoked by abnormal Na^+ entry through mutant channels, also contributes to arrhythmia susceptibility and may account for the greater lethality of this LQTS subtype.[39] Elevated intracellular Ca^{2+} suppresses persistent sodium current associated with LQT3 mutations and may protect cells from delayed repolarization. This finding offers a plausible explanation for the lower arrhythmia risk in LQT3 subjects during fast heart rates when steady-state cytosolic Ca^{2+} concentration is expected to be at its highest levels.[40]

Novel in vitro cellular models of LQT3 have been developed using iPSC technology (see Chapter 57). Five different SCN5A mutations associated with LQTS have been studied in human cardiomyocytes derived from iPSCs.[41-44] These studies generally showed significantly prolonged action potential duration, sometimes with spontaneous EADs, and either greater levels of persistent sodium current or a slower time course of inactivation. Some studies also reported accelerated recovery from inactivation and depolarized steady-state inactivation. These findings offer further evidence for pathogenic human cardiac sodium channel dysfunction and its cellular consequences in LQT3.

Knowledge of the basic mechanisms underlying LQT3 prompted new ideas regarding genotype-specific treatment. Mexiletine and other sodium channel-blocking drugs can reduce persistent sodium current and shorten the QT interval in LQT3 patients.[45-48] In LQT3 mouse models, mexiletine shortens the myocyte action potential and prevents arrhythmias[34,49] mainly during slow pacing rates. Mexiletine also suppressed persistent current and shortened action potential duration in LQT3 patient–derived iPSC-cardiomyocytes.[41,43] Suppression of persistent current by the antianginal drug ranolazine has been demonstrated for LQT3 mutations in vitro,[50] and ranolazine treatment of human subjects with SCN5A mutations shortened the QTc interval significantly[51] or has suppressed ventricular arrhythmia.[52] A more potent and selective inhibitor of persistent sodium current (eleclazine, GS-6615) has entered clinical trials for treatment

of LQT3 subjects (ClinicalTrials.gov identifier NCT02300558). Propranolol, but not other β-adrenergic antagonists, may exhibit sodium channel-blocking effects at high concentrations,[53-55] and certain SCN5A mutations have increased in vitro sensitivity to the drug.[16] There have been conflicting reports regarding the efficacy of propranolol on suppression of arrhythmias in the delKPQ mouse model of LQT3.[38,56]

Perinatal and Neonatal LQT3

SCN5A mutations may cause life-threatening LQTS during gestation (fetal LQTS) and in neonates (neonatal LQTS). Clinical signs suggestive of fetal LQTS include ventricular tachycardia, second-degree atrioventricular (AV) block, and, most commonly, sinus bradycardia,[57] but such findings may go undetected because routine electrocardiographic testing of fetuses is not performed. Certain SCN5A mutations, many of which are de novo,[16,58-61] present with earlier-onset and more severe congenital arrhythmia syndrome than is typical for LQT3. The high rate of reported de novo SCN5A mutations in the perinatal period may reflect low heritability due to a survival disadvantage conferred by severe, life-threatening phenotypes. The functional effects of certain SCN5A mutations associated with fetal LQTS can also be potentiated by a developmentally regulated splice isoform involving alternative forms of exon 6.[6]

There is evidence that occult LQTS can clinically present as the sudden infant death syndrome (SIDS) (see Chapter 98). Cardiac mechanisms including life-threatening arrhythmias have been suspected as risk factors for SIDS, and mutations in genes responsible for LQTS have been identified in approximately 10% of cases.[62,63] SCN5A mutations have accounted for approximately 50% of all LQTS mutations identified in SIDS. SCN5A mutations associated with SIDS exhibit enhanced persistent current overtly or under certain conditions such as intracellular acidosis or in the context of a common splice variant.[62,64-66]

Arrhythmia Susceptibility With Common SCN5A Variants

Common variants within the SCN5A coding region have been identified in certain populations and some of these may confer increased risk of cardiac arrhythmia. One variant common in subjects of African descent (S1103Y, also reported as S1102Y) has been associated with an eight-fold increased risk for ventricular arrhythmia.[67] The functional consequences of S1103Y include increased transient and enhanced persistent current that is sufficient to evoke EADs in a computational model of cardiac action potentials. This variant may also potentiate arrhythmia risk in infants. One study suggested that African-American SIDS victims are more often homozygous for SCN5A-S1103Y when compared with non-SIDS infant deaths.[65] This study further demonstrated that SCN5A-S1103Y channels exhibit a greater level of persistent sodium current when exposed to intracellular acidosis. A subsequent study demonstrated a significantly higher prevalence of heterozygous SCN5A-S1103Y carriers among 71 African-American cases of SIDS as compared with African-American controls.[68]

Impaired Impulse Propagation

Brugada Syndrome

Mutations in SCN5A have been identified in 20%–30% of BrS cases, a genetic form of idiopathic ventricular fibrillation.[69,70] Individuals with BrS have high risk for potentially lethal ventricular arrhythmias typically during sleep, but in the absence of myocardial ischemia, electrolyte abnormalities, or structural heart disease. Elevated risk for atrial fibrillation and intraventricular conduction abnormalities may also occur in BrS. Individuals with the disease may exhibit a characteristic baseline ECG pattern consisting of ST-segment elevation in the right precordial leads, but normal QT intervals.[71] Administration of sodium channel-blocking agents (e.g., procainamide, flecainide, or ajmaline) or fever may expose this ECG pattern in latent cases.[72,73] Inheritance is autosomal dominant, with incomplete, often low, penetrance and a substantial male predominance, but there is recent evidence that BrS may in fact be an oligogenic condition rather than a monogenic disorder.[10] At least 14 other genes have been associated with BrS, and some are proteins that modulate or interact with the cardiac sodium channel. The sudden unexplained death syndrome (SUDS) is clinically similar to BrS and causes sudden death, typically during sleep, in young and middle-aged males in Southeast Asian countries.[74] Additional information about BrS may be found in Chapter 92.

Chen and colleagues first identified three distinct *SCN5A* mutations in two unrelated BrS families and in a third sporadic case.[69] One mutation was missense (T1620M), while the other alleles included a frameshift caused by a single nucleotide deletion and a putative splice-site defect. More than 380 mutations have now been reported in BrS (see Fig. 50.1B). *SCN5A* mutations have also been identified in subjects with SUDS.[75] In contrast to those in LQT3, many mutations in BrS are predicted to cause protein truncation by causing frameshifts, premature stop codons, or aberrant mRNA splicing. These observations provided the first suggestion that sodium channel loss-of-function is responsible for the disorder.

The majority of *SCN5A* mutation–positive BrS subjects are heterozygous, but there have been a few reports of homozygous or compound heterozygous mutation carriers.[76,77] Most *SCN5A* mutation–positive BrS families exhibit low penetrance (i.e., low concordance between genotype and clinical disease). One attractive hypothesis to explain incomplete penetrance in BrS is the existence of genetic modifiers. Genetic variants in the *SCN5A* promoter may influence the clinical expression of heterozygous loss-of-function mutations.[78]

Reduced sodium current is the primary pathophysiological event in BrS, and this is consistent with *SCN5A* mutations predicted to encode nonfunctional channels.[69,79] Some missense mutations are also nonfunctional because of either impaired protein trafficking to the cell membrane or defective ion conductance.[80,81] Trafficking deficient mutants have the potential to exert a dominant-negative effect on the wildtype sodium channel.[82] Other missense mutations are functional but have biophysical defects predicted to reduce channel availability, such as altered voltage dependence of activation, more rapid fast inactivation, and enhanced slow inactivation.[83–85] One mutation (E1053K) disrupts binding of the channel to ankyrin-G, and this alters membrane trafficking and localization in cardiomyocytes.[86] Truncating or nonfunctional missense mutations are generally associated with more severe phenotypes.[87]

Another potential mechanism involves interactions between the wildtype and mutant sodium channel alleles. This idea was first suggested to explain the variable clinical expression of BrS in a family segregating a trafficking defective, missense mutation (R282H) in which an asymptomatic mutation carrier also carried a common variant (H558R) on the opposite allele.[88] In vitro experiments demonstrated that H558R rescued the trafficking defect through interactions between the two variant Na$_V$1.5 proteins.[89] Some *SCN5A* mutations discovered in BrS patients exhibit only minor biophysical defects but exert strong dominant-negative effects on the wildtype allele to cause an overall reduction in sodium current density.[90] Direct or indirect interactions between distinct Na$_V$1.5 subunits are postulated to explain this behavior.[91]

Reduced sodium current may also be the consequence of mutations in other genes that are less frequent causes of BrS including those encoding sodium channel auxiliary subunits (*SCN1B*, *SCN3B*)[92,93] and interacting proteins MOG1,[94] *GPD1L*,[94a] or plakophilin-2 (PKP2).[95] Mutations in *GPD1L* have been suggested to cause suppression of sodium current by a protein kinase C (PKC)–dependent mechanism that is linked with the redox state of the cell.[96,97] Specifically, reduced enzymatic activity of

mutant GPD1L protein is associated with an NADH/NAD$^+$ imbalance that can activate PKC and lead to phosphorylation of a specific serine residue (Ser-1503) in Na$_V$1.5, causing reduced channel activity. PKP2 is a desmosomal protein originally associated with arrhythmogenic cardiomyopathy (see Chapter 87), but it has recently been identified as a component of the sodium channel macromolecular complex (see Chapter 22) that facilitates trafficking of channels to the intercalated disk. Loss-of-function mutations in PKP2 cause diminished sodium current in cardiomyocytes, consistent with a molecular mechanism for BrS.

There have been two proposed mechanisms to explain the cellular and tissue basis of BrS, both implicating electrophysiological defects in the right ventricle.[98,99] In one mechanism, a reduction in myocardial sodium current exaggerates differences in action potential duration between the endocardium and epicardium.[100–102] These differences occur because of unequal distribution of transient outward current (I$_{to}$), a repolarizing current more prominent in the epicardial layer that contributes to the characteristic spike and dome shape of the action potential. Reduced sodium current will cause disproportionate shortening of epicardial action potentials because of unopposed I$_{to}$, leading to an exaggerated transmural voltage-gradient, dispersion of repolarization, and a substrate-promoting phase 2 reentry. This mechanism is supported by elegant work using the arterial-perfused canine ventricular wedge preparation.[100,101] The second hypothesis posits that the main effect of reduced sodium current is a slowing of impulse conduction in the right ventricle and delayed activation of the right ventricular outflow tract (RVOT).[98,103–105] This mechanism has gained support primarily from clinical observations including electroanatomical mapping studies[106,107] and the observed therapeutic benefit of epicardial ablation over the RVOT.[108] It is not clear whether these two hypotheses are mutually exclusive or whether all cases of BrS have the same underlying pathophysiological mechanism.

Heterozygous *Scn5a* knockout mice (*Scn5a$^{+/-}$*) have provided an animal model of BrS.[109–111] Hearts from young *Scn5a$^{+/-}$* mice exhibit conduction slowing in the right ventricle and an increased propensity for ventricular tachycardia, features which are aggravated by flecainide. The arrhythmia has been demonstrated to originate in the RVOT both in vivo and ex vivo. Although data from investigations of *Scn5a$^{+/-}$* mice tend to support the hypothesis of conduction slowing as the primary electrophysiological defect in BrS, mouse ventricular action potentials lack a plateau phase, making this a suboptimal model for testing the alternative mechanism. In older *Scn5a$^{+/-}$* mice, progressive fibrosis and conduction slowing occur in both ventricles, providing a model system with which to understand conduction system disorders associated with *SCN5A* mutations. A novel porcine model of sodium channelopathy was developed on the basis of a truncating *SCN5A* mutation associated with BrS, but the genetically engineered pigs primarily exhibited impaired conduction without ventricular arrhythmia.[112] In vitro studies of intact hearts from this porcine model revealed spontaneous ventricular fibrillation originating in the right ventricle.

Familial Progressive Conduction System Disease

Mutations in *SCN5A* have been associated with a heterogeneous group of disorders that are characterized by impaired cardiac conduction and manifest as abnormal AV conduction (AV block), slowed intraventricular conduction, and/or atrial inexcitability (atrial standstill).[113–116] The degree of impaired cardiac conduction often progresses with advancing age. Inheritance may be autosomal dominant or autosomal recessive, but in rare cases, digenic inheritance has been observed (see the following text).[115,117,118]

Age-related defects in conduction along the His–Purkinje system have been referred to as Lenègre or Lev disease and may be caused by progressive fibrosis of the specialized conducting tissues in the heart.[119] However, clinically similar conditions may be inherited and associated with *SCN5A* mutations.[120] Many names have been applied to this genetic subtype including progressive cardiac conduction disease, familial AV block, and hereditary Lenègre disease. The clinical phenotypes may present in either early childhood or adulthood. In children, progressive AV block is most typical, whereas adults with these disorders usually have intraventricular conduction abnormalities, such as right or left bundle branch block.

More than 30 *SCN5A* mutations have been associated with cardiac conduction diseases such as congenital sick sinus syndrome and atrial standstill (see Fig. 50.1B). The first mutations described by Schott and colleagues were predicted to be complete loss-of-function alleles.[113] Several missense mutations have since been characterized in vitro, and these alleles are either nonfunctional or exhibit complex biophysical abnormalities that are predicted to reduce peak sodium current density at physiological voltages.[114,121] In the case of G514C, a missense mutation segregating with conduction disease in a Dutch family, the mutant sodium channel exhibited unequal depolarizing shifts in the voltage dependence of activation and inactivation such that a smaller number of channels were activated at typical threshold voltages.[121] Computational modeling of these changes supported reduced conduction velocity, but the level of predicted sodium current loss was not sufficient to evoke shortened epicardial action potentials, offering a plausible explanation why these individuals did not manifest BrS. Other missense mutations cause enhanced slow inactivation, a gating process that regulates channel availability over a time course of several seconds to minutes.[114] Lower peak sodium current impairs conduction velocity by slowing the rate of change in membrane potential (dV/dt) during the action potential.

As previously discussed, aging $Scn5a^{+/-}$ mice variably develop progressive conduction system fibrosis and impaired impulse conduction through both ventricles. The molecular basis of fibrosis is unknown but has been correlated with increased expression of transforming growth factor β_1 (TGF-β_1) and reduced expression of the gap junction protein connexin (Cx)40 in heart tissue.[122,123] The degree of fibrosis and severity of impaired conduction in $Scn5a^{+/-}$ mice correlates with the residual level of sodium channel protein, but the underlying mechanism for variable protein levels is unknown.[124] Observations made in $Scn5a^{+/-}$ mice illustrate a continuum of pathophysiological events associated with loss-of-function *SCN5A* mutations and help to explain the co-occurrence of BrS and conduction system diseases, which have been termed "overlap syndromes."

Congenital Sick Sinus Syndrome and Atrial Standstill

Whereas most *SCN5A*-linked disorders manifest clinically with abnormal ventricular excitability or conduction, there are less common syndromes in which mutant sodium channels disproportionately affect atrial electrical activity. In familial atrial standstill and congenital sick sinus syndrome, *SCN5A* mutations cause sinus node dysfunction, which progresses to atrial inexcitability and symptomatic bradycardia in children or young adults. Fetal bradycardia or irregular fetal heart rate may be early signs of the condition during gestation. Surface ECG recordings demonstrate an absence of P waves and a slow AV-junctional rhythm. Electrophysiological studies may reveal prolonged His-ventricular conduction, indicating a more generalized defect in cardiac conduction. In these conditions, the atria, but not the ventricles, are refractory to electrical pacing.

Families with these disorders caused by *SCN5A* mutations may exhibit recessive inheritance. In congenital sick sinus syndrome, affected individuals inherit a nonfunctional or severely dysfunctional *SCN5A* mutation from one parent and a less severely impaired allele from the other.[116] Some of these mutations impair trafficking of the sodium channel protein to the plasma membrane.[125] Heterozygous parents are asymptomatic but may have subclinical first-degree AV block. In addition to compound heterozygous *SCN5A* mutations, similar phenotypes have been associated with homozygous alleles.[117] Familial atrial standstill has also been associated with heterozygous *SCN5A* mutations coinherited with a common promoter variant in the Cx40 gene that is predicted to reduce gene expression.[115,118] In these families, inheritance of the sodium channel mutation alone was not sufficient to evoke a clinical phenotype, a finding consistent with digenic inheritance.

The mechanisms by which *SCN5A* mutations impair sinus node dysfunction have been explored using action potential modeling and studies of $Scn5a^{+/-}$ mice.[126,127] In single-cell action potential simulations, reduced sodium current slows pacing in the peripheral sinoatrial node (SAN) cells but not the central SAN cells, which are primarily responsible for cardiac rhythm and lack sodium channels. In multicellular simulations, reduced sodium current impairs conduction from SAN to surrounding atrial tissue, leading to sinoatrial exit block. These predictions are consistent with observations made in $Scn5a^{+/-}$ mice.[127]

Altered Intracellular Ion Homeostasis

Dilated Cardiomyopathy With Arrhythmia

Mutations affecting cardiac ion channels primarily cause disorders of heart rhythm, whereas familial cardiomyopathy is typically associated with mutations in genes encoding sarcomeric or contractile proteins. An exception to this paradigm is represented by *SCN5A* mutations associated with heart failure, combined variably with atrial and ventricular arrhythmias. McNair and colleagues first reported that a missense mutation, *SCN5A*-D1275N, segregated with a phenotype including dilated cardiomyopathy (DCM), abnormal AV conduction, sinus node dysfunction, and atrial and ventricular arrhythmias in a four-generation kindred.[128] Subsequent studies have revealed additional mutations associated with similar clinical phenotypes described variably as peripartum dilated cardiomyopathy,[129,130] arrhythmic dilated cardiomyopathy,[131] escape capture bigeminy and cardiomyopathy,[132] reversible ventricular ectopy and dilated cardiomyopathy, or multifocal ectopic Purkinje–related premature contractions.[133] Most of these reports emphasized the high burden of ectopic premature ventricular beats (PVBs) and impaired cardiac contractility with the variable presence of atrial tachyarrhythmias.[129–136] Inheritance is most consistent with autosomal dominant with incomplete penetrance except in sporadic cases. Mutation carriers may have frequent, multifocal PVBs that originate in Purkinje fibers.[132,133] Suppression of ventricular ectopy using quinidine or amiodarone has been reported to improve myocardial contractility in some cases.[133,137]

Specific patterns of sodium channel dysfunction have been elucidated for mutations associated with these syndromes. The *SCN5A*-R814W mutation associated with this syndrome exhibited a novel in vitro biophysical phenotype. This mutation, which affects a conserved arginine residue in the D2/S4 voltage-sensing segment, caused a hyperpolarized shift in the voltage dependence of activation (Fig. 50.3A).[138] Subsequently, the same biophysical defect was observed for two other mutations involving different conserved arginine residues in the D1/S4 segment (R222Q, R225P).[132,133,137] These observations led to the prediction that channels might be active at voltages nearing the cardiomyocyte resting membrane potential. Aberrant activation of sodium current nearing the myocyte resting membrane potential can be demonstrated in heterologous cells expressing R814W, R222Q, or R225P subjected to slow voltage ramps (see Fig. 50.3B).[137,138] This phenomenon differs from that observed for LQT3 mutations in that peak current activation during voltage ramps for those mutations occurs at more positive potentials.[139] The tendency for diastolic sodium current activation may predispose

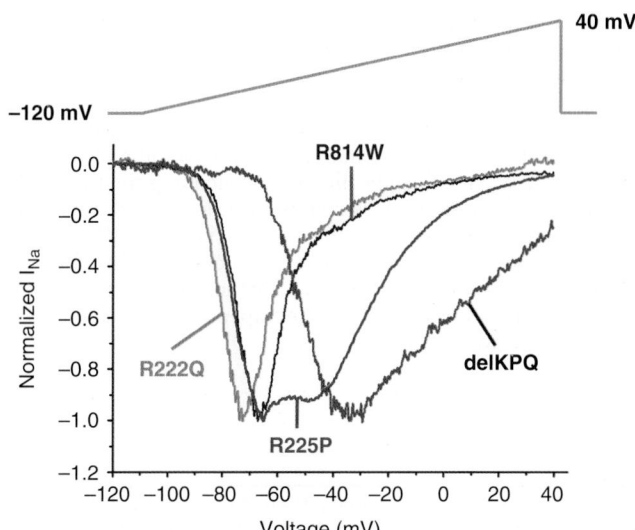

FIGURE 50.3 Aberrant mutant sodium current activation in dilated cardiomyopathy. Activation of sodium current during a voltage ramp from −120 mV to +40 mV for WT-Na$_V$1.5 and mutants associates either with cardiomyopathy (R222Q, R225P, and R814W) or LQT3 (delKPQ). Mutations associated with cardiomyopathy exhibit aberrant activation, with the peak current occurring at voltages nearing the resting membrane potential, suggesting a predisposition to diastolic sodium current. In contrast, peak activation of the LQT3 mutant occurs at −30 mV.

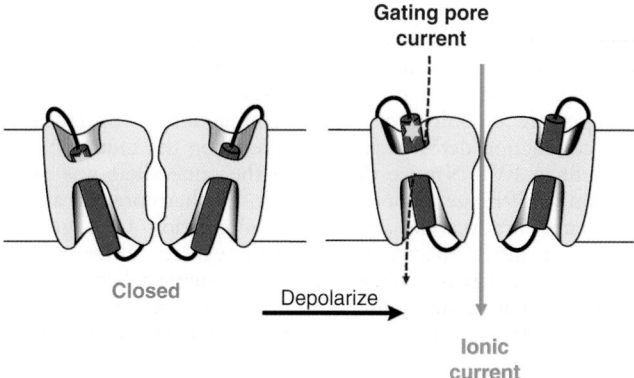

FIGURE 50.4 Sodium channel gating pore current. Cartoon illustrating the different pathways through which ionic current and gating pore current are conducted. *Red cylinders* represent S4 segments, and the *yellow star* represents the approximate location of the SCN5A mutation R219H.

myocytes to disordered intracellular sodium and calcium ion homeostasis, leading to myocardial dysfunction.

Another *SCN5A* mutation associated with DCM (R219H) predisposes to altered intracellular ion homeostasis by a novel mechanism.[135] This mutation replaces the most extracellular arginine residue in the D1/S4 voltage-sensing segment with histidine, but this substitution has no overt effects on channel function. However, cells expressing this mutant sodium channel exhibited rapid internal acidification when exposed to a pH gradient. This finding was explained by the generation of a proton leak current through mutant sodium channels, but the leak does not occur through the normal pathway for sodium ions. Rather, protons are conducted through the "gating pore" consisting of an aqueous channel surrounding the S4 segment (Fig. 50.4). An aberrant proton leak current may create an unstable myocyte membrane potential, possibly evoking PVBs, or may adversely affect contractile proteins through altered intracellular pH. The increased intracellular proton concentration may also stimulate a cascade of ion exchange events (Na$^+$/H$^+$; Na$^+$/Ca^{2+}) that perturb Ca^{2+} homeostasis with long-term deleterious effects on myocardial contractility. Further studies revealed that this mechanism (aberrant gate pore current) may be shared among other *SCN5A* mutations affecting voltage-sensing segments that are associated with cardiomyopathy.[140–142]

One particular *SCN5A* mutation (D1275N) associated with DCM and a variety of conduction disorders, including sinus node dysfunction, causes a complex cardiac phenotype in mice.[143] Mice engineered to be homozygous for the human *SCN5A*-D1275N mutation exhibit bradycardia and impaired atrial and ventricular conduction while young (3–12 weeks) but then progress to develop spontaneous ventricular tachycardia and nonfibrotic DCM when older. Sodium currents in homozygous mutant mice have markedly reduced amplitude and abnormal inactivation gating, including slow kinetics, enhanced persistent current, and depolarized voltage dependence. Interestingly, studies of heterologously expressed *SCN5A*-D1275N channels demonstrated none of these functional abnormalities, prompting speculation

that myocyte-specific factors are required for full expression of the phenotype. Another potential explanation relates to genetic modifiers or environmental factors as suggested by the highly variable nature of the phenotypes associated with this mutation in humans.[115,128,134,144]

Syndromes With Complex Mechanisms

Mutations in *SCN5A* have been associated with complex phenotypes ("overlap syndromes") featuring characteristics of two or more syndromes. Mutant cardiac sodium channels associated with overlap syndromes exhibit more complex functional defects. The in-frame insertion mutation (*SCN5A*-1795insD) identified in a family segregating both LQTS and BrS causes an inactivation defect, resulting in enhanced persistent sodium current typical of LQT3, but also confers enhanced slow inactivation with reduced channel availability that is more consistent with BrS.[145] The combination of enhanced persistent sodium current with enhanced slow inactivation has also been observed with mutation *SCN5A*-E1784K associated with a highly penetrant form of LQT3 and concurrent features of BrS or sinus node dysfunction in some carriers.[146] These distinct biophysical abnormalities have been predicted to predispose to ventricular arrhythmia by different mechanisms at opposite extremes of heart rate.[36] While enhanced persistent current will prolong action potentials especially at slow heart rates, enhanced slow inactivation will predispose to activity-dependent loss of sodium channel availability at fast rates. These findings were confirmed in a mouse model genetically engineered with the *SCN5A*-1795insD mutation[147] and in patient-derived iPSC-cardiomyocytes.[148] In another unusual case, deletion of lysine-1500 in *SCN5A* was associated with the unique combination of LQTS, BrS, and impaired cardiac conduction in the same family.[149] This mutation impairs inactivation, causing enhanced persistent sodium current, but also reduces sodium channel availability by opposite shifts in voltage dependence of inactivation and activation.

A novel *SCN5A* mutation (H1849R), which disrupts the binding site for an interacting protein (fibroblast growth factor homologous factor; see Chapters 18 and 19), causes profound dysfunction of the cardiac sodium channel (dramatic slowing of inactivation) and is associated with autosomal dominant inheritance of atrial and ventricular cardiac arrhythmias.[150] This case illustrates the complexity and severity of arrhythmia phenotypes resulting from impaired interaction between regulatory proteins and cardiac sodium channel.

Certain *SCN5A* mutations may be associated with different clinical manifestations in different families (e.g., D1275N, see previous text),[115,128,134,144] or even among members of the same family,[151] perhaps because of host-specific factors such as modifier genes that influence the final clinical expression. In the mouse model of the *SCN5A*-1795insD mutation, evidence for strain-dependent phenotype severity prompted a search for genetic modifiers of cardiac conduction.[152] Specifically, the conduction defect was less severe when the mutation was present in FVB/N mice than when the same allele was present on a 129P2 genomic background. Furthermore, flecainide worsened bradycardia and QRS prolongation to a greater degree in 129P2 than in FVB/N mutant mice. Differences in functional behavior of cardiac sodium current between the two strains were also observed. Specifically, sodium currents recorded from 129P2 myocytes exhibited a depolarizing shift in the conductance–voltage relationship compared with those recorded from FVB/N myocytes. This finding suggested that insufficient sodium channel activation was the underlying mechanism of impaired conduction velocity, an idea corroborated by computational modeling. Differences in cardiac gene expression between strains may contribute to these differences in sodium currents. Specifically, *Scn4b*, encoding the β_4 sodium channel auxiliary subunit, is expressed at a substantially lower level in right ventricular tissue from 129P2 mice.[152] Several other divergent patterns of gene expression were also observed but the significance was unclear. Further studies to uncover genetic modifiers may yield new therapeutic targets and enable better risk-stratification strategies.

REFERENCES

1. Schroeter A, Walzik S, Blechschmidt S, et al. Structure and function of splice variants of the cardiac voltage-gated sodium channel Na$_V$1.5. *J Mol Cell Cardiol*. 2010;49:16–24.
2. Makielski JC, Ye B, Valdivia CR, et al. A ubiquitous splice variant and a common polymorphism affect heterologous expression of recombinant human SCN5A heart sodium channels. *Circ Res*. 2003;93:821–828.
3. Tan BH, Valdivia CR, Rok BA, et al. Common human SCN5A polymorphisms have altered electrophysiology when expressed in Q1077 splice variants. *Heart Rhythm*. 2005;2:741–747.
4. Tan BH, Valdivia CR, Song C, et al. Partial expression defect for the SCN5A missense mutation G1406R depends upon splice variant background Q1077 and rescue by mexiletine. *Am J Physiol Heart Circ Physiol*. 2006;291:H1822–H1828.
5. Ou SW, Kameyama A, Hao LY, et al. Tetrodotoxin-resistant Na$^+$ channels in human neuroblastoma cells are encoded by new variants of Na$_V$1.5/SCN5A. *Eur J Neurosci*. 2005;22:793–801.
6. Murphy LL, Moon-Grady AJ, Cuneo BF, et al. Developmentally regulated SCN5A splice variant potentiates dysfunction of a novel mutation associated with severe fetal arrhythmia. *Heart Rhythm*. 2011;9:590–597.
7. Atack TC, Stroud DM, Watanabe H, et al. Informatic and functional approaches to identifying a regulatory region for the cardiac sodium channel. *Circ Res*. 2011;109:38–46.
8. Bezzina CR, Shimizu W, Yang P, et al. Common sodium channel promoter haplotype in Asian subjects underlies variability in cardiac conduction. *Circulation*. 2006;113:338–344.
9. Chambers JC, Zhao J, Terracciano CM, et al. Genetic variation in SCN10A influences cardiac conduction. *Nat Genet*. 2010;42:149–152.
10. Bezzina CR, Barc J, Mizusawa Y, et al. Common variants at SCN5A-SCN10A and HEY2 are associated with Brugada syndrome, a rare disease with high risk of sudden cardiac death. *Nat Genet*. 2013;45:1409.
11. van den BM, Wong LY, Tessadori F, et al. Genetic variation in T-box binding element functionally affects SCN5A/SCN10A enhancer. *J Clin Invest*. 2012;122:2519–2530.
12. van den Boogaard M, Smemo S, Burnicka-Turek O, et al. A common genetic variant within SCN10A modulates cardiac SCN5A expression. *J Clin Invest*. 2014;124:1844–1852.
13. Kaufmann SG, Westenbroek RE, Maass AH, et al. Functional protein expression of multiple sodium channel alpha- and beta-subunit isoforms in neonatal cardiomyocytes. *J Mol Cell Cardiol*. 2010;48:261–269.
14. Abriel H. Cardiac sodium channel Na$_V$1.5 and interacting proteins: physiology and pathophysiology. *J Mol Cell Cardiol*. 2010;48:2–11.
15. Wilde AA, Brugada R. Phenotypical manifestations of mutations in the genes encoding subunits of the cardiac sodium channel. *Circ Res*. 2011;108:884–897.
16. Wang DW, Crotti L, Shimizu W, et al. Malignant perinatal variant of long-QT syndrome caused by a profoundly dysfunctional cardiac sodium channel. *Circ Arrhythm Electrophysiol*. 2008;1:370–378.
17. Kapplinger JD, Tester DJ, Salisbury BA, et al. Spectrum and prevalence of mutations from the first 2,500 consecutive unrelated patients referred for the FAMILION long QT syndrome genetic test. *Heart Rhythm*. 2009;6:1297–1303.
18. Horigome H, Nagashima M, Sumitomo N, et al. Clinical characteristics and genetic background of congenital long-QT syndrome diagnosed in fetal, neonatal, and infantile life: a nationwide questionnaire survey in Japan. *Circ Arrhythm Electrophysiol*. 2010;3:10–17.
19. Wang Q, Shen J, Splawski I, et al. *SCN5A* mutations associated with an inherited cardiac arrhythmia, long QT syndrome. *Cell*. 1995;80:805–811.
20. Ben-Johny M, Yang PS, Niu J, et al. Conservation of Ca^{2+}/calmodulin regulation across Na and Ca^{2+} channels. *Cell*. 2014;157:1657–1670.
21. Schwartz PJ, Priori SG, Spazzolini C, et al. Genotype-phenotype correlation in the long-QT syndrome: gene-specific triggers for life-threatening arrhythmias. *Circulation*. 2001;103:89–95.
22. Zhang L, Timothy KW, Vincent GM, et al. Spectrum of ST-T-wave patterns and repolarization parameters in congenital long-QT syndrome: ECG findings identify genotypes. *Circulation*. 2000;102:2849–2855.
23. Zareba W, Moss AJ, Locati EH, et al. Modulating effects of age and gender on the clinical course of long QT syndrome by genotype. *J Am Coll Cardiol*. 2003;42:103–109.
24. Priori SG, Schwartz PJ, Napolitano C, et al. Risk stratification in the long-QT syndrome. *N Engl J Med*. 2003;348:1866–1874.
25. Bennett PB, Yazawa K, Makita N, et al. Molecular mechanism for an inherited cardiac arrhythmia. *Nature*. 1995;376:683–685.
26. Kambouris NG, Nuss HB, Johns DC, et al. Phenotypic characterization of a novel long-QT syndrome mutation (R1623Q) in the cardiac sodium channel. *Circulation*. 1998;97:640–644.
27. Abriel H, Cabo C, Wehrens XH, et al. Novel arrhythmogenic mechanism revealed by a long-QT syndrome mutation in the cardiac Na$^+$ channel. *Circ Res*. 2001;88:740–745.
28. Horne AJ, Eldstrom J, Sanatani S, et al. A novel mechanism for LQT3 with 2:1 block: a pore-lining mutation in Na$_V$1.5 significantly affects voltage-dependence of activation. *Heart Rhythm*. 2011;8:770–777.
29. Medeiros-Domingo A, Kaku T, Tester DJ, et al. *SCN4B*-encoded sodium channel β_4 subunit in congenital long-QT syndrome. *Circulation*. 2007;116:134–142.
30. Vatta M, Ackerman MJ, Ye B, et al. Mutant caveolin-3 induces persistent late sodium current and is associated with long-QT syndrome. *Circulation*. 2006;114:2104–2112.
31. Cheng J, Van Norstrand DW, Medeiros-Domingo A, et al. Alpha1-syntrophin mutations identified in sudden infant death syndrome cause an increase in late cardiac sodium current. *Circ Arrhythm Electrophysiol*. 2009;2:667–676.
32. Ueda K, Valdivia C, Medeiros-Domingo A, et al. Syntrophin mutation associated with long QT syndrome through activation of the nNOS-SCN5A macromolecular complex. *Proc Natl Acad Sci U S A*. 2008;105:9355–9360.
33. Clancy CE, Rudy Y. Linking a genetic defect to its cellular phenotype in a cardiac arrhythmia. *Nature*. 1999;400:566–569.
34. Fabritz L, Kirchhof P, Franz MR, et al. Effect of pacing and mexiletine on dispersion of repolarisation and arrhythmias in DeltaKPQ SCN5A (long QT3) mice. *Cardiovasc Res*. 2003;57:1085–1093.
35. Iyer V, Roman-Campos D, Sampson KJ, et al. Purkinje cells as sources of arrhythmias in long QT syndrome type 3. *Sci Rep*. 2015;5:13287.
36. Clancy CE, Rudy Y. Na$^+$ channel mutation that causes both Brugada and long-QT syndrome phenotypes: a simulation study of mechanism. *Circulation*. 2002;105:1208–1213.
37. Nuyens D, Stengl M, Dugarmaa S, et al. Abrupt rate accelerations or premature beats cause life-threatening arrhythmias in mice with long-QT3 syndrome. *Nature Med*. 2001;7:1021–1027.
38. Fabritz L, Damke D, Emmerich M, et al. Autonomic modulation and antiarrhythmic therapy in a model of long QT syndrome type 3. *Cardiovasc Res*. 2010;87:60–72.
39. Fredj S, Lindegger N, Sampson KJ, et al. Altered Na+ channels promote pause-induced spontaneous diastolic activity in long QT syndrome type 3 myocytes. *Circ Res*. 2006;99:1225–1232.
40. Potet F, Beckermann TM, Kunic JD, et al. Intracellular calcium attenuates late current conducted by mutant human cardiac sodium channels. *Circ Arrhythm Electrophysiol*. 2015;8:933–941.
41. Terrenoire C, Wang K, Tung KW, et al. Induced pluripotent stem cells used to reveal drug actions in a long QT syndrome family with complex genetics. *J Gen Physiol*. 2013;141:61–72.
42. Spencer CI, Baba S, Nakamura K, et al. Calcium transients closely reflect prolonged action potentials in iPSC models of inherited cardiac arrhythmia. *Stem Cell Reports*. 2014;3:269–281.
43. Ma D, Wei H, Zhao Y, et al. Modeling type 3 long QT syndrome with cardiomyocytes derived from patient-specific induced pluripotent stem cells. *Int J Cardiol*. 2013;168:5277–5286.
44. Fatima A, Kaifeng S, Dittmann S, et al. The disease-specific phenotype in cardiomyocytes derived from induced pluripotent stem cells of two long QT syndrome type 3 patients. *PLoS ONE*. 2013;8:e83005.
45. Schwartz PJ, Priori SG, Locati EH, et al. Long QT syndrome patients with mutations of the *SCN5A* and *HERG* genes have differential responses to Na$^+$ channel blockade and to increases in heart rate - Implications for gene-specific therapy. *Circulation*. 1995;92:3381–3386.
46. Wang DW, Yazawa K, Makita N, et al. Pharmacological targeting of long QT mutant sodium channels. *J Clin Invest*. 1997;99:1714–1720.
47. Windle JR, Geletka RC, Moss AJ, et al. Normalization of ventricular repolarization with flecainide in long QT syndrome patients with SCN5A: DeltaKPQ mutation. *Ann Noninvasive Electrocardiol*. 2001;6:153–158.
48. Abriel H, Wehrens XH, Benhorin J, et al. Molecular pharmacology of the sodium channel mutation D1790G linked to the long-QT syndrome. *Circulation*. 2000;102:921–925.
49. Tian XL, Yong SL, Wan X, et al. Mechanisms by which *SCN5A* mutation N1325S causes cardiac arrhythmias and sudden death *in vivo*. *Cardiovasc Res*. 2004;61:256–267.
50. Fredj S, Sampson KJ, Liu H, et al. Molecular basis of ranolazine block of LQT-3 mutant sodium channels: evidence for site of action. *Br J Pharmacol*. 2006;148:16–24.
51. Moss AJ, Zareba W, Schwarz KQ, et al. Ranolazine shortens repolarization in patients with sustained inward sodium current due to type-3 long-QT syndrome. *J Cardiovasc Electrophysiol*. 2008;19:1289–1293.
52. van Den Berg MP, van den Heuvel HF, van Tintelen JP, et al. Successful treatment of a patient with symptomatic long QT syndrome type 3 using ranolazine combined with a beta-blocker. *Int J Cardiol*. 2014;171:90–92.
53. Wang DW, Mistry AM, Kahlig KM, et al. Propranolol blocks cardiac and neuronal voltage-gated sodium channels. *Front Pharmacol*. 2010;1:144.
54. Besana A, Wang DW, George Jr AL, et al. Nadolol block of Na$_V$1.5 does not explain its efficacy in the long QT syndrome. *J Cardiovasc Pharmacol*. 2011;59:249–253.
55. Bankston JR, Kass RS. Molecular determinants of local anesthetic action of beta-blocking drugs: Implications for therapeutic management of long QT syndrome variant 3. *J Mol Cell Cardiol*. 2010;48:246–253.

56. Calvillo L, Spazzolini C, Vullo E, et al. Propranolol prevents life-threatening arrhythmias in LQT3 transgenic mice: implications for the clinical management of LQT3 patients. *Heart Rhythm*. 2014;11:126–132.
57. Hofbeck M, Ulmer H, Beinder E, et al. Prenatal findings in patients with prolonged QT interval in the neonatal period. *Heart*. 1997;77:198–204.
58. Bankston JR, Yue M, Chung W, et al. A novel and lethal de novo LQT-3 mutation in a newborn with distinct molecular pharmacology and therapeutic response. *PLoS ONE*. 2007;2:e1258.
59. Kehl HG, Haverkamp W, Rellensmann G, et al. Images in cardiovascular medicine. Life-threatening neonatal arrhythmia: successful treatment and confirmation of clinically suspected extreme long QT-syndrome-3. *Circulation*. 2004;109:e205–e206.
60. Wedekind H, Smits JP, Schulze-Bahr E, et al. De novo mutation in the SCN5A gene associated with early onset of sudden infant death. *Circulation*. 2001;104:1158–1164.
61. Chang CC, Acharfi S, Wu MH, et al. A novel SCN5A mutation manifests as a malignant form of long QT syndrome with perinatal onset of tachycardia/bradycardia. *Cardiovasc Res*. 2004;64:268–278.
62. Ackerman MJ, Siu BL, Sturner WQ, et al. Postmortem molecular analysis of SCN5A defects in sudden infant death syndrome. *JAMA*. 2001;286:2264–2269.
63. Arnestad M, Crotti L, Rognum TO, et al. Prevalence of long-QT syndrome gene variants in sudden infant death syndrome. *Circulation*. 2007;115:361–367.
64. Schwartz PJ, Priori SG, Dumaine R, et al. A molecular link between the sudden infant death syndrome and the long-QT syndrome. *N Engl J Med*. 2000;343:262–267.
65. Plant LD, Bowers PN, Liu Q, et al. A common cardiac sodium channel variant associated with sudden infant death in African Americans, SCN5A S1103Y. *J Clin Invest*. 2006;116:430–435.
66. Wang DW, Desai RR, Crotti L, et al. Cardiac sodium channel dysfunction in sudden infant death syndrome. *Circulation*. 2007;115:368–376.
67. Splawski I, Timothy KW, Tateyama M, et al. Variant of SCN5A sodium channel implicated in risk of cardiac arrhythmia. *Science*. 2002;297:1333–1336.
68. Van Norstrand DW, Tester DJ, Ackerman MJ. Overrepresentation of the proarrhythmic, sudden death predisposing sodium channel polymorphism S1103Y in a population-based cohort of African-American sudden infant death syndrome. *Heart Rhythm*. 2008;5:712–715.
69. Chen Q, Kirsch GE, Zhang D, et al. Genetic basis and molecular mechanism for idiopathic ventricular fibrillation. *Nature*. 1998;392:293–296.
70. Akai J, Makita N, Sakurada H, et al. A novel SCN5A mutation associated with idiopathic ventricular fibrillation without typical ECG findings of Brugada syndrome. *FEBS Lett*. 2000;479:29–34.
71. Brugada J, Brugada P. Further characterization of the syndrome of right bundle branch block, ST segment elevation, and sudden cardiac death. *J Cardiovasc Electrophysiol*. 1997;8:325–331.
72. Brugada R, Brugada J, Antzelevitch C, et al. Sodium channel blockers identify risk for sudden death in patients with ST-segment elevation and right bundle branch block but structurally normal hearts. *Circulation*. 2000;101:510–515.
73. Keller DI, Huang H, Zhao J, et al. A novel SCN5A mutation, F1344S, identified in a patient with Brugada syndrome and fever-induced ventricular fibrillation. *Cardiovasc Res*. 2006;70:521–529.
74. Nademanee K, Veerakul G, Nimmannit S, et al. Arrhythmogenic marker for the sudden unexplained death syndrome in Thai men. *Circulation*. 1997;96:2595–2600.
75. Vatta M, Dumaine R, Varghese G, et al. Genetic and biophysical basis of sudden unexplained nocturnal death syndrome (SUNDS), a disease allelic to Brugada syndrome. *Hum Mol Genet*. 2002;11:337–345.
76. Cordeiro JM, Barajas-Martinez H, Hong K, et al. Compound heterozygous mutations P336L and I1660V in the human cardiac sodium channel associated with the Brugada syndrome. *Circulation*. 2006;114:2026–2033.
77. Frigo G, Rampazzo A, Bauce B, et al. Homozygous SCN5A mutation in Brugada syndrome with monomorphic ventricular tachycardia and structural heart abnormalities. *Europace*. 2007;9:391–397.
78. Park JK, Martin LJ, Zhang X, et al. Genetic variants in SCN5A promoter are associated with arrhythmia phenotype severity in patients with heterozygous loss-of-function mutation. *Heart Rhythm*. 2012;9:1090–1096.
79. Schulze-Bahr E, Eckardt L, Breithardt G, et al. Sodium channel gene (SCN5A) mutations in 44 index patients with Brugada syndrome: different incidences in familial and sporadic disease. *Hum Mutat*. 2003;21:651–652.
80. Baroudi G, Pouliot V, Denjoy I, et al. Novel mechanism for Brugada syndrome: defective surface localization of an SCN5A mutant (R1432G). *Circ Res*. 2001;88:E78–E83.
81. Valdivia CR, Tester DJ, Rok BA, et al. A trafficking defective, Brugada syndrome-causing SCN5A mutation rescued by drugs. *Cardiovasc Res*. 2004;62:53–62.
82. Clatot J, Ziyadeh-Isleem A, Maugenre S, et al. Dominant-negative effect of SCN5A N-terminal mutations through the interaction of $Na_V1.5$ alpha-subunits. *Cardiovasc Res*. 2012;96:53–63.
83. Dumaine R, Towbin JA, Brugada P, et al. Ionic mechanisms responsible for the electrocardiographic phenotype of the Brugada syndrome are temperature dependent. *Circ Res*. 1999;85:803–809.
84. Wang DW, Makita N, Kitabatake A, et al. Enhanced Na^+ channel intermediate inactivation in Brugada syndrome. *Circ Res*. 2000;87:E37–E43.
85. Rook MB, Alshinawi CB, Groenewegen WA, et al. Human SCN5A gene mutations alter cardiac sodium channel kinetics and are associated with the Brugada syndrome. *Cardiovasc Res*. 1999;44:507–517.
86. Mohler PJ, Rivolta I, Napolitano C, et al. $Na_V1.5$ E1053K mutation causing Brugada syndrome blocks binding to ankyrin-G and expression of $Na_V1.5$ on the surface of cardiomyocytes. *Proc Natl Acad Sci U S A*. 2004;101:17533–17538.
87. Meregalli PG, Tan HL, Probst V, et al. Type of SCN5A mutation determines clinical severity and degree of conduction slowing in loss-of-function sodium channelopathies. *Heart Rhythm*. 2009;6:341–348.
88. Poelzing S, Forleo C, Samodell M, et al. SCN5A polymorphism restores trafficking of a Brugada syndrome mutation on a separate gene. *Circulation*. 2006;114:368–376.
89. Shinlapawittayatorn K, Dudash LA, Du XX, et al. A novel strategy using cardiac sodium channel polymorphic fragments to rescue trafficking-deficient SCN5A mutations. *Circ Cardiovasc Genet*. 2011;4:500–509.
90. Hoshi M, Du XX, Shinlapawittayatorn K, et al. Brugada syndrome disease phenotype explained in apparently benign sodium channel mutations. *Circ Cardiovasc Genet*. 2014;7:123–131.
91. Clatot J, Ziyadeh-Isleem A, Maugenre S, et al. Dominant-negative effect of SCN5A N-terminal mutations through the interaction of $Na_V1.5$ alpha-subunits. *Cardiovasc Res*. 2012;96:53–63.
92. Watanabe H, Koopmann TT, Le SS, et al. Sodium channel beta1 subunit mutations associated with Brugada syndrome and cardiac conduction disease in humans. *J Clin Invest*. 2008;118:2260–2268.
93. Hu D, Barajas-Martinez H, Burashnikov E, et al. A mutation in the beta 3 subunit of the cardiac sodium channel associated with Brugada ECG phenotype. *Circ Cardiovasc Genet*. 2009;2:270–278.
94. Kattygnarath D, Maugenre S, Neyroud N, et al. MOG1: a new susceptibility gene for Brugada syndrome. *Circ Cardiovasc Genet*. 2011;4:261–268.
94a. London B, Michalec M, Mehdi H, et al. Mutation in glycerol-3-phosphate dehydrogenase 1 like gene (GPD1-L) decreases cardiac Na+ current and causes inherited arrhythmias. *Circulation*. 2007;116:2260–2268.
95. Cerrone M, Lin X, Zhang M, et al. Missense mutations in plakophilin-2 cause sodium current deficit and associate with a Brugada syndrome phenotype. *Circulation*. 2014;129:1092–1103.
96. Valdivia CR, Ueda K, Ackerman MJ, et al. GPD1L links redox state to cardiac excitability by PKC-dependent phosphorylation of the sodium channel SCN5A. *Am J Physiol Heart Circ Physiol*. 2009;297:H1446–H1452.
97. Liu M, Sanyal S, Gao G, et al. Cardiac Na^+ current regulation by pyridine nucleotides. *Circ Res*. 2009;105:737–745.
98. Meregalli PG, Wilde AA, Tan HL. Pathophysiological mechanisms of Brugada syndrome: depolarization disorder, repolarization disorder, or more? *Cardiovasc Res*. 2005;67:367–378.
99. Wilde AA, Postema PG, Di Diego JM, et al. The pathophysiological mechanism underlying Brugada syndrome: depolarization versus repolarization. *J Mol Cell Cardiol*. 2010;49:543–553.
100. Antzelevitch C, Yan GX, Shimizu W. Transmural dispersion of repolarization and arrhythmogenicity: the Brugada syndrome versus the long QT syndrome. *J Electrocardiol*. 1999;32(Suppl):158–165.
101. Yan GX, Antzelevitch C. Cellular basis for the Brugada syndrome and other mechanisms of arrhythmogenesis associated with ST-segment elevation. *Circulation*. 1999;100:1660–1666.
102. Antzelevitch C. Ion channels and ventricular arrhythmias: cellular and ionic mechanisms underlying the Brugada syndrome. *Curr Opin Cardiol*. 1999;14:274–279.
103. Tukkie R, Sogaard P, Vleugels J, et al. Delay in right ventricular activation contributes to Brugada syndrome. *Circulation*. 2004;109:1272–1277.
104. Zhang ZS, Tranquillo J, Neplioueva V, et al. Sodium channel kinetic changes that produce Brugada syndrome or progressive cardiac conduction system disease. *Am J Physiol Heart Circ Physiol*. 2007;292:H399–H407.
105. Coronel R, Casini S, Koopmann TT, et al. Right ventricular fibrosis and conduction delay in a patient with clinical signs of Brugada syndrome: a combined electrophysiological, genetic, histopathologic, and computational study. *Circulation*. 2005;112:2769–2777.
106. Postema PG, van Dessel PF, de Bakker JM, et al. Slow and discontinuous conduction conspire in Brugada syndrome: a right ventricular mapping and stimulation study. *Circ Arrhythm Electrophysiol*. 2008;1:379–386.
107. Postema PG, van Dessel PF, Kors JA, et al. Local depolarization abnormalities are the dominant pathophysiologic mechanism for type 1 electrocardiogram in Brugada syndrome a study of electrocardiograms, vectorcardiograms, and body surface potential maps during ajmaline provocation. *J Am Coll Cardiol*. 2010;55:789–797.
108. Nademanee K, Veerakul G, Chandanamattha P, et al. Prevention of ventricular fibrillation episodes in Brugada syndrome by catheter ablation over the anterior right ventricular outflow tract epicardium. *Circulation*. 2011;123:1270–1279.
109. Papadatos GA, Wallerstein PM, Head CE, et al. Slowed conduction and ventricular tachycardia after targeted disruption of the cardiac sodium channel gene Scn5a. *Proc Natl Acad Sci U S A*. 2002;99:6210–6215.
110. Martin CA, Zhang Y, Grace AA, et al. In vivo studies of Scn5a+/- mice modeling Brugada syndrome demonstrate both conduction and repolarization abnormalities. *J Electrocardiol*. 2010;43:433–439.
111. Martin CA, Zhang Y, Grace AA, et al. Increased right ventricular repolarization gradients promote arrhythmogenesis in a murine model of Brugada syndrome. *J Cardiovasc Electrophysiol*. 2010;21:1153–1159.
112. Park DS, Cerrone M, Morley G, et al. Genetically engineered SCN5A mutant pig hearts exhibit conduction defects and arrhythmias. *J Clin Invest*. 2015;125:403–412.
113. Schott JJ, Alshinawi C, Kyndt F, et al. Cardiac conduction defects associate with mutations in SCN5A. *Nature Genet*. 1999;23:20–21.
114. Wang DW, Viswanathan PC, Balser JR, et al. Clinical, genetic, and biophysical characterization of SCN5A mutations associated with atrioventricular conduction block. *Circulation*. 2002;105:341–346.
115. Groenewegen WA, Firouzi M, Bezzina CR, et al. A cardiac sodium channel mutation cosegregates with a rare connexin40 genotype in familial atrial standstill. *Circ Res*. 2003;92:14–22.
116. Benson DW, Wang DW, Dyment M, et al. Congenital sick sinus syndrome caused by recessive mutations in the cardiac sodium channel gene (SCN5A). *J Clin Invest*. 2003;112:1019–1028.
117. Lopez KN, Decker JA, Friedman RA, et al. Homozygous mutation in SCN5A associated with atrial quiescence, recalcitrant arrhythmias, and poor capture thresholds. *Heart Rhythm*. 2011;8:471–473.
118. Makita N, Sasaki K, Groenewegen WA, et al. Congenital atrial standstill associated with coinheritance of a novel SCN5A mutation and connexin 40 polymorphisms. *Heart Rhythm*. 2005;2:1128–1134.
119. Lenègre J. Etiology and pathology of bilateral bundle branch block in relation to complete heart block. *Prog Cardiovasc Dis*. 1964;6:409–444.
120. Wolf CM, Berul CI. Inherited conduction system abnormalities—one group of diseases, many genes. *J Cardiovasc Electrophysiol*. 2006;17:446–455.
121. Tan HL, Bink-Boelkens MT, Bezzina CR, et al. A sodium-channel mutation causes isolated cardiac conduction disease. *Nature*. 2001;409:1043–1047.
122. Hao X, Zhang Y, Zhang X, et al. TGF-beta1-mediated fibrosis and ion channel remodeling are key mechanisms in producing the sinus node dysfunction associated with SCN5A deficiency and aging. *Circ Arrhythm Electrophysiol*. 2011;4:397–406.
123. Royer A, van Veen TA, Le BS, et al. Mouse model of SCN5A-linked hereditary Lenegre's disease: age-related conduction slowing and myocardial fibrosis. *Circulation*. 2005;111:1738–1746.
124. Leoni AL, Gavillet B, Rougier JS, et al. Variable $Na_V1.5$ protein expression from the wild-type allele correlates with the penetrance of cardiac conduction disease in the Scn5a+/- mouse model. *PLoS ONE*. 2010;19:e9298.
125. Gui J, Wang T, Jones RP, et al. Multiple loss-of-function mechanisms contribute to SCN5A-related familial sick sinus syndrome. *PLoS ONE*. 2010;5:e10985.
126. Butters TD, Aslanidi OV, Inada S, et al. Mechanistic links between Na^+ channel (SCN5A) mutations and impaired cardiac pacemaking in sick sinus syndrome. *Circ Res*. 2010;107:126–137.
127. Lei M, Zhang H, Grace AA, et al. SCN5A and sinoatrial node pacemaker function. *Cardiovasc Res*. 2007;74:356–365.
128. McNair WP, Ku L, Taylor MR, et al. SCN5A mutation associated with dilated cardiomyopathy, conduction disorder, and arrhythmia. *Circulation*. 2004;110:2163–2167.
129. Cheng J, Morales A, Siegfried JD, et al. SCN5A rare variants in familial dilated cardiomyopathy decrease peak sodium current depending on the common polymorphism H558R and common splice variant Q1077del. *Clin Transl Sci*. 2010;3:287–294.

130. Morales A, Painter T, Li R, et al. Rare variant mutations in pregnancy-associated or peripartum cardiomyopathy. *Circulation.* 2010;121:2176–2182.

131. McNair WP, Sinagra G, Taylor MR, et al. SCN5A Mutations associate with arrhythmic dilated cardiomyopathy and commonly localize to the voltage-sensing mechanism. *J Am Coll Cardiol.* 2011;57:2160–2168.

132. Nair K, Pekhletski R, Harris L, et al. Escape capture bigeminy: Phenotypic marker of cardiac sodium channel voltage sensor mutation R222Q. *Heart Rhythm.* 2012;9:1681–1688.

133. Laurent G, Saal S, Amarouch MY, et al. Multifocal ectopic Purkinje-related premature contractions: a new SCN5A-related cardiac channelopathy. *J Am Coll Cardiol.* 2012;60:144–156.

134. Olson TM, Michels VV, Ballew JD, et al. Sodium channel mutations and susceptibility to heart failure and atrial fibrillation. *JAMA.* 2005;293:447–454.

135. Gosselin-Badaroudine P, Keller DI, Huang H, et al. A proton leak current through the cardiac sodium channel is linked to mixed arrhythmia and the dilated cardiomyopathy phenotype. *PLoS ONE.* 2012;7:e38331.

136. Rampersaud E, Siegfried JD, Norton N, et al. Rare variant mutations identified in pediatric patients with dilated cardiomyopathy. *Prog Pediatr Cardiol.* 2011;31:39–47.

137. Beckermann TM, McLeod K, Murday V, et al. Novel SCN5A mutation in amiodarone-responsive multifocal ventricular ectopy-associated cardiomyopathy. *Heart Rhythm.* 2014;11:1446–1453.

138. Nguyen TP, Wang DW, Rhodes TH, et al. Divergent biophysical defects caused by mutant sodium channels in dilated cardiomyopathy with arrhythmia. *Circ Res.* 2008;102:364–371.

139. Wang DW, Yazawa K, George AL, et al. Characterization of human cardiac Na$^+$ channel mutations in the congenital long QT syndrome. *Proc Natl Acad Sci U S A.* 1996;93:13200–13205.

140. Moreau A, Gosselin-Badaroudine P, Chahine M. Gating pore currents, a new pathological mechanism underlying cardiac arrhythmias associated with dilated cardiomyopathy. *Channels.* 2015;9:139–144.

141. Moreau A, Gosselin-Badaroudine P, Delemotte L, et al. Gating pore currents are defects in common with two Na$_V$1.5 mutations in patients with mixed arrhythmias and dilated cardiomyopathy. *J Gen Physiol.* 2015;145:93–106.

142. Moreau A, Gosselin-Badaroudine P, Boutjdir M, et al. Mutations in the voltage sensors of domains I and II of Na$_V$1.5 that are associated with arrhythmias and dilated cardiomyopathy generate gating pore currents. *Front Pharmacol.* 2015;6:301.

143. Watanabe H, Yang T, Stroud DM, et al. Striking in vivo phenotype of a disease-associated human SCN5A mutation producing minimal changes in vitro. *Circulation.* 2011;124:1001–1011.

144. Laitinen-Forsblom PJ, Makynen P, Makynen H, et al. SCN5A mutation associated with cardiac conduction defect and atrial arrhythmias. *J Cardiovasc Electrophysiol.* 2006;17:480–485.

145. Bezzina C, Veldkamp MW, van Den Berg MP, et al. A single Na$^+$ channel mutation causing both long-QT and Brugada syndromes. *Circ Res.* 1999;85:1206–1213.

146. Makita N, Behr E, Shimizu W, et al. The E1784K mutation in SCN5A is associated with mixed clinical phenotype of type 3 long QT syndrome. *J Clin Invest.* 2008;118:2219–2229.

147. Remme CA, Verkerk AO, Nuyens D, et al. Overlap syndrome of cardiac sodium channel disease in mice carrying the equivalent mutation of human SCN5A-1795insD. *Circulation.* 2006;114:2584–2594.

148. Davis RP, Casini S, van den Berg CW, et al. Cardiomyocytes derived from pluripotent stem cells recapitulate electrophysiological characteristics of an overlap syndrome of cardiac sodium channel disease. *Circulation.* 2012;125:3079–3091.

149. Grant AO, Carboni MP, Neplioueva V, et al. Long QT syndrome, Brugada syndrome, and conduction system disease are linked to a single sodium channel mutation. *J Clin Invest.* 2002;110:1201–1209.

150. Musa H, Kline CF, Sturm AC, et al. SCN5A variant that blocks fibroblast growth factor homologous factor regulation causes human arrhythmia. *Proc Natl Acad Sci U S A.* 2015;112:12528–12533.

151. Kyndt F, Probst V, Potet F, et al. Novel SCN5A mutation leading either to isolated cardiac conduction defect or Brugada syndrome in a large French family. *Circulation.* 2001;104:3081–3086.

152. Remme CA, Scicluna BP, Verkerk AO, et al. Genetically determined differences in sodium current characteristics modulate conduction disease severity in mice with cardiac sodium channelopathy. *Circ Res.* 2009;104:1283–1292.

51 Genetic, Ionic, and Cellular Mechanisms Underlying the J Wave Syndromes

Charles Antzelevitch and Bence Patocskai

The J wave syndromes, consisting of Brugada syndrome (BrS) and early repolarization syndrome (ERS), have intrigued the cardiology community since the initial delineation of BrS as a clinical entity in 1992.[1] The clinical impact of ERS was not fully realized until 2008, when the publication of the now classical studies of Haissaguerre et al.,[2] Nam et al.,[3] and Rosso et al.[4] appeared. The genetic basis for BrS and ERS has progressed, but the Mendelian nature of their inheritance has been questioned by recent studies. The cellular mechanisms underlying the J wave syndromes have also been a matter of debate. This chapter provides a critical review of the genetic, ionic, and cellular mechanisms underlying the J wave syndromes.

The appearance of prominent J waves in the electrocardiogram (ECG) has long been reported in clinical cases of hypothermia[5–7] and hypercalcemia.[8,9] Accentuation of the J wave has been associated with life-threatening ventricular arrhythmias.[10] Under these circumstances, the accentuated J wave typically may be so broad that it appears as an ST-segment elevation, as in BrS cases. The normal J wave in humans often appears as a J-point elevation, with part of the J wave buried inside the QRS. An ER pattern (ERP) in the ECG, characterized by a distinct J wave, J-point elevation, or a notch or slur of the terminal part of the QRS with and without an ST-segment elevation, has traditionally been viewed as benign.[11,12] In 2000, Gussak and Antzelevitch[13] challenged this view on the basis of experimental data showing that this ECG manifestation predisposes to the development of polymorphic ventricular tachycardia and fibrillation (VT/VF) in coronary-perfused wedge preparations.[10,13–15] This hypothesis was validated 8 years later by Haissaguerre et al.,[2] Nam et al.,[3] and Rosso et al.[4] These formative studies coupled with many additional case control and population-based studies have provided clinical evidence for an increased risk for development of life-threatening arrhythmic events and sudden cardiac death (SCD) among patients presenting with an ERP, particularly in inferior and inferolateral leads. This field has been marred by inconsistent reporting of data due to lack of agreement regarding terminology relative to ER.[16–18] An expert consensus statement recently published by MacFarlane et al. has provided recommendations for measuring and reporting of ER and J waves. The task force recommends that the peak of an end QRS notch and/or the onset of an end

QRS slur should be designated as J_p and that J_p should exceed 0.1 mV in two or more contiguous inferior and/or lateral leads of a standard 12-lead ECG for ER to be present.[19] It was further recommended that the initiation of the end QRS notch or J wave should be designated as J_o and the termination as J_t.

Both BrS and ERS have been associated with vulnerability to the development of polymorphic VT and VF leading to SCD[1–3,10] in young adults and occasionally to sudden infant death syndrome (SIDS).[20–22] The region generally most affected in ERS is the inferior region of the left ventricle (LV), and in BrS it is the anterior right ventricular outflow tract (RVOT).[2,4,23–27] BrS is characterized by accentuated J waves, appearing as a coved-type ST-segment elevation in the right precordial leads V1–V3, whereas ERS is characterized by J waves, J_o elevation, notch, or slur of the terminal part of the QRS and ST-segment or J_t elevation in the lateral (type I), inferolateral (type II), or inferolateral + anterior ventricular or RV leads (type III).[10] ERP is often encountered in healthy individuals, particularly in young black individuals and athletes. ERP is also observed in acquired conditions, including hypothermia and ischemia.[10,28,29] When associated with VT/VF, ERP is referred to as ERS.

The prevalence of type 1 BrS ECG is higher in Asian countries, such as Japan (0.15%–0.27%),[30,31] the Philippines (0.18%),[32] and among Japanese-Americans in North America (0.15%),[33] than in Western countries, including Europe (0–0.017%)[34–36] or North America (0.005%–0.1%).[37,38] The prevalence of ERP in inferior and/or lateral leads with a J_o elevation of ≥0.1 mV ranges between 1% and 24% and that with a J_o elevation of >0.2 mV ranges between 0.6% and 6.4%.[39–41] ERP is significantly more common in blacks than in Caucasians. ER appears to be more common in Aborigine Australians than in Caucasian Australians.[42]

Acquired Brugada Pattern and Syndrome

J waves associated with BrS are often concealed and can be unmasked with a wide variety of drugs and conditions, including a febrile state, vagotonic agents and maneuvers, α-adrenergic agonists, β-adrenergic blockers, tricyclic or tetracyclic antidepressants, hyperkalemia, hypokalemia, and hypercalcemia, as well as by alcohol and cocaine toxicity.[43–53] Chiale et al. were the first to demonstrate that preexcitation of RV can unmask BrS ECG in cases of right bundle branch block (RBBB).[54] An up-to-date list of agents to avoid in BrS can be found at www.brugadadrugs.org.[55]

Similarities and Differences Between Brugada Syndrome and Early Repolarization Syndrome

ERS and BrS display several phenotypic similarities, suggesting similar pathophysiology (Table 51.1).[14,16,56–58] Males predominate in both syndromes: in BrS, presenting in 71%–80% of Caucasians and 94%–96% of Japanese.[59,60] BrS and ERS patients may be totally asymptomatic until they present with sudden cardiac arrest. In both syndromes, the highest incidence of VF or SCD occurs in the third decade of life, perhaps tied to testosterone levels in males.[61] In both syndromes, the appearance of accentuated J waves and ST-segment elevation is generally associated with

TABLE 51.1 Similarities and differences between Brugada syndrome (Brs) and early repolarization syndrome (ERS) and possible underlying mechanisms

	BRS	ERS	POSSIBLE MECHANISM(S)
Similarities Between Brugada Syndrome and Early Repolarization Syndrome			
Male predominance	Yes (>75%)	Yes (>80%)	Testosterone modulation of ion currents underlying the epicardial AP notch
Average age of first event	30–50	30–50	
Associated with mutations or rare variants in *KCNJ8, CACNA1C, CACNB2, CACNA2D, SCN5A, ABCC9, SCN10A*	Yes	Yes	Gain-of-function in outward currents (I_{K-ATP}) or loss of function in inward currents (I_{Ca} or I_{Na})
Relatively short QT intervals in subjects with Ca channel mutations	Yes	Yes	Loss of function of I_{Ca}
Dynamicity of ECG	High	High	Autonomic modulation of ion channel currents underlying early phases of the epicardial AP
VF often occurs during sleep or at a low level of physical activity	Yes	Yes	Higher level of vagal tone and higher levels of I_{to} at slower heart rates
VT/VF trigger	Short-coupled PVC	Short-coupled PVC	Phase 2 reentry
Ameliorative response to quinidine and bepridil	Yes	Yes	Inhibition of I_{to} and possible vagolytic effect
Ameliorative response to isoproterenol, denopamine, and milrinone	Yes	Yes	Increased I_{Ca} and faster heart rate
Ameliorative response to cilostazol	Yes	Yes	Increased I_{Ca}, reduced I_{to} and faster heart rate
Ameliorative response to pacing	Yes	Yes	Reduced availability of I_{to} due to slow recovery from inactivation
Vagally mediated accentuation of ECG pattern	Yes	Yes	Direct effect to inhibit I_{Ca} and indirect effect to increase I_{to} (due to slowing of heart rate)
Effect of sodium channel blockers on unipolar epicardial electrogram	Augmented J waves	Augmented J waves	Outward shift of balance of current in the early phases of the epicardial AP
Fever	Augmented J waves	Augmented J waves (rare)	Accelerated inactivation of I_{Na} and accelerated recovery of I_{to} from inactivation
Hypothermia	Augmented J waves mimicking BrS	Augmented J waves	Slowed activation of I_{Ca}, leaving I_{to} unopposed. Increased phase 2 reentry but reduced pVT due to prolongation of APD[68]
Differences Between Brugada Syndrome and Early Repolarization Syndrome			
Region most involved	RVOT	Inferior LV wall	Higher levels of I_{to} and/or differences in conduction
Leads affected	V1–V3	II, III, aVF V4, V5, V6; I, aVL Both: inferolateral	
Regional difference in prevalence			Europe: BrS = ERS Asia: BrS > ERS
Incidence of late potential in SAECG	Higher	Lower	
Inducibility of VF during an EPS	Higher	Lower	
Prevalence of atrial fibrillation	Higher	Lower	
Effect of sodium channel blockers on the surface ECG	Increased J wave manifestation	Reduced J wave manifestation	Reduction of J wave in the setting of ER is largely considered to be due to prolongation of QRS. Accentuation of repolarization defects predominates in BrS, whereas accentuation of depolarization defects predominates in ERS.

AP, Action potential; *APD*, action potential duration; *ECG*, electrocardiogram; *EPS*, electrophysiological study; *PVC*, premature ventricular contraction; *RVOT*, right ventricular outflow tract; *SAECG*, signal-averaged electrocardiography; *VF*, ventricular fibrillation; *VT*, ventricular tachycardia.
Modified from Antzelevitch C, Yan GX. J wave syndromes. *Heart Rhythm.* 2010;7:549-558.

bradycardia or pauses,[62,63] explaining why VF in both syndromes often occurs during sleep or at a low physical activity level.[64,65] The QT interval is reportedly relatively short in ERS[2,66] and BrS patients who carry mutations in calcium channel genes.[67]

BrS and ERS also show similar responses to pharmacological therapy. In both, electrical storms and associated J wave manifestations can be suppressed using β-adrenergic agonists.[69–72] Chronic oral pharmacological therapy using quinidine,[73,74] cilostazol,[69,71,75–79] denopamine,[69,75] and bepridil[71] has been reported to suppress the development of VT/VF in both syndromes secondary to the inhibition of I_{to} and the augmentation of I_{Ca}, I_{Na}, or both.[3,76,80]

Differences between the two syndromes include (1) the region of the heart most affected (RVOT vs. inferior LV); (2) greater incidence of late potentials (LPs) in signal-averaged ECGs in BrS (60%) versus ERS (7%)[65]; (3) greater inducibility of VF during electrophysiological study in BrS than in ERS; (4) greater elevation of J_o, J_p, or J_t (ST-segment elevation) in response to sodium channel blockers in BrS versus ERS; and (5) higher prevalence of atrial fibrillation in BrS versus ERS.[81] Some early studies suggested a different pathophysiological basis for ERS and BrS because sodium channel blockers were shown to unmask or accentuate J wave manifestation in BrS but reduce J wave amplitude in ERS.[65] Nakagawa et al. recently reported that J waves recorded using unipolar LV epicardial leads introduced into the left lateral coronary vein in ERS patients were indeed augmented, although J waves recorded in the lateral precordial leads were diminished. The latter were principally diminished because of the engulfment of the surface J wave by the widened QRS.[24,65] Furthermore, in support of the thesis that these ECG patterns and syndromes are closely related are reports of cases in which ERS transitions into ERS plus BrS.[58,82]

J waves have been reported to be accentuated or induced by both hypothermia and fever.[83-88] However, the development of arrhythmias in ERS is much more sensitive to hypothermia, and arrhythmogenesis in BrS appears to be exclusively promoted by fever.[83,84] Hypothermia is reported to increase the risk for VF in ERS,[28,29,83,84,89] and fever is well recognized as a major risk factor in BrS.[90,91] It is noteworthy that hypothermia can actually diminish the manifestation of BrS ECG when a prominent J wave or ST-segment elevation is already present.[92,93]

ERP is associated with an increased risk for VF in patients with acute myocardial infarction[94] and hypothermia.[28,95] A concomitant ERP in the inferolateral leads has also been reported to be associated with an increased risk for arrhythmic events in patients with BrS. Kawata et al. reported that the prevalence of ER in inferolateral leads was high (63%) in BrS patients with documented VF.[96]

Genetics

Candidate gene, next-generation, whole genome, and exome sequencing as well as genome-wide association studies (GWAS) have associated variants in 18 different genes in the case of BrS and seven different genes in the case of ERS (Table 51.2). To date, more than 300 BrS-related variants in *SCN5A* have been described.[16,97,98] The available evidence suggests that the presence of a prominent I_{to} determines whether loss-of-function mutations, resulting in a reduction in I_{Na}, will manifest as BrS/ERS or as a conduction disease.[99-102]

Variants in *CACNA1C* (Cav1.2), *CACNB2b* (Cavβ2b), and *CACNA2D1* (Cavα2δ) have been reported in up to 13% of probands.[103-106] Mutations in glycerol-3-phosphate dehydrogenase 1-like enzyme gene (*GPD1L*), *SCN1B* (β1-subunit of Na channel), *KCNE3* (MiRP2), *SCN3B* (β3-subunit of Na channel), *KCNJ8* (Kir 6.1), *KCND3* (Kv4.3), *RANGRF* (MOG1), *SLMAP*, *ABCC9* (SUR2A) (Navβ2), *PKP2* (plakophilin-2), *FGF12* (FHAF1), *HEY2*, and *SEMA3A* (semaphorin) are relatively rare.[107-127] An association of BrS with *SCN10A*, a neuronal sodium channel, was recently reported.[118,128,129] A wide range of yields were reported by the two studies that examined the prevalence of pathogenic *SCN10A* mutations and rare variants (5% vs. 16.7%).[128-130] Mutations in these genes lead to loss of function in sodium (I_{Na}) and calcium (I_{Ca}) channel currents, as well as to a gain-of-function in transient outward potassium current (I_{to}) or adenosine triphosphate (ATP)-sensitive potassium current (I_{K-ATP}).[129]

Recent studies have identified two new susceptibility genes, which await confirmation: transient receptor potential melastatin protein 4 gene (*TRPM4*)[131] and the *KCND2* gene. A *KCND2* variant has been identified in a single patient and has been shown to cause a gain-of-function in I_{to} when heterologously expressed.[132]

Variants in *KCNH2*, *KCNE5*, and *SEMA3A*, although not causative, have been identified as capable of modulating the substrate for the development of BrS.[133-136] Loss-of-function mutations in *HCN4* causing a reduction in pacemaker current I_f can unmask BrS by reducing heart rate.[137]

ERP in the ECG is known to be familial.[138-140] Consistent with the findings that I_{K-ATP} activation can generate ERP in canine ventricular wedge preparations, variants in genes responsible for the pore forming– and ATP-sensing subunits of the I_{K-ATP} channel, *KCNJ8* and *ABCC9*, have been reported in ERS patients.[107,109,141] Loss-of-function variations in the α1-, β2-, and α2δ-subunits of the cardiac L-type calcium channel (*CACNA1C*, *CACNB2*, and *CACNA2D1*) and the α1-subunit of Nav1.5 and Nav1.8 (*SCN5A* and *SCN10A*) have been reported in BRS patients.[66,103,128]

It is important to recognize that very few variants in the genes associated with BrS and ERS have been evaluated using functional expression studies to ascertain causality and establish pathogenicity. Very few have been studied in genetically engineered animal models, native cardiac cells, or in induced pluripotent stem cell–derived cardiomyocytes isolated from ERS and BrS patients. In silico tools developed to predict the functional consequences of mutations are helpful but have not been rigorously tested. The lack of functional validation remains a severe limitation of genetic test interpretation.[142] Recent technological advances have resulted in the expansion of disease-specific panels,[143] which have challenged our understanding of the extent of background genetic variation within cardiac channelopathy susceptibility genes.[144-146] These issues suggest that the results of the genetic test should be treated as probabilistic rather than binary or deterministic. Additional evidence can be obtained from cosegregation, studies,[147] in silico prediction tools,[148-151] and variant frequency in cases and control databases.[144] Despite these aids, a large number of variants remain in "genetic purgatory." Kapplinger et al. recently reported the synergistic use of up to seven in silico tools to help promote or demote a variant's pathogenic status and alter its relegation to genetic purgatory.[152]

Le Scouarnec et al. recently calculated the burden of rare coding variation in arrhythmia susceptibility genes among 167 BrS index patients and compared with 167 individuals aged over 65 years with no history of cardiac arrhythmia.[153] The authors concluded that except for *SCN5A*, rare coding variations in all previously reported BrS susceptibility genes do not significantly contribute to the occurrence of BrS in a population with European ancestry, emphasizing that caution should be taken when interpreting genetic variations in these other genes because rare coding variants are observed to a similar extent in both cases and controls.[153]

These data suggest that in individual cases, BrS and the susceptibility for SCD is not because of a single mutation but rather because of the inheritance of multiple BrS susceptibility variants (oligogenic).[118] The multifactorial nature of the genetics can further be confounded by the fact that expressivity of the syndrome may be multifactorial in that the phenotype can be modulated by hormonal (testosterone, thyroxine) and other environmental factors.

Cellular Mechanisms Underlying Brugada Syndrome and Early Repolarization Syndrome

The J wave syndromes are so named because they involve accentuation of the ECG J wave.[10] The J wave is believed to be inscribed as a consequence of transmural differences in the manifestation of the action potential (AP) notch between the epi- and endocardium secondary to the heterogeneous transmural distribution of the transient outward current (I_{to}).[57]

The ionic and cellular mechanisms underlying J wave syndromes have long been mired in controversy.[154,155] Two principal hypotheses have been advanced to explain BrS: (1) the *repolarization hypothesis* maintains that an outward shift in the balance of currents in the RV epicardium leads to repolarization abnormalities that give rise to phase 2 reentry and the generation of closely coupled premature beats that are capable of precipitating VT/VF and (2) the *depolarization hypothesis* suggests that slow conduction in the RVOT and other regions of RV, secondary to structural defects, including fibrosis and reduced connexin 43 (Cx43), leading to discontinuities in conduction, play a key role in the development of the ECG and arrhythmic manifestations of the syndrome. These theories are not mutually exclusive and may indeed be synergistic.

The most apparently persuasive evidence in support of the depolarization hypothesis comes from the study of Nademanee

TABLE 51.2 Gene defects associated with the early repolarization (ERS) and Brugada (BrS) syndromes

	LOCUS	GENE/PROTEIN	ION CHANNEL	% OF PROBANDS
ERS1	12p11.23	*KCNJ8*, Kir6.1	↑ I_{K-ATP}	
ERS2	12p13.3	*CACNA1C*, $Ca_v1.2$	↓ I_{Ca}	4.1%
ERS3	10p12.33	*CACNB2b*, $Ca_v\beta2b$	↓ I_{Ca}	8.3%
ERS4	7q21.11	*CACNA2D1*, $Ca_v\alpha2\delta$	↓ I_{Ca}	4.1%
ERS5	12p12.1	*ABCC9*, SUR2A	↑ I_{K-ATP}	Rare
ERS6	3p21	*SCN5A*, $Na_v1.5$	↓ I_{Na}	Rare
ERS7	3p22.2	*SCN10A*, $Na_v1.8$	↓ I_{Na}	
BrS1	3p21	*SCN5A*, $Na_v1.5$	↓ I_{Na}	11%–28%
BrS2	3p24	*GPD1L*	↓ I_{Na}	Rare
BrS3	12p13.3	*CACNA1C*, $Ca_v1.2$	↓ I_{Ca}	6.6%
BrS4	10p12.33	*CACNB2b*, $Ca_v\beta2b$	↓ I_{Ca}	4.8%
BrS5	19q13.1	*SCN1B*, $Na_v\beta1$	↓ I_{Na}	1.1%
BrS6	11q13-14	*KCNE3*, MiRP2	↑ I_{to}	Rare
BrS7	11q23.3	*SCN3B*, $Na_v\beta3$	↓ I_{Na}	Rare
BrS8	12p11.23	*KCNJ8*, Kir6.1	↑ I_{K-ATP}	2%
BrS9	7q21.11	*CACNA2D1*, $Ca_v\alpha2\delta$	↓ I_{Ca}	1.8%
BrS10	1p13.2	*KCND3*, $K_v4.3$	↑ I_{to}	Rare
BrS11	17p13.1	*RANGRF*, MOG1	↓ I_{Na}	Rare
BrS12	3p21.2-p14.3	*SLMAP*	↓ I_{Na}	Rare
BrS13	12p12.1	*ABCC9*, SUR2A	↑ I_{K-ATP}	Rare
BrS14	11q23	*SCN2B*, $Na_v\beta2$	↓ I_{Na}	Rare
BrS15	12p11	*PKP2*, Plakophilin-2	↓ I_{Na}	Rare
BrS16	3q28	*FGF12*, FHAF1	↓ I_{Na}	Rare
BrS17	3p22.2	*SCN10A*, $Na_v1.8$	↓ I_{Na}	5%–16.7%
BrS18	6q	*HEY2* (transcriptional factor)	↑ I_{Na}	Rare

Listed in chronological order of their discovery.
Modified from Antzelevitch C, Yan GX. J wave syndromes. *Heart Rhythm*. 2010;7:549-558.

et al.,[156] showing that radiofrequency ablation (RFA) of epicardial sites displaying fractionated bipolar electrograms (EGMs) and LPs in the RVOT of BrS patients reduces the ECG and arrhythmic manifestations of the syndrome. Similar results have been reported by Brugada et al.,[157] and in a case report, Sacher et al.[158] observed that accentuation of the Brugada ECG by ajmaline was associated with increasing area of low-voltage and fractionated EGM activity and a more prominent ST-segment elevation.[157] These authors concluded that the LP and fractionated EGM activities are due to conduction delays within the RVOT and that ablation of the sites of slow conduction is the basis for the ameliorative effect of ablation therapy.[156–158] Szél et al.,[101] in a direct test of this hypothesis, provided strong evidence for an alternative mechanism. Using an experimental model of BrS, they showed that low-voltage and fractionated EGM activity similar to that observed by Nademanee et al. in the RVOT of BrS patients developed because of desynchronization in the appearance of the second AP upstroke, secondary to accentuation of the epicardial AP notch and not because of the slow or delayed conduction (Fig. 51.1). They also found that high-frequency LPs developed in the RV epicardium because of concealed phase 2 reentry. Delayed conduction of the primary beat was never observed in a wide variety of BrS models created by exposing canine RV wedge preparations to drugs mimicking the different genetic defects known to give rise to BrS.[101]

Patocskai et al.[158a] went on to test the hypothesis that ablation ameliorates the BrS phenotype by destroying sites of abnormal conduction. They ablated the epicardial regions displaying fractionated EGMs and LPs in the experimental models of BrS. These manifestations, however, were not because of slow or delayed conduction but rather because of repolarization abnormalities and concealed phase 2 reentry. Ablation of the RV epicardium reduced the manifestation of J waves and ST-segment elevation and abolished all arrhythmic activity, a result identical to that obtained by Nademanee et al. (Fig. 51.2). These observations indicate that ablation can exert an ameliorative effect by destroying the cells with the most prominent AP notch, thus eliminating the cells responsible for the repolarization abnormalities that give rise to phase 2 reentry and VT/VF.[10,159]

In an attempt to create an in vivo model of BrS, Park et al. genetically engineered Yucatan minipigs to heterozygously express a nonsense mutation in *SCN5A* (E558X) originally identified in a child with BrS.[99] Atrial myocytes isolated from the *SCN5A*[E558X/+] pigs showed a loss of function of I_{Na}. Consistent with the loss of function of sodium channel activity, the minipigs displayed conduction abnormalities consisting of prolongation of the P wave, QRS complex, and PR interval. A BrS phenotype was never observed, not even after the administration of flecainide. These observations are expected because of the lack of I_{to} in the pig, which is a prerequisite for the development of repolarization abnormalities associated with BrS. These observations provide strong evidence against the depolarization hypothesis and for the repolarization hypothesis.

These experiments also provide the first test in a large mammal of the hypothesis that a slowly conducting embryonic phenotype is maintained in the adult RVOT and is unmasked when cardiac sodium channel function is reduced.[119] The hypothesis is not supported because conduction in the RVOT of the *SCN5A*[E558X/+] pigs was no different from conduction in the rest of RV. Both were equally depressed by the loss of function of sodium channel activity.[99]

Further evidence in support of the repolarization hypothesis derives from the observation that monophasic APs recorded from the epi- and endocardial surfaces of the RVOT of a BrS patient are nearly identical to transmembrane APs recorded from the epi- and endocardial surfaces of the BrS wedge model.[160,161] In both cases AP displays a prominent accentuation of the notch in epicardium but not in endocardium without any major transmural conduction delays (Fig. 51.3). These differences were not observed in an isolated heart explanted from a BrS patient after

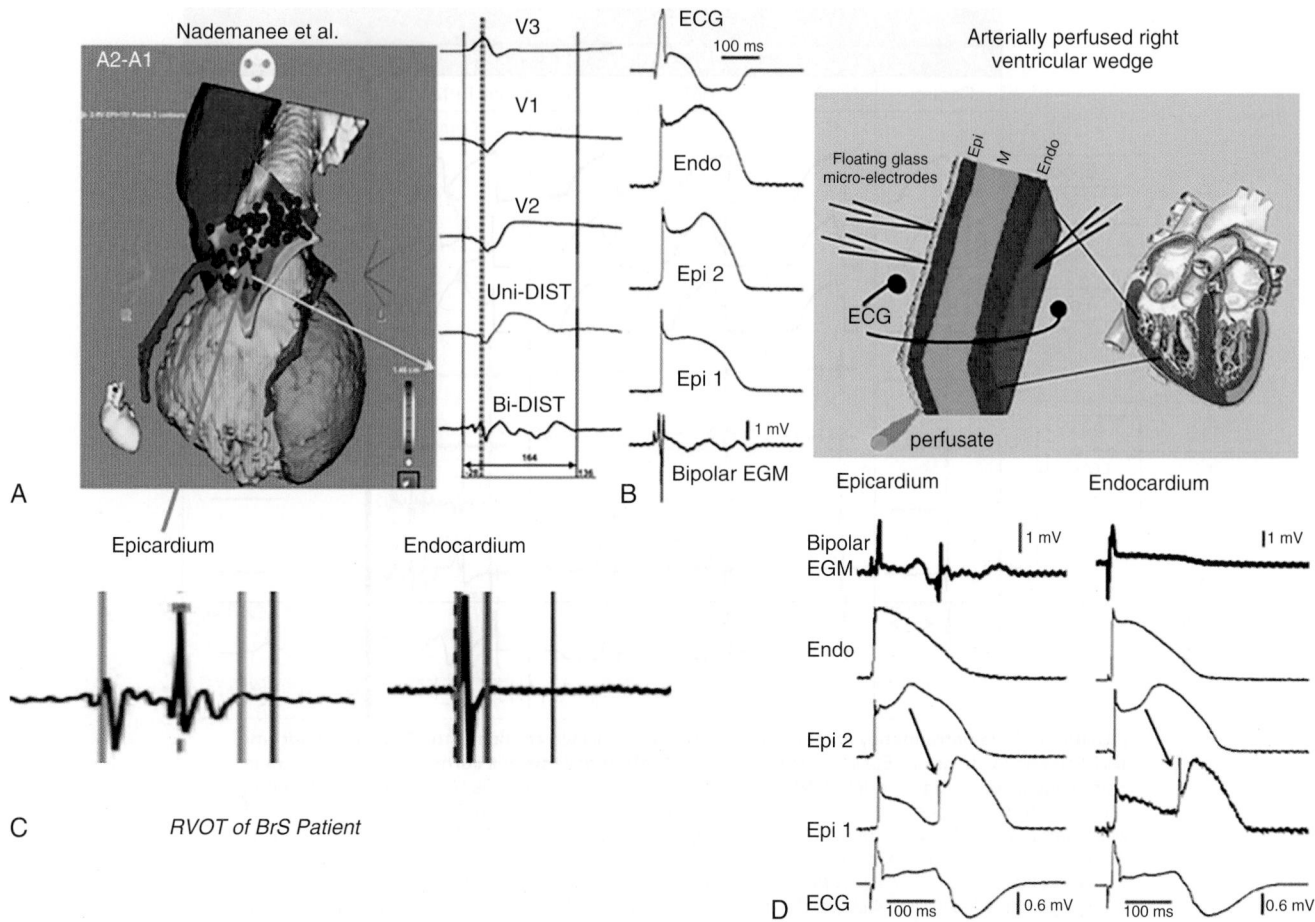

FIGURE 51.1 New interpretation of fractionated electrogram activity and late potentials. Desynchrony in the appearance of the epicardial action potential second upstroke results in fractionated epicardial electrogram (*EGM*) activity, and concealed phase 2 reentry results in high-frequency late potentials in the setting of Brugada syndrome (*BrS*). (A) Shown are the right precordial lead recordings as well as unipolar and bipolar EGMs from the right ventricular outflow tract of a BrS patient. (B) Electrocardiogram (*ECG*), action potentials (*APs*) from the endocardial (*Endo*) and two epicardial (*Epi*) sites, and a bipolar epicardial EGM (*Bipolar EGM*) are all simultaneously recorded from a coronary-perfused right ventricular wedge preparation treated with the I_{to} agonist NS5806 (5 μM) and the calcium channel blocker verapamil (2 μM) to induce the Brugada phenotype. Basic cycle length = 1000 ms. (C) Bipolar EGMs recorded from the epi- and endocardial surfaces of the right ventricular outflow tract (*RVOT*) in a BrS patient. The epicardial EGM displays fractionated EGM activity as well as a high-frequency late potential (130-ms delay). (D) Bipolar EGMs recorded from the epicardium and endocardium of a coronary-perfused wedge model of BrS, together with AP recordings from an endocardial and two epicardial sites and a transmural ECG. Slow or delayed conduction was never observed. *Bi-DIST,* bipolar epicardial EGM; *Uni-DIST,* unipolar epicardial EGM. (Clinical data modified from Nademanee K, Veerakul G, Chandanamattha P, et al. Prevention of ventricular fibrillation episodes in Brugada syndrome by catheter ablation over the anterior right ventricular outflow tract epicardium. *Circulation.* 2011;123:1270-1279; experimental data from Szel T, Antzelevitch C. Abnormal repolarization as the basis for late potentials and fractionated electrograms recorded from epicardium in experimental models of Brugada syndrome. *J Am Coll Cardiol.* 2014;63:2037-2045 with permission.)

transplantation of a new heart. The epicardium of this heart was very depressed, perhaps as a result of the 129 shocks delivered by an implantable cardioverter defibrillator (ICD) in an attempt to control the multiple electrical storms.[27]

Zhang et al. recently reported the results of noninvasive ECG imaging (ECGI) of 25 BrS and 6 RBBB patients.[162] The authors concluded that both slow discontinuous conduction and steep dispersion of repolarization are present in the RVOT of BrS patients. ECGI was able to differentiate between BrS and RBBB. Unlike BrS, RBBB showed delayed activation in the entire RV, without ST-segment elevation, fractionation, or repolarization abnormalities on EGMs. Importantly, in six BrS patients, the response to an increase in rate was studied. The increase in rate increased fractionation of EGM but reduced ST-segment

elevation, indicating that conduction impairment was not the principal cause of BrS ECG.

The strong similarity between BrS and ERS with respect to clinical manifestations and in response to treatment lend further support for the repolarization hypothesis. Using an experimental model of ERS, Koncz et al.[25] provided evidence in support of the hypothesis that, similar to the mechanism operative in BrS, an accentuation of transmural gradients in the LV wall is responsible for the repolarization abnormalities underlying ERS, giving rise to J-point elevation, distinct J waves, or slurring of the terminal part of the QRS. The repolarization defect was shown to be accentuated by cholinergic agonists and reduced by quinidine, isoproterenol, cilostazol, and milrinone, accounting for the ability of these agents to reverse the repolarization abnormalities

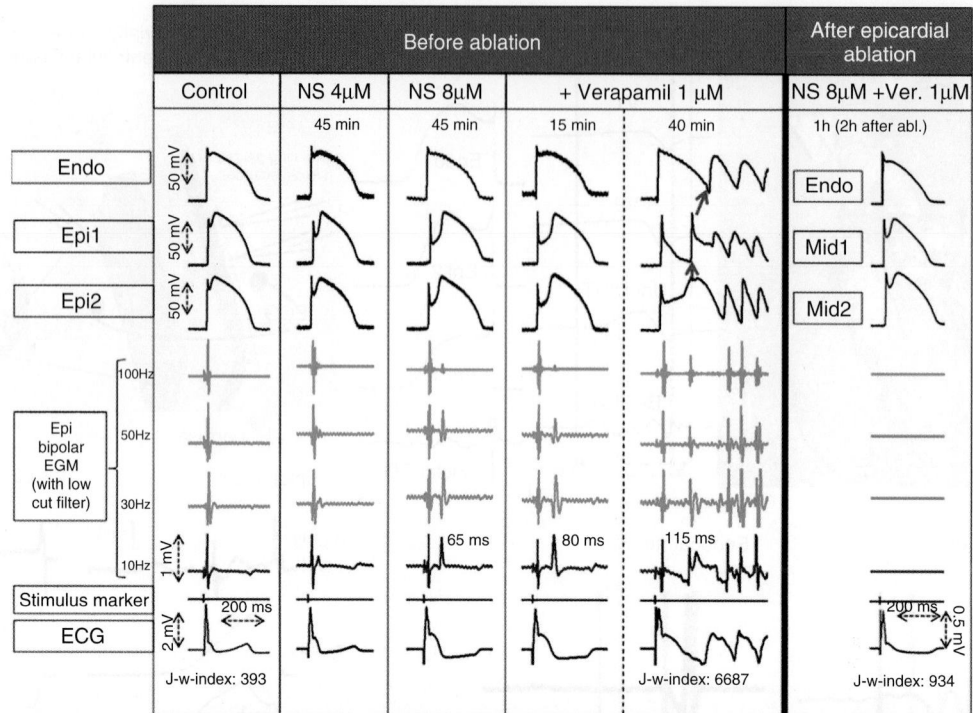

FIGURE 51.2 Radiofrequency ablation of the epicardial surface abolishes the Brugada syndrome (BrS) electrocardiogram (*ECG*) and suppresses arrhythmogenesis in a coronary-perfused canine right ventricular wedge model of BrS. Transmembrane action potentials (APs) were simultaneously recorded from one endocardial (*Endo*) and two epicardial (*Epi*) sites together with epicardial bipolar electrograms (*EGMs*) and a transmural pseudo-ECG. The epicardial bipolar EGMs were recorded at 10–1000-Hz bandwidth (*black trace*) and were simultaneously band-pass filtered at 30–200 Hz, 50–200 Hz, and 100–200 Hz (*green traces*). *Column 1,* Control. *Column 2,* Recorded 45 minutes after the addition of the I_{to} agonist NS5806 (*NS*; 4 µM) to the coronary perfusate. Column 3, Recorded 45 minutes after the concentration of NS5806 was increased to 8 µM. High- and low-frequency late potentials are apparent in the EGM recordings, resulting from progressive delay in the appearance of the second upstroke of the Epi AP secondary to the accentuation of the AP notch. Column 4, Recorded 15 minutes after the addition of the I_{Ca} blocker verapamil (1 µM) to the coronary perfusate. Column 5, Recorded after 40 minutes of exposure to verapamil (1 µM). Loss of the AP dome at Epi1 but not Epi2 results in a phase 2 reentrant beat, which precipitates polymorphic ventricular tachycardia. Column 6, Recorded 2 hours after the radiofrequency ablation of the epicardial surface and 1 hour after the reintroduction of provocative agents to the perfusate (in the same concentration as before ablation). APs are now recorded from the deep subepicardium–midmyocardium (Mid1 and Mid2) instead of the epicardial surface. Ablation markedly suppressed the BrS phenotype and abolished all arrhythmic activity by destroying the cells that exhibit the pronounced repolarization abnormalities. Slow or delayed conduction was not observed at any phase. (Modified from Patocskai B, Antzelevitch C. Novel therapeutic strategies for the management of ventricular arrhythmias associated with the Brugada syndrome. *Expert Opin Orphan Drugs.* 2015;3:633-651.)

responsible for ERS.[25,163] Greater intrinsic levels of I_{to} in the inferior LV were shown to underlie the greater vulnerability of the inferior LV wall to VT/VF.[25] Using ECGI, Rudy et al. provided additional evidence in support of the repolarization abnormalities by identifying abnormally short activation–recovery intervals (ARIs) in the inferior and lateral regions of LV and a marked dispersion of repolarization.[164] Recent ECGI mapping studies performed in an ERS patient during VF demonstrated VF rotors anchored in the inferior-lateral LV wall.[17]

Conduction delays are known to give rise to notching of the QRS complex. When it occurs on the rising phase of the R wave, it can be demonstrated to be due to a conduction defect within the ventricular myocardium. When the notching occurs at the terminal portion of the QRS, thus masquerading as a J wave, it may be due either to a conduction or repolarization defect.[16,165] The response to prematurity or to an increase in rate could differentiate between the two.[100] Delayed conduction invariably becomes more exaggerated at faster rates or during premature beats, thus leading to an accentuation of the QRS notch, whereas repolarization defects are usually moderated, resulting in a diminution of

the J wave at faster rates. Although typical J waves are usually accentuated with bradycardia or long pauses, the opposite has also been described.[166,167] J waves are often seen in young males with no apparent structural heart diseases, whereas intraventricular conduction delay is often observed in older individuals or in cases of postmyocardial infarction or cardiomyopathy.[165,166] The prognostic value of a fragmented QRS has been demonstrated in BrS,[168,169] although QRS fragmentation is not associated with increased risk in the absence of cardiac disease.[170] Factors that may aid in the differential diagnosis of J wave versus intraventricular conduction defect (IVCD)–mediated syndromes are summarized in Table 51.3.

Therapy of Brugada Syndrome and Early Repolarization Syndrome

The only proven effective therapy for the prevention of SCD in high risk BrS and ERS patients is an ICD.[171,172] It is important to appreciate that ICDs are associated with complications, especially in young active individuals.[173,174] Subcutaneous ICDs

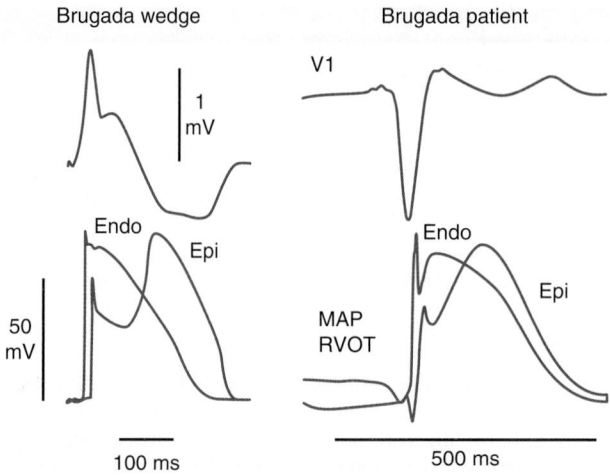

FIGURE 51.3 Comparison of transmembrane and monophasic action potentials (*MAP*) and electrocardiogram recorded from a wedge model of Brugada syndrome (BrS) and a patient diagnosed with BrS. *Left panel* shows a pseudo-electrocardiogram and transmembrane action potentials recorded from the epi- and endocardium of a right ventricular wedge preparation in which the Brugada phenotype was elicited using 5 μM terfenadine to block I_{Na} and I_{Ca}, thus mimicking the genetic variants associated with BrS. *Right panel* shows lead V1 and monophasic action potentials recorded from the epi- (*Epi*) and endocardium (*Endo*) of the right ventricular outflow tract (*RVOT*) of a BrS patient. Note that the apparent notch in the endocardial MAP is an "intrinsic potential" and not a true notch. (Modified from Antzelevitch C, Brugada P, Brugada J, et al. Brugada syndrome: a decade of progress. *Circ Res.* 2002;91:1114-1119; and Kurita T, Shimizu W, Inagaki M, et al. The electrophysiologic mechanism of ST-segment elevation in Brugada syndrome. *J Am Coll Cardiol.* 2002;40:330-334.)

are considered to represent the future for this indication in that they are expected to be associated with fewer complications over a lifetime.[175]

Implantation of an ICD is the first-line therapy for J wave syndrome patients who present with aborted SCD or documented VT/VF with or without syncope (class I recommendation).[171,176] ICDs can be useful (class IIa) in symptomatic BrS patients with type 1 pattern, in whom syncope was likely caused by VT/VF. The Heart Rhythm Society/European Heart Rhythm Association/Asia Pacific Heart Rhythm Society Expert Consensus states that ICD may be considered (class IIb) in asymptomatic patients with inducible VF during programmed electrical stimulation (PES).[177] Some studies suggest that the predictive value of EP studies is improved by limiting the PES protocol to two extrastimuli,[178] but that observation is not supported by other studies.[179,180] Similarly, some studies advocate that PES should be limited to the right ventricular apex and credit this limited PES strategy for a very high positive predictive value found in some series.[181] In addition, that observation is not confirmed by other studies.[178]

Arrhythmic events and SCD in both BrS and ERS generally occur during sleep or at rest and are associated with slow heart rates. These observations notwithstanding, a potential therapeutic role for cardiac pacing remains largely unexplored.[182] A few case reports are available.[183,184]

Nademanee et al.[156] was the first to show that RFA of *epicardial* sites displaying LPs and fractionated bipolar EGMs in the RVOT of BrS patients can significantly reduce the ECG and arrhythmic manifestations of the disease. Additional evidence in support of the effectiveness of epicardial substrate ablation was provided by Shah et al. and Sacher et al.[158,185,186]

More recently, Brugada et al. used flecainide to identify the full extent of low-voltage EGM activity in the anterior RV and RVOT and targeted this region for RFA. In all 14 BrS patients,

RFA eliminated abnormal bipolar EGMs and normalized ST-segment elevation on right precordial leads of ECG, and VT/VF was no longer inducible.[157] Ablation therapy can be life-saving in otherwise uncontrollable cases. RFA is a *class IIa* recommendation in BrS patients with frequent appropriate ICD shocks due to recurrent electrical storms.[187] There are no clinical reports of ablation of the LV substrate in ERS patients.

Pharmacological Approach to Therapy

Brugada Syndrome

The pharmacological approach to therapy stems directly from our understanding of the mechanisms responsible for the ECG and arrhythmic manifestations of BrS. Drug therapy is geared to reversing the substrate responsible for the repolarization abnormalities that underlie the ECG and arrhythmic manifestations of BrS and ERS. The repolarization abnormalities are caused by an outward shift in the balance of current in the early phases of the epicardial AP in the RVOT. Accordingly, the approach to therapy involves an inward shift of the balance of current in the RVOT epicardium. By increasing inward currents such as I_{Ca} or reducing outward currents such as I_{to}, the magnitude of the AP notch is reduced and the AP dome is restored, thus restoring homogeneity within the epicardium and across the ventricular wall. Because the presence of a prominent I_{to} is a prerequisite for the development of both BrS and ERS, the partial inhibition of this current appears to be effective regardless of the ionic or genetic basis for the disease. Unfortunately, cardioselective and I_{to}-specific blockers are not available.

Quinidine is the only agent available in the United States and around the world with significant I_{to}-blocking properties.[14,188] Experimental studies have shown that quinidine is effective in restoring the epicardial AP dome, thus normalizing the ST segment and preventing phase 2 reentry and polymorphic VT in a variety of different experimental models of BrS.[14,101,189-191] A recent experimental study suggests that quinidine, owing to its effect to block I_{to}, can also exert a protective effect against hypothermia-induced VT/VF in a J wave syndrome model.[95] It is noteworthy that, historically, quinidine was used to prevent VF in patients who required hypothermia for surgical procedures.[191]

The effectiveness of quinidine in normalizing ST-segment elevation and/or preventing arrhythmic events in BrS patients has been reported in numerous studies and case reports.[71,73,74,78,192-205] Belhassen et al.[206] reported a 90% efficacy in the prevention of VF induction following treatment with quinidine, despite the use of very aggressive extrastimulation protocols. Furthermore, there were no arrhythmic events among BrS patients treated with quinidine during a mean follow-up period of 10 years.

A prospective registry of empiric quinidine for asymptomatic BrS has been established. The study appears at the National Institutes of Health website (ClinicalTrials.gov) and can be accessed at http://clinicaltrials.gov/ct2/show/NCT00789165?term_bruga da&rank_2. Doses between 600 and 900 mg were recommended, if tolerated.[196]

Agents, such as β-adrenergic agents, including isoproterenol, denopamine, or orciprenaline, that augment I_{Ca} are also useful.[14,71,75,201,207,208] Isoproterenol, at times in combination with quinidine, has been successfully utilized to control VF storms and normalize ST-segment elevation, particularly in children.[46,69-72,193,194,199,205,209-217] Spontaneous VF in BrS patients is often related to increases in vagal tone, and the electrical storm is correspondingly sometimes treatable by increasing the sympathetic tone via isoproterenol administration. Isoprotereonol administration is a class IIa recommendation for BrS patients presenting with electrical storms.[187]

Another promising pharmacological approach for BrS is the administration of the phosphodiesterase (PDE) III inhibitor

TABLE 51.3 Differential diagnosis of J wave versus intraventricular conduction defect (IVCD)-mediated notch syndromes

	J WAVE	IVCD-INDUCED END QRS NOTCH
Male predominance	Yes	No
Average age at initial presentation	Young adults	Older adults
Most common morphology	Dome-like smooth appearance	Relatively sharp appearance
Response to change in heart rate	Bradycardia- and pause-dependent augmentation of J wave that may be accompanied by T wave inversion	Tachycardia and prematurity-dependent augmentation of the notch
Structural heart diseases	Rare	Common
		History of myocardial infarction and/or cardiomyopathy

Modified from Antzelevitch C, Yan GX. J wave syndromes. *Heart Rhythm.* 2010;7:549-558.

cilostazol,[71,75,77] which normalizes the ST segment, most likely by augmenting calcium current (I_{Ca}) as well as by reducing I_{to} secondary to an increase in cAMP and heart rate.[218] Other effects of cilostazol may also contribute (e.g., adenosine, NO, mitochondrial I_{KATP}[219]). Its efficacy in combination with bepridil in preventing VF episodes was recently reported by Shinohara et al.[79] The failure of cilostazol in the treatment of BrS has been described in a single case report.[220]

Milrinone is another PDE III inhibitor recently identified as a more potent alternative to cilostazol in suppressing ST-segment elevation and arrhythmogenesis in an experimental model of BrS.[101,221] No clinical reports have yet appeared.

Wenxin Keli, a traditional Chinese medicine (TCM), has recently been shown to inhibit I_{to} and thus to suppress polymorphic VT in experimental models of BrS when combined with low concentrations of quinidine (5 μM).[190]

Agents that augment peak and late I_{Na}, including bepridil and dimethyl lithospermate B (dmLSB), are suggested to be of value in BrS patients. Bepridil has been reported to suppress VT/VF in several studies of BrS patients.[71,222–224] The actions of the drug are considered to be mediated by (1) inhibition of I_{to}; (2) augmentation of I_{Na} via upregulation of the sodium channels[225]; and (3) prolongation of the QT interval at slow rates, thus increasing the QT/RR slope.[222,224] dmLSB, an extract of Danshen, a traditional Chinese herbal remedy, has been reported to slow inactivation of I_{Na}, thus increasing I_{Na} during the early phases of AP and suppressing arrhythmogenesis in experimental models of BrS.[226]

Because malignant ventricular arrhythmias are infrequent in asymptomatic patients with BrS[227] or ERP[39] and usually unrelated to physical activity, the presence of these patterns does not contraindicate participation in sports.

Early Repolarization Syndrome

It is not surprising that the approach to therapy of ERS is similar to that of BrS because the mechanisms underlying the two syndromes are similar. Quinidine, PDE III inhibitors, and isoproterenol have all been shown to exert an ameliorative effect in preventing or quieting arrhythmias associated with ERS. Isoproterenol has been shown to be effective in quieting electrical storms that develop in patients with either BrS[71,209] or ERS.[141] Isoproterenol has been shown to act by reversing the repolarization abnormalities responsible for the disease phenotype secondary to the restoration of the epicardial AP dome in experimental models of both BrS[14,189] and ERS.[25] This action of the β-adrenergic agonist is expected because of its actions to potently increase I_{Ca}.

The PDE III inhibitor cilostazol has been reported to reduce the ECG and arrhythmic manifestations of ERS.[76] PDE inhibitors are known to activate I_{Ca} secondary to an increase in cAMP.[75,218,228–232] The augmentation of I_{Ca} is considered to prevent arrhythmias associated with J wave syndromes by reversing the repolarization defects and restoring electrical homogeneity across the ventricular wall secondary to the restoration of the epicardial AP dome in both BrS[221] and ERS.[95] Cilostazol has been hypothesized to also block I_{to}. Augmentation of I_{Ca} together with the inhibition of I_{to} are expected to produce an inward shift in the balance of currents active during the early phases of the epicardial AP that should be especially effective in suppressing J wave activity. The effectiveness of bepridil in ERS has been reported in a single patient so far.[233]

No clinical data are available regarding the effectiveness of RFA in the setting of ERS, despite the fact that low-voltage and fractionated EGM activity and high-frequency LPs are observed in LV in ERS patients[234] and in experimental models of ERS (Yoon and Antzelevitch, unpublished observation). Nakagawa et al.[234] reported the results of a study in which they recorded epicardial EGMs directly from LV of patients diagnosed with ERS by introducing a multipolar catheter into the left lateral (marginal) coronary vein, anterior interventricular vein (AIV), and middle cardiac vein (MCV) via the coronary sinus. The authors reported LPs in the bipolar EGMs recorded from the LV epicardium of ERS patients.[234]

Acknowledgments

We acknowledge support from NHLBI (HL47678, CA). Dr. Antzelevitch was a consultant for Gilead Sciences and received grant funding and consulting fees from Gilead Sciences.

REFERENCES

1. Brugada P, Brugada J. Right bundle branch block, persistent ST segment elevation and sudden cardiac death: a distinct clinical and electrocardiographic syndrome: a multicenter report. *J Am Coll Cardiol.* 1992;20:1391–1396.
2. Haissaguerre M, Derval N, Sacher F, et al. Sudden cardiac arrest associated with early repolarization. *N Engl J Med.* 2008;358:2016–2023.
3. Nam GB, Kim YH, Antzelevitch C. Augmentation of J waves and electrical storms in patients with early repolarization. *N Engl J Med.* 2008;358:2078–2079.
4. Rosso R, Kogan E, Belhassen B, et al. J-point elevation in survivors of primary ventricular fibrillation and matched control subjects: incidence and clinical significance. *J Am Coll Cardiol.* 2008;52:1231–1238.
5. Clements SD, Hurst JW. Diagnostic value of ECG abnormalities observed in subjects accidentally exposed to cold. *Am J Cardiol.* 1972;29:729–734.
6. Thompson R, Rich J, Chmelik F, et al. Evolutionary changes in the electrocardiogram of severe progressive hypothermia. *J Electrocardiol.* 1977;10:67–70.
7. Eagle K. Images in clinical medicine. Osborn waves of hypothermia. *N Engl J Med.* 1994;10:680.
8. Kraus F. Ueber die wirkung des kalziums auf den kreislauf 1. *Dtsch Med Wochenschr.* 1920;46:201–203.
9. Sridharan MR, Horan LG. Electrocardiographic J wave of hypercalcemia. *Am J Cardiol.* 1984;54:672–673.
10. Antzelevitch C, Yan GX. J wave syndromes. *Heart Rhythm.* 2010;7:549–558.
11. Wasserburger RH, Alt WJ. The normal RS-T segment elevation variant. *Am J Cardiol.* 1961;8:184–192.
12. Mehta MC, Jain AC. Early repolarization on scalar electrocardiogram. *Am J Med Sci.* 1995;309:305–311.
13. Gussak I, Antzelevitch C. Early repolarization syndrome: clinical characteristics and possible cellular and ionic mechanisms. *J Electrocardiol.* 2000;33:299–309.
14. Yan GX, Antzelevitch C. Cellular basis for the Brugada syndrome and other mechanisms of arrhythmogenesis associated with ST segment elevation. *Circulation.* 1999;100:1660–1666.
15. Shu J, Zhu T, Yang L, et al. ST-segment elevation in the early repolarization syndrome, idiopathic ventricular fibrillation, and the Brugada syndrome: cellular and clinical linkage. *J Electrocardiol.* 2005;38:26–32.
16. Antzelevitch C. J wave syndromes: molecular and cellular mechanisms. *J Electrocardiol.* 2013;46:510–518.
17. Mahida S, Derval N, Sacher F, et al. History and clinical significance of early repolarization syndrome. *Heart Rhythm.* 2015;12:242–249.
18. Wellens HJ, Schwartz PJ, Lindemans FW, et al. Risk stratification for sudden cardiac death: current status and challenges for the future. *Eur Heart J.* 2014;35:1642–1651.

19. Macfarlane P, Antzelevitch C, Haissaguerre M, et al. Consensus Paper- Early Repolarization Pattern. *J Amer Coll Cardiol.* 2015;66:470–477.

20. Kanter RJ, Pfeiffer R, Hu D, et al. Brugada-like syndrome in infancy presenting with rapid ventricular tachycardia and intraventricular conduction delay. *Circulation.* 2012;125:14–22.

21. Antzelevitch C. Molecular biology and cellular mechanisms of Brugada and long QT syndromes in infants and young children. *J Electrocardiol.* 2001;34:177–181.

22. Wedekind H, Smits JP, Schulze-Bahr E, et al. De novo mutation in the *SCN5A* gene associated with early onset of sudden infant death. *Circulation.* 2001;104:1158–1164.

23. Nagase S, Kusano KF, Morita H, et al. Epicardial electrogram of the right ventricular outflow tract in patients with the Brugada syndrome: using the epicardial lead. *J Am Coll Cardiol.* 2002;39:1992–1995.

24. Nakagawa K, Nagase S, Morita H, et al. Left ventricular epicardial electrogram recordings in idiopathic ventricular fibrillation with inferior and lateral early repolarization. *Heart Rhythm.* 2014;11:314–317.

25. Koncz I, Gurabi Z, Patocskai B, et al. Mechanisms underlying the development of the electrocardiographic and arrhythmic manifestations of early repolarization syndrome. *J Mol Cell Cardiol.* 2014;68C:20–28.

26. Antzelevitch C. Brugada syndrome. *Pacing Clin Electrophysiol.* 2006;29:1130–1159.

27. Coronel R, Casini S, Koopmann TT, et al. Right ventricular fibrosis and conduction delay in a patient with clinical signs of Brugada syndrome: a combined electrophysiological, genetic, histopathologic, and computational study. *Circulation.* 2005;112:2769–2777.

28. Bastiaenen R, Hedley PL, Christiansen M, et al. Therapeutic hypothermia and ventricular fibrillation storm in early repolarization syndrome. *Heart Rhythm.* 2010;7:832–834.

29. Federman NJ, Mechulan A, Klein GJ, et al. Ventricular fibrillation induced by spontaneous hypothermia in a patient with early repolarization syndrome. *J Cardiovasc Electrophysiol.* 2013;24:586–588.

30. Sakabe M, Fujiki A, Tani M, et al. Proportion and prognosis of healthy people with coved or saddle-back type ST segment elevation in the right precordial leads during 10 years follow-up. *Eur Heart J.* 2003;24:1488–1493.

31. Tsuji H, Sato T, Morisaki K, et al. Prognosis of subjects with Brugada-type electrocardiogram in a population of middle-aged Japanese diagnosed during a health examination. *Am J Cardiol.* 2008;102:584–587.

32. Gervacio-Domingo G, Isidro J, Tirona J, et al. The Brugada type 1 electrocardiographic pattern is common among Filipinos. *J Clin Epidemiol.* 2008;61:1067–1072.

33. Ito H, Yano K, Chen R, He Q, Curb JD. The prevalence and prognosis of a Brugada-type electrocardiogram in a population of middle-aged Japanese-American men with follow-up of three decades. *Am J Med Sci.* 2006;331:25–29

34. Letsas KP, Weber R, Astheimer K, et al. Tpeak-Tend interval and Tpeak-Tend/QT ratio as markers of ventricular tachycardia inducibility in subjects with Brugada ECG phenotype. *Europace.* 2010;12:271–274.

35. Gallagher MM, Forleo GB, Behr ER, et al. Prevalence and significance of Brugada-type ECG in 12,012 apparently healthy European subjects. *Int J Cardiol.* 2008;130:44–48.

36. Pecini R, Cedergreen P, Theilade S, et al. The prevalence and relevance of the Brugada-type electrocardiogram in the Danish general population: data from the Copenhagen City Heart Study. *Europace.* 2010;12:982–986.

37. Patel SS, Anees SS, Ferrick KJ. Prevalence of a Brugada pattern electrocardiogram in an urban population in the United States. *Pacing Clin Electrophysiol.* 2009;32:704–708.

38. Lee C, Soni A, Tate RB, Cuddy TE. The incidence and prognosis of Brugada electrocardiographic pattern in the Manitoba Follow-Up Study. *Can J Cardiol.* 2005;21:1286–1290.

39. Tikkanen JT, Anttonen O, Junttila MJ, et al. Long-term outcome associated with early repolarization on electrocardiography. *N Engl J Med.* 2009;361:2529–2537.

40. Sinner MF, Reinhard W, Muller M, et al. Association of early repolarization pattern on ECG with risk of cardiac and all-cause mortality: a population-based prospective cohort study (MONICA/KORA). *PLoS Med.* 2010;7:e1000314.

41. Haruta D, Matsuo K, Tsuneto A, et al. Incidence and prognostic value of early repolarization pattern in the 12-lead electrocardiogram. *Circulation.* 2011;123:2931–2937.

42. Brosnan MJ, Kumar S, LaGerche A, et al. Early repolarization patterns associated with increased arrhythmic risk are common in young non-Caucasian Australian males and not influenced by athletic status. *Heart Rhythm.* 2015;12:1576–1583.

43. Shimizu W. Acquired forms of the Brugada syndrome. *J Electrocardiol.* 2005;38l:22–25.

44. Brugada P, Brugada J, Brugada R. Arrhythmia induction by antiarrhythmic drugs. *Pacing Clin Electrophysiol.* 2000;23:291–292.

45. Brugada R, Brugada J, Antzelevitch C, et al. Sodium channel blockers identify risk for sudden death in patients with ST-segment elevation and right bundle branch block but structurally normal hearts. *Circulation.* 2000;101:510–515.

46. Miyazaki T, Mitamura H, Miyoshi S, et al. Autonomic and antiarrhythmic drug modulation of ST segment elevation in patients with Brugada syndrome. *J Am Coll Cardiol.* 1996;27:1061–1070.

47. Babaliaros VC, Hurst JW. Tricyclic antidepressants and the Brugada syndrome: an example of Brugada waves appearing after the administration of desipramine. *Clin Cardiol.* 2002;25:395–398.

48. Goldgran-Toledano D, Sideris G, Kevorkian JP. Overdose of cyclic antidepressants and the Brugada syndrome. *N Engl J Med.* 2002;346:1591–1592.

49. Tada H, Sticherling C, Oral H, et al. Brugada syndrome mimicked by tricyclic antidepressant overdose. *J Cardiovasc Electrophysiol.* 2001;12:275.

50. Ortega-Carnicer J, Bertos-Polo J, Gutierrez-Tirado C. Aborted sudden death, transient Brugada pattern, and wide QRS dysrhythmias after massive cocaine ingestion. *J Electrocardiol.* 2001;34:345–349.

51. Nogami A, Nakao M, Kubota S, et al. Enhancement of J-ST-segment elevation by the glucose and insulin test in Brugada syndrome. *Pacing Clin Electrophysiol.* 2003;26:332–337.

52. Araki T, Konno T, Itoh H, et al. Brugada syndrome with ventricular tachycardia and fibrillation related to hypokalemia. *Circ J.* 2003;67:93–95.

53. Pastor A, Nunez A, Cantale C, et al. Asymptomatic Brugada syndrome case unmasked during dimenhydrinate infusion. *J Cardiovasc Electrophysiol.* 2001;12:1192–1194.

54. Chiale PA, Garro HA, Fernandez PA, et al. High-degree right bundle branch block obscuring the diagnosis of Brugada electrocardiographic pattern. *Heart Rhythm.* 2012;9:974–976.

55. Postema PG, Wolpert C, Amin AS, et al. Drugs and Brugada syndrome patients: review of the literature, recommendations, and an up-to-date website (www.brugadadrugs.org). *Heart Rhythm.* 2009;6:1335–1341.

56. Nam GB. Idiopathic ventricular fibrillation, early repolarization and other J wave-related ventricular fibrillation syndromes. *Circ J.* 2012;76:2723–2731.

57. Yan GX, Antzelevitch C. Cellular basis for the electrocardiographic J wave. *Circulation.* 1996;93:372–379.

58. McIntyre WF, Perez-Riera AR, Femenia F, et al. Coexisting early repolarization pattern and Brugada syndrome: recognition of potentially overlapping entities. *J Electrocardiol.* 2012;45:195–198.

59. Benito B, Sarkozy A, Mont L, et al. Gender differences in clinical manifestations of Brugada syndrome. *J Am Coll Cardiol.* 2008;52:1567–1573.

60. Kamakura T, Kawata H, Nakajima I, et al. Significance of non-type 1 anterior early repolarization in patients with inferolateral early repolarization syndrome. *J Am Coll Cardiol.* 2013;62:1610–1618.

61. Matsumoto AM. Fundamental aspects of hypogonadism in the aging male. *Rev Urol.* 2003;5(suppl 1):S3–S10.

62. Kalla H, Yan GX, Marinchak R. Ventricular fibrillation in a patient with prominent J (Osborn) waves and ST segment elevation in the inferior electrocardiographic leads: a Brugada syndrome variant? *J Cardiovasc Electrophysiol.* 2000;11:95–98.

63. Aizawa Y, Sato A, Watanabe H, et al. Dynamicity of the J-wave in idiopathic ventricular fibrillation with a special reference to pause-dependent augmentation of the J-wave. *J Am Coll Cardiol.* 2012;59:1948–1953.

64. Nademanee K. Sudden unexplained death syndrome in southeast Asia. *Am J Cardiol.* 1997;79(6A):10–11.

65. Kawata H, Noda T, Yamada Y, et al. Effect of sodium-channel blockade on early repolarization in inferior/lateral leads in patients with idiopathic ventricular fibrillation and Brugada syndrome. *Heart Rhythm.* 2012;9:77–83.

66. Watanabe H, Nogami A, Ohkubo K, et al. Electrocardiographic characteristics and SCN5A mutations in idiopathic ventricular fibrillation associated with early repolarization. *Circ Arrhythm Electrophysiol.* 2011;4:874–881.

67. Antzelevitch C, Pollevick GD, Cordeiro JM, et al. Loss-of-function mutations in the cardiac calcium channel underlie a new clinical entity characterized by ST-segment elevation, short QT intervals, and sudden cardiac death. *Circulation.* 2007;115:442–449.

68. Morita H, Zipes DP, Morita ST, et al. Temperature modulation of ventricular arrhythmogenicity in a canine tissue model of Brugada syndrome. *Heart Rhythm.* 2007;4:188–197.

69. Shimizu W, Kamakura S. Catecholamines in children with congenital long QT syndrome and Brugada syndrome. *J Electrocardiol.* 2001;34(suppl):173–175.

70. Suzuki H, Torigoe K, Numata O, et al. Infant case with a malignant form of Brugada syndrome. *J Cardiovasc Electrophysiol.* 2000;11:1277–1280.

71. Ohgo T, Okamura H, Noda T, et al. Acute and chronic management in patients with Brugada syndrome associated with electrical storm of ventricular fibrillation. *Heart Rhythm.* 2007;4:695–700.

72. Watanabe A, Fukushima KK, Morita H, et al. Low-dose isoproterenol for repetitive ventricular arrhythmia in patients with Brugada syndrome. *Eur Heart J.* 2006;27:1579–1583.

73. Hermida JS, Denjoy I, Clerc J, et al. Hydroquinidine therapy in Brugada syndrome. *J Am Coll Cardiol.* 2004;43:1853–1860.

74. Belhassen B, Glick A, Viskin S. Efficacy of quinidine in high-risk patients with Brugada syndrome. *Circulation.* 2004;110:1731–1737.

75. Tsuchiya T, Ashikaga K, Honda T, et al. Prevention of ventricular fibrillation by cilostazol, an oral phosphodiesterase inhibitor, in a patient with Brugada syndrome. *J Cardiovasc Electrophysiol.* 2002;13:698–701.

76. Iguchi K, Noda T, Kamakura S, et al. Beneficial effects of cilostazol in a patient with recurrent ventricular fibrillation associated with early repolarization syndrome. *Heart Rhythm.* 2013;10:604–606.

77. Agac MT, Erkan H, Korkmaz L. Conversion of Brugada type I to type III and successful control of recurrent ventricular arrhythmia with cilostazol. *Arch Cardiovasc Dis.* 2013;107(8-9):476–478.

78. Hasegawa K, Ashihara T, Kimura H, et al. Long-term pharmacological therapy of Brugada syndrome: is J-wave attenuation a marker of drug efficacy? *Intern Med.* 2014;53:1523–1526.

79. Shinohara T, Ebata Y, Ayabe R, et al. Combination therapy of cilostazol and bepridil suppresses recurrent ventricular fibrillation related to J-wave syndromes. *Heart Rhythm.* 2014;11:1441–1445.

80. Haissaguerre M, Sacher F, Nogami A, et al. Characteristics of recurrent ventricular fibrillation associated with inferolateral early repolarization role of drug therapy. *J Am Coll Cardiol.* 2009;53:612–619.

81. Junttila MJ, Tikkanen JT, Kentta T, et al. Early repolarization as a predictor of arrhythmic and nonarrhythmic cardiac events in middle-aged subjects. *Heart Rhythm.* 2014;11:1701–1706.

82. Nam GB, Ko KH, Kim J, et al. Mode of onset of ventricular fibrillation in patients with early repolarization pattern vs. Brugada syndrome. *Eur Heart J.* 2010;31:330–339.

83. Kowalczyk E, Kasprzak JD, Lipiec P. Giant J-wave and Brugada-like pattern in a patient with severe hypothermia. *Acta Cardiol.* 2014;69:66–67.

84. RuDusky BM. The electrocardiogram in hypothermia—the J wave and the Brugada syndrome. *Am J Cardiol.* 2004;93:671–672.

85. Ortega-Carnicer J, Benezet J, Calderon-Jimenez P, et al. Hypothermia-induced Brugada-like electrocardiogram pattern. *J Electrocardiol.* 2008;41:690–692.

86. Bonnemeier H, Mauser W, Schunkert H. Images in cardiovascular medicine. Brugada-like ECG pattern in severe hypothermia. *Circulation.* 2008;118:977–978.

87. Adler A, Topaz G, Heller K, et al. Fever-induced Brugada pattern: how common is it and what does it mean? *Heart Rhythm.* 2013;10:1375–1382.

88. Ansari E, Cook JR. Profound hypothermia mimicking a Brugada type ECG. *J Electrocardiol.* 2003;36:257–260.

89. Noda T, Shimizu W, Tanaka K, et al. Prominent J wave and ST segment elevation: serial electrocardiographic changes in accidental hypothermia. *J Cardiovasc Electrophysiol.* 2003;14:223.

90. Amin AS, Meregalli PG, Bardai A, et al. Fever increases the risk for cardiac arrest in the Brugada syndrome. *Ann Intern Med.* 2008;149:216–218.

91. Rattanawong P, Vutthikraivit W, Charoensri A, et al. Fever-induced Brugada syndrome is more common than previously suspected: a cross-sectional study from an endemic area. *Ann Noninvasive Electrocardiol.* 2016;21:136–141.

92. Tan H.L., Meregalli P.G.. Lethal ECG changes hidden by therapeutic hypothermia. *Lancet.* 2007;369:378.

93. Kurisu S, Inoue I, Kawagoe T, et al. Therapeutic hypothermia after out-of-hospital cardiac arrest due to Brugada syndrome. *Resuscitation.* 2008;79:332–335.

94. Patel RB, Ng J, Reddy V, et al. Early repolarization associated with ventricular arrhythmias in patients with chronic coronary artery disease. *Circ Arrhythm Electrophysiol.* 2010;3:489–495.

95. Gurabi Z, Koncz I, Patocskai B, et al. Cellular mechanism underlying hypothermia-induced VT/VF in the setting of early repolarization and the protective effect of quinidine, cilostazol and milrinone. *Circ Arrhythm Electrophysiol.* 2014;7:134–142.

96. Kawata H, Morita H, Yamada Y, et al. Prognostic significance of early repolarization in inferolateral leads in Brugada patients with documented ventricular fibrillation: a novel risk factor for Brugada syndrome with ventricular fibrillation. *Heart Rhythm.* 2013;10:1161–1168.

97. Antzelevitch C. Genetic, molecular and cellular mechanisms underlying the J wave syndromes. *Circ J.* 2012;76:1054–1065.

98. Kapplinger JD, Tester DJ, Alders M, et al. An international compendium of mutations in the SCN5A encoded cardiac sodium channel in patients referred for Brugada syndrome genetic testing. *Heart Rhythm*. 2010;7:33–46.
99. Park DS, Cerrone M, Morley G, et al. Genetically engineered SCN5A mutant pig hearts exhibit conduction defects and arrhythmias. *J Clin Invest*. 2015;125:403–412.
100. Antzelevitch C, Yan GX. J-wave syndromes: Brugada and early repolarization syndromes. *Heart Rhythm*. 2015;12:1852–1866.
101. Szel T, Antzelevitch C. Abnormal repolarization as the basis for late potentials and fractionated electrograms recorded from epicardium in experimental models of Brugada syndrome. *J Am Coll Cardiol*. 2014;63:2037–2045.
102. Patocskai B, Szel T, Yoon N, et al. Cellular mechanisms underlying the fractionated and late potentials on epicardial electrograms and the ameliorative effect of epicardial radiofrequency ablation in an experimental model of Brugada syndrome. In: *Program and Abstracts of the 24th Annual Upstate New York Cardiac Electrophysiology Society Meeting, November 3, 2014, Buffalo, NY*. 2014:Abstract 006.
103. Burashnikov E, Pfeiffer R, Barajas-Martinez H, et al. Mutations in the cardiac L-type calcium channel associated J wave sydnrome and sudden cardiac death. *Heart Rhythm*. 2010;7:1872–1882.
104. Cordeiro JM, Marieb M, Pfeiffer R, et al. Accelerated inactivation of the L-type calcium due to a mutation in *CACNB2b* underlies Brugada syndrome. *J Mol Cell Cardiol*. 2009;46:695–703.
105. Antzelevitch C, Pollevick GD, Cordeiro JM, et al. Loss-of-function mutations in the cardiac calcium channel underline a new clinical entity characterized by ST segment elevation, short QT intervals, and sudden cardiac death. *Circ Res*. 2006;99:1279.
106. Gurnett CA, De WM, Campbell KP. Dual function of the voltage-dependent Ca2+ channel alpha 2 delta subunit in current stimulation and subunit interaction. *Neuron*. 1996;16:431–440.
107. Barajas-Martinez H, Hu D, Ferrer T, et al. Molecular genetic and functional association of Brugada and early repolarization syndromes with S422L missense mutation in *KCNJ8*. *Heart Rhythm*. 2012;9:548–555.
108. Delaney JT, Muhammad R, Blair MA, et al. A KCNJ8 mutation associated with early repolarization and atrial fibrillation. *Europace*. 2012;14:1428–1432.
109. Medeiros-Domingo A, Tan BH, Crotti L, et al. Gain-of-function mutation S422L in the KCNJ8-encoded cardiac K(ATP) channel Kir6.1 as a pathogenic substrate for J-wave syndromes. *Heart Rhythm*. 2010; 7:1466–1471.
110. Hu D, Barajas-Martinez H, Medeiros-Domingo A, et al. Novel mutations in the sodium channel 2 subunit gene (SCN2B) associated with Brugada syndrome and atrial fibrillation. *Circulation*. 2012;126:A16521.
111. Riuro H, Beltran-Alvarez P, Tarradas A, et al. A missense mutation in the sodium channel β2 subunit reveals *SCN2B* as a new candidate gene for Brugada syndrome. *Hum Mutat*. 2013;34:961–966.
112. Giudicessi JR, Ye D, Tester DJ, et al. Transient outward current (Ito) gain-of-function mutations in the KCND3-encoded Kv4.3 potassium channel and Brugada syndrome. *Heart Rhythm*. 2011;8:1024–1032.
113. Delpón E, Cordeiro JM, Núñez L, et al. Functional effects of *KCNE3* mutation and its role in the development of Brugada syndrome. *Circ Arrhythm Electrophysiol*. 2008;1:209–218.
114. Olesen MS, Jensen NF, Holst AG, et al. A novel nonsense variant in Nav1.5 cofactor MOG1 eliminates its sodium current increasing effect and may increase the risk of arrhythmias. *Can J Cardiol*. 2011;27:523.
115. Kattygnarath D, Maugenre S, Neyroud N, et al. MOG1: a new susceptibility gene for Brugada syndrome. *Circ Cardiovasc Genet*. 2011;4:261–268.
116. Cerrone M, Lin X, Zhang M, et al. Missense mutations in plakophilin-2 cause sodium current deficit and associate with a Brugada syndrome phenotype. *Circulation*. 2013;129:1092–1103.
117. Hennessey JA, Marcou CA, Wang C, et al. FGF12 is a candidate Brugada syndrome locus. *Heart Rhythm*. 2013;10:1886–1894.
118. Bezzina CR, Barc J, Mizusawa Y, et al. Common variants at *SCN5A-SCN10A* and *HEY2* are associated with Brugada syndrome, a rare disease with high risk of sudden cardiac death. *Nat Genet*. 2013;45:1044–1049.
119. Boukens BJ, Sylva M, de Gier-de VC, et al. Reduced sodium channel function unmasks residual embryonic slow conduction in the adult right ventricular outflow tract. *Circ Res*. 2013;113:137–141.
120. Hartman ME, Liu Y, Zhu WZ, et al. Myocardial deletion of transcription factor CHF1/Hey2 results in altered myocyte action potential and mild conduction system expansion but does not alter conduction system function or promote spontaneous arrhythmias. *FASEB J*. 2014;28:3007–3015.
121. Ishikawa T, Takahashi N, Ohno S, et al. Novel *SCN3B* mutation associated with Brugada syndrome affects intracellular trafficking and function of Nav1.5. *Circ J*. 2013;77:959–967.
122. Hu D, Barajas-Martinez H, Burashnikov E, et al. A mutation in the beta 3 subunit of the cardiac sodium channel associated with Brugada ECG phenotype. *Circ Cardiovasc Genet*. 2009;2:270–278.
123. Watanabe H, Koopmann TT, Le Scouarnec S, et al. Sodium channel b1 subunit mutations associated with Brugada syndrome and cardiac conduction disease in humans. *J Clin Invest*. 2008;118:2260–2268.
124. Valdivia CR, Ueda K, Ackerman MJ, et al. GPD1L links redox state to cardiac excitability by PKC-dependent phosphorylation of the sodium channel SCN5A. *Am J Physiol Heart Circ Physiol*. 2009;297:H1446–H1452.
125. Shy D, Gillet L, Abriel H. Cardiac sodium channel NaV1.5 distribution in myocytes via interacting proteins: the multiple pool model. *Biochim Biophys Acta*. 2013;1833:886–894.
126. Weiss R, Barmada MM, Nguyen T, et al. Clinical and molecular heterogeneity in the Brugada syndrome: a novel gene locus on chromosome 3. *Circulation*. 2002;105:707–713.
127. Hu D, Barajas-Martinez H, Medeiros-Domingo A, et al. A novel rare variant in *SCN1Bb* linked to Brugada syndrome and SIDS by combined modulation of Na(v)1.5 and K(v)4.3 channel currents. *Heart Rhythm*. 2012;9:760–769.
128. Hu D, Barajas-Martinez H, Pfeiffer R, et al. Mutations in *SCN10A* are responsible for a large fraction of cases of Brugada syndrome. *J Am Coll Cardiol*. 2014;64: 66–79.
129. Behr ER, Savio-Galimberti E, Barc J, et al. Role of common and rare variants in SCN10A: results from the Brugada syndrome QRS locus gene discovery collaborative study. *Cardiovasc Res*. 2015;106:520–529.
130. Antzelevitch C. Cardiac repolarization. The long and short of it. *Europace*. 2005;7:3–9.
131. Liu H, Chatel S, Simard C, et al. Molecular genetics and functional anomalies in a series of 248 Brugada cases with 11 mutations in the TRPM4 channel. *PLoS One*. 2013;8:e54131.
132. Perrin MJ, Adler A, Green S, et al. Evaluation of genes encoding for the transient outward current (Ito) identifies the *KCND2* gene as a cause of J wave syndrome associated with sudden cardiac death. *Circ Cardiovasc Genet*. 2014;7:782–789.
133. Verkerk AO, Wilders R, Schulze-Bahr E, et al. Role of sequence variations in the human ether-a-go-go-related gene (HERG, KCNH2) in the Brugada syndrome. *Cardiovasc Res*. 2005;68:441–453.
134. Wilders R, Verkerk AO. Role of the R1135H *KCNH2* mutation in Brugada syndrome. *Int J Cardiol*. 2010;144:149–151.
135. Ohno S, Zankov DP, Ding WG, et al. KCNE5 (KCNE1L) variants are novel modulators of Brugada syndrome and idiopathic ventricular fibrillation. *Circ Arrhythm Electrophysiol*. 2011;4:352–361.
136. Boczek NJ, Ye D, Johnson EK, et al. Characterization of SEMA3A-encoded semaphorin as a naturally occurring Kv4.3 protein inhibitor and its contribution to Brugada syndrome. *Circ Res*. 2014;115:460–469.
137. Ueda K, Nakamura K, Hayashi T, et al. Functional characterization of a trafficking-defective *HCN4* mutation, D553N, associated with cardiac arrhythmia. *J Biol Chem*. 2004;279:27194–27198.
138. Noseworthy PA, Tikkanen JT, Porthan K, et al. The early repolarization pattern in the general population clinical correlates and heritability. *J Am Coll Cardiol*. 2011;57:2284–2289.
139. Reinhard W, Kaess BM, Debiec R, et al. Heritability of early repolarization: a population-based study. *Circ Cardiovasc Genet*. 2011;4:134–138.
140. Nunn LM, Bhar-Amato J, Lowe MD, et al. Prevalence of J-point elevation in sudden arrhythmic death syndrome families. *J Am Coll Cardiol*. 2011;58: 286–290.
141. Haissaguerre M, Chatel S, Sacher F, et al. Ventricular fibrillation with prominent early repolarization associated with a rare variant of KCNJ8/K_{ATP} channel. *J Cardiovasc Electrophysiol*. 2009;20:93–98.
142. Schwartz PJ, Ackerman MJ, George Jr AL, et al. Impact of genetics on the clinical management of channelopathies. *J Am Coll Cardiol*. 2013;62:169–180.
143. Raffan E, Semple RK. Next generation sequencing—implications for clinical practice. *Br Med Bull*. 2011;99:53–71.
144. Refsgaard L, Holst AG, Sadjadieh G, et al. High prevalence of genetic variants previously associated with LQT syndrome in new exome data. *Eur J Hum Genet*. 2012;20:905–908.
145. Kapa S, Tester DJ, Salisbury BA, et al. Genetic testing for long-QT syndrome: distinguishing pathogenic mutations from benign variants. *Circulation*. 2009;120:1752–1760.
146. Andreasen C, Refsgaard L, Nielsen JB, et al. Mutations in genes encoding cardiac ion channels previously associated with sudden infant death syndrome (SIDS) are present with high frequency in new exome data. *Can J Cardiol*. 2013;29:1104–1109.
147. Song W, Shou W. Cardiac sodium channel Nav1.5 mutations and cardiac arrhythmia. *Ped Cardiol*. 2012;33:943–949.
148. Ruklisa D, Ware JS, Walsh R, et al. Bayesian models for syndrome- and gene-specific probabilities of novel variant pathogenicity. *Genome Med*. 2015;7:5.
149. Juang JM, Lu TP, Lai LC, et al. Utilizing multiple in silico analyses to identify putative causal SCN5A variants in Brugada syndrome. *Sci Rep*. 2014;4:3850.
150. Walsh R, Peters NS, Cook SA, et al. Paralogue annotation identifies novel pathogenic variants in patients with Brugada syndrome and catecholaminergic polymorphic ventricular tachycardia. *J Med Genet*. 2014;
51:35–44.
151. Kapplinger JD, Giudicessi JR, Tester DJ, et al. Enhanced classification of non-synonymous single nucleotide variants in the SCN5A-encoded Nav1.5 cardiac sodium channel. *Heart Rhythm*. 2012;9:1912.
152. Kapplinger JD, Giudicessi JR, Ye D, et al. Enhanced classification of Brugada syndrome-associated and long-QT syndrome-associated genetic variants in the SCN5A-encoded Nav1.5 cardiac sodium channel. *Circ Cardiovasc Genet*. 2015;8:582–595.
153. Le Scouarnec S, Karakachoff M, Gourraud JB, et al. Testing the burden of rare variation in arrhythmia-susceptibility genes provides new insights into molecular diagnosis for Brugada syndrome. *Hum Mol Genet*. 2015;24:2757–2763.
154. Wilde AA, Postema PG, Di Diego JM, et al. The pathophysiological mechanism underlying Brugada syndrome: depolarization versus repolarization. *J Mol Cell Cardiol*. 2010;49:543–553.
155. Morita H, Zipes DP, Wu J. Brugada syndrome: insights of ST elevation, arrhythmogenicity, and risk stratification from experimental observations. *Heart Rhythm*. 2009;6:S34–S43.
156. Nademanee K, Veerakul G, Chandanamattha P, et al. Prevention of ventricular fibrillation episodes in Brugada syndrome by catheter ablation over the anterior right ventricular outflow tract epicardium. *Circulation*. 2011;123:1270–1279.
157. Brugada J, Pappone C, Berruezo A, et al. Brugada syndrome phenotype elimination by epicardial substrate ablation. *Circ Arrhythm Electrophysiol*. 2015;8:1373–1381.
158. Sacher F, Jesel L, Jais P, et al. Insight into the mechanism of Brugada syndrome: epicardial substrate and modification during ajmaline testing. *Heart Rhythm*. 2014;11:732–734.
158a. Patocskai B, Yoon N, Antzelevitch C, et al. Mechanisms underlying epicardial radiofrequency ablation to suppress arrhythmogenesis in experimental models of Brugada syndrome. *JACC: Clin Electrophysiol*. December 21, 2016, 299;http://dx.doi.org/10.1016/j.jacep.2016.10.011.
159. Patocskai B, Antzelevitch C. Novel therapeutic strategies for the management of ventricular arrhythmias associated with the Brugada syndrome. *Expert Opin Orphan Drugs*. 2015;3:633-651.
160. Antzelevitch C, Brugada P, Brugada J, et al. Brugada syndrome: a decade of progress. *Circ Res*. 2002;91:1114–1119.
161. Kurita T, Shimizu W, Inagaki M, et al. The electrophysiologic mechanism of ST-segment elevation in Brugada syndrome. *J Am Coll Cardiol*. 2002; 40:330–334.
162. Zhang J, Sacher F, Hoffmayer K, et al. Cardiac electrophysiological substrate underlying the ECG phenotype and electrogram abnormalities in Brugada syndrome patients. *Circulation*. 2015;131:1950–1959.
163. Gurabi Z, Koncz I, Patocskai B, et al. Cellular mechanism underlying hypothermia-induced ventricular tachycardia/ventricular fibrillation in the setting of early repolarization and the protective effect of quinidine, cilostazol, and milrinone. *Circ Arrhythm Electrophysiol*. 2014;7:134–142.
164. Ghosh S, Cooper DH, Vijayakumar R, et al. Early repolarization associated with sudden death: insights from noninvasive electrocardiographic imaging. *Heart Rhythm*. 2010;7:534–537.
165. Huikuri HV. Separation of benign from malignant J waves. *Heart Rhythm*. 2015;12:384–385.
166. Aizawa Y, Sato M, Kitazawa H, et al. Tachycardia-dependent augmentation of "notched J waves" in a general patient population without ventricular fibrillation or cardiac arrest: not a repolarization but a depolarization abnormality? *Heart Rhythm*. 2015;12:376–383.
167. Badri M, Patel A, Yan G. Cellular and ionic basis of J-wave syndromes. *Trends Cardiovasc Med*. 2015;25:12–21.
168. Morita H, Kusano KF, Miura D, et al. Fragmented QRS as a marker of conduction abnormality and a predictor of prognosis of Brugada syndrome. *Circulation*. 2008;118:1697–1704.

169. Priori SG, Gasparini M, Napolitano C, et al. Risk stratification in Brugada syndrome: results of the PRELUDE (PRogrammed ELectrical stimUlation preDictive valuE) registry. *J Am Coll Cardiol*. 2012;59:37–45.
170. Terho HK, Tikkanen JT, Junttila JM, et al. Prevalence and prognostic significance of fragmented QRS complex in middle-aged subjects with and without clinical or electrocardiographic evidence of cardiac disease. *Am J Cardiol*. 2014;114:141–147.
171. Brugada J, Brugada R, Brugada P. Pharmacological and device approach to therapy of inherited cardiac diseases associated with cardiac arrhythmias and sudden death. *J Electrocardiol*. 2000;33:41–47.
172. Nademanee K, Veerakul G, Mower M, et al. Defibrillator Versus beta-Blockers for Unexplained Death in Thailand (DEBUT): a randomized clinical trial. *Circulation*. 2003;107:2221–2226.
173. Sacher F, Probst V, Maury P, et al. Outcome after implantation of cardioverter-defibrillator in patients with Brugada syndrome: a multicenter study—part 2. *Circulation*. 2013;128:1739–1747.
174. Conte G, Sieira J, Ciconte G, et al. Implantable cardioverter-defibrillator therapy in Brugada syndrome: a 20-year single-center experience. *J Am Coll Cardiol*. 2015;65:879–888.
175. De Maria E, Olaru A, Cappelli S. The entirely subcutaneous defibrillator (s-icd): state of the art and selection of the ideal candidate. *Curr Cardiol Rev*. 2015;11:180–186.
176. Brugada P, Brugada R, Brugada J, et al. Use of the prophylactic implantable cardioverter defibrillator for patients with normal hearts. *Am J Cardiol*. 1999;83:D98–D100.
177. Priori SG, Wilde AA, Horie M, et al. HRS/EHRA/APHRS expert consensus statement on the diagnosis and management of patients with inherited primary arrhythmia syndromes: document endorsed by HRS, EHRA, and APHRS in May 2013 and by ACCF, AHA, PACES, and AEPC in June 2013. *Heart Rhythm*. 2013;10:1932–1963.
178. Makimoto H, Kamakura S, Aihara N, et al. Clinical impact of the number of extrastimuli in programmed electrical stimulation in patients with Brugada type 1 electrocardiogram. *Heart Rhythm*. 2012;9:242–248.
179. Takagi M, Tatsumi H, Yoshiyama M. Approach to the asymptomatic patients with Brugada syndrome. *Indian Pacing Electrophysiol J*. 2007;7:73–76.
180. Priori SG, Gasparini M, Napolitano C, et al. Risk stratification in Brugada syndrome: results of the PRELUDE (PRogrammed ELectrical stimUlation preDictive valuE) registry. *J Am Coll Cardiol*. 2012;59:37–45.
181. Sieira J, Conte G, Ciconte G, et al. Prognostic value of programmed electrical stimulation in Brugada syndrome: 20 years experience. *Circ Arrhythm Electrophysiol*. 2015;8:777–784.
182. van Den Berg MP, Wilde AA, Viersma TJW, et al. Possible bradycardic mode of death and successful pacemaker treatment in a large family with features of long QT syndrome type 3 and Brugada syndrome. *J Cardiovasc Electrophysiol*. 2001;12:630–636.
183. Bertomeu-Gonzalez V, Ruiz-Granell R, Garcia-Civera R, et al. Syncopal monomorphic ventricular tachycardia with pleomorphism, sensitive to antitachycardia pacing in a patient with Brugada syndrome. *Europace*. 2006;8:1048–1050.
184. Lee KL, Lau C, Tse H, et al. Prevention of ventricular fibrillation by pacing in a man with Brugada syndrome. *J Cardiovasc Electrophysiol*. 2000;11:935–937.
185. Shah AJ, Hocini M, Lamaison D, et al. Regional substrate ablation abolishes Brugada syndrome. *J Cardiovasc Electrophysiol*. 2011;22:1290–1291.
186. Cortez-Dias N, Placido R, Marta L, et al. Epicardial ablation for prevention of ventricular fibrillation in a patient with Brugada syndrome. *Rev Port Cardiol*. 2014;33:305–305.
187. Priori SG, Wilde AA, Horie M, et al. Executive Summary: HRS/EHRA/APHRS Expert Consensus Statement on the Diagnosis and Management of Patients with Inherited Primary Arrhythmia Syndromes. *Heart Rhythm*. 2013;15:1389–1406.
188. Antzelevitch C, Brugada P, Brugada J, et al. *Clinical Approaches to Tachyarrhythmias. The Brugada Syndrome*. Armonk, NY: Futura Publishing Company, Inc; 1999.
189. Minoura Y, Di Diego JM, Barajas-Martinez H, et al. Ionic and cellular mechanisms underlying the development of acquired Brugada syndrome in patients treated with antidepressants. *J Cardiovasc Electrophysiol*. 2012;23:423–432.
190. Minoura Y, Panama BK, Nesterenko VV, et al. Effect of Wenxin Keli and quinidine to suppress arrhythmogenesis in an experimental model of Brugada syndrome. *Heart Rhythm*. 2013;10:1054–1062.
191. Johnson P, Lesage A, Floyd WL, et al. Prevention of ventricular fibrillation during profound hypothermia by quinidine. *Ann Surg*. 1960;151:490–495.
192. Belhassen B, Shapira I, Shoshani D, et al. Idiopathic ventricular fibrillation: inducibility and beneficial effects of class I antiarrhythmic agents. *Circulation*. 1987;75:809–816.
193. Belhassen B, Viskin S, Antzelevitch C. The Brugada syndrome: is an implantable cardioverter defibrillator the only therapeutic option? *Pacing Clin Electrophysiol*. 2002;25:1634–1640.
194. Alings M, Dekker L, Sadee A, et al. Quinidine induced electrocardiographic normalization in two patients with Brugada syndrome. *Pacing Clin Electrophysiol*. 2001;24:1420–1422.
195. Belhassen B, Viskin S. Pharmacologic approach to therapy of Brugada syndrome: quinidine as an alternative to ICD therapy? In: Antzelevitch C, Brugada P, Brugada J, et al., eds. *The Brugada Syndrome: From Bench to Bedside*. Oxford: Blackwell Futura; 2004:202–211.
196. Viskin S, Wilde AA, Tan HL, et al. Empiric quinidine therapy for asymptomatic Brugada syndrome: time for a prospective registry. *Heart Rhythm*. 2009;6:401–404.
197. Belhassen B, Glick A, Viskin S. Excellent long-term reproducibility of the electrophysiologic efficacy of quinidine in patients with idiopathic ventricular fibrillation and Brugada syndrome. *Pacing Clin Electrophysiol*. 2009;32:294–301.
198. Marquez MF, Bonny A, Hernandez-Castillo E, et al. Long-term efficacy of low doses of quinidine on malignant arrhythmias in Brugada syndrome with an implantable cardioverter-defibrillator: a case series and literature review. *Heart Rhythm*. 2013;9:1995–2000.
199. Pellegrino PL, Di Biase M, Brunetti ND. Quinidine for the management of electrical storm in an old patient with Brugada syndrome and syncope. *Acta Cardiol*. 2013;68:201–203.
200. Probst V, Evain S, Gournay V, et al. Monomorphic ventricular tachycardia due to Brugada syndrome successfully treated by hydroquinidine therapy in a 3-year-old child. *J Cardiovasc Electrophysiol*. 2006;17:97–100.
201. Schweizer PA, Becker R, Katus HA, et al. Successful acute and long-term management of electrical storm in Brugada syndrome using orciprenaline and quinine/quinidine. *Clin Res Cardiol*. 2010;99:467–470.
202. Marquez MF, Rivera J, Hermosillo AG, et al. Arrhythmic storm responsive to quinidine in a patient with Brugada syndrome and vasovagal syncope. *Pacing Clin Electrophysiol*. 2005;28:870–873.
203. Viskin S, Antzelevitch C, Marquez MF, et al. Quinidine: a valuable medication joins the list of 'endangered species'. *Europace*. 2007;12:1105–1106.
204. Rosso R, Glick A, Glikson M, et al. Outcome after implantation of cardioverter defribrillator in patients with Brugada syndrome: a multicenter Israeli study (ISRABRU). *Isr Med Assoc J*. 2008;10:435–439.
205. Mok NS, Chan NY, Chi-Suen CA. Successful use of quinidine in treatment of electrical storm in Brugada syndrome. *Pacing Clin Electrophysiol*. 2004;27:821–823.
206. Belhassen B, Rahkovich M, Michowitz Y, et al. Management of Brugada syndrome: a 33-year experience using electrophysiologically-guided therapy with class 1a antiarrhythmic drugs. *Circ Arrhythm Electrophysiol*. 2015;8:1393–1402.
207. Antzelevitch C. The Brugada syndrome: ionic basis and arrhythmia mechanisms. *J Cardiovasc Electrophysiol*. 2001;12:268–272.
208. Kyriazis K, Bahlmann E, van der Schalk H, et al. Electrical storm in Brugada syndrome successfully treated with orciprenaline; effect of low-dose quinidine on the electrocardiogram. *Europace*. 2009;11:665–666.
209. Maury P, Couderc P, Delay M, et al. Electrical storm in Brugada syndrome successfully treated using isoprenaline. *Europace*. 2004;6:130–133.
210. Maury P, Hocini M, Haissaguerre M. Electrical storms in Brugada syndrome: review of pharmacologic and ablative therapeutic options. *Indian Pacing Electrophysiol J*. 2005;5:25–34.
211. Jongman JK, Jepkes-Bruin N, Ramdat Misier AR, et al. Electrical storms in Brugada syndrome successfully treated with isoproterenol infusion and quinidine orally. *Neth Heart J*. 2007;15:151–155.
212. Furniss G. Isoprenaline and quinidine to calm Brugada VF storm. *BMJ Case Rep*. 2012;Aug 13:2012.
213. Shimizu W, Matsuo K, Takagi M, et al. Body surface distribution and response to drugs of ST segment elevation in Brugada syndrome: clinical implication of eighty-seven-lead body surface potential mapping and its application to twelve-lead electrocardiograms. *J Cardiovasc Electrophysiol*. 2000;11:396–404.
214. Tanaka H, Kinoshita O, Uchikawa S, et al. Successful prevention of recurrent ventricular fibrillation by intravenous isoproterenol in a patient with Brugada syndrome. *Pacing Clin Electrophysiol*. 2001;24:1293–1294.
215. Sharif-Kazemi MB, Emkanjoo Z, Tavoosi A, et al. Electrical storm in Brugada syndrome during pregnancy. *Pacing Clin Electrophysiol*. 2011;34:e18–e21.
216. Roten L, Derval N, Sacher F, et al. Heterogeneous response of J wave syndromes to beta-adrenergic stimulation. *Heart Rhythm*. 2012;9:1970–1976.
217. Kaneko Y, Horie M, Niwano S, et al. Electrical storm in patients with Brugada syndrome is associated with early repolarization. *Circ Arrhythm Electrophysiol*. 2014;7:1122–1128.
218. Kanlop N, Chattipakorn S, Chattipakorn N. Effects of cilostazol in the heart. *J Cardiovasc Med (Hagerstown)*. 2011;12:88–95.
219. Bai Y, Muqier, Murakami H, et al. Cilostazol protects the heart against ischaemia reperfusion injury in a rabbit model of myocardial infarction: focus on adenosine, nitric oxide and mitochondrial ATP-sensitive potassium channels. *Clin Exp Pharmacol Physiol*. 2011;38:658–665.
220. Abud A, Bagattin D, Goyeneche R, et al. Failure of cilostazol in the prevention of ventricular fibrillation in a patient with Brugada syndrome. *J Cardiovasc Electrophysiol*. 2006;17:210–212.
221. Szel T, Koncz I, Antzelevitch C. Cellular mechanisms underlying the effects of milrinone and cilostazol to suppress arrhythmogenesis associated with Brugada syndrome. *Heart Rhythm*. 2013;10:1720–1727.
222. Sugao M, Fujiki A, Nishida K, et al. Repolarization dynamics in patients with idiopathic ventricular fibrillation: pharmacological therapy with bepridil and disopyramide. *J Cardiovasc Pharmacol*. 2005;45:545–549.
223. Murakami M, Nakamura K, Kusano KF, et al. Efficacy of low-dose bepridil for prevention of ventricular fibrillation in patients with Brugada syndrome with and without SCN5A mutation. *J Cardiovasc Pharmacol*. 2010;56:389–395.
224. Aizawa Y, Yamakawa H, Takatsuki S, et al. Efficacy and safety of bepridil for prevention of ICD shocks in patients with Brugada syndrome and idiopathic ventricular fibrillation. *Int J Cardiol*. 2013;168:5083–5085.
225. Kang L, Zheng MQ, Morishima M, et al. Bepridil up-regulates cardiac Na+ channels as a long-term effect by blunting proteasome signals through inhibition of calmodulin activity. *Br J Pharmacol*. 2009;157:404–414.
226. Fish JM, Welchons DR, Kim YS, et al. Dimethyl lithospermate B, an extract of danshen, suppresses arrhythmogenesis associated with the Brugada syndrome. *Circulation*. 2006;113:1393–1400.
227. Probst V, Veltmann C, Eckardt L, et al. Long-term prognosis of patients diagnosed with Brugada syndrome: results from the FINGER Brugada Syndrome Registry. *Circulation*. 2010;121:635–643.
228. Kanlop N, Shinlapawittayatorn K, Sungnoon R, et al. Cilostazol attenuates ventricular arrhythmia induction and improves defibrillation efficacy in swine. *Can J Physiol Pharmacol*. 2010;88:422–428.
229. Endoh M, Yanagisawa T, Taira N, et al. Effects of new inotropic agents on cyclic nucleotide metabolism and calcium transients in canine ventricular muscle. *Circulation*. 1986;73:III117–III133.
230. Rapundalo ST, Grupp I, Grupp G, et al. Myocardial actions of milrinone: characterization of its mechanism of action. *Circulation*. 1986;73:III134–III144.
231. Atarashi H, Endoh Y, Saitoh H, et al. Chronotropic effects of cilostazol, a new antithrombotic agent, in patients with bradyarrhythmias. *J Cardiovasc Pharmacol*. 1998;31:534–539.
232. Matsui K, Kiyosue T, Wang JC, et al. Effects of pimobendan on the L-type Ca2+ current and developed tension in guinea-pig ventricular myocytes and papillary muscle: comparison with IBMX, milrinone, and cilostazol. *Cardiovasc Drugs Ther*. 1999;13:105–113.
233. Aizawa Y, Chinushi M, Hasegawa K, et al. Electrical storm in idiopathic ventricular fibrillation is associated with early repolarization. *J Am Coll Cardiol*. 2013;62:1015–1019.
234. Nakagawa K, Nagase S, Morita H, et al. Left ventricular epicardial electrogram recordings in idiopathic ventricular fibrillation with inferior and lateral early repolarization. *Heart Rhythm*. 2013;11:314–317.

52 Inheritable Potassium Channel Diseases

Ahmad S. Amin and Arthur A.M. Wilde

Cardiac potassium (K+) channels are necessary for the proper functioning of atrial and ventricular myocytes by controlling their repolarization during phases 1, 2, and 3 of the action potential and by stabilizing their resting membrane potential during phase 4 of the action potential. In addition, K+ channels can regulate the heart rate by influencing the pacemaker activity in sinoatrial and atrioventricular node cells. In the early 1990s, using both the positional cloning technique and the candidate gene approach, genetic studies first linked mutations in genes encoding cardiac K+ channels to inheritable arrhythmia syndromes.[1,2] The positional cloning technique links a gene to a phenotype by its approximate location on the chromosome and without any earlier knowledge on the molecular basis of the disease. In contrast, the candidate gene approach uses mechanistic hypotheses based on pathophysiology to link certain genes of interest to a specific phenotype. Nowadays, variants in genes coding for cardiac K+ channels or their regulatory subunits have been implicated in the etiology (rare variants: disease-causing mutations) or clinical manifestation (common variants: disease-modifying variants) of various inheritable arrhythmia syndromes. This chapter focuses on the molecular genetics of inheritable arrhythmia syndromes related to cardiac K+ channels, the so-called K+ channelopathies. Clinical features and management of these syndromes and the molecular biology and physiology of cardiac K+ channels are described in detail elsewhere in this book.

Introduction

KVLQ1 (now referred to as *KCNQ1*) and the *human ether-à-go-go related gene* (*hERG*; now referred to as *KCNH2*), each encoding a major cardiac K+ channel, were among the first genes that were linked to an inheritable arrhythmic phenotype (i.e., the long QT syndrome [LQTS]).[1,2] These discoveries stimulated geneticists around the world to search for mutations in families or single affected subjects with an inheritable cardiac phenotype using the positional cloning technique but more often the candidate gene approach. These efforts have resulted in the association of tremendous numbers of variants in several genes encoding cardiac K+ channels or their regulatory subunits with distinct inheritable arrhythmic phenotypes (i.e., LQTS, short QT syndrome, Brugada syndrome [BrS], and familial atrial fibrillation [AF]) (Table 52.1).[3] However, most of these associations do not fulfill the list of criteria necessary to draw a definite conclusion regarding the causative link between a genetic variant and a specific phenotype, including detailed information about the frequency of the variant in the general population, analysis of cosegregation in families, verification of the link in independent cohorts, and experimental evidence for a mechanistic connection between the variant and the phenotype. Fulfilling these criteria has become imperative because many genetic variants previously considered to be rare (mutations) and disease-causing have now appeared to be common and present in healthy subjects with no cardiac history.[4–6] At the same time, it must be noted that complying with these criteria is challenging because acquiring experimental evidence for a mechanistic connection between a variant and a phenotype is a laborious and time-consuming process, while analysis of cosegregation in families is often hampered by small family sizes and low penetrance and variable expressivity of a potential disease-causing variant. Low penetrance indicates that not all carriers of a certain variant develop a phenotype, and variable expressivity refers to the variable degree in which carriers of an identical variant manifest a certain phenotype.[7] Based on these considerations, before continuing this chapter and describing the molecular genetics of K+ channelopathies, it is important to underscore that not all rare variants in K+ channel–encoding genes should automatically be labeled as disease-causing mutations (even if identified in subjects with an inheritable arrhythmic phenotype) and that caution is required while interpreting data from genetic studies and designating a genetic variant as a disease-causing mutation.

Long QT Syndrome

LQTS is a cardiac arrhythmogenic disease that causes syncope and sudden death due to torsades de pointes, a characteristic form of polymorphic ventricular tachycardia (PVT), and ventricular fibrillation (VF). Inheritable (congenital) LQTS is characterized by a prolonged heart rate–corrected QT interval (QTc duration) on a 12-lead electrocardiogram (ECG), due to a delay in the repolarization of the ventricles, in the absence of structural heart diseases or secondary causes of a prolonged QTc duration, such as electrolyte abnormalities, hypothermia, and use of certain drugs. Inheritable LQTS with an autosomal dominant pattern of inheritance has an estimated prevalence of 1:2500 and is traditionally called the Romano-Ward syndrome (first described independently by the Italian pediatrician Cesarino Romano in 1963 and the Irish pediatrician O. Connor Ward in 1964). The very rare autosomal recessive form of LQTS, with concomitant congenital bilateral sensory neural deafness, is called Jervell and Lange-Nielsen syndrome (JLNS; first described by Anton Jervell and his associate Fred Lange-Nielsen in 1957).[3] The autosomal dominant form is subdivided in different subtypes (so far 16 subtypes) according to the affected gene. The subdivision is based on the chronological order in which the subtypes are reported. Based on the underlying molecular genetic and pathophysiological mechanisms, this subdivision is not ideal but is followed in this chapter.

Long QT Syndrome as K+ Channel Disease

Four subtypes of LQTS (LQT1, LQT2, LQT7, and LQT13) are linked to mutations in genes encoding the pore-forming α-subunits of cardiac K+ channels, while three subtypes (LQT5, LQT6, and LQT11) are linked to mutations in genes encoding

TABLE 52.1 Cardiac potassium channel genes related to inheritable arrhythmia syndromes

CURRENT	TISSUE	GENE	SUBUNIT	SUBUNIT	EFFECT OF MUTATION	DISEASE
I_{K1}	Atria Ventricles	KCNJ2	Kir2.1	α-subunit	Loss-of-function	Long QT syndrome type 7[a]
					Gain-of-function	Short QT syndrome type 3[a]
					Gain-of-function	Atrial fibrillation[a]
					Gain-of-function	Catecholaminergic polymorphic ventricular tachycardia
I_{KAch}	Atria SAN, AVN	KCNJ5	Kir3.4	α-subunit	Loss-of-function	Long QT syndrome type
					Loss-of-function	Atrial fibrillation
I_{KATP}	Atria Ventricles	KCNJ8	Kir6.1	α-subunit	Gain-of-function	Brugada syndrome
		ABCC9	SUR2	Regulatory subunit	Gain-of-function	Early repolarization syndrome
					Loss-of-function	Brugada syndrome
					Loss-of-function	Atrial fibrillation
$I_{to,fast}$	Atria Ventricles	KCND2	$K_v4.2$	α-subunit	Gain-of-function	Early repolarization syndrome
		KCND3	$K_v4.3$	α-subunit	Gain-of-function	Brugada syndrome
					Gain-of-function	Atrial fibrillation
		KCNE3	MiRP2	β-subunit	Gain-of-function	Brugada syndrome
		KCNE3	MiRP2	β-subunit	Gain-of-function	Atrial fibrillation
		KCNE5	MiRP4	β-subunit	Gain-of-function	Brugada syndrome
I_{Kur}	Atria	KCNA5	$K_v1.5$	α-subunit	Loss-of-function	Atrial fibrillation
I_{Ks}	Atria Ventricles	KCNQ1	$K_v7.1$	α-subunit	Loss-of-function	Long QT syndrome type 1[a]
					Loss-of-function	Jervell Lange-Nielsen syndrome[a]
					Gain-of-function	Short QT syndrome type 2[a]
					Gain-of-function	Atrial fibrillation[a]
		KCNE1	MinK	α-subunit	Loss-of-function	Long QT syndrome type 5[a]
					Loss-of-function	Jervell Lange-Nielsen syndrome[a]
					Gain-of-function	Atrial fibrillation
		KCNE2	MiRP1	β-subunit	Gain-of-function	Atrial fibrillation
		KCNE3	MiRP2	β-subunit	Loss-of-function	Long QT syndrome
		KCNE5	MiRP4	β-subunit	Gain-of-function	Atrial fibrillation
		AKAP9	Yotiao	Regulatory subunit	Loss-of-function	Long QT syndrome type
I_{Kr}	Atria Ventricles	KCNH2	$K_v11.1$	α-subunit	Loss-of-function	Long QT syndrome type 2[a]
					Gain-of-function	Short QT syndrome type 1[a]
					Gain-of-function	Brugada syndrome
		KCNE2	MiRP1	β-subunit	Loss-of-function	Long QT syndrome type 6[a]
		KCNE3	MiRP2	β-subunit	Gain-of-function	Atrial fibrillation
I_{TASK-1}	Atria, AVN	KCNK3	$K_{2p}3.1$	α-subunit	Loss-of-function	Atrial fibrillation

AVN, Atrioventricular node; *SAN*, sinoatrial node.

[a]Diseases with a strong (causal) association with mutations in the corresponding gene.

one of the regulatory subunits of cardiac K+ channels. Based on the current evidence, mutations in *KCNQ1* (LQT1), *KCNH2* (LQT2), *KCNJ2* (LQT7; also known as Andersen syndrome), *KCNE1* (LQT5), and *KCNE2* (LQT6) can be regarded as causative in the etiology of LQTS. Most mutations involve single nucleotide substitutions in the coding regions (exons) of genes that alter a codon and lead to the replacement of one amino acid by a different one (missense mutations; approximately two-thirds of all mutations) or the creation of an early (premature) stop codon, resulting in the formation of a truncated protein (nonsense mutations). Single nucleotide substitutions in the noncoding regions (introns) also occur and may result in altered gene transcripts. Specific intronic nucleotide sequences at the intron/exon (acceptor site) and exon/intron (donor site) boundaries are crucial for the process whereby introns are excised from gene transcripts to create mature protein-encoding mRNAs (i.e., the splicing process). Mutations within these highly conserved intronic regions may cause aberrant splicing and lead to the deletion of entire exons (or exon parts) or inclusion of entire introns (or intron parts) in the mature mRNA, thereby often altering the open reading frame of translation and generating a new sequence of amino acids in the final product (i.e., frameshift). Mutations also involve the insertion or deletion of one or more nucleotides that may lead to a shift in the open reading frame or (when a multiple of three nucleotides is inserted or deleted) to the addition or removal of one or more amino acids in the final product, without affecting the reading frame.[8]

Pathophysiology of Long QT Syndrome

Experimental investigation of mutated K+ channels (or a normal channel with a mutated regulatory subunit) in heterologous expression systems, such as *Xenopus* oocytes or mammalian cell lines, has unequivocally demonstrated that LQTS-related mutations delay repolarization by reducing the outward K+ current through the affected channel (loss-of-function).[3] Importantly, the loss-of-function effects of LQTS-related mutations in *KCNQ1* and *KCNH2* (causing LQT1 and LQT2, respectively) have also been shown in the much more native environment of cardiomyocytes derived from patient-specific pluripotent stem cells from the members of families affected with these diseases.[9,10] In general, mutations cause a loss-of-function by decreasing the number of functional channels in the sarcolemma (lower expression) or by disrupting the extent or speed of channel opening and closing (altered gating). Because α-subunits of cardiac K⁺ channels assemble as dimers or tetramers to form functional ion channels, it is of functional importance whether mutated channel proteins possess the ability to assemble with normal channel proteins in heterozygous mutation carriers where both normal and mutated channels coexist (a normal allele is inherited from one parent and a mutant allele is inherited from the other parent). When mutated subunits assemble with normal subunits, they can disturb the sarcolemmal expression or gating of the normal channel subunits (i.e., a dominant-negative effect). In this case, the overall loss of the K⁺ current will exceed 50%. In contrast, when mutant subunits do not participate in tetramer assembly, (maximally) 50% reduction of the K⁺ current is anticipated (i.e., haploinsufficiency). As expected, dominant-negative LQTS–linked mutations have a worse clinical outcome than mutations that cause haploinsufficiency.[11,12] In addition, LQTS patients with compound mutations (~8% of all genotyped patients) in the same gene, but particularly in different LQTS-related genes, are also shown to display a more severe phenotype than single mutation carriers.[13] These clinical data indicate that the extent of decrease in cardiac K⁺ currents may determine disease severity in LQTS.

A delicate balance between inward and outward ion currents determines the repolarization of ventricular myocytes. Substantial differences in the expression levels of K⁺ channels among cardiomyocytes in different cardiac regions create a spatial dispersion of repolarization within the healthy ventricular myocardium. In LQTS, K⁺ current reduction leads to prolongation of the action potential plateau phase (reflected as QT interval prolongation on the ECG), and this allows recovery from inactivation and reactivation of L-type Ca^{2+} channels, which produces early afterdepolarizations (EADs). EADs, together with an accentuated spatial dispersion of repolarization, underlie the substrate and the trigger for the development of torsades de pointes in LQTS.[14] There is consensus that EADs initiate torsades de pointes, and EADs are probably the initiating event in LQT2, the second most prevalent type of LQTS. However, in LQT1, the most common type of LQTS, where arrhythmic events usually and predictably start at higher heart rates, the arrhythmogenic mechanism might be different. Delayed afterdepolarizations (DADs), which are spontaneous action potentials during phase 4 of the cardiac action potential, might play a role in this condition. DADs may also trigger ventricular arrhythmias in LQT7 (see further).

Long QT Syndrome Due to I_Ks Loss-of-Function

LQTS type 1 (LQT1), type 5 (LQT5), and type 11 (LQT11) and JLNS are linked to mutations that cause a reduction in the slowly activating delayed rectifier K⁺ current (I_{Ks}) in the heart. The α-subunit of the channel responsible for I_{Ks} ($K_v7.1$) is encoded by *KCNQ1*, and $K_v7.1$ proteins require the presence of their regulatory β-subunit MinK (encoded by *KCNE1*) to conduct I_{Ks}. I_{Ks} is markedly enhanced by β-adrenergic stimulation through the phosphorylation of $K_v7.1$ channels by protein kinase C (PKC), requiring MinK, and protein kinase A (PKA), requiring A-kinase–anchoring proteins (AKAPs). As a result, I_{Ks} enables the physiological response (i.e., abbreviation) of repolarization to fast heart rates during sympathetic nerve activity.[3] In 1991, two linkage studies linked a gene locus on chromosome 11 to LQTS in several unrelated families. Five years later, in 1996, positional cloning techniques established *KCNQ1* as the chromosome 11–linked LQT1 gene.[2] In 1997, targeted mutational analysis of *KCNE1* in two families with LQTS identified two missense mutations in *KCNE1* (LQT5).[15] LQT1 is now known to account for nearly 40% of all LQTS cases. LQT5 is rare, and mutations in *KCNE1*

may be responsible for nearly 3% of all LQTS cases.[16,17] In 2007, targeted mutational analysis of the translated exons of *AKAP9*, encoding AKAP9 (also called Yotiao), identified a missense mutation in one single patient with LQTS (LQT11). So far, only this one mutation in Yotiao has been linked to LQTS.[18]

Long QT Syndrome Type 1

To date, over 300 mutations in *KCNQ1* have been linked to LQT1. Most mutations are missense mutations (~70%), followed by frameshift mutations (~10%), splice site mutations (~10%), nonsense mutations (~5%), and in-frame deletions or insertions (~5%) and large genomic rearrangements (i.e., copy number variants), leading to the complete deletion of one or more exons.[16,17,19] LQT1 mutations in $K_v7.1$ are mostly located in the transmembrane segments (~60%), intracellular C-terminus (~30%), and intracellular N-terminus (~10%).[16,17] A fraction of these mutations have been investigated in experimental settings, and these studies have revealed an array of molecular mechanisms that underlie I_{Ks} loss-of-function (Fig. 52.1). These mechanisms include (1) defective $K_v7.1$ protein synthesis, (2) defective trafficking of mutated $K_v7.1$ proteins to the sarcolemma and their retention in the endoplasmic reticulum, (3) impaired ability of mutated proteins to coassemble into tetrameric channels, (4) altered biophysical properties, (5) disrupted interaction with regulatory proteins, and (6) defective endosomal recycling.[3,20–22] Of note, these mechanisms are not mutually exclusive. Loss-of-function alterations in the biophysical properties of mutated I_{Ks} channels involve a slower rate of channel activation, shift of the voltage dependence of activation toward more depolarized membrane potentials (indicating later channel activation), and accelerated deactivation (indicating faster channel closing). Disrupted interaction of mutated $K_v7.1$ proteins with the key regulatory protein AKAP9 has been demonstrated to reduce $K_v7.1$ phosphorylation by PKA upon β-adrenergic stimulation.[21] Disrupted interaction with phosphatidylinositol-4,5-bisphosphate (PIP2) results in reduced PKC-mediated phosphorylation of $K_v7.1$ proteins. PIP2, a sarcolemmal lipid, increases I_{Ks} activity through phosphorylation.[22] I_{Ks} is also increased by the stress hormone cortisol through the action of serum- and glucocorticoid-inducible kinase 1 (SGK1). Cortisol upregulates SGK1, thereby facilitating the endosomal recycling of $K_v7.1$ channels and stimulating their insertion into the sarcolemma. Mutations in $K_v7.1$ can disturb this process and cause further I_{Ks} reduction upon stimulation of SGK1 by cortisol.[20]

Consistent with the molecular signaling pathways, LQT1-related cardiac events often occur during exercise (swimming in particular) and psychological stress, when the adrenergic tone and plasma cortisol levels are increased.[23] In addition, the QT interval fails to shorten appropriately and might even lengthen (paradoxical QT response) in LQT1 patients upon an increase in heart rate (immediately at standing from supine position or at peak exercise and during the recovery phase of a treadmill exercise testing).[24,25] In healthy subjects, QT intervals shorten at faster heart rates, enabling QTc to remain within normal limits with decreasing RR intervals. Moreover, QTc duration lengthening is also observed in LQT1 patients in response to the intravenous infusion of epinephrine.[26] These clinical features indicate loss of an adequate compensatory response of I_{Ks} to β-adrenergic stimulation and stress hormones, most probably due to reduced phosphorylation and disrupted endosomal recycling of mutated $K_v7.1$ channels. As expected, antiadrenergic therapies, such as β-blockers and left stellate ganglion ablation, have great efficacy in LQT1 patients.[27,28] β-Blockers have been shown to diminish QTc changes during exercise or standing and significantly reduce the rate of cardiac events.[24,27]

Molecular genetics may be useful not only for diagnostic purposes but also for risk stratification in LQT1. In a multicenter study in 600 LQT1 patients, significantly higher rates of cardiac event were found in patients with mutations located in transmembrane segments or with mutations that exert dominant-negative effects on normal I_{Ks} channel subunits.[11] Another large multicenter study associated mutations in highly conserved amino acid residues in $K_v7.1$ with a significant risk for cardiac events.[29] Moreover, a study in 387 LQT1 patients correlated clinical phenotype with changes in biophysical properties of $K_v7.1$ channels caused by different *KCNQ1* mutations. In particular, a slower rate of channel activation was associated with increased risk for events in LQT1.[30] In all these studies, the effects of the mutations were independent of traditional risk factors (i.e., QTc, female gender, and β-blocker therapy). Mutation type and location may also be used to predict whether a *KCNQ1* mutation is pathogenic or an innocuous rare variant.[31] This is clinically relevant because a large overlap of QTc values exists between LQTS patients and healthy subjects. Nonmissense mutations, regardless of location, have an estimated predictive value of more than 99% to be pathogenic, whereas missense mutations have a high predictive value when located in the transmembrane segments, pore loop, and C-terminus of $K_v7.1$ proteins.[31] LQT1 patients with a mutation in the cytoplasmic loops are at higher risk for lethal arrhythmias than patients with a mutation in other regions of $K_v7.1$, probably because of a pronounced reduction in channel activation upon β-adrenergic stimulation.[32]

QT interval duration and risk for cardiac events in LQT1 may be determined not only by the mutation type and location but also by the co-presence of common variants in *KCNQ1*,[33,34] *KCNE1* (encoding MinK),[35] *AKAP9* (encoding yotiao),[36] and *NOS1AP*.[37,38] In particular, single-nucleotide polymorphisms (SNPs) in the nitric oxide synthase 1 adaptor protein gene (*NOS1AP*) have been identified as strong modulators of phenotype in LQT1 (and other LQTS types).[37,38] First, genome-wide association studies associated SNPs in *NOS1AP* with QT interval in the general population. Next, a role for *NOS1AP* SNPs was found in sudden cardiac death in the general population.[39,40] In 2009, a family-based association analysis linked SNPs in *NOS1AP* with QT interval prolongation and a risk for cardiac arrest and sudden death in a large South African cohort of LQT1 patients with the A341V mutation.[37] *NOS1AP* encodes CAPON, an accessory protein of the neuronal NOS, which controls intracellular nitric oxide production. Functional studies indicate that CAPON fastens cardiac repolarization by inhibiting L-type Ca^{2+} channels.[41] This provides a rationale for the association of SNPs in NOS1AP with QT interval duration. SNPs in the 3′ untranslated region (3′UTR) of *KCNQ1* have also been shown to modulate phenotype in LQT. In a study of two independent LQT1 cohorts from the Netherlands and the United States, SNPs in *KCNQ1*'s 3′UTR were associated with QTc duration and symptomatology in an allele-specific manner.[34] Patients with derived SNP variants on their mutated KCNQ1 allele had shorter QTc duration and fewer symptoms, while patients with these variants on their normal KCNQ1 allele had longer QTc duration and more symptoms. Experimental studies showed that the expression of KCNQ1's 3′UTR with the derived SNP variants was lower than the expression of the 3′UTR with the ancestral SNP variants. The 3′UTR plays a crucial regulatory role in gene expression by controlling stability and translation of mRNAs. SNPs in this region were suggested to affect this function of the 3′UTR, thereby altering gene expression in an allele-specific manner.[34] If true, this is expected to be especially relevant when one allele contains a pathogenic mutation. However, these findings await replication in larger LQT1 cohorts before their clinical use is proposed.

Long QT Syndrome Type 5

The *KCNE*-encoded MinK exerts its regulatory effects on $K_v7.1$ via interactions between the transmembrane segments and C-termini of the two proteins. In general, interactions between transmembrane segments are believed to be essential for normal channel activation, while interaction between the C-termini regulate channel assembly and channel deactivation. LQT5 mutations mainly involve missense mutations, although in-frame deletions, nonsense mutations, and frameshift mutations are also found.[16,17] Most mutations impair the ability of MinK to modulate gating properties of $K_v7.1$ and cause a shift of voltage dependence of activation toward more depolarized potentials (particularly mutations in the transmembrane segments) and accelerate deactivation.[42] Other mechanisms include defective trafficking of mutated MinK proteins (and thereby $K_v7.1$ proteins), impaired channel assembly, and reduced sensitivity to PIP2.[22,42] Residues in the C-terminus of MinK are identified as key determinants for sensitivity of $K_v7.1$ to PIP2, and LQT5-linked mutations in these residues are shown to reduce PIP2-mediated phosphorylation of Kv7.1 proteins by PKC.[22] Because of its low prevalence, genotype–phenotype correlations in LQT5 are not available but may resemble those observed in LQT1.

An SNP in *KCNE2*, D85N, located in the C-terminus of MinK, has been associated with QT interval duration in the general population[39,40] and is shown to be more prevalent in (genotype-negative) LQTS patients. Heterologous expression studies revealed significant loss-of-function effects of D85N on *KCNQ1*- and *KCNH2*-encoded currents.[35] Therefore D85N is suggested to be a disease-causing variant in LQTS and, certainly, a modifier of phenotype in LQT1 and LQT2 patients.

Long QT Syndrome Type 11

AKAP9 (yotiao) has an N- and C-terminal–binding domain that interacts with the C-terminus of $K_v7.1$. The only LQT-11 mutation described so far (S1570L) has been found in 1 of 50 genotype-negative unrelated LQTS patients. S1570L is located in the C-terminal–binding domain of AKAP9. It has been shown to disrupt, but not eliminate, the interaction between AKAP9 and $K_v7.1$, leading to reduced cyclic adenosine monophosphate (cAMP)–mediated phosphorylation of $K_v7.1$ by PKA during β-adrenergic stimulation. This is speculated to result in less I_{Ks} enhancement during sympathetic nerve activity.[18] Recently, genetic variations in *AKAP9* have been proposed as modifiers of phenotype in LQT1.[36]

Jervell and Lange-Nielsen Syndrome

JLNS, the autosomal recessive form of LQTS affecting 3 to 5 in one million children, is characterized by QT interval prolongation, congenital bilateral sensory neural deafness, torsades de pointes, and sudden cardiac death from very early in life. JLNS depends on homozygous or compound heterozygous mutations on *KCNQ1* or *KCNE1*. Hearing loss is due to dysfunction of I_{Ks} channels in the inner ear, where they act as K^+ charge carriers for sensory transduction and generation of endocochlear potential in the endolymph. Most JLNS-linked mutations are found in *KCNQ1* (~90%), while mutations in *KCNE1* are associated with a less severe phenotype and are more prevalent in asymptomatic patients. Although exceptions exist, most JLNS-linked mutations are nonsense mutations, frameshift mutations, and splice-site mutations (i.e., mutations that are expected to disrupt channel assembly and lead to haploinsufficiency).[43] This may explain the mild phenotype in heterozygous parents of JLNS patients compared to LQT1 patients. Similar to LQT1, cardiac events are triggered during exercise and emotional stress. However, compared with LQT1, JLNS is associated with longer QTc durations, a higher risk of cardiac events (at younger age), and lower efficacy of β-blocker therapy.[43]

Long QT Syndrome Due to I$_{Kr}$ Loss-of-Function

LQT2 and LQT6 are linked to mutations that cause a reduction of the rapidly activating delayed rectifier K$^+$ current (I$_{Kr}$) in the heart. The α-subunit of the channel responsible for I$_{Kr}$ (K$_v$11.1) is encoded by *KCNH2*, traditionally called *hERG* because of its homology to the *Drosophila ether-à-go-go (eag)* gene. The interaction of K$_v$11.1 with the *KCNE2*-encoded β-subunit (MinK-related peptide 1; MiRP1) is considered to be required for normal gating and pharmacological properties of I$_{Kr}$ channels. In 1994, linkage studies linked a gene locus on chromosome 7 to LQTS in nine families, and in 1995, mutations in *hERG* were found to be responsible for LQT2.[1] In 1999, missense mutations in *KCNE2* were first identified in LQTS patients.[44] LQT2 is now known to account for nearly 30% of all LQTS cases, while mutations in *KCNE2* may be responsible for less than 1% of all LQTS cases.[16,17]

Long QT Syndrome Type 2

The I$_{Kr}$ channel is composed of four α-subunits that are encoded by two transcripts of *KCNH2*: hERG1a or the alternative-spliced transcript of hERG1b.[45] The hERG1b proteins lack the first 376 amino acids of hERG1a. To date, more than 200 LQT2-linked mutations in hERG1a have been reported,[3] while only two missense mutations in hERG1b have been identified in LQT2.[45,46] Most LQT2 mutations are missense mutations (~60%), followed by frameshift mutations (~25%), nonsense mutations (~10%), splice-site mutations, and in-frame deletions or insertions (~5%).[16,17] Large genomic rearrangements (i.e., copy number variants) in *KCNH2* have also been recently found in LQTS patients.[19] LQT2-linked mutations are located in the intracellular C-terminus (~40%), transmembrane segments (~30%), and intracellular N-terminus (~30%) of K$_v$11.1.[16,17] Missense mutations have a predictive value of 100% to be pathogenic when located in the transmembrane segments, linkers, and pore loop of K$_v$11.1 proteins.[31] A multicenter study in 858 LQT2 patients associated missense mutations in the transmembrane pore regions (segment 5, pore loop, and segment 6) and the N-terminus with a significantly higher risk for cardiac events than missense mutations located in the C-terminus or transmembrane nonpore regions (segments 1–4).[12] Moreover, mutations in α-helical domains, where the secondary protein structure may be more highly ordered, were associated with a higher risk than mutations in β-sheet domains or other locations.[12] In contrast, the risk for nonmissense mutations was not location-specific. Of note, an SNP in *KCNH2*, K897T, located in the C-terminus of K$_v$11.1, has been associated with QT interval duration in the general population[39,40] and may modify the phenotype in LQT2.[47] Heterologous expression studies revealed loss-of-function effects of K897T on *KCNH2*-encoded currents.[48]

The underlying mechanisms of I$_{Kr}$ reduction have been experimentally studied for only a fraction of all LQT2 mutations and include (1) defective K$_v$11.1 protein synthesis, (2) nonsense-mediated decay (NMD), (3) impaired intracellular trafficking, (4) abnormal biophysical properties (e.g., slower channel activation, faster inactivation, and/or faster deactivation), and/or (5) reduced K$^+$ selectivity or permeation (see Fig. 52.1).[3,49,50] NMD is an RNA surveillance mechanism that selectively degrades mRNA transcripts containing premature termination codons due to nonsense or frameshift mutations.[49] NMD may have a reciprocal impact on LQT2 phenotype; although NMD may prevent mutated products from exerting a dominant-negative effect on normal K$_v$11.1 proteins, it may also lead to degradation of mutated mRNAs that, if not degraded, can produce partially functional K$_v$11.1 channels. However, defective trafficking of mutated K$_v$11.1 proteins to the sarcolemma is the dominant molecular mechanism of I$_{Kr}$ reduction in LQT2, particularly

for mutations located in highly conserved domains of K$_v$11.1.[50] Normally, K$_v$11.1 proteins are modified through the addition or trimming of sugar moieties in the endoplasmic reticulum (core glycosylation) and in the Golgi apparatus (complex glycosylation). Most LQT2-linked mutations disrupt the trafficking of core-glycosylated ("immature") K$_v$11.1 proteins to the Golgi apparatus, resulting in their retention in the endoplasmic reticulum. Processes suggested to be involved in defective trafficking and intracellular retention of mutated K$_v$11.1 proteins include decreased affinity to heat shock protein 70 (Hsp70; known to promote maturation of K$_v$11.1) and increased affinity to heat shock cognate 70 (Hsc70, which promotes proteasomal degradation of K$_v$11.1),[51] abnormal ubiquitylation of K$_v$11.1 by ubiquitin ligase Nedd4-2,[52] and redistribution of mutated proteins to a microtubule-dependent quality control compartment in the endoplasmic reticulum.[53]

In contrast to I$_{Ks}$, which is significantly enhanced by cAMP-mediated phosphorylation upon β-adrenergic stimulation, cAMP has only a minor effect on I$_{Kr}$ channel gating. The C-terminus of K$_v$11.1 contains a cyclic nucleotide–binding domain (CNBD). Binding of cAMP to the CNBD leads to a small change in the voltage-dependence of channel activation.[54] However, disruption of this minor effect of cAMP on I$_{Kr}$ channel gating in the presence of a mutation may provide a rationale for the characteristic occurrence of arrhythmias in LQT2 upon sudden fright (e.g., unexpected auditory stimuli or other arousal-related stimuli).[23] In agreement with this, QTc duration in LQT2 patients is lengthened immediately at standing from supine position or in response to intravenous injection of an epinephrine bolus, which are conditions associated with an abrupt β-adrenergic stimulation.[25,55] In contrast, QTc changes in LQT2 upon exercise testing or continuous low-dose infusion of epinephrine are variable and transient.[24,26] Accordingly, antiadrenergic therapies (β-blockers and left stellate ganglion ablation) are effective in LQT2 but less so in LQT1.[27,28]

Although mutation-specific therapies for LQT2 are not available in clinical settings, experimental studies have suggested various approaches to restore the effects of a mutation on the expression, trafficking, or gating of K$_v$11.1 channels. Aminoglycoside antibiotics have been shown to partially restore the functional expression of full-length proteins for some *KCNH2* nonsense mutations by permitting read-through of the premature termination codons, created by these mutations.[56] However, how aminoglycoside antibiotics change stop codons at the molecular level and the final effects of read-through on channel level are not yet known. More importantly, it is well established that defective trafficking of mutated K$_v$11.1 proteins may be restored in vitro by culturing cells at lower incubation temperatures or in the presence of high-affinity I$_{Kr}$ channel–blocking drugs (e.g., E4031, cisapride).[50] These interventions may stabilize the mutated proteins in configurations that facilitate normal trafficking. However, the use of such drugs is contraindicated in LQT2 patients because of their potent I$_{Kr}$-blocking properties. Finally, interactions between the N-terminus and pore-forming domains of K$_v$11.1 channels are known to regulate slow deactivation gating. Mutations in the N-terminus disrupt these interactions and cause accelerated deactivation. Application of small molecules containing the N-terminal residues of K$_v$11.1 has been demonstrated to restore the deactivation properties of mutated channels.[57] However, further in vivo studies are required to unravel the possible future clinical benefits of such interventions.

Long QT Syndrome Type 6

Only a few mutations in *KCNE2* have been associated with LQT6. Most of them are missense mutations and are located in the single transmembrane segment of the protein.[16,17] The

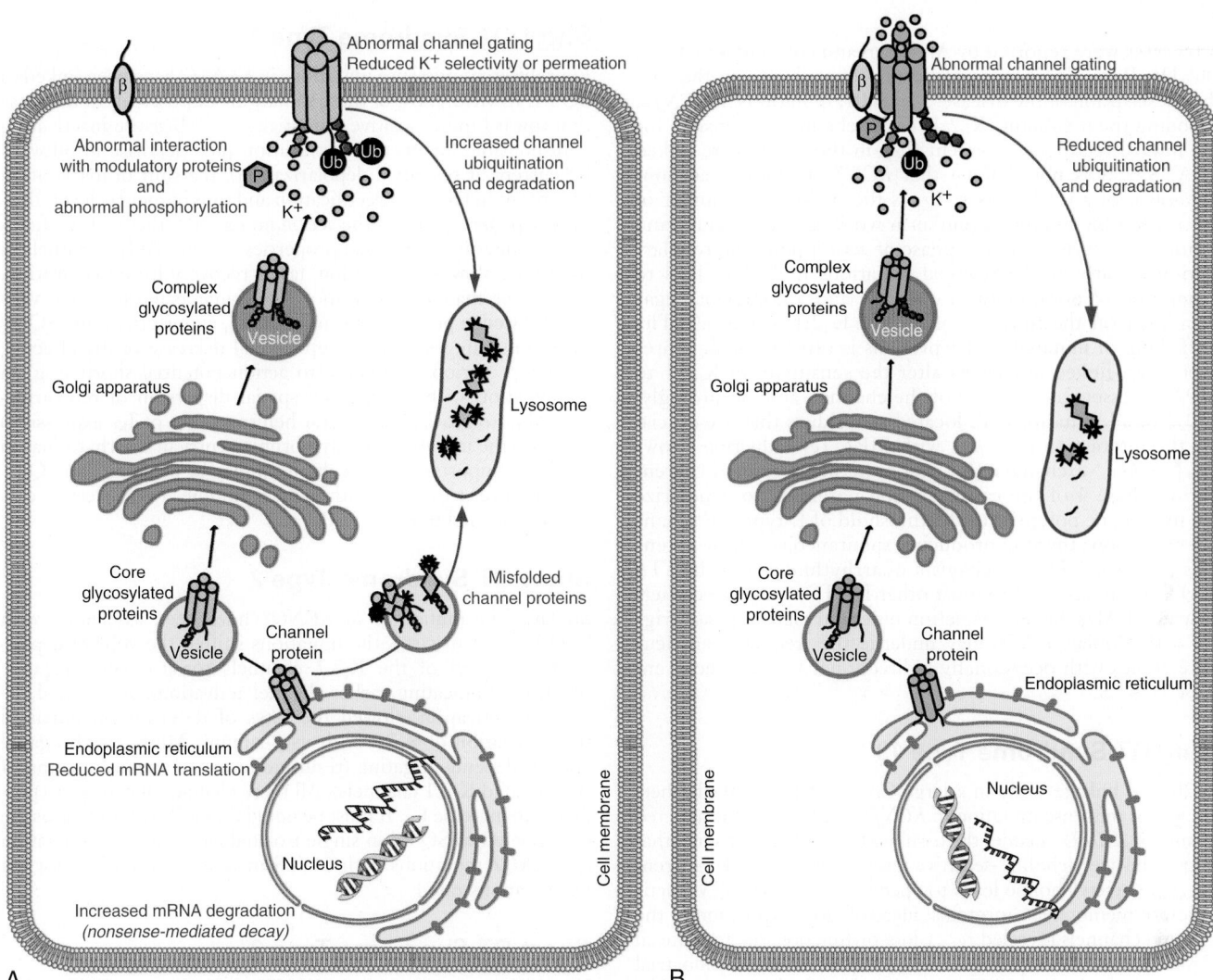

FIGURE 52.1 Common molecular mechanisms for mutations to cause loss- or gain-of-function of the cardiac K⁺ channels in inheritable K⁺ channel diseases. In healthy conditions, mRNA transcripts are processed in the nucleus and translated into proteins in the endoplasmic reticulum (ER). In the ER, translation products (proteins) are folded, core-glycosylated, and coassembled into dimers or tetramers. Next, channel proteins are transported to the Golgi apparatus, where they undergo complex glycosylation. From the Golgi apparatus, channel proteins are transported to the cell membrane where they interact with modulatory proteins (e.g., β-subunits) and undergo additional posttranslational modification (e.g., phosphorylation [*P*] and ubiquitination [*Ub*]). Ubiquitination leads to endocytosis and degradation of channels in the lysosome or proteasome. Modulatory proteins of K⁺ channels are expressed through a similar pathway. (A) displays (in *red*) common mechanisms for mutations that cause loss-of-function. Mutated mRNA transcripts may be degraded through nonsense-mediated decay or miRNA-mediated repression of translation. If misfolded, mutated proteins are directly transported from the ER to the lysosome for degradation. If not misfolded, mutated proteins are transported to the cell membrane. Loss-of-function effects at the cell membrane involve defective interaction with regulatory proteins, abnormal channel phosphorylation, abnormal channel ubiquitination, and/or defective channel gating. (B) displays (in *red*) common mechanisms for mutations to cause gain-of-function. Gain-of-function effects involve changes in channel gating and abnormal (decreased) channel ubiquitination.

presence of mutated MiRP1 subunits leads to reduced current densities and various alterations in the gating properties of $K_v11.1$ channels, including a shift in the voltage-dependent activation toward more positive potentials, faster inactivation, and slower recovery from inactivation.[44–58] Mutated MiRP2 subunits may also change the pharmacological response of $K_v11.1$ channels to drugs.[44] However, the role of MiRP2 in I_{Kr} modulation and ventricular repolarization remains controversial, especially because the expression level of *KCNE2* is very low in the ventricle and only significantly high in pacemaker cells and Purkinje fibers.[59]

Other Long QT Syndrome Subtypes

Long QT Syndrome Type 7

The Andersen-Tawil syndrome (ATS), also called Andersen syndrome, is an uncommon disease associated with ventricular arrhythmias, potassium-sensitive periodic paralysis, and dysmorphic features, including short stature, scoliosis, clinodactyly, hypertelorism, and subtle facial abnormalities.[60] ATS is categorized as LQT7 because of the presence of prominent U waves, which are difficult to distinguish from truly prolonged QT intervals, and mild QT prolongation. The first

ATS cases were reported by Andersen and colleagues in 1971, and Dr. Rabi Tawil has significantly contributed to the further description of the disease.[61] In 2001, mutations in *KCNJ2*, encoding the α-subunit ($K_{ir}2.1$) of the channel responsible for the inward rectifier K^+ current (I_{K1}) in the heart, were linked to ATS.[60] It is now known that *KCNJ2* mutations account for ~60% of all ATS cases. I_{K1} is the major determinant of the resting membrane potential in working myocardium and contributes to the terminal phase of action potential repolarization. Nearly all ATS-linked mutations in *KCNJ2* lead to generation of nonfunctional channels and a dominant-negative effect on the function of normal $K_{ir}2.1$ proteins.[61] The trafficking of mutated $K_{ir}2.1$ proteins is often normal. Moreover, ATS-linked mutations alter the sensitivity of $K_{ir}2.1$ to PIP2, an essential activator of the channel, and, accordingly, ~50% of all mutations are located at residues that are crucial for the interaction of $K_{ir}2.1$ with PIP2. I_{K1} reduction allows the Na^+/Ca^{2+} exchanger ($I_{Na+/Ca2+}$), the major inward current during phase 4 of the cardiac action potential, to depolarize the membrane potential to the threshold of L-type Ca^{2+} channel activation, thereby producing spontaneous action potentials (DADs).[62] This mechanism of arrhythmogenesis in ATS (LQT7) is in contrast to most other LQTS types (see earlier) in which EADs during the action potential plateau phase trigger arrhythmias. DADs may underlie the frequent ventricular ectopies with occasionally bidirectional VT and recurrent PVT in ATS.

Long QT Syndrome Type 13

In 2010, a linkage study in a large Chinese family linked a heterozygous missense mutation in *KCNJ5* to LQTS in the affected members. *KCNJ5* encodes the α-subunit ($K_{ir}3.4$) of a channel that carries the acetylcholine-sensitive inwardly rectifying K^+ current (I_{K-Ach}).[63] Acetylcholine leads to opening of the channel via activation of membrane G proteins. Heterologous expression of the mutated channels revealed I_{K-Ach} loss-of-function due to reduced plasma membrane expression. I_{K-Ach} is present in the sinoatrial node, atria, and atrioventricular node, where it plays a role in the parasympathetic slowing of the heart rate and repolarization of atrial action potentials.[63] However, its precise role in the ventricles remains unclear.

Short QT Syndrome

The short QT syndrome (SQTS) was introduced in 2001 by Gussak and colleagues after the first description of constantly shorter-than-normal QT intervals in one isolated case with syncope and sudden cardiac death at a young age and three familial cases, of whom one suffered from paroxysmal AF.[64] In 2003, Gaita and colleagues associated persistent short QT intervals with syncope, VF, and sudden cardiac death in the absence of cardiac structural abnormalities in several members of two unrelated families.[65] In 2004, SQTS was first linked to missense mutations in *KCNH2*,[66] and in the same year, a missense mutation in *KCNQ1* was associated with the disease.[67] In 2005, a missense mutation in *KCNJ2* was linked to SQTS in a single family.[68] Thus, in a short time, three subtypes of SQTS have been recognized, and each subtype is associated with a mutation in a K^+ channel–encoding gene: *KCNH2* (SQT1), *KCNQ1* (SQT2), and *KCNJ2* (SQT3). All SQTS-linked mutations are missense mutations, and, when studied in heterologous expression systems, they cause gain-of-function of the corresponding K^+ channels by altering the gating properties. The expected increase in I_{Kr} (in SQT1), I_{Ks} (in SQT2), or the outward component of I_{K1} (in SQT3) fastens repolarization and leads to QT interval shortening on ECG.

Short QT Syndrome Type 1

Four different missense mutations in *KCNH2* have been linked to SQT1. In vitro, most of these mutations cause a shift of inactivation toward more positive potentials.[66,69,70] Because inactivation is responsible for inward rectification (i.e., decrease in outward K^+ current at sustained depolarization), the shift of inactivation may result in failure of rectification and thus higher I_{Kr} levels during the plateau phase of the action potential. Other gain-of-function changes in biophysical properties of mutated I_{Kr} channels in SQT1 are slower inactivation, faster recovery from inactivation, and slower channel deactivation. Experiments in canine left ventricular wedge preparations, using an I_{Kr} agonist to mimic SQT1 mutations, suggest that a proportional decrease of the effective refractory period (secondary to action potential shortening) in combination with accentuated spatial dispersion of repolarization (due to spatial transmural heterogeneity of I_{Kr} expression) facilitate the initiation of polymorphic ventricular arrhythmias in SQT1.[71] Importantly, QTc duration may be prolonged in SQT1 patients after treatment with hydroquinidine, a nonselective cardiac K^+ channel blocker.[72]

Short QT Syndrome Type 2

So far, four mutations in *KCNQ1* have been associated with SQT2.[67,73,74] In vitro, the mutations shifted the voltage-dependent activation of the $K_v7.1$ channels toward more negative potentials (indicating earlier channel activation), accelerated the rates of activation, slowed the rates of deactivation, impaired the association of $K_v7.1$ with its β-subunit MinK, or abrogated voltage-dependent gating (resulting in instantaneous opening of the mutated $K_v7.1$ channels). All these changes in gating are predicted to increase I_{Ks}. It must be noted that *KCNQ1* mutations are only related to SQTS in single isolated cases, and cosegregation of *KCNQ1* mutations with SQTS in large families has not yet been demonstrated.

Short QT Syndrome Type 3

Four different mutations in *KCNJ2* are linked to STQ3, often in combination with paroxysmal AF. In vitro, all these mutations carry larger outward I_{K1} at more positive potentials due to changes in gating causing lack of inward rectification, higher channel expression at the cell membrane, and reduced $K_{ir}2.1$ channel degradation.[68,75,76] Larger outward I_{K1} at more positive potentials may result in larger contribution of I_{K1} to the terminal phase of action potential repolarization (because the membrane potential returns from depolarized levels to hyperpolarized levels). Indeed, computer modeling studies showed that increased outward I_{K1} results in shortening of the action potential duration due to abbreviation of the terminal phase of repolarization.[68] These findings are in line with the asymmetrical shape of the T wave in SQT3 patients with a rapid descending limb. In contrast, T waves in SQT1 and SQT2 patients are symmetrical.[66,67]

Other Inheritable Potassium Channel Diseases

Brugada Syndrome and Early Repolarization Syndrome

BrS is associated with typical coved-type ST-segment elevation in the right precordial ECG leads V_1–V_3, often prolonged conduction parameters (PR and QRS), and an increased risk for VT and VF. Early repolarization syndrome (ERS) is characterized by J-point elevation and terminal QRS slurring or notching in at least two contiguous leads.[77] Early repolarization as an ECG sign may be prevalent in the general population but is more often observed in patients who have experienced syncope or an out-of-hospital cardiac arrest due to idiopathic VF. BrS is traditionally linked to loss-of-function mutations in the cardiac Na^+ channel, *SCN5A*. The mutations result in decreased I_{Na} during phase 0 of the cardiac action potential, which may allow the repolarizing transient outward K^+ current (I_{to}; active during action potential phase 0 and 1) to cause loss of the action potential plateau phase by disabling the membrane potential to reach the voltages required for the activation of the L-type Ca^{2+} channels. Because I_{to} is more expressed in subepicardial myocytes compared to subendocardial myocytes, the loss of action potential plateau may mainly occur in the subepicardium, leading to aggravation of transmural voltage gradients and generation of a substrate for reentrant waves.[78] Driven by this hypothesis and the fact that *SCN5A* mutations are identified in only ~20% of all BrS cases, scientists have attempted to find mutations in genes encoding the cardiac K^+ channels that are mainly active during phases 0 and 1 of the action potential. These efforts have led to the identification of a number of variants in genes coding for different subunits of I_{to} (i.e., *KCND2*, *KCND3*, *KCNE3*, and *KCNE5*) and the adenosine triphosphate (ATP)-sensitive K^+ channel I_{K-ATP} (i.e., *KCNJ8* and *ABCC9*), all in single unrelated subjects with BrS or ERS.[3] As expected, all these genetic variants caused I_{to} or I_{K-ATP} gain-of-function when studied in vitro. I_{K-ATP} is active during hypoxia or ischemia when intracellular ATP concentration or ATP/adenosine diphosphate (ADP) ratio declines. However, BrS-linked mutations in *KCNJ8* and *ABCC9* are expected to cause an increase in I_{K-ATP} during "normal" conditions by reducing the sensitivity of mutated channels to intracellular ATP.[3] In addition, missense variants in *KCNH2* with putative gain-of-function effects have also been found in unrelated BrS subjects.[79,80] However, these data have recently been questioned by a large study that searched for the presence of rare coding variants in 45 arrhythmia-susceptibility genes (including *KCND3*, *KCNE3*, *KCNE5*, *KCNJ8*, and *ABCC9*) in 167 BrS patients and 167 healthy controls with no history of cardiac arrhythmia.[5] This study found only an association between BrS and variants in *SCN5A*. In addition, it found that rare variants in most other BrS-susceptibility genes were present in a similar extent among BrS patients and controls. Therefore extreme caution is necessary in denominating variants in genes other than *SCN5A* as disease-causing mutations in BrS or ERS.[5,81]

Atrial Fibrillation

The pathophysiological pathways leading to AF are believed to be multifactorial, involving both environmental and acquired triggers and genetic factors. The latter may play a more dominant role in the case of familial AF.[82] Several mutations in K^+ channel–encoding genes have been found in families or single subjects with AF, including gain-of-function mutations in *KCNJ2* (encoding the α-subunit of I_{K1}), *KCND3* (an α-subunit of I_{to}), *KCNE3* (a β-subunit of I_{to} and I_{Kr}), *KCNQ1* (the α-subunit of I_{Ks}), *KCNE1* (a β-subunit of I_{Ks}), *KCNE2* (a β-subunit of I_{Ks}), *KCNE5* (a β-subunit of I_{Ks}), and loss-of-function mutations in *KCNA5* (encoding the α-subunit of I_{Kur}), *KCNJ5* (the α-subunit of I_{K-Ach}), *ABCC9* (a modulatory subunit of I_{K-ATP}), and *KCNK3* (see later).[3,82] *KCNA5*-encoded $K_v1.5$ channels conduct the ultra-rapidly activating delayed outward rectifier K^+ current (I_{Kur}), a repolarizing current that is only present in the atria. I_{K-Ach} is mainly expressed in the atria (but also in the sinoatrial and atrioventricular nodes) where it accelerates atrial repolarization and shortens atrial refractoriness. *KCNK3* codes for a newly discovered K^+ channel that is responsible for a background K^+ current in the atria. All these AF-associated gain- or loss-of-function mutations in K^+ channel–encoding genes are speculated to shorten or prolong atrial repolarization, thereby facilitating reentry. However, their precise contribution to the complex etiological pathophysiology of AF remains unresolved, and an association

bias as described earlier for BrS and ERS may also account for the association between these mutations and AF.

Catecholaminergic Polymorphic Ventricular Tachycardia

Catecholaminergic PVT (CPVT) is characterized by syncope and sudden death due to exercise-induced (adrenergically mediated) bidirectional VT or PVT and is associated with mutations in the *RyR2*-encoded cardiac ryanodine receptor/Ca^{2+} release channel and *CASQ2*-encoded calsequestrin proteins involved in Ca^{2+} homeostasis and excitation–contraction coupling in cardiomyocytes. Ventricular arrhythmias in CPVT may resemble arrhythmias observed in LQT7 patients. In 2006, a genetic study first identified mutations in *KCNJ2* in 3 of 11 unrelated patients (with normal QT intervals) who were clinically diagnosed with CPVT, suggesting phenotypic mimicry between CPVT and LQT7.[83] However, the mutations were not studied experimentally. In 2009, a *KCNJ2* mutation, which was found in a CPVT patient, was shown to induce loss-of-function of $K_{ir}2.1$ channels by abrogating the increase in I_{K1} upon PKA-dependent phosphorylation (not at baseline).[84] This indicates that at least some *KCNJ2* mutations may cause CPVT by inducing I_{K1} loss-of-function during β-adrenergic stimulation by impairing $K_{ir}2.1$ phosphorylation. However, the role of *KCNJ2* mutations in CPVT should be further clarified.

Sudden Infant Death Syndrome

The term "sudden infant death syndrome" (SIDS), first introduced in 1969, refers to the sudden death of an infant who is younger than 1 year, which is unexpected by clinical history, and in which a thorough postmortem analysis and investigation of the death scene fail to identify an adequate cause of death.[85] SIDS is believed to be a multifactorial disease, with multiple risk factors contributing to its development, including gender, age, and genetic variants (intrinsic), low birth weight and prematurity (developmental), prone sleeping position, mild infections, smoking or drug intake by the parents, and socioeconomic status (extrinsic and/or environmental). Genetic variants associated with the occurrence of SIDS are mutations and polymorphisms in genes encoding for proteins involved in the autonomic nervous system, immune system, fatty acid oxidation, blood glucose regulation, and in genes encoding for the cardiac ion channels or their regulatory subunits.[86]

In 2001, a mutation in *KCNQ1*, previously linked to LQTS, was identified in an infant with SIDS.[87] Ever since, numerous cohort studies and case reports, where mutation screening was performed in cardiac genes that were earlier linked to inheritable arrhythmia syndromes in adults, have related mutations in the following potassium channel encoding genes to SIDS: *KCNQ1*, *KCNH2*, *KCNJ8* (encoding ATP-sensitive K^+ current channels), *KCNE1*, and *KCNE2*.[86] These mutations often cause gating alterations that are expected to result in loss- and/or gain-of-function. Indeed, some of these mutations are also found in adult LQTS or SQTS patients.[86] Although the molecular pathogenesis of SIDS is not well understood, based on the abovementioned findings, it is tempting to speculate that SIDS cases suffer from inheritable arrhythmia syndromes (e.g., LQTS or SQTS), which in conjunction with other intrinsic, developmental, and environmental risk factors, manifest during early childhood.

Acknowledgments

We acknowledge the support from the Netherlands CardioVascular Research Initiative, the Dutch Heart Foundation, Dutch Federation of University Medical Centres, the Netherlands Organisation for Health Research and Development, and the Royal Netherlands Academy of Sciences (PREDICT; AAMW) and the Netherlands Heart Foundation (td/dekk/2388 2013T042; ASA).

REFERENCES

1. Curran ME, Splawski I, Timothy KW, et al. A molecular basis for cardiac arrhythmia: HERG mutations cause long QT syndrome. *Cell.* 1995;8:795–803.

2. Wang Q, Curran ME, Splawski I, et al. Positional cloning of a novel potassium channel gene: *KVLQT1* mutations cause cardiac arrhythmias. *Nat Genet.* 1996;12:17–23.

3. Schmitt N, Grunnet M, Olesen SP. Cardiac potassium channel subtypes: new roles in repolarization and arrhythmia. *Physiol Rev.* 2014;94:609–653.

4. Risgaard B, Jabbari R, Refsgaard L, et al. High prevalence of genetic variants previously associated with Brugada syndrome in new exome data. *Clin Genet.* 2013;84:489–495.

5. Le Scouarnec S, Karakachoff M, Gourraud JB, et al. Testing the burden of rare variation in arrhythmia-susceptibility genes provides new insights into molecular diagnosis for Brugada syndrome. *Hum Mol Genet.* 2015;24:2757–2763.

6. Kapplinger JD, Giudicessi JR, Ye D, et al. Enhanced classification of Brugada syndrome-associated and long-QT syndrome-associated genetic variants in the *SCN5A*-encoded Na$_v$1.5 cardiac sodium channel. *Circ Cardiovasc Genet.* 2015;8:582–595.

7. Amin AS, Pinto YM, Wilde AA. Long QT syndrome: beyond the causal mutation. *J Physiol.* 2013;591:4125–4139.

8. Tester DJ, Ackerman MJ. Genetic testing for potentially lethal, highly treatable inherited cardiomyopathies/channelopathies in clinical practice. *Circulation.* 2011;123:1021–1037.

9. Moretti A, Bellin M, Welling A, et al. Patient-specific induced pluripotent stem-cell models for long-QT syndrome. *N Engl J Med.* 2010;363:1397–1409.

10. Itzhaki I, Maizels L, Huber I, et al. Modelling the long QT syndrome with induced pluripotent stem cells. *Nature.* 2011;471:225–229.

11. Moss AJ, Wataru Shimizu W, Wilde AA, et al. Clinical aspects of type-1 long-QT syndrome by location, coding type, and biophysical function of mutations involving the KCNQ1 gene. *Circulation.* 2007;115:2481–2489.

12. Shimizu W, Moss AJ, Wilde AA, et al. Genotype-phenotype aspects of type 2 long QT syndrome. *J Am Coll Cardiol.* 2009;54:2052–2062.

13. Itoh H, Shimizu W, Hayashi K, et al. Long QT syndrome with compound mutations is associated with a more severe phenotype: a Japanese multicenter study. *Heart Rhythm.* 2010;7:1411–1418.

14. Antzelevitch C. Role of spatial dispersion of repolarization in inherited and acquired sudden cardiac death syndromes. *Am J Physiol Heart Circ Physiol.* 2007;293:H2024–H2038.

15. Splawski I, Tristani-Firouzi M, Lehmann MH, et al. Mutations in the hminK gene cause long QT syndrome and suppress I$_{Ks}$ function. *Nat Genet.* 1997;17:338–340.

16. Splawski I, Shen J, Timothy KW, et al. Spectrum of mutations in long-QT syndrome genes. *KVLQT1, HERG, SCN5A, KCNE1, and KCNE2. Circulation.* 2000;102:1178–1185.

17. Kapplinger JD, Tester DJ, Salisbury BA, et al. Spectrum and prevalence of mutations from the first 2,500 consecutive unrelated patients referred for the FAMILION long QT syndrome genetic test. *Heart Rhythm.* 2009;6:1297–1303.

18. Chen L, Marquardt ML, Tester DJ, et al. Mutation of an A-kinase-anchoring protein causes long-QT syndrome. *Proc Natl Acad Sci U S A.* 2007;104:20990–20995.

19. Barc J, Briec F, Schmitt S, et al. Screening for copy number variation in genes associated with the long QT syndrome. *J Am Coll Cardiol.* 2011;57:40–47.

20. Seebohm G, Strutz-Seebohm N, Ureche ON, et al. Long QT syndrome-associated mutations in KCNQ1 and KCNE1 subunits disrupt normal endosomal recycling of IKs channels. *Circ Res.* 2008;103:1451–1457.

21. Kurokawa J, Motoike HK, Rao J, et al. Regulatory actions of the A-kinase anchoring protein Yotiao on a heart potassium channel downstream of PKA phosphorylation. *Proc Natl Acad Sci U S A.* 2004;101:16374–16378.

22. Li Y, Zaydman MA, Wu D, et al. KCNE1 enhances phosphatidylinositol 4,5-bisphosphate (PIP2) sensitivity of I$_{Ks}$ to modulate channel activity. *Proc Natl Acad Sci U S A.* 2011;108:9095–9100.

23. Schwartz PJ, Priori SG, Spazzolini C, et al. Genotype-phenotype correlation in the long-QT syndrome: gene-specific triggers for life-threatening arrhythmias. *Circulation.* 2001;103:89–95.

24. Wong JA, Gula LJ, Klein GJ, et al. Utility of treadmill testing in identification and genotype prediction in long-QT syndrome. *Circ Arrhythm Electrophysiol.* 2010;3:120–125.

25. Aziz PF, Wieand TS, Ganley J, et al. Genotype- and mutation site-specific QT adaptation during exercise, recovery, and postural changes in children with long-QT syndrome. *Circ Arrhythm Electrophysiol.* 2011;4:867–873.

26. Vyas H, Hejlik J, Ackerman MJ. Epinephrine QT stress testing in the evaluation of congenital long-QT syndrome. *Circulation.* 2006;113:1385–1392.

27. Priori SG, Napolitano C, Schwartz PJ, et al. Association of long QT syndrome loci and cardiac events among patients treated with β-blockers. *JAMA.* 2004;292:1341–1344.

28. Schwartz PJ, Priori SG, Cerrone M, et al. Left cardiac sympathetic denervation in the management of high-risk patients affected by the long-QT syndrome. *Circulation.* 2004;109:1826–1833.

29. Jons C, Moss AJ, Lopes CM, et al. Mutations in conserved amino acids in the KCNQ1 channel and risk of cardiac events in type-1 long-QT syndrome. *J Cardiovasc Electrophysiol.* 2009;20:859–865.

30. Jons C, O-Uchi J, Moss AJ, et al. Use of mutant-specific ion channel characteristics for risk stratification of long QT syndrome patients. *Sci Transl Med.* 2011;3.76ra28.

31. Kapa S, Tester DJ, Salisbury BA, et al. Genetic testing for long-QT syndrome: distinguishing pathogenic mutations from benign variants. *Circulation.* 2009;120:1752–1760.

32. Barsheshet A, Goldenberg I, O-Uchi J, et al. Mutations in cytoplasmic loops of the KCNQ1 channel and the risk of life-threatening events: implications for mutation-specific response to β-blocker therapy in type 1 long-QT syndrome. *Circulation.* 2012;125:1988–1996.

33. Duchatelet S, Crotti L, Peat RA, et al. Identification of a KCNQ1 polymorphism acting as a protective modifier against arrhythmic risk in long-QT syndrome. *Circ Cardiovasc Genet.* 2013;6:354–361.

34. Amin AS, Giudicessi JR, Tijsen AJ, et al. Variants in the 3'untranslated region of the KCNQ1-encoded Kv7.1 potassium channel modify disease severity in patients with type 1 long QT syndrome in an allele-specific manner. *Eur Heart J.* 2012;33:714–723.

35. Nishio Y, Makiyama T, Itoh H, et al. D85N, a KCNE1 polymorphism, is a disease-causing gene variant in long QT syndrome. *J Am Coll Cardiol.* 2009;54:812–819.

36. de Villiers CP, van der Merwe L, Crotti L, et al. AKAP9 is a genetic modifier of congenital long-QT syndrome type 1. *Circ Cardiovasc Genet.* 2014;7:599–606.

37. Crotti L, Monti MC, Insolia R, et al. NOS1AP is a genetic modifier of the long-QT syndrome. *Circulation.* 2009;120:1657–1663.

38. Tomás M, Napolitano C, De Giuli L, et al. Polymorphisms in the NOS1AP gene modulate QT interval duration and risk of arrhythmias in the long QT syndrome. *J Am Coll Cardiol.* 2010;55:2745–2752.

39. Newton-Cheh C, Eijgelsheim M, Rice KM, et al. Common variants at ten loci influence QT interval duration in the QTGEN Study. *Nat Genet.* 2009;41:399–406.

40. Pfeufer A, Sanna S, Arking DE, et al. Common variants at ten loci modulate the QT interval duration in the QTSCD Study. *Nat Genet.* 2009;41:407–414.

41. Chang KC, Barth AS, Sasano T, et al. CAPON modulates cardiac repolarization via neuronal nitric oxide synthase signaling in the heart. *Proc Natl Acad Sci U S A.* 2008;105:4777–8472.

42. Harmer SC, Wilson AJ, Aldridge R, et al. Mechanisms of disease pathogenesis in long QT syndrome type 5. *Am J Physiol Cell Physiol.* 2010;298:C263–C273.

43. Schwartz PJ, Spazzolini C, Crotti L, et al. The Jervell and Lange-Nielsen syndrome: natural history, molecular basis, and clinical outcome. *Circulation.* 2006;113:783–790.

44. Abbott GW, Sesti F, Splawski I, et al. MiRP1 forms I$_{Kr}$ potassium channels with HERG and is associated with cardiac arrhythmia. *Cell.* 1999;97:175–187.

45. Sale H, Wang J, O'Hara TJ, et al. Physiological properties of hERG 1a/1b heteromeric currents and a hERG 1b-specific mutation associated with Long-QT syndrome. *Circ Res.* 2008;103:e81–e95.

46. Crotti L, Tester DJ, White WM, et al. Long QT syndrome-associated mutations in intrauterine fetal death. *JAMA.* 2013;309:1473–1482.

47. Crotti L, Lundquist AL, Insolia R, et al. KCNH2-K897T is a genetic modifier of latent congenital long-QT syndrome. *Circulation.* 2005;112:1251–1258.

48. Gentile S, Martin N, Scappini E, et al. The human ERG1 channel polymorphism, K897T, creates a phosphorylation site that inhibits channel activity. *Proc Natl Acad Sci U S A.* 2008;105:14704–14708.

49. Gong Q, Zhang L, Vincent GM, et al. Nonsense mutations in hERG cause a decrease in mutant mRNA transcripts by nonsense-mediated mRNA decay in human long-QT syndrome. *Circulation.* 2007;116:17–24.

50. Anderson CL, Delisle BP, Anson BD, et al. Most LQT2 mutations reduce Kv11.1 (hERG) current by a class 2 (trafficking-deficient) mechanism. *Circulation.* 2006;113:365–373.

51. Li P, Ninomiya H, Kurata Y, et al. Reciprocal control of hERG stability by Hsp70 and Hsc70 with implication for restoration of LQT2 mutant stability. *Circ Res.* 2011;108:458–468.

52. Albesa M, Grilo LS, Gavillet B, et al. Nedd4-2-dependent ubiquitylation and regulation of the cardiac potassium channel hERG1. *J Mol Cell Cardiol.* 2011;51:90–98.

53. Smith JL, McBride CM, Nataraj PS, et al. Trafficking-deficient hERG K$^+$ channels linked to long QT syndrome are regulated by a microtubule-dependent quality control compartment in the ER. *Am J Physiol Cell Physiol.* 2011;301:C75–C85.

54. Cui J, Melman Y, Palma E, et al. Cyclic AMP regulates the HERG K$^+$ channel by dual pathways. *Curr Biol.* 2000;10:671–674.

55. Hekkala AM, Swan H, Viitasalo M, et al. Epinephrine bolus test in detecting long QT syndrome mutation carriers with indeterminable electrocardiographic phenotype. *Ann Noninvasive Electrocardiol.* 2011;16:172–179.

56. Yao Y, Teng S, Li N, et al. Aminoglycoside antibiotics restore functional expression of truncated HERG channels produced by nonsense mutations. *Heart Rhythm.* 2009;6:553–560.

57. Gianulis EC, Trudeau MC. Rescue of aberrant gating by a genetically encoded PAS (Per-Arnt-Sim) domain in several long QT syndrome mutant human *ether-á-go-go*-related gene potassium channels. *J Biol Chem.* 2011;286:22160–22169.

58. Lu Y, Mahaut-Smith MP, Huang CL, et al. Mutant MiRP1 subunits modulate HERG K$^+$ channel gating: a mechanism for pro-arrhythmia in long QT syndrome type 6. *J Physiol.* 2003;551:253–262.

59. Pourrier M, Zicha S, Ehrlich J, et al. Canine ventricular KCNE2 expression resides predominantly in Purkinje fibers. *Circ Res.* 2003;93:189–191.

60. Plaster NM, Tawil R, Tristani-Firouzi M, et al. Mutations in Kir2.1 cause the developmental and episodic electrical phenotypes of Andersen's syndrome. *Cell.* 2001;105:511–519.

61. Tristani-Firouzi M, Etheridge SP. Kir 2.1. channelopathies: the Andersen-Tawil syndrome. *Pflugers Arch.* 2010;460:289–294.

62. Morita H, Zipes DP, Morita ST, et al. Mechanism of U wave and polymorphic ventricular tachycardia in a canine tissue model of Andersen-Tawil syndrome. *Cardiovasc Res.* 2007;75:510–518.

63. Yang Y, Yang Y, Liang B, et al. Identification of a Kir3.4 mutation in congenital long QT syndrome. *Am J Hum Genet.* 2010;86:872–880.

64. Gussak I, Brugada P, Brugada J, et al. Idiopathic short QT interval: a new clinical syndrome? *Cardiology.* 2000;94:99–102.

65. Gaita F, Giustetto C, Bianchi F, et al. Short QT syndrome: a familial cause of sudden death. *Circulation.* 2003;108:965–970.

66. Brugada R, Hong K, Dumaine R, et al. Sudden death associated with short QT syndrome linked to mutations in HERG. *Circulation.* 2004;109:30–35.

67. Bellocq C, van Ginneken AC, Bezzina CR, et al. Mutation in the KCNQ1 gene leading to the short QT-interval syndrome. *Circulation.* 2004;109:2394–2397.

68. Priori SG, Pandit SV, Rivolta I, et al. A novel form of short QT syndrome (SQT3) is caused by a mutation in the KCNJ2 gene. *Circ Res.* 2005;96:800–807.

69. Sun Y, Quan XQ, Fromme S, et al. A novel mutation in the KCNH2 gene associated with short QT syndrome. *J Mol Cell Cardiol.* 2011;50:433–441.

70. Harrell DT, Ashihara T, Ishikawa T, et al. Genotype-dependent differences in age of manifestation and arrhythmia complications in short QT syndrome. *Int J Cardiol.* 2015;190:393–402.

71. Patel C, Antzelevitch C. Cellular basis for arrhythmogenesis in an experimental model of the SQT1 form of the short QT syndrome. *Heart Rhythm.* 2008;5:585–590.

72. Giustetto C, Schimpf R, Mazzanti A, et al. Long-term follow-up of patients with short QT syndrome. *J Am Coll Cardiol.* 2011;58:587–595.

73. Hong K, Piper DR, Diaz-Valdecantos A, et al. De novo KCNQ1 mutation responsible for atrial fibrillation and short QT syndrome in utero. *Cardiovas Res.* 2005;68:433–440.

74. Moreno C, Oliveras A, de la Cruz A, et al. A new KCNQ1 mutation at the S5 segment that impairs its association with KCNE1 is responsible for short QT syndrome. *Cardiovasc Res.* 2015;107:613–623.

75. Hattori T, Makiyama T, Akao M, et al. A novel gain-of-function KCNJ2 mutation associated with short-QT syndrome impairs inward rectification of Kir2.1 currents. *Cardiovasc Res.* 2012;93:666–673.

76. Ambrosini E, Sicca F, Brignone MS, et al. Genetically induced dysfunction of Kir2.1 channels: implications for short QT3 syndrome and autism-epilepsy phenotype. *Hum Mol Genet.* 2014;23:4875–4886.

77. Junttila MJ, Sager SJ, Tikkanen JT, et al. Clinical significance of variants of J-points and J-waves: early repolarization patterns and risk. *Eur Heart J.* 2012;33:2639–2643.

78. Antzelevitch C, Yan GX. J wave syndromes. *Heart Rhythm.* 2010;7:549–558.

79. Wang Q, Ohno S, Ding WG, et al. Gain-of-function KCNH2 mutations in patients with Brugada syndrome. *J Cardiovasc Electrophysiol.* 2014;25:522–530.

80. Verkerk AO, Wilders R, Schulze-Bahr E, et al. Role of sequence variations in the human ether-a-go-go-related gene (HERG, KCNH2) in the Brugada syndrome. *Cardiovasc Res.* 2005;68:441–453.

81. Kapplinger JD, Giudicessi JR, Ye D, et al. Enhanced classification of Brugada syndrome-associated and long-QT syndrome-associated genetic variants in the SCN5A-encoded Nav1.5 cardiac sodium channel. *Circ Cardiovasc Genet.* 2015;8:582–595.

82. Andrade J, Khairy P, Dobrev D, et al. The clinical profile and pathophysiology of atrial fibrillation: relationships among clinical features, epidemiology, and mechanisms. *Circ Res.* 2014;114:1453–1468.

83. Tester DJ, Arya P, Will M, et al. Genotypic heterogeneity and phenotypic mimicry among unrelated patients referred for catecholaminergic polymorphic ventricular tachycardia genetic testing. *Heart Rhythm.* 2006;3:800–805.

84. Vega AL, Tester DJ, Ackerman MJ, et al. Protein kinase A-dependent biophysical phenotype for V227F-KCNJ2 mutation in catecholaminergic polymorphic ventricular tachycardia. *Circ Arrhythm Electrophysiol.* 2009;2:540–547.

85. Krous HF, Beckwith JB, Byard RW, et al. Sudden infant death syndrome and unclassified sudden infant deaths: a definitional and diagnostic approach. *Pediatrics.* 2004;114:234–238.

86. Tfelt-Hansen J, Winkel BG, Grunnet M, et al. Cardiac channelopathies and sudden infant death syndrome. *Cardiology.* 2011;119:21–33.

87. Schwartz PJ, Priori SG, Bloise R, et al. Molecular diagnosis in a child with sudden infant death syndrome. *Lancet.* 2001;358:1342–1343.

53 Inheritable Phenotypes Associated With Altered Intracellular Calcium Regulation

Francisco J. Alvarado and Héctor H. Valdivia

Calcium (Ca^{2+}) is the most ubiquitous and versatile intracellular messenger. In the heart, it plays an especially remarkable dual role, serving as both a regulator of gene transcription and a triggering signal for contraction. Hence, the cardiac regulation of intracellular $[Ca^{2+}]$ ($[Ca^{2+}]_i$) is a particularly complex process that follows an exquisitely orchestrated sequence of events, ultimately allowing cardiomyocytes to differentiate the global cyclic $[Ca^{2+}]_i$ oscillations required for contraction from the localized, subcellular Ca^{2+} events that regulate gene transcription. Indeed, there is an ~20,000-fold transmembrane $[Ca^{2+}]$ gradient that is essential to endow Ca^{2+} with such versatility.

Since the mid-1990s, hundreds of mutations in Ca^{2+} handling proteins have been linked to inherited cardiac disorders, offering concrete proof that the dysregulation of Ca^{2+} homeostasis has profound pathological relevance. The inherited phenotype most associated with cardiac Ca^{2+} dysregulation is an electrical disturbance (arrhythmia), and catecholaminergic polymorphic ventricular tachycardia (CPVT) is the quintessential example of arrhythmogenic Ca^{2+} disorders of the heart. Nevertheless, as genetic testing becomes more widespread in the clinic and gene panels are extended, new evidence suggests that cardiac Ca^{2+} dysregulation accounts for more than just arrhythmia and leads to structural cardiomyopathy and more complex phenotypes as well. This chapter discusses the current genetic and mechanistic evidence that links mutations in intracellular Ca^{2+}-handling proteins to arrhythmia and structural cardiomyopathy.

Overview of Calcium Homeostasis in the Heart

Calcium Cycling in Excitation–Contraction Coupling

While studying the effect of inorganic salts on several tissues in the late 19th century, physiologist Sidney Ringer realized that Ca^{2+} was an essential ion for cardiac contraction. Working with isolated heart preparations, he noticed that Ca^{2+} removal from the perfusion buffer stopped heart beats, whereas its re-addition restored and maintained contractility.[1] At the time, Ringer almost certainly ignored that external Ca^{2+} only accounted for a small fraction of Ca^{2+} actually needed for the heart to contract. Every action potential (AP) in cardiomyocytes is accompanied by a transient elevation of the free $[Ca^{2+}]_i$, from approximately 100 nM during diastole to nearly 1 µM during systole, activating the myofilaments and producing contraction.[2] This series of events by which membrane depolarization is converted to mechanical contraction is termed excitation–contraction (e–c) coupling (Fig. 53.1A). In adult cardiomyocytes, the amount of extracellular Ca^{2+} entering the cell during AP is insufficient to elicit full contractions. Instead, most of the Ca^{2+} required for contraction (approximately 70% in humans and 90% in mice) flows out of the sarcoplasmic reticulum (SR),[3] an intracellular Ca^{2+} store, through the amplifying mechanism of Ca^{2+}-induced Ca^{2+} release (CICR).[4] In this process, the relatively small inward Ca^{2+} current (I_{CaL}) from L-type Ca^{2+} channels (LTCCs) that occurs during AP activates cardiac ryanodine receptors (RyR2s), which in turn release more Ca^{2+} from SR. Hence, RyR2 acts as a Ca^{2+} sensor and a Ca^{2+} channel, amplifying a small Ca^{2+} signal and potentially turning CICR into a self-sustaining, regenerative process. However, CICR reliably stops in intact cardiomyocytes, and relaxation ensues once Ca^{2+} is removed from the cytosol. Several mechanisms are considered to participate in CICR termination (whose discussion is beyond the scope of this chapter), while two main molecular players work in concert to achieve cytosolic Ca^{2+} removal: the SR Ca^{2+}-ATPase (SERCA2a) refills SR, while the Na^+/Ca^{2+} exchanger (NCX) extrudes Ca^{2+} from the cell. To maintain Ca^{2+} equilibrium, the small inward Ca^{2+} current that triggered CICR (I_{CaL}) must be extruded by NCX, whereas the Ca^{2+} released by RyR2 channels must return to SR. NCX is an electrogenic transporter, which moves three Na^+ in one direction while carrying a single Ca^{2+} in the opposite direction; hence, the extrusion of Ca^{2+} creates an inward depolarizing current that becomes more evident in the late phases of AP.

CICR occurs at specialized regions of the cell where the external membrane is in close proximity to SR, mostly within the T-tubule (TT) network of the myocyte. In these tightly spaced microdomains, clusters of ~20 LTCCs provide the activating Ca^{2+} signal for ~100 RyR2s, forming a calcium release unit (CRU).[3] A Ca^{2+} release event that originates from a single CRU is referred to as a Ca^{2+} spark, while the global cytosolic Ca^{2+} transient results from the temporal and spatial summations of Ca^{2+} sparks coordinated during e–c coupling by AP and I_{CaL}.[5] Isolated Ca^{2+} sparks during diastole are normal and most likely are originated through single CRU activation by the stochastic opening of RyR2 channels.[6] However, the diastolic propagation of Ca^{2+} sparks through the cell as Ca^{2+} waves or synchronization of spontaneous sparks into diastolic Ca^{2+} transients is often observed in pathological conditions (see later).

Adrenergic Regulation of Calcium Homeostasis

The sympathetic branch of the autonomic nervous system increases the dynamic output of the heart in response to increased metabolic demand of the organism. Indeed, this system provides an essential component of the cardiac fight-or-flight response through the activation of β_1-adrenergic receptors (β_1-ARs) by catecholamines: heart rate increase because of a direct effect on the sinus node (positive chronotropic effect), and increase in contractility and rate of relaxation because

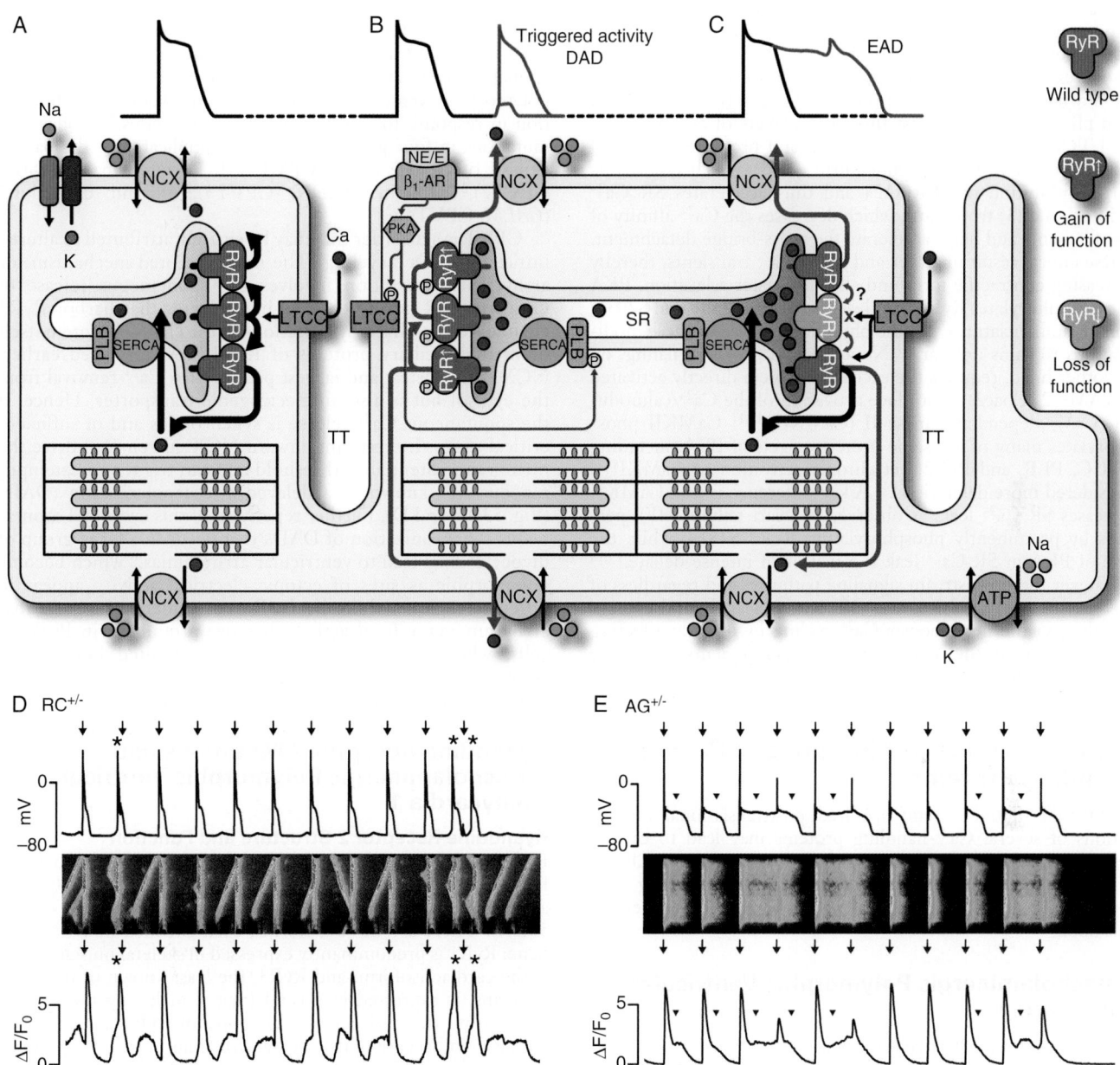

FIGURE 53.1 Cellular mechanisms of catecholaminergic polymorphic ventricular tachycardia (CPVT1). (A) Cardiac excitation–contraction coupling in a normal myocyte. The Ca^{2+} current through the L-type Ca^{2+} channel (*LTCC*) activates ryanodine receptors 2 (*RyR2*), which in turn release Ca^{2+} from the sarcoplasmic reticulum (*SR*), leading to the contraction of myofilaments. Ca^{2+} is then extruded from the cell through the Na^+/Ca^{2+} exchanger (*NCX*) and undergoes reuptake into SR by *SERCA2a*. (B) Stimulation of β_1-adrenergic receptors (β_1-*ARs*) by catecholamines (*NE/E*) promotes the activation of protein kinase A (*PKA*), which phosphorylates (P) several protein targets, including LTCC, RyR2, and phospholamban (*PLB*). During diastole, mutant gain-of-function RyR2 channels spontaneously release Ca^{2+}, which can trigger a delayed afterdepolarization (*DAD*). (C) RyR2 channels that harbor a loss-of-function mutation do not respond to luminal or cytosolic Ca^{2+}. When SR reaches a critical Ca^{2+} load during an action potential (*AP*), both wild-type and hypoactive channels produce a burst of Ca^{2+} that prolongs AP by activating NCX, leading to an early afterdepolarization (*EAD*). (D and E) Representative AP (*top panel*) and Ca^{2+} transient (*middle and lower panels*) traces recorded in cardiomyocytes from heterozygous ($^{+/-}$) RyR2-R4496C (gain-of-function) and RyR2-A4860G (loss-of-function) mice stimulated at 1Hz in the presence of 300 nM isoproterenol. Notice the several Ca^{2+} waves unable to trigger full APs in the RyR2-R4496C$^{+/-}$ traces. *Arrows* indicate the triggered stimuli. *Asterisks* indicate DADs, and *arrowheads* indicate AP prolongation and EADs. ([D] and [E] Data provided by Xi Chen and Yan-Ting Zhao from the University of Michigan Center for Arrhythmia Research.)

of the direct effect on ventricular myocytes (positive inotropic and lusitropic effect, respectively), among others. While the role of Ca^{2+} signaling in sinus node automaticity is emerging,[7] its importance for modulating inotropy and lusitropy has long been established.[2] Canonical β_1-AR signaling in the heart involves an increase in cyclic adenosine monophosphate (cAMP) and the downstream activation of protein kinase A (PKA), which in turn phosphorylates at least three key players of e–c coupling: (1) LTCC, which enhances peak I_{CaL} and promotes increased SR Ca^{2+} content; (2) phospholamban (PLB), which relieves its partial inhibition of SERCA2a and thus accelerates SR Ca^{2+} refilling; and (3) troponin I, which decreases the Ca^{2+} affinity of myofilaments and helps accelerate the cross-bridge detachment. These effects result in larger and faster Ca^{2+} transients, thereby increasing contractile force and allowing faster relaxation. PKA also phosphorylates RyR2 at least two sites (S2808 and S2031, human nomenclature), but the physiological role of these modifications remains unclear.[8,9] Noncanonical β_1-AR signaling, on the other hand, requires the exchange protein directly activated by cAMP 2 (Epac2) to produce activation of the Ca^{2+}/calmodulin (CaM)–dependent kinase II (CaMKII).[10,11] CaMKII phosphorylates many of the same protein targets of PKA, including LTCC, PLB, and RyR2; yet chronic activation of CaMKII is considered more deleterious.[12] A key difference is that CaMKII increases SR Ca^{2+} leak, as observed in heart failure (HF), perhaps by prominently phosphorylating RyR2-S2814, while the role of PKA in SR Ca^{2+} leak is a matter of intense debate.[13,14] Whatever the downstream signaling pathways and regardless of the specific controversies, it is sufficiently clear that adrenergic signaling in the heart boosts Ca^{2+} cycling by directly affecting the sarcolemmal, SR, and myofilament components of the e–c coupling machinery.

Arrhythmia due to Mutations in Calcium-Handling Proteins

Congenital mutations and acquired posttranslational modifications of several Ca^{2+}-handling proteins may lead to cardiac arrhythmias. Here our discussion will be focused on CPVT. Long QT syndrome (LQTS), also in some cases resulting from mutations in Ca^{2+}-handling proteins, is discussed elsewhere in this book.

Catecholaminergic Polymorphic Ventricular Tachycardia

CPVT is a severe inherited syndrome characterized by ventricular tachyarrhythmias triggered by physical or emotional stress in the absence of structural disease or remarkable changes in the resting electrocardiogram.[15–17] The prevalence of the disease in the general population is unknown[18] but is estimated to be 1 in 10,000 in Europe.[16] CPVT primarily affects young patients[17]; however, some do not display symptoms until adulthood.[19] Patients often develop bidirectional tachycardia potentially leading to ventricular fibrillation and sudden cardiac death; however, idiopathic ventricular fibrillation has also been observed.[19] A common feature of a CPVT episode is syncope; therefore many patients are incorrectly diagnosed with epilepsy and accordingly treated.[20] Therefore exercise stress tests, Holter monitoring, and drug challenges with epinephrine or isoproterenol are important tools to establish a correct differential diagnosis of CPVT.[21] If untreated, 60% to 70% of patients may develop severe tachyarrhythmias, and ~30% may undergo cardiac arrest or sudden cardiac death.[17,19]

The study of the genetics of CPVT started when the disease was mapped to chromosome 1q42-43 by Swan and colleagues in 1999.[22] Shortly after, this region was narrowed to the gene that codes for RyR2 when Priori and associates[23] reported four specific mutations in a same number of probands with catecholaminergic VT. One of these mutations, RyR2-R4497C, was later introduced in mice (RyR2-R4496C), and heterozygous animals recapitulated the most relevant clinical signs of CPVT: polymorphic ventricular tachycardia and ventricular fibrillation in response to catecholamines and exercises.[24] Today, the mutations in four genes are currently implicated in the pathogenesis of CPVT: *RYR2* (CPVT1),[23] calsequestrin 2 (*CASQ2*, CPVT2),[25] triadin (*TRDN*, CPVT3),[26,27] and calmodulin (*CALM*, CPVT4).[28]

CPVT is a disorder that may be entirely attributed to altered intracellular Ca^{2+} cycling. The most accepted mechanism for arrhythmia generation involves the spontaneous release of Ca^{2+} from SR during diastole in myocytes that harbor RyR2 channels destabilized by mutations in the channel protein itself or in the ancillary proteins of RyR2.[29] As discussed earlier, NCX is the fastest and largest pathway for Ca^{2+} removal from the cytosol but is also an electrogenic transporter. Hence, if the spontaneous Ca^{2+} release is synchronous and of sufficient critical mass, the resulting inward NCX current can drive the membrane potential to threshold and can trigger an extemporaneous AP, known as a delayed afterdepolarization (DAD) (Fig. 53.1B and D). Further repetition of this cycle and spontaneous synchronization of DADs that occur in a large group of myocytes may lead to ventricular arrhythmias,[6] which become polymorphic as sites of ectopic electrical activity appear in different regions of the heart. Recent evidence suggests that arrhythmogenic focal activity is more prominent in Purkinje cells, where the subcellular structure, limited intercellular connection, and low electrotonicity favor the generation and propagation of DADs.[30]

Ryanodine Receptor 2 Mutations and Catecholaminergic Polymorphic Ventricular Tachycardia 1

Ryanodine Receptor 2 Structure and Function

RyR is the largest ion channel known in nature. Channels are formed by four identical subunits, each containing nearly 5000 amino acids, with a combined molecular mass of >2000 kDa (Fig. 53.2A). There are three isoforms, each encoded by a different gene: RyR1 is predominantly expressed in skeletal muscle; RyR2 is the cardiac isoform; and RyR3, the least known of the three isoforms, is expressed in several tissues, including the brain.[31] Elucidating the molecular architecture of RyR has been difficult, in part because of its colossal size. This hurdle was partially overcome in 2015, when three laboratories published the highest-resolution cryo-EM structures of RyR1 available to date at 3.1 to 6.8 Å.[32–34] More recently, Peng and colleagues elucidated the structure of the closed and open RyR2 at 4.1 Å and 4.2 Å, respectively.[35] Remarkably, both RyR1 and RyR2 share a similar structural hierarchy divided in three levels: (1) a central tower, which forms the protein core and contains the central domain (CD), pore-forming domain (PFD), and the N-terminal domain (NTD); (2) a corona, which tops the central tower and is formed by two helical domains (HD1 and HD2) and a handle domain; and (3) the peripheral region, composed of five smaller domains (SPRY1–3, P1, and P2) that contain phosphorylation sites or anchoring points for accessory proteins. The protein bulk is localized in the cytoplasm, spanning most of the gap between SR and the TT membrane. PFD is made by six transmembrane segments per subunit, where S6 forms the Ca^{2+}-conducting pore. Finally, each subunit has a short luminal loop that protrudes into SR[32,33] and may serve as an interaction site for the SR proteins.

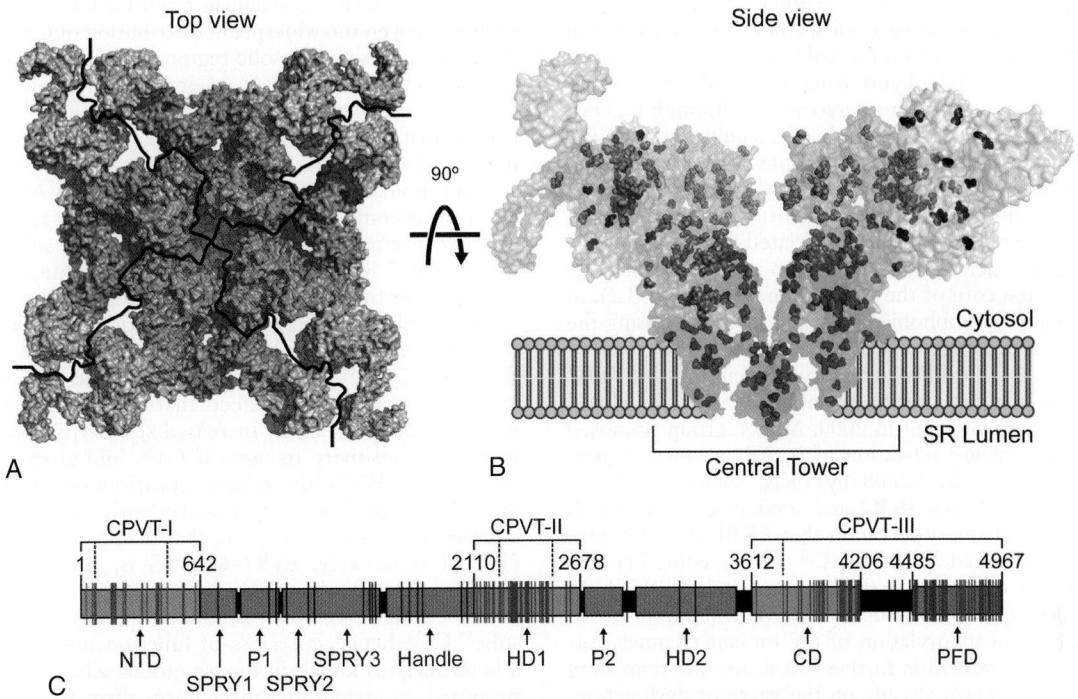

FIGURE 53.2 Ryanodine receptors 2 (*RyR2*) mutations associated with catecholaminergic polymorphic ventricular tachycardia (*CPVT*). The four domains containing the majority of CPVT mutations are color coded in all panels: N-terminal domain (*NTD*), *orange*; helical domain 1 (*HD1*), *green*; central domain (*CD*), *blue*; and pore-forming domain (*PFD*), *magenta*. The peripheral domains (SPRY1-3, P1, and P2), handle domain, and helical domain 2 (*HD2*) are colored *gray*. (A) Single RyR channel observed from the top. *Black lines* delimit the four subunits. (B) Side view of a RyR channel that shows two opposite subunits. The side chain of ~200 residues susceptible to CPVT mutations are identified with *spheres* and *colored* according to the domain. (C) Schematic of a single RyR2 subunit drawn to scale with *superimposed lines*, representing the location of 200 CPVT mutations. The current delimitation of the three CPVT mutation clusters is indicated with *dashed lines*. *Solid lines* indicate our proposed extended delimitation based on specific domains. (Mutation data obtained from the Human Gene Mutation Database [www.hgmd.cf.ac.uk] and from the literature. Atomic coordinates and domain assignment obtained from Peng W, Shen H, Wu J, et al. Structural basis for the gating mechanism of the type 2 ryanodine receptor RyR2. *Science*. 2016 Sep 22 [Epub ahead of print]. PDB ID 5GO9. Images prepared using PyMOL Molecular Graphics software. The atomic coordinates and domains of the porcine RyR2 as reported by Peng and colleagues were used to identify equivalent human RyR2 domains and locate specific residues susceptible to CPVT mutations.)

More than 200 different mutations in *RYR2* (and increasing) have been identified in patients with CPVT; however, only a handful have been fully characterized. Historically, three regions of RyR2 are considered to be canonical clusters of CPVT mutations, arbitrarily defined on the basis of the mutation frequency, location of putative regulatory regions, and overlap with mutation sites in RyR1: CPVT-I (residues 77–466), CPVT-II (2246–2534), and CPVT-III (3778–4967).[36] These regions are often depicted in a linear representation of a RyR2 subunit, oversimplifying the complex three-dimensional structure of the protein. With the recent high-resolution cryo-EM maps, it is possible to limit these sections to four specific structural domains (Fig. 53.2C): 17% of the mutations are localized in NTD (residues 1–642, CPVT-I); ~21% of the mutations occur within HD1 (residues 2110–2678, CPVT-II); and finally, ~55% of the mutations falls within CPVT-III, which corresponds to CD (residues 3612–4206, 27%), PFD (4485–4967, 25%), and the region in between (2%). Intriguingly, only ~7% of the mutations fall in the peripheral domains (residues 643-2109 and 2679-3611), located outside the canonical CPVT regions, whereas the vast majority fall in the central tower of the channel (Fig. 53.2B). If genetic mutations are equally likely to arise anywhere in *RYR2*, those occurring in the peripheral domains are either more deleterious (or perhaps lethal) or they are innocuous compared with those in the canonical sites and thus do not appear in the clinical spectrum.

Arrhythmogenesis Because of Ryanodine Receptor 2 Mutations

The specific molecular mechanism(s) by which RyR2 mutations produce arrhythmias remains unclear. Because arrhythmia episodes in CPVT are induced by stress, and infusion of catecholamines is often used as a diagnostic tool in the clinical arena, the β-adrenergic system must be an important trigger. To date, three specific hypotheses have been proposed to explain arrhythmogenesis because of RyR2 mutations: defective interdomain interaction,[37] enhanced dissociation of the regulatory protein FK506-binding protein (FKBP) 12.6,[38,39] increased sensitivity to activation by luminal Ca^{2+},[15] or a combination thereof.

Normal RyR2 channels are believed to be leak-resistant by interdomain interactions that "zip" various segments of the protein and stabilize the channel in a closed state. Yamamoto and associates[37] suggested that CPVT mutations disrupt the interdomain interactions in RyR2, leading to "domain unzipping" and thus the destabilization of the closed state of the channel. The idea was tested using synthetic peptides with an amino acid sequence similar to small segments of the canonical CPVT domains. The peptides increased RyR activity and evoked Ca^{2+} release, presumably by hybridizing with RyR domains and obstructing native interdomain interactions.[37]Although it is not entirely clear how a synthetic peptide of a significant mass (>2 kDa) may find its way into the tightly apposed domain–domain interspace to "unzip" it, recent cryo-EM data clearly indicate that a significant number of CPVT mutations (and malignant hyperthermia mutations, the RyR1-associated disease of skeletal muscle) alter amino acid residues that form part of the interacting segments in the core of the RyR channel (see Fig. 53.2), in effect destabilizing hydrophobic bonds and likely increasing the magnitude of Ca^{2+} leak from SR.

FKBP12.6 is a 12.6-kDa accessory protein of the RyR2 macromolecular complex that presumably stabilizes the closed state of the channel. Starting in 2000, Marks' group proposed that in HF, the chronic activation of β_1-AR produces hyperphosphorylation of RyR2-S2808 by PKA, leading to dissociation of FKBP12.6 from RyR2 and rendering the channels leaky.[40-43] Following the observation that FKBP12.6 *null* mice developed stress-induced arrhythmias,[38] the preceding hypothesis was expanded to explain arrhythmogenesis in CPVT1. In this scheme, RyR2 mutations destabilize the interaction with FKBP12.6. PKA phosphorylation of the mutant channels following adrenergic stimulation further dissociates the remaining FKBP12.6 from channels already on the verge of dysfunction, hence leading to arrhythmia.[39] However, several laboratories have failed to reproduce key experiments that support the FKBP12.6 dissociation hypothesis in both HF[8,14,44,45] and CPVT.[46,47] Also relevant to this discussion is the fact that the overwhelming majority of the RyR2 mutations occur in regions located far from the FKBP12.6-binding region. Moreover, FKBP interacts with RyR at a site that does not involve CPVT-II, the region where mutations are considered to destabilize the RyR2-FKBP12.6 interaction.[36,48] Thus even if PKA phosphorylation of RyR2 indeed dissociates FKBP12.6, a highly controversial finding, it appears unlikely that this mechanism may be universally applied to CPVT1 because only a few mutations appear in the vicinity of the FKBP12.6-binding site.

The third most prominent hypothesis has been advanced by Chen and colleagues[15] who postulate that RyR2 channels destabilized by CPVT mutations are activated by lower SR luminal $[Ca^{2+}]$ than wild-type channels. The threshold for spontaneous luminal activation is therefore decreased in the mutant channels, making them susceptible to spontaneously release Ca^{2+}, especially during the natural elevation of SR $[Ca^{2+}]$ caused by adrenergic stimulation. This mechanism is called store overload–induced Ca^{2+} release (SOICR)[15] and has been developed predominantly using heterologous expression of RyR2 in HEK293 cells. On loading of the intracellular Ca^{2+} store by increasing extracellular $[Ca^{2+}]$, mutant channels spontaneously release Ca^{2+} more often[47,49] and at lower store load[50] than wild-type channels. On the basis of this observation, most RyR2 mutations are classified as gain-of-function in terms of luminal Ca^{2+} sensitivity.[50] The same group has recently mapped the putative luminal Ca^{2+} sensor of RyR2 to a negatively charged amino acid (RyR2-E4872) in one of the transmembrane regions of RyR2.[51] The mutation of this residue to an alanine (RyR2-E4872A) completely abolished SOICR in vitro. Furthermore, a compound heterozygous mouse for both the CPVT mutation RyR2-R4496C and RyR2-E4872Q does not develop arrhythmia following adrenergic stimulation. These data certainly support the SOICR hypothesis for RyR2-R4496C, a mutation located close to the putative luminal Ca^{2+} sensor; however, as in the FKBP12.6 dissociation hypothesis previously discussed, it seems unlikely that mutations located in other domains of the channel selectively affect the luminal Ca^{2+} sensor, and the general applicability of this mechanism to all CPVT cases appears also unlikely. Given the widespread distribution of CPVT mutations within the massive cytosolic region of RyR2, any of the mechanisms of CPVT mentioned earlier appears narrowly applicable if it does not invoke alterations in multiple aspects of RyR2 function regulated at the cytosolic level (e.g., cytosolic Ca^{2+} sensitivity, phosphorylation).

The molecular heterogeneity associated with RyR2 mutations has become more evident while studying novel mutations, and two examples in the literature provide solid experimental evidence. RyR2-V2475F is a de novo mutation identified during a postmortem study of a young subject that suffered unexplained drowning.[52] This mutation is located in HD1 (CPVT-II), close to other mutations previously studied (e.g., RyR2-R2474S).[39] Interestingly, Loaiza and associates[53] found at least three molecular defects that contribute to the pathogenicity of RyR2-V2475F: increased sensitivity to *cytosolic* Ca^{2+}, increased sensitivity to *luminal* Ca^{2+}, and altered PKA phosphorylation. While the relative contribution of each defect to arrhythmogenesis was not independently assessed, this level of complexity certainly suggests that a universal mechanism for CPVT1 is unlikely. RyR2-A4860G is, perhaps, a more evident example. Distinct from other CPVT1 mutations hitherto described, RyR2-A4860G is not activated by luminal[54] or cytosolic[55] Ca^{2+}; hence, it is a loss-of-function mutation. By studying a heterozygous knock-in mouse model, Zhao and colleagues[55] proposed an arrhythmia mechanism through early afterdepolarizations (i.e., spontaneous depolarizations that occur during the late phases of AP) rather than DADs (Fig. 53.1C and E). In this case, the lack of luminal and cytosolic activation of RyR2-A4860G channels promotes SR overload. Eventually, SR overload, I_{CaL}, and other sympathetically induced activating factors converge to open the hypoactive channels that contain at least one RyR2-A4860G subunit. This extemporaneous release of Ca^{2+} during systole by the mutant channels subsequently activates wild-type channels by CICR, producing a burst of Ca^{2+} that prolongs AP because of the enhanced activation of NCX. The latter may lead to reactivation of other depolarizing currents, producing EADs, focal ectopic activity, and ultimately ventricular fibrillation.

Evidently, as more RyR2 mutations undergo molecular scrutiny, the variety of arrhythmia mechanisms is almost sure to increase. Because of the staggering number of potential alterations, it remains to be seen whether by defining the location of the mutation in the overall structure of RyR2 it will be possible to predict the dominant molecular defects that lead to arrhythmia. This remains challenging, but doing so would allow tailoring therapies for CPVT1, according to the affected RyR2 domain. Obscuring this goal is the fact that the clinical phenotype of CPVT1 is shared by most RyR2 mutations, regardless of the underlying molecular phenotype.

Calsequestrin 2 Mutations and Catecholaminergic Polymorphic Ventricular Tachycardia 2

Calsequestrin 2 (CSQ2) is a 399-amino acid Ca^{2+}–binding protein localized to the lumen of SR in close proximity to RyR2 channels. It works as a moderate-affinity, high-capacity Ca^{2+} buffer,[56] contributing to increase SR Ca^{2+} content while maintaining relatively low free luminal $[Ca^{2+}]$. On the binding of Ca^{2+}, CASQ2 is able to polymerize and hold up to ~40 Ca^{2+} per CASQ2 polymer.[57] Additionally, CASQ2 is able to regulate RyR2 function through its interaction with TRDN and junctin,[58] potentially through effects on the putative luminal Ca^{2+} sensor of RyR2.[59] Shortly after CPVT was mapped to the gene that encodes RyR2, Lahat and associates[25,60] described a missense CASQ2 mutation,

CASQ2-D307H, affecting only homozygous carriers. Thus unlike CPVT1, CPVT2 is an autosomal *recessive* disorder. Since then, a total of 15 CSQ2 mutations have been associated with CPVT.[56] Still, CSQ2 mutations account only for less than 5% of total CPVT cases.[61]

The mechanism that best explains how mutations in CASQ2 cause CPVT involves the altered regulation of RyR2 refractoriness,[62,63] the process that keeps RyR2 channels closed after a regular cycle of Ca^{2+} release. Under normal conditions, RyR2 channels terminate Ca^{2+} release when $[Ca^{2+}]$ inside SR drops below a threshold level, at which point the RyR2 channels stay "refractory" or resistant to opening. RyR2 refractoriness thus avoids premature Ca^{2+} release and allows the SERCA2a pump to refill SR with Ca^{2+} necessary for the next contraction cycle. Because CASQ2 binds and "sequesters" Ca^{2+} (hence the apt name) inside SR, a critical period of time must ensue before SERCA2a may saturate CASQ2 and make Ca^{2+} available for release. It follows therefore that mutations that decrease the Ca^{2+}-binding properties of CASQ2, either by lowering the affinity of its Ca^{2+}-binding sites or by preventing its polymerization, lead to the fast refilling of SR Ca^{2+} and premature termination of RyR refractoriness, causing diastolic Ca^{2+} release.[64] In an alternative but not mutually exclusive scenario, CASQ2 acts as an inhibitor of RyR2 through its interaction with TRDN, which is directly linked to RyR2s.[65] Mutations in CASQ2 may therefore rescind the inhibitory properties of CASQ2 and prompt RyR2 channels to release Ca^{2+} at reduced threshold levels.[64]

Triadin Mutations and Catecholaminergic Polymorphic Ventricular Tachycardia 3

The cardiac isoform of TRDN, also known as Trisk 32, is a 286-amino acid transmembrane protein localized to SR, specifically to CRUs. There it interacts with neighboring proteins, such as CASQ2 and junctin, to modulate RyR2 from the SR lumen.[58] Two reports in the literature described four TRDN mutations with respect to CPVT.[26,27] It is difficult to establish a strong genotype–phenotype association on the basis of current evidence, but both reports described what appeared to be an autosomal recessive form of CPVT. Two of the mutations described in these reports, a 4-bp deletion in exon 2 (TRDN-D18fs*13)[26] and an intronic mutation that produces a putative splice variant (c.22+29 A>G),[27] introduce early termination codons, truncating protein synthesis before the transmembrane domain. A third mutation that occurs in the transmembrane domain, TRDN-T59R, may destabilize the protein and thus lead to early degradation based on in vitro studies.[26] The fourth is a nonsense mutation, TRDN-Q205*, and it is presumed to truncate the protein before the putative TRDN-CASQ2-RyR2 interaction site, located between residues 210 and 224.[65] Therefore Roux-Buisson and colleagues[26] argue that the lack of functional TRDN in affected patients is the underlying cause of CPVT, making CPVT3 a TRDN knockout disorder with *recessive* inheritance. This conclusion is supported by the presence of the CPVT phenotype in patients homozygous for TRDN-D18fs*13 and the observation that TRDN *null* mice develop arrhythmia under acute adrenergic stimulation.[66] Interestingly, some patients had compound heterozygous mutations, in which TRDN-Q205* was present with either TRDN-T59R or c.22+29 A>G. This observation would certainly confirm the hypothesis of CPVT3 being a functional TRDN knockout disorder if TRDN-T59R is shown to produce early protein degradation in vivo. Clearly, more in-depth studies are necessary to elucidate the arrhythmogenic mechanisms because of TRDN mutations. Further complexity is added to this question by the recent description of TRDN mutations in LQTS patients.[67] Interestingly, TRDN-D18fs*13 is one such variant.

Calmodulin Mutations and Catecholaminergic Polymorphic Ventricular Tachycardia 4

Mutations in CaM are perhaps the most recent addition to the CPVT spectrum. CaM is 149-amino-acid 16.7-kDa Ca^{2+}–binding protein that is ubiquitously expressed from three different genes (*CALM1*, *CALM2*, and *CALM3*) that code for the same protein product. The importance of CaM in regulating numerous cellular functions is highlighted by this apparent genetic redundancy. Each terminus of the protein forms a globular domain that contains two Ca^{2+}-binding sites, and these regions are joined by a flexible linker that allows conformational changes following the binding of Ca^{2+}.[68] CaM directly interacts with and regulates RyR2, LTCC, and Nav1.5, the main cardiac sodium channel.[31,69-71] Furthermore, CaM is the Ca^{2+} sensor of the phosphatase calcineurin (CaN) and CaMKII. While both CaN and CaMKII regulate signaling pathways,[72] the latter also modulates several e–c coupling proteins by phosphorylation, including LTCC and RyR2, as previously described. Therefore CaM regulation of cardiac Ca^{2+} handling is at least two-fold: direct, by binding to specific targets, and indirect, through CaMKII.

In 2012, Nyegaard and associates[28] described two missense mutations, CaM-N54I and CaM-N98S, in heterozygous patients with ventricular arrhythmias induced by physical activity, syncope, and sudden cardiac death. Hence, CPVT due to CaM mutations can be further classified as CPVT4, which, as CPVT1, has autosomal dominant inheritance. Interestingly, both mutations affected a single *CALM1* gene, suggesting at first glance either that the other five *CALM* alleles are silent or that a small fraction of affected CaM (as small as one-sixth) is enough to produce a harmful phenotype. Hence, the exact mechanism by which CaM mutations produce arrhythmia is not entirely clear, particularly because recent reports also identified CaM mutations in LQTS patients.[73,74] Among other genetic defects, Makita and colleagues[73] described two LQTS patients with different mutations that affect residue N98 of CaM (CaM-N98S and CaM-N98I). Both mutations were found in *CALM2*, as opposed to *CALM1* in the CPVT cases mentioned earlier. Furthermore, two additional mutations (CaM-D132E and CaM-Q136P) were discovered in patients with a complex phenotype evocative of both CPVT and LQTS: prolonged QT interval together with ventricular arrhythmia induced by physical activity.[73] Hence, CaM-N54I remains as the only mutation strongly related to CPVT.

To establish a mechanistic difference between CPVT and LQTS CaM mutations, Yin and associates studied their effects on sarcolemmal ionic currents.[75] They observed that while three LQTS mutations (CaM-D96V, CaM-D130G, and CaM-F142L) affect the Ca^{2+}-dependent inactivation of I_{CaL}, CaM-N54I does not. Hence, it is likely that defective inactivation of I_{CaL} leads to AP prolongation, which manifests as prolonged QT interval and increased susceptibility to arrhythmia. Søndergaard and colleagues,[76] on the other hand, tried to expand the SOICR mechanism previously discussed to CaM-CPVT mutations. Interestingly, both LQTS mutations and CaM-N54I lowered the SOICR activation and termination thresholds, hence promoting spontaneous Ca^{2+} release. These data suggest that in the case of CaM mutations, SOICR is not a relevant mechanism to define the phenotype produced by a particular amino acid substitution. One last report, however, suggests that in permeabilized myocytes, treatment with CaM-CPVT mutants increased the frequency of Ca^{2+} waves and Ca^{2+} sparks, while CaM-LQTS mutants did not.[77] Additionally, CaM-CPVT mutations increase the open probability of RyR2 channels reconstituted in lipid bilayers, while wild-type CaM produces the opposite effect.[77] Even in this apparently coherent scheme, no study yet has determined how a single mutated allele, among the six encoding for CaM, is able to produce cardiac arrhythmias. The results discussed earlier were obtained in model systems that overexpressed mutant CaM either in myocytes,[75,77] HEK293 cells,[76] or artificial environments of lipid bilayers,[77] hence bearing little resemblance to the human condition. Furthermore, CaM is at the interface of Ca^{2+} signals and cellular functions as it interacts with CaN and CaMKII, both of which are implicated in hypertrophy and HF,[72] with the latter also being involved in cardiac arrhythmia. Therefore the pathogenic mechanisms associated with altered CaM are evidently complex, and more detailed studies are needed to provide a definitive understanding of how CaM mutations affect normal cardiac function.

Inherited Structural Cardiomyopathy

Structural cardiomyopathies are a complex and heterogeneous group of heart diseases that involve the mechanical dysfunction of the heart, often with genetic etiology and involve ventricular hypertrophy or dilation.[78,79] Among them, hypertrophic cardiomyopathy (HCM) is the most common congenital cardiac disease, affecting 1 in every 500 individuals.[18,80] HCM is considered a sarcomeric disease because the vast majority of patients with a positive genetic diagnosis carry a mutation in the genes that encode myosin-binding protein C (*MYPBC2*), β-myosin heavy chain (*MYH7*), or other components of the myofilaments.[81] Nevertheless, approximately half of the patients who undergo genetic testing are negative for mutations in the HCM panel, which screens ~15 associated genes.[81] These are considered idiopathic cases; however, new mutations in several other genes have been recently identified, including in those encoding for Ca^{2+}-handling proteins such as PLB, CASQ2, junctophilin 2, sorcin, and RyR2.[82] It is noteworthy that at least two of these proteins are also involved in CPVT, an entirely electrical disorder.

The first direct evidence that suggested that RyR2 mutations can lead to structural cardiomyopathy came from recent studies of the Meissner laboratory, where they characterized a mouse model that expresses a mutant RyR2 (RyR2-W3587A/L3591D/F3603A) with impaired regulation by CaM.[83-85] Interestingly, mice homozygous for the mutation developed severe hypertrophy and died within 2 weeks of birth, a phenomenon likely associated with increased Erk/p90RSK but not with CaM-CaN-NFAT and CaM-CaMKII-HDAC signaling.[84] The observation that a mutation in RyR2 is enough to induce severe hypertrophy, although it was not a clinically relevant mutation, strongly supported the potential pathogenic role of RyR2-linked cardiomyopathy. To date, three types of cardiomyopathy have been associated with RyR2 mutations in the clinical setting: HCM (RyR2-T1107M),[86] left ventricle noncompaction (LVNC) (in-frame deletion of exon 3),[87-89] and arrhythmogenic right ventricular cardiomyopathy (ARVC) (several mutations).[90,91]

In an effort to determine the pathogenic mechanisms associated with these mutations, Tang and associates[50] measured the activation and termination threshold of SOICR in a heterologous expression system. All CPVT, LVNC, and ARVC mutations studied increased both the activation and termination thresholds of SOICR. Notoriously, RyR2-A1107M, the mouse analog of RyR2-T1107M, behaved differently to all other mutations, showing normal activation but decreased termination threshold, hence being classified as a loss-of-function. Lau and Van Petegem[92] mapped RyR2-A1107 to SPRY2, a small but structurally complex domain. SPRY2 is one of the peripheral domains of RyR2 not considered a hotspot for CPVT mutations (see Fig. 53.2, discussed earlier); however, it might be relevant for intersubunit interactions as it spans the gap between HA and HD2 of two adjacent protomers.[32] Crystallographic data of the isolated SPRY2 further suggest that position 1107 can easily accommodate an alanine or a threonine, while the

bulkier side chain of methionine produces a shift in the amino acid backbone, affecting the interactions of neighboring amino acids.[92] Remarkably, RyR2-T1107M has also been identified in CPVT patients.[36] Together with the crystallographic and functional data previously discussed, this strengthens the pathogenic role of RyR2-T1107M but weakens its role in structural cardiomyopathy.

The in-frame deletion of exon 3, associated with LVNC, showed similar SOICR properties to other CPVT and ARVC mutations studied by Tang and colleagues.[50] Nevertheless, the same group created a mouse with a comparable genetic deletion to characterize the in vivo phenotype.[93] The homozygous mutation was embryonic lethal, but heterozygous mice survived with no evident changes in cardiac structure and normal susceptibility to stress-induced arrhythmia. Remarkably, these mice had decreased cardiac expression of RyR2, similar to the previously characterized RyR2 knockout mice.[94] Because there have been no reports that quantify RyR2 expression in patients who harbor a *RYR2* allele with exon 3 deletion, it is difficult to assess whether the clinical phenotype is associated with decreased RyR2 expression or with the presence of the mutant protein product. Efforts are being made by other groups to determine whether a decrease in RyR2 expression affects cardiac function in an animal model closer to human.[95]

Finally, ARVC is an autosomal dominant congenital cardiomyopathy characterized by progressive fibrofatty replacement of the myocardium that can lead to ventricular arrhythmias and HF. ARVC is more often caused by mutations in genes that encode components of the cardiac desmosome, including plakophilin-2 (*PKP2*) and plakoglobin (*JUP*), but up to 40%–50% of patients do not harbor mutations in the five main desmosomal ARVC genes.[96] Rampazzo and associates[97] first mapped a mutation in a family with the autosomal dominant form of ARVC to chromosome 1q42-q43, and then Tiso and colleagues[90] identified *RYR2* as the gene that harbors the disease-causing mutation (termed ARVC2). Interestingly, the clinical presentation of ARVC2 in these patients resembled CPVT in that arrhythmias could be elicited by exercise, had high penetrance, and equally affected males and females,[90] which are characteristics that do not appear in the typical presentation of ARVC. A clear association between *RYR2* mutations and ARVC remains therefore unproven, but a recent study that analyzed 64 "typical" ARVC patients without desmosomal mutations found six rare missense *RYR2* variants, yielding 9% incidence of rare *RYR2* variants among probands (6/64), clearly higher than those observed in the control population.[98] Thus although the causal association between *RYR2* variants and ARVC was not direct, the study reopened the possibility that RyR2 mutations lead to structural alterations characteristic of ARVC, namely right ventricular dilation, fibrofatty infiltration, and monomorphic VT at rest. Moreover, pertinent to this discussion is the observation that mutations in *PLB*, the gene encoding for the SERCA2a inhibitor PLB, have been linked to classical ARVC.[99] This finding supports the notion that dysfunction of Ca^{2+} regulatory proteins, in addition to desmosomal proteins, may lead to ARVC.

While important steps have been taken to establish a definitive link between mutations in Ca^{2+}-handling proteins and structural cardiomyopathy, all efforts are overshadowed by reports that associate specific variants with both arrhythmogenic disorders and structural cardiomyopathy.[36,91] Hence, the mechanism(s) by which a given mutation in RYR2, PLB, or any other Ca^{2+}-handling gene trigger pathological remodeling instead of a purely arrhythmogenic syndrome (CPVT) remain unknown. It is evident, however, that RyR2 mutations, at least, can produce a wide spectrum of cardiac alterations; yet, the underlying mechanisms that determine the phenotype will remain unknown until novel mutations identified only in patients with structural cardiomyopathy are fully characterized. The most straightforward link between Ca^{2+} dysregulation and structural cardiomyopathy involves activation of the CaM-CaN-NFAT and CaM-CaMKII-HDAC signaling pathways because both are Ca^{2+}-dependent and have been shown to be relevant in hypertrophy and HF.[72] Nevertheless, the apparent disconnection between these pathways and the hypertrophic phenotype of the RyR2-W3587A/L3591D/F3603A mouse discussed earlier foresees a more complex panorama.

Conclusions and Perspectives

Ca^{2+} signaling is pivotal for the control of contractility, AP, gene transcription, mitochondrial activity, and several other important functions of cardiac cells. Today, the role of intracellular Ca^{2+} dysregulation as a trigger of cardiac arrhythmias has been firmly established and is unquestionable. CPVT, caused by mutations in RyR2 and/or their accessory proteins, is the most salient example of intracellular Ca^{2+} signaling gone awry and causing lethal arrhythmias, but as our understanding of the intimate and bidirectional connection between intracellular Ca^{2+}

and membrane potential increases, Ca^{2+}-dependent arrhythmias step ever more firmly beyond CPVT and into the territories of atrial fibrillation, LQTS, and other arrhythmogenic syndromes that will require ample discussion in future editions of this chapter.

Although Ca^{2+}-dependent arrhythmias are known to exacerbate the malignancy of structural diseases, such as HCM and HF, no study has yet established a *direct* causal relationship between intracellular Ca^{2+} dysregulation and pathological structural remodeling. A small number of mutations in genes that encode Ca^{2+} transport proteins have been linked to structural diseases, most notably ARVC and HCM, but the idea that they *directly* cause such diseases remains tantalizing at best. Furthermore, no animal model generated to date harboring such mutations recapitulates the cardinal signs of any structural cardiomyopathy syndrome. Still, it has become increasingly evident that intracellular Ca^{2+} dysregulation may lead to a *spectrum* of cardiac diseases, and the notion that this spectrum is confined to purely arrhythmogenic syndromes is rapidly becoming too narrow. An expanding role for Ca^{2+} disturbances in pathological remodeling may lie ahead, but more studies are needed to ascertain such a role.

REFERENCES

1. Moore B. In memory of Sidney Ringer [1835-1910]: some account of the fundamental discoveries of the great pioneer of the bio-chemistry of crystallo-colloids in living cells. *Biochem J.* 1911;5. i b3-xix.
2. Bers DM. Cardiac excitation-contraction coupling. *Nature.* 2002;415:198–205.
3. Bers DM, *Excitation-Contraction Coupling and Cardiac Contractile Force.* Dordrecht. The Netherlands: Kluwer Academic Publishers; 2001:1–427.
4. Fabiato A, Fabiato F. Calcium release from the sarcoplasmic reticulum. *Circ Res.* 1977;40:119–129.
5. Cheng H, Lederer WJ. Calcium sparks. *Physiol Rev.* 2008;88:1491–1545.
6. Bers DM. Cardiac sarcoplasmic reticulum calcium leak: basis and roles in cardiac dysfunction. *Annu Rev Physiol.* 2014;76:107–127.
7. Lakatta EG, DiFrancesco D. What keeps us ticking: a funny current, a calcium clock, or both? *J Mol Cell Cardiol.* 2009;47:157–170.
8. Benkusky NA, Weber CS, Scherman JA, et al. Intact beta-adrenergic response and unmodified progression toward heart failure in mice with genetic ablation of a major protein kinase A phosphorylation site in the cardiac ryanodine receptor. *Circ Res.* 2007;101:819–829.
9. Houser SR. Role of RyR2 phosphorylation in heart failure and arrhythmias: protein kinase A-mediated hyperphosphorylation of the ryanodine receptor at serine 2808 does not alter cardiac contractility or cause heart failure and arrhythmias. *Circ Res.* 2014;114:1320–1327.
10. Pereira L, Cheng H, Lao DH, et al. Epac2 mediates cardiac beta1-adrenergic-dependent sarcoplasmic reticulum Ca2+ leak and arrhythmia. *Circulation.* 2013;127:913–922.
11. Grimm M, Brown JH. Beta-adrenergic receptor signaling in the heart: role of CaMKII. *J Mol Cell Cardiol.* 2010;48:322–330.
12. Anderson ME, Brown JH, Bers DM. CaMKII in myocardial hypertrophy and heart failure. *J Mol Cell Cardiol.* 2011;51:468–473.
13. Valdivia HH. Ryanodine receptor phosphorylation and heart failure: phasing out S2808 and "criminalizing" S2814. *Circ Res.* 2012;110:1398–1402.
14. Bers DM. Ryanodine receptor S2808 phosphorylation in heart failure: smoking gun or red herring. *Circ Res.* 2012;110:796–799.
15. Priori SG, Chen SR. Inherited dysfunction of sarcoplasmic reticulum Ca2+ handling and arrhythmogenesis. *Circ Res.* 2011;108:871–883.
16. Leenhardt A, Denjoy I, Guicheney P. Catecholaminergic polymorphic ventricular tachycardia. *Circ Arrhythm Electrophysiol.* 2012;5:1044–1052.
17. Leenhardt A, Lucet V, Denjoy I, et al. Catecholaminergic polymorphic ventricular tachycardia in children. A 7-year follow-up of 21 patients. *Circulation.* 1995;91:1512–1519.
18. Mozaffarian D, Benjamin EJ, Go AS, et al. Heart disease and stroke statistics–2015 update: a report from the American Heart Association. *Circulation.* 2015;131:e29–322.

19. Priori SG, Napolitano C, Memmi M, et al. Clinical and molecular characterization of patients with catecholaminergic polymorphic ventricular tachycardia. *Circulation.* 2002;106:69–74.
20. van der Werf C, Wilde AAM. VTs in catecholaminergic cardiomyopathy (catecholaminergic polymorphic ventricular tachycardia). In: Zipes DP, Jalife J, eds. *Cardiac Electrophysiology: from Cell to Bedside.* 6th ed. Philadelphia: Saunders; 2014:895–902.
21. Priori SG, Wilde AA, Horie M, et al. HRS/EHRA/APHRS expert consensus statement on the diagnosis and management of patients with inherited primary arrhythmia syndromes: document endorsed by HRS, EHRA, and APHRS in May 2013 and by ACCF, AHA, PACES, and AEPC in June 2013. *Heart Rhythm.* 2013;(10):1932–1963.
22. Swan H, Piippo K, Viitasalo M, et al. Arrhythmic disorder mapped to chromosome 1q42-q43 causes malignant polymorphic ventricular tachycardia in structurally normal hearts. *J Am Coll Cardiol.* 1999;34:2035–2042.
23. Priori SG, Napolitano C, Tiso N, et al. Mutations in the cardiac ryanodine receptor gene (hRyR2) underlie catecholaminergic polymorphic ventricular tachycardia. *Circulation.* 2001;103:196–200.
24. Cerrone M, Colombi B, Santoro M, et al. Bidirectional ventricular tachycardia and fibrillation elicited in a knock-in mouse model carrier of a mutation in the cardiac ryanodine receptor. *Circ Res.* 2005;96:e77–e82.
25. Lahat H, Pras E, Olender T, et al. A missense mutation in a highly conserved region of CASQ2 is associated with autosomal recessive catecholamine-induced polymorphic ventricular tachycardia in Bedouin families from Israel. *Am J Hum Genet.* 2001;69:1378–1384.
26. Roux-Buisson N, Cacheux M, Fourest-Lieuvin A, et al. Absence of triadin, a protein of the calcium release complex, is responsible for cardiac arrhythmia with sudden death in humans. *Hum Mol Genet.* 2012;21:2759–2767.
27. Rooryck C, Kyndt F, Bozon D, et al. New family with catecholaminergic polymorphic ventricular tachycardia linked to the triadin gene. *J Cardiovasc Electrophysiol.* 2015;26:1146–1150.
28. Nyegaard M, Overgaard MT, Sondergaard MT, et al. Mutations in calmodulin cause ventricular tachycardia and sudden cardiac death. *Am J Hum Genet.* 2012;91:703–712.
29. Valdivia HH. Structural and molecular basis of sarcoplasmic reticulum ion channel function. In: Zipes DP, Jalife J, eds. *Cardiac Electrophysiology: from Cell to Bedside.* 6th ed. Philadelphia: Saunders; 2014:55–69.
30. Herron TJ, Milstein ML, Anumonwo J, et al. Purkinje cell calcium dysregulation is the cellular mechanism that underlies catecholaminergic polymorphic ventricular tachycardia. *Heart Rhythm.* 2010;7:1122–1128.
31. Capes EM, Loaiza R, Valdivia HH. Ryanodine receptors. *Skelet Muscle.* 2011;1:18.
32. Yan Z, Bai XC, Yan C, et al. Structure of the rabbit ryanodine receptor RyR1 at near-atomic resolution. *Nature.* 2015;517:50–55.

33. Zalk R, Clarke OB, des Georges A, et al. Structure of a mammalian ryanodine receptor. *Nature.* 2015;517:44–49.
34. Efremov RG, Leitner A, Aebersold R, et al. Architecture and conformational switch mechanism of the ryanodine receptor. *Nature.* 2015;517:39–43.
35. Peng W, Shen H, Wu J, et al. Structural basis for the gating mechanism of the type 2 ryanodine receptor RyR2. *Science.* 2016 Sep 22. [Epub ahead of print].
36. Medeiros-Domingo A, Bhuiyan ZA, Tester DJ, et al. The RYR2-encoded ryanodine receptor/calcium release channel in patients diagnosed previously with either catecholaminergic polymorphic ventricular tachycardia or genotype negative, exercise-induced long QT syndrome: a comprehensive open reading frame mutational analysis. *J Am Coll Cardiol.* 2009;54:2065–2074.
37. Yamamoto T, Yano M, Xu X, et al. Identification of target domains of the cardiac ryanodine receptor to correct channel disorder in failing hearts. *Circulation.* 2008;117:762–772.
38. Wehrens XHT, Lehnart SE, Huang F, et al. FKBP12.6 deficiency and defective calcium release channel (ryanodine receptor) function linked to exercise-induced sudden cardiac death. *Cell.* 2003;113:829–840.
39. Lehnart SE, Mongillo M, Bellinger A, et al. Leaky Ca2+ release channel/ryanodine receptor 2 causes seizures and sudden cardiac death in mice. *J Clin Invest.* 2008;118:2230–2245.
40. Marx SO, Reiken S, Hisamatsu Y, et al. PKA phosphorylation dissociates FKBP12.6 from the calcium release channel (ryanodine receptor): defective regulation in failing hearts. *Cell.* 2000;101:365–376.
41. Marks AR. Ryanodine receptors, FKBP12, and heart failure. *Front Biosci.* 2002;7:d970–977.
42. Wehrens XH, Lehnart SE, Reiken SR, et al. Protection from cardiac arrhythmia through ryanodine receptor-stabilizing protein calstabin2. *Science.* 2004;304:292–296.
43. Wehrens XH, Lehnart SE, Reiken S, et al. Ryanodine receptor/calcium release channel PKA phosphorylation: a critical mediator of heart failure progression. *Proc Natl Acad Sci U S A.* 2006;103:511–518.
44. MacDonnell SM, Garcia-Rivas G, Scherman JA, et al. Adrenergic regulation of cardiac contractility does not involve phosphorylation of the cardiac ryanodine receptor at serine 2808. *Circ Res.* 2008;102:e65–e72.
45. Zhang H, Makarewich CA, Kubo H, et al. Hyperphosphorylation of the cardiac ryanodine receptor at serine 2808 is not involved in cardiac dysfunction after myocardial infarction. *Circ Res.* 2012;110:831–840.
46. MacLennan DH, Chen SR. Store overload-induced Ca2+ release as a triggering mechanism for CPVT and MH episodes caused by mutations in RYR and CASQ genes. *J Physiol.* 2009;587:3113–3115.
47. Jiang D, Wang R, Xiao B, et al. Enhanced store overload-induced Ca2+ release and channel sensitivity to luminal Ca2+ activation are common defects of RyR2 mutations linked to ventricular tachycardia and sudden death. *Circ Res.* 2005;97:1173–1181.

48. Masumiya H, Wang R, Zhang J, et al. Localization of the 12.6-kDa FK506-binding protein (FKBP12.6) binding site to the NH2-terminal domain of the cardiac Ca2+ release channel (ryanodine receptor). *J Biol Chem.* 2003;278:3786–3792.

49. Jiang D, Xiao B, Yang D, et al. RyR2 mutations linked to ventricular tachycardia and sudden death reduce the threshold for store-overload-induced Ca2+ release (SOICR). *Proc Natl Acad Sci U S A.* 2004;101:13062–13067.

50. Tang Y, Tian X, Wang R, et al. Abnormal termination of Ca2+ release is a common defect of RyR2 mutations associated with cardiomyopathies. *Circ Res.* 2012;110:968–977.

51. Chen W, Wang R, Chen B, et al. The ryanodine receptor store-sensing gate controls Ca2+ waves and Ca2+-triggered arrhythmias. *Nat Med.* 2014;20:184–192.

52. Tester DJ, Kopplin LJ, Creighton W, et al. Pathogenesis of unexplained drowning: new insights from a molecular autopsy. *Mayo Clin Proc.* 2005;80:596–600.

53. Loaiza R, Benkusky NA, Powers PP, et al. Heterogeneity of ryanodine receptor dysfunction in a mouse model of catecholaminergic polymorphic ventricular tachycardia. *Circ Res.* 2013;112:298–308.

54. Jiang D, Chen W, Wang R, et al. Loss of luminal Ca2+ activation in the cardiac ryanodine receptor is associated with ventricular fibrillation and sudden death. *Proc Natl Acad Sci U S A.* 2007;104:18309–18314.

55. Zhao YT, Valdivia CR, Gurrola GB, et al. Arrhythmogenesis in a catecholaminergic polymorphic ventricular tachycardia mutation that depresses ryanodine receptor function. *Proc Natl Acad Sci U S A.* 2015;112:E1669–E1677.

56. Faggioni M, Knollmann BC. Calsequestrin 2 and arrhythmias. *Am J Physiol Heart Circ Physiol.* 2012;302:H1250–H260.

57. Mitchell RD, Simmerman HK, Jones LR. Ca2+ binding effects on protein conformation and protein interactions of canine cardiac calsequestrin. *J Biol Chem.* 1988;263:1376–1381.

58. Gyorke I, Hester N, Jones LR, et al. The role of calsequestrin, triadin, and junctin in conferring cardiac ryanodine receptor responsiveness to luminal calcium. *Biophys J.* 2004;86:2121–2128.

59. Zhang J, Chen B, Zhong X, et al. The cardiac ryanodine receptor luminal Ca2+ sensor governs Ca2+ waves, ventricular tachyarrhythmias and cardiac hypertrophy in calsequestrin-null mice. *Biochem J.* 2014;461:99–106.

60. Lahat H, Eldar M, Levy-Nissenbaum E, et al. Autosomal recessive catecholamine- or exercise-induced polymorphic ventricular tachycardia: clinical features and assignment of the disease gene to chromosome 1p13-21. *Circulation.* 2001;103:2822–2827.

61. Ackerman MJ, Priori SG, Willems S, et al. HRS/EHRA expert consensus statement on the state of genetic testing for the channelopathies and cardiomyopathies: this document was developed as a partnership between the Heart Rhythm Society (HRS) and the European Heart Rhythm Association (EHRA). *Europace.* 2011;13:1077–1109.

62. Knollmann BC, Chopra N, Hlaing T, et al. Casq2 deletion causes sarcoplasmic reticulum volume increase, premature Ca2+ release, and catecholaminergic polymorphic ventricular tachycardia. *J Clin Invest.* 2006;116:2510–2520.

63. Terentyev D, Kubalova Z, Valle G, et al. Modulation of SR Ca release by luminal Ca and calsequestrin in cardiac myocytes: effects of CASQ2 mutations linked to sudden cardiac death. *Biophys J.* 2008;95:2037–2048.

64. Gyorke S. Molecular basis of catecholaminergic polymorphic ventricular tachycardia. *Heart Rhythm.* 2009;6:123–129.

65. Kobayashi YM, Alseikhan BA, Jones LR. Localization and characterization of the calsequestrin-binding domain of triadin 1. Evidence for a charged beta-strand in mediating the protein-protein interaction. *J Biol Chem.* 2000;275:17639–17646.

66. Chopra N, Yang T, Asghari P, et al. Ablation of triadin causes loss of cardiac Ca2+ release units, impaired excitation-contraction coupling, and cardiac arrhythmias. *Proc Natl Acad Sci U S A.* 2009;106:7636–7641.

67. Altmann HM, Tester DJ, Will ML, et al. Homozygous/compound heterozygous triadin mutations associated with autosomal-recessive long-QT syndrome and pediatric sudden cardiac arrest: elucidation of the triadin knockout syndrome. *Circulation.* 2015;131:2051–2060.

68. Babu YS, Sack JS, Greenhough TJ, et al. Three-dimensional structure of calmodulin. *Nature.* 1985;315:37–40.

69. Anderson ME. Calmodulin and the philosopher's stone: changing Ca2+ into arrhythmias. *J Cardiovasc Electrophysiol.* 2002;13:195–197.

70. Meissner G. Regulation of mammalian ryanodine receptors. *Front Biosci.* 2002;7:d2072–d2080.

71. Meissner G. Molecular regulation of cardiac ryanodine receptor ion channel. *Cell Calcium.* 2004;35:621–628.

72. Bers DM. Calcium cycling and signaling in cardiac myocytes. *Annu Rev Physiol.* 2008;70:23–49.

73. Makita N, Yagihara N, Crotti L, et al. Novel calmodulin mutations associated with congenital arrhythmia susceptibility. *Circ Cardiovasc Genet.* 2014;7:466–474.

74. Crotti L, Johnson CN, Graf E, et al. Calmodulin mutations associated with recurrent cardiac arrest in infants. *Circulation.* 2013;127:1009–1017.

75. Yin G, Hassan F, Haroun AR, et al. Arrhythmogenic calmodulin mutations disrupt intracellular cardiomyocyte Ca2+ regulation by distinct mechanisms. *J Am Heart Assoc.* 2014;3:e000996.

76. Sondergaard MT, Tian X, Liu Y, et al. Arrhythmogenic calmodulin mutations affect the activation and termination of cardiac ryanodine receptor-mediated Ca2+ release. *J Biol Chem.* 2015;290:26151–26162.

77. Hwang HS, Nitu FR, Yang Y, et al. Divergent regulation of ryanodine receptor 2 calcium release channels by arrhythmogenic human calmodulin missense mutants. *Circ Res.* 2014;114:1114–1124.

78. Maron BJ, Towbin JA, Thiene G, et al. Contemporary definitions and classification of the cardiomyopathies: an American Heart Association Scientific Statement from the Council on Clinical Cardiology, Heart Failure and Transplantation Committee; Quality of Care and Outcomes Research and Functional Genomics and Translational Biology Interdisciplinary Working Groups; and Council on Epidemiology and Prevention. *Circulation.* 2006;113:1807–1816.

79. Maron BJ. The 2006 American Heart Association classification of cardiomyopathies is the gold standard. *Circ Heart Fail.* 2008;1:72–75.

80. Ommen SR. Hypertrophic cardiomyopathy. *Curr Probl Cardiol.* 2011;36:409–453.

81. Maron BJ, Maron MS, Semsarian C. Genetics of hypertrophic cardiomyopathy after 20 years: clinical perspectives. *J Am Coll Cardiol.* 2012;60:705–715.

82. Landstrom AP, Ackerman MJ. Beyond the cardiac myofilament: hypertrophic cardiomyopathy-associated mutations in genes that encode calcium-handling proteins. *Curr Mol Med.* 2012;12:507–518.

83. Yamaguchi N, Chakraborty A, Huang TQ, et al. Cardiac hypertrophy associated with impaired regulation of cardiac ryanodine receptor by calmodulin and S100A1. *Am J Physiol Heart Circ Physiol.* 2013;305:H86–H94.

84. Yamaguchi N, Chakraborty A, Pasek DA, et al. Dysfunctional ryanodine receptor and cardiac hypertrophy: role of signaling molecules. *Am J Physiol Heart Circ Physiol.* 2011;300:H2187–H2195.

85. Yamaguchi N, Takahashi N, Xu L, et al. Early cardiac hypertrophy in mice with impaired calmodulin regulation of cardiac muscle Ca release channel. *J Clin Invest.* 2007;117:1344–1353.

86. Fujino N, Ino H, Hayashi K, et al. A novel missense mutation in cardiac ryanodine receptor gene as a possible cause of hypertrophic cardiomyopathy: evidence from familial analysis [Abstract]. *Circulation.* 2006;114. II_165.

87. Bhuiyan ZA, van den Berg MP, van Tintelen JP, et al. Expanding spectrum of human RYR2-related disease: new electrocardiographic, structural, and genetic features. *Circulation.* 2007;116:1569–1576.

88. Campbell MJ, Czosek RJ, Hinton RB, et al. Exon 3 deletion of ryanodine receptor causes left ventricular non-compaction, worsening catecholaminergic polymorphic ventricular tachycardia, and sudden cardiac arrest. *Am J Med Genet A.* 2015;167:2197–2200.

89. Ohno S, Omura M, Kawamura M, et al. Exon 3 deletion of RYR2 encoding cardiac ryanodine receptor is associated with left ventricular non-compaction. *Europace.* 2014;16:1646–1654.

90. Tiso N, Stephan DA, Nava A, et al. Identification of mutations in the cardiac ryanodine receptor gene in families affected with arrhythmogenic right ventricular cardiomyopathy type 2 (ARVD2). *Hum Mol Genet.* 2001;10:189–194.

91. d'Amati G, Bagattin A, Bauce B, et al. Juvenile sudden death in a family with polymorphic ventricular arrhythmias caused by a novel RyR2 gene mutation: evidence of specific morphological substrates. *Hum Pathol.* 2005;36:761–767.

92. Lau K, Van Petegem F. Crystal structures of wild type and disease mutant forms of the ryanodine receptor SPRY2 domain. *Nat Commun.* 2014;5:5397.

93. Liu Y, Wang R, Sun B, et al. Generation and characterization of a mouse model harboring the exon-3 deletion in the cardiac ryanodine receptor. *PLoS One.* 2014;9:e95615.

94. Takeshima H, Komazaki S, Hirose K, et al. Embryonic lethality and abnormal cardiac myocytes in mice lacking ryanodine receptor type 2. *EMBO J.* 1998;17:3309–3316.

95. Alvarado FJ, Hernandez JJ, Wang D, et al. Heterozygous knock-out of ryanodine receptor 2 in rabbits produces haploinsufficiency in the absence of compensatory remodeling of the heart [Abstract]. *Circulation.* 2014;130:A19448.

96. Fressart V, Duthoit G, Donal E, et al. Desmosomal gene analysis in arrhythmogenic right ventricular dysplasia/cardiomyopathy: spectrum of mutations and clinical impact in practice. *Europace.* 2010;12:861–868.

97. Rampazzo A, Nava A, Erne P, et al. A new locus for arrhythmogenic right ventricular cardiomyopathy (ARVD2) maps to chromosome 1q42-q43. *Hum Mol Genet.* 1995;4:2151–2154.

98. Roux-Buisson N, Gandjbakhch E, Donal E, et al. Prevalence and significance of rare RYR2 variants in arrhythmogenic right ventricular cardiomyopathy/dysplasia: results of a systematic screening. *Heart Rhythm.* 2014;11:1999–2009.

99. van der Zwaag PA, van Rijsingen IA, Asimaki A, et al. Phospholamban R14del mutation in patients diagnosed with dilated cardiomyopathy or arrhythmogenic right ventricular cardiomyopathy: evidence supporting the concept of arrhythmogenic cardiomyopathy. *Eur J Heart Fail.* 2012;14:1199–1207.

54 Pharmacological Bases of Antiarrhythmic Therapy

Juan Tamargo and Eva Delpón

Treatment of cardiac arrhythmias using antiarrhythmic drugs (AADs) has two main objectives: relieve symptoms and complications (improve quality of life) and reduce mortality directly related to the arrhythmia.[1] A basic principle in pharmacology is that the best treatment is targeted specifically to disease mechanisms. However, in many patients the ultimate underlying mechanisms of the arrhythmia remain incompletely understood. Thus the choice of a given AAD is empiric and based on the characteristics of the arrhythmia, the pharmacological properties of the AAD, and, above all, its safety profile. Moreover, depending on the underlying structural heart disease (i.e., coronary artery disease [CAD], heart failure [HF], left ventricular [LV] hypertrophy, or hypertension), triggers and arrhythmogenic substrates can vary among patients with the same arrhythmia. This variation could explain why AADs produce widely divergent effects, ranging from termination of the arrhythmia to inefficacy, to exacerbation of the treated arrhythmias, or to generation of entirely new ones (proarrhythmia), in different patients. Unfortunately, the risk of life-threatening proarrhythmia increases with chronic treatment and in patients with structural heart diseases who can benefit more from treatment.

Catheter ablation has emerged as an effective alternative therapy for patients with supraventricular (SVT) and ventricular tachycardias (VT), and the implantable cardioverter defibrillator (ICD) has become standard therapy for patients with life-threatening ventricular arrhythmias. Nevertheless, AAD therapy continues to play a key role in preventing recurrences or reducing their frequency in patients with relatively infrequent episodes of benign tachycardias, with recurrences following catheter ablation procedures, and/or with an ICD to decrease the frequency of shocks as an additional therapy to reduce the number of necessary shocks.

Until recently, arrhythmias were primarily considered to be a purely electrophysiological problem. AADs mainly target cardiac Na+, Ca2+, and K+ ion channels (Fig. 54.1). They bind to specific receptor sites within the channel, drug affinity being strongly modulated by the channel state in a time- and voltage-dependent manner. In addition, some AADs modulate the autonomic tone, primarily by antagonizing β1-adrenoceptors (β-blockers) or muscarinic receptors (atropine) or by stimulating adenosine A1 receptors (adenosine) (Table 54.1).

Conventional AADs are most commonly grouped according to the Vaughan-Williams classification into four different groups (see Table 54.1): Na+ channel-blocking drugs (class I), β-adrenoceptor blockers (class II), K+ channel blockers (class III) that prolong action potential (AP) duration (APD) and effective refractory period (ERP), and L-type Ca2+ channel (I_{CaL}) blockers (class IV). However, most AADs are "dirty drugs" that in a narrow range of concentrations can exert simultaneous, multiple direct effects on cardiac channels, receptors, and pumps and operate indirectly by altering hemodynamics, autonomic neural transmissions, or cardiac metabolism. Moreover, some old (adenosine, digoxin) and new AADs (ivabradine, ranolazine, and vernakalant) cannot be listed in any of the original four classes. Table 54.2 shows antiarrhythmic action of AADs on the basis of their respective targets, and Fig. 54.2 shows the main cellular targets for AADs.

Na+ Channel Blockers: Class I Antiarrhythmic Drugs

Na+ channel blockers bind and unbind in a strongly time- and voltage-dependent manner to a receptor site within the pore-forming subunit (Nav1.5) of the channel when channels are in the activated or inactivated state.[2] Na+ channel blockers also slow Na+ channel reactivation (transition from the inactivated to the resting state) upon repolarization, which prolongs refractoriness independently of changes in APD—that is, they increase the ERP/ APD ratio (postrepolarization refractoriness). Consequently, the effects of class I AADs would be expected to increase in the following conditions: (1) at faster rates of stimulation (use-dependent block) because Na+ channels spend more time in activated and inactivated states, and the diastolic time for recovery from drug-induced block is shortened, and (2) in depolarized cardiac tissues (voltage-dependent block) because membrane depolarization inactivates Na+ channels and slows recovery from block.

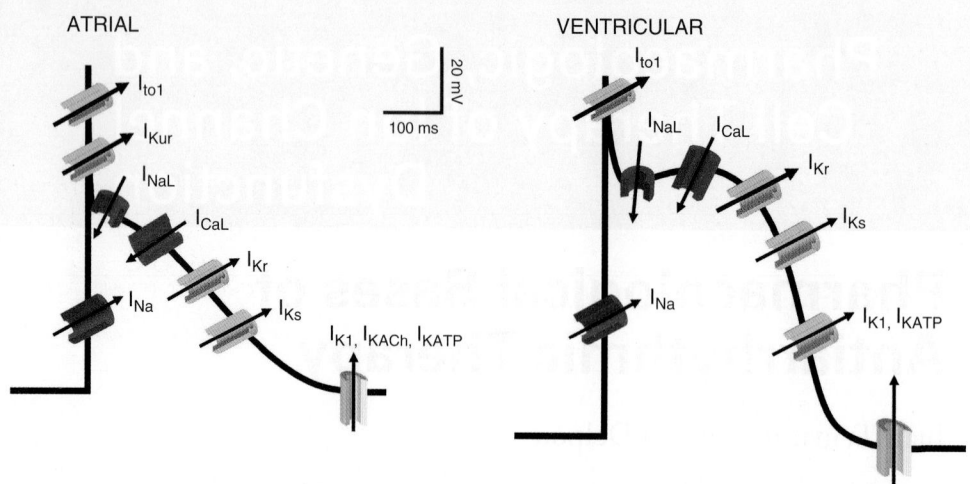

FIGURE 54.1 Ionic currents involved in shaping of human atrial (*left*) and ventricular (*right*) action potentials. The initial upstroke of the action potential is due to the activation of the peak inward Na+ current (I_{Na}). Repolarization is determined by the balance between inward-depolarizing L-type Ca2+ (I_{CaL}) and late Na+ (I_{NaL}) currents and outward-repolarizing K+ currents, including the rapidly activating and inactivating transient current (I_{to1}); ultra-rapid (I_{Kur}), rapid (I_{Kr}), and slow (I_{Ks}) components of the delayed rectifier; the inward rectifier current (I_{K1}); and the ligand-gated currents activated by a decrease in the intracellular concentration of adenosine triphosphate (I_{KATP}) or activated by acetylcholine (I_{KACh}) or adenosine (I_{KAdo}). Some currents are exclusive to the atria (I_{Kur}) or more important (I_{to1}, I_{KACh}) in the atria than in the ventricles and vice versa (I_{Kr}). *Arrows* indicate the ion movement direction.

TABLE 54.1 Antiarrhythmic drug classes

CLASS	MAIN MECHANISM OF ACTION	SUBCLASS	OTHER ACTIONS AND EFFECTS	DRUGS
I	Block Na+ channels Decrease excitability and slow CV Prolong ERP (postrepolarization refractoriness)	IA. Intermediate-offset kinetics (τ_{re} 1–3 s)	Block K+ channels Prolong APD ↑ QRS and QT	Disopyramide, procainamide, quinidine
		IB. Fast-offset kinetics (τ_{re} 300–500 ms)	Shorten APD	Lidocaine, mexiletine
		IC. Slow-offset kinetics (τ_{re} > 5 s)	Markedly slow conduction No effects on ventricular APD ↑ RR, PR, and QRS[a]	Ajmaline, flecainide, propafenone
		Fast atrial selective	Blocks I_{NaL} and K+ channels (I_{Kur}, I_{KACh}) Antianginal drug	Ranolazine
			Blocks K+ channels (I_{Kur}, I_{to1}, I_{Kr}, and I_{KACh})	Vernakalant
II	β-Adrenoceptor antagonists		Reduce sinus rate and AV conduction ↑ RR and PR	Atenolol, carvedilol, metoprolol, propranolol (and others)
III	Pure I_{Kr} inhibitor		Prolong atrial and ventricular APD/ERP	Dofetilide
	I_{Kr} inhibitor, I_{NaL} agonist			Ibutilide
	I_{Kr} inhibitor and β-blocker		↑ QT	D-sotalol
	Block Na+, Ca2+, and several K+ channels and α-/β-adrenoceptors		↑ RR, PR, QRS, and QT	Amiodarone, dronedarone
IV	Block L-type Ca2+ channels		↑ RR and PR	Verapamil, diltiazem
Other	Block I_{KAdo}, inhibit cAMP-induced I_{CaL}		↑ RR and PR	Adenosine
	Block Na+/K+ ATPase, ↑ vagal activity		↑ RR and PR	Digoxin
	Specific I_f inhibitor		↑ RR	Ivabradine

[a]RR and PR intervals of the electrocardiogram

APD, Action potential duration; *cAMP*, cyclic adenosine monophosphate; *CV*, conduction velocity; *ERP*, effective refractory period; ↑, increase.

TABLE 54.2 Drug selection based on the mechanisms underlying cardiac arrhythmias

ARRHYTHMIA MECHANISM	TARGET OR ACTION	DRUGS
Enhanced automaticity	I_f	I_f blockers: adenosine, β-blockers, ivabradine
	I_{CaL}	β-Blockers, diltiazem, verapamil
	I_{NCX}	I_{NCX} blockers, amiodarone, dronedarone
	I_{Na}	Class IA and IC drugs
Abnormal automaticity	I_{CaL}	β-Blockers, diltiazem, verapamil
Early afterdepolarizations	I_{CaL}	β-Blockers, I_{CaL} blockers
	I_{NaL}	I_{NaL} blockers: amiodarone, flecainide, ranolazine
	I_{NCX}	I_{NCX} blockers
	Shorten the APD	I_{Kr}, I_{Ks}, and I_{KATP} (nicorandil) agonists
	I_{Na}	Class IA and IC
	Bradycardia-dependent EADs	Isoproterenol
Delayed afterdepolarizations	Na$^+$-dependent Ca^{2+} overload	I_{Na} (class I drugs) and I_{NaL} blockers
	Ca^{2+}-dependent Ca^{2+} overload	Verapamil, RyR2 stabilizers
	I_{NCX}	I_{NCX} blockers
	Increase threshold potential	Class I drugs
Reentry	Prolong APD, refractoriness	Class I and III drugs
	Improve conduction velocity	Gap junction enhancers: rotigaptide, PUFAs
		Reduce fibrosis
Atrial selective targets	I_{Kur}	I_{Kur} blockers: BMS-394136, XEN-D0103
	I_{KACh}	Disopyramide, NTC-801
	I_{KAChC}	Amiodarone, flecainide
	Atrial I_{Na}	Amiodarone, dronedarone, ranolazine, vernakalant
	I_{NaL}	Amiodarone, ranolazine
Paroxysmal supraventricular tachycardia		Adenosine, β-blockers, diltiazem, verapamil (class I and III AADs)
Abnormalities of Ca^{2+} handling	RyR2	β-Blockers, rycals, flecainide, propafenone, dantrolene, edavarone
	CaMKII	CaMKII inhibitors
Idiopathic VF	Outflow tract arrhythmia due to cAMP-mediated DADs	Adenosine, β-blockers, I_{CaL} blockers
		Verapamil, β-blockers, I_{CaL} blockers
	Left ventricular outflow tract due to His bundle reentry	
Remodeling-induced arrhythmias (upstream therapies)	Fibrosis	β-Blockers, RAAS inhibitors, PUFAs, statins
		TGF-β1 and CTGF inhibitors
	Inflammation	Corticosteroids, PUFAs, statins
	Oxidative stress	Carvedilol, PUFAs, RAAS inhibitors, statins
	Stretch	Stretch-activated channel blockers, PUFAs
Ischemia-induced arrhythmias	Antiischemic drugs	β-Blockers, diltiazem, ivabradine, ranolazine, statins, verapamil
	I_{KATP}	I_{KATP} blockers

AAD, Antiarrhythmic drug; *APD,* action potential duration; *CaMKII,* Ca^{2+}/calmodulin-dependent kinase II; *cAMP,* cyclic adenosine monophosphate; *CTGF,* connective tissue growth factor; *DAD,* delayed afterdepolarization; *EAD,* early afterdepolarization; *PUFA,* polyunsaturated fatty acid; *RAAS,* renin-angiotensin-aldosterone system; *TGF,* transforming growth factor; *VF,* ventricular fibrillation.

Clinical and experimental data suggest that block of atrial Na$^+$ channels can terminate atrial fibrillation (AF). Indeed, propafenone and flecainide are first-choice drugs for AF cardioversion but only in patients without structural heart disease.[3] Conversely, ventricular Na$^+$ channel block is associated with proarrhythmic effects. Class I AADs decrease excitability and slow ventricular conduction and can increase all-cause mortality; therefore they have no role (or are contraindicated) in the primary prevention of sudden cardiac death (SCD) due to the risk of life-threatening ventricular tachyarrhythmias (VT or ventricular fibrillation [VF]) in high-risk, postmyocardial infarction (post-MI) patients.[4,5] In secondary prevention, the use of class I AADs is limited because of their low efficacy and serious adverse effects, including proarrhythmia, multiorgan toxicity, reduced cardiac function, or worsening coexisting diseases, which may offset the therapeutic benefit.[5]

Atrial-Selective Na$^+$ Channel Blockers

Class I drugs are subdivided into drugs with intermediate (IA), fast (IB), and slow (IC) onset/offset kinetics of Na$^+$ channel block (see Table 54.1). Recently, it has been demonstrated experimentally that drugs with very fast offset kinetics of Na$^+$ channel block that in addition display a steep voltage dependence, such as vernakalant and ranolazine, could selectively target atrial versus ventricular Na$^+$ channels.[6,7] This targeting would allow them to exhibit a disease-specific component of atrial selectivity because of the high atrial rate in AF, which enhances the block of atrial over ventricular Na$^+$ channels. Indeed, it has been proposed that the faster the AAD's dissociation kinetics at hyperpolarized potentials, the more selective the atrial effect during AF and the fewer the ventricular proarrhythmic effects because the fast dissociation kinetics allow recovery from block at slower frequencies (e.g., those of the ventricles either at sinus rhythm [SR] or during AF). Moreover, atrial cells exhibit a slightly more depolarized resting membrane potential (RMP) and a more gradual phase 3 of the AP, which at rapid atrial rates results in a less negative take-off potential.[6,7] In addition, compared with ventricular myocytes, atrial cells exhibit a more negative potential for half-maximum inactivation of Na$^+$ channels. Because reactivation depends on the membrane potential, fewer Na$^+$ channels recover from the inactivated state during diastole in atria than in ventricles. Therefore Na$^+$ channel blockers that preferentially bind to the preopen (activated but not open) and open state of the channel and have a fast dissociation rate will exhibit atrial selectivity because steady-state drug binding and

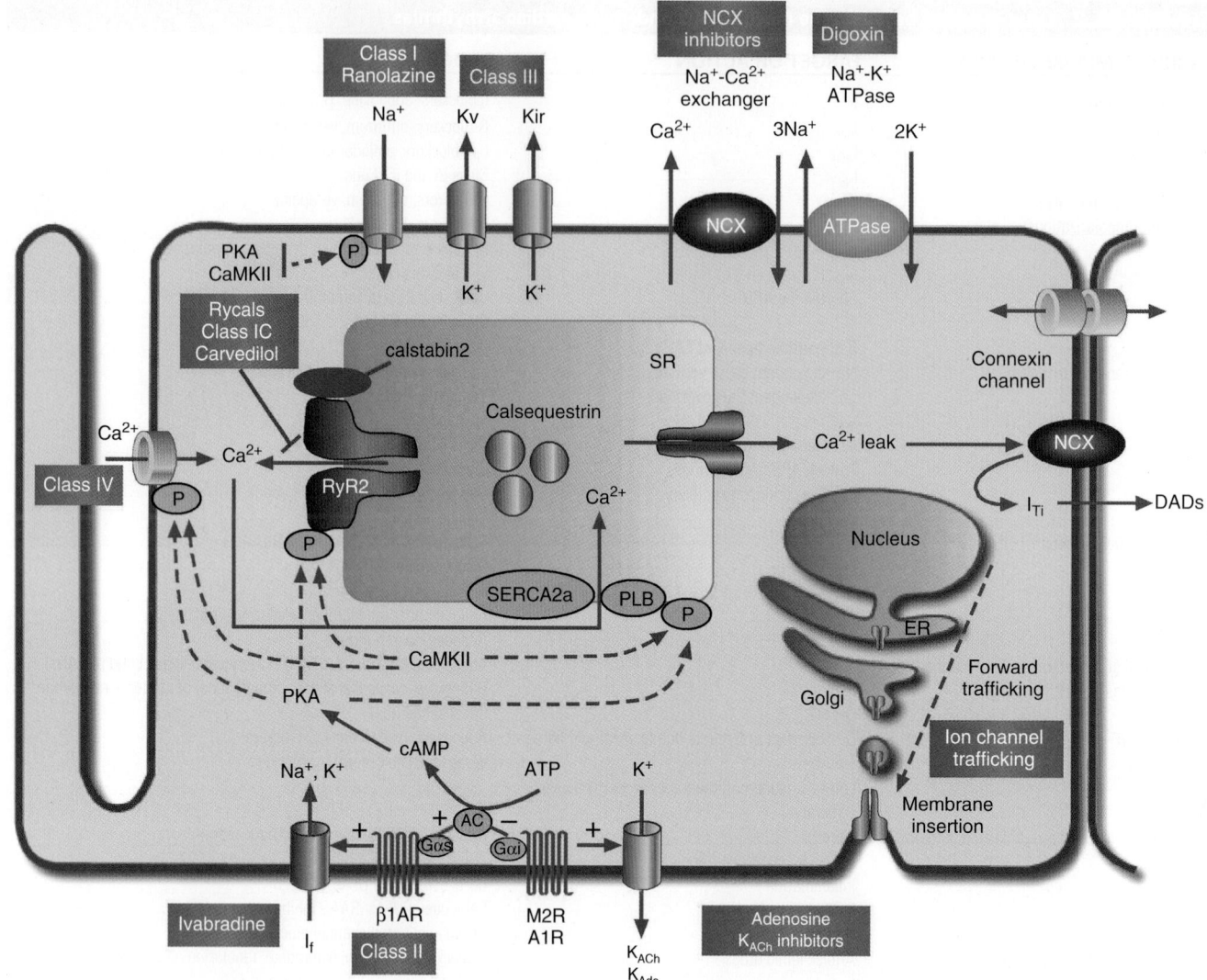

FIGURE 54.2 Cellular targets of antiarrhythmic drugs (AADs). Most available AADs modify the conductance of the Na⁺ (class I), Ca²⁺ (class IV), and K⁺ ion channels (class III) located in the sarcolemma, leading to a decrease or increase in a given ionic current, or they block β-adrenergic (class II), adenosine-A1, and muscarinic-M2 receptors. Some AADs inhibit abnormal persistent Na⁺ entry and diastolic Ca²⁺ release via the ryanodine receptor *RyR2*, with minimal effects on normal channel function. Furthermore, they can inhibit ion exchangers (Na⁺-Ca²⁺ [*NCX*]) or pumps (Na⁺-K⁺ adenosine triphosphatase [*ATPase*]), increase gap junction conductance, and correct ion channel expression within the membrane by modulating trafficking pathways. *A1R,* Adenosine A1 receptor; *AC,* adenylyl cyclase; *ATPase,* Na⁺-K⁺ ATPase; *β1AR,* β₁-adrenergic receptor; *CaMKII,* Ca²⁺/calmodulin kinase II; *CSQ,* calsequestrin; *DADs,* delayed afterdepolarizations; *ER,* endoplasmic reticulum; *Gs,* stimulatory G protein; *M2R,* muscarinic type-2 receptor; *PLB,* phospholamban; *PKA,* protein kinase A; *RyR2,* ryanodine receptor; *SERCA2a,* SR Ca²⁺-ATPase; *SR,* sarcoplasmic reticulum.

consequent channel block will be larger in atria than in ventricles.[7] However, the block of K⁺ channels, particularly those preferentially or exclusively present in the atria, also seems to be required to meet the "class I atrial-selective" profile.

Class IA and IC, like class III AADs, also block several K⁺ channels and prolong ventricular (quinidine) or atrial (propafenone and flecainide) APD depending on the type of K⁺ channel they preferentially block (discussed later). Furthermore, amiodarone, dronedarone, ranolazine, and vernakalant, which produce an atrial-selective I_{Na} block and in animal models suppress AF with minor ventricular effects, also inhibit the rapid component of the delayed rectifier K⁺ current (I_{Kr}) and other K⁺ currents prolonging atrial APD.[7,8] However, I_{Kr} contribution to the APD control is irrelevant at fast rates, which raises doubts whether I_{Kr} inhibitors actually prolong APD and refractoriness during AF episodes.

Late Na⁺ Current Inhibition

Na⁺ channels open for a few milliseconds after membrane depolarization, generating peak I_{Na}, and then most of them undergo fast inactivation. However, some Na⁺ channels either do not inactivate or inactivate but reopen during depolarization, generating the late Na⁺ current (I_{NaL}), which presents slow inactivation and recovery kinetics.[9] I_{NaL} increases under pathological conditions, including myocardial ischemia, LV hypertrophy, HF, AF, and some variants of the long QT syndrome (LQTS).[9-11] In the ventricular wall, M cells present a larger I_{NaL} than that presented by epicardial and endocardial cells, and an increase in I_{NaL} increases transmural dispersion of repolarization (TDR), facilitating reentry. During myocardial ischemia, enhanced I_{NaL} increases Na⁺ influx and, via the Na⁺/Ca²⁺ exchanger (NCX), produces a

Na^+-mediated Ca^{2+} overload that prolongs ventricular APD. APD prolongation enhances triggered activity that can occur during phases 2 or 3 of the AP (early afterdepolarizations [EADs]). Ca^{2+} overload leads to a spontaneous sarcoplasmic reticulum Ca^{2+} leak during diastole that generates a transient inward current (I_{TI}) via the NCX, which depolarizes the RMP and enhances triggered activity after the completion of AP repolarization (delayed afterdepolarizations [DADs]).[9,10]

Several AADs (flecainide, mexiletine, and ranolazine) present a higher selectivity for I_{NaL} than for peak I_{Na}.[9,10] Ranolazine is an antianginal drug that, besides its effects on peak I_{Na} at fast rates, blocks I_{NaL} and suppresses atrial and ventricular arrhythmias in a variety of conditions (e.g., ischemia, reperfusion, HF, AF, or type 3 LQTS).[10,11] During myocardial ischemia, ranolazine reduces intracellular Na^+ and Ca^{2+} overload and improves mechanical dysfunction, but it has no effect on I_{Na}, excitability, or conduction velocity.[10,11] In non–ST-elevation acute coronary syndromes, ranolazine reduces nonsustained VT and SVTs.[12] Small open-label studies suggest that ranolazine converts paroxysmal AF and prevents AF recurrences, but in a randomized trial it did not prolong time to AF recurrence.[13] However, in patients with paroxysmal AF, moderate-dose ranolazine plus reduced-dose dronedarone show synergistic AF burden reduction through atrial-selective depression of Na^+-dependent parameters.[14] Moreover, ranolazine prevents ventricular APD (QT) prolongation, reduces TDR, and suppresses EADs produced by I_{Kr} inhibitors and in patients with type 3 LQTS.[11]

Antiarrhythmic Effects of Class I Antiarrhythmic Drugs

Because of their mechanisms of action, class I AADs (I_{Na} and I_{NaL} inhibitors) are able to terminate arrhythmias generated by both focal ectopic activity and reentry. Class I AADs slow or suppress automatic activity in atrial and ventricular ectopic pacemaker cells that generate Na^+-dependent APs because they slow the spontaneous diastolic depolarization and shift the threshold voltage to less negative potentials. They can also suppress DADs by decreasing Na^+-dependent Ca_i^{2+} overload.

Describing the ultimate mechanisms responsible for the antiarrhythmic effects of class I AADs in reentry is a big challenge. Indeed, the underlying mechanism responsible for reentry itself is a matter of debate. Class I AADs markedly slow conduction and prolong refractoriness. The leading-circle theory of reentry predicts that because Na^+ channel blockers slow conduction, they should, if anything, favor reentry by decreasing the wavelength (product of ERP and conduction velocity), resulting in proarrhythmic effects. The proarrhythmia risk increases with drugs that produce marked conduction slowing in depolarized ischemic cardiac tissues. Experimental and clinical evidence, however, shows that class I AADs can terminate reentrant arrhythmias, such as AF, without increasing the wavelength. The most characteristic electrophysiological change that they produce before AF termination is a widening of the temporal excitable gap.[15] According to the multiple wavelets theory of the origin of AF, this widening will lower the chance that reentrant waves encounter areas of partially refractory tissue so that slowing of conduction and fractionation of wavelets will occur less frequently. This widening decreases the number of fibrillation waves by promoting their fusion, which increases the chance to terminate the arrhythmia.

However, there are clinical and experimental data demonstrating that reentry is maintained by the periodic activity of one or a small number of functional reentrant sources with a wavefront rotating around a central core ("rotor").[16] The waves emerging from the rotors undergo spatially distributed fragmentation and give rise to fibrillatory conduction. The size of the spiral wave is determined by tissue excitability and refractoriness so that the rotor will turn faster and in a more stable position, resulting in higher excitability and shorter refractoriness. In this context, Na^+ channel blockers terminate reentry as they (1) enlarge the center of rotation so that the rotor can no longer be accommodated by the substrate; (2) decrease anchoring to functional obstacles, increasing meander and extinction at boundaries; and (3) reduce the number of daughter waves that could provide new primary rotors.[16]

β-Blockers: Class II Antiarrhythmic Drugs

β-Blockers include a heterogeneous group of drugs that inhibit sympathetic responses mediated through the activation of β-adrenoceptors. Antiarrhythmic effects of β-blockers are the result of their electrophysiological effects (β-adrenoceptor stimulation modulates several ion currents, including hyperpolarization-activated inward current [I_f], I_{Na}, I_{CaL}, I_{K1}, I_{to1}, I_{Kr}, and I_{Ks}); inhibition of neurohumoral activation (and perhaps of sympathetic hyperinnervation and sprouting); and their antiischemic (reduce myocardial oxygen demands, increase subendocardial perfusion, and improve cardiac metabolism), antihypertensive, and antiproliferative effects.[17,18] Indeed, β-blockers exert a beneficial effect on LV remodeling in patients with MI or HF, and in the ischemic myocardium, they decrease dispersion of ventricular repolarization and increase the VF threshold.

Sympathetic hyperactivity is the predominant change in the autonomic tone preceding malignant ventricular arrhythmias and SCD, whereas reduced vagal activity is associated with increased mortality in HF.[4,19,20] β-Blockers are first-line therapy in the management of ventricular arrhythmias and prevention of SCD in different clinical conditions, including acute and chronic myocardial ischemia, congestive HF or LV dysfunction, and hypertrophic cardiomyopathy.[4,5] Thus most patients at risk of developing VT/VF should receive β-blockers because these drugs represent a rational, mechanism-based therapy for the treatment of arrhythmias. β-Blockers decrease the incidence of postoperative AF, which is explained by the role of an increased adrenergic tone in the genesis of this arrhythmia.[3] Moreover, heterogeneous atrial sympathetic hyperinnervation and increased $β_1$-receptor density occur in patients with chronic AF, particularly in the left atria.[21,22] This, in combination with the chronic AF–induced electrical remodeling, explains the further shortening of APD produced by $β_1$-adrenoceptor stimulation in APs recorded in human atrial myocytes.[22]

By inhibiting I_f and I_{CaL}, β-blockers decrease spontaneous activity of the sinoatrial node (SAN), inhibit the ectopic activity of the His–Purkinje system (Purkinje fibers are particularly prone to develop abnormal automaticity during increased sympathetic activation), and suppress abnormal automaticity generated in cardiac cells depolarized to potentials between –60 and –40 mV owing to the activation of I_{CaL}.[18] In the atrioventricular node (AVN), they decrease conduction velocity and prolong refractoriness, being the most effective drugs for ventricular rate control in AF and first-choice drugs in the treatment where the AVN forms a part of the reentrant circuit (AVN reentrant tachycardia [AVNRT] and AV reentrant tachycardia [AVRT]).[1,17] β-Blockers are widely used to treat inappropriate sinus tachycardia as well as exercise-induced and supraventricular and ventricular arrhythmias, where an increase in the sympathetic tone plays a role.[3,5,17] They are also effective in idiopathic right ventricular outflow tract VT and digitalis-induced arrhythmias as well as in controlling the proarrhythmia induced by class I AADs,[17] probably because of their bradycardic effect, which decreases the rate-dependent conduction slowing induced by Na^+ channel blockers.

β-Blockers decrease proarrhythmic actions secondary to the increase in the extracellular Ca^{2+} influx through I_{CaL}, sarcoplasmic reticulum Ca^{2+} release via the ryanodine receptor/Ca^{2+} release channel (RyR2), and intracellular Ca^{2+} overload.[17,18] Thus they suppress EADs and DADs and are the first-choice drugs in drug-induced torsades de pointes (TdP) and in patients with LQTS types 1 and 2 or catecholaminergic polymorphic VT (CPVT).[5,23,24] Surprisingly, even though there are marked pharmacological differences among β-blockers, there are few direct comparator data regarding their efficacy.

K⁺ Channel Blockers: Class III Antiarrhythmic Effects

These drugs prolong cardiac APD and refractoriness effects that, under theoretical bases, can suppress reentry. Some drugs (e.g., dofetilide) are considered pure class III AADs because they selectively block the channels that generate the I_{Kr} (named Kv11.1 or hERG), thus prolonging both atrial and ventricular APD and refractoriness in the absence of effects in conduction velocity.[25] Experimental data have demonstrated that at least at normal SR frequencies, selective I_{Kr} inhibition produces a greater prolongation of APD and refractoriness in atria versus ventricles. Unfortunately, at fast driving frequencies, the relative role of I_{Kr} in atrial and ventricular repolarization diminishes so much that I_{Kr} inhibition is not able to prolong APD during the arrhythmia episodes. This property, known as *reverse use-dependence*, limits the clinical efficacy of these drugs to stop rapid arrhythmias, particularly AF. Moreover, marked I_{Kr} inhibition produces excessive and inhomogeneous ventricular APD prolongation, results in TDR, and predisposes to EADs, which in turn can trigger TdP. Inhibition of I_{Kr}, and hence proarrhythmic risk, increases in the presence of bradycardia, hypokalemia, HF, or other I_{Kr}-inhibiting drugs. Indeed, many other drugs, including antihistamines, antipsychotics, antimicrobials, and diuretics, block Kr channels (https://www.crediblemeds.org), prolong the QT interval (drug-induced LQTS), and increase the incidence of TdP and SCD. It has been proposed that prolongation of APD produced by pure I_{Kr} inhibitors is characterized by a set of four disturbances of repolarization, including triangulation of the AP, reverse use-dependence, instability, and dispersion of APD whose magnitude would help predict drug-induced proarrhythmia risk.[26]

hERG channel blockers gain access through the intracellular side of the membrane to a binding site located within the central cavity of the channel. The inner vestibule of hERG channels is larger than that of other K^+ channels and presents two aromatic residues on each of the four subunits assembled to compose the conducting pore.[27] These topological characteristics explain the marked pharmacological promiscuity of hERG because they allow drugs with rather different chemical structures to establish interactions with the aromatic moieties by π electron stacking and block K^+ efflux through the pore. Finally, it is worth mentioning that besides the "pure Kr blockers" many AADs (see Table 54.1) also block hERG channels at therapeutic concentrations, an effect that could contribute to their antiarrhythmic properties, particularly at the atrial level. However, additional blockade of I_{to}/I_{Kur} restores the effects of I_{Kr} blockers, suggesting that a balanced combination of atrial blockade of Na^+ and K^+ channels (as shown by amiodarone) may be a more effective and safer therapeutic approach in AF.[28] Unfortunately, hERG blockade can also increase the ventricular proarrhythmic effects of such drugs (quinidine).

In healthy human atrial and ventricular myocytes driven at SR frequencies, I_{Ks} seems to be small, and its pharmacological inhibition does not alter APD.[29] Importantly, the role of I_{Ks} in determining APD rises in prominence at increasing beating frequencies or under β-adrenergic stimulation, which causes channel accumulation in closed states that preceded the open state. In addition, I_{Ks} helps terminate the AP when the repolarization reserve is compromised (i.e., I_{Kr} decrease) or inward currents are enhanced (i.e., β-adrenergic stimulation).[30] Chronic AF increases

I_{Ks} density by 100% in myocytes from both the right and left atria.[31] This increase, together with the 30% augmentation in the expression of $β_1$-adrenoceptors, accounts for the APD shortening produced by $β_1$-adrenoceptor stimulation in human atrial myocytes from chronic AF patients.[22]

Mathematical models suggest that this chronic AF–induced remodeling of I_{Ks} density contributes to the atrial APD and refractoriness shortening produced by the arrhythmia, which in turn further enhances reentry, thus favoring AF maintenance. Moreover, there are data indicating that stable fast reentry sources (rotors) occur with significantly higher rotation frequencies, lower conduction velocities, and shorter AP in cells with prominent I_{Ks}.[32] In addition, the frequency-dependent accumulation of I_{Ks} promotes postrepolarization refractoriness and fibrillatory conduction of waves emanating from rotors. Therefore it seems reasonable to propose that I_{Ks} could be an interesting target in the treatment of AF. In fact, some AADs, such as propafenone, quinidine, and amiodarone, inhibit I_{Ks}—an effect that probably contributes to their antiarrhythmic effects.[25] Unfortunately, selective inhibition of I_{Ks} would be difficult to achieve because molecular determinants for channel block are similar to those required for hERG blockade and would not be devoid of ventricular proarrhythmic effects. Indeed, patients carrying mutations in the *KCNQ1* or *KCNE1* genes, which encode the α (Kv7.1)- and β (minK)-subunits that form the channels, present with LQTS types 1 and 5, respectively. This finding suggests that excessive inhibition of I_{Ks} could also lead to a marked prolongation of ventricular APD, particularly under conditions of increased sympathetic tone that promote EADs and TdP.

I_{to1} (4-aminopyridine sensitive component of the transient outward current) determines the amplitude of the phase 1 of early repolarization and thus the height of the AP plateau, which in turn influences the activation of other currents involved in repolarization (mainly I_{CaL}, I_{Kr}, and I_{Ks}).[33] Variations in I_{to1} strongly influence the shape of cardiac AP, intracellular Ca^{2+} transients, and cardiac contractility. Relative I_{to1} density is much higher in atrial, Purkinje, epicardial, and midmyocardial cells than in endocardial cells. I_{to1} densities are also reported to be higher in right ventricular than in LV myocytes. Prominent I_{to1} leads to the "spike and dome" morphology, typical of epicardial (particularly right) and some atrial AP (I_{to1} is also differentially expressed among atrial cells). HF and chronic AF reduce I_{to1} density, with this effect being more marked in the left than in the right atrium. In regions of myocardium exhibiting a prominent I_{to1}, marked accentuation of the AP notch results in a transmural voltage gradient, leading to coved ST-segment elevation diagnostic of Brugada syndrome (BrS).[34] Because accentuation of the AP notch and loss of the dome could be secondary to either a decrease in inward currents (I_{Na} and I_{CaL}) or an increase in outward potassium currents (mainly I_{to1}), Na^+ channel blockers such as procainamide, propafenone, flecainide, ajmaline, and disopyramide can be used to induce or unmask ST-segment elevation in patients with concealed J wave syndromes (BrS and early repolarizing syndromes).[34] Conversely, quinidine, which is a potent I_{to1} inhibitor, reduces the magnitude of the J wave and, being an alternative to ICD in some patients with BrS, is effective in normalizing ST-segment elevation and/or preventing arrhythmic events.[34] In a long-term follow-up (>6 years) study of asymptomatic type 1 BrS patients with inducible VF, 77% of patients were no longer inducible when treated with hydroxyquinidine.[35]

I_{Kur} is carried by Kv1.5 channels; it is detected only in the human atria and not in the ventricles. Therefore I_{Kur} inhibitors would be expected to prolong atrial, but not ventricular, APD and refractoriness.[36] In myocytes from patients with SR, selective I_{Kur} inhibition shifts the plateau phase to more positive potentials at which the I_{Kr} is rapidly activated so that mid to late repolarization is accelerated and APD is slightly shortened.[36] This could explain why selective I_{Kur} inhibitors do not suppress, or even induce, AF in experimental models.[7,37] Indeed, *KCNA5* (the gene encoding Kv1.5) loss-of-function mutations can cause AF. Chronic AF reduces I_{CaL} and markedly shortens atrial APD; thus I_{Kur} blockers increase the plateau potential, over a range (below 0 mV) where the activation of I_{Kr} and I_{Ks} is less pronounced, and prolong atrial APD.[36] Furthermore, mathematical models predict that I_{Kur} or I_{to1} inhibition can induce rotor termination.[38] However, chronic AF also reduces I_{Kur}, particularly in the right atria; this decrease suppresses the endogenous right-to-left gradient of the current.[31] As a result, the relative contribution of I_{Kur} to repolarization in chronic AF can be small, decreasing the atrial sensitivity to I_{Kur} inhibitors. These findings raise serious doubts on the usefulness of "pure" I_{Kur} blockers, and in fact, none of those currently under development have been successfully launched for therapeutics.[37] Conversely, vernakalant, which causes a combined blockade of I_{Kur}, I_{to1}, I_{Kr}, and I_{KACh}, together with a Na+ channel block with slow-onset and very fast-offset kinetics, produces a high conversion rate to SR in patients with recent-onset AF.[39]

I_{K1} contributes to the final phase of repolarization and stabilizes the RMP of atrial and ventricular myocytes.[40] Increase in I_{K1} hyperpolarizes RMP, shortens APD, reduces spontaneous activity, and accelerates and stabilizes arrhythmia-maintaining rotors, playing a role in the genesis of AF and VF.[41] I_{K1} exhibits differential biophysical properties in atrial and ventricular tissues. Moreover, experimental data suggest that the Kir2.1 channel is the major isoform underlying ventricular I_{K1}, whereas the relative contribution of Kir2.2 and 2.3 to atrial I_{K1} seems to be greater. I_{K1} increases in left and right atrial myocytes of patients with chronic AF, an augmentation that is greater in the left than in the right atria in patients with paroxysmal AF. Left-to-right ventricular differences in I_{K1} have been postulated to represent a mechanism for the preferential stabilization of high-frequency rotors in the LV.[41] Moreover, patients carrying gain-of-function Kir2.1 mutations exhibit type 3 short QT syndrome that is characterized by a high incidence of VF and SCD. Furthermore, flecainide and propafenone at therapeutically relevant concentrations selectively increase I_{K1} generated by Kir2.1 homotetramers by binding to a common receptor, an effect that could contribute to their ventricular proarrhythmic effects. Recently, the pharmacophore (i.e., the minimal consensus chemical structure) of drugs that increase I_{K1} generated by Kir2.1 tetramers through binding to Cys311 has been identified.[42] Drug binding to this receptor located at the cytoplasmatic domain decreases channel affinity for polyamines and current rectification, and this can be a mechanism of drug-induced proarrhythmic effects not considered until now. Thus it seems that use of I_{K1} inhibitors could be an efficacious antifibrillatory strategy. Unfortunately, I_{K1} inhibition also results in proarrhythmia. In fact, patients carrying loss-of-function Kir2.1 mutations exhibit congenital LQTS type 7 (Andersen-Tawil syndrome) characterized by APD prolongation, diastolic depolarization, and increased propensity for EAD- and DAD-triggered arrhythmias.[43] Moreover, the development of Kir2.1-based antiarrhythmics is hampered because Kir2.1 channels are expressed in many excitable tissues, which could lead to organ toxicity. The selective blockade of Kir2.3 over Kir2.1 channels for the treatment of AF could be more promising. Kir2.3 channels are indeed preferentially inhibited by several drugs taking advantage of the low affinity of Kir2.3 channels for phosphatidylinositol 4,5-bisphosphate (PIP2), which critically determines the channel function. At high concentrations, propafenone preferentially blocks Kir2.3 over Kir2.2 and Kir2.1 channels by binding to a receptor located at the cytoplasmic domain determined by two arginine residues (R220 and R252).[44] Importantly, this receptor is not located at the pore of the channel, and it does not determine a reduction in the open channel probability but reduces the channel conductance by promoting the occurrence of subconducting states. However, a selective Kir2.3-blocker is not available yet.

Acetylcholine released from vagus nerve terminals activates I_{KACh}. Because I_{KACh} was thought to be exclusively present in the atria, it has been proposed as a target for the development of atrial-selective AADs. I_{KACh} activation slows SAN pacemaker activity; produces a heterogeneous APD and ERP shortening; hyperpolarizes RMP, increasing Na+ channel availability; and promotes EADs toward the end of phase 3 in the AP. These effects create a substrate for reentry, accelerate and stabilize high-frequency rotors, and contribute to the initiation and maintenance of AF.[16,41] Some AADs inhibit I_{KACh} via the blockade of muscarinic receptors (see Table 54.1) and may be useful in vagally mediated AF. Others inhibit I_{KACh} via GTP-binding proteins or the KACh channel itself (propafenone, dronedarone, or NTC-801), an effect that could contribute to their atrial antiarrhythmic properties. NTC-801 inhibits I_{KACh} with a selectivity >1000-fold over other cardiac currents and suppresses AF in several animal models without changes in ventricular APD or QT intervals.[45] However, Kir3.4 channels are also expressed in human ventricle, and their activation hyperpolarizes the RMP and shortens the ventricular APD even in the absence of M2-receptor signaling.[46] Furthermore, a loss-of-function mutation of Kir3.4 is associated with LQTS.[47] This evidence may limit the role of I_{KACh} as a potential target in AF. Furthermore, it has been demonstrated that chronic AF also decreases I_{KACh}, reducing its relative role in atrial repolarization while increasing an I_{KACh} component (I_{KAChC}) with constitutive activity (active in the absence of muscarinic ligands).[48] Ideally, an AAD should selectively inhibit I_{KAChC} (an atrial- and disease-specific therapeutic target) without affecting the I_{KACh} that modulates SAN and AVN and is present in many other tissues. I_{KAChC} is inhibited by flecainide and investigational AADs, but highly selective I_{KAChC} blockers are not currently available.

In up to 80% of cases, VT/VF occurs in the setting of CAD and HF.[4] Attempts to prevent arrhythmic events and SCD with class I and III AADs in the setting of myocardial ischemia have failed. Activation of adenosine triphosphate (ATP)–dependent inwardly rectifying K+ currents (I_{KATP}) during acute myocardial ischemia, as a consequence of the ATP level drop, results in shortening of the APD, accumulation of extracellular K+, membrane depolarization, and slow conduction velocity. These effects render the ischemic heart vulnerable to reentrant arrhythmias.[25] It has been hypothesized that specific I_{KATP} inhibitors, being truly ischemia-selective AADs, prolong ventricular refractoriness in ischemic tissues with little or no effect on normal tissue.[49,50] Conversely, the KATP opener nicorandil shortens the APD, reduces TDR, and suppresses EADs in patients with LQT1.[49,50]

Amiodarone and Dronedarone

Amiodarone is considered the paradigm of class III AADs because, in chronic treatment, it prolongs APD and refractoriness in all cardiac tissues, an effect that is attributable to the blockade of several K+ channels (I_{to1}, I_{Kur}, I_{Kr}, I_{Ks}, I_{K1}, and I_{KACh}). However, as mentioned before, amiodarone also inhibits peak I_{Na} (inhibits inactivated Na+ channels with fast kinetics [class I]), I_{NaL}, and I_{CaL} (class IV) and noncompetitively antagonizes α-/β-adrenergic receptors (class II).[1]

Amiodarone presents a low proarrhythmic risk and is effective against a wide spectrum of supraventricular and ventricular arrhythmias caused by focal activity or reentry. It is the most effective AAD for preventing recurrences of AF,[3] being the last-choice drug in patients with structural heart disease, and in the prophylaxis and treatment of life-threatening ventricular arrhythmias in patients with MI or congestive HF or after cardiac surgery, although it is being replaced by ICDs.[5] Amiodarone is an alternative in post-MI patients who are not eligible for, or who do not have access to, ICD therapy for the prevention of SCD and to inhibit unpleasant ICD shocks.[5,51] However, in patients with HF and an LV ejection fraction of 35% or less, amiodarone has no favorable effect on survival.[5,51]

Because amiodarone presents complex pharmacokinetics, a long half-life, multiple drug interactions, and a high incidence of organ toxicity, new amiodarone-like agents with a better pharmacological profile have been developed. Dronedarone is an amiodarone-like drug without the iodine moieties that exhibit class I, II, III, and IV effects and has a short half-life and less lipophilicity compared with amiodarone. It is approved for the maintenance of SR in patients with atrial flutter (AFl) and AF.[3] Dronedarone has a better safety profile but is less effective than amiodarone in maintaining SR, and unlike amiodarone, it is contraindicated in patients with HF.

Calcium Channel Blockers: Class IV Antiarrhythmic Drugs

Nondihydropyridine Ca^{2+}-channel blockers (e.g., diltiazem, verapamil) inhibit the I_{CaL} and exhibit antiischemic and antihypertensive properties. They stabilize the channel in its inactivated state and prolong its reactivation so that their effects increase at fast rates (use-dependent block) and at depolarized membrane potentials (voltage-dependent block).[1]

In cardiac tissues with RMPs positive to –60 mV (i.e., SAN, AVN, and ischemic tissues), I_{CaL} is responsible for AP depolarization (phase 0) and conduction velocity. Class IV AADs prolong the refractory period and slow conduction through the AVN. The rate-dependent effect of these drugs on the AVN is the basis of their use to terminate or prevent reentrant SVT whose circuit involves the AVN (AVNRT, AVRT), being an alternative to adenosine, and to control the ventricular rate in patients with AF or AFl. At therapeutic concentrations, diltiazem and verapamil decrease the heart rate slightly because their direct negative chronotropic effect is partly counteracted by their peripheral vasodilator effects that produce a sympathetic-mediated reflex response. However, in patients treated with β-blockers, reflex sympathetic stimulation is inhibited, and diltiazem and verapamil slow heart rate and AVN conduction.

Inhibition of I_{CaL} suppresses automaticity generated in depolarized ventricular cells (abnormal automatism) and EADs occurring at the plateau phase of AP because of I_{CaL} reactivation (as marked delay in repolarization allows Ca^{2+} channels to recover from inactivation). Thus class IV AADs and magnesium sulfate (an inorganic Ca^{2+} channel blocker) are effective for the treatment of EAD-triggered arrhythmias. Class IV AADs and AADs that block Ca^{2+} channels at therapeutic concentrations (e.g., amiodarone, β-blockers, dronedarone, or propafenone) suppress DADs by preventing Ca_i^{2+} overload.

Verapamil is a drug of choice in idiopathic LV fascicular VT and drug-induced TdP; it can be an alternative to β-blockers in CPVT and prevents VT related to ischemia.[23] However, class IV drugs have no effect on all-cause mortality in patients with prior MI and are contraindicated in congestive HF.[4,5]

Gap-Junction Coupling Enhancers

Connexins (Cx) are membrane proteins that assemble into hexameric hemichannels, also known as connexons. At the gap junctions, connexons allow electrical flow between cardiomyocytes and thus regulate intercellular coupling. Changes in Cx expression, location (lateralization), and function occur in many forms of heart disease (i.e., ischemia, hypertrophy, HF, or AF) and contribute to arrhythmogenesis as they slow conduction velocity, cause heterogeneities in repolarization, and modulate automaticity. Cx40 has a critical role in mediating atrial conduction, whereas Cx43 seems to be the major ventricular form. Cellular uncoupling owing to dephosphorylation and redistribution of Cx43, together with increased fibrosis[52] and decreased expression of Na^+ channels, is implicated in conduction slowing during ischemia, increasing the risk of fatal ventricular arrhythmias.

Rotigaptide increases gap junction conductance and prevents acute ischemic arrhythmias. However, it partially reverses the loss of Cx43 but does not restore normal conduction or prevent arrhythmias in the healing infarct border zone, such as after a prolonged period of gap junction remodeling.[53] Thus it seems that interventions that are effective in restoring cell-to-cell coupling under conditions of acute ischemia might not be effective in a substrate that has already undergone a prolonged period of gap junction remodeling. Gap junction–enhancing drugs can also reduce AF vulnerability in some models of AF (chronic mitral regurgitation and acute ischemia) but not in others (HF or atrial tachypacing).[53,54] These findings suggest that the role of Cx in AF is disease specific and that gap junction enhancers may be effective only when conduction slowing is due to alterations in gap junctions.

Stretch-Activated Channels

Chronic stretch causes membrane depolarization and heterogeneous conduction, prolongs refractoriness, and induces structural remodeling (dilatation, hypertrophy, and fibrosis), which contributes to both atrial and ventricular arrhythmias. These electrophysiological effects can be explained via the activation of either cation nonselective mechanosensitive transient receptor potential (including canonical [TRPC1,6], vanilloid [TRPV2,4], and melastatin [TRPM4] and Piezo1 channels) or K^+-selective (TREK-1 [$K_2P2.1$], large-conductance Ca^{2+}-activated K^+ [BKCa], and K_{ATP}) channels.[55] In experimental models, nonselective, stretch-activated channel blockers (gadolinium and the tarantula peptide GsMtx-4) suppress AF inducibility. Nowadays, modulation of stretch-activated channels as an antiarrhythmic strategy is limited by the lack of drugs.

Modulation of Ion Channel Trafficking

Structural heart diseases and many mutations associated with channelopathies affect biogenesis, forward trafficking to the surface membrane subdomains, and degradation of cardiac ion channels.[56] Recent evidence demonstrates that AADs inhibit ion conduction and modulate ion channel trafficking or surface density and that channel blockade and trafficking can be targeted independently.[56,57]

Defective trafficking of type 2 LQTS–associated mutant channels can be rescued to the plasma membrane by high- (terfenadine or dofetilide) or low-affinity (fexofenadine) Kv11.1 channel blockers that likely stabilize misfolded protein in the endoplasmic reticulum, although the drug effectiveness depends on the particular mutation present.[58,59] Furthermore, drugs that do not block hERG channel conductance can either decrease (pentamidine or probucol) or increase (fexofenadine) hERG surface density.[58]

Quinidine induces a stereospecific dose-, time-, and subunit-dependent internalization of Kv1.5, concomitant with the classical pore block.[56] The specific expression of Kv1.5 channels in human atria raises the possibility of designing drugs to modulate Kv1.5 channel trafficking.[56] Such drugs, in theory, can cause a rapid and reversible decrease in I_{Kur} and a prolongation of atrial APD, resulting in termination of AF, with minimal risk of ventricular proarrhythmia. However, we need a better understanding of trafficking mechanisms and how chronic decrease in channel expression contributes to arrhythmia-induced remodeling.

Some drugs such as pentamidine and flecainide decrease and increase Kir2.1 channel expression in the membrane, respectively. Flecainide is also able to promote trafficking of some Kir2.1 loss-of-function mutants, increasing the amplitude of the outward K^+ current generated by the channels, if any. This effect could contribute to the empirically observed antiarrhythmic actions produced by flecainide in some patients with Andersen-Tawil syndrome.[57]

Targeting Intracellular Calcium Handling

Abnormal intracellular Ca^{2+} handling can promote both atrial and ventricular arrhythmias; it also has a key role in cardiac electrical and structural remodeling in patients with AF, HF, LV hypertrophy, and CAD.[59-61] Indeed, in a transgenic mice model, RyR2-mediated Ca^{2+} leak, besides increasing atrial ectopy, directly promotes the development of atrial remodeling underlying the AF substrate.[62] Moreover, CPVT associated with mutations in *RyR2* and calsequestrin (*CASQ2*) genes destabilizes the RyR2 channel complex and increases spontaneous Ca^{2+} release, which under certain conditions (e.g., during exercise or β-adrenergic stimulation) facilitates the development of DADs and triggered arrhythmias.[23,60] Thus intracellular Ca^{2+}-handling proteins (Ca^{2+}-ATPase [SERCA2a], phospholamban, RyR2 and its accessory protein calstabin 2, NCX, and CSQ) provide targets for developing new AADs.

Dysregulation of RyR2, characterized by improper sarcoplasmic reticulum Ca^{2+} release and increased diastolic Ca^{2+} leak, is related to the following: (1) RyR2 hyperphosphorylation by protein kinase A (PKA) and Ca^{2+}/calmodulin-dependent kinase II (CaMKII), which transiently dissociates calstabin 2 from the RyR2 complex, increasing open channel probability; (2) increased sensitivity of RyR2 to activation by luminal Ca^{2+}; and (3) reactive oxygen species generated in the diseased heart, which make the channel leaky.[59-61] β-Adrenergic stimulation and activation of the renin-angiotensin-aldosterone system (RAAS) can promote triggered arrhythmias via PKA- and CaMKII-induced RyR2 hyperphosphorylation.[60,63] β-Blockers prevent PKA- and CaMKII-mediated hyperphosphorylation of RyR2, depletion of calstabin 2, and sarcoplasmic reticulum Ca^{2+} leak, being the only effective drugs for improving survival in CPVT.[23] β-Blockers and verapamil act synergistically to prevent stress-induced increase in the sarcoplasmic reticulum Ca^{2+} content by reducing heart rate, Ca^{2+} influx into the cell, and Ca^{2+} uptake into the sarcoplasmic reticulum.[23] However, in patients with CPVT, cardiac events remain considerable even with this combination; thus alternative therapies are needed.

Carvedilol, a nonselective β- and $α_1$-adrenergic antagonist, inhibits several cardiac currents (I_{Kur}, I_{Kr}, I_{CaL}, I_{to1}, and I_{Ks}) and exerts antioxidant and antiproliferative effects. It is the only β-blocker that suppresses sarcoplasmic reticulum Ca^{2+} release by directly reducing RyR2 mean open time, independently of its β- or $α_1$-antagonism or antioxidant activities, which likely contribute to its antiarrhythmic effects in HF patients.[23,60] Carvedilol analogues (VK-II-36) with minimal β-blocking activity retain the ability to suppress Ca^{2+} release and prevent CPVT without causing bradycardia.[64] Interestingly, the combination of these analogues with selective β-blockers (metoprolol or bisoprolol) is more effective compared with each agent alone for preventing CPVT.

Stabilizers of the calstabin 2–RyR2 complex (Rycals) represent a new antiarrhythmic approach. Rycals (JTV519, S44121/Arm036, and S107) increase the binding affinity of calstabin-2 for PKA-hyperphosphorylated RyR2; reduce the channel-opening probability; and prevent arrhythmogenic diastolic Ca^{2+} leak protecting against ventricular tachyarrhythmia, contractile dysfunction, and Ca^{2+} overload.[23,59-61] JTV519 prevents APD alternans and triggered ventricular arrhythmias and reduces Ca^{2+} waves in arrhythmogenic Purkinje fibers following MI. It also reduces ectopic activity and DADs in pulmonary vein cardiomyocytes, decreasing AF inducibility. However, JTV519 also blocks voltage-gated Na^+, I_{CaL}, and K^+ (I_{Kr}, I_{K1}, I_{Kr}, and I_{KAch}) channels, and its effects in patients with AF are uncertain.

Flecainide and propafenone block the open state of RyR2, inhibit arrhythmogenic diastolic Ca^{2+} waves, and suppress DADs and triggered arrhythmias in experimental models and in patients with CPVT.[23,47,65] In addition, their Na^+ channel–blocking properties prevent DADs from reaching threshold potential and triggering premature beats. Recent data suggest that the principal action of flecainide in CPVT is not via a direct interaction with RyR2, but rather via a Na^+-dependent modulation of intracellular Ca^{2+} handling that attenuates RyR2 dysfunction in CPVT.[66] Furthermore, β-blocking activity of propafenone can also contribute to its clinical efficacy in CPVT. Thus class IC AADs can be an alternative to β-blockers in some patients with CPVT.[23]

Some RyR2 mutations can lead to an abnormally tight domain–domain interaction that results in an erroneous activation of the channel and diastolic Ca^{2+} leak.[60] In experimental models, dantrolene stabilizes domain interactions within the RyR2 and prevents aberrant Ca^{2+} release and CPVT.[23] The antioxidant edaravone also ameliorates the defective interdomain interaction of the RyR2 and prevents Ca^{2+} leak and LV remodeling during the development of HF.[61]

β-Adrenergic stimulation, increases in Ca^{2+}_i, or oxidative stress enhances activity and expression of CaMKII. CaMKII, in turn, phosphorylates Na^+, Ca^{2+}, and K^+ channels (increases I_{NaL}, I_{CaL}, I_{to}, and I_{K1} and slows I_{Ca} inactivation) and Ca^{2+} handling proteins (RyR2A, phospholamban). Additionally, it increases APD variability and diastolic Ca^{2+} leak and predisposes to both EADs and DADs while depletion of sarcoplasmic reticulum Ca^{2+} impairs inotropy. Furthermore, CaMKII plays a key role in myocardial inflammation, remodeling, and apoptosis.[67] These findings suggest that CaMKII inhibition might be a potential therapeutic target for the management of cardiac arrhythmias. CaMKII inhibitors, however, might not represent a feasible target because the ubiquitous role of CaMKII in cellular physiology can result in deleterious off-target side effects.[61] Moreover, some CaMKII inhibitors (KN-93) cannot discriminate between CaMKII and CaMKIV and inhibit voltage-gated K^+ and Ca^{2+} channels. Therefore to achieve an effective and safe cardiac effect, drugs with tissue- and isoform-specific actions (CaMKIIδ) are probably required. An alternative strategy is small peptides like autocamtide-2–related inhibitory peptide (AIP) that inhibit CaMKII activation by blocking the binding of calmodulin to CaMKII.

In summary, although abnormal Ca^{2+} handling plays a major role in arrhythmogenesis, the developed drugs have no sufficient specificity, and further optimization of Ca^{2+}-handling targeting is needed. A major challenge is to develop drugs that inhibit diastolic sarcoplasmic reticulum Ca^{2+} leak without compromising systolic RyR2 opening and Ca^{2+} release.

Pharmacological Treatment of Inherited Cardiac Arrhythmia Syndromes

During the past decade, there was an explosion of information that linked mutations in genes encoding ion channel α- and accessory-subunits as well as cytoskeletal molecules to inherited cardiac arrhythmia syndromes, including short QT syndrome, LQTS, BrS, AF, idiopathic VF, and CPVT (Table 54.3).[24,43,47,49,58] Identification of disease-associated genes provides important information on the molecular mechanisms of cardiac arrhythmias and opens the possibility for antiarrhythmic therapies based on genotype and clinical presentation. However, randomized trials have not been conducted because of the rarity of these conditions. Thus use of AADs for inherited primary arrhythmias is an off-label indication.[24] Nevertheless, therapy alleviating the mutation consequences depends on the mutation class, although most AADs lack the desired selectivity for a given channel.

Target Cardiac Remodeling: Upstream Therapies

Upstream therapies to prevent or delay myocardial remodeling are an attractive approach in the prophylaxis and treatment of arrhythmias associated with HF, hypertension, or MI.[3,5,61,68,69]

TABLE 54.3   Pharmacological treatment for inherited arrhythmia syndromes

SYNDROME	GENETIC DISORDER	ALTERATION	SPECIFIC DRUG THERAPY
Long QT syndrome[a]	LQT1, LQT5, LQT11	↓ I_{Ks}	β-Blockers, K+ channel openers (nicorandil, L-364,373)
	LQT2/LQT6	↓ I_{Kr}	β-Blockers, K-sparing agents plus oral K+ supplements, K+ channel openers
	LQT3, LQTS9, LQT10, LQTS12	↑ I_{NaL}	• I_{NaL} inhibitors: flecainide, mexiletine[c], ranolazine
			• β-Blockers are less effective
			• Prevent bradycardia
	LQT7	↓ I_{K1}	β-Blockers, flecainide
	LQT8	↑ I_{CaL}	β-Blockers, ranolazine, verapamil
Short QT syndrome	SQTS1-6	• ↑ I_{Kr}, I_{Ks}, I_{K1}, I_{KATP}	• Hydroquinidine, quinidine
		• ↓ I_{Na}, I_{CaL}	• Blockers of affected K+ channels
CPVT	CPVT1, CPVT2	↑ SR Ca^{2+} leak	• β-Blockers (without ISA) ± verapamil
			• Flecainide plus β-blockers, propafenone
			• RyR2 stabilizers (rycals)[d], dantrolene[d]
J wave syndromes	Brugada syndrome[b]	• ↓ I_{Na}, ↓ I_{CaL}	• I_{to} blockers: hydroquinidine, quinidine
		• ↑ I_{to}, I_{KATP}	• Increase I_{CaL}: cilostazol, denopamine, isoproterenol
	Early repolarization syndromes	• ↑ I_{to}, I_{KAch}, I_{KATP}	• VT/VF storm: Isoproterenol
		• ↓ I_{Na}, I_{CaL}	
Idiopathic VT			• Quinidine, verapamil
			• VT/VF storm: Isoproterenol
Atrial fibrillation		• ↑ I_{Ks}, I_{Kr}, I_{Kur}, I_{to}, I_{K1}, I_{KATP}, I_{Na}	Blockers of affected K+ channels
		• ↓ I_{CaL}, ↓ Cx40	

[a]Avoid QT-prolonging drugs (www.crediblemeds.org).
[b]Avoid drugs that unmask or aggravate BrS (www.brugadadrugs.org/).
[c]Mutation specific.
[d]Based on experimental data.

AF, Atrial fibrillation; *AS*, Andersen-Tawil syndrome; *CPVT*, catecholaminergic polymorphic ventricular tachycardia; *Cx40*, connexin 40; *ISA*, intrinsic sympathomimetic activity; *LQTS/SQTS*, long/short QT syndrome; *RyR2*, ryanodine receptor; *SR*, sarcoplasmic reticulum; *TS*, Timothy syndrome; *VF*, ventricular fibrillation; *VT*, ventricular tachycardia; ↑, increase; ↓, decrease.

Potential drugs in this category include antiinflammatory agents, RAAS inhibitors (angiotensin-converting enzyme inhibitors [ACEIs], angiotensin II receptor antagonists [ARAs], and mineralocorticoid receptor antagonists [MRAs]), omega-3 polyunsaturated fatty acids (PUFAs), statins, and antifibrotic agents.

Antiinflammatory Agents

Increased levels of inflammatory markers (interleukin-6 and high-sensitivity C-reactive protein) are associated with a higher risk of AF and life-threatening ventricular arrhythmias in patients with HF or CAD.[59,61] It has been hypothesized that inflammation contributes to cardiac structural remodeling and might be a target for antiarrhythmic therapies. However, whether inflammation is an initiating event or a consequence in the development of arrhythmias remains controversial. Corticosteroids reduce the risk of postoperative AF,[69] but their potential toxicity restricts their therapeutic value.

Renin-Angiotensin-Aldosterone System Inhibitors

ACEIs and ARAs inhibit angiotensin II AT1 receptor–mediated proarrhythmic effects, including APD shortening, enhanced automaticity, hypokalemia, reduced cell coupling, pressure overload, abnormal Ca^{2+} handling, oxidative stress, neurohumoral activation, and structural remodeling (hypertrophy, fibrosis, and inflammation).[3,5]

In primary prevention, ACEIs and ARAs reduce the risk of AF in patients with HF, hypertension, and LV hypertrophy but not in post-MI patients or those without cardiovascular disease.[3,70] In secondary prevention, they exert a beneficial effect after cardioversion of persistent AF and in the prevention of paroxysmal AF, particularly in patients with significant underlying heart disease (e.g., LV dysfunction or hypertrophy), and when patients have

also received amiodarone.[68,70] However, prospective randomized clinical trials question the value of ARAs in secondary prevention of AF. ACEIs decrease SCD in post-MI patents; in patients with congestive HF, ACEIs reduce all-cause mortality but not SCD.[4,5]

MRAs inhibit cardiac fibrosis, exert direct antiarrhythmic actions, and reduce the risk of hypokalemia; therefore they represent a therapeutic option for patients with HF, LV hypertrophy, and AF. Indeed, preliminary data suggest that MRAs reduce the incidence of recent-onset AF, VT/VF, and SCD in patients with systolic HF.[3,5,68,69]

Statins

Statins exert multiple antiarrhythmic effects, including direct effects on cardiac ion channels; plaque stabilization; and antifibrotic, antiinflammatory, and antioxidant actions.[71] In addition, they suppress triggered activity in preparations of pulmonary veins from canines. Studies of statins for primary or secondary prevention of AF do not support specific recommendations, except for primary prevention of postoperative AF.[3,68,69] Statins do not reduce the risk of ventricular arrhythmias or of cardiac arrest; they produce a modest benefit on SCD in patients with CAD who are treated with an ICD and in patients with nonischemic cardiomyopathy.[4,72]

Omega-3 Polyunsaturated Fatty Acids

Omega-3 polyunsaturated fatty acids modulate ion channels and Cx, reduce fluctuations in Ca^{2+}_i, and exert antiinflammatory and antioxidant actions.[73] However, there is no robust evidence to support their efficacy in primary or secondary prevention of AF or VT/VF.[4,69,73]

Antifibrotic Agents

A variety of stimuli (i.e., fast heart rates, pressure/volume overload, oxidative stress, inflammation, ischemia, cytokines, growth factors, or neurohumoral activation) induce the proliferation of cardiac fibroblasts and their differentiation into myofibroblasts.[74,75] Myofibroblasts when electrotonically coupled to cardiomyocytes cause slow conduction, ectopic activity, and electric remodeling based on paracrine interactions, which generate an arrhythmogenic substrate in fibrotic hearts. Cardiac fibrosis is the final result of multiple signaling pathways that can vary in different cardiac diseases, and many potential therapeutic antifibrotic targets have been identified,[61] although its clinical relevance remains uncertain.

Conclusions

Most positive data with upstream therapies came from experimental models, observational studies, and retrospective analyses of clinical data, whereas prospective randomized trials failed to demonstrate a beneficial effect on secondary prevention of AF burden or cardiovascular outcomes. This can be explained because upstream therapies are effective at the beginning of the remodeling process, but ineffective at later stages when structural remodeling is irreversible, or because remodeling is a disease-specific process presenting important differences with respect to signaling pathways and pharmacological responses among comorbidities. Therefore prospective studies are needed to confirm this hypothesis and to define the populations of patients who are most likely to benefit from upstream therapies.

Other Antiarrhythmic Drugs

Adenosine acting on cardiac A1 receptors activates an outward K^+ current (I_{KAdo}) present in the atria, SAN, and AVN and inhibits I_f and adenylyl cyclase, which indirectly results in a decrease in catecholamine-stimulated I_{CaL} and I_{TI}. As a result, adenosine suppresses the pacemaker activity of SAN and depresses AVN conduction, being the first-line agent for terminating paroxysmal SVTs (AVNRT or AVRT), but does not convert AF/AFl to SR. In addition, adenosine suppresses catecholamine-stimulated EADs and DADs as well as idiopathic right ventricular outflow tract VT due to cyclic adenosine monophosphate (cAMP)–mediated DADs.[5]

Digoxin inhibits Na^+/K^+–ATPase and decreases intracellular Na^+ concentration, which in turn increases both Ca_i^{2+} and contractile force via the NCX. It also enhances vagal tone and reduces sympathetic and RAAS tone. At therapeutic concentrations, digoxin decreases the automaticity of the SAN (vagal stimulation inhibits I_f), slows conduction, and prolongs refractoriness in the AVN. This latter effect is the basis for heart rate control in patients with AF and systolic HF, particularly in unstabilized HF patients in whom β-blockers and calcium antagonists are contraindicated. In permanent AF, the combination of digoxin with these drugs provides a satisfactory rate control both at rest and during exercise.[3] Digoxin has no role in ventricular arrhythmias, does not modify cardiac mortality in patients with congestive HF in SR, and can increase the risk of SCD.[4,5]

Raised resting heart rate is a strong independent risk factor for cardiovascular events. The antianginal drug ivabradine, a selective I_f inhibitor, added as background therapy reduces the risk of hospitalization due to worsening HF in patients with stable, symptomatic HF and an LV ejection fraction of 35% or less with a heart rate of 70 beats/min or greater.[76] The off-label use of ivabradine is effective in patients with inappropriate sinus tachycardia and postural orthostatic tachycardia syndrome.

Experimental data suggest that the atrial expression of several channels might represent novel options for targeted therapy of AF, including two-pore–domain $K_{2P}3.1$ (TASK-1), Ca^{2+}-activated nonselective cation (NSC_{Ca}), small-conductance Ca^{2+}-activated ($SK_{Ca}2.1$-2.3) channels, and mitochondrial large-conductance Ca^{2+}-activated K^+ channels ($KCa1.1$).[8,59] In models of AF, SK_{Ca} blockers (apamin, NS8593, UCL1684, or ICA) increase atrial APD heterogeneity, induce local conduction delay, and promote wave breaks and reentrant arrhythmias; however, other results suggest that SK_{Ca} blockers prevent AF inducibility.[77] Thus the role of these channels in patients with AF remains undefined.

Unresolved Questions and Future Strategies

There are many unresolved questions concerning the pharmacological treatment of cardiac arrhythmias. The bottleneck for the development of AADs is that both the underlying mechanisms of arrhythmias and the mechanisms of action of AADs remain incompletely understood. It is also unclear whether targeting an individual ion channel is better than targeting multiple ion channels. By blocking both inward and outward currents, multichannel blockers can create steady-state conditions that avoid large variations in AP repolarization, thereby preventing the development of electrical instability, although the risk of proarrhythmia may increase. Additionally, there is poor information on effectiveness of combination therapy, including the different combinations of AADs or combinations of AADs with nonpharmacological approaches (catheter ablation or ICD).

As previously mentioned, VT/VF associated with SCD preferentially occurs in the setting of myocardial ischemia. Thus it would be optimal to develop ischemia-selective AADs. Because class I and III AADs failed to prevent ischemia-induced arrhythmias, antiarrhythmic strategy was shifted to drugs commonly prescribed in patients with MI or HF that prevent plaque rupture and reduce myocardial ischemia, such as antianginal drugs (β-blockers, ivabradine, or ranolazine), statins, RAAS inhibitors, and platelet antiaggregants, in an attempt to eliminate potential triggers for ventricular arrhythmias and to prevent the formation of myocardial scars, cardiac remodeling, and SCD in the long term. AF is the most common arrhythmia, and atrial-selective AADs devoid of ventricular proarrhythmic effects based on the identification of atrial-specific targets are under development. Finally, several new putative therapeutic targets (see Table 54.2) have been recently proposed; however, most targets lack sufficient cardiac specificity, and their functional role in humans remains to be determined.

Conclusions

Despite their poor efficacy and adverse effects and the improvements made in the nonpharmacological antiarrhythmic therapies, AADs remain the mainstay of therapy for the majority of patients with cardiac arrhythmias. Nevertheless, there is an unmet need for new drugs that can achieve effective suppression and prevention of life-threatening arrhythmias without exposing the patient to the risk of proarrhythmia. The rational development of these new AADs should be the final result of a better understanding of the molecular and cellular mechanisms involved in the genesis and maintenance of cardiac arrhythmias in different pathological–arrhythmogenic substrates and the mechanisms of action of AADs.

Acknowledgments

The authors thank Ricardo Caballero for comment on the manuscript and Paloma Vaquero for editorial assistance with the manuscript preparation. This work was supported by grants from Instituto de Salud Carlos III [PI16/00398 and CB16/11/00303] and the Ministerio de Economía (SAF2014-58769-P).

REFERENCES

1. Darbar D. Standard antiarrhythmic drugs. In: Zipes D, Jalife J, eds. *Cardiac Electrophysiology: From Cell to Bedside*. 6th ed. Philadelphia: Saunders Elsevier; 2014.
2. Sheets MF, Fozzard HA, Lipkind GM, et al. Sodium channel molecular conformations and antiarrhythmic drug affinity. *Trends Cardiovasc Med*. 2010;20:16–21.
3. January CT, Wann LS, Alpert JS, et al. ACC/AHA Task Force Members. 2014 AHA/ACC/HRS guideline for the management of patients with atrial fibrillation: executive summary: a report of the American College of Cardiology/American Heart Association Task Force on practice guidelines and the Heart Rhythm Society. *Circulation*. 2014;130:2071–2104.
4. Das MK, Zipes DP. Antiarrhythmic and nonantiarrhythmic drugs for sudden cardiac death prevention. *J Cardiovasc Pharmacol*. 2010;55:438–449.
5. Priori SG, Blomström-Lundqvist C, Mazzanti A, et al. 2015 ESC Guidelines for the management of patients with ventricular arrhythmias and the prevention of sudden cardiac death: The Task Force for the Management of Patients with Ventricular Arrhythmias and the Prevention of Sudden Cardiac Death of the European Society of Cardiology (ESC) Endorsed by: Association for European Paediatric and Congenital Cardiology (AEPC). *Eur Heart J*. 2015;36:2793–2867.
6. Hatem SN, Coulombe A, Balse E. Specificities of atrial electrophysiology: clues to a better understanding of cardiac function and the mechanisms of arrhythmias. *J Mol Cell Cardiol*. 2010;48:90–95.
7. Burashnikov A, Antzelevitch C. Novel pharmacological targets for the rhythm control management of atrial fibrillation. *Pharmacol Ther*. 2011;132:300–313.
8. Ravens U. Antiarrhythmic therapy in atrial fibrillation. *Pharmacol Ther*. 2010;128:129–145.
9. Zaza A, Belardinelli L, Shryock JC. Pathophysiology and pharmacology of the cardiac "late sodium current." *Pharmacol Ther*. 2008;119:326–339.
10. Antzelevitch C, Nesterenko V, Shryock JC, et al. The role of late I_{Na} in development of cardiac arrhythmias. *Handb Exp Pharmacol*. 2014;221:137–168.
11. Belardinelli L, Giles WR, Rajamani S, et al. Cardiac late Na^+ current: proarrhythmic effects, roles in long QT syndromes, and pathological relationship to CaMKII and oxidative stress. *Heart Rhythm*. 2015;12:440–448.
12. Scirica BM, Morrow DA, Hod H, et al. Effect of ranolazine, an antianginal agent with novel electrophysiological properties, on the incidence of arrhythmias in patients with non ST-segment elevation acute coronary syndrome: results from the Metabolic Efficiency With Ranolazine for Less Ischemia in Non ST-Elevation Acute Coronary Syndrome Thrombolysis in Myocardial Infarction 36 (MERLIN-TIMI 36) randomized controlled trial. *Circulation*. 2007;116:1647–1652.
13. De Ferrari GM, Maier LS, Mont L, et al. RAFFAELLO Investigators: Ranolazine in the treatment of atrial fibrillation: results of the dose-ranging RAFFAELLO (Ranolazine in Atrial Fibrillation Following An ELectricaL CardiOversion) study. *Heart Rhythm*. 2015;12:872–878.
14. Reiffel JA, Camm AJ, Belardinelli L, et al. The HARMONY trial: combined ranolazine and dronedarone in the management of paroxysmal atrial fibrillation: mechanistic and therapeutic synergism. *Circ Arrhythm Electrophysiol*. 2015;8:1048–1056.
15. Wijffels MC, Dorland R, Mast F, et al. Widening of the excitable gap during pharmacological cardioversion of atrial fibrillation in the goat: effects of cibenzoline, hydroquinidine, flecainide, and d-sotalol. *Circulation*. 2000;102:260–267.
16. Pandit SV, Jalife J. Rotors and the dynamics of cardiac fibrillation. *Circ Res*. 2013;112:849–862.
17. López-Sendón J, Swedberg K, McMurray J, et al. Expert consensus document on beta-adrenergic receptor blockers. *Eur Heart J*. 2004;25:1341–1362.
18. Workman AJ. Cardiac adrenergic control and atrial fibrillation. *Naunyn Schmiedeberg Arch Pharmacol*. 2010;381:235–249.
19. Vaseghi M, Shivkumar K. The role of the autonomic nervous system in sudden cardiac death. *Prog Cardiovasc Dis*. 2008;50:404–409.
20. Triposkiadis F, Karayannis G, Giamouzis G, et al. The sympathetic nervous system in heart failure physiology, pathophysiology, and clinical implications. *J Am Coll Cardiol*. 2009;54:1747–1762.
21. Gould PA, Yii M, McLean C, et al. Evidence for increased atrial sympathetic innervation in persistent human atrial fibrillation. *Pacing Clin Electrophysiol*. 2006;29:821–829.
22. González de la Fuente M, Barana A, Gómez R, et al. Chronic atrial fibrillation up-regulates β1-adrenoceptors affecting repolarizing currents and action potential duration. *Cardiovasc Res*. 2013;97:379–388.
23. van der Werf C, Zwinderman AH, Wilde AA. Therapeutic approach for patients with catecholaminergic polymorphic ventricular tachycardia: state of the art and future developments. *Europace*. 2012;14:175–183.
24. Priori SG, Wilde AA, Horie M, et al. HRS/EHRA/APHRS expert consensus statement on the diagnosis and management of patients with inherited primary arrhythmia syndromes: document endorsed by HRS, EHRA, and APHRS in May 2013 and by ACCF, AHA, PACES, and AEPC in June 2013. *Heart Rhythm*. 2013;10:1932–1963.
25. Tamargo J, Caballero R, Gómez R, et al. Pharmacology of cardiac potassium channels. *Cardiovasc Res*. 2004;62:9–33.
26. Shah RR, Hondeghem LM. Refining detection of drug-induced proarrhythmia: QT interval and TRIaD. *Heart Rhythm*. 2005;2:758–772.
27. Perry M, Sanguinetti M, Mitcheson J. Revealing the structural basis of action of hERG potassium channel activators and blockers. *J Physiol*. 2010;588:3157–3167.
28. Blaauw Y, Schotten U, van Hunnik A, et al. Cardioversion of persistent atrial fibrillation by a combination of atrial specific and non-specific class III drugs in the goat. *Cardiovasc Res*. 2007;75:89–98.
29. Charpentier F, Mérot J, Loussouarn G, et al. Delayed rectifier K^+ currents and cardiac repolarization. *J Mol Cell Cardiol*. 2010;48:37–44.
30. Silva J, Rudy Y. Subunit interaction determines I_{Ks} participation in cardiac repolarization and repolarization reserve. *Circulation*. 2005;112:1384–1391.
31. Caballero R, González de la Fuente M, Gómez R, et al. In humans, chronic atrial fibrillation decreases the transient outward current and ultrarapid component of the delayed rectifier current differentially on each atria and increases the slow component of the delayed rectifier current in both. *J Am Coll Cardiol*. 2010;55:2346–2354.
32. Muñoz V, Grzeda KR, Desplantez T, et al. Adenoviral expression of I_{Ks} contributes to wavebreak and fibrillatory conduction in neonatal rat ventricular cardiomyocyte monolayers. *Circ Res*. 2007;101:475–483.
33. Niwa N, Nerbonne JM. Molecular determinants of cardiac transient outward potassium current (I_{to}) expression and regulation. *J Mol Cell Cardiol*. 2010;48:12–25.
34. Antzelevitch C, Yan GX. J-wave syndromes: Brugada and early repolarization syndromes. *Heart Rhythm*. 2015;12:1852–1866.
35. Bouzeman A, Traulle S, Messali A, et al. Long-term follow-up of asymptomatic Brugada patients with inducible ventricular fibrillation under hydroquinidine. *Europace*. 2014;16:572–577.
36. Ravens U, Wettwer E. Ultra-rapid delayed rectifier channels: molecular basis and therapeutic implications. *Cardiovasc Res*. 2011;89:776–785.
37. Tamargo J, Caballero R, Gómez R, et al. I_{Kur}/Kv1.5 channel blockers for the treatment of atrial fibrillation. *Expert Opin Investig Drugs*. 2009;18:399–416.
38. Pandit SV, Berenfeld O, Anumonwo JM, et al. Ionic determinants of functional reentry in a 2-D model of human atrial cells during simulated chronic atrial fibrillation. *Biophys J*. 2005;88:3806–3821.
39. Savelieva I, Graydon R, Camm AJ. Pharmacological cardioversion of atrial fibrillation with vernakalant: evidence in support of the ESC Guidelines. *Europace*. 2014;16:162–173.
40. Anumonwo JMB, Lopatin AN. Cardiac strong inward rectifier potassium channels. *J Mol Cell Cardiol*. 2010;48:45–54.
41. Jalife J. Inward rectifier potassium channels control rotor frequency in ventricular fibrillation. *Heart Rhythm*. 2009;6:S44–S48.
42. Gómez R, Caballero R, Barana A, et al. Structural basis of drugs that increase cardiac inward rectifier Kir2.1 currents. *Cardiovasc Res*. 2014;104:337–346.
43. Tristani-Firouzi M, Etheridge SP. Kir 2.1 channelopathies: the Andersen-Tawil syndrome. *Pflugers Arch*. 2010;460:289–294.
44. Amorós I, Dolz-Gaitón P, Gómez R, et al. Propafenone blocks human cardiac Kir2.x channels by decreasing the negative electrostatic charge in the cytoplasmic pore. *Biochem Pharmacol*. 2013;86:267–278.
45. Machida T, Hashimoto N, Kuwahara I, et al. Effects of a highly selective acetylcholine-activated K^+ channel blocker on experimental atrial fibrillation. *Circ Arrhythm Electrophysiol*. 2011;4:94–102.
46. Liang B, Nissen JD, Laursen M, et al. G-protein-coupled inward rectifier potassium current contributes to ventricular repolarization. *Cardiovasc Res*. 2014;101:175–184.
47. Obeyesekere MN, Antzelevitch C, Krahn AD. Management of ventricular arrhythmias in suspected channelopathies. *Circ Arrhythm Electrophysiol*. 2015;8:221–231.
48. Dobrev D, Friedrich A, Voigt N, et al. The G protein-gated potassium current $I_{K,ACh}$ is constitutively active in patients with chronic atrial fibrillation. *Circulation*. 2005;112:3697–3706.
49. Terzic A, Alekseev AE, Yamada S, et al. Advances in cardiac ATP-sensitive K^+ channelopathies from molecules to populations. *Circ Arrhythm Electrophysiol*. 2011;4:577–585.
50. Tinker A, Aziz Q, Thomas A. The role of ATP sensitive potassium channels in cellular function and protection in the cardiovascular system. *Br J Pharmacol*. 2014;171:12–23.
51. Piccini JP, Berger JS, O'Connor CM. Amiodarone for the prevention of sudden cardiac death: a meta-analysis of randomized controlled trials. *Eur Heart J*. 2009;30:1245–1253.
52. Severs NJ, Bruce AF, Dupont E, et al. Remodeling of gap junctions and connexin expression in diseased myocardium. *Cardiovasc Res*. 2008;80:9–19.
53. Dhein S, Hagen A, Jozwiak J, et al. Improving cardiac gap junction communication as a new antiarrhythmic mechanism: the action of antiarrhythmic peptides. *Naunyn Schmiedebergs Arch Pharmacol*. 2010;381:221–234.
54. De Vuyst E, Boengler K, Antoons G, et al. Pharmacological modulation of connexin-formed channels in cardiac pathophysiology. *Br J Pharmacol*. 2011;163:469–483.
55. Reed A, Kohl P, Peyronnet R. Molecular candidates for cardiac stretch-activated ion channels. *Glob Cardiol Sci Pract*. 2014;2014:9–25.
56. Schumacher SM, Martens JR. Ion channel trafficking: a new therapeutic horizon for atrial fibrillation. *Heart Rhythm*. 2010;7:1309–1315.
57. Caballero R, Dolz-Gaitón P, Gómez R, et al. Flecainide increases Kir2.1 currents by interacting with cysteine 311, decreasing the polyamine-induced rectification. *Proc Natl Acad Sci U S A*. 2010;107:15631–15636.
58. Sanguinetti MC. HERG1 channelopathies. *Pflugers Arch*. 2010;460:265–276.
59. Wakili R, Voigt N, Kääb S, et al. Recent advances in the molecular pathophysiology of atrial fibrillation. *J Clin Invest*. 2011;121:2955–2968.
60. Venetucci L, Denegri M, Napolitano C, et al. Inherited calcium channelopathies in the pathophysiology of arrhythmias. *Nat Rev Cardiol*. 2012;9:561–575.
61. Tamargo J, López-Sendón J. Novel therapeutic targets for the treatment of heart failure. *Nat Rev Drug Discov*. 2011;10:536–555.
62. Li N, Chiang DY, Wang S, et al. Ryanodine receptor-mediated calcium leak drives progressive development of an atrial fibrillation substrate in a transgenic mouse model. *Circulation*. 2014;129:1276–1285.
63. Dobrev D, Voigt N, Wehrens XH. The ryanodine receptor channel as a molecular motif in atrial fibrillation: pathophysiological and therapeutic implications. *Cardiovasc Res*. 2011;89:734–743.
64. Zhou Q, Xiao J, Jiang D, et al. Carvedilol and its new analogs suppress arrhythmogenic store overload-induced Ca^{2+} release. *Nat Med*. 3020;17:1003–1009.
65. Watanabe H, Chopra N, Laver D, et al. Flecainide prevents catecholaminergic polymorphic ventricular tachycardia in mice and humans. *Nat Med*. 2009;15:380–383.
66. Bannister ML, Thomas NL, Sikkel MB, et al. The mechanism of flecainide action in CPVT does not involve a direct effect on RyR2. *Circ Res*. 2015;116:1324–1335.
67. Swaminathan PD, Purohit A, Hund TJ, et al. Calmodulin-dependent protein kinase II: linking heart failure and arrhythmias. *Circ Res*. 2012;110:1661–1677.
68. Savelieva I, Kakouros N, Kourliouros A, et al. Upstream therapies for management of atrial fibrillation: review of clinical evidence and implications for European Society of Cardiology guidelines. Part I: primary prevention. *Europace*. 2011;13:308–328.
69. Savelieva I, Kakouros N, Kourliouros A, et al. Upstream therapies for management of atrial fibrillation: review of clinical evidence and implications for European Society of Cardiology guidelines. Part II: secondary prevention. *Europace*. 2011;13:610–625.
70. Schneider MP, Hua TA, Bohm M, et al. Prevention of atrial fibrillation by renin-angiotensin system inhibition: a meta-analysis. *J Am Coll Cardiol*. 2010;55:2299–2307.
71. Tamargo J, Caballero R, Gómez R, et al. Lipid-lowering therapy with statins, a new approach to antiarrhythmic therapy. *Pharmacol Ther*. 2007;114:107–126.
72. Rahimi K, Majoni W, Merhi A, et al. Effect of statins on ventricular tachyarrhythmia, cardiac arrest, and sudden cardiac death: a meta-analysis of published and unpublished evidence from randomized trials. *Eur Heart J*. 2012;33:1571–1581.
73. Rizos EC, Ntzani EE, Bika E, et al. Association between omega-3 fatty acid supplementation and risk of major cardiovascular disease events: a systematic review and meta-analysis. *JAMA*. 2012;308:1024–1033.
74. Dzeshka MS, Lip GY, Snezhitskiy V, et al. Cardiac fibrosis in patients with atrial fibrillation: mechanisms and clinical implications. *J Am Coll Cardiol*. 2015;66:943–959.
75. Leask A. Getting to the heart of the matter: new insights into cardiac fibrosis. *Circ Res*. 2015;116:1269–1276.
76. Tardif JC, O'Meara E, Komajda M, et al. SHIFT Investigators: Effects of selective heart rate reduction with ivabradine on left ventricular remodelling and function: results from the SHIFT echocardiography substudy. *Eur Heart J*. 2011;32:2507–2515.
77. Zhang XD, Lieu DK, Chiamvimonvat N. Small-conductance Ca^{2+}-activated K^+ channels and cardiac arrhythmias. *Heart Rhythm*. 2015;12:1845–1851.

55 Pharmacogenomics of Cardiac Arrhythmias

Dan M. Roden

Individuals vary widely in their responses to therapy with most drugs. Indeed, response to cardiovascular drug therapy and anti-arrhythmics in particular is so highly variable that study of the underlying mechanisms has elucidated important lessons for understanding variable responses to drug therapy in general.[1,2]

By disrupting gene product function, single nucleotide changes can produce dramatic changes in physiology: the long QT syndromes and inherited errors of metabolism, such as alkaptonuria, are examples. Indeed, recognition that inborn errors of metabolism arose from defective biotransformation of endogenous substrates led to the suggestion more than a century ago that exogenous substrates (drugs) might similarly be aberrantly metabolized and might produce unusual actions in affected patients. This *pharmacogenetic* paradigm has been validated by the identification of individual patients and families with defects in the genes encoding specific drug-metabolizing enzymes. The term *pharmacogenomics* encompasses the idea that variability in drug responses across individuals or populations reflects the combined influences of many DNA variants across individual genomes.

Principles of Pharmacogenomics

Definitions

The series of events that occur between administration of a drug and the manifestation of its beneficial or adverse effects include two key steps (Fig. 55.1). First, the drug must be delivered to its molecular site of action (e.g., receptor or ion channel). The magnitude of the effect at the target is determined by drug concentration, and study of the time dependence of the drug concentration (and metabolites) achieved in plasma, tissue, or other sites, such as urine or bile, is termed *pharmacokinetics*. The second major process that determines drug action has been termed *pharmacodynamics* and broadly includes the processes that must occur between the interaction of a drug with a specific molecular target and manifestations of drug action at the molecular, cellular, whole-organ, and whole-patient levels. Because drugs act in a complex (and often abnormal) biological milieu, considerable intersubject variability in drug effects can arise from pharmacodynamic mechanisms.

These principles of pharmacokinetics and pharmacodynamics have been recognized for decades, and it is now apparent that they are manifestations of the highly regulated function of individual gene products. Thus metabolism of a drug occurs by the interaction of the drug with specific drug-metabolizing molecules, and the absorption, distribution, and renal and biliary excretion reflect the cellular drug uptake and efflux by specific transporter molecules.[3] It is the variability in the function and expression of metabolizing and transporting molecules, which are regulated by a host of genetic and environmental factors, that determines pharmacokinetic variability. Similarly, variability in the biological milieu in which drugs act can be conceptualized as variability in the function of multiple molecules, including the target molecules with which drugs interact to produce their beneficial and adverse effects.

Some DNA variants are rare, cause specific "monogenic" diseases, and have conventionally been termed *mutations*. More common variants are termed *polymorphisms* and might or might not alter function or expression of the encoded protein. As we begin to understand that each human harbors millions of DNA variants[4]—some common and some extremely rare—the distinction between "mutation" and "rare variant" becomes increasingly unclear, and more generic language, such as rare and common polymorphisms, is being adopted. One critical aspect of modern genomics is that DNA tends to be highly ancestry specific. Variants implicated in traits such as variable drug responses in one ethnic group may be absent in another, or different variants in the same gene may also contribute.

A change in a single nucleotide, a *single-nucleotide polymorphism* (SNP), is the most common type of DNA variant. Others include nucleotide insertions or deletions (*indels*) and duplication or deletion of large stretches of DNA, termed *copy number variations* (CNVs). Only about 1% of the genome is protein-coding (this subset of DNA is termed the *exome*), and protein function can be altered if a polymorphism results in a change in primary amino acid sequence (a *nonsynonymous polymorphism*). In addition, noncoding variants can alter protein abundance through multiple mechanisms (e.g., by changing mRNA stability or by regulating the rate of mRNA transcription). Such regulation can arise because of polymorphisms in the promoter (the region that directly controls gene transcription, often directly upstream of exon 1) or in more distant genomic regions. One emerging view is that polymorphisms may be physiologically silent until an environmental stressor is superimposed: examples of environmental stressors important for arrhythmia pathophysiology include adrenergic stress, acute myocardial ischemia, and drug administration.

Approaches to Identifying Pharmacogenetic Variants

Drugs display variability in both efficacy and toxicity, and pharmacogenomic experiments have addressed both types of responses. Drug efficacy often reflects the combined effects of multiple pharmacokinetic and pharmacodynamic determinants; therefore identifying polymorphisms with large effect sizes contributing to efficacy has been challenging. Similarly, some drug toxicities reflect an extension of the biology of efficacy (e.g., excessive ventricular rate slowing with atrioventricular [AV] nodal blocking drugs), and thus the experimental challenges are similar. However, other toxicities are not predicted by what is known about the efficacy of a drug and seem to occur in a relatively unpredictable fashion; examples include skin rashes, statin-related myopathy, and drug-induced arrhythmias. In some of these apparently

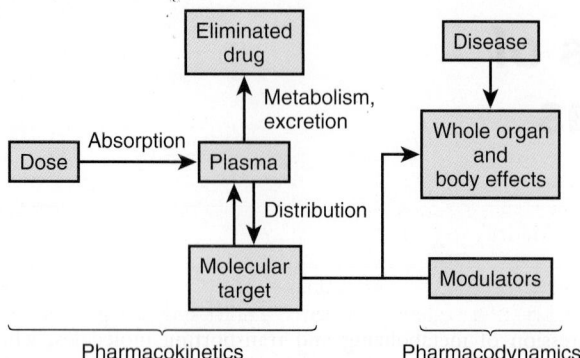

FIGURE 55.1 Mechanisms modulating drug actions. The *left side* illustrates the pharmacokinetic variables that determine absorption, distribution, metabolism, and elimination (often abbreviated ADME). Variability in interactions between drugs and their molecular targets, along with variability in underlying pathophysiologies including disease processes, modulates pharmacodynamic mechanisms (*right*) that contribute to net drug responses. Understanding the molecular determinants of pharmacokinetics and pharmacodynamics is the first step toward identifying genetic variants that contribute to drug responses.

idiosyncratic cases, single variants with relatively large effect sizes have been identified.

Proving that a DNA variant contributes to a specific clinical phenotype (such as an unusual drug response) requires compelling statistical arguments and replication in multiple datasets; demonstration that a variant produces altered biological properties in vitro can also serve as a supporting argument. The rapid proliferation of polymorphism databases has led to a very large number of false-positive associations between polymorphisms and variable human phenotypes—associations that are subsequently not reproduced.[5]

Associating genetic variants with clinical phenotypes, including drug response, in humans has taken one of two broad approaches. The first is predicated on a perceived understanding of the fundamental physiology, pathophysiology, or pharmacology of the phenotype under study; this is termed a *candidate gene* approach (see Fig. 55.1). The second takes advantage of emerging high-throughput technologies by genotyping or direct sequencing of large DNA regions (up to whole exomes and genomes) to then determine whether there is an association between any locus interrogated and the phenotype under study. To date, the most widely used method in this unbiased or hypothesis-free approach is the genome-wide association study (GWAS) paradigm.[6] One clear emerging lesson of these genetic association studies is that any result requires further validation both by replication and by further experiments testing the underlying biology.

Candidate Gene Approaches

Although the candidate gene approach is intuitively very appealing, repeated experience over the past decade has demonstrated that initially identified associations frequently failed to replicate.[5] The reasons for this failure of replication are multiple: (1) the candidate variant may not, in fact, explain a large proportion of the variance in the phenotype under study; (2) the studies generally involve small numbers and so are underpowered; and (3) a publication bias is associated with positive results, so attempts to replicate generally regress to the mean.

A major exception to the general "rule" that candidate gene studies fail to replicate in a robust fashion is seen in pharmacogenomics.[7] Here single variants that alter the function of drug-metabolizing or drug-transporting molecules may confer a very high likelihood of developing aberrantly high (or low) plasma drug concentrations—and thus highly variable drug responses—during treatment. In addition, genetically determined variations

in drug targets (molecules with which drugs interact to achieve their therapeutic or adverse effects) may strongly modulate the outcomes of drug therapy. Specific examples are discussed in the following sections.

Unbiased Approaches: the Genome-Wide Association Study Paradigm

In arrhythmia science, GWASs have been used to identify new genes and pathways involved in physiological traits (such as electrocardiogram [ECG] intervals) and susceptibility to common arrhythmias, including atrial fibrillation (AF) or sudden cardiac death.[8-10] These results, in turn, are being used to explore the role of variants in these genes in variable drug response. In addition, GWASs have been used to directly analyze drug responses, as described later.[11]

A fundamental enabling discovery for the GWAS paradigm is the concept of linkage disequilibrium. Although each human harbors millions of common SNPs, many are "linked" in the sense that knowing the specific genotype at one locus allows an investigator to infer the genotype at a second locus. If an SNP at one genetic locus always informs the genotype at the second SNP site, the two are said to be in complete linkage disequilibrium. Thus a platform that interrogates large numbers of SNPs need only include a few such "tag" SNPs to identify genotypes across an entire linkage disequilibrium block or haplotype.

The GWAS experiment[6] starts by identifying cases and controls for a specific phenotype. These can be categorical (e.g., premature heart disease, breast cancer, drug-induced adverse effect, AF, restless leg syndrome) or continuous (e.g., PR duration, warfarin steady-state dose). High-throughput platforms are then used to determine genotypes at hundreds of thousands or millions of SNP sites in cases and controls, and tests of association are performed at each SNP to identify those associated with the phenotype under study (Fig. 55.2). Evidence that the experiment has yielded a positive result may include very low *p* values (after correction for multiple comparisons), replication, and ultimately biological plausibility. SNPs are chosen because they tag blocks of linkage disequilibrium; therefore there is little expectation that those associated with low *p* values are functional themselves. Rather, they act as signposts within the genome, identifying specific loci at which functional variants may reside.

GWAS analyses of the distribution of normal ECG intervals (e.g., PR, QRS, QT) have been conducted in tens of thousands of patients and have identified genomic loci that contribute to variability in these traits.[12,13] Some of these are familiar from an understanding of underlying physiology. Thus, for example, strong signals are present in the *KCNQ1* and *KCNH2* loci (encoding potassium channels important for cardiac repolarization) in GWAS analyses of variability in the QT interval.[12] Mutations in these genes are the most common causes of the congenital long QT syndrome; the GWAS result demonstrates that common variants in these genes contribute to physiological variability of QT intervals in a normal population. Indeed, common variants have been implicated as modulators of severity of the congenital long QT syndrome.[14]

Other signals identified by GWAS identify genes whose role in the phenotype under study is completely unsuspected. In the QT analyses, the strongest signal has been consistently noted near *NOS1AP*, which encodes an ancillary protein for the neuronal isoform of NOS.[12] Functional studies have implicated *NOS1AP* as a regulator of cardiac potassium and calcium function[15] or of cardiac conduction.[16] Follow-up studies have implicated *NOS1AP* variants in phenotypes beyond normal QT variability: these include the risk for sudden cardiac death in populations,[17] risk for events in patients with congenital long QT syndrome,[18,19] and risk for sudden death during treatment with some drugs.[20] The strongest GWAS signal for variability in PR and QRS is seen in *SCN10A*, which encodes a sodium channel previously implicated

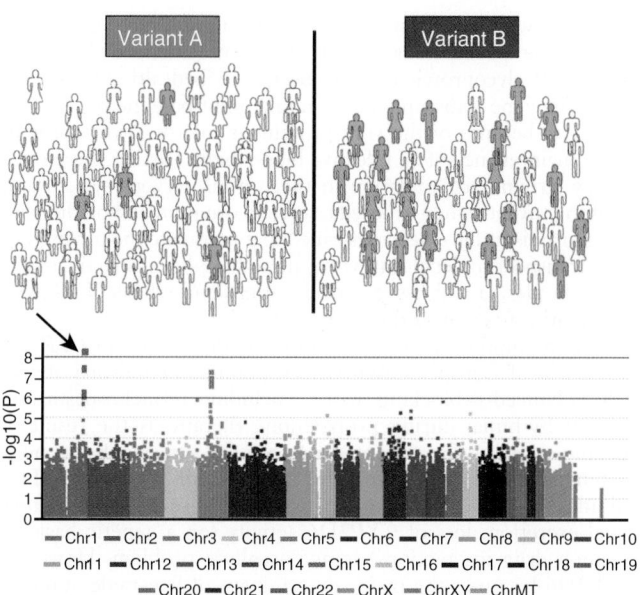

FIGURE 55.2 The genome-wide association study paradigm. The first step (*top panel*) is to assign each subject in a large cohort with either case (*orange*) or control (*white*) status. The entire cohort is then genotyped at hundreds of thousands to millions of common polymorphic sites. The figure illustrates how a hypothetical polymorphism predicting the phenotype in question might segregate: in this case, variant B is associated with the phenotype. A statistical test of association is then performed for each polymorphism, and the results are displayed on a Manhattan plot. *Bottom*, The x-axis is the chromosomal location of the polymorphism, and the y-axis is the negative exponent of the *p* value for the individual statistical test (higher values denote lower *p* values). In the example shown, a cluster of polymorphisms in chromosome 1 (*arrow*) achieves *p* values less than 10^{-8}. The *red horizontal line* denotes an arbitrary level of statistical significance after correction for multiple testing.

only in pain perception and not known to play a role in the heart. Preliminary studies have suggested multiple roles for the gene in the heart: contribution to late sodium current,[21] regulation of the canonical cardiac sodium channel *SCN5A*,[22,23] and a role in neural regulation of conduction.[24]

GWASs of patients with and without AF have consistently implicated SNPs at chromosome 4q25.[9] The nearest gene encodes the transcription factor *PITX2*; initial studies suggest that *PITX2c*, a cardiac-specific isoform, regulates both development of the pulmonary myocardium[25] and expression of other genes (e.g., *NPPA*, *KCNQ1*) that have been implicated in AF susceptibility.[26] These data are also being used to inform additional studies on the variable response to AF therapy. Thus, for example, reports have suggested that SNPs at Chr4q25 predict response to drug[27] or ablation[28] therapy in AF.

In addition to analysis of phenotypes such as ECG intervals or disease susceptibility, the GWAS paradigm has been used to directly study variability in drug response. Here, the problem is that precise definitions of drug response phenotypes are needed, and the numbers of patients that can be accrued is by nature of the experiment much smaller than that by the analyses of ECG intervals or of arrhythmias themselves.[11] Nevertheless, as is described later, initial attempts have been made to analyze phenotypes such as warfarin steady-state dose requirement or susceptibility to drug-induced torsades de pointes (TdP).

Large GWAS analyses have identified incontrovertible statistically significant associations such as those between variants in *NOS1AP* and QT duration or between variants at 4q25 and AF susceptibility. However, the actual size of these effects can be modest, and their contribution to overall heritability of the traits under study is often small, with odds ratios rarely exceeding

2.0; this is not surprising because variants producing very large effects that would alter survival would not be expected to persist in a population. The fact that strong GWAS signals identify common variants with only very modest effect sizes has been a major criticism of the approach. Nevertheless, identification of new physiological pathways in human phenotypes represents the major triumph of the approach and, as has been outlined earlier, can be a starting point for new risk stratifiers in disease settings and with drug exposure.

Other Experimental Approaches

A design intermediate between a single candidate gene interrogation and an unbiased GWAS approach is a multiplexed candidate gene study. In this approach, hundreds of SNPs, chosen because they tag major haplotype blocks within logically chosen candidate genes, are interrogated to identify specific loci that may associate with the phenotype of choice.[29,30] This approach offers the advantage of shifting the focus away from single variants, along with the disadvantage that it remains a candidate gene approach, albeit using candidates chosen often through unbiased approaches. The hypothesis that combinations of genetic variants contribute to a trait can be addressed using this method.[30] Another emerging approach is to combine the results of genomic studies with those of other studies yielding complementary datasets. Examples are expression profiling in cell lines, specific tissues, or human cardiomyocytes derived from induced pluripotent stem cells[31]; informatics approaches[32]; and drug response evaluations in model organisms with known genetic backgrounds, such as mice or zebrafish.[33]

An emerging approach in modern genomics is the direct sequencing of candidate genes, of loci implicated as modulators of a phenotype by GWAS, of large candidate gene sets, and ultimately of the whole genome. New technologies have enabled the development of very high throughput and reasonably accurate genotyping for such experiments. The challenge is that the larger the region of the genome interrogated, the larger the number of genetic variants identified, and the ability to relate specific variants to phenotypes under study remains a major challenge in this area. Nevertheless, these approaches are being explored in genomics and have been applied to electrophysiological phenotypes.[34-36]

Pharmacokinetic Mechanisms

Each drug is a substrate for one or more specific drug-metabolizing enzymes and is transported into and out of cells by specific drug uptake and efflux molecules. When variable drug effects arise because of variability in plasma or tissue drug concentrations, polymorphisms in the genes encoding drug-metabolizing enzymes or transporters are high-priority candidates for explaining variability in drug effects.

Most drug metabolism occurs in the hepatocyte, where drugs are biotransformed to one or more metabolites, usually by oxidation. Drug metabolites are generally more polar than the parent drug and are themselves excreted or conjugated (most commonly as glucuronides) before renal or biliary excretion. Oxidation is usually accomplished by members of the cytochrome P450 (CYP) superfamily, of which the CYP3A family (*CYP3A4* and *CYP3A5*), *CYP2D6*, *CYP2C9*, and *CYP2C19* are the most important members for drug metabolism. Conjugation is accomplished by uridine glucuronyl transferase, *N*-acetyltransferase, or a group of methyltransferases.[7]

High-Risk Pharmacokinetics

The term *high-risk pharmacokinetics* has been used to describe specific clinical settings in which variation in normal metabolism or excretory pathways can confer especially important clinical effects.[37] Such variation most often arises because of genetic polymorphisms in the pathway or because of coadministration

TABLE 55.1 Pharmacogenetics of antiarrhythmic drugs

DRUG	GENES WITH POLYMORPHISMS POSSIBLY AFFECTING RESPONSE	INHIBITOR OF:
Quinidine		CYP2D6, ABCB1
Procainamide	NAT2	
Amiodarone		CYP3A4, ABCB1, CYP2C9
Flecainide	CYP2D6	
Propafenone	CYP2D6	
Sotalol		
Dofetilide		
Dronedarone		ABCB1
Metoprolol, timolol	CYP2D6, ADR1	
β-Blockers	ADR1	
Verapamil		CYP3A4, ABCB1
Diltiazem		CYP3A4, ABCB1
Warfarin	CYP2C9, VKORC1	
Adenosine		
Digoxin	ABCB1	

of drugs that inhibit the pathway. One high-risk setting involves use of a drug that has a narrow margin between effective dose and toxic dose, and that has a single predominant route of elimination. A second setting involves administration of a *prodrug*, a drug that requires a specific metabolic pathway for its bioactivation. Examples of prodrugs whose bioactivation depends on drug metabolism pathways with known polymorphisms include clopidogrel and codeine. Table 55.1 presents examples of antiarrhythmic drugs for which variants in single genes produce large effects.

A spectacular example of high-risk pharmacokinetics was drug interactions involving CYP3A4 substrates, notably the antihistamine terfenadine and the promotility agent cisapride.[38] These compounds are high-potency QT-prolonging agents (resulting from block of the potassium current I_{Kr}) and ordinarily undergo very extensive presystemic metabolism by CYP3A (and no other major pathway) to non-I_{Kr}–blocking metabolites. When drugs that inhibit CYP3A are coadministered, presystemic metabolism is inhibited, terfenadine or cisapride concentrations that enter the systemic circulation can increase by several orders of magnitude, and TdP due to an I_{Kr} block becomes a real risk. These risks led to withdrawal of these drugs from the market.

Although the activity of CYP3A4 varies among individual patients, the reasons for this are not completely understood. Although noncoding SNPs regulating function have been described, no common nonsynonymous SNPs are present in the gene. Functionally important polymorphisms in the coding region of the very closely related gene for CYP3A5 are expressed in enterocytes and hepatocytes. Loss-of-function alleles are more common in white or Asian patients than in African American patients.[39]

Another widely used drug that is eliminated largely by a single molecular mechanism is digoxin, whose hepatic and renal excretion is mediated by the drug efflux transporter P-glycoprotein encoded by *ABCB1*.[3] The well-recognized effects of quinidine, amiodarone, verapamil, and numerous other drugs (erythromycin, itraconazole, and cyclosporine) in elevating digoxin concentrations likely reflect interference with the P-glycoprotein elimination pathway. Similarly, sotalol and dofetilide are largely eliminated by renal excretion of the unchanged drug, so marked QT prolongation is a real risk

in patients with renal dysfunction who are administered usual drug dosages; the specific transporter is unknown. Patients with entirely defective P-glycoprotein have not been described, although mice in which the gene is disrupted have no manifest baseline phenotype. However, because of the very prominent role of P-glycoprotein in the maintenance of an effective blood–brain barrier, these mice display striking accumulation in the central nervous system and resulting toxicity when exposed to certain drugs, including digoxin. Polymorphisms have been described that modulate the function of drug transport molecules in vitro; these have been linked to variability in plasma and tissue concentrations and effects of digoxin, simvastatin, and many other drugs.[3]

Patients homozygous for loss-of-function alleles in *CYP2D6* (5%–10% of European and African populations) display markedly enhanced β-blocking action, including bronchospasm and bradyarrhythmia, during propafenone therapy as the result of accumulation of the parent drug. Similar effects of the poor metabolizer genotype have been reported for metoprolol. Flecainide is also a CYP2D6 substrate, but because it also undergoes renal excretion, loss of CYP2D6 activity (on a genetic basis or through drug interactions) is not usually a problem. However, CYP2D6 becomes the major determinant of flecainide elimination in patients with renal failure, and this is one setting in which flecainide toxicity can occur if CYP2D6 activity is reduced on the basis of genomic variation or drug interactions.

Pharmacodynamic Mechanisms

DNA polymorphisms can result in important functional changes in drug target molecules. One example is the common R389G (substitution of glycine for arginine at position 389) variant in *ADR1* encoding the β₁-adrenergic receptor. The R389 variant demonstrated a two- to four-fold greater increase in myocyte contractility during exposure to β-agonists and predicted a beneficial response of patients with heart failure receiving bucindolol; in fact, clinical response in G389 carriers was no different from response to placebo. Other studies implicate this polymorphism as a modulator of rate control in AF.[40] A variant in the *SCN5A* promoter common in Asian subjects has been described that reduces promoter activity and is associated with longer QRS duration (slower conduction) at baseline,[41] and, as has been discussed, *SCN10A* variants also modulate QRS. The *SCN5A* variant predicted greater QRS prolongation with sodium channel–blocking drug challenge in Asian patients with Brugada syndrome; therefore this becomes a candidate for modulating risk for sudden death seen when conduction is slowed by drugs, disease, or genetic syndromes.

Variable responses to warfarin reveal that this is an example of a drug in which two genes play an important role.[1] One is *CYP2C9*, which is responsible for the bioinactivation of S-warfarin, the active enantiomer of the drug. Patients with *CYP2C9* variants that result in loss of function have higher plasma drug levels, increased drug effects, excessive risk for bleeding at ordinary doses, and decreased steady-state dose requirements. The specific variants and their frequencies vary by ancestry. The second gene is *VKORC1*, which encodes an important component of the warfarin drug target (the vitamin K complex). Very rare patients have *VKORC1* coding region mutations, resulting in warfarin resistance. In addition, however, common variation in the promoter clearly modulates *VKORC1* hepatic mRNA abundance and can be related to warfarin sensitivity. In fact, the initial warfarin dose requirement appears more dependent on *VKORC1* variants than on those in *CYP2C9*. Steady-state warfarin dose requirements vary strikingly across ethnicities, and higher dose requirements in African subjects and lower ones in Asian subjects have been associated with *VKORC1* variation. GWASs of warfarin steady-state doses have confirmed a prominent contribution by common variants in *CYP2C9* and *VKORC1* and have suggested a role for at least one other gene, *CYP4F2*, which is considered to be involved in vitamin K oxidation. Trials evaluating the time to and the therapeutic range during warfarin initiation in subjects randomized to genetically guided and clinical/empiric therapy have yielded contradictory results.[42,43] Rates of bleeding in these initiation trials were very low, and other studies have implicated *CYP2C9* or *CYP4F2* variants in bleeding risk during long-term therapy.[44,45]

The Example of Drug-Induced Long QT Syndrome

A range of genetic approaches have been used to study the potential contributions of DNA variants to risk for drug-induced TdP (diTdP). This serious adverse drug event occurs in 1%–5% of patients treated with QT-prolonging antiarrhythmics, such as sotalol, dofetilide, or quinidine, and to a much lesser extent in patients exposed to noncardiovascular drugs, such as terfenadine, cisapride, erythromycin, haloperidol, and methadone. The mechanism whereby patients receiving antiarrhythmic drugs are at so much higher risk than those receiving noncardiovascular drugs remains unexplained and may reflect a contribution by concomitant disease, notably AF, which is frequently the indication for prescribing QT-prolonging antiarrhythmics. Data suggest that the period of conversion from AF to sinus rhythm is one of high risk for QT interval dysregulation because of mechanisms that are not well understood.[38]

An understanding of normal and abnormal cardiac repolarization informs a set of candidate genes that may modulate QT and diTdP risk. Virtually all drugs that cause TdP are I_{Kr} blockers. The biological context in which I_{Kr} blockers act includes other elements of the action potential (e.g., I_{Kr}, I_{Na}, and I_{Ca}), as well as mechanisms that control normal autonomic function and serum potassium. Another potential contributor to TdP risk is phosphoinositide (PI) 3 kinase inhibition (a property of some anticancer drugs that have been linked to diTdP), which affects multiple ionic currents, suppressing I_{Kr} and I_{Ks} and increasing late sodium current to prolong QT.[46] Hypokalemia, a risk factor for TdP, may act by decreasing I_{Kr}, increasing the potency of I_{Kr} block by drugs, and activating calmodulin kinase, an effect that increases late sodium current.[47] This complexity is consistent with the notion that the mechanisms that maintain a short QT interval vary among individual patients, and patients with reduced repolarization reserve as the result of genetic or environmental factors are at increased risk for developing TdP on challenge with an I_{Kr} blocker. Several studies have implicated variable I_{Ks} as playing an important role in maintaining this reserve.[48] One report indicated that in vitro exposure to an I_{Kr}-blocking drug paradoxically shortened action potentials. The proposed explanation was decreased expression of a microRNA (miRNA), whose ordinary role is to inhibit translation of *KCNQ1*, a key gene in the I_{Ks} complex; the decrease in miRNA thus resulted in increased I_{Ks} expression and unexpectedly shortened action potentials.[49] This experiment highlights the way in which complex regulation of multiple ion currents controls cardiac repolarization, as well as a potential role for miRNAs as modulators of these processes.

Because two common clinical situations in which marked QT prolongation and TdP are observed are diTdP and congenital long QT syndromes, one obvious set of candidate genes for mediating diTdP risk consists of the congenital long QT syndrome disease genes. A second set of candidates are those, such as *NOS1AP*, that have been implicated in variability in normal QT intervals by GWASs. A third set includes genes implicated by physiological studies,[33] informatics approaches,[32] or in silico modeling as modulators of QT; genes involved in autonomic function, potassium homeostasis, or PI3 kinase signaling are examples. A fourth set of candidate genes are those responsible for metabolism and elimination of the QT-prolonging drug; in this case, genetic variants will be specific to individual culprit drugs. For example, the antipsychotic thioridazine is metabolized by *CYP2D6*, and evidence suggests that poor metabolizers are at increased risk for diTdP with this drug.[50]

Individual case reports and series have provided evidence that some patients with previously unrecognized congenital long QT syndrome may present with TdP when challenged with a QT-prolonging drug.[51] In addition, common variants in these genes could contribute; one example is a common nonsynonymous SNP in the cardiac sodium channel gene resulting in S1103Y, which is detected only in African Americans and is reported to modulate the risk for a range of arrhythmias, including diTdP and sudden infant death syndrome.[52] Systematic evaluations of patients with diTdP, which survey increasingly large sets of congenital long QT syndrome and other congenital arrhythmia syndrome genes, have identified potentially contributory variants in patients with diTdP in up to 65% of cases.[51] Another set of candidate variants that might modulate risk are those in the β_1-adrenergic receptor gene, but systematic surveys have not supported this contention.

A large candidate gene survey studied 1424 SNPs in 18 high-priority candidate genes (including congenital long QT syndrome disease genes and *NOS1AP*) in a set of 176 European ancestry patients with diTdP and two sets of controls: 837 population controls and 207 patients exposed to QT-prolonging drugs and who did not develop marked QT interval changes.[29] This study identified a single nonsynonymous SNP (D85N) in *KCNE1* that predicted diTdP with a relatively high odds ratio of 9.0. *KCNE1* encodes a key subunit necessary for physiological I_{Ks} function, and the variant D85N has been implicated as a modulator of normal QT interval and as a risk factor for modulating the phenotype in both congenital and diTdP. GWAS comparing diTdP cases and drug-exposed controls with minimal QT prolongation did not identify common genetic variants with large effect sizes.[53] Exome sequencing in cases and controls replicated the risk associated with *KCNE1* D85N and suggested that variants in *ACN9* (a gene involved in glucose homeostasis) might also play a role.[36] Rare potassium channel variants were somewhat more common in cases (37%) than in controls (21%). Taken together, these genetic studies suggest that *KCNE1* D85N is a risk factor for diTdP, but other single coding variants with large effect sizes probably do not play a major role.

The Future: Using Pharmacogenetic Information in Patient Management

One goal of pharmacogenetic studies is to identify mechanisms leading to large variability with existing drug therapies. These results, in turn, could be used to tailor therapy with existing drugs and to evaluate new drugs to ensure that high-risk situations are avoided. Another possible outcome of pharmacogenomic studies is the development of readily measurable biomarkers to predict individual patient responses. In addition, identification of new pathways to variable physiological and drug responses may be the first clue for the development of new drug targets.

A rapidly increasing knowledge base is relating common and rare polymorphisms to variable drug response and other phenotypes, such as susceptibility to disease. The ultimate hope is that such studies will usher in a new era of personalized medicine, in which an individual patient's polymorphism set will be used to efficiently diagnose disease, determine disease susceptibility, and select optimal therapies. Despite an increasingly compelling body of knowledge linking variable drug effects with genetic variation, adoption in clinical practice has been slow. Many reasons have been proposed to explain this apparent paradox. One is that large randomized clinical trials, with very few exceptions, have not been conducted to demonstrate the value of adding pharmacogenetic information to routine clinical care. A second is that the effects of drug administration are so variable that even factoring out pharmacogenetic contributors still leaves substantial variability in drug responses. A third possible explanation is a logistic one: it is cumbersome to not only prescribe a drug but also at the same time obtain a genetic test whose result (often appearing days later) may require a second patient encounter to adjust the medication dose or change medications. In busy clinical practice environments, it may be simpler to choose different drugs or ignore pharmacogenomic influences altogether.

Rapid advances in genotyping technology are now raising the possibility that testing for pharmacogenomic variation can be accomplished in a "preemptive" fashion; that is, genetic information related to drug response and perhaps to other important pathophysiological phenotypes, such as susceptibility to disease, can be embedded in patients' electronic medical records, to be accessed when a culprit drug is prescribed. Electronic systems would then advise the physician at the point of care whether the drug choice or drug dosage needs to be altered. This potential approach of incorporating genomic variant data into the flow of health care is now being explored at various academic medical centers.[54,55]

REFERENCES

1. Roden DM, Johnson JA, Kimmel SE, et al. Cardiovascular pharmacogenomics. *Circ Res.* 2011;109:807–820.
2. Roden DM, Wilke RA, Kroemer HK, et al. Pharmacogenomics: the genetics of variable drug responses. *Circulation.* 2011;123:1661–1670.
3. DeGorter MK, Xia CQ, Yang JJ, et al. Drug transporters in drug efficacy and toxicity. *Ann Rev Pharmacol Toxicol.* 2012;52:249–273.
4. Consortium TGP. A global reference for human genetic variation. *Nature.* 2015;526:68–74.
5. MacArthur DG, Manolio TA, Dimmock DP, et al. Guidelines for investigating causality of sequence variants in human disease. *Nature.* 2014;508:469–476.
6. Manolio TA. Genome-wide association studies and assessment of the risk of disease. *N Engl J Med.* 2010;363:166–176.
7. Wang L, McLeod HL, Weinshilboum RM. Genomics and drug response. *N Engl J Med.* 2011;364:1144–1153.
8. Bezzina CR, Pazoki R, Bardai A, et al. Genome-wide association study identifies a susceptibility locus at 21q21 for ventricular fibrillation in acute myocardial infarction. *Nat Genet.* 2010;42:688–691.
9. Ellinor PT, Lunetta KL, Albert CM, et al. Meta-analysis identifies six new susceptibility loci for atrial fibrillation. *Nat Genet.* 2012;44:670–675.
10. Milan DJ, Lubitz SA, Kääb S, Ellinor PT. Genome-wide association studies in cardiac electrophysiology: recent discoveries and implications for clinical practice. *Heart Rhythm.* 2010;7:1141–1148.
11. Motsinger-Reif AA, Jorgenson E, Relling MV, et al. Genome-wide association studies in pharmacogenomics: successes and lessons. *Pharmacogenet Genomics.* 2013;23:383–394.
12. Arking DE, Pulit SL, Crotti L, et al. Genetic association study of QT interval highlights role for calcium signaling pathways in myocardial repolarization. *Nat Genet.* 2014;46:826–836.
13. Sotoodehnia N, Isaacs A, de Bakker PI, et al. Common variants in 22 loci are associated with QRS duration and cardiac ventricular conduction. *Nat Genet.* 2010;42:1068–1076.
14. Duchatelet S, Crotti L, Peat RA, et al. Identification of a KCNQ1 polymorphism acting as a protective modifier against arrhythmic risk in long-QT syndrome. *Circ Cardiovasc Genet.* 2013;6:354–361.
15. Chang KC, Barth AS, Sasano T, et al. CAPON modulates cardiac repolarization via neuronal nitric oxide synthase signaling in the heart. *Proc Natl Acad Sci U S A.* 2008;105:4477–4482.
16. Kapoor A, Sekar RB, Hansen NF, et al. An enhancer polymorphism at the cardiomyocyte intercalated disc protein NOS1AP locus is a major regulator of the QT interval. *Am J Hum Genet.* 2014;94:854–869.
17. Kao WH, Arking DE, Post W, et al. Genetic variations in nitric oxide synthase 1 adaptor protein are associated with sudden cardiac death in US white community-based populations. *Circulation.* 2009;119:940–951.
18. Crotti L, Monti MC, Insolia R, et al. NOS1AP is a genetic modifier of the long-QT syndrome. *Circulation.* 2009;120:1657–1663.
19. Tomas M, Napolitano C, De Giuli L, et al. Polymorphisms in the NOS1AP gene modulate QT interval duration and risk of arrhythmias in the long QT syndrome. *J Am Coll Cardiol.* 2010;55:2745–2752.

20. Becker ML, Visser LE, Newton-Cheh C, et al. A common NOS1AP genetic polymorphism is associated with increased cardiovascular mortality in users of dihydropyridine calcium channel blockers. *Br J Clin Pharmacol.* 2009;67:61–67.
21. Yang T, Atack TC, Stroud DM, et al. Blocking Scn10a channels in heart reduces late sodium current and is antiarrhythmic. *Circ Res.* 2012;111:322–332.
22. Arnolds DE, Liu F, Fahrenbach JP, et al. TBX5 drives Scn5a expression to regulate cardiac conduction system function. *J Clin Invest.* 2012;122:2509–2518.
23. van den Boogaard M, Wong LE, Tessadori F, et al. Genetic variation in T-box binding element functionally affects SCN5A/SCN10A enhancer. *J Clin Invest.* 2012;122:2519–2530.
24. Verkerk AO, Remme CA, Schumacher CA, et al. Functional Nav1.8 channels in intracardiac neurons: the link between SCN10A and cardiac electrophysiology. *Circ Res.* 2012;111:333–343.
25. Mommersteeg MTM, Brown NA, Prall OW, et al. (2007). Pitx2c and Nkx2-5 are required for the formation and identity of the pulmonary myocardium. *Circ Res.* 2007;101:902–909.
26. Wang J, Klysik E, Sood S, et al. Pitx2 prevents susceptibility to atrial arrhythmias by inhibiting left-sided pacemaker specification. *Proc Natl Acad Sci U S A.* 2010;107:9753–9758.
27. Parvez B, Vaglio J, Rowan S, et al. Symptomatic response to antiarrhythmic drug therapy is modulated by a common single nucleotide polymorphism in atrial fibrillation. *J Am Coll Cardiol.* 2012;60:539–545.
28. Shoemaker MB, Bollmann A, Lubitz SA, et al. Common genetic variants and response to atrial fibrillation ablation. *Circ Arrhythm Electrophysiol.* 2015;8:296–302.
29. Kaab S, Crawford DC, Sinner MF, et al. A large candidate gene survey identifies the KCNE1 D85N polymorphism as a possible modulator of drug-induced torsades de pointes. *Circ Cardiovasc Genet.* 2012;5:91–99.
30. Lubitz SA, Sinner MF, Lunetta KL, et al. Independent susceptibility markers for atrial fibrillation on chromosome 4q25. *Circulation.* 2010;122:976–984.
31. Wang Y, Liang P, Lan F, et al. Genome editing of isogenic human induced pluripotent stem cells recapitulates long QT phenotype for drug testing. *J Am Coll Cardiol.* 2014;64:451–459.
32. Berger SI, Ma'ayan A, Iyengar R. Systems pharmacology of arrhythmias. *Sci Signal.* 2010;3:ra30.
33. Milan DJ, Kim AM, Winterfield JR, et al. Drug-sensitized zebrafish screen identifies multiple genes, including GINS3, as regulators of myocardial repolarization. *Circulation.* 2009;120:553–559.
34. Olesen MS, Nielsen MW, Haunsø S, et al. Atrial fibrillation: the role of common and rare genetic variants. *Eur J Hum Genet.* 2014;22:297–306.
35. Weeke P, Denny JC, Basterache L, et al. Examining rare and low-frequency genetic variants previously associated with lone or familial forms of atrial fibrillation in an electronic medical record system: a cautionary note. *Circ Cardiovasc Genet.* 2015;8:58–63.
36. Weeke P, Mosley JD, Hanna D, et al. Exome sequencing implicates an increased burden of rare potassium channel variants in the risk of drug-induced long QT interval syndrome. *J Am Coll Cardiol.* 2014;63:1430–1437.

37. Roden DM, Stein CM. Clopidogrel and the concept of high risk pharmacokinetics. *Circulation.* 2009;119:2127–2130.
38. Roden DM. Drug-induced prolongation of the QT interval. *N Engl J Med.* 2004;350:1013–1022.
39. Oetjens M, Bush WS, Birdwell KA, et al. Utilization of an EMR-biorepository to identify the genetic predictors of calcineurin-inhibitor toxicity in heart transplant recipients. *Pac Symp Biocomput.* 2014;19:253–264.
40. Parvez B, Chopra N, Rowan S, et al. A common beta1-adrenergic receptor polymorphism predicts favorable response to rate-control therapy in atrial fibrillation. *J Am Coll Cardiol.* 2012;59:49–56.
41. Bezzina CR, Barc J, Mizusawa Y, et al. Common variants at SCN5A-SCN10A and HEY2 are associated with Brugada syndrome, a rare disease with high risk of sudden cardiac death. *Nat Genet.* 2013;45:1044–1049.
42. Kimmel SE, French B, Kasner SE, et al. A pharmacogenetic versus a clinical algorithm for warfarin dosing. *N Engl J Med.* 2013;369:2283–2293.
43. Pirmohamed M, Burnside G, Eriksson N, et al. A randomized trial of genotype-guided dosing of warfarin. *N Engl J Med.* 2013;369:2294–2303.
44. Kawai VK, Cunningham A, Vear SI, et al. Genotype and risk of major bleeding during warfarin treatment. *Pharmacogenomics.* 2014;15:1973–1983.
45. Roth JA, Boudreau D, Fujii MM, et al. Genetic risk factors for major bleeding in warfarin patients in a community setting. *Clin Pharmacol Ther.* 2014;95:636–643.
46. Yang T, Chun YW, Stroud DM, et al. Screening for acute IKr block is insufficient to detect torsades de pointes liability: role of late sodium current. *Circulation.* 2014;130:224–234.
47. Pezhouman A, Singh N, Song Z, et al. Molecular basis of hypokalemia-induced ventricular fibrillation. *Circulation.* 2015;32:1528–1537.
48. Roden DM, Abraham RL. Refining repolarization reserve. *Heart Rhythm.* 2011;8:1756–1757.
49. Xiao L, Xiao J, Luo X, et al. Feedback remodeling of cardiac potassium current expression: a novel potential mechanism for control of repolarization reserve. *Circulation.* 2008;118:983–992.
50. Llerena A, Berecz R, de la Rubia A, et al. QTc interval lengthening is related to CYP2D6 hydroxylation capacity and plasma concentration of thioridazine in patients. *J Psychopharmacol.* 2002;16:361–364.
51. Roden DM. Long QT syndrome: reduced repolarization reserve and the genetic link. *J Intern Med.* 2006;259:59–69.
52. Plant LD, Bowers PN, Liu Q, et al. A common cardiac sodium channel variant associated with sudden infant death in African Americans, SCN5A S1103Y. *J Clin Invest.* 2006;2006(116):430–435.
53. Behr ER, Ritchie MD, Tanaka T, et al. Genome wide analysis of drug-induced torsades de pointes: lack of common variants with large effect sizes. *PloS ONE.* 2013;8:e78511.
54. Shuldiner AR, Relling MV, Peterson JF, et al. The pharmacogenomics research network translational pharmacogenetics program: overcoming challenges of real-world implementation. *Clin Pharmacol Ther.* 2013;94:207–210.
55. Van Driest SL, Shi Y, Bowton EA, et al. Clinically actionable genotypes among 10,000 patients with preemptive pharmacogenomic testing. *Clin Pharmacol Ther.* 2014;95:423–431.

56 Gene Therapy to Treat Cardiac Arrhythmias

Silvia G. Priori, Marco Denegri, Rossana Bongianino, and Carlo Napolitano

The understanding of the molecular basis of cardiac excitability and the evolution of gene manipulation techniques has grown to a point that it is now conceivable to envisage effective, long-term, and safe antiarrhythmic gene therapies. The need for the search of novel means for the treatment of cardiac arrhythmias and sudden death is based on the evidence of the suboptimal performance of the current pharmacological therapies and the high complication rate of implantable devices.[1–3] This scenario applies particularly to patients with inherited arrhythmogenic diseases who need lifelong treatments and therefore have a long exposure time to the risk of adverse events.

Gene therapy has been initially thought as a way to cure genetic diseases through the direct manipulation of the abnormal gene(s). In a broader definition, gene therapy comprises the use of molecular tools to achieve the correction of a pathological condition caused by genetic mutations or by acquired conditions that alter the normal function of functionally relevant proteins. The strategies used so far to achieve this goal include the delivery of normal copies (wild-type) of the gene of interest, the in situ correction of a mutation (gene editing), the knockdown of a gene involved in the disease pathogenesis (silencing), or the targeted suppression of a mutant allele (allele-specific silencing). These approaches can be used in the whole heart, or they may be administered in specific areas if a local therapeutic effect is desirable.

The efficacy of a gene therapy treatment depends on several factors, including the design of the therapeutic construct, the selection of the vector, and the delivery strategy. An optimal therapy should be effective, specific, and safe.

In the following sections, we will review the vectors available to deliver a therapeutic construct, the molecular strategies adopted so far to manipulate genes for curative purposes, and finally, the state-of-the art of gene therapy to treat cardiac arrhythmias in preclinical studies.

Vectors for Gene Therapy

Several vectors for DNA/RNA transfer have been designed and are being evaluated. Each of them has different pros, cons, and potential area(s) of application. In this section, we will review the most important gene transfer vectors and the techniques available to correct the abnormal gene function.

Naked DNA/Heteroplexes-Polyplexes and Exosomes

A simple injection of nucleic acids (complementary DNA [cDNA] or modified RNA) cloned into a plasmid represents probably the first tested gene therapy approach. The use of naked DNA has some advantages, such as the relatively simple design and the possibility of delivering larger therapeutic molecules, over that of viral vectors. However, important limiting factors are the short duration of the transgene expression and the limited target specificity. One of the first proof-of-concept experiments with naked DNA in the heart was performed in the early 90s by Lin et al.[4] They injected naked DNA in the left ventricular wall of adult rats; the aim was to express a reporter gene, β-galactosidase, under the control of Rous sarcoma virus promoter and to study its persistence in the myocardial tissue. The expression of the transgene was detected until 4 weeks after injection.[4] Thus naked DNA administration does not seem suitable for the therapy of a genetic disease, but it may be considered when an effect is needed for a short duration. Along this line, a multicenter phase I clinical trial demonstrated the safety and efficacy of naked plasmid DNA encoding the human stromal cell–derived factor 1 (SDF1) to periinfarcted areas.[5] The objective was to attract stem cells for repair of myocardial tissue in the first weeks after a myocardial infarction while avoiding the potentially deleterious overgrowth due to long-term persistence of the transgene.

The experience of using naked DNA in the treatment of cardiac arrhythmias is limited. Burton et al.[6] administered a mutant form of the MiRP1 human gene that encodes the β-subunit of the hERG potassium channel. The strategy was to inhibit the rapid component of the cardiac delayed rectifier current (I_{Kr}) using the dominant-negative effect of the Q9E mutation. This approach intended to develop a molecular class III antiarrhythmic therapy. The vector was injected into the right atrium of pigs, and 16% of transfected atrial myocytes were obtained. Patch-clamp experiments demonstrated a significant suppression of I_{Kr} in these cells. However, no data were provided on whether there was an impact on the electrocardiogram in terms of QTc, suggesting the effectiveness of the therapy at the whole organ level.

Several other nonviral strategies are being evaluated to improve the applicability of naked DNA. *Heteroplexes* are multicomponent structures that can package DNA. They are manufactured using cationic elements for DNA condensation, lipidic compounds for enhanced protection and affinity to cell membranes, and additional ligands for cell targeting. In principle, this strategy can improve the specificity, and it can overcome some of the limiting factors of viral vectors (immunogenicity, size limitations, and expensive production). An interesting use of heteroplexes includes the incorporation of proteins (e.g., nuclear localization signal—NLS proteins) to enhance the correct transport of the transgene to its target location. Several NLS proteins have been tested and found to be effective.[7]

Polycations/polyplexes have been also considered as nonviral vectors for gene therapy.[8] Different complexes have been developed including polyethylenimine nanocomplexes (PEIs) used in one study to treat postmyocardial infarction ventricular tachycardia (post-MI VT)[9] (see the following text). These compounds are composed of positively charged amine groups that can bind to the negatively charged molecules of cell membranes to transfer DNA or RNA by endocytosis. Polyplexes have the positive feature of being able to carry large DNA chunks (up to 30 Kb). Unfortunately, polycations and DNA form aggregates that tend to precipitate after repeated exposures (i.e., administrations). This causes toxicity problems, especially with long-term use. Active research is ongoing in an attempt to circumvent this limitation.[8]

Nonviral delivery of therapeutic genes can also be achieved using *exosomes*. Exosomes are small (30–100 nm) membrane vesicles that are secreted by endosomes in almost all types of cell. They are naturally used for transport of genetic materials and for cell-to-cell communication.[10] Exosomes may have advantages over liposomes and other polyplexes given their lower cytotoxicity and the possibility of being designed to target specific cell types.[10] Artificial exosomes can be produced using host cells to overexpress and to package the DNA molecule of interest. The large packaging capacity allows the delivery of different therapeutic molecules, including drugs, small interfering RNA (siRNA), and large cDNAs, into the cytoplasm of target cells. The use of exosomes for cardiac gene therapy is at a very early stage. However, this approach is promising for specific applications, especially when viral vectors cannot be used due to the limited-size DNA inserts they can harbor.

Viral Vectors

Several viral vectors have been investigated for gene delivery in the heart, and among them the adenoviruses (AdVs), lentiviruses (LVs), and adeno-associated viruses (AAVs) have been more extensively tested.

Adenovirus. Adeno viral vectors have been used in gene transfer experiments since the early 90s,[11] and they have been also adopted in many cardiac gene therapy studies. They are medium-sized (90–100 nm) viruses with a double-stranded linear DNA that does not integrate into the host genome. Recombinant modified AdVs for gene therapy[12] have the advantage of showing a large packaging capacity up to 30 Kb, but they also present the limitation of a short-lasting transgene expression that leads to fading of the transgene within 2–4 weeks of administration.[13]

AdVs injected into the coronary circulation can achieve rather diffuse expression,[14] suggesting that intracoronary delivery may be a reasonable option whenever the therapeutic effect is required in the entire organ. In special instances, the time-limited expression of the transgene may be a desirable feature. A typical application is the local delivery of growth factors to promote angiogenesis in patients with coronary artery disease (CAD). In this setting, in fact, the short-term expression of a growth factor may induce a longer-lasting beneficial effect. As an example, Rosengart et al. showed improvement in blood perfusion in the area of vector administration and improvement in the angina symptoms beyond the duration of the transgene expression.[15] The same group showed that in their first study, 31 patients treated using a single direct myocardial injection of AdV-mediated vascular endothelial growth factor 2 (VEGF2) delivery had persistent collateral vascularization in the area distal to the occlusion after a long-term follow-up (median, 11.8 years).[16] Whether or not these effects are directly related to the treatment remains to be definitely established in larger studies.

Concern has been raised about the immunogenic toxicity of AdVs after the death of a young patient enrolled in a clinical trial in the late 90s.[17] Subsequent investigations have highlighted the complex immunogenic response to dVs administration, which involves multiple components of the immune system, and this response is dose dependent.[18] For this reason, the clinical development of AdV has been progressively abandoned.[19]

Lentivirus. LV is a viral species belonging to the family of Retroviridae that include human immunodeficiency virus I (HIV). LVs are RNA viruses with a packaging capacity up to 8 Kb, with the ability to confer long-term transgene expression. Therefore LVs are interesting vectors for cardiac gene therapy. However, there are safety concerns related to the fact that they randomly integrate in the genome and can cause insertional mutagenesis by disrupting other genes, leading to severe adverse events. In a clinical trial on X-linked severe combined immunodeficiency (X-SCID), three out of ten patients developed premalignant

T-cell proliferation that was attributable to dysregulation of a gene at the integration site.[20]

Intense research is ongoing to modify LVs to reduce the risk related to their random integration.[21] An interesting approach, so far applied to hematopoietic disease, is that of collecting and treating in vitro the cells with LV to transfer the gene of interest and injecting back the cells after the treatment. This approach has been recently used in few patients with Wiskott-Aldrich syndrome, with positive clinical results and no adverse events after 28 months of follow-up.[22]

Adeno-Associated Virus. AAVs belong to the Parvoviridae family. AAVs are nonpathogenic DNA viruses that require a helper virus (adenovirus or herpes simplex) to induce reproductive infection and replication. An important property of some AAVs is that they can enter host cells without the helper virus; in such cases they create a sort of "latent infection," either by site-specific integration into the host genome or, most frequently, by persisting in episomal forms. AAVs used for gene therapy have been modified to abate the possibility of integration in the host cell genome (that can cause insertional mutagenesis). On the other hand, the episomal localization can ensure long-term expression of the transgene.[23] This is a very attractive property of AAV vectors.

Extensive investigations on the AAV genome have identified at least 11 serotypes and more than 100 isolates, which are still poorly characterized. They differ in the amino acid sequence of the capsid proteins that confer specific tissue selectivity. The tissue selectivity may differ among species.[19] In rats, AAV1, AAV6, AAV8, and AAV9 have all been shown to transduce the myocardium, with AAV9 being the most cardiotropic. In dogs and monkeys, however, AAV6 and AAV8 were found to be more cardiotropic than AAV9.[24]

The major limitation of AAVs is their small packaging capacity (<5 Kb); larger insert sizes negatively affect the infection efficiency. Therefore AAVs are suitable only for a limited number of gene therapy applications. An alternative strategy, still in its exploratory phase, to allow the use of AAVs for the delivery of large cDNA is to split the therapeutic DNA into two or more independent constructs, one containing the 5′ end and the other the 3′ end of the same transcription cassette, with appropriate splice signals to promote *trans*-splicing inside target cells or with the introduction of overlapping sequence elements to drive homologous recombination.[25] The therapeutic DNA is then reconstructed in the host cell after infection. AAV9-mediated *trans*-splicing has been recently shown to be able to repair a mutant myosin-binding protein C gene (*MYBPC3*) in vitro.[26] Unfortunately, the amount of repaired protein detected in vivo was very low (approximately 0.14%), and the authors speculated (and provided preliminary evidence) that the modification of the *trans*-splicing signals of AAVs could improve the efficiency of repair.

AAVs are currently the most widely used vectors for gene therapy, and there are 137 ongoing or concluded clinical trials including 10 in cardiovascular diseases, mostly heart failure (http://www.wiley.com//legacy/wileychi/genmed/clinical/-update July 2015).

Strategies for Gene Therapy

The therapeutic strategy should be designed based on the pathophysiological mechanisms underlying the disease to be treated and should also aim at minimizing the risk of toxicity.

Gene Transfer

The systemic or local delivery of a wild-type cDNA to compensate for a nonfunctional native gene in the host cell is the aim of this approach. It is particularly useful in genetic diseases where the mutation causes a reduction of the expressed protein. Gene transfer can also be considered when the mutation causes a dominant-negative effect (i.e., the protein produced by the mutant allele impairs the function of protein produced by the wild-type allele). In these cases, it is the abundant production of the normal proteins that limits the consequences of the defective ones. Gene expression can also be used in an acquired disease when the level of a protein is reduced, and therefore the administration of exogenous cDNA of the protein may attenuate the phenotype.

When the therapeutic needs are restricted to a well-identified diseased area, local gene transfer is an interesting alternative to whole-organ delivery. For example, local gene transfer has been used in experimental studies to modify the electrophysiological properties of the atrioventricular node (AVN) in atrial fibrillation (AF) or to treat focal VT (Tables 56.1 and 56.2).

Gene Silencing/Control of Expression

Silencing is a process used by the cells to control gene expression. Physiologically, silencing is controlled by endogenous small RNA molecules (miRNA, 20–25 rt long) that bind with sequence specificity to the 3′ untranslated region of the target transcript(s) to inhibit translation. This process is defined as RNA interference. The control of RNA interference for therapeutic purposes is obtained with the delivery of either chemically synthesized siRNAs or small hairpin inhibitory RNAs (shRNAs). shRNAs are artificially modified siRNAs with a short loop between the two strands; shRNA can be processed into a functional siRNA by Dicer (ribonuclease III). The siRNA antisense strand is designed to be complementary to the target RNA. An siRNA bound to its target sequence forms the so-called RNA-induced silencing complex (RISC), causing translational repression. Experimental data have shown that siRNA can be toxic for the cell, and therefore the use of artificial miRNA may be preferable.[27]

Silencing is a widely used experimental technique to study the functional consequences of specific genes or transcripts. More recently, the approach has been considered for gene therapy. Gene silencing can be useful to treat gain-of-function mutations or to knock down ion channels that may have proarrhythmic effects. For example, AdV-delivered shRNA was used to inhibit the acetylcholine potassium current (I_{KAch}) in AF,[28] and the siRNA-mediated inhibition of the receptor for advanced glycation end-products (RAGE) pathway (a mediator of the ischemia-reperfusion damage) has shown antiarrhythmic effects and preserved connexin (i.e., Cx43) expression as compared with control in an ischemia-reperfusion model[9] (see Table 56.1).

Allele-Specific Silencing

The majority of gene mutations causing inherited arrhythmogenic diseases lead to a loss of function of the mutant protein. Therefore allele-specific silencing allows reducing the expression of the mutant protein, while preserving the expression of the functional one. This approach involves the design of a silencing RNA sequence specific for the mutant allele. The delivery of the allele-specific RNA may be included in a vector that is also harboring the wild-type cDNA of the gene of interest so that the global effect of the therapy is silencing of the mutant allele and increase in the production of the wild-type protein. Allele-specific

---

TABLE 56.1   Gene therapies for atrial fibrillation

AUTHOR (YEAR)	VECTOR	DELIVERY STRATEGY	CLINICAL AND MOLECULAR TARGETS	SPECIES	OUTCOMES
Donahue et al.[40] (2000)	AdV	Injection in AV branch of right coronary artery	Heart rate control in atrial fibrillation—overexpression of inhibitory G protein	Swine	↑ ERP conduction time in AV node; ↓ 20% HR during AF
Bauer et al.[41] (2004)	AdV	Injection in AV branch of right coronary artery	Heart rate control in atrial fibrillation—overexpression of inhibitory gene protein	Swine	↓ HR in persistent AF (conscious)
Perlstein et al.[43] (2005)	Plasmid DNA	Direct injection in right atrial myocardium	Atrial-specific class III antiarrhythmic effect—overexpression of Q9E mutant MiRP	Swine	No APD change at baseline; ↑ APD after clarithromycin administration
Liu et al.[28] (2009)	AdV	Superfusion and culture	Potassium channel blocking effect by shRNA to decrease GIRK4	Human myocytes	↓ 53% of acetylcholine potassium current (I_{KAch})
Amit et al.[44] (2010)	AdV	Epicardial gene painting	Molecular class III effect—increased refractoriness with mutant KCNH2 G628S	Swine	↑ atrial APD; ↓ risk of AF; ↑ atrial ERP
Bikou et al.[50] (2011)	AdV	Injection in atrial appendage and electroporation	Molecular ablation of AF—increased conduction velocity by Cx43 expression	Swine	No AF in treated animals; preserved AF-induced ejection fraction depression
Soucek et al.[47] (2012)	AdV	Direct injection followed by electroporation	Molecular class III effect—increased refractoriness with mutant canine KCNH2 G627S	Swine	↑ atrial APD; ↑ atrial ERP; significant reduction of AF burden
Lugenbiel et al.[42] (2012)	AdV	Injection in AV branch of right coronary artery	Heart rate control in AF—siRNA inhibition of Gs protein	Swine	↓ conduction in AVN; ↓ 20% HR during AF; preserved ejection fraction
Igarashi et al.[51] (2012)	AdV	Epicardial gene painting	Molecular ablation of AF—increased conduction velocity by Cx40 or Cx43 expression	Swine	↑ conduction velocity; ↓ P wave duration; ↓ risk of AF; twofold ↑ increase probability of sinus rhythm in treated animals
Trappe et al.[52] (2013)	AdV	Epicardial injection	AF suppression by reduced apoptosis—siRNA caspase knockdown	Swine	↓ apoptosis; ↑ AF-free time

AdV, Adenovirus; *AF*, atrial fibrillation; *APD*, action potential duration; *AV*, atrioventricular; *AVN*, atrioventricular node; *EAD*, early afterdepolarization; *ERP*, effective refractory period; *HR*, heart rate; *LV*, left ventricle.

TABLE 56.2 Gene therapies for ventricular arrhythmias and electrophysiological substrate

AUTHOR (YEAR)	VECTOR	DELIVERY STRATEGY	CLINICAL AND MOLECULAR TARGETS	CONDITION	SPECIES	OUTCOMES
Brunner et al.[78] (2003)	AdV	Direct injection	Treatment of Long QT syndrome—$K_V1.5$ overexpression	LQTS	Mouse	↓ APD and QT in vivo; ↓ early afterdepolarizations
Mazhari et al.[66] (2002)	AdV	Injection in LV cavity with aortic clamp	Treatment of Long QT syndrome—KCNE3 overexpression	LQTS	Guinea pig	↑ I_{Ks}; ↓ APD; ↓(19%); QT in vivo
Kodirov et al.[64] (2003)	AAV	Direct injection in the LV free wall	Treatment of Long QT syndrome—$K_V1.5$ overexpression	LQTS	Mouse	↑ 4AP-sensitive current (20%); ↓ APD; ↓ EAD
Murata et al.[68] (2004)	AdV	Direct injection in the LV cavity	Molecular calcium antagonist—overexpression of mutant ras-related G-protein	WT	Guinea pig	↓ I_{Ca-L}; ↓ APD and QT in vivo; negative inotropic effect
del Monte et al.[76] (2004)	AdV	Direct injection	Treatment of VT/VF after myocardial infarction—SERCA2a overexpression	CAD	Rat	↓ mortality and VT/VF episodes
Lebeche et al.[79] (2004)	AdV	Injection into aortic root	Hypertrophy-related arrhythmias—Overexpression of Ito ($K_v4.3$)	CPO	Rat	↑ I_{to}; ↓ APD
Sasano et al.[70] (2006)	AdV	Anterograde and retrograde coronary injection	Post MI VT therapy—Dominant-negative hERG variant (G628S mutation)	CAD	Swine	↑ APD; ↑ ERP; ↓ VT INDUCIBILITY
Prunier et al.[80] (2008)	AdV	Anterograde coronary injection	Arrhythmias during ischemia/reperfusion—SERCA2a overexpression	CAD	Swine	↓ VT incidence after reperfusion (not ischemia)
Lau et al.[71] (2009)	AdV	Intramyocardial injection	Post-MI arrhythmias—Overexpression of skeletal sodium channel (SkM1) to increase conduction	CAD	Dog	↓ ECG fragmentation; ↓ inducibility of VTs
Prestia et al.[72] (2011)	AdV	Injection in infarct area	Post-MI arrhythmias—connexin overexpression (Cx32) to avoid gap closure due to Cx43 (sensitive to ischemia)	CAD	Mouse	Larger infarct size; no VT differences
Lyon et al.[81] (2011)	AAV9	Tail vein injection	Post-MI/HF arrhythmias—SERCA2a	CAD	Rat	↓ Ventricular arrhythmias incidence; ↓ isoproterenol triggered VT and PES induced arrhythmias, ↓ SE Ca^{2+} leak
Greener et al.[73] (2012)	AdV	Anterograde and retrograde coronary injection	Post MI monomorphic VT therapy Cx43 overexpression	MI	Swine	↓ EG fragmentation and inducible VT, ↑ CV
Denegri et al.[60] (2012)	AAV9	IP injection	Recessive CPVT arrhythmia therapy—WT CASQ2 administration	CPVT	Mouse (TG)	↓ Triggered activity and ISO-induced arrhythmias, reversal of ultrastructural abnormalities.
Cutler et al.[82] (2012)	AAV9	Injection into aortic root	Arrhythmias in pressure overload HF—SERCA2a overexpression	CHF	Guinea pig	↓ APD alternans; ↓ VT in vivo
Denegri et al.[59] (2014)	AAV9	Tail vein injection	Recessive CPVT arrhythmia therapy—WT CASQ2 administration	CPVT	Mouse (TG)	↓ Triggered activity and ISO-induced arrhythmias, reversal of ultrastructural abnormalities up to 1 year after a single injection
Park et al.[9] (2015)	PEI nano-complex	Injection in the ischemic border zone	Suppress reperfusion arrhythmias by reduction of ischemic damage	CAD	Rat	↑ Conduction velocity and APD in the ischemic area; ↓ arrhythmia inducibility,

AdV, Adenovirus; *AAV*, adeno-associated virus; *APD*, action potential duration; *CAD*, coronary artery disease; *CHF*, congestive heart failure; *CPO*, chronic pressure overload as a model for cardiac hypertrophy; *CPVT*, catecholaminergic polymorphic ventricular tachycardia; *EAD*, early afterdepolarization; *ECG*, electrocardiogram; *EG*, electrogram; *ERP*, effective refractory period; *HF*, heart failure; *ISO*, isoproterenol; *LQTS*, long QT syndrome; *LV*, left ventricle; *MI*, myocardial infarction; *PES*, programmed electrical stimulation; *SERCA*, sarcoendoplasmic reticulum calcium transport adenosine triphosphatase; *VF*, ventricular fibrillation; *VT*, ventricular tachycardia; *WT*, wild-type.

silencing in cardiology has proved to be partially effective in an experimental model of hypertrophic cardiomyopathy.[29]

Gene Editing

Gene editing encompasses a series of molecular technologies that aim at correcting gene mutations in situ. It is a highly attractive strategy for monogenic diseases. The method is based on the use of a DNA-cleavage protein (nuclease) bound to a sequence-specific DNA-binding molecule. This complex induces site-specific DNA double-strand cut that stimulates the endogenous DNA-repair mechanism. Gene repair can be facilitated by providing an exogenous DNA template flanked by homologous sequences to the nuclease target site or by inserting a wild-type copy of the affected gene by homologous recombination. Different methodologies have been developed for gene editing: zinc-finger nucleases, TALEN or CRISPR/Cas9 (for a review, see Bongianino and Priori[19] and Mussolino et al.[30]). However, the use of gene editing to treat cardiac arrhythmias and cardiac diseases, in general, is currently hampered by its limited applicability in nondividing cells.[19]

Pharmacological Gene Therapy

Although it cannot be rigorously classified as a gene therapy approach, the possibility of using chemicals to correct the effects of gene mutations is an interesting possibility. This approach has been considered on the basis of the observation that nonsense mutations (also called PTC, premature termination codon) can undergo "read-through," i.e., a process that enables ribosomes to ignore the stop codon and to produce a full-length protein.[31] PTCs are usually associated with loss of function and variable phenotype as in the case of *SCN5A* mutations causing Brugada syndrome and conduction defects.[32,33] Aminoglycoside (gentamicin, amikacin) and, more recently, Ataluren (formerly PTC124), a small organic molecule with no antibiotic properties, are being studied and preliminarily tested in clinical trials, albeit with conflicting results.[34] Read-through has also been assessed in experimental studies on long QT syndrome (LQTS) to treat *KCNH2* mutations.[35]

Gene Therapy for Cardiac Arrhythmias

Gene therapy for cardiac arrhythmias is a complex task for several reasons. The maintenance of the electrical homeostasis of the myocardium requires a delicate, region-specific regulation of the ion channels and their modulatory proteins. In physiological conditions, regional differences do exist in the atria vs. ventricles, in the apex vs. base, in the epicardium vs. endocardium, and in the right vs. left ventricles.[36,37] For this reason, any gene delivered nonhomogeneously or in an uncontrolled fashion has the potential to disrupt this delicate homeostasis and to be potentially harmful. Thus detailed pathophysiological understanding and effective delivery techniques are crucial steps for the clinical development of antiarrhythmic gene therapies.

In the following paragraphs, we will review the state-of-the-art of gene therapy for atrial and ventricular tachyarrhythmias (brady-arrhythmia and biological pacemaker are the focus of Chapter 26).

Gene Therapy for Atrial Arrhythmias

AF has attracted the interest of several experimental studies. AF is the most common cardiac arrhythmia, and it is a frequent cause of embolic stroke.[3] The current pharmacological armamentarium and radiofrequency ablation are associated with limited efficacy, with high rates of recurrences and frequent transition to chronic AF.[3] For this reason, several investigators have attempted to develop strategies for the genetic manipulation of the atrial electrophysiological substrate (Fig. 56.1).

The standard pharmacological treatments for AF aim at either heart rate control or rhythm control. In a similar fashion, gene therapy studies have attempted to devise ways to control heart rate or to prevent arrhythmia onset. Additionally, other studies have explored the possibility of controlling fibrosis, apoptosis, and inflammation that are important players in the transition from paroxysmal to permanent/chronic AF.[38,39] Table 56.1 summarizes the studies on gene therapy of AF.

Rate Control and the Molecular β-Blockers

Initial studies in the early 2000s focused attention on rate control strategy. The idea was first advanced by Kevin Donhaue, who hypothesized that the genetic modulation of the autonomic signaling in AVN cells could have resulted in a prolongation of AVN refractoriness, with consequent beneficial effects on the control of the heart rate.[40] The endpoint of the study was to overexpress the inhibitory subunit of the G protein (Gαi2) in the AVN. Gαi2 inhibits the G protein pathway, and its overexpression is expected to have an effect similar to that of the activation of the muscarinic receptor. The study was conducted in a porcine model of AF. The animals were injected with AdV-Gαi2 in the AV branch of the right coronary artery (see Fig. 56.1). Forty-five percent of the AVN cells expressed the transgene 7 days after injection, and this resulted in a significant slowing of AV conduction time and prolongation of the AVN refractory period. Electrocardiogram (ECG) analysis showed a 20% reduction in the heart rate during AF episodes. In a subsequent study the same group of investigators provided further support to the effectiveness of this approach in a pig model of persistent AF and heart failure.[41] Lugenbiel et al.[42] followed the opposite strategy: suppression of Gαs, the activating G protein on the protein kinase A (PKA) pathway. This approach was justified with the attempt to avoid the excessive tachycardia response during adrenergic stimulation. They designed a sort of "molecular β-blocker" using AdV-mediated siRNA delivery to the AVN to knock down Gαs in a porcine model of AF. This study showed not only a heart rate reduction and an improved rate control during isoproterenol administration but also the amelioration of AF-dependent reduction of the ventricular ejection fraction.

Taken together, these studies demonstrate that rate control treatment of AF using gene therapy is feasible. However, in line with the expectancy for the use of AdV, these positive electrophysiological effects peak at about 7–10 days and decline thereafter. Follow-up studies with different vectors are not available yet, but it is tempting to speculate that long-term rate control of AF could be achieved using AAVs.

Rhythm Control Strategies

The restoration of normal sinus rhythm or the prevention of AF recurrences is an ambitious goal given the pathophysiological complexity and the tendency for self-maintenance of this arrhythmia. One option under investigation is the development of molecular potassium channel blockers to induce an antiarrhythmic class III effect. The concept was first suggested by in vitro studies showing the possibility of knocking down human potassium channels using AdV-mediated delivery of shRNA.[28] Burton et al. and Perlstein et al.[6,43] hypothesized and demonstrated that the overexpression of a loss-of-function mutation (Q9E) in the potassium channel β-subunit MiRP leads to localized I_{Kr} block and action potential prolongation. Subsequently, Amit et al.[44] further exploited this approach by engineering an AdV vector to carry a mutant *KCNH2* cDNA. *KCNH2* is the gene that causes LQTS type 2 and encodes the I_{Kr}; the engineered mutation (G628S) is a well-characterized loss-of-function variant found in several patients.[45] Therefore the transduced cells are expected to display a typical class III effect with action potential prolongation due to reduced I_{Kr}. To obtain the spatial control of transgene delivery, the authors used the technology of "gene painting," which consists of using a paint brush to cover the epicardium

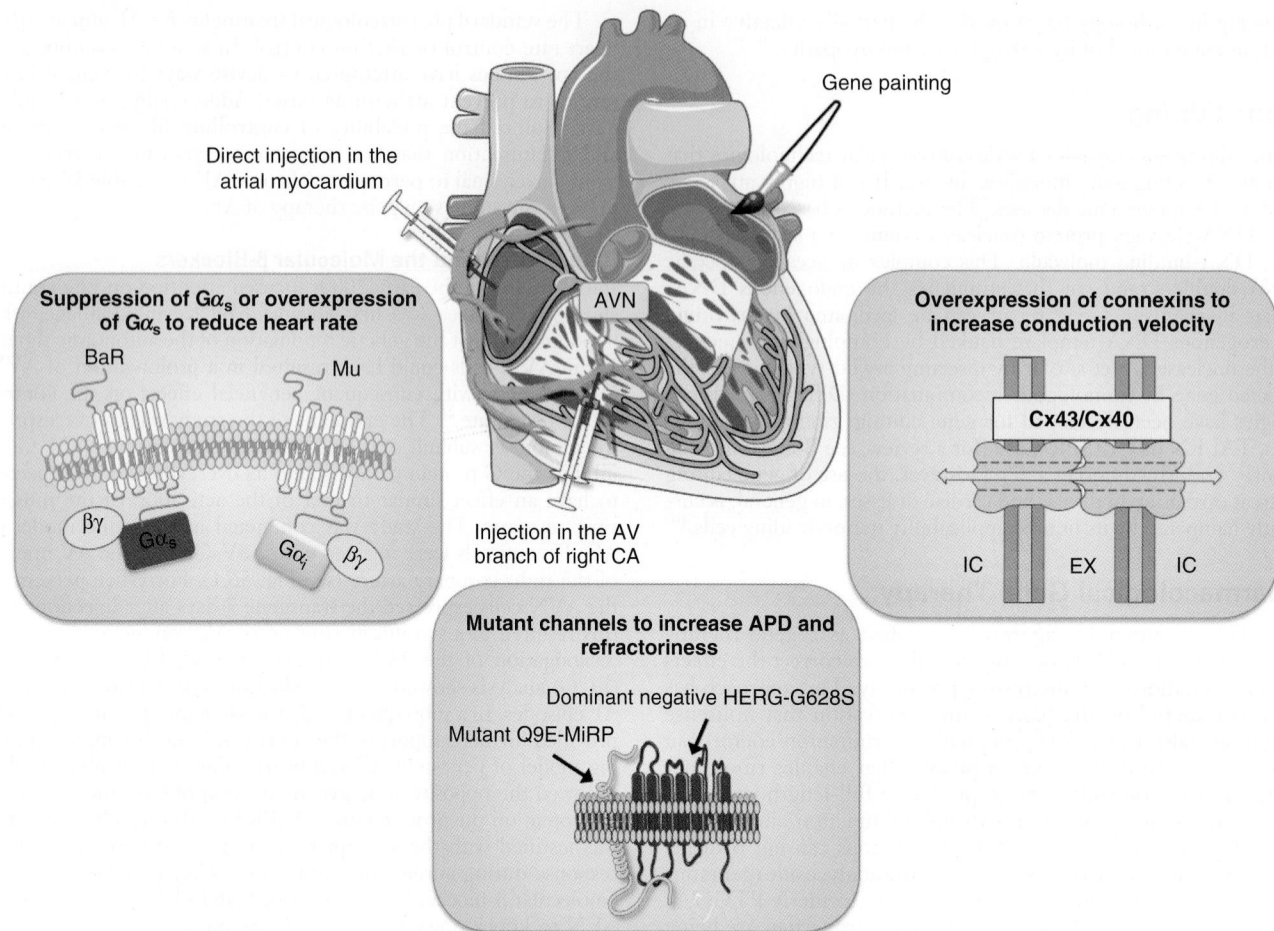

FIGURE 56.1 Gene therapy strategies and delivery approaches that have been tested in experimental studies on atrial fibrillation. See text for the details of the studies. *AV,* Atrioventricular; *AVN,* atrioventricular node; *BaR,* β-adrenergic receptor; *CA,* coronary artery; *EX,* extracellular; *IC,* intracellular; *Mu,* muscarinic receptor.

with a polyoxyethylene/oxypropylene (also known as Pluronic) gel-like material in which the AdV-*KCNH2*-G628S construct was dissolved (before jellification).[46] Open-chest gene painting in pigs with pacing-induced AF resulted in a higher number of animals in sinus rhythm from day 4 to day 10 after painting.[44] This clinical effect was paralleled by increased monophasic action potential duration (APD). The results of Amit et al. have been substantially confirmed by Soucek et al.[47] in a subsequent paper. Together, these studies provide the proof of concept that gene therapy for rhythm control in AF is feasible.

An alternative possibility is the control of conduction velocity. Connexins regulate cell-to-cell electrical coupling. The pathophysiological role of connexins is demonstrated by their downregulation during AF and by the identification of mutations in *GJA5* gene (Cx40) in familial AF.[48,49] Biku et al.[50] and Igarashi et al.[51] assessed the effect of AdV-mediated overexpression of connexins in AF. Igarashi et al.,[51] using atrial gene painting, showed that Cx43 gene transfer is able to reverse the conduction defect and prevent AF induction. Interestingly, Igarashi's study also showed normal conduction velocity during sinus rhythm, suggesting an overall safety of this therapeutic approach.

Control of Inflammation and Apoptosis

The role of inflammation and apoptosis in the maintenance of AF is well known.[38,39] One study has attempted to devise a gene therapy strategy to target this mechanism. Trappe et al. studied a pig model of pacing-induced AF treated with AdV-siRNA-Cas3 to silence caspase, a cysteine protease that is activated specifically

in apoptotic cells.[52] Two weeks after administration (local injections followed by epicardial electroporation), the authors showed significantly increased persistence of sinus rhythm.

In summary, gene therapy studies in AF have attempted to intervene on three vulnerable parameters: refractoriness (APD), conduction velocity, and apoptosis. Robust therapeutic effects have been demonstrated, and the use of localized AVN or atrial delivery avoided proarrhythmic effects at the ventricular level. However, no study has addressed the problem of the short-lasting effects of AdV vectors or attempted the implementation of newer vectors, such as AAVs, to test approaches that may be more suitable for clinical applicability.

Gene Therapy for Ventricular Arrhythmias

The design of gene therapies for ventricular arrhythmias has followed two main strategies (see Table 56.2): to treat the underlying disease that creates the conditions for the onset of the arrhythmias (e.g., ischemia) or to directly treat the specific electrophysiological abnormality (e.g., dysfunctional ion channels) (Fig. 56.2). Gene therapy for both inherited arrhythmogenic disease and acquired arrhythmias, such as those related to CAD, has been considered in the experimental studies.

Inherited Arrhythmias

Inherited arrhythmogenic diseases[45,53] are logical candidates for gene therapy. In these cases the treatment requires a whole-organ administration for widespread infections and at the

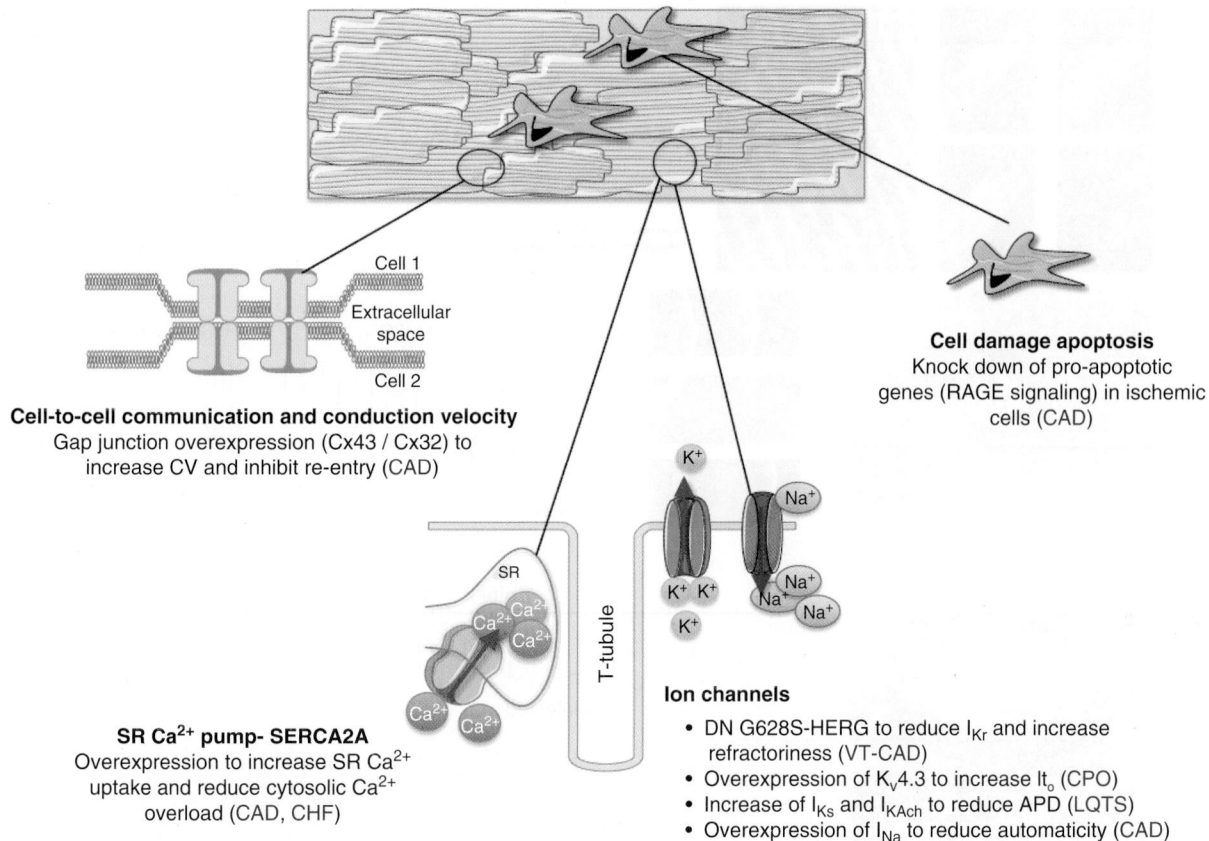

FIGURE 56.2 Strategies for gene therapy of ventricular arrhythmia. See text for the details of the studies. *APD*, Action potential duration; *CAD*, coronary artery disease; *CHF*, congestive heart failure; *CPO*, chronic pressure overload; *CV*, conduction velocity; *DN*, dominant negative; *LQTS*, long QT syndrome; *RAGE*, receptor for advanced glycation end-products; *SR*, sarcoplasmic reticulum; *VT*, ventricular tachycardia.

same time the avoidance of proarrhythmic effects. Therefore the development of effective treatments is very difficult in the absence of reliable animal models reproducing the human disease,[19] as it happens in the case of disorders such as Brugada syndrome and LQTS. On the other hand, we were successful in producing transgenic models of catecholaminergic polymorphic VT (CPVT) that closely reproduce the clinical presentation of the disease.[54–56] The CPVT phenotype is due to altered intracellular calcium handling caused by mutations of two major genes: the cardiac ryanodine receptor (RyR2) and the cardiac calsequestrin (CASQ2).[57,58] These genes are functionally related and, with others, contribute to form the macromolecular complex controlling the sarcoplasmic reticulum (SR) Ca^{2+}-release function. We[55,59,60] and others[61] extensively characterized CASQ2-CPVT mice showing that mutations lead to a reduction of the expressed protein, accompanied by a decrease in the ancillary proteins triadin and junctin (Fig. 56.3A). These abnormalities of gene expression create a series of consequences that are at the origin of the clinical manifestations of the disease: diastolic calcium overload, calcium-wave fragmentation,[62] delayed afterdepolarizations (DADs), adrenergically induced triggered arrhythmias,[56] and ultrastructural abnormalities of the junctional SR (jSR)[60] (see Fig. 56.3). We hypothesized that the restoration of normal CASQ2 protein levels could exert a therapeutic effect in CASQ2-dependent CPVT. We used an AAV9 vector to deliver the *CASQ2* cDNA, and we infected CASQ2-null mice at birth.[60] Five months after infection, we demonstrated a complete normalization of both the electrophysiological and the ultrastructural abnormalities. In subsequent studies, we documented the efficacy of AAV9-*CASQ2* administration in another mouse model harboring a missense

mutation found in a CPVT family (CASQ2-R33Q). Specifically, we confirmed the efficacy of infection at birth, and more importantly, we demonstrated that mice infected at an adult age also showed a complete regression of all the manifestations of the disease, including life-threatening ventricular arrhythmias and ultrastructural abnormalities (see Fig. 56.3A–D). This effect was evident for up to 12 months after the administration of a single dose of the viral construct.[59,62]

From a mechanistic standpoint, it is interesting to observe that the prevention of CPVT arrhythmias was achieved using a relatively limited percentage of infected ventricular myocytes (approximately 40%). We have hypothesized that the apparent discrepancy between the striking therapeutic effect and the relatively low infection rate can be due to the "source–sink" phenomenon.[63] Cell-to-cell propagation is required for a DAD to trigger an action potential. It is only when adjacent myocytes develop synchronous DADs that their summation leads to a triggered action potential spreading to the ventricles. Thus triggered arrhythmias cannot develop unless a sufficient number of the neighboring myocytes develop DADs.[63] Therefore to prevent triggered beats, not all cells are required to be rescued; it is enough that a fraction of them inhibit the propagation of DADs.

Overall, the data on CPVT gene therapy are extremely encouraging for a future clinical development. Few studies focused attention on LQTS. Kodirov et al. used a mouse model of LQTS that they had previously developed using overexpression of a truncated delayed rectifier potassium channel protein (Kv1.1), which has a dominant-negative effect on the 4-aminopyridine (4-AP)–sensitive outward potassium current, I_{Kslow} (encoded by Kv1.5).[64] Although this model does

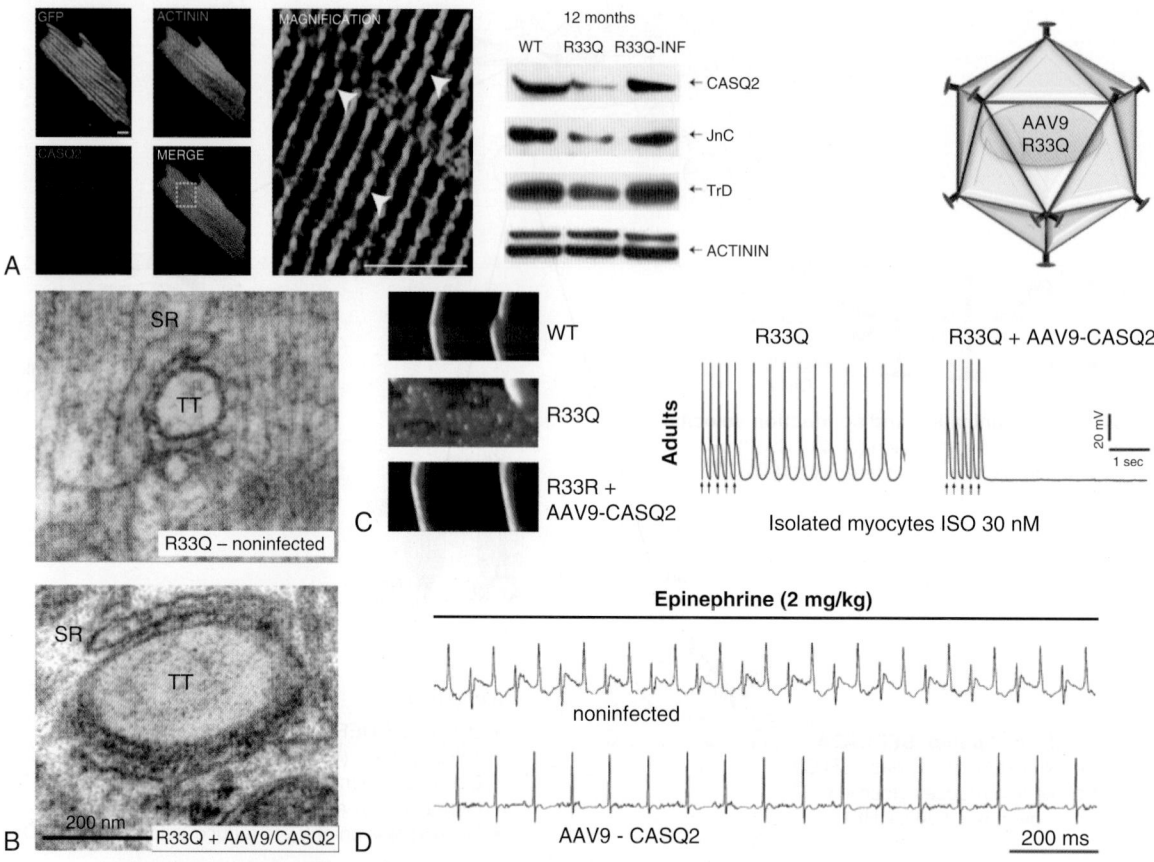

FIGURE 56.3 Gene therapy in catecholaminergic polymorphic ventricular tachycardia. Summary of the effects of administration of AAV9-CASQ2 to transfer wild-type (*WT*) complementary DNA in mice harboring the CASQ2-R33Q mutation. (A) Correct colocalization of calsequestrin (*CASQ2*) (*red*) and actinin (*blue*) in Z lines after gene transfer; the Western blot (*right panel*) shows the restoration of normal calsequestrin levels after gene transfer with AAV9-CASQ2 (R33Q-INF) and normalization of junctin (*JnC*) and triadin (*TrD*) as well. (B) *Upper panel* shows enlarged and fragmented junctional sarcoplasmic reticulum (*SR; yellow*) in untreated mice; *bottom panel*, reappearance of CASQ2 polymers (*small gray spots* into the *SR*) and normalization of the shape of junctional *SR*. (C) Normalization of electrophysiological abnormalities at cellular level: calcium wave fragmentation (*left panel middle*) is reverted to normal (AAV9-CASQ2 *left panel bottom*), and triggered activity is no longer inducible with isoproterenol (*ISO*). *Arrows* indicate stimulated beats. (D) Upper trace shows typical bidirectional ventricular tachycardia that is induced in R33Q mice using epinephrine and is completely prevented after infection with AAV9-CASQ2. All the results presented in the figure have been observed up to 1 year after a single injection of the CASQ2 viral construct. (Modified from Denegri M, Bongianino R, Lodola F, et al. A single delivery of an adeno-associated viral construct to transfer the CASQ2 gene to knock-in mice affected by catecholaminergic polymorphic ventricular tachycardia is able to cure the disease from birth to advanced age. *Circulation.* 2014;129:2673-2681; and Liu N, Denegri M, Dun W, et al. Abnormal propagation of calcium waves and ultrastructural remodeling in recessive catecholaminergic polymorphic ventricular tachycardia. *Circ Res.* 2013;113:142-152.)

not genetically reproduce any of the identified LQTS genetic variants, it is characterized by a very similar phenotype of QT prolongation and ventricular arrhythmias.[65] By direct intramyocardial injection of AAV-Kv1.5, Kodirov et al.[64] showed long-term (6 months) overexpression accompanied by a significant increase in the 4-AP–sensitive current. In parallel, there was a shortening of APD and the suppression of early afterdepolarization. Along the same lines, LQTS gene therapy was attempted by Mazhari et al., who showed a significant action potential and QT shortening with AdV-mediated overexpression of *KCNE3* (a potassium channel β-subunit not normally expressed in the heart). The effect was mediated by increased IKs (slow delayed rectifier) the gene involved in causing the LQT1 variant of LQTS.[66] This proof of concept was obtained in wild-type guinea pigs, and there is no current evidence that the same approach will be effective in transgenic

models of LQT1. Collectively, these data on LQTS-related models prove that it is possible to modify the pattern of ventricular repolarization. Unfortunately, the lack of animal models of LQTS that can fully recapitulate the human phenotype is still a limitation for further development of these approaches.

Acquired Ventricular Arrhythmias

The prevention of ventricular arrhythmias and sudden cardiac death (SCD) in the general population is still a major challenge and one of the most epidemiologically relevant health problems worldwide.[1,45] With the exception of β-blockers, antiarrhythmic drug therapy has largely failed.[67] Thus the availability of more effective strategies to prevent ventricular arrhythmias is a clinically relevant goal. In this context several studies have focused on the development of molecular strategies for the prevention/abolition of ventricular arrhythmias in

CAD models. Four broad therapeutic targets have been identified (see Fig. 56.2):

1. Correction of cellular excitability through the modulation of ion channels
2. Restoration of normal conduction velocity
3. Correction of calcium handling dysfunction
4. Reduction of ischemia-related tissue damage

Ion Channel Modulation. Murata et al.[68] first attempted to create a molecular Ca^{2+}-channel blocker by overexpression of Gem, a GTP-binding protein (RAS superfamily) that suppresses the voltage-gated L-type calcium current (*CACNA1c* gene).[69] AdV-mediated Gem injection in the left ventricular cavity of guinea pigs markedly decreased L-type calcium current density, resulting in the abbreviation of APD and QT interval.[68] Interestingly in the same study, AdV-Gem injection in the AVN successfully reduced heart rate during AF. No direct proofs of an antiarrhythmic effect were reported; furthermore, a negative inotropic effect was noted, thus suggesting that due to the negative hemodynamic consequences, this approach presents substantial limitations.

An interesting alternative was proposed by Sasano et al., who designed an electrophysiologically guided molecular ablation strategy for post-MI VT in pigs.[70] They designed an AdV vector for local delivery of a dominant-negative mutant *KCNH2*-G628S cDNA (the same approach used by Amit et al.[44] for AF). The area of delivery was selected based on the point of origin of the tachycardia mapped using standard clinical electrophysiology techniques. Using this approach, they achieved a complete suppression of inducible VTs accompanied by lengthening of APD and effective refractory period in the injection area.[70] The study by Sasano et al. proves the idea that in cases of a localized arrhythmogenic area (such as the reentrant arrhythmias in the infarct border zone), local gene therapy is a feasible and safe approach. As previously mentioned, in these instances the need for a local antiarrhythmic effect can greatly simplify the choice of the delivery vector and strategy.

Restoration of Conduction Velocity. Other studies have addressed the possibility of treating ischemia-related arrhythmias through the modulation of conduction velocity. The group of Mike Rosen conducted an experimental study targeted to increase conduction velocity in the ischemic tissue to prevent development of reentrant circuits. Accordingly, they explored the use of AdV vectors to express the skeletal muscle sodium channel gene in the infarct border zone.[71] After an average of 6 days postinjection in the infarcted area, the study showed QRS shortening, reduced fragmentation of electrograms, increased Vmax, and increased conduction velocity. Most importantly, there was a 58% absolute risk reduction of VT inducibility during programmed electrical stimulation.[71]

Two additional studies have attempted to increase conduction velocity by overexpressing connexins, the channels controlling the cell-to-cell electrical coupling. Both Cx32[72] and Cx43[73] have been considered as candidates for gene therapy in post-MI VTs. In both cases a significant reduction of inducible VT was observed (see Table 56.2).

Correction of Sarcoplasmic Reticulum Calcium Handling Dysfunction. Gene transfer of the SR adenosine triphosphatase (ATPase) (SERCA) was originally developed as a means to treat heart failure. Based on positive results obtained in an animal study, AAV-mediated gene therapy with SERCA has been clinically tested in the CUPID study.[74] While the CUPID study showed the safety of gene delivery of the SERCA gene in heart failure patients, it failed to demonstrate a beneficial effect on survival.[75] The authors speculated that the lack of reduction in mortality was likely due to a low dose of the therapeutic construct, and they suggested that further studies should be performed to optimize dose finding and delivery strategy. Interestingly, the delivery of the SERCA gene has been successfully used to prevent calcium-overload–induced triggered activity in a model of myocardial infarction followed by reperfusion,[76] supporting the view that this therapy, which has demonstrated safety in the clinical setting, should be further investigated.

Reduction of Ischemia-Related Tissue Damage. An alternative strategy to prevent arrhythmias using a gene therapy approach is acting on the pathways that mediate ischemic cell damage. A recent paper[9] has reported using a nonviral gene delivery approach with PEIs to knock down the RAGE with a specific siRNA. RAGE is a "damage-associated" protein, and its activation is involved in cell migration, proliferation, and inflammatory responses. RAGE is also an important mediator of cardiac ischemic injury.[77] The therapeutic construct containing the siRNA was injected into the infarct border zone in rats. Besides the expected inhibition of inflammation and apoptosis, the authors showed that therapy was able to restore normal action potential amplitude and preserve normal conduction velocity in ischemic cells. Remarkably, this resulted in a significant (71%) reduction in VT inducibility.

In summary, more than one decade of studies has provided important proof of concept that gene therapy is able to modulate the cardiac electrophysiological substrate to achieve an antiarrhythmic effect even in complex substrates such as CAD. However, similar to AF studies, no study has attempted to address the crucial issue of the long-term maintenance of the antiarrhythmic effects. Thus work in this direction is needed before gene therapy may be considered for clinical use.

Conclusions

Historically, the pharmacological therapy of cardiac arrhythmias has been a major challenge for the scientific community. The development of gene therapy for the same targets is revealing itself as a comparably demanding task. Certainly, important proofs of concepts have been obtained, and gene therapy has been revealed to have important "pluses" over standard drug therapy: target selectivity, possibility of localized delivery for focal arrhythmias, and choice of vectors with different expression duration. On the other hand, the precise control of delivery, infection efficiency, and the possibility of toxic/immunogenic side effects are problems that still call for definitive solutions. In recent years, the rapid development of AAV technology that allows for efficient, organ-specific infections and for very long (possibly permanent) transgene expression has paved the way to the clinical applicability of gene therapy for inherited arrhythmogenic diseases. The fundamental studies described in this chapter have identified targets and have proved their feasibility. The next steps of development will require preclinical assessment of safety and dose finding before designing the first clinical study in humans.

REFERENCES

1. Priori SG, Blomstrom-Lundqvist C, Mazzanti A, et al. 2015 ESC Guidelines for the management of patients with ventricular arrhythmias and the prevention of sudden cardiac death: The Task Force for the Management of Patients with Ventricular Arrhythmias and the Prevention of Sudden Cardiac Death of the European Society of Cardiology (ESC). Endorsed by: Association for European Paediatric and Congenital Cardiology (AEPC). *Eur Heart J.* 2015;36:2793–2867.

2. Fabritz L, Guasch E, Antoniades C, et al. Expert consensus document: Defining the major health modifiers causing atrial fibrillation: a roadmap to underpin personalized prevention and treatment. *Nat Rev Cardiol.* 2016;13:230–237.

3. Camm AJ, Lip GY, De Caterina R, et al. 2012 focused update of the ESC Guidelines for the management of atrial fibrillation: an update of the 2010 ESC Guidelines for the management of atrial fibrillation. Developed with the special contribution of the European Heart Rhythm Association. *Eur Heart J.* 2012;33:2719–2747.

4. Lin H, Parmacek MS, Morle G, et al. Expression of recombinant genes in myocardium in vivo after direct injection of DNA. *Circulation.* 1990;82:2217–2221.

5. Penn MS, Mendelsohn FO, Schaer GL, et al. An open-label dose escalation study to evaluate the safety of administration of nonviral stromal cell-derived factor-1 plasmid to treat symptomatic ischemic heart failure. *Circ Res.* 2013;112:816–825.

6. Burton DY, Song C, Fishbein I, et al. The incorporation of an ion channel gene mutation associated with the long QT syndrome (Q9E-hMiRP1) in a plasmid vector for site-specific arrhythmia gene therapy: in vitro and in vivo feasibility studies. *Hum Gene Ther*. 2003;14:907–922.
7. Cartier R, Reszka R. Utilization of synthetic peptides containing nuclear localization signals for nonviral gene transfer systems. *Gene Ther*. 2002;9:157–167.
8. Dincer S, Turk M, Piskin E. Intelligent polymers as nonviral vectors. *Gene Ther*. 2005;12(suppl 1):S139–S145.
9. Park H, Ku SH, Park H, et al. RAGE siRNA-mediated gene silencing provides cardioprotection against ventricular arrhythmias in acute ischemia and reperfusion. *J Control Release*. 2015;217:315–326.
10. Kooijmans SA, Vader P, van Dommelen SM, et al. Exosome mimetics: a novel class of drug delivery systems. *Int J Nanomedicine*. 2012;7:1525–1541.
11. Stratford-Perricaudet LD, Makeh I, Perricaudet M, et al. Widespread long-term gene transfer to mouse skeletal muscles and heart. *J Clin Invest*. 1992;90:626–630.
12. Russell WC. Update on adenovirus and its vectors. *J Gen Virol*. 2000;81:2573–2604.
13. French BA, Mazur W, Geske RS, et al. Direct in vivo gene transfer into porcine myocardium using replication-deficient adenoviral vectors. *Circulation*. 1994;90:2414–2424.
14. Maurice JP, Hata JA, Shah AS, et al. Enhancement of cardiac function after adenoviral-mediated in vivo intracoronary beta2-adrenergic receptor gene delivery. *J Clin Invest*. 1999;104:21–29.
15. Rosengart TK, Lee LY, Patel SR, et al. Angiogenesis gene therapy: phase I assessment of direct intramyocardial administration of an adenovirus vector expressing VEGF121 cDNA to individuals with clinically significant severe coronary artery disease. *Circulation*. 1999;100:468–474.
16. Rosengart TK, Bishawi MM, Halbreiner MS, et al. Long-term follow-up assessment of a phase 1 trial of angiogenic gene therapy using direct intramyocardial administration of an adenoviral vector expressing the VEGF121 cDNA for the treatment of diffuse coronary artery disease. *Hum Gene Ther*. 2013;24:203–208.
17. Assessment of adenoviral vector safety and toxicity. Report of the National Institutes of Health Recombinant DNA Advisory Committee. *Hum Gene Ther*. 2002;13:3–13.
18. Xu ZL, Mizuguchi H, Sakurai F, et al. Approaches to improving the kinetics of adenovirus-delivered genes and gene products. *Adv Drug Deliv Rev*. 2005;57:781–802.
19. Bongianino R, Priori SG. Gene therapy to treat cardiac arrhythmias. *Nat Rev Cardiol*. 2015;12:531–546.
20. Hacein-Bey-Abina S, Von Kalle C, Schmidt M, et al. LMO2-associated clonal T cell proliferation in two patients after gene therapy for SCID-X1. *Science*. 2003;302:415–419.
21. Galimi F, Noll M, Kanazawa Y, et al. Gene therapy of Fanconi anemia: preclinical efficacy using lentiviral vectors. *Blood*. 2002;100:2732–2736.
22. Hacein-Bey Abina S, Gaspar HB, Blondeau J, et al. Outcomes following gene therapy in patients with severe Wiskott-Aldrich syndrome. *JAMA*. 2015;313:1550–1563.
23. Zacchigna S, Zentilin L, Giacca M. Adeno-associated virus vectors as therapeutic and investigational tools in the cardiovascular system. *Circ Res*. 2014;114:1827–1846.
24. Wu Z, Asokan A, Grieger JC, et al. Single amino acid changes can influence titer, heparin binding, and tissue tropism in different adeno-associated virus serotypes. *J Virol*. 2006;80:11393–11397.
25. Ghosh A, Duan D. Expanding adeno-associated viral vector capacity: a tale of two vectors. *Biotechnol Genet Eng Rev*. 2007;24:165–177.
26. Mearini G, Stimpel D, Kramer E, et al. Repair of Mybpc3 mRNA by 5'-trans-splicing in a mouse model of hypertrophic cardiomyopathy. *Mol Ther Nucleic Acids*. 2013;2:e102.
27. Grimm D, Streetz KL, Jopling CL, et al. Fatality in mice due to oversaturation of cellular microRNA/short hairpin RNA pathways. *Nature*. 2006;441:537–541.
28. Liu X, Yang J, Shang F, et al. Silencing GIRK4 expression in human atrial myocytes by adenovirus-delivered small hairpin RNA. *Mol Biol Rep*. 2009;36:1345–1352.
29. Jiang J, Wakimoto H, Seidman JG, et al. Allele-specific silencing of mutant Myh6 transcripts in mice suppresses hypertrophic cardiomyopathy. *Science*. 2013;342:111–114.
30. Mussolino C, Mlambo T, Cathomen T. Proven and novel strategies for efficient editing of the human genome. *Curr Opin Pharmacol*. 2015;24:105–112.
31. Linde L, Boelz S, Nissim-Rafinia M, et al. Nonsense-mediated mRNA decay affects nonsense transcript levels and governs response of cystic fibrosis patients to gentamicin. *J Clin Invest*. 2007;117:683–692.
32. Grant AO, Carboni MP, Neplioueva V, et al. Long QT syndrome, Brugada syndrome, and conduction system disease are linked to a single sodium channel mutation. *J Clin Invest*. 2002;110:1201–1209.
33. Teng S, Gao L, Paajanen V, et al. Readthrough of nonsense mutation W822X in the SCN5A gene can effectively restore expression of cardiac Na+ channels. *Cardiovasc Res*. 2009;83:473–480.
34. Mullard A. EMA reconsiders 'read-through' drug against Duchenne muscular dystrophy following appeal. *Nat Biotechnol*. 2014;32:706.
35. Yao Y, Teng S, Li N, et al. Aminoglycoside antibiotics restore functional expression of truncated HERG channels produced by nonsense mutations. *Heart Rhythm*. 2009;6:553–560.
36. Gaborit N, Le Bouter S, Szuts V, et al. Regional and tissue specific transcript signatures of ion channel genes in the non-diseased human heart. *J Physiol*. 2007;582:675–693.
37. Antzelevitch C, Yan GX. J wave syndromes. *Heart Rhythm*. 2010;7:549–558.
38. Wijffels MC, Kirchhof CJ, Dorland R, et al. Atrial fibrillation begets atrial fibrillation. A study in awake chronically instrumented goats. *Circulation*. 1995;92:1954–1968.
39. Allessie M, Ausma J, Schotten U. Electrical, contractile and structural remodeling during atrial fibrillation. *Cardiovasc Res*. 2002;54:230–246.
40. Donahue JK, Heldman AW, Fraser H, et al. Focal modification of electrical conduction in the heart by viral gene transfer. *Nat Med*. 2000;6:1395–1398.
41. Bauer A, McDonald AD, Nasir K, et al. Inhibitory G protein overexpression provides physiologically relevant heart rate control in persistent atrial fibrillation. *Circulation*. 2004;110:3115–3120.
42. Lugenbiel P, Thomas D, Kelemen K, et al. Genetic suppression of Galphas protein provides rate control in atrial fibrillation. *Basic Res Cardiol*. 2012;107:265.
43. Perlstein I, Burton DY, Ryan K, et al. Posttranslational control of a cardiac ion channel transgene in vivo: clarithromycin-hMiRP1-Q9E interactions. *Hum Gene Ther*. 2005;16:906–910.
44. Amit G, Kikuchi K, Greener ID, et al. Selective molecular potassium channel blockade prevents atrial fibrillation. *Circulation*. 2010;121:2263–2270.
45. Napolitano C, Bloise R, Monteforte N, et al. Sudden cardiac death and genetic ion channelopathies: long QT, Brugada, short QT, catecholaminergic polymorphic ventricular tachycardia, and idiopathic ventricular fibrillation. *Circulation*. 2012;125:2027–2034.
46. Kikuchi K, McDonald AD, Sasano T, et al. Targeted modification of atrial electrophysiology by homogeneous transmural atrial gene transfer. *Circulation*. 2005;111:264–270.
47. Soucek R, Thomas D, Kelemen K, et al. Genetic suppression of atrial fibrillation using a dominant-negative ether-a-go-go-related gene mutant. *Heart Rhythm*. 2012;9:265–272.
48. Delmar M, Makita N. Cardiac connexins, mutations and arrhythmias. *Curr Opin Cardiol*. 2012;27:236–241.
49. Gollob MH, Jones DL, Krahn AD, et al. Somatic mutations in the connexin 40 gene (GJA5) in atrial fibrillation. *N Engl J Med*. 2006;354:2677–2688.
50. Bikou O, Thomas D, Trappe K, et al. Connexin 43 gene therapy prevents persistent atrial fibrillation in a porcine model. *Cardiovasc Res*. 2011;92:218–225.
51. Igarashi T, Finet JE, Takeuchi A, et al. Connexin gene transfer preserves conduction velocity and prevents atrial fibrillation. *Circulation*. 2012;125:216–225.
52. Trappe K, Thomas D, Bikou O, et al. Suppression of persistent atrial fibrillation by genetic knockdown of caspase 3: a pre-clinical pilot study. *Eur Heart J*. 2013;34:147–157.
53. Priori SG, Chen SR. Inherited dysfunction of sarcoplasmic reticulum Ca^{2+} handling and arrhythmogenesis. *Circ Res*. 2011;108:871–883.
54. Cerrone M, Colombi B, Santoro M, et al. Bidirectional ventricular tachycardia and fibrillation elicited in a knock-in mouse model carrier of a mutation in the cardiac ryanodine receptor. *Circ Res*. 2005;96:e77–e82.
55. Rizzi N, Liu N, Napolitano C, et al. Unexpected structural and functional consequences of the R33Q homozygous mutation in cardiac calsequestrin: a complex arrhythmogenic cascade in a knock in mouse model. *Circ Res*. 2008;103:298–306.
56. Liu N, Colombi B, Memmi M, et al. Arrhythmogenesis in catecholaminergic polymorphic ventricular tachycardia: insights from a RyR2 R4496C knock-in mouse model. *Circ Res*. 2006;99:292–298.
57. Eldar M, Pras E, Lahat H. A missense mutation in the CASQ2 gene is associated with autosomal-recessive catecholamine-induced polymorphic ventricular tachycardia. *Trends Cardiovasc Med*. 2003;13:148–151.
58. Priori SG, Napolitano C, Tiso N, et al. Mutations in the cardiac ryanodine receptor gene (hRyR2) underlie catecholaminergic polymorphic ventricular tachycardia. *Circulation*. 2001;103:196–200.
59. Denegri M, Bongianino R, Lodola F, et al. A single delivery of an adeno-associated viral construct to transfer the CASQ2 gene to knock-in mice affected by catecholaminergic polymorphic ventricular tachycardia is able to cure the disease from birth to advanced age. *Circulation*. 2014;129:2673–2681.
60. Denegri M, Avelino-Cruz JE, Boncompagni S, et al. Viral gene transfer rescues arrhythmogenic phenotype and ultrastructural abnormalities in adult calsequestrin-null mice with inherited arrhythmias. *Circ Res*. 2012;110:663–668.
61. Knollmann BC, Chopra N, Hlaing T, et al. Casq2 deletion causes sarcoplasmic reticulum volume increase, premature Ca^{2+} release, and catecholaminergic polymorphic ventricular tachycardia. *J Clin Invest*. 2006;116:2510–2520.
62. Liu N, Denegri M, Dun W, et al. Abnormal propagation of calcium waves and ultrastructural remodeling in recessive catecholaminergic polymorphic ventricular tachycardia. *Circ Res*. 2013;113:142–152.
63. Xie Y, Sato D, Garfinkel A, et al. So little source, so much sink: requirements for afterdepolarizations to propagate in tissue. *Biophys J*. 2010;99:1408–1415.
64. Kodirov SA, Brunner M, Busconi L, et al. Long-term restitution of 4-aminopyridine-sensitive currents in Kv1DN ventricular myocytes using adeno-associated virus-mediated delivery of Kv1.5. *FEBS Lett*. 2003;550:74–78.
65. London B, Jeron A, Zhou J, et al. Long QT and ventricular arrhythmias in transgenic mice expressing the N terminus and first transmembrane segment of a voltage-gated potassium channel. *Proc Natl Acad Sci U S A*. 1998;95:2926–2931.
66. Mazhari R, Nuss HB, Armoundas AA, et al. Ectopic expression of KCNE3 accelerates cardiac repolarization and abbreviates the QT interval. *J Clin Invest*. 2002;109:1083–1090.
67. Preliminary report: effect of encainide and flecainide on mortality in a randomized trial of arrhythmia suppression after myocardial infarction. The Cardiac Arrhythmia Suppression Trial (CAST) Investigators. *N Engl J Med*. 1989;321:406–412.
68. Murata M, Cingolani E, McDonald AD, et al. Creation of a genetic calcium channel blocker by targeted gem gene transfer in the heart. *Circ Res*. 2004;95:398–405.
69. Beguin P, Nagashima K, Gonoi T, et al. Regulation of Ca2+ channel expression at the cell surface by the small G-protein kir/Gem. *Nature*. 2001;411:701–706.
70. Sasano T, McDonald AD, Kikuchi K, et al. Molecular ablation of ventricular tachycardia after myocardial infarction. *Nat Med*. 2006;12:1256–1258.
71. Lau DH, Clausen C, Sosunov EA, et al. Epicardial border zone overexpression of skeletal muscle sodium channel SkM1 normalizes activation, preserves conduction, and suppresses ventricular arrhythmia: an in silico, in vivo, in vitro study. *Circulation*. 2009;119:19–27.
72. Prestia KA, Sosunov EA, Anyukhovsky EP, et al. Increased cell-cell coupling increases infarct size and does not decrease incidence of ventricular tachycardia in mice. *Front Physiol*. 2011;2:1.
73. Greener ID, Sasano T, Wan X, et al. Connexin43 gene transfer reduces ventricular tachycardia susceptibility after myocardial infarction. *J Am Coll Cardiol*. 2012;60:1103–1110.
74. Jessup M, Greenberg B, Mancini D, et al. Calcium Upregulation by Percutaneous Administration of Gene Therapy in Cardiac Disease (CUPID): a phase 2 trial of intracoronary gene therapy of sarcoplasmic reticulum Ca^{2+}-ATPase in patients with advanced heart failure. *Circulation*. 2011;124:304–313.
75. Greenberg B, Butler J, Felker GM, et al. Calcium upregulation by percutaneous administration of gene therapy in patients with cardiac disease (CUPID 2): a randomised, multinational, double-blind, placebo-controlled, phase 2b trial. *Lancet*. 2016;387:1178–1186.
76. del Monte F, Lebeche D, Guerrero JL, et al. Abrogation of ventricular arrhythmias in a model of ischemia and reperfusion by targeting myocardial calcium cycling. *Proc Natl Acad Sci U S A*. 2004;101:5622–5627.
77. Aleshin A, Ananthakrishnan R, Li Q, et al. RAGE modulates myocardial injury consequent to LAD infarction via impact on JNK and STAT signaling in a murine model. *Am J Physiol Heart Circ Physiol*. 2008;294:H1823–H1832.
78. Brunner M, Kodirov SA, Mitchell GF, et al. In vivo gene transfer of Kv1.5 normalizes action potential duration and shortens QT interval in mice with long QT phenotype. *Am J Physiol Heart Circ Physiol*. 2003;285:H194–H203.
79. Lebeche D, Kaprielian R, del Monte F, et al. In vivo cardiac gene transfer of Kv4.3 abrogates the hypertrophic response in rats after aortic stenosis. *Circulation*. 2004;110:3435–3443.
80. Prunier F, Kawase Y, Gianni D, et al. Prevention of ventricular arrhythmias with sarcoplasmic reticulum Ca2+ ATPase pump overexpression in a porcine model of ischemia reperfusion. *Circulation*. 2008;118:614–624.
81. Lyon AR, Bannister ML, Collins T, et al. SERCA2a gene transfer decreases sarcoplasmic reticulum calcium leak and reduces ventricular arrhythmias in a model of chronic heart failure. *Circ Arrhythm Electrophysiol*. 2011;4:362–372.
82. Cutler MJ, Wan X, Plummer BN, et al. Targeted sarcoplasmic reticulum Ca2+ ATPase 2a gene delivery to restore electrical stability in the failing heart. *Circulation*. 2012;126:2095–2104.

57

Highly Mature Human iPSC–Derived Cardiomyocytes as Models for Cardiac Electrophysiology and Drug Testing

Todd J. Herron

Current Guidelines for Cardiotoxicity and Proarrhythmia Screening

Cardiotoxicity is a major reason for drug attrition and is thus a core subject in preclinical and clinical safety testing of new drugs.[1] Cardiac safety testing of new chemical entities that become lead drug candidates is a critical aspect of the drug discovery and development pipeline.[2] A large number of cardiac side effects of cardiac and noncardiac drugs are caused by drug interactions with one or more cardiac ion channels.[1,3] Cardiac ion channels regulate cellular excitability, contractility, and overall cardiac performance, and alteration of cardiac ion channel function can lead to sudden cardiac death[4]; this contributed to the release of International Council on Harmonisation of Technical Requirements for Registration of Pharmaceuticals for Human Use (ICH S7B) guidelines dedicated to the identification of the risk of fatal arrhythmia due to drugs in preclinical testing.[5] Since 2005, cardiac safety of a compound has been determined almost exclusively by its effect or potential effect on the QT interval of the electrocardiogram (ECG) or the action potential duration (APD; Fig. 57.1A and B) and its potential to lead to a life-threatening arrhythmia called torsades de pointes (TdP).[5] QT prolongation, however, is not the ideal indicator for TdP as drugs that prolong QT interval do not always cause TdP.[6] Despite the key role that studies on QT prolongation play in preclinical drug development, it is recognized that this parameter is only a surrogate marker for proarrhythmia.[7] Data from preclinical and clinical trials have shown that there is no fixed relationship between the magnitude of QT prolongation and the risk for development of fatal arrhythmias such as TdP.[8,9] Furthermore, a number of blockbuster drugs have been withdrawn from the market because they were found to cause cardiotoxicity in humans even when they were found to be safe in preclinical animal testing.[10,11] For these reasons, there is a revolution dawning in the cardiotoxicity preclinical testing field and in the search for a more predictive and reliable test.[12]

Current ICH S7B Guidelines for Preclinical Drug Testing: hERG Current Assay

The in vitro surrogate for predicting potential QT prolongation effects of a drug compound involves measurement of single potassium current (I_{Kr}). The human ether-à-go-go–related gene (*hERG* or *KCNH2*) encodes the pore-forming α-subunit of a voltage-gated potassium channel in the heart. hERG (or Kv11.1) (I_{Kr}), which is involved in cardiac repolarization, has become the centerpiece for preclinical in vitro cardiac safety pharmacology.[13] Inhibition of the hERG current is thought to cause cardiac APD prolongation and, by inference, QT interval prolongation resulting in potentially fatal ventricular tachyarrhythmia (TdP). In vitro optical mapping of neonatal rat ventricular cardiomyocytes has revealed that spatial gradients of repolarization caused by hERG activity can lead to arrhythmia phenotypes.[14] Thus altered hERG channel function and spatial dispersion of repolarization are both critical for abnormal cardiac function.[1]

The relationship between the ventricular action potential, hERG channel function, and the ECG is depicted in Fig. 57.1C. hERG channel function contributes to repolarization of the action potential during phases 2–4 of the cardiac action potential. Reduction of the hERG current can cause ventricular cardiomyocyte APD prolongation and is expected to result in QT prolongation in vivo. Fig. 57.1 demonstrates the simple scenario that made it apparent for the drug discovery process to screen drug compounds early in the development phase to determine potential proarrhythmia risk.[15] The dogma followed today is that under normal circumstances, potassium outward current via hERG is a dominant factor in the repolarization phase of the ventricular action potential and thus is a key determinant of the APD. Any inhibitions of this hERG channel activity are presumed to slow repolarization, prolong APD and, by inference, must also prolong the QT interval.[15] This dogma is a gross oversimplification of a complex biological process and does not take into account the potential contributions of other ion channels that compensate for the blockade of the hERG channel. Nevertheless, this paradigm has become the critical element to enable an early in vitro preclinical approach focused on a quantifiable molecular marker (hERG) to predict a potentially fatal adverse drug reaction (TdP).[16]

Limitations of the In Vitro Heterologous Cell–Based hERG Current Assay

The in vitro hERG channel assay is most routinely performed in contract research organizations (CROs) that conduct toxicity studies for pharmaceutical companies.[17] The vast majority

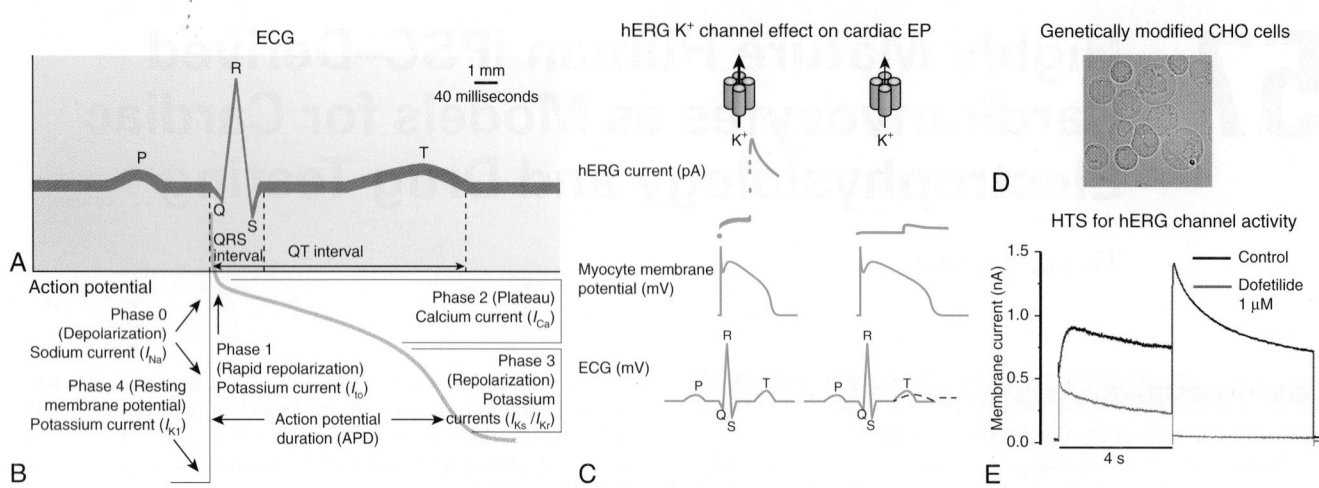

FIGURE 57.1 Current preclinical testing of new drugs focuses on QT prolongation of the electrocardiogram (ECG). (A) Example ECG trace pointing out the QT interval. (B) Cardiac action potential pointing out each phase of the action potential. The action potential duration (APD) determines the duration of the QT interval. Drugs found to prolong the APD are assumed to prolong the QT interval and increase the risk for fatal arrhythmias. (C) hERG channel assay for preclinical proarrhythmia screening of new drugs. The hERG potassium channel is the centerpiece of the current regulatory process. hERG channel function repolarizes the membrane during the action potential. Reduced hERG current (hERG block) prolongs the action potential and is presumed to increase the QT interval on the ECG. (D) The hERG channel assay is performed using Chinese hamster ovary (CHO) cells that are genetically modified to express the human hERG channel. (E) Example recordings of hERG channel function. Dofetilide (*red*) is a standard reagent used to block the hERG channel. ([A and B] Modified from Chi KR. Revolution dawning in cardiotoxicity testing. *Nat Rev Drug Discov.* 2013;12:565-567. [C, D, and E] From Pollard CE, Abi Gerges N, Bridgland-Taylor MH, et al. An introduction to QT interval prolongation and non-clinical approaches to assessing and reducing risk. *Br J Pharmacol.* 2010;159:12-21.)

of hERG channel assays utilize genetically modified animal cells overexpressing just the hERG channel (see Fig. 57.1D and E). In the hERG inhibition assay, Chinese hamster ovary cells transfected with the hERG gene (CHO-hERG) are plated into a high-throughput single-cell planar patch-clamp system.[18] The high-throughput nature of the hERG assay performed in 384 well plates allows recordings of hERG current in up to 384 individual cells within minutes. For this reason, the hERG assay, performed in heterologous cell systems, is currently positioned in lead optimization to eliminate compounds and/or chemically reengineer the compounds early in drug discovery that may have the potential for TdP risk.[19,20] Using this simplified approach to a complex biological process may erroneously label compounds as proarrhythmic and eliminate potentially useful drugs from development and commercialization.

In fact, evidence shows that hERG channel inhibition does not always correlate with APD prolongation, QT prolongation, and risk for proarrhythmia (TdP). For example, Fig. 57.2A demonstrates that not all drugs that block the hERG channel in vitro cause APD prolongation in cardiomyocytes.[7] Fig. 57.2A compares the effects of 10 different drug compounds on hERG current block in the hERG assay, with prolongation of the Purkinje fiber APD in canines. Drugs that block hERG channel activity and clearly increase APD are referred to as overt hERG blockers (e.g., E-4031 and moxifloxacin). On the other hand, there are drugs that block hERG with high potency but have no effect on APD of cardiomyocytes (e.g., haloperidol and fluoxetine). These drugs are called covert hERG blockers. Verapamil is a widely prescribed calcium channel blocker that also blocks the hERG channel in preclinical tests but has not been associated with either QT prolongation or TdP. In fact, verapamil reportedly shortens the QT interval.[21] This effect of verapamil is attributed to concomitant block of L-type calcium current that mitigates effects of hERG channel block.[22] Also, clinically safe drugs such as fluoxetine (Prozac, antidepressant) and citalopram (Celexa, antidepressant) are examples of hERG blocking compounds that do not

affect APD (see Fig. 57.2A) or QT duration and do not lead to clinical TdP.[23] Under the current ICH cardiotoxicity guidelines, the popular and revolutionary antidepressant drug Prozac (Eli Lilly, worldwide exposure of over 54 million patients), which has a low incidence of arrhythmogenic liability, would likely not have been considered for development.[2] Early in the current development pipeline, Prozac would fail under the current guidelines because it is a potent hERG blocker and would be assumed to prolong APD and QT interval. Due to the ubiquitous and nearly exclusive use of the hERG single-cell/single-channel assay early in the drug development process, it is likely that potentially useful drugs have been eliminated wrongfully from development, and potential therapies are not being delivered to patients. A better in vitro testing platform would utilize a cell culture system comprising electrically excitable human cardiomyocytes that contain the full complement of ion channels that make up the cardiac action potential (see Fig. 57.2B).

Human Cardiomyocytes for Preclinical Cardiotoxicity Testing: Primary Cells

The use of human cardiomyocytes that mimic the phenotype of adult cardiomyocytes presents the ideal platform for early preclinical screening for drug cardiotoxicity. Single cardiomyocytes isolated from human hearts have been used to study electrophysiology,[24] intracellular calcium dynamics,[25] and contraction[26]; however, the viability and yield of live cells from these hearts is very low, and studies can only be performed on very small numbers of cells. The availability of usable hearts is limited, and the logistics of obtaining explanted human hearts are complicated and require a team of people on standby to be ready to accept the heart and isolate single cardiomyocytes at any hour. Another limitation of using cardiomyocytes isolated from adult human hearts is the technical challenge of maintaining the cells in culture long term.[24,27] This is due to rapid dedifferentiation of the structural and functional phenotype of adult cardiomyocytes in

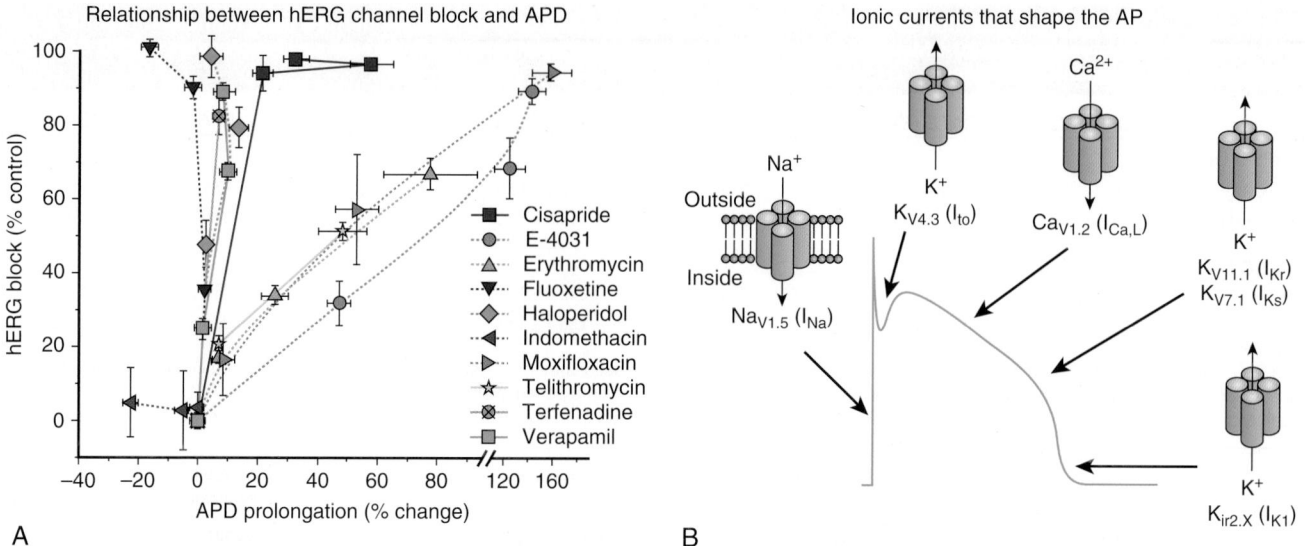

FIGURE 57.2 Comparison of action potential duration (*APD*) prolongation and hERG current inhibition with ten different drugs. (A) Overt hERG blocking drugs increase APD of cardiomyocytes and block the hERG channel. On the other hand, covert hERG blocking drugs do not increase the APD of cardiomyocytes. Exclusive reliance on the hERG assay may falsely label drugs as proarrhythmic. (B) The cardiac action potential (*AP*) is determined by the activity of many ion channels. The hERG channel assay, which relies on a single ion channel (Kv11.1, I_{Kr}) conductance assay, is an oversimplification of a complex biological process. An assay that utilizes cells whose excitability depends on the full complement of cardiac ion channels is required for more accurate drug screening for proarrhythmias. ([A] From Gintant GA. Preclinical torsades-de-pointes screens: advantages and limitations of surrogate and direct approaches in evaluating proarrhythmic risk. *Pharmacol Ther.* 2008;119:199-209. [B] From Pollard CE, Abi Gerges N, Bridgland-Taylor MH, et al. An introduction to QT interval prolongation and non-clinical approaches to assessing and reducing risk. *Br J Pharmacol.* 2010;159:12-21.)

culture.[28] Finally, the low-throughput nature of using human cardiomyocytes obtained from explanted hearts precludes the use of this type of assay for early phases of drug development where high-throughput screens are required.

For study of cardiac electrical impulse propagation, human heart optical mapping is limited to unused donor hearts or explanted diseased hearts available for research at the time of cardiac transplantation.[29] Although in vitro human heart optical mapping has been reported[29,30] and mechanistic insights have been published, the health and availability of the hearts used must be carefully determined and the conclusions that can be drawn based on data collected from clinically unsuitable human hearts must be cautiously made. Here again, the low throughput of this approach precludes utility for drug screening tests, and the unreliable nature of the preparation makes it unattractive for the drug development process. The development of novel approaches for supplying human cardiomyocytes useful in the drug discovery industry is required.

Human Pluripotent Stem Cell–Derived Cardiomyocytes for Cardiotoxicity Testing

Human pluripotent stem cell–derived cardiomyocytes (hPSC-CMs) represent a relatively new alternative model system for the study of human cardiac electrophysiology and arrhythmia mechanisms in vitro.[31–34] hPSC-CMs represent a relatively novel biological system to serve as a pharmacological model for drug testing and for the development of disease-specific models.[35,36] Two types of hPSC-CMs can be used: human embryonic stem cell–derived cardiomyocytes (hESC-CMs) and human induced pluripotent stem cell–derived cardiomyocytes (hiPSC-CMs). hiPSCs can be generated from patient somatic cells through procedures such as a skin punch biopsy or through blood samples and thus obviate the need to utilize embryos for their development.[32,37,38]

The autologous nature of hiPSCs makes them attractive for precision medicine and precision drug testing because the cells are genetically identical to the individual patient.[39] The development of autologous stem cell–based therapies for cardiac regeneration is also possible using hiPSC-CMs. Thus hiPSC-CMs are emerging as an attractive alternative to hESC-CMs.

hESC-CMs have been available since 2001,[34] and hiPSC-CMs were first described in 2009. In 2009, the first report on functional cardiomyocytes derived from hiPSCs was published, and it provided a direct phenotypic comparison with cardiomyocytes derived from hESCs.[40] In this seminal work, Zhang et al. demonstrated that hiPSC-CMs are virtually indistinguishable from hESC-CMs both structurally and functionally.[40] Fig. 57.3 shows the structural similarities between single cardiomyocytes from these two sources of functional human cardiomyocytes. Both hESC-CMs and hiPSC-CMs stain positive for the same cardiac sarcomere markers (cTnT and MLC2v, *green*) and have similar structure. Importantly, this finding was confirmed for multiple hESC (H1 and H9) and hiPSC (IMR90 C4 and Foreskin C1) lines, suggesting that any hPSC line isolated from any source can be utilized to generate human cardiomyocytes. A summary of electrophysiological comparison between hESC-CM and hiPSC-CM by Zhang et al. is presented in Table 57.1.

Fig. 57.3 also demonstrates that three distinct cardiac cell subtypes are present in hiPSC-CMs, including nodal, atrial, and ventricular cardiomyocytes. Using molecular genetic cell sorting approaches, it is possible to generate purified populations of ventricular- and atrial-like cardiomyocytes that recapitulate the chamber-specific electrophysiological and structural phenotype of the adult cardiac chambers.[41] Additionally, Fig. 57.3 shows that hESC- and hiPSC-CMs respond similarly to β-adrenergic receptor stimulation with an increase in spontaneous beating rate and abbreviated APD. The responsiveness to β1-adrenergic receptor activation demonstrates the presence of receptors and

TABLE 57.1 Comparison of action potential properties of ventricular-like cardiomyocytes derived from human embryonic stem cell–derived cardiomyocytes (hESC-CMs) (H9, H1) or human induced pluripotent stem cell–derived cardiomyocytes (hiPSC-CMs) (IMR90 C4, and foreskin C1 cell lines)

	NO. OF CELLS	RATE (BEATS/MIN)	APD50 (ms)	APD90 (ms)	dV/dt^{max} (V/s)	APA (mV)	MDP (mV)
hiPSC-Derived							
IMR90 C4	37	43.8 ± 2.7	240.7 ± 15.0	320.1 ± 17.0	40.5 ± 4.6	87.7 ± 2.6	−63.5 ± 1.7
Foreskin C1	39	44.2 ± 3.5	238.9 ± 10.0	312.5 ± 11.2	27.2 ± 3.7	87.9 ± 2.4	−63.3 ± 1.5
hESC-Derived							
H9	45	44.6 ± 2.8	223.9 ± 13.4	312.6 ± 15.9	33.5 ± 3.7	83.5 ± 2.4	−64.3 ± 3.2
H1	27	33.3 ± 2.3	233.9 ± 11.4	298.7 ± 13.4	17.6 ± 2.6	82.7 ± 3.0	−60.8 ± 2.8

Data are means ± standard error of mean. dV/dt$_{max}$ indicates maximum rate of rise of action potential upstroke; *APA*, action potential amplitude; *APD*, action potential duration; *MDP*, average maximum diastolic potential for action potentials during the time period examined.
Modified from Zhang J, Wilson GF, Soerens AG, et al. Functional cardiomyocytes derived from human induced pluripotent stem cells. *Circ Res*. 2009;104:e30-e41.

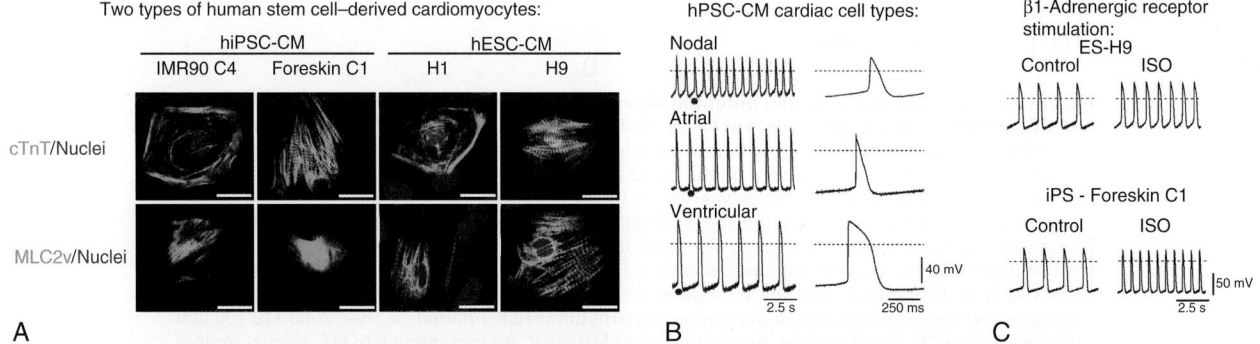

FIGURE 57.3 Human induced pluripotent stem cell–derived cardiomyocytes (*hiPSC-CMs*) are indistinguishable from human embryonic stem cell–derived cardiomyocytes (*hESC-CMs*). (A) Immunolabeling of cardiac-specific markers (cTnT and MLC2v) in hiPSCs and hESC-CMs. Single cardiomyocytes isolated from contracting areas of day 60 embryoid bodies (EBs) from IMR90 C4, Foreskin C1, H1, and H9 were immunolabeled for cTnT, a cardiac-specific myofilament protein, and MLC2v, a ventricular-specific protein. Nuclei were stained with Hoechst (*blue*). Scale bars are 20 μm. (B) Representative action potential recordings demonstrating that each of the three major action potentials types are observed. *Right*, Action potentials shown at an expanded time scale taken from the region indicated on the *left* (•). *Dotted lines* indicate 0 mV. (C) Action potentials recorded from hESC-CM (H9) or hiPSC-CM (foreskin C1) before and during perfusion of isoproterenol (*ISO*). ([A] From Zhang J, Wilson GF, Soerens AG, et al. Functional cardiomyocytes derived from human induced pluripotent stem cells. *Circ Res*. 2009;104:e30-e41. [C] Modified from Zhang J, Wilson GF, Soerens AG, et al. Functional cardiomyocytes derived from human induced pluripotent stem cells. *Circ Res*. 2009;104:e30-e41.)

intracellular mediators of this signaling cascade in hiPSC-CMs. Thus the use of hiPSC-CMs is a viable alternative to the ethically controversial use of hESC-CMs.

Human Induced Pluripotent Stem Cell–Derived Cardiomyocytes Form Electrically and Mechanically Coupled Monolayers for In Vitro Electrophysiological Study

To date, the majority of basic science studies utilizing hiPSC-CMs for modeling of inherited cardiac diseases[42-44] and for drug screening applications[33] have focused on single-cell structure–function relationships. These studies have shown that electrophysiological hallmarks of inherited cardiomyopathies (channelopathies), such as action potential prolongation and abnormal calcium release, can be recapitulated in single hiPSC-CMs.[36,43] Furthermore, drug cardiotoxicity and proarrhythmia risk have been assessed using single hiPSC-CMs.[33] However, fewer data have been generated using electrically and mechanically connected human cardiac two-dimensional (2D) monolayers. The use of syncytia of hiPSC-CMs should mimic the native tissue phenotype more closely compared with that of single cells in culture and also enable the study of electrical impulse propagation. This is important for in vitro modeling of structural heart diseases, such as arrhythmogenic right ventricular cardiomyopathy (ARVC) and hypertrophic cardiomyopathy (HCM).

Human Induced Pluripotent Stem Cell–Derived Cardiomyocyte Two-Dimensional Cardiac Monolayers and Cell Sheets to Study Human Cardiac Arrhythmia Mechanisms

The first report on the development of 2D hiPSC-CM monolayers useful to study human reentrant cardiac arrhythmias was published in 2012.[45] Building upon an hESC monolayer–based cardiac differentiation approach using sequential application of cytokines,[46] it was discovered by Zhang et al. that sequential application of extracellular matrix in the form of matrigel improves efficiency and output of cardiomyocyte production.[45] In this report Zhang et al. replated enriched hiPSC-CMs and hESC-CMs as functional 2D monolayers at a high density (250,000 cells/monolayer). After just 2 days of culture, the monolayers were stained with the voltage-sensitive dye Di-8-ANEPPS, and optical mapping was performed to quantify action potential propagation. Monolayers were spontaneously active, and activation maps

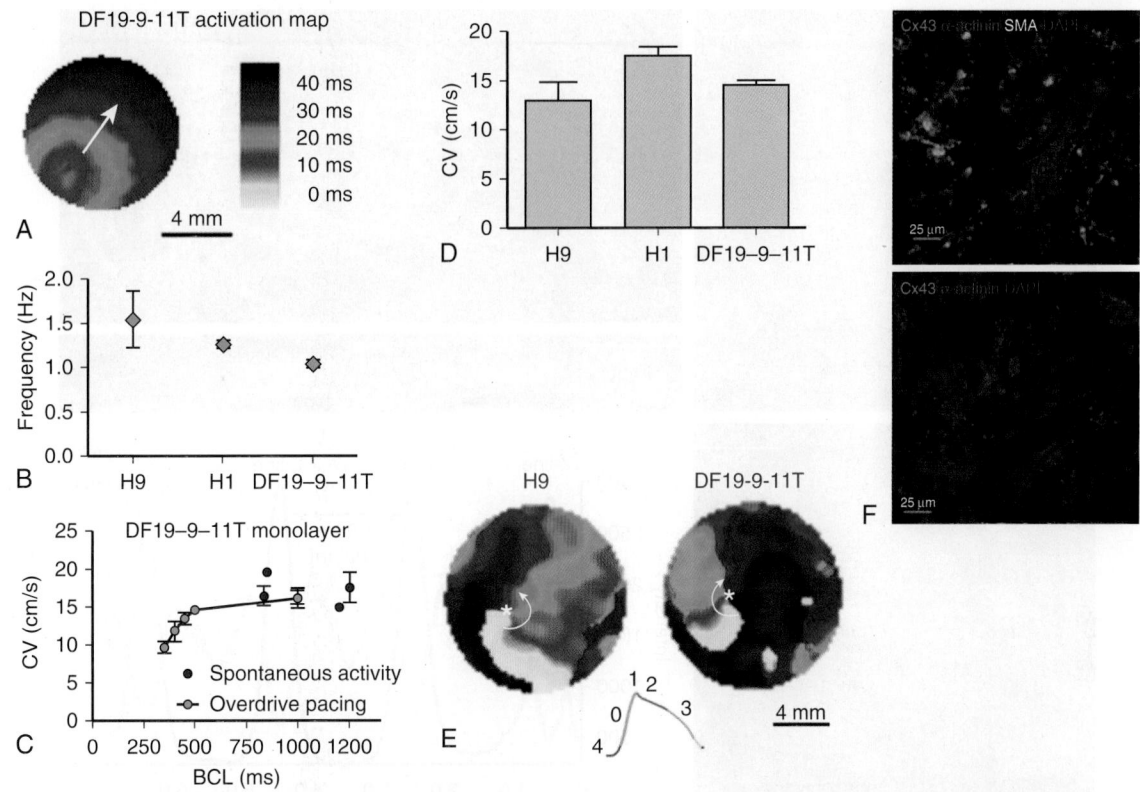

FIGURE 57.4 Optical mapping of human pluripotent stem cell–derived cardiomyocyte (hPSC-CM) membrane voltage (V$_m$). (A) Activation map showing uniform action potential propagation across the monolayer. (B) Spontaneous activation rate for human embryonic stem cell–derived cardiomyocyte (hESC-CM) (H9, H1) and the human induced pluripotent stem cell–derived cardiomyocyte (hiPSC-CM) (DF19-9-11T) monolayers. (C) Spontaneous and electrical pacing average conduction velocities (*CV*) of hiPSC-CM monolayers (basic cycle length [*BCL*]). (D) Average CVs for hESC-CM monolayers and hiPSC-CM monolayers measured at 2-Hz pacing. (E) Representative snapshots from phase movies showing electrical rotors in H9 (hESC-CM) and DF 19-9-11T (hiPSC-CM) monolayers. *Green* represents the depolarization phase of the propagating action potential, phase zero; *red* represents phase 2, or the plateau phase of the action potential; finally, *orange* and *yellow* represent phase 3, repolarization of the action potential. The *white asterisk* indicates the phase singularity, the point where all phases of the action potential converge, which is the organizing center of the arrhythmic reentry. (F) Immunolabeling of the hiPSC-CM monolayer (DF19-9-11T) for sarcomeric protein α-actinin in combination with α-smooth muscle actin (*SMA*) and gap junction protein connexin (*Cx*)43 and Cx40, respectively. Note abundant staining for α-actinin and Cx43 but no staining for SMA or Cx40. Scale bars are 25 µm. Error bars, where shown, represent standard error of mean. (From Zhang J, Klos M, Wilson GF, et al. Extracellular matrix promotes highly efficient cardiac differentiation of human pluripotent stem cells: the matrix sandwich method. *Circ Res.* 2012;111:1125-1136.)

showed uniform spread of the electrical impulse, with conduction velocities (CVs) ranging from 13 to 18 cm s^{-1} (Fig. 57.4A–D). CV was considerably slower than that reported for the mature adult heart and showed a rate-dependent slowing with shorter cycle length (see Fig. 57.4C). Rapid electrical pacing could produce reentrant arrhythmic conduction (see Fig. 57.4E) in both hESC-CM (H9 ESC line) and hiPSC-CM (DF19-9-11T) monolayers. Cardiomyocytes were electrically connected by connexin (Cx)43 gap junctional proteins rather than Cx40, suggesting that ventricular cardiomyocytes were the predominant cardiac cell type (see Fig. 57.4F). The emergence of rotors (see Fig. 57.4E) after rapid electrical stimulation was the first indication that these human stem cell–derived monolayers provide a powerful in vitro tool for studying the mechanisms of fatal cardiac arrhythmias.

In 2013, Kadota et al.[47] developed hiPSC-CM 2D cell sheets to study the functional properties of hiPSC-CMs in complex multicellular networks. Their goal was to study complex arrhythmia phenomena such as reentrant arrhythmias that are caused by spiral wave propagation in whole hearts. These cardiac arrhythmia phenomena cannot be studied in single cells. The cell sheets

were composed of 90% cTnT+ cells, and the identity of the remaining 10% of cells was undefined. Interestingly, the ratio of cTnT+ cells remained unchanged over 50 days after creating the cell sheets, suggesting that the hiPSC-CMs were postmitotic and fully differentiated. Electron microscopy studies over the time course of cell sheet development revealed the formation of gap junctions, adherence junctions, desmosomes, sarcoplasmic reticulum, and intercalated disks. These cell–cell junctions are essential for cardiac electrical and mechanical functions and are absent in single cell studies. Optical mapping of the calcium impulse (using fluo-4) was used to show that the hiPSC-CM–derived cardiac cell sheets generated functional "syncytia." Calcium wave propagation velocity was measured for spontaneous beating as well as for application of electrical stimulation. The CV of calcium wave propagation was reported to increase gradually over 1 month of maturation as gap junctions and other cell–cell adherence structures developed. Additionally, the CV slowed down when the stimulation frequency increased and when the sodium channel blockers lidocaine and tetrodotoxin were applied. This response of CV slowing with increasing pacing and sodium channel

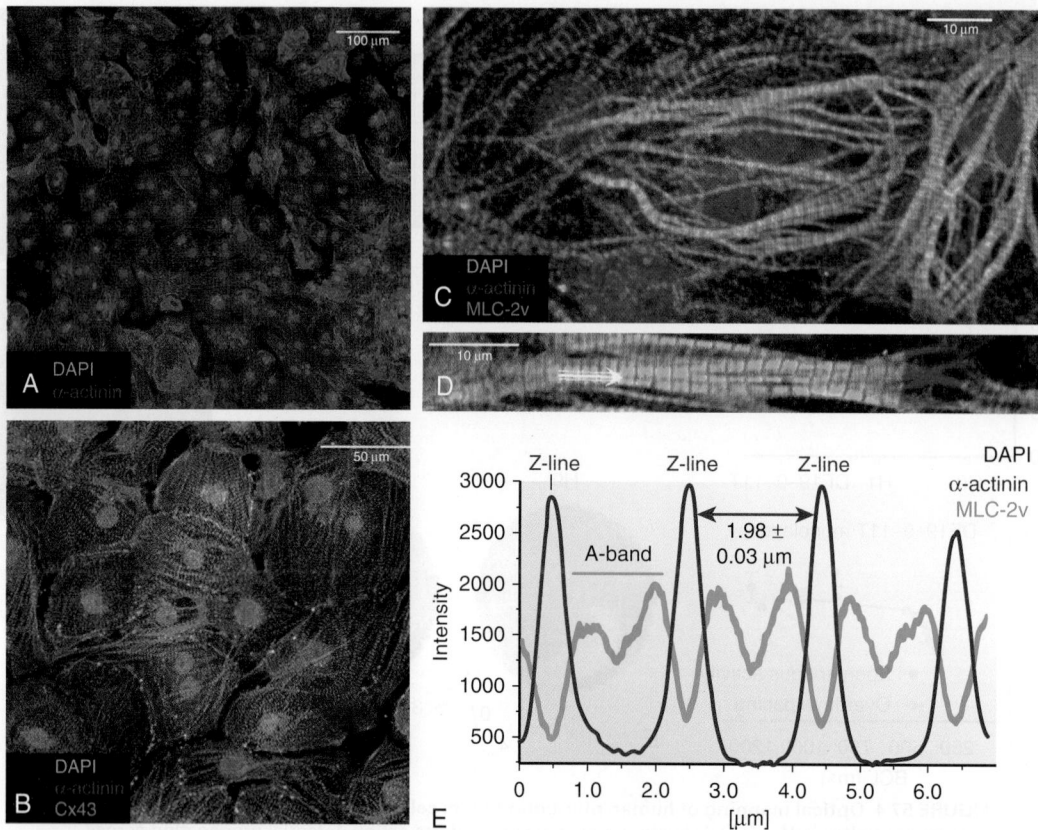

FIGURE 57.5 Genetically purified human induced pluripotent stem cell–derived cardiomyocyte (hiPSC-CM) monolayers. (A) Large field of view shows α-actinin expression in ~100% of hiPSC-CMs, corroborated in (B, 60× magnification). (C) hiPSC-CMs express atrial and ventricular markers (*MLC2v*). (D) and (E) hiPSC-CMs sarcomere organization with MLC2v, making up each half of the A-band, and the Z-line contains α-actinin. (From Lee P, Klos M, Bollensdorff C, et al. Simultaneous voltage and calcium mapping of genetically purified human induced pluripotent stem cell–derived cardiac myocyte monolayers. *Circ Res.* 2012;110:1556-1563.)

blockade is representative of responses of the whole heart. The authors reported the development of rapid pacing–induced reentrant arrhythmias in the cell sheets that were terminated by the application of antiarrhythmic drugs. The results led the authors to propose that the cell sheet platform would be useful for drug testing and for the creation of disease models in vitro. The values of CV during 0.5-Hz pacing were ~5 cm s^{-1}, which is 10× slower than what has been recorded in the whole heart. CV slowing is known to contribute to reentrant arrhythmias in the whole heart, so the reentrant arrhythmias observed by Kadota et al. in their study may be attributed to the relative immature phenotype of the hiPSC-CMs.

Other functional evidence of immaturity of the cell sheets used by Kadota et al.[47] is the very prolonged calcium transient duration values that were around 1 second during 0.5-Hz pacing. The long duration of the calcium transient suggests the absence of major repolarizing currents (i.e., I_{K1}) and calcium removal mechanisms (sarco/endoplasmic reticulum Ca^{2+}–adenosine triphosphatase [ATPase] [SERCA], sodium–calcium exchanger [NCX]). The relative impurity of the cardiomyocyte sheets in this study may also have contributed significantly to the observations of reentrant arrhythmias. This type of optical mapping of the calcium impulse using 2D cell sheets will be important for hiPSC-CM models in which calcium flux dysregulation is thought to underlie disease pathogenesis, such as those for catecholaminergic polymorphic ventricular tachycardia (CPVT).[48,49] Optical mapping of calcium flux and calcium wave propagation will also be important in cardiotoxicity and proarrhythmia testing for early drug discovery projects.

Simultaneous Action Potential and Calcium Impulse Mapping in Purified Two-Dimensional Human Induced Pluripotent Stem Cell–Derived Cardiomyocytes

Every heart beat is a culmination of the action potential that triggers calcium wave propagation throughout the heart, thereby activating the myofilaments. Therefore quantification of each parameter provides important information regarding the excitation–contraction coupling process. The first report on simultaneous recording of membrane voltage and intracellular calcium flux in hiPSC-CM monolayers was published in 2012. Lee et al.[50] reported on the use of genetically purified hiPSC-CM monolayers to study both voltage and calcium impulse propagation. Commercially available cryopreserved hiPSC-CMs (iCell Cardiomyocytes, Cellular Dynamics International, Madison, WI; 95% purity) were thawed and plated as electrically connected monolayers for optical mapping of the electrical impulse. Fig. 57.5 shows the purity and structure of these commercially available hiPSC-CMs. These cardiomyocytes are purified via α-MHC promoter driving antibiotic resistance.

This study utilized a multiparametric imaging system to enable simultaneous quantification of the action potential (membrane voltage, V_m) and the subsequent calcium wave. The authors adapted a previously described light emitting diode (LED) illumination system based on sequential switching between three different LED light sources and a single sensor (charge-coupled device [CCD] camera).[51] hiPSC-CM monolayers demonstrated pacemaker activity, with the pacemaker site consistently located

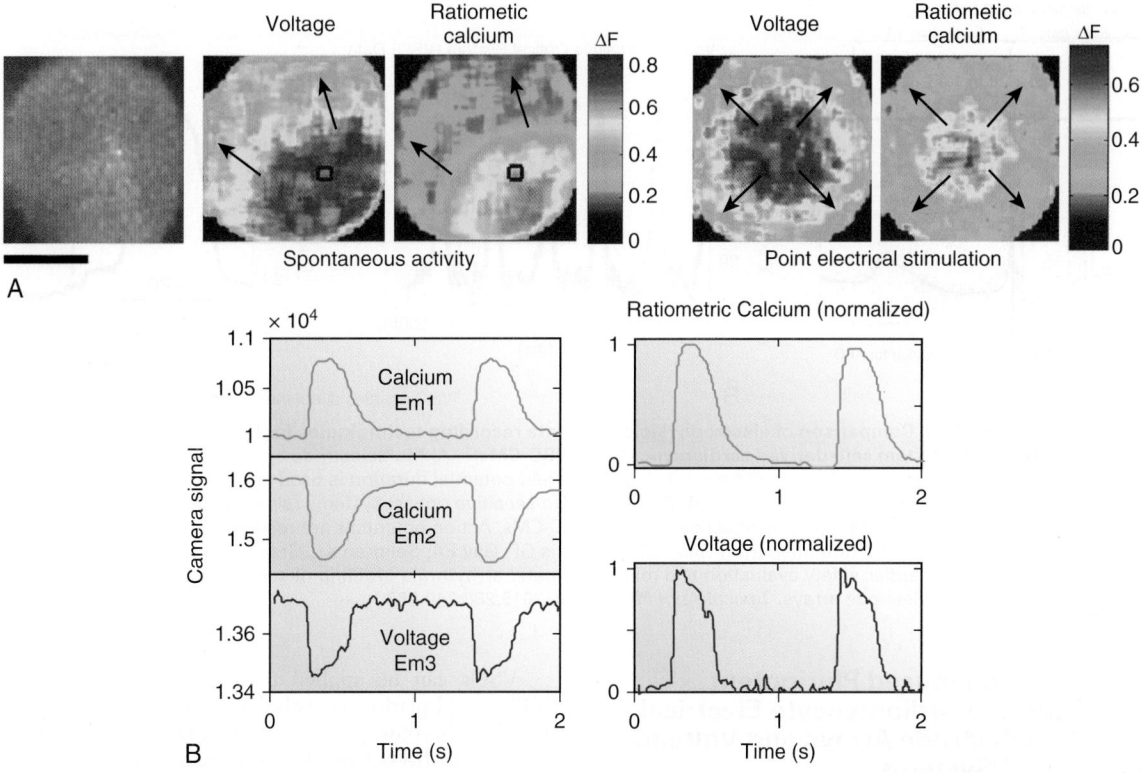

FIGURE 57.6 Simultaneous quantification of V_m and ratiometric $[Ca^{2+}]i$ in human induced pluripotent stem cell–derived cardiomyocyte (hiPSC-CM) monolayers. (A) Normalized fluorescence intensity maps (*color bar* shown) of spontaneous and electrically paced (at the center of the monolayer) activation. *Black arrows* show the direction of activation wave propagation. The *left-most* panel shows a grayscale image of the monolayer. (B) *Left panel*: Camera signals (on a 16-bit scale) of Em1, Em2, and Em3 fluorescence from the blue-squared-region in (A) over the course of 2 seconds. *Right panel*: Normalized ratiometric calcium signal (obtained by dividing Em1 by Em2, followed by normalization) and normalized voltage signal (Em3 normalization). Scale bar is 5 mm. (From Lee P, Klos M, Bollensdorff C, et al. Simultaneous voltage and calcium mapping of genetically purified human induced pluripotent stem cell–derived cardiac myocyte monolayers. *Circ Res.* 2012;110:1556-1563.)

in the same spatial location from beat to beat over the time course of experimentation. The hiPSC-CM monolayers could also be electrically paced using a point stimulator at the center of each monolayer. In Fig. 57.6A, the *black arrows* show the direction of spread of the pacemaker and electrically stimulated beats. The colors in Fig. 57.6A indicate amplitude intensities at a specific frame in the movie acquisition. Panel B shows the calcium and voltage signals obtained in the *blue box* region of panel A. The ratiometric calcium flux and inverted V_m signals are shown for the pacemaker beat. Importantly, the voltage signal occurred before the calcium impulse, indicating normal sequence of activation with an action potential triggering intracellular calcium flux and impulse propagation throughout the monolayer. The conduction velocity of these monolayers was 25 cm s^{-1}, which is faster than that reported in most studies but slower than that recorded in the intact heart.[52–54] The slow conduction velocity was likely due to the immature phenotype of the hiPSC-CMs. The use of hiPSC-CM monolayers like these for multiparametric optical mapping is a platform that may supplant the hERG assay as a front-line proarrhythmia screen for early drug development.

Revolution for Cardiotoxicity Testing: Comprehensive in Vitro Proarrhythmia Assay

Major stakeholders in the regulation of the drug discovery process have now recognized that tests performed on a single channel (hERG assay) using heterologous animal cell systems do not provide a realistic analysis of drug effects on the heart.[12,55] The advent of hiPSC-CM technology and mass production of these purified cells has led these stakeholders to reevaluate the regulatory process for cardiotoxicity screening.[56] In July 2013, a Think Tank cosponsored by the Cardiac Safety Research Consortium (CSRC), the Health and Environmental Sciences Institute (HESI), and the US Food and Drug Administration (FDA) was held to consider new approaches in cardiotoxicity screening. The proposed new paradigm combines in vitro and in silico data for nonclinical assessment of proarrhythmic risk and is now referred to as the Comprehensive in Vitro Proarrhythmia Assay (CiPA). The goal of CiPA is to create an assay or series of assays that provides more accurate electrophysiological and mechanistic understanding of a compound's impact on the heart earlier in the drug discovery process. These assays are likely to replace the current reliance on the hERG channel assay, but the timeline for implementation of CiPA is unclear.

Studies are being conducted to provide support for adoption of CiPA. Currently, nonclinical data are being collected from the examination of multiple ion channels using patch-clamp technologies. In silico models will be built and tested based on these data, leading to standardized computer models for predicting proarrhythmic risk. In parallel, hiPSC-CMs will be tested in vitro using various technologies to determine the proarrhythmic potential of compounds on the basis of their effects on the APD. Finally, nonclinical and first-in-human (FIH) clinical trial ECGs will be assessed and compared against the nonclinical testing approaches.

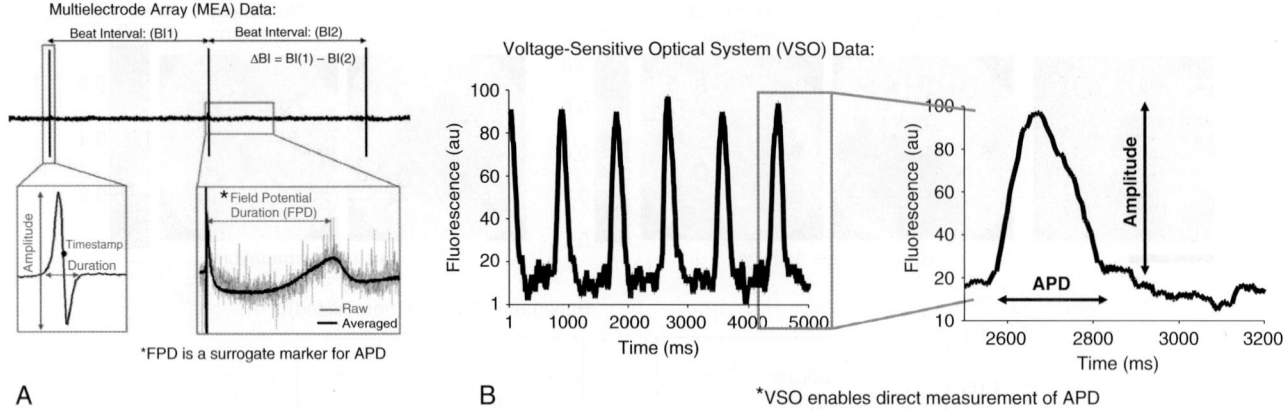

FIGURE 57.7 Comparison of electrophysiological data recording technologies for human induced pluripotent stem cell–derived cardiomyocytes (hiPSC-CMs). (A) Multielectrode array relies on field potential recordings of hiPSC-CM electrical activity. Field potential duration is used as a surrogate marker for action potential duration (*APD*). (B) Voltage-sensitive optical systems rely on optical dyes that report the membrane potential changes of hiPSC-CMs. Action potentials are recorded, and APD is easily calculated. (Modified from Gilchrist KH, Lewis GF, Gay EA, Sellgren KL, Grego S. High-throughput cardiac safety evaluation and multi-parameter arrhythmia profiling of cardiomyocytes using microelectrode arrays. *Toxicol Appl Pharmacol.* 2015;288:249-257.)

Measuring Human Induced Pluripotent Stem Cell–Derived Cardiomyocyte Electrical Function: Multielectrode Arrays and Voltage-Sensitive Optical Systems

Two primary technologies are being considered for the quantification of drug effects on the electrophysiology of hiPSC-CM monolayers: (1) multielectrode arrays (MEAs) and (2) voltage-sensitive optical systems (VSOs). MEA technology involves the plating of hiPSC-CMs on electrodes lined in the center of a multiwell dish. Field potential duration (FPD) is currently being used as a surrogate marker for APD and is quantified using MEA technology.[57] VSO technology involves labeling hiPSC-CMs with a fluorescent reporter that enables visualization of the cardiac action potential. VSOs enable the direct measurement of hiPSC-CM APD and can be used in combination with calcium-sensitive labels and dyes to enable direct examination of excitation–contraction coupling.[50,58] Studies are under way to determine the optimal strategies and technologies to be used for successful implementation in the CiPA initiative.

Comparison of Two Lead Technologies for Cardiotoxicity Screening Using Human Induced Pluripotent Stem Cell–Derived Cardiomyocytes

Each of these in vitro technologies applied to use hiPSC-CMs for drug discovery has its advantages and limitations. MEAs are label free and available for high-throughput screening (HTS) in 96-well formats and thus enable long-term monitoring of drug effects with continuous recording. However, the measurement of FPD is somewhat arbitrary and may not accurately reflect repolarization times. The use of a surrogate marker for human APD is a limitation of MEA technology, just as the surrogate marker of hERG channel block for APD is a limitation. MEA recordings are not readily amenable to direct measurement of drug effects on action potential shape. On the other hand, VSOs enable the quantification of all phases of the action potential as well as the direct measurement of action potential triangulation. Fig. 57.7 shows a comparison of the electrophysiological data obtained from each technology using spontaneously beating hiPSC-CMs. VSOs combined with high-spatiotemporal resolution optical mapping also enable higher resolution quantification of electrical impulse propagation compared to MEA technology.[50,58]

VSOs can be applied to multiple types of bioengineered hiPSC-CM platforms, including three-dimensional (3D) microtissues, spheroids, single cells, and 2D monolayers. MEA recordings are restricted to 2D monolayers plated on the surface of the manufacturer's electrode array; this precludes ease of testing customized cell culture platforms. However, VSOs require a fluorescent label, thus precluding the long-term continuous interrogation of drug effects. Another limitation of VSOs is the potential cytotoxicity associated with dyes. New nontoxic VSO dyes are now commercially available (e.g., FluoVolt from ThermoFisher) and are in continuous development to make the labels more reliable. Also, genetically engineered VSO approaches are being pursued that may circumvent the issues of cytotoxicity and long-term studies.[59,60] Regulatory boards are still testing the efficacy and predictability of each technology to determine proarrhythmia; it is premature to decide which platform will be utilized.

Technological Hurdles for Implementation of Comprehensive in Vitro Proarrhythmia Assay Using Human Induced Pluripotent Stem Cell–Derived Cardiomyocytes: Maturing the Cellular Structural and Functional Phenotypes

There are technological advances that must be made before the use of hiPSC-CM for preclinical drug discovery screening can be implemented.[12,55] First, the Think Tank recognizes that the maturity of the hiPSC-CMs needs to be advanced to create a system that more closely mimics the human heart phenotype. Second is the need for a reliable, robust HTS platform for interrogation of the electrophysiological function of mature hiPSC-CMs. Addressing these two limitations is now a focus of research for many academic, regulatory, and private laboratories to move CiPA closer to implementation.

Currently used hiPSC-CMs have a fetal-like phenotype and structure (Fig. 57.8A) where repolarization of the cells relies almost exclusively on the hERG channel.[61] The immature nature of the electrophysiological function of these hiPSC-CMs is apparent in Table 57.1. For example, dV/dt_{max}, which indicates the maximum rate of rise of the action potential upstroke, ranged from 17 to 45 V/s in the immature human stem cell–derived cardiomyocytes (see Table 57.1), whereas

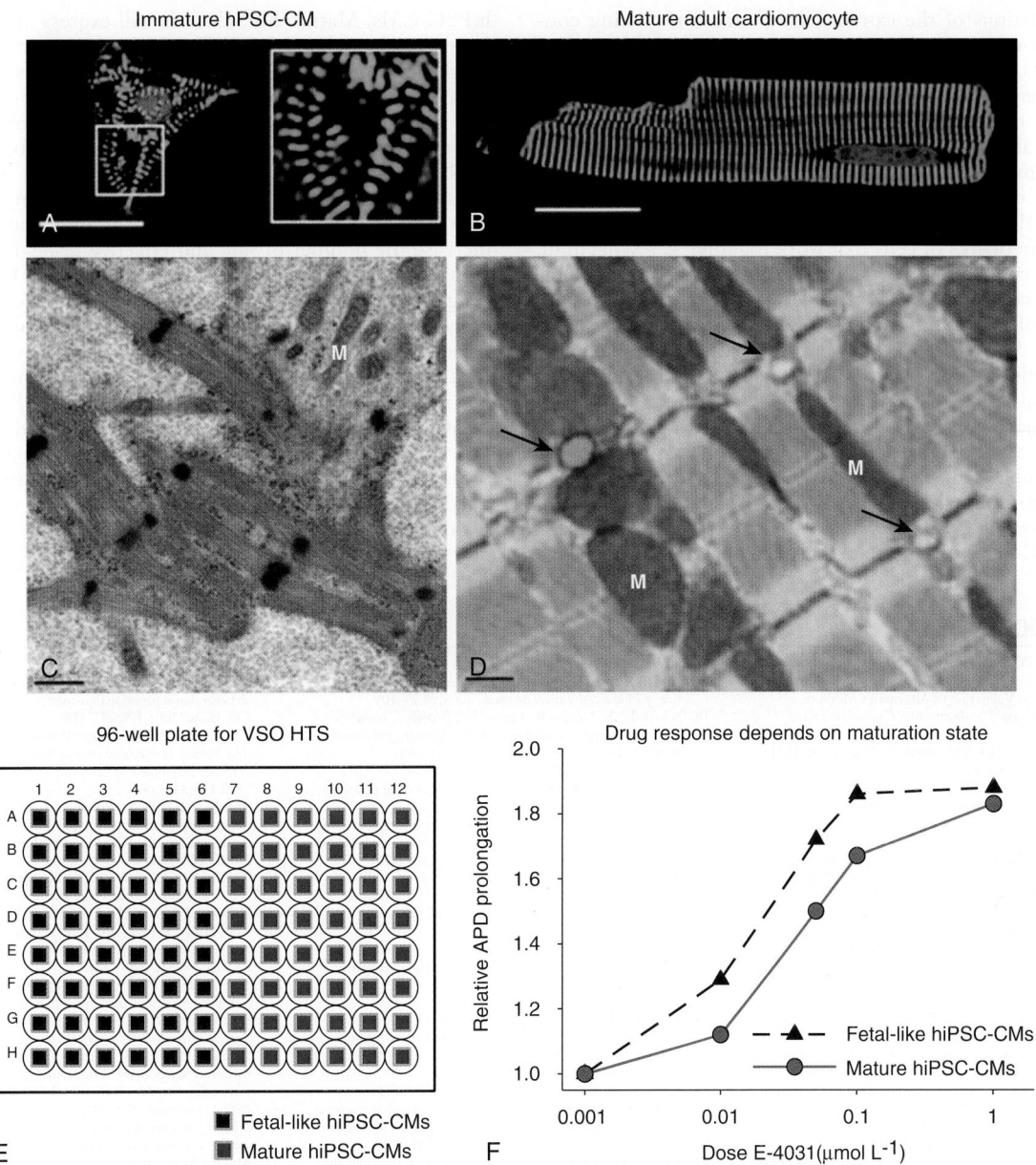

FIGURE 57.8 Morphological differences between an immature human pluripotent stem cell cardiomyocyte (*hPSC-CM*) and adult cardiomyocyte. Overview of contractile cytoskeleton with α-actinin staining (*green*) and blue nuclear counterstain in hPSC-CM (A) and adult rat cardiomyocytes (B). Cellular ultrastructure by electron microscopy in hPSC-CM (C) and adult rat (D). Note that there are significant differences with respect to cell size, length-to-width ratio, mitochondria (*M*) quantity, size and morphology, appearance of T-tubules (*arrows*), and elongated nuclei. Scale bar in (A) and (B) is 25 μm and in (C) and (D) is 0.2 μm. Further development of human induced pluripotent stem cell–derived cardiomyocyte (*hiPSC-CM*) voltage-sensitive optical (*VSO*) technology and maturation will aid with implementation of comprehensive in vitro proarrhythmia assay. (E) Substrate hardness can be fine-tuned in vitro to enable maturation on soft substrates (*red*). This may be difficult to implement using multielectrode arrays, which require direct contact of hiPSC-CMs with the prefabricated electrodes. (F) Mature hiPSC-CMs (*red*) will be less sensitive to hERG channel blockade than immature fetal-like hiPSC-CMs (*black*). Mature hiPSC-CMs will express other ion channels to compensate for the hERG channel block and thus provide a more realistic examination of drug effects on human cardiac electrophysiology. ([A–D] Modified from Yang X, Pabon L, Murry CE. Engineering adolescence: maturation of human pluripotent stem cell-derived cardiomyocytes. *Circ Res.* 2014;114:511-523; [B and C] also courtesy Scott Lundy and Dr. Michael A. Laflamme.)

the dV/dt$_{max}$ of mature adult cardiomyocytes ranges from ~120 V/s to ~200 V/s.[62] Furthermore, the maximal diastolic potential (MDP) of hiPSC-CM (see Table 57.1) was ~–63 mV, but the MDP of mature cardiomyocytes is much more hyperpolarized at ~–86 mV.[62] Fetal-like hiPSC-CMs may not offer

advantages over the hERG channel assay because immature hiPSC-CMs rely almost exclusively on hERG channel function for repolarization.[61] Advancement of the maturation state of hiPSC-CMs is required before this technology can be used as part of the CiPA initiative.

Manipulations of the extracellular matrix and plating conditions can impact on the electrophysiological maturation of hiPSC-CMs, and therefore optimization for maturation may be more feasible in VSO platforms.[63,64] However, the values reported by these groups are still not comparable to the electrophysiological parameters of adult cardiomyocytes. The lack of significant maturation of single hiPSC-CMs may be due to the single-cell culture conditions. Cardiomyocytes do not naturally exist as single cells, but rather as electrically and mechanically connected networks of cells that work together as a syncytium. Therefore compared with single-cell conditions, multicellular culture conditions are more likely to promote maturation. The issue of maturation of the hiPSC-CM phenotype applies to both the MEA and VSO platforms. Further development of the maturation of the electrophysiological and structural phenotype of hiPSC-CM is a focus of much research and is necessary to make this system more useful for drug testing and in vitro disease modeling.[63,65] Mature hiPSC-CMs that express the full complement of ion channels are likely to have distinct sensitivity to drug compounds compared to immature fetal-like hiPSC-CMs. Fig. 57.8 shows the anticipated difference in sensitivity to E-4031 hERG block between mature and fetal-like hiPSC-CMs. Mature hiPSC-CMs will express other repolarizing currents, such as I_{K1} (see Fig. 57.2), that can compensate for blockade of the hERG channel. On the other hand, immature (fetal) hiPSC-CMs rely exclusively on hERG for repolarization and thus are more sensitive to blockade. Mature hiPSC-CMs therefore would be the suitable replacement for the current hERG channel assay.

Implementation of CiPA is expected to streamline the drug discovery process, reduce the cost of preclinical screening, increase the number of safe and effective drugs in the market, and reduce the use of animals and animal cells for preclinical drug screening. Implementation of the CiPA guidelines will indeed represent a revolution in the industry of preclinical drug screening.

The potential of using human cardiac cells that recapitulate the in vivo cardiac function is extraordinary. hiPSC-CMs and hESC-CMs enable the direct examination of the effects of a drug and potential toxins on cardiac function and structure. The use of these incredible cells will transform the way drugs are developed, how medications are prescribed, and how environmental toxins are tested and classified[66] and may lead to revolutionary, new regenerative medicine therapies.

REFERENCES

1. Stummann TC, Beilmann M, Duker G, et al. Report and recommendations of the workshop of the European Centre for the Validation of Alternative Methods for Drug-Induced Cardiotoxicity. *Cardiovasc Toxicol.* 2009;9:107–125.
2. Fermini B, Fossa AA. The impact of drug-induced QT interval prolongation on drug discovery and development. *Nat Rev Drug Discov.* 2003;2:439–447.
3. Pacher P, Kecskemeti V. Cardiovascular side effects of new antidepressants and antipsychotics: new drugs, old concerns? *Curr Pharm Des.* 2004;10:2463–2475.
4. Carmeliet E, Mubagwa K. Antiarrhythmic drugs and cardiac ion channels: mechanisms of action. *Prog Biophys Mol Biol.* 1998;70:1–72.
5. International Conference on Harmonisation; guidance on S7b Nonclinical Evaluation of the Potential for Delayed Ventricular Repolarization (QT interval prolongation) by Human Pharmaceuticals; availability. *Notice. Fed Regist.* 2005;70:61133–61134.
6. Lawrence CL, Pollard CE, Hammond TG, Valentin J-P. Nonclinical proarrhythmia models: predicting torsades de pointes. *J Pharmacol Toxicol Methods.* 2005;52:46–59.
7. Gintant GA. Preclinical torsades-de-pointes screens: advantages and limitations of surrogate and direct approaches in evaluating proarrhythmic risk. *Pharmacol Ther.* 2008;119:199–209.
8. Roden DM. Drug-induced prolongation of the QT interval. *N Engl J Med.* 2004;350:1013–1022.
9. Belardinelli L, Antzelevitch C, Vos MA. Assessing predictors of drug-induced torsade de pointes. *Trends Pharmacol Sci.* 2003;24:619–625.
10. Redfern WS, Carlsson L, Davis AS, et al. Relationships between preclinical cardiac electrophysiology, clinical QT interval prolongation and torsade de pointes for a broad range of drugs: evidence for a provisional safety margin in drug development. *Cardiovasc Res.* 2003;58:32–45.
11. Lasser KE, Allen PD, Woolhandler SJ, Himmelstein DU, Wolfe SM, Bor DH. Timing of new black box warnings and withdrawals for prescription medications. *JAMA.* 2002;287:2215–2220.
12. Chi KR. Revolution dawning in cardiotoxicity testing. *Nat Rev Drug Discov.* 2013;12:565–567.
13. Sanguinetti MC, Jiang C, Curran ME, Keating MT. A mechanistic link between an inherited and an acquired cardiac arrthythmia: hERG encodes the I_{Kr} potassium channel. *Cell.* 1995;81:299–307.
14. Campbell K, Calvo CJ, Mironov S, Herron T, Berenfeld O, Jalife J. Spatial gradients in action potential duration created by regional magnetofection of hERG are a substrate for wavebreak and turbulent propagation in cardiomyocyte monolayers. *J Physiol.* 2012;590:6363–6379.
15. Pollard CE, Abi Gerges N, Bridgland-Taylor MH, Easter A, Hammond TG, Valentin JP. An introduction to QT interval prolongation and non-clinical approaches to assessing and reducing risk. *Br J Pharmacol.* 2010;159:12–21.
16. Priest BT, Bell IM, Garcia ML. Role of hERG potassium channel assays in drug development. *Channels (Austin).* 2008;2:87–93.

17. Lindgren S, Bass AS, Briscoe R, et al. Benchmarking safety pharmacology regulatory packages and best practice. *J Pharmacol Toxicol Methods.* 2008;58:99–109.
18. Schroeder K, Neagle B, Trezise DJ, Worley J, Ionwork HT. A new high-throughput electrophysiology measurement platform. *J Biomol Screen.* 2003;8:50–64.
19. Guth BD, Rast G. Dealing with hERG liabilities early: diverse approaches to an important goal in drug development. *Br J Pharmacol.* 2010;159:22–24.
20. Gintant G. An evaluation of hERG current assay performance: translating preclinical safety studies to clinical QT prolongation. *Pharmacol Ther.* 2011;129:109–119.
21. Aiba T, Shimizu W, Inagaki M, et al. Cellular and ionic mechanism for drug-induced long QT syndrome and effectiveness of verapamil. *J Am Coll Cardiol.* 2005;45:300–307.
22. Zhang S, Zhou Z, Gong Q, Makielski JC, January CT. Mechanism of block and identification of the verapamil binding domain to hERG potassium channels. *Circ Res.* 1999;84:989–998.
23. Fossa AA, Gorczyca W, Wisialowski T, et al. Electrical alternans and hemodynamics in the anesthetized guinea pig can discriminate the cardiac safety of antidepressants. *J Pharmacol Toxicol Methods.* 2007;55:78–85.
24. Bénardeau A, Hatem SN, Rücker-Martin C, et al. Primary culture of human atrial myocytes is associated with the appearance of structural and functional characteristics of immature myocardium. *J Mol Cell Cardiol.* 1997;29:1307–1320.
25. Herron TJ, Devaney E, Mundada L, et al. Ca2+-independent positive molecular inotropy for failing rabbit and human cardiac muscle by α-myosin motor gene transfer. *FASEB J.* 2010;24:415–424.
26. Herron TJ, Rostkova E, Kunst G, Chaturvedi R, Gautel M, Kentish JC. Activation of myocardial contraction by the N-terminal domains of myosin binding protein-C. *Circ Res.* 2006;98:1290–1298.
27. Li R-K, Mickle DAG, Weisel RD, et al. Human pediatric and adult ventricular cardiomyocytes in culture: assessment of phenotypic changes with passaging. *Cardiovasc Res.* 1996;32:362–373.
28. Mitcheson JS, Hancox JC, Levi AJ. Cultured adult cardiac myocytes: future applications, culture methods, morphological and electrophysiological properties. *Cardiovasc Res.* 1998;39:280–300.
29. Boukens BJ, Sulkin MS, Gloschat CR, Ng FS, Vigmond EJ, Efimov IR. Transmural APD gradient synchronizes repolarization in the human left ventricular wall. *Cardiovasc Res.* 2015;108:188–196.
30. Hucker WJ, Fedorov VV, Foyil KV, Moazami N, Efimov IR. Optical mapping of the human atrioventricular junction. *Circulation.* 2008;117:1474–1477.
31. Anson BD, Kolaja KL, Kamp TJ. Opportunities for use of human iPS cells in predictive toxicology. *Clin Pharmacol Ther.* 2011;89:754–758.
32. Kamp TJ, Lyons GE. On the road to iPS cell cardiovascular applications. *Circ Res.* 2009;105:617–619.
33. Liang P, Lan F, Lee AS, et al. Drug screening using a library of human induced pluripotent stem cell–derived cardiomyocytes reveals disease-specific patterns of cardiotoxicity. *Circulation.* 2013;127:1677–1691.

34. Kehat I, Kenyagin-Karsenti D, Snir M, et al. Human embryonic stem cells can differentiate into myocytes with structural and functional properties of cardiomyocytes. *J Clin Invest.* 2001;108:407–414.
35. Harding SE, Ali NN, Brito-Martins M, Gorelik J. The human embryonic stem cell–derived cardiomyocyte as a pharmacological model. *Pharmacol Ther.* 2007;113:341–353.
36. Spencer CI, Baba S, Nakamura K, et al. Calcium transients closely reflect prolonged action potentials in iPSC models of inherited cardiac arrhythmia. *Stem Cell Reports.* 2014;3:269–281.
37. Takahashi K, Yamanaka S. Induction of pluripotent stem cells from mouse embryonic and adult fibroblast cultures by defined factors. *Cell.* 2006;126:663–676.
38. Yu J, Hu K, Smuga-Otto K, et al. Human induced pluripotent stem cells free of vector and transgene sequences. *Science.* 2009;324:797–801.
39. Himmel HM. Drug-induced functional cardiotoxicity screening in stem cell-derived human and mouse cardiomyocytes: effects of reference compounds. *J Pharmacol Toxicol Methods.* 2013;68:97–111.
40. Zhang J, Wilson GF, Soerens AG, et al. Functional cardiomyocytes derived from human induced pluripotent stem cells. *Circ Res.* 2009;104:e30–e41.
41. Bizy A, Guerrero-Serna G, Hu B, et al. Myosin light chain 2-based selection of human iPSC-derived early ventricular cardiac myocytes. *Stem Cell Res.* 2013;11:1335–1347.
42. Moretti A, Bellin M, Welling A, et al. Patient-specific induced pluripotent stem-cell models for long-QT syndrome. *N Engl J Med.* 2010;363:1397–1409.
43. Lan F, Lee Andrew S, Liang P, et al. Abnormal calcium handling properties underlie familial hypertrophic cardiomyopathy pathology in patient-specific induced pluripotent stem cells. *Cell Stem Cell.* 2013;12:101–113.
44. Wang Y, Liang P, Lan F, et al. Genome editing of isogenic human induced pluripotent stem cells recapitulates long QT phenotype for drug testing. *J Am Coll Cardiol.* 2014;64:451–459.
45. Zhang J, Klos M, Wilson GF, et al. Extracellular matrix promotes highly efficient cardiac differentiation of human pluripotent stem cells: the matrix sandwich method. *Circ Res.* 2012;111:1125–1136.
46. Laflamme MA, Chen KY, Naumova AV, et al. Cardiomyocytes derived from human embryonic stem cells in pro-survival factors enhance function of infarcted rat hearts. *Nat Biotech.* 2007;25:1015–1024.
47. Kadota S, Minami I, Morone N, Heuser JE, Agladze K, Nakatsuji N. Development of a reentrant arrhythmia model in human pluripotent stem cell-derived cardiac cell sheets. *Eur Heart J.* 2013;34:1147–1156.
48. Novak A, Barad L, Lorber A, et al. Functional abnormalities in iPSC-derived cardiomyocytes generated from CPVT1 and CPVT2 patients carrying ryanodine or calsequestrin mutations. *J Cell Mol Med.* 2015;19:2006–2018.
49. Zhang XH, Haviland S, Wei H, et al. Ca2+ signaling in human induced pluripotent stem cell-derived cardiomyocytes (iPS-CM) from normal and catecholaminergic polymorphic ventricular tachycardia (CPVT)-afflicted subjects. *Cell Calcium.* 2013;54:57–70.

50. Lee P, Klos M, Bollensdorff C, et al. Simultaneous voltage and calcium mapping of genetically purified human induced pluripotent stem cell–derived cardiac myocyte monolayers. *Circ Res.* 2012;110:1556–1563.

51. Lee P, Bollensdorff C, Quinn TA, Wuskell JP, Loew LM, Kohl P. Single-sensor system for spatially resolved, continuous, and multiparametric optical mapping of cardiac tissue. *Heart Rhythm.* 2011;8:1482–1491.

52. Burridge PW, Thompson S, Millrod MA, et al. A universal system for highly efficient cardiac differentiation of human induced pluripotent stem cells that eliminates interline variability. *PLoS One.* 2011;6:e18293.

53. Mehta A, Chung YY, Ng A, et al. Pharmacological response of human cardiomyocytes derived from virus-free induced pluripotent stem cells. *Cardiovasc Res.* 2011;91:577–586.

54. Nunes SS, Miklas JW, Liu J, et al. Biowire: a platform for maturation of human pluripotent stem cell-derived cardiomyocytes. *Nat Meth.* 2013;10:781–787.

55. Chi KR. Regulatory watch: speedy validation sought for new cardiotoxicity testing strategy. *Nat Rev Drug Discov.* 2013;12:655.

56. Mummery CL, Zhang J, Ng ES, Elliott DA, Elefanty AG, Kamp TJ. Differentiation of human embryonic stem cells and induced pluripotent stem cells to cardiomyocytes: a methods overview. *Circ Res.* 2012;111:344–358.

57. Gilchrist KH, Lewis GF, Gay EA, Sellgren KL, Grego S. High-throughput cardiac safety evaluation and multi-parameter arrhythmia profiling of cardiomyocytes using microelectrode arrays. *Toxicol Appl Pharmacol.* 2015;288:249–257.

58. Herron TJ, Lee P, Jalife J. Optical imaging of voltage and calcium in cardiac cells & tissues. *Circ Res.* 2012;110:609–623.

59. Brinks D, Klein AJ, Cohen E. Two-photon lifetime imaging of voltage indicating proteins as a probe of absolute membrane voltage. *Biophys J.* 2015;109:914–921.

60. Zou P, Zhao Y, Douglass AD, et al. Bright and fast multicolored voltage reporters via electrochromic FRET. *Nat Commun.* 2014;5:4625.

61. Doss MX. Maximum diastolic potential of human induced pluripotent stem cell-derived cardiomyocytes depends critically on I(Kr). *PLoS One.* 2012;7:e40288.

62. Drouin E, Charpentier F, Gauthier C, Laurent K, Le Marec H. Electrophysiologic characteristics of cells spanning the left ventricular wall of human heart: evidence for presence of M cells. *J Am Coll Cardiol.* 1995;26:185–192.

63. Feaster TK, Cadar AG, Wang L, et al. Matrigel mattress: a method for the generation of single contracting human-induced pluripotent stem cell-derived cardiomyocytes. *Circ Res.* 2015;117:995–1000.

64. Ribeiro AJ, Ang Y-S, Fu JD, et al. Contractility of single cardiomyocytes differentiated from pluripotent stem cells depends on physiological shape and substrate stiffness. *Proc Natl Acad Sci U S A.* 2015;112:12705–12710.

65. Yang X, Pabon L, Murry CE. Engineering adolescence: maturation of human pluripotent stem cell–derived cardiomyocytes. *Circ Res.* 2014;114:511–523.

66. Posnack NG, Idrees R, Ding H, et al. Exposure to phthalates affects calcium handling and intercellular connectivity of human stem cell-derived cardiomyocytes. *PLoS One.* 2015;10:e0121927.

58 Cardiac Repair With Human Pluripotent Stem Cell–Derived Cardiovascular Cells and Arrhythmia Risk

Timothy J. Kamp

Introduction to Cardioregenerative Medicine

The human heart has a limited ability for repair after myocardial infarction and other major insults. The remodeling process that occurs in response to major cell loss includes hypertrophy of remaining cardiomyocytes and fibrosis of the myocardium, which provide both triggers and substrate for arrhythmias. Oftentimes continued stress on the myocardium can lead to progressive remodeling and heart failure. Although pharmacological therapies have greatly advanced and can blunt or in some cases partially reverse the remodeling of the failing heart, typically these therapies are only partially effective, with substantial morbidity and mortality remaining, in part, due to arrhythmias.

In the past decade, insights regarding the regenerative capabilities of the heart have offered new hope for the treatment of heart disease. Although the adult human heart was long described as a postmitotic, terminally differentiated organ, new studies have provided evidence that the heart is a dynamic organ with turnover of cells, including cardiomyocytes, throughout life.[1] Like many other organ systems, tissue-specific stem and progenitor cells have recently been identified that provide a source for generation of new cardiomyocytes and other essential cell types in the heart.[2–4] However, endogenous cardiac stem cells are unable to generate adequate numbers of cardiomyocytes to repair the heart after large insults, such as myocardial infarction. Furthermore the capacity of intrinsic repair by cardiac stem cells declines with age.[5] Thus the concept of delivering new, viable cells to the heart for repair and regeneration has been aggressively investigated for treatment following myocardial infarction and in heart failure. Ideally, such cell-based therapy will lead to regenerated myocardium that exhibits normal functional properties and consequently reduces the risk of arrhythmias, as the abnormal substrate is replaced and the conditions that trigger arrhythmias are eliminated. However, the delivery of cells to the myocardium can also potentially introduce conditions that increase the risk for arrhythmias. The purpose of this chapter is to examine the electrophysiological consequences of cell therapy for heart disease based on existing experimental data and early clinical experience.

Cell Sources for Cardiac Repair

A wide variety of different cell sources have been investigated for their ability to repair the heart in animal models and some investigated in clinical trials. Advances in stem cell research over the past two decades have also contributed to the variety of cell types under consideration. Cells from the recipient of the graft (autologous) as well as those isolated from donors (allogeneic) have been tested (Table 58.1). Autologous cell sources hold the possible advantage of not being recognized by the immune system as foreign, but the disadvantages of potentially costly individualized cell processing and the possibility that the underlying disease phenotype will make the transplanted cells dysfunctional. Alternatively, allogeneic cells may be at risk for immune rejection, but the off-the-shelf appeal and ability to optimally engineer the cells could be advantageous. The cell sources vary dramatically in their properties, including proliferative capacity, potency (ability to differentiate into different cell types), ability to survive ischemic and inflammatory insults, and secretion of signaling molecules. Furthermore, it is likely that the different cell sources can differentially impact the electrophysiological properties either acutely or over time.

Initial investigations into cell therapy for the heart sought the goal of remuscularizing the tissue by providing differentiated myocytes. Skeletal myoblasts derived from skeletal muscle satellite cells were the first cell source studied in detail.[6,7] Satellite cells can be isolated from a muscle biopsy and differentiated into myoblasts that can be expanded greatly in culture. Transplanted myoblasts formed viable grafts in animal hearts and improved the functional properties of the hearts[8,9]; however, the transplanted cells formed skeletal muscle grafts, not cardiac muscle, which had consequences, as skeletal muscle lacks connexin expression and gap junctions, so the cells did not electrically integrate into the myocardium.[9,10] Alternatively, transplanted fetal mouse ventricular myocytes were demonstrated to integrate into a recipient mouse heart, forming intercalated disks between donor cells and the recipient myocardium.[11] Treatment of infarcted or cryoinjured myocardium with fetal cardiomyocytes in several animal studies resulted in improved left ventricular function and limited adverse myocardial remodeling compared to sham control animals.[12,13] However, fetal cardiomyocytes are poorly tolerant of acute ischemia with the vast majority not surviving the transplant. Fetal cardiomyocytes are also terminally differentiated, so they do not exhibit significant cell division at the site of engraftment. Thus, it is difficult to obtain adequate cell numbers for larger areas of damage. Finally, the major limitation of applying this strategy to clinical medicine is the ethical objection to the use of human fetal tissue, as well as the very limited supply of such tissue.

The provocative study in 2001 by Orlic, Anversa, and colleagues demonstrated that bone marrow–derived, lineage-negative (lin−), and c-kit+ stem cells injected post–myocardial infarction in a mouse model resulted in remarkable repair of the heart accompanied by functional improvement.[14] The appealing concept that delivering stem cells to the injured heart could

TABLE 58.1   Cell sources for cardiac therapy

AUTOLOGOUS	ALLOGENEIC
Skeletal myoblasts	Fetal cardiomyocytes
Hematopoietic stem cells	Embryonic stem cells and derivatives
• c-kit+ lin−	
• Bone marrow mononuclear cells	
Endothelial progenitor cells	Mesenchymal stem cells[a,b]
• CD34+	
• CD133+	
Cardiac stem/progenitor cells	
• Side population	
• c-kit+	
• Cardiosphere-derived	
• Epicardial progenitors	
Induced pluripotent stem cells (iPSC) and derivatives[a]	
Induced cardiomyocytes (iCM)	
Induced cardiac progenitor cells (iCPC)	

[a]Can be both autologous and allogeneic.
[b]Can be derived from multiple tissues, including bone marrow and adipose.

lead to robust regeneration of functional myocardium was put forward, but soon these results were challenged by others arguing against the ability of hematopoietic stem cells to form cardiac tissue.[15,16] Nevertheless, investigators considered other cell sources, including mesenchymal stem cells (MSCs) derived from bone marrow, to treat the injured heart, likewise suggesting the generation of new myocardium. But this conclusion has also been challenged.[17,18]

The demonstration of rare endogenous cardiac stem and progenitor cells in the heart provided additional possible cell sources for cardiac repair. Investigators have used a number of different techniques and cell surface markers to isolate endogenous cardiac progenitors. In the earliest study, progenitors were suggested based on the ability to expel Hoechst 33342 dye, which was used with fluorescence activated cell sorting (FACS) to identify a rare "side population" of cells in a similar fashion as had previously been used in hematopoietic cells.[19] These side population cells have cardiac potential based on in vitro studies. The cell surface marker c-kit was subsequently used to identify multipotent cardiac stem cells in mouse and human hearts.[20,21] Likewise Sca-1 was identified as a cell surface marker for cardiac progenitors, but this protein is not expressed in humans.[3] The transcription factor Isl-1 has also been used to define a cardiac progenitor cell population in transgenic mouse models and in human hearts.[4,22] Explanted cardiac tissue can be cultured under conditions promoting the migration of cells that can be isolated, cultured, and expanded under nonadherent conditions to form cardiospheres.[23,24] These cardiospheres contain a mixed population of progenitors with the ability to form multiple lineages, including cardiomyocytes. Finally, the epicardium has been reported to contain multipotent epicardial progenitors identified by WT-1 or Tbx-18, which can give rise to multiple cell types in the myocardium.[25,26] The differences between the various progenitor populations is still the subject of intense investigation, and it is possible that different strategies identify related populations at different stages of maturation.[27] Nevertheless, transplanting such progenitor cells holds appeal for cardiac repair, and initial animal studies have shown functional benefit following myocardial infarction.[2,14,28]

The establishment of technologies to produce human pluripotent stem cells (PSCs) provided new considerations for cardiac cell therapy. The successful isolation of human embryonic stem cells (ESCs) from surplus in vitro fertilization embryos

by Thomson and colleagues in 1998 opened up new avenues for cardiac therapeutic applications.[29] Subsequent demonstration that human ESCs could differentiate into functional cardiomyocytes confirmed the potential utility of this cell source for cardiac repair.[30,31] Studies in animal models with mouse ESCs showed that the cells could have beneficial effects post–myocardial infarction and would generate different cell linages following transplantation of undifferentiated ESCs.[32–34] However, transplanting the ESCs without differentiation carries the risk of teratoma tumor formation,[35] so subsequent studies have evaluated differentiated derivatives for repair.[36,37] A limitation of human embryonic stem cells is that they represent an allogeneic cell source likely requiring immunosuppression in the recipient. The recent development of technology to generate ESCs by somatic cell nuclear transfer to oocytes (ntESCs) may overcome this limitation.[38] Alternatively, the breakthrough in cellular reprogramming of somatic cells to induced pluripotent stem cells (iPSCs) provides a remarkable new approach to generate patient-specific therapies that are genetically matched.[39,40] Initial studies using this cell source have shown early promise,[41] but many questions remain regarding the stability of the phenotype, the immune privilege, and the long-term impact of reprogramming. Reprogramming technologies have subsequently identified direct reprogramming approaches to directly generate induced cardiomyocytes (iCM)[42,43] and induced cardiac progenitor cells (iCPC),[44] which may be important tools in cardiac repair and can be autologous cell sources.

As investigators more critically examined cell survival and engraftment after cell delivery, it became progressively clear that many of the functional benefits observed in animal models following cell transplantation in most studies were not due to remuscularization of infarcts. Regardless of the source, the vast majority of transplanted cells did not survive, let alone generate new myocardium. Nevertheless, clear beneficial effects of the therapies were observed based on the functional and structural properties of treated hearts. Thus a number of additional mechanisms of benefit have been proposed (Fig. 58.1). Perhaps most prominent among the potential mechanisms of benefit is the reported paracrine effects of certain cell populations, such as MSCs, which secrete molecules to promote survival of existing heart tissue and blunt adverse remodeling.[18,45] Other potential beneficial effects include activating endogenous stem cells, cell fusion, induction of angiogenesis, antiinflammatory effects, and resynchronizing the myocardium. The exact mechanistic impact likely varies with different cell sources, and these details are far from completely defined in animal studies. Nevertheless, these early animal studies have generated sufficient interest and data to proceed to clinical trials.

Basic Mechanisms by Which Cell Therapy Can Impact Cardiac Electrophysiology

Cellular grafts need to undergo electrical and mechanical integration into the myocardium for optimal benefit. Furthermore, the functional properties of the cells ideally must match those of normal myocardium. In order to investigate and optimize these features of cell therapies, studies have been performed using both in vitro and animal models. Depending on the precise details of the grafts and their integration, the transplanted cells can be either proarrhythmic or antiarrhythmic (Fig. 58.2). Cell therapy can contribute to the genesis of arrhythmias by impacting all three basic mechanisms of arrhythmias: reentry, abnormal automaticity, and triggered activity. Alternatively, cell therapy can blunt arrhythmias by improving the underlying substrate and removing triggers. Careful examination of the integration and functional properties of the cellular grafts is essential for optimizing safe and effective cell therapy approaches.

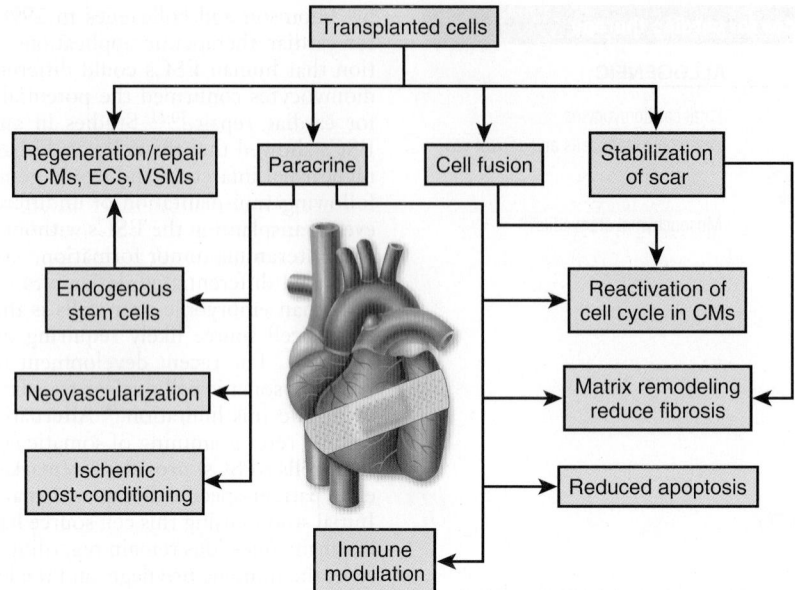

FIGURE 58.1 **Possible mechanisms of benefit from cell therapy for injured myocardium.** *CMs,* cardiomyocytes; *ECs,* endothelial cells; *VSMs,* vascular smooth muscle cells.

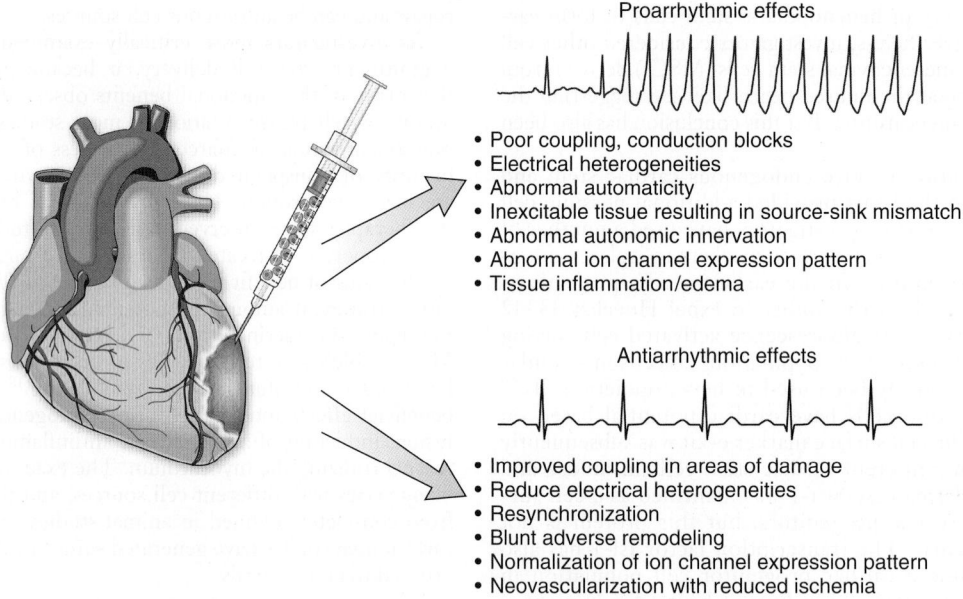

FIGURE 58.2 Potential effects of cardiac cell therapy on arrhythmia risk.

Cell Coupling and Integration

Successful regeneration of myocardium with cell therapy requires electromechanical integration of the new cells into the functional myocardium. However, significant barriers must be overcome in the diseased heart in order for integration to be successful. The presence of scar and fibrosis in the heart requires significant remodeling for integration of transplanted cells with the functional myocardium. Delivering or homing the transplanted cells to the site in the heart in need of repair is likewise a major challenge. Not only must the graft integrate and couple to native myocardium, but it ideally must regenerate tissue with matched anisotropic conduction properties of the heart. The success of graft integration will in part determine the impact on arrhythmia risk. For example, replacing or reducing nonexcitable or slowly conducting tissue at the site of infarction would reduce the substrate for reentrant arrhythmias. Alternatively, if cell therapy produces areas of uncoupled tissue,

poorly coupled tissue, or coupled inexcitable tissue that produces source–sink mismatches, then the delivery of cells could produce wavefront breaks and reentry.

As an initial test of the ability of donor cells to couple with native cardiomyocytes, a number of in vitro coculture experiments have been performed. These cocultures of donor cells with ventricular cardiomyocytes have highlighted different forms of electromechanical coupling. In the case of cocultured human ESC-derived cardiomyocytes, clear coupling with rat neonatal ventricular myocytes has been demonstrated with the formation of connexin 43 (Cx43) gap junctions.[46] Synchronized contractions were observed in the cocultures, suggesting functional coupling. In studies coculturing MSCs with rat ventricular myocytes, formation of Cx43 gap junctions was also observed, and electrotonic conduction occurred via MSCs, as these cells are not electrically excitable.[47,48] In contrast, coculture of skeletal myoblasts with neonatal rat ventricular cardiomyocytes failed to couple, as myotubes do not express Cx43 or form gap junctions.[49] Thus, islands of electrically isolated myotubes provided substrate for reentry involving the surrounding cardiomyocytes. However, genetically engineered expression of Cx43 in myoblasts can lead to functional coupling with neonatal cardiomyocytes.[49] These simple coculture studies highlight key differences in coupling that can occur following cell therapy in the myocardium, but understanding the full complexity of electromechanical coupling resulting from cell therapy requires study in intact hearts.

A wide range of different cell sources have been tested in various animal models of cardiac injury; however, only a small minority of the studies has rigorously investigated the electrophysiological consequences of cell therapy. Transplanted skeletal myoblasts were first examined for their ability to couple to native myocardium. Despite being transplanted into the heart, myoblasts differentiate into skeletal myotubes lacking Cx43 and do not couple to the post–myocardial infarction rat heart,[50,51] which is consistent with the in vitro studies. However, genetically engineered expression of Cx43 in skeletal myotubes can result in coupling to the native heart and reduce risks for ventricular arrhythmias in a mouse infarct model.[52] In the case of bone marrow–derived MSCs, transplantation into a rat myocardial infarction model resulted in improved electrical conduction properties around the borderzone of the infarct, based on voltage optical mapping studies with the MSCs expressing multiple connexins, including Cx43.[53] This finding with MSCs parallels the in vitro studies, suggesting that MSCs can provide electronic coupling of cardiomyocytes.

Mouse fetal cardiomyocytes transplanted into the adult mouse heart have been shown, using a number of different approaches, to electrically couple to the native myocardium. Using GFP-labeled fetal cardiomyocytes transplanted to a native mouse heart, multiphoton microscopy was used to demonstrate synchronized intracellular calcium transients, comparing native adult cardiomyocytes and transplanted fetal cardiomyocytes.[54] Using an alternative imaging approach in which genetically engineered mouse cardiomyocytes expressing a fluorescent calcium indicator protein (GCaMP2) were transplanted to the post–myocardial infarction mouse heart, intracellular Ca^{2+} transients in the transplanted cells entrained with the native cardiac electrical rhythm, indicating coupling of transplanted cells and native heart.[52] Furthermore, conduction in the infarct region improved and inducible ventricular tachycardia decreased significantly in the fetal cardiomyocyte–treated hearts compared with sham or myoblast-treated hearts.[52] In a myocardial cryoinjury mouse model, GFP-labeled fetal cardiomyocytes transplanted to the borderzone were able to couple with native myocardium, as determined by sharp microelectrode recordings of labeled cells, although transplanted cells remote from the border zone in the area of cryoinjury showed spontaneous activity and were not coupled in most cases.[55]

The ability of transplanted PSC-derived cardiomyocytes to couple to native myocardium has also been examined. In one study, transplantation of mouse ESC-derived cardiomyocytes into the post–myocardial infarction mouse heart resulted in an increase in inducible ventricular tachycardia and increased mortality.[37] Another study transplanting human ESC-derived cardiomyocytes into the cryoinjured guinea pig heart suggested a strong antiarrhythmic effect with a reduction in spontaneous ventricular arrhythmias and decreased inducible ventricular tachycardia.[36] In this latter study, the human ESC-derived cardiomyocytes formed Cx43-positive gap junctions with native myocardium, and using the genetically engineered Ca^{2+} reporter construct (GCaMP3), functional coupling of the grafted ESC-cardiomyocytes and native heart was demonstrated.[36] A subsequent study by this same group transplanted human ESC-derived cardiomyocytes with a GCaMP3 reporter to a nonhuman primate (pigtail macaque) heart following

ischemia and reperfusion, and this study, likewise, found evidence of functional coupling between engrafted cardiomyocytes and native myocardium.[56] However, this study raised new concerns about the risk of arrhythmias because all ESC-derived cardiomyocyte–treated animals showed evidence for increased ventricular ectopy in the form of frequent premature ventricular complexes, periods of accelerated idioventricular rhythm, and runs of ventricular tachycardia. However, all of these arrhythmias were tolerated without evidence of mortality or loss of consciousness, and all ventricular arrhythmias were transient, completely resolving after 1 month. In contrast, studies transplanting iPSC-derived cardiomyocytes in sheets or patches to the porcine heart following ischemia and reperfusion found no evidence of an increase in ventricular ectopy, but detailed studies of functional coupling were not performed.[57,58] Thus the few studies exploring PSC-derived cardiomyocytes for cardiac cell therapy have shown conflicting results regarding the arrhythmia risk, but species and model differences, delivery approaches, and cell dose/graft size may help explain the differing results.

Intrinsic Properties of the Transplanted Cells

The impact of cell therapies to the injured heart will depend not only on the integration of the donor cells but also on the functional properties of the transplanted cells. Given the array of different cell types tested, there is a tremendous range of functional properties possible for engrafted cells. Transplantation of stem or progenitor cells may lead to the generation of diverse cellular progeny in the graft (e.g., cardiomyocytes, endothelial cells, and fibroblasts), which can differentially impact the electrophysiological status of the treated heart. Some of the resulting cell types are excitable, whereas others are not. Nonexcitable cells, such as fibroblasts or mesenchymal stem cells, can still exert potent electrophysiological effects by acting to bridge nonconducting areas of myocardium (antiarrhythmic) or to produce current sinks, thereby increasing heterogeneous conduction patterns (proarrhythmic). Transplantation of terminally differentiated cardiomyocytes will lead to cardiomyocyte-dominated grafts. However, a wide range of functional properties of the transplanted cardiomyocyte is possible, given differences in the type and maturity of the engrafted cardiomyocytes. To further complicate the analysis, the functional properties of the transplanted cells can change over time as they adapt and respond to the native cardiac environment. Thus, consideration of the donor cells' functional phenotype requires not only consideration of the cell preparation used for transplantation, but also the resulting cellular phenotype in the cardiac graft. In addition to the presence of new cardiomyocytes in the grafts, cell fusion of donor cells with native heart cells may alter the properties of the native myocardium, which could have important functional consequences.

For transplanted cardiomyocytes or cardiomyocytes that differentiate from transplanted progenitor cells, the functional properties can be put into perspective based on well-known electrophysiological properties seen in healthy and diseased myocardium. PSC-derived cardiomyocytes in culture exhibit features typical of the embryonic heart with cardiomyocytes showing spontaneous automaticity, a more depolarized maximum diastolic potential, and a reduced upstroke velocity.[31] These features all have the potential to be proarrhythmic in the transplanted heart by leading to areas of abnormal automaticity, depolarizing tissue, and slowing conduction, respectively.[59] However, there is evidence that the functional properties of transplanted cardiomyocytes can mature in situ and exhibit more hyperpolarized resting membrane potentials and more rapid upstroke velocities.[55] In addition to manifesting an embryonic phenotype, it is possible that transplanted cardiomyocytes will exhibit differences in repolarization due to the native myocardium creating areas of dispersion of refractoriness and hence substrate for reentry. Because repolarization is finely regulated by multiple ion channels expressed in the cardiomyocytes, altering this delicate balance is possible. Furthermore, if transplanted cardiomyocytes are injured in the transplantation process or respond adversely to the diseased myocardium, they can develop pathological responses, including calcium overload and the propensity to exhibit delayed afterdepolarizations, and the resulting triggered arrhythmias. Despite all of these potential problems, it is encouraging that the slow turnover and replacement of cardiomyocytes in the normal heart results in functionally matched cardiomyocytes based on the similar properties of isolated cardiomyocytes from the adult heart and lack of arrhythmias in normal hearts. Nevertheless, defining the functional properties of engrafted cells remains a critical and currently little-investigated feature of cardiac cell therapy.

Other Cardiac Tissue Effects of Cell Therapy With Arrhythmia Relevance

Cells delivered to the diseased myocardium can exert a number of additional effects that can more generally impact the electrophysiological status of the heart. These effects can be related to the effect of cell therapy on the underlying heart disease pathophysiology, which then secondarily impacts arrhythmia risk. In addition, the method of cell delivery can impact the native myocardium; for example, intramyocardial delivery can disrupt the architecture of the myocardium and introduce areas of impaired conduction. Molecules secreted by the transplanted cells can have powerful paracrine effects on the heart. Likewise cell therapy can impact the status of autonomic innervation of the heart, the burden of ischemia, and cardiac synchronization.

In the setting of the post–myocardial infarction heart, perhaps the most critical impact of cell therapy is the ability to blunt further adverse remodeling of the myocardium, which can progress to LV dysfunction and heart failure with ever-increasing risk of life-threatening ventricular arrhythmias. For many of the cell sources tested to date, the paracrine effects of the transplanted cells are believed to be responsible for the inhibition of adverse remodeling. Potential mechanisms for this beneficial effect include the ability of some stem cell sources to modulate the inflammation present following myocardial infarction and hence improve the remodeling process. Others have suggested that some stem cells can activate endogenous cardiac stem cells and enhance intrinsic cardiac repair.[60] Regardless, if the net result of paracrine signaling is to blunt remodeling and prevent progression to heart failure, then cell therapy will have a long-term antiarrhythmic effect on treated hearts relative to untreated.

Cell therapies that successfully lead to neovascularization and repair of the heart will reduce the ischemia experienced by the myocardium. Eliminating or reducing ischemia as a trigger for arrhythmias can be of obvious benefit. Alternatively, if cell delivery. such as by the intracoronary route, exacerbates ischemia, this could have an adverse effect on arrhythmia risk.

Delivery of MSCs to the injured heart has been associated with areas of cardiac nerve sprouting.[61] The generation of areas of nerve sprouting has previously been associated with an increased risk of sudden cardiac death,[62] so investigators have speculated that MSC cell therapy may likewise generate this risk.

Cardiac resynchronization has become a common therapy to treat heart failure, especially in the presence of impaired conduction. The clinically applied form of resynchronization involves a biventricular pacemaker, but cell therapy may be even more effective in its resynchronization, depending on proper integration and function of the grafts. Potential benefits from this effect may not be evident immediately, but could manifest in longer-term studies.

Clinical Experience With Cell Therapy and Arrhythmias

Starting in 2001, clinical trials have examined the impact of cell therapy for various forms of heart disease. These trials have focused primarily on ischemic heart disease, both following myocardial infarction and in chronic ischemic heart disease with systolic heart failure. In addition, a variety of cell sources have been tested, but autologous bone marrow mononuclear cells have been most commonly used. In addition, allogeneic cells, primarily mesenchymal stem cells, have also been tested. Cell delivery methods have varied, including catheter-based intracoronary, intravenous, and intramyocardial methods, both via epicardial injection at the time of cardiac surgery and via catheter-based endocardial injection. Phase 1 trials have shown that the wide range of cell sources and delivery strategies were safe in the initial analysis. Subsequently a growing number of phase 2 randomized clinical trials have been performed examining both efficacy and safety. While the safety signal continues to be encouraging, the degree of benefit observed by the interventions has been variable with some trials showing a modest improvement in left ventricular remodeling and function and others showing no clear benefit.[63] This first generation of cell therapy for heart disease has raised many questions that will require additional research given the many variables, including marked differences in cell sources, cell processing, delivery strategies, and patient populations. Phase 3 randomized clinical trials are now underway that will provide more clarity with regard to hard clinical endpoints.

The growing body of clinical trial data for cardiac cell therapy is providing a rich dataset on the risk of arrhythmias associated with therapy. All trials monitor for major events during hospitalization, such as death and documented arrhythmias, but follow-up monitoring for arrhythmias has been variable, ranging from no scheduled monitoring to periodic Holter monitoring to loop recorders or mandated implantable cardiodefibrillators. The phase 1 trials to date have found the cell sources tested to be safe, although an early trial delivering skeletal muscle–derived myoblasts at the time of coronary artery bypass surgery provided an initial note of caution, with four of ten patients who were treated with myoblasts experiencing ventricular tachycardia.[64] However, this trial did not use a comparable control group, and the patients were high risk with advanced systolic heart failure. The subsequent phase 2 randomized clinical trials performed for a range of different cell sources and delivery strategies have not identified a statistically increased risk of arrhythmia in any trial to date. Furthermore, careful meta-analysis of 41 randomized trials delivering autologous bone marrow mononuclear cells following myocardial infarction found that 21 trials specifically reported arrhythmia outcomes and found no significant difference between cell-treated and placebo trial subjects.[65] Likewise, a meta-analysis of 23 randomized clinical trials of patients with chronic ischemic heart disease and systolic heart failure found that 19 trials reported arrhythmias and did not find any significant increase in observed arrhythmias in cell-treated patients.[66] So despite very different myocardial substrates in the acute remodeling post–myocardial infarction heart or in the chronic failing ischemic heart, the tested doses of various cell products used to date have not increased arrhythmia risk. Perhaps some of this lack of arrhythmia signal is related to the transient engraftment of most delivered cells tested to date, which are acting primarily by paracrine mechanisms rather than by generating new excitable myocardium.[67] However, new cell types are emerging in clinical trials, including the first-in-man clinical trial of human ESC-derived cardiac progenitor cells.[68] As newer cell sources including excitable cells, such as stem cell–derived cardiomyocytes, transition to clinical applications, the risk of arrhythmias will require continued vigilance. Furthermore, as the patient experience grows with phase 3 trials, the significance of relatively rare adverse events, such as ventricular arrhythmias may become more apparent.

Conclusions and Future Directions

Cell therapy is of growing interest in the treatment of various forms of heart disease, including post–myocardial infarction and heart failure. Basic research and studies in animal models have suggested that the impact of cell therapies on the heart is complex and dependent on the details of cell delivery methodology, donor cell types, and underlying cardiac disease. Multiple mechanisms of benefit on cardiac outcomes have been identified, including a range of paracrine effects, mechanical effects, and, rarely, the generation of new cardiomyocytes. Experimental studies have also identified many potential ways in which cell therapy can be proarrhythmic or antiarrhythmic. The ability of donor cells to couple to the native myocardium via Cx43 gap junctions has been identified in animal studies as a critical variable that can impact whether a cell therapy is proarrhythmic or antiarrhythmic. Although most preclinical animal studies have not identified an increased incidence of ventricular arrhythmias, delivery of large numbers of cardiomyocytes with spontaneous automaticity to the post–myocardial infarction nonhuman primate heart resulted in a clear burst of ventricular arrhythmias in the first weeks after transplantation. Nevertheless, the appealing concept of repairing or regenerating myocardium with stem cells has led to the rapid translation from the research laboratory to clinical trials. A variety of primarily autologous cell preparations have been delivered either intracoronarily or intramyocardially to patients with coronary artery disease in phase 1 and 2 trials. The initial results from the trials have been variable and have shown either an improvement, primarily in ejection fraction, or no effect. The trials have not identified safety concerns to this point, including a lack of proarrhythmia by the cell therapy. Phase 3 trials are under

way, so more definitive clinical data will be available in the next few years.

Future approaches for cardiac cell therapy will undoubtedly evolve. The patient populations most amenable to this therapy are not known, and the optimal cell type for each disease is also unknown. It is likely that different cell preparations will show differences in utility depending on the underlying cardiac disease. Will genetically engineered cells that express proteins that help couple, promote targeting to the area of need, or optimize paracrine signaling be preferable? The revolution in genomic engineering with CRISPR/Cas9 technology makes this option more likely. Tissue engineering applications are under investigation that may allow new delivery strategies using viable patches of myocardial tissue that could greatly impact the substrate for arrhythmias, perhaps creating or removing heterogeneities in conduction. New approaches to directly reprogram fibroblasts into cardiomyocytes (induced cardiomyocytes)[42] or cardiac progenitor cells (induced cardiac progenitors)[44] may also transition to clinical applications with unknown impacts on arrhythmia risk.

Understanding the risk of arrhythmias with the ongoing cell therapy approaches will continue to be of utmost importance to ensure these therapies are safe, as well as effective. Arrhythmia risk may be dynamic, such as an early increase in risk following cell delivery and potentially a decrease later as well. Thus in some cases it may be useful to at least transiently treat with antiarrhythmic drugs to lower the risk of arrhythmias. More detailed monitoring for arrhythmias during the trials is needed to clarify risk and potentially define one form of benefit-reduction in arrhythmias. Routine surveillance for arrhythmias is reasonable using Holter monitors or implantable event recorders. For patients with ICDs, regular interrogations and data analysis pretherapy and posttherapy may be useful. The optimal duration for monitoring is unknown. Consideration of the electrophysiological impacts of cell therapy to the diseased myocardium will continue to be essential to advance this revolutionary new form of treatment.

REFERENCES

1. Bergmann O, Bhardwaj RD, Bernard S, et al. Evidence for cardiomyocyte renewal in humans. *Science.* 2009;324:98–102.
2. Beltrami AP, Barlucchi L, Torella D, et al. Adult cardiac stem cells are multipotent and support myocardial regeneration. *Cell.* 2003;114:763–776.
3. Oh H, Bradfute SB, Gallardo TD, et al. Cardiac progenitor cells from adult myocardium: homing, differentiation, and fusion after infarction. *Proc Natl Acad Sci U S A.* 2003;100:12313–12318.
4. Laugwitz KL, Moretti A, Lam J, et al. Postnatal isl1+ cardioblasts enter fully differentiated cardiomyocyte lineages. *Nature.* 2005;433:647–653.
5. Dimmeler S, Leri A. Aging and disease as modifiers of efficacy of cell therapy. *Circ Res.* 2008;102:1319–1330.
6. Marelli D, Desrosiers C, el Alfy M, et al. Cell transplantation for myocardial repair: an experimental approach. *Cell Transplant.* 1992;1:383–390.
7. Koh GY, Klug MG, Soonpaa MH, et al. Differentiation and long-term survival of c2c12 myoblast grafts in heart. *J Clin Invest.* 1993;92:1548–1554.
8. Taylor DA, Atkins BZ, Hungspreugs P, et al. Regenerating functional myocardium: improved performance after skeletal myoblast transplantation. *Nat Med.* 1998;4:929–933.
9. Scorsin M, Hagege A, Vilquin JT, et al. Comparison of the effects of fetal cardiomyocyte and skeletal myoblast transplantation on postinfarction left ventricular function. *J Thorac Cardiovasc Surg.* 2000;119:1169–1175.
10. Reinecke H, MacDonald GH, Hauschka SD, et al. Electromechanical coupling between skeletal and cardiac muscle. Implications for infarct repair. *J Cell Biol.* 2000;149:731–740.
11. Soonpaa MH, Koh GY, Klug MG, et al. Formation of nascent intercalated disks between grafted fetal cardiomyocytes and host myocardium. *Science.* 1994;264:98–101.
12. Scorsin M, Marotte F, Sabri A, et al. Can grafted cardiomyocytes colonize peri-infarct myocardial areas? *Circulation.* 1996;94:II337–II340.

13. Li RK, Jia ZQ, Weisel RD, et al. Cardiomyocyte transplantation improves heart function. *Ann Thorac Surg.* 1996;62:654–660.
14. Orlic D, Kajstura J, Chimenti S, et al. Bone marrow cells regenerate infarcted myocardium. *Nature.* 2001;410:701–705.
15. Balsam LB, Wagers AJ, Christensen JL, et al. Haematopoietic stem cells adopt mature haematopoietic fates in ischaemic myocardium. *Nature.* 2004;428:668–673.
16. Murry CE, Soonpaa MH, Reinecke H, et al. Haematopoietic stem cells do not transdifferentiate into cardiac myocytes in myocardial infarcts. *Nature.* 2004;428:664–668.
17. Toma C, Pittenger MF, Cahill KS, et al. Human mesenchymal stem cells differentiate to a cardiomyocyte phenotype in the adult murine heart. *Circulation.* 2002;105:93–98.
18. Mirotsou M, Zhang Z, Deb A, et al. Secreted frizzled related protein 2 (sfrp2) is the key akt-mesenchymal stem cell-released paracrine factor mediating myocardial survival and repair. *Proc Natl Acad Sci U S A.* 2007;104:1643–1648.
19. Hierlihy AM, Seale P, Lobe CG, et al. The post-natal heart contains a myocardial stem cell population. *FEBS Lett.* 2002;530:239–243.
20. Beltrami AP, Barlucchi L, Torella D, et al. Adult cardiac stem cells are multipotent and support myocardial regeneration. *Cell.* 2003;114:763–776.
21. Kubo H, Jaleel N, Kumarapeli A, et al. Increased cardiac myocyte progenitors in failing human hearts. *Circulation.* 2008;118:649–657.
22. Bu L, Jiang X, Martin-Puig S, et al. Human isl1 heart progenitors generate diverse multipotent cardiovascular cell lineages. *Nature.* 2009;460:113–117.
23. Messina E, De Angelis L, Frati G, et al. Isolation and expansion of adult cardiac stem cells from human and murine heart. *Circ Res.* 2004;95:911–921.
24. Chimenti I, Smith RR, Li TS, et al. Relative roles of direct regeneration versus paracrine effects of human cardiosphere-derived cells transplanted into infarcted mice. *Circ Res.* 2010;106:971–980.

25. Zhou B, Ma Q, Rajagopal S, et al. Epicardial progenitors contribute to the cardiomyocyte lineage in the developing heart. *Nature.* 2008;454:109–113.
26. Cai CL, Martin JC, Sun Y, et al. A myocardial lineage derives from tbx18 epicardial cells. *Nature.* 2008;454:104–108.
27. Pfister O, Oikonomopoulos A, Sereti KI, et al. Role of the atp-binding cassette transporter abcg2 in the phenotype and function of cardiac side population cells. *Circ Res.* 2008;103:825–835.
28. Smith RR, Barile L, Cho HC, et al. Regenerative potential of cardiosphere-derived cells expanded from percutaneous endomyocardial biopsy specimens. *Circulation.* 2007;115:896–908.
29. Thomson JA, Itskovitz-Eldor J, Shapiro SS, et al. Embryonic stem cell lines derived from human blastocysts. *Science.* 1998;282:1145–1147.
30. Kehat I, Kenyagin-Karsenti D, Snir M, et al. Human embryonic stem cells can differentiate into myocytes with structural and functional properties of cardiomyocytes. *J Clin Invest.* 2001;108:407–414.
31. He JQ, Ma Y, Lee Y, et al. Human embryonic stem cells develop into multiple types of cardiac myocytes: action potential characterization. *Circ Res.* 2003;93:32–39.
32. Behfar A, Zingman LV, Hodgson DM, et al. Stem cell differentiation requires a paracrine pathway in the heart. *FASEB J.* 2002;16:1558–1566.
33. Min JY, Yang Y, Converso KL, et al. Transplantation of embryonic stem cells improves cardiac function in postinfarcted rats. *J Appl Physiol.* 2002;92:288–296.
34. Singla DK, Hacker TA, Ma L, et al. Transplantation of embryonic stem cells into the infarcted mouse heart: formation of multiple cell types. *J Mol Cell Cardiol.* 2006;40:195–200.
35. Nussbaum J, Minami E, Laflamme MA, et al. Transplantation of undifferentiated murine embryonic stem cells in the heart: teratoma formation and immune response. *FASEB J.* 2007;21:1345–1357.
36. Shiba Y, Fernandes S, Zhu WZ, et al. Human ES-cell-derived cardiomyocytes electrically couple and suppress arrhythmias in injured hearts. *Nature.* 2012;489:322–325.

37. Liao SY, Liu Y, Siu CW, et al. Proarrhythmic risk of embryonic stem cell-derived cardiomyocyte transplantation in infarcted myocardium. *Heart Rhythm.* 2010;7(12):1852–1859.

38. Tachibana M, Amato P, Sparman M, et al. Human embryonic stem cells derived by somatic cell nuclear transfer. *Cell.* 2013;153:1228–1238.

39. Takahashi K, Tanabe K, Ohnuki M, et al. Induction of pluripotent stem cells from adult human fibroblasts by defined factors. *Cell.* 2007;131:861–872.

40. Yu J, Vodyanik MA, Smuga-Otto K, et al. Induced pluripotent stem cell lines derived from human somatic cells. *Science.* 2007;318:1917–1920.

41. Nelson TJ, Martinez-Fernandez A, Yamada S, et al. Repair of acute myocardial infarction by human stemness factors induced pluripotent stem cells. *Circulation.* 2009;120:408–416.

42. Ieda M, Fu JD, Delgado-Olguin P, et al. Direct reprogramming of fibroblasts into functional cardiomyocytes by defined factors. *Cell.* 2010;142:375–386.

43. Song K, Nam YJ, Luo X, et al. Heart repair by reprogramming non-myocytes with cardiac transcription factors. *Nature.* 2012;485:599–604.

44. Lalit PA, Salick M, Nelson DO, et al. Lineage reprogramming of fibroblasts to proliferative induced cardiac progenitor cells by defined factors. *Cell Stem Cell.* 2016;18:354–367.

45. Mangi AA, Noiseux N, Kong D, et al. Mesenchymal stem cells modified with Akt prevent remodeling and restore performance of infarcted hearts. *Nat Med.* 2003;9:1195–1201.

46. Kehat I, Khimovich L, Caspi O, et al. Electromechanical integration of cardiomyocytes derived from human embryonic stem cells. *Nat Biotechnol.* 2004;22:1282–1289.

47. Valiunas V, Doronin S, Valiuniene L, et al. Human mesenchymal stem cells make cardiac connexins and form functional gap junctions. *J Physiol.* 2004;555:617–626.

48. Chang MG, Tung L, Sekar RB, et al. Proarrhythmic potential of mesenchymal stem cell transplantation revealed in an in vitro coculture model. *Circulation.* 2006;113:1832–1841.

49. Abraham MR, Henrikson CA, Tung L, et al. Antiarrhythmic engineering of skeletal myoblasts for cardiac transplantation. *Circ Res.* 2005;97:159–167.

50. Leobon B, Garcin I, Menasche P, et al. Myoblasts transplanted into rat infarcted myocardium are functionally isolated from their host. *Proc Natl Acad Sci U S A.* 2003;100:7808–7811.

51. Rubart M, Soonpaa MH, Nakajima H, et al. Spontaneous and evoked intracellular calcium transients in donor-derived myocytes following intracardiac myoblast transplantation. *J Clin Invest.* 2004;114:775–783.

52. Roell W, Lewalter T, Sasse P, et al. Engraftment of connexin 43-expressing cells prevents post-infarct arrhythmia. *Nature.* 2007;450:819–824.

53. Mills WR, Mal N, Kiedrowski MJ, et al. Stem cell therapy enhances electrical viability in myocardial infarction. *J Mol Cell Cardiol.* 2007;42:304–314.

54. Rubart M, Pasumarthi KB, Nakajima H, et al. Physiological coupling of donor and host cardiomyocytes after cellular transplantation. *Circ Res.* 2003;92:1217–1224.

55. Halbach M, Pfannkuche K, Pillekamp F, et al. Electrophysiological maturation and integration of murine fetal cardiomyocytes after transplantation. *Circ Res.* 2007;101:484–492.

56. Chong JJ, Yang X, Don CW, et al. Human embryonic-stem-cell-derived cardiomyocytes regenerate non-human primate hearts. *Nature.* 2014;510:273–277.

57. Kawamura M, Miyagawa S, Miki K, et al. Feasibility, safety, and therapeutic efficacy of human induced pluripotent stem cell-derived cardiomyocyte sheets in a porcine ischemic cardiomyopathy model. *Circulation.* 2012;126:S29–S37.

58. Ye L, Chang YH, Xiong Q, et al. Cardiac repair in a porcine model of acute myocardial infarction with human induced pluripotent stem cell-derived cardiovascular cells. *Cell Stem Cell.* 2014;15:750–761.

59. Zhang YM, Hartzell C, Narlow M, et al. Stem cell-derived cardiomyocytes demonstrate arrhythmic potential. *Circulation.* 2002;106:1294–1299.

60. Hatzistergos KE, Quevedo H, Oskouei BN, et al. Bone marrow mesenchymal stem cells stimulate cardiac stem cell proliferation and differentiation. *Circ Res.* 2010;107:913–922.

61. Pak HN, Qayyum M, Kim DT, et al. Mesenchymal stem cell injection induces cardiac nerve sprouting and increased tenascin expression in a swine model of myocardial infarction. *J Cardiovasc Electrophysiol.* 2003;14:841–848.

62. Cao JM, Chen LS, KenKnight BH, et al. Nerve sprouting and sudden cardiac death. *Circ Res.* 2000;86:816–821.

63. Behfar A, Crespo-Diaz R, Terzic A, et al. Cell therapy for cardiac repair—lessons from clinical trials. *Nat Rev Cardiol.* 2014;11:232–246.

64. Menasche P, Hagege AA, Vilquin JT, et al. Autologous skeletal myoblast transplantation for severe postinfarction left ventricular dysfunction. *J Am Coll Cardiol.* 2003;41:1078–1083.

65. Fisher SA, Zhang H, Doree C, et al. Stem cell treatment for acute myocardial infarction. *Cochrane Database Syst Rev.* 2015;9:CD006536.

66. Fisher SA, Brunskill SJ, Doree C, et al. Stem cell therapy for chronic ischaemic heart disease and congestive heart failure. *Cochrane Database Syst Rev.* 2014;4:CD007888.

67. Tang XL, Li Q, Rokosh G, et al. Long-term outcome of administration of c-kit(POS) cardiac progenitor cells after acute myocardial infarction: transplanted cells do not become cardiomyocytes, but structural and functional improvement and proliferation of endogenous cells persist for at least one year. *Circ Res.* 2016;118:1091–1105.

68. Menasche P, Vanneaux V, Hagege A, et al. Human embryonic stem cell-derived cardiac progenitors for severe heart failure treatment: first clinical case report. *Eur Heart J.* 2015;36:2011–2017.

59 Assessment of the Patient With a Cardiac Arrhythmia

Mithilesh K. Das and Douglas P. Zipes

The evaluation of a patient with a suspected cardiac rhythm disturbance is fundamental to the role of the clinical cardiac electrophysiologist. The approach followed for this evaluation varies from patient to patient and is influenced by the patient's clinical status and symptoms, but a general outline can be established, as presented in this chapter. As always, the initial evaluation begins with a careful history and physical examination.

Taking History of a Patient With Suspected Arrhythmia

Significant overlap exists among the clinical features of various rhythm disturbances, for example, complaints of palpitations or lightheadedness, imparting a degree of imprecision to the interpretation of the patient's history. Despite this, the history often can provide direction and diagnostic clues as the first step in assessing the patient with, or suspected of having, a cardiac arrhythmia. It often is the most important source of information about the arrhythmia.

Symptoms and Signs of Arrhythmia

General

Major symptoms and signs of cardiac arrhythmias are palpitations, shortness of breath, atypical chest pain, lightheadedness, presyncope, syncope, and sudden cardiac death (SCD). In this setting, nonspecific symptoms such as shortness of breath, weakness, and fatigue can be due to compromise in cardiac output impacted by the duration of the arrhythmia or its rate, either very fast or very slow. Older patients with bradycardia owing to sinus node dysfunction or atrioventricular (AV) nodal block can present with altered mental status and dementia.

Palpitations

A palpitation is an awareness of the heartbeat that can be caused by a rapid heart rate, irregularities in heart rhythm, or an increase in the force of cardiac contraction, such as found in a postextrasystolic beat with a greater than normal output. Patients who complain of symptoms most commonly note the palpitations that they experience as sensations of an unpleasant awareness of forceful, irregular, or rapid beating of the heart. Many patients are acutely aware of any cardiac irregularity, whereas others are oblivious even to long runs of a rapid ventricular tachycardia (VT) or atrial fibrillation with a rapid ventricular rate. The latter is particularly noteworthy because it may provoke a stroke or produce a tachycardia-induced cardiomyopathy. Sometimes asymptomatic patients are those referred for evaluation of an arrhythmia noted incidentally during assessment for another reason, such as a preathletic physical examination, a preinsurance physical examination, or a routine preoperative assessment. Patients describe these symptoms in various ways. Most frequently, they use terms such as a *thumping* or *flip-flopping* sensation in the chest; a fullness in the throat, neck, or chest; or a pause in the heartbeat, "as if my heart stopped or skipped a beat." The last most likely results from the compensatory pause after a premature ventricular complex (PVC) or the resetting of sinus rhythm after a premature atrial complex. Usually, the premature beat, particularly if it is a ventricular extrasystole, occurs too early to permit sufficient ventricular filling to cause a sensation when the ventricle contracts. The ventricular systole that ends the compensatory pause is likely responsible for the actual palpitation by a more forceful contraction from prolonged ventricular filling or increased motion of the heart in the chest. Anxiety over such symptoms is commonly the complaint that brings the patient to the physician's office.

Differentiation Between Skipped Beats Versus Sustained Palpitation

Premature atrial or ventricular complexes probably constitute the most common cause of palpitations, and patients often use the term *skipped beat* or *dropped beat* to describe them. If the premature complexes are frequent or particularly if a sustained tachycardia is present, patients are more likely to complain of lightheadedness, syncope or near-syncope, chest pain, fatigue, or shortness of breath. The presence of age and associated cardiovascular problems influences the nature of the symptoms. For example, a supraventricular tachycardia (SVT) at a rate of 180 beats/min can provoke chest pain in a patient with coronary artery disease or syncope in a patient with aortic stenosis, but it may result in only a breathless feeling in an otherwise healthy young person.

It is important to stress that patients with VT, particularly young, otherwise healthy persons, can be completely asymptomatic or experience minimal symptoms during the arrhythmic episode. The lack of significant symptoms should not exclude the diagnosis of important tachycardias such as VT.

Bradyarrhythmias have their own constellation of symptoms. Because of the slow rate, those symptoms usually include light-headedness, syncope, near-syncope, and fatigue.

By careful history-taking, the clinician can obtain information about the arrhythmia, the nature of the beginning and end of the tachycardia, whether the ventricular rhythm is regular or irregular, and the rate of the tachycardia. Knowledge about the typical onset and termination of the tachycardia is helpful. Abrupt, paroxysmal onset is consistent with a tachycardia such as AV nodal reentrant tachycardia (AVNRT; see Chapter 78), whereas gradual speeding and slowing are more in keeping with a sinus tachycardia. Termination by Valsalva maneuver or carotid sinus massage suggests a tachycardia incorporating nodal tissue in the reentrant pathway, such as sinus node reentry, AV reentrant tachycardia (AVRT) or AVNRT (see Chapters 77 and 78), and idiopathic right ventricular outflow tract tachycardia. It often is helpful to have the patient tap out the cadence of the perceived palpitations on his/her knee, from onset to termination.

The rate of the untreated tachycardia often narrows diagnostic possibilities, and patients should be taught to count their radial or carotid pulse rate, noting whether it is regular or irregular. Often blood pressure machines provide such information. Ventricular rates of 150 beats/min should always suggest the potential diagnosis of atrial flutter with 2:1 AV block (see Chapter 75), whereas most SVTs, such as those caused by AVNRT or AVRT, usually occur at rates exceeding 150 beats/min. The rates of VTs overlap those of the SVTs. Palpitations, hot flashes, and sweating in middle-aged women suggest perimenopausal syndrome but can be due to an arrhythmia. Palpitations, dizziness, and shortness of breath on mild exertion, typically in young women with structurally normal hearts, suggest the syndrome of inappropriate sinus tachycardia. Palpitations owing to sinus tachycardia on standing should point toward postural hypotension. Palpitations and presyncope on standing can be symptoms of postural orthostatic tachycardia syndrome. Various possible causes of palpitations are listed in Box 59.1.

Impact of Associated Cardiac or Systemic Diseases

It also is important to establish whether the patient has structural heart disease and, if so, the diagnosis and extent of disease. Certain clinical diagnoses are linked to the presence of specific arrhythmias. For example, the occurrence of mitral stenosis should suggest the possibility of atrial fibrillation, whereas a history of a myocardial infarction or tetralogy of Fallot repair invokes VT as a distinct prospect. Thyrotoxicosis should suggest atrial arrhythmias, including sinus tachycardia. At times it is useful to search for a family history of similar problems and to obtain electrocardiograms (ECGs) of close family members, such as parents, siblings, or children. Family history of palpitations, syncope, or SCD should be investigated carefully for inherited cardiac arrhythmias, including atrial fibrillation, long QT syndrome, short QT syndrome, catecholaminergic polymorphic VT, arrhythmogenic right ventricular dysplasia or cardiomyopathy (ARVD/C), and inherited cardiomyopathy with arrhythmia (see Chapters 86–97).

Signs of Presyncope and Syncope

The diagnosis of presyncope and syncope (see Chapter 103) and its cause requires comprehensive history taking from the patient and witness. The differential diagnosis of syncope is lengthy and can be a warning sign of SCD (see Chapter 103, Table 103.1). It is important to differentiate cardiac versus noncardiac causes of syncope. It is more important to differentiate a benign cause of syncope from a cause that can result in death. Of the reflex syncopes (neurocardiogenic, carotid hypersensitivity, and situational), neurocardiogenic is the most common. It should be differentiated from syncope owing to orthostasis, which is commonly seen in autonomic failure (e.g., due to diabetes) and from syncope resulting from other cardiac causes.

When caused by a cardiac arrhythmia, the onset of syncope is rapid and the duration is brief, with or without preceding aura, and usually is not followed by a postictal confusional state. It can be associated with bodily injury if the patient falls while unconscious. Palpitations preceding syncope also support an arrhythmic

---

BOX 59.1   Differential diagnosis of palpitations

Cardiac Arrhythmias

Sinus Tachycardia
- Physiological
- Inappropriate sinus tachycardia
- Postural orthostatic tachycardia syndrome
- Anxiety disorders, thyrotoxicosis, perimenopausal syndrome, pheochromocytoma

Atrial Arrhythmias
- Atrial premature complexes
- Atrial fibrillation, atrial flutter, atrial tachycardia

Supraventricular Tachycardia
- Atrioventricular nodal reentry tachycardia, orthodromic atrioventricular reciprocating tachycardia in Wolff-Parkinson-White syndrome
- Permanent form of junctional reciprocating tachycardia
- Junctional tachycardia

Ventricular Tachycardia
- Ventricular premature complexes, ventricular couplets, nonsustained VT
- Idiopathic
- Caffeine intake
- Drug-induced: cocaine, QT-prolonging drugs
- Alcohol
- Sustained VT
- Monomorphic VT
- Polymorphic VT and torsades de pointes

Conduction System Disease
- Sinus bradycardia
- Tachycardia-bradycardia syndrome
- Heart block
- Pause-dependent torsades de pointes
- Pacemaker-mediated tachycardia, intermittent ventricular pacing

Familial Arrhythmia Syndrome
- Long QT syndrome: polymorphic VT
- Short QT syndrome: polymorphic VT, AF
- Catecholaminergic polymorphic VT: polymorphic VT, AT/AF
- Brugada syndrome: polymorphic VT, AF
- Inherited cardiomyopathy with ventricular arrhythmias, such as right ventricular cardiomyopathy: monomorphic and polymorphic VT

Metabolic Syndromes
- Hypoglycemia
- Electrolyte imbalance

Structural Heart Disease
- Valvular disease
- Cardiomyopathies
- Primary pulmonary hypertension

Drug Induced
- Proarrhythmia: antiarrhythmic drugs, psychotropic drugs
- Sympathomimetic agents, vasodilators, anticholinergic drugs, β-blocker withdrawal, amphetamine and other antianxiety drugs, nicotine, caffeine

AF, Atrial fibrillation; *AT,* atrial tachycardia; *VT,* ventricular tachycardia.

cause of syncope. Seizure activity is uncommon and occurs mostly after a prolonged asystole or a rapid VT or ventricular fibrillation (VF). Therefore the seizure does not begin with the syncope. However, in epileptic seizures, convulsive movements start within seconds of the onset of syncope. Tongue biting or incontinence is also uncommon in cardiac syncope. The history of syncope should be elicited and interpreted carefully because older people who have fallen might deny loss of consciousness during the event because of brief retrograde amnesia.

To summarize, syncope with early seizure activity is commonly due to epilepsy. Syncope with later seizure is more likely due to a tachyarrhythmia.

With vasodepressor and cardioinhibitory syncope, the episode usually unfolds more slowly and can be preceded by manifestations of autonomic hyperactivity such as nausea, abdominal cramping, diarrhea, sweating, or yawning. On recovery, the patient may be bradycardic, pale, sweaty, and fatigued; this is in contrast with the patient recovering from a Stokes-Adams attack or an episode of VT, who could be flushed and have a sinus tachycardia, usually without persistent mental confusion. Common arrhythmic causes of syncope include bradyarrhythmias caused by sinus node dysfunction or AV block and tachyarrhythmias, most often ventricular but also supraventricular on occasion. Bradycardia can follow tachycardia in patients with the bradycardia–tachycardia syndrome, and the treatment of both may be necessary.

Drug-induced (orthostatic hypotension, bradyarrhythmia) and nonarrhythmic cardiac causes such as aortic stenosis, hypertrophic cardiomyopathy, pulmonary stenosis, pulmonary hypertension, and acute myocardial infarction can be excluded by the history, physical examination, ECG, echocardiography, and other laboratory tests. Noncardiac causes of syncope such as hypoglycemia, transient ischemic attack, and psychogenic often can be excluded by a careful history.

Sudden Cardiac Death (see Chapters 98 and 99)

SCD causes approximately 350,000 to 450,000 deaths annually in the United States. It is responsible for nearly 50% of all cardiovascular-related deaths worldwide. SCD has an incidence of 0.1% to 0.2% per year among adults older than 35 years. Therefore careful evaluation of patients who are resuscitated from SCD is mandatory. SCD occurs in a majority of patients without known heart disease as the first manifestation of underlying coronary artery disease. The life-threatening ventricular arrhythmias, such as sustained VT and VF, are responsible for two-thirds of SCDs, although some data suggest that VT/VF as a cause is decreasing while asystole and pulseless electrical activity are increasing (see Chapter 99). These arrhythmias occur unpredictably, even in high-risk patients. Structural heart diseases, such as coronary artery disease, cardiomyopathy, and congenital heart disease, are responsible for up to 65% to 80% cases of SCD. Approximately 5% to 10% of SCDs occur in people with primary electrical abnormalities of the heart, such as long QT syndrome, Brugada syndrome, idiopathic VF, and Wolff-Parkinson-White syndrome (see relevant chapters). The remaining sudden deaths (15% to 20%) are due to noncardiac causes such as pulmonary embolism, drugs, drowning, and sudden infant death syndrome. Therefore careful questioning to uncover or elucidate a family history of SCD is indicated, and family screening for the suspected cardiac condition should be performed. Genetic screening is recommended for appropriate patients (see Chapter 71).

Arrhythmic Precipitating Factors

Proarrhythmic Drugs

Patients usually cannot indicate a specific inciting event, but the physician should inquire about the use of potentially proarrhythmic drugs such as antiarrhythmic drugs, QT prolonging drugs, bronchodilators, histamine H_1-blocking antihistamines, some decongestants, psychotropic agents, macrolide antibiotics,

or other over-the-counter drugs, illicit drugs such as cocaine or methamphetamines, and the ingestion of alcohol or excessive caffeine-containing foods, energy drinks, and dietary supplements. Patients with long QT syndrome (https://crediblemeds.org/pdftemp/pdf/DrugsToAvoidList.pdf) and Brugada syndrome (http://www.brugadadrugs.org/) are cautioned against taking specific drugs that can affect their disorders.

Exercise, Swimming, Emotions, and Auditory Stimuli

In patients with long QT syndrome (see Chapter 93), exercise such as swimming or acute emotional reactions often precipitate a ventricular arrhythmia in those with the LQT1 variant, whereas exercise, emotional upset, and sleep or rest are culprits of fairly equal frequency in LQT2. Auditory stimuli and events occurring more frequently during rest can precipitate arrhythmias in LQT3.

Exercise also precipitates various benign and malignant arrhythmias; these include idiopathic right ventricular outflow tract tachycardia, catecholamine-induced polymorphic VT, and VT in patients with ARVD/C. Exercise can induce syncope or SCD in patients with outflow tract obstruction and severe pulmonary hypertension.

Physical Examination

The physical examination offers the opportunity to gain important information about the presence of associated structural heart disease, if any, and the nature of the arrhythmia, if present. Although it is well known that patients with normal hearts can have SVTs, it is less commonly appreciated that patients without recognizable structural heart disease can also have VTs that on occasion are life threatening. Thus normal results of a physical examination do not exclude the diagnosis of VT, even in a young person. It is likely that at least some of these patients have unrecognized structural heart disease.

The sex of the patient can be a clue to the nature of the tachycardia because of sex differences in cardiac electrophysiology (see Chapter 107). For example, a young woman who complains of episodes of a regular tachycardia over many years is likely to have AVNRT. In contrast, a young man with a similar history is more likely to have AVRT associated with Wolff-Parkinson-White syndrome. Infants with SVT are more likely to have Wolff-Parkinson-White syndrome, while young adults, particularly females, are likely to have AVNRT. Symptomatic long QT syndrome is more common in females, whereas Brugada syndrome is more common in males.

Physical Manifestations of Atrioventricular Dissociation

If the tachycardia is present during the physical examination, a 12-lead ECG should be obtained, if time and the patient's clinical status permit. If an ECG is not possible, a careful physical examination can yield helpful findings. For example, the presence of regular cannon A waves in the jugular venous pulse would be consistent with a 1:1 retrograde ventriculoatrial relation, as in tachycardias such as AVRT, AVNRT, and some junctional tachycardias and VTs. In contrast, the patient can have physical features indicative of AV dissociation, such as intermittent cannon A waves in the neck, variable intensity of the first heart sound, and variable peak systolic blood pressure. Common arrhythmic causes of AV dissociation include VT and nonparoxysmal AV junctional tachycardia, without retrograde capture of the atria. Ventricular or junctional tachycardias that produce retrograde 2:1 or Wenckebach block cause intermittent cannon A waves that recur at regular intervals.

Atrioventricular Block (see Chapter 106)

In the patient with second-degree AV block, the study of neck veins can reveal the nature of the block, but usually the findings are too subtle to recognize. Patients with type I (Wenckebach) second-degree AV block can exhibit a progressive increase in the A–C jugular venous pulse interval before the nonconducted P wave, a subtle, progressive quickening of the ventricular rate, and a progressive decrease in the intensity of the first heart sound. In type II second-degree heart block, the PR interval remains fixed before the block, and so does the A–C interval and intensity of S_1. The features of AV dissociation noted earlier usually are present during complete AV block.

Carotid Sinus Massage and Valsalva

Modulating autonomic tone by carotid sinus massage during the physical examination can be useful to expose the patient with the hypersensitive carotid sinus reflex. The clinician first needs to listen carefully over both carotids to be certain that no bruit is present, palpate lightly to determine that a normal carotid pulse is present, and then gently depress or rub the carotid sinus. Gentle massage for approximately 10 to 15 seconds or less usually is all that is necessary to produce significant periods of sinus arrest or AV block in susceptible patients.

The response to carotid sinus massage or other vagal maneuvers can be helpful in differentiating one tachycardia from another. In the most definitive responses, carotid sinus massage acutely terminates tachycardias such as AVRT, AVNRT, sinus node reentry, adenosine-sensitive atrial tachycardia, and idiopathic right ventricular outflow tract tachycardia. Carotid sinus massage can gradually slow a sinus tachycardia without termination and will decrease the ventricular response to atrial tachycardia, atrial flutter, and atrial fibrillation without termination, thereby exposing atrial activity. Carotid sinus massage transiently terminates the permanent form of AV junctional reciprocating tachycardia, which then restarts when carotid massage ceases. Carotid sinus massage does not affect reentrant ventricular or junctional tachycardias. Unfortunately, not all presentations of these tachycardias behave in such a predictable fashion, and intermediate or overlapping responses can occur.

A variation to the usual Valsalva maneuver has been proposed during which the individual is semirecumbent with passive leg raising immediately after the Valsalva strain to avoid venous pooling. Such an approach tripled the successful SVT termination rate.[1]

Laboratory Tests

As indicated earlier, the initial assessment of the patient begins with a careful history and physical examination. Several noninvasive and invasive tests add to the physician's ability to obtain information about the arrhythmia. Before any test is ordered, however, it is imperative to decide whether the information provided by the test is sufficiently important to justify its risk or expense. Whenever possible, tests with maximal sensitivity, specificity, and predictive accuracy are chosen. A 12-lead ECG is obtained in all patients, and frequently a 24-hour ECG or 30-day event recording and stress test are helpful in exposing the arrhythmia. A chest roentgenogram and an echocardiogram provide information about the presence of structural heart disease. The hierarchy of steps taken to evaluate and treat a patient suspected of having an arrhythmia generally proceeds from simple, noninvasive, and inexpensive tests to more complex, expensive, and invasive studies.

The nature of the rhythm disturbance and its effects on the patient determine the order in which the tests are performed. Some rhythm disturbances, such as sustained VT or VF, are hazardous in and of themselves, whereas others, such as AVRT or AVNRT, must be evaluated according to the context in which they occur. AVRT or AVNRT occurring at a rate of 180 beats/min in a young patient who complains only of palpitations or mild anxiety is approached differently from such arrhythmias precipitating angina in a patient with coronary artery disease, syncope

in a patient with aortic stenosis, or claudication in a patient with peripheral vascular disease. It is imperative to remember that clinical decision making must be founded on the ECG interpretation of the arrhythmia in concert with the assessment of the patient. Thus the physician evaluates and determines treatment for a patient who has a rhythm disturbance, rather than a rhythm disturbance in isolation.

The principle in diagnosing and treating symptomatic patients with an undocumented cardiac rhythm disturbance is simple and obvious. One needs merely to record the ECG during a symptomatic episode and then document a causal relation between arrhythmia and symptoms. This often is easier said than done, however, and a variety of approaches are used to achieve that result.

Rationale for the Use of Ambulatory Electrocardiography (see Chapter 66)

- Arrhythmia diagnosis and exclusion as a cause of infrequent symptoms
- ST-T changes related to myocardial ischemia

Continuous Ambulatory Electrocardiographic Monitoring

The duration of electrocardiographic monitoring depends on the frequency of symptoms. Rhythm disturbances occurring with great frequency are naturally easier to document than those that occur sporadically. Long-term ECG recordings in the outpatient setting usually constitute one of the early diagnostic choices in the patient without a life-threatening cardiac arrhythmia. The patient with a life-threatening arrhythmia may need to be hospitalized to allow for these recordings. A long-term ECG recording provides the most direct documentation of an infrequent cardiac arrhythmia. Prolonged ECG recordings in patients engaged in normal daily activity provide the methodology to quantitate the frequency and complexity of the rhythm disturbance, to correlate these alterations with symptoms, and to evaluate the effect of appropriate pharmacological therapy on the arrhythmia. In addition, such recordings can document alterations in the QRS-ST and T contour. A 30-day event recorder often is helpful if arrhythmia occurs at least once in a month. The patient can activate these latter devices when symptoms occur, store 30 seconds or more of the ECG rhythm (a memory loop provides ECG information about the arrhythmia that transpired for some seconds before device activation), and transmit it to a central monitoring station over the telephone. Alternatively, some devices automatically record rhythms that exceed preset limits. The automatic recorder is useful in patients who fail to perceive all symptoms associated with the arrhythmia or are unable to activate the recording system because of rapidly progressing syncope or other problems.

1. *24- to 48-hour ambulatory Holter monitoring.* Short-term continuous Holter monitoring may be sufficient for patients with daily symptoms related to arrhythmia such as palpitation, presyncope, or syncope. If the arrhythmia does not occur with sufficient frequency, then a simple 24-hour, or even 48-hour, recording will not be useful. Newer Holter monitors also record a 12-channel ECG. Such studies are helpful in arrhythmia characterization including atrial fibrillation, as well as ST-T wave changes related to ischemia and Brugada syndrome.

2. *Long-term (15-day) Holter monitoring system.* These systems are used for diagnosing arrhythmias occurring once or twice in a week. With these devices, cardiac activity is continuously recorded by chest electrodes that are attached to a pager-sized sensor. The sensor of the pager wirelessly transmits collected data to a portable monitor that analyzes the rhythm data. If an arrhythmia is detected by an arrhythmia algorithm, the monitor automatically transmits recorded data wirelessly via the

Internet to a central monitoring station for subsequent analysis. Patient activated data are also transmitted.

3. *Event recorders (with and without loop capability):*

   a. Trans-telephonic monitoring (TTM) systems are external event recorders without loop; they are noncontinuous ambulatory recording systems.[2] After activation by the patient, an ECG is recorded and directly transmitted by telephone to a receiving center.

   b. Event recorders with looping memory [continuous event recorders (CERs)] make a continuous one-lead recording, but the rhythm strip will only be saved when a patient activates the device. Most devices can be programmed to save preactivation and postactivation rhythm strips.

   c. Autotriggered event monitors with looping memory (auto-triggered CER) devices automatically recognize prespecified high and low heart rates. One such device performs a continuous ECG analysis combined with automatic storage of abnormal events detected in a 20-minute solid-state memory with continuous loop analysis up to 7 days. In addition, it also records patient-trigger events. The most recent advancement in ambulatory arrhythmia monitoring is mobile cardiac outpatient telemetry in which a portable sensor continuously detects asymptomatic, prespecified arrhythmias and transmits the ECG data in real-time to a pocket-sized monitor at the patient's home. If the algorithms in the monitor detect an abnormal heartbeat, the monitor automatically transmits the patient's ECG data to the monitoring center using wireless communications.

4. *Implantable autotriggered and patient-triggered loop recorders.* An implantable loop recorder placed beneath the skin can be used for monitoring of the cardiac rhythm for as long as 12 to 24 months. Therefore it is useful in patients with infrequent symptoms. The device has both autotriggered and patient-activated arrhythmia recording facilities. The devices are also available for recording a specific arrhythmia, such as atrial fibrillation. Use of such devices has been successful in recording tachyarrhythmias and, more commonly, bradyarrhythmias. Arrhythmia recordings can be sent to the analyzing center via the telephone and then to physicians via the Internet.

5. *Pacemakers and implantable cardioverter defibrillators.* Dual-chamber pacemakers can record atrial and ventricular high-rate episodes and can be correlated with the arrhythmia. Apart from diagnosing ventricular arrhythmias, a dual-chamber implantable cardioverter defibrillator also helps in identifying the cycle length, duration, and frequency of atrial arrhythmias. Remote monitoring has been advocated in such patients.

6. *Smart phone technology can be used to record ECGs.* Currently, mobile devices (smartphones, tablets) are an integral part of daily life and could be used as automatic and low cost monitoring solution of the ECG signal. The applications are available for download and can be used for real-time ECG-monitoring in both iPhone as well as Android phones. In a study using an iPhone, atrial fibrillation was detected readily by the software and was also read by cardiologists.[3,4] The overall sensitivity, specificity, and accuracy (95% confidence interval [CI]) for the detection of atrial fibrillation in different study were 98% (89%–100%), 97% (93%–99%), and 97% (94%–99%). The one of the iPhone-based apps also showed good accuracy for premature atrial complex (95.5%) and PVC discrimination (96%). The vast majority of surveyed app users (83%) reported that it was "useful" and "not complex" to use.[4]

Diagnostic Yield of Electrocardiographic Monitoring

For the recording session to be specific, the patient must have both the arrhythmia and symptoms simultaneously. If symptoms occur without an arrhythmia, the latter can be excluded as a cause.

Recording arrhythmias without symptoms precludes a definitive causal relation between symptoms and arrhythmia and reduces the specificity of the test. The sensitivity of the test is highly variable, depending on the prevalence of the arrhythmia.

The diagnostic value of ambulatory monitoring and recording depends on a number of variables, including the frequency and duration of arrhythmia, accurate diary maintenance, and inpatient monitoring versus outpatient monitoring. Approximately 25% to 50% of patients will experience a symptom, but only 2% to 15% will record a causal cardiac arrhythmia, and 35% will log a symptom without a corresponding ECG abnormality.

Correlation With Cardiac Arrhythmias on 24-Hour and Long-Term Electrocardiographic Monitoring

Twenty-Four–Hour Holter Recordings

In an old study of 518 patients, 24-hour Holter recordings were performed for palpitations and other symptoms related to arrhythmia.[5] Two hundred and seventy-four (53%) had significant arrhythmias (41% ventricular, 20% ventricular, and 8% both). No presenting complaint or cardiovascular diagnosis correlated closely with any specific cardiac arrhythmia. Major arrhythmias, including SVTs and VTs, often occurred asymptomatically (in 44 of 54 and 37 of 40 patients, respectively). Among 371 patients with accurate historic logs, only 176 (47%) who had long-term electrocardiographic monitoring had typical symptoms during the monitoring period. Only 50 patients (13%) had concurrence of their presenting complaints with an arrhythmia, whereas 126 patients (34%) had their typical symptoms associated with a normal ECG, which may be helpful in excluding any cardiac arrhythmias as a primary cause for their complaints.

Continuous Event Recording Versus 24- to 48-Hour Holter Monitoring

In a prospective randomized study of 100 patients with syncope and/or presyncope, arrhythmia was either identified or excluded in 63% of patients who had an external loop recorder, as compared to only 24% of patients who were assigned to a Holter monitor ($p < .0001$).[6] Subsequently, 29 patients with negative results with Holter monitoring received a loop recorder and of these, 45% had arrhythmia excluded. The overall probability of obtaining a symptom–rhythm correlation was 56% for loop recorders versus 22% for Holter monitors ($p < .0001$). However, the study showed the major practical limitation these monitoring devices was that, despite patient education and test transmissions, 23% patients who had a recurrence of their symptoms failed to activate their loop recorder properly. In another study, Holter monitoring was performed in 475 octogenarians, and clinical arrhythmia was detected in 11.2% of these patients.[7] These were AV block (n = 13), sinus node dysfunction (n = 13), binodal disease (n = 2), atrial fibrillation with slow or rapid ventricular response (n = 21), VT (n = 3), and SVT (n = 1).

Autotriggered Continuous Event Recording Versus Traditional Continuous Event Recording Versus Holter Recording

In a larger study of 1800 patients, the autotriggered CER was compared with the traditional CER and 24-hour Holter monitoring with 600 patients in each group.[8] The diagnostic yields were 71%, 27%, and 6% in the autotriggered CER, patient-triggered CER, and 24-hour Holter monitoring groups, respectively.

Insertable Loop Recorder

Giada et al. studied 50 patients for the diagnostic yield of the use of an insertable loop recorder (ILR), which was randomly compared with conventional strategy (24-hour Holter recording, a 4-week period of CER, or electrophysiological testing if the previous two strategies yielded negative results).[9] The diagnosis was made in only 5 patients (21%) of 25 patients in the conventional strategy group compared with 19 (73%) of 25 patients in the ILR group (with arrhythmia recordings of up to 1 year). In another study of 100 patients with unexplained syncope and negative electrophysiological as well as neurological workup, the ILR helped to diagnose an arrhythmic etiology in 45% of patients.[10]

Electrophysiological Study

Naturally, in many patients, invasive electrophysiological testing is required to initiate the electrical abnormality. Such studies provide important information when a particular arrhythmia can be initiated that is responsible for the patient's symptoms. In some instances, however, a tachyarrhythmia present clinically cannot be induced in the electrophysiology laboratory. An important point is that failure to demonstrate a rhythm abnormality does not exclude the possibility that it is present on another occasion and is still responsible for the patient's symptoms. Thus the sensitivity of the electrophysiological study may be low, depending on the nature of the rhythm disturbance. Absence of proof is not the same as proof of absence.

Ideally, the electrophysiological study would induce only clinically and prognostically important cardiac arrhythmias in all patients who are at risk for a spontaneous arrhythmia and in no patient without such a risk. Unfortunately, this is not the case, and it is clear that such a study, depending on the number of extra stimuli used, can induce nonspecific tachyarrhythmias, in particular flutter and fibrillation in both the atria and ventricles. With certain arrhythmias, the test can be highly specific. For example, it would be uncommon to induce a sustained AVRT or AVNRT in a patient who does not also have this arrhythmia clinically or is at risk of having it. Furthermore, it would not be likely to induce a sustained monomorphic VT in a patient who is not at risk for a clinical occurrence of such an arrhythmia.

Stress Testing and Other Noninvasive Studies

An exercise stress test can be useful, particularly in patients who experience symptoms when exercising (see Chapter 65). In response to exercise testing, approximately one-third of normal subjects have ventricular ectopy, usually in the form of occasional uniform PVCs. These PVCs are more likely to occur at faster heart rates and are not reproducible from one test to the next. Multiform PVCs, pairs of PVCs, and VT infrequently develop in response to exercise in healthy subjects. Because they can be recorded in normal subjects, their presence does not establish the existence of ischemia or heart disease. Ventricular ectopy generally appears at lower heart rates (<130 beats/min) in patients with coronary artery disease than in a normal population, and it often occurs in the early recovery period. Ventricular arrhythmias are more reproducible from one test to the next in patients with coronary artery disease, and more frequent PVCs (exceeding 10 per minute), polymorphic PVCs, and VT are more likely to occur in patients with coronary artery disease than in persons with normal hearts. PVCs at rest can be suppressed by exercise in patients with documented coronary disease; therefore this observation does not necessarily imply a benign prognosis or the absence of underlying structural heart disease. In normal subjects, results from consecutive exercise tests might not be reproducible, whereas the test results are more reproducible in patients with coronary artery disease, but not dependably so.

Exercise testing also has diagnostic or prognostic value in patients with primary electrical abnormalities such as long QT syndrome (LQTS), catecholaminergic polymorphic VT (CPVT) and Brugada syndrome (BS). Because the QT interval can be normal in 10% to 30% of patients with genetically proven LQTS, exercise testing can be useful to expose ECG abnormalities in these patients. The abnormal response of the QT interval in response to standing is seen in patients with LQTS as compared to normal subjects. In one study the 12-lead ECG of 108 patients with LQTS and 112 healthy subjects were recorded in the supine position.[11] The subjects were then instructed to stand quickly and remain standing for 5 minutes during the continuous ECG recording. The corrected QT interval was measured on three occasions: at baseline (QTc_{base}); when heart rate acceleration without appropriate QT-interval shortening led to maximal QT stretching ($QTc_{stretch}$); and upon the return of heart rate to baseline (QTc_{return}). The study showed that $QTc_{stretch}$ lengthened significantly more in patients with long QTS (103 ± 80 ms vs. 66 ± 40 ms in controls; $p < .001$) and so did QTc_{return} (28 ± 48 ms for patients with long QTS vs. −3 ± 32 ms for controls; $p < .001$). Using a sensitivity cutoff of 90%, the specificity for diagnosing LQTS was 74% for QTc_{base}, 84% for QTc_{return}, and 87% for $QTc_{stretch}$. The study showed an abnormal response of the QT interval in response to standing in patients with LQTS, which persisted even after the heart rate slowed back to baseline.

Exercise testing unmasks arrhythmias in CPVT patients. In patients with Brugada syndrome, ECG showing significant ST segment elevation with coving ST segment during the recovery phase predicts arrhythmic events during follow-up.[12]

A variety of noninvasive tests have been developed in an attempt to identify patients at risk for sudden arrhythmic death. These tests include signal-averaged electrocardiography, heart rate variability QT dispersion testing, T-wave alternans assessment (see Chapter 69), and baroreflex testing. Although these tests can help to identify groups of patients at greater or lower risk for SCD, they all suffer from an inability to predict precisely the occurrence of life-threatening arrhythmias in individual patients

Tests Indicated for Specific Symptoms

Syncope

The underlying disorder can be determined using standardized clinical evaluation in up to three-fourths of patients with syncope. In unselected populations, slightly more than one-third of the patients have neurocardiogenic syncope, one-fourth have orthostatic hypotension, and the remaining patients have miscellaneous conditions. The Task Force for the Diagnosis and The European Society of Cardiology published the guidelines for the management of syncope.[13] Initial evaluation includes careful history taking and an ECG. Evaluation of patients suspected of cardioinhibitory or vasodepressor syncope often includes tilt table testing. If a cardiac cause is suspected, then echocardiography and ambulatory monitoring are indicated. It is important to establish the cause of the syncope, if possible, because patients who have syncope from a noncardiac cause usually have an excellent prognosis, whereas those who have syncope from a cardiac cause have a greater prevalence of SCD.

Postural Orthostatic Tachycardia Syndrome (see Chapter 104)

Postural orthostatic tachycardia syndrome (POTS) or orthostatic intolerance is the inability to tolerate an upright posture and is relieved by recumbence. Patients' symptoms are due to sympathetic nervous system dysfunction and vary from mild to severe and incapacitating. Patients with POTS usually experience presyncope, light-headedness, fatigue, palpitations, and nausea which is most pronounced upon upright posture despite maintained blood pressure. Other symptoms include an inability to concentrate, weakness, anxiety, syncope, chest pain, and bowel motility disorder.

Therefore POTS is often confused with anxiety disorder, inappropriate sinus tachycardia, chronic fatigue syndrome, and fibromyalgia. Twenty-nine percent of these patients have hyperadrenergic POTS with high plasma norepinephrine levels when taken during upright tilt.[14] The tilt table test is helpful for POTS. The majority of these patients improve with autonomic modulation with lifestyle modification, aerobic exercise, and pharmacotherapy.

Bradyarrhythmias

Many patients have asymptomatic bradyarrhythmias, and it is important to establish that the bradycardia produces symptoms in a given patient before assuming that therapy is required. Conversely, if the patient becomes symptomatic when a spontaneous bradyarrhythmia is demonstrated, further diagnostic studies might not be necessary. It is also possible that patients can be minimally symptomatic but have arrhythmias that permit definitive therapeutic decisions. For example, in patients who have type II second-degree AV block, the demonstration of His–Purkinje block, even in the minimally symptomatic or possibly asymptomatic person, can be sufficient evidence to conclude that pacemaker therapy is indicated because of the risk for progression to complete AV block.

The patient with sinus node dysfunction can have syncope or near-syncope but also might complain of symptoms consistent with low cardiac output because of persistent bradycardia, such as fatigue or even manifestations of congestive heart failure. Some patients can have associated tachycardia—producing the aforementioned bradycardia–tachycardia syndrome. Electrophysiological studies of sinus node function have low sensitivity (64%) but relatively high specificity (88%).[15] The correlation of the presence of the bradycardia with the patient's symptoms is of utmost importance. Electrophysiological studies are indicated only when a causal relationship between the appearance of the bradycardia and the patient's symptoms cannot be established despite repeated noninvasive evaluations. It is important to keep in mind that asymptomatic sinus bradycardia with heart rates of 35 to 40 beats/min, sinus arrhythmia with pauses of 2 to 3 seconds, Wenckebach second-degree AV block (particularly during sleep), wandering atrial pacemaker, and junctional escape complexes can be completely normal, especially in young people and in well-conditioned athletes.

In patients with AV block (see Chapter 106), the scalar ECG is the most important laboratory test because the site of block usually dictates the clinical course of the patient and whether a pacemaker is needed, and the site of block usually can be determined from an analysis of the scalar ECG. Only infrequently is an electrophysiological study indicated. Autonomic manipulation can be used to help establish the site of block. Atropine or isoproterenol shorten AV nodal conduction time and refractoriness, whereas vagal maneuvers prolong them. Little change occurs in the normal His–Purkinje conduction. Thus exercise, atropine, or isoproterenol can shorten the PR interval and increase the ratio of conducted P waves during type I (Wenckebach) AV nodal block, whereas these maneuvers can increase the number of blocked P waves in type II second-degree AV block. Of note, however, important overlap between the two responses is possible.

Tachyarrhythmias

As mentioned earlier, a 12-lead ECG should be obtained during tachycardia, as long as the patient's condition is relatively stable. If the QRS is normal and identical to that present during sinus rhythm, the tachycardia must be supraventricular, and the differential diagnosis now relates to its mechanism (see Chapters 73–79). The 12-lead ECG provides many diagnostic clues

in this regard. SVTs can be classified as short RP′ or long RP′ tachycardias, depending on the timing of the P wave in relation to the preceding R wave. When a P wave occurs closer to the preceding R wave (i.e., in the first half of the R-R interval), the tachycardia is called a *short RP′ tachycardia*, whereas if a P wave occurs in the second half of the RR cycle, the arrhythmia is called a *long RP′ tachycardia*. Considerations in the differential diagnosis for a short RP′ tachycardia include AVNRT, AVRT, junctional tachycardia, and atrial tachycardia with a markedly prolonged PR interval. If no P waves or other evidence of atrial activity is apparent, and the R-R interval is regular, AVNRT is most likely. If a retrograde P wave is apparent in the ST segment, AVRT is most probable. Long RP tachycardias include sinus tachycardia, atypical AVNRT, permanent junctional reciprocating tachycardia, and atrial tachycardia. The presence of conduction over an accessory pathway during sinus rhythm or during tachycardia naturally suggests that Wolff-Parkinson-White syndrome with its associated accessory pathway is responsible for the dysrhythmia. During VT, specific QRS contours and the presence of AV dissociation are useful in making the diagnosis (see Chapter 60).

Cryptogenic Stroke Associated With Paroxysmal Atrial Fibrillation

The Cryptogenic Stroke and Underlying AF (CRYSTAL AF) study randomized 441 patients with cryptogenic stroke to long-term monitoring with an ILR compared with conventional follow-up (control) for detecting atrial fibrillation.[16] By 6 months, atrial fibrillation had been detected in 8.9% of patients in the ILR group as compared with 1.4% of patients in the control group (hazard ratio [HR], 6.4; 95% CI, 1.9 to 21.7; $p < .001$). Furthermore, by 12 months, atrial fibrillation had been detected in 12.4% of patients in the ILR group versus 2.0% of patients in the control group (HR, 7.3; 95% CI, 2.6 to 20.8; $p < .001$).

Evaluation of Athletes

Cardiomegaly is often seen in athletes due to endurance training such as long-distance running, which causes a sustained volume load to the heart, resulting in four-chamber enlargement and increased stroke volume at rest and exercise. Strength training such as weight lifting causes a pressure load to the heart accompanied by normal left ventricular wall thickness. Some sports, such as basketball, present a combination of the two types of loads. ECGs may show frequent signs of left ventricular hypertrophy in around 40% of athletes, T-wave inversion in precordial leads V1 to V4 in 14% of African-American athletes, longer QT intervals than in the general population, frequent PVCs, and sinus bradycardia as well as various degrees of AV block due to a high vagal tone. These ECG changes can mimic ARVD/C, Brugada syndrome, or long QT syndrome and may make diagnostic decisions difficult in this population. More importantly, the risk assessment for SCD during athletic activity and permitting them to return to play can be difficult.[17]

Summary

Careful evaluation of the patient who has documented or suspected cardiac arrhythmia is the prime focus of the clinical cardiac electrophysiologist. Much useful information can be gleaned noninvasively, thereby potentially sparing many patients from unnecessary electrophysiological testing. When indicated, however, such studies, particularly when coupled with radiofrequency ablation techniques, provide the most definitive information for appropriate diagnosis and therapy.

REFERENCES

1. Appelboam A, Reuben A, Mann C, et al. Postural modification to the standard Valsalva manoeuvre for emergency treatment of supraventricular tachycardias (REVERT): a randomised controlled trial. *Lancet.* 2015;386:1747–1753.

2. Hoefman E, Bindels PJ, van Weert HC. Efficacy of diagnostic tools for detecting cardiac arrhythmias: systematic literature search. *Neth Heart J.* 2010;18:543–551.

3. Gradl S, Kugler P, Lohmüller C, Eskofier B. Real-time ECG monitoring and arrhythmia detection using Android-based mobile devices. *Conf Proc IEEE Eng Med Biol Soc.* 2012:2452–2455.

4. McManus DD, Chong JW, Soni A, et al. PULSE-SMART: pulse-based arrhythmia discrimination using a novel smartphone application. *J Cardiovasc Electrophysiol.* 2016;27:51–57.

5. Zeldis SM, Levine BJ, Michelson EL, Morganroth J. Cardiovascular complaints. Correlation with cardiac arrhythmias on 24-hour electrocardiographic monitoring. *Chest.* 1980;78:456–461.

6. Sivakumaran S, Krahn AD, Klein GJ, et al. A prospective randomized comparison of loop recorders versus Holter monitors in patients with syncope or presyncope. *Am J Med.* 2003;115:1–5.

7. Kuhne M, Schaer B, Sticherling C, Osswald S. Holter monitoring in syncope: diagnostic yield in octogenarians. *J Am Geriatr Soc.* 2011;59:1293–1298.

8. Reiffel JA, Schwarzberg R, Murry M. Comparison of autotriggered memory loop recorders versus standard loop recorders versus 24-hour Holter monitors for arrhythmia detection. *Am J Cardiol.* 2005;95(9):1055–1059.

9. Giada F, Gulizia M, Francese M, et al. Recurrent unexplained palpitations (RUP) study comparison of implantable loop recorder versus conventional diagnostic strategy. *J Am Coll Cardiol.* 2007;49:1951–1956.

10. Inamdar V, Mehta S, Juang G, Cohen T. The utility of implantable loop recorders for diagnosing unexplained syncope in 100 consecutive patients: five-year, single-center experience. *J Invasive Cardiol.* 2006;18:313–315.

11. Adler A, van der Werf C, Postema PG, et al. The phenomenon of "QT stunning": the abnormal QT prolongation provoked by standing persists even as the heart rate returns to normal in patients with long QT syndrome. *Heart Rhythm.* 2012;9:901–908.

12. Refaat MM, Hotait M, Tseng ZH. Utility of the exercise electrocardiogram testing in sudden cardiac death risk stratification. *Ann Noninvasive Electrocardiol.* 2014;19:311–318.

13. Task Force for the Diagnosis and Management of Syncope, European Society of Cardiology, European Heart Rhythm Association, et al. Guidelines for the diagnosis and management of syncope (version 2009). *Eur Heart J.* 2009;30:2631–2671.

14. Thieben MJ, Sandroni P, Sletten DM, et al. Postural orthostatic tachycardia syndrome: the Mayo clinic experience. *Mayo Clin Proc.* 2007;82:308–313.

15. Subcommittee to Assess Clinical Intracardiac Electrophysiologic Studies. Guidelines for clinical intracardiac electrophysiologic studies. A report of the American College of Cardiology/American Heart Association Task Force on Assessment of Diagnostic and Therapeutic Cardiovascular Procedures. *Circulation.* 1989;80:1925–1939.

16. Gladstone DJ, Spring M, Dorian P, et al. Atrial fibrillation in patients with cryptogenic stroke. *N Engl J Med.* 2014;370:2467–2477.

17. Lawless CE, Olshansky B, Washington RL, et al. Sports and exercise cardiology in the United States: cardiovascular specialists as members of the athlete healthcare team. *J Am Coll Cardiol.* 2014;63:1461–1472.

60 Differential Diagnosis of Narrow and Wide Complex Tachycardias

John M. Miller and Mithilesh K. Das

The differential diagnosis of tachycardias using the electrocardiogram (ECG) remains among the most difficult problems faced by cardiologists in daily practice. Distinguishing supraventricular tachycardias (SVT) from ventricular tachycardia (VT) has obvious importance since treatments are very different. In this chapter, we will explore the tools available to address the diagnosis; after this has been obtained, further evaluation and treatment strategies generally flow naturally. An important distinguishing feature for clinical implications of a tachycardia episode is whether or not structural heart disease (SHD) (prior infarction, cardiomyopathy, prior surgery, etc.) is present: in most cases of SVT, SHD is either absent or unrelated to the tachycardia episode, while in most VT patients, SHD is the basis of, or substrate for, the arrhythmia.

The first major differentiator in correctly diagnosing tachycardias is the width of the QRS complex: narrow (<120 ms) QRS complex tachycardias (NCTs) in adults are almost always supraventricular in origin (involving tissue at or above the His bundle), whereas wide (≥120 ms) QRS complex tachycardias (WCTs) are often, but not always, ventricular in origin.

Narrow QRS Tachycardias

Diagnostic Possibilities

The major categories of NCTs include those that are primarily atrial in origin (atrial tachycardia, flutter, and fibrillation); those that are based in the atrioventricular (AV) junction; and those that incorporate the atrium and the ventricle in a large circuit (accessory pathway-mediated AV reentry). Because of the typical obvious irregularity of ventricular response, atrial fibrillation will not be discussed further in this chapter, but flutter and atrial tachycardias (ATs) deserve consideration. Classic electrocardiographic atrial flutter is now understood to be a continuous wavefront propagating either "clockwise" or "counterclockwise" around the tricuspid annulus, when viewed from a left anterior oblique perspective. Other atrial arrhythmias are termed "flutter" on ECG but are mechanistically distinct; these can be either focal in origin or reentrant (usually large circuits bounded by natural barriers, such as valves or scar tissue). ATs can be focal (a true focus or a microreentry that appears focal in its propagation pattern) or macroreentrant, incorporating significant amounts of atrial tissue in the circuit. The latter are noteworthy in that the P wave comprises a relatively large portion of the tachycardia cycle, as opposed to focal ATs (and all other types of SVTs, during which atrial activation begins at a discrete point as though it were a focus).[1] A major limitation to discerning P-wave morphology is determining what is P wave as distinct from ST segment, T wave, and QRS complex. Helpful aids include finding periods of NCT with 2:1 AV conduction or a spontaneous ventricular premature complex, comparison of the complex in question with a sinus rhythm P-QRS-T cycle, and increasing ECG gain (Fig. 60.1).

History and Physical Examination

Patients with NCTs usually have recurrent episodes of arrhythmia. The age at which episodes began often suggests a diagnosis: episodes from birth onward are likely to be AV reentrant tachycardia (AVRT) using an accessory AV pathway present from birth, or, less commonly, AT. Onset of symptoms during or after puberty is common in AV nodal reentrant tachycardia (AVNRT). While these scenarios are generally true, any type of NCT can occur later in life. Symptoms related to tachycardia include palpitations, lightheadedness, dyspnea, chest pain, and throat fullness. In many, episodes are facilitated by exercise and emotional upset. Physical maneuvers, such as Valsalva or breath holding, can often terminate episodes. Episodes tend to become more common and longer lasting with aging. Physical examination during NCT episodes shows tachycardia in a conscious, often anxious patient. Blood pressure is usually preserved. Bulging of neck veins can sometimes be perceived. In patients with repaired congenital heart disease, scar-based atrial macroreentry should be suspected.

Electrocardiographic Differential Diagnosis

Among NCTs, the differential diagnosis is based on three factors: (1) the A:V ratio; (2) among those with 1:1 AV ratio, the timing of the P wave relative to a QRS complex; and (3) P-wave morphology (Table 60.1). While there is some individual variability, some patterns are relatively constant.

A. A:V ratio:
1. NCTs with A:V ratios >1 include AT and flutter, as well as rare cases of AVNRT with 2:1 block, usually in the His bundle (see Fig. 60.1, far right).
2. NCTs with A:V ratio = 1 comprise a large and diverse group, among which are AVNRT, AVRT, AT, and the uncommon automatic junctional tachycardia. ATs may at times have a 1:1 AV ratio, but the timing relationship between the QRS complex and the subsequent P wave is not fixed.
3. NCTs with A:V ratio <1 are rare and include sinus rhythm with simultaneous conduction over fast and slow AV nodal pathways, nodofascicular pathway–based reentry, and either AVNRT or junctional tachycardia with retrograde block.

B. R-P interval in cases with 1:1 A:V ratio:
1. "No R-P" interval NCTs: Absence of a visible P wave (subsumed in the QRS complex) is common in AVNRT (anterograde slow–retrograde fast pathways) but can occur in AT with a long AV conduction time (PR interval).
2. NCTs with a short R-P interval (P wave in the first one-third of the R-R interval) include AVRT, AVNRT (especially in patients >50 years old) and AT, with junctional tachycardia as a rare cause.

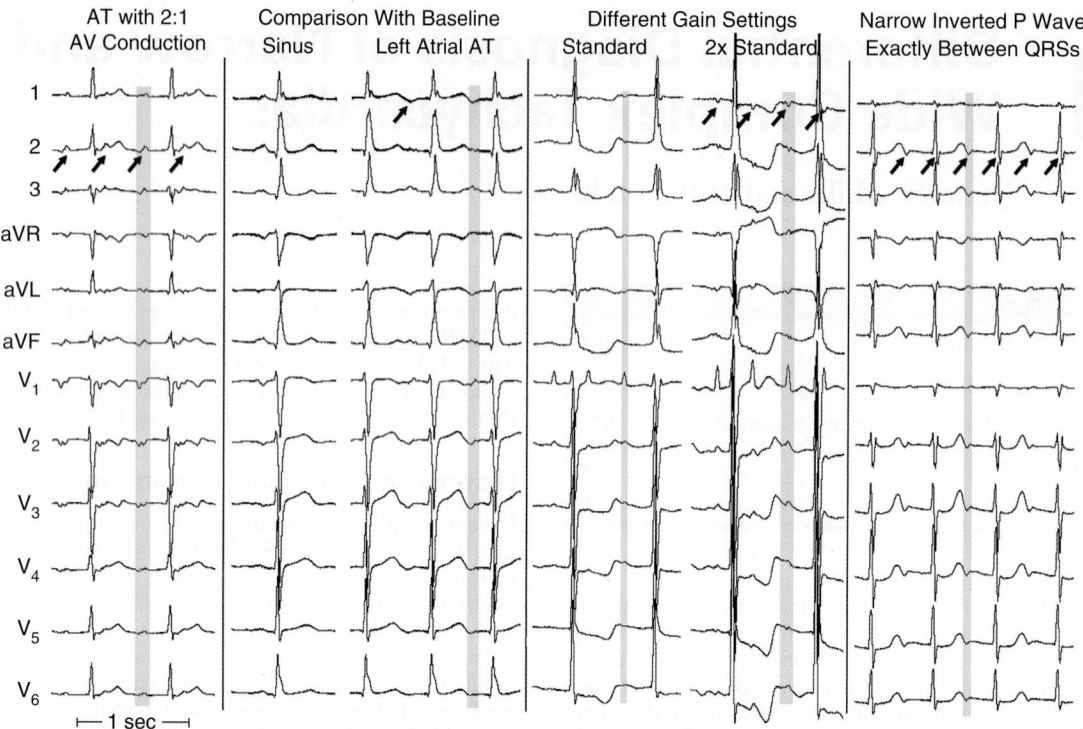

FIGURE 60.1 Determination of P waves during narrow complex tachycardia using a variety of methods. *Vertical blue bands* denote entire width of P wave; *arrows* indicate visible P wave. *AT,* Atrial tachycardia; *AV,* atrioventricular.

TABLE 60.1 Narrow complex tachycardia diagnostic features

	ATRIOVENTRICULAR RATIO			
	>1 (A > V)	**1 (A = V)**	**<1 (A < V)**[A]	**INDETERMINATE (NO CLEAR P)**
Diagnostic possibilities	Atrial tachycardia	AVNRT	Sinus rhythm with 1:2 conduction	AVNRT
	Atrial flutter	AVRT	AVNRT	(Junctional tachycardia)
	(AVNRT)	Atrial tachycardia	Junctional tachycardia	(Atrial tachycardia)
		(Junctional tachycardia)	Nodofascicular tachycardia	

	R-P INTERVAL			
	NO VISIBLE P	**SHORT RP**	**INTERMEDIATE RP**	**LONG RP**
Diagnostic possibilities	AVNRT	AVRT	AVNRT	Atrial tachycardia
	(Atrial tachycardia)	AVNRT	Atrial tachycardia	AVNRT
		Atrial tachycardia	AVRT	AVRT
		(Junctional tachycardia)	(Junctional tachycardia)	(Junctional tachycardia)

	P-WAVE MORPHOLOGY			
	POSITIVE LEADS **II, III, aVF**	**NEGATIVE LEADS** **II, III, aVF**	**NEGATIVE LEAD I**	**POSITIVE ALL PRECORDIAL LEADS**
Diagnostic possibilities	Atrial tachycardia	AVNRT	AVRT (left lateral pathway)	Pulmonary vein ostia
	AVRT	AVRT	Left atrial tachycardia	
		Atrial tachycardia		

[a]All four items in this group are rare.
Diagnostic possibilities are listed in order of frequency.
Terms in parentheses denote rare situations.
AVNRT, Atrioventricular nodal reentrant tachycardia; *AVRT,* atrioventricular reentry tachycardia.

3. Intermediate R-P interval NCTs (P wave in middle one-third of the R-R interval) are of the same types as with short RP NCTs, but AVNRT ("slow–slow") and AT are more common than AVRT.

4. Long R-P NCTs are an interesting group with the same diagnostic possibilities as for the other R-P subsets, but ATs predominate; AVNRT is of the less common antero-grade fast–retrograde slow pathway variety and unusual, slowly conducting accessory pathways.

C. P-wave morphology[2]:

1. Atrial activation in NCTs with positive P waves in the inferior leads begins near the cephalad aspect (top) of the atria, including the upper crista terminalis, superior vena cava and appendage in the right atrium, and the pulmonary veins and appendage in the left atrium, as well as cephalad portions of the tricuspid and mitral annuli. Evaluation of precordial leads (anteroposterior) and lead I (left–right) further refine the site of origin of atrial activation in the other two axes. As such, ATs account for many of these, but AVRT with pathway atrial insertions on the cephalad portions of mitral or tricuspid annuli are also in this group.

2. Negative ("inverted") P waves in the inferior leads denote onset of atrial activation in the lower portion of the atria (low crista terminalis, coronary sinus os, low septum and tricuspid annulus in the right atrium, and low septum or mitral annulus in the left atrium). All varieties of AVNRT, as well as AVRT using posterior AV pathways, fall into this group, as do some ATs.

3. A negative (inverted) P wave in lead I is a reliable indicator of left-to-right atrial activation, either from AT arising in the left atrium or pulmonary veins, or AVRT using a left lateral pathway.

4. When all precordial leads show positive P waves, a left atrial or pulmonary venous source should be suspected.

Special Cases

P-wave morphology is usually a good indicator of the origin of atrial activation; however, there are several situations in which this inference should be made cautiously. These include car-diac malposition (dextrocardia and prior pneumonectomy) and previous extensive atrial ablation or surgery, such as for repair of congenital heart disease. Following catheter or surgical abla-tion, common arrhythmias, such as right atrial cavotricuspid isthmus–dependent flutter can have an unusual appearance (Fig. 60.2), and uncommon arrhythmias (such as left atrial macro-reentry) can masquerade as more common ones (such as right atrial flutter).[3] Finally, very rarely, VT can have a relatively nar-row QRS (<120 ms) and be mistakenly diagnosed as SVT. This occurs in several settings: children (with a narrower baseline QRS in sinus rhythm), adults with VT in the absence of SHD, or either of the aforementioned settings arising in the His–Pur-kinje system or propagating into it very early in the QRS. In almost all of these cases, the prognosis is similar to that of SVT (i.e., benign).

Wide QRS Tachycardias
Diagnostic Possibilities

Although there are several possible causes of WCT (Box 60.1; Fig. 60.3), the vast majority are either VT or SVT with aber-rant interventricular conduction (SVT-A). The remainder of this discussion will concentrate on differentiating between these two entities. Because of the wider diagnostic possibilities and more serious nature of some causes, WCTs evoke more anxiety among health care workers than NCTs. For purposes of classification, WCT with the last portion of V₁ negative are termed *left bundle branch block (LBBB) type QRS*, whereas a right bundle branch

block (RBBB) type QRS pattern is denoted by a positive deflec-tion in the last half of V₁. Some WCTs do not fit well into these descriptions, with "Rs" or "qRs" patterns in V₁; in cases with this degree of ambiguity, the diagnosis is almost always VT.

History and Physical Examination

Patients with SVT-A, like those with NCT, have usually had prior episodes of arrhythmia, whereas in those presenting with

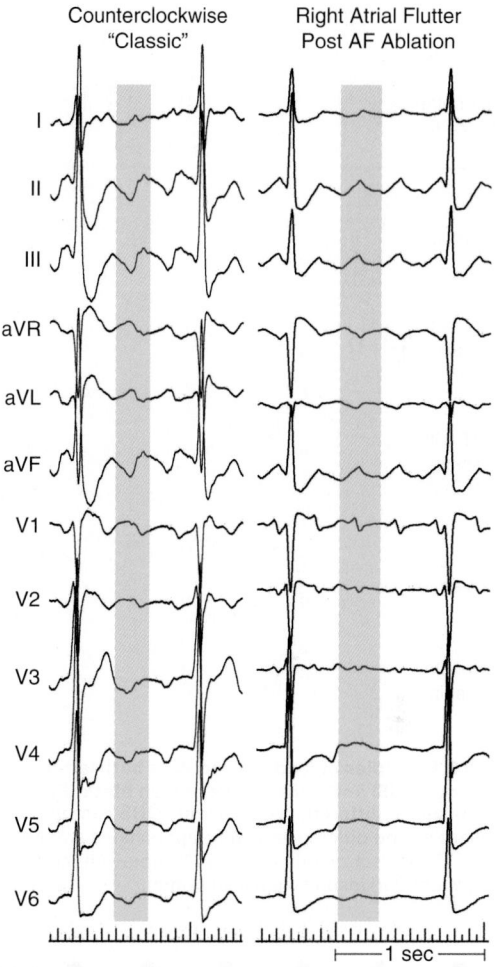

FIGURE 60.2 Two cases of electrophysiological study-proven counterclockwise right atrial flutter. At left is "classic" atrial flutter with inverted flutter waves in inferior leads (*shaded blue*); at right is the same arrhythmia based on endocardial recordings, but occurring after altered atrial conduction and activation following pulmonary vein isolation for treatment of atrial fibrillation (*AF*). Note the flutter waves (*blue shading*) have opposite polarity in most leads to those of "classic" flutter in this setting.

BOX 60.1   Wide complex tachycardia diagnostic possibilities

1. Ventricular tachycardia
2. Supraventricular tachycardia with one of the following:
   a. Aberrant interventricular conduction (His–Purkinje)
   b. Anterograde conduction over accessory pathway
   c. Abnormal baseline QRS configuration
   d. Nonspecific QRS widening due to electrolyte abnormality/drug effect[4]
3. Ventricular pacing
4. Electrocardiographic artifact

VT, it is often their first episode. VT patients tend to have a history of SHD, such as prior myocardial infarction, cardiomyopathy, or significant valvular disease. Symptoms in VT patients include palpitations, lightheadedness or syncope, dyspnea, and chest pain; episodes often begin without apparent provocation. Physical examination during VT episodes shows tachycardia in a patient who may be conscious, but often with marginal blood pressure. Cannon A waves in neck veins and variable intensity of S1 are sometimes present.

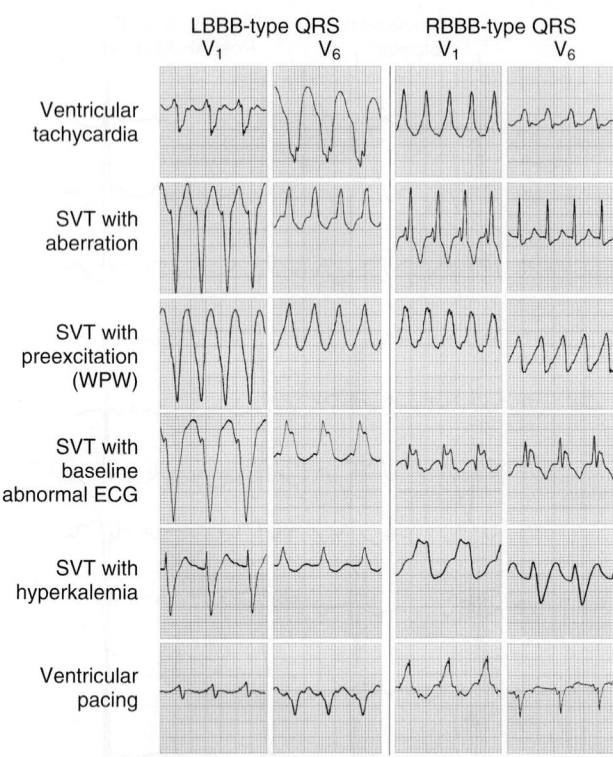

FIGURE 60.3 Examples of leads V₁ and V₆ in both left bundle branch block (*LBBB*) and right bundle branch block (*RBBB*) types of QRS complexes in different types of wide QRS complex tachycardia. Similarities and differences can be appreciated among the various causes. *ECG,* Electrocardiogram; *SVT,* supraventricular tachycardia; *WPW,* Wolff-Parkinson-White (syndrome).

Electrocardiographic Differential Diagnosis

Several features of the 12-lead ECG in WCT have proven diagnostic utility; the more important among these are as follows (Fig. 60.4 shows several examples):

A. QRS duration—In 1978, Wellens found that, among WCTs with QRS duration >140 ms, 95% were VTs. Because some cases of LBBB aberration have QRS >140 ms, this rule was later modified to allow SVT-A with LBBB pattern to have QRS up to 160 ms. This criterion is deceptively simple, in that different observers can measure very different QRS durations, especially when QRS onset or offset are not sharply delineated. For this reason, the widest reproducible QRS duration in several simultaneously recorded leads should always be used.

B. QRS axis—Since aberration patterns are confined to left or right axis deviation (thus –60 degrees to +120 degrees), WCT with a QRS axis outside this range is likely to be VT. This is particularly true for an axis from –90 degrees to 180 degrees (i.e., negative complexes in leads I, II, and III); this criterion has a positive predictive accuracy (PPA) of >95% for VT.

C. AV relationship—It has long been recognized that AV dissociation (ventricular rhythm faster than an independent, regular atrial rhythm) is a reliable indicator of VT, with very rare exceptions. However, it is present (or recognizable) in only one-third of known VT ECGs,[5] thus decreasing its utility. Other AV relationships are also helpful, such as 2:1 retrograde conduction and retrograde Wenckebach conduction (often more difficult to recognize than AV dissociation). The latter forms of non-1:1 retrograde conduction, still diagnostic of VT, are present in about 5% of cases of VT, whereas a 1:1 AV relationship is recognized in about 8% of cases.[5] Uncommonly seen fusion and capture beats are manifestations of a non-1:1 AV relationship during VT.

D. Specific patterns in ECG leads V₁ and V₆ (Fig. 60.5):
   1. RBBB pattern:
      a. Lead V₁: The RBB contributes little to the initial part of the normal QRS; thus when it is blocked, the first 40 ms of the QRS is unchanged. This leads to typical aberration patterns that include rSR′, rSr′, or rR′ in lead V₁; all others, including Rsr′, Rr′, qR, and monophasic R are thus VT patterns.
      b. Lead V₆: A small amount of normal right ventricular voltage is directed away from V₆; in RBBB aberration, this is shifted later in the QRS to enlarge the S wave.

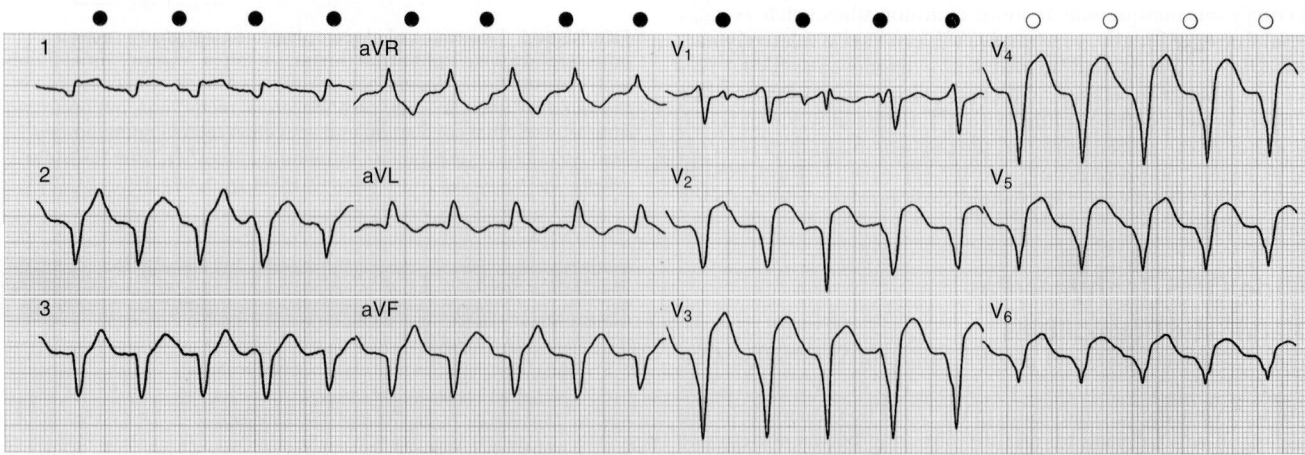

FIGURE 60.4 Electrocardiogram of ventricular tachycardia showing several diagnostic features, including very wide QRS; right superior axis deviation; concordant (negative) precordial R-wave pattern; R-wave duration in V₁ >30 ms; QRS onset to S-wave nadir in V₁ >60 ms; atrioventricular dissociation (*filled black circles* denoting visible P waves, *hollow circles* denoting less visible ones); and fusion beats (third complex in V₁).

Since it is a small vector, the R/S ratio is >1. In left ventricular VT, all of the right ventricular voltage, and some of the left, is directed away from V_6, leading to R/S ratios <1 (rS, QS patterns). In some cases, a monophasic R wave or qR are seen, inconsistent with aberration and thus likely VT.

2. LBBB pattern:
   a. Lead V_1: The LBB determines the initial part of the normal QRS; when blocked, the RBB transmits to the ventricles and although several left ventricular activation patterns may ensue, the initial portion of the QRS is inscribed relatively rapidly. This yields patterns in V_1 (or V_2), such as QS or rS, in which the QRS onset to the S-wave nadir is ≤60 ms and the duration of the r wave, if present, is ≤30 ms. Patterns other than these, such as a QS or an rS with an onset-QRS to S-wave nadir >60 ms or an r wave duration >30 ms, indicate VT.[6] Distinguishing scar-based VT from VT in the absence of SHD (which often resemble SVT-A) can be difficult; R-wave transition after V_4 and, in V_1 or V_2, notching of the downstroke, or an onset of QRS to the nadir of the S wave >90 ms, each indicate scar-based VT.[7]
   b. Lead V_6: In true LBBB, there is no Q wave in the lateral precordial leads; the presence of any Q wave in V_6 during WCT strongly suggests a VT diagnosis.

E. Precordial leads:
   1. Concordance—If all of the precordial leads have the same polarity (all positive or all negative), VT is likely, since aberration patterns fundamentally never have positive concordance; in some cases of LBBB aberration, R waves may not be seen until V_7 or later, leaving a concordant negative pattern. Since concordant patterns are present in <20% of all VTs, this criterion has low sensitivity. A more recent analysis[5] found that a negative concordant pattern had virtually no capacity to distinguish SVT-A from VT, while a positive concordant pattern remained a strong differentiator.
   2. Brugada criteria[8]—In most cases of SVT-A, at least one precordial lead has an "RS" pattern, but this need not be the case in VT; thus if no precordial leads in a WCT have an RS, it is most likely VT. This is the first step of the algorithm by Brugada and colleagues; further, if an RS complex is present, an interval from the onset of R to the nadir of S >100 ms strongly suggests VT. Other steps in the algorithm include evaluation for AV dissociation and the usual V_1 and V_6 patterns.

F. Newer criteria: Two recent algorithms have used single ECG leads (aVR or lead II) to differentiate VT from SVT-A. These have the virtues of simplicity and, with it, easier memorization.
   1. aVR criteria—Vereckei proposed two algorithms incorporating lead aVR. The first had four steps (a positive result at any step makes a VT diagnosis, with the remaining ECGs categorized as SVT-A)[9]: AV dissociation, R wave in aVR, standard criteria in V_1 and V_6, and the ventricular activation velocity index. The latter is the ratio of the vertical amplitude (in tenths of millivolts) traversed in the first 40 ms of the QRS complex, divided by the same amplitude measurement in the last 40 ms, of any lead with a bi- or triphasic QRS complex. Ratios >1 indicate SVT-A, whereas ratios ≤1 indicate VT. This algorithm performed well in initial testing but is somewhat cumbersome, and it is difficult to remember how to make the measurements. The second proposed algorithm[10] involves only aVR and is thus generally simpler; it also has four steps: presence of monophasic R, q or r >40 ms duration, slurred downstroke on Q wave, and the velocity index from the previously-noted algorithm (but applied only to aVR). As with the prior algorithm, a positive result at any step makes a diagnosis of VT with a final default result being SVT-A. This algorithm, like the prior one, had an overall accuracy of 91%. Neither, however, has performed as well when applied to other data sets by different investigators.[11]
   2. R-wave peak time—Pava and colleagues[12] proposed another simple, one-step criterion: the interval from QRS onset to peak amplitude (positive or negative) in lead II. Using a cutoff of 50 ms, almost all WCTs with a shorter time to peak amplitude in lead II were SVTs, whereas almost all WCTs with intervals ≥50 ms were VTs. The sensitivity and specificity were 0.98 and 0.93, respectively. While this criterion appears to have many desirable features (simplicity, ease of application, and accuracy), its performance in the hands of other investigators[11] has been less impressive (sensitivity, 0.60; specificity, 0.83). Examples are shown in Fig. 60.6.

Several studies have compared the relative strengths of various algorithms and criteria for differentiating the cause of WCT; these vary in their conclusions but confirm the general utility of the algorithms in real-world settings.[11,13] Preexisting

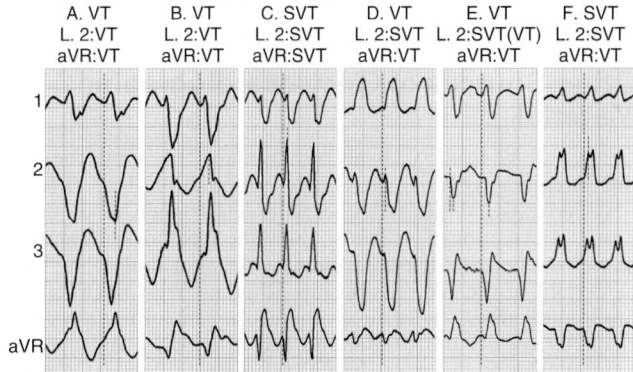

FIGURE 60.6 **Lead II and aVR criteria in supraventricular tachycardia (*SVT*) with aberrant interventricular conduction and ventricular tachycardia (*VT*).** Lead I, II, III, and aVR are shown from several wide QRS complex tachycardias. *Long dashed vertical lines* indicate earliest QRS onset among all leads; *shorter dashed lines* denote peak in lead II. In A and B (VT) and C (SVT), various morphologies of lead II and aVR are shown; both criteria correctly diagnose each rhythm. In D and E (both VT), lead II incorrectly diagnoses SVT while aVR is correct; in E, lead II by itself is incorrect (with an isoelectric segment prior to the QRS downstroke), but when analyzed using the true QRS onset, lead II is correct. In F, SVT is present and correctly diagnosed by lead II, but not aVR (slurred downstroke of Q wave).

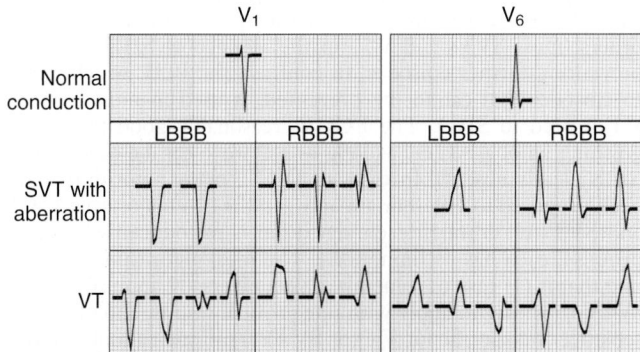

FIGURE 60.5 **Diagrammatic representation of common QRS morphologies encountered in ventricular tachycardia (*VT*) and supraventricular tachycardia (*SVT*) with aberrant interventricular conduction, in leads V_1 and V_6 for both left bundle branch block (*LBBB*) and right bundle branch block (*RBBB*) QRSs.** Note initial portions of the QRS complex in normal and aberrated QRS complexes, contrasted with initial QRS forces in VT complexes.

QRS abnormalities can diminish the diagnostic accuracy of the algorithms.[14]

Special Cases

Several special situations exist in which criteria suggest SVT-A when VT is present:

A. Relatively narrow complex VT—As noted above, these VTs generally (but not always) occur in the absence of SHD and in younger individuals. Correctly identifying these patients is important for therapy, since catheter ablation can be curative in most cases. A more important error is correctly identifying the WCT as VT, but using implantable cardioverter defibrillator (ICD) therapy merely on the basis that the rhythm was VT.

B. Bundle branch reentrant (BBR) VT—In BBR, QRS complexes are identical to either LBBB aberration or, more rarely, RBBB aberration, with either left or right axis deviation. ECG distinction from SVT-A is difficult, in that while most cases have AV dissociation, the heart rate is so rapid that dissociated P waves usually cannot be readily observed. This relatively uncommon arrhythmia is important because of its straightforward treatment with catheter ablation. Most patients with BBR also have other forms of VT for which an ICD is indicated and thus catheter ablation is rarely their sole therapy. If BBR is discovered during electrophysiological testing, ablation can decrease ICD shocks.

C. Irregular VT—Like SVT, almost all VTs have very regular R-R intervals, insofar as can be measured on the standard ECG. A small proportion of VTs are grossly irregular and in these cases, the obvious alternative diagnosis is atrial fibrillation with aberration. In this case, morphology criteria can be quite helpful (as can finding AV dissociation, if atrial fibrillation is not actually present).

Finally, there are situations in which ECG criteria suggest VT in patients with SVT-A. This group includes preexcited SVT (during sinus rhythm, preexcitation is almost always readily apparent) or other typical forms of SVT in patients with significant SHD such as repaired congenital heart disease or severe cardiomyopathy. These populations are relatively small but growing, and for these populations, better methods of distinguishing SVT-A from VT will be increasingly important in the future.

Other Sources of Electrocardiographic Material

Often, full 12-lead ECGs are not available for application of the foregoing criteria, but single- or multiple-lead rhythm strips do exist. While full 12-lead ECGs contain much diagnostic information, they rarely show the onset or termination of tachycardia, and the recording is often not long enough to be certain of the AV relationship. Rhythm strips recorded on hospital telemetry or event or ambulatory monitors, however, characteristically show onset and end of episodes and may be long enough to diagnose the AV relationship. Several criteria for distinguishing SVT-A from VT on such rhythm strips are shown in Table 60.2. Patients with implanted cardiac devices (pacemakers, ICDs, and loop recorders) can have their devices interrogated to obtain valuable diagnostic information about WCT episodes (see elsewhere).

Remaining Problems

Although numerous algorithms have been developed to aid in diagnosis of WCT, none are 100% sensitive and specific; particularly difficult cases include VT in the absence of SHD. In

TABLE 60.2	Electrocardiographic features for diagnosing wide complex tachycardias on monitor strips	
FEATURE	**FAVORS SUPRAVENTRICULAR ORIGIN**	**FAVORS VENTRICULAR ORIGIN**
Initiating event	P wave, with PR ≥ baseline	QRS complex, or P wave with PR < baseline
Initiation sequence	"Long-short"	"Short-long"
Rate of wide vs. contemporaneous narrow QRS complexes	Similar	Disparate
Regularity of wide vs. contemporaneous narrow QRS complexes (AF)	Similar	Disparate (regular wide QRS, irregular narrow QRS)
Fused QRS complexes at onset	Absent	May be present
Last event at termination	QRS complex	P wave or QRS complex
Effect of carotid sinus pressure/adenosine	Slowing or termination; transient AV block (in AF/AFL/AT)	No effect or transient AV dissociation; rare termination (normal heart VT)

AF, atrial fibrillation; *AFL,* atrial flutter; *AV,* atrioventricular; *AT,* atrial tachycardia.

addition, none of the criteria have performed as well in subsequent analysis and "real world" testing as in their original publication. Thus better criteria are necessary, but research is also needed into why the existing criteria are not as robust in practice as they initially seemed to be. Potential causes include (1) misremembering criteria ("was it 130 or 140 ms for QRS duration?"), (2) incorrect application of criteria (i.e., mistaking small irregularities in the ECG baseline for AV dissociation), (3) imperfections of criteria (especially in VT in the absence of SHD, or SVT in patients with severe cardiomyopathy), and (4) unwillingness to believe the results ("all the criteria suggest VT, but I STILL think it's SVT"). Until progress is made on each of these fronts, diagnostic errors will persist.

Summary

Arriving at the correct diagnosis of tachycardias has obvious clinical importance, since current therapies can cure many disorders (most SVTs and VTs in the absence of SHD), thereby preventing further episodes. In contrast, the ICD, which reacts to episodes that cannot be prevented, is used in most cases of VT related to SHD. The ECG is reasonably good for distinguishing among NCTs, as long as a P wave can be clearly seen (or is clearly absent). In cases of WCT, many algorithms have been proposed to differentiate between the two major causes: VT and SVT-A. Although each algorithm is introduced with great promise, each has its limitations. The ideal algorithm would be one that is (1) easy to remember, (2) universally applicable to all WCTs, (3) easy to apply with unequivocal results, and (4) 100% sensitive and specific for VT (or SVT). Until such a tool is developed, when a patient has WCT that cannot be readily classified, it is safest to treat the patient as though the rhythm is VT until proven otherwise.

REFERENCES

1. Shah D, Sunthorn H, Burri H, et al. Narrow, slow-conducting isthmus dependent left atrial reentry developing after ablation for atrial fibrillation: ECG characterization and elimination by focal RF ablation. *J Cardiovasc Electrophysiol*. 2006;17:508–515.

2. Kistler PM, Roberts-Thomson KC, Haqqani HM, et al. P-wave morphology in focal atrial tachycardia: development of an algorithm to predict the anatomic site of origin. *J Am Coll Cardiol*. 2006;48:1010–1017.

3. Gerstenfeld EP, Marchlinski FE. Mapping and ablation of left atrial tachycardias occurring after atrial fibrillation ablation. *Heart Rhythm*. 2007;4:S65–S72.

4. Bhardwaj B, Lazzara R, Stavrakis S. Wide complex tachycardia in the presence of class I antiarrhythmic agents: a diagnostic challenge. *Ann Noninv Electrocardiol*. 2014;19:289–292.

5. Miller JM, Das MK, Yadav AV, Bhakta D, Nair G, Alberte C. Value of the 12-lead ECG in wide QRS tachycardia. *Cardiology Cinics*. 2006;24:439–451.

6. Kindwall KE, Brown J, Josephson ME. Electrocardiographic criteria for ventricular tachycardia in wide complex left bundle branch block morphology tachycardias. *Am J Cardiol*. 1988;61:1279–1283.

7. Wijnmaalen AP, Stevenson WG, Schalij MJ, et al. ECG identification of scar-related ventricular tachycardia with a left bundle-branch block configuration. *Circ Arrhythm Electrophysiol*. 2011;4:486–493.

8. Brugada P, Brugada J, Mont L, Smeets J, Andries EW. A new approach to the differential diagnosis of a regular tachycardia with a wide QRS complex. *Circulation*. 1991;83:1649–1659.

9. Vereckei A, Duray G, Szenasi G, Altemose GT, Miller JM. Application of a new algorithm in the differential diagnosis of wide QRS complex tachycardia. *Eur Heart J*. 2007;28:589–600.

10. Vereckei A, Duray G, Szenasi G, Altemose GT, Miller JM. New algorithm using only lead aVR for differential diagnosis of wide QRS complex tachycardia. *Heart Rhythm*. 2008;5:89–98.

11. Jastrzebski M, Kukla P, Czarnecka D, Kawecka-Jaszcz K. Comparison of five electrocardiographic methods for differentiation of wide QRS-complex tachycardias. *Europace*. 2012;14:1165–1171.

12. Pava LF, Perafan P, Badiel M, et al. R-wave peak time at DII: a new criterion for differentiating between wide complex QRS tachycardias. *Heart Rhythm*. 2010;7:922–926.

13. Kaiser E, Darrieux FC, Barbosa SA, et al. Differential diagnosis of wide QRS tachycardias: comparison of two electrocardiographic algorithms. *Europace*. 2015;17:1422–1427.

14. Datino T, Almendral JM, Avila P, et al. Specificity of electrocardiographic criteria for the differential diagnosis of wide QRS complex tachycardia in patients with intraventricular conduction defect. *Heart Rhythm*. 2013;10:1393–1401.

61 Electroanatomical Mapping for Arrhythmias

Abhishek Deshmukh, Suraj Kapa, and Samuel Asirvatham

The software and hardware related to mapping technologies for cardiac arrhythmias have evolved considerably over the past decades. The history of cardiac mapping dates back to the mid-1900s when Durrer and others used the isolated heart models perfected by Langendorff and colleagues to fully map ventricular wall excitation via handheld and needle electrodes.[1] Since these initial studies, multiple technologies to optimize the mapping of cardiac arrhythmias have been developed. When discussing cardiac mapping, most electrophysiologists immediately think of invasive electroanatomical mapping, involving catheters with electrodes at their tips assuming direct contact with underlying myocardium to acquire local signals and, in turn, to differentiate sites of interest based on abnormalities in voltage, activation, or both. It is via the acquisition, processing, and spatial projection of these points in a three-dimensional (3D) mesh that electrophysiologists may better identify the location and characteristics of substrate for complex arrhythmias and target it for ablation. The most common systems used when discussing cardiac mapping are Carto (Biosense Webster, Diamond Bar, CA), EnSite (St. Jude Medical, St. Paul, MN), and Rhythmia (Boston Scientific, Marlborough, MA). However, cardiac mapping may also be thought of in the context of more basic approaches—such as using the 12-lead electrocardiogram (ECG) to localize arrhythmias—or newer approaches for noninvasive or minimally invasive mapping, such as ECG-I or body surface potential mapping. For the purposes of this chapter, we will focus on electroanatomical mapping in the context of the acquisition and processing of intracardiac signals for creation of 3D electroanatomical maps of cardiac arrhythmias.

Why Do We Use Mapping Systems?

During the formative period of invasive electrophysiology, mapping was performed using multipolar electrode catheters, fluoroscopy to localize the anatomical position within the cardiac chamber of interest, and interpretation of pacing and recorded intracardiac electrograms (EGMs) to define the arrhythmia mechanism, localize the origin or critical components of a tachycardia circuit, and deliver energy. However, as the heart was mapped, there was no way to "take" points, and thus ablation relied on operator recall of the location and approximation of lesions relative to one another.

Each lab had its own unique way of memory tagging the points of interest. This approach to ablation is very effective for arrhythmias such as atrioventricular-nodal reentrant tachycardias (AVNRTs), accessory pathway-mediated tachycardias, or focal outflow tract ventricular arrhythmias, where a single ablation lesion or limited lesion sets may be capable of terminating the arrhythmia. As ablation of more complex arrhythmias such as atrial fibrillation, scar-related atrial flutters, and scar-related ventricular arrhythmias have become more common, the need for systems where regions of abnormal signals (i.e., substrate mapping), tracking sites of ablation, and projection of the generated cardiac anatomy can be used to recognize structures close to one another has become the need of the hour. While modern day mapping systems have improved the efficacy and rapidity with which complex ablations may be performed, they still require an intimate understanding of how they work and their limitations to avoid potential pitfalls. A basic approach to how one may integrate the mapping system into ablation practice is shown in Fig. 61.1.

When Are Mapping Systems Useful?

While modern day mapping systems may also be used for arrhythmias that have traditionally had high success rates even prior to the era of 3D electroanatomical mapping (e.g., accessory pathways, AVNRTs), they hold particular utility for complex arrhythmias where the underlying cardiac substrate is more extensive (e.g., scar-related ventricular arrhythmias, atrial fibrillation, and complex atrial flutters). The ability of the system to "remember" what has been mapped already and reflect it back to the operator can allow the electrophysiologist to (1) recall regions where abnormal substrate exists, (2) recognize sites of prior ablation, (3) better localize subtle differences in local activation via the acquisition of a dense array of points and annotate signals relative to one another, and (4) have an anatomical model for pure anatomically based ablation such as pulmonary vein isolation.

Principles of Electroanatomical Mapping: Point Acquisition

What Do We Map?

There are three principles that underlie all mapping systems: acquiring a signal, projecting that signal within a 3D framework, and accurately projecting signals from different sites relative to one another with a high degree of positional accuracy. The sum of all points, or signals, will generate an electroanatomical shell. Each point is given a position in an x-y-z plane. Accurate projection of signals relative to one another typically requires that a patient not be actively moving. When acquiring a point, the local signal is determined by several factors, including the spacing of electrodes on a given catheter, post-processing of the signal that partly depends on filter characteristics (high pass and low pass frequency) set by the user, contact with the tissue, positioning of the catheter relative to the underlying myocardium (i.e., whether the electrodes are parallel, oblique, or perpendicular to the underlying myocardium), and the rhythm at the time of point acquisition. In this section, we will briefly discuss how points are acquired and considerations that are needed when annotating such points at the time of cardiac mapping.

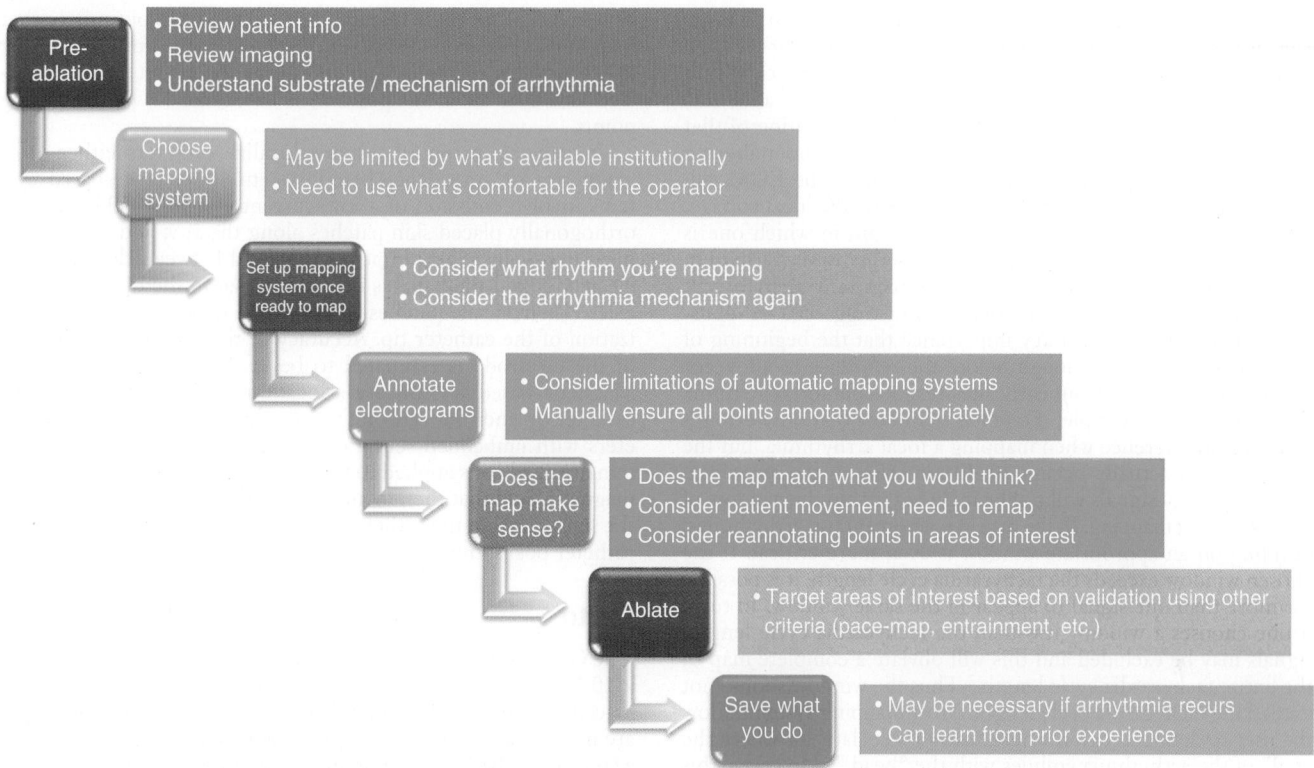

FIGURE 61.1 Approach to workflow in the ablation lab. Shown is how electroanatomical mapping systems may be integrated into ablation practices in the electrophysiology lab. Consideration of the patient's arrhythmia, preoperative imaging, and what mapping systems are either available or which the operator feels comfortable with is necessary prior to starting any case. One value of such systems is the ability to save data and review later to review if the arrhythmia recurs.

How to Acquire an Accurate Point

The fundamental requisite of making an interpretable map is to ensure that all points acquired either as activation points or for identification of substrate are accurate and relevant to each other and to the given case in general. Depending on the arrhythmia mapped, critical considerations include choosing an appropriate reference, establishing a mapping window, and deciding on how an acquired point will be annotated relative to the given reference in terms of activation or voltage. This is discussed in more detail later (Fig. 61.2).

Reference

The prerequisite of a good *reference* is that it should be stable. The reference is meant to be a stable reflection of cardiac electrical activation at that particular site against which relative timing of an acquired local EGM may be compared. The reference may either be a portion of the surface ECG (often used when mapping ventricular arrhythmias) or a local EGM (often used when mapping atrial arrhythmias). When mapping, it is important to ensure that the reference EGM has not shifted, as this may reflect either a shift in the rhythm (in which case local timing may change because of a global shift in activation pattern) or movement of the source from which the reference is being recorded (e.g., the reference catheter or the ECG patch). This can be assessed periodically, especially when the procedure is performed under minimal or no sedation.

Window

After a reference is chosen, the *mapping window* should be set up. Then the duration, onset, and offset of the mapping window

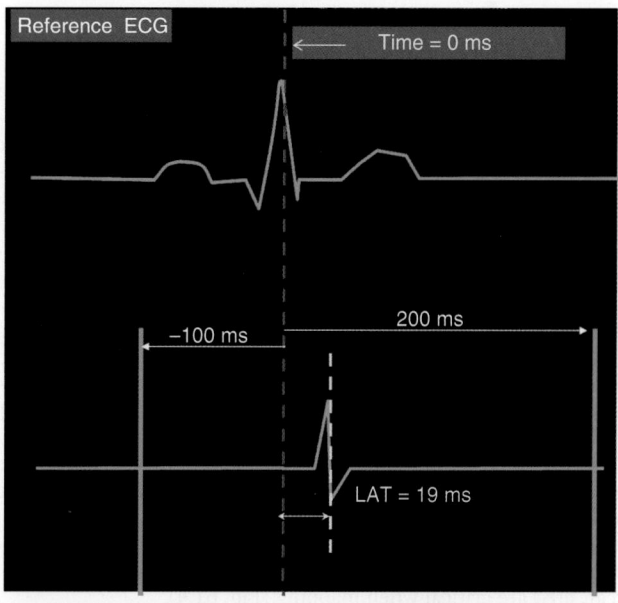

FIGURE 61.2 Example of electrogram annotation. Shown is how a reference, a window, and the timing are set up. A reference (as in this case, the peak of the QRS) is chosen. Then, a window is created based on a certain duration defined prior to the reference and subsequent to the reference (in this case, 100 ms before and 200 ms after). Activation timing of signals occurring within this window is relative to the timing to the reference (in this case, the local electrogram occurs 19 ms after the reference). *ECG,* Electrocardiogram.

relative to the reference signal should be decided upon. This is a critical step that is often overlooked. The mapping window is designed to create a period surrounding the reference within which any recorded EGMs will be acquired. Thus if an EGM (e.g., a late potential) falls outside the window, activation of that excluded portion of the EGM cannot be tagged without altering the window. Voltage of that excluded portion of the EGM will also not be considered when the system reports the local voltage.

It is also important to consider the rhythm in which one is mapping when choosing a window (i.e., whether in sinus rhythm, during a focal arrhythmia, or during a reentrant arrhythmia). When mapping a focal (microreentrant, triggered, or automatic) arrhythmia, it is of key importance that the beginning of the window be set far enough before the reference to allow for acquisition of signals from early sites responsible for arrhythmia propagation. For example, if one has a window that only extends to 10 ms prereference when mapping a focal arrhythmia, but the earliest signal actually occurs 30–40 ms prior to the reference, then these early signals will not be included within the window of interest during mapping. In the case of macroreentrant arrhythmias, deciding on an appropriate window is even more critical. If the chosen window exceeds the tachycardia cycle length, it is possible for more than one signal to appear in the same window. In turn, if one chooses a window less than the tachycardia cycle length, signals may be excluded and this will obviate a complete map of the entire tachycardia cycle length.[2] Thus the window should not exceed the tachycardia cycle length. Most mapping systems allow the user to define a region where "early meets late" or where the "tail" of the arrhythmia collides with the "head."[3] However, this is arbitrary and depends on where the offset and onset of the window are defined relative to the reference. In turn, designation of the activation time of locally acquired signals is generally arbitrary during macroreentrant arrhythmias, and defining critical sites of ablation may require the additional use of entrainment or other maneuvers. The decision to ablate at "early meets late" is fraught with several limitations, and success with such strategy is purely serendipity.[3]

Annotating Points

Before beginning to map, it is helpful to have a detailed plan between the operator and the person acquiring and annotating points. Once the reference and the window are set, accurate annotation of points is critical to appropriate mapping. Specifically, when annotating a point, one has to consider whether the earliest portion of the EGM, the peak of the EGM, the maximum upstroke of the EGM, or the beginning of the maximal downgoing portion of the unipolar EGM will be used to determine local activation (Fig. 61.3). Each of these approaches has its pitfalls. Annotation can become even more complex when considering EGMs at sites of diseased tissue (e.g., split potentials, far-field potentials, or fractionated EGMs).[4] Thus operator considerations of how each individual EGM is annotated during mapping, including differentiating far-field from near-field potentials, recognizing when the annotation of a given point may be impossible given its complexity despite potential relevance to the underlying arrhythmia, and that there may be different considerations about where to annotate the potential when mapping points at different sites (e.g., around sites of anatomical block, within regions of scar, etc.) are critical when mapping (Fig. 61.4).

Mapping Technologies

The fundamental indication for established electroanatomical mapping systems is precise nonfluoroscopic visualization of mapping catheters and reconstruction of 3D volumes of interest. The resulting 3D reconstruction is projected as a shell representing the cardiac chamber or structure of interest (Fig. 61.5). Each

system has proprietary features that are meant to optimize either mapping or ablation. However, the most critical difference that exists between mapping systems is how the catheters are visualized and how their 3D position is determined when acquiring points.

In general, mapping systems localize catheters either via a magnetic- or impedance-based system. Impedance-based systems involve emission of a low-current electrical field via three orthogonally placed skin patches along the x, y, and z axes. The measured voltage and impedance sensed between the catheter's electrodes and the patches is proportional to the distance of the electrode from the patches in 3D space, thus allowing for localization of the catheter tip. Accuracy of the position in the space of the electrode is estimated to be in the range of 0.8–2 mm. Magnetic-based systems use a location sensor embedded in the catheter tip and thus rely on the use of proprietary mapping catheters with embedded sensors for visualization. There are three miniaturized coils applied to the patient that generate a low-level magnetic field that then identifies the location and orientation of the sensor within the catheter, with an estimated range of error in catheter positioning of less than 0.5–0.8 mm (Fig. 61.6).

Carto

The Carto system is based on three active weak magnetic fields (5×10^{-6} to 5×10^{-5} Tesla), generated by a three-coil location pad placed underneath the patient's thorax. Magnetic field strengths are measured with mini-sensors embedded in the catheter tip on a continuous basis providing information about the exact position and orientation of the sensor in space. One sensor attached to the patient's skin within the working space of interest serves as a location reference. Beneath the fluoroscopy table is an electromagnetic location pad that emits a low-intensity series of magnetic fields and allows the system to precisely localize, record, and display in real time the position of the sensors and hence the mapping catheter tip in three dimensions (x, y, and z), as well as orientation (roll, pitch, and yaw).

The Carto mapping system uses a triangulation algorithm similar to that used by a global positioning system (GPS). The magnetic field emitter, mounted under the operating table, consists of three coils that generate a low-intensity magnetic field, approximately 0.05–0.2 gauss, which is a very small fraction of the magnetic field intensity inside a magnetic resonance imaging (MRI) machine. The sensor embedded proximal to the tip of a specialized mapping catheter detects the intensity of the magnetic field generated by each coil and allows for the determination of its distance from each coil. These distances determine the area of theoretical spheres around each coil, and the intersection of these three spheres determines the location of the tip of the catheter. The accuracy of determination of the location is highest in the center of the magnetic field; therefore it is important to position the location pad under the patient's chest. In addition to the x, y, and z coordinates of the catheter tip, the Carto system can determine three orientation determinants—roll, yaw, and pitch—for the electrode at the catheter tip. The position and orientation of the catheter tip can be seen on the screen and monitored in real time as the catheter moves within the electroanatomical model of the chamber mapped. The catheter icon has four color bars (green, red, yellow, and blue), enabling the operator to view the catheter as it turns clockwise or counterclockwise. In addition, because the catheter always deflects in the same direction, each catheter will always deflect toward a single color. Hence, to deflect the catheter to a specific wall, the operator should first turn the catheter so that this color faces the desired wall.

Recent versions of Carto (Carto3) integrate a hybrid of magnetic- and current-based catheter localization technology that enables the visualization of multiple catheters simultaneously without the need for fluoroscopy. This point is critical, given that

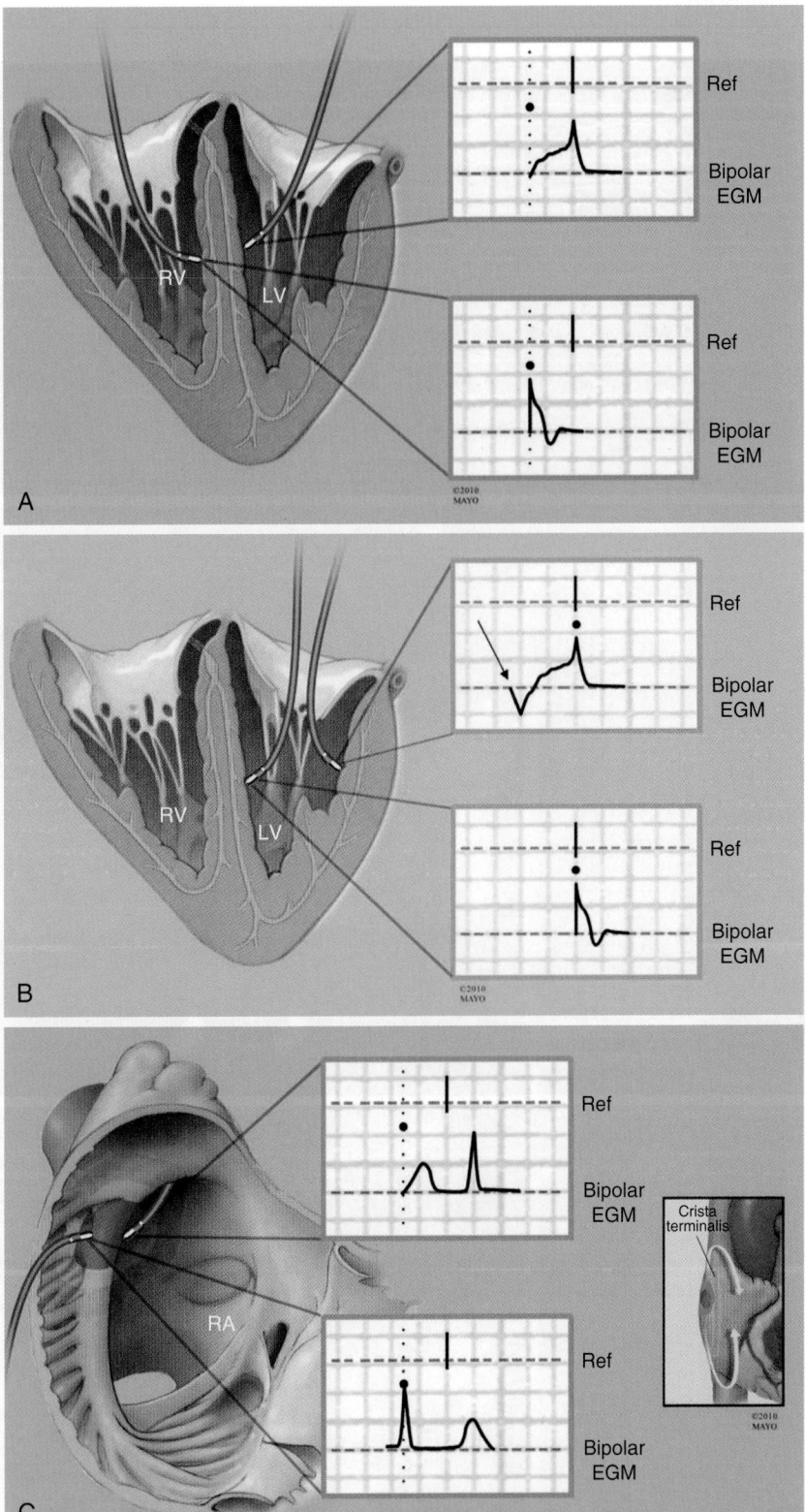

FIGURE 61.3 Annotation of points. Shown are the pitfalls to different methods of annotation. (A) demonstrates annotation according to the electrogram (*EGM*) onset. As shown, mapping is performed from both sides of the septum and each catheter records signals from the ipsilateral and opposite side of the septum. Thus, while the EGM onset from the left ventricular (*LV*) catheter represents right ventricular (*RV*) activation and not local LV activation, the EGM onset from the RV catheter would appropriately reflect local activation. (B) demonstrates the limitation of using the EGM peak. While the septal catheter, which is located in a region of healthy myocardium, is appropriately annotated when using the peak of the EGM, the lateral LV catheter has a multicomponent signal where an earlier part of the signal likely reflects local activation, though automatically annotating the peak may be inaccurate. (C) demonstrates the potential-imposed difficulties when mapping at sites where multiple potentials exist. In this case, the crista terminalis, which reflects a site of anatomical block, may result in double potentials. Annotation at these sites requires close observation of which signal reflects local activation, which may sometimes not be possible without a second catheter located on the other side of the block. (From Del Carpio Munoz F, Buescher T, Asirvatham SJ. Teaching points with 3-dimensional mapping of cardiac arrhythmias: taking points: activation mapping. *Circ Arrhythm Electrophysiol.* 2011;4:e22-e25.

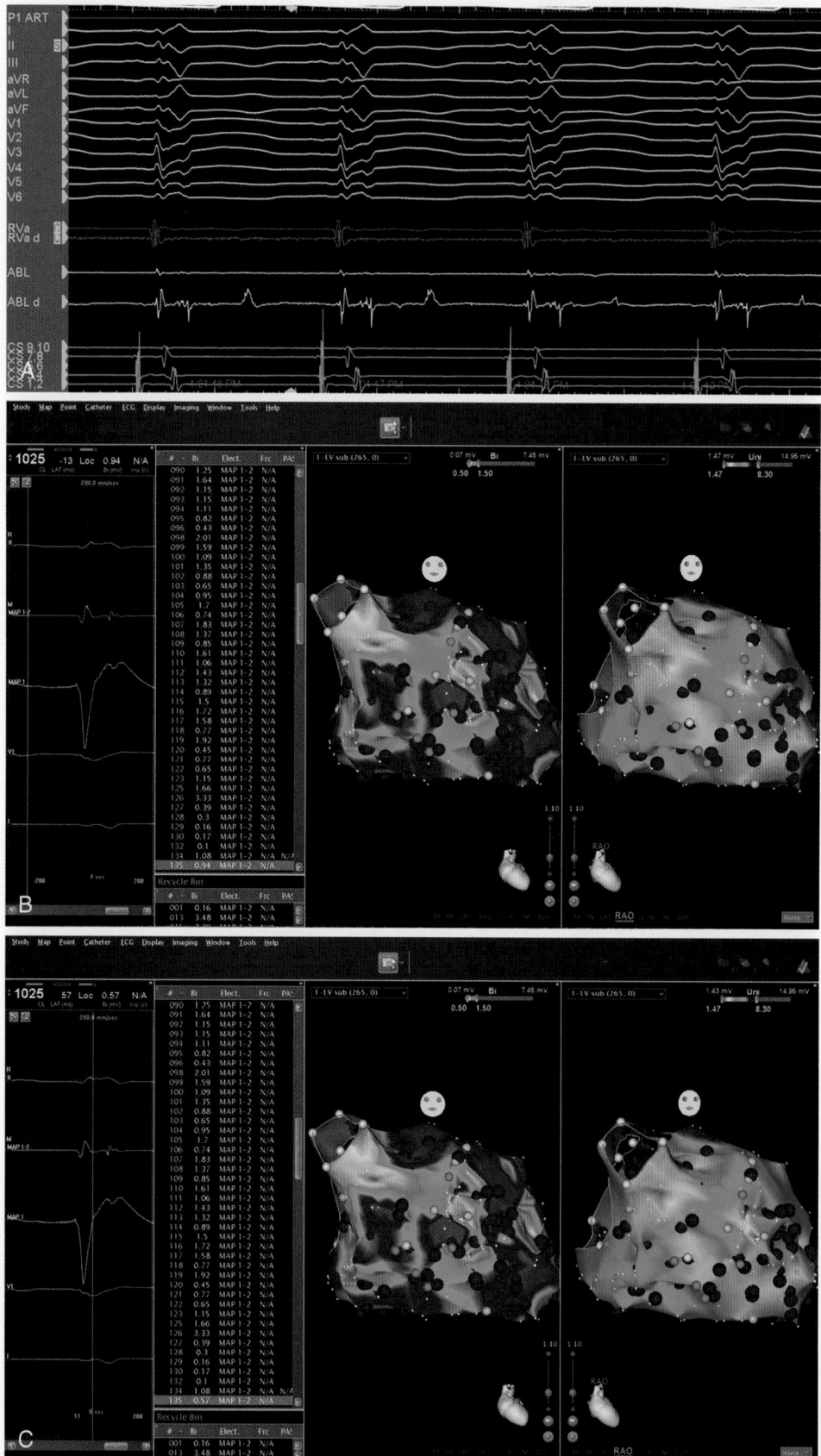

FIGURE 61.4 Limitations in annotation of complex signals. (A) shows a signal acquired from the left ventricular (LV) septum in a patient with nonischemic cardiomyopathy. The multicomponent signal actually reflects both right ventricular (RV) (first component of the signal) and LV (second component of the signal) activation. (B) demonstrates the sensed voltage when both are included in the window of interest (0.94 mV). However, when the initial, far-field signal is excluded, the actual voltage and timing of the near-field LV signal is actually lower (C).

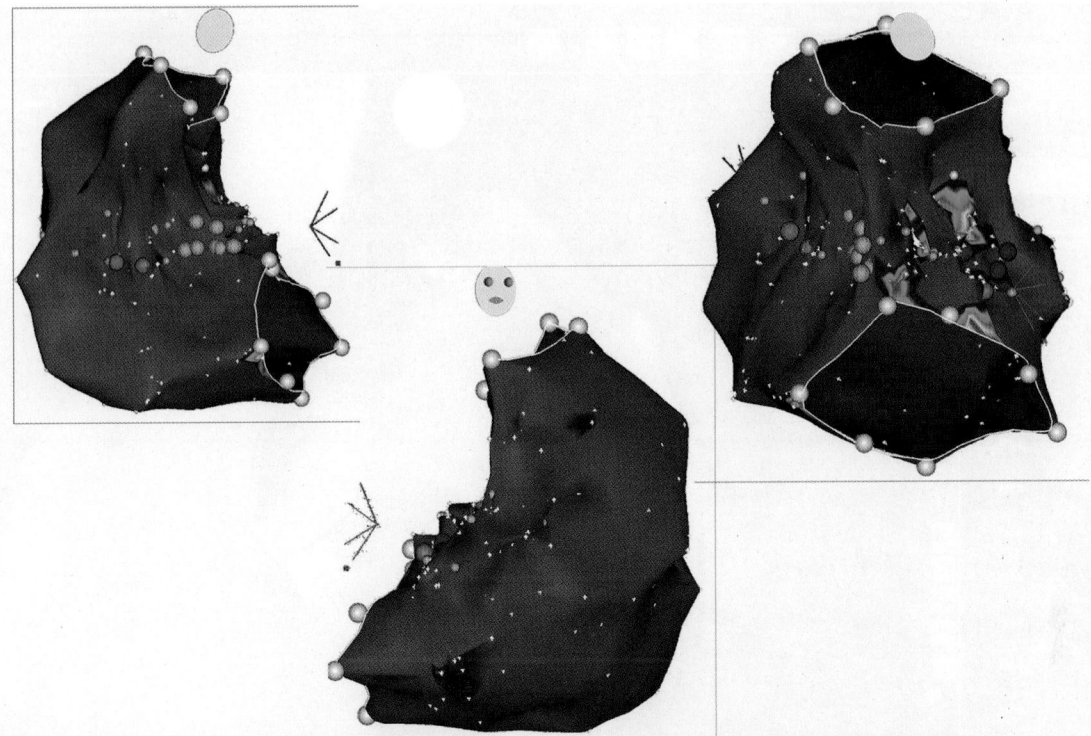

FIGURE 61.5 Example of electroanatomical map. Shown is an example of a voltage map of the right ventricle. *Purple* reflects normal myocardium in this bipolar voltage map. The tricuspid annulus (*bottom*) and pulmonic annulus (*top*) are also shown with valve points tagged. The infundibular region of the right ventricle has sparse abnormal signals as reflected by differences in color (*red* reflecting very low voltage/scar; *shades from orange to indigo* reflecting intermediately abnormal voltage).

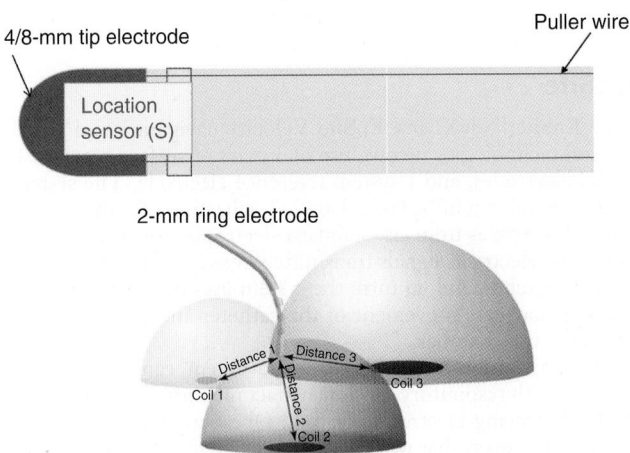

FIGURE 61.6 Magnetic field catheter localization. Shown is a schematic of how the Carto system localizes the sensor-based catheter using magnetic fields. There are three fields generated from separate coils. The catheter is localized based on the intersection of the three magnetic fields. Since the location pad is not attached to the patient and rather located beneath the table, any patient movement will result in a shift in the map. *Coils 1, 2, and 3* represent coils that generate magnetic fields. *Distances 1, 2, and 3* represent the distances from the sensor to the coils.

earlier permutations of the system could only visualize proprietary sensor-based catheters, while the introduction of current (impedance)-based catheter localization technology will allow, in principle, the ability to localize practically all other catheters. For this system, six electrode patches are positioned at the patient's back and chest, and the current emitted at a unique frequency from different catheter electrodes is continuously screened. Localization of the nonmagnetic electrodes can be calibrated by the detection of the magnetic sensor within the coordinate system to overcome distortions from nonuniform intrathoracic resistances. However, one limitation that persists is that visualization of catheters is limited to a 3D volume called a "matrix," which is predefined by the sensor-based catheter localized using the magnetic field. Only catheters within this "matrix" will be visualized, and those beyond the matrix will not.

Another new development in the Carto3 system is fast anatomical mapping (FAM), allowing the creation of detailed shells with multiple simultaneous electrodes of a multipolar mapping catheter by moving it around the chamber of interest. These representations of end-diastolic surfaces provide a better reconstruction than maps in earlier Carto versions. Another development targeting the accuracy of surface reconstructions is accomplished by a unique type of respiratory gating in which varying thoracic impedances are measured throughout the respiratory cycle. Here we review some of the current features that may assist the operator when mapping:

Visitag

The Visitag (Carto) module provides the ability to continuously store, track, and quantify ablation catheter positions along with the electrophysiological parameters acquired during radiofrequency (RF) applications according to user preferences. This module incorporates parameters of lesion formation by assessing contact force, location stability, impedance drop and time at each site and suggests the color-coded quality of lesion. The coloring options could also be represented by total time, impedance drop, median temperature, median power, and average power. The data, however, do not correspond to effectiveness of ablation but add another surrogate. Basing the decision

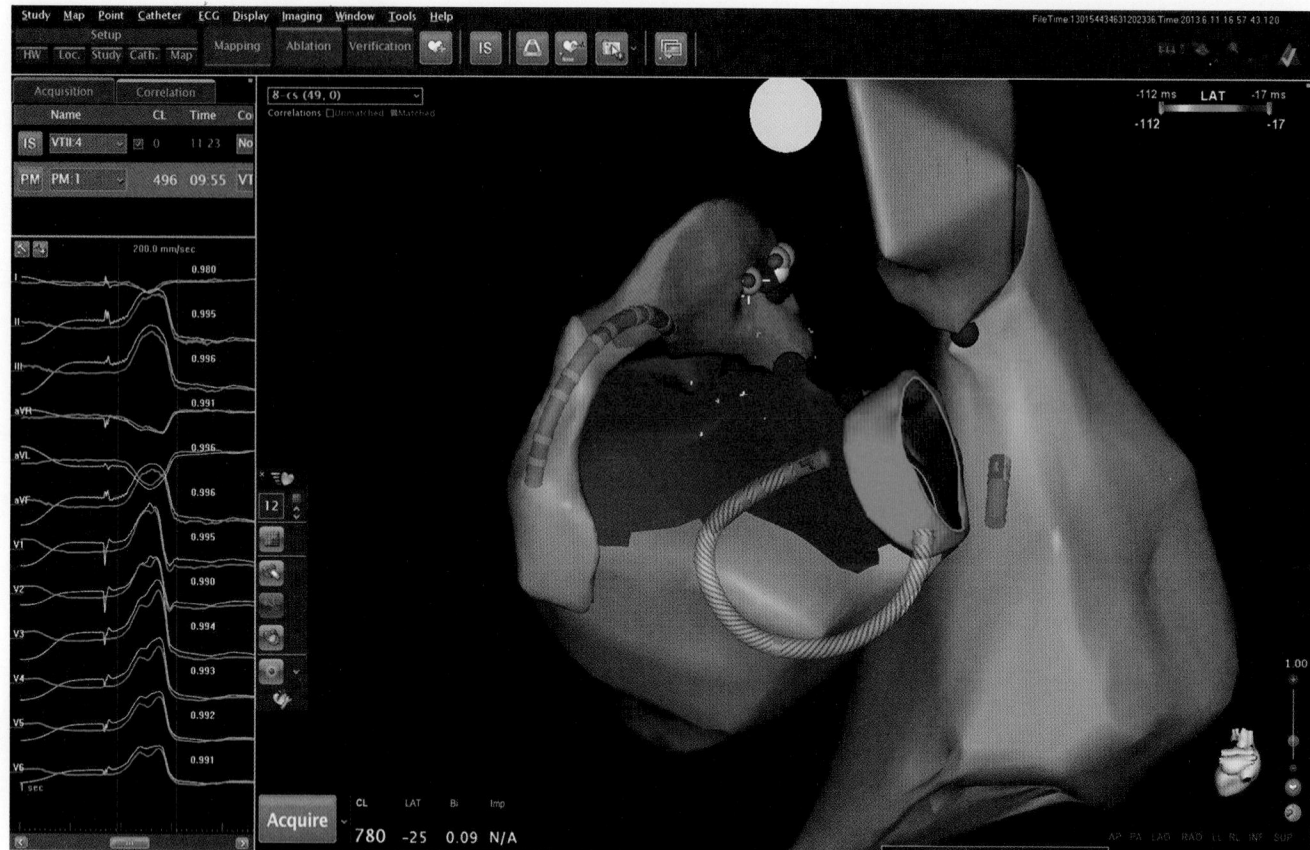

FIGURE 61.7 Passo example. Shown is how a mapping system may be used to determine if local pace mapping reflects the actual arrhythmia based on morphology analysis. A percentage map is generated in each surface electrocardiogram lead to determine the degree of match. The higher the number, the better the match.

of duration of ablation by looking for color change can be extremely dangerous.

UNIVU

This module was developed to allow electroanatomical localization of diagnostic and ablation catheters in prerecorded x-ray images or nongated x-ray videos. The aim of this module was electroanatomical catheter visualization in prerecorded x-ray images or prerecorded nongated fluoroscopy video loops and angiographies. The operator is able to manipulate the catheters, simulating the use of fluoroscopy (optional in two different fluoroscopic views simultaneously) but without the use of further irradiation exposure. The catheter visualization on the prerecorded images or cine-loops is neither ECG nor respiratory movement compensated. This is the most important limitation of this technology. Alignment of the CARTO-UNIVU with fluoroscopy requires only one registration x-ray image of the registration plate. If during the study a map shift of the prerecorded images is recognized, there is a new registration step and recording of new x-ray images. As the image is a snapshot, it does not account for respiratory variation.

Passo

This module streamlines ventricular tachycardia pace mapping and facilitates the approximate area of interest. After a baseline template is created, pacing at each point will give a pacing percentage match to the reference. Assessing match to template is programmable. It does not account for stim-to-QRS, which would be extremely valuable for certain types of tachycardias. In addition, it does not account for pacing match to intracardiac unipolar or bipolar signals (Fig. 61.7).

EnSite

The EnSite, NavX, and EnSite Velocity navigation and visualization technologies involve use of 3 pairs of surface patches, 10 ECG electrodes, and 1 system reference electrode. The systems primarily rely on impedance-based visualization of catheter position.[5] Electrodes from any standard electrophysiological catheter sense the electrical signals transmitted between the three pairs of surface patches, and, in turn, the system uses this information to track or navigate movement of the catheter and construct a 3D model of the chamber.

Compensation for respiratory movement can also be conducted, with respiratory motion artifact measured and subtracted from the roving electrode position. One particular value of the EnSite systems is that while in magnetic-based systems catheters are outside the magnetic field (i.e., the matrix created between the three intersecting magnetic fields), impedance-based systems can visualize nearly any catheter. In part due to the patch location, the observable region for these catheters is much wider (Fig. 61.8). Thus catheters can be visualized from the point of access (e.g., at the femoral vein) and tracked up to the heart with simultaneous acquisition of anatomy. There are reports of use of the system with minimal to no fluoroscopy.[6] Finally, one unique feature of the EnSite systems is the ability to allow for simultaneous pacing and ablation from the tip of the ablation catheter. This may allow for the operator to identify when an adequate lesion has been created based on the loss of local capture.

EnSite: NavX Versus Velocity

One key point is the differences between the older NavX system and the more recently introduced Velocity system.[7] The Velocity system has improved 3D localization accuracy by using a larger current signal for catheter visualization (8.136 kHz rather than the 5.6 kHz used in NavX systems). However, data on the degree of improvement in visualization accuracy are lacking. While both systems have the value of being "open" systems (namely, they can work with any catheter), the NavX system was limited by only being able to visualize 12 catheters with a total of 64 electrodes simultaneously. However, the Velocity system, in principle, can visualize an unlimited number of catheters with up to 128 electrodes.

Rhythmia

The newest system for 3D electroanatomical mapping is Rhythmia. While fewer published clinical data exist with this system compared to the other systems, there are several important differences to note. First, mapping is done with a high resolution, 64-electrode, bidirectional "basket" catheter with eight splines.[8] This catheter is recognized via a magnetic-based system. However, other catheters, including the ablation catheter, are currently mapped via an impedance-based visualization system. Similar to other systems, catheter localization is within 1 mm for the magnetic-based system. However, catheter localization accuracy with the impedance-based system is worse with Rhythmia than with EnSite (<2 mm vs. <1 mm).

One of the key features espoused by the Rhythmia system is the ability of the system to continuously map and to offer automated annotation (Fig. 61.9). Points are acquired and simultaneously annotated in real time. The system automatically ensures that the reference at the time of point acquisition is consistent for all acquired EGMs. For example, if there is a change in QRS

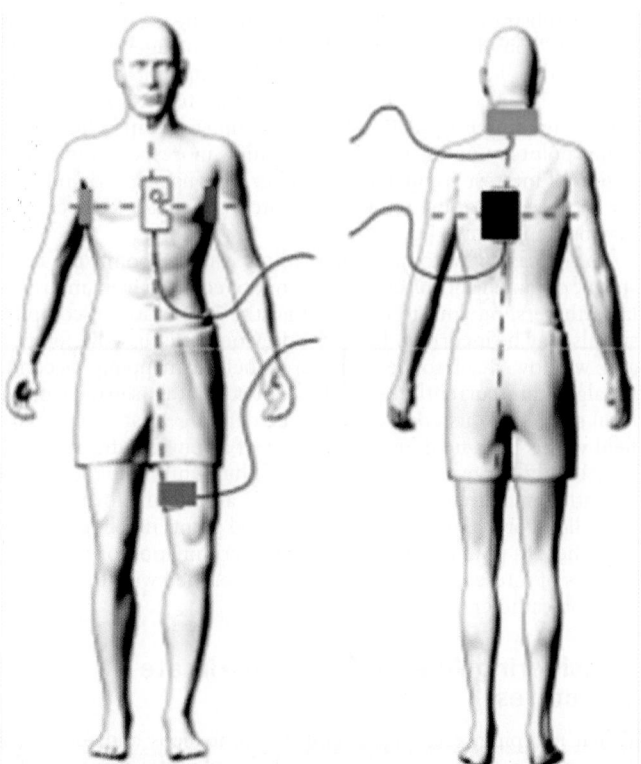

FIGURE 61.8 Patch localization with EnSite. Shown are how the six patches are placed with the EnSite system.

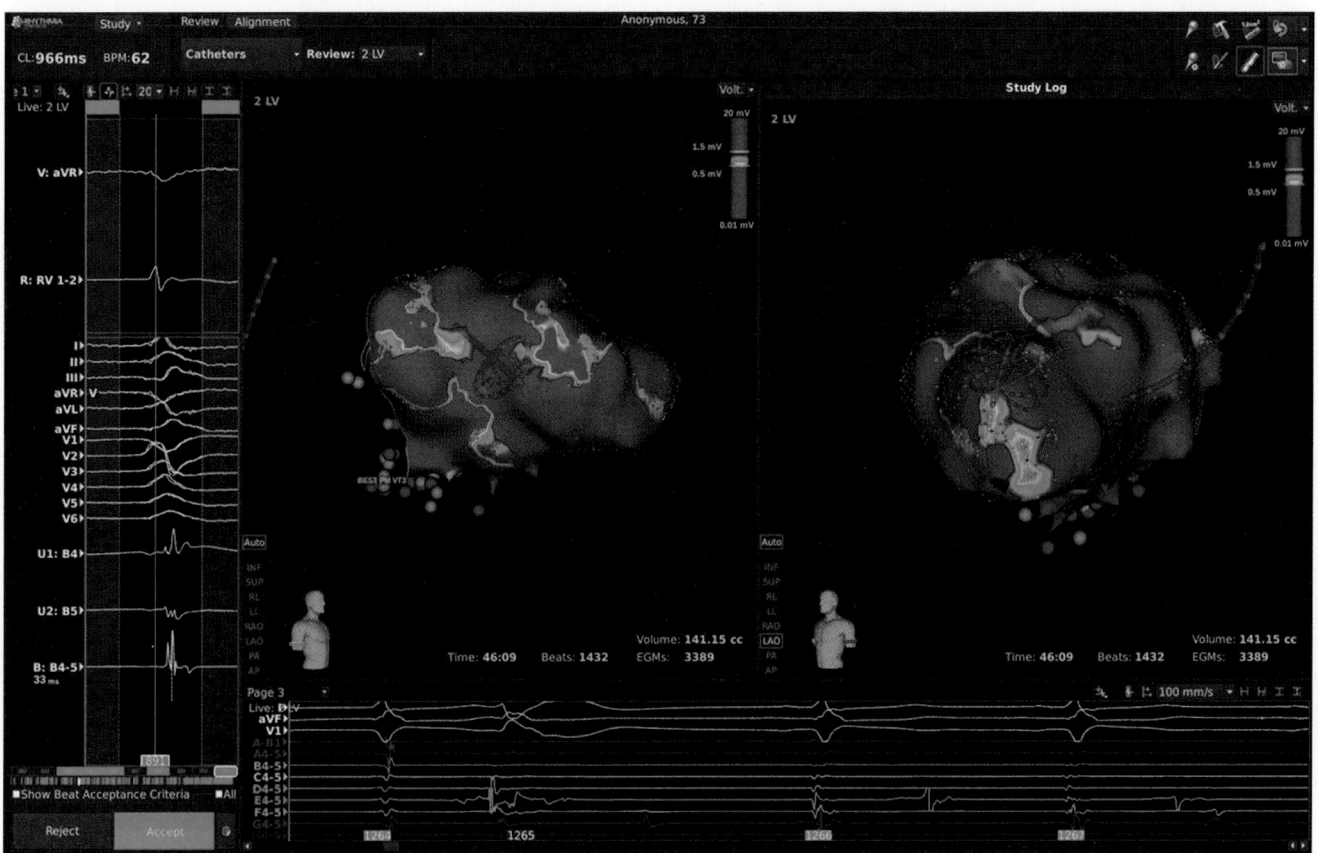

FIGURE 61.9 Rhythmia map of ventricular arrhythmia. Shown is an example of the map generated using the multipolar basket catheter using Rhythmia. Note that during point acquisition, the annotation window on the left is constantly validating the QRS during which the point is acquired against the initial reference QRS.

morphology due to catheter ectopy or a change in rhythm, points will be automatically rejected. Thus this allows for the collection of potentially thousands of points with multipolar catheters much more rapidly than could be achieved with a point-to-point/manual annotation approach.

Principles of Electroanatomical Mapping: Optimizing Creation of a Valid Map

Respiratory Compensation

All mapping systems have modules to allow compensation for respiratory effects on cardiac motion. Depending on the timing in the respiratory cycle (inspiration vs. expiration), catheter shifts may be seen, whether due to changes in blood return (and thus chamber volume) or effects on relative position of the heart within the thoracic cavity. These shifts may be especially pronounced in portions of the atrium, such as the left superior pulmonary vein/left atrial appendage ridge or cavotricuspid isthmus.[9,10] Due to this respiratory variation, if points are acquired at different times in the respiratory cycle, the visualized geometry may be variable. Generally, the way systems determine respiratory motion is based on identification of breathing-dependent changes in transthoracic impedance (NavX/Velocity) or respiratory motion of a sensor-based catheter relative to interpatch current shifts, which is used to correlate with inspiration and expiration (Carto3). While Carto3 has a module to account for respiratory motion, older versions do not.

Use of Multipolar Catheters and Automated Annotation Versus Point-by-Point Mapping

One of the pitfalls to traditional mapping techniques that involved use of point-by-point acquisition is that the process is tedious, requiring meticulous manual annotation. The value, however, is that every point can be assessed and points that may be complex and uninterpretable (e.g., due to the presence of multiple components or potential sensing of surrounding structures) may be labeled differently. When doing a point-by-point map, acquisition of enough points to create a reasonable electroanatomical shell, and in turn, a dense enough array of points to accurately hone in on critical sites to be targeted for ablation (e.g., early sites of activation for focal arrhythmias, or region of scar in the

case of substrate-based ablation) must be done. Whether or not a map is "complete" (i.e., whether the system suggests there are regions that have not been adequately sampled) is defined by user-governed, arbitrary thresholds that may be set for what density of sampling is needed to have a "complete" map. Thus when doing point-by-point mapping, obtaining more points within a region of interest compared with other regions (e.g., when there is a focal region of infarct in scar-related ventricular tachycardia) may be important.

In the case of automated algorithms wherein points are constantly obtained and automatically annotated often from multipolar catheters, one must be aware that the annotation of complex signals may be incorrect. First, the previously discussed reference and window need to be considered before mapping. Second, no algorithm currently exists that can accurately separate out a local signal into its component parts, defining what may be far-field versus near-field, or which point of a complex, fractionated EGM truly suggests local activation. Thus while using multipolar catheters and automated annotation algorithms for mapping may allow for a higher density of acquired points much more rapidly, there is potential for error, and discrimination of signals in regions of interest may have to be reapproached with the bipolar ablation catheter.

Considering Anatomically Proximate Structures

When mapping, creating several different maps and observing relative anatomical proximity may help in achieving successful ablation. In the case of midmyocardial sources of arrhythmia, mapping on either side (i.e., epicardial/endocardial, or right ventricle/left ventricle) may optimize the likelihood of success. In complex regions, such as the outflow tracts, where the coronary sinus, right ventricular outflow tract, and left ventricular outflow tract are close to one another, mapping each site separately may assist in understanding when ablation from more than one approach may be needed (Fig. 61.10).

Map Shifts

One of the principles of map creation is that the map is stable. However, if the patient moves (particularly in magnetic-based

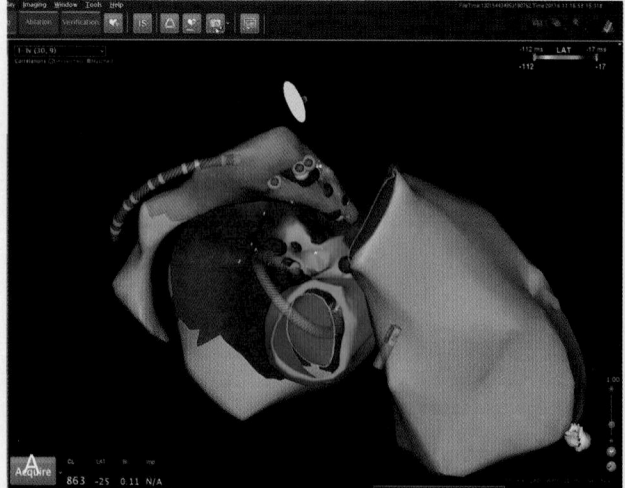
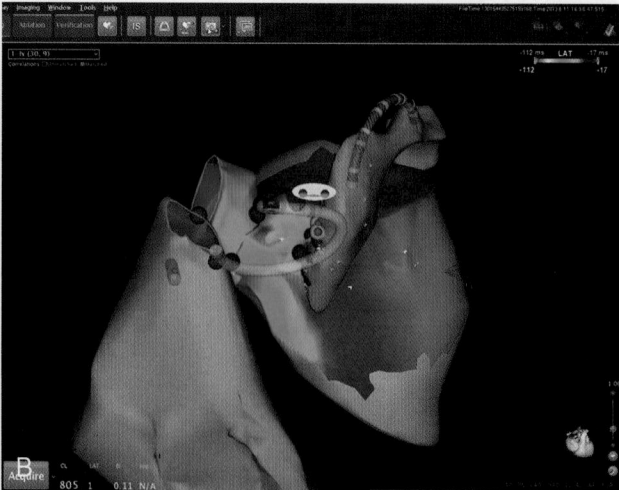

FIGURE 61.10 Mapping anatomical proximity of multiple chambers. (A) and (B) show the anatomical proximity of the right ventricular outflow tract, left ventricular outflow tract, and coronary sinus. While mapping suggested diffuse early sites in the coronary sinus, the opposing region in the left ventricular outflow tract, although having late local signals, required ablation for successful termination of the arrhythmia. Mapping all structures facilitated recognition of anatomically close regions.

systems like Carto, where there is a portion of the localization system not directly affixed to the patient) or the reference moves and/or there is a change in the current parameters that may impact current flow through the patient (particularly in impedance-based systems), the acquired map may no longer be accurate. If this is the case, then the site of interest on the map will no longer be accurate in 3D space, and repeat mapping may be necessary.

Another feature of "map shifts" is the shift due to changes in rhythm. When a catheter is located in a single position in the heart, the actual position of the catheter in 3D space may vary based on how the chamber is activated. For example, during mapping of a premature ventricular contraction (PVC), the earliest point during PVC may lie in a different position in 3D space than during sinus rhythm (Fig. 61.11). Thus if a map is created in a specific rhythm (e.g., an activation map during ablation of a focal PVC), attempts at ablation at that earliest spot while in sinus rhythm may not be accurate spatially due to a map "shift" associated with the change in rhythm.[11]

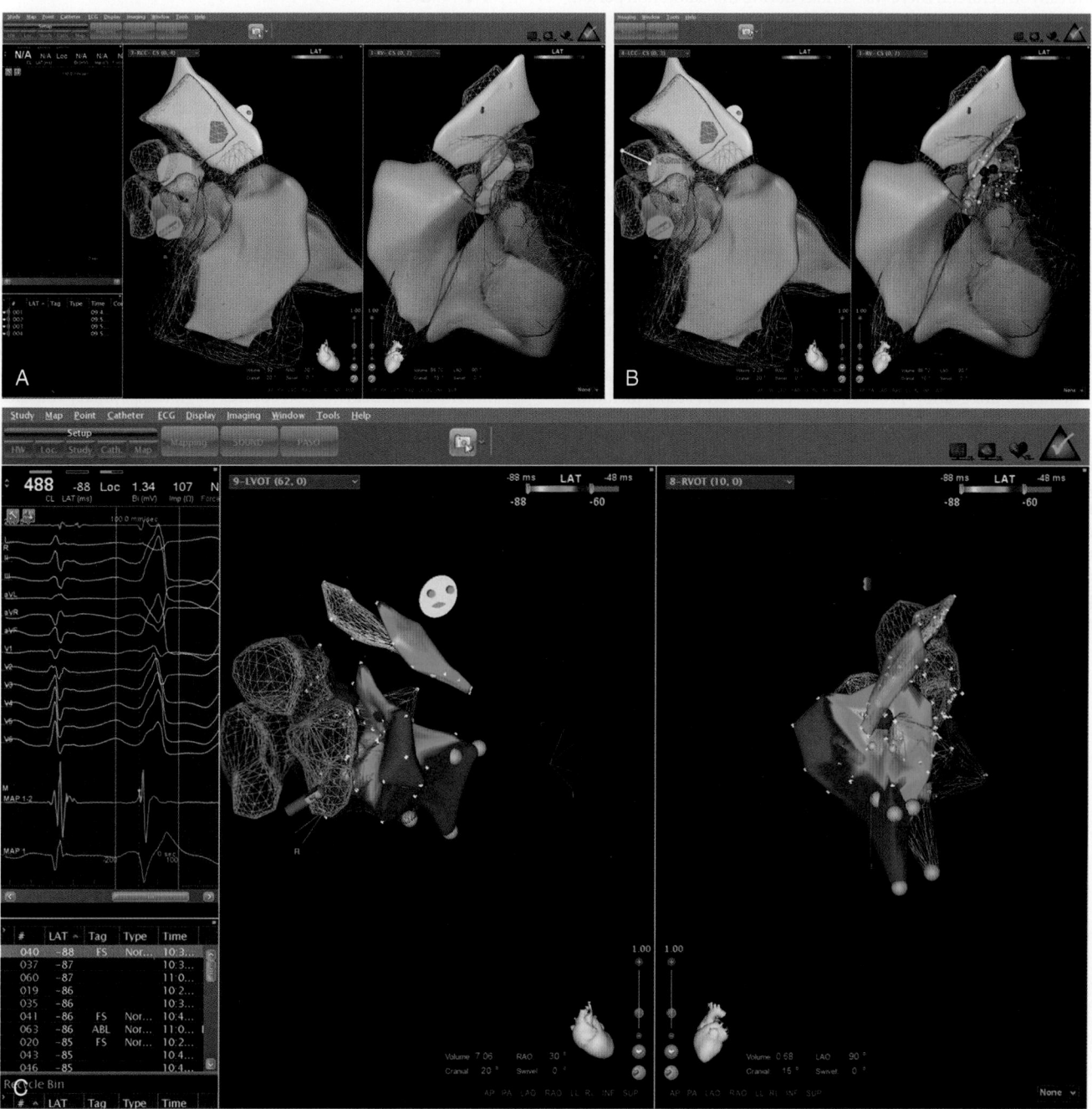

FIGURE 61.11 Map shift while taking points in sinus rhythm versus premature ventricular contraction (PVC). (A) Displayed are CartoSound maps created during both sinus rhythm (structures defined by *hashed lines*) versus during a premature ventricular contraction (*solid colored structures*) of the right ventricle, left ventricle, aortic cusps, and pulmonic artery. (B) Using a fiducial point on the aortic cusps, the displacement during sinus rhythm of the same fiducial anatomic point is ~1.49 cm away than during a PVC. (C) This shift accounts for why the ablation catheter localization during sinus rhythm at the earliest site for the PVC (left hand) is far displaced from the earliest site for the PVC based on the activation map.

Contact Force

Newer technology allows for simultaneous integration of contact force and contact direction with electroanatomical mapping. Thus the system will indicate to the operator the degree of force being exerted on the tip of the catheter to ensure contact. The value of this is both the validation of contact as well as avoiding excessive contact, which may increase risk of perforation. However, use of contact force also has its limitations. First, calibration of the catheter requires the catheter be initially "floating" within the chamber and not in contact with any structure. If there was contact during the calibration period, even if one is in contact with underlying myocardium, the system will not appreciate any force being applied to the tip.

Integration of Computed Tomography and Magnetic Resonance Imaging

The rationale of image integration is the process of combining various imaging techniques to overcome the limitations of each technique. For example, although conventional electroanatomical mapping provides important real-time electrophysiological information, it uses reconstructed anatomy of the left atrium and pulmonary veins. In contrast, computed tomography (CT) or MRI can provide highly detailed information of complex anatomical structures. Image integration is used by many electrophysiologists for catheter ablation, particularly for atrial fibrillation to further increase the understanding of the patient's complex atrial anatomy and to validate the acquired anatomy at the time of ablation. The image integration process consists of several steps, including "field scaling" of the reconstructed geometry, fusion of the structures using fiducial markers (landmarks), and optimization of the integration by adjusting (molding and bending) the reconstructed geometry.[12] CartoMerge and NavX Fusion are two available platforms that facilitate this process. However, differences in breathing during image acquisition and the catheter ablation procedure may affect the image integration process. In general, scanning is performed during an inspiratory or expiratory breath-hold, whereas patients are breathing normally during the ablation procedure. Also, volumes (particularly in the atria) may change due to various

factors between the time of acquisition of image and actual integration. Small observational studies have demonstrated a reduced fluoroscopy and procedure time and an improved outcome with the use of image integration.[13] Larger, randomized studies are needed to fully appreciate the value of image integration in guiding catheter ablation for atrial fibrillation or its use in other types of arrhythmia ablation (e.g., ventricular tachycardia).

Additional Considerations in Modern Mapping Techniques

Integrated Intracardiac Echocardiography With Electroanatomical Mapping

The CartoSound module available in Carto systems allows for real-time integration of acquired anatomical information via intracardiac ultrasound with the electroanatomical map. This is achieved by using a specialized intracardiac echocardiography (ICE) catheter that has an integrated magnetic sensor that can be localized within the 3D magnetic field. Then, depending on the chamber of interest, the ICE catheter is rotated in different planes to acquire multiple two-dimensional (2D) slices of the chamber of interest (Fig. 61.12). The surface of the structure of interest is then manually traced. As one rotates through the structure of interest, a 3D representation is created via the integration of the series of 2D, manually traced slices. Acquisition of a specific slice is done based on a standard reference (generally using the surface ECG). Multiple maps may be created separately for individual endocavitary structures (e.g., the papillary muscles, false tendons, or aortic valve cusps), as well as for the endocardial and/or epicardial surfaces of the chamber of interest. The value of this integration includes the ability to recognize endocavitary structures and create a separate map on these structures (Fig. 61.13). Furthermore, use of the specialized ICE catheter allows for visualization of the tip of the ablation catheter, which may assist the operator in knowing the approximate location of the tip when it is otherwise not quite obvious (Fig. 61.14).

Limitations of this system, however, are several. First, the system depends on manually determining the surface of the

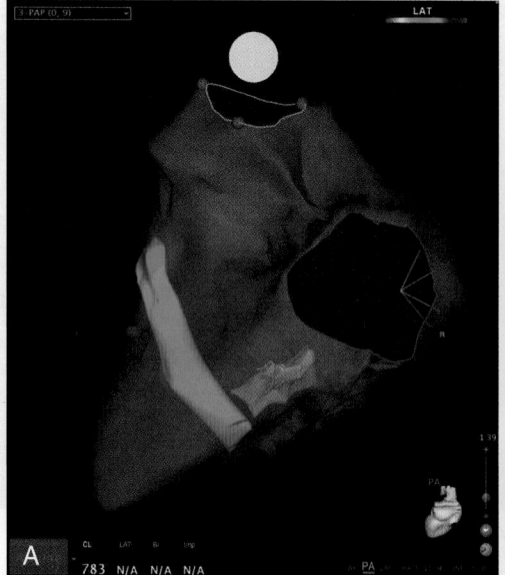
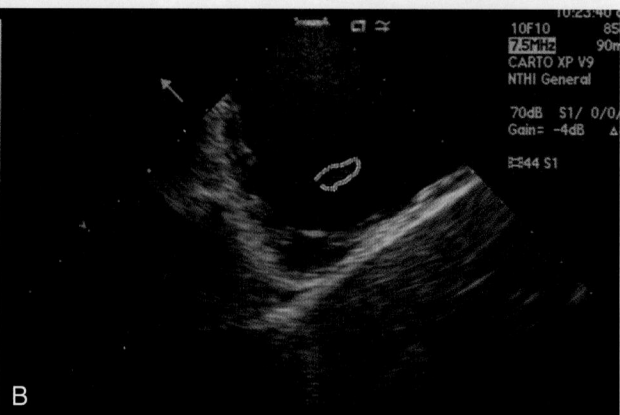

FIGURE 61.12 CartoSound of right ventricle. Shown is an example of how structures are traced in their two-dimensional intracardiac echocardiography (ICE) images to generate the three-dimensional map. (A) shows the green outline around the two-dimensional ICE projection of the moderator band and how that projects into the map. Similarly, (B) shows the same for the right ventricular papillary muscle.

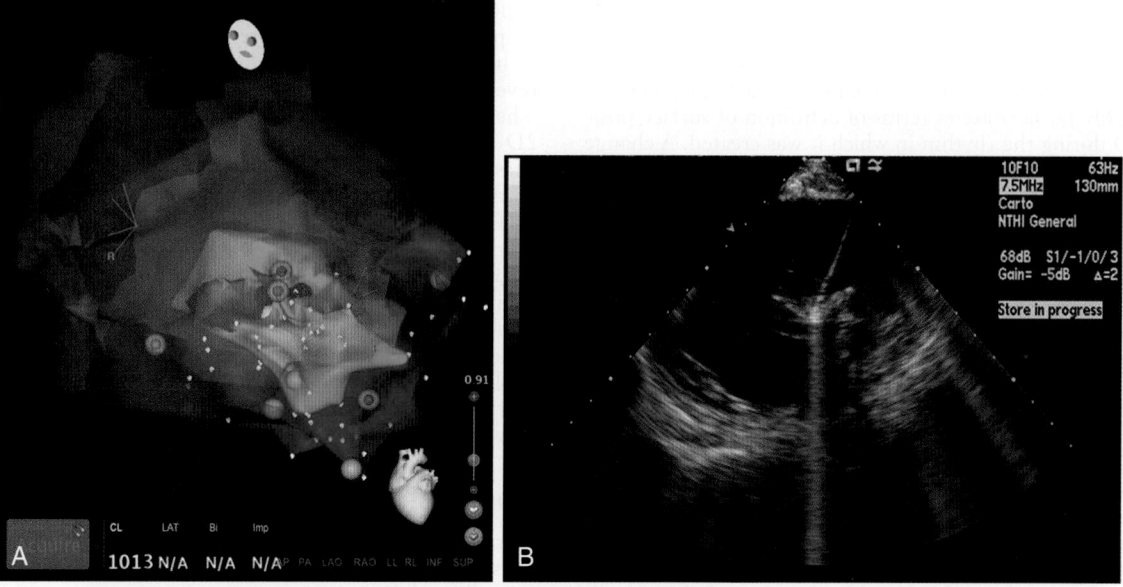

FIGURE 61.13 CartoSound for ablation. Shown in (A) is a CartoSound map of the left ventricle and posteromedial papillary muscle with corresponding ablation and activation mapping. Note that ablation was done in sinus rhythm and thus did not occur at the same projected site of the earliest activation, which was mapped during premature ventricular contractions. (B) shows the endocavitary position of the ablation catheter where successful ablation occurred.

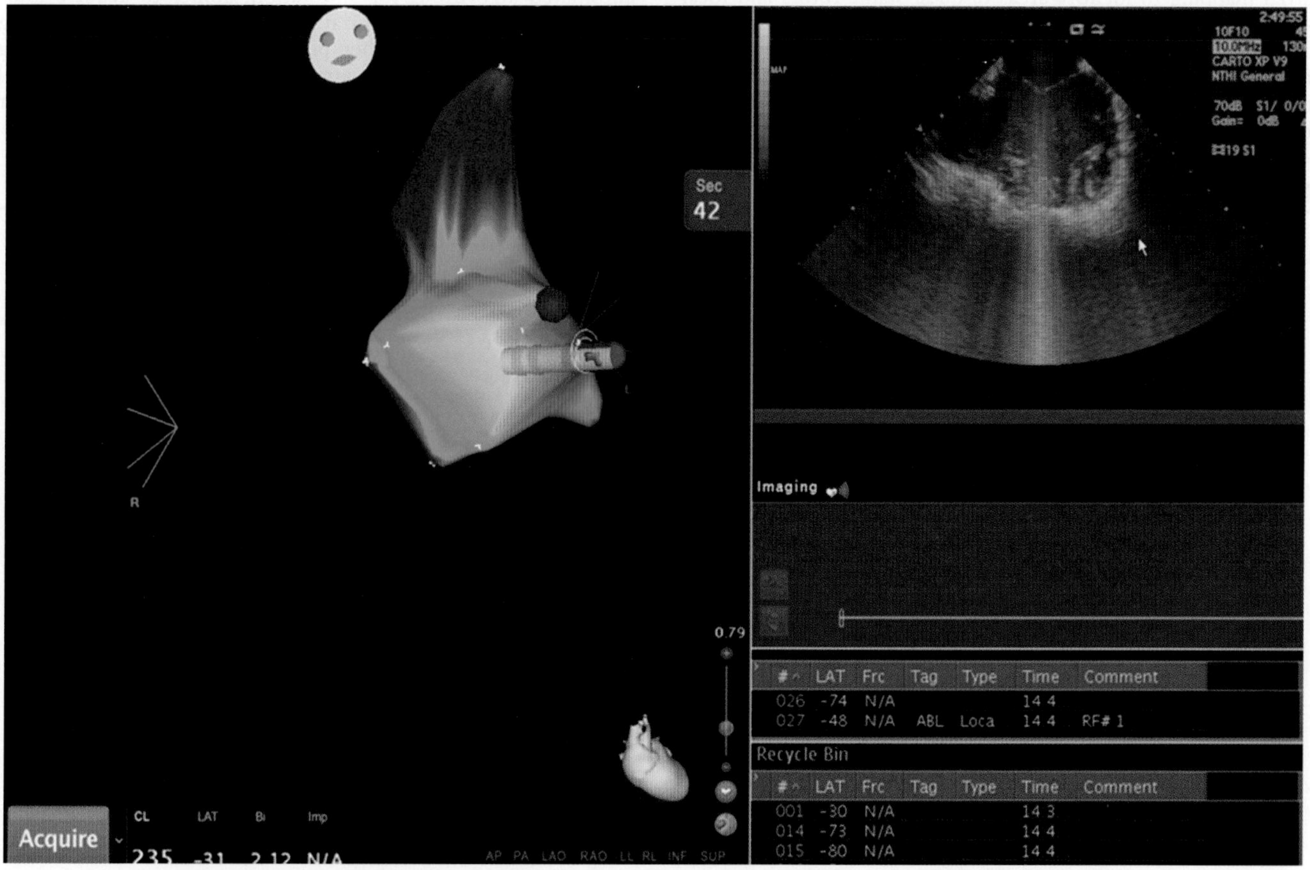

FIGURE 61.14 Catheter tip visualization. Shown here is an example of how the CartoSound system may be used to visualize the ablation catheter tip. While the catheter shaft and tip are not obvious in the intracardiac echocardiography image on the right, the tip is clearly demarcated by a green outline.

structure of interest. However, this may be impossible (e.g., with a highly trabeculated ventricular surface). Furthermore, the accuracy of the map, similar to that obtained via acquisition of signals from mapping catheters, depends on the density of acquired "points." In the case of integrated ICE imaging, the more 2D slices acquired, the more accurate the map. Finally, the map created will only be accurate in terms of definition of surface position in 3D during the rhythm in which it was created. A change in rhythm (e.g., ablating during a PVC vs. a shell created in sinus rhythm) will result in a change in the apparent geometry in 3D space and thus limit accuracy.

Rotor Mapping

Rotors were first reported to drive human atrial fibrillation in 2011 in the Conventional Ablation with or without Focal Impulse and Rotor Modulation (CONFIRM) trial and were previously considered not to exist in humans.[14] There have been extensive developments in mapping to try and define the importance of rotors as ablation targets. During the mapping of rotors, EGMs are analyzed to construct isopotential movies of successive atrial fibrillation cycles, with rotors identified by rotational activity, and focal impulses identified by centrifugal activation from a point of origin. Rotors and focal sources are diagnosed only if stable for thousands of cycles and mapped in time-lapse fashion (multiple epochs) for longer than 10 minutes (≥3000 cycles) to exclude transient pivot points of passive fibrillatory activity. Next, those areas are targeted for catheter ablation.

The RhythmView system (Topera, San Diego, CA)/focal impulse and rotor map (FIRM) involves the use of a 64-pole basket catheter to provide for relatively low-density panoramic atrial mapping to identify areas of quasi-stable rotors and focal sources purported to sustain atrial fibrillation. A commercially available basket catheter is advanced first into the right atrium for mapping and ablation, and then this process is repeated in the left atrium. The system filters EGMs during atrial fibrillation to exclude noise and far-field signals, using the rate dynamics of human atrial action potential duration to estimate the minimum activation time and conduction velocity to identify the physiological propagation paths. The signal processing algorithms filter unipolar EGMs using the previously described rate dependence of biatrial action potential duration and conduction velocity to reveal the primary components of activation at each electrode. The operator then reviews the map, which is represented as a 2D array demonstrating global activation, and tries to identify sites that suggest rotational activity around a fixed site. These perceived rotors are then targeted for ablation.

Despite initial promising clinical reports, the limitations of currently available technology are similar to those leveled at traditional mapping, namely the density of *in contact* points obtained and being able to map a wide enough area of myocardium simultaneously. It is estimated that only 40% of electrodes on currently available basket catheters may be in contact with endocardium at the time of deployment, and this may limit the accuracy of the map. Thus further long-term, multicenter data are required to better understand how best to map rotors and utilize currently available systems.

Conclusion

Current mapping technologies offer multiple features that may assist the electrophysiologist in the ablation of complex arrhythmias. The ability to represent cardiac geometry and EGMs in a saved, 3D projection may optimize recognizing regions of interest for ablation. However, accurate mapping requires one to consider how points are acquired and annotated and the reasons the generated map may not be accurate (e.g., due to map shifts, respiratory shifts, or not considering endocavitary structures). Newer mapping systems may offer additional tools (improved automated algorithms for annotation, ability to acquire multiple simultaneous points, or application of different processing techniques to identify other putative mechanisms underlying certain arrhythmias such as atrial fibrillation), but the potential limitations must still be considered in order to optimize their successful use.

REFERENCES

1. Durrer D, Van Der Twell LH. Spread of activation in the left ventricular wall of the dog. *I. Am Heart J.* 1953;46:683–691.
2. Del Carpio Munoz F, Buescher TL, Asirvatham SJ. Teaching points with 3-dimensional mapping of cardiac arrhythmia: mechanism of arrhythmia and accounting for the cycle length. *Circ Arrhythm Electrophysiol.* 2011;4:e1–e3.
3. Del Carpio Munoz F, Buescher TL, Asirvatham SJ. Three-dimensional mapping of cardiac arrhythmias: what do the colors really mean? *Circ Arrhythm Electrophysiol.* 2010;3:e6–e11.
4. Del Carpio Munoz F, Buescher TL, Asirvatham SJ. Teaching points with 3-dimensional mapping of cardiac arrhythmia: how to overcome potential pitfalls during substrate mapping? *Circ Arrhythm Electrophysiol.* 2011;4:e72–e75.
5. Estner HL, Deisenhofer I, Luik A, et al. Electrical isolation of pulmonary veins in patients with atrial fibrillation: reduction of fluoroscopy exposure and procedure duration by the use of a non-fluoroscopic navigation system (NavX). *Europace.* 2006;8:583–587.
6. Giaccardi M, Del Rosso A, Guarnaccia V, et al. Near-zero x-ray in arrhythmia ablation using a 3-dimensional electroanatomic mapping system: a multicenter experience. *Heart Rhythm.* 2016;13:150–156.
7. Eitel C, Hindricks G, Dagres N, Sommer P, Piorkowski C. EnSite velocity cardiac mapping system: a new platform for 3D mapping of cardiac arrhythmias. *Expert Rev Med Devices.* 2010;7:185–192.
8. Hooks DA, Yamashita S, Capellino S, Cochet H, Jais P, Sacher F. Ultra-rapid epicardial activation mapping during ventricular tachycardia using continuous sampling from a high-density basket (orion(tm)) catheter. *J Cardiovasc Electrophysiol.* 2015;26:1153–1154.
9. de Ruvo E, Dottori S, Sciarra L, et al. Impact of respiration on electroanatomical mapping of the right atrium: implication for cavotricuspid isthmus ablation. *J Interv Card Electrophysiol.* 2013;36:33–40. discussion 40.
10. Noseworthy PA, Malchano ZJ, Ahmed J, Holmvang G, Ruskin JN, Reddy VY. The impact of respiration on left atrial and pulmonary venous anatomy: implications for image-guided intervention. *Heart Rhythm.* 2005;2:1173–1178.
11. Andreu D, Berruezo A, Fernandez-Armenta J, et al. Displacement of the target ablation site and ventricles during premature ventricular contractions: relevance for radiofrequency catheter ablation. *Heart Rhythm.* 2012;9:1050–1057.
12. Tops LF, Schalij MJ, den Uijl DW, Abraham TP, Calkins H, Bax JJ. Image integration in catheter ablation of atrial fibrillation. *Europace.* 2008;10(suppl 3):iii48–56.
13. Martinek M, Nesser HJ, Aichinger J, Boehm G, Purerfellner H. Impact of integration of multislice computed tomography imaging into three-dimensional electroanatomic mapping on clinical outcomes, safety, and efficacy using radiofrequency ablation for atrial fibrillation. *Pacing Clin Electrophysiol.* 2007;30:1215–1223.
14. Narayan SM, Krummen DE, Shivkumar K, Clopton P, Rappel WJ, Miller JM. Treatment of atrial fibrillation by the ablation of localized sources: CONFIRM (Conventional Ablation with or without Focal Impulse and Rotor Modulation) trial. *J Am Coll Cardiol.* 2012;60:628–636.

62 Computed Tomography for Electrophysiology

Alejandro Jimenez Restrepo and Timm M. Dickfeld

Imaging plays a fundamental role in the diagnosis and treatment of cardiac arrhythmias. The increased use of imaging has led to an improved ability to understand and successfully treat complex tachycardia circuits. Traditional imaging methods utilized in the electrophysiology laboratory such as x-ray fluoroscopy, coupled with intracardiac recordings obtained from bipolar electrode catheters, form the basis for the conventional study of electrical conduction inside the human heart. Additionally, the advent of radiofrequency and cryoenergy sources to target specific arrhythmia-enabling structures moved cardiac electrophysiology from a merely diagnostic field to an area of rapidly improved therapeutic success in the management of different arrhythmias. Due to the inherent limitations of fluoroscopy for imaging of cardiac soft tissue structures, the ablation of complex arrhythmias such as scar-mediated ventricular tachycardia (VT) or left atrial (LA) tachycardias proved very challenging. The development of three-dimensional (3D) mapping systems coupled with advanced cardiac imaging allows for detailed tissue characterization and highly refined anatomical delineation,[1] creating an environment for accurate, safe, and effective treatment of complex arrhythmias.

This chapter reviews the technical background and current uses of cardiac computed tomography in the diagnosis and management of atrial and ventricular arrhythmias.

Technical Background of Cardiac Computed Tomography Imaging

The process of computed tomography (CT) imaging of the heart, commonly referred to as cardiac computed tomography (CCT) comprises four main steps: data processing, image acquisition and reconstruction, display, and storage.

CCT is an imaging modality that utilizes x-ray beams that are projected in a fan-shaped configuration and then funneled into a region of interest to encompass the heart and great vessels using a collimator that eliminates the x-ray beams not traveling in parallel to a prespecified direction, thus creating an image within a biplane coordinate system (XY) known as the *imaging plane*. This planar image, although of high resolution, is unable to differentiate contrast differences within an imaging plane due to superimposition of images from multiple adjacent structures. Such images would serve no clinical use, but when combined with the CT capability to provide multiple anatomical cross-sections (stacks of *transverse axial images*), reconstructed CCT dataset can

provide images of very high temporospatial resolution with clear differentiation of adjacent cardiac structures.

For accurate reconstruction of cardiac anatomy, it is important to minimize the time of image acquisition and be able to account for the cardiac movement during respiration and the different phases of the cardiac cycle. *Multislice technology and helical (spiral) scanning* improved the acquisition of image datasets from several minutes to seconds, thus minimizing motion artifact. Coupled with electrocardiography (ECG) and respiratory gating, current CT scanners have multirow detectors (up to 320) with subsecond rotational speeds (gantry rotation) that enable an accurate reconstruction of cardiac structures and assessment of functional parameters. An aluminum beam filter is used to absorb very low energy x-rays, which would not penetrate the body tissue, increasing patient exposure without contributing to image quality. This process, called *beam hardening*, results in uniform average beam energy and can significantly reduce patient radiation exposure.

Synchronization of the x-ray tube and detector movements in the gantry as well as the horizontal table movement where the patient is positioned are essential for spatial resolution and correct reconstruction of the multiplanar images to avoid image overlapping and false spacing. This concept is known as *pitch* in helical CT imaging and is defined as the ratio of the patient's movement through the gantry during one 360-degree beam rotation relative to the beam collimation. Another factor that defines image slices and their relative positions is the distance between reconstructed axial slices in the Z axis. This is known as *increment* and is defined as the distance between axial image slices. The increment can be manipulated, for example, during 3D image reconstruction, to permit some overlap and improve image resolution in specific areas of interest.

Acquisition of correct cardiac imaging dataset (a stack of axial imaging slices of the heart, great vessels, and adjacent structures) requires coordination between scan length, collimation, increment, and the number of slices obtained. During this process, continuous radiation, gantry rotation, imaging table movement, and data transfer from the detector array are occurring. Digital data received from the detectors are transmitted back to a central processing unit using high-speed radiofrequency signals. The computer then synchronizes the gantry and table motion, acquiring data from known positions of the gantry rotation and the imaging table position, allowing for accurate, high-speed data acquisition.[2]

The data acquired from the gantry's helical motion are the projected data representing the attenuated beam of radiation from which a specific algorithm will determine an attenuation coefficient for each pixel inside an image matrix. Once the full volume of the image dataset is obtained, the scan's raw data is reconstructed to obtain images of clinical-diagnostic use. The width of the beam set by the detector size and collimator ultimately determines the maximal resolution of the image dataset.

The process of image reconstruction is complex and requires special algorithms to convert the helical projection data. Reconstructed segments (or *voxels*) are isotopic (equal on the X, Y, and Z axes). The *pixel values*, which are a measure to quantify a grayscale spectrum, are measured in *Hounsfield units* (HU) and essentially represent the amount of x-ray attenuation. They are obtained by calculating the relative difference between the linear attenuation coefficient of tissue and water. As an example, the HU for water is zero, for air is −1000, and for bone varies between 500 and 1000 depending on the bone density. The average HU values for cardiac tissue are between 10 and 60.

Before image reconstruction can be achieved from the acquired raw data, three essential parameters must be defined. The *field of view* (FOV) will determine the area of the image to be reconstructed, and the *matrix* will determine the *pixel size* for each image plane. The following relation is then applied: *Pixel size = FOV/matrix*. In addition, the *kernel* reconstruction defines the degree of smoothing during image reconstruction. Different kernels can be applied depending on the anatomical region or clinical application. Low kernel values provide smoother images, while high values generate sharper images. Ultimately for adequate cardiac image reconstruction, the scan requires adequate ECG and respiratory gating. Held expiration for a few seconds during scanning is usually sufficient to avoid diaphragmatic and chest excursion. The QRS obtained from the ECG determines the boundaries of systole and diastole. Multiple images acquired during consecutive cardiac time intervals can be combined to obtain an image of the heart at the exact same phase of the cardiac cycle, in either a prospective (triggering image acquisition to a specific phase of the cardiac cycle) or retrospective (acquiring images during the complete cardiac cycle and then selecting the specific cardiac timing) fashion. The latter will naturally result in higher radiation exposure.

Finally, CCT images are displayed in a gray scale of 256 intensity values ranging from black to white. Digital image size is measured in *bytes* (each *byte* comprises 8 *bits*). Images can be viewed as slices (bidimensional plane) or volumes (tridimensional reconstruction). 3D images are particularly useful in electrophysiology as they provide accurate anatomical reconstruction of cardiac structures and great vessels. Two techniques for volumetric image reconstruction are *maximum intensity projection* (MIP) and *shaded surface display* (SSD). MIP reconstruction uses a stack of image slices and projects the maximum intensity of the brightest pixel along a specific path. SSD reconstruction uses shading and artificial light sources to create 3D-rendered anatomical images. Once the images are acquired and processed, they are stored and backed up onto a server. Images are stored in standard Digital Imaging and Communications in Medicine (DICOM) format, which allows for the sharing of radiographic image studies across different vendors regardless of the workstation/program utilized for post image processing or reviewing.

Image Integration

Since the mid-2000s, the integration (or fusion) of preprocedural CCT with intraprocedural 3D maps has become a routine practice in many electrophysiology centers for complex arrhythmia ablations, including atrial fibrillation (AF), postprocedural atrial tachycardia, and VT.[3–5] The high temporospatial resolution provided by tomographic scans allows for detailed 3D anatomical reconstruction of the cardiac structures, great vessels, and adjacent relevant structures (esophagus, phrenic nerves, and epicardial coronary arteries). When merged with the electroanatomical information from a 3D mapping system, they provide a very accurate road map of the heart for catheter manipulation and guidance for the mapping and ablation of arrhythmia substrates. Prospective randomized and nonrandomized studies suggest some clinical benefits when image integration imaging is used to guide the ablation of AF. Some of the benefits observed with image integration in AF ablation include long-term AF-free survival,[6–8] reduced fluoroscopy time,[6,9] reduced procedural time,[7,9] and decreased incidence of procedure-related complications.[7] However, other studies have failed to demonstrate a benefit with image integration techniques compared to conventional 3D mapping for ablation of AF in terms of clinical outcomes.[10]

A meta-analysis looking at published studies of image integration for AF ablation showed a trend but no statistically significant improvement in clinical outcomes between image integration and conventional mapping.[11] These discrepant results are likely due to differences in the methodology, image fusion technique used, and center experience with image processing. Two commercially available 3D mapping systems are equipped with image integration or image fusion software models (CARTOMERGE® from Biosense Webster, Inc. [Diamond Bar, CA] and EnSite Verismo for St. Jude Medical [St. Paul, MN]). Both systems allow for 3D reconstruction and registration of preprocedural CCT images with 3D electroanatomical maps. Both imaging software modules continue to be further developed, and integration software continues to improve with newer versions.

Fundamental Concepts of Image Integration

There are three steps involved in any image integration process: preprocedural image acquisition, segmentation of the CCT planar images, and registration of images from the CCT and the 3D mapping system. In order to minimize motion artifact and improve accurate anatomical reconstruction, the CCT image *acquisition* is ECG gated and respiratory gated (although with the current fast acquisition times, current CT scanners can obtain images in end-expiration within a few seconds or even <1 s). Once the preprocedural images are obtained, *segmentation* consists of digital separation of the different cardiac and extracardiac structures using a 3D volume-reconstructed model obtained from biplanar CT slices. The use of iodine-based contrast in CCT allows for the delineation of intravascular (aorta, pulmonary arteries, or coronary arteries) and intracardiac (atria and ventricles) volumes. As the blood pool displays high signal intensity, the striking contrast with adjacent low-intensity structures allows for accurate delineation of endocardial and epicardial contours. The process of segmentation is semiautomatic and utilizes vendor-specific software that employs a combination of signal threshold, boundary detection, and regional identification algorithms. The segmented images are finalized with some degree of visual editing to generate a final CCT volumetric dataset.[12] The final step is *registration*, which is crucial for an accurate fused map. This step requires a thorough understanding of the cardiac anatomy along with the technical expertise for image manipulation within the 3D-merging software environment. An accurate registration will allow for intraprocedural catheter manipulation inside the CCT-generated anatomical 3D images.

Technical Aspects of Image Segmentation and Registration

The most common method for image segmentation is *thresholding*, which consists of separating all pixels of an image on either side of a predetermined threshold value and grouping them into either above or below pixel groups. Once the pixels are divided into the two groups, *boundary extraction methods* are employed to differentiate values between adjacent pixels within a group, which further divides them into regions. These regions represent different chambers depending on their contrast uptake and timing of the contrast bolus respective to image acquisition. For example, a region of high pixel signal intensity after intravenous contrast will represent the left atrium and pulmonary arteries, whereas a region of low pixel signal intensity will correspond to the esophagus, lungs, and phrenic nerves in a CCT obtained for guiding an AF ablation.[13] More advanced algorithms include shape-based assumptions in which the software performs reconstructions using expected geometries extracted from the anatomy of a normal patient cohort (Fig. 62.1).

Registration or fusion of CCT and 3D maps is an *intermodal process*, which means that both image datasets originally reside

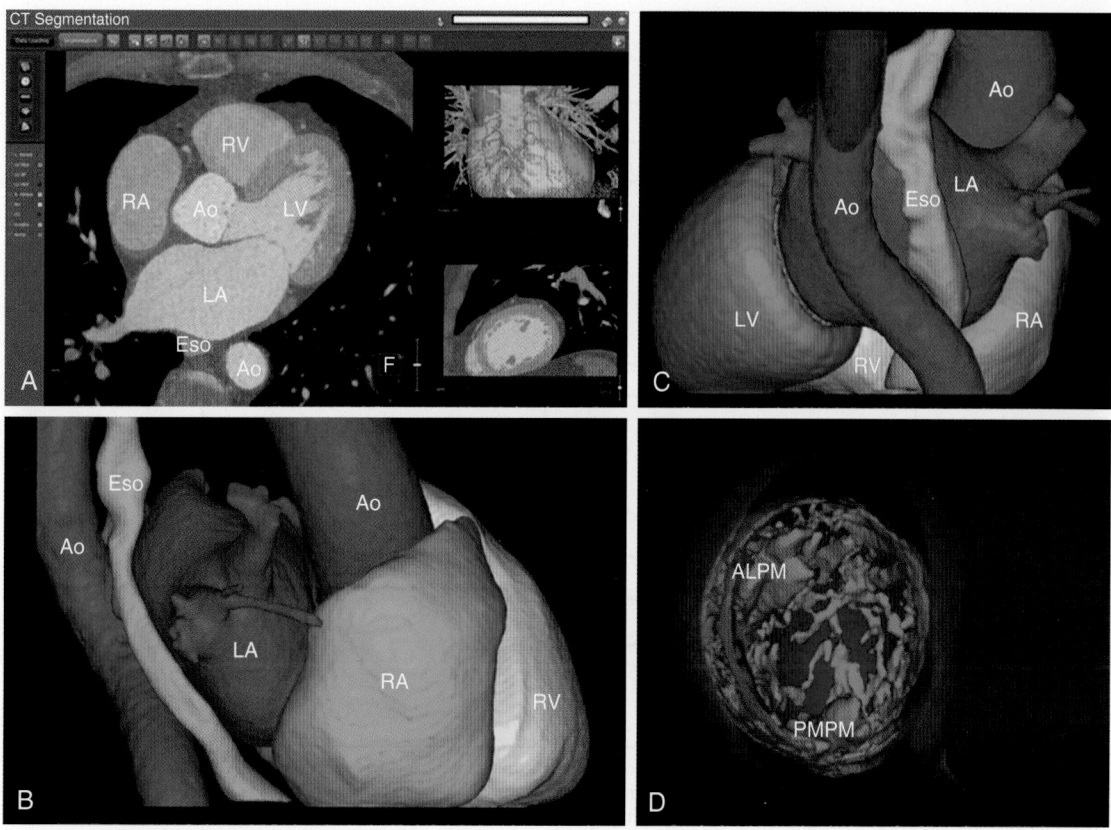

FIGURE 62.1 CARTO® Segmentation Module. Novel CARTO® System computed tomography (CT) segmentation software module for segmentation of radiographic image datasets (Biosense Webster, Inc., Diamond Bar CA). (A) Semiautomatic detection of all four cardiac chambers including endocardial definition of left ventricular (*LV*) trabeculation/papillary muscles and adjacent structures (left atrium [*LA*], *pink*; LV myocardium, *green*; trabeculations/papillary muscles, *blue*; LV blood pool, *orange*; aorta [*Ao*], *very light blue*; right atrium [*RA*], *light blue*; right ventricular [*RV*] blood pool, *yellow*; esophagus [*Eso*], *ocher*). (B) and (C) Unedited semiautomatic reconstruction with excellent delineation of LV epicardium (*green*), LA (*purple*), RA (*light blue*), RV (*yellow*), aorta (*dark blue*), esophagus (*ocher*), and clear demarcation of the pulmonary veins and mitral valve plane. (D) Endoscopic reconstructed cardiac computed tomographic view of the LV endocardium, displaying prominent trabeculations as well as anterolateral and posteromedial papillary muscle (*ocher*) as separately reconstructed structures in addition to LV myocardium (*transparent green*), enabling targeted mapping and ablation. *ALPM,* Anterolateral papillary muscle; *PMPM,* posteromedial papillary muscle.

in separate image spaces, and special registration algorithms are required to transform (*T*) one image space into another. For accurate *linear transformation* of two image datasets residing in different image spaces, six degrees of freedom (three translational and three rotational) are generally employed for accurate image fusion. If the voxel sizes between both image datasets are different, additional calibration parameters in the *XYZ* axis are necessary to reconcile the discrepancy. On the contrary, if *nonlinear transformation* is employed, multiple (often >6) degrees of freedom are necessary to minimize image distortion. A cost function is additionally employed to measure discrepancies or similarities between the reference and transformed images.

Registration methods are mainly geometry or voxel-intensity based. *Geometry-based registration* can be further divided into point-based and surface-based techniques. In *point-based* registration techniques, fiducial points are selected on both images (CCT and 3D map) and are aligned or paired in one single imaging set. The number of fiducial points required for an accurate fusion depends on the available software, chamber of interest, and expertise of the operator. Alignment of fiducial points or superimposed cardiac surfaces can be done by visual estimation or landmark registration (basically the superimposition of all fiducial points between the two images). Fiducial points can be automatically assigned by the fusion software, but usually are

manually selected by the operator. Examples of commonly used fiducial points include atrioventricular valves, the ostium of the pulmonary vein (PV), and the coronary ostia. Once both images (CCT and 3D map) are registered, the difference between each image *centroid* (defined as the central point of an image) is calculated, and it provides an estimation of the translation required to perfectly align all fiducial points in a 3D space. The unified centroid is used as a reference to further align all fiducial points, this time by means of rotation rather than translation, until the sum of the squared distances between each corresponding point pair is minimal. The *fiducial registration error* (FRE) is defined as the square root of the mean squared distance between the point pairs. FRE defines the degree of spatial accuracy of the fused image dataset to be utilized during the procedure.[14] In landmark registration, anatomically distinct endocardial surfaces (the PV ostia, carinas, LA appendage [LAA], and right ventricular [RV] or left ventricular [LV] septum) are used to align both imaging datasets.[13] Any manual registration will inevitably cause an inherent error of alignment for each registered point, known as the *fiducial localization error* (FLE). The FLE represents a vectorial distance from the intended to the actual fiducial point obtained. A similar value known as the *target registration error* (TRE) is obtained from the FLE and is used clinically to quantify the degree of accuracy of the fused images (Fig. 62.2).

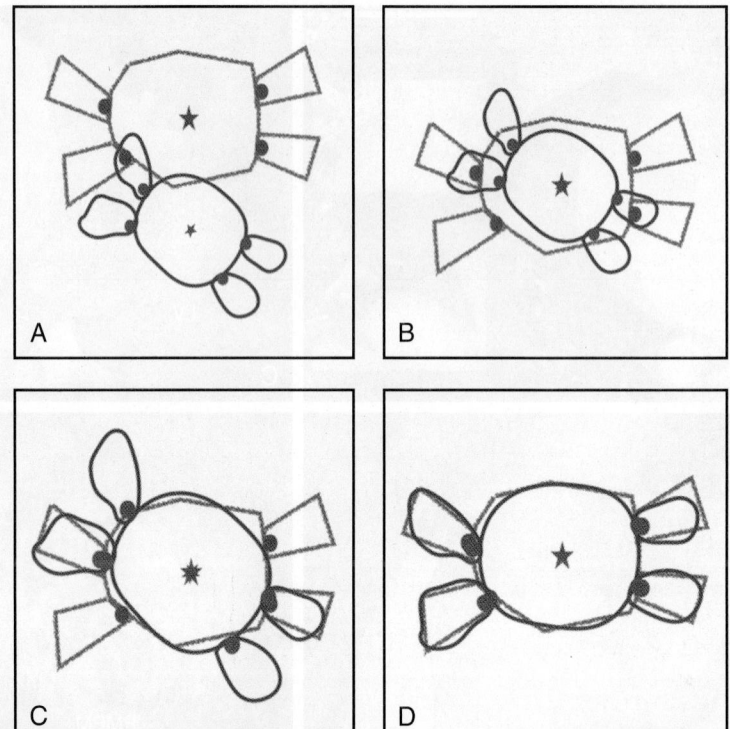

FIGURE 62.2 Registration steps. Schematic representation of a geometry-based point registration process of two image datasets of a left atrium (three-dimensional shell in *red* and cardiac computed tomography [CCT] shell in *purple*). Fiducial points are marked with *dots*, and the centroid (*center point*) for each image is represented with a *star*. (A) Both images are readily available in the merge software environment. (B) First step in the registration process is centroid alignment, irrespective of the size/rotation of the images. (C) Next, scaling and calibrating of the images is performed to essentially make them equal in size. (D) The final step is performed by rotating the images in order to approximate the fiducial points of each image to its corresponding counterpart. The final distance between the fiducial point pairs between both images is known as the *fiducial registration error,* or FRE, and is measured in millimeters.

Surface-based registrations are often the preferred method of image integration between 3D maps and CCT. Similar to point-based registration, both imaging surfaces are delineated, registered, and transformed (*T*). Registration is generally performed using three translations and three rotations. Calibration of each image is performed to determine the image scaling values. Unlike the alignment of fiducial points, the registration of endocardial contours or specific anatomical landmark surfaces is visually easier to achieve.[4] Multiple studies have validated both point and surface registration using CCT, with acceptable registration errors in the range of 2.9 ± 0.7 to 6.9 ± 2.2 mm.[5,6,15,16]

Steps for Image Integration With Commercially Available Mapping Systems

Vendor-specific differences in commonly used 3D mapping systems with image fusion software are as follows:

The CARTO® 3 System uses the image integration software known as CARTOMERGE® Module. The image fusion process begins with the creation of landmark pairs or surface points between the CCT and the 3D map. This is followed by the visual or automated alignment of landmark pairs or surface points between the two images. Finally, the surface registration algorithms are employed to align both image datasets, utilizing three possible registration methods: visual alignment, landmark, and surface registration. The accuracy of the CARTOMERGE® Module was assessed in an animal study where fiducial markers were surgically implanted in the epicardium where radiofrequency ablation lesions were delivered. The offset of an integrated CCT/3D voltage map fusion image to localize the lesion sets was less than 3 mm on average (1.8 ± 1.5 for atrial flutter, 2.2 ± 1.3 for the fossa ovalis, and 2.1 ± 1.2 mm for AF ablations).[17] In

clinical practice, image fusion can be achieved by performing surface registration of an LA posterior wall electroanatomical map with preprocedural CCT images, achieving a mean registration error of 1.27 ± 0.23 (with mean values of 0.03 minimal and 3.9 mm maximal)[18] (Fig. 62.3).

The EnSite NavX and Velocity mapping systems use a fusion registration module (FRM), which consists of three steps. First is the segmentation of a preprocedural CCT–digital image fusion (DIF) model, which is imported into the 3D mapping system environment. Second, field scaling is performed by measuring interelectrode spacing from multiple points collected and adjusting the image volume of the 3D map to approximate that of the preprocedural CCT. Finally, the fusion of both image datasets is accomplished by registration using paired locations (fiducial points). A dynamic registration algorithm locally adjusts the 3D shell geometry and surface to the size and shape of the DIF surface model. Several studies have assessed the registration accuracy of the EnSite system integrating preprocedural CCT with intraprocedural 3D maps for AF ablation. The registration errors range from 1.9 ± 0.4 to 3.2 ± 0.9 mm, and good correlation between PV diameters has been consistently found[19,20] (Fig. 62.4).

Despite the differences in the registration process for both CARTOMERGE® Module (rigid registration using rotational alignment) and EnSite FRM (dynamic registration with both rotation and field scaling), both systems have similar registration accuracy when clinically tested.

During ablation procedures, it is not uncommon to have a sudden change in the patient's heart rhythm, which can possibly affect registration accuracy. A study looking at patients undergoing AF ablation guided by the image integration of CCT and 3D maps found that registration accuracy did not significantly differ between image fusion in sinus rhythm versus AF (surface-to-point

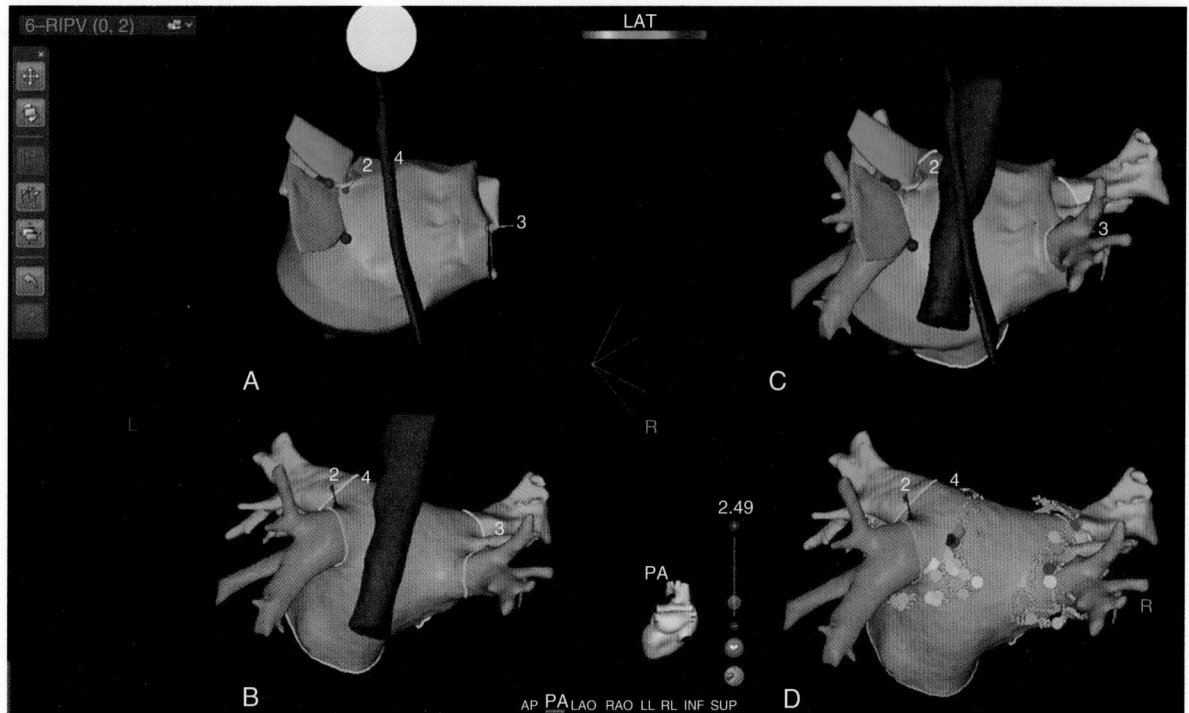

FIGURE 62.3 CARTOMERGE® Module registration. Example of image integration for atrial fibrillation ablation (pulmonary vein [PV] isolation). (A) and (B) Fusion between CARTOSOUND® Module maps of left atrium (LA), PVs, and esophagus shell and preprocedural cardiac computed tomography (CCT). Note landmark point in the left PV carina and fiducial points on all four PV ostia. (C) Fused image showing the alignment of the landmark points. There is a discrepancy in the alignment of the esophagus between the two data-sets, likely due to the real time esophageal position in comparison to when the preprocedural CCT was obtained. This has important safety implications during radiofrequency ablation in the posterior LA wall. (D) Final fused postablation image showing antral PV isolation lesions (esophagus removed).

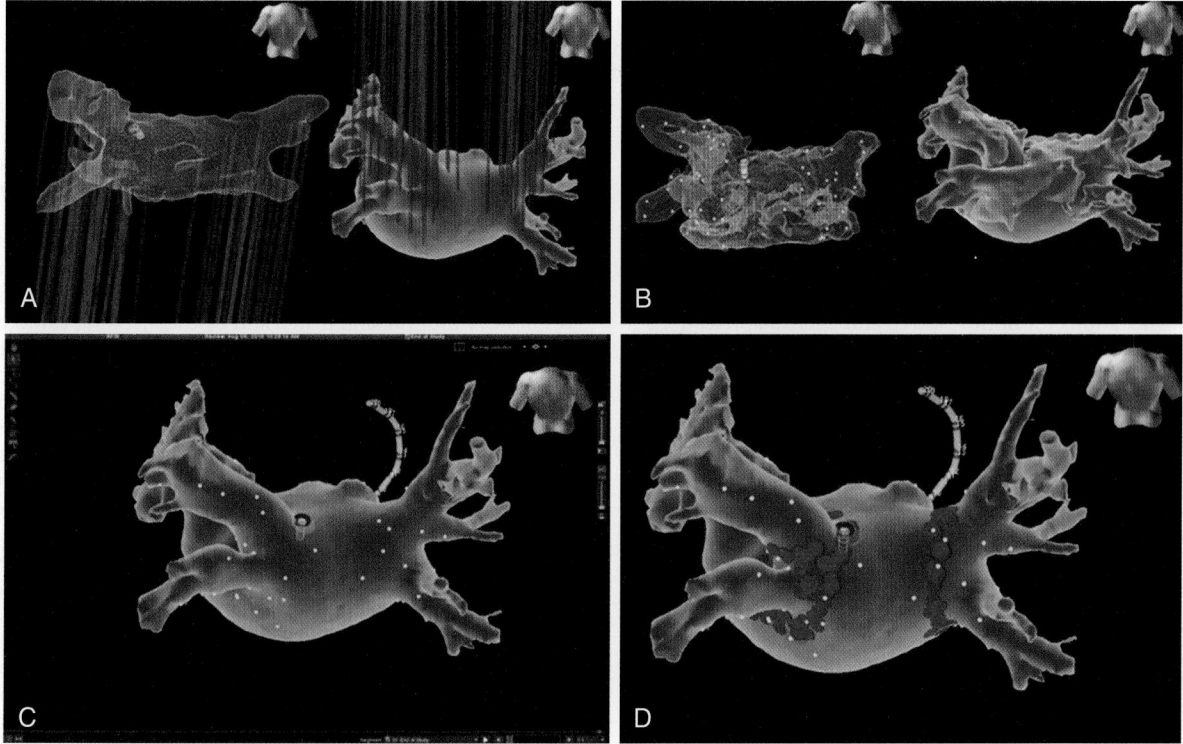

FIGURE 62.4 EnSite Velocity registration. Example of image integration for pulmonary vein (PV) isolation procedure. (A) Fiducial points are obtained on both image datasets (three-dimensional [3D] map on the left and cardiac computed tomography [CCT] shell on the right). (B) Left atrial (LA) shell from the 3D map with fiducial points. Right image is fusion between both datasets (3D map in *green* and LA shell in *blue*). Note that the volume of the CCT LA shell is greater than that of the 3D map. A process called *field scaling* will increase the 3D LA volume to match that of the CCT LA shell. (C) Fused dataset with fiducial points and an ablation catheter positioned near the left superior PV ostium. (D) Final fused image showing the antral circumferential ablation lesions. Additional linear lesions in the left PV carina were required for isolation of the left-sided veins.

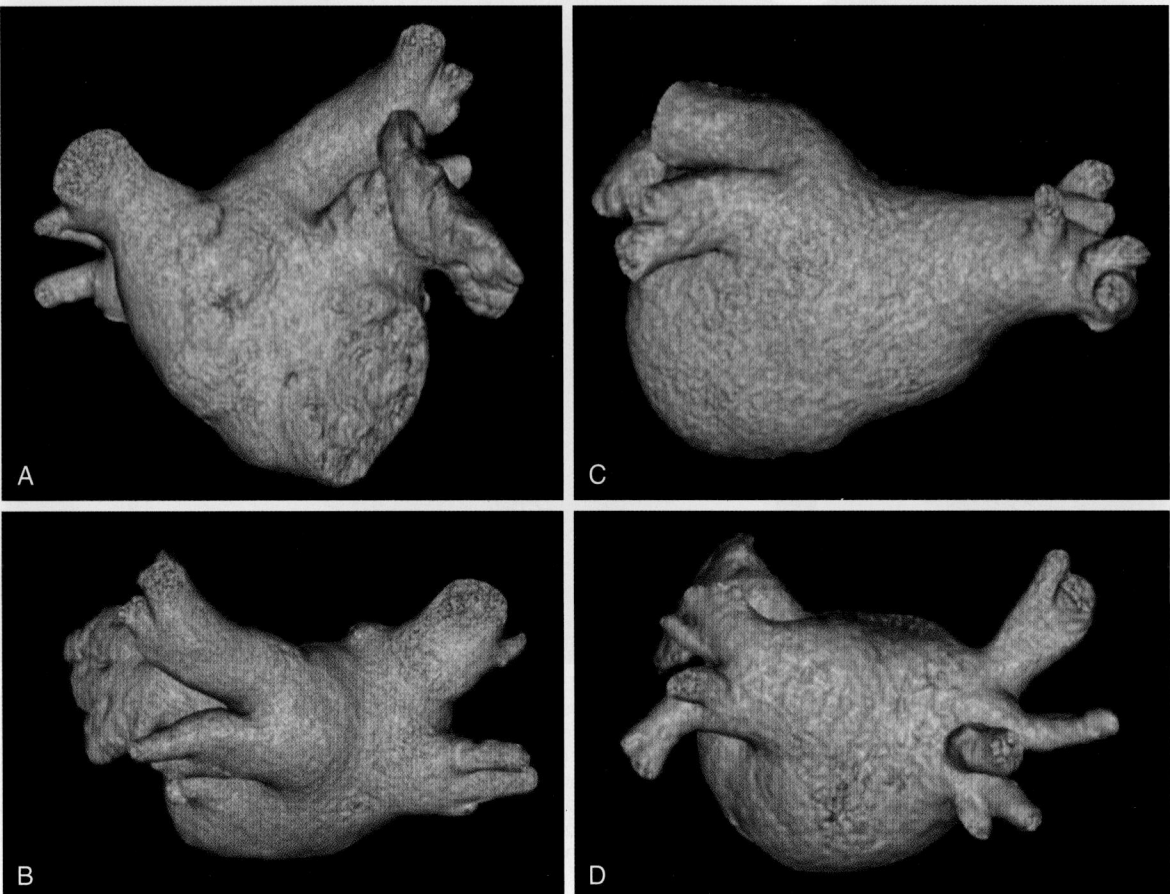

FIGURE 62.5 Pulmonary vein (PV) anatomy. Cardiac computed tomography with a three-dimensional reconstruction of the left atrium and PVs. (A) and (B) Anterior and posterior views, depicting normal PV anatomy (separate ostia, two veins on each side). (C) Anatomical variant with common right PV trunk. (D) Anatomical variant with the right middle vein.

distance of 1.91 ± 0.24 vs. 1.84 ± 0.38 mm, respectively; p = .60); this suggests that reregistration is not required to maintain map accuracy.[21]

In addition to the commercially available image integration algorithms, several research groups in the field of advanced cardiac mapping have developed their own software and image fusion workstations for both research and clinical applications in the field of complex arrhythmia mapping and ablation.[22,23]

Current Applications of Cardiac Computed Tomography in Cardiac Electrophysiology

The clinical uses of CCT in today's electrophysiology practice can be divided into preprocedural, periprocedural, and postprocedural imaging studies and can be further separated depending on the chamber of interest (atrial vs. ventricular).

Pre- and Periprocedural Computed Tomography Imaging for Guiding Atrial and Ventricular Arrhythmia Ablations

Atrial Ablations

Atrial anatomy is a relevant feature for PV isolation procedures. Significant variability exists in the orientation, size, and number of PVs, with various anomalies seen in up to 36% of patients[24–26] (Fig. 62.5). Additional LA characteristics such as the contours of the PV carinas, appendage, ridge, roof, coronary sinus (CS), and septum[27] and the location of adjacent structures such as the

esophagus are some of the important anatomical features that require careful analysis and 3D spatial understanding for complex LA arrhythmias (Fig. 62.6). Fluoroscopy lacks the ability to delineate intracardiac and adjacent soft tissue structures,[4] and 3D electroanatomical maps can have suboptimal spatial resolution as they are affected by mapping density, patient, cardiac and respiratory motion, and distension by the mapping catheter. The information provided by a preprocedural CCT to image the LA provides the electrophysiologist with a better understanding of the patient's unique anatomy. It may also help identify potential hurdles during the procedure and allow selection of the most ideal mapping/ablation tool (diameter of the lasso catheter or cryoballoon according to the size of the PV ostia). The integration of high-resolution CCT images depicting cardiac and extracardiac neighboring structures with 3D maps provides a detailed understanding of patient individual anatomical variations (Table 62.1).

An area of emerging clinical utility is the ability to identify the presence of LAA thrombus using preprocedural CCT. In a recently published study of 320 patients undergoing AF or LA flutter ablation, the sensitivity and negative predictive value of a preprocedural CCT for the detection of LAA thrombus was 100%, using either transesophageal or intracardiac echocardiography as the reference standard.[28] Similarly, a ratio of HU values between the LAA and ascending aorta that was >0.75 had a negative predictive value of 100% for excluding LAA thrombus or dense nonclearing spontaneous echo contrast on transesophageal echocardiogram.[29] However, the most recent expert consensus on AF ablation still advised against the use of CT to rule out

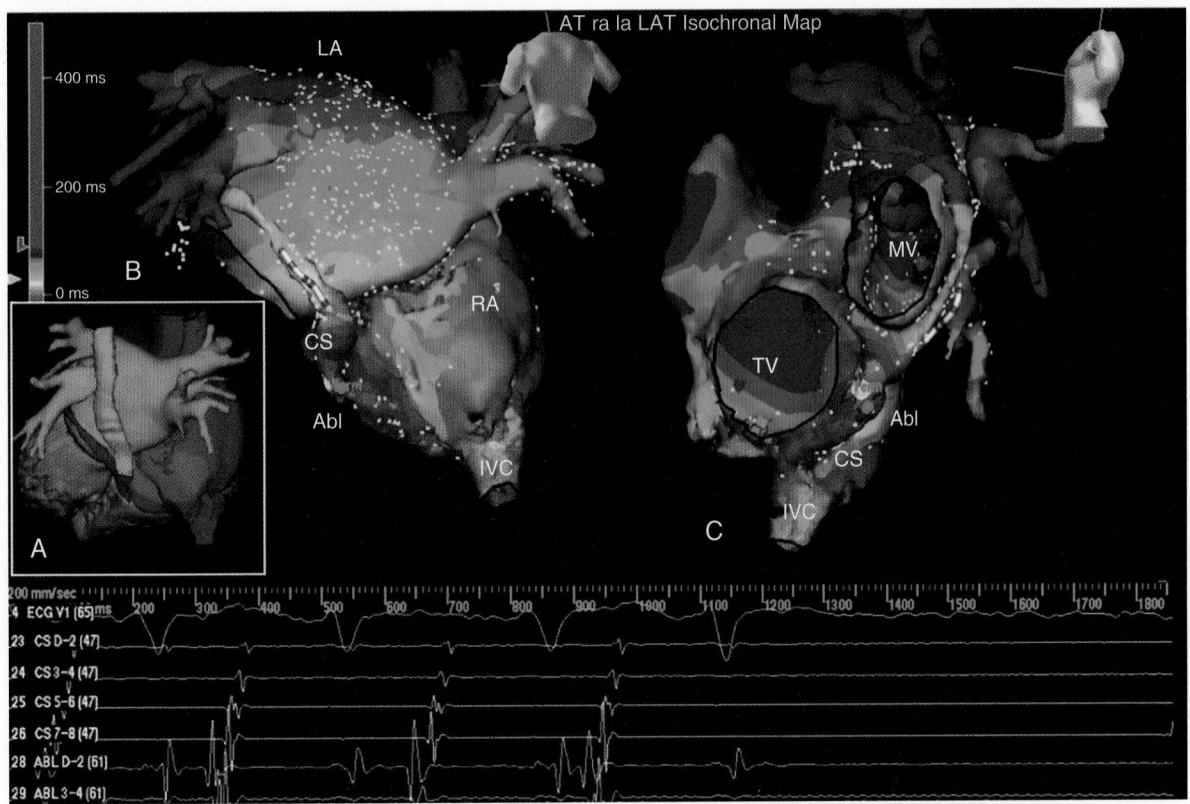

FIGURE 62.6 EnSite Velocity fusion for tachycardia originating in the coronary sinus. Example of image integration using the EnSite Verismo software from the Velocity mapping system. (A) Cardiac computed tomography (CCT) three-dimensional (3D) reconstruction (posterior view) of the left atrium (*LA*) (*gray*), right atrium (*RA*) (*purple*), and esophagus (*yellow*). (B) and (C) Posterior and left lateral views respectively of the CCT-3D fusion for the fluoroless ablation (*Abl*) of atrial tachycardia. The activation map showed the earliest activation in the mid–coronary sinus (*CS*). At this site, the ablation terminated the tachycardia as seen on the intracardiac electrograms. *IVC,* Inferior vena cava; *MV,* mitral valve; *TV,* tricuspid valve. (Courtesy Dr. Vivek Reddy.)

TABLE 62.1 Registration studies using cardiac computed tomography (CCT) and three-dimensional maps for atrial fibrillation ablation

STUDY	N	REGISTRATION METHOD	REGISTRATION ERROR (mm)	COMMENTS
Kistler et al.	60	Fiducial	2.3 ± 0.4	All CCT
Tops et al.	16	Fiducial + surface	2.1 ± 0.2	All CCT
Machine et al.	23	Fiducial	4.7 ± 0.9	13 pts with CCT, 10 pts with CMR
Fahmy et al.	124	Fiducial + surface	5.6 ± 3.2	All CCT
Brooks et al.	55	Field scaling + landmark	1.9 ± 0.4	All CCT
Singh et al.	30	Visual + fiducial + surface (+ ICE)	1.83 ± 0.32 (ICE LA) 2.52 ± 0.58 (ICE RA)	20 pts with CMR, 10 pts with CT
Itoh et al.	108	Visual + fiducial + surface (posterior wall only)	1.37 ± 0.23	All CCT

CMR, cardiovascular magnetic resonance imaging; *ICE,* intracardiac echocardiography; *LA,* left atrium; *pts,* patients; *RA,* right atrium.

LAA thrombus in patients with high stroke risk due to the variability of study results.[30–33] In addition to the ability of CCT to detect LAA thrombi, the morphology of the LAA appears to play a significant role in the risk of stroke. Low left atrial appendage flow velocities (LAAFVs) are known to increase the risk of stroke in patients with AF. In a study of 96 patients undergoing catheter ablation for paroxysmal atrial fibrillation, LAAFVs were classified according to the LAA morphology on CCT (chicken wing, windsock, cactus, and cauliflower shapes). Certain LAA morphologies correlated with lower LAAFV (chicken wing: 73.7 ± 21.9 cm/s, windsock: 61.9 ± 19.6 cm/s, cactus: 55.3 ± 14.1 cm/s,

and cauliflower: 52.7 ± 18.1 cm/s; $p = .008$) and thus presented a higher risk of cardioembolic events.[34]

Ventricular Ablations

In a structurally normal heart, the VT CCT has the potential to visualize relevant endocardial and epicardial structures. Papillary muscles, chordae tendineae, trabeculations, moderator band, coronary arteries, and sinuses of Valsalva have important implications for the ablation of arrhythmogenic foci arising from these intracavitary structures. A recent study of 190 ablations found that endocavitary structures affected the ablations

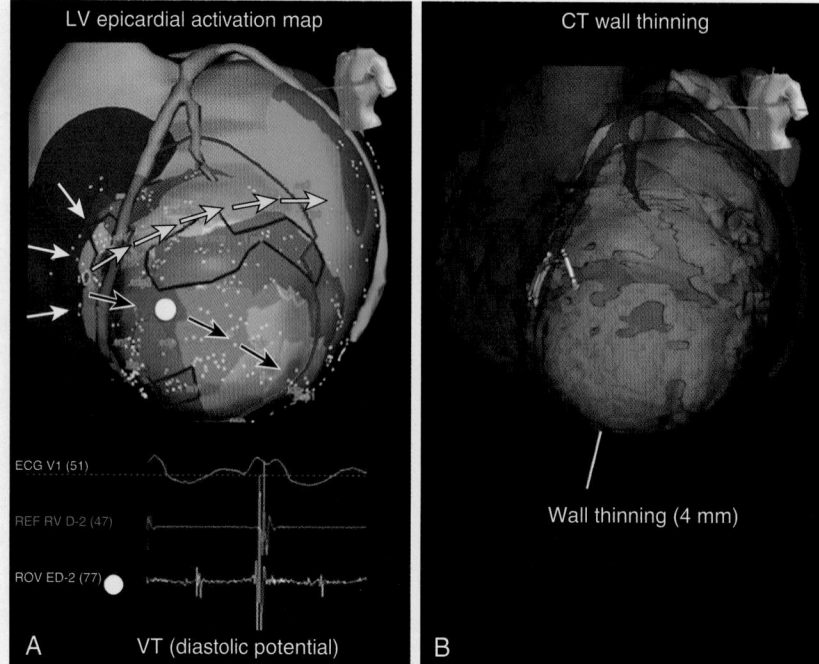

FIGURE 62.7 Epicardial activation map fused with cardiac computed tomography (CCT) for assessment of scar in ischemic ventricular tachycardia (*VT*). (A) EnSite Velocity epicardial activation map with CCT fusion, depicting coronary anatomy and epicardial ventricular activation during VT. There is an anterior VT circuit in an area of existing scar by voltage. Intracardiac electrograms from the anteroapical region show clear mid-diastolic potentials. (B) Reconstructed CCT depicting the left ventricular (*LV*) wall thickness. Note that the areas of scar (decreased wall thickness) correspond to the areas of bipolar scar and mid-diastolic potentials on the prior image. *CT*, Computed tomography. (Courtesy H. Cochet, F. Sacher, and P. Jais [elaborated with the MUSIC software, IHU LIRYC, Bordeaux, France].)

in 24% of cases. Similar to intracardiac echocardiography,[35] segmentation of high-resolution CT image datasets can render accurate reconstruction of these endocavitary structures and facilitate ablation[36] (see Fig. 62.1). It is important to emphasize that although CCT can provide highly detailed anatomical reconstruction of most cardiac structures, the definitive diagnosis of idiopathic tachycardia relies on the presence of a structurally normal heart using cardiac magnetic resonance imaging (MRI).[37]

Identification of fibrosis is particularly relevant in patients with ischemic and nonischemic structural heart disease undergoing VT ablation. Direct assessment of the ventricular scar using delayed enhancement is becoming increasingly possible but is currently still reserved for cardiovascular magnetic resonance imaging (CMRI) in clinical practice given its superior contrast intensity and reproducibility. However, multiple alternative anatomical and functional parameters have been evaluated and correlated with electrophysiological findings.

Due to its exquisite spatial resolution, CCT is able to well delineate wall thickness, intramyocardial fat (arrhythmogenic right ventricular cardiomyopathy [ARVC], post–myocardial infarction) and postischemic myocardial calcium deposits. The reduced end-diastolic/systolic wall thickness correlated with a voltage of <1.5 mV, and wall thinning of <5 mm correlated with local abnormal ventricular activities in 11 and 13 ischemic patients, respectively.[38] Similarly, in 16 ARVC patients, the myocardial fat correlated well with the areas of low voltage and local abnormal ventricular activity[39] and in 22 post–myocardial infarction patients, with decreased uni/bipolar voltage and isolated or fractionated signals.[40]

This preprocedural information can guide a more discrete intracardiac mapping exclusively to the regions of interest where the abnormal electrical substrate is likely to be encountered

(Fig. 62.7). CCT perfusion imaging with the use of intravenous contrast demonstrating low-intensity perfusion defects has been also used to delineate the extent and location of scar substrate,[41,42] incorporating 82% of successful ablation sites. It also provided additional information regarding the intramural location and transmurality of the scar substrate.

Dynamic CCT cine sequences can evaluate wall motion abnormalities and further delineate potentially arrhythmogenic areas within the ventricle. This comprehensive combination of CT-derived anatomical, dynamic, and perfusion data has been shown to be complementary to the 3D mapping data and to help guide successful ablation of clinical VT.[41]

The combination of CCT with positron emission tomography (PET) enables metabolic and anatomical characterization of scar substrate by assessing myocardial viability with 18F-fluorodeoxyglucose (FDG) and perfusion with 82-rubidium (Rb) chloride. Using PET/CT scans, several studies of VT ablation have shown acceptable registration errors (3.7 ± 0.7 to 5.1 ± 2.1 mm) with 3D maps and clinical utility to localize scar and guide ablation therapy.[43–45]

During epicardial ablation, CCT allows for accurate depiction of the coronary epicardial anatomy as well as epicardial fat and its spatial relationship with potential epicardial substrates for ablation (Fig. 62.8). The coronary anatomy and phrenic nerve location identified with CCT was useful to guide the epicardial ablation of the VT substrate in patients with both ischemic and nonischemic heart disease (including ARVC). An important number of patients (18%) could not undergo epicardial ablation due to the close proximity of coronary arteries or phrenic nerve to sites with local abnormal ventricular activities and/or critical targets for ablation.[22]

CCT can also provide information regarding the presence of LV thrombus, often discovered incidentally and prompting confirmation studies such as echocardiography.[46,47] Usually, the presence

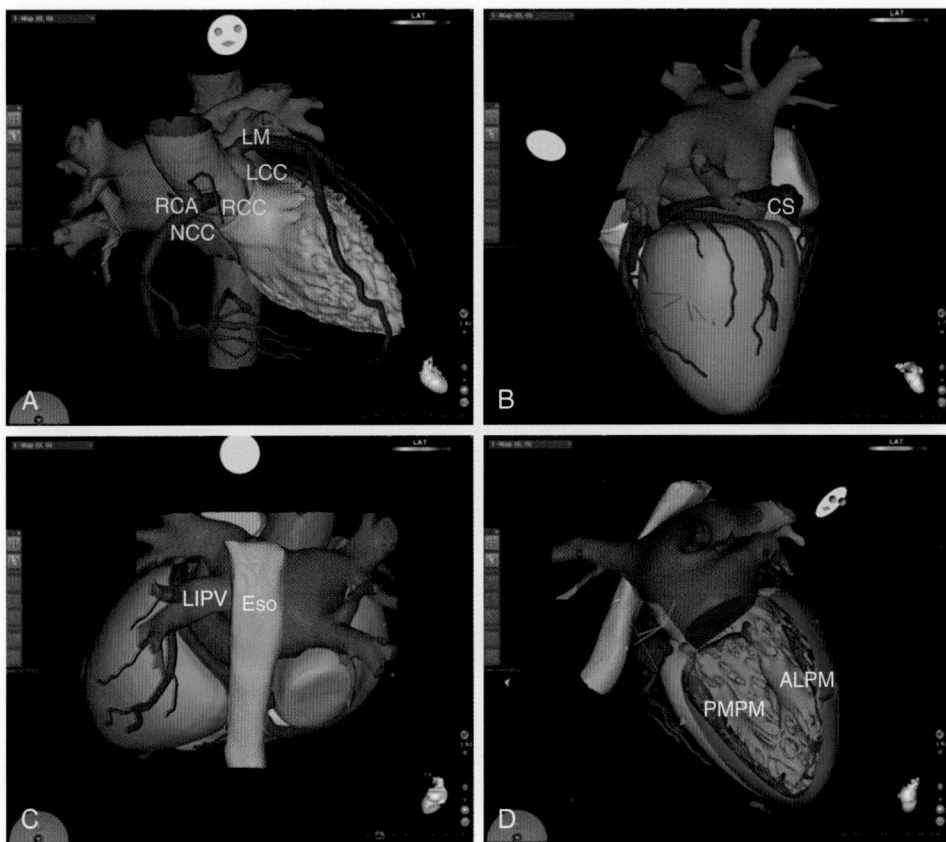

FIGURE 62.8 Cardiac computed tomography (CCT) reconstruction for anatomically guided complex ablations. Reconstructed CCT images (CARTO® Segmentation Module) can provide great anatomical definition, which can safely and effectively guide procedures in specific anatomical areas. (A) Reconstructed images of the aortic cusps and coronary arteries, which can provide crucial information for the safe delivery of ablations near the sinus of Valsalva or left ventricular summit. (B) Reconstruction of the coronary sinus course and ramifications can provide useful preprocedural and intraprocedural information for guiding left ventricular lead placement in cardiac resynchronization therapy implants. (C) The location of the esophagus is crucial when performing pulmonary vein isolation and posterior left atrial lesions for atrial fibrillation, to minimize the risk of atrioesophageal fistula formation. The position of the esophagus can shift throughout the case due to peristalsis. (D) High-resolution reconstruction of the endocardium can provide anatomical information about intracavitary structures such as the moderator band of the right ventricle and the papillary muscles (depicted here) to guide the ablation of idiopathic ventricular tachycardia arising from these structures. *ALPM,* Anterolateral papillary muscle; *CS,* coronary sinus; *Eso,* esophagus; *LCC,* left coronary cusp; *LIPV,* left inferior pulmonary vein; *LM,* left main; *NCC,* noncoronary cusp; *PMPM,* posteromedial papillary muscle; *RCA,* right coronary artery; *RCC,* right coronary cusp.

of intracavitary thrombus will delay an elective procedure until resolution of the thrombus is achieved with systemic anticoagulation and confirmed with further imaging. However, in unstable patients, delaying a potentially lifesaving procedure is not an option. A reported case series of patients with electrical storm and laminated LV thrombus undergoing VT ablation showed an acceptable periprocedural rate of complications (stroke in one out of eight patients) given the critical condition of the patients reported[48] (Fig. 62.9).

Cardiac Computed Tomography for Pacing and Cardiac Resynchronization Therapy

Individual cardiac venous anatomy is relevant for resynchronization therapy. Several anatomical and imaging studies have shown great variability in the size, number orientation, and trajectory of the CS and its tributaries.[49–51] One growing research area with important clinical applicability is the use of preprocedural CT to identify potential posterolateral vein targets for LV lead placement in cardiac resynchronization therapy, either as a standalone technique or utilizing image fusion (with fluoroscopy or 3D mapping overlay).[52–54] In addition to the CS anatomy, the CCT can provide anatomical, dynamic, and perfusion information to

identify scar, thus matching a potential vein target for lead placement with a suitable or unsuitable underlying myocardial substrate. This approach has the potential to improve the response outcomes for cardiac resynchronization therapy by preselecting the optimal cardiac resynchronization therapy candidates. In a study including mostly patients with at least one prior failed LV lead implant (8 of 11 patients) who underwent preprocedural CCT and cardiac MRI, the authors demonstrated that accurate registration between CT- and MRI-derived 3D models with live fluoroscopy can facilitate LV lead implantation (success in 11/12 cases).[55] Another study showed that CT imaging of the CS can successfully facilitate LV lead placement by image fusion between 3D reconstruction of the CS on CT and live fluoroscopy.[54] CCT has also been proposed for the assessment of mechanical dyssynchrony in patients with LV dysfunction. A total of 38 patients were divided into heart failure/wide QRS, heart failure/narrow QRS, and age-matched controls. A higher dyssynchrony index was observed in patients with heart failure (both wide and narrow QRS groups) compared to control subjects, and good correlation was observed between the CCT and echo parameters of dyssynchrony ($r = 0.65$ for two-dimensional and $r = 0.68$ for 3D

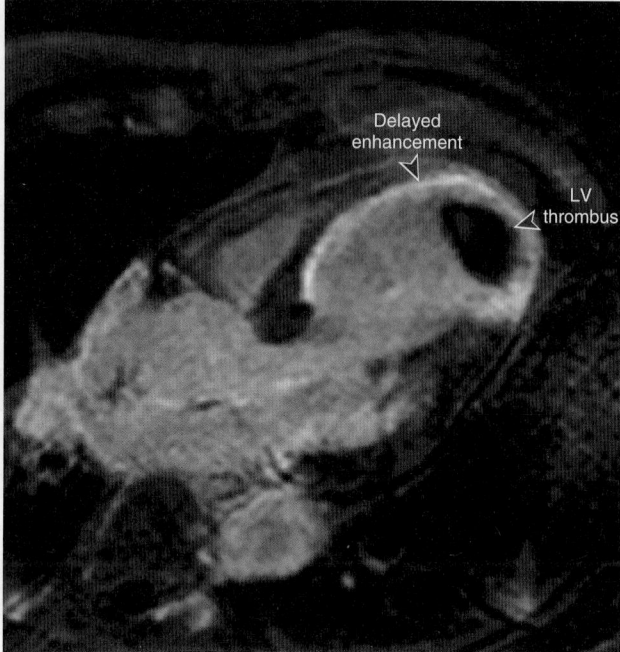

FIGURE 62.9 Evaluation of left ventricular (*LV*) thrombus on cardiac computed tomography (CCT). Patient with ischemic cardiomyopathy and ventricular tachycardia (VT) who underwent CCT prior to VT ablation. Note the areas of delayed hyperenhancement in the anteroseptal wall, wall thinning in the apex, and a large apical thrombus (filling defect inside the LV apex).

echocardiography).[57] Finally, assessment of the RV and LV lead positioning is an important variable in research assessing optimal pacing sites in cardiac resynchronization therapy. A recent study showed that the interobserver agreement regarding actual LV and RV lead positions was poor with fluoroscopy (κ of 0.2 and 0.23) and excellent with CCT (κ of 0.87 and 0.85), using a 16-segment model for the LV and a simplified 8-segment model for the RV.[58]

Two important issues regarding the CT and cardiac implantable electronic devices (CIEDs) are worth mentioning. Metal streak artifacts due to the pulse generator and leads (Fig. 62.10) can potentially affect the image quality of the scan. This has been described for cardiac[59] and noncardiac imaging studies[60] but usually affects only a small portion of the LV septum, allowing diagnostic quality for most of the myocardium. The second one relates to the still active 2008 US Food and Drug Administration advisory reporting the possible interference of CIEDs during diagnostic CT scanning. CT beams positioned directly over the header of the device can lead to current flow, resulting in short-term pacing inhibition or tracking. However, a retrospective study with 516 CIED patients undergoing CT scanning demonstrated no clinical adverse events.[61] Additionally, a MedlinePlus search produced no published reports on CT imaging leading to CIED-related clinically significant events, suggesting that no additional precautions are required for standard CT imaging.

Assessment of Procedural Complications

CCT plays an important role in the assessment of postprocedural complications related to catheter ablation. For complex arrhythmia ablations, up to 6% of patients may suffer procedure-related complications.[62]

Pulmonary Vein Stenosis

PV stenosis is a well-recognized complication of AF ablation that results from thermal injury to the PV structures, including the media, intima, adventitia, and PV musculature, with the published incidence of PV stenosis varying widely from 0% to 38%.[33] CT or MRI of the PVs prior to, and several months following, catheter ablation are the most precise methods for detecting PV stenosis.[63] The severity of PV stenosis is generally defined as mild (<50%), moderate (50%–70%), or severe (>70%) compared to preprocedural imaging. Symptoms of PV stenosis include chest pain, dyspnea, cough, hemoptysis, recurrent lung infections, and symptoms of pulmonary hypertension. It is important to note that even severe PV stenosis can be asymptomatic and that chest imaging is appropriate whenever PV stenosis is suspected. The Worldwide Survey of AF Ablation reported a 0.32% incidence of acute PV stenosis and a 1.3% incidence of persistent PV stenosis. Percutaneous (PV angioplasty ± stenting) or surgical intervention for treatment of PV stenosis was required in 53 cases (0.6%)[63] (Fig. 62.11).

Atrioesophageal Fistula

The exact incidence of atrioesophageal fistulas is unknown, but has been estimated to be 0.01% to 0.2% in percutaneous ablations, with surgical ablation series reporting incidences up to 1.5%.[64,65] A recent meta-analysis of 53 case reports puts the mean interval between procedure and presentation at 20 ± 12 days, ranging from 2 to 60 days with presenting symptoms of fever (83%), neurological deficits (51%), and hematemesis (36%).[64] Chest CT was the preferred diagnostic tool (51%) followed by head CT (28%), with the most common findings of multifocal infarcts consistent with air embolism (23%) or pneumomediastinum (23%). Other specific findings were intracardiac air, hemopericardium, and pneumopericardium. The absence of a fat layer between the LA and the esophagus may increase the risk of atrioesophageal fistula, with CT studies demonstrating, frequently, distances of <5 mm between the esophagus and the LA endocardium.[65] Some reports indicate lateral shifts of the esophagus with intrinsic peristalsis during the course of an AF ablation case, which may limit the value of reconstructed esophagus positions from the previously acquired CT imaging during AF ablations (see Fig. 62.3).

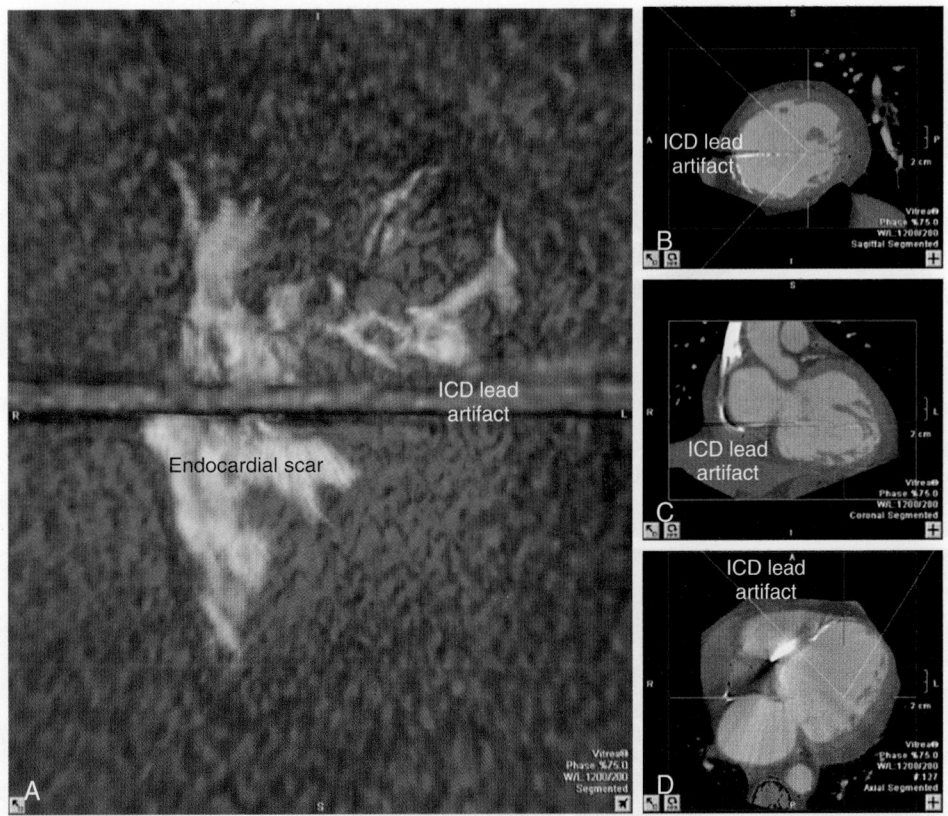

FIGURE 62.10 Implantable cardioverter defibrillator (*ICD*)-lead metal artifact on cardiac computed tomography (CCT). Many patients undergoing CCT for preprocedural and periprocedural guidance have pacemakers or ICDs. This example illustrates linear artifacts or "streaks" caused by the ICD lead, affecting some visualization of tissue characteristics. (A) Endoscopic view of the right ventricular endocardium showing a linear ICD artifact and surrounding scar tissue. (B) (C) and (D) show the sagittal, coronal, and axial segmented CCT images, respectively, with a lineal ICD lead artifact present in all views.

Periesophageal Vagal Injury

During AF ablation, thermal injury of the vagal anterior plexus overlaying the esophagus can result in acute pyloric spasm and gastric hypomotility. Frequently associated symptoms occur within a few hours to a few weeks after ablation and include nausea, vomiting, bloating, or abdominal pain. The incidence may be as high as 1%, and recovery often occurs in the first 2 to 3 weeks but can be protracted.[66] CT imaging can be helpful in demonstrating marked gastric dilatation. Delayed gastric emptying can be demonstrated with technetium-99–labeled studies, while an MRI can demonstrate increased pyloric spasms. The value of an esophageal temperature probe to monitor local temperature and avoid nerve injury has been studied in 359 patients undergoing AF ablation (207 with an esophageal temperature probe). Esophageal temperature monitoring (ETM) was associated with fewer energy requirements to achieve pulmonary vein isolation [6.3 ± 1.9 × 10(4) J vs. 6.8 ± 1.9 × 10(4) J in non-ETM patients, p = .03]. Most notably, gastric hypomotility postprocedure was seen in three patients in the non-ETM group versus none in the ETM group.[67]

Phrenic Nerve Injury

Phrenic nerve injury is an important complication of AF ablation and usually occurs after direct thermal injury to the right phrenic nerve near the right superior PV. In rare circumstances, left phrenic nerve injury can occur during ablation within the LAA.[30] Phrenic nerve injury has been most commonly reported during cryoballoon ablation of the right superior PVs, with an incidence of 4.7% in a large meta-analysis of 1308 patients.[68] When phrenic nerve injury occurs, CT imaging demonstrates an ipsilateral diaphragmatic paralysis with an elevated diaphragmatic "dome." Additionally, a sniff test during fluoroscopy will show lack of diaphragmatic contraction. Most diaphragmatic paralysis cases recover after 6–12 months, with <10% of cases persisting for longer. As discussed previously, CCT has the potential to visualize the phrenic nerve in up to 85% of patients and possibly reduce the rate of nerve injuries.[22]

Stroke and Transient Ischemic Attack

Thromboembolism has been reported in 0%–7% of AF ablations[30] occurring typically within the first 24 hours postprocedure,[69] but with an increased risk throughout the first 2 weeks. Noncontrast CT remains the imaging modality of choice in the acute setting and is able to rule out acute intracranial hemorrhage as the underlying cause of the stroke. With a thromboembolic stroke, a hyperdense segment representing the thrombus may be clearly visible with immediate imaging. During the hyperacute phase (1–3 hours), the loss of gray-white matter differentiation and hypoattenuation of deep nuclei with cortical hypodensity and parenchymal swelling can be seen. In the first week, hypoattenuation and swelling can increase with significant mass effect. During the second and third postprocedure weeks, CT will demonstrate a decrease in edema with cortical petechial hemorrhages. Chronic changes after several months demonstrate reparative gliosis, which appears as a region of low density with negative mass effect and possible hyperdense cortical mineralization.

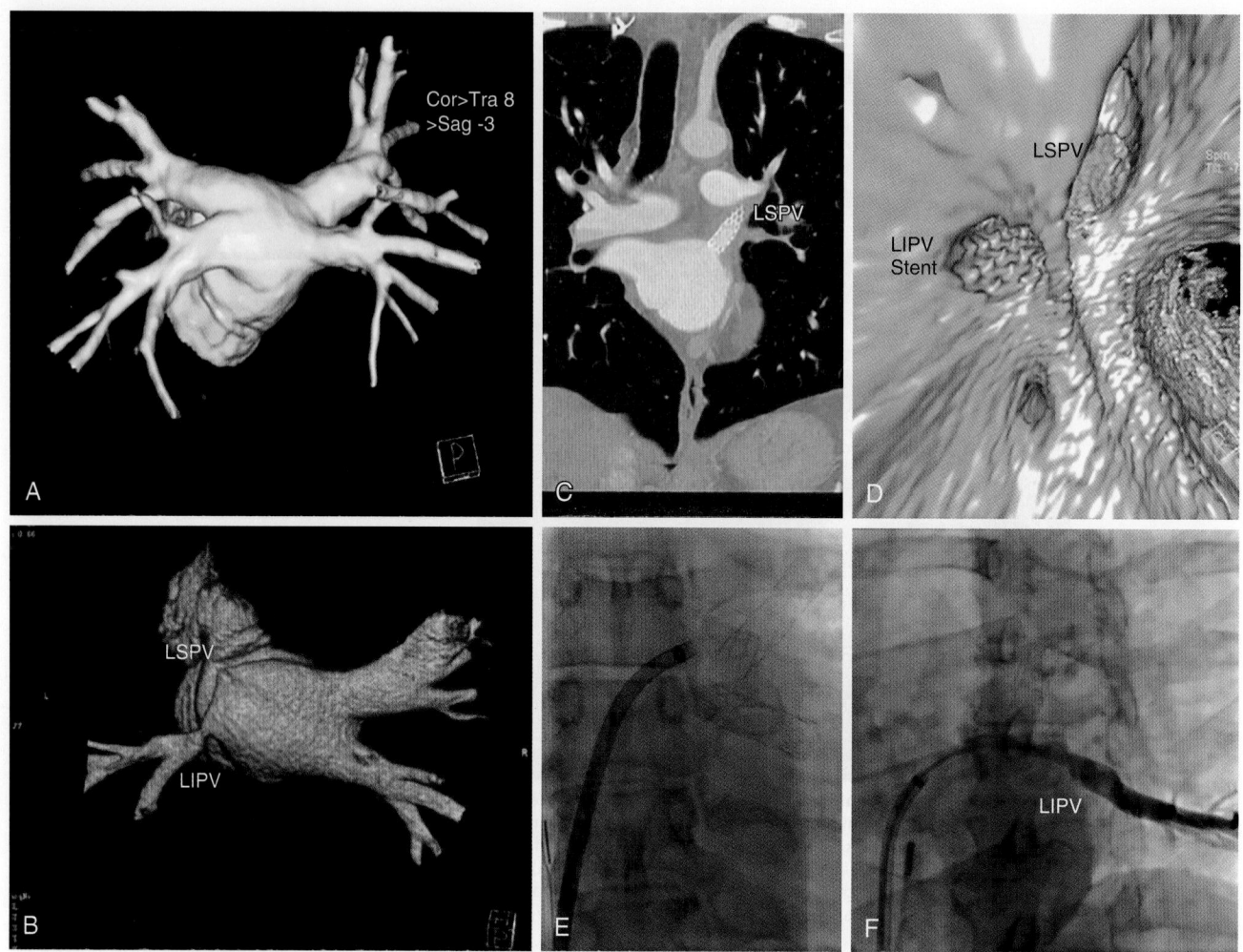

FIGURE 62.11 Pulmonary vein (PV) stenosis after PV isolation (PVI) with stenting. Patient who underwent a PVI for persistent atrial fibrillation. (A) Preprocedural three-dimensional (3D) reconstruction from cardiac magnetic resonance imaging showing normal PV anatomy. (B) 3D left atrial reconstruction of a cardiac computed tomography (CCT) image 1 month after the procedure due to dyspnea on exertion. Note the significant ostial stenosis of left inferior pulmonary vein (*LIPV*) and the lack of contrast entering the left superior pulmonary vein (*LSPV*). The patient underwent successful angioplasty with stenting of both the LSPV and LIPV. (C) and (D) The follow-up CCT 3 months after stenting, showing the coronal view with a patent LSPV stent (contrast is filling the LSPV) and endocardial reconstruction showing patent LSPV and LIPV ostia. The LIPV stent struts can be observed. (E) and (F) 6-month follow-up PV angiography confirming patency of both veins (LIPV angiography shown).

Silent microemboli, which are too small to create clinical symptoms, occur in about 17% of AF ablation procedures and usually require diffusion-weighted MRI for diagnosis. Lesions of <10 mm frequently disappear at 3 months during follow-up scans.[30]

Air embolism is another embolic phenomenon which can occur during a left-sided ablation procedure, most commonly introduced through infusion lines or suction when catheters are removed. If imaged promptly prior to their absorption, a CT may demonstrate multiple serpiginous hypodensities with or without the above-mentioned signs of acute infarction.[30]

Future Applications and Evolving Technology

Assessment of Myocardial Fibrosis and Periinfarct Border Zone

Fibrosis imaging with delayed enhancement is clinically important to evaluate preprocedural scar. Mechanistically, acute disruption of the cellular membrane (e.g., during ischemic injury) as well as increased intracellular fibrosis results in an increased volume of distribution. Together with the decreased wash-in and wash-out kinetics, those histological changes lead to a higher tissue concentration of ionized contrast (CCT) or gadolinium (CMR) (see Fig. 62.9). Several studies have reported the ability of acute infarct and chronic scar imaging in the left ventricle in animal experiments[42,70,71] as well as in human series[70,72] with good correlation (r ≥ 0.90) between CMR and a CCT-delayed enhancement. A recent study reported the ability to visualize myocardial scar in 93% of 42 VT patients with an at least moderate correlation with the electroanatomical map (κ = 0.536) and the ability to determine the endo/epicardial extent in a majority of patients.[72]

Analogously to CMR, CCT has the potential to visualize the periinfarction transition zone containing a possibly proarrhythmic mixture of fibrosis and surviving myocardial cells. This is commonly referred to as *gray zone* or *periinfarct heterogeneous zone* (PIZ) and has been correlated in human CMR studies with mortality, VT inducibility, and appropriate implantable cardioverter defibrillator shocks.[73–75] Animal studies demonstrated an excellent correlation of CCT-defined PIZ with histological transition and less partial volume effect compared to CMR.[71]

However, while clinical LV and RV scar imaging with CMR is well established, delayed enhancement imaging with CCT has so far remained mostly a research tool due to underlying technical limitations and the inability to achieve consistently high-quality images in clinical practice. In a series of 37 patients, the contrast-to-noise ratio of myocardial scar was about four times higher with CMR than with CCT, and an increase in signal intensity was significantly smaller with CCT (+35%) compared with CMR (+45%).[70] Additionally, the best CT imaging parameters (tube current/voltage) as well as contrast administration protocols have not yet been conclusively defined.

In parallel to the ongoing work with ventricular imaging, atrial fibrosis imaging is currently being evaluated using CMR in several highly specialized research centers, but is currently only assessed in ongoing research studies using CCT.[76]

Lesion Imaging

Although cardiac MRI has significant advantages over CCT to accurately depict soft tissue characteristics,[76–81] many patients (e.g., with "Legacy" CIED devices) are often not eligible to undergo cardiac MRI. For such patients, an alternative imaging modality is desirable for assessing tissue changes occurring during and after ablation therapy. As ablation results in fibrotic myocardial remodeling, CCT imaging is feasible in principle and is an area of ongoing research. The typical enhancement pattern of contrast void (during first pass) with delayed peripheral enhancement has been recently described for MRI as well as C-arm CT and likely reflects areas of no-reflow due to the complete tissue destruction of the ablated tissue.[82–84] Using contrast-enhanced CT fluoroscopy, 29 LV lesions in a swine model could be acutely visualized as perfusion defects, with increasing peripheral enhancement in 83% of cases after 5 minutes.[85]

CCT imaging of atrial ablation lesions would have important clinical implications given the increasing number of atrial ablation procedures worldwide; however, due to the low contrast-to-noise ratio and the thin size of the LA wall, CCT imaging of these lesions remains a challenge. Recent studies showed that CT is able to visualize myocardial edema after AF ablation[86] and that low attenuation areas on CCT correlated to low voltage areas in repeat AF ablations.[87]

Real-Time Computed Tomography in the Electrophysiology Laboratory

Given its high spatial and temporal resolutions, real-time CT applications are common for radiological and oncological indications and have been recently evaluated for possible electrophysiology applications. Percutaneous placement of LV pacing leads was feasible in nine swine with stable parameters during a 30-minute follow-up. Radiation times were within the average range for equivalent fluoroscopic studies, and estimated radiation exposure was similar (9.6 mSv) to clinical diagnostic CT imaging procedures.[88] Further research for catheter guidance and CT-guided ablation is ongoing and will determine a possible role for clinical applications.

A logical disadvantage of real-time CT compared to intra-cardiac echocardiography or CMR for purposes of real-time imaging is the use of ionizing radiation required for image acquisition. However, the technological advances in CT technology since the mid-2000s have dramatically reduced the radiation doses used during CT scanning. With prospective gating, iterative reconstruction, and the decrease in tube current and voltage, modern-day scanning protocols using new-generation cardiac CT scanners may offer complementary modalities for advanced image guidance of complex procedures.

REFERENCES

1. Luenberger DG. *Linear and Nonlinear Programming.* 2nd ed. Reading, MA: Addison-Wesley Publishing Co.; 2005.
2. Christian PE, Waterstram-Rich, eds. *Nuclear Medicine and PET/CT: Technologies and Techniques.* 6th ed. St. Louis, MO: Mosby Elsevier; 2007.
3. Sra J, Ratnakumar S. Cardiac image registration of the left atrium and pulmonary veins. *Heart Rhythm.* 2008;5:609–617.
4. Sra J, Narayan G, Krum D, Akhtar M. Registration of 3D computed tomographic images with interventional systems: implications for catheter ablation of atrial fibrillation. *J Interv Card Electrophysiol.* 2006;16:141–148.
5. Solomon SB, Dickfeld T, Calkins H. Real-time cardiac catheter navigation on three-dimensional CT images. *J Interv Card Electrophysiol.* 2003;8:27–36.
6. Kistler PM, Earley MJ, Harris S, et al. Validation of three-dimensional cardiac image integration: use of integrated CT image into electro-anatomic mapping system to perform catheter ablation of atrial fibrillation. *J Cardiovasc Electrophysiol.* 2006;17:341–348.
7. Bertaglia E, Bella PD, Tondo C, et al. Image integration increases efficacy of paroxysmal atrial fibrillation catheter ablation: results from the CartoMerge Italian Registry. *Europace.* 2009;11:1004–1010.
8. Martinek M, Nesser HJ, Aichinger J, Boehm G, Purerfellner H. Impact of integration of multislice computed tomography imaging into three-dimensional electroanatomic mapping on clinical outcomes, safety, and efficacy using radiofrequency ablation of atrial fibrillation. *Pacing Clin Electrophysiol.* 2007;30:1215–1223.
9. Tang K, Ma J, Zhang S, Zhang JY, et al. A randomized prospective comparison of CartoMerge and CartoXP to guide circumferential pulmonary vein isolation for the treatment of paroxysmal atrial fibrillation. *Chin Med J (Engl).* 2008;121:508–512.
10. Brooks AG, Wilson L, Chia NH, et al. Accuracy and clinical outcomes of CT image integration with Carto-Sound compared to electro-anatomical mapping for atrial fibrillation ablation: a randomized controlled study. *Int J Cardiol.* 2013;168:2774–2782.
11. Liu SX, Zhang Y, Zhang XW. Impact of image integration on catheter ablation for atrial fibrillation using three-dimensional electroanatomic mapping: a meta-analysis. *Pacing Clin Electrophysiol.* 2012;35:1242–1247.

12. Dong J, Dickfeld T, Dalal D, et al. Initial experience in the use of integrated electro-anatomical mapping with three-dimensional MR/CT images to guide catheter ablation of atrial fibrillation. *J Cardiovasc Electrophysiol.* 2006;17:459–466.
13. Dong J, Dickfeld T. Image integration in electro-anatomic mapping. *Herzschrittmacherther Elektrophysiol.* 2007;18:122–130.
14. Sonka M, Fitzpatrick JM, eds. *Handbook of Medical Imaging.* Vol. 2. Bellingham, WA: SPIE Press; 2000.
15. Sra J, Krum D, Hare J, et al. Feasibility and validation of registration of three-dimensional left atrial models derived from computed tomography with a noncontact cardiac mapping system. *Heart Rhythm.* 2005;2:55–63.
16. Richmond L, Rajappan K, Voth E, et al. Validation of computed tomography image integration into the EnSite NavX mapping system to perform catheter ablation of atrial fibrillation. *J Cardiovasc Electrophysiol.* 2008;19:821–827.
17. Dong J, Calkins H, Solomon SB, et al. Integrated electro-anatomic mapping with three-dimensional computed tomographic images for real-time guided ablations. *Circulation.* 2006;113:186–194.
18. Itoh T, Sasaki S, Kimura M, et al. Three-dimensional cardiac image integration of electroanatomical mapping of only left atrial posterior wall with CT image to guide circumferential pulmonary vein ablation. *J Interv Card Electrophysiol.* 2010;29:167–173.
19. Richmond L, Rajappan K, Voth E, et al. Validation of computed tomography image integration into the EnSite NavX mapping system to perform catheter ablation of atrial fibrillation. *J Cardiovasc Electrophysiol.* 2008;19:821–827.
20. Martinek M, Nesser HJ, Aichinger J, et al. Accuracy of integration of multislice computed tomography imaging into three-dimensional electro-anatomic mapping for real-time guided radiofrequency ablation of left atrial fibrillation–influence of heart rhythm and radiofrequency lesions. *J Interv Card Electrophysiol.* 2006;17:85–92.
21. Dong J, Dalal D, Scherr D, et al. Impact of heart rhythm status on registration accuracy of the left atrium for catheter ablation of atrial fibrillation. *J Cardiovasc Electrophysiol.* 2007;18:1269–1276.

22. Yamashita S, Sacher F, Mahida S, et al. Role of high-resolution image integration to visualize left phrenic nerve and coronary arteries during epicardial ventricular tachycardia ablation. *Circ Arrhythm Electrophysiol.* 2015;8:371–380.
23. Yamashita S, Sacher F, Mahida S, et al. Image integration to guide catheter ablation in scar-related ventricular tachycardia. *J Cardiovasc Electrophysiol.* 2016;27:699–708.
24. Kato R, Lickfett L, Meininger G, et al. Pulmonary vein anatomy in patients undergoing catheter ablation of atrial fibrillation: lessons learned by use of magnetic resonance imaging. *Circulation.* 2003;107:2004–2010.
25. Ho SY, Sanchez-Quintana D, Cabrera JA, Anderson RH. Anatomy of the left atrium: implications for radiofrequency ablation of atrial fibrillation. *J Cardiovasc Electrophysiol.* 1999;10:1525–1533.
26. Kaseno K, Tada H, Koyama K, et al. Prevalence and characterizaton of pulmonary vein variants in patients with atrial fibrillation determined using 3-dimensional computed tomography. *Am J Cardiol.* 2008;101:1638–1642.
27. Wongcharoen W, Tsao HM, Wu MH, et al. Morphologic characteristics of the left atrial appendage, roof, and septum: implications for the ablation of atrial fibrillation. *J Cardiovasc Electrophysiol.* 2006;17:951–956.
28. Bilchick KC, Mealor A, Gonzalez J, et al. Effectiveness of integrating delayed computed tomography angiography imaging for left atrial appendage thrombus exclusion into the care of patients undergoing ablation of atrial fibrillation. *Heart Rhythm.* 2016;13:12–19.
29. Patel A, Au E, Donegan K, et al. Multidetector row computed tomography for identification of left atrial appendage filling defects in patients undergoing pulmonary vein isolation for treatment of atrial fibrillation: comparison with transesophageal echocardiography. *Heart Rhythm.* 2008;5:253–260.
30. Calkins H, Kuck KH, Cappato R, et al. 2012 HRS/EHRA/ECAS expert consensus statement on catheter and surgical ablation of atrial fibrillation: recommendations for patient selection, procedural techniques, patient management and follow-up, definitions, endpoints, and research trial design: a report of the Heart Rhythm Society (HRS) Task Force on Catheter and Surgical Ablation of Atrial Fibrillation. *Heart Rhythm.* 2012;9:632–696.

31. Hur J, Kim YJ, Lee HJ, et al. Left atrial appendage thrombi in stroke patients: detection with two-phase cardiac CT angiography versus transesophageal echocardiography. *Radiology*. 2009;251:683–690.

32. Shapiro MD, Neilan TG, Jassal DS, et al. Multidetector computed tomography for the detection of left atrial appendage thrombus: a comparative study with transesophageal echocardiography. *J Comput Assist Tomogr*. 2007;31:905–909.

33. Romero J, Husain SA, Kelesidis I, et al. Detection of left atrial appendage thrombus by cardiac computed tomography in patients with atrial fibrillation: a meta-analysis. *Circ Cardiovasc Imaging*. 2013;6:185–194.

34. Fukushima K, Fukushima N, Kato K, et al. Correlation between left atrial appendage morphology and flow velocity in patients with paroxysmal atrial fibrillation. *Eur Heart J Cardiovasc Imaging*. 2016;17:59–66.

35. Abouezzeddine O, Suleiman M, Buescher T, et al. Relevance of endocavitary structures in ablation procedures for ventricular tachycardia. *J Cardiovasc Electrophysiol*. 2010;21:245–254.

36. Gao M, Chen C, Zhang S, et al. Segmenting the papillary muscles and the trabeculae from high resolution cardiac CT through restoration of topological handles. *Inf Process Med Imaging*. 2013;23:184–195.

37. Markowitz SM, Weinsaft JW, Waldman L, et al. Reappraisal of cardiac magnetic resonance imaging in idiopathic outflow tract arrhythmias. *J Cardiovasc Electrophysiol*. 2014;25:1328–1335.

38. Komatsu Y, Cochet H, Jadidi A, et al. Regional myocardial wall thinning at multidetector computed tomography correlates to arrhythmogenic substrate in postinfarction ventricular tachycardia: assessment of structural and electrical substrate. *Circ Arrhythm Electrophysiol*. 2013;6:342–350.

39. Komatsu Y, Jadidi A, Sacher F, et al. Relationship between MDCT-imaged myocardial fat and ventricular tachycardia substrate in arrhythmogenic right ventricular cardiomyopathy. *J Am Heart Assoc*. 2014;3:e000935.

40. Sasaki T, Calkins H, Miller CF, et al. New insight into scar-related ventricular tachycardia circuits in ischemic cardiomyopathy: fat deposition after myocardial infarction on computed tomography–A pilot study. *Heart Rhythm*. 2015;12:1508–1518.

41. Tian J, Jeudy J, Smith MF, et al. Three-dimensional contrast-enhanced multidetector CT for anatomic, dynamic, and perfusion characterization of abnormal myocardium to guide ventricular tachycardia ablations. *Circ Arrhythm Electrophysiol*. 2010;3:496–504.

42. Lardo AC, Cordeiro MA, Silva C, et al. Contrast-enhanced multidetector computed tomography viability imaging after myocardial infarction: characterization of myocyte death, microvascular obstruction, and chronic scar. *Circulation*. 2006;113:394–404.

43. Dickfeld T, Lei P, Dilsizian V, et al. Integration of three-dimensional scar maps for ventricular tachycardia ablation with positron emission tomography-computed tomography. *JACC Cardiovasc Imaging*. 2008;1:73–82.

44. Fahmy TS, Wazni OM, Jaber WA, et al. Integration of positron emission tomography/computed tomography with electro-anatomical mapping: a novel approach for ablation of scar-related ventricular tachycardia. *Heart Rhythm*. 2008;5:1538–1545.

45. Tian J, Smith MF, Chinnadurai P, et al. Clinical application of PET/CT fusion imaging for three-dimensional myocardial scar and left ventricular anatomy during ventricular tachycardia ablation. *J Cardiovasc Electrophysiol*. 2008;20:597–604.

46. Cox M, Balasubramanya R, Hou A, et al. Incidental left atrial and ventricular thrombi on routine CT: outcome and influence on subsequent management at an urban tertiary care referral center. *Emerg Radiol*. 2015;22:657–660.

47. Goldstein JA, Schiller NB, Lipton MJ, Ports TA, Brundage BH. Evaluation of left ventricular thrombi by contrast-enhanced computed tomography and two-dimensional echocardiography. *Am J Cardiol*. 1986;57:757–760.

48. Rao HB, Yu R, Chitnis N, Do D, et al. Ventricular tachycardia ablation in the presence of left ventricular thrombus: safety and efficacy. *J cardiovasc electrophysiol*. 2016;27:453–459.

49. Echeverri D, Cabrales J, Jimenez A. Myocardial venous drainage: from anatomy to clinical use. *J Invasive Cardiol*. 2013;25:98–105.

50. Genc B, Solak A, Sahin N, Gur S, Kalaycioglu S, Ozturk V. Assessment of the coronary venous system by using cardiac CT. *Diagn Interv Radiol*. 2013;19:286–293.

51. Saremi F, Muresian H, Sánchez-Quintana D. Coronary veins: comprehensive CT-anatomic classification and review of variants and clinical implications. *Radiographics*. 2012;32:E1–E32.

52. Catanzaro JN, Makaryus JN, Jadonath R, Makaryus AN. Planning and guidance of cardiac resynchronization therapy-lead implantation by evaluating coronary venous anatomy assessed with multidetector computed tomography. *Clin Med Insights Cardiol*. 2015;8(suppl 4):43–50.

53. Malagò R, Pezzato A, Barbiani C, et al. Noninvasive cardiac vein mapping: role of multislice CT coronary angiography. *Eur J Radiol*. 2012;81:3262–3269.

54. Alikhani Z, Li J, Merchan JA, Nijhof N, Mendel J, Orlov MV. Coronary sinus anatomy by computerized tomography, overlaid on live fluoroscopy can be successfully used to guide left ventricular lead implantation: a feasibility study. *J Interv Card Electrophysiol*. 2013;36:217–222.

55. Duckett SG, Ginks MR, Knowles BR, et al. Advanced image fusion to overlay coronary sinus anatomy with real-time fluoroscopy to facilitate left ventricular lead implantation in CRT. *Pacing Clin Electrophysiol*. 2011;34:226–234.

56. Deleted in review.

57. Truong QA, Singh JP, Cannon CP, et al. Quantitative analysis of intraventricular dyssynchrony using wall thickness by multidetector computed tomography. *JACC Cardiovasc Imaging*. 2008;1:772–781.

58. Sommer A, Kronborg MB, Nørgaard BL, Gerdes C, Mortensen PT, Nielsen JC. Left and right ventricular lead positions are imprecisely determined by fluoroscopy in cardiac resynchronization therapy: a comparison with cardiac computed tomography. *Europace*. 2014;16:1334–1341.

59. Suzuki A, Koshida K, Matsubara K. Effects of pacemaker, implantable cardioverter-defibrillator, and left ventricular leads on CT-based attenuation correction. *J Nucl Med Technol*. 2014;42:37–41.

60. Ay MR, Mehranian A, Abdoli M, Ghafarian P, Zaidi H. Qualitative and quantitative assessment of metal artifacts arising from implantable cardiac pacing devices in oncological PET/CT studies: a phantom study. *Mol Imaging Biol*. 2011;13:1077–1087.

61. Hussein AA, Abutaleb A, Jeudy J, et al. Safety of computed tomography in patients with cardiac rhythm management devices: assessment of the U.S. Food and Drug Administration advisory in clinical practice. *J Am Coll Cardiol*. 2014;63:1769–1775.

62. Dagres N, Hindricks G, Kottkamp H, et al. Complications of atrial fibrillation ablation in a high-volume center in 1,000 procedures: still cause for concern? *J Cardiovasc Electrophysiol*. 2009;20:1014–1019.

63. Cappato R, Calkins H, Chen SA, et al. Prevalence and causes of fatal outcome in catheter ablation of atrial fibrillation. *J Am Coll Cardiol*. 2009;53:1798–1803.

64. Chavez P, Messerli FH, Casso Dominguez A, et al. Atrioesophageal fistula following ablation procedures for atrial fibrillation: systematic review of case reports. *Open Heart*. 2015;2:e000257.

65. Malamis AP, Kirshenbaum KJ, Nadimpalli S. CT radiographic findings: atrio-esophageal fistula after transcatheter percutaneous ablation of atrial fibrillation. *J Thorac Imaging*. 2007;22:188–191.

66. Kuwahara T, Takahashi A, Takahashi Y, et al. Clinical characteristics and management of periesophageal vagal nerve injury complicating left atrial ablation of atrial fibrillation: lessons from eleven cases. *J Cardiovasc Electrophysiol*. 2013;24:847–851.

67. Kuwahara T, Takahashi A, Kobori A, et al. Safe and effective ablation of atrial fibrillation: importance of esophageal temperature monitoring to avoid periesophageal nerve injury as a complication of pulmonary vein isolation. *J Cardiovasc Electrophysiol*. 2009;20:1–6.

68. Andrade JG, Khairy P, Guerra PG, et al. Efficacy and safety of cryoballoon ablation for atrial fibrillation: a systematic review of published studies. *Heart Rhythm*. 2011;8:1444–1451.

69. Liu Y, Zhan X, Xue Y, et al. Incidence and outcomes of cerebrovascular events complicating catheter ablation for atrial fibrillation. *Europace*. 2015 Dec 23. pii: euv356. [Epub ahead of print].

70. Gerber BL, Belge B, Legros GJ, et al. Characterization of acute and chronic myocardial infarcts by multidetector computed tomography: comparison with contrast-enhanced magnetic resonance. *Circulation*. 2006;113:823–833.

71. Schuleri KH, Centola M, George RT, et al. Characterization of peri-infarct zone heterogeneity by contrast-enhanced multidetector computed tomography: a comparison with magnetic resonance imaging. *J Am Coll Cardiol*. 2009;53:1699–1707.

72. Esposito A, Palmisano A, Antunes S, et al. Cardiac CT with delayed enhancement in the characterization of ventricular tachycardia structural substrate: relationship between CT-segmented scar and electro-anatomic mapping. *JACC Cardiovasc Imaging*. 2016;9:822–832.

73. Schmidt A, Azevedo CF, Cheng A, et al. Infarct tissue heterogeneity by magnetic resonance imaging identifies enhanced cardiac arrhythmia susceptibility in patients with left ventricular dysfunction. *Circulation*. 2007;115:2006–2014.

74. Fernandes VR, Wu KC, Rosen BD, et al. Enhanced infarct border zone function and altered mechanical activation predict inducibility of monomorphic ventricular tachycardia in patients with ischemic cardiomyopathy. *Radiology*. 2007;245:712–719.

75. Wu KC, Weiss RG, Thiemann DR, et al. Late gadolinium enhancement by cardiovascular magnetic resonance heralds an adverse prognosis in nonischemic cardiomyopathy. *J Am Coll Cardiol*. 2008;51:2414–2421.

76. Higuchi K, Akkaya M, Akoum N, Marrouche NF. Cardiac MRI assessment of atrial fibrosis in atrial fibrillation: implications for diagnosis and therapy. *Heart*. 2014;100:590–596.

77. Eitel C, Hindricks G, Grothoff M, et al. Catheter ablation guided by real-time MRI. *Curr Cardiol Rep*. 2014;16:511.

78. Longobardo L, Todaro MC, Zito C, et al. Role of imaging in assessment of atrial fibrosis in patients with atrial fibrillation: state-of-the-art review. *Eur Heart J Cardiovasc Imaging*. 2014;15:1–5.

79. Oakes RS, Badger TJ, Kholmovski EG, et al. Detection and quantification of left atrial structural remodeling with delayed-enhancement magnetic resonance imaging in patients with atrial fibrillation. *Circulation*. 2009;119:1758–1767.

80. Spragg DD, Khurram I, Zimmerman SL, et al. Initial experience with magnetic resonance imaging of atrial scar and co-registration with electroanatomic voltage mapping during atrial fibrillation: success and limitations. *Heart Rhythm*. 2012;9:2003–2009.

81. Halbfass PM, Mitlacher M, Turschner O, Brachmann J, Mahnkopf C. Lesion formation after pulmonary vein isolation using the advance cryoballoon and the standard cryoballoon: lessons learned from late gadolinium enhancement magnetic resonance imaging. *Europace*. 2015;17:566–573.

82. Dickfeld T, Kato R, Zviman M, et al. Characterization of radiofrequency ablation lesions with gadolinium-enhanced cardiovascular magnetic resonance imaging. *J Am Coll Cardiol*. 2006;47:370–378.

83. Vergara GR, Marrouche NF. Tailored management of atrial fibrillation using a LGE-MRI based model: from the clinic to the electrophysiology laboratory. *J Cardiovasc Electrophysiol*. 2011;22:481–487.

84. Akoum N, Daccarett M, McGann C, et al. Atrial fibrosis helps select the appropriate patient and strategy in catheter ablation of atrial fibrillation: a DE-MRI guided approach. *J Cardiovasc Electrophysiol*. 2011;22:16–22.

85. Girard EE, Al-Ahmad A, Rosenberg J, et al. Contrast-enhanced C-arm CT evaluation of radiofrequency ablation lesions in the left ventricle. *JACC Cardiovasc Imaging*. 2011;4:259–268.

86. Okada T, Yamada T, Murakami Y, et al. Prevalence and severity of left atrial edema detected by electron beam tomography early after pulmonary vein ablation. *J Am Coll Cardiol*. 2007;49:1436–1442.

87. Ling Z, McManigle J, Zipunnikov V, et al. The association of left atrial low-voltage regions on electroanatomic mapping with low attenuation regions on cardiac computed tomography perfusion imaging in patients with atrial fibrillation. *Heart Rhythm*. 2015;12:857–864.

88. Dickfeld T, Dauer L, Deodhar A, Berger RD, Fleiter T, Solomon S. Real-time CT-guided percutaneous placement of LV pacing leads. *JACC Cardiovasc Imaging*. 2013;6:96–104.

63 Computed Tomography and Magnetic Resonance Imaging for Electrophysiology

Saman Nazarian and Henry R. Halperin

Today's successful electrophysiologist must not only be a competent proceduralist but also a physician who understands the pathophysiology of arrhythmias, new drug targets and developments, complexities of new technologies, and various treatment options. Additionally, an in-depth understanding of cardiac anatomy, common anatomical variations, typical scar patterns, and how anatomical arrhythmia substrates relate to diagnostic and procedural nuances is increasingly important. Advanced imaging modalities, including cardiac computed tomography (CT) and magnetic resonance imaging (MRI), are now important adjuncts for the care of patients with cardiac arrhythmia. In this chapter we will describe the basics of cardiac CT and MRI, diagnostic and prognostic contributions of CT and MRI for common arrhythmia conditions, cardiac MRI safety and advances in the setting of implanted devices, the utility of CT and MRI for interventional electrophysiology, and advantages of each modality in the electrophysiology laboratory.

Basics of Cardiac Computed Tomography

Cardiac CT utilizes postacquisition processing to generate a three-dimensional (3D) image from multiple two-dimensional x-ray projection images taken around the CT gantry's axis of rotation. Use of iodinated contrast is necessary to enable the visualization of cardiac chambers, vascular lumens, and scar substrates. The potential adverse renal effect of iodinated contrast must be considered in many patients referred to the electrophysiology laboratory. Several propensity score–matched studies have suggested that renal effect following administration of typical doses of intravenous contrast for CT scans is probably far lower than previously thought; nevertheless, adequate hydration prior to CT and use of iso-osmolal agents may reduce any potential risk.[1] Notably, the dose of administered contrast may vary depending on the goals of imaging and the body mass index. For example, delayed-enhancement CT for scar identification requires a higher contrast dose than typical perfusion or chamber visualization protocols.[2] The relative timing of scan acquisition from the time of injection is critical depending on the structures of interest. Our preferred approach is the bolus trigger method, whereby a predefined contrast threshold in the ascending aorta is used to trigger image acquisition in the chamber of interest. Breath-holding during acquisition is also of critical importance for generation of quality images. However, potential artifacts are minimized using scanners with multiple detectors, where the gantry rotates around the patient as the scanner bed advances. The "pitch" describes the ratio of distance the scanner bed travels to each rotation of the gantry. A pitch of 1 signifies one detector width advance of the scanner bed for one rotation of the gantry. The commonly utilized pitch of 0.2 allows the acquisition of overlapping data. This methodology can reduce image artifact and allows multiphase image reconstruction for the evaluation of cardiac function, albeit with increased radiation exposure.[3] Depending on the number of detectors in a scanner, multiple heartbeats may be required to complete cardiac imaging. Many electrophysiology patients will have ectopic beats or atrial fibrillation (AF) during scan acquisition. Therefore 256+ slice scanners are optimal to allow~ image acquisition in a single heartbeat. If a scanner with fewer detectors is used, images acquired during ectopic beats should be excluded from the reconstruction dataset to minimize artifacts, and images should be reconstructed from those acquired at a fixed interval relative to the R waves. Techniques such as "tube modulation" or "prospective triggering" can be used to lower the tube current during cardiac phases that are unlikely to be used for image reconstruction.[4] Additionally, heart rate reduction can lead to improved single-heartbeat image acquisition and minimize the radiation exposure.[5] The typical optimal phase for reconstruction of image in the electrophysiology laboratory will be end diastolic, thus allowing improved image registration with electroanatomical mapping systems.

Basics of Cardiac Magnetic Resonance Imaging

To obtain an MR image, a strong static magnetic field is used to orient the magnetic moments of hydrogen nuclei. Radiofrequency pulses are then used to "tip" the magnetic moments in space by applying a resonance frequency equal to the precession frequency of the magnetic moments about the magnetic field lines. After the magnetic moment is tipped, it relaxes and changes the local magnetization, which is measured and used to construct the image. The multitude of available MR pulse sequences, each suited for particular attributes of cardiac function or structure and each with a series of programmable parameters, necessitates significant expertise for appropriate image acquisition. Similarly, due to the multitude of sequence options, it is of paramount importance to accurately communicate the imaging needs for each patient to the scanner operators. If valvular and contractile function and chamber volumes are of interest, cine imaging is required. Inversion recovery (IR) "late gadolinium enhancement" (LGE) imaging 5 to 10 minutes after contrast administration is utilized for scar identification and is routinely performed for ventricles.[6] This technique takes advantage of delayed washout of gadolinium contrast from scar tissue, which results in shortened T1 relaxation and hyperenhancement of scar compared to the surrounding normal myocardium with rapid gadolinium washout.[7] Importantly, a recent US population–based study revealed that up to 6% of individuals have ventricular myocardial scar that remains unrecognized by electrocardiography or clinical evaluation.[8] Atrial LGE imaging requires specialized software for respiratory gating and variations in pulse sequences to visualize the thinner muscular tissue.[9] Such a pulse sequence may not be readily available at all centers and, even when available, is not routinely performed. However, when available, such images allow the integration of preexisting atrial scar into the procedural space. When evaluating the ventricles or atria for fibrosis, focal fibrosis is not always the rule. When the myocardial fibrosis is diffuse rather than focal, after gadolinium contrast injection, and following washout, the contrast may be evenly retained throughout the diffusely fibrotic myocardium. Thus normal myocardium for appropriate selection of the inversion time may be absent. Additionally, compared to the normal tissue, the signal intensity variation in diffusely fibrotic areas may be minimal. As a result, the IR LGE technique may overlook diffuse myocardial fibrosis despite substantial retention of gadolinium. The T1-mapping technique detects diffuse myocardial fibrosis by providing a quantitative measure of the myocardial T1 relaxation times. Diffuse myocardial fibrosis shortens the T1 relaxation time due to retention of gadolinium contrast in increased interstitial spaces. The T1-mapping technique has been successfully utilized to quantify diffuse fibrosis in patients with heart failure, aortic regurgitation, adult congenital heart disease, nonischemic cardiomyopathy (NICM), and myotonic muscular dystrophy.[10-14] It is important to note that histopathological processes other than diffuse myocardial fibrosis, such as fatty infiltration, edema, amyloid protein deposition, and iron deposition, also influence the myocardial T1 relaxation time. Additionally, the postcontrast myocardial T1 time may vary as a function of parameters such as contrast dose, delay time of MRI scan after contrast injection, and patient hematocrit and glomerular filtration rate (GFR). Recently, the native (without contrast) T1 time has been used in multiple clinical scenarios, such as differentiation of hypertrophic cardiomyopathy (HCM) from hypertensive heart disease[15] and characterization of the chronicity of myocarditis.[16]

If an arrhythmia is suspected to be related to myocarditis or active inflammation in the setting of sarcoidosis, visualization of active inflammation may change the management and can be done if T2-weighted imaging is specifically requested.[17] Perhaps, most importantly from an electrophysiology standpoint, magnetic resonance angiography (MRA) protocols are necessary to visualize the end-diastolic dimensions of cardiac chambers and vascular structures of interest. When an MRA is requested, the chambers of interest should be specified to ensure that the field of view and scan timing relative to contrast administration are appropriately set up.

Advantages of Each Imaging Modality in the Electrophysiology Setting

The primary advantage of cardiac MRI over CT is the lack of ionizing radiation. Given the typical length of complex catheter ablation procedures and the potential cumulative radiation exposure to the patient, this is particularly important in women and young patients. Additionally, for imaging myocardial scar as a substrate for arrhythmia, the experience with and the signal-to-noise ratio of cardiac MRI far surpass those with cardiac CT. Cardiac MRI is capable of multiplanar imaging, whereas 3D reconstruction and volume rendering are necessary to visualize unconventional planes when using CT. Finally, when used in patients with GFR >30 mL/min per 1.73 m² to avoid nephrogenic systemic sclerosis, gadolinium-based contrast agents have an improved safety profile compared to the iodinated contrast agents used for cardiac CT.[18] In general, patients with mild renal insufficiency, history of

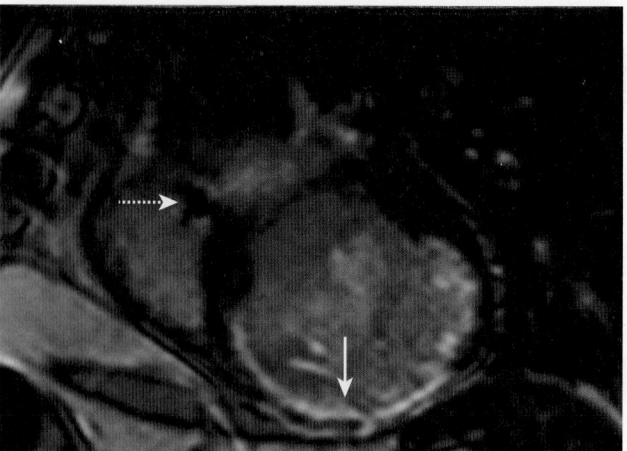

FIGURE 63.1 A short-axis magnetic resonance image that demonstrates the right and left ventricles with an inferior transmural infarction in the left ventricle (*solid arrow*). An implantable cardioverter defibrillator lead artifact is visualized in the right ventricle (*dashed arrow*).

multiple myeloma, risk of contrast-induced nephropathy, recent radioactive iodine therapy, and hyperthyroidism would be better served with cardiac MRI and gadolinium contrast compared to iodinated CT contrast.[4]

In contrast, cardiac CT has a substantially shorter acquisition time than cardiac MRI and may be the preferred alternative for a claustrophobic patient, patients with significant ectopy, and those with breath-holding difficulties. Typical acquisition times for detailed CT images of the entire heart and vasculature are on the order of 15 seconds. In contrast, cardiac MRI requires several minute-long acquisitions that vary in length depending on sequence settings and patient heart rate. Additionally, when evaluating chamber dimensions, the pulmonary vein, the coronary artery, and other vascular boundaries, cardiac CT provides superior resolution. Cardiac CT can acquire images of the esophagus and cardiac chambers in the same sequence, thus allowing incorporation of both structures into the electroanatomical mapping systems without the requirement for "double-registration" techniques. While cardiac CT is easier to perform in the setting of permanent pacemakers and implantable cardioverter defibrillators (ICDs), techniques for safe imaging in this setting are available and will be discussed later in the chapter.[19] Importantly, while the generator artifact is larger on MRI, the artifact due to leads tends to be significantly smaller on MRI than on CT.

Imaging the Arrhythmia Substrate: Implications for Diagnosis and Prognosis
Ischemic Cardiomyopathy

Patients with ischemic cardiomyopathy (ICM) are at risk of ventricular arrhythmia typically due to reentry involving diseased slow-conducting tissue within the infarct scar. The extent and distribution pattern of scar fibrosis is easily recognizable on cardiac MRI (Fig. 63.1). In pioneering work to image the substrate of ventricular tachycardia (VT), Bello and associates showed that measurements of the infarct surface area and mass by cardiac magnetic resonance (CMR) could identify the substrate for inducible monomorphic VT.[20] Later, Yan and colleagues provided evidence for the relationship of the scar substrate to clinical events in a study that revealed a strong association of the extent of the periinfarct zone characterized by CMR to all-cause and cardiovascular mortality.[21] Schmidt and associates later showed that increased "tissue heterogeneity" in the periinfarct zone correlates with inducible VT in an electrophysiology study.[22] Similarly, work with higher-resolution

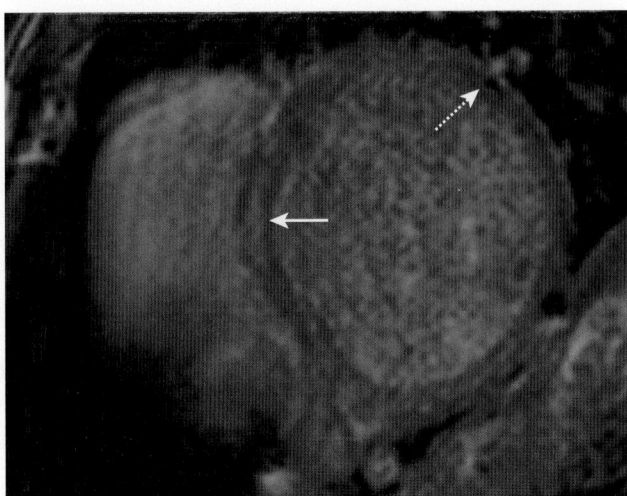

FIGURE 63.2 Short-axis image focusing on the right and left ventricles that demonstrates the atypical and diffuse pattern of scar in nonischemic cardiomyopathy. In this three-dimensional navigator-gated image, the contrast-to-noise ratio is sacrificed to provide greater spatial resolution. The striae of midwall late gadolinium enhancement are readily visualized in the septum (*solid arrow*) and lateral wall (*dashed arrow*).

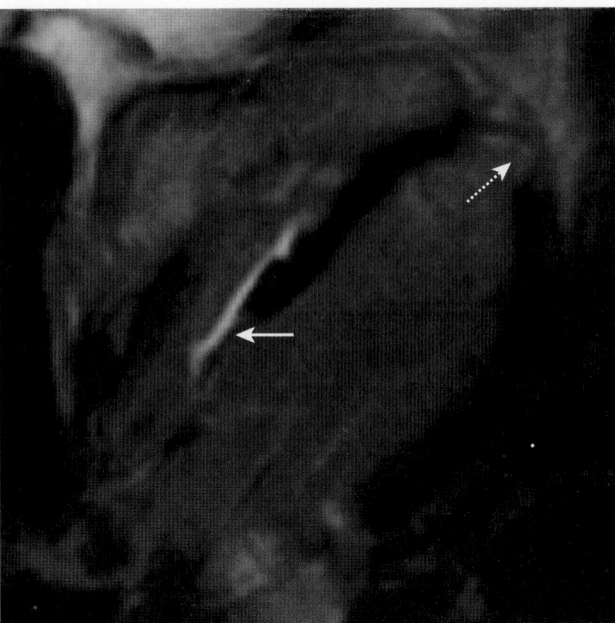

FIGURE 63.3 Four-chamber horizontal long axis image shows basal septal right ventricular endocardial late gadolinium enhancement (*solid arrow*) typical of cardiac sarcoidosis. An area of left ventricular apical aneurysmal change (*dashed arrow*) is also noted, reminding us of the capacity of cardiac sarcoidosis to manifest in many different forms.

MRI in animal models suggested that the reentry isthmus is characterized by a relatively small volume of viable myocardium bound by the scar tissue at the infarct border zone or over the infarct.[23] Recent work also has suggested that CMR-based computer models of ischemic scar substrates may enable the prediction of specific VT circuits resulting from unique infarct architectures.[24]

Nonischemic Cardiomyopathy

The pathogenesis of NICM with ventricular dilatation and reduced cardiac function in the absence of flow-limiting coronary artery disease (CAD) can be genetic, inflammatory, toxic, or viral. However, in the vast majority of cases, the origin is unclear. While syncope and sudden death are rarely the initial manifestations of the disease, NICM is often associated with VT. Cardiac MRI readily assesses the anatomical and functional abnormalities related to NICM. LGE using gadolinium contrast can be used to identify scar in the evaluation of patients with NICM. Although absence of LGE is the most common finding in NICM, midwall striae or patches of enhancement can be identified in up to 42% of cases.[25] Compared to ICM, the pattern and location of delayed enhancement in NICM is often atypical, making it difficult to distinguish artifact from true scar (Fig. 63.2). The presence of scar should therefore be verified using multiple planes. Utilizing CMR to delineate scar distribution, we showed that the VT substrate in NICM is a midwall scar involving greater than 25% of the wall thickness.[26] In a prospective study of patients with NICM, Assomull and colleagues demonstrated that this high-risk midwall fibrosis pattern predicts sudden cardiac death (SCD) and spontaneous VT.[27] In patients with newly diagnosed NICM, the extent of myocardial scar, as quantified by LGE, is independently associated with lack of response to medical therapy, as well as with the combined endpoint of mortality and hospitalizations.[28] The transmural extent of LGE predicts inducibility of VT at the time of electrophysiology study and the composite endpoint of hospitalization for heart failure, appropriate ICD firing, and cardiac death.[25]

Cardiac Sarcoidosis

Sarcoidosis is a multisystem granulomatous disease of unknown origin that is characterized by the presence of noncaseating granulomas in involved organs. Sarcoidosis with cardiac involvement is relatively uncommon (5%), but sudden death due to arrhythmia may be its initial clinical presentation. Techniques for assessment of cardiac involvement, including echocardiography, scintigraphy, and myocardial biopsy, are often inadequate for arrhythmic risk stratification. In patients with systemic sarcoidosis suspected of cardiac involvement, cardiac MRI may provide a diagnostic alternative and a method by which disease activity can be followed. Diagnostic workup of cardiac sarcoidosis also benefits from ^{18}F-fluorodeoxyglucose (FDG)–positron emission tomography (PET) to detect disease activity.[29,30] MRI is sensitive for detection of cardiac involvement, and a positive MRI finding is associated with future adverse events including cardiac death.[31] The pattern of LGE in sarcoidosis can be quite variable; however, the majority of patients have basal septal endocardial right ventricular (RV) involvement (Fig. 63.3). A recent important study has suggested that sarcoidosis patients with LGE are at significant risk for death/VT, even with normal left ventricular (LV) function.[32]

Myocarditis

Severe myocarditis presents as dilated cardiomyopathy (DCM), heart failure, ventricular arrhythmia, and SCD. Cardiac MRI provides valuable clinical information on abnormal tissue characteristics associated with myocarditis,[33] including (1) intracellular and interstitial edema (T2-weighted edema imaging), (2) hyperemia and capillary leakage (myocardial early gadolinium enhancement [EGEr]), and (3) necrosis and fibrosis (LGE).[34] T2-weighted images are optimized for visualization of edema within the myocardium. Myocardial edema has been identified in a variety of disease states, including myocarditis, acute myocardial infarction, sarcoidosis, and HCM.[34–37] Patients with these conditions may present with arrhythmias that bring them to the attention of the electrophysiologist. The identification of active inflammation within the myocardium on T2-weighted MRI may have an impact on treatment decisions. T2-weighted sequences are typically dark blood spin-echo–based techniques that use specialized IR pulses to null the signal from both blood and fat. Due to the use of three separate 180-degree IR pulses, these sequences are occasionally referred to as "triple IR." A drawback of triple IR sequences is their susceptibility to motion artifacts because of long breath-hold requirements that decrease the specificity.[38] LGE also allows visualization of the myocardium with necrosis and fibrosis. In myocarditis, LGE shows two patterns of myocardial damage: (1) an intramural, rim-like pattern in the septal wall and (2) a patchy subepicardial distribution in the free LV lateral wall.[39] However, LGE cannot differentiate between acute and chronic inflammation. The combination of these different MRI techniques provides high sensitivity and specificity.[34,38] Patients with normal CMR findings appear to have a good prognosis independent of their clinical symptoms and other findings.[40]

Hypertrophic Cardiomyopathy

Most individuals with HCM are asymptomatic, and the first manifestation of this condition may be SCD, which is generally related to ventricular arrhythmia triggered by factors such as ischemia, outflow obstruction, or AF.[41] Cardiac MRI is a useful adjunct or alternative to echocardiography for confirmation of the diagnosis or for identification of atypical cases of HCM. In addition, LGE can detect midwall and patchy scar in regions with hypertrophy, most commonly at the RV insertion points. The degree of fibrosis measured by MRI appears to correlate with arrhythmia risk.[42,43] In patients with HCM, LGE involving 15% of the LV myocardium is associated with a two-fold increase in the risk of sudden death in those otherwise considered to be at lower risk. These findings suggest that cardiac MRI improves risk stratification in patients with HCM.[44] Conversely, MRI and CT can be extremely useful for evaluation of resuscitated sudden death substrate in athletes, the most common cause of which is HCM, followed by anomalous origin of the coronary arteries.[45,46]

Arrhythmogenic Right Ventricular Dysplasia/Cardiomyopathy

Arrhythmogenic RV dysplasia/cardiomyopathy (ARVD/C) commonly presents with VT and is associated with SCD. ARVD/C is a genetic disease characterized by fibrofatty infiltration of the RV and, less commonly, the LV. An ICD provides reasonable therapy for patients who have one or more risk factors, including inducible VT, during electrophysiological testing.[47] The diagnosis of ARVD/C has a significant impact not only on the proband with clinical events but also on the family members. Due to its ability to characterize fibrofatty infiltration of the RV, cardiac MRI is an important adjunct diagnostic tool for the identification of ARVD/C in experienced centers. A caveat is that the inversion time for myocardial signal suppression in LGE appears to be different between the LV and RV and must be optimized. The sensitivity of cardiac MRI ranges from 79% to 89% for major criteria and from 68% to 78% for minor criteria, with a specificity of 96%–100%.[47] Substantial normal RV variations, including reduced wall motion near the moderator band, variable trabeculation, and fat deposits surrounding the coronary vessels and epicardium, can lead to reduced specificity. Importantly, assessment of RV dilation and regional function on cine images is essential to establish the correct diagnosis. Independent LV involvement is rare, and the pattern of LV involvement is determined by the underlying genotype. In patients harboring plakophilin mutations (*PKP2*), LV abnormality often occurs in the form of focal epicardial fat infiltration of the LV lateral wall with preserved LV function.[48] On the other hand, mutations in the desmoplakin (*DSP*) gene are associated with LV functional involvement. Minor MRI abnormalities in RV structure, especially in the RV outflow tract, have been reported in up to 60% of mutation

carriers and in none of the noncarriers.[48] RV LGE appears to predict inducible sustained VT in an electrophysiology study[49]; however, the prognostic value of these findings remains unclear.

Surgical Scar

Surgical scar can serve as an anatomical barrier for arrhythmic reentry. Reentrant arrhythmias observed in the postsurgical setting include VT after ventriculotomy or patch repair. CMR is capable of delineating cardiac structure and function postcardiac surgery, a setting where echocardiography is often hindered due to chest wall changes that diminish the acoustic window. RV hypertrophy on CMR is predictive of death and sustained VT in adults with repaired tetralogy of Fallot (TOF).[50] LGE-CMR has been shown to identify fibrous tissue in the postsurgical state. However, the relationship of LGE to postsurgical risk or the electroanatomical mapping substrate of VT has not been assessed.

Chagas Disease

Chagas disease results in ventricular scar and commonly manifests with VT. Importantly, VT due to Chagas disease may develop before cardiomegaly or heart failure is detected. CMR can accurately assess morphological and functional aspects of cardiac involvement in Chagas disease. Chagas disease patients with a previous documented VT event typically have fibrosis detectable by LGE-CMR.[51] The relationship of CMR findings to risk or the electroanatomical mapping substrate of VT in Chagas disease has not been prospectively assessed.

Procedure Guidance

Atrial Fibrillation

The use of cardiac MRI for substrate mapping is not limited to the LV. Techniques for evaluation of delayed enhancement within the left atrium (LA) have recently been developed.[9,52] These utilize high-resolution, thin-section 3D images acquired during free breathing using respiratory and electrocardiogram (ECG) gating to reduce motion artifacts. Images are obtained 15 to 20 minutes after gadolinium administration, and an IR pulse is utilized to null the normal myocardium and maximize the visualization of delayed enhancement. LA imaging is technically challenging as the thin walls of the LA demand very high spatial and contrast resolution that push the boundaries of current MRI technology. Imaging must be performed in sinus rhythm, due to severe gating artifacts that result from arrhythmias, limiting use in some patients. Despite these limitations, there is growing evidence that LA LGE can be reliably identified in patients with AF and that it has important prognostic implications.[53,54] LA LGE has been evaluated in patients both pre- and postablation. In imaging of preablation patients, the increased extent of LA LGE has been associated with greater procedural difficulty in achieving ablation and a higher risk of subsequent recurrence.[54-56] This suggests a role for cardiac MRI in preablation patient selection to reduce the number of ablation procedures performed in patients with a low likelihood of success. Postprocedurally, LGE-MRI has been used to identify ablation lesions in the LA wall and surrounding the pulmonary veins (Fig. 63.4) as well as gaps in circumferential pulmonary vein isolation that are associated with increased risk of recurrence.[9,53,56] In our experience, current MRI techniques lack the resolution to image all gaps in circumferential ablation lines.[57] Despite noting an association between LGE and low voltage, we noted poor diagnostic indices for the identification of scar using typical standard LGE techniques. In a subsequent study, we noted that normalization of the LGE-MRI intensity by the mean blood pool intensity results in a metric that is closely associated with intracardiac voltage as a surrogate of atrial fibrosis.[58] Additionally, we studied the feasibility of measurement and the range

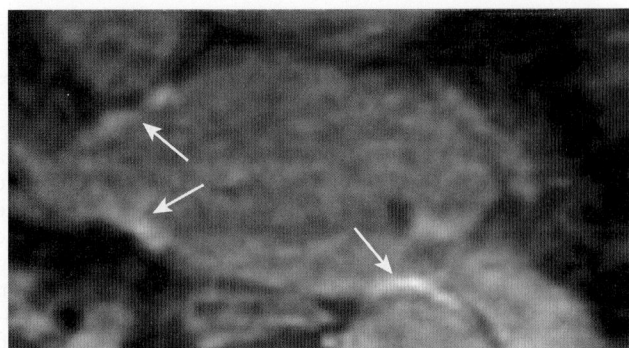

FIGURE 63.4 Postablation late gadolinium enhancement image of the left atrial myocardium. Areas surrounding the pulmonary veins are hyperenhanced following ablation (*arrows*).

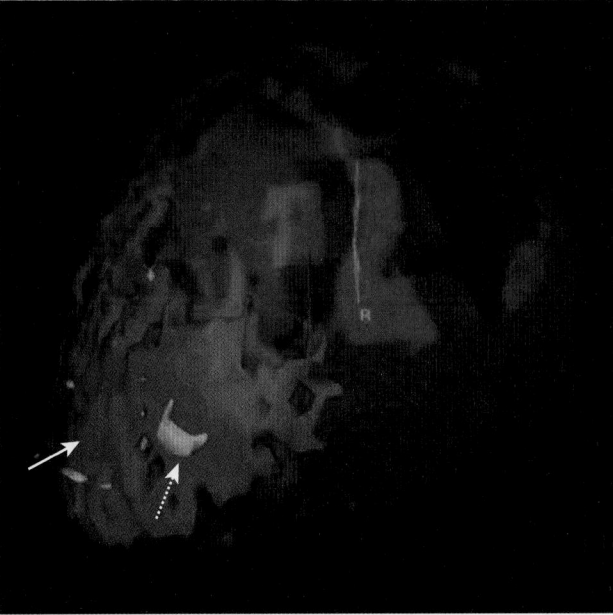

FIGURE 63.5 Segmented computed tomography–delayed enhancement image of the left ventricle shows normal myocardium in *green*, scar as *purple* (*solid arrow*), and areas of calcification as *yellow* (*dashed arrow*).

of T1 relaxation times, for quantification of diffuse LA fibrosis in patients with AF. It had previously been shown that an inverse linear relationship exists between contrast-enhanced LV myocardial T1 time and the burden of global myocardial fibrosis. We applied this technique for the first time to the assessment of myocardial characteristics in the LA. We found shorter median LA T1 relaxation times in AF patients than in healthy volunteers, suggesting an increased diffuse fibrosis in AF patients. Furthermore, AF patients with prior ablation had shorter T1 relaxation times than those without prior ablation. In addition, we established an association between LA T1 relaxation times and intracardiac bipolar LA voltages.[59] A recent study by our group showed that regardless of AF persistence at baseline, patients who undergo AF ablation with baseline LGE 35% or less have favorable outcomes, whereas those with baseline LGE greater than 35% have a higher rate of AF recurrence in the first year after ablation. These findings suggest that LGE extent is useful for patient selection prior to AF ablation. Additionally, patients with LGE extent exceeding >35% may benefit from substrate modification in addition to pulmonary vein isolation.[60]

Ventricular Tachycardia

In patients undergoing catheter ablation of scar-related VT, preprocedural cardiac CT and MRI provide important anatomical information. For example, cardiac CT identifies the locations of myocardial thinning, aneurysm, and calcification, which correspond with the myocardial scar (Fig. 63.5). Moreover, cardiac CT identifies epicardial fat that can mimic scar tissue during epicardial voltage mapping.[61]

The critical advantage of cardiac MRI in VT ablation is its ability to identify the scar regions with abnormal electrophysiology.[62] Another important advantage of cardiac MRI is that it can allow visualization of ablation lesions for prediction of clinical outcomes.[63] MRI scar integration has been applied to VT ablation procedures associated with both ICM[62,64] and NICM.[65,66] The value of MRI scar integration for guiding VT ablation is particularly high in patients with NICM, for whom no information related to the presence or location of the scar is obtained before ablation when a conventional ablation approach is used.[65,66] A significant quantitative association has been noted between local bipolar voltage in the standard electroanatomical mapping system and scar transmurality as quantified by LGE.[62,66] Prior studies have suggested that the size of the border zone between normal myocardium and dense scar associates with ventricular arrhythmia induction,[67] spontaneous ventricular arrhythmia occurrence, and sudden death. On the other hand, invasive studies from our group have suggested that critical slow conduction sites, necessary for VT initiation and maintenance, are observed in regions with nearly transmural scar on cardiac MRI.[62] Critical sites for

maintenance of VT and central common pathways for reentry are associated with >25% and >75% scar transmurality, respectively.[68] A more recent study also noted an association between VT substrate sites identified during an electrophysiology study and sites with high scar transmurality on LGE imaging.[69] Areas adjacent to both transmural scar and scar to border zone transition zones contained the majority of sites where ablation led to VT termination. Recently, infarct transmurality on MRI has been suggested as a useful criterion for the selection of a first-line combined endoepicardial ablation approach for VT in the setting of ischemic cardiomyopthy.[70] These findings are important for the formulation of ablation strategies for VT, especially when the arrhythmia is hemodynamically unstable and a priori identification of the arrhythmia substrate can decrease the procedure time devoted to mapping and substrate identification. Real-time MRI-guided electrophysiological intervention is another emerging application that can be used to take advantage of MRI technology to guide VT ablation.[71]

A potential limitation of cardiac MRI in guiding VT ablation is that most patients who are referred for VT ablation have an ICD, which is traditionally considered as a contraindication for MRI. The potential for movement of the device,[72] programming changes, asynchronous pacing, activation of tachyarrhythmia therapies, inhibition of demand pacing,[73] and induced lead currents leading to heating and cardiac stimulation[74] have led to concerns from device manufacturers and MRI authorities regarding the performance of MRI procedures in cardiac implantable device recipients. However, several studies have reported the safety of MRI in the setting of pacemakers and ICDs.[75,76] At our institution we have developed a protocol including (1) device selection based on previous in vitro and in vivo testing and (2) device programming to minimize inappropriate activation or inhibition of brady/tachyarrhythmia therapies. The protocol is unique in selecting device generators previously tested under worst-case scenario (imaging over the region containing the generator, and specific absorption rate [SAR] up to 3.5 W/kg) MRI conditions.[77] It also describes suggested steps to identify and exclude patients with leads that are more prone to heating. Programming steps to reduce the risk of inappropriate pacemaker inhibition or activation, or inappropriate activation of tachyarrhythmia functions, are also prescribed.[19,78] Using this protocol, we have now safely performed more than 2000 MRI examinations. Image quality is unaffected when the device is outside the field of view. However, thoracic images can be affected with significant susceptibility artifacts. Artifacts can be minimized by using spin-echo sequences or by shortening the echo time.[68]

Mechanical Dyssynchrony and Cardiac Resynchronization Therapy

Cardiac CT and MRI can augment echocardiography and electrocardiography in candidate selection and in preprocedural planning for cardiac resynchronization therapy (CRT). For example, cardiac CT can define the coronary sinus anatomy, which is extremely variable and often lacks an appropriate branch for optimal lead placement.[79] On the other hand, cardiac MRI can quantify myocardial scar distribution with LGE, particularly in patients with ICM. The presence of a posterolateral scar is an independent predictor of major cardiovascular events, and multisite LV pacing may be beneficial in such patients.[80]

A variety of MRI-derived indices have been proposed to quantify mechanical dyssynchrony and to predict the response to CRT. Tissue synchronization index (TSI), which represents the deviation of radial wall motion in LV short-axis cine MRI from an arbitrarily fitted sine function, is a powerful predictor of major cardiovascular events after CRT, particularly when combined with the presence of a posterolateral scar.[81] The circumferential uniformity ratio estimate (CURE), which estimates circumferential mechanical dyssynchrony on the basis of tagged cine MRI, predicts improved function class with 90% accuracy; furthermore, the accuracy improved to 95% when LGE data were added (% total scar <15%).[82] The regional vector of the circumferential strain variance (RVV), based on tagged cine MRI, predicts response to CRT independently of LGE and the origin of heart failure (ICM vs. NICM).[83] A high LGE burden is associated with a poor response to CRT. Diffuse interstitial fibrosis assessment by T1 mapping, however, is not independently predictive of CRT response.[84] Cardiac CT is also used to assess mechanical dyssynchrony on the basis of changes in wall thickness over time, but its ability to predict CRT response remains unclear.[85]

Summary

Cardiac CT and MRI have the ability to significantly augment diagnosis, patient selection, and procedural planning in cardiac electrophysiology. Technical advances in cardiac CT and MRI will continue to expand their role in cardiac electrophysiology. Development of software and hardware to enable real-time MRI guidance of interventional procedures will introduce revolutionary changes to the field of electrophysiology.

REFERENCES

1. Tao SM, Wichmann JL, Schoepf UJ, Fuller SR, Lu GM, Zhang LJ. Contrast-induced nephropathy in CT: incidence, risk factors and strategies for prevention. *Eur Radiol.* 2016;26:3310.
2. Sidhu MS, Ghoshhajra BB, Uthamalingam S, et al. Clinical experiences of delayed contrast enhancement with cardiac computed tomography: case series. *BMC Res Notes.* 2013;6:2.
3. Henzler T, Hanley M., Arnoldi E, Bastarrika G, Schoepf UJ, Becker HC.. Practical strategies for low radiation dose cardiac computed tomography. *J Thorac Imaging.* 2010;25:213–220.
4. Moloo J, Shapiro MD, Abbara S. Cardiac computed tomography: technique and optimization of protocols. *Semin Roentgenol.* 2008;43:90–99.
5. Chen CM, Liu YC, Chen CC, Wen MS, Hung CF, Wan YL. Radiation dose exposure of patients undergoing 320-row cardiac CT for assessing coronary angiography and global left ventricular function. *Int J Cardiovasc Imaging.* 2012;28(suppl 1):1–5.
6. Simonetti OP, Kim RJ, Fieno DS, et al. An improved MR imaging technique for the visualization of myocardial infarction. *Radiology.* 2001;218:215–223.
7. Kim HW, Farzaneh-Far A, Kim RJ. Cardiovascular magnetic resonance in patients with myocardial infarction: current and emerging applications. *J Am Coll Cardiol.* 2009;55:1–16.
8. Turkbey EB, Nacif MS, Guo M, et al. Prevalence and correlates of myocardial scar in a US cohort. *JAMA.* 2015;314:1945–1954.
9. Peters DC, Wylie JV, Hauser TH, et al. Detection of pulmonary vein and left atrial scar after catheter ablation with three-dimensional navigator-gated delayed enhancement MR imaging: initial experience. *Radiology.* 2007;243:690–695.
10. Broberg CS, Chugh SS, Conklin C, Sahn DJ, Jerosch-Herold M. Quantification of diffuse myocardial fibrosis and its association with myocardial dysfunction in congenital heart disease. *Circ Cardiovasc Imaging.* 2010;3:727–734.
11. Iles L, Pfluger H, Phrommintikul A, et al. Evaluation of diffuse myocardial fibrosis in heart failure with cardiac magnetic resonance contrast-enhanced T1 mapping. *J Am Coll Cardiol.* 2008;52:1574–1580.
12. Sparrow P, Messroghli DR, Reid S, Ridgway JP, Bainbridge G, Sivananthan MU. Myocardial T1 mapping for detection of left ventricular myocardial fibrosis in chronic aortic regurgitation: pilot study. *AJR Am J Roentgenol.* 2006;187:W630–W635.
13. Sueyoshi E, Sakamoto I, Uetani M. Contrast-enhanced myocardial inversion time at the null point for detection of left ventricular myocardial fibrosis in patients with dilated and hypertrophic cardiomyopathy: a pilot study. *AJR Am J Roentgenol.* 2010;194:W293–W298.
14. Turkbey EB, Gai N, Lima JA, et al. Assessment of cardiac involvement in myotonic muscular dystrophy by T1 mapping on magnetic resonance imaging. *Heart Rhythm.* 2012;9:1691–1697.
15. Hinojar R, Varma N, Child N, et al. T1 mapping in discrimination of hypertrophic phenotypes: hypertensive heart disease and hypertrophic cardiomyopathy: findings from the International T1 Multicenter Cardiovascular Magnetic Resonance Study. *Circ Cardiovasc Imaging.* 2015;8:e003285.
16. Hinojar R, Foote L, Arroyo Ucar E, et al. Native T1 in discrimination of acute and convalescent stages in patients with clinical diagnosis of myocarditis: a proposed diagnostic algorithm using CMR. *JACC Cardiovasc Imaging.* 2015;8:37–46.
17. Bohnen S, Radunski UK, Lund GK, et al. Performance of T1 and T2 mapping cardiovascular magnetic resonance to detect active myocarditis in patients with recent-onset heart failure. *Circ Cardiovasc Imaging.* 2015;8:e003073.
18. Martin DR, Krishnamoorthy SK, Kalb B, et al. Decreased incidence of NSF in patients on dialysis after changing gadolinium contrast-enhanced MRI protocols. *J Magn Reson Imaging.* 2010;31:440–446.
19. Nazarian S, Hansford R, Roguin A, et al. A prospective evaluation of a protocol for magnetic resonance imaging of patients with implanted cardiac devices. *Ann Intern Med.* 2011;155:415–424.
20. Bello D, Fieno DS, Kim RJ, et al. Infarct morphology identifies patients with substrate for sustained ventricular tachycardia. *J Am Coll Cardiol.* 2005;45:1104–1108.
21. Yan AT, Shayne AJ, Brown KA, et al. Characterization of the peri-infarct zone by contrast-enhanced cardiac magnetic resonance imaging is a powerful predictor of post-myocardial infarction mortality. *Circulation.* 2006;114:32–39.
22. Schmidt A, Azevedo CF, Cheng A, et al. Infarct tissue heterogeneity by magnetic resonance imaging identifies enhanced cardiac arrhythmia susceptibility in patients with left ventricular dysfunction. *Circulation.* 2007;115:2006–2014.
23. Ashikaga H, Sasano T, Dong J, et al. Magnetic resonance-based anatomical analysis of scar-related ventricular tachycardia: implications for catheter ablation. *Circ Res.* 2007;101:939–947.
24. Deng D, Arevalo H, Pashakhanloo F, et al. Accuracy of prediction of infarct-related arrhythmic circuits from image-based models reconstructed from low and high resolution MRI. *Front Physiol.* 2015;6:282.
25. Wu KC, Weiss RG, Thiemann DR, et al. Late gadolinium enhancement by cardiovascular magnetic resonance heralds an adverse prognosis in nonischemic cardiomyopathy. *J Am Coll Cardiol.* 2008;51:2414–2421.
26. Nazarian S, Bluemke DA, Lardo AC, et al. Magnetic resonance assessment of the substrate for inducible ventricular tachycardia in nonischemic cardiomyopathy. *Circulation.* 2005;112:2821–2825.
27. Assomull RG, Prasad SK, Lyne J, et al. Cardiovascular magnetic resonance, fibrosis, and prognosis in dilated cardiomyopathy. *J Am Coll Cardiol.* 2006;48:1977–1985.
28. Leong DP, Chakrabarty A, Shipp N, et al. Effects of myocardial fibrosis and ventricular dyssynchrony on response to therapy in new-presentation idiopathic dilated cardiomyopathy: insights from cardiovascular magnetic resonance and echocardiography. *Eur Heart J.* 2012;33:640–648.
29. Tahara N, Tahara A, Nitta Y, et al. Heterogeneous myocardial FDG uptake and the disease activity in cardiac sarcoidosis. *JACC Cardiovasc Imaging.* 2010;3:1219–1228.
30. Youssef G, Leung E, Mylonas I, et al. The use of 18F-FDG PET in the diagnosis of cardiac sarcoidosis: a systematic review and metaanalysis including the Ontario experience. *J Nucl Med.* 2012;53:241–248.
31. Patel MR, Cawley PJ, Heitner JF, et al. Detection of myocardial damage in patients with sarcoidosis. *Circulation.* 2009;120:1969–1977.
32. Murtagh G, Laffin LJ, Beshai JF, et al. Prognosis of myocardial damage in sarcoidosis patients with preserved left ventricular ejection fraction: risk stratification using cardiovascular magnetic resonance. *Circ Cardiovasc Imaging.* 2016;9:e003738.
33. Kindermann I, Barth C, Mahfoud F, et al. Update on myocarditis. *J Am Coll Cardiol.* 2012;59:779–792.
34. Friedrich MG, Sechtem U, Schulz-Menger J, et al. Cardiovascular magnetic resonance in myocarditis: a JACC White Paper. *J Am Coll Cardiol.* 2009;53:1475–1487.
35. Wright J, Adriaenssens T, Dymarkowski S, Desmet W, Bogaert J. Quantification of myocardial area at risk with T2-weighted CMR: comparison with contrast-enhanced CMR and coronary angiography. *JACC Cardiovasc Imaging.* 2009;2:825–831.
36. Vignaux O, Dhote R, Duboc D, et al. Detection of myocardial involvement in patients with sarcoidosis applying T2-weighted, contrast-enhanced, and cine magnetic resonance imaging: initial results of a prospective study. *J Comput Assist Tomogr.* 2002;26:762–767.
37. Abdel-Aty H, Cocker M, Strohm O, Filipchuk N, Friedrich MG. Abnormalities in T2-weighted cardiovascular magnetic resonance images of hypertrophic cardiomyopathy: regional distribution and relation to late gadolinium enhancement and severity of hypertrophy. *J Magn Reson Imaging.* 2008;28:242–245.
38. Abdel-Aty H, Boye P, Zagrosek A, et al. Diagnostic performance of cardiovascular magnetic resonance in patients with suspected acute myocarditis: comparison of different approaches. *J Am Coll Cardiol.* 2005;45:1815–1822.
39. Mahrholdt H, Wagner A, Deluigi CC, et al. Presentation, patterns of myocardial damage, and clinical course of viral myocarditis. *Circulation.* 2006;114:1581–1590.
40. Schumm J, Greulich S, Wagner A, et al. Cardiovascular magnetic resonance risk stratification in patients with clinically suspected myocarditis. *J Cardiovasc Magn Reson.* 2014;16:14.
41. Maron BJ, Spirito P, Shen WK, et al. Implantable cardioverter-defibrillators and prevention of sudden cardiac death in hypertrophic cardiomyopathy. *JAMA.* 2007;298:405–412.

42. Teraoka K, Hirano M, Ookubo H, et al. Delayed contrast enhancement of MRI in hypertrophic cardiomyopathy. *Magn Reson Imaging*. 2004;22:155–161.

43. Ismail TF, Prasad SK, Pennell DJ. Prognostic importance of late gadolinium enhancement cardiovascular magnetic resonance in cardiomyopathy. *Heart*. 2012;98:438–442.

44. Chan RH, Maron BJ, Olivotto I, et al. Prognostic value of quantitative contrast-enhanced cardiovascular magnetic resonance for the evaluation of sudden death risk in patients with hypertrophic cardiomyopathy. *Circulation*. 2014;130:484–495.

45. Dirksen MS, Bax JJ, Blom NA, et al. Detection of malignant right coronary artery anomaly by multi-slice CT coronary angiography. *Eur Radiol*. 2002;12(suppl 3):S177–S180.

46. White JA, Fine NM, Gula L, et al. Utility of cardiovascular magnetic resonance in identifying substrate for malignant ventricular arrhythmias. *Circ Cardiovasc Imaging*. 2012;5:12–20.

47. Epstein AE, DiMarco JP, Ellenbogen KA, et al. ACC/AHA/HRS 2008 Guidelines for Device-Based Therapy of Cardiac Rhythm Abnormalities: a report of the American College of Cardiology/American Heart Association Task Force on Practice Guidelines (Writing Committee to Revise the ACC/AHA/NASPE 2002 Guideline Update for Implantation of Cardiac Pacemakers and Antiarrhythmia Devices): developed in collaboration with the American Association for Thoracic Surgery and Society of Thoracic Surgeons. *Circulation*. 2008;117:e350–e408.

48. Dalal D, Tandri H, Judge DP, et al. Morphologic variants of familial arrhythmogenic right ventricular dysplasia/cardiomyopathy a genetics-magnetic resonance correlation study. *J Am Coll Cardiol*. 2009;53:1289–1299.

49. Corrado D, Leoni L, Link MS, et al. Implantable cardioverter-defibrillator therapy for prevention of sudden death in patients with arrhythmogenic right ventricular cardiomyopathy/dysplasia. *Circulation*. 2003;108:3084–3091.

50. Valente AM, Gauvreau K, Assenza GE, et al. Contemporary predictors of death and sustained ventricular tachycardia in patients with repaired tetralogy of Fallot enrolled in the INDICATOR cohort. *Heart*. 2014;100:247–253.

51. Rochitte CE, Oliveira PF, Andrade JM, et al. Myocardial delayed enhancement by magnetic resonance imaging in patients with Chagas' disease: a marker of disease severity. *J Am Coll Cardiol*. 2005;46:1553–1558.

52. McGann CJ, Kholmovski EG, Oakes RS, et al. New magnetic resonance imaging-based method for defining the extent of left atrial wall injury after the ablation of atrial fibrillation. *J Am Coll Cardiol*. 2008;52:1263–1271.

53. Badger TJ, Daccarett M, Akoum NW, et al. Evaluation of left atrial lesions after initial and repeat atrial fibrillation ablation: lessons learned from delayed-enhancement MRI in repeat ablation procedures. *Circ Arrhythm Electrophysiol*. 2010;3:249–259.

54. Oakes RS, Badger TJ, Kholmovski EG, et al. Detection and quantification of left atrial structural remodeling with delayed-enhancement magnetic resonance imaging in patients with atrial fibrillation. *Circulation*. 2009;119:1758–1767.

55. Seitz J, Horvilleur J, Lacotte J, et al. Correlation between AF substrate ablation difficulty and left atrial fibrosis quantified by delayed-enhancement cardiac magnetic resonance. *Pacing Clin Electrophysiol*. 2011;34:1267–1277.

56. Akoum N, Marrouche NF. Real-time imaging in electrophysiology: from intracardiac echo to real-time magnetic resonance imaging. *Europace*. 2009;11:539–540.

57. Spragg DD, Khurram I, Zimmerman SL, et al. Initial experience with magnetic resonance imaging of atrial scar and coregistration with electroanatomic voltage mapping during atrial fibrillation: success and limitations. *Heart Rhythm*. 2012;9:2003–2009.

58. Khurram IM, Beinart R, Zipunnikov V, et al. Magnetic resonance image intensity ratio, a normalized measure to enable interpatient comparability of left atrial fibrosis. *Heart Rhythm*. 2014;11:85–92.

59. Beinart R, Khurram IM, Liu S, et al. Cardiac magnetic resonance T1 mapping of left atrial myocardium. *Heart Rhythm*. 2013;10:1325–1331.

60. Khurram IM, Habibi M, Gucuk Ipek E, et al. Left atrial LGE and arrhythmia recurrence following pulmonary vein isolation for paroxysmal and persistent AF. *JACC Cardiovasc Imaging*. 2016;9:142–148.

61. Desjardins B, Morady F, Bogun F. Effect of epicardial fat on electroanatomical mapping and epicardial catheter ablation. *J Am Coll Cardiol*. 2010;56:1320–1327.

62. Sasaki T, Miller CF, Hansford R, et al. Myocardial structural associations with local electrograms: a study of postinfarct ventricular tachycardia pathophysiology and magnetic resonance-based noninvasive mapping. *Circ Arrhythm Electrophysiol*. 2012;5:1081–1090.

63. Ranjan R, Kato R, Zviman MM, et al. Gaps in the ablation line as a potential cause of recovery from electrical isolation and their visualization using MRI. *Circ-Arrhythmia Elec*. 2011;4:279–286.

64. Desjardins B, Crawford T, Good E, et al. Infarct architecture and characteristics on delayed enhanced magnetic resonance imaging and electroanatomic mapping in patients with postinfarction ventricular arrhythmia. *Heart Rhythm*. 2009;6:644–651.

65. Bogun FM, Desjardins B, Good E, et al. Delayed-enhanced magnetic resonance imaging in nonischemic cardiomyopathy utility for identifying the ventricular arrhythmia substrate. *J Am Coll Cardiol*. 2009;53:1138–1145.

66. Sasaki T, Miller CF, Hansford R, et al. Impact of non-ischemic scar features on local ventricular electrograms and scar-related ventricular tachycardia circuits in patients with nonischemic cardiomyopathy. *Circ Arrhythmia Electrophysiol*. 2013;6:1139–1147.

67. Estner HL, Zviman M, Herzka D, et al. The critical isthmus sites of ischemic ventricular tachycardia are in zones of tissue heterogeneity, visualized by magnetic resonance imaging. *Heart Rhythm*. 2011;8:1942–1949.

68. Sasaki T, Hansford R, Zviman MM, et al. Quantitative assessment of artifacts on cardiac magnetic resonance imaging of patients with pacemakers and implantable cardioverter-defibrillators. *Circ Cardiovasc Imaging*. 2011;4:662–670.

69. Piers SR, Tao Q, de Riva Silva M, et al. CMR-based identification of critical isthmus sites of ischemic and nonischemic ventricular tachycardia. *JACC Cardiovasc Imaging*. 2014;7:774–784.

70. Acosta J, Fernandez-Armenta J, Penela D, et al. Infarct transmurality as a criterion for first-line endo-epicardial substrate-guided ventricular tachycardia ablation in ischemic cardiomyopathy. *Heart Rhythm*. 2016;13:85–95.

71. Nazarian S, Kolandaivelu A, Zviman MM, et al. Feasibility of real-time magnetic resonance imaging for catheter guidance in electrophysiology studies. *Circulation*. 2008;118:223–229.

72. Shellock FG, Tkach JA, Ruggieri PM, Masaryk TJ. Cardiac pacemakers, ICDs, and loop recorder: evaluation of translational attraction using conventional ("long-bore") and "short-bore" 1.5- and 3.0-Tesla MR systems. *J Cardiovasc Magn Reson*. 2003;5:387–397.

73. Erlebacher JA, Cahill PT, Pannizzo F, Knowles RJ. Effect of magnetic resonance imaging on DDD pacemakers. *Am J Cardiol*. 1986;57:437–440.

74. Hayes DL, Holmes Jr DR, Gray JE. Effect of 1.5 tesla nuclear magnetic resonance imaging scanner on implanted permanent pacemakers. *J Am Coll Cardiol*. 1987;10:782–786.

75. Martin ET, Coman JA, Shellock FG, Pulling CC, Fair R, Jenkins K. Magnetic resonance imaging and cardiac pacemaker safety at 1.5-Tesla. *J Am Coll Cardiol*. 2004;43:1315–1324.

76. Gimbel JR, Kanal E, Schwartz KM, Wilkoff BL. Outcome of magnetic resonance imaging (MRI) in selected patients with implantable cardioverter defibrillators (ICDs). *Pacing Clin Electrophysiol*. 2005;28:270–273.

77. Roguin A, Zviman MM, Meininger GR, et al. Modern pacemaker and implantable cardioverter/defibrillator systems can be magnetic resonance imaging safe: in vitro and in vivo assessment of safety and function at 1.5 T. *Circulation*. 2004;110:475–482.

78. Nazarian S, Roguin A, Zviman MM, et al. Clinical utility and safety of a protocol for noncardiac and cardiac magnetic resonance imaging of patients with permanent pacemakers and implantable-cardioverter defibrillators at 1.5 Tesla. *Circulation*. 2006;114:1277–1284.

79. Joshi SB, Blum AR, Mansour M, Abbara S. CT applications in electrophysiology. *Cardiol Clin*. 2009;27:619–631.

80. Ginks MR, Duckett SG, Kapetanakis S, et al. Multi-site left ventricular pacing as a potential treatment for patients with postero-lateral scar: insights from cardiac magnetic resonance imaging and invasive haemodynamic assessment. *Europace*. 2012;14:373–379.

81. Leyva F, Foley PW, Stegemann B, et al. Development and validation of a clinical index to predict survival after cardiac resynchronisation therapy. *Heart*. 2009;95:1619–1625.

82. Bilchick KC, Dimaano V, Wu KC, et al. Cardiac magnetic resonance assessment of dyssynchrony and myocardial scar predicts function class improvement following cardiac resynchronization therapy. *JACC Cardiovasc Imaging*. 2008;1:561–568.

83. Petryka J, Misko J, Przybylski A, et al. Magnetic resonance imaging assessment of intraventricular dyssynchrony and delayed enhancement as predictors of response to cardiac resynchronization therapy in patients with heart failure of ischaemic and nonischaemic etiologies. *Eur J Radiol*. 2012;81:2639–2647.

84. Chen Z, Sohal M, Sammut E, et al. Focal but not diffuse myocardial fibrosis burden quantification using cardiac magnetic resonance imaging predicts left ventricular reverse modeling following cardiac resynchronization therapy. *J Cardiovasc Electrophysiol*. 2016;27:203–209.

85. Truong QA, Singh JP, Cannon CP, et al. Quantitative analysis of intraventricular dyssynchrony using wall thickness by multidetector computed tomography. *JACC Cardiovasc Imag*. 2008;1:772–781.

64 Intracardiac Echocardiography for Electrophysiology

Mathew D. Hutchinson and David J. Callans

The rapid growth in the complexity of interventional electrophysiology made the inherent limitation of fluoroscopic imaging quite clear. Although three-dimensional (3D) electroanatomical mapping and preprocedural anatomical imaging have been important in augmenting our intraprocedural understanding of cardiac and extracardiac anatomy, these modalities are potentially limited by their artificially static nature and in difficulties with adequate registration.

Intracardiac echocardiography (ICE) provides real-time imaging of cardiac and extracardiac anatomy. Catheter visualization is also possible with ICE imaging, and most importantly for effective ablation, real-time assessment of catheter contact is easily obtained. ICE imaging provides an important "reality check" for electroanatomical mapping and allows for the understanding of changes in anatomy or complications that can occur during procedures. ICE imaging does have limitations: It is essentially two-dimensional (2D), although it can be incorporated into 3D systems; and its field of view is somewhat narrow. Contemporary electrophysiology procedures require the assimilation of 2D imaging systems into 3D structures. This limitation of ICE can be overcome via integration with electroanatomical mapping systems; however, when used as a stand-alone platform, it requires some expertise in echo imaging. Nonetheless, ICE provides complimentary information to electroanatomical mapping, and vice versa. The combination provides significant improvements in efficacy and safety, particularly in complex, anatomically based ablation procedures.

Intracardiac Echocardiographic Platforms

There are two commercially available types of ICE transducers: mechanical (radial) and phased array systems. The radial ICE transducer is mounted on a 9F, nonsteerable catheter and emits an imaging beam at a 15-degree forward angle, perpendicular to the long axis of the catheter. The transducer rotates at 1800 rpm and has a fixed, 9-MHz frequency; it produces producing a 360-degree imaging plane perpendicular to the axis of the catheter. Due to limited far-field resolution and lack of steerability, the transducer is typically delivered into the chamber of interest using a curved or steerable sheath.

The phased array ICE catheter contains a 64-element transducer with a variable frequency ranging from 5 to 10 MHz, thereby providing greater flexibility to image remote structures (up to 15 cm). The phased array transducer is also capable of full spectral and color Doppler measurements, greatly enhancing the physiological data achievable. The transducer is mounted on a bi- or multidirectional 8–10F catheter. The most commonly used transducer is the AcuNav (Siemens Medical, Mountain View, CA) system, which can be deflected in four directions (anterior, posterior, right, and left) in addition to a 360-degree axial rotation. The ViewFlex Xtra (St. Jude Medical, Mountain View, CA) transducer is another phased array catheter which offers four-way tip deflection and spectral and color Doppler packages as well. Unless otherwise indicated, the remainder of this chapter will describe imaging with the phased array ICE system.

Basic Intracardiac Echocardiographic Imaging Planes

Although imaging with ICE requires a modest learning curve, it is a logical extension for operators with basic catheter manipulation and echocardiography skills. Most new operators find the images somewhat disorienting when taken out of context. Only after an individual echo "view" is integrated mentally with the operator's inherent knowledge of intracardiac anatomy does obtaining and interpreting ICE images become intuitive. It is of paramount importance to realize that the infinite potential orientations of the transducer within the cardiac chambers produce infinite possible imaging planes. To avoid confusion, it is useful to learn a few fiducial imaging planes from which an ICE survey is easily generated. The cardinal imaging plane or "home view" is obtained by placing the ICE catheter in a neutral, mid-right atrial position, at the level of the fossa ovalis. This view naturally allows visualization of the right atrium and the tricuspid valve. Clockwise rotation of the imaging catheter will produce a "survey" from the anterior to posterior atrial images (tricuspid valve, aortic valve, mitral valve/left atrial appendage [LAA], left pulmonary veins, esophagus, right pulmonary veins in sequence). From the home view, anterior deflection of the catheter with continuous imaging of the tricuspid valve allows safe passage into the right ventricle (RV). Clockwise rotation from the RV view allows a sequence of imaging targets (RV, long axis left ventricle [LV] at the level of the papillary muscles, short axis of the LV outflow tract).

Established Clinical Uses

Transseptal Puncture

The position of the fossa ovalis can be appreciated with standard fluoroscopic techniques; however, ICE imaging provides increased safety and flexibility during transseptal puncture. In many labs, transseptal for atrial fibrillation procedures is performed with double anticoagulation (maintained oral anticoagulant plus intravenous heparin), leaving no margin for error. The fossa ovalis is visualized with the ICE catheter in a mid–right atrium position and gently rotating it in a clockwise fashion (approximately 45 to 90 degrees from the home view). Variations in the left atrial "target zone" (e.g., more anterior for balloon ablation devices or LV access, more posterior for approaches to the LAA) are easily appreciated (Fig. 64.1). ICE imaging also facilitates management of anatomical variants, such as lipomatous hypertrophy and atrial septal aneurysms, as well as difficult situations such as navigating around atrial septal closure devices or scarring from prior transseptal procedures.[1,2]

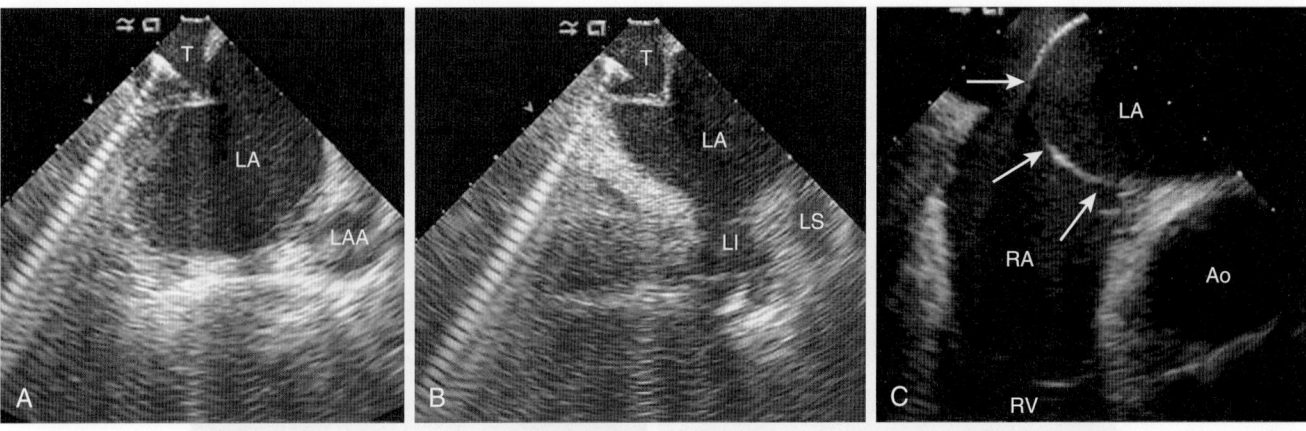

FIGURE 64.1 Using intracardiac echocardiography, the location of the transseptal needle crossing can be optimized. In (A), the transseptal (*T*) needle is directed toward the left atrial appendage (*LAA*). After slight clockwise rotation of the transseptal needle, the apparatus is now directed toward the left pulmonary veins (B). (C) depicts an interatrial septal aneurysm (*arrows*). Often the aneurysm is most prominently visualized in this anterior projection (note the aortic root [*Ao*] is seen as well). *LA,* left atrium; *LI,* Left inferior; *LS,* left superior; *RA,* right atrium; *RV,* right ventricle.

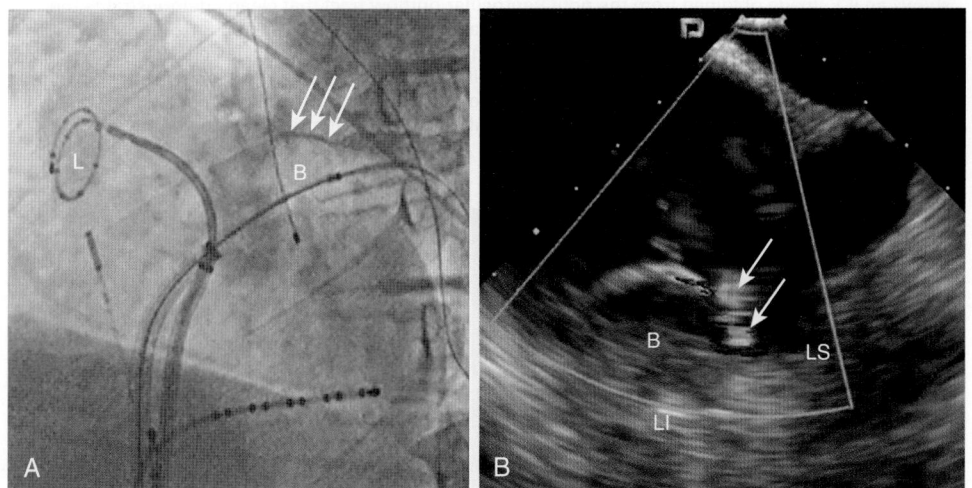

FIGURE 64.2 Intracardiac echocardiography (ICE) allows imaging of both the intracardiac anatomy and catheters and devices, allowing for anatomically accurate positioning. In this example, images are taken during cryoballoon ablation of the left inferior (*LI*) pulmonary vein. (A) is a fluoroscopic image in the left anterior oblique projection that shows the cryoballoon (*B*) placed at the ostium of the left inferior pulmonary vein. Contrast venography through the balloon internal lumen shows a small leak at the superior aspect of the vein (*arrows*). A circular mapping catheter (*L*) is also positioned in the right superior pulmonary vein. ICE can be used as an alternative to contrast angiography in these cases. (B) is a contemporaneous ICE image that shows a high velocity color jet at the superior aspect of the left inferior pulmonary vein (*arrows*). It is important to differentiate the color jet due to the balloon leak from the normal color flow pattern from the adjacent left superior (*LS*) pulmonary vein.

Atrial Fibrillation

ICE imaging is useful in multiple steps during atrial fibrillation (AF) ablation procedures: visualization of the LAA (see later), transseptal puncture, assessment of pulmonary vein anatomy, and positioning of catheters and other ablation devices (Fig. 64.2). The majority of the imaging targets for AF ablation are obtained from the right atrial, fossa ovalis view. The clockwise location discloses the LAA (60 degrees), left pulmonary veins (90 degrees), posterior atrium and adjacent esophagus (135 degrees), and right pulmonary veins (180 degrees). A useful view for visualizing the LAA as well as tracking catheter movements along the ridge between the appendage and the left pulmonary veins is obtained by positioning the imaging catheter within the RV outflow tract (Fig. 64.3).

Atrial Flutter

The majority of ablation procedures for right atrial isthmus–dependent flutter are routine, and imaging is unnecessary. Nonetheless, anatomical variants such as a prominent Eustachian ridge (which can prevent adequate ablation catheter access to the posterior isthmus) or sub-Eustachian atrial pouches (Fig. 64.4).[3] Visualization of these variants with ICE allows alterations in ablation strategy, such as the choice of a more medial or lateral linear lesion set or "doubling back" of the ablation catheter to reach under a guarding Eustachian ridge.[4]

Ventricular Tachycardia

Left Ventricular Outflow Tract. The ablation of ventricular arrhythmias arising from the LV ostium presents unique

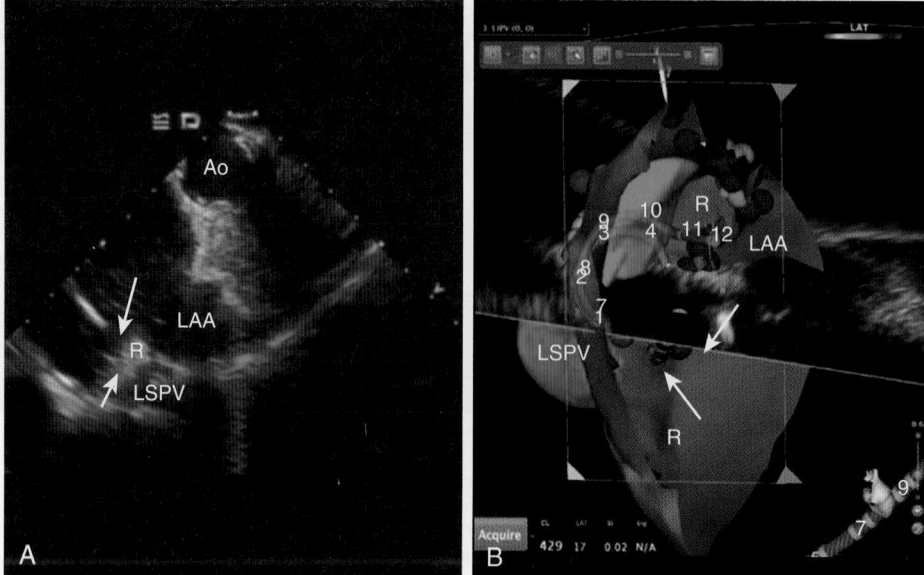

FIGURE 64.3 The integration of intracardiac echocardiography (ICE) with electroanatomical mapping systems can be helpful to guide mapping and ablation of complex or intracavitary structures. (A) shows an ICE image obtained from the right ventricular outflow tract that clearly demonstrates the coumadin ridge separating the left superior pulmonary vein (*LSPV*) from the left atrial appendage (*LAA*). Electrical isolation of the pulmonary veins requires delivering ablation lesions along the ridge, and precise localization of the ablation catheter is critical in this process. In this example, the ablation catheter tip (*arrow*) is seen on the LSPV aspect of the ridge. (B) shows the superimposition of the two-dimensional ICE image on the electroanatomical map of the left atrium. The tip of the ablation catheter (*arrow*) is again visualized within the LSPV. *Ao,* Aortic valve.

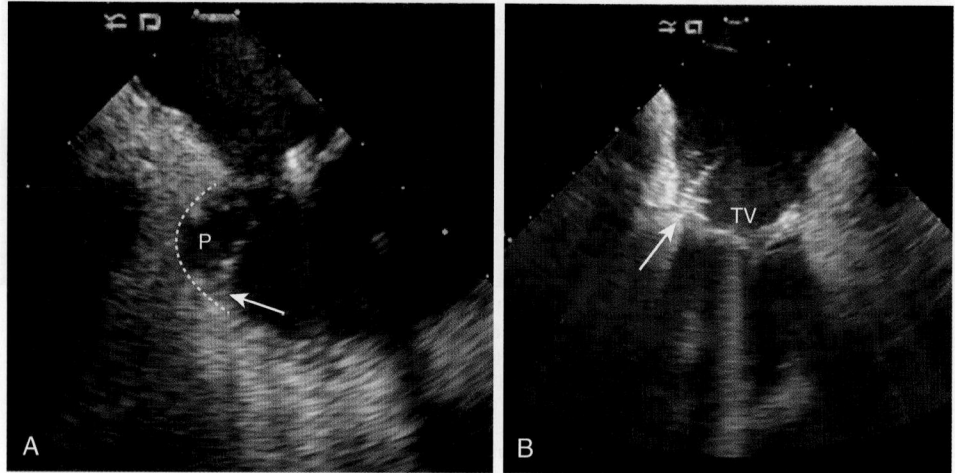

FIGURE 64.4 Intracardiac echocardiography (ICE) can be useful to guide ablation of the cavotricuspid isthmus (CTI) in patients with anatomical variants. (A) depicts a large pouch (*P*) present on the CTI. ICE assists the operator in confirming optimal contact of the ablation catheter (*arrow*) within the pouch. (B) is taken during CTI ablation of a patient with a bioprosthetic tricuspid valve (*TV*). Achieving conduction block across the CTI required ablation of the tissue beneath the valve prosthesis. ICE was used to position the ablation catheter beneath the atrial aspect of the prosthesis (*arrow*).

challenges, due in part to its complex anatomical relationships.[5] Traditional aortic root mapping using a combination of fluoroscopy and intracardiac electrogram characteristics is limited by its variable position and angulation. Since the majority of the arrhythmias targeted from the aortic root actually originate from the LV ostium, it is important to sample the entire surface of the adjacent aortic root. Incorporating ICE into these procedures allows the operator to determine not only which cusp is being sampled but also the precise aspect of the cusp.

The LV outflow tract may be visualized from the right atrium (30-degree clockwise rotation from the "home view") or from the

RV (Fig. 64.5). When imaging from the right atrium, the aortic root is seen in the long axis. This view allows the operator to determine the depth of sampling within the aortic root (e.g., sinotubular junction, cusp nadir), as well as whether the ablation catheter is located above, below, or at the level of the valve plane. The long axis view also allows the operator to determine the vertical distance of the mapping catheter from the coronary arterial ostia. By applying gentle anterior flexion of the ICE probe from the "home" view, the catheter can be easily passed through the tricuspid annulus into the RV. With 180-degree clockwise rotation, a short axis view of the aortic root is obtained. In this position, the

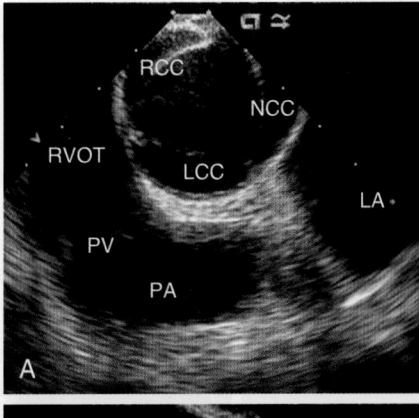

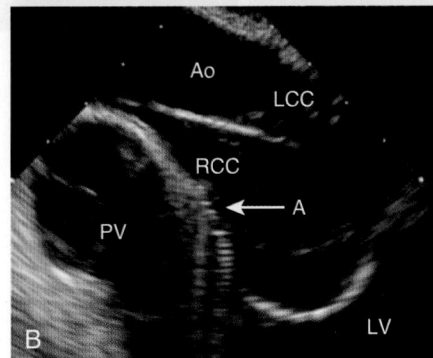

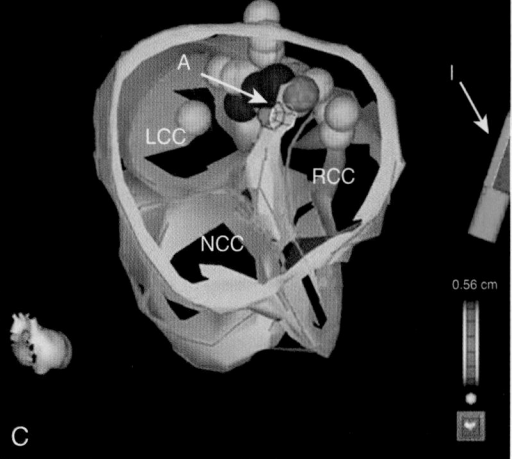

FIGURE 64.5 The aortic root (*Ao*) is viewed with intracardiac echocardiography (ICE) in the short axis from the right ventricular outflow tract (*RVOT*) (A) and in the long axis from the right atrium (B). The close spatial relationship between the right and left ventricular outflow tracts is apparent. The short axis view is used to guide mapping within and between the aortic sinuses. The long axis view demonstrates the vertical position of the mapping catheter. In (B), the ablation catheter is looped into the left ventricle and pulled back against the aortic valve plane. A three-dimensional reconstruction of the aortic sinuses (C) using the CARTO Sound system clarifies its complex anatomical relationships and facilitates catheter mapping. Both the ablation (*A*) and ICE (*I*) catheter positions are displayed in real time. The conventional ICE imaging planes in (A) and (B) are reversed to present the same orientation depicted in the electroanatomical map. *LA,* Left atrium; *LCC,* left coronary cusp; *NCC,* noncoronary cusp; *PA,* pulmonary artery; *PV,* pulmonary vein; *RCC,* right coronary cusp.

ICE probe is positioned at the inferior aspect of the RV outflow tract; the close anatomical relationships between the RV outflow tract and the right and left coronary sinuses are appreciated.

2D ICE images can be incorporated into a 3D (though static), electroanatomical mapping system reality in the CARTO Sound (Biosense Webster, Inc; Diamond Bar, CA) module. This strategy allows for the "building" of 3D chamber representations from individual 2D imaging "slices." This technique is very effective for imaging of the sinuses of Valsalva, but less so for reconstruction of the papillary muscles; because the available imaging planes limit the number of slices, interpolation results in degradation of the complex anatomical detail required for mapping these structures.

Papillary Muscle. The RV and LV papillary muscles are increasingly recognized as an important source of idiopathic ventricular arrhythmias and even triggers for ventricular fibrillation.[6] Traditional electroanatomical mapping of these structures can be challenging due to their complex structure and intracavitary position. Furthermore, since each ventricular arrhythmia originates from a discrete aspect of an individual papillary muscle, precise positioning of the ablation catheter is required to avoid ineffective lesions. Full anatomical characterization of the RV and LV papillary muscles is possible with ICE. This is accomplished from the "home" view by gently flexing the catheter anteriorly and passing it through the tricuspid annulus. From the inferior RV outflow tract, the moderator band and RV papillary apparatus are viewed directly. Counterclockwise rotation of the transducer

demonstrates the insertion of the moderator band into the RV free wall. With slow clockwise rotation from the RV views, the LV anterolateral and posteromedial papillary muscles are seen sequentially.

Visualization of Arrhythmia Substrate. Magnetic resonance imaging with delayed gadolinium enhancement is the primary modality for characterization of arrhythmia substrate.[7] This strategy may be confounded by the artifacts produced by preexisting implantable defibrillators. Since regions of fibrotic and normal myocardium differ in acoustic impedance, it is technically possible to distinguish them with ICE. Patients with postinfarction ventricular tachycardia (VT) characteristically have transmural infarctions, often with aneurysm formation. Similar to transthoracic echocardiography, postinfarct changes can also be visualized with ICE as echo-intense regions with akinesis and wall thinning. Using the CARTO Sound system, diseased myocardial segments can be traced and transposed onto the 3D electroanatomic map, thereby limiting the extent of point-to-point geometry creation. This technique of ICE-guided scar geometry creation has been shown to correlate well with bipolar mapping in postinfarction patients.[8] The detection of epicardial substrate in nonischemic cardiomyopathy can be identified by ICE imaging, as an echo-intense stripe "sandwiched" by normal myocardium.[9] This distinct echocardiographic signature may provide important insight to the presence of VT substrate deep to the endocardium and thus facilitate the decision to pursue percutaneous epicardial mapping (Fig. 64.6).

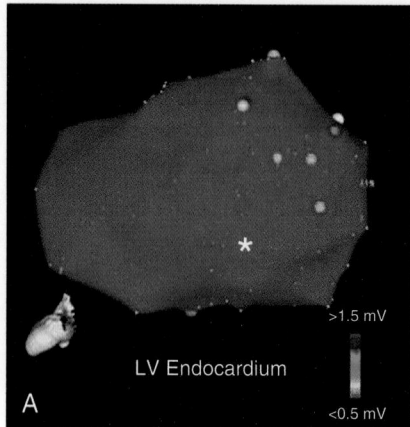
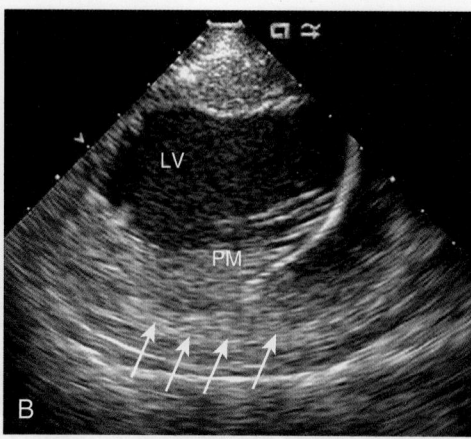
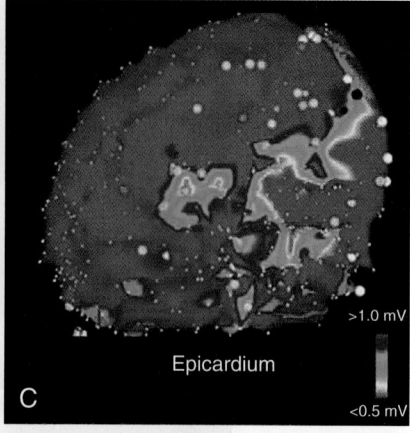

FIGURE 64.6 Images are taken from a 59-year-old man with nonischemic left ventricular (*LV*) cardiomyopathy and recurrent ventricular tachycardia (*VT*). Endocardial voltage mapping of the LV revealed normal bipolar signals (A). The earliest activation time from the endocardium was minimally presystolic (*asterisk*). (B) shows a two-dimensional intracardiac echo image depicting the mapping catheter position at the site of earliest endocardial activation (note that the intracardiac echocardiography [ICE] image orientation is reversed for comparison with voltage maps). Note the tip of the catheter positioned at the basal aspect of the posteromedial papillary muscle (*PM*) (*red arrow*). Ablation at this site produced late VT termination; however, VT remained inducible with programmed stimulation. Heterogeneity in LV echo texture is noted on the ICE image with increased hyperintensity extending from the epicardial surface to the mid myocardium (*white arrows*). This hyperintense region on ICE corresponded spatially to a large region of bipolar voltage abnormality on the epicardium (C). See text for discussion.

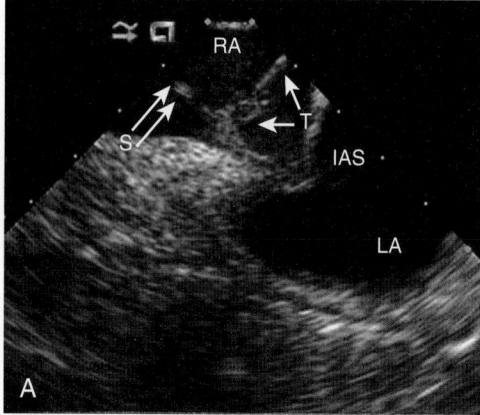
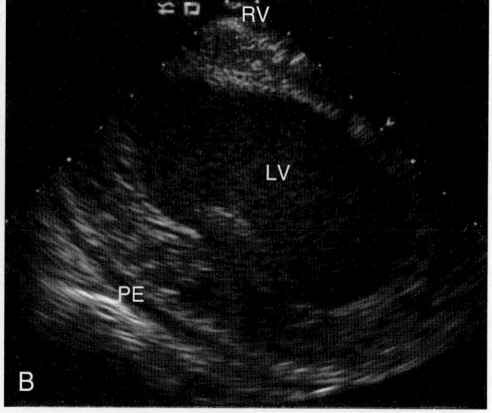

FIGURE 64.7 Procedural complications can be detected early with intracardiac echocardiography (ICE), thereby limiting potential damage. The presence of soft thrombus adherent to vascular sheaths or intracardiac leads can be visualized with ICE. (A) is an ICE image obtained from the right atrium (*RA*) demonstrating a large thrombus (*T*) attached to a transseptal sheath (*S*) that was detected during transseptal puncture; this occurred despite an activated clotting time of 360 seconds and an international normalized ratio of 3.2. The thrombus was cleared prior to left atrial crossing with no clinical sequelae. Routine ICE screening during complex ablation procedures may detect asymptomatic pericardial effusions (*PE*) prior to the development of hemodynamic compromise; this is best accomplished by placing the ICE catheter in the right ventricular outflow tract (B). (B) demonstrates a small effusion that was detected in the asymptomatic state; systemic anticoagulation was reversed thereby avoiding the need for percutaneous drainage. *IAS,* Interatrial septum; *LA,* left atrium; *LV,* left ventricle; *RV,* right ventricle.

Detecting and Preventing Complications

The contribution of ICE toward enhancing the safety of electrophysiology procedures cannot be overstated. The real-time imaging and excellent tissue resolution achieved with ICE provide maximal sensitivity to detect potential complications and to minimize the damage through rapid, early intervention. Early ICE imaging observations of sheath-related thrombus has transformed anticoagulation management during AF ablation procedures (Fig. 64.7).[10] In addition to uninterrupted oral anticoagulation, transseptal procedures are performed only after establishment of therapeutic heparin anticoagulation. Intense intraprocedural anticoagulation increases the risk of pericardial effusion after inadvertent perforation. Intermittent repositioning of the ICE catheter to the RV during AF ablation procedures allows early detection of posterior effusion; prompt reversal of anticoagulation is essential to prevent progressive hemodynamic compromise.

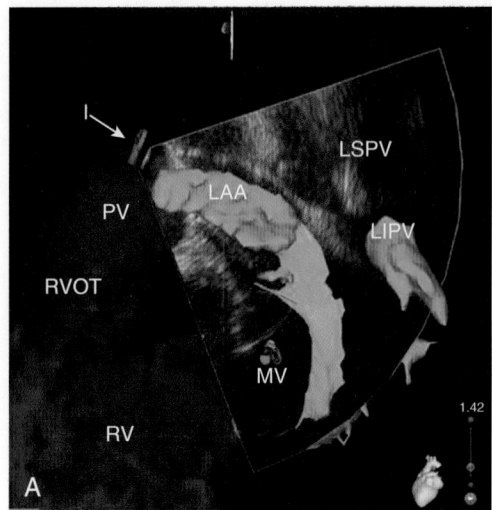
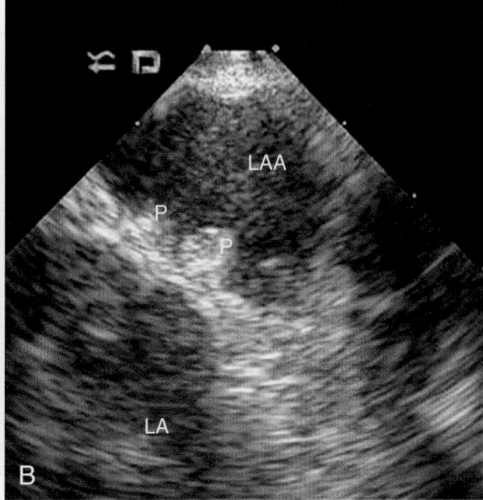

FIGURE 64.8 Systematic imaging of the left atrial appendage (*LAA*) can be reliably achieved with intracardiac echocardiography (ICE) by placing the imaging transducer into the proximal pulmonary artery (PA) (i.e., through the pulmonary valve [*PV*]). (A) shows a coregistered tomographic reconstruction of the right ventricle, proximal PA, and left atrium with the LAA. The tip of the ICE probe (*I*) is visualized within the proximal PA, and the corresponding two-dimensional imaging plane is shown. (B) shows the LAA in the short axis (image slightly enlarged and cropped for demonstration) with prominent pectinate musculature. With the ICE probe thus positioned, the remainder of the LAA is imaged with further rightward rotation of the catheter. *LIPV,* Left inferior pulmonary vein; *LSPV,* left superior pulmonary vein; *MV,* mitral valve; *P,* pectinate muscle; *RV,* right ventricle; *RVOT,* right ventricular outflow tract.

Novel/Clinical Uses in Development

Left Atrial Appendage Visualization

The routine use of ICE imaging in lieu of transesophageal echocardiography (TEE) to exclude the presence of thrombus in the LAA in high risk patients remains controversial. When a full array of imaging locations is utilized (including pulmonary artery and potentially coronary sinus locations), superior, albeit single plane, images of the LAA are possible in the majority of patients. The ICE-CHIP study prospectively compared LAA imaging with transesophageal echo versus phased array ICE. This study found incomplete LAA imaging with ICE in 15% of patients, as well as a lower sensitivity to detect LAA thrombus compared to TEE.[11] The comparative image quality in ICE-CHIP was potentially biased by the exclusive use of a right atrial imaging plane with ICE.

The Action ICE study evaluated 76 patients undergoing ablation for AF with TEE and ICE imaging (with expert echocardiographer analysis) using multiple imaging planes.[12] High quality images of the entire LAA were obtained in 56 of 64 patients (87.5%) with imaging from the pulmonary artery, 13 of 49 (26.5%) from the coronary sinus, and 0 of 76 patients from the right atrium. In all, complete imaging of the LAA was accomplished with ICE in 78% of patients, but it is not clear why all patients were not imaged from all locations. In patients who had complete visualization of the LAA with ICE, there was perfect agreement with TEE in terms of identification of LAA thrombus (2 patients).

A recent report by Anter and colleagues compared contemporaneous TEE and ICE imaging of the right and LAAs in a cohort of 71 patients undergoing atrial ablation.[13] This report differed from ICE-CHIP in that LAA imaging was performed with the ICE probe positioned in the proximal pulmonary artery. The authors found a strong correlation in appendage dimensions between the two modalities, although TEE imaging was not possible in two patients due to a failure to intubate the esophagus. Atrial thrombi were also detected in four ICE studies, compared to one TEE. Importantly, these results were obtained based on image interpretation by expert echocardiographers and may not

be directly translated to most electrophysiological laboratories. Nonetheless, this study highlights the feasibility and safety of ICE as a stand-alone procedure for LA and LAA evaluation (Fig. 64.8).

Considerable interest exists for the potential use of ICE imaging to guide LAA occlusion device procedures. At present, the absence of multiplane imaging is a significant limitation, and most of these procedures are best guided by TEE.

Low/Zero Fluoroscopy Procedures

Several laboratories have devised strategies for low or zero fluoroscopy usage, even for complex ablation procedures such as AF ablation.[14,15] Zero fluoroscopy strategies typically utilize 3D mapping (for chamber reconstruction and lesion delivery; reference is usually to a coronary sinus catheter which is positioned "blindly" using electrograms only) and ICE. In addition to the standard uses of ICE imaging in AF ablation discussed above, ICE imaging of the positioning of wires in the superior vena cava (to ensure safe advancement of transseptal sheaths) is a necessary part of this strategy.

Lesion Assessment

The advantages of lesion visualization are obvious. When delivering lesions during ongoing tachycardia, the failure to terminate the arrhythmia could be due to inadequate lesion delivery or imprecision in mapping; our inability to determine which prevents logical procedural execution. During the creation of more anatomical lesion sets (such as pulmonary vein isolation), the ability to verify that lesions were not only successfully created but also contiguous would greatly facilitate success. The delivery of ablation lesions, even in scarred myocardium, results in changes in near field tissue imaging; most commonly, increased tissue echo density and wall thickness are noted.[16] Near field rotational ICE, positioned within the targeted pulmonary vein, has been demonstrated useful to guide lesion creation in pulmonary vein isolation.[17] The presence of heterogeneous myocardial perfusion with ICE after intracoronary contrast administration has also been correlated with lesion pathology in an animal model.[18] Theoretically, all ablation lesions could be visualized by ICE;

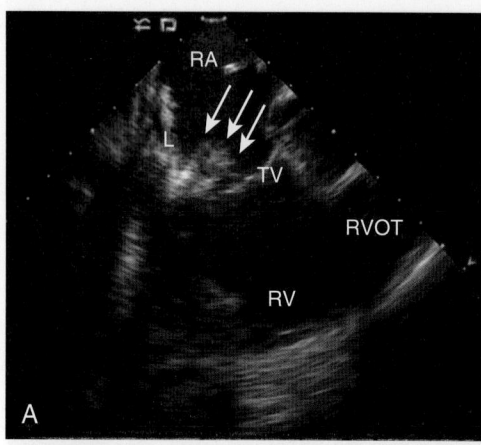
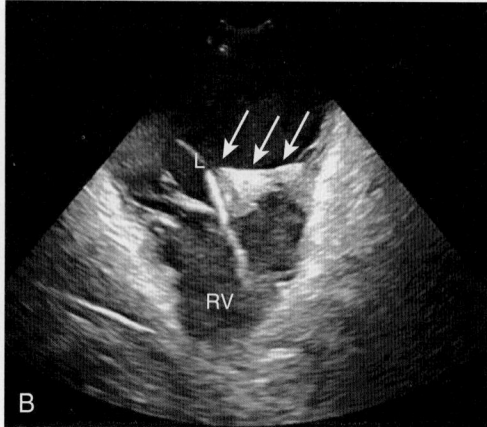

FIGURE 64.9 Images are taken from two patients undergoing laser lead extraction. The patient shown in (A) has large, mobile vegetation (*arrows*) present on the atrial aspect of the right ventricular (*RV*) lead (*L*). Since extraction necessarily produces embolization of these vegetations, an accurate determination of their size and shape has important implications regarding their potential hemodynamic consequences. (B) shows the broad attachment of the RV lead to the subvalvular apparatus of the tricuspid valve (*TV*). *RA,* Right atrium; *RVOT,* right ventricular outflow tract. (Courtesy Robert Schaller, MD.)

however, in clinical practice, this is limited by the narrow slices provided by ICE imaging. "Side-firing" ICE imaging, built into ablation catheters, would provide a more consistent evaluation of lesion creation. In an open chest sheep model, Wright and coworkers demonstrated consistent real-time ICE imaging during the creation of atrial and ventricle lesions in an open chest sheep model.[19] M-mode ICE imaging (changes in tissue brightness) correlated well with pathologically confirmed lesion depth at tissue depths up to 5 mm. Unfortunately, the authors are unaware of the clinical developments for such ICE platforms.

Lead Management

Although certainly not as a matter of routine clinical practice, ICE imaging may prove helpful in some elements of lead management. ICE imaging was demonstrated to be superior to transthoracic echocardiography in detecting lead thrombus on the ICD leads and superior to TEE for imaging to confirm or reject a clinical diagnosis of lead-related endocarditis.[20,21] We use ICE routinely to guide lead extraction, particularly to understand which portions of the lead are the most adherent to the underlying venous or myocardial structures (Fig. 64.9), and to provide rapid detection of complications (such as lead related tricuspid regurgitation or pericardial effusion).

Summary

ICE imaging provides real-time visualization of intracardiac catheters and cardiac as well as extracardiac anatomical structures. In many laboratories, ICE is used routinely in complex ablation procedures to provide an anatomical method of "grounding" 3D mapping systems. It has established and proven benefits for the performance of transseptal puncture, AF, and VT ablation. There is no more immediate method for the detection of intraprocedural complications. There is growing enthusiasm for developing uses of ICE for LAA imaging, ablation lesion assessment, and lead management. Although some degree of experience is required for image interpretation, most operators find the phased array views quite similar in orientation to TEE.

REFERENCES

1. Santangeli P, Di Biase L, Burkhardt JD, et al. Transseptal access and atrial fibrillation ablation guided by intracardiac echocardiography in patients with atrial septal closure devices. *Heart Rhythm.* 2011;8:1669–1675.
2. Arkles J, Zado E, Supple G, et al. Feasibility of transseptal access in patients with previously scarred or repaired interatrial septum. *J Cardiovasc Electrophysiol.* 2015;26:963–996.
3. Asirvatham SJ. Correlative anatomy and electrophysiology for the interventional electrophysiologist: right atrial flutter. *J Cardiovasc Electrophysiol.* 2009;20:113–122.
4. Morton JB, Sanders P, Davidson NC, et al. Phased-array intracardiac echocardiography for defining cavotricuspid isthmus anatomy during radiofrequency ablation of typical atrial flutter. *J Cardiovasc Electrophysiol.* 2003;14:591–597.
5. Yamada T, Litovsky SH, Kay GN. The left ventricular ostium: An anatomic concept relevant to idiopathic ventricular arrhythmias. *Circ Arrhythm Electrophysiol.* 2008;1:396–404.
6. Sadek MM, Benhayon D, Sureddi R, et al. Idiopathic ventricular arrhythmias originating from the moderator band: electrocardiographic characteristics and treatment by catheter ablation. *Heart Rhythm.* 2015;12:67–75.
7. Bogun FM, Desjardins B, Good E, et al. Delayed-enhanced magnetic resonance imaging in nonischemic cardiomyopathy: utility for identifying the ventricular arrhythmia substrate. *J Am Coll Cardiol.* 2009;53:1138–1145.
8. Khaykin Y, Skanes A, Whaley B, et al. Real-time integration of 2D intracardiac echocardiography and

3D electroanatomical mapping to guide ventricular tachycardia ablation. *Heart Rhythm.* 2008;5:1396–1402.
9. Bala R, Ren JF, Hutchinson MD, et al. Assessing epicardial substrate using intracardiac echocardiography during vt ablation. *Circ Arrhythm Electrophysiol.* 2011;4:667–673.
10. Ren JF, Marchlinski FE, Callans DJ, et al. Increased intensity of anticoagulation may reduce risk of thrombus during atrial fibrillation ablation procedures in patients with spontaneous echo contrast. *J Cardiovasc Electrophysiol.* 2005;16:474–477.
11. Saksena S, Jordaens L, Kusumoto F, et al. A prospective comparison of cardiac imaging using intracardiac echocardiography with transesophageal echocardiography in patients with atrial fibrillation: the intracardiac echocardiography guided cardioversion helps interventional procedures study. *Circ Arrhythm Electrophysiol.* 2010;3:571–577.
12. Baran J, Stec S, Pilichowska-Paszkiet E, et al. Intracardiac echocardiography for detection of thrombus in the left atrial appendage: comparison with transesophageal echocardiography in patients undergoing ablation for atrial fibrillation: the Action-ICE Study. *Circ Arrhythm Electrophysiol.* 2013;6:1074–1081.
13. Anter E, Silverstein J, Tschabrunn CM, et al. Comparison of intracardiac echocardiography and transesophageal echocardiography for imaging of the right and left atrial appendages. *Heart Rhythm.* 2014;11:1890–1897.
14. Ferguson JD, Helms A, Mangrum JM, et al. Catheter ablation of atrial fibrillation without fluoroscopy using

intracardiac echocardiography and electroanatomic mapping. *Circ Arrhythm Electrophysiol.* 2009;2:611–619.
15. Reddy VY, Morales G, Ahmed H, et al. Catheter ablation of atrial fibrillation without the use of fluoroscopy. *Heart Rhythm.* 2010;7:1644–1653.
16. Ren JF, Callans DJ, Schwartzman D, et al. Changes in local wall thickness correlate with pathologic lesion size following radiofrequency catheter ablation: an intracardiac echocardiographic imaging study. *Echocardiography.* 2001;18:503–507.
17. Mangrum JM, Mounsey JP, Kok LC, et al. Intracardiac echocardiography-guided, anatomically based radiofrequency ablation of focal atrial fibrillation originating from pulmonary veins. *J Amer Coll Cardiol.* 2002;39:1964–1972.
18. Khoury DS, Rao L, Ding C, et al. Localizing and quantifying ablation lesions in the left ventricle by myocardial contrast echocardiography. *J Cardiovasc Electrophysiol.* 2004;15:1078–1087.
19. Wright M, Harks E, Deladi S, et al. Real-time lesion assessment using a novel combined ultrasound and radiofrequency ablation catheter. *Heart Rhythm.* 2011;8:304–312.
20. Supple GE, Ren JF, Zado ES, Marchlinski FE. Mobile thrombus on device leads in patients undergoing ablation: identification, incidence, location, and association with increased pulmonary artery systolic pressure. *Circulation.* 2011;124:772–778.
21. Narducci ML, Pelargonio G, Russo E, et al. Usefulness of intracardiac echocardiography for the diagnosis of cardiovascular implantable electronic device-related endocarditis. *J Amer Coll Cardiol.* 2013;61:1398–1405.

65 Exercise-Induced Arrhythmias

Antonio B. Fernandez, Eric M. Crespo, and Paul D. Thompson

Exercise and sports participation have increased among the US population over the last few decades.[1] The increase in cardiovascular disease awareness and the multiple initiatives to increase health promotion and disease prevention[2] also encourage exercise and sports participation. The impetus behind these initiatives is to maintain or improve cardiac health. However, several physiological changes that occur during exercise can increase the risk of arrhythmias and sudden cardiac death (SCD) in some individuals with undiagnosed cardiac pathology. Therefore it is important for clinicians to be aware of the most common exercise-induced arrhythmias and their management. We will review some of the exercise-induced physiological changes related to the development and maintenance of arrhythmias in athletes. We will also discuss the salient clinical and electrocardiographic features of exercise-induced atrial and ventricular arrhythmias and their management.

Physiological Changes During Exercise Related to Arrhythmia Development

In humans and in trained animals, anticipation of physical activity inhibits vagus nerve impulses to the heart; this withdrawal of vagus nerve activity underlies the initial increase in heart rate. Subsequently, sympathetic nerve discharge increases. The concerted inhibition of parasympathetic areas and the activation of sympathetic areas of the medulla increase the heart rate and myocardial contractility. The tachycardia and the enhanced contractility increase the cardiac output and systemic blood pressure. Similar to other adrenal hormones, increased secretion of catecholamines is directly related to exercise intensity. Endurance-trained athletes have a higher catecholaminergic response to exercise. This phenomenon is referred to as the "sports adrenal medulla."[3] Long-term endurance training can increase plasma catecholamine concentrations in response to supramaximal exercise.[4] The increase in catecholamine increases automaticity and triggered activity, which may increase the likelihood of arrhythmias during exercise.

The circulatory adjustment to prolonged exercise involves the local formation of vasoactive metabolites and vasodilation of resistance vessels in the active muscle. Potassium (K^+) is one of the substances released by contracting muscle, and it may be responsible, in part, for the decrease in vascular resistance by stimulating the Na^+-K^+ pump and by activation of the inward rectifier K^+ channels.[5] In fact, prolonged exercise can double the plasma concentration of K^+, decrease the plasma pH by up to 0.4 unit, and increase catecholamine levels by 15-fold.[6] These exercise-induced changes are usually well tolerated in the absence of cardiac disease. The mechanism whereby the heart is protected from the chemical stress caused by these changes is not fully understood, but it may be related to a net antiarrhythmic effect of the combination of these changes. Catecholamines can offset the harmful effects of hyperkalemia and acidemia by improving action-potential characteristics in the K^+-depolarized ventricular myocytes. This results from an increase in the inward Ca^{2+} current that is modulated by catecholamines. Conversely, hyperkalemia can reduce or abolish the incidence of norepinephrine-induced arrhythmias. This mutual antagonism is compromised, however, when these changes occur in an infarcted or ischemic myocardium.[6] The volume shifts induced by acute exercise can cause myocardial stretching and baroreceptor activation. These phenomena can also increase arrhythmogenicity during exertion. Exercise can also increase the frequency of premature ventricular complexes, which can lead to reentrant supraventricular and ventricular arrhythmias.[7]

Exercise-Induced Supraventricular Arrhythmias

Exercise-induced supraventricular tachycardias (SVTs) are less common than exercise-induced ventricular arrhythmias. SVTs are not more common in athletes than in the general population, with the exception of atrial fibrillation (AF). In the Baltimore Longitudinal Study of Aging, 1383 asymptomatic, apparently healthy volunteers aged 20 to 94 years underwent maximal treadmill exercise testing. Only 85 men and women developed exercise-induced SVT (6%). The prevalence of exercise-induced SVT increased with age in men but not in women. The majority (98%) of the 141 discrete episodes of exercise-induced SVT were paroxysmal, with heart rates varying from 105 to 290 beats/min. Only 16% were greater than 10 beats in duration, and only 4% were symptomatic. Nearly half (44%) of the SVT episodes occurred at peak effort. Coronary risk factors, left atrial size determined by echocardiography, and the prevalence of exercise-induced ischemia were similar between the participants with and without SVT.[8]

A possible link between AF and the amount of physical activity was first noted in a case-control study in 1998.[9] Another case-control study also reported a higher proportion of sportsmen among patients with "lone AF" than in age- and sex-matched controls.[10] An 11-year follow-up of Barcelona Marathon runners also found that the diagnosis of AF was 8.8-fold higher in the runners than in a sedentary cohort.[11] Similar observations have been reported in elite cyclists[12] and Nordic skiers.[13] Together, these data suggest a three- to eight-fold higher risk of AF in top-level athletes. Epidemiological studies in the general population have also confirmed a higher incidence of AF in individuals with the highest levels of physical activity.[14]

Factors increasing left atrial size or pressure, such as hypertension, left systolic or diastolic heart failure, and mitral stenosis or regurgitation, increase the risk for AF. Increases in preload seen in endurance sports can also increase atrial pressure, shorten the atrial refractory period, and increase the dispersion of atrial refractoriness, all of which increase the risk for AF.[15] Increases in both parasympathetic and sympathetic tone also increase the risk of AF.[16] Increased parasympathetic tone, characteristic of endurance training, shortens the atrial refractory period by decreasing the inward current of the L-type calcium channels.[17] Shortening the atrial refractory period facilitates atrial reentry. Increased sympathetic activity shortens the atrial action potential and produces microreentry atrial circuits, both factors involved in initiating AF.[18] Left atrial size is often increased in endurance athletes, which can also facilitate the initiation and maintenance of AF.[19]

Diagnostic Approach

Athletes with AF should undergo thyroid function tests, be queried about drugs (particularly stimulants) and excessive caffeine and alcohol use, and undergo echocardiography to exclude structural heart disease. An electrocardiogram (ECG) should be obtained and examined for pericarditis, which can provoke new AF.[20] An initial ECG may show persistent AF, but brief or episodic symptoms suggestive of AF generally require longer-term monitoring using a 24-hour ECG, if symptoms are a daily or 30-day event, or implantable devices, if the symptoms are infrequent. AF can also be diagnosed and monitored when infrequent using smartphone-based technology such as AliveCor heart monitor (AliveCor, San Francisco, CA). If symptoms occur during exercise, a treadmill test mimicking the exercise that provokes symptoms may be useful for detecting AF.

Therapeutic Approach in Athletes With Atrial Fibrillation

Treatment of AF in athletes is similar to that in the general population; however, it can often be more challenging. Most athletes desire to continue exercising at high levels, and AF will likely impair their physical performance. Therefore most active individuals require a rhythm control strategy. In endurance athletes (marathon runners, cyclists, etc.), a reduction in exercise intensity or duration may also reduce the AF burden, but many patients, especially competitive athletes, are understandably unwilling to reduce or refrain from exercise. Reduction in exercise intensity is generally not an issue in those who pursue exercise at only a light or moderate intensity; in fact, in less active patients, there is evidence that increasing exercise has beneficial effects on AF burden and symptoms.[21] Any treatment strategy will need to be individualized based on objective data and patient preference.

The most commonly utilized rate control agents are β-adrenergic blockers; however, effective doses are often not tolerated in athletes due to an already low resting heart rate or because the negative chronotropic effects decrease exercise performance. Athletes taking β-blockers often report that a much longer warm-up period is required and the heart rate at peak exertion is reduced. These side effects are generally unacceptable to competitive athletes. We occasionally add digitalis to modest-dose β-blocker therapy to mitigate these issues. Extended-release diltiazem is an alternative that is often better tolerated because it seems to have less negative chronotropy; however, individual responses vary. In the end, there is usually a need to experiment with a variety of agents to find the best regimen for a particular patient.

For patients with rare episodes of AF, we use the "pill-in-the pocket" approach with either flecainide or propafenone.[22] Specifically, when the patient recognizes AF, he/she takes either flecainide 300 mg or 200 mg or propafenone 600 mg or 450 mg depending on body weight greater than or less than 70 kg, respectively. At the same time, a dose of either β-blocker or calcium channel blocker is taken. It is important that this be a short-acting (i.e., rapid onset of action) formulation and not an extended-release form. Concomitant atrioventricular (AV) nodal blockade is mandatory because class I antiarrhythmics

can organize AF into atrial flutter with 1:1 AV conduction (Na$^+$ channel blockade slows the atrial conduction velocity and thus prolongs the flutter cycle length, which in turn leads to less resistance to AV nodal conduction). Some physicians also instruct patients, among those with risk factors, with a high thrombotic risk to take one of the novel oral anticoagulants (NOACs), in case the AF does not resolve and a cardioversion is subsequently needed. Whichever agents are chosen, the patient should be monitored the first time the strategy is utilized. This is generally done in the emergency room or via a brief "observation" in the hospital (usually 6–8 hours following administration). A prescription is then given if the medication is effective and well tolerated. Patients are instructed to rest and avoid driving for at least 4 hours after they take the medication.

For athletes and active individuals with more frequent episodes of AF and a normal heart, we use chronic suppression with a class I antiarrhythmic medication (flecainide or propafenone) and an AV nodal blocking agent. Class I drugs should never be prescribed without concomitant AV nodal blockade. In patients with a resting heart rate less than 50 to 55 beats/min, these agents may not be tolerated, and dofetilide, which is a class III agent and has no effect on heart rate, may be an option. Anticoagulation with warfarin or an NOAC is recommended depending on the individual's risk for thrombosis (CHA2DS2-VASc score). Active subjects who cannot be readily managed with medical therapy should be considered for radiofrequency ablation. Ablation is often preferable to lifelong therapy with pharmacological agents in this population.[20] In athletes with AF, when antithrombotic therapy, other than aspirin, is indicated, it is reasonable to consider the bleeding risk in the specific sport before allowing participation.[20]

Atrial flutter may also be more common in athletes.[12] The evaluation and consideration for anticoagulation is identical to that for AF. However, rate control of atrial flutter is often difficult, and given the high cure rates of ablation and the low complication risk, atrial flutter ablation should be the rhythm control strategy of choice for those with typical cavotriscuspid isthmus–dependent flutter.[20]

Other Supraventricular Arrhythmias

AV nodal reentry tachycardia (AVNRT), AV reciprocating tachycardia (AVRT), and atrial tachycardia share multiple similarities and are considered as a single group. They are discussed in greater detail in other chapters. They present with sudden onset and termination, rates between 150 and 250 beats/min, a regular and narrow QRS, and termination with adenosine. The latter is more likely to be effective in AVRT and ANVRT than in atrial tachycardia. Occasionally, these SVTs can present as a wide-complex tachycardia if a bypass tract is present or if the impulses are aberrantly conducted. Since the ECG appearance of these SVTs can be similar, the definite diagnosis often requires an invasive electrophysiological study (EPS). As with other arrhythmias associated with exercise, the evaluation should include an ECG and echocardiogram. Treatment options can include β-blockers, antiarrhythmic agents, and catheter ablation. However, given the high success and low complication rates, ablation is the treatment of choice in young healthy individuals.[23]

Manifest preexcitation (delta-wave) is found on the 12-lead surface ECG of some athletes. This finding often leads to great consternation due to the association with sudden death. The risk of SCD is due to the possibility of SVT leading to the induction of AF; this can then be rapidly conducted to the ventricles over the accessory pathway, with the subsequent rapid ventricular response degenerating to ventricular fibrillation (VF). While the true number of sudden deaths in athletes due to unrecognized preexcitation is not clear, it appears to be low. In fact, it accounted for less than 1% of the cardiovascular sudden deaths among young athletes in one registry.[24]

While the management of athletes with symptomatic preexcitation (Wolff-Parkinson-White syndrome) is fairly straightforward (catheter ablation), the assessment and treatment of asymptomatic individuals (i.e., those found only through preparticipation screening) is less clear, with the relatively small risk of invasive intervention weighed against the small risk of sudden arrhythmic death. In general, some form of risk stratification is recommended. This begins with an echocardiogram to rule out structural heart disease and a careful history taking to determine whether the symptoms are arrhythmic in nature. This needs to be followed by some assessment regarding whether the pathway is capable of rapid anterograde conduction. The finding of intermittent preexcitation on serial ECGs or on extended monitoring is reassuring. Similarly, the abrupt loss of preexcitation during an exercise treadmill test suggests that the pathway is not capable of rapid conduction. Care needs to be taken to ensure that there is true loss of preexcitation and not simply a reduced preexcitation due to enhanced AV node conduction during exercise. This distinction can sometimes be challenging, and many treadmill tests are nondiagnostic. If a noninvasive assessment is inconclusive or if the patient prefers an invasive approach, an EPS is the gold standard for assessing an accessory pathway. The absence of high-risk findings on an EPS has a negative predictive value of greater than 90%[25] and is very reassuring. The following findings suggest a "high-risk" pathway: (1) shortest preexcited RR interval less than 250 ms during induced AF, (2) accessory pathway effective refractory period less than 240 ms, (3) presence of multiple accessory pathways, (4) ability to induce sustained AVRT, and (5) finding of AVRT precipitating AF. See Chapters 77 and 78 for a more complete description of preexcitation and AV reentry variants.

Exercise-Induced Ventricular Arrhythmias

Premature Ventricular Contractions and Nonsustained Ventricular Tachycardia in Apparently Healthy Subjects

Asymptomatic patients without any evidence of coronary artery disease (CAD) have variable rates of ventricular ectopy. In the Baltimore Longitudinal Study of Aging, 2099 men and women, mean age 52 years, underwent serial stress testing. Only 3.7% (n = 79) of participants free of known cardiovascular disease who completed a symptom-limited treadmill test developed nonsustained ventricular tachycardia (NSVT) with exercise. The mean duration of NSVT was three beats, and the median rate was 175 beats/min. The participants who developed NSVT were older and were more likely to be male and to have baseline ECG abnormalities or ischemic ST-segment changes with exercise. However, over a mean follow-up of 13.5 years, no association was found between NSVT and mortality.[26] Among 1640 healthy military aviators, the prevalence of premature ventricular complexes (PVCs) (other than single or occasional) increased with age from 6.6% for ages 20–29 to 7.6% for ages 30–39 and to 13.1% for ages 40–53. The percentage of patients with three or more consecutive PVCs was 0.8% for ages 20–29, 1.0% for ages 30–39, and 3.5% for ages 40–53.[27] These results support the notion that PVCs and NSVT in asymptomatic individuals are generally benign. The finding of complex ventricular arrhythmias (polymorphic PVCs/VT), however, should spur further investigation.

Outflow Tract Ventricular Tachycardia

Outflow tract ventricular tachycardia should be considered in patients with a structurally normal heart and ventricular tachycardia (VT), with a left bundle branch block (LBBB) morphology and an inferior axis. The majority (close to 80%) of the outflow tract VTs originate from the right ventricular outflow tract (RVOT). Most of the remainder originate from the left ventricular outflow tract (LVOT).[28]

Outflow tract VTs are the product of triggered activity secondary to cyclic adenosine monophosphate–mediated delayed afterdepolarizations. The VT is catecholamine-mediated and is sensitive to perturbations such as adenosine and verapamil, which lower intracellular calcium.[29]

The age at presentation for outflow tract VT is usually 30 to 50 years, and patients generally have a benign clinical course. The most common complaint among patients is palpitations (48%–80%), followed by presyncope or light headedness (28%–50%). Syncope is rare (<10%), and SCD is extremely rare. However, some patients may develop a tachycardia-induced cardiomyopathy from repetitive monomorphic VT or from a high burden of PVCs.[28] Ablation of the focus usually normalizes left ventricular (LV) function in a few months.

The spectrum of outflow tract VT includes three clinical subtypes. Patients may have repetitive monomorphic PVCs, repetitive nonsustained monomorphic VT, or exercise-induced sustained VT. Patients may present with a predominance of one type; however, there is significant overlap, and the subtypes probably share the same cellular mechanism.[30] Generally, outflow tract tachycardias are provoked by exercise, and treadmill testing is useful in reproducing the VT. Approximately 70% of patients who present with sustained VT will have VT induced by exercise testing.[30]

Two responses of outflow tract VT to exercise testing have been reported. In the first case, VT occurs during acceleration of heart rate with exercise. A progression from PVCs to salvos of NSVT and then to sustained VT may occur. In contrast, patients with repetitive monomorphic VT may have suppression of their VT during exercise and development of VT during the recovery phase of exercise.[31] These responses indicate that a critical window of heart rate is required for VT initiation. This cycle-length dependence of ventricular ectopy may also be observed on ambulatory monitoring.[32] Outflow tract morphology VTs may be a manifestation of arrhythmogenic right ventricular cardiomyopathy (ARVC), although the morphology of VT is often varied in ARVC. It is critical to make this distinction because continued exercise in the face of ARVC carries grave consequences (as discussed later). See Chapter 81 for a more complete description of outflow tract VT.

Idiopathic Left Ventricular Tachycardia

Idiopathic VT originating in the LV most commonly represents verapamil-sensitive fascicular VT. This condition should be considered in the differential diagnosis of any right bundle branch block (RBBB)–pattern tachycardia in someone with an otherwise normal heart. In fact, heightened awareness is required since these VTs are often initially mistaken for SVT with aberrant conduction. This form of idiopathic VT was originally recognized by Zipes and colleagues in 1979,[33] with subsequent description of the verapamil sensitivity by Belhassen and coworkers in 1981.[34]

There are three subtypes of fascicular VT, all of which are believed to involve reentry and the left fascicles.[35] The most common form (>80%) is left posterior fascicular VT, which presents with an RBBB and left axis deviation on ECG (mimicking the pattern of RBBB + left anterior fascicular block) (Fig. 65.1). Relatively less common is left anterior fascicular VT, which presents with an RBBB and right axis deviation (mimicking the pattern of RBBB + left posterior fascicular block). Less common still is upper septal fascicular VT, which presents with a relatively narrow QRS with a normal or right axis.

As noted, multiple lines of evidence point to the reentrant nature of this set of VTs, with slow, decremental, anterograde conduction via abnormal Purkinje fibers and retrograde conduction via the fascicle. Intravenous verapamil slows and terminates the VT by prolonging the conduction in the decremental limb of the circuit.[35]

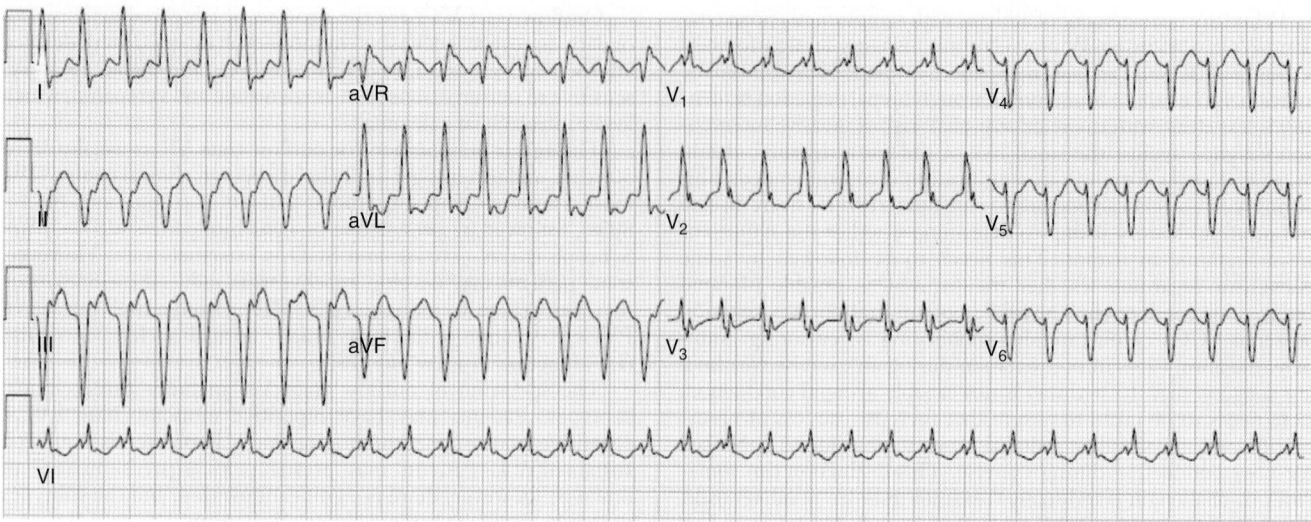

FIGURE 65.1 Left posterior fascicular ventricular tachycardia. Note the right bundle branch block superior axis QRS morphology.

The usual age of presentation of fascicular VT is 15 to 40 years, with a male preponderance. This VT also appears to be somewhat more common in Japan. Although it was first described to occur in patients at rest, it is clearly sensitive to cathecholamines and may be precipitated by exercise or emotional stress. While it is often very sensitive to verapamil, adenosine has no effect.[36]

Patients suspected to have fascicular VT should undergo an evaluation to exclude structural and/or ischemic heart disease. At a minimum, this includes an echocardiogram and a stress test, but in some patients, additional evaluation using cardiac catheterization and/or cardiac magnetic resonance imaging (MRI) may be appropriate.

Therapy for fascicular VT most commonly involves verapamil; however, in some cases, β-blockers and class I/III antiarrhythmic agents may be useful.[35] Catheter ablation is also an excellent option if medical therapy is unsuccessful or is not well tolerated. Athletic patients, in particular, may be better served by ablation because the negative chronotropic effects of medical therapy may prove intolerable. Efficacy of ablation of fascicular VT is on par with ablation of outflow tract VT (80%–90%) and consists of targeting the earliest Purkinje potential during VT and/or linear ablation through the fascicle.[37]

Finally, it should be noted, that although LVOT and fascicular VT are responsible for the vast majority of LV arrhythmias in patients with structurally normal hearts, VT could occasionally originate from a variety of other locations in the LV. These include the mitral annulus, the papillary muscles, and perivascular epicardial sites.[35] These sites should be considered if the presenting VT morphology is not consistent with the more common LVOT and fascicular origins. See Chapter 82 for a more complete description of fascicular VT.

Conditions Associated With Increased Risk of Exercise-Induced Arrhythmias and Sudden Cardiac Death

Patients With Coronary Artery Disease

Exercise treadmill–induced ventricular arrhythmias (ETIVAs) are common in patients with known CAD. The prevalence of any ventricular arrhythmia, including simple PVCs, ranges from 10% to 40% in patients with CAD, with the reported range in most studies being between 20% and 30%.[38] The prevalence of more complex ventricular arrhythmias is lower.[39] In a population of veterans referred for exercise stress testing, the mortality risk in patients

with resting (preexercise) PVCs and ETIVAs was increased.[40] The combination of rest PVCs and ETIVA was associated with the highest cardiovascular mortality independent of other clinical and exercise test variables, including exercise-induced ischemia.[7] These results were not adjusted for LV function or the extent of coronary disease, which might have explained some of the increased mortality. Such results demonstrate that the significance of ETIVA differs depending on the clinical status of the patient. Patients with ETIVA should undergo an evaluation of their LV function and receive appropriate evaluation and therapy if ventricular function is found to be compromised. See Chapter 84 for a more complete description of ischemic heart disease.

Patients With Coronary Anomalies

Congenital coronary anomalies are implicated in 10% to 20% of deaths in young athletes.[41] The right coronary artery arising from the left coronary sinus is more common than the left coronary artery arising from the anterior sinus, although the latter is a more common cause of sudden death. An anomalous coronary course between the pulmonary artery and the aorta is associated with the highest risk for sudden death, especially if the artery courses intramurally within the aortic wall during its initial course. It is hypothesized that the increase in stroke volume during exercise compresses the intramural portion of the artery, which is trapped between the lumen and the adventitia. Alternatively, the artery could be compressed between the pulmonary artery and aorta. Exercise also increases heart rate, which reduces diastole, and this is when there is flow of coronary blood. The increase in systolic compression, coupled with the reduction in diastole, probably explains why SCD most frequently occurs during or shortly after exercise in these subjects.[42] Patients with a single coronary artery that divides into all three major branches are also at risk for SCD during athletic activity.[43] Patients with hypoplasia of portions of the coronary tree or with coronary fistulas, or the small minority of patients (who reached adulthood) with an anomalous left coronary artery arising from the pulmonary artery, are also at risk for exercise-induced arrhythmias.

Arrhythmogenic Right Ventricular Cardiomyopathy

The hallmark of ARVC is a patchy replacement of right ventricular (RV) myocardium by fibrofatty tissue. Generally, this replacement preferentially affects the free wall of the RV; however, the disorder can also affect the outflow tract, the septum, and the LV.

ARVC is an inherited disorder that is more common in males and predominantly affects young adults, with a mean age at diagnosis around 30 years. The disease provides a substrate for reentrant ventricular arrhythmias and is associated with an increased risk of sudden death. It is apparently more prevalent in athletes from the northeastern (Veneto) region of Italy, but this may represent case identification bias.[44]

Ventricular arrhythmias can occur during exercise, and exercise-related SCD with ARVC is thought to result from VT that degenerates into VF. The most common type of arrhythmia is the sustained or nonsustained monomorphic VT from the RV, often manifesting as a left bundle branch with a superior axis. The superior axis helps differentiate this form of VT from the classical RVOT VT, which usually presents with an inferior axis. The isolated RVOT involvement form of ARVC, however, can present with an inferior axis.

The diagnostic criteria of ARVC have recently been revised.[45] ECG findings suggestive of ARVC include the presence of RV conduction delay, precordial T-wave inversions, and epsilon waves. The presence of notching in the QRS complex of the LBBB VT may also suggest ARVC.[46] Exercise is thought to increase stress on the RV by increasing preload and worsening or triggering ventricular arrhythmias and by, possibly, accelerating the manifestation of the ARVC phenotype in susceptible individuals.[47] Exercise testing may induce monomorphic VT in up to 50% to 60% of patients with ARVC and can contribute to the diagnostic evaluation. Nonsustained or sustained VT of LBBB morphology with a superior axis fulfills a major criterion for the diagnosis of ARVC, whereas an inferior axis fulfills a minor criterion.[45] Other corroborative data are needed for the diagnosis of ARVC, and the usual diagnostic work up for ARVC consists of a signal-averaged ECG, echocardiogram, cardiac MRI, a detailed family history, and, if needed, invasive electroanatomical mapping of the RV.

Patients with ARVC should not engage in competitive sports or endurance training and are usually restricted to class 1A sports (bowling, cricket, riflery, billiards, etc.).[48] The treatment also involves an implantable cardioverter defibrillator (ICD) in patients deemed at high risk for arrhythmic events and for the secondary prevention of SCD.[49] Medical management with antiarrhythmics or sotalol may be used in those who are not candidates for ICD therapy and in those with frequent ICD shocks. Radiofrequency ablation can also help reduce the frequency of arrhythmias by ablating the most troublesome foci. See Chapter 87 for a more complete description of ARVC.

Hypertrophic Cardiomyopathy

Hypertrophic cardiomyopathy (HCM) is the most common genetic cardiomyopathy, with a prevalence of 1:500 in the general population. It is also the most common cause of SCD in US athletes. HCM is caused by mutations in genes encoding cardiac sarcomere proteins. The resultant phenotypes are variable and can produce variable degrees of LV hypertrophy and LV outflow obstruction even among subjects with the same mutations. The diagnosis requires an unexplained increase in LV wall thickness (13–60 mm), as determined using echocardiography or cardiac MRI, without LV chamber dilatation.[50] Recurrent syncope, presence of VT or NSVT, exercise-induced hypotension, an LV septum of greater than 30 mm, a family history of SCD, and greater than 15% myocardial scarring shown by late gadolinium enhancement on a cardiac MRI indicate a subgroup at high risk for complications, including SCD.[50]

VT originating from myocardial scarring or from distorted electrophysiological propagation due to disorganized arrangement of cardiac muscle cells in HCM is the probable cause of SCD in most HCM patients. VT/VF events in athletes with

HCM tend to occur during the afternoon hours, and these events are usually preceded by sinus tachycardia, both supporting an exercise-induced mechanism. This is consistent with the general principle that high sympathetic drive is proarrhythmic in abnormal hearts.[51] Among 1380 patients referred to a cardiomyopathy clinic, only 2.0% had NSVT or VF during exercise testing. Nonetheless, exercise-induced NSVT/VF, when present, predicted SCD and appropriate ICD discharge (hazard ratio [HR], 3.14). This suggests that ventricular arrhythmias during symptom-limited exercise are rare in patients with HCM but are associated with an increased risk of SCD.[52]

The prevention of ventricular tachyarrhythmias and SCD in HCM requires the use of ICDs. The risk of SCD may also be reduced with septal myectomy or alcohol septal ablation in patients with symptomatic LVOT obstruction.[53] Pharmacological agents such as antiarrhythmic drugs or negative inotropes have little impact on the incidence of SCD. Patients with HCM should be restricted from most competitive sports and endurance training and are usually restricted to low-intensity, class 1A sports, such as bowling, cricket, riflery, and billiards, because of the potential risk of exercise-associated SCD in HCM.[48] See Chapter 86 for a more complete description of ventricular arrhythmias in HCM.

Long QT Syndrome

Long QT syndrome (LQTS) is a genetic disorder characterized by a prolongation of the QT interval and an increased risk of syncope, life-threatening arrhythmias, and SCD. LQTS has a prevalence of 1 in 2000.[54] The arrhythmias, usually torsades de pointes (TdP) VT, commonly occur during increased sympathetic activity such as that produced by psychological or physical stress, but they can also occur at rest.[54]

LQTS is caused by 16 genes, of which 3 are responsible for approximately 85% to 90% of the cases.[55] A detailed discussion of LQTS is found in other chapters. We will focus on the response of LQTS type 1 (LQT1) to exercise.

The conditions associated with the arrhythmias in LQTS are largely gene-specific.[56] LQT1 is the most common type of LQTS. Arrhythmic events are more often triggered by adrenergic stimuli and exercise in patients with LQT1 than in those with other LQTS subgroups. LQT1 should be considered in patients who have a prolonged corrected QT interval (QTc) and a history of syncope with stress, especially if there is a family history of early SCD or drowning. Swimming, perhaps via the diving reflex, can produce TdP in LQT1 patients. Arrhythmic events in LQT1 generally occur at relatively elevated heart rates. Events in LQT2 patients are more often triggered by sudden auditory stimuli, and those in LQT3 patients usually occur during rest or sleep.[56]

The defect in LQT1 is a loss-of-function mutation in *KCNQ1*, affecting the I_{Ks} current.[57] At fast heart rates, I_{Ks} is the most important current that shortens the action potential. As a result, the QTc is not appropriately shortened in LQT1 patients during exercise. The failure of the QTc to shorten with exercise or with adrenergic stimulation can assist in the diagnosis of LQT1.

LQT1 presents with palpitations, syncope, cardiac arrest, and SCD. Approximately 40% of LQT1 patients are symptomatic by the age of 10, and few develop symptoms after the age of 20. As a result, asymptomatic individuals diagnosed in adulthood are likely at low risk for events.

The ECG of a patient with LQT1 typically shows a broad-based, high-amplitude T-wave. This contrasts with the precordial biphasic T-wave pattern in LQT2 and the long isoelectric ST-T segment in LQT3 (Fig. 65.2). TdP in LQT1 is not pause-dependent, which means that it does not require "long-short" RR interval to initiate the TdP, unlike LQT2.[58] QTc decreases during exercise in patients with LQT2 and LQT3 as well as in normal individuals. In contrast, LQT1 patients essentially have

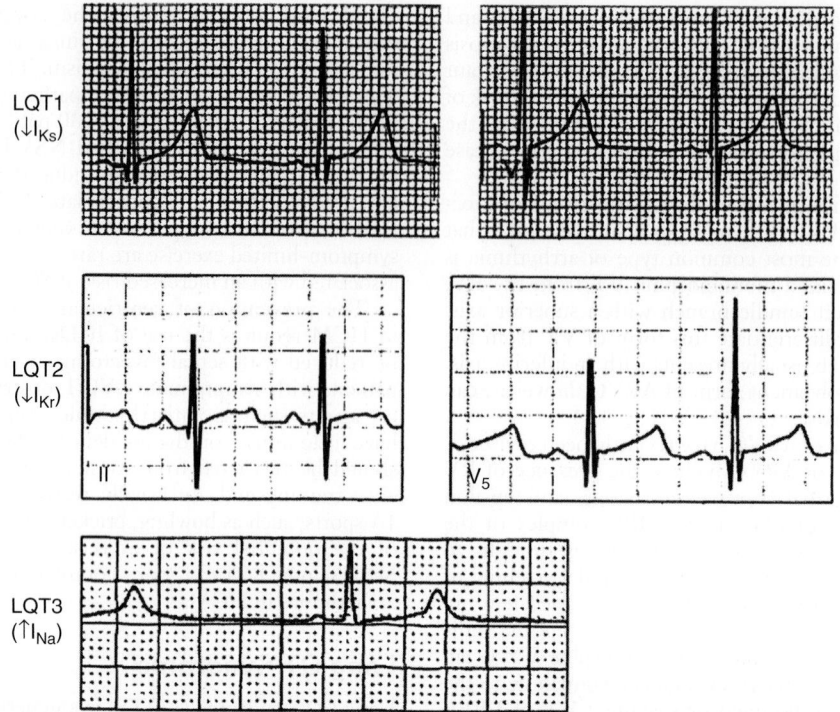

FIGURE 65.2 Electrocardiographic patterns in three types of long QT syndrome. (From Bhatia A, Sra J, Akhtar M. Repolarization syndromes. *Curr Probl Cardiol.* 2012;37:317-362.)

unchanged or even increased QTc durations during exercise (Fig. 65.3). Unapparent or concealed QTc prolongation in patients with LQT1 can be unveiled during exercise or during recovery. A QTc ≥460 ms during the recovery phase or a paradoxical increase in QTc, defined as QTc at 3 minutes of recovery minus the QTc at baseline being ≥30 ms, can reliably help distinguish patients with manifested or concealed LQT1 from those with LQT2 and LQT3.[59] Similarly, a paradoxical prolongation of the uncorrected QT interval by >30 ms during infusion of low-dose epinephrine suggests LQT1.[60] Epinephrine QT stress testing has been demonstrated to have a positive predictive value of 76% and a negative predictive value of 96% for LQT1, even when the baseline ECG shows a normal QTc.[60]

β-Blockers are the treatment of choice and are effective in reducing symptoms and lethal events. Patients who have recurrences despite maximal β-blocker therapy may be considered for ICD implantation or left stellate ganglion ablation.[55] See Chapter 93 for a more complete description of LQTS.

Catecholaminergic Polymorphic Ventricular Tachycardia

Catecholaminergic polymorphic ventricular tachycardia (CPVT) is a rare inherited syndrome that is characterized by adrenergically induced syncope and sudden death.[61] The hallmark of the CPVT is exercise-induced bidirectional VT, where the beat-to-beat axis rotates 180 degrees with each beat (see Fig. 65.3). A minority of patients may also develop polymorphic VT. Although patients usually present with exercise-induced palpitations, dizziness, or syncope, the first presentation may be SCD.[62]

Given that patients have a normal resting ECG and cardiac imaging findings, the exact prevalence of the condition is unknown.[61] CPVT typically manifests in children and adolescents, but its presentation as late as 40 years of age has been reported.[62] A family history of exercise-related syncope, seizures, or sudden death is reported in approximately one-third of patients.[61] Mortality approaches 30% to 40% by age 40.[63]

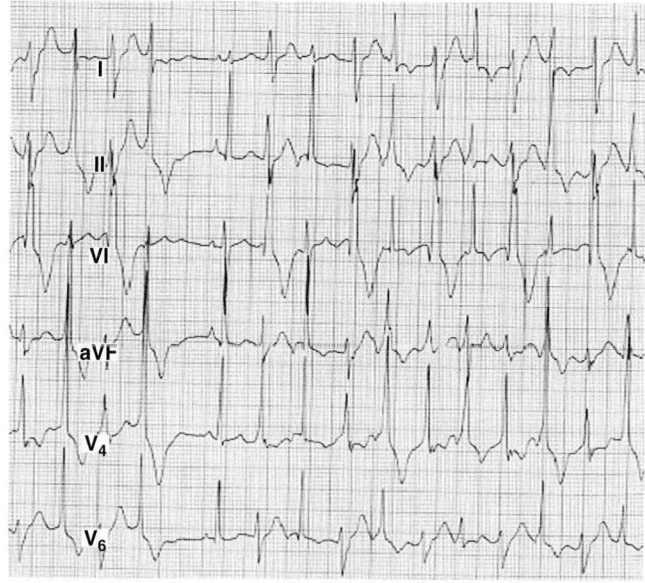

FIGURE 65.3 Catecholaminergic polymorphic ventricular tachycardia. (From Francis J, Sankar V, Nair VK, et al. Catecholaminergic polymorphic ventricular tachycardia. *Heart Rhythm.* 2005;2:550-554.)

CPVT is a disorder of myocardial calcium homeostasis.[4] The majority of cases are inherited in an autosomal dominant fashion and are secondary to a mutation in the cardiac ryanodine receptor (*RyR2*). There is also a less common autosomal recessive form that is secondary to mutations in the gene for cardiac calsequestrin (*CASQ2*). Both *RyR2* and *CASQ2* mutations cause intracellular calcium overload due to an uncontrolled release of calcium from the sarcoplasmic reticulum. This, in turn, results in delayed afterdepolarizations.[35] Mutations in *RyR2* or *CASQ2* are found in approximately 60% of patients with CPVT, which suggests that other genes may be involved.[61]

Exercise testing is the most useful diagnostic test in the evaluation of patients with suspected CPVT. With exercise, there is a progressive increase in both supraventricular and ventricular ectopy. Initially, isolated polymorphic PVCs are noted, but these are soon followed by bigeminy, couplets, and short runs of nonsustained VT. With continued exercise, the classical bidirectional VT or polymorphic VT develops. Supraventricular tachyarrhythmias (including AF) may also develop.[62] EPS is not helpful in the diagnosis of CPVT,[35] but a drug challenge with isoproterenol or epinephrine may be useful in patients who are not able to exercise. The diagnosis of CPVT is made if the patient displays characteristic exercise test findings and has an otherwise normal cardiac work up. Age older than 40 years makes the diagnosis less likely but does not exclude it.[61]

Along with avoidance of strenuous exercise and stressful environments, the primary treatment for CPVT is β-blockade utilizing a nonselective β-blocker that lacks intrinsic sympathomimetic activity. Nadolol is the preferred agent,[61] and fairly high doses are often required. The adequacy of β-blockade can be assessed by performing a repeat exercise test. Patients need to understand that faultless compliance is mandatory as missed doses can provoke lethal arrhythmias.[61,62] There is also evidence that flecainide can be a useful adjunct to β-blockers.[64] Although more studies are needed, there is consensus that flecainide should be considered in patients who have continued symptoms despite adequate β-blockade. In patients who cannot tolerate, or who remain symptomatic despite, β-blockade, left cardiac sympathetic denervation (LCSD) has shown promising results.[65] Studies with longer follow-up periods are needed; furthermore, patient access is limited by the fact that LCSD is available only at a limited number of highly specialized centers. ICD implantation is recommended in patients with CPVT who present with aborted sudden death and in those who remain symptomatic despite optimal medical management.[61] An ICD should not be used as stand-alone therapy because ICD shocks can increase sympathetic tone and trigger further malignant arrhythmias. See Chapter 88 for a more complete description of CPVT.

Antiarrhythmic Medications and Exercise-Induced Ventricular Arrhythmias

Class I antiarrhythmic drugs, such as flecainide and propafenone, can cause exercise-induced arrhythmias and ventricular reentry. Exercise can progressively increase the QRS duration with increasing levels of exercise in patients taking flecainide.[66] A QRS increase of approximately 15% to 20% is consistent with pharmacological effect; however, further increases in QRS duration warrant dose reduction or discontinuation of the drug. Provocation of VT, preceded by excessive QRS widening, has been documented on treadmill exercise testing.[67] The slowing of the ventricular conduction, particularly in the presence of diseased myocardium, could facilitate reentry. Therefore guidelines recommend that the QRS duration should not get prolonged by more than 50% from baseline and that a QRS duration of less than 120 ms should be maintained.[49] To ensure that the QRS duration does not exceed these parameters at higher heart rates, treadmill testing may be employed to determine the degree of maximal QRS prolongation during exercise after the patient is fully loaded with flecainide or propafenone. See Chapter 101 for a more complete description of drug-induced VT.

Conclusion

The neurohormonal and hemodynamic changes caused by acute exercise can induce atrial and ventricular arrhythmias. Most of these arrhythmias are benign in healthy individuals and have no clinical significance. However, in patients with subclinical pathology, exercise could trigger life-threatening arrhythmias. Understanding of these diagnoses is pivotal to guide the management and exercise prescription of the patient.

REFERENCES

1. Running USA. http://www.runningusa.org/statistics. Accessed 05.07.15.
2. Lloyd-Jones DM, Hong Y, Labarthe D, et al. Defining and setting national goals for cardiovascular health promotion and disease reduction: the American Heart Association's strategic Impact Goal through 2020 and beyond. *Circulation.* 2010;121:586–613.
3. Jacob C, Zouhal H, Prioux J, Gratas-Delamarche A, Bentue-Ferrer D, Delamarche P. Effect of the intensity of training on catecholamine responses to supramaximal exercise in endurance-trained men. *Eur J Appl Physiol.* 2004;91:35–40.
4. Zouhal H, Jacob C, Delamarche P, Gratas-Delamarche A. Catecholamines and the effects of exercise, training and gender. *Sports Med.* 2008;38:401–423.
5. Eckman DM, Nelson MT. Potassium ions as vasodilators: role of inward rectifier potassium channels. *Circ Res.* 2001;88:132–133.
6. Paterson DJ. Antiarrhythmic mechanisms during exercise. *J Appl Physiol.* 1985;1996(80):1853–1862.
7. Beckerman J, Wu T, Jones S, Froelicher VF. Exercise test-induced arrhythmias. *Prog Cardiovasc Dis.* 2005;47:285–305.
8. Maurer MS, Shefrin EA, Fleg JL. Prevalence and prognostic significance of exercise-induced supraventricular tachycardia in apparently healthy volunteers. *Am J Cardiol.* 1995;75:788–792.
9. Karjalainen J, Kujala UM, Kaprio J, Sarna S, Viitasalo M. Lone atrial fibrillation in vigorously exercising middle aged men: case-control study. *BMJ.* 1998;316:1784–1785.
10. Mont L, Sambola A, Brugada J, et al. Long-lasting sport practice and lone atrial fibrillation. *Eur Heart J.* 2002;23:477–482.
11. Molina L, Mont L, Marrugat J, et al. Long-term endurance sport practice increases the incidence of lone atrial fibrillation in men: a follow-up study. *Europace.* 2008;10:618–623.
12. Baldesberger S, Bauersfeld U, Candinas R, et al. Sinus node disease and arrhythmias in the long-term follow-up of former professional cyclists. *Eur Heart J.* 2008;29:71–78.
13. Andersen K, Farahmand B, Ahlbom A, et al. Risk of arrhythmias in 52 755 long-distance cross-country skiers: a cohort study. *Eur Heart J.* 2013;34:3624–3631.
14. Drca N, Wolk A, Jensen-Urstad M, Larsson SC. Atrial fibrillation is associated with different levels of physical activity levels at different ages in men. *Heart.* 2014;100:1037–1042.
15. Turagam MK, Velagapudi P, Kocheril AG. Atrial fibrillation in athletes. *Am J Cardiol.* 2012;109:296–302.
16. Guasch E, Benito B, Qi X, et al. Atrial fibrillation promotion by endurance exercise: demonstration and mechanistic exploration in an animal model. *J Am Coll Cardiol.* 2013;62:68–77.
17. Rozmaritsa N, Christ T, Van Wagoner DR, et al. Attenuated response of L-type calcium current to nitric oxide in atrial fibrillation. *Cardiovasc Res.* 2014;101:533–542.
18. Iwasaki YK, Nishida K, Kato T, Nattel S. Atrial fibrillation pathophysiology: implications for management. *Circulation.* 2011;124:2264–2274.
19. Iskandar A, Mujtaba MT, Thompson PD. Left atrium size in elite athletes. *JACC Cardiovasc Imaging.* 2015;8:753–762.
20. Zipes DP, Link MS, Ackerman MJ, Kovacs RJ, Myerburg RJ, Estes 3rd NA. Eligibility and disqualification recommendations for competitive athletes with cardiovascular abnormalities: Task Force 9: arrhythmias and conduction defects: a scientific statement from the American Heart Association and American College of Cardiology. *J Am Coll Cardiol.* 2015;66:2412–2423.
21. Malmo V, Nes BM, Amundsen BH, et al. Aerobic interval training reduces the burden of atrial fibrillation in the short term: a randomized trial. *Circulation.* 2016;133:466–473.
22. Alboni P, Botto GL, Baldi N, et al. Outpatient treatment of recent-onset atrial fibrillation with the "pill-in-the-pocket" approach. *N Engl J Med.* 2004;351:2384–2391.
23. Page RL, Joglar JA, Caldwell MA, et al. 2015 ACC/AHA/HRS Guideline for the management of adult patients with supraventricular tachycardia: a report of the American College of Cardiology/American Heart Association Task Force on Clinical Practice Guidelines and the Heart Rhythm Society. *J Am Coll Cardiol.* 2016;67:e27–e115.
24. Maron BJ, Doerer JJ, Haas TS, Tierney DM, Mueller FO. Sudden deaths in young competitive athletes: analysis of 1866 deaths in the United States, 1980-2006. *Circulation.* 2009;119:1085–1092.
25. Obeyesekere MN, Klein GJ. The asymptomatic Wolff-Parkinson-White patient: time to be more proactive? *Circulation.* 2014;130:805–807.
26. Marine JE, Shetty V, Chow GV, et al. Prevalence and prognostic significance of exercise-induced nonsustained ventricular tachycardia in asymptomatic volunteers: BLSA (Baltimore Longitudinal Study of Aging). *J Am Coll Cardiol.* 2013;62:595–600.
27. Froelicher Jr VF, Allen M, Lancaster MC. Maximal treadmill testing of normal USAF aircrewmen. *Aerosp Med.* 1974;45:310–315.
28. Iwai S, Cantillon DJ, Kim RJ, et al. Right and left ventricular outflow tract tachycardias: evidence for a common electrophysiologic mechanism. *J Cardiovasc Electrophysiol.* 2006;17:1052–1058.
29. Lerman BB. Response of nonreentrant catecholamine-mediated ventricular tachycardia to endogenous adenosine and acetylcholine. Evidence for myocardial receptor-mediated effects. *Circulation.* 1993;87:382–390.
30. Kim RJ, Iwai S, Markowitz SM, Shah BK, Stein KM, Lerman BB. Clinical and electrophysiological spectrum of idiopathic ventricular outflow tract arrhythmias. *J Am Coll Cardiol.* 2007;49:2035–2043.
31. Lerman BB, Stein KM, Markowitz SM, Mittal S, Slotwiner DJ. Ventricular arrhythmias in normal hearts. *Cardiol Clin.* 2000;18:265–291. vii.
32. Josephson M. *Clinical Cardiac Electrophysiology: Techniques and Interpretations.* 4th ed. Baltimore, Lippincott Williams & Wilkins; 2008:912.
33. Zipes DP, Foster PR, Troup PJ, Pedersen DH. Atrial induction of ventricular tachycardia: reentry versus triggered automaticity. *Am J Cardiol.* 1979;44:1–8.
34. Belhassen B, Rotmensch HH, Laniado S. Response of recurrent sustained ventricular tachycardia to verapamil. *Br Heart J.* 1981;46:679–682.
35. Prystowsky EN, Padanilam BJ, Joshi S, Fogel RI. Ventricular arrhythmias in the absence of structural heart disease. *J Am Coll Cardiol.* 2012;59:1733–1744.

36. Okumura K, Tsuchiya T. Idiopathic left ventricular tachycardia: clinical features, mechanisms and management. *Card Electrophysiol Rev.* 2002;6:61–67.

37. Ramprakash B, Jaishankar S, Rao HB, Narasimhan C. Catheter ablation of fascicular ventricular tachycardia. *Indian Pacing Electrophysiol J.* 2008;8:193–202.

38. Marieb MA, Beller GA, Gibson RS, Lerman BB, Kaul S. Clinical relevance of exercise-induced ventricular arrhythmias in suspected coronary artery disease. *Am J Cardiol.* 1990;66:172–178.

39. Elhendy A, Chandrasekaran K, Gersh BJ, Mahoney D, Burger KN, Pellikka PA. Functional and prognostic significance of exercise-induced ventricular arrhythmias in patients with suspected coronary artery disease. *Am J Cardiol.* 2002;90:95–100.

40. Partington S, Myers J, Cho S, Froelicher V, Chun S. Prevalence and prognostic value of exercise-induced ventricular arrhythmias. *Am Heart J.* 2003;145:139–146.

41. Corrado D, Basso C, Rizzoli G, Schiavon M, Thiene G. Does sports activity enhance the risk of sudden death in adolescents and young adults? *J Am Coll Cardiol.* 2003;42:1959–1963.

42. Cheitlin MD, MacGregor J. Congenital anomalies of coronary arteries: role in the pathogenesis of sudden cardiac death. *Herz.* 2009;34:268–279.

43. Mofrad PS, Weigold G, Clavijo LC. Sudden cardiac death in athlete with anomalous single coronary artery. *Cardiovasc Revasc Med.* 2005;6:89–90.

44. Corrado D, Basso C, Pavei A, Michieli P, Schiavon M, Thiene G. Trends in sudden cardiovascular death in young competitive athletes after implementation of a preparticipation screening program. *JAMA.* 2006;296:1593–1601.

45. Marcus FI, McKenna WJ, Sherrill D, et al. Diagnosis of arrhythmogenic right ventricular cardiomyopathy/dysplasia: proposed modification of the Task Force Criteria. *Eur Heart J.* 2010;31:806–814.

46. Hoffmayer KS, Machado ON, Marcus GM, et al. Electrocardiographic comparison of ventricular arrhythmias in patients with arrhythmogenic right ventricular cardiomyopathy and right ventricular outflow tract tachycardia. *J Am Coll Cardiol.* 2011;58:831–838.

47. Perrin MJ, Angaran P, Laksman Z, et al. Exercise testing in asymptomatic gene carriers exposes a latent electrical substrate of arrhythmogenic right ventricular cardiomyopathy. *J Am Coll Cardiol.* 2013;62:1772–1779.

48. Maron BJ, Udelson JE, Bonow RO, et al. Eligibility and disqualification recommendations for competitive athletes with cardiovascular abnormalities: Task Force 3: hypertrophic cardiomyopathy, arrhythmogenic right ventricular cardiomyopathy and other cardiomyopathies, and myocarditis: a scientific statement from the American Heart Association and American College of Cardiology. *Circulation.* 2015;132:e273–e280.

49. Zipes DP, Camm AJ, Borggrefe M, et al. ACC/AHA/ESC 2006 guidelines for management of patients with ventricular arrhythmias and the prevention of sudden cardiac death: a report of the American College of Cardiology/American Heart Association Task Force and the European Society of Cardiology Committee for Practice Guidelines (Writing Committee to Develop Guidelines for Management of Patients with Ventricular Arrhythmias and the Prevention of Sudden Cardiac Death). *J Am Coll Cardiol.* 2006;48:e247–e346.

50. Maron BJ, Ommen SR, Semsarian C, Spirito P, Olivotto I, Maron MS. Hypertrophic cardiomyopathy: present and future, with translation into contemporary cardiovascular medicine. *J Am Coll Cardiol.* 2014;64:83–99.

51. Cha YM, Gersh BJ, Maron BJ, et al. Electrophysiologic manifestations of ventricular tachyarrhythmias provoking appropriate defibrillator interventions in high-risk patients with hypertrophic cardiomyopathy. *J Cardiovasc Electrophysiol.* 2007;18:483–487.

52. Gimeno JR, Tome-Esteban M, Lofiego C, et al. Exercise-induced ventricular arrhythmias and risk of sudden cardiac death in patients with hypertrophic cardiomyopathy. *Eur Heart J.* 2009;30:2599–2605.

53. Vriesendorp PA, Liebregts M, Steggerda RC, et al. Long-term outcomes after medical and invasive treatment in patients with hypertrophic cardiomyopathy. *JACC Heart Fail.* 2014;2:630–636.

54. Schwartz PJ, Stramba-Badiale M, Crotti L, et al. Prevalence of the congenital long-QT syndrome. *Circulation.* 2009;120:1761–1767.

55. Schwartz PJ, Ackerman MJ. The long QT syndrome: a transatlantic clinical approach to diagnosis and therapy. *Eur Heart J.* 2013;34:3109–3116.

56. Schwartz PJ, Priori SG, Spazzolini C, et al. Genotype-phenotype correlation in the long-QT syndrome: gene-specific triggers for life-threatening arrhythmias. *Circulation.* 2001;103:89–95.

57. Swan H, Viitasalo M, Piippo K, Laitinen P, Kontula K, Toivonen L. Sinus node function and ventricular repolarization during exercise stress test in long QT syndrome patients with KvLQT1 and HERG potassium channel defects. *J Am Coll Cardiol.* 1999;34:823–829.

58. Marban E, Robinson SW, Wier WG. Mechanisms of arrhythmogenic delayed and early afterdepolarizations in ferret ventricular muscle. *J Clin Invest.* 1986;78:1185–1192.

59. Horner JM, Horner MM, Ackerman MJ. The diagnostic utility of recovery phase QTc during treadmill exercise stress testing in the evaluation of long QT syndrome. *Heart Rhythm.* 2011;8:1698–1704.

60. Vyas H, Hejlik J, Ackerman MJ. Epinephrine QT stress testing in the evaluation of congenital long-QT syndrome: diagnostic accuracy of the paradoxical QT response. *Circulation.* 2006;113:1385–1392.

61. Priori SG, Wilde AA, Horie M, et al. HRS/EHRA/APHRS expert consensus statement on the diagnosis and management of patients with inherited primary arrhythmia syndromes: document endorsed by HRS, EHRA, and APHRS in May 2013 and by ACCF, AHA, PACES, and AEPC in June 2013. *Heart Rhythm.* 2013;(10):1932–1963.

62. Pflaumer A, Davis AM. Guidelines for the diagnosis and management of catecholaminergic polymorphic ventricular tachycardia. *Heart Lung Circ.* 2012;21:96–100.

63. Mohamed U, Napolitano C, Priori SG. Molecular and electrophysiological bases of catecholaminergic polymorphic ventricular tachycardia. *J Cardiovasc Electrophysiol.* 2007;18:791–797.

64. van der Werf C, Kannankeril PJ, Sacher F, et al. Flecainide therapy reduces exercise-induced ventricular arrhythmias in patients with catecholaminergic polymorphic ventricular tachycardia. *J Am Coll Cardiol.* 2011;57:2244–2254.

65. Wilde AA, Bhuiyan ZA, Crotti L, et al. Left cardiac sympathetic denervation for catecholaminergic polymorphic ventricular tachycardia. *N Engl J Med.* 2008;358:2024–2029.

66. Ranger S, Talajic M, Lemery R, Roy D, Nattel S. Amplification of flecainide-induced ventricular conduction slowing by exercise. A potentially significant clinical consequence of use-dependent sodium channel blockade. *Circulation.* 1989;79:1000–1006.

67. Falk RH. Flecainide-induced ventricular tachycardia and fibrillation in patients treated for atrial fibrillation. *Ann Intern Med.* 1989;111:107–111.

66 Cardiac Monitoring: Short- and Long-Term Recording

Andrew D. Krahn, Raymond Yee, Allan C. Skanes, and George J. Klein

Ambulatory cardiac monitoring to detect arrhythmias became practical with the development of Holter monitoring and its subsequent derivatives. The clinician is currently armed with an array of tools to provide progressively longer durations of electrocardiogram (ECG) monitoring to obtain a rhythm profile and to establish a symptom rhythm correlation in patients with infrequent symptoms (Fig. 66.1).

Clinical trials using traditional skin electrodes, patches, and insertable cardiac monitors have validated a clear role in unexplained syncope and growing utility in a range of conditions including atrial fibrillation, atypical epilepsy, vasovagal syncope, and postmyocardial infarction arrhythmia detection. Advances in design with the potential addition of other physiological sensors have strengthened the capability of external and implantable devices. Sensors and resultant data are poised to transform the nature of health care, evidenced by recent smartphone-based devices and applications that provide a broad range of physiological parameters including the ECG with associated analytics, and imminent access to blood pressure, oxygen saturation, and numerous other traditionally health care facility–based parameters. This chapter will focus on cardiac monitoring as it applies to current practice, recognizing that an explosion of monitoring technologies is in development or validation at present.

Syncope is the prototype condition that is ideally served by long-term ambulatory monitoring. The periodic and unpredictable nature of events and the high spontaneous remission rate are the major obstacles to diagnosis in most patients. Other forms of testing in unexplained syncope usually provide a context for the bedside formulation of a differential diagnosis and prognosis but rarely provide a specific diagnosis. Classic "provocative" testing with tilt and electrophysiological testing may be negative or yield abnormalities of unknown significance, which is reflected in the poor predictive value of both tests. These obvious limitations turn our attention to graduated durations of cardiac monitoring as a step toward the gold standard of comprehensive physiological assessment during spontaneous symptoms. This chapter will discuss the technical aspects and established utility of a monitoring device with a focus on syncope and atrial fibrillation and explore the emerging use of monitoring technologies.

Short-Term Recording

Holter Monitoring

The Holter monitor is a portable battery-operated device that connects to the patient using bipolar electrodes and provides recordings from up to 12 electrocardiographic leads. Data are stored in the device using digital storage media. The data are analyzed using software with technologist and physician editing and reporting. Additional markers for patient-activated events and time correlates are included to allow greater diagnostic accuracy. Continuous electrocardiographic monitoring is possible for 24–72 hours with conventional Holter monitors. Novel extended duration continuous recording technologies will be discussed subsequently. Complete rhythm capture allows documentation of rhythm for symptomatic and asymptomatic events. Holter monitoring is useful if the clinical history is suggestive of an arrhythmic etiology and if the symptoms are frequent enough to be detected within the period of monitoring. Holter monitoring may also provide a rhythm profile to provide evidence of sinus node dysfunction or potentially significant ambient arrhythmias and assess rate control of atrial fibrillation.

Holter monitoring has several drawbacks. Patients may not experience symptoms or cardiac arrhythmias during the usual Holter recording periods. In patients with syncope, the likelihood of another syncopal episode occurring during the monitoring period is the major limiting factor. Presyncope is a more common event during ambulatory monitoring but is less likely to be associated with an arrhythmia.[1] The ubiquity of presyncope as a symptom in the community makes its utility as a surrogate for syncope relatively uncertain. The physical size of the device may hinder the ability of patients to sleep comfortably or engage in activities that precipitate symptoms. Patients are further inconvenienced because the devices have to be removed while showering. The observations on Holter monitoring must be correlated with the clinical context in the absence of symptoms. There is often significant variability in patient documentation of activated events such that the accurate symptom–rhythm correlation is undermined. Lastly, other technologies provide real-time or near real-time analysis (see below), which may be preferred in select clinical situations.

It is not surprising that Holter monitoring has a low diagnostic yield. In several large series utilizing 12 hours or more of ambulatory monitoring for the investigation of syncope, only 4% had a recurrence of symptoms during monitoring. The overall diagnostic yield of ambulatory or Holter monitoring was 19%. These studies reported symptoms that were not associated with arrhythmias in 15% of cases. The causal relationship between the arrhythmia and the syncope was frequently uncertain. Uncommon asymptomatic arrhythmias such as prolonged sinus pauses, atrioventricular block (such as Mobitz type II block), and nonsustained ventricular tachycardia can provide important contributions to the diagnosis instigating further investigations to rule out structural heart disease and other precipitating factors. While these observations necessitate prompt attention, it is important to interpret the results in the clinical context of the clinical presentation, and not unduly exclude common causes of syncope such as neurocardiogenic syncope.

It is also important to understand that a normal Holter monitor does not exclude an arrhythmic cause for syncope. In fact, this is typically the case. If the pretest probability is high for an arrhythmic cause, extended monitoring is often indicated. In a study that evaluated the extension of ambulatory Holter monitoring duration to 72 hours, there was an increase in the number of

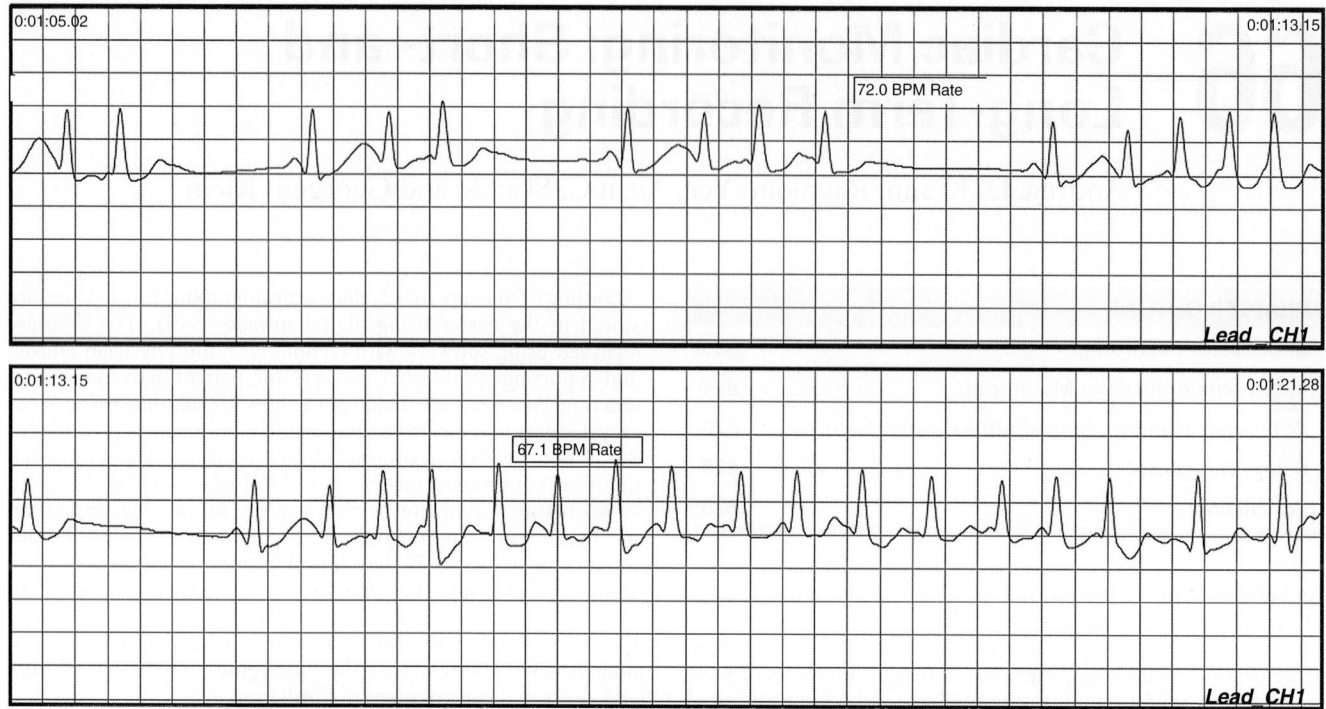

FIGURE 66.1 Ambulatory recording during palpitations and presyncope. Note the burst of atrial tachycardia with associated brief pauses. *BPM,* Beats per minute.

asymptomatic arrhythmias detected but not in the overall diagnostic yield.

In our institution, we typically use Holter monitoring for 24 hours. It is a noninvasive test that provides information to establish a rhythm profile in patients and the diagnosis in those with frequent symptoms. The more frequent the symptoms, the higher the diagnostic yield. The apparent modest yield of Holter monitoring presumably reflects the primary care use of the device in patients with frequent symptoms facilitating a symptom–rhythm correlation. This leads to selection bias in the referral population, leading to an apparent futility in referred patients who, by definition, have failed short-term monitoring.

Intermittent Event Recorders

Transtelephonic monitors are a form of noncontinuous ambulatory recording that are convenient for patient use. During symptomatic episodes, the patient activates the device, which then records the electrocardiographic signals. The recorded event must be directly transmitted to a receiving center (Figs. 66.2 and 66.3). The received signal is then converted to an analog recording that is displayed or printed as a single-lead rhythm strip. The device has solid-state memory capacity allowing the recording and storage of electrocardiographic signals during symptoms. The electrocardiographic signals are collected prospectively for 1–2 minutes upon patient activation. The major disadvantages of such devices include the need for patient activation, missing asymptomatic arrhythmias requiring that the symptoms persist long enough for the device to record the event, and the inability to record the events that surround the onset of symptoms.

Intermediate Duration Monitoring
Patch Recording Devices

Multiple manufacturers now produce a single-lead patch recording device that provide noninvasive intermediate term monitoring without classic electrodes and battery systems, enabling a patch based "all-in-one" system to facilitate 7–14 days of monitoring (Fig. 66.4). Two major forms are in use; one is an extended Holter version that captures data for 7–14 days that is then *subsequently* analyzed. The second device uses Bluetooth technology to transmit real-time data to a smartphone-like device carried by the patient that then transmits data via the Internet to a data monitoring center, where it is analyzed and interpreted by cardiac technologists or nurses with rhythm interpretation expertise. Small studies have validated the recording capabilities but have not evaluated the comparative yield relative to previous technologies beyond that of Holter monitoring.[2]

Hand-Held and Wrist Recorders

Wrist- and mobile phone–based recording devices have emerged as noninvasive recording devices, with rapidly evolving technology. A preliminary report indicated the potential pulse detection capability of a wrist recording device termed the "wriskwatch",[3] which brought attention to alternate means of recording multiple physiological parameters. In addition, these handheld devices have shown remarkable accuracy at generating a high quality single-lead ECG suitable for screening for atrial fibrillation.[4,5]

Extended Holter

Continuous ambulatory monitoring with data transmission to a central monitoring station staffed by health professionals has emerged in the United States as a useful resource to extend traditional Holter monitoring beyond 48 hours (e.g., CardioNet, San Diego, CA). This technique is typically utilized for 7–14 days and has shown incremental benefit to a standard external loop recorder in diagnosing or excluding arrhythmia.[6] This approach also provides the added layer of monitoring center involvement, which enhances responsiveness to changes seen during monitoring. Patch-based versions with the same capability have recently been approved for use (SEEQ; Medtronic,

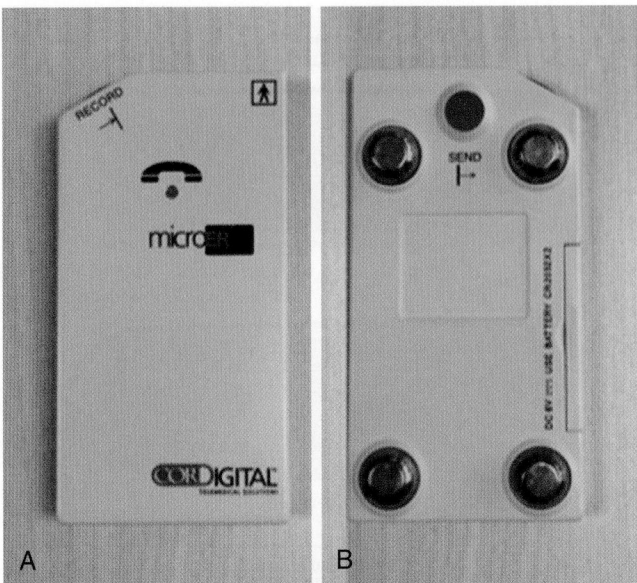

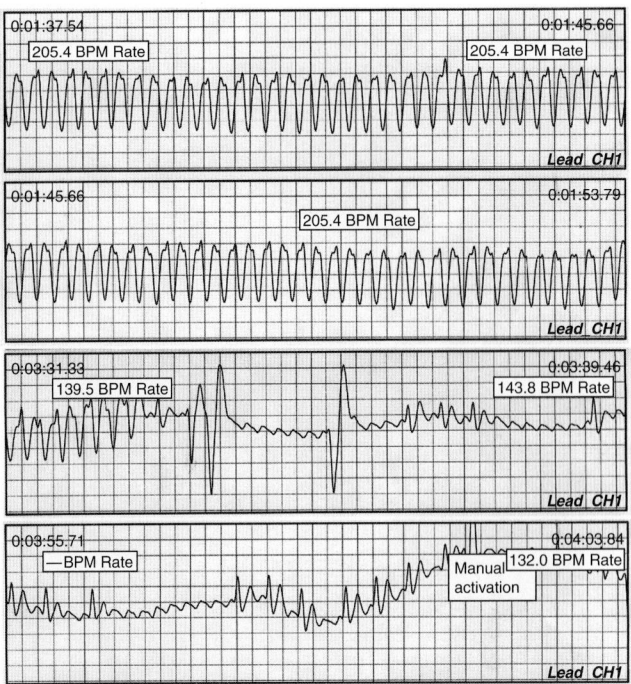

FIGURE 66.3 External loop recording download from a patient with near syncope with palpitations. Wide QRS complex tachycardia is noted at 206 beats/min *(BPM),* which subsequently demonstrates underlying atrial flutter with much slower conduction, and the subsequent patient activation to capture the event. There was no recognized intervention leading to the abrupt reduction in conduction rate.

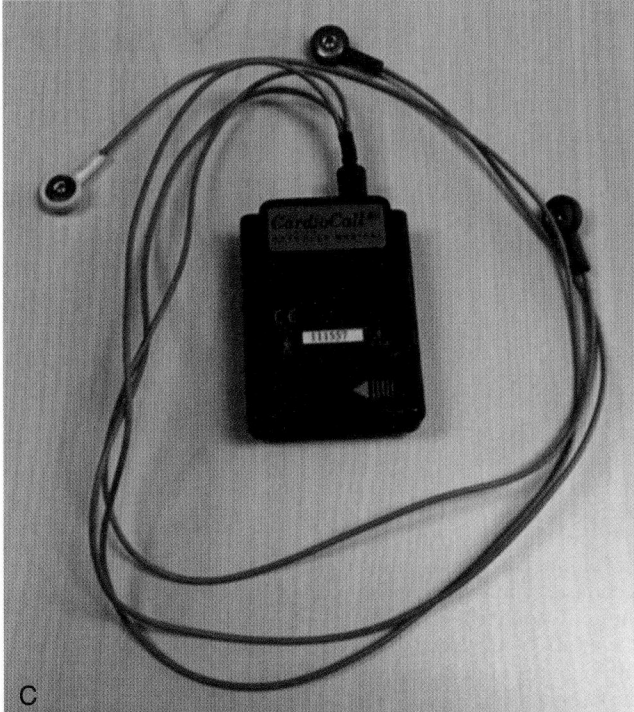

FIGURE 66.2 Photograph of a cardiac event recorder, with the front panel with activation button (A) and the recording electrodes on the back (B). An external loop recorder is illustrated below with recording electrodes (C).

Minneapolis, MN). Unfortunately, real-time monitoring substantially increases cost and is often unnecessary in ambulatory patients, despite the apparent reassurance of constant surveillance. Patch-based systems without active surveillance (i.e., record and analyze) are likely to supplant conventional Holter monitoring because of their ease of use, including lack of changeable batteries, and their moisture and even submersion tolerance. A recent head-to-head comparison demonstrated clear incremental benefit to extending monitoring to 14 days, and 81% of patients preferred the patch to Holter monitoring.[2] They are, however, limited to a single ECG vector, typically lead I, making some rhythm discrimination and p wave identification difficult.

External Loop Recorders

An external loop recorder continuously records and stores a single external modified limb lead electrogram with a 4- to 60-minute memory buffer. After the onset of spontaneous symptoms, the patient activates the device, storing the previous several minutes, and the following 1–4 minutes of recorded information. The captured rhythm strip can subsequently be uploaded and analyzed, often providing critical information regarding the onset and termination of the arrhythmia. This system can theoretically be used indefinitely but in practice is limited to a few weeks in most individuals due to its limitations. The recording device is connected to skin electrodes on the patient's chest wall that need to be removed for bathing or showering, requires weekly battery changes, and can be uncomfortable during sleep.

A randomized trial has shown diagnostic and cost-effective superiority to Holter monitors (22% symptom–rhythm correlation yield for Holter monitoring vs. 56% for the loop recorder, $p < .01$).[7] There is an increment in diagnostic yield when automatic activation is added to patient activation.[8] Automatic detection includes bradycardia, tachycardia, and pauses, as well as atrial fibrillation based on algorithms that detect RR irregularity. There are limited data on the utility of this technology in detecting or excluding atrial fibrillation.

Vest Technology

Multiple vendors now offer wearable monitoring systems that have the potential to acquire and transmit multiple physiological parameters including the ECG. These include vest and shirt technologies using integrated materials for the capture of ECG and respiratory parameters.[4,9,10] Much of this technology falls within the health and fitness sector and does not necessarily pursue health regulatory approval. Thus, though feasible, these devices have not emerged in day-to-day clinical care but promise to revolutionize monitoring technologies. The interested reader

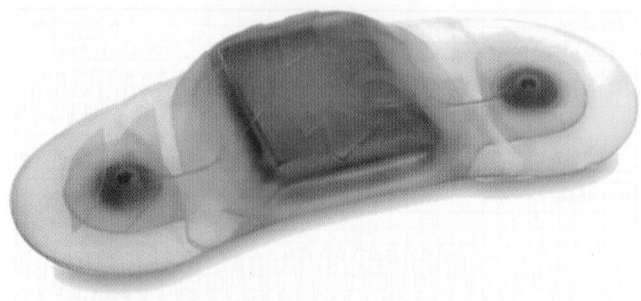

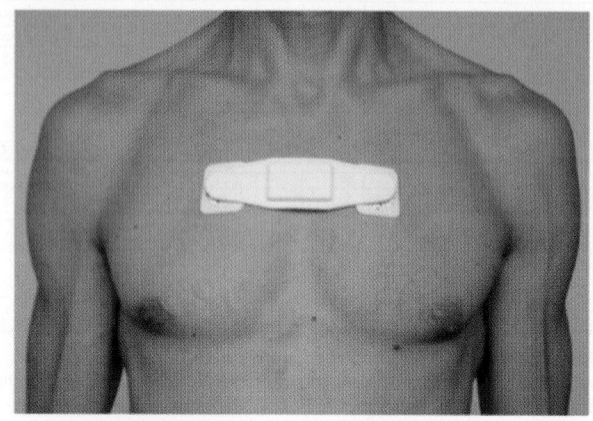

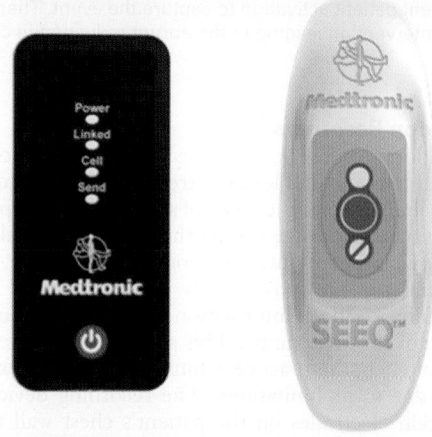

FIGURE 66.4 Sample patch based recording systems that include both acquisition and storage of a single-lead electrocardiogram for 7–14 days. See text for discussion.

is directed to an in-depth review of emerging technologies by Saxon and colleagues.[11]

Prolonged Monitoring: Insertable Cardiac Monitors

The insertable cardiac monitor (ICM) (formerly implantable loop recorder) permits prolonged monitoring without external electrodes. It is ideally suited to patients that require more prolonged monitoring such as those with infrequent recurrent symptoms such as syncope. Similar to the external loop recorder, it is designed to detect arrhythmias and specifically correlate symptoms with the recorded cardiac rhythms. The implanted device obviates surface electrodes and accompanying compliance issues.

ICMs are manufactured by Medtronic (Reveal Linq, Reveal XT Model 9529, DX Model 9538; Minneapolis, MN), St. Jude Medical (Confirm Model DM2100; Minneapolis, MN), and Biotronik Biomonitor (Berlin, Germany) (Fig. 66.5). All

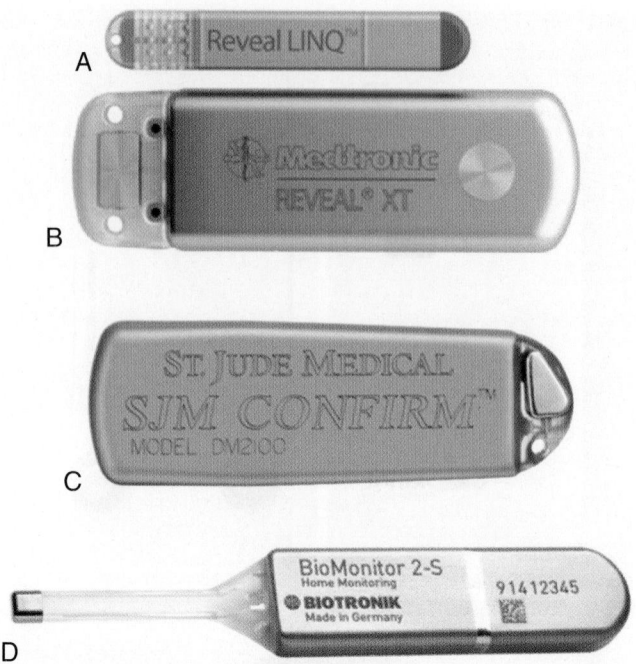

FIGURE 66.5 Implanted loop recorders. The Medtronic Linq (A) and Reveal XT (B). The St. Jude Confirm (C) and the Biotronik Biomonitor (D). See text for discussion.

are smaller than a conventional pacemaker generator, and the most recent release (Reveal Linq) is dramatically smaller than other models. These devices record a single-lead ECG without a transvenous lead, and deliver 3 years of battery life. The device is typically inserted in the left chest using local anesthetic, usually in a high left parasternal or medial pacemaker insertion location. The injectable Linq device has been implanted in a semisterile setting including office-related minor procedure facilities.[12,13] The traditional device implant procedure is similar to fashioning a small pacemaker pocket, with an adequate signal obtained anywhere in the left thorax, without the need for cutaneous mapping. Though mapping is advocated, it is seldom performed, and an adequate signal to assess RR intervals is generally obtained by implanting in the left lower sternal area with an oblique angle analogous to lead II. The patient along with a spouse, family member, or friend is instructed in the use of the activator at the time of implant. Sterile implant technique is essential. Prophylactic antibiotics are generally recommended, although the efficacy in preventing infection has not been rigorously established.

Devices have the ability to automatically detect high and low heart rate and pause events, with irregularity and more recently refined discrimination and detection algorithms demonstrating excellent ability to detect atrial fibrillation.[14,15] Manual activation remains possible if the patient experiences symptoms, typically syncope, presyncope, or palpitations. The recorded bipolar ECG signal is stored in a loop buffer that stores the recorded ECG in several programmable memory bin configurations. Data storage and retrieval are influenced by the manufacturer platform, with the ability to use remote monitoring to obtain alerts for programmed events of interest.

Clinical Studies

Several studies have demonstrated the feasibility of the ICM in establishing a symptom rhythm correlation during long-term monitoring in patients with syncope.[16,17] Pooled data from nine smaller studies summarized in the European Society of Cardiology (ESC) Guidelines summarized 506 patients with unexplained syncope at the end of a complete conventional investigation. A symptom rhythm correlation was found in 176 patients (35%); of these, 56% had asystole (or bradycardia in a few cases) at the time of the recorded event, 11% had tachycardia, and 33% had no arrhythmia.[18]

A study of a "real-world" experience included 570 patients monitored for diagnosis of syncope.[19] The average follow-up time after ICM implant was 10 ± 6 months. Syncope recurred in 19%, 26%, and 36% after 3, 6, and 12 months, respectively. Of 218 events during the follow-up, ICM-guided diagnosis was obtained in 170 cases (78%), of which 128 (75%) were cardiac. The median number of tests performed per patient in the total study population was 13, and patients saw an average of three consultants before the device implantation. This speaks to the immense and misguided industry of evaluation of syncope prior to evaluation by a syncope expert.

Several studies have demonstrated the utility of prolonged cardiac monitoring in select populations. The ISSUE investigators (International Study on Syncope of Uncertain Etiology) assessed 111 patients with presumed vasovagal syncope who underwent tilt testing and loop recorder implants, regardless of tilt result. Syncope recurred in 34% of patients in both the tilt positive and tilt negative group, with marked bradycardia or asystole the most common recorded arrhythmia during follow-up (46% and 62% respectively). Tilt testing failed to predict the recurrence of syncope. Based on promising non randomized results from the ISSUE2 study, Brignole and colleagues implanted ICMs in 511 patients over age 40 with recurrent vasovagal syncope. In the 17% with asystolic recurrence, dual chamber pacemaker therapy was superior to the "pacemaker off" arm in prevention of recurrent syncope (57% reduction: 95% CI, 4%–81%).[20] This suggests that prolonged monitoring with an ICM is useful in patients with frequent vasovagal syncope who are over age 40 if pacemaker therapy is contemplated. This also suggests a diminishing role for tilt testing, which has limited correlation with spontaneous episodes recorded during extended monitoring.

Loop recorders have also shown utility in patients with syncope and bundle branch block with negative electrophysiological testing.[21] Negative electrophysiological testing does not exclude a diagnosis of intermittent complete atrioventricular block, and prolonged monitoring or consideration of permanent pacing is reasonable in this population.[22] A randomized study comparing pacing to ICM monitoring is currently underway.[22] Syncope in the absence of marked reduction in left ventricular function provides grounds to consider an ICM if an ICD is not indicated and noninvasive testing is inconclusive.

Two prospective randomized trials compared early use of the ICM for prolonged monitoring to conventional testing in patients undergoing a cardiac workup for unexplained syncope in patients without significant structural heart disease.[17,23] Conventional testing involved external loop recorders and tilt and electrophysiological testing. Both studies showed a higher diagnostic yield using an ICM. Overall, prolonged monitoring was more likely to result in a diagnosis than conventional testing, with a symptom–rhythm correlation obtained in 55% compared to a 19% diagnostic yield in the RAST Trial (*p* = .0014).[23] Both studies also showed that the apparent upfront cost of an ICM strategy was cost effective compared to conventional testing because of the dramatic improvement in diagnostic yield.[17,24] These data highlight the limitations of conventional diagnostic techniques. In patients with infrequent syncope, the ICM is the diagnostic tool of choice after noninvasive monitoring when an arrhythmia is suspected.

Event Classification

Interrogation of monitoring devices after a recurrence of syncope will often demonstrate rhythm findings that require clinical correlation and considerable judgment to interpret (Fig. 66.6).

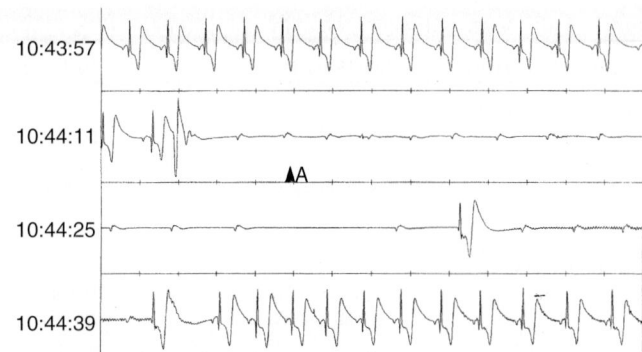

FIGURE 66.6 Rhythm strip from an insertable cardiac monitor from a 77-year-old man with recurrent unexplained syncope and a normal baseline electrocardiogram. Note that a premature ventricular contraction induces persistent complete atrioventricular block without an escape QRS, followed by sinus slowing suggesting a secondary cardioinhibitory vagal reaction.

Nocturnal pauses or atrial fibrillation may have different implications in patients based on their index indication for monitoring. The ISSUE investigators have proposed a useful classification system for symptomatic events in loop recorders applied to patients with syncope,[25] summarized in Table 66.1. This is often helpful in assigning a probable mechanism of syncope.

Emerging Role of Extended Monitoring in Atrial Fibrillation

Given the technical ability to detect atrial fibrillation with excellent sensitivity and specificity, extended monitoring has been employed across the spectrum of potential realms of interest from the detection of occult atrial fibrillation to measuring burden and assuring rate control. Several intervention-based trials have utilized ICMs as a gold standard to detect recurrence of atrial fibrillation after pharmacological or ablative intervention. The wealth of generated data has yet to translate into a clear evidence-based clinical process regarding therapeutic decision making, particularly in the realm of discontinuation of antithrombotic therapy in postablation patients. Several studies are underway utilizing these platforms to determine the best use of the data.

A major emerging role for extended monitoring relates to detection of atrial fibrillation in patients with prior cryptogenic stroke. This draws from evidence that pacemaker- and ICD-detected atrial fibrillation is associated with an incremental risk of stroke, which presumably can be attenuated by antithrombotic therapy.[26] Several modest-sized studies have shown trends in increased detection of atrial fibrillation as duration of monitoring is extended with both external and implanted monitors.[27]

Two recent clinical trials have substantially influenced evidence to support consideration of monitoring in this population. In 572 patients older than 55 years with cryptogenic stroke within 6 months, the EMBRACE trial showed that atrial fibrillation lasting 30 seconds or longer was detected in 45 of 280 patients (16.1%) in a 1-month external monitor group, as compared with 9 of 277 (3.2%) in the control group (absolute difference, 12.9%; number needed to screen, 8).[28] The CRYSTAL-AF trial enrolled 441 patients over age 40 with cryptogenic stroke and a negative 24-hour Holter, randomized to ICM or usual care.[29] By 12 months, atrial fibrillation had been detected in 12.4% versus 2.0% in the usual care arm (*p* < .001) reference. Ongoing divergence in atrial fibrillation detection was noted, although the number of patients with extended follow-up was small. Several recent studies have associated extended monitoring with detection of both atrial fibrillation and frequent supraventricular ectopy with an associated risk of stroke.[30]

TABLE 66.1   ISSUE classification of detected rhythm from the insertable cardiac monitor

CLASSIFICATION	SINUS RATE	AV NODE	COMMENT
Asystole (RR >3 sec)			
1A	Arrest	Normal	Progressive sinus bradycardia until sinus arrest probably vasovagal
1B	Bradycardia	AV block	AV block with associated sinus bradycardia probably vasovagal
1C	Normal or tachycardia	AV block	Abrupt AV block without sinus slowing suggests intrinsic AV conduction disease
Bradycardia			
2A	Decrease > 30%	Normal	Probably vasovagal
2B	HR < 40 for >10 s	Normal	Probably vasovagal
Minimal HR Change			
3A	<10% variation	Normal	Suggests noncardiac cause: unlikely vasovagal
3B	HR increase or decrease 10%–30%, not <40 or >120 beats/min	Normal	Suggests vasovagal
Tachycardia			
4A	Progressive tachycardia	Normal	Sinus acceleration suggests orthostatic intolerance or noncardiac cause
4B	N/A	Normal	Atrial fibrillation
4C	N/A	Normal	Supraventricular tachycardia
4D	N/A	Normal	Ventricular tachycardia

AV, Atrioventricular; *HR,* heart rate; *N/A,* not applicable.
Modified from Brignole M, Moya A, Menozzi C, Garcia-Civera R, Sutton R. Proposed electrocardiographic classification of spontaneous syncope documented by an implantable loop recorder. *Europace.* 2005;7:14-18.

Additional Uses of Extended Monitoring Technologies

Long-term cardiac monitoring is best suited for patients with infrequent intermittent symptoms possibly related to arrhythmia, or those where an infrequent "silent" arrhythmia is sought. Although syncope is a logical first application of this technology, many other clinical disease states stand to benefit from the knowledge gained from prolonged monitoring. This includes atypical epilepsy, where seizures may be evidence of recurrent cerebral hypoperfusion in conjunction with syncope, mistaken as a primary neurological event.

Additional potential uses of the ICM relate to the automatic detection feature of the device in patients for risk stratification after myocardial infarction. The CARISMA study involved implanted ICMs in 297 patients and followed them for 1.9 ± 0.5 years.[31] Predefined arrhythmias were recorded in 137 patients (46%), 86% of which were asymptomatic. The ICM documented a 28% incidence of new-onset atrial fibrillation, a 13% incidence of nonsustained ventricular tachycardia (≥16 beats), a 10% incidence of high-degree atrioventricular block, a 12% incidence of significant sinus node disease, a 3% incidence of sustained ventricular tachycardia, and a 3% incidence of ventricular fibrillation. Regression analysis showed that high-degree atrioventricular block was the most powerful predictor of cardiac death. The implications of this study are not completely understood, and the ability to alter outcomes remains to be established. It certainly demonstrates the incremental detection ability of the ICM in this population, suggesting that historic short-term studies have grossly underestimated the incidence of potentially relevant arrhythmias. Active research in this realm is ongoing.

Finally, strong interest in monitoring of atrial fibrillation to guide treatment of symptomatic atrial fibrillation is underway, but studies have not yet reported data linked to outcomes that influence clinical decision making. Guidelines have not cited ICMs as the gold standard for clinical trials evaluating the efficacy of interventions such as ablation or cardioversion,[32,33] although this is implicit and in use in several ongoing clinical trials. Multiple small studies have evaluated the utility of external monitoring technologies after ablation, and several larger studies with implanted devices measuring both burden of disease and efficacy of an antiarrhythmic intervention are expected to report imminently. While these studies have reported a higher rate of silent atrial arrhythmias than previously suspected, the implication if these findings is speculative.[34,35]

Future Directions

Recent advances in loop recorder design and the presence of multiple manufacturers are indicative of rekindled interest in long-term physiological monitoring for a variety of disease states. Enhanced data capture is providing large-scale, accessible data to analyze potentially contributing novel insights into areas such as risk stratification and arrhythmia burden assessment. Improved onboard and offline diagnostic capabilities may provide an early warning or patient alert mechanism for a range of events, including recurrence of atrial fibrillation or nonsustained ventricular arrhythmia. The notion of detection of catastrophic arrhythmia with a device integrated with an emergency response system has been raised. Of greater interest is the potential to integrate a broader range of physiological sensors in long-term monitoring devices, including but not limited to blood pressure, oxygen saturation, chest impedance, and left atrial pressure. In many respects, the only missing element in this regard is connecting the capabilities in conjunction with acceptable costs and form factor.

Conclusion

Progressively extended monitoring technologies have significantly improved the objective of obtaining ambient or symptomatic physiological data. Long-term monitoring with the ICM is the test of choice in patients with problematic syncope and preserved left ventricular function. Prolonged monitoring with external and implantable monitors has significantly enhanced our ability to diagnose intermittent arrhythmias in a variety of clinical settings. Ongoing clinical trials will undoubtedly expand the use of prolonged monitoring to other disease states.

REFERENCES

1. Olson JA, Fouts AM, Padanilam BJ, Prystowsky EN. Utility of mobile cardiac outpatient telemetry for the diagnosis of palpitations, presyncope, syncope, and the assessment of therapy efficacy. *J Cardiovasc Electrophysiol.* 2007;18:473–477.

2. Barrett PM, Komatireddy R, Haaser S, et al. Comparison of 24-hour Holter monitoring with 14-day novel adhesive patch electrocardiographic monitoring. *Am J Med.* 2014;127:e11–e17.

3. Rickard J, Ahmed S, Baruch M, Klocman B, Martin DO, Menon V. Utility of a novel watch-based pulse detection system to detect pulselessness in human subjects. *Heart Rhythm.* 2011;8:1895–1899.

4. Haberman ZC, Jahn RT, Bose R, et al. Wireless smartphone ECG enables large-scale screening in diverse populations. *J Cardiovasc Electrophysiol.* 2015;26:520–526.

5. McManus DD, Chong JW, Soni A, et al. PULSESMART: pulse-based arrhythmia discrimination using a novel smartphone application. *J Cardiovasc Electrophysiol.* 2016;27:51–57.

6. Rothman SA, Laughlin JC, Seltzer J, et al. The diagnosis of cardiac arrhythmias: a prospective multi-center randomized study comparing mobile cardiac outpatient telemetry versus standard loop event monitoring. *J Cardiovasc Electrophysiol.* 2007;18:241–247.

7. Sivakumaran S, Krahn AD, Klein GJ, et al. A prospective randomized comparison of loop recorders versus Holter monitors in patients with syncope or presyncope. *Am J Med.* 2003;115:1–5.

8. Reiffel JA, Schwarzberg R, Murry M. Comparison of autotriggered memory loop recorders versus standard loop recorders versus 24-hour Holter monitors for arrhythmia detection. *Am J Cardiol.* 2005;95:1055–1059.

9. O'Neil BJ, Hoekstra J, Pride YB, et al. Incremental benefit of 80-lead electrocardiogram body surface mapping over the 12-lead electrocardiogram in the detection of acute coronary syndromes in patients without ST-elevation myocardial infarction: results from the Optimal Cardiovascular Diagnostic Evaluation Enabling Faster Treatment of Myocardial Infarction (OCCULT MI) trial. *Acad Emerg Med.* 2010;17:932–939.

10. Pandian PS, Mohanavelu K, Safeer KP, et al. Smart Vest: wearable multi-parameter remote physiological monitoring system. *Med Eng Phys.* 2008;30:466–477.

11. Konecny T, Saxon LA. Integration of smartphone based monitoring—no modality is an island, entire of itself. *J Cardiovasc Electrophysiol.* 2016;27:58–59.

12. Mittal S, Sanders P, Pokushalov E, et al. Safety profile of a miniaturized insertable cardiac monitor: results from two prospective trials. *Pacing Clin Electrophysiol.* 2015;38:1464–1469.

13. Purerfellner H, Sanders P, Pokushalov E, et al. Miniaturized Reveal LINQ insertable cardiac monitoring system: first-in-human experience. *Heart Rhythm.* 2015;12:1113–1119.

14. Ziegler PD, Rogers JD, Ferreira SW, et al. Real-world experience with insertable cardiac monitors to find atrial fibrillation in cryptogenic stroke. *Cerebrovasc Dis.* 2015;40:175–181.

15. Sanna T, Diener HC, Passman RS. Crystal AF Steering Committee. Cryptogenic stroke and atrial fibrillation. *N Engl J Med.* 2014;371:1261.

16. Brignole M, Sutton R, Menozzi C, et al. Early application of an implantable loop recorder allows effective specific therapy in patients with recurrent suspected neurally mediated syncope. *Eur Heart J.* 2006;27:1085–1092.

17. Farwell DJ, Freemantle N, Sulke N. The clinical impact of implantable loop recorders in patients with syncope. *Eur Heart J.* 2006;27:351–356.

18. Moya A, Sutton R, Ammirati F, et al. Guidelines for the diagnosis and management of syncope (version 2009). *Eur Heart J.* 2009;30:2631–2671.

19. Edvardsson N, Frykman V, van Mechelen R, et al. Use of an implantable loop recorder to increase the diagnostic yield in unexplained syncope: results from the PICTURE registry. *Europace.* 2011;13:262–269.

20. Brignole M, Menozzi C, Moya A, et al. Pacemaker therapy in patients with neurally mediated syncope and documented asystole: Third International Study on Syncope of Uncertain Etiology (ISSUE-3): a randomized trial. *Circulation.* 2012;125:2566–2571.

21. Brignole M, Menozzi C, Moya A, et al. Mechanism of syncope in patients with bundle branch block and negative electrophysiological test. *Circulation.* 2001;104:2045–2050.

22. Krahn AD, Morillo CA, Kus T, et al. Empiric pacemaker compared with a monitoring strategy in patients with syncope and bifascicular conduction block–rationale and design of the Syncope: Pacing or Recording in ThE Later Years (SPRITELY) study. *Europace.* 2012;14:1044–1048.

23. Krahn AD, Klein GJ, Yee R, Skanes AC. Randomized assessment of syncope trial: conventional diagnostic testing versus a prolonged monitoring strategy. *Circulation.* 2001;104:46–51.

24. Krahn AD, Klein GJ, Yee R, Hoch JS, Skanes AC. Cost implications of testing strategy in patients with syncope: randomized assessment of syncope trial. *J Am Coll Cardiol.* 2003;42:495–501.

25. Brignole M, Moya A, Menozzi C, Garcia-Civera R, Sutton R. Proposed electrocardiographic classification of spontaneous syncope documented by an implantable loop recorder. *Europace.* 2005;7:14–18.

26. Healey JS, Connolly SJ, Gold MR, et al. Subclinical atrial fibrillation and the risk of stroke. *N Engl J Med.* 2012;366:120–129.

27. Rizos T, Guntner J, Jenetzky E, et al. Continuous stroke unit electrocardiographic monitoring versus 24-hour Holter electrocardiography for detection of paroxysmal atrial fibrillation after stroke. *Stroke.* 2012;43:2689–2694.

28. Gladstone DJ, Sharma M, Spence JD, Committee ES. Investigators. Cryptogenic stroke and atrial fibrillation. *N Engl J Med.* 2014;371:1260.

29. Sanna T, Diener HC, Passman RS, et al. Cryptogenic stroke and underlying atrial fibrillation. *N Engl J Med.* 2014;370:2478–2486.

30. Larsen BS, Kumarathurai P, Falkenberg J, Nielsen OW, Sajadieh A. Excessive atrial ectopy and short atrial runs increase the risk of stroke beyond incident atrial fibrillation. *J Am Coll Cardiol.* 2015;66:232–241.

31. Bloch Thomsen PE, Jons C, Raatikainen MJ, et al. Long-term recording of cardiac arrhythmias with an implantable cardiac monitor in patients with reduced ejection fraction after acute myocardial infarction: the Cardiac Arrhythmias and Risk Stratification After Acute Myocardial Infarction (CARISMA) study. *Circulation.* 2010;122:1258–1264.

32. January CT, Wann LS, Alpert JS, et al. American College of Cardiology/American Heart Association Task Force on Practice G. 2014 AHA/ACC/HRS guideline for the management of patients with atrial fibrillation: a report of the American College of Cardiology/American Heart Association Task Force on Practice Guidelines and the Heart Rhythm Society. *J Am Coll Cardiol.* 2014;64:e1–e76.

33. Camm AJ, Lip GY, De Caterina R, et al. Guidelines ESCCfP. 2012 focused update of the ESC Guidelines for the management of atrial fibrillation: an update of the 2010 ESC Guidelines for the management of atrial fibrillation. Developed with the special contribution of the European Heart Rhythm Association. *Eur Heart J.* 2012;33:2719–2747.

34. Perez-Castellano N, Fernandez-Cavazos R, Moreno J, et al. The COR trial: a randomized study with continuous rhythm monitoring to compare the efficacy of cryoenergy and radiofrequency for pulmonary vein isolation. *Heart Rhythm.* 2014;11:8–14.

35. Andrade JG, Krahn AD. Is an implantable cardiac monitor the standard of care for determining the success of atrial fibrillation ablation? *J Cardiovasc Electrophysiol.* 2013;24:1083–1085.

67 Head-up Tilt Table Testing

Wayne O. Adkisson and David G. Benditt

Historical Background

Head-up tilt has been used for more than half a century by physiologists and physicians to study cardiovascular adaptation to changes in position, to model responses to hemorrhage, and to evaluate hemodynamic and neuroendocrine responses in congestive heart failure, autonomic dysfunction, and hypertension. During such studies, incidental observations noted that some test subjects experienced total or near-total transient loss of consciousness due to systemic hypotension induced by the head-up tilt procedure.[1-5] Further, in some cases hypotension was associated with unexpected marked bradycardia, including prolonged asystolic periods that terminated spontaneously (Fig. 67.1). By way of example, Hammill and colleagues[5] used 60-degree–head-up posture in an attempt to enhance the diagnostic precision of conventional diagnostic cardiac stimulation studies. In the course of this procedure, a typical vasovagal reaction occurred in 6 of 104 subjects. The investigators noted this result but undertook no formal assessment of the observation.

It was the landmark study by Kenny and colleagues[6] that ultimately led to the concept of using head-up tilt as a diagnostic tool for eliciting the susceptibility to reflex syncope, and in particular vasovagal syncope (VVS). Initially, prolonged periods of head-up tilt at angles of 40 to 60 degrees were used in an attempt to provoke VVS in susceptible individuals. Subsequently, to improve sensitivity of the test, additional interventions were introduced including administration of pharmacological agents (discussed in more detail later) either alone or in conjunction with physical maneuvers such as carotid sinus massage. Several of these additional provocative measures did improve the head-up tilt test sensitivity and remain in use; however, as a rule, their addition has been at the cost of lower specificity. The difficulties in assessing sensitivity and specificity of head-up tilt table testing are discussed in more detail later.

Since its introduction as a clinical diagnostic laboratory tool, the uses of the head-up tilt table testing have expanded. Whereas tilt table testing remains widely accepted for the evaluation of an individual's susceptibility to VVS in selected cases, it has also found a place, albeit less well studied, in the evaluation of (1) orthostatic hypotension (OH), (2) postural orthostatic tachycardia syndrome (POTS), and (3) psychogenic pseudosyncope/pseudoseizures.[7] In this chapter, we review the role of head-up tilt table testing in the evaluation of VVS and OH, discuss limitations of such testing, and review a methodology for its use.

Transient Loss of Consciousness and Syncope

For the most part, patients referred for head-up tilt table testing have previously presented with one or more apparent transient loss of consciousness (TLOC) spells. However, in certain of these cases, the presentation may not have been true loss of consciousness; consequently, the basis for referral may be more broadly viewed as consultation for assessment of self-limited spontaneous collapse (Fig. 67.2). It is the consultant's responsibility to ascertain whether there has been "true" TLOC. If TLOC is deemed to have occurred, then the differential diagnosis primarily includes syncope, epileptic seizures, intoxications, and possibly metabolic disturbances; tilt table testing may be helpful in selected cases for distinguishing among these disorders. On the other hand, if it is determined that TLOC did not occur, then the differential diagnosis principally includes psychogenic pseudosyncope/pseudoseizures, mechanical falls, malingering, and cataplexy (see Fig. 67.2). Tilt table testing may be particularly helpful in identifying pseudosyncope/pseudoseizures. Specifically, the individuals afflicted with this disorder are highly suggestible, and the test may demonstrate normal heart rate and blood pressure despite the patient's head slumping over and seemingly having a loss of consciousness event. Pseudosyncope/pseudoseizure should not be confused with malingering. In our experience, it is exceedingly rare that such patients are trying to mislead by "faking" these events. The episodes are quite real to the sufferer.

Pathophysiology of Loss of Consciousness

Neuronal tissue has limited energy storage capabilities; consequently, maintenance of oxygenated blood flow to the brain is critical. In healthy young individuals, cerebral blood flow (CBF) ranges from 50 to 60 mL/100 g of brain tissue per minute. This represents approximately 12% to 15% of the resting cardiac output. Blood flow of that magnitude can easily supply the minimum oxygen (O_2) requirement needed to maintain consciousness, which is typically 3.0 to 3.5 mL O_2/100 g tissue per minute.[8-10] However, the safety margin for oxygen delivery may be severely

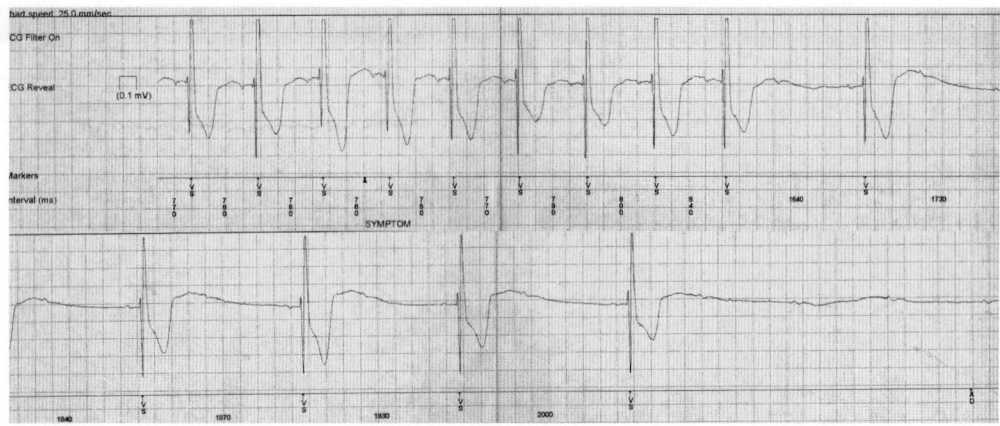

FIGURE 67.1 Electrocardiogram (*ECG*) of a patient during spontaneous episode of vasovagal syncope. The strips are continuous and show the typical sinus rate slowing prior to the event. In this example, sinus arrest did not occur (note P waves remain visible) but progressive AV block results in ventricular asystole. The slowing of the sinus rate helps distinguish a vasovagal event from sinoatrial block or sinus pauses related to sinus node dysfunction.

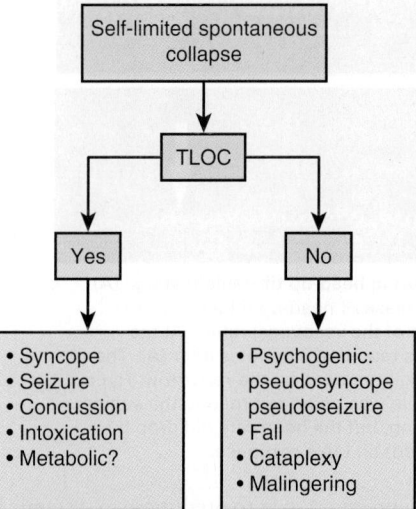

FIGURE 67.2 Schematic diagram illustrating an approach to the patient with self-limited collapse. The first step in the assessment is to determine whether there has been transient loss of consciousness (*TLOC*). For syncope to have occurred, TLOC must have occurred. The use and limitations of head-up tilt table testing to help differentiate among various causes of syncope is discussed in the text.

impaired in the elderly; in persons with hypertension, diabetes mellitus, or heart failure; and in hypoxemic states (e.g., chronic pulmonary disease). In general, a loss of nutrient flow to the brain for 6 to 10 seconds is sufficient to cause a loss of consciousness.[11]

For the most part, CBF remains adequate over perfusion pressures ranging from 50 to 170 mm Hg[12,13] due to cerebral autoregulation.[14] However, abrupt perfusion changes may cause transient CBF inadequacy. In the face of rapid changes in perfusion pressure, cerebral autoregulation may be unable to prevent a drop in CBF, which, if of sufficient magnitude, will result in syncope.

Approach to the Diagnosis of Syncope

Many conditions may cause the physiological disturbances that result in syncope (Table 67.1). Reflex syncope, OH, and cardiac arrhythmias are among the more frequent causes. Of the reflex syncope syndromes, VVS is the most common cause of syncope

across all age groups, and consequently virtually all medical practitioners will encounter VVS patients.

In the case of VVS, the diagnosis can be established in most cases by the medical history without further testing.[7,15] However, when the history surrounding the event is "atypical," even an experienced history-taker may not be able to establish a firm diagnosis. In some cases it may not be possible to obtain an adequate history, especially in the elderly.[16,17] Furthermore, witnesses may not have been present, or they may be unable to provide sufficiently reliable details needed to establish a specific diagnosis. In such cases, availability of diagnostic tests becomes important. Additionally, even when VVS is evident to an experienced clinician, patients who have been subject to several previous unsuccessful evaluations may remain skeptical, and the consultant may reasonably elect to recommend additional testing in an attempt to reproduce the patient's symptoms under controlled and observed conditions. The head-up tilt table test is the most widely available diagnostic intervention for such cases.

Physiological Impact of Upright Posture

Upright posture elicits an orthostatic stress as the effects of gravity result in a redistribution of circulating blood volume in the body.[1,2,4,6–8] As upright posture is achieved; the effects of gravity result in shifting of 500 to 1000 mL of blood to the lower part of the body and in particular to the highly compliant splanchnic bed.[8,18] This initial redistribution is rapid and occurs in the first 10 seconds. If upright posture is maintained, over the course of 10 minutes, an additional 700 mL of protein-free fluid is filtered into the interstitial space. The combined effect of these two shifts is a reduction of venous return and stroke volume.

In humans, diminution of stroke volume upon the assumption of an upright position is compensated for by both an increase in heart rate and by the constriction of both resistance and capacitance blood vessels. An increase in heart rate alone is usually insufficient to maintain cardiac output and CBF. Systemic vasoconstriction is crucial for maintenance of adequate blood pressure. Loss of consciousness can only be prevented if the compensatory mechanisms maintain arterial pressure at a level at least equal to the minimum value needed to ensure adequate CBF.

Short-term cardiovascular responses triggered by orthostatic stress are primarily mediated by the autonomic nervous system via arterial mechanoreceptors (baroreceptors responding to pressure, stretch, or both) located in the aortic arch and carotid

TABLE 67.1 Classification of the causes of syncope

REFLEX SYNDROMES	ORTHOSTATIC HYPOTENSION	CARDIOVASCULAR	
		ARRHYTHMIA	STRUCTURAL
Vasovagal syncope	Secondary autonomic failure (common):	Bradycardia	Valvular stenosis
Carotid sinus syncope	• Drug induced	• Sinus node disease	Cardiomyopathy
Situational:	• Diabetes	• Conduction system disease	Ischemic
• Cough	• Amyloidosis	Tachycardia	• Nonischemic
• Postmicturition	• Alcohol	• Supraventricular	• Hypertrophic
• Others	Primary autonomic failure (rare):	• Ventricular	• Arrhythmogenic
	• Parkinson disease	Ion channel disorders	Pulmonary hypertension
	• Multiple system atrophy		Pulmonary emboli
	• Lewy body dementia		Aortic dissection
	• Pure autonomic failure		
≈60% of cases of syncope	≈15%	≈10%	≈5%
≈10% unknown			

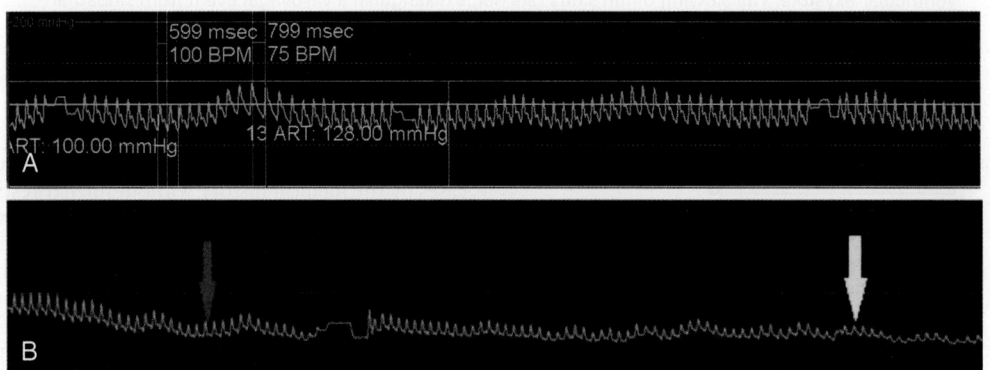

FIGURE 67.3 Beat-to-beat blood pressure recordings obtained during head-up tilt-table testing. (A) and (B) were obtained from the same patient during the passive phase of head-up tilt testing. (A) demonstrates the typical oscillations often seen prior to the onset of the vasovagal reflex. At the time (A) was recorded, the patient reported no symptoms. (B) was recorded 3 minutes after (A). The patient complained of her typical premonitory symptoms at the point marked by the *red arrow*. Hypotension progressed and loss of consciousness occurred as the table was being returned to the supine position (*yellow arrow*). The concomitant bradycardia is not striking, but the heart rate did drop by more than 10%. In the VASIS schema, this would be a type I (mixed) tilt table response.

sinuses. Mechanoreceptors in the heart wall (both atria and ventricles) as well as in the lungs may contribute as well.

Reflex activation of central sympathetic outflow to the systemic vasculature may be augmented by local reflex mechanisms, such as the venoarteriolar reflex. More global mechanisms such as the muscle skeletal pump (active even without overt movement) and the respiratory pump also contribute. All of these mechanisms may play a useful adjunctive role in maintaining cardiac output and arterial pressure, primarily by augmenting venous return.

Failure of compensatory mechanisms during orthostatic stress, assuming no preexisting volume overload, results in impaired venous return and leads to diminished stroke volume, systemic arterial pressure, and CBF. If CBF reduction is of sufficient magnitude, loss of consciousness results. In this setting, loss of consciousness may be principally due to inadequate maintenance of blood pressure in the face of gravitational stress (i.e., "orthostatic hypotension" or "orthostatic syncope") but may additionally be contributed to by an inappropriate reflex response resulting in vasodilation (i.e., vasodepressor response) and severe or relative bradycardia.[7,8,19]

Reflex Faints

Reflex syncope is the preferred term encompassing all conditions in which reflexes modify heart rate (cardioinhibition) and vascular

tone (vasodepression) so as to predispose to systemic hypotension of sufficient severity to cause inadequate cerebral perfusion. Thus reflex syncope incorporates VVS, carotid sinus syndrome, and the situational faints (see later). Other umbrella terms for reflex syncope that have been used, but are less desirable, include neutrally mediated (reflex) syncope and neurocardiogenic syncope.

VVS is the most common reflex syncope, but despite much study, its pathophysiology remains incompletely understood. In any case, systemic hypotension is principally due to vasodilation, mediated by a marked reduction in both the sympathetic vasoconstrictor outflow to skeletal muscle and a substantial increase in venous capacitance, especially in the splanchnic bed. Finally, a parasympathetically mediated bradycardia may also contribute, but usually has a lesser role than vasodilation for producing systemic hypotension.

Head-up Tilt as a Useful Model of Spontaneous Vasovagal Syncope

Several observations suggest that symptomatic hypotension–bradycardia associated with a positive result on head-up tilt table testing is comparable to spontaneous VVS. First, both induced and spontaneous VVS episodes are associated with similar premonitory symptoms (nausea, diaphoresis) and signs (pallor, loss of postural tone). Second, the temporal sequence of blood pressure and heart rate changes during tilt-induced syncope parallels that

BOX 67.1   Utility of head-up tilt testing

1. Assess susceptibility to vasovagal syncope and/or orthostatic hypotension in a controlled and safe environment.
2. Determine whether induced symptoms correspond to spontaneous clinical symptoms.
3. Educate patients regarding warning symptoms so they may take preventive measures.
4. Potentially identify syncope mimics (e.g., psychogenic pseudosyncope).
5. Support the diagnosis in suspected postural orthostatic tachycardia syndrome.
6. Enhance patient confidence that the diagnosis (i.e., vasovagal syncope, orthostatic hypotension, or postural orthostatic tachycardia syndrome) is correct.

TABLE 67.2   Indication for head-up tilt table testing

CLASS	LEVEL OF EVIDENCES	CLINICAL SETTING
I	B	Single episode of unexplained syncope in high-risk setting or occupational implications
		Recurrent in absence of structural heart disease
		Syncope in setting of heart disease when cardiac causes have been excluded
I	C	If there is clinical value in demonstrating susceptibility to reflex syncope to the patient
IIa	C	To discriminate reflex syncope from orthostatic hypotension
IIb	C	To discriminate syncope with jerking movements from epilepsy
		Evaluation of recurrent unexplained falls
		Evaluation of frequent syncope and the possibility of psychiatric illness
III	B	Not recommended to assess efficacy of therapy
III	C	Isoproterenol tilt testing should not be done in patients with ischemic heart diseases

Modified from Moya A, Sutton R, Ammirati F, et al. Guidelines for the diagnosis and management of syncope (version 2009). *Eur Heart J.* 2009;21:2631-2671.

seen in spontaneous events (Fig. 67.3). Finally, plasma catecholamines before and during both spontaneous and tilt-induced syncope exhibit similar patterns. Specifically, there is a premonitory (before hypotension is evident) increase in circulating catecholamines with epinephrine to a greater extent than norepinephrine in both spontaneous as well as tilt-induced VVS.[20,21]

Pathophysiology of Orthostatic Hypotension

A 2011 consensus statement provided a working definition of OH and its several common variants[22]; specifically, OH was defined as a drop in systolic blood pressure of ≥20 mm Hg or a drop in diastolic blood pressure of ≥10 mm Hg that usually occurs within 3 minutes of active standing or passive tilt to a minimum of 60 degrees. In hypertensive patients, a fall of at least 30 mm Hg systolic was deemed more appropriate.

Moving from a supine to upright posture rarely induces syncope in healthy patients. However, a fleeting sensation of "graying out," "dizziness," or "unsteadiness" immediately (usually in the first 15 seconds) upon assuming an upright position is common (so-called "immediate" or "initial" OH), so much so that most individuals do not find it a cause for concern. Symptomatic immediate OH usually requires a blood pressure drop of approximately 40 mm Hg, albeit very brief such that cerebrovascular autoregulation does not have adequate time to respond.[22] "Delayed" or "classical" OH is that which occurs after a period of standing or passive tilt, typically of 3 minutes (an arbitrary cut-off) or somewhat more in duration.[22] Finally and less often, the blood pressure decline occurs very slowly, and the symptoms may not develop for more than 5 minutes after the posture change; this scenario may be termed "progressive" OH and is particularly difficult to recognize as the relationship to recent postural change is at best tenuous. The greater the delay in the onset of symptomatic hypotension, the more likely that the individual has moved away from a chair, bed, or other means of support, and as such has greater propensity for injury.

Orthostatic Provocation for Assessing Susceptibility to Vasovagal Syncope and Orthostatic Hypotension

Several publications address the utility and indications for head-up tilt testing (Box 67.1).[7,23] The next European Society of Cardiology (ESC) guideline update is expected in 2017. In addition, the Heart Rhythm Society recently commented on the staffing requirements for performing head-up tilt table testing.[24] Finally, an American College of Cardiology/American Heart Association Syncope guideline, which will include recommendations related to the use of head-up tilt table testing, is to be published in 2016.

Increasingly, laboratories that undertake head-up tilt table testing are encouraged to include an active standing test component.[7] Active standing, unlike the passive head-up tilt, activates

skeletal muscle pumps. The ESC guidelines[7] recommend active standing as the test of choice for suspected OH. During such testing, we recommend use of noninvasive beat-to-beat blood pressure monitoring. We also prefer a 5- to 10-minute active standing test duration as opposed to the 3-minute test recommended in the ESC guidelines.[7]

Indications for head-up tilt table testing are summarized in Table 67.2.[7] There is general agreement that tilt table testing should be used primarily for confirming a suspected diagnosis. This latter point is important since false-positive tests do occur (especially in young patients); consequently, in the absence of a strong correlation between tilt table–induced and spontaneous symptoms, a positive test should not be assumed to be diagnostic.

The gold standard for VVS diagnosis is the clinical history (including witness observations). A negative tilt study in a patient with a classic history of VVS does not exclude the diagnosis, and a positive study will not alter therapy. However, as noted earlier, head-up tilt table testing is sometimes offered in this circumstance to convince a skeptical patient that the diagnosis is correct (see Box 67.1). Finally, neither head-up tilt table testing nor active standing is considered to be useful in diagnosing or excluding other forms of reflex syncope such as carotid sinus syndrome or situational faints. On the other hand, upright posture may be advantageous to better elicit the hemodynamic consequences of diagnostic interventions such as carotid sinus massage in patients with suspected carotid sinus syndrome.[7] Our view of appropriate current clinical uses of head-up tilt table testing is summarized in Table 67.3.

Protocols for Head-up Tilt Table Testing and Active Standing Test

The first step in the tilt test procedure is a period of rest (typically 10 to 15 minutes) after the instrumentation and monitoring equipment have been attached. Thereafter the patient is passively tilted to a 60- to 70-degree head-up position. The patient is supported by a foot-plate and gently applied body straps to prevent falling. The duration of the tilt varies by laboratory but is typically

TABLE 67.3 Sensitivity, specificity, and diagnostic odds ratio of head-up tilt test protocols (estimates with 95% confidence intervals)

	SENSITIVITY (%)	SPECIFICITY (%)	DIAGNOSTIC ODDS RATIO
Overall passive protocols	37 (29–46)	96 (92–98)	10.14 (6.70–15.34)
Overall isoproterenol protocols	61 (52–69)	86 (79–91)	8.33 (6.38–10.86)
Overall nitroglycerine protocols	66 (60–72)	89 (84–92)	14.40 (11.50–18.05)

Modified from Forleo C, Guida P, Iacoviello M, et al. Head-up tilt testing for diagnosing vasovagal syncope: a meta-analysis. *Int J Cardiol.* 2013;168:27-35.

20 to 45 minutes. If needed, pharmacological provocation may be used in conjunction with a head-up tilt. Various pharmacological agents have been used, but the most common are nitroglycerin and isoproterenol (discussed later). Both increase the sensitivity of the test but at the cost of lower specificity.

As noted earlier, there is no test or laboratory procedure that provides a gold standard for the diagnosis of VVS. VVS is a clinical diagnosis that is primarily based on the medical history including eyewitness observations. The authors consider a head-up tilt study to be positive if the vasovagal reflex is induced *and* reproduces the patient's clinical symptomatology. Induction of VVS that does *not* reproduce the patient's clinical symptoms is problematic. In a patient with little or no doubt regarding the clinical diagnosis of VVS, a tilt test is not usually warranted unless it is being used to educate the patient (see Box 67.1). In this case, a negative study does not exclude the diagnosis and should be considered to be a false negative.

A few laboratories favor a very short tilt test protocol that includes pharmacological provocation from the start. Concerns about adverse drug reactions and the potential for diminished specificity and sensitivity have limited the acceptance of these approaches. Further, a recent report described a shortened tilt protocol that provoked syncope through a painful stimulus.[25] We do not advocate this approach as the deliberate infliction of pain poses, in our opinion, ethical concerns.

Passive Drug-Free Tilt Testing

The 1986 report by Kenny and associates[6] used a 60-degree head-up tilt for up to 60 minutes. The test triggered symptomatic hypotension and bradycardia consistent with a vasovagal reaction in 10/15 patients with syncope of unknown etiology and in only 1/10 control subjects without a history of syncope. Subsequent studies refined the tilt test methodology. By way of example, Fitzpatrick and colleagues[26] investigated the use of a bicycle saddle or seat attached to the tilt table but found that it resulted in an excessive number of positive studies, presumably due to the obstruction of venous return. The saddle tilt configuration has been abandoned. These investigators also demonstrated that the use of tilt angles less than 60 degrees resulted in inadequate test sensitivity. Finally, with respect to conventional 60- or 70-degree tilt angles, these same authors[26] also concluded that given the average time to the onset of syncope (24 ± 10 minutes), a head-up tilt duration of 45 minutes was sufficient. Accordingly, they proposed a protocol utilizing a 60-degre inclination for 45 minutes and observed positive responses for patients with syncope of unknown origin in 75% with a specificity of 93%.

The findings of Fitzpatrick and colleagues[26] were instrumental in defining a practical head-up tilt test protocol. Later, based primarily on reports by Almquist et al.,[27] Natale et al.,[28] and Waxman et al.,[29] the angle of the table was set, in most laboratories, to the 60- to 70-degree angle used today. The 45-minute duration persisted for many years, but the more widespread acceptance of pharmacological provocation (initially isoproterenol in North America but with increasing change to nitroglycerin) allowed for the adoption of shorter tilt duration (the so-called Italian protocol), typically 20 minutes.

Passive Tilt Testing With Pharmacological Provocation

The use of isoproterenol as a provocative agent for tilt table tests in the diagnosis of VVS was introduced in 1989 by both Waxman et al.[29] and Almquist et al.[27] Almquist et al. used a short protocol in which if the initial 10 minutes of passive tilt were not diagnostic, the patient was returned to the supine position and given isoproterenol at a dose of 1 mg/min. After a new steady-state heart rate was achieved, the patient again underwent a head-up tilt. This process was repeated to a maximum dose of 5 mg/min. Using this protocol, 9/11 patients with syncope of unknown origin and negative electrophysiology studies developed hypotension and bradycardia, while only 2/18 control subjects did.

In its use as a provocative agent in tilt table testing, isoproterenol has not been without controversy. In particular, Kapoor and Brant[30] raised concerns over the potentially low specificity (45% to 65%) of isoproterenol provocation. Later, Morillo and colleagues[31] proposed a low-dose isoproterenol protocol, in which after 15 minutes of tilt, incremental doses of isoproterenol (up to 3 mg/min) were administered while the patient remained in a head-up position; they reported a 61% rate of positive responses and a specificity of 93%.

Although isoproterenol is still employed as a provocative agent, its use has waned for several reasons. First, mixing and delivering isoproterenol is time consuming. Second, patients frequently complain of drug-induced anxiety and palpitations. Third, there is the concern of causing ischemia in patients with coronary artery disease. Finally, in the United States at least, the cost of isoproterenol has increased dramatically; this is not due to a shortage of the drug but rather to change in ownership.[32] If for no other reason than to minimize undue expense, the authors suggest that nitroglycerine (see later) be the preferred provocative agent.

In 1994, Raviele and colleagues[33] introduced the use of intravenous nitroglycerin infusion as an alternative to isoproterenol provocation during head-up tilt table testing. Using their nitroglycerin infusion protocol, 21/40 patients (53%) with syncope of unknown origin had a positive head-up tilt test, with a specificity of 92%. Ten of the 40 patients developed progressive hypotension without bradycardia. The latter outcome was not considered a positive result but rather was attributed to the hypotensive effect of the medication and was classified as an "exaggerated" response. Later, Raviele and coworkers[34] demonstrated that sublingual nitroglycerin was a highly effective alternative to intravenous infusion. After 45 minutes of baseline head-up tilt, a 0.3-mg dose of sublingual nitroglycerine was given. With this protocol, the authors reported an overall positive tilt rate of 51% (25% during the baseline tilt and 26% after nitroglycerin provocation). The specificity was 94%. An "exaggerated" response to nitroglycerin was seen in 14% of patients with syncope of unknown origin and in 15% of control patients.

Recently, Forleo and colleagues[35] performed a metaanalysis of 55 studies published prior to March 2012 (see Table 67.3). They included English-only publications involving patients with unexplained syncope and asymptomatic control patients without a history of syncope. Excluding duplicate publications, studies that enrolled fewer than 10 patients, and protocols using tilt angulation of less than 60 degrees or greater than 80 degrees, the resulting selected studies comprised 4361 patients with syncope (mean age, 41 ± 17 years) and 1791 control patients (mean age, 39 ± 17 years). The tilt angle was 60 degrees in 30 studies (2937 patients and 1005 controls), 70 degrees in 15 (991 patients and 485 controls), and 80 degrees in 10 (433 patients and 301 controls). The average overall duration of the tilt was 46 ± 16 minutes (range, 10 to 110 minutes); passive phase, 33 ± 12 minutes, and a provoked stage of 23 ± 12 minutes. In 30 studies, the provocative agent was nitroglycerine; in 22 other studies, it was isoproterenol. The analysis revealed a significant inverse relationship between sensitivity and specificity. The summary receiver-operating curve demonstrated a good overall ability to differentiate between symptomatic patients and asymptomatic controls with an area under the curve of 0.84 (95% confidence interval [CI], 0.81 to 0.87). Not unexpectedly, pharmacological protocols enhanced sensitivity and lowered specificity. Tilt protocols that included nitroglycerin provocation had the highest diagnostic odds ratio (14.40; 95% CI, 11.50 to 18.05) and the greatest sensitivity (66%; 95% CI, 60% to 72%).

Current guidelines[7] recommend a minimum head-up tilt test duration of 20 minutes and a maximum of 45 minutes for the passive component. Forleo and coauthors[35] noted that there was a lack of general agreement regarding the optimal duration of the tilt study. Further, they conceded that their analysis did not "clarify completely" the effect of tilt duration on diagnostic accuracy. They observed that longer passive tilt duration was associated with a higher rate of positivity. Also, an inverse relationship was noted between subject age and sensitivity, while age was associated with an enhanced specificity for the *active* phase of tilt. The authors speculate that a longer duration of passive tilt might be appropriate for younger patients, while a shorter duration of passive tilt might be beneficial in older patients.

Adenosine and Adenosine Triphosphate

It has been postulated that endogenous adenosine release may play a role in some forms of syncope,[36,37] and both adenosine and its precursor adenosine triphosphate (ATP) have been reported to unmask susceptibility to reflex paroxysmal atrioventricular (AV) block.[36-39] It may be that ATP identifies patients at risk for reflex paroxysmal sinus arrest or AV block and thereby identifies patients likely to benefit from pacemakers.[40] However, the US Food and Drug Administration has not approved ATP for injection. That, along with the uncertainty regarding substituting adenosine for ATP, has undermined their use for tilt testing in the United States.

Shifting Patient Patterns in the Tilt Table Testing Laboratory

Insmuch as head-up tilt table testing is not usually warranted in patients with a classic history of VVS (see Box 67.1 for exceptions), we have noted a shift in the type of patient being referred for laboratory evaluation. While the evaluation of TLOC of unknown causes remains important, the trend has been toward the use of tilt studies to assess OH and its subtypes to discriminate between so-called convulsive syncope (VVS associated with jerking movements) versus a true seizure disorder (in these cases with addition of video-electroencephalogram [EEG] monitoring during tilt), POTS, and in patients with possible psychogenic pseudosyncope/pseudoseizures.

The shift in patient referral patterns has led to the frequent inclusion of ancillary tests not associated with traditional head-up tilt table testing. Along with the aforementioned addition of video-EEG monitoring, many of our patients now undergo a basic panel of autonomic tests prior to the head-up tilt table testing. The addition of this autonomic testing has proven useful in

the evaluation of OH, especially in the elderly or patients with conditions such as diabetes mellitus associated with an increased risk of secondary autonomic dysfunction. A review of such testing is available for interested readers.[41]

Autonomic testing is performed prior to head-up tilt, beginning with the patient in a seated position. Noninvasive beat-to-beat blood pressure measurement is used throughout along with continuous ECG monitoring and occasionally with electrical bioimpedance splanchnic blood flow assessment. The Valsalva maneuver is performed in all patients undergoing autonomic testing in our laboratory. Patients over 40 years of age also undergo carotid sinus massage while seated upright. Many patients also undergo assessment of hemodynamic response to volitional cough.[41]

Video-Electroencephalogram Monitoring

In the 2009 ESC syncope practice guidelines,[7] the use of head-up tilt table testing for discriminating convulsive syncope from epilepsy was given a IIb indication (Level of Evidence C). Inasmuch as distinguishing epilepsy from syncope and vice-versa causes considerable diagnostic difficulty,[42] head-up tilt table testing may be helpful[43] especially with the addition of EEG monitoring during the tilt test.[44] Our laboratory has experienced a marked increase in referrals from the neurology service for head-up tilt table testing with EEG monitoring. We provide the tilt table study and its interpretation while the neurologists interpret the video-EEG recording.

Laboratory Environment and Patient Preparation

The laboratory should be quiet, dimly lit, at a comfortable temperature, and as nonthreatening as possible. We ask our patients to fast for 2 to 3 hours prior to testing. Longer periods of fasting may result in dehydration, with the potential to affect testing. Since OH is a consideration in most TLOC patients undergoing study, we direct them to take their antihypertensives, including diuretics, the morning of testing. Medications previously prescribed for the treatment of VVS are held for five half-lives before testing. If patients have been fasting for more than 4 hours, normal saline is given intravenously (250 to 500 mL depending on the duration of fasting status) prior to the tilt. Venous cannulation is done at least 20 minutes prior to testing. If ancillary autonomic testing is to be done, it is completed 15 to 20 minutes prior to initiating the tilt table testing. We forewarn patients that, although we will be monitoring them, we will not be talking with them, and if they experience symptoms they should inform the staff.

Recordings

Three or more simultaneous ECG leads should be recorded continuously, along with beat-to-beat blood pressure monitoring. Arterial access should only rarely be required. If arterial access is needed, at least 20 minutes of quiet rest is required before tilt testing. The use of blood pressure cuffs, whether automated or manual, is discouraged. The process of taking a measurement cannot help but stimulate the patient; such systems can be painful and do provide the beat-to-beat monitoring required.

Tilt Table Design

The table should be capable of smoothly achieving an angle of 60 to 70 degrees within 10 to 15 seconds. Likewise, the table should be capable of quickly being returned to the horizontal position should clinical circumstances require (e.g., syncope, excessive hypotension). A footboard is needed and the patient should be secured gently so as to prevent falling.

Tilt Angle and Duration

Tilt angles of 60 or 70 degrees should be used. Lesser degrees of tilt have been shown to have poor sensitivity. Tilt angles of 80 degrees or higher suffer from a lack of specificity. In terms of duration, current recommendations[7] call for not less than 20 minutes and not greater than 45 minutes. In our laboratory the passive phase of the tilt is 20 minutes. At that time, if the patient has been asymptomatic, 0.4 mg of nitroglycerin is given sublingually. In children, a passive drug-free head-up tilt tends to be favored. In such cases (e.g., in the absence of pharmacological provocation), it may be necessary to extend tilt test duration to 45 or even 60 minutes.

Personnel

The Heart Rhythm Society has published staffing recommendations.[24] In general, tilt table testing requires staffing similar to an exercise stress testing laboratory. The physician does not need to be in immediate attendance but does need to be in close proximity. The relationship of any induced symptoms to the patient's spontaneous symptoms should be documented.

Active Standing Versus Head-up Tilt Test

The active standing test complements head-up tilt table testing and can be undertaken in the laboratory at the same time, or separately in the clinic. In particular, the "initial" and "classic" forms of OH may be diagnosed by active standing (see definitions provided earlier). Beat-to-beat blood pressure recording is desirable during active standing as it is with tilt table testing, and testing may therefore be more suitable for the laboratory setting.

The active standing test has the advantage of corresponding more closely to real-life situations than does tilt table testing. It is simple to perform in the clinic or the laboratory and does not require expensive equipment. However, a medical attendant should remain close to the patient to prevent a fall that could lead to injury. Clearly, active standing may not be possible in some circumstances, such as debilitated patients, patients with severe autonomic dysfunction, patients with muscular dystrophy, and so on.

Reproducibility of Head-up Tilt Table Testing and Active Standing Test

A major issue with assessing reproducibility of a test utilizing orthostatic stress is how to control for variation in volume status prior to testing. Nevertheless, tilt-test reproducibility has been investigated using multiple tilts on the same day, a few days apart, and a few weeks apart. The experience in our laboratory suggests that the reproducibility of tilt-induced VVS is acceptable for use as a diagnostic test.[45] The positivity or negativity of two sequential tests done 30 minutes apart was concordant in 87% of cases. In particular, a negative test has high reproducibility. In one study, none of the patients who were tilt-negative on the initial test developed syncope on repeat testing.[45] The reproducibility of tilt testing with longer interest intervals is similar. Reproducibility with a 3- to 7-day separation was 90% in 21 patients (including isoproterenol provocation), although the level of provocation needed was different in 24%. At intervals of 1 to 6 weeks between testing (including isoproterenol provocation), there was 85% reproducibility in 46 patients who were initially tilt negative and 90% reproducibility in those who were initially tilt positive.[46] Head-up tilt table testing using nitroglycerin for provocation also shows acceptable reproducibility.[47,48] There has not been rigorous examination of the reproducibility of the active standing test.

Risks and Complications

The risks associated with head-up tilt table testing are minimal. A return to the supine position is typically all that is needed to avoid adverse events. As noted above, patients should be gently restrained to avoid falling. With respect to the active standing test, the risk of falling is the primary concern. The technical and nursing staff performing the active standing test should be aware of the "falls risk" possibility and should be authorized to return the patient to a supine or seated position promptly if a fall seems imminent. A chair at hand is usually adequate.

Although none have yet been observed at our institution, there have been reports of ventricular arrhythmias with the use of isoproterenol. The decline in the use of isoproterenol as a provocative agent has reduced that risk even further. To our knowledge, there have been no reports of ventricular arrhythmias with use of nitroglycerine for provocation.

Prolonged asystole has been reported during tilt testing, but long asystolic spells longer than 20 seconds are rare. Nevertheless, recognition of asystole is an important issue for the support staff. They need to be educated that asystole is self-limited and resolves with returning the patient to a supine position and that there is almost never any need for atropine, cardiopulmonary resuscitation, or transcutaneous pacing. It is prudent to warn staff new to tilt table testing that asystolic episodes can be very dramatic, with myotonic jerks and patients who appear to be in extremis. In almost all cases, overreacting to these events is likely to do more harm than good. Finally, we make it a point to warn patients that after a syncopal episode they may continue to feel unwell (fatigue, headache) for several hours. Although, medically, they could return to work or school, we advise against planning significant activity following the tilt study.

Head-up Tilt Testing and Treatment of Vasovagal Syncope

As noted in Table 67.3, the 2009 ESC guidelines[7] do not view head-up tilt table testing as useful for the testing efficacy of therapy for VVS. This use of head-up tilt table testing for defining treatment was given a Class III indication. On the other hand, of interest is the recent observation that a negative tilt study appears to identify a subgroup of syncope patients, who, if found to have significant bradycardia or asystole as part of their clinical syncope picture (usually documented by long-term ambulatory ECG monitoring), are likely to benefit from permanent pacing.[49] If this observation is confirmed, it would suggest a role for head-up tilt table testing for "pacemaker therapy stratification," even if the VVS diagnosis was clear on clinical grounds.

Overview of Uses for Head-up Tilt Table Testing

Established indications for head-up tilt table testing were noted earlier[7] and in Table 67.3. Additionally, head-up tilt table testing has been used (albeit with less supportive evidence) in (1) chronic fatigue syndrome, (2) POTS, (3) recurrent vertigo, (4) recurrent transient ischemic attacks, and (5) conduction system disease that, at electrophysiological testing, does not appear severe enough to explain syncope. With the possible exception of POTS, we do not advocate these other applications, and the existing practice guidelines do not provide support for such use.

Conclusions

Head-up tilt table testing, either drug-free or if necessary with pharmacological provocation (most often nitroglycerine) has

67

proven to be a useful, readily available, and safe modality for identifying susceptibility to VVS and confirming suspected OH. However, tilt testing has not been shown to be a reliable means of testing the efficacy of therapeutic interventions. Additionally, head-up tilt table testing is not known to be helpful in evaluating other forms of reflex syncope, with the possible exception of clarifying the hemodynamic impact of carotid sinus stimulation in patients with suspected carotid sinus syndrome.

Head-up tilt table testing has been the subject of numerous studies, resulting in the development of widely accepted protocols. These protocols offer a level of reproducibility, sensitivity, specificity, and predictive value on par with other widely used cardiovascular tests, such as exercise testing.

Finally, head-up tilt table testing is finding new roles in the evaluation in distinguishing between epilepsy and syncope, detecting psychogenic pseudosyncope/pseudoseizures, and in the assessment of patients initially considered having epilepsy but in whom confirmation of the diagnosis has been elusive. In all of these cases, the tilt test is best combined with ancillary testing, particularly the video-EEG.

Acknowledgment

Dr Benditt is supported in part by a grant in support of heart-brain research from the Dr. Earl E. Bakken family.

REFERENCES

1. Allen SC, Taylor CL, Hall VE. A study of orthostatic insufficiency by the tiltboard method. *Am J Physiol.* 1945;143:11–18.
2. McMicheal J, Sharpey Shafer EP. Cardiac output in man by a direct Fick method: effect of posture, venous pressure change, atropine and adrenalin. *Brit Heart J.* 1944;6:33–40.
3. Sharpey Shafer EP. Syncope. *Brit Med J.* 1956;1:506–509.
4. Davies R, Slater JDH, Forsling ML, Payne N. The response of arginine vasopressin and plasma renin to postural change in normal man, with observations on syncope. *Clin Sci.* 1976;51:267–274.
5. Hammill SC, Holmes DR, Wood DL, et al. Electrographic testing in the upright position: improved evaluation of patients with rhythm disturbances using a tilt table. *J Am Coll Cardiol.* 1984;4:65–71.
6. Kenny RA, Ingram A, Bayliss J, Sutton R. Head-up tilt: a useful test for investigating unexplained syncope. *Lancet.* 1986;1:1352–1355.
7. Moya A, Sutton R, Ammirati F, et al. Guidelines for the diagnosis and management of syncope (version 2009). *Eur Heart J.* 2009;21:2631–2671.
8. Rowell LB. *Human Circulation. Regulation During Physical Stress.* New York: Oxford University Press; 1986.
9. Folino FA. Cerebral autoregulation and syncope. *Prog Cardiovasc Dis.* 2007;50:49–80.
10. Schondorf R, Benoit J, Stein R. Cerebral autoregulation in orthostatic intolerance. *Ann N Y Acad Sci.* 2001;940:514–526.
11. Rossen R, Kabat H, Anderson JP. Acute arrest of cerebral circulation in man. *Arch Neurol Psychiatry.* 1943;50:510–528.
12. Aaslid R, Lindegaard KF, Sorteberg W, Nornes H. Cerebral autoregulation dynamics in humans. *Stroke.* 1989;20:45–52.
13. Paulson OB, Strandgaard S, Edvinsson L. Cerebral autoregulation. *Cerebrovasc Brain Metab Rev.* 1990;2:161–192.
14. Guo H, Tierney N, Schaller F, Raven PB, Smith SA, Shi X. Cerebral autoregulation is preserved during orthostatic stress superimposed with systemic hypotension. *J Appl Physiol.* 2006;100:1785–1792.
15. van Dijk JG, Thijs RD, Benditt DG, Wieling W. A guide to disorders causing transient loss of consciousness: focus on syncope. *Nature Rev Neurosci.* 2009;5:438–448.
16. Shaw FE, Kenny RA. The overlap between syncope and falls in the elderly. *Postgrad Med J.* 1997;73:635–639.
17. McIntosh SJ, Lawson J, Kenny RA. Clinical characteristics of vasodepressor, cardioinhibitory, and mixed carotid sinus syndrome in the elderly. *Am J Med.* 1993;95:203–208.
18. Stewart JM. Postural tachycardia syndrome and reflex syncope: similarities and differences. *J Pediatr.* 2009;154: 481–485.
19. Mathias CJ. Role of autonomic evaluation in the diagnosis and management of syncope. *Clin Auton Res.* 2004;14(suppl 1):45–54.
20. Benditt DG, Lurie KG, Adler SW, et al. Pathophysiology of vasovagal syncope. In: Blanc JJ, Benditt DG, Sutton R, eds. *Neurally Mediated Syncope: Pathophysiology,*

Investigation, and Treatment. Armonk, NY: Futura Publishing; 1996:1–24.
21. Ermis C, Samniah N, Lurie KG, Sakaguchi S, Benditt DG. Adrenal/renal contribution to circulating norepinephrine in posturally induced neurally mediated reflex syncope. *Am J Cardiol.* 2003;91:746–750.
22. Freeman R, Wieling W, Axelord FB, et al. Consensus statement of the definition of orthostatic hypotension, neurally mediated syncope and the postural tachycardia syndrome. *Auton Neurosci.* 2011;161:46–48.
23. Benditt DG, Ferguson DW, Grubb BP, et al. Tilt table testing for assessing syncope. *J Am Coll Cardiol.* 1996;28:263–275.
24. Haines DE, Beheiry S, Akar JG, et al. Heart Rythm Society expert consensus statement on electrophysiology laboratory standards: process, protocols, equipment, personnel, and safety. *Heart Rhythm.* 2014;11:e9–e51.
25. Adamec I, Mismas A, Zaper D, Junakovic A, Hajnsek S, Habek M. Short pain-provoked head-up tilt test for the confirmation of vasovagal syncope. *Neurol Sci.* 2013;34:869–873.
26. Fitzpatrick AP, Theodorakis G, Vardas P, Sutton R. Methodology of head-up tilt testing in patients with unexplained syncope. *J Am Coll Cardiol.* 1991;17: 125–130.
27. Almquist A, Goldenberg IF, et al. Provocation of bradycardia and hypotension by isoproterenol and upright posture in patients with unexplained syncope. *N Engl J Med.* 1989;320:346–351.
28. Natale A, Akhtar M, Jazayeri M, et al. Provocation of hypotension during head-up tilt testing in subjects with no history of syncope or presyncope. *Circulation.* 1995;92:54–58.
29. Waxman MB, Yao L, Cameron DA, Wald RW, Roseman J. Isoproterenol induction of vasodepressor-type reaction in vasodepressor-prone persons. *Am J Cardiol.* 1989;63:58–65.
30. Kapoor WN, Brant N. Evaluation of syncope by upright tilt testing with isoproterenol. A nonspecific test. *Ann Intern Med.* 1992;116:358–363.
31. Morillo CA, Klein GJ, Zandri S, Yee R. Diagnostic accuracy of a low-dose isoproterenol head-up tilt protocol. *Am Heart J.* 1995;129:901–906.
32. Heart Rhythm Society, "*Special Notice Regarding Pricing of Isoproterenol/Isuprel.*" Press release; April 8, 2015.
33. Raviele A, Gasparini G, Di Pede F, et al. Nitroglycerin infusion during upright tilt: a new test for the diagnosis of vasovagal syncope. *Am Heart J.* 1994;127:103–111.
34. Raviele A, Menozzi C, Brignole M, et al. Value of head-up tilt testing potentiated with sublingual nitroglycerin to assess the origin of unexplained syncope. *Am J Cardiol.* 1995;76:267–272.
35. Forleo C, Guida P, Iacoviello M, et al. Head-up tilt testing for diagnosing vasovagal syncope: a meta-analysis. *Int J Cardiol.* 2013;168:27–35.

36. Sinkovec M, Grad A, Rakovec P. Role of endogenous adenosine in vasovagal syncope. *Clin Auton Res.* 2001;11:155–161.
37. Shen WK, Hammill SC, Munger TM, et al. Adenosine: potential modulator for vasovagal syncope. *J Am Coll Cardiol.* 1996;28:146–154.
38. Brignole M; Gaggioli G; Menozzi C; et al. Adenosine-induced atrioventricular block in patients with unexplained syncope: the diagnostic value of ATP testing. *Circulation.* 96:3921–3927.
39. Flammang D, Erickson M, McCarville S, Church T, Hamani D, Donal E. Contribution of head-up tilt testing and ATP testing in assessing vasovagal syndrome: preliminary results and potential therapeutic implications. *Circulation.* 1999;99:2427–2433.
40. Flammang D, Church TR, De Roy L, et al. ATP Multicenter Study. Treatment of unexplained syncope: a multicenter, randomized trial of cardiac pacing guided by adenosine 5′-triphosphate testing. *Circulation.* 2012;125:31–63.
41. Adkisson WO, Benditt DG. Syncope due to autonomic dysfunction: diagnosis and management. *Med Clin North Am.* 2015;99:691–710.
42. Adkisson WO, Benditt DG. Treatment of 'refractory' epilepsy: syncope incognito unmasked by implantable ambulatory electrocardiographical recordings. *Europace.* 2012;14:1540–1542.
43. Rangel I, Freitas J, Correia AS, et al. The usefulness of the head-up tilt test in patients with suspected epilepsy. *Seizure.* 2014;23:367–370.
44. van Dijk JG, Thijs RD, van Zwet E, et al. The semiology of tilt-induced reflex syncope in relation to electroencephalographic changes. *Brain.* 2014;137:576–585.
45. Chen MY, Goldenberg IF, Milstein S, et al. Cardiac electrophysiologic and hemodynamic correlates of neurally mediated syncope. *Am J Cardiol.* 1989;63:66–72.
46. Sheldon R, Splawinski J, Killam S. Reproducibility of isoproterenol tilt-table tests in patients with syncope. *Am J Cardiol.* 1992;69:1300–1305.
47. Del Rosso A, Bartoletti A, Bartoli P, et al. Methodology of head-up tilt testing potentiated with sublingual nitroglycerin in unexplained syncope. *Am J Cardiol.* 2000;85:1007–1011.
48. Foglia-Manzillo G, Giada F, Beretta S, Corrado G, Santarone M, Raviele A. Reproducibility of head-up tilt testing potentiated with sublingual nitroglycerin in patients with unexplained syncope. *Am J Cardiol.* 1999;84:284–288.
49. Brignole M, Donateo P, Tomaino M, et al. International Study on Syncope of Uncertain Etiology 3 (ISSUE-3) Investigators. Benefit of pacemaker therapy in patients with presumed neurally mediated syncope and documented asystole is greater when tilt test is negative: an analysis from the third International Study on Syncope of Uncertain Etiology (ISSUE-3). *Circ Arrhythm Electrophysiol.* 2014;7:10–16.

68 Autonomic Regulation and Cardiac Risk

Marek Malik

The autonomic nervous system is an important contributor to the physiological processes that maintain the homeostasis of the entire organism. Autonomic abnormalities may have a direct basis in autonomopathies, such as autoimmune and metabolic neuropathies, or an indirect basis in autonomopathies, due to the necessity of correcting homeostasis disturbed by pathological processes, such as heart, kidney, or liver failures. Therefore changes in cardiovascular autonomic regulation mirror the global well-being and, when disturbed, may also lead to clinically relevant pathologies in cardiac physiology and function. For this reason, autonomic abnormalities are potent indicators of increased risk of pathological progression and/or all-cause mortality. In cardiac patients, the link between autonomic abnormalities and poor outcome, including not only all-cause mortality but also sudden arrhythmic death, clearly depends on the underlying clinical and pathological conditions. After classifying such conditions into separate categories, research concerning autonomic testing in cardiac patients is orientated mainly toward the assessment of increased risk of different modes of mortality. Among these, particular attention is paid to determining the risk of arrhythmic complications and of sudden cardiac death.

This focus of autonomic testing is not surprising since the present clinical practice of identifying cardiac patients with increased risk of malignant arrhythmias and of sudden cardiac death remains largely suboptimal, as is best seen in reports of real-life experience with the utility of implantable cardioverter defibrillators (ICDs). In a survey of 2349 consecutive cases in the Israeli ICD Registry, Sabbag and colleagues reported the rates of appropriate ICD shock therapy at the 30-month follow-up were only 2.6% and 7.4% among patients who received an ICD for primary or secondary prevention, respectively.[1] This finding agrees well with the report by Lee and colleagues, who investigated the Ontario ICD database.[2] Among 3445 patients with a left ventricular ejection fraction (LVEF) not exceeding 35% who received ICDs for primary prevention, the study reported only 3.6 appropriate ICD shocks per 100 patient-years of follow-up. These incidences of effective ICD utilization appear somewhat fewer compared to previous reports,[3,4] although even the previously reported frequencies of appropriate ICD shocks in primary prevention patients were not too impressive.

The recent data showing low true utilization of ICDs implanted for primary prevention indicate that the strategies used to select patients for primary prophylaxis have low specificity, which is unsurprising since the present guidelines for selecting ICD recipients[5,6] reflect previous seminal trials in which the patient selection was based on the diagnosis of lowered left ventricular performance with depressed LVEF.[7-9] These guidelines remain in place despite repeated observations that reduced LVEF is neither particularly sensitive nor specific in identifying patients at increased risk of arrhythmic complications and sudden cardiac death.[10] The very low utilization of ICDs that have been implanted for primary prophylaxis confirms that only a small proportion of patients with reduced LVEF eventually develop life-threatening arrhythmias, or even arrhythmias that would not necessarily be life terminating but which still trigger an appropriate usage of ICD therapy. Yet many cardiac patients with normal or almost normal LVEF are succumbing to sudden cardiac death.[10] Nevertheless, as discussed further in this text, in the absence of new prospective clinical trials, the calls to reevaluate the ICD guidelines[11] can lead only to an awareness of the need for new investigations; they will not lead to a systematic change of clinical practice regardless of how badly it is needed. However, research aimed at improvement of cardiac risk stratification is still needed and is clinically relevant.

No guidelines should be used blindly, and many risk factors play a role in individual clinical decisions. With the potential harm of prophylactic ICD implantations steadily decreasing,[12] consideration of additional risk factors in decisions concerning patients who are on or beyond the border of present guidelines is not unreasonable. Consequently, a variety of different indices have been tested in terms of risk profiling of cardiac patients, some more[13] and some less[14] successfully.

Assessment of cardiac autonomic regulation and of cardiac autonomic reflexes has a long-standing history of risk stratification.[15] The extent of abnormalities in cardiovascular autonomic regulation does not directly separate the risk of sudden arrhythmic death from the risk of nonarrhythmic and noncardiac death. However, some autonomic indices are more indicative of arrhythmic risk, while others are more indicative of nonarrhythmic risk. Indeed, data available from both experimental and clinical observations suggest that enhanced parasympathetic influence on the heart is generally antiarrhythmic and antifibrillatory,[16] while dominant sympathetic influence is commonly proarrhythmic.[17] Combination of sympathetic dominance with myocardial ischemia and/or other proarrhythmic processes is known to lead to increased probability of ventricular fibrillation and thus higher risk of sudden arrhythmic death.[18] Several recent advances in cardiac risk profiling based on autonomic tests are worth noting.

Heart Rate Variability

The periodicity of the sinus node discharges is controlled by a balance between both autonomic limbs. Any activation of the sympathetic system is accompanied by an inhibition of the parasympathetic system and vice versa. This relationship is driven by peripheral reflex mechanisms with opposing feedback properties (i.e., baroreceptive and vagal afferents with negative feedback characteristics and sympathetic afferents with positive feedback characteristics integrated by the central nervous system). Respiratory modulation of cardiac cycle length and heart rate responses to exercise or mental stressors result from these regulatory processes.[19] Changes of cardiac period can easily be measured and quantified by different expressions of heart rate variability (HRV). The practical utility of HRV assessment for cardiac risk stratification depends largely on the detailed methods used to measure the modulations of cardiac cycles.

The most commonly used methods for HRV assessment are based on statistical analyses of RR interval durations and on spectral analyses of RR interval sequences. The ESC/NASPE Task Force reviewed the technology behind these most common methods in detail in the mid-1990s.[20] Although novel progressive techniques have been proposed, such as the assessment of deceleration capacity (described further in the text), the statistical and spectral analyses have changed little since the time of the ESC/NASPE Task Force review. Still, in populations of contemporarily treated cardiac patients, simple global statistical HRV measurements, such as the SDNN (standard deviation of all normal-to-normal sinus rhythm RR intervals) and SDANN (standard deviation of 5-minute averages of normal-to-normal sinus rhythm RR intervals calculated over a long-term recording) parameters, are not losing their predictive power. In the field of prophylactic ICD implantation, reports have indicated that global HRV measures were among the factors that most powerfully differentiated between patients with and without appropriate ICD shocks.[21] A recent study suggested that this association was made more powerful by ongoing monitoring of HRV in ICD patients.[22] Consistent with what has already been stated, these studies also observed appropriate ICD therapy in only a small proportion of implanted patients. Thus the HRV differences between the patients who do and do not utilize appropriate ICD therapy may contribute to a more focused identification of patients benefiting from primary prophylactic device implantation.

Spectral analysis of HRV, meaning the distinction between modulators of cardiac periodicity operating at different frequencies, was originally seen mainly as a physiological investigative tool. The efferent vagal activity is a major contributor to the so-called high-frequency component of HRV, meaning cardiac cycle modulations appearing at frequencies between 0.15 and 0.4 Hz (modulating waves between approximately 2.5 and 7 seconds). Slightly more controversial is the interpretation of the low frequency component, meaning slower modulations at frequencies between 0.04 and 0.15 Hz (modulating waves between approximately 7 and 25 seconds). These modulations are considered by some to be markers of sympathetic modulation and by others to be parameters that include both sympathetic and vagal influences.[20] While spectral HRV analysis continues to play a role in physiological and population investigations,[23] it has also been reported to improve stratification of the risk of cardiac mortality in contemporarily advanced heart failure patients[24] as well as to provide prognostic characterization in other clinical populations.[25,26]

Deceleration capacity is a nonspectral HRV technique aimed predominantly at addressing the vagal components of RR interval periodicity. The concept of this technique is based on the phase rectified signal averaging method, which is a universal technique capable of processing different medical and biological signals. This method defines moments of interest in a trigger signal (e.g., the beat-to-beat decelerations of cardiac periods); it also averages the surroundings of the moments of interest in an analyzed signal, which might be the same as the trigger signal or it might be a different recording. Of note, in the deceleration capacity assessment, both signals are the same—that is, the cardiac periodograms—but applications triggering on one time series and averaging a different time series have also been reported.[27] The initial observations showing that deceleration capacity is a more powerful risk predictor than conventional HRV measures[28] have recently been independently confirmed, both in postinfarction patients[29] and in a substantial cohort of patients admitted to the medical emergency department among whom the deceleration capacity as a risk predictor outperformed an early warning score model that combined respiratory rate, heart rate, systolic blood pressure, body temperature, and level of consciousness on admission.[30]

The physiological models associating spectral HRV components with different branches of the autonomic nervous system are based on well-established, repeatedly reproduced experiments. Nevertheless, the strictly engineering-based methods

that are used in the spectral assessment of cardiac periodograms cannot possibly reflect all of the autonomic reflexes during the complex dynamic interplay of these reflexes when the underlying autonomic regulations are constantly changing. To address such characteristics of cardiac autonomic status, nonlinear approaches to HRV analysis are frequently advocated. A recent update of the methodological HRV standards concentrated on these nonlinear techniques.[31] This update concluded that, while in some reports nonlinear methods (Fig. 68.1) have been shown to complement risk stratification by standard time-domain and spectral techniques,[32] a clear disconnect exists between high technological complexity and low clinical utility of nonlinear HRV techniques. Further clinical validation of existing nonlinear methods in large multicenter studies is needed. Without such validations, promotion of the development of new nonlinear approaches will be difficult. Signal processing HRV technologies that do not at least partially meet the clinical needs that are unmet by standard techniques are of little practical value, irrespective of the innovation and advancement of their mathematical and technical foundations.

Baroreflex

Arterial baroreflex is an essential component of cardiovascular autonomic regulation that relies on specialized neurons, called the baroreceptors, which are localized in the arterial wall of the aortic arch and, more importantly, of the carotid sinuses. Any rise in arterial pressure above the threshold results in reflex vagal activation with increased discharge from parasympathetic inhibitory neurons leading to chronotropy reduction, which leads to heart rate deceleration and to decreased sympathetic discharge both to the heart (reducing cardiac chronotropy and inotropy) and to peripheral blood vessels (reducing vascular tone). Similarly, any pressure decrease reduces baroreceptor discharge and provokes an increase in sympathetic outflow and vagal inhibition, leading to an increase in heart rate, cardiac contractility, and vascular resistance. Vagal activation leads to an immediate reaction within 200 to 600 ms, while the reaction to cardiac and vasomotor sympathetic activation occurs more slowly (within 2 to 3 seconds). The baroreflex control of the heart rate on a beat-to-beat basis is therefore achieved through vagal, but not sympathetic, mechanisms.

The intensity of the arterial baroreflex can be investigated using different technologies. If blood pressure is changed rapidly by pharmacological agents, the dynamics of induced RR interval changes can easily be measured and expressed in milliseconds of RR interval changes per mm Hg unit change of arterial blood pressure (leading to a measurement in ms/mm Hg units). The correspondence between arterial pressure changes and corresponding RR interval changes can also be addressed by continuous monitoring of spontaneously occurring fluctuations. Different techniques have been reported for this purpose.[27] While some of these techniques might provide more stable baroreflex assessment compared with other possibilities, reported studies that utilized baroreflex to risk-stratify cardiac patients are generally in agreement with each other. Most frequently, levels of RR interval changes versus pressure changes below 3 ms/mm Hg have indicated an increased risk in different cardiac populations.[33]

Baroreflex can also be quantified indirectly by means of heart rate turbulence (HRT) that describes short-term fluctuations in sinus cycle length after spontaneous ventricular ectopic beats.[34] In normal subjects, before the sinus rate returns back to baseline following spontaneous ectopic beats, it initially briefly accelerates and subsequently decelerates compared to the preectopy rate. Similar oscillation in cardiac cycles can also be induced by a paced extrastimulus, delivered either during programmed ventricular stimulation or by an implanted device, such as an ICD. Turbulence onset expresses the initial rate acceleration, while turbulence slope quantifies the subsequent rate deceleration.

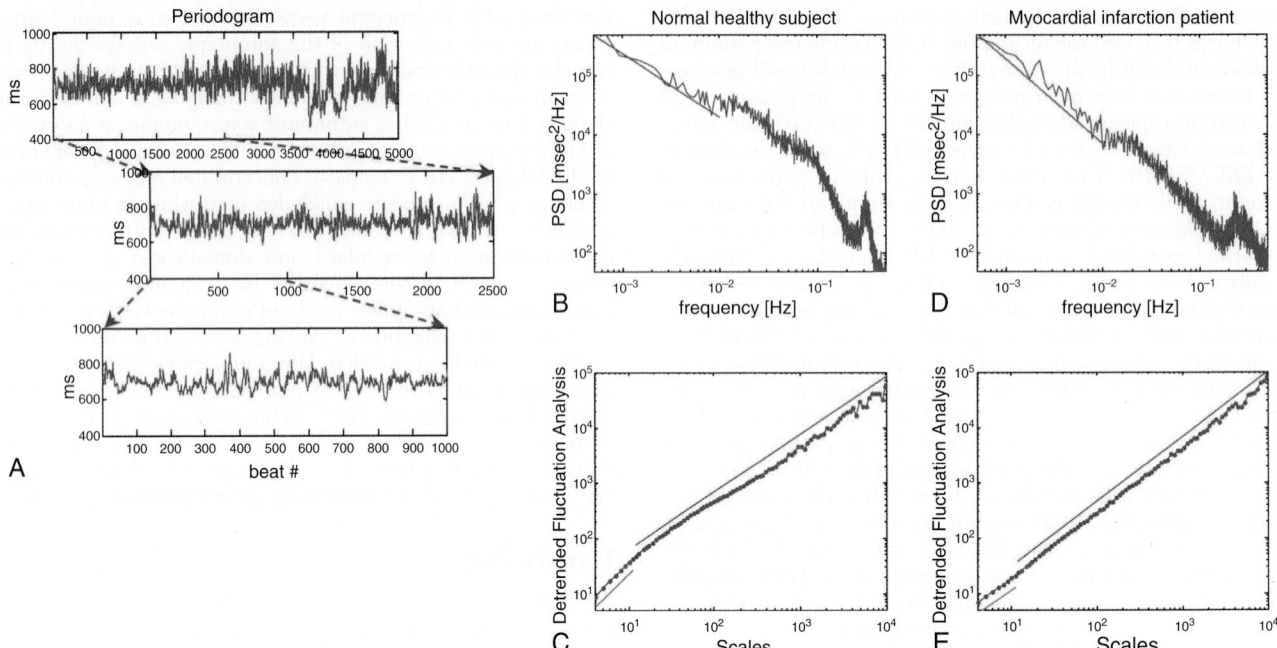

FIGURE 68.1 Example of nonlinear analysis techniques of heart rate variability. (A) Cardiac periodogram in which a common variability pattern is repeated when inspecting the series of RR intervals on different scales. This self-similarity of the sequence translates into a power-law image of power spectral density (*PSD*) in the very low frequency region (B and D), and detrended fluctuation analysis for the long scales (C and E). The scaling does not continue indefinitely as the frequency increases (or as the scale decreases) and breaks down when the other typical heart rate variability spectral components become prevalent. (Note the peak in the PSD around 0.3 Hz, which corresponds to the respiratory frequency.) Self-similarity is influenced by different pathological conditions. A comparison between a healthy subject (B and C) and a patient who survived acute myocardial infarction (D and E) is shown. (Modified from Sassi R, Cerutti S, Lombardi F, et al. Advances in heart rate variability signal analysis: joint position statement by the e-Cardiology ESC Working Group and the European Heart Rhythm Association co-endorsed by the Asia Pacific Heart Rhythm Society. *Europace.* 2015;17:1341-1353.)

The physiology of HRT is reasonably well understood, linking the underlying mechanisms to the arterial baroreflex.[34,35] Systolic blood pressure due to an ectopic beat is considerably lower than that of normal sinus beats for several reasons, including incomplete electrical restitution, reduced diastolic filling, missing atrial kick, reduced myocardial contractility, and less effective ventricular contraction. This lowered blood pressure leads to missed baroreflex afferent input which, through vagal withdrawal, leads to the early heart rate acceleration. Ineffective contraction and compensatory pause also cause diastolic pressure reduction. In subjects with normal left ventricular function, systolic pressure produced by the first postectopic sinus beat is usually lower compared with the preectopic level (this phenomenon appears to have its own risk prediction value[36]). Thus not only the instant hemodynamic effect of the ectopic contraction but also the systolic pressure reduction during the subsequent sinus beat activate aortic and carotid baroreceptors, which leads to the heart rate increase due to vagal inhibition. This relative and transient lowering of the blood pressure stimulates the sympathetic arc of the autonomic nervous system. The postectopic reduction of diastolic blood pressure leads to a surge of muscle sympathetic nerve activity. The magnitude of this sympathetic burst, which occurs simultaneously or slightly delayed compared with the first postectopic sinus beat, provokes noradrenaline release in perivascular sympathetic nerve endings and leads to the increase of peripheral vascular resistance. The latency of the hemodynamic response to this sympathetic nerve stimulation is around 5 seconds. The early HRT rate acceleration is thus not mediated solely by sympathetic efferent arm activation. Both branches of the autonomic nervous system contribute to the late HRT phase, which is characterized by gradual return of systolic blood pressure and heart rate to preectopic levels. Under normal physiological conditions, a significant overshoot of systolic pressure above the baseline level and heart rate reduction below the baseline level occurs around the eighth postectopic sinus beat. This late overcompensation is primarily caused by an early sympathetic activation with delayed vasomotor response together with vagal activation.

HRT assessment is a potent risk predictor. Recent studies using HRT as a risk predictor range from supporting animal studies[37] to investigations in special well-defined clinical populations.[38] When previously combined with deceleration capacity, postinfarction patients who showed abnormalities in both indices were termed as suffering from severe autonomic failure. The seminal study that introduced this concept showed that postinfarction patients with preserved left ventricular function (LVEF >30%) who still suffered from severe autonomic failure had an almost identical risk profile to the patients with an LVEF less than or equal to 30%.[10] Based on previous experience,[39] HRT is also being investigated in the REFINE-ICD trial that aims at evaluating whether, in comparison with usual clinical care, prophylactic ICD implantation reduces total mortality in patients with moderately reduced LVEF (between 36% and 50%) who have, among other symptoms, abnormal HRT and abnormal T-wave alternans.

Because the baroreflex links the arterial pressure to cardiovascular regulation, electronic activation of the carotid sinus baroreceptors might possibly help to lower blood pressure in hypertensive patients, especially those who do not respond

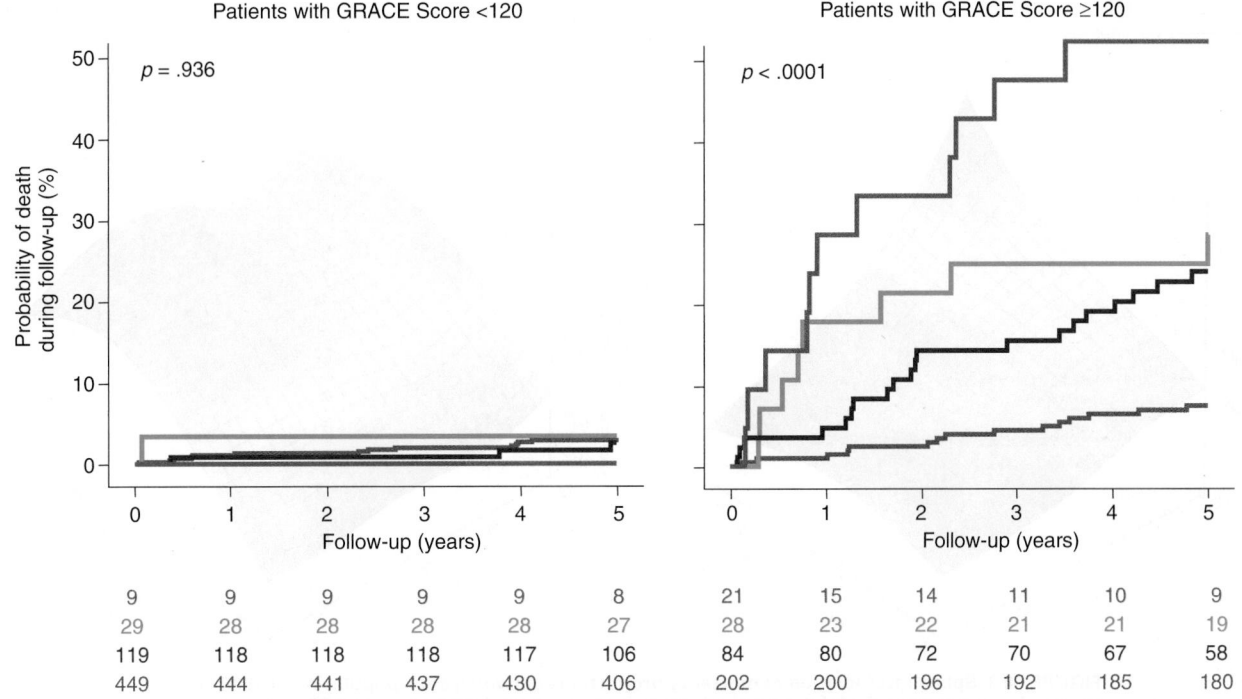

9	9	9	9	9	8	21	15	14	11	10	9
29	28	28	28	28	27	28	23	22	21	21	19
119	118	118	118	117	106	84	80	72	70	67	58
449	444	441	437	430	406	202	200	196	192	185	180

LVEF ≤ 35% and respiratory rate ≥ 20 min⁻¹   LVEF ≤ 35% and respiratory rate < 20 min⁻¹

LVEF > 35% and respiratory rate < 20 min⁻¹   LVEF > 35% and respiratory rate ≥ 20 min⁻¹

FIGURE 68.2 Probabilities of all-cause death in 941 patients who survived the acute phase of myocardial infarction and in whom respiratory frequency was assessed during undisturbed resting position.[45] The patients were stratified by GRACE score (combination of age of the patient, history of past heart failure, history of past myocardial infarction, serum creatinine at admission, cardiac biomarker status at admission, systolic blood pressure at admission, pulse at admission, ST deviation at admission, and in-hospital percutaneous coronary intervention) dichotomized at 120 points, left ventricular ejection fraction (LVEF) dichotomized at 35%, and resting respiratory rate (ReRa) dichotomized at 20 cycles/min. The *red, green, blue,* and *violet lines* correspond to groups of patients with LVEF below 35% and ReRa above 20 cycles/min, LVEF below 35% and ReRa below 20 cycles/min, LVEF above 35% and ReRa above 20 cycles/min, and LVEF above 35% and ReRa below 20 cycles/min, respectively. The numbers of patients involved in the analyses are shown below the graphs; the colors of the numbers correspond to the colors of the lines. (Modified from Barthel P, Wensel R, Bauer A, et al. Respiratory rate predicts outcome after acute myocardial infarction: a prospective cohort study. *Eur Heart J.* 2013;34:1644-1650.)

sufficiently to regular antihypertensive medication.[40] Different safety issues with this possibility have been addressed, including the cross-influence of the stimulating devices with ICDs.[41] At present, the techniques show promising, although potentially conflicting, results.[42,43]

Other Indices

The effects of the autonomic nervous system are universally spread throughout the organism and thus contribute to the manifestation of cardiovascular diseases at the level of other organs, which is reflected in a large variety of autonomic tests that range from simple provocations, such as the Valsalva maneuver, the handgrip test, and the cold face test, to external instrumentation tests, such as carotid massage, neck suction, and the low–body pressure test.[44] While these tests address different reflexes involving distinct aspects of autonomic control, the methodology of all of them is based on the assessment of heart rate (or RR interval) and/or blood pressure responses.

Cardiovascular physiology is also intimately linked to the physiology of respiration in which the pulmonary vagal reflex regulation plays a known role. In addition to affecting ventilatory control, circulation failure also affects the respiration by influencing pulmonary perfusion. A pressure increase during left ventricular filling augments capillary pressure in the lungs, which in turn has an effect on pulmonary compliance and alveolocapillary membrane conductance. These changes lead to the breathing rate increases that are well known in heart failure patients. Recently, Barthel and colleagues[45] rekindled investigations into the value of free breathing rate to predict long-term outcome of contemporarily treated patients who survived the acute phase of myocardial infarction. When stratifying the patients according to the GRACE score[46] (combining age of the patient, history of past heart failure, history of past myocardial infarction, serum creatinine at admission, cardiac biomarker status at admission, systolic blood pressure at admission, pulse rate at admission, ST deviation at admission, and in-hospital percutaneous coronary intervention), they found that increased breathing rate above 20 cycles per minute was a potent stratifier of mortality risk in patients with abnormal GRACE scores, particularly if combined with reduced LVEF (Fig. 68.2).

Subsequently, after solving the problem of detecting undisturbed nocturnal respiratory frequency from long-term Holter recordings,[47] the same investigators reported[48] that in survivors of acute infarction, elevated nocturnal breathing rate combined with reduced LVEF is strongly related to nonsudden cardiac

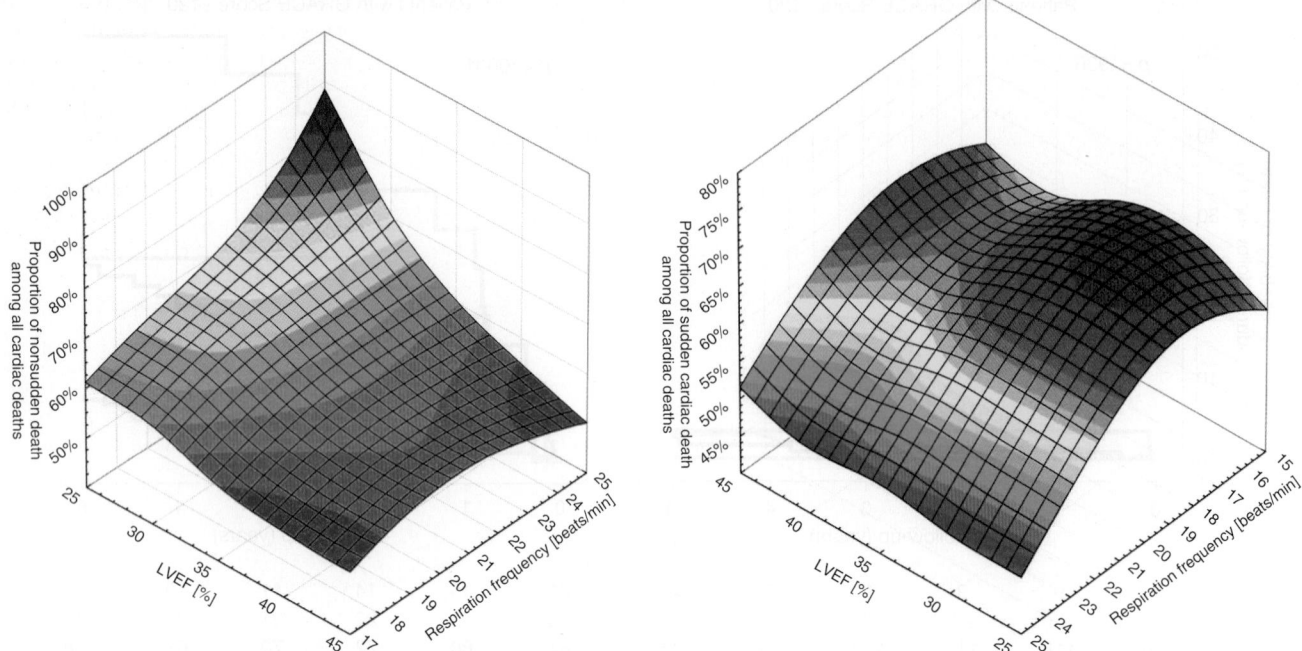

FIGURE 68.3 Spline interpolation of mortality proportions derived from a population of 1538 survivors of acute myocardial infarction in whom average nocturnal (12:00 a.m. to 6:00 a.m.) respiratory rate was derived from in-hospital Holter recordings obtained before hospital discharge. The panels show the proportions of nonsudden deaths (*left panel*) and sudden, presumed arrhythmic deaths (*right panel*) among all cardiac deaths as they relate to left ventricular ejection fraction (*LVEF*) and nocturnal respiratory rate during a follow-up of 5 years after the index infarction. Note that, between the two panels, the numbers of LVEF and respiratory rate axes increase in the opposite directions and that the ranges for the vertical axes are different. Patients with depressed LVEF and increased nocturnal respiratory rate suffer predominantly from nonsudden deaths (the interpolated data in the left panel reach almost a 90% proportion of nonsudden deaths among all cardiac deaths). Patients with depressed LVEF and slower nocturnal respiratory rate suffer from both nonsudden and sudden cardiac death (the interpolated data in the right panel reach above 65% proportion of sudden cardiac deaths among all cardiac deaths). (Partially modified from Dommasch M, Sinnecker D, Barthel P, et al. Nocturnal respiratory rate predicts non-sudden cardiac death in survivors of acute myocardial infarction. *J Am Coll Cardiol.* 2014;63:2432-2433.)

death but not to sudden cardiac death that might perhaps be prevented by prophylactic ICD therapy (Fig. 68.3). This finding indicates a possibility of identifying those patients who are, according to present guidelines, indicated as candidates for prophylactic ICD implantation but who are unlikely to benefit from the ICD therapy.

Conclusion

As already mentioned, guidelines for everyday clinical practice need to be evidence based, reflecting results of available prospective trials. In terms of selection of patients for prophylactic ICD implantation, the present guidelines are not fully satisfactory.[11] Nevertheless, to change these guidelines, new prospective randomized intervention trials are needed. Unfortunately, apart from obvious ethical and legal problems linked to withholding the benefits of ICD from patients who would be eligible based on existing guidelines, the economy of new trials is presently not particularly favorable. Prospective randomized trials of ICD implantation are expensive, and, in the past, their conduct relied heavily on industrial funding. Additionally, prophylactic ICD implantations are also expensive and compete with other health care demands. These economic factors means that even if new trials would substantially improve the accuracy of patient selection for ICD prophylaxis, the overall use of ICDs is unlikely to increase dramatically, which in turn removes the incentive that

the relevant industry might have to conduct new trials. Hence, when the present economic obstacles are overcome, public funding will be needed to advance the ICD guidelines and clinical practice to increase the accuracy of patient selection for prophylactic device treatment. Until that happens, the more accurate cardiac risk predictors offer benefit at the level of the individual patient, particularly in borderline cases and in situations (and health care systems) when the present guidelines are impossible to implement fully because of expenditure limits of health care provision.

Autonomic tests appear well suited to serve both the future trial designs and the present clinical considerations. Of course, this does not mean that further advances in the field of autonomic testing are not needed. In spite of the number of possible autonomic tests, limited comparisons exist on the predictive value of different tests in cardiac patients and on their value in the general population. The predictive power of autonomic tests is generally agreed to increase when studying responses to specific provocations compared with studies of undisturbed baseline conditions. To advance the field further, such provocations need to be standardized together with the environmental conditions under which the tests are performed. Among other confounding factors, the differences in the surrounding to which the autonomic system reacts make analysis of long-term (e.g., 24 hours) cardiac periodograms of little value when obtained in fully ambulating patients. Also, because of the health care provision pressures, short-term (e.g., up to 30 minutes) tests for risk prediction in cardiac patients need to be advanced. Prolonging in-hospital stay for the purposes of maintaining standardized conditions over prolonged monitoring periods of time is presently highly impractical. Studies of the correspondence between RR intervals and noninvasively assessed blood pressure measured on a beat-to-beat basis may be a reasonable target for a standardized autonomic test if involving, not only undisturbed resting period, but also tilting or standardized postural provocations.

Autonomic tests involving RR interval periodicity require physiological sinus nodal rhythm. Little knowledge exists on autonomic tests in cardiac patients with atrial fibrillation[49] or sick sinus syndrome, or in patients who are in a predominantly or permanently paced rhythm or are on drugs that influence the sinus nodal physiology. In these situations, attempts to investigate autonomic influences at ventricular level (e.g., by studying QT interval variability) might be appropriate. Different measurement aspects and issues with the interpretation of results still need to be addressed.[50] Nevertheless, even in patients in sinus rhythm, complementing the RR variability investigations with those of QT interval variability is likely to enhance the assessment of cardiac autonomic status further.

REFERENCES

1. Sabbag A, Suleiman M, Laish-Farkash A, et al. Israeli Working Group of Pacing and Electrophysiology. Contemporary rates of appropriate shock therapy in patients who receive implantable device therapy in a real-world setting: from the Israeli ICD Registry. *Heart Rhythm*. 2015;12:2426–2433.
2. Lee DS, Hardy J, Yee R, et al. Investigators of the Ontario ICD Database. Clinical risk stratification for primary prevention implantable cardioverter defibrillators. *Circ Heart Fail*. 2015;8:927–937.
3. Cheng A, Dalal D, Butcher B, et al. Prospective observational study of implantable cardioverter-defibrillators in primary prevention of sudden cardiac death: study design and cohort description. *J Am Heart Assoc*. 2013;2:e000083.
4. Weeke P, Johansen JB, Jørgensen OD, et al. Mortality and appropriate and inappropriate therapy in patients with ischaemic heart disease and implanted cardioverter-defibrillators for primary prevention: data from the Danish ICD Register. *Europace*. 2013;15:1150–1157.
5. Zipes DP, Camm AJ, Borggrefe M, Buxton AE, Chaitman B, Fromer M, et al. ACC/AHA/ESC 2006 Guidelines for Management of Patients With Ventricular Arrhythmias and the Prevention of Sudden Cardiac Death: a report of the American College of Cardiology/American Heart Association Task Force and the European Society of Cardiology Committee for Practice Guidelines (writing committee to develop Guidelines for Management of Patients With Ventricular Arrhythmias and the Prevention of Sudden Cardiac Death): developed in collaboration with the European Heart Rhythm Association and the Heart Rhythm Society. *Circulation*. 2006;114:e385–e484.
6. Epstein AE, DiMarco JP, Ellenbogen KA, et al. 2012 ACCF/AHA/HRS focused update incorporated into the ACCF/AHA/HRS 2008 guidelines for device-based therapy of cardiac rhythm abnormalities: a report of the American College of Cardiology Foundation/American Heart Association Task Force on Practice Guidelines and the Heart Rhythm Society. *Circulation*. 2013;127:e283–e352.
7. Moss AJ, Zareba W, Hall WJ, et al. Multicenter Automatic Defibrillator Implantation Trial II Investigators. Prophylactic implantation of a defibrillator in patients with myocardial infarction and reduced ejection fraction. *N Engl J Med*. 2002;346:877–883.
8. Bardy GH, Lee KL, Mark DB, et al. Sudden Cardiac Death in Heart Failure Trial (SCD-HeFT) Investigators. Amiodarone or an implantable cardioverter-defibrillator for congestive heart failure. *N Engl J Med*. 2005;352:225–237.
9. Kadish A, Dyer A, Daubert JP, et al. Defibrillators in Non-Ischemic Cardiomyopathy Treatment Evaluation (DEFINITE) Investigators. Prophylactic defibrillator implantation in patients with nonischemic dilated cardiomyopathy. *N Engl J Med*. 2004;350:2151–2158.
10. Bauer A, Barthel P, Schneider R, et al. Improved Stratification of Autonomic Regulation for risk prediction in post-infarction patients with preserved left ventricular function (ISAR-Risk). *Eur Heart J*. 2009;30:576–583.
11. Luermans JG, Mafi Rad M, Vernooy K. A call for re-evaluation of the guidelines for prophylactic ICD implantation. *Neth Heart J*. 2014;22:429–430.
12. Schwab JO, Bonnemeier H, Kleemann T, et al. Reduction of inappropriate ICD therapies in patients with primary prevention of sudden cardiac death: DECREASE study. *Clin Res Cardiol*. 2015;104:1021–1032.
13. Arisha MM, Girerd N, Chauveau S, et al. In-hospital heart rate turbulence and microvolt T-wave alternans abnormalities for prediction of early life-threatening ventricular arrhythmia after acute myocardial infarction. *Ann Noninvasive Electrocardiol*. 2013;18:530–537.
14. Forleo GB, Della Rocca DG, Papavasileiou LP, et al. Predictive value of fragmented QRS in primary prevention implantable cardioverter defibrillator recipients with left ventricular dysfunction. *J Cardiovasc Med*. 2011;12:779–784.
15. Wellens HJ, Schwartz PJ, Lindemans FW, et al. Risk stratification for sudden cardiac death: current status and challenges for the future. *Eur Heart J*. 2014;35:1642–1651.
16. Vanoli E, De Ferrari GM, Stramba Badiale M, Hull Jr SS, Foreman RD, Schwartz PJ. Vagal stimulation and prevention of sudden death in conscious dogs with a healed myocardial infarction. *Circ Res*. 1991;68:1471–1481.
17. Lown B, Verrier RL. Neural activity and ventricular fibrillation. *N Engl J Med*. 1976;294:1165–1170.
18. Schwartz PJ, La Rovere MT, Vanoli E. Autonomic nervous system and sudden cardiac death. Experimental basis and clinical observations for post-myocardial infarction risk stratification. *Circulation*. 1992;85:I77–I91.
19. Chang RB, Strochlic DE, Williams EK, Umans BD, Liberles SD. vagal sensory neuron subtypes that differentially control breathing. *Cell*. 2015;161:622–633.
20. Task Force of the European Society of Cardiology and the North American Society of Pacing and Electrophysiology: heart rate variability—standards of measurement, physiological interpretation, and clinical use. *Circulation*. 1006;93:1043–1065.
21. Battipaglia I, Barone L, Mariani L, et al. Relationship between cardiac autonomic function and sustained ventricular tachyarrhythmias in patients with an implantable cardioverter defibrillators. *Europace*. 2010;12:1725–1731.
22. Ten Sande JN, Damman P, Tijssen JG, et al. Value of serial heart rate variability measurement for prediction of appropriate ICD discharge in patients with heart failure. *J Cardiovasc Electrophysiol*. 2014;25:60–65.
23. Smetana P, Malik M. Sex differences in cardiac autonomic regulation and in repolarisation electrocardiography. *Pflüg Arch Eur J Physiol*. 2013;465:699–717.
24. La Rovere MT, Pinna GD, Maestri R, et al. for the GISSI-HF Investigators. Autonomic markers and cardiovascular and arrhythmic events in heart failure patients: still a place in prognostication? Data from the GISSI-HF trial. *Eur J Heart Fail*. 2012;14:1410–1419.
25. Nicolini P, Ciulla MM, Malfatto G, et al. Autonomic dysfunction in mild cognitive impairment: evidence from power spectral analysis of heart rate variability in a cross-sectional case-control study. *PLoS One*. 2014;9:e96656.
26. Poulikakos D, Banerjee D, Malik M. Repolarisation descriptors and heart rate variability in hemodialysed patients. *Physiol Res*. 2015;64:487–493.
27. Barthel P, Bauer A, Müller A, et al. Spontaneous baroreflex sensitivity: prospective validation trial of a novel technique in survivors of acute myocardial infarction. *Heart Rhythm*. 2012;9:1288–1294.
28. Bauer A, Kantelhardt JW, Barthel P, et al. Deceleration capacity of heart rate as a predictor of mortality after myocardial infarction: cohort study. *Lancet*. 2006;367:1674–1681.
29. Kisohara M, Stein PK, Yoshida Y, et al. Multi-scale heart rate dynamics detected by phase-rectified signal averaging predicts mortality after acute myocardial infarction. *Europace*. 2013;15:437–443.
30. Eick C, Rizas KD, Meyer-Zürn CS, et al. Autonomic nervous system activity as risk predictor in the medical emergency department: a prospective cohort study. *Crit Care Med*. 2015;43:1079–1086.
31. Sassi R, Cerutti S, Lombardi F, et al. Advances in heart rate variability signal analysis: joint position statement by the e-Cardiology ESC Working Group and the European Heart Rhythm Association co-endorsed by the Asia Pacific Heart Rhythm Society. *Europace*. 2015;17:1341–1353.
32. Yeung WT, Reinhall PG, Poole JE, et al. SCD-HeFT: use of R-R interval statistics for long-term risk stratification for arrhythmic sudden cardiac death. *Heart Rhythm*. 2015;12:2058–2066.
33. Gouveia S, Scotto MG, Pinna GD, Maestri R, La Rovere MT, Ferreira PJ. Spontaneous baroreceptor reflex sensitivity for risk stratification of heart failure patients: optimal cut-off and age effects. *Clin Sci (Lond)*. 2015;129:1163–1172.
34. Bauer A, Malik M, Schmidt G, et al. Heart rate turbulence: standards of measurement, physiological interpretation, and clinical use: International Society for Holter and Noninvasive Electrophysiology Consensus. *J Am Coll Cardiol*. 2008;52:1353–1365.
35. Lombardi F, Stein PK. Origin of heart rate variability and turbulence: an appraisal of autonomic modulation of cardiovascular function. *Front Physiol*. 2011;2:95.
36. Sinnecker D, Dirschinger RJ, Barthel P, et al. Postextrasystolic blood pressure potentiation predicts poor outcome of cardiac patients. *J Am Heart Assoc*. 2014;3:e000857.
37. Stöckigt F, Jüngst P, Linhart M, et al. Association of heart rate turbulence with arrhythmia susceptibility and heart disease in mice. *J Cardiovasc Electrophysiol*. 2015. [Epub ahead of print].
38. Schaeffer BN, Rybczynski M, Sheikhzadeh S, et al. Heart rate turbulence and deceleration capacity for risk prediction of serious arrhythmic events in Marfan syndrome. *Clin Res Cardiol*. 2015;104:1054–1063.
39. Exner DV, Kavanagh KM, Slawnych MP, et al. REFINE Investigators. Noninvasive risk assessment early after a myocardial infarction the REFINE study. *J Am Coll Cardiol*. 2007;50:2275–2284.
40. Scheffers IJ, Kroon AA, Schmidli J, et al. Novel baroreflex activation therapy in resistant hypertension: results of a European multi-center feasibility study. *J Am Coll Cardiol*. 2010;56:1254-1248.
41. Madershahian N, Scherner M, Müller-Ehmsen J, et al. Baroreflex activation therapy in patients with pre-existing implantable cardioverter-defibrillator: compatible, complementary therapies. *Europace*. 2014;16:861–865.
42. Victor RG. Carotid baroreflex activation therapy for resistant hypertension. *Nat Rev Cardiol*. 2015;12:451–463.
43. Laffin LJ, Bakris GL. Hypertension and new treatment approaches targeting the sympathetic nervous system. *Curr Opin Pharmacol*. 2015;21:20–24.
44. Malik M, ed. *Clinical Guide to Cardiac Autonomic Tests*. Berlin: Kluwer Academic Publishers; 1998.
45. Barthel P, Wensel R, Bauer A, et al. Respiratory rate predicts outcome after acute myocardial infarction: a prospective cohort study. *Eur Heart J*. 2013;34:1644–1650.
46. Eagle KA, Lim MJ, Dabbous OH, et al. for the GRACE Investigators, A validated prediction model for all forms of acute coronary syndrome: estimating the risk of 6-month postdischarge death in an international registry. *J Am Med Assoc*. 2004;291:2727–2733.
47. Sinnecker D, Dommasch M, Barthel P, et al. Assessment of mean respiratory rate from ECG recordings for risk stratification after myocardial infarction. *J Electrocardiol*. 2014;47:700–704.
48. Dommasch M, Sinnecker D, Barthel P, et al. Nocturnal respiratory rate predicts non-sudden cardiac death in survivors of acute myocardial infarction. *J Am Coll Cardiol*. 2014;63:2432–2433.
49. Sinnecker D, Barthel P, Huster KM, et al. Force-interval relationship predicts mortality in survivors of myocardial infarction with atrial fibrillation. *Int J Cardiol*. 2015;182:315–320.
50. Baumert M, Porta A, Vos MA, et al. QT interval variability in body surface ECG: measurement, physiological basis, and clinical value: position statement and consensus guidance endorsed by the European Heart Rhythm Association jointly with the ESC Working Group on Cardiac Cellular Electrophysiology. *Europace*. 2016;18:925–944.

69

T-Wave Alternans

Stefan H. Hohnloser

History of Cardiac Alternans

Electrical alternans is defined as beat-to-beat alterations in the shape of electrocardiographical waveforms with the occurrence of visible electrical alternans (i.e., "macrovolt" alternans), first described by Hering in 1908.[1] Shortly thereafter, Thomas Lewis noted that alternans could occur in a normal heart following marked accelerations in heart rate and also in diseased or intoxicated myocardium.[2] In 1948, Kalter and Schwartz described an association between macroscopic T-wave alternans (TWA) and an increased mortality among affected patients.[3] Subsequent case reports described the occurrence of visible TWA in various clinical situations such as myocardial ischemia, coronary artery spasm, and electrolyte disturbances, and, particularly, in the setting of congenital long QT syndrome.[4]

Assessment of subtle microvolt TWA (MTWA) was first reported in 1982,[5] utilizing sophisticated computerized analysis. In the 1980s, Cohen and coworkers established a close relationship between MTWA and vulnerability to ventricular fibrillation (VF) in a dog model.[5,6] Similar findings were subsequently reported by Nearing and colleagues.[7] Since the inception of methods for assessment of MTWA, compelling evidence for a mechanistic link between MTWA and occurrence of ventricular tachyarrhythmias exists on the basis of numerous experimental and clinical studies. Clinical studies using implantable cardioverter defibrillator (ICD)–stored electrogram series[8] or recordings from ambulatory monitoring[9] have demonstrated a progressive increase in MTWA shortly before the onset of ventricular tachyarrhythmias.

This chapter reviews the current knowledge regarding MTWA, with particular emphasis on methodological aspects and results of studies on risk stratification for sudden death, utilizing assessment of MTWA.

Mechanisms Underlying T-Wave Alternans

MTWA results from beat-to-beat alternation in the time course of the action potential duration at the cellular level. This was definitively established through detailed measurements of the time course of membrane voltage throughout the ventricle at a time when MTWA was elicited on surface electrocardiogram (ECG) using high-resolution optical mapping techniques in a guinea pig model of pacing-induced MTWA.[10–12] Importantly, in these studies, MTWA was a consistent (in fact requisite) precursor to VF. The mechanism linking action potential alternans (and therefore MTWA) to ventricular arrhythmias involves the development of spatially discordant alternans—that is, action potential alternans that occur in opposite phase between neighboring cells (Fig. 69.1A).[10] When action potential alternans is initiated, action potential duration either prolongs or shortens simultaneously in all cells of a particular region of ventricular myocardium (i.e., concordant alternans; Fig. 69.2A, *left*). As illustrated in Fig. 69.2A (*right*), after a premature impulse (*) or change in pacing rate above a critical heart rate threshold, sequential lengthening and shortening of the action potential, with fluctuations in some regions being 180 degrees out of phase with those in other regions, occur such that some cells undergo a prolongation of action potential duration, while other populations of cells undergo a shortening of action potential duration on the same beat (i.e., discordant alternans).[10,12] During discordant alternans (see Fig. 69.2B, *right*), marked spatial dispersion of action potential duration emerges (*blue bars*), and discordant alternans amplifies physiological heterogeneities of repolarization, present at baseline, into pathophysiological heterogeneities of sufficient magnitude to produce conduction block and reentrant excitation (see Fig. 69.2B).[10–12] Discordant alternans also produces a substrate by which conduction block and reentrant excitation can be easily initiated by a premature stimulus (see Fig. 69.2B). When an impulse (*) propagates (from site A) into the still-depolarized myocardium (i.e., in the wake of enhanced dispersion of repolarization after the long beat, *blue bar* in site B), conduction block, which initiates reentrant excitation, can occur (see Fig. 69.2B, VF). Consequently, discordant alternans is a mechanism that links MTWA to cardiac arrhythmogenesis, and in fact, in experimental models of action potential alternans, VF never occurs without discordant alternans. Thus, under chronotropic or metabolic stress, discordant alternans leads to sufficiently large repolarization gradients that produce unidirectional block and reentry. Without a structural barrier, reentry is functional and manifests as VF or polymorphic ventricular tachycardia (VT). In the presence of structural barriers, reentry can become anatomically fixed, resulting in monomorphic VT.

Cellular Mechanisms of Alternans

Although the cellular mechanism for action potential alternans is not completely elucidated, there is convincing data that indicate a primary role of sarcoplasmic reticulum calcium cycling in its mechanism.[13] Merchant and Armoundas recently provided an in-depth review of cellular mechanisms of alternans.[14] In essence, they emphasized two major hypotheses to explain alternans at the cellular level. The first hypothesis is that alternation in sarcolemmal currents, membrane voltages, and action potential morphologies results in beat-to-beat fluctuations in the intracellular calcium concentration. For example, Shimizu and Antzelevitch used a ventricular wedge preparation in which congenital long QT syndrome physiology was mimicked.[15] In this preparation, alteration of T-wave and action potential duration was elicited during rapid pacing; application of ryanodine or decreasing the extracellular calcium concentration abolished these alterations, implicating intracellular calcium cycling in the maintenance of MTWA. The second major hypothesis is that alternation of intracellular calcium concentration is the initial event that leads in the second step to alternans of membrane voltage and action potential morphology.[10,11,16,17] According to the second hypothesis, alternans of the intracellular calcium concentration may be caused by perturbations of any number of calcium transport processes, which may occur in diseased myocardium.[14]

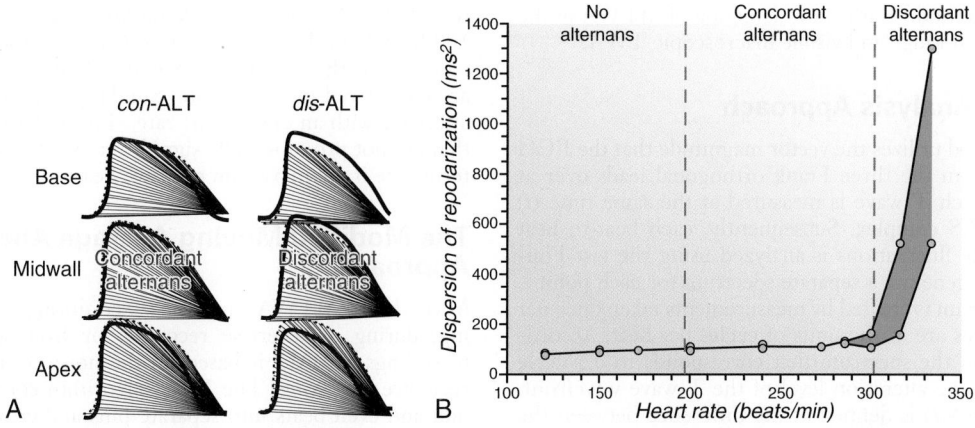

FIGURE 69.1 (A) Action potential assessed by high-resolution optical mapping from epicardial cells on the base, midwall, and apex of the guinea pig left ventricle during two consecutive beats. Above a critical heart rate, concordant alternans is transformed to discordant alternans between the apex and base. (B) Amplification of spatial gradients of repolarization by discordant alternans. (Modified from Pastore JM, Girouard SD, Laurita KR, Akar FG, Rosenbaum DS. Mechanism linking T-wave alternans to the genesis of cardiac fibrillation. *Circulation.* 1999;99:1385-1394.)

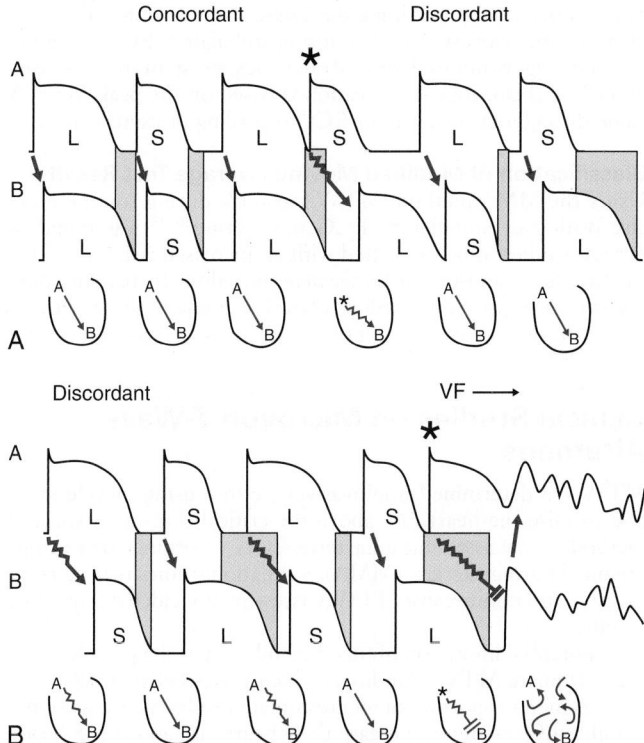

FIGURE 69.2 Concordant and discordant alternans and the induction of ventricular fibrillation (*VF*). (A) Transition of concordant in discordant alternans, following a premature impulse (*asterisk*). (B) Occurrence of conduction block and reentrant excitation, leading to ventricular fibrillation (see text for details). (Modified from Wilson LD, Rosenbaum DS. Mechanisms of arrhythmogenic discordant cardiac alternans. *Europace.* 2007;9:77-82.)

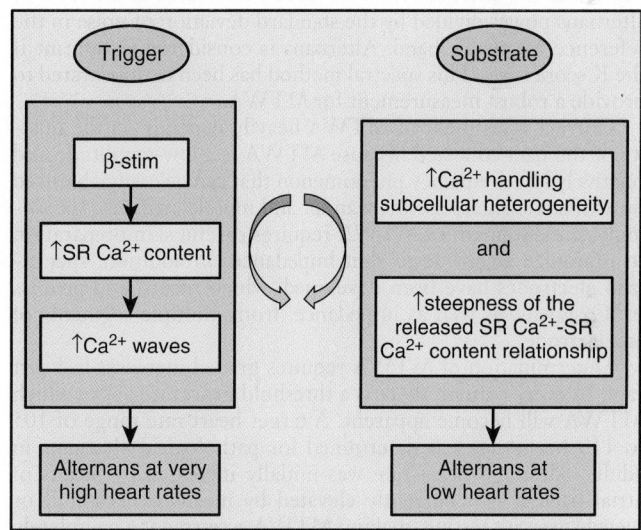

FIGURE 69.3 Different mechanisms of repolarization alternans in normal (*left side*) and diseased hearts (*right side*). See text for details. *SR*, Sarcoplasmic reticulum. (Modified from Merchant FM, Armoundas AA. Role of substrate and triggers in the genesis of cardiac alternans, from myocyte to the whole heart. *Circulation.* 2012;125:539-549.)

an appropriate subcellular substrate to develop. A trigger event may be sufficient to give rise to alternans in the normal heart. However, heart rates should increase above physiological levels to create a heterogeneous (fragmented) subcellular Ca^{2+} release profile.[14,18] On the other hand, in the diseased heart, perturbations in the intracellular calcium cycling machinery can create a sufficiently heterogeneous subcellular substrate to promote the development of alternans at lower (physiological) heart rates and cause predisposition to arrhythmogenesis.[18]

Methodology of T-Wave Alternans Assessment

Two contemporary techniques for the detection and quantification of MTWA have been developed and applied in clinical studies of risk stratification: the spectral method[6] and modified moving

A wealth of recent experimental data supports the second hypothesis, indicating that perturbations of calcium handling processes are fundamental events in the genesis of cellular alternans. As schematically summarized in Fig. 69.3, these findings suggest that in the diseased heart, cellular alternans requires a trigger event (i.e., enhanced adrenergic β-stimulation or Ca^{2+} wave) and

average (MMA) method.[7] Both allow detection of MTWA in the nonvisible microvolt range and visible macroscopic TWA.

The Spectral Analysis Approach

The spectral method utilizes the vector magnitude that the ECG signal recorded from the three Frank orthogonal leads over at least 128 beats. Each T wave is measured at the same time (t) relative to the QRS complex. Subsequently, each beat-to-beat series of amplitude fluctuations is analyzed using the fast Fourier Transform to generate a separate spectrum for each point t. Because this spectrum is created by measurements taken once per beat, its frequencies are in the units of cycles per beat. Accordingly, the point on the spectrum that corresponds to 0.5 cycle per beat indicates the alteration level of the T-wave wavefront. Alternans power ($\mu V2$) is defined as the difference between the power of alternans frequency and that at the noise frequency band (calculated over the reference frequency band between 0.44 and 0.49 cycle per beat). This is a measure of the true physiological alternans level. The alternans voltage (Valt) is simply the square root of alternans power and corresponds to the root mean square difference in the voltage (averaged over the T wave) between the overall mean beats and either the even- or odd-numbered mean beats. A measure of the statistical significance of alternans is defined as the alternans ratio (K score), calculated as the ratio of alternans power divided by the standard deviation of noise in the reference frequency band. Alternans is considered significant if the K score is ≥3. This spectral method has been demonstrated to provide a robust measurement for MTWA.

Correct assessment of MTWA heavily depends on the quality of the data collected because MTWA is a low-amplitude and relatively low-frequency phenomenon that can be easily obscured by artifacts such as baseline wander and muscle artifacts. Accordingly, measurement of MTWA requires careful skin preparation to minimize electrode-to-skin impedance. In addition, specialized electrodes have been developed, which record and process ECG signals, as well as impedance, from multiple segments of an electrode.

Determination of MTWA requires graded increases in heart rate. In every patient, there is a threshold heart rate above which MTWA will become apparent. A target heart rate range of 105 to 110 beats/min was determined for pathological alternans in adults. Although heart rate was initially increased by means of atrial pacing, it is currently elevated by means of treadmill or bicycle exercise testing, making MTWA assessment a completely noninvasive test procedure.

Classification of Spectral Analysis Test Results

The presence of MTWA is defined by its magnitude, the alternans ratio (K score), and the relationship between MTWA and heart rate. Significant MTWA is defined as alternans that has a Valt ≥1.9 μV and a K score ≥3; sustained alternans is defined as significant alternans that has a duration of at least 1 minute and is consistently present above a patient-specific threshold heart rate, which is referred to as the onset heart rate. MTWA tracings are classified as positive, negative, or indeterminate.[19] The classification of MTWA tracing as positive requires only the determination of whether sustained alternans is present at an onset heart rate ≤110 beats/min. The distinction between tracings that are negative or indeterminate is made by determining the maximum negative heart rate and maximum heart rate. The maximum negative heart rate must be ≥105 beats/min to classify a tracing as negative. For example, if a tracing has excessive levels of ectopy or noise above a heart rate of 95 beats/min, one cannot be confident that alternans is not present above a heart rate of 95 beats/min and one cannot consider the tracing to be negative. Accordingly, if the maximum negative heart rate is 95 beats/min, the tracing is classified as indeterminate. Perhaps if ectopy or noise levels

were reduced, alternans would be "unmasked" at the heart rate of 100 beats/min. For this reason, tracings without sustained alternans and with a maximum negative heart rate <105 beats/min are considered indeterminate. Similarly, tracings with sustained alternans with an onset heart rate >110 beats/min (i.e., alternans that are not prognostically significant) are also classified as indeterminate if the maximum negative heart rate is <105 beats/min.

The Modified Moving Average Analysis Approach

MMA-based MTWA can be assessed during exercise stress testing, during postexercise recovery, or from ambulatory ECG recordings.[20] MMA is based on the noise rejection principle of recursive averaging. The MMA algorithm continuously streams odd and even beats into separate bins and creates median complexes for each bin.[7] These complexes are then superimposed, and the maximum difference between the odd and even median complexes at any point within the JT segment is determined as the TWA value, which is averaged every 10 to 15 seconds. The moving average allows control of the influence of new incoming beats on the median templates with an adjustable update factor; that is, the fraction of morphology change that an incoming beat can contribute. Respiration and motion artifacts are reduced by noise reduction software. MMA-based MTWA can be noninvasively assessed from symptom-limited exercise stress testing and during postexercise recovery as well as during ambulatory ECG monitoring. The algorithm excludes extrasystoles, noisy beats, and beats preceding them. Risk stratification is based on the peak MTWA value throughout the 24-hour ECG recording or exercise test.

Classification of Modified Moving Average Test Results

Using the MMA method, MTWA ≥60 μV during routine exercise testing or ambulatory ECG monitoring[20–23] was found in clinical studies to be associated with an increased risk for sudden cardiac death and/or cardiovascular mortality. In patients during the early post–myocardial infarction phase with or without heart failure, a lower cutpoint of ≥47 μV predicted sudden cardiac death.[23,24]

Clinical Studies on Microvolt T-Wave Alternans

MTWA is determined noninvasively, either using bicycle exercise to raise the heart rate above the critical threshold (spectral method) or by assessing long-term ECG recordings or tracings obtained during exercise (MMA). Validation studies revealed that invasive and noninvasive MTWA assessment yielded comparable results.

A potential limitation of this methodology is the prevalence of indeterminate MTWA findings, which varies between 12% and 40%. A high proportion of indeterminate results is because of the inability of patients to increase their heart rate above 105 beats/min (i.e., because of the presence of heart failure) or excessive ventricular ectopy during exercise (patient factors). Other reasons for indeterminate MTWA testing include excessive noise or an exercise protocol that causes an excessively rapid increase in heart rate (technical factors). In terms of prognostic information, however, the current thinking is that an indeterminate test because of patient factors carries similar prognostic information as a positive MTWA test result. Kaufman and associates used data from a large study and specifically examined the prognostic yield of indeterminate MTWA test results. They reported that patients with dilated cardiomyopathy and an indeterminate MTWA test result had a 2-year rate for death or sustained ventricular tachyarrhythmias of 17.8% compared with those with a positive test who had a 2-year rate of 12.3%.[25] Accordingly, newer studies have differentiated "nonnegative" tests (i.e., positive and indeterminate) from negative ones. MTWA cannot be reliably determined in patients who are in atrial fibrillation.

Microvolt T-Wave Alternans Assessment and Results of Invasive Electrophysiological Testing

Rosenbaum and associates conducted the first clinical landmark study on MTWA in 1994.[26] In this study, there was an excellent correlation between the presence of MTWA and the inducibility of VT or VF. During a 20-month observation period, MTWA and inducibility of ventricular arrhythmias were essentially equivalent predictors of arrhythmia-free survival ($p < .001$). Several subsequent studies in patients revealed confirmatory results.[27]

The largest trial to compare invasive electrophysiological (EP) testing to MTWA assessment as a predictor for sudden death is the Alternans Before Cardioverter Defibrillator (ABCD) trial.[28] This study mandated ICD implantation in all patients with either positive MTWA or EP test result. MTWA assessment achieved 1-year positive (9%) and negative (95%) predictive values, which were almost identical to those of EP testing (11% and 95%, respectively). The highest risk was observed in patients with both positive MTWA and EP test results. However, the study failed to predict endpoint events after 2 years, suggesting the potential time dependence of MTWA assessment.

Microvolt T-Wave Alternans Assessment for Noninvasive Risk Stratification

A plethora of studies have evaluated the prognostic power of non-invasively assessed MTWA in an attempt to risk-stratify patients prone to sudden death. The need for better assessment of risk for serious ventricular tachyarrhythmias is driven by the implantable defibrillator, a highly efficacious tool for preventing arrhythmogenic death. However, the use of the ICD has its own risks because of the invasive character of this therapy, and its widespread applicability is limited by high costs and need for trained specialists to apply this therapy. Accordingly, more accurate identification of patients at the highest risk for arrhythmogenic death is of paramount clinical importance.

Utilizing spectral MTWA analysis, at least 32 studies comprising more than 100 patients each have been published, as recently summarized by Verrier and colleagues.[20] As summarized in Table 69.1,[29-58] 25 of 32 studies demonstrated significant predictivity of MTWA; that is, patients with positive or indeterminate test results were found to be at significantly greater risk for sudden death or serious ventricular tachyarrhythmias than those with negative test results. Several reasons for nonpredictability of MTWA have been discussed, including its assessment too early after a cardiac event (myocardial infarction), withholding β-blocker therapy, or the use of ICD therapy as a surrogate endpoint for sudden death (see subsequent text).

Using the MMA method, at least 14 reports were published on the predictive capability of MTWA for cardiovascular or sudden death or serious ventricular arrhythmias (Table 69.2[59-67]).[20] In contrast to studies that utilized the spectral MTWA assessment methodology, these reports used different test conditions for MTWA assessment such as measurement at peak exercise, during exercise recovery, or from ambulatory ECG monitoring. Accordingly, compared with spectral MTWA studies, it is more difficult to directly compare the predictive value of the method between these studies. In general, however,

TABLE 69.1 Clinical studies using the spectral method for MTWA determination in more than 100 patients

STUDY	PATIENT POPULATION (ENROLLMENT, DISEASE)	MEAN LVEF	HAZARD RATIOS FOR TWA
Predictive Studies			
Cardiomyopathy			
Kitamura et al. 2002[29]	104 patients with DCM	37%	11.9 (1.53–92.59)[a] for SCD, VF, or sustained VT at 21 ± 14 months
Hohnloser et al. 2003[30]	137 patients with DCM, LVEF ≤35%	29% ± 11%	3.44 for ventricular tachyarrhythmic events at 14 ± 6 months
Chow et al. 2007[31]	514 patients with ischemic cardiomyopathy, LVEF ≤35%, no previous sustained ventricular arrhythmia and positive or indeterminate TWA test results	26%–29%	2.24 (1.34–3.75) for all-cause mortality; 2.29 (1.00–5.24) for arrhythmic mortality; NS for nonarrhythmic mortality
Salerno-Uriarte et al. 2007 (ALPHA)[32]	446 patients with DCM, LVEF ≤40%	29.5%	4.0 (1.4–11.4) for cardiac death and life-threatening arrhythmias at 18 months
Chow et al. 2006[33]	768 patients with ischemic cardiomyopathy, LVEF ≤35%, no previous sustained ventricular arrhythmia	26%–29%	2.27 (1.22–4.24) for all-cause mortality in patients without an ICD; 2.42 (1.07–5.41) for all-cause mortality or appropriate ICD discharge in patients with an ICD
Chan et al. 2008[34]	768 patients with ischemic cardiomyopathy, LVEF ≤35%, no previous sustained ventricular arrhythmia (same patients as Chow et al. 2007[35])	26%–29%	2.19 (1.1–4.34) for all-cause mortality and appropriate ICD shocks at 1 year; 3.36 (1.28–8.83) at 2 years
Costantini et al. 2009 (ABCD)[28]	566 patients with ischemic cardiomyopathy, LVEF ≤40%, and NSVT	28% ± 8%	2.1 for SCD or appropriate ICD discharge at 1 year
Congenital Heart Disease			
Alexander et al. 2006[36]	304 consecutive pediatric patients with congenital heart disease, myopathy, syncope, or history of cardiac arrest	Not stated	7.9 (2.2–28.1) for ventricular arrhythmia; 6.7 (1.6–28.1) for cardiac arrest at <3 years
Depressed LVEF			
Rashba et al. 2002[35]	108 consecutive patients with CAD and LVEF ≤40%	28% ± 7%	2.2 (1.1–4.7) for death, sustained ventricular arrhythmias, appropriate ICD discharge at 18 ± 13 months in patients with normal QRS segment; NS in patients with prolonged QRS segment
Rashba et al. 2004[37]	144 patients with CAD and LVEF ≤40%	28% ± 7%	2.2 (1.1–4.7) for death, sustained ventricular arrhythmia, or appropriate ICD discharge at 17 ± 13 months; NS in patients with LVEF <30%; ∞ in patients with LVEF >30%

Continued

TABLE 69.1	Clinical studies using the spectral method for MTWA determination in more than 100 patients—cont'd		
STUDY	PATIENT POPULATION (ENROLLMENT, DISEASE)	MEAN LVEF	HAZARD RATIOS FOR TWA
Bloomfield et al. 2006[38]	549 patients with LVEF ≤40%, no history of sustained ventricular arrhythmias	25%	6.5 (2.4–18.1) for all-cause mortality or nonfatal sustained ventricular arrhythmia at 2 years
Cantillon et al. 2006[39]	286 patients with LVEF ≤35%, NSVT, or syncope	26% ± 7%	2.33 (1.44–3.67) for arrhythmia-free survival at 38 ± 11 months
Morin et al. 2007[40]	386 patients with CAD, NSVT, LVEF ≤40%	26%–30%	1.64 for ventricular tachyarrhythmia or death in patients with narrow QRS segment at 40 ± 19 months; NS in patients with wide QRS segment
Merchant et al. 2013[41]	Patient-level data from 3355 patients enrolled in six studies	25%–54% (mostly reduced)	Multivariable model of LVEF, presence of CAD, MTWA: concordance index is 0.817
Molon et al. 2013[42]	178 patients with CAD or DCM, LVEF ≤40%	30%–32%	3.65 for all-cause death
Merchant et al. 2015[43]	651 patients with CAD or DCM, LVEF ≤40%	31%–33%	2.71 for MTWA nonnegative for all-cause death, 7.52 for cardiac mortality
Heart Failure			
Klingenheben et al. 2000[44]	107 consecutive patients with congestive heart failure, LVEF ≤45%, no history of arrhythmia, and no recent MI	28% ± 7%	∞ for SCD, arrhythmias, sustained VT at 14.6 months
Gorodeski et al. 2009[45]	303 consecutive patients with heart failure and LVEF ≤40%	24%	1.89 (1.05–3.39) for total mortality or cardiac transplantation; NS after adjustment for metabolic measures at 2.8 years. Concordance index for time-to-event outcomes is 0.75. C statistic for propensity score is 0.79.
Post–Myocardial Infarction			
Ikeda et al. 2000[46]	102 post-MI patients	20%–40%	16.8 (2.2–127.8) for arrhythmic events
Ikeda et al. 2002[47]	850 post-MI patients	51% ± 13%	5.9 (1.6–21.4) for SCD or resuscitated VF at 25 ± 13 months; 82% were monitored at 2–10 weeks after MI
Bloomfield et al. 2004[48]	177 MADIT-II–like post-MI patients with LVEF ≤30	23% ± 6%	4.8 for all-cause mortality at 2 years
Ikeda et al. 2006[49]	1041 post-MI patients with LVEF >40%	55% ± 10%	23.5 monitored at 48 ± 66 days for SCD or life-threatening arrhythmia at 32 ± 14 months
Exner et al. 2007 (REFINE)[50]	322 post-MI patients with LVEF <50	40% within 1 week and 47% at 8 weeks after MI	2.75 (1.08–7.02) monitored at 10–14 weeks after MI for cardiovascular death or resuscitated cardiac arrest (primary endpoint) at 47 months; NS if monitored at 2–4 weeks after MI. Area under ROC curve for primary endpoint is 0.62; for combination of TWA + HRT, area under ROC curve is 0.70
Referred for Electrophysiological Study			
Gold et al. 2000[27]	313 patients	44% ± 18%	10.9 for SCD, sustained VT, VF, or appropriate ICD discharge at 400 days
Rashba et al. 2002[51]	251 patients with CAD and LVEF	27% ± 8%	2.2 (1.1–4.7) for arrhythmic events (arrhythmic death, VT, aborted VF) at 499 ± 395 days; NS for TWA during atrial pacing at 100–120 beats/min
Nonpredictive Studies			
Schwab et al. 2001[52]	140 post-MI patients	56% ± 14%	NS if monitored at 15 ± 6 days after MI for SCD or sustained VT at 451 ± 210 days
Tapanainen et al. 2001[53]	379 consecutive post-MI patients	45% ± 10%	NS for TWA monitored at ~8 days after MI for all-cause mortality or cardiac death at 14.8 months
Grimm et al. 2003[54]	343 patients with DCM, LVEF ≤45%	31% ± 10%	NS for SCD, VF, or sustained VT at 52 months
Ikeda et al. 2005[55]	124 consecutive subjects with Brugada-type ECG	Not stated	NS for SCD or VT at 40 ± 19 months
Gold et al. 2008 (SCD-HeFT TWA substudy)[56]	490 patients with congestive heart failure	24% ± 7%	NS for SCD, sustained VT/VF, or appropriate ICD discharge at 2.5 years
Chow et al. 2008 (MASTER)[57]	575 post-MI patients with LVEF ≤30%	24% ± 5%	2.04 (1.10–3.78) for total mortality at 2.1 ± 0.9 years; NS for ventricular tachyarrhythmic events
Huikuri et al. 2009 (CARISMA)[58]	312 post-MI patients	31% ± 6%	NS for TWA monitored at 6 weeks after MI for VF or symptomatic, sustained VT at 2 years

[a]Numbers in parentheses are 95% confidence intervals.

ABCD, Alternans before cardioverter defibrillator; *ALPHA*, T-wave alternans in patients with heart failure; *CAD*, coronary artery disease; *CARISMA*, Cardiac Arrhythmias and Risk Stratification After Acute Myocardial Infarction (trial); *CI*, confidence interval; *DCM*, dilated cardiomyopathy; *ECG*, electrocardiogram; *ICD*, implantable cardioverter defibrillator; *LVEF*, left ventricular ejection fraction; *MADIT*, Multicenter Automatic Defibrillator Trial; *MASTER*, Microvolt T-Wave Alternans Testing for Risk Stratification of Post-Myocardial Infarction Patients; *MI*, myocardial infarction; *MTWA*, microvolt T-wave alternans; *NS*, nonsignificant; *NSVT*, nonsustained ventricular tachycardia; *REFINE*, Risk Estimation Following Infarction, Noninvasive Evaluation; *ROC*, receiver operating characteristic; *SCD*, sudden cardiac death; *SCD-HeFT*, Sudden Cardiac Death in Heart Failure Trial; *TWA*, T-wave alternans; *VF*, ventricular fibrillation; *VT*, ventricular tachycardia.

Modified from Verrier RL, Klingenheben T, Malik M, et al. Microvolt T-wave alternans. *J Am Coll Cardiol.* 2011;58:1309-1324.

TABLE 69.2 Clinical studies using the MMA method for MTWA determination

69

TEST SETTING	PATIENT POPULATION (DISEASE, ENROLLMENT CRITERIA, MEAN AGE)	MEAN LVEF	HAZARD RATIOS FOR TWA; NEGATIVE AND POSITIVE PREDICTIVE VALUES
Routine Exercise Testing			
Nieminen et al. 2007 (FINCAVAS)[21]	1037 consecutive patients referred for routine exercise testing; 58 + 13 years (patients included in Leino et al. 2011[60])	Mostly preserved	6.0 (95% CI, 2.8–12.8) for CV death at 44 + 7 months for 65-μV TWA cutpoint; NPV, 97.6; PPV, 12.6
Minkkinen et al. 2009 (FINCAVAS)[61]	2119 consecutive patients referred for routine exercise testing; 57 ± 13 years (patients included in Leino et al. 2011[60])	Mostly preserved (60%–66%)	6.4 (95% CI, 2.0–21.2) for CV death, 4.6 (1.7–12.3) for SCD at 47 months for 60-μV cutpoint; NPV for CV death, 97.4; PPV, 10.2
Leino et al. 2011 (FINCAVAS)[62]	3598 consecutive patients referred for routine exercise testing; 56 ± 13 years	Mostly preserved	1.55 (95% CI, 1.150–2.108, $p < .004$) for CV death; 1.58 (95% CI, 1.041–2.412; $p < .033$) for SCD at 55 months per 20-μV TWA in lead V_5
Exercise Recovery			
Exner et al. 2007 (REFINE)[50]	322 post-MI patients; 62 (interquartile range, 53–70) years	Moderately depressed (38%–48%)	2.94 (1.10–7.87) monitored at 10–14 weeks after event for CV death or resuscitated cardiac arrest (primary endpoint) at 47 months; NS when monitored at 2–4 weeks after MI. For primary endpoint for TWA, area under ROC curve is 0.62; for combination of TWA + HRT, area under ROC curve is 0.71.
Slawnych et al. 2009 (REFINE/FINCAVAS)[22]	322 post-MI patients (from REFINE) and 681 CAD patients (from FINCAVAS); 69 (interquartile range, 57–76) years	Moderately depressed (38%–48%) and preserved (56%–63%) groups	2.5 (1.1–6.0) for CV death at 48 months for 60-μV cutpoint; NPV, 96%; PPV, 13%
Leino et al. 2009 (FINCAVAS)[59]	1972 consecutive patients referred for routine exercise testing; 57 ± 13 years (patients included in Leino et al. 2011[60])	Mostly preserved (60%–66%)	3.5 (1.6–7.9) for CV death at 48 months for 60-μV cutpoint. For CV death, area under ROC curve for TWA is 0.550–0.606; for combination of TWA + HRR, area under ROC curve is 0.671–0.691
Minkkinen et al. 2015[63]	3609 consecutive patients referred for routine exercise testing	Mostly preserved	Combination of low exercise capacity, reduced HRR, and elevated TWA yield concordance index is 0.719
Ambulatory Electrocardiographic Monitoring			
Verrier et al. 2003 (ATRAMI)[23]	Acute post-MI; case-control analysis (15 cases: 29 controls) from 1284 ATRAMI patients, monitored at 15 ± 10 days post-MI; 60–62 years	Moderately depressed (42 ± 3%)	7.9 (1.9–33.1) for cardiac arrest or arrhythmic death at 21 months for 75th %ile cutpoint (47 μV); patients were monitored at 15 ± 10 days post-MI
Stein et al. 2008 (EPHESUS)[24]	Acute post-MI, LVEF ≤40%, and heart failure; case-control analysis (46 cases: 92 controls) from 6632 EPHESUS patients, monitored at 2–10 days post-MI; 68 ± 11 years	Depressed (34 ± 5%)	5.5 (2.2–13.8) for SCD at 16.4 months for 47-μV cutpoint; patients were monitored at 2–10 days post-MI. For SCD, area under ROC curve is 0.73 for V_1 and 0.70 for V_3 ($p < .001$).
Sakaki et al. 2009[64]	295 cardiomyopathy patients with ischemic or nonischemic left ventricular dysfunction; 66 ± 16 years	Depressed (34 ± 6%)	17.1 (6.3–46.6) for CV death, 22.6 (2.6–193.7) for witnessed SCD at 1 year for 65-μV cutpoint; for CV death, NPV is 97% and PPV is 37%
Maeda et al. 2009[65]	63 consecutive patients including 21 controls, 21 post-MI patients without VT, and 21 post-MI patients with VT; 65 ± 11 years	Depressed (36%–43%) for post-MI group	6.1 (1.1–34.0) for sustained VT or VF at 6 years for 65-μV cutpoint
Stein et al. 2010 (CHS)[60]	General population patients ≥65 years old; case-control analysis (49 cases: 98 controls) from 1649 CHS patients	Not tested, assumed preserved	4.8 (1.48–15.81) for SCD at 14 years
Hoshida et al. 2013[66]	313 post-MI patients	47 ± 11%	HR 5.8 for arrhythmic events and SCD
Nieminen et al. 2014[67]	210 patients with ACS (from MERLIN-TIMI 36 trial)	n.a.	4.12 (1.25–13.6) for total mortality if TWA is ≥47 μV

ATRAMI, Autonomic tone and reflexes after myocardial infarction; *CAD*, coronary artery disease; *CHS*, Cardiovascular Health Study; *CI*, confidence interval; *CV*, cardiovascular; *ECG*, electrocardiogram; *EPHESUS*, Eplerenone Post-Acute Myocardial Infarction Heart Failure Efficacy and Survival Study; *FINCAVAS*, Finnish Cardiovascular Study; *HRR*, heart rate recovery; *LVEF*, left ventricular ejection fraction; *MI*, myocardial infarction; *MMA*, modified moving average; *MTWA*, microvolt T-wave alternans; *n.a.*, not available; *NPV*, negative predictive value; *NS*, nonsignificant; *PPV*, positive predictive value; *REFINE*, Risk Estimation Following Infarction, Noninvasive Evaluation; *ROC*, receiver operating characteristic; *SCD*, sudden cardiac death; *VF*, ventricular fibrillation; *VT*, ventricular tachycardia.
Modified from Verrier RL, Klingenheben T, Malik M, et al. Microvolt T-wave alternans. *J Am Coll Cardiol.* 2011;58:1309-1324.

these studies have also reported encouraging predictive power of positive MTWA results. Of particular importance is the Finnish Cardiovascular Study (FINCAVAS) trial because this is one of the largest MTWA studies performed to date, and it enrolled unselected low-risk subjects. This study included 1972 individuals who were referred for routine exercise testing and followed for 4 years. In a multivariate Cox analysis after adjustment for common coronary risk factors, high exercise–based MTWA was associated with a relative risk of 12.3 (95% confidence interval [CI], 2.1–12.2; $p < .01$) for cardiovascular mortality.[59] High recovery–based MTWA had a risk of 8.0 (95% CI, 2.9–22.0; $p < .01$) for cardiovascular mortality. Accordingly, even in this low-risk population, MTWA was a powerful predictor of subsequent mortality.

Microvolt T-Wave Alternans Assessment in Patients After Myocardial Infarction or With Impaired Left Ventricular Function

A number of studies have been conducted to assess the value of MTWA determination after myocardial infarction, utilizing both the spectral and time domain measurement techniques (see Tables 69.1 and 69.2). The studies included between 100 and 1000 patients with follow-up periods of 1 to 2.5 years. In the majority of these investigations, MTWA turned out to be a useful tool to identify patients who were at increased risk for sudden or, at least, cardiovascular mortality or serious ventricular tachyarrhythmias.

One of the most comprehensive studies in this area is the one of Exner and colleagues.[50] These investigators evaluated 322 infarct survivors with a left ventricular ejection fraction (LVEF) <0.50 during the initial week after myocardial infarction who were followed up for a mean of 47 months. Serial assessments of the autonomic tone (heart rate turbulence or baroreflex sensitivity) and electrical substrate (MTWA) were performed. The primary endpoint was cardiac death or resuscitated cardiac arrest. This study is of particular relevance because MTWA was assessed 2 to 4 weeks following the index infarct and again 10 to 14 weeks later. Of note, abnormal MTWA results after 2 to 4 weeks did not significantly predict endpoint events (hazard ratio [HR], 2.42; 95% CI, 0.96–7.71). However, assessment 10 to 14 weeks after the index infarct yielded HR of 2.91 (95% CI, 1.13–7.48; p = .026). When an abnormal autonomic function was combined with positive MTWA findings, predictive accuracy increased, with an HR of 3.27 (95% CI, 1.42–7.00).

Dilated cardiomyopathy is a clinical condition associated with a high incidence of arrhythmogenic death. Unfortunately, the assessment of conventional risk stratifiers, such as spontaneous ventricular arrhythmias, autonomic markers, or EP testing, has yielded insufficient predictive power for future tachyarrhythmic events. On the other hand, recent randomized controlled trials have demonstrated that prophylactic ICD therapy in such patients improves outcome. However, the absolute reduction in mortality was relatively small (i.e., 5.6% over 20 months in the Multicenter Automatic Defibrillator Trial [MADIT] II). Thus routinely implanting defibrillators in this population would be very expensive.

Accordingly, this population has been the focus of intense research activities with respect to the value of MTWA assessment for refining risk prediction in individual patients. A common observation in almost all of these studies was that patients who tested negative for MTWA had very low mortality, particularly low arrhythmic mortality (negative predictive values >95%). In the largest of these trials conducted by Chow and associates,[33] 768 consecutive patients with ischemic cardiomyopathy and an LVEF ≤0.35 were tested and followed up for a mean of 18 months. Patients were classified as MTWA negative or nonnegative (including MTWA-positive and indeterminate patients). After adjusting for important baseline variables, a nonnegative MTWA test was associated with a significantly higher risk for all-cause (HR, 2.24; 95% CI, 1.34–3.75; p = .002) and arrhythmic (HR, 2.29; 95% CI, 1.0–5.25; p = .049) mortalities.

Some studies in patients with ischemic or nonischemic cardiomyopathy, however, did not show the predictive value of MTWA.[52,56,57] On careful examination, there are important differences between these negative and the aforementioned positive studies, particularly as to whether β-blocker therapy was withheld prior to MTWA testing. There is evidence that β-blockers suppress MTWA amplitude and affect the presence of MTWA during testing. Accordingly, a recent meta-analysis of various MTWA studies demonstrated that the predictive power of MTWA was considerably higher in studies in which alternans was measured during continued β-blocker therapy.[68] It seems clear therefore that MTWA should be assessed in a pharmacological environment, consistent with the patient's medical treatment, to ensure that test results reflect the potential benefit of chronic drug therapy.[68]

Risk Prediction for Sudden Death/Ventricular Tachyarrhythmia Versus Prediction of Implantable Cardioverter Defibrillator Therapy by Microvolt T-Wave Alternans

In a substudy of the Sudden Cardiac Death in Heart Failure Trial (SCD-HeFT), MTWA was assessed in 490 patients at 37 sites. There was a high rate of indeterminate tests (41%) by standard criteria.[56] During a mean follow-up of 30 months, no significant differences in event rates (sudden death, VT/VF, or appropriate ICD therapy) were found between MTWA-positive and MTWA-negative patients. The majority of endpoint events consisted of ICD therapies. Similarly, the MASTER study enrolled 575 MADIT-II–like patients and followed them for 2.1 years[57] for the endpoint of sudden death or appropriate ICD discharge. A nonnegative MTWA test was associated with an increased total mortality (HR, 2.04; p = .02), but it did not predict a significant increase in the primary endpoint (HR, 1.26; p = .37).

Given these controversial observations, a recent meta-analysis that comprised 14 clinical trials (including the two above-mentioned negative ones) was conducted to evaluate MTWA as a predictor of ventricular tachyarrhythmic events in primary prevention patients.[69] For the purpose of this specific analysis, nine trials[29,32,33,38,44,47,49,54,70] in which few patients had implanted ICDs (and therefore in which ICD device therapies accounted for ≤15% of all endpoints) were compared with five trials[28,31,39,56,57] in which many patients had implanted ICDs and thus device therapies comprised the majority of endpoints.[69] In the "low ICD group" comprising 3682 patients, the HR for sudden death/cardiac arrest associated with a nonnegative versus negative MTWA test was 13.6 (95% CI, 8.5–30.4), and the annualized event rate among the MTWA-negative patients was 0.3% (95% CI, 0.1–0.5). In contrast, in the "high ICD group" that comprised 2234 patients, the HR was only 1.6 (95% CI, 1.2–2.1), and the annualized event rate among MTWA-negative patients was elevated to 5.4% (95% CI, 4.1–6.7). Therefore these data suggest that MTWA predominantly predicts lethal ventricular tachyarrhythmic events, whereas more benign and often non-sustained ventricular tachyarrhythmias that trigger ICD therapy are not as well predicted. This observation may be attributed to the fact that many "appropriate" device therapies treat arrhythmias that would have self-terminated or that ICDs may induce arrhythmias that they subsequently treat.[71,72]

Microvolt T-Wave Alternans Testing in Patients With Depressed or Preserved Left Ventricular Function

At present, LVEF ≤0.35 is used as the sole risk stratifier for selection of patients for primary preventive ICD therapy. However, a number of studies have demonstrated that only a small percentage of patients who undergo primary prevention ICD implantation actually receive appropriate device therapy during long-term follow-up. Moreover, the majority of all sudden deaths occur in patients with preserved LV function. Some of these issues were recently addressed in a careful patient-level data–based analysis from five prospective studies of MTWA testing in patients with no history of previous ventricular tachyarrhythmias,[73] with further subclassification of patients based on LVEF. Among patients with LVEF ≤35%, annual sudden death event (presumably sustained VT, resuscitated arrest, and sudden death) rates for positive, negative, and indeterminate groups were 4.0%, 0.9%, and 4.6%, respectively. The incidence of sudden death was

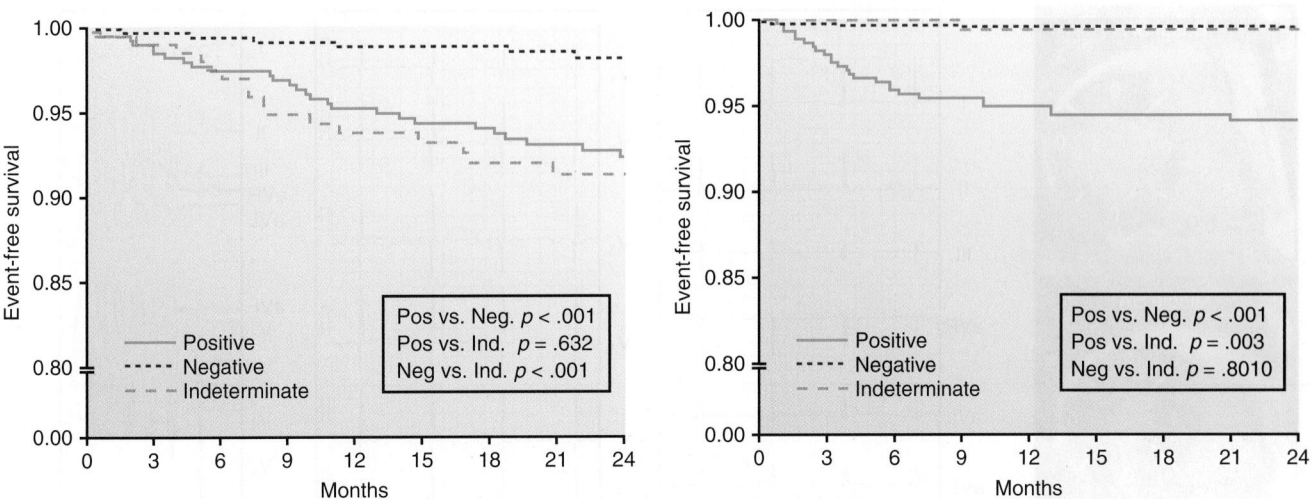

FIGURE 69.4 *Left,* Kaplan-Meier event-free survival (arrhythmic mortality/sudden death) stratified for microvolt T-wave alternans (*MTWA*) test results among patients with a left ventricular ejection fraction (LVEF) ≤0.35. Patients testing positive or indeterminate have significantly lower event-free survival than those testing MTWA negative, with no significant difference between positive or indeterminate patients. *Ind,* Indeterminate; *Neg,* negative; *Pos,* positive. *Right,* Kaplan-Meier event-free survival among patients with LVEF >0.35. Event-free survival is lower in patients with a positive MTWA test than in those from either the negative or indeterminate groups. (From Merchant FM, Ikeda T, Pedretti RFE, et al. Clinical utility of microvolt T-wave alternans testing in identifying patients at high or low risk of sudden cardiac death. *Heart Rhythm.* 2012;9:1256-1264.)

significantly lower among patients with a negative MTWA test than among those with either a positive or indeterminate test (*p* < .001 for both) (Fig. 69.4). There was no significant difference in sudden death event–free survival between positive and indeterminate MTWA test results of patients with LVEF ≤35%.

Among patients with LVEF >35%, sudden death annual event rates, stratified by MTWA test results, were positive (3.0%), negative (0.3%), and indeterminate (0.3%). Among patients in this category, the rate of survival free of sudden death was significantly worse for MTWA-positive patients compared with that for either MTWA-negative (*p* < .001) or MTWA-indeterminate (*p* = .003) patients, whereas event-free survival was not significantly different between negative and indeterminate groups with LVEF >35% (*p* = .801) (see Fig. 69.4). There was only one sudden death event among patients with indeterminate MTWA test result and LVEF >35%; therefore event rates were uniformly low regardless of the cause of indeterminacy. This analysis therefore clearly supports the notion that a negative MTWA test result identifies a population of patients at very low risk for sudden death, irrespective of LV function (annual event rate of 0.9% in patients with LVEF ≤35% and annual event rate of 0.3% in patients with LVEF >35%). This finding suggests that patients with a negative MTWA test, even with LVEF ≤35%, are likely to be at sufficiently low arrhythmic risk that they may not benefit from prophylactic ICD therapy.

A second important finding relates to the population of patients with preserved LV function. Even among patients with LVEF >35%, a positive MTWA test identifies a cohort at significantly increased risk for sudden death for whom device therapy may mitigate arrhythmic risk. Finally, the study shows that the risk for sudden death among patients with indeterminate MTWA results is highly dependent on LV function. Among patients with LVEF ≤35%, an indeterminate MTWA test—particularly among those with an indeterminate test result because of excessive ectopy or inadequate heart rate increase—predicts an increased risk for sudden death similar to that of a positive

test. In contrast, an indeterminate MTWA test in patients with LVEF >35% does not predict an increased risk and therefore these patients should not be grouped with patients who test positive.

Multivariable Risk Prediction Models

Structural heart diseases result in complex anatomical and EP substrates within the myocardium. Similarly, important and complex interactions exist between disease-related risk factors for sudden death. This complexity implies that the risk for arrhythmic death in an individual patient may not be accurately determinable by assessing a single risk factor (i.e., LVEF). Hence, multivariable models that consider different anatomical and EP risk markers may be more helpful in clinical practice. Over the last few years, several such combinations have been tested and are briefly summarized here.

For instance, Sakamoto and associates tested the hypothesis that late gadolinium enhancement (LGE) of cardiac magnetic resonance imaging as a measure of myocardial scar may be linked to MTWA in patients with hypertrophic cardiomyopathy.[74] There was indeed a significant correlation between maximum TWA voltage and scar burden, expressed as total LGE score (r, .59; *p* < .001) (Fig. 69.5). Furthermore, total LGE score and maximum TWA voltage were significantly greater in patients who had spontaneous VT. Of note, LVEF did not distinguish between patients with or without VT. These observations point to a potentially important role of imaging combined with EP measures, but confirmation in future studies is warranted.

The concept of incorporating MTWA into multivariable risk models has been tested in various studies. Exner and associates demonstrated the usefulness of combining MTWA and heart rate turbulence measurements a number of years ago (discussed previously).[50] These observations have recently been

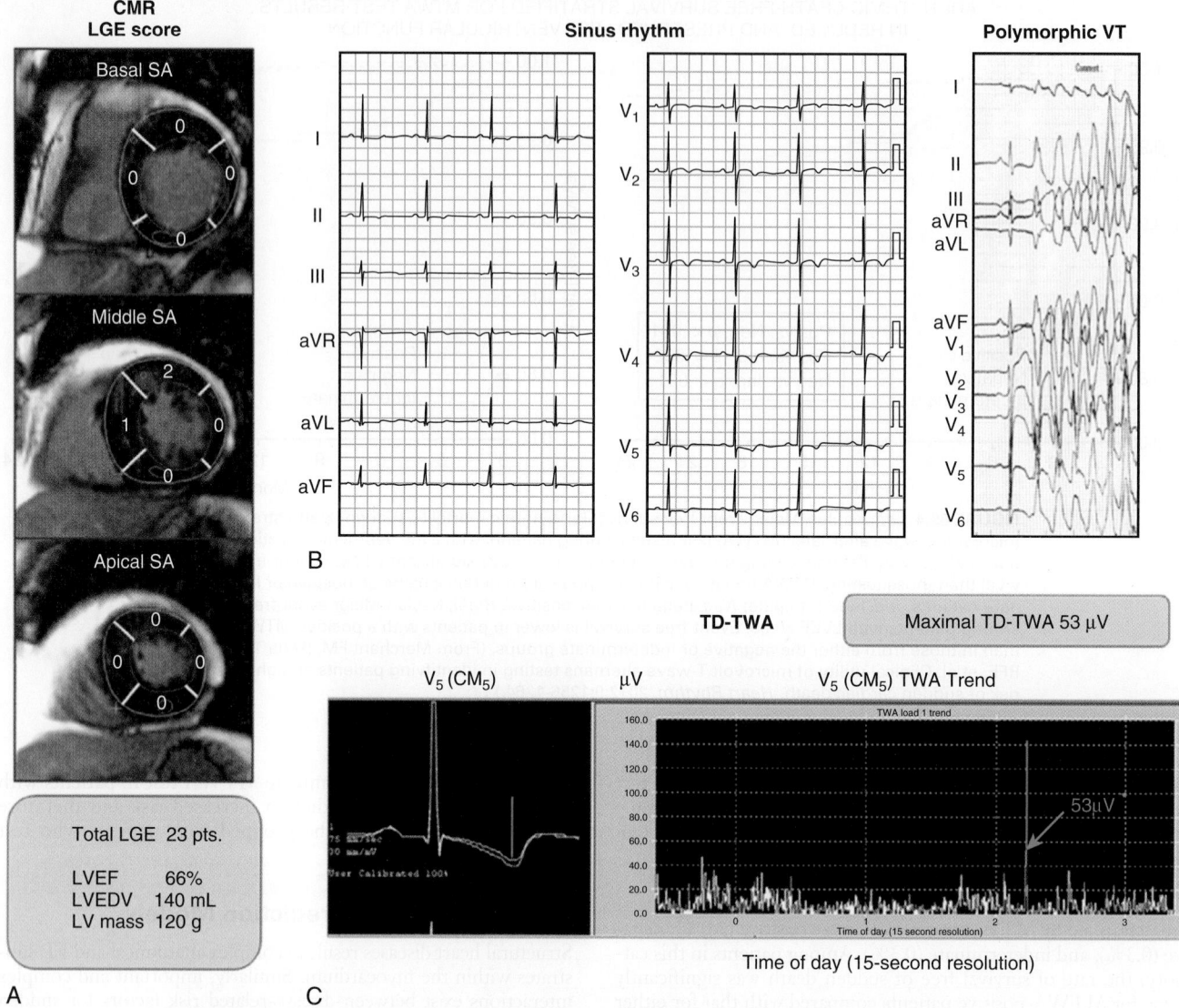

FIGURE 69.5 Cardiac magnetic resonance (*CMR*) images showing significant myocardial scarring (late gadolinium enhancement [*LGE*] score, 23 points [A]) in a patient with polymorphic ventricular tachycardia (*VT*) (B) and a maximum microvolt T-wave alternans (*TWA*) voltage of 87 μV (C). *LV*, Left ventricle; *LVEF*, left ventricular ejection fraction; *LVEDV*, left ventricular end diastolic volume; *SA*, sinoatrial; *TD*, time domain; *VF*, ventricular fibrillation. (Modified from Sakamoto N, Sato N, Oikawa K, et al. Late gadolinium enhancement of cardiac magnetic resonance imaging indicates abnormalities of time-domain T-wave alternans in hypertrophic cardiomyopathy with ventricular tachycardia. *Heart Rhythm.* 2015;12:1747-1755.)

confirmed by Hoshida and colleagues.[66] MTWA as an EP and LVEF marker and the presence of coronary disease as markers of the anatomical substrate have also been carefully evaluated[41] on the basis of an analysis of patient-level data from six studies that comprised 3355 patients. Two-thirds of patients served as a derivation cohort for establishing a multivariable model, which was subsequently retested in 1113 individuals (validation cohort). A model that incorporated LVEF, coronary artery disease, and MTWA status provided optimal sudden death prediction. In both derivation and validation cohorts, the model clearly outperformed the sole analysis of LVEF (c-index of model, .817; Fig. 69.6). Finally, a study of 3609 consecutive patients, referred for routine exercise testing, showed that the prognostic value of such tests was enhanced by the combined analysis of exercise capacity, heart rate recovery, and MTWA determined by the MMA method.[63]

Current Role of Microvolt T-Wave Alternans Testing

There has been significant progress both in understanding cellular and subcellular mechanisms of repolarization alternans and its translation into clinical practice. Despite the sound evidence that MTWA—alone but even more so in combination with other risk markers—may yield a better identification of patients at particularly high risk for arrhythmogenic death, MTWA assessment has still not evolved as a routine method for risk stratification purposes. To convince those who remain uncertain about the prognostic power of MTWA testing in patients with various cardiac diseases, prospective interventional trials based on MTWA test results are urgently warranted. At least one such trial is currently ongoing (NCT 00673842) in which patients will be randomized to ICD or medical therapy based on results of MTWA testing.

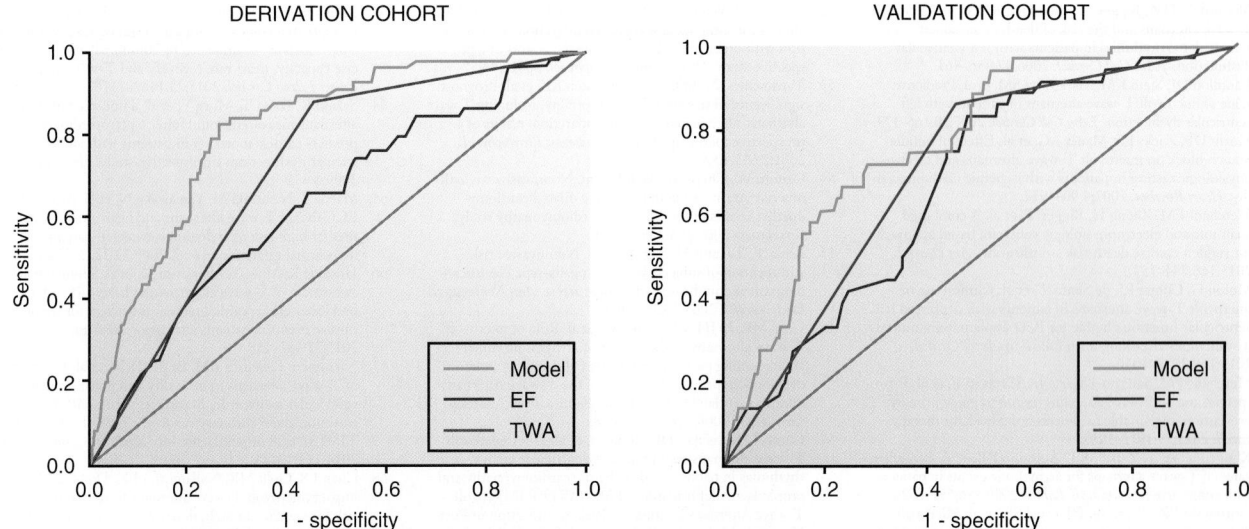

FIGURE 69.6 Receiver operator curves for the prediction of sudden death based on a multivariable model that incorporates coronary disease, left ventricular ejection fraction (*LVEF*), and microvolt T-wave alternans (*MTWA*) versus either LVEF or MTWA as single variables. For patients in the derivation cohort, the concordance index (c-index) is 0.817 and significantly superior to single risk markers ($p < .001$). In the validation cohort, the c-index of the model is 0.774 and better than LVEF ($p < .02$) and nonsignificantly greater than that for MTWA (0.729). (Modified from Merchant FM, Zheng H, Bigger T, et al. A combined anatomic and electrophysiologic substrate based approach for sudden cardiac death risk stratification. *Am Heart J.* 2013;166:744-752.)

Acknowledgment

This chapter is dedicated to the memory of David S. Rosenbaum, MD.

REFERENCES

1. Hering HE. Das Wesen des Herzalternans. *Muenchner Med Wochenschr.* 1908;4:1417–1421.
2. Lewis T. Notes upon alternation of the heart. *Q J Med.* 1910;4:141–144.
3. Kalter HH, Schwartz ML. Electrical alternans. *N Y State J Med.* 1948;1:1164–1166.
4. Schwartz PJ, Malliani A. Electrical alternation of the T wave: clinical and experimental evidence of its relationship with the sympathetic nervous system and with the long-QT syndrome. *Am Heart J.* 1975;89:45–50.
5. Adam DR, Powell AO, Gordon H, et al. Ventricular fibrillation and fluctuations in the magnitude of the repolarization vector. *IEEE Comp Cardiol.* 1982;241–244.
6. Smith JM, Clancy EA, Valeri CR, et al. Electrical alternans and cardiac electrical instability. *Circulation.* 1988;77:110–121.
7. Nearing B, Huang HA, Verrier RL. Dynamic tracking of cardiac vulnerability by complex demodulation of the T wave. *Science.* 1991;252:437–440.
8. Shusterman V, Goldberg A, London B. Upsurge in T-wave alternans and nonalternating repolarization instability precedes spontaneous initiation of ventricular tachyarrhythmias in humans. *Circulation.* 2006;113:2880–2887.
9. Sandhu RK, Constantini O, Cummings JE, et al. Intracardiac alternans compared to surface T-wave alternans as a predictor of ventricular arrhythmias in humans. *Heart Rhythm.* 2008;5:1003–1008.
10. Pastore JM, Girouard SD, Laurita KR, et al. Mechanism linking T-wave alternans to the genesis of cardiac fibrillation. *Circulation.* 1999;99:1385–1394.
11. Pastore JM, Rosenbaum DS. Role of structural barriers in the mechanism of alternans-induced reentry. *Circ Res.* 2000;87:1157–1163.
12. Walker ML, Rosenbaum DS. Repolarization alternans: implications for the mechanism and prevention of sudden cardiac death. *Cardiovasc Res.* 2003;57:599–614.
13. Wilson LD, Rosenbaum DS. Mechanisms of arrhythmogenic discordant cardiac alternans. *Europace.* 2007;9:77–82.
14. Merchant FM, Armoundas AA. Role of substrate and triggers in the genesis of cardiac alternans, from myocyte to the whole heart. *Circulation.* 2012;125:539–549.
15. Shimizu W, Antzelevitch C. Cellular and ionic basis for T-wave alternans under long-QT conditions. *Circulation.* 1999;99:1499–1507.

16. Hüser J, Wang YG, Sheehan KA, et al. Functional coupling between glycolysis and excitation-contraction coupling underlies alternans in cat heart cells. *J Physiol (London).* 2000;524:795–806.
17. Goldhaber JI, Xie LH, Duong T, et al. Action potential duration restitution and alternans in rabbit ventricular myocytes: the key role of intracellular calcium cycling. *Circ Res.* 2005;96:459–466.
18. Merchant FM, Sayadi O, Moazzami K, et al. T-wave alternans as an arrhythmic risk stratifier: state of the art. *Curr Cardiol Rep.* 2013;15:398.
19. Bloomfield DM, Hohnloser SH, Cohen RJ. Interpretation and classification of microvolt T wave alternans tests. *J Cardiovasc Electrophysiol.* 2002;13:502–512.
20. Verrier RL, Klingenheben T, Malik M, et al. Microvolt T-wave alternans. *J Am Coll Cardiol.* 2011;58:1309–1324.
21. Nieminen T, Lehtimäki T, Viik J, et al. T-wave alternans predicts mortality in a population undergoing a clinically indicated exercise test. *Eur Heart J.* 2007;28:2332–2337.
22. Slawnych MP, Nieminen T, Kahonen M, et al. Post-exercise assessment of cardiac repolarization alternans in patients with coronary artery disease using the modified moving average method. *J Am Coll Cardiol.* 2009;53:1130–1137.
23. Verrier RL, Nearing BD, La Rovere MT, et al. Ambulatory electrocardiogram-based tracking of T wave alternans in post-myocardial infarction patients to assess risk of cardiac arrest or arrhythmic death. *J Cardiovasc Electrophysiol.* 2003;14:705–711.
24. Stein PK, Sanghavi D, Domitrovich PP, et al. Ambulatory ECG-based T-wave alternans predicts sudden cardiac death in high-risk post-MI patients with left ventricular dysfunction in the EPHESUS study. *J Cardiovasc Electrophysiol.* 2008;19:1037–1042.
25. Kaufman E, Bloomfield D, Steinman R, et al. "Indeterminate" microvolt T-wave alternans tests predict high risk of death or sustained ventricular arrhythmias in patients with left ventricular dysfunction. *J Am Coll Cardiol.* 2006;48:1399–1404.
26. Rosenbaum DS, Jackson LE, Smith JM, et al. Electrical alternans and vulnerability to ventricular arrhythmias. *N Engl J Med.* 1994;330:235–241.
27. Gold MR, Bloomfield DM, Anderson KP, et al. A comparison of T-wave alternans, signal averaged electrocardiography and programmed ventricular stimulation

for arrhythmia risk stratification. *J Am Coll Cardiol.* 2000;36:2247–2253.
28. Costantini O, Hohnloser SH, Kirk MM, et al. The ABCD (Alternans Before Cardioverter Defibrillator) trial: strategies using T-wave alternans to improve efficiency of sudden cardiac death prevention. *J Am Coll Cardiol.* 2009;53:471–479.
29. Kitamura H, Ohnishi Y, Okajima K, et al. Onset heart rate of microvolt-level T-wave alternans provides clinical and prognostic value in nonischemic dilated cardiomyopathy. *J Am Coll Cardiol.* 2002;39:295–300.
30. Hohnloser SH, Klingenheben T, Bloomfield D, et al. Usefulness of microvolt T-wave alternans for prediction of ventricular tachyarrhythmic events in patients with dilated cardiomyopathy: results from a prospective observational study. *J Am Coll Cardiol.* 2003;41:2220–2224.
31. Chow T, Kereiakes DJ, Bartone C, et al. Microvolt T-wave alternans identifies patients with ischemic cardiomyopathy who benefit from implantable cardioverter-defibrillator therapy. *J Am Coll Cardiol.* 2007;49:50–58.
32. Salerno-Uriarte JA, De Ferrari GM, Klersy C, et al. Prognostic value of T-wave alternans in patients with heart failure due to nonischemic cardiomyopathy: results of the ALPHA study. *J Am Coll Cardiol.* 2007;50:1896–1904.
33. Chow T, Kereiakes DJ, Bartone C, et al. Prognostic utility of microvolt T-wave alternans in risk stratification of patients with ischemic cardiomyopathy. *J Am Coll Cardiol.* 2006;47:1820–1827.
34. Chan PS, Kereiakes DJ, Bartone C, et al. Usefulness of microvolt T-wave alternans to predict outcomes in patients with ischemic cardiomyopathy beyond one year. *Am J Cardiol.* 2008;102:280–284.
35. Rashba EJ, Osman AF, MacMurdy K, et al. Influence of QRS duration on the prognostic value of T wave alternans. *J Cardiovasc Electrophysiol.* 2002;13:770–775.
36. Alexander ME, Cecchin F, Huang KP, et al. Microvolt T-wave alternans with exercise in pediatrics and congenital heart disease: limitations and predictive value. *Pacing Clin Electrophysiol.* 2006;29:733–741.
37. Rashba EJ, Osman AF, Macmurdy K, et al. Enhanced detection of arrhythmia vulnerability using T wave alternans, left ventricular ejection fraction, and programmed ventricular stimulation: a prospective study in subjects with chronic ischemic heart disease. *J Cardiovasc Electrophysiol.* 2004;15:170–176.

38. Bloomfield DM, Bigger JT, Steinman RC, et al. Microvolt T-wave alternans and the risk of death or sustained ventricular arrhythmias in patients with left ventricular dysfunction. *J Am Coll Cardiol.* 2006;47:456–463.

39. Cantillon DJ, Stein KM, Markowitz SM, et al. Predictive value of microvolt T-wave alternans in patients with left ventricular dysfunction. *J Am Coll Cardiol.* 2007;50:166–173.

40. Morin DP, Zacks ES, Mauer AC, et al. Effect of bundle branch block on microvolt T-wave alternans and electrophysiologic testing in patients with ischemic cardiomyopathy. *Heart Rhythm.* 2007;4:904–912.

41. Merchant FM, Zheng H, Bigger T, et al. A combined anatomic and electrophysiologic substrate based approach for sudden cardiac death risk stratification. *Am Heart J.* 2013;166:744–752.

42. Molon G, Cohen RJ, de Santo T, et al. Clinical use of microvolt T-wave alternans in patients with depressed left ventricular function eligible for ICD implantation: mortality outcomes after long term follow up. *Int J Cardiol.* 2013;168:3038–3040.

43. Merchant FM, Salerno-Uriarte JA, Caravati F, et al. Prospective use of T-wave alternans testing to guide primary prevention implantable cardioverter defibrillator therapy. *Circ J.* 2015;79:1912–1919.

44. Klingenheben T, Zabel M, D'Agostino RB, et al. Predictive value of T-wave alternans for arrhythmic events in patients with congestive heart failure. *Lancet.* 2000;356:651–652.

45. Gorodeski EZ, Cantillon DJ, Goel SS, et al. Microvolt T-wave alternans, peak oxygen consumption, and outcome in patients with severely impaired left ventricular systolic function. *J Heart Lung Transplant.* 2009;28:689–696.

46. Ikeda T, Sakata T, Takami M, et al. Combined assessment of T-wave alternans and late potentials used to predict arrhythmic events after myocardial infarction. *J Am Coll Cardiol.* 2000;35:722–730.

47. Ikeda T, Saito H, Tanno K, et al. T-wave alternans as a predictor for sudden cardiac death after myocardial infarction. *Am J Cardiol.* 2002;89:79–82.

48. Bloomfield D, Steinman R, Namerow P, et al. Microvolt T-wave alternans distinguishes between patients likely and patients not likely to benefit from implanted cardiac defibrillator therapy. *Circulation.* 2004;110:1885–1889.

49. Ikeda T, Yoshino H, Sugi K, et al. Predictive value of microvolt T-wave alternans for sudden cardiac death in patients with preserved cardiac function after acute myocardial infarction. *J Am Coll Cardiol.* 2006;48:2268–2274.

50. Exner DV, Kavanagh KM, Slawnych MP, et al. Noninvasive risk assessment early after a myocardial infarction the REFINE study. *J Am Coll Cardiol.* 2007;50:2275–2284.

51. Rashba EJ, Osman AF, MacMurdy K, et al. Exercise is superior to pacing for T wave alternans measurement in subjects with chronic coronary artery disease and left ventricular dysfunction. *J Cardiovasc Electrophysiol.* 2002;13:845–850.

52. Schwab JO, Weber S, Schmitt H, et al. Incidence of T wave alternation after acute myocardial infarction and correlation with other prognostic parameters: results of a prospective study. *Pacing Clin Electrophysiol.* 2001;24:957–961.

53. Tapanainen JM, Still AM, Airaksinen KE, et al. Prognostic significance of risk stratifiers of mortality, including T wave alternans, after acute myocardial infarction: results of a prospective follow-up study. *J Cardiovasc Electrophysiol.* 2001;2:645–652.

54. Grimm W, Christ M, Bach J, et al. Noninvasive arrhythmia risk stratification in idiopathic dilated cardiomyopathy: results of the Marburg cardiomyopathy study. *Circulation.* 2003;108:2883–2891.

55. Ikeda T, Takami M, Sugi K, et al. Noninvasive risk stratification of subjects with a Brugada-type electrocardiogram and no history of cardiac arrest. *Ann Noninvasive Electrocardiol.* 2005;10:396–403.

56. Gold MR, Ip JH, Costantini O, et al. Role of microvolt T-wave alternans in assessment of arrhythmia vulnerability among patients with heart failure and systolic dysfunction: primary results from the T-wave Alternans Sudden Cardiac Death in Heart Failure Trial substudy. *Circulation.* 2008;118:2022–2028.

57. Chow T, Kereiakes DJ, Onufer J, et al. Does microvolt T-wave alternans testing predict ventricular tachyarrhythmias in patients with ischemic cardiomyopathy and prophylactic defibrillators? The MASTER (Microvolt T-wave Alternans Testing for Risk Stratification of Post-Myocardial Infarction Patients) trial. *J Am Coll Cardiol.* 2008;52:1607–1615.

58. Huikuri HV, Raatikainen MJ, Moerch-Joergensen R, et al. Prediction of fatal or near-fatal cardiac arrhythmia events in patients with depressed left ventricular function after an acute myocardial infarction. *Eur Heart J.* 2009;30:689–698.

59. Leino J, Minkkinen M, Nieminen T, et al. Combined assessment of heart rate recovery and T-wave alternans during routine exercise testing improves prediction of total and cardiovascular mortality: the Finnish Cardiovascular Study. *Heart Rhythm.* 2009;6:1765–1771.

60. Stein PK, Sanghavi D, Sotoodehnia N, et al. Association of Holter-based measures including T-wave alternans with risk of sudden cardiac death in the community-dwelling elderly: the Cardiovascular Health Study. *J Electrocardiol.* 2010;43:251–259.

61. Minkkinen M, Kahonen M, Viik J, et al. Enhanced predictive power of quantitative TWA during routine exercise testing in the Finnish Cardiovascular Study. *J Cardiovasc Electrophysiol.* 2009;20:408–415.

62. Leino J, Verrier RL, Minkkinen M, et al. Importance of regional specificity of T-wave alternans in assessing risk for cardiovascular mortality and sudden cardiac death during routine exercise testing. *Heart Rhythm.* 2011;8:385–390.

63. Minkkinen M, Nieminen T, Verrier RL, et al. Prognostic capacity of a clinically indicated exercise test for cardiovascular mortality is enhanced by combined analysis of exercise capacity, heart rate recovery and T-wave alternans. *Europ J Prev Cardiol.* 2015;22:1162–1170.

64. Sakaki K, Ikeda T, Miwa Y, et al. Time-domain T-wave alternans measured from Holter electrocardiograms predicts cardiac mortality in patients with left ventricular dysfunction: a prospective study. *Heart Rhythm.* 2009;6:332–337.

65. Maeda S, Nishizaki M, Yamawake N, et al. Ambulatory ECG-based T-wave alternans and heart rate turbulence predict high risk of arrhythmic events in patients with old myocardial infarction. *Circ J.* 2009;73:2223–2228.

66. Hoshida K, Miwa Y, Myjakoshi M, et al. Simultaneous assessment of T-wave alternans and heart rate turbulence on Holter electrocardiograms as predictors for serious cardiac events in patients after myocardial infarction. *Circ J.* 2013;77:432–438.

67. Nieminen T, Scirica BM, Pegler JRM, et al. Relation of T-wave alternans to mortality and nonsustained ventricular tachycardia in patients with non-ST-segment elevation acute coronary syndrome from the MERLIN-TIMI 36 trial of ranolazine versus placebo. *Am J Cardiol.* 2014;114:17–23.

68. Chan PS, Gold MR, Nallamothu BK. Do beta-blockers impact microvolt T-wave alternans testing in patients at risk for ventricular arrhythmias? A meta-analysis. *J Cardiovasc Electrophysiol.* 2010;21:1009–1014.

69. Hohnloser SH, Ikeda T, Cohen RJ. Evidence regarding clinical use of microvolt T-wave alternans. *Heart Rhythm.* 2009;6:S36–S44.

70. Hohnloser SH, Ikeda T, Bloomfield DM, et al. T-wave alternans negative coronary patients with low ejection fraction and benefit from defibrillator implantation. *Lancet.* 2003;362:125–126.

71. Ellenbogen KA, Levine JH, Berger RD, et al. Are implantable cardioverter defibrillator shocks a surrogate for sudden cardiac death in patients with nonischemic cardiomyopathy? *Circulation.* 2006;113:776–782.

72. Germano JJ, Reynolds M, Essebag V, et al. Frequency and causes of implantable cardioverter-defibrillator therapies: is device therapy proarrhythmic? *Am J Cardiol.* 2006;97:1255–1261.

73. Merchant FM, Ikeda T, Pedretti RFE, et al. Clinical utility of microvolt T-wave alternans testing in identifying patients at high or low risk of sudden cardiac death. *Heart Rhythm.* 2012;9:1256–1264.

74. Sakamoto N, Sato N, Oikawa K, et al. Late gadolinium enhancement of cardiac magnetic resonance imaging indicates abnormalities of time-domain T-wave alternans in hypertrophic cardiomyopathy with ventricular tachycardia. *Heart Rhythm.* 2015;12:1747–1755.

70 Noninvasive Electrocardiographic Imaging of Arrhythmogenic Substrates and Ventricular Arrhythmias in Patients

Yoram Rudy

Ventricular arrhythmia continues to be a major cause of death and disability; however, our understanding of excitation patterns in the human heart during ventricular tachycardia (VT) and ventricular fibrillation (VF) is limited. Such knowledge is essential for improved diagnosis, prevention, and treatment of VT and for prevention of its deterioration to VF. Acquiring this knowledge requires detailed mapping of activation during the arrhythmia, which is often dynamically changing (polymorphic) and unstable. In other words, mapping should be conducted simultaneously over the ventricles with sufficient spatial resolution and continuously in time over a sufficiently long duration. These requirements cannot be met with current invasive, catheter-based mapping techniques. Electrocardiographic imaging (ECGI; also called *electrocardiographic mapping*) is a noninvasive method for electroanatomical mapping developed previously.[1,2] ECGI provides continuous panoramic maps of activation and repolarization on the epicardial surface of the heart. With ECGI, dynamically changing VT can be mapped to capture its evolution in time, and mapping is conducted under real-world conditions, without the need for sedation, surgery, or other invasive procedures. This chapter provides examples of VT patterns mapped noninvasively with ECGI. In many instances, VT is related to abnormal electrophysiological (EP) substrate associated with anatomical scars or with abnormal EP function in the absence of structural heart disease. This chapter provides examples of both through ECGI of the EP substrates of an anatomical scar in patients after myocardial infarction; furthermore, it provides examples of abnormal EP function in patients with hereditary arrhythmic disorders (the long QT and Brugada syndromes). This chapter describes previously published studies[3–8] and covers ventricular substrates and arrhythmias. ECGI applications to atrial arrhythmias have been described elsewhere.[9,10]

Electrocardiographic Imaging and Its Validation

The ECGI methodology has been detailed elsewhere.[1,11] Briefly, body surface electrocardiographic (ECG) potentials are acquired at 1-ms intervals using 250 electrodes mounted in a vest or in strips. The electrode positions and the patient-specific epicardial geometry are simultaneously imaged using an ECG-gated computed tomography (CT) or magnetic resonance imaging (MRI) scan.

ECGI algorithms combine the body surface ECG data and CT anatomical data to noninvasively construct potential maps, electrograms (EGMs), activation sequences (isochrone maps), and repolarization patterns on the epicardial surface of the heart. For imaging EP substrate associated with scar, EGM magnitude maps, EGM deflection maps, and EP scar maps (ESMs) were constructed during sinus rhythm (SR). Low-voltage regions and very-low-voltage regions associated with scar were defined by EGMs with amplitude less than 30% and 15% of the maximum in a given patient's heart, respectively. The "electrical scar" (abnormal EP substrate associated with a scar) was defined as a region with EGMs characterized by low-voltage and multiple deflections (fractionation); it was presented visually as ESM. For studies of repolarization, local recovery time (RT) and activation-recovery interval (ARI; a surrogate for local action potential duration) were determined from each EGM, and epicardial maps of RT and ARI were constructed.

ECGI was validated extensively for reconstruction of EGMs, activation sequences, and repolarization. Validation studies were conducted in animal experiments, in a human-shaped torso-tank containing a beating dog heart placed in the correct anatomical position for humans, and in patients undergoing open-heart surgery and invasive catheter mapping. A summary of the validation studies is provided in the appendix at the end of this chapter.

Electrophysiological Substrate of Post–Myocardial Infarction Scar[5,6]

The substrate of post–myocardial infarction scars is characterized by altered electrical properties because of cellular EP remodeling and structural remodeling that involves gap junction changes and regional fibrosis. As a consequence, conduction of excitation through a heterogeneous scar is slow and discontinuous, a property that is reflected in low voltages and fractionation of local EGMs and delayed local activation (i.e., late potentials).[12–17] These properties have provided the basis for substrate-based ablation strategies in the treatment of VT.[18] ECGI can reconstruct the EGM characteristics associated with a scar, as demonstrated in canine experiments.[19,20]

Fig. 70.1 presents a representative example of an ECGI-reconstructed EP scar substrate in a patient with an anterior myocardial infarction scar (data from 24 patients[5]). The electrical scar reconstructed by ECGI is compared with the anatomical scar imaged with delayed enhanced MRI.[21–23] Fig. 70.1A depicts the electrical scar in *red*. The top image is based on the low-voltage criterion alone; the bottom image combines the low-voltage and EGM fractionation criteria to define the electrical scar. Note that incorporation of the EGM fractionation criterion eliminates the basal part of the scar, which is a low-voltage region in the ECGI potential map and a bright region (suggesting an anatomical scar) in the MRI. It is likely that these characteristics of the ECGI and MRI reflect fat tissue in this region rather than a true scar; the fractionation criterion can remove this artifact. Fig. 70.1B and C shows representative EGMs from the electrical scar region (*red*) and from regions outside the scar (*blue*). The scar EGMs are of low amplitude and long

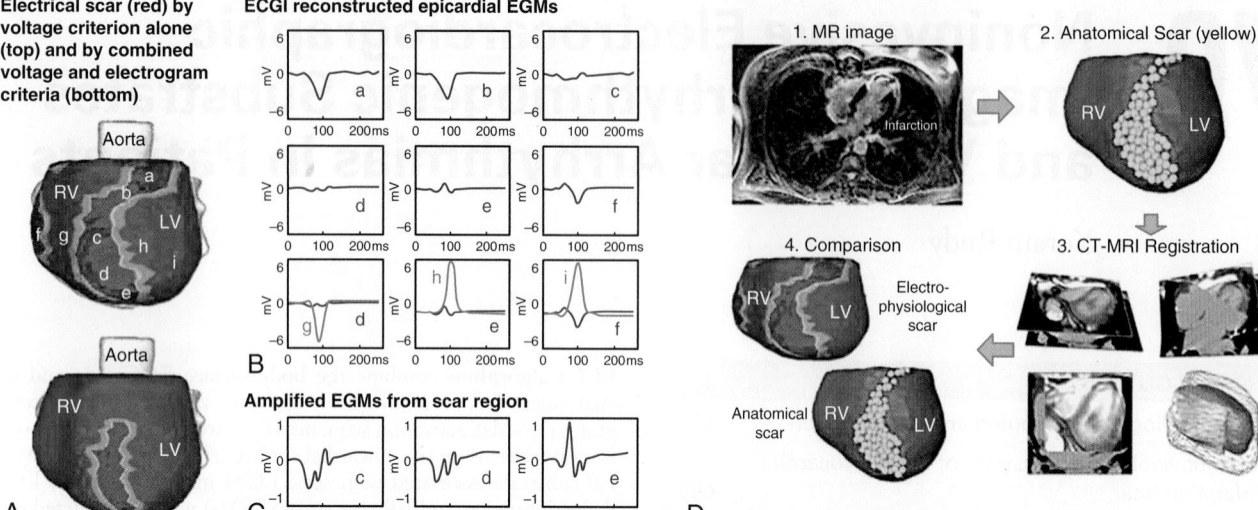

Electrical scar (red) by voltage criterion alone (top) and by combined voltage and electrogram criteria (bottom)

ECGI reconstructed epicardial EGMs

Amplified EGMs from scar region

FIGURE 70.1 Electrocardiographic imaging (*ECGI*)–derived electrical scar and magnetic resonance–imaged anatomical scar. (A) Electrical scar (*red*) in the left anterior oblique view. The *top image* is based on the criterion of low-magnitude electrograms (*EGMs*) only. The *bottom image* adds the criterion of fractionated EGMs. (B) Representative EGMs from the scar region (*red, a–f*) and from outside the scar (*blue, g-i*). EGMs in *a, b,* and *f* are low in amplitude, whereas in *c, d,* and *e* they are both low amplitude and fractionated. The *bottom row* shows EGMs in *d–i* together, on the same scale, to emphasize the magnitude differences. (C) EGMs in *c, d,* and *e* are on an amplified scale to better show fractionation. (D) Comparing electrical scar to anatomical scar. Electrical scar (*red*), based on the low-voltage criterion, is constructed by ECGI. Anatomical scar is imaged with delayed enhanced magnetic resonance imaging (*MRI*) (*1*) and annotated on the epicardial surface of the imaged heart (*2; yellow dots*). Coregistration of the magnetic resonance and the ECGI computed tomography (*CT*) images (*3*) is used to reconstruct the anatomical scar map and to compare (*4*) the electrical scar (*red*) with the anatomical scar (*yellow*). *LV,* Left ventricle; *RV,* right ventricle. (From Cuculich PS, Zhang J, Wang Y, et al. The electrophysiologic cardiac ventricular substrate in patients after myocardial infarction: noninvasive characterization with electrocardiographic imaging. *J Am Col Cardiol.* 2011;58:1893-1902.)

duration, and they exhibit multiple deflections (i.e., fractionation). Fig. 70.1D compares the ECGI-reconstructed electrical scar (*red*) to the anatomical scar imaged with delayed enhanced MRI.

Fig. 70.2 provides a second example of an ECGI scar reconstruction. The ESM is apical, consistent with the magnetic resonance–imaged anatomical scar. The presence of the electrical scar influences the pattern of epicardial activation (AI map). Earliest epicardial breakthrough location (*asterisk*) is normal, but the activation wavefront encounters a line of block along the inferior and apical aspect of the scar. Consequently, left ventricular (LV) activation is from base to apex (*arrows*), with the region near the apical scar activating last. ECGI also reconstructed late potentials that in almost all cases (94%) were within the electrical scar.

Fig. 70.3 shows three examples of scar EGMs with late potentials, reflecting delayed activation in the scar region during SR.

Electrophysiological Substrate of Hereditary Disorders

Congenital Long QT Syndrome[7]

The congenital long QT syndrome (LQTS) is an inherited cardiac channelopathy that causes syncope and sudden death in young adults with structurally normal hearts.[24] Arrhythmias in these patients are classified as polymorphic VT (torsades de pointes). Genetic and molecular studies in humans have provided insight into the molecular basis of the disease.[25,26] However, the arrhythmogenic substrate in the heart of LQTS patients has not been fully defined. ECGI was used to map the EP substrate in 25 patients with genotype-positive, phenotype-positive LQTS.[7] Based on identified mutations, there were nine LQT1 patients (loss-of-function mutations in KCNQ1),

nine LQT2 (loss-of-function mutations in KCNH2), five LQT3 (gain-of-function mutations in SCN5A), and two LQT5 (loss-of-function mutations in KCNE1). Epicardial activation during SR (not shown here; see Vijayakumar and colleagues[7]) was normal in all LQTS patients, with normal right ventricular (RV) breakthrough, uniform spread of the excitation wavefront, and latest activation in the LV base. The total ventricular activation time was around 50 ms, comparable to that in the normal control group (47 ± 9 ms). In contrast to activation, repolarization in LQTS patients of all types was very abnormal, with significant prolongation of the action potential on the ventricular epicardium compared with normal control. This prolongation was spatially heterogeneous, introducing regions with steep dispersion of repolarization. Fig. 70.4 shows representative ARI maps for control, LQT1, LQT2, and LQT3 in superior and inferior views. The ARI values were corrected for heart rate. For example, the maximum ARI in LQT3 was 430 ms compared with only 320 ms in control. Importantly, the regional, heterogeneous prolongation of ARI introduced steep gradients of repolarization in LQTS (shown by *black arrows* in Fig. 70.4). The mean ARI gradient was 92 ± 18 ms/cm in LQT1, 117 ± 29 ms/cm in LQT2, and 129 ± 4 in LQT3, compared with only 2.0 ± 2.0 ms/cm in control ($p < .05$). The presence of regions with steep dispersion of repolarization creates a substrate for asymmetrical conduction (unidirectional block) and reentrant arrhythmias, not detectable by the surface ECG. Interestingly, the location and magnitude of the steep gradient varied between patients, even among patients with the same genetic mutation. However, repolarization gradients were steeper in symptomatic patients (12 patients, gradient = 130 ± 27 ms/cm) than in asymptomatic patients (13 patients, gradient = 98 ± 19 ms/cm), suggesting a possible role for ECGI in arrhythmic risk stratification in LQTS.[27]

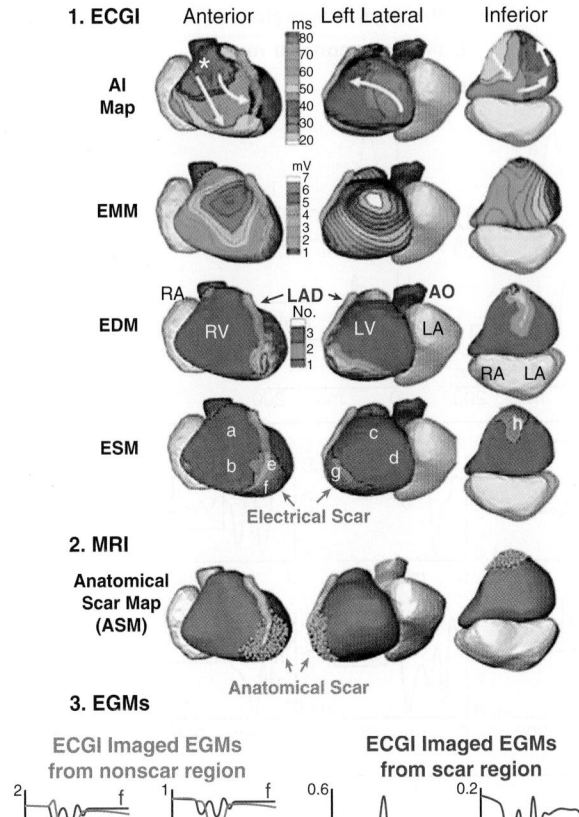

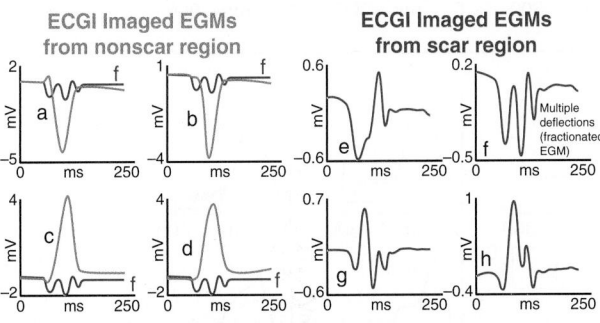

FIGURE 70.2 Electrical and anatomical apical scar. *1,* The *top row* shows epicardial activation (AI map) during sinus rhythm. Earliest activation is at the *asterisk,* and latest activation is in the left ventricular apex *(dark blue)* near the scar. The *bottom row* shows the electrical scar map *(ESM),* with the electrical scar depicted in *red. 2,* Delayed enhanced magnetic resonance–imaged anatomical scar *(gold dots)* corresponds to the electrical scar in 1 (ESM, *red*). *3,* Electrocardiographic imaging *(ECGI)*–reconstructed electrograms *(EGMs)* from the nonscar region *(blue)* and from within the scar *(red).* Note the large magnitude, single-deflection characteristics of nonscar EGMs and the small magnitude and fractionation of scar EGMs. The scar EGMs are amplified on the *right* to show fractionation. *AO,* Aorta; *EDM,* electrogram deflection map; *EMM,* electrogram magnitude map; *LA,* left atrium; *LAD,* left anterior descending coronary artery; *MRI,* magnetic resonance image; *RA,* right atrium. (From Cuculich PS, Zhang J, Wang Y, et al. The electrophysiologic cardiac ventricular substrate in patients after myocardial infarction: noninvasive characterization with electrocardiographic imaging. *J Am Col Cardiol.* 2011;58:1893-1902.)

Brugada Syndrome[8]

Brugada syndrome (BrS) is a highly arrhythmogenic inherited cardiac disorder associated with an increased incidence of sudden death; it affects predominantly men in their forties.[28,29] It presents on the ECG as an atypical right bundle branch block (RBBB) pattern and ST-segment elevation (STE) in leads V1 through V3. BrS is considered a primary electrical cardiac disease, because no structural abnormalities are detected by conventional imaging. About 30% of BrS patients test positive for mutations in SCN5A and loss of sodium channel function.

As with LQTS, the arrhythmogenic substrate of BrS in the intact human heart has not been well defined, with two leading hypotheses about mechanisms that underlie the phenotype: (1) the abnormal repolarization hypothesis (based on a canine wedge preparation)[30] and (2) the abnormal conduction hypothesis.[31-33] Understanding the cardiac EP substrate that determines the phenotype requires high-resolution panoramic EP mapping of the ventricles, which cannot be achieved with invasive catheter mapping. To this end, ECGI was applied in 25 BrS patients to reconstruct epicardial EGMs and to map ventricular activation and repolarization during SR.[8]

In BrS patients, the exclusive localization of the abnormal substrate to the RV outflow tract (RVOT) was a striking difference from LQTS patients, where location of the abnormal substrate (steep repolarization gradients) was highly variable. EGMs in the RVOT (but nowhere else) were characterized by ST-segment elevation and inverted T-wave morphology and by low amplitude and presence of multiple deflections (fractionation); examples can be found in Zhang et al.[8] Fig. 70.5A shows activation isochrone maps from three BrS patients, with a normal control map provided for reference *(left panel).* The BrS patients had normal RV epicardial breakthrough *(asterisk)* on the RV free wall (indicative of a normally functioning conduction system) and normal activation of most of the RV, but delayed activation of the RVOT *(blue),* which was last to activate (in normal hearts, latest activation is in the lateral LV base). The mean time needed for activation of the RVOT among all patients was 36 ± 16 ms, while the RV free wall took 16 ± 3 ms to activate, and the entire RV (including the RVOT) took 40 ± 14 ms, indicating that most of the RV activation duration was taken by slow spread of excitation in the RVOT.

Fig. 70.5B and C shows representative maps of repolarization from the same three patients, together with normal repolarization maps for reference *(left column).* Fig. 70.5B displays ARI maps that reflect local repolarization (local action potential duration), independent of the activation sequence; Fig. 70.5C displays RT maps that are determined by both local repolarization and the activation sequence. That the patterns of the ARI maps and RT maps are similar indicates that local repolarization is the major determinant of the repolarization pattern. ARI prolongation (318 ± 32 vs. 241 ± 27 ms in control) and RT prolongation (381 ± 30 vs. 311 ± 34 ms in control) were observed primarily in the RVOT, but extended somewhat into adjacent regions. This localized prolongation caused steep gradients of ARI and RT at the RVOT-RV free wall or RVOT-LV free wall borders (see *red arrows* in Fig. 70.5B and C).

The results shown in Fig. 70.5 demonstrate the presence of both abnormal repolarization and abnormal conduction in the RVOT of BrS patients. Abnormal repolarization during phase 1 of the action potential can generate potential gradients that give rise to the STE in the EGMs and ECG. Slow discontinuous conduction in the RVOT can give rise to the fractionation and low voltage of RVOT EGMs. Increasing the heart rate should have an effect on both. It diminishes the phase 1 notch of the action potential (by not providing sufficient time for cardiac transient outward potassium current [Ito] recovery from inactivation between beats) and thereby reduces potential gradients and STE. It also compromises conduction further by reducing sodium current (I_{Na}) availability. To examine these hypotheses, we performed ECGI in six BrS patients during increased heart rate through exercise or isoprenaline administration (mean increase from 71 to 133 beats/min). As expected, STE was reduced and fractionation was increased with an increase in heart rate (see Zhang et al.[8]), providing additional supporting evidence for the coexistence of conduction and repolarization abnormalities in the RVOT substrate of BrS patients.

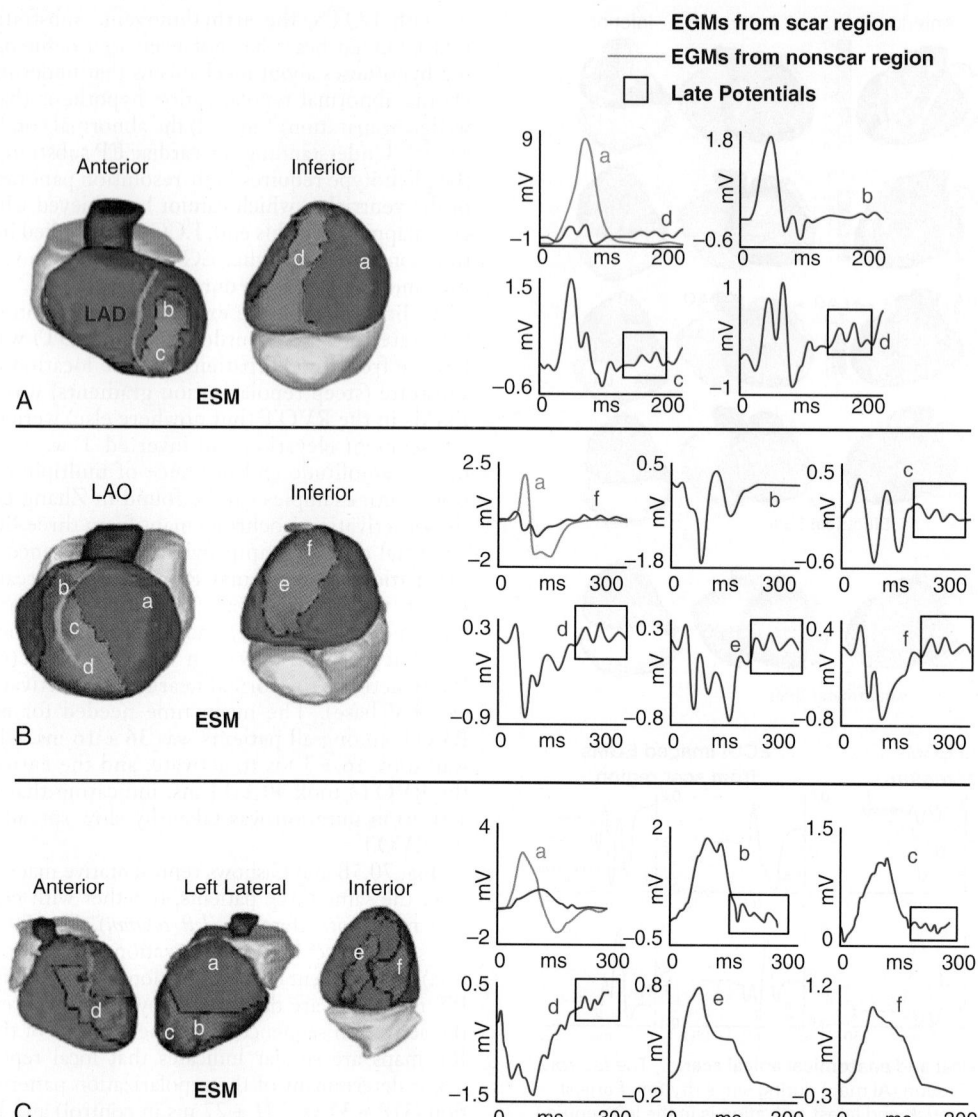

FIGURE 70.3 Late potentials within an electrical scar: examples from three patients. (A) Inferoseptal scar. (B) Anteroapical scar. (C) Complex anterior, apical, and inferior infarction. For each patient, an electrophysiological scar map (*ESM*) is presented on the left and selected electrograms (*EGMs*) on the right (scar EGMs in *red*). *Letters* indicate EGM location. Delayed deflections (late potentials) are highlighted by a box. *LAD,* left anterior descending coronary artery; *LAO,* left anterior oblique. (From Cuculich PS, Zhang J, Wang Y, et al. The electrophysiologic cardiac ventricular substrate in patients after myocardial infarction: noninvasive characterization with electrocardiographic imaging. *J Am Col Cardiol.* 2011;58:1893-1902.)

As stated above, the ECG in BrS is of atypical RBBB pattern. It can be challenging to differentiate BrS from non-BrS right bundle branch (RBB).[34] However, accurate diagnosis is of utmost clinical importance because BrS and RBBB differ greatly in their arrhythmogenicity, with BrS being highly arrhythmogenic. We examined whether ECGI can distinguish between these abnormalities by mapping six non-BrS patients with RBBB, without structural heart disease, during SR. The results (see Zhang et al.[8]) established the ability of ECGI to do so, based on the following: (1) EGMs with the BrS morphology and with low voltage and fractionation were not found in RBBB; (2) normal RV epicardial breakthrough was observed in BrS, reflecting a functioning RBB, but not in RBBB where RBB is defective; (3) delayed activation in BrS was confined to the RVOT, while in RBBB the delay occurred across

the septum; and (4) repolarization abnormalities were not present in RBBB. We concluded that noninvasive substrate mapping with ECGI can assist with a BrS-RBBB differential diagnosis in the clinical setting and with the clinical diagnosis of BrS when it is masked by an RBBB pattern on the body surface ECG.

Examples of Ventricular Tachycardia[3,4]

ECGI was performed in 25 patients with symptomatic VT or premature ventricular contractions who also underwent invasive, catheter-based EP study (EPS). In patients with spontaneous abnormal ventricular rhythms (18 patients), ECGI was performed before EPS. In other patients, ECGI was performed during EPS, where the rhythm was induced.

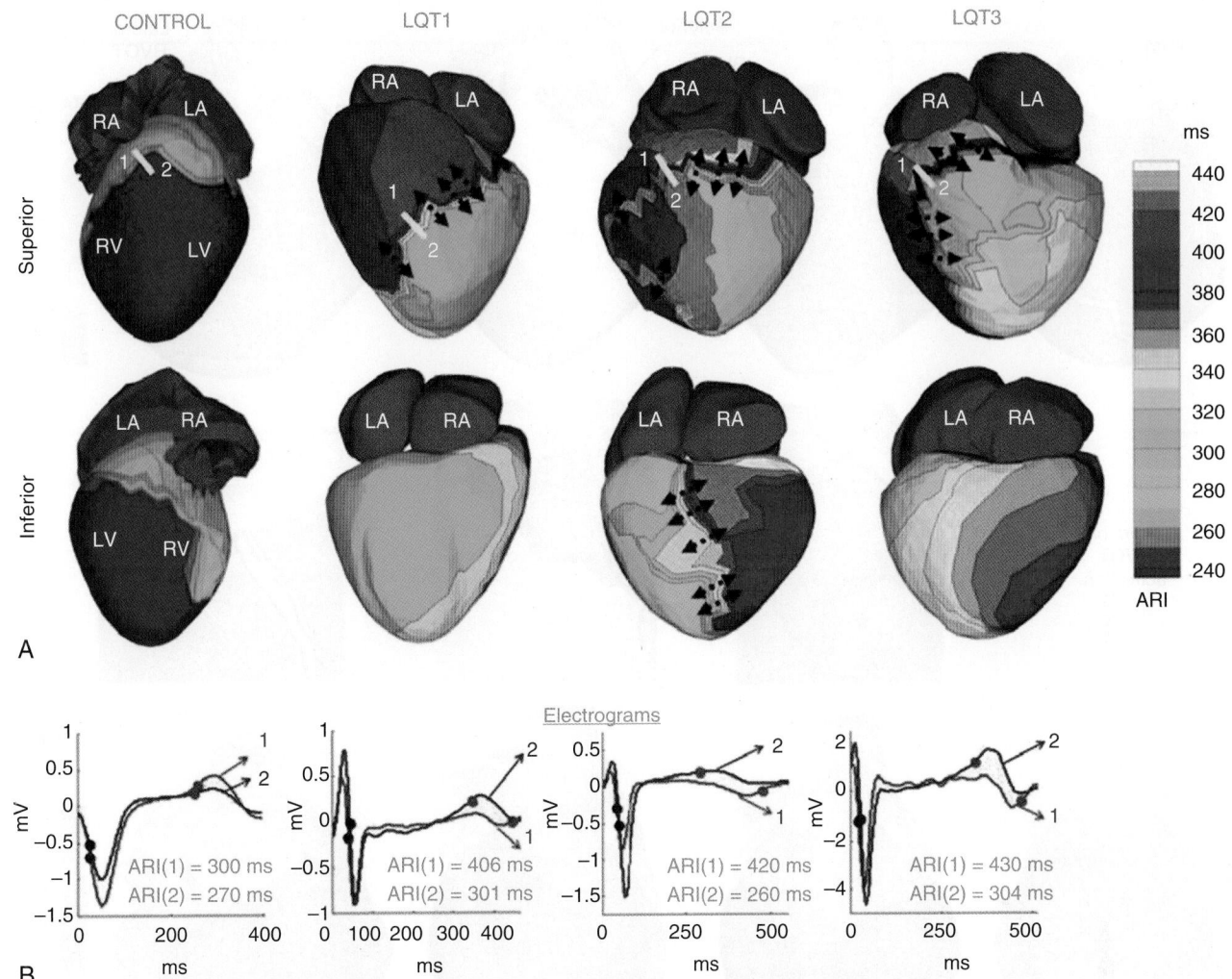

FIGURE 70.4 Activation-recovery interval (*ARI*) maps in long QT syndrome (LQTS) patients. (A) Maps are shown in superior (*top*) and inferior (*bottom*) views. ARI (surrogate for local action potential duration) values were abnormally long (*magenta* and *white* regions) in all three LQTS patients compared with control. The maximum ARI value in LQTS was 450 ms compared with only 340 ms (*green* in the *left column*) in control. The localized prolongation of ARI resulted in steep repolarization gradients in all three LQTS types (*black arrows*). The ARI gradients were two orders of magnitude steeper than control (control, 7 ms/cm; LQT1, 104 ms/cm; LQT2, 146 ms/cm; and LQT3, 140 ms/cm). (B) The electrocardiographic imaging–reconstructed EGMs from locations 1 and 2 in the maps (*top row*) depict the time instances of local activation time (AT; *black dots*) and recovery time (RT; *pink dots*). The corresponding ARI values (RT–AT) are indicated below. *LA*, left atrium; *LV*, left ventricle; *RA*, right atrium; *RV*, right ventricle. (From Vijayakumar R, Silva JN, Desouza KA, et al. Electrophysiologic substrate in congenital long QT syndrome: noninvasive mapping with electrocardiographic imaging (ECGI). *Circulation*. 2014;130:1936-1943.)

Patterns of Ventricular Tachycardia[3]

Based on the invasive EPS, VT in 18 patients was judged to be focal. In all 18 patients, ECGI isochrone maps showed a radial spread of excitation from the site of origin. An example from a patient with nonischemic cardiomyopathy is provided in Fig. 70.6. ECGI was applied in the EP laboratory during induction of VT by programmed electrical stimulation. Fig. 70.6A shows isochrones during baseline pacing (cycle length = 600 ms) from a catheter in the RV apex (marked by a *plus sign*). There is a line of block (*thick black line*) in the lateral LV that is circumvented by the excitation wavefront. Premature pacing (Fig. 70.6B; S1–S2 interval = 280 ms) functionally extends the line

of block (see Fig. 70.6B), forcing the wavefront to make a longer arc around this line and activate a more inferior region of the LV last (indicated by a *minus sign*). The first VT beat is shown in Fig. 70.6C; it originates from the location (marked by an *asterisk*) of latest activation by the S2 premature paced beat in Fig. 70.6B, suggesting that triggered activity is the mechanism of initiation of this focal VT. Note that the local EGM at the site of VT initiation has a pure Q-wave morphology, indicating an epicardial origin. An ECGI movie (Video 70.1) is provided to show the dynamic progression in this case.

Five patients had reentrant VT, as determined during invasive EPS. Noninvasive ECGI maps showed high-curvature rotational

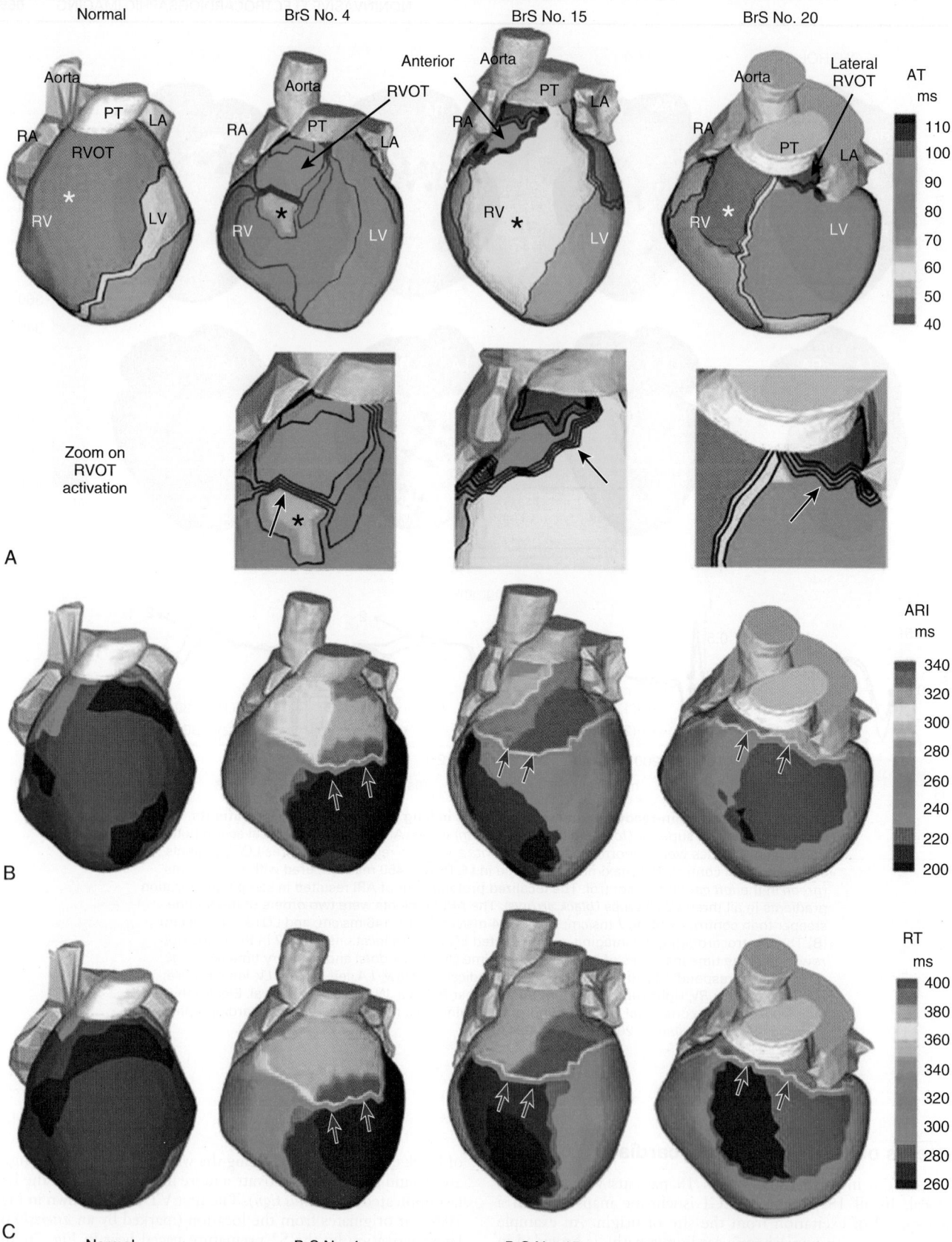

FIGURE 70.5 Activation and repolarization in Brugada syndrome (*BrS*) patients during sinus rhythm. (A) Activation times isochrone maps (*AT*). *Insets,* Zoom on the right ventricular outflow tract (*RVOT*). (B) Activation-recovery interval maps (*ARI*). (C) Recovery time (RT) maps. Epicardial breakthroughs are indicated by *asterisks.* Isochrones are depicted in *thin black lines. Black arrows* in the RVOT zoom maps of (A) point to slow conduction indicated by crowded isochronal lines. *Red arrows* in (B) and (C) point to regions with steep repolarization gradients. *LA,* Left atrium; *LV,* left ventricle; *PT,* pulmonary trunk; *RA,* right atrium; *RV,* right ventricle. (From Zhang J, Sacher F, Hoffmayer K, et al. The cardiac electrophysiologic substrate underlying the ECG phenotype and electrogram abnormalities in Brugada syndrome patients. *Circulation.* 2015;131:1950-1959.)

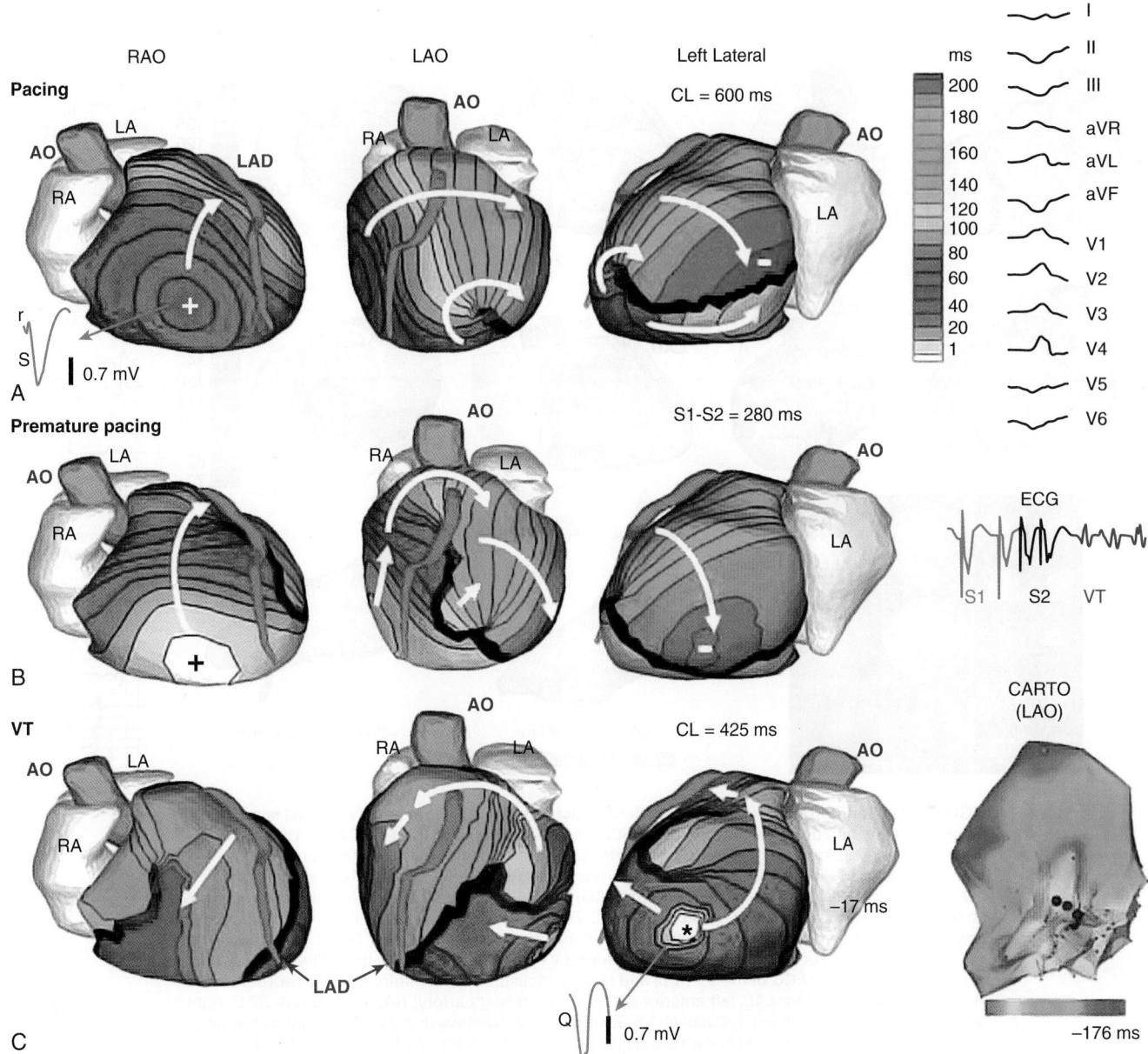

FIGURE 70.6 Focal ventricular tachycardia (*VT*) induced by programmed electrical stimulation. (A) Epicardial activation isochrones during the drive train (*S1*). Site of earliest epicardial activation is marked by a *plus sign* (right anterior oblique [*RAO*] view) and corresponds to the position of the underlying endocardial pacing electrode. The reconstructed electrogram (EGM) at this site (*blue, blue arrow*) is rS in morphology, consistent with endocardial pacing. *White arrows* show direction of wavefront propagation. The *thick black line* (left lateral and left anterior oblique [*LAO*] views) indicates conduction block; the wavefront pivots around this line and terminates at the site indicated by a *minus sign*. Twelve-lead surface electrocardiogram (*ECG*) during VT is shown on the right. (B) Premature paced beat (*S2*). Note functional extension of the line of block. There is some fusion with a transseptal front (*small white arrow*). Trace on the right shows ECG (one lead) during S1 (*blue*), S2 (*black*), and VT (*red*). (C) Epicardial activation during VT. Activation starts from the *asterisk* (the site of latest activation of the previous S2 beat) and spreads radially from this site. EGM at this site is pure Q wave, indicating epicardial origin. Invasive endocardial activation map during VT (*CARTO*) is shown on the *right* (*red* is early). See Video 70.1 for dynamic representation of this VT. *AO,* Aorta; *CL,* cycle length; *LA,* left atrium; *LAD,* left anterior descending coronary artery; *RA,* right atrium. (From Wang Y, Cuculich PS, Zhang J, et al. Noninvasive electroanatomic mapping of human ventricular arrhythmias with electrocardiographic imaging. *Sci Transl Med.* 2011;3:98ra84.)

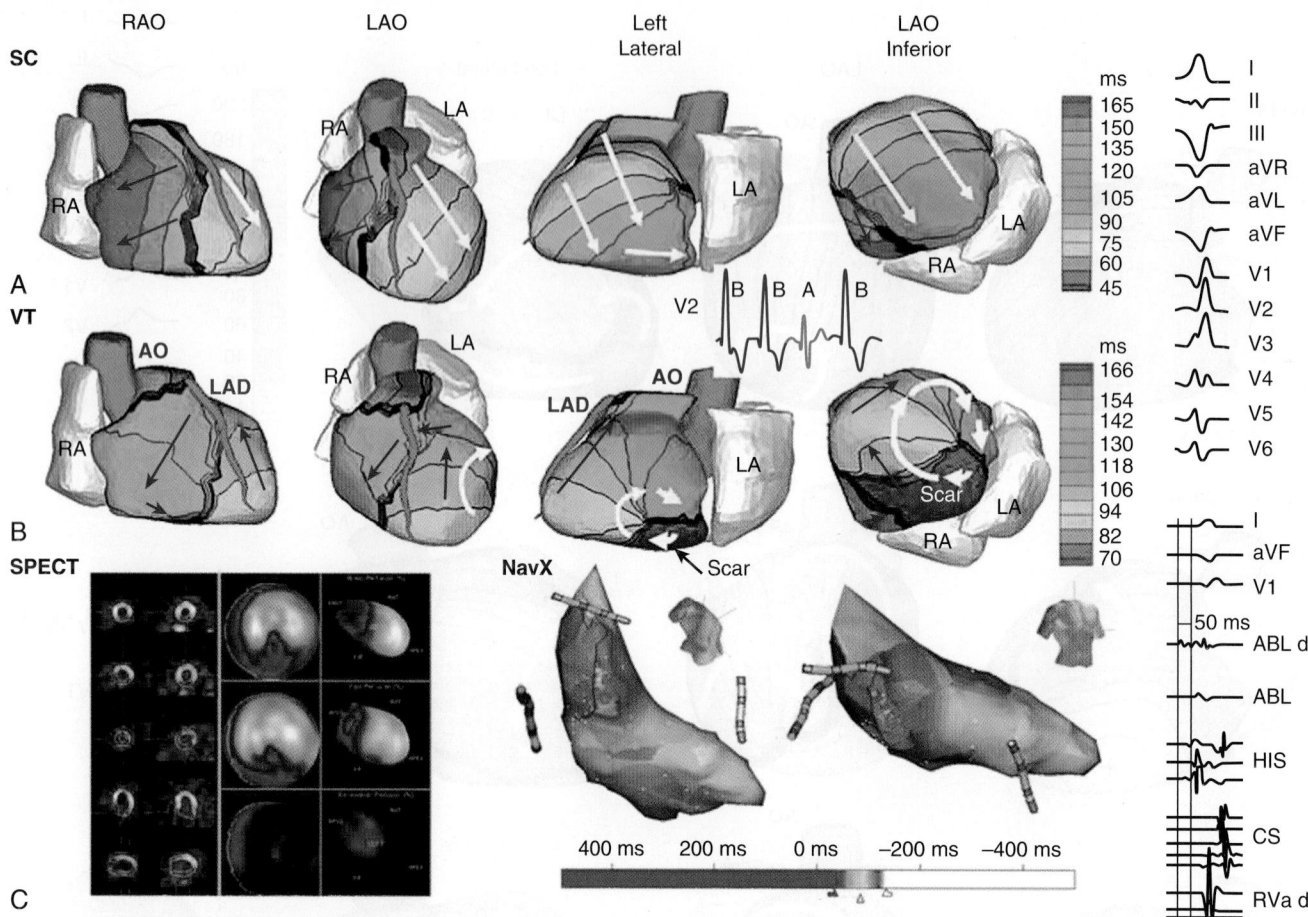

FIGURE 70.7 Spontaneous reentrant ventricular tachycardia (VT) from an inferobasal scar. (A) Epicardial activation during a sinus capture (SC) beat. (B) Activation during a VT beat. *White arrows* (left lateral and left anterior oblique [LAO] inferior views) show a clockwise lateral reentry loop related to the scar. *Pink arrows* show the wavefront propagating counterclockwise into the right ventricle. The *inset* shows electrocardiograph (ECG) lead V2 with two VT beats (*red, B*) interrupted by an SC beat (*blue, A*), followed by another VT beat. Video 70.2 shows this sequence. (C) *Left,* Single-photon emission computed tomography (SPECT) showing an inferobasal scar (*blue*). *Right,* Invasive catheter map (*NavX*) of endocardial activation during VT (*red* is early; *blue* is late). The *right column* shows 12-lead surface ECG of the VT (*top*) and signals measured by the ablation catheter (*bottom*). *AO,* Aorta; *LA,* left atrium; *LAD,* left anterior descending coronary artery; *RA,* right atrium; *RAO,* right anterior oblique. (From Wang Y, Cuculich PS, Zhang J, et al. Noninvasive electroanatomic mapping of human ventricular arrhythmias with electrocardiographic imaging. *Sci Transl Med.* 2011;3:98ra84.)

wavefronts, with the excitation wave returning to its site of initiation. This pattern was consistent in all five patients and related to a ventricular scar in all cases. An example is provided in Fig. 70.7 and Video 70.2. This patient had an extensive inferoseptal scar from a prior inferior wall myocardial infarction (see single-photon emission computed tomography image in Fig. 70.7C). He had a slow, hemodynamically tolerated VT, occasionally interrupted by sinus capture (SC) beats (see ECG lead V2 in inset to Fig. 70.7B; *red [B]* is a VT beat; *blue [A]* is an SC beat). Earliest activation of the VT beat (see Fig. 70.7B) is near the scar border in the inferior basal septum (*red* in the left anterior oblique and left lateral views). The main reentrant wavefront propagates clockwise with a high curvature (*white arrows*) and completes the beat by reentering the area of earliest activation. Immediately before the VT beat, presystolic activation is detected near the inferior scar border where the VT beat begins (the "exit site"; see Video 70.2). A second wavefront (*pink arrows*) propagates toward the base, where it turns slowly counterclockwise into the RV. It then propagates to the inferior base, back toward the scar. In the inferobasal septal region, ECGI-reconstructed EGMs were of low amplitude and highly fractionated,

which is consistent with a scar substrate. Invasive catheter mapping confirmed this ECGI finding. EPS during the VT confirmed its inferior septal origin and, using entrainment criteria, its reentrant mechanism. Ablation in this region terminated the VT.

Initiation and Termination of Spontaneous Ventricular Tachycardia[4]

Fig. 70.8A shows ECGI activation maps during initiation, continuation, and termination by antitachycardia pacing (ATP) of spontaneous VT in a 40-year-old patient with nonischemic cardiomyopathy (LV ejection fraction of 35%). The patient experienced 248 VT episodes terminated by ATP over 14 days. Video 70.3 shows a continuous ECGI reconstruction of one such event, as summarized in Fig. 70.8. The left column of Fig. 70.8A shows the activation pattern during SR, before spontaneous initiation of VT. The following beat (VT1) originated from the inferolateral base (marked by an *asterisk*) and triggered the VT. The next VT beat (VT2) and all VT beats that followed (VT2 to VT14) were monomorphic and started from

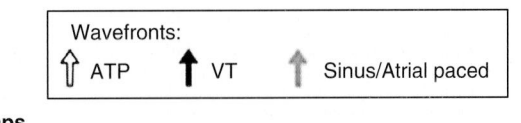

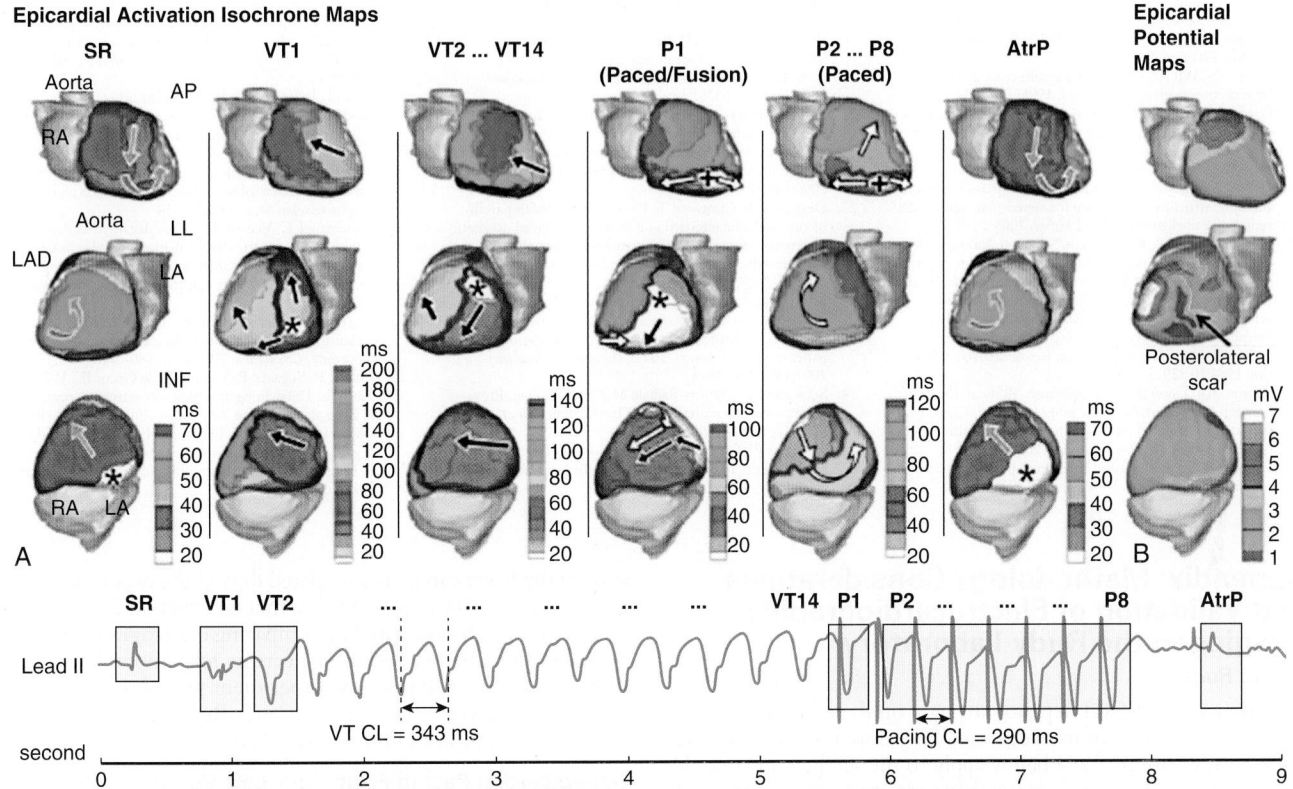

FIGURE 70.8 Continuous electrocardiographic imaging mapping of spontaneous ventricular tachycardia (*VT*) initiation, continuation, and termination by antitachycardia pacing. (A) Epicardial activation maps. (B) Epicardial potential maps showing a posterolateral region of low voltages (scar). See text for a detailed description and Video 70.3 for a dynamic representation of the entire episode. *Asterisk,* Earliest activation site; *plus sign,* right ventricular pacing site; *AP,* anteroposterior view; *AtrP,* atrial paced beat; *CL,* cycle length; *INF,* inferior view; *LA,* left atrium; *LAD,* left anterior descending coronary artery; *LL,* left lateral view; *P,* ventricular paced beat; *RA,* right atrium; *SR,* sinus rhythm. (From Zhang J, Desouza KA, Cuculich PS, et al. Continuous ECGI mapping of spontaneous VT initiation, continuation and termination with antitachycardia pacing. *Heart Rhythm.* 2013;10:1244-1245.)

a different location (superolateral LV base, *asterisk*) versus the triggering beat (VT1). VT cycle length was 343 ms. ATP pacing started after 14 beats of VT, at 85% of the VT cycle length. The first ATP beat (P1) consisted of fusion between the VT wavefront (starting from *) and the wavefront generated by the RV pacing (originated at +). The following ATP beats (P2–P8) successfully captured the myocardium, and the activation was due to RV pacing alone (wavefront originating and spreading from + exclusively). The beat following the last ATP beat (atrial paced [AtrP]; right column of Fig. 70.8A) was identical to the SR beat before VT onset. Video 70.3 provides dynamic images of the entire event. Fig. 70.8B shows ECGI epicardial potential maps with low voltages in the posterolateral region (*dark blue*), indicating the presence of scar where VT originated.

Acknowledgments

This chapter is dedicated to Professor Bruno Taccardi—a scientist, a gentleman, and a dear friend. He will be greatly missed. I am indebted to my outstanding graduate students, research and clinical fellows, and many collaborators who helped make ECGI a reality of great research and clinical promise. Studies presented in this chapter were supported by grants R01-HL33343 and R01-HL49054 from the National Institutes of Health–National Heart, Lung, and Blood Institute.

Y. Rudy co-chairs the scientific advisory board and receives royalties from CardioInsight Technologies (CIT). CIT does not support any research conducted in Y. Rudy's laboratory, including that presented here.

REFERENCES

1. Ramanathan C, Ghanem RN, Jia P, et al. Electrocardiographic imaging (ECGI): a noninvasive imaging modality for cardiac electrophysiology and arrhythmia. *Nat Med.* 2004;10:422–428.
2. Ramanathan C, Jia P, Ghanem RN, et al. Activation and repolarization of the normal human heart under complete physiological conditions. *Proc Natl Acad Sci U S A.* 2006;103:6309–6314.
3. Wang Y, Cuculich PS, Zhang J, et al. Noninvasive electroanatomic mapping of human ventricular arrhythmias with electrocardiographic imaging. *Sci Transl Med.* 2011;3:98ra84.

4. Zhang J, Desouza KA, Cuculich PS, et al. Continuous ECGI mapping of spontaneous VT initiation, continuation and termination with antitachycardia pacing. *Heart Rhythm.* 2013;10:1244–1245.
5. Cuculich PS, Zhang J, Wang Y, et al. The electrophysiologic cardiac ventricular substrate in patients after myocardial infarction: noninvasive characterization with electrocardiographic imaging. *J Am Coll Cardiol.* 2011;58:1893–1902.
6. Rudy Y. Noninvasive electrocardiographic imaging of arrhythmogenic substrates in humans. *Circ Res.* 2013;112:863–874.

7. Vijayakumar R, Silva JN, Desouza KA, et al. Electrophysiologic substrate in congenital long QT syndrome: noninvasive mapping with electrocardiographic imaging (ECGI). *Circulation.* 2014;130:1936–1943.
8. Zhang J, Sacher F, Hoffmayer K, et al. The cardiac electrophysiologic substrate underlying the ECG phenotype and electrogram abnormalities in Brugada syndrome patients. *Circulation.* 2015;131:1950–1959.
9. Cuculich PS, Wang Y, Lindsay BD, et al. Noninvasive characterization of epicardial activation in humans with diverse atrial fibrillation patterns. *Circulation.* 2010;122:1364–1372.

10. Rudy Y, Cuculich PS, Vijayakumar R. Advances in non-invasive electrocardiographic imaging (ECGI): examples of atrial arrhythmias. In: Shenasa M, ed. *Cardiac Mapping*. 4th ed. Oxford, UK: Wiley-Blackwell; 2013.

11. Rudy Y, Ramanathan C, Ghosh S. Noninvasive electrocardiographic imaging (ECGI): methodology and excitation of the normal human heart. In: Zipes DP, Jalife J, eds. *Cardiac Electrophysiology: from Cell to Bedside*. 5th ed. Philadelphia: Elsevier; 2009:467–472.

12. Peters NS, Wit AL. Myocardial architecture and ventricular arrhythmogenesis. *Circulation*. 1998;97:1746–1754.

13. Gardner PI, Ursell PC, Fenoglio Jr JJ, et al. Electrophysiologic and anatomic basis for fractionated electrograms recorded from healed myocardial infarcts. *Circulation*. 1985;72:596–611.

14. de Bakker JM, Stein M, van Rijen HV. Three-dimensional anatomic structure as substrate for ventricular tachycardia/ventricular fibrillation. *Heart Rhythm*. 2005;2:777–779.

15. Klein H, Karp RB, Kouchoukos NT, et al. Intraoperative electrophysiologic mapping of the ventricles during sinus rhythm in patients with a previous myocardial infarction. Identification of the electrophysiologic substrate of ventricular arrhythmias. *Circulation*. 1982;66:847–853.

16. Josephson ME, Wit AL. Fractionated electrical activity and continuous electrical activity: fact or artifact? *Circulation*. 1984;70:529–532.

17. Simson MB, Untereker WJ, Spielman SR, et al. Relation between late potentials on the body surface and directly recorded fragmented electrograms in patients with ventricular tachycardia. *Am J Cardiol*. 1983;51:105–112.

18. Wilber DJ. Substrate-based ablation of postinfarction ventricular tachycardia. In: Wilber DJ, Packer DL, Stevenson WG, eds. *Catheter Ablation of Cardiac Arrhythmias; Basic Concepts and Clinical Applications*. 3rd ed. Oxford, UK: Blackwell-Futura; 2008:326–339.

19. Burnes JE, Taccardi B, MacLeod RS, et al. Noninvasive electrocardiographic imaging of electrophysiologically abnormal substrate in infarcted hearts. *Circulation*. 2000;101:533–540.

20. Burnes JE, Taccardi B, Ershler P, et al. Noninvasive ECG imaging of substrate and intramural ventricular tachycardia in infarcted hearts. *J Am Coll Cardiol*. 2001;38:2071–2078.

21. Yan AT, Shayne AJ, Brown KA, et al. Characterization of the peri-infarct zone by contrast-enhanced cardiac magnetic resonance imaging is a powerful predictor of post-myocardial infarction mortality. *Circulation*. 2006;114:32–39.

22. Desjardins B, Crawford T, Good E, et al. Infarct architecture and characteristics on delayed enhanced magnetic resonance imaging and electroanatomic mapping in patients with postinfarction ventricular arrhythmia. *Heart Rhythm*. 2009;6:644–651.

23. Schmidt A, Azevedo CF, Cheng A, et al. Infarct tissue heterogeneity by magnetic resonance imaging identifies enhanced cardiac arrhythmia susceptibility in patients with left ventricular dysfunction. *Circulation*. 2007;115:2006–2014.

24. Schwartz PJ, Stramba-Badiale M, Crotti L, et al. Prevalence of the congenital long-QT syndrome. *Circulation*. 2009;120:1761–1767.

25. Schwartz PJ, Crotti L, Insolia R. Long-QT syndrome: from genetics to management. *Circ Arrhythm Electrophysiol*. 2012;5:868–877.

26. Roden DM, Balser JR, George Jr AL, Anderson ME. Cardiac ion channels. *Annu Rev Physiol*. 2002;64:431–475.

27. Priori SG, Schwartz PJ, Napolitano C, et al. Risk stratification in the long-QT syndrome. *N Engl J Med*. 2003;348:1866–1874.

28. Antzelevitch C, Brugada P, Borggrefe M, et al. Brugada syndrome: report of the second consensus conference endorsed by the Heart Rhythm Society and the European Heart Rhythm Association. *Circulation*. 2005;111:659–670.

29. Brugada P, Brugada J. Right bundle branch block, persistent ST segment elevation and sudden cardiac death: a distinct clinical and electrocardiographic syndrome. A multicenter report. *J Am Coll Cardiol*. 1992;20:1391–1396.

30. Antzelevitch C. Cellular basis and mechanisms underlying normal and abnormal myocardial repolarization and arrhythmogenesis. *Ann Med*. 2004;36:5–14.

31. Nademanee K, Veerakul G, Chandanamattha P, et al. Prevention of ventricular fibrillation episodes in Brugada syndrome by catheter ablation over the anterior right ventricular outflow tract epicardium. *Circulation*. 2011;123:1270–1279.

32. Frustaci A, Priori SG, Pieroni M, et al. Cardiac histological substrate in patients with clinical phenotype of Brugada syndrome. *Circulation*. 2005;112:3680–3687.

33. Tukkie R, Sogaard P, Vleugels J, de Groot IK, Wilde AA, Tan HL. Delay in right ventricular activation contributes to Brugada syndrome. *Circulation*. 2004;109:1272–1277.

34. Chiale PA, Garro HA, Fernández PA, Elizari MV. High-degree right bundle branch block obscuring the diagnosis of Brugada electrocardiographic pattern. *Heart Rhythm*. 2012;9:974–976.

Appendix: Methodology Considerations and Validation of Electrocardiographic Imaging in the Rudy Laboratory

Yoram Rudy

The accuracy of ECGI depends strongly on the exact methodology used and details of its execution. Therefore the results of the many studies summarized below apply to the method and details of its application in the *Rudy lab*; they cannot be extrapolated and generalized to other laboratories. Moreover, even for the same general approach (e.g., the Boundary Element Method with Tikhonov Zero Order regularization), results depend on details such as measurement noise, signal conditioning (removal of baseline drift; filtering), values of regularization parameter, accuracy and resolution of segmentation and meshing of the heart and torso surfaces, and more. Consequently, one can evaluate accuracy of the ECGI procedure within the same lab, but comparison between labs and generalization of results is limited. This document summarizes many validation studies of ECGI as implemented and practiced in the *Rudy lab* over many years.

Validation in Torso-Tank Experiments

The torso-tank setup consists of an accurate human-shaped torso, with a beating dog heart placed in the correct anatomical position for a human. It allows for precisely controlled experiments. In these experiments, body-surface potentials and epicardial potentials over the entire heart are simultaneously recorded. The body-surface potentials provide the input for the ECGI reconstruction, and the recorded epicardial potentials provide a "gold standard" for evaluation. It represents accurately the geometrical relationship between the heart and torso surfaces in the human anatomy (the proportion of size between the dog heart and the tank that was molded on the torso of a 10-year-old boy are representative of an adult human). This relationship determines the transfer matrix that is used in the ECGI computations. Recordings were conducted with 256 or 384 body-surface electrodes, 490 or 64 electrodes in a nylon sock placed over the heart, and 184 electrodes on rod tips pushed against the heart.[1,2] Advantages of this experimental setup include the following: (1) there is consistency of the torso volume conductor between measurements and computations (homogeneous in both, so the evaluation of the ECGI computation method is not affected by a volume-conductor inconsistency); (2) epicardial electrodes cover the entire heart; and (3) the heart can be manipulated during the experiment—for example, necrosis was produced so that its effect on ECGI reconstruction could be evaluated by comparing electrograms from the same locations before and after necrosis formation. Also, accessibility of the heart during the experiment provides tight control over electrode contact, placement, etc. Results from the torso-tank experiments are summarized below.

Subepicardial Pacing From Four Left Ventricular Sites and One Right Atrial Site Near the Sinoatrial Node[2]

Single-Site Left Ventricular Pacing. An anterior pacing site was reconstructed 7 mm from the measured site and a posterolateral site within 4 mm of the measured site. Two other sites, between these two extreme ones, were reconstructed 0 mm and 10 mm from the measured pacing sites. Average distance between reconstructed and measured sites was 5 mm (range, 0–10 mm). The reconstructed pacing sites were determined from the reconstructed epicardial potential maps (not isochrones). In this method, the initiation site is determined at the center of a quasielliptical negative potential minimum on the epicardium during early activation (this is based on the properties of wavefront propagation in the anisotropic myocardium). **Two simultaneous pacing sites** 52 mm apart (anterior and posterolateral) were reconstructed 7 mm and 4 mm from the actual locations. Two anterior simultaneous sites were reconstructed at their exact positions. Two posterolateral sites only 17 mm apart were reconstructed with 5 mm and 4 mm errors of position.

Electrograms. Correlation coefficients (CCs) between reconstructed and measured EGMs were greater than 0.9 for 72% of all epicardial electrodes (54% with CC greater than 0.95). Some outliers (only 5% of electrodes) had poor CC, smaller than 0.5.

Isochrones. Regions of earliest and latest activation and those of crowded and sparse isochrones were reproduced correctly. Pacing site locations should be determined from the potential pattern, not from isochrones (greater precision).

Intramural Pacing[3]

Anterior Pacing. Errors in positions of reconstructed pacing sites relative to the corresponding sites in the measured maps, determined from the potential pattern, were 4, 6, 2, and 2 mm (average 3.5 mm) for pacing depths increasing from 0 to 9.6 mm. The reconstructed potential pattern was very similar to the measured, capturing its counterclockwise (CCW) rotation in time as the wavefront propagated into deeper myocardium.

Posterolateral Pacing. Errors in determining pacing sites were 6, 6, 4 and 9 mm (average 6.25 mm) for pacing depths of 0, 3.2, 6.4 and 9.6 mm. The reconstructed potential captured correctly the CCW rotation and expansion of the pattern. For all cases, epicardial EGMs and breakthrough times were reconstructed with high accuracy.

Infarct and Ventricular Tachycardia[1]
Based on pure Q-wave epicardial EGMs, ECGI identified the location and extent of an abnormal EP substrate associated with an infarct scar (4-day-old infarction). EGM morphologies were very similar to the measured ones, with attenuation of amplitudes. Nine cycles of VT were reconstructed, accurately depicting the epicardial activation sequence during VT.

Hybrid Dog-Modeling Studies[4,5]
Infarct and Ventricular Tachycardia. Epicardial potentials were recorded from a 490-electrode sock in an open-chest dog. These potentials were used to generate potentials in a human torso model. Realistic geometry errors and measurement noise were added to the torso potentials, which were then used for ECGI input. Infarct was created by left anterior descending coronary artery (LAD) occlusion and ethanol injection. Reconstructed epicardial potential maps captured the pattern and greater than 50% reduction of potentials over the infarct relative to the preinfarct control; CC was 0.90 (control) and 0.91 (infarct) for LV pacing and 0.77 (control) and 0.79 (infarct) for RA pacing. Corresponding CC values for EGMs were 0.89, 0.90, 0.93, and 0.92, respectively. Reduced amplitude, Q-wave morphology and fractionation of EGMs over the infarct were captured correctly. Inverse-estimated region of abnormal EP substrate closely resembled the measured one. During VT, ECGI reconstructed the recorded reentry pathway, including its key components: the central common pathway, VT exit site, lines of block, and regions of slow conduction.

Effects of Torso Inhomogeneities[6]. Amplitudes were affected by assuming a homogeneous torso, but epicardial potential patterns, EGM morphologies, isochrones, and locations of pacing sites were reconstructed with comparable accuracy.

Dependence of Electrocardiographic Imaging Accuracy on Computational and Regularization Methods

As stated in the introduction to this appendix, accuracy of ECGI depends on the choice of methodology and details of its execution, including a choice between numerical methods (e.g., Boundary Element or Finite Element method) segmentation of surfaces, mesh construction, interpolation, signal conditioning (baseline drift correction, filtering, etc.), choice of a regularization method, choice of a regularization parameter, etc. In fact, one can tailor the scheme to the application to optimize accuracy. Examples are provided below.

Generalized Minimal Residual Method versus Tikhonov Regularization[7]
In the same experimental protocol, pacing sites 2.5 cm apart were reconstructed using generalized minimal residual methods (GMRes) with 4 mm and 6 mm localization error; Tikhonov zero order reconstructed only one minimum. CC during repolarization (the T wave) for QRST integral maps was much better for GMRes (0.72) compared with that for Tikhonov regularization (0.57); Tikhonov resulted in much greater smoothing.

L1-Norm Regularization[8]
L1-norm solutions were compared with zero-order and first-order L2-norm Tikhonov solutions and to a measured "gold standard." L1-norm resulted in more accurate solutions (average relative error of 0.36 compared with 0.62) and less smoothing of

potentials, preserving details of patterns and potential gradients. Similar improvement was observed in the presence of an infarct. Morphologies and multiple deflections of postinfarct EGMs were better preserved with L1-norm (CC = 0.97 vs. 0.87).

Quadratic versus Linear Interpolation[9]
Quadratic interpolation improves accuracy. It reduces the average relative error between measured and reconstructed potentials by 25%. Specifically, it dramatically improved preservation of electrogram amplitudes over the entire epicardium, with relative error of 0.38 compared with 0.74 for linear interpolation; EGM morphologies were slightly improved (CC = 0.97 compared with 0.91). For single site pacing, quadratic interpolation reduced the error in locating the pacing site from 4 mm to 2 mm. For dual site pacing (2.5 cm apart), quadratic interpolation was able to differentiate and locate the two pacing sites, while linear interpolation failed to do so.

Method of Fundamental Solutions[10]
This method does not require meshing the heart and torso surfaces, thereby preventing mesh-related artifacts and errors. For single-site pacing (anterior RV), it improves reconstruction of epicardial potentials (CC = 0.92 and relative error = 0.47 relative to measured, compared with CC = 0.85 and relative error = 0.97 with the boundary elements method). Pacing site location was determined with 3 mm error compared with 5 mm error with the boundary elements method. EGMs and isochrones were also reconstructed with high accuracy.

Incorporating Spatial and Temporal Information
Manual editing of directly recorded or inverse-reconstructed maps has always been practiced. Determination of far-field influences, of activation and repolarization times, and of initiation sites involves evaluation of time progression (an example is the rotation and expansion of the epicardial potential pattern generated by focal excitation) as well as spatial relationships between EGMs in neighboring sites. Taking advantage of the fact that the process of cardiac excitation is continuous in time, Oster[11] applied the Twomey technique to incorporate information from the time progression of excitation in the regularization procedure of the inverse solution. This resulted in a marked improvement of accuracy, as quantified by the relative error of reconstruction (relative to measured epicardial potentials). Oster also developed a method to incorporate spatial characteristics of the potentials in the regularization procedure,[12] called *regional regularization*. In a model study, this approach was shown to improve epicardial potential reconstruction by up to 25%.

In reconstruction of repolarization and its spatial dispersion, Ghanem[13] incorporated spatial dependence through the use of Tikhonov second-order regularization. This higher-order regularization scheme constrains the curvature in space of the epicardial potentials rather than their magnitude. With this method, T waves were reconstructed with greater accuracy and preserved amplitudes. Repolarization properties and dispersion introduced by regional myocardial warming and cooling were faithfully reconstructed.

Validation of Electrocardiographic Imaging Reconstructions in Humans

Evaluating Accuracy of Locating Initiation Sites, Based on Known Pacing Site Locations
Ventricular Pacing
Generalized Minimal Residual Methods With Quadratic Interpolation[9]. Patient 1: RV apical pacing site was reconstructed within 10 mm of pacing lead location as determined through CT (based on reconstructed epicardial potentials; from isochrones it was 12 mm, less accurate as expected). Patient 2: error with apical RV pacing = 2 mm; error with LV pacing = 7 mm. Patient 3: error

with LV pacing = 4 mm. Patient 4: error with RV pacing = 2 mm; error with LV pacing = 3 mm. All reconstructions captured the general spread of activation from the pacing site.

Method of Fundamental Solution[10]. RV Pacing: 8 mm error with boundary element method and 5 mm with method of fundamental solutions (MFS). Simultaneous RV and LV pacing during biventricular pacing in CRT: error at the RV pacing site = 5.2 mm; error at the LV pacing site = 7.4 mm.

L-1 Norm[8]. Biventricular pacing from epicardial leads in pediatric patients with congenital heart disease. Patient 1 (6 years old; congenital heart block): error at the RV pacing site = 2 mm; error at the LV pacing site = 6 mm (individual pacing from each lead). Patient 2 (5 years old, corrected transposition of the great arteries and heart block): error at the pulmonary ventricle pacing site = 4 mm; error at the systemic ventricle pacing site = 6 mm. Patient 3 (17 years old, single double-inlet LV post-Fontan and congenital AV block): error at the posterior lead = 3 mm, error at the anterior lead = 5 mm. For five patients with dual lead pacing, the accuracy of L-1 norm was 3.8 ± 1.5 mm and of L-2 norm with zero order Tikhonov 10 ± 2.8 mm.

Early Study Using Tikhonov Zero Order Regularization[14]: Nonsimultaneous Right Ventricular Pacing and Left Ventricular Pacing in the Same Patient. Nonsimultaneous RV pacing and LV pacing in the same patient. Site of earliest activation, as determined from ECGI reconstructed epicardial potential maps, corresponded well with the pacing lead terminal determined from CT for both RV and LV pacing, as did the sequence of epicardial activation. ECGI located the pacing sites to within 7 mm (RV) and 11 mm (LV). The published figure shows translucent views of the heart, allowing the reader to see the pacing lead and potential map simultaneously for comparison of pacing site location.

Atrial Pacing: Atrial Fibrillation Electrocardiographic Imaging Study[15]. In the testing (validation) phase of this study, pacing was performed with a catheter in six patients from 11 different sites, known to be AF initiation sites, providing a total of 37 paced events. Location of pacing site was determined directly by electroanatomical mapping using CARTO. ECGI-determined pacing locations were accurate within 6.3 ± 3.9 mm.

Comparison to Intraoperative Mapping in Patients[16]

Three patients undergoing open-heart surgery were studied during sinus rhythm and right ventricular endocardial and epicardial pacing (total of five datasets). Body surface potentials were acquired preoperatively or postoperatively using a 224-electrode vest. Heart-torso geometry was determined preoperatively using CT. Intraoperative mapping was performed with two 100-electrode epicardial patches. A limitation of this study was the nonsimultaneous acquisition of the surgical and noninvasive ECGI data under different conditions (open vs. closed chest). Because invasive and noninvasive data were not obtained simultaneously, time alignment of the two cardiac sequences was necessary. Noninvasive potential maps captured epicardial breakthrough sites, reflected general activation and repolarization patterns, localized pacing sites to ~1 cm, and distinguished between epicardial and endocardial origin of activation. Noninvasively reconstructed EGM morphologies correlated moderately with their invasive counterparts (cross correlation = 0.72 ± 0.25 [sinus rhythm], 0.67 ± 0.23 [endocardial pacing], and 0.71 ± 0.21 [epicardial pacing]). Noninvasive isochrones captured the sites of earliest activation, areas of slow conduction, and the general excitation pattern.

Validation of Scar Electrophysiological Substrate[17]

The study included 24 subjects with infarct-related myocardial scar. Based on ECGI-reconstructed epicardial EGMs that displayed the characteristics of scar-related EGMs (low voltage and fractionation), the epicardial EP scar was reconstructed. The ECGI-imaged scar matched the anatomical scar (imaged with gadolinium delayed-contrast MRI) in location, size, and morphology. This is an important validation because it is done with a completely independent and well-established method (MRI).

Validation in Clinical Applications

Focal Left Ventricular Tachycardia[18]

ECGI was applied in a young athlete with focal VT. The ECGI-reconstructed isochrones localized the site of origin to the LV apex, in an area of a diverticulum. QS morphology of a reconstructed EGM from this site indicated epicardial origin. These ECGI determinations and the reconstructed activation map precisely correlated with invasive endocardial and epicardial catheter mapping using standard EP mapping techniques.

Wolff-Parkinson-White Syndrome[8,19]

Fourteen Wolff-Parkinson-White pediatric patients undergoing ablation participated in the study. ECGI-localized preexcitation sites were consistent with the successful ablation site with high accuracy, much better than the accuracy with the conventional Arruda algorithm. ECGI distinguished between epicardial and endocardial accessory pathways based on EGM morphology. ECGI also determined the presence and locations of dual pathways, not detectable from the ECG, that were confirmed by invasive EP study and subsequent ablation at the two predicted sites.

Ventricular Arrhythmias Study[20]

Twenty-five patients participated in the study. Compared with invasive EP study, ECGI correctly identified the LV or RV site of origin 100% of the time. Specific locations within each ventricle were in agreement with invasive EP study in 10 of 11 RV sites (91%), and in 11 of 12 LV sites (92%). ECGI-reconstructed reentrant VT patterns were always related to areas of ventricular scar. Entrainment maneuvers confirmed a reentrant mechanism, and when ablation was performed in this region, it terminated the VT. Through comparison with invasive EP studies, ECGI was also evaluated for its ability to determine epicardial or intramural locations (depth) of VT based on EGM morphology. The EP study determined the site of origin to be epicardial in five patients, endocardial in six patients, and midmyocardial in two patients. All five patients with epicardial origin had a reconstructed pure Q-wave EGM (100%) at the site of earliest activation, indicative of epicardial origin. In seven of the eight patients with nonepicardial origin, the EGM had a small r wave (88%) indicative of intramural origin.

Atrial Flutter[14]

ECGI reconstructed the right atrium reentry circuit of typical atrial flutter and the atrial activation pattern driven by this circuit. The maps were consistent with observations from direct mapping of typical atrial flutter using intracardiac catheters.

Focal Atrial Tachycardia[21]

ECGI located the focal source on the roof of the left atrium, between the right superior pulmonary vein and atrial septum. Invasive right and left atrial electroanatomical catheter mapping identified a focal tachycardia originating from the superior left atrium between the right superior pulmonary vein and atrial septum, confirming the ECGI determination. The tachycardia was terminated with application of RF energy to this location.

Normal Excitation[14,22]

ECGI mapping of atrial and ventricular activation was conducted in seven normal subjects under complete physiological conditions. Results are in close agreement with those recorded directly in seven isolated nondiseased human hearts in the classic study by Durrer and colleagues.[23]

APPENDIX REFERENCES

1. Burnes JE, Taccardi B, Ershler P, Rudy Y. Noninvasive electrocardiogram imaging of substrate and intramural ventricular tachycardia in infarcted hearts. *J Amer College Cardiol*. 2001;38:2071–2078.
2. Oster HS, Taccardi B, Lux RL, Ershler PR, Rudy Y. Noninvasive electrocardiographic imaging: reconstruction of epicardial potentials, electrograms, and isochrones, and localization of single and multiple electrocardiac events. *Circulation*. 1997;96:1012–1024.
3. Oster HS, Taccardi B, Lux RL, Ershler PR, Rudy Y. Electrocardiographic imaging: noninvasive characterization of intramural myocardial activation from inverse reconstructed epicardial potentials and electrograms. *Circulation*. 1998;97:1496–1507.
4. Burnes JE, Taccardi B, MacLeod RS, Rudy Y. Noninvasive electrocardiographic imaging of electrophysiologically abnormal substrate in infarcted hearts: a model study. *Circulation*. 2000;101:533–540.
5. Burnes JE, Taccardi B, Rudy Y. A noninvasive imaging modality for cardiac arrhythmias. *Circulation*. 2000;102:2152–2158.
6. Ramanathan C, Rudy Y. Electrocardiographic imaging: I. Effect of torso inhomogeneities on the noninvasive reconstruction of epicardial potentials, electrograms and isochrones. *J Cardiovasc Electrophysiol*. 2001;12:241–252.
7. Ramanathan C, Jia P, Ghanem RN, Calvetti D, Rudy Y. Noninvasive electrocardiographic imaging (ECGI): application of the generalized minimal residual (GMRes) method. *Ann Biomed Eng*. 2003;31:981–994.
8. Ghosh S, Rudy Y. Application of L1-norm regularization to epicardial potential solution of the inverse electrocardiography problem. *Ann Biomed Eng*. 2009;37:902–912.
9. Ghosh S, Rudy Y. Accuracy of quadratic versus linear interpolation in noninvasive electrocardiographic imaging (ECGI). *Ann Biomed Eng*. 2005;33:1187–1201.
10. Wang Y, Rudy Y. Application of the method of fundamental solutions to potential-based inverse electrocardiography. *Ann Biomed Eng*. 2006;34:1272–1288.
11. Oster HS, Rudy Y. The use of temporal information in the regularization of the inverse problem of electrocardiography. *IEEE Trans Biomed Eng*. 1992;39:65–75.
12. Oster HS, Rudy Y. Regional regularization of the electrocardiographic inverse problem: a model study using spherical geometry. *IEEE Trans Biomed Eng*. 1997;44:188–199.
13. Ghanem RN, Burnes JE, Waldo AL, Rudy Y. Imaging dispersion of myocardial repolarization, II. Noninvasive reconstruction of epicardial measures. *Circulation*. 2001;104:1306–1312.
14. Ramanathan C, Ghanem RN, Jia P, Ryu K, Rudy Y. Electrocardiographic imaging (ECGI): a noninvasive imaging modality for cardiac electrophysiology and arrhythmia. *Nat Med*. 2004;10:422–428.
15. Cuculich PS, Wang Y, Lindsay BD, Faddis MN, Schuessler RB, et al. Noninvasive characterization of epicardial activation in humans with diverse atrial fibrillation patterns. *Circulation*. 2010;122:1364–1372.
16. Ghanem RN, Jia P, Ramanathan C, Ryu K, Markowitz A, Rudy Y. Noninvasive electrocardiographic imaging (ECGI): comparison to intraoperative mapping in patients. *Heart Rhythm*. 2005;2:339–354.
17. Cuculich PS, Zhang J, Wang Y, et al. The electrophysiologic cardiac ventricular substrate in patients after myocardial infarction: noninvasive characterization with electrocardiographic imaging. *J Am Col Cardiol*. 2011;58:1893–1902.
18. Intini A, Goldstein RN, Jia P, Ramanathan C, Ryu K, Giannattasio B, Gilkeson R, Stambler BS, Brugada P, Stevenson WG, Rudy Y, Waldo AL. Electrocardiographic imaging (ECGI), a novel diagnostic modality used for mapping of focal left ventricular tachycardia in a young athlete. *Heart Rhythm*. 2005;2:1250–1252.
19. Ghosh S, Rhee EK, Avari JN, Woodard PK, Rudy Y. Cardiac memory in WPW patients: noninvasive imaging of activation and repolarization before and after catheter ablation. *Circulation*. 2008;118:907–915.
20. Wang Y, Cuculich PS, Zhang J, et al. Noninvasive electroanatomic mapping of human ventricular arrhythmias with electrocardiographic imaging. *Sci Transl Med*. 2011;3: 98ra84.
21. Wang Y, Cuculich PS, Woodard PK, Lindsay BD, Rudy Y. Focal atrial tachycardia after pulmonary vein isolation: noninvasive mapping with electrocardiographic imaging (ECGI). *Heart Rhythm*. 2007;4:1081–1084.
22. Ramanathan C, Jia P, Ghanem RN, Ryu K, Rudy Y. Activation and repolarization of the normal human heart under complete physiological conditions. *Proc Natl Acad Sci USA*. 2006;103:6309–6314.
23. Durrer D, Van Dam RT, Freud GE, Janse MJ, Meijler FL, Arzbaecher RC. Total excitation of the isolated human heart. *Circulation*. 1970;41:899–912.

71 Genetic Testing

Christopher Semsarian and Jodie Ingles

Major advances have been made since the mid-1990s that have defined the genetic basis of many medical diseases. There are now over 40 different cardiovascular diseases directly caused by variants in genes that encode cardiac proteins. These cardiovascular diseases include the inherited cardiomyopathies, inherited arrhythmia syndromes, metabolic disorders, and congenital heart diseases. Identification of the genetic causes of cardiovascular disease allows early detection of at-risk asymptomatic family members, and in some cases, helps to guide therapies as well as inform prognosis. This chapter will provide an overview of the current knowledge related to the role of genetic testing in cardiac diseases, with a specific focus on arrhythmogenic diseases.

Basic Genetics

DNA, Genes, and Mutations

With the recent completion of the human genome sequence, and subsequent advances in genetic technologies, we now have a clearer picture of our genetic make-up and how variations in our genome can lead to cardiovascular disease.[1]

Genes

Current estimates suggest our human genome is made up of approximately 3.2 billion base pairs of DNA (composed of four bases—adenine, thymine, guanine, and cytosine), accounting for approximately 22,000 genes. Each gene is defined as a molecular unit that can encode both RNA and protein sequences, which represent functional units in the human body. In cardiovascular disease, these genes can encode both RNA and proteins, and faults in these genes can lead to a disease phenotype. Functionally, disease genes leading to cardiovascular disease encode a range of proteins, including those associated with the sarcomere, ion channels, cytoskeletal structures, and in embryonic heart development.

DNA Variants

Variations, or changes, can occur in the DNA sequence of humans. These variants can be broadly defined as single nucleotide variants (SNVs). SNVs usually occur with a measurable frequency (>0.5% allelic frequency) among a particular ethnic population(s). SNVs can then be subdivided into those that alter the protein sequence (*nonsynonymous*) and those where the protein sequence is unaltered (*synonymous*). Rare variants are seen in everyone, so determining which can cause disease is a significant challenge. The American College of Medical Genetics has developed stringent classification scores for assigning causation to rare variants, and it is expected that these will be further developed to be more disease specific in the near future.[2]

Pathogenic or Likely Pathogenic Variants

Many types of disease-causing variants exist.[3] The vast majority in cardiovascular disease are *missense* mutations, in which a single base pair change results in the change (or replacement) of one amino acid. Other mutations may cause more significant disruptions to the encoded protein, so-called "frameshift" or "truncation" mutations, which can lead to a major change in the protein sequence or a loss of amino acids resulting in a shortened protein. The latter mutations are often caused by deletions or insertions of nucleic acids in the coding region. The terms "pathogenic" or "likely pathogenic" imply there is a level of confidence to pursue cascade genetic testing of asymptomatic relatives (Table 71.1).

Modes of Inheritance

The four major modes of inheritance are summarized in Fig. 71.1. In the majority of cardiovascular genetic diseases, inheritance is autosomal dominant, whereby the disease can be expressed when the mutation is present in just one allele. As a result, the chance of passing on the gene mutation from parent to offspring is 50%. Most primary arrhythmogenic diseases and inherited cardiomyopathies are inherited in this fashion. The other three modes of inheritance in Fig. 71.1 are significantly less common. Autosomal recessive inheritance requires the person to inherit the mutation on both alleles for disease to develop (i.e., one mutation inherited from each parent). The chance of passing on the gene mutation from both parents to offspring is 25%. The Jervell-Lange-Nielsen form of familial long QT syndrome (LQTS) is inherited in an autosomal recessive fashion. X-linked inheritance refers to the situation where the gene mutation is located on the X-chromosome. As such, males develop the phenotype while females are most often asymptomatic gene mutation carriers. Rare forms of dilated cardiomyopathy (DCM) have been shown to have an X-linked pattern of inheritance. Mitochondrial inheritance is a non-Mendelian pattern in which transmission of disease is exclusively via females and involves inheritance of mutant mitochondrial DNA to offspring. While uncommon, this form of inheritance is often seen in mitochondrial diseases that can clinically manifest with a hypertrophic cardiomyopathy (HCM) phenotype (or phenocopy).

Genetic Testing in Cardiovascular Disease

General Principles

Genetic testing is not a simple blood test. There are many considerations that arise with every family. A complete cardiogenetic evaluation is required, which includes a thorough cardiac investigation and a clear diagnosis in the proband, the need for genetic counseling to ensure that the family understands the possible outcomes of genetic testing, and taking a detailed family history to get a sense of disease penetrance and patterns of disease.[1,4]

Importance of Detailed and Accurate Phenotyping

The cornerstone of the utility of genetic testing is accurately defining the clinical phenotype both in the individual patient

TABLE 71.1 Probabilistic Outcomes of Cardiac Genetic Testing

POSSIBLE OUTCOME	CONSEQUENCES FOR THE PROBAND	CONSEQUENCES FOR THE FAMILY
No variants of potential clinical importance identified (benign)	An indeterminate gene result does not exclude a cardiac genetic disease, but reassessment of the phenotype should be considered	Cascade genetic testing cannot be offered to the family; at-risk relatives are advised to be clinically assessed according to current guidelines
Variant of uncertain significance identified	Efforts to delineate pathogenicity of the variant are required, including cosegregation studies involving phenotyped family members	While pathogenicity of a variant is under question, it cannot be used to inform clinical management of family members; cascade genetic testing cannot be offered; at-risk relatives are advised to be clinically assessed according to guidelines
Pathogenic variant identified (pathogenic or likely pathogenic)	Confirm clinical diagnosis, limited therapeutic and prognostic application except in familial long QT syndrome	Cascade genetic testing of asymptomatic family members is available following genetic counseling
Multiple pathogenic variants identified	Confirm clinical diagnosis and potentially explain a more severe clinical phenotype	Complex inheritance risk to first-degree relatives must be discussed; cascade genetic testing of asymptomatic family members is available following genetic counseling
Incidental or secondary pathogenic variant identified	Action regarding incidental or secondary findings must be discussed with the proband pretest	Genetic counseling to determine clinical and genetic impact to family members is available

Modified from Ingles J, Semsarian C. Conveying a probabilistic genetic test result to families with an inherited heart disease. *Heart Rhythm.* 2014;11:1073-1078.

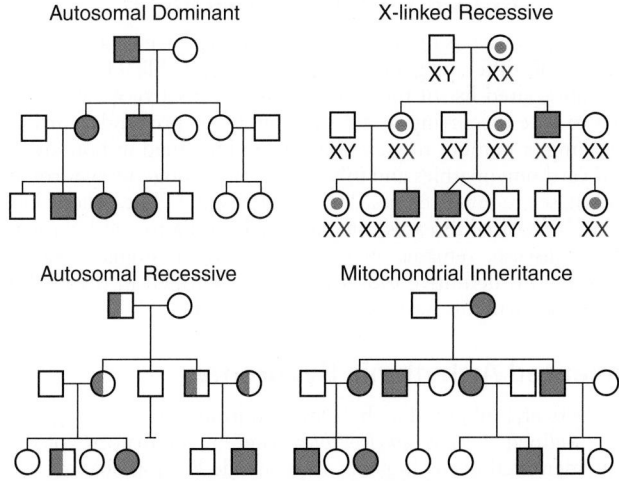

FIGURE 71.1 The four most common modes of inheritance in cardiovascular genetic diseases. Autosomal dominant inheritance accounts for over 90% of genetic heart diseases. *Squares,* males; *circles,* females; *open symbols,* clinically unaffected; *filled-in symbols,* affected; *spot in middle of symbol,* obligate carrier; *half-filled symbol,* heterozygote gene carrier in an autosomal recessive family.

and the family. The highest yields from genetic testing are often based on patient cohorts with confirmed disease. For example, in clinical HCM, careful attention to the family history, clinical symptoms, and defining the extent, distribution, and severity of hypertrophy are all considered essential in clinically distinguishing HCM from other HCM mimickers (or phenocopies), such as Fabry disease or glycogen storage diseases, which have different genetic etiologies.

Genetic Counseling and Informed Consent
In all patients and families with a genetic heart disease, genetic counseling is essential. Genetic testing options span all stages of life, from the preimplanted embryo or fetus, to children and adults. Appropriate pretest and posttest genetic counseling is a vital component of genetic testing. Apart from the diagnostic utility of genetic testing within families, a specific gene result may also guide therapy and provide information about prognosis. The cardiac genetic counselor therefore plays a key role in the testing process, ensuring that the individual understands the clinical and psychosocial implications of every possible result, limitations of the tests including difficulties in interpretation of the results,

as well as the discussion of other issues such as genetic testing of children, prenatal and preimplantation genetic diagnosis, and access to insurance.

Commercially Available Genetic Testing
Since 2006, genetic testing for cardiac diseases was slow, costly, and focused on a handful of cardiac genes. Comprehensive cardiac gene panels including 50 to 100 genes or more are now the norm with a typically turnaround time of 6 to 8 weeks. Due to the advances in the next generation of sequencing technologies, the capability to screen vast numbers of genes has rapidly increased, while the cost continues to decrease. Indeed, the option to perform whole exome sequencing (WES) (the entire coding region of all 22,000 genes) or whole genome sequencing (WGS) (the entire genome, including coding and noncoding regions) at a clinical level now exists.[5]

Proband Genetic Testing

The genetic testing process most frequently begins with testing the proband (or index case). This is often the first person in the family who presents, and the clinical diagnosis is established. Following genetic counseling and informed consent, genetic testing is performed. The outcomes can be divided into (1) those where a variant(s) is identified that is deemed to be pathogenic (disease causing), (2) those where no causative variant is identified (an "indeterminate result"), and (3) those where it is unclear whether the variant is pathogenic or a benign variation in our genetic sequence (variant of uncertain significance).

Determining Pathogenicity
Determining whether a DNA variant is disease-causing is challenging. In most genetic testing reports, evidence will be provided to show the classification of the variant in terms of disease causation. A five-tier system is typically used, grading variants from pathogenic, likely pathogenic, variant of uncertain significance, likely benign, and benign. Evidence that will allow the classification of disease causation (i.e., pathogenic and likely pathogenic status) often includes factors such as the absence or very low frequency in general population databases (i.e., the Exome Aggregation Consortium dataset, ExAC http://exac.broadinstitute.org/); reports of the occurrence of the variant in additional unrelated individuals from the literature or public archives of variant classifications (i.e., ClinVar, http://www.clinvar.com/)[6]; and segregation of the variant to affected relatives in families. Computational tools such as PolyPhen and SIFT that predict the functional consequences of the variant as well as

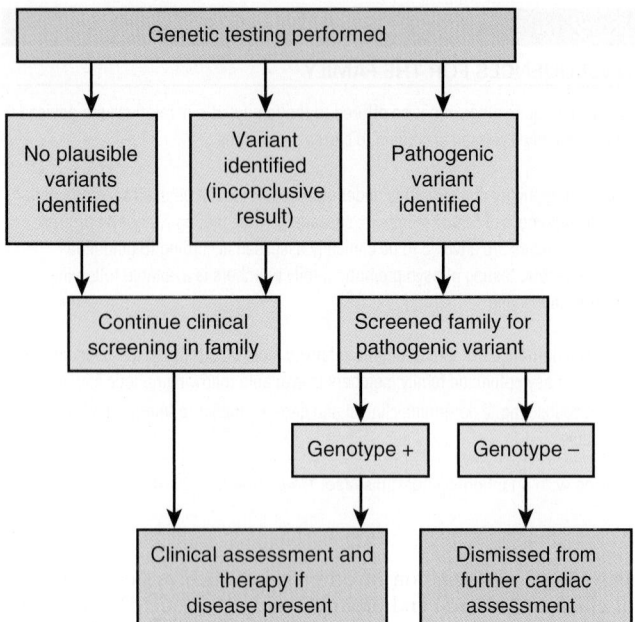

FIGURE 71.2 Flow chart illustrating the role of genetic testing in families with genetic heart disease. Genotype "+" means a positive genetic result; genotype "–" means a negative genetic result.

conservation scores are useful, but are taken together as being supportive and in agreement of pathogenicity, providing only low-level evidence. Stringent and ongoing variant classification is critical in ensuring that the information is used appropriately in the family.

Variants of Uncertain Significance

After applying the criteria listed above, situations arise where the clinical significance and pathogenicity of a variant remains unknown. In these cases, the variant is termed a variant of uncertain significance (VUS). Recent advances in genetic screening technologies have identified that the frequency of VUS is significant among normal populations, and within specific cardiac disease genes. Given this current ambiguity, a VUS is considered an indeterminate result and is not considered reliable for cascade genetic testing in other family members.

Cascade Genetic Testing of Family Members

Genetic Testing in Families

The greatest utility of genetic testing is its diagnostic use in other family members (Fig. 71.2). Once a pathogenic or likely pathogenic variant has been identified in the proband, this information can be used in asymptomatic first-degree relatives and beyond, to identify those people who carry the gene variant and as importantly, those who do not. This process, called *cascade genetic testing*, is the primary utility of performing genetic testing in families. A negative gene test result means the individual no longer requires ongoing clinical screening, eliminating the need for decades of expensive cardiac investigations based on current clinical guidelines. A positive gene result allows a more targeted screening approach, with the goal to prevent serious cardiac events. Just as important, cascade genetic testing can clarify the risk status of *their* first-degree relatives, such as children. Cascade genetic testing of children can be useful; however, it should be approached cautiously in an effort to avoid harm, with expertise from a cardiac genetic counselor imperative. Child psychologists may be useful in this setting to assess the child's capacity to understand a genetic result and to ensure that testing will not have adverse psychosocial effects.

Silent Gene Carriers

As a consequence of the increase in genetic testing in families with inherited heart diseases, a new clinical spectrum of individuals has arisen: those who carry a specific causative gene mutation but have not yet developed a detectable clinical phenotype.[7] These patients are effectively "gene carriers," and very little is known regarding how to best manage these asymptomatic patients (e.g., their participation in competitive sports). For those diseases where clinical tests are the gold standard for disease diagnosis (i.e., inherited cardiomyopathies) it is generally agreed that these individuals should not be considered as patients, but merely presenting a predisposition to developing disease in the future. In HCM, this group presents a fascinating "preclinical" population that is now the target of randomized controlled trials of preventive agents that may prove to one day find an effective "cure" for the disease.[8] In contrast, the inherited arrhythmia syndromes present considerable diagnostic challenges, and diagnosis by genetic testing is a significant step forward in the early detection of disease.

Genes and Cardiovascular Disease

To date, thousands of causative gene variants have been identified in over 40 different genetic heart diseases. Table 71.2 provides an abbreviated list of the most common causative genes identified to date (occurring in ≥5% of genotyped probands). Broadly speaking, a number of genes have been identified in both inherited cardiomyopathies and inherited arrhythmogenic syndromes, and these are inherited in a Mendelian fashion. The genetic basis of multifactorial diseases, such as atrial fibrillation and coronary artery disease, remains an ongoing focus of intense research, although no definitive causative genes identified in over 5% of genotyped patients have been reported to date.

Inherited Arrhythmia Syndromes

Collectively, inherited arrhythmia syndromes have been genetically defined as *ion channelopathies*, whereby the majority of variants identified occur in genes that encode key ion channels and their associated proteins. Specifically, variants in genes that encode potassium, sodium, and calcium channels have predominantly been identified to date. These variants therefore define the genetic basis of familial LQTS, Brugada syndrome (BrS), catecholaminergic polymorphic ventricular tachycardia (CPVT), and short QT syndrome (SQT). While the clinical features of these diseases are detailed elsewhere in this book, there are some important points to be made from a genetic perspective.

The first is the yield from genetic testing. In LQTS and CPVT, the pick-up rates for a pathogenic gene mutation are high at 60% to 75%, with most LQTS mutations identified in three genes (LQT1-3) and one gene (*RYR2*) accounting for the majority of CPVT. In contrast, the pick-up rates for BrS and SQT syndrome are currently low, with only *SCN5A* being a significant cause of BrS in approximately 20% of patients. A second key point is the intriguing overlap in genetic etiology. Mutations in *SCN5A* (see Table 71.2) have been shown to cause LQTS type 3 but also BrS, SQT syndrome, cardiac conduction disease, and some cases of sudden infant death syndrome (SIDS). This commonality may reflect some mechanistic overlap in the development of arrhythmias in these different syndromes.

Most recently, the genetics of inherited J-wave syndromes such as BrS and early repolarization syndrome have shown some progress, although it represents one of the greatest areas of uncertainty in terms of the underlying genetics. The genetics of BrS has become particularly complex, with issues of significant clinical heterogeneity and the suggestion of complex inheritance as shown by large genome-wide association studies.[9] Large families demonstrating autosomal dominant transmission of the clinical

TABLE 71.2 Causative Genes Occurring in ≥5% Tested

GENE	LOCUS	PROTEIN	% OF DISEASE
Long QT Syndrome (LQTS)			
KCNQ1 (LQT1)	11p15.5	I_{Ks} potassium channel alpha subunit (Kv7.1)	30%–35%
KCNH2 (LQT2)	7q35	I_{Kr} potassium channel alpha subunit (Kv11.1 or hERG)	25%–40%
SCN5A (LQT3)	3p21	Cardiac sodium channel alpha subunit (NaV1.5)	5%–10%
Catecholaminergic Polymorphic Ventricular Tachycardia (CPVT)			
RYR2 (CPVT1)	1q42.1	Ryanodine receptor 2	60%
Brugada Syndrome (BrS)			
SCN5A	3p21	Cardiac sodium channel alpha subunit (NaV1.5)	20%–30%
Cardiac Conduction Disease (CCD)			
SCN5A	3p21	Cardiac sodium channel alpha subunit (NaV1.5)	5%
Hypertrophic Cardiomyopathy (HCM)			
MYBPC3	11p11.2	Cardiac myosin-binding protein C	20%–45%
MYH7	14q11.2	β-Myosin heavy chain	15%–20%
TNNT2	1q32	Cardiac troponin T type 2	1%–7%
TNNI3	19q13.4	Cardiac troponin I type 3	1%–7%
Arrhythmogenic Right Ventricular Cardiomyopathy (ARVC)			
PKP2	12p11	Plakophilin 2	25%–40%
DSG2	18q12.1	Desmoglein 2	5%–10%
DSP	6p24	Desmoplakin	2%–12%
DSC2	18q12.1	Desmocollin 2	2%–7%
Dilated Cardiomyopathy (DCM)			
TTN	2q31	Titin	15%–20%
Dilated Cardiomyopathy with Cardiac Conduction Defect (DCM + CCD)			
SCN5A	3p21	Cardiac sodium channel alpha subunit (NaV1.5)	5%–10%
LMNA	1q22	Lamin A/C	5%–10%
Left Ventricular Noncompaction (LVNC)			
LBD3	10q22.2	LIM binding domain 3	~5%
Restrictive Cardiomyopathy (RCM)			
MYH7	14q11.2	β-Myosin heavy chain	~5%
TNNI3	19q13.4	Cardiac troponin I type 3	~5%

Modified from Ackerman MJ, Priori SG, Willems S, et al. HRS/EHRA expert consensus statement on the state of genetic testing for the channelopathies and cardiomyopathies this document was developed as a partnership between the Heart Rhythm Society (HRS) and the European Heart Rhythm Association (EHRA). *Heart Rhythm*. 2011;8:1308-1339.

phenotype of early repolarization syndrome have been shown; however, to date few genes have been implicated.[10]

Inherited Cardiomyopathies

The five main cardiomyopathies have all been identified to have genetic etiologies (see Table 71.2), although the scope and depth of knowledge varies between each. While the clinical features of these diseases are detailed elsewhere in this book, the current knowledge regarding genetic causation is summarized here. The most well studied and prevalent cardiomyopathy is HCM.[11] To date, mutations in at least 13 genes have been identified that encode sarcomere or sarcomere-related proteins.[12] The genetic testing pick-up rate for HCM is approximately 50%.

Arrhythmogenic right ventricular cardiomyopathy (ARVC) has been redefined as a disease of the desmosome, which is important in cell–cell adhesion. While a number of genes have been identified, recent studies suggest significant rates of background DNA variants in these genes, leading to a high "signal-to-noise" ratio. This has complicated the process of determining whether the variants found in these genes are indeed pathogenic. Genetic studies in familial DCM have resulted in over 30 genes being identified that harbor pathogenic mutations. However, to date only three genes have been shown as causative in over 5% of cases (i.e., titin [*TTN*] mutations in DCM, and lamin A/C [*LMNA*] and *SCN5A* mutations in DCM with conduction disease). Left ventricular noncompaction (LVNC) is a cardiomyopathy for which our understanding of the genetic causes is gaining some momentum. Interestingly, isolated LVNC (i.e., not part of a syndrome of features) may be caused by autosomal dominant, X-linked, and mitochondrial gene variants highlighting the complexities underlying the mechanism of disease in this cardiomyopathy.[13]

Clinical Applications of Genetic Testing

The primary clinical application of genetic testing in cardiovascular disease is in diagnosis. Apart from confirming disease in the proband, across all genetic heart diseases, the key application is predictive genetic testing to clarify the risk status of family members. In a proband with an autosomal dominant genetic heart disease, there will be a 50% chance of a first-degree relative having a positive gene result. In those who carry the gene variant, regular

TABLE 71.3	Comparison of Diseases in Terms of Genetic Testing for Diagnosis, Therapy, and Prognosis		
DISEASE	**DIAGNOSTIC**	**THERAPEUTIC**	**PROGNOSTIC**
LQTS	+++	++	+++
CPVT	+++	–	+
BrS	+	–	+
CCD	+	+	+
HCM	+++	+	++
ARVC	+	–	+/–
DCM	+/–	–	–
DCM + CCD	++	+	++
LVNC	+	–	–
RCM	+	+	+

Relative impact of genetic testing (– [negligible] to +++ [strong]).

ARVC, arrhythmogenic right ventricular cardiomyopathy; *BrS*, Brugada syndrome; *CCD*, cardiac conduction disease; *CPVT*, catecholaminergic polymorphic ventricular tachycardia; *DCM*, dilated cardiomyopathy; *HCM*, hypertrophic cardiomyopathy; *LQTS*, long QT syndrome; *LVNC*, left ventricular noncompaction; *RCM*, restrictive cardiomyopathy.

Modified from Ackerman MJ, Priori SG, Willems S, et al. HRS/EHRA expert consensus statement on the state of genetic testing for the channelopathies and cardiomyopathies: this document was developed as a partnership between the Heart Rhythm Society (HRS) and the European Heart Rhythm Association (EHRA). *Heart Rhythm*. 2011;8:1308-1339.

clinical surveillance as per the disease-specific guidelines is followed. In the 50% of people tested who have a negative gene test, no further clinical evaluation is required and the individual can be freed from potentially decades of clinical screening, as can their children (see Fig. 71.2). The health economic impact of genetic testing in such settings has already been shown to be a very cost-effective strategy.

Early Detection of Disease

In some situations, the genetic test result may shed light on optimal therapeutic strategies and prognosis. Table 71.3 summarizes the impact of genetic testing on the index case in terms of diagnosis, prognosis, and in guiding therapy. For example, in LQTS, determining whether the patient's genotype is LQTS1, LQTS2, or LQTS3 may influence whether the patient will benefit from beta blockers, and overall how this might influence prognosis, taking into consideration other clinical factors including gender, symptoms, and severity of QT interval prolongation. It is anticipated that as more patients and families are genotyped, and more genotype-based, long-term clinical follow-up studies are conducted, more will be understood about the impact of genotype on therapeutic responses and prognosis.

Genetic Testing at Different Stages of Life

Comprehensive guidelines exist for genetic testing in children, which take into account many factors related to the child, the parents and family, and the medical circumstances of the underlying genetic heart disease. Genetic testing can be offered in both the prenatal setting (i.e., in early pregnancy), as well as at conception, which is referred to as a preimplantation genetic diagnosis. Such approaches are based on identifying embryos that carry the gene mutation and implanting only those that are unaffected. While available currently, prenatal and preimplantation approaches need to be discussed extensively with families, appropriate counseling provided, and decisions made in an informed manner. Due to the significant clinical heterogeneity that is a hallmark of genetic heart diseases, families do not often utilize these options.

The "Molecular Autopsy"

The genetics of sudden unexplained death is an area gaining a lot of attention. In sudden cardiac death cases where there is no premorbid diagnosis of cardiac disease and no cause of death

identified at postmortem, an inherited arrhythmia syndrome is often suspected.[14] Genetic testing of postmortem DNA (i.e., the "molecular autopsy") may be useful and will provide a genetic diagnosis in 10% to 30% of cases. While the pick-up rate is low, the utility of a genetic diagnosis in this setting—that is, provide a cause of death and a tool for clarification of disease risk for family members—is significant.

Family Management
Multidisciplinary Clinic Approach

A genetic diagnosis in the proband has major implications for family relatives. In all situations where a genetic heart disease is identified, appropriate clinical and, where available, genetic screening is indicated. The clear goal of both clinical and genetic screening of family members is to identify those with clinical evidence of disease or those who may carry the same pathogenic variant as the proband, but do not express a clinical phenotype. As discussed previously, early identification of these at-risk individuals provides opportunities to initiate early therapies aimed at preventing disease complications. For example, gene carriers for LQTS may require the modification of lifestyle activities, avoidance of QT-prolonging medications, initiation of beta-blocker therapy, and, in some, consideration of implantable cardioverter defibrillator therapy.

The management of families with a genetic heart disease is therefore complex. There are many different issues to consider, such as clinical evaluations and management, coordination of services including genetic counseling and testing, patient education and support, and awareness of the psychological, social, and potential legal issues. As a consequence, the ideal model of care is the cardiologist-led specialized multidisciplinary cardiac genetic clinic.[14] Expertise from a number of health professionals is drawn upon, including cardiologists, clinical geneticists, psychologists, and genetic counselors, as well as services such as patient support groups and research centers. This type of multidisciplinary model has been shown to improve psychosocial outcomes of patients with genetic heart diseases, specifically showing less worry and reduced levels of anxiety.

Key Role of Genetic Counseling

A key member of the multidisciplinary team is the cardiac genetic counselor. The cardiac genetic counselor is involved in many aspects of care, of both the individual patient and the wider family.[4] There are many social and emotional consequences of a diagnosis of a genetic heart disease including the possible need for an implantable cardioverter–defibrillator, uncertainty regarding prognosis, restrictions on physical activity, and genetic counseling issues related to the high risk of transmission to children and genetic testing options. One of the key roles of the cardiac genetic counselor is to provide pretest and posttest genetic counseling to all patients undergoing genetic testing, and this is increasingly important as the complexity of the gene results continues to be more difficult to interpret.

Ethical, Legal, and Societal Implications

The broader ethical, legal, and societal implications of genetic testing are beyond the scope of this chapter, and a variety of national regulations and specifications exist. However, there are several common issues surrounding genetic testing for cardiac diseases where ethical, legal, and societal implications must be considered. Many of these relate to the potential for harm from using this technology and shine a light on the importance of multidisciplinary centers with considerable expertise in these areas.

One example relates to the use of genetic information in reproductive decisions. Questions are raised more and more regarding the possibility of genetic testing especially early in life, including the role for preimplantation genetic testing of embryos generated with assisted reproductive technologies. If the attending cardiologist is not equipped to discuss these issues, genetic counseling should be offered in partnership with genetic counselors and/or clinical geneticists. As discussed previously, such a multidisciplinary approach will help serve the needs of the patients and their families more comprehensively, and will facilitate open and informed discussion about the ethical, legal, and societal implications of genetic testing. It is therefore important that pregenetic test counseling, genetic testing, and the interpretation of genetic test results be performed in centers experienced in the genetic evaluation and family-based management of these genetic heart diseases.

Conclusions and the Future

Major advances have been made in our understanding of the genetic causes of heart disease. Currently, the widespread commercial availability of genetic testing has facilitated the steady introduction of genetic testing into clinical cardiology practice. Overall, the greatest utility of genetic testing is in the screening and diagnosis of at-risk relatives through predictive genetic testing. There is also some evidence that the underlying genotype may shed light in guiding therapies and contribute to algorithms that predict prognosis.

As we move forward, the challenges we face will be those relating to interpretation of the vast numbers of variants identified from more comprehensive gene tests. Clearly having the appropriate bioinformatics strategies to identify the key DNA variants from background genetic noise and understanding the functional consequences of these DNA changes will all be essential in developing more comprehensive genetic testing strategies in cardiovascular disease.

REFERENCES

1. Ackerman MJ, Priori SG, Willems S, et al. HRS/EHRA expert consensus statement on the state of genetic testing for the channelopathies and cardiomyopathies this document was developed as a partnership between the Heart Rhythm Society (HRS) and the European Heart Rhythm Association (EHRA). *Heart Rhythm.* 2011;8:1308–1339.
2. Richards S, Aziz N, Bale S, et al. Standards and guidelines for the interpretation of sequence variants: a joint consensus recommendation of the American College of Medical Genetics and Genomics and the Association for Molecular Pathology. *Genet Med.* 2015;17:405–424.
3. Ingles J, Semsarian C. Conveying a probabilistic genetic test result to families with an inherited heart disease. *Heart Rhythm.* 2014;11:1073–1078.
4. Ingles J, Yeates L, Semsarian C. The emerging role of the cardiac genetic counselor. *Heart Rhythm.* 2011;8:1958–1962.
5. Dewey FE, Grove ME, Pan C, et al. Clinical interpretation and implications of whole-genome sequencing. *JAMA.* 2014;311:1035–1045.
6. Landrum MJ, Lee JM, Riley GR, et al. ClinVar: public archive of relationships among sequence variation and human phenotype. *Nucleic Acids Res.* 2014;42:D980–D985.
7. Maron BJ, Semsarian C. Emergence of gene mutation carriers and the expanding disease spectrum of hypertrophic cardiomyopathy. *Eur Heart J.* 2010;31:1551–1553.
8. Olivotto I, Ashley EA. INHERIT (INHibition of the renin angiotensin system in hypertrophic cardiomyopathy and the Effect on hypertrophy-a Randomised Intervention Trial with losartan). *Glob Cardiol Sci Pract.* 2015;2015:7.
9. Bezzina CR, Lahrouchi N, Priori SG. Genetics of sudden cardiac death. *Circ Res.* 2015;116:1919–1936.
10. Haissaguerre M, Chatel S, Sacher F, et al. Ventricular fibrillation with prominent early repolarization associated with a rare variant of KCNJ8/KATP channel. *J Cardiovasc Electrophysiol.* 2009;20:93–98.
11. Gersh BJ, Maron BJ, Bonow RO, et al. 2011 ACCF/AHA Guideline for the Diagnosis and Treatment of Hypertrophic Cardiomyopathy: a report of the American College of Cardiology Foundation/American Heart Association Task Force on Practice Guidelines. *J Am Coll Cardiol.* 2011;58:e212–e260.
12. Maron BJ, Maron MS, Semsarian C. Genetics of hypertrophic cardiomyopathy after 20 years: clinical perspectives. *J Am Coll Cardiol.* 2012;60:705–715.
13. Hussein A, Karimianpour A, Collier P, Krasuski RA. Isolated noncompaction of the left ventricle in adults. *J Am Coll Cardiol.* 2015;66:578–585.
14. Semsarian C, Ingles J, Wilde AA. Sudden cardiac death in the young: the molecular autopsy and a practical approach to surviving relatives. *Eur Heart J.* 2015;36:1290–1296.

72 Sinus Node Abnormalities

Dennis H. Lau, Rajiv Mahajan, Jonathan M. Kalman, and Prashanthan Sanders

Although the sinus node has been recognized as the primary cardiac pacemaker for more than a century, our understanding of its complex anatomy, molecular construct, and pacemaking mechanisms remains incomplete.[1] The cell biology of cardiac impulse initiation and propagation in regard to the sinus node are detailed in Part IV. This chapter explores (1) unique anatomical and physiological features of the sinus node, (2) electrophysiological abnormalities in sinus node disease (SND), (3) the genetic basis for familial SND, and (4) factors predisposing to sinus node remodeling.

The Sinus Node

The sinus node is a crescent-shaped structure that resides subepicardially with its long axis parallel to the terminal groove starting at the junction of the superior vena cava and the right atrial appendage and terminating subendocardially near the inferior vena cava. Histological examination of the sinus node has previously revealed a mean length of 13.5 mm and a width of up to 2 to 3 mm in the adult heart.[2] However, a more recent estimation using a combination of techniques, such as diffusion tensor magnetic resonance imaging and immunohistochemistry, has shown the sinus node to be larger: 29.5 mm in length, 1.8 mm in height, and 6.4 mm in width.[3] The sinus node artery is often found to course centrally along the length of the sinus node, although this can also be eccentric. Of note, the sinus node artery arises from the right coronary artery 55% to 60% of the time and from the left circumflex artery at other times. The sinus node is also well innervated with both adrenergic and cholinergic nerves, as detailed in Chapter 37.

Both the innervation and the complex anatomy of the sinus node are integral to its pacemaking function. The sinus node consists of nodal cells packed in a dense connective tissue matrix. Detailed histological examinations reveal that nodal cells are also found intermingled with ordinary atrial myocytes at the nodal periphery. In addition, nodal extensions are also seen extending toward the superior vena cava, subepicardium, and terminal crest.[2] In addition, a discrete paranodal area with loosely packed myocytes has recently been described in close proximity to, but not contiguous with, the sinus node (Fig. 72.1A).[3–4] The molecular construct of this paranodal area reflects a mixture of sinus node and atrial cells with unique ion channel makeup as well as intermediate cell diameter and connexin 43 and atrial natriuretic peptide expression compared with those at the sinus node and atrial myocardium. This paranodal area is quite extensive with continuation toward the inferior vena cava as shown in the three-dimensional (3D) anatomical model of the human sinus node in Fig. 72.1B. The relatively depolarized state of this paranodal area in comparison to the right atrium could therefore facilitate conduction from the sinus node. Further insights regarding the sinus node can also be derived from high-resolution optical mapping studies. The sinus node appears to be insulated by conduction barriers consisting of coronary arteries and fibrous tissues, with specialized preferential conduction pathways that carry the electrical impulse to the surrounding atrium.[5] Indeed, a high-density noncontact mapping study has also demonstrated these preferential pathways of conduction between the sinus node and the atrial exit site, although none of these insulated tracts have been histologically documented.[2,6]

Further, both the sites of sinus activation and sinoatrial exit have been shown to be highly variable, in keeping with prior epicardial mapping studies, demonstrating a widely distributed atrial pacemaker complex centered about the long axis of the sulcus terminalis.[6] Specifically, the beat-to-beat variation at the site of sinus activation ranged from 0 to 41 mm from the superior vena cava and right atrial junction, while the variation in sinoatrial exit site ranged from 0 to 33 mm. It is also known that changes in heart rate and in neural and hormonal factors can cause a shift in both of these pacemaking and exit sites. For example, sympathetic stimulation results in a superior shift of the dominant pacemaking site and an increase in heart rate, while vagal activation leads to a slower but more caudal pacemaking focus.[7] Taken together, the multicentricity of the sinus node complex, the extensive paranodal area that contains both nodal and atrial tissues, and the preferential conduction pathways may all account for the high incidence of spontaneous P-wave variations seen in normal individuals.

Sinus Node Disease

SND is an abnormality in impulse generation of the sinus node, resulting in a mismatch toward physiological demands. The crude incidence rate of SND was found to be 0.8 per 1000 person-years from recent large prospective cohorts.[8] It affects individuals of all ages, with higher incidence in older individuals, which is in part due to idiopathic degenerative disease. However, causes of SND

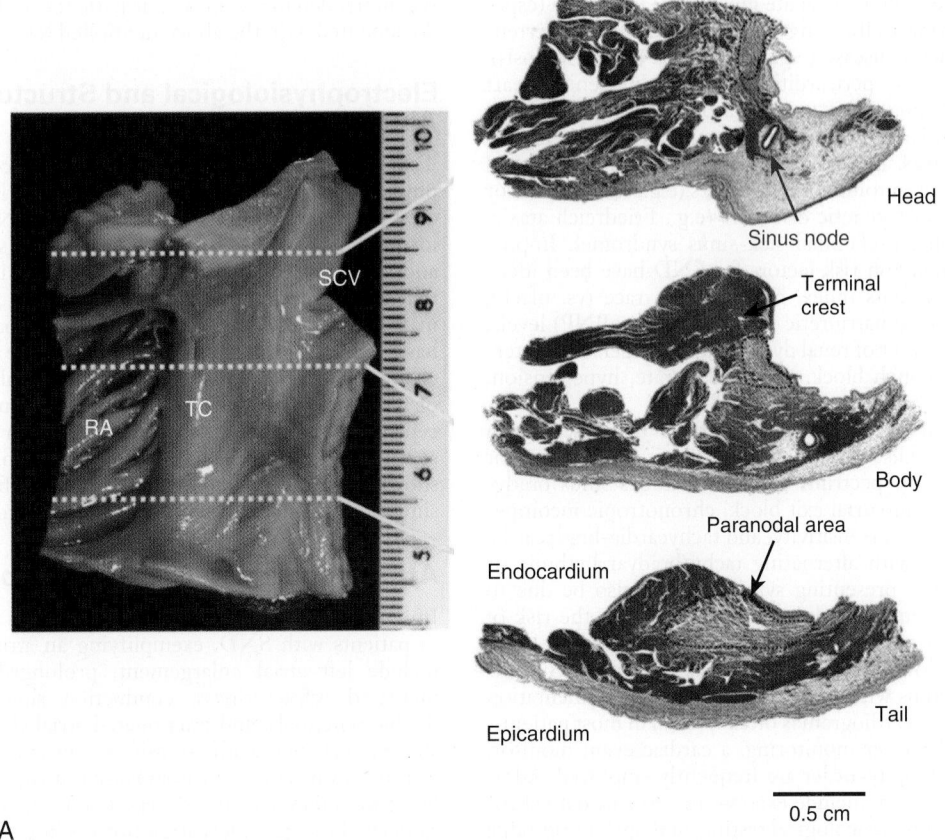

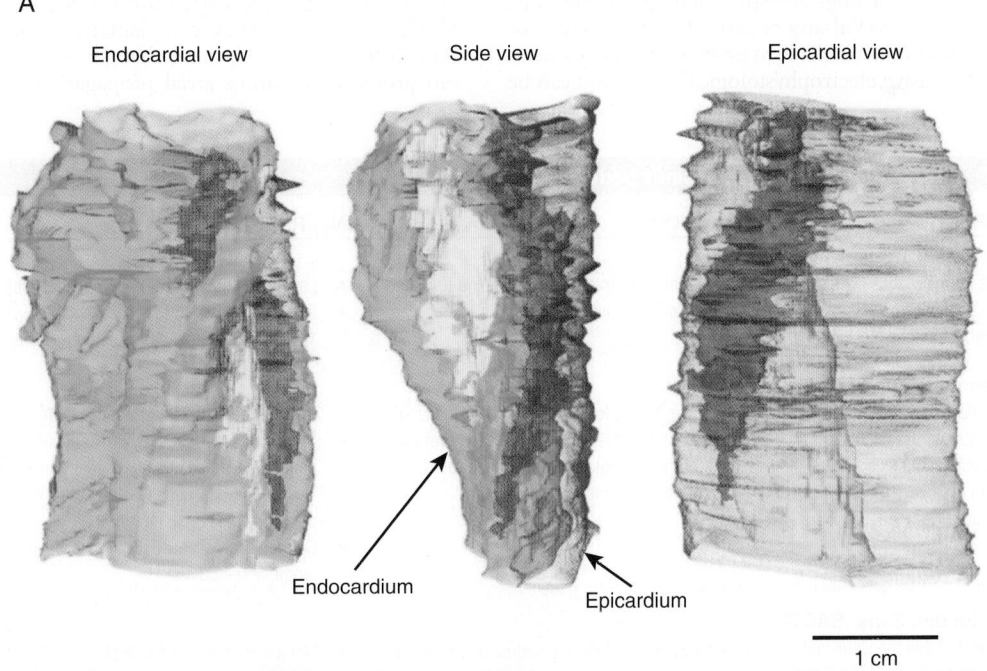

FIGURE 72.1 The sinus node revisited (A) A human sinus node preparation is shown on the left depicting the right atrium (*RA*), terminal crest (*TC*), and superior caval vein (*SCV*). On the right, Masson trichrome sections through the head, body, and tail of the sinus node are shown. These histological specimens demonstrate a paranodal area (*dotted black line*) in close proximity but not contiguous with the sinus node (*dotted red line*). (B) The endocardial, side, and epicardial views of the three-dimensional anatomical model of the human sinus node are shown here with different tissue components marked in different colors (*green*, atrial muscle; *red*, sinus node; *yellow*, paranodal area; and *blue*, adipose tissue). The paranodal area appears quite extensive, with continuation toward the inferior vena cava. (From Chandler N, Aslanidi O, Buckley D, et al. Computer three-dimensional anatomical reconstruction of the human sinus node and a novel paranodal area. *Anat Rec.* 2011;294:970-979.)

can also include the following: acute myocardial infarction (especially of the inferior wall), congestive heart failure, hypertension, infiltrative heart disease (e.g., sarcoidosis or amyloidosis), pericardial disease (e.g., pericarditis or tumor), congenital heart disease, surgical trauma, drugs (e.g., beta-blockers, calcium channel blockers, or antiarrhythmics), autonomic influences, electrolyte imbalance, sepsis, hypothyroidism, hypothermia, increased intracranial pressure, autoimmune disorders (e.g., scleroderma or Reiter syndrome), and genetic disorders (e.g., Friedreich ataxia, myotonic dystrophy, or familial sick sinus syndrome). Importantly, several population risk factors for SND have been identified: greater body mass index, height, white race (vs. black), N-terminal pro b-type natriuretic peptide (NT-proBNP) levels, cystatin C levels (marker of renal dysfunction), longer QRS interval, right bundle-branch block, lower heart rate, hypertension, and past history of cardiovascular events.[8]

Patients with SND can be asymptomatic or present with dizziness, syncope, falls, lethargy, reduced exercise capacity, or dyspnea. The clinical spectrum of SND includes sinus bradycardia, sinus arrest, sinoatrial exit block, chronotropic incompetence, carotid sinus hypersensitivity, and tachycardia-bradycardia syndrome. In those with alternating tachy/bradyarrhythmia or atrial fibrillation, the presenting symptoms can also be due to cerebral vascular events or palpitations. Specifically, the risk of atrial fibrillation in patients with SND is at least one in three with long-term follow-up. The challenge in diagnosing SND is to correlate symptoms with electrocardiographic documentation as the 12-lead electrocardiogram is often normal in most patients. As such, extended Holter monitoring, a cardiac event monitor, or an implantable loop recorder are frequently employed. Additional investigations may include exercise test to elucidate chronotropic response; pharmacological testing; and upright tilt table test, autonomic maneuvers (Valsalva or carotid sinus massage), or pharmacological autonomic blockade to evaluate the role of autonomic influences. Invasive electrophysiological evaluation can be recommended for symptomatic patients in whom SND cannot be documented with the abovementioned tests.

Electrophysiological and Structural Abnormalities

Table 72.1 presents a summary of various conventional electrophysiological measures of sinus node function. These measures of sinus node function in patients with SND can reveal a low intrinsic heart rate as well as prolonged sinus node recovery and sinoatrial conduction times. Of note, it is well established that these tests have their own limitations, with wide variations in their "normal" range. However, electroanatomical mapping has provided further insights regarding the electrophysiological changes in SND with attenuation of the multicentricity property of the sinus node complex, resulting in a more caudal and unicentric pacemaking site close to the region with largest voltage at the crista terminalis.[9] In addition, multiple early studies have shown evidence of atrophy and increased fibrous tissues in the sinus nodes of patients with sick sinus syndrome.[10]

Atrial Abnormalities in Sinus Node Disease

Importantly, significant atrial abnormalities have been described in patients with SND, exemplifying an atrial myopathy. These include left atrial enlargement, prolonged P wave duration, increased refractoriness, conduction slowing with increased double potentials, and fractionated atrial electrograms as well as structural changes with extensive regions of low voltage and scar.[9] Recent advancement in noninvasive imaging of the atria using late-gadolinium–enhanced magnetic resonance imaging has also associated increased left atrial fibrosis in patients with significant SND, requiring pacemaker implantation following atrial fibrillation ablation.[11] Indeed, these changes constitute a substrate that can promote circuitous atrial propagation and perpetuation of

---

TABLE 72.1 Interventional measures of sinus node function

TEST AND DEFINITION	TECHNIQUE	INTERPRETATION
Intrinsic Heart Rate (IHR) • This represents intrinsic sinus node rate sans autonomic influence achieved by pharmacological autonomic blockade	Administration of intravenous atropine (0.04 mg/kg) and propranolol (0.2 mg/kg)	• Low IHR is thought to represent sinus nose disease (SND) • IHR (beats/min) = 118.1 – (0.57 × age), with a range of ± 14 and 18% based on age <45 years and >45 years, respectively
Sinus Node Recovery Time (SNRT) • Test of sinus node automaticity • Longest time interval from the end of overdrive suppression of sinus node activity to return of P wave on surface electrocardiogram	Continuous pacing for 30–60 s is performed in the high right atrium at multiple and progressively shorter cycle lengths in decrements of 50–100 ms, down to 300 ms	• Most widely used test for sinus node automaticity • SNRT can be affected by proximity of pacing site to sinus node and the presence of sinoatrial entrance or exit block • Normal SNRT is usually <1500 ms but varies according to baseline sinus cycle length • Corrected SNRT = SNRT minus baseline cycle length (normal range, 350–550 ms)
Sinoatrial Conduction Time (SACT) • Test of conduction within the sinus node • Time interval from sinus impulse to atrial depolarization	Direct recordings: This is performed with a catheter of close interelectrode spacing (5–15 mm) using high-gain nonfiltered electrograms Indirect methods: Several different methods are used, with each employing different pacing maneuver of atrial premature stimulations and pacing slightly faster than sinus rate	• Not a sensitive test for SND • Direct recordings cannot be obtained in all patients due to technical reasons • In general, for the indirect methods, the intervals between the premature and subsequent sinus beat (A2–A3) and the baseline sinus cycle length (A1–A1) are first measured. The (A2–A3) interval should encompass the (A1–A1) interval plus the time for A2 to enter and exit the sinus node. Therefore the SACT is taken as [(A2–A3) – (A1–A1)]/2. • SACT can be affected by the site of stimulation, rate of premature stimulation (A2), and presence of marked sinus arrhythmia • There is a wide normal range in SACT ~50–120 ms

atrial arrhythmia and may, in part, account for the higher atrial fibrillation recurrence rates in patients with SND following pulmonary vein isolation.[12] This increased vulnerability to atrial fibrillation has also been experimentally shown in a canine model of SND.[13] Recent experimental data also suggest that atrial fibrillation may occur as a result of the competing electrical activations between the sinus node and pulmonary veins when sinus node to pulmonary vein conduction block led to increased pulmonary vein arrhythmogenesis.[14] Furthermore, echocardiographic evaluation of atrial mechanical function has also demonstrated evidence of atrial mechanical dyssynchrony in SND, with lower mitral inflow A velocity and prolonged interatrial dyssynchrony found to be independent predictors for atrial fibrillation.[15]

Familial Sick Node Disease

Despite the advances made in the field of cardiovascular genetics, the familial causes of sick sinus syndrome remain poorly defined. Most of these known mutations were identified from studies investigating family clusters of SND.

SCN5A Mutations

Mutations in the SCN5A gene, which encodes the α subunit of the cardiac sodium channel ($Na_v1.5$), have been associated with SND as well as several heart rhythm disorders, including Brugada syndrome, long QT syndrome type 3, increased susceptibility to atrial fibrillation, and progressive cardiac conduction defect.[16] Familial SND patients with SCN5A gene mutation have been shown to have a male predominance and an earlier age of onset.[17] To date, at least 20 mutations in the SCN5A gene have been identified leading to both loss of function and gain of function of the $Na_v1.5$.[18-19] Loss-of-function mutation of $Na_v1.5$ results in impairment of impulse initiation and impulse propagation both within the SA node and between the SA node and the atrium, whereas gain-of-function mutation of the $Na_v1.5$ results in sinus bradycardia, as seen in patients with long QT syndrome type 3.[20]

Interestingly, given that $Na_v1.5$ was only found in the periphery but not in the center of the murine sinus node, animal studies suggest that $Na_v1.5$ appears to only play a secondary pacemaking role by facilitating action potential propagation without contributing to the sinoatrial node automaticity.[21-22] However, one report suggested the presence of sodium current in human sinoatrial nodal cells.[23] This has since been confirmed by a subsequent study using immunohistochemistry and qualitative polymerase chain reaction, whereby both protein expression and mRNA levels of $Na_v1.5$ were seen in the human sinus node, although these were significantly lower than those in the paranodal area and the right atrium.[4]

The mechanisms underlying SND due to SCN5A mutations are likely to be complex. Insights can be gained from a heterozygous SCN5A knockout model, whereby SCN5A deficiency led to sinus bradycardia and prolonged sinoatrial conduction time, which is indicative of decreased sinoatrial node automaticity and slower conduction.[24] These electrophysiological changes were accompanied by transforming growth factor (TGF)-β_1-mediated fibrosis in the sinoatrial node as well as transcriptional remodeling of ion channels, thereby demonstrating the regulatory role for $Na_v1.5$ in cellular biological process. In addition, recent comprehensive biophysical characterization of mutant $Na_v1.5$ channels linked to familial sick sinus syndrome has revealed multiple molecular mechanisms, including various channel-gating abnormalities and trafficking defects.[25]

HCN4 Mutations

The HCN4 channels are responsible for the hyperpolarization-activated funny current (I_f) essential to sinoatrial node

automaticity. This can be seen in transgenic mice with cardiac specific knockout of the HCN4 gene, whereby there was severe progressive bradycardia.[26] These channels are highly expressed in the sinus node, with mutations in the HCN4 gene also found to be associated with familial SND. These loss-of-function mutations result in reduced I_f in the diastolic depolarization range of sinoatrial cells, thereby contributing to impaired impulse generation together with variable phenotypes. Specifically, more variants have now been identified in different families with (1) sinus bradycardia, chronotropic incompetence, and atrial fibrillation with single base-pair deletion in exon 5 of the HCN4 gene (573X)[27]; (2) sinus node dysfunction, QT prolongation, and polymorphic ventricular tachycardia with a missense mutation in the HCN4 C-linker (D553N)[28]; (3) sinus bradycardia, cardiac arrest, and atrial fibrillation with mutation in the pore region of the HCN4 channel (A485V)[29]; (4) sinus bradycardia with HCN4 mutation near a cyclic AMP binding site (S672R)[30]; (5) sinus bradycardia with point mutation in the HCN4 ion channel pore (G480R)[31]; (6) sinus bradycardia with myocardial noncompaction (with or without atrial fibrillation, mitral valve prolapse, and sudden cardiac arrest) with different mutations in the pore and linker domains of the HCN4 gene (A414G, G482R, Y481H, and 695X)[32-33]; and (7) tachycardia-bradycardia syndrome, sinus pauses, and atrial fibrillation with HCN4 gene mutation (K530N) affecting C-linker oligomerization.[34] While other isoforms of the HCN gene (HCN1 and HCN2) are known to exist in the sinus node with experimental studies demonstrating their potential role in sinus node pacemaking, mutations of these isoforms are yet to be identified.[35-37]

ANK2 Mutations

The ankyrin family of proteins is involved in targeting and membrane stabilization of cardiac ion channels, among its many other functions. Specifically, mutation of the ANK2 gene, which encodes ankyrin-B, has been identified in long QT syndrome type 4 patients who also had increased atrial fibrillation, ventricular arrhythmias, and severe sinus node dysfunction.[38] Experimental study incorporating computational analysis in an ankyrin-B–deficient mouse model has shown a diverse substrate for arrhythmias, including increased atrial fibrosis, slowing of spontaneous pacemaking and action potential shortening due to loss of $Ca_v1.3$, increased variability of sinus node firing and delayed ventricular repolarization due to loss of Na^+/K^+ ATPase, and an overload of calcium in the sarcoplasmic reticulum due to loss of the Na^+/Ca^{2+} exchanger.[39] Recent work has also highlighted that ankyrin-B is present in the human sinoatrial node and plays an important role in targeting ion channels and transporters, calcium homeostasis, and nodal automaticity.[40] Multiple ANK2 loss-of-function variants are known, which can each result in different severities of clinical phenotypes, but the underlying molecular basis remains incompletely understood.

MYH6 Mutations

Genome-wide association study has uncovered a rare missense variant of the MYH6 gene that encodes the alpha heavy chain subunit of cardiac myosin to be associated with high risk of sick sinus syndrome.[41] Normal controls with the R721W variant also demonstrated slower heart rate and longer PR interval. Further, a novel MYH6 delE933 mutation has also been reported in a sick sinus syndrome patient.[42] This mutation was found to impair atrial action potential propagation and disrupt sarcomere integrity when expressed in cardiomyocytes. Taken together, these new findings present a new disease entity of inheritable arrhythmia due to mutations in noncardiac ion channel genes.

Other Mutations

Patients with catecholaminergic polymorphic ventricular tachycardia (CPVT) have been associated with an increased risk of atrial arrhythmias and sinus node dysfunction.[43] Specifically, CPVT patients with mutations in the Calsequestrin 2 (CASQ2) gene are known to exhibit resting bradycardia as in CASQ2-null mice.[44-46] The functional and structural effects of CASQ2 deletion have been detailed in experimental study, with evidence of abnormal sarcoplasmic reticulum calcium release, selective interstitial fibrosis within the sinus node leading to abnormal pacemaking, and increased conduction abnormalities leading to increased atrial fibrillation inducibility.[47]

Emerin is a nuclear envelope protein encoded by the EMD gene. Mutation in the EMD gene (Lys37del) can result in Emery–Dreifuss muscular dystrophy when a coexisting LMNA mutation is present. Emery–Dreifuss muscular dystrophy is an X-linked disorder characterized by muscle contractures, progressive skeletal myopathy, cardiomyopathy, SND in early adulthood, and atrial fibrillation.[48] However, the same EMD gene mutation has also been linked with nonsyndromic X-linked atrial fibrillation and SND.[49]

Sinus Node Remodeling

Subclinical changes in sinus node function have been described in a number of known causative as well as novel risk factors for SND. It is likely that a threshold needs to be reached in each individual before sinus node remodeling manifests clinically as SND, and the presence of multiple such risk factors would likely accelerate this process.

Aging

Sinus node function is known to deteriorate with aging, which can account for the increased incidence of SND and pacemaker implantations in this population.

Electrophysiological Remodeling

Both clinical and basic studies have demonstrated that the intrinsic heart rate decreases, whereas sinoatrial conduction time increases with aging.[7,24,50-53] Specifically, detailed mapping of the sinoatrial region has shown increased conduction time and reduced conduction velocity of the action potential across the sinus node.[51] An inferior shift of the leading pacemaker site has also been shown in the murine aging model.[52] Furthermore, sinus node recovery time was found to be significantly prolonged with aging, together with a global atrial electrical remodeling process.[50,54] The senescent sinus node also exhibited increased action potential duration.[50]

Structural Remodeling

Significant structural changes of the sinus node have been documented with senescence. These include an enlarged sinus node complex with increased collagen content, increased sinoatrial conduction distance, hypertrophy of the sinoatrial cells, and increased area lacking connexin 43.[52,55-56] Aging-related reduction in connexin 43 may be related to long-term activation of C-Jun amino-terminal kinase (JNK), resulting in altered conduction.[51] In addition, extracellular matrix remodeling due to aging has shown variable changes in the murine sinus node, including TGF-β_1–mediated interstitial fibrosis[24] or a decrease in type 1 and 3 collagen, despite a decrease in matrix metalloproteinase 2 and elastin, and increased TGF-β_1 and tumor necrosis factor α in another study.[52] Nevertheless, the signaling cascade underlying aging-related structural remodeling of the sinus node is highly complex and remains incompletely understood.

Ionic Remodeling

While the structural changes may in part account for the electrophysiological manifestations, age-related ionic changes are also important contributors to sinus node remodeling. At present, the molecular mechanisms involved in aging-related ionic remodeling are poorly defined. Initial preclinical study has shown reduced HCN2 and HCN4 expression and function (responsible for the pacemaker current, I_f), which could account for the reduced SA node automaticity in the aging sinus node.[57] In a guinea pig model, the aging sinus node showed a decline in the expression of the $Ca_v1.2$ protein (responsible for $I_{Ca,L}$), with greater sensitivity to calcium channel blockade and reduced amplitude of extracellular potential, which could account for reduced sinus node excitability.[53] However, a myriad of age-dependent changes in the mRNA transcripts of ion channels involved in normal pacemaking has been described with increased $Na_v1.5$ (responsible for I_{Na}), $Ca_v1.2$ ($I_{Ca,L}$), $K_v1.2$ and $K_v4.2$ (I_{to}), K_vLQT1 ($I_{K,s}$), and $K_{ir}6.1$ ($I_{K,ATP}$), together with decreased HCN1 (I_f), $K_v1.5$ ($I_{K,ur}$), and $K_{ir}3.4$ ($I_{K,ACh}$).[50] The same study also demonstrated a significant decrease in ryanodine receptor (RYR2) expression that might contribute to aging-related intrinsic heart rate slowing.[50]

In addition, reduced intrinsic sinoatrial automaticity due to aging can be secondary to deficits in sarcoplasmic reticulum calcium cycling and its response to cAMP-dependent pathway activation, as demonstrated in cellular studies.[58] Altered ion channel activity in the form of reduced L- and T-type calcium currents and I_f, as well as a hyperpolarizing shift in I_f, has also been associated with the depressed excitability of the sinoatrial myocyte that may contribute to the age-dependent decline in maximum heart rate.[59] Age-dependent sinus node dysfunction during physical or mental stress has also been demonstrated in mice with popeye domain–containing gene deficiency.[60] These popeye domain–containing genes are novel membrane-localized cAMP-binding proteins, but the mechanisms by which they impact sinus node function remain to be elucidated.

Congestive Heart Failure

Reduced sinus node reserve has been documented in patients with congestive heart failure, resulting in an increased risk of iatrogenic SND when concurrent negatively chronotropic agents are used to improve the prognosis in such patients.[61-62]

Electrophysiological Remodeling

Prolongation of intrinsic sinus cycle length, sinoatrial conduction time, and sinus node recovery time have been demonstrated in heart failure patients along with a caudal shift in sinus node activity.[61-62] Similar electrophysiological findings were demonstrated in both large and small animal models of ischemic and nonischemic heart failure.[63-66]

Structural Remodeling

Indirect evidence of structural remodeling of the sinus node in patients with heart failure can be gained from electroanatomical mapping findings of reduced bipolar voltage amplitude in the superior region of the crista terminalis, as well as areas of electrical silence, indicating scarring along the crista terminalis.[62]

Ionic Remodeling

Early work in isolated sinoatrial cells from rabbits with volume and pressure overload–induced heart failure showed a reduction in both I_f and $I_{K,s}$.[63] Both HCN2 and HCN4 expressions at the mRNA and protein levels were also significantly reduced in the sinus nodes of dogs with pacing-induced heart failure.[64] Together, these studies suggest the contribution of I_f remodeling to reduced sinus node automaticity. Moreover, there is evidence of impaired rhythmic spontaneous sarcoplasmic reticulum calcium release in the superior sinus node of heart failure dogs.[65] Recent detailed gene expression analysis showed extensive ionic remodeling at the mRNA level in a small animal model of ischemic heart failure.[66] However, differential results were seen with increased HCN2 and HCN4 expression, I_{Na} and $I_{Ca,L}$, $I_{K,r}$ and $I_{K,s}$, and RYR2. Further, in heart failure rabbit sinoatrial nodal cells, only slowed calcium transient decay has been demonstrated without significant changes in sarcoplasmic reticulum calcium content, I_{NCX} density, or calcium transient with β-adrenergic or muscarinic receptor stimulation.[67] This was not likely to have much impact on the pacemaking function. Nevertheless, the reduced late diastolic calcium rise during β-adrenergic stimulation may explain the reduced intrinsic heart rate increase in such situations.[67] Further research will continue to improve our understanding of the mechanisms underlying ionic remodeling due to heart failure.

Atrial Arrhythmias

Patients with SND can sometimes present with tachy/bradyarrhythmic syndrome. Their increased risk of developing atrial fibrillation can be accounted for by the underlying atrial myopathy. On the other hand, it is also known that patients with atrial arrhythmias demonstrate subclinical changes in sinus node function.

Electrophysiological Remodeling

Previous reviews have highlighted in detail the electrophysiological remodeling of the sinus node due to rapid atrial pacing model or atrial fibrillation in a myriad of preclinical and clinical studies.[1,7] In brief, these changes include slowing of intrinsic heart rate, prolonged sinus node recovery time, and increased sinoatrial conduction time.[68-70] Importantly, these changes were evident even following transient exposure of the sinus node to atrial arrhythmia, while reverse remodeling has also been demonstrated following termination of the arrhythmia.[71] Further, in pacemaker patients with atrial arrhythmias, P-wave duration was prolonged, but atrial refractoriness remained unchanged compared with that in patients without atrial arrhythmias.[72] High-density noncontact mapping has shown a caudal shift in sinus node activation with slower conduction along preferential pathways in patients with chronic atrial flutter.[6] In addition, electroanatomical mapping in atrial fibrillation patients with symptomatic bradycardia has shown a lack of cranial shift of the earliest activation site following sympathetic stimulation to indicate superior sinoatrial node dysfunction.[73]

Structural Remodeling

Progressive fibrosis with cell loss and degeneration has been noted in the sinus node of patients with long-standing chronic atrial fibrillation.[74] This was in keeping with recent electroanatomical mapping in patients with atrial arrhythmias demonstrating significantly lower bipolar voltage in the sinus node region near the high lateral right atrium.[6,68] In addition, a significant reduction in the amount of capillaries in the sinus node was seen in chronic atrial fibrillation patients, thereby implicating ischemia as one likely mechanism for sinus node remodeling due to atrial arrhythmias.[75]

Ionic Remodeling

In a rapid-pacing canine model of atrial fibrillation, downregulation of sinus node HCN2 and HCN4 as well as mink subunit expression at the mRNA levels have been reported together with reduced densities of their corresponding I_f and $I_{K,s}$.[69] In the same animal model, downregulation of RYR2 expression was evident in the superior sinus node. Furthermore, there was impairment of isoproterenol-induced late diastolic calcium elevation and reduced heart rate response to caffeine in the superior sinus node, suggesting impaired spontaneous sarcoplasmic reticulum calcium release.[70] Taken together, both abnormal membrane and calcium clocks are implicated in the atrial arrhythmia–related ionic remodeling of the sinus node.

Other Associated Conditions

In addition to the abovementioned factors, several other conditions are also known to affect sinus node function, including atrial septal defects, loss of atrioventricular synchrony due to VVI pacing, pulmonary hypertension with right ventricular hypertrophy, diabetes mellitus, coronary artery disease, and obstructive sleep apnea.[1,10,76,77] Recent experimental work has also uncovered the molecular basis underlying sinus node remodeling with endurance training of HCN4 downregulation.[78] Interestingly, all of these conditions are associated with abnormal atrial substrates that predispose to the development of atrial fibrillation.

Conclusions

Advancements in cardiovascular mapping, molecular biology, and genetics over the last few decades have enhanced our understanding of the complex nature of the sinus node. However, the added knowledge has also highlighted new challenges to further unravel the mechanistic aspects underlying various sinus node abnormalities.

REFERENCES

1. Lau DH, Roberts-Thomson KC, Sanders P. Sinus node revisited. *Curr Opin Cardiol*. 2011;26:55–59.
2. Sanchez-Quintana D, Cabrera JA, Farre J, Climent V, Anderson RH, Ho SY. Sinus node revisited in the era of electroanatomical mapping and catheter ablation. *Heart*. 2005;91:189–194.
3. Chandler N, Aslanidi O, Buckley D, et al. Computer three-dimensional anatomical reconstruction of the human sinus node and a novel paranodal area. *Anat Rec (Hoboken)*. 2011;294:970–979.
4. Chandler NJ, Greener ID, Tellez JO, et al. Molecular architecture of the human sinus node: insights into the function of the cardiac pacemaker. *Circulation*. 2009;119:1562–1575.
5. Fedorov VV, Glukhov AV, Chang R. Conduction barriers and pathways of the sinoatrial pacemaker complex: their role in normal rhythm and atrial arrhythmias. *Am J Physiol Heart Circ Physiol*. 2012;302:H1773–H1783.
6. Stiles MK, Brooks AG, Roberts-Thomson KC, et al. High-density mapping of the sinus node in humans: role of preferential pathways and the effect of remodeling. *J Cardiovasc Electrophysiol*. 2010;21:532–539.
7. Dobrzynski H, Boyett MR, Anderson RH. New insights into pacemaker activity: promoting understanding of sick sinus syndrome. *Circulation*. 2007;115:1921–1932.

8. Jensen PN, Gronroos NN, Chen LY, et al. Incidence of and risk factors for sick sinus syndrome in the general population. *J Am Coll Cardiol*. 2014;64:531–538.
9. Sanders P, Morton JB, Kistler PM, et al. Electrophysiological and electroanatomic characterization of the atria in sinus node disease: evidence of diffuse atrial remodeling. *Circulation*. 2004;109:1514–1522.
10. Monfredi O, Dobrzynski H, Mondal T, Boyett MR, Morris GM. The anatomy and physiology of the sinoatrial node–a contemporary review. *Pacing Clin Electrophysiol*. 2010;33:1392–1406.
11. Akoum N, McGann C, Vergara G, et al. Atrial fibrosis quantified using late gadolinium enhancement MRI is associated with sinus node dysfunction requiring pacemaker implant. *J Cardiovasc Electrophysiol*. 2012;23:44–50.
12. Soga Y, Okabayashi H, Arai Y, et al. Up to 6-year follow-up after pulmonary vein isolation for persistent/permanent atrial fibrillation: importance of sinus node function. *J Thorac Cardiovasc Surg*. 2011;141:1455–1460.
13. Li G, Liu E, Liu T, et al. Atrial electrical remodeling in a canine model of sinus node dysfunction. *Int J Cardiol*. 2011;146:32–36.
14. Chen YC, Lu YY, Cheng CC, Lin YK, Chen SA, Chen YJ. Sinoatrial node electrical activity modulates pulmonary vein arrhythmogenesis. *Int J Cardiol*. 2014;173:447–452.

15. Wang M, Lau CP, Zhang XH, et al. Interatrial mechanical dyssynchrony worsened atrial mechanical function in sinus node disease with or without paroxysmal atrial fibrillation. *J Cardiovasc Electrophysiol*. 2009;20: 1237–1243.
16. Ruan Y, Liu N, Priori SG. Sodium channel mutations and arrhythmias. *Nat Rev Cardiol*. 2009;6:337–348.
17. Abe K, Machida T, Sumitomo N, et al. Sodium channelopathy underlying familial sick sinus syndrome with early onset and predominantly male characteristics. *Circ Arrhythm Electrophysiol*. 2014;7:511–517.
18. Lei M, Zhang H, Grace AA, Huang CL. SCN5A and sinoatrial node pacemaker function. *Cardiovasc Res*. 2007;74:356–365.
19. Lei M, Huang CL, Zhang Y. Genetic Na+ channelopathies and sinus node dysfunction. *Prog Biophys Mol Biol*. 2008;98:171–178.
20. Benson DW, Wang DW, Dyment M, et al. Congenital sick sinus syndrome caused by recessive mutations in the cardiac sodium channel gene (SCN5A). *J Clin Invest*. 2003;112:1019–1028.
21. Protas L, Oren RV, Clancy CE, Robinson RB. Age-dependent changes in Na current magnitude and TTX-sensitivity in the canine sinoatrial node. *J Mol Cell Cardiol*. 2010;48:172–180.

22. Lei M, Jones SA, Liu J, et al. Requirement of neuronal- and cardiac-type sodium channels for murine sinoatrial node pacemaking. *J Physiol.* 2004;559:835–848.
23. Verkerk AO, Wilders R, van Borren MM, Tan HL. Is sodium current present in human sinoatrial node cells? *Int J Biol Sci.* 2009;5:201–204.
24. Hao X, Zhang Y, Zhang X, et al. TGF-beta1-mediated fibrosis and ion channel remodeling are key mechanisms in producing the sinus node dysfunction associated with SCN5A deficiency and aging. *Circ Arrhythm Electrophysiol.* 2011;4:397–406.
25. Gui J, Wang T, Jones RP, Trump D, Zimmer T, Lei M. Multiple loss-of-function mechanisms contribute to SCN5A-related familial sick sinus syndrome. *PLoS One.* 2010;5:e10985.
26. Baruscotti M, Bucchi A, Viscomi C, et al. Deep bradycardia and heart block caused by inducible cardiac-specific knockout of the pacemaker channel gene Hcn4. *Proc Natl Acad Sci U S A.* 2011;108:1705–1710.
27. Schulze-Bahr E, Neu A, Friederich P, et al. Pacemaker channel dysfunction in a patient with sinus node disease. *J Clin Invest.* 2003;111:1537–1545.
28. Ueda K, Nakamura K, Hayashi T, et al. Functional characterization of a trafficking-defective HCN4 mutation, D553N, associated with cardiac arrhythmia. *J Biol Chem.* 2004;279:27194–27198.
29. Laish-Farkash A, Glikson M, Brass D, et al. A novel mutation in the HCN4 gene causes symptomatic sinus bradycardia in Moroccan Jews. *J Cardiovasc Electrophysiol.* 2010;21:1365–1372.
30. Milanesi R, Baruscotti M, Gnecchi-Ruscone T, DiFrancesco D. Familial sinus bradycardia associated with a mutation in the cardiac pacemaker channel. *N Engl J Med.* 2006;354:151–157.
31. Nof E, Luria D, Brass D, et al. Point mutation in the HCN4 cardiac ion channel pore affecting synthesis, trafficking, and functional expression is associated with familial asymptomatic sinus bradycardia. *Circulation.* 2007;116:463–470.
32. Schweizer PA, Schroter J, Greiner S, et al. The symptom complex of familial sinus node dysfunction and myocardial noncompaction is associated with mutations in the HCN4 channel. *J Am Coll Cardiol.* 2014;64:757–767.
33. Milano A, Vermeer AM, Lodder EM, et al. HCN4 mutations in multiple families with bradycardia and left ventricular noncompaction cardiomyopathy. *J Am Coll Cardiol.* 2014;64:745–756.
34. Duhme N, Schweizer PA, Thomas D, et al. Altered HCN4 channel C-linker interaction is associated with familial tachycardia-bradycardia syndrome and atrial fibrillation. *Eur Heart J.* 2013;34:2768–2775.
35. Li N, Csepe TA, Hansen BJ, et al. Molecular mapping of sinoatrial node HCN channel expression in the human heart. *Circ Arrhythm Electrophysiol.* 2015;8:1219–1227.
36. Fenske S, Krause SC, Hassan SI, et al. Sick sinus syndrome in HCN1-deficient mice. *Circulation.* 2013;128:2585–2594.
37. Ludwig A, Budde T, Stieber J, et al. Absence epilepsy and sinus dysrhythmia in mice lacking the pacemaker channel HCN2. *EMBO J.* 2003;22:216–224.
38. Hashemi SM, Hund TJ, Mohler PJ. Cardiac ankyrins in health and disease. *J Mol Cell Cardiol.* 2009;47:203–209.
39. Wolf RM, Glynn P, Hashemi S, et al. Atrial fibrillation and sinus node dysfunction in human ankyrin-B syndrome: a computational analysis. *Am J Physiol Heart Circ Physiol.* 2013;304:H1253–H1266.
40. Le Scouarnec S, Bhasin N, Vieyres C, et al. Dysfunction in ankyrin-B-dependent ion channel and transporter targeting causes human sinus node disease. *Proc Natl Acad Sci U S A.* 2008;105:15617–15622.
41. Holm H, Gudbjartsson DF, Sulem P, et al. A rare variant in MYH6 is associated with high risk of sick sinus syndrome. *Nat Genet.* 2011;43:316–320.

42. Ishikawa T, Jou CJ, Nogami A, et al. Novel mutation in the alpha-myosin heavy chain gene is associated with sick sinus syndrome. *Circ Arrhythm Electrophysiol.* 2015;8:400–408.
43. Sumitomo N, Sakurada H, Taniguchi K, et al. Association of atrial arrhythmia and sinus node dysfunction in patients with catecholaminergic polymorphic ventricular tachycardia. *Circ J.* 2007;71:1606–1609.
44. Lahat H, Pras E, Olender T, et al. A missense mutation in a highly conserved region of CASQ2 is associated with autosomal recessive catecholamine-induced polymorphic ventricular tachycardia in Bedouin families from Israel. *Am J Hum Genet.* 2001;69:1378–1384.
45. Postma AV, Denjoy I, Hoorntje TM, et al. Absence of calsequestrin 2 causes severe forms of catecholaminergic polymorphic ventricular tachycardia. *Circ Res.* 2002;91:e21–e26.
46. Knollmann BC, Chopra N, Hlaing T, et al. Casq2 deletion causes sarcoplasmic reticulum volume increase, premature Ca2+ release, and catecholaminergic polymorphic ventricular tachycardia. *J Clin Invest.* 2006;116:2510–2520.
47. Glukhov AV, Kalyanasundaram A, Lou Q, Hage LT, et al. Calsequestrin 2 deletion causes sinoatrial node dysfunction and atrial arrhythmias associated with altered sarcoplasmic reticulum calcium cycling and degenerative fibrosis within the mouse atrial pacemaker complex1. *Eur Heart J.* 2015;36:686–697.
48. Ben Yaou R, Toutain A, Arimura T, et al. Multitissular involvement in a family with LMNA and EMD mutations: role of digenic mechanism? *Neurology.* 2007;68:1883–1894.
49. Karst ML, Herron KJ, Olson TM. X-linked nonsyndromic sinus node dysfunction and atrial fibrillation caused by emerin mutation. *J Cardiovasc Electrophysiol.* 2008;19:510–515.
50. Tellez JO, McZewski M, Yanni J, et al. Ageing-dependent remodelling of ion channel and Ca2+ clock genes underlying sino-atrial node pacemaking. *Exp Physiol.* 2011;96:1163–1178.
51. Jones SA. Ageing to arrhythmias: conundrums of connections in the ageing heart. *J Pharm Pharmacol.* 2006;58:1571–1576.
52. Yanni J, Tellez JO, Sutyagin PV, Boyett MR, Dobrzynski H. Structural remodelling of the sinoatrial node in obese old rats. *J Mol Cell Cardiol.* 2010;48:653–662.
53. Jones SA, Boyett MR, Lancaster MK. Declining into failure: the age-dependent loss of the L-type calcium channel within the sinoatrial node. *Circulation.* 2007;115:1183–1190.
54. Kistler PM, Sanders P, Fynn SP, et al. Electrophysiologic and electroanatomic changes in the human atrium associated with age. *J Am Coll Cardiol.* 2004;44:109–116.
55. Jones SA, Lancaster MK, Boyett MR. Ageing-related changes of connexins and conduction within the sinoatrial node. *J Physiol.* 2004;560:429–437.
56. Csepe TA, Kalyanasundaram A, Hansen BJ, Zhao J, Fedorov VV. Fibrosis: a structural modulator of sinoatrial node physiology and dysfunction. *Front Physiol.* 2015;6:37.
57. Huang X, Yang P, Du Y, Zhang J, Ma A. Age-related down-regulation of HCN channels in rat sinoatrial node. *Basic Res Cardiol.* 2007;102:429–435.
58. Liu J, Sirenko S, Juhaszova M, et al. Age-associated abnormalities of intrinsic automaticity of sinoatrial nodal cells are linked to deficient cAMP-PKA-Ca(2+) signaling. *Am J Physiol Heart Circ Physiol.* 2014;306:H1385–H1397.
59. Larson ED, St Clair JR, Sumner WA, Bannister RA, Proenza C. Depressed pacemaker activity of sinoatrial node myocytes contributes to the age-dependent decline in maximum heart rate. *Proc Natl Acad Sci U S A.* 2013;110:18011–18016.
60. Froese A, Breher SS, Waldeyer C, et al. Popeye domain containing proteins are essential for stress-mediated modulation of cardiac pacemaking in mice. *J Clin Invest.* 2012;122:1119–1130.

61. Sanders P, Morton JB, Davidson NC, et al. Electrical remodeling of the atria in congestive heart failure: electrophysiological and electroanatomic mapping in humans. *Circulation.* 2003;108:1461–1468.
62. Sanders P, Kistler PM, Morton JB, Spence SJ, Kalman JM. Remodeling of sinus node function in patients with congestive heart failure: reduction in sinus node reserve. *Circulation.* 2004;110:897–903.
63. Verkerk AO, Wilders R, Coronel R, Ravesloot JH, Verheijck EE. Ionic remodeling of sinoatrial node cells by heart failure. *Circulation.* 2003;108:760–766.
64. Zicha S, Fernandez-Velasco M, Lonardo G, L'Heureux N, Nattel S. Sinus node dysfunction and hyperpolarization-activated (HCN) channel subunit remodeling in a canine heart failure model. *Cardiovasc Res.* 2005;66:472–481.
65. Shinohara T, Park HW, Han S, et al. Ca2+ clock malfunction in a canine model of pacing-induced heart failure. *Am J Physiol Heart Circ Physiol.* 2010;299:H1805–H1811.
66. Yanni J, Tellez JO, Maczewski M, et al. Changes in ion channel gene expression underlying heart failure-induced sinoatrial node dysfunction. *Circ Heart Fail.* 2011;4:496–508.
67. Verkerk AO, van Borren MM, van Ginneken AC, Wilders R. Ca2+ cycling properties are conserved despite bradycardic effects of heart failure in sinoatrial node cells. *Front Physiol.* 2015;6:18.
68. Stiles MK, John B, Wong CX, et al. Paroxysmal lone atrial fibrillation is associated with an abnormal atrial substrate: characterizing the "second factor.". *J Am Coll Cardiol.* 2009;53:1182–1191.
69. Yeh YH, Burstein B, Qi XY, et al. Funny current down-regulation and sinus node dysfunction associated with atrial tachyarrhythmia: a molecular basis for tachycardia-bradycardia syndrome. *Circulation.* 2009;119:1576–1585.
70. Joung B, Lin SF, Chen Z, et al. Mechanisms of sinoatrial node dysfunction in a canine model of pacing-induced atrial fibrillation. *Heart Rhythm.* 2010;7:88–95.
71. Hocini M, Sanders P, Deisenhofer I, et al. Reverse remodeling of sinus node function after catheter ablation of atrial fibrillation in patients with prolonged sinus pauses. *Circulation.* 2003;108:1172–1175.
72. Healey JS, Israel CW, Connolly SJ, et al. Relevance of electrical remodeling in human atrial fibrillation: results of the asymptomatic atrial fibrillation and stroke evaluation in pacemaker patients and the atrial fibrillation reduction atrial pacing trial mechanisms of atrial fibrillation study. *Circ Arrhythm Electrophysiol.* 2012;5:626–631.
73. Joung B, Hwang HJ, Pak HN, et al. Abnormal response of superior sinoatrial node to sympathetic stimulation is a characteristic finding in patients with atrial fibrillation and symptomatic bradycardia. *Circ Arrhythm Electrophysiol.* 2011;4:799–807.
74. Hurle A, Climent V, Sanchez-Quintana D. Sinus node structural changes in patients with long-standing chronic atrial fibrillation. *J Thorac Cardiovasc Surg.* 2006;131:1394–1395.
75. Hurle A, Sanchez-Quintana D, Ho SY, Bernabeu E, Murillo M, Climent V. Capillary supply to the sinus node in subjects with long-term atrial fibrillation. *Ann Thorac Surg.* 2010;89:38–43.
76. Medi C, Kalman JM, Ling LH, et al. Atrial electrical and structural remodeling associated with longstanding pulmonary hypertension and right ventricular hypertrophy in humans. *J Cardiovasc Electrophysiol.* 2012;23:614–620.
77. Dimitri H, Ng M, Brooks AG, et al. Atrial remodeling in obstructive sleep apnea: implications for atrial fibrillation. *Heart Rhythm.* 2012;9:321–327.
78. D'Souza A, Bucchi A, Johnsen AB, et al. Exercise training reduces resting heart rate via downregulation of the funny channel HCN4. *Nat Commun.* 2014;5:3775.

73 Atrial Tachycardia

Kenneth A. Ellenbogen and Jayanthi N. Koneru

Atrial tachycardias (ATs) are regular atrial rhythms occurring at a constant rate ≥100 beats/min that originate in the atrium and do not require participation of the atrioventricular node (AVN) for maintenance.[1] ATs constitute an important cause of supraventricular tachycardias. The mechanism of AT can be focal or macroreentrant. Since the 1990s, significant advances in our understanding of AT have occurred. The evolution of advanced mapping tools and their integration with imaging modalities have enabled detailed assessment of the substrate and characteristic anatomical locations of ATs. This chapter reviews information about the classification, mechanisms, electrocardiographic localization, and electrophysiological characterization of ATs.

Classification and Mechanisms

An expert consensus group from the European Society of Cardiology and the North American Society of Pacing and Electrophysiology published a classification of atrial flutter (AFL) and regular ATs based on mechanism and anatomy.[1] ATs were classified as tachycardias with a regular atrial rate arising from the atrium and were further categorized as either focal or macroreentrant. *Focal* ATs may be caused by automatic, triggered, or microreentrant mechanisms. Focal ATs are characterized by centrifugal spread of activation from a single focus or point source and lack of electrical activation spanning the tachycardia cycle length (TCL). *Macroreentrant* ATs are due to reentry through relatively large, potentially well-characterized circuits. Patterns that have been described include a single loop (such as common isthmus-dependent flutter), two reentrant loops creating a figure-of-eight, and reentry through narrow channels adjacent to scars or natural anatomical barriers. Typical AFL, lower loop reentry, double-loop reentry, left atrial macroreentrant AT, scar-related and incisional AT, reverse typical AFL, and right atrial free-wall macroreentry are classified as macroreentrant ATs. ATs occurring in the setting of congenital heart disease are described in Chapter 74 and those occurring after atrial fibrillation ablation in Chapter 125.

Under this classification scheme, a few AT origins are left unclassified. For example, inappropriate sinus tachycardia and sinus node reentry cannot be easily classified. Despite the limitations of this classification scheme and the fact that most clinical arrhythmias are not classified by mechanism, it is useful to think of ATs as being either focal or macroreentrant. This differentiation has important implications for ablative therapy because macroreentrant ATs often require mapping large segments of the circuit using techniques of "entrainment mapping" or "scar mapping" and delivery of multiple radiofrequency (RF) ablation lesions for termination of tachycardia.

Surface electrocardiograms (ECGs) are notoriously inadequate for identifying the mechanism of AT. Techniques that utilize quantitative ECG metrics with computerized signal-averaging techniques have been proposed to differentiate between focal and macroreentrant ATs based on the surface ECG.[2] A short atrial activation time relative to the TCL was used to differentiate focal from macroreentrant ATs based on the principle that macroreentrant ATs have activation throughout the TCL in contrast to focal ATs. The investigators were able to develop algorithms to separate P or F wave duration from overlying T waves by transitions in slope or dV/dT relative to the expected T waves generated from scaling of the sinus T wave. Electrocardiographic P wave duration correlated with the duration of intraatrial activation. Focal ATs had shorter P wave durations and smaller ratios of P wave to cycle length. P waves <160 ms and P wave to cycle length ratios <45% differentiated focal AT from macroreentry with promising accuracy in patients who subsequently underwent invasive catheter mapping and ablation.[2]

Focal Atrial Tachycardias

Sustained, focal ATs almost always arise in the absence of significant, preexisting structural heart disease and can arise at any age, with a greater incidence in middle-aged individuals, with no gender predilection. It originates most commonly from the right atrium (RA), and a second focus can be found in 13% of patients. In one large series, among 345 patients with focal AT who underwent RF ablation, only 4% of patients (*n* = 14) had preexisting structural heart disease.[3] However, incessant or very frequent paroxysmal tachycardia can produce a tachycardia-mediated cardiomyopathy. In the series noted above, about 10% of patients with focal AT developed a tachycardia-mediated cardiomyopathy. A slower incessant tachycardia was more frequently complicated by cardiomyopathy and appendage sites were associated with a higher incidence of incessant tachycardia (84%) and left ventricular (LV) dysfunction (42%). Virtually all patients had restoration of normal LV function after successful ablation at a mean of 3 months.

Pathophysiology

Atrial arrhythmias frequently complicate heart failure and atrial enlargement. In an experimental model, Stambler and colleagues demonstrated that heart failure induced by rapid ventricular pacing provides a substrate that predisposes to focal ATs.[4,5] Sustained ATs could be induced in >90% of animals after an average of 3 weeks of heart failure but in <10% at baseline in the absence of heart failure. The mode of AT induction, responses to pacing maneuvers and Ca^{2+} antagonists, and the presence of delayed afterdepolarizations suggested triggered activity, resulting from intracellular Ca^{2+} overload, as the likely tachycardia mechanism. Strikingly similar to the anatomical distribution of focal ATs in humans, mapping and ablation studies in this heart failure model indicated that the ATs had a focal origin, with sites of earliest activation predominately located along the crista terminalis (CT) and within or near the pulmonary veins (PVs). Rapid, left AT degenerating to atrial fibrillation was localized and ablated inside the PV in this model.

The autonomic nervous system likely plays a critical role in initiating or triggering some ATs. Reports of AT triggered by changes in posture, belching, and swallowing, as well as termination of tachycardia by the Valsalva maneuver, edrophonium, or β-adrenergic blockers, support a probable role of the autonomic nervous system in some patients. A close association between autonomic nervous system activity and paroxysmal atrial arrhythmias in animal models has been documented. In dogs with pacing-induced heart failure, spontaneous paroxysmal ATs are triggered by simultaneous sympathovagal discharges.[6] Likewise in a canine model of intermittent rapid left atrial pacing, autonomic nerve discharge was shown to be an invariable trigger of paroxysmal atrial tachyarrhythmias.[6] All spontaneous AT and atrial fibrillation episodes were preceded (<5 s) by superior left ganglionated plexi nerve activity.

An interaction between respiration and supraventricular arrhythmias has been described in rare cases demonstrating bursts of atrial ectopic beats that emerge after the start of inspiration and cease during expiration. A report described, in detail, respiratory cycle–dependent ATs[7]: among 71 nonreentrant focal ATs in 60 patients, 9 respiratory cycle–dependent ATs (13%) were seen in 7 patients (12%). The arrhythmias were incessant, had irregular TCLs, and emerged in synchrony with respiratory cycles. These ATs converge around the right superior PV (RSPV) and the superior vena cava (SVC) where the anterior right ganglionated plexus is located. They are sensitive to adrenergic stimulation, are suppressed by adenosine, and are believed to be triggered activity–mediated.[7]

Focal ATs may have automaticity, triggered activity, or microreentry as the causative mechanism. Precise characterization of the mechanism of AT might be a difficult exercise, but understanding the principles may help with certain therapeutic decisions.

Abnormal automaticity due to enhanced ionic influx during phase 4 depolarization is the causative mechanism for focal ATs. Clinically, this is associated with a gradual "warm-up" period where the tachycardia rate increases, facilitated by adrenergic surge—either endogenous or exogenous, suppression with vagal maneuvers, beta-blockers, and calcium channel blockers.[8] In the electrophysiology laboratory they are characterized by (1) initiation only by isoproterenol infusion; (2) inability of programmed electrical stimulation to initiate or terminate AT; (3) transient suppression with overdrive pacing, but subsequent resumption with a gradual increase in atrial rate; (4) termination with propranolol; and (5) a "warm-up" and/or "cool-down" phenomenon.

AT due to triggered activity is characterized by one or more of the following: (1) initiation of tachycardia occurs with rapid atrial pacing or atrial extrastimuli, typically dependent on reaching a certain range of atrial pacing cycle lengths; (2) overdrive suppression or termination; (3) delayed afterdepolarizations that can be recorded from a monophasic action potential catheter at the tachycardia site of origin, but cannot be recorded from areas remote from the tachycardia; (4) isoproterenol is typically not required to induce tachycardia; and (5) dipyridamole, propranolol, verapamil, edrophonium, Valsalva maneuvers, and carotid sinus pressure terminate tachycardia.

AT attributed to *microreentry* is characterized by the following: (1) AT was reproducibly initiated and terminated by atrial pacing and extrastimuli, (2) delayed afterdepolarizations were not found on monophasic action potential catheter recordings, (3) pacing during tachycardia fulfilled criteria for manifest and concealed entrainment, and (4) the interval between the initiating premature beat and the first beat of tachycardia were inversely related.

The effects of adenosine on AT have been extensively studied by several groups,[9,10] and these studies are detailed in the previous edition of this textbook. Chiale and associates described the behavior and pharmacological responses of a group of rate-related, repetitive uniform, focal ATs that were highly sensitive to intravenous lidocaine.[11,12] These arrhythmias appear to be rare, show a variable response to intravenous adenosine and verapamil, and are neither consistently induced nor terminated by programmed premature atrial stimulation, suggesting a nonreentrant mechanism. These authors speculated that delayed afterdepolarizations may play a role in these ATs.

Studies attempting to categorize the mechanisms of focal ATs based on their responses to pacing and pharmacological maneuvers in the clinical electrophysiology laboratory are difficult to perform and interpret as most have included small, heterogeneous populations and patients with a variety of ATs and have provided discordant results. Additionally, there is a reluctance to administer pharamacolgical agents, which may make tachycardia induction and ablation more difficult. Thus given the lack of definitive criteria to identify the mechanisms of focal AT in the electrophysiology laboratory, these studies remain largely descriptive and are rarely performed today. Thus pharmacological interventions may not be a reliable means to identify AT mechanism and have largely fallen out of favor.

Further complicating appropriate mechanistic classification of focal ATs, programmed stimulation may initiate and terminate ATs caused by triggered activity and microreentry. Use of newer, multipolar catheters with closely spaced electrodes has allowed for very high-density recordings in a small region of interest. In combination with three-dimensional (3D) electroanatomical mapping, these catheter mapping techniques are shedding new light on the role of microreentry versus nonreentrant mechanisms in focal ATs. Although it may be of academic interest, the clinical significance of identifying the different mechanisms of focal AT is unclear. Discrimination of focal, nonreentrant tachycardia from microreentry may be less important, as both tachycardias can be ablated via focal ablation once tachycardia origin is identified. Therefore knowing the mechanism of focal AT may not predict successful ablation or lack of recurrence after ablation.

Electrocardiography of Focal Atrial Tachycardia

AT foci have a characteristic anatomical distribution. The predominant areas of origin of focal AT include the CT, near or inside the four PVs (superior veins more commonly), around the atrioventricular (AV) annuli, around or inside the coronary sinus (CS), and the para-Hisian region (atrial septum and Koch triangle). Less common sites of origin include the atrial appendages and the SVC[13] (Fig. 73.1).

There is an extensive literature on using the P wave morphology recorded on the 12-lead ECG to identify the site of the atrial focus. The literature on P wave morphology dates back to early studies of differential pacing during electrophysiology studies and during open-heart surgery. Multiple algorithms have been developed and refined over the years. Fig. 73.2 depicts an algorithm that is derived from distilling the results of various studies.[13–19] While limitations exist for identifying the source of AT by electrocardiography, we feel that this algorithm offers a starting point for localization. The limitations of deducing the origin of focal AT with electrocardiography are described in Box 73.1.[20]

Characterization of the mechanism of AT based on electrocardiographic findings is fraught with limitations. Long isoelectric intervals between P waves are not uncommon in macroreentrant ATs when the zone of slow conduction occupies a disproportionate temporal fraction of the TCL while occupying a minute spatial component of the tachycardia circuit. This can cause an erroneous assumption of a tachycardia being focal when it is indeed macroreentrant.

One of the pitfalls of the older algorithms is their inability to differentiate sites of origin that are adjacent to each other (e.g., RSPV vs. SVC). Uhm and colleagues have combined clinical features, including Holter findings to further elucidate the origin of ATs and differentiate adjacent sites of origin. Their algorithm was developed by analyzing data from 194 patients. This algorithm is depicted in Fig. 73.3.[21]

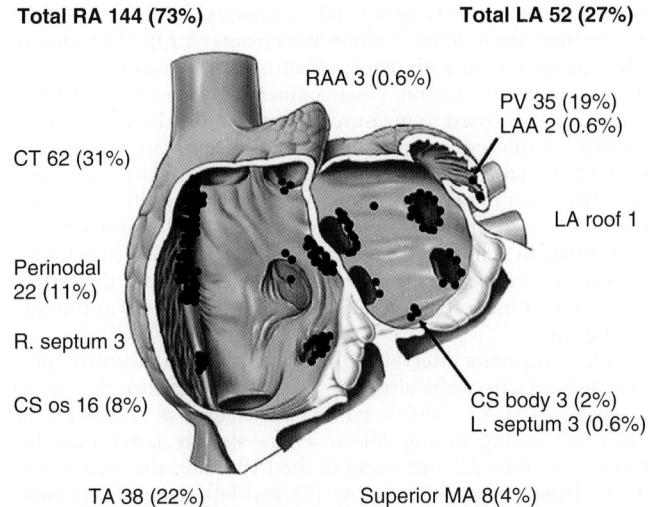

Total RA 144 (73%)   Total LA 52 (27%)

RAA 3 (0.6%)

PV 35 (19%)
LAA 2 (0.6%)

CT 62 (31%)

LA roof 1

Perinodal
22 (11%)

R. septum 3

CS os 16 (8%)

CS body 3 (2%)
L. septum 3 (0.6%)

TA 38 (22%)   Superior MA 8(4%)

FIGURE 73.1 Schematic representation of the anatomical distribution of focal atrial tachycardias. The atrioventricular valvular annuli have been removed. *CS,* Coronary sinus; *CT,* crista terminalis; *LA,* left atrium; *LAA,* left atrial appendage; *MA,* mitral annulus; *PV,* pulmonary vein; *RA,* right atrium; *RAA,* right atrial appendage; *TA,* tricuspid annulus. (From Kistler PM, Roberts-Thompson KC, Haqqani HM, et al. P-wave morphology in focal atrial tachycardia: development of an algorithm to predict the anatomic site of origin. *J Am Coll Cardiol.* 2006;48:1010-1017.)

Noninvasive electrocardiographic imaging or electrocardiographic mapping is a promising tool for diagnosis of tachycardia origin that may potentially be useful in procedure planning prior to catheter ablation.[22] As previously noted, the standard, 12-lead, surface ECG remains a useful tool for providing an initial approximation of the site of origin of AT, but it has numerous limitations. Body surface potential mapping incorporates a much larger number of electrodes, but does not provide anatomical information. The recent development of electrocardiographic imaging represents a further advancement in high-resolution noninvasive mapping by combining body surface electrodes and heart–torso geometric information to produce detailed electroanatomical maps of the epicardial surface through application of inverse solution mathematical algorithms. This technique has permitted accurate localization of focal, microreentrant, and macroreentrant ATs.[23–25]

This work has been extended to clinical practice and 3D electrocardiographic mapping with a vest that comprises 252 electrodes; integration of this information with a computed tomography scan was prospectively validated in 48 patients with outstanding accuracy, both in elucidating the mechanisms (focal vs. reentrant) and in localizing the focus.[26]

Differential Diagnosis of Focal Atrial Tachycardia

Once the diagnosis of AT is suspected, competing diagnoses like AVN reentrant tachycardia and orthodromic reciprocating tachycardia can be systematically excluded by invasive and noninvasive analysis.

We present a distillation of various methods by which the diagnosis of AT can be achieved in Box 73.2.[27–32]

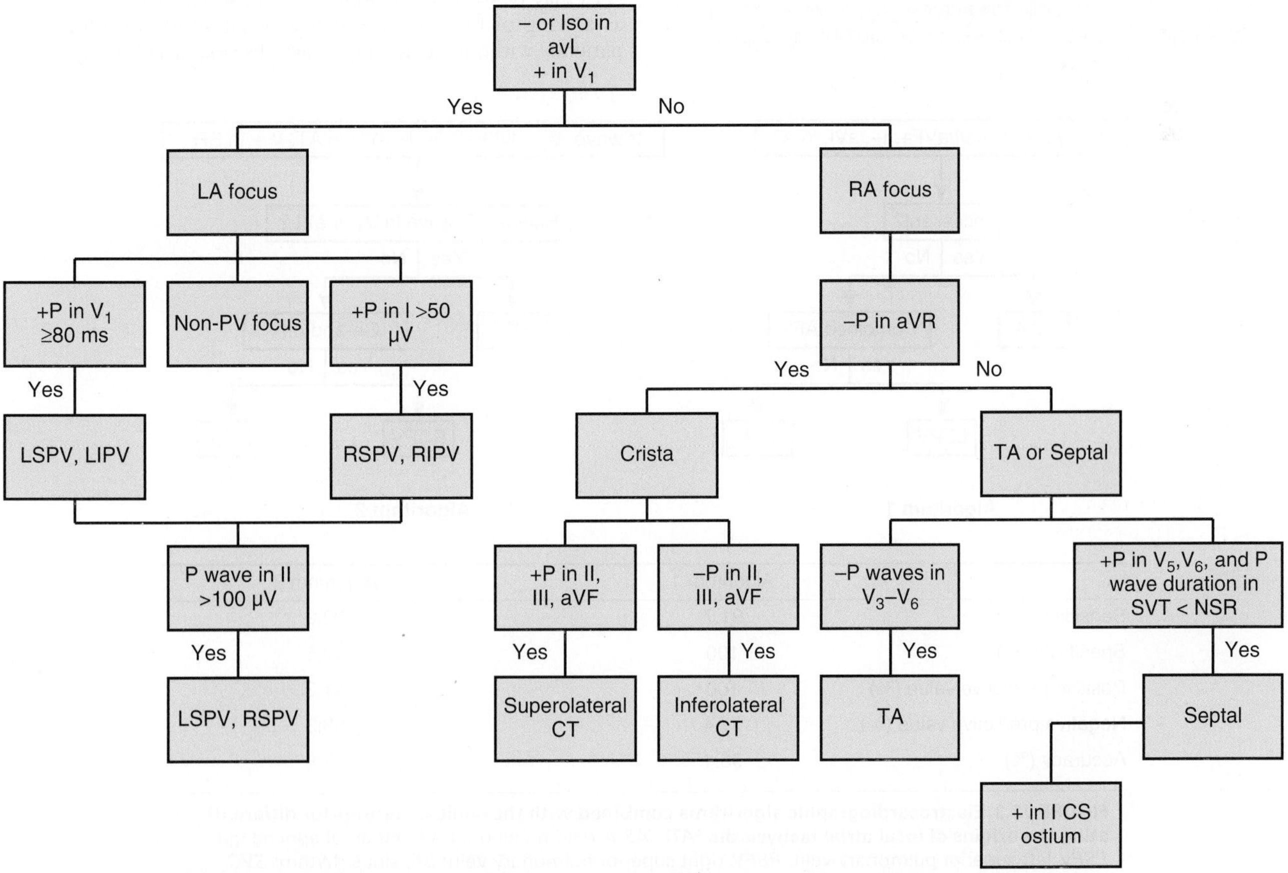

[Algorithm flowchart:]

– or Iso in avL + in V₁

- Yes → LA focus
  - +P in V₁ ≥80 ms → Yes → LSPV, LIPV
  - Non-PV focus → P wave in II >100 µV → Yes → LSPV, RSPV
  - +P in I >50 µV → Yes → RSPV, RIPV
- No → RA focus
  - –P in aVR
    - Yes → Crista
      - +P in II, III, aVF → Yes → Superolateral CT
      - –P in II, III, aVF → Yes → Inferolateral CT
    - No → TA or Septal
      - –P waves in V₃–V₆ → Yes → TA
      - +P in V₅,V₆, and P wave duration in SVT < NSR → Yes → Septal → + in I CS ostium

FIGURE 73.2 Algorithm for localizing the site of origin for focal atrial tachycardias. *CS,* Coronary sinus; *CT,* crista terminalis; *LA,* left atrium; *LIPV,* left inferior pulmonary vein; *LSPV,* left superior pulmonary vein; *NSR,* normal sinus rhythm; *RIPV,* right inferior pulmonary vein; *RSPV,* right superior pulmonary vein; *SVT,* supraventricular tachycardia; *TA,* tricuspid annulus.

Mapping and Ablation of Focal Atrial Tachycardia

Activation mapping is the most commonly used mapping method in ablation of AT. 3D electroanatomical mapping could be valuable in identifying and tagging the earliest site of activation, especially in those instances when the tachycardia is nonsustained. Noncontact mapping with its ability to generate 3000 unipolar electrograms, even with one beat of tachycardia, could be valuable in mapping nonsustained AT and premature atrial contractions. High-density mapping with multipolar or basket shaped catheters has recently led to enhanced understanding of the mechanisms of AT. Very high-density mapping can be performed relatively quickly in an area of interest with excellent spatial and temporal resolution (Fig. 73.4). Typically fractionated bipolar electrograms that precede P waves by 10 to 80 ms are observed at the site of earliest activation (Fig. 73.5). Occasionally,

---

> **BOX 73.1** **Limitations of surface electrocardiography in localizing source of atrial tachycardia**
>
> 1. Obscuration of P wave by QRS complex or T wave and inability to identify an "unencumbered" P wave
> 2. P wave morphology is in large part dependent on left atrial activation. Preferential routes of interatrial conduction causing discordant P wave morphologies despite tachycardia origins being anatomically very close to one another
> 3. Less than 2-cm spatial resolution of surface electrocardiography in localizing P wave origin[20]
> 4. Varying routes of referential interatrial conduction dependent on atrial cycle length (CL) despite originating from the same site will give rise to varying P wave morphologies
> 5. Reentrant tachycardia in "scarred" atria can generate electrocardiograms that resemble focal atrial tachycardia if the zone of slow conduction occupies a very significant portion of the cycle length within a very small anatomical space.

---

unipolar electrograms could reflect cavitary ventricular signals rather than atrial depolarization wavefronts. A QS electrogram, when in agreement with bipolar electrogram characteristics, predicts a successful ablation. Unencumbered P waves in all 12 ECG leads should be used to measure activation time. Premature ventricular complexes or brief bursts of rapid ventricular pacing are useful to visualize a P wave that is not encumbered by ventricular depolarization or repolarization. Ablation is typically performed with RF energy applied using a solid tip electrode, which should be titrated to achieve a tip temperature of 55°C. Abrupt termination and transient acceleration or deceleration are the typical responses within a few seconds of RF energy delivery at the successful site.

The postpacing interval (PPI) response to atrial overdrive pacing during tachycardia also may be useful to localize the site of origin of focal AT. Mohamed and associates[33] performed atrial overdrive pacing during AT at a rate slightly faster than the tachycardia rate. Measurement of the PPI minus the TCL (PPI–TCL) from various sites in the RA and left atrium (LA) localized the tachycardia focus when the PPI–TCL was minimized (e.g., for the successful ablation site, 11 ± 8 ms). The investigators explained this observation by hypothesizing that the difference between the PPI and the TCL was proportional to the distance from the pacing site to the tachycardia focus and conduction time through the surrounding or perifocal tissue. In this study, overdrive suppression of the AT focus was not apparent. The PPI–TCL was never greater than 20 ms at a successful ablation site, suggesting minimal slowing by tissue near the atrial focus.

Specific Sites

Atrial Tachycardia Arising From the Crista Terminalis

ATs may be located all along the CT, which has been described as a "ring of fire" because it is a common location for ATs in patients without structural heart disease, accounting for two

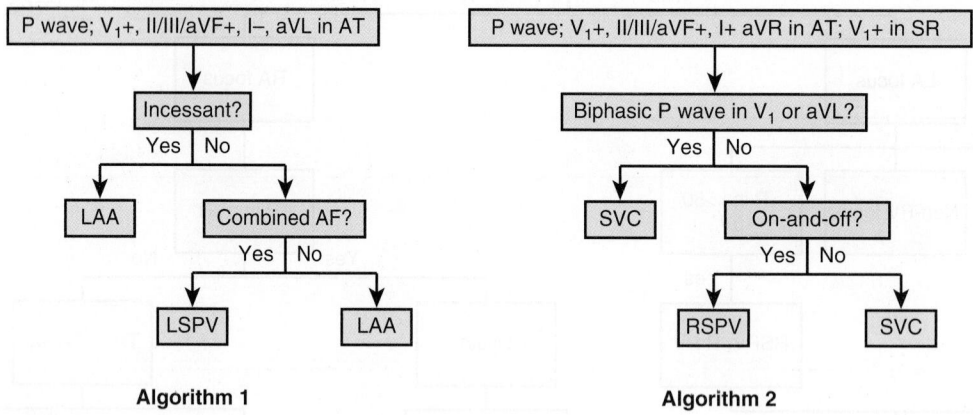

	Algorithm 1	Algorithm 2
Sensitivity (%)	91.7	92.9
Specificity (%)	100	62.5
Positive predictive value (%)	100	81.3
Negative predictive value (%)	71.4	83.3
Accuracy (%)	93.1	81.8

FIGURE 73.3 Electrocardiographic algorithms combined with the clinical features for differentiating the origins of focal atrial tachycardia (AT). *AF,* Atrial fibrillation; *LAA,* left atrial appendage; *LSPV,* left superior pulmonary vein; *RSPV,* right superior pulmonary vein; *SR,* sinus rhythm; *SVC,* superior vena cava. (From Uhm JS, Shim J, Wi J, et al. An electrocardiography algorithm combined with clinical features could localize the origins of focal atrial tachycardias in adjacent structures. *Europace.* 2014;16:1061-1068.)

BOX 73.2   Clinical, electrocardiographic, and electrophysiologic features of atrial tachycardia (AT)

Clinical History

- Gradual onset and offset—typical for automatic mechanisms of tachycardia, thus suggesting AT
- Palpitations especially felt in the neck and throat—suspicious for atrioventricular nodal reentrant tachycardia (AVNRT) due to AV dissociation and simultaneous atrial and ventricular contraction

Electrocardiogram

- Inferiorly directed P wave axis excludes AVNRT
- AV block (more P waves than QRS) excludes orthodromic reciprocating tachycardia (ORT)
- Spontaneous changes in PR and RP intervals but fixed PP intervals suggests AT
- Bundle branch block during tachycardia does not affect PP intervals during AT
- Reproducible termination of tachycardia with a P wave excludes AT
- Reproducible termination of tachycardia with a premature ventricular beat that does not conduct to the atrium excludes AT
- The first P wave that initiates AT is similar to P wave morphology of AT, which suggests automatic AT
- The first P wave that initiates the AT is dissimilar to the P wave morphology of AT, which suggests a premature atrial contraction initiating microreentry or triggered activity as the mechanism of the AT

Induction of Tachycardia

- Induction of tachycardia with ventricular pacing is unlikely to induce AT but is more likely to induce ORT or atypical AVNRT
- Ventriculoatrial (VA) conduction is mandatory for induction of AT with ventricular pacing.
- When induced with ventricular pacing a V-A-A-V pattern of induction is typically observed
- When VA block cycle length (CL) > tachycardia cycle length (TCL), ORT is less likely as the mechanism of tachycardia
- Atrial activation sequence during ventricular pacing is unlikely to be identical to atrial activation during AT

Tachycardia Features

- High to low right activation sequence is incompatible with any form of AVNRT

- AV block during tachycardia excludes ORT
- Changes in HV interval during tachycardia (bundle branch block) does not affect TCL in AT or AVNRT
- If oscillations in TCL are noted, AA intervals predict HH and VV intervals
- When TCL is fixed but VA intervals are not, AT is the likely mechanism

Maneuvers During Tachycardia
Atrial Pacing Maneuvers

- Overdrive pacing and with 1:1 AV relationship:
  - $AH_{SVT} - AH_{TCL} < 20$ ms suggests ORT
  - $AH_{SVT} - AH_{TCL} = 20\text{–}40$ ms suggests AT
  - $AH_{SVT} - AH_{TCL} > 40$ ms suggests AVNRT
- Overdrive suppression and resumption of tachycardia suggests AT as the mechanism
- Overdrive pacing of tachycardia at varying CLs resulting in fixed VA intervals excludes AT
- Overdrive pacing of tachycardia at varying CLs resulting in variable PPIs—suggestive of AT and does not support macroreentry—6 ms-macroreentry vs. 56 ms-focal AT (exceptions occur in structurally abnormal atria)
- Overdrive pacing from two different sites at identical CL, 1:1 AV relationship and resumption of tachycardia after pacing:
  - ΔVA interval between both sites (VA interval at site 1–VA interval at site 2) of first beat of tachycardia postpacing from site <14 ms: AVNRT or ORT
  - ΔVA interval between both sites (VA interval at site 1–VA interval at site 2) of first beat of tachycardia postpacing from site >14 ms: AT

Ventricular Pacing Maneuvers

- Rapid ventricular pacing results in dissociation of atrium with no change in atrial CL—excludes ORT
- Overdrive pacing with entrainment of the atrium:
  - Different atrial activation sequence than tachycardia—excludes ORT
  - The postpacing response of V-A-A-V—excludes ORT and suggests AT (spurious conclusions can be drawn if the last entrained atrial complex is not correctly identified)
  - Fused ventricular beat resets the tachycardia—excludes AT and AVNRT

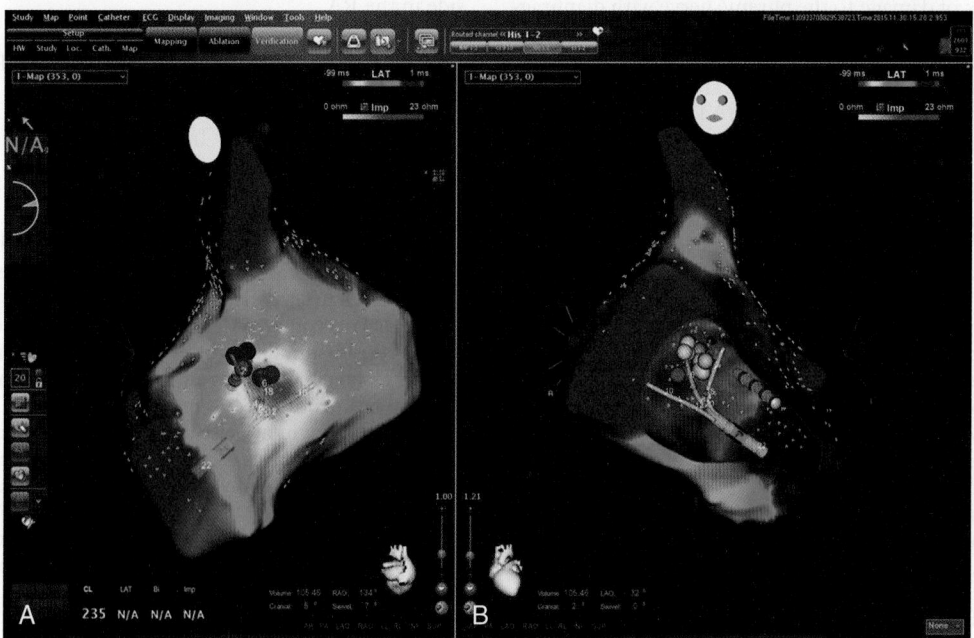

FIGURE 73.4 High-density activation three-dimensional electroanatomical mapping of an atrial tachycardia with particular focus on an area of interest with a Pentaray (Biosense Webster, South Diamond Bar, CA) multipolar catheter. (A) depicts a right posterior view of the right atrium. (B) depicts a left anterior oblique view of the right atrium. Focal ablation at the earliest site of activation terminated the tachycardia.

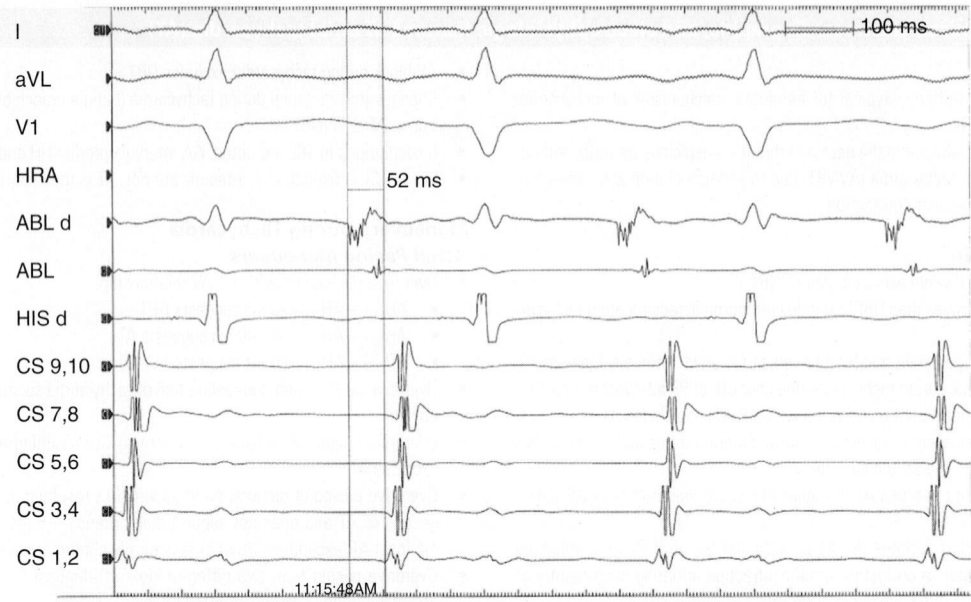

FIGURE 73.5 Example of a fractionated bipolar electrogram seen at the site of successful ablation on ablation distal (*ABL d*). These are characteristic electrograms encountered at the site of successful ablation of focal atrial tachycardias. *CS,* Coronary sinus; *HRA,* high right atrium.

thirds of right ATs in one study. One physiological factor contributing to the clustering of ATs in this area is that the CT demonstrates marked anisotropy due to poor transverse cell-to-cell coupling, which could contribute to slow conduction and microreentry. Another contributory factor is that the CT contains clusters of cells with automaticity. The ECG characteristics of these tachycardias were described earlier and depend on site of origin from the CT (e.g., superior vs. inferior). Intracardiac echocardiography may be particularly useful to demonstrate the close anatomical proximity of the tachycardia focus to the crista during mapping. Ablation of tachycardias arising from the superior CT carries a small risk of damage to the phrenic nerve with diaphragmatic paralysis.

Differentiating ATs originating at the superior CT from sinus tachycardia can be difficult at times. There may be subtle differences in the P wave morphology in AT originating in the superior CT compared with the sinus P wave. Administration of isoproterenol may help differentiate sinus tachycardia from superior crista, focal AT. The origin of earliest activation in sinus tachycardia will move superiorly up the CT with isoproterenol, whereas in focal AT, isoproterenol will increase the AT rate, but the location of earliest atrial activation will not change substantially.

AT originating from high CT can be differentiated from sinus tachycardia, and overdrive pacing at the site of origin of tachycardia will differentiate these two entities. In focal AT, PPI–TCL from the site of origin of the tachycardia is close to zero but during sinus tachycardia, PPI–TCL always exceeds 80 ms due to the presence of perinodal tissue, a unique anatomical and physiological characteristic of the sinus node.[33]

Interatrial conduction time (between high RA [HRA] and distal CS [CSd] recording electrodes) during sinus rhythm compared with AT can be utilized to differentiate tachycardias originating from the superior CT with those from the RSPV. (HRA-CSd $_{NSR}$) – (HRA-CSd $_{AT}$) > 20 ms favors RSPV over SVC and superior CT.[34]

Similarly, *intraatrial conduction* can also facilitate this distinction. Intraatrial conduction time recorded from the HRA to His bundle recording electrodes during sinus rhythm versus during AT, (HRA-HB$_{NSR}$) – (HRA-HB$_{AT}$) < 0 ms, favors SVC and superior CT over right superior pulmonary foci.

3D electroanatomical activation mapping can also be valuable in quickly abandoning the RA, as a site of interest and exploring the LA, especially the RSPV. In one study of 16 patients, right atrial mapping of an RSPV tachycardia revealed double breakthrough sites in 10/16 patients with the initial 10-ms atrial depolarization area averaging 4.3 cm^2.[35]

It is increasingly recognized that posterior connections between the atria via the intercaval bundle play an important role in early transmission of atrial activation to the RA when ATs arise from the RSPV.[36] Such connections occasionally make it impossible to isolate the RSPV without ablating on the contralateral side in the RA.

Atrial Tachycardia Arising From the Tricuspid Atrioventricular Annulus

The tricuspid annulus represents the second most common location of right-sided ATs. In several series, tachycardias arising from the tricuspid annulus accounted for 13% to 22% of right ATs.[37] Tricuspid annular AT has negative or notched P waves in V$_1$ and invariably positive P waves in lead aVL (Figs. 73.6 and 73.7). Reports describe foci from around the entire circumference of the tricuspid annulus. Inferior foci tend to have negative P waves in leads II, III, and aVF, whereas superior foci are usually isoelectric or positive in these leads. Foci from the superior tricuspid annulus and the right atrial appendage (RAA) have similar P wave morphologies, consistent with their close proximity. P waves from the lower tricuspid annulus generally show a negative P wave in at least two consecutive leads of V$_3$–V$_6$. The presence of myocytes with AV nodal–type electrophysiological characteristics around the entire tricuspid annulus has been described in animals.[38] These cells are histologically similar to the atrial cells but resemble nodal cells in their cellular electrophysiology, response to adenosine, and lack of connexin43. They may serve as the substrate for AT originating from around the tricuspid annulus.

Atrial Tachycardia Arising From the Right Atrial Appendage and Superior Vena Cava

The RAA is an uncommon site of origin for AT (<5% of ectopic ATs in several series), although both appendages are a more

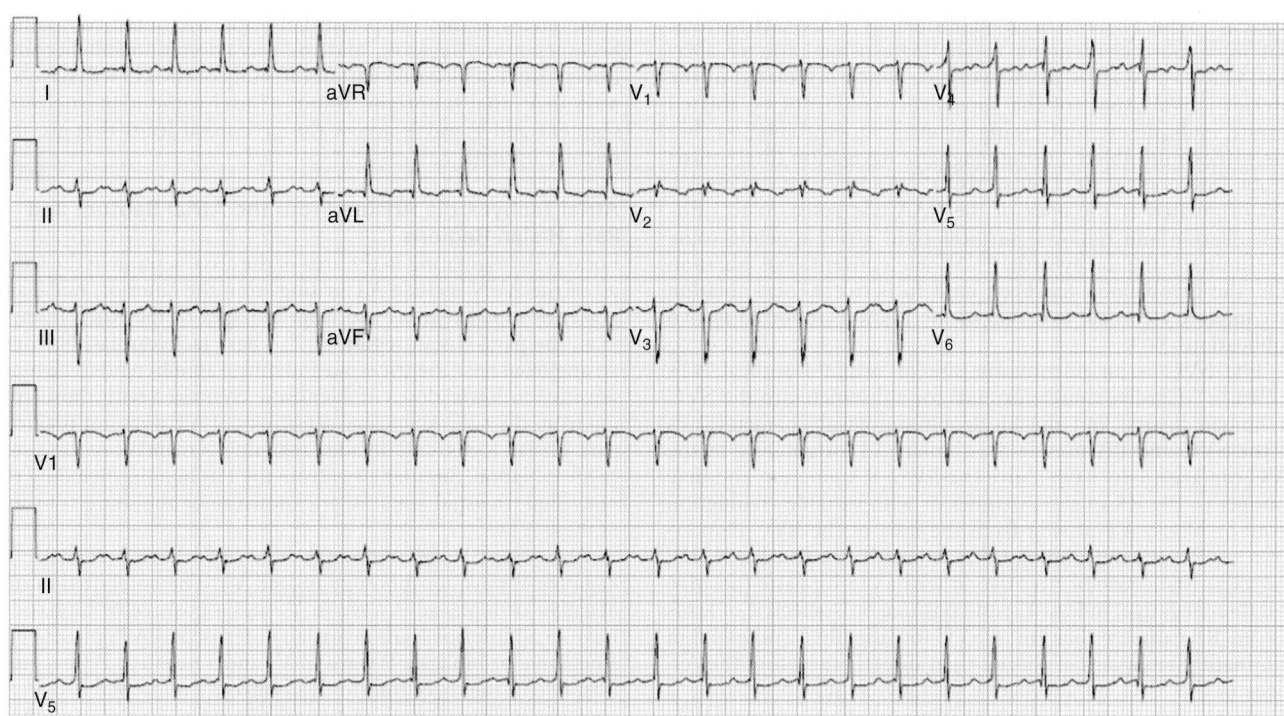

FIGURE 73.6 Low tricuspid annular atrial tachycardia. Note the distinct negative P wave in lead V_1 and positive P waves in lead aVL.

Ablation site

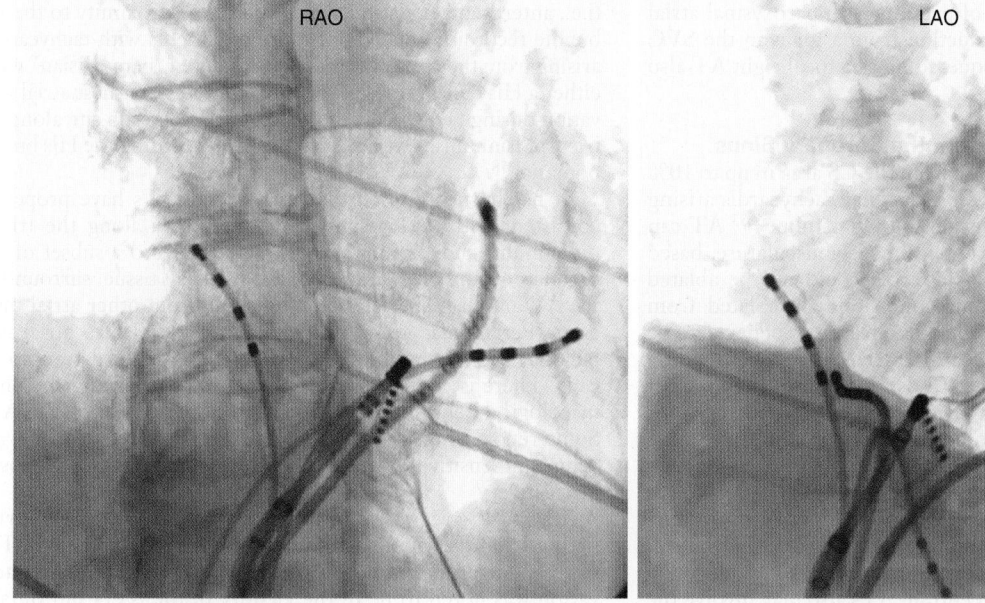
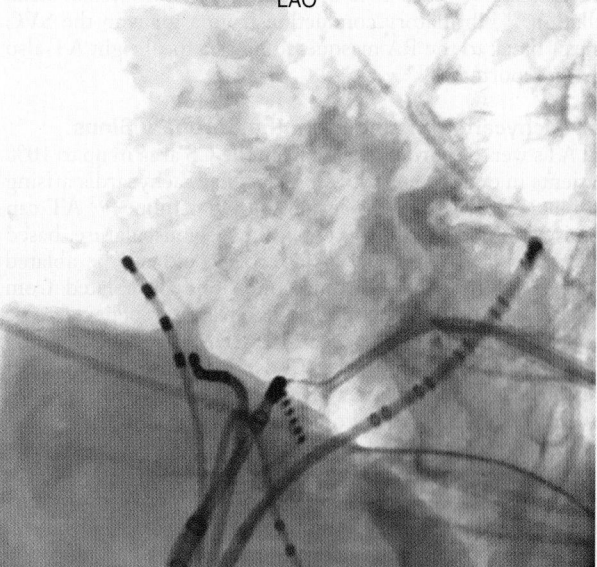

RAO   LAO

FIGURE 73.7 The same tachycardia depicted in Fig. 73.6 was successfully ablated; the representative right and left anterior oblique projections of the heart with the ablation, His bundle, high right atrial, and coronary sinus catheters are depicted. *LAO,* Left anterior oblique; *RAO,* right anterior oblique.

common site for incessant ATs.[39–41] The RAA is composed of ridges formed by pectinate muscles, which arise from the CT. The characteristic electrocardiographic pattern associated with RAA tachycardia shows negative P waves, in lead V_1 due to the anterior location of the RAA, that become progressively more positive across the rest of the precordial leads along with upright P waves in the inferior leads, positive or isoelectric-positive P waves in I, and an inverted P wave in aVR, analogous to AT from

a superior crista origin. As with other right ATs that arise from the superior crista, it can be confused with sinus tachycardia. At least one case series has suggested that RAA tachycardias arise more commonly in younger male patients and can present as an incessant tachycardia, resulting in LV dysfunction secondary to tachycardia-induced cardiomyopathy.[39,42]

Catheter ablation of focal RAA tachycardia is relatively straightforward, with high success rates.[39,42] However, at least two case reports have been published of RAA tachycardias that were more challenging to eliminate using catheter ablation. One case of an RAA tachycardia, which originated in the inferior/lateral aspect of the appendage, could not be ablated despite multiple attempts using manual catheter ablation, but was successfully ablated using magnetic navigation (Stereotaxis Niobe [Stereotaxis, St. Louis, MO]).[43] Another case of an AT that originated at the apex of the RAA was resistant to catheter ablation and required surgical right atrial appendectomy to eliminate the tachycardia.[44] When conventional ablation fails, the cryoballoon has been used to perform focal ablation or complete electrical isolation of the RAA, as reported in two publications.[45,46]

The SVC is an uncommon site of origin for focal ATs (<2%).[47,48] Cardiac muscle extends for a distance into the SVC in human hearts, and the electrophysiological characteristics of the SVC and RA muscle are similar. AT originating in the SVC can arise 1 to 3 cm above the SVC–RA junction and may conduct to the RA in a 1:1 manner or with variable conduction delay or block. AT arising from the area of the SVC demonstrates a P wave morphology that is positive in leads I, II, III, and aVF; isoelectric or negative in lead aVL; biphasic (positive and then negative) in lead V_1; and positive or isoelectric in leads V_2–V_6. RF catheter ablation of SVC foci usually is successful in eliminating tachycardia. Rather than directly targeting the AT focus in the SVC, an alternative strategy employed by some is electrical disconnection of the SVC muscle sleeve at the SVC–RA junction in a circumferential or segmental fashion or isolation of the arrhythmogenic area from the rest of the SVC. Careful attention should be paid to avoid injury to the phrenic nerve during ablation in this region, and complete SVC isolation is best avoided due to the risk of SVC stenosis.[49] The SVC also has been reported to play a role in arrhythmia initiation and maintenance in ~5% to 10% of patients with paroxysmal atrial fibrillation.[50] Fibrillatory conduction from a focus in the SVC with exit block to the RA masquerading as a focal right AT also has been reported.[51]

Atrial Tachycardia Arising From the Coronary Sinus

Focal ATs were reported to arise from the CS area in up to 10% of patients in one study.[13] Most patients had tachycardia arising from outside the CS or just inside the CS ostium.[52,53] AT can also arise from deep within the CS, the CS musculature, based on the observation that the tachycardia could not be ablated from the left atrial endocardium but could be ablated from within the CS.[53] The arrhythmogenic substrate is believed to be the muscular sleeves on the epicardial atrial surface surrounding the CS and extending from the CS ostium to the lateral aspect of the mitral annulus. In human hearts, the CS musculature provides electrical connections to the LA most prominently at the proximal portion, and activation from the RA can conduct to the LA via these electrical connections. A discrete potential is noted after the CS electrogram in sinus rhythm and preceding the surface P wave by 30 to 50 ms during tachycardia. Successful ablation sites typically have activation at least 20 ms before the onset of the P wave.[53] Macroreentrant ATs also may involve the CS and require ablation on the left atrial endocardial surface as well as on the CS.

The electrocardiographic pattern of ATs arising from the CS musculature is fairly typical, with deeply negative P waves in the inferior leads and positive P waves in aVR. As such, the morphology of the ECG during focal AT arising from the CS may be similar to and confused with that of typical counterclockwise AFL, which engages the CS ostium. Notably, tachycardia foci from the CS ostium have characteristic P wave morphologies in the precordial leads. Lead V_1 is biphasic with an initial component that is either isoelectric or mildly inverted (when timed to onset of the P wave in inferior leads) followed by an upright

component. Across the precordial leads, the initial component becomes more negative, and the second component becomes isoelectric. Foci located within the body of the CS will have a P wave in V_1 that is upright from the onset without an isoelectric segment and P waves across the precordial leads that are frequently upright.

Atrial Tachycardia Arising From the Atrial Septum and Para-Hisian Regions

Focal ATs originating in the area of the atrial septum in the vicinity of the AVN include AT arising from the anterior, mid-, and posterior septal regions and from the apex of the Koch triangle (e.g., the para-Hisian region).[54–58] These tachycardias, like ones arising from near the tricuspid and mitral annuli, tend to be more sensitive to lower doses of adenosine compared with those arising from the CT. Adenosine sensitivity of AT does not predict a para-Hisian focus, and detailed mapping is mandatory for a successful ablation. Sites far away from the His bundle, including the nonseptal tricuspid annulus, are known to be the source of some of these ATs.

Anteroseptal and midseptal right ATs have a biphasic or negative P wave morphology in lead V_1. The combination of a negative or biphasic P wave in V_1 and a positive or biphasic P wave in all inferior leads favors an anteroseptal AT; presence of a negative or biphasic P wave in V_1 and a negative P wave in at least two of the three inferior leads favors a midseptal AT. Presence of a positive P wave in V_1 and a negative P wave in all three inferior leads favors a posteroseptal AT. An electrophysiology study is critical for differentiating these tachycardias from atypical AVN reentry or a septal accessory pathway. In several series, 27% to 35% of patients had tachycardias originating from this region.

ATs can originate from near the apex of the Koch triangle (i.e., anteroseptal tricuspid annulus, in close proximity to the His bundle recording) in 10% or more of patients with tachycardias arising from the RA. A location is considered "para-Hisian" when either a His deflection is observed at the site of earliest atrial activation during tachycardia or the successful ablation site along the tricuspid annulus is within 1 cm of a site recording the His bundle potential.[58]

It has been proposed that para-Hisian ATs have properties consistent with AT arising circumferentially along the tricuspid annulus and, as such, should be considered a subset of this broader group of "annular" ATs.[58] Atrial tissue surrounding the AV annuli is specialized and distinct from other atrial myocytes. Periannular cells are histologically similar to atrial cells but may electrophysiologically resemble AV nodal transitional cells. There is controversy in the literature regarding the pharmacological behavior and mechanism of these para-Hisian ATs. Some reports indicate that these tachycardias are adenosine and verapamil sensitive, whereas others report that they are adenosine insensitive.[59]

Recently, a reentrant form of verapamil-sensitive AT originating from the vicinity of the AVN has been described . This study involved 17 patients who had AT where the earliest activation was noted to be in the vicinity of the AVN but outside the Koch triangle.[60] However, manifest entrainment was demonstrated when overdrive pacing was performed from a remote site, suggesting a reentrant mechanism (Figs. 73.8 and 73.9). Additionally, orthodromic capture of the earliest atrial activation site as well as fusion of surface P waves during entrainment indicated the presence of distinct entrance and exit sites for the circuit. AT was terminated by RF energy application at sites that were proximal to the earliest atrial activation signal but in the direction of the rapid pacing wavefront during manifest entrainment. A variant of this form of verapamil-sensitive AT originating from the AV annuli has also been recently reported.[61]

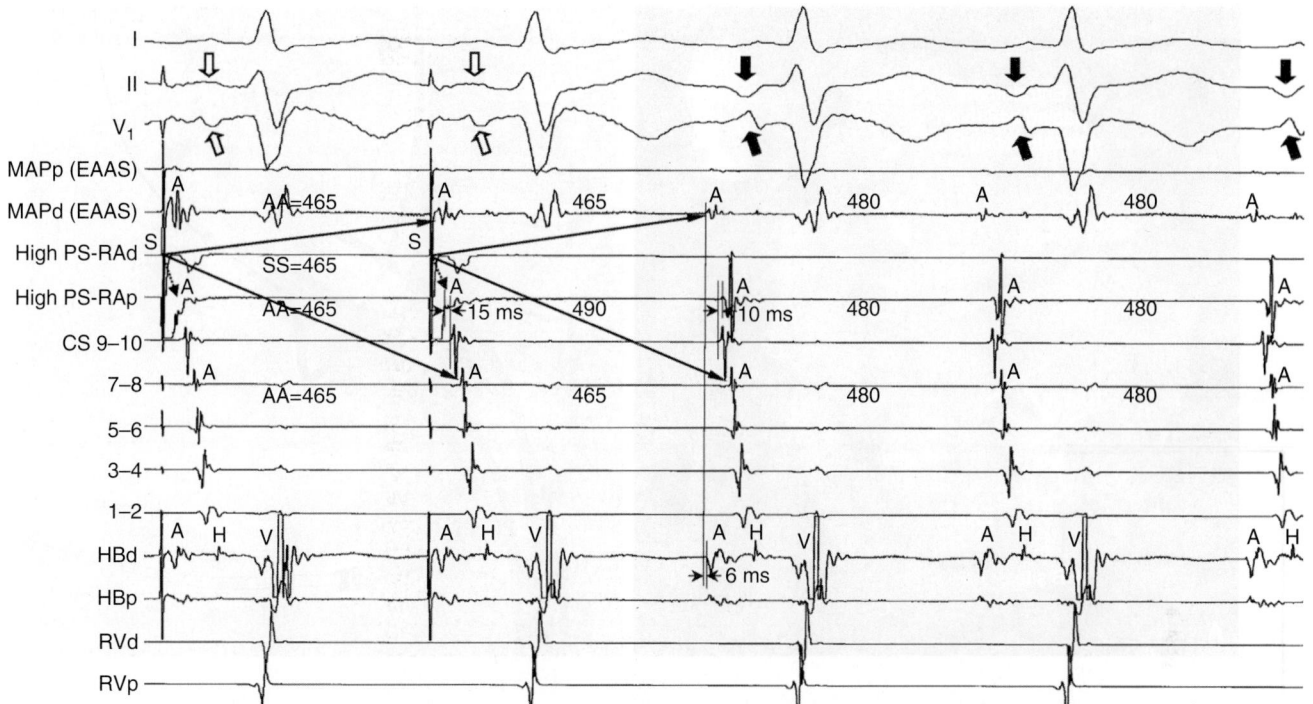

FIGURE 73.8 Tracing during manifest entrainment by rapid atrial pacing delivered during tachycardia from the distal high posteroseptal right atrium (*PS-RAd*). When noting the last captured electrograms at the earliest atrial activation site (*EAAS*) and the coronary sinus (*CS*) 7–8, the cycle lengths were both equal to the pacing interval (465 ms) but shorter than the atrial tachycardia (AT) cycle length (480 ms). Furthermore, the electrogram morphologies were identical to those during AT, indicating the orthodromic capture of the EAAS and the CS 7–8 (*small solid arrows*). On the other hand, the atrial electrograms at proximal high posteroseptal right atrium (*PS-RAp*) occurred 15 ms earlier than those at the CS 9–10 during pacing, but 10 ms later than those at the CS 9–10 during AT. Furthermore, the interval of the atrial electrogram at high PS-RAp just after pacing (490 ms) was longer than the pacing interval, indicating the antidromic capture of the electrogram at high PS-RAp (*dashed arrows*). The surface P wave morphologies during pacing (*open narrow arrows*) are different from the surface P wave morphologies during tachycardia (*closed wide arrows*). (From Yamabe H, Okumura K, Morihisa K, et al. Demonstration of anatomical reentrant tachycardia circuit in verapamil-sensitive atrial tachycardia originating from the vicinity of the atrioventricular node. *Heart Rhythm.* 2012;9:1475-1483.)

ECG findings suggestive of a para-Hisian AT include narrowing of the P wave during AT compared with sinus rhythm, and biphasic P waves in V_1, with the dominant-positive or dominant-negative component having a polarity opposite to that observed in the inferior leads. Some but not all reports suggest that a left-sided para-Hisian AT origin is associated with positive P waves in lead V_1.[56,57] The P waves are consistently positive or isoelectric in leads I and aVL. The P wave morphology in the inferior leads may show two distinct patterns: (1) negative or biphasic with terminal negativity or (2) positive or biphasic P waves and terminal positivity. The P wave morphology in the inferior leads during tachycardia is largely determined by the route of left atrial activation: via the posteroinferior input from the CS versus via the Bachmann bundle.

Analysis of near-field and far-field electrograms can also clue the operator to a right atrial versus left atrial origin for the AT. Representative examples are depicted from study by Traykov and associates[62] (Fig 73.10). Catheter ablation of AT originating in the perinodal region is safe and effective. It is increasingly recognized that these peri-Hisian ATs constitute a broader subset of ATs and can be classified as anterior atrial septal ATs. In most patients, these tachycardias can be ablated without damage to AV nodal conduction. In studies detailing ablation of anterior septal ATs, ablation is quite often "safely" successful in the noncoronary cusp (NCC) of the aorta despite not having the earliest activation times compared to the atrial septal locations. While most people believe that the aortic cusps are devoid of atrial musculature,

anterior atrial septal tachycardias can successfully be targeted from the NCC (majority) and rarely from the other cusps as well as the aortomitral continuity. A strategy for mapping these tachycardias is depicted in Fig. 73.11. In a study by Wang and colleagues, AT was localized to the anterior atrial septum in 47/227 patients. Of these 47 patients, only 8 had successful ablation from the right atrial septum, while 33 were successfully ablated from the NCC.[63] Another study of 34 patients with focal ATs from around the AVN confirmed and extended these findings. It showed that only 7 of 34 were ablated from the RA (with RF or cryoenergy), 7 were ablated from the LA, and the remainder were ablated from the NCC. The authors emphasize the anatomy and point out that the NCC allows access to atrial myocardium between the RA and LA. They emphasize that the NCC provides access and a view of atrial tissue in the septum and a relatively safe site to ablate the origin of this tachycardia.[64]

Transient AV block and PR prolongation has been reported in older reports when ablation has been performed in this region. Cryothermal energy has also been utilized to safely ablate ATs in this location.

ATs successfully ablated from the NCC typically have a negative/positive P wave in lead V_1, isoelectric P wave in lead I, and upright or biphasic (with terminal positivity) P wave morphology in the inferior leads. The NCC is adjacent to the epicardial aspect of the atrial myocardium located between the RA and the LA, immediately anterior to the interatrial septum. The fast pathway input to the AVN is located in close proximity to the anterior

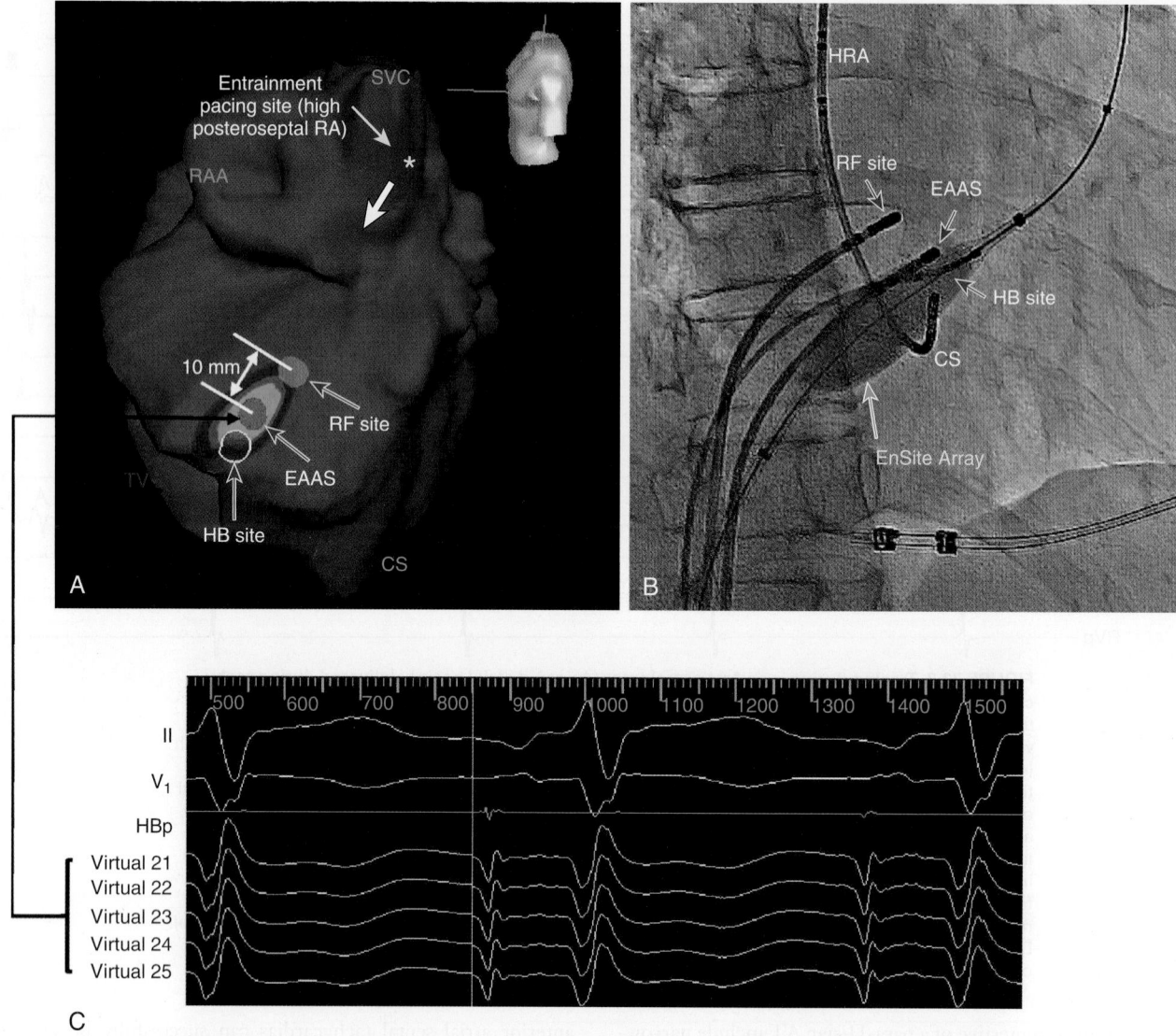

FIGURE 73.9 (A) Isopotential map at the atrial tachycardia onset and (B) fluoroscopic image in the right anterior oblique view. *Asterisk* indicates the pacing site at high posteroseptal right atrium (*RA*) where the manifest entrainment was demonstrated (entrainment pacing site). The radiofrequency (*RF*) site: the successful RF energy application site. (C) Virtual unipolar electrogram at the earliest atrial activation site (*EAAS*) at atrial tachycardia onset. *CS,* Coronary sinus; *HB,* His bundle; *HRA,* high right atrium; *p,* proximal; *RAA,* right atrial appendage; *SVC,* superior vena cava; *TV,* tricuspid annulus. (From Yamabe H, Okumura K, Morihisa K, et al. Demonstration of anatomical reentrant tachycardia circuit in verapamil-sensitive atrial tachycardia originating from the vicinity of the atrioventricular node. *Heart Rhythm.* 2012;9:1475-1483.)

portion of the NCC. RF applications at the NCC result in left atrial lesions located between the floor of the fossa ovalis and the mitral annulus. This is an area in which it can be difficult to position an ablation catheter with sufficient stability and adequate tissue contact using either a retrograde or transseptal approach. Catheter stability within the NCC may allow creation of lesions in the deeper tissues that are otherwise not accessible.

Before performing catheter ablation within the aortic sinuses of Valsalva, if intracardiac echocardiography is not utilized to delineate the origins of the coronary arteries and incorporate the information into the 3D electroanatomical mapping system, coronary angiography or selective angiography of the aortic sinuses should be performed to ensure that the distance between the ablation catheter and coronary ostium is more than 10 mm.

In summary, tachycardias located in the atrial septal region require careful mapping of both sides of the septum, and in

some cases, mapping and ablation in the aortic sinuses of Valsalva. The aortic root occupies a central location between the tricuspid and mitral annulus and in close vicinity to the His bundle. Due to the close proximity of these ATs to the AVN, care needs to be taken to avoid AV block during ablation. However, successful RF ablation is achievable in the majority of cases without complication.

Left Atrial and Pulmonary Vein Tachycardias

Focal tachycardias originating in the LA and PVs not associated with prior catheter ablation for AF form an important subset of all ATs, reportedly constituting ~10% to 40% of all focal ATs.[13,65] These tachycardias may occur in a very wide spectrum of clinical settings, ranging from structurally normal hearts to advanced cardiac disease, and in patients who have undergone a cardiac or lung transplant procedure. Catheter ablation is a generally successful

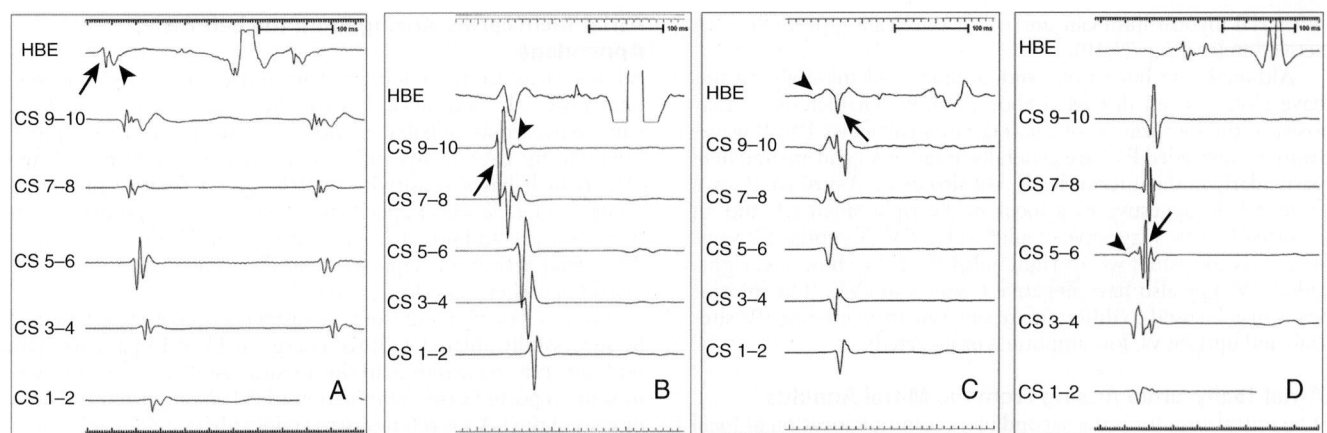

FIGURE 73.10 Representative examples of intracardiac recordings from the focal atrial tachycardia group showing single beats of focal atrial tachycardias successfully ablated in the right atrium (A and B) and in the left atrium (C and D). (A) Earliest activation at the His bundle electrogram (*HBE*) showing (near-field–far-field) N–F sequence. (B) Earliest activation at CS 9–10 with N–F sequence. (C) Earliest activation at the HBE with F–N (far-field–near-field) sequence. (D) Earliest activation at CS 5–6 demonstrating F–N sequence. CS 9–10 is positioned at the ostium. *CS*, Coronary sinus. Paper speed, 300 mm/s. (From Traykov VB, Pap R, Shalganov TN, et al. Electrogram analysis at the His bundle region and the proximal coronary sinus as a tool to predict left atrial origin of focal atrial tachycardias. *Europace.* 2011;13:1022-1027.)

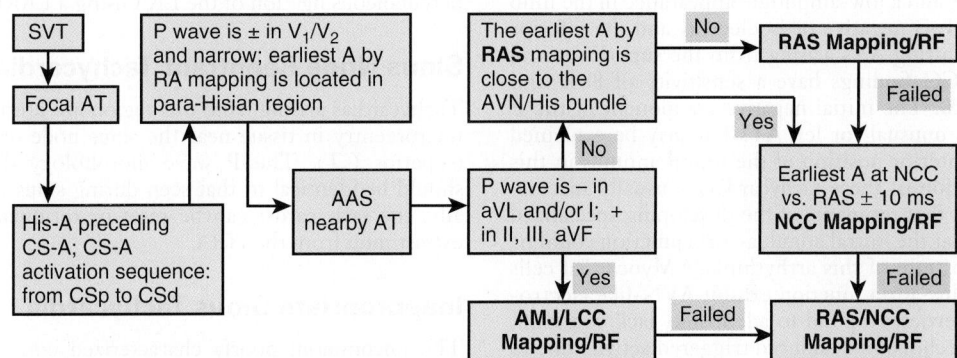

FIGURE 73.11 Flow chart of the strategy for mapping and ablation of anterior atrial septum (*AAS*)– atrial tachycardias (*ATs*). *AMJ,* Aortic mitral junction; *AVN,* atrioventricular node; *CS,* coronary sinus; *LCC,* left coronary cusp; *NCC,* noncoronary cusp; *RAS,* right atrial septum; *RF,* radiofrequency; *SVT,* supraventricular tachycardia. (From Wang Z, Ouyang J, Liang Y, et al. Focal atrial tachycardia surrounding the anterior septum: strategy for mapping and catheter ablation. *Circ Arrhythm Electrophysiol.* 2015;8:575-582.)

treatment for these focal ATs, including those refractory to pharmacological therapy. Left atrial and PV tachycardias may occur in patients following ablation for AF, but will be discussed elsewhere.

The PVs and mitral valve annulus are the main source of focal left ATs. A majority of PV tachycardias originate from the ostium, rather than from deep inside the veins, with a strong propensity for the superior veins. Additionally, it is rare for ATs to recur from different sites in the PVs or for atrial fibrillation to develop after a PV focal ablation.[65–67] Thus unlike patients with PV triggers and atrial fibrillation where there are usually multiple triggers in multiple veins and the pathophysiology involves a diffuse, chronic process often with extensive atrial remodeling, those patients whose sole clinical arrhythmia is AT appear to have an isolated or focal process. As such, patients with focal left-sided AT are curable in the long term with focal ablation.

Superior (Bachmann bundle), inferior (CS), septal (fossa ovalis), and posterior interatrial electrical connections exist between the RA and LA. Additional posterior electrical connections between the right-sided PVs and right atrial posterior walls exist

in human hearts. This may compound the difficulty in differentiating between an AT originating from the PVs and that arising from the posterior RA. Focal AT from the PVs usually has a positive P wave across the precordium, from V_1 to V_6 due to the posterior location of the LA. Careful analysis of the P wave configuration in V_1 may be helpful; the posterior right atrial sites have a biphasic P wave in V_1 with a positive–negative configuration, and the RSPV sites have a positive P wave in V_1. A second differentiating feature is that P waves from the RSPV show notching in lead II in 80% of patients, but are smooth in those coming from the region of the SVC.

Analysis of electrograms recorded from the posterior RA, CS, and His bundle regions during AT often reveals two components: near-field and far-field components, which may assist in determining whether the tachycardia originates in the RA or LA.[62] In the right atrial electrograms, when the amplitude of the first component (near-field electrogram, a sharper electrogram) is higher than that of the second, the AT is likely to originate in the RA. Likewise, analysis of CS electrograms consisting of a near-field component from CS musculature and a far-field component from left atrial myocardium can uncover LA activation preceding RA activation (see Fig. 73.10).

Although the limitations and accuracies of these algorithms have already been discussed above, P wave characteristics may assist in the localization of the focus to a particular PV. P waves from the left-sided PVs are generally broad in V_1 and are notched, particularly in the inferior leads, but also in V_1. A positive P wave in lead I is suggestive of a focus in the right-sided PV and an inverted P wave suggestive of a left-sided PV. An upright P wave in aVL is consistent with a right-sided PV focus; however, right-sided PV may also have negative P waves in aVL. The inferior leads may be used to differentiate superior from inferior PV sites (tall and upright vs. low amplitude or inverted).

Atrial Tachycardia Arising From the Mitral Annulus

The mitral annulus is the second most common location of focal AT in the LA, after the PV region. Interestingly, there appears to be a clustering of these foci around the superior aspect of the mitral annulus in immediate proximity to the region of the left fibrous trigone at the aortic-mitral continuity. A superior mitral annular location (as well as a location along the left side of the atrial septum or at the NCC) should be considered for AT when earliest right atrial activity is recorded in the para-Hisian region (approximately 0–20 ms before P wave onset) and the P wave demonstrates a characteristic morphology consisting of a biphasic (negative followed by positive) appearance in the precordial leads and a low-amplitude appearance in the limb leads.[68,69] Lead aVL is negative or isoelectric, and the inferior leads are positive during ATs arising from the superior mitral annulus. These ECG findings have a sensitivity of 88% and a specificity of 99%. The initial negative component of the P wave in lead V_1 is unusual for left ATs but may be explained by the relatively anterior position of the mitral annulus in this region. Focal ablation of these tachycardias is usually successful. It is speculated that remnants of the developing specialized conduction system at the mitral annulus-aorta junction could be the underlying substrate of this arrhythmia.[68] Myocardial cells at the mitral annulus-aorta junction exhibit AVN-like electrophysiological properties, respond to adenosine, lack connexin, and give rise to catecholamine-induced triggered activity due to delayed afterdepolarizations.[70,71]

Atrial Tachycardia Arising From the Left Atrial Appendage

AT may arise from the left atrial appendage (LAA) (~2% of sustained ATs). LAA tachycardias are often incessant and associated with tachycardia-mediated cardiomyopathy in some cases. The P wave during LAA tachycardias is deeply negative in leads I and aVL (which has a sensitivity of 92% and a positive predictive accuracy of 92% with a specificity of 97%), highly positive in the inferior leads, and broad and positive in lead V_1 (Fig. 73.12).[72,73] The atrial activation sequence typically shows activation in the distal CS earlier than the P wave.

Focal AT originating from the distal portion of the LAA could be successfully ablated with RF energy in 13 of 14 patients, with no long-term recurrences in the 13 successful cases.[74] However, in some reported cases, elimination of AT arising from the body or apex of the LAA is refractory to endocardial catheter ablation.[75] This is similar to what was described earlier for tachycardias arising from the RAA and is likely related to the complex "blind" cul-de-sac, a heavily trabeculated anatomy of the LAA that makes it difficult to manipulate catheters safely or to apply sufficient contact force at the LAA apex. Ancillary imaging modalities like an LAA venogram and intracardiac echocardiography are valuable in placing catheters deep within the LAA.

Rarely, an LAA tachycardia will need to be epicardially ablated, eliminated via surgical left atrial appendectomy, or abolished via thoracoscopic appendage exclusion with an Atriclip device or via percutaneous ligation of the LAA using a LARIAT device.[76–80]

Sinus Node Reentrant Tachycardia

Tachycardias arising from this region are presumed to be due to microreentry in tissue near the sinus node or perinodal region (superior CT). The P wave morphology during tachycardia should be identical to that seen during sinus rhythm. Additionally, the tachycardia can be reset or terminated by premature extrastimuli from the HRA.

Inappropriate Sinus Tachycardia

The uncommon, poorly characterized entity of inappropriate sinus tachycardia is probably a heterogeneous disorder. The

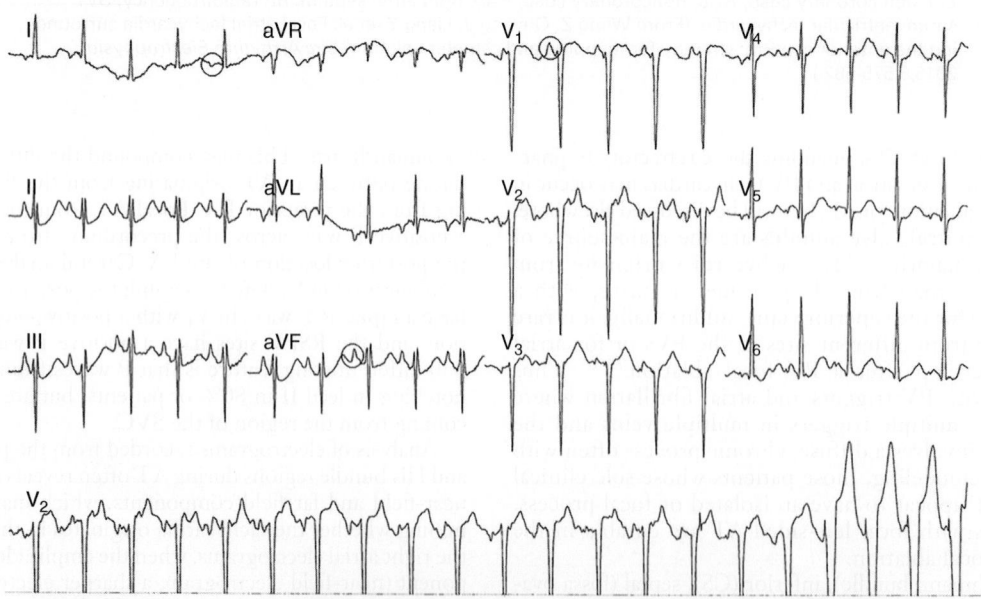

FIGURE 73.12 Representative example of a left atrial appendage tachycardia. Note the distinctly positive P wave in lead V1 due to the posterior location of the left atrium. Another characteristic feature is the markedly negative P waves in I and aVL.

hallmark feature of this syndrome is a consistently elevated resting heart rate (higher than 95 beats/min) and an exaggerated heart rate response to low levels of physical activity. The average sinus rate during 24-hour Holter monitoring is usually greater than 90 beats/min, and a persistent increase of at least 25 beats/min occurs on arising from supine to an upright position, in the absence of orthostatic arterial hypotension. Some affected patients have an elevated intrinsic heart rate, and others have increased responsiveness to infusions of isoproterenol. The ECG characteristics of this tachycardia include an identical P wave configuration in tachycardia and sinus rhythm. It is likely that some patients have primary autonomic abnormalities, including postural orthostatic tachycardia syndrome in some. Some patients may have primary abnormalities of the sinus node. An analysis of 18 patients with inappropriate sinus tachycardia receiving intravenous adenosine (0.1–0.15 mg/kg) showed that these patients demonstrated a blunted response with less sinus cycle length prolongation than age-matched control subjects undergoing electrophysiology studies.[81] The blunted response was seen after pharmacological autonomic blockade as well. These observations suggest that structural abnormalities of the sinus node are responsible for this syndrome. β-adrenergic receptor autoantibodies may be involved in the mechanism of inappropriate sinus tachycardia. In the electrophysiology laboratory, distinction should be made between inappropriate sinus tachycardia and a focal automatic AT with an origin close to the superior CT.[82]

A gain-of-function mutation of the cardiac pacemaker HCN4 channel that results in enhanced cyclic adenosine monophosphate sensitivity is reported as one of the causes of familial inappropriate sinus tachycardia.[83] Neural modulation with stellate ganglion block and renal sympathetic denervation has been employed to successfully treat inappropriate sinus tachycardia.[84,85] Ablation and modification of the sinus node mandates protection of the phrenic nerve. It frequently necessitates an endo-epicardial approach and the use of phrenic nerve displacing maneuvers.[86] Ablation of the sinus node is often frustrating. Extensive ablation with ablation lesions moving inferiorly along the CT is often necessary. Symptom improvement is often only modest, and during follow-up, acceleration of subsidiary pacemakers results in a return of symptoms over time.

Macroreentrant Atrial Tachycardia

Classification

Macroreentrant ATs can be divided into those that are cavotricuspid isthmus (CTI) dependent (dependent on conduction through the tricuspid annulus–inferior vena cava [IVC] isthmus) and nonisthmus dependent.[1] A majority of macroreentrant ATs in the adult population are CTI dependent. A majority of non–CTI-dependent macroreentrant ATs are related to an area of scar, often from a previous surgical incision. Some examples of macroreentrant ATs include typical AFL, lower loop reentry, double-wave reentry, macroreentrant AT from the right atrial free wall, and macroreentrant ATs occurring in the RA or LA related to previous surgery, including atriotomy, surgical scarring, and presence of septal prosthetic patches, suture lines, or other anatomical obstacles. Macroreentrant left ATs are now being seen with increasing frequency after atrial fibrillation ablation. Some unusual causes of macroreentrant tachycardia include reentry at sites of donor recipient anastomosis from either orthotopic heart transplantation or lung transplantation.[87] There has been an increasing recognition of macroreentrant ATs arising from scarring in patients who have not undergone previous atrial surgery or catheter ablation. Such "spontaneous" scarring has been described in the posterior wall of the LA, as well as in the posterolateral and lateral RA, and is now recognized as part of an atrial cardiomyopathy.[88,89] The successful ablation electrogram in these cases is frequently characterized by a long, fractionated signal that is frequently mid-diastolic and broad and fractionated and encompassing much of the TCL (Fig. 73.13).

Diagnostic Maneuvers

Electrophysiological characterization, mapping, and ablation of macroreentrant AT were described by several groups of investigators in the early 1990s, and these classic entrainment principles are described elsewhere in this chapter. Cycle length variability (>15%) is rarely seen with macroreentrant AT, unlike with focal AT. Atrial macroreentrant tachycardias may also occur less commonly in patients without previous cardiac surgery, catheter ablation, or obvious structural heart disease. In these patients, anisotropic conduction resulting in unidirectional block facilitates macroreentry.

Nakagawa and colleagues[90] noted that all macroreentrant postoperative ATs propagated through narrow channels (<2.7 cm) defined by the mapping system as an area of decreased electrogram voltage between two close dense or thin scars. They coined the phrase "no channel–no macroreentry." In their study, electrogram morphology, electrogram amplitude, and electrogram timing did not differentiate between sites within and those outside a narrow channel. Entrainment mapping failed to differentiate sites within the circuit, but was useful for distinction between outer loop sites from sites that were within the circuit and within the channel. Entrainment pacing was not done in many of the patients because it often resulted in induction of a new tachycardia or in termination of the original tachycardia. Additional limitations to entrainment mapping include difficulty measuring PPIs due to low amplitude signals or absence of atrial potentials in scarred atria or inability to pace the tissue. To overcome these limitations, measurements of the PPI-TCL may be made based on the N+1 difference or from recording sites remote from the pacing electrode.[91] Entrainment mapping also can induce atrial fibrillation.

The sensitivity and specificity of classical criteria for concealed entrainment for identification of a critical isthmus were examined by Morton and coworkers.[92] They used the model of typical AFL and performed entrainment mapping from seven sites at four different cycle lengths. Concealed entrainment identified any isthmus site with a flutter cycle length minus pacing cycle length of less than of 10 ms with 100% sensitivity but with a specificity of only 54%. Specificity increased to 98% when the flutter cycle length minus the pacing cycle length was less than 40 ms, but the sensitivity was decreased to 65%. When the flutter cycle length minus the pacing cycle length was less than, sensitivity and specificity were 85% and 90%, respectively. Concealed entrainment was seen from a nonisthmus site in 5 of 10 patients. Another caveat is that pacing at cycle lengths more than 30 ms faster than the tachycardia may give PPIs that are longer than expected due to local pacing latency. Even when pacing at rates slightly below (10–20 ms less than TCL), there could be significant local latency or long local atrial refractory periods that could yield misleadingly long PPI.[93,94] These findings highlight the observation that targeting sites for ablation based solely on entrainment will result in a less than ideal success rate.

In complex atrial arrhythmias quick determination of the mechanism and chamber of interest is mandatory. Recognition of intracardiac electrogram fusion and assessment of stimulus to electrogram times at "upstream sites" indicate that downstream overdrive pacing at sites close to a macroreentrant circuit (PPI-TCL < 40 ms) produced constant fusion demonstrated by a long stimulus to upstream atrial electrogram interval (S – A) >75% TCL and was consistent with orthodromic activation of the upstream site despite its close proximity to the pacing site.[95] In contrast, downstream overdrive pacing during focal AT or remote from the macroreentrant AT circuit (PPI-TCL > 40 ms) always demonstrated a comparatively short S-A <25% of TCL (12% vs.

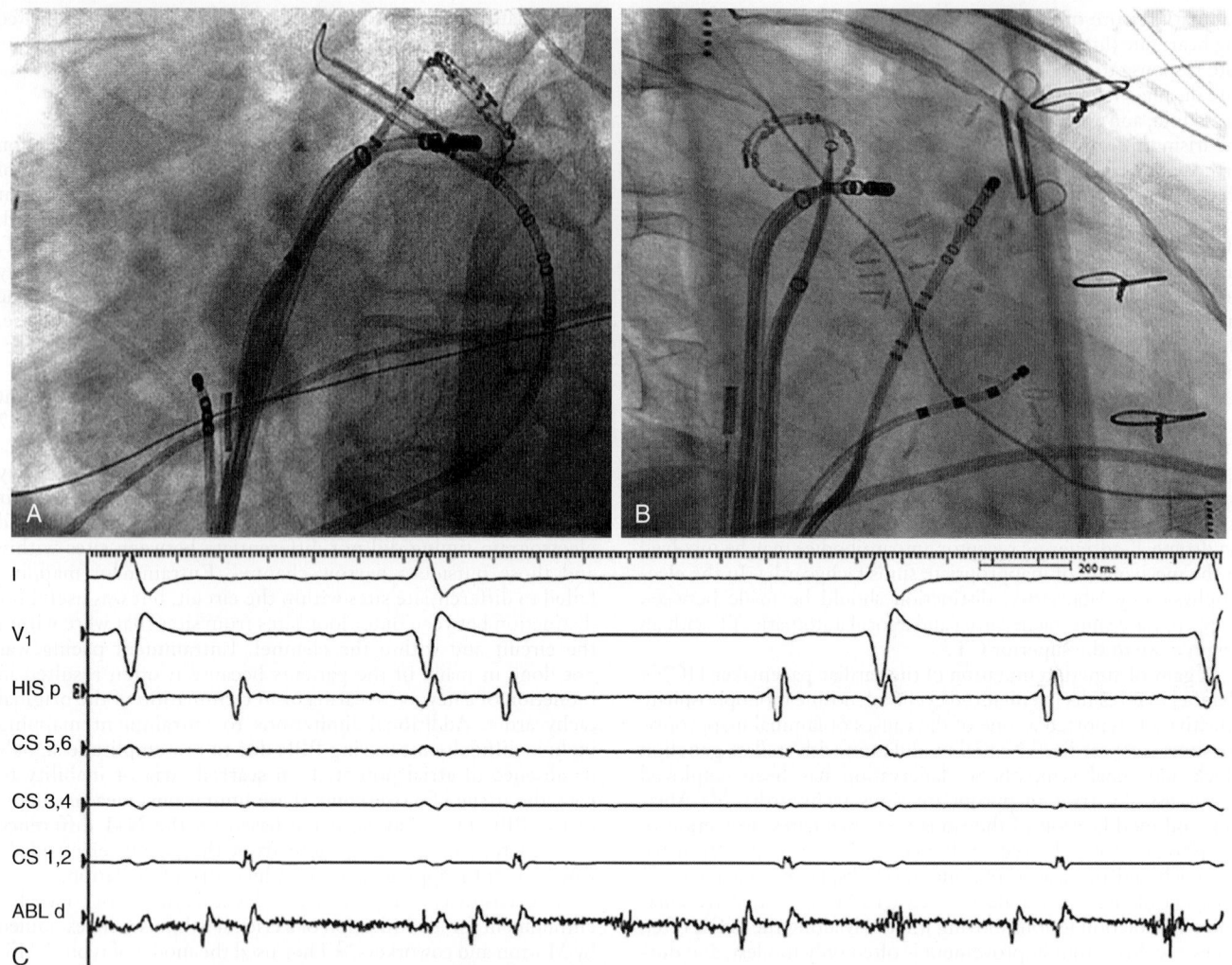

FIGURE 73.13 Representative example of localized reentry where a small area encompasses a large temporal fraction of the tachycardia circuit. (A) Left anterior oblique projection. (B) Right anterior oblique projection. (A) and (B) show the ablation catheter near the junction of the anterosuperior mitral annulus and the anterior ridge tissue abutting the clipped atrial appendage. The circular catheter is positioned in the left superior pulmonary vein. (C) shows that the patient is in atrial tachycardia with Wenckebach conduction through the atrioventricular node and the ablation electrogram records high-frequency, low-amplitude continuous signal that encompasses the majority of the tachycardia cycle length. A single radiofrequency application terminated the tachycardia and rendered it noninducible.

89% of TCL; $p < .001$), consistent with direct (antidromic) activation of sites recorded by the multipolar catheter (Fig. 73.14).

Recently, Linton and associates have described a method to diagnose double-loop reentry versus single-loop reentry.[96] The method involves calculating the time difference in activation recorded between two appropriate stationary positions, and an activation difference of two TCLs usually involves double loop reentry rather than single loop reentry.

$$[T_B\text{-}T_A]_{\text{overdrive 1}} - [T_B\text{-}T_A]_{\text{overdrive 2}}$$
$$\approx \text{TCL (indicates single loop reentry)}$$

$$[T_B\text{-}T_A]_{\text{overdrive 1}} - [T_B\text{-}T_A]_{\text{overdrive 2}}$$
$$\approx 2 \times \text{TCL (indicates double loop reentry)}$$

T_B and T_A represent the time of the first beat of tachycardia at locations B and A, respectively, after cessation of overdrive atrial pacing (Fig. 73.15).

Nevertheless, all the techniques suffer from a lack of spatial fidelity and resolution, which are necessary to identify small areas of the myocardium that can harbor the entire tachycardia circuit or focus. Bipolar voltage is notoriously inaccurate with current mapping modalities and is affected by variables such as contact, angle of contact, interelectrode spacing, size of the electrode, filtering of signals, mapping density, and mapping resolution.[97] Additionally, when electroanatomical mapping is used to create activation maps, uninterpretable maps can be generated, and meticulous attention to detail including determining the "window of interest" is warranted. When an erroneous determination of window of interest is made, a macroreentrant tachycardia may generate an activation map that suggests focal AT and vice versa.[98] Enhancements of existing 3D electroanatomical mapping technologies aim to overcome annotation errors. Ripple mapping is one such promising technology where distinction between functional low-voltage areas and nonfunctional low-voltage areas (scar) is accomplished by incorporating wavefront propagation information into a bipolar voltage map.[99] Ripple mapping helps facilitate localization of ATs. These findings underscore the difficulties of relying on any one criterion for defining sites of ablation of these complex

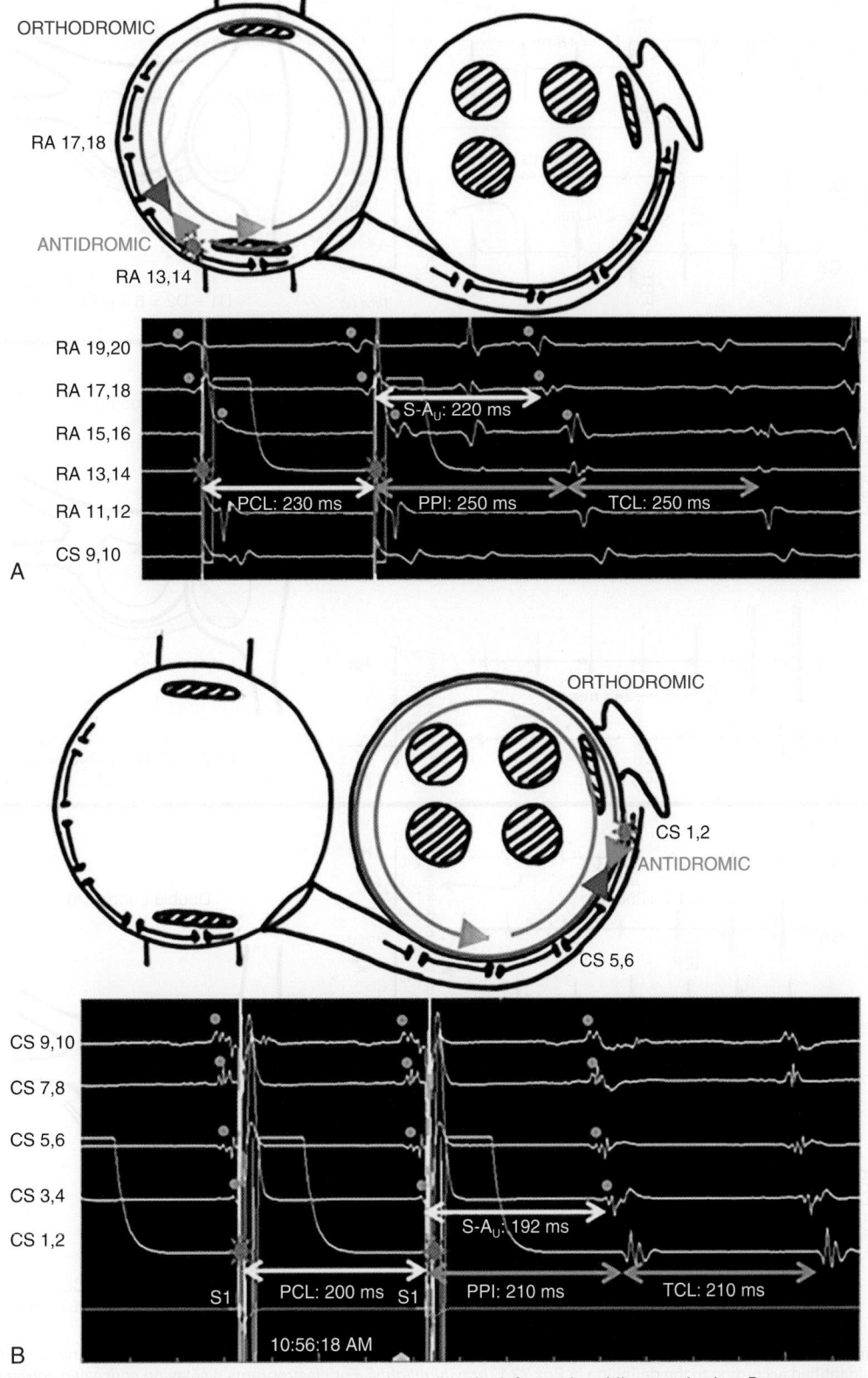

FIGURE 73.14 (A) Schematic representation of tricuspid and mitral annuli in the left anterior oblique projection. Downstream overdrive pacing from the low lateral right atrium (*RA*) (RA 13,14 indicated by the *star*) in cavotricuspid isthmus–dependent atrial tachycardia. Postpacing interval (*PPI*) equals tachycardia cycle length (*TCL*). *Blue dots* indicate each upstream electrode clearly accelerated to the paced cycle length. The stimulus to upstream atrial electrogram (S–A$_u$) interval at RA 17,18 is 220 ms (88% of TCL) and is suggestive of fusion and macroreentry along the multielectrode catheter. Note that RA 15,16 is also an upstream site captured orthodromically but is partially obscured by the pacing stimulus. Therefore RA 17,18 was chosen for S–A$_u$ measurement. Collision of orthodromic (*red arrow*) and antidromic (*green arrow*) wavefronts is likely occurring between RA 13,14 and RA 15,16. (B) Downstream overdrive pacing from the distal coronary sinus (*CS*) in perimitral flutter. Pacing is performed from CS 1,2 (*star*). PPI equals TCL. *Blue dots* indicate each electrogram at upstream electrodes clearly accelerated to the paced cycle length. The S–A$_u$ time is 192 ms (91% of TCL) and is suggestive of fusion and macroreentry along the multielectrode catheter. All orthodromically activated electrograms at upstream electrodes immediately precede pacing stimuli. Collision of antidromic (*green arrow*) and orthodromic (*red arrow*) wavefronts occurs between CS 1,2 and CS 3,4. *PCL,* Paced cycle length. (From Barbhaiya CR, Kumar S, Nq J, et al. Overdrive pacing from downstream sites on multielectrode catheters to rapidly detect fusion and to diagnose macroreentrant atrial arrhythmias. *Circulation.* 2014;129:2503-2510.)

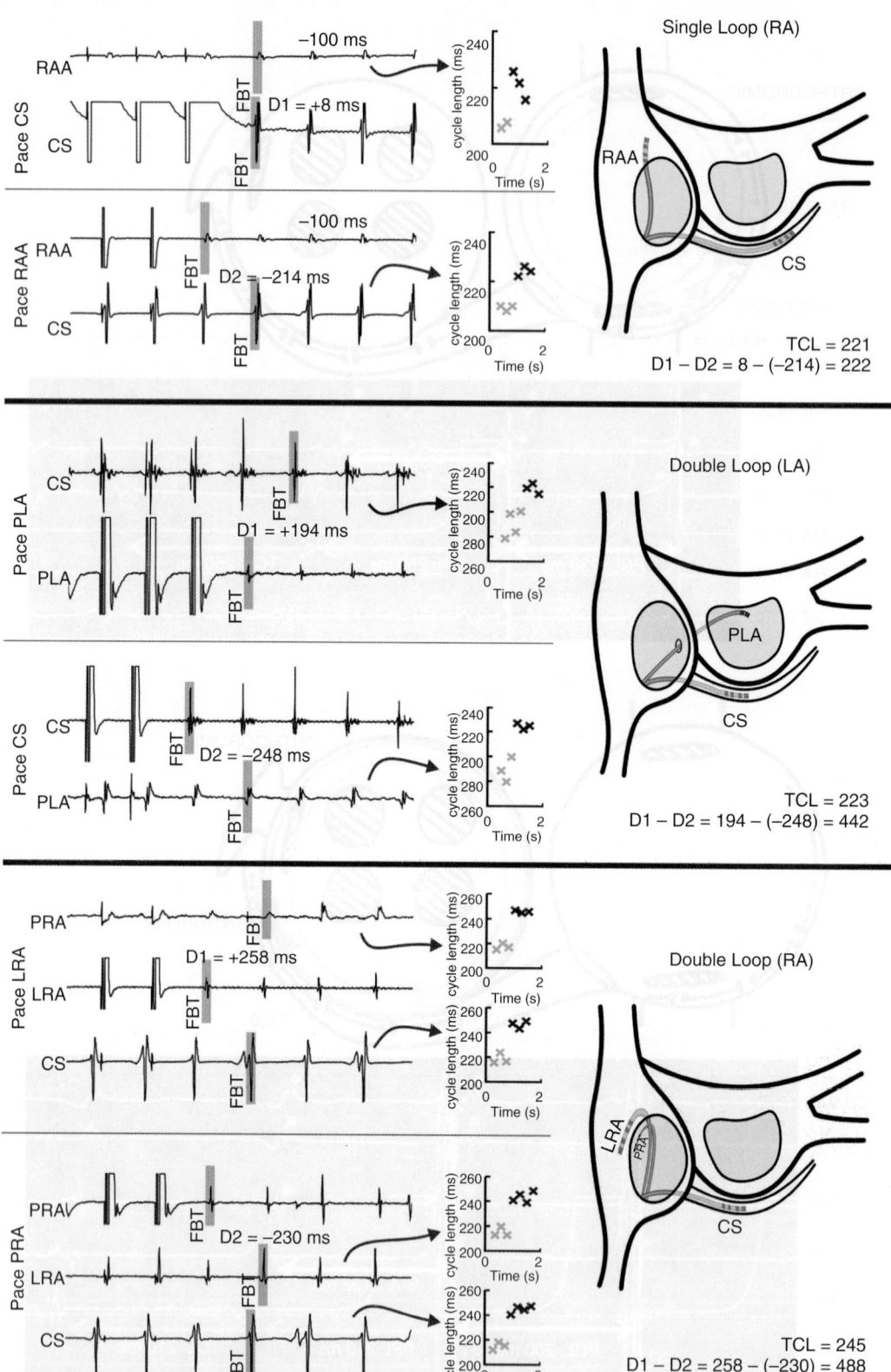

FIGURE 73.15 Examples of the criterion. Two entrainment maneuvers have been performed in three patients. After pacing, first beat of tachycardia (*FBT*) has been identified according to the definition in Box 73.1 (*gray highlights*). For electrograms displaying concealed entrainment, the cycle length has been plotted to confirm a change in cycle length after the cessation of pacing—the *black crosses* represent intervals after FBT and the *gray crosses* prior to FBT. Measurements of activation difference are shown (D1 – D2). Electrode positions are shown in the schematics to the right. *Upper panel:* Common flutter. In the first maneuver, entrainment has been performed from the coronary sinus (*CS*). In the second, the distal bipole of the other catheter was used for entrainment and this was positioned near the right atrial appendage (*RAA*). Artifact rendered the recording from distal bipole unusable. Because the entrainment criterion can be applied to any passive catheter, the recording from the proximal bipole can be used legitimately. The change in activation difference (D1 – D2) was approximately equal to one tachycardia cycle length (*TCL*), confirming reentry. *Middle panel:* Double loop reentry—perimitral and roof dependent tachycardia. Electrodes were placed at the high posterior left atrium (*PLA*) and the mid-CS. The change in activation difference (D1 – D2) was approximately equal to 2 × TCL, indicating double-loop reentry. The diagnosis was confirmed by ablation of the left atrial roof (which caused a change in postpacing interval at the posterior wall) and then termination by ablation at the mitral isthmus. *Lower panel:* Common flutter with a double loop. Electrodes were placed at the anterolateral right atrium (*LRA*), the posterior RA (*PRA*), and the CS. Entrainment was performed from LRA and from PRA. The activation difference between LRA and PRA changed by approximately 2 × TCL, indicating that these electrodes are positioned on different loops. Comparing the activation differences between PRA-to-CS and LRA-to-CS indicated single-loop reentry, confirming that the CS was in continuity with the common isthmus. (From Linton NW, Wilton SB, Scherr D, et al. A practical criterion for the rapid detection of single-loop and double-loop re-entry tachycardias. *J Cardiovasc Electrophysiol.* 2013;24:544-552.)

macroreentrant tachycardias. In general, current approaches that combine definition of anatomy with electrophysiological mapping data are warranted for attempted ablation of these arrhythmias.

Electrocardiographic Characterization of Macroreentrant Atrial Tachycardia

The surface ECG is of limited value for precise anatomical localization of macroreentrant tachycardias. Its use certainly is much less straightforward and has many more limitations than electrocardiographic localization of focal ATs using P wave morphology. The ECG is most useful for establishing a diagnosis of typical counterclockwise AFL. Electrocardiographic localization of the macroreentrant tachycardia circuit is influenced by altered atrial anatomy, previous surgical incisions, and conduction of the atrial wavefront. For example, clockwise and counterclockwise AFLs are characterized by P waves of opposite polarity in the inferior leads. The tachycardia circuit encompassed by these two flutters is the same, but the P wave polarity is affected by the direction in which the atrial wavefront travels (e.g., craniocaudal or reverse direction) and the route of left atrial activation. Macroreentrant circuits near the subeustachian isthmus may result in P wave morphology similar or identical to that seen with typical AFL.

Atypical AFL from the RA or LA has no uniform electrocardiographic characteristics (other than being different from the stereotypic appearance of typical right AFL).[100] An important point is that once the patient has had a previous ablation, the electrocardiographic appearance of the P wave morphology may be altered.[101] Furthermore, a focal AT that arises near an area of previous ablation may electrocardiographically appear like a flutter because of the altered atrial activation sequence caused by the line of block.

Despite the known limitations, a number of studies have attempted to address whether there are general clues from the 12-lead ECG that might assist the clinician in the localization of atrial macroreentrant circuits.[102,103] V_1 is the most useful lead for distinguishing left from right atrial origin, but much overlap exists. A broad-based upright V_1 is predictive of a left-sided flutter. Also, a negative P wave in lead aVL and low amplitude of the P waves in inferior leads are more consistent with left than right AFL. Conversely, when V_1 is deeply inverted, this is suggestive of a right-sided flutter. In addition, right atrial macroreentrant AT tends to have a higher incidence of a negative polarity in at least one precordial lead compared with LA macroreentry.

Left-sided AFL originating from the posterior or lateral wall of the LA and involving the left PVs is characterized by CS activation that usually proceeds from the distal or mid-CS to the proximal CS and demonstrates craniocaudal activation. Miyazaki and colleagues described a simplified approach to the rapid electrophysiological differentiation of left and right ATs.[104] Entrainment was performed at three sites: HRA, proximal CS, and distal CS. PPI-TCL <50 ms versus >50 ms at the HRA distinguished RA from LA reentrant circuits. PPI-TCL was <50 ms for right atrial circuits and >50 ms from the high lateral RA for left atrial circuits. For left atrial circuits, a PPI-TCL difference at the proximal and distal CS >50 ms versus <50 ms differentiated perimitral reentry from reentry involving the right PVs and septum. If the PPI-TCL difference was <50 ms from the proximal CS but >50 ms at the distal CS, the tachycardia was likely to involve the right PVs and septum. Additionally, analysis of stimulus to electrogram intervals and electrogram fusion at upstream sites when pacing from downstream can rapidly delineate the mechanism and circuit characteristics, as previously described.[95]

Specific Types of Macroreentrant Atrial Tachycardia

Right Atrial Macroreentrant Flutters

Right atrial macroreentrant circuits include typical AFL (counterclockwise or clockwise, CTI-dependent) and atypical flutters.

Atypical flutters include right atrial free wall reentry, upper loop reentry, and lower loop reentry. In addition, during some atypical AFLs, the location of the circuit is variable and may involve dual-loop reentry (figure-of-eight) or complex reentrant mechanisms. Atypical reentrant circuits usually are related to surgical scars or electrically silent areas and anatomical obstacles (in the RA: SVC, IVC, CT, and tricuspid annulus). As a general rule, the more complex the surgery, the more arrhythmogenic channels between scars exist, and this produces a larger number of tachycardias. Single and multiple conduction isthmuses bordered by fixed and or functional low-voltage zones are critical for these reentrant circuits.

Right atrial free wall reentry is probably the most common form of right atrial atypical flutter. During right atrial free wall atypical AFL, the activation wavefront circulates around a low-voltage or electrically silent zone in the lateral, posterolateral, or anterior free wall. This low-voltage region may be due to spontaneous scar formation or a prior cardiac surgical procedure. RF ablation of the channel between the IVC or tricuspid annulus and the central obstacle can eliminate this form of macroreentry.

The CT is not always a fixed line of conduction block. Conduction gaps in the CT may provide the substrate for upper loop reentry as well as other double-loop atypical flutters. Upper loop reentry involves the upper portion of the RA with a reentrant circuit that rotates around the SVC and a lower turnaround point located at a conduction gap in the CT. RF linear ablation of the conduction gap in the CT eliminates reentry. An incomplete line of block in the CT during typical AFL may result in double-loop reentry during typical AFL, one circulating around the tricuspid annulus and the other rotating around a part of the CT through the conduction gap. RF ablation of the cavotricuspid isthmus and the gap in the CT eliminates both reentrant loops.

Lower loop reentry (counterclockwise) involves only the lower portion of the RA and depends on conduction through the CTI and usually has a shorter cycle length than typical CTI-dependent AFL. The wavefront rotates around the IVC and tricuspid annulus with a breakthrough site at the low lateral tricuspid annulus. The P wave morphology is dependent on varying degrees of counterclockwise wavefront penetration of the lower RA (antidromic penetration). As such, there is no reliably distinctive P wave morphology that will identify this rhythm prior to invasive electrophysiological analysis. When utilizing multipolar catheters, wavefront collision in adjacent bipoles of the catheter automatically rules out the underlying myocardium participating in the reentrant arrhythmia. Thus vast areas of the RA will automatically be excluded very quickly when such an analysis is undertaken. This arrhythmia is successfully ablated in the CTI.

Left Atrial Macroreentrant Flutters

Left AFL includes mitral annular AFL, PV-related AFL, and left septal AFL. Most of these flutters are iatrogenic and are the result of ablation for atrial fibrillation and incomplete or nondurable linear ablation lines in the LA. In some patients, the LA circuits are complex, with two or three loops rotating concomitantly. These arrhythmias, especially those encountered after PV isolation procedures, are dealt with in more detail elsewhere in this textbook. The left septal AFL macroreentrant circuit rotates around the left septum primum, either counterclockwise or clockwise.[105] The electrocardiographic characteristics are dominant positive P ("F") waves in lead V_1 and low amplitude waves in the other leads. The critical isthmus is located between the septum primum and the PVs (posterior isthmus) or between the septum primum and the mitral annulus ring (anterior isthmus). RF ablation of either the posterior or anterior isthmus can eliminate this left septal AFL.

However, targeting the anterior isthmus may be more effective as the posterior isthmus may be thicker or more difficult to reach with a catheter.

Macroreentrant Atrial Tachycardia Following Cardiac Surgery

The presence of surgical atrial scars (lesion or incisional) provides a substrate for macroreentry. These surgeries may include correction of congenital heart disease or atriotomy scar–related flutter related to the correction of valvular cardiomyopathy or for coronary artery bypass grafting. Following surgery, the reentrant circuit may use the right atriotomy scar as a central obstacle, may rotate around an atrial patch used for atrial septal defect closure, or may be dependent on the CTI. Some circuits may be very complex, using channels between multiple dense scars and lines of fixed conduction block within large areas of low voltage.

Left atrial macroreentrant flutters after surgery are less common than right AFLs; however, they tend to occur more commonly in patients with a history of heart surgery.[106] The mode of atriotomy was noted to be the only independent predictor that determined the mechanism and location of postoperative AT in a study performed by Pap and associates.[107] Demographic and clinical parameters like hypertension, congenital heart disease,

ischemic heart disease, valve surgery, and preprocedural echocardiographic dimensions were not associated with a specific form of AT.

Atrial arrhythmias are common after orthotopic heart transplantation and are most likely due to atrial macroreentry. CTI-dependent donor AFL was noted to be the most common variant in one series.[108] However, due to bicaval anastomosis gaining more widespread acceptance, the incidence of such arrhythmias might decrease in the future. Additionally, recipient-to-donor atrial conduction has been reported to occur either in the right or left atrial anastomotic sites. These arrhythmias are particularly challenging to ablate due to the difficulty in distinguishing between far-field signals and near-field double potentials. Nevertheless, large series have reported acute success in 93% of patients, and 20% needed repeat ablation.[108]

Conclusions

Developments since the 1990s in electrophysiology, including the adoption of sophisticated 3D mapping systems together with the use of classical electrocardiography and electrophysiological maneuvers, have greatly contributed to a better understanding of both focal and macroreentrant ATs. In most cases, these arrhythmias can be successfully cured using catheter ablation with a low risk of complications.

REFERENCES

1. Saoudi N, Cosio F, Waldo A, et al. Classification of atrial flutter and regular atrial tachycardia according to electrophysiologic mechanism and anatomic bases: a statement from a joint expert group from the Working Group of Arrhythmias of the European Society of Cardiology and the North American Society of Pacing and Electrophysiology. *J Cardiovasc Electrophysiol.* 2001;12:852–866.
2. Brown JP, Krummen DE, Feld GK, Narayan SM. Using electrocardiographic activation time and diastolic intervals to separate focal from macro-reentrant atrial tachycardias. *J Am Coll Cardiol.* 2007;49:1965–1973.
3. Medi C, Kalman JM, Haqqani H, et al. Tachycardia-mediated cardiomyopathy secondary to focal atrial tachycardia: long-term outcome after catheter ablation. *J Am Coll Cardiol.* 2009;53:1791–1797.
4. Stambler BS, Fenelon G, Shepard RK, Clemo H, Guiraudon CM. Characterization of sustained atrial tachycardia in dogs with rapid ventricular pacing-induced heart failure. *J Cardiovasc Electrophysiol.* 2003;14:499–507.
5. Fenelon G, Shepard RK, Stambler BS. Focal origin of atrial tachycardia in dogs with rapid ventricular pacing induced heart failure. *J Cardiovasc Electrophysiol.* 2003;14:1093–1102.
6. Ogawa M, Zhou S, Tan AY, et al. Left stellate ganglion and vagal nerve activity and cardiac arrhythmias in ambulatory dogs with pacing-induced congestive heart failure. *J Am Coll Cardiol.* 2007;50:335–343.
7. Yamamoto T, Hayashi M, Miyauchi Y, et al. Respiratory cycle–dependent atrial tachycardia: prevalence, electrocardiographic and electrophysiologic characteristics, and outcome after catheter ablation. *Heart Rhythm.* 2011;8:1615–1621.
8. Chen SA, Chiang CE, Yang CJ, et al. Sustained atrial tachycardia in adult patients: electrophysiological characteristics, pharmacological response, possible mechanisms and effects of radiofrequency ablation. *Circulation.* 1994;90:1262–1278.
9. Markowitz SM, Nemirovsky D, Stein KM, et al. Adenosine-insensitive focal atrial tachycardia. *J Am Coll Cardiol.* 2007;49:1324–1333.
10. De Groot NMS, Schalij MJ. Fragmented, long-duration, low-amplitude electrograms characterize the origin of focal atrial tachycardia. *J Cardiovasc Electrophysiol.* 2006;17:1–7.
11. Chiale PA, Selva HO, Militello CA, Elizari MV. Lidocaine sensitive, rate-related, repetitive atrial tachycardia: a new arrhythmogenic syndrome. *J Am Coll Cardiol.* 2000;36:1637–1645.
12. Chiale PA, Faivelis L, Garro HA, Fernández PA, Herrera Paz JJ, Elizari MV. Distinct pharmacologic substrate in lidocaine-sensitive, rate-related atrial tachycardia. *J Cardiovasc Pharmacol Ther.* 2012;17:146–152.
13. Kistler PM, Roberts-Thompson KC, Haqqani HM, et al. P-wave morphology in focal atrial tachycardia: development of an algorithm to predict the anatomic site of origin. *J Am Coll Cardiol.* 2006;48:1010–1017.

14. Tang CW, Scheinman MM, Van Hare GF, et al. Use of P wave configuration during atrial tachycardia to predict site of origin. *J Am Coll Cardiol.* 1995;26:1315–1324.
15. Tada H, Nogami A, Naito S, et al. Simple electrocardiographic criteria for identifying the site of origin of focal right atrial tachycardia. *Pacing Clin Electrophysiol.* 1998;21:2431–2439.
16. Yamane T, Shah DC, Peng JT, et al. Morphological characteristics of P waves during selective pulmonary vein pacing. *J Am Coll Cardiol.* 2001;38:1505–1510.
17. Hachiya H, Ernst S, Ouyang F, et al. Topographic distribution of focal left atrial tachycardias defined by electrocardiographic and electrophysiologic data. *Circ J.* 2005;69:205–210.
18. Qian ZY, Hou XF, Xu DJ, et al. An algorithm to predict the site of origin of focal atrial tachycardia. *Pacing Clin Electrophysiol.* 2011;34:414–421.
19. Huo Y, Braunschweig F, Gaspar T, et al. Diagnosis of atrial tachycardias originating from the lower right atrium: importance of P-wave morphology in the precordial leads V3-V6. *Europace.* 2013;15:570–577.
20. Man KC, Chan KK, Kovack P, et al. Spatial resolution of atrial pace mapping as determined by unipolar atrial pacing at adjacent sites. *Circulation.* 1996;94:1357–1363.
21. Uhm JS, Shim J, Wi J, et al. An electrocardiography algorithm combined with clinical features could localize the origins of focal atrial tachycardias in adjacent structures. *Europace.* 2014;16:1061–1068.
22. Ramanathan C, Ghanem RN, Jia P, Ryu K, Rudy Y. Noninvasive electrocardiographic imaging for cardiac electrophysiology and arrhythmia. *Nat Med.* 2004;10:422–428.
23. Wang Y, Cuculich PS, Woodard PK, Lindsay BD, Rudy Y. Focal atrial tachycardia after pulmonary vein isolation: noninvasive mapping with electrocardiographic imaging (ECGI). *Heart Rhythm.* 2007;4:1081–1084.
24. Wang Y, Schuessler RB, Damiano RJ, Woodard PK, Rudy Y. Noninvasive electrocardiographic imaging (ECGI) of scar related atypical atrial flutter. *Heart Rhythm.* 2007;4:1565–1567.
25. Roten L, Pedersen M, Pascale P, et al. Noninvasive electrocardiographic mapping for prediction of tachycardia mechanism and origin of atrial tachycardia following bilateral pulmonary transplantation. *J Cardiovasc Electrophysiol.* 2012;23:553–555.
26. Shah AJ, Hocini M, Xhaet O, et al. Validation of novel 3-dimensional electrocardiographic mapping of atrial tachycardias by invasive mapping and ablation: a multicenter study. *J Am Coll Cardiol.* 2013;62:889–897.
27. González-Torrecilla E, Almendral J, Arenal A, et al. Combined evaluation of bedside clinical variables and the electrocardiogram for the differential diagnosis of paroxysmal atrioventricular reciprocating tachycardias in patients without pre-excitation. *J Am Coll Cardiol.* 2009;53:2353–2358.

27a. Knight BP, Ebinger M, Oral H, et al. Diagnostic value of tachycardia features and pacing maneuvers during paroxysmal supraventricular tachycardia. J Am Coll Cardiol. 2000;35:574–582.
28. Knight BP, Zivin A, Souza J, et al. A technique for the rapid diagnosis of atrial tachycardia in the electrophysiology laboratory. *J Am Coll Cardiol.* 1999;33:775–781.
29. Crawford TC, Mukerji S, Good E, et al. Utility of atrial and ventricular cycle length variability in determining the mechanism of paroxysmal supraventricular tachycardia. *J Cardiovasc Electrophysiol.* 2007;18:698–703.
30. Man KC, Niebauer M, Daoud E, et al. Comparison of atrial-His intervals during tachycardia and atrial pacing in patients with long RP tachycardia. *J Cardiovasc Electrophysiol.* 1995;6:700–710.
31. Colombowala IK, Massumi A, Rasekh A, et al. Variability in post-pacing intervals predicts global atrial activation pattern during tachycardia. *J Cardiovasc Electrophysiol.* 2008;19:142–147.
32. Maruyama M, Kobayashi Y, Miyauchi Y, et al. The VA relationship after differential atrial overdrive pacing: a novel tool for the diagnosis of atrial tachycardia in the electrophysiologic laboratory. *J Cardiovasc Electrophysiol.* 2007;18:1127–1133.
33. Mohamed U, Skanes AC, Gula LJ, et al. A novel pacing maneuver to localize focal atrial tachycardia. *J Cardiovasc Electrophysiol.* 2007;8:1–6.
34. Chang KC, Chen JY, Lin YC, Huang SK. Usefulness of interatrial conduction time to distinguish between focal atrial tachyarrhythmias originating from the superior vena cava and the right superior pulmonary vein. *J Cardiovasc Electrophysiol.* 2008;19:1231–1235.
35. Long DY, Salim M, Dong JZ, et al. Electroanatomical mapping of the right atrium during atrial tachycardia originating from right superior pulmonary vein: additional insights on differential diagnosis. *Pacing Clin Electrophysiol.* 2015;38:91–98.
36. Patel PJ, D'Souza B, Saha P, Chik WW, Riley MP, Garcia FC. Electroanatomic mapping of the intercaval bundle in atrial fibrillation. *Circ Arrhythm Electrophysiol.* 2014;7:1262–1267.
37. Morton JB, Sanders P, Das A, Vohra JK, Sparks PB, Kalman JM. Focal atrial tachycardia arising from the tricuspid annulus: electrophysiologic and electrocardiographic characteristics. *J Cardiovasc Electrophysiol.* 2001;12:653–659.
38. McGuire MA, De Bakker JM, Vermeulen JT, et al. Atrioventricular junctional tissue. Discrepancy between histological and electrophysiological characteristics. *Circulation.* 1996;94:571–577.
39. Hillock RJ, Stevenson IH, Morton JB, et al. Focal atrial tachycardias arising from the right atrial appendage: electrocardiographic and electrophysiologic characteristics and radiofrequency ablation. *J Cardiovasc Electrophysiol.* 2007;18:367–372.

40. Freixa X, Berruezo A, Mont L, et al. Characterization of focal right atrial tachycardia. *Europace*. 2008;10:105–109.
41. Zhang T, Li XB, Wang YL, et al. Focal atrial tachycardia arising from the right atrial appendage: electrophysiologic and electrocardiographic characteristics and catheter ablation. *Int J Clin Pract*. 2009;63:417–424.
42. Medi C, Kalman JM, Haqqani H, et al. Tachycardia-mediated cardiomyopathy secondary to focal atrial tachycardia: long-term outcome after catheter ablation. *J Am Coll Cardiol*. 2009;53:1791–1797.
43. Khan MK, Elmouchi D. Ablation of a resistant right atrial appendage tachycardia using a magnetic navigation system. *Pacing Clin Electrophysiol*. 2013;36:e15–e18.
44. Furushima H, Chinushi M, Hosaka Y, Aizawa Y. Focal atrial tachycardia refractory to radiofrequency catheter ablation originating from right atrial appendage. *Europace*. 2009;11:521–522.
45. Amasyali B, Kilic A. Possible role for cryoballoon ablation of right atrial appendage tachycardia when conventional ablation fails. *Tex Heart Inst J*. 2015;42:289–292.
46. Chun KJ, Ouyang F, Schmidt B, Kuck KH. Focal atrial tachycardia originating from the right atrial appendage: first successful cryoballoon isolation. *J Cardiovasc Electrophysiol*. 2009;20:338–341.
47. Dong J, Schreieck J, Ndrepepa G, Schmitt C. Ectopic tachycardia originating from the superior vena cava. *J Cardiovasc Electrophysiol*. 2002;13:620–624.
48. Zhao Z, Li X, Guo J. Electrophysiologic characteristics of atrial tachycardia originating from the superior vena cava. *J Interv Card Electrophysiol*. 2009;24:89–94.
49. Callans DJ, Ren JF, Schwartzman D, Gottlieb CD, Chaudhry FA, Marchlinski FE. Narrowing of the superior vena cava-right atrium junction during radiofrequency catheter ablation for inappropriate sinus tachycardia: analysis with intracardiac echocardiography. *J Am Coll Cardiol*. 1999;33:1667–1670.
50. Tsai CF, Tai CT, Hsieh MH, et al. Initiation of atrial fibrillation by ectopic beats originating from the superior vena cava: electrophysiological characteristics and results of radiofrequency ablation. *Circulation*. 2000;102:67–74.
51. Steven D, Roberts-Thomson KC, Seiler J, Michaud GF, John RM, Stevenson WG. Fibrillation in the superior vena cava mimicking atrial tachycardia. *Circ Arrhythm Electrophysiol*. 2009;2:e4–e7.
52. Badhwar N, Kalman JM, Sparks PB, et al. Atrial tachycardia arising from the coronary sinus musculature. Electrophysiological characteristics and long-term outcome after radiofrequency ablation. *J Am Coll Cardiol*. 2005;46:1921–1930.
53. Kistler PM, Fynn SP, Haqqani H, et al. Focal atrial tachycardia from the ostium of the coronary sinus. Electrocardiographic and electrophysiological characterization and radiofrequency ablation. *J Am Coll Cardiol*. 2005;45:1488–1493.
54. Lai LP, Lin JL, Chen TF, et al. Clinical, electrophysiological characteristics, and radiofrequency catheter ablation of atrial tachycardia near the apex of Koch's triangle. *Pacing Clin Electrophysiol*. 1998;21:367–374.
55. Chen CC, Tai CT, Chiang CE, et al. Atrial tachycardias originating from the atrial septum: electrophysiologic characteristics and radiofrequency ablation. *J Cardiovasc Electrophysiol*. 2000;11:744–749.
56. Frey B, Kreiner G, Gwechenberger M, Gossinger HD. Ablation of atrial tachycardia originating from the vicinity of the atrioventricular node: significance of mapping both sides of the interatrial septum. *J Am Coll Cardiol*. 2001;38:394–400.
57. Marrouche NF, Sippens Groenewegen A, Yang Y, et al. Clinical and electrophysiologic characteristics of left septal atrial tachycardia. *J Am Coll Cardiol*. 2002;40:1133–1139.
58. Iwai S, Badhwar N, Markowitz SM, et al. Electrophysiologic properties of para-hisian atrial tachycardia. *Heart Rhythm*. 2011;8:1245–1253.
59. Zhou Y, Guo J, Xu Y, et al. Electrophysiologic characteristics and radiofrequency ablation of focal atrial tachycardia arising from para-Hisian region. *Int J Clin Pract*. 2007;61:385–391.
60. Yamabe H, Okumura K, Morihisa K, et al. Demonstration of anatomical reentrant tachycardia circuit in verapamil-sensitive atrial tachycardia originating from the vicinity of the atrioventricular node. *Heart Rhythm*. 2012;9:1475–1483.
61. Yamabe H, Okumura K, Koyama J, Kanazawa H, Hoshiyama T, Ogawa H. Demonstration of anatomic reentrant circuit in verapamil-sensitive atrial tachycardia originating from the atrioventricular annulus other than the vicinity of the atrioventricular node. *Am J Cardiol*. 2014;113:1822–1828.
62. Traykov VB, Pap R, Shalganov TN, et al. Electrogram analysis at the His bundle region and the proximal coronary sinus as a tool to predict left atrial origin of focal atrial tachycardias. *Europace*. 2011;13:1022–1027.
63. Wang Z, Ouyang J, Liang Y, et al. Focal atrial tachycardia surrounding the anterior septum: strategy for mapping and catheter ablation. *Circ Arrhythm Electrophysiol*. 2015;8:575–582.
64. Pap R, Makai A, Szilagy J, et al. Should the aortic root be the preferred route for ablation of focal atrial tachycardia from around the AV Node? Support from intracardiac echocardiography. *J Am Coll Cardiol*. 2016;2:193–199.
65. Biviano AB, Bain W, Whang W, et al. Focal left atrial tachycardias not associated with prior catheter ablation for atrial fibrillation: clinical and electrophysiological characteristics. *Pacing Clin Electrophysiol*. 2012;35:17–27.
66. Dong J, Zrenner B, Schreieck J, et al. Catheter ablation of left atrial focal tachycardia guided by electroanatomic mapping and new insights into interatrial electrical conduction. *Heart Rhythm*. 2005;2:578–591.
67. Kistler PM, Sanders P, Fynn SP, et al. Electrophysiological and electrocardiographic characteristics of focal atrial tachycardia originating from the pulmonary veins. Acute and long-term outcomes of radiofrequency ablation. *Circulation*. 2003;108:1968–1975.
68. Teh AW, Kalman JM, Medi C, et al. Long-term outcome following successful catheter ablation of atrial tachycardia originating from the pulmonary veins: absence of late atrial fibrillation. *J Cardiovasc Electrophysiol*. 2010;21:747–750.
69. Gonzalez MD, Contreras LJ, Jongbloed MRM, et al. Left atrial tachycardia originating from the mitral annulus-aorta junction. *Circulation*. 2004;110:3187–3192.
70. Kistler PM, Sanders P, Hussin A, et al. Focal atrial tachycardia arising from the mitral annulus. Electrocardiographic and electrophysiologic characterization. *J Am Coll Cardiol*. 2003;41:2212–2219.
71. Wit AL, Fenoglio Jr JJ, Wagner BM, et al. Electrophysiological properties of cardiac muscle in the anterior mitral valve leaflet and the adjacent atrium in the dog. Possible implications for the genesis of atrial dysrhythmias. *Circ Res*. 1973;32:731–745.
72. Yamada T, Murakami Y, Yoshida Y, et al. Electrophysiological and electrocardiographic characteristics and radiofrequency catheter ablation of focal atrial tachycardia originating from the left atrial appendage. *Heart Rhythm*. 2007;4:1284–1291.
73. Wang YL, Li XB, Quan X, et al. Focal atrial tachycardia originating from the left atrial appendage: electrocardiographic and electrophysiologic characterization and long-term outcomes of radiofrequency ablation. *J Cardiovasc Electrophysiol*. 2007;18:459–464.
74. Yang Qian, Ma Jian, Shu Zhang, Ji-qiang Hu, Liao ZL. Focal atrial tachycardia originating from the distal portion of the left atrial appendage: characteristics and long-term outcomes of radiofrequency ablation. *Europace*. 2012;14:254–260.
75. Hillock RJ, Singarayar S, Kalman JM, Sparks PB. Tale of two tails: the tip of the atrial appendages is an unusual site for focal atrial tachycardia. *Heart Rhythm*. 2006;3:467–469.
76. Phillips KP, Natale A, Sterba R, et al. Percutaneous pericardial instrumentation for catheter ablation of focal atrial tachycardias arising from left atrial appendage. *J Cardiovasc Electrophysiol*. 2008;19:430–433.
77. Raczka F, Granier M, Mathevet L, Davy J. Radiofrequency ablation of a left appendage focal tachycardia using intracardiac ultrasound image integration to guide catheter: minimizing the risk of left appendage perforation. *Europace*. 2009;11:1253–1254.
78. Yamada Y, Ajiro Y, Shoda M, et al. Video-assisted thoracoscopy to treat atrial tachycardia arising from left atrial appendage. *J Cardiovasc Electrophysiol*. 2006;17:895–898.
79. Yamada T, McElderry T, Allison S, Kay N. Focal atrial tachycardia originating from the epicardial left atrial appendage. *Heart Rhythm*. 2008;5:766–767.
80. Pokushalov E, Romanov A, Artyomenko S, Arhipov A, Karaskov A. Left atrial appendectomy after failed catheter ablation of a focal atrial tachycardia originating in the Left Atrial Appendage. *Pediatr Cardiol*. 2010;31:908–911.
81. Still A-M, Huikuri HV, Juhani KE, et al. Impaired negative chronotropic response to adenosine in patients with inappropriate sinus tachycardia. *J Cardiovasc Electrophysiol*. 2002;13:557–562.
82. Chiale PA, Garro HA, Schmidberg J, et al. Inappropriate sinus tachycardia may be related to an immunologic disorder involving cardiac beta andrenergic receptors. *Heart Rhythm*. 2006;3:1182–1186.
83. Baruscotti M, Bucchi A, Milanesi R, et al. A gain-of-function mutation in the cardiac pacemaker HCN4 channel increasing cAMP sensitivity is associated with familial inappropriate sinus tachycardia. *Eur Heart J*. 2015; ehv582. [Epub ahead of print].
84. Huang HD, Tamarisa R, Mathur N, et al. Stellate ganglion block: a therapeutic alternative for patients with medically refractory inappropriate sinus tachycardia? *J Electrocardiol*. 2013;46:693–696.
85. MG1 Kiuchi, Souto HB, Kiuchi T, Chen S. Case report: renal sympathetic denervation as a tool for the treatment of refractory inappropriate sinus tachycardia. *Medicine (Baltimore)*. 2015;94:e2094.
86. Jacobson JT1, Kraus A, Lee R, Goldberger JJ. Epicardial/endocardial sinus node ablation after failed endocardial ablation for the treatment of inappropriate sinus tachycardia. *J Cardiovasc Electrophysiol*. 2014;25:236–241.
87. Sacher F, Vest J, Raymond JM, Stevenson WG. Incessant donor-to-recipient atrial tachycardia after bilateral lung transplantation. *Heart Rhythm*. 2008;5:149–151.
88. Stevenson IH, Kistler PM, Spence SJ, et al. Scar-related right atrial macroreentrant tachycardia in patients without prior atrial surgery: electroanatomic characterization and ablation outcomes. *Heart Rhythm*. 2005;2:594–601.
89. Kottkamp H. Fibrotic atrial cardiomyopathy: a specific disease/syndrome supplying substrates for atrial fibrillation, atrial tachycardia, sinus node disease, AV node disease, and thromboembolic complications. *J Cardiovasc Electrophysiol*. 2012;23:797–799.
90. Nakagawa H, Shah N, Matsudaira K, et al. Characterization of reentrant circuit in macroreentrant right atrial tachycardia after surgical repair of congenital heart disease: isolated channels between scars allow "focal" ablation. *Circulation*. 2001;103:699–709.
91. Derejko P, Szumowski LJ, Sanders P, et al. Clinical validation and comparison of alternative methods for evaluation of entrainment mapping. *J Cardiovasc Electrophysiol*. 2009;20:741–748.
92. Morton JB, Sanders P, Deen V, et al. Sensitivity and specificity of concealed entrainment for the identification of a critical isthmus in the atrium: relationship to rate, anatomic location and antidromic penetration. *J Am Coll Cardiol*. 2002;39:896–906.
93. Koller BS, Karasik PE, Solomon AJ, Franz MR. Prolongation of conduction time during premature stimulation in the human atrium is primarily caused by local stimulus response latency. *Eur Heart J*. 1995;16:1920–1924.
94. Vollmann D, Stevenson WG, Luthje L, et al. Misleading long post-pacing interval after entrainment of typical atrial flutter from the cavotricuspid isthmus. *J Am Coll Cardiol*. 2012;59:819–824.
95. Barbhaiya CR, Kumar S, Ng J, et al. Overdrive pacing from downstream sites on multielectrode catheters to rapidly detect fusion and to diagnose macroreentrant atrial arrhythmias. *Circulation*. 2014;129:2503–2510.
96. Linton NW, Wilton SB, Scherr D, et al. A practical criterion for the rapid detection of single-loop and double-loop reentry tachycardias. *J Cardiovasc Electrophysiol*. 2013;24:544–552.
97. Anter E, Josephson ME. Bipolar voltage amplitude: what does it really mean? *Heart Rhythm*. 2016;13:326–327.
98. Ju W, Yang B, Chen H, et al. Mapping of focal atrial tachycardia with an uninterpretable activation map after extensive atrial ablation: tricks and tips. *Circ Arrhythm Electrophysiol*. 2014;7:598–604.
99. Luther V, Linton NW, Koa-Wing M, et al. A prospective study of ripple mapping in atrial tachycardias: a novel approach to interpreting activation in low-voltage areas. *Circ Arrhythm Electrophysiol*. 2016;9:e003582.
100. Della Bella P, Fraticelli A, Tonod C, et al. Atypical atrial flutter: clinical features, electrophysiological characteristics and response to radiofrequency catheter ablation. *Europace*. 2002;4:241–253.
101. Gerstenfeld EP, Dixit S, Bala R, et al. Surface electrocardiogram characteristics of atrial tachycardias occurring after pulmonary vein isolation. *Heart Rhythm*. 2007;4:1136–1143.
102. Chang SL, Tsao HM, Lin YJ, et al. Differentiating macroreentrant from focal atrial tachycardias occurred after circumferential pulmonary vein isolation. *J Cardiovasc Electrophysiol*. 2011;22:748–755.
103. Medi C, Kalman JM. Prediction of the atrial flutter circuit location from the surface electrocardiogram. *Europace*. 2008;10:786–796.
104. Miyazaki H, Stevenson WG, Stephenson K, et al. Entrainment mapping for rapid distinction of left and right atrial tachycardias. *Heart Rhythm*. 2006;3:516–523.
105. Ouyang F, Ernst S, Vogtmann T, et al. Characterization of reentrant circuits in left atrial macroreentrant tachycardia: critical isthmus block can prevent atrial tachycardia recurrence. *Circulation*. 2002;105:1934–1942.
106. Aktas MK, Khan MN, Di Biase L, et al. Higher rate of recurrent atrial flutter and atrial fibrillation following atrial flutter ablation after cardiac surgery. *J Cardiovasc Electrophysiol*. 2010;21:760–765.
107. Pap R, Kohári M, Makai A, et al. Surgical technique and the mechanism of atrial tachycardia late after open heart surgery. *J Interv Card Electrophysiol*. 2012;35:127–135.
108. Nof E, Stevenson WG, Epstein LM, Tedrow UB, Koplan BA. Catheter ablation of atrial arrhythmias after cardiac transplantation: findings at EP study utility of 3-D mapping and outcomes. *J Cardiovasc Electrophysiol*. 2013;24:498–502.

74 Atrial Tachycardia in Adults With Congenital Heart Disease

Dominic James Abrams

The preoperative, surgical, and long-term management of children who undergo congenital cardiac surgery, leading to an ever expanding population of young patients with adult congenital heart disease (ACHD), has seen major improvements since the 1980s. A regional longitudinal analysis in Quebec demonstrated that between 2000 and 2010, the prevalence of all ACHD and severe ACHD increased by 57% and 55%, respectively, compared with that of all congenital heart disease (CHD) and severe CHD in children, which increased by 11% and 19%, respectively. By 2010, the overall prevalence of ACHD was 6.12 per thousand, and adults accounted for two-thirds of the entire CHD population.[1]

The long-term hemodynamic stress imposed in varying congenital cardiac lesions, coupled with repeated surgical intervention, creates an ideal environment for the genesis of varying tachycardias, specifically reentrant circuits dependent on central fixed obstacles to conduction and variable sites of slow conduction or functional conduction block. As such, the overall prevalence of atrial tachycardias (ATs) in ACHD has been documented at 15% and is higher in more complex congenital lesions, such as Ebstein anomaly (33%), transposition of the great arteries (TGAs; 28%), and Fontan circulations (24.2%). The 20-year risk for developing AT was 7% in a 20-year-old patient and 38% in a 50-year-old patient, such that a 20-year-old ACHD patient has the same arrhythmia risk as a 55-year-old within the normal population. Perhaps most concerning is the finding that AT in ACHD is associated with double the risk for cerebrovascular events and heart failure and a 50% increase in mortality. These findings have led to the apt notion of "young patients with aged hearts."[2]

In many ACHD patients who have been well palliated and lead functionally normal lives, the emergence of AT first indicates the need for an intervention in many years and has major implications on the quality of life in young adults with careers and families. However, in a proportion of patients, perhaps best typified by those with univentricular or Fontan circulation, the onset of arrhythmias may herald the beginning of a gradual hemodynamic decline. As such, prompt recognition and management of AT in all ACHD patients are imperative to prevent the often significant and progressive morbidity.

Atrial Remodeling in Adult Congenital Heart Disease

Congenital cardiac lesions create unique hemodynamic stressors on the developing atrial myocardium, such as chronic volume loading from regurgitant atrioventricular (AV) valves and intracardiac shunts, pressure loading from stenotic AV valves or elevated end-diastolic pressures in noncompliant ventricles, cyanosis, and the often repeated effects of atrial incisions during cardiac surgery and cardiopulmonary bypass. This creates an electrophysiological substrate that satisfies the fundamental criteria of reentry, namely adequate central and lateral boundaries that prevent short circuiting, a path length that exceeds the wavelength determined by the effective refractoriness of the atrial myocardium and the potential for unidirectional block of initiating impulses.[3]

Early animal models of right atrial (RA) enlargement created by the excision of the tricuspid valve septal leaflet via a right atriotomy and pulmonary artery banding demonstrated easily inducible, sustained arrhythmias with electrocardiogram (ECG) and intracardiac electrogram (EGM) morphologies that are consistent with atrial flutter (AFL), which could not be induced in sham animals. Histological analysis demonstrated myocyte hypertrophy and increased intercellular connective tissues, but transmembrane potentials were no different in study animals compared with control animals, suggesting that the effect was independent of the changes in atrial electrophysiological parameters.[4]

Typical AFL is perhaps the best studied atrial arrhythmia, the mechanism for which has been well understood for some time. A reentrant wavefront propagates counterclockwise (or clockwise) around the tricuspid valve that traverses the inferior cavotricuspid isthmus (CTI), sustained by not only RA size but also the presence of conduction block at the crista terminalis (CT) on the posterolateral aspect of the chamber. Initial human mechanistic studies demonstrated that transcristal conduction was possible during sinus rhythm and pacing at longer cycle lengths (CLs) but was prevented during pacing at shorter CL and AFL by the development of functional conduction block, facilitated by the preferential end-to-end distribution of gap junctions within the CT, leading to anisotropic conduction.[5,6] The slowing of transverse conduction across CT and hence the development of a conduction block has been experimentally shown to increase with age.[7,8]

The mechanism by which atrial dilatation may promote typical AFL has been studied in patients with unrepaired atrial septal defects (ASDs), with no prior arrhythmic history that may have facilitated atrial remodeling. Chronic atrial dilatation led to conduction delay at CT as defined by the magnitude of and delay between double potentials recorded at this site. Additionally, there was a trend toward increased atrial effective refractory periods and sinus node dysfunction, but there were no changes in conduction velocity in the RA free wall. These findings were not present in the age-matched controls.

Despite ASD closure, the conduction block at the CT and atrial dilatation were still present at the follow-up evaluation, suggesting that persistent atrial dilatation and conduction delay at the CT support AFL late after ASD closure.[9] Similarly, electrophysiological changes have been documented in the left atrium (LA) of ASD patients, including chamber dilatation and electrical scars with widespread changes in the conduction velocity characterized by fractionated EGMs and double potentials, and similar to RA, an increase in the effective refractory periods. This remodeling was associated with an increased propensity for atrial fibrillation (AF).[10] Atrial remodeling secondary to chronic atrial arrhythmias has also been shown in animal models using an intercaval to RA appendage Y-shaped incision to facilitate AFL induction. Sustained typical AFL led to a significant decrease in both atrial refractoriness and conduction velocity, with the widening of the excitable gap from 13% to 46% of the flutter circuit length. This not only stabilized the AFL circuit but also, with appropriate triggers, facilitated AF induction.[11]

Arrhythmia Mechanisms in Adult Congenital Heart Disease

Arrhythmia mechanisms are highly varied in ACHD. Classically, these lesions are associated with macroreentrant AT (MAT) using sites of fixed and functional conduction block as central obstacles to conduction and narrow channels of viable but slowly conducting myocardium to ensure the reentrant wavefront is always approaching the excitable myocardium. Increasingly, however, other mechanisms have been recognized, including focal ATs (FATs) and common arrhythmias such as AV nodal reentrant tachycardia (AVNRT), which may have different intracardiac activation patterns from that seen in structurally normal hearts because of anatomical and electrophysiological remodeling. As the population ages, AF is increasingly recognized and represents a new challenge in arrhythmia management within this population. Finally, specific lesions may be associated with arrhythmia as part of the underlying pathophysiology rather than as a consequence of remodeling and surgical intervention, perhaps best typified by Ebstein anomaly. In approaching different mechanisms, a simple anatomical categorization, which may be helpful, are those arrhythmias associated with postbiventricular repair, those associated with univentricular repair, and those associated with the underlying cardiac lesion.

Arrhythmia Following Biventricular Repair

In most forms of CHD, the anatomical anomalies permit the surgical creation of a biventricular circulation, including atrial and ventricular septal defects, tetralogy of Fallot variants, anomalous pulmonary venous drainage, truncus arteriosus, and TGA.

Using entrainment mapping and multipolar catheters, initial studies identified two obstacles as key to the arrhythmia mechanism, namely the tricuspid annulus[12] and right atriotomy.[13] In 15 of 21 circuits mapped by Chan, CTI was part of the circuit, with successful ablation achieved in 14 of 15 cases.[12] Conversely, Kalman excluded patients with evidence of CTI-dependent flutter,[13] identifying 11 circuits in nine patients post-ASD closure where the atriotomy was critical to the arrhythmia mechanism, and successful termination could be achieved by the creation of a linear ablation lesion between the atriotomy and tricuspid annulus (5 circuits), the canal veins (5 circuits), and the ASD patch and tricuspid annulus (1 circuit). Subsequent animal studies further demonstrated the MAT mechanism related to atrial incisions. In seven animals, a right "atriotomy" was created in the free wall at 1 to 1.5 cm

anterior and parallel to CT, whereas in six animals, it was positioned more posterior and close to the CT, and the mapping of induced AT was performed using an epicardial multielectrode array. In four cases with an anterior lesion, the wavefront rotated around the atriotomy, whereas in three animals with an anterior lesion and all animals with a posterior lesion, there was a functional extension of the fixed line of block to the caval orifices; this created a posterior line of intercaval block and facilitated CTI-dependent AT,[14] suggesting mechanistic commonality between typical periannular AFL and circuits that are apparently dependent on the atriotomy.

Numerous further studies have documented the arrhythmia mechanism in different ACHD anatomical variants, all supporting the initial mechanistic observations. Typical, CTI-dependent AFL was seen in 14 of 20 patients following detailed mapping after a variety of biventricular repairs, accounting for 46% of successfully mapped MAT.[15] Similarly Delacretaz reported a series of 20 patients, again with differing CHD variants, in whom 47 different MAT circuits were mapped, with 79% dependent on either CTI or the right atriotomy.[16] Subsequent studies have focused on arrhythmia mechanisms in specific congenital lesions, with similar findings (Fig. 74.1). In 20 patients who underwent clinically indicated electrophysiology study (EPS) at 29 ±15 years after surgical ASD closure, CTI-dependent AFL was present in all 20 patients. Additionally, 14 patients had atriotomy-dependent circuits as part of the dual-loop tachycardia mechanism, 2 patients had FAT, and 2 had AVNRT.[17] Dual-loop tachycardias are well recognized following congenital cardiac surgery and typically display an ECG appearance that was consistent with CTI-dependent AFL having a second atriotomy-mediated circuit that was revealed with successful isthmus ablation.[18] In a similar series of 56 patients with tetralogy of Fallot or a double-outlet right ventricle (RV) who underwent EPS between 1997 and 2010, of 95 MAT circuits identified, 85% involved CTI or the lateral RA wall that was consistent with an atriotomy-mediated mechanism.[19]

The atrial switch (Mustard or Senning procedure) was the surgical strategy of choice for TGA prior to the introduction of the arterial switch, although it is still used as part of the "double switch" for the correction of congenitally corrected TGA. Similar to other patients who have undergone postbiventricular repair, CTI-dependent typical AFL remains the most prevalent mechanism, identified in 18 of 24 (75%)[20] and 10 of 13 (77%)[21] MATs in two series. Other MATs may involve sites remote from CTI, including the inferior vena cava (IVC) and pulmonary venous orifices, with other reported mechanisms, including FAT and AVNRT.[20,21]

Specific congenital lesions and associated surgical procedures may generate a unique anatomical substrate and hence arrhythmia mechanism. In total anomalous pulmonary venous connection (TAPVC), the four pulmonary veins drain to a confluence posterior to LA and ultimately to RA via a vertical vein and the superior vena cava (SVC) or IVC. Surgical correction involves the anastomosis of the confluence to the posterior LA, potentially creating a line of conduction block, which may facilitate MAT. AT has been reported after pulmonary lung transplantation, which was shown to be a LA reentrant mechanism in animal models that simulate surgical incisions used in lung transplantation.[22,23] However, the majority of patients with MAT post-TAPVC appear to also have a CTI-dependent mechanism, likely secondary to RA volume loading.[15]

Arrhythmia Following Univentricular Repair

The Fontan procedure has become synonymous with varying different surgical procedures to palliate patients with a functional univentricular circulation, all of which route systemic venous returns directly to the pulmonary vascular bed. Eponymously

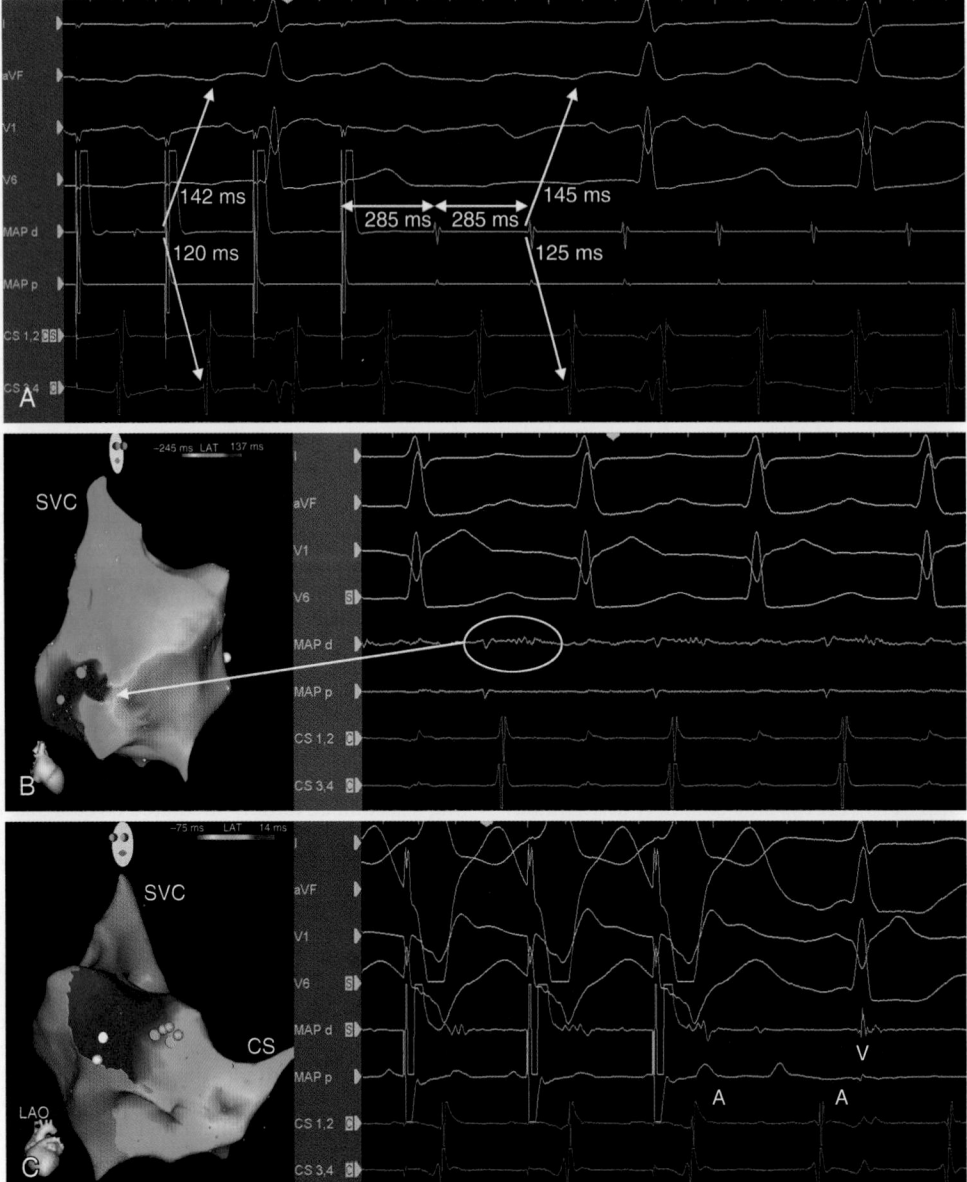

FIGURE 74.1 Arrhythmia mechanisms in tetralogy of Fallot. Three arrhythmias identified in a 50-year-old female with tetralogy of Fallot who presented with asymptomatic atrial tachycardia and a 12-lead electrocardiogram (ECG) appearance consistent with typical atrial flutter. Four surface ECG leads are displayed (I, aVF, V₁, and V₆) with intracardiac electrograms from a mapping catheter with the distal bipole on the cavotricuspid isthmus (CTI) and a quadripolar reference catheter in the coronary sinus (*CS*). (A) Entrainment mapping at CTI demonstrated concealed entrainment, with a postpacing interval equal to the tachycardia cycle length, atrial ECG morphology, and intracardiac activation identical during pacing and atrial flutter, and similar times were recorded from both the mapping pacing spike and mapping electrogram to stable points on surface ECG and CS electrogram. Radiofrequency ablation at CTI terminated tachycardia with a confirmed bidirectional block, and no other arrhythmias were inducible. On a Holter monitor performed 4 weeks later, a further asymptomatic tachycardia was seen, which was spontaneously terminated at night. A second study was performed using the electroanatomical mapping system (Carto [Biosense Webster, Diamond Bar, CA]). A reconstruction of the right atrium is shown with the chamber viewed from a right lateral projection (see cardiac silhouette), with the activation superimposed onto the anatomical shell with *red* denoting the earliest and *purple* denoting the latest sites of activation referenced to a stable catheter in the CS. (B) Clinical tachycardia was identified as a macroreentrant atrial tachycardia with a site of slow conduction characterized by a prolonged, low-amplitude electrogram (*circled*) at the lower crista terminalis, which terminated repeatedly with catheter pressure, and was ultimately successfully ablated. (C) With programmed atrial stimulation, a further tachycardia was induced, with centrifugal activation originating from close to CS os, as displayed on the right atrium reconstruction seen from a left anterior oblique (*LAO*) view. On termination of the ventricular pacing with atrial entrainment, an atrial-atrial-ventricular return sequence was seen, confirming this to be a focal atrial tachycardia, which was successfully ablated. *SVC*, Superior vena cava.

described in 1971, the procedure has undergone numerous surgical modifications, each of which may be associated with different arrhythmia mechanisms. While this was an incredible advance in the management of such patients, Fontan and Baudet recognized the arrhythmic potential and its deleterious effects on hemodynamics, stating

> *"one element remains unpredictable-the hemodynamic consequences of an eventual atrial rhythm disturbance such as an atrial fibrillation or flutter."*[24]

The atriopulmonary Fontan procedure incorporated a surgical anastomosis between the RA roof or appendage and the pulmonary arteries and was the procedure most commonly used over 20 years, generating a large population of such patients with a high incidence of atrial rhythm disturbances.[25] In its adopted role as the subpulmonary chamber, RA in the atriopulmonary Fontan circulation undergoes a severe process of remodeling, characterized by significant chamber dilatation and areas of myocardial scar distant from the sites of surgical intervention. In a series of 26 patients (age, 26.8 ± 8.9 years) who underwent detailed electrophysiological mapping at 18.7 ± 4.4 years after the atriopulmonary Fontan procedure, the median RA surface area was 235 cm^2 (range, 136–455 cm^2), with atrial volumes recorded to be up to 500 mL. The median endocardial surface area covered by the dense scar (bipolar contact EGM or ≤0.05 mV or not identifiable) was 15.07% (1.89%–56.15%), and the additional area of low-voltage endocardium (bipolar contact EGM, ≤0.5 mV) was 25.25% (7.38%–55.11%).[26] While this represents a significant degree of electrical remodeling, it was less than that initially reported by electroanatomical mapping of the Fontan RA, where the viable myocardium was excited only as narrow channels between large, confluent areas of scar, permitting multiple reentrant circuits and a "point ablative" strategy.[27]

Contrary to patients following a biventricular repair, CTI-dependent circuits are rare in the atriopulmonary Fontan, largely because of the fact that a significant proportion of patients who undergo surgery in this era had tricuspid atresia, making such a mechanism much less likely but not impossible. The vast majority of MATs use areas of scar and natural anatomical obstacles as central barriers to conduction, often with the sites of slow conduction seen along CT on the posterolateral wall. Scarring within RA is often primarily distributed on the anterior and lateral surfaces of RA and is almost ubiquitously seen at the inferior aspect of CT on the posterolateral chamber wall. Whether this relates to hemodynamic stress at an anatomically susceptible site or the placement of the inferior bypass cannula at the time of surgery is unclear. This area of scarring combined with a dilated IVC orifice creates a large nonconductive barrier for MAT, with breakthrough sites from the narrow channels seen on the lateral wall, a mechanism that has been termed as pericaval reentry.[15] Detailed mapping of 43 different RA arrhythmias using a combination of electroanatomical and noncontact mapping identified the following mechanisms as MAT (n = 33), FAT (n = 9), and AVNRT (n = 1). MATs were further divided into wavefront propagations that were perpendicular to the vertical axis of RA and dependent on fixed (n = 7) or fixed and functional (n = 8) conduction block on the posterolateral wall of RA at the position of CT (Fig. 74.2), CTI-dependent (n = 5), and scar-related reentry, in which the wavefront propagates around dense scars or sites of fixed conduction block remote from anatomical obstacles (n = 13). The site of FAT origin was from the lateral (n = 4) and anterior (n = 2) walls, CT (n = 1), CTI (n = 1), and para-Hisian location (n = 1).[26]

The concentric spread of activation from an apparently focal source, which can be successfully entrained, thus inferring a microreentrant mechanism, has also been reported.[28,29] In one case, electroanatomical mapping alone failed to identify the mechanism, which was subsequently confirmed by the demonstration of a focal entrained zone that occupies approximately 1% of the mapped surface area on the high lateral wall with the rapid activation of the anterior atrial surface.[29]

In 1978, Björk and colleagues proposed an additional surgical technique, where the rudimentary RV was retained within the subpulmonary circulation, thus contributing to the anterograde pulmonary blood flow.[30] The technique involved the creation of an AV communication using a tissue flap from the RA appendage anastomosed directly to the RV outflow tract, creating a second excitable connection separate from the AV node, thereby permitting a reentrant circuit between the surgically created "accessory pathway" and AV node.[31]

In 1988, de Leval revised the circulation further by creating the total cavopulmonary connection (TCPC), which from an arrhythmic perspective aimed to reduce both the RA size and the degree of atrial myocardium exposed directly to pulmonary vascular loading conditions.[32] Although reduced arrhythmia frequency has been reported in patients following TCPC compared with the atriopulmonary Fontan, the arrhythmia burden at midterm follow-up remains significant.[33,34] The first insight into the potential arrhythmia mechanism came from animal models, where the intraatrial baffle was shown to act as the posterior obstacle within RA akin to CT in the normal heart, and the wavefront propagated around the anterior tricuspid valve via CTI.[35-38] These findings have been supported by studies in human post-TCPC.[39] In 52 patients (age, 18.4 ± 11.8 years) studied between 2006 and 2012, 25 MATs were documented in 17 patients. CTI (or cavomitral isthmus in congenitally corrected TGA [Fig. 74.3]) was critical to 14 circuits with activation maps that demonstrated periannular wavefront propagation. The remaining 11 MATs were located within the intraatrial baffle (n = 8) or the pulmonary venous atrium (n = 3; Fig. 74.4); a further eight FATs were mapped, of which six were within the intracardiac baffle, stressing that the baffle, despite appearing as a mere "conduit" directing IVC blood to the pulmonary circulation, has significant arrhythmogenic potential likely because of the presence of CT, extensive suture lines, and areas of slowly conducting myocardium.

Perhaps most interesting was the finding of 13 arrhythmias in eight patients with a 1:1 AV relationship and either a short (n = 7; 35–65 ms) or long (n = 6; 176–260 ms) ventriculoatrial interval. During tachycardia, it was not possible to reset the atrium, with preexcitation indices ranging from 110 to 180 ms,[40] and an AV response was seen on the cessation of ventricular pacing with atrial entrainment,[41] both strongly supporting AVNRT as the mechanism. In patients with the anatomical triad of atrial isomerism, an AV septal defect, and ventriculoarterial discordance, two AV nodes may be present that permit a reciprocating tachycardia. The diagnosis may be made prior to invasive electrophysiological assessment by the presence of two different QRS morphologies with no evidence of preexcitation or invasively by the finding of two distinct His bundle EGMs, decremental anterograde and retrograde conduction, and regular tachycardia CL with a 1:1 AV relationship anterograde over one AV node and retrograde via the alternate node.[42] These findings highlight the potential for more simple arrhythmia mechanisms despite the anatomical complexity and stress the importance of comprehensive electrophysiological analysis using intracardiac activation patterns, diagnostic maneuvers during tachycardia, and entrainment.

Arrhythmias Associated With Specific Congenital Cardiac Lesions

While many congenital cardiac lesions may have arrhythmias as part of the constellation that underlies anatomical features,[43] this is perhaps best typified by Ebstein anomaly. Eponymously

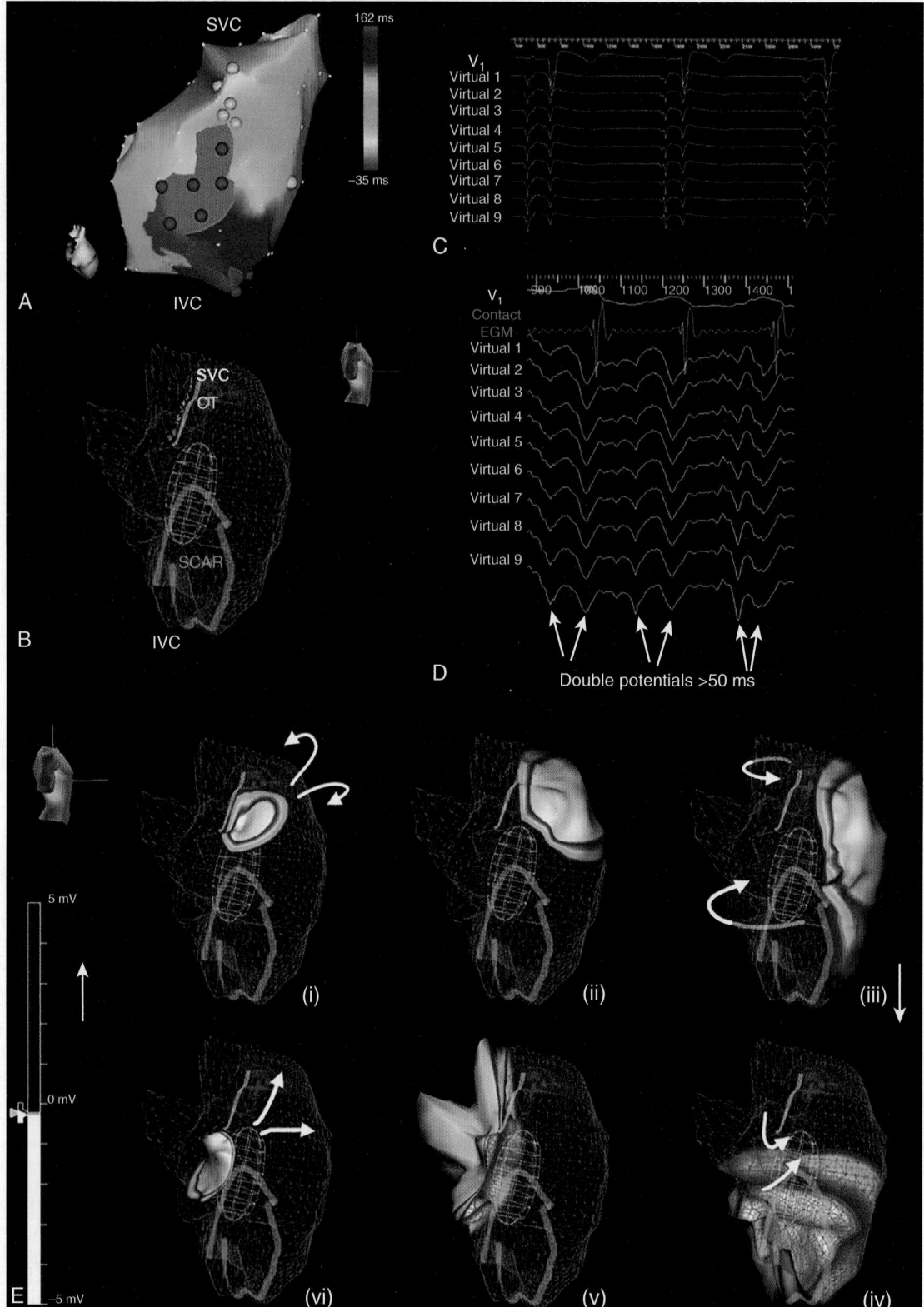

FIGURE 74.2 Functional conduction block at the crista terminalis (*CT*) supporting macroreentry tachycardia in the atriopulmonary Fontan. (A) Right atrial reconstruction is depicted using the electroanatomical system and viewed from the right lateral aspect (see *cardiac silhouette*) recorded during sinus rhythm. An area of dense scar (*gray*) is seen on the posterolateral aspect of the chamber, extending superiorly from the inferior vena cava (*IVC*). Fractionated electrograms (*EGM*s), denoted by *pink spheres*, were seen along the upper section of CT between the scar and superior vena cava (*SVC*). Local endocardial activation is color coded from *red* to *purple* in reference to a stable bipolar catheter. Activation arises immediately posterior to and traverses CT to the lateral wall. (B) The right atrial reconstruction is seen using the noncontact system from the right lateral approach (see *torso*). A *yellow line* denotes the position of the upper section of CT, and the inferior area of the scar identified by electroanatomical mapping has been annotated to the geometry. Noncontact unipolar (*virtual*) EGMs have been recorded along the length of CT, numbered virtual 1 to 9, and are displayed during (C) sinus rhythm with surface ECG lead V_1 and (D) during macroreentry tachycardia with a bipolar right atrial contact EGM and lead V_1. In sinus rhythm, a single atrial EGM is seen followed by a far-field ventricular signal, whereas during tachycardia, widely split double potentials are recorded that denote a functional conduction block. During macroreentry atrial tachycardia, which organized from atrial fibrillation, local activation is denoted by *white* and *colored markings* and wavefront progression by *white arrows*. The wavefront emerges from a gap (*i*) created by a functional conduction block along CT and a fixed block caused by the inferior area of the scar, rotating around the chamber onto the anterior and medial wall perpendicular to the vertical axis of the chambers (*ii*)–(*iv*). Activation is channeled back toward the narrow gap by the two sites of the conduction block (*v*)–(*vi*). Extension of the line of a functional block occluded the gap and terminated tachycardia.

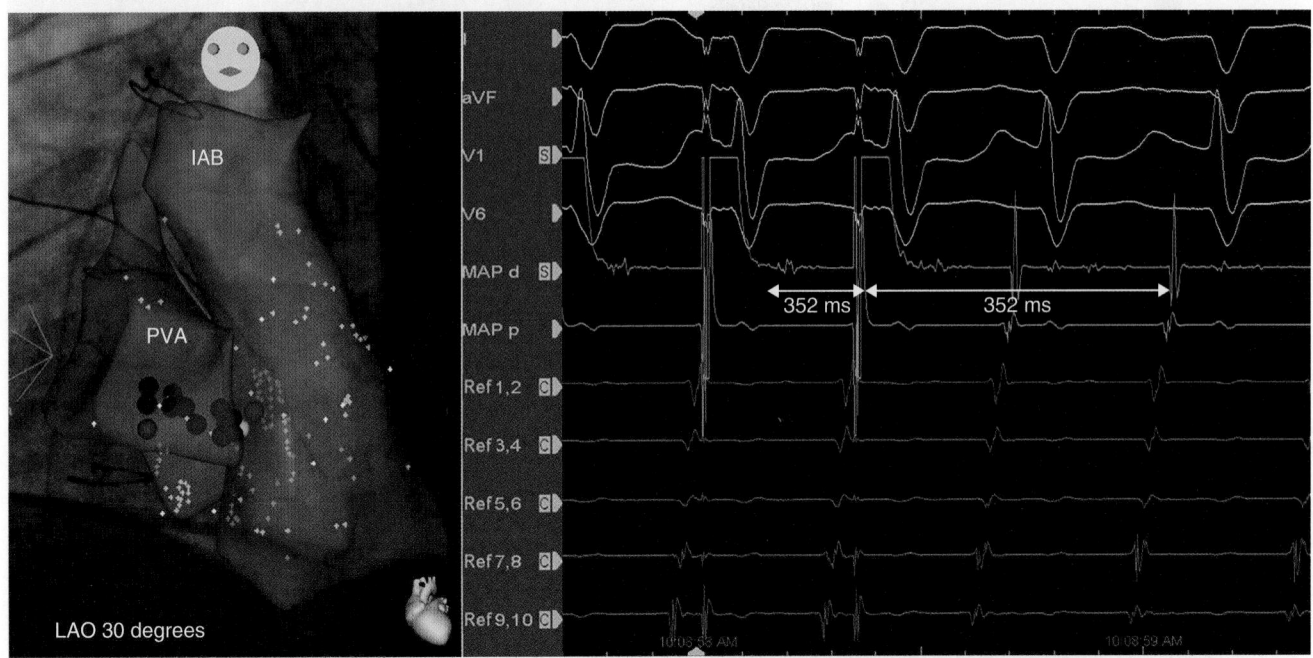

FIGURE 74.3 Entrainment and ablation at the cavomitral isthmus in a patient following total cavopulmonary connection. Images from a patient with right atrial isomerism, congenitally corrected transposition of the great arteries, severe right ventricular hypoplasia, and dextrocardia who underwent a total cavopulmonary connection single ventricular palliation. The *left panel* shows the anatomical reconstructions of the intraatrial baffle (*IAB*) and the pulmonary venous atrium (*PVA*) seen from the left anterior oblique (*LAO*) view created using the electroanatomical mapping system (Carto [Biosense Webster, Diamond Bar, CA]). The *right panel* shows four surface electrocardiographic leads (I, aVF, V$_1$, and V$_6$) with intracardiac electrograms from a mapping catheter and a decapolar reference catheter within the baffle (*Ref*). A transbaffle puncture was performed, and the valvar and posterior ends of the cavomitral isthmus denoted (*light pink spheres*), with entrainment mapping showing a postpacing interval equal to the tachycardia cycle length and an identical intracardiac activation pattern during pacing and tachycardia (*right panel*). A linear set of radiofrequency ablation lesions (*red spheres*) were placed along the cavomitral isthmus with the termination of tachycardia achieved once the line was complete (*blue sphere*).

described in 1866,[44] Ebstein anomaly is characterized by the failure of the posterior and septal leaflets of the tricuspid valve to delaminate from the underlying myocardium to which they are adherent, creating an apical displacement of the leaflets and an "atrialized" portion of RV.[45] The anterior leaflet is often enlarged and fenestrated, which gives the classical echocardiographic "sail-like" appearance. The failure of valve leaflet coaptation leads to varying degrees of tricuspid regurgitation, with the dilatation of the true tricuspid valve annulus and RA, facilitating MAT, most commonly typical AFL via CTI and also AF and FAT[46] (Fig. 74.5). This is often regarded as a consequence of the underlying anatomy, as earlier surgical techniques did not have the same degree of success seen in other lesions, and consequently, intervention was deferred in many patients.

The structural and histological abnormalities around the right AV junction precipitate a high prevalence of right-sided accessory pathways (see Fig. 74.5), are frequently multiple, and display abnormal EGM characteristics because of abnormalities of the underlying myocardium, making an accurate differentiation of the relative atrial, accessory pathway, and ventricular components within a highly complex EGM challenging.[47] During AVRT, the ventriculoatrial timing is often prolonged because of slowed conduction within the atrialized RV, where the vast majority of pathways are located.[48] The normal ECG appearance in Ebstein anomaly is low-amplitude QRS complexes in the anterior precordial leads with a right bundle morphology, indicative of delayed conduction within the right bundle itself or the atrialized portion of RV. The presence of an accessory pathway with anterograde conduction can therefore preexcite the atrialized RV

and "pseudonormalize" ECG, giving a QRS complex of normal morphology and duration[49] (Fig. 74.6).

Surgical intervention in Ebstein anomaly has been recently reinvigorated with the advent of the cone reconstruction of the tricuspid valve, which by its nature limits postoperative access to the true right AV junction.[50] Therefore a preoperative approach for arrhythmia management has been employed by some centers to eliminate the arrhythmia mechanisms that may hinder the postoperative course and be nearly impossible to ablate after the cone reconstruction. The electrophysiological assessment of 42 patients prior to surgery (median age, 13.8 years) identified 56 different arrhythmia mechanisms in 29 patients (69%), including eight with no prior arrhythmic history or ECG features suggestive of an underlying substrate. In 14 of 21 patients with documented accessory pathways, 14 (66%) had a second mechanism identified, including further accessory or atriofascicular fibers, AVNRT, MAT, and AF.[46]

Atrial Fibrillation in Adult Congenital Heart Disease

As the ACHD population ages, it is becoming increasingly apparent that AF will become a significant clinical burden and that it represents the major electrophysiological challenge of the next decade. A comprehensive analysis of 199 patients with a variety of congenital lesions identified that the mean age of onset was 49 ± 17 years, although it could occur at a younger age in those with more complex lesions, and was associated with right- and left-sided valvar disease in 31% of patients.[51]

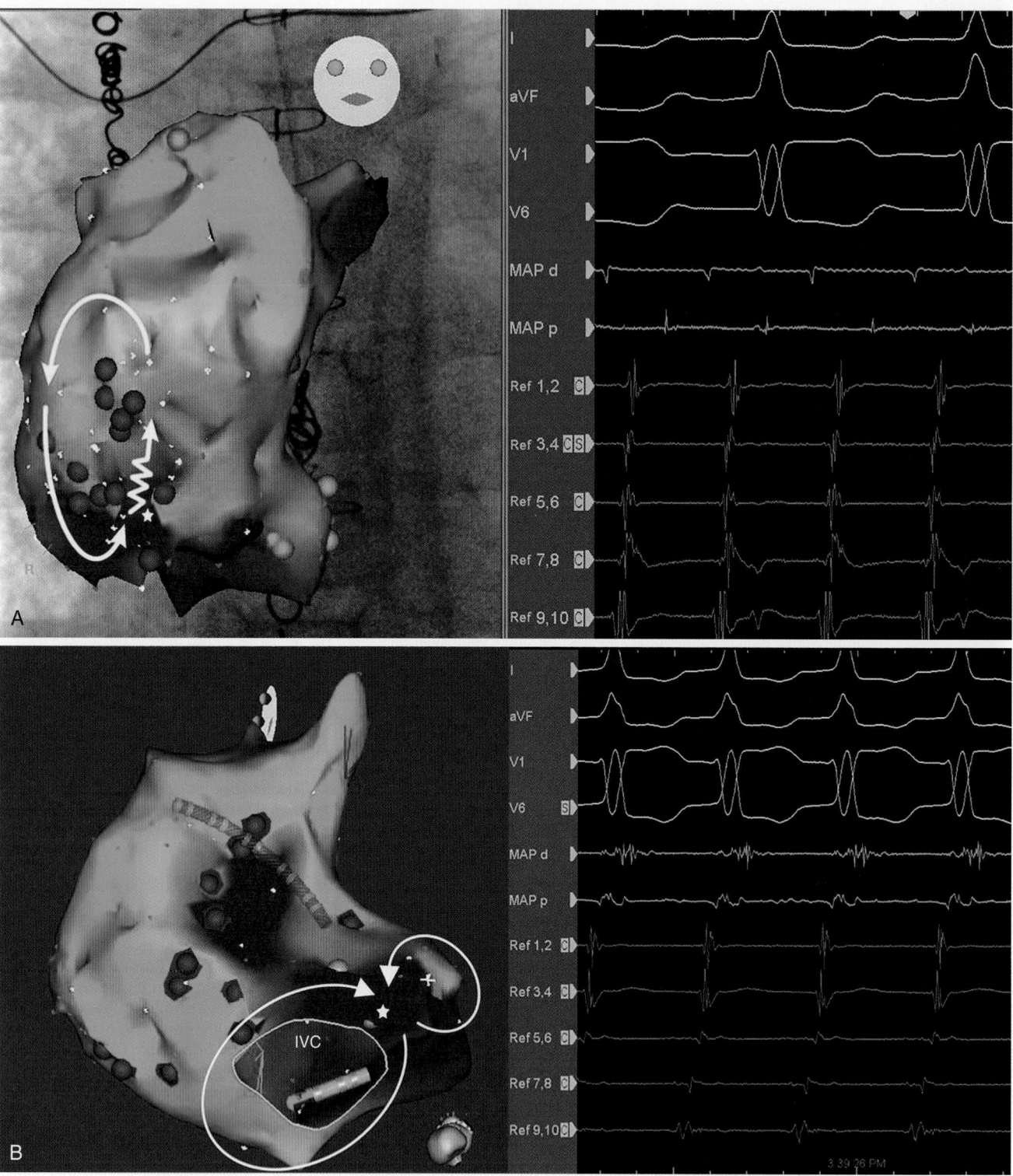

FIGURE 74.4 Scar-based and figure-of-eight macroreentrant atrial tachycardias in a patient following total cavopulmonary connection. Images from a patient with severe tricuspid valve and right ventricular hypoplasia who underwent a total cavopulmonary connection palliation. Both images show four surface electrocardiographic leads (I, aVF, V$_1$, and V$_6$) with intracardiac electrograms from a mapping catheter and a decapolar reference catheter within the baffle (*Ref*), along with the anatomical reconstructions of the intraatrial baffle created using the electroanatomical mapping system (Carto [Biosense Webster, Diamond Bar, CA]). The *upper image* shows the CartoAlara software fusing fluoroscopic and electroanatomical images. Sites of earliest activation are denoted by *red*, and those of the latest activation are denoted by *purple*. (A) The anatomical reconstruction is seen from the anterior projection, displaying a macroreentrant atrial tachycardia that propagates around the anterior wall through an area of scar (*gray spheres*) and an area of slow conduction recorded in a narrow corridor between two areas of the scar (*white star*) characterized by a wide split between the electrogram recorded on the two bipoles of the mapping catheter. Radiofrequency ablation at this site terminated tachycardia. (B) The intraatrial baffle is viewed from below, showing the ostium of the inferior vena cava (*IVC*). A figure-of-eight circuit identified on the inferior aspect of the intraatrial baffle with one limb rotating round IVC and another smaller limb rotating within a discrete area of the baffle without any apparent central obstacle to conduction. At the point of intersection between the two limbs (*white star*), a fractionated, low-amplitude electrogram was recorded as shown on the intracardiac mapping channel. Entrainment mapping demonstrated concealed entrainment, and radiofrequency ablation at this point terminated tachycardia.

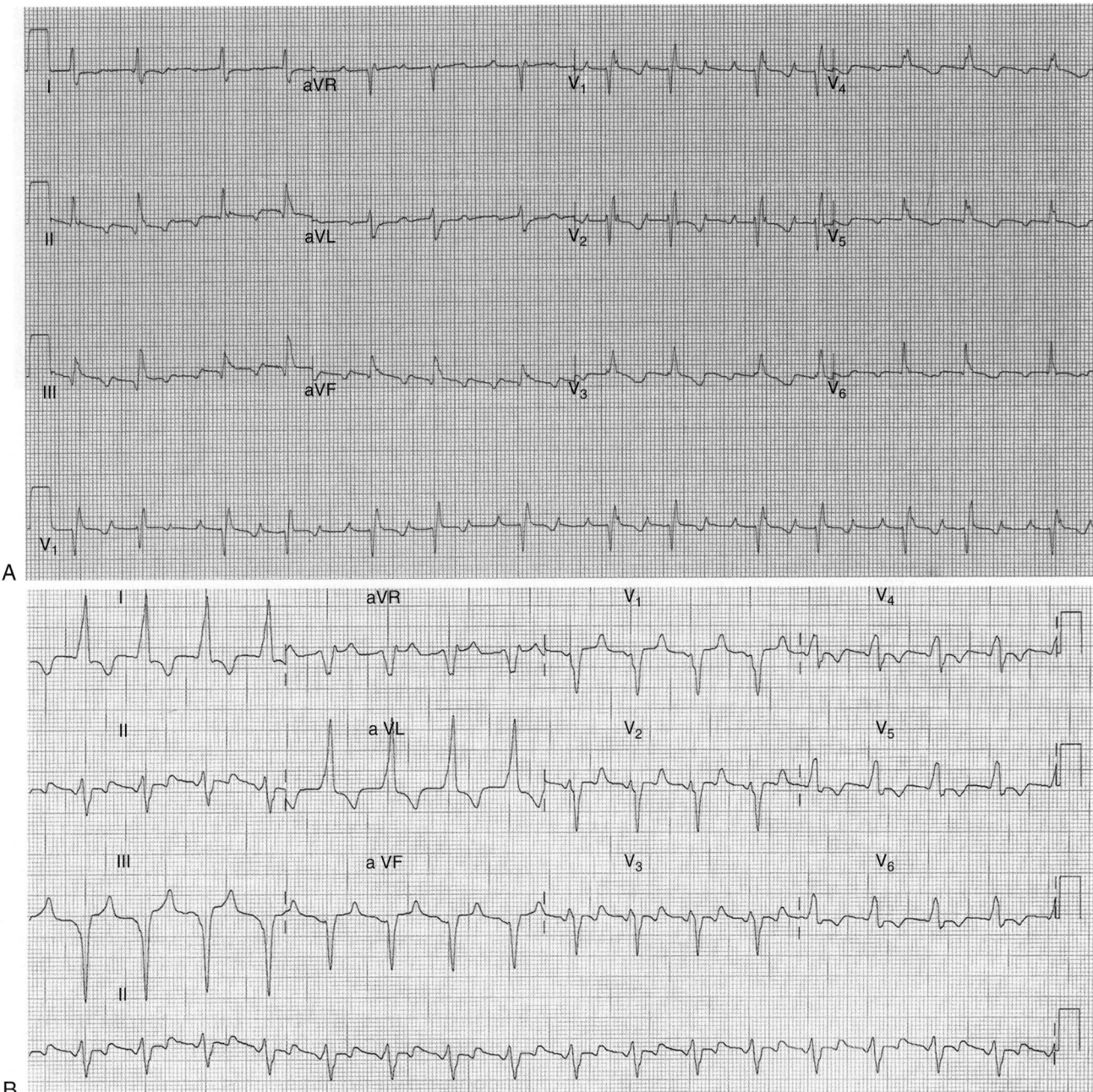

FIGURE 74.5 Electrocardiograms (ECGs) in Ebstein anomaly demonstrating atrial flutter. Twelve-lead ECGs from two patients with Ebstein anomaly. (A) A 40-year-old patient who underwent a prior tricuspid valve replacement and who presented with palpitations. The ECG appearance is consistent with typical atrial flutter (AFL) that propagates around the tricuspid valve via the cavotricuspid isthmus. Note the relative isoelectric interval between discrete AFL waves and cycle lengths of >200 ms. (B) A 38-year-old patient with no prior surgery who presented with mild lethargy and exercise intolerance and an ECG appearance of preexcited AFL, with inverted AFL waves best seen in lead II.

Cerebral thromboembolic complications were reported in 13%, occurring in the majority prior to the onset of AF, suggesting that the presence of AF as an underlying etiology should be actively pursued in patients with apparent isolated stroke. Additionally, it appears there is frequent and rapid progression from paroxysmal to permanent AF, supporting the notion that AF begets AF[52] in ACHD as well as other forms of cardiovascular disease.

The AF mechanism in ACHD is not well understood. One important question is whether in many patients with advanced RA remodeling, the pulmonary veins can be implicated in the AF etiology and if so, will an ablative strategy that primarily incorporates pulmonary vein isolation be successful? Supporting evidence for this comes from a series of 559 patients with tetralogy of Fallot, 41 of whom were found to have AF, the onset of which was associated with an increased age and LA size, reduced left ventricular function, and a number of prior surgeries.[53] Similarly LA remodeling has been demonstrated in patients with a chronic left-to-right shunting via ASD, with LA enlargement, areas of abnormal bipolar voltage and reduced conduction

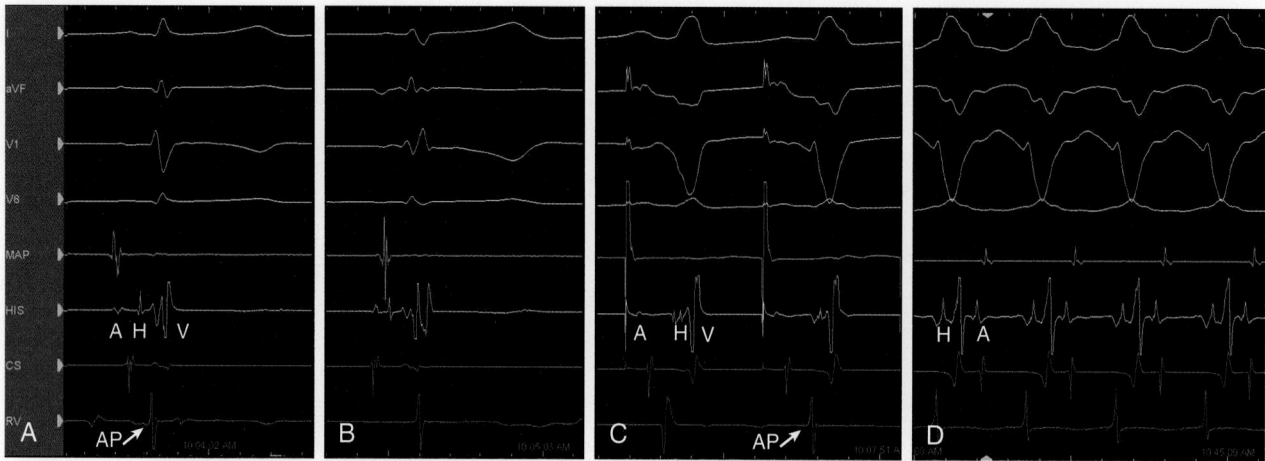

FIGURE 74.6 Variable QRS morphologies in Ebstein anomaly resulting from an atriofascicular fiber. Four electrocardiographic (ECG) leads (I, aVF, V_1, and V_6) and intracardiac electrograms from a teenage patient with Ebstein anomaly who presented with an irregular broad complex tachycardia, necessitating cardioversion. A four-wire electrophysiology study was performed with catheters positioned in the high right atrium, His bundle, coronary sinus, and on the lateral wall of the right ventricle (RV). (A) At baseline, the QRS morphology and duration and sinus intervals are normal. A sharp deflection can be seen on the RV catheter immediately prior to the local ventricular electrogram, suggestive of an accessory pathway (AP) potential, with anterograde conduction via both the atrioventricular node and AP, preexciting the atrialized portion of RV and creating a pseudonormalized ECG appearance. (B) A premature atrial beat from the left atrium (note coronary sinus atrial electrogram lead) preferentially engages the atrioventricular node and gives a right bundle branch block ECG morphology in V_1, as is typically seen in Ebstein. (C) Pacing from the lateral right atrium demonstrates long AH and negative HV intervals and a left bundle branch block ECG morphology because of the preferential engagement of the accessory pathway, with the AP potential and RV electrogram ahead of surface QRS. (D) Induction of tachycardia demonstrated an identical left bundle morphology on ECG, and the RV catheter leading the His bundle potential. Introduction of a premature atrial beat coincidental with low right atrial activation preexcited the ventricle, confirming the antidromic atrioventricular reentry via an atriofascicular fiber. *(For further details see Sherwin and colleagues.[49])*

velocity, and an increased propensity to AF induction despite no reduction in atrial refractoriness.[10] However, a temporal relationship between AF and organized MAT is well recognized and documented to coexist in 33% and 31% in two studies in 199 and 149 patients, respectively, suggesting a mechanistic relationship[51,54] (see Fig. 74.2).

In the presence of diffuse atrial electrophysiological remodeling as may be encountered in ACHD, rapid activation from a focal or localized reentrant source with fibrillatory conduction to the remainder of the atria has always been an attractive mechanism. RA foci identified in patients without structural heart disease include the SVC, sinus node, and coronary sinus os.[55,56] This phenomenon has also been described in two ACHD patients with AF on surface ECG.[57] In one patient after the Fontan procedure, large parts of the atrium were activated in a regular manner, although one small area was found to display continuous local electrical activity. Ablation at this point terminated AF into an organized AT. In a second case, AF originated from a focal area of the myocardium surrounded by dense scars with a narrow gap that connects the site of onset to the remaining myocardium.

Organized rotors have been a major focus of research attention as an AF mechanism over the last few years, initially demonstrated in animal models[58] and also in the structurally normal heart[59,60] using electroanatomical and noncontact mapping, respectively. Although the majority of rotors locate to LA, using noncontact mapping and high-frequency spectral analysis, Lin found paroxysmal AF in a small proportion of patients was driven by organized reentrant circuits dependent on the conduction block at CT that could drive fibrillatory conduction to large areas of the atrial myocardium that acts as a bystander. Ablation of gaps within CT terminated tachycardia.[60] In animal models, Ortiz and colleagues[61] demonstrated that the length of a line functional conduction block in the RA free wall was

fundamental in determining fibrillation or stable reentry. A longer line of block creates a circuit of sufficient length to support a stable macroreentry rhythm. Reduction in tachycardia CL coupled with changes in length and position of the line of block generates one or two unstable reentry circuits, which change shape, disappear, and reform, ultimately generating fibrillation. Ultimately, the AF mechanisms in the ACHD population require further investigation to determine optimal ablative strategies.

Management of Atrial Tachycardia in Adult Congenital Heart Disease

Recognition and Diagnosis

Because of their young age and relatively preserved AV nodal conduction, many ACHD patients who develop arrhythmias will present with symptomatic palpitations and varying degrees of hemodynamic compromise. However, many patients may be incidentally found to have AT or present with nonspecific symptoms of exercise intolerance and lethargy. A bundle branch morphology and abnormal repolarization patterns are common to many lesions, such that the identification of atrial activity can be difficult, especially at higher rates.

Pharmacological Therapies

The pharmacological management of atrial arrhythmias in ACHD with drug therapy has produced largely disappointing results.[62–64] β-Blockers and calcium channel antagonists may provide rate control, either acutely during AT or when combined with other agents on a preventive basis but alone exert little antiarrhythmic effect. The potent negative ino- and chronotropic properties shown by many commonly used antiarrhythmic medications may exacerbate ventricular dysfunction and sinus node dysfunction or may be proarrhythmic. A study of 70 patients treated with antiarrhythmic agents after a first episode of AT showed only 45% were free from recurrence after 2.5 ± 1.4 years,[65] although the most prevalent mechanism was AF and 25% of patients had residual left-sided lesions or had not undergone primary repair; therefore this may not be reflective of a typical population. Sotalol appears to be safe and moderately effective, although it has again been associated with significant side effects during arrhythmia management in other settings. Amiodarone is associated with significant side effects, specifically thyroid dysfunction,[66] which significantly limits its use in a relatively young population.

Anticoagulation is an important component of arrhythmia management as thromboembolic cerebrovascular accidents (CVA) are prevalent in ACHD patients, with age–sex standardized incidence rates of ischemic stroke at 9 to 12 times that for the general population aged below 55 years.[67] The peak incidence is around 30 years of age, with a high prevalence in patients with uncorrected cyanotic ACHD (23.3%), Eisenmenger physiology (5.1%), open ASD (4%), and the Fontan circulation (4.1%), all significantly associated with the loss of sinus rhythm.[68] As the population ages, the onset of acquired cardiovascular diseases, including ventricular failure, diabetes, and myocardial infarction secondary to coronary artery disease, becomes ever prevalent; these risk factors have been recently shown to be important predictors of stroke.[67]

While it appears reasonable that the majority of ACHD patients can have anticoagulation strategies similar to those employed for other variants of structural heart disease, namely the CHA2DS2-VASc risk factor–based approach,[69] specific patients, such as those with the Fontan circulation where venous and systemic atrial flow patterns may be significantly altered, or those with persistent (or the potential for) right-to-left intracardiac shunts, may benefit from formal anticoagulation at the onset of arrhythmias, although other nonarrhythmic indications may exist. Practically, given the unique needs and heterogeneity of the ACHD population, antiarrhythmic and anticoagulant pharmacological treatments should be employed on a highly individualized basis.

Invasive Electrophysiological Assessment

Vascular and Intracardiac Access

Vascular access to the heart may be limited in a significant proportion of patients, relating to either anatomical or acquired etiologies. Patients with LA isomerism have azygous continuation of IVC, draining to the SVC, that makes accurate and safe catheter manipulation highly challenging. Prolonged postoperative stays in childhood requiring repeated femoral access for intravenous infusions or catheter-based interventions frequently lead to femoral venous occlusion. In both of these scenarios, access from the internal jugular and subclavian veins is necessary.

In postatrial switch procedures and TCPC, access to CTI for ablation of typical AFL is limited because the intraatrial baffle bisects the isthmus, and ablation in both the systemic and pulmonary venous atrium is typically necessary to achieve tachycardia termination. Access to the pulmonary venous chamber can be achieved via a fenestration within the baffle, by transbaffle puncture, or a retrograde approach, using either conventional catheters or robotic magnetic resonance navigation.[70] A study of 74 patients who required baffle punctures postatrial switch or TCPC using either standard or radiofrequency (RF) transseptal needles showed a high success rate (96%) with no complications directly attributable to the puncture,[71] and although a single puncture is typically employed,

this allows the definition of arrhythmia mechanism and successful ablation.[38,71]

Case-Specific Anatomical and Surgical Information

Given that the anatomical location of the cardiac conduction system varies with different lesions, precise knowledge of these locations is imperative prior to defining an ablative strategy. In tricuspid atresia and AV septal defects, the compact AV node and penetrating conduction bundles are located posteroseptally close to the coronary sinus os, which accounts for the superior QRS access on surface ECG. This assumes great importance in patients who undergo slow pathway modification for AVNRT,[72] ablation of a posteroseptal accessory pathway, or ablation of typical AFL. Conversely, in congenitally corrected TGA, the compact node assumes a more superior position on the mitral valve annulus because of the malalignment of the interatrial and interventricular septa and the deep position of the pulmonary artery that overrides the midportion of the interventricular septum. This causes the conducting bundles to take a circuitous course around the pulmonary artery, a factor considered to contribute to the high rate of AV nodal condition disease associated with this lesion.[73]

In light of the anatomical variations, the use of integrated three-dimensional reconstructions appears attractive. Recreation and segmentation of computed tomography or magnetic resonance images using software integrated with mapping technologies and registration with fluoroscopic landmarks during the procedure allows for the superimposition of activation and specific points directly onto the integrated image. Such an approach has been employed with success for the ablation of AF using empiric lesson sets, initially demonstrating a reduction in AF recurrence,[74] although this has not been confirmed by a prospective, randomized study.[75] While this technique has been validated for LA ablation, where it is facilitated by the proximity of the pulmonary venous landmarks to the atrial myocardium and the use of an empiric ablative strategy, neither of these are applicable to ACHD, where ablation is performed typically with comprehensive RA mapping and EGM characteristics, and suitable anatomical landmarks are remote from the chamber, reducing the fidelity of the registration. Other technologies, such as intracardiac echo (ICE)–guided real-time anatomical acquisition, offer promise for the future, but to date, no study has demonstrated improved acute procedural success or long-term arrhythmia freedom via the incorporation of anatomical images.

Mapping and Ablative Strategies

Mapping Technologies

Electroanatomical mapping (Carto [Biosense Webster, Diamond Bar, CA]) using a three-dimensional anatomical reconstruction has become the modality of choice for mapping and ablation in ACHD, combining the high-resolution reconstruction of atrial activation (or voltage) with the annotation of natural and surgical barriers to conduction. Early studies demonstrated that electroanatomical mapping was a positive predictor of a positive long-term outcome, as defined by a 12-point clinical arrhythmia severity score, subdivided into four categories: arrhythmia detection, arrhythmia severity, cardioversion frequency, and antiarrhythmic medication.[76] However, electroanatomical mapping is best suited to hemodynamically stable, sustained arrhythmias, although it allows for detailed substrate mapping and empiric ablation if the circuits are nonsustained or noninducible.

Given the potential for multiple interchanging circuits and hemodynamic instability of rapidly conducted atrial arrhythmias, noncontact mapping is an attractive option and provides additional information regarding arrhythmia onset, termination, or changes between circuits. Noncontact mapping uses >3000 simultaneously and continuously recorded, reconstructed, unipolar EGMs to provide real-time assessments of global atrial activation and may therefore overcome the limitations of sequential contact mapping afforded by electroanatomical mapping. However, in a situation where its advantages were most applicable, the atriopulmonary Fontan, its inherent limitations of increasing the distance of the multielectrode array (MEA) from the endocardium and its inability to identify scars were exposed. In a comparative analysis of both systems, electroanatomical mapping was shown to be a superior modality[26] and provided fascinating insights into arrhythmia mechanism, although the noncontact MEA naturally sits close to the posterolateral aspect of the RA and hence the CT. More recent advances enable the use of previously acquired fluoroscopic and angiographic images in the electroanatomical mapping system (CartoAlara [Biosense Webster, Diamond Bar, CA]), which facilitates the creation of three-dimensional anatomical shells with real-time fluoroscopic landmarks, without exposing the patient or operator to excessive radiation.

Voltage Mapping

The definition of an endocardial scar using EGM amplitude remains uncertain, largely because of the absence of any comparative electrophysiological–histological study that examines the human atrial myocardium in ACHD. A myocardial scar is traditionally defined using bipolar EGMs, although accurate recordings may be affected by the electrode configuration, distance between electrodes, and direction of the wavefront with respect to the recording catheter. Conversely, unipolar EGMs are more susceptible to far-field interference, potentially limiting their use in a low-voltage substrate; this is a notion supported by the findings of a comparative study of unipolar and bipolar signals in ACHD, which found that only bipolar EGMs permit voltage-based scar delineation.[77] Therefore in a myocardial substrate where accurate circuit mapping may be dependent on the identification of areas of scars interspersed by narrow corridors of the viable myocardium critical to reentrant circuits, bipolar EGMs are most effective in ACHD.[78–80] The EGM amplitude used to define scar varies. A comparative study between ACHD patients and controls found no bipolar EGM amplitude of <0.1 mV in normal subjects, whereas 16% of sampled points were below this value in the congenital group, leading the authors to propose this figure as a cut-off for scars in the congenital population.[77] However, Nakagawa considered scars to be the only areas with no discernible EGM above background noise, reaching EGM amplitudes as low as 0.03 mV, an approach supported by the identification of an EGM amplitude of <0.1 mV at 7 of 15 successful ablation sites.[27] Alternative methods include the patch index, a factor of local impedance, and EGM amplitude.[81]

Entrainment Mapping

Despite the resolution and fidelity of current activation maps on three-dimensional mapping technologies, entrainment mapping remains integral for the confirmation of tachycardia mechanisms and the identification of candidate sites for ablation. This is especially true if reentrant circuits locate to a small area of the endocardium with the vast majority of the chamber activated passively, or if the intraatrial conduction time is longer than the tachycardia CL.[82] Certainly if activation maps do not accurately define an arrhythmia mechanism, entrainment mapping should be superimposed, and after biventricular repair with ECG features consistent with typical AFL, entrainment from the CTI alone is frequently enough to confirm the mechanism. In more complex substrates, it

has been shown that sites with diastolic potentials, concealed entrainments, and postpacing intervals that are equal to the tachycardia CL can be identified both within and outside of the protected channels identified by electroanatomical mapping.[78] Detailed entrainment of reentrant circuits has demonstrated that large areas (~30%) of the endocardial surface may be "in circuit," and entrainable wavefronts are broad, supporting the low positive predictive value of identifying sites for ablation using entrainment alone. Importantly, protected corridors identified using detailed electroanatomical activation maps were not found to be critical to the intraarterial reentrant tachycardia circuit following entrainment pacing, supported by the finding that in 9 of 18 circuits, successful ablation was achieved at sites distant from the protected channel. This suggested that in a number of circuit fusions of activation and entrainment data were necessary for successful mechanistic determination and ablation.[29]

Ablation Technologies

Irrigated RF ablation (RFA) catheters have become the standard for ablation in ACHD, as in many other variants of structural heart disease.[83,84] Early studies, using conventional ablation in the atriopulmonary Fontan where atrial hypertrophy may reach 15 mm, showed no visual evidence of RF lesions in patients undergoing conversion surgery who had previously undergone extensive ablation.[85] Historical data analysis in a large cohort of patients undergoing RFA identified irrigated RFA with a positive outcome using multivariate analysis,[76] supported further by the findings of a prospective, randomized control trial that found the overall success to be significantly higher with irrigated as opposed to conventional RFA.[86]

Outcomes and Complications

As in many complex substrates, the success of ablation in most variants of ACHD is high, enhanced over the last decade by operator and institutional experience, mapping and ablative technologies, and a better understanding of the electroanatomical substrate and arrhythmia mechanisms (Table 74.1). However, a proportion of patients develop further arrhythmia because of the continual process of atrial remodeling, and as the population ages, AF emerges as an important clinical problem. Although complications undoubtedly exist, including thromboembolism, complete heart block, cardiac tamponade, and coronary artery injury, these can be limited by procedures performed by appropriately trained personnel in institutions that specialize in the care of ACHD patients.[87] However, specific complications have greater ramifications for ACHD patients; for example, in patients with a Fontan circulation, phrenic nerve injury in a circulation, where negative pressure ventilation drives pulmonary blood flow, could have major implications for the patient's overall hemodynamic status, and complete heart block necessitates a surgically implanted epicardial pacemaker, which can be a major procedure with significant morbidity.

Conclusions

Atrial arrhythmias are a major cause of morbidity in the ACHD population and are associated with an increased risk for stroke, heart failure, and mortality. However, the last decade has led to a greater understanding of arrhythmia mechanisms in different circulations, which coupled with technological advances has led to a greater success in the care of these patients. Nevertheless, as the population ages, it is likely that AF will become an ever-increasing burden that will need to be addressed.

TABLE 74.1   Outcome of electrophysiology study and radiofrequency ablation in adult congenital heart disease

	YEAR	NO.	ACUTE SUCCESS	RECURRENCE RATE	FOLLOW-UP (MONTHS)
Biventricular Repair					
Triedman et al.[76]	2002	71	79%	36%	25 ± 11
Kannankeril et al.[88]	2003	25	93%	31%	38
Paul et al.[28]	2001	7	100%	14%	7
de Groot et al.[77]	2003	17	85%	18%	18 ± 6
Delacretaz et al.[16]	2001	20	83%	20%	19 ± 14
Nakagawa et al.[27]	2001	10	100%	10%	13.5
Akar et al.[89]	2001	16	92%	8%	24 ± 12
Anné et al.[90]	2002	28	95%	30%	24 ± 18
Mah et al.[19]	2011	58	90%	34%	36
Teh et al.[17]	2011	20	100%	25%	13 ± 8
Mustard/Senning					
Zrenner et al.[21]	2005	12	86%	30%	19 ± 8
Kriebel et al.[91]	2002	13	93%	17%	20
Wu et al.[20]	2013	26	85%	30%	34 ± 24
Univentricular Repair					
Triedman et al.[76]	2002	63	—	52%	25 ± 11
Kannankeril et al.[88]	2003	15	—	55%	38
Paul et al.[28]	2001	7	83%	0%	7
Nakagawa et al.[27]	2001	6	100%	33%	13.5
Abrams et al.[26]	2007	28	88%	48%	48
Correa et al.[39]	2015	52	80%	50%	18

REFERENCES

1. Marelli AJ, Ionescu-Ittu R, Mackie AS, et al. Lifetime prevalence of congenital heart disease in the general population from 2000 to 2010. *Circulation.* 2014;130:749–756.
2. Bouchardy J, Therrien J, Pilote L, et al. Atrial arrhythmias in adults with congenital heart disease. *Circulation.* 2009;120:1679–1686.
3. The Sicilian gambit. A new approach to the classification of antiarrhythmic drugs based on their actions on arrhythmogenic mechanisms. Task Force of the Working Group on Arrhythmias of the European Society of Cardiology. *Circulation.* 1991;84:1831–1851.
4. Bowden PA, Hoffman BF. The effects on atrial electrophysiology and structure of surgically induced right atrial enlargement in dogs. *Circ Res.* 1981;49:1319–1331.
5. Shumacher B, Jung W, Schmidt H, et al. Transverse conduction capabilities of the crista terminalis in patients with atrial flutter and atrial fibrillation. *J Am Coll Cardiol.* 1999;34:363–373.
6. Arenal A, Almendral J, Alday J, et al. Rate-dependent conduction block of the crista terminalis in patients with typical atrial flutter. Influence on evaluation of cavotricuspid isthmus block. *Circulation.* 1999;99:2771–2778.
7. Spach MS, Dolber PC. Relating extracellular potentials and their derivatives to anisotropic propagation at a microscopic level in human cardiac tissue: evidence for electrical uncoupling of side-to-side fiber connection with increasing age. *Circ Res.* 1986;58:356–371.
8. Koura T, Hara M, Takeuchi S, et al. Anisotropic conduction properties in canine atria analyzed by high-resolution optical mapping. Preferential direction of conduction block changes from longitudinal to transverse with increasing age. *Circulation.* 2002;105:2092–2098.
9. Morton JB, Sanders P, Vohra JK, et al. Effect of chronic right atrial stretch on atrial electrical remodeling in patients with an atrial septal defect. *Circulation.* 2003;107:1775–1782.
10. Roberts-Thomson KC, John B, Worthley SG, et al. Left atrial remodeling in patients with atrial septal defects. *Heart Rhythm.* 2009;6:1000–1006.
11. Morton JB, Byrne MJ, Power JM, et al. Electrical remodeling of the atrium in an anatomic model of atrial flutter. Relationship between substrate and triggers for conversion to atrial fibrillation. *Circulation.* 2002;102:1283–1289.
12. Chan DP, van Hare GF, Mackall JA, et al. Importance of atrial flutter isthmus in post-operative intra-atrial re-entry. *Circulation.* 2000;102:1283–1289.
13. Kalman JM, Van Hare GF, Olgin JE, et al. Ablation of 'incisional' reentrant atrial tachycardia complicating surgery for congenital heart disease. Use of entrainment to define a critical isthmus of conduction. *Circulation.* 1996;93:502–512.

14. Tomita Y, Matsuo K, Sahadevan J, et al. Role of functional block extension in lesion-related atrial flutter. *Circulation.* 2001;103:1025–1030.
15. Mandapati R, Walsh EP, Triedman JK. Pericaval and periannular intra-atrial reentrant tachycardias in patients with congenital heart disease. *J Cardiovasc Electrophysiol.* 2003;14:119–125.
16. Delacretaz E, Ganz LI, Soejima K, et al. Multi atrial macro-re-entry circuits in adults with repaired congenital heart disease: entrainment mapping combined with three-dimensional electroanatomic mapping. *J Am Coll Cardiol.* 2001;37:1665–1676.
17. Teh AW, Medi C, Lee G, et al. Long-term outcome following ablation of atrial flutter occurring late after atrial septal defect repair. *Pacing Clin Electrophysiol.* 2011;34:431–435.
18. Shah D, Jaïs P, Takahashi A, et al. Dual-loop intra-atrial reentry in humans. *Circulation.* 2000;101:631–639.
19. Mah DY, Alexander ME, Cecchin F, et al. The electroanatomic mechanisms of atrial tachycardia in patients with tetralogy of Fallot and double outlet right ventricle. *J Cardiovasc Electrophysiol.* 2011;22:1013–1017.
20. Wu J, Deisenhofer I, Ammar S, et al. Acute and long-term outcome after catheter ablation of supraventricular tachycardia in patients after the Mustard or Senning operation for D-transposition of the great arteries. *Europace.* 2013;15:886–891.
21. Zrenner B, Dong J, Schreieck J, et al. Delineation of intra-atrial reentrant tachycardia circuits after Mustard operation for transposition of the great arteries using biatrial electroanatomic mapping and entrainment mapping. *J Cardiovasc Electrophysiol.* 2003;14:1302–1310.
22. Gandhi SK, Bromberg BI, Mallory GB, et al. Atrial flutter: a newly recognized complication of pediatric lung transplantation. *J Thorac Cardiovasc Surg.* 1996;112:984–991.
23. Gandhi SK, Bromberg BI, Schuessler RB, et al. Left-sided atrial flutter: characterization of a novel complication of pediatric lung transplantation in an acute canine model. *J Thorac Cardiovasc Surg.* 1996;112:992–1001.
24. Fontan F, Baudet E. Surgical repair of tricuspid atresia. *Thorax.* 1971;26:240–248.
25. Kreutzer G, Galindez E, Bono H, et al. An operation for the correction of tricuspid atresia. *J Thorac Cardiovasc Surg.* 1973;66:613–621.
26. Abrams DJ, Earley MA, Sporton SC, et al. Comparison of non-contact and electroanatomic mapping to identify scar and arrhythmia late after the modified Fontan procedure. *Circulation.* 2007;115:1738–1746.
27. Nakagawa H, Shah N, Matsudaira K, et al. Characterization of reentrant circuits in macroreentrant right atrial

tachycardia after surgical repair of congenital heart disease. Isolated channels between scars allow "focal" ablation. *Circulation.* 2001;103:699–709.
28. Paul T, Windhagen-Mahnert B, Kriebel T, et al. Atrial reentry tachycardia after surgery for congenital heart disease. Endocardial mapping and radiofrequency catheter ablation using a novel, noncontact mapping system. *Circulation.* 2001;103:2266–2271.
29. Triedman JK, Alexander ME, Berul CI, et al. Electroanatomic mapping of entrained and exit zones in patients with repaired congenital heart disease and intra-atrial reentrant tachycardia. *Circulation.* 2001;103:2060–2065.
30. Björk VO, Olin CL, Bjarke BB, et al. Right atrial-right ventricular anastomosis for correction of tricuspid atresia. *J Thorac Cardiovasc Surg.* 1978;77:452–458.
31. Hager A, Zrenner B, Brodherr-Heberlein S, et al. Congenital and surgically acquired Wolff-Parkinson-White syndrome in patients with tricuspid atresia. *J Thorac Cardiovasc Surg.* 2004;130:48–53.
32. De Leval MR, Kilner P, Gewillig M, et al. Total cavopulmonary connection: a logical alternative to the atriopulmonary connection for complex Fontan operations. Experimental studies and early clinical experience. *J Thorac Cardiovasc Surg.* 1988;96:682–695.
33. Gardiner HM, Dhillon R, Bull C, et al. Prospective study of the incidence and determinants of arrhythmia after total cavopulmonary connection. *Circulation.* 1996;94:17–21.
34. d'Udekem Y, Iyengar AJ, Cochrane AD, et al. The Fontan procedure: contemporary techniques have improved long-term outcomes. *Circulation.* 2007;116:I157–I164.
35. Rodefeld MD, Bromberg BI, Shuessler RB, et al. Atrial flutter after lateral tunnel construction in the modified Fontan operation. A canine model. *J Thorac Cardiovasc Surg.* 1996;111:514–526.
36. Ghandi SK, Bromberg BI, Rodefeld MD, et al. Spontaneous atrial flutter in a chronic canine model of the modified Fontan procedure. *J Am Coll Cardiol.* 1997;30:1095–1103.
37. Ghandi SK, Bromberg BI, Rodefeld MD, et al. Lateral tunnel suture line variation reduces atrial flutter after the modified Fontan operation. *Ann Thorac Surg.* 1996;61:1229–1309.
38. Rodefeld MD, Ghandi SK, Huddlestone CB, et al. Anatomically based ablation of atrial flutter in an acute canine model of the Fontan operation. *J Thorac Cardiovasc Surg.* 1996;112:898–907.
39. Correa R, Sherwin ED, Kovach J, et al. Mechanism and ablation of arrhythmia following total cavopulmonary connection. *Circ Arrhythm Electrophysiol.* 2015;8:318–325.

40. Miles WM, Yee R, Klein GJ, et al. The preexcitation index: an aid in determining the mechanism of supraventricular tachycardia and localizing accessory pathways. *Circulation.* 1986;74:493–500.

41. Knight BP, Zivin A, Souza J, et al. A technique for the rapid diagnosis of atrial tachycardia in the electrophysiology laboratory. *J Am Coll Cardiol.* 1999;33:775–781.

42. Epstein MR, Saul JP, Weindling SN, et al. Atrioventricular reciprocating tachycardia involving twin atrioventricular nodes in patients with complex congenital heart disease. *J Cardiovasc Electrophysiol.* 2001;12:671–679.

43. Chetaille P, Walsh EP, Triedman JK. Outcomes of radiofrequency catheter ablation of atrioventricular reciprocating tachycardia in patients with congenital heart disease. *Heart Rhythm.* 2004;1:168–173.

44. van Son JA, Konstantinov IE, Zimmermann V. Wilhelm Ebstein and Ebstein's malformation. *Eur J Cardiothorac Surg.* 2001;20:1082–1085.

45. Attenhofer Jost CH, Connolly HM, Dearani JA, et al. Ebstein's anomaly. *Circulation.* 2007;115:277–285.

46. Shivapour JK, Sherwin ED, Alexander ME, et al. Utility of preoperative electrophysiologic studies in patients with Ebstein's anomaly undergoing the Cone procedure. *Heart Rhythm.* 2014;11:182–186.

47. Cappato R, Schlüter M, Weiss C, et al. Radiofrequency current catheter ablation of accessory atrioventricular pathways in Ebstein's anomaly. *Circulation.* 1996;94:376–383.

48. Smith WM, Gallagher JJ, Kerr CR, et al. The electrophysiologic basis and management of symptomatic recurrent tachycardia in patients with Ebstein's anomaly of the tricuspid valve. *Am J Cardiol.* 1982;49:1223–1234.

49. Sherwin ED, Walsh EP, Abrams DJ. Variable QRS morphologies in Ebstein's anomaly: what is the mechanism? *Heart Rhythm.* 2013;10:933–937.

50. da Silva JP, Baumgratz JF, da Fonseca L, et al. The cone reconstruction of the tricuspid valve in Ebstein's anomaly. The operation: early and midterm results. *J Thorac Cardiovasc Surg.* 2007;133:215–223.

51. Teuwen CP, Ramdjan TT, Götte M, et al. Time course of atrial fibrillation in patients with congenital heart defects. *Circ Arrhythm Electrophysiol.* 2015;8:1065–1072.

52. Wijffels MC, Kirchhof CJ, Dorland R, et al. Atrial fibrillation begets atrial fibrillation. A study in awake chronically instrumented goats. *Circulation.* 1995;92:1954–1968.

53. Khairy P, Aboulhosn J, Gurvitz MZ, et al. Alliance for Adult Research in Congenital Cardiology (AARCC). Arrhythmia burden in adults with surgically repaired tetralogy of Fallot: a multi-institutional study. *Circulation.* 2010;122:868–875.

54. Kirsh JA, Walsh EP, Triedman JK. Prevalence of and risk factors for atrial fibrillation and intra-atrial reentrant tachycardia among patients with congenital heart disease. *Am J Cardiol.* 2002;90:338–340.

55. Haïssaguerre M, Jaïs P, Shah DC, et al. Spontaneous initiation of atrial fibrillation by ectopic beats originating in the pulmonary veins. *N Engl J Med.* 1998;339:659–666.

56. Jaïs P, Haïssaguerre M, Shah DC, et al. A focal source of atrial fibrillation treated by discrete radiofrequency ablation. *Circulation.* 1997;95:572–576.

57. De Groot NM, Zeppenfeld K, Wijffels MC, et al. Ablation of focal atrial tachycardia in patients with congenital heart defects after surgery: role of circumscribed areas with heterogeneous conduction. *Heart Rhythm.* 2006;3:526–535.

58. Mandapati R, Skanes A, Chen J, et al. Stable microreentrant sources as the mechanism of atrial fibrillation in the isolated sheep heart. *Circulation.* 2000;101:194–199.

59. Sanders P, Berenfeld, Hocini M, et al. Spectral analysis identifies sites of high frequency activity maintaining atrial fibrillation in humans. *Circulation.* 2005;112:789–797.

60. Lin Y-J, Tai C-T, Kao T, et al. Electrophysiological characteristics and catheter ablation in patients with paroxysmal right atrial fibrillation. *Circulation.* 2005;112:1692–1700.

61. Ortiz J, Niwano S, Abe H, et al. Mapping the conversion of atrial flutter to atrial fibrillation and atrial fibrillation to atrial flutter: insights into mechanisms. *Circ Res.* 1994;74:882–894.

62. Koyak Z, Kroon B, de Groot JR, et al. Efficacy of antiarrhythmic drugs in adults with congenital heart disease and supraventricular tachycardias. *Am J Cardiol.* 2013;112:1461–1467.

63. Balaji S, Johnson TB, Sade RM, et al. Management of atrial flutter after the Fontan procedure. *J Am Coll Cardiol.* 1994;23:1209–1215.

64. Coumel P, Leclercq JF, Assayag P. European experience with the antiarrhythmic efficacy of propafenone for supraventricular and ventricular arrhythmias. *Am J Cardiol.* 1984;54:60D–66D.

65. Garson A, Gillette PC, McVey P, et al. Amiodarone treatment of critical arrhythmias in children and young adults. *J Am Coll Cardiol.* 1984;4:749–755.

66. Thorne SA, Barnes I, Cullinan P, et al. Amiodarone-associated thyroid dysfunction risk factors in adults with congenital heart disease. *Circulation.* 1999;100:149–154.

67. Lanz J, Brophy JM, Therrien J, et al. Stroke in adults with congenital heart disease: incidence, cumulative risk, and predictors. *Circulation.* 2015;132:2385–2394.

68. Hoffmann A, Chockalingam P, Balint OH, et al. Cerebrovascular accidents in adult patients with congenital heart disease. *Heart.* 2010;96:1223–1226.

69. Lip GY, Nieuwlaat R, Pisters R, et al. Refining clinical risk stratification for predicting stroke and thromboembolism in atrial fibrillation using a novel risk factor-based approach: the Euro Heart Survey on atrial fibrillation. *Chest.* 2010;137:263–272.

70. Ernst S, Babu-Narayan SV, Keegan J, et al. Remote-controlled magnetic navigation and ablation with 3D image integration as an alternative approach in patients with intra-atrial baffle anatomy. *Circ Arrhythm Electrophysiol.* 2012;5:131–139.

71. Correa R, Walsh E, Alexander M, et al. Transbaffle mapping and ablation for atrial tachycardias after Mustard, Senning or Fontan operations. *J Am Heart Assoc.* 2013;2:e000325.

72. Abrams DJ, Earley M, Sporton C, et al. Successful ablation of atrioventricular nodal reentry tachycardia following the modified Fontan procedure. *Europace.* 2006;8:907–910.

73. Anderson RH, Becker AE, Arnold R, et al. The conducting tissues in congenitally corrected transposition. *Circulation.* 1974;50:911–923.

74. Kistler PM, Rajappan K, Jahngir M, et al. The impact of CT image integration into an electroanatomic mapping system on clinical outcomes of catheter ablation of atrial fibrillation. *J Cardiovasc Electrophysiol.* 2006;17:1093–1101.

75. Kistler PM, Rajappan K, Harris S, et al. The impact of image integration on catheter ablation of atrial fibrillation using electroanatomic mapping. a prospective randomized study. *Eur Heart J.* 2008;29:3029–3036.

76. Triedman JK, Alexander ME, Love BA, et al. Influence of patient factors and ablative technologies on outcomes of radiofrequency ablation of intra-atrial re-entrant tachycardia in patients with congenital heart disease. *J Am Coll Cardiol.* 2002;39:1827–1835.

77. De Groot N, Schalij M, Zeppenfeld K, et al. Voltage and activation mapping: how the recording technique affects the outcome of catheter ablation procedures in patients with congenital heart disease. *Circulation.* 2003;108:2099–2106.

78. Deleted in review.

79. Love BA, Collins KK, Walsh EP, et al. Electroanatomic characterization of conduction barriers in sinus/atrially paced rhythm and association with intra-atrial reentrant tachycardia circuits following congenital heart disease surgery. *J Cardiovasc Electrophysiol.* 2001;12:17–25.

80. Mandapati R, Walsh EP, Triedman JK. Pericaval and periannular intraatrial reentrant tachycardias in patients with congenital heart disease. *J Cardiovasc Electrophysiol.* 2003;14:119–125.

81. Dorotskar P, Cheng J, Scheinman M. Electroanatomical mapping and ablation of the substrate supporting intraatrial reentrant tachycardia after palliation of complex congenital heart disease. *PACE.* 1998;21:1810–1819.

82. Ikeguchi S, Peters NS. Novel use of postpacing interval mapping to guide radiofrequency ablation of focal atrial tachycardia with long intra-atrial conduction time. *Heart Rhythm.* 2004;1:88–93.

83. Jais P, Shah DC, Haissaguerre M, et al. Prospective randomised comparison irrigated-tip versus conventional-tip catheters for ablation of common flutter. *Circulation.* 2000;101:772–776.

84. Soejima K, Delacretaz E, Suzuki M, et al. Saline-cooled versus standard radiofrequency catheter ablation for infarct-related ventricular tachycardia. *Circulation.* 2001;103:1858–1867.

85. Betts TR, Roberts PR, Allen SA, et al. Electrophysiological mapping and ablation of intra-atrial reentry tachycardia after Fontan surgery with the use of a noncontact mapping system. *Circulation.* 2000;102:419–425.

86. Triedman JK, DeLucca JM, Alexander ME, et al. Prospective trial of electroanatomically guided, irrigated catheter ablation of atrial tachycardia in patients with congenital heart disease. *Heart Rhythm.* 2005;2:700–705.

87. Khairy P, Van Hare GF, Balaji S, et al. PACES/HRS Expert Consensus Statement on the Recognition and Management of Arrhythmias in Adult Congenital Heart Disease: developed in partnership between the Pediatric and Congenital Electrophysiology Society (PACES) and the Heart Rhythm Society (HRS). Endorsed by the governing bodies of PACES, HRS, the American College of Cardiology (ACC), the American Heart Association (AHA), the European Heart Rhythm Association (EHRA), the Canadian Heart Rhythm Society (CHRS), and the International Society for Adult Congenital Heart Disease (ISACHD). *Heart Rhythm.* 2014;11:e102–e165.

88. Kannankeril PJ, Anderson ME, Rottman JN, et al. Frequency of late recurrence of intra-atrial reentry tachycardia after radiofrequency catheter ablation in patients with congenital heart disease. *Am J Cardiol.* 2003;92:879–881.

89. Akar JG, Kok LC, Haines DE, et al. Coexistence of type I atrial flutter and intra-atrial re-entrant tachycardia in patients with surgically corrected congenital heart disease. *J Am Coll Cardiol.* 2001;38:377–384.

90. Anné W, van Rensburg H, Adams J, et al. Ablation of post-surgical intra-atrial reentrant tachycardia. Predilection target sites and mapping approach. *Eur Heart J.* 2002;23:1609–1616.

91. Kriebel T, Tebbenjohanns J, Janousek J, et al. Intraatrial reentrant tachycardias in patients after atrial switch procedures for d-transposition of the great arteries: endocardial mapping and radiofrequency catheter ablation primarily targeting protected areas of atrial tissue within the systemic venous atrium. *Z Kardiol.* 2002;9:806–817.

75 Typical and Atypical Atrial Flutter: Mapping and Ablation

Chrishan Joseph Nalliah, Saurabh Kumar, Prashanthan Sanders, and Jonathan M. Kalman

Atrial flutter (AFL) is one of the most common cardiac arrhythmias in humans, afflicting ~0.19 million people in the United States in 2005; its prevalence is expected to increase to 0.44 million by 2050 because of the aging population.[1] AFL often occurs in the context of structural heart disease (e.g., valvular, ischemic heart disease, cardiomyopathy) and may also manifest during acute disease process (e.g., sepsis, myocardial infarction). In this chapter, we will review recent advances in our understanding of AFL mechanisms, its heterogeneous nature, and treatment. We define AFL as an arrhythmia with a macroreentrant circuit (>2 cm) distinct from focal atrial tachycardias (or small circuit reentry) with subsequent centrifugal spread.

Mechanisms of Atrial Flutter

Reentry as the mechanism of AFL was first suspected in the canine heart. Though AFL was difficult to induce and sustain in the normal atria, a linear lesion between the superior vena cava (SVC) and inferior vena cava (IVC) facilitated AFL inducibility and sustainability. A line of block enabled reentry around an electrically inert obstacle without short-circuiting. These fundamental principles can be extrapolated such that the line of block need not be located at the intercaval region and may be functional as well as anatomical in nature. Thus a right atrial (RA) lesion, as in the case of an atriotomy scar, can form the obstacle around which a wavefront circulates (incisional reentry).

However, the functional extension of a fixed line of block as described in an animal model may result in a circuit similar to typical AFL, where the extended line of block forms a posterior barrier. In the absence of the functional extension of the anatomical line of block, reentry was noted to occur around the lesion alone.[2] These findings explain the mechanism for the coexistence of classical cavotricuspid isthmus (CTI)-dependent AFL and incisional reentrant AFL, and the conversion from one arrhythmia to the other after development of CTI block with catheter ablation.

Atrial Fibrillation and Atrial Flutter: Two Sides of the Same Coin

Animal and human studies of induced and spontaneous AFL have shown that AFL is usually preceded by a transitional period of atrial fibrillation (AF).[2] It appears that AF provides the necessary line of intercaval block for flutter reentry. Absence of the line of block results in AF persistence or termination without transition to AFL, and shortening of the line of block converts AFL to AF. This is clinically evidenced by the conversion of AF to AFL by antiarrhythmic drugs that slow atrial conduction, by creating a posterior or intercaval functional line. Because of the dependence of flutter on fibrillation, the two arrhythmias commonly coexist clinically, with documented AF in up to 75% of AFL patients.

Though AF and AFL frequently coexist, one arrhythmia usually dominates. The predominance of AFL may be explained by more advanced RA remodeling with slowed conduction and regional conduction block, particularly in the posterior RA. This distribution of remodeling may facilitate the stabilization of AFL and its persistence as the dominant clinical arrhythmia.[3] When episodes of AFL are remotely studied, atria demonstrate atrial structural changes, conduction abnormalities, and sinus node dysfunction and may explain a predisposition to AFL and the subsequent development of AF.[4]

Clinical data that demonstrate the high rate of incident AF in AFL patients highlight the close pathophysiological relationship of the two arrhythmias.[5-7] Some clinical scores have been developed to predict the risk for developing AF following AFL ablation (e.g., HATCH score).[8] AFL patients in whom AF was inducible were also at a higher risk for clinical AF.[9] Among AFL patients, concomitant CTI ablation and pulmonary vein isolation (PVI) decrease the recurrence of AFL.[10,11] The elimination of PV triggers prevents the development of AF, which may be viewed as the initiating rhythm for AFL. In a separate study, incident AF was decreased in flutter patients who underwent prophylactic PVI versus CTI ablation alone.[12]

There is emerging evidence of a genetic basis for AFL and AF. The rs2200733 allele (4q25) increases the risk for AFL by twofold and implies that the AFL phenotype results from a complex interaction between genetic and clinical factors.[13]

Cavotricuspid Isthmus-Dependent Flutter

These circuits may be characterized as RA with a broad activation wavefront rotating between the tricuspid annulus (TA) as the anterior barrier and crista terminalis–eustachian ridge/IVC as the posterior barrier in either a counterclockwise or clockwise direction. The CTI provides the narrowest segment of the circuit (Fig. 75.1A and B).[14] Although these are critical barriers, significant variations in the leading edge or active region of the reentrant loop have been described. In an entrainment study, Santucci and colleagues demonstrated that only approximately one-third of typical AFL cases had an active circuit adjacent to the TA.[15] In others, the circuit took an oblique course between the anterior and posterior barriers, with the upper circuit off the annulus and posterior to the RA appendage (RAA) base. Of these, some coursed anterior to the SVC and others behind the SVC (across the crista terminalis). In others, bifurcation of the upper circuit was seen around the RAA, SVC, or both.[15]

Counterclockwise-typical AFL is the most common form of macroreentrant AFL. The classical inferior lead flutter waves

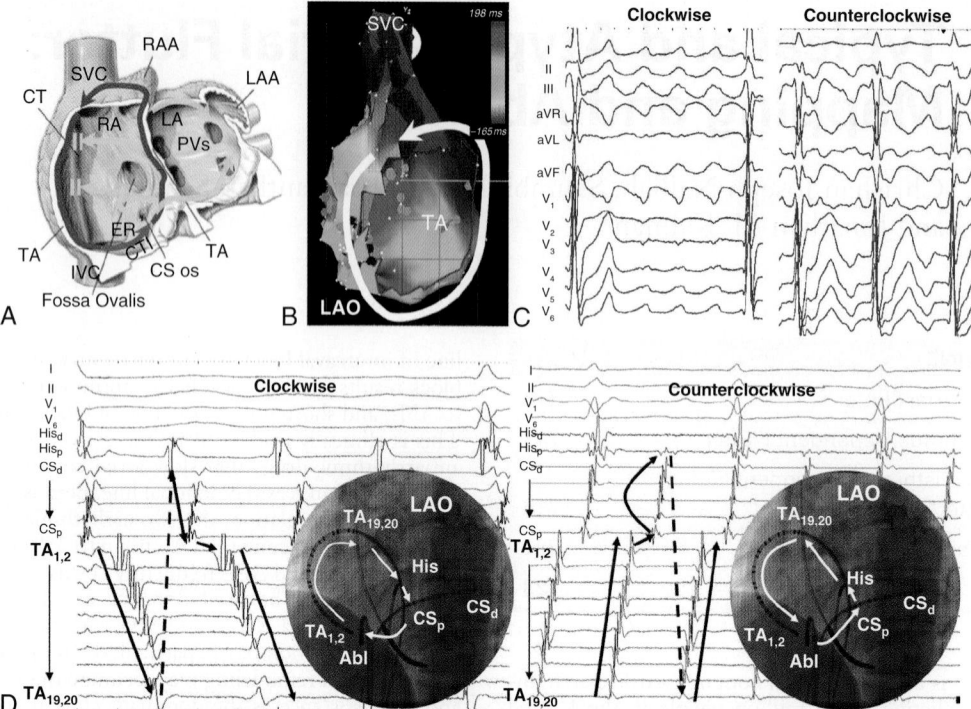

FIGURE 75.1 Cavotricuspid isthmus (*CTI*)-dependent flutter. (A) Schematic representation of the circuit of typical counterclockwise atrial flutter (AFL). Right atrium (*RA*) is seen anterior-posterior with the anterior surface removed. *Arrows* represent the atrial activation sequence during AFL. *Red arrows* identify components that are part of the circuit, and *yellow arrows* mark regions activated passively outside the circuit. Areas of conduction block are marked with *double lines* (//; crista terminalis [*CT*], eustachian ridge), providing the adequate path length for the flutter reentry circuit and preventing its short-circuiting. (B) Three-dimensional electroanatomical activation map of the RA during counterclockwise AFL shows "early" to late activation around the tricuspid annulus using a color spectrum from *red* (*marking early*) to *purple* (*marking late*) using an arbitrary reference. (C) Characteristic P-wave morphology of clockwise and counterclockwise AFL, which are best observed during periods of atrioventricular block or during ventricular pacing to unencumber the P waves. (D) Intracardiac electrograms and fluoroscopic left anterior oblique (*LAO*) view of multipolar catheters (*insets*), documenting the circuit of clockwise and counterclockwise AFL. *Arrows* depict the direction of atrial activation during AFL. *Abl*, Ablation; *CS*, coronary sinus; *d*, distal; *His*, His bundle electrogram; *IVC*, inferior vena cava; *LA*, left atrium; *p*, proximal; *PVs*, pulmonary veins; *RAA*, right atrial appendage; *SVC*, superior vena cava; *TA*, tricuspid annulus. ([A–C] From Medi C, Kalman JM. Prediction of the atrial flutter circuit location from the surface electrocardiogram. *Europace.* 2008;10:786-796.)

("saw-tooth" pattern) demonstrate an initial gradual downsloping segment followed by a deeply inverted component with a terminal positive component (of variable amplitude) (Fig. 75.1C). Although the flutter wave typically appears inverted in inferior leads, variations in the amplitude of both the negative and positive components can create atypical patterns. In the precordial leads, V_1 classically demonstrates an initial isoelectric component followed by an upright component. With progression across the precordial leads, the initial component becomes inverted and the second component becomes isoelectric such that V_5 and V_6 demonstrate an inverted flutter wave.[16] Lead I is low amplitude/isoelectric and aVL usually upright (see Fig. 75.1C). Unusual flutter wave morphologies may be seen with counterclockwise AFL, and a left AFL may mimic the counterclockwise AFL appearance.

Clockwise AFL comprises 10% of cases with its boundaries identical to counterclockwise AFLs but with a reversal of the wavefront activation. Surface electrocardiogram (ECG) is less predictable but retains some characteristic features. Flutter waves in the inferior leads are usually broadly positive, with the upright component preceded by an inverted component of variable amplitude. There is characteristic notching on the upright component, which has a bifid appearance. V_1 is characterized by a broad negative and usually notched deflection with a transition

to an upright deflection in V_6. Lead I is usually upright and aVL is low amplitude negative, giving an overall appearance that is the reverse of counterclockwise AFL (see Fig. 75.1C).

Diagnosis in the Laboratory

Notwithstanding typical ECG patterns, the mapping of AFL by activation and entrainment techniques remains critical prior to ablation. Activation sequences demonstrate clockwise or anticlockwise RA activation during flutter, with a multipolar catheter positioned in the coronary sinus (CS) and around the TA and His bundle positions (Fig. 75.1D). When patients present in sinus rhythm, atrial pacing can be utilized to initiate AFL, although there is an inherent risk for inducing AF. Onset typically occurs during burst atrial pacing, leading to unidirectional block within the CTI.

Electrophysiological testing of typical AFL is primarily aimed at confirming that the circuit is macroreentrant and that the CTI is integral. At a minimum, entrainment should be performed within the CTI to confirm that it is within the circuit (postpacing interval–tachycardia cycle length [PPI–TCL] <20 ms). We use entrainment pacing with a CL of 10 to 20 ms less than the TCL. Entrainment should be performed with synchronization to the entraining electrode to avoid the initial introduction of a tight-coupled stimulus that may terminate or change the circuit. Where the entraining CL is short, decrement can be introduced into the circuit that produces an erroneous result by prolonging PPI. Entrainment should be performed at multiple sites that are anticipated to lie within (i.e., around the TA) and outside the circuit (mid- and distal CS) to confirm the AFL mechanism. Furthermore, only a few extrastimuli are required to entrain the large AFL circuit in the RA.[17,18] When entrainment is "in" at two sites more than 2 cm apart, the presence of macroreentry is confirmed.

During transient entrainment of a tachycardia with a pacing CL of 10 to 20 ms shorter than the flutter CL, the wavefront from each pacing impulse propagates in both the ortho- and antidromic directions. The antidromic wavefront will collide with the preceding orthodromic wavefront as it exits the critical isthmus. Entrainment will result in acceleration of the atrium to the pacing CL with each antidromic wavefront colliding with the orthodromic wavefront of the preceding pacing stimulus (constant fusion). When pacing stops, CL of the orthodromic wavefront of the last pacing stimulus is equal to that of the entrainment, but as it does not encounter a further pacing-induced antidromic wavefront, it is not fused (the last entrained but not fused beat). When the pacing rate is further increased, the collision site between the ortho- and antidromic wavefronts is shifted farther from the pacing site so that more of the ECG complex appears paced (progressive ECG fusion), and more electrogram (EGM) sites are antidromically captured (progressive EGM fusion). When entrainment is performed in a narrow isthmus, the extent of antidromic capture is limited within the isthmus and fusion will not be evident on surface ECG (concealed entrainment). When outside a protected isthmus, antidromic atrial capture or penetration is more extensive and therefore manifest on surface ECG (manifest fusion) (Fig. 75.2).

However, while the presence of concealed entrainment can be an extremely useful tool for mapping ventricular arrhythmias, in practice it is of limited utility for atrial arrhythmias. The flutter wave morphology is of relatively low amplitude and is frequently obscured by an overlap with QRS complexes and T waves, making it difficult or impossible to detect changes in morphology. Distortion of the stimulus artifact may render it difficult to detect subtle degrees of fusion. Thus while entrainment remains one of the cornerstone tools for the evaluation of atrial arrhythmias, the focus is on PPI–TCL to determine which sites are within the circuit.

High-density three-dimensional (3D) electroanatomical mapping (contact or noncontact mapping) is able to delineate the RA circuit during typical AFL with the use of activation maps represented as a continuous progression of colors (see Fig. 75.1B). A key point with activation mapping using electroanatomical mapping systems in macroreentrant circuits is that early activation is not applicable to any specific point in the circuit as activation is continuous and the origin of activation is always arbitrary with respect to the particular reference chosen for illustration. Activation timing should span the entire CL of a macroreentrant circuit. Where "earliest" meets "latest" activation in a continuous circuit ("head meets tail") is again an arbitrary anatomical point determined by the choice of the zero point.

Using 3D mapping, the activation wavefront in counterclockwise AFL will most typically appear as a broad wavefront that exits the medial CTI, ascends the septum, passes anterior to the SVC, and descends the anterolateral RA to laterally enter the CTI (see Fig. 75.1B). Passive wavefronts will activate the left atrium (LA) and posterior RA where conduction delay or block at the crista terminalis will prevent a "short circuiting" of the TA (see Fig. 75.1).[14] In addition to entrainment and noncontact mapping, 3D mapping can characterize tissue voltage of the CTI, which may be useful in planning ablation as lower voltage may predict an

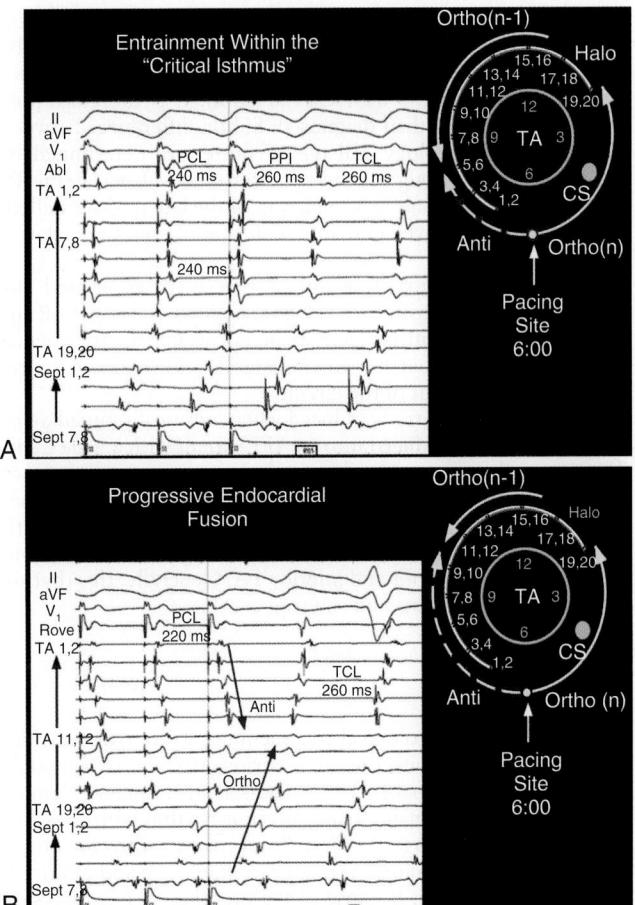

FIGURE 75.2 Entrainment of typical flutter within the critical isthmus. (A) Entrainment of typical counterclockwise atrial flutter from within the cavotricuspid isthmus. Almost the complete circuit is recorded on the septal catheter and the tricuspid annulus (*TA*) catheter. Entrainment from the ablation (*Abl*) catheter within the cavotricuspid isthmus results in some concealed antidromic penetration (note that electrograms on the distal TA catheter are marginally altered in morphology and sequence). The 12-lead electrocardiogram panel demonstrates that this is concealed on surface electrocardiogram (*next panel*). The postpacing interval (*PPI*) equals the tachycardia cycle length (*TCL*) and hence is in the circuit. (B) With an increase in the entraining rate (CL 220 ms), there is now obvious antidromic penetration from TA 1,2 to approximately TA 9,10 (the region of collision with the n-1 orthodromic beat). Antidromic capture of upstream electrograms with demonstration of the collision point with the n-1 orthodromic electrograms proves that this is atrial macroreentry. The last orthodromic beat (*Ortho/arrow*) is entrained at the pacing rate but not fused (as it is not met by another paced antidromic wavefront). Progressive fusion is demonstrated as the extent of antidromic capture is greater when pacing at the faster rate compared with the first panel. *PCL,* Paced cycle length.

easier ablation path. Delineation of regions amenable to simple ablation may be facilitated by magnetic resonance imaging (MRI) in the future.

Other Cavotricuspid Isthmus-Dependent Flutters

Lower loop reentry is also a CTI-dependent flutter but has a shorter circuit confined to the lower RA, with clockwise or counterclockwise rotation around the IVC. It is created by the presence of a posterior breakthrough at the crista terminalis and often coexists with typical AFL around the TA.[19] The circuit exits the medial CTI, with activation proceeding across the posterior RA.

Clockwise variants of lower loop reentry have also been described. The true prevalence of lower loop reentry is uncertain as the ECG morphology may be indistinguishable from typical flutter and termination occurs with CTI ablation. It is therefore possibly more common than diagnosed. Subtle differences between flutter wave morphology and typical flutter are determined by the level of breakthrough at the crista terminalis. Low lateral RA breakthrough will result in attenuation of the late positive deflection of the flutter wave compared with that of counterclockwise typical AFL.

Intraisthmus reentry is a circuit that revolves around the medial CTI and CS ostium; the lateral isthmus is not part of the circuit. Concealed entrainment is demonstrable in the medial CTI or CS ostium but not in the lateral CTI, and other sites around the TA are out of the circuit.[20]

Double wave reentry is induced when a critically timed atrial extrastimulus is introduced into an AFL circuit with a wide excitable gap resulting in a second excitation wavefront such that two wavefronts simultaneously coexist within the circuit.[21] The phenomenon manifests as acceleration of the flutter CL with identical surface and intracardiac EGM morphology and simultaneous activation of the superior and inferior TA. Generally, this rhythm lasts for only a few beats and can trigger AF.

Treatment

Pharmacological

Principles of pharmacological treatment are to control ventricular rate during AFL with the use of atrioventricular (AV) nodal–blocking agents (β-blockers or cardiac-selective calcium channel blockers) and/or the maintenance of sinus rhythm with class I or III antiarrhythmic drugs. Class 1c drugs may stabilize the flutter by slowing the rate and increasing the excitable gap and can result in 1:1 AV conduction. Because of the presence of postreversion atrial stunning (whether this be pharmacological or electrical), it is mandatory to follow anticoagulation guidelines for the reversion of AF. Because of the high late incidence of AF after successful flutter ablation coupled with the documented late risk for stroke,[22] it is our practice to make decisions regarding ongoing anticoagulation (with Coumadin or an equivalent) on the basis of the CHADS$_2$ score. In the absence of supporting data, an alternate approach is to continue to closely monitor for the development of late AF, particularly in patients with stroke risk factors.

Catheter Ablation

Pharmacological treatments result in the long-term maintenance of sinus rhythm in only 36% to 73% of AFL patients; moreover, complete arrhythmia suppression can be difficult. Evidence from randomized studies has demonstrated the superiority of catheter ablation over antiarrhythmic drugs in the treatment of AFL, with higher rates of maintenance of sinus rhythm, improvement in quality of life, and reduction in the recurrence of future AF.[23] Thus catheter ablation is a class I recommendation for AFL if it is recurrent, is poorly tolerated, or reemerges after treatment with a class I antiarrhythmic or amiodarone. Some clinical series have observed that AFL ablation is independently associated with a lower risk for stroke and/or thromboembolic events and death of any cause, whether a history of AF is present or not.[24] Evolving technology that utilizes novel imaging systems and new generation catheters may also render catheter ablation easier, faster, and safer.[25–27] Real-world evidence also indicates that flutter ablation decreases hospital resource utilization.[28]

Catheter ablation may be performed in either the septal or mid aspects of the CTI and will be determined by the stability of catheter access and anatomical variation (see Fig. 75.1D). It is important to be aware that inadvertent AV block has rarely been reported during ablation at the septal aspect of the CTI because of the proximity posterior extensions of the AV node. The lateral isthmus is generally longer and is not usually the primary ablation target. Ablation may be performed during AFL or proximal coronary pacing (in sinus rhythm). The latter allows the identification of a change in the activation sequence on the tricuspid annular catheter, signifying the slowing of CTI conduction or block.

The usual approach is for ablation to commence at the annular end with either continuous pullback or focal point-by-point ablation across the CTI to the eustachian ridge at the anterior margin of the IVC. The adequacy of lesion formation is confirmed by the diminution of the local EGM signal and the emergence of the local double potentials on the ablation catheter. The ablation endpoint is the demonstration of a complete bidirectional conduction block across the isthmus.

An alternative approach is to use the maximum voltage-guided technique, which is based on the premise that there are only discrete muscle bundles in the CTI that participate in the flutter circuit; these can be identified by the presence of large EGM voltages, which are selectively targeted for ablation. In this technique, peak-to-peak bipolar EGMs are measured during pullback along the CTI and the largest amplitude signal ablated regardless of the location along the line. The next largest EGM is sequentially mapped and targeted for ablation until block is achieved.

The advent of contact force–sensing ablation technology has demonstrated that dormant CTI conduction is related to insufficient contact force during ablation delivery. Nearly half of all lesions delivered at the CTI line had low contact force, despite other surrogate markers, suggesting satisfactory contact. There was also marked region-specific variability of contact force, with the lowest contact force observed at the annular region.[29] Other indices of tissue contact, such as the electrical coupling index, have also been shown to have some utility in improving ablation efficacy.[30] Use of this technology may potentially result in lower recurrence rates, but this is yet to be shown. Anatomical variations can pose considerable challenges in achieving successful CTI ablation. These may include a prominent subeustachian pouch or prominent and deep pectinate muscles that crisscross the isthmus.[31]

The efficacy of radiofrequency (RF) lesion application has been investigated. In a recent study, Pambrun and colleagues demonstrated that the complete elimination of the unipolar negative component during flutter ablation was an indicator of tissue transmurality.[32,33] Future directions include MRI-guided electrophysiology studies, which hold the promise of visualizing lesion formation and even confirming transmurality.[34]

Demonstration of bidirectional CTI block is the key endpoint in AFL ablation, and neither termination of AFL during ablation nor noninducibility can be considered as reliable endpoints (Fig. 75.3). Adenosine administration following CTI line completion may unmask dormant conductions that can be targeted for further ablation to improve long-term results.[35]

A meta-analysis including more than 10,000 patients (158 studies) showed that the acute procedural success rate of CTI-dependent AFL ablation was approximately 91%, with a complication rate of 2.6%.[36] The most common complications were vascular. The incidence of complete heart block was 0.2% and that of other major complications, including cerebrovascular events, myocardial infarctions, and ventricular arrhythmias, was 0.1%. There were no deaths reported. Recurrence rate was low with the use of 8- to 10-mm non-irrigated or 4-mm irrigated catheters (6.3%).

Noncavotricuspid Isthmus-Dependent Flutter ("Atypical Flutter")

General Principles

Atypical AFL encompasses a range of macroreentrant arrhythmias that are not dependent on the CTI. They have varied ECG characteristics, and the flutter wave morphology is generally not particularly useful for determining the circuit location. Occasionally,

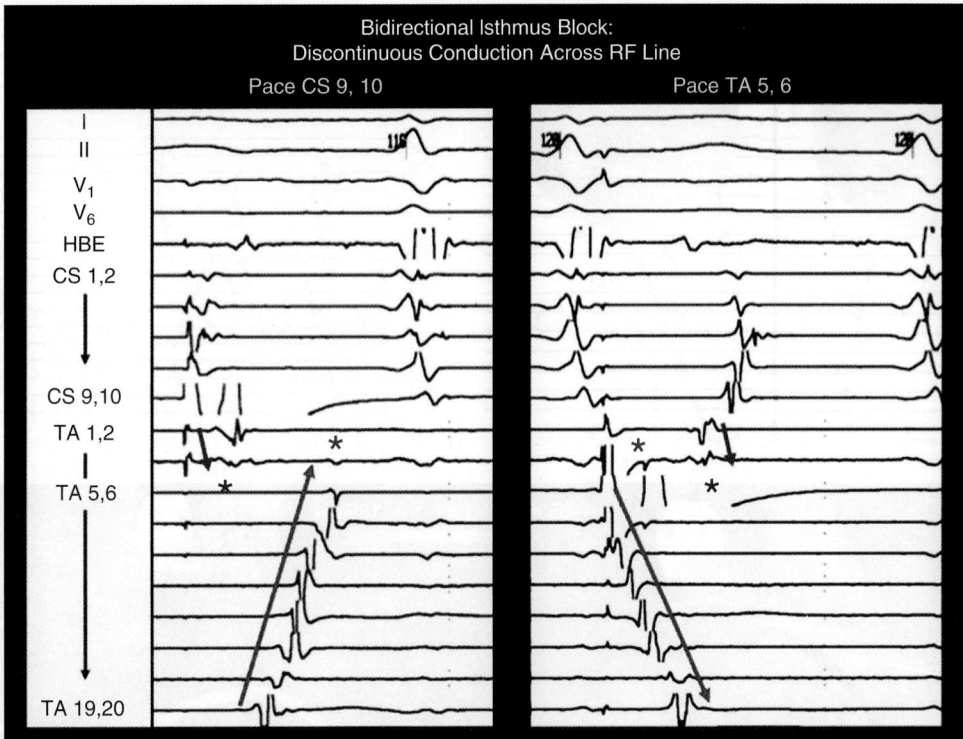

FIGURE 75.3 Demonstration of bidirectional conduction block across the cavotricuspid isthmus. The tricuspid annulus (*TA*) catheter is positioned such that it crosses the ablation line of block in the cavotricuspid isthmus. Pacing from the coronary sinus ostium (*CS* os; *CS* 9,10) septum to the line in the *left panel* demonstrates linear activation around the TA to TA 3,4 where low-amplitude split potentials are seen; this indicates that this bipole is straddling the line of block. Pacing from TA 5,6 immediately lateral to the ablation line in the *right panel* demonstrates linear activation around the TA with the reversal of the activation on the distal TA catheter (TA 1,2 precedes TA 3,4). The CS catheter is positioned distally at this time and so is activated late. *HBE,* His bundle electrogram; *RF,* radiofrequency.

atypical flutter may present ECG characteristics, suggesting an isthmus-dependent mechanism. Broadly, these AFLs can occur (1) in the absence of prior atrial surgery or intervention, (2) in the context of prior corrective atrial surgery (congenital heart disease, valvular heart disease, postmaze procedure, or cardiac transplantation), or (3) with previous AF ablation.[37–39] Reentry occurs around a central barrier (e.g., AV annulus, venous ostia, scar, or a functional line of block). Macroreentry can exist in either atrium, and multiple circuits can coexist. Dual-loop or figure-of-eight reentry has been described where one circuit may involve the CTI. It is important to note that in patients with macroreentry, "focal" sources with early activation and centrifugal spread may coexist.

Atypical AFL is best mapped using a combination of activation mapping and entrainment mapping. Both techniques should be considered complementary, each with its advantages and disadvantages. Multipolar catheters can rapidly detect atrial activation patterns, double potentials, low amplitude, and fractionated signals. They are particularly useful for right-sided circuits (Fig. 75.4A and B).

Entrainment mapping remains a cornerstone technique for the evaluation of non-CTI dependent flutter mechanism. Initial entrainment from a number of widely separated right and LA sites will provide rapid clues to both the general circuit location and the likely anatomical isthmus sites. For example, entrainment that is "in" the circuit in the mitral isthmus will suggest that the linear ablation of this isthmus may be necessary. The risk for terminating tachycardia or converting one form of AFL to another can be minimized by ensuring synchronization to the entraining electrode and pacing at just 10 to 20 ms below the TCL. In our experience, when using these precautions in a stable circuit with an excitable gap, termination or alteration of the tachycardia

is unusual. In circuits with significant decremental conduction, entrainment within the circuit may be erroneously associated with a long PPI, particularly at higher pacing rates. Perhaps the most significant limitation of entrainment is at sites where signal amplitude is very low, rendering capture and EGM marking difficult or impossible.

Rapid assessment of circuit proximity can also be performed by entraining from a "downstream" electrode (i.e., an electrode that is activated later than neighboring electrodes). A short PPI accompanied by a long stimulus to atrial EGM on an "upstream" electrode indicates circuit proximity.[40]

3D mapping will allow definition of the tachycardia activation sequence along with the definition of substrate and anatomical barriers, such as low-voltage areas that represent scars and their relationship to natural barriers to conduction such as the tricuspid and mitral annuli, venae cavae, and pulmonary venous ostia (Fig. 75.4C). The generated atrial activation sequence can be superimposed on atrial images segmented from a preprocedural computed tomography (CT) or MRI scan to facilitate correlation of electrical substrate with anatomical detail.

3D mapping allows detailed anatomical characterization of the sites of double potentials representing lines of conduction block and fractionated EGMs that may potentially represent regions of slow conduction critical to arrhythmia maintenance (see Fig. 75.4C). Voltage maps will allow identification of electrical scar (amplitude <0.05 mV) and low-voltage zones (atrial amplitude <0.5 mV), which may identify lines of block critical to the reentrant mechanism but which may also serve as boundaries for the design of ablation strategies. In these circumstances, linear ablation connecting two anatomically defined structures (e.g., from scar to vena cava or scar to scar) may be necessary for tachycardia

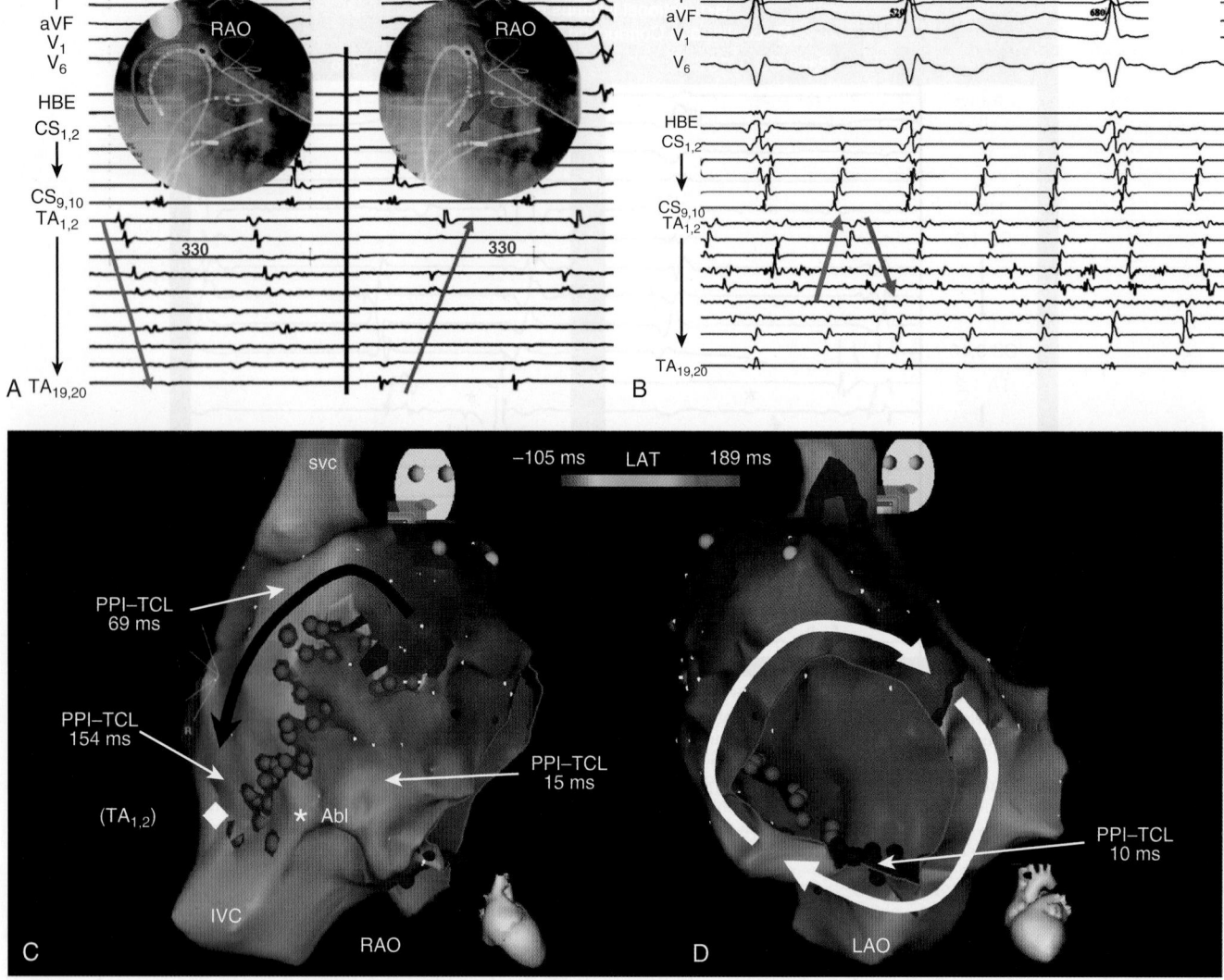

FIGURE 75.4 Atypical atrial flutter. (A) Atypical free wall right atrial flutter in a patient with a prior history of atrial septal defect repair. In the *left panel*, there is an ascending wavefront in the posterior right atrium. In the *right panel*, there is a descending wavefront in the anterior right atrium. This simple mapping approach rapidly indicates the probable circuit location that rotates around the scar in the free wall. Between these two catheter positions, signals were unrecordable because of the presence of a broad scar. (B) In this patient with free wall flutter after an atrial septal defect repair, the narrow scar allowed the recording of the entire circuit on a single multipolar catheter. (C) and (D) Three-dimensional electroanatomical activation maps of another patient with a history of atrial septal defect repair. The electroanatomical map suggests the presence of dual-loop reentry with one circuit that rotates around the free wall scar (*gray region*) in the counterclockwise direction (*left panel*) and a simultaneous circuit with clockwise rotation around the tricuspid annulus (*TA*). Although this is a commonly observed pattern after atrial septal defect repair, in this case, entrainment showed that sites around the TA had postpacing interval–tachycardia cycle length (*PPI–TCL*) of <20 ms ("in the circuit") but that sites posterior to the scar showed progressively longer PPI and were out of the circuit. In this case, the appearance on the electroanatomical map was misleading as the free wall scar was contiguous with the inferior vena cava (*IVC*), preventing a second loop. The region posterior to the scar was thus akin to a "blind loop." This was confirmed with pacing maneuvers after termination of this circuit with ablation in the cavotricuspid isthmus. *Abl*, Ablation; *CS*, coronary sinus; *HBE*, His bundle electrogram; *LAO*, left anterior oblique; *RAO*, right anterior oblique; *SVC*, superior vena cava.

termination. Although linear ablation between two anatomical sites is frequently required for the termination of these circuits, many atypical circuits can be ablated at a single critical site of slow conduction.

A key point to note is that in atria with significant scarring and conduction slowing, the electroanatomical map can provide a misleading picture, even creating the appearance of a circuit with head-meets-tail that ultimately is remote from the tachycardia circuit (see Fig. 75.4C and D). For this reason, entrainment as

described earlier can rapidly identify the region of interest. One approach is to only include sites within the activation map where PPI–TCL is <40 ms. An alternative approach is to create an electroanatomical map of PPI, which may allow the precise definition of the active reentrant circuit versus passively activated regions of the atrial chamber.[15] Here sites in the atrium with PPI–TCL ≤20 ms (within the circuit) are differentiated from sites where PPI–TCL is >40 ms (well outside the circuit) using color coding. Sites with PPI–TCL of 20 to 40 ms are intermediate.

Right Atrial Atypical Flutter

Although ECG is generally unhelpful for the localization of atypical flutter, a completely negative flutter wave in lead V_1 will generally indicate an RA circuit.

RA free wall flutter has been described in the context of spontaneous scar. This is characterized by areas of electrical silence, low voltage, and/or presence of double potentials in the RA free wall in the absence of previous cardiac surgery. The scar has a characteristic lateral to posterolateral anatomical location. There is often evidence of coexistent sinus node dysfunction, suggesting an underlying global RA myopathic process. Patients frequently demonstrate more than one tachycardia mechanism, including (1) a circuit around the scar, which forms the central obstacle; (2) a CTI-dependent typical flutter; and (3) a circuit that involves a channel between two scar regions. The ablation strategy targets the narrowest part of the circuit, which may include an ablation line from the scar to the IVC (most common), SVC, or TA with a bidirectional block. A channel between two scar regions may be targeted with focal ablation.[41] High-output pacing maneuvers should be employed to check for phrenic nerve capture before ablation in the posterolateral RA. Reported acute success rates have been approximately 90%.[42] Regardless of the presence of CTI-dependent flutter, it is advisable to perform CTI ablation to reduce the long-term occurrence of this arrhythmia. Focal atrial tachycardias may also occur in this population that has a significant atrial pathology.

Upper Loop Reentry

This arrhythmia is characterized by reentry around a central obstacle, including the SVC and the crista terminalis, which forms a region of functional conduction block. The lower turnaround point is a region of slow conduction where the wavefront propagates across the crista terminalis.[43] Rotation may be either counterclockwise or clockwise around these anatomical structures. Ablation of the conduction gap in the crista terminalis often requires relatively focal ablation.

Left Atrial Atypical Flutter

These tachycardias are characterized by reentry around anatomical structures such as the mitral annulus, PV ostia, and regions of electrical silence or scar.[44] Anterior wall reentry has also recently been described.[44] Characteristically, scar can be observed at the LA posterior wall, roof, and anterior wall. It can facilitate reentry around anatomical structures or may form the obstacle around which reentry occurs.

Single-loop, double-loop, and multiple circuit left AFLs (two or three loops simultaneously rotating) have been described.[44] Dual- and multiple-loop flutters should be considered when disparate LA regions are all "in the circuit" by entrainment (Fig. 75.5). Perimitral flutters may show clockwise or counterclockwise rotation with the posterior wall scar serving as a posterior boundary. Scars may also anchor circuits around the ipsilateral PV pairs. Left septal AFLs are characterized by reentry around the left septum primum with a critical isthmus located between PVs posteriorly and/or mitral annulus anteriorly and the septum primum.

Although surface ECG is generally unhelpful, a broad-based upright flutter wave in V_1 is highly suggestive of an LA origin.[16] Flutter wave morphologies in other leads are highly variable but frequently of low amplitudes and may erroneously suggest AF. An LA circuit should also be considered when less than 50% of the TCL is mapped within the RA and when RA entrainment demonstrates all regions to be out of the circuit (PPI−TCL >40 ms). Further evidence for an LA circuit is passive conduction in the RA via the earliest septal activation.

The general approach to the ablation of left AFLs involves the identification of a critical isthmus using both entrainment and 3D activation mapping. In addition, the voltage map is very useful in

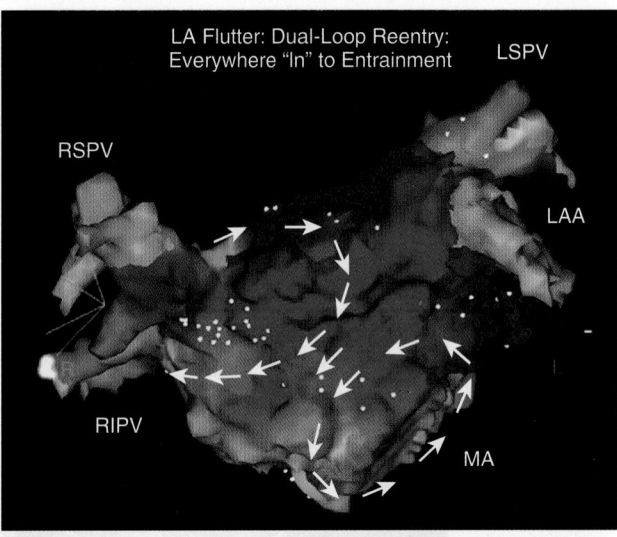

FIGURE 75.5 Left atrial (*LA*) activation map from a patient with dual-loop reentry. There is a counterclockwise circuit around the mitral annulus (*MA*) and a simultaneous clockwise circuit around the right pulmonary veins. Again, there is no narrow circuit point, and linear ablation to transect both circuits simultaneously was performed from the MA to the right superior pulmonary vein (*RSPV*). *LAA*, Left atrial appendage; *LSPV*, left superior pulmonary vein; *RIPV*, right inferior pulmonary vein.

planning an ablation line through low-amplitude tissue. Recent reports have utilized MRI to define the substrate that sustains AFL and to strategically plan ablation at critical sites.[45,46] Common linear ablation targets include (1) the mitral isthmus (from the left inferior or right superior PV to the mitral annulus); (2) a "roof line" between the left and right superior PVs, usually with circumferential isolation of these veins to "anchor" the line to a region of conduction block; and (3) electrically silent areas connected by an ablation line (Fig. 75.6). However, circuits are very variable, and lesion sets may be required between any of these anatomical structures and a region of scarring. It is generally feasible to demonstrate the presence of complete conduction block as an endpoint to linear ablation in the LA. In one novel series, investigators reported a transthoracic epicardial approach to perimitral flutter ablation in patients refractory to endocardial ablation.[47]

Common Flutters Following Cardiac Surgery/Procedures

Congenital Heart Disease

These AFLs occur in the context of surgical repair of congenital heart defects, including atrial septal defect, tetralogy of Fallot, Mustard or Senning repair for d-transposition, and patients with Fontan repair for single ventricular physiology.[48] In general, these arrhythmias develop many years after the initial surgery, and the complexity and number of circuits mirror the complexity of the underlying condition and the surgical repair. They consist primarily of macroreentrant circuits that involve atriotomy incisions, cannulation sites, prosthetic material, and anatomical structures (Fig. 75.7). Barriers that border the critical isthmus of conduction can be identified on anatomical grounds by the presence of areas of electrical silence or by the demonstration of split potentials that signify a line of block. Mapping will involve multipolar activation, entrainment, and 3D electroanatomical maps.[49] Ablation is targeted to a narrow isthmus between anatomical structures and/or electrically silent areas and may require either linear or focal ablation dependent on isthmus width. CTI flutter frequently coexists (70% of cases), and the CTI should in general always be an ablation target Because dual-loop reentry may be present, during

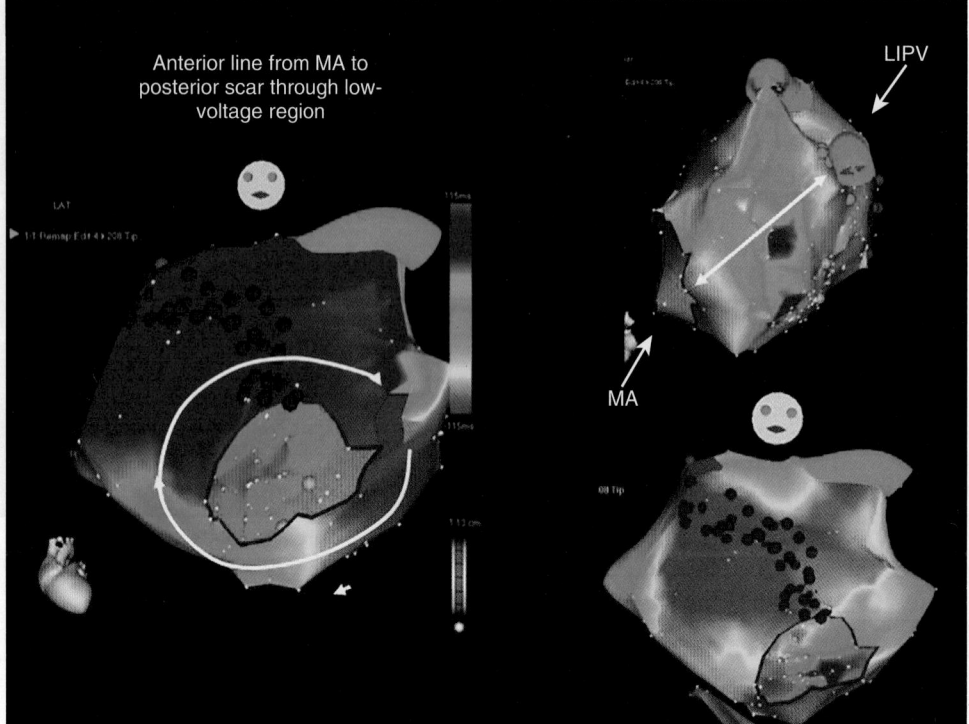

FIGURE 75.6 Clockwise perimitral flutter. *Left panel*, Carto images from this case show perimitral flutter with activation proceeding from *red* to *yellow* to *green*, *blue*, and *purple* before the "head meets tail" at the *dark red band*. The *right superior panel* shows the voltage map of the mitral isthmus. The line is very long at approximately 4 cm (*white arrow*), and the voltages are high (*blue and green*). The *right inferior panel* shows the voltage map of the anterior atrium, which is also a long line from the mitral annulus (*MA*) back to a posterior scar; however, this is all low voltage. Ablation was performed from the MA to the posterior scar through this low-voltage zone to terminate flutter. It can also be seen that the circuit is a very broad wavefront, and there is no narrow isthmus. A narrow isthmus is not always present during atrial macroreentry, and when absent, it is often wise to join an ablation line between two anatomical obstacles that traverses the low-voltage atrium. *LIPV*, Left inferior pulmonary vein.

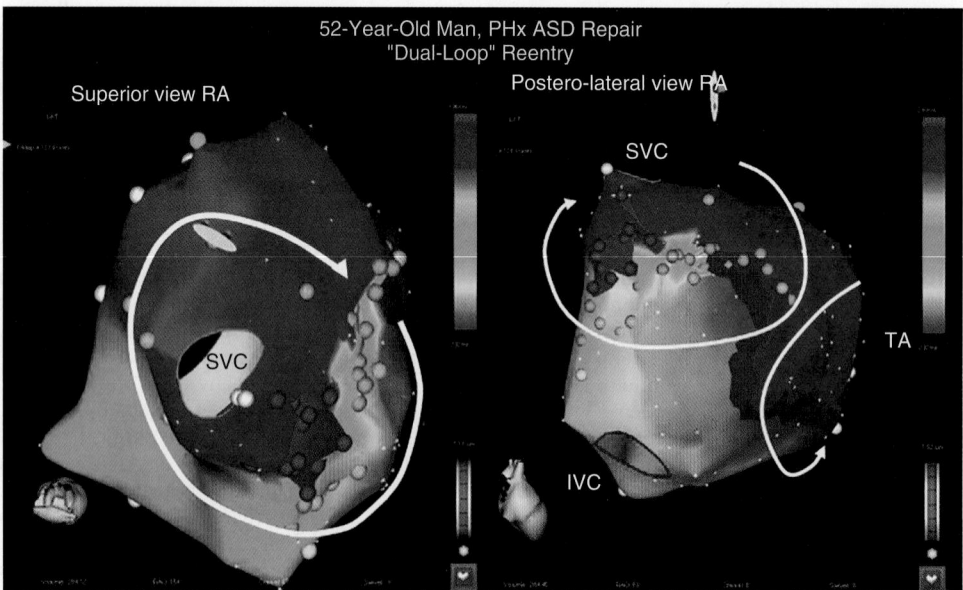

FIGURE 75.7 Dual-loop atrial flutter postatrial septal defect (*ASD*) repair. A 52-year-old man with a past history of ASD repair presents with an atrial flutter. The *right panel* shows the region of the scar marked both by the *gray area* (*silent*) and the *blue dots*, which mark a zone of double potentials. The *pink dots* mark fractionated signals. There are two simultaneous wavefronts: one around the tricuspid annulus (*TA*) and one around the superior vena cava (*SVC*). After ablation in the cavotricuspid isthmus, the circuit around the SVC ("upper loop reentry") persisted. Linear ablation from the scar to the inferior vena cava (*IVC*) terminated the tachycardia. *RA*, Right atrium.

RA Lesional Tachycardias in MV Surgery

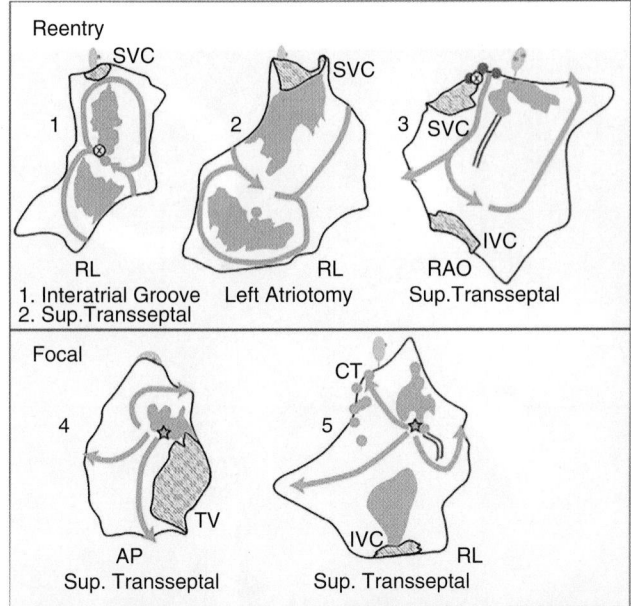

FIGURE 75.8 Common flutter circuits following mitral valve surgery. Possible different flutter circuits following mitral valve surgery depends on the different surgical access approaches. *AP,* Anteroposterior; *CT,* crista terminalis; *IVC,* inferior vena cava; *RA,* right atrium; *RAO,* right anterior oblique; *RL,* right lateral; *SVC,* superior vena cava. (From Markowitz SM, Brodman RF, Stein KM, et al. Lesional tachycardias related to mitral valve surgery. *J Am Coll Cardiol.* 2002;39:1973-1983.)

ablation, it is important to be vigilant for subtle changes in the flutter wave morphology, CL, and endocardial activation pattern to determine whether the circuit has changed.[50] Periodically repeating entrainment if flutter has not terminated will rapidly identify when a region is no longer critical to the circuit. AFL after surgery or in structural heart disease has a high acute success rate but carries significant risk for arrhythmia recurrence and AF.[51]

Mitral Valve Surgery
The majority of AFL circuits in patients who have undergone mitral valve surgery occur in relation to surgical incisions, which provide a substrate for late macroreentrant atrial arrhythmias. Three commonly described approaches include (1) right lateral approach to the LA, (2) incision through the interatrial (Waterston) groove, and (3) superior transseptal approach. The circuits described included single and figure-of-eight circuits constrained by regions of surgical scar that correspond to sites of atriotomy scars and anatomical boundaries. Depending on the surgical approach, it is frequently possible to identify a critical isthmus within the RA. Circuits have been described around septal and free wall scars, and there may be simultaneous peritricuspid reentry, creating a dual loop (Fig. 75.8). In the LA, circuits may occur around the incision as a central obstacle, or the scar may facilitate reentry around PVs or the mitral annulus. Dual-loop reentry is commonly present.

An incision in the Waterston groove may create the substrate for reentry in the LA or RA. A recent report described the presence of an upper loop (peri-SVC) circuit stabilized by slow conduction at the site of the surgical incision (see Fig. 75.8). The approach to all of these circuits is as previously described, with the use of 3D activation mapping and entrainment to define a critical isthmus between anatomical barriers and/or scar.

Other Cardiac Surgery: Maze Procedures and Cardiac Transplantation
AFLs post maze are most commonly because of gaps in surgical or ablative lesions.[52] A variety of circuits have been described,

including perimitral reentry and circuits around ipsilateral pairs of PVs in addition to those circuits that use the surgical scar as the central obstacle. Focal atrial tachycardias or AF may occur because of PV reconnection.

CTI-dependent AFL is the most common macroreentrant arrhythmia reported in the cardiac transplant population.[53] P-wave morphology of this flutter is rarely typical (seen in only 20% of cases)[53] given the lack of contribution of the electrically isolated recipient posterior atria to the P-wave morphology. In contrast to CTI-dependent AFL in nontransplanted hearts, the donor-to-recipient atrioatrial suture line forms the posterior boundary of the flutter circuit rather than the crista terminalis/eustachian ridge, resulting in narrowing of the isthmus boundaries. Successful ablation can be achieved by creating a line of electrical block, extending from the tricuspid valve to the surgical atrial anastomosis, with no requirement to extend the line back to the IVC. This represents elimination of the electrically active component of the isthmus (donor region) that is narrower than the anatomical isthmus (donor plus recipient region).

A perimitral flutter circuit restricted to the donor atrium has been successfully described to be treated with an ablation line from the mitral annulus to the left inferior PV and from the mitral annulus to the LA roof surgical anastomosis with the recipient atria. AFL that involves the donor RA posterior wall with a circuit that incorporates the surgical incision as a boundary has been described, which was treated by an ablation line from the midposterior RA to the incision line at the IVC surgical anastomosis.

A unique feature of the transplanted heart is the occurrence of one or more isolated areas of recipient-to-donor conduction along the otherwise inert anastomotic suture line that serves as a putative line of conduction block, thus creating the substrate for reentry. AFL occurring in the recipient atria may conduct with variable block in the donor atrium. The approach to these arrhythmias in general is to identify and ablate the site or sites of electrical connection between donor and recipient atrium.

Atrial Fibrillation Ablation
Left AFLs that complicate catheter ablation for AF are well recognized. These circuits are unusual following simple antral PVI in patients without structural heart disease. However, they are much more commonly observed when linear ablation and extensive ablation of fractionated signals are undertaken. Circuits may be single or dual loop that use gaps in previous ablation lines as a critical region of slowed conduction. In addition, small reentrant circuits have been described, particularly in the setting of prior ablation of regions of complex fractionated EGMs. In addition, reentrant circuits may arise around PVs, particularly if two gaps are present in the circumferential ring. The most commonly described circuits are perimitral, roof-dependent, and reentry that involves the interatrial septum. Catheter ablation using the mapping principles described earlier can yield initial success rates of approximately 90%.

High-Density Mapping

Standard mapping technologies have traditionally been limited by their poor spatial resolution and time-intensive nature. Wide interelectrode spacing and/or low-point density can fail to capture important mechanistic details of an activation wavefront and thereby mischaracterize the underlying reentry circuit or fail to delineate critical aspects of the flutter circuit (such as an isthmus). These limitations are compounded where AFL is not sustained.

The evolution of technology has sought to address these weaknesses by enabling rapid high-density atrial mapping by utilizing a combination of catheters with multiple closely spaced electrodes and data processing platforms capable of complex computation[54] (Fig. 75.9). Appreciation of the circuit's nuances is

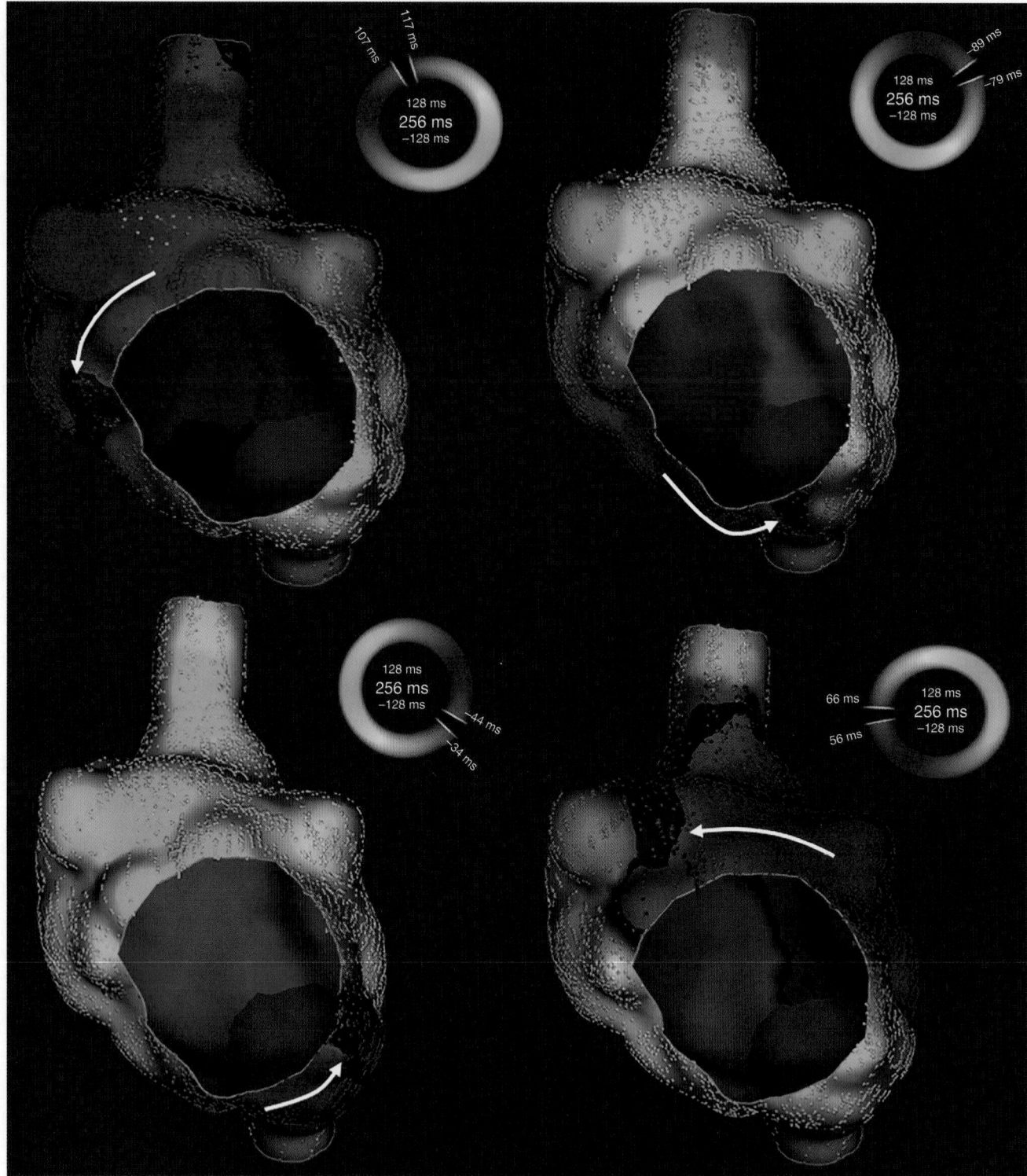

FIGURE 75.9 High density activation mapping of typical atrial flutter. Use of the Rhythmia mapping system to create high-density maps of the atrium. This is a 20,000-point map of typical cavotricuspid isthmus–dependent counterclockwise flutter. The *dark red band* represents the amount of atrium activated over that 10-ms window. Conduction velocity in this case is relatively uniform around the tricuspid annulus. This system creates very high-density automated maps within 5 to 10 minutes with very high accuracy.

enhanced by improved spatial resolution that is better placed to delineate multiple wavefronts, regions of breakthrough, and critical isthmus, decreasing but not entirely eliminating the potential for misinterpretation of the circuit's critical aspects. Although high-density mapping systems have been validated in both animal[55] and human hearts[56] for rapid, accurate atrial mapping and evaluation of conduction block, prior to ablation, all putative flutter circuits should be corroborated by standard entrainment techniques.

Conclusions

The field of mapping and ablation of typical and atypical flutter circuits has advanced to the point where the vast majority can be successfully treated with catheter ablation. The principles are to use a combination of multipolar activation, entrainment, and 3D electroanatomical mapping as complementary approaches to identify the critical narrow isthmus where catheter ablation will eliminate the circuit.

REFERENCES

1. Naccarelli GV, Varker H, Lin J, et al. Increasing prevalence of atrial fibrillation and flutter in the United States. *Am J Cardiol.* 2009;104:1534–1539.
2. Waldo AL, Feld GK. Inter-relationships of atrial fibrillation and atrial flutter mechanisms and clinical implications. *J Am Coll Cardiol.* 2008;51:779–786.
3. Medi C, Teh AW, Roberts-Thomson K, et al. Right atrial remodeling is more advanced in patients with atrial flutter than with atrial fibrillation. *J Cardiovasc Electrophysiol.* 2012;23:1067–1072.
4. Stiles MK, Wong CX, John B, et al. Characterization of atrial remodeling studied remote from episodes of typical atrial flutter. *Am J Cardiol.* 2010;106:528–534.
5. Mittal S, Pokushalov E, Romanov A, et al. Long-term ECG monitoring using an implantable loop recorder for the detection of atrial fibrillation after cavotricuspid isthmus ablation in patients with atrial flutter. *Heart Rhythm.* 2013;10:1598–1604.
6. Voight J, Akkaya M, Somasundaram P, et al. Risk of new-onset atrial fibrillation and stroke after radiofrequency ablation of isolated, typical atrial flutter. *Heart Rhythm.* 2014;11:1884–1889.
7. Seara JG, Roubin SR, Gude Sampedro F, et al. Risk of atrial fibrillation, stroke, and death after radiofrequency catheter ablation of typical atrial flutter. *Clin Res Cardiol.* 2014;103:543–552.
8. Chen K, Bai R, Deng W, et al. HATCH score in the prediction of new-onset atrial fibrillation after catheter ablation of typical atrial flutter. *Heart Rhythm.* 2015;12:1483–1489.
9. Joza J, Filion KB, Eberg M, et al. Prognostic value of atrial fibrillation inducibility after right atrial flutter ablation. *Heart Rhythm.* 2014;11:1870–1876.
10. Schneider R, Lauschke J, Tischer T, et al. Pulmonary vein triggers play an important role in the initiation of atrial flutter: initial results from the prospective randomized Atrial Fibrillation Ablation in Atrial Flutter (Triple A) trial. *Heart Rhythm.* 2015;12:865–871.
11. Steinberg JS, Romanov A, Musat D, et al. Prophylactic pulmonary vein isolation during isthmus ablation for atrial flutter: the PReVENT AF Study I. *Heart Rhythm.* 2014;11:1567–1572.
12. Mohanty S, Natale A, Mohanty P, et al. Pulmonary vein isolation to reduce future risk of atrial fibrillation in patients undergoing typical flutter ablation: results from a randomized pilot study (REDUCE AF). *J Cardiovasc Electrophysiol.* 2015;26:819–825.
13. Roberts JD, Hsu JC, Aouizerat BE, et al. Impact of a 4q25 genetic variant in atrial flutter and on the risk of atrial fibrillation after cavotricuspid isthmus ablation. *J Cardiovasc Electrophysiol.* 2014;25:271–277.
14. Teh AW, Kalman JM. Electrophysiological evaluation of atrial tachycardia and atrial flutter. In: Saksena S, Camm AJ, eds. *Electrophysiological Disorders of the Heart.* 2nd ed. Philadelphia: Saunders; 2012:345–355.
15. Santucci PA, Varma N, Cytron J, et al. Electroanatomic mapping of postpacing intervals clarifies the complete active circuit and variants in atrial flutter. *Heart Rhythm.* 2009;6:1586–1595.
16. Medi C, Kalman JM. Prediction of the atrial flutter circuit location from the surface electrocardiogram. *Europace.* 2008;10:786–796.
17. Kaiser DW, Hsia HH, Dubin AM, et al. The precise timing of tachycardia entrainment is determined by the post-pacing interval, the tachycardia cycle length, and the pacing rate: theoretical insights and practical applications. *Heart Rhythm.* 2016;13:695–703.
18. Maruyama M, Yamamoto T, Abe J, et al. Number needed to entrain: a new criterion for entrainment mapping in patients with intra-atrial reentrant tachycardia. *Circ Arrhythm Electrophysiol.* 2014;7:490–496.
19. Zhang S, Younis G, Hariharan R, et al. Lower loop reentry as a mechanism of clockwise right atrial flutter. *Circulation.* 2004;109:1630–1635.
20. Allamsetty S, Chang SL, Lin YJ, et al. Intra-isthmus reentry flutter localizing at pouch of cavotricuspid isthmus. *J Cardiovasc Electrophysiol.* 2015;26:1383–1384.
21. Yang Y, Mangat I, Glatter KA, et al. Mechanism of conversion of atypical right atrial flutter to atrial fibrillation. *Am J Cardiol.* 2003;91:46–52.
22. Tomson TT, Kapa S, Bala R, et al. Risk of stroke and atrial fibrillation after radiofrequency catheter ablation of typical atrial flutter. *Heart Rhythm.* 2012;9:1779–1784.
23. Da Costa A, Thevenin J, Roche F, et al. Results from the Loire-Ardeche-Drome-Isere-Puy-de-Dome (LADIP) trial on atrial flutter, a multicentric prospective randomized study comparing amiodarone and radiofrequency ablation after the first episode of symptomatic atrial flutter. *Circulation.* 2006;114:1676–1681.
24. Clementy N, Desprets L, Pierre B, et al. Outcomes after ablation for typical atrial flutter (from the Loire Valley Atrial Fibrillation Project). *Am J Cardiol.* 2014;114:1361–1367.
25. Iwasawa J, Miyazaki S, Takagi T, et al. Cavotricuspid isthmus ablation using a catheter equipped with mini electrodes on the 8 mm tip: a prospective comparison with an 8 mm dumbbell-shaped tip catheter and 8 mm tip cryothermal catheter. *Europace.* 2016;18:868–872.
26. Schoene K, Rolf S, Schloma D, et al. Ablation of typical atrial flutter using a non-fluoroscopic catheter tracking system vs. conventional fluoroscopy—results from a prospective randomized study. *Europace.* 2015;17:1117–1121.
27. Muser D, Magnani S, Santangeli P. Ablation of typical atrial flutter using the novel MediGuide 3D catheter tracking system: a review of the literature. *Expert Rev Cardiovasc Ther.* 2014;12:799–802.
28. Dewland TA, Glidden DV, Marcus GM. Healthcare utilization and clinical outcomes after catheter ablation of atrial flutter. *PLoS One.* 2014;9:e100509.
29. Kumar S, Morton JB, Lee G, et al. High incidence of low catheter-tissue contact force at the cavotricuspid isthmus during catheter ablation of atrial flutter: implications for achieving isthmus block. *J Cardiovasc Electrophysiol.* 2015;26:826–831.
30. Jones MA, Webster D, Wong KC, et al. The benefit of tissue contact monitoring with an electrical coupling index during ablation of typical atrial flutter—a prospective randomised control trial. *J Interv Card Electrophysiol.* 2014;41:237–244.
31. Asirvatham SJ. Correlative anatomy and electrophysiology for the interventional electrophysiologist: right atrial flutter. *J Cardiovasc Electrophysiol.* 2009;20:113–122.
32. Piorkowski C, Grothoff M, Gaspar T, et al. Cavotricuspid isthmus ablation guided by real-time magnetic resonance imaging. *Circ Arrhythm Electrophysiol.* 2013;6:e7–e10.
33. Pambrun T, Roig J, Bouzeman A, et al. Modification of the unipolar atrial electrogram as a local endpoint during common atrial flutter ablation. *J Cardiovasc Electrophysiol.* 2015;26:1196–1203.
34. Hilbert S, Sommer P, Gutberlet M, et al. Real-time magnetic resonance-guided ablation of typical right atrial flutter using a combination of active catheter tracking and passive catheter visualization in man: initial results from a consecutive patient series. *Europace.* 2016;18:572–577.
35. Morales GX, Macle L, Khairy P, et al. Adenosine testing in atrial flutter ablation: unmasking of dormant conduction across the cavotricuspid isthmus and risk of recurrence. *J Cardiovasc Electrophysiol.* 2013;24:995–1001.
36. Perez FJ, Schubert CM, Parvez B, et al. Long-term outcomes after catheter ablation of cavo-tricuspid isthmus dependent atrial flutter: a meta-analysis. *Circ Arrhythm Electrophysiol.* 2009;2:393–401.
37. Huo Y, Schoenbauer R, Richter S, et al. Atrial arrhythmias following surgical AF ablation: electrophysiological findings, ablation strategies, and clinical outcome. *J Cardiovasc Electrophysiol.* 2014;25:725–738.
38. Scaglione M, Caponi D, Ebrille E, et al. Very long-term results of electroanatomic-guided radiofrequency ablation of atrial arrhythmias in patients with surgically corrected atrial septal defect. *Europace.* 2014;16:1800–1807.
39. Mikhaylov EN, Mitrofanova LB, Vander MA, et al. Biatrial tachycardia following linear anterior wall ablation for the perimitral reentry: incidence and electrophysiological evaluations. *J Cardiovasc Electrophysiol.* 2015;26:28–35.
40. Barbhaiya CR, Kumar S, Ng J, et al. Overdrive pacing from downstream sites on multielectrode catheters to rapidly detect fusion and to diagnose macroreentrant atrial arrhythmias. *Circulation.* 2014;129:2503–2510.
41. Nakagawa H, Shah N, Matsudaira K, et al. Characterization of reentrant circuit in macroreentrant right atrial tachycardia after surgical repair of congenital heart disease: isolated channels between scars allow "focal" ablation. *Circulation.* 2001;103:699–709.
42. Stevenson IH, Kistler PM, Spence SJ, et al. Scar-related right atrial macroreentrant tachycardia in patients without prior atrial surgery: electroanatomic characterization and ablation outcome. *Heart Rhythm.* 2005;2:594–601.
43. Tai CT, Huang JL, Lin YK, et al. Noncontact three-dimensional mapping and ablation of upper loop re-entry originating in the right atrium. *J Am Coll Cardiol.* 2002;40:746–753.
44. Fukamizu S, Sakurada H, Hayashi T, et al. Macroreentrant atrial tachycardia in patients without previous atrial surgery or catheter ablation: clinical and electrophysiological characteristics of scar-related left atrial anterior wall reentry. *J Cardiovasc Electrophysiol.* 2013;24:404–412.
45. Wieczorek M, Hoeltgen R. Right atrial tachycardias related to regions of low-voltage myocardium in patients without prior cardiac surgery: catheter ablation and follow-up results. *Europace.* 2013;15:1642–1650.
46. Bisbal F, Andreu D, Berruezo A. Simplified mapping and ablation of a scar-related atrial tachycardia using magnetic resonance imaging tissue characterization. *Europace.* 2015;17:186.
47. Berruezo A, Bisbal F, Fernandez-Armenta J, et al. Transthoracic epicardial ablation of mitral isthmus for treatment of recurrent perimitral flutter. *Heart Rhythm.* 2014;11:26–33.
48. Wasmer K, Kobe J, Dechering DG, et al. Isthmus-dependent right atrial flutter as the leading cause of atrial tachycardias after surgical atrial septal defect repair. *Int J Cardiol.* 2013;168:2447–2452.
49. Coffey JO, d'Avila A, Dukkipati S, et al. Catheter ablation of scar-related atypical atrial flutter. *Europace.* 2013;15:414–419.
50. Bowers RW, Yue AM. Careful observation of changes in the cycle length in the evaluation of atrial tachycardia mechanism. *J Cardiovasc Electrophysiol.* 2015;26:1385–1387.
51. Anguera I, Dallaglio P, Macias R, et al. Long-term outcome after ablation of right atrial tachyarrhythmias after the surgical repair of congenital and acquired heart disease. *Am J Cardiol.* 2015;115:1705–1713.
52. Wazni OM, Saliba W, Fahmy T, et al. Atrial arrhythmias after surgical maze: findings during catheter ablation. *J Am Coll Cardiol.* 2006;48:1405–1409.
53. Nof E, Stevenson WG, Epstein LM, et al. Catheter ablation of atrial arrhythmias after cardiac transplantation: findings at EP study utility of 3-D mapping and outcomes. *J Cardiovasc Electrophysiol.* 2013;24:498–502.
54. Bollmann A, Hilbert S, John S, et al. Initial experience with ultra high-density mapping of human right atria. *J Cardiovasc Electrophysiol.* 2016;27:154–160.
55. Nakagawa H, Ikeda A, Sharma T, et al. Rapid high resolution electroanatomical mapping: evaluation of a new system in a canine atrial linear lesion model. *Circ Arrhythm Electrophysiol.* 2012;5:417–424.
56. Anter E, Tschabrunn CM, Contreras-Valdes FM, et al. Pulmonary vein isolation using the Rhythmia mapping system: verification of intracardiac signals using the Orion mini-basket catheter. *Heart Rhythm.* 2015;12:1927–1934.

76 Atrial Fibrillation: Mechanisms, Clinical Features, and Management

Saurabh Kumar and Gregory F. Michaud

Atrial fibrillation (AF) is responsible for significant impairment in quality of life, can result in thromboembolism, and contributes to substantial morbidity and health care expenditure. AF is the most common arrhythmia in humans and, as such, is heterogeneous in its mechanism, presentation, and clinical course and therefore requires individualized treatment. This chapter will discuss the epidemiology, nomenclature, current mechanistic insights, and contemporary treatment strategies for the management of AF.

Epidemiology

AF is a health problem of epidemic proportions, with a projected prevalence of 5.6 million by 2050 in the United States alone.[1] Population studies have shown that AF confers a significant impairment in quality of life, with a four- to five-fold increase in the risk of stroke, a doubling of the risk of dementia, a tripling of the risk of heart failure, and a 40% to 90% increased risk of mortality.[2] AF is an age-dependent disease, and its prevalence doubles with each decade above the age of 55, independently of known preexisting conditions. Its prevalence is 0.1% in those under 55 years of age but increases to 9.0% for those aged above 80 years.[3] The lifetime risk of developing AF is ~25% in those who have reached the age of 40.[4] Men are more frequently affected than women. Moreover, AF is acknowledged to be a costly public health problem at a global level, with hospitalization as the primary cost driver.[5] Annual health care expenditures resulting from AF were over $7 billion in 2001.[6] Unsurprisingly, costs are strongly influenced by the number of arrhythmia recurrences, with one to two recurrences of paroxysmal AF, for example, costing $6331 and more than three recurrences costing $10,312.[7] In response to the rising "tide" of AF and related hospitalizations, there has been an exponential increase in the number of AF ablations being performed (Fig. 76.1).[8]

Classification

Following initial presentation, AF can be categorized according to the 2014 American Heart Association (AHA)/American College of Cardiology (ACC)/Heart Rhythm Society (HRS) guidelines on AF management[9]:

- *Paroxysmal AF*: episodes that terminate spontaneously or with intervention within 7 days of onset

- *Persistent AF*: episodes that fail to self-terminate within 7 days and often require pharmacological or electrical cardioversion to restore sinus rhythm
- *Longstanding persistent AF*: persistent AF that has lasted longer than 12 months
- *Permanent AF*: a term used to identify individuals with persistent AF for whom a combined decision has been made by the patient and clinician to no longer pursue a rhythm control strategy

The above definitions apply to recurrent episodes of AF that last longer than 30 seconds. The term "lone AF" refers to patients with paroxysmal, persistent, or permanent AF who have no structural heart disease, but emerging consensus is that this term does not enrich either the understanding of the mechanism or patient management.[10] Finally, it is apparent that these terms are not mutually exclusive and are insufficient to describe the complexity of the clinical spectrum of AF.

Pathophysiology

A detailed discussion on AF mechanisms and the role of autonomic and genetic factors in AF is presented in detail in earlier chapters (see Part VII); a brief overview is provided here as it is of particular relevance to AF management.

The wide range of clinical presentation of AF is fundamentally governed by the variable extent of interaction between AF triggers (or drivers) and the necessary "substrate" created by electrophysiologically and structurally remodeled atrial tissue capable of supporting and maintaining AF.[11] Haissaguerre and colleagues in 1998 made the observation that spontaneous initiation of AF occurred by focal ectopy originating within the pulmonary veins.[12] Such pulmonary vein "triggers" are thought to be primarily responsible for paroxysmal AF episodes, and pulmonary vein isolation has since become the cornerstone of contemporary AF ablation strategies.

In contrast to the proposed mechanism of paroxysmal AF, there is much debate and controversy on the mechanism of persistent and permanent AF, specifically related to factors that promote its sustenance. The conventional paradigm is that persistent and permanent forms of AF are associated with atrial electrical and structural remodeling predicated by underlying atrial fibrosis and maintained by spatially disorganized mechanisms.[11,13] More recently, however, Narayan and colleagues have reported that persistent and permanent AF may be maintained by highly localized drivers or organized sources of reentry.[14,15] These localized "rotors" and focal sources are not necessarily constrained to the pulmonary veins, may be biatrially distributed, and can be targeted with focal ablation in an attempt to improve outcomes.[15] In contrast, other investigators have failed to demonstrate the presence of stable reentrant foci during mapping of patients undergoing cardiac surgery.[16,17] Allesie and colleagues have shown that endo-epicardial electrical dissociation between the complex three-dimensional myocardial bundle architecture of the atria, rather than ectopic focal discharges, are responsible for the appearance of apparent "drivers."[16-19] Work from Waldo and colleagues suggests that persistent or long-standing persistent AF are maintained

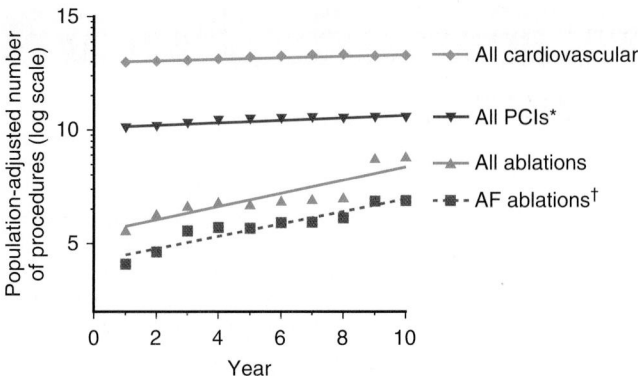

FIGURE 76.1 Population adjusted trends in cardiovascular procedures in Australia from 2000/2001 to 2009/2010. Fitted trend line showing the population-adjusted number of procedures over 10 years in Australia. Compared to percutaneous coronary interventions (*PCIs;**), atrial fibrillation (*AF*) ablations (†) and all-ablation procedures had a significantly higher growth rate (*p* < .001). (From Kumar S, Walters TE, Halloran K, et al. Ten-year trends in the use of catheter ablation for treatment of atrial fibrillation vs. the use of coronary intervention for the treatment of ischaemic heart disease in Australia. *Europace.* 2013;15:1702-1709.)

by continuous collision and merging of activation wavefronts that create the appearance of foci and breakthrough sites that demonstrate no evidence of reentry.[17] The lack of consensus may come in part because there is no single model of AF that accurately represents the marked heterogeneity of patients represented in these studies. Much further work is necessary to elucidate the mechanisms of AF, and it is likely that high-fidelity mapping tools are required to clarify the complex electrical activation patterns during AF.

A well-accepted concept is that atrial remodeling is necessary for AF perpetuation. Electrical and structural remodeling are fundamental components. Electrical remodeling constitutes reduction in atrial effective refractory periods, increased spatial heterogeneity of refractoriness, and conduction slowing. These changes are governed by shortening of the atrial action potential duration, changes in ion channel expression associated with atrial repolarization abnormalities, alteration in cellular coupling mediated by changes in connexin protein expression, changes in atrial conductivity, and the development of fibrosis.[11] Electrical remodeling, however, likely only contributes to short-term changes and can reverse quickly. It is thought that the presence of structural remodeling is fundamental to the stability and progression of AF to persistent and permanent forms. These changes can be self-perpetuating, hence the concept of "AF begets AF" as proposed by Wijfells and colleagues in their seminal study in awake instrumented goats.[20] An increase in AF duration can promote atrial dilatation, myocyte hypertrophy, sarcomere loss, glycogen accumulation, mitochondrial abnormalities, and the development of atrial fibrosis. Atrial fibrosis is thought to be a fundamental component of AF sustenance.[21]

Detailed electrophysiological and electroanatomical studies have documented that many disease processes known to be associated with AF contribute to atrial structural remodeling, including aging, sinus node dysfunction, conditions of chronic atrial stretch (e.g., atrial septal defects, mitral stenosis, heart failure, and forced ventricular pacing), systemic and pulmonary hypertension, obesity, and obstructive sleep apnea.[13,22] The common paradigm that emerges is that these conditions are associated with atrial remodeling manifesting as global and regional conduction slowing and the development of atrial fibrosis. More recently, there has been recognition of patients who have advanced fibrotic atrial cardiomyopathy even before

the advent of AF, proposing that this disease entity has a pathophysiological mechanism that may be distinct from the situation where the presence of AF itself promotes fibrosis. Such patients with "fibrotic atrial cardiomyopathy" possess a specific disease/syndrome that supplies substrates for AF, atrial tachycardia, sinus node disease, atrioventricular (AV) node disease, and thromboembolic complications.[23]

The autonomic nervous system also plays an important role in AF initiation and maintenance.[24] The pulmonary veins and the pulmonary vein–left atrial junction are richly innervated by autonomic nerves. A dynamic relationship between the parasympathetic and sympathetic nervous system plays a critical role in the initiation of AF from the pulmonary veins. AF onset can be preceded by altered autonomic activity or change in autonomic balance. Autonomic neural remodeling contributes to positive feedback loops that are thought to be essential for AF persistence and recurrence; remodeling of this sort may be a major reason AF maintains itself in the first few hours.[25] Simultaneous sympathovagal discharges may also contribute to the mechanism of AF associated with heart failure.[26]

There is also increasing appreciation of a large genetic contribution to AF. History of AF in a family member is associated with a 40% increased risk for AF.[27] The majority of monogenic causes of AF are attributed to a gain-of-channel function mutation in potassium channels or their subunits, with an expected shortening of atrial refractory periods. Variations in sodium channel subunits, gap junction proteins, and several developmentally related transcription factors also play an important role in the development of familial AF. Genome-wide association studies have identified several genetic loci containing single-nucleotide polymorphisms throughout the genome that are associated with AF.[28] These studies have yielded novel insights into mechanisms of AF in different populations and may ultimately provide novel therapeutic targets.

Clinical Features

The most common symptom of AF is palpitations. AF leads to loss of coordinated atrial contraction and can acutely cause a 5% to 15% drop in cardiac output, leading to symptoms of weakness, fatigue, lightheadedness, reduced exercise tolerance, or dyspnea. Rapid ventricular response to AF can reduce ventricular filling time, which is poorly tolerated in patients with reduced left ventricular compliance, such as the elderly, hypertensive patients with left ventricular hypertrophy, and those with hypertrophic cardiomyopathy or coronary disease. In such patients, AF can precipitate angina, flash pulmonary edema, or syncope. In the presence of rate-related bundle branch block, further ventricular dysfunction may be provoked via dyssynchrony of ventricular contraction. Heart rate irregularity can lead to deleterious hemodynamic effects.[29,30] If left uncontrolled, a persistently rapid heart rate can lead to tachycardia-induced cardiomyopathy.[30] Restoration of sinus rhythm or rate control will usually reverse the ventricular dysfunction.[31] Heart failure and AF often coexist, and one condition can lead to and/or precipitate the other. Restoration of sinus rhythm or adequate ventricular rate control can reverse tachycardia-induced cardiomyopathy and improve heart failure symptoms. In some patients, stroke or a thromboembolic event may be the first presentation of AF, which may be otherwise asymptomatic.[32] Indeed, a third of patients may remain asymptomatic, and the discovery of AF is incidental during a routine examination, even when the ventricular response is rapid.[33]

Key points to note when taking a patient history are the initial onset of symptoms of AF, the typical and longest episode duration, whether episodes require electrical or pharmacological conversion, the putative behavioral or physical triggers (e.g., excessive alcohol consumption), the severity of symptoms, and

BOX 76.1 Conditions commonly associated with and potentially reversible causes of atrial fibrillation

Conditions Commonly Associated With Atrial Fibrillation

Older age
Congestive heart failure
Hypertension
Obesity
Obstructive sleep apnea
Coronary artery disease
Valvular heart disease, particularly mitral valve stenosis and regurgitation
Hypertrophic cardiomyopathy
Congenital heart disease

Potentially Reversible Causes of Atrial Fibrillation

Pericarditis
Thyrotoxicosis
Alcohol intoxication
Stimulant drugs, such as pseudoephedrine
Supraventricular tachycardia, such as that associated with the presence of an accessory pathway
Infection
Obstructive sleep apnea

TABLE 76.1 Investigations and their focus in the assessment of a patient with atrial fibrillation (AF)

TYPE OF EXAMINATION OR INVESTIGATION	KEY POINTS OF FOCUS
History and physical examination	Identify hypertension, hyperthyroidism, congestive heart failure, valvular disease
Electrocardiogram	Measure resting ventricular response; identify associated cardiac conditions, such as left ventricular hypertrophy, prior myocardial infarction, sinus node dysfunction, QT prolongation, or presence of an accessory pathway
Exercise testing	Identify coronary artery disease, measure ventricular response to exertion
Ambulatory monitoring	Identify suspected AF if symptoms infrequent or sporadic; correlate symptoms to arrhythmia; calculate ambulatory ventricular response and AF burden
Echocardiogram	Identify valvular disease, left atrial size, ventricular function, associated left ventricular hypertrophy
Electrophysiology study	Identify triggers for atrial fibrillation such as supraventricular tachycardias or atrial tachycardias
Chemistries	Measure thyroid and renal function, ensure electrolytes (especially potassium and magnesium) are in the normal range

a search for reversible and irreversible underlying conditions associated with AF (Box 76.1), such as hyperthyroidism, alcoholism, or pericarditis. There is dramatic variability in the types and degrees of symptoms related to AF, yet a significant number of patients may have at least minor symptoms that are not easily described, such as fatigue or exercise intolerance. A physical examination should focus on contributing factors, such as the presence of valvular heart disease, obesity, and obstructive sleep apnea or on the impact of AF, such as heart failure.

Investigations

An outline of potential investigations is shown in Table 76.1. AF is readily detected on electrocardiography (ECG) as fibrillatory waves. More importantly, however, the ECG may give clues to etiology, such as left ventricular hypertrophy (hypertension), associated conditions such as conduction disease (bundle branch block, slow ventricular response in the absence of AV nodal blocking agents), or sinus node dysfunction and anticipated problems with drug therapy, such as QT interval prolongation (proarrhythmia risk).

Ambulatory monitoring can play a critical role in the diagnosis of AF, especially if events are sporadic or associated with thromboembolic events in the absence of documented AF. Monitoring may be continuous, symptom driven, or autotriggered. Such devices can be placed externally for extended periods, often 30 days. Internally placed miniature autotriggered monitors can allow prolonged monitoring (up to several years) and allow rapid wireless data transmissions. Since AF may be silent, autotriggered or continuous monitoring for several weeks may be necessary to detect arrhythmia paroxysms and calculate the burden of AF. In patients with cryptogenic stroke, implantable monitors detected AF in 12% of patients at a 1-year follow-up versus detection of AF in only 2% of patients with periodic monitoring.[32]

When AF is newly diagnosed, transthoracic echocardiography is necessary to look for valvular and structural heart disease, ventricular hypertrophy, and ventricular dysfunction and to evaluate left atrial size, which may indicate the degree of AF chronicity. Transesophageal echocardiography is also useful for exclusion of left atrial appendage (LAA) thrombi when the duration of AF is unknown and external cardioversion is planned.

To exclude coronary artery disease in association with AF, exercise testing (with or without imaging as indicated) should be considered. Although coronary artery disease rarely is a direct cause of AF, its presence limits suitability for class I antiarrhythmic drugs (AADs) (discussed later). Exercise testing may also be useful to evaluate the proarrhythmic potential of antiarrhythmic medications, assess heart rate control with exertion, and unmask a potential trigger for AF.

The role of formal electrophysiology study in AF is limited, and electrophysiology is usually performed in the context of catheter ablation. Nevertheless, in young patients it is useful to exclude supraventricular tachycardia, such as AV nodal reentry or AV reentry, which are identified during electrophysiology study in 4% to 10% of patients with AF referred for pulmonary vein isolation.[34] Ablation of supraventricular tachycardia without attempting pulmonary vein isolation may prevent AF recurrences in the majority of these patients. This, however, is uncommon, and the yield for supraventricular tachycardia as the main driver for recurrent AF is likely to be low in the general population and should only be reserved for when AF symptoms are recurrent and drug refractory and when catheter ablation is anticipated.

Treatment

Key issues in AF management are control of symptoms through rate or rhythm control using medications or catheter ablation, management of thromboembolism risk, and identification of associated conditions that can exacerbate AF. Furthermore, treatment can be divided into acute and long-term management. It is well appreciated that common disorders such as hypertension, obesity, obstructive sleep apnea, valvular or infiltrative heart disease, diabetes, thyroid disorders, drug use (smoking and alcohol), and acute illnesses (e.g., electrolyte abnormalities and infection) can trigger AF and worsen control. Risk factor management probably plays an underappreciated role in determining AF burden and severity as well as arrhythmia control. There is increasing recognition of this in the literature. Multiple risk factors probably have a cumulative effect on promoting substrate for AF.[13] Importantly, weight loss, improvement in cardiac fitness, and risk factor management in patients with AF have been demonstrated to meaningfully improve AF-free survival.[35–37] An integrated care model involving multiple health care members may be necessary to aggressively achieve targets for risk factor control.[13,22]

Treatment of Acute Atrial Fibrillation

Rate Control

The first treatment priority for an acute episode of AF is to control the ventricular response. This may not be an issue if the patient is already on AV nodal blocking drugs or has concurrent AV nodal disease. AV nodal blocking agents may be intravenously or orally administered, unless compromised hemodynamics mandate immediate direct current cardioversion to restore sinus rhythm. If AF exists in the presence of ventricular preexcitation via a rapidly conducting accessory pathway, AV nodal blocking agents should be avoided, and ibutilide or procainamide are suggested to block conduction over the accessory pathway. This is because pure AV nodal blocking agents have little direct effect on the accessory pathway conduction and may paradoxically accelerate conduction over the pathway.

Acute Anticoagulation

For patients in whom cardioversion is being considered for AF lasting longer than 48 hours, anticoagulation is necessary due to a high risk of thromboembolic events (mainly stroke[38]). This risk is also significant for patients treated with warfarin for more than 3 weeks prior to cardioversion if the international normalized ratio (INR) is <2.5.[39] The risk of stroke is also high after conversion of atrial flutter by pharmacological cardioversion or ablation in the absence of appropriate anticoagulation. Patient history may be unreliable for symptom onset because symptomatic and asymptomatic AF episodes coexist. When uncertainty exists, it is wise to prescribe oral anticoagulation for a minimum of 4 weeks before attempting cardioversion. Alternatively, transesophageal echocardiography can be used to exclude atrial thrombus prior to cardioversion.[40,41] It is critical to appreciate that full anticoagulation is required during and after cardioversion for 3 to 4 weeks due to the presence of atrial mechanical stunning, regardless of the type of arrhythmia (AF or atrial flutter) and the mode of termination (pharmacological or external cardioversion, catheter ablation).[41–43]

Rhythm Control

There are few data on the best treatment strategy for a first episode of persistent AF; however, it may be prudent to consider cardioversion if the duration of AF is unknown or is less than 1 year. New onset AF often spontaneously reverts to normal sinus rhythm, with the incidence of reversion related to the duration of the arrhythmia; patients with spontaneous reversion often have episodes that last less than 24 hours.[44] In some patients, AADs can be given prior to cardioversion to increase the chances of successful reversion and to prevent recurrence. Cardioversion may be attempted via pharmacological or electrical methods; however, the latter has a higher success rate.

Acute reversion with pharmacological agents is most successful if the AF has persisted for a short duration. Commonly recommended drugs are flecainide, dofetilide, propafenone, or intravenous ibutilide, provided there are no contraindications to their use.[9] Dofetilide and ibutilide should be administered under medical supervision given the potential for excessive QT prolongation and torsades de pointes. Amiodarone may be beneficial for use on an outpatient basis in patients with paroxysmal or persistent AF when rapid restoration of sinus rhythm is not

deemed necessary.[9] Outpatient use of propafenone or flecainide (as a "pill-in-the-pocket" approach) in addition to a β-blocker or nondihydropyridine calcium channel antagonist is also reasonable.[9] Ibutilide, a class III AAD that prolongs the QT interval, can be expected to convert approximately 60% of patients, with a mean AF duration of 21 days compared to 18% converted with procainamide.[45]

It is important to note that AF recurrence after cardioversion can be high; in one study, after a single cardioversion, only 23% of patients maintained sinus rhythm after 1 year and only 16% after 2 years.[46] When antiarrhythmic therapy is administered after cardioversion, AF recurrence after 1 year for any form of AF was 67% for sotalol and 65% for quinidine plus verapamil versus 83% for placebo.[47] One must be cognizant of the modest rates of AF recurrence after cardioversion against potential hazards of AADs, such as proarrhythmia and poor tolerance. AF recurrence is higher in the first few weeks after cardioversion due to atrial electrical remodeling, and one study found that 6 months versus 4 weeks of flecainide prevented midterm AF recurrences to a greater extent.[48]

Long-Term Management of Atrial Fibrillation

Recurrence of AF is common; hence long-term strategies for management are necessary. In patients presenting with paroxysmal AF and no associated comorbidities or heart disease, 60% of patients will not have a recurrence over the next 5 years.[49] In a systematic review on the progression of paroxysmal AF to persistent or permanent forms, studies reported an incidence of 10% to 20% at 1 year and 50% to 77% after 12 years.[50] Progression is seen more frequently in older patients and in those with cardiac disease.[51] In these patients, early treatment may help to prevent progression of AF to persistent forms if rhythm control strategies are warranted. Although guidelines are available based on large randomized trials, treatment strategies need to be individualized and involve the patient's input to be effective. Furthermore, data are lacking concerning the best treatment strategy in the era of catheter ablation. The discussion will focus on strategies for rate and rhythm control in addition to strategies for long-term anticoagulation.

Rate Control

Rate control is critical for long-term AF management, as poor rate control can lead to congestive heart failure.[31] Based on the RACE 2 study, the 2014 ACC/AHA/ESC guidelines for AF management suggest that a target resting heart rate goal of less than 80 beats/min is reasonable to control symptoms in symptomatic patients, but that lenient rate control (<110 beats/min) may be adequate in asymptomatic patients with stable left ventricular ejection fraction (left ventricular ejection fraction >0.4).[9] In symptomatic patients where the symptoms can be directly attributed to poor rate control of AF, the adequacy of rate control should be assessed during exertion to allow adjustment of pharmacological dosing to control ventricular rate within the physiological range.

Rate control is best achieved with a β-blocker or nondihydropyridine calcium channel antagonist. Common drugs used for rate control are shown in Table 76.2. A prospective randomized study of five different rate control regimens demonstrated that combination of a β-blocker and digoxin was most effective for ventricular rate control during daily activities.[52] β-Blockers are particularly useful for rate control in situations with high adrenergic tone and in the presence of myocardial ischemia. Diltiazem and verapamil have the potential for myocardial depression and hence are best avoided in patients with systolic heart failure. Digoxin is useful when a β-blocker or nondihydropyridine calcium blocker alone fails to control heart rate adequately. The main limitation of digoxin is that its effects are easily overdriven by sympathetic

TABLE 76.2 Commonly used medications for the rate control of atrial fibrillation

	INTRAVENOUS ADMINISTRATION	USUAL ORAL MAINTENANCE DOSE
β-Blockers		
Metoprolol tartrate	2.5–5 mg bolus over 2 min; up to three doses	25–100 mg twice daily
Metoprolol XL (succinate)	N/A	50–400 mg once daily
Atenolol	N/A	25–100 mg once daily
Esmolol	500 µg/kg bolus over 1 min then 50–300 µg/kg/min	N/A
Propranolol	1 mg over 1 min, up to 3 doses at 2-min intervals	10–40 mg three times a day, or four times a day
Nadolol	N/A	10–240 mg once daily
Carvedilol	N/A	3.125–25 mg twice daily
Bisoprolol	N/A	2.5-10 mg once daily
Nondihydropyridine Calcium Channel Antagonists		
Verapamil	0.075–0.15 mg/kg bolus over 2 min; may give additional 10 mg after 30 min if no response, then 0.005 mg/kg/min infusion	180–480 mg once daily (extended release)
Diltiazem	0.25 mg/kg bolus over 2 min, then 5–15 mg/h	120–360 mg once daily (extended release)
Digitalis Glycosides		
Digoxin	0.25 mg with repeat dosing with a maximum of 1.5 mg over 24 h	0.125–0.25 mg once daily
Others		
Amiodarone	300 mg over 1 h, then 10–50 mg/h over 24 h	100–200 mg once daily

N/A, not applicable.
Modified from January CT, Wann LS, Alpert JS, et al. 2014 AHA/ACC/HRS guideline for the management of patients with atrial fibrillation: a report of the American College of Cardiology/American Heart Association Task Force on Practice Guidelines and the Heart Rhythm Society. *J Am Coll Cardiol.* 2014;64:e1-76.

stimulation; hence the drug does little to control excessive tachycardia related to exercise. Recent studies have found an increased risk of mortality with digoxin used for rate control, which needs to be confirmed by prospective trials.[52a,52b] None of these drugs is particularly effective in preventing recurrent AF except in the context of thyrotoxicosis or exercise-induced AF where β-blockers can be effective. Oral dosing for rate control is usually sufficient, except in the acute setting where it may be intravenously administered in the absence of preexcitation. Acute cardioversion may be best form of rate control in a true emergency where a patient is hemodynamically decompensated. Intravenous amiodarone may be useful for rate control in critically ill patients without evidence for preexcitation, particularly if AF keeps recurring after electrical cardioversion. Lastly, AV nodal ablation with permanent ventricular pacing forms a reasonable strategy for rate control when pharmacological therapy is inadequate and rhythm control is not achievable.[53] However, right ventricular pacing can induce ventricular dyssynchrony and create or aggravate ventricular dysfunction, leading to heart failure symptoms. In a randomized study, patients with medically refractory AF who underwent AV nodal ablation and who were assigned biventricular pacing versus right ventricular pacing had preservation of ventricular function, whereas it was reduced in the right ventricular pacing group.[54] A recent meta-analysis evaluating the outcomes of biventricular versus right ventricular pacing after AV nodal ablation reported increased left ventricular ejection fraction and improved symptoms with biventricular pacing among patients with a depressed ventricular function.[55] Direct His bundle pacing may also be a superior mode of pacing after AV node ablation.[56] Rhythm control, however, with pulmonary vein isolation may be superior to AV node ablation with biventricular pacing in some patients, such as those with heart failure.[57,58]

It is important to note that on an individual basis, however, heart rate control can be challenging and needs to be considered as part of both rate and rhythm control strategies because no rhythm control strategy to date has been completely successful in eliminating recurrent episodes of AF. Often the limiting factor with rate control is the presence of concurrent sinus node dysfunction and symptomatic sinus bradycardia, which may prevent adequate doses of AV nodal blocking agents from controlling rapid rates during AF. Atrial pacing can be used as concomitant therapy when drug therapy alone is not tolerated.

Rhythm Control

A number of studies have evaluated the relative benefit of rate versus rhythm control to treat recurrent AF.[59–63] Uniformly, no differences in major endpoints could be found in any of these studies, including serious endpoints such as stroke and all-cause mortality in a meta-analysis of all the major trials.[64] This held true even in patients with left ventricular dysfunction, heart failure, and AF where a rhythm control strategy did not appear to confer a benefit compared with rate control.[65,66] A recent exploratory subanalysis within a meta-analysis found that patients younger than 65 years demonstrated an advantage of rhythm control over rate control in the prevention of all-cause mortality, but this needs to be studied further.[67] In a large population-based study, crude mortality rates were similar in the rate versus rhythm control groups; however, in patients surviving more than 5 years, mortality was lower in the rhythm control group.[68] The benefits of rate versus rhythm control with percutaneous catheter ablation in specific populations such as the young, highly symptomatic; those with drug intolerance; or those with heart failure have not been examined appropriately. In these instances, treatment should remain highly patient focused.

The choice of rate versus rhythm control therapy should be individualized with flexibility in modifying the strategy according to the clinical situation. Rate control in patients older than 65 years appears safe and appropriate as an initial therapy; however, in patients with ongoing symptoms, a rhythm control strategy should be considered, being cognizant of the fact that symptoms can be subtle in the form of fatigue or exercise intolerance. For younger patients, it may well be that sinus rhythm has distinct advantages over rhythm control in the absence of any clear randomized data. Whether a rhythm control strategy by catheter ablation will be associated with a survival benefit remains to be determined in large-scale, prospective randomized studies with long-term follow-up and is currently being investigated in an ongoing multicenter, randomized clinical trial.[69]

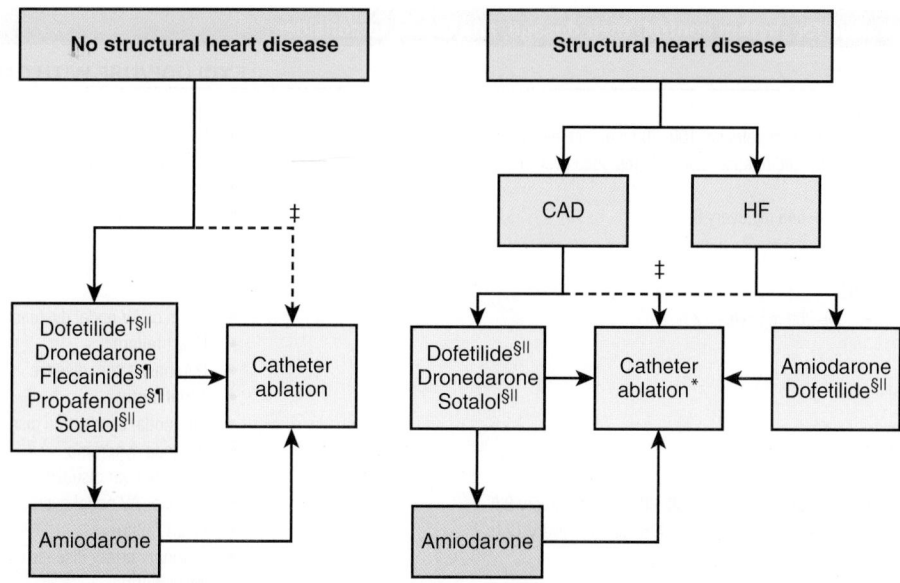

FIGURE 76.2 Strategies for rhythm control in patients with paroxysmal and persistent atrial fibrillation.

*Catheter ablation is only recommended as first-line therapy for patients with paroxysmal atrial fibrillation (class IIa recommendation).

†Drugs are listed alphabetically.

‡Depending on patient preference when performed in experienced centers.

§Not recommended with severe left ventricular hypertrophy (wall thickness >1.5 cm).

∥Should be used with caution in patients at risk for torsades de pointes ventricular tachycardia.

¶Should be combined with atrioventricular nodal blocking agents.

CAD, Coronary artery disease; *HF*, heart failure. (From January CT, Wann LS, Alpert JS, et al. 2014 AHA/ACC/HRS guideline for the management of patients with atrial fibrillation: a report of the American College of Cardiology/American Heart Association Task Force on Practice Guidelines and the Heart Rhythm Society. *J Am Coll Cardiol.* 2014;64:e1-76.)

Antiarrhythmic Drugs for Rhythm Control

AADs should be tailored to the specific disease states (Fig. 76.2). Common drugs used for rhythm control, their doses, and issues to consider are shown in Table 76.3. The incidence of AF recurrence at 1 year after electrical cardioversion is very high (71%–84%).[70] AADs are only modestly effective in maintaining sinus rhythm; a recent meta-analysis has found that several class IA, IC, and III drugs reduced the risk of AF recurrence by 19% to 70% compared with placebo, rate control drugs, or no treatment.[70] For the majority of patients, it is unrealistic to expect complete elimination of all AF episodes, and the treatment goal should instead be a marked reduction in the frequency and duration of AF episodes, with an acceptable side effect profile compatible with an overall improvement in quality of life.[71] The majority of AADs have extracardiac and cardiac side effects, and safety rather than efficacy primarily should guide choice. In the presence of significant sinus node or AV conduction disease, cardiac pacing should be considered before using drugs as a part of a rhythm or rate control strategy. AADs may play a critical role in maintaining sinus rhythm in patients who have tachycardia-induced cardiomyopathy, especially when rate control is problematic.[9]

AADs are broadly grouped according to the Vaughan Williams classification. The most commonly used drugs are: (1) class IA drugs that have mixed sodium and potassium blocking properties (procainamide, quinidine, and disopyramide); (2) class IC drugs, predominantly sodium channel blockers (flecainide and propafenone); and (3) class III drugs that prolong the QT interval predominantly by potassium channel blockade (sotalol, amiodarone, dofetilide, and dronedarone).

Class IA drugs have limited efficacy and potentially significant adverse effects. As such, their use for AF has been largely abandoned, except in patients with hypertrophic obstructive cardiomyopathy where they can reduce outflow tract obstruction[72] or in AF provoked by hypervagotonia.[73]

Class IC drugs, such as flecainide and propafenone, are sodium channel blockers and significantly increase the chances of maintaining sinus rhythm.[70] These drugs exhibit "use-dependence," which is characterized by slow binding and unbinding kinetics that translates to progressive conduction-slowing effects at faster heart rates. This manifests in the form of QRS widening during tachycardia. In the presence of structural heart disease, especially coronary artery disease and prior myocardial infarction, class IC drugs are proarrhythmic and should not be used.[74] Class IC drugs are recommended for use only in patients with normal ventricular function and intact His–Purkinje conduction. Another potential proarrhythmic property is their ability to convert AF to atrial flutter with 1:1 AV conduction, resulting in rapid wide complex tachycardia due to use-dependent QRS widening. It is thus recommended that a concomitant AV nodal blocker be used to prevent this complication. Therefore class IC AADs are often the initial choice in patients with preserved left ventricular function, no ischemia, and no significant left ventricular hypertrophy, and they can be administered daily to prevent AF or as needed in patients with infrequent, reasonably well-tolerated, and longer episodes of AF to shorten the duration of the arrhythmia ("pill in the pocket" approach).

Class III drugs including sotalol and dofetilide have efficacy similar to flecainide and propafenone, albeit with the additional benefits of safety in patients with coronary artery disease and lack of increase in mortality in heart failure (in the case of dofetilide).[75] However, class III drugs prolong the QT interval and predispose to torsades de pointes. For this reason, initiation is usually in the hospital setting. Patients at highest risk for proarrhythmia are

TABLE 76.3	Drugs used for rhythm control, their dosage, and issues to consider	
DRUG	**DOSE**	**EXCLUDE/USE WITH CAUTION**
Vaughan Williams Class IA		
Disopyramide	• Immediate release: 100–200 mg once every 6 h • Extended release: 200–400 mg once every 12 h	• Heart failure • QT prolongation • Prostatism, glaucoma
Quinidine	• 324–648 mg every 8 h	• QT prolongation • Diarrhea
Vaughan Williams Class IC		
Flecainide	• 50–200 mg every 12 h	• Sinus or AV nodal dysfunction • Heart failure • Coronary artery disease • Atrial flutter • Infranodal conduction disease • Brugada syndrome • Renal or liver disease
Propafenone	• Immediate release: 150–300 mg once every 8 h • Extended release: 225–425 mg once every 12 h	• Sinus or AV nodal dysfunction • Heart failure • Coronary artery disease • Atrial flutter • Infranodal conduction disease • Brugada syndrome • Liver disease • Asthma
Vaughan Williams Class III		
Amiodarone	• Oral: 400–600 mg daily in divided doses for 2–4 wk; maintenance typically 100–200 mg once daily • IV: 150 mg over 10 min; then 1 mg/min for 6 h; then 0.5 mg/min for 18 h or change to oral dosing; after 24 h, consider decreasing dose to 0.25 mg/min	• Sinus or AV node dysfunction • Infranodal conduction disease • Lung disease • Prolonged QT interval
Dofetilide	• 125–500 µg once every 12 h	• Prolonged QT interval • Renal disease • Hypokalemia • Hypomagnesemia • Diuretic therapy • Avoid other QT interval–prolonging drugs
Dronedarone	• 400 mg once every 12 h	• Bradycardia • Heart failure • Long-standing persistent atrial fibrillation/flutter • Liver disease • Prolonged QT interval
Sotalol	• 40–160 mg once every 12 h	• Prolonged QT interval • Renal disease • Hypokalemia • Hypomagnesemia • Diuretic therapy • Avoid other QT interval–prolonging drugs • Sinus or AV nodal dysfunction • Heart failure • Asthma

AV, atrioventricular.
Modified from January CT, Wann LS, Alpert JS, et al. 2014 AHA/ACC/HRS guideline for the management of patients with atrial fibrillation: a report of the American College of Cardiology/American Heart Association Task Force on Practice Guidelines and the Heart Rhythm Society. *J Am Coll Cardiol*. 2014;64:e1-76.

women and patients with marked left ventricular hypertrophy, QT prolongation at baseline, severe bradycardia, renal dysfunction, hypokalemia, and hypomagnesemia.[76] As previously mentioned, ibutilide, another class III agent, is useful in intravenous form for acute conversion of AF and atrial flutter. Although the efficacy of ibutilide for the acute conversion of AF is limited (40%–70%), atrial flutter responds more frequently[77,78] and ibutilide is thus very useful in facilitating external cardioversion for atrial flutter.[79]

The most effective drug for the prevention of AF episodes is amiodarone, which is a class III drug. Amiodarone has emerged as the most effective drug for preventing recurrent AF[70] in analyses of pooled data on AADs and is superior to propafenone and sotalol for preventing AF recurrence.[65] Amiodarone has activity on multiple ion channels (beyond the action anticipated by a class III drug). Although it can cause significant QT prolongation, the risk of torsades de pointes is lower than that with dofetilide and sotalol. Amiodarone has the distinct advantage of safety in patients with structural heart disease including coronary artery disease.[80] The main problem with amiodarone is its potential for multiple end-organ toxic side effects that limit its utility in many patients with AF. Specifically, monitoring of liver, thyroid, and lung function is necessary. Furthermore, it has the potential to worsen bradyarrhythmias and conduction disease.

Dronedarone is a drug that is similar to amiodarone in structure, except that it is devoid of an iodine moiety. Despite multichannel blocking properties, its efficacy is inferior to that of amiodarone for maintenance of sinus rhythm.[81] Additionally, unlike amiodarone, dronedarone is contraindicated in patients with severe heart failure and left ventricular systolic dysfunction, in whom treatment with dronedarone was associated with increased early mortality related to the worsening of heart failure.[82] Compared with placebo, dronedarone aids in the maintenance of sinus rhythm.[83] In permanent AF with pre-existing cardiovascular disease, there was an increase in mortality associated with the drug.[84] Dronedarone is recommended only in patients with nonpermanent AF and no structural heart disease.

Long-Term Management of Thromboembolic Risk

AF is associated with a fivefold increase in thromboembolic risk.[85] The proclivity to thromboembolic events can be attributed to left atrial mechanical dysfunction and stasis that promote LAA thrombus formation. Moreover, AF has been associated with an intrinsically hypercoagulable and proinflammatory state characterized by platelet and endothelial dysfunction and with increased expression of prothrombotic factors, such as thromboglobulin, and platelet factor 4, fibrinogen, and C-reactive protein levels.[86,87] Furthermore, there is evidence that AF-associated hypercoagulability may play an integral role in AF initiation and progression.[13] Hence anticoagulation may carry atrial electrical and structural protective effects to reduce AF burden in addition to preventing thromboembolic complications.

The management of AF-associated thromboembolic risk involves a complex evaluation of thromboembolic and bleeding risk interposed with selection of the most appropriate thromboembolic agent. Thromboembolic risk is present in patients with paroxysmal, persistent, or permanent AF and is determined by the presence of readily identifiable factors. Previously, an algorithm that incorporated a composite score, called the CHADS$_2$ score, estimated annual stroke risk on the basis of five clinical risk factors (1 point each except 2 points for stroke): heart failure, hypertension, age, diabetes, and previous stroke (Table 76.4).[88,89] Although readily applied in the clinical setting, low-risk patients in this scoring system still had an event rate of 1% to 2% per year, and 62% of patients fall within an intermediate risk category, where recommendations for oral anticoagulation therapy are more ambiguous.

This has been replaced by the revised CHA$_2$DS$_2$-VASc score[90] (see Table 76.4) that places age older than 74 years as a high risk factor (2 points) and recognizes additional risk factors of **V**ascular disease, **A**ge from 65 to 74 years, and **S**ex **c**ategory (female gender). Many patients considered low risk in the classical CHADS$_2$ system guidelines are considered intermediate or high risk in the CHA$_2$DS$_2$-VASc system. For instance, a 65-year-old female patient with paroxysmal AF and coronary artery disease would receive 0 points in the CHADS$_2$ scoring system but 3 points in the revised CHA$_2$DS$_2$-VASc system, which more accurately reflects her risk. For patients with nonvalvular AF and a CHA$_2$DS$_2$-VASc score of 0, it is reasonable to omit antithrombotic therapy. For patients with nonvalvular AF and a CHA$_2$DS$_2$-VASc score of 1, no antithrombotic therapy or treatment with an oral anticoagulant or aspirin may be considered. With prior stroke, TIA, or CHA$_2$DS$_2$-VASc score ≥2, oral anticoagulation is strongly recommended.[9]

In addition to assessment of thromboembolic risk, a patient's individualized bleeding risk can be evaluated through a number

TABLE 76.4 Definition for CHADS$_2$ and CHA$_2$DS$_2$-VASc scores and adjusted stroke rate

DEFINITION AND SCORES FOR CHADS$_2$ AND CHA$_2$DS$_2$-VASc		STROKE RISK STRATIFICATION WITH THE CHADS$_2$ AND CHA$_2$DS$_2$-VASc SCORES	
	SCORE	SCORE	ADJUSTED STROKE RATE (% PER YEAR)
CHADS$_2$		**CHADS$_2$**	
Congestive heart failure	1	0	1.9
Hypertension	1	1	2.8
Age ≥75 years	1	2	4
Diabetes mellitus	1	3	5.9
Stroke/TIA/TE	2	4	8.5
Maximum score	6	5	12.5
		6	18.2
CHA$_2$DS$_2$-VASc		**CHA$_2$DS$_2$-VASc**	
Congestive heart failure	1	0	0
Hypertension	1	1	1.3
Age ≥75 years	2	2	2.2
Diabetes mellitus	1	3	3.2
Stroke/TIA/TE	2	4	4
Vascular disease (prior MI, PAD, or aortic plaque)	1	5	6.7
Age 65–74 years	1	6	9.8
Sex category (meaning female sex)	1	7	9.6
Maximum score	9	8	6.7
		9	15.2

MI, myocardial infarction; *PAD*, peripheral arterial disease; *TE*, thromboembolism; *TIA*, transient ischemic attack.

Data from Kumar S, Walters TE, Halloran K, et al. Ten-year trends in the use of catheter ablation for treatment of atrial fibrillation vs. the use of coronary intervention for the treatment of ischaemic heart disease in Australia. *Europace*, 2013;15:1702-1709; and Gage BF, Waterman AD, Shannon W, et al. Validation of clinical classification schemes for predicting stroke: results from the National Registry of Atrial Fibrillation. *JAMA*. 2001;285:2864-2870.

of algorithms, of which the HAS-BLED score is the most simple and readily applicable in clinical practice and has a high predictive value for the identification of at risk patients.[91] The score is a composite of points given for uncontrolled hypertension, abnormal renal or liver function, stroke, bleeding history or predisposition (anemia), labile INR, elderly, and use of drugs or alcohol concomitantly (Table 76.5).[92,93] The HAS-BLED score is useful to individualize patient therapy, for prompt regular follow-up and vigilance for potential bleeding complications, and to address reversible risk factors for bleeding; it is not designed to deter anticoagulation as patients at higher risk of bleeding are often at high thromboembolic risk. A HAS-BLED score of ≥3 indicates that caution is warranted when prescribing oral anticoagulation, and regular review is recommended.

Owing to recent advancements, there are now many drug choices for long-term anticoagulation in AF. Warfarin had been the drug of choice until recently. Indeed, it is highly efficacious with a meta-analysis showing that adjusted-dose warfarin (INR of 2–3) reduces stroke risk by 64%.[94] Absolute risk reductions for primary and secondary prevention were 2.7% and 8.4% per year, respectively. Warfarin conferred a 0.3% absolute increase in the risk of major extracranial bleeding.[95] Comparatively, aspirin reduced stroke by 22% with absolute risk reduction for primary

TABLE 76.5 HAS-BLED scoring system

ACRONYM	RISK FACTOR	POINT(S)
H	Hypertension: systolic BP >160 mm Hg	1
A	Abnormal renal or liver function[a]	1 point each
S	Stroke	1
B	Major bleeding history[b]	1
L	Labile INRs: within therapeutic range <60%[c]	1
E	Elderly: age >65 years	1
D	Antiplatelet agents or alcohol use[d]	1 point each

[a]This was defined as the presence of chronic dialysis, renal transplantation, or serum creatinine ≥200 mmol/L; abnormal liver function was defined as chronic hepatic disease or biochemical evidence of significant hepatic derangement.
[b]This was defined as a patient history of bleeding or predisposition (anemia).
[c]This was defined as a time in therapeutic INR range of less than 60%.
[d]This includes concomitant antiplatelets, nonsteroidal antiinflammatory drugs, or excess alcohol.
BP, blood pressure; *INRs,* international normalized ratios.
Modified from Lane DA, Lip GY. Use of the CHA$_2$DS$_2$-VASc and HAS-BLED scores to aid decision making for thromboprophylaxis in nonvalvular atrial fibrillation. *Circulation.* 2012;126:860-865.

and secondary prevention of 1.5% and 2.5% per year, respectively. Adjusted-dose warfarin is substantially more efficacious than antiplatelet therapy, with a relative risk reduction of 39%.[94] Aspirin plus clopidogrel was inferior to oral anticoagulation with warfarin in the prevention of vascular events including stroke and systemic embolism.[96] However, in patients with contraindication to oral anticoagulation, aspirin plus clopidogrel reduced the risk of major vascular events, especially stroke, at the cost of increased risk of major hemorrhage.[97]

A number of direct oral anticoagulants (DOACs) that are non–vitamin K antagonists have been evaluated in clinical trials and have received US Food and Drug Administration (FDA) approval for prevention of thromboembolism in nonvalvular AF. They are either direct thrombin inhibitors (dabigatran) or activated factor Xa inhibitors (rivaroxaban, apixaban, and edoxaban). Key advantages of DOACs are fixed dosing that eliminates the need for blood tests, lack of significant dietary restrictions, and full anticoagulation effect that occurs within 1 to 4 hours of ingestion of a dose. DOACs also carry the potential advantage that patients may spend more time in the therapeutic range with proper compliance, especially since patients taking warfarin might not be in the optimal therapeutic anticoagulation range 59% to 68% of the time.[98] However, there are potential disadvantages for DOACs that include the lack of adequate testing to indicate patient compliance and the lack of a reversal agent with the factor Xa inhibitors. Idarucizumab, a reversal agent for dabigatran, has just received FDA approval in the United States, but reversal agents for the Xa agents will soon be available. DOACs are generally avoided when creatinine clearance falls below 15 mg/dL and in pregnancy.

It is important to note that the presence of a mechanical prosthetic valve is currently considered to be a contraindication to the use of DOACs. This is because DOAC clinical trials excluded patients with valvular AF; one study found dabigatran was inferior to warfarin early after prosthetic valve implantation.[99]

Dabigatran is a direct thrombin inhibitor that is mainly excreted by the kidneys. When given at a dose of 110 mg, dabigatran demonstrated similar rates of embolism but with lower rates of hemorrhage; when given at a dose of 150 mg, it was associated with lower rates of thromboembolism but similar rates of major hemorrhage compared with warfarin.[100]

Rivaroxaban, apixaban, and edoxaban are oral inhibitors of activated factor Xa. All three drugs were compared with warfarin in randomized double blind trials.[101–103] Rivaroxaban at a dose of 20 mg daily was noninferior to warfarin and had similar bleeding rates.[103] Edoxaban at a dose of 60 mg daily was found to be noninferior to warfarin, with lower bleeding risk.[101] Apixaban at dose of 5 mg twice a day proved to be superior to warfarin in reducing stroke and systemic embolism and had a significantly lower incidence of major bleeding. The predominant positive effect on stroke was by reduction of hemorrhagic stroke.[102] In the study, if two or more of the following were present, the dose of apixaban was reduced to 2.5 mg twice daily without loss in efficacy in stroke prevention but with lower bleeding rate: age >80, body weight <60 kg, and serum creatinine ≥1.5 mg/dL.[102]

LAA occlusion or removal is a potential treatment alternative to oral anticoagulation, given that 90% of observed thrombi are within the LAA.[104] LAA occlusion approaches include a percutaneous endocardial approach or a percutaneous epicardial approach. There are two main types of percutaneously deployed LAA devices; the first is the WATCHMAN device, which is essentially a nitinol plug with fenestrated fabric, and the second is the LARIAT system, which is an epicardially deployed suture that snares the LAA closed.[105] The current ACC/AHA/HRS guideline for the management of patients with AF does not include recommendations for the use of LAA occlusion devices because of the lack of adequate data and the fact that at the time of writing of that document, the FDA had not approved LAA closure devices for stroke prevention, approval of which has been granted recently.[9]

In a randomized study, the WATCHMAN device was noninferior to warfarin for the composite endpoint of ischemic or hemorrhagic stroke, cardiovascular or unexplained death, or systemic embolus; however, the rate of adverse safety events (e.g., serious pericardial effusion, device embolization, or procedure related stroke) was 4.4%.[106] A "learning curve," however, was noted, with a decline in acute complications with increasing procedural experience. Long-term follow-up data (mean, 45 months) from PROTECT AF showed that WATCHMAN patients had significantly lower rates of hemorrhagic stroke and cardiovascular death than did patients receiving anticoagulation therapy.[107] One major issue is that the study excluded patients who had contraindications to long-term anticoagulation and enrolled a majority of patients with relatively low estimated stroke risk (i.e., CHADS$_2$ scores of 1 and 2). Outcomes in patients undergoing LAA occlusion with the LARIAT are only reported in the context of an uncontrolled case series. The published literature is focused on outcomes of functional LAA occlusion, and none have included longitudinal outcomes; hence the long-term efficacy in stroke reduction or its safety relative to other approaches remains unknown.[105] The LAA occlusion devices offer an alternative to OAC, although more data are needed to demonstrate long-term efficacy for ischemic stroke prevention.

Catheter Ablation for Atrial Fibrillation

A detailed discussion on the rationale, methods, advantages, and disadvantages of contemporary catheter ablation techniques is described in other chapters; an overview is provided here. Catheter ablation for AF should be considered for patients with symptomatic paroxysmal or persistent AF refractory or intolerant to at least one class I or III antiarrhythmic medication when a rhythm control strategy is desired.[9,108] Catheter ablation can be considered first-line therapy in some patients who wish to avoid or cannot take antiarrhythmic medications after a detailed discussion of the risks and benefits.[9,108] There are a number of factors that should be weighed carefully against the long-term efficacy and risk of complications associated with catheter ablation. These include patient age, functional status, symptoms, long-term thromboembolic risk, extent of structural remodeling associated with AF, long-term risk of anticoagulant therapy, presence of structural heart disease (including tachycardia-mediated cardiomyopathy), left atrial size, duration of AF, and the availability of effective and tolerable pharmacological therapy. AF ablation should not be performed in patients who cannot be treated with anticoagulant therapy during and after the procedure.[9]

In the majority of paroxysmal AF cases, targeting triggers of AF, which primarily emanate from pulmonary veins, can successfully prevent recurrent arrhythmia. The pulmonnary veins can be targeted with a variety of techniques, including segmental ostial ablation, circumferential pulmonary vein ablation, wide-area circumferential ablation, and antral pulmonary vein isolation. The beneficial effects extend by elimination of arrhythmogenic sites within the pulmonary veins and their antra, atrial "debulking," potential elimination of anchor points of rotors, coincidental ablation of ganglionic plexuses, and ablation of the ligament of Marshall.[108]

Randomized controlled trials have reported that the success of pulmonary vein isolation in maintaining sinus rhythm is between 66% and 89% at a 12-month follow-up.[108] In a meta-analysis of all randomized and nonrandomized studies, the single-procedure success rate of catheter ablation off AAD therapy was 57%; multiple-procedure success rate off AADs was 71%.[109] In each trial, catheter ablation was superior to AADs, which had an efficacy of 9% to 58%. In a meta-analysis, the mean success rate for AADs was 52%.[109] Furthermore, catheter ablation has been found to be superior to AADs in reducing AF symptoms and in improving quality of life.[108] Patients with recurrence of AF after ablation are almost always found to have recovered conduction in one or more pulmonary veins.[110,111] One of the key challenges is obtaining transmural lesions and having reliable intraprocedural markers to identify incomplete lesions. A number of factors have been investigated, such as pacing along the ablation line and reablating at the sites of pace capture,[112] systematic use of impedance,[113] catheter stability,[114] use of unipolar electrogram markers of transmurality,[115] or use of force sensing.[116] The common paradigm that emerges is that procedural success can be improved if prospectively defined markers of lesion transmurality, tissue contact, and catheter stability can be achieved with the majority of lesions.[117] For example, freedom from AF was much higher if operators followed predefined contact forces for ≥90% of lesions than those who did not in a randomized study using the novel contact force-sensing catheters.[116]

AF-free survival after catheter ablation is significantly lower for patients with persistent AF. A systematic review of outcomes following ablation found an approximately 20% AF-free survival at 12 months with pulmonary vein isolation alone.[118] Although pulmonary vein isolation has reasonably good success in curing patients with paroxysmal AF, its efficacy has been found to be limited in patients with persistent AF. Focus has been directed to deciphering AF mechanisms, including targeting nonpulmonary vein triggers, rotors, complex fractionated atrial electrograms, and cardiac autonomic ganglia activity.[71,108] A number of ablation strategies have been proposed, including linear ablation, ablation of complex fractionated atrial electrograms, a "stepwise" approach of incremental extent of atrial ablation until AF terminates, targeting rotors using proprietary software, and abolishment of autonomic ganglia.[108] Although some methods reported an initially high success rate, enthusiasm has been tempered by randomized controlled trials showing no incremental benefit over pulmonary vein isolation alone[119,120] or lack of reproducibiltity of proprietary software–guided approaches.[121] Furthermore, extensive ablation beyond

pulmonary vein isolation often leads to recurrent atrial tachycardia, repeat ablation procedures, and/or antiarrhythmic medications. There is no consensus on an overall optimal strategy for ablation of persistent AF, but antral pulmonary vein isolation remains a critical component. Adjunctive strategies can be tailored to the individual patient and depend on operator preference. Clearly, a better understanding of basic AF mechanisms needs to be elucidated before critical substrate can be identifed during catheter ablation procedures.

Catheter ablation procedures for AF are associated with uncommon but potentially life-threatening adverse events. A systematic review found that the pooled estimate for death was 0.06%.[122] Other severe or life-threatening complications include atrioesophageal fistula formation (0.08%), pulmonary vein stenosis (0.5%), stroke or transient ischemic attack (0.6%), cardiac tamponade (1%), and phrenic nerve paralysis (0.4%).[122] The pooled estimate for vascular complications is 1.6%.[122] Atrioesophageal fistula usually occurs within the first 2 to 4 weeks after the procedure. It is important to recognize that complication still occurs, albeit rarely, despite precautionary measures taken to visualize and monitor the esophagus during the procedure.[123] Pooled estimates for significant periprocedural complication is 2.9%.[122] Performing the AF procedure with a therapeutic INR or uninterrupted novel anticoagulation agents is safe and appears to reduce the risk of symptomatic and asymptomatic thromboembolic events.[124,125]

Catheter ablation has undoubtedly had a significant beneficial effect on the perceived quality of life for patients living with AF, chiefly by reducing symptomatic episodes more effectively than antiarrhythmic medications. It has beneficial effect in patients with left ventricular systolic dysfunction, especially when performed early in the course of AF and heart failure.[126] Retrospective analyses have also suggested that maintenance of sinus rhythm may translate to a reduction in stroke or death compared with patients who are managed medically[127,128] or may reduce progression of AF to persistent or permanent forms.[50] Whether stroke reduction and improved survival are additional benefits of catheter ablation awaits results of pivotal trials such as the NIH-NLBI sponsored trial CABANA,[69] which will compare these outcomes between an ablation strategy versus a medical strategy. Another study, the ongoing Early Treatment of Atrial Fibrillation for Stroke Prevention Trial (EAST), is designed to answer whether the early use of rhythm control (ablation, AADs, or both) can improve end points.[129]

Catheter ablation as a first-line therapy for AF has been addressed by two recent studies: the first study showed a higher 1-year freedom from AF in the ablation group,[130] while the other showed no significant differences between the groups for the cumulative burden of AF during a period of 2 years; however, symptomatic AF was significantly lower in the ablation group than in the drug therapy group.[131]

Conclusions and Future Directions

Our understanding of the mechanisms underlying AF has improved substantially since the late 1990s, but much remains to be learned. Technological advances in mapping and ablation systems have made ablation a safe and effective alternative to medical therapy, which has seen no significant recent advances. Future goals of treatment lie in prevention and modification of risk factors for AF, including possible genetic modification. Once we decipher mechanisms for the perpetuation of AF, novel therapeutic targets for drug therapy and ablation can be developed to help the large number of patients with this troublesome arrhythmia.

REFERENCES

1. Go AS, Hylek EM, Phillips KA, et al. Prevalence of diagnosed atrial fibrillation in adults: national implications for rhythm management and stroke prevention: the anticoagulation and risk factors in atrial fibrillation (atria) study. *JAMA*. 2001;285:2370–2375.
2. Benjamin EJ, Chen PS, Bild DE, et al. Prevention of atrial fibrillation: report from a national heart, lung, and blood institute workshop. *Circulation*. 2009;119:606–618.
3. Benjamin EJ, Levy D, Vaziri SM, et al. Independent risk factors for atrial fibrillation in a population-based cohort. The Framingham Heart Study. *JAMA*. 1994;271:840–844.
4. Lloyd-Jones DM, Wang TJ, Leip EP, et al. Lifetime risk for development of atrial fibrillation: The Framingham Heart Study. *Circulation*. 2004;110:1042–1046.
5. Le Heuzey JY, Paziaud O, Piot O, et al. Cost of care distribution in atrial fibrillation patients: the COCAF study. *Am Heart J*. 2004;147:121–126.
6. Coyne KS, Paramore C, Grandy S, et al. Assessing the direct costs of treating nonvalvular atrial fibrillation in the United States. *Value Health*. 2006;9:348–356.
7. Reynolds MR, Essebag V, Zimetbaum P, Cohen DJ. Healthcare resource utilization and costs associated with recurrent episodes of atrial fibrillation: the FRACTAL registry. *J Cardiovasc Electrophysiol*. 2007;18:628–633.
8. Kumar S, Walters TE, Halloran K, et al. Ten-year trends in the use of catheter ablation for treatment of atrial fibrillation vs. the use of coronary intervention for the treatment of ischaemic heart disease in Australia. *Europace*. 2013;15:1702–1709.
9. January CT, Wann LS, Alpert JS, et al. 2014 AHA/ACC/HRS guideline for the management of patients with atrial fibrillation: a report of the American College of Cardiology/American Heart Association Task Force on Practice Guidelines and the Heart Rhythm Society. *J Am Coll Cardiol*. 2014;64:e1–e76.
10. Wyse DG, Van Gelder IC, Ellinor PT, et al. Lone atrial fibrillation: does it exist? *J Am Coll Cardiol*. 2014;63:1715–1723.
11. Kumar S, Teh AW, Medi C, et al. Atrial remodeling in varying clinical substrates within beating human hearts: relevance to atrial fibrillation. *Prog Biophys Mol Biol*. 2012;110:278–294.
12. Haissaguerre M, Jais P, Shah DC, et al. Spontaneous initiation of atrial fibrillation by ectopic beats originating in the pulmonary veins. *N Engl J Med*. 1998;339:659–666.
13. Lau DH, Schotten U, Mahajan R, et al. Novel mechanisms in the pathogenesis of atrial fibrillation: practical applications. *Eur Heart J*. 2016;37:1573–1581.
14. Narayan SM, Baykaner T, Clopton P, et al. Ablation of rotor and focal sources reduces late recurrence of atrial fibrillation compared with trigger ablation alone: extended follow-up of the CONFIRM trial (Conventional Ablation for Atrial Fibrillation With or Without Focal Impulse and Rotor Modulation). *J Am Coll Cardiol*. 2014;63:1761–1768.
15. Narayan SM, Krummen DE, Shivkumar K, et al. Treatment of atrial fibrillation by the ablation of localized sources: CONFIRM (Conventional Ablation for Atrial Fibrillation With or Without Focal Impulse and Rotor Modulation) trial. *J Am Coll Cardiol*. 2012;60:628–636.
16. Lee G, Kumar S, Teh A, et al. Epicardial wave mapping in human long-lasting persistent atrial fibrillation: transient rotational circuits, complex wavefronts, and disorganized activity. *Eur Heart J*. 2014;35:86–97.
17. Lee S, Sahadevan J, Khrestian CM, et al. Simultaneous biatrial high-density (510-512 electrodes) epicardial mapping of persistent and long-standing persistent atrial fibrillation in patients: new insights into the mechanism of its maintenance. *Circulation*. 2015;132:2108–2117.
18. Allessie MA, de Groot NM, Houben RP, et al. Electropathological substrate of long-standing persistent atrial fibrillation in patients with structural heart disease: longitudinal dissociation. *Circ Arrhythm Electrophysiol*. 2010;3:606–615.
19. de Groot NM, Houben RP, Smeets JL, et al. Electropathological substrate of longstanding persistent atrial fibrillation in patients with structural heart disease: epicardial breakthrough. *Circulation*. 2010;122:1674–1682.
20. Wijffels MC, Kirchhof CJ, Dorland R, Allessie MA. Atrial fibrillation begets atrial fibrillation. A study in awake chronically instrumented goats. *Circulation*. 1995;92:1954–1968.
21. Kalman JM, Kumar S, Sanders P. Markers of collagen synthesis, atrial fibrosis, and the mechanisms underlying atrial fibrillation. *J Am Coll Cardiol*. 2012;60:1807–1808.
22. Miller JD, Aronis KN, Chrispin J, et al. Obesity, exercise, obstructive sleep apnea, and modifiable atherosclerotic cardiovascular disease risk factors in atrial fibrillation. *J Am Coll Cardiol*. 2015;66:2899–2906.
23. Kottkamp H. Human atrial fibrillation substrate: towards a specific fibrotic atrial cardiomyopathy. *Eur Heart J*. 2013;34:2731–2738.
24. Chou CC, Chen PS. New concepts in atrial fibrillation: neural mechanisms and calcium dynamics. *Cardiol Clin*. 2009;27:35–43. viii.
25. Yu L, Scherlag BJ, Sha Y, et al. Interactions between atrial electrical remodeling and autonomic remodeling: how to break the vicious cycle. *Heart Rhythm*. 2012;9:804–809.
26. Tan AY, Zhou S, Ogawa M, et al. Neural mechanisms of paroxysmal atrial fibrillation and paroxysmal atrial tachycardia in ambulatory canines. *Circulation*. 2008;118:916–925.
27. Lubitz SA, Yin X, Fontes JD, et al. Association between familial atrial fibrillation and risk of new-onset atrial fibrillation. *JAMA*. 2010;304:2263–2269.
28. Tucker NR, Ellinor PT. Emerging directions in the genetics of atrial fibrillation. *Circ Res*. 2014;114:1469–1482.
29. Clark DM, Plumb VJ, Epstein AE, Kay GN. Hemodynamic effects of an irregular sequence of ventricular cycle lengths during atrial fibrillation. *J Am Coll Cardiol*. 1997;30:1039–1045.
30. Ling LH, Kistler PM, Kalman JM, Schilling RJ, Hunter RJ. Comorbidity of atrial fibrillation and heart failure. *Nat Rev Cardiol*. 2016;13:131–147.
31. Packer DL, Bardy GH, Worley SJ, et al. Tachycardia-induced cardiomyopathy: a reversible form of left ventricular dysfunction. *Am J Cardiol*. 1986;57:563–570.
32. Sanna T, Diener HC, Passman RS, et al. Cryptogenic stroke and underlying atrial fibrillation. *N Engl J Med*. 2014;370:2478–2486.
33. Savelieva I, Camm AJ. Clinical relevance of silent atrial fibrillation: prevalence, prognosis, quality of life, and management. *J Interv Card Electrophysiol*. 2000;4:369–382.
34. Sauer WH, Alonso C, Zado E, et al. Atrioventricular nodal reentrant tachycardia in patients referred for atrial fibrillation ablation: response to ablation that incorporates slow-pathway modification. *Circulation*. 2006;114:191–195.
35. Pathak RK, Elliott A, Middeldorp ME, et al. Impact of cardiorespiratory fitness on arrhythmia recurrence in obese individuals with atrial fibrillation: the CARDIO-FIT study. *J Am Coll Cardiol*. 2015;66:985–996.
36. Pathak RK, Middeldorp ME, Lau DH, et al. Aggressive risk factor reduction study for atrial fibrillation and implications for the outcome of ablation: the ARREST-AF cohort study. *J Am Coll Cardiol*. 2014;64:2222–2231.
37. Pathak RK, Middeldorp ME, Meredith M, et al. Long-term effect of goal-directed weight management in an atrial fibrillation cohort: a long-term follow-up study (LEGACY). *J Am Coll Cardiol*. 2015;65:2159–2169.
38. Bjerkelund CJ, Orning OM. The efficacy of anticoagulant therapy in preventing embolism related to D.C. electrical conversion of atrial fibrillation. *Am J Cardiol*. 1969;23:208–216.
39. Gallagher MM, Hennessy BJ, Edvardsson N, et al. Embolic complications of direct current cardioversion of atrial arrhythmias: association with low intensity of anticoagulation at the time of cardioversion. *J Am Coll Cardiol*. 2002;40:926–933.
40. Manning WJ, Silverman DI, Gordon SP, Krumholz HM, Douglas PS. Cardioversion from atrial fibrillation without prolonged anticoagulation with use of transesophageal echocardiography to exclude the presence of atrial thrombi. *N Engl J Med*. 1993;328:750–755.
41. Black IW, Fatkin D, Sagar KB, et al. Exclusion of atrial thrombus by transesophageal echocardiography does not preclude embolism after cardioversion of atrial fibrillation. A multicenter study. *Circulation*. 1994;89:2509–2513.
42. Fatkin D, Kuchar DL, Thorburn CW, Feneley MP. Transesophageal echocardiography before and during direct current cardioversion of atrial fibrillation: evidence for "atrial stunning" as a mechanism of thromboembolic complications. *J Am Coll Cardiol*. 1994;23:307–316.
43. Irani WN, Grayburn PA, Afridi I. Prevalence of thrombus, spontaneous echo contrast, and atrial stunning in patients undergoing cardioversion of atrial flutter. A prospective study using transesophageal echocardiography. *Circulation*. 1997;95:962–966.
44. Danias PG, Caulfield TA, Weigner MJ, Silverman DI, Manning WJ. Likelihood of spontaneous conversion of atrial fibrillation to sinus rhythm. *J Am Coll Cardiol*. 1998;31:588–592.
45. Volgman AS, Carberry PA, Stambler B, et al. Conversion efficacy and safety of intravenous ibutilide compared with intravenous procainamide in patients with atrial flutter or fibrillation. *J Am Coll Cardiol*. 1998;31:1414–1419.
46. Lundstrom T, Ryden L. Chronic atrial fibrillation. Long-term results of direct current conversion. *Acta Med Scand*. 1988;223:53–59.
47. Fetsch T, Bauer P, Engberding R, et al. Prevention of atrial fibrillation after cardioversion: results of the PAFAC trial. *Eur Heart J*. 2004;25:1385–1394.
48. Kirchhof P, Andresen D, Bosch R, et al. Short-term versus long-term antiarrhythmic drug treatment after cardioversion of atrial fibrillation (Flec-SL): a prospective, randomised, open-label, blinded endpoint assessment trial. *Lancet*. 2012;380:238–246.
49. Pappone C, Radinovic A, Manguso F, et al. Atrial fibrillation progression and management: a 5-year prospective follow-up study. *Heart Rhythm*. 2008;5:1501–1507.
50. Proietti R, Hadjis A, AlTurki A, et al. A systematic review on the progression of paroxysmal to persistent atrial fibrillation: shedding new light on the effects of catheter ablation. *JACC: Clinical Electrophysiology*. 2015;1:105–115.
51. Kerr CR, Humphries KH, Talajic M, et al. Progression to chronic atrial fibrillation after the initial diagnosis of paroxysmal atrial fibrillation: results from the Canadian Registry of Atrial Fibrillation. *Am Heart J*. 2005;149:489–496.
52. Farshi R, Kistner D, Sarma JS, Longmate JA, Singh BN. Ventricular rate control in chronic atrial fibrillation during daily activity and programmed exercise: a crossover open-label study of five drug regimens. *J Am Coll Cardiol*. 1999;33:304–310.
52a. Chao TF, Liu CJ, Tuan TC. et al. Rate-control treatment and mortality in atrial fibrillation. *Circulation*. 2015;132:1604–1612.
52b. Vamos M, Erath JW, Hohnloser SH. Digoxin-associated mortality: a systematic review and meta-analysis of the literature. *Eur Heart J*. 2015;36:1831–1838.
53. Manolis AG, Katsivas AG, Lazaris EE, Vassilopoulos CV, Louvros NE. Ventricular performance and quality of life in patients who underwent radiofrequency AV junction ablation and permanent pacemaker implantation due to medically refractory atrial tachyarrhythmias. *J Interv Card Electrophysiol*. 1998;2:71–76.
54. Doshi RN, Daoud EG, Fellows C, et al. Left ventricular-based cardiac stimulation post AV nodal ablation evaluation (the PAVE study). *J Cardiovasc Electrophysiol*. 2005;16:1160–1165.
55. Chatterjee NA, Upadhyay GA, Ellenbogen KA, et al. Atrioventricular nodal ablation in atrial fibrillation: a meta-analysis and systematic review. *Circ Arrhythm Electrophysiol*. 2012;5:68–76.
56. Deshmukh P, Casavant DA, Romanyshyn M, Anderson K. Permanent, direct His-bundle pacing: a novel approach to cardiac pacing in patients with normal His-Purkinje activation. *Circulation*. 2000;101:869–877.
57. Hsieh MH, Tai CT, Lee SH, et al. Catheter ablation of atrial fibrillation versus atrioventricular junction ablation plus pacing therapy for elderly patients with medically refractory paroxysmal atrial fibrillation. *J Cardiovasc Electrophysiol*. 2005;16:457–461.
58. Khan MN, Jais P, Cummings J, et al. Pulmonary-vein isolation for atrial fibrillation in patients with heart failure. *N Engl J Med*. 2008;359:1778–1785.
59. Hohnloser SH, Kuck KH, Lilienthal J. Rhythm or rate control in atrial fibrillation—Pharmacological Intervention in Atrial Fibrillation (PIAF): a randomised trial. *Lancet*. 2000;356:1789–1794.
60. Wyse DG, Waldo AL, DiMarco JP, et al. A comparison of rate control and rhythm control in patients with atrial fibrillation. *N Engl J Med*. 2002;347:1825–1833.
61. Carlsson J, Miketic S, Windeler J, et al. Randomized trial of rate-control versus rhythm-control in persistent atrial fibrillation: the Strategies of Treatment of Atrial Fibrillation (STAF) study. *J Am Coll Cardiol*. 2003;41:1690–1696.
62. Opolski G, Torbicki A, Kosior DA, et al. Rate control vs rhythm control in patients with nonvalvular persistent atrial fibrillation: the results of the Polish How to Treat Chronic Atrial Fibrillation (HOT CAFE) Study. *Chest*. 2004;126:476–486.
63. Van Gelder IC, Hagens VE, Bosker HA, et al. A comparison of rate control and rhythm control in patients with recurrent persistent atrial fibrillation. *N Engl J Med*. 2002;347:1834–1840.
64. de Denus S, Sanoski CA, Carlsson J, Opolski G, Spinler SA. Rate vs rhythm control in patients with atrial fibrillation: a meta-analysis. *Arch Intern Med*. 2005;165:258–262.
65. Roy D, Talajic M, Nattel S, et al. Rhythm control versus rate control for atrial fibrillation and heart failure. *N Engl J Med*. 2008;358:2667–2677.
66. Talajic M, Khairy P, Levesque S, et al. Maintenance of sinus rhythm and survival in patients with heart failure and atrial fibrillation. *J Am Coll Cardiol*. 2010;55:1796–1802.
67. Chatterjee S, Sardar P, Lichstein E, Mukherjee D, Aikat S. Pharmacologic rate versus rhythm-control strategies in atrial fibrillation: an updated comprehensive review and meta-analysis. *Pacing Clin Electrophysiol*. 2013;36:122–133.

68. Ionescu-Ittu R, Abrahamowicz M, Jackevicius CA, et al. Comparative effectiveness of rhythm control vs rate control drug treatment effect on mortality in patients with atrial fibrillation. *Arch Intern Med*. 2012;172:997–1004.

69. Mayo Clinic. Catheter ablation vs anti-arrhythmic drug therapy for atrial fibrillation trial (CABANA). <https://clinicaltrials.gov/ct2/show/NCT00911508>; 2009 Accessed 28.09.16.

70. Lafuente-Lafuente C, Valembois L, Bergmann JF, Belmin J. Antiarrhythmics for maintaining sinus rhythm after cardioversion of atrial fibrillation. *Cochrane Database Syst Rev*. 2015;3: CD005049.

71. Prystowsky EN, Padanilam BJ, Fogel RI. Treatment of atrial fibrillation. *JAMA*. 2015;314:278–288.

72. Sherrid MV, Barac I, McKenna WJ, et al. Multicenter study of the efficacy and safety of disopyramide in obstructive hypertrophic cardiomyopathy. *J Am Coll Cardiol*. 2005;45:1251–1258.

73. Scheinman MM, Morady F. Nonpharmacological approaches to atrial fibrillation. *Circulation*. 2001;103: 2120–2125.

74. Preliminary report. effect of encainide and flecainide on mortality in a randomized trial of arrhythmia suppression after myocardial infarction. The Cardiac Arrhythmia Suppression Trial (CAST) Investigators. *N Engl J Med*. 1989;321:406–412.

75. Torp-Pedersen C, Moller M, Bloch-Thomsen PE, et al. Dofetilide in patients with congestive heart failure and left ventricular dysfunction. Danish Investigations of Arrhythmia and Mortality on Dofetilide Study Group. *N Engl J Med*. 1999;341:857–865.

76. Roden DM. Drug-induced prolongation of the QT interval. *N Engl J Med*. 2004;350:1013–1022.

77. Ellenbogen KA, Stambler BS, Wood MA, et al. Efficacy of intravenous ibutilide for rapid termination of atrial fibrillation and atrial flutter: a dose-response study. *J Am Coll Cardiol*. 1996;28:130–136.

78. Stambler BS, Wood MA, Ellenbogen KA, et al. Efficacy and safety of repeated intravenous doses of ibutilide for rapid conversion of atrial flutter or fibrillation. Ibutilide Repeat Dose Study Investigators. *Circulation*. 1996;94:1613–1621.

79. Oral H, Souza JJ, Michaud GF, et al. Facilitating transthoracic cardioversion of atrial fibrillation with ibutilide pretreatment. *N Engl J Med*. 1999;340:1849–1854.

80. Malik M, Camm AJ. Amiodarone after myocardial infarction: EMIAT and CAMIAT trials. *Lancet*. 1997;349:1767–1768.

81. Le Heuzey JY, De Ferrari GM, Radzik D, et al. A short-term, randomized, double-blind, parallel-group study to evaluate the efficacy and safety of dronedarone versus amiodarone in patients with persistent atrial fibrillation: the DIONYSOS study. *J Cardiovasc Electrophysiol*. 2010;21:597–605.

82. Kober L, Torp-Pedersen C, McMurray JJ, et al. Increased mortality after dronedarone therapy for severe heart failure. *N Engl J Med*. 2008;358:2678–2687.

83. Singh BN, Connolly SJ, Crijns HJ, et al. Dronedarone for maintenance of sinus rhythm in atrial fibrillation or flutter. *N Engl J Med*. 2007;357:987–999.

84. Hohnloser SH, Crijns HJ, van Eickels M, et al. Dronedarone in patients with congestive heart failure: insights from ATHENA. *Eur Heart J*. 2010;31:1717–1721.

85. Wolf PA, Abbott RD, Kannel WB. Atrial fibrillation as an independent risk factor for stroke: the Framingham Study. *Stroke*. 1991;22:983–988.

86. Aviles RJ, Martin DO, Apperson-Hansen C, et al. Inflammation as a risk factor for atrial fibrillation. *Circulation*. 2003;108:3006–3010.

87. Sohara H, Amitani S, Kurose M, Miyahara K. Atrial fibrillation activates platelets and coagulation in a time-dependent manner: a study in patients with paroxysmal atrial fibrillation. *J Am Coll Cardiol*. 1997;29:106–112.

88. Gage BF, Waterman AD, Shannon W, et al. Validation of clinical classification schemes for predicting stroke: results from the National Registry of Atrial Fibrillation. *JAMA*. 2001;285:2864–2870.

89. van Walraven C, Hart RG, Wells GA, et al. A clinical prediction rule to identify patients with atrial fibrillation and a low risk for stroke while taking aspirin. *Arch Intern Med*. 2003;163:936–943.

90. Lip GY, Nieuwlaat R, Pisters R, Lane DA, Crijns HJ. Refining clinical risk stratification for predicting stroke and thromboembolism in atrial fibrillation using a novel risk factor-based approach: the Euro Heart Survey on atrial fibrillation. *Chest*. 2010;137:263–272.

91. Pisters R, Lane DA, Nieuwlaat R, et al. A novel user-friendly score (HAS-BLED) to assess 1-year risk of major bleeding in patients with atrial fibrillation: the Euro Heart Survey. *Chest*. 2010;138:1093–1100.

92. Camm AJ, Lip GY, De Caterina R, et al. 2012 focused update of the ESC Guidelines for the management of atrial fibrillation: an update of the 2010 ESC Guidelines for the management of atrial fibrillation. Developed with the special contribution of the European Heart Rhythm Association. *Eur Heart J*. 2012;33:2719–2747.

93. Lane DA, Lip GY. Use of the CHA(2)DS(2)-VASc and HAS-BLED scores to aid decision making for thromboprophylaxis in nonvalvular atrial fibrillation. *Circulation*. 2012;126:860–865.

94. Hart RG, Pearce LA, Aguilar MI. Meta-analysis: antithrombotic therapy to prevent stroke in patients who have nonvalvular atrial fibrillation. *Ann Intern Med*. 2007;146:857–867.

95. Hart RG, Benavente O, McBride R, Pearce LA. Antithrombotic therapy to prevent stroke in patients with atrial fibrillation: a meta-analysis. *Ann Intern Med*. 1999;131:492–501.

96. ACTIVE writing Group of the ACTIVE Investigators, Connolly S, Pogue J, et al. Clopidogrel plus aspirin versus oral anticoagulation for atrial fibrillation in the Atrial fibrillation Clopidogrel Trial with Irbesartan for prevention of Vascular Events (ACTIVE W): a randomised controlled trial. *Lancet*. 2006;367:1903–1912.

97. ACTIVE Investigators, Connolly SJ, Pogue J, et al. Effect of clopidogrel added to aspirin in patients with atrial fibrillation. *N Engl J Med*. 2009;360:2066–2078.

98. Amouyel P, Mismetti P, Langkilde LK, et al. INR variability in atrial fibrillation: a risk model for cerebrovascular events. *Eur J Intern Med*. 2009;20:63–69.

99. Eikelboom JW, Connolly SJ, Brueckmann M, et al. Dabigatran versus warfarin in patients with mechanical heart valves. *N Engl J Med*. 2013;369:1206–1214.

100. Connolly SJ, Ezekowitz MD, Yusuf S, et al. Dabigatran versus warfarin in patients with atrial fibrillation. *N Engl J Med*. 2009;361:1139–1151.

101. Giugliano RP, Ruff CT, Braunwald E, et al. Edoxaban versus warfarin in patients with atrial fibrillation. *N Engl J Med*. 2013;369:2093–2104.

102. Granger CB, Alexander JH, McMurray JJ, et al. Apixaban versus warfarin in patients with atrial fibrillation. *N Engl J Med*. 2011;365:981–992.

103. Patel MR, Mahaffey KW, Garg J, et al. Rivaroxaban versus warfarin in nonvalvular atrial fibrillation. *N Engl J Med*. 2011;365:883–891.

104. Blackshear JL, Odell JA. Appendage obliteration to reduce stroke in cardiac surgical patients with atrial fibrillation. *Ann Thorac Surg*. 1996;61:755–759.

105. Masoudi FA, Calkins H, Kavinsky CJ, et al. 2015 ACC/HRS/SCAI Left Atrial Appendage Occlusion Device Societal Overview: a professional societal overview from the American College of Cardiology, Heart Rhythm Society, and Society for Cardiovascular Angiography and Interventions. *J Am Coll Cardiol*. 2015;66:1497–1513.

106. Holmes DR, Reddy VY, Turi ZG, et al. Percutaneous closure of the left atrial appendage versus warfarin therapy for prevention of stroke in patients with atrial fibrillation: a randomised non-inferiority trial. *Lancet*. 2009;374:534–542.

107. Reddy VY, Sievert H, Halperin J, et al. Percutaneous left atrial appendage closure vs warfarin for atrial fibrillation: a randomized clinical trial. *JAMA*. 2014;312:1988–1998.

108. Calkins H, Kuck KH, Cappato R, et al. 2012 HRS/EHRA/ECAS expert consensus statement on catheter and surgical ablation of atrial fibrillation: recommendations for patient selection, procedural techniques, patient management and follow-up, definitions, endpoints, and research trial design: a report of the Heart Rhythm Society (HRS) Task Force on Catheter and Surgical Ablation of Atrial Fibrillation. Developed in partnership with the European Heart Rhythm Association (EHRA), a registered branch of the European Society of Cardiology (ESC) and the European Cardiac Arrhythmia Society (ECAS); and in collaboration with the American College of Cardiology (ACC), American Heart Association (AHA), the Asia Pacific Heart Rhythm Society (APHRS), and the Society of Thoracic Surgeons (STS). Endorsed by the governing bodies of the American College of Cardiology Foundation, the American Heart Association, the European Cardiac Arrhythmia Society, the European Heart Rhythm Association, the Society of Thoracic Surgeons, the Asia Pacific Heart Rhythm Society, and the Heart Rhythm Society. *Heart Rhythm*. 2012;9:632–696. e21.

109. Calkins H, Reynolds MR, Spector P, et al. Treatment of atrial fibrillation with antiarrhythmic drugs or radiofrequency ablation: two systematic literature reviews and meta-analyses. *Circ Arrhythm Electrophysiol*. 2009;2:349–361.

110. Nanthakumar K, Plumb VJ, Epstein AE, et al. Resumption of electrical conduction in previously isolated pulmonary veins: rationale for a different strategy? *Circulation*. 2004;109:1226–1229.

111. Verma A, Kilicaslan F, Pisano E, et al. Response of atrial fibrillation to pulmonary vein antrum isolation is directly related to resumption and delay of pulmonary vein conduction. *Circulation*. 2005;112:627–635.

112. Steven D, Sultan A, Reddy V, et al. Benefit of pulmonary vein isolation guided by loss of pace capture on the ablation line: results from a prospective 2-center randomized trial. *J Am Coll Cardiol*. 2013;62:44–50.

113. Reichlin T, Lane C, Nagashima K, et al. Feasibility, efficacy, and safety of radiofrequency ablation of atrial fibrillation guided by monitoring of the initial impedance decrease as a surrogate of catheter contact. *J Cardiovasc Electrophysiol*. 2015;26:390–396.

114. Anter E, Tschabrunn CM, Contreras-Valdes FM, Buxton AE, Josephson ME. Radiofrequency ablation annotation algorithm reduces the incidence of linear gaps and reconnection after pulmonary vein isolation. *Heart Rhythm*. 2014;11:783–790.

115. Bortone A, Appetiti A, Bouzeman A, et al. Unipolar signal modification as a guide for lesion creation during radiofrequency application in the left atrium: prospective study in humans in the setting of paroxysmal atrial fibrillation catheter ablation. *Circ Arrhythm Electrophysiol*. 2013;6:1095–1102.

116. Reddy VY, Dukkipati SR, Neuzil P, et al. Randomized, controlled trial of the safety and effectiveness of a contact force-sensing irrigated catheter for ablation of paroxysmal atrial fibrillation: results of the tacticath contact force ablation catheter study for atrial fibrillation (TOCCASTAR) study. *Circulation*. 2015;132:907–915.

117. Kumar S, Michaud GF. Unipolar electrogram morphology to assess lesion formation during catheter ablation of atrial fibrillation: successful translation into clinical practice. *Circ Arrhythm Electrophysiol*. 2013;6:1050–1052.

118. Brooks AG, Stiles MK, Laborderie J, et al. Outcomes of long-standing persistent atrial fibrillation ablation: a systematic review. *Heart Rhythm*. 2010;7:835–846.

119. Verma A, Jiang CY, Betts TR, et al. Approaches to catheter ablation for persistent atrial fibrillation. *N Engl J Med*. 2015;372:1812–1822.

120. Vogler J, Willems S, Sultan A, et al. Pulmonary vein isolation versus defragmentation: the CHASE-AF clinical trial. *J Am Coll Cardiol*. 2015;66:2743–2752.

121. Benharash P, Buch E, Frank P, et al. Quantitative analysis of localized sources identified by focal impulse and rotor modulation mapping in atrial fibrillation. *Circ Arrhythm Electrophysiol*. 2015;8:554–561.

122. Gupta A, Perera T, Ganesan A, et al. Complications of catheter ablation of atrial fibrillation: a systematic review. *Circ Arrhythm Electrophysiol*. 2013;6:1082–1088.

123. Barbhaiya CR, Kumar S, John RM, et al. Global survey of esophageal and gastric injury in atrial fibrillation ablation: incidence, time to presentation, and outcomes. *J Am Coll Cardiol*. 2015;65:1377–1378.

124. Wazni OM, Beheiry S, Fahmy T, et al. Atrial fibrillation ablation in patients with therapeutic international normalized ratio: comparison of strategies of anticoagulation management in the periprocedural period. *Circulation*. 2007;116:2531–2534.

125. Santangeli P, Di Biase L, Horton R, et al. Ablation of atrial fibrillation under therapeutic warfarin reduces periprocedural complications: evidence from a meta-analysis. *Circ Arrhythm Electrophysiol*. 2012;5:302–311.

126. Anselmino M, Matta M, D'Ascenzo F, et al. Catheter ablation of atrial fibrillation in patients with left ventricular systolic dysfunction: a systematic review and meta-analysis. *Circ Arrhythm Electrophysiol*. 2014;7:1011–1018.

127. Hunter RJ, McCready J, Diab I, et al. Maintenance of sinus rhythm with an ablation strategy in patients with atrial fibrillation is associated with a lower risk of stroke and death. *Heart*. 2012;98:48–53.

128. Bunch TJ, May HT, Bair TL, et al. Atrial fibrillation ablation patients have long-term stroke rates similar to patients without atrial fibrillation regardless of CHADS2 score. *Heart Rhythm*. 2013;10:1272–1277.

129. German Atrial Fibrillation Network. Early treatment of atrial fibrillation for stroke prevention trial (EAST). <https://clinicaltrials.gov/ct2/show/NCT01288352#wrapper>; 2011 Accessed 28.09.16.

130. Morillo CA, Verma A, Connolly SJ, et al. Radiofrequency ablation vs antiarrhythmic drugs as first-line treatment of paroxysmal atrial fibrillation (RAAFT-2): a randomized trial. *JAMA*. 2014;311:692–700.

131. Cosedis Nielsen J, Johannessen A, Raatikainen P, et al. Radiofrequency ablation as initial therapy in paroxysmal atrial fibrillation. *N Engl J Med*. 2012;367:1587–1595.

77 Preexcitation, Atrioventricular Reentry, and Variants

Aman Chugh and Fred Morady

Definitions

Atrioventricular (AV) reentry is the second most common cause of paroxysmal supraventricular tachycardia (PSVT) among patients referred for catheter ablation. In most cases of AV reentrant tachycardia (AVRT), the reentrant circuit involves the AV node as the anterograde limb and the accessory pathway (AP) as the retrograde limb. The electrocardiogram (ECG) typically shows a regular, narrow complex rhythm referred to as orthodromic reciprocating tachycardia (ORT). Less commonly, a wide complex rhythm may be observed when anterograde conduction occurs over the AP and retrograde conduction over the AV node or another AP, referred to as antidromic reciprocating tachycardia (ART).

If the AP is capable of anterograde conduction, the baseline ECG reveals a short PR interval and a slurred upstroke of the QRS complex referred to as a delta wave, the hallmark of ventricular preexcitation. The AP is thus considered to be *manifest* (Fig. 77.1A). In approximately 50% of AVRT patients, the AP is capable of only retrograde conduction. The ECG during sinus rhythm shows a normal QRS complex, and the accessory connection is referred to as *concealed*. Patients with evidence of preexcitation on resting ECG and symptomatic tachycardia are said to have Wolff-Parkinson-White (WPW) syndrome. An asymptomatic patient who is incidentally found to have preexcitation on ECG is said to have a WPW "pattern."

Accessory Pathways

APs are anomalous bypass tracts that are typically composed of working myocardial cells. Most APs insert along the mitral or tricuspid valve and are referred to as AV APs. Approximately 60% of APs insert along the mitral valve and are referred to as left free wall pathways. About one-fourth insert along the septal aspect of

the tricuspid or mitral valve and are classified as septal pathways. The remaining 15% are right free wall pathways.

Occasionally, one may encounter APs that do not insert along the AV valves. Examples include atriofascicular, nodoventricular, nodofascicular, and atrionodal pathways. Atriofascicular pathways connect the right atrium to the distal ramifications of the right bundle branch and are capable of only anterograde conduction. Nodoventricular and nodofascicular pathways connect the AV node to the right ventricular myocardium or the specialized conduction system, respectively. Atriofascicular and nodoventricular/nodofascicular connections are also notable for their decremental conduction properties. Atrionodal pathways are rare and connect the right atrial myocardium to the AV node. The fact that these unusual pathways do not insert along the AV annulus calls for a mapping approach that is different than that for typical AV pathways. Conduction over fasciculoventricular pathways is mediated by a connection between the His–Purkinje system and the ventricular myocardium. They may serve as bystanders but have not been shown to be responsible for reentrant arrhythmias, and hence do not require ablation. The presence of left ventricular hypertrophy in a patient with a fasciculoventricular AP should raise suspicion of a glycogen storage cardiomyopathy caused by a mutation in the *PRKAG2* gene.[1]

Presentation and Evaluation

Clinical presentation of patients with ORT is similar to those with PSVT due to other mechanisms. Symptoms commonly include rapid palpitations, chest discomfort, dizziness/lightheadedness, dyspnea, weakness, neck pulsations, and presyncope. Syncope is an uncommon symptom of AVRT. Occasionally, AVRT patients develop atrial fibrillation (AF) that may lead to hemodynamic deterioration because of rapid anterograde conduction over the AP (Fig. 77.1B). This may cause syncope, cardiac arrest, or sudden death.

Although AVRT may occur at any age, it usually occurs in young patients without evidence of structural heart disease. As such, patients typically do not require an extensive cardiac evaluation. Nonetheless, frequent or incessant episodes of AVRT, such as may occur with permanent junctional reciprocating tachycardia (PJRT) (see later) may be associated with tachycardia-related cardiomyopathy. Rarely, AVRT may be associated with other cardiac conditions such as hypertrophic cardiomyopathy or Ebstein anomaly. Physical examination and resting ECG are helpful in screening for these unusual associations. Although ECG during AVRT (or other causes of SVT) may reveal ST-segment depression, such changes are usually related to tachycardia and are not indicative of myocardial ischemia. Thus, barring symptoms consistent with angina, coronary angiography is usually not required. Compared with AV nodal reentrant tachycardia (AVNRT) patients, AVRT patients are more likely to be male and develop symptoms at a younger age.

Electrocardiographic Characterization

In patients referred for an electrophysiological evaluation for PSVT, the ECG during sinus rhythm and during tachycardia may be helpful in identifying the mechanism of the tachycardia.

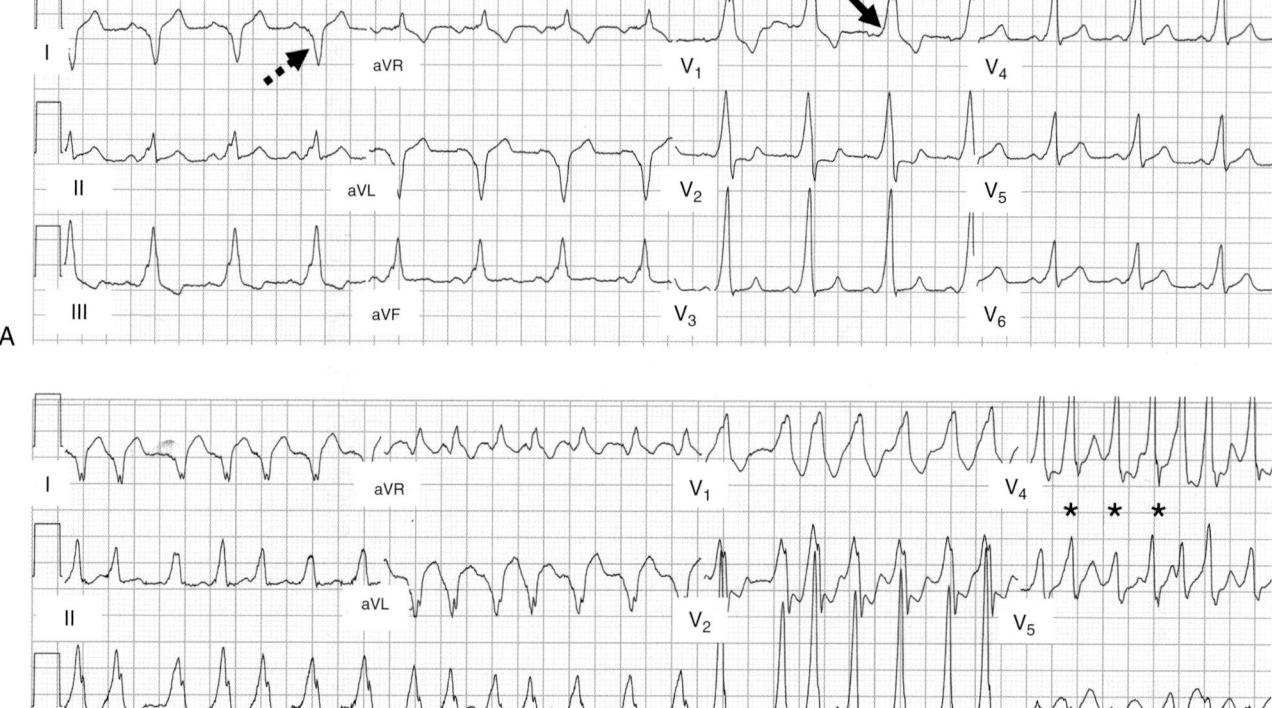

FIGURE 77.1 (A) Ventricular preexcitation. The electrocardiogram shows sinus rhythm, a short PR interval, and a slurred upstroke of QRS (delta waves, *arrow*), compatible with a left free wall accessory pathway (AP). Paper speed = 25 mm/s. (B) Preexcited atrial fibrillation. This electrocardiogram was recorded from the same patient as in (A) who presented to the hospital with near-syncope. The ventricular rate is irregular and at times is as short as 200 ms (300 beats/min). The QRS morphology is not uniform (*asterisks*), reflecting a varying degree of fusion of ventricular activation over the AP and the specialized conduction system. The AP was successfully ablated at the lateral mitral annulus.

Evidence of preexcitation during sinus rhythm in a patient with a history of tachycardia makes AVRT very likely. The degree of preexcitation may be subtle, especially in patients with a left free wall or slowly conducting AP. In the former, it is helpful to analyze the QRS morphology in the lateral precordial leads. In patients with subtle preexcitation because of a left free wall AP, a "septal" q wave is not inscribed in the lateral precordial leads (Fig. 77.2). The left-sided location of the pathway allows ventricular activation to proceed more so over the AV node than would be possible with right-sided pathways. Right-sided APs are associated with a greater degree of preexcitation. In patients with an equivocal ECG, administration of adenosine is helpful in unmasking preexcitation.

In most ORT patients, the ECG shows a regular, narrow QRS complex tachycardia. The timing of the P wave with respect to QRS is a useful clue. During ORT, atrial activation can occur only after ventricular activation, and therefore the P wave is shortly inscribed after the QRS complex, frequently within the ST segment. This feature is suggestive but not diagnostic of ORT as it may be seen with AVNRT or atrial tachycardia. During typical ("slow-fast") AVNRT, the atrium and ventricle are activated nearly simultaneously. The P wave is inscribed within or at the end of the QRS complex, resulting in a pseudo R′ in lead V_1 and a pseudo S wave in lead II. These features help to rule out ORT as the mechanism.

In PJRT patients, the AP is usually located in the posteroseptal region and has decremental conduction properties. As a result, the ECG shows a long RP tachycardia, with inverted P waves in the inferior leads. PJRT may be incessant and can result in a tachycardia-induced cardiomyopathy that generally resolves after AP ablation.

The mode of tachycardia initiation and termination is also helpful. If the tachycardia is initiated with anterograde conduction block in the AP, the mechanism is very likely to be ORT. If the tachycardia persists despite AV block, ORT is ruled out because the ventricle is an obligatory component of the reentrant circuit. If the tachycardia reliably terminates with AV block, atrial tachycardia is unlikely.

Beat-to-beat alternation of the QRS amplitude is more common in ORT than in AVNRT and atrial tachycardia. However, the QRS alternans is not specific for ORT and is probably related to a higher heart rate during ORT compared with other mechanisms. Although the ECG is a helpful guide, it frequently does not provide unambiguous diagnostic features. In fact, approximately 20% of tachycardias are misclassified when the diagnosis is based on only the ECG.

Analysis of the P-wave morphology during ORT may be helpful in localizing the AP. For example, negative P waves in the inferior leads are consistent with an atrial insertion at the inferoposterior aspect of the AV valves. Upright P waves in the

Pre-RFA   Post-RFA

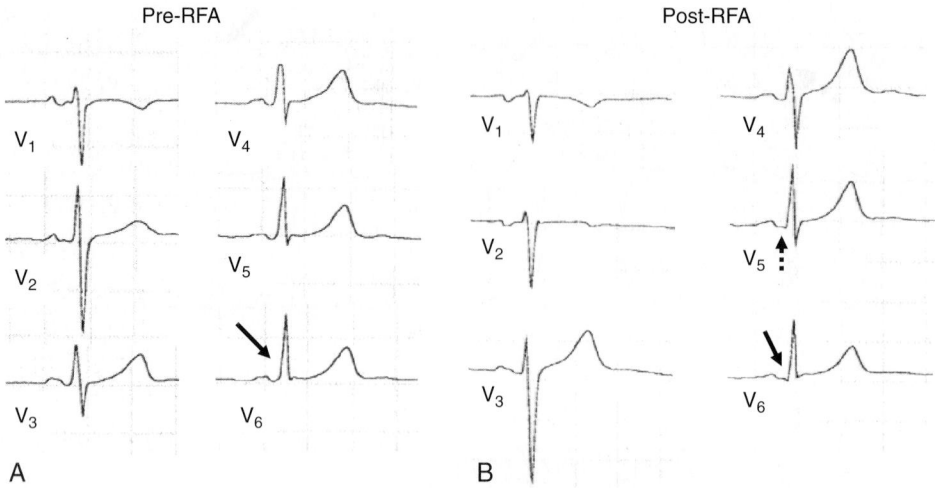

FIGURE 77.2 (A) An example of subtle preexcitation. There is slight slurring of the QRS complex upstroke (*arrow*) and a short PR interval, consistent with ventricular preexcitation. In addition, note that the QRS complex in the lateral precordial leads lacks a "septal" q wave. *RFA*, Radiofrequency ablation. (B) A postablation electrocardiogram obtained from the same patient as in (A). After elimination of the left lateral accessory pathway, the delta wave is no longer present, and the PR interval is longer (*dashed arrow*). Furthermore, now there is a small q wave in lead V$_6$ (*solid arrow*), reflecting normal septal activation.

inferior leads are associated with craniocaudal activation from the anterosuperior aspect of the AV valves. Relatively narrow P waves are typically inscribed during ORT, utilizing a septal AP, whereas broad P waves are consistent with activation over a free wall AP. However, the P wave is often obscured by the ST segment or T wave during tachycardia, making it difficult to discern the morphologies.

ECG during ART that utilizes a typical AV AP reveals a broad QRS complex tachycardia that does not resemble a typical bundle branch block pattern and may be mistaken for VT. The QRS morphology during ART is a fully preexcited version of the preexcitation pattern observed during sinus rhythm.

The ECG in patients with an atriofascicular bypass tract is notable for several reasons. During sinus rhythm, the ECG usually does not reveal preexcitation because conduction preferentially occurs over the AV node as a result of the long conduction time over the bypass tract. The ECG during ART shows a wide complex tachycardia that resembles a typical left bundle branch block pattern. In addition, the precordial transition occurs relatively late, typically at lead V$_5$.

Electrocardiogram Localization of Accessory Pathways

Resting ECG that shows preexcitation can be very helpful in approximating the location of the AP. This is important as it gives the operator a head start in mapping of the AP. It also allows the electrophysiologist to effectively counsel the patient regarding the risk of AV block when the ECG suggests the presence of a septal AP. Although there are a number of detailed algorithms available to localize the AP, the following simple approach usually suffices. Left free wall APs are associated with positive delta waves in lead V$_1$ and negative delta waves in leads I and aVL. The ECG in a patient with a manifest right-sided AP shows a negative delta wave in lead V$_1$ and positive delta waves in leads I and aVL. The polarity of the delta waves in leads III and aVF is helpful in localizing the AP on the AV annulus. Positive delta waves in these leads indicate an insertion at the anterior, anterolateral, or lateral aspect of the tricuspid or mitral annulus. Conversely, negative delta waves in these leads are consistent with an insertion at the inferior aspect of the AV

valves (e.g., posterior, posterolateral, or posteroseptal aspect of the tricuspid or mitral annulus).

For anteroseptal and midseptal APs, a few additional observations are helpful. Typically, a negative delta wave is present in lead V$_1$ in patients with anteroseptal and midseptal APs. Septal APs may be distinguished from right free wall pathways if the precordial QRS transition (negative to positive) occurs at or before lead V$_3$. If the transition occurs between V$_3$ and V$_4$, then the amplitude of the delta wave in lead II is examined. An amplitude ≥1.0 mV is consistent with a septal AP, whereas an amplitude <1.0 mV suggests a right free wall connection. In a patient whose ECG is consistent with a posteroseptal AP, a steeply negative delta wave in lead II is suggestive of an epicardial connection.

Management

The acute treatment of SVT in the emergency room is straightforward. Patients without hemodynamic instability can be treated with intravenous adenosine, a highly effective agent with an extremely short half-life. Although the risks for adenosine and other AV nodal–blocking agents in preexcited AF patients are well known, caution should also be exercised in patients with narrow QRS complex tachycardia. Adenosine can induce AF in about 10% of patients undergoing electrophysiological evaluation for SVT. If a patient presenting to the emergency room with a narrow QRS complex tachycardia also has manifest preexcitation during sinus rhythm (which may not be known until sinus rhythm is restored), adenosine administration may result in AF with a very rapid ventricular response and hemodynamic deterioration. Therefore, when administering adenosine in this situation, emergency resuscitation equipment and appropriately trained personnel should be available. Patients presenting with narrow QRS complex tachycardia who have a history of asthma should not receive adenosine and should be treated with intravenous calcium blockers. Patients with preexcited AF who are hemodynamically stable may be treated with intravenous procainamide or ibutilide. Patients who present with hemodynamic instability should undergo urgent direct current cardioversion.

Long-term treatment of SVT patients should be individualized. In a patient with a first episode or infrequent, well-tolerated episodes of tachycardia and no evidence of preexcitation on the

ECG, abortive maneuvers and reassurance are reasonable options. Alternatively, these patients may be offered a "pill-in-the-pocket" approach, which involves self-administration of oral AV nodal agents at the onset of symptoms. If the patient prefers, an electrophysiological procedure also is a reasonable option. Patients with recurrent SVT should be considered for an electrophysiological evaluation and catheter ablation.

SVT in association with ventricular preexcitation is considered a class I indication for an electrophysiological evaluation and catheter ablation.[2] Catheter ablation is highly effective in eliminating AP conduction, thereby eliminating symptoms caused by SVT and the small risk for sudden death associated with WPW syndrome. WPW syndrome patients in whom ablation would likely result in a high-grade AV block should be treated with a combination of rhythm- and rate-controlling medications.

An observational study suggested that the outcome of patients with their initial presentation of WPW syndrome was benign as long as there was no history of syncope or malignant arrhythmias (syncope, preexcited AF with an RR interval ≤250 ms, or ventricular fibrillation [VF]). These patients (369 of 8575 patients) underwent an electrophysiological study but declined catheter ablation.[3] The investigators identified high-risk features, including a short AP effective refractory period, inducible AVRT triggering preexcited AF, and the presence of multiple APs. In the absence of high-risk clinical or electrophysiological features, patients with an initial manifestation of AP-mediated arrhythmias seem to fare well during long-term follow-up.

Asymptomatic Individuals

Because the risk for a malignant presentation in asymptomatic patients with a WPW pattern has been considered to be low, many clinicians recommended a conservative approach. In fact, the previous guidelines for the management of SVT patients considered "no treatment" as a class I recommendation in people with asymptomatic preexcitation. However, recent studies have led to a modification of recommendations for such individuals. A randomized study from Italy showed that prophylactic catheter ablation among "high-risk" individuals (defined as <35 years old with inducible AVRT or AF) was associated with a reduction in adverse arrhythmic outcomes.[4] A more recent observational study also suggested that an electrophysiological evaluation in asymptomatic preexcitation patients is useful.[5] Among 2169 patients with WPW pattern/syndrome, 1001 patients (550 patients without symptoms) did not undergo catheter ablation. The incidence of VF was 1.5% in these patients and occurred mostly (13/15 patients) in children (median age, 11 years). The likelihood of experiencing VF was associated with a short AP effective refractory period and AVRT initiating AF. Patients who underwent catheter ablation (N = 1168, including 206 asymptomatic individuals) remained free of malignant arrhythmias. The investigators concluded that the prognosis of patients with WPW pattern/syndrome depends on the conduction properties of the AP as opposed to the presence or absence of symptoms and that risk stratification by electrophysiological study is helpful in optimizing outcomes.

In the absence of large, randomized studies, it is difficult to formulate definitive recommendations in this challenging population. Prior to considering invasive risk stratification, exercise testing should be performed. The abrupt loss of preexcitation during exercise implies that the AP is incapable of rapid conduction during AF and thus confers a lower risk of VF. Such patients usually do not require further evaluation. Patients in whom an abrupt loss of preexcitation cannot be definitively documented may be considered for an electrophysiological evaluation (class IIa).[2] Catheter ablation is also reasonable in such patients if high-risk features (AP effective refractory period <240 ms, shortest preexcited RR interval <250 ms, inducible AF or AVRT, presence of multiple APs, or AVRT leading to preexcited AF) are identified. However, this decision has to be considered in the context of the AP location. For example, if the risk for an AV block is deemed to be high in patients with a midseptal or para-Hisian AP, catheter ablation should probably not be performed.

After discussing the risk for sudden death and the possibility of an electrophysiology procedure and potential ablation, the patient and/or physician may elect to take a conservative approach. In other words, the current guidelines recognize the fact that the vast majority of asymptomatic preexcitation patients have a benign prognosis and that the majority of adverse outcomes occur in children. Thus adult patients without symptoms may be observed without medical therapy or invasive risk stratification (class IIa).[2] Lastly, catheter ablation is also considered reasonable (class IIa) in individuals in whom the presence of an AP is an obstacle in procuring or continuing employment (e.g., in pilots).

Electrophysiological Findings During Sinus Rhythm

In patients referred for an electrophysiological evaluation for PSVT, one may observe several findings during sinus rhythm that support the diagnosis of ORT (Table 77.1). Evidence of preexcitation (HV <35 ms) strongly suggests that the mechanism of the tachycardia is ORT. If the delta wave is subtle, atrial pacing is helpful in accentuating the preexcitation. In a patient with

---

TABLE 77.1 Positive predictive value and prevalence of baseline observations and tachycardia features for the tachycardia mechanism during an electrophysiology study for paroxysmal supraventricular tachycardia

BASELINE OBSERVATIONS AND TACHYCARDIA FEATURES	PREVALENCE (%)	POSITIVE PREDICTIVE VALUE (%)		
		AVNRT	ORT	AT
Preexcitation present during sinus rhythm	15	10	86	3
Extranodal response to para-Hisian pacing	18	17	83	0
VA block cycle length >600 ms at baseline	11	41	5	55
Septal VA interval >70 ms	53	17	59	24
Eccentric atrial activation	31	0	76	24
Spontaneous AV block during tachycardia	10	60	0	40
Spontaneous termination with AV block	28	66	34	0
Development of LBBB	12	4	92	4
Increase in VA interval >20 ms with BBB	7	0	100	0

AT, Atrial tachycardia; *AV,* atrioventricular; *AVNRT,* atrioventricular nodal reentrant tachycardia; *BBB,* bundle branch block; *LBBB,* left bundle branch block; *ORT,* orthodromic reciprocating tachycardia; *VA,* ventriculoatrial.

an atriofascicular or a nodoventricular connection, atrial pacing results in a gradual increase in preexcitation that is accompanied by a progressive increase in the stimulus delta wave and atrial-His (AH) intervals, which are hallmarks of a decrementally conducting AP (Fig. 77.3).

Evidence of eccentric atrial activation during ventricular pacing also supports the diagnosis of ORT. The absence of ventriculoatrial (VA) conduction makes ORT extremely unlikely. Rarely, isoproterenol may facilitate retrograde AP conduction in patients with VA dissociation at baseline.

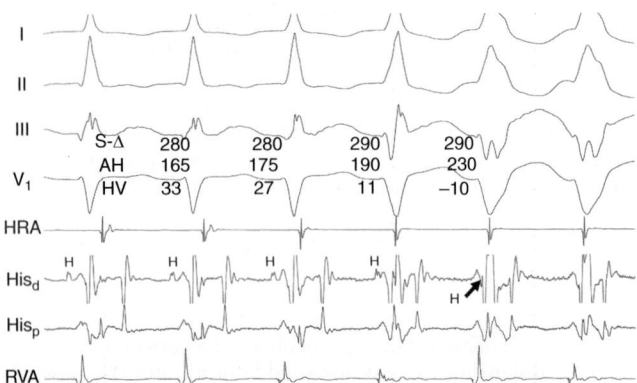

FIGURE 77.3 Example of decremental conduction properties of an atriofascicular accessory pathway. During atrial pacing at 330 ms, there is evidence of progressive prolongation in the stimulus-delta (S-Δ) and atrial-His (AH) intervals. Concomitantly, there is a gradual increase in the degree of ventricular preexcitation as evidenced by widening of the QRS complex and a decrease in the HV interval. *HRA,* High right atrium; *RVA,* right ventricular apex.

Para-Hisian pacing is very helpful for determining whether retrograde conduction is occurring over the AV node versus a septal AP.[6] A minimum of two catheters is required for this maneuver—one at the His bundle position and another in the atrium. High-output pacing is performed, and the stimulus-atrial time is analyzed with and without His bundle capture. A relatively narrow QRS complex is inscribed when both the specialized conduction system and the basal right ventricular myocardium are captured (Fig. 77.4). At a lower output, only the ventricular myocardium is captured because of the higher capture threshold of the His bundle, yielding a relatively wide QRS. If the stimulus-atrial time is the same irrespective of the His bundle capture, it indicates retrograde conduction over a septal AP. In an "AV nodal" response to para-Hisian pacing, the stimulus-atrial interval is longer when the His bundle is not captured. In the absence of a septal AP, the atria can only be activated after depolarization of the right ventricular myocardium, followed by engagement of the His–Purkinje system, the His bundle, and finally, the AV node. During His bundle capture, atrial activation occurs earlier because the wavefront travels to the atrium from the very proximal aspect of the specialized conduction system (as opposed to originating from the RV apical pacing site). Para-Hisian pacing is also helpful for determining whether a septal pathway has been successfully ablated (see Fig. 77.4).

Occasionally, the response to para-Hisian pacing can be confusing. If the stimulus-atrial electrogram interval is extremely short, one should suspect direct atrial capture with high-output pacing. The catheter should be advanced further across the tricuspid annulus, and the maneuver should be repeated. It is also worth noting that high-output pacing may result in "pure" His capture. As a result, the paced QRS complex will be narrow, and the stimulus to a ventricular electrogram interval will approximate the HV interval.[7]

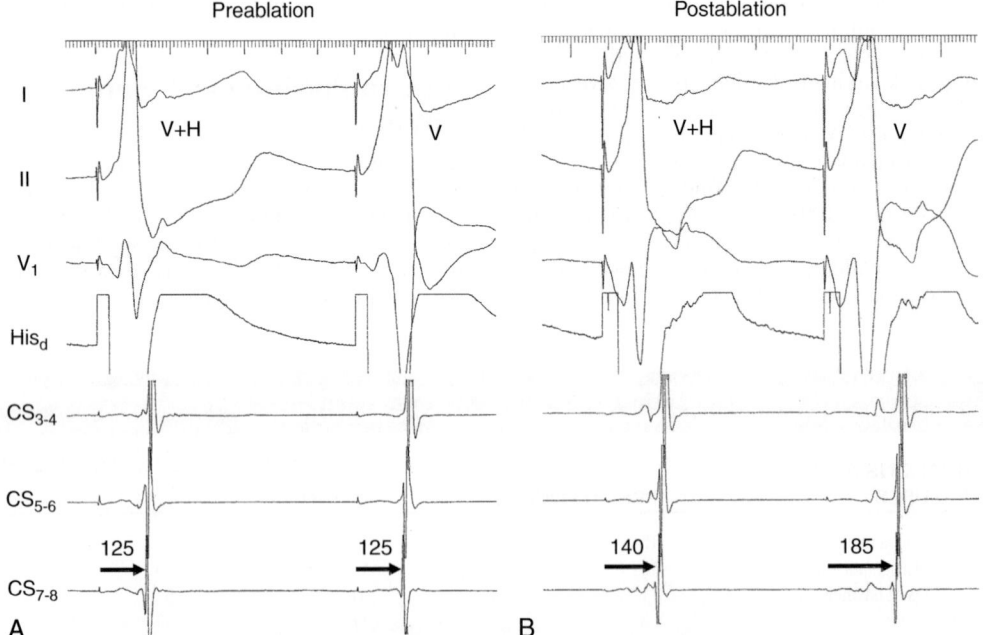

FIGURE 77.4 Response to para-Hisian pacing in a patient with a concealed anteroseptal accessory pathway (AP). (A) The QRS complex is narrower when both the ventricular myocardium and His bundle (*V+H*) are captured. The stimulus-atrial (S-A) electrogram interval is 125 ms irrespective of whether the ventricle (*V*) or the ventricle and His bundle are captured, consistent with retrograde activation over the AP. *CS,* Coronary sinus. (B) Para-Hisian pacing in the same patient as in (A) after ablation of the anteroseptal AP. The S-A interval during the ventricular plus His bundle (*V+H*) capture is 140 ms, which is shorter than when there is ventricular capture only (185 ms). This observation is consistent with retrograde conduction over the atrioventricular node and confirms that AP conduction has been eliminated.

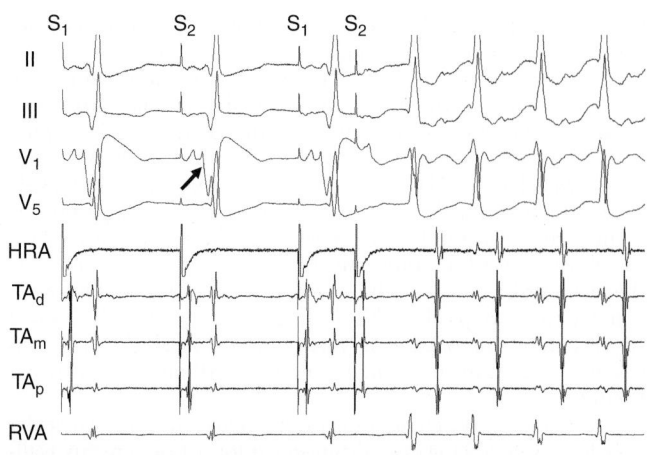

FIGURE 77.5 Initiation of orthodromic reciprocating tachycardia during programmed atrial stimulation. During the drive train (S_1 = 700 ms), there is a short PR interval and slurred QRS complex (*arrow*), consistent with ventricular preexcitation. With the introduction of S_2 (330 ms), there is a block in the accessory pathway and conduction over the specialized conduction system, initiating tachycardia. *HRA,* High right atrium; *RVA,* right ventricular apex; *TA,* tricuspid annulus.

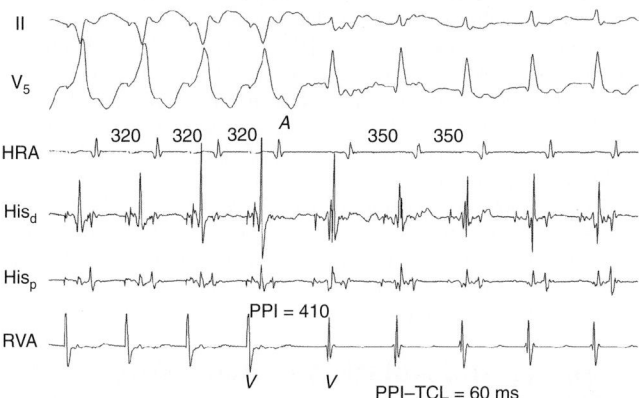

FIGURE 77.6 Value of the postpacing interval (*PPI*). Ventricular overdrive pacing accelerates the tachycardia (cycle length, 350 ms) to the paced cycle length (320 ms). An atrioventricular response, on the cessation of pacing, rules out atrial tachycardia. Furthermore, PPI–tachycardia cycle length (*PPI–TCL*) is 60 ms (i.e., <115 ms), ruling out atrioventricular nodal reentrant tachycardia and supporting the diagnosis of orthodromic reciprocating tachycardia. *HRA,* High right atrium; *RVA,* right ventricular apex.

Electrophysiological Findings During Tachycardia

Induction of tachycardia that is dependent on anterograde conduction block in the AP is very suggestive of ORT as the mechanism (Fig. 77.5). A change in the atrial cycle length that is predicted by a change in the preceding ventricular cycle length favors the diagnosis of ORT or typical AVNRT, as opposed to atrial tachycardia or atypical AVNRT.[8] Entrainment of SVT during ventricular overdrive pacing is very helpful for elucidating the mechanism of tachycardia.[9] An atrial-ventricular (A-V) response after cessation of pacing that has entrained the tachycardia rules out atrial tachycardia, leaving AVNRT (or automatic junctional tachycardia) and ORT as possibilities (Fig. 77.6). Thereafter, one may employ a number of other observations/ maneuvers to distinguish between these possibilities. If the high right atrial electrogram is recorded within or at the end of the QRS complex, ORT may be ruled out because atrial activation can only occur following ventricular activation during

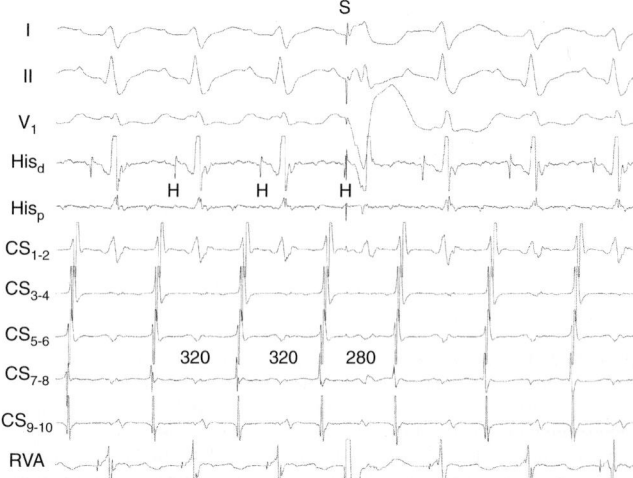

FIGURE 77.7 Introduction of a His (*H*)-synchronous ventricular extrastimulus during supraventricular tachycardia. The atrial electrogram following the ventricular extrastimulus (*S*) is advanced by 40 ms, consistent with the presence of an accessory pathway. *CS,* Coronary sinus; *RVA,* right ventricular apex.

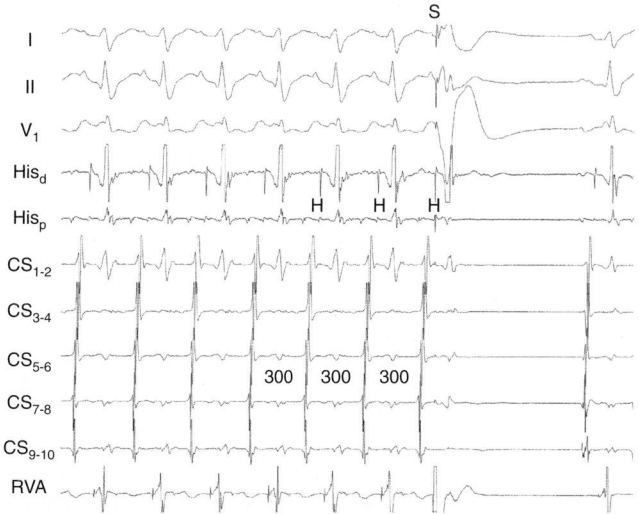

FIGURE 77.8 Termination of a supraventricular tachycardia with a His (*H*)-synchronous ventricular complex (*S*), without affecting the atrial electrogram. This observation is diagnostic of orthodromic reciprocating tachycardia. *CS,* Coronary sinus; *RVA,* right ventricular apex.

ORT. More precisely, a VA time less than 70 ms measured in the His-bundle electrogram is an argument against ORT.[10] If atrial activation is not simultaneous with ventricular activation, a His-synchronous ventricular extrastimulus is delivered during tachycardia. If the timing of the atrial electrogram following the extrastimulus is altered, an extranodal AP is present, consistent with the diagnosis of ORT. A number of responses are possible. The atrial electrogram may be advanced (Fig. 77.7) or delayed, or the tachycardia may be terminated in the retrograde limb without affecting the atrial electrogram (Fig. 77.8). The latter finding is diagnostic of ORT. Failure to affect the tachycardia with a His-synchronous ventricular extrastimulus does not rule out ORT in a patient with an AP located remote from the right ventricular pacing site (e.g., a left free wall pathway).

An intermittent bundle branch block during SVT may provide important clues regarding the mechanism of the tachycardia. Prolongation of the VA interval during bundle branch block is diagnostic of ORT, utilizing an AP that is ipsilateral to the bundle

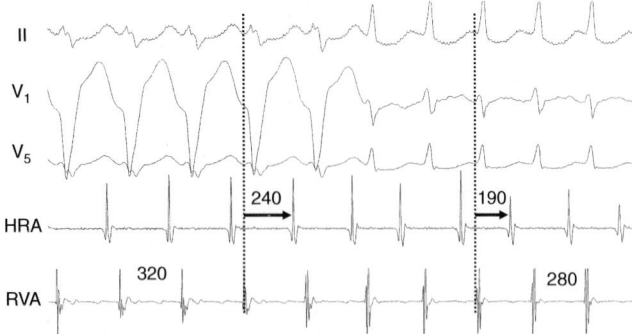

FIGURE 77.9 Change in ventriculoatrial time with a left bundle branch block during supraventricular tachycardia. This tachycardia occurred during catheter placement in a patient undergoing electrophysiological testing. The ventriculoatrial interval during left bundle branch block (240 ms) is longer than when the QRS complex is narrow (190 ms), which is diagnostic of orthodromic reciprocating tachycardia, utilizing a left free wall accessory pathway. *HRA,* High right atrium; *RVA,* right ventricular apex.

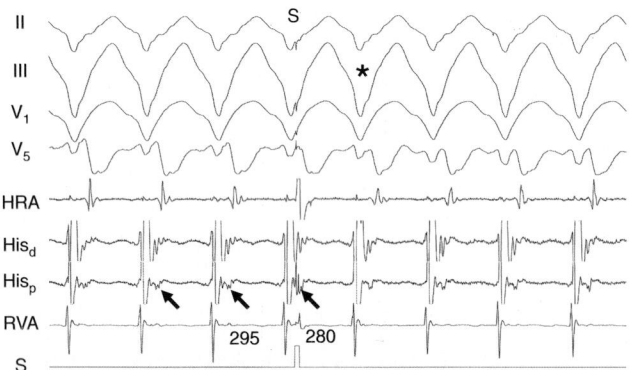

FIGURE 77.10 Antidromic reciprocating tachycardia. There is no evidence of activation of the His bundle, consistent with anterograde activation over an accessory pathway. An atrial extrastimulus is introduced at a time when the atrioventricular node should be refractory (*arrows* indicate the atrial electrogram recorded by the catheter at the His position). The following QRS complex (*asterisk*) is advanced with no change in the QRS morphology, consistent with the diagnosis of antidromic reciprocating tachycardia. *HRA,* High right atrium; *RVA,* right ventricular apex; *S,* stimulus.

branch block (Fig. 77.9). Specifically, if the VA time prolongs by more than 30 ms during the bundle branch block, the tachycardia is using a free wall AP. Prolongation of the VA interval less than 30 ms is consistent with a left posteroseptal tract when there is a left bundle branch block and an anteroseptal pathway when there is a right bundle branch block.

Several clues are helpful in making the diagnosis of ART. First, ECG during tachycardia shows a wide-complex rhythm in which the QRS does not resemble a typical left or right bundle branch block pattern and is identical to the maximally preexcited QRS during atrial pacing. Second, because ventricular activation occurs only over the AP and not through the His bundle, an anterograde His bundle potential is not inscribed prior to the local ventricular electrogram in the His bundle electrogram. Further, because in most cases of ART retrograde atrial activation occurs over the AV node, the His bundle is activated in a retrograde fashion. The most helpful maneuver is to insert an atrial extrastimulus at the time when the AV node should be refractory. If the subsequent ventricular electrogram is advanced with a QRS morphology identical to that during tachycardia, anterograde conduction over an AP is assured (Fig. 77.10). Resetting of the

tachycardia indicates that the AP is part of the tachycardia circuit and is not an "innocent bystander."

In distinguishing atypical AVNRT ("fast/slow") from ORT using a septal AP, the postpacing interval after the cessation of ventricular pacing that has entrained the tachycardia is helpful. If the difference between the postpacing interval and the tachycardia cycle length is less than 115 ms, the diagnosis is very likely to be ORT (see Fig. 77.6).[11] Because the ventricle is a part of the reentry circuit in ORT, the return cycle should be shorter than that during AVNRT. Alternatively, if the postpacing interval less the tachycardia cycle length is greater than 115 ms, the diagnosis is likely to be atypical AVNRT. In some cases of ORT using a slowly conducting AP, the difference may be greater than 115 ms because of decremental conduction in the AP during ventricular pacing.

Occasionally, the tachycardia may terminate during ventricular overdrive pacing. However, diagnostic information remains available in this setting that can help distinguish ORT from atypical ("fast-slow") AVNRT. During ventricular overdrive pacing, the operator observes how readily the tachycardia can be reset with respect to the degree of QRS fusion.[12] If the tachycardia is reset with the first fixed morphology QRS complex, the mechanism is very likely to be ORT. If resetting occurs after ≥2 beats of the fixed RV–paced QRS morphology, the mechanism is atypical AVNRT.

Alternatively, one may also compare the atrial-His intervals during tachycardia and atrial pacing (ΔAH) to distinguish between various causes of a long RP tachycardia. If the AH interval during atrial pacing at the tachycardia cycle length exceeds that during tachycardia by more than 40 ms, atypical AVNRT is much more likely than ORT (using a slow conduction AP) or atrial tachycardia. In contrast, a ΔAH of 10 to 20 ms favors either ORT or atrial tachycardia.

Ventricular burst pacing during tachycardia may also provide some insight into the mechanism of the tachycardia. Dissociation of the atrial electrogram during ventricular pacing rules out ORT. Termination of the tachycardia without affecting the timing of the atrial electrogram makes atrial tachycardia very unlikely.

Mapping and Ablation of Accessory Pathways

Mapping in patients with a concealed AP is best performed during ORT. One may also map the pathway during ventricular pacing. However, ventricular pacing in a patient with a septal AP is not helpful because the operator is unable to distinguish between retrograde AV nodal and AP conduction. In patients with a manifest AP, mapping may be performed in sinus rhythm, atrial pacing, or ORT.

One must be aware of the fact that many APs have an oblique course along the AV annulus.[6] In other words, the earliest atrial activation during ORT or ventricular pacing and the earliest ventricular activation during sinus rhythm may not occur at the same point along the annulus. Confusion is avoided in most cases by targeting the earliest atrial activation when the mapping catheter is on the atrial side of the annulus and mapping for earliest ventricular activation when the ablation catheter is on the ventricular side of the annulus. If radiofrequency (RF) current is being delivered during ORT, it is helpful to do so during ventricular pacing at a similar cycle length as that of the tachycardia. This helps prevent sudden catheter dislodgement as the tachycardia terminates to sinus rhythm.

Patients who undergo catheter ablation of septal bypass tracts may be at a risk for developing AV block. In a patient with an anteroseptal AP, this risk may be minimized by targeting the pathway at the noncoronary cusp of the aortic valve (Fig. 77.11). An aortogram and/or coronary angiography is helpful for delineating the relevant anatomy. Analysis of the local electrogram can also help distinguish between the noncoronary and the right and left coronary cusps. Because there is no direct relationship

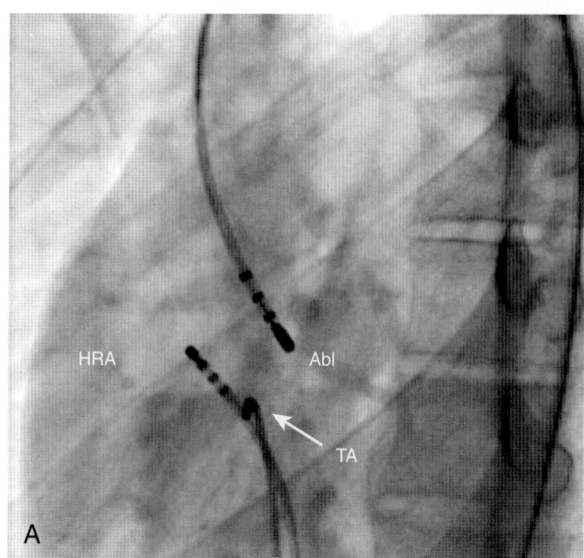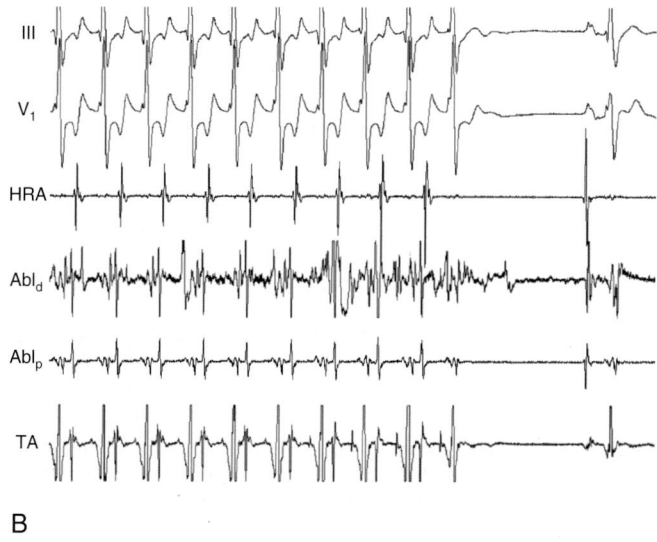

FIGURE 77.11 (A) Cinefluoroscopic view (left anterior oblique) that shows the position of the ablation catheter (*Abl*) during radiofrequency ablation of a concealed anteroseptal accessory pathway at the noncoronary cusp of the aortic valve. (B) Termination of orthodromic reciprocating tachycardia during radiofrequency energy delivery at the noncoronary cusp in the same patient as in (A). Note that there is no junctional ectopy during energy delivery. *HRA*, High right atrium; *TA*, catheter at the anterior tricuspid annulus, near the His bundle.

between the noncoronary cusp and the ventricular myocardium, the electrode records a large atrial electrogram and only a far-field ventricular electrogram. Cryoablation is another option in patients with septal APs. If a septal AP cannot be eliminated without an AV block, it may be best to defer ablation and treat the patient with antiarrhythmic therapy.

Catheter ablation of right free wall APs may be challenging for a variety of reasons. Catheter stability is often suboptimal at the lateral, anterolateral, and anterior tricuspid annulus. A deflectable sheath can overcome this limitation. In addition, general anesthesia is associated with enhanced catheter stability and higher contact force at the target site. Occasionally, the atrial insertion of these pathways may be found a few centimeters from the tricuspid annulus or even in the right atrial appendage. Using a three-dimensional mapping system may be helpful in these cases.[13]

The mapping technique for an atriofascicular bypass tract is different than for typical AV APs. Atriofascicular bypass tracts are best mapped during sinus rhythm by seeking a high-frequency atriofascicular potential between the atrial and ventricular electrograms. The effective target site typically lies between 7 and 11 o'clock in the left anterior oblique view on the tricuspid annulus. Atriofascicular potentials are present during sinus rhythm even when there is no ventricular preexcitation and also during antidromic tachycardia. Ablation at the site of an atriofascicular potential is often accompanied by pathway automaticity.

Ablation of Left-Sided Accessory Pathways

For mapping and ablation of left-sided APs, two approaches are available to the operator: either an anterograde transseptal or a retrograde aortic approach. For anterolateral, lateral, and posterolateral left-sided APs, the transseptal approach is preferable because of the ease of catheter manipulation. For posteroseptal and posterior left-sided APs, the retrograde aortic approach may be preferred because of catheter stability in this region. The main disadvantage of the retrograde approach is a longer vascular recovery time. Occasionally (<5% of cases), one may encounter the need for an epicardial approach to ablation of a challenging AP. If endocardial mapping does identify a suitable target in a patient with a posteroseptal, left posterior, or left

lateral AP, the coronary sinus (CS) and its branches should be mapped. Prior to delivering RF energy within the CS, coronary angiography should be performed to delineate the relationship between the AP and the branch of the coronary artery. If the insertion site of the AP lies within 5 mm of a coronary artery branch, there is a significant risk for injury to the coronary artery.[14] In this setting, cryoablation may be safer, albeit less effective. Repeat angiography should be performed in this setting to verify the integrity of the coronary arteries after ablation. If an appropriate target site cannot be identified in the CS venous system, mapping and ablation within the pericardial space may be required.

Patients With Prior Procedures

Not uncommonly, patients may be referred for a repeat session in case of a challenging procedure. As has been shown in a number of studies, suboptimal mapping is probably the major reason that an AP ablation procedure is unsuccessful. Some pathways that are considered to be "anteroseptal" in location may actually insert at the anterior tricuspid annulus (12 o'clock on the tricuspid annulus) (i.e., lateral to the bundle of His) and thus can be safely ablated without injury to the conduction system.

Prior to embarking on a repeat session in a patient who has previously undergone ablation of a septal AP, it is important to document the presence of AV nodal conduction. The presence of ORT on an event monitor or ECG is sufficient in this regard. Otherwise, it is critical to do so during an electrophysiological study prior to the delivery of RF current. If the AV node was injured during the prior procedure, ablation of the pathway can result in complete AV block (Fig. 77.12) and the need for a permanent pacemaker. It is important to discuss this possibility with the patient and family, especially because most WPW syndrome patients are young. A permanent pacemaker in these patients can have important long-term ramifications.

Although catheter ablation of left free wall APs is usually straightforward, occasionally patients may experience recurrence of AP conduction or may have "multiple" APs. During the repeat procedure, one may observe findings that suggest ORT using a septal AP; for example, proximal-to-distal activation of the CS,

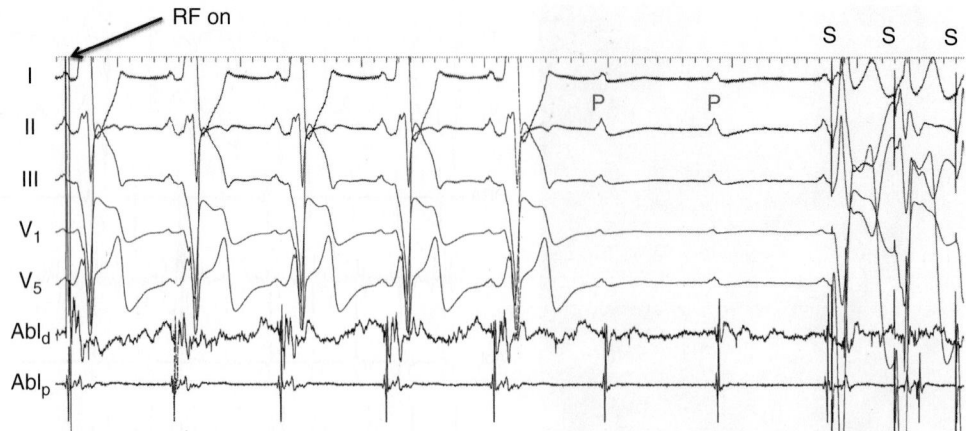

FIGURE 77.12 Atrioventricular (AV) block following ablation (*Abl*) of a posteroseptal accessory pathway (AP) in a patient who previously underwent three ablation procedures at another facility for Wolff-Parkinson-White syndrome. He presented to the hospital with preexcited atrial fibrillation and syncope. The electrocardiogram during rapidly conducted atrial fibrillation showed no evidence of fusion, and hence it was suspected that the AV node had been injured during the prior attempts. Prior to the procedure at our institution, we had discussed the possibility of a permanent pacemaker in case of the lack of AV nodal conduction after elimination of the AP. As shown in this tracing, radiofrequency (*RF*) energy delivery outside the ostium of the coronary sinus quickly eliminated AP conduction without junctional ectopy. Elimination of the AP unmasked the underlying AV block related to the prior procedure. *S*, Ventricular pacing.

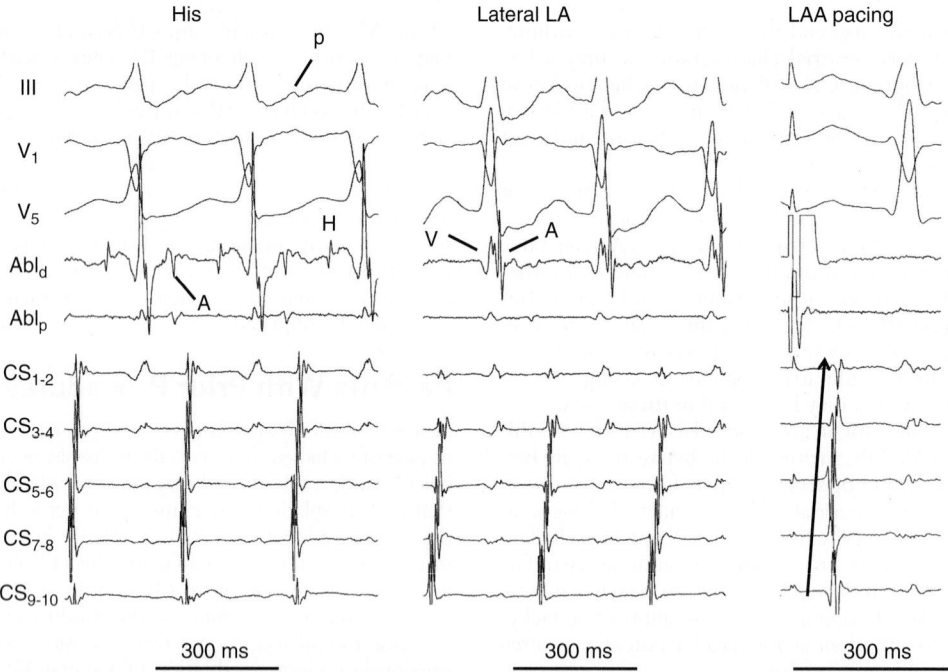

FIGURE 77.13 Orthodromic reciprocating tachycardia (ORT) using a left lateral accessory pathway (AP), masquerading as ORT using a septal AP. This patient underwent catheter ablation (*Abl*) of a concealed lateral AP at another institution and was referred for a "septal" pathway. The *first panel* shows tachycardia (diagnostic maneuvers had confirmed ORT as the mechanism) with concentric activation, consistent with ORT using a septal AP. Prior to ablation at the septum, the lateral left atrium (*LA*) was mapped (*second panel*), which showed a much earlier site immediately below the lateral aspect of the LA appendage (*LAA*). Pacing from LAA (*third panel*) showed proximal-to-distal activation of the coronary sinus (*CS*), consistent with slow conduction instead of the expected distal-to-proximal activation (see Fig. 77.14). *p*, P wave.

and septal atrial electrogram preceding CS activation (Fig. 77.13). However, prior to attempting to ablate a "septal" AP, it is critical to rule out the presence of a left free wall AP. Mapping of the lateral mitral annulus may reveal that the local atrial electrogram is much earlier than the septal or CS electrogram (see Fig.

77.13). RF current delivery at this site is successful in eliminating conduction over the AP (Fig. 77.14). The reason that one observes concentric as opposed to the expected eccentric activation of the CS is that prior ablation at the lateral mitral annulus ("isthmus") results in slow conduction into the lateral left atrium/

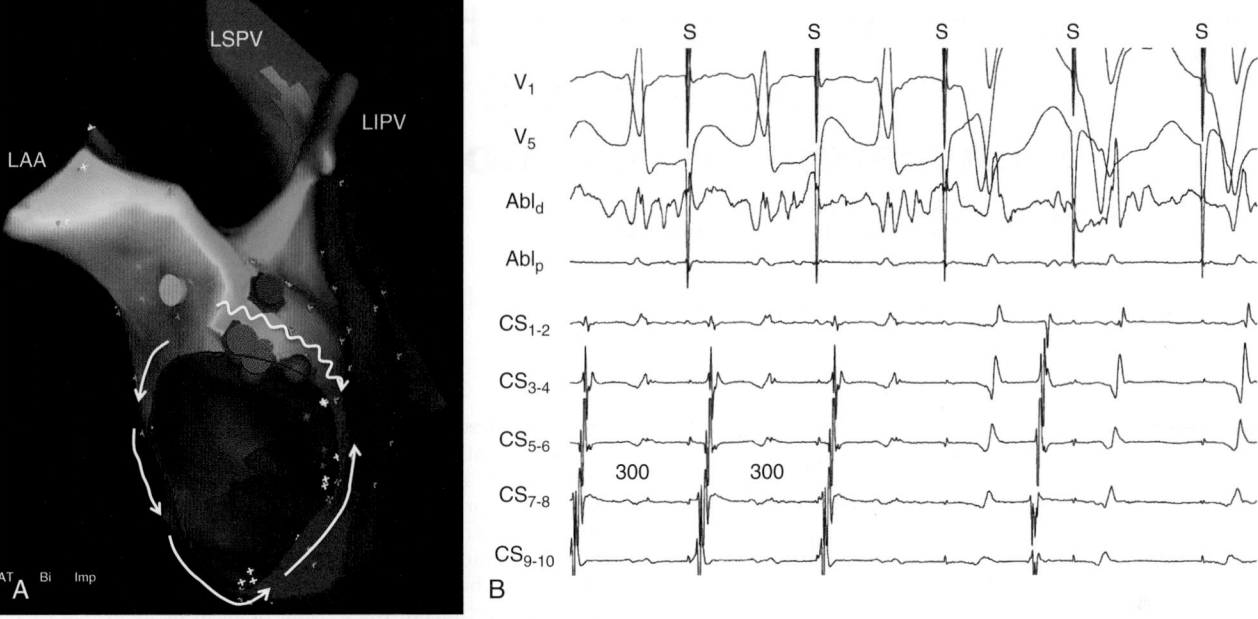

FIGURE 77.14 (A) A three-dimensional activation map of the left atrium during orthodromic reciprocating tachycardia (ORT) in the same patient as in Fig. 77.13. The *yellow tag* denotes the pathway insertion site where radiofrequency (RF) energy delivery eliminated the accessory pathway conduction and ORT. Note the presence of scar at the lateral annulus because of a prior ablation, which results in proximal-to-distal activation of the coronary sinus (*CS*), instead of the expected distal-to-proximal activation. (B) Termination of ORT during RF energy delivery. To enhance catheter stability, RF energy was delivered during ventricular pacing (*S*). There is ventriculoatrial dissociation after termination of ORT. *Abl*, Ablation; *LAA*, left atrial appendage; *LSPV/LIPV*, left superior/left inferior pulmonary vein.

distal CS complex, such that the CS is activated in a proximal-to-distal fashion (see Figs. 77.13 and 77.14). Being prepared for this possibility may help avoid AV block while attempting to target a "septal" AP.

Outcome of Ablation

Catheter ablation of APs has been shown to be highly effective and is associated with a low risk for complications. Among 6065 patients pooled from several electrophysiology laboratories, catheter ablation resulted in a successful long-term outcome in 98% of patients.[15] A repeat procedure was required in about 2% of patients. A serious complication (e.g., tamponade, AV block, coronary artery injury, retroperitoneal hemorrhage, or stroke) occurred in 0.6% of patients. There was one fatality (0.02%) in this series. Therefore the one-time risk for an ablation procedure compares favorably with the cumulative risk for sudden death in WPW syndrome patients (3%–4%).

Summary

AV reentry is the most common arrhythmia in WPW syndrome patients. It also accounts for approximately one-third of the cases among patients referred for electrophysiological evaluation for PSVT. AVRT utilizes both the specialized conduction system and the AP, which typically inserts at the AV annulus. Catheter ablation of APs is highly effective and is associated with a low risk of complications. Catheter ablation is the treatment of choice in patients with WPW syndrome and in those with recurrent SVT mediated by a concealed AP.

REFERENCES

1. Sternick EB, Oliva A, Gerken LM, et al. Clinical, electrocardiographic, and electrophysiologic characteristics of patients with a fasciculoventricular pathway: the role of PRKAG2 mutation. *Heart Rhythm.* 2011;8:58–64.
2. Page RL, Joglar JA, Caldwell MA, et al. 2015 ACC/AHA/HRS Guideline for the Management of Adult Patients With Supraventricular Tachycardia: a Report of the American College of Cardiology/American Heart Association Task Force on Clinical Practice Guidelines and the Heart Rhythm Society. *J Am Coll Cardiol.* 2016;67:e27–e115.
3. Pappone C, Vicedomini G, Manguso F, et al. Risk of malignant arrhythmias in initially symptomatic patients with Wolff-Parkinson-White syndrome: results of a prospective long-term electrophysiological follow-up study. *Circulation.* 2012;125:661–668.
4. Pappone C, Santinelli V, Manguso F, et al. A randomized study of prophylactic catheter ablation in asymptomatic patients with the Wolff-Parkinson-White syndrome. *N Engl J Med.* 2003;349:1803–1811.
5. Pappone C, Vicedomini G, Manguso F, et al. Wolff-Parkinson-White syndrome in the era of catheter ablation:

insights from a registry study of 2169 patients. *Circulation.* 2014;130:811–819.
6. Nakagawa H, Jackman WM. Catheter ablation of paroxysmal supraventricular tachycardia. *Circulation.* 2007;116:2465–2478.
7. Takatsuki S, Mitamura H, Tanimoto K, et al. Clinical implications of "pure" Hisian pacing in addition to para-Hisian pacing for the diagnosis of supraventricular tachycardia. *Heart Rhythm.* 2006;3:1412–1418.
8. Crawford TC, Mukerji S, Good E, et al. Utility of atrial and ventricular cycle length variability in determining the mechanism of paroxysmal supraventricular tachycardia. *J Cardiovasc Electrophysiol.* 2007;18:698–703.
9. Knight BP, Morady F. Atrioventricular reentry and variants. In: Zipes DP, Jalife J, eds. *Cardiac Electrophysiology: from Cell to Bedside.* 4th ed. WB Saunders; 2004: 528–536.
10. Knight BP, Ebinger M, Oral H, et al. Diagnostic value of tachycardia features and pacing maneuvers during paroxysmal supraventricular tachycardia. *J Am Coll Cardiol.* 2000;36:574–582.

11. Michaud GF, Tada H, Chough S, et al. Differentiation of atypical atrioventricular node re-entrant tachycardia from orthodromic reciprocating tachycardia using a septal accessory pathway by the response to ventricular pacing. *J Am Coll Cardiol.* 2001;38:1163–1167.
12. Dandamudi G, Mokabberi R, Assal C, et al. A novel approach to differentiating orthodromic reciprocating tachycardia from atrioventricular nodal reentrant tachycardia. *Heart Rhythm.* 2010;7:1326–1329.
13. Long DY, Dong JZ, Liu XP, et al. Ablation of right-sided accessory pathways with atrial insertion far from the tricuspid annulus using an electroanatomical mapping system. *J Cardiovasc Electrophysiol.* 2011;22:499–505.
14. Stavrakis S, Jackman WM, Nakagawa H, et al. Risk of coronary artery injury with radiofrequency ablation and cryoablation of epicardial posteroseptal accessory pathways within the coronary venous system. *Circ Arrhythm Electrophysiol.* 2014;7:113–119.
15. Morady F. Catheter ablation of supraventricular arrhythmias: state of the art. *J Cardiovasc Electrophysiol.* 2004;15: 124–139.

78

Electrophysiological Characteristics of Atrioventricular Nodal Reentrant Tachycardia: Implications for the Reentrant Circuits

Deborah J. Lockwood, Hiroshi Nakagawa, and Warren M. Jackman

Atrioventricular (AV) nodal reentrant tachycardia (AVNRT) was originally proposed to result from reentry confined within the compact AV node. However, AVNRT is now thought to involve the AV node, at least two atrionodal connections, and a component of the atrial myocardium. Much of our current understanding about the components of the reentrant circuits has evolved from the development of ablation procedures in which one of the atrionodal connections, remote from the compact AV node, is destroyed, eliminating AVNRT without producing AV block.

The multiple forms of AVNRT use different atrionodal connections ("AV nodal pathways") for the anterograde and retrograde limbs of the tachycardia. Traditionally, variants of AVNRT have been distinguished based on the site of earliest retrograde atrial activation and the relative duration of the H-A and A-H intervals into Slow/Fast, Fast/Slow, and Slow/Slow AVNRT. Slow/Fast AVNRT was identified by earliest retrograde atrial activation at the interatrial septum behind the tendon of Todaro (ToT), with long A-H and short H-A intervals. Slow/Slow and Fast/Slow AVNRT were distinguished from Slow/Fast AVNRT by recognizing earliest retrograde activation at the inferior triangle of Koch (ToK) or coronary sinus (CS). Slow/Slow and Fast/Slow AVNRT were then differentiated by the relative duration of the H-A and A-H intervals. In our experience of 734 patients referred for catheter ablation of AVNRT, by this definition, 515 patients (77%) had Slow/Fast AVNRT, 80 patients (11%) had Slow/Slow AVNRT, and 89 patients (12%) had Fast/Slow AVNRT.

Because more is now known about the anatomical substrate for the various forms of AVNRT, the different forms of AVNRT can be distinguished anatomically by the atrionodal connections forming the anterograde and retrograde pathways used in the tachycardia. For greater depth and full bibliography please refer to the fifth edition of this text.[1]

Anatomical Correlates to the Atrionodal Connections

Evidence that the fast pathway (FP) and slow pathways (SPs) involved in the reentrant circuits of AVNRT represent conduction over different atrionodal connections, rather than functional longitudinal dissociation within the compact AV node, includes the following: (1) different sites of earliest atrial activation during retrograde conduction over the FP and each of the SPs, as originally described by Sung and colleagues[2] (Fig. 78.1); (2) the ability of a late extrastimulus delivered to the atrium outside the compact AV node to advance the timing in an anterograde SP (advancing or sometimes delaying the next His bundle potential) and reset the various forms of AVNRT; and (3) the selective elimination of FP or SP conduction by catheter or surgical ablation in the atrium, remote from the compact AV node. The atrial connections of the FP and SPs can be identified by locating the site of earliest atrial activation during selective retrograde conduction over each pathway. These sites are located far from the compact AV node.

Fast Atrioventricular Nodal Pathway

During retrograde FP conduction, right atrial mapping using closely spaced electrodes (1 mm edge-to-edge) records the earliest right atrial activation posterior to the ToT at a level approximately 10 mm inferior to the level recording the proximal His bundle potential (Fig. 78.2). The position posterior to the ToT is confirmed radiographically by leftward deviation of the mapping catheter in the left anterior oblique (LAO) projection (*RA septum* in Fig. 78.2B), indicating that the mapping catheter was not constrained by the tricuspid annulus (TA) and ToT. If the mapping catheter had been positioned across the ToT, the catheter would have been oriented parallel to the His bundle catheter.

During retrograde FP conduction (ventricular pacing or Slow/Fast AVNRT), right atrial activation, beginning posterior to the ToT (outside the ToK), propagates away in the posterior, superior, and inferior directions (*green arrows No. 2* in Fig. 78.3A). Activation propagating inferiorly along the posterior aspect of the eustachian ridge produces an early far-field atrial potential recorded from the inferior aspect of the ToK (A_{Far} in Fig. 78.4). Atrial activation within the ToK (adjacent to the TA) occurs relatively late and proceeds in an inferior-to-superior direction, beginning just outside the CS ostium (*blue arrows No. 6* in Fig. 78.3A and A_{SP} potential in Fig. 78.4) and propagates superiorly, producing a second late atrial potential near the apex of the ToK, occurring 50 to 115 ms after the earliest atrial activation (*2nd A* in Figs. 78.2C and 78.5). The two wavefronts, propagating in opposite directions on either side of the ToT (*green arrow No. 2* and *blue arrow No. 6* in Fig. 78.3A), suggest conduction block across the ToT and eustachian ridge. The timing of the second atrial potential near the apex of the ToK is later than the timing of atrial activation in the inferior ToK (A_{SP} potential recorded between the CS ostium and the TA), which is later than the timing of activation within the proximal CS (see Figs. 78.2C and 78.4). This suggests that the tissue within the ToK is activated by the CS myocardium (*brown arrows* in Fig. 78.3A).

If only the second of the two potentials is recorded on the His bundle electrogram during Slow/Fast AVNRT (see Fig. 78.2C), this may lead to the erroneous impression that activation is earliest at the inferior ToK or in the CS (retrograde SP conduction)

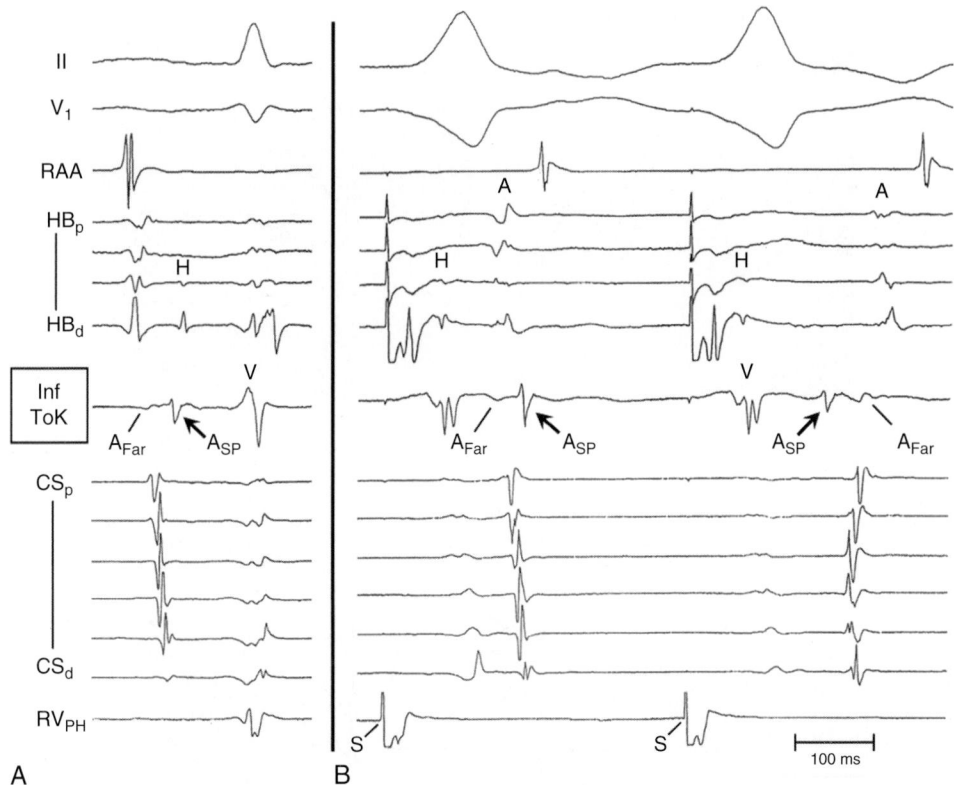

FIGURE 78.1 Different atrial activation sequence during retrograde conduction over the fast pathway (FP) and a slow pathway (SP) formed by the rightward inferior extension (RIE) of the atrioventricular (AV) node. The catheters are in similar positions to those in Fig. 78.4. Recordings from the top are electrocardiography (ECG) leads II and V_1 and electrograms recorded from the right atrial appendage (*RAA*), the His bundle region (proximal to distal, HB_p to HB_d), the inferior triangle of Koch (*Inf ToK*), the coronary sinus (*CS*) (proximal to distal, CS_p to CS_d), and the superior basal aspect of the right ventricle (*RV*) septum close to the proximal right bundle branch (para-Hisian RV, RV_{PH}). (A) During sinus rhythm the anterograde A_{SP} potential was recorded after activation in the proximal CS electrograms (CS_p) and long after septal activation recorded in the His bundle electrogram. (B) Ventricular pacing (*S*) from the para-Hisian RV (RV_{PH}). During retrograde conduction over the FP (first beat), early atrial activation (*A*) is appreciated in the His bundle electrograms (proximal two *HB* electrograms recorded from behind the tendon of Todaro [ToT]). Activation propagates inferiorly behind the eustachian ridge to produce an early far-field potential (A_{Far}) in the *Inf ToK* electrogram. Late activation of the inferior ToK is represented by the sharper A_{SP} potential. Note that the A_{SP} potential is recorded after the timing of activation of the proximal CS myocardium, suggesting that the inferior ToK is activated from the CS. A similar pattern of activation is seen in the *Inf ToK* electrogram during sinus rhythm (A), with an early far-field atrial potential (A_{Far}) followed by a later A_{SP} potential. In the second beat of (B), recorded during retrograde conduction over the SP formed by the RIE, the sharp A_{SP} potential is earliest, with later activation behind the eustachian ridge (A_{Far}) and behind the ToT (*A* potential in the HB_p electrogram). Note that basal septal ventricular pacing from the para-Hisian position, combined with closely spaced bipolar electrodes on the His bundle catheter, results in early completion of the local ventricular potential recorded in the His bundle electrograms and late retrograde activation of the His bundle, allowing visualization of the entire retrograde His bundle potential (*H*).

and may suggest the incorrect diagnosis of Slow/Slow AVNRT. This error can be avoided by mapping behind the ToT as well as along the TA and in the CS to identify the true site of earliest activation during AVNRT (see Fig. 78.2).

Animal studies suggest that the FP may be formed by transitional cells (with action potentials having features intermediate between those of atrial cells and AV nodal cells), which begin in both atria, cross the right and left sides of the ToT, and insert into the AV bundle relatively close to the central fibrous body (i.e., His bundle). As a result, retrograde conduction over the FP results in almost simultaneous activation of both the left and right sides of the interatrial septum.[1,3] The left atrial wavefront propagates around the inferior mitral annulus in the counterclockwise direction, as viewed in the LAO projection (*green arrows No. 3* in Fig. 78.3A), activating the CS myocardium at

the roof, 1 to 2 cm from the CS ostium. CS activation propagates in both lateral and septal directions (*brown arrows No. 4* in Fig. 78.3A). The septally oriented CS wavefront activates the inferior ToK (*brown arrows No. 5* in Fig. 78.3A), resulting in activation in the superior direction in the ToK (*blue arrow No. 6*, A_{SP} in Fig. 78.3A).

A study in isolated perfused canine hearts found that anterograde conduction block in the FP occurred posterior to the ToT.[1] As the atrial pacing rate was increased, block occurred at progressively more proximal locations (i.e., closer to the anterior limbus of the fossa ovalis). Anterograde FP block may therefore occur outside the ToK, which may prevent retrograde invasion of the SP, allowing anterograde conduction over one of the SPs and thus facilitating initiation of Slow/Fast AVNRT and possibly other forms, such as Slow/Slow AVNRT.

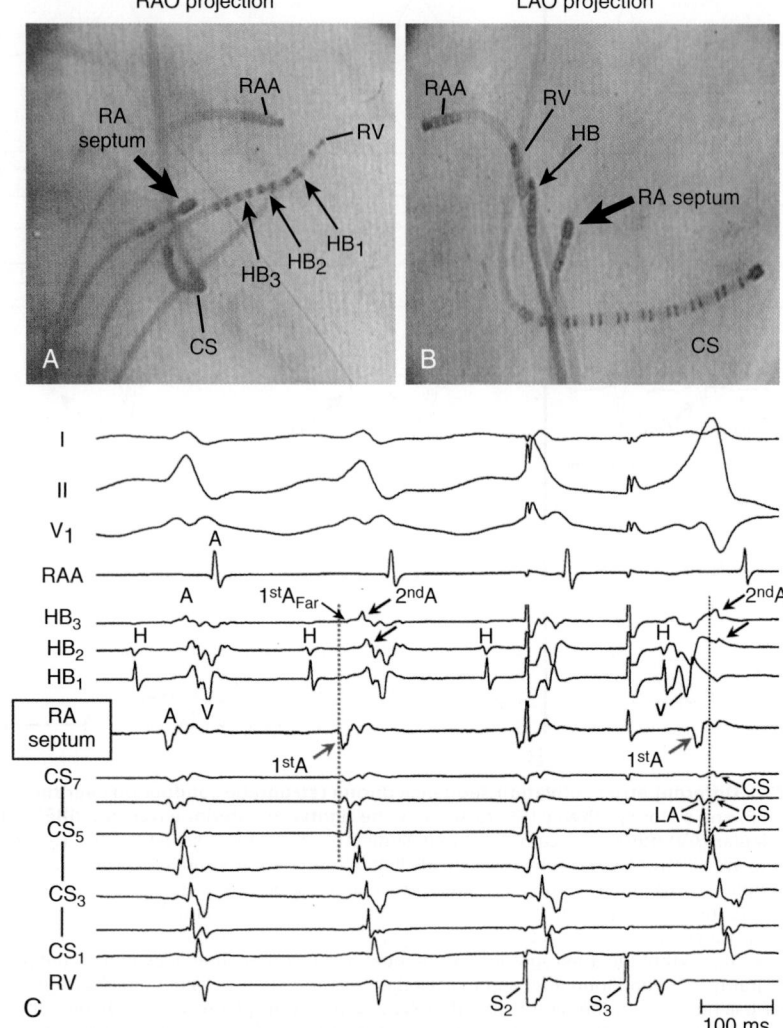

FIGURE 78.2 Pattern of atrial activation during Slow/Fast atrioventricular nodal reentrant tachycardia (AVNRT). (A) and (B) Radiographs in the right anterior oblique (*RAO*) and left anterior oblique (*LAO*) projections, showing the relationship between the His bundle catheter electrodes (*HB* and *HB₁–HB₃*) and catheter electrodes on the right side of the interatrial septum (*RA septum*) at the site recording earliest retrograde atrial activation during Slow/Fast AVNRT. The octapolar His bundle catheter (*HB*) was positioned across the tendon of Todaro (ToT) and tricuspid annulus (TA). The angle for the *LAO projection* was selected to be parallel with the His bundle catheter (looking straight at the tip). The mapping catheter, *RA septum*, was positioned at the site of the earliest retrograde right atrial activation during Slow/Fast AVNRT, approximately 1.5 cm posterior and inferior to the site recording the most proximal His bundle activation (*HB₂*). In the LAO projection, the mapping catheter (*RA septum*) is deviated leftward of the His bundle catheter, confirming a location posterior to the ToT, not constrained by the tricuspid annulus. (C) Bipolar electrograms (filter 30–500 Hz) recorded with closely spaced electrodes. There are two potentials recorded from the His bundle–RA septum region. The first potential (*1ˢᵗ A, arrows*) was recorded behind the ToT (*RA septum*). This was the site of earliest activation found during mapping of the right atrium and coronary sinus (*CS*). A far-field first potential was recorded in the *HB₃* electrogram (*1ˢᵗ A_Far, small arrow*). The second potential (*2ⁿᵈ A*) was recorded near the apex of the ToK (electrograms *HB₃* and *HB₂*). Note that *2ⁿᵈ A* propagates in the inferior-to-superior direction (*HB₃* then *HB₂, arrows*) and is recorded after CS myocardial activation (electrograms *CS₅–CS₇*) and 40 ms after earliest atrial activation recorded behind the ToT (*1ˢᵗ A*).

Rightward Inferior Extension

At least four atrionodal connections other than the FP participate in various forms of AVNRT, and these atrionodal connections have generally been labeled as SPs. The SP most commonly used in either the anterograde or retrograde direction is formed by the rightward inferior extension (RIE) of the AV node (Fig. 78.6).[4] Detailed mapping during retrograde conduction over the RIE suggests that this structure extends over a long length (*blue arrows* in Fig. 78.3B) and connects selectively to

the *floor of the CS ostium* (to connect with the left atrium via the CS myocardium, *brown arrows No. 3* in Fig. 78.3B). The eustachian ridge forms a complete line of block to prevent the right atrium from being activated from the ToK (*green line* parallel to the eustachian ridge [*ER*] in *RAO projection* of Fig. 78.3B). The earliest retrograde high-frequency potential (A_SP potential) is recorded at the inferior ToK between the TA and the CS ostium (second complex in Figs. 78.1B and 78.7B, *blue arrow No. 2* in Fig. 78.3B). Activation is then recorded at the *floor* of the CS

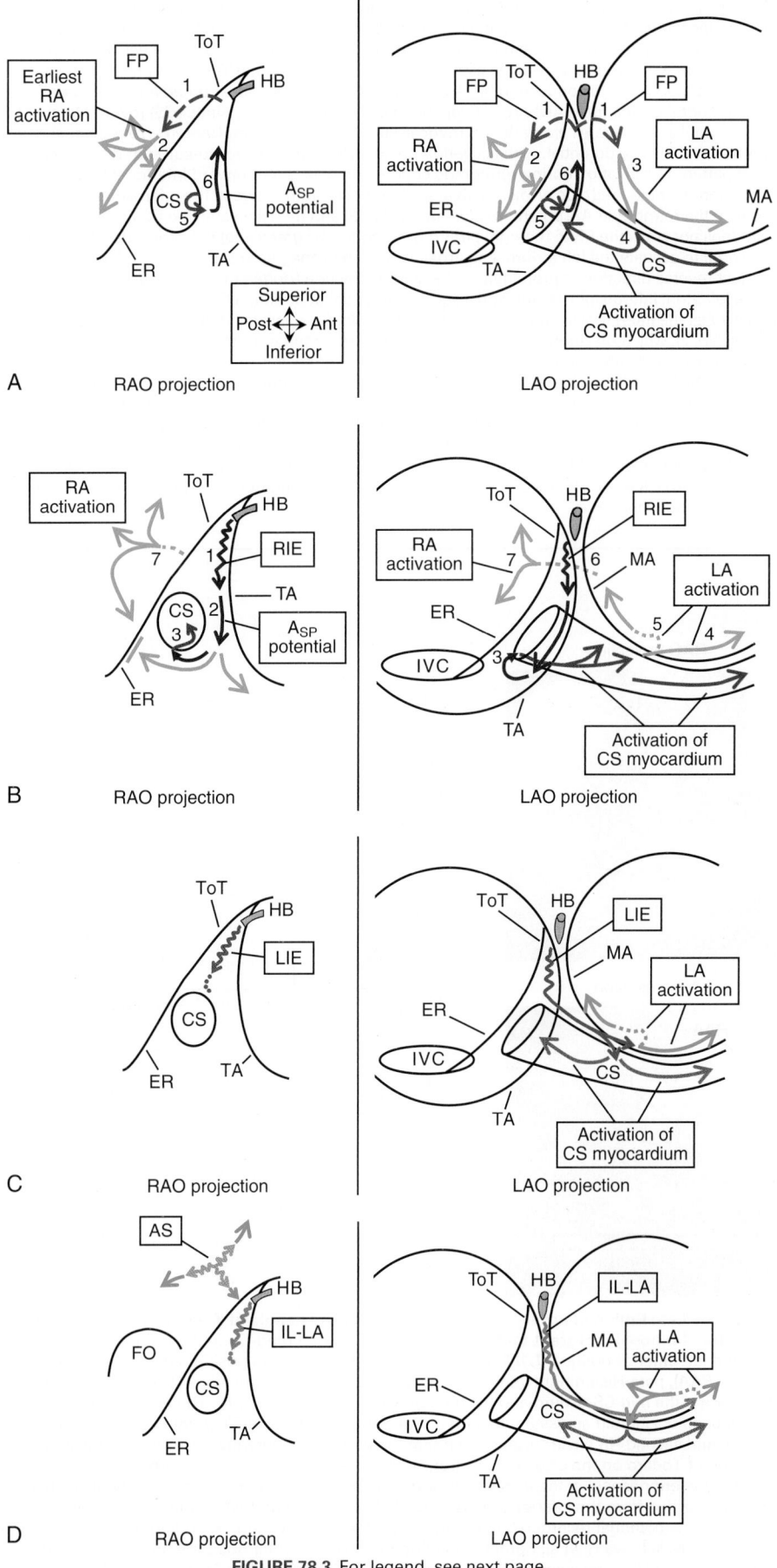

FIGURE 78.3 For legend, see next page.

Continued

FIGURE 78.3, cont'd (A) Proposed pattern of atrial activation during retrograde conduction over the fast pathway (*FP*). Retrograde FP conduction (*dotted red arrows, No. 1*) activates the right and left atrium at the interatrial septum, posterior to the tendon of Todaro (*ToT*) outside the triangle of Koch (*ToK*). Right atrial activation propagates away in the posterior, superior, and inferior directions (*RA activation, green arrows, No. 2*). This results in superior-to-inferior right atrial activation along the eustachian ridge (*ER*) outside the ToK. This right atrial wavefront is unable to cross the ER and ToT to enter the ToK, presumably due to conduction block at the ER (*short perpendicular green line*). Left atrial activation propagates inferiorly (*green arrows, No. 3 in left anterior oblique [LAO] projection*) and activates the coronary sinus (*CS*) myocardium, 1 to 3 cm from the ostium (*brown arrows*). The reentrant impulse propagates along the CS myocardium to the CS ostium (*brown arrows, No. 4*) where it activates the inferior ToK (*brown arrow, No. 5*), producing the A_{SP} potential, with activation proceeding in the inferior-to-superior direction along the inferior ToK (*blue arrows, No. 6*). (B) Postulated pattern of activation during retrograde conduction over the rightward inferior extension (*RIE*) of the atrioventricular (AV) node. Retrograde conduction over the RIE (*blue arrows*) activates the myocardium between the inferoseptal tricuspid annulus (*TA*) and the CS ostium (inferior ToK) to produce the retrograde A_{SP} potential (*blue arrow, No. 2*) and then activates the CS at the floor of the ostium (*brown arrows, No. 3*). Activation in the ToK does not cross the ER to the right atrium (*perpendicular green line*) but proceeds leftward along the CS myocardium (*brown arrows in LAO projection*) to activate the left atrium. Left atrial activation propagates rapidly in the leftward direction (*solid green arrow in LAO projection, No. 4*) but must reverse direction to propagate in the septal direction (*dotted green line, No. 5*). The reversal of direction produces late left atrial activation at the left atrial inferoseptal region and a second potential in proximal CS electrograms (recorded from the CS roof). This septal left atrial wavefront activates the interatrial septum (*dotted green line, No. 6*), which is followed by activation of the right atrium posterior to the ToT and ER (*green arrows, No. 7*), which produces a late far-field potential recorded from the inferior ToK. (C) Postulated pattern of activation during retrograde conduction over the leftward inferior extension (*LIE*) of the AV node. It is unknown whether retrograde conduction over the LIE (*purple arrows*) initially activates the left atrial myocardium close to the inferoseptal mitral annulus (*MA; top purple arrowhead in LAO projection*) or the CS myocardium at the roof of the proximal CS (*lower purple arrowhead in LAO projection*). During retrograde conduction over the LIE, CS activation (*brown arrows*) is recorded earliest at the CS roof, 1.5 to 4 cm from the ostium. (D) Postulated pattern of activation during retrograde conduction over the inferolateral left atrial SP (*IL-LA*) and the anterior superior SP (*AS*). Retrograde conduction over the IL-LA SP (*orange arrows*) activates the left atrium close to the inferolateral MA at 4:30 to 5 o'clock, as viewed in the LAO projection (*green arrows*). Right atrial mapping during retrograde conduction over the AS (*pink arrows*) records earliest activation at the anterior-superior aspect of the septum or medial right atrial free-wall. *FO*, Fossa ovalis; *IVC*, inferior vena cava.

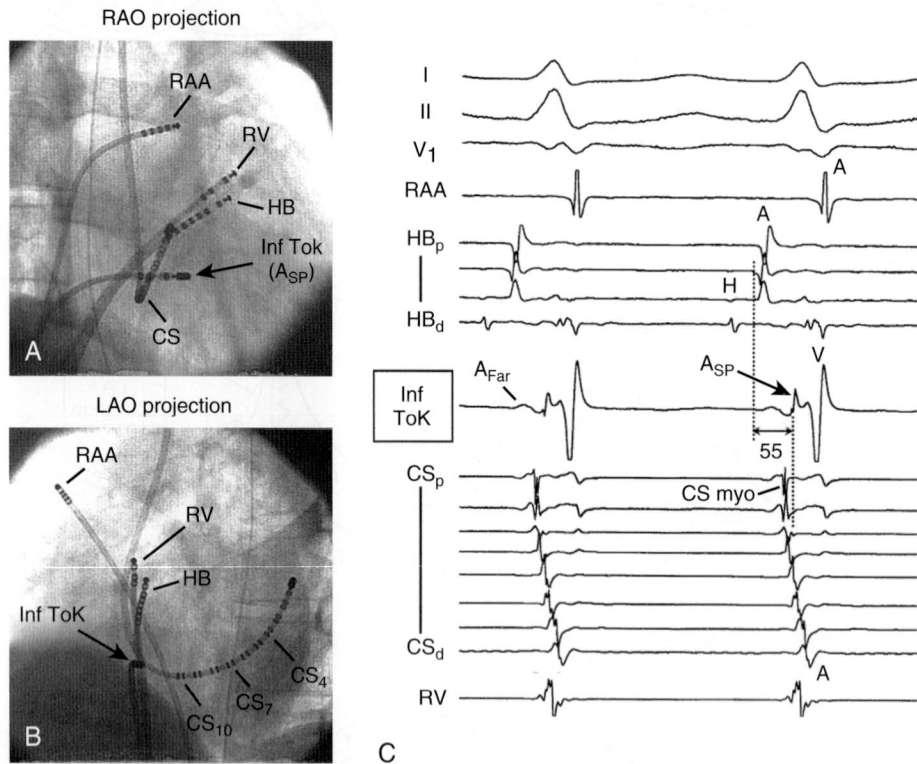

FIGURE 78.4 Late timing of atrial activation at the inferior triangle of Koch (*ToK*) during Slow/Fast atrioventricular nodal reentrant tachycardia. (A) and (B) Radiographs in the right anterior oblique (*RAO*) and left anterior oblique (*LAO*) projections show the catheters positioned in the right atrial appendage (*RAA*), para-Hisian right ventricular pacing site (*RV*), coronary sinus (*CS*), and at the inferior ToK, between the mid-CS ostium and the tricuspid annulus (TA) (*Inf ToK*). The His bundle catheter (*HB*) has been positioned across the tendon of Todaro, with a His bundle potential recorded only on the distal and second HB electrograms, such that the early atrial potentials are recorded from behind the tendon of Todaro on the proximal electrograms. (C) Right atrial activation propagating inferiorly along the posterior aspect of the eustachian ridge (outside the ToK) produces an early far-field atrial potential recorded from the inferior ToK (A_{Far}) while local activation (within the ToK) is represented as a late sharp A_{SP} potential recorded 55 ms after earliest atrial activation. (Modified from Jackman WM, Lockwood D, Nakagawa H, et al. Catheter ablation of atrioventricular nodal reentrant tachycardia. In: Wilber DJ, Packer DL, Stevenson WG, eds. *Catheter Ablation of Cardiac Arrhythmias: Basic Concepts and Clinical Applications*. 3rd ed. Hoboken, NJ: Blackwell Futura; 2008:120-148.)

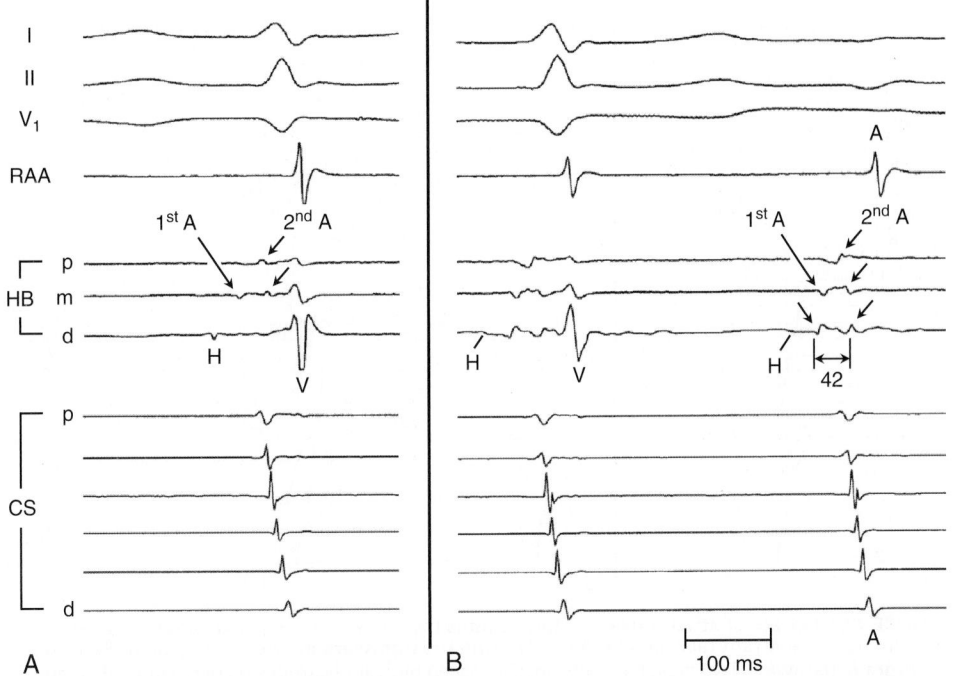

FIGURE 78.5 Two distinct sets of atrial potentials recorded in the proximal His bundle (*H*) electro-grams during Slow/Fast atrioventricular nodal reentrant tachycardia. (A) The His-bundle catheter was positioned to record the proximal His bundle potential from the distal pair of electrodes (HB_d electrogram). Two distinct sets of atrial potentials were recorded in the proximal two His bundle electrograms (HB_m and HB_p electrograms). The first set of potentials originate posterior to the tendon of Todaro, outside the triangle of Koch (*1st A*). The second set (*2nd A*) is generated close to the tricuspid annulus, inside the triangle of Koch. (B) The His bundle catheter was withdrawn proximally, such that only a tiny, far-field His bundle potential was recorded in the first complex (*H* on HB_d electrogram). AV block occurred during the second complex, allowing clear identification of the two sets of atrial potentials in the absence of the ventricular potentials. The first set of potentials (*1st A*) was activated in the distal-to-proximal direction (inferior-to-superior, *left arrows* in HB_d and HB_m electrograms). The second set of potentials (*2nd A*) propagated in the proximal-to-distal direction (superior-to-inferior, *right arrows* in HB_p to HB_d electrograms). The time between the first and second atrial potentials in HB_d was 42 ms. This delay supports the concept of conduction block across the eustachian ridge and tendon of Todaro.

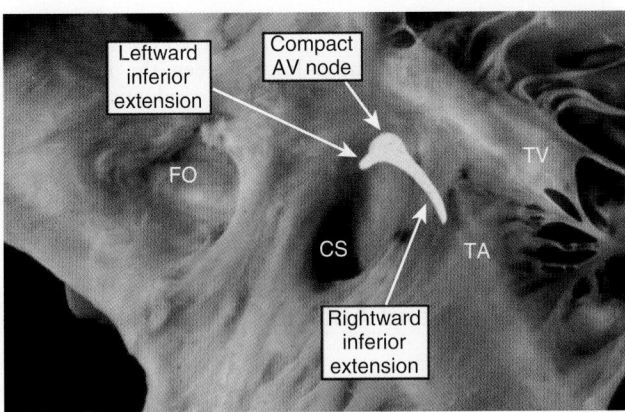

FIGURE 78.6 Representation of the locations of the rightward and leftward inferior extensions of the atrioventricular (*AV*) node. Photograph (right-sided view) of the AV septal junction of a human heart showing the locations of the rightward and leftward inferior extensions of the AV node and the compact node, as identified from detailed histological study. *CS,* Coronary sinus; *FO,* fossa ovalis; *TA,* tricuspid annulus; *TV,* tricuspid valve. (Modified from Inoue S, Becker AE. Posterior extensions of the human compact atrioventricular node: a neglected anatomic feature of potential clinical significance. *Circulation.* 1998;97:188-193.)

ostium (*brown arrow No. 3* in Fig. 78.3B and *CS myo arrow* in CS *floor_p* electrogram in Fig. 78.7B). The CS myocardium propagates the impulse leftward and superiorly, activating the left atrial myocardium approximately 2 to 3 cm from the CS ostium. Left atrial activation proceeds rapidly leftward (*green arrow No. 4* in Fig. 78.3B), while slowly reversing direction to propagate rightward toward the septum (*dotted green arrow No. 5* in Fig. 78.3B). Activation then propagates across the interatrial septum to activate the right atrium behind the ToT (*green arrows No. 6 and No. 7* in Fig. 78.3B). Right atrial activation proceeds superiorly (behind the ToT) to create the atrial potential in the His bundle electrogram and inferiorly (behind the eustachian ridge and CS ostium) to create the late, far-field potential recorded at the inferior ToK (A_{Far} in the second complex of Figs. 78.1B and 78.7B). Late right atrial extrastimuli will advance the atrial potential behind the ToT, without advancing the A_{Sp} potential, supporting the presence of conduction block across the ToT and eustachian ridge.

Conduction block across the eustachian ridge may also account for the late timing of activation within the ToK during sinus rhythm (A_{Sp} potential in Figs. 78.1A and 78.7A). The two most likely explanations for the late A_{Sp} potential during sinus rhythm are that the inferior ToK is activated by either (1) the CS musculature, which is activated from the left atrium (Fig. 78.8A) or (2) the crista terminalis (see Fig. 78.8B). Observations that the CS myocardium propagates in a distal-to-proximal direction in the proximal 1 to 2 cm of the CS (*CS myo* in Fig. 78.7A) and that

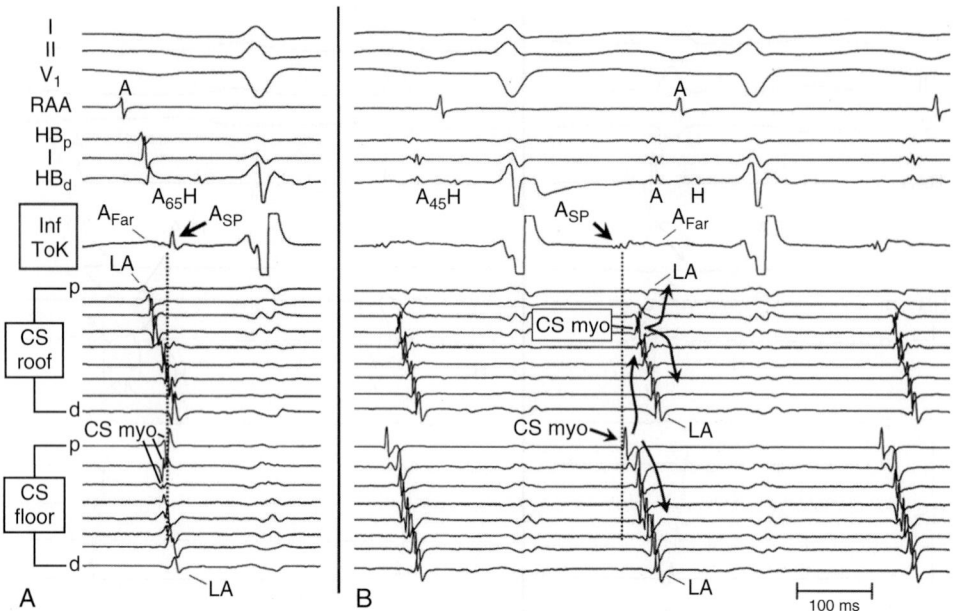

FIGURE 78.7 Pattern of atrial activation during sinus rhythm and during Fast/Slow atrioventricular nodal reentrant tachycardia (AVNRT) using the rightward inferior extension (RIE) for the retrograde pathway. Two catheters with closely spaced bipolar electrodes were positioned along the roof (femoral vein approach) and floor (right subclavian vein approach) of the coronary sinus (*CS*) (similar to Fig. 78.10). (A) During sinus rhythm, atrial activation at the inferior triangle of Koch (*Inf ToK*) (*A_SP* potential, *arrow*) was recorded later than atrial activation in the His bundle electrograms and the roof of the proximal CS (*vertical dotted line*). (B) During Fast/Slow (leftward inferior extension [LIE]/RIE) AVNRT, earliest retrograde activation (*A_SP*) was recorded at the inferior ToK region, followed by activation of the floor of the CS ostium (*arrow, CS myo* in proximal *CS floor* electrogram). Activation propagates laterally along the CS myocardium (proximal to distal *CS floor* electrograms) and superiorly (to the roof of the CS). The left atrium is activated by the CS myocardium (*CS myo* in the *CS roof* electrograms). Left atrial activation (*LA*) then propagates septally and laterally (*curved arrows*). The late far-field potential (*A_Far*) following the *A_SP* potential in the inferior ToK electrogram results from right atrial activation, posterior to the eustachian ridge, with timing similar to atrial activation recorded in the His bundle electrograms (*A*). Note that the A-H interval is shorter during Fast/Slow (LIE/RIE) AVNRT (45 ms) than during sinus rhythm (65 ms). (Modified from Jackman WM, Lockwood D, Nakagawa H, et al. Catheter ablation of atrioventricular nodal reentrant tachycardia. In: Wilber DJ, Packer DL, Stevenson WG, eds. *Catheter Ablation of Cardiac Arrhythmias: Basic Concepts and Clinical Applications*. 3rd ed. Hoboken, NJ: Blackwell Futura; 2008:120-148.)

the A_{SP} potential is recorded after CS activation in the proximal CS (see Figs. 78.1A and 78.7A) suggest that the inferior ToK is activated from the CS myocardium (see Fig. 78.8A).

Leftward Inferior Extension

The leftward inferior extension (LIE) of the AV node is the second most commonly observed SP. During retrograde conduction over the LIE, earliest activation is recorded at the roof of the CS, 1.5 to 4 cm from the ostium (see Figs. 78.3C and 78.9B and the first beat of Fig. 78.10B), and the H-A interval is usually shorter than when retrograde conduction is occurring over the RIE (see Fig. 78.10B). The LIE can often be ablated from the roof of the CS but may require ablation from the inferior or inferior paraseptal left atrium, close to the mitral annulus.

Evidence of conduction over more than one SP includes the observation of multiple, abrupt increases of 50 ms or more ("jumps") in the A_2-H_2 interval in some patients during atrial extrastimulus testing. Additionally, during programmed ventricular stimulation, two distinct retrograde atrial activation sequences with different H-A intervals are sometimes seen, representing retrograde conduction over two separate SPs (RIE and LIE). The two retrograde SPs can best be distinguished using two CS catheters with closely spaced bipolar electrodes, one positioned to record activation at the roof and the other at the floor of the CS (see Fig. 78.10). Evidence of conduction

over more than one SP is also often observed during ablation. For example, ablation along a line between the inferoseptal TA and the CS ostium often eliminates conduction over the SP (RIE) participating in Slow/Fast AVNRT. However, atrial extrastimulus testing continues to show a jump in the A_2-H_2 interval (often with a single Slow/Fast nodal reentrant atrial echo beat) in approximately 75% of patients, consistent with conduction over the LIE or another SP.

Other Slow Pathways: Inferolateral Left Atrial Slow Pathway and Anterior Superior Slow Pathway

We are aware of the existence of at least two other SPs. Retrograde conduction over these SPs is occasionally seen during Slow/Slow and Fast/Slow AVNRT, but is only rarely observed during ventricular pacing. Earliest retrograde atrial activation over the inferolateral left atrial SP is located in the left atrium close to the mitral annulus at 4:30 to 5 o'clock in the LAO projection (Fig. 78.11 and *green arrows* in the second panel of Fig. 78.3D), while retrograde conduction over the anterior superior SP results in earliest atrial activation superiorly in the anterior atrial septum, slightly superior and posterior to the site recording proximal His bundle activation and 1.5 to 2 cm superior to the site of retrograde FP activation (*pink arrows* in the first panel of Fig. 78.3D). There may be additional SPs that have not been described.

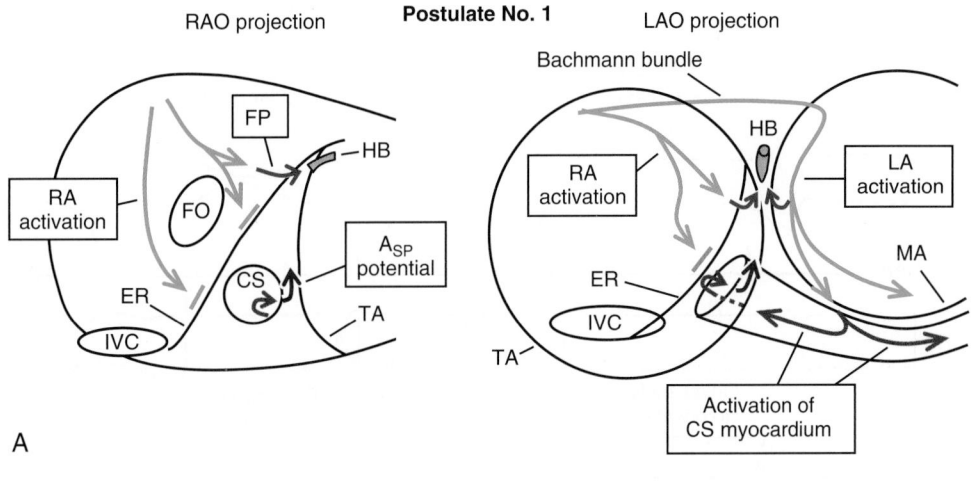

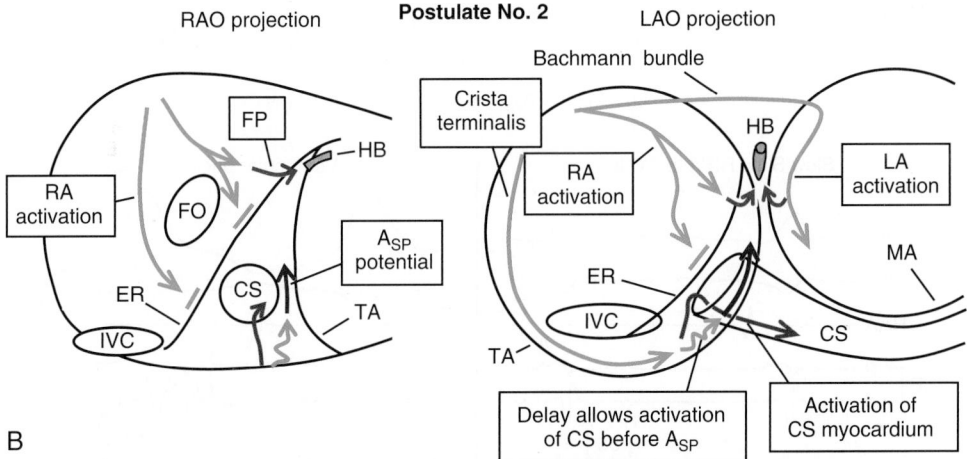

FIGURE 78.8 Schematic representation of two possible patterns of activation during sinus rhythm that may explain the late A$_{SP}$ potential in the inferior triangle of Koch (ToK). (A) Postulate No. 1: Right atrial (*RA*) activation does not penetrate the ToK due to conduction block across the eustachian ridge (*ER; green arrows* and *short perpendicular green lines*). The left atrium is activated rapidly over the Bachmann bundle (*horizontal green arrow* in left anterior oblique [*LAO*] projection). Left atrial (*LA*) activation proceeds inferiorly and laterally along the mitral annulus (*MA; green arrows*), activating the coronary sinus (*CS*) myocardium (*brown arrows*). Activation propagates in the septal direction along the CS myocardium to the CS ostium (*brown arrows*) and activates the inferior region of the ToK to generate the late A$_{SP}$ potential (*blue arrows*). (B) Postulate No. 2: Septal RA activation does not cross the ER to activate the ToK (similar to Postulate No. 1). Activation propagating inferiorly along the crista terminalis activates the region between the tricuspid annulus (*TA*) and ER (subeustachian isthmus, *long green arrow* in LAO projection). Continued RA activation in the septal and superior direction (*short squiggly green arrows*) activates the inferior ToK to generate the late A$_{SP}$ potential (*blue arrows*) and the CS ostium (*brown arrows*). This postulate does not explain the usual findings that the A$_{SP}$ potential is recorded later than activation at the roof of the proximal CS during sinus rhythm or the distal-to-proximal direction of activation along the roof of the proximal CS. *FP*, Fast pathway; *FO*, fossa ovalis; *HB*, His bundle; *IVC*, inferior vena cava; *RAO*, right anterior oblique.

Presence of Slow Pathway Conduction in Individuals Without Atrioventricular Nodal Reentrant Tachycardia

The atrionodal connections which form the FP and SPs are present in normal hearts. This suggests that conduction over the FP and at least one SP (*dual-pathway physiology*) should be demonstrable in most people. In a series of 200 consecutive patients in our laboratory who underwent radiofrequency catheter ablation of an accessory pathway (without a history of AVNRT or inducible AVNRT during the procedure), evidence of dual-pathway physiology in either the anterograde or retrograde direction was present in 168 (84%). The ability to demonstrate anterograde or retrograde SP conduction in a high percentage of patients was probably related to heavy sedation or general anesthesia, which depressed anterograde and retrograde

FP conduction. Small doses of isoproterenol (0.25–0.5 μg/min) enhanced FP conduction to a greater extent than SP conduction and often obscured anterograde and retrograde SP conduction. These low doses of isoproterenol in heavily sedated or anesthetized patients probably mimic normal resting sympathetic tone, which explains the low incidence of dual-pathway physiology observed in nonsedated patients without AVNRT. Other reasons may include a similar conduction time over the FP and an SP just before block in the FP (smooth transition). A smooth transition from FP to SP conduction may also be seen in the retrograde direction. There is no specific value of H-A interval that identifies retrograde SP conduction. However, the transition from retrograde FP conduction to retrograde SP conduction is easy to recognize because of the shift in retrograde atrial activation sequence (see Fig. 78.1).

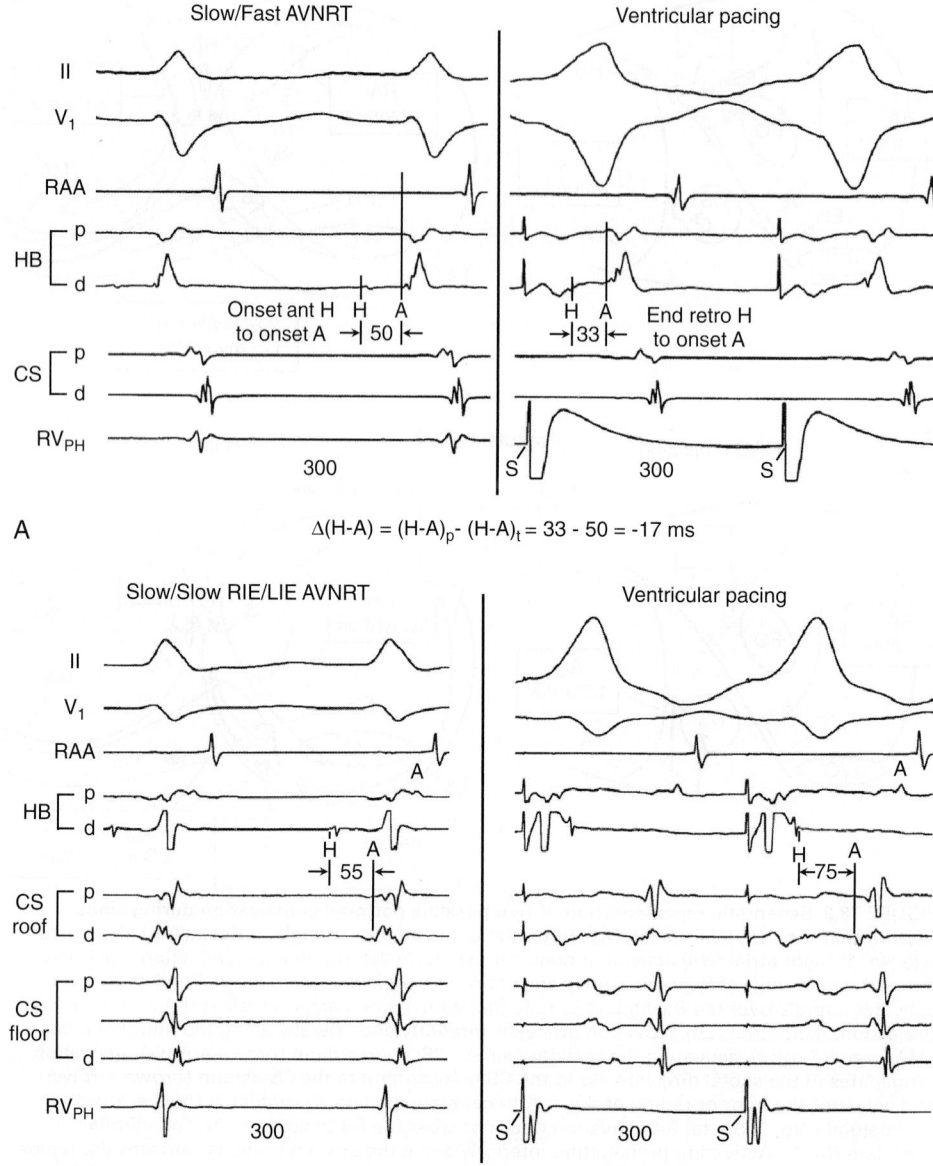

FIGURE 78.9 Comparison of the H-A interval during tachycardia and during ventricular pacing for Slow/Fast atrioventricular nodal reentrant tachycardia (*AVNRT*) and Slow/Slow (rightward inferior extension [*RIE*]/leftward inferior extension [*LIE*]) AVNRT. (A) *Left panel:* During Slow/Fast AVNRT at cycle length 300 ms, the H-A interval, *(H-A)$_t$*, was 50 ms, measured from the onset of the most proximal anterograde His bundle potential (*H, left panel*) to the onset of the atrial potential. *Right panel:* Para-Hisian right ventricular pacing at cycle length 300 ms (*S* in *RV$_{PH}$* electrogram) was initiated immediately after termination of the tachycardia. The H-A interval during ventricular pacing (H-A)$_p$, measured from the end of the retrograde His bundle potential (*H, right panel*), was 33 ms, 17 ms shorter than the H-A interval during tachycardia (H-A)$_t$, resulting in a negative Δ(H-A) of −17 ms. Note that para-Hisian ventricular pacing resulted in very early ventricular activation recorded in the His bundle electrogram and delayed retrograde activation of the His bundle, allowing identification of the end of the retrograde His bundle potential. (B) *Left panel:* During Slow/Slow (RIE/LIE) AVNRT, the atrial and ventricular potentials were overlapping in the His bundle (*HB*) and coronary sinus (*CS*) electrograms. (H-A)$_t$ was 55 ms. *Right panel:* Para-Hisian right ventricular pacing at the same cycle length as tachycardia (300 ms), instituted immediately upon terminating the tachycardia, separated the atrial and ventricular potentials, showing that earliest activation was recorded at the roof of the CS approximately 2 cm from the CS ostium (distal *CS roof* electrogram). (H-A)$_p$ was 75 ms. The Δ(H-A) during Slow/Slow (RIE/LIE) AVNRT was a positive value, 75 − 55 ms = 20 ms.

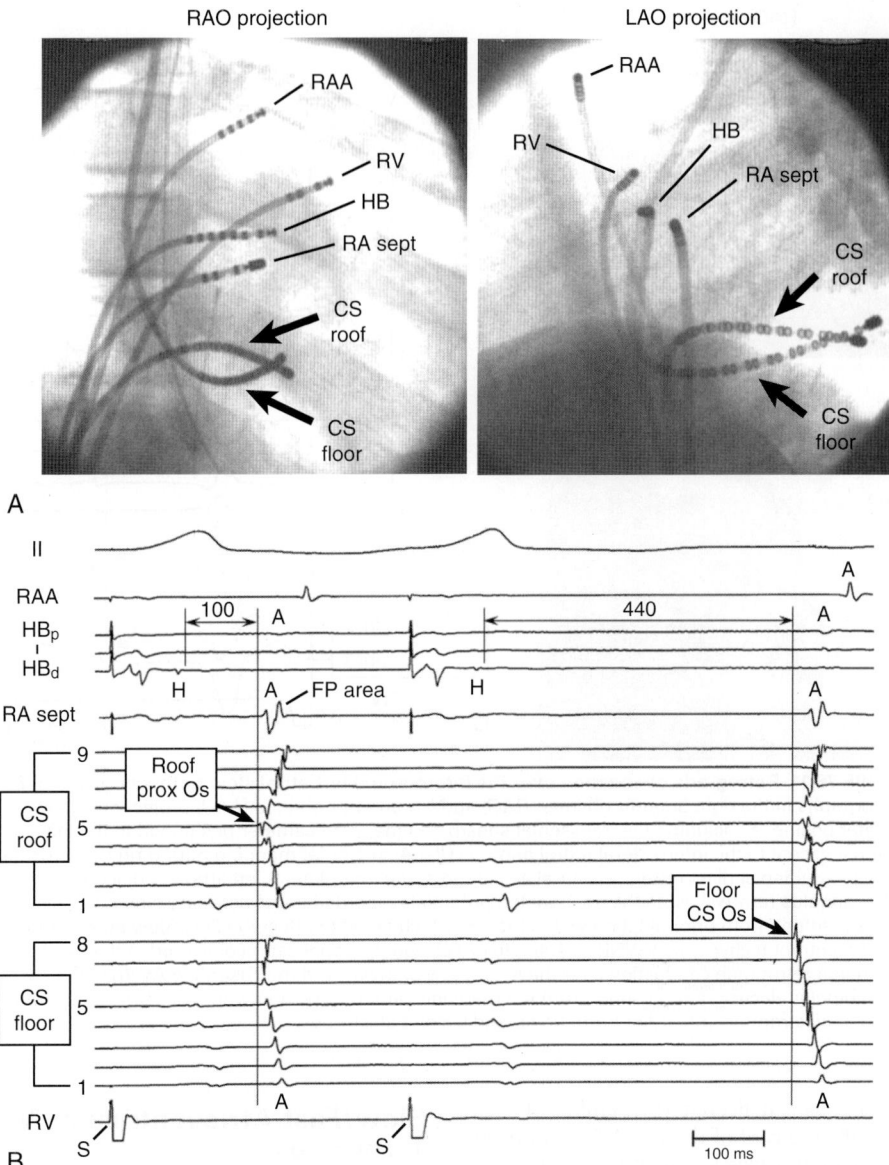

FIGURE 78.10 Two retrograde atrial activation sequences following retrograde conduction over the rightward inferior extension (RIE) and leftward inferior extension (LIE) (two different slow pathways [SPs]). (A) Radiographs in the right anterior oblique (*RAO*) and left anterior oblique (*LAO*) projections show two catheters positioned in the coronary sinus (*CS*): one inserted via the right subclavian vein and positioned along the floor of the CS (*CS floor*) and one inserted via the right femoral vein and positioned along the roof of the CS (*CS roof*). A mapping catheter (*RA sept*) is positioned on the right atrial septum, posterior to the tendon of Todaro where earliest right atrial activation had been previously recorded during retrograde fast pathway (*FP*) conduction. (B) Electrograms recorded following two paced ventricular complexes. Retrograde atrial activation following the first ventricular complex has an H-A interval of 100 ms, measured from the end of the retrograde His bundle (*HB*) potential to earliest atrial activation, which was recorded from the roof of the CS approximately 3 cm from the CS ostium (*arrow* in *CS roof 5* electrogram), consistent with retrograde activation over the LIE. Activation in the FP area (*FP area* in *RA sept* electrogram) was recorded later, excluding retrograde conduction over the FP. Atrial activation following the second ventricular complex had a longer H-A interval (440 ms) and a different retrograde atrial activation sequence. Earliest CS activation was recorded at the floor of the CS ostium (*arrow* in *CS floor 8* electrogram), consistent with retrograde conduction over the RIE. *RAA,* Right atrial appendage; *RV,* right ventricle.

Variants of Atrioventricular Nodal Reentrant Tachycardia

The different forms of AVNRT can now be distinguished based on the anatomical substrate forming the anterograde and retrograde pathways used in the tachycardia. The retrograde pathway is identified by mapping during AVNRT and by locating the site of earliest retrograde atrial activation. The anterograde limb of the tachycardia can be identified using the resetting response to late atrial extrastimuli. If an atrial extrastimulus is delivered close to or within the atrial component of the reentrant circuit (close enough to capture the anterograde pathway of the circuit), the extrastimulus will advance (or delay) the timing of the next His bundle potential and reset the tachycardia. For this

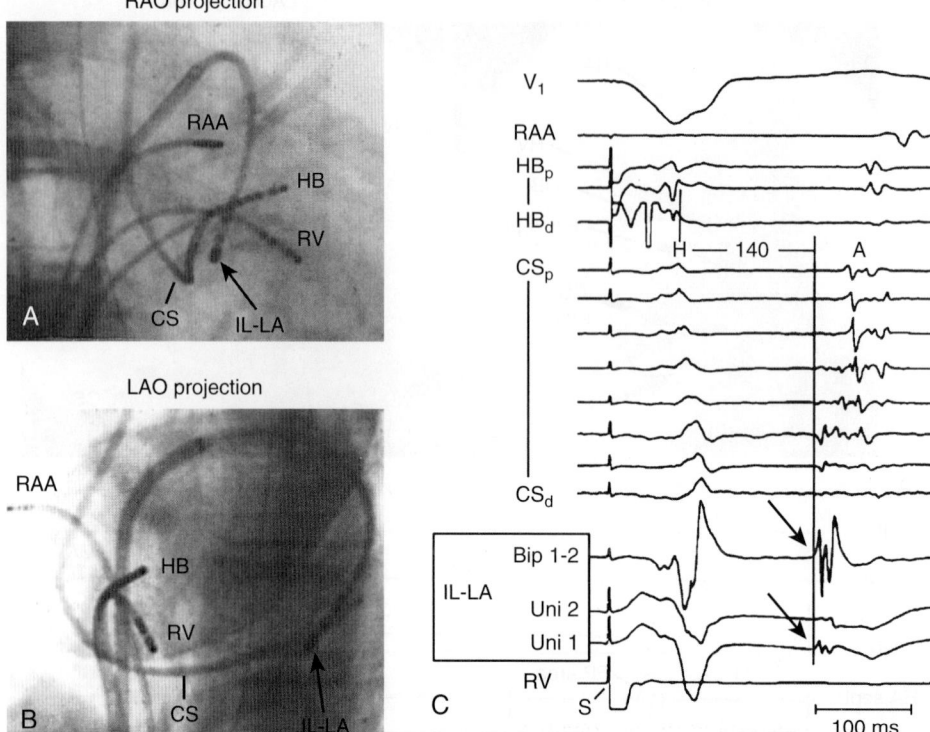

FIGURE 78.11 Retrograde conduction over the inferolateral left atrial slow pathway. (A) and (B) Radiographs in the right anterior oblique (*RAO*) and left anterior oblique (*LAO*) projections show catheter positions, including the transseptal sheath and mapping catheter positioned in the left atrium adjacent to the inferolateral mitral annulus (*IL-LA*). (C) Atrial mapping during right ventricular pacing identified earliest retrograde atrial activation at the inferolateral left atrium, adjacent to the mitral annulus (*arrows*). Note the fractionated potentials recorded in the coronary sinus (*CS*) electrograms resulting from prior ablation within the CS, which failed to affect the Fast/Slow atrioventricular nodal reentrant tachycardia (AVNRT). A single radiofrequency application delivered at the IL-LA site eliminated retrograde conduction over the IL-LA slow pathway and the Fast/Slow AVNRT. *Bip 1-2*, Distal bipolar electrogram recorded from the mapping catheter; *RV*, right ventricle; *Uni 1* and *Uni 2*, unipolar electrograms recorded from the tip and second electrodes.

approach, a late extrastimulus is delivered at a number of sites including the inferior ToK, the roof of the CS (1.5–5 cm from the ostium) and, if resetting is not achieved at either of these two sites, at the inferolateral left atrium, close to the mitral annulus (4:30–5 o'clock in the LAO projection). The atrial extrastimulus coupling interval (A-S_2) is shortened by 2- to 5-ms decrements until the timing of the next His bundle potential (H-H_2 interval) is changed (usually shortened, but may be lengthened due to decremental conduction properties within the anterograde pathway or AV node). The anterograde limb is identified by the site where the latest extrastimulus (relative to a reference atrial or ventricular potential) advances or delays the next His bundle potential *and resets the tachycardia*. For example, the RIE is identified as the anterograde pathway of the reentrant circuit when the latest extrastimulus to advance the next His bundle potential is located at the inferior ToK. The LIE is identified when the roof of the CS (1.5–4 cm from the ostium) allows the latest extrastimulus to advance the next His bundle potential. The inferolateral left atrial SP is identified as the anterograde limb of the circuit when the latest extrastimulus to advance the next His bundle potential is at the inferolateral left atrium, close to the mitral annulus. An important technical consideration is that the extrastimulus must be delivered sufficiently late to prevent the paced atrial impulse from reaching the site of earliest retrograde atrial activation before normal retrograde activation occurs. This prevents the extrastimulus from reaching the AV node over the retrograde pathway.

Slow/Fast Atrioventricular Nodal Reentrant Tachycardia

Slow/Fast AVNRT is identified by the long A-H interval, short H-A interval, and mapping during tachycardia, which identifies the earliest atrial activation posterior to the ToT and eustachian ridge at a height approximately 1 cm inferior to the level recording the most proximal His bundle potential. The short H-A interval usually results in superimposition of the P wave onto the QRS complex in the electrocardiogram, obscuring most of the P wave. However, the terminal portion of the P wave may be distinguishable at the end of the QRS complex, producing a characteristic late positive component in lead V_1 (*pseudo r′* wave) or a negative component in the inferior leads (*pseudo S* wave).

The induction of Slow/Fast AVNRT by programmed atrial stimulation typically occurs with an abrupt (≥50 ms) increase in the A-H interval, confirming that anterograde conduction occurs over an SP. However, in some patients, the induction of tachycardia may occur following a smooth increase in the A-H interval (without a ≥50 ms "jump") because of similar conduction times over the two pathways at the time of transition.

The distance between the atrial connections of the FP and the three most common SPs suggests that the reentrant circuit in Slow/Fast AVNRT may contain a relatively large atrial component (without an upper common pathway) in which the reentrant impulse propagates from the atrial end of the FP to the atrial end of the SP. The traditional hypothesis in which the reentrant circuit is confined within the ToK (providing an upper common pathway between the circuit and the atrium) does not explain the ability to reset the tachycardia by late atrial extrastimuli delivered to the CS or left atrium or by successful ablation of AVNRT when radiofrequency current is delivered to the atrial connection to the SP away from the compact AV node. Atrial extrastimuli delivered behind the eustachian ridge, at the level of the middle of the CS ostium, usually fail to reset the tachycardia without first advancing the timing of the atrial potential in the His bundle electrogram, dissociating this region from the reentrant circuit.

The distal junction of the FP and SPs in Slow/Fast AVNRT has traditionally been considered to be located in the AV node, with a region of AV nodal tissue extending between the distal junction of the two pathways and the His bundle (i.e., the lower common pathway). The presence of a lower common pathway comprised of AV nodal tissue would predict the occasional occurrence of spontaneous block proximal to the His bundle without terminating or even resetting Slow/Fast AVNRT. However, a tiny, proximal His bundle potential is almost always recorded during Slow/Fast AVNRT with 2:1 block, and AV block proximal to the His bundle potential is exceedingly rare. More recent evidence, using late para-Hisian ventricular extrastimuli during tachycardia, suggests a very short or minimal lower common pathway in Slow/Fast AVNRT.[1] A late ventricular extrastimulus begins to advance the timing of atrial activation as soon as the proximal His bundle potential is activated in the retrograde direction (Fig. 78.12B). There is generally a linear relationship between the degree of advance in timing of the retrograde His bundle potential (H-H_2 interval) and the advance in timing of atrial activation (A-A_2 interval) (see Fig. 78.12), suggesting relatively little decrement in conduction in the lower common pathway and the retrograde FP.

Similar evidence of a minimal lower common pathway is obtained by comparing the H-A intervals during Slow/Fast AVNRT and during ventricular pacing at the same cycle length. The H-A interval during tachycardia (measured from the *beginning of the anterograde His bundle potential* to the onset of atrial activation) should be equal to the retrograde conduction time over the FP *minus* the anterograde conduction time over the lower common pathway (from the distal junction of the two pathways to the His bundle). The H-A interval during ventricular pacing, measured from the *end of the retrograde His bundle potential* to the onset of atrial activation, should be equal to the retrograde conduction time over the FP *plus* the retrograde conduction time over the lower common pathway (from the proximal end of the His bundle to the FP). Given the two assumptions that the retrograde FP is the same anatomical structure during tachycardia and during ventricular pacing and that the FP has the same retrograde conduction time during tachycardia and during ventricular pacing, subtracting the H-A interval during tachycardia from the H-A interval during ventricular pacing would equal the sum of the anterograde and retrograde conduction times over the lower common pathway. To measure this correctly, the most proximal His bundle potential must be recorded because recording more distally will erroneously increase the H-A interval during ventricular pacing and shorten the H-A interval during tachycardia, incorrectly suggesting a longer lower common pathway. To record the *end* of the most proximal retrograde His bundle potential, ventricular pacing must be performed at a site that separates the activation times of the His bundle and the local ventricular myocardium. This can be accomplished by pacing at the superior-basal right ventricular septum, very close to the proximal right bundle branch, but not capturing the proximal right bundle branch (para-Hisian pacing). This results in retrograde activation of the His bundle long after completion of the local ventricular potential (see Figs. 78.1 and 78.9–78.11). The most accurate comparison is obtained when a sustained episode of Slow/Fast AVNRT (>3 min) is terminated by a three- to four-beat burst of

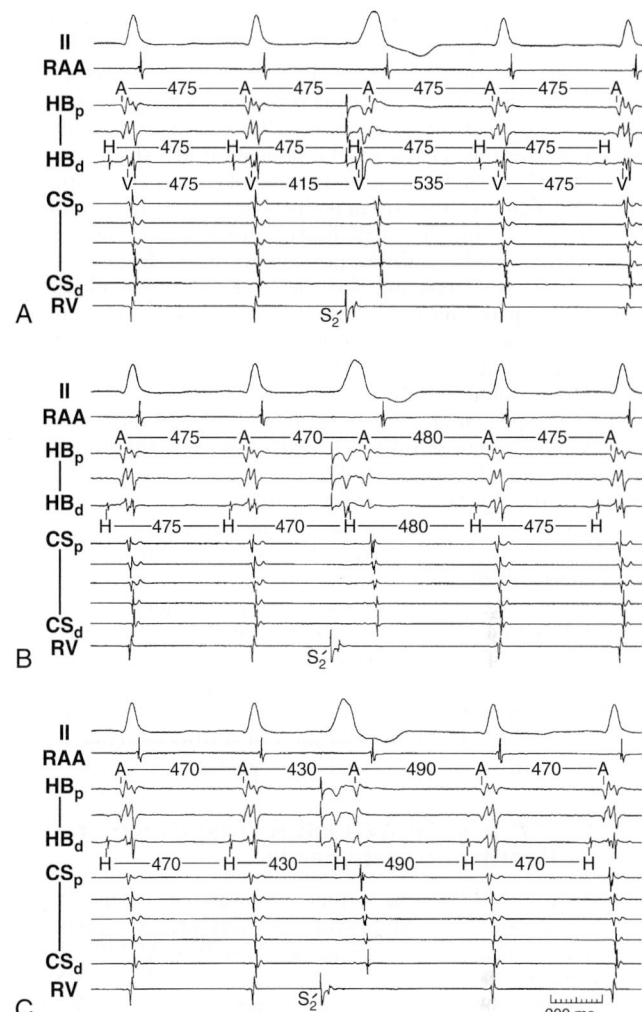

FIGURE 78.12 Use of ventricular extrastimuli to verify the diagnosis of Slow/Fast atrioventricular nodal reentrant tachycardia (AVNRT). (A) During tachycardia, a single extrastimulus (S_2) was delivered to the superior-basal right ventricular septum (para-Hisian region), close to the site of earliest atrial activation. This advanced the timing of ventricular activation in the electrograms recording earliest atrial activation (*HB* electrograms) by 60 ms (V-V = *415* ms, compared with 475 ms). S_2 did not advance the timing of His bundle activation (*H*) or the timing of retrograde atrial activation (A-A remained *475* ms). This indicates that the timing of atrial activation during tachycardia is independent of local ventricular activation, excluding retrograde conduction over an accessory pathway and orthodromic atrioventricular reentrant tachycardia. (B) An earlier ventricular extrastimulus (S_2) resulted in retrograde activation of the His bundle. The end of the retrograde His bundle potential occurred 5 ms before anterograde His bundle activation would have occurred (H-H = *470* ms, compared with 475 ms). This was associated with a 5-ms advance in the timing of the retrograde atrial activation (A-A = *470* ms, compared with 475 ms) without a change in the atrial activation sequence, indicating that atrial activation was dependent on retrograde His bundle activation, excluding an atrial tachycardia and confirming the diagnosis of AVNRT. (C) Further shortening of the extrastimulus coupling interval resulted in earlier retrograde activation of the His bundle. This was associated with an identical advance in the timing of retrograde atrial activation (H-H = A-A = *430* ms).

rapid atrial pacing, and ventricular pacing at the tachycardia cycle length is initiated immediately after termination of the tachycardia. This technique minimizes any change in the autonomic tone between pacing and tachycardia. Using this methodology, the H-A interval during pacing is a mean of 9 ms *shorter* than the H-A interval during Slow/Fast AVNRT (see Fig. 78.9A).[1] This seemingly paradoxical finding (an H-A interval longer during tachycardia than during ventricular pacing), implying minimal lower common pathway in Slow/Fast AVNRT, has several possible explanations. One is that the retrograde FP arises from the His bundle (i.e., no lower common pathway), but this is unlikely for several reasons. Histological examination in a small number of explanted human hearts with documented dual-pathway physiology revealed no atrio-Hisian pathway and no evident anatomical differences from "normal" hearts.[5] Because we now believe that dual AV nodal pathway physiology results from multiple atrionodal connections and that these are present in all hearts, atrio-Hisian pathways would have to be present in a large number of people to explain the dual-pathway physiology. However, a histological study of 687 autopsy hearts identified a possible true atrio-Hisian connection in only 2 (0.3%) hearts.[6]

Likely explanations for a longer H-A interval during Slow/Fast AVNRT than during ventricular pacing, either singly or in combination, include the following: (1) the recording of activation of the AV bundle proximal to the central fibrous body (before the junction of the FP and SP) and misinterpreting this as activation of the His bundle, which would artificially increase the H-A interval during tachycardia and shorten it during ventricular pacing; (2) a true increase in the H-A interval during tachycardia produced by a delay associated with the change in direction of the wavefront at the junction of the two pathways, decreasing the amount of current available to activate the FP, decreasing the initial conduction velocity, and lengthening the conduction time over the FP; and (3) different routes of retrograde conduction during AVNRT and during ventricular pacing.

Three Forms of Slow/Fast Atrioventricular Nodal Reentrant Tachycardia

Slow/Fast AVNRT can be further subdivided into at least three forms, based on which SP provides the anterograde limb of the circuit: (1) rightward inferior extension Slow/Fast AVNRT (most common); (2) leftward inferior extension Slow/Fast AVNRT (uncommon); or (3) inferolateral left atrial Slow/Fast AVNRT (rare).

Rightward Inferior Extension Slow/Fast Atrioventricular Nodal Reentrant Tachycardia

This is the most common form of AVNRT and uses the RIE of the AV node for anterograde conduction (SP) and the FP for retrograde conduction. The A-H interval during RIE Slow/Fast AVNRT is relatively long (usually more than 200 ms) and in our experience has been as long as 550 ms (median, 290 ms). The H-A interval measured in the His bundle electrogram is relatively short, usually 25 to 90 ms (median, 50 ms; see Figs. 78.2, 78.4, and 78.9A). The timing of activation (earliest outside and latest inside the ToK; see Figs. 78.2, 78.3A, and 78.4) suggests the hypothesis for the reentrant circuit in Slow/Fast AVNRT shown in Fig. 78.13A. In this hypothesis, retrograde activation over the FP activates both the right and left sides of the interatrial septum (dotted red arrows in Fig 78.13A), but it is only the left atrial activation that participates in the reentrant circuit. Propagation in the left atrium adjacent to the mitral annulus activates the CS myocardium, approximately 1 to 3 cm from the ostium (green and brown arrows in Fig. 78.13A). The reentrant impulse propagates along the CS myocardium to the CS ostium. Activation at the floor of the CS ostium (bottom brown arrow in Fig. 78.13A) activates fibers that connect with the rightward inferior extension of the AV node, initiating propagation along the SP. The role of the RIE as the anterograde SP is confirmed during resetting testing by finding the inferior ToK as the site of the latest extrastimulus to reset Slow/Fast AVNRT.

The delivery of radiofrequency current to the inferior aspect of the ToK, between the TA and the CS ostium (at the level of

the middle of the CS ostium or even lower), at a site recording a large, sharp A_{SP} potential (on the unipolar tip electrogram), usually results in an immediate accelerated junctional rhythm with retrograde conduction over the FP. In some patients, junctional rhythm is preceded by one to three atrial extrasystoles with an activation pattern consistent with retrograde activation over the RIE. The occurrence of an accelerated junctional rhythm during the application of radiofrequency current indicates heating of tissue connected to the RIE and is usually associated with modification or elimination of anterograde and retrograde SP conduction, without depressing FP conduction. Histological studies in dogs and in one patient with AVNRT who underwent SP ablation at the inferior ToK showed that the radiofrequency lesions involved the RIE of the AV node while leaving the compact AV node intact.

After ablation along a line between the inferoseptal TA and the CS ostium, the A_{SP} potential during sinus rhythm is eliminated superior to the ablation line, but remains present inferior to the ablation line. This suggests that the A_{SP} potential recorded during sinus rhythm in the inferior ToK represents activation in the inferior-to-superior direction (blue arrows in Fig. 78.8). The high success rate of eliminating Slow/Fast AVNRT by ablation procedures targeting tissue in the inferior ToK, outside of the CS, provides strong evidence that the majority of Slow/Fast AVNRTs use the RIE for the anterograde limb (SP) of the reentrant circuit.

Leftward Inferior Extension Slow/Fast Atrioventricular Nodal Reentrant Tachycardia

The failure to eliminate Slow/Fast AVNRT by ablation of the RIE (despite junctional automaticity during ablation at the inferior ToK) in a small percentage of patients supports the role of other anatomical substrates for the SP in these patients. In approximately 5% of patients with Slow/Fast AVNRT, the anterograde limb of the circuit (SP) appears to be formed by the leftward inferior extension of the AV node (LIE, Fig. 78.13B). This can be confirmed by testing the resetting response at the roof of the CS and inferior ToK. In patients with LIE Slow/Fast AVNRT, the His bundle potential is advanced (and the tachycardia reset) by a later extrastimulus delivered at the roof of the proximal CS (1.5–4 cm from the CS ostium) than at the inferior ToK. A circuit using the LIE for the SP has been most frequently identified by the response to ablation.[7] In these patients, ablation across the inferior ToK, between the TA (at the level of the middle of the CS ostium) and the apical edge of the CS ostium, produces vigorous accelerated junctional rhythm (indicating injury to the RIE) but fails to affect the tachycardia. Elimination of tachycardia may be achieved in one approach by delivering energy at progressively more superior sites adjacent to the TA, presumably near the junction of the leftward and rightward inferior extensions and closer to the compact AV node. We prefer to target the atrial end of the LIE at the roof of the proximal CS, either empirically (1.5–4 cm from the ostium) or, ideally, at the site where the latest extrastimulus resets the tachycardia (see Figs. 78.13B and 78.14).[1] This approach reduces the risk of causing complete AV nodal conduction block.

Inferolateral Left Atrial Slow/Fast Atrioventricular Nodal Reentrant Tachycardia

In a rare variant of Slow/Fast AVNRT, the SP participating in the reentrant circuit cannot be ablated from the inferior ToK or from the roof of the CS (see Fig. 78.13C).[1] In 12 such patients, the tachycardia could only be reset by a late atrial extrastimulus, which was delivered in the left atrium, close to the inferolateral mitral annulus at 4:30 to 5 o'clock as viewed in the LAO projection (Fig. 78.15C). In 10 of these 12 patients, the SP was eliminated by left atrial ablation close to the inferolateral mitral annulus at the site of resetting. Radiofrequency current at these

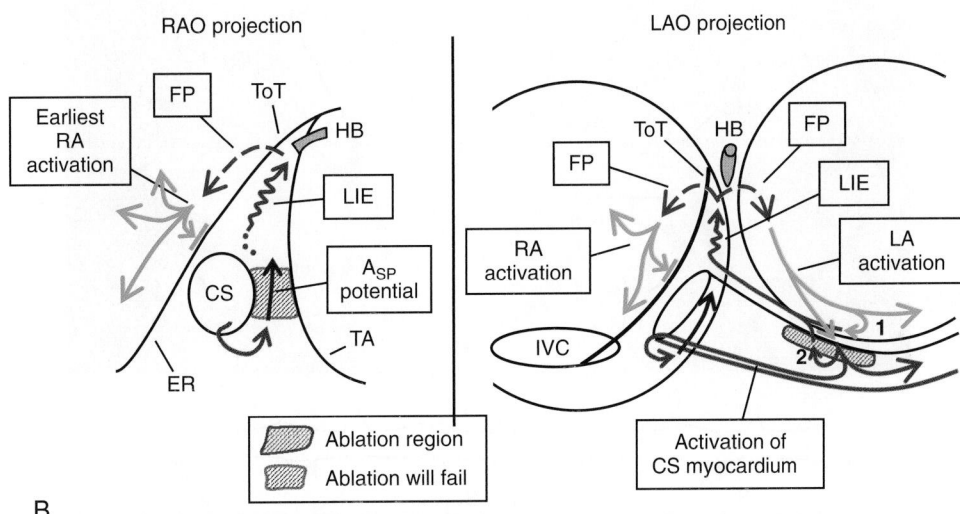

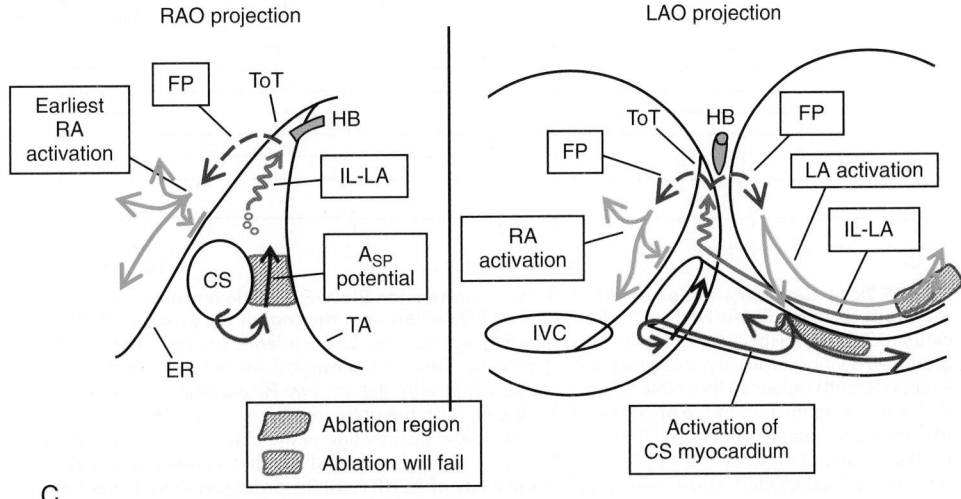

FIGURE 78.13 Schematic representation of the circuit and ablation sites for three forms of Slow/Fast atrioventricular nodal reentrant tachycardia (AVNRT). (A) Rightward inferior extension (*RIE*) Slow/Fast AVNRT. Retrograde conduction over the fast pathway (*FP*) (*dotted red arrows*) activates the right and left sides of the interatrial septum, posterior to the tendon of Todaro (*ToT*), at a level slightly inferior to the level of the His bundle (*HB*). The right atrial (*RA*) and left atrial (*LA*) activation pattern (*green arrows*) is the same as that shown in Fig. 78.3A. The left atrium activates the coronary sinus (*CS*) myocardium (*brown arrows*). The CS myocardium (*brown arrows*) activates the floor of the CS ostium, followed by activation of the inferior triangle of Koch (ToK), generating the A_{SP} potential (*straight blue arrows*) and anterograde

Continued

FIGURE 78.13, cont'd conduction over the RIE (*blue arrows, RIE*). Ablation across the inferior ToK, between the inferoseptal tricuspid annulus (*TA*) and the anterior (apical) margin of the CS ostium (*red crosshatched area* and *black dots*), interrupts anterograde conduction over the RIE and eliminates RIE Slow/Fast AVNRT. (B) Leftward inferior extension (*LIE*) Slow/Fast AVNRT. Retrograde FP conduction (*dotted red arrows*) and atrial activation (*green arrows*) same as (A). The left atrium activates the CS myocardium (*brown arrows*) and the proximal end of the LIE of the atrioventricular node (*LIE, purple arrows*), either directly (*1*) or via the CS myocardium (*2*). Activation propagates along the LIE of the atrioventricular node in the anterograde direction (*squiggly purple arrows*) forming the slow pathway (SP) and completing the reentrant circuit. The CS myocardium activates the inferior ToK generating the A_{SP} potential (*blue arrows*), but this tissue is not involved in the circuit. For ablation of the atrial end of the LIE (anterograde SP in this tachycardia) we target the roof of the proximal CS, beginning the ablation 3 to 4 cm from the CS ostium and continuing proximally toward the superior-anterior edge of the CS ostium (*red crosshatched area*). The *gray crosshatched area* indicates that ablation of the RIE will fail to eliminate the tachycardia, despite producing junctional automaticity. (C) Inferolateral left atrial (*IL-LA*) Slow/Fast AVNRT. FP conduction (*dotted red arrows*) and atrial activation (*green arrows*) same as (A) and (B). The left atrium activates the atrial end of the IL-LA SP (*orange arrows*) originating close to the inferolateral mitral annulus (*red crosshatched area*). The left atrium also activates the CS myocardium (*brown arrows*), which activates the inferior ToK (*blue arrows*) generating an A_{SP} potential. However, ablation of the RIE at the inferior ToK (*gray crosshatched area* in the right anterior oblique [*RAO*] projection) and the LIE at the roof of the proximal CS (*gray crosshatched area* in the left anterior oblique [*LAO*] projection) will fail to eliminate the tachycardia. Ablation at the inferolateral mitral annulus (*red crosshatched area*) is required to eliminate the tachycardia. *IVC,* Inferior vena cava.

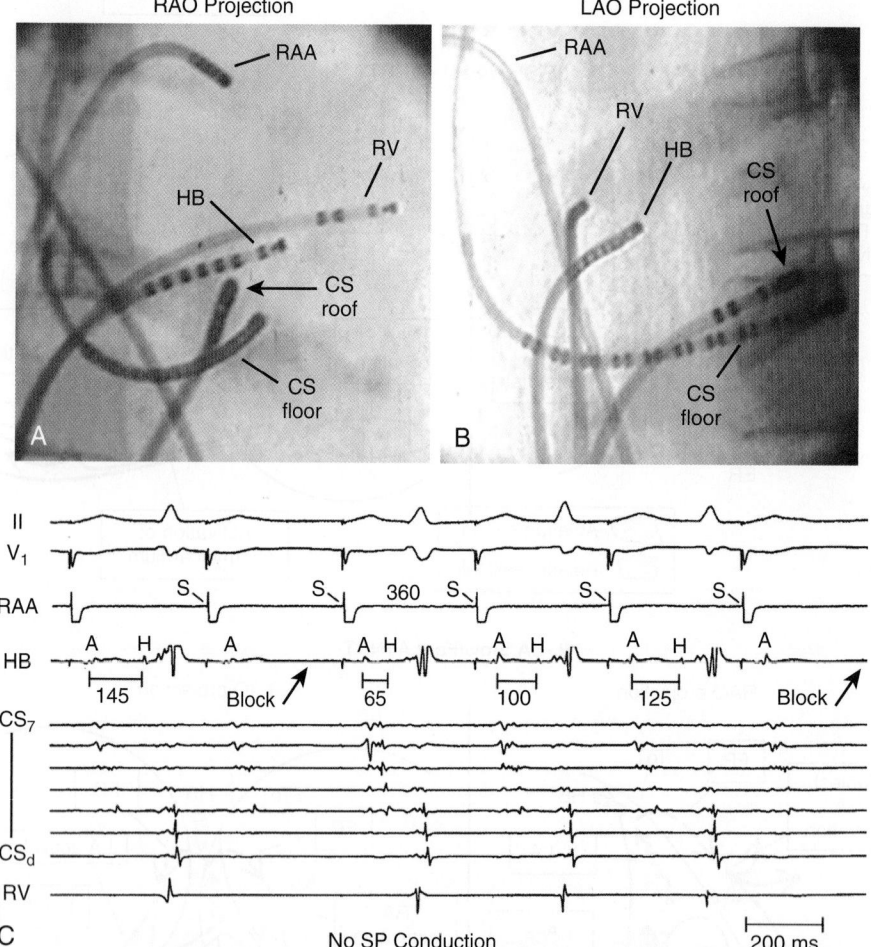

FIGURE 78.14 Catheter ablation of leftward inferior extension Slow/Fast atrioventricular nodal reentrant tachycardia (AVNRT) by radiofrequency (RF) ablation at the roof of the proximal coronary sinus (*CS*). Prior to this figure, five RF applications were delivered to the inferior triangle of Koch. They produced a vigorous accelerated junctional rhythm, but sustained Slow/Fast AVNRT (with no change in cycle length) remained inducible by programmed atrial stimulation. Two RF applications were then delivered along the roof of the proximal CS. Radiographs in the right anterior oblique (*RAO*) projection (A) and the left anterior oblique (*LAO*) projection (B) show the position of the ablation catheter (*CS roof*) for the second of these two RF applications (RF No. 7), which eliminated all residual anterograde slow pathway (*SP*) conduction and eliminated the inducibility of AVNRT. (C) Recordings during decremental atrial pacing from the right atrial appendage (pacing stimuli *S,* in the right atrial appendage [*RAA*] electrogram) following RF No. 7. A decrease in atrial pacing cycle length to 360 ms was associated with Wenckebach block in fast pathway conduction with longest A-H interval of only 145 ms, suggesting complete absence of anterograde conduction over any SP. It is likely that ablation at the inferior triangle of Koch eliminated conduction over the rightward inferior extension and ablation at the roof of the proximal CS eliminated conduction over the leftward inferior extension of the atrioventricular node, eliminating all SP conduction. *HB,* His bundle; *RV,* right ventricle.

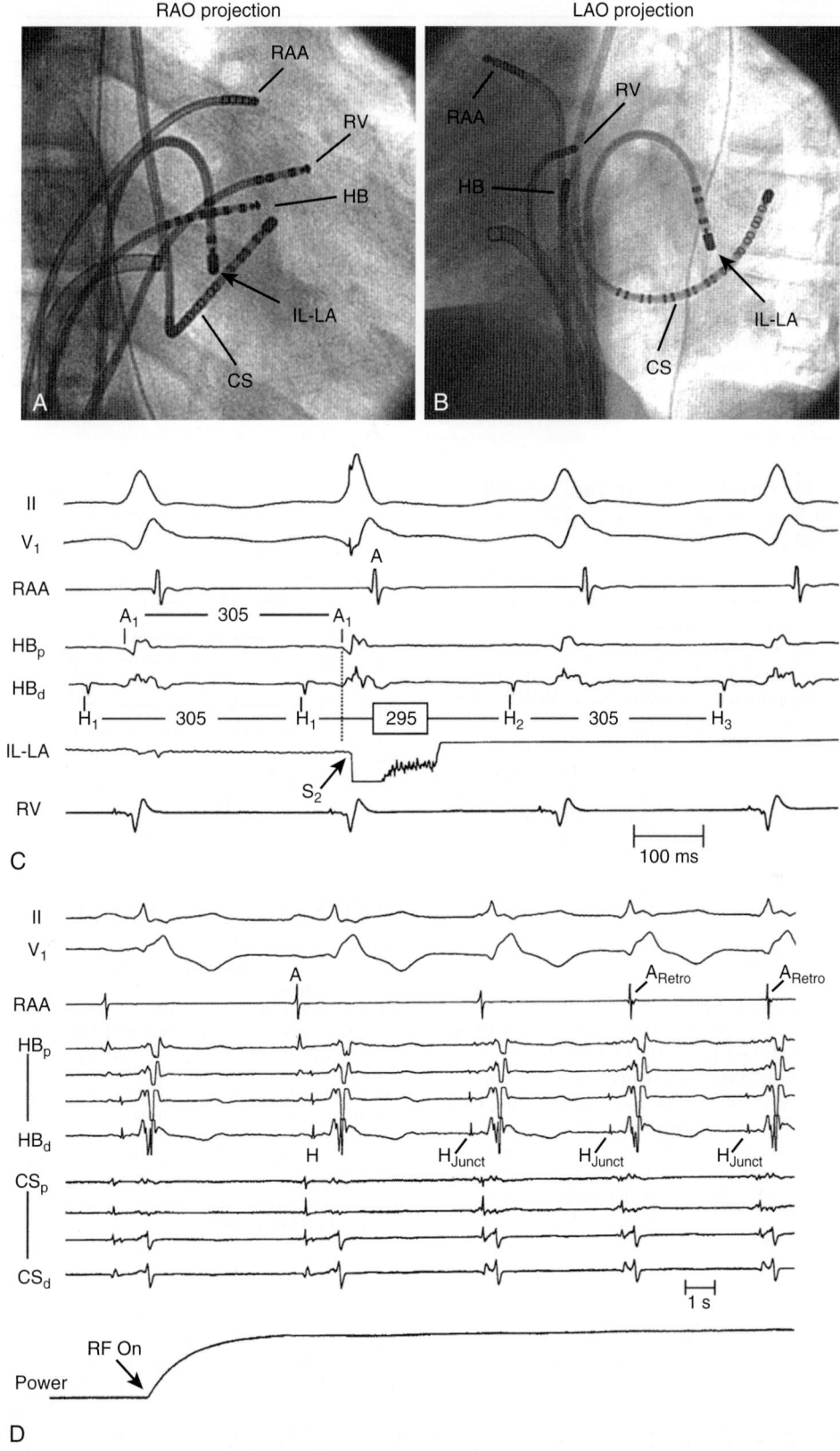

FIGURE 78.15 Localization of the inferolateral left atrial (*IL-LA*) slow pathway using the resetting technique followed by catheter ablation of IL-LA Slow/Fast atrioventricular nodal reentrant tachycardia (AVNRT) in the left atrium close to the inferolateral mitral annulus. (A) and (B) Radiographs in the right anterior oblique (*RAO*) and left anterior oblique (*LAO*) projections show catheter positions, including the mapping catheter in the left atrium (transseptal technique), positioned close to the inferolateral mitral annulus (*IL-LA*). (C) During Slow/Fast AVNRT with a constant cycle length of 305 ms, an atrial extrastimulus was delivered to the mapping catheter in the left atrium close to the inferolateral mitral annulus (*arrow, S_2 in IL-LA* electrogram) after retrograde atrial activation had occurred (A_1-A_1 = 305 ms in the *HB_p* electrogram). The atrial extrastimulus advanced the next His bundle (*HB*) potential (H_2) by 10 ms (H_1-H_2 = 295 ms). H_2 was followed by an interval equal to the tachycardia cycle length (H_2-H_3 = 305 ms), completing the resetting response. The resetting of the tachycardia suggests the site where the left atrial extrastimulus was delivered was located close to an atrial connection with the slow pathway forming the anterograde limb of the reentrant circuit (IL-LA slow pathway). (D) An application of radiofrequency (*RF*) current was delivered to the resetting site in the left atrium (*arrow, RF On* in the RF power tracing). This produced an immediate accelerated junctional rhythm. Each His bundle potential of the accelerated junctional rhythm (H_{Junct}) was followed by retrograde conduction over the fast atrioventricular nodal pathway (A_{Retro}), consistent with heating-induced automaticity of the IL-LA slow pathway. *CS,* Coronary sinus; *RAA,* right atrial appendage; *RV,* right ventricle.

sites produced accelerated junctional rhythm with 1:1 retrograde FP conduction (see Fig. 78.15D), identical to that observed during radiofrequency current delivery to the inferior ToK in patients with RIE Slow/Fast AVNRT, indicating heating of the inferolateral atrial SP. In the remaining two patients, AVNRT was eliminated by complete isolation of the CS myocardium from the left and right atria. These observations suggest that the SP participating in this form of Slow/Fast AVNRT has an atrial connection located in the left atrium. Two unusual features were found in some of these patients: (1) a very short H-A interval during tachycardia (15 ms or less) and (2) the occurrence of the "2-for-1 phenomenon" during programmed atrial stimulation in which an atrial extrastimulus produces two His bundle potentials, presumably resulting from conduction over both an FP and SP. The "2-for-1" response suggests an absence of retrograde penetration of the SP during anterograde FP conduction and may be a useful marker for this type of circuit.

Atrioventricular Nodal Reentrant Tachycardia Using Two Slow Pathways (RIE/LIE AVNRT and LIE/RIE AVNRT)

Short H-A Interval

Both RIE anterograde/LIE retrograde (RIE/LIE) AVNRT and LIE anterograde/RIE retrograde (LIE/RIE) AVNRT may present with a relatively long A-H interval (up to 485 ms in our experience; median, 240 ms) and short H-A interval, representing the tachycardias traditionally referred to as Slow/Slow AVNRT (see Figs. 78.9B and 78.16–78.19). These tachycardias often mimic Slow/Fast AVNRT; however, they are differentiated from Slow/Fast AVNRT by the presence of earliest retrograde activation recorded at the roof of the CS, 1.5 to 4 cm from the ostium (see Figs. 78.9B and 78.16B)[8] representing retrograde conduction over the LIE, or at the inferior ToK (see Fig. 78.17) representing retrograde conduction over the RIE, rather than posterior to the ToT (FP area, see Fig. 78.2). RIE/LIE AVNRT accounts for the majority of these tachycardias. When induced by programmed atrial stimulation, the initiation is associated with an abrupt increase in the A-H interval. These patients often exhibit multiple jumps in the A_2-H_2 interval during atrial extrastimulus testing, consistent with multiple SPs.

Compared with Slow/Fast AVNRT (the other "Short H-A" form of AVNRT), RIE/LIE and LIE/RIE AVNRT have a much wider range of H-A interval, in our experience, ranging from –35 to 260 ms (median, 120 ms). Unlike Slow/Fast AVNRT, the H-A interval can be very short or even negative (see Fig. 78.17), despite retrograde conduction over an SP, because of the presence of a lower common pathway. Short H-A intervals can be explained by retrograde conduction over the LIE (or RIE) with simultaneous bystander conduction over a lower common pathway from the distal junction of the two SPs to the His bundle. The longer the conduction time over the lower common pathway, the shorter the H-A interval. The short HA interval produces simultaneous atrial and ventricular activation, simulating Slow/Fast AVNRT (see Figs. 78.9B, 78.16, and 78.17), and has sometimes been considered a variant of Slow/Fast AVNRT with an inferior exit for the retrograde FP (formerly described as "posterior type" AVNRT). However, approximately half of the patients with this form of AVNRT also have retrograde conduction over the FP with earliest atrial activation recorded posterior to the ToT. The shift in the retrograde atrial activation sequence during programmed ventricular stimulation from retrograde FP to retrograde SP confirms that retrograde conduction is not occurring over the FP during tachycardia (see Figs. 78.1 and 78.17). In patients with simultaneous atrial and ventricular activation during tachycardia, identification of the retrograde atrial activation sequence is facilitated by the use of para-Hisian late ventricular extrastimuli, which separate the atrial and ventricular potentials (see Fig. 78.16B).

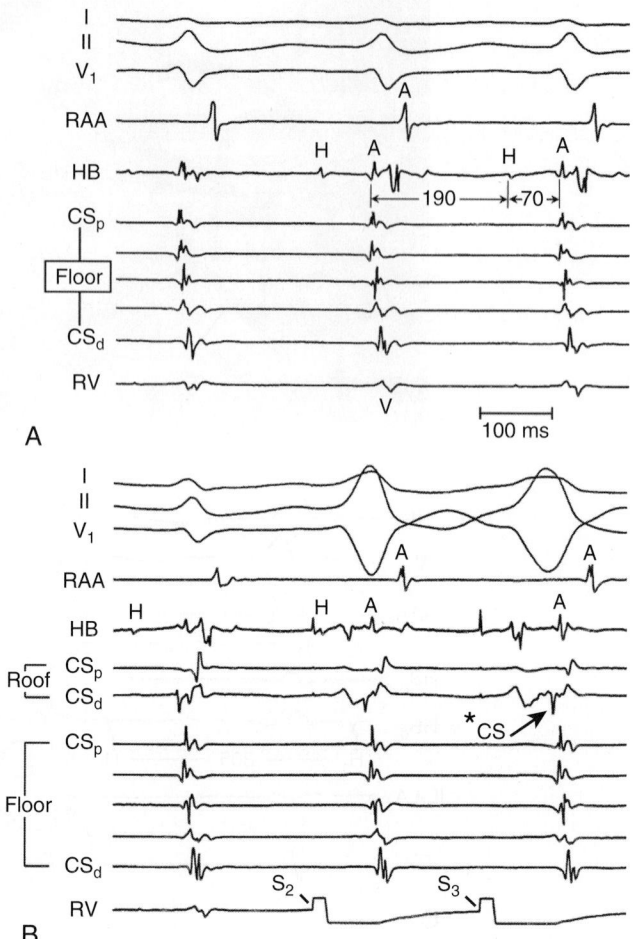

FIGURE 78.16 Rightward inferior extension anterograde/leftward inferior extension retrograde (RIE/LIE) atrioventricular nodal reentrant tachycardia (AVNRT) (Slow/Slow AVNRT) with a short H-A interval mimicking Slow/Fast AVNRT. (A) During RIE/LIE AVNRT, a short H-A interval (*70 ms* in *HB* electrogram) resulted in simultaneous atrial and ventricular activation, which obscures the retrograde atrial activation sequence and mimics Slow/Fast AVNRT. (B) Two right ventricular extrastimuli were delivered to the para-Hisian right ventricular septum. The second ventricular extrastimulus (S_3) advanced the timing of local ventricular activation, revealing the retrograde atrial activation sequence with earliest activation recorded at the roof of the proximal coronary sinus (*CS*) (**CS* potential in *roof* CS_d electrogram), consistent with retrograde conduction over the slow pathway (SP) formed by the LIE, with activation propagating away in both directions in the floor CS electrograms. *HB*, His bundle; *RAA*, right atrial appendage.

Cycle length changes and changes in H-A interval during tachycardia are much more common in RIE/LIE and LIE/RIE AVNRT than in Slow/Fast AVNRT. In addition, during RIE/LIE or LIE/RIE AVNRT, the H-A interval is consistently shorter (by a mean of 30 ms) than during ventricular pacing at the tachycardia cycle length (see Fig. 78.9B), whereas in Slow/Fast AVNRT, the H-A interval is usually slightly longer (mean, 9 ms) than during ventricular pacing at the tachycardia cycle length (see Fig. 78.9A).[1] The longer H-A interval during ventricular pacing in patients with RIE/LIE and LIE/RIE AVNRT results from conduction over the relatively long lower common pathway. In patients with AVNRT exhibiting a short H-A interval, an H-A interval during ventricular pacing at the tachycardia cycle length (measured from the *end* of the most proximal retrograde His bundle potential) exceeding the H-A interval during tachycardia (ΔHA) by ≥15 ms is probably diagnostic of RIE/LIE or

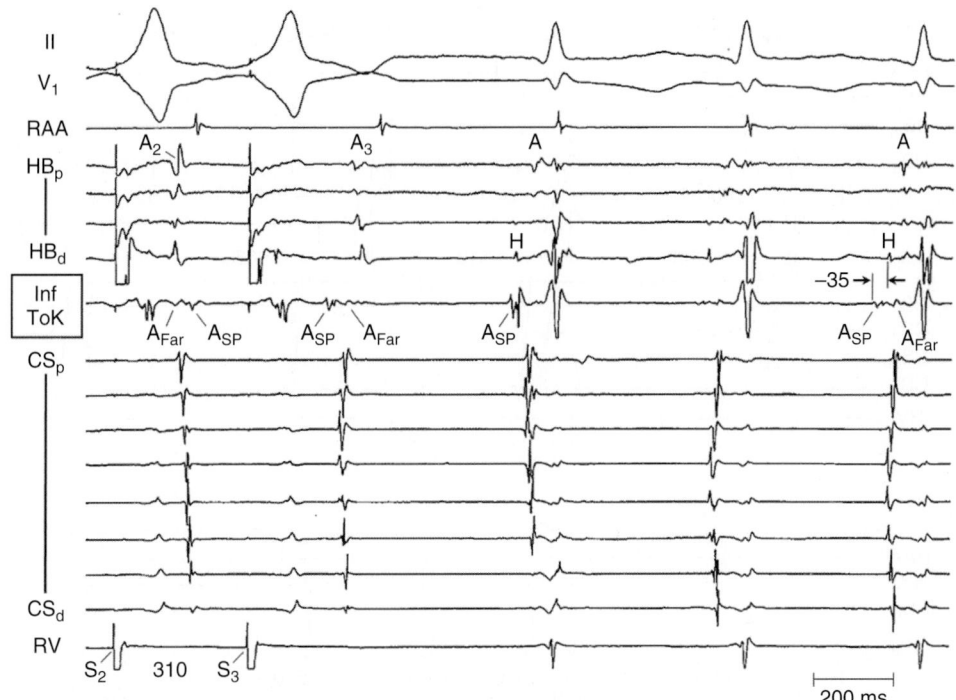

FIGURE 78.17 Induction by ventricular extrastimuli of leftward inferior extension anterograde/ rightward inferior extension retrograde (LIE/RIE) atrioventricular nodal reentrant tachycardia (AVNRT) (Slow/Slow AVNRT) with negative H-A interval. In the first complex of the tracing, a ventricular extrastimulus (S_2) resulted in a retrograde atrial activation sequence consistent with retrograde conduction over the fast atrioventricular nodal pathway. Note the retrograde A_{SP} potential follows the timing of atrial activation in the proximal coronary sinus (*CS*), as well as the far-field atrial potential (A_{Far}) from behind the eustachian ridge. The second ventricular extrastimulus (S_3) resulted in retrograde block in fast pathway conduction and selective retrograde conduction over a slow pathway, with an activation sequence consistent with conduction over the RIE (A_{SP} potential precedes atrial activation at other sites), initiating sustained LIE/RIE AVNRT (Slow/Slow AVNRT). During tachycardia, atrial activation in the His bundle electrograms (*A* potential) followed His bundle activation, simulating Slow/Fast AVNRT. However, the retrograde A_{SP} potential in the inferior triangle of Koch (*Inf ToK*) electrogram preceded His-bundle activation by 35 ms (negative H-A interval). *RAA,* Right atrial appendage; *RV,* right ventricle.

LIE/RIE AVNRT (Slow/Slow AVNRT), excluding Slow/Fast AVNRT (see Fig. 78.9).[1]

The long lower common pathway in AVNRT using two SPs is also demonstrated by the response to ventricular extrastimuli during tachycardia. Atrial activation is not advanced until the ventricular extrastimulus retrogradely advances the proximal His bundle potential by 30 to 60 ms (see Fig. 78.18). This contrasts with Slow/Fast AVNRT wherein any advance in the timing of retrograde His bundle activation by a ventricular extrastimulus usually results in an equal advance in the timing of retrograde atrial activation (see Fig. 78.12). The longer lower common pathway during reentry between the two SPs suggests that the junction between the anterograde and retrograde limbs of this tachycardia is located more inferiorly in the ToK than during Slow/Fast AVNRT.[9]

It is important to differentiate RIE/LIE and LIE/RIE AVNRT from Slow/Fast AVNRT for at least two reasons. First, the technique of FP ablation, now only rarely used for ablation of Slow/Fast AVNRT, does not eliminate RIE/LIE or LIE/RIE AVNRT. In fact, RIE/LIE and LIE/RIE AVNRT with a short H-A interval, mimicking Slow/Fast AVNRT, probably accounts for the 5% to 10% incidence of "atypical AVNRT" reported after FP ablation in patients *thought to have* Slow/Fast AVNRT. Second, in our experience, the recurrence rate after SP ablation is greater for RIE/LIE or LIE/RIE AVNRT than for Slow/Fast AVNRT (8.3% vs. 0.5%, respectively) and therefore ablation targeting both RIE and LIE (inferior ToK and the roof of the CS) may be justified. Of 650 consecutive patients with AVNRT

exhibiting a short H-A interval (<120 ms) referred for ablation in our laboratory, the earliest retrograde activation was recorded behind the ToT (Slow/Fast AVNRT) in 541 (83%), while 109 (17%) had RIE/LIE or LIE/RIE AVNRT.

Rarely, short H-A AVNRT using two SPs is seen using the anterior superior SP for retrograde conduction and the RIE or LIE for anterograde conduction. This tachycardia is identified by recording earliest retrograde activation at the anterior-superior atrial septum, slightly superior and posterior to the site recording His bundle activation and 1.5 to 2 cm superior to the site of earliest activation during retrograde FP conduction (*pink arrows* in Fig. 78.3D).

Long H-A Interval
AVNRT with a relatively short A-H interval and long H-A interval usually represents LIE/RIE AVNRT, formed by anterograde conduction over the LIE and retrograde conduction over the RIE (see Fig. 78.19B), with the earliest retrograde activation recorded at the inferior ToK. The RP interval is longer than the PR interval, with a wide inverted P wave in the inferior electrocardiographic leads (see Fig. 78.7B) due to activation of the left atrium by the CS. This circuit probably accounts for almost all of the tachycardias traditionally classified as Fast/Slow AVNRT.

In the more usual manifestation of this tachycardia (long H-A), the short A-H interval may be even shorter than during sinus rhythm (see Fig. 78.7). The short A-H (and PR) interval may be explained by the following mechanism. Retrograde activation of the RIE (*blue arrow* in Fig. 78.19D) activates the

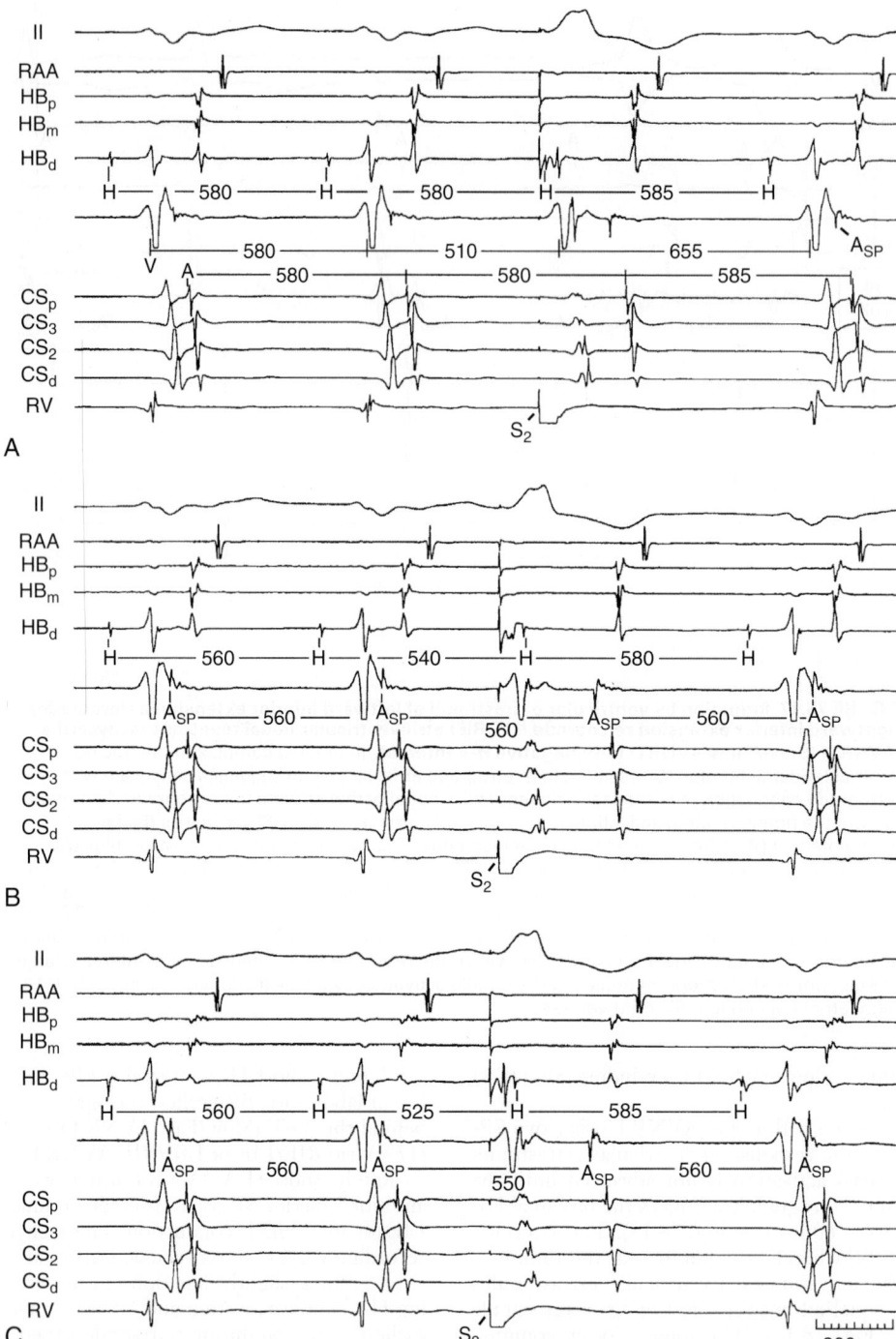

FIGURE 78.18 Use of ventricular extrastimuli to verify the diagnosis of leftward inferior extension anterograde/rightward inferior extension retrograde (LIE/RIE) (Slow/Slow) atrioventricular nodal reentrant tachycardia (AVNRT). (A) During tachycardia, a single extrastimulus (S_2) was delivered to the para-Hisian right ventricular septum. S_2 advanced the timing of local ventricular activation near the site of earliest retrograde atrial activation (inferior triangle of Koch electrogram) by 70 ms (V-$V = 510$ ms, compared with 580 ms). *However, S_2 did not* advance the timing of His bundle activation (H) or atrial activation, excluding retrograde conduction over an inferoseptal accessory pathway and orthodromic atrioventricular reentrant tachycardia. Note that the ventricular extrastimulus provided further separation of the ventricular and atrial potentials, allowing clear identification of the retrograde atrial activation sequence, including the early retrograde A_{SP} potential. (B) An earlier S_2 resulted in retrograde activation of the His bundle. The end of the retrograde His bundle potential occurred 20 ms before anterograde His bundle activation would have occurred (H-$H = 540$ ms, compared with 560 ms). This failed to advance the timing of retrograde atrial activation (A_{SP}-$A_{SP} = 560$ ms), consistent with either AVNRT with a long lower common pathway or atrial tachycardia. (C) *Further shortening of the extrastimulus coupling interval* (an earlier S_2) resulted in earlier retrograde activation of the His bundle. The end of the retrograde H potential occurred 35 ms before the anterograde H potential would have occurred (H-$H = 525$ ms, compared with 560 ms). This resulted in a 10 ms advance in the timing of retrograde atrial activation without a change in the atrial activation sequence (A_{SP}-$A_{SP} = 550$ ms, compared with 560 ms), indicating that the timing of atrial activation was dependent on the timing of His-bundle activation, excluding an atrial tachycardia and confirming AVNRT.

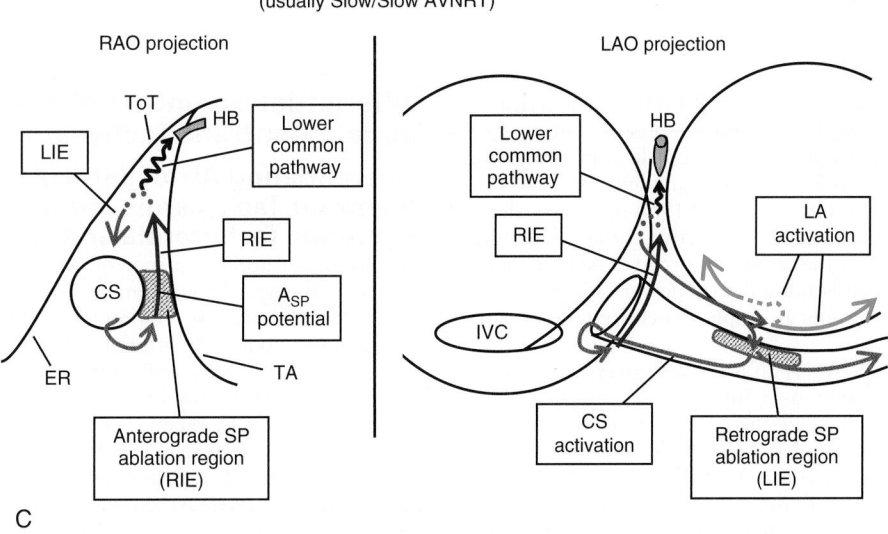

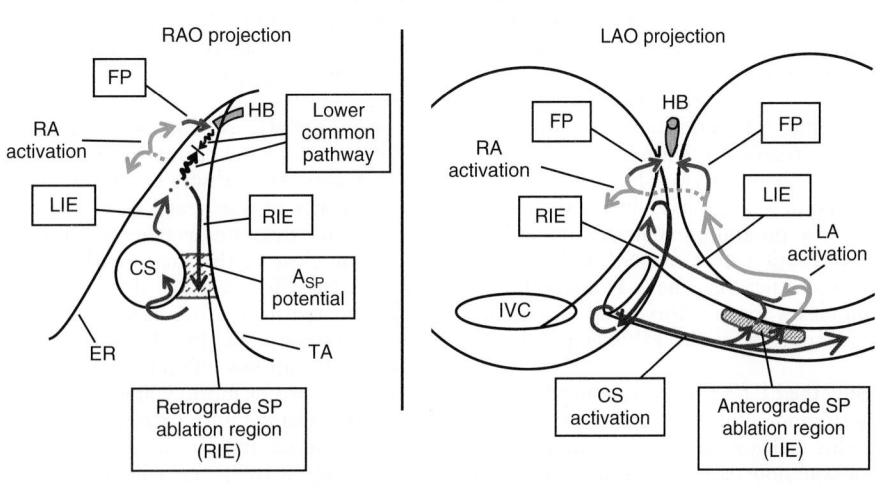

FIGURE 78.19 Hypothesis that Slow/Slow atrioventricular nodal reentrant tachycardia (*AVNRT*) and Fast/Slow AVNRT result from reentry between the rightward and leftward inferior extensions (*RIE* and *LIE*, respectively) of the atrioventricular (*AV*) node and schematic representations for the proposed circuits for these tachycardias. (A) Reentry using the RIE in the anterograde direction (*blue arrow*) and the LIE in the retrograde direction (*purple arrow*) with earliest activation in the roof of the proximal coronary sinus (*CS*) often produces a long A-H interval and

Continued

FIGURE 78.19, cont'd shorter H-A interval typical of Slow/Slow AVNRT. (B) Reentry using the LIE for anterograde conduction (*purple arrow*) and the RIE for retrograde conduction (*blue arrow*) with earliest activation at the inferior triangle of Koch (ToK) (A_{SP} potential) often produces a short A-H (left atrium activates the fast pathway [*FP*]) and long H-A, typical of Fast/Slow AVNRT. (C) Schematic representation of reentry between the RIE and LIE postulated by the authors to be the reentrant circuit in most cases of Slow/Slow AVNRT. Activation propagates in the anterograde direction along the slow pathway (*SP*) formed by the RIE (*blue arrows*) to activate the lower common pathway in the anterograde direction (*squiggly black arrows*) and the SP formed by the LIE in the retrograde direction (*purple arrows*). The LIE activates the roof of the CS myocardium (*brown arrows*), which propagates the impulse to the floor of the CS ostium (*brown arrows*) to activate the inferior ToK and RIE (*blue arrows* and A_{SP} potential) to complete the circuit. The FP does not participate in the circuit, even though the H-A interval is often short. The conduction time over the lower common pathway delays His bundle (*HB*) activation, shortening the H-A interval during tachycardia mimicking Slow/Fast AVNRT. Our approach to ablation is to target the atrial end of the retrograde limb of the circuit (usually the LIE at the roof of the CS, *red crosshatched area* in left anterior oblique [*LAO*] projection) followed by ablation of the atrial end of the anterograde limb (usually the RIE at the inferior ToK, *red crosshatched area* in right anterior oblique [*RAO*] projection). (D) Schematic representation of the proposed circuit for LIE/RIE AVNRT (accounting for the majority of Fast/Slow AVNRT and some Slow/Slow AVNRT). Activation propagates in the anterograde direction along the SP formed by the LIE (*purple arrows*) to activate the lower common pathway in the anterograde direction (*lower squiggly black arrows* in RAO projection) and the retrograde SP formed by the RIE in the retrograde direction (*blue arrows*). The RIE activates the floor of the CS ostium (*brown arrow* in RAO projection). The CS myocardium propagates the impulse laterally (*brown arrows* in LAO projection) to activate the left atrium (*green arrow*) and the LIE in the anterograde direction (*purple arrows*) to complete the circuit. Left atrial activation propagates rapidly (*green arrows* in LAO projection) to the atrial septum to activate the FP (*red arrows*), producing a short A-H interval, and across the atrial septum to activate the right atrium (*dotted green lines* and *green arrows*). The FP serves as a bystander. Ablation is targeted to the atrial end of the retrograde SP at the inferior ToK at a site recording a sharp retrograde A_{SP} potential (*red crosshatched area* in RAO projection), followed by the atrial end of the anterograde SP at the roof of the coronary sinus (*red crosshatched area* in LAO projection). *ER*, Eustachian ridge; *IVC*, inferior vena cava; *TA*, tricuspid annulus; *ToT*, tendon of Todaro. ([A] and [B] Modified from Inoue S, Becker AE. Posterior extensions of the human compact atrioventricular node: a neglected anatomic feature of potential clinical significance. *Circulation.* 1998;97:188–193.)

CS myocardium (*brown arrows* in Fig. 78.19D), which activates the left atrium (*green arrows* in Fig. 78.19D) and the LIE (*purple arrows* in Fig. 78.19D). Relatively rapid conduction along the left atrium (*green arrows* in Fig. 78.19D) and anterograde conduction over the FP (*red arrows* in Fig. 78.19D) produce a short A-H interval. In this mechanism, the FP activates the His bundle but does not participate in the reentrant circuit (bystander activation). The H-A interval is not a direct measure of any of the components of the circuit, but is simply the entire cycle length minus the AH interval.

Traditionally, Fast/Slow AVNRT was given this label because the relatively short A-H interval was interpreted as indicating that the FP formed the anterograde limb of the tachycardia circuit. This label suggested that the circuit was the same as that used in Slow/Fast AVNRT, but in the reverse direction. However, several findings suggest the presence of a long lower common pathway, which would not be present if the circuit was using the same anatomical substrate as RIE Slow/Fast AVNRT. First, the H-A interval during ventricular pacing at the tachycardia cycle length is much longer than the H-A interval during tachycardia (compared with the slightly shorter H-A interval during ventricular pacing in Slow/Fast AVNRT). Second, unlike Slow/Fast AVNRT, ventricular extrastimuli during tachycardia must advance His bundle activation by 30 to 60 ms before resetting the tachycardia (see Fig. 78.18). Another observation supporting reentry between two SPs is the frequent occurrence of a >50-ms jump in A-H interval during the initiation of Fast/Slow AVNRT by programmed atrial stimulation, suggesting anterograde conduction over one SP, followed by retrograde conduction over another SP. The A-H interval then shortens over several complexes to the short value during the established tachycardia, presumably as the FP is engaged as a bystander.

Fast/Slow AVNRT using the FP for the anterograde limb and one of the SPs for the retrograde limb may occur, but appears to be very uncommon. This tachycardia would be expected to have a very short lower common pathway (as for Slow/Fast AVNRT). As a result, ventricular extrastimuli during tachycardia that advance the His bundle potential by 5 to 10 ms would be expected to change the timing of the next atrial potential and reset the tachycardia. This finding is rarely, if ever, encountered in long H-A AVNRT.

Differential Diagnosis of Atrioventricular Nodal Reentrant Tachycardia

Differentiating Atrioventricular Nodal Reentrant Tachycardia From Atrioventricular Reentrant Tachycardia and Atrial Tachycardia

The atrial activation sequence of the various forms of AVNRT may be indistinguishable from the atrial activation sequence of either orthodromic AV reentrant tachycardia (using an anteroseptal, inferoseptal, left inferior, or left inferolateral accessory pathway) or atrial tachycardia arising from the septum or region surrounding the CS. Any form of AVNRT can be differentiated from orthodromic AV reentrant tachycardia and atrial tachycardia by the use of ventricular extrastimuli, which establishes whether the reentrant circuit incorporates ventricular myocardium. The extrastimuli are best delivered to the base of the ventricle, close to the site of earliest retrograde atrial activation. An advance in the timing of atrial activation without first retrogradely activating the His bundle establishes the presence of an accessory AV pathway. If the atrial activation sequence of the advanced complex is identical to the other tachycardia complexes and if a slight advance in the timing of atrial activation results in a change in the timing of the next His bundle activation (resetting the tachycardia), then an accessory pathway is being activated during the tachycardia and it forms part of the reentrant circuit, respectively. Conversely, an accessory AV pathway is unlikely to be present if the timing and sequence of retrograde atrial activation are unchanged by a ventricular extrastimulus that advances the timing of ventricular activation close to the site of earliest atrial activation by 50 ms or more (see Figs. 78.12A, 78.16B, and 78.18A). AVNRT can be differentiated from atrial tachycardia by the use of earlier ventricular extrastimuli. In AVNRT, ventricular extrastimuli that significantly advance the timing of retrograde His bundle activation (30–60 ms or more) will alter the timing of atrial activation (without a change in the atrial activation sequence) or will produce V-A block and terminate the tachycardia (see Figs. 78.12B and C and 78.18C), but will have no effect on the timing or sequence of atrial activation in atrial tachycardia. This degree of advance in His bundle activation often requires the use of multiple ventricular extrastimuli or continuous ventricular pacing at a cycle length slightly shorter than tachycardia cycle length. Atrial tachycardia is diagnosed if ventricular extrastimuli or ventricular pacing during tachycardia retrogradely advances His bundle activation by more than 60 to 80 ms without changing the timing or sequence of atrial activation. A long advance in His-bundle activation is required to differentiate AVNRT using two SPs from atrial tachycardia due to the long lower common pathway between the RIE and LIE and the His bundle.

REFERENCES

1. Lockwood D, Nakagawa H, Jackman WM. Electrophysiologic characteristics of atrioventricular nodal reentrant tachycardia: implications for reentrant circuits. In: Zipes DP, Jalife J, eds. *Cardiac Electrophysiology: from Cell to Bedside.* 5th ed. Philadelphia: Saunders Elsevier; 2009:615–646.
2. Sung RJ, Waxman HL, Saksena S, Juma Z. Sequence of retrograde atrial activation in patients with dual atrioventricular nodal pathways. *Circulation.* 1981;64:1059–1067.
3. Katritsis DG, Ellenbogen KA, Becker AE. Atrial activation during atrioventricular nodal reentrant tachycardia: studies on retrograde fast pathway conduction. *Heart Rhythm.* 2006;3:993–1000.
4. Inoue S, Becker AE. Posterior extensions of the human compact atrioventricular node: a neglected anatomic feature of potential clinical significance. *Circulation.* 1998;97:188–193.
5. Ho SW, McComb JM, Scott CD, Anderson RH. Morphology of the cardiac conduction system in patients with electrophysiologically proven dual atrioventricular nodal pathways. *J Cardiovasc Electrophysiol.* 1993;4:504–512.
6. Brechenmacher C. Atrio-His bundle tracts. *Br Heart J.* 1975;37:853–855.
7. Jackman WM, Lockwood D, Nakagawa H, et al. Catheter ablation of atrioventricular nodal reentrant tachycardia. In: Wilber DJ, Packer DL, Stevenson WG, eds. *Catheter Ablation of Cardiac Arrhythmias: Basic Concepts and Clinical Applications.* 3rd ed. Hoboken, NJ: Blackwell Futura; 2008:120–148.
8. Otomo K, Okamura H, Noda T, et al. "Left variant" atypical atrioventricular nodal reentrant tachycardia: electrophysiological characteristics and effect of SP ablation within CS. *J Cardiovasc Electrophysiol.* 2006;17:1177–1183.
9. Yamabe H, Tanaka Y, Morihisa K, Uemura T, et al. Electrophysiologic delineation of the tachycardia circuit in the slow-slow form of atrioventricular nodal reentrant tachycardias. *Heart Rhythm.* 2007;4:713–721.

79 Junctional Tachycardia

Christopher F. Liu, James E. Ip, Steven M. Markowitz, and Bruce B. Lerman

Junctional tachycardia (JT), alternatively known as junctional ectopic tachycardia (JET), originates from the atrioventricular (AV) junction—encompassing the AV node and His bundle. JT is rarely encountered, especially in the adult population, and its pathogenesis remains incompletely understood. Furthermore, its presentation can be variable, and the diagnosis and therapy can be challenging. This chapter will focus on the tachycardic forms of junctional arrhythmia, although escape rhythms that arise from the AV junction in the setting of severe bradycardia and AV block may also occur.

Electrocardiographic Features and Diagnosis

The surface electrocardiographic findings of JET can be variable depending on whether the tachycardia is paroxysmal or incessant and whether there is ventriculoatrial (VA) conduction during tachycardia. An incessant JT with a 1:1 VA conduction presents as a regular narrow QRS tachycardia with short RP interval and retrograde P waves, mimicking typical AV nodal reentrant tachycardia (AVNRT). In contrast, in paroxysmal JET without VA conduction, the electrocardiogram (ECG) will show an irregular narrow QRS tachycardia with intermittent sinus capture beats. During periods of frequent irregular junctional ectopy without obvious P waves or with variable distortion of the sinus P waves, the surface ECG can mimic the appearance of multifocal atrial tachycardia or atrial fibrillation. Finally, JT with bundle branch block can mimic ventricular tachycardia that involves the specialized conduction system, particularly if VA conduction is absent. Because of its relative rarity in the adult population, JET may not always be considered in the differential diagnosis and therefore may be underdiagnosed.

To differentiate JET from AVNRT based on the surface ECG, the pattern of tachycardia initiation can be informative—that is, whether there is critical prolongation of the PR interval on the initiating beat (which would suggest AVNRT). Bursts of short RP tachycardia without initiating premature atrial contractions (PACs) or PR prolongation suggest that JET is more likely. Finally, the complete absence of VA conduction also favors the diagnosis of JET because AVNRT with complete block of the upper common pathway is less likely.

Differentiation During Electrophysiological Study

The electrophysiological hallmark of JT is the presence of a His bundle electrogram that precedes the QRS complex. The HV interval is either normal or prolonged (in the setting of infra-Hisian conduction system disease). A short HV interval in association with a narrow QRS complex (<35 ms) should prompt suspicion for fascicular tachycardia. The differentiation of JET with aberrant conduction from myocardial ventricular tachycardia is primarily based on the presence of a normal HV interval. When VA conduction is present, the differentiation of JET from atrial tachycardia can be based on the observation of the HH interval variability driving the AA interval variability. Ventricular overdrive pacing yields a V-A-H-V response, also ruling out atrial tachycardia.

As indicated earlier, the most challenging differential diagnosis is between JET and AVNRT, as the two arrhythmias present with similar HV intervals recorded during tachycardia and sinus rhythm. Each arrhythmia may also be associated with VA block.[1] Several maneuvers can help differentiate JT from AV nodal reentry, but these require the presence of VA conduction. Atrial overdrive pacing yields an A-H-H-A response in JET and an A-H-A response in AVNRT (Fig. 79.1).[2] In the case of JET, overdrive pacing advances His bundle activation to the pacing cycle length (A-H). JET resumes after the cessation of pacing, with the first return beat of the tachycardia characterized by an H-A sequence. Therefore the general response to atrial overdrive pacing in JET is A-H-H-A. In a typical slow–fast AVNRT, atrial entrainment proceeds via the slow pathway (same anterograde limb as the reentrant circuit); therefore the final entrained His has a long A-H interval and results in the immediate return of atrial activation via the retrograde fast pathway (A-H-A response). Alternatively, atrial overdrive pacing may terminate AVNRT by causing an anterograde block in the slow pathway as well as a block in the retrograde fast pathway. Another useful maneuver involves the introduction of PACs during tachycardia. A late-coupled PAC delivered during His refractoriness does not affect the continuation of JET because it does not reset the JET focus but can preexcite or delay the subsequent ventricular beat in AVNRT by engaging the anterograde slow AV nodal pathway (Fig. 79.2A and B). An early coupled PAC that captures the His bundle and ventricle advances JET for one cycle with subsequent continuation of the tachycardia, whereas an early PAC often terminates AVNRT because it anterogradely engages the fast pathway to advance His bundle activation, thus preventing retrograde activation of the fast pathway from propagation that emerges from the slow pathway (Fig. 79.2C and D).[3] A similar response to PACs can also be demonstrated in the absence of a His bundle recording (Fig. 79.3).

Mechanisms

There is a dearth of data regarding the electrophysiological mechanism of JET. However, its lack of dependence on a critical coupling interval for tachycardia initiation, the often irregular tachycardia rate, and the inability to entrain the arrhythmia suggest a focal nonreentrant mechanism. With regard to cellular mechanism, most published case series of JET have postulated that enhanced automaticity is responsible for the arrhythmia.[4-6] However, recent evidence suggests at least two other mechanisms that may be responsible for JET cases: abnormal automaticity and triggered activity.[7]

In contrast to enhanced automaticity, tissue with abnormal automaticity generally does not demonstrate overdrive

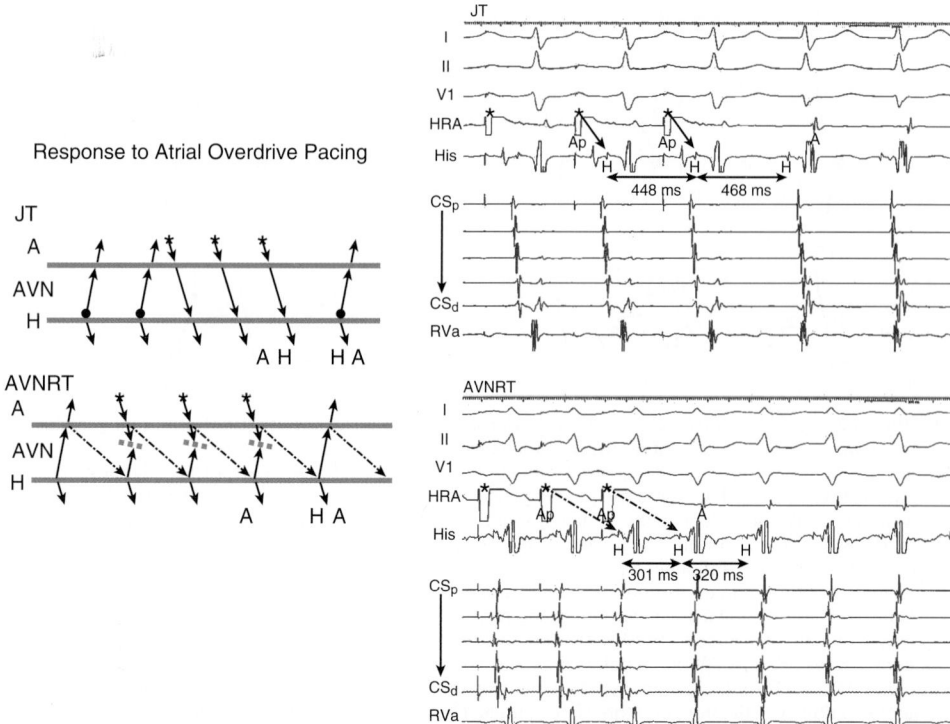

FIGURE 79.1 Atrial overdrive pacing to differentiate junctional tachycardia (*JT*) from atrioventricular nodal reentrant tachycardia (*AVNRT*). *Left side*, Ladder diagrams that illustrate the response to atrial overdrive pacing. *Top*, During JT, the earliest return signal is an H followed by an A, resulting in an A-H-H-A response. *Bottom*, During AVNRT, the earliest return signal is an A, resulting in an A-H-A response. *Asterisk* represents atrial pace (*Ap*). *Solid arrows* represent conduction through the atrium (*A*), fast AV nodal (*AVN*) pathway, and His (*H*). *Interrupted arrows* represent conduction through the slow AV nodal pathway. *Right side*, Intracardiac electrograms. *Top*, During JT, the tachycardia cycle length is 468 ms. Atrial overdrive pacing is performed at 448 ms. After the cessation of pacing, an A-H-H-A response is observed. *Solid arrows* represent conduction down the fast AV nodal pathway. *Bottom*, During AVNRT, the tachycardia cycle length is 320 ms. Atrial overdrive pacing is performed at 300 ms. After the cessation of pacing, an A-H-A response is observed. *Interrupted arrows* represent slow pathway conduction. *CS*, Coronary sinus; *HRA*, high right atrium; *RVa*, right ventricular apex. (From Fan R, Tardos JG, Almasry I, et al. Novel use of atrial overdrive pacing to rapidly differentiate junctional tachycardia from atrioventricular nodal reentrant tachycardia. *Heart Rhythm*. 2011;8:840-844.)

suppression because of its reduced resting membrane potential (typically ≤–60 mV) and inactivated state of the sodium current and electrogenic sodium pump. Abnormal automaticity is then dependent on the slow inward calcium current and is therefore sensitive to calcium channel blockers.[8] Adenosine has no effect on abnormal automaticity, whereas it transiently suppresses enhanced normal automaticity (Fig. 79.4).[9] Therefore sensitivity of an automatic tachycardia to calcium channel blockade and insensitivity to adenosine are consistent with abnormal automaticity (rather than enhanced "normal" automaticity; Fig. 79.5).

A second mechanism—triggered activity—has also been shown to be responsible for JET in some patients. In contrast to JET because of abnormal automaticity, in the triggered subset, the arrhythmia can be induced and terminated with programmed stimulation and can be terminated with adenosine (Fig. 79.6).[10–12]

Clinical Features

Primary JET typically occurs in two clinical settings: in infants, usually shortly after birth, and in children and adults as sporadic cases. The presentation and clinical outcomes are very different in these two settings.

The "congenital" form, which was first described by Coumel and colleagues, manifests at birth or within the first 6 months of age.[13] There is a strong familial association, with up to 50% reported in multiple series. A significant minority of cases occur in association with a structural congenital cardiac abnormality such as an atrial or ventricular septal defect.[14,15] The congenital form of JET is usually incessant and rapid, with mean ventricular rates of 200 to 250 beats/min. Prenatal cases may present with fetal tachycardia and hydrops. The congenital form of JET is associated with a high incidence of ventricular systolic dysfunction and clinical heart failure, and despite intervention, mortality is high—reported to be 35% in an older series (although some deaths were because of procedural complications)[14] and 9% in a more recent series.[16] Documented spontaneous causes of death include ventricular fibrillation, AV block, and refractory heart failure. Because of the frequent requirement for multiple antiarrhythmic drugs, proarrhythmia is suspected to play a role in some cases of sudden death. Limited autopsy data of JT patients have shown focal degeneration and fibroelastosis involving the AV node region and His bundle.[14,17]

In cases of spontaneous JET that present after 6 months of age in the pediatric population, the clinical course is usually benign. Spontaneous JET is extremely rare in adults, and reported series have also suggested a mostly benign course,

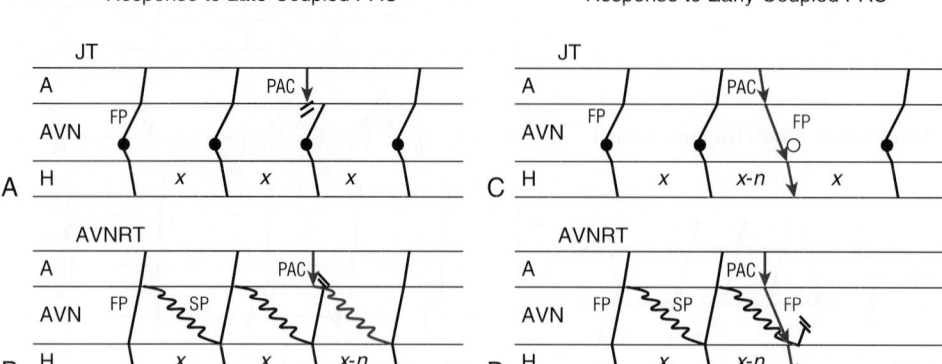

FIGURE 79.2 Premature atrial contraction (*PAC*) response to differentiate junctional tachycardia (*JT*) from atrioventricular nodal reentrant tachycardia (*AVNRT*). *Left*, Response to PAC delivered when the junction is refractory (local atrial activation from PAC occurs at or after His activation). (A) During JT, PAC delivered at a time the junction focus has already depolarized blocks at the AV node (*AVN*) and is unable to influence the immediate or next junction beat. *Solid circles* represent junction focus. *Black lines* show conduction through AVN, His (*H*), and atrium (*A*). (B) During AVNRT, a similarly timed PAC can influence the next beat of AVNRT by early engagement of the slow pathway. *Black lines* show conduction through AVN, His, and atrium, and *red lines* show PAC and its response. Although this figure shows advancement of the next beat (*x-n*), delay of the next beat or termination of tachycardia are also specific to AVNRT. *Red arrow* indicates PAC and its response. *FP*, Fast AV nodal pathway; *SP*, slow AV nodal pathway; *x* and *x-n*, H-H intervals. *Right*, Response to earlier-coupled PACs. (C) During JT, an early PAC advances the immediate JT beat and His timing by the AV nodal fast pathway activation, and the JT continues. *Open circle* represents the anticipated JT beat timing if no PAC were delivered. (D) During AVNRT, an early PAC may advance the immediate His by activation of the AV nodal fast pathway. However, that makes the fast pathway refractory and unavailable for retrograde conduction, thus terminating the AVNRT circuit. (From Padanilam BJ, Manfredi JA, Steinberg LA, et al. Differentiating junctional tachycardia and atrioventricular node re-entry tachycardia based on response to atrial extrastimulus pacing. *J Am Coll Cardiol.* 2008;52:1711-1717.)

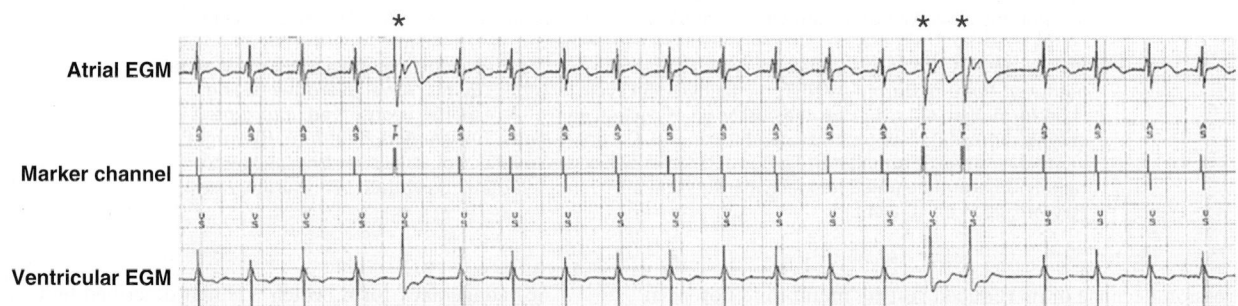

FIGURE 79.3 Dual-chamber pacemaker recording of tachycardia with nearly simultaneous atrioventricular timing. Early coupled premature atrial contractions are delivered at several time points during tachycardia (*asterisks*), each time with the immediate advancement of ventricular activation, followed by the resumption of tachycardia. This response is diagnostic of junctional tachycardia (rather than atrioventricular node reentry). *Top*, Right atrial electrogram (*EGM*); *middle*, marker channels; *bottom*, right ventricular EGM. *AS*, Atrial sensed event; *TP*, atrial pacing in response to tachycardia; *VS*, ventricular sensed event.

similar to other forms of supraventricular tachycardia in adults.[5,6,12] The typical presentation is symptomatic tachycardia, usually exacerbated by exercise or stress; occasionally, JET may cause syncope. As in pediatric patients, congenital cardiac anomalies, such as atrial or ventricular septal defects, can present with JET in the adult population. Similar to other forms of supraventricular tachycardia, tachycardia-mediated cardiomyopathy is a potential concern when there is a high arrhythmia burden.

JT can present in the postoperative setting after cardiac surgery, usually in children after the correction of congenital cardiac defects. Hoffman and associates identified postoperative JET in 5.6% of 594 pediatric patients after cardiac surgery; the vast majority occurred within the first 48 hours.[18] Multivariate

analysis showed that an age of less than 6 months and the postoperative use of dopamine were associated with the occurrence of JET. Moak and colleagues reported a 15.3% incidence of JET following cardiac surgery in 750 patients.[19] Multivariate analysis in this series found that the total surgical time and the postoperative use of milrinone were independent predictors for JET, whereas the use of nitroprusside was associated with a reduced incidence of JET. Another study reported that patients who manifest JET after surgery had a longer requirement for mechanical ventilation, a longer stay in the cardiac intensive care unit, and a higher mortality rate.[20] Although the cause of postoperative JET was historically considered to be mechanical injury to the AV junction, additional mechanisms and associations (such as

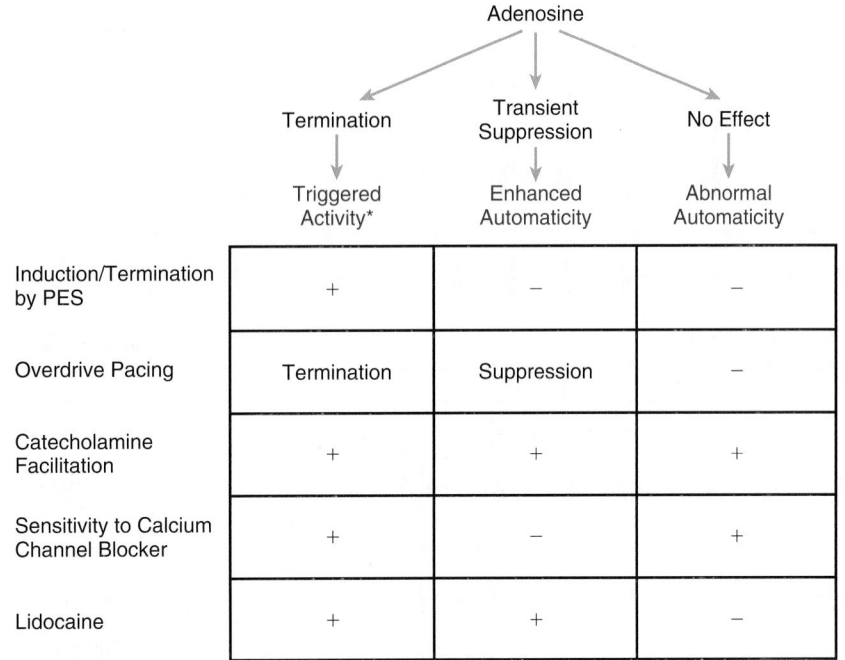

	Triggered Activity*	Enhanced Automaticity	Abnormal Automaticity
Induction/Termination by PES	+	−	−
Overdrive Pacing	Termination	Suppression	−
Catecholamine Facilitation	+	+	+
Sensitivity to Calcium Channel Blocker	+	−	+
Lidocaine	+	+	−

FIGURE 79.4 Electrophysiological mechanism of arrhythmia based on the response to adenosine (*top*) **as well as electrophysiological and pharmacological maneuvers (***left***).** "*+*" denotes that a relationship or response exists; "*–*" denotes that the maneuver has no effect on arrhythmia. *PES,* Programmed electrical stimulation. *Cyclic adenosine monophosphate–mediated delayed afterdepolarization. (From Liu CF, Ip JE, Lin AC, et al. Mechanistic heterogeneity of junctional ectopic tachycardia in adults. *Pacing Clin Electrophysiol.* 2013;36:e7-e10.)

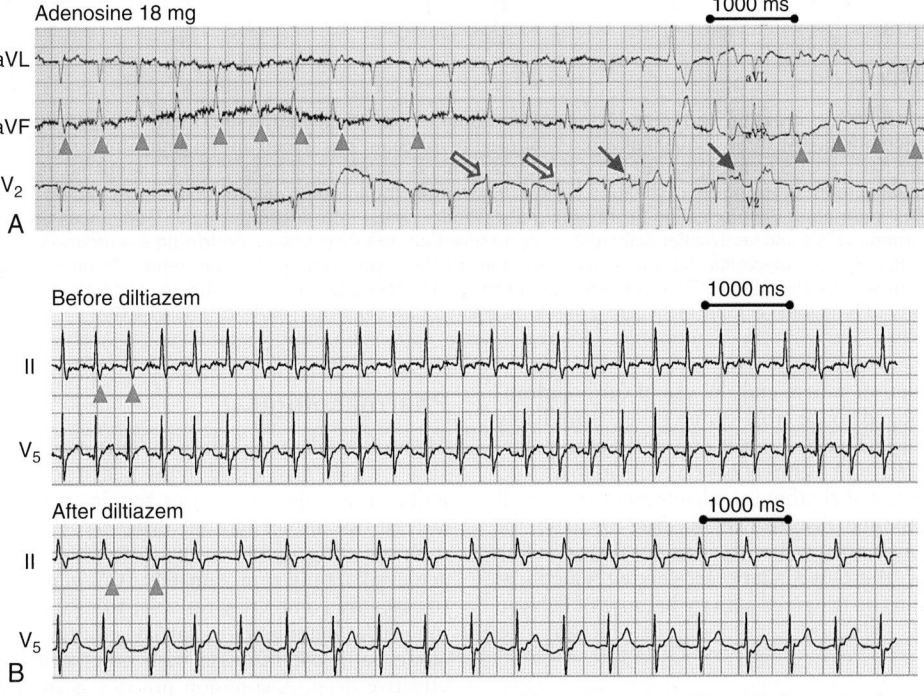

FIGURE 79.5 Adenosine and diltiazem responses in junctional ectopic tachycardia because of abnormal automaticity. (A) Surface electrocardiographic recording (leads as labeled) immediately after the administration of adenosine during short-RP tachycardia (retrograde P waves denoted by *arrowheads*) results in transient ventriculoatrial block followed by dissociated sinus rhythm P waves (*hollow arrows*) with intermittent capture beats (*solid arrows*), but the tachycardia continues. (B) Electrocardiogram of the tachycardia response to diltiazem. The tachycardia rate is 158 beats/min before diltiazem is administered (*top*) and slows to 113 beats/min after diltiazem is administered (*bottom*). Note pseudo–S waves in lead II (*arrowheads*). This arrhythmia was demonstrated to be junctional tachycardia in an electrophysiological study (not shown). (From Liu CF, Ip JE, Lin AC, et al. Mechanistic heterogeneity of junctional ectopic tachycardia in adults. *Pacing Clin Electrophysiol.* 2013;36:e7-e10.)

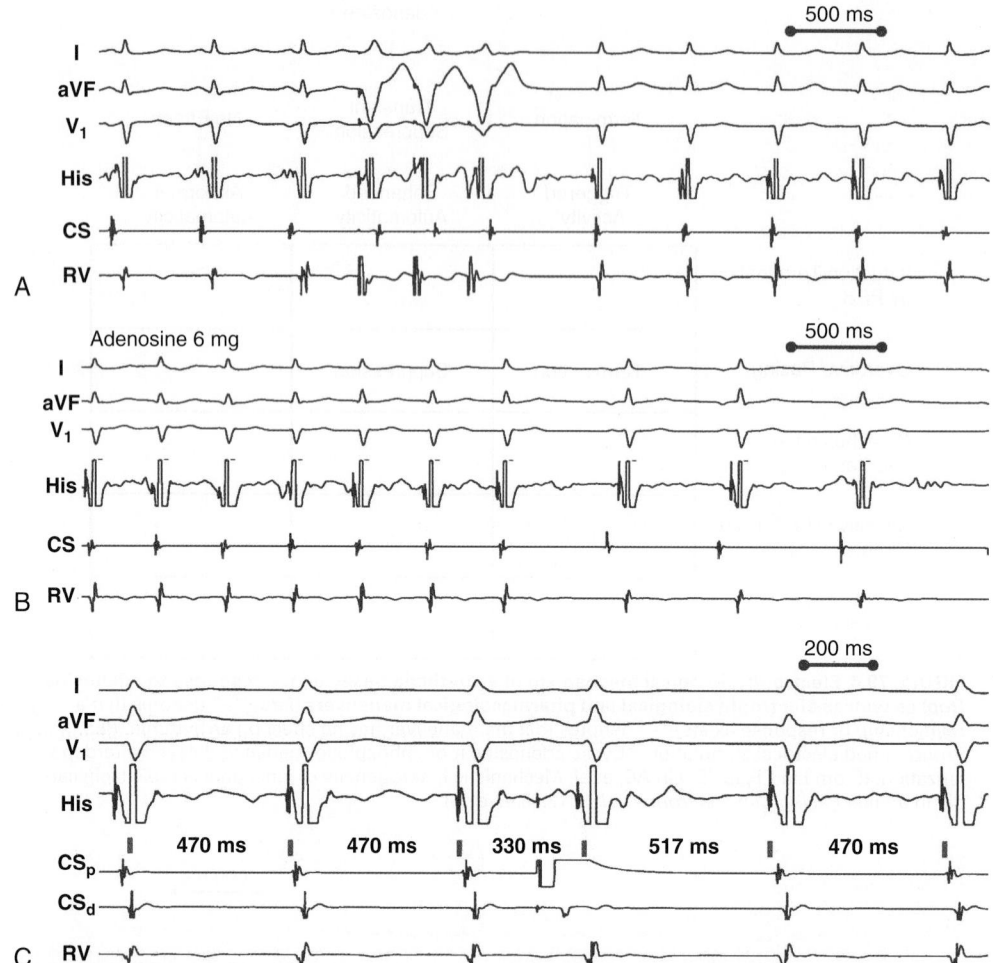

FIGURE 79.6 Initiation and termination of junctional ectopic tachycardia (JET) with a triggered mechanism. (A) Three sequential ventricular premature beats introduced during sinus rhythm initiates narrow QRS tachycardia. (B) JET abruptly terminates with a bolus dose of 6 mg adenosine. (C) Advancement of His bundle activation during tachycardia. Intracardiac recording of early coupled atrial premature depolarization (from proximal coronary sinus) introduced during JET advances the immediate His and ventricular activation without terminating tachycardia, confirming the diagnosis of JET. Surface electrocardiographic leads as labeled; *CS*, coronary sinus (*p* = proximal; *d* = distal bipoles); *His*, His bundle; *RV*, right ventricle. (From Liu CF, Ip JE, Lin AC, et al. Mechanistic heterogeneity of junctional ectopic tachycardia in adults. *Pacing Clin Electrophysiol.* 2013;36:e7-e10.)

ischemia to the conduction system and the use of cardiopulmonary bypass and prolonged aortic cross-clamp times[19]) are likely to be involved because JET occurs in patients without intracardiac surgery. Postoperative JT is rarely observed in adults.

An accelerated junctional rhythm can also present as a result of metabolic or autonomic disturbance or drug toxicity; for example, myocardial ischemia and with digitalis toxicity. The likely mechanism for these secondary accelerated junctional rhythms is considered to be triggered activity because of delayed afterdepolarizations.[21]

Management

The treatment of JET remains a vexing clinical problem. Options include pharmacological suppression, selective catheter ablation of the JET focus, and His bundle ablation with the implantation of a permanent pacemaker. Indications for treatment include symptoms (including syncope), signs of hemodynamic compromise, evidence of cardiac dilatation or decline in ventricular function, congestive heart failure, and in fetal cases, evidence of hydrops.

Pharmacological

Most of the data regarding the pharmacological management of JET have been reported in the pediatric literature. In this population, the majority of cases require combination therapy with at least two antiarrhythmic drugs to achieve efficacy. Even with multiple drug combinations, complete suppression of JET is achieved in only approximately 10% of patients, and almost 20% of cases are completely resistant to medical therapy (the remaining 70% demonstrate partial efficacy).[16] Amiodarone—used alone or in combination with other drugs—is the single most effective drug. A common practice is to add a second agent to reduce the dose of amiodarone and its potential long-term toxicity. Although digoxin is ineffective in suppressing tachycardia when used alone, it is frequently used as part of a combination regimen in the pediatric population, likely because of its safety and tolerability profile. In addition, digoxin is often used in the congenital form of JET to control the symptoms and signs of congestive heart failure.[15] A recent case report documented the efficacy of the I_f current inhibitor ivabradine, achieving complete suppression of JET in an infant.[22] Almost all other antiarrhythmic drugs have had limited reported efficacy. There is limited literature regarding the efficacy of medical therapy for JET in adults, but in general, similar agents to those used in the pediatric population are employed. As part of its more malignant clinical course, the congenital form of JET is more resistant to therapy and is associated with a higher incidence of proarrhythmia.[4,14–16] Cases of ventricular fibrillation have been documented during intravenous digoxin loading, and sudden death is often suspected to be due to the sequelae of heart failure and/or proarrhythmia of medical therapy in this sicker population.

Because postoperative JT in the pediatric population is associated with hemodynamic compromise and higher morbidity and mortality, aggressive management should be pursued to maintain AV synchrony and avoid excessive tachycardia. The mainstays of management involve a typical sequence of rapid weaning of catecholaminergic agents, correction of fever, maintenance of deep sedation, and correction of electrolyte disturbance (particularly of serum magnesium). Most cases of postoperative JET resolve with these initial measures. However, a significant minority of patients will require active therapy, including atrial overdrive pacing, amiodarone, procainamide, or hypothermia (core temperature of 33–35°C).[23,24] A recent randomized study reported efficacy for the α₂ agonist dexmedetomidine, which reduced the incidence and duration of JET after corrective surgery for tetralogy of Fallot.[25] For refractory cases of postsurgical JET, a combination of antiarrhythmic drugs and hypothermia appears to be synergistically effective.[18]

Ablation

Prior to the advent of catheter ablation, surgical dissection and cautery of the AV junction were performed for rare refractory forms of JET associated with severe manifestations.[14] In these cases, successful suppression of JET was uniformly associated with permanent AV block. Once catheter ablation became available, the goal was to achieve tachycardia suppression while preserving AV conduction. However, the challenge in this regard has been two-fold: the lack of a well-defined electrophysiological method to precisely map the JET focus and the significant risk for a permanent AV block from ablation in close proximity to the normal conduction system. Nevertheless, the initial published experience with radiofrequency catheter ablation showed that selective ablation of the JET focus is feasible. In the presence of VA conduction during JET, the site of earliest atrial activation can be mapped and initially targeted for ablation.[12,26] If this approach is ineffective or if there is absence of VA conduction during JET, sequential empirical lesions can be applied in the posterior septum (the slow AV nodal pathway region), midseptum, and then anterior septum, incurring a higher risk for permanent AV block. In cases where a clear His bundle electrogram is difficult to ascertain, para-Hisian pacing may be helpful to localize proximity to the His bundle, where ablation is likely to result in complete heart block (Fig. 79.7). In most reported series, successful suppression of JET during the ablation procedure has been an excellent predictor of long-term freedom from recurrence. In cases where the JET focus cannot be selectively suppressed, ablation of the AV junction and His bundle with implantation of a permanent pacemaker is another option to achieve ventricular rate control.

In recent years, the advent of three-dimensional mapping systems and cryothermal ablation has dramatically improved the risk profile of JET ablation with regard to reducing the risk for permanent AV block.[27] Cryoablation is particularly well suited for this arrhythmia because of its ability to ablate in the "mapping mode" (–30°C), which enables reversible

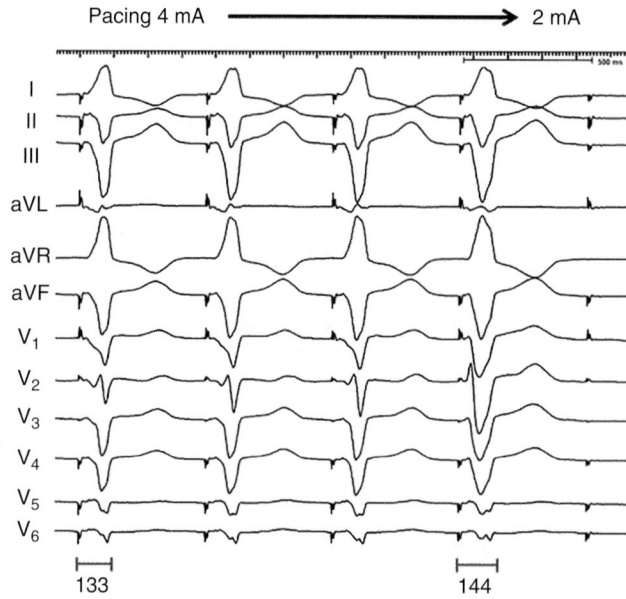

Pacing 4 mA ⟶ 2 mA

I
II
III
aVL
aVR
aVF
V₁
V₂
V₃
V₄
V₅
V₆

133   144

FIGURE 79.7 Para-Hisian pacing to detect the proximity of the His bundle. In this patient with atrial fibrillation undergoing atrioventricular junction ablation, a clear His bundle potential was not identified. The mapping/ablation catheter was positioned at the anatomical region of the His bundle. Pacing was initially performed at high output, with capture of His. Reducing the pacing output below 4 to 2 mA results in loss of His capture and prolongation of QRS duration from 133 to 144 ms. The variation in QRS duration suggests proximity to the His bundle, and ablation at this site resulted in complete atrioventricular block. This maneuver may be helpful for identifying sites that should be avoided during ablation of junctional tachycardia.

injury. Thus both efficacy with regard to tachycardia suppression and the advent of AV block can be assessed at an ablation site prior to full ablation (–70°C) and more permanent cryothermal injury. In experienced centers, cryoablation has been reported to achieve success rates (approximately 80%–85%) similar to those achieved with radiofrequency ablation but with a much lower risk for inadvertent permanent AV block (close to 0%).[16,28] As a result, cryoablation is now considered the preferred method of ablative therapy, especially in pediatric cases.

With regard to electrophysiological targets, Eizmendi and associates described a novel method of mapping the focal site of origin of junctional ectopy from the His bundle.[29] The mapping catheter is moved along the His bundle from proximal to distal. At more proximal His bundle sites (where ablation was unsuccessful and caused transient AV block), the HV interval was shorter during ectopy than during sinus rhythm, and the local unipolar His bundle recording showed an "RS" morphology (Fig. 79.8A and C). Once the mapping catheter reached the more distal successful ablation site, the HV interval during ectopy was noted to be identical to the HV interval during sinus rhythm, and unipolar recording of the His bundle electrogram showed a "QS" morphology during ectopy (Fig. 79.8B and D).

Conclusions

JT presents in a variety of clinical settings. It can occur in a congenital form, which is poorly tolerated and causes significant morbidity and mortality if not adequately controlled. Postoperative JT is associated with longer recovery time and poor outcomes, and therefore aggressive intervention with medical

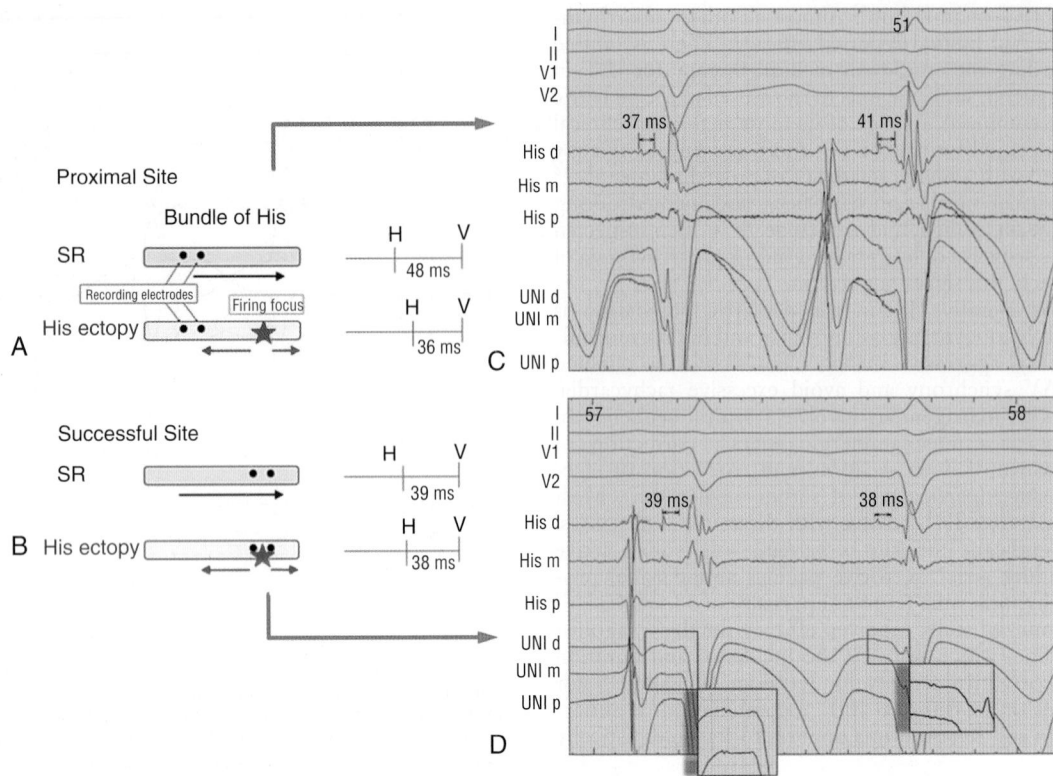

FIGURE 79.8 *Left side*, Schematic representation of the proposed method to map the focal origin of His bundle ectopy. (A) When the recording site is proximal to the focus, the local HV interval is longer in the sinus than in the ectopic beat (because the ectopic beat activation wavefront simultaneously proceeds retrogradely and to the ventricles). (B) Recording at the focus site yields an identical HV interval in sinus and ectopic beats. *Right side*, (C) Bi- and unipolar recordings at a site proximal to the ectopy focus. The first complex corresponds to a Hisian ectopy, whereas the second one corresponds to a sinus beat. (D) Bi- and unipolar recordings at the successful cryoablation site. The first complex corresponds to a sinus beat, and the second complex corresponds to a Hisian ectopy. The unipolar recordings of the His bundle have been magnified to show morphology. The HV interval at the distal His bundle is almost identical in the sinus (39 ms) and ectopic (38 ms) beats. The unipolar His bundle recording shows an "RS" pattern during the sinus beat and a "QS" pattern during the ectopic beat. *UNI d, m, p*, Unipolar recordings from the distal, mid-, and proximal His bundle. (From Eizmendi I, Almendral J, Hadid C, et al. Successful catheter cryoablation of Hisian ectopy using 2 new diagnostic criteria based on unipolar and bipolar recordings of the His electrogram. *J Cardiovasc Electrophysiol.* 2011;23:325-329.)

therapy and hypothermia is often warranted. The spontaneous form of JET is uncommon in children and rare in adults. Recent data suggest that this enigmatic arrhythmia can occur because of abnormal automaticity or triggered activity. Treatment is aimed at the suppression of symptoms and the prevention of tachycardia-associated cardiomyopathy and hemodynamic compromise. With the advent of cryothermal ablation and additional insights into electrophysiological targets for ablation, catheter-based ablative therapy is increasingly utilized for both children and adults.

REFERENCES

1. Hamdan MH, Kalman JM, Lesh MD, et al. Narrow complex tachycardia with VA block: diagnostic and therapeutic implications. *Pacing Clin Electrophysiol.* 1998;21:1196–1206.
2. Fan R, Tardos JG, Almasry I, et al. Novel use of atrial overdrive pacing to rapidly differentiate junctional tachycardia from atrioventricular nodal reentrant tachycardia. *Heart Rhythm.* 2011;8:840–844.
3. Padanilam BJ, Manfredi JA, Steinberg LA, et al. Differentiating junctional tachycardia and atrioventricular node reentry tachycardia based on response to atrial extrastimulus pacing. *J Am Coll Cardiol.* 2008;52:1711–1717.
4. Garson Jr A, Gillette PC. Junctional ectopic tachycardia in children: electrocardiography, electrophysiology and pharmacologic response. *Am J Cardiol.* 1979;44:298–302.
5. Ruder MA, Davis JC, Eldar M, et al. Clinical and electrophysiologic characterization of automatic junctional tachycardia in adults. *Circulation.* 1986;73:930–937.

6. Kumagai K, Yamato H, Yamanouchi Y, et al. Automatic junctional tachycardia in an adult. *Clin Cardiol.* 1990;13:813–816.
7. Liu CF, Ip JE, Lin AC, et al. Mechanistic heterogeneity of junctional ectopic tachycardia in adults. *Pacing Clin Electrophysiol.* 2013;36:e7–e10.
8. Dangman KH, Hoffman BF. Effects of nifedipine on electrical activity of cardiac cells. *Am J Cardiol.* 1980;46:1059–1067.
9. Rosen MR, Danilo Jr P, Weiss RM. Actions of adenosine on normal and abnormal impulse initiation in canine ventricle. *Am J Physiol.* 1983;244:H715–H721.
10. Lerman BB, Wesley Jr RC, DiMarco JP, et al. Antiadrenergic effects of adenosine on His-Purkinje automaticity. Evidence for accentuated antagonism. *J Clin Invest.* 1988;82:2127–2135.
11. Lerman BB, Belardinelli L. Cardiac electrophysiology of adenosine. Basic and clinical concepts. *Circulation.* 1991;83:1499–1509.

12. Scheinman MM, Gonzalez RP, Cooper MW, et al. Clinical and electrophysiologic features and role of catheter ablation techniques in adult patients with automatic atrioventricular junctional tachycardia. *Am J Cardiol.* 1994;74:565–572.
13. Coumel P, Fidelle JE, Attuel P, et al. Congenital bundle-of-His focal tachycardias. Cooperative study of 7 cases. *Arch Mal Coeur Vaiss.* 1976;69:899–909.
14. Villain E, Vetter VL, Garcia JM, et al. Evolving concepts in the management of congenital junctional ectopic tachycardia. A multicenter study. *Circulation.* 1990;81:1544–1549.
15. Sarubbi B, Musto B, Ducceschi V, et al. Congenital junctional ectopic tachycardia in children and adolescents: a 20 year experience based study. *Heart.* 2002;88:188–190.
16. Collins KK, Van Hare GF, Kertesz NJ, et al. Pediatric nonpost-operative junctional ectopic tachycardia medical management and interventional therapies. *J Am Coll Cardiol.* 2009;53:690–697.

17. Bharati S, Moskowitz WB, Scheinman M, et al. Junctional tachycardias: anatomic substrate and its significance in ablative procedures. *J Am Coll Cardiol*. 1991;18:179–186.

18. Hoffman TM, Bush DM, Wernovsky G, et al. Postoperative junctional ectopic tachycardia in children: incidence, risk factors, and treatment. *Ann Thorac Surg*. 2002;74:1607–1611.

19. Moak JP, Arias P, Kaltman JR, et al. Postoperative junctional ectopic tachycardia: risk factors for occurrence in the modern surgical era. *Pacing Clin Electrophysiol*. 2013;36:1156–1168.

20. Dodge-Khatami A, Miller OI, Anderson RH, et al. Impact of junctional ectopic tachycardia on postoperative morbidity following repair of congenital heart defects. *Eur J Cardiothorac Surg*. 2002;21:255–259.

21. Bigger Jr JT. Digitalis toxicity. *J Clin Pharmacol*. 1985;25:514–521.

22. Al-Ghamdi S, Al-Fayyadh MI, Hamilton RM. Potential new indication for ivabradine: treatment of a patient with congenital junctional ectopic tachycardia. *J Cardiovasc Electrophysiol*. 2013;24:822–824.

23. Raja P, Hawker RE, Chaikitpinyo A, et al. Amiodarone management of junctional ectopic tachycardia after cardiac surgery in children. *Br Heart J*. 1994;72:261–265.

24. Walsh EP, Saul JP, Sholler GF, et al. Evaluation of a staged treatment protocol for rapid automatic junctional tachycardia after operation for congenital heart disease. *J Am Coll Cardiol*. 1997;29:1046–1053.

25. Rajput RS, Das S, Makhija N, et al. Efficacy of dexmedetomidine for the control of junctional ectopic tachycardia after repair of tetralogy of Fallot. *Ann Pediatr Cardiol*. 2014;7:167–172.

26. Hamdan M, Van Hare GF, Fisher W, et al. Selective catheter ablation of the tachycardia focus in patients with nonreentrant junctional tachycardia. *Am J Cardiol*. 1996;78:1292–1297.

27. Emmel M, Sreeram N, Brockmeier K. Catheter ablation of junctional ectopic tachycardia in children, with preservation of atrioventricular conduction. *Z Kardiol*. 2005;94:280–286.

28. Law IH, Von Bergen NH, Gingerich JC, et al. Transcatheter cryothermal ablation of junctional ectopic tachycardia in the normal heart. *Heart Rhythm*. 2006;3:903–907.

29. Eizmendi I, Almendral J, Hadid C, et al. Successful catheter cryoablation of Hisian ectopy using 2 new diagnostic criteria based on unipolar and bipolar recordings of the His electrogram. *J Cardiovasc Electrophysiol*. 2011;23:325–329.

80   Premature Ventricular Complexes

Frank Bogun and Rakesh Latchamsetty

Premature ventricular complexes (PVCs) are increasingly recognized not only as a marker of structural cardiac disease but also often as a potential cause; more recently, they have been associated with increased mortality.[1] The decisions of when to pursue therapy to suppress PVCs and whether to utilize pharmacotherapy or catheter ablation can be challenging. This chapter discusses the diagnosis and prognosis of frequent PVCs in the presence or absence of other structural heart disease and describes a treatment strategy for idiopathic frequent PVCs.

Mechanism

The initiation of PVCs is dependent on the underlying cardiac substrate and, similar to other arrhythmias, can be explained by reentry, automaticity, or triggered activity. The most likely mechanism of PVCs in patients without structural heart disease is triggered activity. Reentry has primarily been found and described in postinfarction animal models.[2] In postinfarction patients, PVCs usually originate in scar tissue, and in the presence of inducible ventricular tachycardia (VT), the VT exit site often corresponds to the PVC origin site.[3] Even in nonischemic cardiomyopathy patients, scars may be identified by magnetic resonance imaging (MRI) and can often harbor PVC origin sites.

The potential for frequent idiopathic PVCs to result in cardiomyopathy has been established on the basis of the reversibility of cardiomyopathy with the successful elimination of PVCs, as demonstrated in observational studies. However, the mechanisms responsible for the development of cardiomyopathy remain under investigation. On the basis of short-term animal studies, a fibrotic process seems unlikely.[4] PVC-induced chronic left ventricular (LV) dyssynchrony is the most plausible mechanism for ventricular dysfunction similar to other forms of dyssynchrony, including right ventricular pacing or left bundle branch block.

Epidemiology

History

Irregularities in pulse and their association with poor outcomes have been hypothesized for centuries. The Chinese physician Pien

Ts'Io, who lived approximately in the 6th century BC, taught that occasional pulse irregularities did not predict an adverse outcome; however, frequent irregularities (1 in 10 beats) were linked with an ominous prognosis (often resulting in death within 1 year).[5] Reliable differentiation of PVCs from other arrhythmias became possible only since the early 20th century. An investigation in patients with minimal or no structural heart disease demonstrated that the risk for death in patients with frequent PVCs was low.[6] This study is often cited as showing that PVCs are benign arrhythmias. More recently, however, frequent idiopathic PVCs have been linked with the development of cardiomyopathy, a higher incidence of congestive heart failure, and increased mortality.[1]

Prevalence and Frequency

Interpreting the prevalence and frequency of PVCs is dependent on the patient population studied and the duration of monitoring. Prevalence in the normal healthy population can range from less than 1% in healthy populations monitored for just 48 seconds[7] to 62% when monitored for 6 hours.[8] Different definitions have been used to describe the prevalence of PVCs. In patients with prior myocardial infarction, a PVC burden greater than 10 PVCs per hour was defined as frequent and was associated with increased mortality.[9] A much higher PVC burden is required for PVC-induced cardiomyopathy. The prevalence of PVCs depends on the presence or absence of structural heart disease, and in healthy subjects, they have been reported to occur in up to 75% of the general population. However, in most healthy subjects, the burden is fewer than 100 PVCs per day.[10] A higher burden of 60 PVCs or more per hour has been described in 1% to 4% of the population.[6] The definition of *high-frequency* PVCs is therefore variable and depends on the context of the patient and the purpose of evaluation.

Prognosis

Factors used to determine cardiac prognosis in patients with frequent PVCs include the presence of underlying cardiac disease and the nature of the PVCs. In postinfarction patients, predischarge documentation of more than 10 PVCs per hour correlated with increased 6-month mortality.[11] A direct link between postinfarction VT and PVCs was established in a mapping study of patients with previous myocardial infarctions.[3] PVCs were mapped to the scar, and the PVC origin site was often correlated with the VT exit site of an inducible VT. The elimination of PVCs often permanently eliminated VTs with the shared exit site.

Frequent PVCs (>30/h) have been associated with increased mortality in men without coronary disease.[12] The primary risk in patients with idiopathic frequent PVCs seems to be progression to cardiomyopathy. Factors associated with increased risk for cardiomyopathy include the frequency of PVCs, duration of PVCs, lack of symptoms, interpolation of PVCs, epicardial origin, increased PVC–QRS width, lack of circadian PVC variability,[13] and male gender.[14–18]

While a PVC burden greater than 24% has been associated with impaired LV function (sensitivity, 79%; specificity, 78%),[17] it is important to note that cardiomyopathy has also developed with considerably less frequent PVCs and has been reported with a burden as low as 4%.[19] Furthermore, about 20% of patients with a PVC burden greater than 24% do not develop cardiomyopathy.[17] Therefore factors other than the PVC burden affect the development of cardiomyopathy. Longer duration of PVCs is believed to be contributory to the development of LV dysfunction, and patients who are asymptomatic and seek medical attention later may fall victim to this scenario. Two other factors—epicardial location and an increased QRS duration (>150 ms) of PVCs[16]—are associated with a greater likelihood of causing a cardiomyopathy, supporting that ventricular dyssynchrony may indeed be the mechanism that results in LV dysfunction. Constant exposure to PVCs throughout the day and night has also been found to correlate with a higher risk for the development of PVC-induced cardiomyopathy.[13]

Overall, data have consistently challenged the previously held tenet that PVCs constitute a generally benign finding. A recent population sample followed for more than 13 years showed that a higher frequency burden (even at overall low burdens) was associated with decreased LV ejection fraction, congestive heart failure, and even mortality.[1] Underlying cardiac substrate needs to be carefully considered in establishing a patient's risk profile. In addition to ischemia, the presence of other underlying cardiac disorders, such as sarcoidosis or arrhythmogenic right ventricular dysplasia, should be investigated in appropriate patients. A recent study suggests that mitral valve prolapse may be an underestimated cause of sudden cardiac death due to ventricular arrhythmia, particularly in patients with bileaflet involvement[20] and those with evidence of fibrosis or scarring at or near the papillary muscles.[21]

Diagnosis

Clinical Presentation

Patients with frequent PVCs can present asymptomatically with PVCs discovered incidentally or can suffer from debilitating symptoms. Presenting complaints may include palpitations, chest pain, dyspnea, fatigue, lightheadedness, or dizziness. Symptoms related to other cardiac comorbidities such as coronary artery disease may prompt initial workup; however, particularly with idiopathic PVCs, clinical presentation may be late and may often occur after the development of a cardiomyopathy. Several clinical scenarios are important to recognize:

- *Congestive heart failure and frequent PVCs:* PVCs can cause or worsen an existing cardiomyopathy. Treatment of PVCs in this scenario can improve ventricular function and heart failure symptoms.
- *Ventricular fibrillation (VF) triggered by PVCs:* PVCs can trigger VF in the setting of idiopathic VF or after acute myocardial infarction. Elimination of these PVCs can prevent recurrence of sustained ventricular arrhythmias.
- *Insufficient biventricular pacing:* Frequent PVCs can diminish the frequency of biventricular pacing and curtail its clinical benefit. Elimination of PVCs can enhance resynchronization therapy.

Electrocardiography

Advances in and increased availability of home monitoring have enhanced PVC detection and characterization. Twenty-four-hour and 48-hour Holter monitors can assess PVC frequency and correlate symptoms; 30-day event monitors increase sensitivity when symptoms or arrhythmias occur less frequently. In particular, 12-lead Holter monitors have the ability to quantify different PVC morphologies and can be used to approximate PVC location. This information is extremely valuable for clinicians in deciding when and how to treat frequent PVCs.

Idiopathic ventricular arrhythmias most often originate from outflow tracts, and 12-lead electrocardiographic morphology helps in identifying the PVC origin. Left bundle branch block morphology with an inferior axis indicates an outflow tract origin of the PVCs, with a late precordial transition (>V_3) marking an origin in the right ventricular outflow tract, and an early transition (≤V_3), suggesting an origin from the aortic cusps, LV outflow tract, or the basal LV epicardium. Right bundle branch block PVC morphologies indicate an LV origin, with a positive concordance that indicates a basal origin and precordial transition to an R/S complex, suggesting origin in the papillary muscle.[22] Epicardial origins have a slower initial QRS upstroke, also called pseudo-delta wave,[23] compared with endocardial origins. Intramural arrhythmias are more difficult to localize, and a specific pattern has not yet been described.

Clinical Management

Decision to Treat

Treatment to decrease or eliminate PVCs should be considered in patients when an expected benefit in terms of symptoms or cardiac function exists. The categories of patients who should undergo treatment that targets PVCs can be summarized as follows:

- Patients with PVCs believed to be causing or contributing to LV dysfunction or dilatation
- Patients with symptomatically limiting PVCs
- Patients with VT or VF for which a PVC trigger can be identified (Fig. 80.1)
- Patients in whom response to cardiac resynchronization therapy is limited by frequent PVCs
- Patients in whom the deterioration of the LV function may be expected, such as those with very frequent PVCs (>24%), may also be considered for therapy to reduce PVCs

Although clinical data regarding the last category are not yet definitive, PVC frequency in this range has been shown to often result in LV dysfunction, and a decision must be made on an individual basis between close follow-up of cardiac function versus prophylactic treatment to eliminate or suppress PVCs.

Initial management of PVCs should focus on identifying triggers or potentially reversible causes. Abnormalities in electrolytes, active ischemia, significant valvular disease, hypoxia, or other metabolic processes should be investigated and treated when appropriate. If clinical triggers (including caffeine, stress, recreational drugs, stimulants, and alcohol) are identified, they should also be modified.

Pharmacotherapy

Medical management of frequent PVCs will depend on the underlying cause as well as comorbidities. In the absence of contraindications, initial therapy with β-blockers or calcium channel blockers can be attempted. Particularly with β-blockers, the benefit to be derived in patients with cardiomyopathy, heart failure, and ischemic disease is well established. Effective PVC suppression with β-blockers and calcium channel blockers is only modest, with reported rates near 20%, although a higher percentage may experience symptom improvement. If this treatment does not provide adequate clinical benefit, antiarrhythmic medication can be attempted. Abnormalities in cardiac function, renal function, and baseline QTc interval, as well as potential side effects and patient age, may limit the selection

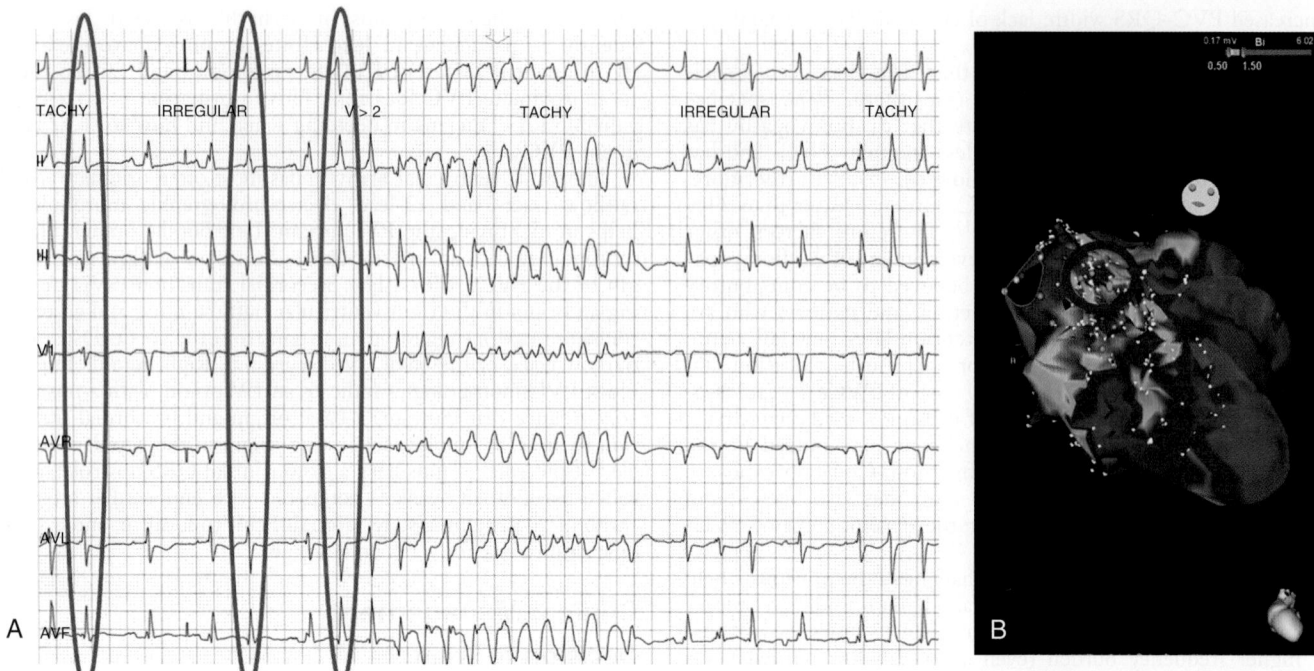

FIGURE 80.1 *Encircled* in the electrocardiogram in (A) is a recurrent premature ventricular complex that triggers an episode of self-terminating ventricular fibrillation. The Carto (Biosense Webster, Diamond Bar, CA) three-dimensional electroanatomical map in (B) shows the successfully ablated premature ventricular complex site of origin circled in *blue* at the left anterior fascicle.

of some of these agents; however, in appropriate patients, a decrease in arrhythmia burden and improvement in LV function have been observed.[24] A mortality benefit has not been established.

Catheter Ablation

Catheter ablation has emerged as a favorable option for many patients with PVCs who are refractory or intolerant to pharmacotherapy or even as a first-line therapy in selected patients. Catheter ablation has been found to be superior to medical management for PVCs that originate from the right ventricular outflow tract.[25] The goal of catheter ablation of PVCs is to ameliorate symptoms, improve or curtail deterioration of LV function or dimensions, or prevent sustained ventricular arrhythmias.

Techniques

Advances in mapping technology, signal analysis, catheter design, and ablation techniques have evolved to establish catheter ablation of PVCs as an effective and safe alternative to pharmacological management of frequent PVCs. Activation and pace mapping are techniques predominantly used for localization of PVCs (Fig. 80.2), with activation mapping being more accurate than pace mapping.

The main challenges for ablation include a low PVC prevalence during mapping and the presence of pleomorphic PVCs. Some anatomical sites of origin are more challenging than others, and the reported success rates are variable depending on the inclusion of these patients. PVCs that originate from the right ventricular outflow tract have the highest success rates, whereas those that originate from papillary muscles or the epicardium have lower success rates.[18,26] PVCs that originate from the epicardium pose a particular challenge but often can be approached via a percutaneous approach to the pericardial space. However, proximity to coronary arteries and the basal

location of epicardial fat can lead to an ineffective ablation.[27] An approach via the coronary venous system, alone or in combination with adjacent anatomical sites, may be necessary to eliminate epicardial PVCs. The latter approach is the currently favored approach for epicardial PVCs given the lower success rate and higher potential for periprocedural complications with the subxiphoid epicardial approach.[28,29] Intramural PVCs represent a particular challenge with respect to diagnosis, localization, and ablation. Recently, PVC suppression with injection of cold saline within the coronary venous system has been demonstrated to be particularly useful for identifying intramural PVCs that originate from the interventricular septum.[30] A new dual-site pacing technique has also been proposed that may help to better detect intramural PVC origins.[31]

Outcomes

Catheter ablation in patients with frequent and symptomatic PVCs has been shown to improve both symptoms and quality of life.[32,33] Results are favorable and often signify an improvement over those produced by pharmacotherapy.[34] In a recent multicenter survey, acute procedural success was reported in 84% of all patients undergoing ablation for idiopathic PVCs. Continued success defined as an 80% decrease in PVC burden off antiarrhythmic drugs was maintained in 71% of patients (Fig. 80.3). Right ventricular outflow tract location was predictive of procedural success, while epicardial location and multiple PVC morphologies were predictive of failure.[18]

With regard to patients with cardiomyopathy and frequent PVCs, ablation has been shown to restore LV function in patients who underwent successful procedures. Bogun and colleagues observed normalization of ejection fraction in 82% of patients ablated for frequent idiopathic PVCs, with an average change in ejection fraction from 34% to 59% within 6 months after ablation (Fig. 80.4).[35] Latchamsetty and colleagues reported that in 245 cardiomyopathy patients undergoing PVC ablation, mean ejection fraction improved from 38% to 50%, with 85% of

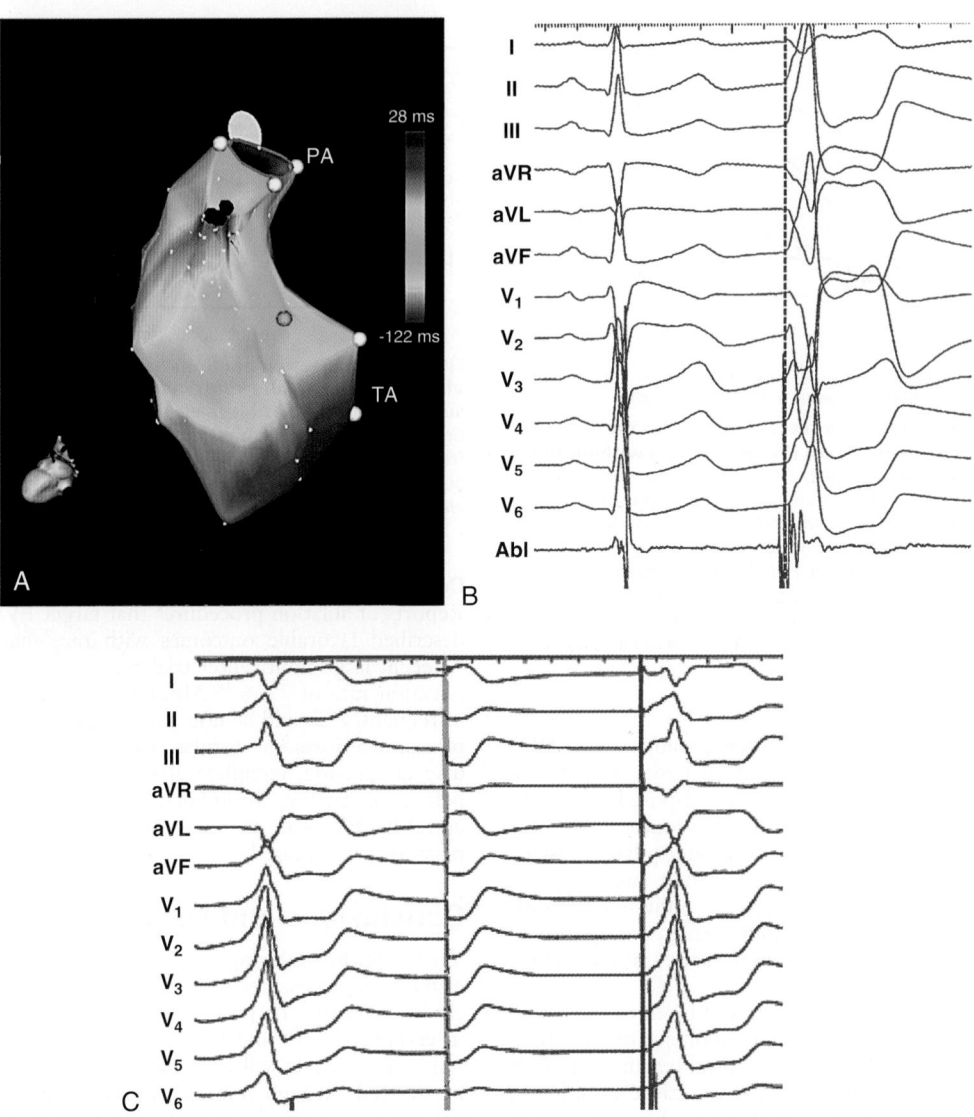

FIGURE 80.2 (A) An activation map with a three-dimensional electroanatomical mapping system shows the origin of the clinical premature ventricular complex (PVC). The site of origin is the posterior right ventricular outflow tract. Ablation points are in *red* at the site of earliest activation. The pulmonary artery (*PA*) valve and the tricuspid annulus (*TA*) are indicated. (B) Twelve-lead electrocardiogram of PVC depicted in (A), with intracardiac recordings from the site of origin (*Abl*) preceding the PVC–QRS complex by 25 ms. (C) Twelve-lead electrocardiogram of an epicardial PVC (*left*). Pacing from the site of origin within the great cardiac vein shows a morphology (*right*) similar to that of the spontaneous PVC.

patients experiencing some improvement in ejection fraction.[18] In addition to improvement in ejection fraction, other parameters such as LV size, mitral regurgitation, B-type natriuretic peptide levels, and New York Heart Association class have been shown to improve in patients after effective ablation.[36,37] In patients with preexisting cardiomyopathy, ablation of PVCs has also been shown to improve LV function. In 15 postinfarct patients with frequent PVCs, Sarrazin and associates demonstrated that ablation of frequent PVCs resulted in an improvement in ejection fraction from 38% to 51%.[38] Three patients in this study who qualified for implantable cardioverter defibrillators (ICDs) for primary prevention of sudden cardiac death on the basis of ejection fraction no longer qualified for ICD implantation postablation. Among patients in whom the ejection fraction improved, scar size as assessed using MRI was out of proportion to LV dysfunction compared with a control group. This might help clinicians to identify patients who will benefit from an ablation

procedure. These data were recently confirmed in a prospective study by Penela and colleagues, who investigated 66 patients with frequent PVCs who also met the criteria for ICD implantation for primary prevention. At 6 to 12 months postablation, the majority of patients (64%) no longer met the ICD implant criteria, and no patients experienced sudden cardiac death during follow-up.[36] However, MRIs were not routinely performed in this study, and the extent of preexisting structural heart disease may have been underestimated in some patients. Furthermore, programmed stimulation for risk stratification was also not performed in the latter study.

El Kadri and associates further demonstrated improvement of LV function and symptoms in patients with nonischemic cardiomyopathy in the presence of LV scarring.[39] The success rate of eliminating PVCs was lower than that in patients with idiopathic PVCs, most likely because of the higher prevalence of intramural scarring.

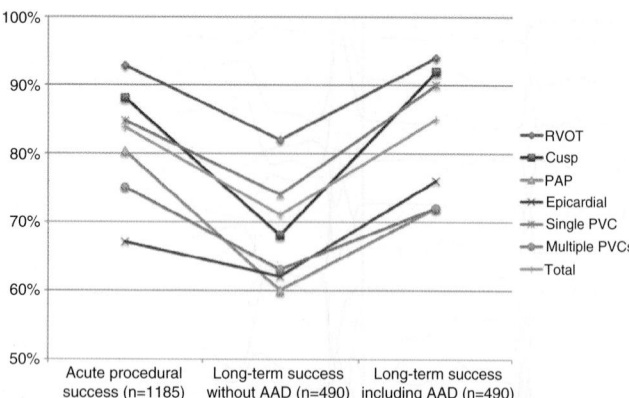

FIGURE 80.3 Acute and long-term success rates after the ablation of premature ventricular complexes (*PVCs*) with and without the use of antiarrhythmic drugs (*AADs*). Acute procedural success data are for the entire cohort of 1185 patients, whereas long-term success data are for 490 patients at centers where Holter monitoring was performed routinely after ablation. Results are shown by PVC location and single versus multiple PVCs. *PAP,* Papillary muscle; *RVOT,* right ventricular outflow tract. (From Latchamsetty RY, Morady M, Kim F, et al. Multicenter outcomes for catheter ablation of idiopathic premature ventricular complexes. *JACC Clin Electrophysiol.* 2015;1:116-123.)

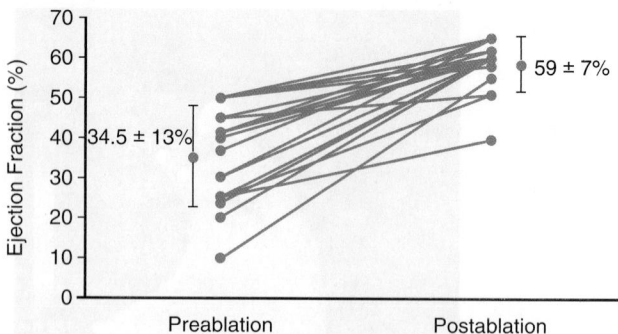

FIGURE 80.4 Ejection fractions before and after catheter ablation of frequent premature ventricular complexes in patients with a successful outcome. Mean ejection fractions and standard deviations are indicated. (From Bogun F, Crawford T, Reich S, et al. Radiofrequency ablation of frequent, idiopathic premature ventricular complexes: comparison with a control group without intervention. *Heart Rhythm.* 2007;4:863-867.)

Reemergence of frequent PVCs after resolution of PVC-induced cardiomyopathy, however, puts patients at risk for recurrent cardiomyopathy.[40] Patients predisposed to PVC recurrence are patients who have frequent pleomorphic PVCs and those who have PVCs that originate from papillary muscles because of the inherent difficulty in adequately mapping and eliminating PVCs that originate from papillary muscles. Because of the risk for the recurrence of cardiomyopathy, asymptomatic patients should be followed up even after successful PVC ablation procedures.

Patients with congestive heart failure and biventricular pacemakers or defibrillators in whom the amount of biventricular pacing is less than 93%[41] may derive less clinical benefit and often have adverse outcomes. Frequent PVCs may cause insufficient biventricular pacing.[42] Elimination of PVCs in this scenario can produce improvement in heart failure symptoms and ejection fraction.[43]

Lastly, PVCs can trigger VF in patients with channelopathies, idiopathic VF, or ongoing ischemia. Often the triggering PVCs originate from the Purkinje fiber system or papillary muscles, and ablation of the triggering PVCs minimizes or even eliminates VF recurrences.[44,45]

Complications

Reports of ablation procedures that target PVCs have generally described favorable outcomes with rare major complications. A recent large multicenter trial reported an overall major complication rate of 2.4%.[18] Although complications are relatively infrequent, it should be noted that they can include groin hematomas, arteriovenous fistulas, pseudoaneurysm formation, cardiac tamponade, complete atrioventricular block that requires permanent pacing, thromboembolic events, or, rarely, death. If epicardial PVCs are targeted for ablation, the potential for complications is increased.[28,29]

Conclusions and Future Directions

Treatment for reducing or eliminating PVCs can improve associated symptoms, recover cardiac function in PVC-induced cardiomyopathy, or prevent malignant ventricular arrhythmias in certain patients and may even improve survival. Prospective randomized trials will be critical for confirming the benefit to be derived through nonrandomized observational reports and will reveal specific indications for therapy, particularly among asymptomatic patients with frequent PVCs without evidence of cardiomyopathy.

Identification of the mechanism of PVC-induced cardiomyopathy will allow clinicians to better identify patients with frequent PVCs who are at higher risk for development of cardiomyopathy. Advances in mapping and catheter technology are required to further improve mapping accuracy and results of ablation.

REFERENCES

1. Dukes JW, Dewland TA, Vittinghoff E, et al. Ventricular ectopy as a predictor of heart failure and death. *J Am Coll Cardiol.* 2015;66:101–109.
2. El-Sherif N, Scherlag BJ, Lazzara R, et al. Re-entrant ventricular arrhythmias in the late myocardial infarction period. 1. Conduction characteristics in the infarction zone. *Circulation.* 1977;55:686–702.
3. Bogun F, Crawford T, Chalfoun N, et al. Relationship of frequent postinfarction premature ventricular complexes to the reentry circuit of scar-related ventricular tachycardia. *Heart Rhythm.* 2008;5:367–374.
4. Huizar JF, Kaszala K, Potfay J, et al. Left ventricular systolic dysfunction induced by ventricular ectopy: a novel model for premature ventricular contraction-induced cardiomyopathy. *Circ Arrhythm Electrophysiol.* 2011;4:543–549.
5. Lüderitz B. *History of the Disorders of Cardiac Rhythm.* Armonk, NY: Futura Publishing Company; 1998.
6. Kennedy H, Witlock J, Sprague M, et al. Long-term follow-up of asymptomatic healthy subjects with frequent and complex ventricular ectopy. *N Engl J Med.* 1985;312:193–198.
7. Hiss RG, Lamb LE. Electrocardiographic findings in 122,043 individuals. *Circulation.* 1962;25:947–961.

8. Hinkle LE, Carver ST, Stevens M. The frequency of asymptomatic disturbances of cardiac rhythm and conduction in middle-aged men. *Am J Cardiol.* 1969;24:629–650.
9. Hallstrom AP, Bigger Jr JT, Roden D, et al. Prognostic significance of ventricular premature depolarizations measured 1 year after myocardial infarction in patients with early postinfarction asymptomatic ventricular arrhythmia. *J Am Coll Cardiol.* 1992;20:259–264.
10. Kostis JB, McCrone K, Moreyra AE, et al. Premature ventricular complexes in the absence of identifiable heart disease. *Circulation.* 1981;63:1351–1356.
11. Maggioni AP, Zuanetti G, Franzosi MG, et al. Prevalence and prognostic significance of ventricular arrhythmias after acute myocardial infarction in the fibrinolytic era. Gissi-2 results. *Circulation.* 1993;87:312–322.
12. Bikkina M, Larson MG, Levy D. Prognostic implications of asymptomatic ventricular arrhythmias: the Framingham Heart Study. *Ann Intern Med.* 1992;117:990–996.
13. Bas HD, Baser K, Hoyt J, et al. Effect of circadian variability in frequency of premature ventricular complexes on left ventricular function. *Heart Rhythm.* 2016;13:98–102.
14. Yokokawa M, Kim HM, Good E, et al. Relation of symptoms and symptom duration to premature ventricular

complex-induced cardiomyopathy. *Heart Rhythm.* 2012;9:92–95.
15. Olgun H, Yokokawa M, Baman T, et al. The role of interpolation in PVC-induced cardiomyopathy. *Heart Rhythm.* 2011;8:1046–1049.
16. Yokokawa M, Kim HM, Good E, et al. Impact of QRS duration of frequent premature ventricular complexes on the development of cardiomyopathy. *Heart Rhythm.* 2012;9:1460–1464.
17. Baman TS, Lange DC, Ilg KJ, et al. Relationship between burden of premature ventricular complexes and left ventricular function. *Heart Rhythm.* 2010;7:865–869.
18. Latchamsetty RY, Morady M, Kim F, et al. Multicenter outcomes for catheter ablation of idiopathic premature ventricular complexes. *JACC Clin Electrophysiol.* 2015;1:116–123.
19. Shanmugam N, Chua TP, Ward D. 'Frequent' ventricular bigeminy—a reversible cause of dilated cardiomyopathy. How frequent is 'frequent'? *Eur J Heart Fail.* 2006;8:869–873.
20. Sriram CS, Syed FF, Ferguson ME, et al. Malignant bileaflet mitral valve prolapse syndrome in patients with otherwise idiopathic out-of-hospital cardiac arrest. *J Am Coll Cardiol.* 2013;62:222–230.

21. Basso C, Perazzolo Marra M, Rizzo S, et al. Arrhythmic mitral valve prolapse and sudden cardiac death. *Circulation.* 2015;132:556–566.

22. Good E, Desjardins B, Jongnarangsin K, et al. Ventricular arrhythmias originating from a papillary muscle in patients without prior infarction: a comparison with fascicular arrhythmias. *Heart Rhythm.* 2008;5:1530–1537.

23. Berruezo A, Mont L, Nava S, et al. Electrocardiographic recognition of the epicardial origin of ventricular tachycardias. *Circulation.* 2004;109:1842–1847.

24. Singh SN, Fletcher RD, Fisher SG, et al. Amiodarone in patients with congestive heart failure and asymptomatic ventricular arrhythmia. Survival trial of antiarrhythmic therapy in congestive heart failure. *N Engl J Med.* 1995;333:77–82.

25. Ling Z, Liu Z, Su L, et al. Radiofrequency ablation versus antiarrhythmic medication for treatment of ventricular premature beats from the right ventricular outflow tract: Prospective randomized study. *Circ Arrhythm Electrophysiol.* 2014;7:237–243.

26. Yokokawa M, Good E, Desjardins B, et al. Predictors of successful catheter ablation of ventricular arrhythmias arising from the papillary muscles. *Heart Rhythm.* 2010;7:1654–1659.

27. Desjardins B, Morady F, Bogun F. Effect of epicardial fat on electroanatomical mapping and epicardial catheter ablation. *J Am Coll Cardiol.* 2010;56:1320–1327.

28. Nagashima K, Choi EK, Lin KY, et al. Ventricular arrhythmias near the distal great cardiac vein: challenging arrhythmia for ablation. *Circ Arrhythm Electrophysiol.* 2014;7:906–912.

29. Santangeli P, Marchlinski FE, Zado ES, et al. Percutaneous epicardial ablation of ventricular arrhythmias arising

from the left ventricular summit: outcomes and electrocardiogram correlates of success. *Circ Arrhythm Electrophysiol.* 2015;8:337–343.

30. Yokokawa M, Morady F, Bogun F. Injection of cold saline for diagnosis of intramural ventricular arrhythmias. *Heart Rhythm.* 2016;13:78–82.

31. Yokokawa M, Yon Jung D, Hero 3rd AO, et al. Single- and dual-site pace mapping of idiopathic septal intramural ventricular arrhythmias. *Heart Rhythm.* 2016;13:72–77.

32. Zhu DW, Maloney JD, Simmons TW, et al. Radiofrequency catheter ablation for management of symptomatic ventricular ectopic activity. *J Am Coll Cardiol.* 1995;26:843–849.

33. Huang CX, Liang JJ, Yang B, et al. Quality of life and cost for patients with premature ventricular contractions by radiofrequency catheter ablation. *Pacing Clin Electrophysiol.* 2006;29:343–350.

34. Stec S, Sikorska A, Zaborska B, et al. Benign symptomatic premature ventricular complexes: short- and long-term efficacy of antiarrhythmic drugs and radiofrequency ablation. *Kardiol Pol.* 2012;70:351–358.

35. Bogun F, Crawford T, Reich S, et al. Radiofrequency ablation of frequent, idiopathic premature ventricular complexes: comparison with a control group without intervention. *Heart Rhythm.* 2007;4:863–867.

36. Penela D, Acosta J, Aguinaga L, et al. Ablation of frequent PVC in patients meeting criteria for primary prevention ICD implant. Safety of withholding the implant. *Heart Rhythm.* 2015;12:2434–2442.

37. Takemoto M, Yoshimura H, Ohba Y, et al. Radiofrequency catheter ablation of premature ventricular complexes from right ventricular outflow tract improves left ventricular

dilation and clinical status in patients without structural heart disease. *J Am Coll Cardiol.* 2005;45:1259–1265.

38. Sarrazin JF, Labounty T, Kuhne M, et al. Impact of radiofrequency ablation of frequent post-infarction premature ventricular complexes on left ventricular ejection fraction. *Heart Rhythm.* 2009;6:1543–1549.

39. El Kadri M, Yokokawa M, Labounty T, et al. Effect of ablation of frequent premature ventricular complexes on left ventricular function in patients with nonischemic cardiomyopathy. *Heart Rhythm.* 2015;12:706–713.

40. Baser K, Bas HD, LaBounty T, et al. Recurrence of PVCs in patients with PVC-induced cardiomyopathy. *Heart Rhythm.* 2015;12:1519–1523.

41. Koplan BA, Kaplan AJ, Weiner S, et al. Heart failure decompensation and all-cause mortality in relation to percent biventricular pacing in patients with heart failure: is a goal of 100% biventricular pacing necessary? *J Am Coll Cardiol.* 2009;53:355–360.

42. Mullens W, Verga T, Grimm RA, et al. Persistent hemodynamic benefits of cardiac resynchronization therapy with disease progression in advanced heart failure. *J Am Coll Cardiol.* 2009;53:600–607.

43. Lakkireddy D, Di Biase L, Ryschon K, et al. Radiofrequency ablation of premature ventricular ectopy improves the efficacy of cardiac resynchronization therapy in nonresponders. *J Am Coll Cardiol.* 2012;60:1531–1539.

44. Haissaguerre M, Shah DC, Jais P, et al. Role of Purkinje conducting system in triggering of idiopathic ventricular fibrillation. *Lancet.* 2002;359:677–678.

45. Haissaguerre M, Shoda M, Jais P, et al. Mapping and ablation of idiopathic ventricular fibrillation. *Circulation.* 2002;106:962–967.

81 Outflow Tract Ventricular Tachyarrhythmias: Mechanisms, Clinical Features, and Management

Zian H. Tseng and Edward P. Gerstenfeld

Idiopathic ventricular tachycardias (VTs) typically occur in the absence of structural heart disease and can originate from multiple anatomical regions, including the left ventricular outflow tract (LVOT) and right ventricular outflow tract (RVOT), the left fascicular system, the mitral and tricuspid annuli, and the papillary muscles, or they can develop perivascularly in the epicardial space. More than half of all idiopathic VTs originate from the outflow tracts (OTs), and of these, approximately 80% originate from the RVOT.[1] The remainder originate from the LVOT, which is located immediately posterior to the RVOT and includes the aortic sinuses of Valsalva, the ventricular myocardium just inferior to the aortic valve, the aortomitral continuity (AMC), the superior basal septum (ventricular summit), and the epicardial OT surface.[2] OT arrhythmias can present as isolated premature ventricular complexes (PVCs), as nonsustained VTs, or as sustained VTs.[3] Symptoms of OT VTs vary widely and may include palpitations, presyncope, and syncope. Since OT VTs were initially described, advances in understanding of their mechanism and pathophysiology have been significant. This chapter reviews the anatomy, epidemiology, mechanisms, diagnosis, prognosis, and management of OT PVCs and VTs.

Anatomy

Right Ventricular Outflow Tract

The RVOT is generally divided into free wall and septal regions and then subdivided within each region into anterior, mid, and posterior (Fig. 81.1).[4] The RVOT courses anterior and leftward of the LVOT, with the distal RVOT and pulmonic valve located leftward of the distal LVOT and aortic valve, respectively. The pulmonary valve is superior to the aortic valve, such that the posteroseptal RVOT is immediately anterior and adjacent to the aortic valve, specifically the right and left coronary cusps (RCCs and LCCs, respectively).[4] Its inferior and most rightward portion is continuous with the tricuspid annulus and the interventricular septum, where the bundle of His and the proximal right bundle branch are located, whereas its most superior and leftward portion is above the anterior pulmonary valve leaflet (Fig. 81.2). Although the RVOT is muscular throughout, it is relatively thin in the free wall and immediate subpulmonary valve portions and thicker in the proximal posterior portion, where it is directly opposite the LVOT and the anterior interventricular septum.

Relationship to Coronary Arteries

The left main coronary artery arises from the LCC, adjacent and immediately posterior to the RVOT below the pulmonary valve; therefore the potential for left main arterial damage exists during ablation in the LCC, in the septal and posterior regions of the RVOT (see Fig. 81.1), or during ablation within the pulmonary artery (PA) itself. The left main coronary artery courses laterally relative to the RVOT as it branches into the left circumflex and left anterior descending arteries. Because the RVOT courses leftward, the right coronary artery, arising from the RCC, is closest to the proximal RVOT near the tricuspid annulus.

Left Ventricular Outflow Tract

Unlike the entirely muscular RVOT, part of the LVOT is muscular and part is fibrous. Most of the RCC and the anterior aspect of the LCC lie above the muscular (anterior) portion of the LVOT. The junction between the RCC and the noncoronary cusp overlies the membranous interventricular septum, where the bundle of His and the proximal left bundle branch are located. The noncoronary cusp and the posterior aspect of the LCC are continuous with the fibrous AMC in the posterior portion of the LVOT.

Aortic and Pulmonary Valve Cusps

The ventricular myocardium extends beyond the semilunar valves into the proximal PA and the aortic valve cusps[5] and can be found both between and within the cusps.[6] Some cases of myocardial sleeves in the region of the coronary artery have also been reported.[7,8] Because the pulmonary valve is superior and leftward of the aortic valve, the RVOT beneath the pulmonary valve is at the same level as the aortic cusps. The RCC and the junction between the LCC and RCC lie immediately adjacent to the posterior RVOT, beneath the pulmonary valve. Myocardial sleeves are found most often in the RCC and less commonly in the LCC.[5] The noncoronary cusp lies posterior and immediately adjacent to the interatrial septum; therefore its myocardial sleeves may be a site of origin for atrial tachycardias but not for idiopathic VTs.[9]

Epicardial and Perivascular Sites

Approximately 9% of idiopathic VTs originate epicardially, most often near coronary venous sites: the great cardiac vein (GCV), the anterior interventricular vein (AIV), and the middle cardiac vein (MCV).[10] Immediately distal (in the retrograde direction to blood flow) to the coronary sinus ostium, the coronary sinus gives rise to the MCV, which courses in the posterior interventricular sulcus. The coronary sinus courses in the inferior aspect of the atrioventricular groove parallel to the mitral valve annulus and ends at the valve of Vieussens in the region of obtuse marginal arteries. Beyond the valve of Vieussens, the vein continues as the GCV, coursing epicardially directly overlying the lateral mitral annulus. The junction of the AIV and the GCV is immediately lateral to the LCC. Proximal to distal, the AIV is adjacent to the posterolateral subvalvar RVOT, or the epicardial lateral RVOT, and to the anterior epicardial space. Transpericardial mapping of the origin of epicardial idiopathic VTs has confirmed their propensity for origin near these perivascular structures.[10]

Left Ventricular Summit

OT VTs may also originate from the region of the left ventricular (LV) summit, the most superior LV epicardial region at the top of the interventricular septum. The LV summit lies between the left anterior descending and left circumflex arteries, near the junction of the GCV and the AIV, and superior to the aortic valve cusps.[11] One series reported that 12% of idiopathic LV VTs originate from the LV summit.[11] The superior-most region of the LV summit is close to the left anterior descending and left circumflex arteries, along with prominent overlying epicardial fat, and thus is often inaccessible to epicardial catheter ablation; the lateral region is accessible via the GCV.

Epidemiology

OT VTs have accounted for approximately 10% of all patients referred for evaluation of VT.[12] OT VTs may present from the spectrum of PVCs, nonsustained VT, and sustained monomorphic VT.[3] OT VT typically occurs in young to middle-aged patients, with mean age at presentation lower than that of patients with VT secondary to structural heart disease.[13,14] Although some have noted a higher incidence in women,[2] others have reported no gender predominance.[3]

Symptoms

Palpitations, chest pain, dyspnea, and light-headedness during episodes are common, and, rarely, syncope can occur; some patients may have only fatigue or may be entirely asymptomatic.[13]

Triggers

Episodes are often triggered by caffeine, emotional stress, or exercise, typically during the recovery period after exercise.[13,15,16] In women, hormonal flux (e.g., premenstrual or perimenopausal) may be a particular trigger.[16] Circadian variation with morning and late afternoon peaks of occurrence of OT PVCs has also been reported.[17] These suggest the importance of sympathetic activity and circulating catecholamines in the mechanism of OT VTs.

Mechanism

The mechanism of OT VTs is triggered activity due to cyclic adenosine monophosphate (cAMP)-mediated delayed

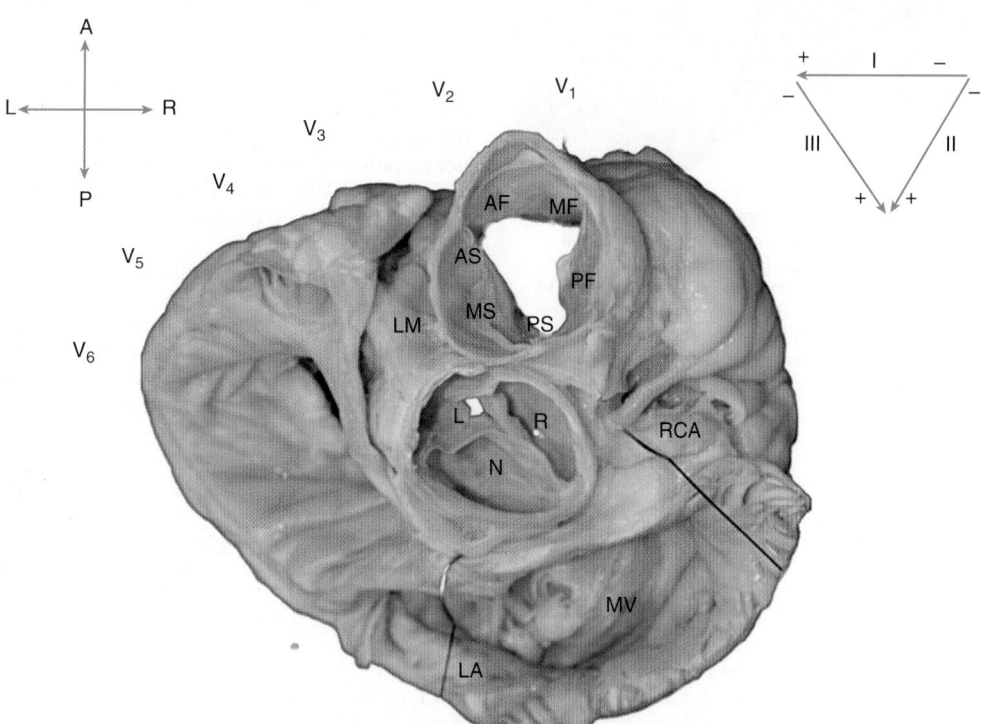

FIGURE 81.1 Superior view of the human heart with the atria, pulmonary artery, and aorta cut away. The heart is oriented with the anterior (*A*) aspect of the chest at the top, the posterior (*P*) aspect at the bottom, and the right (*R*) and left (*L*) sides in the appropriate orientations. The location of the electrocardiographic leads on the chest is shown. The most anterior and superior part of the ventricles is the right ventricular free wall just below the pulmonic valve, which is separated into anterior (*AF*), mid (*MF*), and posterior (*PF*) free-wall regions. Just posterior to the free wall is the septal aspect of the right ventricular outflow tract (RVOT), separated into anterior (*AS*), mid (*MS*), and posterior (*PS*) septal regions. Immediately posterior and slightly inferior to the RVOT septum lies the aortic root. The right coronary cusp (*R*) lies immediately posterior to the PS RVOT, and the left coronary cusp (*L*) lies posterior to the AS RVOT. The noncoronary cusp (*N*) overlies the atrial septum and therefore is a useful location for mapping atrial tachycardia but not outflow tract ventricular tachycardias. Posterior to the aortic root lies the mitral annulus, below the left atrium (*LA*). *LM,* Left main coronary artery; *MV,* mitral valve; *RCA,* right coronary artery.

afterdepolarizations.[1,18] Increased cAMP can occur with beta-adrenergic receptor stimulation (e.g., during exercise), resulting in increased intracellular calcium and delayed afterdepolarizations, triggering OT VT.

Consistent with this mechanism, in the electrophysiology laboratory OT PVCs and VTs typically are induced by burst atrial or ventricular pacing rather than by programmed stimulation (which would be more characteristic of monomorphic VT due to reentrant mechanism) and are facilitated by isoproterenol or epinephrine infusion.[13,19] OT VTs cease with adenosine, verapamil, and β-blockers, all of which interfere with the cAMP-mediated calcium flux.[20,21]

Diagnosis

Recognition and localization of OT arrhythmias are ideally suited to the 12-lead electrocardiogram (ECG)[13] because they originate from a focal source and usually occur in a structurally normal heart. The classic ECG pattern consists of left bundle branch block morphology in V_1 with a marked inferior axis (Fig. 81.3). This occurs because the PVC/VT originates from the superior-most aspect of the ventricle, just at or below the level of the semilunar valves. Recognizing the typical ECG pattern is important for establishing the correct diagnosis and for discussing the prognosis with the patient. More detailed ECG localization is helpful when treatment options and the risks of catheter ablation are discussed and when a starting point is identified from which more detailed intracardiac mapping can be performed in the electrophysiology laboratory.

Right Ventricular Outflow Tract

The most common origin of OT VT is the septal aspect of the RVOT, just inferior to the pulmonic valve (see Fig. 81.2). Because the PVC/VT exits from the superior-most region of the right ventricle, the inferior leads in stereotypical ECG morphology are markedly positive and narrow (see Fig. 81.3). Leads aVR and aVL are markedly negative with a QS pattern. All RVOT PVCs/VT have left bundle branch block morphology in lead V_1 (rS or QS; see Fig. 81.3). The precordial lead transition from net negative to net positive (from r<S to R>s) is critical for distinguishing RVOT from LVOT origin. The later the precordial transition, the more likely the PVC originates from the RVOT; the earlier the transition, the more likely the PVC exits from the LVOT. The transition for PVCs of right ventricular (RV) origin typically occurs at or later than lead V_3. Lead I is typically of low amplitude and is useful for differentiating posteroseptal (positive) from midseptal (multiphasic) or anteroseptal (negative) origin (Fig. 81.4). The more leftward location of the anterior RVOT compared with the posterior RVOT accounts for

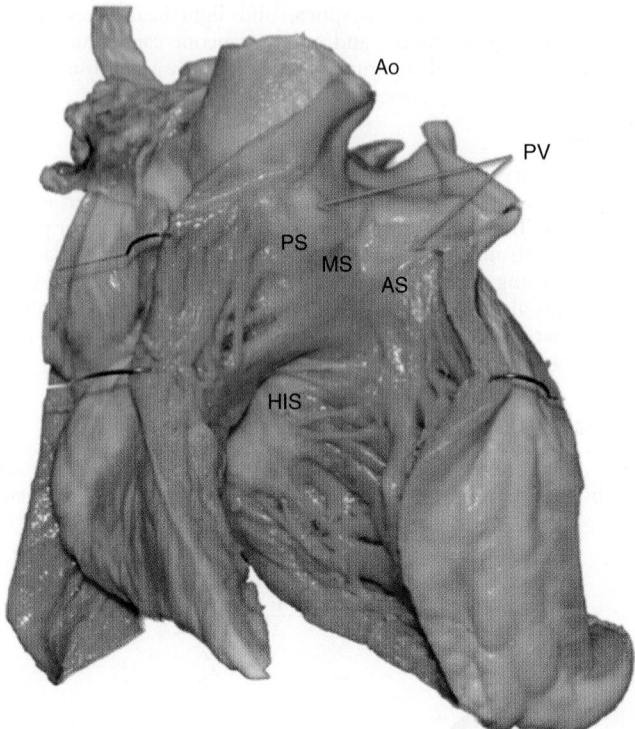

FIGURE 81.2 Anterior view of the human heart, with the free wall of the right ventricle cut open. This view shows the anteroseptal (*AS*), midseptal (*MS*), and posteroseptal (*PS*) aspects of the right ventricular outflow tract (RVOT) just below the pulmonic valve (*PV*). Immediately posterior to the RVOT lies the aortic root (*Ao*). Inferior and posterior to the RVOT lies the para-Hisian region (*HIS*), a less common site of origin of idiopathic premature ventricular complexes. This region at the superior aspect of the tricuspid valve has been termed the tricuspid "inflow tract."

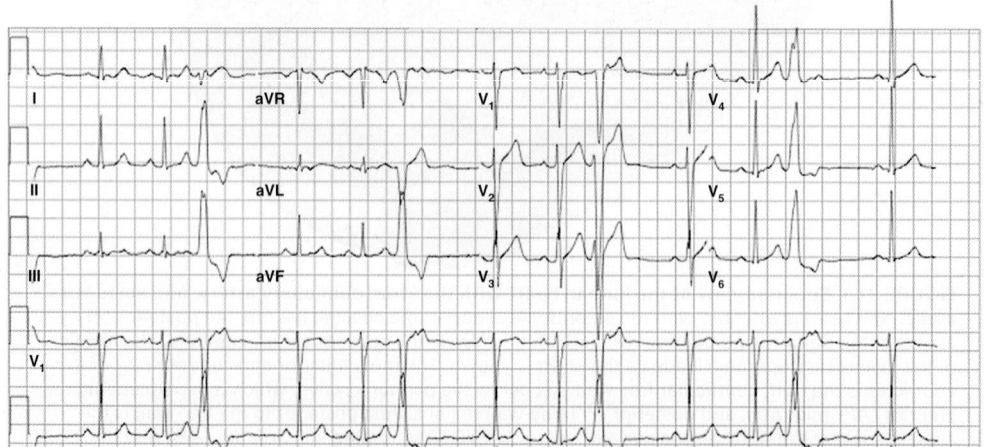

FIGURE 81.3 12-lead electrocardiogram of a patient with a typical right ventricular outflow tract premature ventricular complex (PVC). The PVC has a left bundle branch block pattern in V_1 with an rS—a transition at lead V_4 that is typical of right ventricular outflow tract PVCs. The PVC has a marked inferior axis and is multiphasic in lead I, suggesting a midseptal origin. Although notching in the inferior leads is more commonly seen in PVCs of free-wall origin, it can also be seen in PVCs of septal origin.

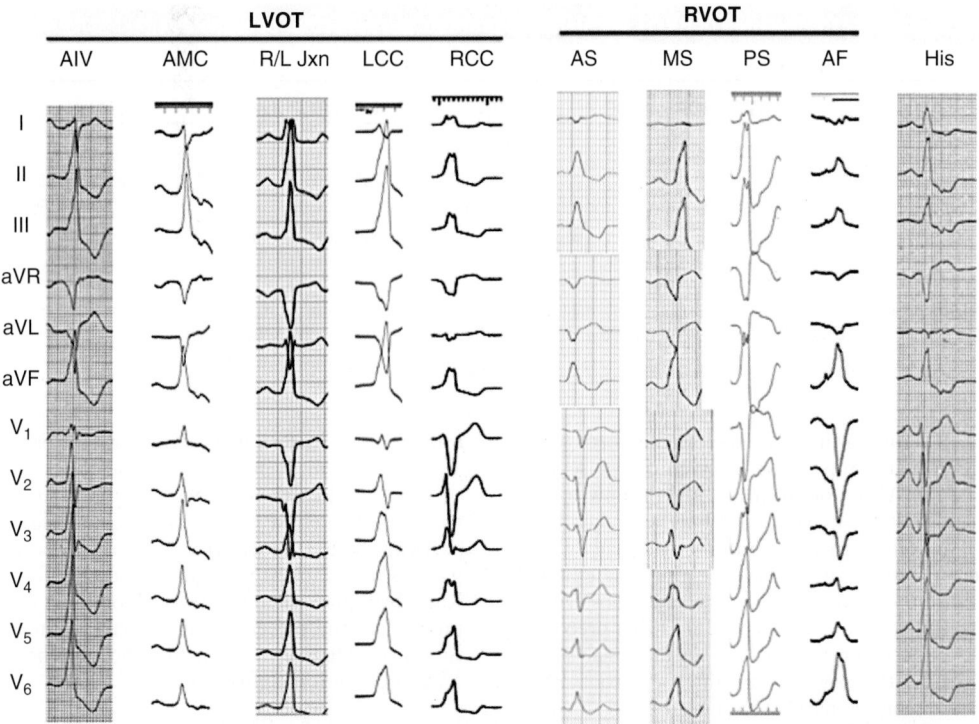

FIGURE 81.4 Typical 12-lead electrocardiographic morphologies of outflow tract ventricular tachycardias, all from patients with the origin confirmed with intracardiac mapping and ablation. From right to left, para-Hisian premature ventricular complexes (PVCs) are not really located in the outflow tract but do have a left bundle inferior axis; the hallmark is the isoelectric or "W" pattern in lead aVL and the more positive R wave in lead I. Next, an anterior free-wall (*AF*) PVC is shown, with the characteristic lower amplitude and notched inferior leads and a late precordial transition. The more typical septal PVCs originating just under the pulmonic valve are shown next; lead I distinguishes anteroseptal (*AS*, negative) from midseptal (*MS*, multiphasic) or posteroseptal (*PS*, positive) origin. The coronary cusp PVCs all have left bundle branch block morphology in V_1 with an earlier precordial transition. More posteriorly located is the region of aortomitral continuity (*AMC*), which has an inferior axis and a signature qR pattern in lead V_1. The leftmost panel shows a PVC from the left ventricular summit with a slurred positive r wave in V_1 and rS in lead I that was ablated from within the anterior interventricular vein (*AIV*). See text for a more detailed discussion. *LCC,* Left coronary cusp; *LVOT,* left ventricular outflow tract; *R/L Jxn,* right/left cusp junction; *RCC,* right coronary cusp; *RVOT,* right ventricular outflow tract.

the differences in lead I polarity (see Figs. 81.1 and 81.4). The most common site of PVC origin is the anteroseptal or midseptal region. Fewer than 10% of RVOT PVCs originate from the RV free wall.[22] For free-wall RVOT PVCs, the QRS remains inferiorly directed but is wider and notched compared with those of septal origin (see Fig. 81.4). In the study by Dixit and colleagues,[23] no QRS width cutoff clearly separated free wall from septal origin; however, relative QRS widening with free wall compared with septal origin was clearly noted within each patient. Because the RV free wall is more anteriorly located, the precordial transition is seen later than that of VT with septal origin, nearly always at or later than lead V_4 (see Fig. 81.4). Similar to septal PVCs, lead I is useful for differentiating anterior (negative) from posterior (positive) free-wall origin. Because a free-wall origin is very uncommon in patients with a structurally normal heart, the presence of PVCs of free-wall morphology should elicit a more thorough search for underlying structural heart disease, in particular arrhythmogenic right ventricular cardiomyopathy (ARVC).

PVCs may also originate lower in the OT, beneath the pulmonic valve. As the origin becomes more inferior, a series of changes to the ECG occurs: The inferior leads become less positive (first lead III, then lead aVF, and finally lead II), lead aVL becomes less negative, and lead I becomes more positive (as the origin becomes more posterior toward the tricuspid valve; see Fig. 81.2). An ECG morphology that is slightly inferiorly

directed (positive in II and aVF and biphasic or positive in III), flat, or W-shaped in lead aVL and is more positive in lead I than in the typical posteroseptal PVC is typical for a PVC that originates from the RV inflow tract at the level of the His bundle[24] (see Fig. 81.4). These para-Hisian PVCs are less common than OT PVCs but do occur in structurally normal hearts. The origin may be just superior or free wall to the His bundle region, or from the left side of the septum; careful mapping is critical to avoid heart block during ablation.

PVCs may also originate superior to the pulmonic valve from myocardial fibers that extend above the pulmonary valve.[25] Few ECG features are helpful in distinguishing PA from RVOT PVCs, other than a markedly inferior axis, earlier precordial transition (>R/S ratio in lead V_2), and the presence of a small atrial and ventricular potential on the mapping catheter at the site of successful ablation.[26] Recent data using detailed electroanatomical mapping together with intracardiac echocardiography (ICE) suggest that PVC origin from the PA just superior to the pulmonic valve may be more common than that previously described.[27]

Left Ventricular Outflow Tract

Recognition that OT PVCs can also originate from the LVOT is increasing.[28] The most common origin is from myocardial fibers within or adjacent to the aortic root,[29,30] but PVCs may also

TABLE 81.1 Distinguishing ECG features of RVOT versus LVOT premature ventricular complexes

	RVOT				LVOT	
ECG LEAD	**ANTERIOR**	**POSTERIOR**	**LCC**	**RCC**	**LCC/RCC Jxn**	**Epi/AIV**
I	rS or QS	r (notch)	rS	r (notch)	rS	rS or QS
aVR, aVL	QS	QS	QS	QS	QS	QS, QaVL <1.5*QaVR
Precordial transition	≥V$_3$ or >SR	≥V$_3$ or >SR	≤V$_2$ or <SR	≤V$_3$ or <SR	≤V$_3$ or <SR	≤V$_2$, MDI >0.55, "pattern break" in V$_1$–V$_3$
V$_1$	rS or qS	rS or qS	qS or "W"	rS	qrS; notch on downstroke	rS
V$_5$, V$_6$	R or Rs	R	R	R	R	R

AIV, anterior interventricular vein; *ECG,* electrocardiogram; *Epi,* epicardial; *Jxn,* junction; *LCC,* left coronary cusp; *LVOT,* left ventricular outflow tract; *MDI,* maximal deflection index; *RCC,* right coronary cusp; *RVOT,* right ventricular outflow tract; *SR,* sinus rhythm precordial transition.
See text for discussion.

originate from the LV myocardium just below the aortic valve, from the LV summit at the top of the interventricular septum, from the region of the AMC, or from the LV outflow epicardium.[31] Most LVOT PVCs also have a left bundle branch block pattern in lead V$_1$ (usually rS) with an inferior axis; PVCs from the AMC or superior mitral annulus have a right bundle branch block pattern. Because the aortic root is immediately posterior to the RVOT (see Fig. 81.1), LVOT PVCs have an earlier precordial transition, typically at or before lead V$_3$.[6,32] Further analysis can be performed to identify the origin within the aortic root. PVCs from the LCC region typically have an rS in lead I and an earlier precordial transition (lead V$_1$ or V$_2$) than those from the RCC (see Fig. 81.4). PVCs from the RCC typically are positive and notched in lead I, with a precordial transition at lead V$_2$ or V$_3$.[33] The region at the junction of the RCC and LCC is a common site of muscular fiber extension; PVC origin from this location has a signature initial "notch" or qrS pattern in lead V$_1$ or V$_2$[34,35] (see Fig. 81.4).

As was already mentioned, PVCs with a precordial transition before lead V$_3$ typically originate in the LVOT, and those with a transition after V$_3$ typically originate in the RVOT. PVCs with a transition at lead V$_3$ are therefore challenging to localize.[36] In addition, cardiac rotation or precordial lead misplacement can confound most ECG localization algorithms. One study found that comparing the precordial transition of the PVC with that in sinus rhythm can be helpful in localizing PVCs with a V$_3$ transition. If the PVC transition occurs after the sinus rhythm transition, the origin is RVOT with 93% specificity.[37] Other algorithms are available for distinguishing RVOT from LVOT arrhythmias[38–40] (Table 81.1).

Rarely, PVCs can originate just below the aortic valve at the AMC—the region between the aortic and mitral valves. These PVCs have a marked inferior axis with a "signature" qR pattern in lead V$_1$, an rS in lead I, and a positive QRS complex in all precordial leads (see Fig. 81.4).[41]

Recognition of an epicardial PVC origin is important, as the risks of ablation are higher and success rates lower than those for typical endocardial RV or LVOT PVC origin. Several criteria can be used to identify an epicardial exit to OT PVCs. The typical morphology is a left bundle branch block/inferior axis with an early precordial transition, a delayed or "slurred" intrinsicoid deflection, and a QS pattern in lead I. A criterion called the *maximal deflection index* (MDI) takes advantage of the slower intrinsicoid deflection for arrhythmias of epicardial origin.[10] The MDI measures the time from onset to the latest R wave peak in any precordial lead divided by the QRS duration; an MDI greater than 0.55 suggests an epicardial origin that is best approached via the coronary venous system or epicardium rather than via the aortic cusps. The typical PVC morphology originating closest to the GCV or the AIV has an early transition (V$_1$ or V$_2$) with a slurred initial r wave in V$_1$ and an rS or QS in lead I.[42] Another common morphology for an epicardial OT PVC is a right bundle

branch block pattern in V$_1$, where a "pattern break" occurs from V$_1$ to V$_3$ (i.e., an R in V$_1$ and V$_3$ and an Rs or rS in V$_2$).

One should always be aware of the location of the ECG electrodes on the chest when analyzing a 12-lead ECG of OT VT, particularly in the electrophysiology laboratory, where other patches on the chest may affect usual ECG electrode placement. Limb lead placement in the anterior chest during a stress test or precordial lead placement at the wrong interspace may lead to a significant change in ECG morphology that may confound any PVC localization algorithm.[43]

Prognosis

In contrast to many ventricular arrhythmias that occur in the setting of structural heart disease, OT PVCs and VTs are generally considered benign, with long-term studies demonstrating that a vast majority of patients do not develop structural heart disease or sudden cardiac death.[13] Of course, OT VT can also occur in patients with underlying structural heart disease—it is important to identify the typical OT morphology in these patients, as the presence of VT does not have the same implications as the presence of ventricular arrhythmias that are associated with scar. Two notable instances when OT VT may have more serious implications involve patients with "short-coupled" PVCs triggering polymorphic VT and patients with a PVC-induced cardiomyopathy.

A malignant variant of "short-coupled" PVCs triggering torsades de pointes VT was first described in the 1990s.[44] Initial reports identified a high mortality risk in these patients, despite medical treatment with traditional β-blockers or calcium channel blockers. Noda and Viskin then reemphasized the phenomenon of short-coupled OT PVCs that triggered torsades de pointes VT and resulted in syncope or sudden death.[45,46] Although no absolute coupling interval cutoff identifies potentially "malignant" PVCs, the coupling interval that triggered polymorphic VT was generally shorter than that of benign OT PVCs, even within the same patient.[47] Catheter ablation should be strongly considered in patients with short-coupled OT PVCs with syncope or runs of torsades de pointes VT,[45] and an implanted cardioverter defibrillator (ICD) may be required if the PVC trigger cannot be completely eliminated or if the patient has a history of cardiac arrest.

The syndrome of PVC-triggered torsades should be differentiated from inherited arrhythmia syndromes, such as catecholaminergic polymorphic VT (CPVT). Both may be triggered by exercise. CPVT has a younger age of onset, a more malignant clinical history with frequent syncope, a family history of sudden death, and may manifest as sustained bidirectional VT. Genetic testing for CPVT should be considered if the diagnosis is unclear. In some patients, PVCs triggering runs of polymorphic VT during extreme exertion may present in older adulthood. The prognosis in these patients has not been clearly defined but may be better compared with those with younger onset.[48]

Some patients with very frequent OT PVCs and VT may develop a tachycardia-mediated cardiomyopathy.[49] The PVC burden appears to be the best predictor of those patients who may develop a cardiomyopathy. In retrospective studies, the PVC burden required to produce LV dysfunction has ranged from 10,000 to 30,000 PVCs/day,[50] or 10% to 30% of daily heartbeats. Patients with fewer than 10% PVCs will rarely develop a cardiomyopathy. In a prospective study of 1139 patients undergoing Holter monitoring, those in the upper quartile versus the lowest quartile of PVC frequency had a 48% increased risk of congestive heart failure and a 31% increased risk of death during a median follow-up of greater than 13 years. The population-level risk for incident congestive heart failure attributed to PVCs was 8.1%, similar in magnitude to the risk attributed to hypertension. Therefore PVCs may be an underappreciated cause of cardiomyopathy and congestive heart failure in the general population. Importantly, Bogun and colleagues described a group of patients with cardiomyopathy and frequent PVCs who had near-complete resolution of the cardiomyopathy after PVC ablation.[51] Multiple subsequent studies have demonstrated significant improvement in LV function after PVC ablation in this cohort of patients.[1,52] Therefore early recognition and treatment are essential. The mechanism of PVC-induced cardiomyopathy is not well understood, but other predictors of cardiomyopathy beyond PVC burden include PVC QRS width[53,54] and epicardial PVC origin.[54–56] Among patients with residual PVCs after ablation, those with a burden reduced to less than 5% generally fared well, with LV ejection fraction improvement of 10% to 15%.[52]

Even in some patients with underlying structural heart disease, a significant improvement in LV function can still be noted after PVC ablation. Therefore in nearly any patient with frequent PVCs (>10% or 10,000/day) and reduced LV function, medical or catheter-based treatment of PVCs should be considered. Patients who are asymptomatic with normal LV size and function should undergo yearly echocardiograms and are often treated with β-blockers, although limited data support this. At the first sign of LV dilatation or decreased LV function, more aggressive treatment with antiarrhythmic medication or catheter ablation should be undertaken. It should be noted that even after complete resolution of a tachycardia-mediated cardiomyopathy, some residual LV structural changes and risk of malignant arrhythmias may occur, particularly with any recurrent PVCs or tachycardia.[57]

A common inherited arrhythmia syndrome that is also associated with OT PVCs is ARVC. This inherited disorder of the myocardial desmosome leads to fibrofatty replacement of the RV myocardium and is associated with syncope, left bundle branch morphology PVCs/VT, and sudden death. Screening tests for ARVC include genetic testing, echocardiography, and magnetic resonance imaging. Treatment of PVCs associated with ARVC is different from treatment of idiopathic PVCs as an implantable defibrillator is nearly always required and ablation typically requires an epicardial approach. Therefore distinguishing patients with benign OT PVCs from those with ARVC is important. In general, young patients with a single-morphology PVC of typical origin from the RV anteroseptum or the LVOT and no family history of sudden death do not require screening beyond transthoracic echocardiography. Patients with multiple PVC morphologies or with PVCs originating from an unusual location, such as the RV free wall, may require a screening magnetic resonance image. ECG criteria have been developed that help to distinguish PVCs/VT in ARVC from benign idiopathic VT.[58] These include a late precordial transition at or beyond lead V_5 (suggesting an RV free-wall origin), QRS notching in multiple leads, and a lead I QRS duration of 120 ms or longer.

Finally, in the inherited arrhythmia syndromes such as Brugada syndrome or long QT syndrome, OT PVCs can serve as initiators of life-threatening arrhythmias by creating long-short coupling intervals that may predispose to torsades de pointes VT. Ablation of PVCs in patients with these inherited syndromes and frequent ICD shocks has been associated with a marked reduction in ICD therapy.[59]

Management

Given its generally benign prognosis, treatment decisions for patients with OT VTs largely depend on the severity of symptoms. More aggressive therapy may be warranted in patients with severe symptoms, syncope, short-coupled PVCs, or PVCs triggering torsades de pointes VT and in those with frequent PVCs believed to be contributing to a cardiomyopathy or worsening of preexisting LV dysfunction. Therefore in all patients who present for PVC evaluation, we typically take a careful symptoms-based history, perform a continuous 24-hour outpatient telemetric monitoring to quantify PVC burden, and obtain an echocardiogram with careful attention to RV and LV size and function. In patients with infrequent PVCs (<5%), mild to no symptoms, and normal LV function, reassurance of the benign prognosis with no specific therapy is sufficient. For patients with bothersome PVCs or frequent PVCs and abnormal LV function, treatment options include medical therapy or catheter ablation.

Medical Therapy

OT VTs generally respond well to β-blockers or calcium channel blockers. These medications are typically first-line treatment because they have mild side effect profiles as compared with other antiarrhythmic medications, along with success rates in the range of 65%.[13] Side effects such as fatigue may limit patient adherence. Calcium channel blockers may be tried in patients with asthma or intolerance to β-blockers but are typically less effective.

For patients who do not respond to β-blockers or calcium channel blockers, the addition or substitution of a class IC antiarrhythmic drug (flecainide or propafenone) may be useful.[14,60] In refractory patients, class III drugs (sotalol or amiodarone) may also be considered.[60] Because class I medications are contraindicated in the setting of ischemic heart disease, coronary artery disease should be excluded in patients with intermediate or higher risk before considering the administration of such medications. The efficacy of drug therapy can be monitored by patient symptoms, Holter monitoring, or stress testing to detect exertional PVs/VT. We typically perform a routine stress test every other year in patients on class IC antiarrhythmic drugs to exclude coronary artery disease.

Mapping and Catheter Ablation

Catheter ablation is now considered an alternative first-line option for treatment of symptomatic OT PVCs and is detailed here. For patients with recurrent syncope due to rapid VT- or PVC-induced torsades de pointes VT, catheter ablation should be strongly considered early in the course of therapy. In some patients who suffer cardiac arrest caused by short-coupled PVC-induced torsades, an ICD may be recommended. In general, though, ICD therapy is not warranted for most OT PVCs because they are typically associated with a benign prognosis and frequently can be cured with catheter ablation.

Mapping of PVCs in the electrophysiology laboratory requires fluoroscopy and an electrophysiological recording system that is typically coupled with an electroanatomical mapping system. For

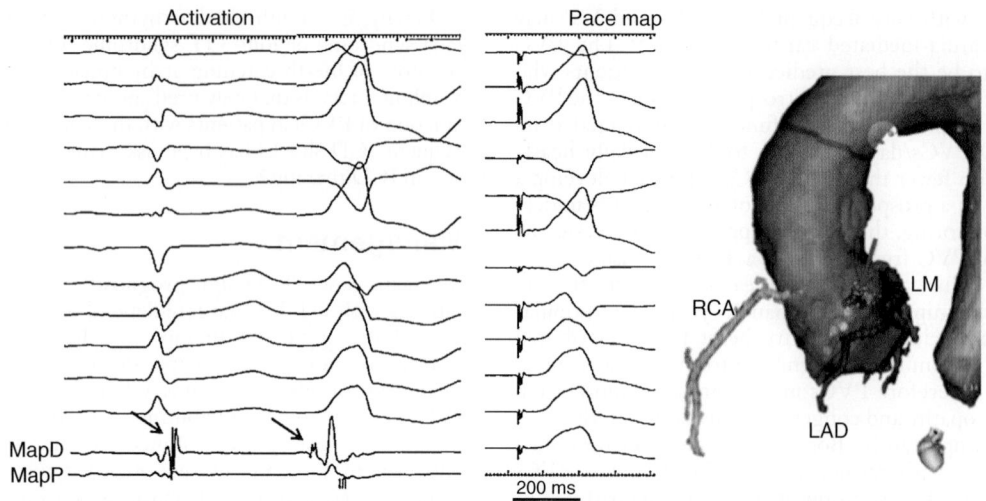

FIGURE 81.5 *Left panel,* Surface electrocardiographic leads and intracardiac electrograms recorded from the distal (*MapD*) and proximal (*MapP*) mapping electrodes in a patient with premature ventricular complex (PVC) originating from the left sinus of Valsalva. Note the rS in lead I, the notch in lead V$_1$, and early precordial transition. There is a small potential on the bipolar MapD catheter that is late during sinus rhythm but precedes the QRS during the PVC by 22 ms (*black arrow*). *Middle panel,* A perfect pace map from this location is shown. Reversal of potentials with the catheter in the aortic cusps confirms a supraaortic valve PVC origin, and ablation at this site was successful in eliminating the PVC. *Right panel,* Registration of a computed tomographic image with the electroanatomical mapping system allows delineation of the proximal coronary arteries so that ablation can be performed without a coronary angiogram (as long as registration is confirmed to be accurate). Here the ablation sites are denoted by red tags (*arrow*) in the left coronary cusp, near the junction of the left and right cusps—a safe distance from the left main ostium (*LM*) and the left anterior descending coronary artery (*LAD,* colored *purple*). The right coronary artery (*RCA*) is colored *yellow.* The *yellow tags* represent sites of pace mapping.

cases of aortic root or LVOT arrhythmia, phased-array ICE can be invaluable. PVCs can be mapped with pace mapping or activation mapping. If PVCs occur spontaneously and frequently, activation mapping can be used to identify the earliest bipolar electrogram preceding the surface QRS. For typical OT PVCs, a bipolar activation time longer than 20 to 25 ms before QRS is usually sufficient for successful ablation. A QS pattern on the unipolar electrogram can also be recorded at the site of origin of the PVC/VT. Pace mapping in the RVOT should also be performed at the earliest site—recording of a pace map that does not match the clinical PVC at the earliest recorded site suggests that the PVC may originate from an adjacent cardiac chamber (e.g., LVOT when recording from posterior RVOT or epicardium). In cases of infrequent RVOT PVCs, pace mapping alone can be used to localize PVC origin. Pacing output should be set to twice diastolic threshold to avoid far-field or anodal capture. Pace mapping should begin in the area of suspected VT origin based on the 12-lead ECG, and the catheter should be manipulated to achieve a 12/12 lead pace-map match with clinic VT (Fig. 81.5). The first beat of sustained VT can sometimes have a slightly different morphology than the sustained run as the result of repolarization changes during initiation; therefore the morphology during sustained VT should be targeted. In addition, sometimes a pace map can appear similar over a sizable distance (1–3 cm^2).[61,62] Attempts to match notching and QRS amplitude in all 12 leads will yield better ablation success.

For nearly all patients, mapping of the RVOT should occur first, given the low risk and high prevalence of RVOT origin PVCs. When the RVOT is mapped, positioning a catheter at the RV apex helps to delineate septal from free-wall RVOT locations in the left anterior oblique projection. Typically the site of earliest activation will also have a perfect 12-lead pace-map match; if activation is longer than 20 ms before QRS with qS on

the unipolar electrogram, the radiofrequency energy should be applied. A standard nonirrigated 4-mm radiofrequency energy ablation catheter can be used in the RVOT. Because the origin of these PVCs is superficial, powers of 25 to 30 watts are usually sufficient. An early "flurry" of PVCs during ablation is often considered a good sign, although this may occur with catheter ablation in any myocardial region. Very high-power lesions should be used cautiously, given the proximity of the superior RVOT, and particularly the proximal PA, to the coronary arteries.[63] If the earliest activation is less than 20 ms before QRS, if a small initial r wave is present on the unipolar electrogram at the earliest site, and/or if the pace map has a later precordial transition than the clinical PVC, mapping of the LVOT should be performed. Because the aortic valve plane is inferior to the plane of the pulmonic valve, when PVC activation is diffusely early in the low posterior RVOT and is less than 20 ms before QRS, an LVOT origin should be suspected. Typically the RCC is directly posterior to the inferoposterior RVOT, and the LCC is posterior to the anterior RVOT (see Fig. 81.1). Unsuccessful ablation in these RVOT regions should lead to exploration of the corresponding aortic sinus regions. If a PVC has a marked inferior axis or if a change in PVC morphology after ablation is noted to a more inferior axis, the septal aspect of the PA should be explored (Fig. 81.6).[64] Coronary angiography should be performed prior to ablation if the catheter is advanced into the PA more than 2 cm beyond the pulmonic valve. Cryoablation of RVOT and of PA PVCs has been described but offers few advantages over radiofrequency ablation unless one is close to the His bundle.[65] Cryoablation may be useful in para-Hisian PVCs, although the RCC should be explored before performing ablation in the para-Hisian region because this region lies just above the His region and may serve as a safer location for catheter ablation (Fig. 81.7).[66]

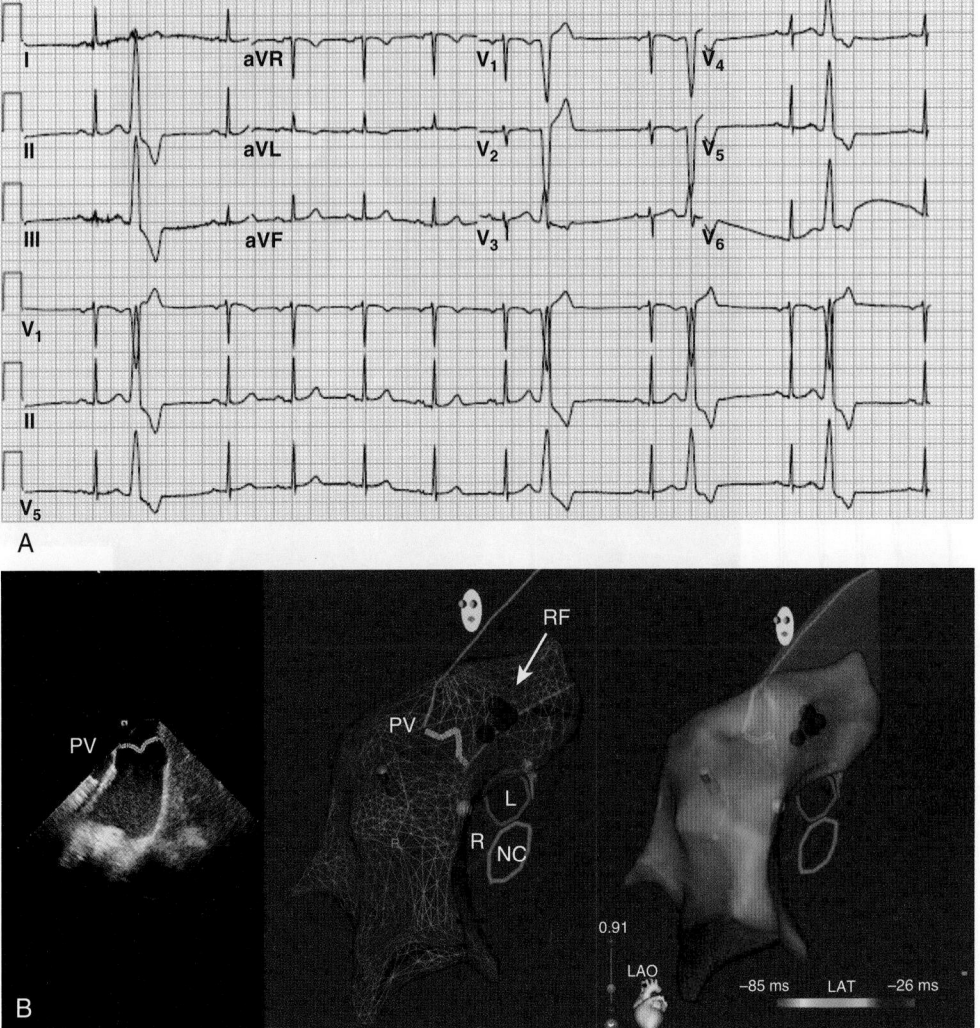

FIGURE 81.6 Integration of electrocardiographic, intracardiac echocardiography, and electroanatomical mapping to identify a pulmonary artery premature ventricular complex (PVC) origin. (A) A 12-lead electrocardiogram recorded from a patient with frequent PVCs mapped to the pulmonary artery. Note the marked inferior axis of the PVCs compared with sinus rhythm. (B) The left panel shows an intracardiac echocardiographic view of the pulmonary artery, with the pulmonic valve (*PV*) outlined in *orange*. In the middle panel, the PV is superimposed on a transparent electroanatomical map of the right ventricular outflow tract. Ablation lesions are shown (*red tags*) to be clearly above the PV in the pulmonary artery. The aortic cusps outlined on the intracardiac echocardiography are also shown (*L*, left cusp; *NC*, noncoronary cusp; *R*, right cusp). The rightmost panel shows the right ventricular outflow tract activation map, with earliest activation during the PVC (*red*) located above the PV in the pulmonary artery. *LAO*, Left anterior oblique; *LAT*, local activation time; *RF*, radiofrequency ablation lesions.

For LVOT mapping catheter localization, unless the operator has experience with aortography for identifying the coronary cusps, ICE is extremely useful for identifying the aortic cusps and the catheter position within the cusps (Fig. 81.8). Fluoroscopy alone can often be misleading. The aortic root is typically mapped using the retrograde aortic approach, and it should be mapped as a separate cardiac chamber, with multiple activation points and pace maps taken throughout each coronary cusp at the valve level and up to 2 cm above the valve (staying below the left main coronary ostium). The noncoronary cusp overlies the left atrium and has not been associated with PVC origin in our experience. However, sites throughout the RCC, RCC/LCC junction, and LCC have been described. In contrast to the RVOT, activation mapping is always preferable in the aortic root because pace maps are often unreliable due to capture of adjacent structures rather than the thin sleeves of myocardium that may be the source of LVOT PVCs.

Therefore, while a poor LVOT pace map should not dissuade ablation, a perfect pace map remains a useful guide for suggesting an aortic root origin.

Early LVOT sites recorded with activation mapping are typically greater than 20 ms before the surface ECG QRS onset. In the aortic root, "reversal" of a sharp potential, from late (during sinus rhythm) to early (during a PVC), confirms the origin as aortic root and often suggests a successful ablation site[67] (see Fig. 81.5). Because of the proximity of the aortic valve region to the coronary arteries, coronary angiography is recommended before ablation is performed in the aortic root. If ICE is being used by an experienced operator, coronary angiography may be omitted if the site of earliest activation is at the RCC/LCC junction or at the LCC farther than 1 cm from the left main coronary artery.[68] Registering an electroanatomical map with another imaging modality such as computed tomography angiography can also facilitate identification of the proximal

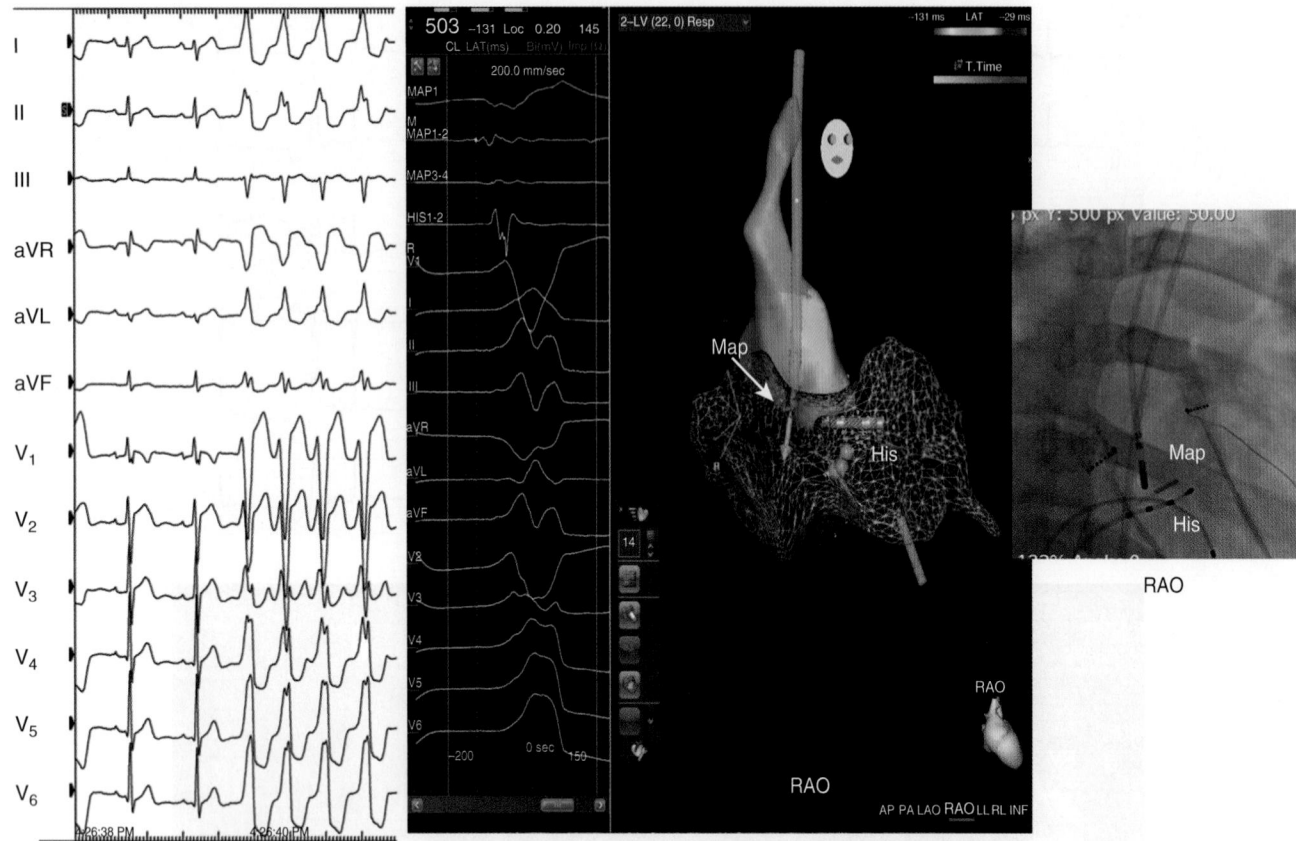

FIGURE 81.7 *Left panel:* A 12-lead electrocardiogram in a patient with para-Hisian premature ventricular complex (PVC) exit. Note that leads II and aVF are positive while lead III is negative, suggesting an origin lower on the septum. Lead aVR is negative; however, lead aVL is positive, suggesting a para-Hisian exit site. Earliest activation in the right ventricle during the PVC was mapped to a site with a sharp His deflection recorded during sinus rhythm. An electroanatomical map (*middle panel*) and fluoroscopy (*right panel*) show that retrograde aortic mapping in the right coronary cusp revealed equally early activation with only a far-field His signal. This PVC was successfully ablated using a 6-mm cryoablation catheter in the right aortic sinus. *Map,* Mapping catheter; *RAO,* right anterior oblique.

coronary arteries (see Fig. 81.5) and may be useful in patients with suspected coronary anomalies. Visualizing the right coronary artery with ICE is difficult; therefore coronary angiography should be performed before ablation within the right cusp. If ablation at an early site is ineffective, changing the angle of the catheter or looping the catheter into the LV cavity and back up into the aortic root can sometimes help. Mapping in the aortic root should be performed under systemic heparinization, and ablation should be performed using irrigated ablation catheters because any thrombus can potentially embolize to a coronary artery. Power during ablation is typically initiated at 15 to 20 watts and is slowly titrated up to 30 watts. Higher powers usually are not needed, although for an intramyocardial or epicardial focus, powers of up to 50 watts may be used. The impedance drop should be carefully observed and power discontinued at any sign of a rise in impedance.

While the aortic cusps are the most common sites of LVOT PVCs, other sites include the LVOT myocardium just beneath the aortic valve and the LVOT epicardium (LV summit), which can be approached via the aortic root or the coronary venous system or by subxiphoid epicardial access. Mapping and ablation of the LVOT endocardium beneath the aortic valve can be undertaken using conventional activation and pace mapping as described for the RVOT, although catheter stability is often challenging. For LV summit PVCs with a suggested epicardial exit by ECG or mapping, we often first explore the coronary venous system (GCV or AIV) and the left aortic sinus before considering epicardial access because epicardial fat and proximity to the coronary arteries often limit the ability to perform successful epicardial ablation. A coronary sinus venogram can be performed to delineate the caliber and anatomy of the distal AIV. We also place a small coronary sinus catheter as far distally as possible in the AIV for all LVOT PVCs to compare activation timing during the PVC with that recorded from catheters in the RVOT and the aortic root (see Fig. 81.8). The main limitations of ablation within the GCV/AIV include the following: (1) the small size may not allow access with the ablation catheter; (2) low flow within a small vein may limit the power delivered, even with irrigated radiofrequency ablation; and (3) the proximity to the left main and left anterior descending coronary arteries (see Fig. 81.8). Coronary angiography should always be performed before ablation is begun in the GCV/AIV so that proximity to the left anterior descending coronary artery may be noted and ablation avoided if the catheter tip is less than 5 mm away. If activation is noted to be similarly early in AIV and LCC, ablation in the LCC can be safer and more effective because higher power can be delivered.[69] In some cases, the AIV has been the only site in which PVC elimination has occurred.[42,70]

Percutaneous subxiphoid access can also be used to gain transpericardial access to map the epicardial free-wall surface of the OT. Although this is often limited by epicardial fat and proximity

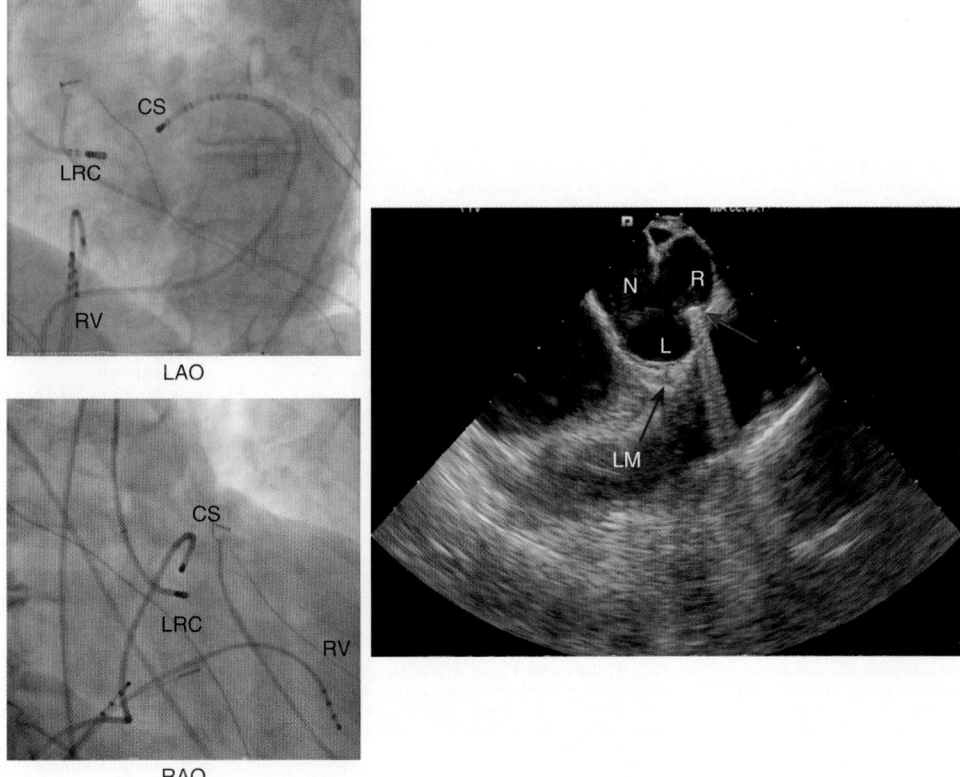

FIGURE 81.8 The *left panels* demonstrate fluoroscopic views of catheter positions in the right anterior oblique (*RAO*) and left anterior oblique (*LAO*) projections during an ablation procedure. The coronary sinus catheter (*CS*) has been advanced distally to the anterior interventricular vein for mapping purposes. The ablation catheter is taking a retrograde aortic route to the junction of the right and left coronary cusps (*LRC*). The exact location of the ablation catheter tip is difficult to confirm using fluoroscopy. In the *right panel*, a phased-array intracardiac echocardiographic image is shown, confirming the catheter tip location at the junction of the left (*L*) and right (*R*) coronary cusps (*red arrow*). Ablation was performed at this site without coronary angiography, as the location of the left main coronary artery (*LM, blue arrow*) can also be seen on intracardiac echocardiography at a safe distance from the tip of the ablation catheter. *N,* Noncoronary cusp; *RV,* right ventricular catheter.

to the epicardial coronary arteries, a safe site that results in PVC elimination can occasionally be identified. It should be emphasized that even in expert hands, some PVCs of epicardial or intramyocardial origin near a major coronary artery cannot be eliminated with catheter ablation. Cryoablation has been performed for lesions near epicardial coronary arteries.[71] In theory, the warm blood pool should protect the coronary arteries, making cryoablation safer than radiofrequency energy when near a

coronary vessel. However, animal studies have demonstrated that chronic coronary artery damage can occur after cryoablation directly on top of coronary arteries.[72] In cases of unsuccessful ablation, treatment with drug therapy, including 1C agents, sotalol, ranolazine, dronedarone, or, if necessary, amiodarone, can then be undertaken. Minimally invasive surgical cryoablation under direct visualization has also been described for malignant PVCs originating near a coronary artery.[73]

REFERENCES

1. Iwai S, Cantillon DJ, Kim RJ, et al. Right and left ventricular outflow tract tachycardias: evidence for a common electrophysiologic mechanism. *J Cardiovasc Electrophysiol.* 2006;17:1052–1058.
2. Gerstenfeld E, Tseng Z. Outflow tract ventricular tachyarrhythmias: mechanisms, clinical features, and management. In: Zipes DP, Jalife J, eds. *Cardiac Electrophysiology: From Cell to Bedside.* 6th ed. Philadelphia: Saunders; 2013:815–825.
3. Kim RJ, Iwai S, Markowitz SM, et al. Clinical and electrophysiological spectrum of idiopathic ventricular outflow tract arrhythmias. *J Am Coll Cardiol.* 2007;49:2035–2043.
4. Asirvatham SJ. Correlative anatomy for the invasive electrophysiologist: outflow tract and supravalvar arrhythmia. *J Cardiovasc Electrophysiol.* 2009;20:955–968.
5. Hasdemir C, Aktas S, Govsa F, et al. Demonstration of ventricular myocardial extensions into the pulmonary artery and aorta beyond the ventriculo-arterial junction. *Pacing Clin Electrophysiol.* 2007;30:534–539.
6. Asirvatham SJ. Correlative anatomy and electrophysiology for the interventional electrophysiologist: right atrial flutter. *J Cardiovasc Electrophysiol.* 2009;20:113–122.

7. Kanagaratnam L, Tomassoni G, Schweikert R, et al. Ventricular tachycardias arising from the aortic sinus of Valsalva: an under-recognized variant of left outflow tract ventricular tachycardia. *J Am Coll Cardiol.* 2001;37:1408–1414.
8. Srivathsan KS, Bunch TJ, Asirvatham SJ, et al. Mechanisms and utility of discrete great arterial potentials in the ablation of outflow tract ventricular arrhythmias. *Circ Arrhythm Electrophysiol.* 2008;1:30–38.
9. Yamada T, Huizar JF, McElderry HT, et al. Atrial tachycardia originating from the noncoronary aortic cusp and musculature connection with the atria: relevance for catheter ablation. *Heart Rhythm.* 2006;3:1494–1496.
10. Daniels DV, Lu YY, Morton JB, et al. Idiopathic epicardial left ventricular tachycardia originating remote from the sinus of Valsalva: electrophysiological characteristics, catheter ablation, and identification from the 12-lead electrocardiogram. *Circulation.* 2006;113:1659–1666.
11. Yamada T, McElderry HT, Doppalapudi H, et al. Idiopathic ventricular arrhythmias originating from the left ventricular summit: anatomic concepts relevant to ablation. *Circ Arrhythm Electrophysiol.* 2010;3:616–623.

12. Brooks R, Burgess JH. Idiopathic ventricular tachycardia. A review. *Medicine (Baltimore).* 1988;67:271–294.
13. Buxton AE, Waxman HL, Marchlinski FE, et al. Right ventricular tachycardia: clinical and electrophysiologic characteristics. *Circulation.* 1983;68:917–927.
14. Mont L, Seixas T, Brugada P, et al. The electrocardiographic, clinical, and electrophysiologic spectrum of idiopathic monomorphic ventricular tachycardia. *Am Heart J.* 1992;124:746–753.
15. Lemery R, Brugada P, Bella PD, et al. Nonischemic ventricular tachycardia: clinical course and long-term follow-up in patients without clinically overt heart disease. *Circulation.* 1989;79:990–999.
16. Marchlinski FE, Deely MP, Zado ES. Sex-specific triggers for right ventricular outflow tract tachycardia. *Am Heart J.* 2000;139:1009–1013.
17. Hayashi H, Fujiki A, Tani M, et al. Circadian variation of idiopathic ventricular tachycardia originating from right ventricular outflow tract. *Am J Cardiol.* 1999;84:99–101. A108.
18. Yamawake N, Nishizaki M, Hayashi T, et al. Autonomic and pharmacological responses of idiopathic ventricular tachycardia arising from the left ventricular outflow tract. *J Cardiovasc Electrophysiol.* 2007;18:1161–1166.

19. Niroomand F, Carbucicchio C, Tondo C, et al. Electrophysiological characteristics and outcome in patients with idiopathic right ventricular arrhythmia compared with arrhythmogenic right ventricular dysplasia. *Heart.* 2002;87:41–47.

20. Lerman BB, Stein K, Engelstein ED, et al. Mechanism of repetitive monomorphic ventricular tachycardia. *Circulation.* 1995;92:421–429.

21. Sung RJ, Keung EC, Nguyen NX, et al. Effects of beta-adrenergic blockade on verapamil-responsive and verapamil-irresponsive sustained ventricular tachycardias. *J Clin Invest.* 1988;81:688–699.

22. Tada H, Ito S, Naito S, et al. Prevalence and electrocardiographic characteristics of idiopathic ventricular arrhythmia originating in the free wall of the right ventricular outflow tract. *Circulation.* 2004;68:909–914.

23. Dixit S, Gerstenfeld EP, Callans DJ, et al. Electrocardiographic patterns of superior right ventricular outflow tract tachycardias: distinguishing septal and free-wall sites of origin. *J Cardiovasc Electrophysiol.* 2003;14:1–7.

24. Yamauchi Y, Aonuma K, Takahashi A, et al. Electrocardiographic characteristics of repetitive monomorphic right ventricular tachycardia originating near the His-bundle. *J Cardiovasc Electrophysiol.* 2005;16:1041–1048.

25. Timmermans C, Rodriguez LM, Medeiros A, et al. Radiofrequency catheter ablation of idiopathic ventricular tachycardia originating in the main stem of the pulmonary artery. *J Cardiovasc Electrophysiol.* 2003;13:281–284.

26. Sekiguchi Y, Aonuma K, Takahashi A, et al. Electrocardiographic and electrophysiologic characteristics of ventricular tachycardia originating within the pulmonary artery. *J Am Coll Cardiol.* 2005;45:887–895.

27. Liu CF, Cheung JW, Thomas G, Ip JE, Markowitz SM, Lerman BB. Ubiquitous myocardial extensions into the pulmonary artery demonstrated by integrated intracardiac echocardiography and electroanatomic mapping changing the paradigm of idiopathic right ventricular outflow tract arrhythmias. *Circ Arrhythm Electrophysiol.* 2014;7:691–700.

28. Callans DJ, Menz V, Schwartzman D, et al. Repetitive monomorphic tachycardia from the left ventricular outflow tract: electrocardiographic patterns consistent with a left ventricular site of origin. *J Am Coll Cardiol.* 1997;29:1023–1027.

29. Kanagaratnam L, Tomassoni G, Schweikert R, et al. Ventricular tachycardias arising from the aortic sinus of Valsalva: an under-recognized variant of left outflow tract ventricular tachycardia. *J Am Coll Cardiol.* 2001;37:1408–1414.

30. Ouyang F, Fotuhi P, Ho SY, et al. Repetitive monomorphic ventricular tachycardia originating from the aortic sinus cusp: electrocardiographic characterization for guiding catheter ablation. *J Am Coll Cardiol.* 2002;39:500–508.

31. Tada H, Nogami A, Naito S, et al. Left ventricular epicardial outflow tract tachycardia: a new distinct subgroup of outflow tract tachycardia. *Japanese Circulation J.* 2001;65:723–730.

32. Hachiya H, Aonuma K, Yamauchi Y, et al. How to diagnose, locate, and ablate coronary cusp ventricular tachycardia. *J Cardiovasc Electrophysiol.* 2002;13:551–556.

33. Lin D, Ilkhanoff L, Gerstenfeld E, et al. Twelve-lead electrocardiographic characteristics of the aortic cusp region guided by intracardiac echocardiography and electroanatomic mapping. *Heart Rhythm.* 2008;5:663–669.

34. Yamada T, Yoshida N, Murakami Y, et al. Electrocardiographic characteristics of ventricular arrhythmias originating from the junction of the left and right coronary sinuses of Valsalva in the aorta: the activation pattern as a rationale for the electrocardiographic characteristics. *Heart Rhythm.* 2008;5:184–192.

35. Bala R, Garcia FC, Hutchinson MD, et al. Electrocardiographic and electrophysiologic features of ventricular arrhythmias originating from the right/left coronary cusp commissure. *Heart Rhythm.* 2010;7:312–322.

36. Tanner H, Hindricks G, Schirdewahn P, et al. Outflow tract tachycardia with r/s transition in lead V3: six different anatomic approaches for successful ablation. *J Am Coll Cardiol.* 2005;45:418–423.

37. Betensky BP, Park RE, Marchlinski FE, et al. The v(2) transition ratio: a new electrocardiographic criterion for distinguishing a left from right ventricular outflow tract tachycardia origin. *J Am Coll Cardiol.* 2011;57:2255–2262.

38. Yang Y, Saenz LC, Varosy PD, et al. Using the initial vector from surface electrocardiogram to distinguish the site of outflow tract tachycardia. *Pacing Clin Electrophysiol.* 2007;30:891–898.

39. Kumagai K, Fukuda K, Wakayama Y, et al. Electrocardiographic characteristics of the variants of idiopathic left ventricular outflow tract ventricular tachyarrhythmias. *J Cardiovasc Electrophysiol.* 2008;19:495–501.

40. Yoshida N, Yamada T, McElderry HT, et al. A novel electrocardiographic criterion for differentiating a left from right ventricular outflow tract tachycardia origin: the V2S/V3R index. *J Cardiovasc Electrophysiol.* 2014;25:747–753.

41. Shimoike E, Ohba Y, Yanagi N, et al. Radiofrequency catheter ablation of left ventricular outflow tract tachycardia: report of two cases. *J Cardiovasc Electrophysiol.* 1998;9:196–202.

42. Hirasawa Y, Miyauchi Y, Iwasaki YK, et al. Successful radiofrequency catheter ablation of epicardial left ventricular outflow tract tachycardia from the anterior interventricular coronary vein. *J Cardiovasc Electrophysiol.* 2005;16:1378–1380.

43. Anter E, Frankel DS, Marchlinski FE, et al. Effect of electrocardiographic lead placement on localization of outflow tract tachycardias. *Heart Rhythm.* 2012;9:697–703.

44. Leenhardt A, Glaser E, Burguera M, et al. Short-coupled variant of torsade de pointes: a new electrocardiographic entity in the spectrum of idiopathic ventricular tachyarrhythmias. *Circulation.* 1994;89:206–215.

45. Noda T, Shimizu W, Taguchi A, et al. Malignant entity of idiopathic ventricular fibrillation and polymorphic ventricular tachycardia initiated by premature extrasystoles originating from the right ventricular outflow tract. *J Am Coll Cardiol.* 2005;46:1288–1294.

46. Viskin S, Rosso R, Rogowski O, et al. The "short-coupled" variant of right ventricular outflow ventricular tachycardia: a not-so-benign form of benign ventricular tachycardia? *J Cardiovasc Electrophysiol.* 2005;16:912–916.

47. Shimizu W. Arrhythmias originating from the right ventricular outflow tract: how to distinguish "malignant" from "benign"? *Heart Rhythm.* 2009;6:1507–1511.

48. Tan JH, Scheinman MM. Exercise-induced polymorphic ventricular tachycardia in adults without structural heart disease. *Am J Cardiol.* 2008;101:1142–1146.

49. Baman TS, Lange DC, Ilg KJ, et al. Relationship between burden of premature ventricular complexes and left ventricular function. *Heart Rhythm.* 2010;7:865–869.

50. Yarlagadda RK, Iwai S, Stein KM, et al. Reversal of cardiomyopathy in patients with repetitive monomorphic ventricular ectopy originating from the right ventricular outflow tract. *Circulation.* 2005;112:1092–1097.

51. Bogun F, Crawford T, Reich S, et al. Radiofrequency ablation of frequent, idiopathic premature ventricular complexes: comparison with a control group without intervention. *Heart Rhythm.* 2007;4:863–867.

52. Mountantonakis SE, Frankel DS, Gerstenfeld EP, et al. Reversal of outflow tract ventricular premature depolarization-induced cardiomyopathy with ablation: effect of residual arrhythmia burden and preexisting cardiomyopathy on outcome. *Heart Rhythm.* 2011;8:1608–1614.

53. Carballeira Pol L, Deyell MW, Frankel DS, et al. Ventricular premature depolarization QRS duration as a new marker of risk for the development of ventricular premature depolarization-induced cardiomyopathy. *Heart Rhythm.* 2014;11:299–306.

54. Yokokawa M, Kim HM, Good E, et al. Impact of QRS duration of frequent premature ventricular complexes on the development of cardiomyopathy. *Heart Rhythm.* 2012;9:1460–1464.

55. Yokokawa M, Good E, Crawford T, et al. Recovery from left ventricular dysfunction after ablation of frequent premature ventricular complexes. *Heart Rhythm.* 2013;10:172–175.

56. Sadron Blaye-Felice M, Hamon D, Sacher F, et al. Premature ventricular contraction-induced cardiomyopathy: related clinical and electrophysiologic parameters. *Heart Rhythm.* 2016;13:103–110.

57. Nerheim P, Birger-Botkin S, Piracha L, et al. Heart failure and sudden death in patients with tachycardia-induced cardiomyopathy and recurrent tachycardia. *Circulation.* 2004;110:247–252.

58. Hoffmayer KS, Machado ON, Marcus GM, et al. Electrocardiographic comparison of ventricular arrhythmias in patients with arrhythmogenic right ventricular cardiomyopathy and right ventricular outflow tract tachycardia. *J Am Coll Cardiol.* 2011;58:831–838.

59. Haissaguerre M, Extramiana F, Hocini M, et al. Mapping and ablation of ventricular fibrillation associated with long-QT and Brugada syndromes. *Circulation.* 2003;108:925–928.

60. Ritchie AH, Kerr CR, Qi A, et al. Nonsustained ventricular tachycardia arising from the right ventricular outflow tract. *Am J Cardiol.* 1989;64:594–598.

61. Azegami K, Wilber DJ, Arruda M, et al. Spatial resolution of pacemapping and activation mapping in patients with idiopathic right ventricular outflow tract tachycardia. *J Cardiovasc Electrophysiol.* 2005;16:823–829.

62. Bogun F, Taj M, Ting M, et al. Spatial resolution of pace mapping of idiopathic ventricular tachycardia/ectopy originating in the right ventricular outflow tract. *Heart Rhythm.* 2008;5:339–344.

63. Vaseghi M, Cesario DA, Mahajan A, et al. Catheter ablation of right ventricular outflow tract tachycardia: value of defining coronary anatomy. *J Cardiovasc Electrophysiol.* 2006;17:632–637.

64. Tada H, Tadokoro K, Miyaji K, et al. Idiopathic ventricular arrhythmias arising from the pulmonary artery: prevalence, characteristics, and topography of the arrhythmia origin. *Heart Rhythm.* 2008;5:419–426.

65. Kurzidim K, Schneider HJ, Kuniss M, et al. Cryocatheter ablation of right ventricular outflow tract tachycardia. *J Cardiovasc Electrophysiol.* 2005;16:366–369.

66. Yamada T, McElderry HT, Doppalapudi H, et al. Catheter ablation of ventricular arrhythmias originating in the vicinity of the His bundle: significance of mapping the aortic sinus cusp. *Heart Rhythm.* 2008;5:37–42.

67. Srivathsan KS, Bunch TJ, Asirvatham SJ, et al. Mechanisms and utility of discrete great arterial potentials in the ablation of outflow tract ventricular arrhythmias. *Circ Arrhythm Electrophysiol.* 2008;1:30–38.

68. Hoffmayer KS, Dewland TA, Hsia HH, et al. Safety of radiofrequency catheter ablation without coronary angiography in aortic cusp ventricular arrhythmias. *Heart Rhythm.* 2014;11:1117–1121.

69. Jauregui Abularach ME, Campos B, Park KM, et al. Ablation of ventricular arrhythmias arising near the anterior epicardial veins from the left sinus of Valsalva region: ECG features, anatomic distance, and outcome. *Heart Rhythm.* 2012;9:865–873.

70. Obel OA, d'Avila A, Neuzil P, et al. Ablation of left ventricular epicardial outflow tract tachycardia from the distal great cardiac vein. *J Am Coll Cardiol.* 2006;48:1813–1817.

71. Di Biase L, Al-Ahamad A, Santangeli P, et al. Safety and outcomes of cryoablation for ventricular tachyarrhythmias: results from a multicenter experience. *Heart Rhythm.* 2011;8:968–974.

72. D'Avila A, Aryana A, Thiagalingam A, et al. Focal and linear endocardial and epicardial catheter-based cryoablation of normal and infarcted ventricular tissue. *Pacing Clin Electrophysiol.* 2008;31:1322–1331.

73. Frey B, Kreiner G, Fritsch S, et al. Successful treatment of idiopathic left ventricular outflow tract tachycardia by catheter ablation or minimally invasive surgical cryoablation. *Pacing Clin Electrophysiol.* 2000;23:870–876.

82 Fascicular Ventricular Arrhythmias

Akiko Ueda and Kyoko Soejima

Various types of ventricular tachycardia (VT) are known to arise from the His-Purkinje network in patients with or without structural heart diseases (SHDs). In this chapter, we describe the clinical manifestation, mechanism, diagnosis, and therapeutic option for each VT. We first focus on the basic concept of the most common reentrant fascicular VT, which is known as verapamil-sensitive fascicular VT. Recent findings on the VT circuit and characteristics of the rare form are also addressed. We then describe focal Purkinje VT and ventricular premature contractions (VPCs) arising from the Purkinje system that could trigger ventricular fibrillation (VF). We also briefly describe bundle branch reentrant VT (BBRVT) and interfascicular reentrant VT (IFVT).

Verapamil-Sensitive Fascicular Ventricular Tachycardia

Clinical Manifestation

Although most VTs are related to SHDs, 10% are identified in patients with no apparent structural abnormalities. Following right ventricular (RV) outflow tract VTs, left ventricular (LV) fascicular VT is the second most common form, comprising 7% to 12% of such "idiopathic" VTs.[1,2] In 1979, Zipes and colleagues first described the diagnostic characteristics of this type of VT, which included (1) induction by atrial pacing, (2) VT configuration of the right bundle branch block (RBBB) and left axis, and (3) manifestation in patients with no apparent SHD.[3] Belhassen and associates reported verapamil sensitivity of this VT in 1981,[4] currently known as the fourth feature. This VT typically presents in young adulthood, and there is a slight male predominance.

Classification

Following the initial report by Zipes,[3] two additional QRS morphologies have been reported.[5,6] At present, idiopathic verapamil-sensitive fascicular VT is classified into three forms according to the QRS morphologies: (1) RBBB pattern with left axis deviation (common form, left posterior fascicular [LPF] VT, 90%), (2) RBBB pattern with right axis deviation (uncommon form, left anterior fascicular [LAF] VT, 10%), and (3) narrow QRS morphology with normal axis (rare form, upper septal [US] VT, <1%) (Fig. 82.1).

Mechanism and Ventricular Tachycardia Circuit

The mechanism of verapamil-sensitive fascicular VT is reentry as ventricular or atrial programmed stimulation can induce, entrain, and terminate VT. A multitude of studies investigating the role of the Purkinje system in the VT circuit has been conducted. Several groups demonstrated that the Purkinje network at the LPF region is a critical component of the most common VT circuit on the basis of the high success rate of ablation at this site. Nakagawa and coworkers first reported the importance of Purkinje potentials at the successful ablation site.[7] Ablation sites were at the apical inferior septum of the LV. Tsuchiya and associates reported the significance of a late diastolic potential (DP) and emphasized the role of late DPs and presystolic potentials (PPs) in the VT circuit.[8] Their successful ablation sites were located at the basal septal region close to the main trunk of the left bundle (LB) branch.

In 2000, Nogami and colleagues first demonstrated the macroreentrant circuit of this verapamil-sensitive fascicular VT using a multielectrode catheter placed at the LV midseptal area.[9] During sinus rhythm, Purkinje potentials preceding the QRS complex were recorded along the septal wall from proximal to distal electrodes (basal to apical direction) (Fig. 82.2A). During VT, two distinct types of potentials were recorded: DPs and PPs. DP indicated the propagation of excitation in the basal to apical direction, but PP showed propagation from apical to basal direction, which is the reverse of the activation sequence during sinus rhythm (Fig. 82.2B). Entrainment mapping at the exit site where PP and the earliest ventricular activation were fused demonstrated orthodromic DP capture with a postpacing interval identical to the VT cycle length. When entrainment pacing was performed with a shorter cycle length, DP was antidromically captured and VT was terminated. Furthermore, the administration of verapamil during VT significantly prolonged both the DP-PP and PP-DP intervals but not the PP-QRS interval, suggesting that the location of slow conduction was from DP to PP. From the abovementioned findings, it was concluded that DP arose from abnormal Purkinje fibers with verapamil sensitivity and were a critical component of the VT circuit. In contrast, PP, representing the activation of LPF or Purkinje fibers adjacent to LPF, might not be involved in the VT circuit. Recent reports electrophysiologically demonstrated that LPF was more likely to be a bystander as PP could be captured by a sinus beat without affecting the VT cycle length.[10,11] These authors advocated the hypothesized VT circuit shown in Fig. 82.3A.

Endocardial mapping during the uncommon type of verapamil-sensitive fascicular VT, namely LAF VT, exhibits DP in the LV midseptum and PP near the LAF region. The VT activation is considered to antegradely propagate over the midseptal area similar to the common type of LPF VT and then retrogradely propagate over the area near the LAF. Kottkamp and associates reported a patient who had two VTs with left and right axis QRS configurations.[12] Radiofrequency (RF) energy delivered to the area between the LPF and the LAF successfully eliminated both VTs, suggesting that both LPF and LAF VT shared the midseptal area as an antegrade limb of the circuit. Fig. 82.3B depicts a schema of the hypothesized LAF VT circuit.

Details of the reentrant circuit of the rare form of verapamil-sensitive fascicular VT, USVT, were unclear until recently. Ahmed and coworkers reported that the VT activation propagated antegradely in the LAF or the LPF and then retrogradely in abnormal Purkinje tissue in the LV septum, which is the reverse direction of propagation as observed for LPF and LAF VT[13] (Fig. 82.3C). USVT is known to develop following ablation of other types of verapamil-sensitive fascicular VTs. Ahmed and

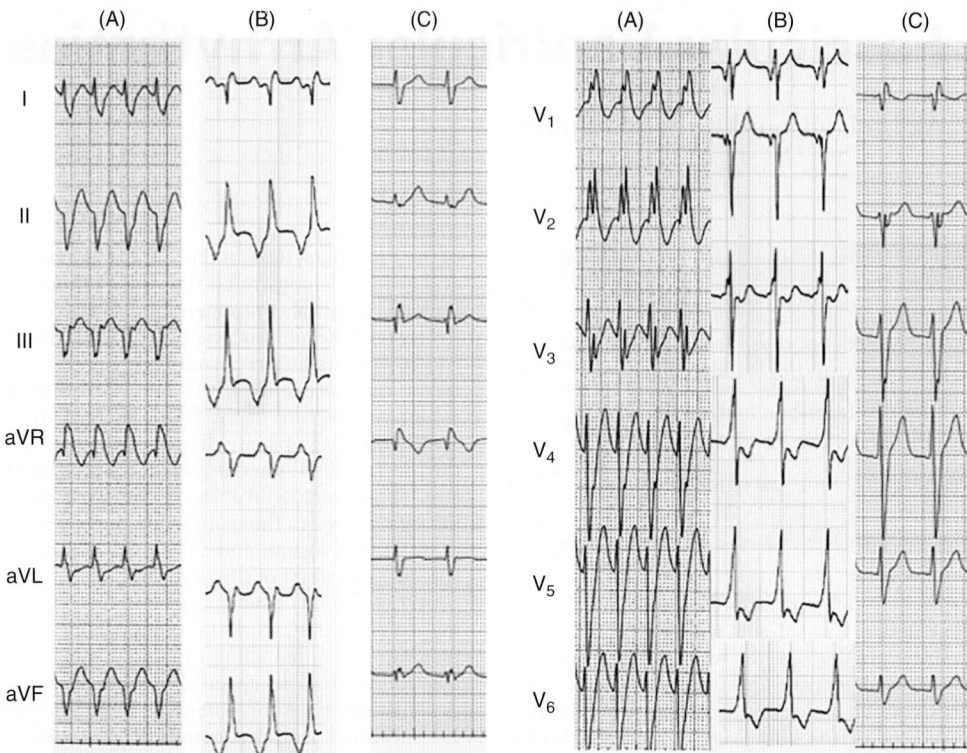

FIGURE 82.1 Twelve-lead electrocardiograms of verapamil-sensitive fascicular ventricular tachycardia (VT). (A) Common form (left posterior fascicular VT) shows right bundle branch block (RBBB) with left axis configuration. (B) Uncommon form (left anterior fascicular VT) shows RBBB with right axis configuration. (C) Rare form (upper septal VT) shows narrow QRS with normal axis.

colleagues reported that half of their USVT cohort previously underwent LPF region ablation. Conduction delay in the fascicular region created by ablation seems to provide a new substrate of USVT. However, the remaining half of their cohort had no previous ablation but presented with minor electrocardiogram (ECG) abnormalities, such as small Q waves in the inferior leads and/or S waves in leads I and/or aVF. Regardless of iatrogenic or idiopathic causes, the presence of conduction abnormalities in the midseptum could be a substrate for USVT.

Anatomical Substrate

Verapamil-sensitive fascicular VT is idiopathic and is not usually associated with an abnormal low-voltage area. However, there have been reports of fascicular VT in ischemic cardiomyopathy. Earlier studies using canine infarct models showed that Purkinje fibers over the infarcted region remain almost structurally intact but present abnormal electrophysiological (EP) properties, such as decreased resting potential, lower action potential amplitude, and increased action potential duration. These properties may lead to both triggered and reentrant mechanisms of VT.[14,15] Hayashi and associates reported four cases with acute or chronic phase of ischemic cardiomyopathy, who developed VT with similar EP properties.[16] The VTs were reproducibly induced by programmed stimulation and entrained by atrial pacing. DP and PP were sequentially recorded along the LV posterior septum during the VT, and ablation at either site successfully terminated the tachycardia in all patients. Verapamil sensitivity was confirmed in only one patient in this study because of unstable hemodynamics. A case of reentrant LAF VT associated with healed myocardial infarction was also reported.[17] These VTs present several characteristic differences compared with the usual scar-related VT in patients with ischemic cardiomyopathy: (1) relatively narrow QRS morphology during VT, (2) verapamil sensitivity, (3) PPs or DPs during VT, and (4) VT termination by a few RF energy applications to the site.[14]

A controversy remains regarding the involvement of false tendons or fibromuscular bands in LV verapamil-sensitive fascicular VT. Several reports have suggested the anatomical or EP involvement of false tendons. Thakur and colleagues reported that false tendons were observed more frequently in patients with fascicular VT (100%) compared with those without VT (5%).[18] Maruyama and associates reported that an electrode catheter positioned at the LV mid- to inferoapical septum along a false tendon recorded sequential DPs that encompassed the entire VT cycle length.[19] In contrast, Lin and coworkers reported a similar prevalence of a fibromuscular band in patients with or without the fascicular VTs.[20] Although small fibromuscular bands or trabeculae not detectable by echocardiography could play roles in reentrant circuits, this has not yet been fully elucidated.

Differential Diagnosis

Other types of idiopathic VTs arising from the posterior papillary muscle (PPM) or cardiac crux can present with a similar QRS morphology. Kawamura and associates described a stepwise ECG algorithm to differentiate these VTs that have an RBBB and a superior axis.[21] A lower maximum deflection index (MDI) of <0.55 and a shorter QRS duration of <150 ms diagnosed verapamil-sensitive LPF VTs with high sensitivity and specificity. VT originating from the PPM is not typically induced by programmed stimulation and is catecholamine sensitive, suggesting a nonreentrant mechanism.[22] Crux VT has also a nonreentrant mechanism and catecholamine sensitivity.[23]

Therapy

Catheter ablation can be a first-line therapy for verapamil-sensitive fascicular VT as both the acute and long-term success rates are high.[7-9,24] As the DP is recorded at a critical part of the VT circuit, identification of the potential during the VT is

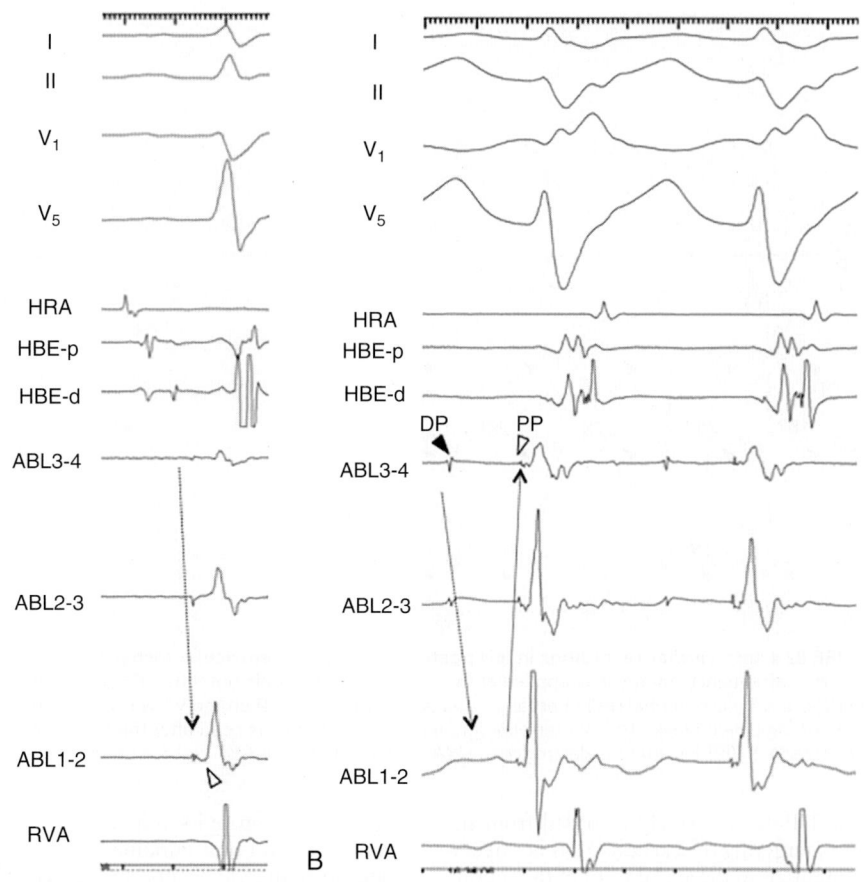

FIGURE 82.2 Intracardiac recordings in a patient with left posterior fascicle-ventricular tachycardia. Ablation catheter is placed at the left ventricular midseptum. The distal electrode (*ABL1*) is located most apically and the proximal electrode (*ABL4*) is located more basal. (A) During sinus rhythm, Purkinje potentials preceding the QRS complex are recorded along the septal wall from proximal to distal electrodes (basal to apical direction). (B) During ventricular tachycardia, two distinct potentials, middiastolic potentials (DP) and Purkinje potentials at the presystolic timing (PP), are recorded. While DP shows propagation in the basal to apical direction, PP shows propagation in the apical to basal direction, which is the reverse of the direction during sinus rhythm. The *black triangle* indicates DP. The *white triangle* indicates Purkinje potentials that propagate from proximal to distal during sinus rhythm and from distal to proximal during the ventricular tachycardia. *ABL*, Ablation; *d*, distal; *DP*, diastolic potential; *HBE*, His bundle electrogram; *HRA*, high right atrium; *PP*, presystolic potential; *RVA*, right ventricular apex.

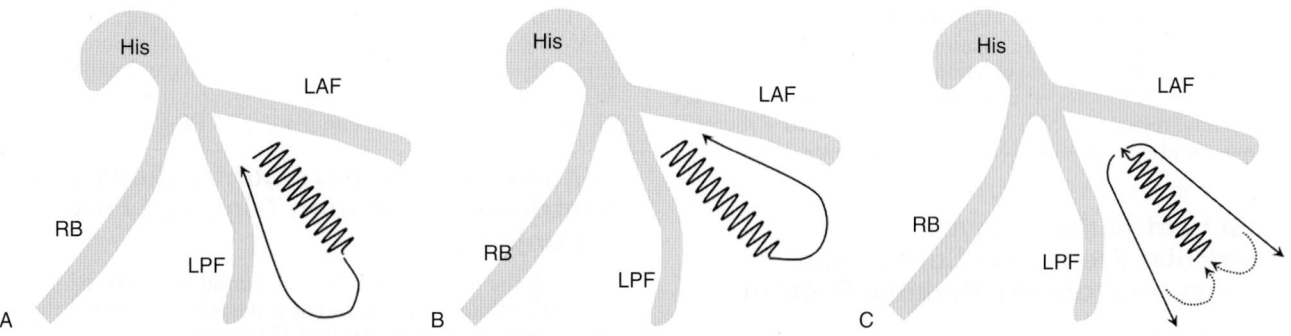

FIGURE 82.3 Schematic representation of macroreentrant circuits of three types of verapamil-sensitive fascicular ventricular tachycardia (VT). (A) In left posterior fascicle (*LPF*)-VT, activation propagates antegradely in the midseptum where abnormal Purkinje tissue distributes and conducts retrogradely near the LPF. In the past, LPF was considered as part of the circuit, but recent reports suggest the LPF is a bystander. (B) In left anterior fascicle (*LAF*)-VT, activation propagates antegradely in the midseptum and conducts retrogradely near the LAF. (C) In USVT, activation propagates antegradely in the LPF or LAF and then conducts retrogradely in the midseptum. *RB*, Right bundle.

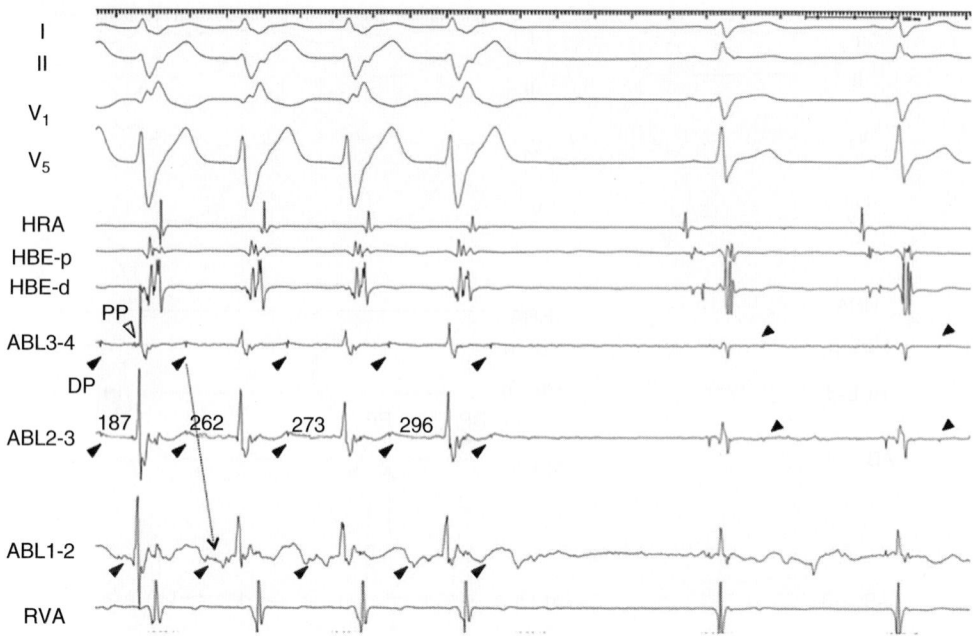

FIGURE 82.4 Intracardiac recordings in left posterior fascicular ventricular tachycardia (VT). Radiofrequency energy was applied at the site where a diastolic potential (*DP*) was identified. The DP-presystolic potential (*PP*) interval gradually prolonged, and then the VT was terminated at the timing of the DP-PP block. After VT termination, a delayed potential is seen after the QRS complex. *ABL*, Ablation; *HBE*, His bundle electrogram; *HRA*, high right atrium; *RVA*, right ventricular apex.

important. Although the DP can be widely recorded from the basal to apical LV septum, targeting the earliest DP is not necessary; rather, targeting potentials in the apical third of the septum is advisable, as the RF application to the proximal portion of the LV septum could result in LBBB or atrioventricular (AV) block. When RF is applied during the VT, the DP-PP interval gradually prolongs, and DP to PP block terminates the VT. Following successful ablation, the DP is recorded after the QRS complex during sinus rhythm (Fig. 82.4). If no DP is identified, the earliest PP at the VT exit is an alternative target.

Verapamil-sensitive fascicular VT can sometimes be noninducible or self-terminating during the EP study. Catheter contact during mapping can mechanically suppress the conduction over the VT circuit (so-called "bump" phenomenon).[25] On such occasions, activation mapping can still be performed if a ventricular echo beat with the same QRS morphology as the VT is observed. If no echo beat is inducible, anatomical linear ablation through the inferior mid-LV septum perpendicular to its long axis can be successful. Following the ablation, DPs could be observed after the QRS complex if the ablation line crosses the antegrade limb of the VT circuit. The ablation target for LAF VT is also the region of DPs recorded in the midseptum or PPs in the LV anterolateral region.[26] USVT can be eliminated by RF delivery to the upper midseptum where DPs appear during the VT.[13]

Focal Ventricular Tachycardia and Ventricular Premature Contraction Originating From the Purkinje System

Mechanism

Focal Purkinje VT arising from the LV demonstrates RBBB morphology with either left or right axis deviation on the 12-lead ECG. Lopera and colleagues reported that 2 (0.8%) of 234 SHD-associated VTs were focal Purkinje VT.[27] This type of VT is mainly seen in patients with SHD but can also be seen in patients with structurally normal hearts. Although its surface ECG configuration is very

similar to verapamil-sensitive VT, the mechanism is considered nonreentrant. Focal Purkinje VT can be induced with infusion of catecholaminergic agents, such as isoproterenol, but not usually with programmed ventricular stimulation. In addition, β-blockers, but not verapamil, are effective for terminating the VT. On the basis of these characteristics, the mechanism of focal Purkinje VT is considered to be automaticity or triggered activity.[28] As the distal Purkinje network is anatomically linked to PMs, PM has been recognized as a major source of VPCs that can be targeted for ablation.[21]

Therapy

Catheter ablation for this VT should target the earliest Purkinje activation during the tachycardia. Pace mapping at the successful ablation site shows the identical QRS morphology with the S-QRS interval identical to the Purkinje potential to the QRS onset during the VT.[28,29] When the target ablation site is located at a relatively proximal portion, there is a potential risk for LBBB or AV block.[27] For VPCs from the PM, real-time imaging with intracardiac echo is very useful.[30] The contact and stability of the catheter on the PM can be challenging, and sometimes multiple RF lesions are required to eliminate the VPCs.

Ventricular Premature Contractions and Ventricular Fibrillation Triggered From the Purkinje System

Although the majority of VPCs are considered to be benign and with little clinical impact, recent reports demonstrated that the VPCs originating from RV or LV fascicles can trigger VF (see Chapter 129).[31,32] VF triggered by the fascicular-origin VPC has been reported in ischemic cardiomyopathy, long QT syndrome,[33] early repolarization,[34] and catecholaminergic polymorphic VT.[35] Elimination of the VPC by ablation successfully prevents recurrent VF. Mapping and ablation strategies are similar to those of the focal Purkinje VT.

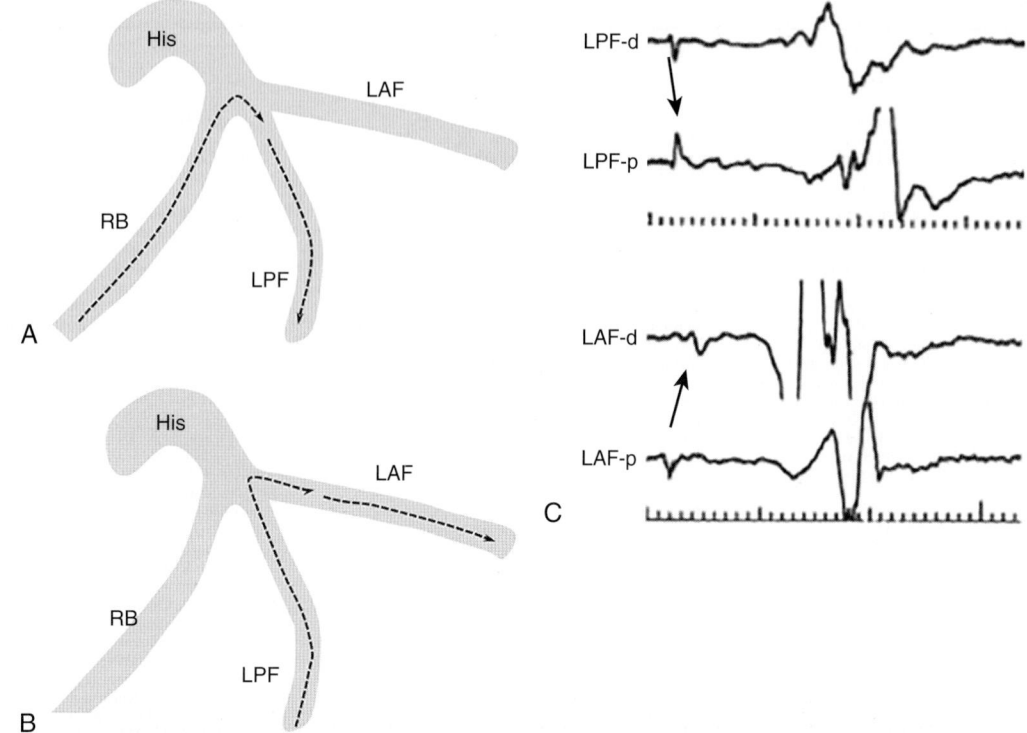

FIGURE 82.5 Schematic representation of the bundle branches and interfascicular ventricular tachycardia (VT). (A) Bundle branch reentrant VT includes the right and left bundle (*RB* and *LB*) in the circuit. In this schema, activation propagates the RB from distal to proximal and the LB from proximal to distal, but the VT propagating the opposite direction is also possible. (B) Interfascicular VT (IFVT) involves the left anterior and posterior fascicles (*LAF* and *LPF*) in the circuit. Both fascicles can be antegrade and retrograde limbs of the circuit. (C) Intracardiac recordings during IFVT. *Upper panel* shows recording from the catheter placed along LPF. Activation propagates from distal to proximal direction. *Lower panel* shows a recording from the catheter placed along the LAF. Activation propagates from proximal to distal direction. *RB*, Right bundle.

Bundle Branch Reentry and Interfascicular Reentry

BBRVT (see Chapter 83) is a macroreentrant tachycardia involving RBs and LBs as essential components of the circuit (Fig. 82.5A). Purkinje system conduction disturbances, usually associated with dilated cardiomyopathy,[36] valvular diseases,[37] ischemic cardiomyopathy, or myotonic dystrophy,[38] provide a substrate for BBRVT. However, BBRVT has also been reported in patients with isolated conduction system disease and no apparent structural heart abnormalities.[39]

The surface ECG during sinus rhythm characteristically shows intraventricular conduction delay: nonspecific or typical bundle branch block patterns with prolonged QRS duration. The surface ECG of BBRVT has an LBBB or RBBB configuration. The HV interval during sinus rhythm is usually prolonged. BBRVT is usually inducible by ventricular programmed stimulation. The diagnosis of BBRVT can be made by demonstrating that the His and RB or LB potentials precede the ventricular activation, and HH and RB-RB or LB-LB interval oscillations precede VV oscillations. An HV interval during the VT is usually longer than that during sinus rhythm but can be equal or shorter depending on the His recording site and upper turnaround point of BBRVT or the balance between antegrade and retrograde conduction times from the upper turnaround point.[40] RF ablation is regarded as the first-line therapy and usually targets the RB. Ablation of LB has been proposed in patients with underlying LBBB pattern to reduce the chance of complete AV block.

IFVT is less common compared with BBRVT but is also a macroreentrant tachycardia through the branches of the LV Purkinje system[41] (Fig. 82.5B). IFVT has a relatively narrow QRS complex with an RBBB pattern with superior or inferior axis deviation. EP study demonstrates that the LAF or the LPF precedes the ventricular activation, and analysis of oscillations shows that LAF-LAF or LPF-LPF intervals drive the VV intervals. As opposed to BBRVT, the His potential follows the LAF or LPF potential, and the HV interval during the VT is shorter than that during sinus rhythm. Ablation of the IFVT is guided by fascicular potentials and targets either the left anterior or posterior fascicle.

Conclusions

VTs arising from the fascicles or the Purkinje network include a wide spectrum of substrates and mechanisms. The ECG morphologies can mimic each other and sometimes be misleading despite different mechanisms. Careful consideration of the patient's underlying heart disease and understanding of the ECG and EP characteristics are required for differential diagnosis and appropriate therapy.

REFERENCES

1. Tada H, Ito S, Naito S, et al. Idiopathic ventricular arrhythmia arising from the mitral annulus: a distinct subgroup of idiopathic ventricular arrhythmias. *J Am Coll Cardiol*. 2005;45:877–886.

2. Lin D, Hsia HH, Gerstenfeld EP, et al. Idiopathic fascicular left ventricular tachycardia: linear ablation lesion strategy for noninducible or nonsustained tachycardia. *Heart Rhythm*. 2005;2:934–939.

3. Zipes DP, Foster PR, Troup PJ, et al. Atrial induction of ventricular tachycardia: reentry versus triggered automaticity. *Am J Cardiol*. 1979;44:1–8.

4. Belhassen B, Rotmensch HH, Laniado S. Response of recurrent sustained ventricular tachycardia to verapamil. *Br Heart J*. 1981;46:679–682.

5. Ohe T, Shimomura K, Aihara N, et al. Idiopathic sustained left ventricular tachycardia: clinical and electrophysiologic characteristics. *Circulation*. 1988;77:560–568.

6. Shimoike E, Ueda N, Maruyama T, et al. Radiofrequency catheter ablation of upper septal idiopathic left ventricular tachycardia exhibiting left bundle branch block morphology. *J Cardiovasc Electrophysiol*. 2000;11:203–207.

7. Nakagawa H, Beckman KJ, McClelland JH, et al. Radiofrequency catheter ablation of idiopathic left ventricular tachycardia guided by a Purkinje potential. *Circulation*. 1993;88:2607–2617.

8. Tsuchiya T, Okumura K, Honda T, et al. Significance of late diastolic potential preceding Purkinje potential in verapamil-sensitive idiopathic left ventricular tachycardia. *Circulation*. 1999;99:2408–2413.

9. Nogami A, Naito S, Tada H, et al. Demonstration of diastolic and presystolic Purkinje potentials as critical potentials in a macroreentry circuit of verapamil-sensitive idiopathic left ventricular tachycardia. *J Am Coll Cardiol*. 2000;36:811–823.

10. Morishima I, Nogami A, Tsuboi H, et al. Negative participation of the left posterior fascicle in the reentry circuit of verapamil-sensitive idiopathic left ventricular tachycardia. *J Cardiovasc Electrophysiol*. 2012;23:556–559.

11. Maeda S, Yokoyama Y, Nogami A, et al. First case of left posterior fascicle in a bystander circuit of idiopathic left ventricular tachycardia. *Can J Cardiol*. 2014;30:1460. e11–e13.

12. Kottkamp H, Chen X, Hindricks G, et al. Idiopathic left ventricular tachycardia: new insights into electrophysiological characteristics and radiofrequency catheter ablation. *Pacing Clin Electrophysiol*. 1995;18:1285–1297.

13. Talib AK, Nogami A, Nishiuchi S, et al. Verapamil-sensitive upper septal idiopathic left ventricular tachycardia: prevalence, mechanism, and electrophysiological characteristics. *JACCC: Clin Electrophysiol*. 2015;1:369–380.

14. Friedman PL, Stewart JR, Wit AL. Spontaneous and induced cardiac arrhythmias in subendocardial Purkinje fibers surviving extensive myocardial infarction in dogs. *Circ Res*. 1973;33:612–626.

15. Sugi K, Karagueuzian HS, Fishbein MC, et al. Spontaneous ventricular tachycardia associated with isolated right ventricular infarction, one day after right coronary artery occlusion in the dog: studies on the site of origin and mechanism. *Am Heart J*. 1985;109:232–244.

16. Hayashi M, Kobayashi Y, Iwasaki YK, et al. Novel mechanism of postinfarction ventricular tachycardia originating in surviving left posterior Purkinje fibers. *Heart Rhythm*. 2006;3:908–918.

17. Morishima I, Nogami A, Tsuboi H, Sone T. Verapamil-sensitive left anterior fascicular ventricular tachycardia associated with a healed myocardial infarction: changes in the delayed Purkinje potential during sinus rhythm. *J Interv Card Electrophysiol*. 2008;22:233–237.

18. Thakur RK, Klein GJ, Sivaram CA, et al. Anatomic substrate for idiopathic left ventricular tachycardia. *Circulation*. 1996;93:497–501.

19. Maruyama M, Tadera T, Miyamoto S, et al. Demonstration of the reentrant circuit of verapamil-sensitive idiopathic left ventricular tachycardia: direct evidence for macroreentry as the underlying mechanism. *J Cardiovasc Electrophysiol*. 2001;12:968–972.

20. Lin FC, Wen MS, Wang CC, et al. Left ventricular fibromuscular band is not a specific substrate for idiopathic left ventricular tachycardia. *Circulation*. 1996;93:525–528.

21. Kawamura M, Hsu JC, Vedantham V, et al. Clinical and electrocardiographic characteristics of idiopathic ventricular arrhythmias with right bundle branch block and superior axis: comparison of apical crux area and posterior septal left ventricle. *Heart Rhythm*. 2015;12:1137–1144.

22. Doppalapudi H, Yamada T, McElderry HT, et al. Ventricular tachycardia originating from the posterior papillary muscle in the left ventricle: a distinct clinical syndrome. *Circ Arrhythm Electrophysiol*. 2008;1:23–29.

23. Doppalapudi H, Yamada T, Ramaswamy K, et al. Idiopathic focal epicardial ventricular tachycardia originating from the crux of the heart. *Heart Rhythm*. 2009;6:44–50.

24. Nogami A. Purkinje-related arrhythmias part ii: polymorphic ventricular tachycardia and ventricular fibrillation. *Pacing Clin Electrophysiol*. 2011;34:1034–1049.

25. Blomstrom-Lundqvist C, Blomstrom P, Beckman-Suurkula M. Incessant ventricular tachycardia with a right bundle-branch block pattern and left axis deviation abolished by catheter manipulation. *Pacing Clin Electrophysiol*. 1990;13:11–16.

26. Nogami A, Naito S, Tada H, et al. Verapamil-sensitive left anterior fascicular ventricular tachycardia: results of radiofrequency ablation in six patients. *J Cardiovasc Electrophysiol*. 1998;9:1269–1278.

27. Lopera G, Stevenson WG, Soejima K, et al. Identification and ablation of three types of ventricular tachycardia involving the His-Purkinje system in patients with heart disease. *J Cardiovasc Electrophysiol*. 2004;15:52–58.

28. Rodriguez LM, Smeets JL, Timmermans C, et al. Radiofrequency catheter ablation of idiopathic ventricular tachycardia originating in the anterior fascicle of the left bundle branch. *J Cardiovasc Electrophysiol*. 1996;7:1211–1216.

29. Nogami A. Purkinje-related arrhythmias part I: monomorphic ventricular tachycardias. *Pacing Clin Electrophysiol*. 2011;34:624–650.

30. Crawford T, Mueller G, Good E, et al. Ventricular arrhythmias originating from papillary muscles in the right ventricle. *Heart Rhythm*. 2010;7:725–730.

31. Haissaguerre M, Shoda M, Jais P, et al. Mapping and ablation of idiopathic ventricular fibrillation. *Circulation*. 2002;106:962–967.

32. Knecht S, Sacher F, Wright M, et al. Long-term follow-up of idiopathic ventricular fibrillation ablation: a multicenter study. *J Am Coll Cardiol*. 2009;54:522–528.

33. Haissaguerre M, Extramiana F, Hocini M, et al. Mapping and ablation of ventricular fibrillation associated with long-QT and Brugada syndromes. *Circulation*. 2003;108:925–928.

34. Haissaguerre M, Derval N, Sacher F, et al. Sudden cardiac arrest associated with early repolarization. *N Engl J Med*. 2008;358:2016–2023.

35. Kaneshiro T, Naruse Y, Nogami A, et al. Successful catheter ablation of bidirectional ventricular premature contractions triggering ventricular fibrillation in catecholaminergic polymorphic ventricular tachycardia with RyR2 mutation. *Circ Arrhythm Electrophysiol*. 2012;5:e14–e17.

36. Cohen TJ, Chien WW, Lurie KG, et al. Radiofrequency catheter ablation for treatment of bundle branch reentrant ventricular tachycardia: results and long-term follow-up. *J Am Coll Cardiol*. 1991;18:1767–1773.

37. Narasimhan C, Jazayeri MR, Sra J, et al. Ventricular tachycardia in valvular heart disease: facilitation of sustained bundle-branch reentry by valve surgery. *Circulation*. 1997;96:4307–4313.

38. Merino JL, Carmona JR, Fernandez-Lozano I, et al. Mechanisms of sustained ventricular tachycardia in myotonic dystrophy: implications for catheter ablation. *Circulation*. 1998;98:541–546.

39. Blanck Z, Jazayeri M, Dhala A, et al. Bundle branch reentry: a mechanism of ventricular tachycardia in the absence of myocardial or valvular dysfunction. *J Am Coll Cardiol*. 1993;22:1718–1722.

40. Tchou P, Jazayeri M, Denker S, et al. Transcatheter electrical ablation of right bundle branch. A method of treating macroreentrant ventricular tachycardia attributed to bundle branch reentry. *Circulation*. 1988;78:246–257.

41. Crijns HJ, Smeets JL, Rodriguez LM, et al. Cure of interfascicular reentrant ventricular tachycardia by ablation of the anterior fascicle of the left bundle branch. *J Cardiovasc Electrophysiol*. 1995;6:486–492.

83 Bundle Branch Reentry Tachycardia

Akihiko Nogami and Brian Olshansky

Bundle branch reentrant ventricular tachycardia (BBRVT), first elucidated by Guerot and colleagues in 1974, is a unique, fast (200–300 beats/min), monomorphic tachycardia associated with hemodynamic collapse, syncope, and/or cardiac arrest.[1] It has also been described as a mechanism for nonsustained VT and coupled ventricular ectopy.[2] It is caused by a macroreentrant circuit involving the right and left bundle branches (RBBs and LBBs), an upper common pathway, and septal ventricular muscle.[1–5] BBR occurs in patients who have dilated cardiomyopathy[3] and in those with coronary artery disease,[3] valvular heart disease,[3,6,7] muscular dystrophy,[8–10] congenital heart disease,[11] left ventricular noncompaction,[12] arrhythmogenic right ventricular cardiomyopathy,[13] Brugada syndrome,[14] or even no heart disease with associated His-Purkinje system disease.[15–17] The incidence was reported to be 3.5% and 6% of VTs in separate series and 20% in a series of patients with nonischemic cardiomyopathy alone undergoing evaluation for ablation.[18–20] Likely, BBR is underrecognized as a clinical problem.

Surface Electrogram and Classification

The morphology of the tachycardia can have a typical LBB block (LBBB)[21] pattern (Fig. 83.1A) or RBB block (RBBB) pattern (Fig. 83.1B). Some patients have both counterclockwise and clockwise BBR, causing an LBBB and RBBB morphology, respectively.[22] It is possible for LBBB morphology BBR to have several morphologies presumably as the result of extensive RBB disease in patients with dilated hearts.[21] Multiple monomorphic morphologies can occur, as anterograde conduction via the left anterior fascicle (LAF) or left posterior fascicle (LPF) can be present along with retrograde activation of the RBB.[23] BBRVT with multiple morphologies has also been described in Ebstein anomaly.[11] A narrow QRS complex BBR has been postulated to occur via bystander longitudinal dissociation of the His-RBB system.[24]

Tchou and colleagues described three categories of BBRVT (Table 83.1; Fig. 83.2).[25] Types A and C are the classic counterclockwise and clockwise BBRVT circuits, respectively. Type B is reentry within the LBB fascicles (interfascicular reentry). BBR can present with a similar or identical QRS complex morphology to that present in normal sinus rhythm. Although the QRS complex morphology in VT can be identical to that in sinus rhythm in all 12 electrocardiographic (ECG) leads,[26] not all such VTs are BBR.[27] An RBBB and left hemiblock pattern is more consistent with interfascicular tachycardia (Fig. 83.1C).

Pathophysiology

Attempts have been made to model the His-Purkinje system and to define the reentrant circuit(s) responsible for BBR.[28] Under normal conditions, sustained reentry cannot occur, but under conditions of slowed conduction in the His-Purkinje system and ventricular muscle, the path length can be increased such that sustained anatomical reentry does occur using these structures and with an excitable gap (Fig. 83.3).

Patients with BBR generally have a prolonged PR interval, QRS duration, and HV interval. For BBR to occur, there must be a delay or a complete anterograde block in at least one bundle branch. An LBBB, most commonly, or an RBBB, present on the surface 12-lead ECG, is more indicative of conduction slowing than of complete block in LBB or the RBB, respectively. If complete anterograde block is present in one bundle branch, there must be conduction (likely slow) retrograde in that bundle branch for BBRVT to occur.

During type A BBRVT, activation proceeds anterograde via the RBB and then through the septum. Following this, retrograde conduction via the LBB activates the septal summit/His bundle and sequentially reactivates the RBB ("counterclockwise" reentry). The ECG morphology of counterclockwise BBR (type A) is a typical LBBB with an R-wave transition between leads V_4 and V_5. Type A BBRVT with an LBBB morphology is the cause of 98% of BBRVT episodes.[29] The LBB may be the preferred retrograde route of activation.[30]

Alternatively, activation can anterogradely proceed via the LBB and then through the septum. Retrograde activation can proceed via the RBB, creating an RBBB morphology ("clockwise" reentry, type C).[18,30] Anterograde activation via the RBB and retrograde via the LPF or the LAF alone is another possibility. Fig. 83.4 demonstrates the spontaneous change from interfascicular reentrant VT (type B BBRVT) to type A BBRVT. Anterograde activation during interfascicular reentrant VT is via the LPF and during type A BBRVT is via the RBB; retrograde activation during both tachycardias is via the LAF.

Conduction delay, which is critical for initiation and perpetuation of BBR, may be present in connections between the bundles and even within the His bundle itself. Anisotropic conduction in the common His bundle, potentially critical for initiation and maintenance of BBR,[31] may explain the greater degree of HV delay often noted during tachycardia than in sinus rhythm. Other mechanisms potentially explaining the observed HV prolongation during tachycardia could be because of the progressive distal Purkinje system conduction delay in diseased bundles, whose slowing is more apparent at rapid rates (phase 3 block).

Although rate-related conduction delay between the His bundle and the RBB and/or the LBB during tachycardia may explain a greater HV delay than that present during sinus rhythm, it is not clear that the common His bundle is required for BBR propagation. Although the upper common pathway responsible for reentry between the right and left bundles is not understood completely, the His bundle or another septal connection is necessary for reentry to occur. BBR has not been described in patients with infra-Hisian block. Nevertheless, a shorter HV interval during VT indicates that tachycardia is not consistent with BBR (Fig. 83.5).

BBR can occur in patients who have apparently normal His-Purkinje conduction during sinus rhythm but who have evidence of functional conduction impairment at faster rates.[32] Li and colleagues reported a series of 178 patients with VT, of whom 13 had BBRVT.[32] Of those 13, 6 had an HV interval ≤55 ms during sinus rhythm (i.e., normal). In those BBRVT patients with a normal HV interval at baseline, the HV interval was prolonged during BBRVT (73 ± 18 vs. 47 ± 7 ms; $p = .007$). Functional His-Purkinje delay was present with rapid atrial pacing or premature extrastimuli in patients of this group but not in those with prolonged HV intervals in sinus rhythm who had BBRVT. The explanation for BBRVT in these patients may be the higher turnaround point in the BBR circuit in the proximal portion of the His bundle or in the NH region of the atrioventricular (AV) node. Additionally, functional block initiating BBR may be perpetuated by persistent "linking."[33] A successive impulse entering a BBR circuit preferentially propagates along one limb because of functional block in the contralateral limb, resulting from the effects of the prior impulse.

Even in otherwise normal individuals, occasional spontaneous BBR beats are common. This is seen as a normal response to premature ventricular extrastimuli in patients undergoing programmed electrical stimulation who do not have BBRVT or even known His-Purkinje disease (Fig. 83.6). This finding is known as

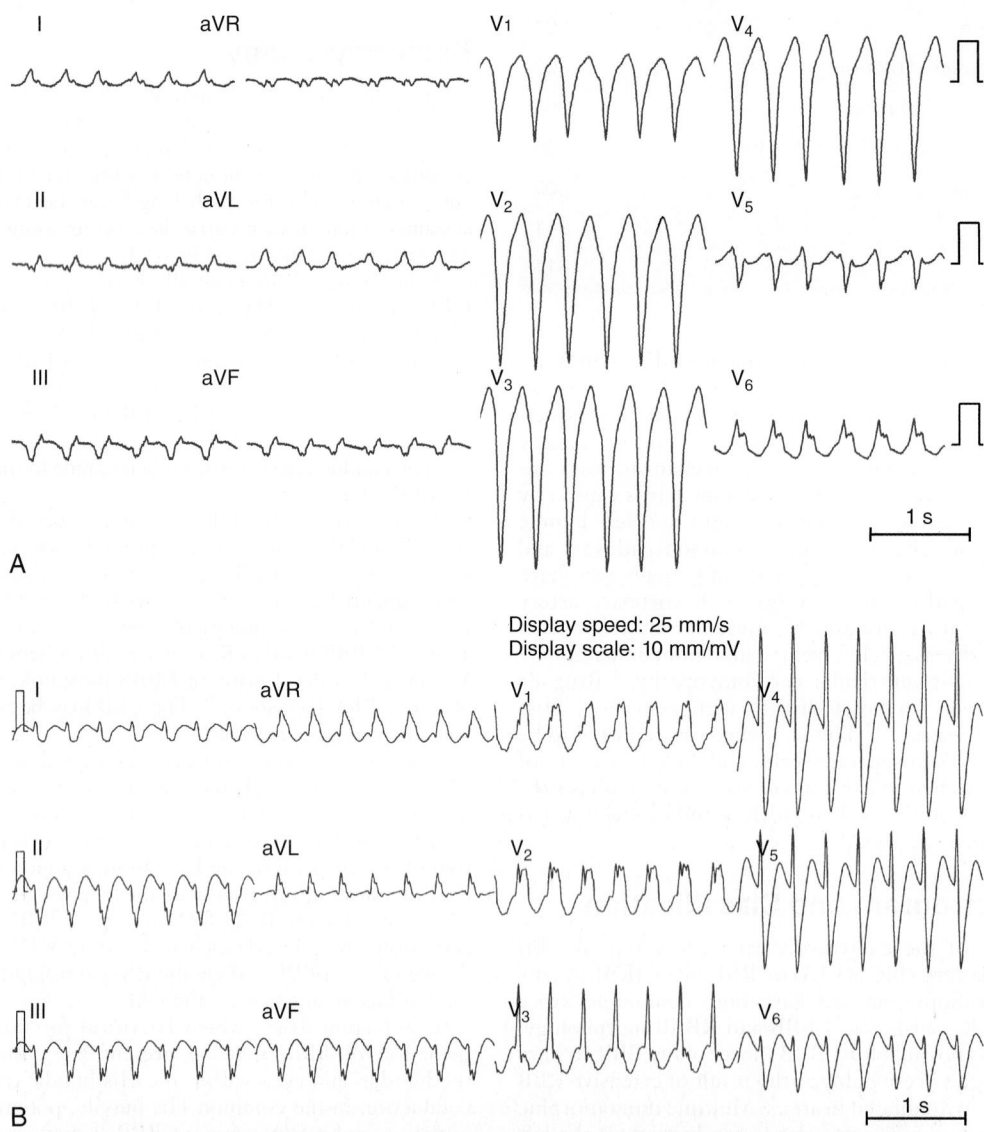

FIGURE 83.1 Twelve-lead electrocardiograms (ECGs) during bundle branch reentry tachycardias. (A) ECG of bundle branch reentry with left bundle branch block morphology (type A). (B) ECG of bundle branch reentry with right bundle branch block morphology and left-axis deviation (type C). (C) ECG of an interfascicular reentry with right bundle branch block morphology and right-axis deviation (type B). (D) ECG during sinus rhythm of the patient with interfascicular reentry in (C), showing PR prolongation, right bundle branch block, and right-axis deviation. Note that QRS morphology in tachycardia is identical to that in sinus rhythm.

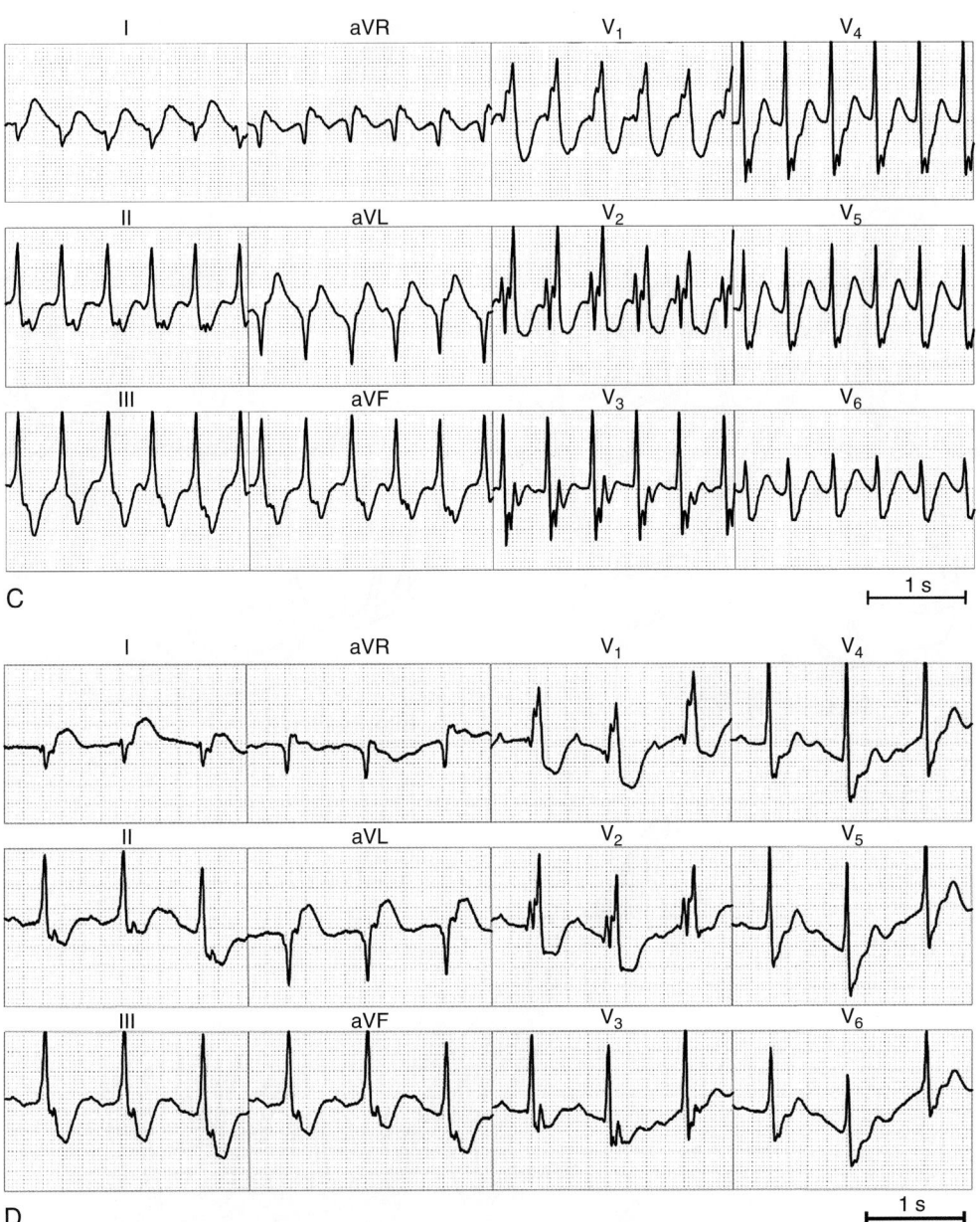

FIGURE 83.1, cont'd For legend, see opposite page.

TABLE 83.1	Types of bundle branch reentry tachycardia		
	TYPE A	**TYPE B (INTERFASCICULAR TACHYCARDIA)**	**TYPE C**
ECG morphology	LBBB pattern	RBBB pattern	RBBB pattern
Anterograde limb	RBB	LAF or LPF	LBB
Retrograde limb	LBB	Contra-left fascicle	RBB

ECG, Electrocardiogram; *LAF,* left anterior fascicle; *LBB,* left bundle branch; *LBBB,* left bundle branch block; *LPF,* left posterior fascicle; *RBB,* right bundle branch; *RBBB,* right bundle branch block.

V_3 phenomenon.[2,34] The premature stimulus (S2) produces an impulse that blocks retrogradely in the RBB system but propagates through the septum to the LV, where it conducts retrogradely via the LBB system, causing a prolongation of the S-H2 interval that is followed by V_3 from anterograde conduction down the RBB.

During interfascicular tachycardia, the morphology is an RBBB with right- or left-axis deviation (see Figs. 83.1C and 83.4). Right BBR has been reported.[35]

Initiation of Tachycardia

BBRVT has several modes of spontaneous initiation. Ventricular premature beats are often the trigger. Occasionally, premature atrial beats or atrial fibrillation[36] can initiate BBR. Bradycardia-dependent LBBB initiation of BBR, without obvious intramyocardial conduction delay, is possible spontaneously during sinus bradycardia.[37] BBR has also been described in a patient with cycles of AV block and in association with bradycardia-dependent phase 4 bundle branch block.[38] BBRVT storm has been related to ventricular pacing that causes retrograde activation through the His-Purkinje system.[39]

In the electrophysiology laboratory, ventricular extrastimuli delivered with short–long–short coupling intervals (pacing

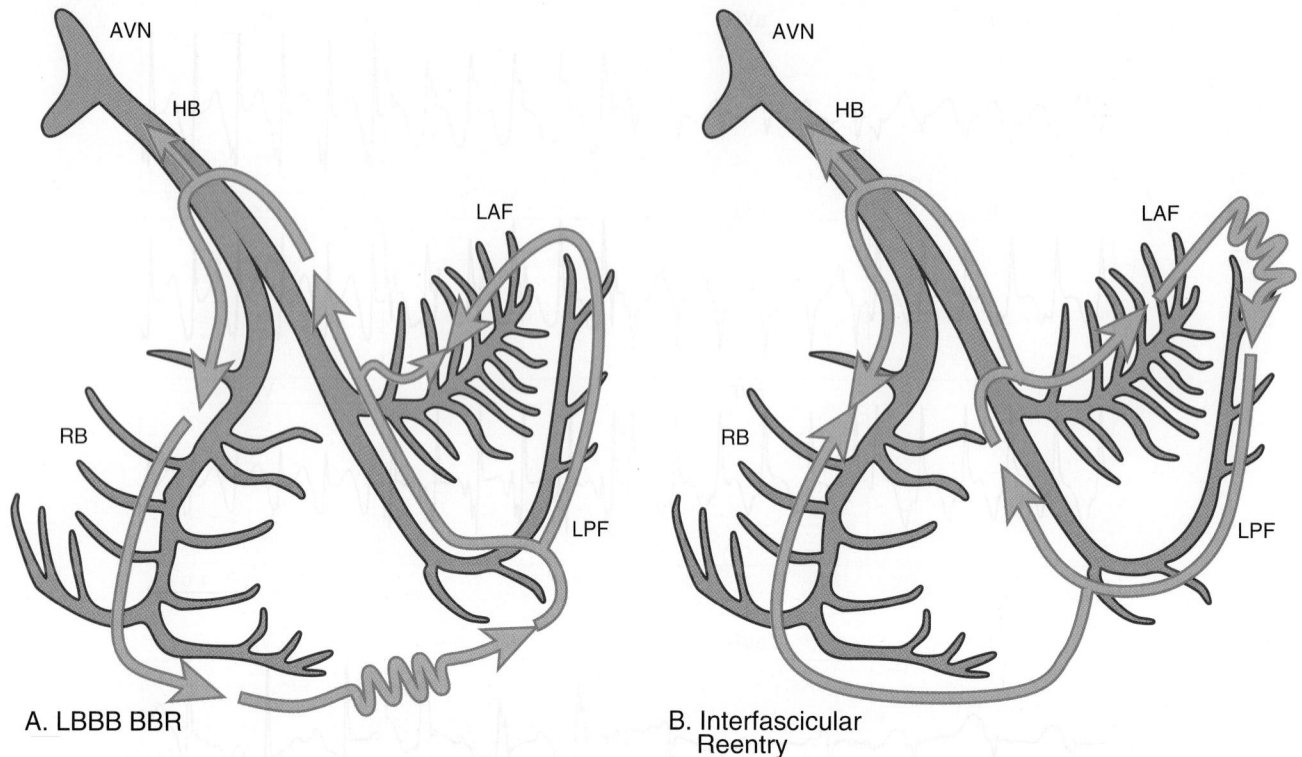

A. LBBB BBR

B. Interfascicular Reentry

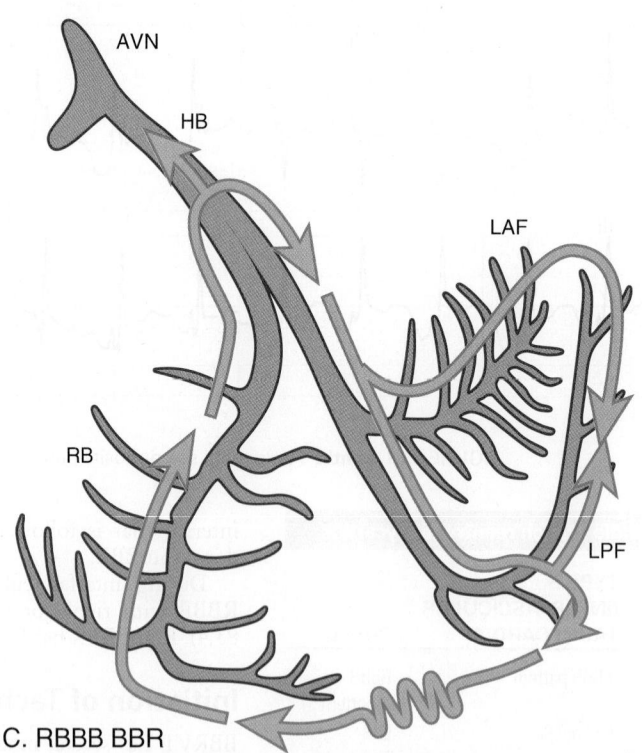

C. RBBB BBR

FIGURE 83.2 Schematic illustrations of reentrant circuits for bundle branch reentry (BBR) and interfascicular reentry. (A) A typical type of BBR in which retrograde conduction occurs via the left bundle branch (LBB) and anterograde conduction over the right bundle branch (RBB). (B) Interfascicular reentry with anterograde and retrograde conduction over opposing fascicles of the LBB. (C) Reversal of the circuit depicted in (A). *AVN,* Atrioventricular node; *HB,* His bundle; *LAF,* left anterior fascicle; *LBBB,* left bundle branch block; *LPF,* left posterior fascicle; *RB,* right bundle; *RBBB,* right bundle branch block. (Modified from Nogami A. Purkinje-related arrhythmias. Part I: monomorphic ventricular tachycardias. *Pacing Clin Electrophysiol.* 2011;34:624-650.)

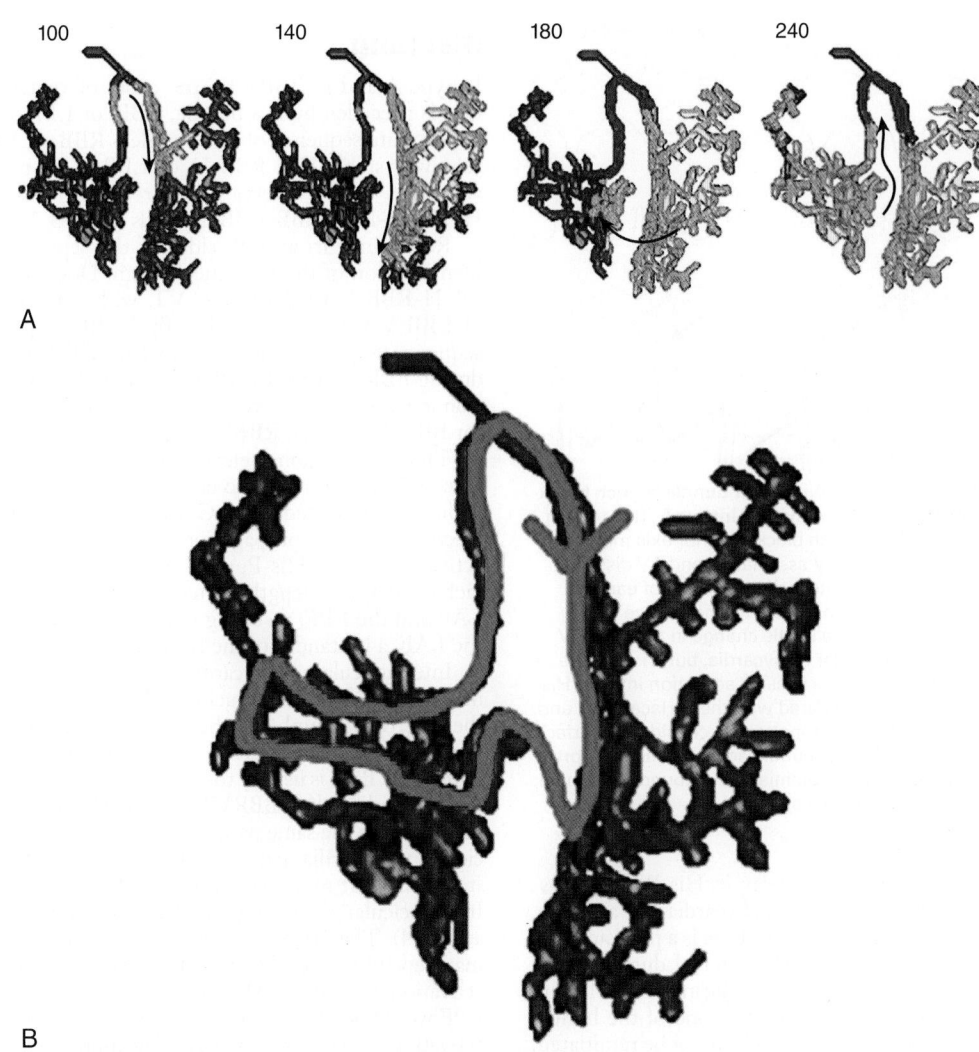

A

B

FIGURE 83.3 Successful attempt to stimulate bundle branch reentry in a model of ventricular conduction system. Activation sequence in the Purkinje system under simulated temporal conduction block in the right Purkinje branch. (A) *Arrows* indicate the direction of wave propagation. Excitation goes from the left bundle branch to the septum, up the right bundle branch, toward the left bundle branch, where it runs into the previous excitation wave. (B) To attain sustained bundle branch reentrant ventricular tachycardia, the effective path length of the reentrant circuit needs to be increased (or the conduction must be slowed sufficiently). (Modified from Tusscher KH, Panfilov AV. Modeling of the ventricular conduction system. *Prog Biophys Mol Biol.* 2008;96:152-170.)

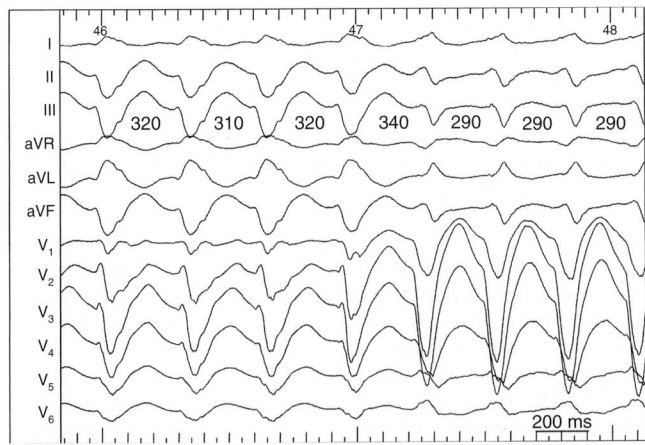

FIGURE 83.4 Change from interfascicular ventricular tachycardia (type B) to bundle branch reentry (type A). Anterograde activation during the interfascicular reentrant ventricular tachycardia (first four beats) was via the left posterior fascicle and that during type A bundle branch reentrant ventricular tachycardia (last four beats) was via the right bundle branch. Retrograde activation during both tachycardias was via the left anterior fascicle.

train of 400 ms with a delay of 600 or 800 ms before the short-coupled premature coupling intervals are introduced) tend to cause unidirectional block or sufficient conduction delay in a bundle branch to initiate BBR. Long–short coupling intervals are specific for initiation of BBR.[40]

Atrial pacing and/or isoproterenol may be required.[41] In one report, incremental atrial pacing during isoproterenol infusion initiated BBR with an RBBB pattern in four of six patients with inducible BBRVT.[42] Class IA or IC antiarrhythmic drugs may sufficiently slow conduction in one of the bundles to allow BBR to occur (and thus may be proarrhythmic for this condition[43]). Rarely are such drugs used to initiate BBR in the clinical context.

Initiation of interfascicular reentry occurs when an atrial or ventricular premature depolarization conducts over the healthy fascicle, giving rise to a QRS identical to that in sinus rhythm, and then reenters the blocked fascicle in the retrograde direction to induce and sustain reentrant VT.

Diagnosis

Several criteria help in the diagnosis of BBRVT (Box 83.1). The 12-lead ECG morphology during tachycardia is a typical LBBB

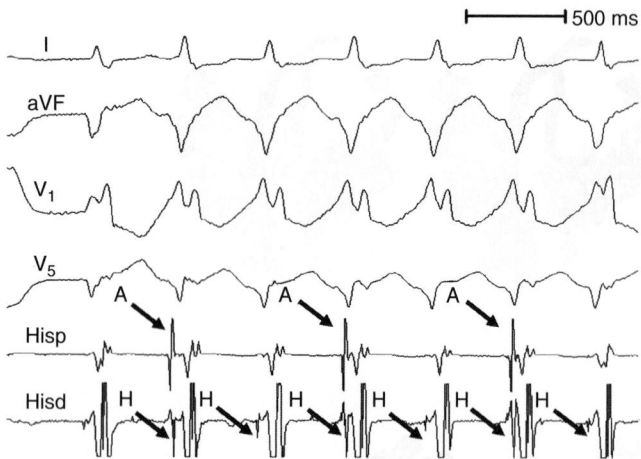

⊢————⊣500 ms

FIGURE 83.5 Wide QRS tachycardia with right bundle branch block configuration, superior axis, and negative HV interval. This tracing shows a wide QRS, right bundle branch block superior axis morphology ventricular tachycardia with 1:1 HV association and AV dissociation (atrial activation labeled "*A*"). Note the His to onset of earliest ventricular activation is negative (compared with the surface electrocardiogram [ECG] leads). There is a subtle change in the local HV relationship consistent with ventricular tachycardia, but it is *not* due to bundle branch reentry. Instead, there is passive activation into the His-Purkinje system. The HV interval compared with the surface lead I and V₅ may appear to be positive, but it is important to consider all surface ECG recordings to determine if the His bundle activation actually precedes ventricular activation. *A*, Atrial potential; *H*, His bundle potential; *Hisd*, His bundle distal; *Hisp*, His bundle proximal.

or RBBB morphology, and a critical delay in His-Purkinje system conduction is needed to initiate tachycardia. In addition, although AV dissociation may be present, there is a persistent 1:1 His bundle/QRS activation with the HV interval during tachycardia that is equal to or longer than that during sinus rhythm (and no HV dissociation),[31] If conduction in one of the bundle branches is disrupted, tachycardia stops and cannot be reinitiated. In some instances, a temporary disruption of conduction via one bundle may occur purposefully or unintentionally with a catheter bump.[44] Furthermore, during BBR, the His bundle, RBB, and LBB activation sequences during an LBBB morphology tachycardia or those during an RBBB morphology tachycardia remain stable. If rate fluctuations exist, a predictable change in the VV interval occurs after the HH interval. The HH interval timing changes before the VV interval timing. The HV timing remains constant. If no perturbation in the HH interval is present, atrial pacing may advance atrial followed by ventricular activation with a similar QRS complex morphology and similar HV interval. Moreover, entrainment with constant fusion (manifest entrainment) is present during pacing from the right ventricular apex.[45] However, pacing from the right ventricular apex during BBRVT results in a postpacing interval that is similar to the tachycardia cycle length and is never longer than 30 ms.[46] These findings serve as evidence of macroreentry within the His-Purkinje system.[47] During resetting, when pacing from the right ventricular apex, an increasing reset response is noted (i.e., return cycle length is progressively longer), whereas recordings with respect to the HV interval show a flat response consistent with a reentrant circuit that has an excitable gap and involves the bundle branches but not the ventricular muscles.[48] Finally, entrainment with concealed fusion is present during atrial pacing if AV nodal conduction allows faster pacing than that seen with tachycardia.

Interfascicular reentry similarly demonstrates variations in the VV interval preceded by changes in the HH interval. In contrast to BBRVT, the HV interval in the interfascicular reentry is shorter than that in sinus rhythm (see Box 83.1).

Mapping

In type A and C BBRVTs, the onset of ventricular depolarization is preceded by His bundle, RBB, or LBB potentials with an appropriate sequence of His bundle > RBB > LBB activation and relatively stable HV, RBB-V, or LBB-V intervals. Spontaneous variations in VV intervals are preceded by similar changes in HH/RBB-RBB/LBB-LBB intervals (Fig. 83.7).

Recordings from both sides of the septum may help in the identification of the BBR mechanism. Documentation of a typical H-RBB-V-LBB (during VT with LBBB morphology) or H-LBB-V-RBB (during VT with RBBB morphology) activation sequence would further support a BBRVT diagnosis. In addition, during BBRVT with LBBB morphology, right ventricular excitation must precede left ventricular excitation. The opposite is true for BBRVT with an RBBB morphology.[25]

Three-dimensional electroanatomical mapping is also valuable in demonstrating the entire reentrant circuit. Machino and colleagues reported type C BBRVT using three-dimensional electroanatomical propagation mapping (Fig. 83.8).[49] Sequential activation of the His-Purkinje system accounted for the entire tachycardia cycle length. Anterograde activation occurred via the LAF and the LPF, resulting in collision at the middle portion of the LAF, a bystander of the reentrant circuit.

Interfascicular tachycardia has been reported less commonly.[3,39,41,50–52] In this tachycardia, one of the fascicles serves as the anterograde limb and the other as the retrograde circuit. The distal link between fascicles occurs through ventricular myocardium. The LAF is usually the anterograde limb, and the LPF is the retrograde limb.[16,52] BBRVT and interfascicular tachycardia may be present in the same patient (see Fig. 83.4),[2,39,53] or the interfascicular tachycardia may be inducible after ablation of the RBB to stop BBR.[52] It may even become incessant after RBB ablation.[54] Interfascicular VT usually has RBBB morphology (see Figs. 83.2C and 83.4). The orientation of the frontal plain axis is variable and may depend on the direction of the reentrant circuit. Anterograde activation over the LAF and retrograde activation through the LPF would be associated with right axis deviation and the reverse activation sequence with left axis deviation. In contrast to BBR, the HV interval during interfascicular tachycardia is usually shorter by more than 40 ms than that recorded in sinus rhythm.[55] This occurs because the upper turnaround point of the circuit (the left bundle branching point) is relatively far from the His bundle activated in the retrograde direction. During interfascicular tachycardia, the LBB potential is inscribed before the His potential.[55]

Differential Diagnosis

It is important to recognize BBRVT and interfascicular tachycardia because they can be cured with catheter ablation. The differential diagnosis for BBR includes (1) VT because of a myocardial reentry, (2) idiopathic left intrafascicular VT, (3) supraventricular mechanism with aberrant conduction in the presence of a 1:1 ventriculoatrial relationship, and (4) atriofascicular reentry.

VT as a result of myocardial reentry needs to be excluded in every case because most patients with BBR also have the clinical substrate for developing myocardial VT. VT originating from the myocardium with passive conduction into the His-Purkinje system can have a 12-lead QRS complex morphology similar to a supraventricular conducted rhythm.[27] With myocardial reentry, however, the His potential usually does not precede the QRS complex, and variations in the HH interval follow changes in the VV interval as there is retrograde passive activation of the His-Purkinje system. The postpacing interval after entrainment of tachycardia from the right ventricular apex may differentiate BBR from myocardial VT.[3,46] The difference between the postpacing interval and the tachycardia cycle length with BBR is short (<30 ms) because the RBB inserts into the ventricular apex. For

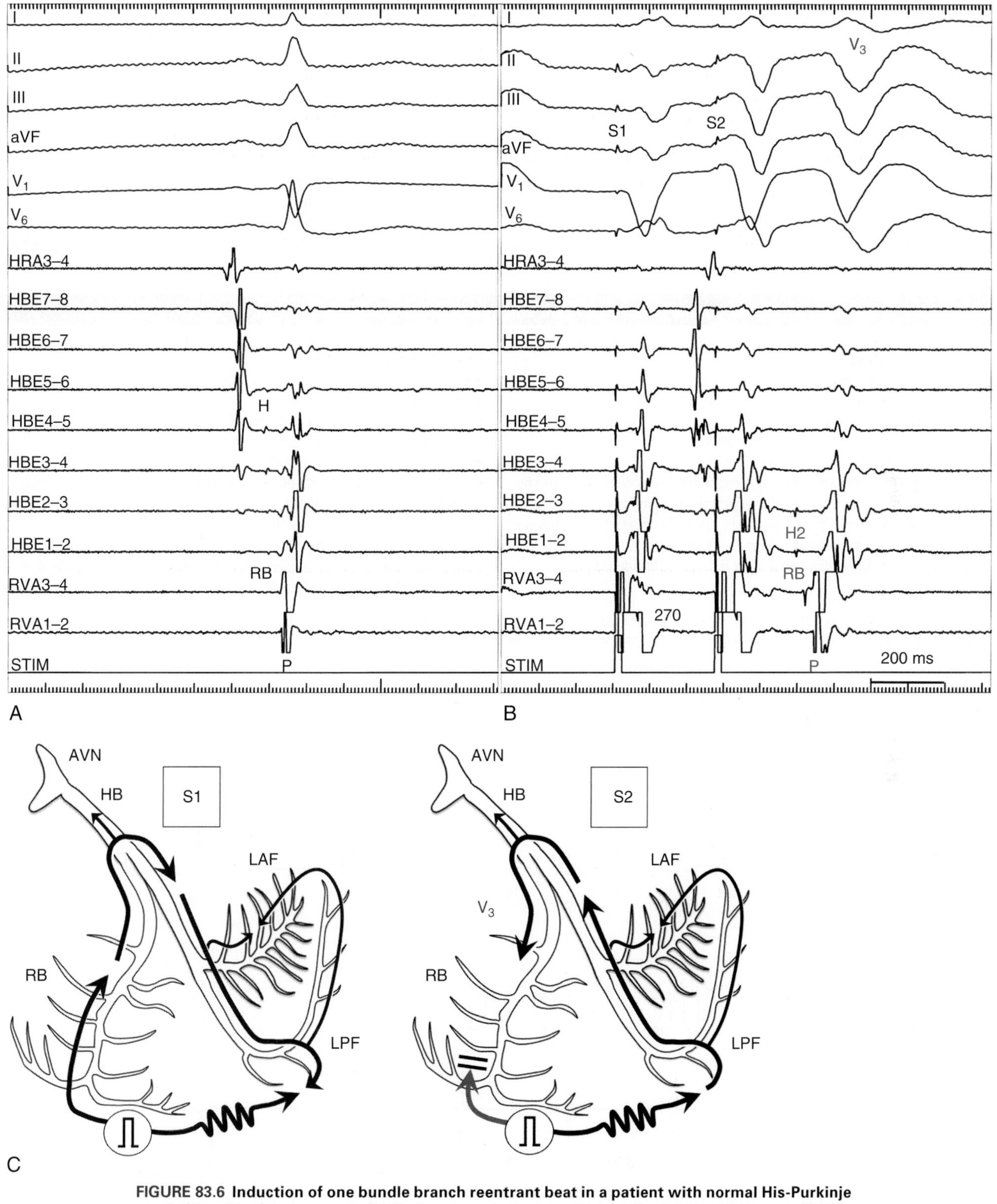

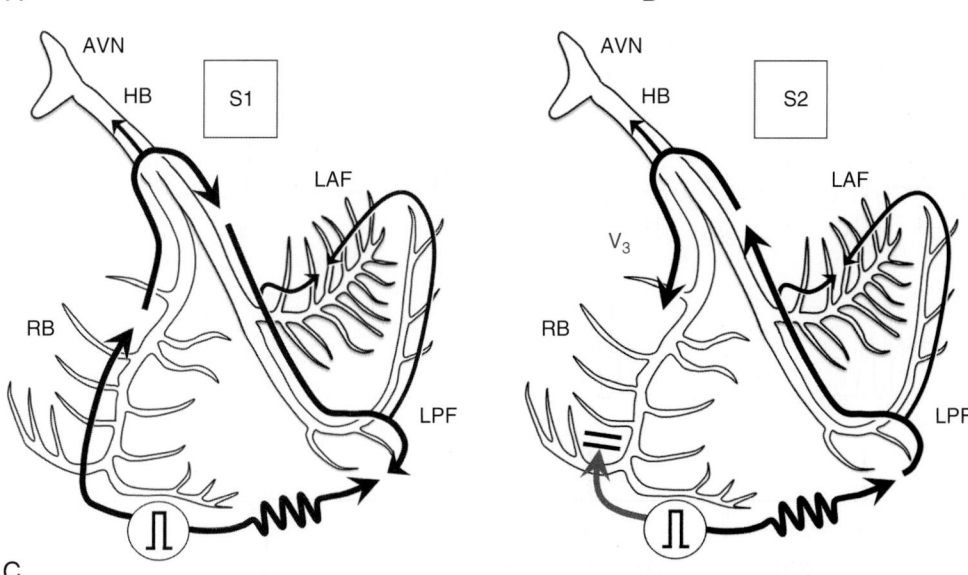

FIGURE 83.6 Induction of one bundle branch reentrant beat in a patient with normal His-Purkinje conduction (V₃ phenomenon). (A) During sinus rhythm, the His bundle, right bundle branch (RBB), and fused Purkinje potentials were recorded. There was no infra-Hisian conduction disturbance. (B) Programmed ventricular stimulation repeatedly induced repetitive ventricular responses with the left bundle branch (LBB) block configuration and superior axis. Before the ventricular response, His bundle, RBB, and Purkinje potentials were recorded. This finding is called a V₃ phenomenon. (C) Schema of V₃ phenomenon. The S2 premature impulse initially blocked in the RBB system and conducted retrogradely via the LBB system as manifested by sudden prolongation of S2H2 interval and the appearance of V₃. *AVN,* Atrioventricular node; *HB,* His bundle; *HBE,* His bundle electrogram; *HRA,* high right atrium; *LAF,* left anterior fascicle; *LPF,* left posterior fascicle; *RB,* right bundle; *RVA,* right ventricular apex; *STIM,* stimulus artifact.

myocardial VT (unless originating in the apex), the difference greatly exceeds 30 ms.

The possibilities of Purkinje-related VTs,[56] such as idiopathic fascicular VT,[57] fascicular VT postmyocardial infarction,[58,59] automatic His-Purkinje VT, focal Purkinje VT,[60] and AV node/His-Purkinje reentry,[61] should also be considered. Intrafascicular VT has a negative or short HV interval during tachycardia and a normal baseline QRS and HV interval.[56] VT arising from myocardial foci rarely produces entirely typical RBBB or LBBB patterns on the surface 12-lead ECG, as is expected with BBR. In addition, His activation usually occurs late in the QRS complex and may be dissociated from the tachycardia.

Exclusion of supraventricular tachycardia is particularly important because the QRS morphology during BBRVT is a typical bundle branch block pattern and may be similar to that seen in sinus rhythm. AV dissociation is typically present during BBR. However, AV nodal reentry tachycardia with an upper common pathway block, junctional tachycardia, intra-Hisian reentry, and orthodromic tachycardia using a retrograde nodofascicular (ventricular) pathway are other possibilities in which VA dissociation or block can occur.

When 1:1 ventriculoatrial conduction is present, the diagnoses of orthodromic AV reciprocating tachycardia, tachycardia using an anterograde atriofascicular accessory pathway, and atrial tachycardia with aberrant ventricular conduction need to be considered.

BOX 83.1 Diagnostic criteria for bundle branch reentrant and interfascicular tachycardias

Bundle Branch Reentry

- VT morphology is a typical LBBB or RBBB
- Induction is dependent on HP conduction delay
- His potential precedes each QRS complex.
- HV during VT usually ≥ HV during sinus rhythm
- Terminates with block in HP system
- His, RBB, and LBB activation sequences during an LBBB morphology tachycardia or His, LBB, and RBB activation sequences during an RBBB morphology tachycardia
- Variations in the VV interval are preceded by similar changes in the HH interval
- PPI–TCL < 30 ms with entrainment from the RV apex
- QRS morphology during atrial entrainment is similar to that during VT

Interfascicular Reentry

- VT morphology is an RBBB with left anterior or posterior fascicular hemiblock
- Induction is dependent on left fascicular conduction delay
- His potential precedes each QRS complex
- HV during VT usually < HV during sinus rhythm
- Terminates with block in left fascicular system
- LAF, ventricle, and LPF activation sequences during a left posterior hemiblock morphology tachycardia or LPF, ventricle, and LAF activation sequences during a left anterior hemiblock morphology tachycardia
- Variations in the VV interval are preceded by similar changes in the HH interval
- Atrial entrainment exhibits a similar left fascicular hemiblock morphology; however, RBBB configuration might be changed

LAF, Left anterior fascicle; *LBB,* left bundle branch; *LBBB,* left bundle branch block; *LPF,* left posterior fascicle; *PPI–TCL,* postpacing interval minus the tachycardia cycle length; RBB, right bundle branch; *RBBB,* right bundle branch block; *VT,* ventricular tachycardia.

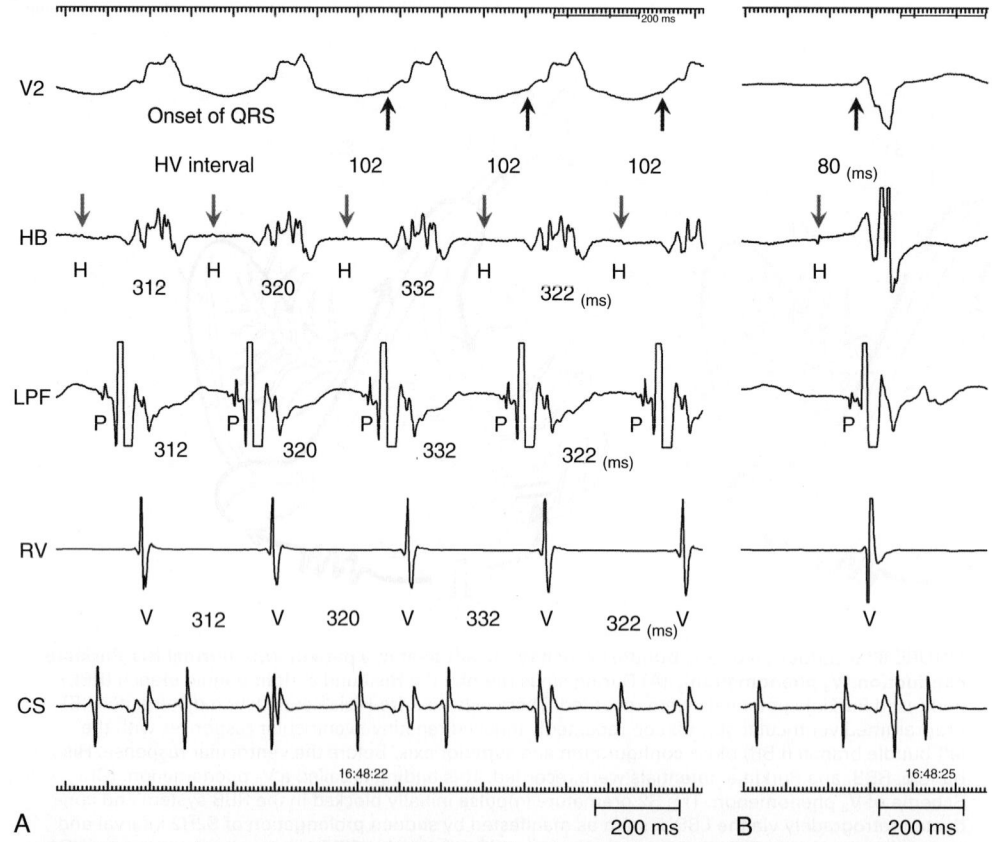

FIGURE 83.7 Intracardiac recording during bundle branch reentry (BBR; type C). (A) During BBR, each His (*H*) activation precedes the ventricular (*V*) depolarization. Changes in the HH interval precede any changes in the VV interval. The HV interval during BBR was longer than the HV interval during sinus rhythm (B). *CS,* Coronary sinus; *HB,* His bundle; *LPF,* left posterior fascicle; *RV,* right ventricle. (Modified from Machino T, Tada H, Sekiguchi Y, Aonuma K. Three-dimensional visualization of the entire reentrant circuit. *Heart Rhythm.* 2013;10:459-460.)

Entrainment with manifest QRS fusion during ventricular pacing and the ability to terminate or reset the tachycardia with a ventricular extrastimulus introduced when the His bundle is refractory will rule out atrial tachycardia, AV nodal reentry tachycardia, junctional tachycardia, and intra-Hisian reentry.

A negative HV interval at the onset of tachycardia is observed in Mahaim tachycardia using an anterograde atriofascicular pathway. AV nodal reentrant and AV reciprocating tachycardias commonly stop with adenosine; BBR rarely stops with adenosine, but adenosine has been reported to affect BBR in a case report.[62]

Catheter Ablation

Elimination of BBRVT and interfascicular tachycardia would decrease the need for pharmacological antiarrhythmic therapy and the frequency of defibrillator shocks. It may also improve the amount of biventricular pacing in those with cardiac resynchronization therapy (CRT) pacing devices[63] and prevent VT storm with ventricular pacing.[40] Pharmacological antiarrhythmic therapy, either empirical or electrophysiologically guided, is usually ineffective. Radiofrequency (RF) catheter ablation of a bundle branch can cure BBRVTs and is currently regarded as first-line therapy. Box 83.2 shows the targets for ablation of BBRVTs.

Right Bundle Branch Ablation

The technique of choice is ablation of the RBB.[3,53,64] BBRVT may be prevented by ablation of the right or left main bundle branch.[15,25] Even though most patients demonstrate increased conduction system disease in the LBB, the RBB is typically the target for ablation. This is so because of the technical ease of ablation of the RBB, which is in contrast to the difficulties involved in ablation of the LBB. With this technique, the catheter is initially placed at the His bundle area and then is gradually advanced toward the anterosuperior ventricular septum. To ensure catheter stability, slight clockwise torque is applied to improve contact with the RBB (Fig. 83.9).

The RBB potential is identified by the following characteristics: (1) a sharp deflection inscribed 10 to 15 ms after the typical His potential and (2) the absence of an atrial electrogram on the same recording. The RBB-V interval value of less than 30 ms may not be a reliable marker of RBB potential in these patients because of His-Purkinje system disease that can cause prolongation of the RBB-V conduction time (Fig. 83.10A).[53,64,65] If any RBB conduction delay is present, the RBB potential may be obscured by local ventricular activation in sinus rhythm. Electroanatomical mapping with multipolar catheters may help map the

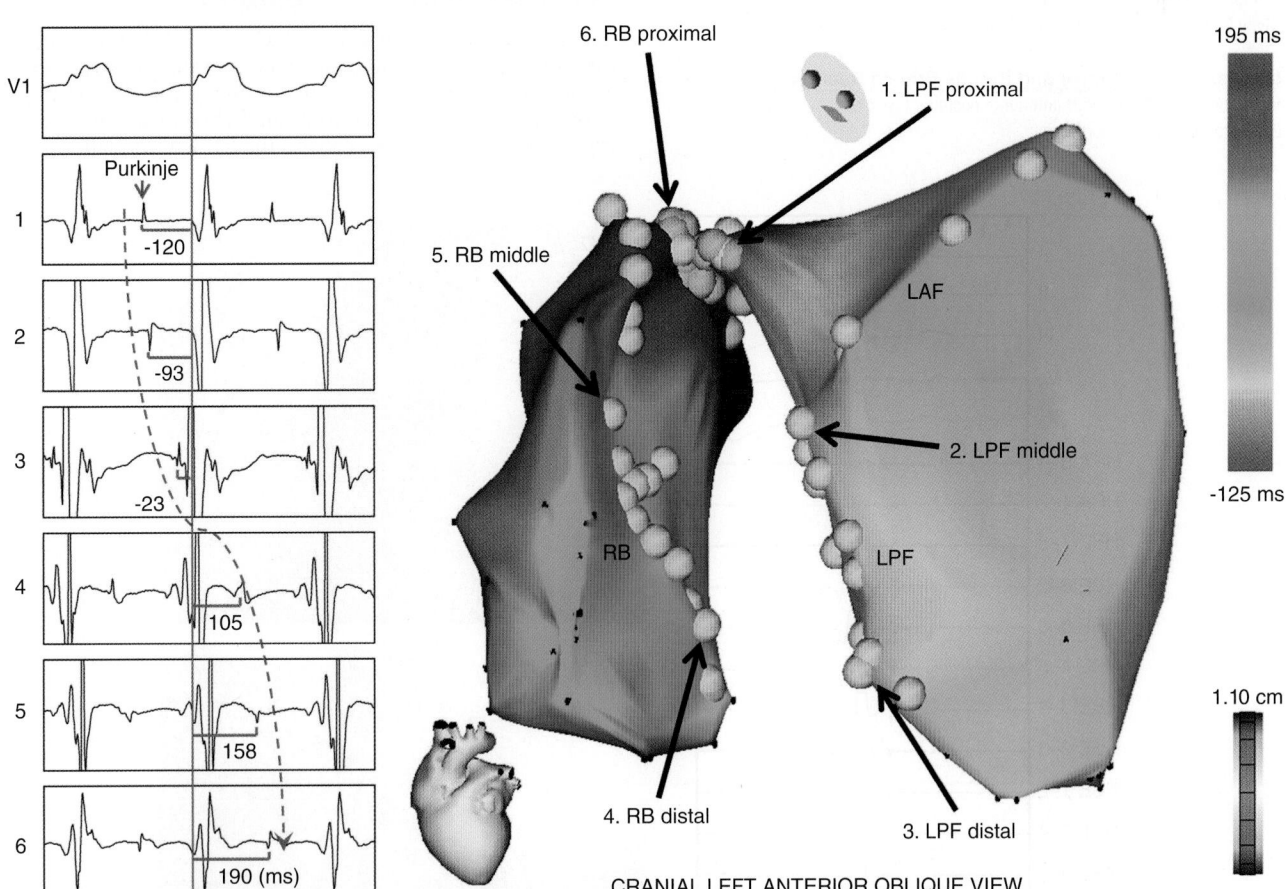

CRANIAL LEFT ANTERIOR OBLIQUE VIEW

FIGURE 83.8 Three-dimensional electroanatomical mapping during bundle branch reentry (BBR). The activation map of the bundle branch reentrant ventricular tachycardia (BBRVT) descending the left posterior fascicle (*LPF*) and ascending the right bundle branch (RBB), with the earliest activation displayed in *red* (LPF proximal) and the latest in *violet* (RBB proximal). The *yellow dots* and the *numbered sites with arrows* indicate fascicular potentials and local activations of the His-Purkinje system (*left boxes*), respectively. Sequential activations of the local His-Purkinje system accounted for the entire tachycardia cycle length. The propagation map of BBRVT also demonstrated that anterograde activation through the left anterior fascicle and LPF resulted in a collision at the middle portion of the left anterior fascicle—a bystander of the reentrant circuit (see the Online Supplemental Movie: http://dx.doi.org/10.1016/j.hrthm.2011.11.001). *LAF,* Left anterior fascicle; *RB,* right bundle. (From Machino T, Tada H, Sekiguchi Y, Aonuma K. Three-dimensional visualization of the entire reentrant circuit. *Heart Rhythm.* 2013;10:459-460.)

conduction system in better detail and allow for catheter stability and location during initial and subsequent RF energy applications. Temporary interruption of RBB conduction may interrupt BBRVT and prove the mechanism, but it may also occur with trauma and catheter manipulation. While it may be inadvertent, if RF energy is not delivered, it may not necessarily be permanent.[44] The use of electroanatomical mapping may therefore enhance the delivery of additional lesions near the proper spot in the Purkinje system.

Although it is important to obtain a stable catheter position to minimize the risk of AV block, in some cases, the RBB potential may not be identifiable in sinus rhythm and may be evident only during retrograde conduction during sustained BBRVT or BBR echo beats. If the RBB is not well recorded at the basilar septum,

BOX 83.2 Targets for ablation

Bundle Branch Reentry
Right bundle branch, usual primary target
Left bundle branch

Interfascicular Reentry
Left anterior or posterior fascicle
Distal Purkinje network between the fascicles

Interfascicular Reentry and Bundle Branch Reentry
Right bundle branch and [left anterior or posterior fascicle]
Left anterior and posterior fascicle

mapping of the apical course of the RBB may be effective. Energy settings of 20 to 60 W are reported effective with a 4 mm–tipped catheter.[3,52] In sinus rhythm, complete RBB or LBB develops with successful ablation (Fig. 83.10B), although QRS changes may be subtle in patients with preexisting conduction abnormalities. Electrical axis changes may be the only manifestation of fascicular ablation. Elimination of retrograde VH conduction has been used as a marker of successful ablation.[3]

After successful RBB ablation, programmed electrical stimulation is performed at baseline and with isoproterenol infusion. This should include pacing from two different sites at two different cycle lengths and with the use of extrastimuli with a short–long–short sequence. In patients with complete anterograde block in the LBB, RBB ablation necessitates subsequent permanent pacing. The reported incidence of clinically significant conduction system impairment requiring implantation of a permanent pacemaker varies from 0% to 30%.[3,6,8,32,40,52,53] In patients with His-Purkinje disease, it is important to ascertain the need for permanent pacing by atrial stimulation (Fig. 83.10C and D). It is advisable to stress the His-Purkinje system with an intravenous class IA antiarrhythmic drug to ensure that the anterograde conduction is preserved.

Left Bundle Branch Ablation

For many patients with BBRVT who have LBBB during sinus rhythm, anterograde slow conduction over the LBB is present[49,66] or the LBB is activated retrograde (transseptal).[16] In patients with a complete LBBB pattern during sinus rhythm, anterograde ventricular activation occurs solely via the RBB. These latter patients

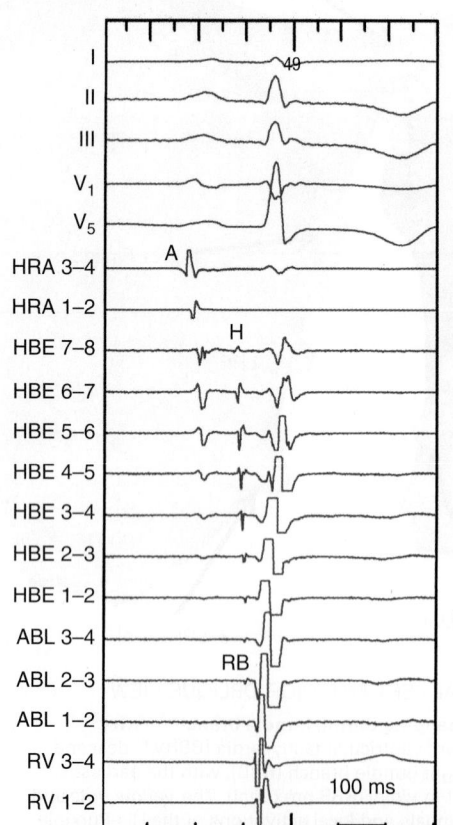
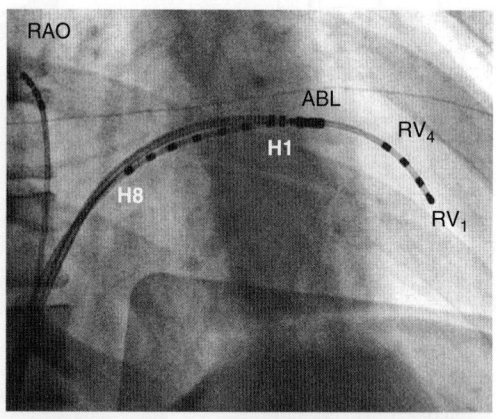
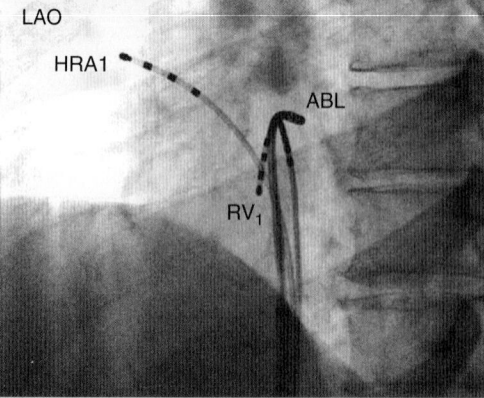

FIGURE 83.9 Recording of the right bundle branch (RBB). Right and left anterior oblique (*RAO* and *LAO*) views of the eight-polar His and ablation (*ABL*) catheters are shown. His and RBB potentials are recorded continuously. The RBB recording occurs more than 10 ms later than the typical His potential with a large atrial electrogram, and no atrial electrogram is recorded at the RBB recording site. *HBE*, His bundle electrogram; *HRA*, high right atrium; *RV*, right ventricle.

are at risk of developing complete AV block with RBB ablation. To avoid this potential complication, the LBB might be targeted in such patients with LBBB during sinus rhythm, with BBRVT as an alternative approach (Fig. 83.11).[16,66] However, LBB ablation is technically difficult because it is a broad structure and usually requires arterial access; a catheter placed at the left ventricular septum may be unstable when the transseptal approach is used, even with a deflectable sheath. The risk for procedural complications (e.g., damage to the femoral, coronary, and carotid arteries) is increased.

The LBB arises as a broad band of fibers directed inferiorly from the His bundle. The left main bundle is typically 1 to 3-cm long and 1-cm wide but shows great individual variation. For LBB ablation, the ablation catheter is advanced across the aortic valve and is positioned in the left ventricle along the interventricular septum. The LBB potential is recorded beneath the aortic valve, typically 1 to 1.5 cm inferior to the optimal His bundle recording site.[25,64] The LBB potential is identified by a potential-to-ventricular electrogram interval of ≤20 ms and an A/V electrogram ratio of ≤1:10.[25] Delivery of RF energy at this level results in complete LBBB and successfully interrupts the tachycardia circuit. However, LBB ablation usually requires more extensive ablation to transect this broad structure.

In patients with an LBBB during sinus rhythm, slow conduction over the LBB is often present.[66] In patients with a relatively narrow QRS duration, the left ventricle is activated by a slow propagation through the LBB and Purkinje network, with earliest activation occurring at the site of the latest Purkinje activation during sinus rhythm (see Fig. 83.11A).[66] In patients with a wider QRS duration, the earliest left ventricular activation site is located far from the site with the latest Purkinje potential, which indicates passive activation via the transseptal route from the RBB (see Fig. 83.11B).[66] In such patients, the anterograde LBB potential can be targeted instead of the intact RBB.

After LBB ablation, follow-up for progression to AV block is recommended even if the anterograde conduction via the RBB appears preserved.

Ablation of Interfascicular Tachycardia

In interfascicular reentry, RBB ablation will not cure the tachycardia because the RBB is a bystander. Similarly, ablation of the main LBB would not be expected to terminate the tachycardia because the circuit is distal to this point. Catheter ablation of the LAF or the LPF will result in termination of the tachycardia (Fig. 83.12).[39,51,52,67] Limited data suggest that elimination of interfascicular tachycardia should be attempted by targeting the distal Purkinje network around the fascicle instead of ablation of the proximal fascicle to avoid the development of a complete fascicular block.[39] Ablation of one of the left-sided fascicles would not be expected to prevent BBRVT in a patient with both interfascicular VT and BBRVT. In this situation, both of the left-sided fascicles and the RBB must be ablated.

Clinical Outcomes

In the two largest series reported, acute success rates for BBRVT and interfascicular reentry were 100%.[3,52] After ablation, BBRVT

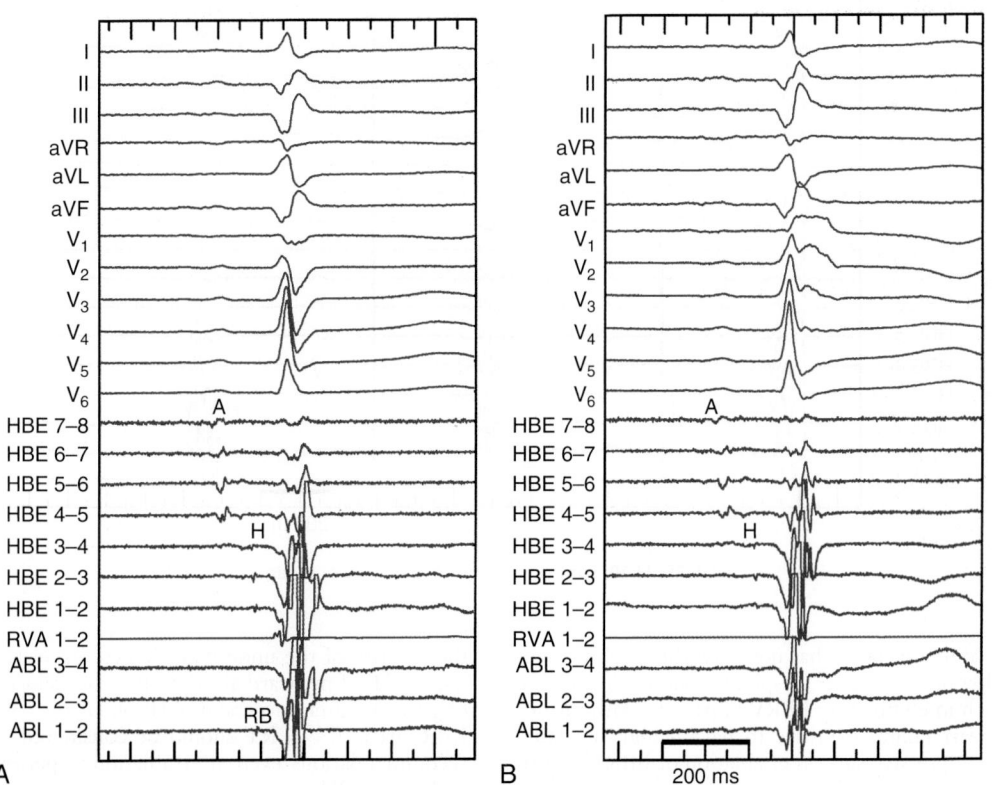

FIGURE 83.10 Recordings before and after right bundle ablation during sinus rhythm and atrial pacing. (A) Before the ablation of the right bundle branch (RBB). The RBB recording occurs more than 10 ms later than the His potential, and no atrial electrogram is recorded at the RBB recording site. The RBB-V interval is 32 ms. (B) After ablation of the RBB, the surface electrocardiogram shows complete RBB block, and the RBB potential at the ablation site has disappeared. (C) Before ablation, burst atrial pacing at a cycle length of 400 ms exhibits a complete left bundle branch block configuration that is identical to clinical tachycardia. (D) After ablation of the RBB, burst atrial pacing shows 2:1 H-V block. *ABL,* Ablation; *HBE,* His bundle electrogram; *RVA,* right ventricular apex.

Continued

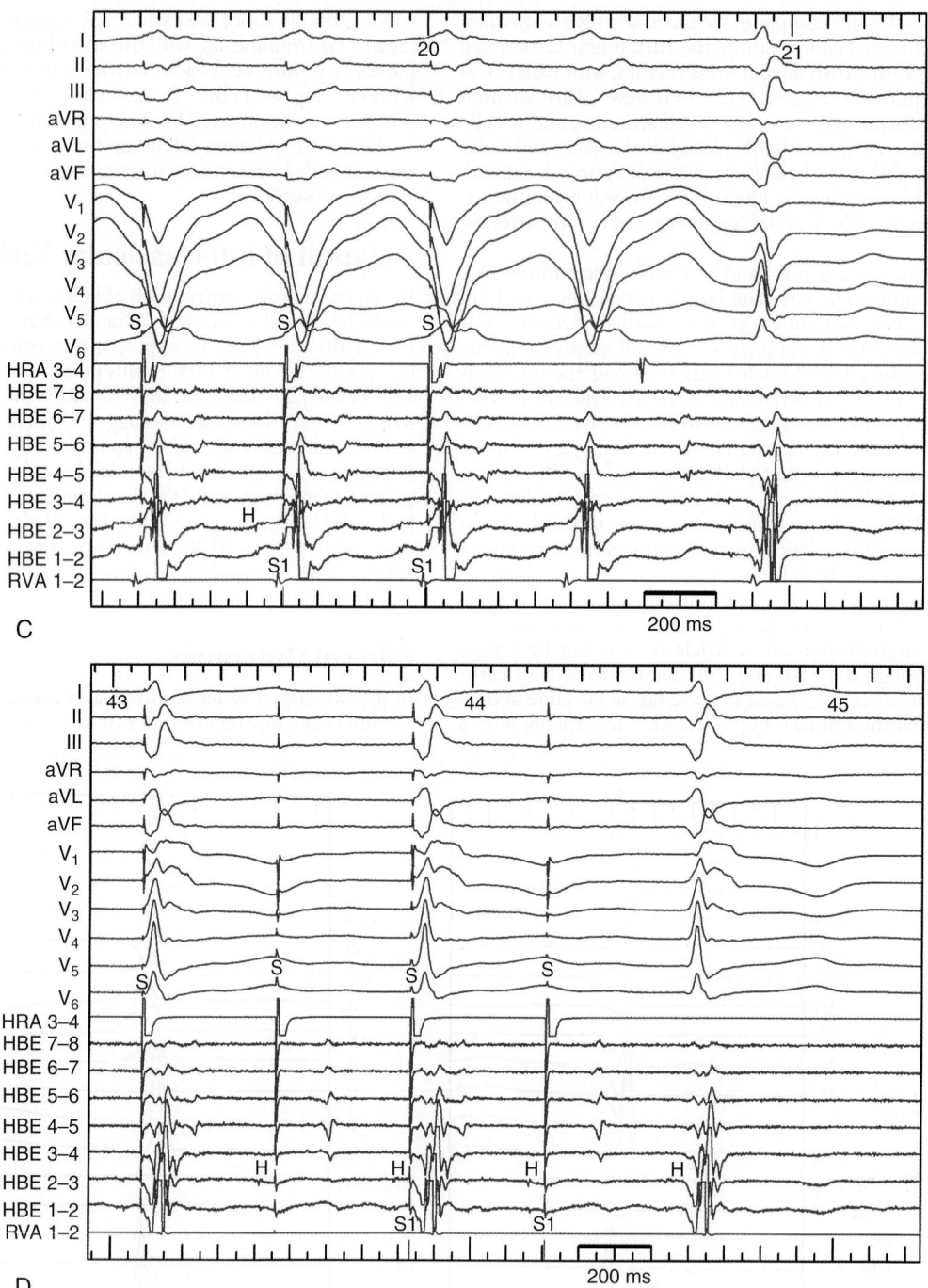

FIGURE 83.10, cont'd For legend, see previous page.

recurrence is uncommon, but it has not been thoroughly documented with follow-up testing.[3,52] Despite the success of ablation of the RBB branch in eliminating BBRVT, patients with cardiomyopathy and heart failure continue to have a high mortality rate. Despite the impressive success of ablation of BBRVT, progressive heart failure is a common cause of death.[3,6,18,29,32,53,64,65] Furthermore, patients with cardiomyopathy remain at high risk for sudden cardiac death. A small risk of progressive AV block is present as well.

Therefore, after ablation, the need for a permanent pacemaker or an implantable cardioverter defibrillator (ICD), with or without cardiac resynchronization capabilities, should be considered based on the status of the residual conduction system and the severity of the underlying structural heart disease. Furthermore, VT of myocardial origin may be induced in 36% to 60% of patients after successful ablation of one of the limbs of the BBR circuit.[29,52] CRT should be considered based on standard recommendations even after ablation is performed for patients with severe left ventricular dysfunction and an intraventricular conduction disturbance.

The management strategy for patients with BBRVT and preserved left ventricular function who have no other risk markers for sudden death is less clear. Very limited data suggest that these patients have a favorable long-term prognosis after successful ablation of the RBB to cure BBRVT.[3,15,53] However, they still have long-term risks of complete heart block and progressive

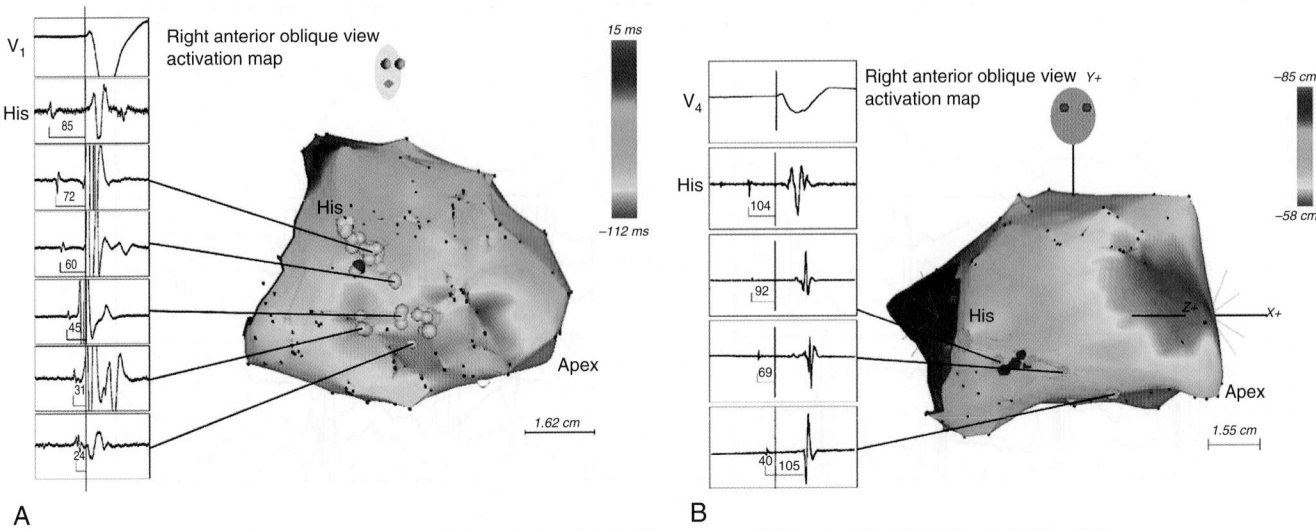

FIGURE 83.11 Electroanatomical map of the left ventricle during sinus rhythm in patients with an electrocardiogram pattern of complete left bundle branch block. (A) A patient with QRS duration of 135 ms due to slow conduction in the left bundle system. Note there is no Purkinje activation in the area of the left anterior fascicular Purkinje fiber. The interval from His bundle activation to the latest Purkinje activation in the left posterior fiber was 61 ms with slow conduction over the left bundle branch and posterior fascicular fiber, and earliest activation (*red*) of the left ventricle around the sites with latest Purkinje activation. *Dark brown tag* indicates site of successful ablation. (B) A patient with QRS duration of 225 ms. Note no Purkinje activation was recorded in the area of the left anterior fascicular Purkinje fiber. The interval from His bundle activation to the latest Purkinje activation was 64 ms with slow conduction over the left bundle branch and posterior fascicular fiber, and the interval from latest Purkinje activation to local ventricular action was 105 ms, with earliest activation (*red*) of the left ventricle at the apical portion of the left septum approximately 3 cm away from the sites with latest Purkinje potentials; this indicates left ventricular activation via a transseptal route. *Dark brown tags* indicate site of successful ablation. *ABL,* Ablation; *HBE,* His bundle electrogram; *HRA,* high right atrium; *RVA,* right ventricular apex. (From Schmidt B, Tang M, Chun KJ, et al. Left bundle branch-Purkinje system in patients with bundle branch reentrant tachycardia: lessons from catheter ablation and electroanatomic mapping. *Heart Rhythm.* 2009;6:51-58.)

heart failure when undergoing LBB ablation to cure BBRVT. After ablation, patients with Mobitz II second- or third-degree AV block at physiological heart rates or a markedly prolonged HV interval (>100 ms) but with preserved ventricular function and no inducible tachycardia should be considered for a dual-chamber pacemaker. Patients with myotonic dystrophy should be considered for prophylactic permanent pacemaker (or ICD) implantation because of the progressive nature of their conduction system disease.[16]

Complications

The most common complication of the ablation of BBRVT is high-grade AV block, which is reported to occur in 0% to 30% of patients after a successful ablation.[3,6,16,32,40,52,53] In most of these patients, the RBB was ablated to cure BBRVT. In a series of 20 patients with BBRVT, 15 had permanent pacemakers or ICDs at the time of the ablation, and two of the remaining five patients had indications for ICD implantation after the ablation as the result of myocardial VT.[52] Only two patients underwent pacemaker implantation for impaired AV conduction. Incessant interfascicular tachycardia after successful RBB ablation for the treatment of BBRVT has been reported.[44] The long-term risk

of complete heart block and progressive heart failure after LBB ablation remains uncertain, although in a recent report of nine patients with BBRVT having RBB ablations, three developed complete heart block within 2 months of ablation (two had pre-existing LBBBs and one had RBBB and LAFB).[68]

Conclusions

BBRVT, a unique form of reentrant VT involving the His-Purkinje system, occurs in patients with cardiomyopathy and His-Purkinje conduction disease. Several criteria distinguish supraventricular and myocardial VTs from BBRVT. Detailed mapping on both sides of the septum and electrophysiological analyses facilitate an appropriate diagnosis.

It is important to recognize BBRVT because it responds poorly to pharmacological therapy and can be cured effectively with catheter ablation. Even after ablation, however, patients may remain at risk for total mortality and sudden cardiac death and may require further therapies, including, but not limited to, CRT or an ICD. Elimination of BBRVT will reduce associated episodic hemodynamic collapse and syncope, decrease the need for pharmacological antiarrhythmic therapy, and curtail the frequency of ICD shocks.

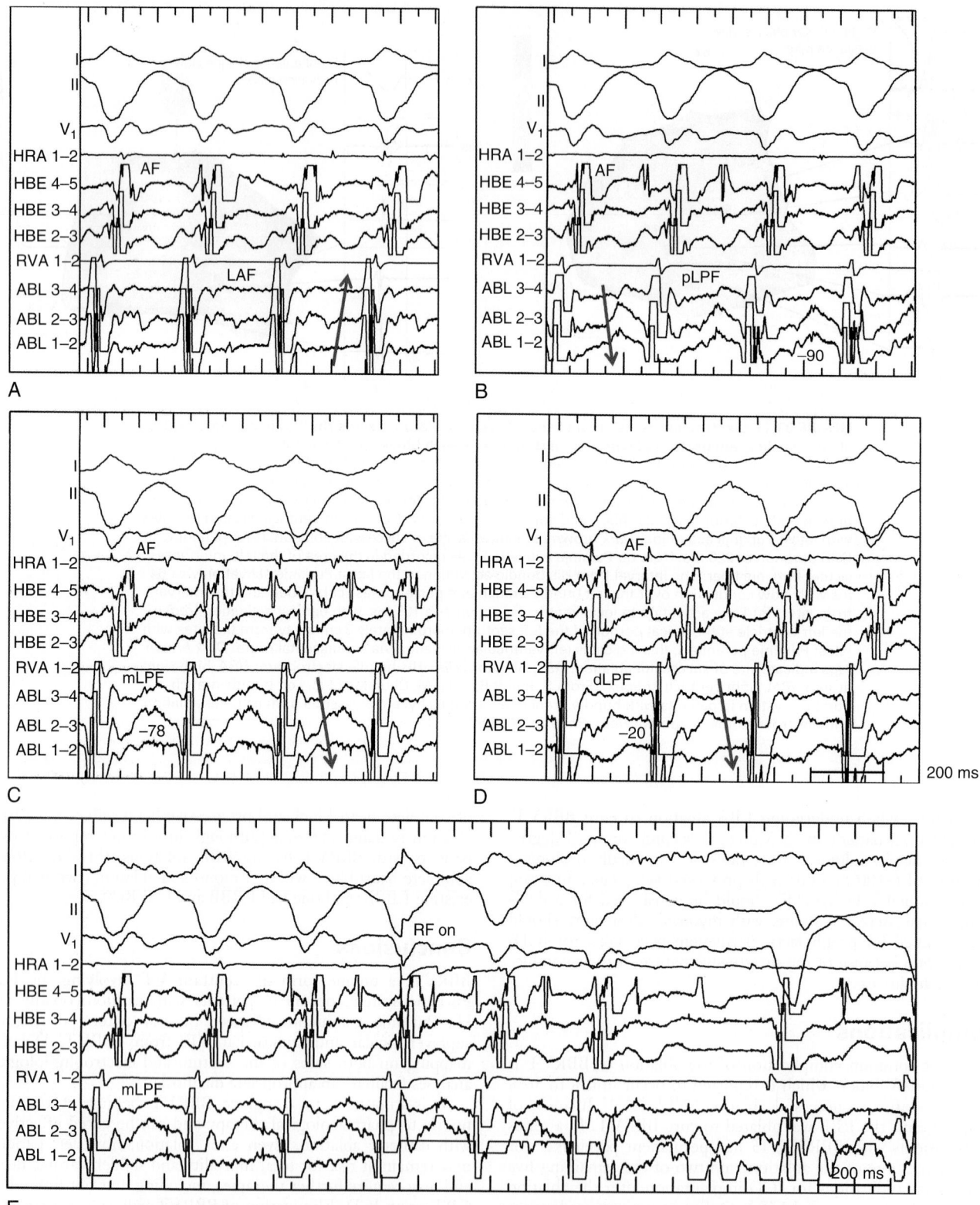

FIGURE 83.12 Radiofrequency catheter ablation of the distal left Purkinje network in a patient with interfascicular ventricular tachycardia. (A) During an interfascicular ventricular tachycardia, His potentials are not seen before the QRS. Activation sequences of the left anterior fascicle are from distal to proximal. (B) Activation sequences of proximal LPF (*pLPF*) are from distal to proximal. (C) Activation sequences of middle LPF (*mLPF*) are from distal to proximal. (D) Activation sequences of distal LPF (*dLPF*) are from distal to proximal, and the distal LPF electrogram fused with the ventricular electrogram. (E) Catheter ablation to mLPF terminated the tachycardia. The QRS configuration after the ablation is the same as that before the ablation (incomplete left bundle branch block). *ABL*, Ablation; *AF*, atrial fibrillation; *HB*, His bundle; *HBE*, His bundle electrogram; *HRA*, high right atrium; *RF*, radiofrequency; *RVA*, right ventricular apex.

REFERENCES

1. Guerot C, Valere PE, Castillo-Fenoy A, et al. Tachycardia by branch-to-branch reentry. *Arch Mal Coeur Vaiss*. 1974;67:1–11.
2. Akhtar M, Damato AN, Batsford WP, et al. Demonstration of re-entry within the His-Purkinje system in man. *Circulation*. 1974;50:1150–1162.
3. Blanck Z, Dhala A, Deshpande S, et al. Bundle branch reentrant ventricular tachycardia: cumulative experience in 48 patients. *J Cardiovasc Electrophysiol*. 1993;4:253–262.
4. Lloyd EA, Zipes DP, Heger JJ, et al. Sustained ventricular tachycardia due to bundle branch reentry. *Am Heart J*. 1982;104:1095–1097.
5. Touboul P, Kirkorian G, Atallah G, et al. Bundle branch reentry: a possible mechanism of ventricular tachycardia. *Circulation*. 1983;67:674–680.
6. Narasimhan C, Jazayeri MR, Sra J, et al. Ventricular tachycardia in valvular heart disease: facilitation of sustained bundle-branch reentry by valve surgery. *Circulation*. 1997;96:4307–4313.
7. Eckart RE, Hruczkowski TW, Tedrow UB, et al. Sustained ventricular tachycardia associated with corrective valve surgery. *Circulation*. 2007;116:2005–2011.
8. Merino JL, Carmona JR, Fernandez-Lozano I, et al. Mechanisms of sustained ventricular tachycardia in myotonic dystrophy: implications for catheter ablation. *Circulation*. 1998;98:541–546.
9. Negri SM, Cowan MD. Becker muscular dystrophy with bundle branch reentry ventricular tachycardia. *J Cardiovasc Electrophysiol*. 1998;9:652–654.
10. Takeda K, Takemoto M, Mukai Y, et al. Bundle branch re-entry ventricular tachycardia in a patient with myotonic dystrophy. *J Cardiol*. 2009;53:463–466.
11. Andress JD, Vander Salm TJ, Huang SK. Bidirectional bundle branch reentry tachycardia associated with Ebstein's anomaly: cured by extensive cryoablation of the right bundle branch. *Pacing Clin Electrophysiol*. 1991;14:1639–1647.
12. Barra S, Moreno N, Providência R, et al. Incessant slow bundle branch reentrant ventricular tachycardia in a young patient with left ventricular noncompaction. *Rev Port Cardiol*. 2013;32:523–529.
13. Dora SK, Valaparambil A, Namboodiri N, et al. Bundle branch reentry ventricular tachycardia in arrhythmogenic right ventricular dysplasia. *J Interv Card Electrophysiol*. 2008;21:215–218.
14. Rodríguez-Mañero M, Sacher F, Asmundis C, et al. Monomorphic ventricular tachycardia in patients with Brugada syndrome: a multicenter retrospective study. *Heart Rhythm*. 2016;13:669–682.
15. Blanck Z, Jazayeri M, Dhala A, et al. Bundle branch reentry: a mechanism of ventricular tachycardia in the absence of myocardial or valvular dysfunction. *J Am Coll Cardiol*. 1993;22:1718–1722.
16. Blanck Z, Deshpande S, Jazayeri MR, et al. Catheter ablation of the left bundle branch for the treatment of sustained bundle branch reentrant ventricular tachycardia. *J Cardiovasc Electrophysiol*. 1995;6:40–43.
17. Phlips T, Ramchurn H, De Roy L. Reverse BBRVT in a structurally normal heart. *Acta Cardiol*. 2012;67:603–607.
18. Caceres J, Jazayeri M, McKinnie J, et al. Sustained bundle branch reentry as a mechanism of clinical tachycardia. *Circulation*. 1989;79:256–270.
19. Delacretaz E, Stevenson WG, Ellison KE, et al. Mapping and radiofrequency catheter ablation of the three types of sustained monomorphic ventricular tachycardia in nonischemic heart disease. *J Cardiovasc Electrophysiol*. 2000;11:11–17.
20. Cantillon DJ, Bianco C, Wazni OM, et al. Electrophysiologic characteristics and catheter ablation of ventricular tachyarrhythmias among patients with heart failure on ventricular assist device support. *Heart Rhythm*. 2012;9:859–864.
21. Wang CW, Sterba R, Tchou P. Bundle branch reentry ventricular tachycardia with two distinct left bundle branch block morphologies. *J Cardiovasc Electrophysiol*. 1997;8:688–693.
22. Wang PJ, Friedman PL. "Clockwise" and "counterclockwise" bundle branch reentry as a mechanism for sustained ventricular tachycardia masquerading as supraventricular tachycardia. *Pacing Clin Electrophysiol*. 1989;12:1426–1432.
23. Enjoji Y, Mizobuchi M, Shibata K, et al. Bundle brunch reentrant ventricular tachycardia with two distinct conduction patterns in a patient with complete right bundle branch block. *Pacing Clin Electrophysiol*. 2006;29:1438–1441.
24. Kusa S, Taniguchi H, Hachiya H, et al. Bundle branch reentrant ventricular tachycardia with wide and narrow QRS morphology. *Circ Arrhythm Electrophysiol*. 2013;6:e87–e91.
25. Tchou P, Mehdirad AA. Bundle branch reentry ventricular tachycardia. *Pacing Clin Electrophysiol*. 1995;18:1427–1437.
26. Olshansky B. Ventricular tachycardia masquerading as supraventricular tachycardia: a wolf in sheep's clothing. *J Electrocardiol*. 1988;21:377–384.
27. Guo H, Hecker S, Levy S, et al. Ventricular tachycardia with QRS configuration similar to that in sinus rhythm and a myocardial origin: differential diagnosis with bundle branch reentry. *Europace*. 2001;3:115–123.
28. Tusscher KH, Panfilov AV. Modelling of the ventricular conduction system. *Prog Biophys Mol Biol*. 2008;96:152–170.
29. Blanck Z, Akhtar M. Ventricular tachycardia due to sustained bundle branch reentry: diagnostic and therapeutic considerations. *Clin Cardiol*. 1993;16:619–622.
30. Mehdirad AA, Keim S, Rist K, et al. Asymmetry of retrograde conduction and reentry within the His-Purkinje system: a comparative analysis of left and right ventricular stimulation. *J Am Coll Cardiol*. 1994;24:177–184.
31. Fisher JD. Bundle branch reentry tachycardia: why is the HV interval often longer than in sinus rhythm? The critical role of anisotropic conduction. *J Interv Card Electrophysiol*. 2001;5:173–176.
32. Li YG, Gronefeld G, Israel C, et al. Bundle branch reentrant tachycardia in patients with apparent normal His-Purkinje conduction: the role of functional conduction impairment. *J Cardiovasc Electrophysiol*. 2002;13:1233–1239.
33. Lehmann MH, Denker S, Mahmud R, et al. Linking. A dynamic electrophysiologic phenomenon in macroreentry circuits. *Circulation*. 1985;71:254–265.
34. Reddy CP, Harris B. Gap phenomenon in "the right and left bundle branch systems" during retrograde conduction in man. *Am Heart J*. 1979;97:216–224.
35. Littmann L, Tenczer J, Svenson RH. Demonstration of reentry within the right bundle branch in man. *Pacing Clin Electrophysiol*. 1984;7:861–866.
36. Blanck Z, Jazayeri M, Akhtar M. Facilitation of sustained bundle branch reentry by atrial fibrillation. *J Cardiovasc Electrophysiol*. 1996;7:348–352.
37. Morgera T, Zecchin M, Camerini F. Bundle-branch reentry ventricular tachycardia induced by sinus beat. *G Ital Cardiol*. 1996;26:1295–1301.
38. Fedgchin B, Pavri BB, Greenspon AJ, et al. Unique self-perpetuating cycle of atrioventricular block and phase IV bundle branch block in a patient with bundle branch reentrant tachycardia. *Heart Rhythm*. 2004;1:493–496.
39. Reithmann C, Hahnefeld A, Oversohl N, et al. Reinitiation of ventricular macroreentry within the His-Purkinje system by back-up ventricular pacing: a mechanism of ventricular tachycardia storm. *Pacing Clin Electrophysiol*. 2007;30:225–235.
40. Akhtar M, Denker S, Lehmann MH, et al. Macro-reentry within the His Purkinje system. *Pacing Clin Electrophysiol*. 1983;6:1010–1028.
41. Simons GR, Sorrentino RA, Zimerman LI, et al. Bundle branch reentry tachycardia and possible sustained interfascicular reentry tachycardia with a shared unusual induction pattern. *J Cardiovasc Electrophysiol*. 1996;7:44–50.
42. Mizusawa Y, Sakurada H, Nishizaki M, et al. Characteristics of bundle branch reentrant ventricular tachycardia with a right bundle branch block configuration: feasibility of atrial pacing. *Europace*. 2009;11:1208–1213.
43. Chalvidan T, Cellarier G, Deharo JC, et al. His-Purkinje system reentry as a proarrhythmic effect of flecainide. *Pacing Clin Electrophysiol*. 2000;23:530–533.
44. Gössinger HD, Siostrzonek P, Wagner L, et al. Inadvertent catheter-induced right bundle branch block in a patient with preexistent left bundle branch block and recurrent macroreentrant ventricular tachycardia. *Pacing Clin Electrophysiol*. 1989;12:1857–1862.
45. Merino JL, Peinado R, Fernandez-Lozano I, et al. Transient entrainment of bundle-branch reentry by atrial and ventricular stimulation: elucidation of the tachycardia mechanism through analysis of the surface ECG. *Circulation*. 1999;100:1784–1790.
46. Merino JL, Peinado R, Fernandez-Lozano I, et al. Bundle-branch reentry and the postpacing interval after entrainment by right ventricular apex stimulation: a new approach to elucidate the mechanism of wide-QRS-complex tachycardia with atrioventricular dissociation. *Circulation*. 2001;103:1102–1108.
47. Kitazawa H, Washizuka T, Uchiyama H, et al. Fusion with postpaced return cycle identical to tachycardia cycle length during transient entrainment of ventricular tachycardia and its implications. *Jpn Heart J*. 1997;38:369–378.
48. Sarter BH, Schwartzman D, Callans DJ, et al. Bundle branch reentry ventricular tachycardia: an investigation of the circuit with resetting. *J Cardiovasc Electrophysiol*. 1996;7:1082–1085.
49. Machino T, Tada H, Sekiguchi Y, et al. Three-dimensional visualization of the entire reentrant circuit of bundle branch reentrant tachycardia. *Heart Rhythm*. 2013;10:459–460.
50. Berger RD, Orias D, Kasper EK, et al. Catheter ablation of coexistent bundle branch and interfascicular reentrant ventricular tachycardias. *J Cardiovasc Electrophysiol*. 1996;7:341–347.
51. Crijns HJ, Smeets JL, Rodriguez LM, et al. Cure of interfascicular reentrant ventricular tachycardia by ablation of the anterior fascicle of the left bundle branch. *J Cardiovasc Electrophysiol*. 1995;6:486–492.
52. Lopera G, Stevenson WG, Soejima K, et al. Identification and ablation of three types of ventricular tachycardia involving the His-Purkinje system in patients with heart disease. *J Cardiovasc Electrophysiol*. 2004;15:52–58.
53. Cohen TJ, Chien WW, Lurie KG, et al. Radiofrequency catheter ablation for treatment of bundle branch reentrant ventricular tachycardia: results and long-term follow-up. *J Am Coll Cardiol*. 1991;18:1767–1773.
54. Blanck Z, Sra J, Akhtar M. Incessant interfascicular reentrant ventricular tachycardia as a result of catheter ablation of the right bundle branch: case report and review of the literature. *J Cardiovasc Electrophysiol*. 2009;20:1279–1283.
55. Crijns HJ, Kingma JH, Gosselink AT, et al. Comparison in the same patient of aberrant conduction and bundle branch reentry after dofetilide, a new selective class III antiarrhythmic agent. *Pacing Clin Electrophysiol*. 1993;16:1006–1016.
56. Nogami A. Purkinje-related arrhythmias part I: monomorphic ventricular tachycardias. *Pacing Clin Electrophysiol*. 2011;34:624–650.
57. Nogami A. Idiopathic left ventricular tachycardia: assessment and treatment. *Card Electrophysiol Rev*. 2002;6:448–457.
58. Morishima I, Nogami A, Tsuboi H, et al. Verapamil-sensitive left anterior fascicular ventricular tachycardia associated with a healed myocardial infarction: changes in the delayed Purkinje potential during sinus rhythm. *J Interv Card Electrophysiol*. 2008;22:233–237.
59. Hayashi M, Kobayashi Y, Iwasaki YK, et al. Novel mechanism of postinfarction ventricular tachycardia originating in surviving left posterior Purkinje fibers. *Heart Rhythm*. 2006;3:908–918.
60. Metzner A, Ouyang F, Wissner E, et al. Monomorphic and polymorphic ventricular tachycardias arising from the His-Purkinje system: what do we know? *Future Cardiol*. 2011;7:835–846.
61. Markowitz SM, Stein KM, Engelstein ED, et al. AV nodal-His-Purkinje reentry: a novel form of tachycardia. *J Cardiovasc Electrophysiol*. 1995;6:400–409.
62. Rubenstein DS, Burke MC, Kall JG, et al. Adenosine-sensitive bundle branch reentry. *J Cardiovasc Electrophysiol*. 1997;8:80–88.
63. Barra S, Fynn S. Bundle branch reentry beats, Hisian ectopics, or dual AV nodal physiology? Ablating to achieve 100% biventricular pacing. *Pacing Clin Electrophysiol*. 2015;38:768–771.
64. Mehdirad AA, Keim S, Rist K, et al. Long-term clinical outcome of right bundle branch radiofrequency catheter ablation for treatment of bundle branch reentrant ventricular tachycardia. *Pacing Clin Electrophysiol*. 1995;18:2135–2143.
65. Tchou P, Jazayeri M, Denker S, et al. Transcatheter electrical ablation of right bundle branch: a method of treating macroreentrant ventricular tachycardia attributed to bundle branch reentry. *Circulation*. 1988;78:246–257.
66. Schmidt B, Tang M, Chun KR, et al. Left bundle branch-Purkinje system in patients with bundle branch reentrant tachycardia: lessons from catheter ablation and electroanatomic mapping. *Heart Rhythm*. 2009;6:51–58.
67. Okishige K, Sakurada H, Mizusawa Y, et al. The radio frequency catheter ablation of inter-fascicular reentrant tachycardia: new insights into the electrophysiological and anatomical characteristics. *J Interv Card Electrophysiol*. 2014;41:39–54.
68. Reithmann C, Herkommer B, Huemmer A, et al. The risk of delayed atrioventricular and intraventricular conduction block following ablation of bundle branch reentry. *Clin Res Cardiol*. 2013;102:145–153.

84 Ischemic Heart Disease

David S. Frankel and Francis E. Marchlinski

Electroanatomical Substrate

If not promptly revascularized, coronary artery occlusion leads to infarction with subsequent scarring of the ventricular myocardium. During the infarct healing process, necrotic myocardium is replaced by fibrous tissue that surrounds surviving myocytes.[1–3] These bundles of surviving, diseased myocytes are the key substrate for reentrant, monomorphic ventricular tachycardia (VT). With a reduced number and altered distribution of gap junctions, cellular coupling is poor, resulting in slow, heterogeneous, anisotropic conduction and allowing reentry to occur.[1,4]

This substrate develops within days of myocardial infarction and once established, persists indefinitely.[5,6] Nevertheless, it is only the minority of myocardial infarctions that support reentrant monomorphic VT.

Abnormalities of conduction can be described in terms of electrogram amplitude and morphology. Endocardial recordings from sites of VT origin during sinus rhythm consistently demonstrate low amplitude, prolonged duration, and multicomponent potentials frequently occurring after the end of the QRS complex (Fig. 84.1). In addition to infarct size, the degree of signal abnormality and conduction delay can distinguish patients with sustained VT from those with prior myocardial infarction and no tachycardia.[7]

Early lessons regarding the arrhythmogenic substrate were learned during surgical VT ablation. It was observed that resecting the transmurally infarcted aneurysm would render many (though not all) VTs noninducible. Therefore it became clear that some VT circuits were contained within the border of the aneurysm. With the addition of encircling endocardial ventriculotomy, in which the border zone was resected in full thickness, all VTs were typically rendered noninducible.[8] However, mortality due to worsened heart failure was unacceptably increased by resecting large amounts of viable myocardium. The addition of subendocardial resection of the border zone to aneurysmectomy, with supplemental targeted cryoablation at the mapped VT site of origin, resulted in good arrhythmia control without worsening heart failure.[9]

Using recordings from multiple plunge electrodes, Miller and colleagues further demonstrated that the conduction abnormalities observed during sinus rhythm before resection normalized following resection, again supporting the notion that the diseased, slowly conducting bundles of myocytes are the necessary substrate for reentrant VT.[10]

In attempts to replicate the surgical experience with catheter ablation, the development of three-dimensional mapping systems has allowed detailed spatial characterization of the anatomical substrate. The amplitude of electrograms is proportional to the number of viable muscle fibers under the recording electrode.

Cassidy and coworkers validated this concept using bipolar electrogram characteristics (voltage and duration) to identify the underlying substrate at individual endocardial sites.[11] With the use of a 4-mm tip electrode attached to a second pole 2 mm proximally (filtered at 10 and 400 Hz), statistical analysis of recordings in humans demonstrated that 95% of bipolar signals are ≥1.67 mV in the left ventricle and ≥1.42 mV in the right ventricle. As a result, 1.5 mV has been used as the standard voltage cutoff for defining bipolar endocardial voltage abnormalities. These data were further validated in human and porcine models of infarction and in isolated human autopsy studies.[12–14] A bipolar electrogram amplitude of 0.5 mV or less represents dense scar, and areas with bipolar amplitude between 0.5 and 1.5 mV represent the border zone (see Figs. 84.1 and 84.2). These voltage definitions correlate well to scar as defined by other imaging modalities, particularly delayed gadolinium enhancement on cardiac magnetic resonance imaging.[15,16] The "protected isthmus" of reentrant VT circuits is typically found within the dense scar, whereas exit sites to the normal endocardium are consistently located at the scar border zone. Voltage mapping may also facilitate identification of "channels" within the infarct. Channels are corridors of preferential conduction through dense scar that can serve as an isthmus during VT. They are indicated by relatively preserved voltage within the dense scar containing late potentials. They may be visualized on the electroanatomical map by lowering the voltage cutoffs on the color isopotential display (see Fig. 84.2).[17–19] It is important to note that a voltage cutoff of 1.5 mV is not absolute; occasionally this cutoff must be increased to incorporate areas of conduction abnormality containing VT circuitry. This is particularly true when the scar is patchy, as in reperfused infarctions. Thus attention must be paid to not only electrogram amplitude but also morphology.

Analogous to endocardial resection, elimination of the VT substrate by catheter ablation during sinus rhythm can be a highly successful strategy. Jais and colleagues identified local abnormal ventricular activities (LAVAs) using a multipolar catheter during sinus rhythm.[20] They then targeted these abnormal potentials with radiofrequency ablation. While LAVAs cannot be eliminated in all patients, those in whom LAVAs are eliminated have better long-term survival, free of VT. Another approach to eliminating the VT substrate is "scar dechanneling."[21] Conducting channels are identified during sinus rhythm, containing delayed electrograms. As one progresses from the scar border zone into the dense scar, the late component of electrograms within the chain becomes more delayed. By ablating the entrance to these conducting channels, the authors describe eliminating entire chains of late potentials, which serve as the protected corridors during VT. We have described core isolation as another way to eliminate the VT substrate without requiring extensive ablation.[22] After identifying components of the VT circuit or surrogates of the VT circuitry recorded in sinus rhythm, a core of endocardium containing these abnormalities is isolated with circumferential ablation. Following core isolation, exit block is demonstrated by pacing within the core and failing to generate a QRS complex with or without evidence of local capture (Fig. 84.3).

As our management of myocardial infarction has improved, with earlier revascularization and better medications to reduce adverse remodeling, infarctions have become smaller and patchier, with less extensive scarring and conduction

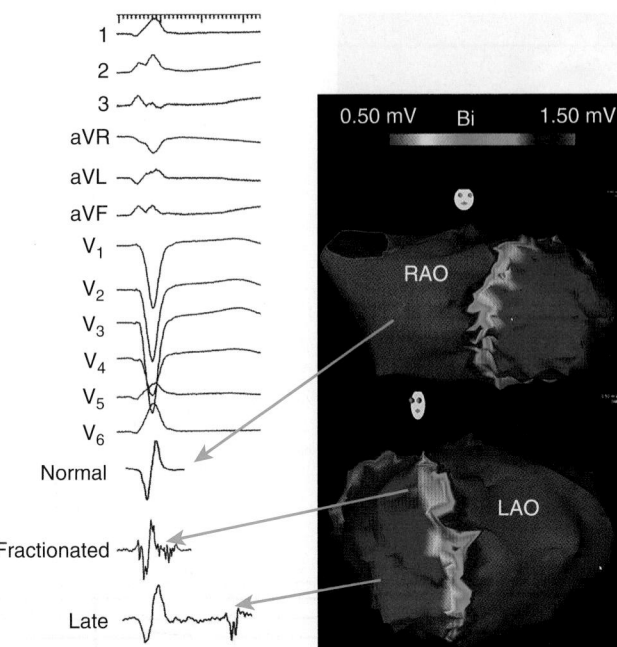

FIGURE 84.1 Electroanatomical map and electrogram morphologies recorded during sinus rhythm in a patient with healed anteroapical myocardial infarction. The surface electrocardiogram demonstrates q waves in leads 1 and aVL, as well as poor R wave progression across the precordium, suggestive of a sizable myocardial infarction. Bipolar voltage mapping confirmed a large area of anteroapical scar, consistent with occlusion of the left anterior descending coronary artery. Bipolar electrogram amplitude of 0.5 mV or less represents dense scar (*red*), and areas with bipolar amplitude between 0.5 and 1.5 mV (*yellow, green,* and *blue*) represent the border zone. Healthy myocardium (>1.5 mV) is colored *purple*. Examples are provided of a normal electrogram recorded from the basal septum as well as fractionated and late electrograms recorded within the dense, apical scar. *LAO,* Left anterior oblique; *RAO,* right anterior oblique.

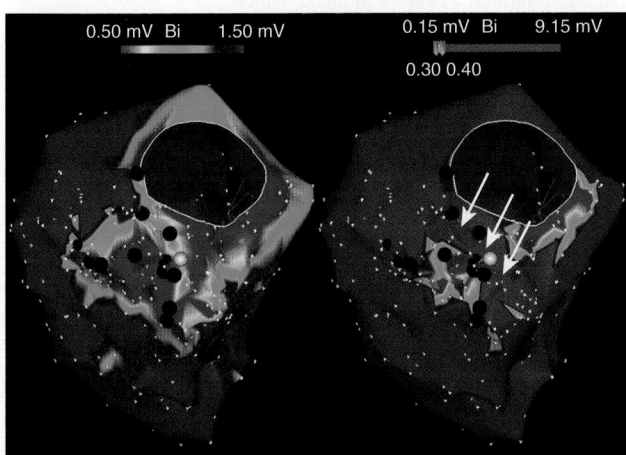

FIGURE 84.2 Electroanatomical map with voltage channel in a patient with healed inferior myocardial infarction. The maps are color coded to represent bipolar electrogram voltage. On the *left* are the standard settings, with *red* representing dense scar (≤0.5 mV), *purple* representing normal voltage (≥1.5 mV), and the intervening colors representing the border zone. This patient had a moderate-sized basal, inferior scar containing late potentials (*black dots*). By lowering the voltage cutoff from 1.5 to 0.4 mV, a channel emerges in the map on the *right* (*white arrows*). This voltage channel contained an isthmus site for the clinical ventricular tachycardia (VT), defined by entrainment (*white dot*). Ablation at this location terminated the clinical VT. Voltage channels that contain late potentials often contain VT isthmuses.

abnormality. Shorter time to reperfusion of myocardial infarction has been associated with lower incidence of acutely inducible VT and of spontaneous VT in follow-up.[23] Furthermore, given less extensive conduction abnormality, the VTs that do occur have shorter cycle lengths and are less tolerated hemodynamically.

Catheter ablation of ischemic VT typically focuses on the endocardium. However, the VT circuit may involve deeper layers of myocardium including the epicardium. This may be particularly relevant in patients with inferior infarction.[24,25] However, even though components of the reentrant circuit may be located on the epicardium, ischemic VT can usually be rendered noninducible with endocardial ablation alone in contrast to nonischemic VT.

Ventricular Tachycardia Mechanisms

Initiation

The predominant mechanism of postinfarction VT is macroreentry, utilizing a protected corridor of slow conduction within the dense scar, which serves as the critical isthmus. The critical isthmus is bounded by two approximately parallel conduction barriers.[26] These conduction barriers can either be anatomical, and therefore present in sinus or paced rhythm, or functional, and thus absent at slower rates.[27]

Evidence for reentry includes the mode of initiation and response to pacing maneuvers during tachycardia. In the majority of cases, VT can be reproducibly initiated with programmed stimulation. In fact, persistent inducibility of VT with programmed stimulation at the conclusion of ablation or during noninvasive programmed stimulation performed several days later portends a high risk of subsequent VT recurrence.[28,29] Pacing adjacent to or within the scar increases the likelihood of induction.[30] There is an inverse relationship between the coupling interval of the extrastimulus and the first tachycardia beat, which results from decrement in the protected zone of slow conduction. While certain anesthetic agents can lengthen refractory periods either directly or by slowing the resting heart rate, induction of reentrant VT is generally not catecholamine dependent, and inducibility of VT does not seem to be impaired by the administration of general anesthesia.[31]

The reentrant circuit has several components, including entrance, isthmus, exit, and outer loop (Fig. 84.4). The wavefront enters the reentrant circuit at the entrance site and then propagates through the critical isthmus during electrical diastole. Because the critical isthmus usually is composed of a small amount of myocardial tissue and is bounded by anatomical or functional barriers preventing spread of the electrical signal, except in the orthodromic direction, propagation of the wavefront in the protected isthmus is silent on the surface electrocardiogram. The wavefront leaves the protected isthmus at the exit site to depolarize the remainder of the ventricles, producing the QRS complex. The reentrant wavefront returns to the entrance site via an outer loop.

Resetting and Entrainment

Pacing during VT can establish reentry as the tachycardia mechanism and can also be used to define the location of the reentrant circuit and thereby identify ablation targets. A premature paced beat can enter the excitable gap of the tachycardia circuit and propagate orthodromically through the entrance, isthmus, and exit sites, thereby advancing the next tachycardia beat (resetting the tachycardia). The paced wavefront simultaneously collides antidromically with the previous tachycardia wavefront. The ability to reset VT with fusion is diagnostic of reentry. Entrainment is the continuous resetting of the reentrant circuit by a train of extrastimuli.[32] Constant fusion when pacing at a fixed

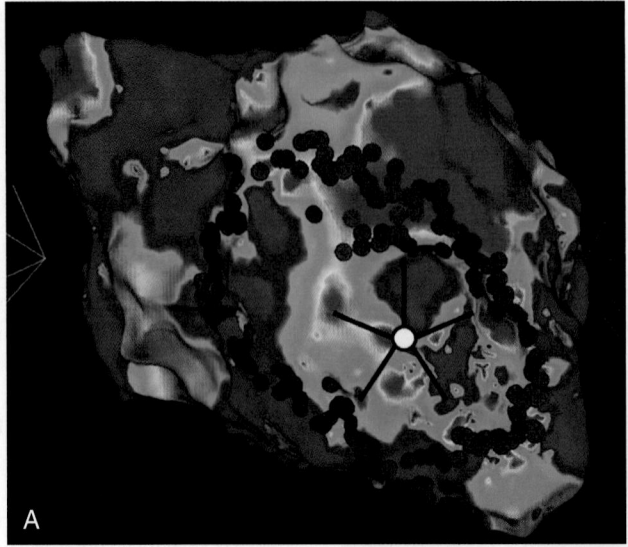

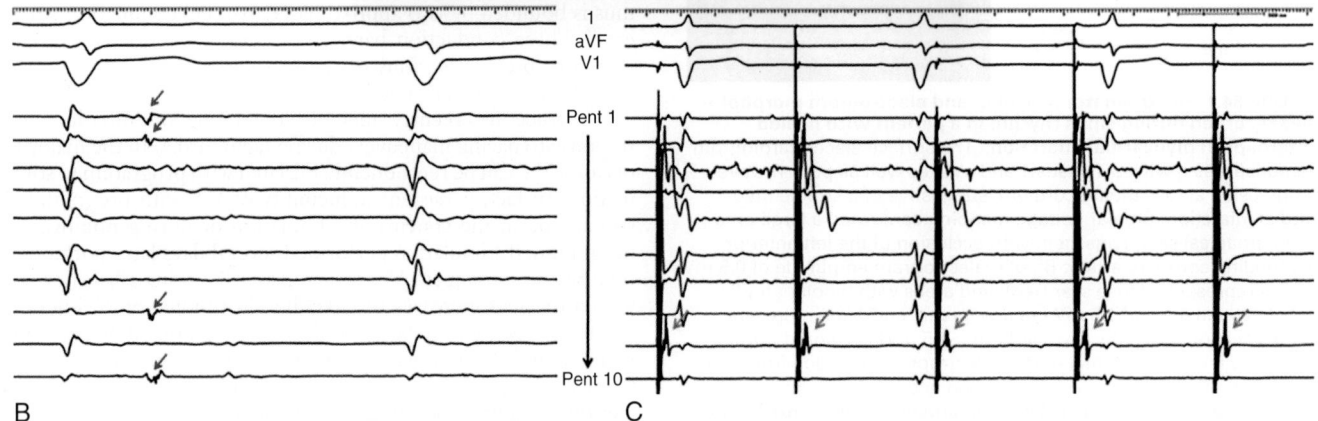

FIGURE 84.3 **Isolation of the ventricular tachycardia (VT) core.** (A) The electroanatomical map demonstrates a patchy anteroseptal infarction. Two rapid, nontolerated VTs were induced, which matched the clinical VTs stored by implantable cardioverter defibrillator electrograms. Perfect pace maps with long stimulus-to-QRS intervals were obtained within the scar. A box lesion was then delivered surrounding the core of low-voltage tissue containing the sites of presumed VT circuitry. The Pentaray catheter (*Pent*) was positioned within the core. (B) Entrance block was achieved with loss of the sharp, local potentials recorded by the Pentaray following the first beat (*red arrows*). (C) Pacing within the core was then performed, capturing the local tissue (*blue arrows*), but not exiting to the ventricle. The VTs were rendered noninducible following core isolation. (Modified from Tzou WS, Frankel DS, Hegeman T, et al. Core isolation of critical arrhythmia elements for treatment of multiple scar-based ventricular tachycardias. *Circ Arrhythm Electrophysiol.* 2015;8:353-361.)

cycle length and progressive fusion when pacing at shorter cycle lengths again are diagnostic of reentry. These maneuvers can be performed quickly and easily and are worthwhile to exclude focal tachycardia mechanisms.

Resetting or entrainment with concealed fusion is defined as orthodromic capture resulting in a surface QRS complex identical to that of tachycardia. Entrainment with concealed fusion suggests that the paced wavefront exits the protected corridor via the VT exit site. Although entrainment with concealed fusion can occur when pacing from critical parts of the VT circuit, it can also occur with pacing from adjacent bystanders. Hence, the positive predictive value of entrainment with concealed fusion in identifying effective ablation sites is only 50% to 60%.[33]

Therefore in addition to concealed fusion, one must also compare the postpacing interval to the tachycardia cycle length. When concealed fusion is present and the postpacing interval is within 30 ms of the tachycardia cycle length, the pacing site is confirmed to be an entrance, isthmus, or exit, rather than an adjacent bystander (see Fig. 84.4). If the postpacing interval is within

30 ms of the tachycardia cycle length, the interval between the pacing stimulus and paced QRS complex should be divided by the tachycardia cycle length. By convention, if this ratio is <0.3, the pacing site is defined as an exit site in the VT circuit.[34] If this ratio is between 0.3 and 0.7, the pacing site is considered an isthmus site. If this ratio is >0.7, the pacing site is an entrance site. To avoid rate-related slowing of the paced wavefront and thereby prolongation of the postpacing interval, the pacing cycle length should be ≤30 ms faster than the VT cycle length. When pacing within the narrow, protected corridor of the tachycardia circuit, the paced wavefront occasionally collides both with the refractory tail of the VT wavefront in the orthodromic direction and the head of the VT wavefront in the antidromic direction, thereby extinguishing the tachycardia without activating the rest of the ventricle. This so-called nonpropagated extrastimulus is highly predictive of a successful ablation site (Fig. 84.5).[35]

Others have described strategies for locating the VT circuitry in the setting of prior infarction by pacing during sinus rhythm.[12] When pacing at the VT exit site, a perfect pace map results in a

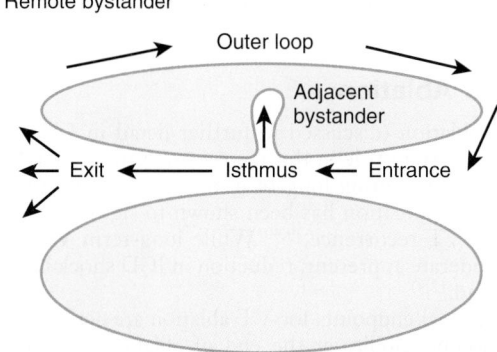

Entrainment site	Concealed	PPI	S-QRS/TCL
Entrance	Y	=TCL	>70%
Isthmus	Y	=TCL	30–70%
Exit	Y	=TCL	<30%
Outer loop	N	=TCL	<30%
Adjacent bystander	Y	>TCL	Variable
Remote bystander	N	>TCL	<30%

FIGURE 84.4 The reentrant ventricular tachycardia (VT) circuit and response to entrainment. The reentrant VT wavefront enters the protected corridor at an entrance site, passes through the isthmus, and exits via an exit site to activate the healthy myocardium and generate the VT QRS complex. While the wavefront slowly traverses the protected corridor, the surface electrocardiogram is electrically silent. The wavefront then returns to the entrance site via an outer loop. Adjacent bystanders branch off the isthmus and dead end; they are not part of the VT circuit. The response to entrainment at each site is provided in the table. *PPI*, Post pacing interval; *S-QRS*, interval from the pacing stimulus to the QRS complex; *TCL*, tachycardia cycle length.

QRS that matches VT and a short stimulus-to-QRS interval. As the pacing site moves toward the isthmus, the stimulus-to-QRS interval increases, but the pace-map QRS morphology remains similar. Importantly, this mapping strategy requires fixed conduction barriers when the pacing rate is slow. Alternatively, pacing can be performed at the tachycardia cycle length. As the pacing site approaches the entrance, the paced wavefront exits antidromically, producing a QRS morphology that differs from VT. de Chillou and colleagues utilized this phenomenon to identify the VT isthmus.[36] When the pace map transitions from an excellent to a poor QRS match over a small distance, the pacing sites likely span the mid-isthmus and are therefore an excellent region to target with transecting ablation. Tung and colleagues described "multiple exit sites," where pacing during sinus rhythm generates alternating QRS morphologies.[37] These sites have access to multiple exits from the dense scar and are therefore likely to be within one or more VT circuits. The authors reported improved outcomes when multiple exit sites were detected from identical or closely approximated pacing sites and then ablated.

Nonreentrant Ventricular Tachycardia Mechanisms

Focal VT mechanisms, including triggered activity and enhanced automaticity, are encountered less commonly (<10%).[38] It is important to recognize these tachycardias because mapping and ablation strategies will differ. Clues to a focal mechanism include initiation by maneuvers that increase cyclic adenosine monophosphate, including straight pacing and infusion of catecholamines. As the pacing cycle length decreases, the interval between the last paced beat and first tachycardia beat shortens in contrast to reentry. Often there is a warm-up period, during which the rate of triggered activity accelerates before reaching a stable cycle length. Most importantly, focal VTs cannot be entrained, only overdriven; constant QRS fusion will not be observed when pacing just faster than VT.

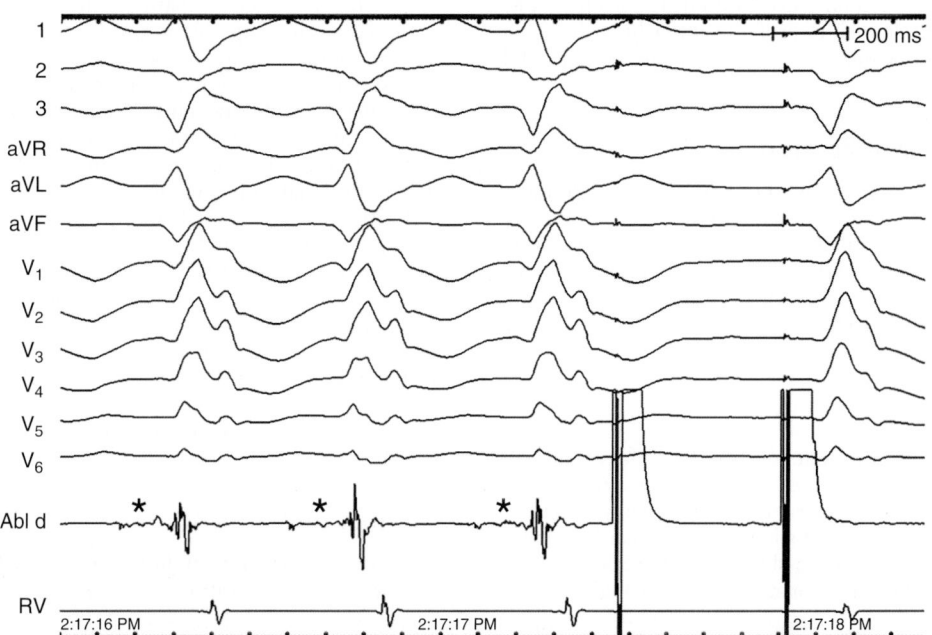

FIGURE 84.5 Nonpropagated extrastimulus. There is an early potential recorded by the ablation catheter (annotated with stars). The first pacing stimulus terminates ventricular tachycardia (VT) without generating a QRS complex (nonpropagated extrastimulus). The second pacing stimulus produces a very close pace map for the VT. A nonpropagated extrastimulus occurs when pacing inside the narrow, protected corridor of the tachycardia circuit. The paced wavefront collides with the refractory tail of the VT wavefront in the orthodromic direction and with the head of the VT wavefront in the antidromic direction, thereby extinguishing the tachycardia.

Clinical Presentation and Acute Management

Only a minority of patients surviving myocardial infarction develop VT, particularly with contemporary advances in prompt revascularization and pharmacotherapy. Nevertheless, with the population aging and more patients surviving myocardial infarction, the total number of patients with ischemic VT continues to increase. While men comprise the large majority of ablation study populations, it is unclear whether this is related to differences in the electroanatomical substrate or referral patterns.[39–42] The time from infarction to first episode of VT is highly variable, ranging from days to many years.

The hemodynamic consequence of VT depends on arrhythmia cycle length and duration, as well as underlying ventricular function. Symptom severity ranges from palpitations and angina to syncope and sudden cardiac death. VT that is poorly tolerated should be promptly treated with direct current cardioversion. For VT that is better tolerated, intravenous amiodarone, lidocaine, and procainamide are the most commonly used medications. One randomized trial found procainamide to be more likely than amiodarone to terminate VT and less likely than amiodarone to exacerbate heart failure, lower blood pressure, or accelerate VT.[43] Also, if catheter ablation is planned, amiodarone administration should be limited to avoid altering the electrophysiological milieu, thereby inhibiting the ability to induce all relevant VTs during ablation. Induction of general anesthesia can be helpful in temporizing VT storm.

Chronic Management and Areas of Uncertainty

Implantable Cardioverter Defibrillator

Implantable cardioverter defibrillators (ICDs) are well established to decrease mortality in appropriately selected patients with ischemic cardiomyopathy, in both primary and secondary prevention settings.[44–48] However, ICD shocks themselves may increase mortality and certainly decrease quality of life.[49] Thus ICDs should be programmed to promote antitachycardia pacing over shocks whenever possible. Further, treatment to reduce ICD therapies is important.

Antiarrhythmic Medications

Amiodarone[50] and sotalol[51] have both been demonstrated to reduce risk of VT recurrence in patients with ICDs. Amiodarone was more effective than sotalol in direct comparison.[52] Chronic amiodarone use can be limited by multiple organ toxicities.[53] Whether amiodarone can be safely reduced or discontinued following apparently successful ablation needs to be defined.

Neuromodulation

Reduction of cardiac sympathetic tone can be useful in the acute management of VT storm, most commonly by induction of general or thoracic epidural anesthesia. Additionally, interest is emerging in chronic spinal cord stimulation and cardiac sympathetic denervation for long-term shock reduction. A case series of patients undergoing left or bilateral stellate ganglionectomy

reported encouraging results,[54] and a multicenter trial is in planning (PREVENT VT).

Catheter Ablation

Catheter ablation (discussed in further detail in Chapter 127) plays an important role in the acute management of VT storm, as well as in preventing long-term recurrences. In randomized trials, catheter ablation has been shown to significantly reduce the risk of VT recurrence.[39,40] While long-term VT-free survival is moderate at present, reduction in ICD shock burden can be profound.[12,41]

The optimal endpoints for VT ablation are actively debated. Clearly noninducibility at the end of ablation of clinical VT, and ideally all VT, is necessary for achieving optimal long-term results.[55] Unfortunately, even when noninducibility of all VT is achieved at the end of ablation, VT may recur during follow-up. Therefore additional endpoints beyond noninducibility at the end of ablation are needed. We and others have demonstrated that noninducibility of VT during noninvasive programmed stimulation performed several days following ablation is a powerful predictor of VT-free survival during follow-up.[29] It has therefore become our practice to repeat ablation when clinical VT is induced during noninvasive programmed stimulation. Achieving other endpoints beyond noninducibility at the end of ablation has also been shown to improve VT-free survival, including elimination of LAVA or late potentials, scar homogenization, and VT core isolation.[20,22,56,57]

ICD shocks are associated with increased mortality, and VT ablation reduces ICD shocks.[39,40,49] Whether VT ablation reduces mortality remains to be proven. Bogun and colleagues pooled data from 1064 patients with ischemic VT undergoing ablation. They found that VT noninducibility at the end of ablation was associated with lower rates of VT recurrence during follow-up and, more importantly, improved survival.[28] Tung and colleagues combined data from 2061 patients with structural heart disease undergoing VT ablation, including 1095 with ischemic cardiomyopathy. Those without VT recurrence in the year following ablation were significantly more likely to survive compared with those with VT recurrence. It could be argued that VT is merely a marker of more advanced heart failure rather than an important cause of death. Arguing for causality, the improvement in survival was observed within each New York Heart Association heart failure class and remained robust after multivariate adjustment.

Lastly, the timing of ablation is likely important. Reddy and colleagues demonstrated that compared with standard care, VT ablation at the time of ICD implant reduces ICD therapies during follow-up.[39] We and others have demonstrated in an observational fashion that earlier ablation is associated with improved outcomes compared with later ablation.[58,59] To confirm the effect of ablation timing on VT-free survival, and ultimately, the impact of ablation on mortality, adequately powered randomized trials are needed. The results of the PARTITA and BERLIN trials are eagerly awaited.

Acknowledgment

The authors wish to thank Jeffrey Stiffler, CCDS, CEPS, for his assistance with preparation of figures.

REFERENCES

1. de Bakker JM, van Capelle FJ, Janse MJ, et al. Slow conduction in the infarcted human heart. 'Zigzag' course of activation. *Circulation*. 1993;88:915–926.
2. Josephson ME, Wit AL. Fractionated electrical activity and continuous electrical activity: fact or artifact? *Circulation*. 1984;70:529–532.
3. Fenoglio Jr JJ, Pham TD, Harken AH, Horowitz LN, Josephson ME, Wit AL. Recurrent sustained ventricular tachycardia: structure and ultrastructure of subendocardial regions in which tachycardia originates. *Circulation*. 1983;68:518–533.
4. de Bakker JM, Coronel R, Tasseron S, et al. Ventricular tachycardia in the infarcted, Langendorff-perfused human heart: role of the arrangement of surviving cardiac fibers. *J Am Coll Cardiol*. 1990;15:1594–1607.
5. Roy D, Marchand E, Theroux P, et al. Long-term reproducibility and significance of provokable ventricular arrhythmias after myocardial infarction. *J Am Coll Cardiol*. 1986;8:32–39.
6. Marchlinski FE, Waxman HL, Buxton AE, Josephson ME. Sustained ventricular tachyarrhythmias during the early postinfarction period: electrophysiologic findings and prognosis for survival. *J Am Coll Cardiol*. 1983;2:240–250.
7. Haqqani HM, Kalman JM, Roberts-Thomson KC, et al. Fundamental differences in electrophysiologic and electroanatomic substrate between ischemic cardiomyopathy patients with and without clinical ventricular tachycardia. *J Am Coll Cardiol*. 2009;54:166–173.
8. Guiraudon G, Fontaine G, Frank R, Escande G, Etievent P, Cabrol C. Encircling endocardial ventriculotomy: a new surgical treatment for life-threatening ventricular tachycardias resistant to medical treatment following myocardial infarction. *Ann Thorac Surg*. 1978;26:438–444.
9. Josephson ME, Harken AH, Horowitz LN. Endocardial excision: a new surgical technique for the treatment of recurrent ventricular tachycardia. *Circulation*. 1979;60:1430–1439.
10. Miller JM, Tyson GS, Hargrove 3rd WC, Vassallo JA, Rosenthal ME, Josephson ME. Effect of subendocardial resection on sinus rhythm endocardial electrogram abnormalities. *Circulation*. 1995;91:2385–2391.
11. Cassidy DM, Vassallo JA, Miller JM, et al. Endocardial catheter mapping in patients in sinus rhythm: relationship to underlying heart disease and ventricular arrhythmias. *Circulation*. 1986;73:645–652.
12. Marchlinski FE, Callans DJ, Gottlieb CD, Zado E. Linear ablation lesions for control of unmappable ventricular tachycardia in patients with ischemic and nonischemic cardiomyopathy. *Circulation*. 2000;101:1288–1296.
13. Callans DJ, Ren JF, Michele J, Marchlinski FE, Dillon SM. Electroanatomic left ventricular mapping in the porcine model of healed anterior myocardial infarction. Correlation with intracardiac echocardiography and pathological analysis. *Circulation*. 1999;100:1744–1750.
14. Koa-Wing M, Ho SY, Kojodjojo P, Peters NS, Davies DW, Kanagaratnam P. Radiofrequency ablation of infarct scar-related ventricular tachycardia: correlation of electroanatomical data with post-mortem histology. *J Cardiovasc Electrophysiol*. 2007;18:1330–1333.
15. Codreanu A, Odille F, Aliot E, et al. Electroanatomic characterization of post-infarct scars comparison with 3-dimensional myocardial scar reconstruction based on magnetic resonance imaging. *J Am Coll Cardiol*. 2008;52:839–842.
16. Gupta S, Desjardins B, Baman T, et al. Delayed-enhanced MR scar imaging and intraprocedural registration into an electroanatomical mapping system in post-infarction patients. *JACC Cardiovasc Imaging*. 2012;5:207–210.
17. Arenal A, del Castillo S, Gonzalez-Torrecilla E, et al. Tachycardia-related channel in the scar tissue in patients with sustained monomorphic ventricular tachycardias: influence of the voltage scar definition. *Circulation*. 2004;110:2568–2574.
18. Hsia HH, Lin D, Sauer WH, Callans DJ, Marchlinski FE. Anatomic characterization of endocardial substrate for hemodynamically stable reentrant ventricular tachycardia: identification of endocardial conducting channels. *Heart Rhythm*. 2006;3:503–512.
19. Mountantonakis SE, Park RE, Frankel DS, et al. Relationship between voltage map "channels" and the location of critical isthmus sites in patients with post-infarction cardiomyopathy and ventricular tachycardia. *J Am Coll Cardiol*. 2013;61:2088–2095.

20. Jais P, Maury P, Khairy P, et al. Elimination of local abnormal ventricular activities: a new end point for substrate modification in patients with scar-related ventricular tachycardia. *Circulation*. 2012;125:2184–2196.
21. Berruezo A, Fernandez-Armenta J, Andreu D, et al. Scar dechanneling: new method for scar-related left ventricular tachycardia substrate ablation. *Circ Arrhythm Electrophysiol*. 2015;8:326–336.
22. Tzou WS, Frankel DS, Hegeman T, et al. Core isolation of critical arrhythmia elements for treatment of multiple scar-based ventricular tachycardias. *Circ Arrhythm Electrophysiol*. 2015;8:353–361.
23. Kumar S, Sivagangabalan G, Thiagalingam A, et al. Effect of reperfusion time on inducible ventricular tachycardia early and spontaneous ventricular arrhythmias late after ST elevation myocardial infarction treated with primary percutaneous coronary intervention. *Heart Rhythm*. 2011;8:493–499.
24. Schmidt B, Chun KR, Baensch D, et al. Catheter ablation for ventricular tachycardia after failed endocardial ablation: epicardial substrate or inappropriate endocardial ablation? *Heart Rhythm*. 2010;7:1746–1752.
25. Yoshiga Y, Mathew S, Wissner E, et al. Correlation between substrate location and ablation strategy in patients with ventricular tachycardia late after myocardial infarction. *Heart Rhythm*. 2012;9:1192–1199.
26. de Chillou C, Lacroix D, Klug D, et al. Isthmus characteristics of reentrant ventricular tachycardia after myocardial infarction. *Circulation*. 2002;105:726–731.
27. Josephson M, Anter E. Substrate mapping for ventricular tachycardia: assumptions and misconceptions. *JACC Clin Electrophysiol*. 2015;1:342–352.
28. Yokokawa M, Kim HM, Baser K, et al. Predictive value of programmed ventricular stimulation after catheter ablation of post-infarction ventricular tachycardia. *J Am Coll Cardiol*. 2015;65:1954–1959.
29. Frankel DS, Mountantonakis SE, Zado ES, et al. Noninvasive programmed ventricular stimulation early after ventricular tachycardia ablation to predict risk of late recurrence. *J Am Coll Cardiol*. 2012;59:1529–1535.
30. Morady F, Hess D, Scheinman MM. Electrophysiologic drug testing in patients with malignant ventricular arrhythmias: importance of stimulation at more than one ventricular site. *Am J Cardiol*. 1982;50:1055–1060.
31. Nof E, Reichlin T, Enriquez AD, et al. Impact of general anesthesia on initiation and stability of VT during catheter ablation. *Heart Rhythm*. 2015;12:2213–2220.
32. Josephson M. *Clinical Cardiac Electrophysiology: Techniques and Interpretations*. 5th ed. Philadelphia: Lippincott Williams & Wilkins; 2015.
33. Morton JB, Sanders P, Deen V, Vohra JK, Kalman JM. Sensitivity and specificity of concealed entrainment for the identification of a critical isthmus in the atrium: relationship to rate, anatomic location and antidromic penetration. *J Am Coll Cardiol*. 2002;39:896–906.
34. Stevenson WG, Khan H, Sager P, et al. Identification of reentry circuit sites during catheter mapping and radiofrequency ablation of ventricular tachycardia late after myocardial infarction. *Circulation*. 1993;88:1647–1670.
35. Altemose GT, Miller JM. Termination of ventricular tachycardia by a nonpropagated extrastimulus. *J Cardiovasc Electrophysiol*. 2000;11:125.
36. de Chillou C, Groben L, Magnin-Poull I, et al. Localizing the critical isthmus of postinfarct ventricular tachycardia: the value of pace-mapping during sinus rhythm. *Heart Rhythm*. 2014;11:175–181.
37. Tung R, Mathuria N, Michowitz Y, et al. Functional pace-mapping responses for identification of targets for catheter ablation of scar-mediated ventricular tachycardia. *Circ Arrhythm Electrophysiol*. 2012;5:264–272.
38. Das MK, Scott LR, Miller JM. Focal mechanism of ventricular tachycardia in coronary artery disease. *Heart Rhythm*. 2010;7:305–311.
39. Reddy VY, Reynolds MR, Neuzil P, et al. Prophylactic catheter ablation for the prevention of defibrillator therapy. *N Engl J Med*. 2007;357:2657–2665.
40. Kuck KH, Schaumann A, Eckardt L, et al. Catheter ablation of stable ventricular tachycardia before defibrillator implantation in patients with coronary heart disease (VTACH): a multicentre randomised controlled trial. *Lancet*. 2010;375:31–40.
41. Stevenson WG, Wilber DJ, Natale A, et al. Irrigated radiofrequency catheter ablation guided by electroanatomic mapping for recurrent ventricular tachycardia after myocardial infarction: the multicenter thermocool ventricular tachycardia ablation trial. *Circulation*. 2008;118:2773–2782.

42. Calkins H, Epstein A, Packer D, et al. Catheter ablation of ventricular tachycardia in patients with structural heart disease using cooled radiofrequency energy: results of a prospective multicenter study. Cooled RF Multi Center Investigators Group. *J Am Coll Cardiol*. 2000;35:1905–1914.
43. Ortiz M, Martín A, Arribas F, et al. PROCAMIO Study Investigators. Randomized comparison of intravenous procainamide vs. intravenous amiodarone for the acute treatment of tolerated wide QRS tachycardia: the PROCAMIO study. *Eur Heart J*. 2016 Jun 28. pii: ehw230. [Epub ahead of print].
44. A comparison of antiarrhythmic-drug therapy with implantable defibrillators in patients resuscitated from near-fatal ventricular arrhythmias. The Antiarrhythmics versus Implantable Defibrillators (AVID) Investigators. *N Engl J Med*. 1997;337:1576–1583.
45. Connolly SJ, Gent M, Roberts RS, et al. Canadian implantable defibrillator study (CIDS): a randomized trial of the implantable cardioverter-defibrillator against amiodarone. *Circulation*. 2000;101:1297–1302.
46. Kuck KH, Cappato R, Siebels J, Ruppel R. Randomized comparison of antiarrhythmic drug therapy with implantable defibrillators in patients resuscitated from cardiac arrest: the Cardiac Arrest Study Hamburg (CASH). *Circulation*. 2000;102:748–754.
47. Moss AJ, Zareba W, Hall WJ, et al. Prophylactic implantation of a defibrillator in patients with myocardial infarction and reduced ejection fraction. *N Engl J Med*. 2002;346:877–883.
48. Buxton AE, Lee KL, DiCarlo L, et al. Electrophysiologic testing to identify patients with coronary artery disease who are at risk for sudden death. Multicenter Unsustained Tachycardia Trial Investigators. *N Engl J Med*. 2000;342:1937–1945.
49. Moss AJ, Schuger C, Beck CA, et al. Reduction in inappropriate therapy and mortality through ICD programming. *N Engl J Med*. 2012;367:2275–2283.
50. Kowey PR, Crijns HJ, Aliot EM, et al. Efficacy and safety of celivarone, with amiodarone as calibrator, in patients with an implantable cardioverter-defibrillator for prevention of implantable cardioverter-defibrillator interventions or death: the ALPHEE study. *Circulation*. 2011;124:2649–2660.
51. Pacifico A, Hohnloser SH, Williams JH, et al. Prevention of implantable-defibrillator shocks by treatment with sotalol. d,l-Sotalol Implantable Cardioverter-Defibrillator Study Group. *N Engl J Med*. 1999;340:1855–1862.
52. Connolly SJ, Dorian P, Roberts RS, et al. Comparison of beta-blockers, amiodarone plus beta-blockers, or sotalol for prevention of shocks from implantable cardioverter defibrillators: the OPTIC Study: a randomized trial. *JAMA*. 2006;295:165–171.
53. Vassallo P, Trohman RG. Prescribing amiodarone: an evidence-based review of clinical indications. *JAMA*. 2007;298:1312–1322.
54. Vaseghi M, Gima J, Kanaan C, et al. Cardiac sympathetic denervation in patients with refractory ventricular arrhythmias or electrical storm: intermediate and long-term follow-up. *Heart Rhythm*. 2014;11:360–366.
55. Ghanbari H, Baser K, Yokokawa M, et al. Noninducibility in postinfarction ventricular tachycardia as an end point for ventricular tachycardia ablation and its effects on outcomes: a meta-analysis. *Circ Arrhythm Electrophysiol*. 2014;7:677–683.
56. Silberbauer J, Oloriz T, Maccabelli G, et al. Noninducibility and late potential abolition: a novel combined prognostic procedural end point for catheter ablation of postinfarction ventricular tachycardia. *Circ Arrhythm Electrophysiol*. 2014;7:424–435.
57. Di Biase L, Santangeli P, Burkhardt DJ, et al. Endoepicardial homogenization of the scar versus limited substrate ablation for the treatment of electrical storms in patients with ischemic cardiomyopathy. *J Am Coll Cardiol*. 2012;60:132–141.
58. Frankel DS, Mountantonakis SE, Robinson MR, Zado ES, Callans DJ, Marchlinski FE. Ventricular tachycardia ablation remains treatment of last resort in structural heart disease: argument for earlier intervention. *J Cardiovasc Electrophysiol*. 2011;22:1123–1128.
59. Dinov B, Arya A, Bertagnolli L, et al. Early referral for ablation of scar-related ventricular tachycardia is associated with improved acute and long-term outcomes: results from the Heart Center of Leipzig ventricular tachycardia registry. *Circ Arrhythm Electrophysiol*. 2014;7:1144–1151.

85 Ventricular Tachycardia in Patients With Dilated Cardiomyopathy

Borislav Dinov, Arash Arya, and Gerhard Hindricks

Definition, Etiology, and Genetics of Dilated Cardiomyopathy

Dilated cardiomyopathy (DCM) is a disease of the heart muscle that is characterized by heart chamber dilation and usually progressive decrease of heart contractility. It most typically affects the left ventricle, but the right ventricle can be involved as well.[1] DCM can present with symptoms of heart failure and is the most frequent reason for heart transplantation. However, ventricular and supraventricular arrhythmias can also be the first manifestation of DCM. Sudden cardiac death (SCD) is an important cause of mortality in DCM. The Olmsted County Study estimated DCM prevalence at 35.5/100,000 inhabitants.

The current understanding recognizes that DCM is not a distinct clinical entity and distinguishes between primary and secondary DCM on the basis of etiology. The most frequent causes of secondary DCM are as follows: toxins (ethanol, heavy metals, anthracyclines, cocaine, and amphetamine); nutrition (tiamin and carnitin deficiency and starvation); infections (viral and Chagas disease); systemic diseases (sarcoidosis, systemic sclerosis, lupus erythematosus, and vasculitis); valvular diseases (mitral and aortic regurgitation); endocrine disorders (diabetes mellitus, hyper- and hypothyroidism, and hyper- and hypoparathyroidism); and peripartum DCM, infiltrative DCM (amyloidosis and glycogen storage disease), burned-out hypertrophic cardiomyopathy, and hypertension. Moreover, multiple causes can be responsible for each individual case. Usually, DCM as a consequence of myocardial infarction or significant coronary artery disease is regarded as a separate clinical entity. However, overlap between ischemic and "nonischemic" DCM can be observed as well. To find a specific cause for DCM is often difficult but important for successful treatment of a potentially reversible condition. Patients without an identifiable cause are classified as having primary DCM. A careful screening of the family history and genetic makeup can identify distinct genetic mutations in up to 48% of primary DCM patients.[2]

The rapid evolution of genetics in the last decades changed the understanding about the molecular pathophysiology of DCM. Mutations in genes encoding different cytoskeletal and sarcomeric proteins cause DCM in most familial forms of DCM. Genetic testing is becoming increasingly available for confirmation of the diagnosis and for screening of patient's relatives. However, the diagnostic yield of genetic testing in DCM remains relatively low. The most frequently identified gene in DCM associated with atrioventricular (AV) block is *laminin A/C*.[3] Other frequently identified genes are *TAZ*,[4] *ZASP*,[5] *β-sarcoglycan*,[6] *β-myosin heavy chain*, *myosin-binding protein C*, *actin*, *cardiac troponin T and C*,[7,8] *desmin*[9] and in men, *dystrophin*.[10] Autosomal-dominant inheritance is the predominant pattern of transmission in familial DCM, with X-linked, autosomal-recessive, and mitochondrial inheritance being less common.

Familial Forms of Dilated Cardiomyopathy Associated With Arrhythmias or Conduction Disturbances

LMNA-Associated Dilated Cardiomyopathy

LMNA-associated DCM is a form of DCM associated with mutations in the *LMNA* gene, which encodes the nuclear envelope protein laminin A/C.[3,11] This cardiolaminopathy has an autosomal-dominant inheritance pattern with high (almost 100%) penetrance.[12] The initial manifestation of the disease is AV block that progresses to complete AV block. Heart failure symptoms usually follow conduction disturbances by several years. Patients with severely reduced contractile function have higher risk of ventricular tachycardias (VTs) and SCD. Premature supraventricular beats and eventually atrial fibrillation are a frequent presentation of *LMNA*-associated DCM. The genetic screening for *LMNA* mutation is widely available.

TTN-Associated Dilated Cardiomyopathy

TTN-associated DCM is a form of DCM associated with mutations in the *TTN* (*titin*) gene. Furthermore, it is a common form of familial DCM that is usually not accompanied by conduction disturbances of the heart or by skeletal muscle abnormalities.[13]

X-Linked Forms of Dilated Cardiomyopathy

Two distinct forms of X-linked DCM are well described: the X-linked DCM, which presents in adolescence, and Barth syndrome.[14] The first one is caused by mutation in the dystrophin gene and affects young males. Death usually occurs due to end-stage heart failure or ventricular arrhythmias. Mutations in the dystrophin gene are also responsible for Duchenne and Becker muscular dystrophy, in which DCM can occur along with skeletal muscular dystrophy.[15] In Barth syndrome, mutations in the

TAZ (*tafazzin*) gene cause DCM, presenting with heart failure, neutropenia, and acidosis.[16] Arrhythmias are also a frequent presentation.

Dilated Cardiomyopathy Associated With Mutations in the Genes Encoding Ion Channels

Mutations in the *PLN* (*phospholamban*) gene, which encodes a protein that inhibits the cardiac sarcoplasmic reticulum Ca^{2+}-adenosine triphosphatase (SERCA2a) pump, can cause a phenotype of DCM or arrhythmogenic right ventricular cardiomyopathy.[17] In a study, *PLN* R14del mutation was found in up to 15% of patients with "idiopathic" DCM that was associated with an early onset of SCD.[18,19] Lately, missense sodium voltage-gated channel alpha subunit 5 (*SCN5A*) mutations have been identified in members of families with DCM.[20] *SCN5A* mutation carriers show a high prevalence of ventricular and supraventricular arrhythmias and conduction disturbances.

Ventricular Arrhythmias in Nonischemic Dilated Cardiomyopathy

Different types of ventricular arrhythmias have been observed in patients with DCM. Holter electrocardiogram (ECG) studies reported premature ventricular beats (PVBs) in up to 90% of patients with DCM.[20a] Although nonsustained VT is observed in 40% to 60% of patients with DCM, occurrence of sustained VT is described in only 5% of patients with this disease.[21] Most of the monomorphic sustained VTs are caused by a reentry mechanism and are scar related. Polymorphic ventricular arrhythmias are also frequently observed and are likely caused by triggered activity.

Bundle Branch Reentry Ventricular Tachycardia

Bundle branch reentry VT (BBRVT) is a macroreentry VT involving the His–Purkinje system, usually with antegrade conduction over the right bundle branch and retrograde conduction over the left bundle branch. This tachycardia, although rare in the general population, is described in up to 41% of patients with idiopathic DCM. It is usually rapid, and patients frequently present with syncope due to hemodynamic deterioration. Typically, the surface ECG presents a wide complex tachycardia with left bundle branch block QRS morphology that resembles the QRS morphology in sinus rhythm. BBRVT must be differentiated from supraventricular tachycardia with aberrancy, from antidromic tachycardia using Mahaim tract, and from myocardial VT.

A stable intracardiac signal from His bundle potential is crucial for confirming the diagnosis. Characteristically, a His deflection precedes every QRS complex during BBRVT (a positive HV interval VT), and the HV interval during BBRVT exceeds the HV interval in sinus rhythm. Additionally, in BBRVT with left bundle branch block pattern, the right bundle potentials will precede the His deflection; in BBRVT with right bundle branch block pattern, the right bundle potential will occur after the His deflection. Importantly, spontaneous tachycardia cycle length variations are preceded by similar H-H interval variations. The recognition of BBRVT is important because ablation of the right bundle branch is curative for this type of VT. However, BBRVT is rarely the sole inducible and clinically relevant VT in patients with DCM.

Tachycardia-Induced Dilated Cardiomyopathy

Ventricular arrhythmias, particularly PVBs, can be not only a consequence but also the primary cause of DCM. A PVB-induced cardiomyopathy can be suspected in patients with high arrhythmia

burden after exclusion of other causes of DCM.[22] Programmed ventricular stimulation (PVS)-associated ventricular asynchrony, neurohumoral changes, and alterations in intracellular Ca^{2+} handling have been proposed as explanations for the development of PVS-induced cardiomyopathy. Although, PVB burden and symptom duration are the most important predictors of tachycardiomyopathy, many patients with high arrhythmia burden retain a normal left ventricular (LV) function over time. In a recent report of 45 patients with frequent premature ventricular complexes (PVCs) (defined as >10% PVC burden), cardiomyopathy developed in 38% of the cases.[23] In this study, patients in whom cardiomyopathy developed had a broader PVC-QRS complex (>150 ms) and a broader sinus rhythm QRS duration. Obviously, the ventricular arrhythmia burden is not the only determinant of the PVB-induced cardiomyopathy. Numerous experimental and clinical data suggest that PVB-QRS duration, site of origin, and coupling intervals can also contribute to the worsening of the cardiac function.[24] There were two patient series that related frequent PVCs originating from the ventricular outflow tracts to LV dilatation.[25,26] Yarlagadda and colleagues demonstrated that patients with frequent right ventricular outflow tract (RVOT) PVBs can develop cardiomyopathy, which can be reversed by an effective ablation procedure.[27]

Sudden Cardiac Death Risk Stratification in Nonischemic Dilated Cardiomyopathy

Nonischemic DCM (NIDCM) is associated with up to 20% estimated mortality in 3 years, with advanced heart failure and SCD accounting for most mortality cases.[28] In a meta-analysis of implantable cardioverter defibrillator (ICD) trials in patients with NIDCM, there was a 31% reduction in mortality with ICD therapy, indicating that VT/ventricular fibrillation (VF) is an important cause of death in this disease.[29] In contrast with ischemic cardiomyopathy, the arrhythmogenesis in NIDCM is less well understood and is likely multifactorial. A complex interaction between structural abnormalities, such as fibrosis and LV dilatation, and electrophysiological alterations may play a role in the occurrence of VT/VF. As a consequence, multiple structural parameters, arrhythmia characteristics, depolarization and repolarization abnormalities, and autonomic disturbances have been studied as predictors for SCD in NIDCM.

In a retrospective study of 137 children with NIDCM, repolarization abnormalities were a common finding. Prolongation of the JTc interval ≥390 ms and the QTc interval ≥510 ms as well as abnormal T wave inversion were associated with life-threatening arrhythmic events.[30] A recent meta-analysis of 45 studies enrolling 6088 patients with NIDCM evaluated the association between SCD and different predictive tests such as baroreflex sensitivity, heart rate variability, heart rate turbulence, signal-averaged ECG, QRS duration, QRS fragmentation, LV ejection fraction (LVEF), LV end-diastolic dimension, nonsustained VT, electrophysiology study, T-wave alternans, and QRS–T wave angle. Altogether, the sensitivity and specificity of these tests for prediction of SCD were modest, with T-wave alternans having the highest sensitivity but low specificity for prediction of SCD: 91% and 36%, respectively. On the other hand, the induction of VT/VF during an electrophysiology study had a poor sensitivity but a high specificity for arrhythmic events and SCD: 29% and 87% respectively. The odds ratio (OR) was the highest for QRS fragmentation (OR 6.73; 95% confidence interval [CI], 3.85–11.76) and T-wave alternans (OR, 4.66; 95% CI, 2.55–8.53) and the lowest for QRS duration (OR, 1.51; 95% CI, 1.13–2.01). None of the autonomic parameters (heart rate variability, baroreflex sensitivity, and heart rate turbulence) was predictive for SCD in NIDCM. These findings suggest that disturbances in autonomic tone do not appear promising for SCD risk stratification in DCM.[31] Some novel parameters can be useful for predicting the probability of death in patients with DCM. In a recent study of 55 patients with NIDCM who underwent catheter ablation, the size of the endocardial unipolar voltage area (cutoff >145 cm^2) was associated with an increased probability for cardiac death (area under the curve [AUC] 0.89, $p < .0001$; 83% sensitivity and 78% specificity) after adjustment for the LVEF.[32]

Left Ventricular Ejection Fraction and New York Heart Association Functional Class

Current guidelines for ICD implantation in patients with DCM rely on imprecise parameters of depressed LVEF and New York Heart Association (NYHA) functional class. These criteria are neither specific nor sensitive enough to adequately identify the patients at risk for SCD.[33] Indeed, epidemiological observations imply that many SCDs occur in patients with an LVEF >35%. Moreover, in patients with DCM and ICD implanted for primary prevention of SCD, less than one-third receive an appropriate shock.[34] Measurement of the LV longitudinal strain using speckle tracking is a promising echocardiographic tool to identify patients at high risk for malignant VT/VF. Recently, we showed in 20 patients with NIDCM that LV mechanical dispersion was significantly greater in patients with VT/VF than in those without arrhythmias (84 ± 31 ms vs. 53 ± 16 ms, $p = .017$). Furthermore a mechanical dispersion >50 ms was associated with 12 times higher risk of VT/VF in patients with NIDCM (OR, 12.5; 95% CI, 1.1–143.4).[35]

The prevalence of complex ventricular arrhythmias has been shown to increase from 15%–20% in NYHA class I–II to 50%–70% in NYHA IV. Although the likelihood of SCD increases with the NYHA functional class as well, ventricular arrhythmias are not the only cause of SCD in patients with NIDCM. In a small observational study, bradycardia or electromechanical dissociation were the most common initial presentations leading to SCD in patients with NIDCM.[36] Other nonarrhythmic causes can be precipitators of sudden death in NIDCM as well.

Role of Cardiac Magnetic Resonance Imaging in Risk Stratification for Sudden Cardiac Death

There is growing evidence demonstrating the value of cardiac magnetic resonance (CMR) in identifying patients at risk for SCD. One of the greatest achievements of CMR is the ability to visualize myocardial scar using the late gadolinium enhancement (LGE) technique. Among patients with DCM, up to 71% have a scar with a mid-wall pattern and, less commonly, an epicardial scar. Unlike with ischemic cardiomyopathy, subendocardial LGE is infrequently observed in DCM. Several studies with different endpoints evaluated the role of CMR in risk stratifying for SCD in DCM. Although these studies have different endpoints, they demonstrate that presence of LGE was independently associated with increased likelihood for major adverse events.[37–41] Moreover, the scar size (cutoff >5% of the LV mass) and transmurality are strong predictors for SCD or for ICD therapy in DCM patients.[42] In patients with postinflammatory DCM, CMR can visualize scar on LGE in the chronic phase or tissue edema using T2 mapping in the acute phase. In the study by Grun and colleagues, none of the patients without LGE experienced SCD, irrespective of LVEF and LV volumes.[43] In patients with Chagas disease and a history of VT, LGE might be present in up to 69%.[44] However, in a small study, an LVEF of <40%, but not LGE, was the only predictor of SCD.[45]

Along with areas of dense scar, diffuse myocardial fibrosis can be frequently observed in DCM and may serve as a substrate for VT. An accurate assessment of diffuse LV fibrosis is not possible using conventional LGE-CMR since it relies on an arbitrary scale of the relative signal intensity difference between regions of dense scar and regions of user-defined "normal" tissue. Myocardial

tissue characterization using T1 mapping has the potential to overcome the limitations of the conventional contrast-enhanced CMR. Several studies have shown a good correlation between the T1-derived extracellular volume and quantitative histological measurements.[46–48] A recent study showed that native myocardial T1 is independently associated with appropriate ICD therapy in patients with DCM.[49]

Sarcoidosis is a frequently unrecognized cause of DCM, and LGE-CMR can be extremely sensitive in detecting cardiac involvement. Patel and colleagues showed that patients with sarcoidosis and LGE in CMR had an 11.5-fold higher unadjusted rate of cardiac death than those without LGE.[50] Although LGE allows earlier detection of cardiac involvement, the association with SCD beyond LVEF remains ill-defined. Moreover, LGE areas may disappear after treatment, suggesting that risk assessment on the basis of single CMR might be inappropriate. However, patients with histologically proven sarcoidosis and VT inducible with PVS had a greater likelihood of spontaneous VT or death.[51] The current practice is to implant an ICD in patients with cardiac sarcoidosis who exhibit sustain VTs, irrespective of the scar observed via CMR.

Although CMR provides a unique opportunity to visualize and quantify the myocardial scar, its implementation for risk stratification requires a greater level of evidence and uniform endpoints. Furthermore, application of CMR in patients with devices remains, in general, contraindicated. However, CMR (1.5 T) may be performed in patients with magnetic resonance imaging (MRI)-compatible devices as long as patients are not device dependent and receive appropriate device interrogation before and after CMR.[52,53]

Electroanatomical Substrate for Ventricular Tachycardia in Patients With Dilated Cardiomyopathy

Consistent with older pathological findings from necropsy studies, CMR detects fibrosis in 40%–50% of patients with idiopathic DCM. It is usually patchy, midmyocardial or epicardial, does not correspond to specific coronary territory, and commonly affects the basal segments of the LV.[39,40,54,55] Increased fibrosis in the heart predisposes to both atrial and ventricular arrhythmias. Myocardial fiber disarray, loss of gap junctions, and slow longitudinal and transmural myocardial conduction play a role in the initiation and perpetuation of VT. In DCM, VT inducibility by PVS was associated with transmurality of the visible LGE in CMR scans.[39] Furthermore, patients with a larger scar and larger border zones are at a higher risk for VT.[56] In addition to fibrosis, several other factors such as increased dispersion of refractoriness, alterations in action potential duration, and increased sympathetic activity further enhance the susceptibility for ventricular arrhythmias.

Areas of fibrosis in DCM can be visualized indirectly using bipolar and unipolar electroanatomical voltage mapping. Similar to ischemic cardiomyopathy, low-amplitude and fragmented electrograms can be recorded in the scar regions. However, the VT substrate in NIDCM exhibits some peculiarities in the special distribution and electrophysiological properties. Hsia and colleagues described that low-amplitude areas having voltage <1.8 mV were typically confined to basal and lateral aspects of the left ventricle.[57] Subsequent studies demonstrated that in a significant proportion of patients with NIDCM, the arrhythmogenic substrate is located entirely intramurally or epicardially.[58,59] In such cases, the scar may remain undetected during endocardial bipolar voltage mapping, and its visualization would require unipolar voltage mapping or epicardial mapping (Fig. 85.1). Unipolar voltage mapping with low-amplitude definition (<8.3 mV for the left ventricle and <5.5 mV for the right ventricle) might be useful to predict the

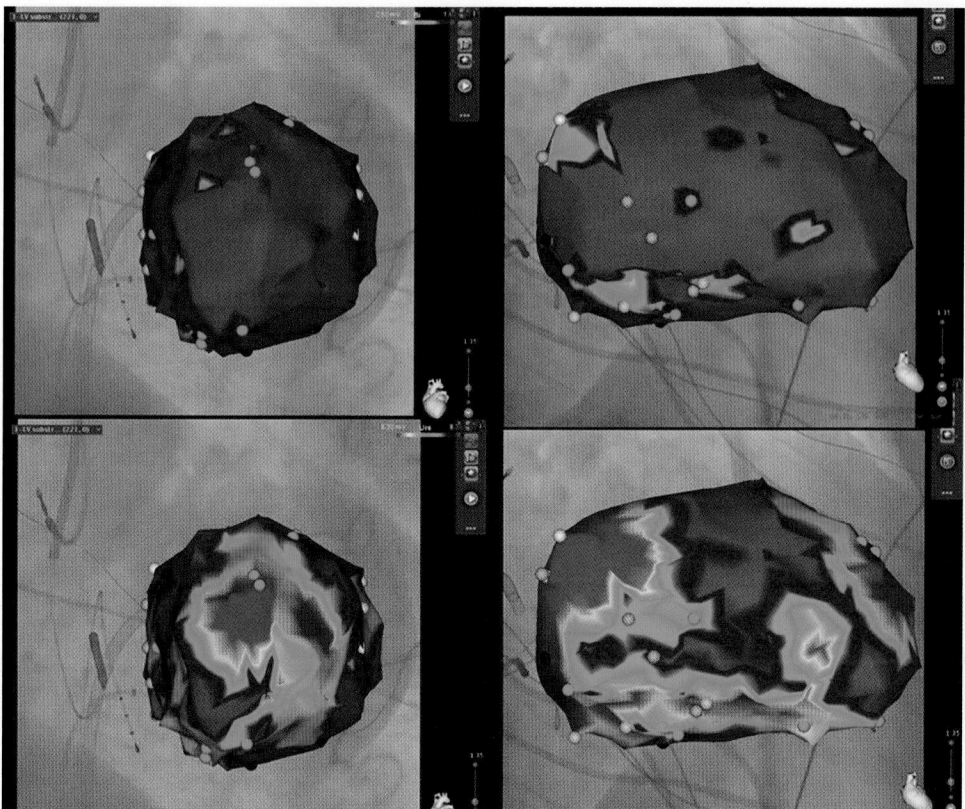

FIGURE 85.1 Examples of bipolar voltage maps of the endocardium of a patient with nonis-chemic dilated cardiomyopathy in left lateral oblique view (*left top*) and right lateral view (*right top*). There is no evidence of low-amplitude areas endocardially with the usual thresholds of 0.5 to 1.5 mV. Both panels at the bottom present unipolar voltage maps of the same patient with a threshold of 5.5 to 8.3 mV, suggesting the presence of a patchy epicardial scar in basal, septal, and apical left ventricular segments.

presence of nonendocardial scars.[60] Cano and colleagues studied the epicardial substrate in patients with DCM and demonstrated that the epicardial low-amplitude areas were larger in size compared with the endocardial fibrotic areas. However, the low-amplitude signals are not always consistent with epicardial scars because they can be the result of epicardial fat or underlying coronary vessels. Only low-voltage areas harboring fragmented, split, or late potentials should be considered scars.[59] Additionally, information about the distribution of the epicardal fat derived from computer tomography scans and the path of the great coronary vessels may be helpful in preventing misinterpretation of electrograms and avoiding coronary injury during ablation.

Ablation Targets and Outcomes of Ventricular Tachycardia Ablation in Patients With Dilated Cardiomyopathy

Because of the high prevalence of nonendocardial substrate for VT, epicardial mapping and ablation is frequently performed in patients with DCM. The 12-lead ECG can provide clues for epicardial exit of a VT. The presence of a Q wave in lead I during VT can predict an epicardial origin in the basolateral aspect of the LV with 88% sensitivity and specificity. The absence of Q waves in inferior leads also suggests an epicardial VT with sensitivity of 94% and specificity of 63%. Additionally, the presence of a pseudo delta-wave in V3–4 ≥34 ms and shortest precordial RS of ≥121 ms indicate epicardial VT exit (Fig. 85.2).[61] Using entrainment and pace mapping, Soejima and colleagues demonstrated that in patients with DCM, the reentry circuit can be confined

to the epicardial substrate and epicardial ablation can successfully treat VT in cases of failed endocardial ablation.[62] Using CMR before ablation to assess the function and anatomy of the ventricles as well as to visualize the substrate may be helpful in planning the procedure. Three-dimensional reconstruction of scar based on the LGE-CMR scans is already possible and provides detailed information about scar size, spatial distribution, inhomogeneity, and conduction channels.[63] Eventually, these high-resolution, three-dimensional scar maps can be matched with electroanatomical voltage maps to facilitate the mapping and ablation (Fig. 85.3).

There is no universally recommended strategy to ablate a VT in DCM. Detailed electroanatomical mapping in sinus rhythm helps delineate the underlying arrhythmogenic substrate (Fig. 85.4). Based on the growing evidence that epicardial ablation may increase the procedural success, many centers routinely perform both endo- and epicardial mapping in all patients with VT in NIDCM.[64] However, epicardial access and ablation may be associated with risk of serious complications, such as heart peroration and coronary artery or phrenic nerve injuries. A high-output pacing can be performed to identify capture of the phrenic nerve, and when necessary, it can be displaced away from the ablation site by inflating a percutaneous transluminal angioplasty (PTA) balloon in the epicardial space. Coronary angiography is indispensable for avoiding coronary artery injury during ablation.

In ongoing and hemodynamically tolerated VT, activation mapping to localize the sites of presystolic activity and entrainment can be performed. Entrainment can be useful for determining the position of the ablation catheter in respect to the

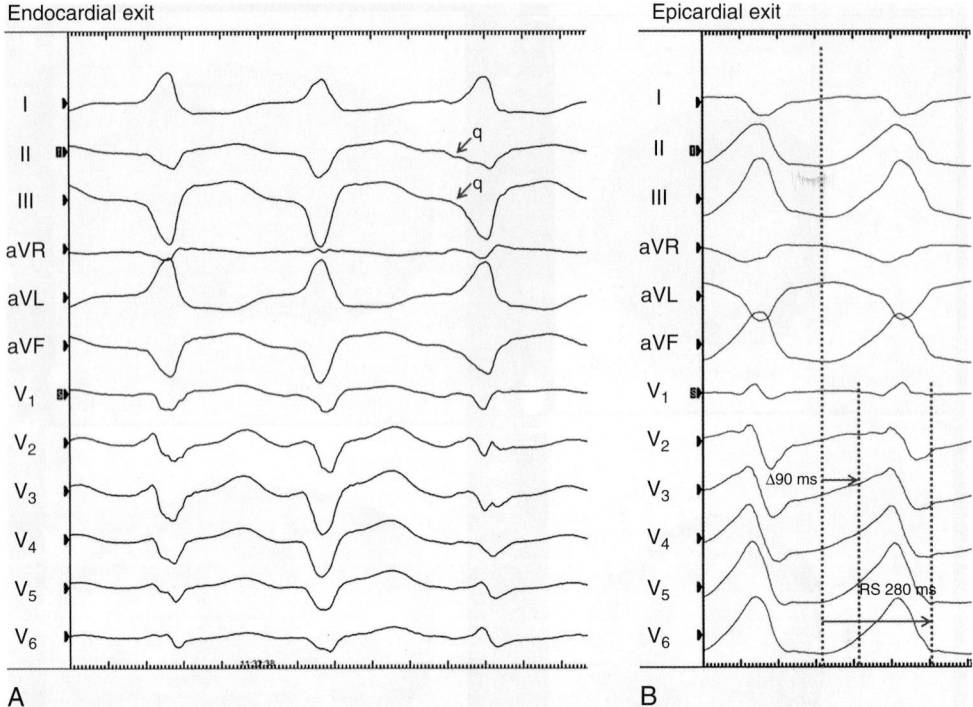

FIGURE 85.2 The *left panel* (A) is an example of ventricular tachycardia in a patient with dilated cardiomyopathy. The absence of q in I and presence of q in II and III suggests endocardial exit of the ventricular tachycardia (VT). The *right panel* (B) is an example of VT with an epicardial exit. Note the wide QRS during VT, a pseudo-delta in V3–4 of 90 ms, and a shortest RS of 280 ms.

reentry circuit. Demonstration of entrainment with a concealed fusion and a postpacing return cycle <30 ms from the tachycardia cycle length proves the exit site of the VT. For unstable VT, pacing from sites of late and fractionated potentials can be useful for delineating the VT circuit. Sites with good ECG match and long stimulus-to-QRS intervals suggest the site of origin of the VT.[21]

At present, inducibilty of VT by PVS is widely used to evaluate the procedural success, although there is no consensus whether the ablation of the clinical VT or of all inducible VT is the appropriate endpoint. Recently, we demonstrated that complete VT noninducibility after ablation was associated with the reduction of VT recurrence and cardiac mortality in patients with DCM (Fig. 85.5).[65] Although the acute success rates after VT ablation in patients with DCM are comparable to those in patients with ischemic cardiomyopathy, the long-term VT-free survival in patients with DCM is worse (Fig. 85.6).[66] The heterogeneity of NIDCM, progressive myocardial degeneration, and collagen accumulation may explain the poorer outcomes in patients with DCM and VT than in those with postinfarction cardiomyopathy.

Outcome data on catheter ablation of VT in NIDCM are limited to mostly single-center studies with relatively low numbers of patients. Differences in the ablation approaches (endocardial vs. epicardial ablation), the baseline characteristics, procedural endpoints, postprocedural antiarrhythmic drug usage, and technical equipment may explain the variability in the published clinical outcomes for NIDCM. Despite these differences, the available data suggest a VT-free survival ranging from 41% to 71% at 1-year follow-up (Table 85.1).[59,62,66–69] In the International VT Ablation Center Collaborative Group Study, a retrospective analysis of 2601 patients with structural heart disease found a 68% 1-year freedom from VT recurrence in patients with NIDCM.[69]

Management of Ventricular Tachycardia in Patients With Dilated Cardiomyopathy and Left Ventricular Assist Devices

Portable LV assist devices (LVADs) have been approved as a bridge to transplantation or as a destination therapy for patients with DCM and severe heart failure. Patients who receive an LVAD can experience recurrent VT. Observational studies suggested that LV wall suction and mechanical effects of the LVAD cannula inserted in an area of scar may play roles in VT arrhythmogenesis. With the hemodynamic support of the LVAD, even fast, sustained VT can be hemodynamically tolerable. However, recurrent intractable VT can precipitate ICD shocks as well as further deterioration of DCM. Recently, catheter ablation for VT has been demonstrated to be feasible and safe even in LVAD patients.[70] Ultimately, heart transplantation is recommended as the definitive solution in patients with symptomatic VT that is refractory to all therapies.

Specific Pharmacological Therapy for Ventricular Tachycardia in Dilated Cardiomyopathy

In earlier trials the use of antiarrhythmic drugs for suppression of VT in heart failure patients was associated with excess mortality attributed mainly to arrhythmia. However, the use of specific antiarrhythmic drugs is an indispensable part of management in patients with DCM who present with incessant or recurrent VT precipitating ICD shocks. Since electrical storm (ES) is frequently caused by an increase in sympathetic tone, the β-blockade of both β1- and β2-receptors remains an important ES treatment. Additionally, β-blockers are known to increase the ventricular fibrillation threshold, an effect that is thought to be due to inhibition of the β1-receptors.

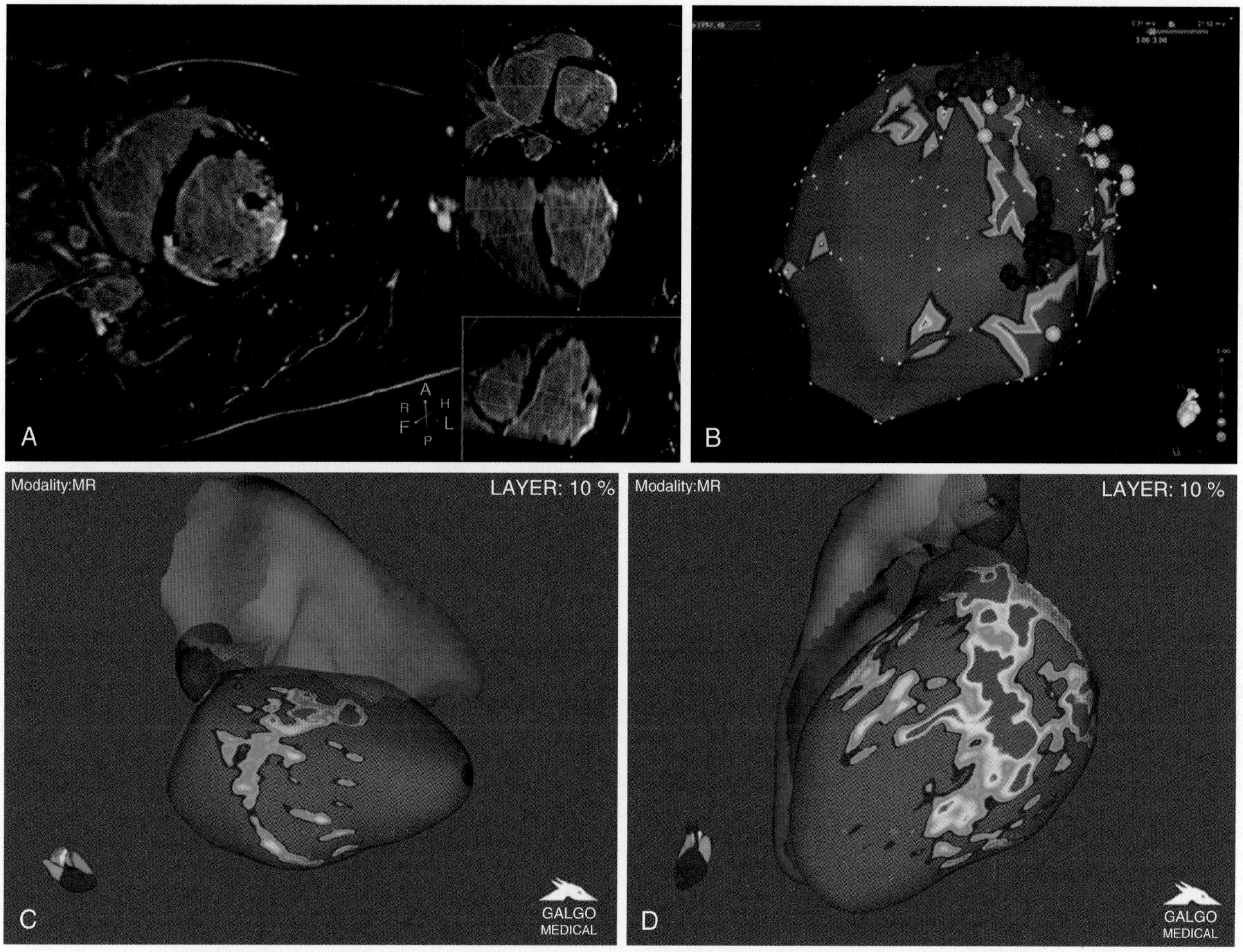

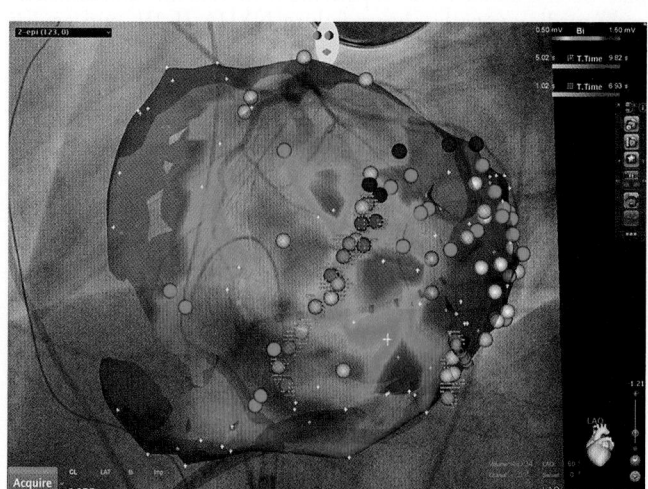

FIGURE 85.3 (A) presents a late gadolinium-enhanced (LGE) cardiovascular magnetic resonance (CMR) image of the heart of a patient with nonischemic dilated cardiomyopathy with visible scar areas in the inferior, inferoseptal, and anterolateral basal left ventricular segments. (B) is an example of an endocardial voltage map (left anterior oblique view) of the same patient with an evidence of patchy low-amplitude areas corresponding to the scar areas in LGE-CMR. The panels at the bottom represent three-dimensional CMR signal intensity reconstruction images of the inhomogeneous scar in the inferior view (C) and left lateral view (D). (Courtesy Luis Serra and I. Paetch.)

FIGURE 85.4 An example of epicardial voltage map in a patient with dilated cardiomyopathy showing vast low-voltage epicardial areas. Coronary artery angiography was integrated into the epicardial electroanatomical voltage map, which allowed the differentiation of the areas of real scar from the low-voltage areas along the epicardial coronary arteries.

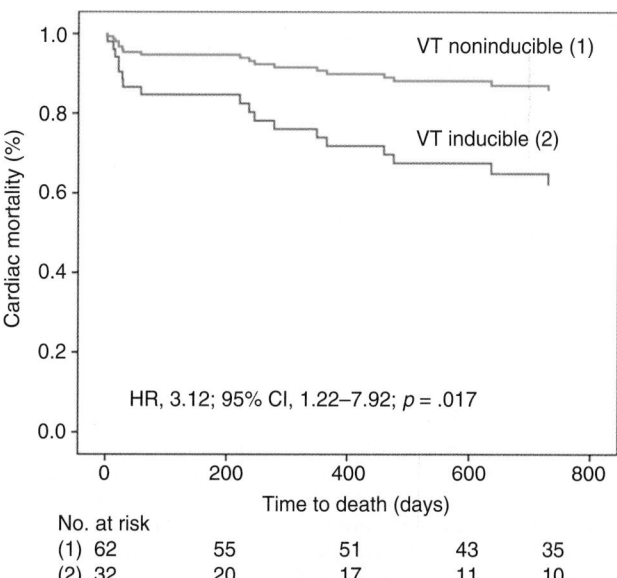

FIGURE 85.5 Kaplan–Meier curves for cardiac mortality in patients with inducible and noninducible ventricular tachycardia (*VT*) after catheter ablation of VT. Patients with persistently inducible VT after catheter ablation had a significantly higher likelihood for death than those with noninducible VT (adjusted hazard ratio [*HR*] = 3.12; *p* = .017). (From Dinov B, Arya A, Schratter A, et al. Catheter ablation of ventricular tachycardia and mortality in patients with nonischemic dilated cardiomyopathy: can noninducibility after ablation be a predictor for reduced mortality? *Circ Arrhythm Electrophysiol.* 2015;8:598-605.)

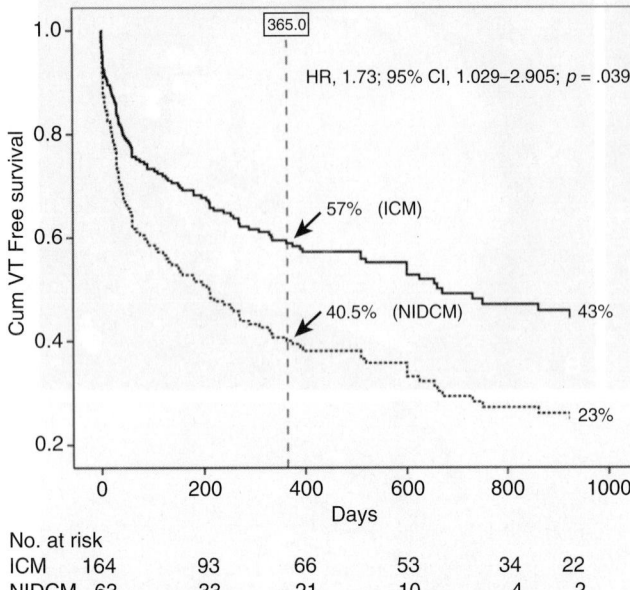

No. at risk

ICM	164	93	66	53	34	22
NIDCM	63	33	21	10	4	2

FIGURE 85.6 Kaplan–Meier curves for the freedom of ventricular tachycardia (*VT*) in patients with ischemic cardiomyopathy (*ICM*) and nonischemic dilated cardiomyopathy (*NIDCM*) after catheter ablation of VT. The likelihood for VT recurrence after ablation was significantly higher in patients with nonischemic DCM (hazard ratio [*HR*] = 1.73; *p* = .039). (From Dinov B, Fiedler L, Schönbauer R, et al. Outcomes in catheter ablation of ventricular tachycardia in dilated nonischemic cardiomyopathy compared with ischemic cardiomyopathy: results from the Prospective Heart Centre of Leipzig VT (HELP-VT) Study. *Circulation.* 2014;129:728-736.)

TABLE 85.1 Outcomes of ventricular tachycardia ablation in patients with nonischemic cardiomyopathy

STUDY	SIZE	ACUTE COMPLETE SUCCESS	FOLLOW-UP	FREEDOM OF VENTRICULAR TACHYCARDIA
Delacretaz et al.,[67] 2000	26	53%	15 ± 12 months	77%
Soejima et al.,[62] 2004	28	55%	1 year	54%
Cano et al.,[59] 2009	22	67%	18 ± 7 months	71%
Piers et al.,[68] 2013	45	38%	25 ± 15 months	47%
Dinov et al.,[66] 2014[a]	63	67%	1 year	41%
Tung et al.,[69] 2015[a]	966	67%	1 year	68%

[a]Data relate only to dilated cardiomyopathy patients.

Amiodarone is a potent class III potassium channel blocker that also exhibits features of class I use-dependent sodium channel blockade, as well as class II nonselective sympathetic blockade. It effectively suppresses VT even when other medications are unsuccessful. In the OPTIC trial, a combination of amiodarone and β-blocker significantly reduced the risk of shock compared with β-blocker alone (hazard ratio [HR], 0.27; 95% CI, 0.14–0.52; *p* < .001) and sotalol (HR, 0.43; 95% CI, 0.22–0.85; *p* = .02). However, its long-term use was associated with considerable side effects, and discontinuation of the medication occurred in 23.5% of patients within 1 year of initiation of therapy.[71] Nevertheless, intravenous

amiodarone and β-blockers are the preferred antiarrhythmic medications for acute management of ES.[72] In the AMIOVIRT trial comprising only patients with NIDCM, there was no significant difference in 3-year mortality, quality of life, or arrhythmia-free survival between patients treated with prophylactic ICDs or amiodarone therapy; however, amiodarone therapy was cost-saving as compared with ICD therapy.[73] The experience with newer class III drugs and with aldosterone blockade for VT/VF suppression is limited to small and retrospective studies.[74,75]

In July 2015 the US Food and Drug Administration (FDA) approved a sacubitril/valsartan combination for the treatment of heart failure, which was followed by marketing authorization in the European Union in September 2015. Sacubitril is the first in a new class of drugs for the treatment of heart failure and works through inhibition of neprilysin, an enzyme responsible for the degradation of the natriuretic peptides. In the PARADIGM-HF trial, 8442 patients with ischemic (60%) and nonischemic cardiomyopathy (40%), heart failure (71% NYHA Class II), and an ejection fraction <40% were randomized to either sacubitril/valsartan (twice daily) or enalapril (10 mg twice daily). The study was terminated prematurely after the interim analysis demonstrated a survival benefit with sacubitril/valsartan. In the PARADIGM-HF trial, the primary endpoint, which is death due to cardiovascular causes or hospitalization due to heart failure, occurred in 914 patients (21.8%) in the sacubitril/valsartan group and in 1117 patients (26.5%) in the enalapril group (HR, 0.80; 95% CI, 0.73–0.87; *p* < .001.[76] It also reduced the risk for SCD (HR, 0.80; 95% CI, 0.68–0.94; *p* = .008).[77]

Defibrillator Therapy for Prevention of Sudden Cardiac Death in Dilated Cardiomyopathy

Current guidelines recommend ICD therapy for secondary prevention of SCD in DCM and hemodynamically relevant VT. Concerning the primary prevention of SCD, randomized studies have demonstrated mortality benefit of ICD over optimal medical therapy in patients with NIDCM. The DEFINITE study randomized patients with NIDCM, NYHA class I–III, an LVEF ≤35%, and complex ventricular arrhythmias (VPBs and nonsustained VT) to ICD therapy in addition to standard medical therapy (including both angiotensin-converting enzyme inhibitors and β-blockers) or to standard medical therapy alone. In this trial, ICD therapy significantly reduced arrhythmic death and was associated with a trend toward reduction of all-cause mortality.[78] The multicenter Sudden Cardiac Death in Heart Failure (SCD-HeFT) trial confirmed the benefit of ICD over placebo and amiodarone in patients with ischemic and nonischemic cardiomyopathy, heart failure NYHA II–III, and an EF ≤35%. However, in the prespecified subgroup analysis, ICD was associated with a trend toward survival benefit in NIDCM (HR, 0.73; 97.5% CI, 0.50–1.07; *p* = .06) that was explained by the lower event rate observed in patients with NIDCM when compared with ischemic cardiomyopathy (5-year event rate with ICD therapy: ischemic 0.359 vs. nonischemic 0.214).[79] Based on the evidence from these two randomized trials, the current guidelines recommend ICD implantation for primary prevention of SCD in patients with NIDCM, heart failure NYHA II–III, and an LVEF ≤35% who have reasonable expectation of survival for at least 1 year. However, the median age of patients enrolled in DEFINITE and SCD-HeFT was 58 and 60 years, respectively, with only a minority of them aged >75 years. On the other hand, in routine clinical practice, the percentage of ICD recipients for primary prevention aged ≥75 years is increasing. However, the life prolongation by ICD is significantly less in elderly compared with younger patients, which can be explained by the higher incidence of comorbid illnesses in the elderly.[80] In a recent meta-analysis combining data from five major studies (MUSTT, MADIT I and II, DINAMITE, and SCD-HeFT), the benefit of ICD for primary prevention of SCD was demonstrated in all age groups but was attenuated with increasing age.[81] Therefore the decision for ICD implantation for primary prevention of SCD in elderly patients should be taken after careful evaluation of the comorbid illnesses and consideration of the higher complication rate in this population. The decision to abstain from ICD frequently necessitates a careful discussion with the patient.

The decision of whether or when to implant an ICD is challenging in patients who have recently been diagnosed with NIDCM. The initiation and titration of optimal medical therapy, including angiotensin-converting enzyme inhibitors and β-blockers, often improves LVEF to the extent where a primary ICD implantation is no longer needed. Data from several cohort studies emphasize the dynamic nature of LV function in patients with recently diagnosed DCM. In the IMAC-2 study comprising 373 patients with new-onset DCM (LVEF <40% and duration <6 months) the mortality was 4% at 4-year follow-up. Notably, at 6 months, 70% of patients had an absolute increase in LVEF of 10%, and 39% of patients demonstrated an increase of at least 20%. Furthermore, 40% of patients had an LVEF of 45% or more, and 25% of patients had complete or near-complete (LVEF >0.50) resolution of their cardiomyopathy at 6 months.[82] Similarly, in a cohort of 245 patients with newly identified DCM who met the SCD-HeFT criteria for ICD implantation, only 31% met the criteria for primary prevention ICD implantation after reevaluation at 9 months.[83] Therefore the most recent position statement of the Heart Rhythm Society/American College of Cardiology/American Heart Association (HRS/ACC/AHA) does not recommend implantation of an ICD for primary prevention within the first 3 months after initial diagnosis of NIDCM. However, prophylactic ICD implantation can be useful between 3 and 9 months after initial diagnosis if recovery of LV function is unlikely. Furthermore, the guideline recognizes the higher risk for subsequent events in patients with DCM and sustained VT and recommends ICD implantation in patients less than 9 months from the initial diagnosis of NIDCM with sustained (or hemodynamically significant) ventricular tachyarrhythmia. Additionally, implantation of an ICD can be useful in patients with recently diagnosed nonischemic cardiomyopathy who present with syncope that is thought to be due to a VT (by clinical history or documented nonsustained VT).[84]

Wearable Cardioverter Defibrillators in Patients With Dilated Cardiomyopathy and at High Risk for Sudden Cardiac Death

Recently, the FDA has approved the wearable cardioverter defibrillator (WCD) for use in patients who are at increased risk for sudden cardiac arrest and who do not meet the recommendations for ICD implantation. Currently, LifeVest (Zoll, Pittsburgh, PA) is the only commercially available and approved WCD. The device weighs 1.5 kg, has four sensing electrodes, and is capable of detecting and storing ECG signals. In cases of detectable VTs, the device alerts the patient and delivers a shock, typically within 60 seconds of arrhythmia onset. Based on the earlier WEARIT/BIROAD study, WCDs were approved for selected patients at high risk of SCD.[85] The recent WEARIT-II registry enrolled 2000 patients, of whom 927 (46%) had NIDCM. In this registry, the rate of VT/VF in the NIDCM population was lower (1%) than that in patients with ischemic cardiomyopathy and congenital heart disease (3%). At the end of WCD use, an ICD was implanted in 36% of patients with NIDCM. The most frequent reason not to implant ICD was improvement of the LVEF. The rate of inappropriate WCD shocks in the registry was very low (0.5%).[86] The current consensus statement from HRS/ACC/AHA 2014 recommends the use of WCD in patients with expected reversible arrhythmic conditions, such as myocarditis or newly diagnosed nonischemic cardiomyopathy during the first 3 to 6 months after initiation of optimal medical therapy.[87] Furthermore, the usage of a WCD is justified in patients with other secondary forms of NIDCM due to transient causes such as alcoholic cardiomyopathy, tachycardia-induced cardiomyopathy, or chemotherapy-induced cardiomyopathy, who usually have a good prognosis after recovery.

Conclusion

The occurrence of VT in NIDCM is associated with an increased hospitalization rate and mortality. The widespread use of ICDs and cardiac resynchronization therapy significantly improved the prognosis in these patients. However, the renin-angiotensin-aldosterone system blockers and β-blockers remain the mainstay of the therapy preventing further LV remodeling. A new drug that inhibits the degradation of the natriuretic peptides has been shown effective in reducing SCD in patients with DCM and heart failure. Recent advances in mapping and catheter ablation have led to a significant increase in the use of this technique in NIDCM. However, because of frequent midmyocardial and epicardial involvement and the progressive nature of NIDCM, catheter ablation is associated with poorer procedural outcomes than ischemic cardiomyopathy. Epicardial mapping and ablation is frequently necessary to achieve long-term success. CMR can be helpful in visualization of the arrhythmia substrate and has an increasing importance in catheter ablation as well as for the risk stratification of patients with DCM and VT.

REFERENCES

1. Elliot P, Andersson B, Arbustini E, et al. Classification of the cardiomyopathies: a position statement from the European Society of Cardiology Working Group for Myocardial and Pericardial Diseases. Eur Heart J. 2008;29:270–276.
2. Michels VV, Moll PP, Miller FA, et al. The frequency of familial dilated cardiomyopathy in series of patients with idiopathic dilated cardiomyopathy. N Engl J Med. 1992;326:77–82.
3. van Tintelen JP, Hofstra RM, Katerberg H, et al. High yield of LMNA mutations in patients with dilated cardiomyopathy and/or conduction disease referred to cardiogenetics outpatient clinics. Am Heart J. 2007;154:1130–1139.
4. Bione S, D'Adamo P, Maestrini E, Gedeon AK, Bolhuis PA, Toniolo D. A novel X-linked gene, G4.5 is responsible for Barth syndrome. Nat Genet. 1996;12:385–389.
5. Vatta M, Mohapatra B, Jimenez S, et al. Mutations in Cypher/ZASP in patients with dilated cardiomyopathy and left ventricular non-compaction. J Am Coll Cardiol. 2003;42:2014–2027.
6. Barresi R, Di Blasi C, Negri T, et al. Disruption of heart sarcoglycan complex and severe cardiomyopathy caused by beta sarcoglycan mutations. J Med Genet. 2000;37:102–107.
7. Chang AN, Potter JD. Sarcomeric protein mutations in dilated cardiomyopathy. Heart Fail Rev. 2005;10:225–235.
8. Kamisago M, Sharma SD, De Palma SR, et al. Mutations in sarcomere protein genes as a cause of dilated cardiomyopathy. N Engl J Med. 2000;343:1688–1696.
9. Taylor MR, Slavov D, Ku L, et al. Prevalence of desmin mutations in dilated cardiomyopathy. Circulation. 2007;115:1244–1251.
10. Feng J, Yan J, Buzin CH, Towbin JA, Sommer SS. Mutation in the dystrophin gene are associated with sporadic dilated cardiomyopathy. Mol Genet Metab. 2002;77:119–126.
11. Fatkin D, MacRae C, Sasaki T, et al. Missense mutations in the rod domain of the lamin A/C gene as causes of dilated cardiomyopathy and conduction-system disease. N Engl J Med. 1999;341:1715–1724.
12. Pasotti M, Klersy C, Pilotto A, et al. Long-term outcome and risk stratification in dilated cardiolaminopathies. J Am Coll Cardiol. 2008;52:1250–1260.
13. Herman D, Lam L, Taylor M, et al. Truncations of titin causing dilated cardiomyopathy. N Engl J Med. 2012;366:619–628.
14. Berko BA, Swift M. X-linked dilated cardiomyopathy. N Engl J Med. 1987;316:1186–1191.
15. Towbin JA, Hejtmanchik JF, Brink P, et al. X-linked dilated cardiomyopathy. Molecular genetic evidence of linkage to the Duchenne muscular dystrophy (dystrophin) gene at the Xp21 locus. Circulation. 1993;87:1854–1865.
16. Barth PG, Valianpour F, Bowen VM, et al. X-linked cardioskeletal myopathy and neutropenia (Barth syndrome): an update. Am J Med Genet A. 2004;126A:349–354.
17. Schmitt JP, Kamisago M, Asahi M, et al. Dilated cardiomyopathy and heart failure caused by mutation in phospholamban. Science. 2003;299:1410–1413.
18. van der Zwaag PA, van Rijsingen IA, Asimaki A, et al. R14del mutation in patients diagnosed with dilated cardiomyopathy or arrhythmogenic right ventricular cardiomyopathy: evidence supporting the concept of arrhythmogenic cardiomyopathy. Eur J Heart Fail. 2012;14:1199–1207.
19. van Rijsingen IA, van der Zwaag PA, Groeneweg JA, et al. Outcome in phospholamban R14del carriers: results of a large multicentre cohort study. Circ Cardiovasc Genet. 2014;7:455–465.
20. McNair WP, Sinagra G, Taylor MR, et al. SCN5A mutations associate with arrhythmic dilated cardiomyopathy and commonly localize to the voltage-sensing mechanism. J Am Coll Cardiol. 2011;57:2160–2168.

20a. Singh SN, Fisher SG, Carson PE, Fletcher RD. Prevalence and significance of nonsustained ventricular tachycardia in patients with premature ventricular contractions and heart failure treated with vasodilator therapy. Department of Veterans Affairs CHF STAT Investigators. *J Am Coll Cardiol*. 1998;32:942–947.

21. Liuba I, Marchlinksi F. The substrate and ablation of ventricular tachycardia in patients with nonischemic cardiomyopathy. *Circ J*. 2013;77:1957–1966.

22. Baman TS, Lange DC, Ilg KJ, et al. Relationship between burden of premature ventricular complexes and left ventricular function. *Heart Rhythm*. 2010;7:865–869.

23. Carballeira Pol L, Deyell MW, Frankel DS, et al. Ventricular premature depolarization QRS duration as a new marker of risk for the development of ventricular premature depolarization-induced cardiomyopathy. *Heart Rhythm*. 2014;11:299–306.

24. Potfay J, Kaszala K, Tan AY, et al. Abnormal left ventricular mechanics of ventricular ectopic beats: insights into origin and coupling interval in premature ventricular contraction-induced cardiomyopathy. *Circ Arrhythm Electrophysiol*. 2015;8:1194–1200.

25. Takemoto M, Yoshimura H, Ohba Y, et al. Radiofrequency catheter ablation of premature ventricular complexes from right ventricular outflow tract improves left ventricular dilation and clinical status in patients without structural heart disease. *J Am Coll Cardiol*. 2005;45:1259–1265.

26. Sekiguchi Y, Aonuma K, Yamauchi Y, et al. Chronic hemodynamic effects after radiofrequency catheter ablation of frequent monomorphic ventricular premature beats. *J Cardiovasc Electrophysiol*. 2005;16:1057–1063.

27. Yarlagadda RK, Iwai S, Stein KM, et al. Reversal of cardiomyopathy in patients with repetitive monomorphic ventricular ectopy originating from the right ventricular outflow tract. *Circulation*. 2005;112:1092–1097.

28. Strickberger SA, Hummel JD, Bartlett TG, et al. Amiodarone versus implantable cardioverter-defibrillator: randomized trial in patients with nonischemic dilated cardiomyopathy and asymptomatic nonsustained ventricular tachycardia—AMIOVIRT. *J Am Coll Cardiol*. 2003;41:1707–1712.

29. Desai AS, Fang JC, Masisel WH, Baughman KL. Implantable defibrillators for the prevention of mortality in patients with nonischemic cardiomyopathy: a meta-analysis of randomized controlled trials. *JAMA*. 2004;292:2874–2879.

30. Chen S, Motonaga K, Hollander S, et al. Electrocardiographic repolarization abnormalities and increased risk of life-threatening arrhythmias in children with dilated cardiomyopathy. *Heart Rhythm*. 2016;13:1289–1296.

31. Goldberger JJ, Subacius H, Patel T, Cunnane R, Kadish A. Sudden cardiac death risk stratification in patients with nonischemic dilated cardiomyopathy. *J Am Coll Cardiol*. 2014;63:1879–1889.

32. Dinov B, Schratter A, Schirripa V, et al. Procedural outcomes and survival after catheter ablation of ventricular tachycardia in relation to electroanatomical substrate in patients with nonischemic-dilated cardiomyopathy: the role of unipolar voltage mapping. *J Cardiovasc Electrophysiol*. 2015;26:985–993.

33. Buxton AE, Lee KL, Hafley GE, et al. Limitations of ejection fraction for prediction of sudden death risk in patients with coronary artery disease: lessons from the MUSTT study. *J Am Coll Cardiol*. 2007;50:1150–1157.

34. Bardy GH, Lee KL, Mark DB, et al. Sudden Cardiac Death in Heart Failure Trial (SCD-HeFT) Investigators. Amiodarone or an implantable cardioverter-defibrillator for congestive heart failure. *N Engl J Med*. 2005;352:225–237.

35. Kosiuk J, Dinov B, Bollmann A, et al. Association between ventricular arrhythmias and myocardial mechanical dispersion assessed by strain analysis in patients with nonischemic cardiomyopathy. *Clin Res Cardiol*. 2015;104:1072–1077.

36. Luu M, Stevenson WG, Stevenson LW, Baron K, Walden J. Diverse mechanisms of unexpected cardiac arrest in advanced heart failure. *Circulation*. 1989;80:1675–1680.

37. Gao P, Gula L, Yee R, et al. Prediction of arrhythmic events in ischemic and dilated cardiomyopathy patients referred for implantable cardiac defibrillator evaluation of multiple scar quantification measures for late gadolinium enhancement magnetic resonance imaging. *Circ Cardiovasc Imaging*. 2012;5:448–456.

38. Assomull RG, Prasad SK, Lyne J, et al. Cardiovascular magnetic resonance, fibrosis, and prognosis in dilated cardiomyopathy. *J Am Coll Cardiol*. 2006;48:1977–1985.

39. Nazarian S, Bluemke DA, Lardo AC, et al. Magnetic resonance assessment of the substrate for inducible ventricular tachycardia in nonischemic cardiomyopathy. *Circulation*. 2005;112:2821–2825.

40. Illes L, Pfluger H, Lefkovitz L, et al. Myocardial fibrosis predicts appropriate device therapy in patients with implantable cardioverter-defibrillators for primary prevention of sudden cardiac death. *J Am Coll Cardiol*. 2011;57:821–828.

41. Wu KC, Weiss RG, Thiemann DR, et al. Late gadolinium enhancement by cardiovascular magnetic resonance heralds an adverse prognosis in nonischemic cardiomyopathy. *J Am Coll Cardiol*. 2008;51:2414–2421.

42. Klem I, Weinsaft JW, Bahnson TD, et al. Assessment of myocardial scarring improves risk stratification in patients evaluated for cardiac defibrillator implantation. *J Am Coll Cardiol*. 2012;60:408–420.

43. Grun S, Schumm J, Greunlich S, et al. Long-term follow-up of biopsy-proven viral myocarditis: predictors of mortality and incomplete recovery. *J Am Coll Cardiol*. 2012;59:1604–1615.

44. Rochitte CE, Oliveira PF, Andrade JM, et al. Myocardial delayed enhancement by magnetic resonance imaging in patients with Chagas' disease. A marker of disease severity. *J Am Coll Cardiol*. 2005;46:1553–1558.

45. Sarabanda AV, Marin-Neto JA. Predictors of mortality in patients with Chagas' cardiomyopathy and ventricular tachycardia not treated with implantable cardioverter-defibrillators. *Pacing Clin Electrophysiol*. 2011;34:54–62.

46. Illes L, Pfluger H, Phromminitikul A, et al. Evaluation of diffuse myocardial fibrosis in heart failure with cardiac magnetic resonance contrast-enhanced T1 mapping. *J Am Coll Cardiol*. 2008;52:1574–1580.

47. Fleu AS, Hayward MP, Ashwort MT, et al. Equilibrium contrast cardiovascular magnetic resonance for the measurement of diffuse myocardial fibrosis: preliminary validation in humans. *Circulation*. 2010;122:138–144.

48. Sibley CT, Nouredin RA, Gai N, et al. T1 mapping in cardiomyopathy at cardiac MR: comparison with endomyocardial biopsy. *Radiology*. 2012;265:724–732.

49. Chen Z, Sohal M, Voigt T, et al. Myocardial tissue characterization by cardiac magnetic resonance imaging using T1 mapping predicts ventricular arrhythmia in ischemic and non-ischemic cardiomyopathy patients with implantable cardioverter-defibrillators. *Heart Rhythm*. 2015;12:792–801.

50. Patel MR, Cawley PJ, Heitner JF, et al. Detection of myocardial damage in patients with sarcoidosis. *Circulation*. 2009;120:1969–1977.

51. Mehta D, Mori N, Goldbarg SH, et al. Primary prevention of sudden cardiac death in silent cardiac sarcoidosis: role of programmed ventricular stimulation. *Circ Arrhythm Electrophysiol*. 2011;4:43–48.

52. Junttila MJ, Fishmann JE, Lopera GA, et al. Safety of serial MRI in patients with implantable cardioverter defibrillators. *Heart*. 2011;97:1852–1856.

53. Naele CP, Kreuz J, Strach K, et al. Safety, feasibility, and diagnostic value of cardiac magnetic resonance imaging in patients with cardiac pacemakers and implantable cardioverters-defibrillators at 1.5 T. *Am Heart J*. 2011;161:1096–1105.

54. McCrohon JA, Moon JC, Prasad SK, et al. Differentiation of heart failure related to dilated cardiomyopathy and coronary artery disease using gadolinium-enhanced cardiovascular magnetic resonance. *Circulation*. 2003;108:54–59.

55. Masci PG, Barison A, Aquaro GD, et al. Myocardial delayed enhancement in paucisymptomatic nonischemic dilated cardiomyopathy. *Int J Cardiol*. 2012;157:43–47.

56. Fernandez- Armenta J, Beruezzo A, Mont L, et al. Use of myocardial scar characterization to predict ventricular arrhythmia in cardiac resynchronization therapy. *Europace*. 2012;14:1578–1586.

57. Hsia HH, Calans DJ, Marchlinski FE. Characterization of endocardial electrophysiological substrate in patients with nonischemic cardiomyopathy and monomorphic ventricular tachycardia. *Circulation*. 2003;108:704–710.

58. Haqqani HM, Tschabrunn CM, Tzou WS, et al. Isolated septal substrate for ventricular tachycardia in nonischemic dilated cardiomyopathy: incidence, characterization, and implications. *Heart Rhythm*. 2011;8:1169–1176.

59. Cano O, Hutchinson M, Lin D, et al. Electroanatomical substrate and ablation outcome for suspected epicardial ventricular tachycardia in left ventricular nonischemic cardiomyopathy. *J Am Coll Cardiol*. 2009;54:799–808.

60. Hutchinson MD, Gerstenfeld EP, Desjardins B, et al. Endocardial unipolar voltage mapping to detect epicardial ventricular tachycardia substrate in patients with nonischemic left ventricular cardiomyopathy. *Circ Arrhythm Electrophysiol*. 2011;4:49–55.

61. Valles E, Bazan V, Marchlinski FE. ECG criteria to identify epicardial ventricular tachycardia in nonischemic cardiomyopathy. *Circ Arrhythm Electrophysiol*. 2012;3:63–71.

62. Soejima K, Stevenson WG, Sapp JL, et al. Endocardial and epicardial radiofrequency ablation of ventricular tachycardia associated with dilated cardiomyopathy: the importance of low-voltage scars. *J Am Coll Cardiol*. 2004;43:1834–1842.

63. Bogun F, Desjardin B, Good E, et al. Delayed-enhanced magnetic resonance imaging in nonischemic dilated cardiomyopathy: utility for identifying the ventricular arrhythmia substrate. *J Am Coll Cardiol*. 2009;53:1138–1145.

64. Della Bella P, Brugada J, Zeppenfeld K, et al. Epicardial ablation for ventricular tachycardia: a European multicenter study. *Circ Arrhythm Electrophysiol*. 2011;4:653–659.

65. Dinov B, Arya A, Schratter A, et al. Catheter ablation of ventricular tachycardia and mortality in patients with nonischemic dilated cardiomyopathy: can noninducibility after ablation be a predictor for reduced mortality? *Circ Arrhythm Electrophysiol*. 2015;8:598–605.

66. Dinov B, Fiedler L, Schönbauer R, et al. Outcomes in catheter ablation of ventricular tachycardia in dilated nonischemic cardiomyopathy compared with ischemic cardiomyopathy: results from the prospective Heart Centre of Leipzig VT (HELP-VT) Study. *Circulation*. 2014;129:728–736.

67. Delacretaz E, Stevenson WG, Ellison KE, et al. Mapping and radiofrequency ablation of the three types of sustained monomorphic ventricular tachycardia in nonischemic heart disease. *J Cardiovasc Electrophysiol*. 2000;11:11–17.

68. Piers SR, Leong DP, van Huls, van Taxis CF, et al. Outcome of ventricular tachycardia ablation in patients with nonischemic cardiomyopathy: the impact of noninducibility. *Circ Arrhythm Electrophysiol*. 2013;6:513–521.

69. Tung R, Vaseghi M, Frankel DS, et al. Freedom from recurrent ventricular tachycardia after catheter ablation is associated with improved survival in patients with structural heart disease: an International VT Ablation Center Collaborative Group Study. *Heart Rhythm*. 2015;12:1997–2007.

70. Sacher F, Reichlin T, Zado ES, et al. Characteristics of ventricular tachycardia ablation in patients with continuous flow left ventricular assist devices. *Circ Arrhythm Electrophysiol*. 2015;8:592–597.

71. Connolly SJ, Dorian P, Roberts RS, et al. Comparison of beta-blockers, amiodarone plus beta-blockers, or sotalol for prevention of shocks from implantable cardioverter defibrillators: the OPTIC study: a randomized trial. *JAMA*. 2006;295:165–171.

72. Sorajja D, Munger T, Shen WK. Optimal antiarrhythmic drug therapy for electrical storm. *J Biomed Res*. 2015;29:20–34.

73. Kadish A, Dyer A, Daubert JP, et al. Prophylactic defibrillator implantation in patients with nonischemic dilated cardiomyopathy. *N Engl J Med*. 2004;350:2151–2158.

74. Baquero GA, Banchs JE, Depalma S, et al. Dofetilide reduces the frequency of ventricular arrhythmias and implantable cardioverter defibrillator therapies. *J Cardiovasc Electrophysiol*. 2012;23:296–301.

75. Zaraga IG, Dougherty CM, MacMurdy KS, Raitt M. The effect of spironolactone on ventricular tachyarrhythmias in patients with implantable cardioverter-defibrillators. *Circ Arrhythm Electrophysiol*. 2012;5:739–747.

76. McMurray JJ, Packer M, Desai A, et al. Angiotensin-neprilysin inhibition versus enalapril in heart failure. *N Engl J Med*. 2014;371:993–1004.

77. Desai AS, McMurray JJ, Packer M, et al. Effect of the angiotensin-receptor-neprilysin inhibitor LCZ696 compared with enalapril on mode of death in heart failure patients. *Eur Heart J*. 2015;36:1990–1997.

78. Bardy GH, Lee KL, Mark DB, et al. Amiodarone or an implantable cardioverter–defibrillator for congestive heart failure. *N Engl J Med*. 2005;352:225–237.

79. Bristow M, Saxon L, Boehmer J, et al. Cardiac-resynchronization therapy with or without an implantable defibrillator in advanced chronic heart failure. *N Engl J Med*. 2004;350:2140–2150.

80. van Rees JB, Borleffs CJ, Thijssen J, et al. Prophylactic implantable cardioverter-defibrillator treatment in the elderly: therapy, adverse events, and survival gain. *Europace*. 2012;14:66–73.

81. Hess PL, Al-Khatib SM, Han JY, et al. Survival benefit of the primary prevention implantable cardioverter-defibrillator among older patients: does age matter? An analysis of pooled data from 5 clinical trials. *Circ Cardiovasc Qual Outcomes*. 2015;8:179–186.

82. McNamara DM, Starling RC, Cooper LT, et al. Clinical and demographic predictors of outcomes in recent onset dilated cardiomyopathy: results of the IMAC (Intervention in Myocarditis and Acute Cardiomyopathy)-2 study. *J Am Coll Cardiol*. 2011;58:1112–1118.

83. Zecchin M, Merlo M, Pivetta A, et al. How can optimization of medical treatment avoid unnecessary implantable cardioverter-defibrillator implantations in patients with idiopathic dilated cardiomyopathy presenting with "SCD-HeFT criteria"? *Am J Cardiol*. 2012;109:729–735.

84. Kusumoto F, Calkins H, Boehmer J, et al. HRS/ACC/AHA expert consensus statement on the use of implantable cardioverter-defibrillator therapy in patients who are not included or not well represented in clinical trials. *Circulation*. 2014;130:94–125.

85. Feldman AM, Klein H, Tchou P, et al. Use of wearable defibrillator in terminating tachyarrhythmias in patients at high risk for sudden death: results of the WEARIT/BIROAD. *Pacing Clin Electrophysiol*. 2004;27:4–9.

86. Kutyifa V, Moss A, Klein H, et al. Use of the wearable cardioverter defibrillator in high-risk cardiac patients: data from the Prospective Registry of Patients Using the Wearable Cardioverter Defibrillator (WEARIT-II Registry). *Circulation*. 2015;132:1613–1619.

87. Kusutomo FM, Calkins H, Boehmer J, et al. HRS/ACC/AHA expert consensus statement on the use of implantable cardioverter defibrillator therapy in patients who are not included or not well represented in clinical trials. *J Am Coll Cardiol*. 2014;64:1143–1177.

86 Ventricular Arrhythmias in Hypertrophic Cardiomyopathy: Sudden Death, Risk Stratification, and Prevention With Implantable Defibrillators

Barry J. Maron and Martin S. Maron

Hypertrophic cardiomyopathy (HCM) is a genetic cardiac disease with heterogeneous clinical presentation.[1] Although the clinical course is diverse and compatible with normal longevity, unexpected sudden cardiac death (SCD) has been recognized as a devastating consequence of HCM since the initial description of this disease over 55 years ago. Ventricular tachyarrhythmias have been regarded as a prominent feature and source of concern in this disease because of the perceived causal relationship with SCD.[2,3] Indeed, introduction and penetration of the implantable cardioverter defibrillator (ICD) into HCM practice since 2000[2] and the reality of device-mediated prevention of SCD by effective termination of life-threatening ventricular tachyarrhythmias has made the science of risk stratification a much higher priority.[4] As a result, identification of those patients who would benefit most from ICD therapy has evolved considerably.[2–7] This comprehensive chapter presents a contemporary accounting of the profile of ventricular tachyarrhythmias, the linkage with SCD, and contemporary risk stratification and strategies for prevention of SCD, which have altered the natural history of this complex genetic disease for many patients.

Clinical Presentation and Sudden Cardiac Death

HCM is the most common cause of SCD in young people, including competitive athletes.[1,4–8] However, it should be underscored that HCM-related SCD events occur in only a small minority of patients (about 5%), notably much less common than other adverse disease consequences in this disease, such as atrial fibrillation (AF) or heart failure, and the vast majority of affected individuals probably experience an uncomplicated if not benign clinical course compatible with normal or extended longevity, even into their 80s or 90s (Fig. 86.1).[1,4,6–9] Nevertheless, the relatively high prevalence of HCM in the general population (with

estimates of 1:500 or possibly as high as 1:200)[10] suggests that there could be one million affected Americans, including a significant minority at SCD risk, of whom only a small proportion are recognized clinically.

The clinical profile of SCD risk in HCM is predominantly asymptomatic (or mildly symptomatic) in patients younger than 30 to 35 years old.[1–8] However, the likelihood of SCD events does not increase linearly with aging and in fact appears to be low for clinically stable patients who achieve 60 years of age or older. This observation translates to higher thresholds for prophylactic ICDs in this older age group (Fig. 86.2).[1,11] No difference has been reported for SCD risk between the genders or with respect to race.[12]

Historically, mortality rates in HCM have evolved considerably over time, from 6% per year reported from hospital-based cohorts in the older HCM literature (now regarded as overestimates due to the skewed referral of higher-risk patients to tertiary centers). Thereafter, reports from less selected cohorts, in the pre-ICD era, placed HCM-related mortality (largely due to SCD) at 1.5% per year.[13]

Myocardial Substrate

Triggers for potentially lethal ventricular tachyarrhythmias are incompletely understood, although rapid sinus tachycardia is frequently a preceding rhythm, suggesting that high sympathetic drive can be proarrhythmic in some patients.

The underlying left ventricular (LV) myocardial substrate (Fig. 86.3) consists of extensive areas of myocyte disarray with cardiac muscle cells characteristically arranged at oblique and perpendicular angles, creating a chaotic architecture most marked in younger SCD victims studied at autopsy.[1] In addition, a "small vessel disease" is likely responsible for altered myocardial blood flow,[1] with numerous intramural coronary arterioles with thickened media and narrowed lumen producing bursts of silent microvascular ischemia and subsequent myocyte death. Ultimately, a repair process of replacement fibrosis and scarring is triggered. Myocardial scars are detectable in vivo with quantitative contrast-enhanced cardiovascular magnetic resonance (CMR) and late gadolinium enhancement (LGE). When extensive, these areas of myocardial fibrosis are the source of ventricular tachyarrhythmias[14] and constitute a novel sudden death risk marker.[15]

Ventricular Tachyarrhythmias

Utilizing the monitoring capability of ICDs, data assembled from stored electrograms in HCM patients documented that aborted SCD events are caused by ventricular fibrillation (VF) and rapid monomorphic ventricular tachycardia (VT).[2,3] To date, there is no evidence that bradyarrhythmias play a role in HCM-related SCD.

The frequency of ambulatory asymptomatic ventricular tachyarrhythmias in HCM is disproportionate to the relatively

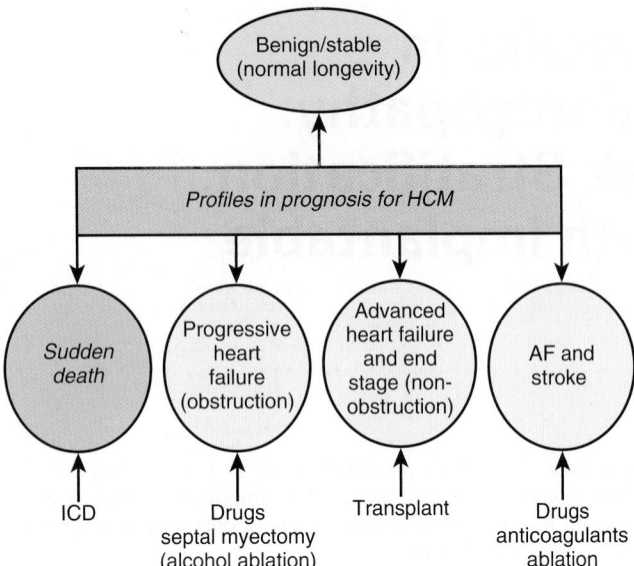

FIGURE 86.1 Profiles in prognosis for the hypertrophic cardiomyopathy (HCM) disease spectrum. *AF,* Atrial fibrillation; *ICD,* implantable cardioverter defibrillator.

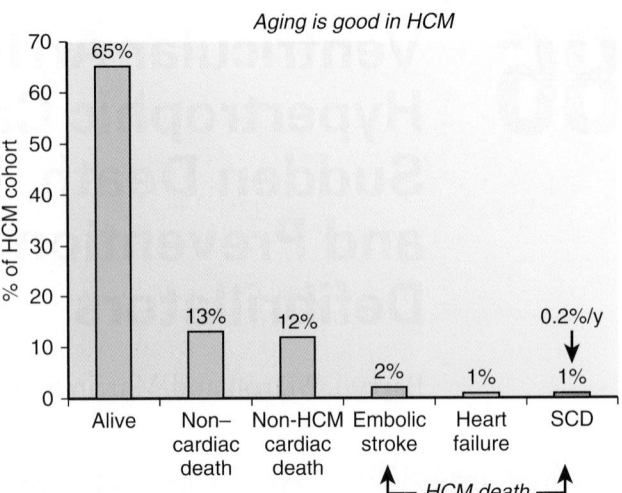

FIGURE 86.2 Clinical outcome in hypertrophic cardiomyopathy (*HCM*) patients evaluated at ≥60 years of age. Risk of HCM-related sudden cardiac death (*SCD*) is very low in this age group. (From Maron BJ, Rowin EJ, Casey SA, et al. Risk stratification and outcome of patients with hypertrophic cardiomyopathy ≥60 years of age. *Circulation.* 2013;127:585-593.)

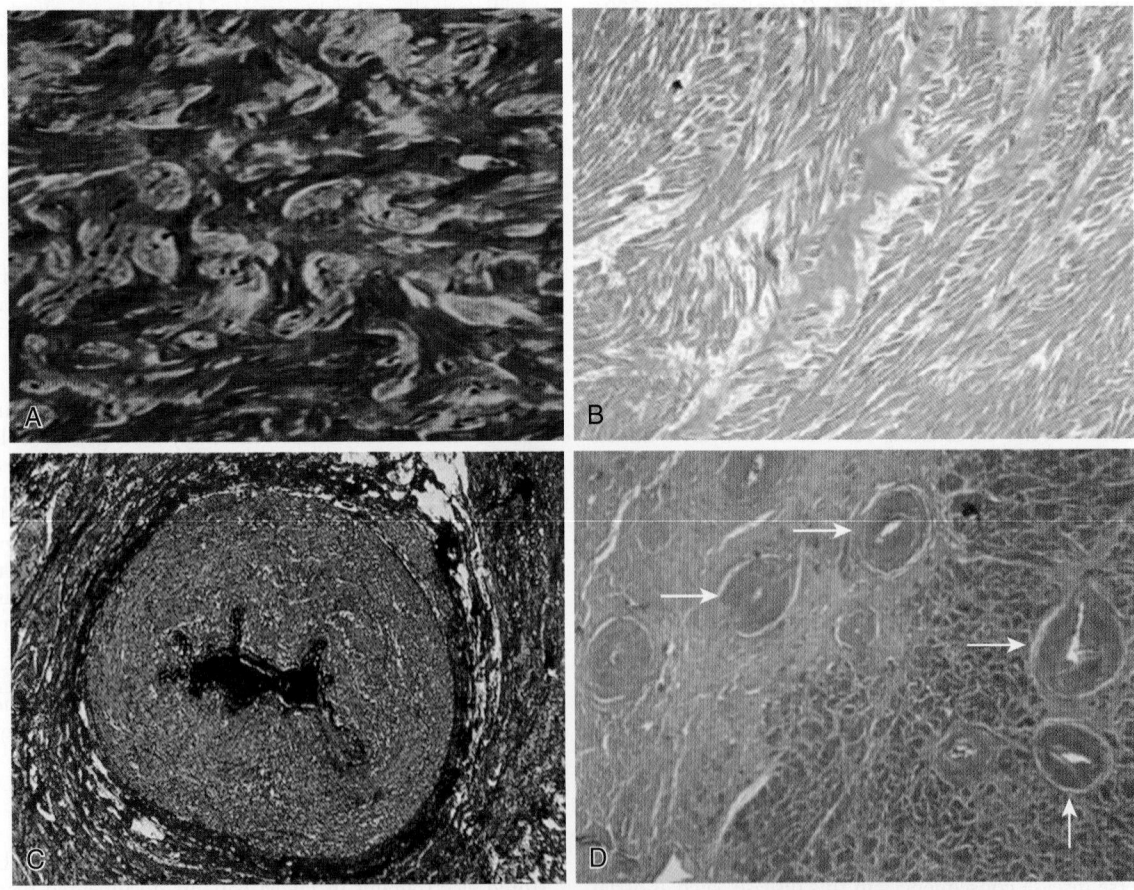

FIGURE 86.3 Arrhythmogenic myocardial substrate in hypertrophic cardiomyopathy. (A) Disorganized myocardial architecture. Marked disarray of hypertrophied myocytes arranged at oblique and perpendicular angles. (B) Myocytes encased within a dense network of matrix (interstitial) collagen. (C) Small vessel disease; remodeled intramural coronary arteriole with thickened media and narrowed lumen. (D) Numerous intramural coronary arteries (*arrows*) within and adjacent to replacement fibrosis, a consequence of silent microvascular ischemia and cell death.

low prevalence of SCD in this patient population.[1,7,14] On 24- to 48-hour ambulatory (Holter) electrocardiogram (ECG) monitoring, 90% of HCM patients demonstrate ventricular tachyarrhythmias, which not uncommonly are frequent and complex, including premature ventricular depolarizations, ventricular couplets, and, most importantly, bursts of nonsustained ventricular tachycardia (NSVT) in 20% to 30%, which have proven to be a risk marker in HCM. Indeed, about 10% of patients show particularly substantial ambulatory ectopy, including combinations of frequent premature ventricular depolarizations, couplets, and ≥1 NSVT bursts in a 24-hour monitoring period.

Initiatives for Sudden Death Prevention

Drugs

During the early pre-ICD history of HCM, strategy for SCD prevention included a variety of empiric pharmacological interventions, such as β-blockers, procainamide, quinidine, verapamil, and amiodarone,[1,7] all of which are now regarded as obsolete for this purpose. While such approaches were popular as the only available treatment options in the pre-ICD era, drugs failed to demonstrate absolute protection from SCD or ventricular tachyarrhythmias and in some cases, may have been proarrhythmic. In one series of high-risk HCM patients treated only pharmacologically, including with amiodarone, there was failure to prevent SCD.[1] In addition, ICD trials in HCM have demonstrated that a substantial proportion of patients experience appropriate shocks for VT/VF while taking β-blockers and/or antiarrhythmic drugs.[2,3]

Introduction and Evolution of the Implantable Cardioverter Defibrillator

The ICD was introduced into cardiovascular medicine for SCD prevention in the 1980s due to the vision and work of Dr. Michel Mirowski with Dr. Morton Mower at the Sinai Hospital (Baltimore)[16] initially despite antagonism from the cardiology establishment. Clinical development of the ICD ultimately created a paradigm shift from ineffective drug strategies to sophisticated and permanently implanted devices which recognize and automatically terminate potentially lethal ventricular tachyarrhythmias.[17]

Notably, of the first three ICD patients studied successfully in the laboratory setting in 1980 at Johns Hopkins Hospital to determine whether the device would reliably and spontaneously terminate VF, two had HCM. Each had previously survived two cardiac arrests due to recruitment restrictions of the US Food and Drug Administration.[16] However, application of the ICD to patients with genetic heart disease (including HCM) was largely ignored for the next 20 years, as device therapy was developed in clinical practice for patients with ischemic heart disease and ultimately tested in randomized secondary and primary prevention trials.[17]

Implantable Cardioverter Defibrillators in the Hypertrophic Cardiomyopathy Population

ICDs were employed sparingly in cases of HCM until the *New England Journal of Medicine* report in 2000 demonstrated efficacy of ICD therapy, with absolute protection from SCD for the first time in a series of patients.[2] Thereafter, greater numbers of HCM patients as well as patients with other genetic heart diseases, such as arrhythmogenic right ventricular cardiomyopathy, were implanted prophylactically.

Since the ICD was initially designed for coronary artery disease (CAD), there are certain distinctions between high-risk HCM and CAD patients that deserve consideration. ICD candidates with CAD average about 65 years at implant, usually with systolic dysfunction and compromised LV substrate following myocardial infarction, as well as with extracardiac organ comorbidities.[17] Because of the relatively advanced age of the patients,

the future time period for postimplant device interventions is relatively shorter, with some prolongation of life as the aspiration. High-risk HCM patients are generally at least 25 years younger than CAD patients at the time of prophylactic ICD implant (commonly in adolescents and young adults), usually with an intact myocardial substrate unencumbered by multisystem disease.[2,3] Younger HCM patients have potentially expansive risk periods with the aspiration for achieving substantial longevity with the ICD, although with greater likelihood of incurring device-related complications. Due to the low HCM-related SCD rate in clinically stable patients over 60 years of age (even in the presence of risk markers),[11] a higher threshold for primary prevention implants for most patients in this age group is prudent, with ICD decisions often made on a case-by-case basis.

Implantable Cardioverter Defibrillator Efficacy in Hypertrophic Cardiomopathy

ICDs have created a new strategy within the HCM armamentarium and are the most effective means available for preventing SCD and changing disease course for many patients.[2–4,6,18–22] Data from large patient cohorts assembled over the last decade have documented that appropriate ICD interventions not uncommonly occur in high-risk HCM patients and are highly effective in terminating potentially lethal ventricular tachyarrhythmias.[2,3,6,7,18–22] Furthermore, the ICD is effective despite the complex HCM phenotype, which may include extreme LV hypertrophy, a variety of patterns and locations of wall thickening, LV outflow obstruction, microvascular ischemia, and diastolic dysfunction.

The largest single dedicated series of high-risk patients with ICDs is the International Multicenter Registry ("ICD in HCM").[3] Important principles regarding ICD therapy in HCM have been derived from this registry of more than 500 patients (Figs. 86.4 and 86.5). Over an average follow-up of 3.7 years, 20% of patients experienced appropriate device therapy for VT/VF (see Fig. 86.3). Discharge rates were 5.5% per year overall, 11% per year for secondary prevention implants after cardiac arrest, and 4% per year for primary prevention (implant based on ≥1 major risk factors) (see Fig. 86.5). Primary prevention-appropriate discharge rates of 4% per year have now been consistently reported from populations in Europe, Australia, and Canada.[18–22] The primary prevention discharge rate does not differ significantly for patients implanted for 1, 2, or ≥3 risk factors, and about one-third of patients with appropriate interventions were implanted for only one major risk marker (most commonly for unexplained syncope) (see Fig. 86.4).[3] Of note, this ICD intervention rate is similar to that reported for SCD in the pre-ICD era from tertiary HCM centers with referral patterns skewed to highest-risk patients.[1]

In a multicenter international registry comprising 224 high-risk children and adolescents with HCM implanted less than 20 years old, ICD interventions terminating life-threatening ventricular tachyarrhythmias were also frequent (see Fig. 86.5).[22] Defibrillators were activated to abolish VT/VF in 19% of patients over 4.3 ± 3.3 years. Intervention rates were: 4.5% per year overall, 12% per year for secondary prevention after cardiac arrest, and 3% per year for primary prevention on the basis of risk factors. Mean time from implant to first appropriate discharge was 3.0 years with a range up to 11 years. The primary prevention discharge rates did not differ significantly for patients implanted for 1, 2, or ≥3 risk factors. In young patients, extreme LV hypertrophy (maximum wall thickness ≥30 mm) was the most common risk factor associated with an appropriate intervention, either alone or in combination with other markers.[22] The frequency of ICD-related complications, particularly inappropriate shocks and lead malfunction, was high, occurring in 40% of patients at 17 ± 5 years of age.[22] This rate of device complications adds a measure of complexity to ICD decision-making in this age group, in which preservation of life must unavoidably be measured against

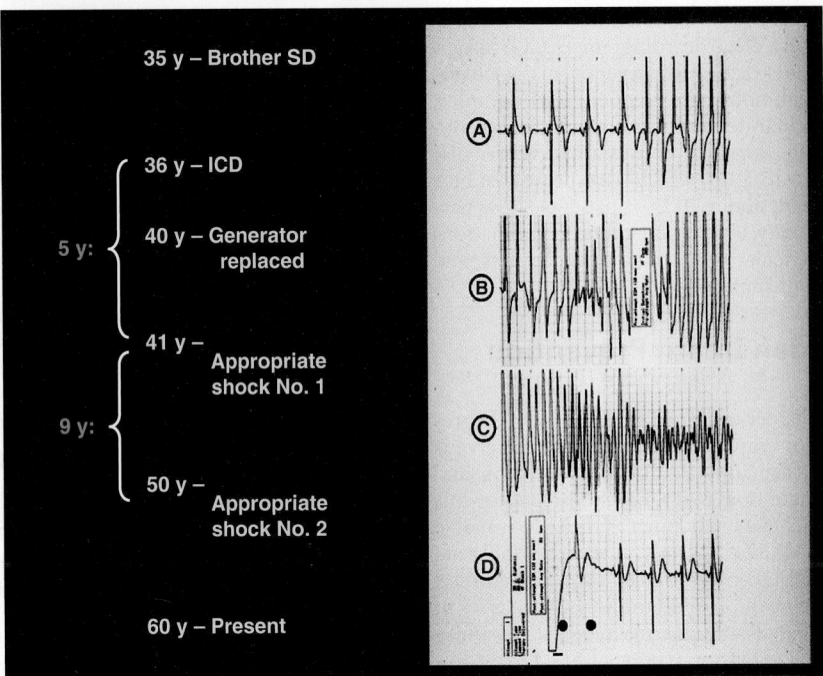

FIGURE 86.4 Primary prevention of sudden cardiac death in hypertrophic cardiomyopathy (HCM). Stored ventricular electrogram from an asymptomatic 35-year-old man who received an implantable cardioverter defibrillator (*ICD*) prophylactically due to a family history of HCM-related sudden death (*SD*) and marked ventricular septal hypertrophy (i.e., wall thickness, 31 mm). Intra-cardiac electrogram was triggered 4 years and 8 months after the defibrillator implant (at 1:20 a.m. during sleep). Continuous recording at 25 mm/s, shown in four contiguous panels, with the tracing recorded continuously left-to-right in each segment. (A) Four beats of sinus rhythm and thereafter, ventricular tachycardia (VT) begins abruptly (at 200 beats/min). (B) Device senses VT and charges. (C) VT deteriorates into ventricular fibrillation (VF). (D) Defibrillator discharges appropriately (20-J shock) during VF and restores sinus rhythm. (From Maron BJ, Spirito P, Shen W-K, et al. Implantable cardioverter-defibrillators and prevention of sudden cardiac death in hypertrophic cardiomyopathy. *JAMA.* 2007;298:405-412.)

the risk for device-related problems over long periods of time. An exception to the efficacy of ICDs in young patients with marked LV hypertrophy has been *LAMP2* cardiomyopathy, an X-linked lysosomal storage disease and HCM phenocopy, which has proved largely refractory to device therapy[24] (Fig. 86.6).

Cohort Survival With Implantable Cardioverter Defibrillators

The potential of the ICD initiative for altering clinical course in HCM is underscored in a 1000-patient hospital-based cohort (30–59 years at presentation) followed for over 20 years.[4] In these patients, appropriate ICD interventions were largely responsible for reducing HCM-related mortality to 0.5% per year, equivalent to that in an age- and gender-matched general population (Fig. 86.7). Notably, 80% of patients who died suddenly had either declined a formal recommendation for an ICD based on standard criteria or were evaluated in the era prior to translation of primary prevention transvenous device therapy to HCM.

The number of ICDs required to generate one implant that will eventually intervene appropriately is about 9:1 in adults (7:1 in children and young adults), similar to that in randomized trials of high-risk and clinically compromised patients with CAD, myocardial infarction, and systolic dysfunction[17] or with nonischemic cardiomyopathy. However, such cross-sectional study designs in HCM do not exclude the possibility that additional appropriate ICD interventions will continue to occur in additional patients.

An important principle related to ICD decisions in HCM patients is the unpredictable nature of the underlying arrhythmic substrate (i.e., timing of life-threatening ventricular tachyarrhythmias). This principle translates to the highly variable periods of dormancy for implanted devices,[2,3,25] with delays not uncommon for up to 10 or more years between implant and initial appropriate ICD intervention (Fig. 86.8).[2,3] In addition, circadian patterns of defibrillator-terminated events have been reported,[26] showing an afternoon peak[27] or absence of a discrete hourly predilection,[26] while SCD in the pre-ICD era showed an early morning peak similar to CAD, and patients have been reported with long-term survival following single episodes of VT/VF (for up to 30 years) without event recurrence.[25] Notably, in contrast to CAD,[28] the development of disabling heart failure symptoms following appropriate ICD interventions appear to be rare in HCM, without evidence that the mechanism of demise shifts from SCD to progressive heart failure.

Some ICD interventions triggered by ventricular tachyarrhythmias may occur relatively early after implant (within the first 12–18 months) (see Fig. 86.8),[2,3] suggesting that the device itself may have proarrhythmic effects generated locally by the leads embedded within the ventricular myocardium.[28] However, independent evidence in HCM suggests that such events are likely not proarrhythmic, but more likely driven by patient subgroups at higher arrhythmic risk, such as those with prior cardiac arrest or systolic dysfunction.[29] Observations from CAD-randomized trials in which appropriate interventions in the ICD arms substantially exceeded expected SCD rates in control patients have suggested that many arrhythmic episodes may be self-terminating and not truly lifesaving.[28] However, at present, there is no evidence specifically in HCM that VT episodes that trigger ICDs are irrelevant to SCD risk.

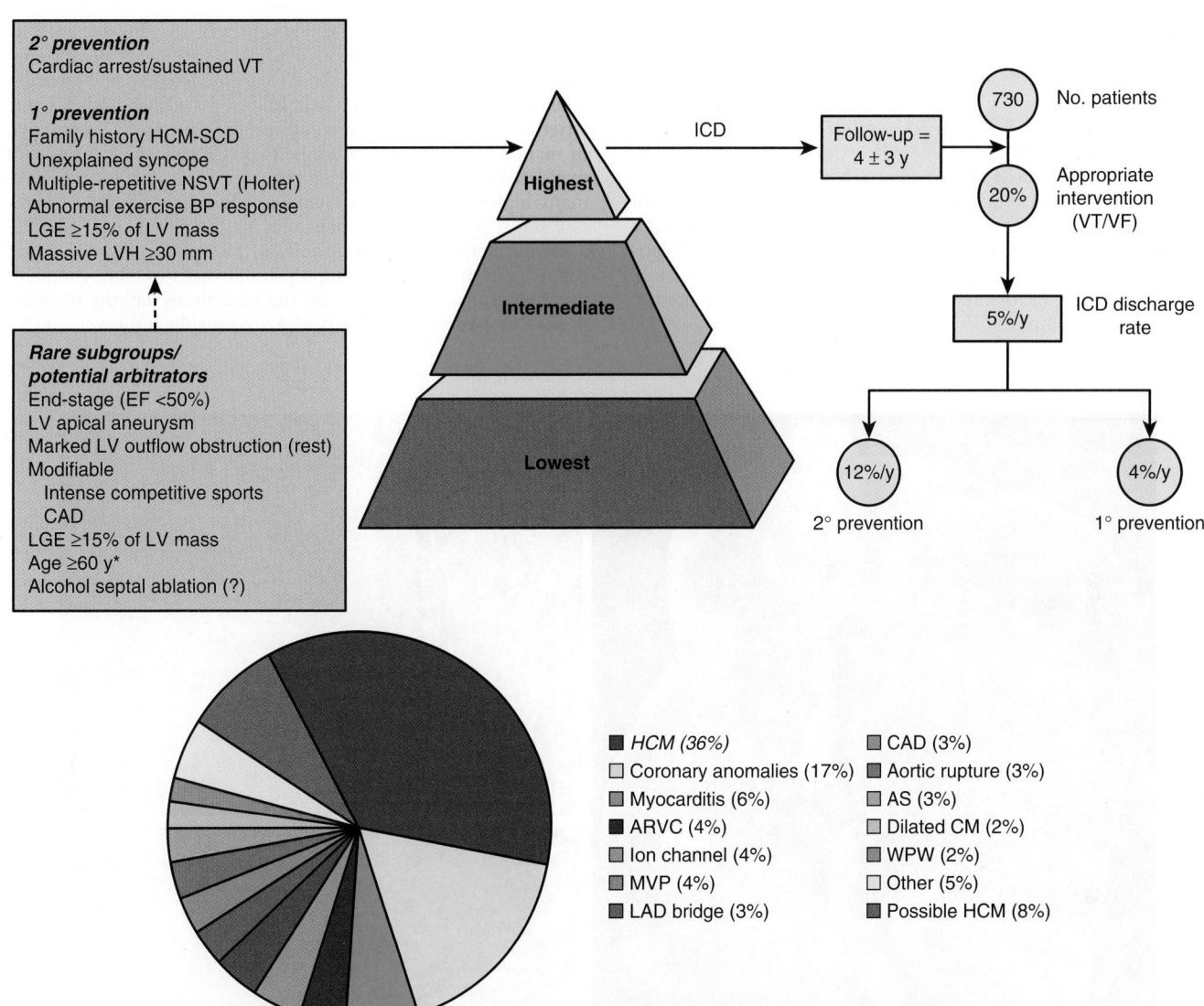

FIGURE 86.5 Risk stratification and sudden cardiac death (*SCD*). *Top,* Risk stratification model used to identify highest risk patients who may be candidates for SCD prevention with implantable cardioverter defibrillator (*ICD*). At right is outcome of ICD therapy in 730 adults and children reported from registry studies.[8,23] *SCD events uncommon after age 60. *Bottom,* Hypertrophic cardiomyopathy (*HCM*) is the single most common cause of SCD in young competitive athletes in the United States. *ARVC,* Arrhythmogenic right ventricular cardiomyopathy; *AS,* aortic stenosis; *BP,* blood pressure; *CAD,* coronary artery disease; *CM,* cardiomyopathy; *EF,* ejection fraction; *LAD,* left anterior descending; *LGE,* late gadolinium enhancement; *LV,* left ventricular; *LVH,* left ventricular hypertrophy; *MVP,* mitral valve prolapse; *NSVT,* nonsustained ventricular tachycardia; *VF,* ventricular fibrillation; *VT,* ventricular tachycardia; *WPW,* Wolff-Parkinson-White. (*Top,* From Maron BJ, Ommen SR, Semsarian C, Spirito P, Olivotto I, Maron MS. Hypertrophic cardiomyopathy: present and future, with translation into contemporary cardiovascular medicine. *J Am Coll Cardiol.* 2014;64:83-99. *Bottom,* From Maron BJ, Doerer JJ, Haas TS, Tierney DM, Mueller FO. Sudden deaths in young competitive athletes: analysis of 1866 deaths in the United States, 1980-2006. *Circulation.* 2009;119:1085-1092.)

Selecting Patients for Implantable Cardioverter Defibrillators

Conventional Risk Markers

There is universal agreement that HCM patients should be afforded secondary prevention ICDs following cardiac arrest or sustained VT episodes.[7,17,30] However, selection of patients most likely to benefit from primary prevention ICD therapy has been the source of considerable investigation and even controversy.[7,27,30,31]

By virtue of numerous retrospective and observational studies over 20 years,[1,4,6,7,30] a risk stratification algorithm has emerged

that is effective in identifying many high-risk patients who have benefited from prophylactic ICD therapy.[2,3,18–22] *The predominant strategy to anticipate these important but relatively uncommon SCD events utilizes one or more conventional noninvasive risk markers judged to be of major significance within the clinical profile of individual HCM patients, thereby justifying consideration for a primary prevention ICD* (see Fig. 86.8). This strategy has proved effective and has achieved general acceptance and standardization with incorporation into HCM guidelines and expert consensus panels: American College of Cardiology (ACC)/American Heart Association (AHA),[7] ACC/European Society of Cardiology (ESC),[30] and ACC/AHA/ESC.[17] Notably, selection of patients for ICDs in HCM differs from that in CAD, which is based largely on a predominant quantitative marker of systolic dysfunction with an ejection fraction ≤30%–35%,[17] derived from prospective randomized trials.

Conventional risk factors used to select patients deserving of primary prevention ICDs[6,7,27,30,31] are as follows : (1) family history of ≥1 HCM-related SCD in close relatives, (2) ≥1 recent episode of unexplained syncope, (3) massive LV hypertrophy (wall thickness ≥30 mm), (4) multiple repetitive or prolonged episodes of NSVT on ambulatory 24-hour (Holter) ECG, and (5) a hypotensive or attenuated blood pressure response to exercise (see Fig. 86.5). These risk factors assume greater weight as SCD predictors in younger patients.[4,11,21,22]

While a single risk marker is sufficient to consider an ICD in HCM, multiple risk factors in a given patient intuitively suggest higher risk status, greater arrhythmic burden, and stronger consideration for a prophylactic ICD.[2,3,7,30] On the other hand, strict adherence to simple counting and arithmetic summation of markers, using a minimum of two risk factors as an implant mandate (once popular in Europe), is not sustainable and leaves many high-risk patients vulnerable.[5] Initial recognition of high-risk status in an HCM patient may be fortuitous (e.g., SCD in a family member or first episode of unexplained syncope) and removed in time from the unpredictable onset of a life-threatening arrhythmia, which explains the sometimes lengthy dormant period in patients for ICDs.[2,3] Unavoidably, however, at the

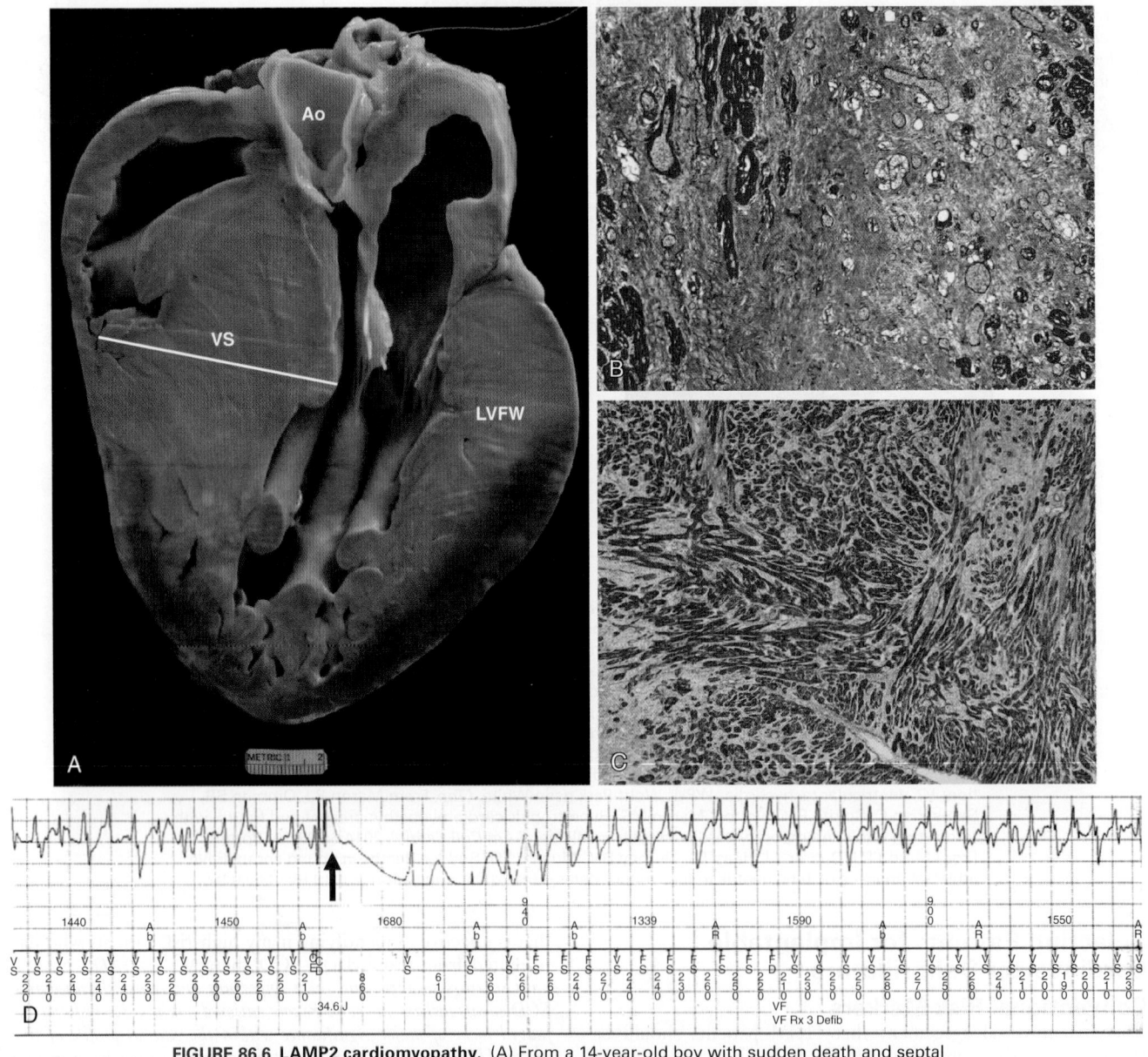

FIGURE 86.6 LAMP2 cardiomyopathy. (A) From a 14-year-old boy with sudden death and septal thickness of 65 mm (heart weight, 1425 g). *Ao,* Aorta; *LVFW,* left ventricular free wall; *VS,* ventricular septum. (B) Clusters of myocytes with vacuolated sarcoplasm (stained *red*) embedded in area of scarring (stained *blue;* Masson trichrome). (C) Disorganized arrangement of myocytes, most typical of sarcomeric hypertrophic cardiomyopathy. (D) Intracardiac electrogram. Implantable cardioverter defibrillator elicited five defibrillation shocks that failed to interrupt ventricular fibrillation (280 beats/min). (From Maron BJ, Roberts WC, Arad M, et al. Clinical outcome and phenotypic expression in LAMP2 cardiomyopathy. *JAMA.* 2009;301:1253-1259.)

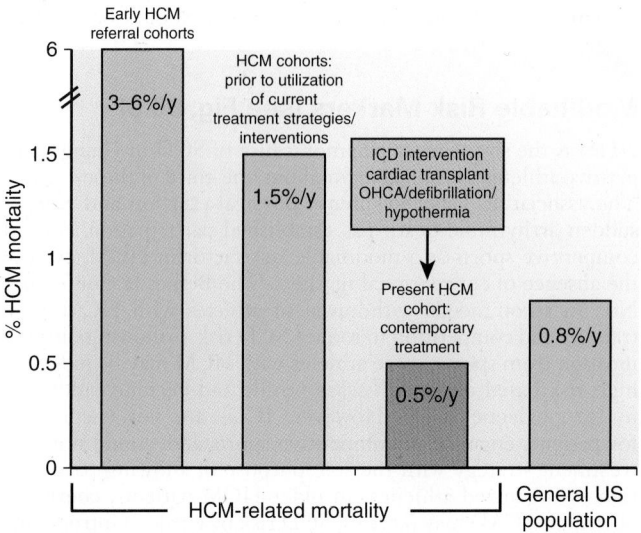

FIGURE 86.7 Evolution of hypertrophic cardiomyopathy (*HCM*)-related mortality. Contemporary cardiovascular strategies, including advanced risk stratification and implantable cardioverter defibrillators (*ICD*s) have decreased HCM mortality substantially (to 0.5% per year), similar to that expected in an age- and gender-matched US population. (From Maron BJ, Rowin EJ, Casey SA, et al. Hypertrophic cardiomyopathy in adulthood associated with low cardiovascular mortality with contemporary management strategies. *J Am Coll Cardiol.* 2015;65:1915-1928.)

time increased SCD risk is recognized, the managing cardiologist and patient are obligated to consider an ICD through shared decision-making.

Laboratory electrophysiological testing with programmed ventricular stimulation, once a popular risk stratification strategy many years ago, has been abandoned in the clinical risk stratification practice of HCM. Invasive testing is impractical and nonspecific, expensive, irrelevant to the clinical arrhythmia environment as well as without an advantage over noninvasive risk stratification.

Patients Lacking Current Conventional Risk Markers

Despite the intensive series of investigations involved in creating the present HCM risk stratification algorithm, several investigations have identified a relatively small subset of patients without conventional risk markers who nevertheless may be at risk for SCD events (0.5% per year in one report).[32] This important observation underscores the need for additional markers to complete the clinical risk algorithm in HCM.

Recently, risk stratification was improved by introducing extensive distribution of LGE by quantitative contrast-CMR.[15] Risk of SCD increases in a linear fashion with respect to %LGE in the LV myocardium, with 15% conveying a two-fold increase in SCD risk, while absent or focal LGE is associated with lower risk (Fig. 86.9) Extensive LGE acts as an independent risk factor even in the absence of conventional markers and can also

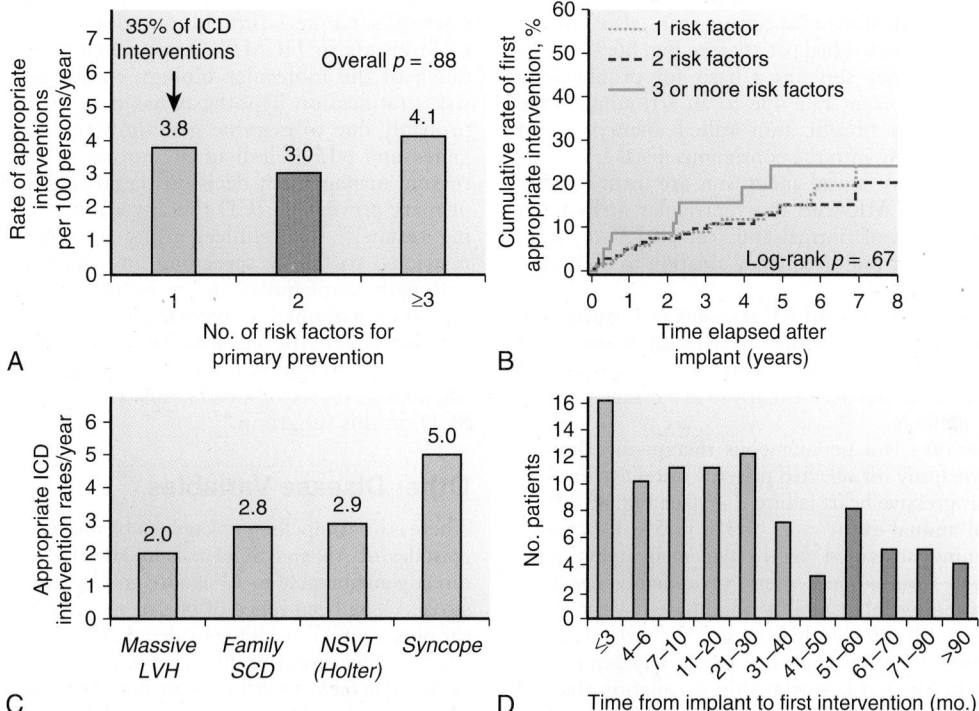

FIGURE 86.8 Strategies for risk stratification and prevention of sudden cardiac death (*SCD*) in hypertrophic cardiomyopathy. (A) Implantable cardioverter defibrillator (*ICD*) intervention rates do not differ significantly with respect to implants for 1, 2, or ≥3 conventional risk factors; 35% of ICD interventions are in patients with only one major risk factor. (B) Cumulative rates for first device intervention with respect to 1, 2, or ≥3 risk markers. (C) ICD intervention rates in patients implanted for only one risk factor. (D) Time interval between implant and first appropriate intervention varies, with some device discharges delayed for 5 to 11 years. *LVH,* Left ventricular hypertrophy; *NSVT,* nonsustained ventricular tachycardia. (From Maron BJ, Spirito P, Shen W-K, et al. Implantable cardioverter-defibrillators and prevention of sudden cardiac death in hypertrophic cardiomyopathy. *JAMA.* 2007;298:405-412.)

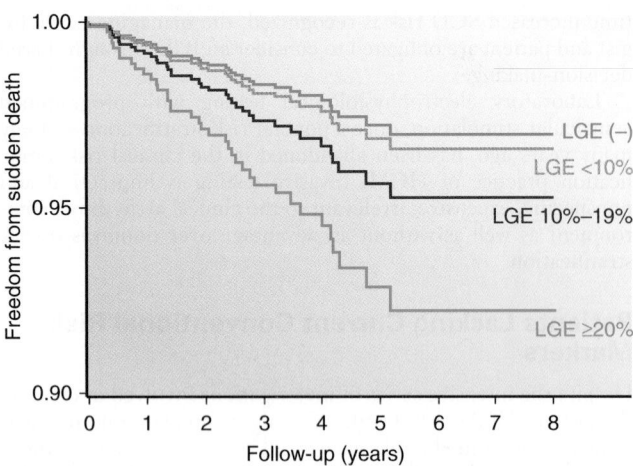

FIGURE 86.9 Relation between percent of late gadolinium enhancement (LGE) and sudden cardiac death events in 1293 hypertrophic cardiomyopathy patients. (From Chan RH, Maron BJ, Olivotto I, et al. Prognostic value of quantitative contrast-enhanced cardiovascular magnetic resonance for the evaluation of sudden death risk in patients with hypertrophic cardiomyopathy. *Circulation.* 2014;130:484-495.)

represent an arbitrator when ICD decision-making remains ambiguous based on established risk markers (see Fig. 86.3). Therefore extensive LGE alone can identify at-risk patients who otherwise would not be considered candidates for primary prevention ICDs.[15]

Also, relatively uncommon disease features or subgroups within the broad HCM disease spectrum can also convey increased SCD risk in an individual patient (see Fig. 86.9).

LV apical aneurysms may serve as a basis for prophylactic ICDs with a 5% annual event rate due to an arrhythmogenic substrate created by the fibrotic thin-walled aneurysm and regional scarring extending into the contiguous distal LV myocardium[33] (Fig. 86.10). LV apical aneurysms are most reliably recognized by contrast CMR with the ventricular arrhythmia focus at the border zone of normal and scarred LV myocardium, which is the site for radiofrequency ablation to obliterate arrhythmogenicity.

End-stage phase with widespread LV scarring and irreversible systolic dysfunction (ejection fraction <50%) is often associated with LV remodeling with wall thinning and cavity enlargement[34] (see Fig. 86.10). The ICD has been employed as a bridge to heart transplant in such patients.

Alcohol septal ablation is a percutaneous therapeutic alternative to surgical myectomy for selected patients to relieve outflow obstruction and progressive heart failure[7,35,36] (see Fig. 86.10). Postprocedural annual event rates of 3% to 5% for potentially life-threatening sustained ventricular tachyarrhythmias have been reported from some centers, presumably resulting from an electrophysiological instability potentiated by the myocardial scar.[31,37] A multicenter study from the Netherlands comparing percutaneous therapy to surgical myectomy reported a two-fold increase in SCD risk attributable to ablation (hazard ratio, 2.1; 95% CI, 1.0–44).[37] Furthermore, appropriate ICD interventions for VT/VF were eight-fold more frequent postablation than after myectomy. Based on a prudent measure of concern that alcohol-imposed infarcts could compound preexisting electrophysiological instability, some practitioners have implanted ICDs in selected patients after alcohol ablation. However, routine prophylactic ICD implants following alcohol septal ablation appear to be an unsubstantiated strategy, particularly in the absence of a risk stratification formula for this

patient subset. Therefore implant decisions should be resolved on a case-by-case basis.

Modifiable Risk Markers (see Fig. 86.3)

HCM is the single most common cause of SCD in young competitive athletes, responsible for about one-third of these events.[8] The association between intense physical exertion and risk for sudden arrhythmic death has established participation in most competitive sports as a modifiable risk factor in HCM, even in the absence of conventional markers. The Bethesda Conference No. 36 recommends withdrawal of athletes with HCM from training and competition to reduce SCD risk. Following disqualification from sports, some athletes with HCM may be judged at high risk based on their disease profile and become candidates for prophylactic ICDs. However, ICDs are not encouraged for patients engaged in competitive sports and should not be a treatment strategy with the sole purpose of allowing participation in organized athletics. In older HCM patients, coexistent obstructive CAD may increase SCD risk by virtue of introducing myocardial ischemia but is potentially modifiable by coronary intervention.

LV outflow obstruction with high intraventricular pressures has been promoted as a risk marker in HCM by some investigators[38] but disputed by others.[39,40] There is some evidence that surgical septal myectomy, by abolishing LV outflow obstruction and normalizing intraventricular pressures, reduces SCD risk.[41] However, surgical reduction of outflow gradients is not a primary strategy to mitigate SCD risk, and the muscular resection itself does not reduce risk in patients with massive hypertrophy by virtue of changing basal septal thickness to <30 mm.[27]

There is no evidence that specific pathogenic (disease-causing) sarcomere protein mutations are predictive of future SCD events in HCM.[42] Despite being heavily promoted by much of the molecular biology community, the gene-based risk stratification hypothesis has not proved clinically viable, probably due to extreme genetic heterogeneity now with 11 genes and >1500 individual mutations reported.[42] For this reason, management decisions regarding high-risk status and primary prevention ICD therapy are never based on genotyping results.[42] The clinical utility of genotyping is currently restricted to family screening and identification of relatives with pathogenic mutations in the absence of the HCM phenotype (i.e., without LV hypertrophy).[42] While these genotype-positive/phenotype-negative family members are theoretically at risk for developing LV hypertrophy, there is little evidence for increased risk of adverse disease-related events (including SCD) in this subgroup.[42]

Other Disease Variables

There is no compelling linkage established between clinically overt episodes of AF and SCD risk in HCM,[1,9] and HCM-mortality directly attributable to AF is rare and largely confined to embolic stroke.[1] The occurrence of one or more paroxysmal AF episodes (or persistent AF) is not considered an indication for prophylactic ICDs.[7,9] Occasionally, this arrhythmia has acted as a trigger for ventricular tachyarrhythmias in the electrophysiology laboratory or provoked ICD interventions in high-risk patients. There is insufficient evidence to consider either coronary arterial bridging[23] or 12-lead ECG patterns as specific risk markers in HCM.

Clinical Decision-Making
Ambiguous Zones

Not uncommonly, decision-making dilemmas concerning prophylactic ICDs inevitably arise when the level of risk cannot be

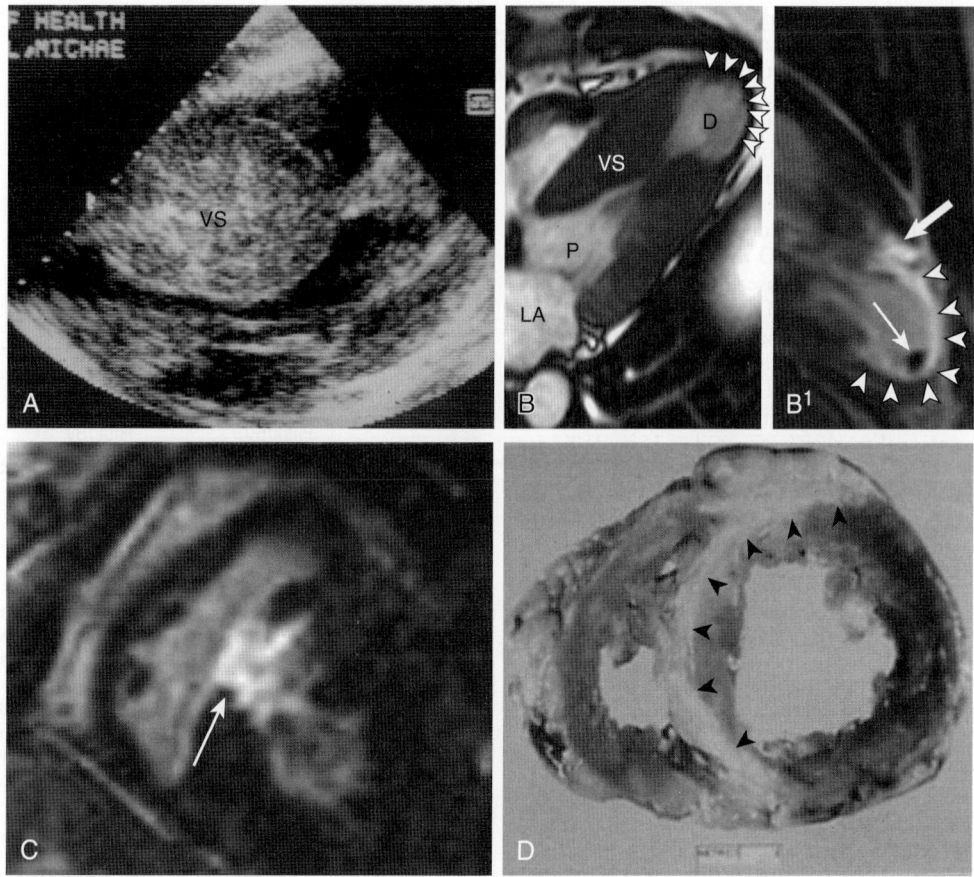

FIGURE 86.10 Subgroups with risk for sustained ventricular tachyarrhythmias and sudden cardiac death. (A) Massive thickening (i.e., 33 mm) confined to anterolateral left ventricular wall, greatly underestimated by echocardiography and prompting implantable cardioverter defibrillator recommendation. *VS,* Ventricular septum. (B) Akinetic thin-walled left ventricular apical aneurysm (*arrowheads*), with mid-cavity muscular apposition. *D,* Distal (cavity); *LA,* left atrium; *P,* proximal (cavity). (B[1]) Late gadolinium enhancement (i.e., scar) involving aneurysm rim (*arrowheads*) and contiguous myocardium (*thick arrow*); small apical thrombus is evident (*thin arrow*). (C) Large transmural ventricular septal scar (*arrow*) from alcohol ablation. (D) "End-stage" (ejection fraction = 35%); extensive scarring with transmural late gadolinium enhancement in lateral wall (*small arrowheads*) and septum extending into right ventricle and biatrial enlargement and dilated left ventricular cavity. ([B[1]] From Maron MS, Finley JJ, Bos JM, et al. Prevalence, clinical significance and natural history of left ventricular apical aneurysms in hypertrophic cardiomyopathy. *Circulation.* 2008;118:1541-1549. [D] From Maron BJ. Contemporary insights and strategies for risk stratification and prevention of sudden death in hypertrophic cardiomyopathy. *Circulation.* 2010;121:445-456.)

determined with precision.[1,5,6] This is largely due to the heterogeneity of HCM in which some patients do not easily fall into clear-cut high- or low-risk subgroups based solely on the conventional risk marker algorithm.

Potentially contributing to this uncertainty is the prevailing but unavoidable imprecision in defining some of the risk markers used in HCM risk stratification—for example, the literature records multiple versions for the family history of SCD, including in 1 first-degree relative, ≥2 relatives <40 years old, ≥1 first-degree relative <40 years old, or ≥1 relative <50 years old.[1,7,30] This may be further encumbered by small pedigree size or adoption, as well as frequent ambiguity regarding the precise cause of death in relatives without autopsy confirmation or clinical diagnosis of HCM, or when events occurred many years ago. When risk level cannot be assigned with a sufficient degree of certainty due to gaps in knowledge and data, a measure of individual clinical judgment and experience, as well as full transparency within the shared decision-making model, is most appropriate.

Primary prevention ICD decision-making is generally more difficult in young children and adolescents, particularly when the risk criteria are borderline or less than definitive.[6,7,22,43] A measure of hesitancy toward lifelong ICDs often arises in young patients when confronting the clinical paradox of active and healthy-appearing patients exposed to greatest SCD risk not only by age but also with the highest device complication rates over long time periods (including potential problems with vascular access).[3,20,44] Also, some risk stratification markers that are useful in adults cannot be easily extrapolated to young children with HCM, including the uncertainty often encountered in defining massive degrees of LV hypertrophy with respect to differences in age and body size.

Counting Risk Factors

While it is a reasonable intuition that patients with multiple risk factors are at greater SCD risk, the ICD in HCM Registry demonstrated that an important proportion of ICD interventions for

VT/VF occurred in patients implanted for only one risk factor (i.e., 35%)[8] and appropriate device therapy was not significantly more common in patients with two or three risk markers than in those patients with only one risk factor.

Rigid adherence to the strategy of simple arithmetic summing of risk markers, with a minimum of two of these considered mandatory before recommending a primary prevention ICD (an approach once favored by European investigations),[38] unavoidably creates the possibility that some deserving one-risk-factor patients will not be considered for ICD therapy and will be left unprotected from SCD. However, based on US guidelines, a single strong and established marker of increased risk within the clinical profile of an individual HCM patient can be sufficient to identify unacceptably increased SCD risk.

However, the one-risk-factor model is complicated by recognition that the proportion of patients in tertiary center cohorts with only one conventional marker (estimated at 15%–35%) far exceeds the number of HCM patients that may be expected to die suddenly. Indeed, not all patients with one marker have the same magnitude of risk, and universal implantation of devices in this patient subgroup is not sustainable. For example, many clinically stable patients who survive >60 years are, in fact, one-risk-factor patients with a lower risk by virtue of uncomplicated survival and disease tolerance over decades.[11]

It should also be underscored that risk level can potentially change over time (always toward higher levels), emphasizing the importance of ongoing clinical surveillance on an annual basis, optimally carried on in multidiscipline, dedicated HCM centers.[45] For example, in young patients, LV wall thickness can increase abruptly, unexplained syncope may occur for the first time, a family member may unexpectedly experience an SCD event, or nonsustained bursts of VT can appear on routine ambulatory (Holter) ECGs.

Implantable Cardioverter Defibrillator Complications

The decision to implant an ICD prophylactically in HCM patients is also measured against consideration for potential complications and inconvenience incurred by permanently implanted devices. Clearly, these two scenarios are not of equal weight, given the capability of the ICD for terminating lethal arrhythmias and preserving life.

In addition to the occasional infection, pocket hematoma, pneumothorax, and venous thrombosis,[3,18,19,20,44] about 25% of HCM patients experience inappropriate shocks (5% per year)[44] resulting from lead fracture or dislodgement, oversensing, or double-counting and programming malfunctions, or when triggered inadvertently by sinus tachycardia or AF with rapid ventricular response. Reports of multiple shock "storms" are exceedingly uncommon in HCM. Device complications, including inappropriate shocks, are most common in young patients due largely to heightened activity levels and accelerated body growth, placing continual and sometimes excessive strain on the leads, generally considered the weakest link in this system.[21,22,43,44,46]

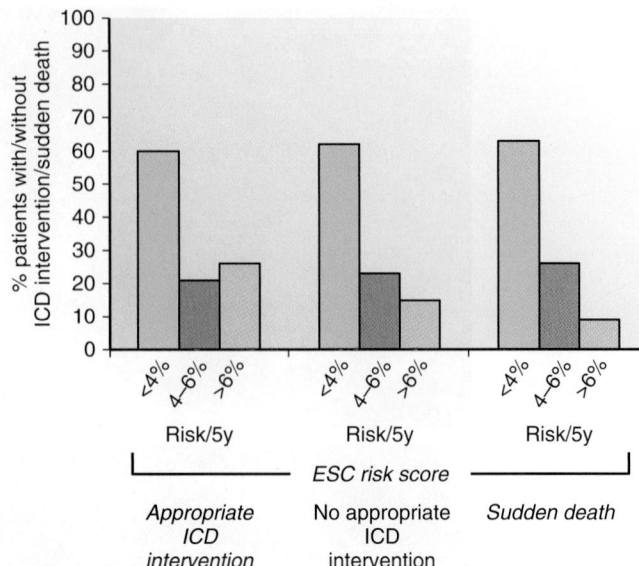

FIGURE 86.11 Assessment of European Society of Cardiology (*ESC*) prognostic score for sudden cardiac death in hypertrophic cardiomyopathy. With the ESC risk score applied retrospectively to a large US cohort, only 20% of patients with sudden cardiac death or appropriate implantable cardioverter defibrillator (*ICD*) interventions were considered sufficiently high risk by ESC to justify consideration for a primary prevention ICD (with scores >6% per 5 years).[47] (From Maron BJ, Casey SA, Garberich RF, Rowin EJ, Maron MS. Independent assessment of the European Society of Cardiology sudden death risk model for hypertrophic cardiomyopathy. *Am J Cardiol.* 2015;116:757-764.)

Statistically Based Risk Predictors

The ESC advanced a risk stratification strategy to identify high-risk HCM patients, employing mathematical and statistical methods to weight the relative effects and interactions of specific risk markers.[38] This approach has been validated with respect to the C-statistic, but not in terms of clinical decision-making regarding ICDs for individual HCM patients.[38]

However, when the ESC risk model and score was tested against a large (*n* = 1629) diverse and independent HCM cohort (previously risk-stratified based on US guidelines), it proved to be generally unreliable for predicting future SCD events in individual patients (Fig. 86.11).[47] Most HCM patients with SCD or appropriate ICD interventions are misclassified by low-risk scores and therefore would have remained unprotected from lethal ventricular tachyarrhythmias. For example, of patients in the cohort with SCD or appropriate ICD discharges, only about 20% had a prognostic risk score (>6% per 5 years) that would justify a primary prevention ICD, leaving 65 individual patients vulnerable to SCD. Furthermore, most of these patients (about 60%) were misclassified by the lowest calculated risk scores of <4% per 5 years, which excluded prophylactic ICDs that theoretically would have prevented SCD.[47]

REFERENCES

1. Maron BJ, Ommen SR, Semsarian C, Spirito P, Olivotto I, Maron MS. Hypertrophic cardiomyopathy: present and future, with translation into contemporary cardiovascular medicine. *J Am Coll Cardiol.* 2014;64:83–99.
2. Maron BJ, Shen W-K, Link MS, et al. Efficacy of implantable cardioverter-defibrillators for the prevention of sudden death in patients with hypertrophic cardiomyopathy. *N Engl J Med.* 2000;342:365–373.
3. Maron BJ, Spirito P, Shen W-K, et al. Implantable cardioverter-defibrillators and prevention of sudden cardiac death in hypertrophic cardiomyopathy. *JAMA.* 2007;298:405–412.
4. Maron BJ, Rowin EJ, Casey SA, et al. Hypertrophic cardiomyopathy in adulthood associated with low cardiovascular mortality with contemporary management strategies. *J Am Coll Cardiol.* 2015;65:1915–1928.

5. Nishimura RA, Ommen SR. Hypertrophic cardiomyopathy, sudden death, and implantable cardiac defibrillators: how low the bar? *JAMA.* 2007;298:452–454.
6. Maron BJ. Contemporary insights and strategies for risk stratification and prevention of sudden death in hypertrophic cardiomyopathy. *Circulation.* 2010;121:445–456.
7. Gersh BJ, Maron BJ, Bonow RO, et al. 2011 ACCF/AHA guidelines for the diagnosis and treatment of hypertrophic cardiomyopathy: a report of the American College of Cardiology Foundation/American Heart Association Task Force on Practice Guidelines. *Circulation.* 2011;124:2761–2796. *J Am Coll Cardiol.* 2011;58:e212-e60; *J Thorac Cardiovasc Surg.* 2011;142:e153–e203.

8. Maron BJ, Doerer JJ, Haas TS, Tierney DM, Mueller FO. Sudden deaths in young competitive athletes: analysis of 1866 deaths in the United States, 1980-2006. *Circulation.* 2009;119:1085–1092.
9. Olivotto I, Cecchi F, Casey SA, Dolara A, Traverse JH, Maron BJ. Impact of atrial fibrillation on the clinical course of hypertrophic cardiomyopathy. *Circulation.* 2001;104:2517–2524.
10. Semsarian C, Ingles J, Maron MS, Maron BJ. New perspectives on the prevalence of hypertrophic cardiomyopathy. *J Am Coll Cardiol.* 2015;65:1249–1254.
11. Maron BJ, Rowin EJ, Casey SA, et al. Risk stratification and outcome of patients with hypertrophic cardiomyopathy ≥60 years of age. *Circulation.* 2013;127:585–593.

12. Olivotto I, Maron MS, Adabag AS, et al. Gender-related differences in the clinical presentation and outcome of hypertrophic cardiomyopathy. *J Am Coll Cardiol*. 2005;46:480–487.

13. Maron BJ, Casey SA, Poliac LC, Gohman TE, Almquist AK, Aeppli DM. Clinical course of hypertrophic cardiomyopathy in a regional United States cohort. *JAMA*. 1999;281:650–655.

14. Adabag AS, Maron BJ, Appelbaum E, et al. Occurrence and frequency of arrhythmias in hypertrophic cardiomyopathy in relation to delayed enhancement on cardiovascular magnetic resonance. *J Am Coll Cardiol*. 2008;51:1369–1374.

15. Chan RH, Maron BJ, Olivotto I, Pencina MJ, Assenza GE, Haas TS, et al. Prognostic value of quantitative contrast-enhanced cardiovascular magnetic resonance for the evaluation of sudden death risk in patients with hypertrophic cardiomyopathy. *Circulation*. 2014;130:484–495.

16. Mirowski M, Reid PR, Mower MM, et al. Termination of malignant ventricular arrhythmias with an implanted automatic defibrillator in human beings. *N Engl J Med*. 1980;303:322–324.

17. Zipes DP, Camm AJ, Borggrefe M, et al. ACC/AHA/ESC 2006 guidelines for management of patients with ventricular arrhythmias and the prevention of sudden cardiac death. *Circulation*. 2006;114:e385–e484.

18. Woo A, Monakier D, Harris L, et al. Determinants of implantable defibrillator discharges in high-risk patients with hypertrophic cardiomyopathy. *Heart*. 2007;93:1044–1045.

19. Schinkel AF, Vriesendorp PA, Sijbrands EJ, Jordaens LJ, ten Cate FJ, Michels M. Outcome and complications after implantable cardioverter defibrillator therapy in hypertrophic cardiomyopathy: systematic review and meta-analysis. *Circ Heart Fail*. 2012;5:552–559.

20. Vriesendorp PA, Schinkel AF, Van Cleemput J, et al. Implantable cardioverter-defibrillators in hypertrophic cardiomyopathy: patient outcomes, rate of appropriate and inappropriate interventions, and complications. *Am Heart J*. 2013;166:496–502.

21. Maron BJ, Rowin EJ, Casey SA, et al. Hypertrophic cardiomyopathy in children, adolescents and young adults associated with low cardiovascular mortality with contemporary management strategies. *Circulation*. 2016;133:62–73.

22. Maron BJ, Spirito P, Ackerman MJ, et al. Prevention of sudden cardiac death with implantable cardioverter-defibrillators in children and adolescents with hypertrophic cardiomyopathy. *J Am Coll Cardiol*. 2013;61:1527–1535.

23. Basso C, Thiene G, Mackey-Bojack S, Frigo AC, Corrado D, Maron BJ. Myocardial bridging: a frequent component of the hypertrophic cardiomyopathy phenotype lacks systematic association with sudden cardiac death. *Eur Heart J*. 2009;30:1627–1634.

24. Maron BJ, Roberts WC, Arad M, et al. Clinical outcome and phenotypic expression in LAMP2 cardiomyopathy. *JAMA*. 2009;301:1253–1259.

25. Maron BJ, Haas TS, Shannon KM. Long-term survival after cardiac arrest in hypertrophic cardiomyopathy. *Heart Rhythm*. 2009;6:993–997.

26. Maron BJ, Semsarian C, Shen W-K, et al. Circadian patterns in the occurrence of malignant ventricular tachyarrhythmias triggering defibrillator interventions in patients with hypertrophic cardiomyopathy. *Heart Rhythm*. 2009;6:599–602.

27. Spirito P, Bellone P, Harris KM, Bernabo P, Bruzzi P, Maron BJ. Magnitude of left ventricular hypertrophy predicts the risk of sudden death in hypertrophic cardiomyopathy. *N Engl J Med*. 2000;342:1778–1785.

28. Tung R, Zimetbaum P, Josephson ME. A critical appraisal of implantable cardioverter-defibrillator therapy for the prevention of sudden cardiac death. *J Am Coll Cardiol*. 2008;52:1111–1121.

29. Alsheikh-Ali AA, Link MS, Semsarian C, et al. Ventricular tachycardia/fibrillation early after defibrillator implantation in patients with hypertrophic cardiomyopathy is explained by a high-risk subgroup of patients. *Heart Rhythm*. 2013;10:214–218.

30. Maron BJ, McKenna WJ, Danielson GK, et al. American College of Cardiology/European Society of Cardiology clinical expert consensus document on hypertrophic cardiomyopathy: a report of the American College of Cardiology foundation task force on clinical expert consensus documents and the European Society of Cardiology committee for practice guidelines. *J Am Coll Cardiol*. 2003;42:1687–1713. and *Eur Heart J*. 2003;24:1965–1991.

31. Spirito P, Autore C, Rapezzi C, et al. Syncope and risk of sudden death in hypertrophic cardiomyopathy. *Circulation*. 2009;119:1703–1710.

32. Spirito P, Autore C, Formisano F, et al. Risk of sudden death and outcome in patients with hypertrophic cardiomyopathy with benign clinical presentation and without risk factors. *Am J Cardiol*. 2014;113:1550–1555.

33. Maron MS, Finley JJ, Bos JM, et al. Prevalence, clinical significance and natural history of left ventricular apical aneurysms in hypertrophic cardiomyopathy. *Circulation*. 2008;118:1541–1549.

34. Harris KM, Spirito P, Maron MS, et al. Prevalence, clinical profile, and significance of left ventricular remodeling in the end-stage phase of hypertrophic cardiomyopathy. *Circulation*. 2006;114:216–225.

35. Noseworthy PA, Rosenberg MA, Fifer MA, et al. Ventricular arrhythmia following alcohol ablation for obstructive hypertrophic cardiomyopathy. *Am J Cardiol*. 2009;104:128–132.

36. Sorajja P, Ommen SR, Holmes Jr DR, et al. Survival after alcohol septal ablation for obstructive hypertrophic cardiomyopathy. *Circulation*. 2012;126:2374–2380.

37. Vriesendorp PA, Liebregts M, Steggerda RC, et al. Long-term outcomes after medical and invasive treatment in patients with hypertrophic cardiomyopathy. *JACC Heart Fail*. 2014;2:630–636.

38. Elliott PM, Anastasakis A, Borger MA, et al. 2014 ESC Guidelines on diagnosis and management of hypertrophic cardiomyopathy: the Task Force for the Diagnosis and Management of Hypertrophic Cardiomyopathy of the European Society of Cardiology (ESC). *Eur Heart J*. 2014;35:2733–2779.

39. Efthimiadis GK, Pacharidou DG, Giannakoulas G, et al. Left ventricular outflow tract obstruction as a risk factor for sudden cardiac death in hypertrophic cardiomyopathy. *Am J Cardiol*. 2009;104:695–699.

40. Maron MS, Olivotto I, Betocchi S, et al. Effect of left ventricular outflow tract obstruction on clinical outcome in hypertrophic cardiomyopathy. *N Engl J Med*. 2003;348:295–303.

41. Ommen SR, Maron BJ, Olivotto I, et al. Long-term effects of surgical septal myectomy on survival in patients with obstructive hypertrophic cardiomyopathy. *J Am Coll Cardiol*. 2005;46:470–476.

42. Maron BJ, Maron MS, Semsarian C. Genetics of hypertrophic cardiomyopathy after 20 years: clinical perspectives. *J Am Coll Cardiol*. 2012;60:705–715.

43. Berul CI, Van Hare GF, Kertesz NJ, et al. Results of a multicenter retrospective implantable cardioverter-defibrillator registry of pediatric and congenital heart disease patients. *J Am Coll Cardiol*. 2008;51:1685–1691.

44. Lin G, Nishimura RA, Gersh BJ, Ommen S, Ackerman M, Brady PA. Device complications and inappropriate implantable cardioverter-defibrillator shocks in patients with hypertrophic cardiomyopathy. *Heart*. 2009;95:709–714.

45. Maron BJ. Hypertrophic cardiomyopathy centers. *Am J Cardiol*. 2009;104:1158–1159.

46. Hauser RG, Kallinen LM, Almquist AK, Gornick CC, Katsiyiannis WT. Early failure of a small-diameter high-voltage implantable cardioverter-defibrillator lead. *Heart Rhythm*. 2007;4:892–896.

47. Maron BJ, Casey SA, Garberich RF, Rowin EJ, Maron MS. Independent assessment of the European Society of Cardiology sudden death risk model for hypertrophic cardiomyopathy. *Am J Cardiol*. 2015;116:757–764.

87 Ventricular Tachycardias in Arrhythmogenic Right Ventricular Dysplasia/Cardiomyopathy

Harikrishna Tandri and Hugh Calkins

Arrhythmogenic right ventricular dysplasia/cardiomyopathy (ARVD/C) is an inherited cardiomyopathy that is characterized by ventricular arrhythmias, an increased risk of sudden death, and abnormalities of right ventricular (RV) structure and function.[1-4] Although structural involvement of the right ventricle predominates, a left-dominant form of ARVD/C has been described.[5-8] In most patients in the United States, structural abnormalities of the right ventricle predominate. The pathologic hallmark of ARVD/C is RV myocyte loss with fibrofatty replacement (Fig. 87.1). Since the first detailed clinical description of the disorder in 1982,[1] significant advances have been made in our understanding of all aspects of this disease. Since the beginning of the 21st century, mutations in most desmosomal proteins and also some nondesmosomal proteins have been identified as the genetic basis of ARVD/C. Since a pathogenic mutation can be identified in more than 50% of affected individuals, genetic testing has emerged as an important diagnostic tool.[8-10] The purpose of this chapter is to provide a concise and up-to-date review of the current state of knowledge regarding the natural history, clinical presentation, pathogenesis, diagnosis, and treatment of patients with ARVD/C. Specific emphasis will be placed on exploring the relationship between ARVD/C and exercise.

Clinical Presentation and Natural History

ARVD/C is an unusual condition with an estimated prevalence of 1 per 5000 in the general population. This is roughly 10-fold less common than hypertrophic cardiomyopathy, which occurs in about 1 per 500 of the general population.

Patients usually present during the second to fifth decade of life with palpitations, lightheadedness, syncope, or sudden death[1,2,4] (Figs. 87.2 and 87.3A and B). In our experience, it is extremely rare to manifest clinical signs or symptoms of ARVD/C prior to the age of 12 years or after the age of 60 years.

Although ARVC/D is predominantly a disease of the right ventricle, it is now well established that involvement of the left ventricle is not uncommon, particularly when magnetic resonance (MR) imaging is used to detect subtle abnormalities in left ventricular (LV) function and also in patients with advanced disease.[5-8] Left-dominant arrhythmogenic cardiomyopathy also occurs and is defined by early disease of the LV, often affecting the posterolateral wall, in the absence of significant RV systolic dysfunction. Left-dominant disease is more commonly seen in patients with desmoplakin mutations.[8]

Etiology

In most cases, ARVD/C is inherited in an autosomal dominant pattern with significantly variable penetrance and expressivity. Among probands diagnosed with this disease, screening of first-degree relatives identifies other affected individuals in approximately 50% of cases. In a minority of cases, ARVD/C is inherited in an autosomal recessive pattern as part of a cardiocutaneous syndrome, such as Naxos disease or Carvajal syndrome, which is also characterized by wooly hair and palmoplantar keratodermia.[9,10]

Linkage mapping and candidate gene evaluation studies performed on patients with the autosomal dominant form of ARVD/C was not initially productive due to significant variability in the penetrance and expressivity of the disease. It was the evaluation of patients with Naxos syndrome, a disease with 100% penetrance by adolescence, that identified a disease causing mutation: a homozygous deletion of two base pairs found in the plakoglobin gene located in the 17q21 locus.[10] The gene encodes a key component of desmosomes, which are complex intercellular adhesion structures found in stratified epithelial cells of the skin as well as in myocytes. Desmosomes are composed of three major groups of proteins: cadherins are transmembrane proteins that provide the actual mechanical coupling between individual cells and include desmoglein and desmocollin. Desmoplakin is a plakin-family protein that serves to anchor the desmosomal structure to the intermediate filaments of the cell. Lastly, armadillo proteins, including plakoglobin and plakophillin, link desmoplakin and the cadherin tails.

The identification of defective desmosomal proteins in Naxos syndrome led to studies investigating their role in other arrhythmogenic cardiomyopathies. Carvajal syndrome, another cardiocutaneous syndrome that has left-dominant arrhythmogenic cardiomyopathy, was shown to be associated with a recessive mutation in desmoplakin. Other genetic mutations were subsequently identified in the autosomal-dominant form of ARVC/D and include desmoplakin, desmoglein-2, desmocollin-2, and plakophillin-2 (PKP2) genes. Mutations in several extradesmosomal genes, such as those encoding transforming growth factor β3 (TGFβ3), the cardiac ryanodine receptor (RyR2), Titin, and transmembrane protein 43 (TMEM43), have also been implicated in specific types of atypical forms of ARVC/D. In the United States, a desmosomal protein mutation can be identified in approximately 50% of ARVD/C patients.[8] The most commonly mutated genes are PKP2 (45%) and desmoglein-2 (9%). Importantly, while 86% of patients in this series had a single heterozygous gene mutation, 7% showed compound heterozygosity and another 7% showed digenic heterozygosity. This is important as clinicians need to be aware that some individuals with ARVD/C may have more than one mutation in one or more of the many desmosomal proteins. Other candidate genes are likely to be identified in the future. Thus it is possible that the affected individual (the proband) will have more than one defective gene.

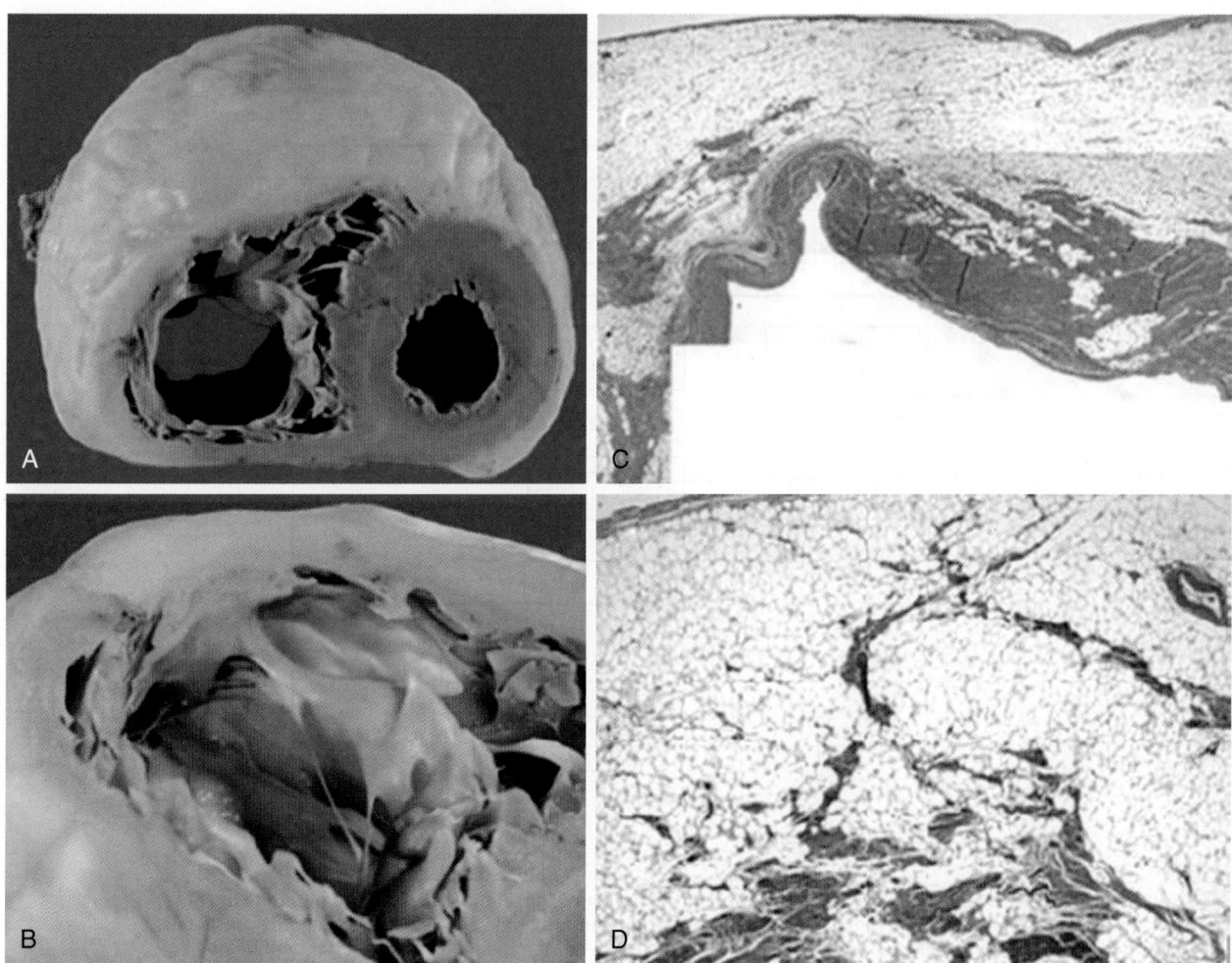

FIGURE 87.1 (A) Gross specimen of an explanted heart showing a massive right ventricle (RV) with extensive fat that replaced the entire RV epicardium, leaving a thin rim of fibrotic endocardium. Also note the relative sparing of the left ventricle and the interventricular septum. (B) Near-total fatty replacement of the RV wall with loss of myocytes renders the RV translucent. (C) Transmural low-resolution histopathological image shows the fat replacement extending from epicardium to the endocardium. (D) Trichrome staining reveals fibrous tissue interspersed with fat tissue, characteristic of this disease. (From Tandri H, Asimaki A, Dalal D, Saffitz JE, Halushka MK, Calkins H. Gap junction remodeling in a case of arrhythmogenic right ventricular dysplasia due to plakophilin-2 mutation. *J Cardiovasc Electrophysiol.* 2008;19:1212-1214.)

Since all the genetic abnormalities have not yet been identified, the first-degree relatives may not have the known gene but could have inherited the unknown gene mutation. Therefore finding a pathogenic gender mutation in the proband but not in the first-degree relative does not completely exclude the possibility of desmosomal mutation in the first-degree relative. It is also important to recognize that not all variants identified in a desmosomal protein are causal mutations.

Pathogenesis

Initial attempts to explain the pathogenesis of ARVC/D produced several hypotheses including the dysplastic theory, which held that the atrophy and fibrofatty replacement of the RV myocardium in ARVD/C was a congenital, developmental defect. This led to the original description of the syndrome as ARVD. It is now clear, however, that the structural defects in ARVD/C are not present at birth but actually develop progressively throughout childhood and early adulthood.

The genetics of ARVD/C has provided support for the hypothesis that the disease may be caused by desmosomal dysfunction. The pathogenic mechanisms are not fully clear, but

several theories have been posited.[12–15] Defective desmosomal proteins may lead to impaired mechanical coupling between individual cells, leading to myocyte uncoupling especially under conditions that increase myocardial strain. The resulting inflammation, fibrosis, and adipocytosis may be a nonspecific response to injury similar to that seen in other forms of myocardial damage. This pathogenic model can explain the observation that prolonged strenuous exertion, which increases myocardial strain, significantly increases the risk of an earlier clinical onset of the disease and augments the risk of sudden death. It also explains why the RV, which is more distensible than the LV due to its thinner wall and asymmetric shape, is more often involved in ARVC/D, especially in its early stages. Furthermore, defects in mechanical coupling of myocytes may also lead to impairment in electrical coupling. Ultrastructural evaluation of the myocardium of patients with ARVC/D has shown reduced expression of several intercalated disk proteins, including connexin-43, a key component of gap junctions.[13,15] This finding may account for the development of conduction delay and arrhythmias even in the absence of significant structural defects in the early "concealed" phase of the disease. Recent studies have also shown that PKP2 haploinsufficiency leads to sodium current (I_{Na}) deficit in murine

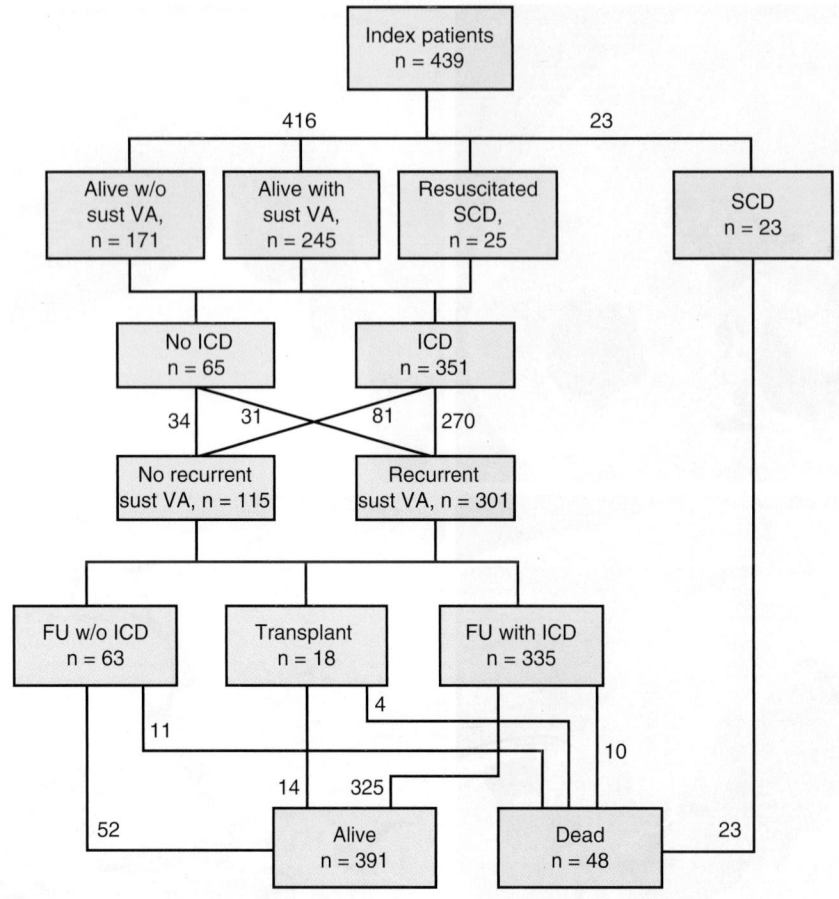

FIGURE 87.2 Schematic representation of the presentation, clinical course, and outcome in arrhythmogenic right ventricular dysplasia/cardiomyopathy index patients. The majority presented with sustained ventricular arrhythmias (*VA*) and received an implantable cardioverter defibrillator (*ICD*) during follow-up. *FU,* Follow-up; *SCD,* sudden cardiac death; *sust,* sustained. (From Groeneweg J, Bhonsale A, James C, et al. Clinical presentation, long-term follow-up, and outcomes of 1001 arrhythmogenic right ventricular dysplasia/cardiomyopathy patients and family members. *Circ Genetics.* 2015;8:437-446.)

hearts. The results of this study suggest that there is cross-talk between the desmosome and sodium channel complex. The resultant sodium channel dysfunction may contribute to the development of ventricular arrhythmias in patients with ARVD/C.

The mechanisms that lead to the variability in penetrance and expressivity of disease are still not fully understood. Family members with identical genotypes and even monozygotic twins show significant differences in symptomatology, presence and distribution of structural changes, and rate of disease progression. This observation has led to the "second hit" hypothesis, which suggests that modifier genes and/or environmental factors are likely responsible for phenotypic heterogeneity.

Relationship Between Arrhythmogenic Right Ventricular Dysplasia/ Cardiomyopathy and Exercise

The observation that there is a disproportionate number of athletes among patients with ARVD/C led to the hypothesis that exercise is an environmental factor in the pathogenesis of this disease.[16] A series of recent studies has proven beyond a doubt that this hypothesis is correct. Exercise has now been demonstrated to be the single most powerful environmental factor that impacts both the development and the clinical course of the disease.

One of the first studies to highlight the relationship between exercise and ARVD/C was by Corrado et al.[16] who reported that young athletes had a five-fold risk of dying of ARVD/C

compared with nonathletes. A subsequent study confirmed this finding when they found that implementing a preparticipation screening declined the incidence of sudden cardiovascular death in competitive athletes.[17]

Since then, many studies followed, and their aim has been to determine the role of exercise as a disease modifier in ARVD/C. La Gerche and colleagues[18] are credited with recognizing that the ARVD/C phenotype can be acquired through intense exercise. They studied 47 athletes with definite or probable ARVD/C. The majority (*n* = 41) practiced endurance sports (cyclists, 72%; distance runners, 6%; triathletes, 6%; and kayakers, 2%). They identified desmosomal mutations in only six athletes, and only two patients in the group had family history of ARVD/C. They found that the group that performed the most exercise had lower rates of desmosomal mutations, yet many of them met diagnostic criteria for definite or probable ARVD/C. On the basis of these results they concluded that high-intensity endurance exercise may be sufficient to evoke an ARVD/C phenotype, even in mutation-negative individuals. Saverniak and associates[19] investigated the impact of exercise on myocardial function. The study included 110 patients, 65 of them with ARVD/C and 45 mutation-positive family members. Exercise participation was measured by metabolic equivalent (MET)-minutes per week. Athletes were classified as those participating in vigorous exercise (≥6 METs) for ≥ 4 hours per week. The authors found that athletes were more likely to meet diagnostic criteria, they had a lower biventricular function, and earlier onset of life-threatening ventricular arrhythmias

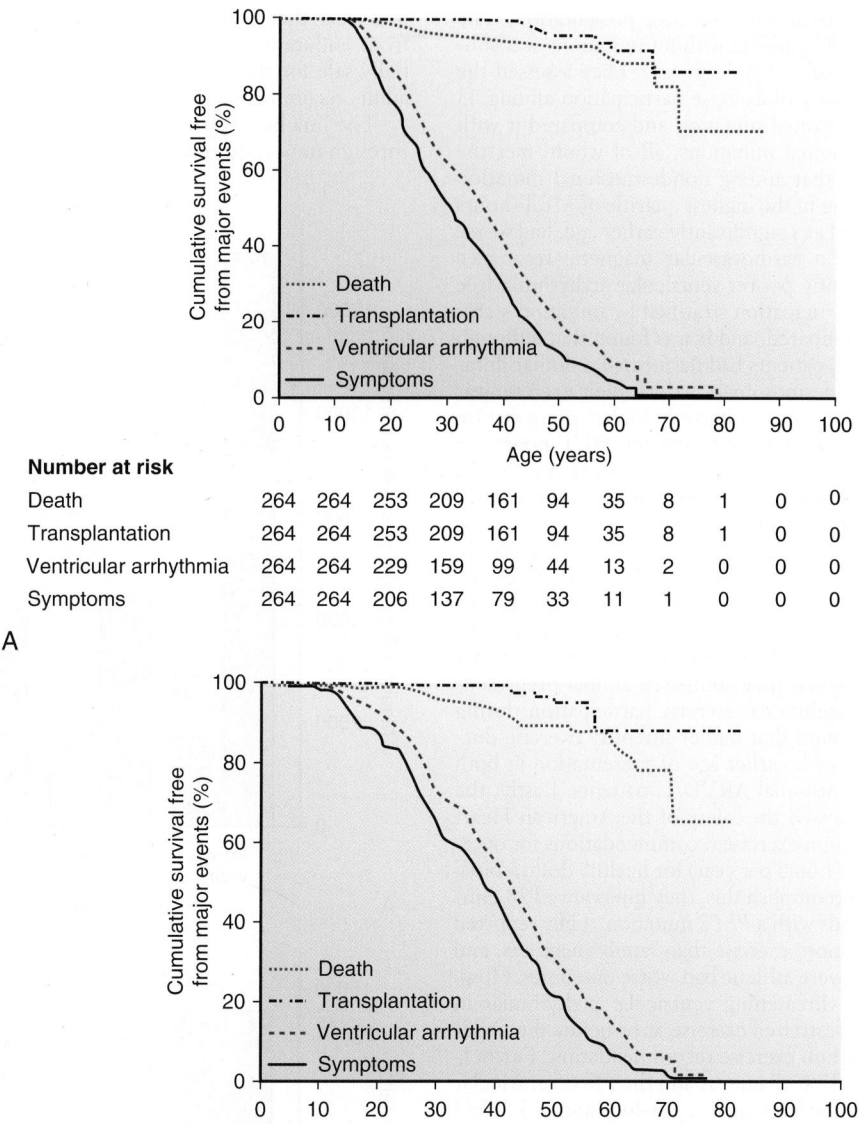

Number at risk											
Death	264	264	253	209	161	94	35	8	1	0	0
Transplantation	264	264	253	209	161	94	35	8	1	0	0
Ventricular arrhythmia	264	264	229	159	99	44	13	2	0	0	0
Symptoms	264	264	206	137	79	33	11	1	0	0	0

FIGURE 87.3 Survival free from any arrhythmogenic right ventricular dysplasia/cardiomyopathy (ARVD/C)–related symptoms, sustained ventricular arrhythmias (VAs), cardiac death, and cardiac transplantation in ARVD/C index patients with (A) pathogenic mutations and (B) without identified mutations. Symptoms ($p = .005$) and sustained VA ($p = .020$) occurred more often at a younger age in index patients with mutations. Survival free from cardiac death ($p = .644$) and transplantation ($p = .704$) was similar in both groups. (From Groeneweg J, Bhonsale A, James C, et al. Clinical presentation, long-term follow-up, and outcomes of 1001 arrhythmogenic right ventricular dysplasia/cardiomyopathy patients and family members. *Circ Genetics.* 2015;8:437-446.)

when compared with nonathletes. Ruwald and colleagues[20] studied 108 probands that met Task Force Criteria (TFC) for ARVD/C diagnosis; they assessed the effects of competitive and recreational sports on age of onset and risk of ventricular arrhythmias or death. Via a questionnaire, patients self-reported the age at which they initiated the sport and the commonly practiced sport. They found that the patients who engaged in competitive exercise had an earlier presentation of the disease and also had a two-fold increase in the risk of life-threatening arrhythmias and death when compared with inactive patients and those practicing recreational sports.

The Johns Hopkins ARVD Program has contributed three important manuscripts that have helped define the link between exercise and ARVD in patients with and without mutations, as well as examining the important question of a safe exercise threshold. James and associates[21] were the first to study the role of exercise in ARVD/C patients who had inherited a pathogenic

desmosomal mutation (Fig. 87.4). They evaluated 87 probands and family members from the Johns Hopkins ARVD/C Registry. All patients participated in an exercise interview detailing their exercise history for leisure/recreation, work, and transportation. Participants were classified as an endurance athlete if they performed 50 hours per year or more of vigorous intensity sports with a high dynamic demand as defined by the 36th Bethesda Conference Classification of Sports (Task Force 8).[22] The study had several key findings. First, ARVD/C patients who were endurance athletes became symptomatic at an earlier age. Furthermore, endurance exercise and higher duration of exercise participation were both associated with increased likelihood of developing manifest ARVD/C. Endurance exercise was also associated with worse survival from a ventricular arrhythmia and heart failure. Lastly, those individuals who continued to participate in the top quartile for hours of annual exercise after presentation had worse survival from first ventricular arrhythmia compared with individuals who reduced their exercise after presentation. The role of exercise in ARVD/C patients without mutations was subsequently studied by Sawant and colleagues.[23] They assessed the role of duration and intensity of exercise participation among 43 probands without a desmosomal mutation and compared it with 39 probands with desmosomal mutations, all of whom met the 2010 TFC. It was found that among nondesmosomal mutation patients, those participating in the highest quartile of MET-hours per year exercise presented at a significantly earlier age, had worse structural abnormalities on cardiovascular magnetic resonance (CMR), and had significantly poorer ventricular arrhythmia-free survival. Next, exercise participation stratified by mutation status and family history was compared, and it was found that although nondesmosomal ARVD/C patients had performed a similar duration of annual exercise as desmosomal carriers, their exercise was significantly more intense, with significantly higher participation in endurance sports and expenditure of greater MET-hours per year of exercise compared with desmosomal patients (Fig. 87.5). Lastly, ARVD/C nondesmosomal mutation patients with no family history performed the highest MET-hours per year exercise compared with nondesmosomal mutation patients with family history and desmosomal mutation carriers (Fig. 87.6). Since the nondesmosomal mutation patients without family history did the highest intensity exercise, they concluded that exercise may be the key environmental factor driving disease pathogenesis in that subgroup. Interestingly, when they compared annual prepresentation MET-hours and endurance exercise participation during youth (age ≤25), it was found that higher-intensity exercise during youth was associated with earlier age of presentation in both desmosomal and nondesmosomal ARVD/C patients. Lastly, the Johns Hopkins group assessed the safety of the American Heart Association (AHA) minimum exercise recommendations for overall health (390–690 MET-hours per year) for healthy desmosomal mutation carriers.[24] To accomplish this, they interviewed 28 family members of 10 probands with a *PKP2* mutation. They reported that probands had done more exercise than family members, and the family members that were athletic had worse outcomes. However, there were no life-threatening ventricular arrhythmias in the healthy carriers that restricted exercise at or below the upper bound of the AHA minimum exercise recommendation. Furthermore, at the time of ARVD/C diagnosis and their first ventricular arrhythmia, patients had accumulated a 2.8-fold and a 3.5-fold greater MET-hours exercise, respectively, than that recommended by the AHA (Fig. 87.7). Their conclusion was that while

it is clear that unaffected *PKP2* mutation carriers should refrain from endurance and high-intensity exercise, it might be potentially safe for them to practice the minimum exercise for healthy adults recommended by the AHA.

The link between exercise and ARVD has also been advanced through important research in animal models. The production of

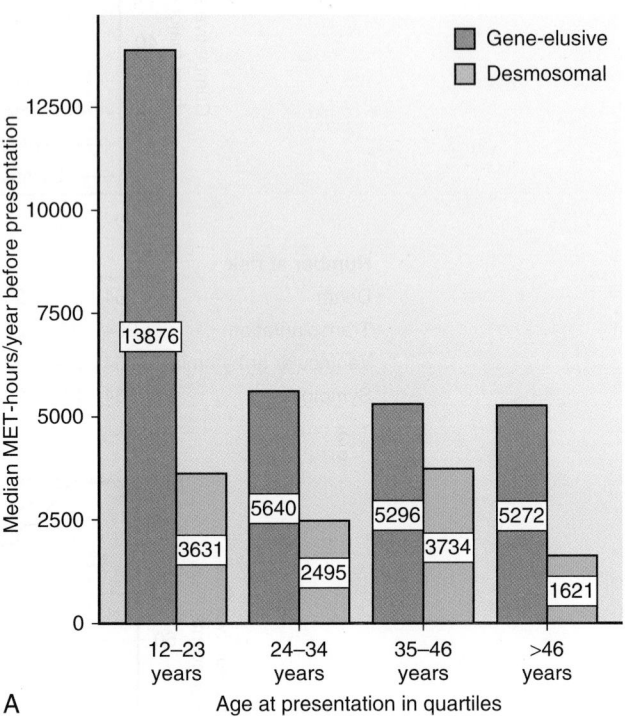

A Age at presentation in quartiles

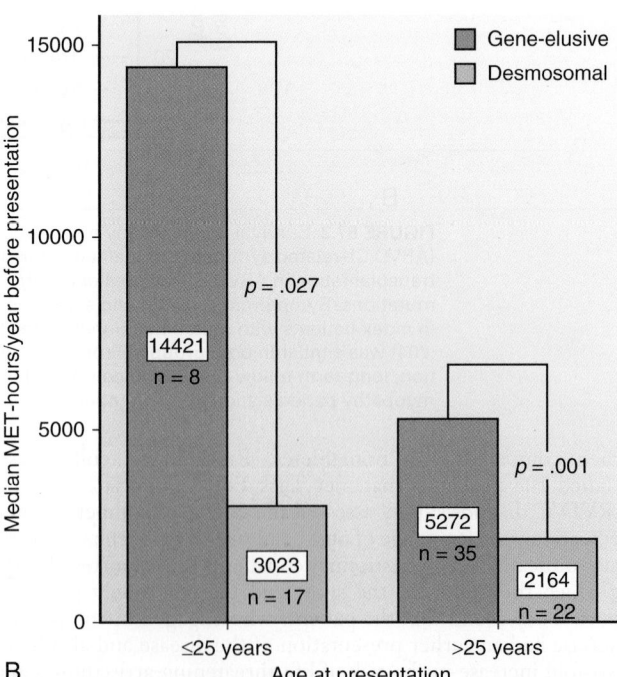

B Age at presentation

FIGURE 87.5 Exercise intensity (median metabolic equivalent hours [*MET-hours*] per year) stratified by (A) quartiles of age of clinical presentation and (B) age of clinical presentation before and after age 25. Gene-elusive patients had done more intense exercise regardless of age of presentation. Among patients presenting by age 25 there is a five-fold difference in intensity. (From Sawant AC, Bhonsale A, Te Riele AS, et al. Exercise has a disproportionate role in the pathogenesis of arrhythmogenic right ventricular dysplasia/cardiomyopathy in patients without desmosomal mutations. *J Am Heart Assoc.* 2014;3:e001471.)

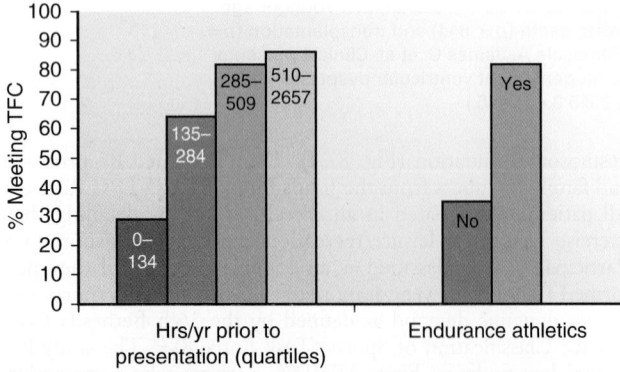

FIGURE 87.4 Association of exercise history with the likelihood of a diagnosis of arrhythmogenic right ventricular dysplasia/cardiomyopathy (ARVD/C). The likelihood of meeting the ARVD/C diagnostic criteria at last follow-up is associated with increasing hours per year (*Hrs/yr*) of exercise ($p < .001$) and participation in endurance athletics ($p < .001$)., *TFC*, 2010 Task Force (diagnostic) Criteria. (From James CA, Bhonsale A, Tichnell C, et al. Exercise increases age-related penetrance and arrhythmic risk in arrhythmogenic right ventricular dysplasia/cardiomyopathy–associated desmosomal mutation carriers. *J Am Coll Cardiol.* 2013;62:1290-1297.)

transgenic animals is a very important tool that has been used to understand ARVD/C. They have helped us not only to understand how desmosomal mutations produce the ARVD/C phenotype but also provided more evidence of the relationship between exercise and the disease. In 2006, Kirchhof and associates[25] used heterozygous plakoglobin-deficient mice and their wild-type siblings to study whether plakoglobin and training have a functional role in the development of ARVD/C. Endurance training with 8 weeks of daily swimming was used to test the hypothesis. Using

murine echocardiography, electrocardiogram (ECG), magnetic resonance imaging (MRI), and positron-emission tomography, they measured cardiac dimensions and function as well as myocardial glucose uptake. They found that plakoglobin deletion is sufficient to produce an ARVD/C-like phenotype. Furthermore, endurance training produced altered RV contractile and electrophysiological function in plakoglobin-deficient mice, manifested by increased RV volume, reduced RV function, spontaneous ventricular arrhythmias, and prolonged conduction times when compared with their wild-type counterparts. Another group evaluated the impact of exercise on ARVD/C cardiac manifestations.[26] To accomplish this they used an adeno-associated virus (AAV)-mediated *PKP2* mutant gene to produce an ARVC/D-causing mutation in the cardiac tissue of wild-type mice. Subsequently, the mice were divided in two groups, trained and sedentary, and they were euthanized to obtain heart sampling. Left and right end-diastolic volume, end-systolic volume, ejection fraction, and wall motion abnormalities were assessed via CMR. They found that sedentary mice did not have any sign of RV dysfunction. On the contrary, endurance exercise training resulted in RV dysfunction that was similar to the ARVD/C phenotype. Recently, Chelko and coworkers[27] analyzed disease progression in a mouse model with ARVD/C. They compared desmoglein-2 homozygous, heterozygous, and wild-type mice by examining the effects that exercise had on the disease. This was done by making mice swim 90 minutes per day, 5 days per week. This resulted in 6/12 homozygous mutant mice surviving to 16 weeks of age, with 6 dying during exercise. With the help of echocardiography and electrocardiography they observed that the homozygous mice had reduced ejection fraction, longer QRS duration and isovolumetric relaxation, and an increased risk of dying from a cardiac arrhythmia when compared with the heterozygous and wild-type mice. In the most recent study using animal models, the investigators generated transgenic mice with overexpression of desmoplakin, both wild type and mutant, and compared them to a nontransgenic model.[28] The mice were divided into two groups, sedentary or those exposed to a 12-week running regimen. Their results showed that exercise accelerated the development of the disease, manifested by RV dilation and focal fat infiltration in the mutant mice when compared with the wild-type and nontransgenic mice. LV function was not affected in either of the models.

These data raise a critical question of how much exercise can be considered safe in these patients. The answer is that more

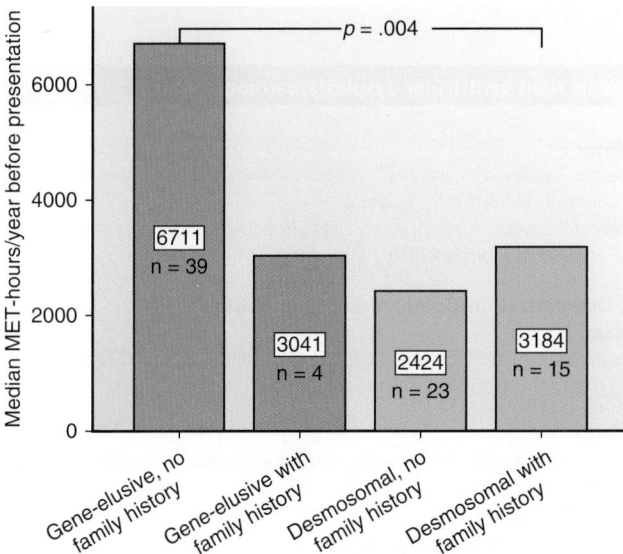

FIGURE 87.6 Exercise intensity among patients stratified by genotype and 2010 family history Task Force Criteria. Gene-elusive, nonfamilial patients participated in significantly higher-intensity exercise than those with family history or desmosomal mutations ($p = .004$, Kruskal–Wallis one-way analysis of variance). *MET-hours*, Metabolic equivalent hours. (From Sawant AC, Bhonsale A, Te Riele AS, et al. Exercise has a disproportionate role in the pathogenesis of arrhythmogenic right ventricular dysplasia/cardiomyopathy in patients without desmosomal mutations. *J Am Heart Assoc.* 2014;3:e001471.)

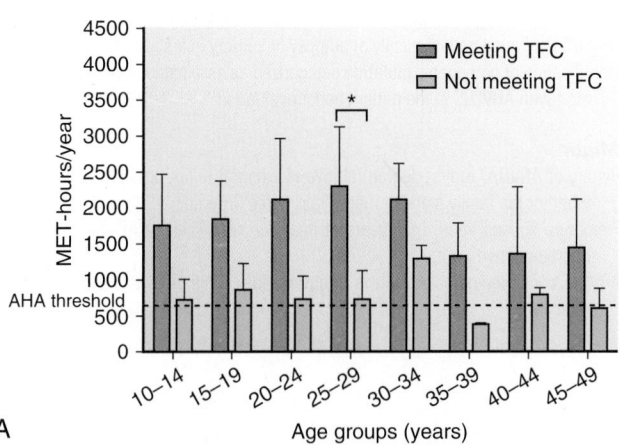

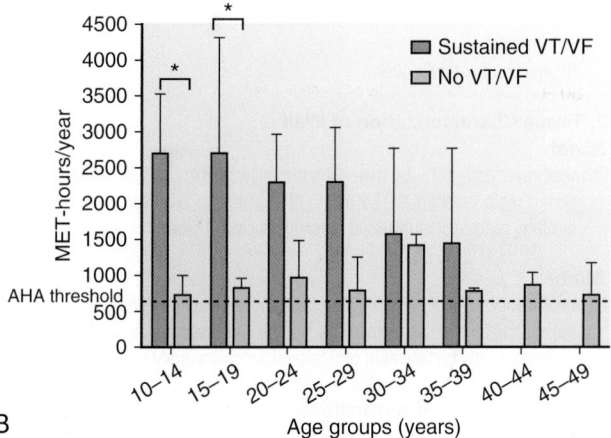

FIGURE 87.7 Median exercise intensity (metabolic equivalent hours [*MET-hours*] per year) before diagnosis in 5-year age increments compared with the American Heart Association (AHA)-recommended minimum stratified by diagnosis by 2010 Task Force Criteria (*TFC*) (A) and ventricular tachycardia/ventricular fibrillation (*VT/VF*) history (B). *Dotted black line* represents the upper bound of the AHA-recommended minimum exercise (650 MET-hours per year). *Error bars* depict interquartile range. *Statistically significant $p < .05$. (From Sawant AC, Te Riele AS, Tichnell C, et al. Safety of American Heart Association-recommended minimum exercise for desmosomal mutation carriers. *Heart Rhythm.* 2015;13:199-207.)

research is required to evaluate the threshold needed to trigger the onset of ARVD/C. Understanding of the interaction of genotype and exercise, as well as other environmental factors with the potential of triggering the disease, is also required. Furthermore, the improved understanding of the molecular mechanisms through which exercise causes the pathological features of ARVD/C is key to the improvement of patient care.

Management

Management of patients with ARVD/C has four components. The first is getting the diagnosis correct. The second component involves accurate risk stratification for sudden cardiac death and deciding whether to place an implantable cardioverter defibrillator (ICD). The third component of management is minimizing ICD therapies. The final component of management is preventing progression of the disease. Each of these will be examined in detail.

Establishing an Accurate Diagnosis

As previously noted, the first step in management is making the diagnosis. Misdiagnosis of ARVD/C is common due to lack of awareness of the 2010 TFC and misinterpretation of MRI[29,30] (Box 87.1).

BOX 87.1   2010 Task Force Criteria for the diagnosis of arrhythmogenic right ventricular dysplasia/cardiomyopathy

1. Global or Regional Dysfunction and Structural Alterations
Major
Two-Dimensional Echo Criteria
Regional RV akinesia, dyskinesia, or aneurysm *and* one of the following measured at end diastole:
   PLAX RVOT ≥ 32 mm or
   PSAX RVOT ≥ 36 mm,
   Fractional area change ≤ 33%

MRI Criteria
Regional RV akinesia or dyskinesia or dyssynchronous RV contraction *and* one of the following:
   Ratio of RV end-diastolic volume to BSA ≥ 100, 110 mL/m² (male) or ≥ 100 mL/m² (female)
   RV ejection fraction > 40% ≤ 45%

RV Angiography Criteria
Regional RV akinesia, dyskinesia, or aneurysm

Minor
Two-Dimensional Echo Criteria
Regional RV akinesia or dyskinesia or dyssynchronous RV contraction *and* one of the following measured at end diastole:
   PLAX RVOT ≥ 29 < 32 mm or
   PSAX RVOT ≥ 32 < 36 mm
   Fractional area change > 33% ≤ 40%

MRI Criteria
Regional RV akinesia or dyskinesia or dyssynchronous RV contraction *and* one of the following:
   Ratio of RV end-diastolic volume to BSA ≥110 mL/m² (male) or ≥100 mL/m² (female)
   RV ejection fraction ≤ 40%

2. Tissue Characterization of Wall
Major
Residual myocytes <60% by morphometric analysis (or <50% if estimated), with fibrous replacement of the RV free wall myocardium in ≥1 sample, with or without fatty replacement of tissue on endomyocardial biopsy

Minor
Residual myocytes 60%–75% by morphometric analysis (or 50%–65% if estimated), with fibrous replacement of the RV free wall myocardium in ≥1 sample with or without fatty replacement of tissue on endomyocardial biopsy

3. Repolarization Abnormalities
Major
Inverted T waves in right precordial leads (V₁, V₂, and V₃) or beyond in individuals >14 years of age (in the absence of complete RBBB QRS ≥ 120 ms)

Minor
Inverted T waves in V₁ and V₂ in individuals >14 years of age (in the absence of complete RBBB) or in V₄, V₅, and V₆
Inverted T waves in leads V₁, V₂, V₃, and V₄ in individuals >14 years of age in the presence of a complete RBBB

4. Depolarization/Conduction Abnormalities
Major
Epsilon wave (reproducible low-amplitude signals between end of QRS complex to onset of T wave) in the right precordial leads (V₁–V₃)

Minor
Late potentials by SAECG in ≥1 of 3 parameters in the absence of a QRSd ≥110 ms on standard ECG
Filtered QRS duration (fQRS) ≥ 114 ms
Duration of terminal QRS < 40 µV ≥ 38 ms
Root-mean-square voltage of terminal 40 ms ≤ µV
Terminal activation duration ≥ 55 ms measured from the nadir of the end of the QRS, including R′, in V₁, V₂, or V₃ in absence of complete RBBB

5. Arrhythmias
Major
Nonsustained or sustained VT of LBBB morphology with superior axis

Minor
Nonsustained or sustained VT of RVOT configuration, LBBB morphology with inferior axis or of unknown axis > 500 PVCs per 24-hour (Holter) monitoring

6. Family History
Major
ARVD/C in first-degree relative who meets Task Force Criteria
ARVD/C confirmed pathologically at autopsy or surgery in first-degree relative
Identification of pathogenic mutation categorized as associated or probably associated with ARVD/C in the patient under evaluation

Minor
History of ARVD/C in first-degree relative in whom it is not possible to determine whether the family member meets Task Force Criteria
Premature sudden death (<35 years of age) due to suspected ARVD/C in a first-degree relative
ARVD/C confirmed pathologically or by current Task Force Criteria in second-degree relative

---

ARVD/C, Arrhythmogenic right ventricular dysplasia/cardiomyopathy; *BSA*, body surface area; *ECG*, electrocardiogram; *LBBB*, left bundle branch block; *MRI*, magnetic resonance imaging; *PLAX*, parasternal long axis; *PSAX, parasternal short axis*; *PVC*, premature ventricular contraction; *RBBB*, right bundle branch block; *RV*, right ventricular; *RVOT*, right ventricular outflow tract; *SAECG*, signal-averaged electrocardiogram; *VT*, ventricular tachycardia.
Modified from Marcus FI, McKenna WJ, Sherrill D, et al. Diagnosis of arrhythmogenic right ventricular cardiomyopathy/dysplasia: proposed modification of the task force criteria. *Circulation*. 2010;121:1533-1541.

Due to the significant heterogeneity in the manifestation of disease, there is no single gold-standard diagnostic test for ARVD/C. Instead, the diagnosis relies upon a scoring system with major and minor criteria based on the demonstration of a combination of defects in RV morphology and function, characteristic depolarization/repolarization ECG abnormalities, characteristic tissue pathology, typical arrhythmias, family history, and the results of genetic testing. Thus the initial evaluation of all patients suspected of having ARVD/C should include a physical exam and a clinical history including family history of arrhythmias or sudden death, ECG, signal averaged–ECG (SAECG) (if available), 24-hour Holter monitoring, and comprehensive noninvasive imaging of both ventricles. If this noninvasive workup is suggestive but not diagnostic of ARVD/C, further testing should be considered to establish a diagnosis, including electrophysiological testing with or without electroanatomical mapping, and endomyocardial biopsy. Although right ventriculography was commonly used in the past, in our experience ventriculography is rarely needed due to the availability of high-quality echocardiography and MRI.

The diagnosis of ARVD/C should be considered in any patient who does not have known heart disease and who presents with frequent premature ventricular complexes (PVCs) or symptomatic ventricular tachycardia (VT), especially if there is left bundle branch block (LBBB) morphology with superior axis, the LBBB VT ECG pattern is not typical of idiopathic RV outflow tract VT (RVOT-VT), or the VT occurs in a patient with T wave inversion in the right precordial leads. The most common conditions that must be considered in the differential diagnosis include idiopathic RVOT-VT and cardiac sarcoidosis. Of note, ARVD/C can be very difficult to distinguish from RVOT-VT in the absence of structural changes during early disease. They can both present with LBBB-type VT with inferior axis. The differential diagnosis is based on the fact that RVOT-VT is nonfamilial, and patients do not have the characteristic ECG/SAECG abnormalities of ARVD/C and do not usually have inducible arrhythmias on programmed electrical stimulation. This diagnostic distinction is important to make because RVOT-VT carries a benign prognosis and generally can be cured or effectively treated with antiarrhythmic drugs or catheter ablation. Several studies have recently compared the morphology of VT or PVCs with an LBBB inferior axis morphology between patients with idiopathic RVOT-VT and those with ARVC/D. The first study reported that an algorithm combining lead I QRS duration for sensitivity and axis for specificity is useful for differentiating the two tachycardia substrates. A lead I QRS duration ≥120 ms had a sensitivity of 100%, specificity 46%, positive predictive value 61%, and negative predictive value 100% for ARVD/C. The addition of a mean QRS axis <30 degrees (R < S in lead III) to the above criterion increased specificity for ARVD/C to 100%. A more recent study examining patients with PVCs or VT with an LBBB inferior axis morphology confirmed that a QRSd >120 ms in lead V1 during VT or with PVCs favors the diagnosis of ARVD/C as compared with idiopathic RVOT-VT.[28] Although it is important to consider the diagnosis of ARVD/C in a patient with LBBB inferior (LBI) axis PVCs or VT, we do not recommend that each of these patients undergo a complete evaluation to exclude a possible diagnosis of ARVD/C. If the ECG and echocardiogram is normal and there is no family history of premature sudden death, we do not advise an exhaustive evaluation for ARVD/C. If the patient prefers a curative ablative strategy, an electrophysiological study (EPS) and possible ablation would be the next step. Only if at the time of EP testing, multiple forms of VT are induced would the potential diagnosis of ARVD/C be reconsidered.

Cardiac sarcoidosis should be suspected in patients who have evidence of conduction system abnormalities, especially in the presence of other extracardiac symptoms. In rare situations, an endomyocardial biopsy may become necessary to differentiate between the two disorders. The infrequency with which endomyocardial biopsy is required reflects the fact that cardiac sarcoidosis can usually be suspected based on the presence of conduction system abnormalities, mediastinal lymphadenopathy, tissue diagnosis of extracardiac sarcoidosis, or the presence of septal scar.

A minority of ARVD/C patients first present with symptoms of RV systolic heart failure. The differential diagnosis in such patients includes RV infarction or pulmonary hypertension. Dilated cardiomyopathy must be considered if there is evidence of biventricular failure. Patients with dilated cardiomyopathy who have early significant ventricular ectopy should be evaluated for possible biventricular arrhythmogenic cardiomyopathy.

Risk Stratification and Deciding When to Implant an Implantable Cardioverter Defibrillator

Prevention of sudden cardiac death is the primary goal of management. Several studies of ARVD/C patients who received an ICD have reported appropriate interventions during follow-up in more than 50% of patients.[31,32] Predictors of appropriate therapy included a prior sustained ventricular arrhythmia, syncope, and the extent of structural heart disease.

The incidence of appropriate ICD therapy among 84 patients who had an ICD implanted for primary prevention was recently reported.[31] Over a mean follow-up of 4.7 ± 3.4 years, appropriate ICD therapy was experienced by 40 patients (48%), of whom 16 (19%) received interventions for rapid VT/ventricular fibrillation (VF). Proband status, inducibility at electrophysiological study (EPS), presence of nonsustained ventricular tachycardia (NSVT), and a PVC count > 1000 per 24 hours were identified as significant predictors of appropriate ICD therapy (see Fig. 87.6). Survival rates free from appropriate ICD therapy for patients with one, two, three, and four risk factors were 100%, 83%, 21%, and 15%, respectively. Inducibility at EPS and NSVT remained significant predictors on multivariable analysis. These findings are important as they demonstrate that nearly half of the ARVD/C patients treated with an ICD for primary prevention experienced appropriate ICD interventions. Inducibility at EPS and NSVT are independent strong predictors of appropriate ICD therapy. More frequent ventricular ectopy is associated with progressively more common ICD therapy. Incremental risk of ventricular arrhythmias and ICD therapy was observed in the presence of multiple risk factors.

At present, ICD placement is recommended in all probands who meet TFC, especially if they have a history of sudden death, sustained VT, or arrhythmogenic syncope or have a high degree of ventricular ectopy and/or NSVT. Clinicians should be more circumspect about recommending implantation of an ICD in a family member who has been diagnosed with ARVD/C as a result of cascade screening. These individuals are being identified at a much earlier stage in their disease than was previously possible. With exercise restriction and the use of a β-blocker, their risk of sudden death appears to be reduced to a level below which placement of an ICD should be routinely advised. If a decision is made not to implant an ICD, close monitoring and follow-up are emphasized.

Minimizing Symptoms and Preventing Implantable Cardioverter Defibrillator Therapies

Pharmacological Therapy

Pharmacological therapy plays an important role in the management of patients with ARVD/C. This is the case despite the fact that few studies have been performed to define the safety and efficacy of pharmacological therapy. β-Blockers are recommended for almost all patients with ARVD/C, which reflects several lines of evidence. First, β-blockers are the only pharmacological agents that have been shown to reduce risk of sudden cardiac death in populations of patients without ARVD/C. Second, the great majority of ventricular arrhythmias and sudden death episodes are triggered by exercise. And third, high-dose isoproterenol results in the triggering of VT in patients with ARVD/C. Angiotensin-converting-enzyme (ACE) inhibitors are also used in most patients with ARVD/C and especially those with evidence of significant ventricular dysfunction. There are no published trials in patients with ARVD/C, but there is a wealth of data supporting the role of ACE inhibitors in a broader population of patients with cardiomyopathy. When it comes to membrane-active antiarrhythmic agents, sotalol and amiodarone are most commonly used. In rare cases, flecainide, propafenone, or dofetilide can be used. For most patients with ARVD/C and symptomatic ventricular arrhythmias and/or ICD therapies, we will attempt therapy with at least one antiarrhythmic medication before considering VT ablation.

Catheter Ablation

Catheter ablation is another important option for treatment of patients with ARVD/C who have ventricular tachycardia. It is important to recognize that unlike in patients with idiopathic VT in whom catheter ablation is curative, the role of catheter ablation in patients with ARVD/C is to improve quality of life by decreasing the frequency of episodes of VT.

A number of studies have evaluated the outcomes of catheter ablation of VT in patients with ARVD/C.[33–35] One study reported on a cohort of 24 patients with ARVD/C who underwent VT ablation.[33] These 24 patients underwent 48 ablation procedures at 29 different electrophysiology centers. The cumulative VT-free survival was 75% at 1.5 months, 50% at 5 months, and 25% at 14 months. The immediate success of the procedure had no bearing on recurrence; nor did the use of assisted mapping techniques or repetition of the procedure.[33] A second study reported on an expanded series of 83 patients who underwent a total of 175 VT ablation procedures.[34] Over a follow-up of 88 ± 66 months, the freedom from VT was 47%, 21%, and 15% at 1, 5, and 10 years, respectively. The cumulative freedom from VT following epicardial VT ablation was 64% and 45% at 1 and 5 years, respectively. Importantly, the burden of VT decreased following ablation from a median of 0.16 VT episodes per month preablation to 0.08 episodes per month postablation. Most recently, a single-center experience with epicardial VT ablation in patients with ARVD/C has been published.[35] It included 30 ARVD/C patients who underwent endo-/epicardial mapping and epicardial catheter ablation of VT. ICD interrogations were evaluated for VT recurrence. Eight patients (27%) experienced VT recurrence after epicardial radiofrequency ablation (RFA), and the VT-free survival was 83%, 76%, and 70% at 6, 12, and 24 months, respectively. A significant reduction of the VT burden was observed. No complications occurred. The majority of VT recurrences occurred during the first year after RFA, during exercise, had fast cycle lengths, and required ICD shock for termination.

Exercise Restriction

An important recommendation for patients with ARVD/C is exercise restriction. The association of exercise stems from the observation that sudden cardiac death in ARVD/C patients often occurs during exertion and that there is a large number of athletes among patients with ARVD/C. There is enough evidence that supports the hypothesis that repeated strenuous exercise is an important factor that could increase the chance of development of ARVD/C, especially in patients with a mutation.

Recently, an update to the 36th Bethesda Conference Eligibility Recommendations for Competitive Athletes with Cardiovascular Abnormalities has been published by the AHA and the American College of Cardiology.[36] The current recommendation is to avoid all competitive activities for patients with probable, borderline, or definite diagnosis of ARVD/C except for class I-A sports with a low cardiovascular demand (Class III, Level of Evidence C). A recent ARVD consensus, published by Corrado and colleagues, concluded that healthy gene carriers should be restricted only from competitive sports (Class IIa).

Multiple studies show that patients with overt disease or who are at risk for development of ARVD/C and who participate in high-intensity exercise can develop the disease earlier and have a more severe clinical course manifested by earlier onset arrhythmias, structural dysfunction, heart failure, and need for transplant. Therefore patients should refrain from practicing high-intensity endurance exercise. More research is needed to establish recommendations for at-risk family members.

Prevent Progression

The final consideration in patients with ARVD/C is preventing disease progression.

It is important to note that no studies have examined the extent and rate of progression of ARVD/C. Exercise restriction is a very important tool in preventing disease progression. Evidence supporting this statement was provided in the section on exercise and ARVD/C in this chapter.

Cardiac Transplantation

It is rare that patients with ARVD require cardiac transplantation.[37] The details of 18 ARVD/C patients who underwent cardiac transplantation for ARVD/C have been recently reported. The average age at first ARVD symptoms was 24 ± 13 years, and the average age at cardiac transplant was 40 ± 14 years. These patients often had clinical onsets of the disease at a relatively young age. One year after transplantation, survival was 94%, and 88% were alive at an average posttransplant follow-up of 6.2 ± 4.8 years.

Summary

ARVD/C is an inherited cardiomyopathy characterized clinically by ventricular arrhythmias, sudden death, and structural abnormalities of the right ventricle. Due to significantly variable penetrance and expressivity, the diagnosis of ARVD/C is challenging and requires a multifaceted approach to patient evaluation. Exercise has been widely described as an important environmental factor that contributes to the development of the disease. The observation that there is a disproportionate number of athletes with ARVD/C has led to extensive research in this area in animal models and humans. Multiple studies have shown that among patients with overt disease or at risk for development of ARVD/C, those who participate in high-intensity exercise can develop the disease earlier and have a more severe clinical course manifested by earlier onset arrhythmias, structural dysfunction, heart failure, and a need for transplantation.

The management of patients with ARVD/C is primarily aimed at reducing the burden of symptomatic arrhythmias and decreasing the incidence of sudden cardiac death. An important consideration in patients with ARVD/C is preventing disease progression, and this can be accomplished by exercise restriction. In conclusion, there is enough evidence to say that regardless of their genotype, patients with ARVD/C should be restricted from competitive, frequent, high-intensity exercise.

REFERENCES

1. Marcus FI, Fontaine GH, Guiraudon G, Frank R, Laurenceau JL, Malergue C, et al. Right ventricular dysplasia: a report of 24 adult cases. *Circulation*. 1982;65:384–398.
2. den Haan AD, Tan BY, Zikusoka MN, Lladó LI, Jain R, Daly A, et al. Comprehensive desmosome mutation analysis in North Americans with arrhythmogenic right ventricular dysplasia/cardiomyopathy. *Circ Cardiovasc Genet*. 2009;2:428–435.
3. Groeneweg J, Bhonsale A, James C, te Riele A, Dooijes D, Tichnell C, et al. Clinical presentation, long-term follow-up, and outcomes of 1001 arrhythmogenic right ventricular dysplasia/cardiomyopathy patients and family members. *Circ Genetics*. 2015;8:437–446.
4. Dalal D, Nasir K, Bomma C, Prakasa K, Tandri H, Piccini J, et al. Arrhythmogenic right ventricular dysplasia: a United States experience. *Circulation*. 2005;112:3823–3832.
5. Jain A, Tandri H, Calkins H, Bluemke DA. Role of cardiovascular magnetic resonance imaging in arrhythmogenic right ventricular dysplasia. *J Cardiovasc Magn Reson*. 2008;10:10–32.
6. Rastegar N, Burt JR, Corona-Villalobos CP, Te Riele AS, James CA, Murray B, et al. Cardiac MR findings and potential diagnostic pitfalls in patients evaluated for arrhythmogenic right ventricular cardiomyopathy. *Radiographics*. 2014;34:1553–1570.
7. Rastegar N, Zimmerman SL, Te Riele AS, James C, Burt JR, Bhonsale A, et al. Spectrum of biventricular involvement on CMR among carriers of ARVD/C-associated mutations. *JACC Cardiovasc Imaging*. 2015;8:863–864.
8. Bhonsale A, Groeneweg JA, James CA, Dooijes D, Tichnell C, Jongbloed JD, et al. Impact of genotype on clinical course in arrhythmogenic right ventricular dysplasia/cardiomyopathy-associated mutation carriers. *Eur Heart J*. 2015: ehu509.
9. McCoy G, Protonotarios N, Crosby A, Tsatsopoulou A, Anastasakis A, Coonar A, et al. Identification of a deletion in plakoglobin in arrhythmogenic right ventricular cardiomyopathy with palmoplantar keratoderma and woolly hair (Naxos disease). *Lancet*. 2000;355:2119–2124.
10. Norgett EE, Hatsell SJ, Carvajal-Huerta L, Cabezas JC, Common J, Purkis PE, et al. Recessive mutation in desmoplakin disrupts desmoplakin-intermediate filament interactions and causes dilated cardiomyopathy, woolly hair and keratoderma. *Hum Mol Genet*. 2000;9:2761–2766.
11. Deleted in review.
12. Chen SN, Gurha P, Lombardi R, Ruggiero A, Willerson JT, Marian AJ. The hippo pathway is activated and is a causal mechanism for adipogenesis in arrhythmogenic cardiomyopathy. *Circ Res*. 2014;114:454–468.
13. Asimaki A, Kleber AG, Saffitz JE. Pathogenesis of arrhythmogenic cardiomyopathy. *Can J Cardiol*. 2015;31:1313–1324. Review.
14. Kim C, Wong J, Wen J, et al. Studying arrhythmogenic right ventricular dysplasia with patient-specific iPSCs. *Nature*. 2013;494:105–110.
15. Cerrone M, Delmar M. Desmosomes and the sodium channel complex: implications for arrhythmogenic cardiomyopathy and Brugada syndrome. *Trends Cardiovasc Med*. 2014;24:184–190. Review.
16. Corrado D, Basso C, Rizzoli G, Schiavon M, Thiene G. Does sports activity enhance the risk of sudden death in adolescents and young adults? *J Am Coll Cardiol*. 2003;42:1959–1963.
17. Corrado D, Basso C, Pavei A, Michieli P, Schiavon M, Thiene G. Trends in sudden cardiovascular death in young competitive athletes after implementation of a preparticipation screening program. *JAMA*. 2006;296:1593–1601.
18. La Gerche A, Burns AT, Mooney DJ, et al. Exercise-induced right ventricular dysfunction and structural remodeling in endurance athletes. *Eur Heart J*. 2012;33:998–1006.
19. Saberniak J, Hasselberg NE, Borgquist R, et al. Vigorous physical activity impairs myocardial function in patients with arrhythmogenic right ventricular cardiomyopathy and in mutation positive family members. *Eur J Heart Fail*. 2014;16:1337–1344.
20. Ruwald AC, Marcus F, Estes 3rd NA, et al. Association of competitive and recreational sport participation with cardiac events in patients with arrhythmogenic right ventricular cardiomyopathy: results from the North American multidisciplinary study of arrhythmogenic right ventricular cardiomyopathy. *Eur Heart J*. 2015;36:1735–1743.
21. James CA, Bhonsale A, Tichnell C, Murray B, Russell SD, Tandri H, et al. Exercise increases age-related penetrance and arrhythmic risk in arrhythmogenic right ventricular dysplasia/cardiomyopathy-associated desmosomal mutation carriers. *J Am Coll Cardiol*. 2013;62:1290–1297.
22. Maron BJ, Zipes DP. 36th Bethesda Conference: eligibility recommendations for competitive athletes with cardiovascular abnormalities. *J Am Coll Cardiol*. 2005;45:2–64.
23. Sawant AC, Bhonsale A, Te Riele AS, Tichnell C, Murray B, Russell SD, et al. Exercise has a disproportionate role in the pathogenesis of arrhythmogenic right ventricular dysplasia/cardiomyopathy in patients without desmosomal mutations. *J Am Heart Assoc*. 2014;16(3):e001471.
24. Sawant AC, Te Riele AS, Tichnell C, et al. Safety of American Heart Association–recommended minimum exercise for desmosomal mutation carriers. *Heart Rhythm*. 2016;13:199–207.
25. Kirchhof P, Fabritz L, Zwiener M, et al. Age- and training-dependent development of arrhythmogenic right ventricular cardiomyopathy in heterozygous plakoglobin-deficient mice. *Circulation*. 2006;114:1799–1806.
26. Cruz FM, Sanz-Rosa D, Roche-Molina M, et al. Exercise triggers ARVC phenotype in mice expressing a disease-causing mutated version of human plakophilin-2. *J Am Coll Cardiol*. 2015;65:1438–1450.
27. Chelko S, Asimaki A, Wei A-C, et al. Abstract 20589: exercise and mitochondrial respiration in mice with arrhythmogenic cardiomyopathy. *Circulation*. 2014;130:A20589.
28. Martherus R, Jain R, Takagi K, et al. Accelerated cardiac remodeling in desmoplakin transgenic mice in response to endurance exercise is associated with perturbed Wnt/β-catenin signaling. *Am J Physiol Heart Circ Physiol*. 2016;310:H174–H187.
29. Bomma C, Rutberg J, Tandri H, Nasir K, Tichnell C, James C, et al. Misdiagnosis of arrhythmogenic right ventricular dysplasia (ARVD). *J Cardiovasc Electrophysiol*. 2004;15:300–306.
30. Marcus FI, McKenna WJ, Sherrill D, Basso C, Bauce B, Bluemke DA, et al. Diagnosis of arrhythmogenic right ventricular cardiomyopathy/dysplasia: proposed modification of the task force criteria. *Circulation*. 2010;121:1533–1541.
31. Bhonsale A, James CA, Tichnell C, Murray B, Gagarin D, Philips B, et al. Incidence and predictors of implantable cardioverter-defibrillator therapy in patients with arrhythmogenic right ventricular dysplasia/cardiomyopathy undergoing implantable cardioverter-defibrillator implantation for primary prevention. *J Am Coll Cardiol*. 2011;58:1485–1496.
32. Piccini JP, Dalal D, Roguin A, Bomma C, Cheng A, Prakasa K, et al. Predictors of appropriate implantable defibrillator therapies in patients with arrhythmogenic right ventricular dysplasia. *Heart Rhythm*. 2005;2:1188–1194.
33. Dalal D, Jain R, Tandri H, Dong J, Eid SM, Prakasa K, et al. Long-term efficacy of catheter ablation of ventricular tachycardia in patients with arrhythmogenic right ventricular dysplasia/cardiomyopathy. *J Am Coll Cardiol*. 2007;50:432–440.
34. Philips B, Madhavan S, James C, Tichnell C, Murray B, Dalal D, et al. Outcomes of catheter ablation of ventricular tachycardia in arrhythmogenic right ventricular dysplasia/cardiomyopathy (ARVD/C). *Circ Arrhythm Electrophysiol*. 2012;5:499–505.
35. Philips B, Te Riele AS, Sawant A, Kareddy V, James CA, Murray B, et al. Outcomes and VT recurrence characteristics after epicardial ablation of ventricular tachycardia in arrhythmogenic right ventricular dysplasia/cardiomyopathy. *Heart Rhythm*. 2015;12:716–725.
36. Maron BJ, Udelson JE, Bonow RO, et al. Eligibility and Disqualification Recommendations for Competitive Athletes With Cardiovascular Abnormalities: Task Force 3: Hypertrophic Cardiomyopathy, Arrhythmogenic Right Ventricular Cardiomyopathy and Other Cardiomyopathies, and Myocarditis: A Scientific Statement From the American Heart Association and American College of Cardiology. *Circulation*. 2015;132:e273–e280.
37. Tedford RJ, James C, Judge DP, Tichnell C, Murray B, Bhonsale A, et al. Cardiac transplantation in arrhythmogenic right ventricular dysplasia/cardiomyopathy. *J Am Coll Cardiol*. 2012;59:289–290.

88 Ventricular Tachycardias in Catecholaminergic Cardiomyopathy (Catecholaminergic Polymorphic Ventricular Tachycardia)

Christian van der Werf and Arthur A.M. Wilde

Catecholaminergic polymorphic ventricular tachycardia (CPVT) is an inherited arrhythmia syndrome that is characterized by adrenergically mediated polymorphic ventricular tachyarrhythmias in patients with no structural heart disease and a normal electrocardiogram (ECG) at rest. The prevalence of CPVT in the general population is unknown but is estimated to be 1 in 10,000. Although the clinical course is very diverse, mortality in severely affected untreated CPVT patients in early series was up to 50% before the age of 20.[1] Accordingly, CPVT is a significant cause of sudden infant death syndrome (see Chapter 98), sudden arrhythmic death syndrome or sudden unexplained death syndrome in the young,[2] and unexplained cardiac arrest.[3]

In this chapter, we review the present knowledge on CPVT with a focus on clinical manifestation, diagnosis, therapy, and prognosis. The pathophysiological mechanisms through which the genetic determinants of CPVT lead to the clinical phenotype are discussed in Chapter 53.

Historical Background

The first patients with the clinical characteristics of CPVT were described in 1960 by Berg, who reported three young sisters with cardiac events and polymorphic ventricular arrhythmias without structural heart disease, of whom one died suddenly.[4] In 1975, Reid et al. described another typical CPVT patient: a 6-year-old girl with bidirectional ventricular tachycardia (VT) precipitated by exercise or emotional stress.[5] Thereafter, the Paris group (Lariboisierre Hospital) of Philippe Coumel published two important clinical articles in 1978[6] and 1995,[1] including 4 and 21 patients, respectively, resulting in the definite recognition of CPVT as a distinct primary arrhythmia syndrome (instead of a subtype of the long QT syndrome). The genetic background of CPVT was first discovered in 2001: mutations in the cardiac ryanodine receptor gene (RYR2) were found to underlie the majority of CPVT cases,[7] while mutations in cardiac calsequestrin (CASQ2) were identified in rare, autosomal recessively inherited CPVT cases.[8]

Diagnosis

A definite clinical diagnosis of CPVT requires the presence of reproducible unexplained exercise- or emotion-induced polymorphic VT or bidirectional VT in the absence of structural heart disease and resting ECG abnormalities, particularly a normal heart rate–corrected QT (QTc) interval.[9,10] In individuals aged over 40 years, current recommendations require the exclusion of (significant) coronary artery disease.[9] The hallmark of CPVT is the presence of bidirectional VT, characterized by a beat-to-beat 180-degree alternating QRS axis, but this is only observed in a minority of patients.[11]

In addition, CPVT is diagnosed in patients who are carriers of a pathogenic mutation in the two genes that traditionally have been associated with CPVT: RYR2 and CASQ2.[9,10] A number of other genes have also been linked to patients with a CPVT-like phenotype, but whether these cases represent "true" CPVT or a CPVT phenocopy remains debatable (see Genetic Basis).

According to the current Heart Rhythm Society/European Heart Rhythm Association/Asia Pacific Heart Rhythm Society expert consensus recommendations, CPVT is also diagnosed in patients with physical or emotional stress–related polymorphic or bidirectional ventricular premature beats (VPBs), although the minimally required ventricular arrhythmia burden is not further specified.[9] In patients with possible CPVT (e.g., with little or nonreproducible polymorphic ventricular ectopy), genetic testing is critical to make a definite diagnosis of CPVT. In genotype-negative cases with a possible CPVT phenotype, it may be challenging to distinguish CPVT from other resembling conditions (see Differential Diagnosis), and it may not be possible to make a definite diagnosis.

Clinical Manifestations

Clinical Presentation

The typical clinical presentation of CPVT is the occurrence of syncope, aborted cardiac arrest, or sudden cardiac death in the circumstances of physical or emotional stress in normally developed children or young adolescents. Swimming seems a particular important trigger.[12] In two large series, the age of onset was 10.8 (interquartile range, 6.8–13.2)[13] and 12 ± 8 years.[14] Some patients are initially diagnosed with epilepsy because CPVT-related syncope may include convulsive movements and urinary or fecal incontinence.[13] If these symptomatic patients receive antiepileptic or no treatment, further cardiac events can occur and eventually prove fatal in some cases. Classically, the family history of these young patients includes relatives with syncope, aborted cardiac arrest, sudden cardiac death, or "epilepsy" under similar conditions.

Today, however, numerous patients and families with a different clinical presentation and a more benign course have been recognized.[15] On the contrary, RYR2 mutations have been identified

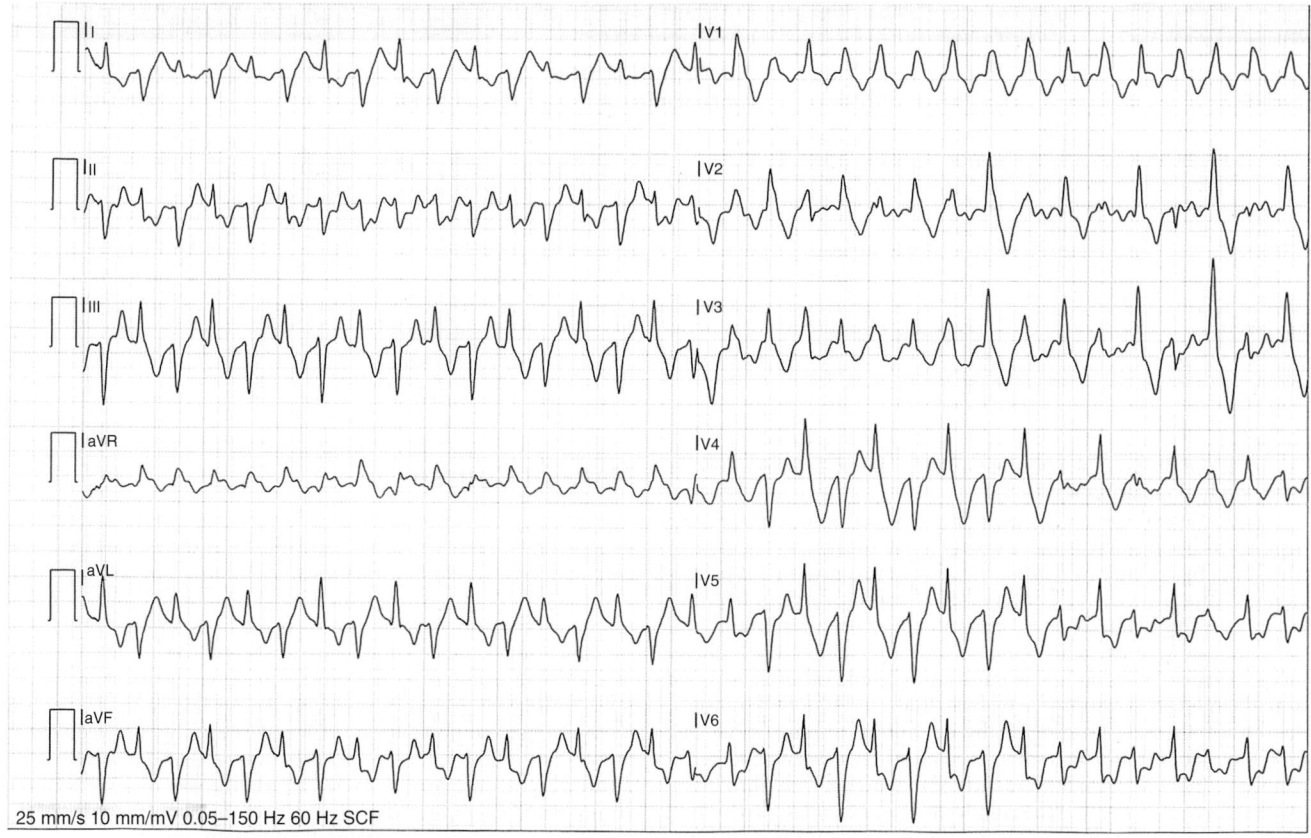

FIGURE 88.1 An electrocardiographic strip that shows typical bidirectional ventricular tachycardia in a patient with catecholaminergic polymorphic ventricular tachycardia during exercise testing.

in victims of sudden infant death syndrome (see Chapter 98), suggesting a wide range of phenotype severity among *RYR2* mutation carriers.

Cardiologic Examination

Most CPVT patients have an unremarkable 12-lead resting ECG, including a normal QTc interval. However, sinus bradycardia and prominent U waves on resting ECG have been associated with CPVT (see Supraventricular Disease Manifestations).

The gold standard for the diagnosis of CPVT is provocative testing, preferably using exercise testing. Typically, a gradual increase of ventricular arrhythmia burden and complexity is observed, starting with isolated VPBs at a heart rate of approximately 110 to 130 beats/min. In the absence of important therapeutic modifications, the ventricular arrhythmia threshold heart rate is accurately reproducible in an individual patient. VPBs are late coupled with a coupling interval of approximately 400 ms.[16] Left bundle branch inferior axis and right bundle branch block superior axis morphologies have been consistently shown to be predominant in CPVT,[11,16] and VPB morphologies are usually reproducible in an individual patient. Further exercise causes the number of isolated VPBs to increase to bigeminal VPBs, and eventually, polymorphic couplets or nonsustained VTs, including bidirectional VT, may be induced (Fig. 88.1). In very rare cases, this may further escalate to polymorphic sustained VT or ventricular fibrillation. When exercise testing is terminated, ventricular arrhythmias rapidly recede in most patients, whereas VPBs recorded for more than 1 minute during the recovery are very uncommon.[16] In some patients with ventricular arrhythmias who reach a high maximum heart rate, arrhythmias are paradoxically suppressed as the heart rates

increase further with continued exercise.[17] This phenomenon was also observed in CPVT mice models when intrinsic sinus rates were increased with atropine and after atrial overdrive pacing.[17]

Holter monitoring, during which a patient should be encouraged to exercise, can be used as an alternative test in selected cases, although its sensitivity is considered to be lower. It may, for example, be useful in young children or other patients who are unable to perform an adequate exercise test, patients suspected with emotion-related rather than exercise-related ventricular arrhythmias, and patients who report possible CPVT-related symptoms but have an unremarkable exercise test.

The use of an adrenaline infusion (initiated at a dose of 0.05 μg/kg/min and then titrated at 5-minute intervals to a maximum dose of 0.2 μg/kg/min) in CPVT has also been advocated. For example, in patients with unexplained cardiac arrest (i.e., normal left ventricular function, coronary arteries, and QT interval), the adrenaline challenge for CPVT was positive in 7% and borderline in 5%.[3] Interestingly, adrenaline infusion–provoked ventricular arrhythmias consistent with CPVT have been reported in patients who did not have any ventricular arrhythmia during the exercise testing or Holter monitoring. Whether these patients represent "true" CPVT based on a similar pathophysiological mechanism as in patients with classical CPVT remains to be determined. One study that compared the diagnostic value of adrenaline infusion and exercise testing in 36 CPVT patients (including 25 *RYR2* mutation carriers and 11 genotype-negative patients) and 45 unaffected relatives showed a low sensitivity of adrenaline infusion, probably because the maximum heart rate achieved following adrenaline challenge was markedly lower than that following exercise testing.[18] Among 25 CPVT patients with a positive exercise test, only 7 had a positive adrenaline test

TABLE 88.1 Genetics of catecholaminergic polymorphic ventricular tachycardia

GENE	LOCUS	INHERITANCE	NO. OF MUTATIONS IDENTIFIED	PHENOTYPE	FREQUENCY
RYR2	1q42-43	Autosomal dominant	>130	CPVT (exon 3 deletion: sinoatrial node, atrioventricular node dysfunction, atrial fibrillation, atrial standstill, dilated cardiomyopathy)	≈60%
CASQ2	1p13.3-p11	Autosomal recessive	12	CPVT	<5%
TRDN	6q22-23	Autosomal recessive	3	CPVT	<5%
Unknown	7p14-22	Autosomal recessive	Not applicable	CPVT, mild QTc interval prolongation	Unknown
KCNJ2	17q24.3	Autosomal dominant		CPVT phenocopy	<5%

CPVT, Catecholaminergic polymorphic ventricular tachycardia.

(sensitivity of 28%). The specificity of adrenaline infusion in the entire study population was 98%.

Electrophysiology studies generally have no role in diagnosing CPVT because ventricular arrhythmias cannot be triggered other than by adrenergic stimulation. However, prominent postpacing changes of the QT interval in mutation carriers from a family with the M4109R *RYR2* mutation have been reported.[10]

In an index patient who presents with a possible CPVT phenotype, cardiac imaging is mandatory to exclude other causes of exercise-induced polymorphic tachyarrhythmias (see Differential Diagnosis). Cardiac imaging is, by definition, unremarkable in CPVT patients. However, some exceptions have been reported. Mutations in *RYR2* have been identified in patients with fibrofatty myocardial replacement in the right ventricle, mimicking arrhythmogenic cardiomyopathy, and intracellular calcium deposits.[11] In a recent series of 64 patients diagnosed with arrhythmogenic cardiomyopathy according to the Task Force Criteria and without desmosomal gene mutations, 6 (9%) *RYR2* rare missense variants were identified.[19] However, because of inconclusive segregation analyses and the absence of functional studies, definite conclusions on the causal role of these variants could not be reached.

Members from two separate families with a large genomic deletion in *RYR2*, involving exon 3, showed sinoatrial node and atrioventricular node dysfunction, atrial fibrillation, atrial standstill, and left ventricular dysfunction and dilatation, in addition to the classic CPVT phenotype.[12] A recent study reported a possible association between *RYR2* exon 3 deletion to (left ventricular) noncompaction cardiomyopathy in addition to the aforementioned complex phenotype.[20]

Supraventricular Disease Manifestations

The most common supraventricular manifestation of CPVT is sinus bradycardia and/or sinus node dysfunction. In one study, *RYR2* mutation carriers had a lower average resting heart rate compared with nonmutation carriers.[13] Heart rates tended to be lowest in males and *RYR2* mutation carriers with a CPVT phenotype. In a large series that included 116 relatives from 15 families who were identified by cascade screening for the *RYR2* mutation that caused CPVT in the proband, sinus bradycardia was observed in 19%.[14] In addition, other supraventricular dysrhythmias were present in 16% and mainly included intermittent ectopic atrial rhythm identified by Holter monitoring. In another study, paroxysmal supraventricular arrhythmias were observed in 7 of 27 (26%) patients with CPVT.[11] In one study in which electrophysiological analysis was performed in eight CPVT patients, four demonstrated evidence of sinus node dysfunction.[15]

The occurrence of exercise-induced supraventricular tachyarrhythmias in CPVT patients has been reported but is not commonly observed.[14]

Natural Course

The natural course of CPVT is diverse and ranges from a phenotype that causes sudden infant death syndrome to the classical phenotype, including fatalities in children and young adults, and to carriers of a pathogenic CPVT-associated mutation who remain asymptomatic for their entire lives in the absence of therapy. One study provided more insight into the natural course of CPVT by comparing the mortality of past generations of the *RYR2* p.R420W Dutch founder mutation family to the mortality of the general population.[21] Overall, mortality between family members and the general population was similar. However, in the 20-to 30-year age group, excess mortality was observed among family members. These data may reflect the clinical course of this specific mutation and is potentially different in patients and families with different CPVT-associated mutations.

Genetic Basis

Although the familial nature of CPVT was already observed in the first reports, critical steps for unrevealing the genetic basis of CPVT have been taken in the past 15 years (Table 88.1).

Cardiac Ryanodine Receptor (CPVT 1)

In 1999, the CPVT phenotype was linked to a disease locus on chromosome 1q42-q43, and an autosomal dominant inheritance pattern of this CPVT form was suggested.[20] The disease-causing gene residing on this locus, the cardiac ryanodine receptor gene (*RYR2*), was identified in 2001.[7] RYR2 governs the release of calcium from the sarcoplasmic reticulum, which initiates cardiac muscle contraction. Nowadays, over 170 unique, mostly missense mutations in *RYR2* have been identified.[22] Approximately 20% of *RYR2* mutations are de novo in origin, and in one study, multiple *RYR2* mutations were identified in 4 of 73 patients (5.5%).[23] Mutations in *RYR2* cluster in three hotspots: the N-terminal domain (codons 44–466; ~16% of mutations), central domain (codons 2246–2534; ~20% of mutations), and C-terminal channel–forming domain (codons 3778–4959; ~50% of mutations). Several *RYR2* founder mutations have been identified, including the p.G357S mutation in approximately 180 family members from the Canary Islands[24] and the p.R420W mutation in over 60 family members from the Netherlands[15] (see Natural Course and Risk Stratification).

Mutations in *RYR2* are identified in approximately 60% of patients with a strong CPVT phenotype.[23,25] The yield of *RYR2* genetic testing decreases to 5%–38% of patients with a possible clinical diagnosis of CPVT, 31% of patients with exertional syncope, and 15% of relatives of victims of exercise- or emotion-related aborted cardiac arrest or sudden cardiac death with no signs of other inherited cardiac disease.[23,25]

Rare missense mutations in *RYR2* are, however, also identified in control populations. In one study, six different rare variants were identified in 200 control subjects (3%).[23] Another important study analyzed the prevalence of previously reported CPVT-associated *RYR2* variants.[22] These variants were identified in 41 of 6131 (6.7%) control subjects, yielding a prevalence of up to 1:150, which is much higher than the estimated prevalence of clinically diagnosed CPVT. It is therefore likely that many of the *RYR2* variants identified in this study are not the major or monogenic cause of CPVT. These data indicate that extreme caution needs to be taken before classifying a novel *RYR2* variant as pathogenic, in particular when the variant resides outside of the three regional hot spots. In addition, these data highlight the need for further research on the role of *RYR2* variants in apparently healthy individuals (so-called genetic background noise).

Cardiac Calsequestrin (CPVT 2)

In 2001, mutations in the gene that encodes cardiac calsequestrin (*CASQ2*) were found to underlie a malignant autosomal recessive inherited form of CPVT in seven related Bedouin families.[7] *CASQ2* is located within the sarcoplasmic reticulum and also plays a pivotal role in calcium homeostasis. Mutations in *CASQ2* are identified in less than 5% of CPVT index cases. At present, 14 CPVT-associated *CASQ2* variants have been reported, and recent data classify the vast majority of these variants as disease causing.[22] Although *CASQ2* mutations are typically identified in consanguineous families, compound heterozygosity in nonconsanguineous families has been observed. It is unclear whether some *CASQ2* mutations, such as the R33X[26] and K206N[27] mutations, also cause autosomal dominant transmission of the phenotype.

Triadin

In 2012, triadin (*TRDN*) was reported as a new gene responsible for an autosomal recessive form of CPVT.[28] Triadin is a transmembrane sarcoplasmic reticulum protein and is another component of sarcoplasmic reticulum calcium release during cardiac contraction. In the initial report, three *TRDN* mutations were identified in 2 of 97 (2%) CPVT probands without mutations in *RYR2* or *CASQ2*.[28] In addition, three related children who carry two heterozygous *TRDN* mutations and display significant ventricular arrhythmias during isoproterenol infusion testing have been reported.[29] Importantly, skeletal muscle weakness has been observed in some patients and may thus be an associated feature of this CPVT form.

Calmodulin

Mutations in two of the three genes that encode the identical calcium-signaling protein calmodulin have been identified in patients with CPVT,[30] with congenital long QT syndrome with exertion-induced ventricular arrhythmia-phenotypes,[31] and with idiopathic ventricular fibrillation[32] phenotypes.

A heterozygous *CALM1* missense mutation was identified in a large family with a classical CPVT phenotype.[30] Subsequently, another *CALM1* missense mutation was identified in 63 *RYR2* mutation–negative individuals.[30] In another study, five de novo *CALM2* mutations were identified in patients with markedly prolonged QTc intervals in all patients and the development of a CPVT-like phenotype in one of these patients.[31] At present, the exact pathophysiology of arrhythmia susceptibility in the setting of *CALM1* and *CALM2* mutations, resulting in very diverse phenotypes, is largely unknown.

Other Catecholaminergic Polymorphic Ventricular Tachycardia Types and Phenocopies

Another CPVT form, inherited as an autosomal recessive trait, was mapped to a 25-Mb interval on chromosome 7p14-p22 in a report that included four children from an inbred Arabic family.[33] All children presented before the age of 12 years, showed mild QTc interval prolongation, and three children eventually succumbed because of this condition. Recently, a homozygous mutation in the trans-2,3-enoyl-CoA reductase-like (*TECRL*) gene was identified in this family.[33a]

Patients with a CPVT phenotype and associated mutations in genes that suggest another underlying pathophysiology than intracellular calcium handling dysfunction are considered to represent CPVT phenocopies.

Mutations in the gene that encodes the potassium inwardly rectifying channel Kir2.1 (*KCNJ2*) are generally associated with Andersen-Tawil syndrome but may also cause CPVT phenocopies, including the typical bidirectional VT (see Differential Diagnosis).

Multiple series have described a phenotype with polymorphic ventricular ectopy in carriers of gain-of-function mutations in the gene that encodes the pore-forming subunit of the cardiac sodium channel, $Na_v1.5$ (*SCN5A*),[34,35] including families in which these arrhythmias were apparently exercise induced.[34]

Loss-of-function mutations in the membrane adaptor protein ankyrin-B (*ANK2*) are associated with type 4 congenital long QT syndrome. Some patients, however, display exercise-induced ventricular arrhythmias in the absence of QTc interval prolongation.[36]

Genetic Testing

In CPVT, genetic testing has a diagnostic value but not a therapeutic or prognostic value. The results of genetic testing may help confirm the diagnosis in patients with a possible clinical diagnosis of CPVT. According to the 2011 Heart Rhythm Society/European Heart Rhythm Association consensus statement on genetic testing in inherited arrhythmia syndromes and cardiomyopathies, comprehensive CPVT genetic testing is indicated in probands in whom "a cardiologist has established a clinical index of suspicion for CPVT based on examination of the patient's clinical history, family history, and expressed electrocardiographic phenotype during provocative stress testing with cycle, treadmill, or catecholamine infusion."[37]

In addition, it is stated that *RYR2* mutations may be regarded as a cause of adrenergically mediated idiopathic ventricular fibrillation, which may justify genetic testing in such instances.[9] This recommendation is based on several case reports that described patients with idiopathic ventricular fibrillation (i.e., those who experienced ventricular fibrillation with no abnormalities during a thorough cardiologic evaluation [including no ventricular arrhythmias during exercise testing]), in whom mutations in *RYR2* were identified.[38] An *RYR2* mutation was also associated with a clinical phenotype of short-coupled polymorphic VT at rest.[39] It has been proposed that loss-of-function *RYR2* mutations increase the propensity for calcium and electromechanical alternans, which could result in alternans-associated ventricular fibrillation rather than exercise-induced polymorphic VT.[40]

In the past, *RYR2* mutational analyses were performed in a tiered fashion, starting with exons in which mutations were mostly identified.[23] Nowadays, with next generation gene sequencing techniques, all exons in *RYR2* are sequenced at once (usually in addition to many other genes that are part of the "arrhythmia panel"). *CASQ2* and *TRDN* have also been added to these "arrhythmia panels" and should mainly be screened in consanguineous families. KCNJ2, the genes encoding calmodulin, and *SCN5A* will also be frequently screened simultaneously with *RYR2* and may help identify CPVT phenocopies.

In relatives, genetic testing is critically important for identifying asymptomatic mutation–carrying relatives of a mutation-positive proband (see later). Predictive genetic testing of relatives with a 50% risk for carriership (cascade screening) is fairly straightforward.[41] Genetic testing should be performed even in young children, possibly even at birth, because of the young age of CPVT manifestation and its association with sudden infant death syndrome.[37] Among *RYR2* mutation–carrying relatives identified by cascade screening, approximately 50% have a CPVT phenotype.[15] Relatives who are noncarriers of the familial CPVT–causing mutation can be reassured and dismissed from further cardiologic evaluation.

When both parents of a mutation-carrying proband have a negative genetic test, the possibility of mosaicism should be considered. Otherwise, the mutation in the proband may be incorrectly considered de novo, and siblings (who have a 50% chance of being mutation carriers) might not be tested.[42]

Differential Diagnosis

The differential diagnosis of CPVT will often include long QT syndrome, Andersen-Tawil syndrome and other aforementioned inherited phenocopies of CPVT, and concealed structural heart disease, particularly arrhythmogenic cardiomyopathy.

When both long QT syndrome and CPVT are considered likely in a patient with nondiagnostic resting ECG, exercise testing is usually helpful. The QTc interval in the recovery phase of the exercise test is accurate for identifying long QT syndrome patients with a normal or borderline QTc interval at rest.[43] The presence of exercise-induced ventricular ectopy beyond isolated VPBs favors a diagnosis of CPVT.[44]

The classical phenotypic triad of Andersen-Tawil syndrome, which is caused by the loss of function mutations in *KCNJ2* in approximately 60% of cases, consists of ventricular arrhythmia, periodic paralysis, and facial and limb dysmorphism (see Chapter 94). Common cardiac manifestations are mild QTc interval prolongation, prominent U waves, and ventricular arrhythmias, which may range from frequent VPBs to bidirectional VT or polymorphic VT. In patients who lack the classical triad of Andersen-Tawil syndrome, the phenotype may very much mimic CPVT. Genetic testing may guide the distinction with other forms of CPVT, which is important because patients with Andersen-Tawil syndrome show a much more benign course. In a series of 24 *KCNJ2* mutation carriers, two individuals (8%) displayed a CPVT phenotype.[45] These two patients had their first syncope after the age of 30 years and also had ventricular arrhythmias at rest.

In (adult) patients with exercise-induced ventricular arrhythmias, initially concealed structural heart disease, such as arrhythmogenic or hypertrophic cardiomyopathy, mitral valve prolapse or ischemic heart disease may be alternate diagnoses. Cardiac imaging techniques and genetic testing may help in making a specific diagnosis. However, in some cases, the underlying condition may be revealed only after close follow-up.

Clinical Management

The clinical management of patients with CPVT is summarized in Fig. 88.2.

Risk Stratification

At present, very little is known about risk stratification for the occurrence of arrhythmic events in CPVT, particularly in comparison with other inherited arrhythmia syndromes such as

PHENOTYPE-POSITIVE PATIENTS

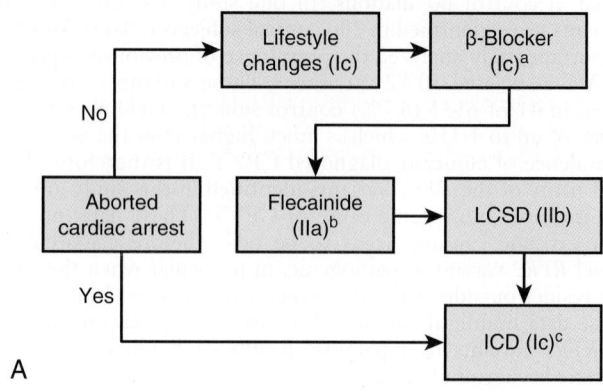

GENOTYPE-POSITIVE PHENOTYPE-NEGATIVE PATIENTS

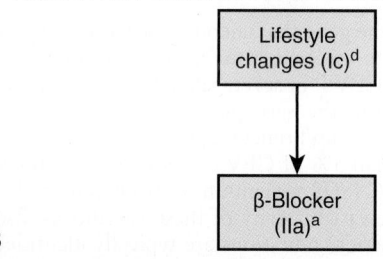

FIGURE 88.2 Therapeutic approach to patients with catecholaminergic polymorphic ventricular tachycardia (CPVT) according to current recommendations.[9,10]
Class of recommendation and level of evidence are indicated in parentheses. (A) Therapeutic approach to patients with a CPVT phenotype. The initial approach depends on the presence or absence of aborted cardiac arrest. (B) Therapeutic approach to genotype-positive patients with no CPVT phenotype. When a patient develops ventricular arrhythmias during follow-up, the therapeutic approach outlined in (A) becomes applicable. *LCSD,* Left cardiac sympathetic denervation.
a Nadolol is the first choice β-blocker. β-Blockers should be titrated to the highest tolerable dosage.
b The optimal daily flecainide dosage is 2 to 3 mg/kg.
c Patients with an implantable cardioverter defibrillator (*ICD*) should also receive a β-blocker, and the addition of flecainide should be considered (class IIa recommendation) [10] to reduce appropriate and inappropriate shocks.
d Recommendations on lifestyle changes are more lenient than in patients with a CPVT phenotype (see text for details).[46]

congenital long QT and Brugada syndromes. In general, most *CASQ2* mutation–related CPVT patients seem to display a more severe phenotype compared with *RYR2* mutation carriers. In a large CPVT series, including *RYR2* and *CASQ2* mutation carriers as well as nongenotyped patients and including both probands and relatives, young age at diagnosis and a history of aborted cardiac arrest were associated with future arrhythmic events.[14] Among asymptomatic *RYR2* or *CASQ2* mutation–carrying relatives who are identified by cascade screening, having a CPVT phenotype at the first exercise test may increase the risk for future cardiac events.[46] Relatives with a *RYR2* mutation in the C-terminal channel–forming domain have increased odds of nonsustained VT compared with those with a *RYR2* N-terminal mutation,[15] but whether this translates into an increased risk for arrhythmic events is unknown.

Altogether, current advice is to actively treat all clinically or genetically diagnosed CPVT patients until markers become available that allow adequate identification of patients at high and low risk.[9,10] Larger patient populations and longer follow-up durations are needed to identify these risk markers.

Lifestyle

All patients with CPVT are recommended to limit or avoid competitive sports, strenuous exercise, and exposure to stressful environments.[9,10] However, very recent recommendations are more lenient concerning genotype-positive phenotype-negative athletes by stating that they may participate in all competitive sports with appropriate precautionary measures, including the acquisition of a personal automatic external defibrillator and establishment of an emergency action plan.[47] Arrhythmic events during sexual intercourse have been described but are rare.[48]

β-Adrenoceptor Blockade

β-Blockers in the highest tolerable dosage are the first choice therapy in CPVT. β-Blockers are recommended in all patients with a clinical diagnosis of CPVT (class Ic recommendation) and should be considered in genotype-positive phenotype-negative individuals (class IIa recommendation).[9,10]

β-Blockers significantly reduce the risk for cardiac events, and nadolol may be superior to other β-blockers.[14,49] The β-blocker dose should be titrated to the highest dose tolerated. In a meta-analysis regarding the efficacy of β-blockers in the first eleven CPVT patient series published, the estimated overall 4- and 8-year arrhythmic event rates were 18.0% (95% confidence interval [CI], 7.7–28.9) and 35.9% (95% CI, 15.3–56.5), respectively.[50] Four- and eight-year fatal or near-fatal arrhythmic event rates were 7.2% (95% CI, 3.1–11.3) and 14.3% (95% CI, 6.1–22.5), respectively (Fig. 88.3). In a large series of 211 mostly symptomatic children with CPVT, syncopal events or cardiac arrest occurred in 25% of patients on β-blockers.[13] However, nonoptimal dosing and poor adherence contributed to 40% and 48% of all events, respectively. In a study that included 98 *RYR2* mutation–carrying relatives, only two asymptomatic relatives experienced exercise-induced syncope during a median follow-up of 4.7 years (range, 0.3–19 years).[15]

Thus β-blocker therapy is sufficiently protective in the vast majority of CPVT patients, in particular relatives who are identified through cascade screening. In addition, a significant proportion of events may not be because of β-blocker inefficacy but because of nonadherence. CPVT patients should therefore be well informed about the lifesaving importance of drug compliance, and the presence of side effects (reported in approximately a quarter of CPVT patients)[15] should be seriously addressed as these may hamper drug compliance.

β-Blocker therapy is considered insufficiently effective when arrhythmic events occur or couplets or more successive VPBs are documented during provocative testing. The presence of couplets or VT during exercise testing has been shown to be significantly associated with future arrhythmic events, with a moderate sensitivity and specificity of 0.62 and 0.67, respectively.[14]

Flecainide

On the basis of an increasing body of evidence, adding flecainide (2–3 mg/kg/day) to β-blocker therapy is considered an effective second step (class IIa recommendation).[14,49] First, flecainide was discovered to have a possible direct RYR2-blocking effect in a CPVT mouse model,[51] although this is questioned by others.[52] In an international study that included 33 severely affected patients, flecainide (1.5–4.5 mg/kg body weight) partially or completely suppressed exercise-induced ventricular arrhythmias in 76% of patients.[53] Arrhythmic events were prevented during a median follow-up of 20 (range, 12–40) months, except for one patient who received

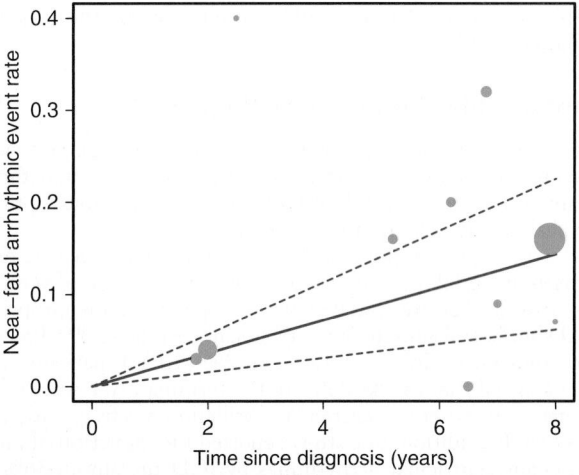

FIGURE 88.3 Near-fatal and fatal cardiac event curves of 360 patients with catecholaminergic polymorphic ventricular tachycardia on β-blocker therapy from ten studies.

The *red line* and *its corresponding area* indicate the proportion of patients with near-fatal or fatal cardiac events and its corresponding 95% confidence interval on the basis of a random-effect meta-analysis model. The *blue-green data points* represent the near-fatal and fatal cardiac event rates of individual studies. The area of each data point is proportional to its number of patients and statistical weight. (Modified from van der Werf C, Zwinderman AH, Wilde AA. Therapeutic approach for patients with catecholaminergic polymorphic ventricular tachycardia: state of the art and future developments. *Europace.* 2012;14:175-183. With permission of Oxford University Press.)

appropriate implantable cardioverter defibrillator (ICD) shocks after noncompliance. Importantly, proarrhythmia as a result of flecainide was not observed in this relatively young patient population. A similar ventricular arrhythmia suppression by flecainide was observed in a series of 12 patients with genotype-negative CPVT.[54] Flecainide was associated with a complete suppression of exercise-induced ventricular arrhythmias in 10 insufficiently controlled CPVT patients who carried a *CASQ2* mutation.[55] However, two patients experienced a VT storm with recurrent ICD shocks. In 51 children treated with flecainide, eight (16%) experienced an arrhythmic event. Importantly, seven events occurred on a suboptimal dose and six in the context of nonadherence. A small case series reported favorable ventricular arrhythmia–suppressing effects of flecainide monotherapy in patients,[56] but at present, this is only recommended in patients who are intolerant to β-blocker therapy.

Left Cardiac Sympathetic Denervation

When ventricular arrhythmias cannot be controlled by drug therapy, left cardiac sympathetic denervation (LCSD), usually using video-assisted thoracoscopic surgery, may be considered (class IIb recommendation).[14,49] In this procedure, the lower half of the left stellate ganglion and thoracic ganglia T2–T4 are removed, thereby largely preventing norepinephrine release in the heart. Among 63 severely symptomatic patients who underwent LCSD, the 2-year cumulative event-free survival rate was 81%.[57] LCSD was associated with a significant reduction of major arrhythmic events from 100% to 32%. Patients with an incomplete LCSD were more likely to experience major arrhythmic events. It is unknown which pharmacological regimen should be followed after a successful procedure, so it is recommended to continue β-blocker therapy.

The quality of life of CPVT patients who underwent LCSD has been well studied and reported to be favorable, despite minor side effects that were reported by the majority of patients.[58,59]

Implantable Cardioverter Defibrillator

According to current guidelines, ICD is indicated in patients with previous aborted cardiac arrest and in patients with arrhythmic events or polymorphic VT or bidirectional VT, despite optimal medical therapy (class Ic recommendation).[9,10]

Two early case reports demonstrated that ICDs may be proarrhythmic in CPVT and may even be fatal because of ventricular storms that are initiated by appropriate or inappropriate ICD shocks and subsequent catecholamine release.[60,61] Indeed, two studies that included 13[62] and 24[63] CPVT patients with ICD showed that shocks delivered to terminate VT were often unsuccessful, whereas ventricular fibrillation was frequently terminated. In addition, one study reported the induction of more malignant ventricular arrhythmias by ICD therapy in 36% of patients, including an electrical storm in 29% and 8.5% of total shocks.[62] In a large series of children with CPVT, appropriate and inappropriate shocks occurred in 46% and 22% of 94 children with ICD.[13] A number of these children (43%) received a cumulative sum of six or more shocks. An electrical storm occurred in 18%, and ICD-related complications occurred in 23%. In a meta-analysis regarding ICD harm in young patients with inherited cardiac diseases, the annual rate of inappropriate shocks in patients with CPVT was 7.6% (95% CI, 2.8–12.4), which was higher than that in patients with other conditions.[64]

In addition, CPVT patients had the highest rate of other ICD–related complications (annual rate of 21.2%).

Altogether, these data indicate that among patients who did not have an aborted cardiac arrest, ICD implantation should be restricted to CPVT patients who do not sufficiently respond to an aggressive therapeutic strategy, including β-blockers, flecainide, and LCSD. Some may implant ICDs in symptomatic patients at an earlier stage, but in any case, additional therapy with β-blockers and flecainide should also be intensified, and LCSD may be considered to minimize the number of appropriate and inappropriate ICD shocks. In addition, careful ICD programming, e.g., with one ventricular fibrillation zone with a detection interval of 240 beats/min and (exceptionally) long detection intervals, is important.

Other and Future Therapies

Additional pharmacological therapies that may play a role in the future include propafenone[65] and dantrolene,[66] which is already used for treating malignant hyperthermia, a disorder caused by mutations in the skeletal ryanodine receptor (*RYR1*). In addition, small molecules that stabilize RyR2, such as S107,[67] are being studied. Finally, the first step on the road toward gene therapy for CPVT was recently made. A viral gene transfer of wild-type CASQ2 into the heart of *CASQ2* mutant mice showed a long-lasting efficiency in mice infected at birth as well as a reversal of the CPVT phenotype in the adult mice.[68]

REFERENCES

1. Leenhardt A, Lucet V, Denjoy I, et al. Catecholaminergic polymorphic ventricular tachycardia in children. A 7-year follow-up of 21 patients. *Circulation*. 1995;91:1512–1519.
2. van der Werf C, Hofman N, Tan HL, et al. Diagnostic yield in sudden unexplained death and aborted cardiac arrest in the young: the experience of a tertiary referral center in The Netherlands. *Heart Rhythm*. 2010;7:1383–1389.
3. Krahn AD, Healey JS, Chauhan VS, et al. Epinephrine infusion in the evaluation of unexplained cardiac arrest and familial sudden death: from the cardiac arrest survivors with preserved ejection fraction registry. *Circ Arrhythm Electrophysiol*. 2012;5:933–940.
4. Berg K. Multifocal ventricular extrasystoles with Adams-Stokes syndrome in children. *Am Heart J*. 1960;60:965–970.
5. Reid DS, Tynan M, Braidwood L, et al. Bidirectional tachycardia in a child. A study using His bundle electrography. *Br Heart J*. 1975;37:339–344.
6. Coumel P, Fidelle J, Lucet V, et al. Catecholamine-induced severe ventricular arrhythmias with Adam-Stokes in children: report of four cases. *Br Heart J*. 1978;40:28–37.
7. Priori SG, Napolitano C, Tiso N, et al. Mutations in the cardiac ryanodine receptor gene (hRyR2) underlie catecholaminergic polymorphic ventricular tachycardia. *Circulation*. 2001;103:196–200.
8. Lahat H, Pras E, Olender T, et al. A missense mutation in a highly conserved region of CASQ2 is associated with autosomal recessive catecholamine-induced polymorphic ventricular tachycardia in Bedouin families from Israel. *Am J Hum Genet*. 2001;69:1378–1384.
9. Priori SG, Wilde AA, Horie M, et al. HRS/EHRA/APHRS expert consensus statement on the diagnosis and management of patients with inherited primary arrhythmia syndromes. *Heart Rhythm*. 2013;10:1932–1963.
10. Authors/Task Force Members, Priori SG, Blomström-Lundqvist C, et al. 2015 ESC Guidelines for the management of patients with ventricular arrhythmias and the prevention of sudden cardiac death: the task force for the management of patients with ventricular arrhythmias and the prevention of sudden cardiac death of the European Society of Cardiology (ESC). Endorsed by: Association for European Paediatric and Congenital Cardiology (AEPC). *Eur Heart J*. 2015;36:2793–2867.
11. Sy RW, Gollob MH, Klein GJ, et al. Arrhythmia characterization and long-term outcomes in catecholaminergic polymorphic ventricular tachycardia. *Heart Rhythm*. 2011;8:864–871.

12. Tester DJ, Medeiros-Domingo A, Will ML, et al. Unexplained drownings and the cardiac channelopathies: a molecular autopsy series. *Mayo Clin Proc*. 2011;86:941–947.
13. Roston TM, Vinocur JM, Maginot KR, et al. Catecholaminergic polymorphic ventricular tachycardia in children: an analysis of therapeutic strategies and outcomes from an international multicenter registry. *Circ Arrhythm Electrophysiol*. 2015;8:633–642.
14. Hayashi M, Denjoy I, Extramiana F, et al. Incidence and risk factors of arrhythmic events in catecholaminergic polymorphic ventricular tachycardia. *Circulation*. 2009;119:2426–2434.
15. van der Werf C, Nederend I, Hofman N, et al. Familial evaluation in catecholaminergic polymorphic ventricular tachycardia: disease penetrance and expression in cardiac ryanodine receptor mutation-carrying relatives. *Circ Arrhythm Electrophysiol*. 2012;5:748–756.
16. Blich M, Marai I, Suleiman M, et al. Electrocardiographic comparison of ventricular premature complexes during exercise test in patients with CPVT and healthy subjects. *Pacing Clin Electrophysiol*. 2015;38:398–402.
17. Faggioni M, Hwang HS, van der Werf C, et al. Accelerated sinus rhythm prevents catecholaminergic polymorphic ventricular tachycardia in mice and in patients. *Circ Res*. 2013;112:689–697.
18. Marjamaa A, Hiippala A, Arrhenius B, et al. Intravenous epinephrine infusion test in diagnosis of catecholaminergic polymorphic ventricular tachycardia. *J Cardiovasc Electrophysiol*. 2012;23:194–199.
19. Roux-Buisson N, Gandjbakhch E, Donal E, et al. Prevalence and significance of rare RYR2 variants in arrhythmogenic right ventricular cardiomyopathy/dysplasia: results of a systematic screening. *Heart Rhythm*. 2014;11:1999–2009.
20. Ohno S, Omura M, Kawamura M, et al. Exon 3 deletion of RYR2 encoding cardiac ryanodine receptor is associated with left ventricular non-compaction. *Europace*. 2014;16:1646–1654.
21. Nannenberg EA, Sijbrands EJG, Dijksman LM, et al. Mortality of inherited arrhythmia syndromes: insight into their natural history. *Circ Cardiovasc Genet*. 2012;5:183–189.
22. Jabbari J, Jabbari R, Nielsen MW, et al. New exome data question the pathogenicity of genetic variants previously associated with catecholaminergic polymorphic ventricular tachycardia. *Circ Cardiovasc Genet*. 2013;6:481–489.

23. Medeiros-Domingo A, Bhuiyan ZA, Tester DJ, et al. The RYR2-encoded ryanodine receptor/calcium release channel in patients diagnosed previously with either catecholaminergic polymorphic ventricular tachycardia or genotype negative, exercise-induced long QT syndrome: a comprehensive open reading frame mutational analysis. *J Am Coll Cardiol*. 2009;54:2065–2074.
24. Wangüemert F, Bosch Calero C, Pérez C, et al. Clinical and molecular characterization of a cardiac ryanodine receptor founder mutation causing catecholaminergic polymorphic ventricular tachycardia. *Heart Rhythm*. 2015;12:1636–1643.
25. Bai R, Napolitano C, Bloise R, et al. Yield of genetic screening in inherited cardiac channelopathies: how to prioritize access to genetic testing. *Circ Arrhythm Electrophysiol*. 2009;2:6–15.
26. Postma AV, Denjoy I, Hoorntje TM, et al. Absence of calsequestrin 2 causes severe forms of catecholaminergic polymorphic ventricular tachycardia. *Circ Res*. 2002;91:e21–e26.
27. Kirchhefer U, Wehrmeister D, Postma AV, et al. The human CASQ2 mutation K206N is associated with hyperglycosylation and altered cellular calcium handling. *J Mol Cell Cardiol*. 2010;49:95–105.
28. Roux-Buisson N, Cacheux M, Fourest-Lieuvin A, et al. Absence of triadin, a protein of the calcium release complex, is responsible for cardiac arrhythmia with sudden death in humans. *Hum Mol Genet*. 2012;21:2759–2767.
29. Rooryck C, Kyndt F, Bozon D, et al. New family with catecholaminergic polymorphic ventricular tachycardia linked to the triadin gene. *J Cardiovasc Electrophysiol*. 2015;26:1146–1150.
30. Nyegaard M, Overgaard MT, Søndergaard MT, et al. Mutations in calmodulin cause ventricular tachycardia and sudden cardiac death. *Am J Hum Genet*. 2012;91:703–712.
31. Makita N, Yagihara N, Crotti L, et al. Novel calmodulin mutations associated with congenital arrhythmia susceptibility. *Circ Cardiovasc Genet*. 2014;7:466–474.
32. Marsman RF, Barc J, Beekman L, et al. A mutation in CALM1 encoding calmodulin in familial idiopathic ventricular fibrillation in childhood and adolescence. *J Am Coll Cardiol*. 2014;63:259–266.
33. Bhuiyan ZA, Hamdan MA, Shamsi ETA, et al. A novel early onset lethal form of catecholaminergic polymorphic ventricular tachycardia maps to chromosome 7p14-p22. *J Cardiovasc Electrophysiol*. 2007;18:1060–1066.

33a. Devalla HD Gélinas R, Aburawi EH, et al. TECRL, a new life-threatening inherited arrhythmia gene associated with overlapping clinical features of both LQTS and CPVT. *EMBO Mol Med*. 2016;8:1390–1408.

34. Swan H, Amarouch MY, Leinonen J, et al. Gain-of-function mutation of the SCN5A gene causes exercise-induced polymorphic ventricular arrhythmias. *Circ Cardiovasc Genet*. 2014;7:771–781.

35. Laurent G, Saal S, Amarouch MY, et al. Multifocal ectopic Purkinje-related premature contractions: a new SCN5A-related cardiac channelopathy. *J Am Coll Cardiol*. 2012;60:144–156.

36. Mohler PJ, Splawski I, Napolitano C, et al. A cardiac arrhythmia syndrome caused by loss of ankyrin-B function. *Proc Natl Acad Sci U S A*. 2004;101:9137–9142.

37. Ackerman MJ, Priori SG, Willems S, et al. HRS/EHRA expert consensus statement on the state of genetic testing for the channelopathies and cardiomyopathies: this document was developed as a partnership between the Heart Rhythm Society (HRS) and the European Heart Rhythm Association (EHRA). *Heart Rhythm*. 2011;8:1308–1339.

38. Paech C, Gebauer RA, Karstedt J, et al. Ryanodine receptor mutations presenting as idiopathic ventricular fibrillation: a report on two novel familial compound mutations, c.6224T>C and c.13781A>G, with the clinical presentation of idiopathic ventricular fibrillation. *Pediatr Cardiol*. 2014;35:1437–1441.

39. Cheung JW, Meli AC, Xie W, et al. Short-coupled polymorphic ventricular tachycardia at rest linked to a novel ryanodine receptor (RyR2) mutation: leaky RyR2 channels under non-stress conditions. *Int J Cardiol*. 2015;180:228–236.

40. Jiang D, Chen W, Wang R, et al. Loss of luminal Ca2+ activation in the cardiac ryanodine receptor is associated with ventricular fibrillation and sudden death. *Proc Natl Acad Sci U S A*. 2007;104:18309–18314.

41. Hofman N, Tan HL, Alders M, et al. Active cascade screening in primary inherited arrhythmia syndromes: does it lead to prophylactic treatment? *J Am Coll Cardiol*. 2010;55:2570–2576.

42. Roux-Buisson N, Egéa G, Denjoy I, et al. Germline and somatic mosaicism for a mutation of the ryanodine receptor type 2 gene: implication for genetic counselling and patient caring. *Europace*. 2011;13:130–132.

43. Sy RW, van der Werf C, Chattha IS, et al. Derivation and validation of a simple exercise-based algorithm for prediction of genetic testing in relatives of LQTS probands. *Circulation*. 2011;124:2187–2194.

44. Horner JM, Ackerman MJ. Ventricular ectopy during treadmill exercise stress testing in the evaluation of long QT syndrome. *Heart Rhythm*. 2008;5:1690–1694.

45. Kimura H, Zhou J, Kawamura M, et al. Phenotype variability in patients carrying KCNJ2 mutations. *Circ Cardiovasc Genet*. 2012;5:344–353.

46. Hayashi M, Denjoy I, Hayashi M, et al. The role of stress test for predicting genetic mutations and future cardiac events in asymptomatic relatives of catecholaminergic polymorphic ventricular tachycardia probands. *Europace*. 2012;14:1344–1351.

47. Ackerman MJ, Zipes DP, Kovacs RJ, et al. Eligibility and disqualification recommendations for competitive athletes with cardiovascular abnormalities: task force 10: the cardiac channelopathies: a scientific statement from the American Heart Association and American College of Cardiology. *J Am Coll Cardiol*. 2015;132:e326–e329.

48. Loar RW, Bos JM, Cannon BC, et al. Sudden cardiac arrest during sex in patients with either catecholaminergic polymorphic ventricular tachycardia or long-QT syndrome: a rare but shocking experience. *J Cardiovasc Electrophysiol*. 2015;26:300–304.

49. Leren IS, Saberniak J, Majid E, et al. Nadolol decreases the incidence and severity of ventricular arrhythmias during exercise stress testing compared with β1-selective β-blockers in patients with catecholaminergic polymorphic ventricular tachycardia. *Heart Rhythm*. 2016;13:433–440.

50. van der Werf C, Zwinderman AH, Wilde AAM. Therapeutic approach for patients with catecholaminergic polymorphic ventricular tachycardia: state of the art and future developments. *Europace*. 2012;14:175–183.

51. Watanabe H, Chopra N, Laver D, et al. Flecainide prevents catecholaminergic polymorphic ventricular tachycardia in mice and humans. *Nat Med*. 2009;15:380–383.

52. Bannister ML, Thomas NL, Sikkel MB, et al. The mechanism of flecainide action in CPVT does not involve a direct effect on RyR2. *Circ Res*. 2015;116:1324–1335.

53. van der Werf C, Kannankeril PJ, Sacher F, et al. Flecainide therapy reduces exercise-induced ventricular arrhythmias in patients with catecholaminergic polymorphic ventricular tachycardia. *J Am Coll Cardiol*. 2011;57:2244–2254.

54. Watanabe H, van der Werf C, Roses-Noguer F, et al. Effects of flecainide on exercise-induced ventricular arrhythmias and recurrences in genotype-negative patients with catecholaminergic polymorphic ventricular tachycardia. *Heart Rhythm*. 2013;10:542–547.

55. Khoury A, Marai I, Suleiman M, et al. Flecainide therapy suppresses exercise-induced ventricular arrhythmias in patients with CASQ2-associated catecholaminergic polymorphic ventricular tachycardia. *Heart Rhythm*. 2013;10:1671–1675.

56. Padfield GJ, AlAhmari L, Lieve KVV, et al. Flecainide monotherapy is an option for selected patients with catecholaminergic polymorphic ventricular tachycardia intolerant of β-blockade. *Heart Rhythm*. 2016;13:509–613.

57. De Ferrari GM, Dusi V, Spazzolini C, et al. Clinical management of catecholaminergic polymorphic ventricular tachycardia: the role of left cardiac sympathetic denervation. *Circulation*. 2015;131:2185–2193.

58. Waddell-Smith KE, Ertresvaag KN, Li J, et al. Physical and psychological consequences of left cardiac sympathetic denervation in long-QT syndrome and catecholaminergic polymorphic ventricular tachycardia. *Circ Arrhythm Electrophysiol*. 2015;8:1151–1158.

59. Antiel RM, Bos JM, Joyce DD, et al. Quality of life after videoscopic left cardiac sympathetic denervation in patients with potentially life-threatening cardiac channelopathies/cardiomyopathies. *Heart Rhythm*. 2016;13:62–69.

60. Pizzale S, Gollob MH, Gow R, et al. Sudden death in a young man with catecholaminergic polymorphic ventricular tachycardia and paroxysmal atrial fibrillation. *J Cardiovasc Electrophysiol*. 2008;19:1319–1321.

61. Mohamed U, Gollob MH, Gow RM, et al. Sudden cardiac death despite an implantable cardioverter-defibrillator in a young female with catecholaminergic ventricular tachycardia. *Heart Rhythm*. 2006;3:1486–1489.

62. Roses-Noguer F, Jarman JWE, Clague JR, et al. Outcomes of defibrillator therapy in catecholaminergic polymorphic ventricular tachycardia. *Heart Rhythm*. 2014;11:58–66.

63. Miyake CY, Webster G, Czosek RJ, et al. Efficacy of implantable cardioverter defibrillators in young patients with catecholaminergic polymorphic ventricular tachycardia: success depends on substrate. *Circ Arrhythm Electrophysiol*. 2013;6:579–587.

64. Olde Nordkamp LRA, Postema PG, Knops RE, et al. Implantable cardioverter-defibrillator harm in young patients with inherited arrhythmia syndromes: a systematic review and meta-analysis of inappropriate shocks and complications. *Heart Rhythm*. 2016;13:443–454.

65. Hwang HS, Hasdemir C, Laver D, et al. Inhibition of cardiac Ca2+ release channels (RyR2) determines efficacy of class I antiarrhythmic drugs in catecholaminergic polymorphic ventricular tachycardia. *Circ Arrhythm Electrophysiol*. 2011;4:128–135.

66. Penttinen K, Swan H, Vanninen S, et al. Antiarrhythmic effects of dantrolene in patients with catecholaminergic polymorphic ventricular tachycardia and replication of the responses using iPSC models. *PLoS One*. 2015;10:e0125366.

67. Lehnart SE, Wehrens XHT, Laitinen PJ, et al. Sudden death in familial polymorphic ventricular tachycardia associated with calcium release channel (ryanodine receptor) leak. *Circulation*. 2004;109:3208–3214.

68. Denegri M, Bongianino R, Lodola F, et al. Single delivery of an adeno-associated viral construct to transfer the CASQ2 gene to knock-in mice affected by catecholaminergic polymorphic ventricular tachycardia is able to cure the disease from birth to advanced age. *Circulation*. 2014;129:2673–2681.

89 Ventricular Arrhythmias in Heart Failure

Lynne Warner Stevenson, Roy M. John, and Neal K. Lakdawala

This chapter addresses the consideration of ventricular arrhythmias in the setting of heart failure (HF) with reduced ejection fraction (EF). HF with preserved EF accounts for approximately half of all patients and hospitalizations with HF diagnoses and is complicated by atrial fibrillation as frequently as HF with reduced EF, but it is rarely associated with ventricular arrhythmias and will not be discussed in this chapter. Some causes of HF such as sarcoidosis or inherited lamin mutations can cause ventricular arrhythmias prior to or simultaneously with the first diagnosis of cardiac dysfunction. More commonly, ventricular arrhythmias associated with HF arise within a substrate of myocyte hypertrophy and chronic myocardial remodeling with diffuse or focal fibrosis, the common pathway of response to various causes of cardiac injury. The combination of ventricular arrhythmias and HF focuses on special consideration of both etiology and therapies, but the initial approach to any patient with HF includes systematic assessment of contributing causes and need for hemodynamic stabilization prior to further intervention (Table 89.1).[1]

Etiology

Patients Presenting With Ventricular Arrhythmias and Reduced Ejection Fraction Without Prior Heart Failure Diagnosis

General Evaluation

Ventricular arrhythmia or sudden cardiac death may be the initial manifestation of cardiac disease. After acute initial stabilization, the focus is on diagnosis of the underlying cause and any aggravating factors, with emphasis on spontaneously resolving or treatable conditions (Fig. 89.1). An estimation of the duration of ventricular dysfunction helps to guide initial evaluation. It is crucial to recognize that a new presentation of HF often does not reflect new-onset disease as many patients have gradual deterioration of left ventricular (LV) function without obvious clinical symptoms. Superimposed infection or arrhythmias often exacerbate previously unrecognized cardiac dysfunction. Structural clues to chronic disease include marked ventricular and/or atrial dilation, but the chronic course is often revealed through a detailed clinical history probing for progressive limitation of specific activity, often highlighted by comparing summer vacations, winter snow shoveling, holidays, or the routine of household errands from previous years. On the other hand, prolonged tachycardia or a recent cardiac arrest in a heart with otherwise normal function may cause a transient reduction of LV ejection fraction (LVEF), which should be reassessed about a week later.

The electrocardiogram often provides the first clue to structural heart disease, and it is rarely completely normal in patients with cardiomyopathy (CM). Cardiac enzymes may be slightly elevated following a prolonged arrhythmia and are often slightly elevated in chronic HF, but higher levels suggest either acute major cardiac injury, inflammation, or a condition affecting skeletal muscle as well. Elevations in B-type natriuretic peptide (BNP) or N-terminal-pro-BNP (NT-proBNP) suggest disease of at least several days' duration, and very high levels suggest severe chronic disease, although these levels are also very high in individuals with renal dysfunction. Echocardiography is usually the first imaging step taken to determine LV function, right ventricular (RV) function, and possible primary valvular disease, congenital heart disease, or regional abnormalities consistent with prior infarction. Echocardiography prior to electrophysiological procedures should also inform hemodynamic assessment for triage (see below). In patients with low EF and extensive wall motion abnormalities, nuclear imaging may not be sensitive enough to exclude diffuse coronary artery disease. Hence, cardiac catheterization with coronary angiography should be performed to exclude or define coronary artery disease in patients for whom revascularization would be considered.[2] Concomitant endomyocardial biopsy will be discussed in relation to inflammatory myocardial diseases. Cardiac magnetic resonance (CMR) imaging is emerging as a valuable tool for detection of intramyocardial disease not readily evident on echocardiography, such as inflammation or focal scarring.

Inflammatory Myocarditis

The first diagnosis to consider when ventricular arrhythmias and HF present simultaneously is an inflammatory myocarditis. These disorders are associated with a high incidence of life-threatening repetitive ventricular tachycardia (VT)/ventricular fibrillation (VF) but may also demonstrate some response to immunosuppression. Cardiac sarcoidosis can occur with or without pulmonary sarcoidosis and is often first suspected after presentation with ventricular arrhythmias or a new conduction block.[3] Sarcoidosis can be associated with vague symptoms of fevers or arthralgias and also with uveitis or iritis. Fewer than half of patients with evidence of cardiac sarcoid at autopsy will have had clinically apparent cardiac involvement. Patchy noncaseating granulomas tend to involve the basal ventricular septum, often with AV conduction abnormalities. A normal LVEF may be falsely reassuring as sarcoidosis has a predilection for the right ventricle and the clinical presentation is frequently confused with arrhythmogenic RV dysplasia.

Presentation with atrioventricular (AV) block should prompt a search for cardiac sarcoidosis. In a review of unexplained heart block in patients younger than 55 years of age, cardiac sarcoid or giant cell myocarditis accounted for 25% of cases, and these patients had a high incidence of sudden death or VT or the need for cardiac transplantation.[4] Left bundle branch block occurs commonly in CM, sometimes years before HF develops, but in sarcoidosis right bundle branch block is often the pattern. Prior to implantable cardioverter-defibrillators (ICDs), sudden cardiac death accounted for up to two-thirds of terminal events in patients with overt cardiac sarcoidosis.[4]

Although endomyocardial biopsy provides a definitive diagnosis, sensitivity is low, at 10% to 20%, because of the patchy

TABLE 89.1 Initial assessment of the patient with heart failure

1.	Etiology of heart failure and exacerbating factors	New or chronic ventricular dysfunction?	Coronary artery disease or other structural heart disease?	Inflammatory, genetic, or possibly reversible cardiomyopathy?	Exacerbating factors (e.g., recent viral infection, medication change, thyroid disease)
2.	Hemodynamic profiles requiring stabilization	Clinical assessment for elevated cardiac filling pressures and adequacy of cardiac output	Cardiac reserve as evidenced by baseline patient functional capacity	Consider also pulmonary hypertension and right heart function	
3.	Beats and clots	Contribution of arrhythmias or abnormal conduction to heart failure profile	Targets for therapy and prevention of arrhythmias	Risk of thromboembolic events	Considerations for anticoagulation therapy
4.	Disease trajectory	Milestones of heart failure progression	Frailty and other comorbidities influencing prognosis	Triage for heart transplant or left ventricular assist devices for highly selected patients	Discussions of patient goals and preferences and "what if" in light of competing risks for heart failure death, sudden death, and noncardiac death or disability

Modified from Stevenson L. Management of acute decompensated heart failure. In: Mann DL, Felker GM, eds. *Heart Failure: A Companion to Braunwald's Heart Disease*. 3rd ed. Philadelphia: Saunders; 2015.

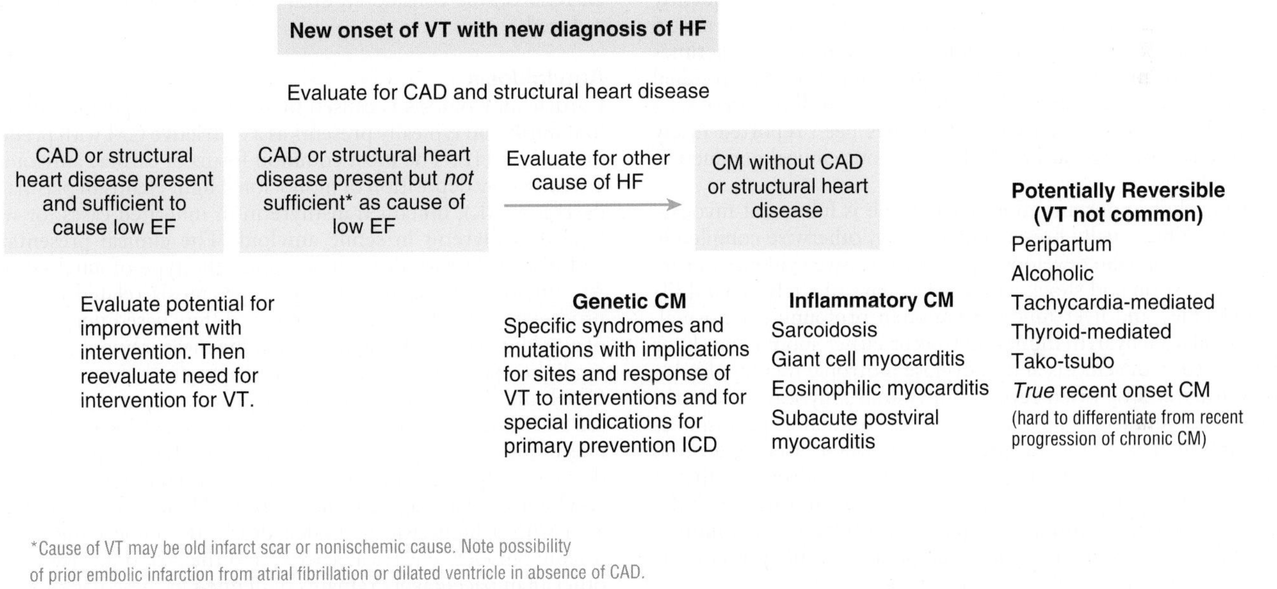

FIGURE 89.1 **Examples of causes of cardiomyopathy (*CM*) with particular relevance for those associated with ventricular arrhythmias.** *CAD,* Coronary artery disease; *EF,* ejection fraction; *HF,* heart failure; *ICD,* implantable cardioverter defibrillator; *VT,* ventricular tachycardia.

distribution of the granulomas. CMR with gadolinium enhancement and positron emission tomography (PET) scanning for areas of active glucose uptake are becoming valuable aids in diagnosis.[5] There is interest in using CMR, PET, and endocardial voltage mapping to guide endomyocardial biopsy to increase its yield,[6] which may be increased with LV endomyocardial biopsy as performed in some centers. A recent consensus statement recommended an ICD for patients with cardiac sarcoidosis who have sustained ventricular arrhythmias or depressed ventricular function (LVEF ≤0.35) and stated that it can be useful for patients who have had syncope, inducible VT at electrophysiology study, or those who need a permanent pacemaker for bradyarrhythmias.[7] An ICD is not recommended for patients with no evidence of ventricular scarring on CMR imaging with relatively preserved ventricular function and no arrhythmia symptoms. For patients with active inflammation and arrhythmias, immunosuppressive therapy is more likely to improve AV block than sustained monomorphic VT. Once the LVEF is below 30%, it is not common to see major improvement in LV function with immunosuppression unless some of the dysfunction was related to tachyarrhythmias.

Large areas of active inflammation are likely to subside to leave a heavy scar burden. If treatment is initiated prior to extensive scarring, sarcoidosis often "burns out" such that immunosuppression can be weaned and modestly impaired LV function remains stable, although the right ventricle should continue to be monitored carefully. The risk of ventricular arrhythmias remains, however, as the scars provide foci for reentrant arrhythmias even after the inflammation has resolved.

Giant cell myocarditis is generally characterized by a more fulminant course with worse outcomes than sarcoidosis. The granulomas are accompanied by a diffuse inflammatory infiltrate that usually includes lymphocytic infiltrates as well as granulomas, so the biopsy is generally positive. Although generally considered as distinct entities on the basis of biopsy and presentation, sarcoidosis and giant cell myocarditis may represent different levels along a spectrum of inflammation with giant cells. Hearts showing sarcoidosis on endomyocardial biopsy have occasionally been found to have areas consistent with giant cell myocarditis after removal at the time of transplantation. Cases of patients in whom giant cell myocarditis has been stabilized for a year or longer by high-dose combination immunosuppressive therapy have been reported, but the most favorable outcome in eligible patents is usually from transplantation.[8,9]

Eosinophilic myocarditis can also be associated with ventricular arrhythmias at the time of presentation. Most cases are related to an allergic reaction to long-term administration of a drug, but idiopathic eosinophilic syndromes may also cause eosinophilic myocarditis. Arrhythmias and systolic dysfunction generally respond well to steroid treatment and withdrawal of the offending drug, although patients may be left with restrictive physiology.

Postviral myocarditis is probably more common than recognized, and in most cases, it resolves without detection. (As previously mentioned, it is often assumed to be the cause for idiopathic "recent onset CM," but many of these are actually chronic CMs with recent exacerbation due to overlaid viral symptoms.) The prevalence of lymphocytic infiltrates on endomyocardial biopsy diminishes rapidly with time after presentation, and often endomyocardial biopsy later shows mild hypertrophy without evidence of cellular inflammation or significant fibrosis. Although premature ventricular contractions (PVCs) may occur, sustained VT or VF is uncommon in early stages of presumed postviral myocarditis. When it is diagnosed, postviral myocarditis will frequently improve substantially to an LVEF of at least 40% in the next 6 to 12 months.[9] However, the clinical improvement is sometimes less than that predicted by the EF improvement because residual diastolic dysfunction and RV dysfunction may limit exercise.[10] It should be noted that Lyme disease has been reported rarely to cause clinical myocarditis with or without clinical conduction system disease.

A rare but important clinical syndrome is fulminant myocarditis.[11,12] This usually presents in a young, otherwise completely healthy person who develops rapidly progressive evidence of cardiac congestion and shock within a few days of a febrile viral illness. Kidney and liver function are often profoundly abnormal. Ventricular tachyarrhythmias may occur either spontaneously or in the setting of acidosis and high-dose inotropic therapy. Endomyocardial biopsy often reveals only intense myocardial edema, but it may reveal lymphocytic infiltrates. Immunosuppression is not indicated in the acute presentation, when viral replication may be intensified. The importance of this syndrome is that it often resolves completely within days to weeks, during which the patient may require intensive support with high doses of inotropic therapy and sometimes with temporary mechanical circulatory assist devices.

Genetic Cardiomyopathy

Familial CMs account for 30% to 40% of disease originally categorized as idiopathic dilated CM (DCM).[12–14] Most cases are transmitted in an autosomal dominant pattern with age-dependent penetrance and variable clinical expression. X-linked, autosomal recessive, and mitochondrial inheritance patterns are also recognized but are substantially less common. More than 50 genes have been implicated as a cause of DCM; however, mutations in these genes account for no more than half of the reported cases.[15,16]

Truncating mutations in *TTN*, the gene that encodes the giant protein titin, are the most common identifiable cause of DCM and underlie approximately 20% of familial, peripartum, and sporadic DCM, which typically presents in adulthood. However, truncating mutations in titin are also present in 1% to 3% of controls, complicating the distinction of which *TTN* variants are pathogenic.[17] Titin plays a role in sarcomeric structure and function, and DCM-causing *TTN* mutations usually affect the A-band region. Mutations in other sarcomere genes (e.g., *MYH7*, *TNNT2*, and *TPM1*) account for ~10% of DCM which may clinically present from infancy to late adulthood. Mutations in *LMNA*, the gene coding for structural proteins of the nuclear lamina (lamin A and C), are particularly associated with conduction system disease and with atrial and ventricular arrhythmias,

which may supersede or precede the associated CM.[18] Due to the high burden of ventricular tachyarrhythmia and sudden death seen with *LMNA*-associated CM, primary prevention ICD implantation is reasonable when CM is evident in a family member even if the LVEF is higher than 0.35.[15,19]

Arrhythmogenic RV cardiomyopathy (ARVC) due to mutations in genes encoding for cardiac desmosomal proteins (e.g., *PKP2*, *DSP*, *DSC2*, and *JUP*) predominantly affects the RV, but LV involvement is common, especially with *DSP* mutations, and can precede RV manifestations.[20] Approximately 50% of cases are familial and are characterized by autosomal dominant inheritance, with clinical expression apparently worsened by endurance exercise training. Sudden death and ventricular arrhythmias are often the initial presentation. RV failure due to progressive myocardial loss is seen in later stages of the disease and may progress to a phase of biventricular failure that can mimic DCM. However, less than 10% of cases progress to end-stage HF. Autosomal recessive forms of ARVC due to defects in plakoglobin or desmoplakin result in cardiocutaneous syndromes with abnormalities of hair and skin, such as is seen in Naxos disease and Carvajal syndrome.[21] As with other familial ventricular arrhythmia/CM, an ICD can be considered even when the LVEF is not severely reduced.

Amyloidosis

Cardiac amyloidosis is caused by myocardial deposition of amyloid fibrils and typically presents as a restrictive CM with predominant right HF. The most common forms of cardiac amyloidosis are caused by deposition of monoclonal light chains in plasma cell dyscrasia (AL), mutant transthyretin in inherited cases, or wild-type transthyretin in senile amyloid. The clinical presentation and natural history differ based upon the type of amyloid, with AL amyloid associated with worse prognosis related to rapidly progressive HF. Similarly, diagnosis differs based upon the type of amyloid. Recent developments in the measurement of circulating light chains and contemporary imaging techniques (especially CMR and Tc99 single photon emission computed tomography [SPECT]) may enable diagnosis without need for endomyocardial biopsy. Therapy specific to the underlying type of amyloidosis has improved the outlook for AL and mutant transthyretin amyloidosis. Although advanced HF in AL amyloidosis is associated with a high risk of sudden death, the underlying cause is usually pulseless electrical activity and the role of device therapy other than pacemakers remains undefined in these patients.[22,23]

Potentially Reversible Causes of Cardiomyopathy

Most potentially reversible causes of CM are not typically associated with clinically significant ventricular tachyarrhythmia. Takotsubo CM, which is an exception, may present with VT or cardiac arrest. Peripartum CM is rarely associated with clinical arrhythmias, except in the setting of severe hypoxia or acidosis early after delivery. Alcoholic CM or other cardiac dysfunction with a superimposed alcoholic component may improve markedly within months of complete abstention from alcohol. Truly new onset HF without identifiable cause improves spontaneously to normal or near-normal EF in almost half of patients.[23] (When EF shows major clinical improvement by 3 to 6 months, but not yet to 0.35, it may be reasonable to wait longer before placement of a primary prevention ICD.)

Tachycardia Causing Cardiomyopathy. Prolonged periods of all forms of tachycardia, including frequent PVCs (see Chapter 80), are well recognized as a cause of reversible CM. Ventricular arrhythmia is uncommon in tachycardia-related CM unless it is the causative tachycardia. The diagnosis of tachycardia CM is often a retrospective one based on recovery of ventricular function after treatment of the arrhythmia. In one retrospective analysis of 174 patients with idiopathic PVCs referred for catheter ablation, LV dysfunction was present in 33%.[24] The smallest

PVC burden resulting in LV dysfunction was 10% over a 24-hour period, but a 24% PVC burden best differentiated the group that demonstrated CM from the group with preserved LV function. Data also suggest that the probability of LV dysfunction is related to QRS duration of the PVCs; frequent PVCs with a wider QRS (>150 ms) are associated with greater risk of CM.[24,25] Frequent runs of nonsustained VT, PVCs, or supraventricular arrhythmias should also be considered a potential cause of CM or of deteriorating LV function in cases of previously stable CM of another origin.

Evaluation of New Ventricular Arrhythmias in Patients With Known Heart Failure

The onset of ventricular arrhythmias in a previously stable HF patient may result from electrolyte abnormalities, ischemia, drug effects, or intercurrent illness but often heralds the progression of underlying cardiac disease. Most patients with a known LVEF <35% and chronic HF symptoms will have an ICD in place to prevent premature sudden death unless they have competing risks that render anticipated survival with good quality of life to be less than a year.[26] Thus an ICD shock is often the first presentation of ventricular arrhythmias in known HF. In the SCD-Heft trial, implantation of an ICD for primary prevention was followed by therapies for a ventricular arrhythmia in 16% of patients over a mean follow-up of 45 months.[27] ICD therapies are more common in patients who receive an ICD for secondary prevention. Several studies have shown an association of ICD shocks with reduced survival, with HF being the dominant cause of mortality.[27,28] Whether the arrhythmia is a marker of hemodynamic deterioration or progression of underlying disease, or actually contributes to the deterioration is not clear.

Ventricular arrhythmia in a patient with an ICD should prompt careful patient reassessment, even though the ICD promptly restored sinus rhythm. The original diagnosis should be reviewed and may need to be reevaluated. New evidence may have arisen, implicating genetic CM either in the patient or in other family members. In HF with known coronary artery disease, ischemia and infarction can contribute to hemodynamic deterioration and arrhythmias may develop without recognized angina. Baseline abnormalities of CM may mask typical diagnostic features of coronary artery disease progression; therefore perfusion stress imaging or coronary angiography is often required. In a significant proportion of patients who receive an ICD shock, progressive ventricular remodeling may emerge evidenced by ventricular enlargement and declining LVEF.[29] Development of bundle branch block and dyssynchronous contraction can further contribute to adverse ventricular remodeling.

Identifying the type of ventricular arrhythmia is helpful in determining the cause. Monomorphic VT usually represents reentry involving regions of scar from prior infarction, inflammation, replacement fibrosis, or surgery. A syncytium of fibrosis and surviving strands of myocardium allow for reentrant VTs that have a high recurrence rate, exceeding 20% per year.[30] Polymorphic VT does not require a fixed arrhythmia substrate, although migratory circuits around scars can be a cause. Acute myocardial ischemia and electrolyte disturbances should be major considerations and require correction. Ventricular hypertrophy; predisposition to potassium, magnesium, and calcium loss; and diminished drug excretion increase susceptibility to drug-induced QT prolongation and torsades de pointes. Sotalol and dofetilide are important causes (see Chapter 101). Treatment is discontinuation of the offending drug, intravenous administration of magnesium, correction of electrolyte derangements, and, occasionally, pacing to increase the heart rate.

Infrequently, implanted devices themselves may exert proarrhythmic effects. Pacing algorithms designed to minimize ventricular pacing can induce VT/VF through induction of long–short intervals.[31] Sinus tachycardia or supraventricular tachycardia detected in the VT zone of an ICD can trigger unnecessary

antitachycardia pacing that can induce VT or VF. The appearance of ventricular arrhythmia in close temporal proximity to the implementation of LV epicardial pacing should raise the possibility of related proarrhythmia, possibly due to the change in activation sequence.[32] Inactivation of LV pacing may be necessary. If loss of cardiac resynchronization therapy (CRT) results in hemodynamic deterioration, cautious reinstitution of LV pacing after control of the arrhythmia with drugs or ablation is a possibility. Rarely, RV leads can trigger PVCs or sustained VT or VF through a mechanical effect or change in activation sequence. Repositioning of the lead has occasionally resulted in resolution of VT in such patients.[33]

Hemodynamic Triage and Management Prior to Procedures

Before undertaking any invasive evaluation or attempted therapy for new onset ventricular arrhythmias, it is important to carefully evaluate the hemodynamic status and consider the overall disease trajectory.

Hemodynamic Profiles: Filling and Flow

Careful consideration of HF hemodynamics is key to initial stabilization, preparation for smooth procedures and progress to discharge, and to the design of therapy after discharge, whether that is guided by the electrophysiologist or a cardiology colleague. Bedside assessment allows broad triage into four hemodynamic profiles based on whether clinical evidence reveals the presence of elevated filling pressures (wet or dry) and whether cardiac output is adequate or critically low for the support of peripheral perfusion and vital organ function (warm or cold) (Fig. 89.2).[34] In the setting of chronic HF, rales and peripheral edema are frequently

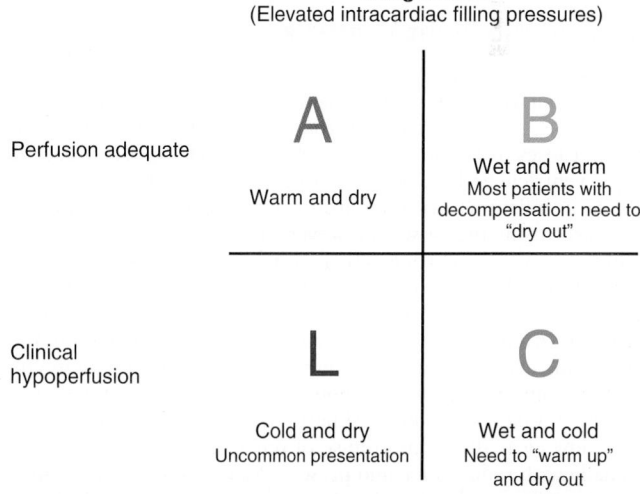

FIGURE 89.2 Simple 2 × 2 table to indicate the general hemodynamic profiles of patients with low ejection fraction. Most are able to maintain good perfusion without evidence of elevated intracardiac filling pressures—"warm and dry." Profile B is the most common profile of decompensation—"warm and wet"—which requires thorough diuresis. The patient presenting with profile C—"cold and wet"—usually requires major intervention before procedures can be performed safely and in some cases may require triage for assessment of potential candidacy for transplantation or mechanical circulatory support. Very few patients present with profile L—"cold and dry"—unless they have recently been treated aggressively. Such patients generally do not have resting symptoms but may have very limited cardiac reserve. (From Nohria A, Tsang SW, Fang JC, et al. Clinical assessment identifies hemodynamic profiles that predict outcomes in patients admitted with heart failure. *J Am Coll Cardiol.* 2003;41:1797-1804.)

absent despite severely elevated filling pressures, which should be suspected in patients with orthopnea or dyspnea on minimal exertion, such as that associated with getting dressed.[35] High pressures in chronic HF are best detected through experienced evaluation of jugular venous pressure, symptoms of orthopnea, and immediate dyspnea on light exertion and may also be identified from echocardiographic findings of dilated inferior vena cava, tricuspid regurgitation, and elevated pulmonary artery pressures. The presence of rales or ascites usually indicates more severe congestion, while peripheral edema often indicates central fluid overload but may also result from peripheral venous disease.

HF decompensation is typically characterized by congestion and much less commonly by clinically significant hypoperfusion at rest, although measured cardiac output is often slightly below the normal range. Because congestion is often present without hypoperfusion, it is important to consider these two hemodynamic abnormalities as distinct. On the other hand, hypoperfusion occurring without congestion is rare and in general is underappreciated because the patient usually has no resting symptoms. Serious hypoperfusion should be suspected in patients with a narrow pulse pressure (even if the systolic blood pressure is not markedly low) and in patients with vague or fluctuating mental status.[35] Many patients with hypoperfusion will have been intolerant of attempts to uptitrate angiotensin-converting enzyme inhibitors (ACEIs) or β-blockers due to hypotension or declining renal function. When assessing perfusion at the bedside, one should assess the skin temperature of calves and forearms (rather than hands and feet which are often cold) and auscultate the blood pressure with a manual cuff, particularly in the presence of irregular heartbeats due to atrial fibrillation or frequent PVCs. The automated blood pressure machines will frequently give falsely reassuring measurements due to detection of an occasional higher beat after a long pause. Patients with frequent PVCs are often revealed to have an effective pulse only during the regular beats.

Look at the Right Ventricle

The role of the right ventricle in the progression of HF has been underrecognized and remains difficult to track because of the challenges associated with routine imaging of this chamber. Some causes of HF such as sarcoidosis and ARVC can affect the right ventricle early. The causes of HF in younger patients, particularly inflammatory myocarditis, often affect both ventricles similarly from the onset. However, the main challenge to the right ventricle in chronic HF is usually presented by progressive left-sided congestion because worsening mitral regurgitation and higher LV filling pressures contribute to secondary pulmonary hypertension and subsequent right HF. RV dilatation and tricuspid regurgitation then contribute to renal dysfunction and further fluid retention, commonly termed the cardiorenal syndrome.[36] Once attributed primarily to reduced cardiac output, it is now clear that compromise of renal function in HF occurs equally with reduced EF and preserved EF.[37] The hemodynamic parameter most closely related to progressive renal dysfunction is elevated right atrial pressure, which is further aggravated by worsening tricuspid regurgitation.

Progressive RV dysfunction represents a "tipping point" after which compensation despite low LVEF becomes increasingly fragile. Diuretic resistance requires increasing diuretic doses, often resulting in labile potassium levels, which themselves trigger more arrhythmias. Inotropic infusions may more commonly be initiated in the attempt to clear fluid accumulation. Chronic congestion of the liver and intestinal tract system leads to malnutrition, translocation of gut flora antigens, and increased inflammatory mediators in late-stage disease.

RV dysfunction predicts significantly worse survival in patients after cardiac resynchronization.[38] RV dysfunction assessed by echocardiography also identifies a group with significantly higher

mortality after VT ablation. For 320 patients with an LVEF ≤40% at the time of VT ablation, annualized mortality overall was only 10%.[39] However, moderate or greater RV dysfunction, particularly with moderate or greater tricuspid regurgitation, predicted at least a two-fold higher mortality at 2 years after VT ablation (Fig. 89.3). Elevated pulmonary pressure on echocardiography identifies higher risk both as a passive reflection of elevated left-sided filling pressure and as a measurement of the elevated RV afterload that leads to RV failure. By 5 years after VT ablation in this group with reduced LVEF, mortality was 90% in patients who had the combination of pulmonary artery systolic pressure ≥45 mm Hg and moderate or worse RV dysfunction and tricuspid regurgitation.[39]

The details of RV dysfunction with focused echocardiographic quantitation should be carefully assessed prior to procedures in high-risk patients for whom there is concern that prolonged mechanical circulatory support might be required. RV failure restricts emergency "bail-out" options for such procedures. The LV support devices approved for "destination" therapy do not support the right ventricle and in fact often further overload and distort it. Durable devices to support the right ventricle are only approved as "bridges" for patients who are candidates for cardiac transplantation. Thus neither the pairing of current LV assist devices (LVADs) to provide biventricular support nor the implantation of a total artificial heart are durable options for patients not awaiting cardiac transplantation.

Initial Hemodynamic Optimization

In general, even patients transferred for therapy of recurrent or incessant arrhythmias should be as stabilized as possible before undergoing procedures. It is rare that patients cannot be stabilized briefly in the intensive care unit using intravenous vasoactive agents, antiarrhythmic therapy, generous sedation, and sometimes general anesthesia. Even after transfer with VT storm, a cooling-off period is highly desirable both to render ablation procedures safer and to review the disease trajectory with a view to "bail-out" options if adverse events occur in the periprocedural period. When there is major concern about hemodynamic stability, particularly uncertainty regarding volume status or cardiac output, a pulmonary artery catheter can often provide unexpected information about the degree of elevated filling pressures, vasoconstriction, and decreased cardiac output, as well as the relationship between right- and left-sided filling pressures.[2]

Congestion should be relieved at least to the point when the patient can recline comfortably, if not intubated. Ideally, there should be an adequate margin such that oxygenation is not compromised even if there is a brief need for intravenous fluid with anesthesia during the procedure. When organ function appears to be compromised or lactate levels are elevated, cardiac output must be supported, even if it requires the cautious use of low doses of intravenous inotropic agents. However, there is a consistent absence of benefit of cardiac resynchronization therapy when initiated as "rescue" therapy in patients who have recently required intravenous inotropic therapy.[40]

It is important to recognize that neurohormonal antagonist therapy is not only ineffective but also deleterious for rapid hemodynamic stabilization. By limiting the sympathetic stimulation support and angiotensin potentiation of cardiac output and diuresis, the addition or uptitration of neurohormonal therapy can acutely worsen the situation. Their beneficial impact is to decrease remodeling and improve long-term prognosis for patients who have already been stabilized. β-Blockers as antiarrhythmic agents are generally not effective until they can be titrated to doses higher than can be tolerated by patients with severely elevated filling pressures or compromised perfusion. Note also that rapid loading with amiodarone can also worsen hemodynamic status early after admission, although cautious use may be necessary to stabilize serious ventricular arrhythmias.

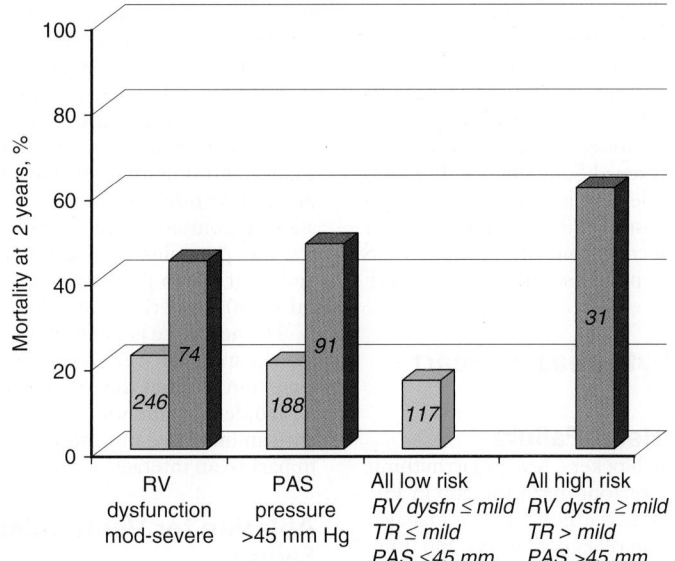

FIGURE 89.3 Bar graph showing 2-year mortality after ventricular tachycardia ablation in relation to initial echocardiographic assessment of right heart function and pulmonary artery pressures in 320 patients with a left ventricular ejection fraction <0.40.[39] Mortality is doubled for patients who have moderate or severe right ventricular (RV) dysfunction (*dysfn*) or estimated pulmonary artery systolic pressure (*PAS*) greater than 45 mm Hg. Patients who had no more than mild RV dysfunction, no more than mild tricuspid regurgitation (*TR*), and pulmonary artery systolic pressure ≤45 mm Hg had a 2-year mortality of 16% compared with 61% for patients with all three of these risk factors for poor survival. *Purple and blue bars* indicate patients with and without risk features on echocardiography, respectively.

If inotropic therapy has been initiated to treat hypoperfusion and to improve diuretic response, neurohormonal antagonists should be initiated only after successful weaning of the inotropic therapy. Initial doses should be small and escalated gradually. Careful uptitration over weeks to months is required to individualize "optimal" dosing, which frequently is lower than that in trial populations, particularly for elderly patients.[41]

If hemodynamic stability cannot be achieved with pharmacological measures, temporary hemodynamic support with an intraaortic balloon pump, percutaneous ventricular assist, or even extracorporeal membrane oxygenation may be required. Definition of options for longer-term support with transplantation or destination ventricular assist devices (VADs) should be clarified, ideally before these measures are implemented, as they may be required if the arrhythmia cannot be controlled or if control of the arrhythmia fails to improve the hemodynamic profile.

Limited Role of Cardiac Transplantation

At one time, cardiac transplantation was considered an attractive option for patients presenting with refractory ventricular arrhythmias and severe chronic HF. The outcomes of transplantation for HF are excellent for the few patients who can undergo this procedure, with median survival now 11 years, limited primarily by allograft vascular disease and malignancy.[42]

Cardiac transplantation, however, is not feasible as a rescue strategy for patients needing control of ventricular arrhythmias. The number of recipients is limited by the fixed donor supply to about 2200 adult candidates per year in the United States. The current waiting list for cardiac transplantation contains over three times as many patients as will undergo transplantation this year.[43] Each year almost 50% more patients are listed for transplantation than will actually undergo the procedure. This has led to waiting times that are often over 6 months and sometimes up to 2 years even for the most urgently ill candidates with or without VADs. Affluent patients can consider traveling to regions of the country where the donor supply is most favorable, which raises serious concern regarding equitable allocation of a national resource. This crisis will continue to worsen in the near future until

candidate-listing practices are constrained to better match the anticipated donor supply.[44] There is wide variation in decisions regarding relative contraindications such as obesity, severity of diabetes, requirements for family support, and duration of smoking cessation. Although there has been relaxation of the upper age limit, which was at one time 55 years, frailty is increasingly a focus of assessment as an integrating condition that precludes good outcome with aggressive surgical intervention.

Consideration of Implantable Circulatory Assist Devices

Mechanical circulatory support devices are being implanted as "bridges" to transplantation in almost half of patients (in some regions over 90% of patients) who eventually undergo transplantation in the United States and Germany. The majority of these devices, however, are being used in patients who are not listed for transplantation.[45] While some may become eligible for transplantation in the future, the most common intent at the time of device implantation is now the expectation of lifetime "destination" therapy. Two-year survival with the currently implanted continuous-flow devices for destination therapy is now over 70%, with a cerebrovascular event rate of about 1 in 12 and higher rates of drive-line infection and gastrointestinal bleeding.[45] Early experience has demonstrated worse outcomes when the major surgery currently required for implantation of durable assist devices is performed on an urgent basis in INTERMACS profile 1 ("crash and burn") patients.[46] Initial device "rescue" of these patients is generally attempted instead with short-term extracorporeal devices or in some cases ECMO (extracorporeal membrane oxygenation) that can be easily instituted as temporary support and subsequently removed without major surgery. In some cases this support may be initiated electively at the start of an electrophysiological or other catheter-based procedure with ongoing or anticipated hemodynamic instability.

Whenever possible, the long-term options for advanced HF should be reviewed before embarking upon procedures that could precipitate the need for urgent support.[47] Eligibility for transplantation influences other options, even though it is not itself an option for urgent "rescue" or "bail-out" procedure for patients with life-threatening circulatory collapse during arrhythmias or arrhythmia procedures. This is particularly important with the regard to the assessment and severity of RV dysfunction, as described above. The cost of the device, the hospitalizations, and the infrastructure required for perioperative and long-term support often exceed $200,000 per life-year gained.[48] Although the supply of devices is not as constrained as that of donor hearts, the high cost of this care mandates that device candidates be carefully selected from the estimated US population of more than 150,000 patients with advanced HF who might benefit.[49]

Treatment of Tachyarrhythmias in Heart Failure

Antiarrhythmic Drugs in Heart Failure

With the exception of β-adrenergic blockers, few antiarrhythmic drugs have been shown to be safe for long-term therapy in HF. However, β-blockers alone have limited efficacy in the management of arrhythmias based on scar-related reentry, and their negative inotropic effects may not be tolerated for management in unstable patients. Suppression of VT or VF often requires specific antiarrhythmic agents. Sodium channel blockade (a class I antiarrhythmic drug effect) has a negative inotropic effect and tends to worsen HF. Hence, drugs such as flecainide, propafenone, procainamide, disopyramide, and mexiletine are best avoided. Quinidine may be an exception because its prolongation of the action potential, which allows for longer calcium flux and vasodilatory effects, may offset the negative inotropic effects of sodium channel blockade. Apart from their effects on contractility, class I drugs can also exert significant proarrhythmic effects by virtue of conduction slowing. Hence, use of these drugs is limited to patients with implanted defibrillators to control ventricular or atrial arrhythmias when class III drugs are not an option.

Amiodarone. Amiodarone has been most extensively studied in patients with HF. Apart from one study that showed increased noncardiac mortality in class III HF, most studies have described neutral effects on mortality or benefit in reducing arrhythmia-related deaths.[50,51] Amiodarone in combination with a β-blocker is the most effective pharmacological intervention for reducing ICD shocks.[50] Bradycardia remains a limitation. In patients with sinus node or AV nodal disease, this drug has the potential for marked bradycardia and worsening HF symptoms. In addition, amiodarone may lead to ventricular pacing in patients with implanted defibrillators, thereby provoking ventricular dyssynchrony.

In stable patients, loading doses of amiodarone 600 to 800 mg daily are usually well tolerated. However, in patients with decompensated HF, high doses can potentially worsen clinical status by slowing heart rate without allowing for increased stroke volume. Slow titration can often avoid this initial negative inotropic effect. The noncardiac toxicities of amiodarone can adversely impact the course of HF. Hyperthyroidism can lead to acute hemodynamic instability, often with onset of atrial fibrillation with rapid ventricular rates and intractable ventricular arrhythmias. In one study, amiodarone-induced thyrotoxicosis was associated with a 2.7-fold increase in major adverse cardiac events, driven primarily by higher rates of ventricular arrhythmia requiring hospitalization.[52,53] Amiodarone lung toxicity occurs at a rate of 1% per year, and risk increases with daily doses that exceed 300 mg. Differentiation from pulmonary congestion may require right-heart catheterization and/or bronchoalveolar lavage.

Other Class III Drugs. Sotalol has modest efficacy in reducing ICD shocks and is a reasonable initial choice in younger patients to avoid the cumulative organ toxic effects of amiodarone.[52] It is a nonselective β-blocker with approximately one-fifth the potency of propranolol. Its use as a substitute for β-blockers in HF is controversial. Dofetilide is a class III antiarrhythmic agent approved for the management of AF that does not increase mortality in HF when precautions to minimize the risk of torsades de pointes are taken.[52] It has been used to reduce ventricular arrhythmias in patients with ICDs but experience is limited. Both sotalol and dofetilide prolong the QT interval by blocking the delayed rectifier potassium (Ikr) channel and can provoke torsades de pointes VT. This risk is increased in HF patients (3%–5%), as previously discussed. These drugs are excreted renally, and their use in patients with reduced glomerular filtration (<30 mL/min) is not recommended.

Dronedarone is a newer antiarrhythmic drug approved for the management of AF. Despite its structural similarity to amiodarone (but without the iodine moiety), it is less effective. It should be avoided in patients with HF because its use has been associated with an increased mortality in this population that may be related in part to an interaction with digoxin.[54]

Ablation for Ventricular Arrhythmias in Heart Failure

Catheter ablation is an important therapy for controlling incessant VT or very frequent ventricular ectopy that is causing or aggravating HF (see Chapters 127 and 80) and for reducing VT episodes requiring termination by an ICD, particularly ICD shocks.[55] Catheter ablation for VT generally requires significant expertise, and epicardial ablations carry higher risks.[56] Nevertheless, catheter ablation can be life-saving in patients with incessant VT and in those presenting with electrical storm.[57] In experienced centers, catheter ablation is now an early consideration in the course of management of recurrent monomorphic VT to avoid exposing patients to toxic drugs and multiple ICD shocks with associated posttraumatic stress disorder.[58] Catheter ablation reduces VT episodes in over 70% of patients with recurrent sustained monomorphic VT and depressed ventricular function.[59] Most of these patients have scar-related VT. The location of the scar is related to the underlying disease, and hence the approach and efficacy varies with the type of disease. Ablation is more effective for patients with prior myocardial infarction than for patients with nonischemic CM, who often require percutaneous epicardial mapping and ablation due to the subepicardial scar location. Procedure-related mortality for VT ablation is 1% to 3%, but most deaths are due to continued VT when ablation attempts have failed to control VT. Minor complications, most commonly related to vascular access, occur in 3% to 12% of patients. Risks are greater for epicardial ablation procedures.

In patients with advanced HF, prolonged procedure times, fluid load, and arrhythmias associated with ablation for VT can precipitate acute decompensation. In one series, decompensation occurred in 11% of patients and was associated with advanced age, ischemic CM, more severe HF, chronic lung disease, diabetes mellitus, and VT storm.[60]

Circulatory support can allow mapping during VT without hemodynamic deterioration.[61] In most patients, however, the arrhythmia substrate can be identified and targeted during stable sinus or paced rhythm, reducing the risk imposed by frequent induction of VT (see Chapter 127). Strategies for management of hemodynamic deterioration and uncommon but known complications such as ventricular perforation and damage to coronary arteries should be anticipated. Temporary support device use should be tempered by considerations of overall prognosis in end-stage HF. In patients with HF and severe hemodynamic compromise, expedited review of potential eligibility for transplantation or long-term mechanical circulatory support before the procedure is performed may simplify difficult decisions if the ablation procedure fails to control recurrent or incessant VT or precipitates hemodynamic deterioration.

Ventricular Arrhythmias in Patients With Ventricular Assist Devices

The use of VADs as a bridge to transplantation and as destination "lifetime" therapy has become more common and successful. As a result, ventricular arrhythmias have gained greater importance in this patient population (see Chapter 111). The overall prevalence of ventricular arrhythmia in LVAD patients is similar to that in a population with comparable LV dysfunction and HF, but after LVAD, ventricular arrhythmias can resolve, persist, or appear for the first time.[62–65] Patients with a prior history of ventricular arrhythmia and atrial fibrillation are at the greatest risk. Ventricular arrhythmias do not appear to contribute to worse outcomes in patients with LVADs. Most patients who are candidates for LVADs will have an ICD already in place. Immediately after LVAD placement, the ICD settings should be reviewed and adjusted to minimize shocks for rhythms that are unlikely to be lethal during LVAD support. Even hours of tolerated VT is preferable to ICD shocks for most patients. When ventricular arrhythmias appear for the first time or have a markedly different pattern after LVAD placement, the possible cause may be mechanical stimulation from cannula suction events that can relate to intravascular volume depletion or high LVAD flow rates. There is a characteristic pattern in some patients of very frequent nonsustained VT of varying morphology, which can resemble torsades de pointes. Lowering the LVAD speed can often be helpful in reducing nonsustained VT that precipitates sustained arrhythmias.

As most device configurations only support the left ventricle (LVAD), the RV output is vulnerable to ventricular arrhythmias, which thus can compromise LV inflow. Although rarely lethal, ventricular arrhythmias can cause syncope and injury in patients, particularly in the upright position. Management of ventricular arrhythmias in LVAD patients includes the use of antiarrhythmic drugs, such as amiodarone, mexiletine, and quinidine. Catheter ablation can be accomplished safely and is useful in refractory cases but is technically more difficult because of the collapsed ventricle (see Chapter 111).

Occasionally, patients with a precipitous course after an acute event such as myocarditis or acute myocardial infarction or in relation to peripartum CM progress to LVAD therapy without an ICD. In the absence of observed ventricular arrhythmias, implantation of an ICD as a prophylaxis against adverse effects of VT/VF is not routine and practices vary among centers.[65]

Tracking the Heart Failure Journey

Enhanced Survival With Current Therapies

The journey for patients with HF and reduced EF has been dramatically extended since the mid-1980s. From a disease that was rapidly fatal, unless transplantation could be performed, it has evolved to a chronic condition requiring long-term team management (Fig. 89.4). Many patients have a good quality of life with apparently stable disease for many years.[66] A population of patients with "HF better EF" has emerged, in whom LVEFs below 25% have improved to over 40%, often within months after initiation of β-blocker therapy, or earlier with responders to CRT.[67,68] In large populations with symptomatic HF (stage C), improved survival has been documented in symptomatic HF from outpatient populations,[69–71] in patients discharged from hospitalization,[72,73] and for patients after referral for advanced therapies.[66,74]

The threat of sudden death has diminished markedly, associated most directly with increasing penetrance of early β-blocker therapy. This was shown in a large registry from a United Kingdom population of patients with mild-moderate ambulatory HF,

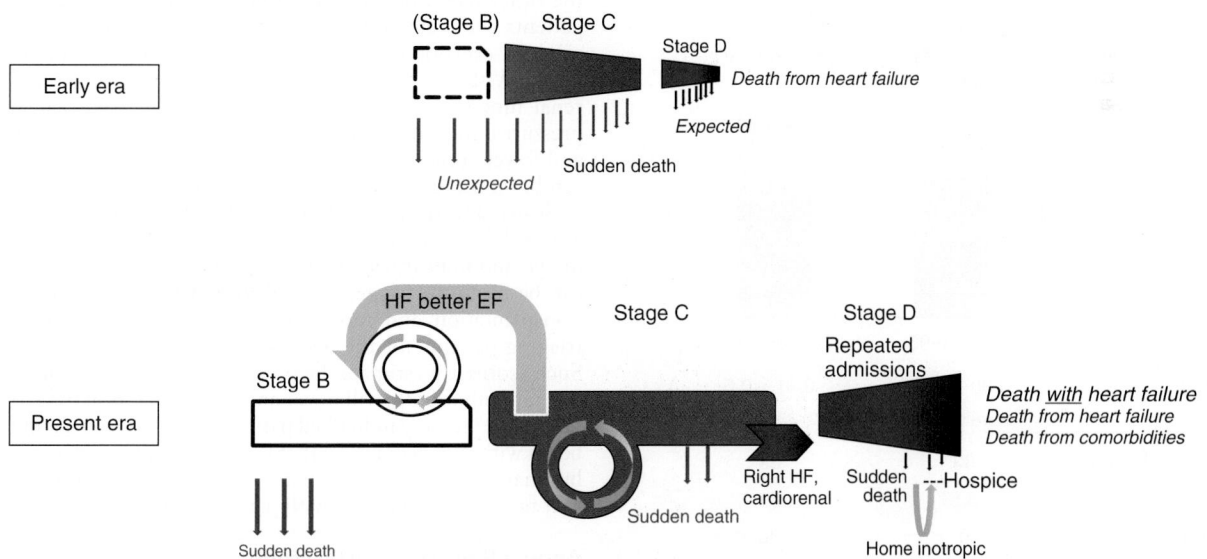

FIGURE 89.4 Diagram contrasting the duration of disease stages for heart failure with low ejection fraction, between the previous era from the early days of heart transplantation and the contemporary era with high prevalence of β-blocker use and inhibition of the renin-angiotensin system. There was limited recognition at that time of asymptomatic left ventricular dysfunction, subsequently defined in 2001 as stage B. With modern therapies to prevent or delay disease progression, many patients in stage B and stage C appear to remain stable for many years. There is increasing recognition that many patients with previously stage C symptomatic heart failure can return to a stage B, defined as "HF (heart failure) better EF (ejection fraction)" for patients who have enjoyed substantial improvement in both EF and functional capacity. In the previous era, sudden death often occurred early in the clinical disease of HF with reduced EF, incurred with increasing frequency as heart failure progressed, and usually intervention occurred before symptoms of class IV HF became persistent. Dramatic reduction of sudden death by current intervention has averted the premature deaths during good quality of life, but also leads to more survivors reaching advanced symptomatic limitations. In the current era, right HF and the cardiorenal syndrome frequently herald progression to stage D heart failure, with increasing referral to hospice.

in whom sudden death decreased by 75% from before 2000 to after 2005 even in patients without ICDs (Fig. 89.5).[71] The large proportional decrease in sudden death in this population was accompanied, but not canceled out, by an increase in noncardiovascular death. The increasing penetrance of ICDs results in further decrease of the sudden-death rate in the target population of patients with mild-moderate HF, thus further prolonging the extension of good quality of life with HF.

The impact of ICD on the decrease of sudden death has also resulted in an increased rate of survival into advanced HF. This flux is harder to document, but familiar to those who have seen the field evolve since 1983, when the availability of cyclosporin led to a burgeoning of heart transplant centers to which many patients with HF were attracted and then diverted onto a trajectory of medical therapy. At that time, for those who did not experience clinical improvement on medical therapy, the misery of refractory class IV was mercifully short before patients died peacefully in their sleep, and there was rarely time for consideration of hospice.

Increasing Prevalence of End-Stage Heart Failure

Stage D HF is now a major cause of repeated hospital admissions.[75] For a majority of this population, cardiac transplantation and LVADs are not appropriate, due to comorbidities and general frailty. As we have prolonged life with HF, we have also prolonged death[76] (see Fig. 89.4). An interesting development is the increased use of chronic inotropic therapy. Abandoned at the end of the last century due to the evidence of increased mortality, the survival with continuous intravenous inotropic therapy with

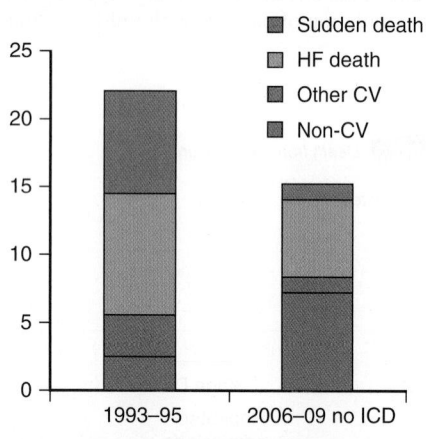

	1993–95	2006–09 no ICD
LVEF	0.30 ± 0.5	0.31 ± 0.5
Age	62 ± 1	66 ± 1
% on ACEI/ARB	83	89
% on β-blocker	8.5	80
% on aldo. antag.	0	36

FIGURE 89.5 Decrease in sudden death and mortality at 2 years for patients in the United Kingdom Heart Studies, comparing 281 patients registered in 1993–1995 to 300 patients registered in 2006–2009. (This analysis excludes 57 patients with implantable cardioverter-defibrillators [*ICD*], which represented 16% of patients in the newer cohort.) The major change in therapy is the increasing use of β-blocker therapy, with a smaller increase in the use of aldosterone antagonists (*aldo. antag.*). Total mortality declined by 31%, although there was an increase in noncardiovascular death. *ACEI,* Angiotensin-converting enzyme inhibitor; *ARB,* angiotensin receptor blocker; *CV,* cardiovascular; *HF,* heart failure; *LVEF,* left ventricular ejection fraction. (From Cubbon RM, Gale CP, Kearney LC, et al. Changing characteristics and mode of death associated with chronic heart failure due to left ventricular systolic dysfunction: a study across therapeutic eras. *Circ Heart Fail.* 2011;4:396-403.)

low doses of milrinone and dobutamine is now frequently seen at a year or longer.[77,78] This better outcome has been attributed to the frequent presence of ICDs, as well as to much lower doses of inotropic agents, and may lead to a resurgence of interest in the oral forms that do not require chronic indwelling lines.[78]

In contrast to the early days of HF experience, most deaths due to HF are now heralded by evidence of inexorable disease progression and often by refractory symptoms. Even the deaths that are termed sudden are rarely unexpected, at least by the medical team providing ongoing care, unless they are due to some event other than HF.

Patients surviving longer with HF also survive to develop more comorbidities, such as cancer and dementia. As the proportion of sudden deaths diminishes, there is an increase not only in deaths termed as hemodynamic or "HF" deaths but also in deaths attributed to noncardiac comorbidities in patients who have HF. Of 14,000 patients identified at the time of their first HF hospitalization in a Canadian province, over half of deaths were attributed to noncardiac causes, two-thirds of cardiac deaths occurred in-hospital, and only 7.6% of the overall mortality in this HF patient population was attributed to cardiac deaths occurring out-of-hospital in patients living independently at home.[79]

Shared Decision-Making

Risk Scores and Uncertainty

Clinical status and recent course remain the most robust predictors of outcomes, although extensive efforts have been devoted to more objective stratification of risk for patients with HF.[80] Early in the disease, when few symptoms are noted, the reduction in LVEF is a significant risk factor, but annual mortality is generally <10% for patients with stable New York Heart Association (NYHA) class I or II symptoms, even if the LVEF is <25%. On the other hand, death at any time would not be unexpected in patients with refractory symptoms of congestion at rest or with minimal exertion (stage D), and most patients will die within 2 years. Within a given clinical status, risk factors include worse renal function, lower blood pressure, higher ventricular filling pressures, and worse RV function. High natriuretic peptide levels and lower serum sodium predict worse outcome, although they can be separately influenced by some therapies. Risk scores such as Seattle Heart Failure, ESCAPE Discharge, and Heart Failure Survival Scores reflect trial populations in whom the contribution of age and noncardiac factors are not well represented, but they can be useful to trigger referral for advanced therapies, such as transplantation, and, more importantly, may be one approach to triaging patients for the discussion about disease trajectory.[80–82] Such scores can estimate the proportion of a population that may die, but importantly will never answer the question of "How long do I have?" for any individual patient. All discussion should in fact begin with the recognition that this question cannot be answered, but that discussion must nonetheless take place in order to ensure that future care will align with patient goals and preferences.[47]

Annual Review and Milestones

An annual review of current status and recent trajectory has been recommended for all patients with advanced HF,[47] generally patients having persistent symptoms that limit daily life (classes III and IV) despite standard medical therapy and patients who often have had at least two HF hospitalizations in the past year. To diminish apprehension in the patient, such a review could be scheduled routinely, perhaps at the time of the annual influenza vaccine visit. It would include medical summary of the current therapies and possible new therapies that could be appropriate, including whether or not cardiac transplantation or LVADs might be an option in the future. This review would provide the opportunity for the patient and family to consider the major goals and preferences that would guide decisions that might arise in the future, particularly for events that would involve the health care proxy. Such a review could then be updated after an increase in ICD activity or another milestone as in Box 89.1. Ideally, the discussion should be initiated before the end of life is anticipated within the year. However, there is increasing agreement that the discussion becomes urgent as soon as the clinician would answer "yes" to the question "Would you be surprised if your patient died within the next 6 months?"

Procedures and the Implantable Cardioverter-Defibrillator in Advanced Heart Failure

Requests are frequently made regarding management of the ICD during noncardiac procedures. As part of the care team of a patient with advanced HF, it is always appropriate to query the indications and benefit:risk considerations for any invasive procedure. This is particularly relevant for procedures that are being performed primarily to reduce a future risk, such as a screening colonoscopy or resection of an asymptomatic pulmonary nodule.[47] On the other hand, most patients who do not have resting symptoms or evidence of hemodynamic decompensation can safely undergo procedures necessary to preserve or improve quality of life, such as indicated for orthopedic injury, as long as fluid status, blood pressure, and renal function are closely maintained.

A majority of patients who reach advanced stages of HF in the United States already have an ICD in place. In the rare consideration of a patient who does not, it is important to review the competing risks of sudden cardiac death and other death[26] before considering implantation. The major benefit of ICD for primary prevention is in those patients who are neither too well nor too sick, as demonstrated from the MADIT analyses.[83] The ICD is not indicated in patients who have class IV symptoms of HF or who for other reasons do not have an expected survival of over a year with good quality of life.[84,85] Within the Medicare population, the benefit of ICDs is not evident for patients undergoing implantation during an HF hospitalization, whereas those undergoing elective implantation without multiple prior HF hospitalizations appear to derive substantial benefit similar to that observed during the pivotal primary prevention trials.[86,87]

ICD generator replacement currently accounts for over 25% of all ICD procedures and is more common than initial implantation in the elderly population. As this procedure may be associated with up to 5% complication rates, the routine replacement has been questioned, particularly for patients with progressive HF.[88] For patients with advanced HF, imminent end of life for the battery should trigger a review of remaining life expectancy for the patient, with particular focus on if and when deactivation of defibrillation would be considered.

The inactivation of ICDs at the end of life with HF remains a challenge. A recent study of 150 patients with ICD inactivation revealed that most occurred within 2 days of death, and over half of the decisions were made by surrogates because the issue had never been discussed with the patient.[89] Surveys of physicians reveal that the majority describe discomfort around ICD deactivation, although almost all describe comfort around withdrawal of life-sustaining care in an intensive care unit. The ethical basis and importance of patient autonomy for decisions about device deactivation have been well established in the Heart Rhythm Society (HRS) consensus statement,[90] which deserves more attention as part of continuing education programs.

Patients and families often have an unrealistic perception of the actual function and benefit of the ICD and will rarely broach this subject. Many do not know that ICDs can be deactivated without an invasive procedure. This discussion seems to be easier for patients who received initial ICD teaching that included the possibility, feasibility, and rationale of deactivation[85] with specific wording that "the time may come when..." It is then possible to reintroduce the subject later: "Remember when we talked about how the time might come...this could be that time." Although it is strongly recommended, deactivation of the ICD is not mandatory for a peaceful death with dignity. Only a small number of deaths from terminal HF in ICD recipients are accompanied by painful shocks. The patients most likely to suffer repeated shocks while dying are those who have previously experienced repeated shocks. The most common terminal rhythm is progressive bradycardia with pulseless electrical activity that does not trigger defibrillation.

Summary

The combination of ventricular arrhythmias and HF carries special implications for etiology, treatment, and prognosis of each. Thoughtful assessment of hemodynamic compensation, RV function, and the clinical trajectory is crucial for effective management of ventricular arrhythmias at all stages of HF. Cardiac transplantation and durable mechanical circulatory support devices influence triage for a small but important minority of patients with HF. Shared decision-making in advanced HF should encompass ICD implantation, generator replacement, and deactivation after review of the prognosis of HF and comorbidities, with elicitation of the patient goals and preferences (Box 89.2).

BOX 89.1   Milestones for recognition of limited survival with heart failure

- Repeated (≥2) hospitalizations or emergency room visits for heart failure in the last year
- Persistent symptoms at rest or with minimal activities of daily living
- Frequent systolic blood pressure <90 mm Hg
- Progressive deterioration in renal function (rise in creatinine and/or blood urea nitrogen)
- Progressive decline in serum sodium, usually to <133 mEq/L
- Intolerance to angiotensin-converting enzyme inhibitors or β-blockers caused by hypotension and/or worsening renal function
- Intolerance to β-blockers as a result of worsening heart failure symptoms or hypotension
- Recent need to escalate diuretics to maintain volume status, often reaching a daily furosemide equivalent dose of over 160 mg a day and/or use of supplemental metolazone therapy
- Development of malnutrition and cardiac cachexia

BOX 89.2   Ventricular arrhythmias in heart failure: key points

- Simultaneous new diagnosis of heart failure and ventricular tachyarrhythmias should raise concern for inflammatory heart disease.
- Multiple genes can cause cardiomyopathy with ventricular arrhythmias and affect family members with either or both.
- Hemodynamic status should be assessed carefully and stabilized before arrhythmia procedures are undertaken.
- Treatment with neurohormonal antagonists and amiodarone can worsen decompensated heart failure acutely despite long-term benefit in stable patients.
- Right ventricular dysfunction heralds worse outcome with heart failure and shorter survival after ventricular tachycardia ablation.
- Severe right ventricular dysfunction is a contraindication to durable mechanical circulatory support except in patients who are candidates for cardiac transplantation.
- Cardiac transplantation cannot be performed urgently, but eligibility should be considered to define intermediate options in the event of rapid deterioration.
- Consider competing risks of death from pump failure or comorbidities when planning interventions to treat or prevent life-threatening arrhythmic events.
- Shared decision-making in advanced heart failure should encompass implantable cardioverter-defibrillator implantation, generator replacement, and deactivation after consideration of prognosis with heart failure and comorbidities as well as patient goals and preferences

REFERENCES

1. Stevenson L. Management of acute decompensated heart failure. In: Mann DL, Felker GM, eds. *Heart Failure: A Companion to Braunwald's Heart Disease*. 3rd ed. Philadelphia: Saunders; 2015.
2. Yancy CW, Jessup M, Bozkurt B, et al. 2013 ACCF/AHA Guideline For The Management of Heart Failure: Executive Summary: A Report of the American College of Cardiology Foundation/American Heart Association Task Force on Practice Guidelines. *Circulation*. 2013;128:810–852.
3. Sekhri V, Sanal S, Delorenzo LJ, Aronow WS, Maguire GP. Cardiac sarcoidosis: a comprehensive review. *Arch Med Sci*. 2011;7:546–554.
4. Kandolin R, Lehtonen J, Kupari M. Cardiac sarcoidosis and giant cell myocarditis as causes of atrioventricular block in young and middle-aged adults. *Circ Arrhythm Electrophysiol*. 2011;4:303–309.
5. Blankstein R, Osborne M, Naya M, et al. Cardiac positron emission tomography enhances prognostic assessments of patients with suspected cardiac sarcoidosis. *J Am Coll Cardiol*. 2014;63:329–336.
6. Casella M, Pizzamiglio F, Dello Russo A, et al. Feasibility of combined unipolar and bipolar voltage maps to improve sensitivity of endomyocardial biopsy. *Circ Arrhythm Electrophysiol*. 2015;8:625–632.
7. Birnie DH, Sauer WH, Bogun F, et al. HRS expert consensus statement on the diagnosis and management of arrhythmias associated with cardiac sarcoidosis. *Heart Rhythm*. 2014;11:1305–1323.
8. Cooper Jr LT, Hare JM, Tazelaar HD, et al. Usefulness of immunosuppression for giant cell myocarditis. *Am J Cardiol*. 2008;102:1535–1539.
9. Kindermann I, Barth C, Mahfoud F, et al. Update on myocarditis. *J Am Coll Cardiol*. 2012;59:779–792.
10. Semigran M, Thaik CM, Fifer MA, Boucher CA, Palacios IF, Dec GW. Exercise capacity and systolic and diastolic ventricular function after recovery from acute dilated cardiomyopathy. *J Am Coll Cardiol*. 1994;24:462–470.
11. McCarthy 3rd RE, Boehmer JP, Hruban RH, et al. Long-term outcome of fulminant myocarditis as compared with acute (nonfulminant) myocarditis. *N Engl J Med*. 2000;342:690–695.
12. Mahon NG, Murphy RT, MacRae CA, Caforio AL, Elliott PM, McKenna WJ. Echocardiographic evaluation in asymptomatic relatives of patients with dilated cardiomyopathy reveals preclinical disease. *Ann Intern Med*. 2005;143:108–115.
13. Watkins H, Ashrafian H, Redwood C. Inherited cardiomyopathies. *N Engl J Med*. 2011;364:1643–1656.
14. Hershberger RE, Hedges DJ, Morales A. Dilated cardiomyopathy: the complexity of a diverse genetic architecture. *Nat Rev Cardiol*. 2013;10:531–547.
15. Ackerman MJ, Priori SG, Willems S, et al. HRS/EHRA expert consensus statement on the state of genetic testing for the channelopathies and cardiomyopathies. *Europace*. 2011;13:1077–1087.
16. Hershberger RE, Lindenfeld J, Mestroni L, et al. Genetic evaluation of cardiomyopathy—Heart Failure Society of America practice guideline. *J Card Fail*. 2009;15:2009–2020.
17. Herman DS, Lam L, Taylor MR, et al. Truncations of titin causing dilated cardiomyopathy. *N Engl J Med*. 2012;366:619–628.
18. van Rijsingen IA, Arbustini E, Elliott PM, et al. Risk factors for malignant ventricular arrhythmias in lamin a/c mutation carriers: a European cohort study. *J Am Coll Cardiol*. 2012;59:493–500.
19. Epstein AE, DiMarco JP, Ellenbogen KA, et al. ACC/AHA/HRS 2008 Guidelines for Device-Based Therapy of Cardiac Rhythm Abnormalities: a report of the American College of Cardiology/American Heart Association Task Force on Practice Guidelines (Writing Committee to Revise the ACC/AHA/NASPE 2002 Guideline Update for Implantation of Cardiac Pacemakers and Antiarrhythmia Devices): developed in collaboration with the American Association for Thoracic Surgery and Society of Thoracic Surgeons. *Circulation*. 2008;117:e350–e408.
20. Bhonsale A, Groeneweg JA, James CA, et al. Impact of genotype on clinical course in arrhythmogenic right ventricular dysplasia/cardiomyopathy-associated mutation carriers. *Eur Heart J*. 2015;36:847–855.
21. Groeneweg JA, Bhonsale A, James CA, et al. Clinical presentation, long-term follow-up, and outcomes of 1001 arrhythmogenic right ventricular dysplasia/cardiomyopathy patients and family members. *Circ Cardiovasc Genet*. 2015;8:437–446.
22. Sayed RH, Rogers D, Khan F, et al. A study of implanted cardiac rhythm recorders in advanced cardiac AL amyloidosis. *Eur Heart J*. 2015;36:1098–1105.
23. Steimle AE, Stevenson LW, Fonarow GC, Hamilton MA, Moriguchi JD. Prediction of improvement in recent onset cardiomyopathy after referral for heart transplantation. *J Am Coll Cardiol*. 1994;23:553–559.
24. Yokokawa M, Good E, Crawford T, et al. Recovery from left ventricular dysfunction after ablation of frequent premature ventricular complexes. *Heart Rhythm*. 2013;10:172–175.
25. Yokokawa M, Kim HM, Good E, et al. Impact of QRS duration of frequent premature ventricular complexes on the development of cardiomyopathy. *Heart Rhythm*. 2012;9:1460–1464.
26. Epstein AE, Dimarco JP, Ellenbogen KA, et al. ACC/AHA/HRS 2008 guidelines for device-based therapy of cardiac rhythm abnormalities. *Heart Rhythm*. 2008;5:e1–e62.
27. Poole JE, Johnson GW, Hellkamp AS, et al. Prognostic importance of defibrillator shocks in patients with heart failure. *N Engl J Med*. 2008;359:1009–1017.
28. Daubert JP, Zareba W, Cannom DS, et al. Inappropriate implantable cardioverter-defibrillator shocks in MADIT II: frequency, mechanisms, predictors, and survival impact. *J Am Coll Cardiol*. 2008;51:1357–1365.
29. St John Sutton M, Lee D, Rouleau JL, et al. Left ventricular remodeling and ventricular arrhythmias after myocardial infarction. *Circulation*. 2003;107:2577–2582.
30. Kuch KH, Schaumann A, Eckhardt L, et al. Catheter ablation of stable ventricular tachycardia before defibrillator implantation in patients with coronary heart disease (VTACH): a multicentre randomised controlled trial. *Lancet*. 2010;375:31–40.
31. Sweeney MO, Ruetz LL, Belk P, et al. Bradycardia pacing-induced short-long-short sequences at the onset of ventriculat tachyarrhythmias: a possible mechanism of proarrhythmia? *J Am Coll Cardiol*. 2007;50:614–622.
32. Turitto G, El-Sherif N. Cardiac resynchronization therapy: a review of proarrhythmic and antiarrhythmic mechanisms. *Pacing Clin Electrophysiol*. 2007;30:115–122.
33. Lee JC, Epstein LM, Huffer LL, et al. ICD lead proarrhythmia cured by lead extraction. *Heart Rhythm*. 2009;6:613–618.
34. Nohria A, Tsang SW, Fang JC, et al. Clinical assessment identifies hemodynamic profiles that predict outcomes in patients admitted with heart failure. *J Am Coll Cardiol*. 2003;41:1797–1804.
35. Stevenson LW, Perloff JK. The limited reliability of physical signs for estimating hemodynamics in chronic heart failure. *JAMA*. 1989;261:884–888.
36. Mullens W, Abrahams Z, Francis GS, et al. Importance of venous congestion for worsening of renal function in advanced decompensated heart failure. *J Am Coll Cardiol*. 2009;53:589–596.
37. Forman DE, Butler J, Wang Y, et al. Incidence, predictors at admission, and impact of worsening renal function among patients hospitalized with heart failure. *J Am Coll Cardiol*. 2004;43:61–67.
38. Tedrow UB, Kramer DB, Stevenson LW, et al. Relation of right ventricular peak systolic pressure to major adverse events in patients undergoing cardiac resynchronization therapy. *Am J Cardiol*. 2006;97:1737–1740.
39. Ujeyl A, Inada K, Hillmann K, et al. Right heart function prediction of outcome in heart failure patients after catheter ablation for recurrent ventricular tachycardia. *JACC Heart Fail*. 2013;1:281–289.
40. Bhattacharya S, Abebe K, Simon M, Saba S, Adelstein E. Role of cardiac resynchronization in end-stage heart failure patients requiring inotrope therapy. *J Card Fail*. 2010;16:931–937.
41. Nohria A, Lewis E, Stevenson LW. Medical management of advanced heart failure. *JAMA*. 2002;287:628–640.
42. Lund LH, Edwards LB, Kucheryavaya AY, et al. The registry of the International Society for Heart and Lung Transplantation: thirty-first official adult heart transplant report—2014; focus theme: retransplantation. *J Heart Lung Transplant*. 2014;33:996–1008.
43. Stevenson LW. Crisis awaiting heart transplantation: Sinking the lifeboat. *JAMA Intern Med*. 2015;175:1406–1409.
44. Stevenson LW. The urgent priority for transplantation is to trim the waiting list. *J Heart Lung Transplant*. 2013;32:861–867.
45. Kirklin JK, Naftel DC, Pagani FD, et al. Seventh INTERMACS annual report: 15,000 patients and counting. *J Heart Lung Transplant*. 2015;34:1495–1504.
46. Stevenson LW, Pagani FD, Young JB, et al. INTERMACS profiles of advanced heart failure: the current picture. *J Heart Lung Transplant*. 2009;28:535–541.
47. Allen LA, Stevenson LW, Grady KL, et al. Decision making in advanced heart failure: a scientific statement from the American Heart Association. *Circulation*. 2012;125:1928–1952.
48. Rogers JG, Bostic RR, Tong KB, Adamson R, Russo M, Slaughter MS. Cost-effectiveness analysis of continuous-flow left ventricular assist devices as destination therapy. *Circ Heart Fail*. 2012;5:10–16.
49. Stewart GC, Stevenson LW. Keeping left ventricular assist device acceleration on track. *Circulation*. 2011;123:1559–1568. discussion 1568.
50. Packer DL, Prutkin JM, Hellkamp AS, et al. Impact of implantable cardioverter-defibrillator, amiodarone, and placebo on the mode of death in stable patients with heart failure: analysis from the sudden cardiac death in heart failure trial. *Circulation*. 2009;120:2170–2176.
51. Connolly SJ, Dorian P, Roberts RS, et al. Comparison of beta blockers, amiodarone plus beta blockers or sotalol for prevention of shocks from implantable cardioverter defibrillators. The OPTIC study: a randomized trial. *JAMA*. 2006;295:165–171.
52. Schleifer JW, Sorajja D, Shen WK. Advances in the pharmacologic treatment of ventricular arrhythmias. *Expert Opin Pharmacother*. 2015;16:2637–2651.
53. Yiu KH, Jim MH, Siu CW, et al. Amiodarone induced thyrotoxicosis is a predictor of adverse cardiovascular outcome. *J Clin Endocrinol Metab*. 2009;94:109–114.
54. Hohnloser SH, Kuck KH, Dorian P, et al. Prophylactic use of an implantable cardioverter-defibrillator after acute myocardial infarction. *N Engl J Med*. 2004;351:2481–2488.
55. Chik WW, Marchlinski FE. Ablation of ventricular arrhythmia in patients with heart failure. *Heart Fail Clin*. 2015;11:319–336.
56. Bohnen M, Stevenson WG, Tedrow UB, et al. Incidence and predictors of major complications from contemporary catheter ablation to treat cardiac arrhythmias. *Heart Rhythm*. 2011;8:1661–1666.
57. Carbucicchio C, Santamaria M, Trevisi N, et al. Catheter ablation for the treatment of electrical storm in patients with implantable cardioverter-defibrillators: short and long term outcomes in a prospective single center study. *Circulation*. 2008;117:462–469.
58. Aliot EM, Stevenson WG, Almendral-Garrote JM, et al. EHRA expert consensus on catheter ablation for ventricular arrhythmias. *Heart Rhythm*. 2009;6:886–893.
59. Tung RVM, Frankel DS, Vergara P, et al. Freedom from recurrent ventricular tachycardia after catheter ablation is associated with improved survival in patients with structural heart disease: an International VT Ablation Center Collaborative Group study. *Heart Rhythm*. 2015;12:1997–2007.
60. Santangeli P, Muser D, Zado ES, et al. Acute hemodynamic decompensation during catheter ablation of scar-related ventricular tachycardia: incidence, predictors, and impact on mortality. *Circ Arrhythm Electrophysiol*. 2015;8:68–75.
61. Reddy YM, Chinitz L, Mansour M, et al. Percutaneous left ventricular assist devices in ventricular tachycardia ablation: multicenter experience. *Circ Arrhythm Electrophysiol*. 2014;7:244–250.
62. Yoruk A, Sherazi S, Massey HT, et al. Predictors and clinical relevance of ventricular tachyarrhythmias in ambulatory continuous flow left ventricular assist device patients. *Heart Rhythm*. 2016;13:1052–1056.
63. Garan AR, Levin AP, Topkara V, et al. Early post-operative ventricular arrhythmias in patients with continuous-flow left ventricular assist devices. *J Heart Lung Transplant*. 2015;34:1611–1616.
64. Sacher F, Reichlin T, Zado ES, et al. Characteristics of ventricular tachycardia ablation in patients with continuous flow left ventricular assist devices. *Circ Arrhythm Electrophysiol*. 2015;8:592–597.
65. Enriquez AD, Calenda B, Miller MA, Anyanwu AC, Pinney SP. The role of implantable cardioverter-defibrillators in patients with continuous flow left ventricular assist devices. *Circ Arrhythm Electrophysiol*. 2013;6:668–674.
66. Stevenson LW, Pande R. Witness to progress. *Circ Heart Fail*. 2011;4:390–392.
67. Punnoose LR, Givertz M, Lewis EF, Pratibhu P, Stevenson LW, Desai AS. Heart failure with recovered ejection fraction: a distinct clinical entity. *J Card Fail*. 2011;17:527–532.
68. Stevenson LW. Heart failure with better ejection fraction: a modern diagnosis. *Circulation*. 2014;129:2364–2367.
69. Levy D, Kenchaiah S, Larson MG, et al. Long-term trends in the incidence of and survival with heart failure. *N Engl J Med*. 2002;347:1397–1402.
70. Owan TE, Hodge DO, Herges RM, Jacobsen SJ, Roger VL, Redfield MM. Trends in prevalence and outcome of heart failure with preserved ejection fraction. *N Engl J Med*. 2006;355:251–259.
71. Cubbon RM, Gale CP, Kearney LC, et al. Changing characteristics and mode of death associated with chronic heart failure due to left ventricular systolic dysfunction: a study across therapeutic eras. *Circ Heart Fail*. 2011;4:396–403.
72. MacIntyre K, Capewell S, Stewart S, et al. Evidence of improving prognosis in heart failure: trends in case fatality in 66,547 patients hospitalized between 1986 and 1995. *Circulation*. 2000;102:1126–1131.
73. Shafazand M, Schaufelberger M, Lappas G, Swedberg K, Rosengren A. Survival trends in men and women with heart failure of ischaemic and non-ischaemic origin: data for the period 1987-2003 from the Swedish Hospital Discharge Registry. *Eur Heart J*. 2009;30:671–678.
74. Loh JC, Creaser J, Rourke DA, et al. Temporal trends in treatment and outcomes for advanced heart failure with reduced ejection fraction from 1993-2010: findings from a university referral center. *Circ Heart Fail*. 2013;6:411–419.
75. Desai AS, Stevenson LW. Rehospitalization for heart failure: predict or prevent? *Circulation*. 2012;126:501–506.

76. Stevenson LWLN. Ventricular arrhythmias in heart failure. In: Zipes D, Jalife J, eds. *Cardiac Electrophysiology: From Bench to Bedside*. Philadelphia: Elsevier; 2016.

77. Hashim T, Sanam K, Revilla-Martinez M, et al. Clinical characteristics and outcomes of intravenous inotropic therapy in advanced heart failure. *Circ Heart Fail*. 2015;8:880–886.

78. Pinney SP, Stevenson LW. Chronic inotropic therapy in the current era: old wines with new pairings. *Circ Heart Fail*. 2015;8:843–846.

79. Setoguchi S, Stevenson LW, Schneeweiss S. Repeated hospitalizations predict mortality in the community population with heart failure. *Am Heart J*. 2007;154:260–266.

80. Levy WC, Mozaffarian D, Linker DT, et al. The Seattle Heart Failure Model: prediction of survival in heart failure. *Circulation*. 2006;113:1424–1433.

81. O'Connor CM, Hasselblad V, Mehta RH, et al. Triage after hospitalization with advanced heart failure: the ESCAPE (Evaluation Study of Congestive Heart Failure and Pulmonary Artery Catheterization Effectiveness) risk model and discharge score. *J Am Coll Cardiol*. 2010;55:872–878.

82. Aaronson KD, Schwartz JS, Chen TM, Wong KL, Goin JE, Mancini DM. Development and prospective validation of a clinical index to predict survival in ambulatory patients referred for cardiac transplant evaluation. *Circulation*. 1997;95:2660–2667.

83. Goldenberg I, Vyas AK, Hall WJ, et al. Risk stratification for primary implantation of a cardioverter-defibrillator in patients with ischemic left ventricular dysfunction. *J Am Coll Cardiol*. 2008;51:288–296.

84. Yancy CW, Jessup M, Bozkurt B, et al. 2013 ACCF/AHA guideline for the management of heart failure: a report of the American College of Cardiology Foundation/American Heart Association Task Force on Practice Guidelines. *J Am Coll Cardiol*. 2013;62:e147–e239.

85. Stevenson LW, Desai AS. Selecting patients for discussion of the ICD as primary prevention for sudden death in heart failure. *J Card Fail*. 2006;12:407–412.

86. Chen CY, Stevenson LW, Stewart GC, et al. Real world effectiveness of primary implantable cardioverter defibrillators implanted during hospital admissions for exacerbation of heart failure or other acute co-morbidities: cohort study of older patients with heart failure. *BMJ*. 2015;351: h3529.

87. Chen CY, Stevenson LW, Stewart GC, et al. Impact of baseline heart failure burden on post-implantable cardioverter-defibrillator mortality among Medicare beneficiaries. *J Am Coll Cardiol*. 2013;61:2142–2150.

88. Kramer DB, Buxton AE, Zimetbaum PJ. Time for a change—a new approach to ICD replacement. *N Engl J Med*. 2012;366:291–293.

89. Buchhalter LC, Ottenberg AL, Webster TL, Swetz KM, Hayes DL, Mueller PS. Features and outcomes of patients who underwent cardiac device deactivation. *JAMA Int Med*. 2014;174:80–85.

90. Lampert R, Hayes DL, Annas GJ, et al. HRS Expert Consensus Statement on Management of Cardiovascular Implantable Electronic Devices (CIEDs) in patients nearing end of life or requesting withdrawal of therapy. *Heart Rhythm*. 2010;7:1008–1026.

90 Arrhythmias and Conduction Disturbances in Noncompaction Cardiomyopathy

Luc Jordaens and Jeffrey A. Towbin

In this chapter, the form of cardiomyopathy known as left ventricular noncompaction cardiomyopathy (LVNC) will be discussed, with a specific focus on the arrhythmias associated with LVNC. This presentation of heart disease carries a substantial risk of heart failure, stroke, metabolic derangement, arrhythmias, and sudden cardiac death (SCD). It can occur at any age and appears often because of mutations in genes identified to encode primarily for cytoskeletal or sarcomeric proteins. It seems to be a continuum with other cardiomyopathies.

Characterized by excessive and unusual trabeculation of the mature left ventricle (LV), LVNC has been considered to occur because of arrest of the final phase of cardiac development, the compaction phase, where the compact myocardium fully forms. Clinically and pathologically, LVNC is characterized by a spongy morphological appearance of the myocardium, with abnormal trabeculations and intertrabecular recesses typically being most evident in the apical portion of the LV. [1,2]

In 2006, the American Heart Association Scientific Statement on the classification of cardiomyopathies formally classified LVNC as its own disease entity.[3] The European Working Group on Myocardial Disease, however, continues to consider LVNC to be a trait rather than a specific disease, but recommends genetic analysis when a diagnosis is made.[4,5] Indeed, multiple forms of LVNC occur, including dilated and hypertrophic cardiomyopathy (DCM and HCM, respectively) and noncompaction associated with congenital heart diseases (CHDs) such as atrial or ventricular septal defects, pulmonic stenosis, and hypoplastic left heart syndrome, among others.[6–9] In all forms, metabolic derangements may be notable.[10,11]

Pathology of Left Ventricular Noncompaction

In the early embryo, the heart is a loose interwoven mesh of muscle fibers.[12] The developing myocardium gradually condenses, and the large spaces within the trabecular meshwork disappear, condensing and compacting the ventricular myocardium and solidifying the endocardial surfaces. Trabecular compaction is normally more complete in the LV than in the right ventricular (RV) myocardium. The situations in which this compacting pathway fails are thought to be due to an arrest in endomyocardial morphogenesis and result in postnatal LV noncompaction.[6,12] The gross pathological appearance of LVNC is characterized by numerous, excessively prominent trabeculations and deep intratrabecular recesses resembling RV endomyocardial morphology. Histologically, the recesses and their troughs are lined with endothelium, indicating that these recesses are not sinusoids. In some cases, zones of fibrous and elastic tissue are found scattered on the endocardial surfaces with extension into the recesses. The coronary arterial circulation is usually normal, and extramural myocardial blood supply is not believed to play a role in these abnormalities. Intramural perfusion could be adversely affected by the prominent trabeculations and intratrabecular recesses, particularly in the subendocardium. The abnormal endocardial fibrous and elastic tissue will result in abnormal mechanics, causing the apex and basis to rotate in the same direction, without the normal twisting contraction of the heart.[13,14] The endomyocardial morphology of LVNC lends itself to the development of mural thrombi within the recesses, which can embolize and cause a stroke.[11,15,16] Arrhythmias can also occur because of associated pathology or can be acquired.[17–19] The precise substrate for malignant ventricular arrhythmias in LVNC patients is not known. Histological examination shows myocardium around deep intratrabecular recesses that can serve as slow conducting zones with reentry. Furthermore, impaired flow reserve, causing intermittent ischemia, has been proposed as having a role.

Incidence of Left Ventricular Noncompaction

Although LVNC is considered rare by some authors, the incidence and prevalence of LVNC is uncertain because of changing diagnostic criteria as well.[20–23] Further, it has been realized that many patients are asymptomatic, making it almost impossible to describe the real incidence if no data from population studies are available.[24] In the 1990s, the reported prevalence of isolated LVNC was 0.05% of all adult echocardiographic examinations in a large institution, whereas more recently the prevalence was reported as less than 0.14% of all adults referred for echocardiograms. In contrast, Sandhu et al.[20] demonstrated a 3.7% prevalence of definite or probable LVNC by echocardiography in adults with LV ejection fraction (LVEF) less than or equal to 45% and a 0.26% prevalence for all patients referred for echocardiography. Among heart failure patients, the prevalence of LVNC has been reported as 3%–4%.[23] A registry of pediatric cardiomyopathy discovered noncompaction in 5% of registered children.[25] Overdiagnosis of LVNC has been described; African Americans and athletes may show a high prevalence of LV hypertrabeculation.[26–28]

Clinical Features and Diagnosis of Left Ventricular Noncompaction

The clinical presentation of LVNC is highly variable, ranging from asymptomatic to end-stage heart failure, lethal arrhythmias, or thromboembolic events.[2,3,15-19] LVNC may exist as isolated disease, but may also be a trait or a continuum with hypertrophic and dilated cardiomyopathies (HCMs and DCMs, respectively).

In infancy, LVNC commonly develops with signs and symptoms of heart failure.[2,6,9] Childhood LVNC can occur with heart failure, rhythm abnormalities, or sudden death.[15,16,22,24] Ichida et al.[9] found good survival and limited symptoms in their childhood patients, whereas Chin et al.[6] reported three deaths in the eight children studied. Pignatelli and associates[2] demonstrated poor outcomes in neonates but excellent outcomes in those outside the neonatal period. All the neonates who died had systemic disease (mitochondrial and other metabolic disorders); they demonstrated a 5-year survival rate of 86%. When patients receiving transplants were added, the 5-year survival free of death or transplantation was 75%.

The same specter (arrhythmia, heart failure, and thrombosis) is described in adults. However, a high percentage of patients are asymptomatic and identified serendipitously on echocardiography, with deep trabeculations and intertrabecular recesses noted in the LV apex and lateral wall. It might be advisable to use multimodality imaging (validated echocardiographic criteria, speckle tracking, and cardiac magnetic resonance imaging [MRI]) to confirm the diagnosis based on the ratio of compacted and noncompacted layers and on the nontrabeculated mass.[8,29]

Patients with LVNC are known to develop ventricular arrhythmias (ventricular tachycardia [VT] and ventricular fibrillation [VF]), atrial fibrillation, or conduction abnormalities (sinus bradycardia and complete heart block). Wolff-Parkinson-White (WPW) syndrome is common (>10%).[2,6,9,30] Reports of survival have been inconsistent.

Adult clinical studies have consistently described a high risk of ventricular tachyarrhythmias and SCD in LVNC,[1,16,18] with as high as 47% of adults (and 75% of symptomatic patients) dying within 6 years of presentation. More recent reports, however, have shown a more benign natural history.[31] Bhatia et al.[32] reviewed published studies of 241 adults with isolated LVNC diagnosed by echocardiographic criteria followed for a mean duration of 39 months. The annualized event rate was 4% for cardiovascular deaths, 6.2% for cardiovascular death and its surrogates (heart transplant and appropriate implantable cardioverter defibrillator [ICD] shocks), and 8.6% for all cardiovascular events (death, stroke, ICD shocks, and transplantation). Familial LVNC occurrence was identified in first-degree relatives screened using echocardiography in 30% of index cases.[32] This was confirmed by Caliskan and colleagues,[24] who also showed that the majority of these patients were asymptomatic, in spite of mild to moderate LV dysfunction. Inducibility of sustained VT during electrophysiological studies has demonstrated little value as a tool for risk stratification in LVNC.[17,33] An electrocardiographic sign suggestive of reentry is the presence of QRS notches (QRS fragmentation) or the presence of J waves (early repolarization), which have been frequently reported.[17,18,34] Additionally, a high proportion of patients without previously documented arrhythmia have the same amount of spontaneous arrhythmias (premature ventricular complexes [PVCs] or nonsustained VT) on the Holter as those who survived an arrest, suggesting that this might be a trigger for more serious events.

Subtypes of Left Ventricular Noncompaction

One of the important issues in the diagnosis and outcomes of these patients, particularly in childhood, is the specific LVNC phenotype, as this may have different outcomes (Fig. 90.1). A special feature is that the phenotype may vary between dilated and hypertrophic forms (the "undulating phenotype" in which the heart finally often reverts to the original morphology).[2]

The subtypes include the following types:

1. *Isolated LVNC*, in which abnormal trabeculations are associated with normal LV size, thickness, and systolic and diastolic function in the absence of other structural heart diseases with no evidence of arrhythmias. Clinically, this subgroup appears to be benign during childhood and affects approximately 25% of all subjects. These individuals do well unless they exhibit ventricular arrhythmias. This subgroup usually undergoes yearly follow-ups in the outpatient clinic, and patients are not treated with medication or restricted from activities.[6,8,9,35]

2. In *isolated LVNC with arrhythmias*, there are predominant arrhythmias (usually runs of tachyarrhythmias). These patients appear to have an elevated risk of sudden events and require closer follow-up and therapeutic intervention. The arrhythmias noted include VT, VF, atrioventricular block, supraventricular tachycardia, WPW, and atrial fibrillation.[36,37]

3. The *dilated form of LVNC* clinically mimics DCM, with a dilated trabeculated LV with depressed systolic function, and it likely has similar outcomes. The follow-up for these patients is similar to those with pure DCM.

4. The *hypertrophic form of LVNC* mimics HCM with LV hypertrophy (commonly with asymmetrical septal hypertrophy) and a small, trabeculated LV cavity. Hypercontractile systolic function and diastolic dysfunction appear to have similar outcomes as in pure HCM.

5. The *hypertrophic and dilated form of LVNC* appears to be the worst form of LVNC clinically and, in many cases, is associated with neuromuscular disease and hypotonia. These young children, particularly infants, can succumb to heart failure or arrhythmias, especially if they have metabolic derangement.[2,11] The electrocardiograms (ECGs) of these patients have the same abnormalities as the other forms.

6. The *restrictive form of LVNC* is rare and is clinically challenging because it mimics the clinical behavior of restrictive cardiomyopathy (RCM), with dilated atria and diastolic dysfunction associated with a trabeculated LV with normal dimension, thickness, and systolic function.[38] Like children with RCM, this subgroup is typically considered a transplant candidate early after diagnosis.

7. In *LVNC with congenital heart disease*, any form of CHD can occur in conjunction with LVNC, but right heart obstructive forms are most typical.[21] The most common simple forms of CHD include septal defects and pulmonic stenosis. However, LVNC has been identified in subjects with severe CHD, including Ebstein anomaly, pulmonary atresia, tricuspid atresia, hypoplastic left heart syndrome, and heterotaxy syndrome. Outcomes depend on the specific CHD but can be worse than the postoperative outcomes of the same CHD without LVNC.

Imaging of Left Ventricular Noncompaction

The diagnostic criteria for LVNC are based on imaging. Echocardiography has been the most commonly used modality to diagnose and describe LVNC. The diagnostic criteria were recently revisited by some of the original authors, and they suggested the use of multimodality imaging (the validated echocardiographic criteria, speckle tracking, and cardiac MRI) to confirm the diagnosis. The initial echocardiographic criteria were based on the ratio of noncompacted and compacted layers (which should be more than 2 in LVNC) and on measurement of the nontrabeculated mass versus the mass of the global LV with cardiac MRI.[8] Speckle tracking may reveal rigid body rotation, in an objective way, with absence of the normal twist.[39] It was present in children and their family members and is associated with lower functional status.[13,40,41]

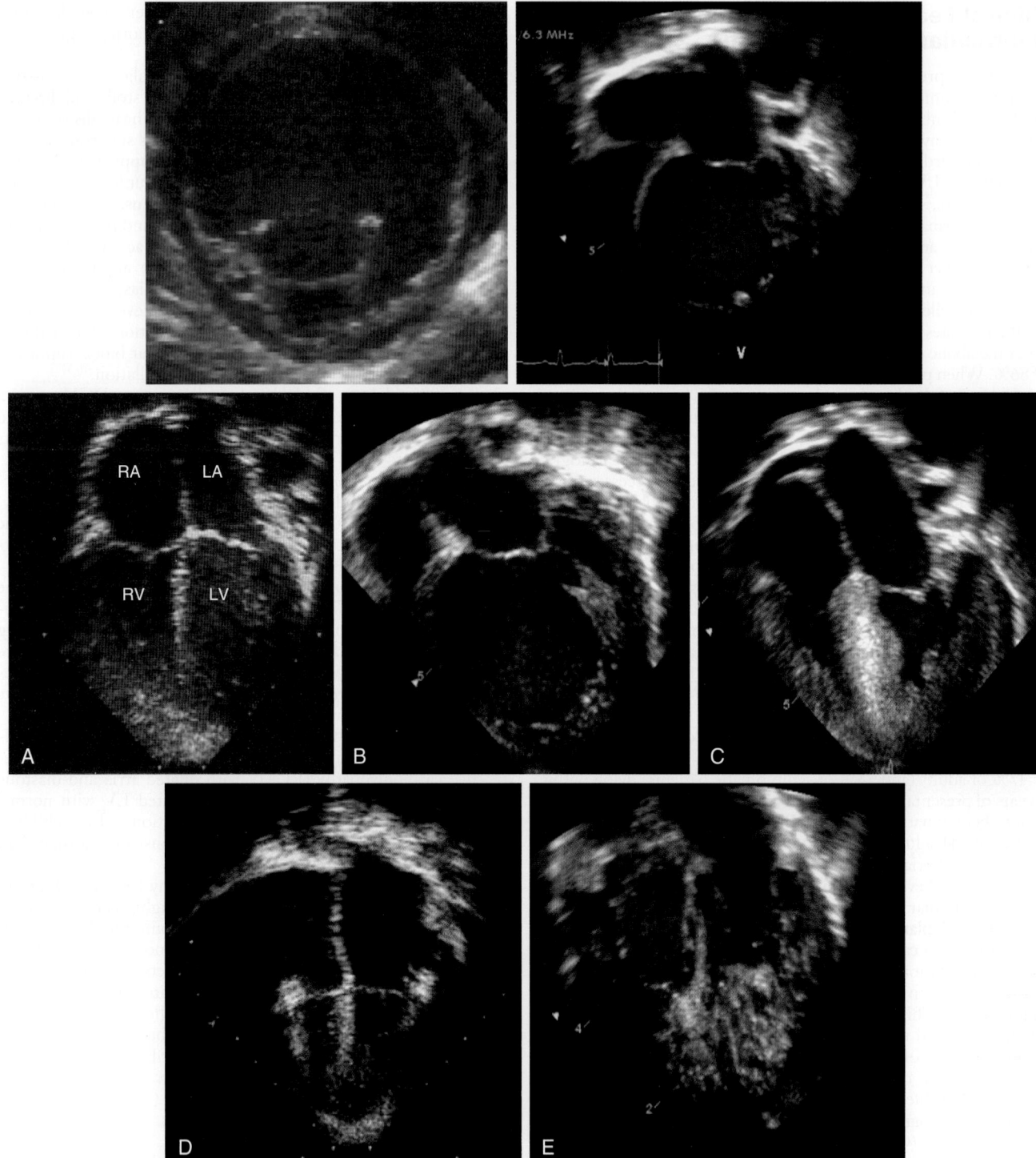

FIGURE 90.1 Echocardiographic pictorial of heterogeneous forms of left ventricular noncompaction (LVNC). The *top panel* shows a parasternal short axis view of a dilated form of LVNC. Apical trabeculations are noted at the apex. An apical four-chamber view at the right side of the figure demonstrates the same findings. The *lower panel* shows heterogeneous phenotypes associated with LVNC. (A) LVNC with normal left ventricle size, thickness, and function. (B) Dilated form of LVNC. (C) Hypertrophic form of LVNC. (D) Restrictive form of LVNC. (E) Biventricular LVNC.

Thuny et al.[29] compared two-dimensional echocardiography images obtained at end-diastole and end-systole with the images obtained using cardiovascular magnetic resonance imaging (CMR) at end-diastole to validate the diagnosis of LVNC. Sixteen adults (48 ± 17 years) with LVNC underwent echocardiography and CMR within the same week and were compared to assess noncompaction in 17 anatomical segments. All segments were analyzed using CMR, but only 87% could be analyzed using echocardiography. A two-layered structure was observed in 54% of patients by CMR and in 43% by echocardiography. Therefore CMR was thought to be superior to standard echocardiography in assessing the extent of noncompaction and providing

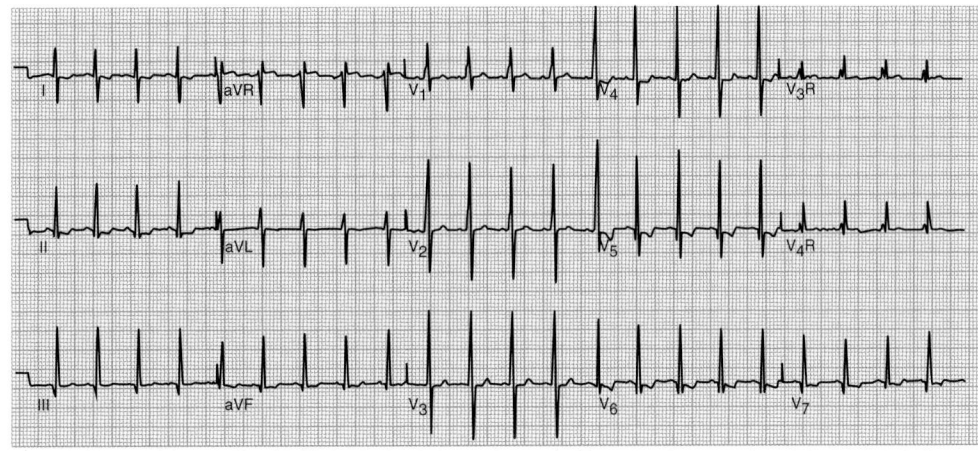

All leads ¹/₄ standard

FIGURE 90.2 Electrocardiographic features of left ventricular noncompaction. Note the excessive midprecordial voltages (one-fourth of standard).

supplemental morphological information beyond that obtained with conventional echocardiography; however, this has not been validated in children. Furthermore, the presence of extensive fibrosis correlates with late gadolinium enhancement, also when a normal function is detected.[42]

Electrocardiography in Left Ventricular Noncompaction

The ECG for patients with LVNC is typically abnormal and, in infants and young children, commonly shows excessive voltage (Fig. 90.2).[2,9] In fact, approximately 30% of these young subjects with LVNC have extreme midprecordial voltages that mimic the ECG seen in Pompe disease. The childhood forms of LVNC may be associated with preexcitation as well (Fig. 90.3).

Adult patients often also have left ventricular hypertrophy and atrioventricular and intraventricular conduction delay. Left bundle branch block (LBBB) is often present (Fig. 90.4).[17,18] Arrhythmias, including supraventricular tachycardia, atrial fibrillation, and VT are common and dangerous accompaniments to all subtypes of LVNC. Early repolarizations as described by Haissaguerre and colleagues were more often present in those who had a history of VT or VF, but also occurred in 23% of patients without such history.[18,43] The same finding was reported by Steffel.[17]

Arrhythmias in Left Ventricular Noncompaction

Bradycardia, including heart block and sinus node disease, may require pacing. Cardiac resynchronization therapy might be necessary as many patients have a combination of a low LVEF and a wide QRS complex. Supraventricular arrhythmias, including accessory pathways, can often be ablated.[30]

Life-threatening ventricular arrhythmias, which are among the most frequent causes of death in subjects with LVNC, can be treated with ICDs. Secondary prevention is generally accepted after cardiac arrest, VT, or syncope. The fact that LVNC often presents as superimposed upon another cardiomyopathy or in combination with heart failure suggests the use of at least the guidelines for primary prevention of those conditions.[44,45] It seems logical to also treat patients having preserved or moderately depressed ejection fraction with a family history, a syncope, or nonsustained VT with a prophylactic ICD (in line with the task force for hypertrophic cardiomyopathy).[46] Whether fibrosis

on MRI in the presence of normal LV function is enough to consider prophylactic ICD implantation remains a question, certainly in the presence of a family history.[42]

Ventricular tachyarrhythmias, including cardiac arrest owing to VF, are reported in 38%–47% and sudden death in 13%–18% of adult patients with LVNC.[18,19,33,37] Caliskan and coworkers[47] recently investigated ICD therapy indications and outcomes in 77 patients with LVNC (mean age, 40 ± 14 years), 44 (57%) of whom had an ICD implanted using standard ICD guidelines for nonischemic cardiomyopathy. Implantation for secondary prevention occurred in 12 patients (7 with VF, 5 with sustained VT) and for primary prevention (heart failure or severe LV dysfunction) in 32 patients.[47] During a mean follow-up of 33 ± 24 months, eight patients presented with appropriate ICD shocks owing to sustained VT after a median of 6.1 months (range, 1–16 months), including 4 of 32 (13%) patients in the primary prevention group and 4 of 12 (33%) in the secondary prevention group (p = .04). At a median follow-up of 4 months (range, 2–23 months), an additional nine patients had received inappropriate ICD therapy: six (19%) in the primary group and three (25%) in the secondary prevention group. The relatively high percentage of appropriate shocks for sustained VT in this population suggests that patients with LVNC are at high risk for SCD and that implanting an ICD in these adult patients is appropriate, although no patients with LVNC were included in the previous trials that were the basis of the current guidelines.[46] All the appropriate ICD interventions in this patient cohort were due to fast VTs, although it is not certain that the initial rhythm in those SCD and VF patients was also started with a VT trigger. In patients with LVNC and sustained VT or VF, there was a 33% risk of recurrent, sustained VT followed by appropriate ICD shocks after a median follow-up period of 26 months. Similarly, Kobza et al.[48] reported 37% appropriate shocks during a mean follow-up of 40 months among 30 patients with LVNC and an ICD. These observations support the current guidelines to implant an ICD for primary prevention based on the presence of heart failure or severe LV dysfunction in combination with other (presumed) high-risk factors in patients with LVNC.[45]

In the cohort reported by Caliskan and associates,[47] severe LV dysfunction or dilation were not prominent in the secondary prevention group with a history of sustained VT or VF, making it difficult to rely on the severity of the LV dysfunction for SCD risk stratification. There were more PVCs in the patients treated with ICDs than in those without one, with a trend toward higher numbers of PVCs in the secondary prevention group with VT or VF versus those receiving an ICD for

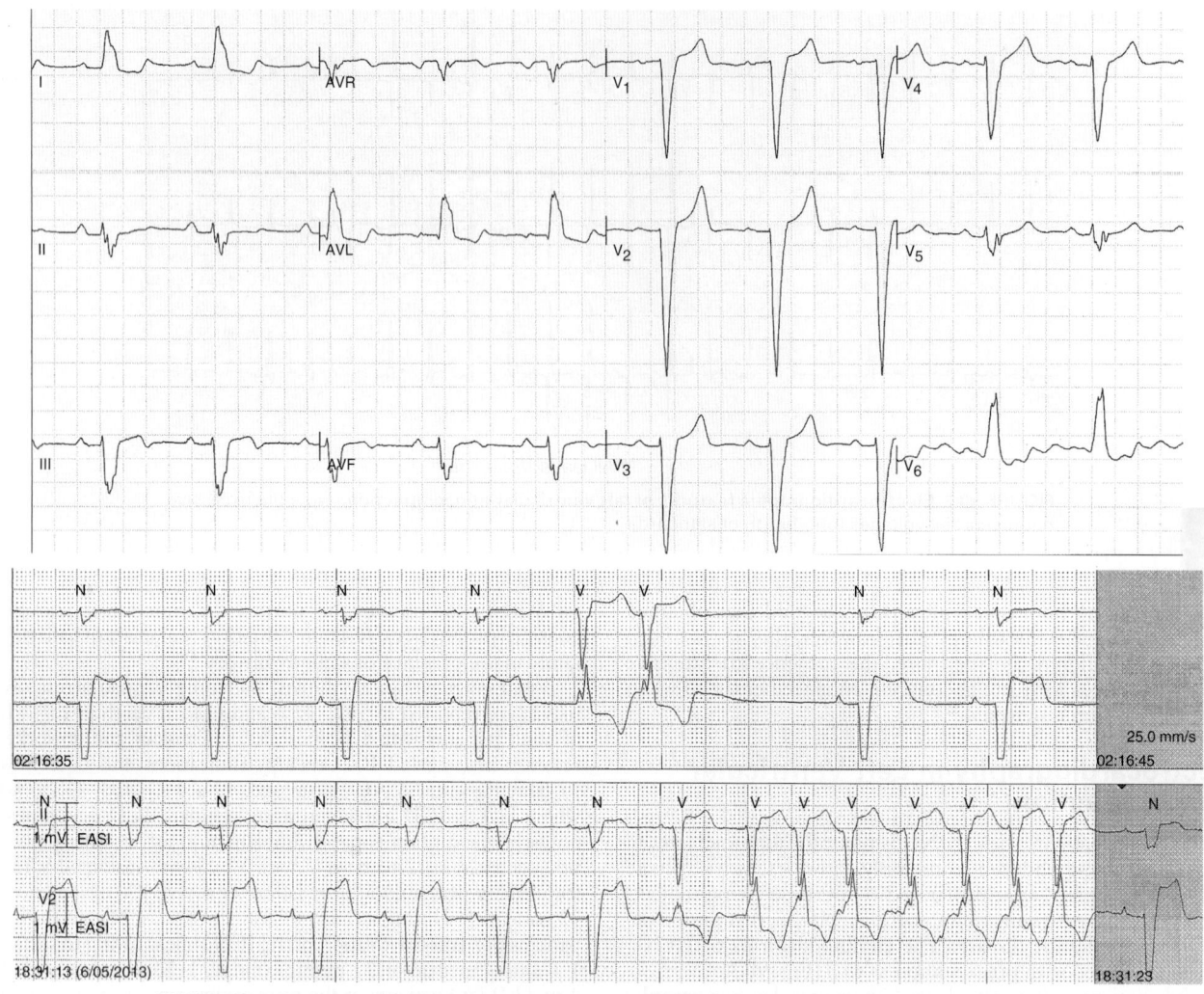

FIGURE 90.3 Complete left bundle branch block in a 48-year-old female patient, with evident left ventricular noncompaction on magnetic resonance imaging. During monitoring the patient shows bradycardia as well as nonsustained ventricular tachycardia. She has a left ventricular ejection fraction of 45% and is a responder to cardiac resynchronization.

primary prevention. Nonsustained VT was also more frequent on 24-hour Holter recording in the VT/VF group versus both the primary prevention patients and those without ICD.

Clinical Genetics of Left Ventricular Noncompaction

Ichida and colleagues[9] reported that 44% of isolated LVNC patients had inherited LVNC, with 70% having autosomal dominant and 30% having X-linked inheritance. This was confirmed by Hoedemakers and coworkers[49] who showed by cardiological screening that in 194 family members from 50 LVNC probands, two-thirds of families had a familial cardiomyopathy; however, not only LVNC but HCM and DCM were also detected. This pleiomorphism was confirmed by Arbustini.[50] Nonpenetrance of the detected genetic defects was high, which means that affected family members have to be followed over time.[49,50]

In X-linked recessive LVNC, female carriers have not been found to develop frank clinical disease and are echocardiographically normal.[35] Consistent with X-linked inheritance, no male-to-male transmission of the disease occurs. Autosomal dominant inheritance occurs in some familial cases of LVNC without CHD and in most, if not all, cases associated with CHD.[9,31,35,51] In

some families with autosomal dominant LVNC associated with CHD, affected members can be identified in whom no CHD can be identified at the time of evaluation because their cardiac defects include minor forms of CHD, such as small atrial or ventral septal defects or patent ductus arteriosus that have spontaneously closed, along with other individuals with severe CHD, such as hypoplastic left heart syndrome. Autosomal recessive and mitochondrial inheritance is seen in cases dominated by mitochondrial and metabolic derangement.[11,35]

Molecular Genetics of Left Ventricular Noncompaction

Barth syndrome is a clinical association of myocardial dysfunction, neutropenia, skeletal myopathy, abnormal mitochondria, organic aciduria (primarily 3-methylglutaconic aciduria), growth retardation, and cholesterol abnormalities.[52] It is an X-linked disorder and has been thought to be allelic to several phenotypically different disorders on Xq28,[35,52] such as LVNC and DCM. Mutations in the G4.5 or tafazzin (*TAZ*) gene were among the first to be identified in male patients and carrier females with isolated LVNC and with Barth syndrome, but not in the adult population with dominant transmission. This gene encodes a novel protein family (tafazzins) that participate in the metabolism of

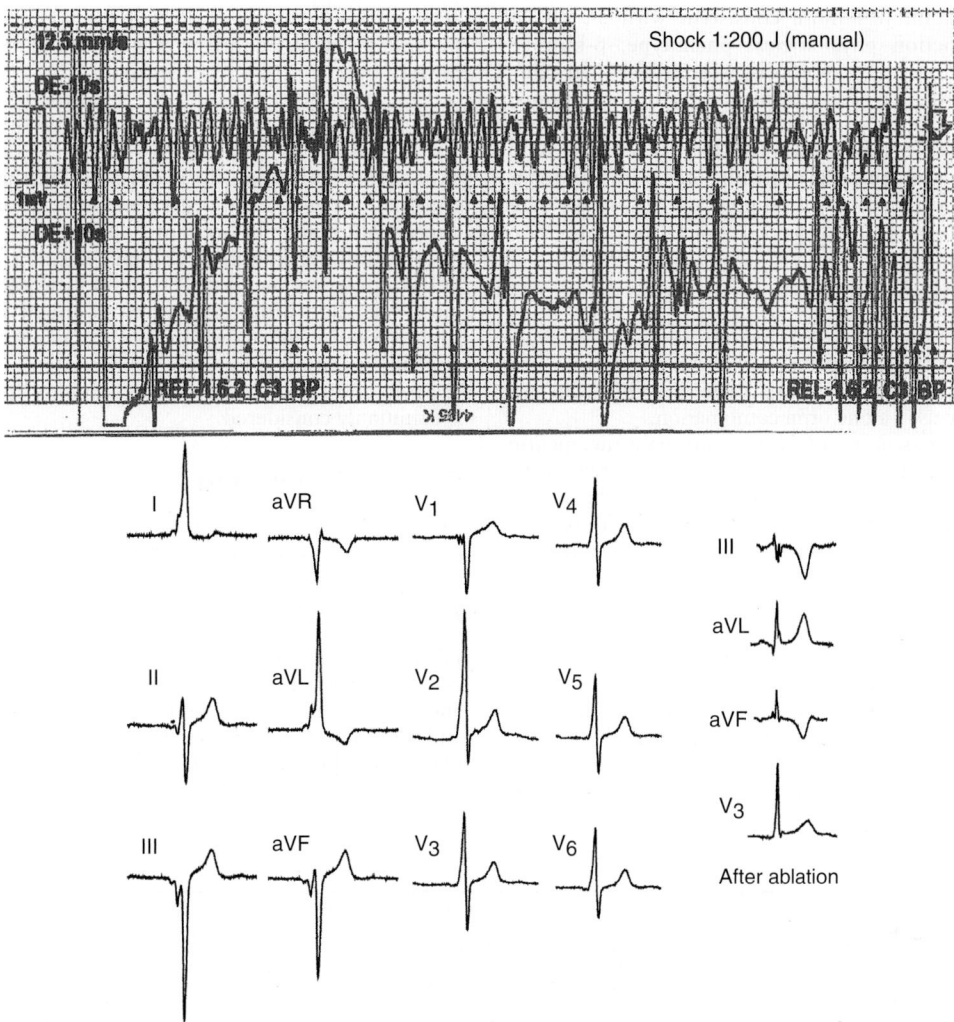

FIGURE 90.4 Automated external defibrillation of a collapsing young female who later showed left ventricular noncompaction. After the first shock (*upper tracing*), sinus rhythm is restored, but in the *lower strip,* the patient has recurrence of ventricular fibrillation. After two more shocks, she is admitted to the hospital, demonstrates right posteroseptal Wolff-Parkinson-White syndrome (*lower left panel*) with short effective refractory period (ERP), and is ablated. In the tracings after ablation (*below, at the right*), fragmentation is observed in III; a QRS notch is observed in aVL and AVF, while early repolarization is seen in V₃. The T wave inversion in III is due to cardiac memory after the ablation.

cardiolipin, the signature phospholipid of mitochondria, and is also responsible for other forms of infantile cardiomyopathy.[35,52]

In autosomal dominant LVNC, multiple genes have been identified. Ichida et al.[10] identified mutations in α-dystrobrevin as causative in children and young adults with LVNC with or without CHD. Subsequently, mutations in sarcomere protein– and Z-line protein–encoding genes were identified, with mutations in β-myosin heavy chain (*MYH7*), α-cardiac actin (*ACTC*), cardiac troponin T (*TNNT2*), and ZASP.[35,51,53,54] Sarcomeric gene mutations in the LVNC population imply that LVNC is part of a broader spectrum of cardiomyopathies including HCM, RCM, and DCM.[8,51] In addition to sarcomere-encoding genes and cytoskeletal genes, mutations in the sodium channel gene *SCN5A* have been shown to cause LVNC and rhythm disturbance.[55]

Dystrophin is another cytoskeletal protein that has been associated with LVNC in boys with Duchenne and Becker muscular dystrophy.[56] Skeletal muscle biopsy has, in some patients, identified mitochondrial abnormalities, suggesting a nuclear import protein as the primary abnormality. Mutation analysis of the mitochondrial genome has identified mutations

as well.[57] Consideration of other potential genetic causes needs to account for the known molecular defects resulting in congenital heart anomalies, as well as those molecular abnormalities resulting in diseases of the myocardium itself.

In general, genetic heterogeneity is found, and the same mutation can result in different phenotypes (DCM, HCM, or RCM). Pedigree analysis, family study, and genetic counseling are necessary, in collaboration with a cardiologist. Genetic testing is recommended when a mutation is identified in the proband.[58]

Therapy and Outcome
Heart Failure

The specific therapy depends on the clinical and echocardiographic findings. In patients with systolic dysfunction and heart failure, anticongestive therapies identical to those used in patients with DCM are appropriate. In particular, angiotensin-converting enzyme inhibitors and β-adrenergic blocking agents are useful. Diuretics may also be needed; however, among patients exhibiting findings more consistent with an HCM or diastolic dysfunction physiological phenotype, β-blocker therapy alone may be more appropriate in children. In children and adults with the HCM form and having symptoms, myectomy may be appropriate. Cardiac resynchronization therapy can be helpful, certainly for LBBB with septal flash.[59] Finally, in patients with heart failure associated with any form of LVNC, mechanical circulatory support and transplant may be necessary.[8]

Specific Conditions

In patients having LVNC with associated mitochondrial or metabolic dysfunction, some investigators add a "vitamin cocktail" to the cardiac therapy, with coenzyme Q_{10}, carnitine, riboflavin, and thiamine commonly used alone or in combination.

In patients having associated CHD, appropriate therapeutic approaches can include simple pharmacological therapy with diuretics for volume overload associated with left to right shunts, more complex pharmacological therapy for patients with restrictive physiology and pulmonary hypertension, or invasive therapy with catheter intervention or surgical repairs, depending on the lesions.

Antithrombotic Therapy

Anticoagulation is needed in depressed LV function and in the presence of AF. The CHADS2-VASC score might be helpful in decision making, also when AF is not present.[60] When there is evidence of thrombi in the LV, oral anticoagulation with anti–vitamin K antagonists or heparin seems to be necessary, as we have no evidence for the efficacy of the newer anticoagulant drugs.[61]

Arrhythmias

In patients who have any form of LVNC and have arrhythmias or syncope, prolonged ambulatory monitoring or an electrophysiological study may be warranted. Pacing or cardiac resynchronization can be indicated. Catheter ablation is appropriate for WPW syndrome and probably as well for other atrial arrhythmias, including atrial fibrillation. It might be challenging to address ventricular arrhythmias with catheter ablation as well. ICD implantation is typically appropriate as mentioned before. In adults and a small cadre of at-risk children, primary prevention is commonly considered.

Genetic Counseling

Finally, genetic counseling is difficult and may impose a heavy psychological stress upon patients and their families.[62]

Acknowledgments

J.A.T. is funded, in part, by the National Institutes of Health; the National Heart, Lung and Blood Institute (grants R01 HL53392 and R01 HL087000, for the Pediatric Cardiomyopathy Registry and Pediatric Cardiomyopathy Specimen Repository, respectively); and the Cincinnati Children's Kindervelt-Samuel Kaplan Chair in Cardiology and Cardiac Research.

REFERENCES

1. Engberding R, Yelbuz TM, Breithardt G. Isolated noncompaction of the left ventricular myocardium: a review of the literature two decades after the initial case description. *Clin Res Cardiol*. 2007;96:481–488.
2. Pignatelli RH, McMahon CJ, Dreyer WJ, et al. Clinical characterization of left ventricular noncompaction in children. A relatively common form of cardiomyopathy. *Circulation*. 2003;108:2672–2678.
3. Maron BJ, Towbin JA, Thiene G, et al. Contemporary definitions and classification of the cardiomyopathies: An American Heart Association Scientific Statement from the Council on Clinical Cardiology, Heart Failure and Transplantation Committee; Quality of Care and Outcomes Research and Functional Genomics and Translational Biology Interdisciplinary Working Groups; and Council on Epidemiology and Prevention. *Circulation*. 2006;113:1807–1816.
4. Elliott P, Andersson B, Arbustini E, et al. Classification of the cardiomyopathies: a position statement from the European Society of Cardiology Working Group on Myocardial and Pericardial Diseases. *Eur Heart J*. 2008;29:270–276.
5. Rapezzi C, Arbustini E, Caforio AL, et al. Diagnostic work-up in cardiomyopathies: bridging the gap between clinical phenotypes and final diagnosis. A position statement from the ESC Working Group on Myocardial and Pericardial Diseases. *Eur Heart J*. 2013;34:1448–1458.
6. Chin TK, Perloff JK, Williams RG, et al. Isolated noncompaction of left ventricular myocardium. A study of eight cases. *Circulation*. 1990;82:507–513.
7. Finsterer J, Stöllberger C, Fazio G. Neuromuscular disorders in left ventricular hypertrabeculation/noncompaction. *Curr Pharm Des*. 2010;16:2895–2904.
8. Oechslin E, Jenni R. Left ventricular non-compaction revisited: a distinct phenotype with genetic heterogeneity? *Eur Heart J*. 2011;32:1446–1456.
9. Ichida F, Hamamichi Y, Miyawaki T, et al. Clinical features of isolated noncompaction of the ventricular myocardium: long-term clinical course, hemodynamic properties and genetic background. *J Am Coll Cardiol*. 1999;34:233–240.
10. Ichida F, Tsubata S, Bowles KR, et al. Novel gene mutations in patients with left ventricular noncompaction or Barth syndrome. *Circulation*. 2001;103:1256–1263.
11. Scaglia F, Towbin JA, Craigen WJ, et al. Clinical spectrum, morbidity, and mortality in 113 pediatric patients with mitochondrial disease. *Pediatrics*. 2004;114:925–931.
12. Sedmera D, McQuinn T. Embryogenesis of the heart muscle. *Heart Fail Clin*. 2008;4:235–238.

13. Kauer F, Geleijnse ML, van Dalen BM. Role of left ventricular twist mechanics in cardiomyopathies, dance of the helices. *World J Cardiol*. 2015;7:476–482.
14. Peters F, Khandheria BK, Libhaber E, et al. Left ventricular twist in left ventricular noncompaction. *Eur Heart J Cardiovasc Imaging*. 2014;15:48–55.
15. Stöllberger C, Blazek G, Dobias C, et al. Frequency of stroke and embolism in left ventricular hypertrabeculation/noncompaction. *Am J Cardiol*. 2011;108:1021–1023.
16. Greutmann M, Mah ML, Silversides CK, et al. Predictors of adverse outcome in adolescents and adults with isolated left ventricular noncompaction. *Am J Cardiol*. 2012;109:276–281.
17. Steffel J, Kobza R, Oechslin E, et al. Electrocardiographic characteristics at initial diagnosis in patients with isolated left ventricular noncompaction. *Am J Cardiol*. 2009;104:984–989.
18. Caliskan K, Ujvari B, Bauernfeind T, et al. The prevalence of early repolarization in patients with noncompaction cardiomyopathy presenting with malignant ventricular arrhythmias. *J Cardiovasc Electrophysiol*. 2012;23:938–944.
19. Celiker A, Ozkutlu S, Dilber E, et al. Rhythm abnormalities in children with isolated ventricular noncompaction. *Pacing Clin Electrophysiol*. 2005;28:1198–1202.
20. Sandhu R, Finkelhor RS, Gunawardena DR, et al. Prevalence and characteristics of left ventricular noncompaction in a community hospital cohort of patients with systolic dysfunction. *Echocardiography*. 2008;25:8–12.
21. Hughes ML, Carstensen B, Wilkinson JL, et al. Angiographic diagnosis, prevalence and outcomes for left ventricular noncompaction in children with congenital cardiac disease. *Cardiol Young*. 2007;17:56–63.
22. Aras D, Tufekcioglu O, Ergun K, et al. Clinical features of isolated ventricular noncompaction in adults: long-term clinical course, echocardiographic properties, and predictors of left ventricular failure. *J Card Fail*. 2006;12:726–733.
23. Kovacevic-Preradovic T, Jenni R, Oechslin EN, et al. Isolated left ventricular noncompaction as a cause for heart failure and heart transplantation: a single center experience. *Cardiology*. 2009;112:158–164.
24. Caliskan K, Michels M, Geleijnse ML, et al. Frequency of asymptomatic disease among family members with noncompaction cardiomyopathy. *Am J Cardiol*. 2012;110:1512–1527.
25. Jefferies JL, Wilkinson JD, Sleeper LA, et al. Pediatric Cardiomyopathy Registry Investigators. Cardiomyopathy phenotypes and outcomes for children with left ventricular myocardial noncompaction: results from the Pediatric Cardiomyopathy Registry. *J Card Fail*. 2015;21:877–884.

26. Kohli SK, Pantazis AA, Shah JS, et al. Diagnosis of left-ventricular non-compaction in patients with left-ventricular systolic dysfunction: time for a reappraisal of diagnostic criteria? *Eur Heart J*. 2008;29:89–95.
27. Gati S, Rajani R, Carr-White GS, Chambers JB. Adult left ventricular noncompaction: reappraisal of current diagnostic imaging modalities. *JACC Cardiovasc Imaging*. 2014;7:1266–1275.
28. Gati S, Chandra N, Bennett RL, et al. Increased left ventricular trabeculation in highly trained athletes: do we need more stringent criteria for the diagnosis of left ventricular non-compaction in athletes? *Heart*. 2013;99:401–408.
29. Thuny F, Jacquier A, Jop B, et al. Assessment of left ventricular non-compaction in adults: side-by-side comparison of cardiac magnetic resonance imaging with echocardiography. *Arch Cardiovasc Dis*. 2010;103:150–159.
30. Yaksh A, Haitsma D, Ramdjan T, Caliskan K, Szili-Torok T, de Groot NM. Unexpected finding in an adult with ventricular fibrillation and an accessory pathway: non-compaction cardiomyopathy. *Neth Heart J*. 2014;22:182–185.
31. Murphy RT, Thaman R, Blanes JG, et al. Natural history and familial characteristics of isolated left ventricular non-compaction. *Eur Heart J*. 2005;26:187–192.
32. Bhatia NL, Tajik AJ, Wilansky S, et al. Isolated noncompaction of the left ventricular myocardium in adults: a systematic overview. *J Card Fail*. 2011;17:771–778.
33. Caliskan K, Kardos A, Szili-Torok T. Empty handed: a call for an international registry of risk stratification to reduce the "sudden-ness" of death in patients with non-compaction cardiomyopathy. *Europace*. 2009;11:1138–1139.
34. Das MK, Maskoun W, Shen C, et al. Fragmented QRS on twelve-lead electrocardiogram predicts arrhythmic events in patients with ischemic and nonischemic cardiomyopathy. *Heart Rhythm*. 2010;7:74–80.
35. Towbin JA. Left ventricular noncompaction: a new form of heart failure. *Heart Fail Clin*. 2010;6:453–469.
36. Stöllberger C, Blazek G, Wegner C, et al. Heart failure, atrial fibrillation and neuromuscular disorders influence mortality in left ventricular hypertrabeculation/noncompaction. *Cardiology*. 2011;119:176–182.
37. Steffel J, Duru F. Rhythm disorders in isolated left ventricular noncompaction. *Ann Med*. 2012;44:101–108.
38. Martinez HR, Niu MC, Sutton VR, et al. Coffin-Lowry syndrome and left ventricular noncompaction cardiomyopathy with a restrictive pattern. *Am J Med Genet A*. 2011;155A:3030–3034.

39. van Dalen BM, Caliskan K, Soliman OI, et al. Diagnostic value of rigid body rotation in noncompaction cardiomyopathy. *J Am Soc Echocardiogr*. 2011;24:548–555.

40. Nemes A, Havasi K, Forster T. "Rigid body rotation" of the left ventricle in hypoplastic right-heart syndrome: a case from the three-dimensional speckle-tracking echocardiographic MAGYAR-Path Study. *Cardiol Young*. 2015;25:768–772.

41. Udink ten Cate FE, Schmidt BE, Lagies R, Brockmeier K, Sreeram N. Reversed apical rotation and paradoxical increased left ventricular torsion in children with left ventricular non-compaction. *Int J Cardiol*. 2010;145:558–559.

42. Wan J, Zhao S, Cheng H, et al. Varied distributions of late gadolinium enhancement found among patients meeting cardiovascular magnetic resonance criteria for isolated left ventricular non-compaction. *J Cardiovasc Magn Reson*. 2013;15:20.

43. Roten L, Derval N, Maury P, et al. Benign vs malignant inferolateral early repolarization: Focus on the T wave. *Heart Rhythm*. 2015;13:894–902.

44. Elliott PM, Anastasakis A, Borger MA, et al. 2014 ESC guidelines on diagnosis and management of hypertrophic cardiomyopathy: The Task Force for the Diagnosis and Management of Hypertrophic Cardiomyopathy of the European Society of Cardiology (ESC). *Eur Heart J*. 2014;35:2733–2779.

45. Smith T, Theuns DA, Caliskan K, Jordaens L. Long-term follow-up of prophylactic implantable cardioverter-defibrillator-only therapy: comparison of ischemic and nonischemic heart disease. *Clin Cardiol*. 2011;34:761–767.

46. Zipes DP, Camm AJ, Borggrefe M, et al. ACC/AHA/ESC 2006 guidelines for management of patients with ventricular arrhythmias and the prevention of sudden cardiac death: a report of the American College of Cardiology/American Heart Association Task Force and the European Society of Cardiology Committee for Practice Guidelines (writing committee to develop Guidelines for Management of Patients with Ventricular Arrhythmias and the Prevention of Sudden Cardiac Death): Developed in collaboration with the European Heart Rhythm Association and the Heart Rhythm Society. *Circulation*. 2006;114:e385–e484.

47. Caliskan K, Szili-Torok T, Theuns DA, et al. Indications and outcome of implantable cardioverter-defibrillators for primary and secondary prophylaxis in patients with noncompaction cardiomyopathy. *J Cardiovasc Electrophysiol*. 2011;22:898–904.

48. Kobza R, Steffel J, Erne P, et al. Implantable cardioverter defibrillator and cardiac resynchronization therapy in patients with left ventricular noncompaction. *Heart Rhythm*. 2010;7:1545–1549.

49. Hoedemaekers YM, Caliskan K, Michels M, et al. The importance of genetic counseling, DNA diagnostics, and cardiologic family screening in left ventricular noncompaction cardiomyopathy. *Circ Cardiovasc Genet*. 2010;3:232–239.

50. Arbustini E, Weidemann F, Hall JL. Left ventricular noncompaction: a distinct cardiomyopathy or a trait shared by different cardiac diseases? *J Am Coll Cardiol*. 2014;64:1840–1850.

51. Hoedemaekers YM, Caliskan K, Majoor-Krakauer D, et al. Cardiac beta-myosin heavy chain defects in two families with non-compaction cardiomyopathy: linking non-compaction to hypertrophic, restrictive, and dilated cardiomyopathies. *Eur Heart J*. 2007;28:2732–2737.

52. Aprikyan AA, Khuchua Z. Advances in the understanding of Barth syndrome. *Br J Haematol*. 2013;161:330–338.

53. Teekakirikul P, Kelly MA, Rehm HL, et al. Inherited cardiomyopathies: molecular genetics and clinical genetic testing in the postgenomic era. *J Mol Diagn*. 2013;15:158–170.

54. Klaassen S, Probst S, Oechslin E, et al. Mutations in sarcomere protein genes in left ventricular noncompaction. *Circulation*. 2008;117:2893–2901.

55. Shan L, Makita N, Xing Y, et al. SCN5A variants in Japanese patients with left ventricular noncompaction and arrhythmia. *Mol Genet Metab*. 2008;93:468–474.

56. Finsterer J, Stöllberger C. Primary myopathies and the heart. *Scand Cardiovasc J*. 2008;42:9–24.

57. Tang S, Batra A, Zhang Y, et al. Left ventricular noncompaction is associated with mutations in the mitochondrial genome. *Mitochondrion*. 2010;10:350–357.

58. Ackerman MJ, Priori SG, Willems S, et al. Heart Rhythm Society (HRS); European Heart Rhythm Association (EHRA). HRS/EHRA expert consensus statement on the state of genetic testing for the channelopathies and cardiomyopathies: this document was developed as a partnership between the Heart Rhythm Society (HRS) and the European Heart Rhythm Association (EHRA). *Europace*. 2011;13:1077–1109.

59. Bertini M, Ziacchi M, Biffi M, et al. Effects of cardiac resynchronisation therapy on dilated cardiomyopathy with isolated ventricular non-compaction. *Heart*. 2011;97:295–300.

60. Stöllberger C, Wegner C, Finsterer J. CHADS2- and CHA2DS2VASc scores and embolic risk in left ventricular hypertrabeculation/noncompaction. *J Stroke Cerebrovasc Dis*. 2013;22:709–712.

61. Lip GY, Piotrponikowski P, Andreotti F, et al. Heart Failure Association (EHFA) of the European Society of Cardiology (ESC) and the ESC Working Group on Thrombosis. Thromboembolism and antithrombotic therapy for heart failure in sinus rhythm: an executive summary of a joint consensus document from the ESC Heart Failure Association and the ESC Working Group on Thrombosis. *Thromb Haemost*. 2012;108:1009–1022.

62. Brouwers C, Caliskan K, Bos S, et al. Health status and psychological distress in patients with non-compaction cardiomyopathy: the role of burden related to symptoms and genetic vulnerability. *Int J Behav Med*. 2015;22:717–725.

91 Ventricular Arrhythmias in Takotsubo Cardiomyopathy

Abhiram Prasad

Takotsubo cardiomyopathy (TC), also known as *apical ballooning syndrome* or *stress cardiomyopathy*, is a reversible cause of left ventricular dysfunction that is frequently precipitated by an emotionally or physically stressful event.[1-5] Dote and colleagues first reported the occurrence of an unusual systolic left ventricular configuration in patients suspected of an acute myocardial infarction (MI).[6] They coined the term "takotsubo cardiomyopathy" due to the resemblance of the left ventricle in systole to a Japanese octopus trapping pot (takotsubo) that has a round bottom and narrow neck. Tsuchihashi and associates, also from Japan, published the first multicenter study and called the condition "left ventricular apical ballooning syndrome"[7]; it was following this paper that the cardiomyopathy started being recognized across the world.[8,9] The pathophysiology of TC is not well understood, but catecholamine-mediated myocardial toxicity and accompanying microvascular dysfunction are believed to play a major role.[1,10-12] The electrocardiographic (ECG) abnormalities of TC resemble those seen in acute coronary syndromes. ST-segment elevation is present in a significant proportion of patients,[13,14] most commonly involving the precordial leads. Some patients have widespread deep T wave inversion (TWI) and prolongation of the corrected QT interval at presentation on the ECG; in others the repolarization abnormalities develop over the first 2–3 days of hospitalization, especially in the precordial leads.[15-17] Thus TC may be considered among the causes of acquired long QT syndrome (LQTS),[18,19] a syndrome associated with sudden cardiac death (SCD) due to reentrant polymorphic ventricular tachyarrhythmia and torsades de pointes (TdP), which can degenerate to ventricular fibrillation (VF). However, the risk factors and potential mechanism of life-threatening arrhythmias in TC remain incompletely understood.

Clinical Characteristics of Takotsubo Cardiomyopathy

The incidence of TC is estimated at 1%–2% of patients initially suspected of an acute coronary syndrome,[1,8,20] although its diagnosis is increasing over time.[21] TC patients are predominantly females, accounting for 80%–100% of cases in different series.[2,4,5] The women are typically postmenopausal, with peak incidence in the seventh and eighth decades of life.[21] Chest pain, similar to that experienced with angina, and dyspnea are the most common presenting symptoms. The symptoms and signs are similar to those seen in other acute cardiac conditions characterized by acute myocardial ischemia or heart failure and hence do not help in the differential diagnosis.[22]

TC is characterized by decreased left ventricular ejection fraction on presentation, and generally, recovery of normal systolic function occurs over a period of days to weeks. The typical wall motion abnormality (hypokinesis to dyskinesis) involves the apical and mid-ventricular segments, with the distribution extending beyond a single epicardial coronary distribution (Fig. 91.1). Other patterns of regional wall motion abnormalities include the mid-ventricular and reverse variants.[1] Transient right ventricular systolic dysfunction may coexist in approximately 30%–50% of patients and is associated with lower left ventricular ejection fraction, greater likelihood of acute heart failure, and longer hospitalization.[23,24] The right ventricular apex is most frequently involved, and the regional wall motion abnormalities resolve over time. Acute heart failure occurs in approximately 40% of patients, and cardiogenic shock necessitating intraaortic balloon counterpulsation occurs in up to 10%–20% of cases.[22,25] Other complications include dynamic left ventricular outflow tract obstruction and acute mitral regurgitation due to transient valve dysfunction. Rare complications include thrombus formation in the ventricle and cardiac rupture.[1,4,5] The lack of a diagnostic test and the heterogeneity in clinical presentations necessitate the use of diagnostic criteria that encompass the broadest defining features of TC. The Mayo Clinic diagnostic criteria have been widely utilized and are based on an expert consensus.[1]

Virtually all patients have elevated blood levels of cardiac troponin, and the great majority have an elevation of creatine kinase–MB fraction. The troponin T levels peak over the first 24 hours followed by a gradual fall, although the peak levels are significantly lower than those seen in ST-segment elevation MI.[1] TC patients usually have either normal coronary arteries or nonobstructive coronary artery disease; however, obstructive disease may coexist in a small proportion of patients.[26,27] Cardiac magnetic resonance imaging is helpful in differentiating TC from acute MI and myocarditis because, typically, the TC patients do not demonstrate delayed gadolinium enhancement.[28] The vast majority of patients with TC have good prognosis. In-hospital mortality in older studies has been reported to be approximately 2%,[5,29] but more recent studies have found rates closer to 4%,[22,30] similar to that of an acute MI. Among those who make a recovery and are discharged, long-term survival has been reported to be similar to that for the age- and gender-matched population in one study.[29] In another study, increased mortality in the first year after the index event was noted; however, all the deaths were noncardiac (mostly due to cancer).[5] Recurrence rates have been estimated at 1%–2% per year.[5,29]

Electrocardiographic Changes

The ECG findings at presentation are often those associated with myocardial ischemia or an injury pattern. ST-segment elevation occurs in approximately 30%–50% of cases. Other findings include deep TWI, ST-segment depression, anterior Q waves, bundle branch block, and minor nonspecific abnormalities; furthermore, in some patients the ECG may be normal.[5,13,14,16,17,28] TC is associated with less ST-segment elevation compared with

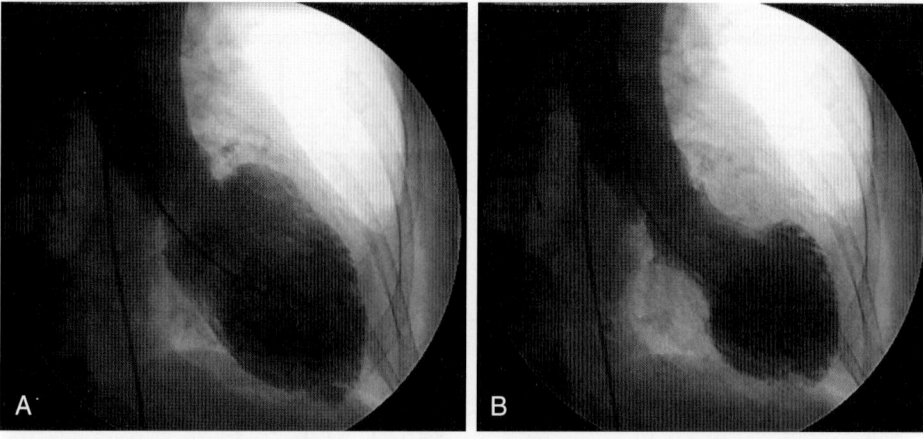

FIGURE 91.1 The left ventriculogram in a patient with takotsubo cardiomyopathy in the right anterior oblique projection: (A) end-diastole; (B) end-systole. An extensive area of akinesis involving the apical and mid-ventricular segments with hyperkinesis of the base results in a balloon-like appearance of the left ventricle.

anterior MI, but with involvement of a greater number of leads and a greater frequency of involvement of limb leads. Abnormal Q waves and reciprocal changes are less frequent and transient.[31] Various ECG criteria have been proposed to differentiate ST-segment elevation MI from TC, but none have sufficient accuracy to be used in clinical practice.[32,33]

In the subacute phase (days 2–3), if present, the ST-segment elevation resolves. TWI is frequently observed and is more widespread and deeper when compared with that in patients who sustain anterior MI. The TWI often progresses and deepens over time, with the negative peak usually occurring 2–3 days following admission. The TWI subsequently diminishes; however, in some patients, a second phase of TWI may develop that lasts for days to weeks, even after systolic function has recovered.[15–17]

QT interval prolongation, which can be extreme, is also a common finding, and it follows a time course similar to that of the TWI, with a peak occurring at 2–3 days following admission.[15–17,34] The frequency ranges from 50% to as high as 100% in various case series.[1–5,19] The QT interval recovers over days in conjunction with resolution of the TWI. In patients with a biphasic pattern of TWI, the QT interval lengthens again, but not to the extent seen during the subacute phase. The precise time course of QT interval recovery is not well defined, but repolarization changes can persist for weeks and beyond the period of wall motion recovery.[16,17]

Migliore and colleagues have proposed that myocardial edema, which occurs frequently in TC, may be the cause of the subacute ECG repolarization abnormalities.[28,35] They cite the following facts: (1) there is a parallel time course for the development and resolution of ventricular repolarization abnormalities and myocardial edema, (2) a correlation is present between the extent of ECG changes and the magnitude of edema, and (3) in some cases there is colocalization of the repolarization abnormalities on the ECG and regional distribution of myocardial edema.

The ECG patterns described above relate to the common apical ballooning variant of TC. Whether the same is true for other less frequently occurring variants is not clear, although some studies suggest that differences may exist.[36]

Ventricular Arrhythmias

Supraventricular arrhythmias such as atrial fibrillation and supraventricular tachycardia, as well as bradycardia and heart block, have been reported in TC. However, this chapter will limit the discussion to ventricular arrhythmias, which are increasingly recognized as an important clinical entity in TC.[37] The reported

prevalence of ventricular arrhythmias in TC has varied between publications. Early single-center studies found relatively low rates, with Syed and associates reporting a sustained VT or VF frequency of 3.4% in their comprehensive literature review.[37] A similar rate of 4.2% was found in a more recent analysis from the National Inpatient Sample administrative database which analyzed 16,450 patients.[38] However, other publications suggest that the frequency may be higher, with a figure of 8.9% reported by Madias and colleagues,[15] and 9.6% from a single-center German registry of 178 patients.[39] The latter study was unique in that it provided follow-up data for patients with ventricular arrhythmias. The occurrence of VT or VF was associated with a higher 1-year mortality in a univariate analysis, with a separation in the survival within the first 2 months.

The clinical manifestations of TC often follow a time course that can be broadly divided into acute (day 1), subacute (days 2–3), and recovery (>day 3) phases,[16,17,34] with the arrhythmic risk, and potentially the mechanisms, changing over time.[15] The most common mechanism of ventricular arrhythmia during the subacute phase appears to be pause-dependent TdP or VF associated with QT interval prolongation (Fig. 91.2).[15,40] Even though TWI may be present at presentation, the arrhythmic risk appears to be greatest in the subacute phase, when QT interval prolongation is maximal.[16,17,34]

The earliest report of TdP in the setting of TC was published in 2005,[18] and several subsequent reports and series have confirmed the association. In a case series of 93 TC patients, there were 8 who developed sustained ventricular arrhythmias; 2 patients had VF in the acute phase and 6 had pause-dependent TdP or VF in the subacute phase, associated with substantial QT interval prolongation.[15] The QTc interval at presentation was longer in patients with VF and TdP than in those without ventricular arrhythmias. The QTc increased further in the subacute phase in both groups and by the fifth hospital day, resolved to a similar extent (Fig. 91.3). Patients with ventricular arrhythmias had longer maximal QT intervals (581 [568–679] vs. 488 [465–519] ms; p = .0003).[15] This pattern of arrhythmic risk and QT interval prolongation has also been described by Behr and Mahida.[40] In a literature review, these authors identified 11 cases of TdP associated with TC and found a mean QTc interval at presentation of 595 ms and a mean maximal QTc interval of 706 ms. In another retrospective literature review, Samuelov-Kinori et al. identified 15 cases of TdP associated with TC.[19] Again, the mean maximal QTc interval was longer among patients with TdP than in those without (679.9 ± 230.6 vs. 555.9 ± 63.8 ms; p = .06).

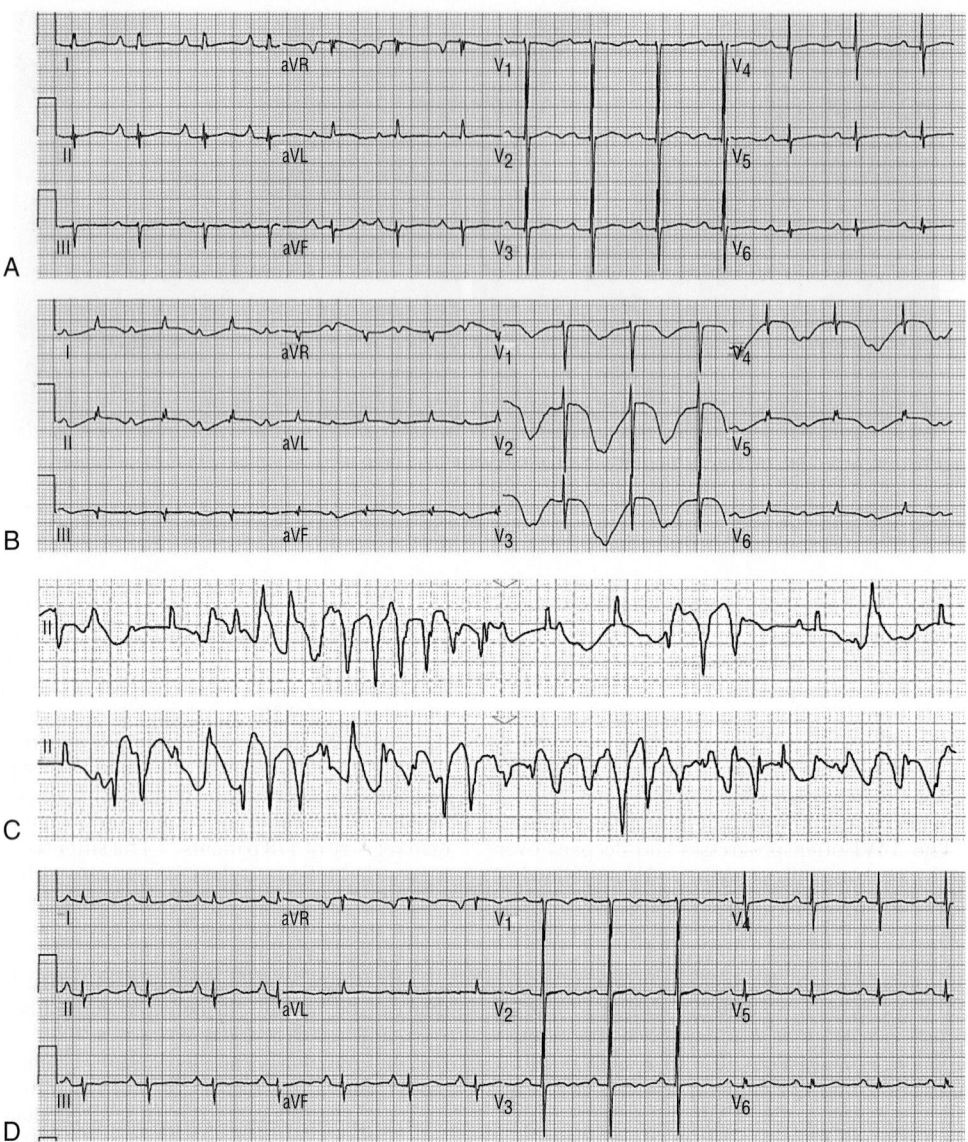

FIGURE 91.2 Electrocardiograms (ECGs) and telemetry strips from a patient with takotsubo cardiomyopathy and torsades de pointes (TdP). The patient experienced takotsubo cardiomyopathy secondary to sepsis and epinephrine infusion for hypotension. (A) Admission ECG shows first-degree atrioventricular block with QT interval prolongation and diffuse nonspecific T wave abnormalities. (B) ECG 24 hours after epinephrine infusion shows long first-degree atrioventricular block with diffuse T wave inversions and marked QT interval prolongation. (C) Telemetry strips show heart block and junctional escape rhythm with premature ventricular contractions triggering runs of torsades de pointes. The patient was managed with temporary pacing. (D) ECG several months later shows resolution of T wave inversions and normalization of PR- and QT intervals.

In comparison, ventricular arrhythmias appear to be rare during the acute phase. VT or VF is an infrequent mode of presentation of TC.[5,15,37] Thus there are two possibilities regarding ventricular arrhythmias in the acute phase. First, the mechanism is distinct from that in the subacute phase. Second, TC may not be the arrhythmic trigger but rather a consequence of the stress associated with a major cardiac arrhythmia/arrest and the subsequent resuscitation.[15] A study by Singh and associates provides some insights into these hypotheses.[41] In a literature review, they found 77 published cases of cardiac arrest associated with TC. These were predominantly due to ventricular arrhythmia. Patients in whom the cardiac arrest occurred prior to the diagnosis of TC were younger (49.5 ± 16 vs. 64.9 ± 11 years) and had a shorter QTc interval (530 ± 16 vs. 616 ± 140 ms) at the time of the cardiac arrest. Hypotension appeared to be a mediating factor in TC-related cardiac arrest in the acute phase. Syed and associates have reported in their review article that ventricular arrhythmia–related cardiac arrest occurred in 1.1% of TC cases during the index hospitalization.[37] However, a word of caution is required regarding the estimation of the frequency of life-threatening arrhythmias in the acute phase of TC. It is possible that the actual incidence of SCD due to TC is higher, as some patients with out-of-hospital arrests may not survive to reach a hospital for a diagnosis to be made. Autopsies are infrequently performed, and even when conducted, TC hearts may have a relatively normal appearance. It is worth noting that SCD is not a feature of TC during long-term follow-up.[5,29,42]

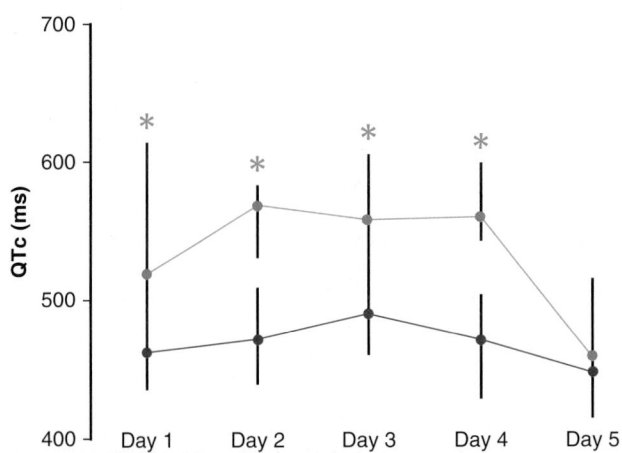

FIGURE 91.3 Time course of QT prolongation in patients with takotsubo cardiomyopathy and ventricular arrhythmias. Patients with takotsubo cardiomyopathy and ventricular arrhythmias *(blue)* show longer QTc intervals on presentation than those with takotsubo cardiomyopathy without ventricular arrhythmias *(red)*. During the subacute phase (days 2–3), QTc intervals are further prolonged significantly in patients with ventricular arrhythmias. By day 5, QTc intervals return to similar levels in both groups. Data shown are median QTc intervals with interquartile range (*p < .05). (From Madias C, Fitzgibbons TP, Alsheikh-Ali AA, et al. Acquired long QT syndrome from stress cardiomyopathy is associated with ventricular arrhythmias and torsades de pointes. *Heart Rhythm.* 2011;8:555-561.)

Pathogenesis of Ventricular Arrhythmias

The mechanisms of life-threatening ventricular arrhythmia in TC remain incompletely understood. The pathogenesis likely involves a complex interaction and dysfunction of the autonomic system, myocardial structure and function, electrical remodeling, and potentially genetic factors.

In the more common scenario of acute MI, TdP is also infrequent, but when it occurs, it is also in the subacute phase (>48 hours). In a series of eight patients with acute MI who developed pause-dependent TdP, diffuse TWI and severe QT interval prolongation were observed in each case.[43] The timing of QT interval prolongation was similar to that observed in TC, peaking in the subacute phase. Although obstructive coronary disease is not a feature of TC, the similarities between the clinical findings and arrhythmias in TC and MI-associated TdP suggest the potential for shared mechanisms. In contrast, reentry is unlikely to be a factor in TC since scar formation is not a feature of the cardiomyopathy.

Catecholamine-mediated myocardial toxicity is the leading hypothesis for the pathophysiology of TC. Plasma catecholamine levels have been shown to be substantially elevated in some studies of TC.[1,3,10] Iatrogenic precipitation of TC has been reported to occur as a consequence of excessive administration of catecholamines.[11] Decreased ventricular iodine-metaiodobenzylguanidine uptake in TC patients also suggests impaired cardiac sympathetic innervation.[1] Further support for the neurogenic basis of myocardial stunning includes the presence of contraction band necrosis in biopsy specimens from TC patients. Contraction band necrosis is a unique form of myocardial injury that is characterized by hypercontracted sarcomeres and has been described in clinical states of catecholamine excess.[44]

Catecholamines induce calcium overload in cardiomyocytes via receptor-dependent calcium channels. Excessive local and circulating catecholamines might also induce repolarization abnormalities.[44] Moreover, similarities exist with regard to myocardial stunning and repolarization abnormalities seen in other hyperadrenergic states, such as pheochromocytoma and subarachnoid hemorrhage.[2] The sympathetic nervous system is a recognized

modulator of arrhythmic risk in the pathophysiology of LQTS. Stimulation of the left stellate ganglion has been shown to prolong the QT interval, and left cardiac sympathetic denervation is a potential treatment for recurrent arrhythmias in congenital LQTS. In pathological states associated with reduced repolarization reserve (e.g., heart failure and channelopathies such as LQTS), sympathetic stimulation can serve as a potent trigger for the generation of arrhythmia by enhancing dispersion of repolarization or by inducing after-depolarizations—the arrhythmic stimuli for TdP. When the action potential is prolonged, intracellular calcium overload can further augment ionic currents underlying after-depolarizations.[45] Early after-depolarizations may be represented by giant T-U waves in patients with TdP, and this has been observed before initiation of TC-associated TdP.[15]

SCD is an important cause of mortality in adults and is frequently associated with MI and coronary artery disease. Evidence suggests that a genetic predisposition might increase the risk of arrhythmic death in acute coronary events.[46] The incidence of TdP in the setting of MI was estimated to be 1.8% in one series.[43] A genetic basis for TdP in MI has been reported in the presence of deep TWI and QT interval prolongation.[47] Among 13 such patients who developed TdP in the subacute phase of an MI, 2 were found to carry long QT mutations (*KCNH2-R744X* and *SCN5A-E446K*). Of the remaining 11 patients, 9 carried the *KCNH2-K897T* polymorphism, which was present in only 35% of the controls (*p* = .0035). The polymorphism was associated with an eight-fold increased risk of TdP.[47] The *KCNH2-K897T* polymorphism also modulates the arrhythmic risk of sudden death in congenital LQTS.[48]

The concept of an abnormal repolarization reserve has been used to describe the impact of QT interval–prolonging drugs in susceptible individuals who may carry clinically silent or unexpressed mutations implicated in congenital LQTS.[49] The previously described studies suggest that such polymorphisms also reduce repolarization reserve and increase arrhythmic risk in the subacute phase of MI. Thus subclinical genetic predispositions may become clinically significant in the setting of ischemic events or pharmacological therapies.[47] There is a distinct possibility that this is relevant to TC, as is suggested by cases in which there is persistent QT interval prolongation following TdP.[40,50,51] In one such case, congenital LQTS was uncovered when genetic testing revealed a mutation in the *KCNH2* gene.

Management

Telemetry monitoring is recommended through the first 48–72 hours following presentation. A longer duration of monitoring may be indicated if QT interval prolongation persists. A QTc interval of >500 ms may be a useful cutoff for predicting the arrhythmic risk for TdP,[40] together with the presence of bradycardia, atrioventricular block, and perhaps male sex.[19] TdP should be treated by eliminating the associated bradycardia and ventricular pauses using temporary pacing. Isoproterenol is rarely used in current practice and would be inappropriate in TC given the role of catecholamines in inducing the cardiomyopathy.

Long-term β-blocker therapy is used on an empiric basis.[1,5,28] Combined α- and β-receptor antagonists may be preferred. Therapy should be initiated cautiously in the presence of bradycardia or severe QT interval prolongation[3,15] and should be withheld if TdP occurs until the bradycardia and QT interval prolongation have resolved. It is unknown whether β-blockers modify the acute risk for ventricular arrhythmia or the likelihood of recurrence.[5]

Hypokalemia may occur due to catecholamine excess or diuretic use, and it is advisable to maintain serum potassium levels in the high-normal range. With this in mind, urgent potassium supplementation should be considered in patients who develop TdP or VF and in those with severe QT interval prolongation. Magnesium supplementation to maintain levels at the upper end of the normal range also seems reasonable. Medications that potentially prolong the QT interval should be avoided.

The long-term risk among those who suffer SCD or life-threatening ventricular arrhythmia remains unclear. Women who have recovered from TC have augmented sympathetic activation in response to acute mental stress.[52] Whether this impacts the risk for recurrent arrhythmia is unknown, and hence it is not possible to make definitive recommendations regarding device therapy. The decision needs to be individualized, with implantation of a permanent pacemaker or defibrillator being considered for patients with persistent bradycardia or QT interval prolongation.[15,37]

Conclusions

TC is generally associated with a good prognosis, but life-threatening ventricular arrhythmias may occur in approximately 5% of cases. The mechanism for the arrhythmias may vary during the acute and subacute phases, the latter being associated with QT interval prolongation and pause-dependent TdP. Thus TC may be considered a cause for acquired LQTS, and patients with a prolonged QT interval should be monitored on a telemetry unit until there is recovery of the repolarization abnormality. Further research is required to understand the mechanisms and risk of arrhythmias in TC.

REFERENCES

1. Prasad A, Lerman A, Rihal CS. Apical ballooning syndrome (tako-tsubo or stress cardiomyopathy): a mimic of acute myocardial infarction. *Am Heart J*. 2008;155:408–417.
2. Bybee K, Prasad A. Stress-related cardiomyopathy syndromes. *Circulation*. 2008;118:397–409.
3. Akashi YJ, Goldstein DS, Barbaro G, et al. Takotsubo cardiomyopathy: a new form of acute, reversible heart failure. *Circulation*. 2008;118:2754–2762.
4. Gianni M, Dentali F, Grandi AM, et al. Apical ballooning syndrome or takotsubo cardiomyopathy: a systematic review. *Eur Heart J*. 2006;27:1523–1529.
5. Sharkey SW, Windenburg DC, Lesser JR, et al. Natural history and expansive clinical profile of stress (tako-tsubo) cardiomyopathy. *J Am Coll Cardiol*. 2010;55:333–341.
6. Dote K, Sato H, Tateishi H, Uchida T, Ishihara M. [Myocardial stunning due to simultaneous multivessel coronary spasms: a review of 5 cases]. *J Cardiol*. 1991;21:203–214.
7. Tsuchihashi K, Ueshima K, Uchida T, et al. Transient left ventricular apical ballooning without coronary artery stenosis: a novel heart syndrome mimicking acute myocardial infarction. Angina Pectoris-Myocardial Infarction Investigations in Japan. *J Am Coll Cardiol*. 2001;38:11–18.
8. Bybee KA, Prasad A, Barsness G, et al. Clinical characteristics, outcomes, and impaired myocardial microcirculation in patients with transient left ventricular apical ballooning syndrome: a case-series from a US medical center. *Am J Cardiol*. 2004;94:343–346.
9. Desmet WJ, Adriaenssens BF, Dens JA. Apical ballooning of the left ventricle: first series in white patients. *Heart*. 2003;89:1027–1031.
10. Wittstein IS, Thiemann DR, Lima JA, et al. Neurohumoral features of myocardial stunning due to sudden emotional stress. *N Engl J Med*. 2005;352:539–548.
11. Abraham J, Mudd JO, Kapur N, et al. Stress cardiomyopathy after intravenous administration of catecholamines and beta-receptor agonists. *J Am Coll Cardiol*. 2009;53:1320–1325.
12. Paur H, Wright PT, Sikkel MB. High levels of circulating epinephrine trigger apical cardiodepression in a β2-adrenergic receptor/Gi-dependent manner: a new model of takotsubo cardiomyopathy. *Circulation*. 2012;126:697–706.
13. Sharkey SW, Lesser JR, Menon M, et al. Spectrum and significance of electrocardiographic patterns, troponin levels, and thrombolysis in myocardial infarction frame count in patients with stress (tako-tsubo) cardiomyopathy and comparison to those in patients with ST-elevation anterior wall myocardial infarction. *Am J Cardiol*. 2008;101:1723–1728.
14. Dib C, Asirvatham S, Elesber A, et al. Clinical correlates and prognostic significance of electrocardiographic abnormalities in apical ballooning syndrome (takotsubo/stress-induced cardiomyopathy). *Am Heart J*. 2009;157:933–938.
15. Madias C, Fitzgibbons TP, Alsheikh-Ali AA, et al. Acquired long QT syndrome from stress cardiomyopathy is associated with ventricular arrhythmias and torsades de pointes. *Heart Rhythm*. 2011;8:555–561.
16. Kurisu S, Inoue I, Kawagoe T, et al. Time course of electrocardiographic changes in patients with tako-tsubo syndrome: comparison with acute myocardial infarction with minimal enzymatic release. *Circ J*. 2004;68:77–81.
17. Mitsuma W, Kodama M, Ito M, et al. Serial electrocardiographic findings in women with tako-tsubo cardiomyopathy. *Am J Cardiol*. 2007;100:106–109.

18. Denney SD, Lakkireddy DR, Khan IA. Long QT syndrome and torsade de pointes in transient left ventricular apical ballooning syndrome. *Int J Cardiol*. 2005;100:499–501.
19. Samuelov-Kinori L, Kinori M, Kogan Y, et al. Takotsubo cardiomyopathy and QT interval prolongation: who are the patients at risk for torsades de pointes? *J Electrocardiol*. 2009;42:353–357.
20. Parodi G, Del Pace S, Carrabba N, et al. Incidence, clinical findings, and outcome of women with left ventricular apical ballooning syndrome. *Am J Cardiol*. 2007;99:182–185.
21. Minhas AS, Hughey AB, Kolias TJ. Nationwide trends in reported incidence of takotsubo cardiomyopathy from 2006 to 2012. *Am J Cardiol*. 2015;116:1128–1131.
22. Templin C, Ghadri JR, Diekmann J, et al. Clinical features and outcomes of takotsubo (stress) cardiomyopathy. *New Engl J Med*. 2015;373:929–938.
23. Elesber AA, Prasad A, Bybee KA, et al. Transient cardiac apical ballooning syndrome: prevalence and clinical implications of right ventricular involvement. *J Am Coll Cardiol*. 2006;47:1082–1083.
24. Haghi D, Athanasiadis A, Papavassiliu T, et al. Right ventricular involvement in takotsubo cardiomyopathy. *Eur Heart J*. 2006;27:2433–2439.
25. Madhavan M, Rihal CS, Lerman A, Prasad A. Acute heart failure in apical ballooning syndrome (takotsubo/stress cardiomyopathy): clinical correlates and Mayo Clinic risk score. *J Am Coll Cardiol*. 2011;57:1400–1401.
26. Hoyt J, Lerman A, Lennon RJ, Rihal CS, Prasad A. Left anterior descending artery length and coronary atherosclerosis in apical ballooning syndrome (takotsubo/stress induced cardiomyopathy). *Int J Cardiol*. 2010;145:112–115.
27. Gaibazzi N, Ugo F, Vignali L, et al. Tako-Tsubo cardiomyopathy with coronary artery stenosis: a case-series challenging the original definition. *Int J Cardiol*. 2009;133:205–212.
28. Eitel I, von Knobelsdorff-Brenkenhoff F, Bernhardt P, et al. Clinical characteristics and cardiovascular magnetic resonance findings in stress (takotsubo) cardiomyopathy. *JAMA*. 2011;306:277–286.
29. Elesber AA, Prasad A, Lennon RJ, et al. Four-year recurrence rate and prognosis of the apical ballooning syndrome. *J Am Coll Cardiol*. 2007;50:448–452.
30. Brinjikji W, El-Sayed AM, Salka S. In-hospital mortality among patients with takotsubo cardiomyopathy: a study of the National Inpatient Sample 2008 to 2009. *Am Heart J*. 2012;164:215–221.
31. Kosuge M, Ebina T, Hibi K, et al. Simple and accurate electrocardiographic criteria to differentiate takotsubo cardiomyopathy from anterior acute myocardial infarction. *J Am Coll Cardiol*. 2010;55:2514–2516.
32. Bybee KA, Motiei A, Syed IS, et al. Electrocardiography cannot reliably differentiate transient left ventricular apical ballooning syndrome from anterior ST-segment elevation myocardial infarction. *J Electrocardiol*. 2007;40:38. e1-e6.
33. Scantlebury D, Prasad A. Diagnosis of takotsubo cardiomyopathy. *Circ J*. 2014;78:2129–2139.
34. Matsuoka K, Okubo S, Fujii E, et al. Evaluation of the arrhythmogenicity of stress-induced "takotsubo cardiomyopathy" from the time course of the 12-lead surface electrocardiogram. *Am J Cardiol*. 2003;92:230–233.

35. Migliore F, Zorzi A, Perazzalo M, et al. Myocardial edema as a substrate of electrocardiographic abnormalities and life-threatening arrhythmias in reversible ventricular dysfunction of takotsubo cardiomyopathy: imaging evidence, presumed mechanisms, and implications for therapy. *Heart Rhythm*. 2015;12:1867–1877.
36. Hahn JY, Gwon HC, Park SW, et al. The clinical features of transient left ventricular nonapical ballooning syndrome: comparison with apical ballooning syndrome. *Am Heart J*. 2007;154:1166–1173.
37. Syed FF, Asirvatham SJ, Francis J. Arrhythmia occurrence with takotsubo cardiomyopathy: a literature review. *Europace*. 2011;13:780–788.
38. Pant S, Deshmukh A, Mehta K, et al. Burden of arrhythmias in patients with takotsubo cardiomyopathy (apical ballooning syndrome). *International J Cardiol*. 2013;170:64–68.
39. Stiermaier T, Eitel C, Denef S, et al. Prevalence and clinical significance of life-threatening arrhythmias in takotsubo cardiomyopathy. *J Am Coll Cardiol*. 2015;65:2148–2150.
40. Behr ER, Mahida S. Takotsubo cardiomyopathy and the long-QT syndrome: an insult to repolarization reserve. *Europace*. 2009;11:697–700.
41. Singh K, Carson K, Hibbert B, Le May M. Natural history of cardiac arrest in patients with takotsubo cardiomyopathy. *Am J Cardiol*. 2015;115:1466–1472.
42. Liang J, Cha YM, Oh JK, Prasad A. Sudden cardiac death: an increasingly recognized presentation of apical ballooning syndrome (takotsubo cardiomyopathy). *Heart Lung*. 2013;42:270–272.
43. Halkin A, Roth A, Lurie I, et al. Pause-dependent torsade de pointes following acute myocardial infarction: a variant of the acquired long QT syndrome. *J Am Coll Cardiol*. 2001;38:1168–1174.
44. Samuels MA. The brain-heart connection. *Circulation*. 2007;116:77–84.
45. Zipes DP, Rubart M. Neural modulation of cardiac arrhythmias and sudden cardiac death. *Heart Rhythm*. 2006;3:108–113.
46. Bezzina CR, Pazoki R, Bardai A, et al. Genome-wide association study identifies a susceptibility locus at 21q21 for ventricular fibrillation in acute myocardial infarction. *Nat Genet*. 2010;42:688–691.
47. Crotti L, Hu D, Barajas-Martinez H, et al. Torsades de pointes following acute myocardial infarction: evidence for a deadly link with a common genetic variant. *Heart Rhythm*. 2012;9:1104–1112.
48. Crotti L, Lundquist AL, Insolia R, et al. KCNH2-K897T is a genetic modifier of latent congenital long-QT syndrome. *Circulation*. 2005;112:1251–1258.
49. Roden DM. Long QT syndrome: reduced repolarization reserve and the genetic link. *J Intern Med*. 2006;259:59–69.
50. Grilo LS, Pruvot E, Grobety M, et al. Takotsubo cardiomyopathy and congenital long QT syndrome in a patient with a novel duplication in the Per-Arnt-Sim (PAS) domain of hERG1. *Heart Rhythm*. 2010;7:260–265.
51. Gupta A, Lawrence AT, Krishnan K, et al. Current concepts in the mechanisms and management of drug-induced QT prolongation and torsade de pointes. *Am Heart J*. 2007;153:891–899.
52. Martin EA, Prasad A, Rihal CS, et al. Endothelial function and vascular response to mental stress are impaired in patients with apical ballooning syndrome. *J Am Coll Cardiol*. 2010;56:1840–1846.

92

Brugada Syndrome

Pedro Brugada

In 1992, a manuscript titled "Right bundle branch block, persistent ST segment elevation and sudden cardiac death: a distinct clinical and electrocardiographical syndrome" was published in the *Journal of the American College of Cardiology*.[1] This publication described eight individuals with a common phenotype: all had a structurally normal heart and had been resuscitated from sudden cardiac death (SCD) caused by documented ventricular fibrillation (VF). All of them had a characteristic ST-segment elevation in the right precordial leads (Fig. 92.1). It looked like a scientific curiosity; however, after all these years, this syndrome, now known as Brugada syndrome (BrS), is recognized as a major disease that integrated previous syndromes such as idiopathic VF, sudden unexplained death syndrome, and some forms of sudden infant death syndrome. Nowadays, the overlapping syndromes with BrS and long or short QT interval bring all these syndromes into a clear pathophysiological background: alteration of ionic currents leading to depolarization and for repolarization abnormalities and ventricular arrhythmias. At least 19 different genetic variants of BrS are known nowadays, with more than 300 mutations reported and most of them only located in the *SCN5A* gene. The extremely wide genetic heterogeneity of BrS and other inherited cardiac disorders makes this new arena of genetic arrhythmology an interesting one. In this chapter, we will review the present knowledge, progress made, and future research directions on BrS.

Electrocardiographical Features

The diagnosis of BrS is based on clinical and electrocardiographical features. Patients present with syncope or (aborted) SCD due to malignant ventricular arrhythmias; however, others are completely asymptomatic. Per definition, apparent structural heart disease can be found. The hallmark of BrS is the transient or persistent appearance of typical electrocardiogram (ECG) changes in the right precordial leads. The second Brugada Syndrome Consensus Report of 2005 (endorsed by the Heart Rhythm Society and the European Heart Rhythm Association)[2] stated the current recommendations regarding the diagnostic criteria. Three different ECG patterns (see Fig. 92.1), all featuring ST-segment elevation in the right precordial leads, have been recognized: type

I is the only pattern that is diagnostic for BrS. It consists of a coved-type ST-segment elevation greater than 2 mm, followed by a descending negative T wave in at least one right precordial lead (V_1–V_3). Types II and III are saddleback-shaped patterns, with a high initial augmentation followed by an ST-segment elevation greater than 2 mm for type II and less than 2 mm for type III. Both patterns are suggestive of, but not diagnostic for, BrS.

Whenever a large number of baseline ECGs were available during follow-up, the diagnostic pattern could be documented in only approximately 25% of the tracings. Almost every individual with a type I ECG will show normalization of the ECG during follow-up. Because the presence of the spontaneous coved-type (type I) ECG pattern is a useful predictor of future arrhythmic events in asymptomatic patients, this variation of the ECG pattern is of great clinical importance. The class IC antiarrhythmic drug test provided a tool to unmask these concealed forms. Intravenous administration of ajmaline, flecainide, or procainamide is able to elicit the diagnostic coved-type BrS ECG pattern (Fig. 92.2). On the basis of the results of comparative studies, ajmaline, in a dose of 1 mg/kg, appears to be the best drug. The full stomach test was proposed as an alternative tool in diagnosing BrS.[3] Here, the ST segment changes appear to be provoked by an enhanced vagal tone. Adrenergic stimulation decreases the ST-segment elevation, whereas vagal stimulation increases it. Obviously, it is important to exclude other causes of ST-segment elevation before making the diagnosis of BrS (Table 92.1).

Genetics

BrS is a familial disease with an autosomal dominant pattern of inheritance. To date, nearly 300 pathogenic variants in 19 genes have been published (Table 92.2). The first gene associated with BrS was *SCN5A*, which encodes the α-subunit of the cardiac sodium channel.[4] The *SCN5A* gene is responsible for phase 0 of the cardiac action potential. Mutations in *SCN5A* result in loss of function of the sodium channel. Twenty percent to 25% of patients with BrS have a mutation in the *SCN5A* gene, classified as BrS type 1.[5] Recently, an individual diagnosed with BrS and concomitant conduction system disease had a large-scale deletion of the *SCN5A* gene.[6] This copy number variation (CNV) is the only rearrangement identified as a cause of the disease to date. Despite these ongoing developments in understanding the genetic causes of BrS, only 30%–35% of clinically diagnosed cases are genetically diagnosed, and most of these (25%–30%) result from pathogenic alterations in *SCN5A*.[5] In a recent study, a comprehensive genetic evaluation of main BrS-susceptibility genes and CNV in a Spanish BrS cohort has been published. Selga and colleagues report that the mean pathogenic variation discovery yield is higher than that described for other European BrS cohorts (32.7% vs. 20%–25%, respectively) and is even higher for patients in the age range of 30–50 years.[7]

There have also been published mutations in sodium channel beta-1 subunit (*SCN1B*),[8] sodium channel beta-2 subunit (*SCN2B*), and sodium channel beta-3 subunit (*SCN3B*),[9] which modify the function of the channel (increasing or decreasing I_{Na}).[8–10] Recently, the *SCN10A* gene (neuronal sodium channel $Na_V1.8$) has been shown to modulate *SCN5A* expression and the electrical function of the heart.[11] Another gene reported as

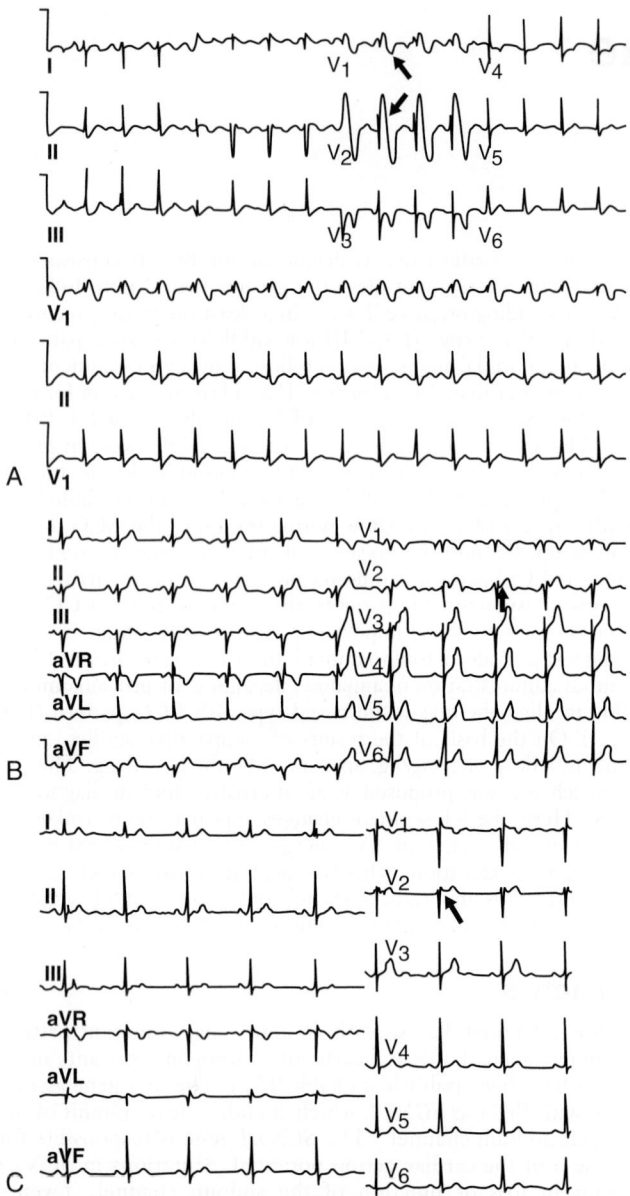

FIGURE 92.1 Brugada electrocardiogram (ECG) patterns. (A) A diagnostic coved-type (type I) Brugada ECG pattern documented in a 9-year-old girl who presented with syncope and positive family history of Brugada syndrome. Note the pattern resembles a right bundle branch block (*arrows*) in leads V_1 and V_2, with typical ST-segment elevation. (B) Baseline ECG of a 58-year-old asymptomatic man with a positive family history of Brugada syndrome. Example of a type II saddleback Brugada ECG pattern. Genetic analysis revealed a mutation in the *SCN5A* gene. Note the saddleback-shaped patterns, with a high initial augmentation followed by ST-segment elevation greater than 2 mm in lead V_2. (C) Example of a baseline type III saddleback Brugada ECG pattern (*arrow*) documented in a 61-year-old asymptomatic man who was diagnosed based on a positive result on class IC antiarrhythmic drug testing.

responsible for BrS was *GPD1-L*. Mutations in *GPD1-L* reduce both the surface membrane expression and inward sodium current.[12] Recently, Kattygnarath and associates published a study supporting that *RANGRF* can impair the trafficking of $Na_V1.5$ to the membrane, leading to I_{Na} reduction and clinical manifestation of BrS.[13] In 2012, Ishikawa and coworkers reported pathogenic variations in the sarcolemmal membrane–associated protein (*SLMAP*) gene, a gene of unknown function that is found at T-tubules and the sarcoplasmic reticulum. SLMAP

causes BrS by modulating the intracellular trafficking of the $Na_V1.5$ channel.[14] Recently, pathogenic variations in the plakophilin-2 (*PKP2*) gene were reported to be associated with BrS.[15,16] *PKP2* is the primary gene responsible for arrhythmogenic right ventricular cardiomyopathy (ARVC), a desmosomal disease characterized by fibrofatty replacement of myocardium, leading to SCD in young men, mainly during exercise. Correlation between the loss of expression of PKP2 and reduced I_{Na} has been identified in BrS patients. Apart from sodium channels, several potassium channels have also been related to BrS. The first one described was *KCNE3*, which codifies MiRP2 protein (β-subunit that regulates the potassium channel I_{to}) and modulates some potassium currents in the heart.[17] Another gene associated with BrS is *KCNJ8*, also previously related to early repolarization syndrome (ERS).[18] *KCNJ8* was described as a novel J-wave susceptibility gene and a marker gain-of-function in the cardiac $K_{(ATP)}$ Kir6.1 channel.[19] In 2011, Giudicessi and coworkers provided the first molecular and functional evidence implicating novel *KCND3* gain-of-function mutations (Kir4.3 protein) in the pathogenesis and phenotypic expression of BrS, with enhanced I_{to} current gradient within the right ventricle where *KCND3* gene expression is the highest.[20] Furthermore, in 2011, novel variants in *KCNE5* appeared to cause gain-of-function effects on I_{to}. The *KCNE5* gene is located in the X chromosome and encodes an auxiliary β-subunit for K channels.[21] Similar is the role of sulfonylurea receptor subunit 2A (SUR2A), encoded by the ATP-binding cassette, subfamily C member 9 (*ABCC9*) gene.[22] Gain-of-function pathogenic variants in *ABCC9* induce changes in ATP-sensitive potassium (K-ATP) channels, and, when coupled with loss-of-function pathogenic variants in *SCN5A*, these pathogenic variants may underlie the severe arrhythmic phenotype of BrS. BrS was also associated with *HCN4*, which codes for HCN4 channel or If channel (hyperpolarization-activated cyclic nucleotide-gated potassium channel 4). Its mutations also predispose to inherited sick sinus syndrome (SSS) and long QT syndrome associated with bradycardia.[23] Calcium channels have also been associated with BrS. Mutations in the *CACNA1C* gene are responsible for a defective unit of the L-type calcium channel. Mutation of the *CACNB2B* gene leads to a defect in the L-type calcium channel. Both induce a loss of channel function.[24] In 2010, the *CACNA2D1* gene was reported to be responsible for BrS. The α_2/δ-subunit of voltage-dependent calcium channels regulates current density and activation/inactivation kinetics of the calcium channel.[25] Finally, pathogenic variations have also been reported in the transient receptor potential melastatin protein number 4 (*TRPM4*) gene, a calcium-activated nonselective cation channel that is a member of a large family of transient receptor potential genes.[26] This gene is involved in conduction blocks, and the consequences of pathogenic variations are diverse. Thus reduction or increase in TRPM4 channel function may reduce the availability of the sodium channel and lead to BrS.

Genetic and Environmental Modulators

In recent years, several genetic and environmental modulators of the phenotype have been described. It is well known that environment may play a role in the predisposition to arrhythmias in patients with BrS. The identification of several triggering factors of the Brugada ECG pattern and of SCD, such as fever, cocaine, electrolyte disturbances, class I antiarrhythmic medications, and a number of other noncardiac medications,[27] some of them with a genetic predisposition, has brought the need to adopt preventive measures in patients with the diagnostic ECG pattern.[28] In addition, the incomplete penetrance of the disease, as well as the variable expressivity, has brought into question the role of additional genetic factors in the final phenotype. Single nucleotide polymorphisms (SNPs) became one

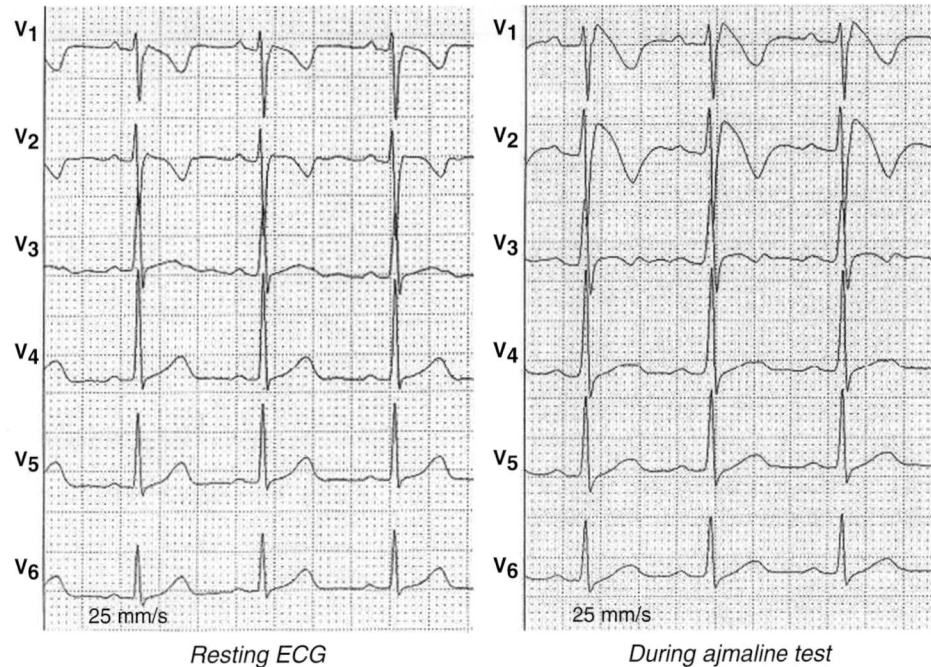

Resting ECG   During ajmaline test

FIGURE 92.2 Induction of a diagnostic coved-type (type I) electrocardiogram (*ECG*) by the administration of a sodium channel–blocking agent.

TABLE 92.1   Acquired Brugada syndrome: differential diagnosis of ST-segment elevation in electrocardiogram leads V$_1$ and V$_2$

Drugs	
Antiarrhythmic drugs	• Class 1C sodium channel blockers (e.g., flecainide, pilsicainide, propafenone)
	• Class 1A sodium channel blockers (e.g., procainamide, disopyramide, cibenzoline)
	• Verapamil (L-type calcium channel blocker)
	• β-Blockers (inhibit I$_{Ca,L}$)
Antianginal drugs	• Nitrates
	• Calcium channel blockers (e.g., nifedipine, diltiazem)
Psychotropic agents	• Tricyclic antidepressants (e.g., amitriptyline, desipramine, clomipramine, nortriptyline)
	• Tetracyclic antidepressants (e.g., maprotiline)
	• Phenothiazines (e.g., perphenazine, cyamemazine)
	• Selective serotonin uptake inhibitors (e.g., fluoxetine)
	• Cocaine intoxication
Antiallergic agents	• Histamine H1 antihistaminics. First generation (dimenhydrinate)
Acute ischemia in RVOT	
Electrolyte disturbances	• Hyperkalemia
	• Hypercalcemia
Hyperthermia and hypothermia	
Elevated insulin level	
Mechanical compression of RVOT	

RVOT, Right ventricular outflow tract.

of the first players to be studied in defining this variability. The *SCN5A* polymorphism p.H558R is present in 20% of the population. This polymorphism has been shown to partially restore the sodium current impaired by other simultaneous BrS causing mutations in *SCN5A*.[29] Thus this common variant is a genetic modulator of BrS among carriers of an *SCN5A* mutation, in whom the presence of the less common allele makes BrS less severe.[30] Genetic variants in the *SCN5A* promoter region may also play a pathophysiological role in BrS. A haplotype of six polymorphisms in the *SCN5A* promoter has been identified and functionally linked to a reduced expression of the sodium current in the Japanese population.[31] Other studies have shown the role of double mutants in causing a more severe phenotype.[32,33] The role of genetic mutation in risk stratification remains to be

clearly defined. Recent data proposed the type of genetic mutation as a tool for risk stratification in BrS. In this study, patients and relatives with a truncated protein had a more severe phenotype and more severe conduction disorders. This is the proof of concept that some of the mutations appear to confer a worse prognosis, but the use of these data in the clinical setting is not yet sufficient to make clinical decisions.[34]

Overlapping Syndromes

Several of the families studied show several phenotypes among its members. These so-called overlapping syndromes represent a tremendous challenge to physicians for diagnosis and risk stratification.

TABLE 92.2	Brugada syndrome types		
INHERITANCE	**LOCUS**	**GENE**	**PROTEIN**
(Sodium)	3p21-p24	SCN5A	Na$_V$1.5
Autosomal dominant	3p22.3	GPD1-L	Glycerol-3-P-DH-1
	19q13.1	SCN1B	Na$_V$β1
	11q24.1	SCN3B	Na$_V$β3
	11q23.3	SCN2B	Na$_V$β2
	3p22.2	SCN10A	Na$_V$1.8
	17p13.1	RANGRF	RAN-G-release factor (MOG1)
	3p14.3	SLMAP	Sarcolemma-associated protein
	12p11.21	PKP2	Plakofilin-2
(Potassium)	12p12.1	ABCC9	Adenosine triphosphate–sensitive
Autosomal dominant	11q13-q14	KCNE3	MiRP2
Chromosome X	12p12.1	KCNJ8	Kv6.1 Kir6.1
	15q24.1	HCN4	Hyperpolarization cyclic nucleotide–gated 4
	1p13.2	KCND3	Kv4.3 Kir4.3
	Xq22.3	KCNE5	Potassium voltage–gated channel subfamily E member 1
(Calcium)	2p13.3	CACNA1C	Cav1.2
Autosomal dominant	10p12.33	CACNB2B	Voltage-dependent β-2
	7q21-q22	CACNA2D1	Voltage-dependent α2/δ1
	19q13.33	TRPM4	Transient receptor potential M4

Early Repolarization Syndrome

ERS is a common ECG variant characterized by J-point elevation, ST-segment elevation with upper concavity, and prominent T waves in at least two contiguous leads.[35] ERS and BrS share cellular, ionic, and ECG similarities (appearance of J waves), representing parts of a phenotypic spectrum called "J-wave syndromes," although the degree to which ERS and BrS may overlap remains undetermined.[36] In last 5 years, reports have been published on patients with BrS and ERS.[37] ERS has been linked to mutations in CACNA1C, CACNB2, CACNA2D1, and KCNJ8.[38]

Lev-Lenègre Syndrome

Lev-Lenègre syndrome (also called progressive cardiac conduction disease [PCCD]) is a rare entity characterized by disruption of the conduction system through the His-Purkinje system, associated with syncope and even SCD. The presence of PCCD in BrS families is not uncommon as they both result from a reduction in the sodium current, and it has been described as a different expression of the same genetic phenotype. The first mutations associated with PCCD were described on SCN5A[39,40] and in its B1 subunit.[8]

Sick Sinus Syndrome

SSS is characterized by persistent inappropriate sinus bradycardia, sinus arrest, atrial standstill, and tachycardia–bradycardia syndrome, all of which are associated with dysfunction of the sinoatrial node (SAN). Patients may exhibit varied symptoms, including syncope, and even SCD. The course of SSS can be intermittent and unpredictable and is related to the severity of the underlying heart disease.[41] So far, both autosomal recessive and dominant forms have been described. In 2003, the association between SCN5A mutations and congenital SSS was reported.[42] In 2005, a novel SCN5A mutation was identified in patients presenting with both SSS and BrS,[43] showing that in the same family, both diseases may be related to the expression of a loss-of-function mutation in I_{Na}.

Atrial Fibrillation

Atrial fibrillation (AF) is the most common atrial arrhythmia found in BrS.[44] It is of extreme clinical importance to realize that AF can be the first manifestation of BrS. Administration of antiarrhythmic drugs in these cases can lead to VF and sudden death. BrS should be excluded by drug challenge in young individuals with atrial flutter or AF and a normal heart and normal ECG. Approximately 15%–20% of patients with BrS develop supraventricular arrhythmias.[45] Some studies have reported prolongation of His atrial and His ventricular (HV) interval; these changes occur principally in patients with SCN5A mutations[46] and are consistent with a decreased excitability in the conduction system secondary to the loss-of-function of sodium channel activity.[47]

Long QT Syndrome Type 3

Long QT syndrome (LQTS) is an inherited arrhythmogenic disease characterized by prolongation of the QT interval and susceptibility to ventricular tachyarrhythmias. Among all described subtypes of LQTS, type 3 (LQT3) has a relative prevalence of 7%–10%.[48] LQT3 occurs because of mutations in the SCN5A gene. The most intriguing situation arises from the fact that some family members may display the ECG pattern of LQT3, while others display the pattern of BrS.[49] The overlap between the LQT3 and BrS phenotypes was also reported in other SCN5A mutations.[50] However, it remains unclear whether development of the BrS phenotype in a patient with LQT3 is solely determined by the biophysical properties of the mutant channel or by coinherited genetic variations, gender, ethnicity, or other environmental factors.[51]

Epilepsy

Cardiac arrhythmias are associated with abnormal channel function due to mutations in ion channel genes. Epilepsy is a disorder of neuronal function also involving abnormal channel function. It is increasingly demonstrated that the etiologies of BrS and epilepsy may partly overlap. It has been reported that SCN5A mutations may confer susceptibility for recurrent seizure activity, supporting the emerging concept of a genetically determined cardiocerebral channelopathy.[52,53]

Myotonic Phenotypes

To date, except for nonspecific cardiac arrhythmias described in two SCN4A-associated case reports,[54] no overlapping phenotypes between muscular and cardiac sodium channelopathies have been reported. In a recent study, Bissay and colleagues reported a high number of patients with coexisting BrS and sodium channel myotonia, suggesting a possible impact of *SCN4A* variants on the pathophysiological mechanism underlying the development of a type 1 ECG pattern and of malignant arrhythmia symptoms in some patients with BrS.[55]

Risk Stratification

After the diagnosis of BrS is made, the next step is risk stratification, of which the main objective is the accurate identification and treatment of individuals at high risk for SCD. To date, some markers of high risk in BrS patients have been clearly identified and accepted by all groups, but the issue of risk stratification of asymptomatic BrS patients remains controversial.[56] The reported annual rate of events has decreased from the first patients initially reported to the most recent published series; the change probably reflects the inherent bias during the first years following the description of a novel disease, in which particularly severe forms of the disease are most likely to be diagnosed.[57] A recent study by Sieira and associates shows that arrhythmic events in asymptomatic BrS patients are not insignificant (0.5% annual incidence rate). In this cohort, the inducibility of ventricular arrhythmias, spontaneous type I ECG, and presence of SAN dysfunction might be considered as risk factors and used to drive long-term management.[58] A recently published meta-analysis also showed that asymptomatic subjects with either a spontaneous diagnostic ECG pattern or inducible ventricular arrhythmias on programmed ventricular stimulation are at increased risk.[59] Several clinical variables have been demonstrated to predict a worse outcome in patients with BrS. In almost all the analyses, the presence of symptoms before diagnosis, a spontaneous type-1 ECG at baseline, and male gender have consistently shown to be related to the occurrence of cardiac events in follow-up.[60,61] Little controversy exists on the value of a previous cardiac arrest as a risk marker for future events (between 17% and 62% of patients will have a new arrhythmic event within 48 and 84 months of follow-up). Similarly, the presence of syncope identifies patients with a high risk for events (6%–19% at 24–39-month follow-up); thus there is general agreement that these patients should be protected with an ICD irrespective of the presence of other risk factors. Spontaneous ECG type 1 has been identified as an independent predictor of ventricular arrhythmias in multivariate analysis of the largest cohort of BrS patients published to date[62] (hazard ratio [HR], 1.8; 95% confidence interval [CI], 1.03–3.33; *p* = .04) and in the majority of series by others.

Male sex has consistently shown a trend to present more arrhythmic events in all the studies and has even been defined as an independent predictor for a worse outcome in a meta-analysis.[63]

Spontaneous AF, which can appear in 10%–53% of cases, has been shown to have prognostic significance, and spontaneous AF was associated with higher incidence of syncopal episodes (60.0% vs. 22.2%, *p* < .03) and documented VF (40.0% vs. 14.3%, *p* < .05).[64]

The risk of lethal or near-lethal arrhythmic episodes among previously asymptomatic patients with BrS varies according to the series: 8% recurrence rate at 33 ± 39 months of follow-up reported by Brugada and colleagues[65]; 6% recurrence rate at 34 ± 44 months by Priori and colleagues[66]; 1% recurrence rate after 40 ± 50 months and 30 ± 21 months of follow-up by Eckardt and associates [67] and Giustetto and coworkers,[68] respectively; and finally, Probst and coworkers reported a 1.5% recurrence rate at 31 months of follow-up.[62]

Although large registries agree that electrophysiological study (EPS) inducibility is greatest among BrS patients with previous sudden death or syncope,[65] there is no consensus on the value of the EPS in predicting outcome. The results published by Brugada and colleagues[65] indicate that inducibility during EPS is an independent predictor for cardiac events, and Giustetto and associates[68]

stressed the negative predictive value (none of the patients with a negative EPS developed arrhythmic events vs. 15% of patients with a positive EPS result during 30 ± 21 months of follow-up); however, the rest of the registries failed to demonstrate this.[62] The largest series of BrS patients published so far found that inducibility of sustained ventricular arrhythmias was significantly associated with a shorter time to first arrhythmic event in the univariate analysis; however, when performing the multivariable analysis, inducibility did not predict arrhythmic events,[62] as confirmed by the results in a recent prospective study in previously asymptomatic patients. In 2015, a single center study has been recently published that shows the results of a cohort of 96 BrS patients with various clinical presentations and who had an inducible VF using an aggressive programmed ventricular stimulation protocol. The authors reported an excellent protective effect of class 1 AAD (mainly quinidine) during EP testing and an excellent clinical outcome in drug-treated patients.[69] In addition, Sieira and colleagues published a series of 403 BrS cases. The authors concluded that programmed ventricular stimulation of the heart was a good predictor of outcome in individuals with BrS. It might be of special value to guide further management when performed in asymptomatic individuals. The overall accuracy of the test makes it a suitable screening tool to reassure noninducible asymptomatic individuals.[70]

A family history of sudden death or the presence of an *SCN5A* mutation have not been proven to be risk markers in any of the large studies conducted thus far.[63] However, recent data suggest that other genetic findings, like the presence of mutations leading to a truncated protein, or the presence of common polymorphisms located in *SCN5A*, might have some prognostic implications.[34] A recent publication by Meregelli of 147 BrS patients with identified *SCN5A* mutations showed a significantly higher rate of syncope among patients carrying *SCN5A* truncation mutations (caused by a premature stop codon) and those with *SCN5A* missense mutations, resulting in a decrease of more than 90% of the I_{Na} (nonfunctional Na^+ channels) compared with patients with *SCN5A* missense mutations that produce a decrease of I_{Na} (≤90%). They could not demonstrate a higher rate of more serious arrhythmic events (SCD or VF) in those patients with mutations encoding nonfunctional Na^+ channels. The first two groups of patients also presented longer PR interval in basal ECG and showed a greater increase of PR and QRS intervals after the class I AAD test. This is the first study that proposed the use of genetics in risk stratification for BrS. The recent finding that common polymorphisms located in *SCN5A* may modulate the effect of mutations causing, resulting in a counterbalance of its deleterious consequences with improvement of the BrS phenotype, opens the possibility of identifying polymorphisms as risk stratification tools as well as suggests that polymorphisms may be possible targets for therapeutic interventions.

In summary, few things are clear from the risk stratification data: symptomatic patients are at higher risk than asymptomatic ones, sudden death survivors are at higher risk than patients with syncope, males are at higher risk than females, patients with type I ECG at baseline have a higher risk than those who require class I antiarrhythmics, and asymptomatic patients may also die suddenly. This latter statement is based on the fact that all symptomatic patients with BrS have remained asymptomatic for decades. Thus at present the biggest challenge is the detection of these few asymptomatic patients who will develop symptoms.

Postulated Noninvasive Markers of Arrhythmic Risk in Brugada Syndrome

In an effort to solve the complex issue of risk stratification in BrS, several noninvasive methods have been postulated as markers of arrhythmic events among these patients: a decreased nocturnal standard deviation of the 5 minute–averaged NN intervals (SDANNs), measured in Holter recordings; an S-wave width in V_1 ≥ 80 msec and ST-segment elevation ≥ 0.18 mV in V_2; spontaneous changes in ST segment, a corrected QT interval (QTc) higher than 460 ms in V_2, prolonged T peak–T end (Tp-e) interval, and T p-e dispersion; the "aVR sign" (R wave ≥ 0.3 mV or R/q ≥ 0.75 in lead aVR); prolonged QRS duration in precordial leads (r-J interval in V_2 ≥ 90 ms and QRS ≥ 90 ms in V_6; QRS ≥ 120 ms in V_2); even an indicator of interventricular mechanical dyssynchrony has been recently found to be associated with high risk for fatal or near-fatal arrhythmias in BrS. The usefulness of late potentials (LPs), assessed by signal-averaged ECG (SAECG) as a marker of high risk has been extensively studied by various groups; a recent prospective study showed that positive LP was an independent marker of high risk in BrS patients, with a hazard ratio of 10.9 (95% CI, 1.1–104.3; p = .038), sensitivity of 95.7%, specificity of 65%, positive predictive value of 75.9%, negative predictive value of 92.9%, and predictive accuracy of 81.4%. Before including LP as a marker for risk, there is the need of more prospective studies, including more patients and with a longer follow-up, evaluating the value of different noninvasive markers of risk in BrS.

In conclusion, risk stratification is really the most controversial issue so far. Looking at the literature, there are two types of series: ones with almost no events at all during follow-up and in which obviously the lack of events brings a negative value of any studied factor. Others have a reasonable number of events during follow-up, and different factors have been studied; some of them have shown a value for stratification. The discussion is not which factor is more efficient to stratify patients, but why there is this big and so far unexplained difference among series. Certainly, some international consensus will have to be done, basically on how to make the diagnosis based on the new and updated studies that have been published since the last one.

Therapeutic Options and Recommendations for Brugada Syndrome Patients

Implantable Cardioverter Defibrillator

To date, the only proven effective therapeutic strategy for the prevention of SCD in BrS patients is the ICD. This fact is supported by a recent study of Conte and associates that showed the treatment of potentially lethal arrhythmias in 17% of patients during a follow-up period of nearly 85 months. Appropriate shocks were significantly associated with the presence of aborted SCD.[71] It is important to remark that ICDs are not free from several disadvantages, especially in this group of patients sharing a particular profile: active young individuals, facing a long-lasting coexistence with the device and multiple device replacements, and a long life expectancy (especially since device implantation). Some series have reported low rates of appropriated shocks (8%–15%; median follow-up, 45 months) and a high rate of complications, such as inappropriate shocks (20%–36% at 21–47 months of follow-up).[72–74] In a recent study, Rodriguez-Mañero and coworkers found that T-wave oversensing was a potential reason for inappropriate shocks in patients with BrS who received ICDs. In the vast majority, it can be solved by reprogramming. However, in some patients, it still requires invasive intervention. Importantly, incidence is significantly lower using an integrated bipolar lead system than when using a dedicated bipolar lead system, and hence the latter should be routinely used in BrS cases.[75]

Pharmacological Treatment in Brugada Syndrome

With the objective of rebalancing ionic currents affected in BrS during cardiac action potential, drugs that inhibit the Ito current or increase the Na^+ and Ca^{2+} currents have been tested in BrS:
- Isoproterenol (which increases the Ica L current) has proved to be useful for treatment of electrical storm in BrS.[76]
- Quinidine, a class Ia AAD with Ito and I-Kr blocker effects, has been shown to prevent induction of VF and suppress spontaneous ventricular arrhythmias in a clinical setting, being currently used in patients with ICD and multiple shocks, cases in which ICD implantation is contraindicated, or for the

treatment of supraventricular arrhythmias. It has been suggested that it could be also useful in children with BrS as a bridge to ICD or as an alternative to it.[77]

Radiofrequency Catheter Ablation in Brugada Syndrome

After demonstrating that VF events were triggered by similar ventricular ectopy, radiofrequency catheter ablation (RFCA) of ventricular ectopy has been postulated as a therapeutic approach in BrS patients. Few anecdotal cases in high-risk BrS patients implanted with an ICD have shown no short-term recurrence of VF, syncope, or SCD.[78,79] Nademanee presented the first series showing that electrical disconnection of the right ventricular outflow tract can prevent VF inducibility in a high-risk population.[80] In 2014, a BrS case of an ablation of the epicardial substrate in the right ventricular outflow tract was published.[81] In 2015, Forkmann and coworkers reported a BrS case in which an epicardial ventricular tachycardia ablation was performed, and noninducibility of any VT during programmed ventricular stimulation was identified. During the 9 months of follow-up, device interrogation showed no recurrence of any VT episodes.[82] Recently, a study focused on epicardial ablation has been published showing an apparent elimination of the BrS phenotype. However, this technique is a current matter of argument, and further studies should be performed to corroborate these preliminary results.[83]

External Factors and Brugada Syndrome

It is important to underline that ECG typically fluctuates over time in BrS patients and thus can change between the three patterns or even be transiently normal.[84] Based on this, it seems that repetitive ECG recordings may be mandatory in patients with or suspected of having the syndrome. It is worth noting that some factors can account for an ECG abnormality that can closely resemble the Brugada ECG (see Table 92.1). Importantly, some of them are conditions different from the syndrome and should be carefully excluded during the differential diagnosis, whereas others may induce ST-segment elevation probably when an underlying genetic predisposition is present.

Modulating factors play a major role in the dynamic nature of the ECG and may also be responsible for the ST-segment elevation in genetically predisposed patients. Sympathovagal balance, hormones, metabolic factors, and pharmacological agents, by means of specific effects on transmembrane ionic currents, are considered to modulate not only the ECG morphology but also to explain the development of ventricular arrhythmias under certain conditions. Indeed, bradycardia and vagal tone may contribute to ST-segment elevation and arrhythmia initiation by decreasing calcium currents.[85] This explains the greater ST-segment elevation recorded in vagal settings,[86] and the notorious incidence of cardiac arrhythmias and sudden death at night in patients with BrS.[87]

The role of sex hormones is currently being established. Published data suggest that they also play a role in the phenotypic manifestations of BrS.[88] For example, regression of typical ECG features has been reported in castrated men,[89] and levels of testosterone seem to be higher in Brugada male patients compared with those in control males.[90] Two main hypotheses have been proposed for sex distinction, perhaps interacting with each other: the sex-related intrinsic differences in ionic currents and the hormonal influence. Consequently, with the hormonal hypothesis, the few available data existing thus far regarding BrS in children have not shown a difference in phenotypic presentation between boys and girls.[91] Temperature may be an important modulator in some patients with BrS. Premature inactivation of the sodium channel has been shown to be accentuated at higher temperatures in some *SCN5A* mutations, suggesting that febrile states may unmask certain BrS patients or temporarily increase the risk of arrhythmias.[92] It seems that fever would be a particularly important trigger factor among the pediatric population.[91] Thus temperature control is crucial in BrS patients.

Brugada Syndrome and Pregnancy

The gender-related differences in the phenotypic expression of BrS have been widely reported, but the basis for gender distinction is not yet fully understood.[93] During pregnancy, autonomic and hemodynamic alterations occur, and estrogen and progesterone blood levels are reduced at peripartum. The largest study of pregnant women with BrS has been recently published by Rodríguez-Mañero and colleagues.[94] This study describes a relatively benign course of pregnancy and peripartum period among women with BrS. In addition, only a few cases exhibiting syncope were found, and the presence of syncope during pregnancy did not seem to be related to a worse outcome of the disease, in neither the postpartum nor the peripartum periods. Nevertheless, the management of pregnant women affected by BrS should be very strict and multidisciplinary in cooperation with a cardiologist and an anesthesiologist.[95] Further clinical assessment and follow-up during the pregnant, postpartum, and peripartum periods should be performed, considering the favorable maternal and fetal outcome of disease.

Brugada Syndrome in Children

SCD accounts for approximately 20% of sudden deaths in the pediatric age group. Inherited arrhythmias are increasingly known to be responsible for these deaths. The prevalence of BrS in children is variable among different studies, accounting for up to 0.0098% in a Japanese series.[96] Despite massive progress in characterizing BrS, little is known about this disease in the pediatric population. In the initial description of the disease, three out of eight patients were children.[1] Since then, several authors have reported isolated cases.[97,98] Finally, in 2007 Probst and colleagues published a study with 30 affected individuals aged less than 16 years from 13 European institutions,[91] the largest series of pediatric BrS patients.

Diagnostic and Clinical Presentation

Brugada ECG pattern in children remains the same as in adults, considering its transiency. Moreover, there are no standardized data for optimal positioning of the right precordial leads in children, and the shape of the chest in a growing body can lead to confusion. With all these characteristics, symptoms of syncope associated with typical ECG pattern should alert to the possibility of BrS.

From asymptomatic patients (mainly discovered in routine ECG screening or familial screening) to sudden death, in children as in adults, the whole spectrum of clinical presentation is possible. In contrast to adults, no male predominance in symptomatic patients is found. This could be related to lower levels of testosterone in prepubertal children.[91] Several case reports have demonstrated the importance of fever as a precipitating factor for ventricular arrhythmias in children, probably not because of special predisposition of children. Interestingly, as the febrile state can unmask Brugada ECG pattern, performing a 12-lead ECG test during fever is recommended. Moreover, as febrile convulsions are a relatively common occurrence in childhood, one wonders if ECG should be part of the diagnostic routine when a febrile seizure occurs.[91]

Drug Challenge Test

Sodium channel blocker test (ajmaline 1 mg/kg or flecainide 2 mg/kg over 10 minutes)[99] should be restricted to children with normal baseline ECGs and typical symptoms with a positive family history. As in adults, a spontaneous type I ECG pattern is enough to establish the diagnosis, and performing a drug challenge can be dangerous. The existence of an age-dependent response to the ajmaline challenge is an intriguing recent finding and might have relevant clinical implications.[100] Thus, in a recent study, Conte and associates showed that repeat ajmaline challenge after puberty unmasked BrS in 23% of relatives with a previously negative drug test performed during childhood. The ECG phenotype does not appear during childhood in most cases but may develop later in response to hormonal, autonomic, or genetic factors.[101] However, repeating the ajmaline challenge after puberty in patients with an initial negative drug test remains controversial and should be further investigated. Thus controversy exists whether to practice drug challenge for relatives in asymptomatic resting ECG children and when it should be performed. Moreover, considering that a false-negative result can be seen in up to 30%, depending on the drug, the question is whether the second test should be performed some years later.

Electrophysiological Study in Children

If controversy exists about whether to perform EPS testing or not in the adult population, even more conflict appears if children should undergo programmed extrastimulation techniques to test malignant arrhythmia inducibility.[65] When indicated, protocol remains the same as in the adult population.

Therapeutic Implications and Implantable Cardioverter Defibrillator Implantation

As seen in other parts of this chapter, BrS can overlap with other entities such as LQT3 or Lev-Lenègre syndrome. Bradyarrhythmias can be a cause of death in these patients; thus pacemaker implantation is mandatory in certain cases.[91] Hydroquinidine has been shown to be a good alternative to ICD implantation at a short follow-up in children who are at risk for developing malignant arrhythmias, but further studies are required.[91]

Patients presenting with aborted sudden death and syncope with spontaneous type I ECG are clearly at high risk for malignant arrhythmias; therefore an ICD should be considered, irrespective of age. Special approaches for ICD implantation have been described for small children when needed (Fig. 92.3).

Familial Screening

First-degree affected relatives should be screened by clinical examination, interrogation, and performance of a 12-lead ECG (basal and upper intercostal space recording). Genetic tests should be performed in index cases, and when there is a positive result, mutations should be identified in children, whatever age they are, to follow the recommendations on fever control and avoidance of listed drugs. Mutation carriers should be annually screened with an ECG when asymptomatic, taking into account that a symptom of dizziness should require a 12-lead ECG.

In the era of personalized medicine, using high-throughput tools (next generation sequencing [NGS]) is the best cost-effective approach to identify the cause of the disease. The main problems in using NGS technologies are the large amount of data provided and the insufficient experience to translate this information into clinical practice.[102,103] One of the crucial elements for the correct interpretation of pathogenicity is the genotype–phenotype correlation in families. This leads to the need for each family to be studied separately, analyzing the variations in each relative and correlating clinical–genetic information. Final decisions should be made by a group consensus based on the experience of each member of the working group in each institution dedicated to this purpose.

Brugada Syndrome in Older Individuals

The fourth decade of life is the mean age of clinical manifestations of BrS, mainly in men. Thus the clinical course and prognosis of BrS in older individuals is unknown. Recently, Conte and colleagues published a systematic analysis of BrS in the aging population, reporting a benign prognosis and lower risk category of BrS patients in comparison to younger patients. Consequently, older

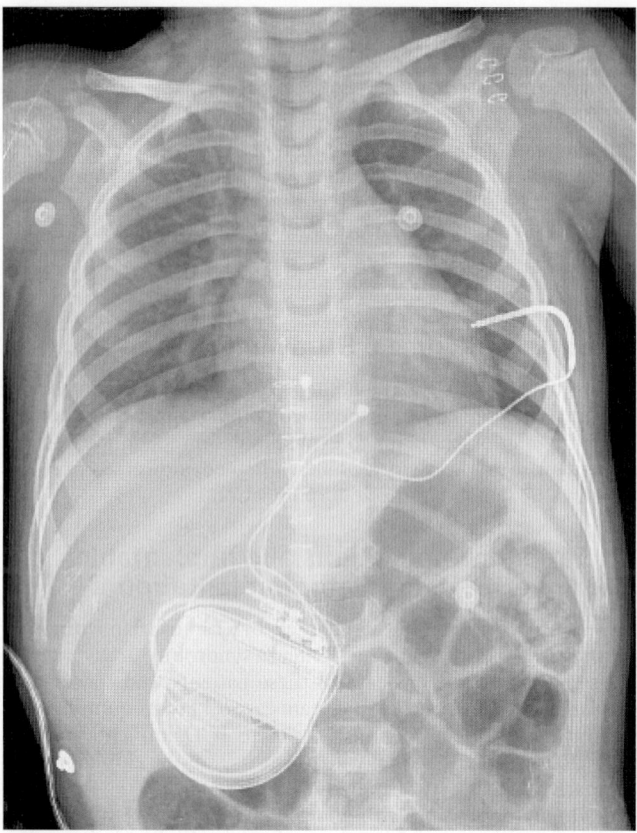

FIGURE 92.3 X-ray after implantable cardioverter defibrillator implantation in a small child: epicardial electrode on the epicardial right ventricle free wall and defibrillation electrode tunneled to the left thoracic wall. Note generator in a subcutaneous infrasternal region.

patients presented fewer ventricular arrhythmias and less family history of SCD. However, two main challenges remain controversial: use of drug-induced tests and device-guided management. Thus despite Conte and colleagues reporting in the abovementioned study that "BrS was diagnosed after ajmaline challenge in 86% of elderly patients," the value of unmasking a type I ECG as well as its safety has not been methodically assessed.[104] Regarding the use of an ICD, a consensus conference reported that older BrS patients with syncope should undergo ICD implantation if life expectancy is at least 6 months.[105] Recently, Kamakura and associates reported that long-term follow-up of high-risk BrS patients

with ICD showed a low incidence of VF in those aged >70 years. Considering the increasing risk of inappropriate shocks because of the relatively late onset of supraventricular tachycardia and lead failures, avoidance of ICD implantation or replacement may be considered in elderly BrS patients who remain free from VF until 70 years of age.[106] However, clinical decisions regarding both controversies should be analyzed on a case-by-case basis.

The Future

In recent years, cardiovascular studies have been focused on personalizing risk assessment and determining optimal therapy individually. BrS has also benefited from these advances, although there remain several key points to elucidate. Future genetics, epigenetics, transcriptomics, proteomics, metabolomics, and animal model approaches can help us understand the complexity of BrS-like diseases through the establishment and use of more reliable models at in silico, in vitro, and in vivo levels.

The genetic revolution in cardiac diseases was initiated with the knowledge of the human genome and has advanced exponentially linked to the development of new genomic technologies, such as NGS.[107] These new genetic technologies will allow performance of comprehensive genetic analysis in BrS patients, improving the identification of pathogenic variations.

Research in stem cells is one of the last fields that has been incorporated into the cardiac arrhythmia scenario. It has improved the identification, derivation, and characterization of human stem or progenitor cells, containing embryonic stem cells (ESCs) and the recently described induced pluripotent stem (iPS) cells. The human iPS cells from patients diagnosed with LQTS can differentiate to cardiomyocytes, allowing electrophysiological and molecular improvement of arrhythmic mechanisms.[108,109] However, BrS has not yet benefited from these advances.

Another interesting point is the use of animal models. They constitute useful tools for addressing the role of genetic and environmental modifiers on cardiac electrical activity. The only genetic model of the BrS to date is the SCN5A knockout mouse. The heterozygous SCN5A null allele results in impaired atrioventricular conduction, delayed intramyocardial conduction, increased ventricular refractoriness, and ventricular tachycardia.[110]

Computational power allows molecular modeling and molecular dynamics simulations of complex proteins. A full in silico model of potassium channel has been developed based on the available structures of channels, which includes all transmembrane segments.[111]

Altogether, there is still a long way to go toward the future of cardiac diseases associated with SCD, supporting the need to use the new emerging tools in the field of biomedicine.

REFERENCES

1. Brugada P, Brugada J. Right bundle branch block, persistent ST segment elevation and sudden cardiac death: a distinct clinical and electrocardiographic syndrome. A multicenter report. *J Am Coll Cardiol.* 1992;20:1391–1396.
2. Antzelevitch C, Brugada P, Borggrefe M, et al. Brugada syndrome: report of the second consensus conference. *Heart Rhythm.* 2005;2:429–440.
3. Ikeda T, Abe A, Yusu S, et al. The full stomach test as a novel diagnostic technique for identifying patients at risk of Brugada syndrome. *J Cardiovasc Electrophysiol.* 2006;17:602–607.
4. Chen Q, Kirsch GE, Zhang D, et al. Genetic basis and molecular mechanism for idiopathic ventricular fibrillation. *Nature.* 1998;392:293–296.
5. Kapplinger JD, Tester DJ, Alders M, et al. An international compendium of mutations in the SCN5A-encoded cardiac sodium channel in patients referred for Brugada syndrome genetic testing. *Heart Rhythm.* 2010;7:33–46.
6. Eastaugh LJ, James PA, Phelan DG, et al. Brugada syndrome caused by a large deletion in SCN5A only detected by multiplex ligation-dependent probe amplification. *J Cardiovasc Electrophysiol.* 2011;22:1073–1076.
7. Selga E, Campuzano O, Pinsach-Abuin ML, et al. Comprehensive genetic characterization of a Spanish Brugada syndrome cohort. *PLoS ONE.* 2015;10:e0132888.

8. Watanabe H, Koopmann TT, Le Scouarnec S, et al. Sodium channel beta1 subunit mutations associated with Brugada syndrome and cardiac conduction disease in humans. *J Clin Invest.* 2008;118:2260–2268.
9. Hu D, Barajas-Martinez H, Burashnikov E, et al. A mutation in the beta 3 subunit of the cardiac sodium channel associated with Brugada ECG phenotype. *Circ Cardiovasc Genet.* 2009;2:270–278.
10. Riuro H, Beltran-Alvarez P, Tarradas A, et al. A missense mutation in the sodium channel beta2 subunit reveals SCN2B as a new candidate gene for Brugada syndrome. *Hum Mutat.* 2013;34:961–966.
11. Hu D, Barajas-Martinez H, Pfeiffer R, et al. Mutations in SCN10A are responsible for a large fraction of cases of Brugada syndrome. *J Am Coll Cardiol.* 2014;64:66–79.
12. London B, Michalec M, Mehdi H, et al. Mutation in glycerol-3-phosphate dehydrogenase 1 like gene (GPD1-L) decreases cardiac Na+ current and causes inherited arrhythmias. *Circulation.* 2007;116:2260–2268.
13. Kattygnarath D, Maugenre S, Neyroud N, et al. MOG1: a new susceptibility gene for Brugada syndrome. *Circ Cardiovasc Genet.* 2011;4:261–268.
14. Ishikawa T, Sato A, Marcou CA, et al. A novel disease gene for Brugada syndrome: sarcolemmal membrane-associated protein gene mutations impair intracellular trafficking of hNav1.5. *Circ Arrhythm Electrophysiol.* 2012;5:1098–1107.

15. Cerrone M, Delmar M. Desmosomes and the sodium channel complex: implications for arrhythmogenic cardiomyopathy and Brugada syndrome. *Trends Cardiovasc Med.* 2014;24:184–190.
16. Cerrone M, Lin X, Zhang M, et al. Missense mutations in plakophilin-2 cause sodium current deficit and associate with a Brugada syndrome phenotype. *Circulation.* 2014;129:1092–1103.
17. Delpon E, Cordeiro JM, Nunez L, et al. Functional effects of KCNE3 mutation and its role in the development of Brugada syndrome. *Circ Arrhythm Electrophysiol.* 2008;1:209–218.
18. Haissaguerre M, Chatel S, Sacher F, et al. Ventricular fibrillation with prominent early repolarization associated with a rare variant of KCNJ8/KATP channel. *J Cardiovasc Electrophysiol.* 2009;20:93–98.
19. Medeiros-Domingo A, Tan BH, Crotti L, et al. Gain-of-function mutation S422L in the KCNJ8-encoded cardiac K(ATP) channel Kir6.1 as a pathogenic substrate for J-wave syndromes. *Heart Rhythm.* 2010;7:1466–1471.
20. Giudicessi JR, Ye D, Tester DJ, et al. Transient outward current (i(to)) gain-of-function mutations in the KCND3-encoded Kv4.3 potassium channel and Brugada syndrome. *Heart Rhythm.* 2011;8:1024–1032.

21. Ohno S, Zankov DP, Ding WG, et al. KCNE5 (KCNE1L) variants are novel modulators of Brugada syndrome and idiopathic ventricular fibrillation. *Circ Arrhythm Electrophysiol.* 2011;4:352–361.

22. Hu D, Barajas-Martinez H, Terzic A, et al. ABCC9 is a novel Brugada and early repolarization syndrome susceptibility gene. *Int J Cardiol.* 2014;171:431–442.

23. Ueda K, Hirano Y, Higashiuesato Y, et al. Role of HCN4 channel in preventing ventricular arrhythmia. *J Hum Genet.* 2009;54:115–121.

24. Antzelevitch C, Pollevick GD, Cordeiro JM, et al. Loss-of-function mutations in the cardiac calcium channel underlie a new clinical entity characterized by ST-segment elevation, short QT intervals, and sudden cardiac death. *Circulation.* 2007;115:442–449.

25. Burashnikov E, Pfeiffer R, Barajas-Martinez H, et al. Mutations in the cardiac L-type calcium channel associated with inherited J-wave syndromes and sudden cardiac death. *Heart Rhythm.* 2010;7:1872–1882.

26. Stallmeyer B, Zumhagen S, Denjoy I, et al. Mutational spectrum in the Ca^{2+}-activated cation channel gene TRPM4 in patients with cardiac conductance disturbances. *Hum Mutat.* 2012;33:109–117.

27. Junttila MJ, Gonzalez M, Lizotte E, et al. Induced Brugada-type electrocardiogram, a sign for imminent malignant arrhythmias. *Circulation.* 2008;117:1890–1893.

28. Barajas-Martinez HM, Hu D, Cordeiro JM, et al. Lidocaine-induced Brugada syndrome phenotype linked to a novel double mutation in the cardiac sodium channel. *Circ Res.* 2008;103:396–404.

29. Poelzing S, Forleo C, Samodell M, et al. SCN5A polymorphism restores trafficking of a Brugada syndrome mutation on a separate gene. *Circulation.* 2006;114:368–376.

30. Lizotte E, Junttila MJ, Dube MP, et al. Genetic modulation of Brugada syndrome by a common polymorphism. *J Cardiovasc Electrophysiol.* 2009;20:1137–1141.

31. Bezzina CR, Shimizu W, Yang P, et al. Common sodium channel promoter haplotype in Asian subjects underlies variability in cardiac conduction. *Circulation.* 2006;113:338–344.

32. Makita N, Mochizuki N, Tsutsui H. Absence of a trafficking defect in R1232W/T1620M, a double SCN5A mutant responsible for Brugada syndrome. *Circ J.* 2008;72:1018–1019.

33. Cordeiro JM, Barajas-Martinez H, Hong K, et al. Compound heterozygous mutations P336L and I1660V in the human cardiac sodium channel associated with the Brugada syndrome. *Circulation.* 2006;114:2026–2033.

34. Meregalli PG, Tan HL, Probst V, et al. Type of SCN5A mutation determines clinical severity and degree of conduction slowing in loss-of-function sodium channelopathies. *Heart Rhythm.* 2009;6:341–348.

35. Miyazaki S, Shah AJ, Haissaguerre M. Early repolarization syndrome—a new electrical disorder associated with sudden cardiac death. *Circ J.* 2010;74:2039–2044.

36. Antzelevitch C, Yan GX. J wave syndromes. *Heart Rhythm.* 2010;7:549–558.

37. McIntyre WF, Perez-Riera AR, Femenia F, et al. Coexisting early repolarization pattern and Brugada syndrome: recognition of potentially overlapping entities. *J Electrocardiol.* 2011;45:195–198.

38. Antzelevitch C, Yan GX. J-wave syndromes. From cell to bedside. *J Electrocardiol.* 2011;44:656–661.

39. Schott JJ, Alshinawi C, Kyndt F, et al. Cardiac conduction defects associate with mutations in SCN5A. *Nat Genet.* 1999;23:20–21.

40. Wang DW, Viswanathan PC, Balser JR, et al. Clinical, genetic, and biophysical characterization of SCN5A mutations associated with atrioventricular conduction block. *Circulation.* 2002;105:341–346.

41. Brignole M. Sick sinus syndrome. *Clin Geriatr Med.* 2002;18:211–227.

42. Benson DW, Wang DW, Dyment M, et al. Congenital sick sinus syndrome caused by recessive mutations in the cardiac sodium channel gene (SCN5A). *J Clin Invest.* 2003;112:1019–1028.

43. Smits JP, Koopmann TT, Wilders R, et al. A mutation in the human cardiac sodium channel (E161K) contributes to sick sinus syndrome, conduction disease and Brugada syndrome in two families. *J Mol Cell Cardiol.* 2005;38:969–981.

44. Yamada T, Watanabe I, Okumura Y, et al. Atrial electrophysiological abnormality in patients with Brugada syndrome assessed by P-wave signal-averaged ECG and programmed atrial stimulation. *Circ J.* 2006;70:1574–1579.

45. Letsas KP, Sideris A, Efremidis M, et al. Prevalence of paroxysmal atrial fibrillation in Brugada syndrome: a case series and a review of the literature. *J Cardiovasc Med (Hagerstown).* 2007;8:803–806.

46. Smits JP, Eckardt L, Probst V, et al. Genotype-phenotype relationship in Brugada syndrome: electrocardiographic features differentiate SCN5A-related patients from non-SCN5A-related patients. *J Am Coll Cardiol.* 2002;40:350–356.

47. Francis J, Antzelevitch C. Atrial fibrillation and Brugada syndrome. *J Am Coll Cardiol.* 2008;51:1149–1153.

48. Kramer DB, Zimetbaum PJ. Long-QT syndrome. *Cardiol Rev.* 2011;19:217–225.

49. Bezzina C, Veldkamp MW, van Den Berg MP, et al. A single Na⁺ channel mutation causing both long-QT and Brugada syndromes. *Circ Res.* 1999;85:1206–1213.

50. Grant AO, Carboni MP, Neplioueva V, et al. Long QT syndrome, Brugada syndrome, and conduction system disease are linked to a single sodium channel mutation. *J Clin Invest.* 2002;110:1201–1209.

51. Makita N. Phenotypic overlap of cardiac sodium channelopathies: individual-specific or mutation-specific? *Circ J.* 2009;73:810–817.

52. Parisi P, Oliva A, Coll Vidal M, et al. Coexistence of epilepsy and Brugada syndrome in a family with SCN5A mutation. *Epilepsy Res.* 2013;105:415–418.

53. Camacho Velasquez JL, Rivero Sanz E, Velazquez Benito JA, et al. Epilepsy and Brugada syndrome. *Neurologia.* 2015; pii:S0213-4853(15) 00062–6.

54. Pereon Y, Lande G, Demolombe S, et al. Paramyotonia congenita with an SCN4A mutation affecting cardiac repolarization. *Neurology.* 2003;60:340–342.

55. Bissay V, Van Malderen SC, Keymolen K, et al. SCN4A variants and Brugada syndrome: phenotypic and genotypic overlap between cardiac and skeletal muscle sodium channelopathies. *Eur J Hum Genet.* 2016;24:400–407.

56. Adler A, Rosso R, Chorin E, et al. Risk stratification in Brugada syndrome: clinical characteristics, electrocardiographic parameters, and auxiliary testing. *Heart Rhythm.* 2016;13:299–310.

57. Kamakura S, Ohe T, Nakazawa K, et al. Long-term prognosis of probands with Brugada-pattern ST-elevation in leads V₁-V₃. *Circ Arrhythm Electrophysiol.* 2009;2:495–503.

58. Sieira J, Ciconte G, Conte G, et al. Asymptomatic Brugada syndrome: clinical characterization and long-term prognosis. *Circ Arrhythm Electrophysiol.* 2015;8:1144–1150.

59. Letsas KP, Liu T, Shao Q, et al. Meta-analysis on risk stratification of asymptomatic individuals with the Brugada phenotype. *Am J Cardiol.* 2015;116:98–103.

60. Brugada J, Brugada R, Brugada P. Right bundle-branch block and ST-segment elevation in leads V1 through V3: a marker for sudden death in patients without demonstrable structural heart disease. *Circulation.* 1998;97:457–460.

61. Benito B, Sarkozy A, Mont L, et al. Gender differences in clinical manifestations of Brugada syndrome. *J Am Coll Cardiol.* 2008;52:1567–1573.

62. Probst V, Veltmann C, Eckardt L, et al. Long-term prognosis of patients diagnosed with Brugada syndrome: results from the finger Brugada syndrome registry. *Circulation.* 2010;121:635–643.

63. Gehi AK, Duong TD, Metz LD, et al. Risk stratification of individuals with the Brugada electrocardiogram: a meta-analysis. *J Cardiovasc Electrophysiol.* 2006;17:577–583.

64. Kusano KF, Taniyama M, Nakamura K, et al. Atrial fibrillation in patients with Brugada syndrome: relationships of gene mutation, electrophysiology, and clinical backgrounds. *J Am Coll Cardiol.* 2008;51:1169–1175.

65. Brugada J, Brugada R, Brugada P. Determinants of sudden cardiac death in individuals with the electrocardiographic pattern of Brugada syndrome and no previous cardiac arrest. *Circulation.* 2003;108:3092–3096.

66. Priori SG, Napolitano C, Gasparini M, et al. Natural history of Brugada syndrome: insights for risk stratification and management. *Circulation.* 2002;105:1342–1347.

67. Eckardt L, Probst V, Smits JP, et al. Long-term prognosis of individuals with right precordial ST-segment-elevation Brugada syndrome. *Circulation.* 2005;111:257–263.

68. Giustetto C, Drago S, Demarchi PG, et al. Risk stratification of the patients with Brugada type electrocardiogram: a community-based prospective study. *Europace.* 2009;11:507–513.

69. Belhassen B, Rahkovich M, Michowitz Y, et al. Management of Brugada syndrome: a 33-year experience using electrophysiologically-guided therapy with class 1a antiarrhythmic drugs. *Circ Arrhythm Electrophysiol.* 2015;8:1393–1402.

70. Sieira J, Conte G, Ciconte G, et al. Prognostic value of programmed electrical stimulation in Brugada syndrome: 20 years experience. *Circ Arrhythm Electrophysiol.* 2015;8:777–784.

71. Conte G, Sieira J, Ciconte G, et al. Implantable cardioverter-defibrillator therapy in Brugada syndrome: A 20-year single-center experience. *J Am Coll Cardiol.* 2015;65:879–888.

72. Sarkozy A, Boussy T, Kourgiannides G, et al. Long-term follow-up of primary prophylactic implantable cardioverter-defibrillator therapy in Brugada syndrome. *Eur Heart J.* 2007;28:334–344.

73. Rosso R, Glick A, Glikson M, et al. Outcome after implantation of cardioverter defibrillator [corrected] in patients with Brugada syndrome: a multicenter Israeli study (ISRABRU). *Isr Med Assoc J.* 2008;10:435–439.

74. Zipes DP, Camm AJ, Borggrefe M, et al. [Guidelines for management of patients with ventricular arrhythmias and the prevention of sudden cardiac death. Executive summary]. *Rev Esp Cardiol.* 2006;59:1328.

75. Rodriguez-Manero M, de Asmundis C, Sacher F, et al. T-wave oversensing in patients with Brugada syndrome: true bipolar versus integrated bipolar implantable cardioverter defibrillator leads: multicenter retrospective study. *Circ Arrhythm Electrophysiol.* 2015;8:792–798.

76. Maury P, Hocini M, Haissaguerre M. Electrical storms in Brugada syndrome: review of pharmacologic and ablative therapeutic options. *Indian Pacing Electrophysiol J.* 2005;5:25–34.

77. Schweizer PA, Becker R, Katus HA, et al. Successful acute and long-term management of electrical storm in Brugada syndrome using orciprenaline and quinine/quinidine. *Clin Res Cardiol.* 2010;99:467–470.

78. Nakagawa E, Takagi M, Tatsumi H, et al. Successful radiofrequency catheter ablation for electrical storm of ventricular fibrillation in a patient with Brugada syndrome. *Circ J.* 2008;72:1025–1029.

79. Morita H, Zipes DP, Morita ST, et al. Epicardial ablation eliminates ventricular arrhythmias in an experimental model of Brugada syndrome. *Heart Rhythm.* 2009;6:665–671.

80. Nademanee K, Veerakul G, Chandanamattha P, et al. Prevention of ventricular fibrillation episodes in Brugada syndrome by catheter ablation over the anterior right ventricular outflow tract epicardium. *Circulation.* 2011;123:1270–1279.

81. Szeplaki G, Ozcan EE, Osztheimer I, et al. Ablation of the epicardial substrate in the right ventricular outflow tract in a patient with Brugada syndrome refusing implantable cardioverter defibrillator therapy. *Can J Cardiol.* 2014;30: 1249.e9-1249.e11.

82. Forkmann M, Tomala J, Huo Y, et al. Epicardial ventricular tachycardia ablation in a patient with Brugada ECG pattern and mutation of PKP2 and DSP genes. *Circ Arrhythm Electrophysiol.* 2015;8:505–507.

83. Brugada J, Pappone C, Berruezo A, et al. Brugada syndrome phenotype elimination by epicardial substrate ablation. *Circ Arrhythm Electrophysiol.* 2015;8:1373–1381.

84. Veltmann C, Schimpf R, Echternach C, et al. A prospective study on spontaneous fluctuations between diagnostic and non-diagnostic ECGs in Brugada syndrome: implications for correct phenotyping and risk stratification. *Eur Heart J.* 2006;27:2544–2552.

85. Yan GX, Antzelevitch C. Cellular basis for the Brugada syndrome and other mechanisms of arrhythmogenesis associated with ST-segment elevation. *Circulation.* 1999;100:1660–1666.

86. Tatsumi H, Takagi M, Nakagawa E, et al. Risk stratification in patients with Brugada syndrome: analysis of daily fluctuations in 12-lead electrocardiogram (ECG) and signal-averaged electrocardiogram (SAECG). *J Cardiovasc Electrophysiol.* 2006;17:705–711.

87. Matsuo K, Kurita T, Inagaki M, et al. The circadian pattern of the development of ventricular fibrillation in patients with Brugada syndrome. *Eur Heart J.* 1999;20:465–470.

88. Benito B, Brugada R, Brugada J, et al. Brugada syndrome. *Prog Cardiovasc Dis.* 2008;51:1–22.

89. Matsuo K, Akahoshi M, Seto S, et al. Disappearance of the Brugada-type electrocardiogram after surgical castration: a role for testosterone and an explanation for the male preponderance. *Pacing Clin Electrophysiol.* 2003;26:1551–1553.

90. Shimizu W, Matsuo K, Kokubo Y, et al. Sex hormone and gender difference—role of testosterone on male predominance in Brugada syndrome. *J Cardiovasc Electrophysiol.* 2007;18:415–421.

91. Probst V, Denjoy I, Meregalli PG, et al. Clinical aspects and prognosis of Brugada syndrome in children. *Circulation.* 2007;115:2042–2048.

92. Dumaine R, Towbin JA, Brugada P, et al. Ionic mechanisms responsible for the electrocardiographic phenotype of the Brugada syndrome are temperature dependent. *Circ Res.* 1999;85:803–809.

93. Tadros R, Ton AT, Fiset C, et al. Sex differences in cardiac electrophysiology and clinical arrhythmias: epidemiology, therapeutics, and mechanisms. *Can J Cardiol.* 2014;30:783–792.

94. Rodriguez-Manero M, Casado-Arroyo R, Sarkozy A, et al. The clinical significance of pregnancy in Brugada syndrome. *Rev Esp Cardiol (Engl Ed).* 2014;67:176–180.

95. Giambanco L, Incandela D, Maiorana A, et al. Brugada syndrome and pregnancy: highlights on antenatal and prenatal management. *Case Rep Obstet Gynecol.* 2014;2014:531648.

96. Yamakawa Y, Ishikawa T, Uchino K, et al. Prevalence of right bundle-branch block and right precordial ST-segment elevation (Brugada-type electrocardiogram) in Japanese children. *Circ J.* 2004;68:275–279.

97. Probst V, Allouis M, Sacher F, et al. Progressive cardiac conduction defect is the prevailing phenotype in carriers of a Brugada syndrome SCN5A mutation. *J Cardiovasc Electrophysiol.* 2006;17:270–275.

98. Probst V, Evain S, Gournay V, et al. Monomorphic ventricular tachycardia due to Brugada syndrome successfully treated by hydroquinidine therapy in a 3-year-old child. *J Cardiovasc Electrophysiol.* 2006;17:97–100.

99. Sorgente A, Sarkozy A, De Asmundis C, et al. Ajmaline challenge in young individuals with suspected Brugada syndrome. *Pacing Clin Electrophysiol.* 2011;34:736–741.

100. Conte G, Brugada P. The challenges of performing ajmaline challenge in children with suspected Brugada syndrome. *Open Heart*. 2014;1:e000031.

101. Conte G, de Asmundis C, Ciconte G, et al. Follow-up from childhood to adulthood of individuals with family history of Brugada syndrome and normal electrocardiograms. *JAMA*. 2014;312:2039–2041.

102. Allegue C, Coll M, Mates J, et al. Genetic analysis of arrhythmogenic diseases in the era of NGS: the complexity of clinical decision-making in Brugada syndrome. *PLoS One*. 2015;10:e0133037.

103. Di Resta C, Pietrelli A, Sala S, et al. High-throughput genetic characterization of a cohort of Brugada syndrome patients. *Hum Mol Genet*. 2015;24:5828–5835.

104. Conte G, De Asmundis C, Sieira J, et al. Clinical characteristics, management, and prognosis of elderly patients with Brugada syndrome. *J Cardiovasc Electrophysiol*. 2014;25:514–519.

105. Antzelevitch C, Brugada P, Borggrefe M, et al. Brugada syndrome: report of the second consensus conference: endorsed by the Heart Rhythm Society and the European Heart Rhythm Association. *Circulation*. 2005;111:659–670.

106. Kamakura T, Wada M, Nakajima I, et al. Evaluation of the necessity for cardioverter-defibrillator implantation in elderly patients with Brugada syndrome. *Circ Arrhythm Electrophysiol*. 2015;8:785–791.

107. Desai AN, Jere A. Next-generation sequencing: ready for the clinics? *Clin Genet*. 2012;81:503–510.

108. Itzhaki I, Maizels L, Huber I, et al. Modelling the long QT syndrome with induced pluripotent stem cells. *Nature*. 2011;471:225–229.

109. Moretti A, Bellin M, Welling A, et al. Patient-specific induced pluripotent stem-cell models for long-QT syndrome. *N Engl J Med*. 2010;363:1397–1409.

110. Derangeon M, Montnach J, Baro I, et al. Mouse models of SCN5A-related cardiac arrhythmias. *Front Physiol*. 2012;3:210.

111. Subbotina J, Yarov-Yarovoy V, Lees-Miller J, et al. Structural refinement of the hERG1 pore and voltage-sensing domains with rosetta-membrane and molecular dynamics simulations. *Proteins*. 2010;78:2922–2934.

93 Long and Short QT Syndromes

Peter J. Schwartz and Lia Crotti

Long QT Syndrome

Congenital long QT syndrome (LQTS), a leading cause of sudden death in the young, is characterized by a prolongation of the QT interval in the standard electrocardiogram (ECG) and by syncopal episodes, which often result in cardiac arrest (CA) and sudden death and usually occur under physical or emotional stress in otherwise healthy young individuals.[1] The availability of very effective therapies for this otherwise highly lethal disorder among symptomatic and untreated patients makes the existence of symptomatic and undiagnosed patients unacceptable. The genetic findings have made LQTS a unique paradigm for genetically mediated sudden cardiac death (SCD), which allows a tight correlation between genotype and phenotype and provides a direct bridge between molecular biology and clinical cardiology, with a direct impact on patients' management.[2]

Genetic Basis of Long QT Syndrome

So far, 17 genes have been associated with LQTS (Table 93.1), but the first three identified in 1995–96 (*KCNQ1*, *KCNH2*, and *SCN5A*) remain responsible for the vast majority of genotype-positive cases.[2,3] Of note, the so-called LQT4 and LQT7 (Andersen-Tawil syndrome) are complex clinical disorders in which a modest prolongation of the QT interval is only a secondary epiphenomenon and should not be regarded as part of LQTS.[3] For other variants (LQT9–LQT13), there are only preliminary descriptions.[3] These 17 genes can be classified into three major groups: those reducing potassium outward currents, those increasing sodium inward current, and those increasing calcium inward current. The consistent outcome, however, is a prolongation of the action potential duration at the cellular level and of the QT interval on the standard ECG with an increased risk of life-threatening arrhythmias.

Potassium-Related Long QT Syndrome: The Most Common Forms

The delayed rectifier potassium current (I_K) is a major determinant of phase 3 of the cardiac action potential. It comprises two independent components: one rapid (I_{Kr}) and one slow (I_{Ks}). The *KCNQ1* and *KCNE1* genes encode, respectively, α-(KvLQT1) and β-(MinK) subunits of the potassium channel conducting the I_{Ks} current. *KCNQ1* mutations produce the LQT1 variant of LQTS, which is also the most prevalent.

Homozygous or compound heterozygous mutations in *KCNQ1* and *KCNE1* cause the recessive Jervell and Lange-Nielsen (JLN) variants of LQTS (JLN1 and JLN2, respectively). LQT5 is an uncommon variant (2%–3%) caused by mutations in the *KCNE1* gene.

The *KCNH2* and *KCNE2* genes encode, respectively, the α-(hERG) and β-(MIRP) subunits of the potassium channel conducting the I_{Kr} current and are responsible for the LQT2 and LQT6 variants of LQTS, respectively. LQT2 is the second most prevalent variant of LQTS, accounting for 35%–40% of LQTS genotype-positive patients.

Mutations in these genes causing LQTS provoke a loss of I_{Ks} or I_{Kr} current through different mechanisms. Defective proteins may coassemble with wild-type protein and exert a dominant-negative effect. Other mutations lead to defective proteins that do not assemble with wild-type peptides, resulting in a loss of function that reduces the I_{Ks} current by 50% or less (haploinsufficiency). Finally, defective peptides may not even reach the membrane of the cardiac cell because the mutations interfere with intracellular protein trafficking.

The I_{Ks} current is augmented by sympathetic activation and heart rate increases and is essential for QT adaptation. If I_{Ks} is defective, the QT interval will fail to shorten appropriately during tachycardia, thus creating a highly arrhythmogenic condition.

Other very rare genetic subtypes caused by mutations inducing a reduced potassium outward current are LQT7 or Andersen-Tawil syndrome (due to mutations in the *KCNJ2* gene), LQT11 (due to mutation in the *AKAP9* gene encoding for yotiao, a protein modulating I_{Ks} current), and LQT13 (due to mutation in *KCNJ5* gene, causing a reduced acetylcholine-dependent inward rectifier current [I_{KACh}])[2,3] (see Table 93.1).

Sodium-Related Long QT Syndrome: The Most Eclectic Forms

The *SCN5A* gene encodes the protein of the cardiac sodium channel. In vitro expression studies[4] have shown that LQTS-*SCN5A* mutations produce the LQTS phenotype by inducing a "gain-of-function," leading to an increase in the sodium inward current, which prolongs action potential duration. The prevalence of LQT3 among genotype-positive LQTS patients is 10%–15%. Other, less common genetic subtypes of LQTS are related to proteins that are part of the so-called sodium channel macromolecular complex. Specifically, mutations in *ANK4* (LQT4), *CAV3* (LQT9), *SCN4B* (LQT10), and *SNTA1* (LQT12) have been associated with the disease, and they act by directly or indirectly increasing the sodium current[3] (see Table 93.1). Mutations in *SCN5A* are also associated with overlapping phenotypes (LQTS, Brugada syndrome, and cardiac conduction defects). The most common and best studied mutations associated with overlapping phenotypes are *SCN5A*-E1784K, 1795insD, ΔKPQ,

TABLE 93.1   Long QT syndrome (LQTS) genes

GENE	SYNDROME	FREQUENCY	LOCUS	PROTEIN (FUNCTIONAL EFFECT)
KCNQ1 (LQT1)	RWS, JLN	40–55	11p15.5	Ik ($\downarrow$)
KCNH2 (LQT2)	RWS	30–45	7q35-36	Ik ($\downarrow$)
SCN5A (LQT3)	RWS	5–10	3p21-p24	NaV1.5 ($\uparrow$)
ANKB (LQT4)	RWS	<1%	4q25-q27	NaV1.5 ($\uparrow$)
KCNE1 (LQT5)	RWS, JLN	<1%	21q22.1	Ik ($\downarrow$)
KCNE2 (LQT6)	RWS	<1%	21q22.1	Ik ($\downarrow$)
KCNJ2 (LQT7)	AS	<1%	17q23	Kir2.1 ($\downarrow$)
CACNA1C (LQT8)	TS	<1%	12p13.3	L-type calcium channel ($\uparrow$)
CAV3 (LQT9)	RWS	<1%	3p25	NaV1.5 ($\uparrow$)
SCN4B (LQT10)	RWS	<1%	11q23.3	NaV1.5 ($\uparrow$)
AKAP9 (LQT11)	RWS	<1%	7q21-q22	Ik ($\downarrow$)
SNTA1 (LQT12)	RWS	<1%	20q11.2	NaV1.5 ($\uparrow$)
KCNJ5 (LQT13)	RWS	<1%	11q24	Kir3.4 ($\downarrow$)
CALM1 (LQT14)	RWS	?	14q32.11	L-type calcium channel ($\uparrow$)
CALM2 (LQT15)	RWS	?	2p21	L-type calcium channel ($\uparrow$)
CALM3 (LQT16)	RWS	?	19q13.32	L-type calcium channel ($\uparrow$)
TRDN (LQT17)	Recessive LQTS	?	6q22.31	L-type calcium channel ($\uparrow$)

AS, Andersen syndrome; *JLN*, Jervell and Lange-Nielsen syndrome; *RWS*, Romano-Ward syndrome; *TS*, Timothy syndrome.
Functional effect: ($\downarrow$) loss-of-function or ($\uparrow$) gain-of-function at the cellular in vitro level.

and ∆K1500; it would appear that a negative shift of steady-state sodium channel inactivation and enhanced tonic block by class IC drugs represent the common biophysical mechanisms underlying the phenotypic overlap of LQT3 and Brugada syndrome.[5]

Another peculiarity of sodium-related LQTS is that, despite being less frequent than potassium-related LQTS in adulthood, it constitutes the most common genetic form associated with LQTS-related perinatal mortality, including life-threatening arrhythmias in the first year of life, sudden infant death syndrome (SIDS), and sudden unexplained intrauterine fetal demise (IUFD)[6] (Fig. 93.1). This opposite pattern between perinatal life and adulthood is likely due to a negative selection for *SCN5A* carriers in the perinatal and early-infancy period.

The genetic variants identified on *SCN5A* in SIDS, IUFD, and neonatal LQT3 have different topological distributions. Indeed, mutations located in the transmembrane and linker regions are significantly more present in neonatal LQT3 cases than in SIDS/IUFD (86% vs. 22%; *p* = .002),[6] while the variants located in the N-terminal and interdomain linkers (the regions where variants present in controls are more frequently observed) are 9.5% in neonatal LQT3 vs 44.4% in SIDS/IUFD (*p* = .01).[6] Furthermore, while none of the mutations identified in severe neonatal LQT3 cases are present in the publicly available control databases, 47% of functional variants associated with SIDS/IUFD are also observed in the general population. These considerations support the concept that severe neonatal LQT3 cases are caused by mutations able *per se* to cause a phenotype unlikely to be compatible with survival to adulthood. Indeed, the mutations identified in this subgroup of patients are mainly *de novo*. By contrast, the genetic variants identified in SIDS and IUFD cases have a wider range of clinical severity, and some of them, identified also in the general population, are probably not able *per se* to cause SCD, while they can act as favoring factors. In further support of this view, we have observed that the *SCN5A* rare variants with a functional effect identified in SIDS and IUFD, also present in the publicly available databases, are significantly more prevalent in the SIDS/IUFD cohorts than in the general population (12/634, 1.9% vs. 45/6261, 0.7%; *p* = .0019).[6]

Calcium-Related Long QT Syndrome: The Most Complex and Dangerous Forms

In the heart, prolonged calcium current delays cardiomyocyte repolarization and increases the risk of arrhythmia. Five major genetic forms of LQTS linked to this mechanism have been described.

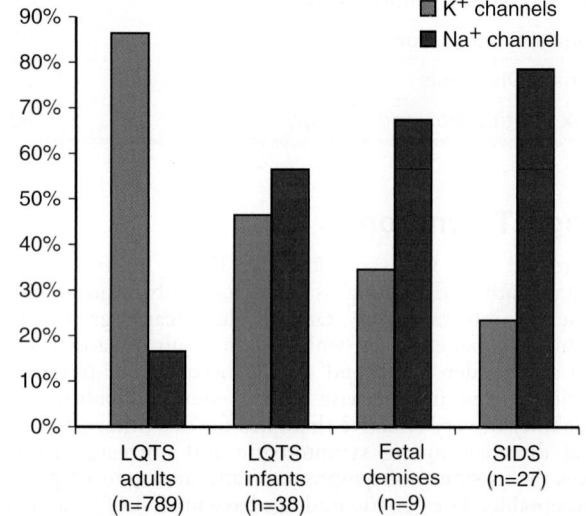

FIGURE 93.1 Distribution of mutation carriers in the two main potassium (*K⁺*) channel genes (*KCNQ1* and *KCNH2*; in *blue*) and in the sodium (*Na⁺*) channel gene (*SCN5A*; in *red*), for four different populations: long QT syndrome (*LQTS*) adult patients, LQTS infants with life-threatening arrhythmias in utero or within the first year of life, intrauterine fetal demises (*IUFDs*), and sudden infant death syndrome (*SIDS*) victims. The distribution of variants between the potassium and sodium channel genes is similar in SIDS, IUFD, and LQTS infant populations, all significantly different from the adults (*p* < .0005). (From Crotti L, Ghidoni A, Insolia R, Schwartz PJ. The role of the cardiac sodium channel in perinatal early infant mortality. *Card Electrophysiol Clin.* 2014;6:749-759.)

***CACNA1c* (LQT8)—Timothy Syndrome.** LQT8 is a rare variant characterized by marked QT interval prolongation, often presenting with 2:1 functional atrioventricular block, macroscopic T wave alternans, and syndactyly. LQT8 is highly malignant, and 10 (59%) of the 17 children reported by Splawski and colleagues[7] died at a mean age of 2.5 years. Some children with Timothy syndrome also had congenital heart diseases, immune deficiency, intermittent hypoglycemia, cognitive abnormalities, and autism.

Molecular screening identified a missense mutation (G406R) in the voltage-gated calcium channel gene (*CACNA1c*) in all probands analyzed. G406R produces sustained inward calcium currents by causing nearly complete loss of voltage-dependent inactivation.[7] In the ClinVar database (http://www.ncbi.nlm.nih.gov/clinvar/?term=Timothy+Syndrome) three amino acid substitutions have been so far reported in association with Timothy syndrome: G406R, G402S, and A1473G.

CALM1-3 **(LQT14–16)—Calmodulinopathy.** The small calcium-binding protein calmodulin (CaM) is an important modulator of different ion channels, such as the L-type calcium channel, the sodium channel, potassium channels, and ryanodine receptor. The evolutionary importance of this protein is highlighted by the presence of three different genes located in three different chromosomes (14q32.11, 2p21, and 19q13.32) encoding the same protein, a unique example in the human genome. Until recently, mutations in CaM genes were thought to probably be incompatible with survival, but during the last few years several cases were reported showing severe cases of LQTS, catecholaminergic polymorphic ventricular tachycardia (CPVT), or idiopathic ventricular fibrillation (IVF), all due to mutations on CaM genes.[8–14] In 2013 we reported on four infants and very young children presenting with major QT prolongation, recurrent CA, and poor response to therapy. They were all genotype negative and had unaffected parents. Using exome sequencing in parents-child trios, we identified *de novo* mutations in either *CALM1* or *CALM2*, two of the three human genes encoding CaM.[8] More recently, mutations on *CALM3* were also identified.[12] All mutation carriers were infants with recurrent ventricular fibrillation (VF) usually triggered by sympathetic activation, major QT prolongation (corrected QT interval [QTc] >600 ms), intermittent 2:1 atrioventricular block, and the presence of T wave alternans.[8] The mutations altered residues in or adjacent to critical calcium-binding loops in the CaM carboxyl-terminal domain and exhibited major reductions in calcium binding affinity.[8] The overexpression of these mutations in heterologous systems showed that the LQTS phenotype was mainly due to a reduction in the calcium-dependent inactivation of L-type calcium channels, causing an increase in inward calcium and a prolongation of the plateau phase of action potential duration.[15,16] However, in heterologous systems, the overexpression of the mutated allele does not take into account the native allelic balance, specifically important for CaM in which six alleles are expressed. Indeed, all mutations so far identified are in heterozygosity, and therefore a mutated allele is expressed with five normal ones. We have generated patient-specific induced pluripotent stem cells (iPS) from skin fibroblasts of one of the identified mutation carriers (*CALM1*-F142L) and have differentiated them into cardiomyocytes.[17] This approach allowed testing the mutation in the context of the physiological allelic balance, including potential adaptive transcriptional or posttranscriptional remodeling. Our results confirm the derangement of L-type Ca^{2+} current (I_{CaL}) inactivation as the dominant mutation consequence and suggest the resulting repolarization delay as the most likely arrhythmogenic effect.[17] Recently, an international calmodulinopathy registry has been established and as of February 2017 enrolls more than 50 patients with a *CALM* mutation and a wide range of phenotypic manifestations.[18]

TRDN **(LQT17)—Triadin Knockout Syndrome.** Cardiac triadin is a protein critical to the structure and functional regulation of cardiac muscle calcium release units and excitation–contraction coupling. Through whole-exome sequencing (WES), a homozygous frameshift mutation (D18fs13) was recently identified in a 10-year-old girl with LQTS, with a QTc of 500 ms and life-threatening arrhythmias occurring since the age of 1 year.[19] Subsequent targeted screening of the *TRDN* gene allowed the identification of either homozygous or compound heterozygous frameshift mutations in 4/33 unrelated LQTS cases.[19] All these cases had exercise-induced CA in early childhood and T wave inversion in V_1–V_4 (but their ages ranged from 2 to 6 years) together with QTc prolongation.[19] Despite the lack of functional data, the role of triadin is supported by sympathetically mediated arrhythmias and cardiomyocyte calcium overload due to slower calcium-dependent inactivation of the L-type calcium channel in *TRDN* null mice.[19]

Prevalence

At variance with all other cardiac diseases of genetic origin for which only estimates exist, the prevalence of LQTS has been established on the basis of hard data provided by the largest prospective study of neonatal electrocardiography ever performed,[20] which involved 44,596 infants aged 3–4 weeks and was complemented by genetic screening. Among these infants, 1.4% had a QTc between 440 and 469 ms and 0.7/1000 had a QTc ≥470 ms, regarded as markedly prolonged by the European Task Force on Neonatal Electrocardiography.[21] In the latter group (n = 31), more than 90% of infants underwent molecular screening, and LQTS disease-causing mutations were found in 13 of 28 (46%).[20] As almost 50% of the infants with QTc ≥470 ms (0.7/1000) are affected by LQTS, and as some of those infants with a QTc between 440 and 469 ms are also affected (unpublished), it follows that the prevalence of LQTS must be close to 1/2000 live births. This does not include the "silent mutation carriers" (QTc <440 ms), a group ranging between 10% and 36% according to genotype[22] that escapes ECG diagnosis and is usually identified using cascade screening.

Clinical Presentation

Over the years, cardiologists have progressively become more aware of LQTS and now tend more easily to suspect it. This has contributed to the realization that a relatively large number of LQTS patients may remain asymptomatic even off therapy. The typical clinical presentation of LQTS years ago, when only the more serious cases were diagnosed, was the occurrence of syncope or CA, precipitated by emotional or physical stress, in a young individual with a prolonged QT interval on ECG. If these symptomatic patients were left untreated, the syncopal episodes would recur and eventually prove fatal in most cases.[1] Nowadays, the majority of patients are identified before symptoms occur, largely because of ECG screening either before practicing sports or for other reasons, and it is clear that many affected patients have a very benign course.

The clinical history of repeated episodes of loss of consciousness under emotional or physical stress, in a subject with a prolonged QT interval, is so typical as to be almost unmistakable, provided that the physician is aware of LQTS. However, the clinical presentation is not always so clear.

Cardiac Events and Their Relation to Genotype

The syncopal episodes are due to torsades de pointes (TdP) ventricular tachycardia (VT) often degenerating into VF. Most patients develop their symptoms under stress, but these life-threatening cardiac events can also occur at rest. These different patterns remained puzzling until molecular biology allowed the differentiation among different genotypes. In 670 LQTS patients of known genotype who had all experienced symptoms (syncope, CA, or sudden death), we examined possible relations between the three major genotypes and the conditions ("triggers") associated with the events.[23] As predicted by the impairment of the I_{Ks} current in LQT1 patients (essential for QT shortening during increases in heart rate), most of their events occurred during exercise or stress. Conversely, most of the events in LQT2 patients occurred during emotional stress such as auditory stimuli (sudden noises and telephone ringing, especially occurring while at rest), and most of the events among LQT3 patients occurred while they were asleep or at rest. LQT2 and LQT3 are at low risk during exercise because they have a well-preserved I_{Ks} current and are therefore able to shorten their QT interval whenever heart rate increases. The practical implication is that LQT2 and LQT3 youngsters should be allowed to play (no competitive sports) rather freely, with significant psychological benefits.

Even in the postpartum period, genotype is important because the risk is higher for LQT2 than for LQT1 patients.[3] The higher

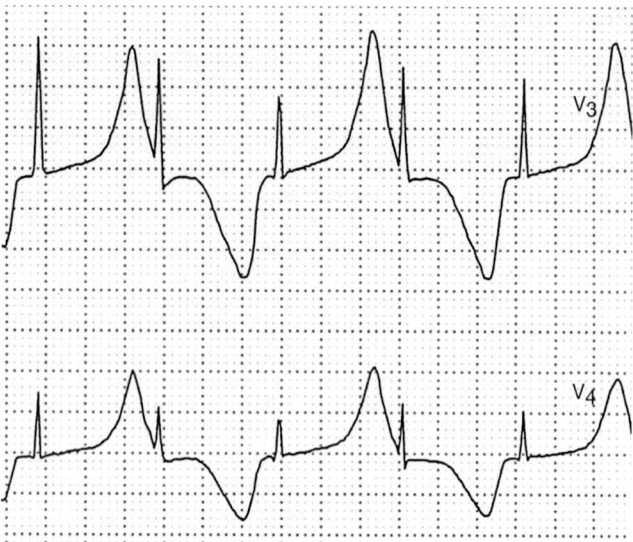

FIGURE 93.2 Example of T wave alternans from a 3-year-old long QT syndrome patient with multiple episodes of cardiac arrest and carrying the *CALM*1-D1306 mutation. Tracings are from a 24-hour Holter recording.

risk for LQT2 women is probably partly related to sleep disruption, but hormonal changes could play a role as well. Indeed, LQT2 women have an increased risk of cardiac events during the menopause transition and postmenopausal periods (hazard ratio [HR] of 3.38 and 8.10, respectively), whereas for LQT1 women, the onset of menopause is associated with a reduction in the risk for cardiac events (HR 0.19).[24]

Electrocardiographic Aspects

The bizarre ECG of many LQTS patients should be easily recognized. Besides QT prolongation, the T wave has several morphological patterns easily recognizable with clinical experience, which are difficult to quantify but useful for diagnosis.

QT Interval Duration

The Bazett's correction for heart rate remains very useful despite unrelenting criticism and the recognized hyper- and undercorrection at slow and fast rates, respectively. Upper limits of normal QTc values are 440 ms for males and up to 460 ms for females. Given the frequency of measurement errors, it is wise to use repeated measurements. In general, the longer the QT, the greater the risk for malignant arrhythmias, and when QTc exceeds 500–550 ms, the risk is definitely high.

The unorthodox proposal, made in the 1980s, that some patients might be affected by LQTS and nonetheless have a normal QT interval on the surface ECG was proved correct by our demonstration of low penetrance[25] and by the existence of a previously unexpected number of mutation carriers with a normal QT interval.[3,22] This concept has important practical and medicolegal implications because, for example, it no longer allows a cardiologist to define the sibling of an affected patient with a normal QTc as "definitely not affected by LQTS."

T Wave Morphology

The T wave is often biphasic or notched. These abnormalities are particularly evident in the precordial leads and contribute to the diagnosis of LQTS; they often are more immediately striking than the sheer prolongation of the QT interval. Following cessation of exercise, major repolarization changes often appear, and they are useful for the diagnosis.

Notched T waves are more frequent in symptomatic patients (81% vs. 19%; $p < .005$).[3] They probably reflect the presence of subthreshold early afterdepolarizations (EADs). Their appearance following exercise is markedly more frequent (85% vs. 3%; $p < .0001$) among LQTS patients than among healthy controls. Among children, notched T waves are not necessarily abnormal. Gene-specific ECG patterns do exist. LQT1 patients tend to have smooth, broad-based T waves, whereas LQT2 patients frequently have low-amplitude and notched T waves; LQT3 patients have a more distinctive pattern characterized by a late onset of the T wave. However, even within families, extreme heterogeneity of T wave morphology may be observed.

T Wave Alternans

Since 1975,[26] macroscopic T wave alternans has been regarded as a characteristic ECG feature of LQTS. Beat-to-beat alternation of the T wave, in polarity or amplitude, may be present at rest for brief moments but usually appears during emotional or physical stress and may precede TdP (Fig. 93.2). This is a rather gross phenomenon that should not go unnoticed, when present, because it is a marker of major electrical instability, and it identifies patients at particularly high risk. Its transient nature limits the possibility of its observation. The observation of T wave alternans in a LQTS patient on therapy should prompt reassessment of therapy.

Heart Rate and Its Reflex Control

Studies in a large South African LQT1 founder population in which all the affected members carried the *KCNQ1*-A341V mutation provided the novel evidence that faster basal heart rates and brisk autonomic responses are associated with a greater probability of being symptomatic.[27,28] Whereas among patients with a major arrhythmogenic substrate (QTc >500 ms), basal heart rate is rather unimportant, among patients with a QTc ≤500 ms, those in the lower tertile of heart rate were more frequently asymptomatic. Furthermore, relatively low values of baroreflex sensitivity (BRS), an index of the ability to respond with brisk increases in either vagal or sympathetic activity, were associated with a reduced probability of being symptomatic.[28] This likely depends on the fact that LQT1 patients have an impaired ability to shorten their QT interval during heart rate increases because of the mutation-dependent impairment in I_{Ks}. The lack of QT shortening during sudden heart rate increases favors the R-on-T phenomenon and initiation of VT/VF, while sudden pauses elicit EADs in LQTS patients, which can trigger TdP. Blunted autonomic responses, revealed by relatively low values of BRS, imply a reduced ability to change heart rate suddenly, which appears to be a protective mechanism for LQT1 patients.

As BRS is seldom used in clinical practice, the same concept was reassessed with another and simpler marker of reflex vagal activation, i.e., the heart rate reduction during the first minute of recovery from an exercise stress test.[29] This is a parameter strongly correlated with BRS ($r = .64$; $p = .001$).[29] Symptomatic LQT1 patients reduced their heart rate significantly more than asymptomatic patients during the first minute of recovery, and those with marked heart rate reductions had a three times greater risk of suffering cardiac events (odds ratio [OR] 3.28, 95% confidence interval [CI] 1.3–8.3; $p = .012$). The phenomenon so clearly evident among LQT1 patients is totally absent among LQT2 and LQT3 patients; this difference was expected, given that LQT2 and LQT3 patients have a normal I_{Ks} current, and therefore they are less prone to the onset of life-threatening arrhythmias related to rapid changes in heart rate, especially increases in heart rate. In LQTS patients, an exercise stress test should be always performed, not only to analyze repolarization changes useful for the diagnosis but also to help with risk stratification in LQT1 subjects. Another practical implication is that intense exercise training, which potentiates vagal reflexes, should be discouraged in LQT1 patients.

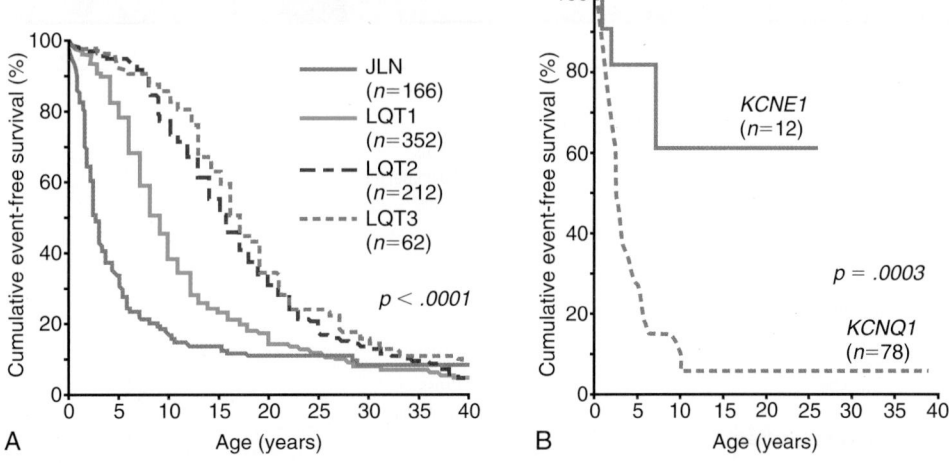

FIGURE 93.3 (A) Kaplan-Meier curves of event-free survival comparing Jervell Lange-Nielsen (*JLN*) syndrome patients vs. long QT type 1 (*LQT1*), LQT2, and LQT3 symptomatic patients. (B) Kaplan-Meier curve of event-free survival in JLN patients with mutations in *KCNQ1* or *KCNE1* genes. ([A and B] From Schwartz PJ, Spazzolini C, Crotti L, et al. The Jervell and Lange-Nielsen syndrome. Natural history, molecular basis, and clinical outcome. *Circulation.* 2006;113:783-790.)

Recently, the hypothesis that vagal and sympathetic control, as assessed from spectral analysis of spontaneous beat-to-beat variability of RR and QT intervals from standard 24-hour ECG Holter recordings, could modulate the clinical severity of LQT1 was tested in 46 members of the South African LQT1 founder population. It was found that a "normal" autonomic control increases risk, whereas patients with higher sympathetic control of the QT interval and reduced vagal control of heart rate are at lower risk.[30] This differential "autonomic makeup," likely under genetic control, allows refinement of risk stratification within LQT1 families by the use of clinically quantifiable autonomic parameters, thus leading to more targeted management.

Echocardiographic Abnormalities

In the early 1990s, we reported for the first time the presence of mechanical abnormalities in the contraction pattern of LQTS patients, showing both the presence of rapid early contraction and of an extended "plateau" phase, well visible at M-mode Doppler, before rapid relaxation.[31] These abnormalities were almost absent in controls and more prevalent among symptomatic than asymptomatic patients (77% vs. 19%, relative risk [RR], 2.75), suggesting their potential value for diagnosis and risk stratification of LQTS patients. These abnormalities were abolished by calcium blockers[32] and could represent the mechanical counterparts of EADs, thus being markers of arrhythmic propensity. After confirmation of these findings through a large Norwegian study,[33] the era in which LQTS was considered a pure electrical disease ended.[34] A recent study indicated the presence of a negative "electromechanical window" in LQTS patients and reported a strong association between a markedly negative value and arrhythmic events.[35] It looks like the time has come to start using echocardiographic indexes in addition to QTc in the risk stratification of patients with LQTS.[36]

Jervell and Lange-Nielsen Syndrome

JLN syndrome,[37] characterized by congenital deafness, is due to the presence of two homozygous or compound heterozygous mutations on either the *KCNQ1* or *KCNE1* gene.[3]

Data from 187 JLN patients[37] have shown clear differences versus the other types of LQTS including LQT1, the variant which shares with JLN impairment in the I_{Ks} current. JLN is a very severe variant of LQTS. Almost 90% of the patients have cardiac events and 50% become symptomatic by the age of 3 years; their average QTc is markedly prolonged (557 ± 65 ms), and they become symptomatic much earlier than any other major genetic subgroup of LQTS (Fig. 93.3A). Within JLN patients, there are subgroups at lower risk, i.e., those with a QTc <500 ms, those without syncope in the first year of life, and especially those with *KCNE1* mutations (see Fig. 93.3B). The latter point makes it important to genotype all JLN patients because the smaller group with *KCNE1* mutations has a markedly less severe clinical course.

The therapeutic approach to JLN patients is made complex by the early age at which most of them become symptomatic and especially by the fact that β-blockers appear to have limited efficacy; furthermore, left cardiac sympathetic denervation (LCSD), while useful, may also be less effective in JLN patients than in other LQTS patients. Thus for many JLN patients, an implantable cardioverter defibrillator (ICD) should be seriously considered in addition to the traditional therapies. For the subgroups at lower risk, it may be reasonable to postpone a decision about an ICD implant until the age of 8–10 years.

Clinical Diagnosis

Typical cases of LQTS are so characteristic that they present no diagnostic difficulty for the physician who is aware of the disease. However, as time progresses, more and more borderline cases raise the suspicion of LQTS, and sometimes the diagnosis is objectively complex. Some of the diagnostic issues have been recently reviewed.[38]

There are established diagnostic criteria[39] that have been updated[3] and validated.[40] These diagnostic criteria are listed in Table 93.2. Based on our experience, we have arbitrarily divided the point score into three probability categories: (1) ≤1 point = low probability of LQTS, (2) >1–3.0 points = intermediate probability of LQTS, and (3) ≥3.5 points = high probability of LQTS. Whenever a patient receives a score of 2–3 points, serial ECGs and especially several 24-hour Holter recordings should be obtained because the QTc value in LQTS patients may vary from time to time and from day to night. Indeed, 12-lead 24-hour Holter recordings provide very useful diagnostic information. In the group with intermediate probability of LQTS, the presence of additional morphological abnormalities may help in the diagnostic decisions. Often precordial leads are more informative. The Heart Rhythm Society/European Heart Rhythm Association/

TABLE 93.2   1993–2011 long QT syndrome (LQTS) diagnostic criteria

			POINTS
Electrocardiographic Findings[a]			
A	QTc[b]	≥480 ms	3
		460–479 ms	2
		450–459 (male) ms	1
B	QTc[b] 4th minute of recovery from exercise stress test ≥ 480 ms		1
C	Torsades de pointes[c]		2
D	T wave alternans		1
E	Notched T wave in three leads		1
F	Low heart rate for age[d]		0.5
Clinical History			
A	Syncope[c]	With stress	2
		Without stress	1
B	Congenital deafness		0.5
Family History			
A	Family members with definite LQTS[e]		1
B	Unexplained sudden cardiac death below age 30 among immediate family members[e]		0.5

[a]In the absence of medications or disorders known to affect these electrocardiographic features.
[b]QTc calculated by Bazett's formula where QTc = QT/√RR.
[c]Mutually exclusive.
[d]Resting heart rate below the 2nd percentile for age.
[e]The same family member cannot be counted in A and B.
SCORE:
  ≤1 point: low probability of LQTS
  1.5–3 points: intermediate probability of LQTS
  ≥3.5 points: high probability
From Schwartz PJ, Crotti L. QTc behavior during exercise and genetic testing for the long-QT syndrome. *Circulation*. 2011;124:2181–2184.

Asia Pacific Heart Rhythm Society (HRS/EHRA/APHRS) Expert Consensus document[41] indicates a score of ≥3.5 points as one of the three major ways to reach a diagnosis of LQTS, the other being the presence of an unequivocally pathogenic mutation in one of the LQTS genes and/or the presence of a QTc ≥500 ms in repeated 12-lead ECGs.

These diagnostic criteria, usually referred to as "Schwartz criteria," were conceived in the premolecular era and, clearly, they cannot be useful for identifying the "silent mutation carriers." For these subjects, molecular screening is essential. The main value of these criteria is during a first contact with a patient and in clinical studies when uniformity in diagnosis is essential.

Molecular Diagnosis in Long QT Syndrome

Who Should Be Screened for Long QT Syndrome and Medicolegal Implications

Molecular diagnosis should always be attempted whenever the diagnosis of LQTS has either been made or suspected on sound clinical grounds. When successful (75%–80% of cases in our laboratory), it allows the rapid screening of all family members and the identification of all "silent mutation carriers," thus allowing the institution of preventive measures and the essential recommendation to avoid QT prolonging drugs by consulting https://www.crediblemeds.org.

This concept has clinical and medicolegal implications. Physicians who do not attempt to genotype their LQTS probands are willfully choosing to ignore the possibility that other family members, even those with a borderline-normal QT interval, might be mutation carriers who would become at risk for sudden death should they receive one of the many drugs that prolong the QT interval. Once the proband has been genotyped, it is simple, inexpensive, and fast to identify the other mutation carriers in the family.

Molecular Genetics and Risk Stratification

Molecular genetics undoubtedly contribute to risk stratification in LQTS. However, clinical decisions based on laboratory results should be made by experts to avoid disquieting mistakes, as happened when too many asymptomatic LQT3 patients were implanted with an ICD just because of a *SCN5A* mutation.[42]

In 2003,[22] data on 647 patients of known genotype and from 193 families indicated that the incidence of life-threatening events was lower among LQT1 patients, but largely because of the high prevalence of "silent mutation carriers"; the risk was higher among LQT2 females vs. males as well as LQT3 males vs. females. However, independently of genotype, a large number of individuals were asymptomatic without therapy as well, and the risk of cardiac events was strongly correlated with a QTc >500 ms. Despite no systematic studies, the available data suggest that whenever the mutations affect the calcium current, the phenotype tends to be more complex and severe.[7,8,17]

Also, the location of the mutation across the protein matters. Location in the pore region of *hERG* for LQT2 patients,[43] the transmembrane location, and dominant-negative effect for LQT1 patients[44] are independent risk factors for cardiac events. *KCNQ1* missense mutations located in the cytoplasmic loops connecting S2–S3 and S4–S5[27] were reported to be particularly severe, but a further analysis concluded that this was true only among women.[45]

Mutation-specific risk stratification became a reality when it was documented that the hot spot *KCNQ1*-A341V is associated with unusually high clinical severity, independently of the ethnic background, and this is explained neither by the location (transmembrane) nor by the functional consequence of the mutation (mild dominant negative).[27,46] Somewhat similarly, *SCN5A*-E1784K, a common LQT3 mutation, is also associated with Brugada syndrome and sinus node dysfunction.[5] Thus when managing families with this mutation, the possibility of an overlap syndrome should be considered (e.g., family members with a normal QT interval should undergo a flecainide/ajmaline test).

The evidence that even within families a very different clinical outcome can be observed among siblings carrying the same mutation has stimulated the search for modifier genes, those relatively common genetic variants that may be associated with increased or decreased arrhythmic risk.[47] The first modifier of the clinical severity in LQTS, the common polymorphism KCNH2-K897T, was identified in 2005.[48] Cellular electrophysiology showed that K897T accentuated the I_{Kr} current loss produced by the disease-causing mutation, thus unmasking a clinically latent C-terminal LQT2 mutation.[48] This finding has already been validated.[49]

Genome-wide association (GWA) studies aimed at the identification of single nucleotide polymorphisms (SNPs) influencing the QT interval in the general population contributed to the search for modifier genes in LQTS.[50-52] Among the SNPs recognized to have an influence on QT interval, those on the NOS1AP gene consistently appeared to give the strongest signal and therefore represented optimal candidate genes. Indeed, in the LQT1-A341V founder population, two common variants of this gene, encoding a nitric oxide synthase adaptor protein, almost double the risk of life-threatening arrhythmias.[53] The modifier role of NOS1AP was subsequently validated in a heterogeneous population of LQTS patients.[54] More recently, the major role played by NOS1AP was confirmed in a multicenter analysis on more than 600 LQT2 patients testing all major SNPs identified by GWA studies for being associated with the QT interval.[55] Thus NOS1AP consistently appears as a strong modifier factor of the clinical severity in LQTS. Other modifier genes so far identified in different studies are SNPs in the 3′ UTR region of KCNQ1,[56] not validated in an independent cohort,[57] a protective SNP in an intronic region of KCNQ1 (rs2074238),[58] and SNPs in AKAP9, the gene encoding yotiao, a prominent protein in the regulation of the KCNQ1-KCNE1 channel.[59] Conceptually important is the fact that modifier genes with a protective effect have also been identified.[58]

The search for modifier genes represents one of the most exciting current endeavors, but some time will be necessary before they enter clinical practice. Nonetheless, the strength of the NOS1AP data is such that the presence of these deleterious SNPs should already suggest a more aggressive therapeutic strategy.

Drug-Induced Torsades de Pointes and Other Types of a "Forme Fruste" of Long QT Syndrome

In 1982 Moss and Schwartz[60] proposed that a significant number of drug-induced LQTS might occur in individuals with a "forme fruste" of LQTS. Their hypothesis, initially confirmed by the evidence[61] of a LQT1 disease-causing mutation in a patient with normal QTc at baseline and prolonged QT with VF while on therapy with cisapride, is now fully validated. The problem of drug-induced LQTS and TdP is a major one, and the identification of the subjects at risk is complex.[62]

Under the more comprehensive heading of acquired LQTS (aLQTS) are currently included all cases in which QT prolongation, often accompanied by TdP, is caused by drugs, hypokalemia, or bradycardia. The most recent data,[63] based on 188 aLQTS patients and on 2379 members of 1010 families with congenital LQTS, including 1938 mutation carriers and 441 noncarriers, provide novel and clinically relevant information. The baseline QTc of the aLQTS (453 ± 39 ms) is intermediate between that of the congenital LQTS and the controls (478 ± 46 ms vs. 406 ± 26 ms; $p < .001$). LQTS-causing mutations were found in 28% of the aLQTS subjects, a percentage higher than that previously reported. At variance with congenital LQTS, among aLQTS, LQT2-causing mutations are significantly more frequent than LQT1-causing

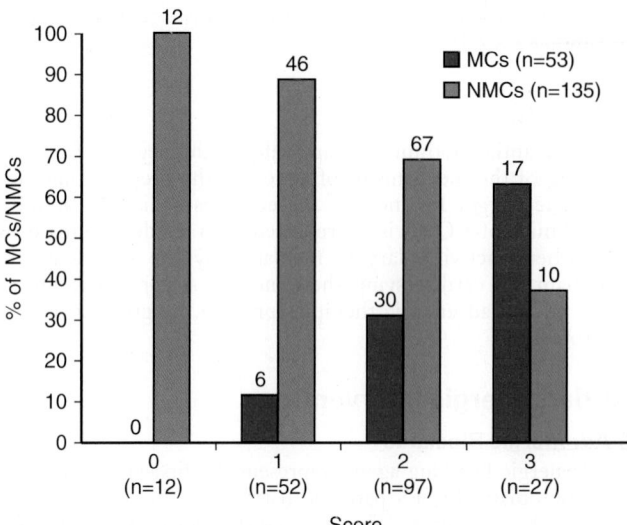

FIGURE 93.4 Proportions of mutation carriers/nonmutation carriers (*MCs/NMCs*) among the 188 patients according to increasing score values. Score 0 = age ≥40 years + asymptomatic + QTc ≤440 ms; score 3 = age <40 years + symptomatic + QTc >440 ms; scores 1 and 2 represent the presence of one or two factors. The figure shows that the number of mutation carriers increases with increasing score values (from 0 in the group with a score of 0) and indicates that 89% of mutation carriers (47 of 53) are found within the scores 2 and 3. Conversely, among the 52 patients with a score of 1, which represent 28% of the entire population, there were six mutation carriers; this means that while within the group with a score of 1 there are 11% mutation carriers, when looking at the entire population, this percentage drops to 3%. This would be the percentage of mutation carriers missed if genetic screening was limited to the groups with a score of 2 and 3. (From Itoh H, Crotti L, Aiba T, et al. The genetics underlying acquired long QT syndrome. Impact on management. *Eur Heart J.* 2016;37:1456-1464.)

mutations (64% vs. 20%; $p < .001$). These data were used to develop a score, based on simple clinical parameters such as QTc, age, and symptoms, which allows the identification of aLQTS subjects who are more likely to carry LQTS-causing mutations (Fig. 93.4).

Sudden Infant Death Syndrome and Neonatal Electrocardiogram Screening

SIDS remains the leading cause of sudden death during the first year of life in the Western world, but its causes are still largely unknown. Following the 1976 hypothesis by Schwartz[64] that an undefined number of SIDS victims might die because of an arrhythmic death akin that of LQTS, a series of studies confirmed the validity of the concept and provided evidence that a definite percentage of SIDS victims indeed carry a LQTS-causing mutation. The largest such study,[65] based on 201 SIDS victims and 187 controls, identified genetic variants in LQTS genes in 9.5% (95% CI, 5.8%–14.4%) of the victims and in none of the controls. More recently, in 161 European SIDS infants, variants with likely functional effects in genes associated with channelopathies were identified in 9% of the cases.[66] Therefore, a number of currently labeled "SIDS deaths" are actually due to LQTS; as such, these are preventable deaths.

These data clearly support the controversial concept of neonatal ECG screening[67] to prevent those sudden deaths due to unrecognized LQTS, which may occur during the first few months of life or later on. Such a screening is clearly cost effective in Europe.[68]

Following the hypothesis that as any disease that causes death during the first months of life, LQTS could also do the same shortly before birth,[69] a genetic study was performed in 97 stillbirths: an LQTS-causing mutation was found in 3.3% of the cases and a rare missense variant with a favoring arrhythmic role in another 8.8%.[70]

Therapy

Effective antiarrhythmic therapy reflects the degree of understanding of the mechanisms of action of the precipitating factors. The trigger for most of the episodes of life-threatening arrhythmias of LQTS is represented by a sudden increase in sympathetic activity, largely mediated by the quantitatively dominant left cardiac sympathetic nerves. Accordingly, and as expected, antiadrenergic therapies provide the greatest degree of protection.

Antiadrenergic Interventions

β-Adrenergic Blockade

β-Adrenergic blocking agents represent the first-choice therapy in symptomatic LQTS patients, barring specific contraindications such as asthma. The first nonanecdotal demonstration of their efficacy came in 1985 by a study on 233 symptomatic patients, which allowed a comparison between patients treated with β-blockers and patients either left untreated or treated with nonantiadrenergic interventions.[38]

Propranolol is still the most widely used drug, at 2–3 mg/kg per day; sometimes the dosage is increased to 4 mg/kg or even more. Nadolol is used very often, as its longer half-life allows twice-a-day administration, usually at 1–1.5 mg/kg per day. Atenolol and, especially, metoprolol have been associated with clinical failures more often than propranolol or nadolol; specifically, a multicenter study has indicated a four times greater risk of recurrences with metoprolol.[71] Accordingly, we now strongly recommend not using metoprolol for symptomatic LQTS patients. No solid data are available for other β-blockers. β-Blockers seldom result in excessive bradycardia, especially if the dosage is very gradually increased over several weeks.

In a large number of patients of unknown genotype, mortality while on β-blocker therapy was 2%, and it was 1.6% when limited to patients with syncope (no CA) without events in the first year of life.[38] β-Blockers are extremely effective in LQT1 patients. Data from two large studies[38] indicate that mortality is around 0.5%, and sudden death combined with CA reaches 1%. The impairment in the I_{Ks} current makes these patients particularly sensitive to catecholamines and quite responsive to β-blockade. These patients seldom need more than antiadrenergic therapy. Compared with LQT1 patients, LQT2 patients are more likely to have life-threatening events despite β-blockers, but most of these are resuscitated CA (6%–7%).[38]

Among LQT3 patients, the initial studies, based on very small numbers, reported a high incidence (10%–15%) of major events despite β-blockers[38] and contributed to the incorrect notion that β-blockers are of limited or no value for LQT3 patients and are potentially proarrhythmic. A less superficial analysis indicated that β-blocker failure was almost entirely due to those LQT3 patients who had suffered a cardiac event during the first year of life[72]; by contrast, the remaining LQT3 patients responded very well to antiadrenergic therapy. This conclusion is supported by the largest study ever performed in LQT3 patients, which involved over 400 subjects and showed that mortality for patients taking β-blockers and without cardiac events in the first year of life was <3% and was largely related to the patients with a QTc >600 ms.[73] β-Blockers are less effective in protecting JLN patients,[37] Timothy syndrome patients, and, in general, all patients with CA during the first year of life. Compliance is essential for LQTS patients treated with β-blockers. Most of the so-called failures of β-blocker therapy are due to incomplete compliance.[38]

Left Cardiac Sympathetic Denervation

LCSD requires ablation of the first four thoracic ganglia (T1–T4). The cephalic portion of the left stellate ganglion should be left intact to avoid Horner syndrome, which is expected in 1%–2% of patients.[74] The traditional retroclavicular approach[74] has been largely superseded by the thoracoscopic approach.[75] The latter is easier but seems to be associated with a higher incidence of transient postoperative neuralgic pain. The rationale for LCSD has recently been reviewed in detail[76] and is largely based on its antifibrillatory effect,[76] on the major reduction of norepinephrine release at the ventricular level in the absence of postdenervation supersensitivity,[76] and on the lack of reduction in heart rate.

The latest data already published in 2004 include 147 LQTS patients who underwent LCSD during the last 35 years.[77] They were a very high-risk group, in that 99% were symptomatic, their mean QTc was very long (563 ± 65 ms), 48% had a CA, and, especially, 75% continued to have syncope despite full-dose β-blockers. The data most relevant to current clinical decisions are those regarding patients without CA (these should receive an ICD) who suffer syncope despite being treated with a full dose of β-blockers. During a mean follow-up of 8 years, there was a 91% reduction in cardiac events. LCSD produced a mean QTc shortening of 39 ms, pointing to an action on the substrate as well as on the trigger (i.e, attenuation of localized norepinephrine release). Mortality was 3% in this high-risk group. A postsurgery QTc of <500 ms predicted a very favorable outcome. Importantly, this series included five patients who underwent LCSD due to multiple ICD shocks and electrical storms: in this group, over a 4-year follow-up, there was a 95% decrease in the number of shocks (from an average of 29 shocks/year), with a dramatic improvement in the quality of life of the patients and their families.[78] The striking antifibrillatory efficacy of LCSD has recently been confirmed by the impressive results obtained in a large cohort of a related channelopathy, the CPVT.[79]

LCSD is obviously indicated when β-blockers are contraindicated (e.g., for asthma or excessive bradycardia). Whenever syncopal episodes recur despite a full-dose β-blocking therapy, LCSD should be considered and implemented whenever possible, either as an alternative or in conjunction with an ICD. In the latter cases, LCSD is used to prevent life-threatening arrhythmias and the ICD, which cannot prevent arrhythmias, is used as a safety net.

The current indications for LCSD include patients with appropriate VF-terminating ICD shocks, patients with LQTS-triggered breakthrough cardiac events while on adequate drug therapy, patients with a failure to tolerate β-blocker therapy because of unacceptable side effects or because of asthma, and high-risk young patients where primary drug therapy may not be sufficiently protective, with hopes to serve as a "bridge to an ICD."[38]

Cardiac Pacing

The LQTS patients for whom cardiac pacing is indicated are few. The fact that the onset of TdP is often preceded by a pause justifies consideration for a pacemaker as an adjunct to the therapy of selected LQTS patients and to allow increases in β-blocker dosages. However, if a pacemaker is being considered, nowadays it is more logical to implant an ICD with pacing modes. One possible exception might be represented by very small infants for whom atrial pacing may represent a transient bridge to an ICD. It is important to remember that fast heart rates, while having sometimes an antiarrhythmic effect, may produce a tachycardia-mediated cardiomyopathy and thus should be used sparingly and transiently.

Implantable Cardioverter Defibrillators

The usage of ICDs in LQTS patients has increased significantly, but it is often unjustified. There is a consensus for immediately implanting an ICD in case of a documented CA, either on or off therapy.[80] By contrast, opinions strongly differ regarding the use of ICDs in patients without CA.

Many cardiologists quickly opt for ICD implantation. In the case of appropriate shocks, he/she will have saved the life of the patient; in case of no shocks and possibly of complications, he/she will have "done the best" for the patient's protection. No one could argue against such positive goals. Conversely, without the support of a very strong rationale, the decision of not implanting an ICD could carry medicolegal consequences in the case of a tragic outcome. In the era of "defensive medicine," these considerations unfortunately do affect medical decisions. Currently, there is a major mismatch in ICD utilization for patients with LQTS, with some programs in the USA implanting an ICD in 80% of their patients, while among two of the largest LQTS referral centers in the world (Mayo Clinic and Milano) the ICD utilization rate is 15% and 3%, respectively.[38]

The European ICD-LQTS Registry,[42] based on 233 patients, has provided disquieting information. The majority of implanted patients had not suffered a CA and, moreover, many had not even failed β-blocker therapy! Asymptomatic patients, almost absent among LQT1 and LQT2 patients, represent a staggering 45% of LQT3 patients, reflecting the misconception that LQT3 patients are not adequately protected by β-blockers.[72] During a mean follow-up of almost 5 years, at least one appropriate shock was received by 28% of patients and adverse events occurred in 31%, including a 6% rate of inappropriate shocks. Appropriate ICD therapies were independently predicted by four main variables: (1) age <20 years at implantation, (2) a QTc >500 ms, (3) a prior CA, and (4) cardiac events despite therapy. Indeed, within 7 years, appropriate shocks occurred in no patients with none of these factors and in 70% of those with all factors.[42]

Gene-Specific Therapy and Management

The rather amazing progress in understanding the genotype–phenotype correlation[23] has allowed LQTS to become the first disease for which initial steps for gene-specific management have become possible and are already usefully implemented.

LQT1 patients are at higher risk during sympathetic activation (e.g., during exercise and emotional stress). In our opinion, they should absolutely not participate in competitive sports, even though some dissenting respectable opinions have been expressed.[81] Swimming is particularly dangerous as 99% of the arrhythmic episodes associated with swimming occur in LQT1 patients.[23]

In LQT2 patients, some of whom have a tendency to lose potassium, it is essential to preserve adequate potassium levels. Oral potassium supplements in combination with potassium-sparing agents are a reasonable approach. As these patients are at higher risk, especially when aroused from sleep or rest by a sudden noise,[23] we recommend to remove telephones and alarm clocks from their bedrooms and, especially with children, whenever they have to be awakened in the morning, to do it gently without yelling. This combines good parenting and gene-specific management. Women with LQT2,[82] but not with LQT1,[83] are at increased risk during the postpartum period, and compliance with LQT2-directed therapy, adequate rest, and avoidance of QT-prolonging medications is important, particularly during this time. If LQT2 mothers choose not to breastfeed, we recommend that their male partners take care of nighttime feeding for the first 3–4 months postpartum.

The realization that *SCN5A* mutations producing LQT3 have a "gain-of-function" effect[4] has lent support to our early suggestion[84] to test sodium channel blockers, certainly mexiletine and possibly ranolazine, as possible adjuvants in the management of LQT3 patients. We routinely test the effectiveness of mexiletine in all LQT3 patients with a QTc >500 ms using the acute oral drug test technique (half the daily dose during continuous ECG monitoring). Within 90 minutes, the peak plasma concentration is reached, and if the QTc is shortened by more than 40 ms, we add mexiletine to the β-blocker therapy. In most LQT3 patients, mexiletine shortens QTc by more than 70–80 ms. Even though there is no conclusive evidence for a beneficial effect and definite failures have occurred, there is also growing evidence of significant benefit in a number of individual cases.

Asymptomatic Long QT Syndrome Patients and Patients With a Normal QTc

As the first manifestation of LQTS in approximately 13% of cases is sudden death,[22] β-blocker treatment should be initiated in all patients including those still asymptomatic. Among these, reasonable exceptions appear to be LQT1 males with a QTc <500 ms and age above 40 years because they very seldom have a first event beyond this age. LQT2 women seem to remain at risk throughout life, and we always recommend treating them.

Patients with a normal QTc (<440 ms) have a significantly lower risk for life-threatening events than phenotypically affected patients; however, their risk for CA/SCD is 10-fold greater compared with family members with a negative genetic test.[85] The decision on whether to initiate therapy in an asymptomatic mutation carrier with a normal QTc should probably be based on considerations specific for the individual patient. It is important to keep in mind that once β-blocker therapy has been initiated for a "LQTS patient," it is always difficult to discontinue it because of potential medicolegal considerations as well.

What really matters is that cardiac and noncardiac drugs that block the I_{Kr} current and thereby prolong the QT interval should always be avoided by LQTS patients.[61] A list of drugs that block the I_{Kr} should be given to all LQTS patients because their physicians may not be aware of these electrophysiological actions. Additionally, all patients should be encouraged to take potassium supplements in case of vomiting, diarrhea, and excessive sweating. Potassium levels should be maintained above 4 mEq/L. Finally, concerns have recently been raised for the use of energy drinks by young asymptomatic patients.[86,87]

Short QT Syndrome

The description of the short QT syndrome (SQTS) as a new clinical entity dates back to 2000[88] but, despite rapid advances in the recognition of its genetic bases,[89–91] clinical information remains scant as very few patients and families have been identified worldwide. The explanation that SQTS is so highly malignant that most patients die before transmitting the disease, and thus it represents a self-extinguishing condition seems unlikely. The same goes for the absence of clear diagnostic criteria and QTc cutoff values to suspect/diagnose the disease that would favor the diagnosis of only the most severe cases. It seems more likely that this is a very rare disease.

Genetic Basis of Short QT Syndrome

Three main genetic variants have been described so far in SQTS, and they all involve potassium channel genes, specifically *KCNH2*, *KCNQ1*, and *KCNJ2*. While mutations on these genes causing LQTS are loss-of-function, those observed in SQTS are gain-of-function, which shorten the action potential duration.[89–91]

Also mutations in genes encoding calcium channel subunits have been associated with a short QT interval, mainly observed with a coexisting Brugada phenotype, and the functional consequence of these mutations is a loss of function in calcium channel activity.[92]

At variance with LQTS, in familial cases with an identified genetic defect, the penetrance of the disease is almost complete, but the probability of identifying a disease-causing mutation in affected probands is significantly lower than that in LQTS, ranging from 11% to 22% according to the cohort investigated.[93-95] Molecular screening for SQTS is recommended (class I indication) only for family members of probands with a known disease-causing mutation, while the screening in probands is a class IIb recommendation.[96]

Clinical Presentation

The clinical presentation of SQTS in the available cohorts[93-95] tends to be quite severe, with a high incidence of CA and SCD. This could be due to the real malignancy of the condition or could simply be a consequence of the criteria used for the diagnosis. Indeed, the criteria used in the two major cohorts described so far were either a QTc ≤340 ms or a QTc between 341 and 360 but with an associated history of CA, SCD, or syncope of arrhythmic origin or, as an alternative, a family history for SQTS or SCD below the age of 40 years.[93,95] Atrial fibrillation has been observed in several patients and is probably related to short atrial refractory periods.

The age of onset of symptoms is highly variable, ranging from the first manifestations in utero or at the age of 70 years.[93] Sometimes SQTS manifests as SIDS.[65] However, the peak occurrence of life-threatening arrhythmias seems to be during the first year of life and then between the ages of 14 and 40 years.[93,95]

SQTS is an autosomal dominant disease, and it should be equally prevalent in male and female patients. However, there is an overwhelming predominance of male patients in the cohorts so far described, suggesting a sex-dependent penetrance.[93,95] In the European Short QT Registry[93] despite the male overrepresentation (75% of the entire cohort), CA had a similar prevalence in males and females (35% vs. 30%; *p* = .15). In both genders, episodes before 1 year of life were reported, but whereas in males more than 90% of CAs occurred between 14 and 40 years of age, in females the events were spread across the entire lifespan.[93] No specific triggers for the arrhythmic episodes have been identified[93] in the European Short QT Registry, but one report[95] indicated that the majority (83%) of CAs occurred under resting conditions or during sleep, and only few major cardiac events were related to sympathetic activation.

Clinical Diagnosis

The diagnosis of SQTS is still a matter of debate as there is no consensus on the QTc value to be used as a cutoff for the diagnosis after exclusion of acquired causes of short QT such as digitalis toxicity, acidosis, hypercalcemia, androgen use, and increased vagal tone. There is a considerable overlap between the QTc of affected and healthy individuals. Indeed, the SQTS patients described so far had a QTc in the range of 250–380 ms,[93-95] and large studies in normal populations (all >10,000 individuals) showed that QTc in the lowest 0.5 percentile of the normal distribution (QTc ≤330 ms)[97] or below 340, 330, and 320 ms[98,99] were not associated with an increased risk of SCD.

Both the European Short QT Registry[93] and another cohort[95] considered those patients to be affected who had a QTc ≤340 ms or a QTc between 341 and 360 ms in the presence of symptoms (SCD, CA, or syncope of arrhythmic origin) or of a family history for SQTS or for SCD below age 40. Gollob and associates[94] proposed a diagnostic scoring system, rather similar to the Schwartz criteria for LQTS, in which the

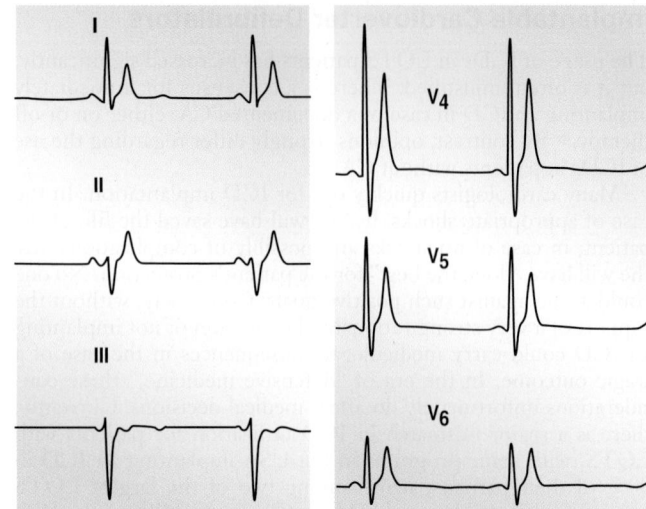

FIGURE 93.5 Example of short QT syndrome. Twelve-lead electrocardiography (25 mm/s paper speed) of a patient in sinus rhythm, with a heart rate of 52 beats/min, left-axis deviation, and QTc of 280 ms. (Modified from Gaita F, Giustetto C, Bianchi F, et al. Short QT syndrome: a familial cause of sudden death. *Circulation.* 2003;108:965-970.)

QTc and Jpoint-Tpeak interval were considered together with the clinical and family history and the genotype, if available. Regarding the QTc cutoff, in the Gollob score, a QTc <370 ms received 1 point, QTc <350 ms 2 points, and QTc <330 ms 3 points.[94] Recently, the HRS/EHRA/APHRS expert consensus statement on the diagnosis and management of patients with inherited primary arrhythmia syndromes[41] reduced the cutoff value for a certain diagnosis of SQTS to 330 ms, whereas when the QTc is between 330 and 360 ms, a SQTS can be diagnosed only in the presence of at least one additional criterion among a pathogenic mutation, family history of SQTS, family history of SCD below the age of 40 years, or survival of a VT/VF episode in the absence of heart disease.

Beside QTc values, other ECG characteristics can be useful to suspect or diagnose the disease. For instance, the morphology of the T wave can be informative. Affected patients also have a short or absent ST segment, with the T wave immediately initiating from the S wave. In SQT1 patients (those with a mutation in *KCNH2*), T waves in the precordial leads are often tall, narrow, and symmetrical, with an increased Tpeak–Tend ratio (Fig. 93.5). In SQT2 patients (those with a mutation in *KCNQ1*) and in most nongenotyped patients, T waves are still tall and symmetrical, but not as sharp. In SQT3 patients (those with a mutation in *KCNJ2*), the T wave appears peaked but asymmetrical, with a normal ascending component and a rapid descending terminal phase.

An additional helpful element for the diagnosis of SQTS is the analysis of the QT behavior during 24-hour ECG recordings and stress test.[100] The QT interval does not shorten physiologically in response to heart rate increases; therefore the slope of the QT–RR relationship is usually less steep.[100] Indeed, with a similar heart rate at rest and at the peak of exercise, the QT shortening in SQTS patients was only 48 ± 14 ms compared with 120 ± 20 ms in the control group.[100] Of course, a ceiling effect cannot be ruled out. Also, the analysis of the PQ interval could provide some useful insights. Indeed, most SQTS patients have a PQ depression ≥0.05 mV, rarely observed in healthy individuals, which may be due to the heterogeneous abbreviation of atrial repolarization.[101] A careful echocardiographic evaluation showed that SQTS patients have a higher probability to show a slightly reduced ejection fraction compared with controls and present a significant dispersion of myocardial contraction through tissue

Doppler imaging (TDI) as a consequence of a dispersion of repolarization.[102]

Risk Stratification and Therapy

The optimal strategy for primary prevention of CA in SQTS is unclear, given the lack of independent risk factors for CA. The electrophysiological study was found ineffective for predicting CA,[93,95] with a sensitivity of only 37% and a negative predictive value of 58%.[93] Genetic screening does not help in risk assessment of the proband, but it is useful to identify "silent mutation carriers" whose arrhythmic risk is still unknown.[96]

Villafañe and colleagues modified the SQTS diagnostic score by removing clinical events and tried to correlate the score with the risk of life-threatening arrhythmias.[103] In their cohort, asymptomatic SQTS patients with a modified Gollob score <5 remained event free, while a score of 5 or more was associated with the likelihood of clinical events.[103] However, when this score was tested in an independent cohort, the incidence of CA was similar in high- and low-risk groups ($p = .73$) during a follow-up of 55 months.[95]

There is still uncertainty on the therapy of SQTS. Given the high incidence of SCD, an ICD represents the therapy of choice in patients symptomatic for sustained VT with or without syncope and CA (class I).[41] An ICD has also been proposed for asymptomatic subjects with a strong family history of SCD (class IIb).[41] This suggestion is probably premature as the European Short QT Registry has shown a dreadfully high incidence of complications (58%) among the patients implanted, mainly related to inappropriate shocks due to T wave oversensing or episodes of supraventricular arrhythmias.[93]

Several antiarrhythmic drugs have been tested in the attempt to correct action potential duration and prevent arrhythmic risk. Gaita and associates[104] tried flecainide, ibutilide, sotalol, and quinidine in six SQT1 patients. Only quinidine normalized the QT interval, T wave morphology, and ventricular effective refractory period and made VF noninducible. In vitro studies showed that the $KCNH2$-N588K mutation produced only a 5.8-fold decrease in the I_{Kr} channel-blocking effect of quinidine in contrast to the 20-fold decrease in the effect of sotalol.[104] Further studies of the same mutation and data in two SQT1 patients also suggested the efficacy of disopyramide on ECG features,[105] while amiodarone had an opposite effect in the two patients in whom it was tested.[93] The major limitation of all these studies is the very small number of patients and the lack of follow-up data showing a reduction of the arrhythmic episodes. Data from the European Short QT Registry are partially overcoming these limitations, at least for hydroquinidine, which was tested in 41% of the patients; this agent normalized the QT interval and refractory periods in SQT1 patients, with a weaker and variable effect in the non-SQT1 patients. Interestingly, during the follow-up period, the incidence of arrhythmic events was 4.9% per year in patients without pharmacological prophylaxis, whereas no arrhythmic events occurred in those treated with hydroquinidine, even in the previously symptomatic ones.[93] Drug tolerability was also acceptable as only 9% of the patients interrupted therapy because of side effects (gastroenteric intolerance or dermatitis).[93]

Given these promising data, quinidine is a class IIb indication in asymptomatic patients with a diagnosis of SQTS and a family history of SCD.[41] Despite less supportive data, sotalol is a class IIb indication in the same category of patients.[41]

REFERENCES

1. Schwartz PJ, Periti M, Malliani A. The long Q-T syndrome. *Am Heart J.* 1975;89:378–390.
2. Schwartz PJ, Ackerman MJ, George Jr AL, Wilde AM. Impact of genetics on the clinical management of channelopathies. *J Am Coll Cardiol.* 2013;62:169–180.
3. Schwartz PJ, Crotti L, Insolia R. Arrhythmogenic disorders of genetic origin: long QT syndrome: from genetics to management. *Circ Arrhythm Electrophysiol.* 2012;5:868–877.
4. Bennett PB, Yazawa K, Makita N, George Jr AL. Molecular mechanism for an inherited cardiac arrhythmia. *Nature.* 1995;376:683–685.
5. Makita N, Behr E, Shimizu W, et al. The E1784K mutation in *SCN5A* gene is associated with mixed clinical phenotype of type 3 long QT syndrome. *J Clin Invest.* 2008;118:2219–2229.
6. Crotti L, Ghidoni A, Insolia R, Schwartz PJ. The role of the cardiac sodium channel in perinatal early infant mortality. *Card Electrophysiol Clin.* 2014;6:749–759.
7. Splawski I, Timothy KW, Sharpe LM, et al. Ca$_V$1.2 calcium channel dysfunction causes a multisystem disorder including arrhythmia and autism. *Cell.* 2004;119:19–31.
8. Crotti L, Johnson CN, Graf E, et al. Calmodulin mutations associated with recurrent cardiac arrest in infants. *Circulation.* 2013;127:1009–1017.
9. Nyegaard M, Overgaard MT, Søndergaard MT, et al. Mutations in calmodulin cause ventricular tachycardia and sudden cardiac death. *Am J Hum Genet.* 2012;91:703–712.
10. Marsman RF, Barc J, Beekman L, et al. A mutation in CALM1 encoding calmodulin in familial idiopathic ventricular fibrillation in childhood and adolescence. *J Am Coll Cardiol.* 2014;63:259–266.
11. Makita N, Yagihara N, Crotti L, et al. Novel calmodulin mutations associated with congenital arrhythmia susceptibility. *Circ Cardiovasc Genet.* 2014;7:466–474.
12. Reed GJ, Boczek NJ, Etheridge SP, Ackerman MJ. CALM3 mutation associated with long QT syndrome. *Heart Rhythm.* 2015;12:419–422.
13. Boczek NJ, Gomez-Hurtado N, Ye D, et al. Spectrum and prevalence of CALM1-, CALM2-, and CALM3-encoded calmodulin variants in long QT syndrome and functional characterization of a novel long QT syndrome-associated calmodulin missense variant, E141G. *Circ Cardiovasc Genet.* 2016;9:136–146.
14. Pipilas DC, Johnson CN, Webster G, et al. Novel calmodulin mutations associated with congenital long QT syndrome affect calcium current in human cardiomyocytes. *Heart Rhythm.* 2016;13:2012–2019.

15. Limpitikul WB, Dick IE, Joshi-Mukherjee R, et al. Calmodulin mutations associated with long QT syndrome prevent inactivation of cardiac L-type Ca^{2+} currents and promote proarrhythmic behavior in ventricular myocytes. *J Mol Cell Cardiol.* 2014;74:115–124.
16. Yin G, Hassan F, Haroun AR, et al. Arrhythmogenic calmodulin mutations disrupt intracellular cardiomyocyte Ca^{2+} regulation by distinct mechanisms. *J Am Heart Assoc.* 2014;3:e000996.
17. Rocchetti M, Sala L, Dreizehnter L, et al. Elucidating arrhythmogenic mechanisms of long-QT syndrome CALM1-F142L mutation in patient-specific induced pluripotent stem cell-derived cardiomyocytes. *Cardiovasc Res.* 2017 Feb 2. http://dx.doi.org/10.1093/cvr/cvx006. [Epub ahead of print]
18. Crotti L, Spazzolini C, Boczek NJ, et al. International Calmodulinopathy Registry (ICaMR). *Circulation.* 2016;134:A14840.
19. Altmann HM, Tester DJ, Will ML, et al. Homozygous/compound heterozygous triadin mutations associated with autosomal-recessive long QT Syndrome and pediatric sudden cardiac arrest: elucidation of the triadin knockout syndrome. *Circulation.* 2015;131:2051–2060.
20. Schwartz PJ, Stramba-Badiale M, Crotti L, et al. Prevalence of the congenital long-QT syndrome. *Circulation.* 2009;120:1761–1767.
21. Schwartz PJ, Garson Jr A, Paul T, et al. Guidelines for the interpretation of the neonatal electrocardiogram. *Eur Heart J.* 2002;23:1329–1344.
22. Priori SG, Schwartz PJ, Napolitano C, et al. Risk stratification in the long-QT syndrome. *N Engl J Med.* 2003;348:1866–1874.
23. Schwartz PJ, Priori SG, Spazzolini C, et al. Genotype-phenotype correlation in the long-QT syndrome: gene-specific triggers for life-threatening arrhythmias. *Circulation.* 2001;103:89–95.
24. Buber J, Mathew J, Moss AJ, et al. Risk of recurrent cardiac events after onset of menopause in women with congenital long-QT syndrome types 1 and 2. *Circulation.* 2011;123:2784–2791.
25. Priori SG, Napolitano C, Schwartz PJ. Low penetrance in the long QT syndrome. Clinical impact. *Circulation.* 1999;99:529–533.
26. Schwartz PJ, Malliani A. Electrical alternation of the T wave: clinical and experimental evidence of its relationship with the sympathetic nervous system and with the long QT syndrome. *Am Heart J.* 1975;89:45–50.

27. Brink PA, Crotti L, Corfield V, et al. Phenotypic variability and unusual clinical severity of congenital long QT Syndrome in a founder population. *Circulation.* 2005;112:2602–2610.
28. Schwartz PJ, Vanoli E, Crotti L, et al. Neural control of heart rate as an arrhythmia risk modifier in long QT syndrome. *J Am Coll Cardiol.* 2008;51:920–929.
29. Crotti L, Spazzolini C, Porretta AP, et al. Vagal reflexes following an exercise stress test: a simple clinical tool for gene-specific risk stratification in the long QT syndrome. *J Am Coll Cardiol.* 2012;60:2515–2524.
30. Porta A, Girardengo G, Bari V, et al. Autonomic control of heart rate and of QT interval variability influences arrhythmic risk in long QT syndrome Type 1. *J Am Coll Cardiol.* 2015;65:367–374.
31. Nador F, Beria G, De Ferrari GM, et al. Unsuspected echocardiographic abnormality in the long QT syndrome: diagnostic, prognostic, and pathogenetic implications. *Circulation.* 1991;84:1530–1542.
32. De Ferrari GM, Nador F, Beria G, et al. Effect of calcium channel block on the wall motion abnormality of the idiopathic long QT syndrome. *Circulation.* 1994;89:2126–2132.
33. Haugaa KH, Edvardsen T, Leren TP, et al. Left ventricular mechanical dispersion by tissue Doppler imaging: a novel approach for identifying high-risk individuals with long QT syndrome. *Eur Heart J.* 2009;30:330–337.
34. De Ferrari GM, Schwartz PJ. Long QT syndrome, a purely electrical disease? Not anymore. *Eur Heart J.* 2009;30:253–255.
35. ter Bekke RMA, Haugaa KH, van den Wijngaard A, et al. Electromechanical window negativity in genotyped long-QT syndrome patients: relationship to arrhythmia risk. *Eur Heart J.* 2015;36:179–186.
36. De Ferrari GM, Schwartz PJ. Vox clamantis in deserto. We spoke but nobody was listening: echocardiography can help risk stratification of the long QT syndrome. *Eur Heart J.* 2015;36:148–150.
37. Schwartz PJ, Spazzolini C, Crotti L, et al. The Jervell and Lange-Nielsen syndrome. Natural history, molecular basis, and clinical outcome. *Circulation.* 2006;113:783–790.
38. Schwartz PJ, Ackerman MJ. The long QT syndrome: a transatlantic clinical approach to diagnosis and therapy. *Eur Heart J.* 2013;34:3109–3116.
39. Schwartz PJ, Moss AJ, Vincent GM, Crampton RS. Diagnostic criteria for the long QT syndrome: an update. *Circulation.* 1993;88:782–784.

40. Hayashi K, Konno T, Fujino N, et al. Impact of updated diagnostic criteria for long QT syndrome on clinical detection of diseased patients: results from study of patients carrying gene mutations. *J Am Coll Cardiol.* 2016;2:279–287.

41. Priori SG, Wilde AA, Horie M, et al. HRS/EHRA/APHRS Expert consensus statement on the diagnosis and management of patients with inherited primary arrhythmia syndromes. *Heart Rhythm.* 2013;10:1932–1963.

42. Schwartz PJ, Spazzolini C, Priori SG, et al. Who are the long-QT syndrome patients who receive an implantable cardioverter defibrillator and what happens to them? Data from the European Long-QT Syndrome Implantable Cardioverter-Defibrillator (LQTS ICD) Registry. *Circulation.* 2010;122:1272–1282.

43. Moss AJ, Zareba W, Kaufman ES, et al. Increased risk of arrhythmic events in long-QT syndrome with mutations in the pore region of the human ether-a-go-go-related gene potassium channel. *Circulation.* 2002;105:794–799.

44. Moss AJ, Shimizu W, Wilde AA, et al. Clinical aspects of type-1 long-QT syndrome by location, coding type, and biophysical function of mutations involving the KCNQ1 gene. *Circulation.* 2007;115:2481–2489.

45. Costa J, Lopes CM, Barsheshet A, et al. Combined assessment of sex- and mutation-specific information for risk stratification in type 1 long QT syndrome. *Heart Rhythm.* 2012;9:892–898.

46. Crotti L, Spazzolini C, Schwartz PJ, et al. The common long QT syndrome mutation KCNQ1/A341V causes unusually severe clinical manifestations in patients with different ethnic backgrounds: toward a mutation-specific risk stratification. *Circulation.* 2007;116:2366–2375.

47. Schwartz PJ. Sudden cardiac death, founder populations and mushrooms. What is the link with gold mines and modifier genes? *Heart Rhythm.* 2011;8:548–550.

48. Crotti L, Lundquist AL, Insolia R, et al. KCNH2-K897T is a genetic modifier of latent congenital long QT syndrome. *Circulation.* 2005;112:1251–1258.

49. Nof E, Cordeiro JM, Pérez GJ, et al. A common single nucleotide polymorphism can exacerbate long-QT type 2 syndrome leading to sudden infant death. *Circ Cardiovasc Genet.* 2010;3:199–206.

50. Newton-Cheh C, Eijgelsheim M, Rice KM, et al. Common variants at ten loci influence QT interval duration in the QTGEN Study. *Nat Genet.* 2009;41:399–406.

51. Pfeufer A, Sanna S, Arking DE, et al. Common variants at ten loci modulate the QT interval duration in the QTSCD Study. *Nat Genet.* 2009;41:407–414.

52. Arking DE, Pulit SL, Crotti L, et al. Genetic association study of QT interval highlights role for calcium signaling pathways in myocardial repolarization. *Nat Genet.* 2014;46:826–836.

53. Crotti L, Monti MC, Insolia R, et al. NOS1AP is a genetic modifier of the long-QT syndrome. *Circulation.* 2009;120:1657–1663.

54. Tomas M, Napolitano C, De Giuli L, et al. Polymorphisms in the NOS1AP gene modulate QT interval duration and risk of arrhythmias in the long QT syndrome. *J Am Coll Cardiol.* 2010;55:2745–2752.

55. Kolder IC, Tanck MW, Postema PG, et al. Analysis for genetic modifiers of disease severity in patients with long-QT syndrome type 2. *Circ Cardiovasc Genet.* 2015;8:447–456.

56. Amin AS, Giudicessi JR, Tijsen AJ, et al. Variants in the 3' untranslated region of the KCNQ1-encoded Kv7.1 potassium channel modify disease severity in patients with type 1 long QT syndrome in an allele-specific manner. *Eur Heart J.* 2012;33:714–723.

57. Crotti L, Lahtinen AM, Spazzolini C, et al. Genetic modifiers for the long QT syndrome. How important is the role of variants in the 3' untranslated region of KCNQ1? *Circ Cardiovasc Genet.* 2016;9:330–339.

58. Duchatelet S, Crotti L, Peat R, et al. Identification of a KCNQ1 polymorphism acting as a protective modifier against arrhythmic risk in the long QT syndrome. *Circ Cardiovasc Genet.* 2013;6:354–361.

59. de Villiers CP, van der Merwe L, Crotti L, et al. AKAP9 is a genetic modifier of congenital long-QT syndrome type 1. *Circ Cardiovasc Genet.* 2014;7:599–606.

60. Schwartz PJ, Moss AJ. QT interval prolongation. What does it mean? *J Cardiovasc Med.* 1982;7:1317–1330.

61. Napolitano C, Schwartz PJ, Brown AM, et al. Evidence for a cardiac ion channel mutation underlying drug-induced QT prolongation and life-threatening arrhythmias. *J Cardiovasc Electrophysiol.* 2000;11:691–696.

62. Schwartz PJ, Woosley RL. Predicting the unpredictable: drug-induced QT prolongation and torsades de pointes. *J Am Coll Cardiol.* 2016;67:1639–1650.

63. Itoh H, Crotti L, Aiba T, et al. The genetics underlying acquired long QT syndrome. Impact on management. *Eur Heart J.* 2016;37:1456–1464.

64. Schwartz PJ. Cardiac sympathetic innervation and the sudden infant death syndrome. A possible pathogenetic link. *Am J Med.* 1976;60:167–172.

65. Arnestad M, Crotti L, Rognum TO, et al. Prevalence of long QT syndrome gene variants in sudden infant death syndrome. *Circulation.* 2007;115:361–367.

66. Neubauer J, Lecca MR, Russo G, et al. Post-mortem whole-exome analysis in a large sudden infant death syndrome cohort with a focus on cardiovascular and metabolic genetic diseases. *Eur J Hum Genet.* 2017;25:404–409.

67. Saul JP, Schwartz PJ, Ackerman MJ, Triedman JK. Rationale and objectives for ECG screening in infancy. *Heart Rhythm.* 2014;11:2316–2321.

68. Quaglini S, Rognoni C, Spazzolini C, et al. Cost-effectiveness of neonatal ECG screening for the long QT-syndrome. *Eur Heart J.* 2006;15:1824–1832.

69. Schwartz PJ. Stillbirths, sudden infant deaths, and long QT syndrome. Puzzle or mosaic, the pieces of the jigsaw are being fitted together. *Circulation.* 2004;109:2930–2932.

70. Crotti L, Tester DJ, White WM, et al. Long QT syndrome-associated mutations in intrauterine fetal death. *JAMA.* 2013;309:1473–1482.

71. Chockalingam P, Crotti L, Girardengo G, et al. Not all beta-blockers are equal in the management of long QT syndrome types 1 and 2: Higher recurrence of events under metoprolol. *J Am Coll Cardiol.* 2012;60:2092–2099.

72. Schwartz PJ, Spazzolini C, Crotti L. All LQT3 patients need an ICD. True or false? *Heart Rhythm.* 2009;6:113–120.

73. Wilde AAM, Moss AJ, Kaufman ES, et al. Clinical aspects of type 3 long QT syndrome: an international multicenter study. *Circulation.* 2016;134:872–882.

74. Odero A, Bozzani A, De Ferrari GM, Schwartz PJ. Left cardiac sympathetic denervation for the prevention of life-threatening arrhythmias. the surgical supraclavicular approach to cervico-thoracic sympathectomy. *Heart Rhythm.* 2010;7:1161–1165.

75. Collura CA, Johnson JN, Moir C, Ackerman MJ. Left cardiac sympathetic denervation for the treatment of long QT syndrome and catecholaminergic polymorphic ventricular tachycardia using video-assisted thoracic surgery. *Heart Rhythm.* 2009;6:752–759.

76. Schwartz PJ. Cardiac sympathetic denervation to prevent life-threatening arrhythmias. *Nat Rev Cardiol.* 2014;11:346–353.

77. Schwartz PJ, Priori SG, Cerrone M, et al. Left cardiac sympathetic denervation in the management of high-risk patients affected by the long QT syndrome. *Circulation.* 2004;109:1826–1833.

78. Schwartz PJ. When the risk is sudden death, does quality of life matter? *Heart Rhythm.* 2016;13:70–71.

79. De Ferrari GM, Dusi V, Spazzolini C, et al. Clinical management of catecholaminergic polymorphic ventricular tachycardia: the role of left cardiac sympathetic denervation. *Circulation.* 2015;131:2185–2193.

80. Schwartz PJ, Dagradi F. Management of survivors of arrhythmic cardiac arrest—the importance of genetic investigation. *Nat Rev Cardiol.* 2016;13:560–566.

81. Johnson JN, Ackerman MJ. Competitive sports participation in athletes with congenital long QT syndrome. *JAMA.* 2012;308:764–765.

82. Khositseth A, Tester DJ, Will ML, et al. Identification of a common genetic substrate underlying postpartum cardiac events in congenital long QT syndrome. *Heart Rhythm.* 2004;1:60–64.

83. Heradien MJ, Goosen A, Crotti L, et al. Does pregnancy increase cardiac risk for LQT1 patients? *J Am Coll Cardiol.* 2006;48:1410–1415.

84. Schwartz PJ, Priori SG, Locati EH, et al. Long QT syndrome patients with mutations of the SCN5A and HERG genes have differential responses to Na+ channel blockade and to increases in heart rate. Implications for gene-specific therapy. *Circulation.* 1995;92:3381–3386.

85. Goldenberg I, Horr S, Moss AJ, et al. Risk for life-threatening cardiac events in patients with genotype-confirmed long-QT syndrome and normal-range corrected QT intervals. *J Am Coll Cardiol.* 2011;57:51–59.

86. Gray B, Ingles J, Medi C, Driscoll T, Semsarian C. Cardiovascular effects of energy drinks in familial long QT syndrome: a randomized cross-over study. *Int J Cardiol.* 2017;231:150–154.

87. Schwartz PJ, Dagradi F. Red Bull®: red flag or red herring? *Int J Cardiol.* 2017;231:179–180.

88. Gussak I, Brugada P, Brugada J, et al. Idiopathic short QT interval: a new clinical syndrome? *Cardiology.* 2000;94:99–102.

89. Brugada R, Hong K, Dumaine R, et al. Sudden death associated with short-QT syndrome linked to mutations in HERG. *Circulation.* 2004;109:30–35.

90. Hong K, Piper DR, Diaz-Valdecantos A, et al. De novo KCNQ1 mutation responsible for atrial fibrillation and short QT syndrome in utero. *Cardiovasc Res.* 2005;68:433–440.

91. Hattori T, Makiyama T, Akao M, et al. A novel gain-of-function KCNJ2 mutation associated with short-QT syndrome impairs inward rectification of Kir2.1 currents. *Cardiovasc Res.* 2012;93:666–673.

92. Antzelevitch C, Pollevick GD, Cordeiro JM, et al. Loss-of-function mutations in the cardiac calcium channel underlie a new clinical entity characterized by ST-segment elevation, short QT intervals, and sudden cardiac death. *Circulation.* 2007;115:442–449.

93. Giustetto C, Schimpf R, Mazzanti A, et al. Long-term follow-up of patients with short QT syndrome. *J Am Coll Cardiol.* 2011;58:587–595.

94. Gollob MH, Redpath CJ, Roberts JD. The short QT syndrome: proposed diagnostic criteria. *J Am Coll Cardiol.* 2011;57:802–812.

95. Mazzanti A, Kanthan A, Monteforte N, et al. Novel insight into the natural history of short QT syndrome. *J Am Coll Cardiol.* 2014;63:1300–1308.

96. Ackerman MJ, Priori SG, Willems S, et al. HRS/EHRA expert consensus statement on the state of genetic testing for the channelopathies and cardiomyopathies. *Europace.* 2011;13:1077–1109.

97. Gallagher MM, Magliano G, Yap YG, et al. Distribution and prognostic significance of QT intervals in the lowest half centile in 12,012 apparently healthy persons. *Am J Cardiol.* 2006;98:933–935.

98. Anttonen O, Junttila MJ, Rissanen H, et al. Prevalence and prognostic significance of short QT interval in a middle-aged Finnish population. *Circulation.* 2007;116:714–720.

99. Dhutia H, Malhotra A, Parpia S, et al. The prevalence and significance of a short QT interval in 18,825 low-risk individuals including athletes. *Br J Sports Med.* 2016;50:124–129.

100. Giustetto C, Scrocco C, Schimpf R, et al. Usefulness of exercise test in the diagnosis of short QT syndrome. *Europace.* 2015;17:628–634.

101. Tülümen E, Giustetto C, Wolpert C, et al. PQ segment depression in patients with short QT syndrome: a novel marker for diagnosing short QT syndrome? *Heart Rhythm.* 2014;11:1024–1030.

102. Frea S, Giustetto C, Capriolo M, et al. New echocardiographic insights in short QT syndrome: more than a channelopathy? *Heart Rhythm.* 2015;12:2096–2105.

103. Villafañe J, Atallah J, Gollob MH, et al. Long term follow-up of a pediatric cohort with short QT syndrome. *J Am Coll Cardiol.* 2013;61:1183–1191.

104. Gaita F, Giustetto C, Bianchi F, et al. Short QT syndrome: pharmacological treatment. *J Am Coll Cardiol.* 2004;43:1494–1499.

105. Schimpf R, Veltmann C, Giustetto C, et al. In vivo effects of mutant HERG K+ channel inhibition by disopyramide in patients with a short QT-1 syndrome: a pilot study. *J Cardiovasc Electrophysiol.* 2007;18:1157–1160.

94

Andersen-Tawil Syndrome

Martin Tristani-Firouzi

This chapter summarizes Andersen-Tawil syndrome (ATS), an ion channelopathy. This clinically pleiotropic disorder results from mutations in an ion channel gene that modulates the most terminal portion of cardiac repolarization. ATS is fundamentally a disorder of ventricular repolarization, although the clinical manifestations are distinct from classic long QT syndrome (LQTS). The degree of repolarization derangement observed in this entity is directly related to the contribution of the disordered ion channel to the repolarization phase of the cardiac action potential. This chapter discusses the most recent genetic, cellular, and clinical data underlying this unique ion channelopathy.

Andersen-Tawil Syndrome

In 1971, Andersen reported a series of patients with periodic skeletal muscle paralysis, ventricular ectopy, and dysmorphic features, the triad of clinical manifestations known as Andersen's syndrome.[1] Prolongation of the QT interval was incorporated as an important cardiac manifestation in subsequent larger studies of this disorder.[2] The syndrome was renamed "Andersen-Tawil syndrome" in recognition of the exceptional contributions of the clinical neurologist Dr. Rabi Tawil. Within the cardiovascular field, this disorder remained obscure until mutations in the K+ channel gene *KCNJ2* were identified as a cause of ATS.[3] *KCNJ2* encodes the inward rectifier K+ channel Kir2.1, a component of the inward rectifier current I_{K1}. I_{K1} provides substantial repolarizing current during the most terminal repolarization phase of the cardiac action potential and is the primary conductance controlling the diastolic membrane potential.[4]

Clinical Manifestations

The clinical features of ATS represent a spectrum of phenotypic manifestations encompassing the skeletal muscle and cardiac systems, in addition to craniofacial and skeletal anomalies (Fig. 94.1). A major obstacle in the clinical diagnosis of ATS is the high degree of phenotypic variability and nonpenetrance. The full triad of clinical features (ventricular arrhythmias, periodic paralysis, and characteristic dysmorphic features) is present in 58%–78% of mutation-positive patients,[5] while between 32% and 81% manifest involvement of two of the three organ systems.[3,5,6] Nonpenetrance ranges from 6%–20% of mutation-positive individuals.[5,6] In an interesting report, a large ATS family presented with sex-specific clinical manifestations. In this kindred,

females manifested ventricular arrhythmias, while affected males had periodic paralysis. None of the 41 mutation carriers expressed the complete triad of ATS features.[6] These sex-specific clinical findings, however, appear to be unique to this particular family in that the same mutation was reported in other individuals who manifested the typical ATS triad.[7] Recently, the ATS phenotype was expanded to include several consistent craniofacial features and dental and skeletal anomalies that were observed in all members of a small cohort, irrespective of cardiac or neuromuscular findings.[8] These new findings help to clinch the clinical diagnosis when cardiac or skeletal muscle findings are absent.

ATS is an autosomal dominant or sporadic disorder of ventricular repolarization manifested by mild QTc-interval prolongation, but marked prolongation of the QUc-interval[5,9] (Fig. 94.2). Prominent U waves are commonly described. Zhang and colleagues reported distinct electrocardiographic (ECG) findings unique to ATS that included prolongation of the T wave downslope, wide T-U junction and high amplitude, and broad U waves.[9] Arrhythmias in ATS patients include frequent premature ventricular complexes (PVCs), bigeminy, and polymorphic ventricular tachycardia (VT).[5] Typically, VT is nonsustained and bidirectional in nature with heart rates in the 130–150 beats/min range. The degree of ventricular ectopy is quite variable between subjects, but up to 50% of all beats may be ventricular in origin.[8] While tachycardia burden is often high in ATS subjects,[10] degeneration into lethal ventricular arrhythmias is relatively uncommon.[11] For example, torsades de pointes was documented in only 3 of 96 *KCNJ2* mutation–positive individuals.[9]

In skeletal muscle, *KCNJ2* mutations can cause intermittent muscle membrane inexcitability, leading to episodic weakness that can last several hours.[11] These episodes are clinically identical to those observed in other forms of periodic paralysis and are most frequently triggered by rest following exercise. While other forms of periodic paralysis are clinically defined by serum potassium levels during an episode of paralysis, ictal serum potassium levels in ATS are commonly low, but can be normal or elevated in some patients.[11] Episodes of periodic paralysis can be as infrequent as once a year to once a day. In addition to the episodic weakness, some ATS patients can develop fixed, progressive weakness.

A number of craniofacial and skeletal anomalies are described in ATS, the most common of which are low-set ears, ocular hypertelorism, broad nasal root, small mandible, clinodactyly in the hands, and syndactyly in the toes.[2,5] Dental anomalies reported in ATS include persistent primary dentition, multiple missing teeth, and crowded dentition.[8] Because of the phenotypic variability in ATS, the clinical diagnosis can be easily missed. Cardiologists should consider the diagnosis of ATS in patients presenting with otherwise unexplained ventricular arrhythmias or LQTS, and neurologists should screen all patients presenting with periodic paralysis for cardiac involvement.

Phenotypic Overlap Between Andersen-Tawil Syndrome and Catecholaminergic Polymorphic Ventricular Tachycardia

In general, bidirectional VT (BVT) is rarely observed in clinical medicine, but is the hallmark of a handful of disease states,

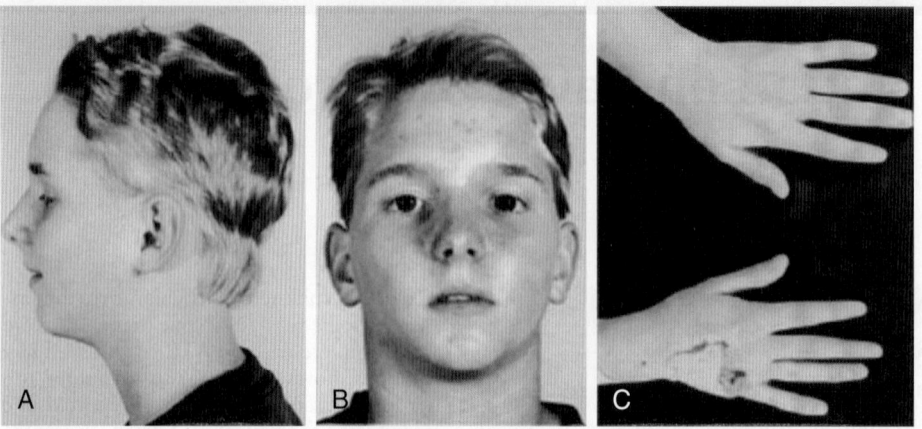

FIGURE 94.1 Typical dysmorphic features in a patient with Andersen-Tawil syndrome. Note the low-set ears, hypertelorism (wide interpupillary distance), micrognathia (small jaw) (A and B), and clinodactyly of the fifth digits (C). (From Plaster NM, Tawil R, Tristani-Firouzi M, et al. Mutations in Kir2.1 cause the developmental and episodic electrical phenotypes of Andersen's syndrome. *Cell.* 2001;105:511-519.)

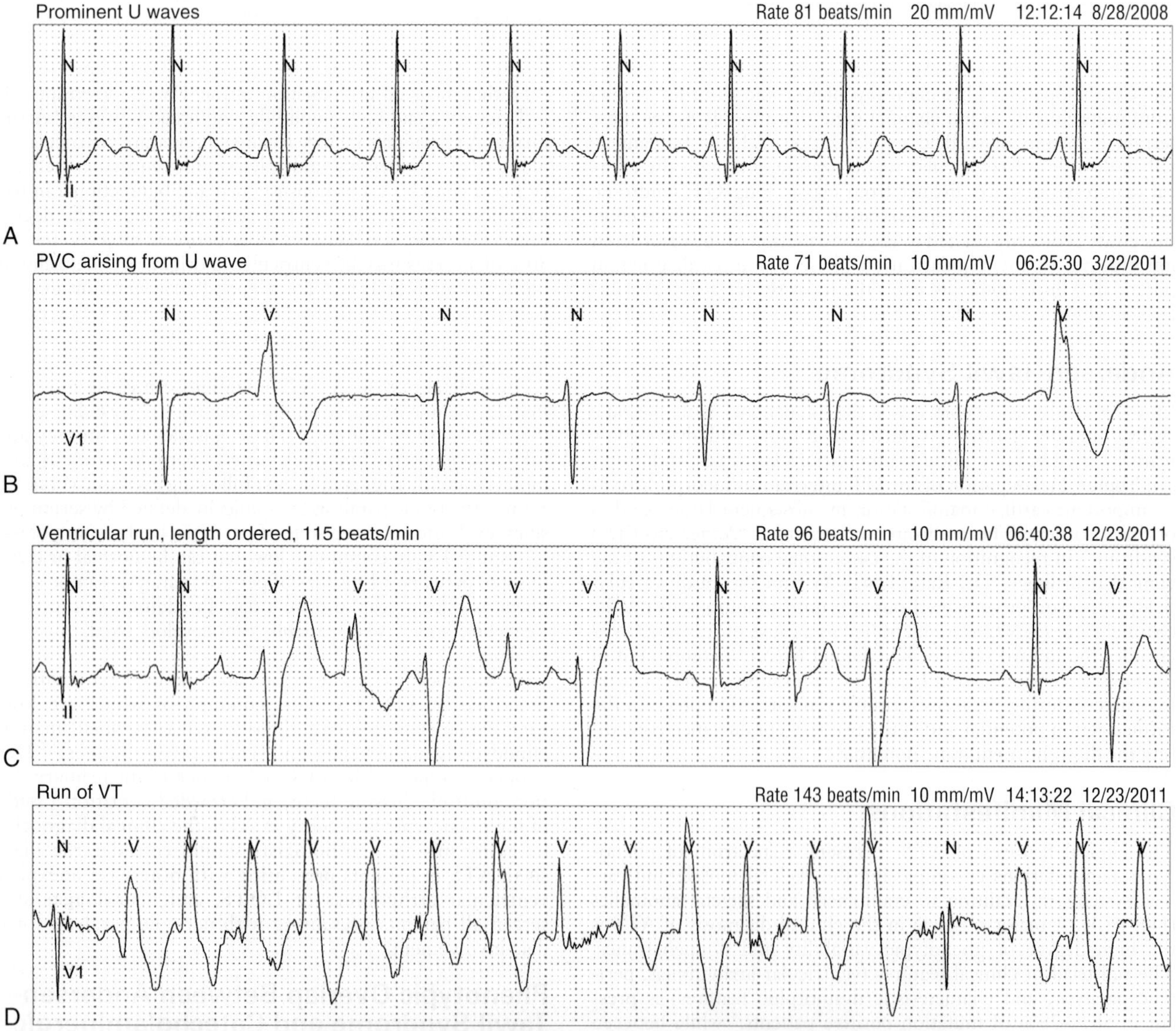

FIGURE 94.2 Representative electrocardiogram traces from patients with Andersen-Tawil syndrome. (A) Rhythm strip demonstrating pathological U waves at a heart rate of 81 beats/min. (B) It is not unusual to observe premature ventricular complexes (*PVC*) arising from the prominent U waves. (C) A short run of nonsustained bidirectional ventricular tachycardia (note alternating QRS axis polarity). Unlike catecholaminergic polymorphic ventricular tachycardia (CPVT), bidirectional ventricular tachycardia in Andersen-Tawil syndrome patients is typically slow (rates 110–150 beats/min). (D) A run of nonsustained polymorphic ventricular tachycardia (*VT*) is demonstrated in this rhythm strip.

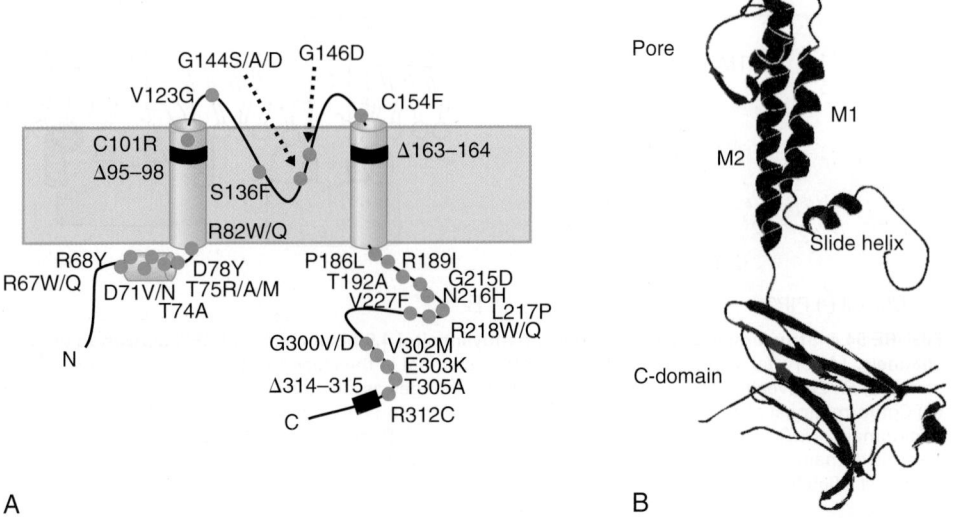

FIGURE 94.3 Locations of selected Andersen-Tawil syndrome (ATS) mutations mapped to Kir2.1 channel topology. (A) Topology of the Kir2.1 channel subunit demonstrating position of selected ATS-associated mutations in *KCNJ2*. (B) Homology model of the Kir2.1 channel subunit based on the crystal structure of the bacterial inward rectifier KirBac1.1.[19] Amino acids associated with ATS missense mutations are depicted in *red*. The majority of ATS mutations are located on the N-terminal slide helix and the C-terminal cytoplasmic domain (*C-domain*) and localize to residues involved in PIP2 binding or PIP2-induced conformational changes.

including ATS, catecholaminergic polymorphic VT (CPVT), and digitalis toxicity. Each of these clinical entities shares a common underlying abnormality in calcium homeostasis that can trigger delayed after-depolarization (DAD)-dependent arrhythmias. CPVT is characterized by sympathetic-mediated BVT and/or polymorphic VT and is due to mutations in the calcium-handling genes *RYR2* (cardiac ryanodine receptor) and *CASQ2* (calsequestrin-2).[12] In a minority of *KCNJ2* mutation-positive patients, BVT is enhanced by exercise, suggesting a clinical diagnosis of CPVT, especially in patients that lack other typical ATS features. Indeed, several patients have been reported with clinical manifestations that overlap ATS and CPVT, including patients submitted for commercial CPVT genetic testing.[13–16] The *KNCJ2* mutation V227F results in channels that function normally under basal conditions, but fail to increase current in response to protein kinase A stimulation, suggesting a clinical link between adrenergic stimulation and arrhythmia in ATS patients harboring this mutation.[16] However, in most ATS cases of exercise-induced ventricular arrhythmia, careful inspection of the ECG will reveal either a prominent U wave or ventricular ectopy at rest, thereby distinguishing the ATS patient from the CPVT patient. In addition, the rates of BVT in ATS patients tend to be slower (~150 beats/min) than those observed in CPVT patients.

Molecular Correlate of I_{K1}

The inward rectifier potassium current I_{K1} is the major determinant of the resting membrane potential in the heart and participates in the most terminal phase of action potential repolarization.[4] I_{K1} is conducted by homo- and/or heterotetrameric channels formed by coassembly of the Kir2.x subfamily of proteins (Kir2.1, Kir2.2, and Kir2.3). Message and protein expression studies indicate that Kir2.1 is the most abundant subfamily member in ventricular tissue.[17,18] The finding that mutations in *KNCJ2* cause human disease (but not in the genes encoding Kir2.2 and 2.3) further underscores the pivotal role of Kir2.1 as a primary component of I_{K1}.

Cellular Basis

Nearly all the *KCNJ2* mutations described to date cause dominant-negative suppression of Kir2.1 channel function (Fig. 94.3[19]). A minority of mutations alter channel assembly and trafficking, with resultant accumulation of subunits within the endoplasmic reticulum and Golgi apparatus.[14,20,21] Most mutant subunits coassemble with wild-type subunits and traffic appropriately to the cell surface, but fail to function normally. The mechanism underlying this abnormal function is an altered sensitivity of the mutant channel to the membrane-delimited second messenger phosphatidylinositol 4,5-bisphosphate (PIP$_2$), an essential activator of most inward rectifier K$^+$ channels.[22] Nearly one-half of all reported *KCNJ2* mutations occur at residues known to be important for PIP$_2$-channel interaction, supporting the idea that reduced PIP$_2$ binding is critical to the pathogenesis of ATS.[7] Recently, the effects of ATS mutations were studied at the atomic level by crystallizing the N-terminal and C-terminal cytoplasmic domains of Kir2.1. Arg218 and Glu303 in the C-terminus form charged and polar interactions with neighboring residues Thr309 and Arg312.[23,24] ATS mutations at Arg218 and Glu303 destabilize these interactions and likely render the channel insensitive to the activating effects of PIP$_2$.[23,24] The mechanism of PIP2 activation of Kir channels was elucidated recently by crystallizing the related Kir2.2 channel in the absence or presence of PIP2. PIP2 binds to the interface between the transmembrane and cytoplasmic domains and induces large conformational changes that open the ion conduction pathway[25] (Fig. 94.4). In light of this complex mechanism of PIP2 activation, one can imagine that ATS mutations that localize to non-PIP2 binding sites can disrupt the transduction of PIP2 binding to channel opening, while mutations at PIP2 binding sites can alter PIP2 binding directly.

How does reduced Kir2.1 channel function lead to arrhythmia susceptibility? Selective I_{K1} blockade in feline Purkinje fibers results in action potential prolongation and an increased frequency of spontaneous action potentials.[26] In an elegant in vivo study, gene transfer of a Kir2.1 dominant-negative construct resulted in QT-interval prolongation in adenoviral-transfected guinea pigs as well as spontaneous action potentials in isolated ventricular myocytes.[27] Both studies support the idea that a reduction in I_{K1} leads to the

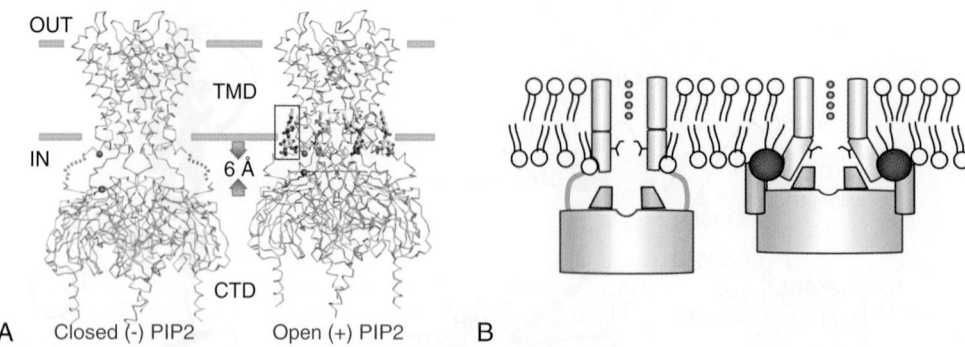

FIGURE 94.4 Structural mechanism of phosphatidylinositol 4,5-bisphosphate (PIP2) activation of Kir channels. (A) Crystal structure of the related Kir2.2 channel in the closed state (*[–] PIP2*) and the open state (*[+] PIP2*) revealing long-range conformational changes associated with PIP2 channel activation. (B) Conformational changes induced by PIP2 that open the ion conduction pathway. *CTD,* Cytoplasmic domain; *TMD,* transmembrane domain. (Modified from Pegan S, Arrabit C, Zhou W, et al. Cytoplasmic domain structures of Kir2.1 and Kir3.1 show sites for modulating gating and rectification. *Nat Neurosci.* 2005;8:279-287.)

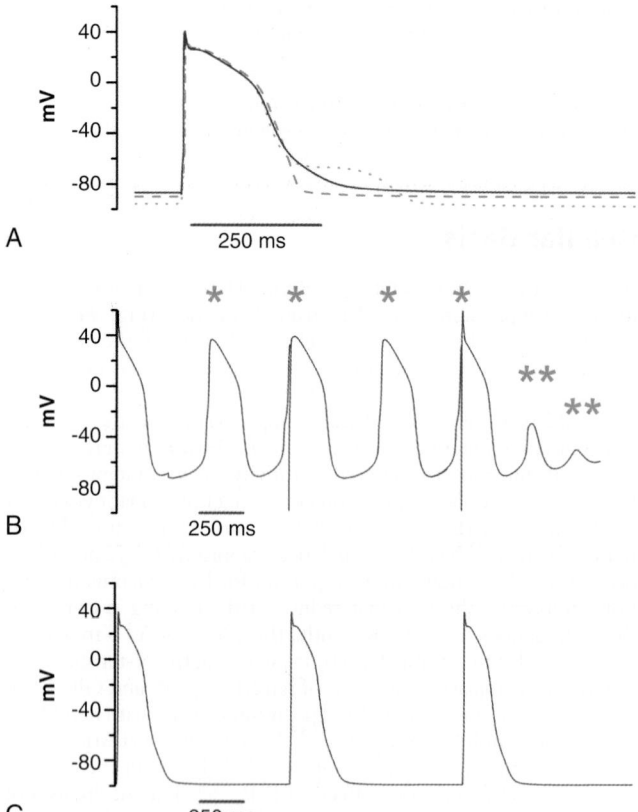

FIGURE 94.5 Simulated effect of reduced I_{K1} on cardiac action potentials. (A) Model of rabbit ventricular action potential under baseline conditions. *Dashed line,* $[K^+]_o$ = 4.5 mEq/L; *solid line,* 50% reduction in I_{K1} conductance; *dotted line,* 50% reduction in I_{K1} conductance and $[K^+]_o$ = 2.9 meq/L. (B) Reduction in $[K^+]_o$ and I_{K1} conductance resulted in spontaneous action potentials (*) and delayed after-depolarizations (**) that did not reach threshold for action potential generation. Basic cycle length of stimulation was 1000 ms. (C) Spontaneous action potentials and delayed after-depolarizations seen in (B) were eliminated by a reduction in the amplitude of the Na^+/Ca^{2+} exchanger. (From Tristani-Firouzi M, Jensen JL, Donaldson MR, et al. Functional and clinical characterization of KCNJ2 mutations associated with LQT7 (Andersen syndrome). *J Clin Invest.* 2002;110:381-388.)

generation of spontaneous ventricular activity. The cellular consequences of reduced I_{K1} have been studied using in silico approaches. Reductions in I_{K1} initially cause mild prolongation of the most terminal foot of the cardiac action potential[28] (Fig. 94.5), which is consistent with intracardiac recordings in ATS patients[29] (Fig. 94.6). Greater reductions in I_{K1} result in the generation of spontaneous action potentials that are triggered by the Na^+/Ca^{2+} exchanger.[5,28,30] This is unlike the traditional forms of LQTS whereby prolongation of the plateau phase results in L-type Ca^{2+}-channel–triggered early after-depolarizations. Computer simulations of reduced I_{K1} in virtual left ventricular tissue reveal an increase in action potential duration across the ventricular wall, without an increase in transmural dispersion of repolarization.[28] Thus the low frequency of torsades de pointes arrhythmia in ATS patients may be a consequence of the lack of transmural dispersion of repolarization in the setting of reduced I_{K1}, despite the fact that action potential duration is prolonged. The in silico data are consistent with data from the isolated canine wedge preparation using $BaCl_2$ as a model of ATS.[31] Interestingly, the contribution of I_{Kr} to phase 3 repolarization increased dramatically in the setting of computer-simulated I_{K1} reductions.[28] The consequences of this observation are that patients with ATS may be particularly susceptible to arrhythmias in the setting of reduced I_{Kr} (such as hERG channel blockers or decreased $[K^+]_o$), given the baseline reduced repolarization reserve and the dependence upon I_{Kr} as a substitute for reduced I_{K1}.

Precisely how reduced I_{K1} predisposes to BVT remains speculative, in large part, because the mechanism of BVT remains unclear. In ATS, BVT involves alternating right- and left-axis QRS deviations in the setting of a right bundle branch pattern and is frequently associated with stable periods of ventricular bigeminy and frequent PVCs. A conceptually intuitive mechanism, coined the "ping-pong" mechanism, was recently proposed and tested in silico to explain the phenomenon of BVT based on the idea of reciprocating bigeminy.[32] Computer modeling revealed that DAD-triggered activity in the left anterior or posterior fascicles sets the stage for ventricular bigeminy. As different regions of the ventricle have different heart rate thresholds for DAD-triggered activity, bigeminy can trigger DADs within the opposite fascicle by a "ping pong" mechanism that maintains reciprocating activation of the anterior and posterior fascicles. Thus this "ping pong" mechanism results in an alternating QRS axis with a right bundle branch block pattern, as observed in ATS patients. Interestingly, computer simulations of rate-related activation of a third DAD-triggered site induced ECG tracings consistent with polymorphic VT.[32]

Treatment Options

The frequent ventricular ectopy typical of ATS is notoriously difficult to suppress with pharmacological therapy.[10,33] In our database, the majority of subjects are prescribed β-blocking agents, but in most cases the frequency of ventricular ectopy does not change (unpublished data and Delannoy et al.[34]). A single case

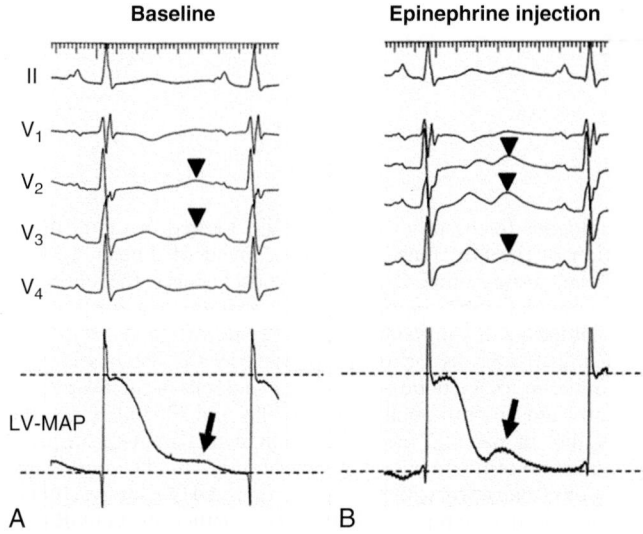

Baseline   **Epinephrine injection**

II

V₁

V₂

V₃

V₄

LV-MAP

A   B

FIGURE 94.6 Comparison of surface electrocardiogram (ECG) leads and monophasic action potentials (*MAP*) recorded from the left ventricle (*LV*) in a patient with Andersen-Tawil syndrome.
(A) LV-MAP recording demonstrates prolongation of the most terminal portion of the MAP, resulting in a small secondary depolarization or "hump" (*arrow*). The position of the hump corresponds to the position of the U wave on the surface ECG leads (*arrowheads*). (B) Epinephrine infusion accentuates the secondary depolarization and magnitude of U waves on surface ECGs. In silico simulations suggest that the secondary depolarization is due to depolarizing current generated by the Na⁺/Ca²⁺ exchanger.[5] (From Seemann G, Sachse FB, Weiss DL, et al. Modeling of IK1 mutations in human left ventricular myocytes and tissue. *Am J Physiol Heart Circ Physiol.* 2007;292:H549-H559.)

report documented the efficacy of verapamil in suppressing BVT in a patient with ATS.[35] However, in a subsequent report, verapamil was documented to induce runs of torsades de pointes arrhythmia and syncope.[34,36] Recently, efficacy of flecainide therapy in suppressing ventricular arrhythmias in ATS patients has been reported.[36,37] Finally, an interesting case report described two unrelated ATS patients with incessant ventricular ectopy that was refractory to verapamil and flecainide, but successfully controlled with a combination of pyridostigmine and imipramine.[38]

Given that many patients with frequent ventricular ectopy are entirely asymptomatic, the question arises as to whether therapy is indicated in most patients. While therapy may be debatable, there remains the difficult task of identifying the subset of ATS patients at risk for life-threatening arrhythmias.[10,33] In light of the absence of published criteria for therapy, any patient with runs of rapid polymorphic VT or symptoms such as syncope should be considered a candidate for placement of an implantable cardioverter defibrillator (ICD).

Treatment for attacks of periodic paralysis in ATS depends on attack frequency, duration, and severity. For infrequent attacks in patients with demonstrated hypokalemia during attacks, oral potassium taken at the onset of an attack may suffice. In patients with frequent, disruptive attacks of weakness, prophylactic daily treatment is necessary.[39] The carbonic anhydrase inhibitors, such as acetazolamide and dichlorphenamide, are effective in reducing the frequency and severity of paralytic attacks in other forms of periodic paralysis and are also effective in treating periodic paralysis in ATS.[40] Some patients also report a benefit on attack frequency from daily supplementation with potassium. The latter may also help reduce the QT interval, potentially lessening the predilection for ventricular ectopy. As some antiarrhythmic agents can potentially cause skeletal muscle weakness, treatment plans for patients with ATS should be closely coordinated between the treating cardiologist and neurologist.

REFERENCES

1. Andersen ED, Krasilnikoff PA, Overvad H. Intermittent muscular weakness, extrasystoles, and multiple developmental anomalies. A new syndrome? *Acta Paediatr Scand.* 1971;60:559–564.
2. Sansone V, Griggs RC, Meola G, et al. Andersen's syndrome: a distinct periodic paralysis. *Ann Neurol.* 1997;42:305–312.
3. Plaster NM, Tawil R, Tristani-Firouzi M, et al. Mutations in Kir2.1 cause the developmental and episodic electrical phenotypes of Andersen's syndrome. *Cell.* 2001;105:511–519.
4. Sanguinetti MC, Tristani-Firouzi M. Delayed and inward rectifier potassium channels. In: Zipes DP, Jalife J, eds. *Cardiac Electrophysiology: From Cell to Bedside.* 3rd ed. Philadelphia: WB Saunders; 2000:79–86.
5. Tristani-Firouzi M, Jensen JL, Donaldson MR, et al. Functional and clinical characterization of KCNJ2 mutations associated with LQT7 (Andersen syndrome). *J Clin Invest.* 2002;110:381–388.
6. Andelfinger G, Tapper AR, Welch RC, Vanoye CG, George Jr AL, Benson DW. KCNJ2 mutation results in Andersen syndrome with sex-specific cardiac and skeletal muscle phenotypes. *Am J Hum Genet.* 2002;71:663–668.
7. Donaldson MR, Jensen JL, Tristani-Firouzi M, et al. PIP2 binding residues of Kir2.1 are common targets of mutations causing Andersen syndrome. *Neurology.* 2003;60:1811–1816.
8. Yoon G, Oberoi S, Tristani-Firouzi M, et al. Andersen-Tawil syndrome: prospective cohort analysis and expansion of the phenotype. *Am J Med Genet A.* 2006;140:312–321.
9. Zhang L, Benson DW, Tristani-Firouzi M, et al. Electrocardiographic features in Andersen-Tawil syndrome patients with KCNJ2 mutations: characteristic T-U-wave patterns predict the KCNJ2 genotype. *Circulation.* 2005;111:2720–2726.
10. Chun TU, Epstein MR, Dick 2nd M, et al. Polymorphic ventricular tachycardia and KCNJ2 mutations. *Heart Rhythm.* 2004;1:235–241.
11. Venance SL, Cannon SC, Fialho D, et al. The primary periodic paralyses: diagnosis, pathogenesis and treatment. *Brain.* 2006;129:8–17.
12. Venetucci L, Denegri M, Napolitano C, Priori SG. Inherited calcium channelopathies in the pathophysiology of arrhythmias. *Nat Rev Cardiol.* 2012;9:561–575.
13. Barajas-Martinez H, Hu D, Ontiveros G, et al. Biophysical and molecular characterization of a novel de novo KCNJ2 mutation associated with Andersen-Tawil syndrome and catecholaminergic polymorphic ventricular tachycardia mimicry. *Circ Cardiovasc Genet.* 2011;4:51–57.

14. Kimura H, Zhou J, Kawamura M, et al. Phenotype variability in patients carrying KCNJ2 mutations. *Circ Cardiovasc Genet.* 2012;5:344–353.
15. Tester DJ, Arya P, Will M, et al. Genotypic heterogeneity and phenotypic mimicry among unrelated patients referred for catecholaminergic polymorphic ventricular tachycardia genetic testing. *Heart Rhythm.* 2006;3:800–805.
16. Vega AL, Tester DJ, Ackerman MJ, Makielski JC. Protein kinase A-dependent biophysical phenotype for V227F-KCNJ2 mutation in catecholaminergic polymorphic ventricular tachycardia. *Circ Arrhythm Electrophysiol.* 2009;2:540–547.
17. Wang Z, Yue L, White M, Pelletier G, Nattel S. Differential distribution of inward rectifier potassium channel transcripts in human atrium versus ventricle. *Circulation.* 1998;98:2422–2428.
18. Zobel C, Cho HC, Nguyen TT, et al. Molecular dissection of the inward rectifier potassium current (IK1) in rabbit cardiomyocytes: evidence for heteromeric co-assembly of Kir2.1 and Kir2.2. *J Physiol.* 2003;550:365–372.
19. Kuo A, Gulbis JM, Antcliff JF, et al. Crystal structure of the potassium channel KirBac1.1 in the closed state. *Science.* 2003;300:1922–1926.
20. Bendahhou S, Donaldson MR, Plaster NM, Tristani-Firouzi M, Fu YH, Ptacek LJ. Defective potassium channel Kir2.1 trafficking underlies Andersen-Tawil syndrome. *J Biol Chem.* 2003;278:51779–51785.
21. Ma D, Taneja TK, Hagen BM, et al. Golgi export of the Kir2.1 channel is driven by a trafficking signal located within its tertiary structure. *Cell.* 2011;145:1102–1115.
22. Lopes CM, Zhang H, Rohacs T, Jin T, Yang J, Logothetis DE. Alterations in conserved Kir channel-PIP2 interactions underlie channelopathies. *Neuron.* 2002;34:933–944.
23. Pegan S, Arrabit C, Slesinger PA, Choe S. Andersen's syndrome mutation effects on the structure and assembly of the cytoplasmic domains of Kir2.1. *Biochemistry.* 2006;45:8599–8606.
24. Pegan S, Arrabit C, Zhou W, et al. Cytoplasmic domain structures of Kir2.1 and Kir3.1 show sites for modulating gating and rectification. *Nat Neurosci.* 2005;8:279–287.
25. Hansen SB, Tao X, MacKinnon R. Structural basis of PIP2 activation of the classical inward rectifier K⁺ channel Kir2.2. *Nature.* 2011;477:495–498.
26. Sanchez-Chapula JA, Salinas-Stefanon E, Torres-Jacome J, Benavides-Haro DE, Navarro-Polanco RA. Blockade of currents by the antimalarial drug chloroquine in feline ventricular myocytes. *J Pharmacol Exp Ther.* 2001;297:437–445.

27. Miake J, Marban E, Nuss HB. Biological pacemaker created by gene transfer. *Nature.* 2002;419:132–133.
28. Seemann G, Sachse FB, Weiss DL, Ptacek LJ, Tristani-Firouzi M. Modeling of IK1 mutations in human left ventricular myocytes and tissue. *Am J Physiol Heart Circ Physiol.* 2007;292:H549–H559.
29. Nagase S, Kusano KF, Yoshida M, Ohe T. Electrophysiologic characteristics of an Andersen syndrome patient with KCNJ2 mutation. *Heart Rhythm.* 2007;4:512–515.
30. Silva J, Rudy Y. Mechanism of pacemaking in I(K1)-downregulated myocytes. *Circ Res.* 2003;92:261–263.
31. Tsuboi M, Antzelevitch C. Cellular basis for electrocardiographic and arrhythmic manifestations of Andersen-Tawil syndrome (LQT7). *Heart Rhythm.* 2006;3:328–335.
32. Baher AA, Uy M, Xie F, Garfinkel A, Qu Z, Weiss JN. Bidirectional ventricular tachycardia: ping pong in the His-Purkinje system. *Heart Rhythm.* 2011;8:599–605.
33. Tristani-Firouzi M. Polymorphic ventricular tachycardia associated with mutations in KCNJ2. *Heart Rhythm.* 2004;1:242–243.
34. Delannoy E, Sacher F, Maury P, et al. Cardiac characteristics and long-term outcome in Andersen-Tawil syndrome patients related to KCNJ2 mutation. *Europace.* 2013;15:1805–1811.
35. Kannankeril PJ, Roden DM, Fish FA. Suppression of bidirectional ventricular tachycardia and unmasking of prolonged QT interval with verapamil in Andersen's syndrome. *J Cardiovasc Electrophysiol.* 2004;15:119.
36. Bokenkamp R, Wilde AA, Schalij MJ, Blom NA. Flecainide for recurrent malignant ventricular arrhythmias in two siblings with Andersen-Tawil syndrome. *Heart Rhythm.* 2007;4:508–511.
37. Pellizzon OA, Kalaizich L, Ptacek LJ, Tristani-Firouzi M, Gonzalez MD. Flecainide suppresses bidirectional ventricular tachycardia and reverses tachycardia-induced cardiomyopathy in Andersen-Tawil syndrome. *J Cardiovasc Electrophysiol.* 2008;19:95–97.
38. Bigelow AM, Khalifa MM, Clark JM. Imipramine for incessant ventricular arrhythmias in 2 unrelated patients with Andersen-Tawil syndrome. *Heart Rhythm.* 2015;12:1654–1657.
39. Sansone V, Tawil R. Management and treatment of Andersen-Tawil syndrome (ATS). *Neurotherapeutics.* 2007;4:233–237.
40. Venance SL, Cannon SC, Fialho D, et al. CINCH investigators. The primary periodic paralyses: diagnosis, pathogenesis and treatment. *Brain.* 2006;129:8–17.

95 Timothy Syndrome

Silvia G. Priori and Carlo Napolitano

Timothy syndrome (TS) is a rare inherited arrhythmogenic disorder with cardiac and extracardiac abnormalities. It is generally considered a long QT syndrome (LQTS) variant (LQT8), but its clinical presentation is remarkably more complex, and it involves skeletal abnormalities and structural cardiac disease as well as central nervous system and metabolic abnormalities. The first reported case of TS dates back to 1992, when Reichenbach[1] reported a child who died suddenly at the age of 5 years with severe QT prolongation, bradycardia, second-degree atrioventricular (AV) block, and hand and foot syndactyly. Anecdotal reports followed,[2] all including life-threatening arrhythmias and similar extracardiac abnormalities. Interestingly, no familial distribution of the phenotype was noted (all clinically sporadic cases). Thanks to the work of Katherine Timothy who coordinated an international collaboration aimed at creating a registry of TS cases, the clinical features of the disease were defined and the discovery of the TS gene (*CACNA1c*) became possible.[3] *CACNA1c* encodes for the voltage-dependent cardiac L-type calcium channel, also called CaV1.2. CaV1.2 generates the I_{Ca} current, the major player during the plateau phase of the cardiac action potential. Recently, *CACNA1c* mutations have been associated with a larger spectrum of clinical manifestations. Here we will outline the most recent advancement of the clinical and pathophysiological knowledge on this disorder.

Pathophysiology

Genetics of Timothy Syndrome

The electrocardiograms (ECGs) of the initially reported TS patients were characterized by a peculiar ST-T pattern with straight, long ST segments and small T waves similar to that of LQT3 (Fig. 95.1). This immediately suggested the involvement of an inward current with prolongation of phase 2 of the action potential. In 2004[3] we reported the first *CACAN1c* mutations as a result of a common DNA sequencing effort led by the group of Mark Keating. The same nucleotide transition (G1216A) in exon 8A (an alternatively spliced exon) was identified in all patients with available DNA.[3] A few months later, Igor Splawski and coworkers[4] identified two *CACNA1c* mutations in the alternatively spliced exon 8: G406R (homologous with the mutation identified in exon 8A) and G402S. Interestingly, both cases presented the entire spectrum of clinical manifestations but no syndactyly. For this reason, the disorder was classified as a new variant, namely TS2. In 2011[5] a fourth *CACNA1c* mutation was found in association with a typical and severe phenotype (C4418G), leading to the missense mutation A1473G in exon 38. This mutation occurs in the transmembrane segment 6 of domain IV (i.e., in a position

homologous to the other three that are located in the terminal portion of the 6th transmembrane segment of domain I) (Fig. 95.2), suggesting similar biophysical consequences. In addition to the common features reported in the previous TS subjects, cortical blindness and joint contractions were noted.

Familial transmission of the phenotype was not observed in the initial series. Genetic cosegregation analysis in the relatives of TS probands in both publications of 2004 and 2005 identified the possibility of parental mosaicism leading to parent-to-offspring transmission of the mutation. More recently,[6] mild clinical manifestations (syndactyly with borderline corrected QT interval [QTc] prolongation) were reported in the mosaic father of a G406R proband. Because of the technical complexity of detecting genetic mosaics (the mutation can be randomly distributed in various tissues), the rate of TS cases actually explained by parental mosaicism is not known; this possibility should always be carefully considered.

Novel *CACNA1c* Mutations and Nonsyndromic Timothy Syndrome

Growing evidence shows that the spectrum of genetic mutations of *CACNA1c* is larger than previously thought.[7] As a consequence, the variability of the associated clinical manifestations is expanding. As of today, 22 mutations have been reported and seven of them are associated with QTc prolongation accompanied by one or more of the distinguishing traits of TS (Table 95.1; also see Fig. 95.2). Fourteen mutations are associated with variable degree of QTc prolongation and are also borderline prolonged in the absence of other pathological findings (see Table 95.1). For this reason, it seems indicated to include the cardiac calcium channel in the genetic testing of nonsyndromic LQTS subjects when the analysis of the most frequently mutated genes turns out to be negative, especially in the presence of a typical ST-T morphology. Familial distribution of the phenotype is also more likely in these less severe clinical presentations. Overall, it is appropriate to include neurological, musculoskeletal, and metabolic assessments when assessing subjects/families with prolonged QTc and *CACNA1c* mutations.

Functional Characterization of *CACNA1c* Mutations in Timothy Syndrome

Calcium Channel Structure and Function

The L-type calcium channel is a macromolecular complex constituted by an ion-conducting protein (the α_1-subunit) and several ancillary proteins, with regulatory function, called $\alpha_2\delta$-, β_{1-4}-, and γ-subunits.[7] *CACNA1c* encodes the α_1-subunit, CaV1.2. The gene spans >500 kb, and it undergoes extensive alternative splicing with at least 34 known splice variants.[19,20] Some of these splice variants are expressed in the heart and have been associated with a diversity of biophysical properties, including inactivation kinetic, drug sensitivity, and phosphorylation sensitivity.[7]

The structure of the α_1-subunit is similar to that of the sodium channel, and it consists of four homologous domains (I–IV), each one formed by transmembrane-spanning segments (S1–S6) and a membrane-associated loop between S5 and S6 that forms the pore (see Fig. 95.2).[21] CaV1.2 conducts the inward calcium current (I_{Ca}) that maintains the plateau (phase 2) of the cardiac action potential and participates in the calcium-induced calcium release process.

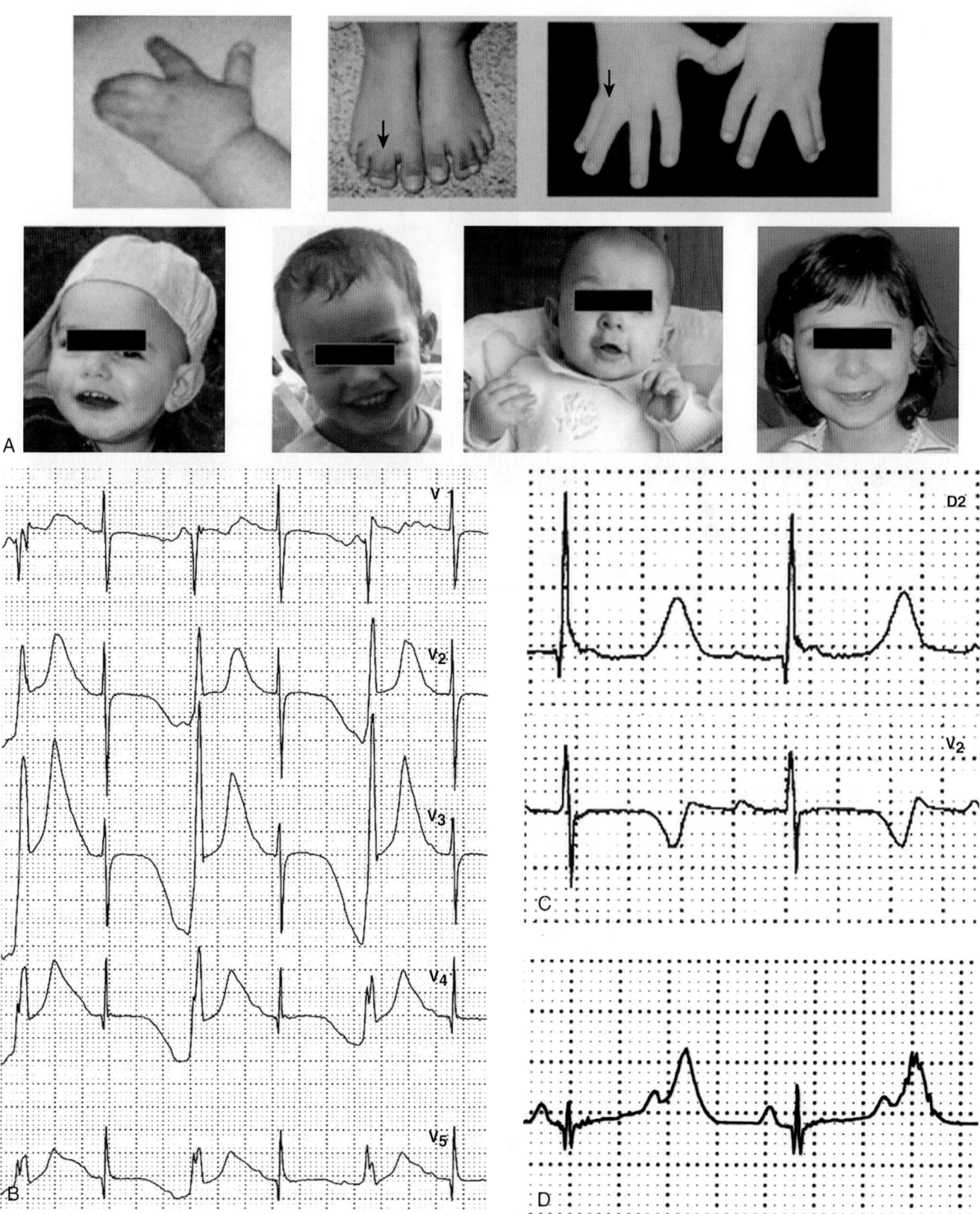

FIGURE 95.1 Clinical manifestation of Timothy syndrome (TS): the most relevant phenotypical features of TS are shown in the figure. (A) Examples of syndactyly of hand and toes and of TS facial dysmorphisms. (B) Precordial leads (V$_1$–V$_5$) from a TS patient during macroscopic T wave alternans. The extreme prolongation of repolarization creates an intermittent intraventricular conduction delay. (C) The ST–T segment in TS is often "straight," with a small and regular T wave. (D) An example of 2:1 atrioventricular block due to the extreme QT prolongation.

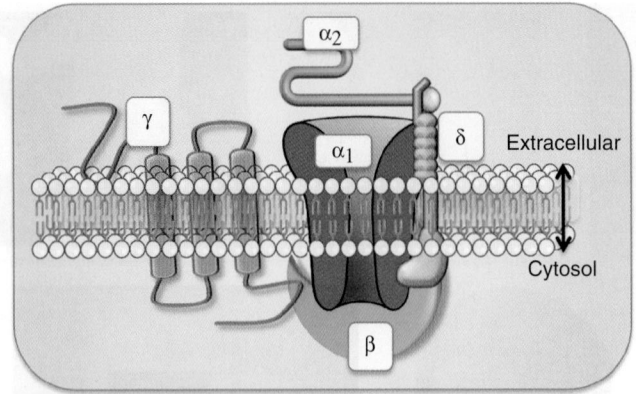

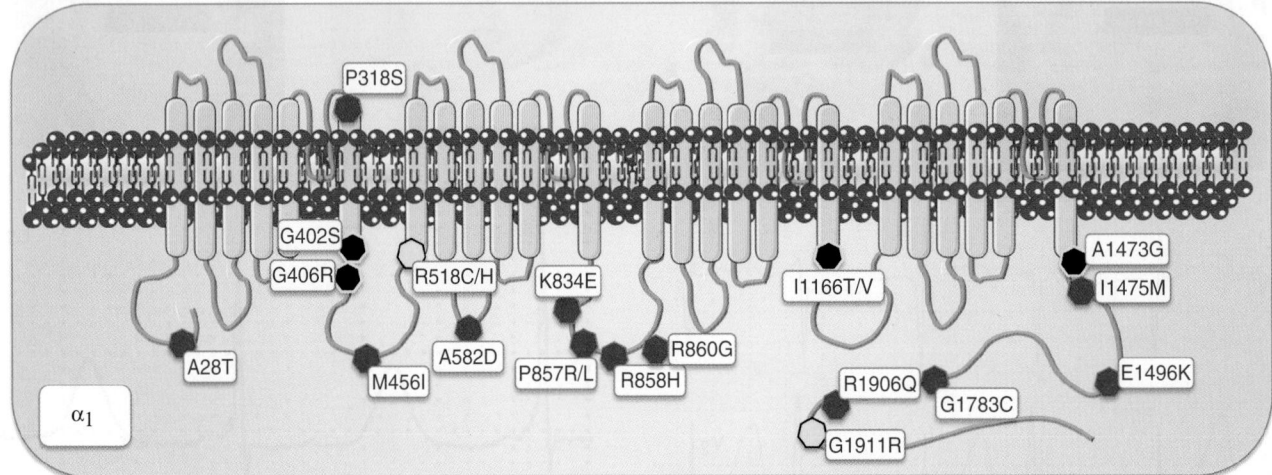

FIGURE 95.2 *Upper panel:* Schematic representation of the macromolecular complex forming the L-type cardiac calcium channel, showing the calcium-conducting subunit (α_1) and the localizations of the regulatory subunits. The β-subunit, important for channel inactivation, interacts with L-type calcium channel from the intracellular side. *Lower panel* shows a two-dimensional representation of the cardiac calcium channel with the four homologous domains. The position of the mutations associated with Timothy syndrome (TS) or isolated QT prolongation is reported. The mutations associated with fully penetrant TS are depicted with *black* symbols; mutations associated with incomplete TS phenotype are depicted in *yellow*, and mutations found in subjects with isolated QTc prolongation in *red*. The mutation G406R can occur both in exons 8 and 8A.

The accessory subunits modulate gating, trafficking, and responses to neurohormonal stimuli. The β-subunit has an important role as it increases I_{Ca} density by enhancing single channel open probability and slowing inactivation.[22,23]

Functional Consequences of Timothy Syndrome Mutations and Arrhythmogenesis

The first identified CaV1.2 mutation G406R in exon 8A[3] was expressed in Chinese hamster ovary (CHO) cells and revealed a remarkable slowing of current inactivation (Fig. 95.3). Of note, the inactivation process of L-type calcium channels includes two major components: voltage- (VDI) and Ca^{2+} (CDI)-dependent inactivation. In normal channels, VDI is stronger at membrane potentials positive to +0 mV[24] where it causes almost complete channel inactivation. The Ca^{2+}-mediated component of inactivation is modulated by the intracellular (cytosolic) concentration of calcium ([Ca^{2+}]i). The current–voltage relationship of the TS-G406R mutant channels showed that as much as 60% of the current remains activated at 0 mV. Further characterization using barium as a charge carrier (that allows to distinguish the relative contribution of VDI and CDI) confirmed that the slow inactivation in TS is due to the loss of the voltage-dependent component.[3] Computer action potential modeling including the biophysical properties of

G406R channels predicts significant prolongation, consistent with the extremely prolonged QTc observed in the clinical setting. Similar, but even more prominent, impairment of VDI is observed for G406R in exon 8 and for G402S,[4] as described in TS2.

The impairment of VDI is present in the majority of TS mutant channels so far functionally characterized (see Table 95.1). Additional abnormalities include the presence of increased window current, faster voltage-dependent activation, and increased current density. Thus the mutants associated with TS produce a gain-of-function effect (driven by the loss of VDI) that increases the amount of available current during phase 2 of the action potential (plateau) and causes action potential prolongation. Using computer simulation, Splawski and colleagues[4] showed that the increased cytosolic calcium (determined by the increase of I_{Ca}) led to an increase of the sarcoplasmic reticulum (SR) calcium release (calcium transients) with subsequent activation of the sodium–calcium exchanger (NCX) and an increased propensity for triggered arrhythmias (see Fig. 95.3). The role of triggered activity and the presence of both early and delayed afterdepolarizations (EADs and DADs, respectively) was also experimentally observed by Sung and associates[25] and confirmed in a mouse model of TS.[26] In the same paper, Sung and colleagues reported the presence of an altered subcellular localization of CaV1.2 characterized by increased expression in the intercalated

TABLE 95.1   Timothy syndrome mutations and phenotypes

MUTATION	QTc (ms)[a]	CH/CONG	SYNDACTYLY	AUTISM/ DEV. DELAY	IMMUNO	OUTCOME	FAM. HISTORY	IN VITRO	REFERENCE
A28T	450	No	No	No	No	Asymptomatic	LQTS	↑Density; ↓inactivation	8
P381S	548	No	No	No	No	Asymptomatic	Syncope	=	9
G402S	650	No	No	Yes	Yes	Cardiac arrest	None	NA	4,10–12
G406R (8A)	570	Yes	Yes	Yes	Yes	SCD < 2 months	Syndactyly, dev. delay	NA	4,13
G406R (8)	>700	No	No	Yes	No	Cardiac arrest / SCD	None	↓VDI	3,12,14
M456I	568	No	No	No	No	Asymptomatic	None	=	9
R518C/H[b]	520	Yes	No	No	No	Asymptomatic	SCD, HCM	↓Inactivation; ↓trafficking; ↑window current	15
A582D	560	No	No	No	No	Asymptomatic	Parox AF, LQTS, stillbirth	↓VDI	9
K834E	475	No	No	No	No	Syncope	None	NA	15
R857L	514	No	No	No	No	None	SCD	NA	15
P857R	500	No	No	No	No	Asymptomatic	SCD/LQTS	↑Density	15
R858H	567	No	No	No	No	Cardiac arrest/ bradycardia	SCD/LQTS	↑Density	9
R860G	498	No	No	No	No	Cardiac arrest	None	↑Density; ↓inactivation	8
I1166V	450	No	No	No	NA	Syncope	LQTS	↑Voltage-dependent activation; ↓inactivation	8
I1166T	550	Yes	Yes	Yes	Yes	Sudden death (age 1)	None	↑Density; ↓inactivation	8,16,17
A1473G	640	Yes	Yes	Yes	No	Cardiac arrest	None	NA	5,5
I1475M	473	No	No	No	NA	Cardiac arrest	LQTS	↑Voltage-dependent activation; ↓inactivation	8
E1496K	480	No	No	No	NA	Cardiac arrest	None	↓VDI; ↑voltage-dependent activation	8
G1783C	720	No	No	No	No	Cardiac arrest	SCD/LQTS	=	9
R1906Q	513	No	No	No	No	Syncope	None	NA	15
G1911R	520	No	No	Yes	Yes	Polymorphic VTs	None	↑Window current; ↓VDI	18

[a]Longest QTc reported.
[b]Two probands with mutations at the same codon were found in the same study.
=, Not different from wild type.
AF, Atrial fibrillation; *CDI*, calcium-dependent inactivation; *CH*, cardiac hypertrophy; *CONG*, congenital cardiac defects *HCM*, hypertrophic cardiomyopathy; *LQTS*, long QT syndrome; *NA*, not available; *QTc*, corrected QT interval; *SCD*, sudden cardiac death; *VDI*, voltage-dependent inactivation.

disks and multiple clusters near the nuclear envelope, suggesting a possible interference of TS mutations on the calcium-induced calcium release process. The development of DADs and abnormal calcium handling was confirmed in cardiomyocytes derived from induced pluripotent stem cells (iPSCs) of TS subjects.[27]

Other authors have linked the calcium handling abnormality and calcium overload with the propensity to cardiac hypertrophy observed in some TS patients.[28] This electrically unstable substrate can be worsened through a calcium-calmodulin kinase II (CaMKII)–mediated mechanism (see Fig. 95.3). Thiel and associates[29] found that loss of VDI is accompanied by abnormally increased CaMKII activity. This effect may be due to the loss of inactivation that leads to local increase of cytosolic [Ca²⁺] with

consequent activation of CaMKII. Further CaMKII activation is observed specifically with R406G that creates a CaMKII consensus site at Ser-409; the consequent increased phosphorylation leads to an increased channel activity ("mode 2" gating).[30] Finally, the presence of R406G homolog mutation in rabbits makes the protein more sensitive to CaMKII and less prone to dephosphorylation. Interestingly, the inhibition of CaMKII activity reversed the proarrhythmic phenotype,[29] thus suggesting that the inhibition of the CaMKII pathway is a sound therapeutic target for TS. The role of CaMKII has also been confirmed in cardiomyocytes derived from TS patients using iPSCs.

Finally, an important role for the variability of the severity of TS mutations can be played by the extensive alternative splicing

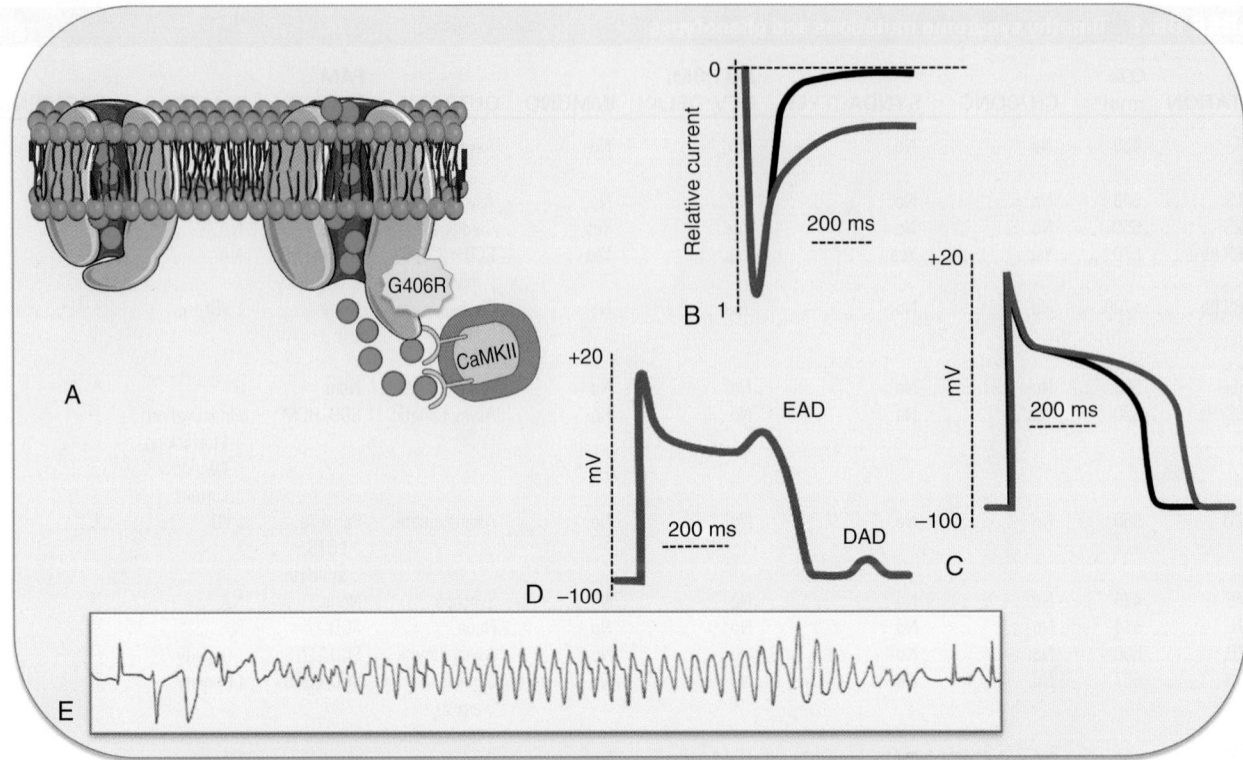

FIGURE 95.3 Electrophysiological abnormalities observed in Timothy syndrome. (A) Representation of a wild-type channel (*left*) with normal inactivation and a mutant channel *(right)* with loss of inactivation. The noninactivating current (B—*red line*) as compared with wild-type channel (*black line*) leads to action potential prolongation (C—*red line*), with an increased propensity for both delayed and early after-depolarizations (*DAD* and *EAD*, respectively) (D). The excess of calcium in close proximity with the channel pore activates Ca^{2+}/calmodulin-dependent kinase II (*CaMKII*) and further promotes triggered activity, leading to malignant ventricular arrhythmias (E).

of *CACNA1c*, which may influence the level of organ-specific expression pattern of the mutant channels.[7]

Pathophysiology of the Extracardiac Manifestations of Timothy Syndrome

The heterogeneous phenotypic consequences of TS mutations reflect the complexity of regulation and distribution of tissue expression of *CACNA1c*. The gene is widely expressed in the heart, brain, kidney, gastrointestinal tract, immune system, smooth muscle, testis, and pituitary and adrenal glands.[3,4] At least 22 splicing variants are expressed at high levels in the heart with marked interindividual variability.[19] This condition is replicated in other tissues where the gene is expressed. The mechanisms underlying this variability are largely unknown at present. Therefore the severity of the extracardiac manifestations also can be determined in a similar fashion as the cardiac ones. As of today, very few studies have specifically addressed the functional consequence of TS mutations in tissues different from those of the heart. A study has observed that variations of CaV1.2 activity are associated with the loss of control over proliferation of kidney epithelium and may play a role in the development of cystic kidney disease.[31]

The neurological consequences are somewhat better investigated. The appearance of a bipolar disorder in a TS patient has been associated with increased expression of mutant CaV1.2 protein in the cerebellum,[32] and mice harboring the G406R in exon 8 (TS2)[33] recapitulate some of the features of the autism spectrum disorder observed in TS patients; these features include repetitive and preservation behavior, reduced social memory, and increased contextual fear memory (of note, these mice do not present cardiac abnormalities). Neurons differentiated from iPSCs of TS patients revealed a spectrum of abnormalities[28] of action potentials

(prolonged), calcium transients (prolonged), and cytosolic [Ca^{2+}] (increased). Gene expression analysis showed upregulation of several calcium-related pathways, including that of CaMKII, suggesting a relevant pathophysiological role of increased CaMKII activity not only in the heart but also in the central nervous system. Furthermore, the same study showed a significant increase of tyrosine hydroxylase activity linked to increased catecholamine secretion.

Clinical Presentation

The rapid progression of the knowledge on the genetic mutations of the cardiac calcium channel has modified the approach to the clinical assessment of TS. We may recognize the existence of the typical, rare, and severe phenotypes as described in the initial reports,[3,4] and other cases (of still unknown prevalence) presenting with milder cardiac abnormalities and with mild or absent extracardiac manifestations.

Clinical Phenotype of Typical Timothy Syndrome

In typical cases, the diagnosis is generally made within the first few days of life and often earlier due to fetal bradycardia. The bradycardia is due to functional 2:1 AV block that is caused by the extreme prolongation of refractory periods (manifesting as QT prolongation on the ECG). In these instances, the T wave offset occurs later than the blocked P wave, and it is often juxtaposed to the subsequent QRS (see Fig. 95.1D).

When completely expressed, TS is lethal within the first years of life, and few patients survive after puberty. In these instances, TS is a multisystem disorder with more evident cardiac, hand/foot, facial, and neurodevelopmental features. The complete list

TABLE 95.2   Comparison of clinical features of Timothy syndrome variants

SYSTEM	PHENOTYPE
Cardiac	QT prolongation
	Cardiac hypertrophy
	Congenital cardiac defects (PDA, PFO, and TOF)
	First- and second-degree atrioventricular block
	Ventricular tachycardia/ventricular fibrillation
Musculoskeletal	Syndactyly hands/feet[a]
	Joint contracture or hypermobility
	Depressed nasal bridge
	Sparse hypoplastic teeth
	Short neck
	Hypotonia
	Low-set ears
	Dislocated hips
	Nemaline myopathy
Neurological	Autism/mental retardation/delayed development
	Seizures
	Bipolar disorder
Metabolic	Hypoglycemia
	Hypocalcemia
	Reduced immunological response
Skin/facies	Round face
	Low-set ears
	Flat nasal bridge
	Mandibular hypoplasia
	Sparse hair
	Downturned lip corners, thin upper lips

[a]It may involve all fingers but more frequently the second and third ones.
PDA, Patent ductus arteriosus; *PFO*, patent foramen ovale; *TOF*, Tetralogy of Fallot.

of all signs associated with the disease is reported in Table 95.2. The high lethality implies that TS patients are usually sporadic; multiple affected children from a mosaic parent constitute anecdotal reports.[11] The typical TS phenotype is more often associated with the G406R and G402R mutations, even if with the latter the lack of syndactyly[4] and possibility of relatively mild extracardiac manifestations are possible.[10,11] Other *CACNA1c* mutations have been associated with extracardiac phenotypes typical for TS, namely: I1166T, A1473G, and G1911R.

Cardiac Manifestations

Repolarization is remarkably prolonged in most TS patients, and the QTc often exceeds 550–600 ms.[3] Besides the abnormal duration of repolarization, the morphology of the T wave is characterized by a set of abnormalities ranging from a prolonged ST segment followed by a small T wave to giant negative T waves and macroscopic T wave alternans (see Fig. 95.1B). Congenital cardiac defects (patent ductus arteriosus, patent foramen ovale, ventricular septal defect, and tetralogy of Fallot) are present in approximately 60% of the patients; cardiac hypertrophy and ventricular dilatation are reported in more than 50% of patients.[3,4,34] Ventricular arrhythmias and ventricular fibrillation (VF) are the most frequent causes of death. Therefore the prevention of arrhythmias is the primary goal of the clinical management.

Facial, Skeletal, and Muscular Findings

Skeletal and hand/foot findings are the unilateral or bilateral cutaneous syndactyly variably involving up to all five fingers and the bilateral cutaneous syndactyly of toes two and three (see Fig. 95.1A). Facial findings include a depressed nasal bridge, low-set ears, a thin vermilion border of the upper lip, and a round face. Additional features have been inconstantly reported: microcephaly, short stature, lower extremity weakness and atrophy with

hyperreflexia, spastic diplegia, multiple dental caries, and episodes of rhabdomyolysis. as well as nemaline myopathy and dislocated hips.

Neurological

Neuropsychiatric involvement occurs in approximately 80% of individuals and consists of autism spectrum disorder; developmental delays; and language, motor, and generalized cognitive impairment. Children can be impaired in all areas of adaptive function, including communication, socialization, and daily living skills. Some children do not produce speech sounds (babbling) during infancy, and others have significant problems in articulation as well as receptive and expressive language. Profound developmental delay, intractable seizures, stroke, cortical blindness, and myopathy were reported in one individual.[5]

Metabolic

Recurrent infections and hypoglycemia are present in approximately 40% of typical TS subjects.

Timothy Syndrome and LQTS

Accumulating evidence is suggesting that *CACNA1c* can also cause a phenotype indistinguishable from the typical form of LQTS (i.e., QT prolongation and a propensity to ventricular arrhythmias in the absence of structural cardiac abnormalities and extracardiac manifestations). As shown in Table 95.1, there are several calcium channel mutations that cause isolated LQTS.[8,9] In other cases, "mild"[15] or nontypical[5] extracardiac manifestations may occur, suggesting that there is a continuum of the clinical manifestations. Furthermore, the possibility of mild manifestations due to the presence of mosaicism has been reported.[6,35] Thus the identification of a *CACNA1c* mutation in a patient with apparently isolated QT prolongation requires careful investigations to exclude the possibility of mild or subclinical immunological, neurological, or skeletal muscle involvement. In this context, it is important to consider that the combination of syndactyly, QT prolongation, and facial dysmorphisms may also occur in Andersen-Tawil syndrome (ATS).[36] Differential diagnosis is very important because ATS is rarely a lethal condition.

Overall, these data suggest that the initial distinction between TS1 and TS2 based on the presence/absence of syndactyly could be probably abandoned for a more comprehensive concept of "cardiac calcium channel disease" with a continuum of manifestations. This concept is particularly evident when one considers the possibility of CaV1.2 loss-of-function mutations associated with short QT syndrome and Brugada syndrome (see Chapters 92 and 93).

Cardiac Events and Mortality

Due to the limited size of TS cohorts studied so far, the natural history is poorly characterized. A mortality rate of 59%, with a mean age at death of 2.5 years, has been reported in the initial series. In 2006 we reported data from our population of 21 patients with TS[37] and showed that ventricular tachyarrhythmias, including ventricular tachycardia (VT) and VF, occurred in approximately 80% of patients and constituted the most frequent cause of death. Functional AV block leading to bradycardia has been documented in 85% of our patients. However, bradyarrhythmias do not seem to play a major role in TS-related mortality. The initial reports depicting remarkably severe manifestations and high mortality included only typical TS cases (TS1 or TS2). It is very well possible that the outcome associated with genetic mutations with reduced expressivity and borderline-prolonged QTc (see Table 95.1) may be less malignant and similar to that of Romano-Ward LQTS.[38] No specific trigger for cardiac arrhythmias has been reported. Anecdotal reports have described the occurrence of life-threatening arrhythmias during anesthesia, but no information is available on specific anesthetics that may be dangerous to these patients.[39] Nonarrhythmia-related deaths include sepsis and malignant hypoglycemia.

Therapy

There are no systematic studies assessing the best therapeutic strategy for TS or isolated QT prolongation due to *CACNA1c* mutations. Thus the approach to drug therapy is unavoidably empirical. Life-threatening ventricular tachyarrhythmia is the leading cause of death; therefore the stabilization of the electrophysiological substrate represents a primary endpoint of the treatment.

β-Blockers were initially used based on their efficacy in LQTS.[40] A computer modeling study[25] showed that adrenergic activation increases the transmural dispersion of repolarization, DADs, and EADs. As previously outlined, the hyperactivation of CaMKII pathways (an important component of the intracellular adrenergic signaling) is another arrhythmogenic factor in TS.[29] Taken together, these evidences provide a pathophysiological justification to the use of β-blockers.

Other authors have suggested that the block of the sodium current (I_{Na}) can significantly shorten repolarization in TS. Gao and colleagues[41] empirically treated a TS patient (R406R mutation) with 12.5 mg/kg per day of mexiletine, demonstrating a consistent QTc shortening of approximately 70 ms. In vitro assessment showed that the clinical effect was due to the block of both early (fast) and late components of the current. Along the same line, ranolazine (500 mg bid) abolished nonsustained VTs and implantable cardioverter defibrillator (ICD) shocks in another TS case[42] and was found to counteract the electrophysiological abnormalities in a wedge preparation in which TS was pharmacologically

induced (with BayK8644).[43] Taken together, these results suggest that the block of late sodium current can be beneficial in TS and support the use of mexiletine or ranolazine over β-blockers. Finally, verapamil has been reported to be effective in a single TS2 (G402S mutation) patient,[44] but it was not effective in TS1.

In summary, the available evidence supports the use of β-blockers and late sodium blockers (mexiletine or ranolazine); still the use of ICDs even for primary prevention of VT/VF appears indicated in fully blown typical TS. Importantly, however, other causes of death should be considered when managing TS patients: recurrent infections (secondary to altered immune responses), severe hypoglycemia, or recurrent sepsis.[3] Close monitoring of glucose levels, especially in patients receiving β-blockers, is essential because these drugs may mask the symptoms of hypoglycemia.

Summary

TS is a rare and severe disease. While the earlier discoveries portrayed remarkably homogeneous clinical manifestations and genetic backgrounds, the recent accumulating knowledge supports the idea of a multifaceted phenotype. Indeed, human calcium channel mutations can cause a spectrum of phenotypes from a fully expressed severe TS phenotype to a mild and isolated QT prolongation (indistinguishable from Romano-Ward syndrome). The long-term outcome of typical TS is extremely severe, and aggressive treatment is warranted. At the moment, the prognosis and response to therapy of subjects with *CACNA1c* mutations and isolated QT prolongation are superficially known and further studies are warranted.

REFERENCES

1. Reichenbach H, Meister EM, Theile H. The heart-hand syndrome. A new variant of disorders of heart conduction and syndactylia including osseous changes in hands and feet. *Kinderarztl Prax.* 1992;60:54–56.
2. Marks ML, Trippel DL, Keating MT. Long QT syndrome associated with syndactyly identified in females. *Am J Cardiol.* 1995;76:744–745.
3. Splawski I, Timothy KW, Sharpe LM, et al. Ca(V)1.2 calcium channel dysfunction causes a multisystem disorder including arrhythmia and autism. *Cell.* 2004;119:19–31.
4. Splawski I, Timothy KW, Decher N, et al. Severe arrhythmia disorder caused by cardiac L-type calcium channel mutations. *Proc Natl Acad Sci U S A.* 2005;102:8089–8096.
5. Gillis J, Burashnikov E, Antzelevitch C, et al. Long QT, syndactyly, joint contractures, stroke and novel CACNA1C mutation: expanding the spectrum of Timothy syndrome. *Am J Med Genet A.* 2012;158A:182–187.
6. Etheridge SP, Bowles NE, Arrington CB, et al. Somatic mosaicism contributes to phenotypic variation in Timothy syndrome. *Am J Med Genet A.* 2011;155A:2578–2583.
7. Napolitano C, Antzelevitch C. Phenotypical manifestations of mutations in the genes encoding subunits of the cardiac voltage-dependent L-type calcium channel. *Circ Res.* 2011;108:607–618.
8. Wemhoner K, Friedrich C, Stallmeyer B, et al. Gain-of-function mutations in the calcium channel CACNA1C (Cav1.2) cause non-syndromic long-QT but not Timothy syndrome. *J Mol Cell Cardiol.* 2015;80:186–195.
9. Fukuyama M, Wang Q, Kato K, et al. Long QT syndrome type 8: novel CACNA1C mutations causing QT prolongation and variant phenotypes. *Europace.* 2014;16:1828–1837.
10. Hiippala A, Tallila J, Myllykangas S, et al. Expanding the phenotype of Timothy syndrome type 2: an adolescent with ventricular fibrillation but normal development. *Am J Med Genet A.* 2015;167A:629–634.
11. Frohler S, Kieslich M, Langnick C, et al. Exome sequencing helped the fine diagnosis of two siblings afflicted with atypical Timothy syndrome (TS2). *BMC Med Genet.* 2014;15:48.
12. Diep V, Seaver LH. Long QT syndrome with craniofacial, digital, and neurologic features: is it useful to distinguish between Timothy syndrome types 1 and 2? *Am J Med Genet A.* 2015;167:2780–2785.
13. Corona-Rivera JR, Barrios-Prieto E, Nieto-Garcia R, et al. Unusual retrospective prenatal findings in a male newborn with Timothy syndrome type 1. *Eur J Med Genet.* 2015;58:332–335.
14. Ergul Y, Ozyilmaz I, Haydin S, et al. A rare association with suffered cardiac arrest, long QT interval, and syndactyly: Timothy syndrome (LQT-8). *Anatol J Cardiol.* 2015;15:672–674.
15. Boczek NJ, Ye D, Jin F, et al. Identification and functional characterization of a novel CACNA1C-mediated cardiac disorder characterized by prolonged QT intervals with hypertrophic cardiomyopathy, congenital heart defects, and sudden cardiac death. *Circ Arrhythm Electrophysiol.* 2015;8:1122–1132.
16. Boczek NJ, Miller EM, Ye D, et al. Novel Timothy syndrome mutation leading to increase in CACNA1C window current. *Heart Rhythm.* 2015;12:211–219.
17. Papineau SD, Wilson S. Dentition abnormalities in a Timothy syndrome patient with a novel genetic mutation: a case report. *Pediatr Dent.* 2014;36:245–249.
18. Hennessey JA, Boczek NJ, Jiang YH, et al. A CACNA1C variant associated with reduced voltage-dependent inactivation, increased CaV1.2 channel window current, and arrhythmogenesis. *PLoS One.* 2014;9:e106982.
19. Wang D, Papp AC, Binkley PF, et al. Highly variable mRNA expression and splicing of L-type voltage-dependent calcium channel alpha subunit 1C in human heart tissues. *Pharmacogenet Genomics.* 2006;16:735–745.
20. Tang ZZ, Liang MC, Lu S, et al. Transcript scanning reveals novel and extensive splice variations in human l-type voltage-gated calcium channel, Cav1.2 alpha1 subunit. *J Biol Chem.* 2004;279:44335–44343.
21. Catterall WA. Structure and regulation of voltage-gated Ca²⁺ channels. *Annu Rev Cell Dev Biol.* 2000;16:521–555.
22. Tang Y, Tian X, Wang R, et al. Abnormal termination of Ca²⁺ release is a common defect of RyR2 mutations associated with cardiomyopathies. *Circ Res.* 2012;110:968–977.
23. Chen X, Zhang X, Kubo H, et al. Ca²⁺ influx-induced sarcoplasmic reticulum Ca²⁺ overload causes mitochondrial-dependent apoptosis in ventricular myocytes. *Circ Res.* 2005;97:1009–1017.
24. Barrett CF, Tsien RW. The Timothy syndrome mutation differentially affects voltage- and calcium-dependent inactivation of CaV1.2 L-type calcium channels. *Proc Natl Acad Sci U S A.* 2008;105:2157–2162.
25. Sung RJ, Wu YH, Lai NH, et al. Beta-adrenergic modulation of arrhythmogenesis and identification of targeted sites of antiarrhythmic therapy in Timothy (LQT8) syndrome: a theoretical study. *Am J Physiol Heart Circ Physiol.* 2010;298:H33–H44.
26. Cheng EP, Yuan C, Navedo MF, et al. Restoration of normal L-type Ca²⁺ channel function during Timothy syndrome by ablation of an anchoring protein. *Circ Res.* 2011;109:255–261.
27. Yazawa M, Hsueh B, Jia X, et al. Using induced pluripotent stem cells to investigate cardiac phenotypes in Timothy syndrome. *Nature.* 2011;471:230–234.
28. Pasca SP, Portmann T, Voineagu I, et al. Using iPSC-derived neurons to uncover cellular phenotypes associated with Timothy syndrome. *Nat Med.* 2011;17:1657–1662.
29. Thiel WH, Chen B, Hund TJ, et al. Proarrhythmic defects in Timothy syndrome require calmodulin kinase II. *Circulation.* 2008;118:2225–2234.
30. Erxleben C, Liao Y, Gentile S, et al. Cyclosporin and Timothy syndrome increase mode 2 gating of CaV1.2 calcium channels through aberrant phosphorylation of S6 helices. *Proc Natl Acad Sci U S A.* 2006;103:3932–3937.
31. Jin X, Muntean BS, Aal-Aaboda MS, et al. L-type calcium channel modulates cystic kidney phenotype. *Biochim Biophys Acta.* 2014;1842:1518–1526.
32. Gershon ES, Grennan K, Busnello J, et al. A rare mutation of CACNA1C in a patient with bipolar disorder, and decreased gene expression associated with a bipolar-associated common SNP of CACNA1C in brain. *Mol Psychiatry.* 2014;19:890–894.
33. Bader PL, Faizi M, Kim LH, et al. Mouse model of Timothy syndrome recapitulates triad of autistic traits. *Proc Natl Acad Sci U S A.* 2011;108:15432–15437.
34. Lo-A-Njoe SM, Wilde AA, van Erven L, et al. Syndactyly and long QT syndrome (CaV1.2 missense mutation G406R) is associated with hypertrophic cardiomyopathy. *Heart Rhythm.* 2005;2:1365–1368.
35. Dufendach KA, Giudicessi JR, Boczek NJ, et al. Maternal mosaicism confounds the neonatal diagnosis of type 1 Timothy syndrome. *Pediatrics.* 2013;131:e1991–e1995.
36. Plaster NM, Tawil R, Tristani-Firouzi M, et al. Mutations in Kir2.1 cause the developmental and episodic electrical phenotypes of Andersen's syndrome. *Cell.* 2001;105:511–519.
37. Bloise R, Napolitano C, Timothy KW, et al. Clinical profile and risk of sudden death in children with Timothy syndrome. *Circulation.* 2007;114(suppl II):502–502.
38. Priori SG, Schwartz PJ, Napolitano C, et al. Risk stratification in the long-QT syndrome. *New Engl J Med.* 2003;348:1866–1874.
39. Joseph-Reynolds AM, Auden SM, Sobczyzk WL. Perioperative considerations in a newly described subtype of congenital long QT syndrome. *Paediatr Anaesth.* 1997;7:237–241.
40. Priori SG, Napolitano C, Schwartz PJ, et al. Association of long QT syndrome loci and cardiac events among patients treated with beta-blockers. *JAMA.* 2004;292:1341–1344.
41. Gao Y, Xue X, Hu D, et al. Inhibition of late sodium current by mexiletine: a novel pharmotherapeutical approach in Timothy syndrome. *Circ Arrhythm Electrophysiol.* 2013;6:614–622.
42. Shah DP, Baez-Escudero JL, Weisberg IL, et al. Ranolazine safely decreases ventricular and atrial fibrillation in Timothy syndrome (LQT8). *Pacing Clin Electrophysiol.* 2012;35:e62–e64.
43. Sicouri S, Timothy KW, Zygmunt AC, et al. Cellular basis for the electrocardiographic and arrhythmic manifestations of Timothy syndrome: effects of ranolazine. *Heart Rhythm.* 2007;4:638–647.
44. Jacobs A, Knight BP, McDonald KT, et al. Verapamil decreases ventricular tachyarrhythmias in a patient with Timothy syndrome (LQT8). *Heart Rhythm.* 2006;3:967–970.

96

J-Wave Syndromes

Sami Viskin and Raphael Rosso

The term *J-wave syndromes* denotes a clinical spectrum consisting of diseases that differ from each other in terms of etiology and clinical characteristics, but share similar electrocardiographic (ECG) features and arrhythmogenic mechanisms.[1,2] The etiologies of these disorders include genetic disorders (like Brugada syndrome), acquired disorders (myocardial ischemia and hypothermia), and diseases of unclear etiology (like "idiopathic ventricular fibrillation [VF] with early repolarization") (Table 96.1). The common arrhythmogenic mechanism shared by these diseases is a marked abbreviation of the action potential, affecting some myocardial areas more than others. The resulting increase in dispersion of ventricular repolarization underlies the ECG hallmark of these disorders: elevation of the J-point—also termed "J-wave"—followed by different degrees of ST-segment elevation. When dispersion of ventricular repolarization reaches a certain threshold (that is, when areas of markedly different action-potential duration coexist in contiguous myocardial areas), malignant reentrant polymorphic ventricular tachyarrhythmias occur. This common arrhythmogenic mechanism explains why disorders with fundamentally different etiologies, like an inborn malfunction of cardiac sodium channels in Brugada syndrome versus acute coronary occlusion in the case of acute myocardial infarction, cause ventricular arrhythmias of identical morphology and mode of onset. As shown in Fig. 96.1, arrhythmias in the various J-wave syndromes are polymorphic and invariably start with a ventricular extrasystole preceded by a short-coupling interval.

Three points are noteworthy: First, while some J-wave syndromes (e.g., idiopathic VF[2] or hypothermia[3]) appear to be entirely due to *repolarization* abnormalities, *depolarization delay* is important in others. Specifically, conduction delays to the right ventricular outflow tract (RVOT) and through ischemic myocardial zones contribute to the arrhythmias of Brugada syndrome[4,5] and ischemic VF,[6] respectively. Second, although the J-wave syndromes are classified as "congenital" *or* "acquired" (see Table 96.1), both characteristics may coexist. For example patients with congenital Brugada syndrome are predisposed to develop the drug-induced form of this disease when challenged with specific drugs (http://www.brugadadrugs.org); patients with genetic mutations causing loss of function of the sodium channel not severe enough to manifest the Brugada syndrome,[7] as well as seemingly healthy patients who have J-waves in their baseline ECG,[8] appear to be at increased risk for ischemic VF during acute myocardial infarction, whereas patients with idiopathic VF may develop recurrent VF as a result of J-wave augmentation during therapeutic hypothermia.[9,10] Finally, it is important to emphasize that J-waves are often observed in healthy individuals who have the "early repolarization" ECG pattern.[11–13] Although this ECG pattern has long been considered benign, case-controlled series recently demonstrated a significant association between the early repolarization pattern and idiopathic VF.[11] It is therefore imperative to distinguish the very common and benign "early repolarization" pattern from the rare and malignant ECG of the J-wave syndromes.[13] In this regard, it is important to note the following: the early repolarization pattern has conventionally been defined as the combination of J-waves (in the form of "J-point elevation" or "slurred R-waves") with ST-segment elevation. However, each of these components may have different diagnostic and prognostic significance.[14] As explained below, the pattern of early repolarization most strongly associated with idiopathic VF includes *tall J-waves, flat ST-segment,* and *low-amplitude T-waves.*[15] This chapter summarizes the main clinical and ECG features of the J-wave syndromes with an emphasis on the morphology of the J-wave and the contour of the ST-segment.

Acquired J-Wave Syndromes: Hypothermia and Ischemic Ventricular Fibrillation

The prototypical arrhythmogenic J-wave was described by Osborn in the setting of experimental hypothermia[16]: dogs subjected to worsening degrees of hypothermia and metabolic acidosis developed increasingly taller J-waves and eventually VF.[16] This ECG hallmark of impending VF involves giant J-waves *without* ST-segment elevation (Fig. 96.2A), and the same applies to clinically significant hypothermia in humans[17,18] (see Fig. 96.2B). Experiments involving differential cooling of cardiac-wedge preparations[19] or cooling of preparations mimicking early repolarization[3] demonstrated that hypothermia-related J-waves are the ECG reflection of increased dispersion of repolarization caused by disproportionate abbreviation of the epicardial action potential, eventually leading to phase 2 reentry and VF (see Fig. 96.1A).[3,19] Quinidine is extremely effective for preventing hypothermia-induced VF in tissue[3] and animal studies,[20] an interesting finding considering that quinidine is the most effective drug for preventing VF in clinical J-wave syndromes, including idiopathic VF[21] and Brugada syndrome.[22]

The mechanisms underlying ischemic arrhythmias (described in Chapter 84) are more complex.[6] Yet, phase 2 reentry appears to be the cause of VF occurring shortly after the onset of acute ST-elevation myocardial infarction.[6] In the setting of acute coronary occlusion, the fall in the action potential dome in the ischemic zone occurs principally because of activation of the adenosine triphosphate (ATP)-sensitive potassium current (I_{K-ATP}) secondary to a reduction in intracellular ATP levels and an increase in adenosine diphosphate (ADP) levels as a result of tissue ischemia. Phase 2 reentry occurs secondary to propagation of the action-potential dome from the normal zone (where it is normally present) to the ischemic region.[6] This translates in

TABLE 96.1 J-wave syndromes

	CONGENITAL J-WAVE SYNDROMES[a]		ACQUIRED J-WAVE SYNDROMES[a]		
	CONGENITAL BRUGADA SYNDROME	IDIOPATHIC VF WITH J-WAVES	ACQUIRED BRUGADA SYNDROME	MYOCARDIAL ISCHEMIA	HYPOTHERMIA
Etiology	Genetic mutations leading to malfunctioning ion channels (SCN5A, CACNA1C, CACNB2b, GPD1L, SCN1B, KCNE3, SCN3B, SCN10A).	Unknown in most cases. Genetic mutations in some (KCNJ8, CACNA1C, CACNB2b, CACNA2D1, ABCC9).	Medications blocking sodium channels www.brugadadrugs.org	Acute coronary vessel obstruction with transmural myocardial ischemia	Experimental or clinical lowering of body temperature
Site of J-wave and ST-segment elevation[c]	Right precordial leads	Inferior and inferolateral leads	As in congenital Brugada syndrome	Depending on the occluded coronary artery	Inferolateral leads
Clinical arrhythmias	VF at rest, mainly in adult males, sometimes triggered by fever and drugs[b]	VF at rest, mainly in young adults of both genders, sometimes triggered by fever	VF may rarely occur during drug exposure	VF during the hyperacute phase of ST-elevation myocardial infarction	VF during clinical or experimental hypothermia
Effective therapy	Intravenous isoproterenol and oral quinidine	Intravenous isoproterenol and oral quinidine. Reports of bepridil and cilostazol	Discontinuation of the culprit drug. Intravenous isoproterenol intuitively effective	Myocardial revascularization. Quinidine intuitively effective	Quinidine, cilostazol, milrinone effective in experimental hypothermia

[a]The distinction between "congenital" and "acquired" forms is not always straightforward. For example, some data suggest that individuals with inborn "J-waves" are at increased risk for ischemic VF in the event of acute coronary occlusion (see text).
[b]Drugs causing the "acquired Brugada syndrome" by blocking sodium channels may provoke arrhythmias in patients with the congenital form.
[c]Type I Brugada in the *inferolateral* leads and nontype-I J-waves in the right precordial leads also associated with arrhythmic risk (see text).
VF, Ventricular fibrillation.

the clinical setting as the distinctive VF initiation, with short-coupled extrasystoles, during ST-segment elevation myocardial infarction[25] (see Fig. 96.1B).

Congenital J-Wave Syndromes: Brugada Syndrome and Idiopathic Ventricular Fibrillation With Early Repolarization

Brugada syndrome is a genetic disease (described in detail in Chapters 51 and 92), whereas genetic mutations are identified in only a minority of cases with idiopathic VF[26,27] (Chapter 97). In both diseases, VF results from phase 2 reentry made possible by an abnormal increase in ventricular repolarization dispersion (Fig. 96.3). In the case of Brugada syndrome, genetic mutations leading to reduced sodium or calcium depolarizing currents lead to a loss of the action potential dome within the RVOT epicardium, where I_{To} repolarizing currents are generally prominent.[2] Delayed conduction in the RVOT undeniably contributes to the ECG manifestations of the disease (see Fig. 96.3A and D), but controversy continues regarding the role of conduction delay in arrhythmogenesis, specifically for spontaneous VF initiation[4,28] (see Fig. 96.3C and E). In idiopathic VF with early repolarization, areas of early repolarization in the left ventricular epicardium probably allow the very premature Purkinje-fiber ectopy to trigger the reentrant polymorphic arrhythmias.[26]

Both diseases present as syncope or cardiac arrest in young adults (mean age of 43 ± 14 years in Brugada syndrome[31] and 35 ± 10 years in idiopathic VF).[32] The baseline ECG is characteristic in Brugada syndrome (right bundle branch pattern with ST-segment elevation in the right precordial leads) and, by definition, is considered normal in idiopathic VF, albeit with a QT-interval in the low-normal range.[33,34] Moreover, a higher than expected prevalence of J-waves in the inferior and inferolateral leads has been described in idiopathic VF[32,35] and Brugada syndrome.[31] Among idiopathic VF patients, those with J-waves in the inferior leads are more often male, have shorter QT-intervals, and have a more malignant course.[32,36] A worse

prognosis has also been described in Brugada syndrome patients who also have J-waves in the inferior leads.[31] In both conditions, VF is initiated by ventricular extrasystoles with a short coupling interval (particularly short in the case of idiopathic VF) (see Fig. 96.1C and D). These extrasystoles originate in the RVOT in Brugada syndrome and in left ventricular Purkinje fibers or the RVOT in 85% and 15% of idiopathic VF patients, respectively.[37] Arrhythmic storms with frequent VF episodes occur in 18% of patients with Brugada syndrome[31] and in 27% of patients with idiopathic VF and early repolarization.[36] It is important to emphasize that these VF storms are refractory to conventional antiarrhythmic drugs, including amiodarone, but respond extremely well to intravenous isoproterenol and oral quinidine.[21,36,38]

By convention,[1,2] the congenital J-wave syndromes have been defined as *either* Brugada syndrome or early repolarization syndrome based on the presence of J-waves in the right precordial or the inferolateral leads, respectively. However, this dichotomization may not be as strict as originally conceived. J-waves in the right precordial leads but *without* the type-I Brugada pattern of ST-segment elevation are also associated with increased arrhythmic risk,[39] and the same is true for type-I Brugada ECG pattern in the *inferolateral* leads.[40]

Early Repolarization in Healthy Individuals and J-Waves in Idiopathic Ventricular Fibrillation

The presence of J-waves and ST-segment elevation on the ECG, jointly termed "the early repolarization pattern," is present in 2%–14% of healthy individuals and is more prevalent in young males, particularly if athletic and of African American origin.[14,41] The normal-variant early repolarization pattern characteristically includes marked ST-segment elevation, to the point that, for decades, investigations of this phenomenon focused exclusively on how to distinguish this normal variant from clinically important causes of ST-segment elevation, most notably, acute myocardial infarction.[14]

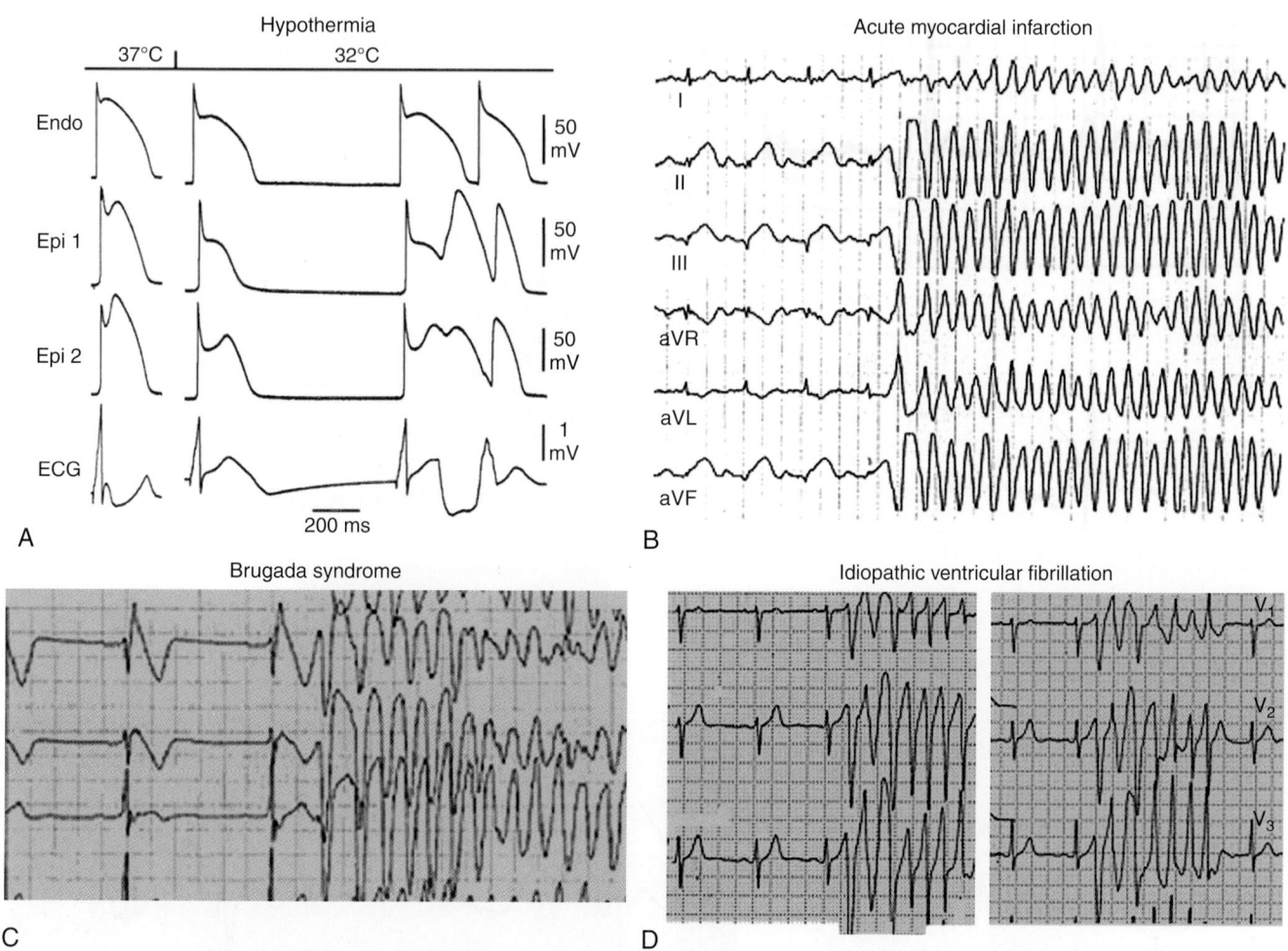

FIGURE 96.1 Arrhythmias in the J-wave syndromes. (A) Experimental hypothermia in the wedge-preparation model.[3] At baseline, the action potential is slightly shorter in the epicardium than in the epicardium because the former normally has larger I_{To} currents; however, the dispersion of repolarization (i.e., the difference between the shortest and longest action potential duration) is small. Cooling of the preparation leads to shortening of the action potential; moreover, this action-potential shortening is disproportionately accentuated in epicardial layers, leading to loss of the action potential dome. Note that the action potential dome is still present in the endocardium at a time when the epicardium is no longer refractory. This allows for propagation of the action potential dome from endocardium to epicardium (phase 2 reentry). In a setting mimicking inborn early repolarization, polymorphic arrhythmias occur.[3] (B), (C), and (D), Spontaneous initiations of ventricular fibrillation (VF) in a patient with acute inferior myocardial infarction. Note the ST-segment elevation in leads II, III, and aVF (B), in a patient with Brugada syndrome (C), and in a patient with idiopathic VF (D). Note that in all cases VF is initiated by a ventricular extrasystole with a very short coupling interval (on the T-wave of the last sinus complex). ([A] From Gurabi Z, Koncz I, Patocskai B, et al. Cellular mechanism underlying hypothermia-induced ventricular tachycardia/ventricular fibrillation in the setting of early repolarization and the protective effect of quinidine, cilostazol, and milrinone. *Circ Arrhythm Electrophysiol.* 2014;7:134-142.)

Given the fact that early repolarization is more prevalent in the young and the fittest, and predominates at slower heart rates, it was generally viewed as an ECG marker of "good health." This view was first challenged based on experimental models where early repolarization is proarrhythmic.[42] Subsequently, case reports (summarized elsewhere)[41] highlighted the fact that some patients with idiopathic VF not only have obvious J-waves but also demonstrate augmentation of the J-wave amplitude immediately prior to the onset of malignant arrhythmias,[36,43,44] the latter phenomenon suggesting cause and effect. As opposed to the "normal" early repolarization pattern, ECGs in idiopathic VF generally show marked J-waves without ST-segment elevation.[14,34] Finally, case-control series have consistently shown that J-waves and early repolarization

are more prevalent among patients with idiopathic VF than among matched healthy controls.[32,35,45–47] J-waves followed by horizontal (rather than rapidly ascending) ST-segments are strongly associated with idiopathic VF.[48] In one study, the presence of J-waves correlated with a history of idiopathic VF with an odds ratio of 4.0 (95% confidence intervals 2.0–7.9) and having both J-waves with horizontal/descending ST-segment yielded an odds ratio of 13.8 (95% confidence intervals 5.1–37.2) for having idiopathic VF.[48] Importantly, even though association was confirmed in subsequent studies,[11] the absolute risk is low because idiopathic VF is a rare disease. For an individual 35–45 years old, the risk of developing idiopathic VF is only 3.4 in 100,000; this risk increases to 1 in 10,000 in the presence of J-waves and rises to 1 in 3000 if the J-waves are

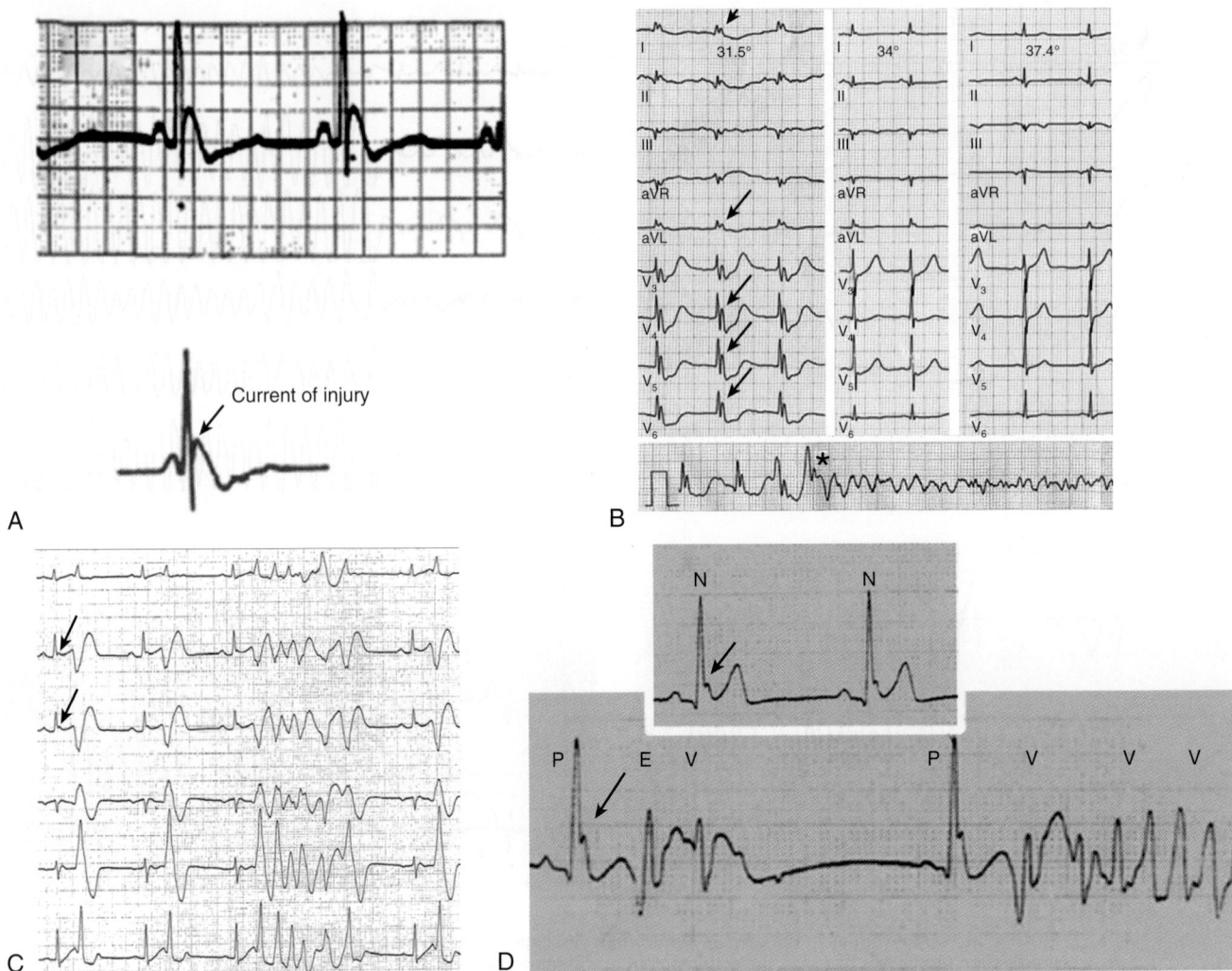

FIGURE 96.2 The arrhythmogenic J-wave. (A) Shows the J-waves recorded by Osborn during his experiments of hypothermia in dogs, including his original annotation: "current of injury."[16] Dogs with this injury current went on to develop spontaneous ventricular fibrillation (VF). Note that the marked J-waves of hypothermia are *not* accompanied by ST-segment elevation in experimental hypothermia (A) or in clinically significant hypothermia in humans (B).[18] (C) and (D) show examples of spontaneous initiation of polymorphic ventricular tachycardia/fibrillation in patients with idiopathic VF.[23,24] Note the absence of ST-segment elevation in both cases. In (D) the J-wave amplitude increases after pauses and immediately prior to the onset of VF; however J-wave augmentation is *not* accompanied by ST-segment elevation. ([A] From Osborn JJ. Experimental hypothermia; respiratory and blood pH changes in relation to cardiac function. *Am J Physiol.* 1953;175:389-398. [B] Modified from Richter S, Ehrlich JR, Fassbender S, et al. Malignant Osborn waves during therapeutic hypothermia. *Europace.* 2009;11:668-669. [C] From Kawata H, Morita H, Yamada Y, et al. Prognostic significance of early repolarization in infero-lateral leads in Brugada patients with documented ventricular fibrillation: a novel risk factor for Brugada syndrome with ventricular fibrillation. *Heart Rhythm.* 2013;10:1161-1168. [D] From Shinohara T, Takahashi N, Saikawa T, et al. Characterization of J wave in a patient with idiopathic ventricular fibrillation. *Heart Rhythm.* 2006;3:1082-1084.)

coupled with a horizontal ST-segment.[48] These data should be considered judiciously in the management of asymptomatic patients with J-waves (see the following text).

Arrhythmic Risk for Patients With Early Repolarization in Large Prospective Population Studies

Large population-based studies provide conflicting evidence concerning the long-term prognostic implication of early repolarization.[49] The conflicting results may be due in part to differences in definitions, and attempts have been made to unify the terminology used to describe the ECG.[13] Some data suggest that the long-term arrhythmic risk associated with early repolarization is limited only to those patients who have J-waves followed by a horizontal ST-segment.[50] However, in a recent study of >20,000 initially asymptomatic adults aged 20–55 years (90% males and 16% African Americans), cardiac death was *not* higher among patients with early repolarization, even if prominent J-waves were followed by descending ST-segments.[12] Idiopathic VF is a very rare disease, and it is unrealistic to expect prospective identification of the few patients prone to developing this disease by population-based studies. Furthermore, the survival curves of patients with and without J-waves in the

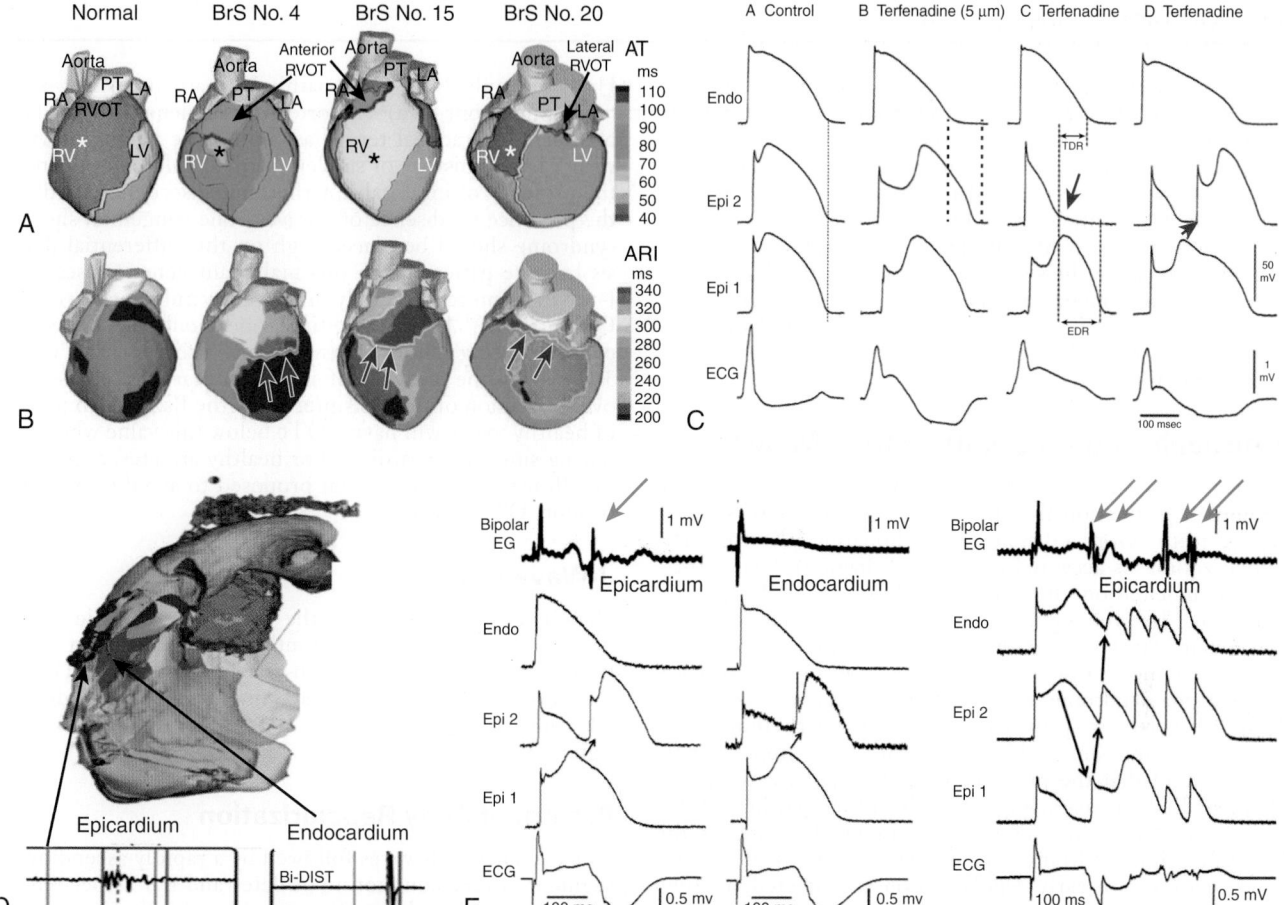

FIGURE 96.3 Clinical and experimental data supporting depolarization and repolarization mechanisms in Brugada syndrome (*BrS*). (A) and (B) show high-resolution panoramic electrophysiological data recorded with noninvasive electrocardiographic imaging for a healthy control and for three patients with BrS[5]: (A) shows activation time (*AT*) isochrones with the color coding referenced to the onset of the QRS complex shown on the *right* (red areas are activated within 40 ms of the QRS onset as opposed to *blue* areas, which are activated 110 ms after the onset of QRS). Note that in the control (marked "*normal*") the entire right ventricle, including the right ventricular outflow tract (*RVOT*) is activated early (shown in *red*) and before the left ventricle (shown in *yellow* and *green*). In contrast, the three patients with BrS show delayed activation of the RVOT (depicted as *blue* areas). (B) shows the activation recovery interval (*ARI*), used as a surrogate for action potential duration at the given zones. Again, the color coding is on the *right*, with areas with the shortest ARI (200-ms duration) shown in *blue* and areas with the longest ARI (340-ms duration) shown in *red*. Note that in the healthy control the repolarization is fairly homogeneous and the entire heart (left and right ventricles) repolarizes within 240 ms. In contrast, in patients with BrS, there are areas with steep repolarization gradients in the RVOT (areas with prolonged action potentials in *red* contiguous to areas with shorter action potentials in *green* and *yellow*). (C) shows the wedge-preparation model using terfenadine to block sodium and calcium currents to mimic BrS: Transmembrane action potentials from one endocardial (*top*) and two epicardial sites, together with a transmural electrocardiogram (*ECG*) recorded from a canine arterially perfused right ventricular wedge preparation are shown.[29] At baseline (*control*) the action potentials recorded at two epicardial sites (*Epi 1* and *Epi 2*) show the normal epicardial repolarization notch hardly visible at the endocardium (*Endo*). Following heart rate acceleration under terfenadine (sodium channel blockade), accentuation of the action potential notch leads to *prolongation* of the action potential that is prominent at some epicardial sites (*Epi 2*), leading to a marked dispersion of repolarization (end of repolarization at epicardial site 2 versus end of repolarization at endocardium; *red* and *blue* dotted lines, respectively). *This experimental recording from the wedge preparation is similar to the clinical recordings presented in (B).* It is only during further heart rate acceleration that terfenadine leads to calcium channel blockade, which causes loss of the action potential dome (*red arrow*), increasing the total dispersion of repolarization (*TDR* in figure) as well as the epicardial dispersion of repolarization (*EDR* in figure) eventually leading to phase 2 reentry (*red arrowhead*). (D) shows the electroanatomical mapping recorded at the time of epicardial ablation in a patient with BrS as reported by Nademanee.[30] Note the fractionation of the local bipolar electrograms recorded from the ablation catheter in the RVOT epicardium, and note that the fractionated electrograms are not visible at the bipolar electrograms recording at the same RVOT site from the endocardium.[30] These clinical recordings are presented as evidence of delayed conduction in the RVOT in BrS. However, (E) shows that in the wedge preparation model of BrS, concealed phase 2 reentry may appear in bipolar recordings from the epicardium as "late potential" (*green arrow*) or as a fractionation of the local epicardial recording (*orange arrows*), while being absent in bipolar recordings from the endocardium.[28] ([A] and [B] From Zhang J, Sacher F, Hoffmayer K, et al. Cardiac electrophysiological substrate underlying the ECG phenotype and electrogram abnormalities in Brugada syndrome patients. *Circulation.* 2015;131:1950-1959. [C] Modified from Fish JM, Antzelevitch C. Role of sodium and calcium channel block in unmasking the Brugada syndrome. *Heart Rhythm.* 2004;1:210-217. [D] Modified from Nademanee K, Veerakul G, Chandanamattha P, et al. Prevention of ventricular fibrillation episodes in Brugada syndrome by catheter ablation over the anterior right ventricular outflow tract epicardium. *Circulation.* 2011;123:1270-1279. [E] Modified from Szél T, Antzelevitch C. Abnormal repolarization as the basis for late potentials and fractionated electrograms recorded from epicardium in experimental models of Brugada syndrome. *J Am Coll Cardiol.* 2014;63:2037-2045.)

positive studies (by Tikkanen[51] and Sinner[52]) began to diverge at approximately 60 years of age, an age above that of the typical idiopathic VF patient. A plausible explanation for these findings is that patients with J-waves have increased dispersion of repolarization to some degree that places them at increased risk for arrhythmic death only when additional proarrhythmic triggers occur. Such triggers could be Purkinje-extrasystoles with a short coupling interval (in the very rare case of idiopathic VF) or, far more commonly, myocardial ischemia. Indeed, patients with J-waves on their baseline ECG who subsequently develop acute myocardial infarction have been reported to be at increased risk for ischemic VF.[8,53]

Approach to the Patient With J-Waves

Cardiac arrest survivors who have J-waves should undergo a complete evaluation for all potential etiologies of sudden cardiac death before a diagnosis of "idiopathic VF with early repolarization" is accepted as the final diagnosis. Nevertheless, documentation of recurrent VF preceded by pause-dependent J-wave augmentation and VF initiation by a ventricular extrasystole with very short coupling interval is pathognomonic of a J-wave syndrome; once coronary disease and Brugada syndrome are excluded, the diagnosis of idiopathic VF is certain, provided the recurrent arrhythmias did not occur during therapeutic hypothermia. It is important to keep in mind that the presence of early repolarization, just like many ECG features, is a hereditable trait regardless of the presence of arrhythmic disease.[54] Consequently, one should be careful about defining asymptomatic relatives of cardiac arrest victims with early repolarization as "affected" merely because they have a similar ECG.

The approach to a patient with syncope and early repolarization should be mainly guided by the clinical characteristics of the event, keeping in mind that both vagal syncope and early repolarization are common and do not necessarily justify extensive evaluation. As for asymptomatic patients with early repolarization, the following clinical and ECG characteristics should be taken into consideration.

Gender

Although male gender predominates among idiopathic VF patients with J-waves, the same is true for controls.[32,35]

History of Familial Sudden Death

In the study by Haissaguerre, a history of familial sudden death was significantly more frequent among idiopathic VF patients with J-waves than among those without J-waves.[32]

However, only 22% of idiopathic VF patients in that series[32] (and none in our own)[35] reported the sudden death of a family member. In practical terms, asymptomatic young individuals with a family history of sudden death should be evaluated for the presence of inheritable arrhythmic disorders regardless of the presence or absence of J-waves. The congenital short QT syndrome should be placed high on this differential diagnosis because patients with this malignant genetic disease have J-waves far more frequently than healthy individuals with short QT-interval.[55] At the same time, one should be careful about overdiagnosing "short QT syndrome" using a cutoff value of 360 ms[56] in the presence of sinus bradycardia. Because of the overcorrection of the QT-interval by the Bazett formula, 20% of healthy males will have a QTc below this value when tested during sinus bradycardia.[57] For healthy athletes, a QTc value of 320 ms has recently been proposed to avoid overdiagnosis of short QT syndrome.[58]

J-Wave Amplitude

Haissaguerre[32] reported that the J-wave amplitude in the idiopathic VF patients was significantly larger than that in the controls, and a similar trend was observed in our study.[35] However, the absolute differences in J-wave amplitude between idiopathic VF patients and controls were too small to be of real clinical significance.

Pattern of Early Repolarization

The presence of J-waves followed by a rapidly ascending ST-segment is very common in athletes and not associated with arrhythmic risk and therefore considered a "benign pattern." In contrast, J-waves followed by a horizontal ST-segment are relatively less common in healthy individuals and are more strongly associated with arrhythmic risk and are therefore considered a potentially malignant pattern (Fig. 96.4).[11] However, according to present estimates, the risk of idiopathic VF following the incidental finding of "malignant early repolarization" in an asymptomatic individual is only 1:3000. Also, as opposed to the athlete population, where the "benign" ascending ST-segment pattern is quasi-universal, the "potentially malignant" horizontal ST-segment pattern is not at all rare among healthy adults,[11] where the long-term prognostic value of its presence is now controversial.[49] Nevertheless, the concept that prominent J-waves *without* ST-segment elevation are potentially proarrhythmic is supported by a study showing that "high-amplitude J-waves followed by *low* amplitude T-waves" are strongly associated with idiopathic VF (see Fig. 96.4D).[15] At the time of this writing, these promising results remain unconfirmed.[34]

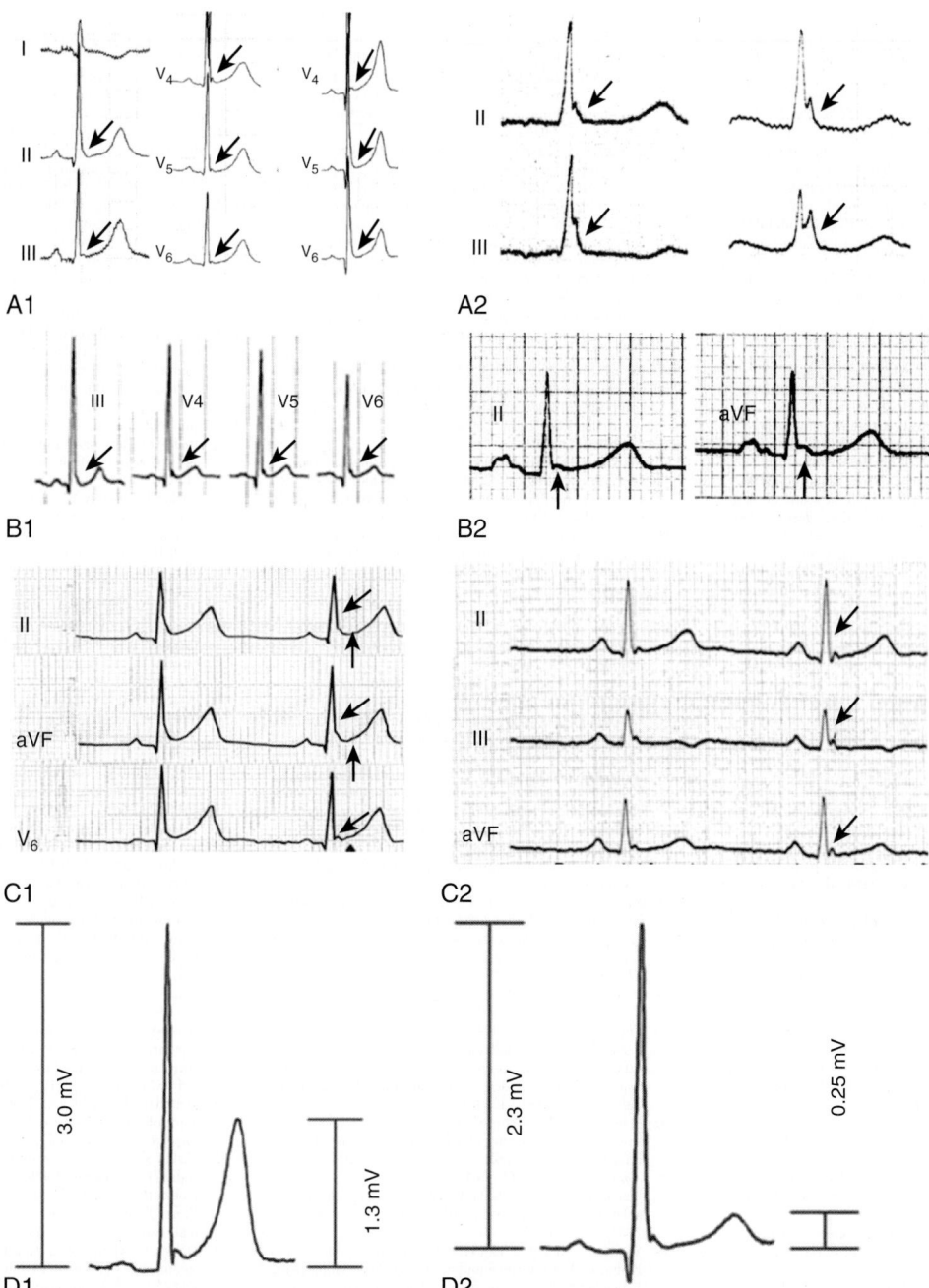

FIGURE 96.4 Benign (A1–D1; *left*) and "potentially malignant" (A2–D2; *right*) early repolarization patterns. (A) shows examples of early repolarization with "rapidly ascending" (A1) and "horizontal" (A2) ST-segment as reported by Tikkanen.[50] The first pattern (A1) was quasiuniversal in athletes and had no adverse prognostic significance for the general population, whereas subjects with a horizontal pattern (A2) had an increased hazard-ratio of arrhythmic death.[50] (B) demonstrates our findings in a case-control series of idiopathic VF. Using Tikkanen's criteria, we found that almost all the controls with early repolarization had upsloping ST-elevation (B1), whereas almost 70% of idiopathic VF patients with J-waves had horizontal ST-elevation (B2). (C) is a reproduction of the figure published by Cappato.[59] (C1) shows J-waves with upsloping ST-elevation in a healthy athlete, whereas (C2) shows J-waves with horizontal ST-elevation in a young soccer player with cardiac arrest.[59] (D) shows recently published data suggesting that low amplitude T-waves best discriminate between benign and malignant early repolarization.[15] ([A] [B] and [C] Modified from Viskin S, Rosso R, Halkin A. Making sense of early repolarization. *Heart Rhythm.* 2012;9:566-568; [D] Modified from Roten L, Derval N, Maury P, et al. Benign versus malignant inferolateral early repolarization: focus on the T wave. *Heart Rhythm.* 2016;13:894-902.)

REFERENCES

1. Antzelevitch C, Yan GX. J wave syndromes. *Heart Rhythm.* 2010;7:549–558.
2. Antzelevitch C, Yan GX. J-wave syndromes: Brugada and early repolarization syndromes. *Heart Rhythm.* 2015;12:1852–1866.
3. Gurabi Z, Koncz I, Patocskai B, Nesterenko VV, Antzelevitch C. Cellular mechanism underlying hypothermia-induced ventricular tachycardia/ventricular fibrillation in the setting of early repolarization and the protective effect of quinidine, cilostazol, and milrinone. *Circ Arrhythm Electrophysiol.* 2014;7:134–142.
4. Wilde AA, Postema PG, Di Diego JM, et al. The pathophysiological mechanism underlying Brugada syndrome: depolarization versus repolarization. *J Mol Cell Cardiol.* 2010;49:543–553.
5. Zhang J, Sacher F, Hoffmayer K, et al. Cardiac electrophysiological substrate underlying the ECG phenotype and electrogram abnormalities in Brugada syndrome patients. *Circulation.* 2015;131:1950–1959.
6. Di Diego JM, Antzelevitch C. Ischemic ventricular arrhythmias: experimental models and their clinical relevance. *Heart Rhythm.* 2011;8:1963–1968.
7. Hu D, Viskin S, Oliva A, et al. Novel mutation in the SCN5A gene associated with arrhythmic storm development during acute myocardial infarction. *Heart Rhythm.* 2007;4:1072–1080.
8. Naruse Y, Tada H, Harimaura Y, et al. Concomitant early repolarization increases occurrences of ventricular fibrillation in patients with acute myocardial infarctions. *Circulation.* 2011;124:A9945.
9. Bastiaenen R, Hedley PL, Christiansen M, Behr ER. Therapeutic hypothermia and ventricular fibrillation storm in early repolarization syndrome. *Heart Rhythm.* 2010;7:832–834.
10. Takahiro T, Kou S, Toshinobu Y, Yuichi H. Accidental hypothermia-induced electrical storm successfully treated with isoproterenol. *Heart Rhythm.* 2015;12:644–647.
11. Adler A, Rosso R, Viskin D, Halkin A, Viskin S. What do we know about the "malignant form" of early repolarization? *J Am Coll Cardiol.* 2013;62:863–868.
12. Pargaonkar VS, Perez MV, Jindal A, Mathur MB, Myers J, Froelicher VF. Long-term prognosis of early repolarization with J-wave and QRS slur patterns on the resting electrocardiogram: a cohort study. *Ann Intern Med.* 2015;163:747–755.
13. Macfarlane PW, Antzelevitch C, Haissaguerre M, et al. The early repolarization pattern: a consensus paper. *J Am Coll Cardiol.* 2015;66:470–477.
14. Viskin S, Rosso R, Halkin A. Making sense of early repolarization. *Heart Rhythm.* 2012;9:566–568.
15. Roten L, Derval N, Maury P, et al. Benign versus malignant inferolateral early repolarization: focus on the T wave. *Heart Rhythm.* 2016;13:894–902.
16. Osborn JJ. Experimental hypothermia; respiratory and blood pH changes in relation to cardiac function. *Am J Physiol.* 1953;175:389–398.
17. Kanna B, Wani S. Giant J wave on 12-lead electrocardiogram in hypothermia. *Ann Noninvasive Electrocardiol.* 2003;8:262–265.
18. Richter S, Ehrlich JR, Fassbender S, Fichtlscherer S. Malignant Osborn waves during therapeutic hypothermia. *Europace.* 2009;11:668–669.
19. Fish JM, Antzelevitch C. Link between hypothermia and the Brugada syndrome. *J Cardiovasc Electrophysiol.* 2004;15:942–944.
20. Johnson P, Lesage A, Floyd WL, Young Jr WG, Sealy WC. Prevention of ventricular fibrillation during profound hypothermia by quinidine. *Ann Surg.* 1960;151:490–495.
21. Viskin S, Belhassen B. Idiopathic ventricular fibrillation. *Am Heart J.* 1990;120:661–671.
22. Belhassen B, Rahkovich M, Michowitz Y, Glick A, Viskin S. Management of Brugada Syndrome: 33-year experience using electrophysiologically-guided therapy with class 1A antiarrhythmic drugs. *Circ Arrhythm Electrophysiol.* 2015;8:1393–1402.
23. Shinohara T, Takahashi N, Saikawa T, Yoshimatsu H. Characterization of J wave in a patient with idiopathic ventricular fibrillation. *Heart Rhythm.* 2006;3:1082–1084.
24. Kawata H, Morita H, Yamada Y, et al. Prognostic significance of early repolarization in infero-lateral leads in Brugada patients with documented ventricular fibrillation: a novel risk factor for Brugada syndrome with ventricular fibrillation. *Heart Rhythm.* 2013;10:1161–1168.
25. Wolfe CL, Nibbley C, Bhandari A, Chatterjee K, Scheinman MM. Polymorphous ventricular tachycardia associated with acute myocardial infarction. *Circulation.* 1991;84:1543–1551.
26. Xiao L, Koopmann TT, Ordog B, et al. Unique cardiac Purkinje fiber transient outward current beta-subunit composition: a potential molecular link to idiopathic ventricular fibrillation. *Circ Res.* 2013;112:1310–1322.
27. Marsman RF, Barc J, Beekman L, et al. A mutation in CALM1 encoding calmodulin in familial idiopathic ventricular fibrillation in childhood and adolescence. *J Am Coll Cardiol.* 2014;63:259–266.
28. Szel T, Antzelevitch C. Abnormal repolarization as the basis for late potentials and fractionated electrograms recorded from epicardium in experimental models of Brugada syndrome. *J Am Coll Cardiol.* 2014;63:2037–2045.
29. Fish JM, Antzelevitch C. Role of sodium and calcium channel block in unmasking the Brugada syndrome. *Heart Rhythm.* 2004;1:210–217.
30. Nademanee K, Veerakul G, Chandanamattha P, et al. Prevention of ventricular fibrillation episodes in Brugada syndrome by catheter ablation over the anterior right ventricular outflow tract epicardium. *Circulation.* 2011;123:1270–1279.
31. Adler A, Rosso R, Chorin E, Havakuk O, Antzelevitch C, Viskin S. Risk stratification in Brugada syndrome: clinical characteristics, electrocardiographic parameters, and auxiliary testing. *Heart Rhythm.* 2016;13:299–310.
32. Haissaguerre M, Derval N, Sacher F, et al. Sudden cardiac arrest associated with early repolarization. *N Engl J Med.* 2008;358:2016–2023.
33. Viskin S, Zeltser D, Ish-Shalom M, et al. Is idiopathic ventricular fibrillation a short QT syndrome? Comparison of QT intervals of patients with idiopathic ventricular fibrillation and healthy controls. *Heart Rhythm.* 2004;1:587–591.
34. Viskin S, Havakuk O, Antzelevitch C, Rosso R. Malignant early repolarization: it's the T-waves, stupid. *Heart Rhythm.* 2016;13:903–904.
35. Rosso R, Kogan E, Belhassen B, et al. J-point elevation in survivors of primary ventricular fibrillation and matched control subjects: incidence and clinical significance. *J Am Coll Cardiol.* 2008;52:1231–1238.
36. Haissaguerre M, Sacher F, Nogami A, et al. Characteristics of recurrent ventricular fibrillation associated with inferolateral early repolarization role of drug therapy. *J Am Coll Cardiol.* 2009;53:612–619.
37. Haissaguerre M, Shoda M, Jais P, et al. Mapping and ablation of idiopathic ventricular fibrillation. *Circulation.* 2002;106:962–967.
38. Viskin S, Wilde AA, Tan HL, Antzelevitch C, Shimizu W, Belhassen B. Empiric quinidine therapy for asymptomatic Brugada syndrome: time for a prospective registry. *Heart Rhythm.* 2009;6:401–404.
39. Kamakura T, Kawata H, Nakajima I, et al. Significance of non-type 1 anterior early repolarization in patients with inferolateral early repolarization syndrome. *J Am Coll Cardiol.* 2013;62:1610–1618.
40. Rollin A, Sacher F, Gourraud JB, et al. Prevalence, characteristics, and prognosis role of type 1 ST elevation in the peripheral ECG leads in patients with Brugada syndrome. *Heart Rhythm.* 2013;10:1012–1018.
41. Rosso R, Adler A, Halkin A, Viskin S. Risk of sudden death among young individuals with J waves and early repolarization: putting the evidence into perspective. *Heart Rhythm.* 2011;8:923–929.
42. Gussak I, Antzelevitch C. Early repolarization syndrome: clinical characteristics and possible cellular and ionic mechanisms. *J Electrocardiol.* 2000;33:299–309.
43. Aizawa Y, Sato A, Watanabe H, et al. Dynamicity of the J-wave in idiopathic ventricular fibrillation with a special reference to pause-dependent augmentation of the J-wave. *J Am Coll Cardiol.* 2012;59:1948–1953.
44. Haissaguerre M, Sacer F, Derval N, et al. Early repolarization in the inferolateral leads: a new syndrome associated with sudden cardiac death [abstract]. *J Interv Card Electrophysiol.* 2007;18:281.
45. Abe A, Ikeda T, Tsukada T, et al. Circadian variation of late potentials in idiopathic ventricular fibrillation associated with J waves: insights into alternative pathophysiology and risk stratification. *Heart Rhythm.* 2010;7:675–682.
46. Merchant FM, Noseworthy PA, Weiner RB, Singh SM, Ruskin JN, Reddy VY. Ability of terminal QRS notching to distinguish benign from malignant electrocardiographic forms of early repolarization. *Am J Cardiol.* 2009;104:1402–1406.
47. Nam GB, Kim YH, Antzelevitch C. Augmentation of J waves and electrical storms in patients with early repolarization. *N Engl J Med.* 2008;358:2078–2079.
48. Rosso R, Glikson E, Belhassen B, et al. Distinguishing "benign" from "malignant early repolarization": the value of the ST-segment morphology. *Heart Rhythm.* 2012;9:225–229.
49. Wu SH, Lin XX, Cheng YJ, Qiang CC, Zhang J. Early repolarization pattern and risk for arrhythmia death: a meta-analysis. *J Am Coll Cardiol.* 2013;61:645–650.
50. Tikkanen JT, Junttila MJ, Anttonen O, et al. Early repolarization: electrocardiographic phenotypes associated with favorable long-term outcome. *Circulation.* 2011;123:2666–2673.
51. Tikkanen JT, Anttonen O, Junttila MJ, et al. Long-term outcome associated with early repolarization on electrocardiography. *N Engl J Med.* 2009;361:2529–2537.
52. Sinner MF, Reinhard W, Muller M, et al. Association of early repolarization pattern on ECG with risk of cardiac and all-cause mortality: a population-based prospective cohort study (MONICA/KORA). *PLoS Med.* 2010;7:e1000314.
53. Rudic B, Veltmann C, Kuntz E, et al. Early repolarization pattern is associated with ventricular fibrillation in patients with acute myocardial infarction. *Heart Rhythm.* 2012;9:1295–1300.
54. Noseworthy PA, Tikkanen JT, Porthan K, et al. The early repolarization pattern in the general population: clinical correlates and heritability. *J Am Coll Cardiol.* 2011;57:2284–2289.
55. Watanabe H, Makiyama T, Koyama T, et al. High prevalence of early repolarization in short QT syndrome. *Heart Rhythm.* 2010;7:647–652.
56. Viskin S. The QT interval: too long, too short or just right. *Heart Rhythm.* 2009;6:711–715.
57. Kobza R, Roos M, Niggli B, et al. Prevalence of long and short QT in a young population of 41,767 predominantly male Swiss conscripts. *Heart Rhythm.* 2009;6:652–657.
58. Dhutia H, Malhotra A, Parpia S, et al. The prevalence and significance of a short QT interval in 18 825 low-risk individuals including athletes. *Br J Sports Med.* 2016;50:124–129.
59. Cappato R, Furlanello F, Giovinazzo V, et al. J wave, QRS slurring, and ST elevation in athletes with cardiac arrest in the absence of heart disease: marker of risk or innocent bystander? *Circ Arrhythm Electrophysiol.* 2010;3:305–311.

97 Idiopathic Ventricular Fibrillation

Christian Steinberg, Zachary W.M. Laksman, and Andrew D. Krahn

The definition of the clinical syndrome of idiopathic ventricular fibrillation (IVF) has evolved over time and continues to do so. Historically, the term IVF was used to describe polymorphic ventricular tachycardia (VT)/ventricular fibrillation (VF) in the absence of structural heart disease (SHD) or reversible metabolic-toxicological conditions. As our ability to clinically and genetically characterize, diagnose, and manage inherited arrhythmia syndromes has improved, the proportion of cases that are labeled as IVF has declined. IVF has historically been an inclusive term for unexplained episodes of VF or sudden death, but we have moved toward defining IVF as a distinct primary arrhythmogenic syndrome that has unique clinical and molecular features. This confounds the interpretation and applicability of the previous literature related to IVF, as the populations described were heterogeneous and ultimately found to have cases with other primary electrical conditions such as Brugada syndrome or early repolarization (ER) syndrome.

A detailed characterization and in-depth understanding of IVF has been difficult because it is an uncommon condition.[1] IVF accounts for less than 10% of all VF episodes; however, IVF plays a major role in the context of unexplained cardiac arrest in otherwise healthy individuals.[2]

Definition

The 2013 Heart Rhythm Society/European Heart Rhythm Association/Asia Pacific Heart Rhythm Society (HRS/EHRA/APHRS) Expert Consensus on inherited arrhythmia defined IVF as "a resuscitated cardiac arrest victim, preferably with documentation of VF, in whom known cardiac, respiratory, metabolic, and toxicological etiologies have been excluded through clinical evaluation."[3] To help differentiate this arrhythmogenic disorder from pause-dependent polymorphic VT/VF or torsades de pointes, some authors have put forth the term short-coupled IVF (SCIVF). This description also reflects a typical electrocardiogram (ECG) feature that characterizes the onset of IVF (see the following text).

Phenotype and Triggers of Idiopathic Ventricular Fibrillation

The majority of patients with IVF have a normal resting ECG with an unremarkable corrected QT (QTc) interval. Nevertheless, subtle repolarization abnormalities may be present, with a variable degree of overlap of IVF, short QT syndrome (SQTS), ER, and SCIVF in our current understanding (Fig. 97.1). For example, the ER pattern is overrepresented in IVF patients[4,5]; these patients have subsequently been "hived off" into a category called ER *syndrome* (ER pattern and symptoms).[3] Similarly, evidence supports a weak male preponderance and shorter QTc intervals in IVF compared with the normal population. The most extreme of these have been defined as what we now formally call SQTS. One study reported QTc intervals of ≤360 ms in 35% of male patients with IVF compared with only 10% in healthy controls, with no patient meeting the formal criteria for SQTS.[6] A substudy of the Japan Idiopathic Ventricular Fibrillation Study (J-IVFS) registry found mild PR and QRS prolongation in 22.5% of a small IVF cohort without signs of ER. The findings were unrelated to clinical endpoints or the recurrence of VF.[7] This is discussed in more detail under "Interaction With Other Inherited Arrhythmias."

Electrocardiogram Phenomenology

A hallmark of IVF is the initiation: typically short-coupled premature ventricular complexes (PVCs).[8] In one study, initiating PVCs had a mean coupling interval of 302 ± 52 ms, and it occurred within 40 ms of the peak of the preceding T-wave.[8] The mode of onset of IVF is not bradycardia or pause dependent.[8] In contrast to classic torsades de pointes in the context of QT prolongation, IVF is not associated with an electrical prodrome of T wave alternans or giant T-U waves (Fig. 97.2).[9]

Triggering PVCs typically arise from the His–Purkinje system or from the right ventricular outflow tract (RVOT).[8,10–12] PVCs from the RVOT need to be distinguished from the benign forms of idiopathic RVOT tachycardia, which are more common and usually associated with an excellent prognosis. The largest series of malignant RVOT-PVCs triggering IVF was published by Noda and colleagues.[10] In their cohort of 101 patients with documented RVOT arrhythmia (monomorphic VT and VF), they identified 16 patients (15.8%) who presented with RVOT-PVCs initiating polymorphic VT/VF. The ECG morphology of the malignant trigger PVCs was similar to that of the PVCs of benign RVOT-VT, and there was no difference in the coupling interval. The coupling interval of malignant PVCs was 409 ± 62 ms. The strongest predictors of malignant arrhythmias were a shorter tachycardia cycle length (245 ± 28 ms vs. 328 ± 65 ms; *p* < .001) and a history of syncope that was present in 69% of patients with IVF. The latter speaks to varying mechanisms in IVF because apparently benign RVOT-PVCs triggering VF speak to a predominantly substrate-based vulnerability in contrast to short-coupled IVF, which argues that the short coupling interval is integral to the initiation of VF in the susceptible patient.

The role of the His–Purkinje system in the initiation of IVF has been described in a large series by Haissaguerre and colleagues.[12] Triggering PVCs from the His–Purkinje system can arise from both ventricles, with a short coupling interval of 260–320 ms. Intracardiac mapping of His–Purkinje PVCs in the study of Haissaguerre and associates typically showed a relatively narrow QRS (126 ± 17 ms) and a preceding Purkinje potential.

Unlike with Brugada and ER syndromes, there is currently no functional model suggesting the existence of an electroanatomical substrate for IVF.[13,14]

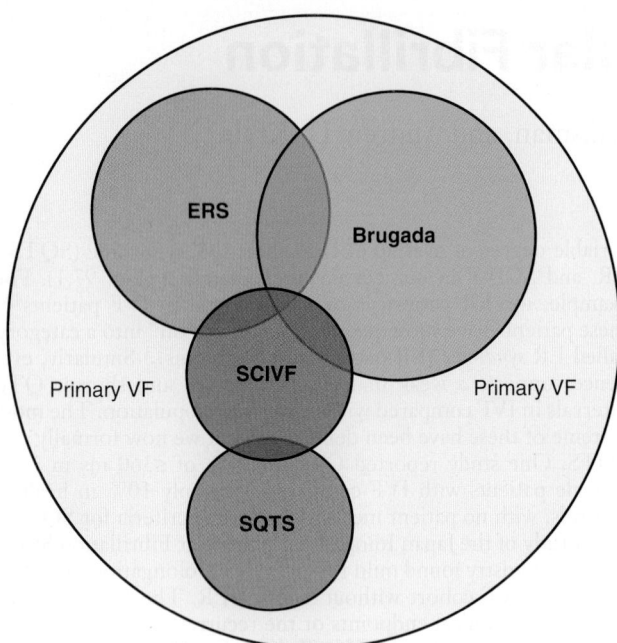

FIGURE 97.1 Schematic overlap between electrical disorders presenting with primary ventricular fibrillation (*VF*). *ERS,* Early repolarization syndrome; *SCIVF,* short-coupled idiopathic ventricular fibrillation; *SQTS,* short QT syndrome.

Arrhythmic events in IVF typically occur at rest or during sleep, which is similar to Brugada and ER syndromes, suggesting a contributory role of increased vagal tone.[10,15,16]

Molecular Mechanisms

The pathophysiology of IVF is largely speculative. Approximately 20% of patients with IVF have a positive family history of sudden cardiac death (SCD), suggesting a genetic contribution in at least a subset of cases. Recent studies identified several genetic mutations that could be linked to familial forms of IVF (Table 97.1).

Dipeptidyl-aminopeptidase–like protein 6 (DPP6) is a serine-protease without enzymatic activity that is expressed in the brain and myocardium.[17] The gene locus for DPP6 is chromosome 7q36. Functional studies suggest that DPP6 is a putative regulatory β-subunit of the rapidly recovering cardiac transient outward K$^+$ current ($I_{to,f}$) that contributes to the ER of the action potential (phase 1).[18] The role of DPP6 in IVF was first reported by Alders and associates, who performed a genome-wide haplotype analysis among members of three unrelated families from the same area in the Netherlands.[19] They identified a disease-causing DPP6 mutation (c.1-340C>T) within a noncoding, regulatory sequence of the gene. The mutation results in myocardial DPP6 overexpression in haplotype carriers who have a poor prognosis, with 50% experiencing SCD before the age of 58 years. In the Dutch population, the DPP6 mutation was not associated with structural features or ECG differences between gene carriers and noncarriers. A subsequent study looking at the regional variation of the prevalence of the DPP6 mutation across the Dutch population revealed a distribution pattern typical for a genetic founder effect.[20] Further insight into molecular mechanisms of DPP6-related IVF comes from a recent study that described a gain-of-function mutation with increased I_{to} currents in the Purkinje fibers of individuals with the Dutch DPP6 mutation.[21] These data support the concept of trigger PVCs arising from the His–Purkinje system.[12] Recently, a second DPP6 mutation was identified in a single individual with IVF.[22] The H332R variant is the first known coding DPP6 mutation, which results in

the translation of a truncated version of the protein (DPP6-T). The DPP6-T p.H332R variant is a dominant isoform of DPP6 and is characterized by an increased binding affinity to Kv4.3 (KCND3), one of the pore-forming α-subunits of $I_{to,f}$.[22,23] The result is a significant increase in $I_{to,f}$ current compared with that of the wild-type DPP6 form.[22]

Another familial form of IVF was linked to calmodulin1 (CALM1). CALM1 is a cytoplasmic, calcium-binding protein with ubiquitous expression that has a regulatory function for numerous calcium-dependent processes including cardiac ion channels.[24,25] CALM1 mutations have been previously described in long QT syndrome type 14 and catecholaminergic polymorphic VT type 5 (CPVT5).[26,27] A pathogenic IVF-related CALM1 mutation with autosomal dominant transmission was recently described in a family of Moroccan descent with four affected and two unaffected individuals.[28] The CALM1 c.268T>C (p.F90L) variant affects a highly conserved amino acid position. In F90L carriers, VF and SCD occur in childhood and adolescence. Cardiac events in the index family included two SCDs and two aborted VF arrests. All affected individuals were younger than 17 years. Cardiac events in CALM1 F90L carriers seem partially related to a hyperadrenergic state, but stress testing failed to induce ventricular arrhythmias in all the evaluated index patients. The phenotype of CALM1 F90L carriers is otherwise characterized by mild, subclinical QT prolongation during exercise and recovery.

A central role of abnormal calcium homeostasis is also suggested by another recent study that identified two novel ryanodine receptor (RYR2) mutations in a family with multiple IVF victims.[29] In seven affected family members with a likely diagnosis of IVF, two different heterozygous mutations were identified: c.6224T>C (p.IIe2075Thr, exon 41) and c.13781A>G (p.Lys4594Arg, exon 94). Cardiac events in gene carriers occurred at any age between 5 and 55 years. Although adrenergic triggers were associated with some events, clinical testing failed to induce PVCs or ventricular arrhythmia. The results of this study suggest that the two novel mutations result in a distinct phenotype that would not fit with classic RYR2-related CPVT.[30,31] The recent genetic discoveries of familial IVF also highlight the utility of whole exome sequencing.[22,28,29] Clearly, we lack a refined phenotype in many of these emerging rare causes of IVF, and further follow-up data with invasive and surface arrhythmia recording capability will inform the apparent phenotype. The current inability to reproduce a phenotype supports the concept of broad genetic screening of IVF survivors, despite the immense limitations of complex interpretation.

Diagnostic Evaluation

As growing evidence suggests features of a distinct entity, the term IVF should be used carefully and only after a systematic and comprehensive assessment eliminating SHD, other primary electrical heart disorders, and metabolic-toxicological conditions (see Chapter 99).

The Cardiac Arrest Survivors With Preserved Ejection Fraction Registry (CASPER) is a Canadian registry that attempts to provide a more inclusive population strategy to enroll and follow unexplained cardiac arrest including IVF patients. The CASPER registries identified a specific diagnosis in 56% of victims of unexplained cardiac arrest and established a final diagnosis of IVF in the remaining 44%.[4,32] A stepwise diagnostic approach such as the CASPER algorithm (Fig. 97.3) is recommended.[32] Cardiac evaluation should always start with a detailed history, with special focus on the clinical circumstances surrounding the episode of VF (resting state/sleep vs. nonspecific or adrenergic state), preceding episodes of syncope or seizure, and family history. Cardiac magnetic resonance imaging (MRI) is helpful in eliminating SHD in most cases if performed in experienced centers. A normal

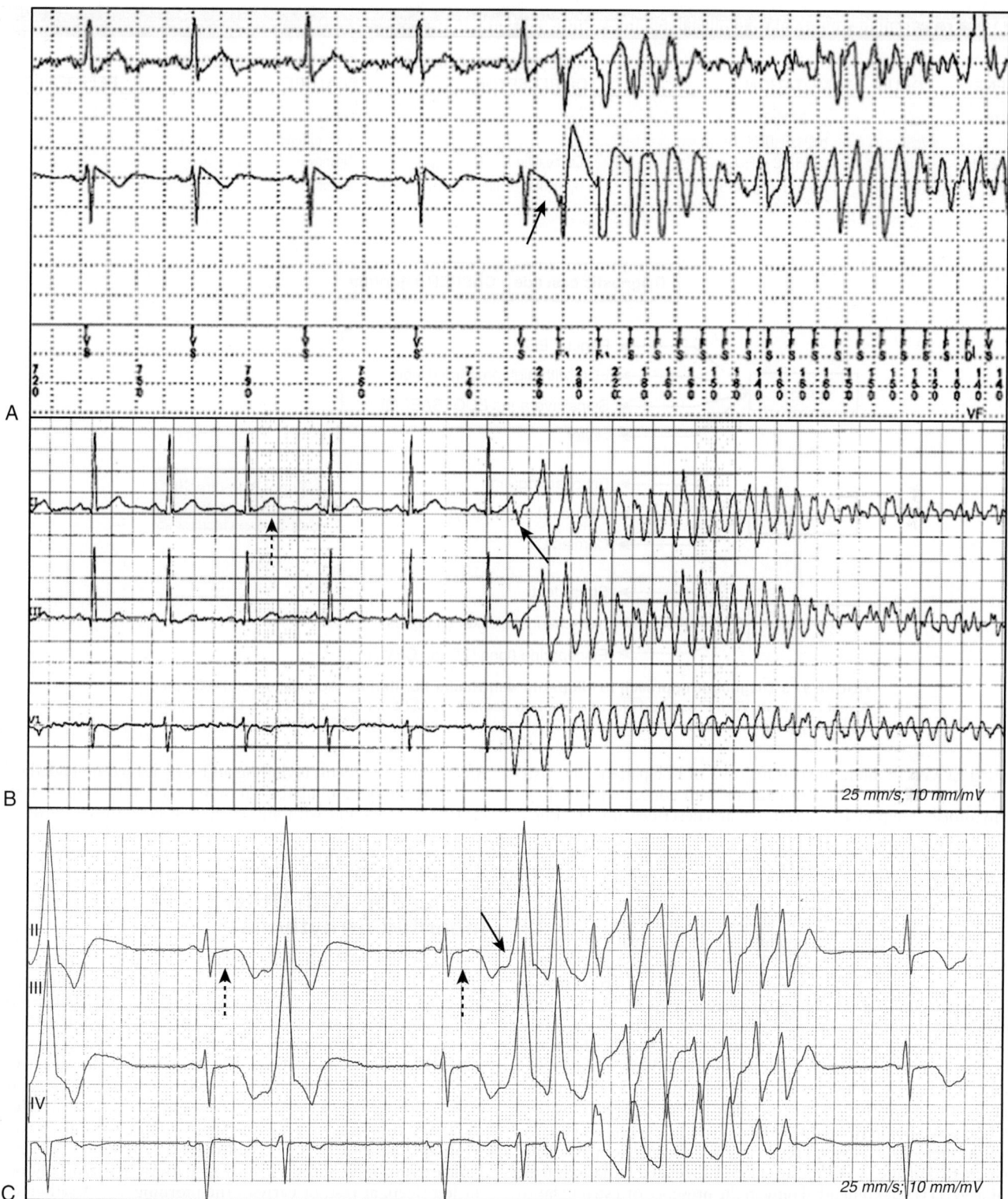

25 mm/s; 10 mm/mV

25 mm/s; 10 mm/mV

FIGURE 97.2 Short-coupled idiopathic ventricular fibrillation (SCIVF) in comparison to torsades de pointes. (A) Episode of recurrent ventricular fibrillation (*VF*) in a patient with SCIVF and implantable cardioverter defibrillator for secondary prevention. VF is initiated by a short-coupled premature ventricular contraction (PVC) (*arrow*). (B) Electrocardiogram recording of VF in a patient with SCIVF. Hallmark is the VF initiation by a short-coupled PVC (*solid arrow*). There is no preceding bradycardia or sinus pause (heart rate around 80 beats/min), and the corrected QT (QTc) interval is normal (*dashed arrow*). Absence of T-wave alternans or giant T-U waves. (C) Electrocardiogram recording of nonsustained torsades de pointes from a patient with hereditary long QT syndrome. Note the preceding sinus bradycardia with marked QTc prolongation (*dashed arrow*) and ventricular bigeminy. In contrast to SCIVF, torsades de pointes are typically initiated by late-coupled PVCs (*solid arrow*) and arise based on the underlying QT prolongation. Other characteristics include inducibility by bradycardia or pauses triggering ventricular ectopy with late coupling intervals that might fall in the vulnerable period of ventricular excitability.

TABLE 97.1		Genetic mutations in familial idiopathic ventricular fibrillation			
GENE	LOCUS	MUTATION	AFFECTED ION CHANNEL OR RECEPTOR	ELECTROPHYSIOLOGICAL FEATURE	REFERENCE
DPP6	7q36	c.1-340C>T	$I_{to,f}$	Gain of function	19–21
	7q36	pH332R (DPP6-T)	$I_{to,f}$	Gain of function	22
CALM1	14q32.11	c.268T>C: p.F90L	Calmodulin 1	Unknown	28
RYR2	1q43	c.6224T>C: p.Ile2075Thr, exon 41	Ryanodine receptor 2	Unknown	29
		c.13781A>G: p.Lys4594Arg, exon 94			

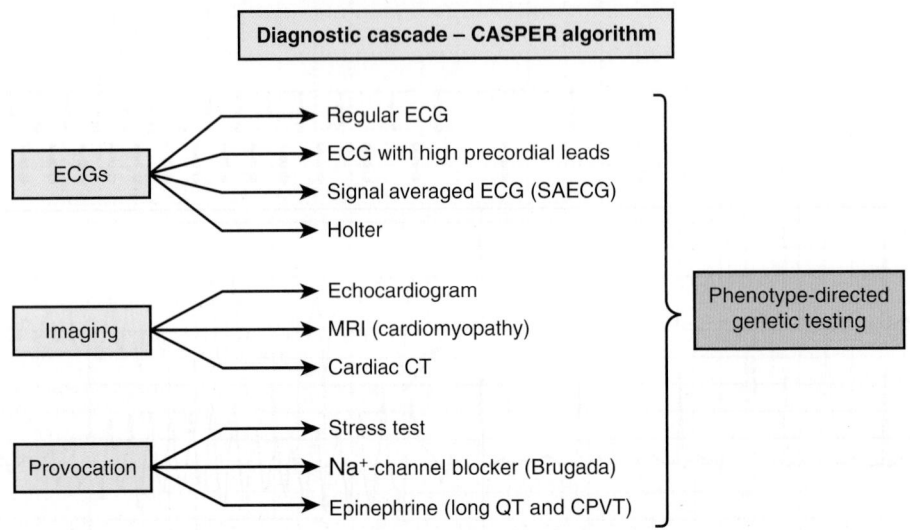

FIGURE 97.3 Diagnostic approach to idiopathic ventricular fibrillation. Application of the Cardiac Arrest Survivors With Preserved Ejection Fraction Registry (*CASPER*) algorithm. *CPVT*, Catecholaminergic polymorphic ventricular tachycardia; *CT*, computed tomography; *ECG*, electrocardiogram.

resting ECG is found in the vast majority of IVF patients but also in a substantial proportion of patients with concealed inherited arrhythmias. Helpful ECG features are described under "Phenotype and Triggers of Idiopathic Ventricular Fibrillation." Spontaneous PVCs with a short coupling interval and RVOT or His–Purkinje morphology might be suggestive but are in no way pathognomonic, or predictive, for IVF.

Unlike Brugada syndrome, signal-averaged ECG (SAECG) and resting ECG with high precordial leads are usually normal in patients with IVF. Extended ECG analysis and complementary functional tests (exercise testing, pharmacological provocation) are useful to unmask subclinical primary electrical disorders and distinguish them from IVF.[33–35] Routine invasive electrophysiology studies are not currently recommended for the diagnosis and risk stratification of IVF given the overall low inducibility rate and poor predictive values. In one study, VF was inducible in 39% (sensitivity 43%, specificity 64%), and the positive and negative predictive value over a mean follow-up of 41 ± 27 months was 43% and 64%, respectively.[36] Given the sparse data on genetic linkage in IVF, testing for IVF-related mutations (see Table 97.1) is recommended only in the presence of a strong family history of IVF or unexplained cardiac death.

Once established, the diagnosis of IVF should periodically be reevaluated because phenotypic findings of other inherited arrhythmia might fluctuate and manifest over time. This was demonstrated by a study from the CASPER registry reporting an evolving diagnosis in 21% of patients with an initial diagnosis of IVF over a follow-up period of 30 ± 17 months. The most useful test was a repeat resting ECG.[35] Therefore repeat clinical reassessment including history, physical exam, and ECG testing with or without repeat functional tests and/or cardiac imaging should be performed in all patients with a final diagnosis of IVF.

An annual assessment, including an ECG, is recommended using repeat imaging, ambulatory monitoring, and exercise testing every 2–3 years and with any change in arrhythmia burden. As for other inherited arrhythmias, a thorough and complete family screening is an integral part of a complete diagnostic workup.

Interaction With Other Inherited Arrhythmias

Short-coupled IVF displays remarkable clinical and electrophysiological overlap with other primary electrical disorders (see Fig. 97.1 and Table 97.2). Brugada and ER syndromes represent the so-called primary J-wave syndromes.[37] Unlike IVF, the resting ECG in Brugada and ER syndromes is characterized by marked J-point abnormalities.[37,38] Arrhythmogenesis of J-wave syndromes and IVF is characterized by repolarization abnormalities implicating I_{to}, I_{Na}, and, to some extent, cardiac calcium channels, resulting in polymorphic VT/VF, typically initiated by short-coupled PVCs.[37,38] Ventricular arrhythmias in IVF and J-wave syndromes show a circadian pattern and typically occur during sleep, at rest, or early in the morning.[15,16] Another striking feature is the excellent response to oral quinidine and intravenous isoproterenol for the treatment of electrical storm and the prevention of VF recurrence that was first documented in classical J-wave syndromes, suggesting common pathways of arrhythmogenesis.[39–41] Despite the clinical and electrophysiological overlap between IVF and J-wave syndrome, there are significant differences with respect to genetic factors. The strongest genetic basis has been documented in Brugada syndrome, with causal mutations in up to 25%–30% of patients.[37,38] In contrast, data on genetic mutations linked to ER syndrome or IVF are currently limited to case reports or isolated familial forms. At present, it is

TABLE 97.2 Overlap between short-coupled idiopathic ventricular fibrillation (IVF) and other electrical disorders with primary ventricular fibrillation (VF)

	SHORT-COUPLED IVF	EARLY REPOLARIZATION SYNDROME	BRUGADA SYNDROME	SHORT QT SYNDROME
J-point abnormalities on resting ECG	–	+	+	–
QTc on resting ECG	Normal; 330 ms < QTc ≤ 360 ms in up to 35%	Usually normal	Usually normal	≤330 ms
Ventricular arrhythmia				
Morphology	Polymorphic VT/VF	Polymorphic VT/VF	Polymorphic VT/VF[a]	Polymorphic VT/VF
Initiation by short-coupled PVCs	+	+	+	+
Electroanatomical substrate	–	Inferolateral LV epicardium	RVOT epicardium	–
Origin of triggering PVCs	RVOT, His–Purkinje system	?	RVOT and other RV sites	?
Clinical circumstances of events	Predominantly at sleep/rest	Predominantly at sleep/rest	Predominantly at sleep/rest	Predominantly at sleep/rest
Strength of genetic linkage	Rare familial forms	Rare familial forms	25%–30% of cases	Rare familial forms
Efficacy of isoproterenol for acute treatment	+	+	+	+
Efficacy of quinidine for acute treatment and chronic prevention	+	+	+	+

[a]Rare cases of monomorphic VT reported.

ECG, Electrocardiogram; *IVF,* idiopathic ventricular fibrillation; *LV,* left ventricle; *PVC,* premature ventricular complex; *QTc,* corrected QT interval; *RV,* right ventricle; *RVOT,* right ventricular outflow tract; *VT,* ventricular tachycardia.

still controversial if IVF without signs of ER represents a variant J-wave syndrome or a distinct entity.

Remarkable overlap also exists between IVF and short QT syndrome, a rare channelopathy with less than 200 published cases. To date, only a small proportion of short QT cases have been linked to familial mutations.[42,43] Similar to IVF and J-wave syndromes, short QT syndrome is characterized by accelerated repolarization with abbreviated duration of the cardiac action potential. The resulting transmural dispersion of repolarization represents the substrate for malignant arrhythmia. Ventricular arrhythmias in short QT syndrome also occur more commonly during sleep or at rest and are typically initiated by short-coupled PVCs.[42,43] Interestingly, a QTc duration of ≤360 ms occurs more often in patients with IVF compared with healthy controls.[6] Similar to IVF and J-wave syndromes, quinidine is the therapy of choice for prevention and treatment of ventricular arrhythmia in short QT syndrome.[43]

Management and Follow-up

The insertion of an implantable cardioverter defibrillator (ICD) is the standard treatment for all IVF patients with an aborted cardiac arrest or documented polymorphic VT/VF.[3] As patients with IVF are unlikely to benefit from antitachycardia pacing (ATP) and most of them will not need cardiac pacing, the selection of a subcutaneous ICD (S-ICD) may be an attractive alternative compared with a standard transvenous ICD system.[44] Most patients with IVF are relatively young and physically active, which should be taken into account during ICD programming to avoid inappropriate shocks. Appropriate strategies include programming to a single-therapy zone with a high cutoff rate (>210–220 beats/min) and a long detection interval as demonstrated in patients with Brugada and other inherited arrhythmia syndromes.[45]

Recurrence of IVF with appropriate ICD therapies occurs in 18%–39% of patients over a median follow-up of 41–63 months, with a median delay to the first recurrence of 4–12 months.[36,46] These patients may well present with a ventricular storm with a series of appropriate shocks. Adjunct pharmacological treatment is indicated for patients with frequent IVF recurrence or those who refuse ICD implantation. The preferred medication is quinidine, a class IA antiarrhythmic agent, which is a potent inhibitor of I$_{to}$.[47–49] Long-term treatment with oral quinidine has

demonstrated freedom from recurrent VF over a mean follow-up period of 9.1 ± 5.6 years.[49] The mean effective quinidine dose is usually between 1000–2000 mg per day, which corresponds to a therapeutic serum quinidine level of 3.4 ± 1.6 mg/L. A major challenge of quinidine therapy is currently the limited worldwide accessibility.[50] The drug is also typically difficult to tolerate at high doses, with frequent gastrointestinal side effects.

β-Blockers and other standard antiarrhythmic drugs including class III agents are ineffective in IVF. Selected medications might be useful for specific types of IVF, but data are limited to case reports or small series. For example, the combination of dalfampridine/cilostazol seemed to be effective in a patient with IVF and DPP6-T mutation.[22]

Electrical storm (≥3 VF episodes in 24 hours) has been reported in up to 13% of patients with IVF. A multicenter study by Haissaguerre and associates showed that oral quinidine or continuous infusion of isoproterenol are effective therapies to terminate electrical storms in patients with IVF or ER syndrome when added to standard intensive care treatment (airway protection, sedation, and mechanical circulatory support if needed).[41] Given its rapid onset of action and greater availability, isoproterenol is the medication of choice for electrical storm in the context of IVF. Isoproterenol infusions in this setting are usually initiated at rates of 1–5 μg/min and subsequently uptitrated according to the clinical response, targeting a sinus rate of 100–120 beats/min.

Mapping and catheter ablation of triggering PVCs from the RVOT or His–Purkinje system are the emerging therapies with promising results, but the limited data do not support their role as routine first-line treatment (Fig. 97.4). At present, catheter ablation should be considered as adjunct therapy in selected patients with failure or unavailability of quinidine and frequent VF recurrence. The feasibility of elimination of triggering PVCs has been demonstrated in several small studies.[10,46,51] A Japanese study by Noda and associates targeted RVOT-triggered PVCs in 16 patients with IVF. Successful ablation was achieved in 13 patients (81.3%), with no VF recurrence over a mean follow-up period of 54 ± 39 months. A multicenter study by Haissaguerre and associates targeted triggering PVCs from the RVOT and His–Purkinje system and reported short- and long-term success rates of 89% and 82%, respectively.[46,51] However, it is important to emphasize that studies focusing on the impact of interventions such as ablation or antiarrhythmic drugs typically consist of highly selected

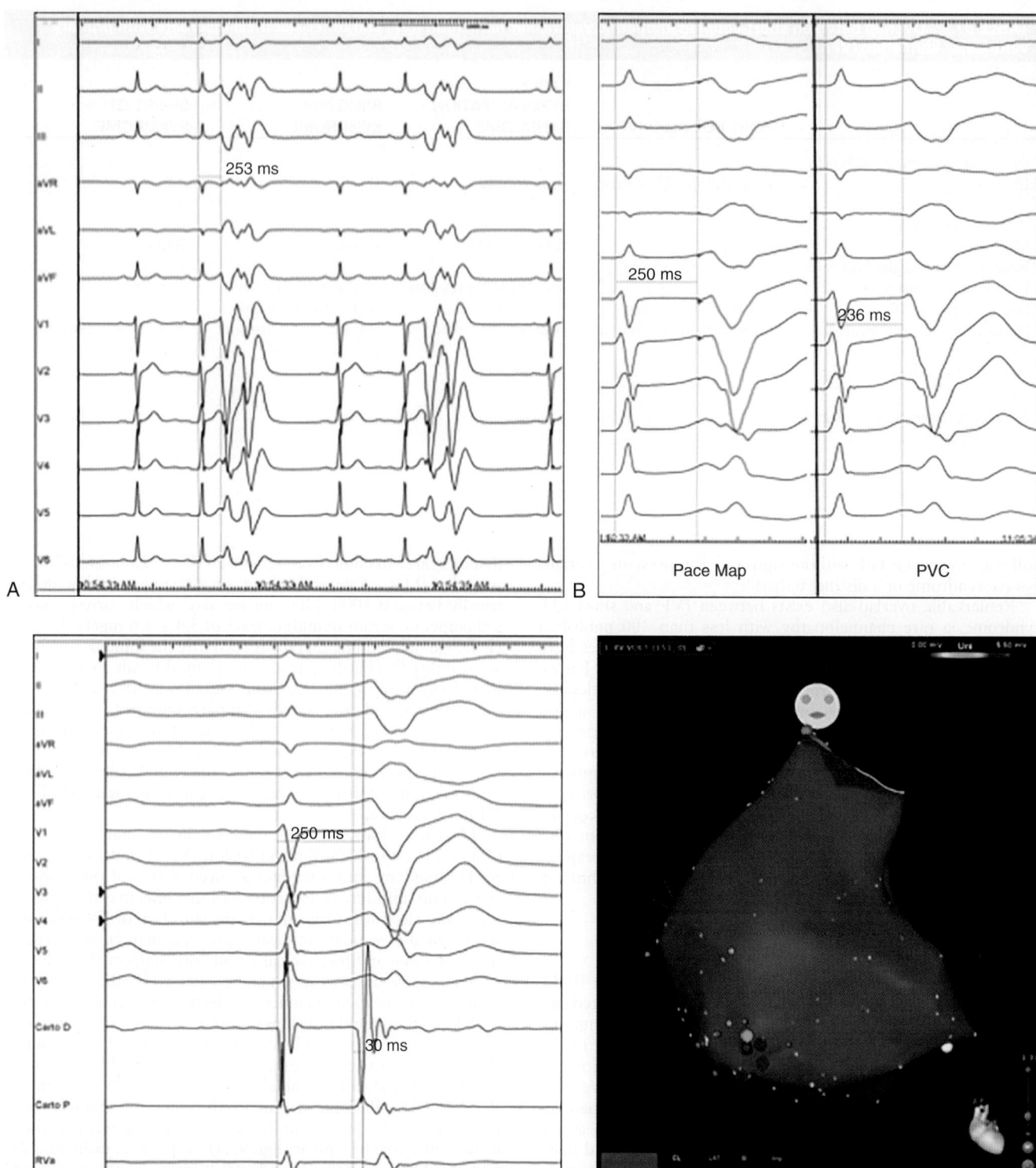

FIGURE 97.4 Key findings from a successful ablation of culprit premature ventricular complexes (*PVC*) triggering idiopathic ventricular fibrillation in a 27-year-old otherwise healthy female with previous unexplained cardiac arrest. (A) 12-lead electrocardiogram recording of nonsustained polymorphic ventricular tachycardia. Note the short-coupled triggering PVC with a stereotypical morphology in two bursts, which was seen repeatedly by telemetry and reproduced when compared with implantable cardioverter defibrillator–stored signals. (B) Pace mapping demonstrates the best pace map in the right ventricle near a moderator band. (C) Activation mapping at the site of a successful ablation shows a sharp, high-amplitude signal that precedes the surface QRS complex, also illustrated on the accompanying Carto map. (D) Note the normal voltage map and localization at the right ventricular papillary muscle/moderator band. (Courtesy Dr. David Callans.)

refractory patients referred to international specialty centers. Those cohorts are not representative of rare, community-based IVF patients that may have a different presentation and natural history.

Future Directions

Our current understanding of SCIVF is still very limited, and further research is required to characterize this entity and its relationship to other electrical disorders that present with primary VF. Initial steps could include the creation of registries with the goal of a better characterization of the SCIVF patients and their clinical evolution. Registries would also be useful to address practical clinical questions including response to medical treatment, comparison of local practices, and optimal device management in this particular population. Functional in vitro models or molecular imaging techniques for SCIVF are still at the early stage of development.

REFERENCES

1. Viskin S, Belhassen B. Idiopathic ventricular fibrillation. *Am Heart J.* 1990;120:661–671.
2. Survivors of out-of-hospital cardiac arrest with apparently normal heart. Need for definition and standardized clinical evaluation. Consensus Statement of the Joint Steering Committees of the Unexplained Cardiac Arrest Registry of Europe and of the Idiopathic Ventricular Fibrillation Registry of the United States. *Circulation.* 1997;95:265–272.
3. Priori SG, Wilde AA, Horie M, et al. HRS/EHRA/APHRS expert consensus statement on the diagnosis and management of patients with inherited primary arrhythmia syndromes: document endorsed by HRS, EHRA, and APHRS in May 2013 and by ACCF, AHA, PACES, and AEPC in June 2013. *Heart Rhythm.* 2013;10:1932–1963.
4. Derval N, Simpson CS, Birnie DH, et al. Prevalence and characteristics of early repolarization in the CASPER registry: cardiac arrest survivors with preserved ejection fraction registry. *J Am Coll Cardiol.* 2011;58:722–728.
5. Haissaguerre M, Derval N, Sacher F, et al. Sudden cardiac arrest associated with early repolarization. *New Engl J Med.* 2008;358:2016–2023.
6. Viskin S, Zeltser D, Ish-Shalom M, et al. Is idiopathic ventricular fibrillation a short QT syndrome? Comparison of QT intervals of patients with idiopathic ventricular fibrillation and healthy controls. *Heart Rhythm.* 2004;1:587–591.
7. Sekiguchi Y, Aonuma K, Takagi M, et al. New clinical and electrocardiographic classification in patients with idiopathic ventricular fibrillation. *J Cardiovasc Electrophysiol.* 2013;24:902–908.
8. Viskin S, Lesh MD, Eldar M, et al. Mode of onset of malignant ventricular arrhythmias in idiopathic ventricular fibrillation. *J Cardiovasc Electrophysiol.* 1997;8:1115–1120.
9. Leenhardt A, Glaser E, Burguera M, Nurnberg M, Maison-Blanche P, Coumel P. Short-coupled variant of torsades de pointes. A new electrocardiographic entity in the spectrum of idiopathic ventricular tachyarrhythmias. *Circulation.* 1994;89:206–215.
10. Noda T, Shimizu W, Taguchi A, et al. Malignant entity of idiopathic ventricular fibrillation and polymorphic ventricular tachycardia initiated by premature extrasystoles originating from the right ventricular outflow tract. *J Am Coll Cardiol.* 2005;46:1288–1294.
11. Viskin S, Rosso R, Rogowski O, Belhassen B. The "short-coupled" variant of right ventricular outflow ventricular tachycardia? A not-so-benign form of benign ventricular tachycardia? *J Cardiovasc Electrophysiol.* 2005;16:912–916.
12. Haissaguerre M, Shah DC, Jais P, et al. Role of Purkinje conducting system in triggering of idiopathic ventricular fibrillation. *Lancet.* 2002;359:677–678.
13. Koncz I, Gurabi Z, Patocskai B, et al. Mechanisms underlying the development of the electrocardiographic and arrhythmic manifestations of early repolarization syndrome. *J Mol Cell Cardiol.* 2014;68:20–28.
14. Szel T, Antzelevitch C. Abnormal repolarization as the basis for late potentials and fractionated electrograms recorded from epicardium in experimental models of Brugada syndrome. *J Am Coll Cardiol.* 2014;63:2037–2045.
15. Matsuo K, Kurita T, Inagaki M, et al. The circadian pattern of the development of ventricular fibrillation in patients with Brugada syndrome. *Eur Heart J.* 1999;20:465–470.
16. Aizawa Y, Sato M, Ohno S, et al. Circadian pattern of fibrillatory events in non-Brugada-type idiopathic ventricular fibrillation with a focus on J waves. *Heart Rhythm.* 2014;11:2261–2266.
17. Niwa N, Nerbonne JM. Molecular determinants of cardiac transient outward potassium current (I$_{to}$) expression and regulation. *J Mol Cell Cardiol.* 2010;48:12–25.
18. Radicke S, Cotella D, Graf EM, Ravens U, Wettwer E. Expression and function of dipeptidyl-aminopeptidase-like protein 6 as a putative beta-subunit of human cardiac transient outward current encoded by Kv4.3. *J Physiol.* 2005;565:751–756.
19. Alders M, Koopmann TT, Christiaans I, et al. Haplotype-sharing analysis implicates chromosome 7q36 harboring DPP6 in familial idiopathic ventricular fibrillation. *Am J Hum Genet.* 2009;84:468–476.
20. Postema PG, Christiaans I, Hofman N, et al. Founder mutations in the Netherlands: familial idiopathic ventricular fibrillation and DPP6. *Neth Heart J.* 2011;19:290–296.
21. Xiao L, Koopmann TT, Ordog B, et al. Unique cardiac Purkinje fiber transient outward current beta-subunit composition: a potential molecular link to idiopathic ventricular fibrillation. *Cir Res.* 2013;112:1310–1322.
22. Sturm AC, Kline CF, Glynn P, et al. Use of whole exome sequencing for the identification of Ito-based arrhythmia mechanism and therapy. *J Am Heart Assoc.* 2015;4:e001762.
23. Nerbonne JM, Kass RS. Molecular physiology of cardiac repolarization. *Physiol Rev.* 2005;85:1205–1253.
24. Halling DB, Aracena-Parks P, Hamilton SL. Regulation of voltage-gated Ca2+ channels by calmodulin. *Sci STKE.* 2005;2005:re15.
25. Saimi Y, Kung C. Calmodulin as an ion channel subunit. *Annu Rev Physiol.* 2002;64:289–311.
26. Crotti L, Johnson CN, Graf E, et al. Calmodulin mutations associated with recurrent cardiac arrest in infants. *Circulation.* 2013;127:1009–1017.
27. Nyegaard M, Overgaard MT, Sondergaard MT, et al. Mutations in calmodulin cause ventricular tachycardia and sudden cardiac death. *Am J Hum Genet.* 2012;91:703–712.
28. Marsman RF, Barc J, Beekman L, et al. A mutation in CALM1 encoding calmodulin in familial idiopathic ventricular fibrillation in childhood and adolescence. *J Am Coll Cardiol.* 2014;63:259–266.
29. Paech C, Gebauer RA, Karstedt J, Marschall C, Bollmann A, Husser D. Ryanodine receptor mutations presenting as idiopathic ventricular fibrillation: a report on two novel familial compound mutations, c.6224T>C and c.13781A>G, with the clinical presentation of idiopathic ventricular fibrillation. *Pediatr Cardiol.* 2014;35:1437–1441.
30. Laitinen PJ, Brown KM, Piippo K, et al. Mutations of the cardiac ryanodine receptor (RyR2) gene in familial polymorphic ventricular tachycardia. *Circulation.* 2001;103:485–490.
31. Priori SG, Napolitano C, Tiso N, et al. Mutations in the cardiac ryanodine receptor gene (hRyR2) underlie catecholaminergic polymorphic ventricular tachycardia. *Circulation.* 2001;103:196–200.
32. Krahn AD, Healey JS, Chauhan V, et al. Systematic assessment of patients with unexplained cardiac arrest: Cardiac Arrest Survivors With Preserved Ejection Fraction Registry (CASPER). *Circulation.* 2009;120:278–285.
33. Krahn AD, Healey JS, Chauhan VS, et al. Epinephrine infusion in the evaluation of unexplained cardiac arrest and familial sudden death: from the cardiac arrest survivors with preserved Ejection Fraction Registry. *Circ Arrhythm Electrophysiol.* 2012;5:933–940.
34. Somani R, Krahn AD, Healey JS, et al. Procainamide infusion in the evaluation of unexplained cardiac arrest: from the Cardiac Arrest Survivors with Preserved Ejection Fraction Registry (CASPER). *Heart Rhythm.* 2014;11:1047–1054.
35. Vittoria Matassini M, Krahn AD, Gardner M, et al. Evolution of clinical diagnosis in patients presenting with unexplained cardiac arrest or syncope due to polymorphic ventricular tachycardia. *Heart Rhythm.* 2014;11:274–281.
36. Champagne J, Geelen P, Philippon F, Brugada P. Recurrent cardiac events in patients with idiopathic ventricular fibrillation, excluding patients with the Brugada syndrome. *BMC Med.* 2005;3:1.
37. Antzelevitch C, Yan GX. J-wave syndromes: Brugada and early repolarization syndromes. *Heart Rhythm.* 2015;12:1852–1866.
38. Antzelevitch CJ. Wave syndromes: molecular and cellular mechanisms. *J Electrocardiol.* 2013;46:510–518.
39. Belhassen B, Glick A, Viskin S. Efficacy of quinidine in high-risk patients with Brugada syndrome. *Circulation.* 2004;110:1731–1737.
40. Belhassen B, Rahkovich M, Michowitz Y, Glick A, Viskin S. Management of Brugada syndrome: a 33-year experience using electrophysiologically-guided therapy with class 1A antiarrhythmic drugs. *Circ Arrhythm Electrophysiol.* 2015;8:1393–1402.
41. Haissaguerre M, Sacher F, Nogami A, et al. Characteristics of recurrent ventricular fibrillation associated with inferolateral early repolarization role of drug therapy. *J Am Coll Cardiol.* 2009;53:612–619.
42. Patel C, Yan GX, Antzelevitch C. Short QT syndrome: from bench to bedside. *Circ Arrhythm Electrophysiol.* 2010;3:401–408.
43. Mazzanti A, Kanthan A, Monteforte N, et al. Novel insight into the natural history of short QT syndrome. *J Am Coll Cardiol.* 2014;63:1300–1308.
44. Bardy GH, Smith WM, Hood MA, et al. An entirely subcutaneous implantable cardioverter-defibrillator. *N Engl J Med.* 2010;363:36–44.
45. Sacher F, Probst V, Maury P, et al. Outcome after implantation of a cardioverter-defibrillator in patients with Brugada syndrome: a multicenter study-part 2. *Circulation.* 2013;128:1739–1747.
46. Knecht S, Sacher F, Wright M, et al. Long-term follow-up of idiopathic ventricular fibrillation ablation: a multicenter study. *J Am Coll Cardiol.* 2009;54:522–528.
47. Belhassen B, Shapira I, Shoshani D, Paredes A, Miller H, Laniado S. Idiopathic ventricular fibrillation: inducibility and beneficial effects of class I antiarrhythmic agents. *Circulation.* 1987;75:809–816.
48. Belhassen B, Viskin S, Fish R, Glick A, Setbon I, Eldar M. Effects of electrophysiologic-guided therapy with Class IA antiarrhythmic drugs on the long-term outcome of patients with idiopathic ventricular fibrillation with or without the Brugada syndrome. *J Cardiovasc Electrophysiol.* 1999;10:1301–1312.
49. Belhassen B, Glick A, Viskin S. Excellent long-term reproducibility of the electrophysiologic efficacy of quinidine in patients with idiopathic ventricular fibrillation and Brugada syndrome. *Pacing Clin Electrophysiol.* 2009;32:294–301.
50. Viskin S, Wilde AA, Guevara-Valdivia ME, et al. Quinidine, a life-saving medication for Brugada syndrome, is inaccessible in many countries. *J Am Coll Cardiol.* 2013;61:2383–2387.
51. Haissaguerre M, Shoda M, Jais P, et al. Mapping and ablation of idiopathic ventricular fibrillation. *Circulation.* 2002;106:962–967.

98 Sudden Infant Death Syndrome

Jonathan C. Makielski and Jianding Cheng

Sudden infant death syndrome (SIDS) ranks third as a cause of infant mortality.[1] SIDS is defined as the sudden, unexpected death of an infant (before the age of 1 year) for which no cause is apparent.[2] *Sudden unexpected death syndrome* refers to the unexpected death of a person older than 1 year but younger than 35 or 40 years.[3] This chapter addresses only SIDS, but the age demarcation of 1 year is somewhat arbitrary, and overlap surely exists for the two syndromes. Depending on the precise definition of SIDS, the historical era, demographics, and ethnic status of the population, SIDS affects approximately 0.1–2 infants per 1000 live births, with a peak incidence between the ages of 2 and 5 months.[2,3] The etiological basis for SIDS can be neurological, endocrine, metabolic, pulmonary, immune, or cardiac, with a genetic basis implicated for each.[4,5] This chapter reviews the evidence that cardiac arrhythmia has a role in SIDS, with a focus on genetic predisposition to fatal arrhythmia.[4] The literature on SIDS, in general, and on the role for arrhythmia and SIDS, in particular, is vast, with numerous studies, reviews, editorials, and commentaries highlighting the controversies. The focus of this chapter is on more recent studies and review articles that will lead the interested reader to this rich literature.

Arrhythmia as a Cause of Sudden Infant Death Syndrome

By definition, SIDS occurs in infants without diagnosed or suspected disease ante mortem and with no clear cause of death on routine postmortem examination. This lack of antemortem data has been an obstacle for the field overall and particularly for establishing a link to arrhythmia. Techniques to investigate the etiology of SIDS include analyses of epidemiological data, studies of the parents and relatives of SIDS victims, and studies of infants who were considered to be at high risk for SIDS. Infants who came to medical attention before death or who were resuscitated from an event (called *survivors of SIDS* or designated as having *near-miss SIDS*) also have been studied. These cases provide valuable insights into and proof of principle for etiological factors in SIDS. The near-miss cases, however, do not fit the clinical and epidemiological definition of SIDS because the affected patients either had clinical manifestations detected antemortem or did

not die. Mutations in the ion channels and associated proteins cause a number of inherited arrhythmia syndromes (IAS) such as long QT syndrome (LQTS; see Chapters 50 and 93), Brugada syndrome (BrS; see Chapters 50 and 92), and catecholaminergic polymorphic ventricular tachycardia (CPVT; see Chapter 53). As susceptibility genes were identified for IAS, it became possible to perform a "molecular autopsy"[3] for SIDS victims by screening candidate genes for mutations.

A study of cohorts of true SIDS cases that meet the rigorous definition of SIDS can give an estimate of how many cases might be explained by mutations in ion channels or related proteins (channelopathies) that cause IAS. A certain semantic paradox occurs, however, because once a cause is established, an individual case should no longer be considered SIDS. This chapter focuses on recent studies showing that some cases previously considered to be SIDS can be explained by IAS channelopathies, and it discusses the extent to which these discoveries and undiscovered channelopathies will lead to reclassification of SIDS cases as early deaths due to channelopathies. The importance of making the diagnosis extends well beyond reclassification because it leads to elucidation of mechanism, prevention, and possible therapy in individual patients.

It also is important to recognize that the presence of a mutation in a susceptible gene does not necessarily imply a link to causation because mutations without functional significance occur as common polymorphisms (affecting greater than 0.5% of the population) or as rare variants (affecting less than 0.5% of the population). The absence of the mutation in control panels provides supporting evidence for pathogenicity, but the possibility of discovering an incidental rare variant in SIDS increases with increase in the number of genes screened. Traditional linkage studies in family kindreds are used to connect the genotype to the phenotype, but such studies are not possible in SIDS because the phenotype is death in infancy, and mutations can be de novo, that is, not present in the parents. When a mutation is found, biophysical function of the mutation can be investigated by expressing the mutated protein in heterologous expression systems or in myocytes to demonstrate an abnormality consistent with known pathogenetic mechanisms for LQTS, BrS, CPVT, or other arrhythmia syndromes. If such a mutation is present, it provides strong, but not conclusive, evidence for pathogenicity. If it is absent, however, it does not prove nonpathogenicity because the mutation might not have been studied under the conditions necessary to elicit the dysfunction (e.g., reduced pH)[6,7] or that the presence of the complete macromolecular complex present in myocytes, but not heterologous cells, is required to manifest dysfunction. To support the conclusion of a link between a genotype and an arrhythmic SIDS clinical phenotype, a mutation should cause biophysical dysfunction of an ion current under relevant environmental conditions that result in a cellular phenotype supporting an arrhythmogenic phenotype at the tissue and organ level.

Sudden Infant Death Syndrome, Long QT Syndrome, and Environmental Factors

In the 1970s, Schwartz suggested that abnormalities of cardiac sympathetic innervation caused a disorder of the heart's electrical rhythm known as LQTS and that this can also cause SIDS.

TABLE 98.1   Frequency of channelopathies in cohort studies of sudden infant death syndrome (SIDS)

SYNDROME AND GENE	INCIDENCE	FREQUENCY IN SIDS (%)	RELATIVE FREQUENCY IN SIDS (%)	FREQUENCY IN IAS GROUP (%)
LQT1 *KCNQ1*	5/418	1.2	10.9	30–35
LQT2 *KCNH2*	4/418	1.0	8.9	25–30
LQT3 *SCN5A*	25/577	4.3	39.4	5–10
LQT5 *KCNE1*	0/437	0.0	0	1
LQT6 *KCNE2*	1/437	0.2	2.0	Rare
LQT7 *KCNJ2*	0/303	0.0	0	Rare
LQT9 *CAV3*	7/401	1.7	15.9	1
LQT10 *SCN4B*	1/358	0.3	2.5	Rare
LQT12 *SNTA1*	8/358	2.2	20.4	Rare
Total for LQTS		10.9	100	
BrS *SCN5A*	7/577	1.2	32.3	20
BrS *GPD1L*	4/370	1.1	28.9	Rare
BrS *SCN1B*	1/358	0.3	7.4	Rare
BrS *SCN3B*	3/358	0.8	22.3	Rare
BrS *KCND3*	1/292	0.3	9.1	
Total for BrS		3.8	100	
CPVT1 *RYR2*	2/134	1.5		
SQT1 *KCNQ1*	1/201	0.5		
Other *GJA1*	2/292	0.7		
Other *KCNJ8*	2/292	0.7		
Other *HCN4*	2/46	4.3		
Other *HCN2*	0/46	0.0		
Total for all groups		22.4		

Frequency was derived from data from the cohort studies.[12–17,19–21,25–29] Not every gene listed was tested for every cohort. The S1103Y polymorphism study was not included.[4] Relative frequency in the IAS citations has been reported in Lehnart et al.[20] The frequency estimates given for IAS include cases that were not genotyped in the denominator.

IAS, Inherited arrhythmia syndromes.

Maron and colleagues[8] showed a longer QT interval in parents of SIDS victims and provided evidence for a role of LQTS in SIDS. In a prospective trial of electrocardiogram (ECG) screening in more than 34,000 infants that produced 24 SIDS cases,[9] a long QT interval increased the risk of SIDS by a factor of 41. The proof of principle that congenital LQTS could cause SIDS came from two cases: a near-miss case[10] in which the infant survived and a case in which the patient died in infancy but LQTS was recognized antemortem.[11] In both cases, a mutation in the gene *SCN5A* encoding the voltage-dependent cardiac sodium channel was found, and it had the characteristic biophysical phenotype of increased late sodium current associated with LQTS type 3 (LQT3). These cases, however, did not meet the formal epidemiological definition of SIDS.

In 2001, Ackerman and associates[12] screened a cohort of 93 patients with defined SIDS for mutations in *SCN5A* and found two novel mutations that on expression in heterologous cells showed the increased late sodium current of LQT3. Additional studies in SIDS cohorts have found additional mutations in *SCN5A* associated with LQT3.[6,13–17] Most of these mutations were rare and novel, but one, S1103Y, was a common polymorphism with an allelic frequency of approximately 10% in the black population. S1103Y had previously been associated with ventricular arrhythmia in adults.[18] Plant and coworkers[6] showed that homozygosity for S1103Y increased the risk of SIDS by 24-fold. Moreover, the biophysical abnormality of increased late sodium current depended on acidosis, linking the interaction of environmental influences with the genotype to produce the pathological phenotype. Subsequently, two other mutations were shown to require acidosis to produce the abnormal phenotype.[7] Three novel mutations in caveolin-3 (encoded by *CAV3*), a channel accessory protein, were found in a SIDS cohort and were shown to cause late sodium current characteristic of LQTS.[19] Four novel mutations in α-syntrophin (encoded by *SNTA1*),

a scaffolding protein associated with SCN5A, were found in a SIDS cohort and were shown to cause increased late sodium current by a nitrosylation-dependent mechanism.[20] Novel mutations in the sodium channel–associated β-subunits β3 (encoded by *SCN3B*) and β4 (encoded by *SCN4B*) were found in the same SIDS cohort and shown to cause increased late sodium current.[21] Thus the abnormality of sodium current in LQTS as a cause of SIDS is not restricted to mutations in *SCN5A*.

Mutations in potassium channel genes *KCNQ1*[14–16,22] (LQT1), *KCNH2*[14–16,23] (LQT2), and *KCNE2*13 (LQT6), which cause loss of function in potassium currents, have also been described in SIDS cohorts. The common KCNH2 polymorphism K897T was found to be strongly associated with two cases of SIDS in a singular family.[24] Two other LQTS potassium channel genes, *KCNJ2* (LQT7) and *KCNE1* (LQT5), were screened in 303 SIDS cases,[13,16] but no pathological mutations were found. Currently, approximately 80% of all genetic LQTS can be accounted for by mutations in the known genes (for LQT1–LQT13),[25] with the majority of cases being caused by *KCNQ1* (LQT1) and *KCNH2* (LQT2). In SIDS, however, mutations in *SCN5A* (in LQT3), *CAV3* (LQT9), *SCN4B* (LQT10), and *SNTA1* (LQT12) predominate, and in the cohort studies to date they account for 78% of cases of LQTS in SIDS and for 8.6% of SIDS cases overall (Table 98.1).

Sudden Infant Death Syndrome and Other Inherited Arrhythmia Syndromes

BrS manifests clinically with ventricular arrhythmia, sudden death, and a characteristic resting or provoked ECG pattern of ST-segment elevation in precordial leads. BrS was suggested as the underlying disorder in a child with a near miss, and a mutation in *SCN5A* showed characteristic decreased sodium current. *SCN5A* mutations cause approximately 20% of cases of BrS[25] but appear to

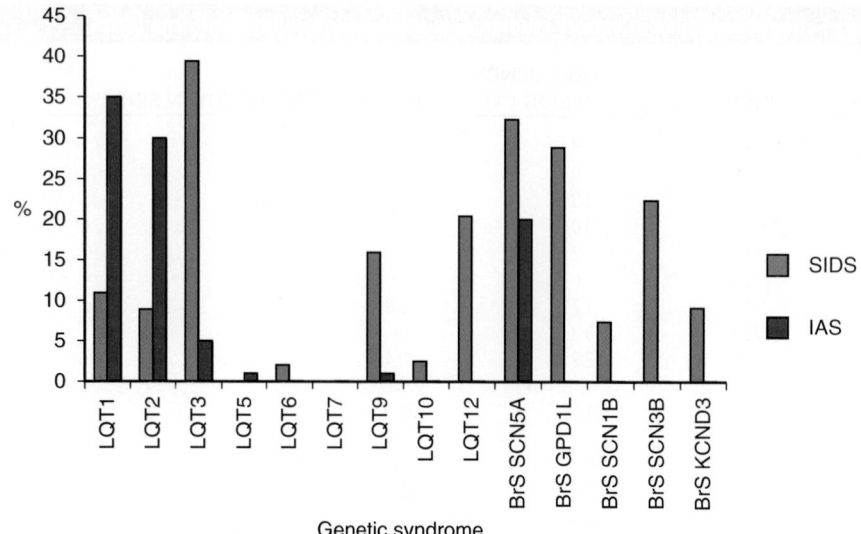

FIGURE 98.1 Comparison of the relative frequencies of long QT (*LQT*) and Brugada syndrome (*BrS*) in sudden infant death syndrome (*SIDS*) versus inherited arrhythmia syndrome (*IAS*). The values are taken from Table 98.1.

be a rare cause of SIDS because only seven likely pathogenic variants (including BrS causing variant R1193Q in six cases[16,17]) were found in 577 cases of SIDS in cohort studies (see Table 98.1).[6,13–17] Four separate mutations in *GPD1L*, a known BrS susceptibility gene, were found in cases of SIDS at an early age[17,30] and could account for 1% of SIDS cases overall. In addition, mutations in the β_3-subunit[17,21] and the β_1-subunit[17,31] were found in SIDS cases and caused a loss of sodium current consistent with BrS. Interestingly, the mutation in the β_1-subunit also caused a gain of function for transient outward current[31] when coexpressed with $K_V4.3$, which is also consistent with BrS. In a SIDS cohort study, two mutations in the ryanodine receptor 2 (RyR2) were found to be associated with the characteristic biophysical phenotype for CPVT[32] and accounted for 1.5% of cases (see Table 98.1). Proof of principle that short QT syndrome can cause SIDS was provided by an early pediatric diagnosis in a child who did not die,[33] and subsequently a mutation in *KCNQ1* was discovered in a SIDS cohort that had the characteristic biophysical phenotype of gain of function found in short QT syndrome (see Table 98.1)[13] and accounted for 0.5% of cases. Mutations in the gap junction protein connexin43 (encoded by *GJA1*) identified in two SIDS cases and causing a loss of function could plausibly cause death by arrhythmia.[26] Mutations in the adenosine triphosphate–sensitive potassium current pore Kir6.1 (encoded by *KCNJ8*) found in two cases of SIDS caused a loss of function,[27] but the link to arrhythmia is less certain than that for the other mutations described here.

Unlike the cardiac-specific channels associated with LQTS, BrS, and CPVT, HCN channels are responsible for generating spontaneous rhythmic activity in both cardiac pacemaker cells and neurons in the brain. Human genetic and animal studies have highlighted the involvement of HCN channels in the pathophysiology of arrhythmias.[28] Two potentially pathogenic nonsynonymous variants in HCN4 were identified in two SIDS cases out of a cohort of 46 SIDS cases, and they may have contributed to the SIDS event.[29] The role of HCN4 should be considered speculative, as the dysfunction, if any, caused by these mutations is unknown.

Sudden Infant Death Syndrome and Channelopathies: Frequency and Spectrum

A comprehensive study[13] investigating seven LQTS genes found mutations in 26 of 201 SIDS cases (12.9%) and, on the basis of molecular phenotype, concluded that 19 of these (9.5%)

were pathogenic. Table 98.1 summarizes data from the cohort studies.[12–17,19–21,25–29] Adding BrS, CPVT, short QT syndrome, and "other" to LQTS brings the total incidence of putative channelopathies in SIDS to 22.4%. More studies are necessary to verify this number in additional, larger, and diverse cohorts. This number may represent a minimum because new gene discoveries for IAS could increase it. In 2007 it was estimated that 75% of cases of LQTS, 50%–60% of CPVT cases, and 20% of cases of BrS could be attributed to the known arrhythmia genes.[25] As new arrhythmia genes are discovered for IAS, they will become candidates for SIDS as well. Moreover, channel-opathies unique to SIDS may be discovered. The pattern for the incidence of certain genes in SIDS already diverges sharply from that in non-SIDS congenital arrhythmia syndromes (Fig. 98.1). For example, *GPD1L* mutations are rare compared with *SCN5A* mutations as a cause of BrS but are prominent BrS mutations for SIDS. *CAV3* and *SNTA1* mutations are rare causes of LQTS in inherited arrhythmia syndromes but are relatively common in SIDS. *SCN5A* mutations cause only 5%–10% of cases of LQTS; however, in SIDS, *SCN5A* accounts for 39.4% of the LQTS-type mutations identified so far (see Fig. 98.1). Thus the relative frequency of genetic defects in non-SIDS inherited arrhythmia syndromes appears to be a poor predictor of their relative frequency in SIDS. Finally, a novel gene discovery in SIDS has the potential to dramatically increase the percentage of SIDS cases that could be potentially explained by channelopathies.

Sudden Infant Death Syndrome: Channelopathies and the Triple Risk Hypothesis

Are channelopathies in SIDS fundamentally different from those in non-SIDS? What accounts for their early lethality? The triple risk hypothesis[34] for SIDS states that (1) a vulnerable infant (genetically predisposed), (2) a critical development period, and (3) an environmental trigger or stressor come together to cause SIDS. The explanation for increased and early lethality could be pertinent at each level of risk. A point of interest is that abnormalities in the sodium current through mutations in *SCN5A*, *GPD1L*, and *CAV3* account for approximately 50% of channelopathies in SIDS (Fig. 98.2) and for nearly 8% of SIDS cases overall (see Table 98.1). What implication does this finding have for the early lethality of SIDS? At the genetic level, the severity or character of the biophysical

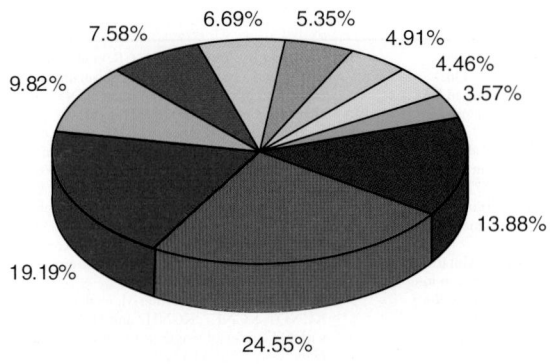

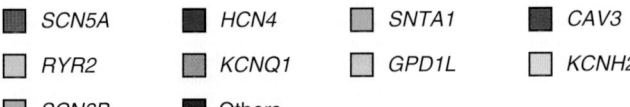

- ■ *SCN5A*
- ■ *HCN4*
- ■ *SNTA1*
- ■ *CAV3*
- □ *RYR2*
- ■ *KCNQ1*
- □ *GPD1L*
- □ *KCNH2*
- ■ *SCN3B*
- ■ Others

FIGURE 98.2 Frequency of genes with mutations as putative causes of sudden infant death syndrome (SIDS). The proposed mechanism for SIDS involves dysfunction of the sodium current for up to 51% of SIDS (mutations in *SCN5A, SNTA1, CAV3, GPD1L, SCN3B, SCN1B,* and *SCN4B*). The percentage of 9.8% for HCN4 may be overrepresented because of the small numbers (*n* = 46) in the cohort studied. The values are taken from Table 98.1.

phenotype itself could account for the early lethality. For example, common LQT3 mutations such as ΔKPQ and R1623Q show slow inactivation of the late sodium current, which accumulates at more rapid rates, thereby mitigating QT prolongation and predisposing to arrhythmia at slower rates, when the QT is longest. Two mutations unique to SIDS, A997S and R1826H,[12] did not show this slow inactivation. Perhaps this feature accounts for the early lethality. A unique interaction with the environment could account for a more severe biophysical phenotype, as for the mutations in *SCN5A* such as S1103Y,[6] R680H, and Δ586[7] that result in an augmented late sodium current at low pH. The magnitude of the dysfunction in low pH, however, was not more severe than that for defects described in non-SIDS arrhythmia mutations. Although this is an attractive hypothesis for the interaction of genetic background and environment (see Fig. 98.1), it alone might not account for early lethality. Overall, the studies to date suggest that the severity of the biophysical phenotypes for SIDS mutations appears to be similar to that for non-SIDS mutations. Why such early deaths in SIDS with channelopathies? Does this effect merely represent the leading edge of the non-SIDS cases? The epidemiology of SIDS (deaths concentrated in months 3–5) and the different distribution of channelopathies and genetic defects between SIDS and non-SIDS suggest otherwise. Nevertheless, the mechanism for early lethality at the level of biophysical dysfunction remains unknown.

The early lethality could come from other genetic interactions. The common *SCN5A* polymorphism H558R markedly affects wild-type *SCN5A*[35] and modifies the function of other mutations in *SCN5A*,[36,37] and it has been associated with atrial fibrillation, BrS, and long QTc.[38–40] The allelic frequency of H558R was two-fold higher than that expected (44% vs. 21%) in SIDS cases with *SCN5A* mutations,[13] suggesting a "double hit," but the allelic frequency of H558R was no greater in SIDS cases overall when patients without an *SCN5A* mutation were considered. The S1103Y mutation is a common polymorphism in the black population,[41] with homozygosity associated with SIDS.[6] Three common polymorphisms in potassium channel genes (K897T in *KCNH2*, R1047L in *KCNH2*, and G38S in *KCNE1*) either were no different in SIDS or, in one instance (R1047L), were actually lower in SIDS cases.[13] However, as

noted earlier, K897T in *KCNH2* was associated with SIDS in a single family.[24]

In addition to channelopathies, genes for serotonin transporter, the autonomic nervous system, nicotine metabolism, inflammation, metabolism, and thermoregulation[4,42,43] all have been implicated in SIDS in accordance with hypotheses generated by clinical and epidemiological data. These data support the common view that SIDS is likely to be a heterogeneous disorder, but they also suggest that lethality associated with arrhythmia in infancy could involve an intersection of several genetic factors causing predisposition to SIDS and contributing to the development of arrhythmia. Finally, early death by arrhythmia could be influenced by environmental factors such as respiratory acidosis. This association provides a rationale for the apparent success of the move to supine sleeping in the "Back to Sleep" campaign.[44] The so-called triple risk hypothesis involving the complex interaction of genetic background, developmental state, and environmental triggers remains an important model for the etiology of SIDS and can link disorders of different systems in causing SIDS.

Implications for Screening, Therapy, and Further Research

Primary genetic screening of all infants for channelopathies is not yet practical. Not only do issues of expense and low yield need to be addressed, but such screening would uncover many rare variants of unknown significance. For example, in healthy populations of different racial and ethnic backgrounds, approximately 3% of screened subjects have been found to harbor a mutation in *SCN5A*.[41] The possible significance of these variants in asymptomatic populations is not immediately apparent. On the other hand, a screen for channelopathies would appear to be useful for SIDS victims and their families, especially as next-generation sequencing (NGS)–based genetic screening becomes common.[45] An important unanswered question is how often channelopathies in SIDS are sporadic or de novo in the affected infant and not present in the parents. This consideration has important implications for inheritance and recurrence in siblings.

Primary ECG screening in neonates for LQTS, as suggested by Schwartz,[46] can be a practical and cost-effective measure.[47] Issues of sensitivity and specificity as well as cost effectiveness have been raised, but with the increasing evidence for the importance of channelopathies in SIDS and the prominent role of LQTS in these channelopathies, the impetus for neonatal screening is increasing.[48]

Besides, LQTS-associated ion channel gene variants were identified in 8.8% of intrauterine fetal death cases. This is supported by the development of fetal magnetocardiography (fMCG) technology, which allows detection of fetal arrhythmias in utero during development.[49] fMCG is an accurate technology for identification of fetuses with LQTS and for prediction of a severe phenotype; thus it may also be able to play a role in the diagnosis and management of infants at risk of SIDS after birth.

With the predominance of *SCN5A* LQTS mutations in SIDS, the possible effectiveness of blocking of the late sodium current[50,51] in treating the primary biophysical abnormality suggests a potential pharmacological therapy in addition to other therapies such as β-blockade and use of implanted defibrillators.

This chapter has focused on ion channelopathies as a cause or contributing factor to SIDS, and such channelopathies appear to occur in 15%–20% of defined SIDS cases, with the possibility that more channelopathies and a higher frequency of channelopathies in SIDS will be discovered as research continues. The possibility also exists that arrhythmia unrelated to channelopathies but related to other genetic or developmental factors contribute to SIDS. How these channelopathies contribute to such early death compared with the non-SIDS channelopathies requires further study. Investigation of the overall contribution of channelopathies and arrhythmia in SIDS is a part of the wider search into causes for SIDS.

REFERENCES

1. Hamilton BE, Hoyert DL, Martin JA, et al. Annual summary of vital statistics: 2010-2011. *Pediatrics*. 2013;131:548.

2. Kinney HC, Thach BT. The sudden infant death syndrome. *N Engl J Med*. 2009;361:795-805.

3. Tester DJ, Ackerman MJ. The molecular autopsy: should the evaluation continue after the funeral? *Pediatr Cardiol*. 2012;33:461-470.

4. Van Norstrand DW, Ackerman MJ. Genomic risk factors in sudden infant death syndrome. *Genome Med*. 2010;2:86.

5. Rubens D, Sarnat HB. Sudden infant death syndrome: an update and new perspectives of etiology. *Handb Clin Neurol*. 2013;112:867-874.

6. Plant LD, Bowers PN, Liu Q, et al. A common cardiac sodium channel variant associated with sudden infant death in African Americans, SCN5A S1103Y. *J Clin Invest*. 2006;116:430-435.

7. Wang DW, Desai RR, Crotti L, et al. Cardiac sodium channel dysfunction in sudden infant death syndrome. *Circulation*. 2007;115:368-376.

8. Maron BJ, Clark CE, Goldstein RE, et al. Potential role of QT interval prolongation in sudden infant death syndrome. *Circulation*. 1976;54:423-430.

9. Schwartz PJ, Stramba-Badiale M, Segantini A, et al. Prolongation of the QT interval and the sudden infant death syndrome. *N Engl J Med*. 1998;338:1709-1714.

10. Schwartz PJ, Priori SG, Dumaine R, et al. A molecular link between the sudden infant death syndrome and the long-QT syndrome. *N Engl J Med*. 2000;343:262-267.

11. Wedekind H, Smits JP, Schulze-Bahr E, et al. De novo mutation in the SCN5A gene associated with early onset of sudden infant death. *Circulation*. 2001;104:1158-1164.

12. Ackerman MJ, Siu BL, Sturner WQ, et al. Postmortem molecular analysis of SCN5A defects in sudden infant death syndrome. *JAMA*. 2001;286:2264-2269.

13. Arnestad M, Crotti L, Rognum TO, et al. Prevalence of long-QT syndrome gene variants in sudden infant death syndrome. *Circulation*. 2007;115:361-367.

14. Otagiri T, Kijima K, Osawa M, et al. Cardiac ion channel gene mutations in sudden infant death syndrome. *Pediatr Res*. 2008;64:482-487.

15. Millat G, Kugener B, Chevalier P, et al. Contribution of long-QT syndrome genetic variants in sudden infant death syndrome. *Pediatr Cardiol*. 2009;30:502-509.

16. Glengarry JM, Crawford J, Morrow PL, et al. Long QT molecular variation in sudden infant death syndrome. *Arch Dis Child*. 2014;99:635-640.

17. Winkel BG, Yuan L, Olesen MS, et al. The role of the sodium current complex in a nonreferred nationwide cohort of sudden infant death syndrome. *Heart Rhythm*. 2015;12:1241-1249.

18. Splawski I, Timothy KW, Tateyama M, et al. Variant of SCN5A sodium channel implicated in risk of cardiac arrhythmia. *Science*. 2002;297:1333-1336.

19. Cronk LB, Ye B, Kaku T, et al. Novel mechanism for sudden infant death syndrome: Persistent late sodium current secondary to mutations in caveolin-3. *Heart Rhythm*. 2007;4:161-166.

20. Cheng J, Van Norstrand DW, Medeiros-Domingo A, et al. Alpha1-syntrophin mutations identified in sudden infant death syndrome cause an increase in late cardiac sodium current. *Circ Arrhythm Electrophysiol*. 2009;2:667-676.

21. Tan BH, Pundi KN, Van Norstrand DW, et al. Sudden infant death syndrome-associated mutations in the sodium channel beta subunits. *Heart Rhythm*. 2010;7:771-778.

22. Schwartz PJ, Priori SG, Bloise R, et al. Molecular diagnosis in a child with sudden infant death syndrome. *Lancet*. 2001;358:1342-1343.

23. Christiansen M, Tonder N, Larsen LA, et al. Mutations in the HERG K⁺ ion channel: A novel link between long QT syndrome and sudden infant death syndrome. *Am J Cardiol*. 2005;95:433-434.

24. Nof E, Cordeiro JM, Perez GJ, et al. A common single nucleotide polymorphism can exacerbate long-QT type 2 syndrome leading to sudden infant death. *Circ Cardiovasc Genet*. 2010;3:199-206.

25. Lehnart SE, Ackerman MJ, Benson DW, et al. Inherited arrhythmias: A National Heart, Lung, and Blood Institute and Office of Rare Diseases workshop consensus report about the diagnosis, phenotyping, molecular mechanisms, and therapeutic approaches for primary cardiomyopathies and gene mutations affecting ion channel function. *Circulation*. 2007;116:2325-2345.

26. Van Norstrand DW, Asimaki A, Rubinos C, et al. Connexin43 mutation causes heterogeneous gap junction loss and sudden infant death. *Circulation*. 2012;125:474-481.

27. Tester DJ, Tan BH, Medeiros-Domingo A, et al. Loss-of-function mutations in the KCNJ8-encoded Kir6.1 K(ATP) channel and sudden infant death syndrome. *Circ Cardiovasc Genet*. 2011;4:510-515.

28. Herrmann S, Hofmann F, Stieber J, et al. HCN channels in the heart: lessons from mouse mutants. *Br J Pharmacol*. 2012;166:501-509.

29. Evans A, Bagnall RD, Duflou J, et al. Postmortem review and genetic analysis in sudden infant death syndrome: an 11-year review. *Hum Pathol*. 2013;44:1730-1736.

30. Van Norstrand DW, Valdivia CR, Tester DJ, et al. Molecular and functional characterization of novel glycerol-3-phosphate dehydrogenase 1 like gene (GPD1-L) mutations in sudden infant death syndrome. *Circulation*. 2007;116:2253-2259.

31. Hu D, Barajas-Martinez H, Medeiros-Domingo A, et al. A novel rare variant in SCN1Bb linked to Brugada syndrome and SIDS by combined modulation of Na(v)1.5 and K(v)4.3 channel currents. *Heart Rhythm*. 2012;9:760-769.

32. Tester DJ, Dura M, Carturan E, et al. A mechanism for sudden infant death syndrome (SIDS): Stress-induced leak via ryanodine receptors. *Heart Rhythm*. 2007;4:733-739.

33. Giustetto C, Di Monte F, Wolpert C, et al. Short QT syndrome: clinical findings and diagnostic-therapeutic implications. *Eur Heart J*. 2006;27:2440-2447.

34. Filiano JJ, Kinney HC. A perspective on neuropathologic findings in victims of the sudden infant death syndrome: the triple-risk model. *Biol Neonate*. 1994;65:194-197.

35. Makielski JC, Ye B, Valdivia CR, et al. A ubiquitous splice variant and a common polymorphism affect heterologous expression of recombinant human SCN5A heart sodium channels. *Circ Res*. 2003;93:821-828.

36. Ye B, Valdivia CR, Ackerman MJ, et al. A common human SCN5A polymorphism modifies expression of an arrhythmia causing mutation. *Physiol Genomics*. 2003;12:187-193.

37. Viswanathan PC, Benson DW, Balser JR. A common SCN5A polymorphism modulates the biophysical effects of an SCN5A mutation. *J Clin Invest*. 111:341-346.

38. Chen LY, Ballew JD, Herron KJ, et al. A common polymorphism in SCN5A is associated with lone atrial fibrillation. *Clin Pharmacol Ther*. 2007;81:35-41.

39. Gouas L, Nicaud V, Berthet M, et al. Association of KCNQ1, KCNE1, KCNH2 and SCN5A polymorphisms with QTc interval length in a healthy population. *Eur J Hum Genet*. 2005;13:1213-1222.

40. Chen JZ, Xie XD, Wang XX, et al. Single nucleotide polymorphisms of the SCN5A gene in Han Chinese and their relation with Brugada syndrome. *Chin Med J (Engl)*. 2004;117:652-656.

41. Ackerman MJ, Splawski I, Makielski JC, et al. Spectrum and prevalence of cardiac sodium channel variants among black, white, Asian, and Hispanic individuals: implications for arrhythmogenic susceptibility and Brugada/long QT syndrome genetic testing. *Heart Rhythm*. 2004;1:600-607.

42. Rognum IJ, Tran H, Haas EA, et al. Serotonin metabolites in the cerebrospinal fluid in sudden infant death syndrome. *J Neuropathol Exp Neurol*. 2014;73:115-122.

43. Blackwell C, Moscovis S, Hall S, et al. Exploring the risk factors for sudden infant deaths and their role in inflammatory responses to infection. *Front Immunol*. 2015;6:44.

44. Mitchell EA, Hutchison L, Stewart AW. The continuing decline in SIDS mortality. *Arch Dis Child*. 2007;92:625-626.

45. Hertz CL, Christiansen SL, Larsen MK, et al. Genetic investigations of sudden unexpected deaths in infancy using next-generation sequencing of 100 genes associated with cardiac diseases. *Eur J Hum Genet*. 2016;24:817-822.

46. Schwartz PJ. Pro: Newborn ECG screening to prevent sudden cardiac death. *Heart Rhythm*. 2006;3:1353-1355.

47. Quaglini S, Rognoni C, Spazzolini C, et al. Cost-effectiveness of neonatal ECG screening for the long QT syndrome. *Eur Heart J*. 2006;27:1824-1832.

48. Berul CI, Perry JC. Contribution of long-QT syndrome genes to sudden infant death syndrome: is it time to consider newborn electrocardiographic screening? *Circulation*. 2007;115:294-296.

49. Cuneo BF, Strasburger JF, Yu S, et al. In utero diagnosis of long QT syndrome by magnetocardiography. *Circulation*. 2013;128:2183-2191.

50. Nagatomo T, January CT, Makielski JC. Preferential block of late sodium current in the LQT3 (KPQ) mutant by the class I(C) antiarrhythmic flecainide. *Mol Pharmacol*. 2000;57:101-107.

51. Makielski JC. SIDS: genetic and environmental influences may cause arrhythmia in this silent killer. *J Clin Invest*. 2006;116:297-299.

99 Sudden Cardiac Death in Adults

Robert J. Myerburg and Jeffrey J. Goldberger

Sudden cardiac death (SCD) is defined as death following a sudden cardiac arrest (SCA) in a patient with either known or previously undetected cardiac abnormalities, in whom the mode and time of death are unexpected. In addition, transient endogenous influences on cardiac physiology, such as electrolyte, metabolic, or respiratory disturbances, or exogenous factors, such as drug effects or chest wall trauma (as in *commotio cordis*), can contribute to unanticipated risk. Although *unexpectedness* is a key feature of the SCD definition, clinical markers that cause enhanced predisposition to SCA, such as heart failure or transient ischemia, have been identified. However, despite knowledge of these predictors, a large proportion of SCDs occur as the first clinically recognized expressions of cardiac issues, as in patients with previously unrecognized ischemic heart disease or inherited arrhythmogenic disorders.

The generally accepted temporal definition is an interval of up to 1 hour between the onset of an abrupt change in clinical status and loss of consciousness.[1] This time period defines the onset of SCA, but the absolute definition of biological death, which could be delayed for days to a month or more by life-support interventions after central nervous system injury resulting from the SCA, should be used in population studies and clinical analyses.

Sudden Cardiac Death as a Public Health Burden

For the last 30 years of the 20th century, the incidence of SCD in the United States was estimated at 300,000 to 350,000 events per year. These estimates were derived from a broad-based accumulation of clinical and population data available at the time, rather than from direct epidemiological studies providing national statistics that included representation from various regions of the country. During the first decade of the 21st century, conflicting statements have been put forward regarding the current incidence of SCD (Fig. 99.1A). These newer estimates were derived from retrospective death certificate analyses and extrapolations from SCD incidences identified in specific communities. For example, an estimate from the statistical handbook of the American Heart Association (AHA),[2] based on data from the National Center for Health Statistics (NCHS) and the National Heart, Lung, and Blood Institute, suggested an annual incidence of fewer than 250,000 SCDs. An additional analysis from the Seattle, Washington emergency medical system (EMS) database, extrapolated to total US population numbers, calculated 184,000 cardiac arrests nationwide in the year 2000,[3] which is a significant decrease compared with 1980 statistics. Another community-based study from Oregon, based on prospective medical examiner data plus other sources of data, also yielded a national extrapolation of fewer than 200,000 cardiac arrests.[4] In contrast, a death certificate–based study, also from the NCHS, has suggested that more than 50% of all cardiac deaths are sudden and estimated the total annual incidence of SCD to be in the range of 460,000.[5] In the most recent statistical update from the AHA,[6] the estimated annual number of EMS-assessed sudden cardiac arrests in adults in the United States is 347,322. Other sources suggest >400,000 EMS responses to cardiac arrest.[7] Combining statistics from several sources, in addition to accounting for actual deaths by subtracting survivors, this figure returns to the rate of 300,000 to 350,000 SCDs annually, with somewhat lower numbers in specific locations as cited above. Despite these various estimates, an accurate count of the SCD burden in the United States will require reporting of all cardiac arrests in a national registry, which should include data on sites, causes, responses, and outcomes.[7]

The large discrepancy between the two estimates from NCHS death certificate data stems from differences between the definitions of SCD used and between population sources. The AHA restricted its application of the NCHS data solely to coronary heart disease–related deaths, based only on International Classification of Diseases–Ninth Revision codes 410 to 414 (Fig. 99.1B), whereas the cumulative NCHS data included almost all causes of SCD (Fig. 99.1C). The much broader range of inclusion in the latter study resulted in the much larger estimate, perhaps overestimating the true incidence. The Seattle data include only SCDs involving emergency rescue responses, whereas the Oregon study population is not necessarily representative of the incidence variations within the entire US population. National estimates remain uncertain because of the hazards of relying on death certificate classification and on extrapolations from a few large population centers of excellence that might not be representative of smaller metropolitan statistical areas constituting the majority of the US population. This limitation could affect appropriateness of regional response strategies and outcomes, in addition to knowledge of the true population burden.

The strongly emphasized continuous reduction in age-adjusted risk of coronary heart disease mortality in the United States beginning in the 1970s, when translated to total number of events and size of populations at risk for future events, cannot be interpreted to mean that the absolute burden of SCD events has decreased.[8] General preventive therapies and lifestyle modifications for controlling risk factors for coronary heart disease, plus interventions in acute coronary syndromes, have likely contributed to a population effect on evolution of disease and

SUDDEN CARDIAC DEATH Conflicting Incidence Estimates

Source	Incidence
Conventional U.S. Estimate (Derived from clinical and epidemiological studies)	300,000-350,000
AHA Statistical Update, 2001 (Derived from death certificate data – ICD9:410-414)	250,000
National Center for Health Statistics, 2001 (Derived from death certificate data – all cause)	456,000
Seattle Emergency Rescue Data, 2002 (Derived from large EMS system data) Oregon Community Population Study, 2004 (Prospective, multi-source design)	<200,000
AHA Statistical Update, 2012 (Estimate extrapolated from CAD-SCD and ROC data)	>300,000

A

Reported 1° Cause		Reported 2° Cause		Edited 1° Cause		Adjudication
ICD-9	Condition	ICD-9	Condition	ICD-9	Condition	SCD Count
410-414	ASHD	427.5	SCA	ICD-9	----	YES
427.5	SCA	410-414	ASHD	410-414	ASHD	YES
427.5	SCA	–None Provided–		----	----	NO
425	CM	427.5	SCA	----	----	NO
428	HF	427.5	SCA	----	----	NO
427.5	SCA	425	CM	425	CM	NO

B

ATTRIBUTED CAUSE (ICD-9)	DEATHS (%) [N = 456,076]
Acute ischemic HD (410-411)	26.9 } 62
Chronic ischemic HD (412-414)	35.3
Cardiovascular disease, unspecified (429.2)	12.1
Cardiomyopathy/arrhythmias (425-427)	9.3
Hypertensive HD (402, 404)	5.1
Heart failure (428)	6.7
Carditis, valvular HD (420-424, 429.1-.2)	2.2
Pulmonary HD (415-417)	1.0
All others (390-398, 429.3-.9)	1.4

C

FIGURE 99.1 Conflicting estimates on the incidence of sudden cardiac death (*SCD*) in the United States. Recent estimates range from less than 185,000 to more than 450,000 SCDs annually. (A) Estimates over time. Most of the estimates are derived from retrospective analysis of death certificate data and none is based on a prospective analysis of a population representative of the entire country. Each study used different inclusion criteria. (B) The data available in the American Heart Association (*AHA*) Statistical Handbook are limited to out-of-hospital cardiac arrest with a diagnosis of coronary heart disease, using specific International Classification of Diseases (*ICD-9*) codes (410 to 414). This source estimated 250,000 SCDs annually in 2001 and in the range of 300,000 to 350,000 in 2012. (C) Using a broader range of etiological definitions for SCD (note the ICD-9 codes used), the National Center for Health Statistics demonstrated that only 62% of all SCDs have a primary diagnosis using the ICD-9 codes on which the AHA estimates are based and reported an annual frequency of more than 450,000 SCDs. A prospective study using uniform criteria is desirable for clarifying the actual incidence of SCD in the United States. *ASHD,* Arteriosclerotic heart disease; *CM,* cardiomyopathy; *HD,* heart disease; *HF,* heart failure; *SCA,* sudden cardiac arrest. ([A] and [B] Modified and updated from Myerburg RJ. Scientific gaps in the prediction and prevention of sudden cardiac death. *J Cardiovasc Electrophysiol.* 2002;13:709-723. [C] Modified from Zheng ZJ, Croft JB, Giles WH, Mensah GA. Sudden cardiac death in the United States 1989 to 1998. *Circulation.* 2001;104:2158-2163.)

the reduction in age-adjusted mortality rates. However, these therapies, lifestyle modifications, and interventions have not had a proportional effect on SCD incidence, especially in low-risk subsets with large denominators and high absolute numbers of events. Based on existing data, it appears that the total numerical burden of SCD has not changed significantly over the past 30 years, although underlying disease burden has, and SCD accounts for an increasing proportion of cardiovascular deaths, constituting 50% of cardiac deaths in the United States and Northern Europe.[9,10] The limitations of the various sources

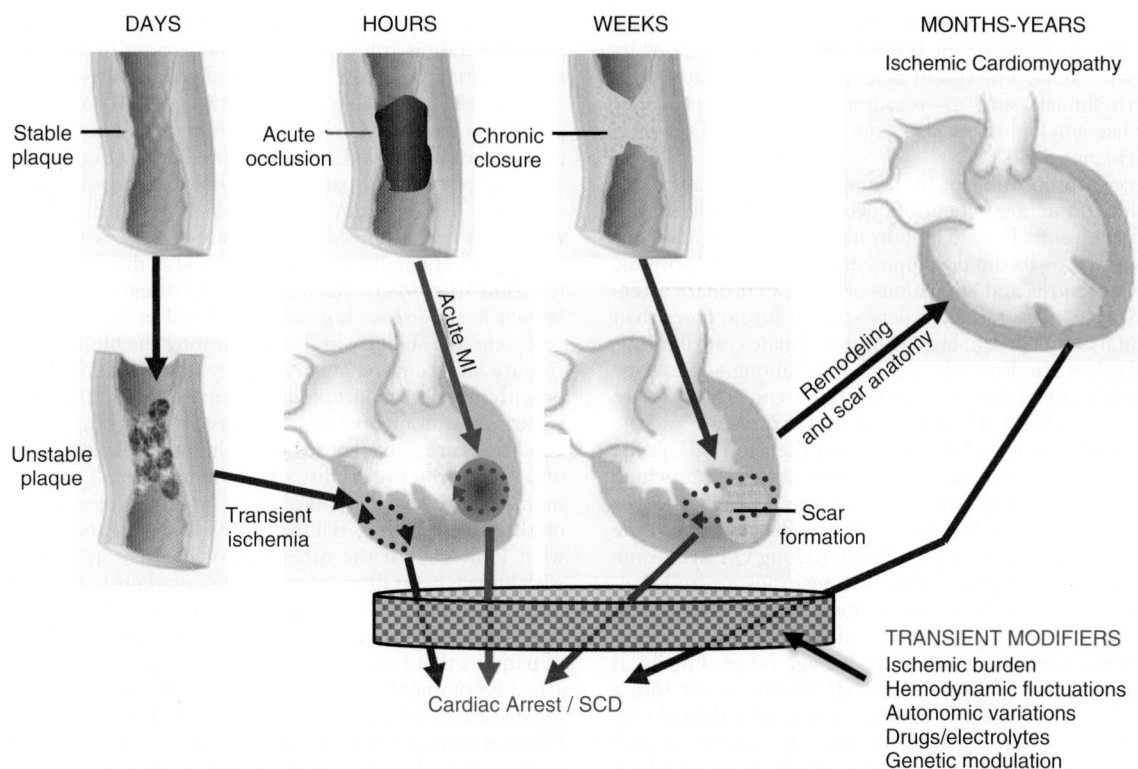

FIGURE 99.2 Pathophysiology of cardiac arrest caused by coronary heart disease. Four pathophysiological substrates contribute to arrhythmic risk and sudden cardiac death (*SCD*) in coronary artery disease. These include transient ischemia, acute coronary syndromes, scar-related pathophysiology, and ischemic cardiomyopathy. The pathophysiology, clinical implications, and long-term risk of each are described in the text. (Modified from Myerburg RJ. Implantable cardioverter-defibrillators after myocardial infarction. *New Engl J Med*. 2008;359:2245-2253, with permission of the publisher. Copyright Massachusetts Medical Society, 2008.)

and the reliability of currently available data[11] suggest that a prospective epidemiological study, designed to provide accurate counts of SCDs and its specific mechanisms, including proportional representation from metropolitan statistical areas of different sizes, would be a wise investment to help future health needs planning, community response system designs, and clinical research targets.

The foregoing statements are limited to the specific problem of out-of-hospital cardiac arrest (OHCA) and related SCDs. Another large group of SCAs, estimated at approximately 200,000 per year in the United States, occur in-hospital (IHCA), with ~75% resulting in death.[12]

Structural Substrates and Clinical Expressions Associated With Sudden Cardiac Death

The etiological basis for SCD can be analyzed in the context of two general categories: substrate-based causes and expression-based triggers. *Substrate-based causation* refers to the presence of vascular, myocardial, or molecular substrates that associate with SCD. In parallel, *expression risk* refers to the identification of mechanisms that contribute to the clinical expression of the risk predisposed by the substrate. In the case of SCD owing to coronary heart disease, these are suggested by the plaque transition and acute syndrome modules in Fig. 99.2 (plaque disruption and thrombogenesis) and their subsequent expression as an arrhythmic event (arrhythmogenic module) in the susceptible individual. The arrhythmogenic category of pathophysiology can also be viewed to include modifiers of molecular-based risk that drive individual expression.

Among the general population in the Western hemisphere, coronary heart disease is the most common substrate for SCD. Although estimates vary, approximately 75% to 80% of all SCDs in the United States and Western Europe are associated with this underlying substrate.[1] Cardiomyopathies compose the second most common category of disorders associated with SCD. Most definitions of this category include both dilated cardiomyopathy (DCM) and hypertrophic cardiomyopathy (HCM), but the hypertrophic form is more appropriately counted among the rare genetic syndromes associated with SCD risk, for both clinical and epidemiological reasons. DCMs collectively account for 10% to 15% of all SCDs. Many studies of SCD risk and interventions fail to distinguish between DCM as an etiology and congestive heart failure (CHF) as a clinical expression.

Various infiltrative, inflammatory, and valvular diseases constitute the underlying causes in most of the remaining SCDs. Viral or autoimmune myocarditis, whether manifest clinically or silent, can be associated with SCD. The frequency of this disorder is uncertain because of the difficulty validating its presence, even histopathologically. It has been considered to be among the more common causes of SCD in adolescents and young adults,[13] but its incidence is debated because many of the estimates are derived from studies that predated the consistent definitions established by the Dallas criteria. More recently, the recognition of persistence of viral DNA fragments in myocytes of SCD victims, even without inflammatory markers, further confounds the issue.[14]

SCD can be sporadically associated with virtually all of the less common systemic conditions that can have cardiac involvement. These include chronic granulomatous diseases, autoimmune disorders, infiltrative diseases, various cardiac tumors, and protozoan infestations. Among the granulomatous diseases, sarcoidosis is the most prominent because of the frequency of its association with SCD. The risk of SCD has been associated with ambient arrhythmias, such as nonsustained ventricular tachycardia. Cardiac amyloidosis is also associated with SCD, with a reported incidence of 30%.

Only a small proportion of SCDs in middle-aged and older adults are due to the rare genetically determined disorders, such as long QT syndrome, Brugada syndrome, HCM, and right ventricular dysplasia, or to the developmental congenital disorders, such as aortic stenosis and anomalous origins of coronary arteries. Cumulatively, these rare disorders account for no more than 1% of the total SCD burden, but the proportionate contributions of these disorders are distinctly age related. Among adolescents and young adults, these disorders (in addition to myocarditis), are dominant causes of SCD, whereas coronary heart disease and the dilated cardiomyopathies dominate beyond the age of 35 years. A transition occurs in the age range of 30 to 45 years, in which the rare disorders comingle with increasing prevalence of coronary heart disease (Fig. 99.3). Entities such as Brugada syndrome and right ventricular dysplasia, in addition to long QT syndrome with expression owing to proarrhythmic drug exposures and electrolyte disturbances, are those that are most likely to blend with the progressively increasing prevalence of coronary heart disease and nonischemic cardiomyopathies in this age range. Finally, it is becoming increasingly apparent that HCM may evolve into a more general cardiomyopathy, having features of a dilated cardiomyopathy, with advancing age. An increasing number of such cases are being recognized in later years of life, many of which had not been diagnosed earlier in life.

For the general population older than 35 years, the average mortality rate is subgrouped into pockets of higher- and lower-risk densities, based on numbers and power of risk factors. However, currently available profiling strategies do not have sufficient power to identify small groups with high-risk density that would permit meaningful individual risk prediction (Fig. 99.4).

The spectrum of patterns of clinical expression of the SCD syndrome ranges from anticipated events in high-risk patients with identified advanced heart disease to those with unrecognized or new-onset conditions in which SCD is the first clinical manifestation (Fig. 99.5). An intermediate category of patients have known heart disease but are considered to be at low risk based on extent and stability of disease. Among the highest-risk categories are subgroups characterized by low ejection fractions, with or without heart failure, following myocardial infarction or nonischemic cardiomyopathies. Various other myocardial or valvular conditions are also associated with high risk. Among these groups of patients, the probability of a potentially fatal cardiac arrest is high, but the positive and negative predictive accuracies of most methods of profiling risk for individual patients are still somewhat limited.[15] At the other end of the risk spectrum, patients with known heart disease but low-risk markers (e.g., ejection fractions greater than 40%, no heart failure, no arrhythmias) contribute a large absolute number of SCDs because of the vast number of patients that reside in this low-risk group. In addition, cardiac arrest is commonly the first clinical manifestation of the underlying disease in subjects without previously identified heart disease. Postmortem studies of cardiac arrest victims have shown that previously silent disease in such subjects is often advanced. The last two categories account for approximately two-thirds of all SCDs.

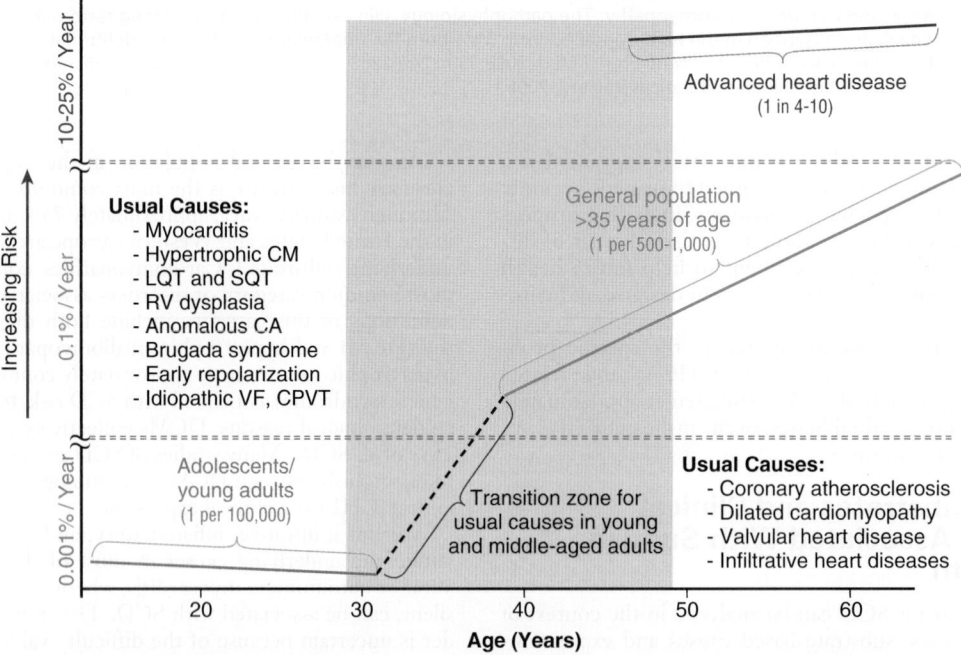

FIGURE 99.3 Age-related risk for sudden cardiac death. For the general population 35 years of age and older, the risk of sudden cardiac death is 0.1% to 0.2% per year (1 per 500 to 1,000 population), and the age-risk curve is steep (*middle curve*). For the same population, subgrouped for advanced heart disease, the latter blunts the age–risk relationship (*top curve*). Among adolescents and young adults, the risk is 1 per 100,000 population, or 0.001% per year, and the age–risk relationship is inverse (*bottom curve*), with a higher risk at the younger end of the range because of enhanced expression of inherited disorders after puberty. In the age range of 30 to 45 years, a transition occurs in both incidence and usual causes in younger adults to those in middle-aged adults and those in older adults; evaluation for causes should account for this. *CA,* Coronary artery; *CM,* cardiomyopathy; *CPVT,* catecholaminergic polymorphic ventricular tachycardia; *LQT,* long QT; *SQT,* short QT; *VF,* ventricular fibrillation. (Modified from Myerburg RJ, Castellanos A. Cardiac arrest and sudden cardiac death. In: Zipes D, Libby P, Bonow RO, Braunwald E, eds. *Heart Disease: A Textbook of Cardiovascular Medicine.* 7th ed. Philadelphia: Saunders; 2004:865-908.)

Pathological Substrates in Sudden Cardiac Death Victims

Much of the information available on the pathological anatomy in SCD victims reflects the predominance of coronary heart disease as the major underlying etiological disorder. Both the extent of coronary artery disease and the resulting abnormalities in ventricular myocardium have been well described. Extensive coronary atherosclerosis has been recognized for many years as the primary anatomical hallmark of coronary heart disease–related SCDs.[1] Also, SCD closely associates with the presence of plaque

fissuring or erosion, platelet aggregation, and acute thrombosis within the matrix of coronary atherosclerosis. This feature of coronary artery anatomy, superimposed on chronic lesions, does not differ among the three primary expressions of acute coronary syndromes—SCD, acute myocardial infarction, and unstable angina pectoris. Various studies have demonstrated the presence of one or more active coronary lesions in up to 90% of SCD victims.[16] The active plaque state and its consequences (plaque disruption with hemorrhage into the plaque or intraluminal thrombosis) are more important than simply the degree of chronic occlusion in the pathophysiology of acute coronary syndromes, apparently including SCD. Active plaques are not restricted to the apparent culprit vessel in acute coronary syndromes, including SCD. Thus a 70% to 80% obstruction without a fresh thrombus might not be the true culprit when it coexists with lesser lesions in an active state.[17] One precaution regarding postmortem studies is the apparent severity of stenosis in a vessel in the absence of the intravascular filling pressure present during life. Overestimation of the severity of stenosis has to be kept in mind.[18]

Myocardial pathology reflects the presence and extent of chronic coronary atherosclerosis, in that myocardial scars owing to healed myocardial infarction are common.[1] Clinically recognized and unrecognized scars are both associated with SCD risk, and the magnitude of risk associated with each appears equivalent, based on a recent cardiac magnetic resonance imaging study.[19] This observation has implications for potential screening techniques for victims in the category of SCDs that are first clinical events. Evidence of acute myocardial infarction is far less common, probably because the pathophysiological mechanism leading to the anatomical and histopathological expression is interrupted by the fatal arrhythmia. However, even among cardiac arrest survivors studied during the prethrombolytic or percutaneous coronary intervention era, evolution to acute transmural myocardial infarction was less common. An association between the number of involved coronary arteries and the extent of ventricular hypertrophy in SCD victims has also been recognized. A correlation between extensive coronary artery disease and left ventricular hypertrophy might be a consequence of long-standing hypertension as a risk factor in coronary heart disease patients or of postmyocardial infarction remodeling. Regardless

99

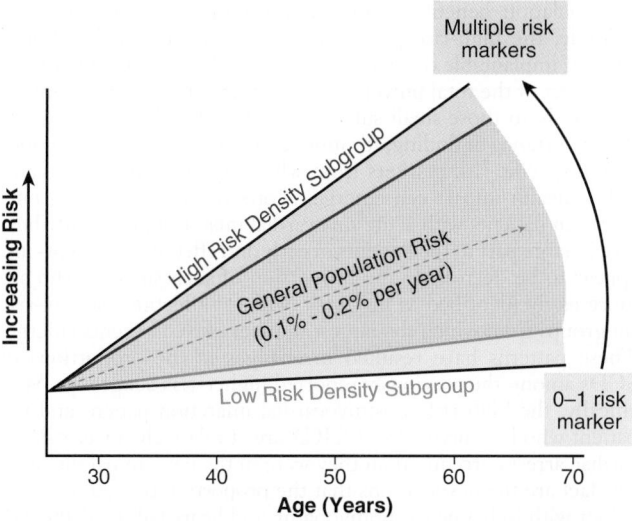

FIGURE 99.4 Stratified risk density curves for the general population older than 35 years of age. The commonly cited average risk in the range of one to two SCDs per 1000 patient years reflects the cumulative effects of higher- and lower-risk strata. Identification of the discriminating risk factors would allow for more accurate risk profiling for individual patients within the general population, but current markers of risk do not have sufficient power to yield effect sizes sufficient to significantly improve individual risk prediction. (From Myerburg RJ, Junttila MJ. Sudden cardiac death caused by coronary heart disease. *Circulation.* 2012;125:1043-1052.)

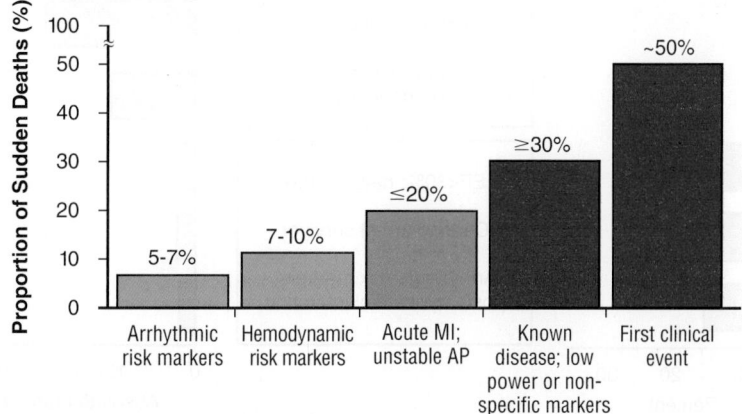

FIGURE 99.5 Clinical status of sudden cardiac death victims. Effectively predicting cardiac arrest among a high percentage of potential victims is difficult because approximately 80% of cardiac arrests occur as the first clinically manifested events (50%) or in the clinical setting of known disease in the absence of strong risk predictors. Less than 20% of the victims have high-risk markers based on arrhythmic or hemodynamic parameters. Persons at high risk constitute a proportionately smaller segment of the population base. The total exceeds 100% because of overlap between the first event and low-risk categories within the acute coronary syndrome group. *AP,* Angina pectoris; *MI,* myocardial infarction. (Modified and updated from Myerburg RJ. Sudden cardiac death: exploring the limits of our knowledge. *J Cardiovasc Electrophysiol.* 2001;12:369-381.)

of the mechanism, myocardial scars and left ventricular hypertrophy are considered factors in arrhythmogenesis during transient ischemia.[1,7]

Among the less common structural causes of SCD, pathological anatomy reflects the underlying etiology. In DCMs, the pathological findings are nonspecific and are characterized by interstitial fibrosis and myocyte degeneration. In HCMs, the anatomy depends on the specific form of the disease. Obstructive, nonobstructive, apical, and concentric hypertrophy patterns are all observed. Although risk is increased in all forms of HCM, it is greater in the obstructive pattern and the least in the apical HCM subgroup. One common feature observed in HCM is myocyte disarray, which is common to most, but not all, genetic forms of the disease. The association between HCM expression and SCD risk is complex because of patterns of inheritance involving multiple gene loci and variable expression. Because of the large number of candidate genes for HCM and the high proportion of family-specific variants, the challenge of interpreting findings of previously unreported variants of uncertain significance is a particular problem in HCM.

Prediction and Strategies for Prevention of Sudden Cardiac Death

The landscape of SCD risk prediction is complex. Risk analysis should be divided into two general categories: population-based risk prediction and individual risk prediction. Conventional epidemiological markers provide insight into probabilities for the development of coronary heart disease within a general class of subjects, but the limitations of individual risk prediction constrict the ability to profile risk and apply preventive strategies to the specific individual in the clinical setting. The inverse relationship between the incidence of SCD and absolute numbers of events in the various epidemiological or clinical categories is important (Fig. 99.6), especially when the intent is to use therapeutic interventions.[20] Among the general population aged 35 years and older, the estimated SCD incidence of 0.1% to 0.2% per year incorporates all the sudden deaths that occur annually in the United States. However, the low individual event rate among the general population, unselected except for age, limits the range of applicable therapeutic approaches. If patients who fall into categories of high risk for development of coronary atherosclerosis and unselected patients with established coronary heart disease are included, event rates are higher but still have limited power for specific individual risk prediction. In contrast, patients with heart failure or ejection fractions less than 35%, cardiac arrest survivors, and the specific high-risk post–myocardial infarction patients have higher event rates, but constitute decreasing absolute numbers of events and a much smaller component of the total population burden of SCD.[7] The importance of recognizing this principle relates to the magnitude of population benefit for various preventive interventions. For example, the high-risk patient categories studied in the clinical trials of implantable defibrillators (see Fig. 99.6) constitute only a small part of the total universe of SCDs, and the reported benefits apply only to those small subgroups. This observation highlights the importance of finding, for more general segments of the population, specific risk markers from which the potential for greater public health impact can emerge. Moreover, the improving outcomes in patients with acute myocardial infarction, likely attributable in large part to the benefits of early and effective interventions, appear to be decreasing the proportion of such subjects who are more easily identified as high risk, without affecting the low-risk subgroups from which the largest number of SCD events emerge. These patterns have resulted in changes in the proportions of SCDs among the previously reported higher-risk subgroups. Specifically, the high-risk, postmyocardial infarction patient and the patient who has survived an OHCA are at relatively lower risk for cardiac arrest currently than they were in the past. In parallel with this fact are the observations that the proportion of victims in the subset with ischemic cardiomyopathy and heart failure as the risk basis for SCD has increased (see Fig. 99.6). In addition, in long-term studies, a pattern suggests that a prior history of heart disease is becoming less common among victims of OHCA, while a history of risk factors is increasing.[21]

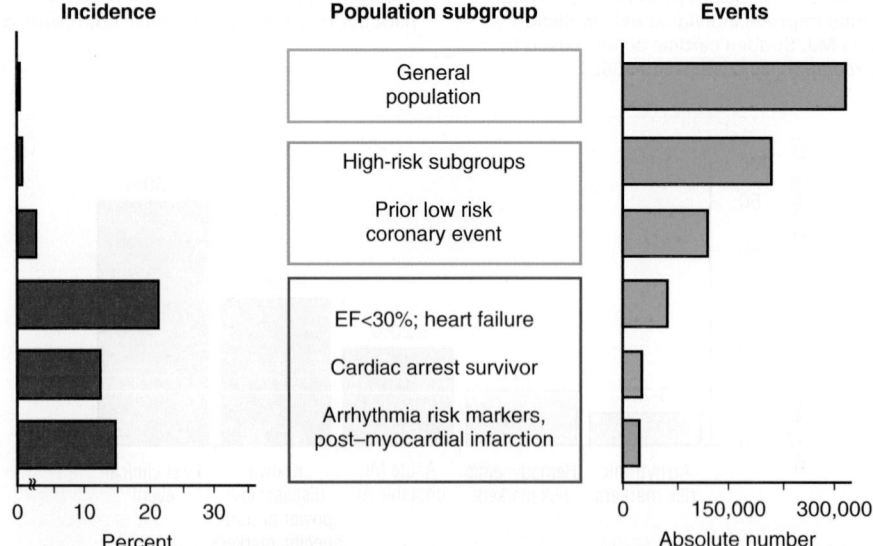

FIGURE 99.6 Relationship among population subsets, incidence of sudden cardiac death, and total population burden for each group. With increasing incidence, based on subgroup profiling, a decrease in proportion of the total sudden death burden is seen. This effect relates to the population impact of known evidence-based outcomes of various prevention therapies, and it highlights the challenge of the low-risk, high-numbers subsets. The incidence statistics cited in the original versions of this descriptor have changed over time because of changes in medical care. (Modified from Myerburg RJ, Junttila MJ. Sudden cardiac death caused by coronary heart disease. *Circulation.* 2012;125:1043-1052; and Myerburg RJ, Interian A Jr, Mitrani RM, et al. Frequency of sudden cardiac death and profiles of risk. *Am J Cardiol.* 1997;80:10F-19F.)

The foregoing concepts can be viewed in the context of clinical patterns preceding cardiac arrest in patients with coronary heart disease. A number of studies suggest that up to 50% of all OHCAs and consequent SCDs resulting from coronary heart disease occur as the first clinical event and that up to 30% more are associated with clinical markers suggesting a low risk for an event (see Fig. 99.5). A major effect on the population burden of SCD will require the development of strategies to identify very high-risk subgroups among small clusters in the general population.

Magnitude of risk of SCD is a complex epidemiological and clinical function, even within subgrouped categories of risk (see Fig. 99.3). Among the adult population, increasing age is a powerful risk predictor that becomes blunted in the presence of advanced heart disease, when it is overwhelmed by higher-risk clinical factors. The general population can be viewed as composed of a gradient of risk, depending on the number of risk factors present (see Fig. 99.4). However, the risk gradient based on current methods is still insufficient, and it is anticipated that pockets of increased risk density will eventually be identifiable with better profiling methods.[8,22]

Prediction of Risk of Sudden Cardiac Death in Coronary Heart Disease

The evolution and expression of SCD resulting from coronary heart disease involve a multitiered cascade of pathophysiology operating in different time domains[8,16] (see Fig. 99.6). This cascade includes the elements of initiation and progression of disease in the coronary arteries, development of myocardial scarring/fibrosis, transition of vascular lesions from quiescent to active states, initiation of acute coronary syndromes, and, finally, acute arrhythmogenesis. In the early years of attention to the epidemiology of SCD, the conventional risk factors for coronary artery disease were the major focus of SCD risk prediction (Table 99.1; see also Fig. 99.6). From a statistical and public health standpoint, this approach remains reasonable because of the large proportion and numbers of SCDs that are attributable to coronary artery disease.

This concept is limited, however, by the fact that these risk factors largely predict the evolution of the substrate-based risk over time and identify orders of magnitude of risk that are too low for specific drug or device antiarrhythmic interventions. Furthermore, these risk factors do not provide a specific marker of risk for arrhythmic deaths. Other methods for identifying the presence of structural abnormalities in coronary arteries have been suggested as potential strategies to provide greater sensitivity

and specificity (see Table 99.1). For example, anatomical disease screening using calcium scoring and coronary computed tomographic angiography have been suggested as methods for large-scale screening to identify abnormal coronary arteries. Although this technology identifies structural changes in coronary arteries with an acceptable degree of accuracy, its value is limited by the fact that identification of the structural abnormality does not reveal the vulnerability of plaques or specific markers of arrhythmic risk. Repeated exposure to radiation over time is also considered a limitation of this as a screening approach.

Much of the progress that has been made to date in profiling risk of SCD has been based on clinical markers, which primarily identify the extent of disease either at a myocardial or a vascular level (see Table 99.1). Ischemic cardiomyopathy identifies high risk for SCD, which is particularly notable when accompanied by a history of clinical heart failure. The use of LV ejection fraction as the primary indicator of risk is regarded as less specific than previously thought. Other indicators, such as myocardial scarring revealed by cardiac magnetic resonance (CMR) imaging and left ventricular volumes, are emerging as markers of potential interest.

To achieve better profiling of arrhythmic risk, two approaches appear promising for application in future studies. One approach is prediction of transient risk, which is intended to identify patients who are at risk for the events that trigger fatal arrhythmias in a shorter time frame[8,20,23] (see Table 99.1). Pathophysiological elements that may contribute to transient risk include control mechanisms mediated through autonomic nervous system functions (such as heart rate variability or baroreceptor sensitivity), measures of repolarization alterations (such as T-wave alternans), and inflammatory markers that are being evaluated as a predictor of risk for plaque destabilization.[22] Whereas the inflammatory markers for plaque disruption can generally provide higher resolution of risk for acute coronary syndromes,[24,25] individual risk predictors, such as familial or genetic profiling, can potentially provide even greater resolution for SCD risk in specific persons. Because of the general principle of variable expression of many genetic risk markers, any likely future model for individual risk prediction incorporating genetic markers will have to be integrated with other methods of risk profiling, based on population or individual clinical factors.[8,26]

The ability to identify the individual patient at risk for plaque disruption, in advance of an acute coronary syndrome, could provide a powerful method for identifying individuals at potential risk of SCD. In retrospective studies of men[27] and women[28] in whom both cholesterol levels and indices of

TABLE 99.1 Indicators of risk for arrhythmic sudden cardiac death (SCD)

TARGET	EXAMPLES	GOAL	SENSITIVITY
ASHD risk factors	Framingham risk index	Predict evolution of disease	Very low
Anatomical screening	Calcium scoring; CT angiography	Identify CAD	Very low
Clinical markers	EF; angiography; AM; EPS	Define extent of disease	Variable with extent of disease; low specificity
	AM/EPS combined with EF	Identify arrhythmia markers	Low to intermediate for screening
		Define high-risk subgroups	High for specific groups
			Primary predictive value unknown
Transient risk predictors	T-wave alternans; QT dispersion	Identify ECG markers of risk	Unknown, potentially high
	Pathophysiological controls (e.g., HRV, BRS)	Quantify autonomic regulation	
	Inflammatory markers	Predict unstable plaques	
Individual risk predictors	Familial/genetic profiles	Predict specific SCD risk before disease expression	High potential for future profiling
			Uncertain at present; some measures useful (?)

The conventional risk factors and anatomical disease screening have some general use for predicting risk, but sensitivity is very low and nonspecific for arrhythmic deaths. Transient risk predictors and individual risk predictors offer the hope for more powerful individual prediction of SCD.
AM, ambulatory monitor; *ASHD*, arteriosclerotic heart disease; *BRS*, baroreflex sensitivity; *CAD*, coronary artery disease; *ECG*, electrocardiogram; *EF*, ejection fraction; *EPS*, electrophysiological studies; *HRV*, heart rate variability; *QT*, QT interval
From Myerburg RJ. Sudden cardiac death: exploring the limits of our knowledge. *J Cardiovasc Electrophysiol.* 2001:12:369-381.

inflammation could be correlated with risk of coronary events, each risk factor appeared to provide an independent predictive value and this combination had the strongest power of prediction of relative risk increase. However, because the outcomes were expressed as relative increases of a baseline risk among the subjects in the lowest tertiles of cholesterol and inflammatory marker concentration, the absolute contribution of inflammatory markers compared with cholesterol markers remains to be determined. A recent observation demonstrating that complex plaques are multiple suggests a generalized or systemic susceptibility to plaque disruption (rather than plaque-specific risk) and a higher recurrent event rate after myocardial infarction.[17] This observation supports the notion of inflammation-based susceptibility. Other direct and indirect markers of the risk of plaque destabilization from inflammatory processes could also contribute to this theory of risk prediction.

Sudden Cardiac Death Risk in Nonischemic Dilated Cardiomyopathy

Sudden cardiac death is more difficult to predict among patients with nonischemic cardiomyopathies, including those with familial dilated cardiomyopathies.[29] Although LV ejection fraction is a general risk predictor among patients who have DCM, a better association with functional capacity has been proposed.[30] For example, among patients with DCM who are functional class I, the risk of dying is low, but the proportional probability that a death will be sudden is relatively high. As this category encompasses a large number of patients at relatively low risk, the predictive power for benefit from interventions is limited. At the other end of the spectrum, functional class III and class IV patients are at a higher risk of death generally and at a higher risk for SCD in terms of absolute numbers of deaths,[30] although the proportional risk of SCD is lower. Moreover, among patients in this category who experience OHCA, many have nonshockable rhythms, and some shockable rhythms are secondary to the hemodynamic state and are resistant to defibrillation, possibly limiting the practical benefit of implantable cardioverter defibrillators (ICDs) in this group as well.

For this etiological category of SCD, discriminators of risk across the entire spectrum of disease expression, from early to advanced, are inconsistent. The importance of this limitation resides in the fact that the absolute number of SCDs counted among the relatively low-risk subgroups, which do not justify advanced interventions on a statistical basis, is disturbingly high. Future research must focus on discrimination of risk within the larger lower-risk population subsets,[31] as well as SCDs that occur in the familial forms of DCM.[29]

Cardiac Arrest Mechanisms: Tachyarrhythmic, Pulseless Electrical Activity, and Asystole

Ventricular tachyarrhythmias, including ventricular fibrillation and pulseless ventricular tachycardia, are no longer the most common electrophysiological mechanisms of cardiac arrest leading to SCD.[32] Estimates for the proportions of tachyarrhythmic and nontachyarrhythmic mechanisms in the out-of-hospital environment vary according to specific sites (e.g., home versus public sites),[33] but the overall statistics suggest that initial ventricular fibrillation or pulseless ventricular tachycardia account for 25% and 50%, respectively.[32,34,35] The proportion is somewhat higher in public sites and lower in the home environment. In addition, there are data suggesting that ICD therapy has contributed to a portion of the decline of ventricular tachycardia and ventricular fibrillation–associated SCDs.[36] Nontachyarrhythmic mechanisms include pulseless electrical activity (PEA), asystole, and bradycardia severe enough to result in loss of adequate cerebral and other organ perfusion. The proportions of these mechanisms are in the range of 50% for asystole and 25% for PEA.[32–35]

The distinction between tachyarrhythmic mechanisms and the other (nonshockable) mechanisms is important both clinically and epidemiologically. The probability that an event will be tachyarrhythmic has an effect on the potential value of antitachycardia strategies, such as ICDs and automated external defibrillators. Moreover, survival statistics are far more encouraging for tachyarrhythmic events in all clinical settings (i.e., both IHCA and OHCA). However, outcomes after asystolic arrest and PEA vary according to specific clinical circumstances. The worst outcomes occur with PEA or asystole following defibrillation (i.e., secondary PEA–asystole), and the best outcomes occur among those with PEA or asystole associated with noncardiac causes, such as acute respiratory insufficiency and acute severe volume loss. There is new evidence suggesting that longer durations of life support efforts provide better outcomes in nontachyarrhythmic events than previously thought.[37]

Defining the initial rhythm can be difficult because of spontaneous changes between ventricular fibrillation/ventricular tachycardia and the nontachyarrhythmic mechanisms. This difficulty can confound attempts to correlate primary electrophysiological mechanisms with outcome. For example, the time between onset of a ventricular tachyarrhythmia and deterioration to asystole or PEA can be brief, limiting the potential benefit of interventions. Conversely, an initial bradyarrhythmic event can change to ventricular fibrillation/ventricular tachycardia with or without therapy, and this circumstance appears to reduce the probability of successful defibrillation.[38] Finally, data from emergency rescue responses to OHCA can be misleading in regard to initial mechanisms. Higher proportions of asystole and PEA at initial contact could reflect delayed 911 calls by witnesses, and shortening such delays could yield higher proportions of victims found in ventricular tachycardia at initial contact. Even among IHCA patients, a differential survival benefit has been reported for early defibrillation, defined as occurring at 2 minutes or less after onset of the arrhythmia, compared with delayed defibrillation, defined as occurring beyond 2 minutes (39% versus 22%).[39]

Inherited Basis of Sudden Cardiac Death Risk in Adults

Familial clustering of SCD risk has been observed across the entire list of causative diseases and the spectrum of age, ranging from infancy through late adulthood. Across the age range, there is a transition from direct causation by inherited disorders that directly affect arrhythmogenesis to indirect influences of genetic variants that influence how diseases present. Regarding SCD as the initial manifestation of coronary heart disease, two population-based studies[40,41] and two clinical and pathological studies[42,43] suggest that SCD is a patient-specific response to acute coronary syndromes. Each of these studies demonstrated a pattern of familial clustering of SCD, with an excess risk of cardiac arrest as the initial manifestation of an acute coronary syndrome when a family history was positive for SCD in one parent, and an even higher risk when both sides of the family were affected.[41,42] Although familial clustering could be environmental in part, as hinted in a study suggesting exogenous/endogenous effects on QTc interval patterns,[44] ongoing studies are seeking mutations or polymorphisms that can predispose an individual to abnormal electrophysiological function in the presence of acute ischemia, even if the affected person is phenotypically normal at baseline. Support has been emerging for the general concept of genetic variations that do not affect the baseline phenotype but are associated with expression of effects during a transient event.[45]

BOX 99.1 Epidemiological paradigms for population and individual risk prediction of sudden cardiac death

Conventional Epidemiology
- Population risk and primary prevention (e.g., atherogenesis)
- Secondary and tertiary prevention

Transient Risk Prediction
- Acute coronary syndrome, hemodynamic changes, electrical instability, autonomic predictors

Interventional Epidemiology
- Predictors derived from clinical trials
- Long-term surveillance observations for safety

Genetic Epidemiology
- Individual (personalized) risk
- Prediction of specific expression

BOX 99.2 Genetic epidemiology of risk for sudden cardiac death (SCD)

Genetically Based Primary Arrhythmia Disorders
- Congenital long QT syndrome
- Brugada syndrome
- Idiopathic (catecholaminergic) ventricular tachycardia–fibrillation

Inherited Structural Disorders With Risk of Arrhythmic SCD
- Hypertrophic cardiomyopathy
- Right ventricular dysplasia/cardiomyopathy

Genetic Predisposition to Drug- and Electrolyte-Induced Arrhythmias and SCD
- Acquired long QT syndrome

Genetic Modulation of Complex Acquired Diseases
- Coronary artery disease, acute coronary syndromes
- Congestive heart failure, dilated cardiomyopathies

Epidemiological Paradigms for Sudden Cardiac Death Prediction

Limited ability to identify individuals at risk of SCD from among the general population is a major reason why SCD remains an important public health burden. Variations in definitions of SCD, pathophysiological mechanisms, and outcomes from cardiac arrest in various sites (OHCA versus IHCA; home versus public sites), all result in persisting questions about the balance between population-attributable risk and individual risk prediction. Inconsistency in access to data is another major limitation that may be addressed by national reporting policies for uniform reporting of cardiac arrest.[7] To further address these limitations, conventional epidemiological concepts must be supplemented by the integration of new epidemiological paradigms (Box 99.1), including the emerging fields of transient risk markers and genetic epidemiology (Box 99.2), and by interventional epidemiology, which is a term coined to define the population dynamics of clinical trial design and outcomes.

The most prominent paradigm shift has occurred in perceptions of the epidemiology of coronary heart disease. The conventional model describes a cascade progressing sequentially from coronary atherogenesis to plaque destabilization to initiation of acute coronary syndromes and, finally, to triggering of fatal arrhythmias (Fig. 99.7). These elements can be viewed as modules, each containing defined pathophysiological pathways that interact with one another. Furthermore, each pathway appears to be under unique genetic controls. Genetic factors in atherogenesis, plaque destabilization, and the thrombotic cascade, added to the genetics of ion channel function, potentially have definable effects on individual risks and responses to pathophysiological states.[8] The notion that a few common genetic variants would have the power to predict SCD with some degree of sensitivity and accuracy came and went quickly. Although variants influencing molecular electrophysiology might make significant contributions to risk profiling, the remainder of the cascade depends on major interactions with conventional risk factors, such as diabetes mellitus, hypertension, cigarette smoking, and hyperlipidemias. Genetic markers for these basic risk factors are evolving, but the genetic contribution to lesion initiation, progression, and transition from stable to active states is not yet clear.

As an expanded epidemiological approach evolves, it will initiate a conceptual transformation of the sequential pathophysiological cascade (see Fig. 99.7) into a complex system analysis model.[46] The need for this approach derives from the fundamentally limited ability of conventional risk factors to identify specific persons at high risk for SCD (or other manifestations of coronary

artery disease) from among the general population. Because a majority of SCDs occur in people without easily identifiable high absolute risks for cardiovascular or total mortality (see Fig. 99.6) and because risk is multifactorial (see Fig. 99.7), more precise predictors of single-patient probabilities of risk of coronary heart disease generally, and of SCD in particular, must be sought. This information will have to come from mathematical analyses of the interactions between multiple risk factors or from complex system analysis.

Despite impressive relative risks identified by some single markers, small effect sizes result in limited power for individual risk prediction. In parallel, the relative benefits of some interventions targeting specific risk factors studied in controlled interventions are impressive for select groups of patients, but they provide limited predictive power for absolute risk reduction in individual patients. The study groups from most of the primary prevention clinical trials, such as the 3-hydroxy-3-methylglutaryl–coenzyme A reductase (i.e., statin) trials for cholesterol lowering, and from studies of the prophylactic use of aspirin, are instructive of these limitations. When the absolute mortality outcomes among the aspirin- or statin-treated and control groups in primary prevention studies are analyzed, the absolute reduction in mortality risk for persons in the treatment groups is modest. The reported outcomes of such studies emphasize group effect (relative risk reduction) rather than individual effect (absolute benefit).[20] Among three major primary prevention statin trials,[47] total mortality rates fell over 5 years from 3.7% to 2.8%, indicating a 5-year reduction of approximately 0.9%. Cardiovascular mortality benefit was 0.5% over 5 years. These figures derive from the fact that the absolute mortality risk in the placebo groups is relatively low (3.7% over 5 years, or 0.72% per year), even though the beneficial effect in a relative sense is impressively high. However, because of the absolute magnitude of the numerators and denominators in these lower-risk groups, the potential benefit of identifying persons at risk with a higher degree of precision is very large. These studies were not powered to identify SCD benefit. In order to do so, the epidemiological mission becomes much more complex, but the potential yield in clinical and economic terms is huge.[48]

When viewed from the perspective of a complex system containing voluminous bioinformation, both the difficulty and the opportunity become evident. Genetic, environmental, and acquired pathophysiological states can all have roles. The value of genetically based analysis of risk is the fact that it has the potential to provide predetermined predictors in advance of

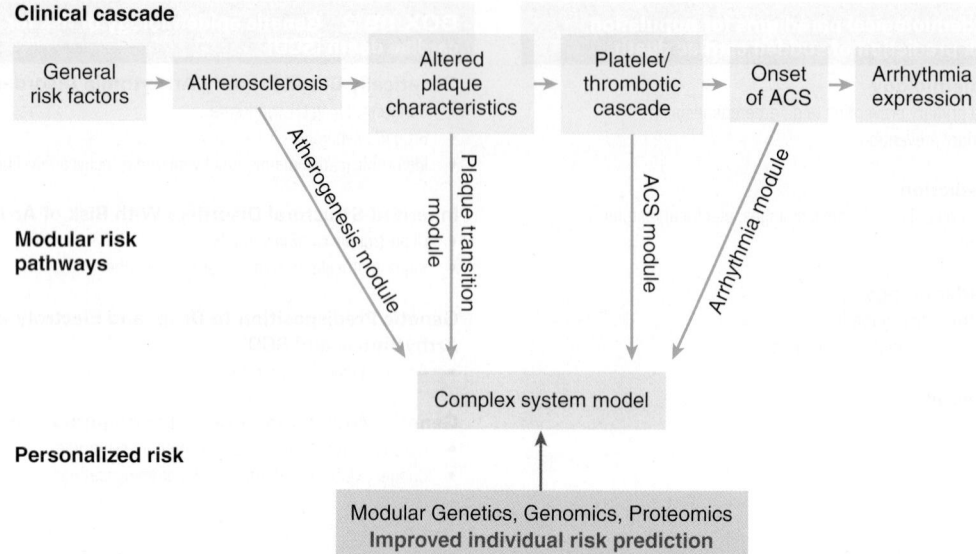

FIGURE 99.7 Genetic imprints on the coronary heart disease–sudden cardiac death cascade. Genetic influences have been identified for multiple inheritance modules along the cascade from general risk factors for atherosclerosis to arrhythmic expression leading to sudden cardiac death. Individual risk based on genetic profiles has been identified for atherogenesis, plaque evolution, the thrombotic cascade, and arrhythmia expression, but few of the markers identified thus far have sufficient individual predictive power to be clinically useful. Genomic and proteomic strategies can lead to stepwise integration of these modules through complex analytic methods, permitting better individual applications. Ultimately, treatment of these concepts as a biological system may offer even greater power to the field of genetic epidemiology, leading to higher-order single-patient probabilities for predicting sudden cardiac death. *ACS,* Acute coronary syndrome. (Modified from Myerburg RJ, Junttila MJ. Sudden cardiac death caused by coronary heart disease. *Circulation.* 2012;125:1043-1052.)

clinical events. Acquired characteristics may be more difficult to identify with sufficient lead-time for practical interventions.

The components of a complex biological system leading to genetic and genomic epidemiological models include polymorphisms or mutations along multiple steps of the clinical expression cascade, which together can provide information that can enhance the power of risk prediction (see Fig. 99.7). First on the list of complexities is the study of interactions among genes, which can be directly related, functionally related, or integrated with remotely related functions. The genes that control ion channel pore structure (e.g., *KCNQ1, KCNH2,* and *SCN5A*) and those that control their associated modulating peptides (e.g., *KCNE1, KCNE2,* and *SCN1B*) provide examples of direct relationships.[31] Interactions between the expression of ion channel gene variants and genes that modulate or modify calcium handling are examples of indirect but related interactions between products of multiple genes. Identified mutations of the latter (e.g., *RYR2* and *CASQ2*) are associated with arrhythmias. In addition, KcLQT-1/MinK can interact with *RYR2* or *CASQ2* variations, resulting in an association between control of repolarization and calcium handling, a relationship suggested as a mechanism for arrhythmogenesis. Finally, a genetically determined influence on β-adrenergic receptor function,[49] interacting with the ion channel–calcium handling complex,[50] is an example of a remote but integrated gene–gene relationship. A second component in the complex system for control of ion channel function is the interaction between genetic influences and pathophysiological functions. Examples include the relationships between genetic channelopathies and β-adrenergic control or between benign polymorphisms and transient pathophysiological modifiers.[31] The interaction between outcomes in a large LQT kindred with a potentially genetically controlled autonomic interaction at the myocyte level[51] is another conceptual level of the effects of genetic modification.[26]

The third, and most challenging, component in the system leading to genetic and genomic epidemiological models is the construct of the pathophysiological cascade itself, leading from atherogenesis to plaque characteristics to the thrombotic cascade and then to specific arrhythmic expression. Within each module of the cascade reside evolving clusters of information on genetic influences, potentially contributing to risk prediction. These features offer the opportunity for the cascade to evolve into a complex system for simultaneous interactive analysis of multiple gene influences, rather than a sequence of independent variables. Complex system analyses can then be used to integrate genetics into epidemiology, providing a stepwise amplification of risk prediction based on individual probability profiles. Within each element in the cascade—atherogenesis risk undergoing transition to risk for an active plaque state, followed by genetic properties of the thrombotic cascade, and finally triggering of arrhythmias—genetic influences feed into an integrated pool of characteristics that determine individual probabilities.

Higher-order or personalized single-patient probabilities (for example, 1 in 10 versus 1 in 1000 annual risk), derived from the integration of properties at multiple levels of pathophysiology, will complement the power of risk expression for specific components of the SCD cascade. The ultimate goal is to profile individual risk at multiple steps in the SCD cascade, generating probability figures that are powerful enough to be useful for preventive strategies far in advance of clinical events.

Interventional Epidemiology of Sudden Cardiac Death Risk

The outcomes of randomized clinical trials and observational interventional studies and the results of epidemiological surveys all contribute to the development of strategies for the management of risk for SCD.[8] However, the application of the knowledge gained from each of these data sources differs in regard to

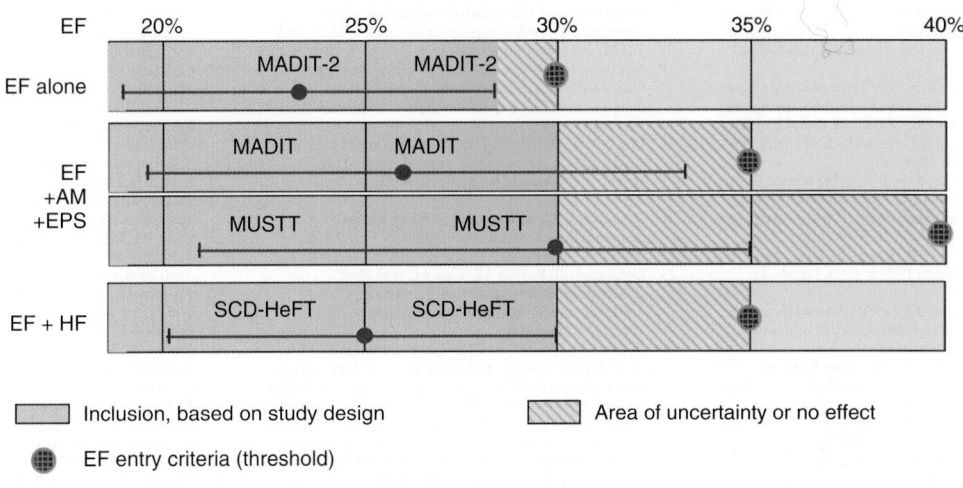

PRIMARY PREVENTION ICD TRIALS
Entry Criteria versus Enrollment

| | Inclusion, based on study design | | Area of uncertainty or no effect |

EF entry criteria (threshold)

EF of enrolled subjects (means ± SD [MADIT, MADIT-2] or median and 25th, 75th percentile [MUSTT, SCD-HeFT])

FIGURE 99.8 Evidence-based indications for implantable cardioverter defibrillator (ICD) after surviving myocardial infarction. Each of these four primary prevention trials had a qualifying ejection fraction (*EF*) cutoff (*green circle*) above which patients were not randomized (*gray box*). The EFs of enrolled patients create uncertainties for subgroups within the study populations, despite overall benefits of ICD therapy in the studies. In each study, the EF subgroup that dominated enrollment (*shown with red dots and bars*; mean ± SD [*MADIT, MADIT-2*] or median and 25th, 75th percentile [*MUSTT, SCD-HeFT*]) achieved a clear benefit from ICD therapy, whereas those that extended back to the upper limit of entry criterion for EF (*blue cross-hatched boxes*) were underrepresented, achieved no benefit, or were indeterminate. *AM,* Ambulatory monitor; *EPS,* electrophysiological study; *HF,* heart failure. (From Myerburg RJ. Implantable cardioverter-defibrillators after myocardial infarction. *N Engl J Med.* 2008;359:2245-2253, with permission of the publisher. Copyright Massachusetts Medical Society, 2008.)

population effects and individual clinical effects. For example, mining of existing databases can identify risk factors or strong associations. Observations generally are expressed in terms of relative risk statements, which can be derived from low absolute event rates. Low event rates with large relative differences identify effects, but usually with limited individual patient impact. In contrast, randomized clinical trials with large absolute differences in outcome are better able to define individual patient benefits. Observational studies are often limited by their dependence on data compared with historical controls or the absence of control groups.

SCD in an unselected adult population includes victims whose cardiac arrests occur as a first cardiac event, as well as those whose events can be predicted with greater accuracy because they are included in higher-risk subgroups. Based on a cumulative incidence of 1 to 2 per 1000 population (0.1% to 0.2%) per year in the United States (see Fig. 99.6), any intervention designed for the general population must be applied to the 999 in 1000 persons who will not have an event, in order to reach and possibly influence the 1 in 1000 who will have an event. Cost- and risk-benefit uncertainties limit the nature of broad-based interventions and demand a higher resolution of risk identification. With each group-specific escalation of risk, the probability of an event increases, whereas the corresponding absolute number of deaths becomes progressively smaller,[1] limiting the population effect of interventions in high-risk subgroups yet magnifying the individual benefit.

All studies of group outcomes of therapy for complex pathophysiological states must consider four factors: (1) relative risk reduction, (2) absolute risk reduction, (3) residual risk, and (4) cumulative benefits of multiple interventions. The primary endpoint reports for all clinical trials of ICD therapy, and for most

other large clinical trials, focus largely on reduction in relative risk[20] because this measure identifies the effect of the intervention. Relative risk reduction, however, does not quantify the benefit for the individual patient. To do so, a measure of absolute risk reduction is required, such as the number of patients that need to be treated in order to save a life or the absolute numerical difference in risk observed in the test and control groups.

Residual risk and cumulative benefit are other measures of group effects that do not commonly receive attention. *Residual risk,* referring to the absolute outcome among the treated group or test group in a clinical trial population, identifies the component of total mortality risk that does not respond to the tested therapy. If residual risk is high, the absolute and relative risk reduction benefits are correspondingly limited. *Cumulative benefit* refers to the increment in benefit from integration of multiple interventions; despite its importance,[20,52] this is rarely stratified in clinical trial designs because it requires larger study populations, and it has not been used prospectively in any of the ICD or antiarrhythmic trials. Post hoc subgroup analysis can be used to suggest added benefit of a secondary strategy, but this does not replace stratifying the multiple interventions.

A final consideration in the epidemiology of interventions is the comparison of entry criteria against actual enrollment (Fig. 99.8). In many of the ICD trials, the ranges of ejection fractions and functional classifications were unintentionally biased toward certain values, thereby limiting the interpretation and proper application of the outcomes. Ejection fraction entry criteria were largely in the range of 30% to 40% or less, but individuals with ejection fraction in the lower ranges dominated enrollment.[15] Therefore the benefit to patients with ejection fraction values at the higher end of the range is not clear.

REFERENCES

1. Myerburg RJ, Castellanos A. Cardiac arrest and sudden cardiac death. In: Bonow RO, Mann DL, Zipes DP, et al, eds. *Braunwald's Heart Disease: A Textbook of Cardiovascular Medicine.* 9th ed. Oxford, UK: Elsevier; 2012:845–884. [chapter 41].

2. American Heart Association. *2001 Heart and Stroke Statistical Update.* Dallas, TX: American Heart Association; 2000.

3. Cobb LA, Fahrenbruch CE, Olsufka M, et al. Changing incidence of out-of-hospital ventricular fibrillation, 1980-2000. *JAMA.* 2002;288:3008–3013.

4. Chugh SS, Jui J, Gunson K, et al. Current burden of sudden cardiac death: multiple source surveillance versus retrospective death certificate–based review in a large U.S. community. *J Am Coll Cardiol.* 2004;44:1268–1275.

5. Zheng ZJ, Croft JB, Giles WH, et al. Sudden cardiac death in the United States, 1989 to 1998. *Circulation.* 2001;104:2158–2163.

6. Mozaffarian D, Benjamin EJ, Go AS, Arnett DK, et al. on behalf of the American Heart Association Statistics Committee and Stroke Statistics Subcommittee. AHA Statistical Update: Heart Disease and Stroke Statistics—2016 Update: A Report From the American Heart Association. *Circulation.* 2016;133:e38–60.

7. IOM (Institute of Medicine) Committee on the Treatment of Cardiac Arrest. *Current Status and Future Directions: Strategies to Improve Cardiac Arrest Survival: A Time to Act.* Washington, DC: The National Academies Press; 2015.

8. Myerburg RJ, Junttila MJ. Sudden cardiac death caused by coronary heart disease. *Circulation.* 2012;125:1043–1052.

9. Gerber Y, Jacobsen SJ, Frye RL, et al. Secular trends in deaths from cardiovascular diseases: a 25-year community study. *Circulation.* 2006;113:2285–2292.

10. Dudas K, Lappas G, Stewart S, et al. Trends in out-of-hospital deaths due to coronary heart disease in Sweden (1991 to 2006). *Circulation.* 2011;123:46–52.

11. Kong MH, Fonarow GC, Peterson ED, et al. Systematic review of the incidence of sudden cardiac death in the United States. *J Am Coll Cardiol.* 2011;57:794–801.

12. Girotra S, Nallamothu BK, Spertus JA, Li Y, Krumholz HM, Chan PS. For the American Heart Association Get with the Guidelines–Resuscitation Investigators. Trends in survival after in-hospital cardiac arrest. *N Engl J Med.* 2012;367:1912–1920.

13. Wisten A, Forsberg H, Krantz P, et al. Sudden cardiac death in 15–35-year olds in Sweden during 1992–99. *J Intern Med.* 2002;252:529–536.

14. Pauschinger M, Bowles NE, Fuentes-Garcia FJ, et al. Detection of adenoviral genome in the myocardium of adult patients with idiopathic left ventricular dysfunction. *Circulation.* 1999;99:1348–1354.

15. Myerburg RJ. Implantable cardioverter-defibrillators after myocardial infarction. *New Engl J Med.* 2008;359:2245–2253.

16. Mehta D, Curwin J, Gomes A, et al. Sudden death in coronary artery disease: acute ischemia versus myocardial substrate. *Circulation.* 1997;96:3215–3223.

17. Goldstein JA, Demetriou D, Grines CL, et al. Multiple complex coronary plaques in patients with acute myocardial infarction. *N Engl J Med.* 2000;343:915–922.

18. Mann JM, Davies MJ. Assessment of the severity of coronary artery disease at postmortem examination. Are the measurements clinically valid? *Br Heart J.* 1995;74:528–530.

19. Schelbert EB, Cao JJ, Sigurdsson S, et al. Prevalence and prognosis of unrecognized myocardial infarction determined by cardiac magnetic resonance in older adults. *JAMA.* 2012;308:890–896.

20. Myerburg RJ, Mitrani R, Interian A, et al. Interpretation of outcomes of antiarrhythmic clinical trials: design features and population impact. *Circulation.* 1998;97:1514–1521.

21. Wong MK, Morrison LJ, Qiu F, et al. Trends in short- and long-term survival among out-of-hospital cardiac arrest patients alive at hospital arrival. *Circulation.* 2014;130:1883–1890.

22. Huikuri HV, Castellanos A, Myerburg RJ. Sudden death due to cardiac arrhythmias. *N Engl J Med.* 2001;345:1473–1482.

23. Goldberger JJ, Buxton AE, Cain M, et al. Risk stratification for arrhythmic sudden cardiac death: identifying the roadblocks. *Circulation.* 2011;123:2423–2430.

24. Ridker PM, Danielson E, Fonseca FA, et al. JUPITER Study Group. Rosuvastatin to prevent vascular events in men and women with elevated C-reactive protein. *N Engl J Med.* 2008;359:2195–2207.

25. Heart Protection Study Collaborative Group. C-reactive protein concentration and the vascular benefits of statin therapy: an analysis of 20,536 patients in the Heart Protection Study. *Lancet.* 2011;377:469–476.

26. Myerburg RJ. Physiological variations, environmental factors, and genetic modifications in inherited LQT syndromes. *J Am Coll Cardiol.* 2015;65:375–377.

27. Ridker PM, Cushman M, Stampfer MJ, et al. Inflammation, aspirin, and the risk of cardiovascular disease in apparently healthy men. *N Engl J Med.* 1997;336:973–979.

28. Ridker PM, Hennekens CH, Buring JE, et al. C-reactive protein and other markers of inflammation in the prediction of cardiovascular disease in women. *N Engl J Med.* 2000;342:836–843.

29. Burkett EL, Hershberger RE. Clinical and genetic issues in familial dilated cardiomyopathy. *J Am Coll Cardiol.* 2005;45:969–981.

30. Merit-HF Study Group. Effect of metoprolol CR/XL in chronic heart failure: Metoprolol CR/XL Randomised Intervention Trial in Congestive Heart Failure (MERIT-HF). *Lancet.* 1999;353:2001–2007.

31. Myerburg RJ. Scientific gaps in the prediction and prevention of sudden cardiac death. *J Cardiovasc Electrophysiol.* 2002;13:709–723.

32. Nichol G, Thomas E, Callaway CW, et al. Regional variation in out-of-hospital cardiac arrest incidence and outcome. *JAMA.* 2008;300:1423–1431.

33. Weisfeldt ML, Everson-Stewart S, Sitlani C, et al. Resuscitation Outcomes Consortium Investigators. Ventricular tachyarrhythmias after cardiac arrest in public versus at home. *N Engl J Med.* 2011;364:313–321.

34. Teodorescu C, Reinier K, Dervan C, et al. Factors associated with pulseless electric activity versus ventricular fibrillation: The Oregon Sudden Unexpected Death Study. *Circulation.* 2010;122:2116–2122.

35. Vaillancourt C, Everson-Stewart S, Christenson J, et al.; the Resuscitation Outcomes Consortium Investigators. The impact of increased chest compression fraction on return of spontaneous circulation for out-of-hospital cardiac arrest patients not in ventricular fibrillation. *Resuscitation.* 2011;82:1501–1507.

36. Hulleman M1, Berdowski J, de Groot JR, et al. Implantable cardioverter-defibrillators have reduced the incidence of resuscitation for out-of-hospital cardiac arrest caused by lethal arrhythmias. *Circulation.* 2012;126:815–821.

37. Goldberger ZD, Chan PS, Berg RA, et al. For the American Heart Association Get With The Guidelines—Resuscitation (formerly the National Registry of Cardiopulmonary Resuscitation) Investigators. Duration of resuscitation efforts and survival after in-hospital cardiac arrest: an observational study. *Lancet.* 2012;380:1473–1481.

38. Kudenchuk PJ, Cobb LA, Copass MK, et al. Amiodarone for resuscitation after out-of-hospital cardiac arrest due to ventricular fibrillation. *N Engl J Med.* 1999;341:871–878.

39. Chan PS, Krumholz HM, Nichol G, et al. Delayed time to defibrillation after in-hospital cardiac arrest. *N Engl J Med.* 2008;358:9–17.

40. Friedlander Y, Siscovick DS, Weinmann S, et al. Family history as a risk factor for primary cardiac arrest. *Circulation.* 1998;97:155–160.

41. Jouven X, Desnos M, Guerot C, et al. Predicting sudden death in the population: the Paris Prospective Study I. *Circulation.* 1999;99:1978–1983.

42. Kaikkonen KS, Kortelainen ML, Linna E, et al. Family history and the risk of sudden cardiac death as a manifestation of an acute coronary event. *Circulation.* 2006;114:1462–1467.

43. Dekker LR, Bezzina CR, Henriques JP, et al. Familial sudden death is an important risk factor for primary ventricular fibrillation: a case-control study in acute myocardial infarction patients. *Circulation.* 2006;114:1140–1145.

44. Friedlander Y, Vatta M, Sotoodehnia N, et al. Possible association of the human KCNE1 (minK) gene and QT interval in healthy subjects: evidence from association and linkage analyses in Israeli families. *Ann Hum Genet.* 2005;69:645–656.

45. Spooner PM, Albert C, Benjamin EJ, et al. Sudden cardiac death, genes, and arrhythmogenesis: consideration of new population and mechanistic approaches from a National Heart, Lung, and Blood Institute Workshop, Part I. *Circulation.* 2001;103:2361–2364.

46. Bonow R, Clark EB, Curfman GD, et al. Task Force on Strategic Research Direction. Clinical Science Subgroup key science topics report. *Circulation.* 2002;106:e162–e166.

47. Hebert PR, Gaziano JM, Chan KS, et al. Cholesterol lowering with statin drugs, risk of stroke, and total mortality: an overview of randomized trials. *JAMA.* 1997;278:313–321.

48. Myerburg RJ, Ullmann SG. Alternative research funding to improve clinical outcomes: the model of prediction and prevention of sudden cardiac death. *Circ Arrhythm Electrophysiol.* 2015;8:492–498.

49. Podlowski S, Wenzel K, Luther HP, et al. β1-adrenoceptor gene variations: a role in idiopathic dilated cardiomyopathy? *J Mol Med (Berl).* 2000;78:87–93.

50. Pogwizd SM, Schlotthauer K, Li L, et al. Arrhythmogenesis and contractile dysfunction in heart failure: roles of sodium-calcium exchange, inward rectifier potassium current, and residual beta-adrenergic responsiveness. *Circ Res.* 2001;88:1159–1167.

51. Porta A, Girardengo G, Bari V, George Jr AL, et al. Autonomic control of heart rate and of QT variability influences arrhythmic risk in long QT syndrome type 1. *J Am Coll Cardiol.* 2015;65:367–674.

52. Califf RM, DeMets DL. Principles from clinical trials relevant to clinical practice: part I. *Circulation.* 2002;106:1015–1021.

100 Arrhythmia in Neurological Disease

Tarek Zghaib and Saman Nazarian

Electrophysiologists are routinely tasked with the management of arrhythmia in the setting of an underlying acute or chronic neurological disturbance. The underlying neurological diagnosis often carries important implications regarding the permanence, rate of progression, and prognosis of the arrhythmic manifestations. This chapter will review neurological disorders that commonly present with arrhythmia manifestations.

Neurological Disorders With Transient Arrhythmia Manifestations

Neurogenic Heart Disease

Transient electrocardiogram (ECG) abnormalities and arrhythmias may arise after acute neurological stress and independent of any preexisting heart disease. The main neurological precipitants of transient cardiac injury are acute central nervous system (CNS) disease (subarachnoid hemorrhage [SAH], ischemic stroke, traumatic brain injury (TBI), epilepsy, and even meningitis) or emotional stress (fear, anger, grief).[1,2] This phenomenon, referred to as neurogenic heart disease (NHD), is characterized by a spectrum of cardiac disorders ranging from isolated rhythm disturbance or conduction abnormalities to stress-induced cardiomyopathy, also known as Takotsubo cardiomyopathy (TTC) or transient left ventricular (LV) apical ballooning.[3] Sudden cardiac death (SCD) is the most feared outcome of NHD.[4]

Autonomic Nervous System and Neuronal Networks

The key link between neurological stress and secondary cardiac dysfunction is the autonomic nervous system (ANS). By sending regulatory signals from brain centers to the heart through the sympathetic and/or parasympathetic nervous systems (SNS and PNS), the ANS drives the cardiac response to neurogenic stress. The appropriate balance between SNS and PNS is fundamental for desired physiological responses. The complex organization of the ANS allows for fine-tuning of physiological responses via feedback inhibition. The actual ANS pathways are highly complex, and their description goes beyond the scope of this chapter.[5,6] Briefly, a loop including the insular cortex, amygdala, and hypothalamic nuclei regulates the autonomic response.[7,8] Evidence has also been found for lateralization of the cardiac function, with the SNS thought to be established at the right insular cortex and the PNS by the left insula.[9,10] In addition to its role in visceral motor regulation, the insular cortex is integral to the response to emotional stressors such as fear or anxiety through dense connections with the limbic/paralimbic system. The insular cortex has a direct influence on the cardiac response to physiological, environmental, and emotional stressors triggering fear or anxiety. Clinically, this close relationship is seen in patients suffering from middle cerebral artery strokes involving the insula. Such patients were indeed found to have autonomic dysregulation, rhythm disturbance, and arrhythmias, leading to SCD.[11] The hypothalamus has also been shown to be an integration center of autonomic stimuli as well as a regulator of cardiovascular response, especially at the posterolateral and paraventricular nuclei.[12–15] At the subcortical level, postganglionic fibers exit the spine via upper thoracic roots to the stellate and superior cervical ganglia, ending in the cardiac muscle where the ANS regulates heart rhythm, blood pressure (BP), and contractility and excitability of the heart.

Pathophysiology of Neurogenic Heart Disease

Several theories regarding the pathophysiology of cardiac injury in the setting of neurological stress have been hypothesized. Multivessel coronary spasm and microvascular dysfunction have been proposed as mediators for ST-segment elevations and cardiac enzyme level elevations seen in NHD, which mirror ischemic manifestations. However, in the face of normal coronary arteries as well as normal myocardial perfusion seen on contrast echocardiography,[3] the "catecholamine toxicity hypothesis" has gained traction in explaining the underlying source of cardiac damage in NHD. Neurological, physiological, and emotional stresses are all associated with a systemic elevation in plasma catecholamine levels, which persists beyond the acute insult.[16–19] The concentration of epinephrine and norepinephrine was positively correlated with serum cardiac enzyme levels, and sympathetic blockade was shown to be cardioprotective in the setting of stress.[20] However, mild stress-induced myocardial injury still occurs despite bilateral adrenalectomy; furthermore, a complete denervation of the heart in models subjected to artificially produced intracranial hypertension prevented myocardial injury.[21] This suggests that neurogenic myopathy is at least partially incurred by norepinephrine released locally at the sympathetic myocardial nerve terminals rather than by circulating catecholamines.

Pathology

The classic pathology observed in patients with NHD is myofibrillary degeneration, also referred to as coagulative myocytolysis or contraction band necrosis.[18,22–24] On light microscopy, mononuclear infiltrates are seen. The heart tissue changes range from increased eosinophilia with preservation of cross bands to complete distortion of the cell structure with dense eosinophilic transverse bands. Myocardial fibers are in a hypercontracted state. At the cellular level, hypercalcification is common and may explain the cytotoxicity of catecholamines. Increased binding of norepinephrine causes opening of the calcium channel, leading to excessive entry of calcium and release of potassium from the cardiac cell, hence the hyperkalemic pattern seen on ECG (peaked T waves). Actin is continuously bound to myosin under the effect of calcium, causing hypercontraction of the sarcomeres. Eventually, this leads to cell death with leakage of the cell content and cardiac enzymes into the blood. In addition, the metabolism of catecholamines is known to produce reactive oxygen species contributing to cell membrane disruption.[24,25] These changes occur within 2–4 μm from the nerve ending, reinforcing the cytolytic role of locally released norepinephrine.[26] In addition, these lesions are predominantly seen in the endocardium close to the conduction system. The location of these abnormalities, in addition to the high level of catecholamines, may explain the propensity for arrhythmia, conduction disturbances, and SCD in these patients. Of note, myocytolysis is distinguished from ischemic coagulation necrosis by the relaxed fibers, relative absence of contraction bands, elicited polymorphonuclear response, and delayed calcification seen in the latter.[27]

Acute Cerebrovascular Disease

Cardiac Manifestations

Cardiac injury in the setting of neurological insult is common, especially after acute stroke, SAH, and intracranial hemorrhage (ICH). It manifests as repolarization abnormalities, arrhythmias, or sudden death. The typical ECG pattern described consists of large inverted "cerebral" T waves, prolonged QT intervals, and large U waves.[28–30] In addition, ST-segment changes, ectopic ventricular beats, and variable atrioventricular (AV) block can also be seen in the absence of preexisting heart disease.[31,32] LV hypertrophy (LVH), diagnosed by ECG criteria, has been reported in 14% of patients after SAH. The prevalence of these abnormalities is variable among observational studies, but a recent systematic review has reported higher occurrence of ECG changes in SAH (75%) than in ischemic stroke and ICH (30%–50%). The incidence of ECG changes in patients with SAH has been shown to correlate with the amount of intracranial blood.[33] ECG changes indicate a worse outcome after cerebrovascular disease, especially when the insular cortex is involved, pointing to the role of ANS dysregulation in NHD.[34]

Arrhythmias are well known to occur in the setting of acute cerebrovascular disease, with a reported incidence of 20%–40% in the setting of ischemic stroke or ICH and reaching 100% in some series of patients with SAH.[35] The most common of these arrhythmias are sinus bradycardia and tachycardia, atrial flutter (AFL), atrial fibrillation (AF), supraventricular tachycardia, premature ventricular complexes, multifocal ventricular tachycardia (VT), torsades de pointes, and ventricular fibrillation (VF). AF, with a reported incidence of 14%, is the most common arrhythmia secondary to stroke.[36] It is certainly possible, however, that some AF diagnoses after stroke actually represent a new diagnosis of an asymptomatic, but preexisting arrhythmia that actually led to the stroke. Life-threatening ventricular arrhythmias occur in 5% of patients after SAH,[37] while sudden death has been reported in 12% of patients with SAH.[38]

Management

Arrhythmias in these patients should be managed according to the appropriate clinical guidelines. Neurogenic ECG changes do not warrant any primary intervention. However, appropriate investigations should be made to detect and correct any coexistent conditions with similar ECG manifestations, such as hereditary long QT syndromes, electrolyte disturbances (particularly hypokalemia and hypomagnesemia), medication side effects, and acute myocardial infarction. β-Blockers may have a cardioprotective role in the setting of neurogenic cardiac injury given the role of the SNS in the disease, but further studies are needed to demonstrate a benefit in these patients. As to the prognosis of the NHD, ECG changes and arrhythmias dictate a poor outcome after cerebrovascular events.[39,40]

Traumatic Brain Injury

Cardiac Manifestations

TBI, in the absence of obvious cerebral bleed on imaging, can lead to neurogenic cardiac injury secondary to ANS impairment. The most commonly reported ECG abnormality is transient ST-segment elevation or depression, reflecting myocardial injury in the absence of coronary abnormalities or preexisting structural heart disease.[41,42] These changes were seen even in the pediatric population, ruling out the possibility of ischemic coronary disease as a possible etiology.[43] Other electrical abnormalities reported in TBI are peaked P and T waves, short PR intervals,

sinus tachycardia, ventricular premature beats, and VTs.[44] Of note, these changes are often accompanied by transient, mild to moderate elevation of cardiac enzymes, such as creatine kinase-MB (CK-MB) and troponin T.[45] Global or local impairment of ventricular mechanical function can be seen affecting the ejection fraction (EF) on echocardiography.[42] TBI can also cause TTC in typical or atypical forms.[46] On autopsy, contraction band necrosis has been reported and confirms the neurogenic etiology of cardiac injury.[47] In most cases, cardiac changes are reversible within 48 hours of intensive care and close monitoring.

Another manifestation of dysautonomia in TBI occurs in up to 15% of patients who develop a sudden onset of severe and paroxysmal episodes of sympathetic hyperactivity.[48] Symptoms are typical of catecholamine excess and consist of paroxysms of increased BP, respiratory rate, and heart rate. Hyperthermia, decreased level of consciousness, diaphoresis, and sympathetic overreactivity to normally nonpainful stimuli are also seen.[49] These clinical features persist for at least 2 weeks and have been reported to last up to a year after TBI.[48] Pathophysiology is based on ANS dysfunction with an imbalance between SNS and PNS. Although associated with poor outcomes, this condition is treatable with opioids, gabapentin, benzodiazepines, centrally acting α-agonists, and β-antagonists.[50]

Migraines

Cardiac Manifestations

The prevalence of migraine is estimated at 30 million individuals in the United States alone.[51] Most of the common symptoms experienced during a migraine episode are related to dysfunction of the ANS.[52] The cardiac conduction system is closely interrelated with the ANS. Hence, during migraine episodes, a wide array of electrophysiological abnormalities are reported, including bradycardia, AV block, bundle branch block, ST and T wave changes, AF, premature ventricular beats, and VTs.[53–56] In addition, PR and QTc interval dispersion, predictors of AF and ventricular arrhythmia, respectively, tends to increase during migraine episodes compared with pain-free periods.[57–59] In a case of sudden death after migraine, the autopsy showed contraction band necrosis, the hallmark of neurogenic cardiac injury from excessive SNS activation.[60] Migraines can also lead to TTC. Furthermore, some medications commonly prescribed for the treatment of migraine (such as triptans and ergotamine) have been reported to cause serious arrhythmias, including VT and VF, but epidemiological data do not show a definite risk.[61–64]

Stress-Induced Cardiomyopathy

Cardiac Manifestations

Stress-induced cardiomyopathy, also known as apical ballooning syndrome or TTC, overlaps significantly with NHD and is included in the spectrum of manifestations of cardiac disease secondary to neurological stress.[65,66] It is most common among postmenopausal women above the age of 50 years.[67,68] Common triggers are acute emotional stress; physical stress; exposure to a surge of catecholaminergic agents, such as cocaine, dobutamine, and epinephrine; and acute neurological events, such as SAH, epilepsy, intracerebral hemorrhage, encephalitis/meningitis, head trauma, and acute ischemic stroke.[69–71] Although a catecholamine "storm" and an exaggerated hyperadrenergic response to stress were documented in this condition, the susceptibility of individual patients remains unexplained. A recent study in women with a history of TTC showed that these patients, long after their initial episode, still exhibit the characteristic dysautonomia of excessive sympathetic response as well as reduced parasympathetic and cardiovagal modulation of the heart.[72] This could potentially constitute a predisposing substrate for the disease, but more studies are necessary to replicate the findings in larger populations.

Clinically, the presentation mimics that of acute coronary syndrome, namely chest pain, dyspnea on exertion, or syncope. ECG abnormalities typical of myocardial ischemia are characteristically detected, with ST-elevation seen in virtually all the cases, mostly in the precordial leads but less commonly in the inferior leads, which is usually accompanied by T wave inversion and QTc prolongation. New bundle branch blocks, pathological Q waves, and prolonged QTc are also reported.[3,73–75] Mild to moderate elevations in CK-MB and troponin T are seen but at levels much lower than those in myocardial ischemia.[74,75] On echocardiography, the syndrome is characterized by reversible wall-motion abnormalities that extend beyond the distribution of a single coronary artery. The LV apex and mid-ventricular segment show moderate to severe impaired function with apparent hypercontractility of the base. Atypical presentations can manifest as inverted TTC (hypokinesis of the base and/or the mid-ventricle with sparing of the apex) or as a biventricular cardiomyopathy.[3,46,74,76] Often, there is the absence of significant coronary artery obstruction or plaque rupture on angiography. Autopsy typically shows mononuclear interstitial infiltrates and contraction band necrosis.[3]

As to the burden of arrhythmias, a large study reported a 26% incidence in patients with TTC, including supraventricular tachycardia, AF/AFL, and VT/fibrillation.[77] Sudden cardiac arrest was reported at 2% among these patients, and in-hospital mortality was increased in patients who developed arrhythmias.

Management

The management of the disease itself is primarily supportive and dependent upon the occurrence of complications. Abnormalities on echocardiography are expected to revert spontaneously to baseline within days to weeks. The prognosis is favorable, with an in-hospital mortality rate of 1%–4%.[65,68] Potential complications include acute left heart failure (HF), pulmonary edema, cardiogenic shock, mitral regurgitation, ventricular mural thrombus, ventricular free-wall rupture, arrhythmias, and SCD.[67,70] The pathogenesis of the disease is related to the sympathetic "storm" resulting from the acute stress, and therefore adrenergic blockers (α- and β-blockers) are the most appropriate first-line medications.[78] In addition, estrogen was shown to partially attenuate the cardiac effects of neurogenic stress.[79] Aggressive diuresis, angiotensin inhibitors, and hemodynamic support with intraaortic balloon pump or ventricular assist device may be required in cases of acute LV dysfunction. As the presentation mimics acute coronary syndrome, coronary angiography is commonly performed in the acute setting to rule out plaque or thrombus rupture along with the administration of aspirin, heparin, and β-blockers. Short-term anticoagulation with vitamin K antagonists should be considered to prevent the development of mural thrombi due to apical akinesis. Close monitoring in a hospital setting is favored to detect fatal arrhythmias and hemodynamic collapse, and patients should be monitored even after complete resolution as TTC may recur in some cases.

Meningitis/Encephalitis

Cardiac Manifestations

Arrhythmia in the setting of meningitis/encephalitis is rare and has been presented as case reports in the literature. ECG changes that have been described include sinus bradycardia, AV block, VT, QTc prolongation, ST-segment changes, and sick sinus syndrome.[80–83] These are usually temporary and resolve with treatment of the underlying infection.

Central Sleep Apnea

Cardiac Manifestations

Central sleep apnea (SA), mediated by respiratory control dysregulation, may be caused by a variety of diseases, including Rett syndrome, Prader-Willi syndrome, myotonic dystrophy, Arnold-Chiari malformation, HF, and ischemic stroke. Arrhythmias are common cardiovascular complications of SA. Potential mediators are thought to include repetitive hypoxemia, hypercapnia, and changes in intrathoracic pressure, leading to increases in sympathetic activation and circulating catecholamines, potentiation of peripheral chemoreceptor sensitivity, spikes of BP creating mechanical stress on the heart and vessels, inflammation, oxidative stress, and atrial remodeling.[84–87] The most commonly reported arrhythmia is AF, but nonsustained VT, AV block, bradyarrhythmias, and asystole have also been described.[88,89] It has been reported that more than 60% of patients with a high burden of AF have sleep-disordered breathing, and patients with SA were less likely to respond to antiarrhythmic medication.[90] The risk of nocturnal SCD is higher in patients with SA than in the general population.[91]

Management

Continuous positive airway pressure (CPAP) can reduce the burden of pauses and bradycardia and significantly reduce AF recurrence after cardioversion or catheter ablation.[92–94] In patients with severe HF, treatment of coexisting SA with CPAP improves cardiac function and reduces the frequency of ventricular premature beats during sleep, potentially reducing the incidence of fatal ventricular arrhythmias.[95,96] In patients with congenital SA syndromes like Prader-Willi, oxygen therapy has been efficacious.[97] In contrast, in patients with Cheyne-Stokes respiration in HF, adaptive seroventilation has failed to show definite benefit in survival and remains a controversial treatment modality.[98,99]

Epilepsy

Cardiac Manifestations

Epilepsy is the most common serious neurological disease. Patients with epilepsy were found to have a 24-fold increase in the risk of sudden death compared with the general population.[100] The occurrence of sudden unexplained/unexpected death in patients with epilepsy (SUDEP) has been reported during or shortly after seizures.[101] The incidence of SUDEP is reported to be between 0.1 and 9.3 per 1000 patient-years depending on the population studied.[102] Although potential mechanisms of SUDEP are numerous, the occurrence of arrhythmia in the setting of epilepsy is commonly reported to increase mortality and morbidity.

ECG abnormalities were found both during and after seizure episodes. ST-segment depression can be found in 40% of cases. QT prolongation and T wave inversion are significant predictors of sudden death.[103–105] In addition, patients with generalized tonic-clonic seizures were more likely to show ECG changes than patients with complex partial seizures.[106]

Sinus tachycardia is universally present during seizures. Periictal asystole, bradycardia, AV block, AF, AFL, and VF were all reported in the literature.[107] Ictal asystole, bradycardia, and AV block were self-limiting, and no SUDEP was reported. Such events occurred predominantly during focal dyscognitive seizures (formerly known as complex partial seizures) with a temporal or, less commonly, frontal lobe focus. In contrast, postictal asystole, AF, and VF occurred after convulsive seizures and were frequently associated with SUDEP. Epilepsy is associated with a three-fold increase in the risk of sudden cardiac arrest, and most postictal asystole episodes were preceded by apnea; however, the exact mechanism remains elusive.[108,109] Activation of carotid chemoreceptors due to hypercapnia and hypoxia may lead to vagal stimulation, bradycardia, and asystole.

The previously mentioned structure of the ANS and its direct connections with the cardiac conduction system could potentially explain the disturbance in rhythm observed in epilepsy. In fact, a direct stimulation of autonomic centers in the brain located in the limbic circuit including the insula, amygdala, and cingulate gyrus may cause high-grade AV block, asystole, and supraventricular tachycardia.[110-113] This is supported by dysfunction of the ANS in epileptic patients, especially in those with a higher burden of seizures and a longer duration of the disease.[114,115] In addition, both ECG and biochemical markers of direct cardiac injury, such as QTc prolongation, ST-segment changes, and elevated troponin levels, were found in greater proportions in epileptic patients.[104,116-118] Seizure duration was longer in patients with electrical abnormalities than in those without, possibly reflecting increased cardiac damage due to greater autonomic stress.[106,119] Pathological changes in the heart were seen in SUDEP cases as interstitial myocardial fibrosis, cardiomyocyte atrophy, myofibrillar degeneration, leukocytic infiltration, and edema of the conduction system tissue.[120,121] This picture converges with the abovementioned SNS-triggered myocardial injury, suggesting a common pathophysiology with similar manifestations. In fact, generalized seizures are the second most frequent neurological disorder triggering TTC.[70] Other potential mechanisms for arrhythmias in seizures are myocardial ischemia, metabolic changes, electrolyte abnormalities, conduction system abnormalities, arrhythmogenic antiepileptic drugs like carbamazepine, and structural heart disease.[122,123]

Management

Since most periictal arrhythmias are reversible, the first-line management in these patients is close observation, optimization of antiepileptic regimen, epilepsy surgery, and discontinuation of proarrhythmic and conduction-slowing drugs.[124] If asystole or conduction block does not remit, pacing is indicated, and it has been shown to reduce morbidity and falls.[125]

Cardiac-induced syncope and seizures can be clinically indistinguishable. Cerebral hypoxia induced by VF or asystole may trigger tonic-clonic jerking movements mimicking convulsive seizures.[126] Hence, long QT syndrome, arrhythmogenic right ventricular (RV) dysplasia, AV nodal reentry tachycardia, bradycardia, and sinus node disease can be misdiagnosed as epilepsy. This underscores the importance of a comprehensive personal and family history, 12-lead ECGs or continuous rhythm monitoring, and checking prior ECGs when available.[127]

Guillain-Barré Syndrome

Pathophysiology and Clinical Presentation

Guillain-Barré syndrome (GBS), also known as acute inflammatory demyelinating polyneuropathy, presents with an estimated incidence of 1–2 per 100,000 individuals per year.[128] It is an autoimmune disorder in which an aberrant immune response develops against the motor, sensory, or autonomic peripheral nerves due to antigen cross-reactivity, leading to demyelination.[129] It is often preceded by a respiratory or gastrointestinal infection that triggers the immune response. The most common organism observed in GBS is *Campylobacter jejuni*, but viral infections with cytomegalovirus (CMV), Epstein-Barr virus (EBV), and human immunodeficiency virus (HIV) have all been reported. It presents as a symmetrical, progressive ascending weakness accompanied by loss of reflexes, variable sensory loss, and paresthesias. Presentation can be acute or subacute and can lead to respiratory failure despite treatment.[130]

Cardiac Manifestations

Dysregulation of the PNS and SNS is known to occur in GBS and is attributed to autonomic neuropathy.[131] Vasomotor changes are responsible for the fluctuations in BP and heart rate seen in these patients and reflect an increased risk of arrhythmias.[132]

ECG manifestations of cardiac involvement in GBS are various and nonspecific. Reported changes include large T waves, ST-T changes, prolonged QT interval, U waves, and AV blocks.[133,134]

As seen in other conditions involving the ANS, this pattern in ECG changes may reflect myocardial stunning due to the sympathetic "storm" associated with the condition. Transient LV hypokinesis and reduced EF have been reported in this setting.[135]

Several patterns of rhythm disturbance may be encountered in GBS, with sinus tachycardia being the most common abnormality reported. Various atrial tachycardias and VTs have also been reported.[132] Bradyarrhythmias are well described in GBS and may be related to vagal nerve overactivity, leading to bradycardia, severe conduction block, sinus pauses, or even asystole.

Management

In addition to early initiation of plasmapheresis or intravenous immunoglobulins, GBS patients with dysautonomia and fluctuating BPs require close hemodynamic monitoring, preferentially in an intensive care setting, until the condition resolves. These patients are at risk of severe hypo- or hypertension and life-threatening brady- or tachyarrhythmias. Dysrhythmias in GBS are temporary in most cases and resolve with treatment of the condition, but severe conduction disturbance may require temporary or even permanent pacemakers.

Parkinson Disease: Cardiac Manifestations

In Parkinson disease (PD), cardiac involvement manifests mainly as dysautonomia and orthostatic hypotension.[136] QTc prolongation has been reported in these patients and correlates with the stage of PD and the level of dysautonomia.[137-139] Numerous QT-prolonging medications are routinely prescribed for movement disorders, such as domperidone, escitalopram, and antimicrobials such as macrolides, azoles, and fluoroquinolones.[140] Iatrogenic and pathological repolarization abnormalities should be factored into the care of these patients, and screening for dysautonomia and QT-segment abnormalities should be performed to prevent sudden death.

Neuromuscular Diseases

Muscular Dystrophies

Myotonic Muscular Dystrophy (Type 1 and 2)

Genetics and Pathophysiology. Myotonic muscular dystrophy (MMD) is the most common inherited muscular dystrophy presenting in adulthood, with an incidence of 1:8000 births and a prevalence of 3–15 per 100,000.[141-143] It is transmitted in an autosomal dominant fashion with incomplete penetrance and displays somatic mosaicism and anticipation and commonly presents in two forms.[144] MMD type 1, also known as Steinert disease, is caused by a mutation in the 3′ untranslated region of the myotonic dystrophy protein kinase (MDPK) gene (*DMPK*) on chromosome 19q13.3, leading to the expansion of CTG repeats beyond the normal range of 5–35 repeats.[145] There is a correlation between the size of the repeats and the age of onset, severity, and rate of progression of the disease. MMD type 2 arises from an expansion mutation in a CCTG repeat on the zinc finger protein 9 gene on chromosome 3.[146] The pathophysiology is related to the toxicity of the mutant *DMPK* mRNA in the nucleus, where it causes abnormal slicing of pre-mRNA transcripts of major proteins, such as the skeletal muscle chloride (Cl⁻) ion channels, cardiac gap junctions, and calcium channels, resulting in disease manifestations such as myotonia and conduction system disease.[147-150]

Clinical Presentation. MMD type 1 has four different phenotypes based on the age at onset and number of CTG repeats: mild, classical, childhood-onset, and congenital MMD. Repeat size in each of these is 50–150, 50–1000, >800, and >1000 CTG repeats with an age at onset of 20–70 years, 10–30 years, 1–10 years, and in the neonatal period, respectively. Age at death is positively correlated with age at onset of the disease. MMD patients have a reduced life expectancy, with a mean age at death of 53 years and a mortality rate seven times that of an age-matched individual.[151] The most common cause of death is respiratory failure in 40% followed by cardiac disease in 30%, with sudden death attributed to a fatal arrhythmia occurring in 10%.

Patients with congenital MMD have the most severe manifestations and present with feeding difficulties, respiratory failure, hypotonia, and developmental delays. Myotonia in these patients typically appears in the second decade of life. Mortality is high in the neonatal period; however, the prognosis improves beyond it, and the average age at death is 45 years. Childhood-onset MMD is milder than the congenital form and manifests as psychosocial and intellectual disabilities. The classical form of MMD has varied and multisystemic manifestations that are typically more severe in type 1 and occur at an earlier age. Significant weakness, wasting, and myotonia characterize skeletal muscle involvement. As the disease progresses, patients develop a typical facial appearance consisting of ptosis, temporal muscle atrophy, early hair loss, and face "drop." Patients may experience weakness in the jaw and the tongue as well as swallowing difficulties. Weakness in the ankles and the long fingers leads to frequent falls and functional disabilities. Respiratory muscle weakness constitutes a major source of morbidity and mortality in the MMD population.[151] It can manifest as respiratory failure with poor coughing reflex and reduced vital capacity, leading to recurrent aspiration pneumonia.[152] These patients are particularly sensitive to general anesthesia, which can lead to prolonged respiratory depression after surgery.[153] Endocrine abnormalities are common in MMD patients and include thyroid and parathyroid dysfunction, diabetes/insulin resistance, and hypogonadism.[154,155] Gastrointestinal (dysphagia, gallstones, pseudo-bowel obstruction), CNS (cognitive impairment, attention disorders), ophthalmological (cataracts), and cardiovascular manifestations have all been reported in MMD patients.

In contrast, MMD type 2 patients typically present in their third decade and complain mainly of proximal muscle weakness, stiffness, and fatigue, although they are not spared from the other manifestations.[156]

Cardiac Manifestations. MMD commonly involves the cardiac conduction system at an early stage, with pathological studies showing diffuse interstitial fibrosis, fatty infiltration, and focal vacuolar degeneration.[157,158] Conduction abnormalities are the most common cardiac manifestations in MMD patients and predict cardiac events and sudden death. Both conduction disease and cardiac events are correlated with the length of CTG repeats and the age of the patient.[159,160] In fact, the QRS interval has been reported to increase by 0.54 ms/year.[161] Patients with >1000 repeats seem to be at a higher risk for a rapid progression of conduction system disease.[159] MMD most commonly affects the His–Purkinje system but may involve the sinoatrial and AV nodes. Sixty-five percent of MMD patients are reported to have abnormalities on ECG, including prolonged PR, QRS, and QTc; nonspecific ST-T changes; AV blocks; bundle branch block; and premature ventricular beats.[162] Studies have shown that surface ECG changes are important markers of sudden death and all-cause mortality.[163] Patients with conduction defects may be asymptomatic or may experience shortness of breath, dizziness, syncope, and, in more severe cases, sudden death.[164]

The most commonly reported tachyarrhythmias are AF and AFL, likely promoted by atrial wall fibrosis and fatty infiltration.[165] The possible mechanisms leading to VT are varied and include triggered activity, reentry around fibrofatty infiltrates, fascicular VT, and torsades de pointes induced by prolonged QT and bundle branch reentrant VT.[166,167] Recognition of the latter is essential as its induction requires specific pacing protocols (long-short–coupled extra stimuli), infusion of drugs (isoproterenol or procainamide), or both and is readily amenable to ablation.[168]

LV dysfunction occurs in MMD patients to a lesser extent and at later disease stages than conduction disturbances; nonetheless, it increases all-cause as well as cardiovascular death rates (relative risk [RR] of 3.9 and 5.7, respectively).[169,170] LVH and LV dilation as well as systolic dysfunction were reported to have a prevalence of 15%–20%, correlating with patient age and CTG repeats.[170] Clinical HF occurs at a lower rate of approximately 2%–6%. Other structural abnormalities reported in MMD include ischemic heart disease, LV dyssynchrony, LV relaxation dysfunction (or myocardial myotonia), HF with preserved EF, left atrial dilation, mitral valve prolapse, and RV dysfunction.[171–173]

Management. Initial cardiac screening should include a 12-lead ECG and echocardiogram regardless of symptom status. Abnormal findings on tissue Doppler, speckle tracking for ventricular strain, and measurement of myocardial performance index all correlate with disease progression even when findings are not apparent on two-dimensional (2D) echocardiography.[174–176] In addition, 24-hour ambulatory Holter monitoring has been shown to detect abnormalities in up to 32% of patients with normal ECG.[161] Implanted loop monitors have been used in small series and have led to device implantation for asymptomatic asystole and VT.[177] The His bundle is the most prevalent target of conduction disease in MMD, and H-V measurement during an electrophysiology study (EPS) can be useful for management. The invasiveness of the procedure, combined with the higher risk associated with anesthesia in MMD patients and the need for follow-up investigations due to the progressive nature of the disease, justifies the reluctance of physicians to rely on EPS for monitoring. In addition, the prognostic implication of inducible VT in the absence of spontaneous VT is uncertain in MMD. In the presence of structural heart disease, however, VT induction on EPS likely warrants implantable cardioverter defibrillator (ICD) implantation.[178]

Cardiac magnetic resonance imaging (MRI) is an accurate tool to measure cardiac structure, fibrosis, and function. Hence it constitutes an important tool to detect early cardiac involvement.[173,179] Both focal and patchy patterns of fibrosis have been observed in MMD and constitute a substrate for VTs.[179] Techniques to examine diffuse myocardial fibrosis appear to be associated with QRS prolongation and may have a role for identification of those at highest risk for sudden death.[180]

Management of MMD patients with symptomatic bradyarrhythmia and high-grade AV block should not differ from that of non-MMD patients, and permanent pacemakers should be implanted.[181] Despite the use of pacemakers, a significant number of sudden deaths have been attributed to VT, hence the ongoing trend to implant prophylactic ICDs in patients with significant cardiac involvement.[167,182] Despite the lack of properly randomized trials for the management of asymptomatic patients with documented conduction system disease, an aggressive strategy with early device implantation seems to be widely supported based on reduction of sudden death and overall mortality.[183–185] To screen for conduction abnormalities, a yearly ECG is appropriate. Groh and colleagues developed a set of criteria to predict the risk of sudden death.[186] The criteria include a rhythm other than sinus, PR >240 ms, QRS >120 ms, and second- or third-degree AV block. An EPS, Holter monitoring, or cardiac MRI to further evaluate the extent of cardiac disease is appropriate in the presence of any of these abnormalities in addition to nonsustained VT, LV or RV dysfunction, and any symptom suggestive of arrhythmias.[187] The latest guidelines suggest permanent pacemaker implantation for any degree of AV block (including first degree) or fascicular block, regardless of symptoms.[181] The rationale for the recommendation is based on the unpredictable progression of the disease to complete heart block and sudden death. An H-V interval >70 ms on EPS reflects severe His-bundle disease and warrants a pacemaker. The life expectancy of the patient, reflected by the overall disease burden, as well as cardiac and respiratory comorbidities should be considered prior to implanting a device.

Emery-Dreifuss Muscular Dystrophy

Genetics and Pathophysiology. The hallmark of Emery-Dreifuss muscular dystrophy (EDMD) is early and debilitating joint contractures. Three genetic forms exist. X-linked recessive EDMD has a prevalence of 1 in 100,000 males and affects the *STA* gene located at the Xq28 chromosome, leading to the complete absence of the nuclear protein emerin.[188] Emerin is a component of the inner nuclear membrane linking filamentous actin to the nuclear lamina or chromatin.[189,190] Autosomal dominant and the rare autosomal recessive EDMDs result from a mutation in the lamin A/C gene (*LMNA*) on chromosome 1q21 and are part of the so-called laminopathies.[191,192] The pathophysiology of EDMD is thought to be related to the sensitivity of the cells lacking emerin or lamin A/C to the mechanical stress of contraction, which leads to loss of integrity of the nuclear membrane, abnormal gene expression, and early apoptosis of muscle fibers.[193]

Clinical Presentation. The phenotype of EDMD has three main features. First, early contractures appear, selectively affecting the Achilles tendons, elbows, and posterior cervical extensor muscles. This may lead to the rigid spine syndrome as a result of lumbar and cervicodorsal contractures.[194] Second, muscle atrophy and weakness arise in a characteristic humeroperoneal distribution. As the disease evolves in a slowly progressive manner in the first three decades, scapular and proximal limb-girdle musculatures are also affected. Unlike the myotonic dystrophies, severe respiratory muscle impairment is not a common finding. Third, cardiac manifestations arise, typically after the second decade of life, and are the main source of morbidity and mortality in EDMD due to sudden death or progressive HF.

Cardiac Manifestations. Typically, EDMD leads to sinus bradycardia and conduction disease.[195] Atrial paralysis with loss of electrical and mechanical activity is characteristic of the disease. Absence of P wave, loss of impulse generation by the sinus node, and a junctional escape rhythm are common signs of atrial paralysis, which predispose patients to future embolic events.[196] Adipose and fibrous tissue are seen in atrial and ventricular myocardia (but not in the conduction system), resulting in a substrate for arrhythmias.[197] Similar to other muscular dystrophies, both atrial tachycardia and VT are frequently encountered and can lead to sudden death despite pacemaker placement.[198] Dilated cardiomyopathy with systolic dysfunction has also been reported in this patient group, especially in the autosomal dominant form.[196,199] Symptoms include syncope, shortness of breath, dizziness, poor exercise tolerance, palpitations, and signs of congestive HF.[195] Sudden death is the most common cause of mortality in these patients, and it can arise prior to any cardiac or muscular symptom, mostly in young healthy adults.[200,201] A large meta-analysis reported a mean age at death of 46 years.[198] Female carriers of the X-linked mutation may be spared from muscle disease but are nonetheless at risk of arrhythmias and sudden death, typically occurring at an older age.[202,203]

Management. Due to the high risk of sudden death, patients with EDMD should be closely monitored for conduction disease with yearly ECG or Holter monitoring. Pacemaker implantation is needed in severe sinus or AV nodal disease.[204] There are no specific guidelines on the optimal age for device implantation, but most patients receive a pacemaker by the age of 30.[205] However, prophylactic pacemakers may not protect patients from sudden death due to ventricular arrhythmias.[198,204,206] Risk factors for sudden death and appropriate ICD therapy include nonsustained VT on Holter monitoring, an LVEF <45%, male sex, and nonmissense mutations (ins-del/truncating or mutations affecting splicing) of lamin A/C.[207] Monitoring for dilated cardiomyopathy and HF with regular echocardiograms is indicated as these patients may benefit from medical therapy. Anticoagulation with vitamin K antagonists is appropriate in patients with atrial standstill due to the risk of stroke.[204]

Limb-Girdle Muscular Dystrophy

Genetics and Pathophysiology. Limb-girdle muscular dystrophies (LGMDs) are characterized by varying genetic and clinical presentations. At least 27 different muscular diseases are currently classified as LGMDs. Classically, LGMDs are grouped into autosomal dominant LGMD (LGMD1) and autosomal recessive LGMD (LGMD2), and the estimated overall prevalence of LGMD ranges from 1:23,000 to 1:150,000.[208] Protein defects can arise from any component of the muscle fiber, including cell signaling, sarcolemmal repair, and structural proteins related to the dystrophin–glycoprotein complex, the nuclear lamina, or the sarcomere.[209]

Clinical Presentation. LGMD universally presents with muscle weakness, particularly in the pelvic and proximal limb musculature. Onset is early, usually by the age of 30 years. Autosomal dominant forms are rare and generally less severe than recessive types.

Cardiac Manifestations. Cardiac involvement is common in the autosomal dominant LGMD1B. This disorder is caused by a mutation in the lamin A/C and has a similar phenotype as the previously described autosomal dominant EDMD. In brief, it is characterized by a high prevalence of conduction defects and AV blocks, atrial paralysis, arrhythmias, and sudden death despite pacemaker implantation.[198] Dilated cardiomyopathy may also be seen at a later stage possibly leading to HF. LGMD1E is a rare disease with phenotype similar to that of LGMD1B.[210] Cardiac involvement in the remaining LGMDs is clustered mainly in the autosomal recessive subtypes (LGMD2B-F and 2I). The hallmark of cardiac disease in these patients is dilated cardiomyopathy and ventricular dysfunction, although overt cardiac dysfunction is rare and no correlation between skeletal muscle and cardiac involvement is seen.[211,212] ECG manifestations include left or right bundle branch blocks, LVH, RV hypertrophy, and Q waves in the lateral leads.[213,214] The significantly impaired LV systolic function is associated with life-threatening arrhythmias.[212] Echocardiography can range from normal to severely dilated cardiomyopathy depending on the subtype. Regional wall abnormalities can be seen with a slight increase in the end-diastolic volume and a decrease in EF. In a study of LGMD2I cases, cardiac MRI showed early functional and morphological ventricular impairment along with increased wall fibrosis and fatty replacement.[214]

Management. The recommendations for cardiac monitoring in patients with LGMD depend on the subtype as various genotypes show variable cardiac involvement. As such, cardiac surveillance is not indicated in LGMD2A-B,G,H,J and LGMD1A,C.[204] Patients with LGMD2B-F and 2I should receive ECG and echocardiography as standard initial assessment as well as for follow-up. Any rhythm or conduction abnormality should prompt further investigation with Holter monitoring. In patients with severe dilated cardiomyopathy, cardiac transplant can be therapeutic. Regarding patients with LGMD1B, management is similar to that in patients with the aforementioned EDMD as the phenotype and disease history of the two disorders are nearly identical.

Duchenne Muscular Dystrophy and Becker Muscular Dystrophy

Genetics and Pathophysiology. Duchenne muscular dystrophy (DMD) and Becker muscular dystrophy (BMD) are X-linked recessive disorders of the Dystrophin gene located at Xp21. The affected protein, dystrophin, is part of a large multimeric protein complex, the dystrophin–glycoprotein complex, located in the sarcolemma. It acts as a link between the actin cytoskeleton and the muscle membrane. Disruption of this protein complex leads to membrane fragility, making muscle cells susceptible to contraction-induced damage.[215] As the disease advances, regenerative processes cannot adequately sustain the ongoing muscle damage, yielding progressive degeneration of skeletal and cardiac myocytes, and replacement with fibrofatty tissue, resulting in muscle weakness.[216] Dystrophin is completely absent in DMD due to a frameshift mutation. In BMD, dystrophin is reduced in amount or size since the mutation conserves the reading frame, making BMD a milder variant of DMD with a better prognosis.[217]

Clinical Presentation. DMD is the most common muscular dystrophy with an incidence of 1 in 3500 male newborns and a prevalence of 6 in 100,000 in the male population.[218] The onset of DMD occurs in early childhood, and most boys present before the age of 5 years. DMD manifests as proximal weakness in the leg, shoulder, and pelvic girdle muscles, resulting in difficulties in running and climbing stairs. Affected children display the Gower maneuver due to weakness in the knees and hip extensors. Most patients have pseudo-hypertrophy of the calves due to fibrofatty replacement of the muscle tissue. Weakness is progressive, and patients become wheelchair-bound by the age of 12 in most cases. Respiratory muscles become compromised, and cardiomyopathy typically develops in the second decade. Symptoms associated with cardiac defects may be masked by the progressive muscle weakness and reduced physical activity. Pneumonia in the setting of respiratory failure and cardiac disease is the most frequent cause of death. The improved accessibility to invasive ventilation has significantly delayed the mortality of DMD patients from the late teens to the late 20s.[219] Mental impairment is present in some cases, and about 20% have an IQ of less than 70.

BMD has a later onset (12 years on average) and a more benign course. It has an incidence of approximately 1 in 18,450 males and a prevalence of 2.4 per 100,000.[220] Distribution of muscle weakness is similar to that in DMD, but mortality occurs between the fourth and fifth decades.[221]

In female carriers of the DMD or BMD mutation, some level of muscle weakness and enlarged calves is seen in 5%–10% of the cases. Onset of symptoms ranges from childhood to adulthood, and the disease can be progressive or remain static.

Cardiac Manifestations. In DMD, cardiac involvement is first evident after 10 years of age and is ubiquitous after 18.[222,223] Typical ECG findings include sinus tachycardia, short PR, a tall R wave in V1, inferolateral Q waves, and complete or incomplete bundle branch blocks.[224] Arrhythmias are commonly reported in DMD, and their incidence increases with age and impaired ventricular function. Sinus or AV node dysfunction, AFL, premature atrial and ventricular beats, and ventricular arrhythmias may all occur.[225] Cardiomyopathy in DMD progresses from hypertrophy and dilation to frank systolic dysfunction.[223] Echocardiography (2D) shows LV dysfunction and wall motion abnormalities at 10–15 years, but tissue Doppler shows ongoing myocardial damage in earlier age groups.[226] Cardiac MRI is an important screening tool as it can reveal early and subclinical myocardial fibrosis.[227] Positron emission tomography (PET) metabolic imaging shows a predilection for the posterobasal and posterolateral walls of the left ventricle.

An acute form of accelerated myocardial cell damage may transiently occur and mimics myocardial ischemia in presentation (acute chest pain), ECG (ST-elevation, T wave inversion), echocardiography (regional akinesia and decreased EF), and chemical markers (troponin I elevation).[228] However, the mechanism of such an acute event has not been elucidated. Cardiac disease causes death in 10%–20% of DMD patients, either by progressive congestive HF or by sudden death due to arrhythmia. However, with advances in invasive respiratory support of these patients, primary cardiac death is expected to rise.

BMD patients invariably suffer from cardiomyopathy, albeit at a later age than DMD patients.[229,230] Cardiac involvement is often out of proportion to the level of skeletal muscle impairment. A subset of BMD patients experience severe dilated cardiomyopathy at an early age, requiring early medical therapy or transplant.[231] Primary cardiac death in BMD is estimated at 50% of cases due to the lower respiratory muscle impairment as compared with DMD.

Up to 40% of female carriers of the BMD or DMD mutation may experience arrhythmias or hypertrophic or dilated cardiomyopathy, with an equal distribution among BMD and DMD carriers.[232,233] A larger percentage of patients bear subclinical myocardial involvement, and this percentage increases significantly with age. However, the burden of cardiac disease on life expectancy or cardiac death is still unclear.[234]

Management. The number of DMD patients reaching adulthood is significantly increasing, owing to advancements in respiratory support, emphasizing the importance of proper cardiac screening and management. Initial evaluation at diagnosis of DMD or BMD consists of ECG, echocardiography, and possibly Holter monitoring. Cardiac MRI is able to detect early changes in cases where echocardiography is still normal and thus guide clinicians on the appropriate timing to start cardioprotective treatment.[235] Screening is recommended every 2 years until the age of 10 in DMD patients and annually thereafter.[204] In BMD patients, screening is recommended at least every 5 years. ICDs are appropriate in patients presenting with ventricular arrhythmias, but their implantation may be challenging in cases of severe kyphoscoliosis.

Therapy for skeletal muscle disease consists of glucocorticoids starting at the age of 5, and there is no evidence of detrimental effect on the heart.[236] Cardiac management with early, preventive angiotensin-converting enzyme (ACE) inhibitors has been shown to be effective in maintaining a ventricular function after 5 years of therapy, with a proven 10-year mortality benefit in DMD patients.[237] The combination of ACE inhibitor/angiotensin II receptor blocker (ARB) with β-blocker in DMD and BMD patients seems to impart significant beneficial effects.[238] Cardiac transplantation was successful in cases of BMD.[239]

Because of the unclear burden of cardiomyopathy in carriers of BMD and DMD, cardiac screening is recommended at diagnosis or after the age of 16 years and at least every 5 years thereafter to detect early cardiac disease and initiate ACE inhibitor therapy. Additional studies are needed in this patient group to confirm the mortality benefit of early treatment.

Facioscapulohumeral Muscular Dystrophy

Genetics and Pathophysiology. Facioscapulohumeral muscular dystrophy (FSHD) is an autosomal dominant muscular dystrophy with a prevalence of 1 in 20,000.[240] It is caused by a deletion in the D4Z4 repeat elements at 4q35.[241] This gain-of-function mutation leads to decreased DNA methylation, opening of the chromatin structure, and inappropriate expression of the *DUX4* gene.[242]

Clinical Presentation. FSHD typically appears in the first or second decade but may appear in older individuals.[243] It is characterized by asymmetric and often descending weakness in the face, shoulder girdle, and proximal arms followed by the lower extremities and pelvic girdle.[240] Progression of the disease is slow, but its severity correlates with the residual fragment size.[243] It is estimated that 20% of patients above the age of 50 will be wheelchair bound, but patients with greater D4Z4 contractures suffer earlier functional impairment during the second decade.[244] Respiratory impairment is seen in 10% of the cases, mostly in those with the most severe muscular manifestations. Similarly, patients with greater D4Z4 contractures suffer from extramuscular involvement, including retinal vascular disease, hearing loss, cognitive impairment, or seizures.[245,246]

Cardiac Manifestations. Cardiac involvement in FSHD is rare and, in many cases, unrelated to the disease itself.[247] Reported arrhythmias in FSHD are AV block, intraventricular conduction delay, and supraventricular tachycardias.[248–250]

Management. Due to the low incidence of cardiac disease, echocardiography and ECG are only recommended at diagnosis and upon signs of cardiac disturbance.[204]

Friedreich Ataxia

Genetics and Pathophysiology
Friedreich ataxia (FA) is an autosomal recessive degenerative disease with a prevalence of 1:50,000 in the United States. It is the most common form of inherited ataxia. The mutated locus on chromosome 9q13 codes for the mitochondrial protein frataxin, which is involved in oxidative metabolism.[251] The mutation, a GAA trinucleotide expansion with 120–1700 repeats, must be found on both alleles to manifest the disease. Lower levels of frataxin are found in FA as the triplet expansion is thought to induce silencing of the gene.[252] Frataxin deficiency is associated with mitochondrial iron accumulation and abnormalities of adenosine triphosphate (ATP) synthesis, which lead to the production of reactive oxygen species in nervous, cardiac, and pancreatic tissues. FA is associated with degeneration of neurons in the cerebellum and dorsal root ganglion, leading to ataxia and loss of proprioception.

Clinical Presentation
Onset of the disease occurs typically around the teenage years, but symptoms may appear earlier.[253] Presenting symptoms usually are difficulty in walking, dysarthria, and loss of coordination and proprioception.[254,255] FA is a multisystem disorder leading to eclectic manifestations such as hypertrophic cardiomyopathy, diabetes, insulin resistance, and scoliosis. Studies have shown that larger GAA expansions correlate with earlier onset of the disease as well as a higher frequency of cardiomyopathy and functional impairment.[254] The disease has a slow progression with an average time from onset to death of 36 years, and most patients are wheelchair-bound by the third decade.

Cardiac Manifestations
Cardiac involvement in FA occurs in more than 90% of the cases and does not correlate with the degree of neurological deficit.[256] Heart disease typically follows neurological manifestations and is often clinically silent due to the restricted physical activity of the patients. Classically, concentric LVH is seen on ultrasound. Later stages are characterized by myocardial atrophy and fibrosis, leading to dilated cardiomyopathy.[257,258] Occasionally, an asymmetric LV septal hypertrophy occurs, leading to outflow obstruction.

ECG abnormalities are found in the vast majority of patients and reflect the hypertrophic process in the ventricle.[259] The most commonly reported changes are nonspecific ST-T wave changes, LVH or RVH patterns, axis deviation, and PR shortening or prolongation, reflecting atrial disease.[260,261] Impulse formation and conduction is intact in all reports. Atrial and ventricular tachyarrhythmias have been reported in FA, especially in patients with dilated cardiomyopathy, and predict a worse prognosis.[262-264] Cardiac disease, including HF and sudden death, is the most common cause of mortality.[262]

Management
Once cardiac disease is documented in FA, physicians should perform a close follow-up of patients for monitoring of symptoms or ECG findings of arrhythmias that warrant the need for a pacemaker or an ICD. Screening ECGs, echocardiography, and Holter monitoring should be done routinely due to the progressive but unpredictable nature of cardiac disease. Current guidelines on device placement in the setting of HF, neuromuscular diseases, and ventricular arrhythmias should be followed.[181,265]

Routinely used agents for FA cardiomyopathy are ACE inhibitors, ARB, digoxin, calcium channel blockers, and β-blockers in the setting of symptomatic hypertrophic/congestive HF; however, there is little evidence on the benefit of initiating treatment in the presymptomatic phases. Select patients may benefit from heart transplantation.[266]

Mitochondrial Diseases

Genetics and Pathophysiology
Mitochondrial diseases (MitDs) are a heterogeneous group of inherited anomalies in oxidative phosphorylation due to mutations in the mitochondrial (70%) or nuclear DNA (30%). Mitochondrial DNA mutations behave recessively and exhibit strict maternal inheritance, whereas nuclear DNA anomalies are inherited in an autosomal fashion. Sporadic mutations have also been reported. Reactive oxygen species, promoted by the absence of functional mitochondria, are known to play a role in the cytotoxicity of MitD.[267] As organ involvement in MitD is wide and varied across genotypes, tissue specificity of mutation load is an important factor in generating the clinical picture.[268]

Clinical Presentation
MitDs are common, with an estimated prevalence of clinical disease of 9.2 per 100,000 adults <65 years of age and a mutation prevalence of 16.5 per 100,000 adults <65 years of age.[269] The disease may present at any age and involve any organ, particularly those with high energy-requirements like the brain, heart, eye, and skeletal muscle.[270] Disease manifestations may be restricted to one organ or may have multisystemic features. Mortality in these patients is most commonly attributed to neurological and cardiac disease.

Cardiac Manifestations
Cardiac involvement in MitD is progressive and affects morbidity and mortality.[271,272] The most reported pattern in MitD is hypertrophic cardiomyopathy, occurring in 40% of patients.[272] Hypertrophic disease often progresses to LV dilatation and impaired systolic function but rarely causes outflow tract obstruction.[271] In rare cases, dilated or restrictive cardiomyopathies can be the primary manifestation. LV noncompaction or hypertrabeculation is increasingly being recognized as a manifestation of MitD, commonly in the setting of a multisystem disease.[273]

Arrhythmias can be reported in any MitD with cardiomyopathy but are more common in certain subtypes, such as Kearns-Sayre syndrome (KSS), mitochondrial encephalomyopathy lactic acidosis and stroke-like episode syndrome (MELAS), Leber hereditary optic neuropathy (LHON), myoclonic epilepsy with ragged-red fibers syndrome (MERRF), and Leigh syndrome (LS). Conduction defects, such as advanced AV block, are typically reported in KSS along with progressive ophthalmoplegia and atypical pigment retinopathy. Ventricular preexcitation and Wolff-Parkinson-White syndrome are frequently seen in MitDs, such as MELAS, MERRF, and LHON. There is a reported association between MitDs and prolonged QT.[274] Other reported electrical abnormalities include bundle blocks, premature ventricular beats, bradyarrhythmias, AF, and VTs.[275] Sudden death, attributed to severe conduction disease or arrhythmias, is a well-recognized cause of mortality, with varying contribution to all-cause deaths depending on the syndrome.[276]

Management
Baseline cardiac assessment at diagnosis should include 12-lead ECG and echocardiography. Cardiac MRI permits the early detection of cardiac involvement using late gadolinium enhancement and may identify patients at risk of developing cardiomyopathy.

Standard optimal therapy for hypertrophy and HF, including medical treatment and ICD implantation, is used in MitD.[277] Heart transplant has been successful in MitD patients with lower extracardiac disease burden.[278] Progression to high-grade AV block is unpredictable, and it is recommended that a pacemaker be implanted in patients with neuromuscular disease displaying third- or advanced second-degree AV block (class I recommendation) or any degree of AV or fascicular block (class IIb recommendation).[181] Similar to other muscular dystrophies with conduction disease, significant H-V interval prolongation (>70 ms) may warrant device implantation. Primary prevention ICD implantation is less clear in

MitDs. Ventricular preexcitation is successfully treated with radio-frequency ablation of the accessory pathways.

Periodic Paralysis

Genetics and Pathophysiology

The familial periodic paralyses (PPs) are caused by autosomal dominant mutations in ion channels and are characterized by episodic flaccid paralysis triggered in most cases by variations in potassium (K^+) levels. Three genetic forms are recognized in this disease family. Hyperkalemic PP is caused by a gain-of-function mutation in the voltage-gated sodium (Na^+) channel involved in generating muscle action potentials. It leads to an increased influx of Na^+ and a sustained membrane depolarization, driving K^+ extracellularly and causing muscle paralysis.[279] Hypokalemic PP is associated with a loss-of-function mutation in either the L-type dihydropyridine Ca^+ receptor located on the T-tubules or the voltage-gated Na^+ channel. These mutations favor the inactivated state of the Na^+ channels, producing lasting membrane depolarization and fiber inexcitability.[280,281] Patients with Andersen-Tawil syndrome (ATS) have a mutation in the gene encoding the inward rectifier K^+ channel in both skeletal and cardiac muscles.[282] The function of these channels is to promote repolarization of the membrane, and mutation in the gene encoding these leads to membrane inexcitability, causing paralysis and arrhythmias.

Clinical Presentation

Hyperkalemic PP, with a prevalence of 1:200,000, is provoked by an increase in serum K^+ (e.g., after the ingestion of K^+-rich food), rest after exercise, stress, fasting, or pregnancy. Glucose intake is a remedy. In between the episodes, patients may experience transient and mild myotonia. In contrast, hypokalemic PP, with a prevalence of 1:100,000, is triggered by low K^+ levels and is particularly sensitive to carbohydrate- and sodium-rich food. K^+ improves patient condition, and myotonia has not been reported in these cases. The attacks in the hypokalemic subtype are generally longer and more severe than hyperkalemic PP. During an attack, respiratory insufficiency may be fatal. In both conditions, disturbances of K^+ can be severe enough to cause arrhythmias. As patients get older, they can develop a chronic progressive myopathy, typically in the fifth decade. It affects mostly the pelvic girdle and lower limbs and is due to fatty replacement of the muscles. Patients with ATS present with a characteristic triad of PP, cardiac dysrhythmias, and dysmorphic features, including hypertelorism, mandibular hypoplasia, low-set ears, syndactyly, clinodactyly, cleft palate, and scoliosis.[283] ATS is rare, with a prevalence of 1:1,000,000 and displays phenotypic variability. The paralytic attacks can occur in hypo-, hyper- or normokalemic conditions with an unpredictable response to K^+.

Cardiac Manifestations

Patients with ATS may present with ECG abnormalities, including prominent U waves on anterior precordial leads, prolonged QT and QU intervals, premature ventricular contractions, and ventricular bigeminy. Reported arrhythmias in PP are polymorphic VTs (including torsades de pointes) and bidirectional VTs.[284] Ventricular arrhythmias in ATS occur independently of the paralytic attacks or the K^+ level and are rarely life threatening. Ventricular arrhythmias in the hypo- and hyperkalemic PP include torsades de pointes and may cause syncope or sudden death.

Management

Hyperkalemic PP responds to carbohydrate ingestion, inhalation of salbutamol, or correction of K^+ levels. First-line medications given for prophylaxis in all three types of PP are carbonic anhydrase inhibitors (acetazolamide or dichlorphenamide). Stabilizing the K^+ level is an essential component of paralysis and arrhythmia prevention. In ATS, propranolol and verapamil reduce the burden of PVCs and VTs.[285] When added to β-blockers, amiodarone and flecainide have been observed to reduce polymorphic and bidirectional VTs, respectively.[286–288] Recurrent polymorphic VTs resistant to drug therapy, prior cardiac arrest, and a high overall risk profile warrant ICD implantation, although the efficacy of ICDs is debatable in lower risk ATS patients.

Myasthenia Gravis

Pathophysiology and Presentation

Myasthenia gravis (MG) is an autoimmune disorder caused by antibodies to the nicotinic acetylcholine receptors at the neuromuscular junction. Prevalence of this disease is estimated to be 20 per 100,000 in the United States.[289] Women younger than 40 years of age are three times more likely to be affected by MG than men of the same age group, whereas men are more likely to suffer from MG above the age of 50.[290] The triggering mechanism is unknown, but thymus gland abnormalities as well as genetic predisposition seem to play a determining role.[291,292] MG is typically associated with hyperplasia of the thyroid or an epithelial neoplasia (thymoma). Clinically, fluctuating weakness that worsens with activity and improves with rest is characteristic of the disease. Patients present initially with ocular weakness manifesting as ptosis and diplopia. Other common symptoms are dysarthria, dysphagia, facial weakness, or limb or axial weakness. MG can progress to generalized weakness where respiratory impairment can be life threatening.[290]

Cardiac Manifestations

Myocarditis is a rare complication of MG, with important prognostic implications due to its potentially fatal manifestations. It was more commonly found in patients with thymoma than those without thymoma. The pathophysiology is unclear as the typical antinicotinic receptor autoantibodies do not bind to the heart. In fact, other antibodies commonly found in these patients seem to be responsible for the myocardial inflammation.[293] Symptoms range from dyspnea and chest pain to cardiogenic shock and sudden death due to arrhythmias.[293] The true prevalence of cardiac involvement may be underestimated due to the physical restriction of patients with MG. Pathological specimens range from simple lymphocytic invasion to frank myofibrillar necrosis and edema.[294] ECG abnormalities are widely reported in MG patients, both with and without evidence of myocarditis, and include ST and T wave abnormalities; QT prolongation; and conduction abnormalities, such as second- or third-degree AV block, bundle branch blocks, and sinus arrest.[293,294] Arrhythmias are recorded in approximately 10% of MG cases and include supraventricular tachycardia, AF, and VT (including torsades de pointes). SCD, typically attributed to arrhythmia, is a common cause of death in MG.

Management

The treatment of MG consists of immune and supportive therapy. Cardiac screening at diagnosis has been recommended in all patients. Due to the masking of cardiac symptoms by MG, physicians should maintain a low threshold for patients to undergo cardiac monitoring with ECG and/or echocardiography during MG exacerbations, even after thymectomy. Pacemaker implantation is warranted in severe conduction disease.

Concluding Remarks

This chapter has provided a basic overview of neurological disorders that commonly present with arrhythmic manifestations. The fascinating and essential interaction between the CNS, ANS, myocardium, and cardiac conduction system is easily perturbed and can lead to devastating complications in the setting of neurological disorders. The appropriate management of arrhythmia in patients with primary neurological disease is best achieved by close collaboration between neurology and cardiology.

REFERENCES

1. Banki NM, Zaroff JG. Neurogenic cardiac injury. *Curr Treat Options Cardiovasc Med*. 2003;5:451–458.
2. Oehmichen M, Pedal I, Hohmann P. Diagnostic significance of myofibrillar degeneration of cardiocytes in forensic pathology. *Forensic Sci Int*. 1990;48:163–173.
3. Wittstein IS, Thiemann DR, Lima JA, et al. Neurohumoral features of myocardial stunning due to sudden emotional stress. *N Engl J Med*. 2005;352:539–548.
4. Leor J, Poole WK, Kloner RA. Sudden cardiac death triggered by an earthquake. *N Engl J Med*. 1996;334:413–419.
5. Benarroch EE. The central autonomic network: functional organization, dysfunction, and perspective. *Mayo Clin Proc*. 1993;68:988–1001.
6. Verberne AJM, Owens NC. Cortical modulation of the cardiovascular system. *Prog Neurobiol*. 1998;54:149–168.
7. Napadow V, Dhond R, Conti G, Makris N, Brown EN, Barbieri R. Brain correlates of autonomic modulation: combining heart rate variability with fMRI. *Neuroimage*. 2008;42:169–177.
8. Lane RD, McRae K, Reiman EM, Chen K, Ahern GL, Thayer JF. Neural correlates of heart rate variability during emotion. *Neuroimage*. 2009;44:213–222.
9. Zhang ZH, Dougherty PM, Oppenheimer SM. Characterization of baroreceptor-related neurons in the monkey insular cortex. *Brain Res*. 1998;796:303–306.
10. Zamrini EY, Meador KJ, Loring DW, et al. Unilateral cerebral inactivation produces differential left/right heart rate responses. *Neurology*. 1990;40:1408–1411.
11. Christensen H, Boysen G, Christensen AF, Johannesen HH. Insular lesions, ECG abnormalities, and outcome in acute stroke. *J Neurol Neurosurg Psychiatry*. 2005;76:269–271.
12. Allen GV, Cechetto DF. Functional and anatomical organization of cardiovascular pressor and depressor sites in the lateral hypothalamic area: I. Descending projections. *J Comp Neurol*. 1992;315:313–332.
13. Allen GV, Cechetto DF. Functional and anatomical organization of cardiovascular pressor and depressor sites in the lateral hypothalamic area. II. Ascending projections. *J Comp Neurol*. 1993;330:421–438.
14. Fernandes KB, Tavares RF, Pelosi GG, Correa FM. The paraventricular nucleus of hypothalamus mediates the pressor response to noradrenergic stimulation of the medial prefrontal cortex in unanesthetized rats. *Neurosci Lett*. 2007;426:101–105.
15. Tavares RF, Pelosi GG, Correa FM. The paraventricular nucleus of the hypothalamus is involved in cardiovascular responses to acute restraint stress in rats. *Stress*. 2009;12:178–185.
16. Naredi S, Lambert G, Eden E, et al. Increased sympathetic nervous activity in patients with nontraumatic subarachnoid hemorrhage. *Stroke*. 2000;31:901–906.
17. Masuda T, Sato K, Yamamoto S, et al. Sympathetic nervous activity and myocardial damage immediately after subarachnoid hemorrhage in a unique animal model. *Stroke*. 2002;33:1671–1676.
18. Elrifai AM, Bailes JE, Shih SR, Dianzumba S, Brillman J. Characterization of the cardiac effects of acute subarachnoid hemorrhage in dogs. *Stroke*. 1996;27:737–741. discussion 741–742.
19. Shivalkar B, Van Loon J, Wieland W, et al. Variable effects of explosive or gradual increase of intracranial pressure on myocardial structure and function. *Circulation*. 1993;87:230–239.
20. Kawahara E, Ikeda S, Miyahara Y, Kohno S. Role of autonomic nervous dysfunction in electrocardiographic abnormalities and cardiac injury in patients with acute subarachnoid hemorrhage. *Circ J*. 2003;67:753–756.
21. Novitzky D, Wicomb WN, Cooper DK, Rose AG, Reichart B. Prevention of myocardial injury during brain death by total cardiac sympathectomy in the Chacma baboon. *Ann Thorac Surg*. 1986;41:520–524.
22. Reichenbach D, Benditt EP. Myofibrillar degeneration: a common form of cardiac muscle injury. *Ann N Y Acad Sci*. 1969;156:164–176.
23. Karch SB, Billingham ME. Myocardial contraction bands revisited. *Hum Pathol*. 1986;17:9–13.
24. Fineschi V, Michalodimitrakis M, D'Errico S, et al. Insight into stress-induced cardiomyopathy and sudden cardiac death due to stress. A forensic cardio-pathologist point of view. *Forensic Sci Int*. 2010;194:1–8.
25. Singal PK, Kapur N, Dhillon KS, Beamish RE, Dhalla NS. Role of free radicals in catecholamine-induced cardiomyopathy. *Can J Physiol Pharmacol*. 1982;60:1390–1397.
26. Jacob WA, Van Bogaert A, De Groodt-Lasseel MH. Myocardial ultrastructure and haemodynamic reactions during experimental subarachnoid haemorrhage. *J Mol Cell Cardiol*. 1972;4:287–298.
27. Rona G. Catecholamine cardiotoxicity. *J Mol Cell Cardiol*. 1985;17:291–306.
28. Burch GE, Meyers R, Abildskov JA. A new electrocardiographic pattern observed in cerebrovascular accidents. *Circulation*. 1954;9:719–723.
29. Sommargren CE, Zaroff JG, Banki N, Drew BJ. Electrocardiographic repolarization abnormalities in subarachnoid hemorrhage. *J Electrocardiol*. 2002;35(suppl):257–262.
30. Di Pasquale G, Pinelli G, Andreoli A, Manini G, Grazi P, Tognetti F. Holter detection of cardiac arrhythmias in intracranial subarachnoid hemorrhage. *Am J Cardiol*. 1987;59:596–600.
31. Kono T, Morita H, Kuroiwa T, Onaka H, Takatsuka H, Fujiwara A. Left ventricular wall motion abnormalities in patients with subarachnoid hemorrhage: neurogenic stunned myocardium. *J Am Coll Cardiol*. 1994;24:636–640.
32. Stead LG, Gilmore RM, Bellolio MF, et al. Prolonged QTc as a predictor of mortality in acute ischemic stroke. *J Stroke Cerebrovasc Dis*. Nov-Dec 2009;18:469–474.
33. Manninen PH, Ayra B, Gelb AW, Pelz D. Association between electrocardiographic abnormalities and intracranial blood in patients following acute subarachnoid hemorrhage. *J Neurosurg Anesthesiol*. 1995;7:12–16.
34. Hjalmarsson C, Bergfeldt L, Bokemark L, Manhem K, Andersson B. Electrocardiographic abnormalities and elevated cTNT at admission for intracerebral hemorrhage: predictors for survival? *Ann Noninvasive Electrocardiol*. 2013;18:441–449.
35. Brouwers PJ, Wijdicks EF, Hasan D, et al. Serial electrocardiographic recording in aneurysmal subarachnoid hemorrhage. *Stroke*. 1989;20:1162–1167.
36. Goldstein DS. The electrocardiogram in stroke: relationship to pathophysiological type and comparison with prior tracings. *Stroke*. 1979;10:253–259.
37. Solenski NJ, Haley Jr EC, Kassell NF, et al. Medical complications of aneurysmal subarachnoid hemorrhage: a report of the multicenter, cooperative aneurysm study. Participants of the Multicenter Cooperative Aneurysm Study. *Crit Care Med*. 1995;23:1007–1017.
38. Schievink WI, Wijdicks EF, Parisi JE, Piepgras DG, Whisnant JP. Sudden death from aneurysmal subarachnoid hemorrhage. *Neurology*. 1995;45:871–874.
39. van der Bilt IA, Hasan D, Vandertop WP, et al. Impact of cardiac complications on outcome after aneurysmal subarachnoid hemorrhage: a meta-analysis. *Neurology*. 2009;72:635–642.
40. Coghlan LA, Hindman BJ, Bayman EO, et al. Independent associations between electrocardiographic abnormalities and outcomes in patients with aneurysmal subarachnoid hemorrhage: findings from the intraoperative hypothermia aneurysm surgery trial. *Stroke*. 2009;40:412–418.
41. Greenspahn BR, Barzilai B, Denes P. Electrocardiographic changes in concussion. *Chest*. 1978;74:468–469.
42. Wittebole X, Hantson P, Laterre PF, et al. Electrocardiographic changes after head trauma. *J Electrocardiol*. 2005;38:77–81.
43. Dash M, Bithal PK, Prabhakar H, Chouhan RS, Mohanty B. ECG changes in pediatric patients with severe head injury. *J Neurosurg Anesthesiol*. 2003;15:270–273.
44. McLeod AA, Neil-Dwyer G, Meyer CH, Richardson PL, Cruickshank J, Bartlett J. Cardiac sequelae of acute head injury. *Br Heart J*. 1982;47:221–226.
45. Bhagat H, Narang R, Sharma D, Dash HH, Chauhan H. ST elevation—an indication of reversible neurogenic myocardial dysfunction in patients with head injury. *Ann Card Anaesth*. 2009;12:149–151.
46. Riera M, Llompart-Pou JA, Carrillo A, Blanco C. Head injury and inverted Takotsubo cardiomyopathy. *J Trauma*. 2010;68:E13–E15.
47. Baroldi G, Di Pasquale G, Silver MD, Pinelli G, Lusa AM, Fineschi V. Type and extent of myocardial injury related to brain damage and its significance in heart transplantation: a morphometric study. *J Heart Lung Transplant*. 1997;16:994–1000.
48. Fernandez-Ortega JF, Prieto-Palomino MA, Garcia-Caballero M, Galeas-Lopez JL, Quesada-Garcia G, Baguley IJ. Paroxysmal sympathetic hyperactivity after traumatic brain injury: clinical and prognostic implications. *J Neurotrauma*. 2012;29:1364–1370.
49. Baguley IJ, Nott MT, Slewa-Younan S, Heriseanu RE, Perkes IE. Diagnosing dysautonomia after acute traumatic brain injury: evidence for overresponsiveness to afferent stimuli. *Arch Phys Med Rehabil*. 2009;90:580–586.
50. Perkes I, Baguley IJ, Nott MT, Menon DK. A review of paroxysmal sympathetic hyperactivity after acquired brain injury. *Ann Neurol*. 2010;68:126–135.
51. Lipton RB, Stewart WF, Diamond S, Diamond ML, Reed M. Prevalence and burden of migraine in the United States: data from the American Migraine Study II. *Headache*. 2001;41:646–657.
52. Melek IM, Seyfeli E, Duru M, Duman T, Akgul F, Yalcin F. Autonomic dysfunction and cardiac repolarization abnormalities in patients with migraine attacks. *Med Sci Monit*. 2007;13:RA47–49.
53. Jhee SS, Salazar DE, Ford NF, Fulmor IE, Sramek JJ, Cutler NR. Monitoring of acute migraine attacks: placebo response and safety data. *Headache*. 1998;38:35–38.
54. Pitarokoili K, Dahlhaus S, Hellwig K, et al. Ventricular tachycardia during basilar-type migraine attack. *Ther Adv Neurol Disord*. 2013;6:35–40.
55. Peterson J, Scruton D, Downie AW. Basilar artery migraine with transient atrial fibrillation. *Br Med J*. 1977;2:1125–1126.
56. Russell D, Storstein L. Chronic paroxysmal hemicrania: heart rate changes and ECG rhythm disturbances. A computerized analysis of 24 h ambulatory ECG recordings. *Cephalalgia*. 1984;4:135–144.
57. Aygun D, Altintop L, Doganay Z, Guven H, Baydin A. Electrocardiographic changes during migraine attacks. *Headache*. 2003;43:861–866.
58. Duru M, Melek I, Seyfeli E, et al. QTc dispersion and P-wave dispersion during migraine attacks. *Cephalalgia*. 2006;26:672–677.
59. May LJ, Millar K, Barlow KM, Dicke F. QTc Prolongation in acute pediatric migraine. *Pediatr Emerg Care*. 2015;31:409–411.
60. Monroe DJ, Meehan JT, Schandl CA. Sudden cardiac death in a young man with migraine-associated arrhythmia. *J Forensic Sci*. 2015;60:1633–1636.
61. Hill SE, Kirsten L. Triptan-induced torsades de pointes and ventricular fibrillation cardiac arrest: case report and review of the literature. *Curr Drug Saf*. 2014;9:236–239.
62. Velez Roa S, Preumont N, Mols P, Stoupel E, Renard M. Ventricular fibrillation secondary to ergotamine in a healthy young woman. *Acta Cardiol*. 1999;54:283–286.
63. Laine K, Raasakka T, Mantynen J, Saukko P. Fatal cardiac arrhythmia after oral sumatriptan. *Headache*. 1999;39:511–512.
64. Hall GC, Brown MM, Mo J, MacRae KD. Triptans in migraine: the risks of stroke, cardiovascular disease, and death in practice. *Neurology*. 2004;62:563–568.
65. Tsuchihashi K, Ueshima K, Uchida T, et al. Transient left ventricular apical ballooning without coronary artery stenosis: a novel heart syndrome mimicking acute myocardial infarction. Angina Pectoris-Myocardial Infarction Investigations in Japan. *J Am Coll Cardiol*. 2001;38:11–18.
66. Connelly KA, MacIsaac AI, Jelinek VM. Stress, myocardial infarction, and the "tako-tsubo" phenomenon. *Heart*. 2004;90:e52.
67. Bybee KA, Kara T, Prasad A, et al. Systematic review: transient left ventricular apical ballooning: a syndrome that mimics ST-segment elevation myocardial infarction. *Ann Int Med*. 2004;141:858–865.
68. Brinjikji W, El-Sayed AM, Salka S. In-hospital mortality among patients with takotsubo cardiomyopathy: a study of the National Inpatient Sample 2008 to 2009. *Am Heart J*. 2012;164:215–221.
69. Lee VH, Connolly HM, Fulgham JR, Manno EM, Brown Jr RD, Wijdicks EF. Tako-tsubo cardiomyopathy in aneurysmal subarachnoid hemorrhage: an underappreciated ventricular dysfunction. *J Neurosurg*. 2006;105:264–270.
70. Finsterer J, Wahbi K. CNS disease triggering Takotsubo stress cardiomyopathy. *Int J Cardiol*. 2014;177:322–329.
71. Abraham J, Mudd JO, Kapur NK, Klein K, Champion HC, Wittstein IS. Stress cardiomyopathy after intravenous administration of catecholamines and beta-receptor agonists. *J Am Coll Cardiol*. 2009;53:1320–1325.
72. Norcliffe-Kaufmann L, Kaufmann H, Martinez J, Katz SD, Tully L, Reynolds HR. Autonomic findings in Takotsubo cardiomyopathy. *Am J Cardiol*. 2016;117:206–213.
73. Abe Y, Kondo M, Matsuoka R, Araki M, Dohyama K, Tanio H. Assessment of clinical features in transient left ventricular apical ballooning. *J Am Coll Cardiol*. 2003;41:737–742.
74. Bybee KA, Prasad A, Barsness GW, et al. Clinical characteristics and thrombolysis in myocardial infarction frame counts in women with transient left ventricular apical ballooning syndrome. *Am J Cardiol*. 2004;94:343–346.
75. Desmet WJ, Adriaenssens BF, Dens JA. Apical ballooning of the left ventricle: first series in white patients. *Heart*. 2003;89:1027–1031.
76. Shoukat S, Awad A, Nam DK, et al. Cardiomyopathy with inverted tako-tsubo pattern in the setting of subarachnoid hemorrhage: a series of four cases. *Neurocrit Care*. 2013;18:257–260.
77. Pant S, Deshmukh A, Mehta K, et al. Burden of arrhythmias in patients with Takotsubo cardiomyopathy (apical ballooning syndrome). *Int J Cardiol*. 2013;170:64–68.
78. Liang CW, Chen R, Macri E, Naval N. Preadmission beta-blockers are associated with decreased incidence of neurogenic stunned myocardium in aneurysmal subarachnoid hemorrhage. *J Stroke Cerebrovasc Dis*. 2013;22:601–607.
79. Ueyama T, Ishikura F, Matsuda A, et al. Chronic estrogen supplementation following ovariectomy improves the emotional stress-induced cardiovascular responses by indirect action on the nervous system and by direct action on the heart. *Circ J*. 2007;71:565–573.

80. Lee YS, Han SW, Kim KS, Kim YN, Cho YW. Incessant monomorphic ventricular tachycardia associated with pneumococcal meningitis: a case report. *J Cardiol*. 2007;50:135–139.
81. Etherington J, Salmon J, Ratcliffe G. Atrio-ventricular dissociation in meningococcal meningitis. *J R Army Med Corps*. 1995;141:169–171.
82. Gach O, Lancellotti P, Pierard LA. Acute ST-segment elevation in *Neisseria* meningitis. *Acta Cardiol*. 2001;56:327–329.
83. Pollock S, Reid H, Klapper P, Metcalfe RA, Ahmed N. Herpes simplex encephalitis presenting as the sick sinus syndrome. *J Neurol Neurosurg Psychiatry*. 1986;49:331–332.
84. Narkiewicz K, van de Borne PJ, Pesek CA, Dyken ME, Montano N, Somers VK. Selective potentiation of peripheral chemoreflex sensitivity in obstructive sleep apnea. *Circulation*. 1999;99:1183–1189.
85. Trombetta IC, Maki-Nunes C, Toschi-Dias E, et al. Obstructive sleep apnea is associated with increased chemoreflex sensitivity in patients with metabolic syndrome. *Sleep*. 2013;36:41–49.
86. Dumitrascu R, Heitmann J, Seeger W, Weissmann N, Schulz R. Obstructive sleep apnea, oxidative stress and cardiovascular disease: lessons from animal studies. *Oxid Med Cell Longev*. 2013;2013:234631.
87. Iwasaki YK, Kato T, Xiong F, et al. Atrial fibrillation promotion with long-term repetitive obstructive sleep apnea in a rat model. *J Am Coll Cardiol*. 2014;64:2013–2023.
88. Sano K, Watanabe E, Hayano J, et al. Central sleep apnoea and inflammation are independently associated with arrhythmia in patients with heart failure. *Eur J Heart Fail*. 2013;15:1003–1010.
89. Mehra R, Benjamin EJ, Shahar E, et al. Association of nocturnal arrhythmias with sleep-disordered breathing: The Sleep Heart Health Study. *Am J Respir Crit Care Med*. 2006;173:910–916.
90. Monahan K, Brewster J, Wang L, et al. Relation of the severity of obstructive sleep apnea in response to anti-arrhythmic drugs in patients with atrial fibrillation or atrial flutter. *Am J Cardiol*. 2012;110:369–372.
91. Gami AS, Howard DE, Olson EJ, Somers VK. Day-night pattern of sudden death in obstructive sleep apnea. *N Engl J Med*. 2005;352:1206–1214.
92. Simantirakis EN, Schiza SI, Marketou ME, et al. Severe bradyarrhythmias in patients with sleep apnoea: the effect of continuous positive airway pressure treatment: a long-term evaluation using an insertable loop recorder. *Eur Heart J*. 2004;25:1070–1076.
93. Kanagala R, Murali NS, Friedman PA, et al. Obstructive sleep apnea and the recurrence of atrial fibrillation. *Circulation*. 2003;107:2589–2594.
94. Fein AS, Shvilkin A, Shah D, et al. Treatment of obstructive sleep apnea reduces the risk of atrial fibrillation recurrence after catheter ablation. *J Am Coll Cardiol*. 2013;62:300–305.
95. Nakao YM, Ueshima K, Yasuno S, Sasayama S. Effects of nocturnal oxygen therapy in patients with chronic heart failure and central sleep apnea: CHF-HOT study. *Heart Vessels*. 2016;31:165–172.
96. Javaheri S. Effects of continuous positive airway pressure on sleep apnea and ventricular irritability in patients with heart failure. *Circulation*. 2000;101:392–397.
97. Cohen M, Hamilton J, Narang I. Clinically important age-related differences in sleep related disordered breathing in infants and children with Prader-Willi Syndrome. *PloS One*. 2014;9:e101012.
98. Correia S, Martins V, Sousa L, Moita J, Teixeira F, Dos Santos JM. Clinical impact of adaptive servoventilation compared to other ventilatory modes in patients with treatment-emergent sleep apnea, central sleep apnea and Cheyne-Stokes respiration. *Rev Port Pneumol (2006)*. 2015;21:132–137.
99. Cowie MR, Woehrle H, Wegscheider K, et al. adaptive servo-ventilation for central sleep apnea in systolic heart failure. *N Engl J Med*. 2015;373:1095–1105.
100. Ficker DM, So EL, Shen WK, et al. Population-based study of the incidence of sudden unexplained death in epilepsy. *Neurology*. 1998;51:1270–1274.
101. Nashef L, Brown S. Epilepsy and sudden death. *Lancet*. 1996;348:1324–1325.
102. Devinsky O. Sudden, unexpected death in epilepsy. *N Engl J Med*. 2011;365:1801–1811.
103. Tavernor SJ, Brown SW, Tavernor RM, Gifford C. Electrocardiograph QT lengthening associated with epileptiform EEG discharges—a role in sudden unexplained death in epilepsy? *Seizure*. 1996;5:79–83.
104. Lamberts RJ, Blom MT, Novy J, et al. Increased prevalence of ECG markers for sudden cardiac arrest in refractory epilepsy. *J Neurol Neurosurg Psychiatry*. 2015;86:309–313.
105. Zijlmans M, Flanagan D, Gotman J. Heart rate changes and ECG abnormalities during epileptic seizures: prevalence and definition of an objective clinical sign. *Epilepsia*. 2002;43:847–854.
106. Opherk C, Coromilas J, Hirsch LJ. Heart rate and EKG changes in 102 seizures: analysis of influencing factors. *Epilepsy Res*. 2002;52:117–127.
107. Espinosa PS, Lee JW, Tedrow UB, Bromfield EB, Dworetzky BA. Sudden unexpected near death in epilepsy: malignant arrhythmia from a partial seizure. *Neurology*. 2009;72:1702–1703.
108. Bardai A, Lamberts RJ, Blom MT, et al. Epilepsy is a risk factor for sudden cardiac arrest in the general population. *PloS One*. 2012;7:e42749.
109. Ryvlin P, Nashef L, Lhatoo SD, et al. Incidence and mechanisms of cardiorespiratory arrests in epilepsy monitoring units (MORTEMUS): a retrospective study. *Lancet Neurol*. 2013;12:966–977.
110. Pool JL, Ransohoff J. Autonomic effects on stimulating rostral portion of cingulate gyri in man. *J Neurophysiol*. 1949;12:385–392.
111. Oppenheimer SM, Gelb A, Girvin JP, Hachinski VC. Cardiovascular effects of human insular cortex stimulation. *Neurology*. 1992;42:1727–1732.
112. Altenmuller DM, Zehender M, Schulze-Bonhage A. High-grade atrioventricular block triggered by spontaneous and stimulation-induced epileptic activity in the left temporal lobe. *Epilepsia*. 2004;45:1640–1644.
113. Devinsky O, Pacia S, Tatambhotla G. Bradycardia and asystole induced by partial seizures: a case report and literature review. *Neurology*. 1997;48:1712–1714.
114. Ansakorpi H, Korpelainen JT, Suominen K, Tolonen U, Myllyla VV, Isojarvi JI. Interictal cardiovascular autonomic responses in patients with temporal lobe epilepsy. *Epilepsia*. 2000;41:42–47.
115. Mukherjee S, Tripathi M, Chandra PS, et al. Cardiovascular autonomic functions in well-controlled and intractable partial epilepsies. *Epilepsy Res*. 2009;85:261–269.
116. Surges R, Adjei P, Kallis C, et al. Pathologic cardiac repolarization in pharmacoresistant epilepsy and its potential role in sudden unexpected death in epilepsy: a case-control study. *Epilepsia*. 2010;51:233–242.
117. Tigaran S, Molgaard H, McClelland R, Dam M, Jaffe AS. Evidence of cardiac ischemia during seizures in drug refractory epilepsy patients. *Neurology*. 2003;60:492–495.
118. Schneider F, Kadel C, Pagitz M, Sen S. Takotsubo cardiomyopathy and elevated troponin levels following cerebral seizure. *Int J Cardiol*. 2010;145:586–587.
119. Nei M, Ho RT, Sperling MR. EKG abnormalities during partial seizures in refractory epilepsy. *Epilepsia*. 2000;41:542–548.
120. Natelson BH, Suarez RV, Terrence CF, Turizo R. Patients with epilepsy who die suddenly have cardiac disease. *Arch Neurol*. 1998;55:857–860.
121. Falconer B, Rajs J. Post-mortem findings of cardiac lesions in epileptics: a preliminary report. *Forensic Sci*. 1976;8:63–71.
122. Lamberts RJ, Blom MT, Wassenaar M, et al. Sudden cardiac arrest in people with epilepsy in the community: circumstances and risk factors. *Neurology*. 2015;85:212–218.
123. Timmings PL. Sudden unexpected death in epilepsy: is carbamazepine implicated? *Seizure*. 1998;7:289–291.
124. Strzelczyk A, Cenusa M, Bauer S, et al. Management and long-term outcome in patients presenting with ictal asystole or bradycardia. *Epilepsia*. 2011;52:1160–1167.
125. Moseley BD, Ghearing GR, Munger TM, Britton JW. The treatment of ictal asystole with cardiac pacing. *Epilepsia*. 2011;52:e16–19.
126. Linzer M, Grubb BP, Ho S, Ramakrishnan L, Bromfield E, Estes NM. Cardiovascular causes of loss of consciousness in patients with presumed epilepsy: a cause of the increased sudden death rate in people with epilepsy? *Am J Med*. 1994;96:146–154.
127. Venkataraman V, Wheless JW, Willmore LJ, Motookal H. Idiopathic cardiac asystole presenting as an intractable adult onset partial seizure disorder. *Seizure*. 2001;10:359–364.
128. McGrogan A, Madle GC, Seaman HE, de Vries CS. The epidemiology of Guillain-Barré syndrome worldwide. A systematic literature review. *Neuroepidemiology*. 2009;32:150–163.
129. Hartung HP, Pollard JD, Harvey GK, Toyka KV. Immunopathogenesis and treatment of the Guillain-Barré syndrome—part I. *Muscle Nerve*. 1995;18:137–153.
130. Teitelbaum JS, Borel CO. Respiratory dysfunction in Guillain-Barré syndrome. *Clin Chest Med*. 1994;15:705–714.
131. Ahmad J, Kham A, Siddiqui M. Estimation of plasma and urinary catecholamines in Guillain-Barré syndrome. *Jpn J Med*. 1985;24:24–29.
132. Winer JB, Hughes RA. Identification of patients at risk of arrhythmia in the Guillain-Barré syndrome. *Q J Med*. 1988;68:735–739.
133. Yoshii F, Kozuma R, Haida M, et al. Giant negative T waves in Guillain-Barré syndrome. *Acta Neurol Scand*. 2000;101:212–215.
134. Tonelli AR, Khasnis A, Abela GS. Peaked T-waves and sinus arrhythmia before prolonged sinus pauses and atrioventricular block in Guillain-Barré syndrome. *Indian Pacing Electrophysiol J*. 2007;7:249–252.
135. Bernstein R, Mayer SA, Magnano A. Neurogenic stunned myocardium in Guillain-Barré syndrome. *Neurology*. 2000;54:759–762.
136. Oka H, Mochio S, Inoue K. Relation between autonomic dysfunction and progression of Parkinson's disease. *Rinsho Shinkeigaku*. 2001;41:283–288.
137. Ishizaki F, Harada T, Yoshinaga H, Nakayama T, Yamamura Y, Nakamura S. Prolonged QTc intervals in Parkinson's disease—relation to sudden death and autonomic dysfunction. *No To Shinkei*. 1996;48:443–448.
138. Deguchi K, Sasaki I, Tsukaguchi M, et al. Abnormalities of rate-corrected QT intervals in Parkinson's disease—a comparison with multiple system atrophy and progressive supranuclear palsy. *J Neurol Sci*. 2002;199:31–37.
139. Oka H, Mochio S, Sato H, Katayama K. Prolongation of QTc interval in patients with Parkinson's disease. *Eur Neurol*. 1997;37:186–189.
140. Malek NM, Grosset KA, Stewart D, Macphee GJ, Grosset DG. Prescription of drugs with potential adverse effects on cardiac conduction in Parkinson's disease. *Parkinsonism Relat Disord*. 2013;19:586–589.
141. Harper PS. Gene mapping and the muscular dystrophies. *Prog Clin Biol Res*. 1989;306:29–49.
142. Mathieu J, De Braekeleer M, Prevost C. Genealogical reconstruction of myotonic dystrophy in the Saguenay-Lac-Saint-Jean area (Quebec, Canada). *Neurology*. 1990;40:839–842.
143. Yotova V, Labuda D, Zietkiewicz E, et al. Anatomy of a founder effect: myotonic dystrophy in northeastern Quebec. *Hum Genet*. 2005;117:177–187.
144. Lavedan C, Hofmann-Radvanyi H, Shelbourne P, et al. Myotonic dystrophy: size- and sex-dependent dynamics of CTG meiotic instability, and somatic mosaicism. *Am J Hum Genet*. 1993;52:875–883.
145. Brook JD, McCurrach ME, Harley HG, et al. Molecular basis of myotonic dystrophy: Expansion of a trinucleotide (CTG) repeat at the 3′ end of a transcript encoding a protein kinase family member. *Cell*. 1992;68:799–808.
146. Liquori CL, Ricker K, Moseley ML, et al. Myotonic dystrophy type 2 caused by a CCTG expansion in intron 1 of ZNF9. *Science*. 2001;293:864–867.
147. Mankodi A, Takahashi MP, Jiang H, et al. Expanded CUG repeats trigger aberrant splicing of ClC-1 chloride channel pre-mRNA and hyperexcitability of skeletal muscle in myotonic dystrophy. *Mol Cell*. 2002;10:35–44.
148. Wheeler TM, Thornton CA. Myotonic dystrophy: RNA-mediated muscle disease. *Curr Opinion Neurol*. 2007;20:572–576.
149. Lee JE, Cooper TA. Pathogenic mechanisms of myotonic dystrophy. *Biochem Soc Trans*. 2009;37:1281–1286.
150. Rau F, Freyermuth F, Fugier C, et al. Misregulation of miR-1 processing is associated with heart defects in myotonic dystrophy. *Nat Struct Mol Biol*. 2011;18:840–845.
151. Mathieu J, Allard P, Potvin L, Prevost C, Begin PA. 10-year study of mortality in a cohort of patients with myotonic dystrophy. *Neurology*. 1999;52:1658–1662.
152. Bogaard JM, van der Meche FG, Hendriks I, Ververs C. Pulmonary function and resting breathing pattern in myotonic dystrophy. *Lung*. 1992;170:143–153.
153. Mathieu J, Allard P, Gobeil G, Girard M, De Braekeleer M, Begin P. Anesthetic and surgical complications in 219 cases of myotonic dystrophy. *Neurology*. 1997;49:1646–1650.
154. Orngreen MC, Arlien-Soborg P, Duno M, Hertz JM, Vissing J. Endocrine function in 97 patients with myotonic dystrophy type 1. *J Neurol*. 2012;259:912–920.
155. Savkur RS, Philips AV, Cooper TA. Aberrant regulation of insulin receptor alternative splicing is associated with insulin resistance in myotonic dystrophy. *Nat Genet*. 2001;29:40–47.
156. Day JW, Ricker K, Jacobsen JF, et al. Myotonic dystrophy type 2: molecular, diagnostic and clinical spectrum. *Neurology*. 2003;60:657–664.
157. Uemura N, Tanaka H, Niimura T, et al. Electrophysiological and histological abnormalities of the heart in myotonic dystrophy. *Am Heart J*. 1973;86:616–624.
158. Thomson AM. Dystrophia cordis myotonica studied by serial histology of the pacemaker and conducting system. *J Pathol Bacteriol*. 1968;96:285–295.
159. Clarke NR, Kelion AD, Nixon J, Hilton-Jones D, Forfar JC. Does cytosine-thymine-guanine (CTG) expansion size predict cardiac events and electrocardiographic progression in myotonic dystrophy? *Heart*. 2001;86:411–416.
160. Melacini P, Villanova C, Menegazzo E, et al. Correlation between cardiac involvement and CTG trinucleotide repeat length in myotonic dystrophy. *J Am Coll Cardiol*. 1995;25:239–245.
161. Merlevede K, Vermander D, Theys P, Legius E, Ector H, Robberecht W. Cardiac involvement and CTG expansion in myotonic dystrophy. *J Neurol*. 2002;249:693–698.
162. Petri H, Vissing J, Witting N, Bundgaard H, Køber L. Cardiac manifestations of myotonic dystrophy type 1. *Int J Cardiol*. 2012;160:82–88.
163. Mörner S, Lindqvist P, Mellberg C, et al. Profound cardiac conduction delay predicts mortality in myotonic dystrophy type 1. *J Int Med*. 2010;268:59–65.

164. Pelargonio G, Dello Russo A, Sanna T, De Martino G, Bellocci F. Myotonic dystrophy and the heart. *Heart*. 2002;88:665–670.

165. Olofsson BO, Forsberg H, Andersson S, Bjerle P, Henriksson A, Wedin I. Electrocardiographic findings in myotonic dystrophy. *Br Heart J*. 1988;59:47–52.

166. Nageh MF. Recurrent fascicular ventricular tachycardia in myotonic dystrophy. *Europace*. 2006;8:336–337.

167. Merino JL, Carmona JR, Fernández-Lozano I, Peinado R, Basterra N, Sobrino JA. Mechanisms of sustained ventricular tachycardia in myotonic dystrophy: implications for catheter ablation. *Circulation*. 1998;98:541–546.

168. Blanck Z, Dhala A, Deshpande S, Sra J, Jazayeri M, Akhtar M. Bundle branch reentrant ventricular tachycardia: cumulative experience in 48 patients. *J Cardiovasc Electrophysiol*. 1993;4:253–262.

169. Bhakta D, Groh MR, Shen C, Pascuzzi RM, Groh WJ. Increased mortality with left ventricular systolic dysfunction and heart failure in adults with myotonic dystrophy type 1. *Am Heart J*. 2010;160:1137–1141.

170. Bhakta D, Lowe MR, Groh WJ. Prevalence of structural cardiac abnormalities in patients with myotonic dystrophy type I. *Am Heart J*. 2004;147:224–227.

171. Child JS, Perloff JK. Myocardial myotonia in myotonic muscular dystrophy. *Am Heart J*. 1995;129:982–990.

172. Lindqvist P, Mörner S, Olofsson BO, et al. Ventricular dysfunction in type 1 myotonic dystrophy: electrical, mechanical, or both? *Int J Cardiol*. 2010;143:378–384.

173. De Ambroggi L, Raisaro A, Marchianò V, Radice S, Meola G. Cardiac involvement in patients with myotonic dystrophy: characteristic features of magnetic resonance imaging. *Eur Heart J*. 1995;16:1007–1010.

174. Wahbi K, Ederhy S, Bécane HM, et al. Impaired myocardial deformation detected by speckle-tracking echocardiography in patients with myotonic dystrophy type 1. *Int J Cardiol*. 2011;152:375–376.

175. Di Cori A, Bongiorni MG, Zucchelli G, et al. Early left ventricular structural myocardial alterations and their relationship with functional and electrical properties of the heart in myotonic dystrophy type 1. *J Am Soc Echocardiogr*. 2009;22:1173–1179.

176. Vinereanu D, Bajaj BPS, Fenton-May J, Rogers MT, Mädler CF, Fraser AG. Subclinical cardiac involvement in myotonic dystrophy manifesting as decreased myocardial Doppler velocities. *Neuromuscul Disord*. 2004;14:188–194.

177. Stöllberger C, Steger C, Gabriel P, Finsterer J. Implantable loop recorders in myotonic dystrophy 1. *Int J Cardiol*. 2011;152:249–251.

178. Kumar S, Sivagangabalan G, Zaman S, et al. Electrophysiology-guided defibrillator implantation early after ST-elevation myocardial infarction. *Heart Rhythm*. 2010;7:1589–1597.

179. Verhaert D, Richards K, Rafael-Fortney JA, Raman SV. Cardiac involvement in patients with muscular dystrophies magnetic resonance imaging phenotype and genotypic considerations. *Circ Cardiovasc Imaging*. 2011;4:67–76.

180. Nazarian S, Bluemke DA, Wagner KR, et al. QRS prolongation in myotonic muscular dystrophy and diffuse fibrosis on cardiac magnetic resonance. *Magn Reson Med*. 2010;64:107–114.

181. Epstein AE, DiMarco JP, Ellenbogen KA, et al. ACC/AHA/HRS 2008 Guidelines for Device-Based Therapy of Cardiac Rhythm Abnormalities: American College of Cardiology/American Heart Association Task Force on Practice Guidelines (Writing Committee to Revise the ACC/AHA/NASPE 2002 Guideline Update for Implantation of Cardiac Pacemakers and Antiarrhythmia Devices) Developed in Collaboration With the American Association for Thoracic Surgery and Society of Thoracic Surgeons. *Heart Rhythm*. 2008;5:e1–e62.

182. Bhakta D, Shen C, Kron J, Epstein AE, Pascuzzi RM, Groh WJ. Pacemaker and implantable cardioverter-defibrillator use in a US myotonic dystrophy type 1 population. *J Cardiovasc Electrophysiol*. 2011;22:1369–1375.

183. Wahbi K, Meune C, Porcher R, et al. Electrophysiological study with prophylactic pacing and survival in adults with myotonic dystrophy and conduction system disease. *JAMA*. 2012;307:1292–1301.

184. Lazarus A, Varin J, Babuty D, Anselme F, Coste J, Duboc D. Long-term follow-up of arrhythmias in patients with myotonic dystrophy treated by pacing: a multicenter diagnostic pacemaker study. *J Am Coll Cardiol*. 2002;40:1645–1652.

185. Laurent V, Pellieux S, Corcia P, et al. Mortality in myotonic dystrophy patients in the area of prophylactic pacing devices. *Int J Cardiol*. 2011;150:54–58.

186. Groh WJ, Groh MR, Saha C, et al. Electrocardiographic abnormalities and sudden death in myotonic dystrophy type 1. *N Engl J Med*. 2008;358:2688–2697.

187. Lau JK, Sy RW, Corbett A, Kritharides L. Myotonic dystrophy and the heart: a systematic review of evaluation and management. *Int J Cardiol*. 2015;184:600–608.

188. Bione S, Maestrini E, Rivella S, et al. Identification of a novel X-linked gene responsible for Emery-Dreifuss muscular dystrophy. *Nat Genet*. 1994;8:323–327.

189. Manilal S, Nguyen TM, Sewry CA, Morris GE. The Emery-Dreifuss muscular dystrophy protein, emerin, is a nuclear membrane protein. *Hum Mol Genet*. 1996;5:801–808.

190. Manilal S, Recan D, Sewry CA, et al. Mutations in Emery-Dreifuss muscular dystrophy and their effects on emerin protein expression. *Hum Mol Genet*. 1998;7:855–864.

191. Bonne G, Di Barletta MR, Varnous S, et al. Mutations in the gene encoding lamin A/C cause autosomal dominant Emery-Dreifuss muscular dystrophy. *Nat Genet*. 1999;21:285–288.

192. Raffaele Di Barletta M, Ricci E, Galluzzi G, et al. Different mutations in the LMNA gene cause autosomal dominant and autosomal recessive Emery-Dreifuss muscular dystrophy. *Am J Hum Genet*. 2000;66:1407–1412.

193. Lammerding J, Hsiao J, Schulze PC, Kozlov S, Stewart CL, Lee RT. Abnormal nuclear shape and impaired mechanotransduction in emerin-deficient cells. *J Cell Biol*. 2005;170:781–791.

194. Bonne G, Quijano-Roy S. Emery–Dreifuss muscular dystrophy, laminopathies, and other nuclear envelopathies. In: Olivier Dulac ML, Harvey BS, eds. *Handbook of Clinical Neurology*. Vol. 113. Amsterdam: Elsevier; 2013:1367–1376.

195. Waters DD, Nutter DO, Hopkins LC, Dorney ER. Cardiac features of an unusual X-linked humeroperoneal neuromuscular disease. *N Engl J Med*. 1975;293:1017–1022.

196. Voit T, Krogmann O, Lenard HG, et al. Emery-Dreifuss muscular dystrophy: disease spectrum and differential diagnosis. *Neuropediatrics*. 1988;19:62–71.

197. Fishbein MC, Siegel RJ, Thompson CE, Hopkins LC. Sudden death of a carrier of X-linked Emery-Dreifuss muscular dystrophy. *Ann Int Med*. 1993;119:900–905.

198. Van Berlo JH, De Voogt WG, Van Der Kooi AJ, et al. Meta-analysis of clinical characteristics of 299 carriers of LMNA gene mutations: do lamin A/C mutations portend a high risk of sudden death? *J Mol Med (Berl)*. 2005;83:79–83.

199. Bonne G, Mercuri E, Muchir A, et al. Clinical and molecular genetic spectrum of autosomal dominant Emery-Dreifuss muscular dystrophy due to mutations of the lamin A/C gene. *Ann Neurol*. 2000;48:170–180.

200. Merlini L, Granata C, Dominici P, Bonfiglioli S. Emery-Dreifuss muscular dystrophy: report of five cases in a family and review of the literature. *Muscle Nerve*. 1986;9:481–485.

201. Becane HM, Bonne G, Varnous S, et al. High incidence of sudden death with conduction system and myocardial disease due to lamins A and C gene mutation. *Pacing Clin Electrophysiol*. 2000;23:1661–1666.

202. Sakata K, Shimizu M, Ino H, et al. High incidence of sudden cardiac death with conduction disturbances and atrial cardiomyopathy caused by a nonsense mutation in the STA gene. *Circulation*. 2005;111:3352–3358.

203. Bialer MG, McDaniel NL, Kelly TE. Progression of cardiac disease in Emery-Dreifuss muscular dystrophy. *Clin Cardiol*. 1991;14:411–416.

204. Bushby K, Muntoni F, Bourke JP. 107th ENMC International Workshop: the management of cardiac involvement in muscular dystrophy and myotonic dystrophy. 7th–9th June 2002, Naarden, The Netherlands. *Neuromuscul Disord*. 2003;13:166–172.

205. Boriani G, Gallina M, Merlini L, et al. Clinical relevance of atrial fibrillation/flutter, stroke, pacemaker implant, and heart failure in Emery-Dreifuss muscular dystrophy: a long-term longitudinal study. *Stroke*. 2003;34:901–908.

206. Meune C, Van Berlo JH, Anselme F, Bonne G, Pinto YM, Duboc D. Primary prevention of sudden death in patients with lamin A/C gene mutations. *N Engl J Med*. 2006;354:209–210.

207. van Rijsingen IA, Arbustini E, Elliott PM, et al. Risk factors for malignant ventricular arrhythmias in lamin A/C mutation carriers a European cohort study. *J Am Coll Cardiol*. 2012;59:493–500.

208. van der Kooi AJ, Barth PG, Busch HF, et al. The clinical spectrum of limb girdle muscular dystrophy. A survey in The Netherlands. *Brain*. 1996;119:1471–1480.

209. Wicklund MP, Kissel JT. The limb-girdle muscular dystrophies. *Neurol Clin*. 2014;32:729–749. ix.

210. Messina DN, Speer MC, Pericak-Vance MA, McNally EM. Linkage of familial dilated cardiomyopathy with conduction defect and muscular dystrophy to chromosome 6q23. *Am J Hum Genet*. 1997;61:909–917.

211. Fanin M, Melacini P, Boito C, Pegoraro E, Angelini C. LGMD2E patients risk developing dilated cardiomyopathy. *Neuromuscul Disord*. 2003;13:303–309.

212. Politano L, Nigro V, Passamano L, et al. Evaluation of cardiac and respiratory involvement in sarcoglycanopathies. *Neuromuscul Disord*. 2001;11:178–185.

213. Melacini P, Fanin M, Duggan DJ, et al. Heart involvement in muscular dystrophies due to sarcoglycan gene mutations. *Muscle Nerve*. 1999;22:473–479.

214. Wahbi K, Meune C, Hamouda EH, et al. Cardiac assessment of limb-girdle muscular dystrophy 2I patients: an echography, Holter ECG and magnetic resonance imaging study. *Neuromuscul Disord*. 2008;18:650–655.

215. Petrof BJ, Shrager JB, Stedman HH, Kelly AM, Sweeney HL. Dystrophin protects the sarcolemma from stresses developed during muscle contraction. *Proc Natl Acad Sci U S A*. 1993;90:3710–3714.

216. Wallace GQ, McNally EM. Mechanisms of muscle degeneration, regeneration, and repair in the muscular dystrophies. *Annu Rev Physiol*. 2009;71:37–57.

217. Monaco AP, Bertelson CJ, Liechti-Gallati S, Moser H, Kunkel LM. An explanation for the phenotypic differences between patients bearing partial deletions of the DMD locus. *Genomics*. 1988;2:90–95.

218. Emery AE. Population frequencies of inherited neuromuscular diseases—a world survey. *Neuromuscul Disord*. 1991;1:19–29.

219. Eagle M, Baudouin SV, Chandler C, Giddings DR, Bullock R, Bushby K. Survival in Duchenne muscular dystrophy: improvements in life expectancy since 1967 and the impact of home nocturnal ventilation. *Neuromuscul Disord*. 2002;12:926–929.

220. Bushby KM, Thambyayah M, Gardner-Medwin D. Prevalence and incidence of Becker muscular dystrophy. *Lancet*. 1991;337:1022–1024.

221. Bushby KM, Gardner-Medwin D. The clinical, genetic and dystrophin characteristics of Becker muscular dystrophy—I. Natural history. *J Neurol*. 1993;240:98–104.

222. Perloff JK. Cardiac rhythm and conduction in Duchenne's muscular dystrophy: a prospective study of 20 patients. *J Am Coll Cardiol*. 1984;3:1263–1268.

223. Nigro G, Comi LI, Politano L, Bain RJ. The incidence and evolution of cardiomyopathy in Duchenne muscular dystrophy. *Int J Cardiol*. 1990;26:271–277.

224. Thrush PT, Allen HD, Viollet L, Mendell JR. Re-examination of the electrocardiogram in boys with Duchenne muscular dystrophy and correlation with its dilated cardiomyopathy. *Am J Cardiol*. 2009;103:262–265.

225. Yanagisawa A, Miyagawa M, Yotsukura M, et al. The prevalence and prognostic significance of arrhythmias in Duchenne type muscular dystrophy. *Am Heart J*. 1992;124:1244–1250.

226. Bahler RC, Mohyuddin T, Finkelhor RS, Jacobs IB. Contribution of Doppler tissue imaging and myocardial performance index to assessment of left ventricular function in patients with Duchenne's muscular dystrophy. *J Am Soc Echocardiogr*. 2005;18:666–673.

227. Silva MC, Meira ZM, Gurgel Giannetti J, et al. Myocardial delayed enhancement by magnetic resonance imaging in patients with muscular dystrophy. *J Am Coll Cardiol*. 2007;49:1874–1879.

228. Ramaciotti C, Iannaccone ST, Scott WA. Myocardial cell damage in Duchenne muscular dystrophy. *Pediatr Cardiol*. 2003;24:503–506.

229. Nigro G, Comi LI, Politano L, et al. Evaluation of the cardiomyopathy in Becker muscular dystrophy. *Muscle Nerve*. 1995;18:283–291.

230. Kirchmann C, Kececioglu D, Korinthenberg R, Dittrich S. Echocardiographic and electrocardiographic findings of cardiomyopathy in Duchenne and Becker-Kiener muscular dystrophies. *Pediatr Cardiol*. 2005;26:66–72.

231. Kaspar RW, Allen HD, Ray WC, et al. Analysis of dystrophin deletion mutations predicts age of cardiomyopathy onset in becker muscular dystrophy. *Circ Cardiovasc Genet*. 2009;2:544–551.

232. Politano L, Nigro V, Nigro G, et al. Development of cardiomyopathy in female carriers of Duchenne and Becker muscular dystrophies. *JAMA*. 1996;275:1335–1338.

233. Hoogerwaard EM, van der Wouw PA, Wilde AA, et al. Cardiac involvement in carriers of Duchenne and Becker muscular dystrophy. *Neuromuscul Disord*. 1999;9:347–351.

234. Holloway SM, Wilcox DE, Wilcox A, et al. Life expectancy and death from cardiomyopathy amongst carriers of Duchenne and Becker muscular dystrophy in Scotland. *Heart*. 2008;94:633–636.

235. Yilmaz A, Gdynia HJ, Baccouche H, et al. Cardiac involvement in patients with Becker muscular dystrophy: new diagnostic and pathophysiological insights by a CMR approach. *J Cardiovasc Magn Reson*. 2008;10:50.

236. Dubrovsky AL, Angelini C, Bonifati DM, Pegoraro E, Mesa L. Steroids in muscular dystrophy: where do we stand? *Neuromuscul Disord*. 1998;8:380–384.

237. Duboc D, Meune C, Pierre B, et al. Perindopril preventive treatment on mortality in Duchenne muscular dystrophy: 10 years' follow-up. *Am Heart J*. 2007;154:596–602.

238. Jefferies JL, Eidem BW, Belmont JW, et al. Genetic predictors and remodeling of dilated cardiomyopathy in muscular dystrophy. *Circulation*. 2005;112:2799–2804.

239. Piccolo G, Azan G, Tonin P, et al. Dilated cardiomyopathy requiring cardiac transplantation as initial manifestation of Xp21 Becker type muscular dystrophy. *Neuromuscul Disord*. 1994;4:143–146.

240. Mostacciuolo ML, Pastorello E, Vazza G, et al. Facioscapulohumeral muscular dystrophy: epidemiological and molecular study in a north-east Italian population sample. *Clin Genet*. 2009;75:550–555.

241. van Deutekom JC, Wijmenga C, van Tienhoven EA, et al. FSHD associated DNA rearrangements are due to deletions of integral copies of a 3.2 kb tandemly repeated unit. *Hum Mol Genet.* 1993;2:2037–2042.

242. Yao Z, Snider L, Balog J, et al. DUX4-induced gene expression is the major molecular signature in FSHD skeletal muscle. *Hum Mol Genet.* 2014;23:5342–5352.

243. Lunt PW. 44th ENMC International Workshop: Facioscapulohumeral Muscular Dystrophy: Molecular Studies: 19–21 July 1996, Naarden, The Netherlands. *Neuromuscul Disord.* 1998;8:126–130.

244. Statland JM, Tawil R. Risk of functional impairment in Facioscapulohumeral muscular dystrophy. *Muscle Nerve.* 2014;49:520–527.

245. Statland JM, Sacconi S, Farmakidis C, Donlin-Smith CM, Chung M, Tawil R. Coats syndrome in facioscapulohumeral dystrophy type 1: frequency and D4Z4 contraction size. *Neurology.* 2013;80:1247–1250.

246. Lutz KL, Holte L, Kliethermes SA, Stephan C, Mathews KD. Clinical and genetic features of hearing loss in facioscapulohumeral muscular dystrophy. *Neurology.* 2013;81:1374–1377.

247. de Visser M, de Voogt WG, la Riviere GV. The heart in becker muscular dystrophy, facioscapulohumeral dystrophy, and bethlem myopathy. *Muscle Nerve.* 1992;15:591–596.

248. Laforêt P, De Toma C, Eymard B, et al. Cardiac involvement in genetically confirmed facioscapulohumeral muscular dystrophy. *Neurology.* 1998;51:1454–1456.

249. Trevisan CP, Pastorello E, Armani M, et al. Facioscapulohumeral muscular dystrophy and occurrence of heart arrhythmia. *Eur Neurol.* 2006;56:1–5.

250. Stevenson WG, Perloff JK, Weiss JN, Anderson TL. Facioscapulohumeral muscular dystrophy: Evidence for selective, genetic electrophysiologic cardiac involvement. *J Am Coll Cardiol.* 1990;15:292–299.

251. Pandolfo M, Pastore A. The pathogenesis of Friedreich ataxia and the structure and function of frataxin. *J Neurol.* 2009;256:9–17.

252. Herman D, Jenssen K, Burnett R, Soragni E, Perlman SL, Gottesfeld JM. Histone deacetylase inhibitors reverse gene silencing in Friedreich's ataxia. *Nat Chem Biol.* 2006;2:551–558.

253. Filla A, DeMichele G, Caruso G, Marconi R, Campanella G. Genetic data and natural history of Friedreich's disease: a study of 80 Italian patients. *J Neurol.* 1990;237:345–351.

254. Dürr A, Cossee M, Agid Y, et al. Clinical and genetic abnormalities in patients with Friedreich's ataxia. *N Engl J Med.* 1996;335:1169–1175.

255. Campuzano V, Montermini L, Molto MD, et al. Friedreich's ataxia: autosomal recessive disease caused by an intronic GAA triplet repeat expansion. *Science.* 1996;271:1423–1427.

256. Child JS, Perloff JK, Bach PM, Wolfe AD, Perlman S, Kark RA. Cardiac involvement in Friedreich's ataxia: a clinical study of 75 patients. *J Am Coll Cardiol.* 1986;7:1370–1378.

257. Casazza F, Morpurgo M. The varying evolution of Friedreich's ataxia cardiomyopathy. *Am J Cardiol.* 1996;77:895–898.

258. Hewer R. The heart in Friedreich's ataxia. *Br Heart J.* 1969;31:5–14.

259. Alboliras ET, Shub C, Gomez MR, et al. Spectrum of cardiac involvement in Friedreich's ataxia: clinical, electrocardiographic and echocardiographic observations. *Am J Cardiol.* 1986;58:518–524.

260. Schadt KA, Friedman LS, Regner SR, Mark GE, Lynch DR, Lin KY. Cross-sectional analysis of electrocardiograms in a large heterogeneous cohort of Friedreich ataxia subjects. *J Child Neurol.* 2012;27:1187–1192.

261. Panas M, Gialafos E, Spengos K, et al. Prevalence of interatrial block in patients with Friedreich's ataxia. *Int J Cardiol.* 2010;145:386–387.

262. Hewer RL. Study of fatal cases of Friedreich's ataxia. *Br Med J.* 1968;3:649–652.

263. Asaad N, El-Menyar A, Al Suwaidi J. Recurrent ventricular tachycardia in patient with Friedreich's ataxia in the absence of clinical myocardial disease. *Pacing Clin Electrophysiol.* 2010;33:109–112.

264. Lee JM, Turner I, Agarwal A, Fynn SP. An unusual atrial tachycardia in a patient with Friedreich ataxia. *Europace.* 2011;13:1660–1661.

265. Zipes DP, Camm AJ, Borggrefe M, et al. ACC/AHA/ESC 2006 guidelines for management of patients with ventricular arrhythmias and the prevention of sudden cardiac death: a report of the American College of Cardiology/American Heart Association Task Force and the European Society of Cardiology Committee for Practice Guidelines (Writing Committee to Develop Guidelines for Management of Patients With Ventricular Arrhythmias and the Prevention of Sudden Cardiac Death). *J Am Coll Cardiol.* 2006;48:e247–e346.

266. Sedlak TL, Chandavimol M, Straatman L. Cardiac transplantation: a temporary solution for Friedreich's ataxia-induced dilated cardiomyopathy. *J Heart Lung Transplant.* 2004;23:1304–1306.

267. Esposito LA, Melov S, Panov A, Cottrell BA, Wallace DC. Mitochondrial disease in mouse results in increased oxidative stress. *Proc Natl Acad Sci U S A.* 1999;96:4820–4825.

268. Muller-Hocker J, Jacob U, Seibel P. The common 4977 base pair deletion of mitochondrial DNA preferentially accumulates in the cardiac conduction system of patients with Kearns-Sayre syndrome. *Mod Pathol.* 1998;11:295–301.

269. Schaefer AM, McFarland R, Blakely EL, et al. Prevalence of mitochondrial DNA disease in adults. *Ann Neurol.* 2008;63:35–39.

270. Tuppen HA, Blakely EL, Turnbull DM, Taylor RW. Mitochondrial DNA mutations and human disease. *Biochim Biophys Acta.* 2010;1797:113–128.

271. Wahbi K, Larue S, Jardel C, et al. Cardiac involvement is frequent in patients with the m.8344A>G mutation of mitochondrial DNA. *Neurology.* 2010;74:674–677.

272. Scaglia F, Towbin JA, Craigen WJ, et al. Clinical spectrum, morbidity, and mortality in 113 pediatric patients with mitochondrial disease. *Pediatrics.* 2004;114:925–931.

273. Tang S, Batra A, Zhang Y, Ebenroth ES, Huang T. Left ventricular noncompaction is associated with mutations in the mitochondrial genome. *Mitochondrion.* 2010;10:350–357.

274. Khatami M, Houshmand M, Sadeghizadeh M, et al. Accumulation of mitochondrial genome variations in Persian LQTS patients: a possible risk factor? *Cardiovas Pathol.* 2010;19:e21–e27.

275. Zhang LH, Fang LG, Cheng ZW, Fang Q. Cardiac manifestations of patients with mitochondrial disease. *Zhonghua Xin Xue Guan Bing Za Zhi.* 2009;37:892–895.

276. Majamaa-Voltti K, Turkka J, Kortelainen M-L, Huikuri H, Majamaa K. Causes of death in pedigrees with the 3243A>G mutation in mitochondrial DNA. *J Neurol Neurosurg Psychiatry.* 2008;79:209–211.

277. Maron BJ, McKenna WJ, Danielson GK, et al. American College of Cardiology/European Society of Cardiology Clinical Expert Consensus Document on Hypertrophic Cardiomyopathy. A report of the American College of Cardiology Foundation Task Force on Clinical Expert Consensus Documents and the European Society of Cardiology Committee for Practice Guidelines. *J Am Coll Cardiol.* 2003;24:1965–1991.

278. Bonnet D, Rustin P, Rötig A, et al. Heart transplantation in children with mitochondrial cardiomyopathy. *Heart.* 2001;86:570–573.

279. Fontaine B, Khurana TS, Hoffman EP, et al. Hyperkalemic periodic paralysis and the adult muscle sodium channel alpha-subunit gene. *Science.* 1990;250:1000–1002.

280. Jurkat-Rott K, Mitrovic N, Hang C, et al. Voltage-sensor sodium channel mutations cause hypokalemic periodic paralysis type 2 by enhanced inactivation and reduced current. *Proc Natl Acad Sci U S A.* 2000;97:9549–9554.

281. Jurkat-Rott K, Uetz U, Pika-Hartlaub U, et al. Calcium currents and transients of native and heterologously expressed mutant skeletal muscle DHP receptor alpha1 subunits (R528H). *FEBS Lett.* 1998;423:198–204.

282. Plaster NM, Tawil R, Tristani-Firouzi M, et al. Mutations in Kir2.1 cause the developmental and episodic electrical phenotypes of Andersen's syndrome. *Cell.* 2001;105:511–519.

283. Sansone V, Griggs RC, Meola G, et al. Andersen's syndrome: a distinct periodic paralysis. *Ann Neurol.* 1997;42:305–312.

284. Tristani-Firouzi M, Jensen JL, Donaldson MR, et al. Functional and clinical characterization of KCNJ2 mutations associated with LQT7 (Andersen syndrome). *J Clin Invest.* 2002;110:381–388.

285. Kannankeril PJ, Roden DM, Fish FA. Suppression of bidirectional ventricular tachycardia and unmasking of prolonged QT interval with verapamil in Andersen's syndrome. *J Cardiovasc Electrophysiol.* 2004;15:119.

286. Bokenkamp R, Wilde AA, Schalij MJ, Blom NA. Flecainide for recurrent malignant ventricular arrhythmias in two siblings with Andersen-Tawil syndrome. *Heart Rhythm.* 2007;4:508–511.

287. Fox DJ, Klein GJ, Hahn A, et al. Reduction of complex ventricular ectopy and improvement in exercise capacity with flecainide therapy in Andersen-Tawil syndrome. *Europace.* 2008;10:1006–1008.

288. Delannoy E, Sacher F, Maury P, et al. Cardiac characteristics and long-term outcome in Andersen–Tawil syndrome patients related to KCNJ2 mutation. *Europace.* 2013;15:1805–1811.

289. Phillips 2nd LH. The epidemiology of myasthenia gravis. *Ann N Y Acad Sci.* 2003;998:407–412.

290. Grob D, Brunner N, Namba T, Pagala M. Life-time course of myasthenia gravis. *Muscle Nerve.* 2008;37:141–149.

291. Berrih S, Morel E, Gaud C, Raimond F, Le Brigand H, Bach JF. Anti-achr antibodies, thymic histology, and T cell subsets in myasthenia gravis. *Neurology.* 1984;34:66–71.

292. Giraud M, Beaurain G, Yamamoto AM, et al. Linkage of HLA to myasthenia gravis and genetic heterogeneity depending on anti-titin antibodies. *Neurology.* 2001;57:1555–1560.

293. Suzuki S, Baba A, Kaida K, et al. Cardiac involvements in myasthenia gravis associated with anti-Kv1.4 antibodies. *Eur J Neurol.* 2014;21:223–230.

294. Hofstad H, Ohm OJ, Mork SJ, Aarli JA. Heart disease in myasthenia gravis. *Acta Neurol Scand.* 1984;70:176–184.

101 Drug-Induced Ventricular Tachycardia

Lars Eckardt and Günter Breithardt

Overview

Drug-induced proarrhythmia represents a challenge for clinicians as well as those involved in the development of novel pharmaceuticals. It may be a predictor of sudden cardiac death and thus the risks and benefits of the suspect medication need to be critically reevaluated. Drug-induced ventricular tachyarrhythmias can be caused by cardiovascular drugs, noncardiovascular drugs, and, even, nonprescription agents. They can also result in arrhythmic emergencies and sudden cardiac death.[1,2] Development of a new arrhythmia, or aggravation of an existing arrhythmia, during therapy with a drug at a concentration usually considered not to be toxic is defined as *proarrhythmia*. This condition occurs in patients with or without structural heart disease. Major causes of proarrhythmia include direct pharmacological effects on ion channels of the heart. Cardiac glycosides, QT-prolonging agents, and sodium channel–blocking drugs have all been implicated in this proarrhythmic category. In addition, certain drugs can cause a cardiomyopathy that ultimately leads to ventricular tachyarrhythmias, specifically ventricular tachycardia (VT). Others can cause coronary vasoconstriction and acute myocardial ischemia.

The proportion of patients with proarrhythmia that initially manifests as sudden death and the extent to which proarrhythmia contributes to the overall problem of sudden death are unknown. Nevertheless, the experience with terfenadine or cisapride and the Cardiac Arrhythmia Suppression Trial (CAST)[3] has illustrated the potential for drugs to result in unusual severe adverse effects, which can be difficult to detect. General treatment guidelines focus on avoidance of drug therapy in high-risk patients, recognition of the syndromes of drug-induced proarrhythmia, and withdrawal of the culprit agents.[1]

Pharmacokinetic Risk Factors

The arrhythmogenic potential can manifest in patients who are particularly sensitive to the electrophysiological effects of a particular drug (i.e., pharmacodynamic sensitivity).[4] This phenomenon can be the result of a drug overdose or of drug interactions in such highly sensitive patients in whom usual drug dosages lead to extreme elevations in plasma drug concentration. The latter most commonly occurs when the culprit drug is eliminated by a single metabolizing pathway. If this pathway is susceptible to inhibition by the administration of a second drug or is inhibited by coadministration of other drugs or by genetic factors, marked elevation of drug concentrations and electrophysiological toxicity can result. This was the case with terfenadine[5] and cisapride, both of which are eliminated as noncardioactive metabolites by the intestinal and hepatic P-450 system, CYP3A4. Many commonly used drugs, such as erythromycin, ketoconazole, and some calcium channel blockers, are potent CYP3A4 inhibitors. Of note, grapefruit juice markedly inhibits the activity of intestinal but not hepatic CYP3A4. Although CYP3A4 is the most important drug-metabolizing enzyme expressed in the liver and elsewhere, some drugs use other pathways. Among other members of the CYP superfamily, genetically determined polymorphisms have been described in three: CYP2D6, CYP2C9, and CYP2C19. A subset of the population absolutely lacks catalytic activity, and thus plasma concentrations of substrate drugs are much higher in these "poor metabolizer" patients. The activity of the P-450 CYP2D6, for example, is absent in approximately 7% of whites and in persons of African heritage. In a situation in which CYP2D6 is the sole eliminating pathway, patients with this "poor metabolizer" trait can display markedly aberrant drug concentrations.

Genetic Predisposition

Administration of a drug can unmask a subclinical (forme fruste) monogenic arrhythmia syndrome. Mutations in genes (e.g., *KCNQ1*, *KCNH2*, or *SCN5A*) causing congenital forms of long QT syndrome have been identified in patients with acquired forms of long QT syndrome. The exact contribution and mutation frequency cannot be estimated. Mutations in the relevant genes have only a minor role, and rare variations in genes responsible for congenital long QT syndrome seem to be frequent in drug-induced long QT syndrome.[6] A subclinical form of Brugada syndrome can similarly predispose affected patients to the development of drug-induced forms of Brugada syndrome (see www.brugadadrugs.org)[7] as a consequence of polymorphisms or mutations in *SCN5A* or other genes. In these monogenic syndromes, penetrance of the electrocardiographic phenotype can be highly variable, an effect often attributed to unidentified modifier genes. In addition, genetic polymorphisms can increase the risk for drug-induced sudden cardiac death. For example, approximately 10% of African-Americans carry a variant in their sodium channel gene that results in a tyrosine (Y) rather than a serine (S) at position 1103 of the protein.[8] Study of this variant protein in vitro indicates that it confers changes consistent with the sodium channel–linked variant of long QT syndrome. Similarly, the polymorphisms resulting in T8A and Q9E in the *KCNE2* gene have been associated with unusual in vitro characteristics and a higher incidence of proarrhythmia during drug therapy.

Drug-Induced Long QT Syndrome

Drug effects are the most common cause of acquired long QT syndrome (Table 101.1). Although syncope occurring soon after the initiation of quinidine therapy was recognized as early as the 1920s, it was not until the advent of continuous electrocardiographic monitoring that "quinidine syncope" was recognized to be due to polymorphic VT. In recent years, it has become apparent that in addition to antiarrhythmic drugs, a large spectrum of noncardiac drugs (see Table 101.1) can cause QT prolongation and torsades de pointes. In addition, drug–drug interaction may be of major relevance for proarrhythmia. The combination of inhibitors of the renin-angiotensin system and antibiotics, such as cotrimoxazole, with unrecognized hyperkalemia has been associated recently with an increased risk of death.[9] The incidence of drug-induced torsades de pointes in the general population is unknown. Dessertenne[10] used the term *torsades de pointes* initially to describe this characteristic undulating pattern of tachycardia in 1966. It is characterized by a polymorphic, usually nonsustained, pause-dependent VT that almost always only develops in association with an excessively prolonged QT interval. It can be associated with syncope or degenerate into a sustained VT or ventricular fibrillation (VF). An electrocardiogram (ECG) recorded just before or after termination of a polymorphic VT helps distinguish torsades from other polymorphic VTs mainly occurring in patients with structural heart disease. Features that are diagnostic for torsades de pointes include a prolonged QT interval, presence of U waves before the onset or after the termination of the arrhythmia, relatively long coupling intervals, and a typical initiating sequence. In drug-induced long QT syndrome, short-long-short cycle-length changes constitute the typical pattern of initiation of torsades de pointes and can be regarded as a warning sign of an impending episode of torsades. Premature ventricular beats are often found to arise from exaggerated T/U waves after longer intervals, such as after extrasystolic pauses (Fig. 101.1).

Torsades de pointes is a major safety concern with drugs submitted for regulatory approval. Of concern is that the proarrhythmic risk for many of the drugs that can prolong repolarization, thereby causing torsades de pointes, is not detected during the developmental phase and is recognized only after such drugs have been on the market for many years. In larger case series of torsades de pointes, the death rate was as high as 16%. In a survey in the United Kingdom and Italy, noncardiovascular drugs that have proarrhythmic potential (i.e., an official warning regarding risk for QT prolongation or torsades de pointes or with published data on QT prolongation, VT, or class III effect) represented 3% and 2% of total prescriptions in both countries, respectively.[11] The growing awareness of drug-induced long QT syndrome over the past several years has resulted in a marked increase in the number of spontaneous reports. However, the spontaneous reporting most likely underestimates the true incidence of serious adverse reactions, so that the true incidence of drug-induced torsades de pointes remains uncertain. Although torsades de pointes typically occurs shortly after initiation of therapy, it can also develop during long-term treatment. The late occurrence has been linked to changes in dose, reinitiation of the drug after short discontinuation, and transient electrolyte disorders, such as hypokalemia or hypomagnesemia. The incidence of torsades de pointes associated with sotalol has been estimated to range between 1.8% and almost 5%.

The torsadogenic potential of drugs is extremely variable, even within the same class of drugs.[12] Some drugs can provoke torsades de pointes only in the setting of overdose, with concomitant administration of other QT-prolonging drugs, or in the presence of risk factors such as hypokalemia, whereas others can induce torsades de pointes when used alone, even at therapeutic levels, and in the absence of additional risk factors.

Risk Factors for Torsades de Pointes

Drug-induced torsades de pointes is a complicated phenomenon related not only to a particular drug and its dose but also

TABLE 101.1	Drugs that can cause QT prolongation or torsades de pointes
DRUG CLASS	**DRUG**
Antiarrhythmic	Amiodarone, ajmaline, azimilide, bretylium, disopyramide, d,l-sotalol, dofetilide, dronedarone, flecainide, ibutilide, propafenone, tedisamil
Anticancer	Arsenic trioxide, lapatinib, nilotinib, tamoxifen, vandetanib
Antifungal	Fluconazole, itraconazole, ketoconazole, voriconazole
Antimicrobial	Azithromycin, clarithromycin, erythromycin, spiramycin, telithromycin, levofloxacin, moxifloxacin, sparfloxacin, gatifloxacin, grepafloxacin, gemifloxacin, ofloxacin, trimethoprim-sulfamethoxazole, pentamidine, quinine, chloroquine, mefloquine, halofantrine, amantadine
Antiviral	Foscarnet
Antihistamine	Astemizole, diphenhydramine, ebastine, terfenadine, hydroxyzine, loratadine
Antidepressant	Citalopram, clomipramine, desipramine, doxepin, escitalopram, fluoxetine, imipramine paroxetine, sertraline, venlafaxine
Antipsychotic	Chlorpromazine, chloral hydrate, droperidol, felbamate, fluphenazine, haloperidol, lithium, maprotiline, mesoridazine, pericycline, pimozide, prochlorperazine, quetiapine, risperidone, sertindole, sultopride, thioridazine, tiapride, trifluoperazine, zimelidine, ziprasidone
Antimigraine	Naratriptan, sumatriptan, zolmitriptan
Bronchodilators	Albuterol, salmeterol
Diuretics	Indapamide, furosemide, thiazide
Gastrointestinal stimulants	Cisapride, domperidone, metoclopramide
Hormones	Octreotide, vasopressin
Immunosuppressives	Tacrolimus
Vasodilators	Bepridil, lidoflazine, prenylamine
Miscellaneous	Aconitine, amantadine, budipine, cesium, cocaine, methadone, probucol, terodiline, tizanidine, veratridine, vincamine

Data derived from nonrandomized studies of the literature and modified from reference 15. This list is not comprehensive; rather, it gives examples. Please see also http://www.crediblemeds.org. Accessed July 28, 2016 and http://www.sads.org. Accessed July 28, 2016.

to drug–drug interactions and a variety of patient factors, including age, sex, presence of structural heart disease, and genetic predisposition. Patients who developed drug-related torsades de pointes were found to have a borderline or prolonged (more than 0.44 second) QTc before drug administration. The fact that the QT interval is shorter in men than in women has been suggested to account for the two- to three-fold higher incidence of abnormal QT prolongation and torsades de pointes in females. The potential mechanisms are significant differences in ion-channel subunit composition. Besides, QT prolongation and torsades de pointes are more frequent in older patients who are also often exposed to polypharmacy.

One hypothesis to explain the development of torsades de pointes is that normal repolarization is accomplished by multiple ion channels, providing a safety reserve for repolarization (Fig. 101.2). In the presence of an otherwise subclinical impairment in the repolarization mechanisms (i.e., reduced repolarization reserve), patients can have a certain propensity for the development of torsades de pointes. Patients with a history of drug-related torsades de pointes are highly likely to experience additional episodes on exposure to any other QT-prolonging

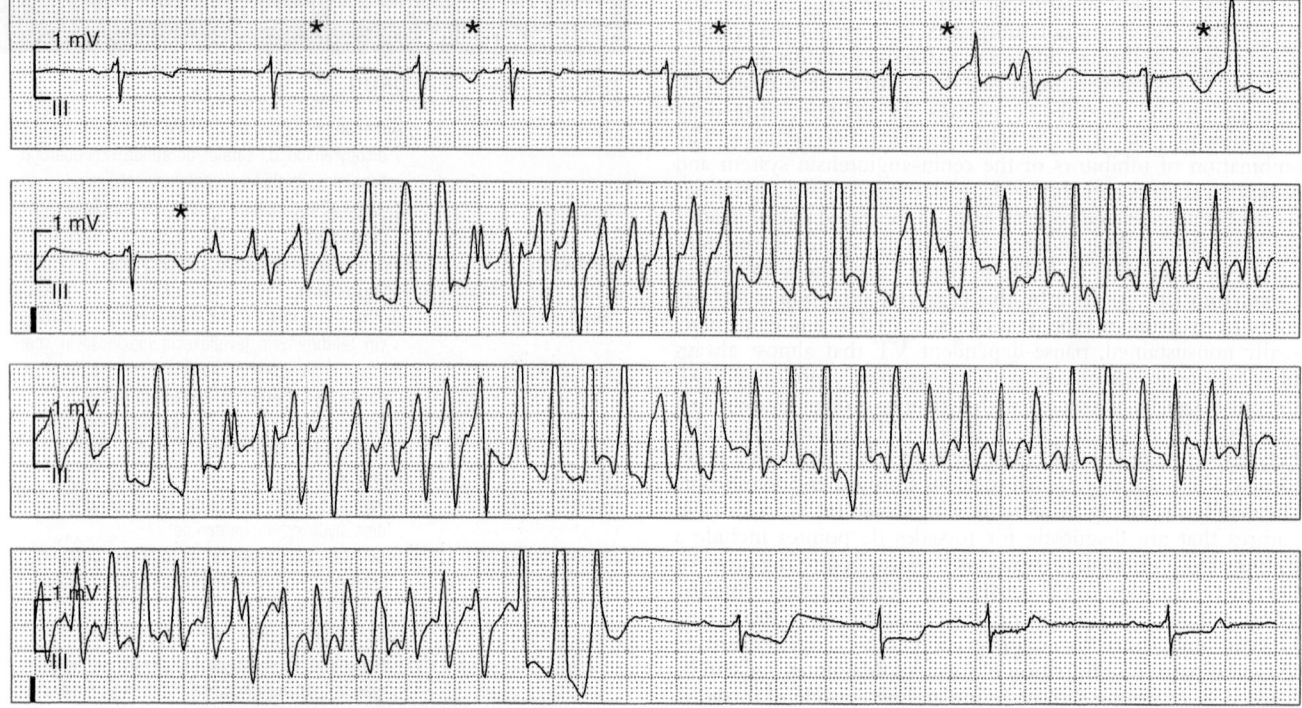

FIGURE 101.1 Monitor strip showing long-short ventricular cycle, pause-dependent QT prolongation with abnormal and gradually augmented T/U waves (*asterisk*) leading to a self-terminating episode of torsades de pointes demonstrating the typical "twisting" morphology. Ventricular premature beats are followed by a postextrasystolic pause. The initial beat starts from the peak of the U wave. This patient was taking a combination of clarithromycin and ketoconazole.

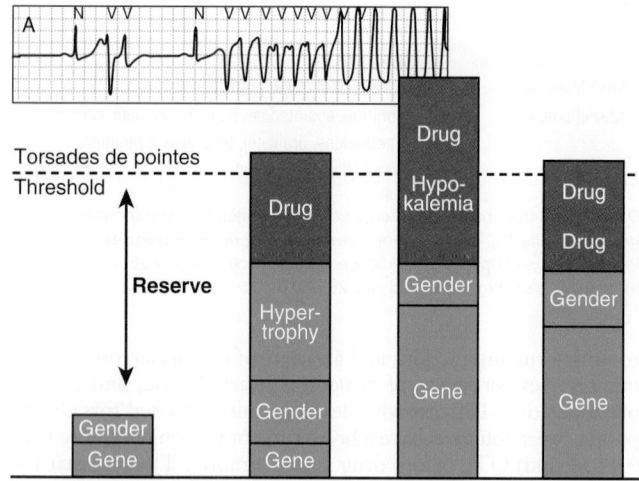

FIGURE 101.2 The concept of repolarization reserve. In healthy hearts (*left*) the repolarization reserve is large. Several factors (e.g., drugs, hypokalemia, gender, genetic predisposition/polymorphisms, and structural heart disease) can reduce the reserve so that the threshold for the occurrence of torsades de pointes is reached.

drug.[12] Thus the need for prophylactic implantable cardioverter defibrillator (ICD) implantation should be considered based on an individual evaluation of the future risk of life-threatening ventricular arrhythmias (class IIa recommendations).[1] Controlled exposure to sotalol successfully identified patients with normal QTc intervals but altered myocardial repolarization. Hypokalemia and hypomagnesemia prolong repolarization. An occasionally overlooked cause for hypokalemia can be ingestion of licorice.

Clinical as well as experimental data suggest that potassium channel downregulation or aberrant intracellular calcium handling predispose patients to the development of arrhythmias when a QT interval–prolonging drug is superimposed. The importance of underlying structural heart disease as a potential risk factor for torsades de pointes is not clear. Acquired abnormal QT prolongation and torsades de pointes have been observed in patients with various types of heart disease and in patients without detectable heart disease. In larger series, arterial hypertension was present in a significant proportion of patients. In addition, there is experimental evidence that heart failure is a risk factor for drug-induced torsades de pointes.[13] Any combination of risk factors will additionally reduce the repolarization reserve and thereby prolong the action potential and the QT interval. In addition, therapies used in heart failure can increase the risk. Diuretics, for example, can decrease serum potassium and potentiate QT prolongation by directly blocking potassium channels. Other risk factors that can affect repolarization and reduce the repolarization reserve, apart from the congenital long QT syndrome and drugs, are listed in Box 101.1. Knowledge of the clinical risk factors that identify patients with an increased propensity for development of drug-induced torsades de pointes and of the drugs known to provoke such arrhythmias can help prevent the occurrence of drug-induced proarrhythmia.

Mechanisms of Drug-Induced Torsades de Pointes

A large number of experimental and molecular studies have resulted in a better understanding of the mechanisms of torsades de pointes.[2,14] Acquired forms of QT prolongation and proarrhythmia are frequently related to drug effects on the same ion channels involved in genetic forms of long QT syndrome.

Prolongation of the action potential can be achieved by a reduction of the outward currents, particularly the outward delayed rectifier potassium currents I_{Kr} and I_{Ks}, or by enhancement of the inward currents during phases 2 and 3 of the action potential. Among the potassium currents, I_{Kr} is most susceptible to pharmacological influence. In all known cases of drug-related acquired long QT syndrome, the blockade of I_{Kr} current is at least, in part, responsible for action potential prolongation and proarrhythmia. Blockade of I_{Kr} results in a reduction in the net outward current, a prolongation of the action potential, and the possible development of T/U wave abnormalities. The prolongation of repolarization can allow subsequent activation of an inward depolarization current ($I_{Ca,L}$ and I_{Na}), which may generate early afterdepolarizations and promote triggered activity at the end of repolarization. Other mechanisms for drug-induced QT prolongation include blockade of both I_{Kr} and I_{Ks} by, for example, azimilide or inhibition of hERG trafficking to the cell membrane by pentamidine and arsenic trioxide. Of note, fluoxetine, an antidepressant, has been found to prolong QT by two mechanisms: direct block of I_{Kr} and disruption of hERG trafficking to the cell membrane. It has also been demonstrated that some, but not all, arrhythmogenic I_{Kr} blockers can generate arrhythmias by augmenting I_{Na-L} (late sodium current) through the phosphoinositide 3-kinase pathway.[15]

Boulasksil and colleagues[16] showed that focal activity may be the dominant mechanism involved in the perpetuation of drug-induced torsades de pointes in chronic atrioventricular (AV) block dog models. Prolongation of phase 2 repolarization, rather than phase 3 repolarization, by augmenting the I_{Na} current could reduce the propensity to induce early afterdepolarizations and torsades de pointes. The cardiac membrane is relatively inexcitable during phase 2 compared with phase 3, which is the phase prolonged by most drugs causing torsades de pointes. Prolongation of phase 3 allows a longer time interval for the development of early afterdepolarizations and triggered activity. In an in vitro model of torsades de pointes, it could be demonstrated that QT prolongation mainly by phase 3 prolongation (triangulation of the action potential) corresponded to the occurrence of torsades de pointes, whereas "rectangulation" of the action potential had no proarrhythmic effects and even suppressed torsades de pointes.[11] Calcium channel blockade also can diminish the induction of early afterdepolarizations and torsades de pointes,[13] a property that helps explain the low torsadogenic potential of quinidine in a fixed combination with verapamil and most likely also explains the same low potential of amiodarone. In the case of amiodarone (which is associated with an incidence of torsades de pointes of <1%), the ability to diminish or eliminate dispersion of repolarization could also be important. It has also been postulated that beat-to-beat variability in repolarization may be particularly relevant and may even discriminate between safe and unsafe drugs.[14]

Prevention of Acquired Torsades de Pointes

Prevention of drug-related torsades de pointes, especially by noncardiovascular drugs, is a major challenge for physicians, researchers engaged in the development of new drugs, and regulatory agencies. In general, available strategies for reducing the risk of drug-induced proarrhythmia include the exclusion by regulatory agencies of drugs with unfavorable risk-to-benefit profiles. Early identification of a potentially adverse response of the QT interval to a drug requires careful and regular observation of the ECG.[1] Apart from the analysis of QT intervals, special attention should be directed to excessive QT prolongation, QT dispersion, and developing changes in T wave morphology (e.g., negative, notched, or biphasic T waves and appearance of prominent U waves). According to the most recent European Society of Cardiology (ESC) Guidelines, withdrawal of offending agents is recommended whenever drug-induced arrhythmias are suspected and the presence of other arrhythmogenic substrates has been excluded (class IB recommendation).[1] Intravenous magnesium, isoproterenol, or temporary pacing are highly effective in managing torsades de pointes. Of note, inhibition of the Na^+/Ca^{2+} exchanger (NCX)[17] has been shown to reduce action potential duration, early afterdepolarizations, and torsades de pointes in the setting of both hERG-blocking and SCN5A-activating drugs (mimicking LQT2 and LQT3, respectively) and heart failure.[18] Genetic inhibition of NCX has recently been demonstrated to protect against afterdepolarizations in a murine model.[19]

Sodium Channel Blocker–Related Toxicity

Compared with torsades de pointes, which is related to abnormalities in repolarization, sodium channel–related toxicity is related to slowing of conduction.[20] Antiarrhythmic drugs are the most common precipitants, although other agents (e.g., antidepressants and cocaine) can produce some of their toxic effects through sodium channel–blocking properties. Sodium channel–blocking drugs with slower rates of dissociation from the sodium channel (e.g., flecainide, propafenone, and quinidine) tend to generate these adverse effects more commonly. These drugs tend to prolong QRS duration even at normal heart rates because of their slow dissociation rates. The drug dose does not have to be toxic, but it must be large enough to slow conduction velocity. In a large, nationwide cohort of atrial fibrillation patients, propafenone therapy was found to be associated with new-onset ventricular arrhythmias. Old age, presence of J waves in inferior leads, and wider QRS on ECG were found to be the significant risk factors.[21]

In contrast with the occurrence of torsades de pointes, which is promoted by a slow heart rate, induction of VT by class IC drugs is promoted by a fast heart rate, which can aggravate a preexisting slowing of conduction. In the CAST study,[3] the mortality rate was higher among patients receiving flecainide for frequent ventricular ectopy after a myocardial infarction than among patients receiving placebo. Subgroup analyses of CAST data suggested that the lack of β-blocker therapy, which avoids high rates, was accompanied by a higher mortality. Among patients in whom the index myocardial infarction was a non–Q wave event and who therefore have a high incidence of recurrent ischemia, an 8.7-fold increase in mortality was observed compared with a 1.7-fold increase in patients with transmural infarctions. Based on the CAST findings,[3] class I antiarrhythmic drugs are contraindicated in patients with a history of previous myocardial infarction, but this has largely been extended to other forms of structural heart disease.[1] There is also some concern about using flecainide or propafenone in patients with significant left ventricular (LV) hypertrophy (LV wall thickness > 1.4 cm).[1]

Genetic factors can also have a role. An SCN5A promoter polymorphism common in Asians was found to modulate the duration of the PR and QRS intervals. The extent of QRS widening after challenge with sodium channel–blocking drugs is genotype dependent.

Sodium channel blockers can also convert atrial fibrillation to slow atrial flutter, which can show 1:1 AV conduction with wide QRS complexes. This drug-induced arrhythmia can be confused with a VT; therefore, when used for atrial fibrillation, an AV node–blocking drug should be coadministered with a sodium channel blocker to prevent rapid ventricular rates in case atrial flutter occurs.

In some patients receiving sodium channel–blocking drugs (particularly flecainide and propafenone), mostly a slow, incessant VT can develop that occasionally is resistant to cardioversion (Fig. 101.3). These tachyarrhythmias may be hemodynamically tolerated because of the slow heart rate; they can also degenerate into a hemodynamically significant VT or VF that can be lethal. They usually are observed with high or toxic doses of the drug or in the setting of other pathophysiological conditions that exaggerate the effects of the drug on conduction (e.g., acidosis, hyperkalemia, and concomitant sodium channel blockade); however, they also can occur with tricyclic antidepressant overdose. In such instances, the antiarrhythmic drug should be discontinued immediately. Hypertonic saline or sodium bicarbonate can reverse the conduction slowing and terminate or accelerate the arrhythmia (see Fig. 101.3). Rate slowing also can be beneficial because the magnitude of conduction slowing is less at slower heart rates.

Drug-Induced Brugada Syndrome

There are two principal hypotheses concerning the pathophysiological basis of Brugada syndrome: the "depolarization hypothesis," namely right ventricular conduction delay, and the "repolarization hypothesis." The latter argues that a prominent transient outward current (I_{to})-mediated action potential notch and a subsequent loss of action potential dome in the right ventricular outflow tract epicardium, but not in the endocardium, give rise to a transmural voltage gradient, resulting in ST-segment elevation in surface ECG leads V_1–V_3 and the possible induction of subsequent VT through the mechanism of phase 2 reentry. Because the maintenance of the action potential dome is determined by the balance of currents active at the end of phase 1 of the action potential, any intervention that increases outward currents (e.g., I_{to}, adenosine triphosphate–sensitive potassium current [I_{KATP}], I_{Kr}, and I_{Ks}) or decreases inward currents (e.g., $I_{Ca,L}$ and I_{Na}) at the end of phase 1 of the action potential can accentuate or unmask ST-segment elevation similar to that found in Brugada syndrome. A number of drugs and conditions that cause an outward shift in the current active at the end of phase 1 have been reported to induce transient Brugada-like ST-segment elevation (see www.brugadadrugs.org).[7] Whether

this drug-induced form of Brugada syndrome unmasks clinically inapparent Brugada syndrome (forme fruste) or merely represents one end of a broad spectrum of responses to sodium channel–blocking drugs is not known. In a majority of reported cases of acquired Brugada syndrome, however, the characteristic type I Brugada ECG pattern disappeared after withdrawal of the drugs and could not be reproduced with subsequent flecainide testing in these patients (Table 101.2).

Among antiarrhythmic drugs, class IC drugs most effectively amplify or unmask ST-segment elevation secondary to their strong effect in blocking I_{Na} and are therefore used as a diagnostic tool in Brugada patients with transient ECG abnormalities. Among the class IC drugs, pilsicainide, a pure class IC drug developed in Japan, is thought to induce ST-segment elevation more strongly than flecainide. Class IA antiarrhythmic drugs (e.g., ajmaline, procainamide, disopyramide, and cibenzoline), which exhibit less use-dependent blocking of I_{Na} owing to faster dissociation of the drug from the sodium channels, show weaker ST-segment elevation than that caused by class IC drugs. Of note, quinidine, another class IA drug, generally normalizes ST-segment elevation because of its relatively strong I_{to}-blocking effect, and its use has been proposed for the pharmacological treatment of Brugada syndrome.

Several psychotropic drugs, including tricyclic antidepressants (e.g., amitriptyline, nortriptyline, desipramine, and clomipramine), tetracyclic antidepressants (e.g., maprotiline), phenothiazine (e.g., cyamemazine), and selective serotonin reuptake inhibitors (e.g., fluoxetine) have been reported to unmask Brugada-like ST-segment elevation, secondary to block of fast I_{Na} associated with overdose of these drugs. It has been postulated that this could be an important mechanism for drug-related sudden cardiac death in patients receiving continued treatment with antidepressants and neuroleptics. One study of intoxication with tricyclic antidepressants (defined by a plasma concentration greater than 1 μm/L) in a series of consecutive patients reported a Brugada electrocardiographic pattern in 15 of 98 cases (15.3%).[22] The mortality rate was slightly higher among patients with the Brugada ECG pattern (6.7%) than among those without it (2.4%), but the difference did not reach statistical significance.[22] Of note, the ECG pattern disappeared when plasma concentrations of tricyclic antidepressants were less than 1 μm/L. Cocaine intoxication (discussed later) also has been reported to unmask the characteristic Brugada ECG pattern. In addition, a number of case reports have demonstrated that fever (hyperthermia) can unmask Brugada-like ST-segment elevation and provoke VF as a result of reduced I_{Na} at high temperature.

Digitalis Toxicity

Digitalis has a narrow therapeutic window, and the mortality associated with unrecognized digitalis intoxication is high and often unacknowledged. Digitalis inhibits Na^+/K^+-ATPase, thereby interfering with the sodium pump; as a result, Na^+ accumulates within the cell, which in turn alters the Na^+–Ca^{2+} exchange. The result is an increase in Ca^{2+} concentration within the cell, which explains the positive inotropic effect of the drug. To reduce calcium transient, an electrogenic Na^+–Ca^{2+} exchange occurs. This Na^+–Ca^{2+} exchange can mediate delayed afterdepolarizations, resulting in triggered activity, which can cause the characteristic tachycardias. Many factors determine whether a given blood level of digitalis is actually toxic and causes arrhythmias. Therefore the serum concentrations should not be used as the only determinant for evaluating toxicity. The ECG-related and gastrointestinal (e.g., nausea and abdominal pain), visual (changes in color vision and reduced vision secondary to diminished accommodation), neuropsychiatric (hallucinations, nightmares, and depression), and muscular (fatigue and weakness) complaints are clues

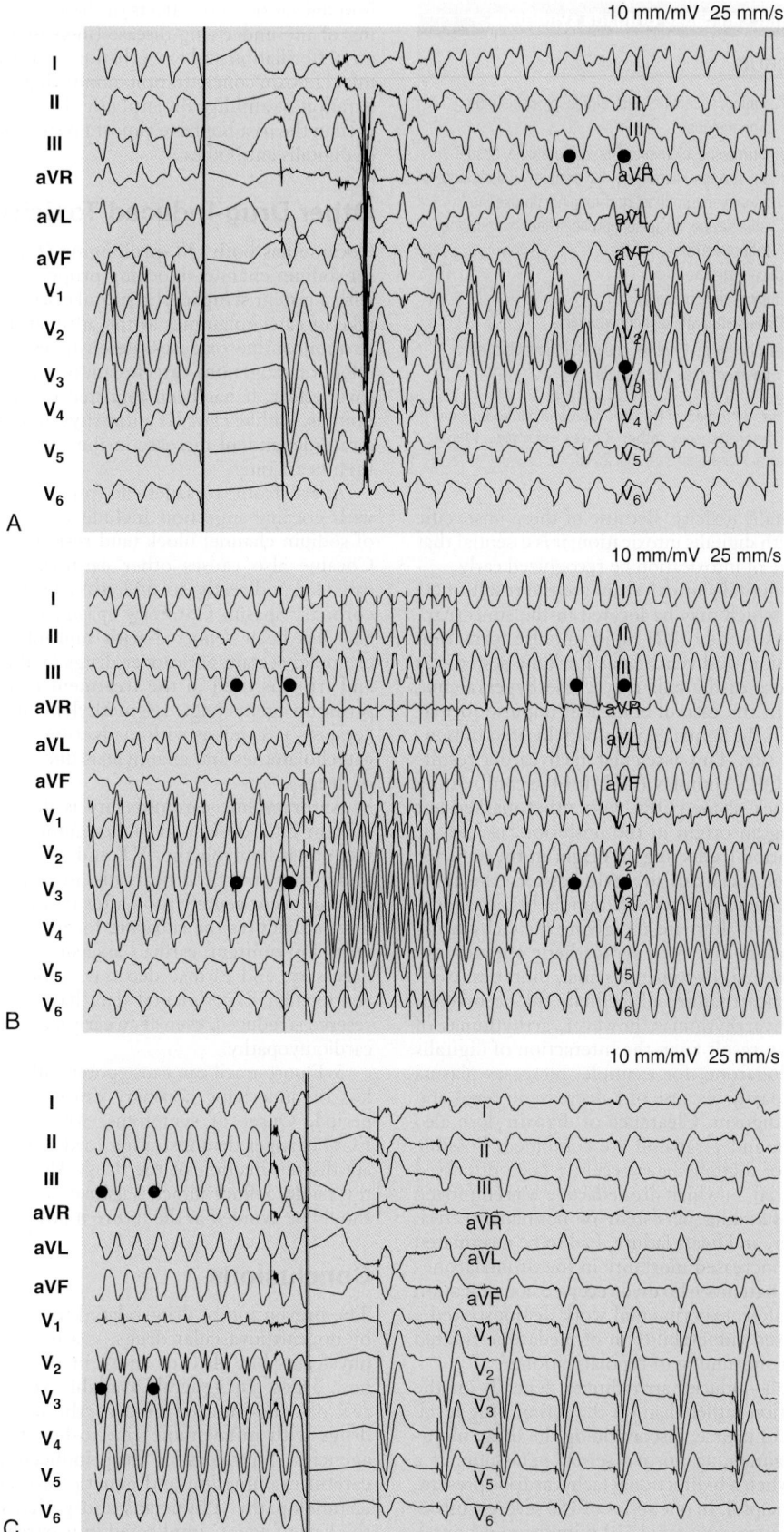

FIGURE 101.3 (A) Hemodynamically stable, incessant monomorphic ventricular tachycardia (VT) in a 61-year-old man with a history of an inferior myocardial infarction 12 years earlier. Because of a recurrent monomorphic VT, an implantable cardioverter defibrillator had been implanted 10 months previously and amiodarone therapy was started (loading dose of 1 g/day for 10 days, then 400 mg for 8 weeks, followed by 200 mg daily). Five days before the onset of the incessant VT, a cluster of VTs occurred; an additional 5 g of amiodarone was given, and continuous ajmaline infusion was started because of numerous recurrent VT episodes. Thereafter, the incessant VT began. (B) The VT immediately recurred after cardioversion or overdrive pacing. (C) After administration of 10 mL of sodium chloride (20%), overdrive pacing converted the incessant VT into a different rapid, hemodynamically not tolerated VT, which was successfully converted into a stable sinus rhythm. Sodium chloride was given to overcome sodium channel blockade.

TABLE 101.2 Drugs that can cause Brugada syndrome

DRUG CLASS	DRUG
Antiarrhythmic	Ajmaline, flecainide, pilsicainide, procainamide, propafenone
Antidepressant	Amitriptyline, clomipramine, desipramine, dosulepin, doxepin, fluoxetine, fluvoxamine, imipramine, lithium, maprotiline, nortriptyline, paroxetine
Antipsychotic	Cyamemazine, loxapine, perphenazine, thioridazine, trifluoperazine
Antiepileptic	Oxcarbazepine
Anesthetics/analgetics	Bupivacaine, propofol
Antihistamines	Dimenhydrinate, diphenhydramine
Miscellaneous	Alcohol, acetylcholine, cocaine, ergonovine, edrophonium, metoclopramide,

Data derived from nonrandomized studies of the literature and modified from reference 14. This list is not comprehensive; rather, it gives examples. Please see also http://brugadadrugs.org. Accessed July 28, 2016.

to the detection of digitalis toxicity. Because of these unspecific symptoms in patients with digitalis intoxication, it is essential that ECG findings suggestive of intoxication be recognized early.

The arrhythmias of digitalis intoxication are the result of (1) a block in conduction, which may be located in the sinus (e.g., sinus bradycardia) or AV node or (2) rapid impulse formation in the atrium, AV junction, and ventricular Purkinje system. In addition, severe overdose of digitalis may cause hyperkalemia and cardiac standstill. In the case of abnormal impulse formation, the site of origin in the ventricle is usually located in bundle branch Purkinje tissue. This fascicular tachycardia results in a relatively narrow QRS complex (0.12–0.14 second) and a right bundle branch block–shaped QRS with either marked left axis deviation (denoting an origin in the posterior fascicle) or marked right axis deviation (reflecting an origin in the anterior fascicle). In addition, the focus can alternate between the anterior and the posterior fascicles of the left bundle branch, causing the frontal plane axis to alternate and giving the tachycardia a bidirectional appearance. Increased sympathetic stimulation, hypokalemia, hypercalcemia, hypomagnesemia, diuretics, ischemia, reperfusion, and heart failure all facilitate the occurrence of digitalis-related tachyarrhythmias; however, arrhythmias of digitalis toxicity also can result from the interaction of digitalis with other drugs. Amiodarone, for example, increases plasma digoxin concentration partly because of a decrease in renal and nonrenal clearance of digoxin. Clearance of digoxin dose also decreases when digoxin and verapamil are combined. Possible proarrhythmic effects of digitalis have recently been discussed because the PALLAS trial, in which dronedarone was employed in patients with long-standing persistent or permanent atrial fibrillation, atrial flutter, and heart failure, had to be terminated prematurely due to an increased mortality in the dronedarone-group. The majority of patients who died received comedication with digitalis.[21] Thereafter, experimental work demonstrated a digitalis-related increased vulnerability in dronedarone-treated hearts and a significant shortening of repolarization.[22]

Treatment of digitalis-induced arrhythmias depends on the patient's clinical condition rather than on the serum drug level. Management includes, of course, discontinuing the drug, monitoring rhythm, and maintaining normal serum potassium. If a VT occurs, especially when a bidirectional tachycardia is present, digoxin antibodies are helpful. In one series of 150 severely intoxicated patients, the response was rapid (30 minutes to 4 hours). Approximately half of the patients with a cardiac arrest survived

hospitalization. Side effects of these antibodies included worsening of the underlying disease (increased ventricular rate during atrial fibrillation and exacerbation of heart failure) and hypokalemia. Digoxin concentration monitoring is unreliable after administration of antidigoxin antibody. Lidocaine and phenytoin were used in the past but have almost no role today with the availability of digitalis antibodies.

Other Drug-Induced Toxicity

Cocaine has both QT-prolonging (I_{Kr}-blocking) and slow-offset sodium channel–blocking properties. It is a local anesthetic with a potent sympathetic stimulatory effect. It blocks the reuptake of catecholamines at the adrenergic nerve endings, inhibits monoamine oxidases, desensitizes peripheral organs to the effect of exogenous catecholamines, and exerts a direct cardiotoxic effect. It has been reported to cause VF and torsades de pointes. Unlike class III antiarrhythmic drugs, cocaine produces a rate-dependent increase in the QT interval that is greatest at high heart rates.

Apart from torsades de pointes, arrhythmias associated with cocaine ingestion include monomorphic VT suggestive of sodium channel block (and responding to sodium infusion). Cocaine also causes other cardiovascular complications that can lead indirectly to arrhythmias, notably myocarditis, and coronary spasm. Coronary spasm, which can manifest as VF, also has been reported with multiple other medications; for example, certain anticancer drugs (5-fluorouracil, capecitabine, and triptans used in the treatment of migraines) and nonprescription agents (e.g., 3,4-methylenedioxymethamphetamine or "ecstasy") as well as with inadvertent vascular administration of catecholamines and anaphylaxis due to any one of a wide range of drugs.

Anthracycline cardiotoxicity is dose dependent, with intermittent high doses and higher cumulative doses increasing the risk of cardiomyopathy. VT and VF can arise secondary to the underlying structural heart disease. This form of cardiomyopathy can occur acutely soon after treatment, within a few months of treatment (as the subacute form), or many years later. Long-term intermittent cardiac assessment of patients is therefore necessary, and cardiac decompensation should be treated conventionally. Experimental data have shown that repolarization reserve is reduced, even at an early stage of anthracycline-induced cardiomyopathy.

5-Fluorouracil can cause potentially fatal arrhythmias regardless of underlying coronary disease during the acute infusion period. Onset of symptoms, with or without corresponding ECG changes demonstrating cardiac ischemia, dictates immediate discontinuation of the drug. Although this cardiotoxicity is reversible, 5-fluorouracil sensitizes the patient to such effects and should be avoided in the future if possible.

Conclusions

The prevention of drug-related torsades de pointes, especially by noncardiovascular drugs, is a major challenge not only for physicians but also for those involved in the development of new drugs. In general, available strategies for reducing the risk of drug-induced proarrhythmia include the exclusion of drugs with unfavorable risk-to-benefit profiles by regulatory agencies. Survivors of drug-induced proarrhythmia require careful examination and genetic testing for the presence of a channelopathy. Physicians and patients are advised to follow the lists of agents implicated in proarrhythmia to minimize the risk of arrhythmias.

REFERENCES

1. Priori SG, Blomström-Lundqvist C, Mazzanti A, et al. 2015 ESC Guidelines for the management of patients with ventricular arrhythmias and the prevention of sudden cardiac death. The Task Force for the Management of Patients with Ventricular Arrhythmias and the Prevention of Sudden Cardiac Death of the European Society of Cardiology (ESC) Endorsed by: Association for European Paediatric and Congenital Cardiology (AEPC). *Europace*. 2015;17:1601–1687.

2. Frommeyer G, Eckardt L. Drug-induced proarrhythmia: risk factors and electrophysiologic mechanisms. *Nat Rev Cardiol*. 2016;13:36–47.

3. Preliminary report: Effect of encainide and flecainide on mortality in a randomized trial of arrhythmia suppression after myocardial infarction. Cardiac Arrhythmia Suppression Trial (CAST) Investigators. *N Engl J Med*. 1989;321:406–412.

4. Hondeghem LM, Dujardin K, Hoffmann P, et al. Drug-induced QTc prolongation dangerously underestimates proarrhythmic potential: lessons from terfenadine. *J Cardiovasc Pharmacol*. 2011;57:589–597.

5. Lin YL, Hsiao CL, Wu YC, et al. Electrophysiologic, pharmacokinetic, and pharmacodynamic values indicating a higher risk of torsades de pointes. *J Clin Pharmacol*. 2011;51:819–829.

6. Ramirez AH, Shaffer CM, Delaney JT, et al. Novel rare variants in congenital cardiac arrhythmia genes are frequent in drug-induced torsades des pointes. *Pharmacogenomics*. 2013;13:325–329.

7. Postema PG, Wolpert C, Amin AS, et al. Drugs and Brugada syndrome patients: review of the literature, recommendations, and an up-to-date website (www.brugadadrugs.org). *Heart Rhythm*. 2009;6:1335–1341.

8. Splawski I, Timothy KW, Tateyama M, et al. Variant of SCN5A sodium channel implicated in risk of cardiac arrhythmia. *Science*. 2002;297:1333–1336.

9. Fralick M, Macdonald EM, Gomes T, et al. Canadian drug safety and effectiveness research network (CDSERN). Co-trimoxazole and sudden cardiac death in patients receiving inhibitors of renin-angiotensin system: population based study. *BMJ*. 2014;359:g6196.

10. Dessertenne F. La tachycardia ventriculaire a deux foyers opposes variables. *Arch Mal Coeur*. 1966;59:263–272.

11. De Ponti F, Poluzzi E, Montanaro N, et al. QTc and psychotropic drugs. *Lancet*. 2000;356:75–76.

12. Frommeyer G, Milberg P, Witte P, et al. A new mechanism preventing proarrhythmia in chronic heart failure: rapid phase III depolarization explains the low proarrhythmic potential of amiodarone in contrast to sotalol in a model of pacing-induced heart failure. *Eur J Heart Fail*. 2011;13:1060–1069.

13. Milberg P, Fink M, Pott C, et al. Blockade of I(Ca) suppresses early afterdepolarizations and reduces transmural dispersion of repolarization in a whole heart model of chronic heart failure. *Br J Pharmacol*. 2012;166:557–568.

14. Konstantopoulou A, Tsikrikas S, Asvestas D, et al. Mechanisms of drug-induced proarrhythmia in clinical practice. *World J Cardiol*. 2013;5:175–185.

15. Yang T, Chun YW, Stroud DM, et al. Screening for acute I_{Kr} block is insufficient to detect torsades de pointes liability-role of late sodium current. *Circulation*. 2014;130:224–234.

16. Boulaksi M, Jungschleger JG, Antoons G, et al. Drug-induced torsade de pointes arrhythmias in the chronic AV block dog are perpetuated by focal activity. *Circ Arrhythm Electrophysiol*. 2011;4:566–576.

17. Bögeholz N, Eckardt L, Pott C. Advantages and limitations of transgenic mice: the role of the Na^+/Ca^{2+} exchanger in cardiac electrophysiology and arrhythmia. *Curr Med Chem*. 2014;21:1330–1335.

18. Milberg P, Pott C, Frommeyer G, et al. Acute inhibition of the Na^+/Ca^{2+} exchanger reduces proarrhythmia in an experimental model of chronic heart failure. *Heart Rhythm*. 2012;9:570–578.

19. Bögeholz N, Pauls P, Bauer K, et al. Suppression of early and late afterdepolarisations by heterozygous knockout of the Na^+/Ca^{2+} exchanger in a murine model. *Circ Arrhythm Electrophysiol*. 2015;8:1210–1218.

20. Roden DM. Pharmacology and toxicology of Nav1.5-Class 1 anti-arrhythmic drugs. *Card Electrophysiol Clin*. 2014;6:695–704.

21. Lin CY, Lin YJ, Lo LW, et al. Factors predisposing to ventricular proarrhythmia during antiarrhythmic drug therapy for atrial fibrillation in patients with structurally normal hearts. *Heart Rhythm*. 2015;12:1490–1500.

22. Goldgran-Toledano D, Sideris G, Kevorkian JP. Overdose of cyclic antidepressants and the Brugada syndrome. *N Engl J Med*. 2002;346:1591–1592.

102 Ventricular Arrhythmias in Congenital Heart Disease

Katja Zeppenfeld, Monique Jongbloed, and Martin Jan Schalij

The reported incidence of congenital heart disease (CHD) depends on the number of trivial lesions included. For moderate to severe CHD that will require specialized care, numbers are stable, with 6 per 1000 live births.[1] The prevalence of CHD is 5.8 per 1000 people, with 11.9 per 1000 children and 4.1 per 1000 adults being affected. The prevalence of severe defects, including tetralogy of Fallot (TOF), is 1.45 per 1000 children and 0.38 per 1000 adults. Of importance, between 1985 and 2000, the prevalence of severe CHD increased by 85% in adults but only by 22% in children.[2] A clear change in mortality in CHD has been observed, with better survival in infancy and a trend toward death at older age.[3] Survival to adulthood increased from 81% for individuals born between 1970 and 1974 to 88.6% for those born in 1990–92.[4] Improvements in survival are driven by a decreased mortality in moderate and severe forms of CHD in childhood, including TOF, truncus arteriosus, atrioventricular septal defect (AVSD), transposition of the great arteries (TGA), and univentricular hearts. For individuals born in 1990–92, survival to the age of 18 was 78.1% for TOF, 76.5% for AVSD, 70.7% for TGA, and 49.1% for univentricular hearts.[4] This is likely the result of earlier surgical interventions and improved surgical techniques and outcomes. However, improved survival is not exclusively a function of lower mortality in infancy.[4] The increasing number of patients with repaired CHD joining the adult population requires the training of electrophysiologists with a special interest in adult CHD, because potentially life-threatening ventricular arrhythmias (VAs) and sudden cardiac deaths (SCDs) can still occur late after surgery.

The leading cause of mortality in contemporary adults with CHD is chronic heart failure (42%), followed by pneumonia (10%) and SCD, which still accounts for 7% of all deaths, despite a more liberal use of implantable defibrillators in the current era.[5,6] The incidence of SCD in repaired CHD is 0.9–2.6 per 1000 patient-years, which is 25- to 100-fold higher than that for the general population.[5,7,8] In a population-based series of CHD patients who underwent surgery between 1958 and 1996, 90% of all sudden deaths occurred in the following four main categories: aortic stenosis, aortic coarctation, d-TGA, and TOF.[7] Similarly, a single-center cohort study of CHD patients with a reparative or palliative intervention before the age of 20 years reported the highest incidence of SCD in patients with TGA, univentricular hearts, aortic coarctation, and TOF.[8] If nonoperated patients were also included in a large, multicenter case-control study, cyanotic Eisenmenger syndrome accounted for 19% of all SCDs, followed by TGA (19%), repaired TOF (16%), and left-sided outflow lesions.[9] An apparent time-dependent incremental risk for SCD has been observed in patients with left heart obstructions and TOF. Six percent to 9% of patients who underwent repair of TOF died suddenly after 21–35 years of follow-up (2%–3% per decade), accounting for up to 50% of all deaths in this group.[7,10,11] The highest incidence of SCD was found in patients with aortic stenosis, with SCD rates between 10% and 13% after 15–20 years of follow-up.[7,12] The majority of CHD-related SCD is presumably due to VAs, either hemodynamically not tolerated sustained monomorphic ventricular tachycardia (SMVT), with a higher prevalence in patients who have undergone ventricular incision and patch closure of a ventricular septal defect (VSD), or monomorphic and polymorphic VT and ventricular fibrillation (VF) in the absence of surgical scars. Although data are lacking, the latter arrhythmia mechanisms may be similar to those observed in other cardiac diseases with pathological hypertrophy, fibrosis, impairment of cardiac function, and, ultimately, heart failure. Impairment of right and left ventricular (RV and LV, respectively) function is likely to result in altered ion channel and transporter function. Downregulation of K^+ currents and action potential duration (APD) prolongation, which is a consistent finding in ventricular myocytes from subjects with cardiac dysfunction, promote early afterdepolarization. In addition, changes in Ca^{2+}-handling proteins, which are also observed in heart failure, can cause diastolic Ca^{2+} leak from the sarcoplasmic reticulum, resulting in delayed afterdepolarization and triggered activity. Advanced hypertrophy can be due to chronic pressure overload in left heart obstructions and unrepaired TOF. Ventricular dysfunction occurs if the RV serves as the systemic ventricle after an atrial switch operation for TGA or in congenitally corrected TGA (ccTGA). LV dysfunction may be due to longstanding cyanosis if the TOF repair is performed at an older age or if chronic volume overload after palliative shunting has occurred. Furthermore, long-lasting volume overload owing to chronic pulmonary regurgitation after initial correction contributes to ventricular dysfunction. In unselected populations of adults with CHD, moderate to severe systemic ventricular dysfunction is a dominant predictor for SCD.[8,9] However, two-thirds of patients who die suddenly or experience life-threatening ventricular tachycardia (VT), typically early to middle-aged adults, have a preserved cardiac function before the first event.[9,13] Understanding of the different mechanisms of ventricular arrhythmogenesis in CHD is therefore crucial for both risk stratification and treatment. Current data on late morbidity and mortality are based on patients who underwent repair as adolescents. Early surgical intervention and changes in the surgical strategy in particular for TOF and TGA might not only influence early mortality but also affect the incidence and the potential mechanism of arrhythmias and perhaps late morbidity and mortality in adult CHD patients in the future. Detailed descriptions of the most common forms of CHD related to VAs are provided in the following sections.

Ventricular Arrhythmias as Related to Specific Types of Congenital Heart Disease

Tetralogy of Fallot

Developmental and Anatomical Aspects

TOF affects approximately 7.5% of all children born with a congenital heart defect. It is characterized by subpulmonary stenosis, a subaortic VSD, dextroposition of the aortic orifice, and RV hypertrophy, the latter being a feature secondary to the volume

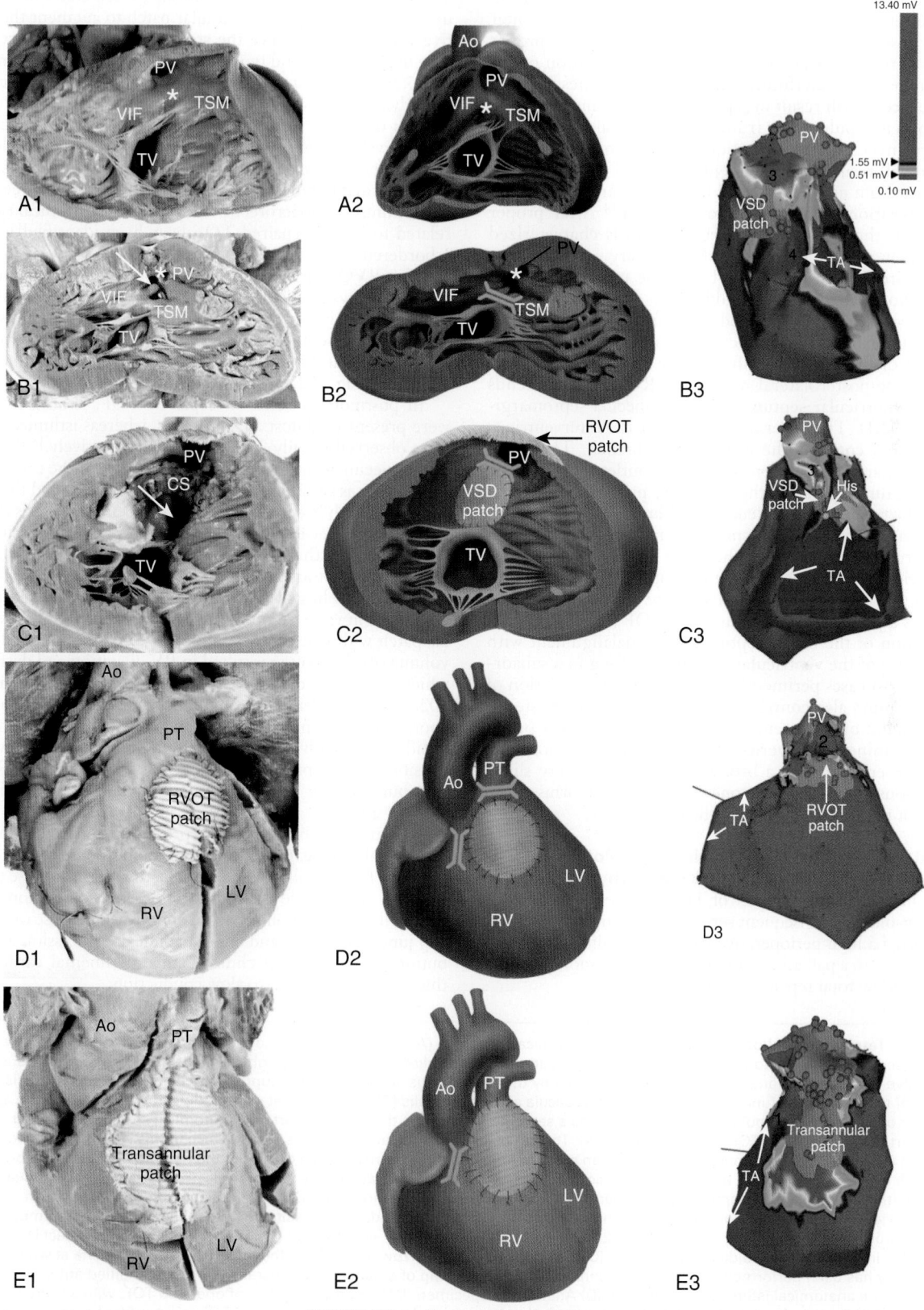

FIGURE 102.1 For legend, see next page.

and pressure overload of the VSD and subpulmonary stenosis, respectively.

During normal development, the outlet portion of the heart needs to evolve from a single myocardial tube to a situation where the separated aorta and pulmonary trunk achieve their definitive positional relationship. This process requires proper septation of the outlet portion of the heart. Formation of the aortopulmonary septum (future outlet septum), orchestrated by neural crest cells, will result in separation of the common trunk into an aorta and pulmonary trunk. Asymmetrical, mainly subpulmonary, myocardial contributions from the so-called second heart field will result in marked lengthening of the subpulmonary myocardium and will "push" the pulmonary trunk to its definitive position, left anterior to the aorta.[14] After proper development, the RV outflow tract (RVOT) is characterized by the presence of a muscular subpulmonary infundibulum forming a circular muscular tube below the pulmonary valve. The posterior wall of the infundibulum, also known as the *crista supraventricularis*, is situated between the tricuspid valve and the pulmonary valve. The crista supraventricularis forms the summit of the ventriculoinfundibular fold, a fold of myocardium at the posterolateral wall of the RVOT, and extends toward the ventricular septum into the trabecula septomarginalis (Fig. 102.1). The latter continues over the interventricular septum and contains the right bundle branch. The crista supraventricularis also encompasses the outlet septum (the muscular septum separating the aortic and pulmonary outlets), situated in between the ventriculoinfundibular fold and trabecula septomarginalis, which is small and not recognizable as a separate structure in the normal heart. In TOF, however, there is an anterior deviation of the outlet septum that, in contrast to normal, can be recognized as a separate structure, which is regarded as a pathognomonic feature of TOF (see Fig. 102.1). The deviation of the outlet septum causes malalignment with the remainder of the ventricular septum, resulting in a subaortic, and in most cases perimembranous, VSD. The deviation of the outlet septum also contributes to the subpulmonary stenosis. The amount of displacement and hypertrophy of the outlet septum determines the severity of the stenosis. The morphology of TOF encompasses a broad spectrum, with very slight malformations and cyanosis on one end and severe forms of the disease with pulmonary atresia on the other.

Type and Timing of Surgical Repair and Its Potential Relation to Risk Factors for Ventricular Arrhythmias

After the first intracardiac repair of TOF in 1954 by Lillehei in a 10-month-old boy, subsequent series of early surgical interventions reported a high perioperative mortality, leading to a "two-stage repair," with a palliative shunt to augment pulmonary blood flow, followed by total repair later in childhood.

Total repair included (patch) closure of the perimembranous or muscular VSD and relief of the infundibular or valvular RVOT obstruction. This repair was initially performed through a vertical or transverse right ventriculotomy, often combined with the use of an RVOT or a transannular patch to augment the restrictive RVOT or to relieve the stenosis of the pulmonary orifice. The malformation and type of repair are important determinants of potential reentrant tachycardia circuits, which is a common underlying mechanism of VT in repaired TOF.[15] Areas of dense fibrosis owing to surgical incisions, as well as the patch material and valve annuli, can form regions of conduction block that define reentry circuit borders and create intervening isthmuses of myocardial bundles that might contain the critical reentry circuit isthmus of a macroreentrant VT. Four anatomical isthmuses related to VT in repaired TOF have been identified[15]: isthmus 1 bordered by the tricuspid annulus and the scar or patch in the anterior RVOT, isthmus 2 between the pulmonary annulus and the RV free wall incision or RVOT patch sparing the pulmonary valve annulus, isthmus 3 between the pulmonary annulus and the VSD patch or septal scar, and isthmus 4 between the VSD patch or septal scar and the tricuspid annulus in patients with muscular VSDs (see Fig. 102.1).

In postmortem series of repaired TOF, isthmuses 3 and 1 were present in almost all specimens, whereas isthmuses 2 and 4 were observed in only 25% and 13%, respectively.[15,16] Of interest, in specimens from patients aged ≥5 years at the time of death, isthmus 1 was significantly wider (3.9 ± 1.08 cm) and thicker (1.5 ± 0.29 cm) with less interstitial and replacement fibrosis than isthmus 3 (width, 1.4 ± 0.77 cm; wall thickness, 0.6 ± 0.25 cm).[16] Not all anatomical isthmuses are related to VT.[17] Specific characteristics of the anatomical isthmuses may be one decisive factor for further remodeling over time, forming the substrate for late VTs.

The right ventriculotomy and the frequent use of a transannular patch with consecutive pulmonary regurgitation and chronic volume overload often resulted in RV dilatation and dysfunction, which is associated with VT and SCD in the long term (Table 102.1). Consequently, a combined transatrial–transpulmonary approach has been introduced. Currently, patch augmentation is avoided or usually limited to the pulmonary annulus whenever possible. This approach does not only positively affect RV function but also can prevent the development of anatomical isthmuses 1 and 2.

Reentrant tachycardias are promoted by slow conduction. Interstitial fibrosis owing to longstanding cyanosis and pressure overload functionally prolongs the pathway for impulse propagation and can provide the substrate for slow conduction. In addition, cell-to-cell coupling can be diminished because of decreased gap junction density and altered connexin expression and distribution, as observed in clinical and experimental cardiomyopathies also contributing to slow conduction.

FIGURE 102.1 Tetralogy of Fallot (TOF) isthmus. (A) Anatomical specimen (A1) and drawing (A2) of the normal heart, right ventricular view. The heart is sectioned parallel to the interventricular septum and opened to allow a view into the right ventricle (*RV*). The fibrous tissues of the tricuspid valve (*TV*) and pulmonary valve (*PV*) are separated by the muscular tissues of the crista supraventricularis (*CS*), which consists of the continuum of the ventriculoinfundibular fold (*VIF*) and trabecula septomarginalis (*TSM*). The outlet septum (location indicated by the *asterisk*) is also a part of the continuum but cannot be identified as a separate structure in the normal heart. (B) Anatomical specimen (B1) and drawing (B2) of a heart with unoperated TOF, same view as in (A). The outlet septum (indicated by the *asterisk*), which in this case is small and fibrous, has deviated from the other components of the CS in an anterior direction, thus narrowing the ostium of the *PV*. The dextroposed aorta can be seen through the ventricular septal defect (*arrow*), which has a muscular rim (substrate for the anatomical isthmus 4). (B3) Electroanatomical voltage map (three-dimensional mapping system, CartoXP, Biosense Webster, Diamond Bar, CA) for a patient with operated TOF in a modified left posterior view. Voltages are color coded according to the color bar; *gray tags* indicate unexcitable tissue. The anatomical isthmus 4 is indicated. (C) Anatomical specimen (C1) and drawing (C2) of operated TOF, same view as in (A) and (B). The ventricular septal defect (*VSD*) patch drawn in place in (C2) has been folded to the right in (C1) to expose the *VSD* (*arrow* in C1). Note the hypertrophic *CS*, the site at which an infundibulectomy has been performed (C1). (C3) Electroanatomical voltage map of a patient with operated TOF in a modified anterior view (*same color coding*). The anatomical isthmus 3 is indicated. (D) Anatomical specimen (D1) and drawing (D2) of operated TOF, with a right ventricular outflow tract (*RVOT*) patch, frontal view. (D3) Electroanatomical voltage map of a patient with operated TOF in a modified anterior view (*same color coding*). The anatomical isthmuses 1 and 2 are indicated. (E) Anatomical specimen (E1) and drawing (E2) of operated TOF, with a transannular patch, frontal view. (E3) Electroanatomical voltage map of a patient with operated TOF in a modified anterior view (*same color coding*). Anatomical isthmus 1 is indicated. *Ao,* Aorta; *PT,* pulmonary trunk; *TA,* tricuspid annulus.

TABLE 102.1 Risk factors for ventricular tachycardia, sudden cardiac death, and adverse events in tetralogy of Fallot				
RISK FACTOR	**VT**	**SCD**	**VT + SCD**	**AE**
Symptoms of (pre)syncope	Yes[1]	Yes[8]		
History of SMVT		Yes[8]		
History of atrial arrhythmias				Yes[28]
Age at total repair		Yes[6,17,21]		Yes[9,11,20]
Presence of transannular patch	Yes[6]	Yes[6]		No[11,14]/Yes[13,20]
QRS-duration ≥180 ms	Yes[1,6,7]	Yes[6,7,8]	Yes[2]	Yes[28]
QRS-duration increase per year	Yes[6]	Yes[6]		
QRS-dispersion	Yes[5]			
QT-duration	Yes[5]			
QT-dispersion	Yes[5]			Yes[22]
JT(c)-dispersion	Yes[5]		Yes[2]	
PVC on ECG		Yes[16,17]		
VA on Holter (PVC >30/min and/or nsVT)	Yes[15,27]	No[3,6]	Yes[26]	Yes[12,28]
LV longitudinal strain on echo				Yes[4]
LV reduced systolic function		Yes[8]		Yes[18,28]
RV reduced systolic function			Yes[25]	Yes[28]
RV LGE				Yes[23]/No[24]
RV akinetic region length			Yes[25]	
RV dimensions (cm)	Yes[1]		Yes[22]	Yes[4,18,19]
RV end systolic pressure (mm Hg)		Yes[16,17,21]		
RV mass/volume ratio ≥0.3 g/mL				Yes[28]
Moderate or severe PVR	Yes[6]	Yes[6,8]		
Inducible for SMVT or SPVT			Yes[10]	

AE, Adverse events; *nsVT,* nonsustained VT; *PVC,* premature ventricular contraction; *PVR,* pulmonary valve regurgitation; *SCD,* sudden cardiac death; *SMVT,* sustained monomorphic VT; *SPVT,* sustained polymorphic VT; *VA,* ventricular arrhythmias; *VT,* ventricular tachycardia.

AE[4], SCD + LTA (sustained VT, resuscitated SCD or appropriate ICD discharge); AE[9/11], mortality; AE[12], appropriate ICD therapy; AE[13], all-cause mortality; AE[14], survival; AE[18], death + sustained VT + increase to NYHA III of IV; AE[19], death + VT; AE[20], late death; AE[23], RV dysfunction + clinical arrhythmias (SVT+VT); AE[24], clinical arrhythmias; AE[28], all-cause mortality + aborted SCD + sustained VT.

1: Balaji et al. *Am J Cardiol.* 1997;80:160-163. (n = 135)
2: Berul et al. *J Cardiovasc Electrophysiol.* 1997;8:1349-1356. (n = 101)
3: Cullen et al. *J Am Coll Cardiol.* 1994;23:1151-1155. (n = 86)
4: Diller et al. *Circulation.* 2012;125:2440-2446. (n = 413)
5: Gatzoulis et al. *Circulation.* 1997;95:401-404. (n = 99)
6: Gatzoulis et al. *Lancet.* 2000;356:975-981. (n = 793)
7: Gatzoulis et al. *Circulation.* 1995;92:231-237. (n = 178)
8: Ghai et al. *J Am Coll Cardiol.* 2002;40:1675-1680. (n = 125)
9: Karamlou et al. *Ann Thorac Surg.* 2006;81:1786-1793; discussion 1793. (n = 249)
10: Khairy et al. *Circulation.* 2004;109:1994-2000. (n = 252)
11: Murphy et al. *N Engl J Med.* 1993;329:593-599. (n = 163)
12: Khairy et al. *Circulation.* 2008;117:363-370. (n = 68)
13: Nollert et al. *J Am Coll Cardiol.* 1997;30:1374-1383. (n = 490)
14: Nollert et al. *Thorac Cardiovasc Surg.* 1997;45:178-181. (n = 71)

15: Harrison et al. *J Am Coll Cardiol,* 1997;30:1368-1373. (n = 210)
16: Garson et al. *Circulation.* 1979;59:1232-1240. (n = 207)
17: Garson et al. *J Am Coll Cardiol.* 1985;6:221-227. (n = 488)
18: Knauth et al. *Heart.* 2008;94:211-216. (n = 88)
19: Ortega et al. *J Am Coll Cardiol.* 2011;107:1535-1540. (n = 39)
20: Jonsson et al. *Scand J Thorac Cardiovasc Surg.* 1995;29:43-51. (n = 165)
21: Jonsson et al. *Scand J Thorac Cardiovasc Surg.* 1995;29:131-139. (n = 141)
22: Daliento et al. *Heart.* 1999;81:650-655. (n = 66)
23: Babu-Narayan et al. *Circulation.* 2006;113:405-413. (n = 92)
24: Preim et al. *Cardiology in the Young.* 2015;25:1268-1275 (n = 53)
25: Bonello et al. *Int J Cardiol.* 2013;168:3280-3286. (n = 154)
26: Czosek et al. *Am J Cardiol.* 2013;111:723-730. (n = 101)
27: Koyak et al. *Int J Cardiol.* 2013;167:1532-1535. (n = 36)
28: Valente et al. *Heart.* 2014;100:247-253. (n = 873)

Myocardial histopathological changes, in particular interstitial fibrosis of the muscular tissue of the crista supraventricularis, are more pronounced in patients who were operated on at an older age, specifically beyond the age of 4 years, and are thus subjected to longstanding cyanosis (SaO$_2$ < 80%) and higher end-diastolic RV pressure (>12 mm Hg).[18]

The current clinical gold standard to detect ventricular fibrosis is late gadolinium enhancement (LGE) on cardiac magnetic resonance (CMR). Myocardial RV LGE was present in almost all adult patients (age, 32.2 ± 1 years) repaired at a median age of 5 years (interquartile range [IQR], 2–8) at the anterior RVOT (99%), septal patch region (98%), and, frequently, RV insertion points (79%). Patients with more extensive fibrosis also involving the RV trabeculations and/or the LV were older and had a later repair. A supramedian RV LGE score and LV LGE were related to adverse clinical effects such as ventricular dysfunction; specifically, RV LGE was associated with atrial arrhythmia and VA.[19] In a younger cohort of patients (age, 20 ± 12 years) with earlier repair at a median age of 2 years, LGE was less frequently detected in the RVOT (15%) and LV and was not associated with adverse events. Patients without LGE were repaired at a median age of 12 months, suggesting that earlier repair and refined surgical techniques may prevent fibrosis detectable by CMR.[20]

Histopathological changes can contribute to the occurrence of complex ventricular ectopy, which has been considered a risk factor for fatal VAs. In particular, older age at repair has been associated with a higher grade of ventricular ectopy.[18,21] Only 11% of patients in whom repair was performed between the ages of 4 and 15 years showed complex ectopy on Holter monitoring 6–12 months after operation compared with 39.4% of patients who underwent surgery beyond the age of 15 years.[18] The age dependency of the occurrence of complex ventricular ectopy could also be demonstrated in uncorrected patients. No significant ventricular ectopy (defined as Lown ≥2, <30 uniform premature ventricular complexes [PVCs]/h) was observed in patients 0–7 years old. In contrast, 58% of patients 16 years or older had complex ectopy, with 21% having runs of nonsustained VT. Of interest, in corrected patients, the relationship between complex ventricular ectopy and time of repair persisted and was independent of the duration of follow-up or of the postoperative hemodynamic status.[22] Although a higher grade of ectopy and nonsustained VT have been associated with VT inducibility, data regarding their association with SCD are inconsistent.[10,21] In a large multicenter cohort asymptomatic complex ectopy and nonsustained VTs were not predictive for SCD.[10] A small, retrospective, single-center study analyzing Holter recordings reported only a weak association between nonsustained VT and sudden cardiac events, including aborted SCD and appropriate implantable cardioverter defibrillator (ICD) therapy.[21] Accordingly, treatment of asymptomatic complex ventricular ectopy is not recommended.[23] In selected patients who received an ICD for primary prevention, nonsustained VT independently predicted ICD therapy,[24] and in a cohort of 36 patients implanted for primary prevention, symptomatic, but not asymptomatic, nonsustained VTs were the only factor associated with appropriate ICD shocks.[25] However, as in other nonischemic cardiomyopathies, ICD therapy may not be a reliable surrogate for SCD. Longer episodes of rapid, nonsustained VTs are more likely to cause symptoms and may prompt inappropriate ICD activation, if short detection times are programmed, with potential adverse effects.[26]

Primary repair in infancy before the age of 18 months has been a common practice since the early 1990s and can be performed with low perioperative mortality. Avoiding long-standing prolonged hypoxemia and pressure overload can reduce the histopathological changes and substrate for slow conduction, complex ventricular ectopy, and fatal VA.

Despite early operation, progressive pulmonary regurgitation occurs in almost all patients after transannular patch repair and is an important reason for reintervention. Although often tolerated, pulmonary regurgitation ultimately leads to RV dilatation and dysfunction, which can be further aggravated by residual RVOT obstruction. Moderate to severe pulmonary regurgitation and abnormal RV hemodynamics in particular and increased RV end-systolic pressure have been associated with VT and SCD.

In addition, a wide QRS (≥180 ms) and an increase in QRS duration (QRSd) have consistently been reported as risk factors for SMVT and SCD.[10] In particular, RV dilatation, but not restrictive RV physiology, has been associated with QRS prolongation, referred to as *mechanoelectrical interaction*.[27]

Impairments of RV function and LV hemodynamics have important roles. A moderate to severe LV systolic dysfunction—defined as ejection fraction (EF) of less than 39% and 20%, respectively—was also more common in patients with TOF and (aborted) SCD.[28] In addition, an LV end-diastolic pressure (LVEDP) ≥12 mm Hg was a strong and independent predictor of appropriate ICD shocks in patients with TOF who received an ICD for primary prevention.[24]

Effect of Pulmonary Valve Replacement and Intraoperative Cryoablation on QRS Duration and Ventricular Arrhythmias

Although surgical pulmonary valve replacement (PVR) has been associated with a reduction in RV end-diastolic volume in selected patients, a consistent reduction in QRSd after surgery has not been demonstrated.[29,30] A QRSd greater than 180 ms 6 months after PVR or no reduction in the postoperative QRSd was, however, a strong predictor of adverse events defined as all-cause mortality, reoperation for pulmonary regurgitation, heart failure, or VT.[31] In particular, patients with severely prolonged QRSd that did not change postoperatively had the highest incidence of adverse events. Prolonged QRSd may reflect global conduction delay in a dilated RV and may serve as one surrogate marker for the changes in mechanical forces that trigger changes at cellular and subcellular levels, also known as mechanoelectrical coupling associated with arrhythmogenesis. QRS prolongation can also be the result of right bundle branch damage, which can occur at different levels (proximal, distal, and terminal) during the initial repair or as a consequence of pressure or volume overload.[32] QRS

prolongation may, however, also more specifically reflect morphological and functional changes of the RVOT beyond the conduction system. In patients with a QRS ≥155 ms, a strong correlation between QRSd and echocardiographic delay in RVOT motion was reported, which was outside the normal range in all patients with a QRSd >165 ms.[33]

QRSd also correlated with morphological abnormalities like the akinetic area length on CMR. In a single-center study following 154 TOF patients over a median of 5.6 years (IQR, 4.6–7.0), the RVOT akinetic region length remained the only independent predictor for VAs.[34]

Localized conduction delay may have effects beyond mechanical dyssynchrony of the RVOT. Slow-conducting anatomical isthmuses identified using electroanatomical mapping during sinus rhythm (calculated conduction velocity index of <0.5 m/s) were related to 37 of 41 VTs that could be induced in 26 TOF patients.[34a] In particular, the slow-conducting anatomical isthmus 3 bordering the infundibular septum may further delay activation of the lateral RVOT and basal RV in those with a preexisting terminal right bundle branch block (RBBB). This finding may provide an important link between a prolonged QRSd ≥180 ms and VT (unpublished data).

Despite the remarkable reduction of RV volumes and hemodynamic improvement of RV function after PVR,[35] simply replacing the valve might not eliminate the substrate for reentrant VTs; reentry was the underlying mechanism of all VTs that were associated with a QRS greater than 180 ms in one series.[27] After a late PVR performed in 98 patients 20 ± 9 years after TOF repair, VT occurred in 11 and death occurred in 6 patients after a mean follow-up of 2.8 ± 4.3 years; the 5- and 10-year measures of freedom of the composite outcome of death and VT were 80% and 41%, respectively, which were not different from those of the control group (*n* = 77) matched for age, pulmonary regurgitation, RV dilatation, and QRSd and who did not undergo PVR.[36] These data suggest that either PVR was performed too late, not leading to a favorable reverse remodeling despite a reduction in RV size, or VTs are the result of a fixed substrate not influenced by hemodynamic improvements. Of interest, five of seven patients who underwent PVR and concomitant (not further specified) intraoperative cryoablation experienced VT during follow-up. In contrast, map-guided intraoperative ablation was more effective in controlling VT recurrence. Of 44 patients with documented SMVT, 31 underwent cryoablation applied to the macroreentry site, as assessed using the combined endocardial and epicardial mapping during cardioplegic arrest. VT recurred in only three (10%) patients after ablation, with a 96% freedom from VT after 7.5 years.[37]

Based on the observation that VTs often depend on four anatomically defined isthmuses, a surgical cryoablation lesion connecting the boundaries may be a reasonable alternative to mapping-guided ablation at the time of PVR. In 22 patients (history of VT in 4 and inducible at EPS in 10), the superior aspect of the VSD and the pulmonary annulus (isthmus 3) were connected during PVR. In selected patients, an additional lesion grounding the ventriculotomy to the pulmonary (isthmus 2) or tricuspid annulus (isthmus 1) was performed. Only a single event occurred 7 years after PVR.[38] Achieving bidirectional conduction block is an accepted endpoint for linear lesions. Whether intraoperative cryoablation without endpoint confirmation is sufficient for patients with isthmus-dependent VTs and not potentially proarrhythmogenic in those with normal conduction properties before surgery requires further study.

Role of Programmed Electrical Stimulation

A positive programmed electrical stimulation (PES), usually defined as inducibility of an SMVT, provides an important tool to prove the presence of a substrate for reentrant VT, although VT based on triggered activity may also be inducible in the electrophysiology laboratory. Accordingly, only 16% of patients who had documented sustained VT were not inducible by PES in one series.[39] Inducibility of the clinical or presumed clinical VT could, however, be achieved in all patients referred for VT ablation if PES was also performed from a site close to the infundibular septum.[17]

Consequently, PES has also been used to identify patients with TOF who are at risk of potential fatal VAs. Inducibility of sustained VT is high in patients with presyncope and complex PVCs on Holter monitoring and is more likely in patients repaired at older age and when PES is performed late after surgery.[40,41] Importantly, inducibility strongly depends on the applied induction protocol; SMVT induction required three extrastimuli in 70% and isoproterenol in 11% of the patients in two series.[39,40] Using a complete PES protocol (two RV sites, three cycle lengths [CLs], triples, and isoproterenol), the diagnostic value (sensitivity, 77.4%; specificity, 79.5%) and the prognostic significance (relative risk, 5.0 for clinical VT or SCD) of PES in TOF patients are comparable with those of the postinfarct population.[39] Of interest, the highest event rate (SCD, VT, or both) was observed in patients inducible for sustained polymorphic VT (SPVT). Although derived from a small number of patients, induction of SPVT may not be an unspecific finding and may reflect a different but potentially fatal arrhythmogenic substrate.

Type of Ventricular Arrhythmias and the Underlying Substrate: Impact on Treatment and Risk Stratification

The majority of VA documented in TOF patients is monomorphic VT. The prevalence of SMVT was 14.2% in a recently conducted multicenter study comprising 556 TOF patients and was markedly increased after the age of 45 years; in contrast, VF could be documented in only 0.5% of the population.[3] The incidence of VF in TOF patients may be underestimated, as patients in the cohort are survivors. However, in 121 TOF patients who received an ICD for primary or secondary prevention, 81.5% of all appropriately delivered therapy was for monomorphic VT. Of importance, VTs were fast with a median heart rate of 213 beats/min (182–264).[24] There are no available data on the efficacy of antiarrhythmic drugs, and only limited data exist on dosage and toxicity in different age groups. In general, antiarrhythmic drugs initiated to prevent recurrence of reentrant VT in structural heart disease have disappointing efficacy, and the use of antiarrhythmic drugs is hampered by potentially serious side effects.

The feasibility of catheter ablation of VT in CHD, with the majority performed in TOF patients, has been reported (Table 102.2). In most of the earlier series and case reports, the targeted VTs were slow, hemodynamically tolerated, and therefore approachable through conventional mapping techniques, such as activation and entrainment mapping during ongoing VT. An intention-to-treat analysis was published by the group from the Boston Children's Hospital.[42] In this study, acute ablation failure was 50% because of noninducibility or hemodynamic instability or due to anatomical reasons. Three recently published studies used substrate mapping techniques to target all inducible and, in particular, fast and poorly tolerated VTs, which are common.

Using a noncontact mapping system consisting of a multielectrode balloon array that allows simultaneous acquisition of virtual unipolar electrograms, the activation sequence of 13 fast or nonsustained VTs in 10 patients could be obtained.[43] Of the 13 induced VTs, 11 were due to macroreentrant circuits, whereas 2 were due to microreentrant circuits. The anatomical location of the isthmus could be identified in all patients and was successfully targeted by a linear ablation lesion in eight patients. In two patients, radiofrequency delivery was withheld because of the proximity of the His bundle. An alternative approach applies point-by-point electroanatomical voltage and activation

mapping during stable sinus rhythm to obtain a three-dimensional (3D) reconstruction of all potential isthmuses by identifying the anatomical boundaries (see Fig. 102.1).[15] Peak-to-peak bipolar electrogram amplitudes can be displayed color coded and projected on a 3D shell of the RV. Electrograms greater than 1.5 mV are considered as having normal voltage. At sites with amplitudes less than 0.5 mV, high output pacing (10 mA, 2 ms) can be performed to identify unexcitable tissue, which is consistent with patch material or surgical scars. The critical reentry circuit isthmus of each induced VT can be determined by activation and entrainment mapping for tolerated VT or by pace mapping for poorly tolerated ones. If the critical isthmus is located within an anatomically defined isthmus (Fig. 102.2), the "critical isthmus" can be transected by connecting the adjoining anatomical boundaries by linear radiofrequency lesions. A systematic approach (Fig. 102.3) has been highly effective in the treatment of all VTs, in particular poorly tolerated ones, with promising long-term results.[15,17] A demonstration of conduction block after isthmus transection by radiofrequency catheter ablation or cryoablation provides a defined procedural endpoint similar to that for achieving block in the common cavotricuspid isthmus.[17]

In the largest series to date that reported on VT ablation in 34 adults with CHD (82% TOF; median VTCL, 295 ms; and IQR, 242–346), complete procedural success was defined as noninducibility of any VT and transection of the critical anatomical isthmus. This endpoint was achieved in 25 adults (74%). None of the patients in whom complete procedural success was achieved had recurrence of a monomorphic VT during 46 ± 29 months of follow-up, whereas one patient with poor RV function experienced appropriate ICD discharge for VF.[17] These data suggest that macroreentrant VTs based on an anatomical substrate can be effectively treated using catheter ablation and that isthmus ablation with confirmed conduction block may be considered curative in patients with preserved cardiac function and no competing arrhythmia mechanism; however, other VAs can occur in patients with impaired RV function.[17] Anatomical isthmuses are present in almost all tetralogy patients but not all are related to VT. Specific characteristics of an anatomical isthmus may be required to constitute the substrate for reentry VT.

Detailed electroanatomical mapping during sinus rhythm performed in a cohort of 74 consecutive TOF patients with at least one risk factor for VA, including 13 with prior documented VT, could demonstrate that narrow and slow conducting anatomical isthmuses (calculated conduction velocity <0.5 m/s) were the substrate for all documented and induced VT in patients with *preserved* cardiac function (unpublished data). Of interest, the most prevalent arrhythmogenic anatomical isthmus was isthmus 3, which was narrower with thinner walls in postmortem specimens.[16] These specific characteristics may facilitate further arrhythmogenic remodeling. Direct identification of the substrate for VT in an individual patient is appealing, could overcome the problem of lacking clinical arrhythmia predictors, and could allow personalized risk stratification and tailored treatment.

Of importance, inducibility of the clinical arrhythmia and hemodynamic tolerance is no longer a prerequisite for successful ablation. The strong association between anatomically defined isthmuses and macroreentrant VT might also be helpful to guide intraoperative ablation in patients who require reoperation for PV regurgitation.

Implantable Cardioverter Defibrillator

As discussed earlier, the risk of SCD in patients with surgically corrected TOF is estimated to be 1.2%–1.8% 10 years after surgery and 2.5% 20 years after surgery. The SCD risk increases to 4% and 6% 25 and 30 years after surgery, respectively, with a risk between 6% and 10% per decade 25 years

| TABLE 102.2 | Published data on ventricular tachycardia ablation in congenital heart disease | | | | | | | |

AUTHOR, YEAR	CHD	METHOD	PATIENT (N)	SUS-VT (N)	VTCL MEAN (MS)	ACUTE SUCCESS	RECURRENCE
Burton, 1993	TOF	PM	2	2	270	2/2	0/2
Biblo, 1994	TOF	AM	1	2	430	1/1	0/1
Goldner, 1994	TOF	PM	1	1	240	1/1	0/1
Cinushi, 1995	TOF	AM + LL	1	2	420	2/2	0/1
Gonska, 1996[c]	TOF 7, VSD 1, TGA + VSD 1, PS 2	AM	11	11	377	9/11	2/11
Horton, 1997	TOF	AM + LL	2	2	430	2/2	0/2
Baral, 2004	ccTGA + Ebstein + TVR	AM (NC) + ENT	1	1	380	1/1	0/1
Rostock, 2004	TOF	AM + LL	1	1	340	1/1	0/1
Morwood, 2004	TOF 8, VSD 3, Others 3	—	14 Patients 20 Procedures	—	—	10/20	4/10
Furushima, 2005	TOF/DORV	AM + LL	7	14 Targeted 8	346	4/7	6/7
Kriebel, 2007	TOF	SSM + LVA (NC) + LL	10	13	269	8/10	2/8
Zeppenfeld, 2007	TOF 9, AVSD 1, TGA + VSD 1	SSM + EUS + LL + IMG (1/11, CT)	11	15	276	11/11	1/11
Nair, 2011	TGA + VSD + sPS	SSM + PM + IMG (CT)	1	1	350	1/1	0/1
Piers, 2012	TGA + sPS	SSM + AM + IMG (CT, CMR)	1	1	340	1/1	0/1
Kapel, 2015	TOF 28, TGA + sPS 1, TGA + VSD 1 VSD + sPS 1, PS 1 VSD + bAV 1, AVSD 1	SSM +EUS + LL + IMG	34	61	295 (242–346)[a]	25/34[b]	0/25[c]

[a]Median, IQR.
[b]Acute success defined as noninducibility and transection of anatomical isthmus.
[c]One patient had ICD shock for VF.
AM, Activation mapping; *AVSD,* atrioventricular septal defect; *CMR,* cardiac magnetic resonance imaging; *(cc)TGA,* (congenitally corrected) transposition of the great arteries; *CHD,* congenital heart disease; *CT,* computed tomography; *DORV,* double outlet right ventricle; *ENT,* entrainment; *EUS,* electrically unexcitable scar; *IMG,* image integration; *LL,* linear lesions; *LVA,* low voltage areas; *NC,* noncontact; *PM,* pace mapping; *(s)PS,* (sub)pulmonary stenosis; *SSM,* substrate mapping; *sus-VT,* sustained ventricular tachycardia; *TOF,* tetralogy of Fallot; *TVR,* tricuspid valve replacement; *VSD,* ventricular septal defect; *VTCL,* ventricular tachycardia cycle length.

Sources:
Burton et al. *Pacing Clin Electrophysiol.* 1993;16:2319-2325.
Biblo et al. *Pacing Clin Electrophysiol.* 1994;17:1556-1560.
Goldner et al. *Pacing Clin Electrophysiol.* 1994;17:1441-1446.
Chinushi et al. *Pacing Clin Electrophysiol.* 1995;18:1713-1716.
Gonska et al. *Circulation.* 1996;94:1902-1908.
Horton et al. *J Cardiovasc Electrophysiol.* 1997;8:432-435.
Baral et al. *J Interv Card Electrophysiol.* 2004;11:211-215.
Rostock et al. *Pacing Clin Electrophysiol.* 2004;27:801-804.
Morwood et al. *Heart Rhythm.* 2004;1:301-308.
Furushima et al. *J Electrocardiol.* 2006;39:219-224.
Kriebel et al. *J Am Coll Cardiol.* 2007;50:2162-2168.
Zeppenfeld et al. *Circulation.* 2007;116:2241-2252.
Nair et al. *Indian Pacing Electrophysiol J.* 2011;11:120-125.
Piers et al. *Circ Arrhythm Electrophysiol.* 2012;5:e38-e40.
Kapel et al. *Circ Arrhythm Electrophysiol.* 2015;8:102-109.

after surgery.[44] Several factors associated with SCD in patients with TOF have been identified (see Table 102.1); however, the prognostic value of each factor is limited. According to the Pediatric and Congenital Electrophysiology Society/Heart Rhythm Society (PACES/HRS) expert consensus statement and the European Society of Cardiology (ESC) guidelines, an ICD should be implanted in SCD survivors after exclusion of a reversible etiology.[23,45] Furthermore, an ICD is indicated in patients with spontaneous sustained VT. Considering the recent reports, catheter ablation or surgery may offer a reasonable alternative to ICD therapy in carefully selected patients.[17,38] ICD implantation can be considered in patients after unexplained syncope without a defined and reversible cause. However, if symptoms of presyncope or syncope are reported, an induction protocol for both VT and supraventricular tachycardias (SVTs) may be helpful. Prophylactic implantation of ICDs is still under debate. In patients with CHD and a systemic LVEF ≤35% as well as New York Heart Association (NYHA) class II–III symptoms, an ICD is indicated. Primary prevention ICD implantation is considered reasonable in selected adults with TOF and multiple risk factors for

sudden cardiac death, such as LV systolic or diastolic dysfunction, nonsustained VT, QRS greater than 180 ms, extensive RV scarring, or inducible sustained VT at electrophysiological study.[23,45] In high-risk patients with TOF, ICD implantation has been shown to be effective for both primary and secondary prevention, with appropriate and effective shocks in more than 30% of patients.[24] Of importance, more than 80% of the treated VAs in the Fallot population were monomorphic VT and fast VT (median heart rate, 212 beats/min), but 70% of the patients required ICD shocks to terminate the first arrhythmia. Even if antitachycardia pacing was programmed and appropriately delivered, it failed in 81% of patients with CHD.[46] These fast VTs are currently approachable by substrate-based ablation techniques, which should be considered as an adjunct to ICD therapy. Although long-term efficacy data of catheter ablation of fast VT are lacking, results from a recent series are promising.[17] Important device-related complications are inappropriate shocks, which were observed in 25%–30% of all patients[24,46] (actuarial rate, 5.8% of patients per year) and are often due to supraventricular arrhythmias and late lead-related complications occurring in 20%.[17,24]

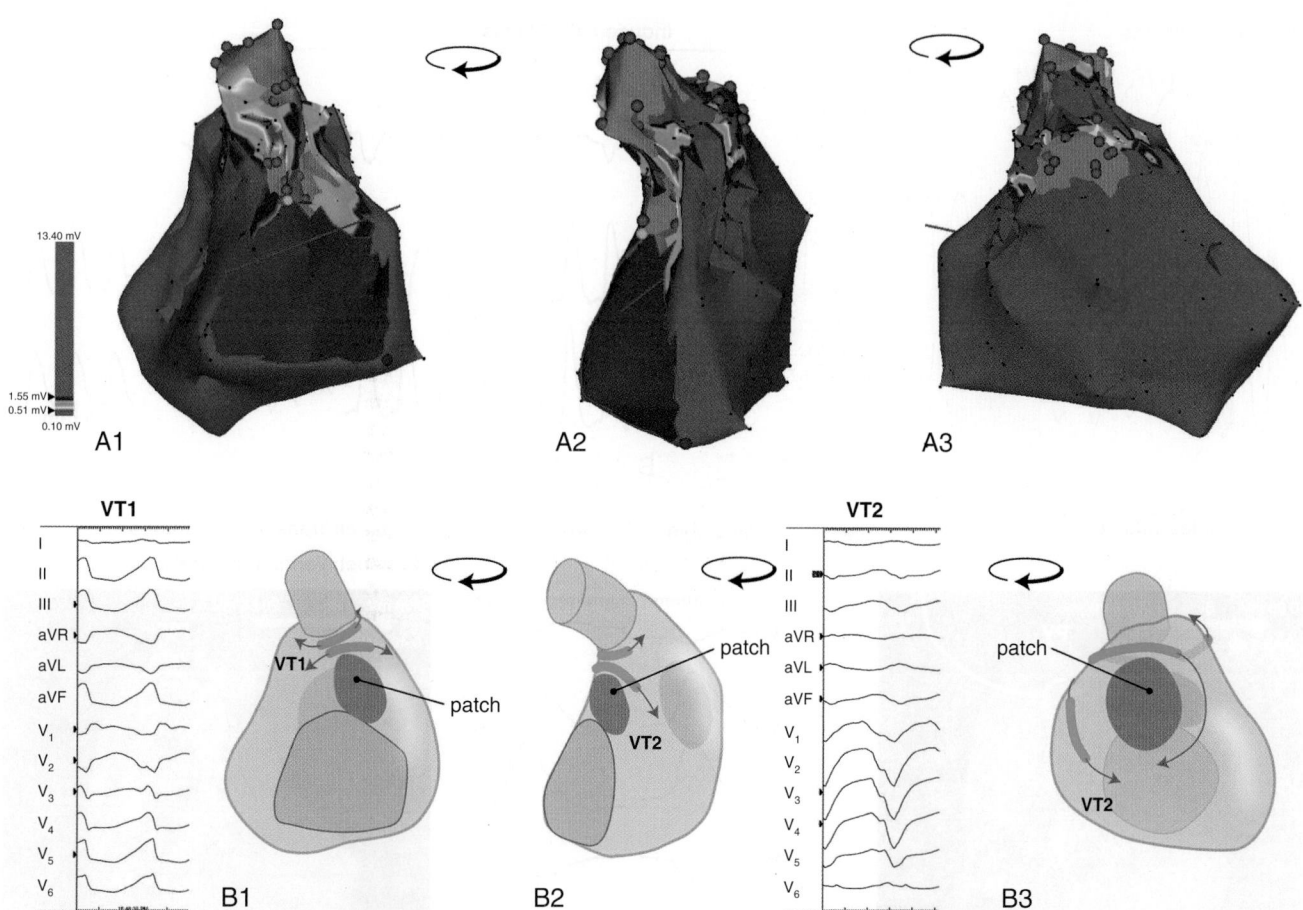

FIGURE 102.2 Potential anatomical isthmuses for reentry. (A) Electroanatomical voltage map of a patient with operated tetralogy of Fallot (closure of a perimembranous ventricular septal defect, a right ventricular outflow tract patch sparing the pulmonary vein, and the resection of infundibular muscle). Bipolar voltages are color coded according to the color bar; *gray* indicates inexcitable tissue; *yellow tag* indicates the position of the His bundle. The map is turned counterclockwise from a posterior (A1) through a right lateral (A2) to an anterior view (A3). (B) Schematic of panel (A). Potential anatomical isthmuses are indicated, as are potential directions of wavefront propagation during ventricular tachycardia (*VT*). Schematic drawings in panels (B1)–(B3) correspond with the electroanatomical voltage maps in (A1)–(A3). Note that activation of the same isthmus in a counterclockwise or clockwise direction results in a different 12-lead electrocardiogram. Example provided for the isthmus 3: counterclockwise activation results in VT1 and clockwise activation in VT2.

Transposition of the Great Arteries

Developmental and Anatomical Aspects

TGA (Fig. 102.4) is the most common cyanotic heart disease in newborns, comprising 5% of all CHDs. It can occur isolated (simple TGA) or in association with other congenital malformations (complex TGA). In TGA, there is a concordant atrioventricular (AV) connection in combination with ventriculoarterial discordance, with the aorta connecting to the morphological RV and the pulmonary trunk to the morphological LV. There is often a parallel course of the great arteries, with a right anterior position of the aorta with respect to the pulmonary orifice.[47] From a developmental point of view, the abnormal position of the great arteries in TGA might be related to a deficient lengthening of the outflow tract during development, for which contributions from the so-called second heart field are necessary.[14]

Complex TGA is most commonly associated with VSDs (in approximately 40%) and LV outflow tract (LVOT) or RVOT obstruction. In cases with infundibular VSDs, the outlet septum can often be recognized as a separate structure. Obstruction of the RVOT and LVOT are usually caused by rightward and leftward deviations of the outlet septum, respectively, and can become more pronounced by hypertrophy of the outlet septum. In addition, muscle bundles, subvalvular fibrous tissues, or abundant AV valve tissues can contribute to the narrowing of RVOT and LVOT.[47]

Type and Timing of Surgical Repair and Its Potential Relation to Risk Factors for Ventricular Arrhythmias

Before the 1980s, most patients underwent a two-stage repair surgical intervention. The Blalock-Hanlon atrial septectomy, introduced in 1950 and replaced by the Raskind balloon atrial septostomy after 1966, is usually performed acutely after birth. This is followed by an atrial switch operation—either the Senning or the Mustard procedure—within the first year of life. The Senning procedure, first performed in 1959, used the atrial septum to create a baffle to redirect the blood flow from the caval veins to the LV. The Mustard procedure, introduced in 1964, used a baffle from pericardium or synthetic material.

Currently, most of the patients seen at the adult outpatient clinic have been treated with the atrial switch operation. SCD is the leading cause of late mortality and seems to be constant over time, with an estimated incidence of 4% ± 7% at 10 years and 9% ± 4% at 20 years of follow-up.[7] In a retrospective study of

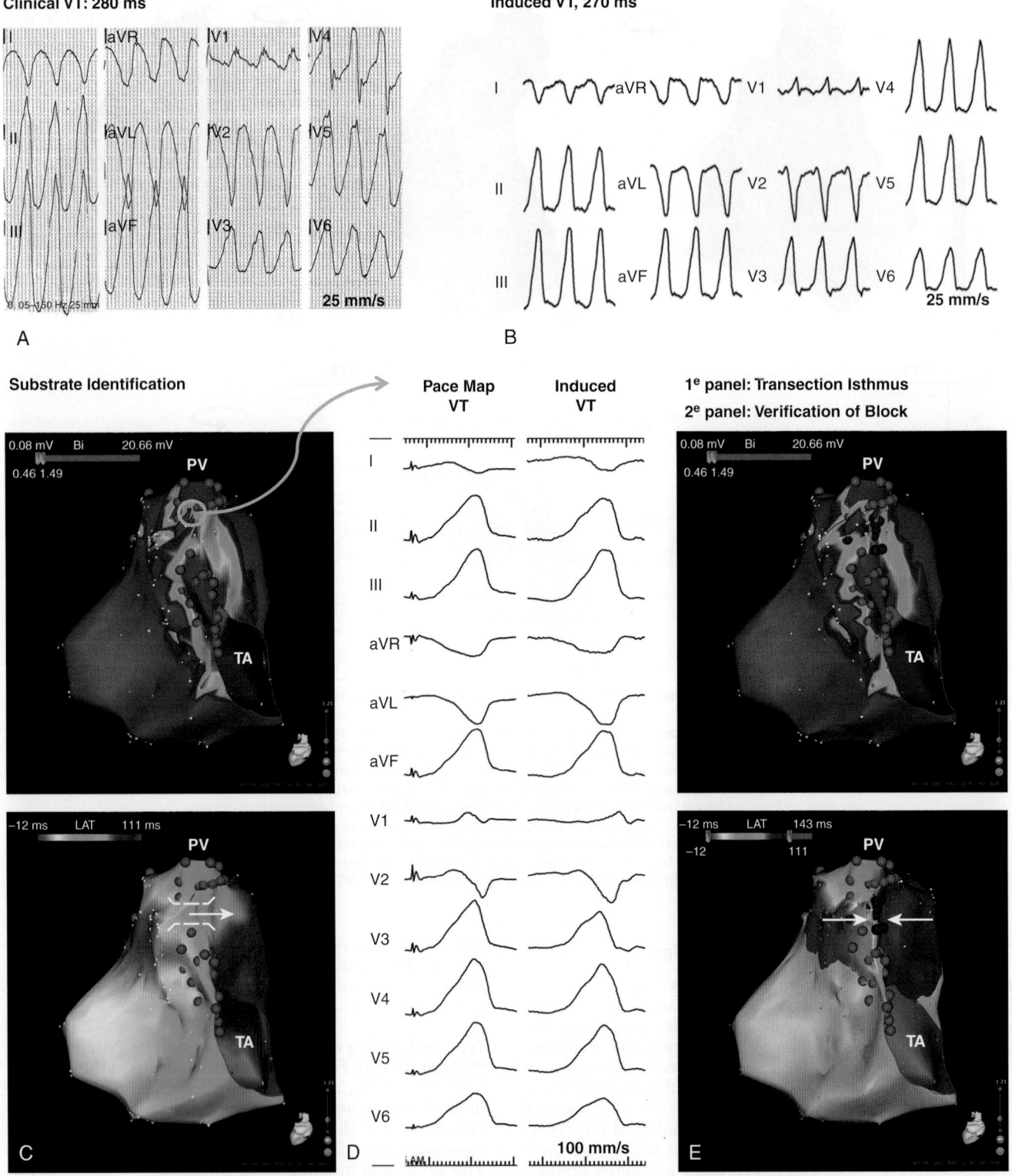

FIGURE 102.3 Systematic approach for hemodynamically untolerated ventricular tachycardia (*VT*). (A) 12-lead VT-electrocardiogram of the clinical VT during resuscitation. (B) Induced clinical VT. (C) Bipolar voltage and activation map during sinus rhythm (*modified posteroanterior view*). Voltage and activation time is color coded according to the bar, and the *gray tags* indicate unexcitable tissue. Anatomical isthmus 3 (*white dashed brackets*) is present between the ventricular septal defect patch and the pulmonary valve (*PV*) with continuous but slow conduction during sinus rhythm. (D) VT isthmus site within the anatomical isthmus 3 is identified by pace mapping. (E) Voltage and activation map after ablation. *Red tags* indicate ablation sites. After a linear radiofrequency lesion through isthmus 3, the activation sequence has changed (*white arrows*), consistent with a block across the line. *TA*, Tricuspid annulus. (From Kapel GF, Reichlin T, Wijnmaalen AP, et al. Re-entry using anatomically determined isthmuses: a curable ventricular tachycardia in repaired congenital heart disease. *Circ Arrhythm Electrophysiol.* 2015;8:102-109.)

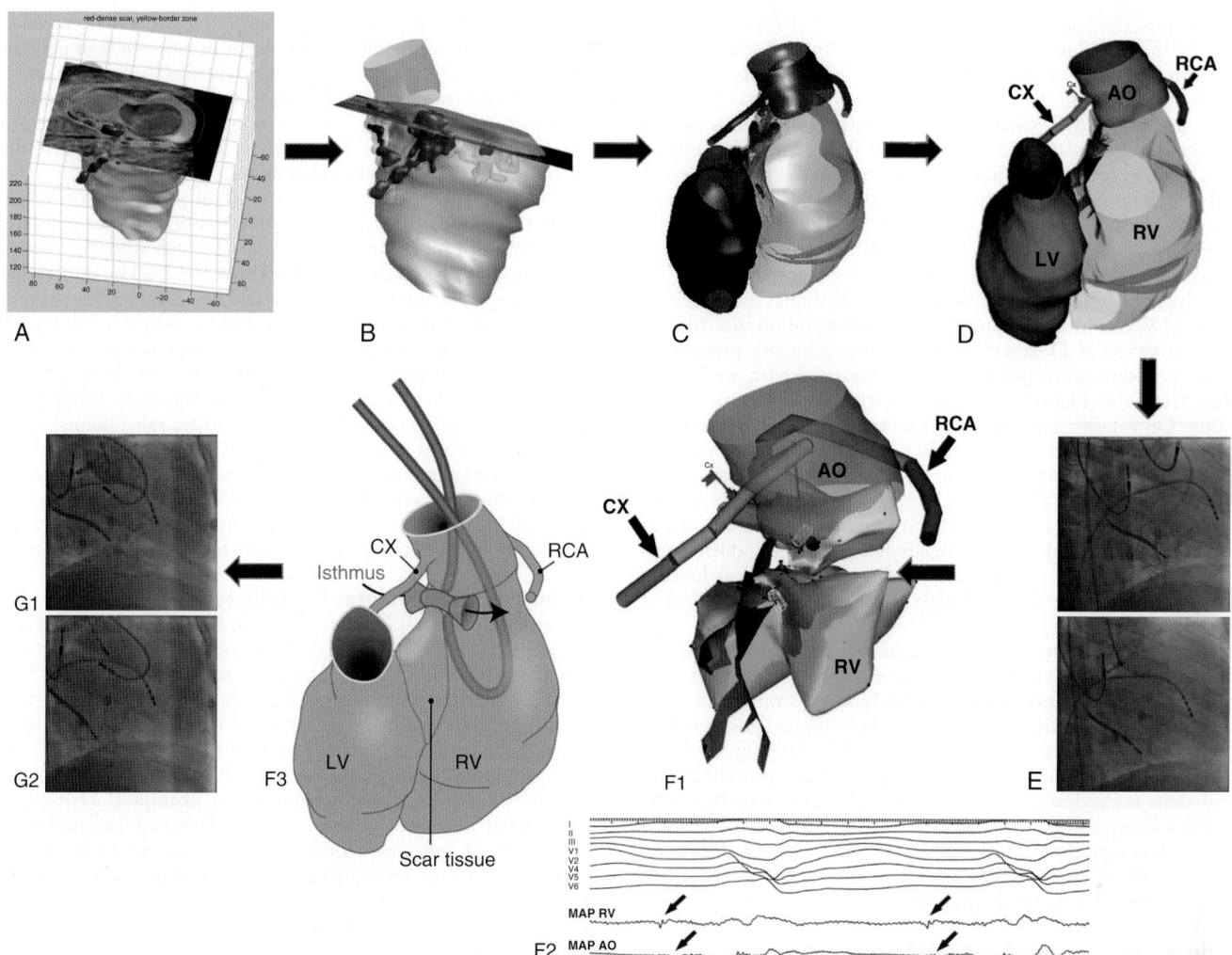

FIGURE 102.4 Transposition of the great arteries (TGA; including image integration). Ventricular tachycardia ablation in a patient with Mustard baffle and resection of a subpulmonary stenosis for complex TGA. Preprocedure contrast-enhanced (CE) cardiac magnetic resonance imaging (MRI) (A) was followed by image processing to reconstruct the anatomy and scar distribution based on signal intensity. *Red areas* indicate dense scar, and *yellow areas* indicate the scar border zone (B and C). (D) Integration of MRI-derived scar projected on the endocardial surface of the right ventricle (*RV*) was performed using the position of the ostium of the right coronary artery (*RCA*) and circumflex branch of the left coronary artery (*CX*) determined using contrast injection through the mapping catheter (E). (C), (D), and (F) demonstrate the same posterior view. After two-point image integration, limited activation mapping from the aorta (*AO*) and *RV* restricted to the area of interest showed a macro-reentrant tachycardia (*red* indicates early activation and *purple* late activation ([F1] with middiastolic activity recorded from *RV* and *AO* [F2]). The schematic illustrates the identified anatomical isthmus on the basis of CE-MRI, which was bordered by the septal scar tissue and the aortic root. Transection of the isthmus required bipolar ablation delivered between two ablation catheters, one placed in the aortic root and the other opposite in the *RV,* as indicated on the map (F1), the schematic (F3), and the fluoroscopic image (G2). Radiofrequency delivery terminated ventricular tachycardia after 3 seconds (not shown). Before radiofrequency delivery, the distance between the catheter and the ostium of the RCX was estimated based on a contrast injection in the aortic root and was considered safe (G1). *LV,* Left ventricle.

47 patients with sudden death (34 SCD; 13 aborted), the event occurred at a median age of 9.7 years (range, 0.3–32 years) and 7.9 years (range, 0.3–28.8 years) after surgery.[48] A longitudinal, single-center study following 81 hospital survivors after a Mustard repair reported 17 late deaths; 9 died suddenly at a median age of 10 years without evidence of prior heart failure or arrhythmias in 8 patients.[49] Similarly, sudden death was the most common cause, accounting for 8 of 14 deaths at a median age of 10.5 years, in 108 patients with a Mustard repair for simple TGA who survived the first postoperative year.[50]

Of importance, more than 80% of SCDs occurred during exercise, likely because of an inability to increase cardiac output as a response to the increased demand, leading to low output cardiac failure. The latter can be worsened by coexisting conditions such as baffle obstruction, pulmonary vein stenosis, or ventricular dysfunction.[48] Atrial arrhythmias that preceded SCD in 7% of the patients further impaired AV transport and decreased RV filling. RV dysfunction may also lead to VA as a consequence of RV dilatation and tricuspid regurgitation, resulting in hemodynamic compromise and mechanoelectrical interaction (i.e., a relation of mechanical and electrical properties of the RV due to which RV dilation and life-threatening arrhythmias may occur).[27] Ischemia of the systemic RV may further contribute to ventricular arrhythmogenesis.[51] Late-enhancement CMR studies have indicated the occurrence of myocardial fibrosis in the systemic RV in patients after physiological correction, which may be relevant in the occurrence of VAs.[52] Although risk stratification is generally limited, symptoms of arrhythmias and heart failure and documented atrial flutter or fibrillation have been identified as predictors of SCD in patients after a Mustard or Senning procedure.[48]

The implication of supraventricular arrhythmias in the occurrence of VAs is further supported by the observation that 50% of all appropriate ICD shocks in primary or secondary prevention ICD recipients were preceded by or coexisted with an SVT.[53] Risk factors as identified in patients with TOF are of limited value. Only 1 of 23 patients who received an ICD for primary prevention experienced appropriate ICD therapy. Implantation was prompted by presyncope in 48% of patients, nonsustained VT in 48%, QRSd ≥180 ms in 30%, RVEF ≤35% in 35%, and inducible VT in 30.4%. However, in a single-center review of 149 adults, the combined endpoint of sustained VT and sudden death was more likely in patients with additional anatomical lesions, impaired RV function, NYHA class III or greater, and a QRSd of 140 ms or greater.

Since 1975, anatomical correction with the arterial switch operation has become the treatment of choice. During this procedure, the aorta and pulmonary trunk are disconnected from their arterial roots (that will remain in their original position) and "switched" to connect to the proper ventricle. This approach not only reduces the incidence of postoperative atrial arrhythmias and sinus node dysfunction, it is also likely to reduce fatal VAs as the LV supports the systemic circulation. In complex cases of TGA, modification of these operations or other operation techniques, such as the Rastelli operation for treatment of TGA with LVOT obstruction, may be necessary.

Role of Programmed Electrical Stimulation
There are few data regarding the role of PES in adult patients with TGA. In one series, 17 patients underwent PES before ICD implantation (10 of 17 patients for primary prevention).[53] Nine patients (six of nine primary prevention patients) were inducible, but with only three for monomorphic VT and six for SPVT. During follow-up, none of the inducible but three of the noninducible patients, all receiving implants after a spontaneous VA event, experienced appropriate ICD therapy. These data suggest that different substrates and underlying mechanisms occur in patients with TGA.

Types of Ventricular Arrhythmias and the Underlying Substrate: Effect on Treatment
The Senning and Mustard procedures result in physiological repair, after which the morphological RV supports the systemic circulation, with the risk of right heart failure and related VAs over time. Accordingly, more than 50% of all VAs prompting ICD therapy in TGA among patients receiving implants for primary or secondary prevention were polymorphic VT or VF.[53] SMVT is relatively uncommon, with an estimated incidence rate of 0.5% per year.[7]

Simple TGA does not require surgical incisions of the ventricles or patch material, which has been associated with monomorphic VT in the TOF population. Surgical incisions or patch material are, however, necessary in complex TGA, which is usually defined as the additional presence of a VSD requiring patch closure or other lesions like outflow tract obstruction requiring surgical intervention.[48,54] Surgical scars and patch material can serve as anatomical boundaries facilitating macroreentrant VT, as in TOF (see Fig. 102.2). In an adult cohort of 149 patients of whom 107 (72%) had simple transposition, sustained VT was documented in

7 patients. Four of these seven had complex TGA. VT occurred in 9.5% of patients with complex TGA but in only 2.8% of patients with simple TGA.[54] Sustained VT is rarely observed during childhood. The deterioration of RV function over time with electrical and structural remodeling, which is more often observed in complex TGA (42% vs. 2% at 20 years),[55] is likely to contribute to the late occurrence of VT and sudden death.

There are no specific data on medical treatment of VA in TGA, and there are only four case reports on catheter mapping and ablation of monomorphic VT, all of which were performed in patients with complex TGA (see Table 102.2). The underlying mechanism was reentry, and the critical reentrant circuit isthmus was located in an anatomical isthmus bordered by the VSD patch and aortic valve in three patients and in an area of septal transmural scar and at the aortic valve in one patient. In the latter patient, preprocedural imaging of the 3D scar architecture using LGE CMR and its spatial relationship to the aortic valve helped identify the anatomical isthmus (see Fig. 102.3). Integration of the CMR-derived anatomical information with the electroanatomical mapping data was applied to guide and facilitate ablation.[56] Substrate imaging and image integration should be considered in all patients with CHD with complex anatomy and surgical scars.[56]

Implantable Cardioverter Defibrillator
The risk of SCD in TGA is reported to be 4% after 10 years and 9% after 20 years (5–8 per 1000 patient-years). In the majority of patients who have undergone an atrial switch operation, VAs are the underlying cause of SCD. It is important to note that VF can be preceded by atrial arrhythmias in a significant number of these patients.[53] Other reported risk factors for SCD are RV dysfunction, venous obstruction, and a QRSd of 140 ms or greater[54]; however, specific criteria that prompt ICD implantation have not been defined. An ICD should be implanted after an SCD episode and may be reasonable in adults with a systemic RVEF of <35%, particularly in the presence of additional risk factors such as unexplained syncope, NYHA class II or III symptoms, QRSd ≥140 ms, or severe systemic AV valve regurgitation.[23,57]

In TGA patients after atrial switch, ICD implantation has been shown to be effective for secondary prevention. However, the effectiveness of ICD implantation for primary prevention could not be demonstrated, and inducible VT on electrophysiological testing did not predict future events, suggesting that risk stratification is limited.[53] It is important to recognize that implantation of an ICD can be technically challenging because of the presence of intraatrial baffles and implantation of the lead in a morphological LV. In addition, after ICD implantation, the number of inappropriate shocks (6.6% per year) and late lead-related complications are high.[53,58]

Other

In this section, a miscellaneous group of VAs associated with congenital heart malformations will be discussed. Although several congenital malformations are associated with an increased risk of SCD, not much is known about the substrate of these events. Accordingly, risk stratification is limited.

Left Ventricular Outflow Tract Obstruction
Despite surgical repair, aortic stenosis has the highest incidence of SCD (5.4 per 1000 patient-years).[7] LVOT obstruction comprises a variable group of patients with obstruction at subvalvular, valvular, or supravalvular levels. Valvular stenosis, which constitutes the largest group in CHD patients, is usually attributable to a bicuspid aortic valve. Congenital cases of subvalvular aortic stenosis are usually the result of a subaortic valvular membrane. Supravalvular aortic stenosis is less common and is often associated with other congenital malformations or syndromes, such as Williams

syndrome, or related to previous surgery (e.g., the suture site in the ascending aortic wall after arterial switch for TGA).

The risk of sudden death in patients with aortic stenosis seems time dependent. Etiologies of sudden death were variable and included arrhythmic sudden death (often in the presence of significant residual valve dysfunction), cerebral and coronary complications (often related to aortic valve endocarditis), and low cardiac output failure secondary to acute ventricular failure.[7] Other suggested mechanisms for the high occurrence of sudden cardiac death in this group include ventricular dysfunction and ventricular hypertrophy. Longstanding pressure overload may play an important role. Of the 44 cardiac deaths reported in a cohort of 462 patients with congenital aortic valve stenosis (cAS) followed for 15 years, 25 were sudden and occurred almost exclusively in those with a gradient of >50 mm Hg.[12] Symptoms (angina, dyspnea on exertion, and two or more episodes of syncope) were a strong predictor of mortality. In contrast, in a more recent cohort of 528 patients with cAS who underwent balloon valvuloplasty at a median age of 1.9 years, only 6 of the 49 cardiac deaths during a median follow-up of 12 years were sudden and unexpected. Of importance, only one SCD occurred late, beyond the age of 4, suggesting that early intervention may prevent the substrate for late VA.[59]

Deficient coronary perfusion during exercise can play a role in patients with unoperated severe aortic stenosis. In asymptomatic patients with aortic stenosis, QRSd and morphology were independently associated with the risk of SCD.[60]

Coarctation of the Aorta

The reported incidence of SCD in patients after repair of coarctation of the aorta is 1.3 per 1000 patient-years.[7] Coarctation of the aorta can occur at different levels, but it is classically found at the so-called isthmus, just below the branching of the left subclavian artery. One-third of patients have a bicuspid aortic valve. Even after surgical resection of the coarctation, patients may remain prone to hypertension and concomitant LV hypertrophy that can contribute to the increased incidence of SCD in this group.

Atrioventricular Septal Defect

In patients with AVSD, the reported incidence of SCD is 0.9 per 1000 patient-years.[7] AVSD is part of a broad morphological spectrum that includes complete AVSD and partial AVSD. Extreme disbalance of the ventricles can result in hypoplastic right or left heart syndrome. AVSD can occur isolated or in association with other CHDs, such as LVOT obstruction. AV conduction disorders can occur because of an abnormal position and morphology of the AV conduction system. VAs and SCD are less common and can be related to LVOT obstruction, amount and duration of left AV valve regurgitation, amount of ventricular disproportion, complete AV block, and association with complex cardiac anomalies, although data are limited.

Congenitally Corrected Transposition of the Great Arteries

In ccTGA, there is discordance at both the AV and ventriculoarterial levels. In the absence of AVSDs or VSDs or an open ductus arteriosus, patients will not exhibit shunting or cyanosis, and late complications of the disease are largely associated with the fact that the RV is the systemic ventricle, predisposing for right heart failure, and regurgitation of the often abnormal (Ebstein-like) tricuspid valve. Data on the occurrence of VAs in this group are limited. VT and SCD can be related to ventricular dysfunction, AV valve regurgitation, or AV block. In a cross-sectional study examining the mode of death in patients with CHD, 40% of all deaths in patients with ccTGA were sudden death.[61] Of interest, in a multicenter case-control study 9 of 12 ccTGA patients who died suddenly had associated

defects (7 with VSD + pulmonary stenosis; 2 with Ebstein-like malformation), and 6 patients underwent VSD closure, perhaps facilitating reentry VTs like those described in TOF patients.[9]

Univentricular Hearts

The univentricular heart comprises a highly heterogeneous group of malformations that include hypoplastic right and left heart syndromes, extreme forms of Ebstein anomaly, and (rarely) true univentricular hearts. Incidence numbers of SCD in this group as a whole are unknown. Surgical palliation in most cases includes either partial or total cavopulmonary connections. Arrhythmias are usually of atrial origin because of right atrial scarring, dilatation, or hypertrophy. Usually, high ventricular rates are poorly tolerated.

There is also an increased risk of VAs that might be attributed to the morphology, function, and myocardial quality of the systemic ventricle (e.g., dilatation and presence of advanced ventricular hypertrophy of the systemic ventricle) and associated anomalies (e.g., noncompaction cardiomyopathy of the systemic ventricle). Myocardial fibrosis that was detected on CMR using LGE was associated with dilatation, hypertrophy, and dysfunction of the systemic ventricle, with a higher prevalence of nonsustained VT, compared with that detected without LGE on CMR.[62]

Eisenmenger Syndrome

Patients with Eisenmenger syndrome are at increased risk of SCD. In a multicenter case-control study of 25,790 adults with CHD, cyanotic Eisenmenger syndrome was associated with 19% of the 171 SCDs. However, VA could be documented in only 31 of 171 SCDs; therefore other acute cardiac or noncardiac events cannot be excluded.[9] In one series of 77 patients, SCD occurred in 63% of patients but were not related to arrhythmias.[63] Nonsustained VTs were frequently present in this group, but they did not result in SCD. Cardiac deaths are probably related to progressive heart failure and hypoxemia. Administration of drugs is problematic because many drugs are not tolerated and can cause adverse events.

Implanted Cardioverter Defibrillator Therapy

Only small studies evaluating the cause of SCD in patients with ICDs are available; however, patients with LVOT obstruction, aortic coarctation, or univentricular heart are at a higher risk of SD. The incidence of SCD remains high in postoperative patients with congenital aortic stenosis (3% after 10 years, 13% after 20 years, and 20% after 30 years). Although VA as the underlying cause of SCD is likely, only limited data are available. An ICD should be implanted after an aborted SCD only after the exclusion of reversible etiologies. Primary prevention ICD implantation is indicated in those with a systemic LVEF of ≤35%, biventricular physiology, and NYHA class II or III symptoms and may be reasonable in adults with a single ventricular EF of <35%.[23,57] Complex anatomy and altered venous access (e.g., implantation of lead in an anatomical LV and cavopulmonary connections) can hamper ICD implantation. Although potentially lifesaving, significant adverse effects on the quality of life have been reported in these often young patients, especially after ICD shocks.[64] In addition, lead failure is relatively high, possibly because of a more active lifestyle in young patients.[65]

Acknowledgments

The authors thank Margot M. Bartelings for support and useful comments while preparing the anatomy embryology part of the manuscript, and for her help in making the morphological photographs, and Ron Slagter for help in preparing the figures.

REFERENCES

1. Hoffman JI, Kaplan S. The incidence of congenital heart disease. *J Am Coll Cardiol.* 2002;39:1890–1900.
2. Marelli AJ, Mackie AS, Ionescu-Ittu R, Rahme E, Pilote L. Congenital heart disease in the general population: changing prevalence and age distribution. *Circulation.* 2007;115:163–172.
3. Khairy P, Ionescu-Ittu R, Mackie AS, Abrahamowicz M, Pilote L, Marelli AJ. Changing mortality in congenital heart disease. *J Am Coll Cardiol.* 2010;56:1149–1157.
4. Moons P, Bovijn L, Budts W, Belmans A, Gewillig M. Temporal trends in survival to adulthood among patients born with congenital heart disease from 1970 to 1992 in Belgium. *Circulation.* 2010;122:2264–2272.
5. Verheugt CL, Uiterwaal CS, van der Velde ET, et al. Mortality in adult congenital heart disease. *Eur Heart J.* 2010;31:1220–1229.
6. Diller GP, Kempny A, Alonso-Gonzalez R, et al. Survival prospects and circumstances of death in contemporary adult congenital heart disease patients under follow-up at a large tertiary centre. *Circulation.* 2015;132:2118–2125.
7. Silka MJ, Hardy BG, Menashe VD, Morris CD. A population-based prospective evaluation of risk of sudden cardiac death after operation for common congenital heart defects. *J Am Coll Cardiol.* 1998;32:245–251.
8. Gallego P, Gonzalez AE, Sanchez-Recalde A, et al. Incidence and predictors of sudden cardiac arrest in adults with congenital heart defects repaired before adult life. *Am J Cardiol.* 2012;110:109–117.
9. Koyak Z, Harris L, de Groot JR, et al. Sudden cardiac death in adult congenital heart disease. *Circulation.* 2012;126:1944–1954.
10. Gatzoulis MA, Balaji S, Webber SA, et al. Risk factors for arrhythmia and sudden cardiac death late after repair of tetralogy of Fallot: a multicentre study. *Lancet.* 2000;356:975–981.
11. Murphy JG, Gersh BJ, Mair DD, et al. Long-term outcome in patients undergoing surgical repair of tetralogy of Fallot. *N Engl J Med.* 1993;329:593–599.
12. Keane JF, Driscoll DJ, Gersony WM, et al. Second natural history study of congenital heart defects. Results of treatment of patients with aortic valvar stenosis. *Circulation.* 1993;87:I16–I27.
13. Diller GP, Kempny A, Liodakis E, et al. Left ventricular longitudinal function predicts life-threatening ventricular arrhythmia and death in adults with repaired tetralogy of fallot. *Circulation.* 2012;125:2440–2446.
14. Scherptong RW, Jongbloed MR, Wisse LJ, et al. Morphogenesis of outflow tract rotation during cardiac development: the pulmonary push concept. *Dev Dyn.* 2012;241:1413–1422.
15. Zeppenfeld K, Schalij MJ, Bartelings MM, et al. Catheter ablation of ventricular tachycardia after repair of congenital heart disease: electroanatomic identification of the critical right ventricular isthmus. *Circulation.* 2007;116:2241–2252.
16. Moore JP, Seki A, Shannon KM, Mandapati R, Tung R, Fishbein MC. Characterization of anatomic ventricular tachycardia isthmus pathology after surgical repair of tetralogy of Fallot. *Circ Arrhythm Electrophysiol.* 2013;6:905–911.
17. Kapel GF, Reichlin T, Wijnmaalen AP, et al. Re-entry using anatomically determined isthmuses: a curable ventricular tachycardia in repaired congenital heart disease. *Circ Arrhythm Electrophysiol.* 2015;8:102–109.
18. Chowdhury UK, Sathia S, Ray R, Singh R, Pradeep KK, Venugopal P. Histopathology of the right ventricular outflow tract and its relationship to clinical outcomes and arrhythmias in patients with tetralogy of Fallot. *J Thorac Cardiovasc Surg.* 2006;132:270–277.
19. Babu-Narayan SV, Kilner PJ, Li W, et al. Ventricular fibrosis suggested by cardiovascular magnetic resonance in adults with repaired tetralogy of Fallot and its relationship to adverse markers of clinical outcome. *Circulation.* 2006;113:405–413.
20. Preim U, Sommer P, Hoffmann J, et al. Delayed enhancement imaging in a contemporary patient cohort following correction of tetralogy of Fallot. *Cardiol Young.* 2015;25:1268–1275.
21. Czosek RJ, Anderson J, Khoury PR, Knilans TK, Spar DS, Marino BS. Utility of ambulatory monitoring in patients with congenital heart disease. *Am J Cardiol.* 2013;111:723–730.
22. Deanfield JE, McKenna WJ, Presbitero P, England D, Graham GR, Hallidie-Smith K. Ventricular arrhythmia in unrepaired and repaired tetralogy of Fallot. Relation to age, timing of repair, and haemodynamic status. *Br Heart J.* 1984;52:77–81.
23. Baumgartner H, Bonhoeffer P, De Groot NM, et al. ESC Guidelines for the management of grown-up congenital heart disease (new version 2010). *Eur Heart J.* 2010;31:2915–2957.
24. Khairy P, Harris L, Landzberg MJ, et al. Implantable cardioverter-defibrillators in tetralogy of Fallot. *Circulation.* 2008;117:363–370.

25. Koyak Z, de Groot JR, Bouma BJ, et al. Symptomatic but not asymptomatic non-sustained ventricular tachycardia is associated with appropriate implantable cardioverter therapy in tetralogy of Fallot. *Int J Cardiol.* 2013;167:1532–1535.
26. Moss AJ, Schuger C, Beck CA, et al. Reduction in inappropriate therapy and mortality through ICD programming. *N Engl J Med.* 2012;367:2275–2283.
27. Gatzoulis MA, Till JA, Somerville J, Redington AN. Mechanoelectrical interaction in tetralogy of Fallot. QRS prolongation relates to right ventricular size and predicts malignant ventricular arrhythmias and sudden death. *Circulation.* 1995;92:231–237.
28. Ghai A, Silversides C, Harris L, Webb GD, Siu SC, Therrien J. Left ventricular dysfunction is a risk factor for sudden cardiac death in adults late after repair of tetralogy of Fallot. *J Am Coll Cardiol.* 2002;40:1675–1680.
29. van Huysduynen BH, van Straten A, Swenne CA, et al. Reduction of QRS duration after pulmonary valve replacement in adult Fallot patients is related to reduction of right ventricular volume. *Eur Heart J.* 2005;26:928–932.
30. Cheung EW, Wong WH, Cheung YF. Meta-analysis of pulmonary valve replacement after operative repair of tetralogy of Fallot. *Am J Cardiol.* 2010;106:552–557.
31. Scherptong RW, Hazekamp MG, Mulder BJ, et al. Follow-up after pulmonary valve replacement in adults with tetralogy of Fallot: association between QRS duration and outcome. *J Am Coll Cardiol.* 2010;56:1486–1492.
32. Horowitz LN, Alexander JA, Edmunds Jr LH. Postoperative right bundle branch block: identification of three levels of block. *Circulation.* 1980;62:319–328.
33. Uebing A, Gibson DG, Babu-Narayan SV, et al. Right ventricular mechanics and QRS duration in patients with repaired tetralogy of Fallot: implications of infundibular disease. *Circulation.* 2007;116:1532–1539.
34. Bonello B, Kempny A, Uebing A, et al. Right atrial area and right ventricular outflow tract akinetic length predict sustained tachyarrhythmia in repaired tetralogy of Fallot. *Int J Cardiol.* 2013;168:3280–3286.
34a. Kapel GF, Sacher F, Dekkers OM, et al. Arrhythmogenic anatomical isthmuses identified by electroanatomical mapping are the substrate for ventricular tachycardia in repaired tetralogy of Fallot. *Eur Heart J.* 2017;38:268–276.
35. Vliegen HW, van Straten A, de Roos A, et al. Magnetic resonance imaging to assess the hemodynamic effects of pulmonary valve replacement in adults late after repair of tetralogy of Fallot. *Circulation.* 2002;106:1703–1707.
36. Harrild DM, Berul CI, Cecchin F, et al. Pulmonary valve replacement in tetralogy of Fallot: impact on survival and ventricular tachycardia. *Circulation.* 2009;119:445–451.
37. Karamlou T, Silber I, Lao R, et al. Outcomes after late reoperation in patients with repaired tetralogy of Fallot: the impact of arrhythmia and arrhythmia surgery. *Ann Thorac Surg.* 2006;81:1786–1793.
38. Sabate RA, Connolly HM, Warnes CA, et al. Ventricular arrhythmia risk stratification in patients with tetralogy of Fallot at the time of pulmonary valve replacement. *Circ Arrhythm Electrophysiol.* 2015;8:110–116.
39. Khairy P, Landzberg MJ, Gatzoulis MA, et al. Value of programmed ventricular stimulation after tetralogy of Fallot repair: a multicenter study. *Circulation.* 2004;109:1994–2000.
40. Lucron H, Marcon F, Bosser G, Lethor JP, Marie PY, Brembilla-Perrot B. Induction of sustained ventricular tachycardia after surgical repair of tetralogy of Fallot. *Am J Cardiol.* 1999;83:1369–1373.
41. Chandar JS, Wolff GS, Garson Jr A, et al. Ventricular arrhythmias in postoperative tetralogy of Fallot. *Am J Cardiol.* 1990;65:655–661.
42. Morwood JG, Triedman JK, Berul CI, et al. Radiofrequency catheter ablation of ventricular tachycardia in children and young adults with congenital heart disease. *Heart Rhythm.* 2004;1:301–308.
43. Kriebel T, Saul JP, Schneider H, Sigler M, Paul T. Noncontact mapping and radiofrequency catheter ablation of fast and hemodynamically unstable ventricular tachycardia after surgical repair of tetralogy of Fallot. *J Am Coll Cardiol.* 2007;50:2162–2168.
44. Nollert G, Fischlein T, Bouterwek S, Bohmer C, Klinner W, Reichart B. Long-term survival in patients with repair of tetralogy of Fallot: 36-year follow-up of 490 survivors of the first year after surgical repair. *J Am Coll Cardiol.* 1997;30:1374–1383.
45. Khairy P, Van Hare GF, Balaji S, et al. PACES/HRS expert consensus statement on the recognition and management of arrhythmias in adult congenital heart disease: developed in partnership between the Pediatric and Congenital Electrophysiology Society (PACES) and the Heart Rhythm Society (HRS). Endorsed by the governing bodies of PACES, HRS, the American College of Cardiology (ACC), the American Heart Association (AHA), the European Heart Rhythm Association (EHRA), the Canadian Heart Rhythm Society (CHRS), and the International Society for Adult Congenital Heart Disease (ISACHD). *Can J Cardiol.* 2014;30:e1–e63.

46. Koyak Z, de Groot JR, Van Gelder IC, et al. Implantable cardioverter defibrillator therapy in adults with congenital heart disease: who is at risk of shocks? *Circ Arrhythm Electrophysiol.* 2012;5:101–110.
47. Bartelings MM, Gittenberger-de Groot AC. Morphogenetic considerations on congenital malformations of the outflow tract. Part 2: Complete transposition of the great arteries and double outlet right ventricle. *Int J Cardiol.* 1991;33:5–26.
48. Kammeraad JA, van Deurzen CH, Sreeram N, et al. Predictors of sudden cardiac death after Mustard or Senning repair for transposition of the great arteries. *J Am Coll Cardiol.* 2004;44:1095–1102.
49. Cuypers JA, Eindhoven JA, Slager MA, et al. The natural and unnatural history of the Mustard procedure: long-term outcome up to 40 years. *Eur Heart J.* 2014;35:1666–1674.
50. Wilson NJ, Clarkson PM, Barratt-Boyes BG, et al. Long-term outcome after the Mustard repair for simple transposition of the great arteries. 28-year follow-up. *J Am Coll Cardiol.* 1998;32:758–765.
51. Millane T, Bernard EJ, Jaeggi E, et al. Role of ischemia and infarction in late right ventricular dysfunction after atrial repair of transposition of the great arteries. *J Am Coll Cardiol.* 2000;35:1661–1668.
52. Babu-Narayan SV, Goktekin O, Moon JC, et al. Late gadolinium enhancement cardiovascular magnetic resonance of the systemic right ventricle in adults with previous atrial redirection surgery for transposition of the great arteries. *Circulation.* 2005;111:2091–2098.
53. Khairy P, Harris L, Landzberg MJ, et al. Sudden death and defibrillators in transposition of the great arteries with intra-atrial baffles: a multicenter study. *Circ Arrhythm Electrophysiol.* 2008;1:250–257.
54. Schwerzmann M, Salehian O, Harris L, et al. Ventricular arrhythmias and sudden death in adults after a Mustard operation for transposition of the great arteries. *Eur Heart J.* 2009;30:1873–1879.
55. Roubertie F, Thambo JB, Bretonneau A, et al. Late outcome of 132 Senning procedures after 20 years of follow-up. *Ann Thorac Surg.* 2011;92:2206–2213.
56. Piers SR, Dyrda K, Tao Q, Zeppenfeld K. Bipolar ablation of ventricular tachycardia in a patient after atrial switch operation for dextro-transposition of the great arteries. *Circ Arrhythm Electrophysiol.* 2012;5:e38–e40.
57. Khairy P, Van Hare GF, Balaji S, et al. PACES/HRS Expert Consensus Statement on the Recognition and Management of Arrhythmias in Adult Congenital Heart Disease: developed in partnership between the Pediatric and Congenital Electrophysiology Society (PACES) and the Heart Rhythm Society (HRS). Endorsed by the governing bodies of PACES, HRS, the American College of Cardiology (ACC), the American Heart Association (AHA), the European Heart Rhythm Association (EHRA), the Canadian Heart Rhythm Society (CHRS), and the International Society for Adult Congenital Heart Disease (ISACHD). *Heart Rhythm.* 2014;11:e102–e165.
58. Khanna AD, Warnes CA, Phillips SD, Lin G, Brady PA. Single-center experience with implantable cardioverter-defibrillators in adults with complex congenital heart disease. *Am J Cardiol.* 2011;108:729–734.
59. Brown DW, Dipilato AE, Chong EC, et al. Sudden unexpected death after balloon valvuloplasty for congenital aortic stenosis. *J Am Coll Cardiol.* 2010;56:1939–1946.
60. Greve AM, Gerdts E, Boman K, et al. Impact of QRS duration and morphology on the risk of sudden cardiac death in asymptomatic patients with aortic stenosis: the SEAS (Simvastatin and Ezetimibe in Aortic Stenosis) Study. *J Am Coll Cardiol.* 2012;59:1142–1149.
61. Oechslin EN, Harrison DA, Connelly MS, Webb GD, Siu SC. Mode of death in adults with congenital heart disease. *Am J Cardiol.* 2000;86:1111–1116.
62. Rathod RH, Prakash A, Kim YY, et al. Cardiac magnetic resonance parameters predict transplantation-free survival in patients with Fontan circulation. *Circ Cardiovasc Imaging.* 2014;7:502–509.
63. Niwa K, Perloff JK, Kaplan S, Child JS, Miner PD. Eisenmenger syndrome in adults: ventricular septal defect, truncus arteriosus, univentricular heart. *J Am Coll Cardiol.* 1999;34:223–232.
64. Sears SF Jr., Conti JB. Quality of life and psychological functioning of ICD patients. *Heart.* 2002;87:488–493.
65. Alexander ME, Cecchin F, Walsh EP, Triedman JK, Bevilacqua LM, Berul CI. Implications of implantable cardioverter defibrillator therapy in congenital heart disease and pediatrics. *J Cardiovasc Electrophysiol.* 2004;15:72–76.

103 Syncope

J. William Schleifer, Dan Sorajja, and Win–Kuang Shen

Definitions and Scope

Definitions

Syncope is a symptom of transient loss of consciousness caused by a temporary reduction in cerebral perfusion.[1,2] This definition excludes trauma, seizure, metabolic derangements, and psychiatric conditions, which cause loss of consciousness by different mechanisms.[1] In true syncope, changes in cardiac output, vascular tone, and cardiac rhythm or a combination of these factors reduce cerebral perfusion, triggering reflexive loss of consciousness and control of muscular tone and posture. Confirmation of cerebral perfusion at the time of syncope is usually not feasible, but presumably once cerebral perfusion normalizes, consciousness recovers rapidly.

Significance of Syncope

Syncope is common; an estimated 28% of males and 41% of females experience at least one episode of syncope during their lives.[3] Syncope is responsible for approximately 1% of emergency room visits, 27%–35% of which result in hospitalizations.[4] Syncope evaluation is estimated to cost 2.4–5.4 billion US dollars per year.[5] In a study of the Framingham population, syncope was reported with an incidence of 6.2 per 1000 person-years. When stratified by type of syncope, patients who experienced syncope due to cardiac, neurological, or unknown causes had an increased mortality risk compared with that of the general population, whereas those who experienced vasovagal syncope had a prognosis no different from that of the general population.[6]

Etiologies and Pathophysiology

Pathophysiology of Neurally Mediated Syncope

Reflex or neurally mediated syncope includes vasovagal syncope, situational syncope, and carotid sinus hypersensitivity. The vasovagal reflex involves a trigger causing a sympathetic surge, followed by a sudden withdrawal of cardiac and vascular sympathetic tone and unopposed parasympathetic activation.[1] This reflex results in transient profound vasodilation, transient asystole, or profound bradycardia or a combination of these. The trigger can be a noxious stimulus, as in vasovagal syncope; baroreceptor activation, as in carotid sinus hypersensitivity; or other vagal stimuli in situational syncope, such as micturition or cough. The relative contributions of acute changes in cardiac contractility, reduced cardiac output, reduced preload, and peripheral vasodilation are debated. Studies of patients with recurrent vasovagal syncope show that significantly abnormal cardiac autonomic function,[7] impaired baroreceptor function,[8,9] sudden reduction in cardiac output,[10] and abnormal endothelial function[11] all have a role in vasovagal syncope. Conflicting studies regarding muscle sympathetic nerve activity during vasovagal syncope[8,12] may indicate that more than one type of physiological response is possible. While family history and twin studies indicate that syncope often affects family members,[13] genomic studies for markers of recurrent vasovagal syncope have yet to yield significant genetic associations.[14]

Orthostatic Hypotension

Upon standing, 500–800 mL of blood is displaced to the lower extremities. This results in a significant reduction in blood pressure if compensatory baroreceptor responses and venoconstriction are impaired. Volume depletion, antihypertensive medications, and endocrine abnormalities in the pituitary–adrenal axis exacerbate orthostatic hypotension. Baroreflex impairment is also associated with autonomic neuropathy, multiple system atrophy, and Parkinson disease and may occur in up to 30% of the elderly.[15] Orthostatic hypotension is diagnosed clinically by a drop in systolic blood pressure >20 mm Hg 2 minutes after standing.[16]

Carotid Hypersensitivity

Carotid hypersensitivity is more common in older adults. It is associated with autonomic abnormalities including elevated sympathetic tone and a dysregulated autonomic response to baroreceptor stimulation, resulting in profound bradycardia or hypotension, or both upon mechanical pressure placed on the carotid sinus.[17] It is diagnosed by carotid sinus massage.

Cardiac Etiologies of Syncope

Arrhythmias

Arrhythmias result in syncope by suddenly reducing cardiac output with reductions in diastolic filling during tachycardias or reduction in diastolic pressure during bradyarrhythmias. Pauses related to sinus node dysfunction, complete heart block, and self-terminating tachyarrhythmias are important causes of syncope potentially associated with an increased risk of sudden death. Features suggesting an arrhythmic syncope include an unpredictable onset that is independent of position or noxious trigger and an absent or short (only a few seconds) prodrome usually limited to palpitations. The management of particular arrhythmias is described elsewhere in this book.

Structural Heart Disease

Fixed or dynamic cardiac obstructions, such as aortic valvular stenosis or hypertrophic cardiomyopathy, can reduce cardiac output to the point that hypotension and syncope ensue. Syncope can also occur because of low cardiac output in heart failure with a reduced ejection fraction or pulmonary arterial hypertension. Syncope related to hemodynamic considerations is often reproducible after a certain degree of exertion or a certain change in loading conditions. In each case, syncope necessitates an intervention to improve hemodynamic status. Acute cardiovascular events, such as myocardial infarction, pulmonary embolism, and aortic dissection, may cause syncope because of reduced cardiac output, hypoxemia, vascular occlusion, or arrhythmia.

Distinguishing Seizure From Syncope

In the absence of witnesses to the event, seizures may be difficult to distinguish from syncope. Seizure is more likely if tongue biting, buccal mucosa injury, and head turning to one side occurred during the episode; if abnormal behavior, déjà vu, or jamais vu sensation preceded the episode; or if postictal confusion followed the episode. Seizure is unlikely to be preceded by an autonomic prodrome.[18]

Psychiatric Etiologies of Syncope

Psychogenic pseudosyncope, or the apparent abrupt loss of consciousness without hemodynamic change, reduction in cerebral perfusion, or alteration in cerebral activity, occurs in approximately 5% of patients presenting with syncope. It is characterized by an abrupt closing of the eyes, loss of muscle tone, and collapse in the setting of normal or slightly increased heart rate and blood pressure[19] and normal cerebral activity on electroencephalography.[20] Its diagnosis is confirmed using video monitoring during head-up tilt-table testing and electroencephalography.

Clinical Evaluation

Acute Considerations

In most cases, the loss of consciousness with syncope is so short in duration that recovery is usually complete by the time of medical evaluation. If not, the patient should be kept supine and treated supportively until normotensive and fully conscious. If loss or marked alteration of consciousness continues despite normalization of vital signs, other nonsyncopal conditions should be promptly considered.

Goals of Clinical Evaluation

Once the patient has recovered from the syncopal episode, the two questions to answer during clinical evaluation are: (1) what caused the episode and (2) what is the risk of future episodes and other adverse events? As suggested by the Framingham study,[6] answering the first question often helps with answering the second question, but even if syncope is uncertain in cause, risk stratification is important to determine the urgency and extent of evaluation, including whether patients require hospitalization. Because patients with structural heart disease are at a higher risk for adverse events, a thorough evaluation is required to determine multiple potential contributors to syncope. In patients with no known cardiac disease or cardiac risk factors who have a history consistent with vasovagal syncope with a normal cardiac exam and electrocardiogram (ECG), little further testing is required.[2]

History and Physical Examination

The history and physical examination seek to identify triggering factors, associated symptoms, and other medical comorbidities to determine the etiology of syncope. Factors that indicate arrhythmia or structural heart disease are associated with an increased risk of future cardiovascular adverse events and death, and these should prompt a more extensive cardiac work-up. Occurrence of the episode during exertion or while supine is associated with arrhythmias, as are a lack of a prodrome, associated palpitations, chest discomfort, or dyspnea. The strongest predictor of cardiac syncope is the presence of structural heart disease; the strongest predictor of noncardiac syncope is age <40 years. A model that combines structural heart disease; syncope during effort; age ≥60 years; male gender; supine posture during episode; less than three spells; and absence of a prodrome with diaphoresis, blurred vision, and nausea has a sensitivity of 73%–92% and a specificity of 52%–68% for cardiac syncope.[21] While helpful, symptom scores appear to have reduced specificity when applied clinically.[22]

Diagnostic Testing

While many diagnostic tests are available, testing should be carefully selected with consideration of the anticipated yield. Table 103.1 lists potential diagnostic tests, situations in which they are useful, and abnormalities that lead to specific treatment.

An ECG, blood chemistries to identify anemia and metabolic abnormalities, and orthostatic vital signs are important diagnostic studies in most patients. An exercise ECG is valuable in selected patients, particularly if ischemia is suspected or syncope occurs during exertion.

An echocardiogram can identify structural and hemodynamic abnormalities; it can also confirm that the heart is structurally normal if arrhythmias are suspected.

Neurological testing and cerebrovascular imaging such as carotid duplex ultrasound, computed tomography, magnetic resonance imaging, or electroencephalography are of very limited value to determine the cause of syncope. In the absence of carotid bruits or other contraindications (such as recent stroke), carotid sinus massage can be performed in older patients presenting with unexplained syncope to evaluate for pauses or asystole indicative of carotid sinus hypersensitivity. A causal relationship between carotid sinus hypersensitivity and syncope can be challenging to establish in the elderly patients where multiple causes of syncope can be present.[23]

Ambulatory monitoring is useful in identifying arrhythmias in the outpatient setting. As the duration of monitoring increases, the sensitivity for identifying arrhythmias improves. A 24-hour Holter monitoring may be useful in identifying asymptomatic nonsustained ventricular tachycardia or AV block, but the likelihood that a symptomatic episode will occur during the 24-hour period is small. Duration of monitoring should be commensurate with the anticipated frequency of the episodes, and an implantable loop recorder can be considered for very rare and symptomatic episodes.

Head-up tilt-table testing is useful for identifying vasovagal syncope. Medications (isoproterenol or nitroglycerin) can be used to increase sensitivity at the expense of specificity. The primary role of head-up tilt-table testing is to identify vasovagal syncope in patients where the history is unclear and to help the patient identify prodromal symptoms so that he or she understands the syncopal prodrome better. Vasovagal syncope induced by head-up tilt-table testing does not rule out arrhythmic syncope; it only demonstrates that the individual is prone to reflex syncope. The three types of vasovagal syncope responses reproduced on head-up tilt-table testing are shown in Fig. 103.1.

103

TABLE 103.1   Diagnostic testing, indications, and findings suggestive of neurally mediated (vasovagal) syncope versus arrhythmic or other cardiac causes of syncope

TEST	CIRCUMSTANCE	FINDINGS SUGGESTIVE OF NEURALLY MEDIATED SYNCOPE	FINDINGS SUGGESTIVE OF ARRHYTHMIC OR CARDIAC SYNCOPE
ECG	All patients	Normal	AV block, Q waves, ST segment abnormalities, delta waves, epsilon waves, Brugada pattern, or QT interval prolongation
Exercise ECG	Exertional syncope Ischemic symptoms or chest discomfort	Symptoms during recovery	Increasing PVCs, AV block, or QT prolongation with exertion ST segment abnormalities suggestive of ischemia
Echocardiogram	History, signs or symptoms of structural heart disease	Normal	Reduced ejection fraction, stenotic valvular disease, pulmonary hypertension
Carotid sinus massage	Syncope with shaving or head turning	Profound bradycardia or syncopal symptoms	
Ambulatory ECG monitor or implantable loop recorder	History suggestive of arrhythmia	Bradycardia during syncopal symptoms	Arrhythmias correlating with symptoms
Head-up tilt-table testing	Etiology unknown or history unclear	Vasodepressor, cardioinhibitory, or mixed response	Arrhythmias correlating with symptoms
Electrophysiological study	Strong suspicion of arrhythmia	Not recommended if ECG is normal and the heart is structurally normal	Easily inducible arrhythmias associated with hypotension Induction of sustained monomorphic ventricular tachycardia Corrected sinus node recovery time >525 ms HV interval >70 ms; infra-His or intra-His block

AV, Atrioventricular; *ECG,* electrocardiogram; *HV,* His bundle electrogram to ventricular activation interval; *PVCs,* premature ventricular contractions.

Electrophysiological study is an invasive study to evaluate for sinus node dysfunction, abnormal atrioventricular conduction, or inducible atrial or ventricular arrhythmias. Electrophysiological study can be useful when an arrhythmic etiology is suspected based on history, physical examination, and initial evaluation. It is not recommended if the ECG is normal and the heart is structurally normal.[2] Interpretation of electrophysiological findings must be put in the context of the overall clinical presentation. Aggressive induction protocols may induce incidental atrial or ventricular arrhythmias that may be clinically irrelevant. Patients may display normal conduction properties that under other physiological conditions may have abnormal responses. Also, an abnormal electrophysiological study does not rule out vasovagal syncope as a potential etiology of the patient's syncope.

Risk Stratification Approaches

Because the risk of morbidity and mortality determines the extent and urgency of evaluation, many risk stratification approaches have been developed. Inclusion of potential risk factors increases not only the sensitivity of identifying patients at increased risk but also the likelihood of unnecessary hospitalization and utilization of resources.[24] Risk factors from various decision rules are compared in Table 103.2.[25-30] However, risk scores do not consistently perform better than clinical judgment in having better sensitivity, specificity, or diagnostic yield.[31] For patients who do not have high-risk features, but yet cannot be confirmed to be low risk, a randomized trial showed that observation within an emergency department syncope unit with evaluation by a cardiologist or electrophysiologist within 72 hours was a safe, cost-effective, efficient method of evaluating intermediate-risk patients presenting with syncope.[25]

Syncope While Driving

Vasovagal syncope is the most common cause of syncope while driving. An episode of syncope carries approximately 1% per year risk of recurrent syncope while driving and does not necessarily affect the patient's risk of future adverse outcome.[32]

Difficulties With Syncope Evaluation

The evaluation of syncope is beset with a number of difficulties. First, the possible causes of syncope range from benign vasovagal reflex syncope to aborted sudden death; however, by the time the patient is evaluated, both the precipitant and the symptom of syncope have subsided. The spontaneous recovery leaves both the patient and clinician often uncertain about the cause, risk of recurrence, and risk of more serious consequences with the next event. Second, historical details that help to differentiate arrhythmic syncope from other causes of syncope may be difficult to determine depending on the patient's and witnesses' recollection of the incident. Third, multiple causes of syncope may be possible. Because patients with multiple potential causes of syncope are at even higher risk of adverse outcomes, all potential causes should be considered in patients presenting with transient loss of consciousness.[23]

Treatment of Vasovagal Syncope

Because the treatment of specific arrhythmias, conduction disturbances, and autonomic syndromes including postural orthostatic tachycardia syndrome is discussed elsewhere in this book, what follows is a discussion of treatment for vasovagal syncope.

Conservative Treatment

In all cases, patients' medications should be evaluated for antihypertensives, diuretics, or medications that affect heart rate, and these should be discontinued if possible. Salt and fluid intake should be liberalized. Compression hose improve orthostatic symptoms by preventing pooling of blood in the lower extremity veins. Isometric exercises (physical counterpressure maneuvers) increase venous return and increase peripheral resistance to abort the vasovagal reflex in patients with sufficient prodrome. When patients were taught these maneuvers, they experienced a 36% relative risk reduction in recurrent syncope.[33]

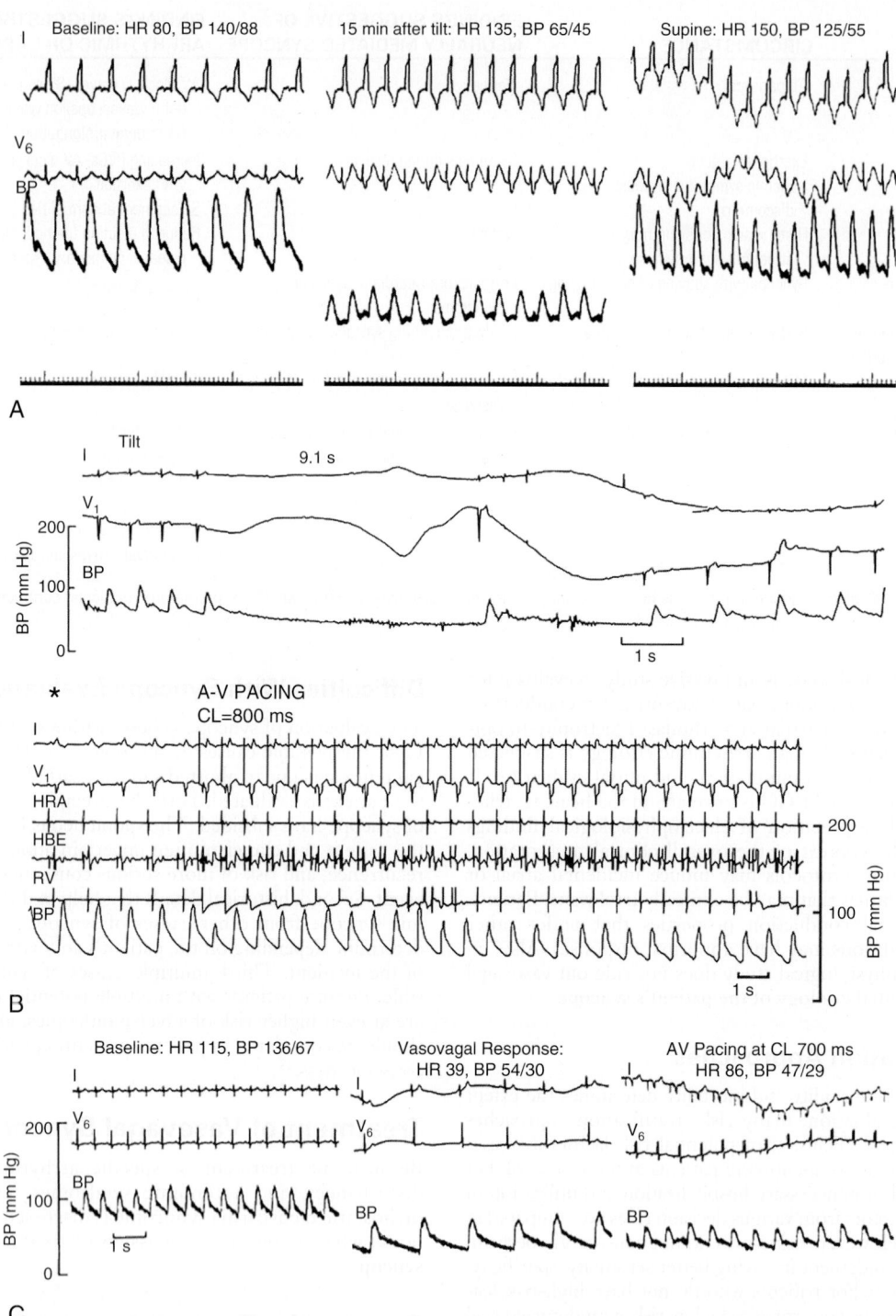

FIGURE 103.1 Three types of vasovagal response. (A) Vasodepressor syncope is characterized by a decreased blood pressure (*BP*) with no reduction in heart rate (*HR*); (B) pure cardioinhibitory syncope is characterized by bradycardia or asystole without vasodilation (this example shows normalization of BP once cardiac pacing is performed); (C) mixed syncope is characterized by bradycardia with vasodilation and a reduction of *BP* that occurs whether or not pacing is performed. *AV pacing,* Atrioventricular pacing; *CL,* cycle length; *HBE,* His bundle electrogram; *HRA,* high right atrial electrogram; *RV,* right ventricle. (From Chen LY, Shen WK. Neurocardiogenic syncope: latest pharmacologic therapies. *Expert Opin Pharmacother.* 2006;7:1151-1162.)

TABLE 103.2 Common factors among risk stratification scores for syncope

	OESIL SCORE[26]	SAN FRANCISCO SYNCOPE RULE[27]	SEEDS HIGH RISK CRITERIA[25]	EGSYS SCORE[28]	ROSE STUDY[29]	BOSTON SYNCOPE CRITERIA[30]
Abnormal ECG	Includes: • Any arrhythmia • Second- or third-degree AVB, BBB or IVCD • LVH or RVH • Left axis deviation • Old MI • Ischemia	Includes: • Any arrhythmia • Any changes from previous	Includes: • Ischemia • QTc >500 ms • Trifascicular block or pauses >2 s • Sinus bradycardia <60 beats/min • Atrial fibrillation • Nonsustained ventricular tachycardia	Includes: • Any arrhythmia • Sinus bradycardia • Second- or third-degree AVB or BBB • Acute or old MI • LVH or RVH • Preexcitation • Prolonged QTc • Brugada pattern	Includes: • Bradycardia ≤50 beats/min • Q waves (except in lead III)	Includes: • Ischemia • Q waves • QTc >500 ms • AVB or IVCD • Sinus bradycardia <50 beats/min • Atrial fibrillation • Ventricular arrhythmias
Cardiac history	History of heart disease		Moderate to severe valvular disease History of ventricular arrhythmias Cardiac device with possible dysfunction	History of heart disease		History of coronary heart disease History of ventricular arrhythmia, pacemaker, defibrillator, or antiarrhythmic use Murmur on examination
Heart failure		History or symptoms of heart failure	History or symptoms of heart failure		BNP ≥300 pg/mL	History of heart failure
History suggests arrhythmia		Syncope without prodrome			Syncope without prodrome or precipitating emotional factors Syncope during exertion or while supine Palpitations preceding syncope	Syncope during exercise
Other signs or symptoms of cardiopulmonary disease		Shortness of breath Systolic blood pressure <90 mm Hg	Chest pain		Chest pain Oxygen saturation ≤94%	Chest pain Shortness of breath Oxygen saturation <90% Respiratory rate >24/min Systolic blood pressure <90 mm Hg
Anemia		Hematocrit <30%			Fecal occult blood present Hemoglobin ≤9 g/dL	Fecal occult blood present Hematocrit <30%
Other	Age >65 years					Family history of sudden death Recent primary neurological event Multiple episodes within 6 months

AVB, Atrioventricular block; *BBB*, bundle branch block; *BNP*, brain natriuretic peptide; *ECG*, electrocardiography; *IVCD*, interventricular conduction delay; *LVH*, left ventricular hypertrophy; *MI*, myocardial infarction; *RVH*, right ventricular hypertrophy.

Tilt training is a method of using repetitive head-up tilt-table tests or standing against a wall for 30–60 minutes a day to enable patients to recognize the prodrome and resist the vasovagal reflex. While it is effective in preventing syncope in compliant patients,[34] tilt training is cumbersome and not recommended routinely.[1]

Pharmacological Treatment

Midodrine

An α-adrenergic receptor agonist, midodrine increases peripheral resistance and is an established therapy for orthostatic hypotension. It causes downregulation of the sympathetic receptors, reducing cardiac sensitivity to a sympathetic surge. Nonpressor doses are useful in recurrent vasovagal syncope and significantly reduced syncope recurrence in a randomized, placebo-controlled trial of 61 patients.[35] However, a small placebo-controlled, randomized, blinded study showed no difference in comparison with placebo after 3 months of follow-up in 23 patients.[36] Midodrine may be considered in patients with recurrent syncope despite conservative treatment, but it should be avoided in patients with supine hypertension or urinary retention.

β-Blockers

Despite earlier studies that suggested benefit, a large placebo-controlled, randomized, blinded study (Prevention of Syncope Trial) has shown that β-blockers cause similar reductions in syncope as caused by placebo.[37] A subsequent analysis of the Prevention of Syncope Trial showed that patients older than 42 years may benefit from β-blockers to prevent the recurrence of vasovagal syncope[38]; therefore β-blockers may be considered in such patients.[1]

Fludrocortisone

Fludrocortisone is a mineralocorticoid that is well established in the treatment of orthostatic hypotension because it causes sodium retention. A benefit was seen in children with recurrent vasovagal syncope in a randomized, placebo-controlled trial.[39] Therefore it may be used, particularly in patients with orthostatic symptoms.

Other Medications

The vasovagal reflex is thought to involve the serotonergic neurons within the central nervous system; therefore selective serotonin reuptake inhibitors may affect the vasovagal reflex directly. Paroxetine and fluoxetine showed symptomatic improvements compared with placebo in small studies.[40,41] Other medications such as octreotide, sibutramine, theophylline, and clonidine have been evaluated only in small case series. Fig. 103.2 summarizes the mechanisms of action of different medications as they target different aspects of the vasovagal reflex.

Nonpharmacological Treatment

Permanent Pacemaker Implantation

Several trials have assessed the impact of pacing on vasovagal syncope. Two large controlled trials that were not blinded to treatment approach showed that pacing significantly reduced syncope recurrence in patients with cardioinhibitory syncope on tilt testing.[42,43] Later, two randomized, double-blinded, placebo-controlled trials (VPS II and SYNPACE) failed to show a significant benefit from pacemakers programmed to DDD mode compared to a sensing-only ODO mode, indicating a significant placebo effect.[44,45] The Third International Study on Syncope of Uncertain Etiology (ISSUE-3), a double-blinded, randomized, placebo-controlled trial of pacing for patients with neurally mediated syncope and asystole documented on implantable loop recorder, indicated benefit in patients with a cardioinhibitory response who are more than 40 years old.[46] This benefit was greatest in patients with a negative head-up tilt-table test.[47] Guidelines support the consideration of dual-chamber pacing in patients >40 years of age with neurally mediated syncope and asystole.[2]

Advanced pacing algorithms have been developed with the goal of more effectively treating cardioinhibitory syncope. Rate hysteresis algorithms sense sudden reductions in heart rate (even reductions that do not go below the lower rate limit) and intervene with pacing at a faster rate. Closed-loop stimulation is another algorithm that senses the intracardiac impedance. Sudden changes in intracardiac impedance would be associated with changes in cardiac contractility and filling conditions. Sensed changes in intracardiac impedance then trigger increases in pacing rates with a goal of anticipating cardiac inhibition and aborting syncope. In a retrospective assessment of closed-loop stimulation versus rate hysteresis algorithms, the former appears to significantly reduce the recurrence of vasovagal syncope, with recurrence in 4% of patients compared with that in 38% of patients with the latter,[48] but this will need to be validated in a randomized, controlled trial.

Autonomic Modulation

Ablation for atrial fibrillation has stimulated interest in modifying the autonomic ganglia, through either endocardial or epicardial ablation. At this point, ablation has been attempted only in small numbers of patients with recurrent vasovagal syncope in unblinded studies.[49,50] In each case, the autonomic ganglia were identified differently: one with a fast Fourier transform and one with high-frequency stimulation protocols. As with the pharmacological and pacing therapies, these interventions will need to be tested in placebo-controlled, randomized, double-blinded trials before they have widespread acceptance.

Conclusion

Despite many advances in the understanding of the pathophysiology and risk stratification of syncope, evaluation remains predominantly based on history, with vasovagal syncope being the most frequent cause. The prognosis for vasovagal syncope is generally benign, but structural heart disease and arrhythmic etiologies should be considered in the appropriate context and would require further evaluation. For most patients with vasovagal syncope, conservative lifestyle measures (education, salt and fluid liberalization, and counterpressure maneuvers) are adequate, but some patients require pharmacological therapy such as fludrocortisone or midodrine. Targeted therapy for other specific etiologies should be given.

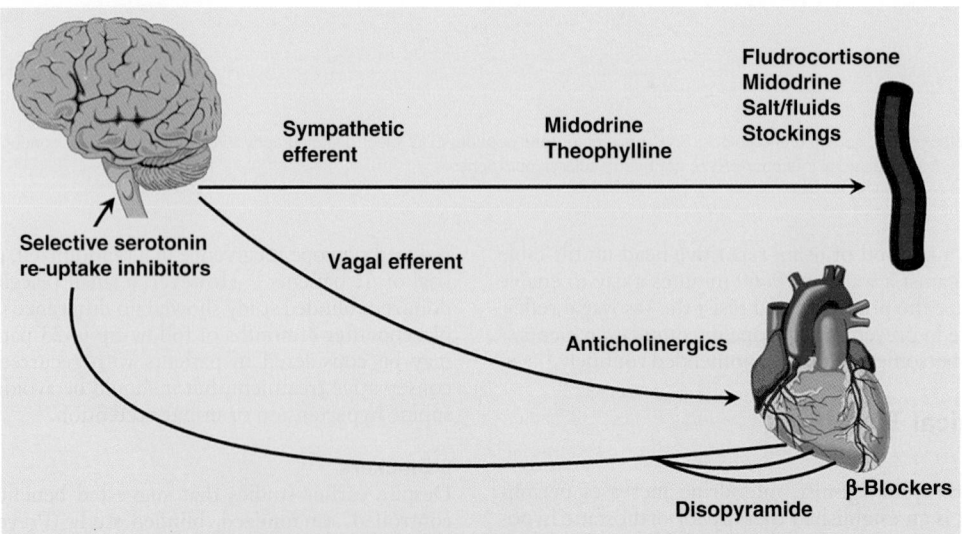

FIGURE 103.2 Medications to prevent syncope and their putative autonomic targets. (From Chen LY, Shen WK. Neurocardiogenic syncope: latest pharmacologic therapies. *Expert Opin Pharmacother.* 2006;7:1151-1162.)

REFERENCES

1. Sheldon RS, Grubb BP, Olshansky B, et al. 2015 Heart Rhythm Society expert consensus statement on the diagnosis and treatment of postural tachycardia syndrome, inappropriate sinus tachycardia, and vasovagal syncope. *Heart Rhythm.* 2015;12:e41–e63.

2. Moya A, Sutton R, Ammirati F, et al. Guidelines for the diagnosis and management of syncope (version 2009): The Task Force for the Diagnosis and Management of Syncope of the European Society of Cardiology (ESC). *Eur Heart J.* 2009;30:2631–2671.

3. Ganzeboom KS, Mairuhu G, Reitsma JB, et al. Lifetime cumulative incidence of syncope in the general population: a study of 549 Dutch subjects aged 35–60 years. *J Cardiovasc Electrophysiol.* 2006;17:1172–1176.

4. Probst MA, Kanzaria HK, Gbedemah M, et al. National trends in resource utilization associated with ED visits for syncope. *Am J Emerg Med.* 2015;33:998–1001.

5. Sun BJ, Emond JA, Camargo CA. Direct medical costs of syncope-related hospitalizations in the United States. *Am J Cardiol.* 2005;95:668–671.

6. Soteriades ES, Evans JC, Larson MG, et al. Incidence and prognosis of syncope. *N Engl J Med.* 2002;347:878–885.

7. Shinohara T, Ebata Y, Ayabe R, et al. Cardiac autonomic dysfunction in patients with head-up tilt test-induced vasovagal syncope. *Pacing Clin Electrophysiol.* 2014;37:1694–1701.

8. Morillo CA, Eckberg DL, Ellenbogen KA, et al. Vagal and sympathetic mechanisms in patients with orthostatic vasovagal syncope. *Circulation.* 1997;96:2509–2513.

9. Iacoviello M, Forleo C, Guida P, et al. Independent role of reduced arterial baroreflex sensitivity during head-up tilt testing in predicting vasovagal syncope recurrence. *Europace.* 2010;12:1149–1155.

10. Verheyden B, Liu J, van Dijk N, et al. Steep fall in cardiac output is main determinant of hypotension during drug-free and nitroglycerine-induced orthostatic vasovagal syncope. *Heart Rhythm.* 2008;5:1695–1701.

11. Galetta F, Franzoni F, Plantinga Y, et al. Endothelial function in young subjects with vaso-vagal syncope. *Biomed Pharmacother.* 2006;60:448–452.

12. Vaddadi G, Esler MD, Dawood T, Lambert E. Persistence of muscle sympathetic nerve activity during vasovagal syncope. *Eur Heart J.* 2010;31:2027–2033.

13. Klein KM, Xu SS, Lawrence K, et al. Evidence for genetic factors in vasovagal syncope: a twin-family study. *Neurology.* 2012;79:561–565.

14. Sorrentino S, Forleo C, Iacoviello M, et al. Lack of association between genetic polymorphisms affecting sympathetic activity and tilt-induced vasovagal syncope. *Auton Neurosci.* 2010;155:98–103.

15. Low PA, Tomalia VA. Orthostatic hypotension: mechanisms, causes, management. *J Clin Neurol.* 2015;11:220–226.

16. Atkins D, Hanusa B, Sefcik T, Kapoor W. Syncope and orthostatic hypotension. *Am J Med.* 1991;91:179–185.

17. Tan MP, Kenny RAM, Chadwick TJ, et al. Carotid sinus hypersensitivity: disease state or clinical sign of ageing? Insights from a controlled study of autonomic function in symptomatic and asymptomatic subjects. *Europace.* 2010;12:1630–1636.

18. Sheldon R, Rose S, Ritchie D, et al. Historical criteria that distinguish syncope from seizures. *J Am Coll Cardiol.* 2002;40:142–148.

19. Tannemaat MR, van Niekerk J, Reijntjes RH, et al. The semiology of tilt-induced psychogenic pseudosyncope. *Neurology.* 2013;81:752–758.

20. Benbadis SR, Chichkova R. Psychogenic pseudosyncope: an underestimated and provable diagnosis. *Epilepsy Behav.* 2006;9:106–110.

21. Berecki-Gisolf J, Sheldon A, Wieling W, et al. Identifying cardiac syncope based on clinical history: a literature-based model tested in four independent datasets. *PLoS One.* 2013;8:e75255.

22. Romme JJCM, van Dijk N, Boer KR, et al. Diagnosing vasovagal syncope based on quantitative history-taking: validation of the Calgary Syncope Symptom Score. *Eur Heart J.* 2009;30:2888–2896.

23. Chen LY, Gersh BJ, Hodge DO, et al. Prevalence and clinical outcomes of patients with multiple potential causes of syncope. *Mayo Clin Proc.* 2001;78:414–420.

24. Serrano LA, Hess EP, Bellollo MF, et al. Accuracy and quality of clinical decision rules for syncope in the emergency department: a systematic review and meta-analysis. *Ann Emerg Med.* 2010;56:362–373.

25. Shen WK, Decker WW, Smars PA, et al. Syncope Evaluation in the Emergency Department Study (SEEDS): a multidisciplinary approach to syncope management. *Circulation.* 2004;110:3636–3645.

26. Colivicchi F, Ammirati F, Melina D, et al. Development and prospective validation of a risk stratification system for patients with syncope in the emergency department: the OESIL risk score. *Eur Heart J.* 2003;24:811–819.

27. Quinn JV, Stiell IG, McDermott DA, et al. Derivation of the San Francisco syncope rule to predict patients with short-term serious outcomes. *Ann Emerg Med.* 2004;43:224–232.

28. Ungar A, Del Rosso A, Giada F, et al. Early and late outcome of treated patients referred for syncope to emergency department: the EGSYS 2 follow-up study. *Eur Heart J.* 2010;31:2021–2026.

29. Reed MJ, Newby DE, Coull AJ, et al. The ROSE (Risk Stratification of Syncope in the Emergency Department) Study. *J Am Coll Cardiol.* 2010;55:713–721.

30. Grossman SA, Fischer C, Lipsitz LA, et al. Predicting adverse outcomes in syncope. *J Emerg Med.* 2007;33:233–239.

31. Costantino G, Casazza G, Reed M, et al. Syncope risk stratification tools vs clinical judgment: an individual patient data meta-analysis. *Am J Med.* 2014;127:1126e13–1126e25.

32. Sorajja D, Nesbitt GC, Hodge DO, et al. Syncope while driving: clinical characteristics, causes, and prognosis. *Circulation.* 2009;120:928–934.

33. Van Dijk N, Quartieri F, Blanc JJ, et al. Effectiveness of physical counterpressure maneuvers in preventing vasovagal syncope: the Physical Counterpressure Manoeuvres Trial (PC-Trial). *J Am Coll Cardiol.* 2006;48:1652–1657.

34. Di Girolamo E, Di Iorio C, Leonzio L, et al. Usefulness of a tilt training program for the prevention of refractory neurocardiogenic syncope in adolescents: a controlled study. *Circulation.* 1999;100:1798–1801.

35. Perez-Luogones A, Schweikert R, Pavia S, et al. Usefulness of midodrine in patients with severely symptomatic neurocardiogenic syncope: a randomized control study. *J Cardiovasc Electrophysiol.* 2001;12:935–938.

36. Romme JJCM, van Dijk N, Go-Schön IK, et al. Effectiveness of midodrine treatment in patients with recurrent vasovagal syncope not responding to non-pharmacological treatment (STAND-trial). *Europace.* 2011;13:1639–1647.

37. Sheldon R, Connolly S, Rose S, et al. Prevention of syncope trial (POST): a randomized, placebo-controlled study of metoprolol in the prevention of vasovagal syncope. *Circulation.* 2006;113:1164–1170.

38. Sheldon RS, Morillo CA, Klingenheben T, et al. Age-dependent effect of beta-blockers in preventing vasovagal syncope. *Circ Arrhythm Electrophysiol.* 2012;5:920–926.

39. Salim MA, Di Sessa TG. Effectiveness of fludrocortisone and salt in preventing syncope recurrence in children: a double-blind, placebo-controlled, randomized trial. *J Am Coll Cardiol.* 2005;45:484–488.

40. Di Girolamo E, Di Iorio C, Sabatini P, et al. Effects of paroxetine hydrochloride, a selective serotonin reuptake inhibitor, on refractory vasovagal syncope: a randomized, double-blind, placebo-controlled study. *J Am Coll Cardiol.* 1999;33:1227–1230.

41. Theodorakis GN, Leftheriotis D, Livanis EG, et al. Fluoxetine vs. propranolol in the treatment of vasovagal syncope: a prospective, randomized, placebo-controlled study. *Europace.* 2006;8:193–198.

42. Connolly SJ, Sheldon R, Roberts RS, Gent M. The North American Vasovagal Pacemaker Study (VPS): a randomized trial of permanent cardiac pacing for the prevention of vasovagal syncope. *J Am Coll Cardiol.* 1999;33:16–20.

43. Sutton R, Brignole M, Menozzi C, et al. Dual-chamber pacing in the treatment of neurally mediated tilt-positive cardioinhibitory syncope: pacemaker versus no therapy: a multicenter randomized study. *Circulation.* 2000;102:294–299.

44. Connolly SJ, Sheldon R, Thorpe KE, et al. Pacemaker therapy for prevention of syncope in patients with recurrent severe vasovagal syncope: second Vasovagal Pacemaker Study (VPS II): a randomized trial. *JAMA.* 2003;289:2224–2229.

45. Raviele A, Giada F, Menozzi C, et al. A randomized, double-blind, placebo-controlled study of permanent cardiac pacing for the treatment of recurrent tilt-induced vasovagal syncope: the vasovagal syncope and pacing trial (SYNPACE). *Eur Heart J.* 2004;25:1741–1748.

46. Brignole M, Menozzi C, Moya A, et al. Pacemaker therapy in patients with neurally mediated syncope and documented asystole: Third International Study on Syncope of Uncertain Etiology (ISSUE-3): a randomized trial. *Circulation.* 2012;125:2566–2571.

47. Brignole M, Donateo P, Tomaino M, et al. Benefit of pacemaker therapy in patients with presumed neurally mediated syncope and documented asystole is greater when tilt test is negative: an analysis from the Third International Study on Syncope of Uncertain Etiology (ISSUE-3). *Circ Arrhythm Electrophysiol.* 2014;7:10–16.

48. Palmisano P, Zaccaria M, Luzzi G, et al. Closed-loop cardiac pacing versus conventional dual-chamber pacing with specialized sensing and pacing algorithms for syncope prevention in patients with refractory vasovagal syncope: results of a long-term follow-up. *Europace.* 2012;14:1038–1043.

49. Pachon MJC, Pachon MEI, Cunha Pachon MZ, et al. Catheter ablation of severe neurally mediated reflex (neurocardiogenic or vasovagal) syncope: cardioneuroablation long-term results. *Europace.* 2011;13:1231–1242.

50. Yao Y, Shi R, Wong T, et al. Endocardial autonomic denervation of the left atrium to treat vasovagal syncope: an early experience in humans. *Circ Arrhythm Electrophysiol.* 2012;5:279–286.

104 Postural Orthostatic Tachycardia Syndrome

Blair P. Grubb and Beverly Karabin

Since the mid-1980s there has been a tremendous increase in our knowledge concerning illnesses that result from disturbances in the normal functioning of the autonomic nervous system (ANS). Initially, many of these investigations were principally focused on neurocardiogenic (or vasovagal) syncope, primarily as a consequence of the development of head-upright tilt-table testing as a method for uncovering a predisposition to the condition. During the course of these investigations, it became evident that a distant subgroup of patients experienced a related, while at the same time distinct, autonomic disturbance that resulted in persistent orthostatic tachycardia and orthostatic intolerance.[1] This disorder has come to be known as postural orthostatic tachycardia syndrome (POTS) and seems to consist of a heterogeneous group of disorders that share similar clinical characteristics. This chapter will present a review of the pathophysiology, diagnosis, and management of this disorder.

Autonomic Nervous System

In order to survive in the world, all organisms must possess the ability to make rapid alterations that stably maintain their internal environments despite significant changes in their external environments. This encompasses not only changes in environmental temperature, barometric pressure, and humidity but also the capability to quickly respond to sources of possible danger. The major natural processes through which this "homeostasis" is sustained and regulated are controlled by the hypothalamus and its effects on two systems: the ANS and the endocrine system.

While the assumption of upright posture was one of the truly defining moments in the process of human evolution, it had the effect of placing the organ that most defines our humanity, the brain, in a somewhat precarious position in regard to the maintenance of constant oxygenation, as the blood pressure–regulating system had evolved principally to meet the needs of an animal in a dorsal position. The ANS is the principal modality for both short- and long-term changes in position. While the renin-angiotensin-aldosterone system also plays a role, it does so over a much longer period of time.

In a normal individual, close to 25%–30% of the body's blood volume is in the thorax while supine.[2] Upon standing, the effect of gravity is to displace approximately 300–800 mL of blood downward to the abdomen and lower extremities. This is a volume drop of roughly 25%–30% in the thorax, and it occurs in the first few moments of standing, resulting in a decline in the venous return to the heart. Because the heart can only pump the blood that it receives, this produces an approximately 40% decline in the stroke volume as well as a decline in the arterial blood pressure. The area around which these changes occur is referred to as the venous hydrostatic indifference point (HIP) and represents the point in the vascular system where blood pressure is independent of position. The arterial HIP is near the level of the left ventricle, and the venous HIP is around the diaphragm.

Standing also results in a substantial rise in the transmural capillary pressure that is present in the dependent areas of the body, resulting in a rise in fluid filtration into the tissue spaces. This process arrives at a steady state after around 30 minutes of upright posture and can result in close to 10% decline in the plasma volume.

Adequate maintenance of cerebral perfusion during upright posture is the product of the interaction of several cardiovascular regulatory systems. The exact changes that occur with standing (an active process) differ somewhat from those seen during head-up tilt (a more passive process). Wieling and van Lieshout[2] have described three phases of orthostatic response: (1) the initial response (in the first 30 seconds), (2) the early steady-state alteration (at 1–2 minutes), and finally (3) the prolonged orthostatic period (after at least 5 minutes upright).

In the first moments following head-up tilt, cardiac stroke volume remains constant despite the decline in venous rhythm (possibly due to the blood in the pulmonary circulation). Afterward, there is a gradual fall in both cardiac filling and arterial pressure. This results in actuation in two distinct sets of pressure receptors compressed by high-pressure receptors in the carotid sinus and aortic arch as well as low-pressure receptors in the heart and lungs. In the heart mechanoreceptors connected by vagal afferents in each of the four cardiac chambers are present. These mechanoreceptors have a tonic inhibitory effect on the cardiovascular regulatory centers of the medulla (especially the nudeus tractus solitarii). The baroreceptive neurons located here can directly activate the cardiovagal neurons of the nucleus ambiguous and dorsal vagal nucleus while at the same time inhibiting the sympathoexcitatory neurons of the rostral ventrolateral medulla.

The reduced venous return and fall in filling pressure that occur during upright posture reduce the stretch on these receptors. As their firing rates decrease, there is a change in not only the systemic resistance vessels but also the splanchnic capacitance vessels. In addition, there is a local axon reflex (the venoarteriolar axon reflex) that can constrict flow to the skin, muscle, and adipose tissue. This may contribute up to 50% of the increase in limb vascular resistance seen during upright posture.

During head-up tilt, there is also activation of the high-pressure receptors in the carotid sinus. The carotid sinus contains a group of baroreceptors and nerve endings located in the enlarged area of the internal carotid artery, just after its origin from the common carotid artery. Here, the mechanoreceptors are located in the adventitia of the arterial wall. The afferent impulses generated by stretch on the arterial wall are then transmitted via the sensory fibers of the carotid sinus nerve that travels with the glossopharyngeal nerve. These afferent pathways terminate in the nucleus tractus solitarii in the medulla, near the dorsal and ambiguous nuclei. The initial increase in heart rate seen during tilt is thought to be modulated by a decline in carotid artery pressure. The slow rise in diastolic pressure seen during upright tilt is believed to be more closely related to a progressive increase in peripheral vascular resistance.

The circulatory changes seen during standing are somewhat different from those seen during tilt. Standing is a much more active process that is accompanied by contractions of muscles of both the legs and abdomen, which produces a compression of both capacitance and resistance vessels and results in an elevation in peripheral vascular resistance. This increase is sufficient to cause a transient increase in both right atrial pressure and cardiac output, which in turn cause an activation of the low-pressure receptors of the heart. This provokes an increase in neural traffic to the brain, with a subsequent decrease in peripheral vascular resistance, which can fall as much as 40%. This can allow a fall in mean arterial pressure of up to 20 mm Hg that can last for up to 6–8 seconds. The decline in pressure is then compensated for by the same mechanisms as during head-up tilt.

The early steady-state adjustments to upright posture consist of an increase in the heart rate of ≈10–15 beats/min, an increase in diastolic blood pressure of ≈10 mm Hg, and little or no change in systolic blood pressure. At this point, compared with supine posture, the blood volume of the thorax has fallen by 30%, cardiac output has increased by 30%, and heart rate is 10–15 beats/min higher.

At any given moment, ≈5% of the body's blood is in the capillaries, 8% in the heart, 12% in the pulmonary vasculature, 15% in the arterial system, and 60% in the venous system. The inability of any one of these mechanisms to operate adequately (or in a coordinated manner) may result in a failure of the body to compensate for either an initial or prolonged orthostatic challenge. This, in turn, would result in systemic hypotension, which, if sufficiently profound, could lead to cerebral hypoperfusion and subsequent loss of consciousness.

Historical Perspective

By the middle of the 19th century, physicians had begun to report on a group of patients who had developed a disorder characterized by exercise intolerance, severe fatigue, and palpitations.[3] These symptoms would often appear suddenly without a discernible cause (such as prolonged immobility, blood loss, or dehydration). At the time of the American Civil War, DeCosta described patients suffering from postural tachycardia and orthostatic intolerance, a condition he referred to as "irritable heart syndrome."[4]

Around the time of the First World War, a condition referred to as "neurocirculatory asthenia" began to be reported. The most remarkable of such reports was a study by Thomas Lewis, who described a condition he referred to as "the effort syndrome."[5] In the paper, he stated that fatigue was "an almost universal complaint" among these patients, as well as exercise intolerance in conjunction with symptoms such as palpitations, chest pain, syncope, and near syncope. In addition, Lewis reported that these patients demonstrated a significant postural tachycardia, with heart rates changing from 85 beats/min while supine to 120 beats/min while upright. In some of these patients there was a significant decline in blood pressure while upright, while others demonstrated only a modest decline.[5] Lewis concluded that in these patients "the potential reservoir in the veins takes up the blood, the supply to the heart falls away, and the arterial pressure falls rapidly," often accompanied by a compensatory tachycardia. Lewis further wrote that the reduction in blood flow "may be sufficient to produce cerebral anemia."

Over the ensuing years additional reports appeared.[6,7] This condition was later expanded on by Schondorf and Low, who performed extensive evaluations in 16 patients who suffered from extreme fatigue, exercise intolerance, bowel hypomotility, and lightheadedness.[8] During head-upright tilt-table testing, these individuals displayed distinctly abnormal cardiovascular responses to upright posture, with heart rate elevations to as high as 120–170 beats/min within the first 2–5 minutes of upright tilt. While some of these patients became hypotensive, the majority remained normotensive (and a small percentage became hypertensive). In describing the condition, Schondorf and Low used the term "postural orthostatic tachycardia syndrome" (POTS).[9]

Later investigations have found that POTS is not a single entity but rather a heterogeneous group of disorders with similar clinical characteristics.[9–11]

Definitions

The hallmark of these disorders is orthostatic intolerance, the definition of which is the occurrence of symptoms upon standing, which are generally relieved by becoming supine. As noted earlier, these patients will complain of symptoms such as palpitations, fatigue, exercise intolerance, lightheadedness, nausea, headache, near syncope, and syncope. As the amount of autonomic failure that these patients exhibit is not severe and the physical findings are often subtle, they may be misdiagnosed as having chronic anxiety or a panic disorder.[12]

Some patients can be so severely affected that the regular activities of daily life, such as housework, bathing, and even eating, can greatly exacerbate symptoms. Studies have shown that some patients with POTS can suffer from the same degree of functional impairment as patients with congestive heart failure or chronic obstructive pulmonary disease. Interestingly, the severity of symptoms may be greater in patients with POTS than in those with more severe autonomic failure syndromes, such as pure autonomic failure. A grading system to classify the severity of orthostatic intolerance has been developed (similar to that used in congestive heart failure) as noted in Box 104.1.

The impact of the disorder is substantial. It is presently estimated that between one-half million and one million people suffer from POTS in the United States alone. Of these, at least 25% are disabled and unable to work or attend school. Especially tragic is the fact that the majority of these patients are young and

---

BOX 104.1   The grading of orthostatic intolerance

Grade 0
Normal orthostatic tolerance

Grade I
Orthostatic symptoms are infrequent or occur only under conditions of increased orthostatic stress.
Subject is able to stand >15 minutes on most occasions.
Subject typically has unrestricted activities of daily living.

Grade II
Orthostatic symptoms are frequent, developing at least once a week. Orthostatic symptoms commonly develop with orthostatic stress.
Subject is able to stand >5 minutes on most occasions.
Some limitation in activities of daily living is typical.

Grade III
Orthostatic symptoms develop on most occasions and are regularly unmasked by orthostatic stress.
Subject is able to stand >1 minute on most occasions.
Patient is seriously incapacitated, being bed- or wheelchair-bound because of orthostatic intolerance.
Syncope/presyncope is common if patient attempts to stand.

Symptoms may vary with time and state of hydration and circumstances. Orthostatic stresses include prolonged standing, a meal, exertion, and head stress.
Modified from Kanjwal K, Saeed B, Karabin B, et al. Erythropoietin in the treatment of postural tachycardia syndrome. *Am J Ther.* 2012;19:92–95.

are most symptomatic during what is usually the most productive part of a person's life.

POTS is currently defined as the presence of symptoms of orthostatic intolerance associated with a postural change of 30 beats/min in the heart rate (or a rate that exceeds 120 beats/min that occurs within the first 10 minutes of standing or upright tilt). This should occur in the absence of other chronic debilitating conditions, such as prolonged bed rest or medications that impair vascular tone. It has been suggested that in children a more appropriate cutoff would be an increase of 40 beats/min. It should be kept in mind that many patients with orthostatic intolerance may not display orthostatic hypotension (a drop of >20/10 mm Hg upon standing). Indeed, they may have only a small decline in blood pressure, have no change at all, or even have an increase in blood pressure upon standing. Some investigators have noted that the focus on heart rate may cause many of the other autonomic symptoms to be overlooked, such as alterations in thermoregulatory, sudomotor, bowel, and bladder function. For many patients these complaints are often more troubling than the orthostatic issues.

Classification

In some ways POTS is best thought of as an abnormal physiological state (somewhat akin to the term "heart failure") that can be brought about by a wide range of different disorders. While differing ways of classifying POTS have been proposed, the system that follows is both clinically useful and conforms to the current scientific knowledge.[11,12]

We presently classify POTS as being either primary or secondary. The primary forms are not associated with other illnesses, while the secondary forms occur in association with another known disease or disorder. Proper recognition of subtypes is often important in management. The primary forms are divided into two major subtypes. The first and largest of these is referred to as the partial dysautonomia (also called "neurogenic") form. These patients are afflicted with a mild form of peripheral autonomic neuropathy, one of the principal manifestations of which appears to be an inability of the peripheral vasculature to initiate and/or maintain an adequate degree of peripheral vasoconstriction in the face of orthostatic stress. This inability results in a much greater than normal degree of blood pooling in the dependent areas of the body while upright, which in turn provokes a compensatory increase in both the heart rate and myocardial contractility in an attempt to maintain an adequate degree of cerebral perfusion. While these responses may initially be compensatory, the degree of peripheral vascular pooling may increase over time and exceed the compensatory effect. Many of these patients will become increasingly dependent on this peripheral skeletal muscle pump to maintain adequate blood pressure until further degrees of peripheral venous pooling occur in the mesenteric vasculature. One of the more striking features that these patients may display is the development of a deep, mottled (almost blue colored) discoloration in the lower extremities upon standing (a finding referred to as acral cyanosis). This excessive degree of peripheral vascular pooling may result in a state of "functional hypovolemia." Some studies have suggested that the vascular dysregulation extends to the cerebral vasculature's autoregulatory functions as well, a finding that may help explain the frequent complaint of cognitive impairment that many patients report.

There is a female predominance in this form of POTS (with a 5:1 female-to-male ratio), suggesting a possible causative role for female reproductive hormones. The majority of patients report that their symptoms appeared abruptly after a febrile illness (presumed to be viral). Surgery and pregnancy are also frequently related to the onset of symptoms. Trauma (most often from motor vehicle accidents) and electrical injuries have also been known to precipitate symptoms. Patients will present with complaints of extreme fatigue, syncope, near syncope, palpitations, exercise intolerance, and blurred vision as well as a generalized sense of weakness. As was mentioned previously, many patients will complain of cognitive impairment. A significant number of patients will also report nausea, bloating, altered bowel habits, abnormal sweating, pain in the extremities, and a sensation of always feeling cold. The severity of the symptoms often waxes and wanes. Many women will relate that their symptoms increase in the 4–5 days prior to their menstrual cycles.[13]

Most researchers feel that this form of POTS is often immune mediated in nature. Several studies have demonstrated that patients with postviral POTS have serum autoantibodies to α3-acetylcholine receptors in the peripheral autonomic ganglia.[14] Other autoantibodies to α1-adrenergic receptors have also been identified.[15] Recent studies have suggested a link with mitochondrial disorders (which may also be immune mediated); other etiologies most likely exist as well.

One subtype of the partial dysautonomic form of POTS appears to affect adolescents, a group that we have labeled as "developmental." The usual age of onset is around 14 years and often follows a period of very rapid growth.[16] Symptoms reach their peak at around 16 years. Symptoms of orthostatic intolerance, and often migraines, may be of such intensity that the patient is disabled. Symptoms will often fade over the ensuing years, so that by young adulthood (19–20 years of age) approximately 80% will have experienced a significant recovery. The etiology here remains unclear but is felt to reflect a transient period of autonomic imbalance that can occur in rapidly growing adolescents.

A second and much less common type of primary POTS is referred to as the "hyperadrenergic" form.[17] Here patients tend to report a more gradual and progressive onset of symptoms. They will often present complaining of persistent tachycardia, tremor, hyperhidrosis, and anxiety. Patients frequently complain of always feeling "too hot." The distinguishing characteristic of this group is an orthostatic hypertension that occurs in addition to a postural tachycardia. A large number of these patients complain of migraines, and some will report a significant increase in urinary output after only brief periods of upright posture. Most will display an exaggerated response to isoproterenol infusion. Many of the hyperadrenergic POTS patients will have significantly elevated serum norepinephrine levels (>600 ng/mL) during upright posture.

There is sometimes a family history of the disorder. We believe that there may be two forms of this disorder. The best understood subtype is a genetic disorder in which a single point mutation causes a dysfunction in the norepinephrine reuptake transport protein that cleans (and recycles) norepinephrine spillover in response to a wide range of sympathetic stimuli, resulting in a "hyperadrenergic" state that can mimic the state caused by a pheochromocytoma.[18] A second type of hyperadrenergic POTS appears to be autoimmune in nature and is characterized by an abrupt onset following an acute febrile illness (presumed to be viral). This form may overlap with inappropriate sinus tachycardia syndrome. Investigators have isolated autoantibodies to β1 cardiac receptors that stimulate the sites without producing a tachyphylaxis.

The term "secondary POTS" is employed to describe the wide variety of conditions that result in varying degrees of peripheral autonomic denervation with relative sparing of cardiac innervation.[19] The most frequent cause of secondary POTS is diabetes mellitus. It can also be seen as a result of multiple sclerosis, amyloidosis, sarcodosis, lupus, Sjögren's syndrome, alcoholism, and Lyme disease and following chemotherapy (with the vinca alkaloids in particular).[20]

A particularly noteworthy form of secondary POTS occurs in conjunction with the connective tissue disorder known as joint hypermobility syndrome (JHS), a condition also referred to as type III Ehlers-Danlos syndrome.[21] An inherited condition, JHS is characterized by joint hypermobility, soft velvety skin with variable hyperextensibility, and connective tissue fragility. Patients will also demonstrate easy bruising, premature varicose veins, diffuse joint and muscle pain, and orthostatic acrocyanosis. Patients with JHS may develop orthostatic intolerance due to the presence of abnormally elastic tissue in the vasculature, resulting in an increased vessel elasticity in response to the increase in hydrostatic pressure that occurs during orthostatic stress. This can allow for an excessive degree of peripheral venous pooling with a resultant compensatory tachycardia. Gazit and colleagues reported that up to 70% of patients with JHS may suffer from some degree of orthostatic intolerance.[21] Many adolescents with the developmental form of POTS will have features of JHS.

At times, POTS may be the presenting sign of a more severe form of autonomic disorder such as pure autonomic failure or multiple system atrophy. In addition, POTS may be the presenting sign of a paraneoplastic syndrome that can occur in association with adenocarcinomas of the lung, breast, pancreas, and ovary. It has been found that some of these tumors produce autoantibodies against postganglionic acetylcholine receptors in the autonomic ganglia, not dissimilar to those that have been found in the postviral autonomic neuropathies.[22]

Evaluation and Management

The first and most critical step is to obtain a detailed history followed by a thorough physical examination (which should include a complete neurological examination). It is important to identify conditions that may cause orthostatic intolerance (such as anemia, dehydration, and other chronic debilitating illnesses). Also any medications that could cause or worsen the condition (e.g., vasodilators, tricyclic antidepressants, or monoamine oxidase inhibitors) or consumption of alcohol should be identified.

A careful physical exam is paramount. Blood pressure and heart rate should be obtained in the supine, sitting, and standing positions and after 2 and 5 minutes of standing. It is helpful to be able to watch the lower extremities for the appearance of acral cyanosis, reflecting venous pooling. As the results obtained during standing are quite variable, we usually perform tilt-table testing on most patients as this setting is more controlled with fewer variables and with more reproducible results (in our experience better than those seen with neurocardiogenic syncope). Other tests of ANS function may be useful in select POTS patients as a way of measuring the degree of systemic autonomic involvement. Sudomotor function can be determined using thermoregulatory sweat testing or by assessment of skin conductance, skin resistance, or sympathetic skin potentials. Serum catecholamine levels, both in the supine and upright positions, should be obtained in patients suspected of having the hyperadrenergic form of POTS. Bowel motility studies are useful in ascertaining the degree of gastrointestinal involvement. More detailed descriptions of autonomic testing can be found elsewhere.[11,22]

An important differential diagnosis is with inappropriate sinus tachycardia. There are several similarities between inappropriate sinus tachycardia and POTS, particularly the hyperadrenergic form of POTS. Clinical presentations are much the same, and inappropriate sinus tachycardia is seen more frequently in women. Increased heart rate responsiveness to isoproterenol is seen in both conditions, suggesting that they represent different points on the spectrum of the same disease process. The major differences are that POTS patients seem to display a greater degree of postural change in heart rate, and their resting (supine) heart rates infrequently exceed 100 beats/min (as opposed to inappropriate sinus tachycardia, where resting heart rates >100 beats/min are more common).

It should also be remembered that POTS may occur due to some other disorder. While such patients present with symptoms of POTS, they often also have signs and symptoms of the primary disorder. While some degree of weight loss may be seen in POTS patients, extreme cachexia is uncommon and should prompt a search for other disorders (such as a malignancy or diabetes). In some patients with secondary POTS, the underlying disorder may not be evident at first and will only become apparent over time.

Treatments must be individualized to meet the particular needs of each patient. Any medication that the patient is taking that could contribute to the problem should be discontinued when possible (Box 104.2). Also, underlying conditions that may be causing a POTS-like state should be identified and treated (e.g., sarcoidosis, malignancy, etc.). Patient and family education regarding the nature of the problem is critical, particularly in relation to avoidance of aggravating factors, such as extreme heat, dehydration, and alcohol consumption. Patients with the partial dysautonomic form of POTS are encouraged to increase their fluid and sodium intake (at least 2 L of fluid and 3–5 g of salt per day). Compression stockings are sometimes helpful but must provide 30 mm Hg of counterpressure and be waist high to be effective.

One of the most important aspects of treatment is reconditioning,[23] as this augments venous return through enhancement of the skeletal muscle pump. Many patients are often quite deconditioned and find that aquatic activities are better tolerated as a place to begin. Recumbent bikes are also useful, as are rowing machines. Our initial goal is to have the patient perform 20–30 minutes of continuous aerobic activity at least three times per week as well as interspersed periods of resistance training.

In regard to pharmacotherapy, treatment must be individualized and is initiated with the goal of getting patients well enough to pursue reconditioning. No drug is currently approved by the US Food and Drug Administration (FDA) for the treatment of POTS; therefore any use of pharmacotherapy is done "off label." Knowing the POTS subtype is important in choosing the appropriate pharmacotherapy (Table 104.1).

In the partial dysautonomic POTS patients, therapies are oriented toward increasing fluid volume and augmenting peripheral vesicular resistance. We often begin with the mineralocorticoid agent fludrocortisone as it promotes both sodium and fluid retention as well as sensitizing peripheral α-receptors to the patients' own catecholamines. Oral desmopressin is also used as a volume-expanding agent. The next step is to use a vasoconstrictor such as midodrine, starting at a dosage of 5 mg orally three times a day (usually with meals). Dosages can be titrated up to 15–20 mg orally four times a day, if necessary.[22,23]

BOX 104.2   Drugs that may cause or worsen postural tachycardia syndrome

Calcium channel blockers
α-Receptor blockers
Angiotensin-converting enzyme inhibitors
Tricyclic antidepressants
Ethanol
Opiates
Diuretics
Phenothiazines
Nitrates
Sildenafil
Monoamine oxidase inhibitors
β-Blockers

TABLE 104.1	Therapeutic options in postural tachycardia syndrome		
TREATMENT	**APPLICATION**	**EFFECTIVE IN**	**PROBLEMS**
Reconditioning	Aerobic exercise 20 min three times/wk	PD, H	If too vigorous, may worsen symptoms
Hydration	2 L qd	PD	Edema
Salt	2–4 g/d	PD	Edema
Bupropion	150–300 mg qd	PD, H	Tremor, agitation, insomnia
Clonidine HCl	0.1–0.3 mg bid	H	Dry mouth, blurred vision
Catapres	0.1–0.3 mg patch/wk		
Desmopressin acetate (DDAVP)	0.1–0.2 mg qhs	PD	Hyponatremia, headache
Duloxetine HCl	20–30 mg qd	PD, H	Nausea, sleep disturbance
Erythropoietin	10,000–20,000 U SC/wk	PD	Pain at injection site, expensive
Escitalopram oxalate	10 mg qd	PD, H	Tremor, agitation, sexual problems
Fludrocortisone	0.1–0.2 mg qd	PD	Hypokalemia, acetate edema, hypomagnesemia,
Labetalol HCl	100–200 mg bid	H	Fatigue
Methylphenidate	5–10 mg tid	PD	Anorexia, insomnia, dependency
Midodrine	5–10 mg tid	PD	Nausea, itching scalp, supine hypertension
Octreotide acetate	50–200 μg SC tid	PD	Nausea, diarrhea, gallstones
Pyridostigmine bromide	30–60 mg qd	PD	Nausea, diarrhea
Venlafaxine HCl	75 mg qd or bid	PD, H	Nausea, anorexia, tremor
Ivabradine	5–7.5 mg bid	PD, H	Nausea, headache
Intravenous saline	1 L	PD	Infection at infusion site

bid, Twice a day; *H,* hyperadrenergic; *PD,* partial dysautonomic; *qd,* daily; *qhs,* every night at bedtime; *SC,* subcutaneous; *tid,* three times a day.
Note: The US Food and Drug Administration has not approved any drug for treating postural tachycardia syndrome.

Since patients are most symptomatic early in the morning, we often advise them to take their midodrine dose approximately 15 minutes prior to getting out of bed. We also advise patients that they can take an extra 5 mg dose as needed if severe breakthrough symptoms occur. The most common problems encountered with midodrine are nausea, "goose bumps," and scalp itching. If midodrine is not tolerated, methylphenidate can be an effective alternative, especially because it comes in several long-acting preparations. Some investigators have also advocated the use of yohimbine.

A very useful agent in managing this form of POTS is pyridostigmine, an acetyl cholinesterase inhibitor that facilitates neural transmission at the ganglionic level in both the sympathetic and parasympathetic nerves.[24] Several studies have suggested a greater than 50% response rate with the agent. Dosages range from 60–120 mg orally three times daily. Principal side effects include nausea and diarrhea.

In some patients, small doses of a β-blocker, such as propranolol, may be effective in controlling excessive heart rate responses to upright posture.[25,26]

If patients continue to be symptomatic, we add either a serotonin reuptake inhibitor (SSRI) or a norepinephrine reuptake inhibitor. While the SSRIs are very useful in the prevention of neurocardiogenic syncope, the norepinephrine reuptake inhibitors are somewhat more helpful in POTS patients. We usually employ bupropion in the XL form starting at 150 mg orally each day and titrating to 300 mg XL daily, if necessary.

In patients who have proved refractory to the aforementioned agents, we often try therapy with injected octreotide.[27] A potent vasoconstrictor of the mesenteric vasculature, it is administered by subcutaneous injection. Dosages range from 50–200 μg twice daily. A long-acting form lasting 28 days is also available. Another agent employed in refractory patients is erythropoietin (EPO). It not only augments vascular volume by causing an increase in red cell mass but also seems to have direct vasoconstrictive effects. As EPO must be administered by subcutaneous injection and is expensive, its use is normally reserved for refractory patients.[28]

Prior to starting EPO, a complete serum blood count (CBC) as well as serum iron, total iron-binding capacity, and ferritin level should be obtained. EPO can be employed as long as the hematocrit (HCT) is less than 50. The usual starting dose is 10,000 units injected subcutaneously once weekly. It usually takes 4–6 weeks to see the full effect of a particular dose. While the red cell augmentation and hemodynamic effects are independent, they tend to rise in parallel. Patients appear to achieve the best hemodynamic effect when the HCT does not exceed 50. If the HCT in a patient under EPO therapy goes above this value, the patient is usually asked to skip doses until it drops below 50 and then asked to restart EPO at a lower dose (in a manner not dissimilar to the way warfarin is managed with respect to the international normalized ratio [INR]).

The most common complaint of patients under EPO therapy is pain at the injection site. This can be minimized by allowing the EPO (which is kept refrigerated) to warm prior to injection. One way to do this is to roll the vial between the hands until it becomes warm. An additional way to minimize injection discomfort is to place an ice cube on the injection site 3–5 minutes before use; alternatively, a lidocaine patch or cream can be applied 15–30 minutes before use.

Many patients will require supplemental oral iron for EPO to have its best effect. If no clinical improvement is seen from the starting EPO dose till after 4–6 weeks, the weekly dose can be increased to 20,000 units. We have rarely had to exceed this dose in POTS patients. A rare complication of EPO therapy is that the patient can develop a "serum sickness"-like reaction to EPO, characterized by fever, chills, nausea, and a general sense of malaise. We have only seen this occur in a handful of patients over the last 12 years; it resolves promptly after the agent is discontinued.

In patients refractory to all other forms of therapy, we have employed intermittent intravenous saline therapy. The usual dose is 1 L of normal saline solution one to three times a week. While effective, problems with obtaining intravenous access often require a permanent subcutaneous port placement.[29] Long-term port use exposes the patient to potentially life-threatening infections.

With respect to patients suffering from the hyperadrenergic form of POTS, therapies are directed at release or receptor effects of norepinephrine. β-Adrenergic blocking agents are useful, but they tend to work best when combined with an α receptor–blocking effect. Labetalol and carvedilol are useful, as is the agent nebivolol. Clonidine is an α2-receptor agonist that produces a central sympatholytic effect and is a very useful agent in treating patients. Some investigators have reported that methyldopa can be useful, while other groups have suggested that phenobarbital can help in refractory patients.[17] A new agent, ivabradine, may be useful in the treatment of both forms of POTS.[30]

It should be remembered that patients suffering from POTS may experience an inability to pursue normal employment or educational opportunities and often suffer significant psychological disruption. Patients frequently require the services of psychologists, social workers, and lawyers to address these aspects of their illness. The attitude of the treating physician is crucial. Hope is a powerful medicine that should be encouraged by all.

Conclusions

POTS represents a pathophysiological state affecting the ANS, the most prominent features of which are postural tachycardia, palpitations, fatigue, weakness, and exercise intolerance. These disorders are not new; rather, what has changed is our ability to recognize and treat them. Continuing research will be required to improve our understanding of these disorders and uncover further therapeutic modalities.

REFERENCES

1. Low P, Sandroni P. Postural tachycardia syndrome. In: Robertson D, Biaggioni I, Burnstock G, Low P, Paton JFR, eds. *Primer on the Autonomic Nervous System*. 3rd ed. London, UK: Academic Press/Elsevier; 2012:517–519.
2. Wieling W, van Lieshout J. Maintenance of postural normotension in humans. In: Low P, Benarroch E, eds. *Clinical Autonomic Disorders*. 3rd ed. Baltimore: Lippincott Williams and Wilkins; 2008:57–67.
3. Streeten DH. Orthostatic intolerance: a historical introduction to the pathophysiological mechanisms. *Am J Med Sci*. 1999;317:78–87.
4. DaCosta JM. An irritable heart. *Am J Med Sci*. 1871;27:145–163.
5. Lewis T. *The Soldier's Heart and the Effort Syndrome*. London, UK: Shaw & Sons; 1919.
6. MacLean AR, Allen EV, Magath TB. Orthostatic tachycardia and orthostatic hypotension: defects in the return of venous blood to the heart. *Am Heart J*. 1944;27:145–163.
7. MacLean AR, Allen EV. Orthostatic hypotension and orthostatic tachycardia: treatment with the "head-up" bed. *JAMA*. 1940;115:2162–2167.
8. Schondorf R, Low P. Idiopathic postural orthostatic tachycardia syndrome: an attenuated form of acute pandysautonomia? *Neurology*. 1993;43:132–137.
9. Khurana RK. Orthostatic intolerance and orthostatic tachycardia: a heterogeneous disorder. *Clin Auton Res*. 1995;5:12–18.
10. Low P, Opfer-Gehrking T, Textor S, et al. Postural tachycardia syndrome. *Neurology*. 1995;45:519–525.
11. Grubb BP, Calkins H, Rowe P. Postural tachycardia, orthostatic intolerance and the chronic fatigue syndrome. In: Grubb BP, Olshansky B, eds. *Syncope, Mechanisms and Management*. Malden, MA: Blackwell Publishing; 2005:225–244.
12. Sheldon R, Grubb B, Olshansky B, et al. 2015 Heart Rhythm Society Expert Consensus Statement on the Diagnosis and Treatment of Postural Tachycardia Syndrome, Inappropriate Sinus Tachycardia, and Vasovagal Syncope. *Heart Rhythm*. 2015;12:e41–e60.
13. Karas B, Grubb B, Boehm K, et al. The postural orthostatic tachycardia syndrome: a potentially treatable cause of chronic fatigue, exercise intolerance, and cognitive impairment in adolescents. *Pacing Clin Electrophysiol*. 2000;23:344–351.
14. Vernino S, Low P, Fealey RD, et al. Autoantibodies to ganglionic acetylcholine receptors in autoimmune autonomic neuropathies. *N Engl J Med*. 2000;343:847–855.
15. Li H, Yu X, Liles C, et al. Autoimmune basis for postural tachycardia syndrome. *J Am Heart Assoc*. 2014;3:e000755.
16. Grubb BP. The postural tachycardia syndrome: when to consider it in adolescents. *Fam Pract Recertification*. 2006;28:19–30.
17. Kanjwal K, Saeed B, Karabin B, et al. Clinical presentation and management of patients with hyperadrenergic postural tachycardia syndrome: a single center experience. *Cardiol J*. 2011;18:527–531.
18. Shannon JR, Flatten NL, Jordan J, et al. Orthostatic intolerance and tachycardia associated with norepinephrine-transporter deficiency. *N Engl J Med*. 2000;342:541–549.
19. Nankiewicz K, Somers V. Chronic orthostatic intolerance: part of a spectrum of dysfunction in orthostatic cardiovascular homeostasis? *Circulation*. 1998;98:2105–2107.
20. Kanjwal K, Karabin B, Kanjwal Y, et al. Postural tachycardia syndrome following Lyme disease. *Cardiol J*. 2011;18:63–66.
21. Kanjwal K, Saeed B, Karabin B, et al. Comparative clinical profile of postural orthostatic tachycardia patients with and without joint hypermobility syndrome. *Indian Pacing Electrophysiol J*. 2010;10:173–178.
22. Grubb BP, Kanjwal Y, Kosinski D. The postural tachycardia syndrome: a concise guide to diagnosis and management. *J Cardiovasc Electrophysiol*. 2006;17:108–112.
23. Grubb BP. The postural tachycardia syndrome. *Circulation*. 2008;117:2814–2817.
24. Kanjwal K, Sheikh M, Karabin B, et al. Pyridostigmine in the treatment of postural orthostatic tachycardia: a single center experience. *Pacing Clin Electrophysiol*. 2011;34:750–755.
25. Fu Q, VanGundy T, Shibata S, et al. Exercise training versus propranolol in the treatment of postural tachycardia syndrome. *Hypertension*. 2011;58:167–175.
26. Raj S, Black B, Biaggioni I, et al. Propranolol decreases tachycardia and improves symptoms in the postural tachycardia syndrome. *Circulation*. 2009;120:725–734.
27. Kanjwal K, Saeed B, Karabin B, et al. Use of octreotide in the treatment of refractory orthostatic intolerance. *Am J Ther*. 2012;19:7–10.
28. Kanjwal K, Saeed B, Karabin B, et al. Erythropoietin in the treatment of postural tachycardia syndrome. *Am J Ther*. 2012;19:92–95.
29. Moak J, Leong D, Fabian R, et al. Intravenous hydration for management of medication-resistant orthostatic intolerance in the adolescent and young adult. *Pediatr Cardiol*. 2016;37:278–282.
30. McDonald C, Frith J, Newton J. Single centre experience of ivabradine in postural tachycardia syndrome. *Europace*. 2011;13:427–430.

105 Progressive Conduction System Disease

Demosthenes G. Katritsis

Progressive conduction system disease is a slow, degenerative process that affects the cardiac conduction system at any level and manifests itself as sinoatrial exit block, atrioventricular (AV) block at the nodal or Hisian level, or bundle branch block of varying severity. It was initially described by Lev and Lenegre as a progressive AV block of unknown origin with myocardial sclerosis and loss of conduction fibers that develops over decades.

Patients may present with bradycardia, a long P wave, prolonged PR and/or QRS intervals, fascicular blocks, or AV block of various types. Clinical and echocardiographic examination is otherwise unremarkable in isolated conduction system disease. Progressive conduction disease may be also seen in the context of other disorders, with symptoms and signs of the associated condition being present (Box 105.1). Subjects with prolonged QRS duration, even without bundle branch block, are at increased risk for future pacemaker implantation and may warrant monitoring for progressive conduction disease.[1] The severity of progressive conduction disease is independently associated with hospitalization and cardiovascular mortality.[2]

Etiology and Pathophysiology

Progressive myocardial degeneration with increased myocardial collagen turnover and fibrosis of the conduction system are the main histopathological findings in patients with Lev and Lenegre disease.[3] Lev and Lenegre hypothesized that progressive conduction defects were due to a primary degenerative disease of unknown origin that was exaggerated by aging. However, fibrosis of the conduction system may also be seen in the elderly in the absence of conduction defects, and there has been evidence that progressive conduction system disease has genetic and autoimmune origins (see Box 105.1).[4–7]

The most common cause of isolated AV conduction disease are mutations in the gene SCN5A that encodes for the pore-forming α-subunit of the cardiac sodium channel (Nav1.5) and affects depolarization phase 0 (Table 105.1 and Fig. 105.1). There is also evidence for a regulatory role of Nav1.5 in cellular biological processes in addition to its electrophysiological function.[8] These mutations result in slowing of conduction and fibrosis, and the cardiac conduction defect deteriorates progressively with age, leading to life-threatening conduction blocks only in the elderly. Most of the described mutations in the SCN5A gene are autosomal dominant, but recessive mutations have also been described.

Loss- and gain-of-function mutations of SCN5A, as well as mutations in genes encoding other ion channels, may also result in isolated or overlapping phenotypes of sick sinus syndrome, AV conduction defects, and other conditions such as Brugada syndrome, long QT syndrome (LQTS), dilated cardiomyopathy, and multifocal ectopic Purkinje–related premature contractions.[9–14] The same SCN5A gene mutation can lead to conduction disease, Brugada syndrome, or LQTS 3, although LQTS 3 mutations induce a gain-of-function of the sodium channel, whereas conduction disease or Brugada syndrome mutations induce loss-of-function of this channel. Functional analysis has also demonstrated that hereditary conduction disease may be caused by a haploinsufficiency mechanism (i.e., the single functional copy of the gene does not produce enough protein), which in combination with aging leads to progressive alteration in conduction velocity and results in AV block only in elderly carriers.[15] Why haploinsufficiency leads to Brugada syndrome in some families and to hereditary conduction disease in others is not known. Modifier genes, allele penetrance, specific promoter variants, truncation mutations that potentially reduce the sodium current more than missense mutations, and/or environmental factors and sex may also influence both the severity and the phenotype induced by an SCN5A mutation.[16,17]

Other gene families affecting ionic currents as well as the structure or coupling of conducting myocytes may also result in conduction defects and arrhythmias in the context of congenital heart disease or Wolff-Parkinson-White (WPW) syndrome (see Table 105.1).

Progressive conduction disease may also be seen with neuromuscular disorders, infective and autoimmune disorders (due to chronic inflammation and fibrosis), the osteoblast phenotype of calcific aortic stenosis, and other conditions that may involve the conduction system at any level (see Box 105.1).

Idiopathic Isolated Conduction Disease (Progressive Familial Heart Block Type IA and IB)

In the 1960s, Lev noticed progressive AV block and left bundle branch block (LBBB) in the elderly population, while Lenegre reported defects in the middle and distal portions of both bundle branches in relatively young patients. Familial investigations of patients with bifascicular or complete AV block had suggested that genetic factors could be involved in the pathogenesis of the disease, and in 1995 a locus for progressive familial heart block was mapped to chromosome 19q13.2-13.3 (gene TRPM4).[18] Subsequently, loss-of-function mutations of the cardiac sodium channel SNC5A gene in chromosome 3p21 were identified.[19] Thus in the Online Mendelian Inheritance in Man database of the US National Center for Biotechnology Information, progressive

BOX 105.1	Causes of progressive conduction disease

Inherited
  Isolated (progressive familial heart block type IA and IB)
  Genetic arrhythmia syndromes (Brugada syndrome, long QT syndrome 3, arrhythmia-prone cardiomyopathy)
  Congenital cardiac defects (Holt-Oram syndrome, nonsyndromic cardiac defects such as atrial septal defect, tetralogy of Fallot, ventricular septal defect, pulmonary atresia, and subvalvular aortic stenosis)
  Wolff-Parkinson-White syndrome and cardiomyopathy
  Neuromuscular disorders (myotonic dystrophy type 1, Emery-Dreifus muscular dystrophy, limb-girdle muscular dystrophy, desmin myopathy)
  Anderson-Fabry disease
  Familial amyloidosis
  Mucopolysaccharidosis IV
Calcific valve disease (aortic stenosis and mitral annulus calcification)
Dilated cardiomyopathy (ischemic and nonischemic)
Autoimmune and infective disorders
  Sarcoidosis
  Rheumatoid arthritis
  Ankylosing spondylitis (HLA B27)
  Systemic sclerosis
  Systemic lupus erythematosus
  Sjögren syndrome
  Wegener granulomatosis
  Behçet disease
  Chagas disease
  Anti-Ro/SSA, anti-LA/SSA antibodies
Kearns-Sayre syndrome

familial heart block (PFHB) type IA or Lenegre-Lev disease is classified as a disorder due to *SCN5A* mutations on locus 3p21. PFHB type IB is due to mutations in the gene *TRPM4* on locus 19q13.33 that encodes the calcium-activated nonselective cation channel of the transient receptor potential melastatin.

Specific loss-of-function *SCN5A* mutations demonstrate varied competing gating effects that reduce sodium current density and enhance slow inactivation with selective slowing of conduction velocity in a way that may result in isolated conduction system disease without provoking tachyarrhythmias.[5,20] Histological examination of the hearts of patients with *SCN5A* mutations has also revealed severe degenerative changes in the conduction system, and Nav1.5 deficiency has been found to cause tissue degeneration via transforming growth factor-β_1 (TGF-β_1)-mediated fibrosis.[8] *SNC5A* mutations cause the majority of isolated conduction disease and are usually autosomal dominant but with reduced penetrance and variable expressivity. Initial electrophysiology studies in mutation carriers with AV block revealed prolonged HV but normal AH intervals, thus suggesting infra-Hisian block, but progressive AV block due to *SCN5A* mutations can be both supra- and infra-Hisian.

The *TRPM4* gene encodes the transient receptor potential cation channel, subfamily M, member 4 (melastatin-4). The *TRPM4* channel is highly expressed in cardiac Purkinje fibers, and gain-of-function mutations at chromosomal locus 19q13.3 have been associated with isolated progressive cardiac conduction block.[21] Described families with *TRPM4* mutations exhibit conduction blocks transmitted via an autosomal dominant inheritance and incomplete penetrance. Usually, patients present with right bundle branch block (RBBB) and prominent R waves in right precordial leads. These mutations may account for a significant portion of inherited forms of RBBB (25%) or AV block (10%).[22]

Overlapping Genetic Arrhythmia Syndromes

Both loss- and gain-of-function *SCN5A* mutations may slow normal automaticity and affect conduction to the surrounding atrial

tissue.[8,23] Cases of *congenital sick sinus syndrome* have been ascribed to recessive *SCN5A* mutations that may also lead to bradycardia in the fetus or infants. It seems that tissue degeneration triggered by Nav1.5 deficiency, causing TGF-β_1–mediated fibrosis, accompanied by sinus node dysfunction associated with *SCN5A* disruption or aging may be the cause.[8] The pacemaker or funny current (I_f) is generated by the hyperpolarization-activated cyclic nucleotide-gated (*HCN*) channel. Familial sinus bradycardia has been linked to *HCN4* mutations, but clinical cases are usually benign with intact chronotropic competence and do not necessitate pacemaker implantation.[24] Genome-wide association studies have also demonstrated an association between *MYH6*, the gene encoding α-myosin heavy chain (α-MHC), and sinus node function in the general population.[25] Sinus bradycardia has also been noted in other genetic syndromes, such as catecholaminergic polymorphic ventricular tachycardia (VT) (see Table 105.1).

Mutations of the *SCN10A* gene that encodes for the channel Nav1.8 have also been associated with conduction disease but usually in the context of *Brugada syndrome*.[14,26,27] SCN10A may affect AV conduction through a cardiac enhancer that interacts with and regulates the promoter of SCN5A.[28]

Sodium channel β_1-subunit (*SCN1B*) gene mutations that have been associated with Brugada syndrome may also cause phenotypes of isolated progressive conduction disturbances mainly by affecting Purkinje fibers. *SCN1B* encodes for a modulatory β-subunit of the sodium channel (Scn1b) and also affects phase 0 of the action potential. Mutations are located either in β_1 or in the newly described transcript β_1B, and coexpression of mutant β-subunits with Nav1.5 results in diminished sodium current.[29]

Disruption of the gap junction protein connexin40 (Cx40), which is predominantly expressed in the atria and His–Purkinje system, results in prolonged AV conduction.[30] A novel germ-like mutation in *GJA5*, the gene encoding Cx40, has been recently described as a cause of *familial progressive heart block*, *slow heart rate*, and *malignant ventricular arrhythmias*. The disease has an early onset and is associated with sudden cardiac death.[31]

Mutations in *KCNJ2* are found in the autosomal dominant *Andersen-Tawil* or *long QT 7 syndrome*. *KCNJ2* encodes for the inward rectifier potassium channel (Kir2.1) and affects phases 3 and 4, i.e., terminal repolarization and resting potential. Inactivation of Kir2.1 results in action potential prolongation and slowing of heart rate and conduction.[32] Besides QT interval prolongation, potassium-sensitive paralysis, and hypoplastic mandibles, patients may present with conduction abnormalities, such as AV block, bundle branch block, or nonspecific intraventricular conduction delay.

In a small percentage of cases, *WPW syndrome* is familial. Mutations in the gene *PRKAG2*, which encodes the regulatory γ-subunit of adenosine monophosphate (AMP)-activated protein kinase (AMPK), are transmitted as an autosomal dominant disorder and are associated with glucogen storage cardiomyopathy.[33,34] The annulus fibrosis, which normally insulates the ventricles from inappropriate excitation by the atria, is thinned and disrupted by glycogen-filled myocytes, and these anomalous microscopic AV connections, rather than morphologically distinct bypass tracts, appear to provide the anatomical substrate for ventricular preexcitation. Patients present with a variable combination of glycogen storage cardiomyopathy, progressive conduction system disease (including sinus bradycardia and AV block), ventricular preexcitation, arrhythmias, and sudden death.[34] Particular mutations have been associated with nodoventricular and fasciculoventricular accessory pathways.[33,34] Prognosis is unfavorable because there is a high risk of atrial arrhythmias and complete infra-Hisian block, and early pacemaker implantation may be considered.[34] Recently, exome analysis of a family with WPW syndrome identified a novel disease locus on gene *MYH6*.[35] Another novel form of WPW syndrome is associated with microdeletion in the region of the gene *BMP2* that encodes the bone

TABLE 105.1 Genetic causes of conduction system disease

GENE	PROTEIN	CONDUCTION DEFECT AND ASSOCIATED CONDITIONS	MECHANISM(S)
Ion Channels			
SCN5A	Nav1.5	AV conduction defect, sick sinus syndrome, bundle branch block	Slowing of conduction velocity and pacemaking rate, tissue degeneration via TGF-β_1
		Brugada syndrome, LQTS 3, AF, dilated cardiomyopathy	
SCN10A	Nav1.8	Conduction defects, sick sinus syndrome, RBBB	Slowing of conduction velocity and pacemaking rate
		Brugada syndrome, early repolarization syndrome, AF, VT/VF	
TRPM4	TRPM4	AV conduction defect, RBBB	Possibly elevated density of TRPM4 channels disables action potential propagation down the Purkinje fibers.
		Brugada syndrome	
SCN1B	Scn1b	Bundle branch block	Slowing of conduction velocity, mainly in Purkinje fibers
		Brugada syndrome, AF	
KCNJ2	Kir2.1	AV block, bundle branch block	Prolongation of action potential and slowing of pacemaking rate
		Andersen-Tawil syndrome (LQTS 7)	
HCN4	HCN4	Sick sinus syndrome	Reduction of pacemaker current I_f
		Brugada syndrome, AF	
		Noncompaction cardiomyopathy	
		Mitral valve prolapse	
Structural Proteins			
GJA5	Connexin40	AV block, bradycardia	Defective coupling of conducting myocytes
		Ventricular arrhythmias	
ANK2	Ankyrin-B	Sick sinus syndrome	Abnormal sinoatrial electrical activity due to dysfunction in ankyrin B–based trafficking pathways
		LQTS 4, AF, CPVT	
DES	Desmin	AV block	Desmin-positive aggregates and inability of mutated desmin to interact with cellular structures
		VT/VF, cardiomyopathy	
		Skeletal myopathy	Mitochondrial dysfunction
MYH6	α-Myosin heavy chain	Sick sinus syndrome	Unknown
		AF, thoracic aortic aneurysm	Possibly interference with connexin40 and microRNA involved in conduction
		WPW syndrome?	
Protein Kinases			
PRKAG2	γ2-Subunit of AMP-activated protein kinase (AMPK)	Sinus bradycardia, AV block	Disruption of annulus fibrosus by glycogen-filled myocytes
		WPW syndrome	
		Glycogen storage cardiomyopathy	
DMPK	Myotonic dystrophy protein kinase	AV block, bundle branch block, VT/VF, cardiomyopathy	Toxic mutant RNA impairs conduction with various mechanisms
		Myotonic dystrophy type I	
TGF-β Superfamily			
BMP2	Bone morphogenetic protein 2	AV block	Disruption of annulus fibrosus
		WPW syndrome, cognitive defects, dysmorphic features	
Transcription Factors			
TBX5	Tbx5	Sinus bradycardia, AV block, bundle branch block	Defective development and coupling of conducting myocytes
		Holt-Oram syndrome, AF, Ischemic stroke	
NKX2-5	Nkx2-5	AV block, bundle branch block	Defective development and coupling of conducting myocytes
		VSD, Fallot, subvalvar AS, pulmonary atresia	
Nuclear Membrane Proteins			
LMNA	Lamin A/C	AV block,	Possibly, hyperactivation of mitogen-activated protein kinase, and interference with nucleus integrity and gap junctions
		VT/VF, cardiomyopathy	
		Emery-Dreifuss muscular dystrophy	
		Limb-girdle muscular dystrophy	
EMD	Emerin	AV block	Mechanism poorly understood
		VT/VF	
		Emery-Dreifuss muscular dystrophy	
Lysosomal Enzymes			
GLA	α-Galactosidase (α-GALA)	AV block	Accumulation of glycosphingolipids
		Anderson-Fabry disease	
Ca^{2+}-Handling Proteins			
RYR2	Ryanodine receptor	Sick sinus syndrome, AV block	Altered calcium handling
		CPVT	Mechanism of bradycardia and block unknown
		AF, dilated cardiomyopathy	
CASQ2	Calsequestrin	Sinus bradycardia	Altered calcium handling
		CPVT	Mechanism of bradycardia and block unknown

AF, Atrial fibrillation; *AMP*, adenosine monophosphate; *AV*, atrioventricular; *CPVT*, catecholaminergic polymorphic ventricular tachycardia; *LQTS*, long QT syndrome; *Nav1.5*, cardiac sodium channel; *RBBB*, right bundle branch block; *TGF-β_1*, transforming growth factor-β_1; *VF*, ventricular fibrillation; *VSD*, ventricular septal defect; *VT*, ventricular tachycardia; *WPW*, Wolff-Parkinson-White.

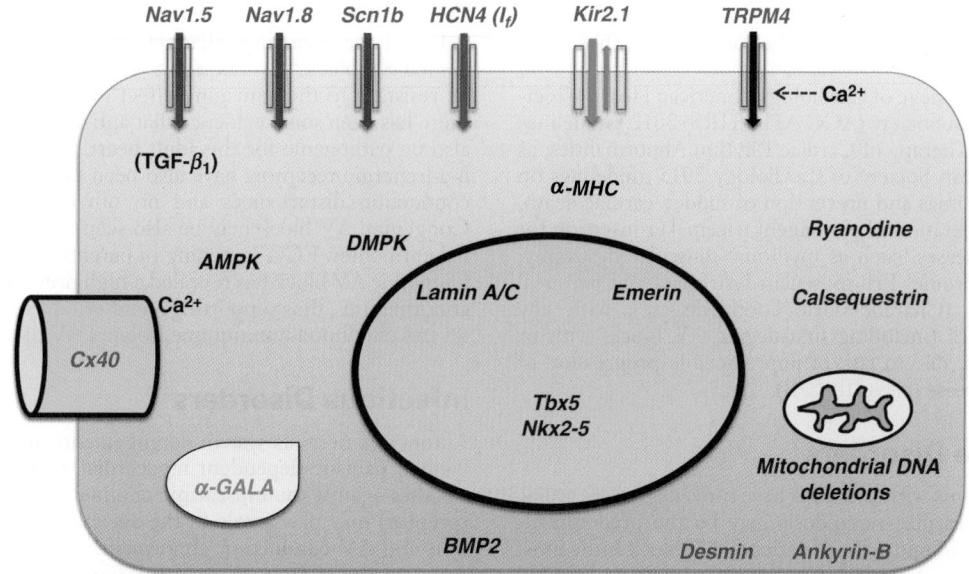

FIGURE 105.1 Proteins and mechanisms related to cardiac conduction system disease. Please see text and Table 105.1 for details.

morphogenetic protein-2, a member of the transforming growth factor-β (*TGF-β*) gene *superfamily*, and affects the development of the annulus fibrosus. It is characterized by variable cognitive deficits, dysmorphic features, and prolonged AV conduction on atrial pacing.[35]

Congenital Heart Deformities

Mutations affecting *transcription factor 5 (Tbx5)* and *homeobox factor* Nkx2-5, which facilitate the development of the conduction lineage, result in defective expression of gap junction connexin proteins, such as Cx40, and incomplete development of the entire AV conduction system.[8] Mutations in the TBX5 gene cause *Holt-Oram syndrome*. Patients with Holt-Oram syndrome exhibit variable degrees of progressive conduction system dysfunction, such as sinus bradycardia and AV block, even in the absence of atrial septal defects (ASDs) or other overt structural heart disease. Mutations in the gene encoding factor NKX2-5 cause nonsyndromic, congenital heart disease, mainly *secundum ASDs*, as well as *tetralogy of Fallot, ventricular septal defects (VSDs), pulmonary atresia, subvalvular aortic stenosis*, and *hypoplasia of the conduction system*.[36,37] These mutations are associated with progressive AV node dysfunction and other diffuse conduction system abnormalities. The absence of heart block in the presence of other major structural heart defects, as well as the presence of AV block in the absence of other malformations in mutation carriers, suggests that both Nkx2-5 and *TBx5* have specific roles in conduction system development and integrity, independent of their roles in structural heart development.

Neuromuscular Disorders

Several different types of muscular dystrophies, such as Emery-Dreifuss muscular dystrophy, limb girdle muscular dystrophy (Erb muscular dystrophy), myotonic dystrophy type 1 (Steinert disease), and desmin-related myopathy, are associated with cardiac conduction defects. Patients typically present with sinus bradycardia, first- or higher-degree AV block or bundle branch block, and vulnerability for sudden cardiac death.

Mutations in the nuclear envelope proteins such as lamin A/C (*LMNA*) or emerin (*EMD*) that maintain nuclear envelope integrity cause Emery-Dreifuss muscular dystrophy and limb

girdle muscular dystrophy. Individuals with muscular dystrophies develop progressive skeletal muscle weakness in the first decade of life and cardiac involvement, such as progressive AV block and dilated cardiomyopathy with propensity to lethal ventricular arrhythmias, in later decades.[38,39] Whereas heart failure is a common feature in families with neuromuscular and cardiac manifestations of LMNA disease, structural and functional abnormalities as determined using echocardiography may be absent in mutation carriers, with conduction disease as the only apparent abnormality. Thus if conventional polymerase chain reaction–based direct sequencing approaches for LMNA analysis are negative in suggestive pedigrees, mutation detection techniques capable of detecting gross genomic lesions involving deletions and insertions (genome-wide linkage approach) should be considered.[38] Independent risk factors for malignant arrhythmias in *LMNA* mutation carriers are nonsustained VT (NSVT), a left ventricular ejection fraction (LVEF) <45% at the first clinical contact, male sex, and nonmissense mutations (ins/del/truncating or mutations affecting splicing). Patients with specific mutations have rapid progression of AV conduction abnormalities, and sudden death may be the presenting feature.[40] They should be considered for early implantation of an implantable cardioverter defibrillator (ICD) rather than a pacemaker alone.

Desmin-related myopathy is an autosomally inherited skeletal and cardiac myopathy, mainly caused by dominant mutations in the *desmin* gene. Up to 50% of carriers of any one of the described mutations have cardiomyopathy, and around 60% have cardiac conduction disease or arrhythmias, with AV block as an important hallmark. Progression to AV block is rapid and ICD backup to pacing may be needed for malignant ventricular arrhythmias.[41]

Mutations in the gene *DMPK* encoding myotonic dystrophy protein kinase result in nuclear entrapment of "toxic" mutant RNA and cause myotonic dystrophy type 1, left ventricular (LV) dysfunction, and AV conduction block.[42] Myotonic dystrophy type 1 is an autosomal dominant disorder that represents the most common muscular dystrophy in adults. Conduction system dysfunction is seen in 70% of patients with the disease, and bundle branch block or AV block that is progressive and infra-Hisian block are the most common conduction system defects. In patients with myotonic dystrophy type I and PR interval >200 ms, QRS interval >100 ms, or both, pacing is indicated when HV interval is >70 ms, and it improves survival.[43] However, patients may suddenly die from VT/ventricular fibrillation (VF), and ICDs rather than pacemakers should be considered in those with conduction disturbances.[44]

The American College of Cardiology/American Heart Association/Heart Rhythm Society (ACC/AHA/HRS) 2012 Guidelines for Device-Based Therapy of Cardiac Rhythm Abnormalities, as well as the European Society of Cardiology 2015 guidelines on ventricular arrhythmias and prevention of sudden cardiac death, recommend consideration of permanent pacemaker insertion for neuromuscular diseases, such as myotonic muscular dystrophy, Kearns-Sayre syndrome, Erb muscular dystrophy, and peroneal muscular atrophy (Charcot-Marie-Tooth disease), with any degree of AV block (including first-degree AV block) with or without symptoms, due to risk of unpredictable progression of AV conduction disease (class IIb-C/B).

Autoimmune Disorders

Up to 50% of patients with *sarcoidosis* have some degree of cardiac involvement, and cardiac sarcoidosis may be the predominant form of the disease in up to 5% of patients. AV block is the most common clinical manifestation. Cardiac sarcoidosis and a mild form of giant cell myocarditis were diagnosed in 25% of initially unexplained AV block in young and middle-aged adults.[44] Up to 14% of patients with high-degree AV block had cardiac sarcoidosis. Thus cardiac sarcoidosis may represent a cause of progressive AV conduction disease, especially in women, and should be considered in adults aged <55 years who present with unexplained high-degree AV block. In cardiac sarcoidosis, the conduction disease, as opposed to VT, might improve with steroids.[45]

In rheumatoid disorders, rhythm and conduction defects are usually mild but may progress, although rarely, to complete heart block. Conduction defects occur frequently in patients with spondyloarthropathies and in those with various forms of vasculitis. All degrees of AV block have been described in *rheumatoid arthritis* (RA) patients, and RBBB is found in up to 35% of them. AV blocks in RA patients do not respond to immunosuppressive treatment.[6] Cardiac conduction defects occur in about 5% of all *systemic lupus erythematosus* (SLE) patients, more frequently in young women, and include all degrees of AV block, intraventricular conduction defects, and sick sinus syndrome. In adults, complete heart block is rare. Arrhythmias in SLE may respond to immunosuppressive therapy.[6] Up to 20% of patients with *systemic sclerosis* have LBBB or first-degree block in their electrocardiograms (ECGs), although at electrophysiology studies, detectable conduction abnormalities are considerably higher.[6] RBBB is less common, and complete AV block occurs in <2% of patients. It is estimated that one-third of *ankylosing spondylitis* patients experience conduction abnormalities. AV block is the most common conduction defect in *HLA B27* gene carriers, and the level of the block is usually at the AV node rather than infra-Hisian. First-degree AV block as well as complete heart block have been described in *Sjögren syndrome* patients, and an association between disease activity and the presence of anti-Ro/SSA and anti-La/SSB antibodies has been described.[6] Left anterior hemiblock and RBBB have also been described in *polymyositis*, but complete AV block is rare.[6] *Wegener granulomatosis* is associated with conduction disturbances of various forms that may require permanent pacing.[6] Rapidly progressive AV conduction disease may, although rarely, be an early manifestation of *Behçet disease*.[46] Drugs that are used in rheumatic diseases may also affect the conduction system. *Methotrexate* may induce RBBB, whereas *chloroquine* (but not hydrochloroquine) is associated with a high incidence of cardiac conduction disorders, including bundle branch blocks and incomplete or complete AV blocks.[47,48]

Transplacental penetration of *anti-Ro/SSA and anti-La/SSB ribonucleoprotein antibodies* from the mother, who may have SLE, systemic sclerosis, or Sjögren syndrome or may be entirely asymptomatic, may cross-react with T- and L-type calcium channels and the potassium channel, hERG, and may induce congenital AV block.[49,50] The adult AV node is generally thought to be resistant to the damaging effect of these autoantibodies, but there has been some evidence that anti-Ro/SSA antibodies might also be pathogenic for the adult heart.[49] Autoantibodies against β-adrenergic receptors have also been observed in patients with conduction disturbances and no other cardiac abnormalities. Congenital AV block may be also seen in the absence of maternal antibodies. ECG screening in parents of children affected by idiopathic AV block has revealed a high prevalence of conduction abnormalities, thus supporting an inheritable trait in the congenital and childhood nonimmune isolated AV block.

Infectious Disorders

Autonomic nervous system derangements, microvascular disturbances, parasite-dependent myocardial aggression, and autoantibodies against the muscarinic cholinergic type 2 receptor (M2 receptor) may play a role in the associated sinus nodal dysfunction and AV conduction abnormalities seen in chronic *Chagas heart disease*.[51] Chagas disease may be seen in the Western world because of immigration patterns. Cardiac involvement in chronic disease develops gradually, with ECG abnormalities, such as fascicular blocks, preceding changes in LV function. Sinus bradycardia, atrial fibrillation, and high-grade AV block usually accompany LV remodeling with pathological Q waves and increased risk of death from brady- or tachyarrhythmias. Antiprotozoal therapy with benznidazole may modify the progression of cardiac disease.[52]

Lyme borreliosis is caused by *Borrelia burgdorferi*, which is transmitted by the tick genus *Ixodes*.[53] However, although Lyme borreliosis is the most common tick-borne infectious disease in North America and in countries with moderate climates in Eurasia, Lyme carditis is rare. AV block may be seen during the acute course of the disease that involves the heart, with a clinical picture similar to that in acute rheumatic fever, and this AV block responds to antibiotics.

Although *Borrelia* antibodies may be sought with Western blot in cases of otherwise unexplained acute AV block, there is no convincing evidence for progressive conduction disease with late Lyme disease or post–Lyme borreliosis syndrome.[54]

Calcific Valve Disease

Calcific aortic stenosis and mitral annulus calcification are progressive processes that involve the conduction system and may result in conduction block at any level. Calcific AV stenosis has characteristic pathological features of an osteoblast phenotype with cell proliferation and atherosclerosis.[55] The HV interval is typically prolonged in calcific aortic stenosis, and the progressive conduction disease may need permanent pacing, particularly after surgical or transcatheter valve replacement. Aortic sclerosis is an age-related process, but recent data have demonstrated a familial aggregation for this disease.[56]

Other Disorders

Myocardial ischemia modifies conduction by depressing membrane excitability and promoting electrical uncoupling at gap junctions. Myocardial ischemia and infarction usually result in acute heart block. Progressive conduction disease due to stable ischemic heart disease may be seen in the context of ischemic or nonischemic cardiomyopathy and heart failure and may constitute an indication of cardiac pacing or resynchronization therapy.

Many other forms of *dilated cardiomyopathy* that may be seen at late stages of arrhythmogenic right ventricular cardiomyopathy, cardiac iron overload, hypertrophic cardiomyopathy, and LV noncompaction are associated with progressive conduction disease.[57] In most of these conditions, ventricular arrhythmias are the main concern.

Mitochondrial DNA deletions are also associated with AV conduction disorders, albeit through undefined mechanisms, in the context of *Kearns-Sayre syndrome* (chronic progressive external ophthalmoplegia and retinal degeneration with onset before age 20). Patients with Kearns-Sayre syndrome and conduction defects display an accelerated and unpredictable rate of progression to infra-Hisian AV block with a considerable associated mortality, and early pacemaker insertion is recommended in patients who develop initial signs of conduction disease, such as bifascicular block.[58]

Anderson-Fabry disease is a rare X-linked lysosomal storage disorder caused by mutations of the *GLA* gene that encodes α-galactosidase A, and this disorder results in intracellular accumulation of neutral glycosphingolipids. Neurological, gastrointestinal, renal, ophthalmological, and dermatological manifestations start in childhood and adolescence. Increasing age is associated with PR and QRS interval prolongation and left QRS axis deviation, and patients with QRS interval ≥110 ms should be monitored for bradyarrhythmias.[59]

Cardiac involvement is primarily encountered in immunoglobulin- and transthyretin-associated amyloidosis (i.e., *hereditary/familial and senile amyloidosis*).[60] Familial amyloidosis may be indolent and, especially in the rare form that presents with polyneuropathy, is associated with sinoatrial and AV progressive conduction abnormalities. Conduction disturbances are not related to the thickness of the intraventricular septum, indicating that the distribution and extent of infiltration into the heart by amyloid are heterogeneous and related to gender and age of onset. In patients with familial amyloid polyneuropathy and conduction disturbances, early prophylactic pacing should be considered.[61]

Cardiac involvement that emerges silently has been reported in all *mucopolysaccharidoses*, and conduction abnormalities are seen particularly with form VI (Maroteaux-Lamy) in which patients may survive to middle age.[62]

Hypoxia during *sleep apnea* has been associated with nocturnal paroxysmal asystole, bradyarrhythmias, and AV nodal block.[63] These patients should be treated with continuous positive airway pressure (CPAP) therapy, and in the absence of symptoms, pacing is not recommended (class III-B, by the ACC/AHA/HRS 2012 Guidelines for Device-Based Therapy of Cardiac Rhythm Abnormalities).

Other conditions such as myocarditis, endocarditis, electrolyte abnormalities, drug toxicity, cardiac valve or congenital surgery, heart transplantation, sleep apnea, transcatheter aortic valve implantation, and catheter ablation procedures may affect the conduction system and cause permanent or paroxysmal AV block. Usually, conduction system disease secondary to these processes does not have a delayed, progressive course.

Management

Patients with progressive conduction disease should be followed up and considered for permanent pacing according to standard indications. In addition, certain conditions such as muscular dystrophies and variants of LMNA may require early pacing, usually with an ICD, due to accelerated but unpredictable progression of conduction disease and malignant arrhythmias. Patients with WPW syndrome due to mutations in the gene *PRKAG2* may also require careful follow-up and early implantation of a pacemaker due to high incidence of complete AV block.

Genetic testing plays an important role in identifying patients at risk because young individuals presenting with a normal ECG may be at risk of arrhythmia and sudden death as they get older. Genetic testing may be considered as a part of the diagnostic evaluation for patients with either isolated cardiac conduction disease or conduction disease with concomitant congenital heart disease, especially when there is documentation of a positive family history of conduction disease. Mutation-specific genetic testing is recommended for family members and appropriate relatives following the identification of the cardiac conduction disease–causing mutation in an index case.

REFERENCES

1. Cheng S, Larson MG, Keyes MJ, et al. Relation of QRS width in healthy persons to risk of future permanent pacemaker implantation. *Am J Cardiol.* 2010;106:668–672.
2. Kawaguchi T, Hayashi H, Miyamoto A, et al. Prognostic implications of progressive cardiac conduction disease. *Circ J.* 2013;77:60–67.
3. Bozkaya YT, Aydin HH, Celik HA, et al. Increased myocardial collagen turnover in patients with progressive cardiac conduction disease. *Pacing Clin Electrophysiol.* 2008;31:1284–1290.
4. Munshi NV. Gene regulatory networks in cardiac conduction system development. *Circ Res.* 2012;110:1525–1537.
5. Baruteau AE, Probst V, Abriel H. Inherited progressive cardiac conduction disorders. *Curr Opin Cardiol.* 2015;30:33–39.
6. Eisen A, Arnson Y, Dovrish Z, Hadary R, Amital H. Arrhythmias and conduction defects in rheumatological diseases—a comprehensive review. *Semin Arthritis Rheum.* 2009;39:145–156.
7. Lee HC, Huang KT, Wang XL, Shen WK. Autoantibodies and cardiac arrhythmias. *Heart Rhythm.* 2011;8:1788–1795.
8. Hao X, Zhang Y, Zhang X, et al. TGF-β1-mediated fibrosis and ion channel remodeling are key mechanisms in producing the sinus node dysfunction associated with SCN5A deficiency and aging. *Circ Arrhythm Electrophysiol.* 2011;4:397–406.
9. Kanter RJ, Pfeiffer R, Hu D, et al. Brugada-like syndrome in infancy presenting with rapid ventricular tachycardia and intraventricular conduction delay. *Circulation.* 2012;125:14–22.
10. Olesen MS, Yuan L, Liang B, et al. High prevalence of long QT syndrome associated SCN5A variants in patients with early-onset lone atrial fibrillation. *Circ Cardiovasc Genet.* 2012;5:450–459.
11. Nakaya H. SCN5A mutations associated with overlap phenotype of long QT syndrome type 3 and Brugada syndrome. *Circ J.* 2014;78:1061–1062.
12. Hothi SS, Ara F, Timperley JP. Y1449C SCN5A mutation associated with overlap disorder comprising conduction disease, Brugada syndrome, and atrial flutter. *J Cardiovasc Electrophysiol.* 2015;26:93–97.
13. Laurent G, Saal S, Amarouch MY, et al. Multifocal ectopic Purkinje-related premature contractions: a new SCN5A-related cardiac channelopathy. *J Am Coll Cardiol.* 2012;60:144–156.
14. Bezzina CR, Barc J, Mizusawa Y, et al. Common variants at SCN5A-SCN10A and HEY2 are associated with Brugada syndrome, a rare disease with high risk of sudden cardiac death. *Nat Genet.* 2013;45:1044–1049.
15. Probst V, Kyndt F, Potet F, et al. Haploinsufficiency in combination with aging causes SCN5A-linked hereditary Lenègre disease. *J Am Coll Cardiol.* 2003;41:643–652.
16. Park JK, Martin LJ, Zhang X, Jegga AG, Benson DW. Genetic variants in SCN5A promoter are associated with arrhythmia phenotype severity in patients with heterozygous loss-of-function mutation. *Heart Rhythm.* 2012;9:1090–1096.
17. Meregalli PG, Tan HL, Probst V, et al. Type of SCN5A mutation determines clinical severity and degree of conduction slowing in loss-of-function sodium channelopathies. *Heart Rhythm.* 2009;6:341–348.
18. Brink PA, Ferreira A, Moolman JC, et al. Gene for progressive familial heart block type I maps to chromosome 19q13. *Circulation.* 1995;91:1633–1640.
19. Schott JJ, Alshinawi C, Kyndt F, et al. Cardiac conduction defects associate with mutations in SCN5A. *Nat Genet.* 1999;23:20–21.
20. Wang DW, Viswanathan PC, Balser JR, et al. Clinical, genetic, and biophysical characterization of SCN5A mutations associated with atrioventricular conduction block. *Circulation.* 2002;105:341–346.
21. Kruse M, Pongs O. TRPM4 channels in the cardiovascular system. *Curr Opin Pharmacol.* 2014;15:68–73.
22. Ackerman MJ, Priori SG, Willems S, et al. HRS/EHRA expert consensus statement on the state of genetic testing for the channelopathies and cardiomyopathies: this document was developed as a partnership between the Heart Rhythm Society (HRS) and the European Heart Rhythm Association (EHRA). *Heart Rhythm.* 2011;8:1308–1339.
23. Wu J, Zhang Y, Zhang X, Cheng L, et al. Altered sinoatrial node function and intra-atrial conduction in murine gain-of-function Scn5a+/ΔKPQ hearts suggest an overlap syndrome. *Am J Physiol Heart Circ Physiol.* 2012;302:H1510–H1523.
24. Nof E, Luria D, Brass D, et al. Point mutation in the HCN4 cardiac ion channel pore affecting synthesis, trafficking, and functional expression is associated with familial asymptomatic sinus bradycardia. *Circulation.* 2007;116:463–470.
25. Ishikawa T, Jou CJ, Nogami A, et al. Novel mutation in the α-myosin heavy chain gene is associated with sick sinus syndrome. *Circ Arrhythm Electrophysiol.* 2015;8:400–408.
26. Chambers JC, Zhao J, Terracciano CM, et al. Genetic variation in SCN10A influences cardiac conduction. *Nat Genet.* 2010;42:149–152.
27. Hu D, Barajas-Martinez H, Pfeiffer R, et al. Mutations in SCN10A are responsible for a large fraction of cases of Brugada syndrome. *J Am Coll Cardiol.* 2014;64:66–79.
28. van den Boogaard M, Smemo S, Burnicka-Turek O, et al. A common genetic variant within SCN10A modulates cardiac SCN5A expression. *J Clin Invest.* 2014;124:1844–1852.
29. Watanabe H, Koopmann TT, Le Scouarnec S, et al. Sodium channel beta1 subunit mutations associated with Brugada syndrome and cardiac conduction disease in humans. *J Clin Invest.* 2008;118:2260–2268.
30. Bevilacqua LM, Simon AM, Maguire CT, et al. A targeted disruption in connexin40 leads to distinct atrioventricular conduction defects. *J Interv Card Electrophysiol.* 2000;4:459–467.
31. Makita N, Seki A, Sumitomo N, et al. A connexin40 mutation associated with a malignant variant of progressive familial heart block type I. *Circ Arrhythm Electrophysiol.* 2012;5:163–172.
32. Zhang L, Benson DW, Tristani-Firouzi M, et al. Electrocardiographic features in Andersen-Tawil syndrome patients with KCNJ2 mutations: characteristic T-U-wave patterns predict the KCNJ2 genotype. *Circulation.* 2005;111:2720–2726.

33. Tan HL, van der Wal AC, Campian ME, et al. Nodo-ventricular accessory pathways in PRKAG2-dependent familial preexcitation syndrome reveal a disorder in cardiac development. *Circ Arrhythm Electrophysiol*. 2008;1:276–281.

34. Sternick EB, Oliva A, Gerken LM, et al. Clinical, electrocardiographic, and electrophysiologic characteristics of patients with a fasciculoventricular pathway: the role of PRKAG2 mutation. *Heart Rhythm*. 2011;8:58–64.

35. Lalani SR, Thakuria JV, Cox GF, et al. 20p12.3 Microdeletion predisposes to Wolff-Parkinson-White syndrome with variable neurocognitive deficits. *J Med Genet*. 2009;46:168–175.

36. Chowdhury R, Ashraf H, Melanson M, et al. A mouse model of human congenital heart disease: progressive atrioventricular block induced by a heterozygous Nkx2-5 homeodomain missense mutation. *Circ Arrhythm Electrophysiol*. 2015;8:1255–1264.

37. McElhinney DB, Geiger E, Blinder J, et al. NKX2.5 mutations in patients with congenital heart disease. *J Am Coll Cardiol*. 2003;42:1650–1655.

38. Marsman RF, Bardai A, Postma AV, et al. A complex double deletion in LMNA underlies progressive cardiac conduction disease, atrial arrhythmias, and sudden death. *Circ Cardiovasc Genet*. 2011;4:280–287.

39. van Rijsingen IA, Arbustini E, Elliott PM, et al. Risk factors for malignant ventricular arrhythmias in lamin a/c mutation carriers: a European cohort study. *J Am Coll Cardiol*. 2012;59:493–500.

40. Antoniades L, Eftychiou C, Kyriakides T, Christodoulou K, Katritsis DG. Malignant mutation in the lamin A/C gene causing progressive conduction system disease and early sudden death in a family with mild form of limb-girdle muscular dystrophy. *J Interv Card Electrophysiol*. 2007;19:1–7.

41. van Spaendonck-Zwarts K, van Hessem L, Jongbloed JD, et al. Desmin-related myopathy: a review and meta-analysis. *Clin Genet*. 2010;80:354–366.

42. Mahadevan MS, Yadava RS, Yu Q, et al. Reversible model of RNA toxicity and cardiac conduction defects in myotonic dystrophy. *Nat Genet*. 2006;38:1066–1070.

43. Wahbi K, Meune C, Porcher R, et al. Electrophysiological study with prophylactic pacing and survival in adults with myotonic dystrophy and conduction system disease. *JAMA*. 2012;307:1292–1301.

44. Bhakta D, Shen C, Kron J, et al. Pacemaker and implantable cardioverter-defibrillator use in a US myotonic dystrophy type 1 population. *J Cardiovasc Electrophysiol*. 2011;22:1369–1375.

45. Kandolin R, Lehtonen J, Kupari M. Cardiac sarcoidosis and giant cell myocarditis as causes of atrioventricular block in young and middle-aged adults. *Circ Arrhythm Electrophysiol*. 2011;4:303–309.

46. Yu JS, Cho EJ, Ji EH, et al. Rapidly progressive cardiac manifestation of Behçet's disease involving conduction system and aortic valve. *J Cardiovasc Ultrasound*. 2011;19:199–202.

47. Thonhofer R, Kriessmayr M, Thonhofer U, et al. Right bundle branch block induced by low-dose methotrexate in a patient with rheumatoid arthritis. *Scand J Rheumatol*. 2007;36:241–242.

48. Costedoat-Chalumeau N, Hulot JS, Amoura Z, et al. Heart conduction disorders related to antimalarials toxicity: an analysis of electrocardiograms in 85 patients treated with hydroxychloroquine for connective tissue diseases. *Rheumatology (Oxford)*. 2007;46:808–810.

49. Lazzerini PE, Capecchi PL, Laghi-Pasini F. Anti-Ro/SSA antibodies and cardiac arrhythmias in the adult: facts and hypotheses. *Scand J Immunol*. 2010;72:213–222.

50. Izmirly PM, Saxena A, Kim MY, et al. Maternal and fetal factors associated with mortality and morbidity in a multi-racial/ethnic registry of anti-SSA/Ro-associated cardiac neonatal lupus. *Circulation*. 2011;124:1927–1935.

51. Marin-Neto JA, Cunha-Neto E, Maciel BC, Simões MV. Pathogenesis of chronic Chagas heart disease. *Circulation*. 2007;115:1109–1123.

52. Morillo CA, Marin-Neto JA, Avezum A, et al. BENEFIT Investigators. Randomized Trial of Benznidazole for Chronic Chagas' Cardiomyopathy. *N Engl J Med*. 2015;373:1295–1306.

53. Stanek G, Wormser GP, Gray J, Strle F. Lyme borreliosis. *Lancet*. 2012;379:461–473.

54. Dubrey SW, Mehta PA, O'Connell S. Lyme disease and the heart in the UK. *Br J Hosp Med (Lond)*. 2011;72:621–622, 624–625.

55. Rajamannan NM, Evans FJ, Aikawa E, et al. Calcific aortic valve disease: not simply a degenerative process: A review and agenda for research from the National Heart and Lung and Blood Institute Aortic Stenosis Working Group. Executive summary: Calcific aortic valve disease-2011 update. *Circulation*. 2011;124:1783–1791.

56. Probst V, Le Scouarnec S, Legendre A, et al. Familial aggregation of calcific aortic valve stenosis in the western part of France. *Circulation*. 2006;113:856–860.

57. Lakdawala NK, Givertz MM. Dilated cardiomyopathy with conduction disease and arrhythmia. *Circulation*. 2010;122:527–534.

58. Kabunga P, Lau AK, Phan K, et al. Systematic review of cardiac electrical disease in Kearns-Sayre syndrome and mitochondrial cytopathy. *Int J Cardiol*. 2015;181:303–310.

59. O'Mahony C, Coats C, Cardona M, et al. Incidence and predictors of anti-bradycardia pacing in patients with Anderson-Fabry disease. *Europace*. 2011;13:1781–1788.

60. Kapoor P, Thenappan T, Singh E, et al. Cardiac amyloidosis: a practical approach to diagnosis and management. *Am J Med*. 2011;124:1006–1015.

61. Algalarrondo V, Dinanian S, Juin C, et al. Prophylactic pacemaker implantation in familial amyloid polyneuropathy. *Heart Rhythm*. 2012;9:1069–1075.

62. Braunlin EA, Harmatz PR, Scarpa M, et al. Cardiac disease in patients with mucopolysaccharidosis: presentation, diagnosis and management. *J Inherit Metab Dis*. 2011;34:1183–1197.

63. Jaffe LM, Kjekshus J, Gottlieb SS. Importance and management of chronic sleep apnoea in cardiology. *Eur Heart J*. 2013;34:809–815.

106 Atrioventricular Block

Roy M. John

The atrioventricular (AV) node is the only connection between the atria and ventricles in the normal heart. It modulates the AV conduction to provide enough delay between atrial and ventricular conduction to allow for ventricular filling. In addition, its decremental conduction properties limit ventricular rates during atrial arrhythmias, such as atrial flutter and fibrillation (AFL and AF, respectively). The AV node also has the capability to serve as a subsidiary pacemaker.

AV conduction is dependent on distinct types of myocardial tissue and includes atrial inputs into the AV node, the various components of the AV node, and the His–Purkinje conduction system. Disorders of AV conduction may be due to defects in impulse transmission at any of these levels with varying prognostic and therapeutic implications. In general, conduction disturbances above the His bundle are seldom life threatening, and the presence of symptoms is the predominant driver for therapeutic intervention with cardiac pacing. Intermittent or persistent conduction block at or below the His bundle has graver consequences and generally warrants permanent pacing.

AV block may be reversible and recognition of temporary causes of AV block is critical to avoid long-term commitment to cardiac pacing. In a quarter of patients who present with heart block before the age of 50, genetic or inflammatory conditions may be present.[1] Assessment for the associated cardiomyopathy and risk of sudden cardiac death, which require the consideration of additional therapies such as the use of an implantable cardioverter defibrillator (ICD), is essential.

Types and Levels

On the basis of electrocardiogram (ECG) characteristics, AV block is classified as first-, second-, and third-degree AV block. Anatomically, block can occur at various levels in the AV conduction system; above the His bundle (supra-His), within the His bundle (intra-His), and below the His bundle within the bundle branches (infra-His).

First-degree AV block is defined as abnormal prolongation of the PR interval to greater than 200 ms and is commonly due to a delay in the AV node irrespective of the QRS width. Intracardiac recordings show an AH interval greater than 130 ms in the presence of a normal HV interval. Occasionally, a transition of AV nodal conduction from a fast to slow AV nodal pathway can manifest as first-degree AV block. Less commonly, first-degree AV block can also occur at or below the His bundle; in such cases the HV interval is prolonged beyond 55 ms (or 65 ms in the presence of left bundle branch block [LBBB]). First-degree AV block with a relatively narrow QRS due to His–Purkinje conduction delay is

not an uncommon finding in cardiac amyloidosis, where diffuse amyloid infiltration into the myocardium can delay conduction equally in both right and left bundles (Fig. 106.1).[2]

Type I second-degree heart block on ECG refers to progressive PR prolongation before a nonconducted beat and a shorter PR interval for the next conducted beat (Fig. 106.2). This is the classical Wenckebach-type AV block, usually in conjunction with narrow QRS complexes, implying a more proximal level of block, usually in the AV node. Less commonly, Wenckebach-type AV block can also occur in a diseased His–Purkinje system. Intra-His Wenckebach phenomenon is manifested as a prolonged His electrogram (>30 ms) with splitting and progressive prolongation of the split before block (Fig. 106.3). Unlike Wenckebach block at the AV nodal level, intra-His AV block tends to worsen with exercise or with atropine. Rarely, Wenckebach block can be demonstrated below the His bundle, with progressive delay in the HV interval and with block and resumption of conduction with the shorter HV interval.

Type II second-degree heart block (Mobitz type II block) is characterized by fixed PR intervals before and after blocked beats (see Fig. 106.2). It is usually associated with a wider QRS complex, indicating distal levels of block in the conduction system with progression to complete AV block. Type II block cannot be diagnosed if the PR interval following a pause is shorter than the PR immediately preceding the nonconducted P wave. The PP interval remains constant, and the pause incorporating the nonconducted P wave is twice the PP interval. True Mobitz type II block is rare with normal QRS complexes, and atypical Wenckebach should be considered. This is particularly true during sleep when sinus slowing precedes nonconducted P waves due to vagotonia. When Mobitz type II block occurs in conjunction with a narrow QRS, the block is usually within the His bundle.

AV conduction in a 2:1 pattern can be due to proximal or distal block. Differentiation between proximal and distal levels of block can be difficult. In general, a narrow QRS implies block at the AV nodal level, whereas a wide QRS makes it more likely to be below the AV node. Fixed 2:1 AV block with a constant normal or relatively short PR interval suggests infranodal block, whereas a prolonged PR (>300 ms) or a preceding Wenckebach-type AV conduction implies block at the level of the AV node. Atropine and exercise tend to improve AV nodal block.

Advanced second-degree block (or "high-grade" AV block) refers to two or more nonconducted sinus P waves but with resumption of normal AV conduction in between. It is important to exclude retrograde invasion into the AV conduction system by ventricular or junctional beats. In the setting of AF or AFL, a prolonged pause (e.g., greater than 5 s) is often due to advanced second-degree AV block.

Third-degree AV block is defined as the complete absence of AV conduction, with P waves dissociated from the QRS. The atrial rate is always faster than the ventricular. In the case of AF, complete AV block is manifested as a regularized slow ventricular rate.

Functional Delay of Atrioventricular Conduction

Premature atrial contractions (PACs) that occur early, so as to find the AV node refractory, can simulate 2:1 AV block (Fig. 106.4).

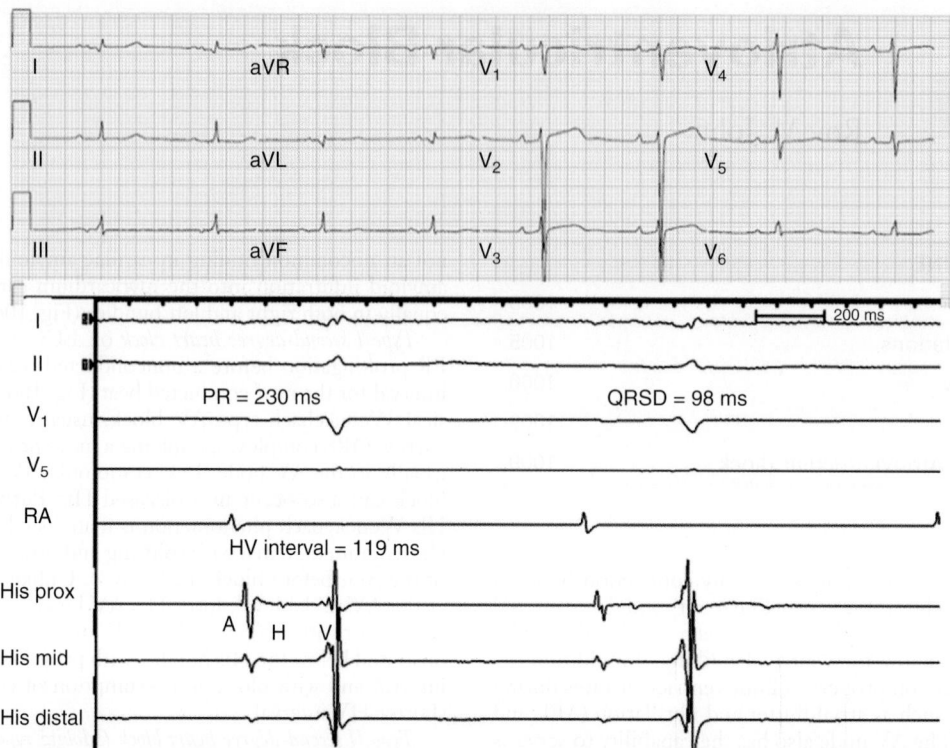

FIGURE 106.1 12-lead electrocardiogram (*top*) and intracardiac recordings (*bottom*) in a patient with senile cardiac amyloidosis. There is first-degree atrioventricular block with narrow QRS complexes. The first-degree atrioventricular block is due to prolongation of the HV interval to 119 ms. *RA*, Right atrium.

Mobitz type I block (Wenckebach)

A-A	800	800	800	800	800	800	
Atrium							
	20	20	20	20	20	20	
AV node	140	260 (+120)	340 (+80)	380 (+40)			
His	15	15	15	15			
Ventricle							
	25	25	25	25			
V-V	800	920	880	840	1360		
P-R	200	200	320	400	440		200

A

Mobitz type II block

A-A	800	800	800	800	800	800	
Atrium							
	20	20	20	20	20	20	
AV node	140	140	140	140	140		
His	35	35	35	35			
Ventricle							
	45	45	45	45			
V-V	800	800	800	800	1600		
P-R	240	240	240	240	240		240

B

FIGURE 106.2 Ladder diagram demonstrating type I and type II second-degree atrioventricular (*AV*) block in Mobitz type I or Wenckebach block (A); progressive delay of the atrial impulse occurs in the AV node proximal to the His bundle. The greatest increment occurs in the second beat (+120 ms) and becomes less in subsequent beats (+80 ms and +40 ms), leading to gradual shortening of the RR interval (920 ms–880 ms–840 ms). The pause measures less than the sum of two PP intervals (1360 ms). Mobitz type II AV block (B) is not preceded by PR interval lengthening, and the pause equals two PP intervals. The site of block is usually distal to the AV node. Activation times in the diagrams are given in milliseconds (ms); *double bars* indicate conduction block. *A*, Atrium; *V*, ventricle.

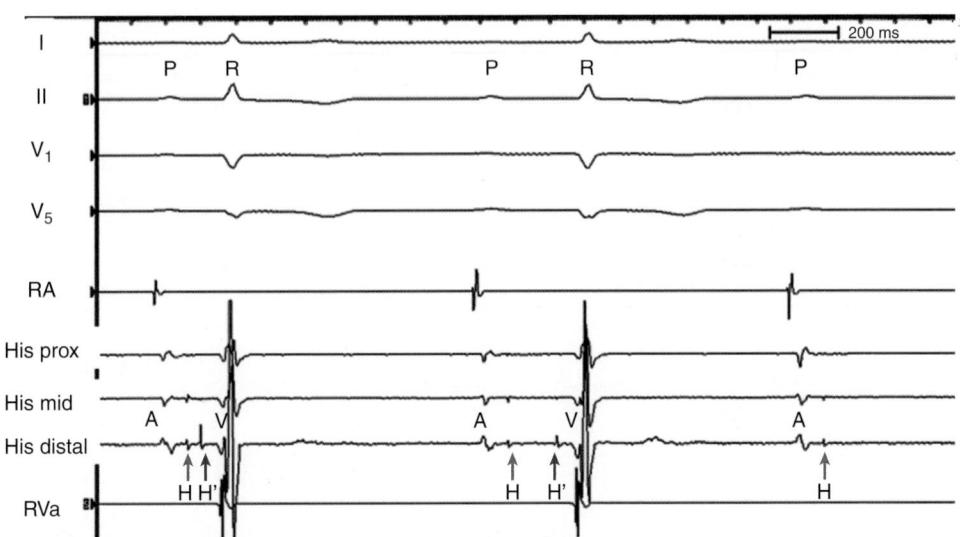

FIGURE 106.3 Intracardiac recording showing Wenckebach atrioventricular block at the level of the His bundle in a patient with exertional dyspnea. There is progressive PR prolongation before nonconduction of the third P wave. His bundle recordings show splitting of the His (H and H′). There is widening of the split with intra-His block accounting for the nonconducted beat. *RA*, Right atrium; *RVa*, right ventricular apex.

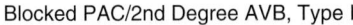
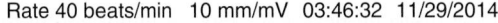

Blocked PAC/2nd Degree AVB, Type I   Rate 40 beats/min   10 mm/mV 03:46:32 11/29/2014

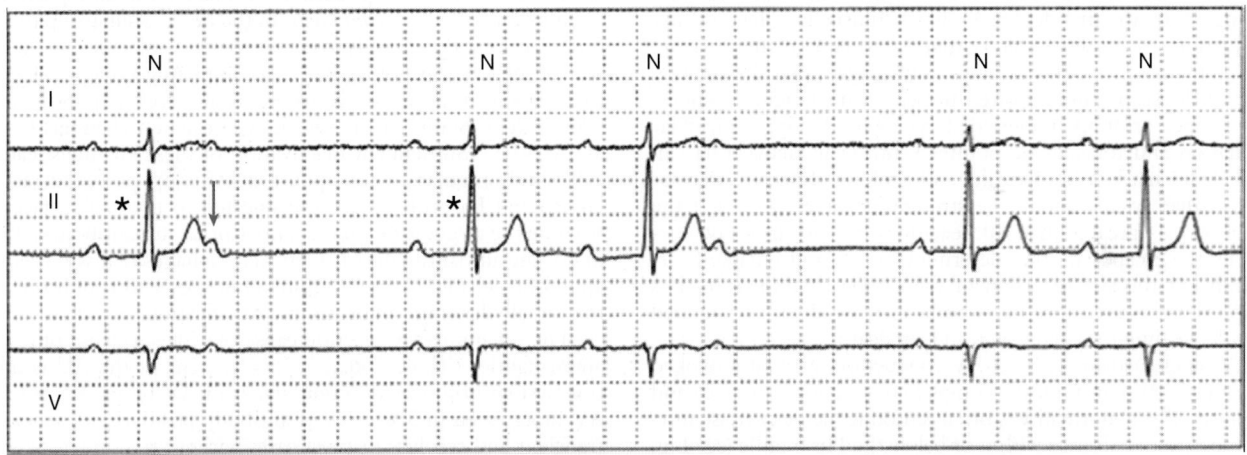

FIGURE 106.4 Blocked atrial extrasystole simulating Mobitz type II atrioventricular block (*AVB*). The second P wave is premature (*arrow*) and fails to conduct to the ventricle. The PR interval in the beats before and after the atrial ectopic is identical (*asterisk*). If the prematurity of the blocked beat is not recognized, this sequence could be misinterpreted as Mobitz type II block. *PAC*, Premature atrial contraction.

These nonconducted P waves are distinguished by their prematurity and a morphology that is likely to be different from sinus P waves. Occasionally, they are buried within a T wave, making this distinction difficult. Concealed junctional ectopics arising from the His bundle that fail to conduct to the atria or ventricles and invade the AV node to induce refractoriness to the subsequent sinus beat can mimic Mobitz type II block.[3] Differentiation can be difficult and often requires an electrophysiological study, unless obvious junctional extrasystoles are evident elsewhere on the patient's ECGs. In patients with first-degree or type 1 second-degree block due to AV nodal disease, occurrence of atrial fibrillation may paradoxically cause slow heart rate due to concealment into the AV node. With restoration of sinus mechanism, heart rate usually improves due to restoration of 1:1 AV conduction.

Marked prolongation of the QT interval can lead to a pseudo 2:1 AV block when the sinus interbeat intervals are shorter than the ventricular refractory period (Fig. 106.5).

Clinical Manifestations

There is considerable variation in the symptomatic manifestation of AV block, ranging from an asymptomatic status to syncope and sudden death. First-degree AV block and asymptomatic type I second-degree AV block are, in general, benign and infrequently associated with symptoms. However, rarely, first-degree block with marked PR prolongation can potentially cause atrial systole to occur in close proximity to the preceding ventricular systole and give rise to symptoms similar to a pacemaker syndrome.[4] Prolongation of the PR interval is particularly important in patients with left ventricular (LV) dysfunction when marked PR prolongation in excess of 250–300 ms can lead to impaired LV filling, increased pulmonary capillary wedge pressure, and decreased cardiac output.[5] Similar consequences can ensue with type I second-degree AV block even in the absence of symptoms related to bradycardia.

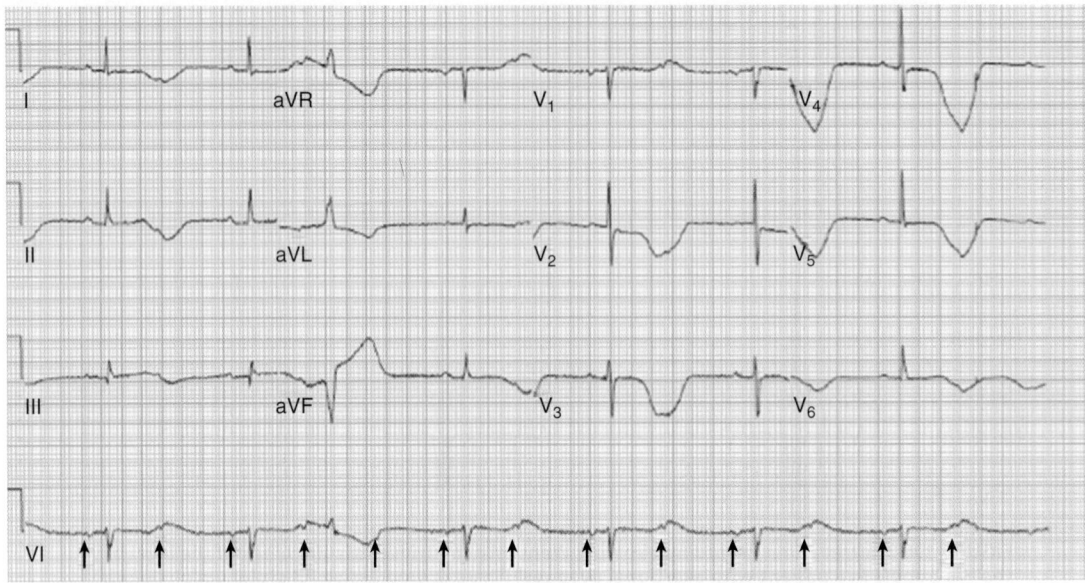

FIGURE 106.5 Marked drug-induced QT prolongation associated with 2:1 atrioventricular response due to the sinus rhythm intervals being shorter than the refractory period of the ventricle. There is one ventricular response for two P waves (P waves denoted by *arrows*) except the fourth P wave that depolarizes the ventricle with aberration.

Type II second-degree AV block is important for its high rate of progression to third-degree AV block. It usually reflects diffuse conduction system disease and often warrants permanent pacing even in the absence of symptoms. Third-degree AV block with a wide QRS escape rhythm often presents with fatigue, dyspnea, presyncope, or frank unheralded syncope. Rarely, ventricular fibrillation and torsades de pointes ventricular tachycardia can result from marked bradycardia and prolonged pauses. Permanent cardiac pacing should be strongly considered even if the escape rate is greater than 40 beats/min because it is not necessarily the escape rate that determines a safe and reliable heart rhythm but the site of origin of the escape rhythm. Infra-His escape rhythms are more likely to be associated with prolonged asystole, leading to syncope and sudden death.

AV block, usually with 2:1 AV conduction, may be provoked by exercise. Patients typically complain of exertional dyspnea and dizziness. The abnormality is often reproducible by exercise testing and is due to disease within or below the His bundle (see Fig. 106.3). It is rarely due to ischemia or disease in the AV node. Permanent pacing is remarkably effective for symptom relief.

Pathophysiology

Congenital Atrioventricular Block

A modern definition of congenital AV block (CAVB) requires its diagnosis in utero or during the first month of life.[6] About one-third of cases have concomitant complex structural heart defects (i.e., congenitally corrected transposition of the great arteries or left isomerism). Two-thirds of cases have no or only minor structural defects.

Isolated complete CAVB is associated in approximately 90% of cases with the presence of maternal autoantibodies against intracellular ribonucleoproteins SS-A/Ro (especially Ro52) and SS-B/La. AV block diagnosed later in life (>1 month) is less commonly associated with maternal autoantibodies.[7,8] Autoantibodies are frequently found in mothers with overt autoimmune disease, as well as in apparently healthy mothers (although less frequently). The exact mechanism by which commonly found autoantibodies can cause a rare disease such as CAVB is not yet fully elucidated. Fig. 106.6 depicts a recent pathophysiological model from Ambrosi and Wahren-Herlenius.[6] Maternal autoantibodies cross the placenta and are deposited in various fetal tissues, producing a syndrome called *neonatal lupus*. In the heart, a subgroup of antibodies against Ro52 binds to cross-reactive molecules on the surface of the fetal cardiomyocytes. Accumulating evidence suggests that among these cross-reactive molecules are the pore-forming protein α_1-subunits of the two L-type calcium channels Cav1.2 and Cav1.3.[9] Subsequent inactivation of these channels leads to calcium dysregulation and apoptosis. After apoptosis, intracellular Ro and La proteins are translocated to the cell surface and become the target for maternal anti-Ro/La autoantibodies. Binding of the autoantibodies attracts macrophages that will clear the apoptotic cells and secrete proinflammatory and profibrotic factors, finally leading to fibrosis and calcification.[9,10]

The inflammatory reaction causes a wide spectrum of cardiac abnormalities (Table 106.1).[11] Involvement of the AV conduction system produces different stages of AV block. First-degree AV block, seen in 3%–25% of antibody-positive pregnancies, is transient and resolves in most cases without treatment. Second-degree AV block reverses only very rarely, whereas complete AV block is always irreversible.[12] The level of block in most cases of isolated AV block tends to be at the AV node.

Acquired Atrioventricular Block

Progressive Cardiac Conduction Disease

Primary degenerative disease of the conduction system or Lev-Lenègre disease accounts for approximately 50% of cases of acquired AV block. Although Lev and Lenègre described sclerotic changes principally affecting the conduction system, the initiating and underlying processes in the disease may be multifactorial. Some may have chronic ischemia or autoimmune processes, and several patients may have a genetic basis (see Chapter 105). The disease usually progresses through bundle branch blocks eventually to complete AV block that is symptomatic.

Although the term *progressive cardiac conduction disease* (PCCD) has been used to encompass all forms of progressive conduction disease, recent consensus recommended its use in the presence of unexplained progressive conduction abnormalities in young patients (aged <50 years) with normal hearts and no skeletal myopathies.[13] Early onset PCCD with a family history of pacemakers or sudden death merits the consideration of genetic

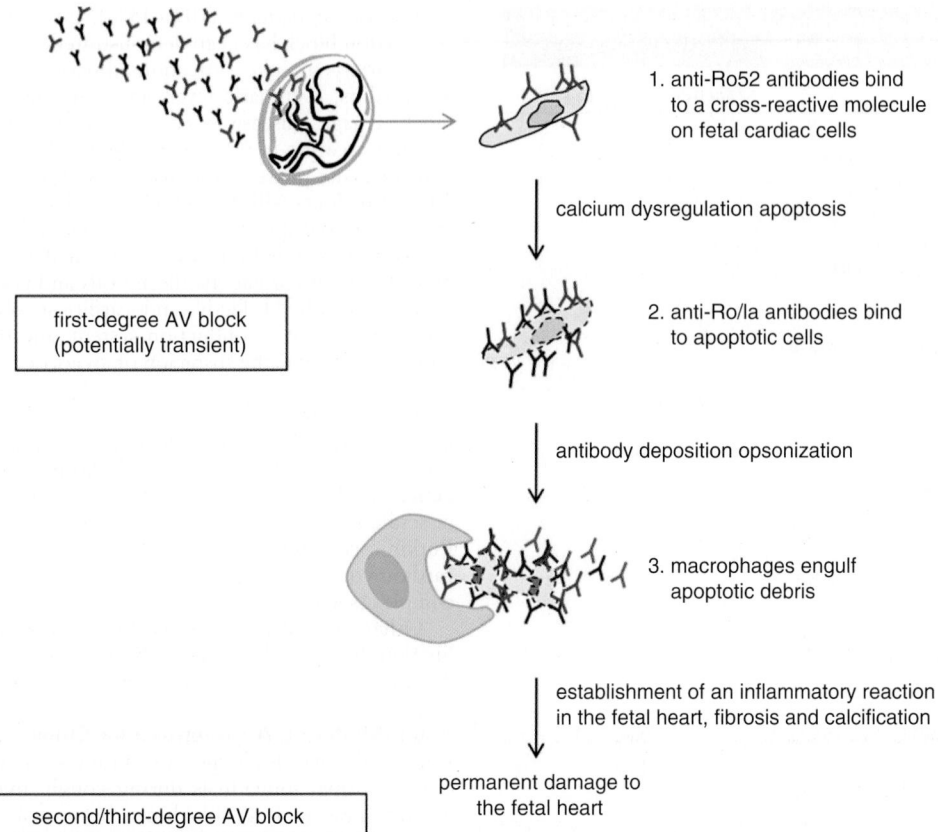

1. anti-Ro52 antibodies bind
to a cross-reactive molecule
on fetal cardiac cells

calcium dysregulation apoptosis

first-degree AV block
(potentially transient)

2. anti-Ro/la antibodies bind
to apoptotic cells

antibody deposition opsonization

3. macrophages engulf
apoptotic debris

establishment of an inflammatory reaction
in the fetal heart, fibrosis and calcification

second/third-degree AV block

permanent damage to
the fetal heart

FIGURE 106.6 Pathophysiological model for the development of congenital atrioventricular (*AV*) block. (From Ambrosi A, Wahren-Herlenius M. Congenital heart block: evidence for a pathogenic role of maternal autoantibodies. *Arthritis Res Ther.* 2012;14:208-218.)

testing.[13] Mutations in the *SCN5A* gene cause the majority of familial PCCD and may have a common phenotype with Brugada syndrome.[13–15] Mutations in *TRPM4*, a Ca^{2+}-activated channel gene, is estimated to account for 25% of inherited forms of right bundle branch block (RBBB) and 10% of inherited AV block.[16]

PCCD may precede the development of overt ventricular dysfunction in the genetic cardiomyopathies. Recognition of these cardiomyopathies is critical to determine the associated risk of sudden tachyarrhythmia–related death. A typical example is mutations in the *LMNA* gene encoding Lamin A/C.[17] These mutations are highly penetrant, with most carriers demonstrating some evidence of cardiac involvement by 65 years of age. Initial manifestations may be first-degree AV block with gradual progression to compete heart block. Associated atrial arrhythmias are common. Cardiomyopathy usually follows the development of conduction system disease by several years, and risk of ventricular arrhythmias is highest when significant systolic dysfunction is present.[17] The risk of sudden death is also more frequent in the PCCD patients who carry loss-of-function *SCN5A* mutations.[18]

Several of the genetic muscular dystrophies are associated with PCCD and are discussed in Chapter 100. Sclerodegenerative processes that do not begin in the conduction system can secondarily affect the conduction system. Extension of aortic and, less commonly, mitral annular calcification has been shown to produce AV block.

Ischemic Heart Disease

In the postthrombolytic era, AV block in relation to an acute ST-segment elevation myocardial infarction (MI) occurs in approximately 7% of patients.[19] Lesser degrees of AV block that manifest as first-degree or type I second-degree AV block are more common following inferior MI. Vagotonia is the common mechanism and is associated with other signs of vagal stimulation, such as sinus bradycardia, and prompt response to atropine and catecholamine stimulation. Wenckebach block that appears late following an inferior MI may not respond to atropine and may relate to ischemia of the AV nodal tissue or local release of adenosine. The block is usually at the level of the AV node and resolves spontaneously; in the current era of revascularization, temporary pacing is rarely necessary.

High-grade AV block complicating an anterior wall infarction is due to ischemia or infarction of the His–Purkinje system. The transition from the first nonconducted P wave to high-grade AV block is often abrupt, and the resulting escape rhythm is typically slow and unreliable. Conducted beats usually have a wide QRS complex. In general, an interruption of the blood supply to the anterior wall and the interventricular septum severe enough to cause AV block usually causes severe LV dysfunction and results in high mortality. Emergency temporary pacing and prophylactic pacing are indicated, although survival may not be significantly improved because of associated extensive myocardial damage.

New bundle branch block is three times more likely during anterior infarction than during inferior infarction because the left anterior descending coronary artery provides the major blood supply to the His bundle and the bundle branches. New bundle branch block reflects extensive myocardial damage and is associated with a four-fold increase in risk of progression to high-grade AV block (an increase from 4% to 18%).[20] Both in-hospital and out-of-hospital mortality are higher for patients presenting with bundle branch block during acute infarction. Development of RBBB tends to carry a worse prognosis than LBBB.[20]

TABLE 106.1   Spectrum of cardiac abnormalities in neonatal lupus and associated mortality rates

CARDIAC DEFECT	MORTALITY RATE
Electrophysiological	
Children with isolated congenital AV block	4%–6%
Infants with isolated congenital AV block	4%–8%
Adults with isolated congenital AV block who were previously asymptomatic	5%
First-, second-, and third-degree AV block	
Atrial and ventricular ectopic beats	
Atrial flutter	
Ventricular and junctional ectopic tachycardia	
Sinus node dysfunction	
Long QT interval	
Myocardial/Functional	80%
Myocarditis	
Cardiomyopathy	
Can develop before birth, after infancy, or in adults	
Can occur with or without conduction abnormalities	
Endocardial fibroelastosis	
Pericarditis/pericardial effusion	
Structural	
Infants with congenital AV block and structural disease	29%
Children with congenital AV block and structural disease	10%
Semilunar and AV valve dysplasia, stenosis, and regurgitation	
Patent ductus arteriosus	
Atrial septal defects	
Ventricular septal defects	

AV, Atrioventricular.
From Capone C, Buyon JP, Friedman DM, Frishman WH. Cardiac manifestations of neonatal lupus: a review of antibody associated congenital heart block and its impact in an adult population. *Cardiol Rev.* 2012;20:72-76 and Hornberger LK, Al Rajaa N. Spectrum of cardiac involvement in neonatal lupus. *Scand J Immunol.* 2010;72:189-197.

Occasionally, chronic ischemia to the AV node can result in AV block. Heart block is known to occur in conjunction with angina and acute coronary spasm.

Inflammatory and Infectious Diseases

Sarcoidosis is a relatively common disorder characterized by formation of noncaseating granulomas in various organs, including the myocardium. Cardiac involvement is common in autopsy studies but infrequently recognized clinically.[21] Approximately 5% will have cardiac-predominant disease without evidence for other organ involvement. Granulomas typically involve the basal septum, resulting in conduction disease. Although heart block is a common cardiac presentation, the risk of ventricular arrhythmia is high, and if the diagnosis of sarcoidosis is suggested by imaging or biopsy, it is common to consider an ICD.[21]

Several collagen vascular diseases have been recognized to cause conduction system disease that includes heart block. Fibrosis of the conduction system has been demonstrated, particularly in Wegener's granulomatosis and systemic sclerosis.[22]

Heart block is a common manifestation of carditis associated with Lyme disease; one-third of patients may need temporary pacing. Typically, AV conduction abnormalities reverse within 1–6 weeks following appropriate antibiotic treatment. The most common site of involvement is the AV node, but in a small proportion of patients (10%–15%), intra-His or His–Purkinje conduction block has been demonstrated.[23]

A variety of other infectious diseases, including acute viral myocarditis, rheumatic fever, and tuberculosis, can cause heart block. Chagas disease, a chronic inflammatory disease that is endemic to areas in Central and South America, is important in that the acute phase of the disease often goes unrecognized, but 20% of patients will develop chronic disease later (10–20 years) after the initial infection. Cardiac conduction system disease in the form of bundle branch block, fascicular block, and AV block precedes other cardiac manifestations and is associated with risk of sudden death.[24] Infective endocarditis involving the aortic root can invade the AV conduction system, and the presence of AV block should raise the suspicion of an aortic root abscess.

Infiltrative Processes

Cardiac amyloidosis results in deposition of extracellular amyloid proteins (light chains, in AL amyloidosis, or transthyretin). Evidence for His–Purkinje conduction delay is particularly common in senile amyloidosis and tends to progress to heart block. His–Purkinje conduction times are prolonged in advanced amyloid cardiomyopathy despite the presence of a relatively narrow QRS complex (see Fig. 106.1).[2,25]

Other infiltrative cardiomyopathies associated with AV conduction block include hemochromatosis, lymphomas, Fabry's disease, and glycogen storage diseases (Danon disease).

Vagal-Mediated Atrioventricular Block

Enhanced vagal discharge can cause transient AV block in otherwise normal individuals during cough, micturition, or swallowing. Transient AV block can be provoked by carotid sinus massage and in individuals with hypersensitive carotid sinus and neurocardiogenic syncope. The AV block is typically paroxysmal, at the level of the AV node, and benign. Type 1 second-degree AV block may be seen in athletes due to hypervagotonia and resolves after physical deconditioning.

A distinct form of paroxysmal AV block associated with syncope has been described in patients without structural heart disease or evidence for conduction disturbance on ECG.[26] Patients present with abrupt syncope associated with abrupt onset of high-grade AV block and prolonged asystole, with recovery of normal AV conduction soon afterward. Electrophysiological studies do not indicate the presence of His–Purkinje disease.[26] The majority tends to have an exaggerated response to intravenous adenosine, raising the possibility of a variant of reflex syncope, as discussed in the following text. However, the classical sinus slowing prior to onset of AV block that is typical of vagally mediated AV block is usually absent in this group of patients. Pacemaker implantation is highly effective for relief of symptoms.

Iatrogenic Atrioventricular Block

Drug-induced AV block might not always resolve after discontinuation of the potentially offending drug. In one series, approximately half of patients who developed heart block in the context of therapy with an AV nodal blocking agent required permanent pacing for persistent or recurrent AV block.[27] Cessation of digoxin therapy has the best chance of recovery of AV nodal conduction, whereas β-adrenergic blocker therapy often unmasks underlying conduction disease.

Approximately 3%–5% of patients will develop persistent bradyarrhythmias after open-heart surgery, with a higher incidence following repeat surgery. In adults, persistent AV block is most common after valvular surgery, particularly tricuspid valve replacement. Risk is higher with multivalvular surgery.[28] In one large retrospective study, preexisting RBBB was more predictive than LBBB, but preoperative PR prolongation, repeat surgery, and age above 70 years were all predictors for the need for permanent pacing.[28] In patients with congenital heart disease, postoperative heart block complicates 1%–3% of corrective surgeries, the risk being greatest for repair of ventricular septal defects.[29] Because the majority of patients who develop bradyarrhythmias following cardiac surgery recover, it is customary to wait 7–10 days before consideration of permanent pacing. Patients who ultimately undergo permanent cardiac pacing tend to have a good prognosis. More than 65% of patients who undergo pacing for AV block remain dependent on pacing in the longer term.[30,31]

Transcatheter aortic valve replacement (TAVR) is rapidly evolving as an effective alternative to valve surgery for nonsurgical patients with aortic stenosis. Unlike in the surgical procedure where the valve is excised prior to replacement, the calcified valve remains in situ in TAVR. Transcatheter placement of a valve prosthesis and balloon dilatation within this calcified valve produce a mass effect in the region of the membranous septum and adjoining conduction system. This potential mechanism leads to persistent heart block requiring cardiac pacing in 15%–20% of patients.[32–33] New LBBB occurs in 5%–6% of patients but does not necessarily progress to heart block.[34] One-third of new AV block cases may be related to acute balloon dilatation during the procedure and may recover during the first 24 hours. A QRS duration less than 120 ms was predictive of recovery.[35] The risk of persistent AV block appears to be specific to the type of prosthetic valve used (27%–33% with the CoreValve system and 4%–12% with the Edwards SAPIEN valve). The incidence of persistent AV block is lower when close attention is paid to the optimal placement of the CoreValve relative to the native annulus.[36] Preexisting RBBB and oversized valve prosthesis for the native annulus are other risk factors for persisting AV block.

Rarely, heart block may occur late after mediastinal radiation therapy for Hodgkin's disease. Diffuse fibrotic changes and vascular compromise to the conduction tissue has been described in autopsy studies in such patients.[37]

Prognosis

The prognosis of AV block depends on the level of AV block and associated structural heart disease. First-degree AV block carries a good prognosis. In the absence of symptoms, even the presence of bifascicular block associated with first-degree AV block has a low rate of progression to third-degree AV block. Similarly, type I second-degree AV block is a benign condition. However, when it is associated with a wide QRS, bifascicular block, or worsens with exercise (see Fig. 106.3), there is a possibility that the level of block may be more distal with a higher risk of complete AV block. True Mobitz type II block is often associated with symptoms and, in conjunction with a wide QRS, has a high risk of progression to complete AV block. Symptomatic complete AV block has a poor prognosis without cardiac pacing. Wide complex escape rhythms associated with complete AV block are commonly unstable, resulting in prolonged asystole with a risk of syncope and sudden death. After successful pacing, the prognosis of these patients is dependent on the underlying structural heart disease. In cases of idiopathic fibrotic conduction system disease without other cardiac abnormalities, the prognosis is usually good.

The management of complete CAVB has changed significantly in recent years on the basis of the recognition that Stokes-Adams attacks and heart failure may develop at any age and that there is a risk of sudden cardiac death. In canine models of chronic complete AV block, ventricular remodeling that occurs over time increased susceptibility to torsades de pointes VT due to downregulation of cardiac rapidly and slowly activating delayed rectifier potassium currents (I_{Kr} and I_{Ks}, respectively).[38] Unnecessary delay of pacemaker implantation in patients with high-risk features should be avoided.[29] In the present era, more than 90% of patients below age 15 years with congenital heart block (CHB) undergo permanent pacemaker implantation.[39] Syncope, presyncope, heart failure, or exercise limitation due to chronotropic incompetence indicate the need for cardiac pacing. In asymptomatic patients, the risk of syncope or sudden death is predicted by the presence of a wide QRS, marked bradycardia with pauses greater than three times the cycle length of the escape rhythm, prolonged QT interval, presence of LV dilation or dysfunction, or complex ectopy.[29,39] A subset of patients (6%–11%) paced for isolated complete CAVB develop dilated cardiomyopathy, the risk being higher for the antibody-mediated CHB.[40] Cardiac resynchronization therapy improves LV function in these patients.[41]

Management of Atrioventricular Block

Cardiac pacing is the mainstay of treatment for symptomatic, persistent AV block. Pharmacological therapy with atropine (for block at the level of the AV node) or isoproterenol may be helpful in increasing heart rate pending pacing. Transcutaneous or temporary transvenous pacing is necessary in the event of hemodynamically important bradycardia. The most important consideration in the decision to proceed to permanent cardiac pacing is whether the AV block is reversible. Permanent pacemakers are generally a lifetime commitment with need for periodic generator replacements and risk of infection and hardware malfunction. These morbidities associated with long-term permanent pacing are particularly pertinent to the younger patients. Withdrawal of offending drugs, correction of electrolyte and metabolic abnormalities, treatment of inflammatory conditions, and correction of ischemia are essential prior to consideration of permanent pacemaker implant. Indications and appropriate choice of pacing modalities are discussed in Chapter 119.

The recognition of progressive cardiomyopathy resulting from ventricular dyssynchrony created by right ventricular pacing has raised interest in alternative pacing sites and cardiac resynchronization with biventricular pacing. Biventricular pacing is well established, but implantation is associated with more complications. His bundle pacing has shown early promise in maintaining normal ventricular activation.[42] Direct His bundle pacing can normalize QRS duration in some patients and is an alternative to biventricular pacing.[43]

Acknowledgment

The author would like to acknowledge Drs. A. Christian Blank, Peter Loh, and Marc A. Vos for their contribution of this chapter in the previous (sixth) edition of this book.

REFERENCES

1. Kandolin R, Lehtonen J, Kupari M. Cardiac sarcoidosis and giant cell myocarditis as cause of atrio-ventricular block in young and middle aged adults. *Circ Arrhythm Electrophysiol.* 2011;4:303–309.
2. Barbhaiya CR, Kumar S, Baldinger SH, et al. Electrophysiologic assessment of conduction abnormalities and atrial arrhythmias associated with amyloid cardiomyopathy. *Heart Rhythm.* 2016;13:383–390.
3. Kasaoka Y, Ajiki K, Hayami N, Murakawa Y. His bundle parasystole masquerading as exercise-induced 2:1 atrio-ventricular block. *J Cardiovasc Electrophysiol.* 2001;12:965–967.
4. Laurent G, Eicher J, Wolf J. First degree atrioventricular block and pseudopacemaker syndrome. *Arch Cardiovasc Dis.* 2013;106:690–693.
5. Kutyifa V, Stockburger M, Daubert JP, et al. P-R interval identifies clinical response in patients with non-LBBB: a MADIT-CRT sub-study. *Circ Arrhythmia Electrophysiol.* 2014;7:645–651.
6. Ambrosi A, Wahren-Herlenius M. Congenital heart block: evidence for a pathogenic role of maternal autoantibodies. *Arthritis Res Ther.* 2012;14:208–218.
7. Eliasson H, Sonesson SE, Salomonsson S, Skog A, Wahren-Herlenius M, Gadler F. Outcomes in young patients with isolated complete atrioventricular block and permanent pacemaker treatment: a nationwide study of 127 patients. *Heart Rhythm.* 2015;12:2278–2284.
8. Baruteau AE, Fouchard S, Behaghel A, et al. Characteristics and long-term outcome of non-immune isolated atrioventricular block diagnosed in utero or early childhood: a multicentre study. *Eur Heart J.* 2012;33:622–629.

9. Karnabi E, Qu Y, Mancarella S, et al. Rescue and worsening of congenital heart block–associated electrocardiographic abnormalities in two transgenic mice. *J Cardiovasc Electrophysiol.* 2011;22:922–930.

10. Capone C, Buyon JP, Friedman DM, et al. Cardiac manifestations of neonatal lupus: a review of antibody associated congenital heart block and its impact in an adult population. *Cardiol Rev.* 2012;20:72–76.

11. Hornberger LK, Rajaa Al. Spectrum of cardiac involvement in neonatal lupus. *Scand J Immunol.* 2010;72:189–197.

12. Friedman DM, Kim MY, Copel JA, et al. Prospective evaluation of fetuses with autoimmune-associated congenital heart block followed in the PR Interval and Dexamethasone Evaluation (PRIDE) study. *Am J Cardiol.* 2009;103:1102–1106.

13. Priori SG, Wilde AA, Horie M. Executive summary: HRS/EHRA/APHRS expert consensus statement on the diagnosis and management of patients with inherited primary arrhythmia syndromes. *Europace.* 2013;15:1389–1406.

14. Probst V, Kyndt F, Potet F, et al. Haploinsufficiency in combination with aging causes SCN5A-linked hereditary Lenègre disease. *J Am Coll Cardiol.* 2003;41:643–652.

15. Kyndt F, Probst V, Potet F, et al. Novel SCN5A mutation leading either to isolated cardiac conduction defect or Brugada syndrome in a large French family. *Circulation.* 2001;104:3081–3086.

16. Kruse M, et al. Impaired endocytosis of the ion channel TRPM4 is associated with human progressive familial heart block type I. *J Clin Invest.* 2009;119:2737–2744.

17. Lakdawala NH, Givertz MM. Dilated cardiomyopathy with conduction disease and arrhythmia. *Circulation.* 2010;122:527–534.

18. Ackerman MJ, Prior SG, Willems S, et al. HRS/EHRA expert consensus statement on the state of genetic testing for the channelopathies and cardiomyopathies. *Europace.* 2011;13:1077–1109.

19. Meine TJ, Al-Khatib SM, Alexander JH, et al. Incidence, predictors, and outcomes of high-degree atrioventricular block complicating acute myocardial infarction treated with thrombolytic therapy. *Am Heart J.* 2005;149:670–674.

20. O'Gara PT, Kushner FG, Ascheim DD, et al. 2013 ACCF/AHA guideline for the management of ST-elevation myocardial infarction. *Circulation.* 2013;127:e362–e425.

21. Birnie DH, Sauer W, Bogun F, et al. HRS expert consensus statement on the diagnosis and management of arrhythmias associated with cardiac sarcoidosis. *Heart Rhythm.* 2014;11:1304–1323.

22. Roman M, Salmon JE. Cardiovascular involvement in general medical conditions: cardiovascular manifestations of rheumatological diseases. *Circulation.* 2007;116:2346–2355.

23. Forrester JD, Mead P. Third degree heart block associated with Lyme carditis. *Clin Infec Dis.* 2014;59:996–1000.

24. Bern C, Montgomery SP, Herwaldt BL, et al. Evaluation and treatment of Chagas disease in the United States: a systematic review. *JAMA.* 2007;298:2171–2181.

25. Falk RH. Cardiac amyloidosis: a treatable disease, often overlooked. *Circulation.* 2011;124:1079–1085.

26. Brignole M, Deharo J, De Roy L, et al. Syncope due to idiopathic paroxysmal atrioventricular block: long term follow-up of a distinct form of atrioventricular block. *J Am Coll Cardiol.* 2011;58:167–173.

27. Osmonov D, Erdinler I, Ozcan KS, et al. Management of patients with drug-induced atrioventricular block. *Pacing Clin Electrophysiol.* 2012;35:804–810.

28. Koplan BA, Stevenson WG, Epstein LM, Aranki SF, Maisel WH. Development and validation of a simple risk score to predict the need for permanent pacing after cardiac valve surgery. *J Am Coll Cardiol.* 2003;41:795–801.

29. Auricchio A, Baron-Esquivias G, Bordachar P, et al. 2013 ESC guidelines on cardiac pacing and cardiac resynchronization therapy. *Eur Heart J.* 2013;34:2281–2329.

30. Merin O, Ilan M, Oren A, et al. Permanent pacemaker implantation following cardiac surgery: indications and long-term follow-up. *Pacing Clin Electrophysiol.* 2009;32:7–12.

31. Riaza SS, Li JM, John R, et al. Long-term mortality and pacing outcomes of patients with permanent pacemaker implantation after cardiac surgery. *Pacing Clin Electrophysiol.* 2011;34:331–338.

32. Siontis GC, Jüni P, Pilgrim T, et al. Predictors of permanent pacemaker implantation in patients with severe aortic stenosis undergoing TAVR: a meta-analysis. *J Am Coll Cardiol.* 2014;64:129–140.

33. Bleiniffer S, Ruge H, Horer J, et al. Predictors of new-onset complete heart block after transcatheter aortic valve implantation. *J Am Coll Cardiol.* 2010;3:525–530.

34. Sinhal A, Altwegg L, Pasupati S, et al. Atrioventricular block after transcatheter balloon expandable aortic valve implantation. *J Am Coll Cardiol Interv.* 2008;1:305–309.

35. Roten L, Stortecky S, Scarcia F, et al. Atrioventricular conduction after transcatheter aortic valve implantation and surgical valve replacement. *J Cardiovasc Electrophysiol.* 2012;23:1115–1122.

36. Petronio AD, Sinning J, Van Mieghem N, et al. Optimal implantation depth and adherence to guidelines on permanent pacing to improve the results of transcatheter aortic valve replacement with the Medtronic Core Valve system. *JACC Cardiovasc Interv.* 2015;8:837–846.

37. Bovelli D, Plataniotis G, Roila F. Cardiotoxicity of chemotherapeutic agents and radiotherapy-related disease: ESMO clinical practice guidelines. *Ann Oncol.* 2010;21:v277–v282.

38. Boulaksil M, Jungschleger JG, Antoons G, et al. Drug induced torsade de pointes arrhythmias in the chronic AV-block dog are perpetuated by focal activity. *Circ Arrhythm Electrophysiol.* 2011;4:566–576.

39. Villain E, Coastedoat-Chalumeau N, Marijon E, Boudjemline Y, Piette JC, Bonnet D. Presentation and prognosis of complete atrioventricular block in childhood, according to maternal antibody status. *J Am Coll Cardiol.* 2006;48:1682–1687.

40. Moak JP, Barron KS, Hougen TJ, et al. Congenital heart block: development of late-onset cardiomyopathy, a previously underappreciated sequela. *J Am Coll Cardiol.* 2001;37:238–242.

41. Moak JP, Hasbani K, Ramwell C, et al. Dilated cardiomyopathy following right ventricular pacing for AV block in young patients: resolution after upgrading to biventricular pacing systems. *J Cardiovasc Electrophysiol.* 2006;17:1068–1071.

42. Sharma PS, Dandamudi G, Naperkowski A, et al. Permanent His-bundle pacing is feasible, safe and superior to right ventricular pacing in routine clinical practice. *Heart Rhythm.* 2015;12:305–312.

43. Lustgarten DL, Crespo EM, Arkhipova-Jenkins I, et al. His-bundle pacing versus biventricular pacing in cardiac resynchronization therapy patients: a crossover design comparison. *Heart Rhythm.* 2015;12:1548–1557.

107 Sex Differences in Arrhythmias

Cevher Ozcan and Anne B. Curtis

Understanding and recognition of sex-based differences, with respect to both normal cardiac electrophysiology and the pathophysiology of arrhythmias, are important for the diagnosis and treatment of heart rhythm disorders in women. There are cellular and clinical electrophysiological differences that have been identified between men and women. Although genetics and the sex hormones partially explain the morphological differences in cardiovascular systems, the mechanisms of the sex-specific variations in the incidence and prevalence of arrhythmias, in addition to the clinical presentation and prognosis of rhythm disorders, are not well characterized. This chapter reviews current knowledge of sex differences in cellular and clinical electrophysiology.

Basic Electrophysiology

Since the observation of higher resting heart rates (HRs) and longer rate-corrected QT (QTc) intervals in women by Bazett in the early twentieth century, sex differences in the electrical properties of cardiomyocytes and the myocardial conduction system have been extensively studied. As summarized here, sex-based differences in clinical arrhythmias could potentially be explained by changes in ion channel function, expression patterns, ionic currents, action potential (AP) morphology, intercellular conduction, autonomic tone, hemodynamics, and the effects of sex hormones and genetics.

Cellular Electrophysiology

Significant differences in female cardiomyocyte electrical properties from those in males have been documented in various species, including humans. In addition to other factors, genetics and sex hormones modify cardiomyocyte structure, function, and ionic currents. Alteration of cellular ionic hemostasis and AP morphology increases susceptibility to arrhythmias by causing abnormal depolarization and repolarization as well as changes in conduction intervals. Sex-based differences in clinical arrhythmias are essentially based on these cellular dissimilarities.

Ion Channels

Several sex-based differences in function, structure, quantity, and currents of cardiomyocyte ion channels, including sodium (Na^+), potassium (K^+), and calcium (Ca^{2+}) channels and their components, have been defined (Fig. 107.1).

Sex hormones affect Na^+ channel function and the transmural distribution of Na^+ channel current (I_{Na}).[1] In the canine left ventricle (LV), I_{Na} amplitude is smaller in female epicardial and endocardial layers. Testosterone decreases the transmural dispersion in amplitude of I_{Na} in females, causing similar amplitudes as in males. Transmural dispersion of I_{Na} increases the risk of ventricular arrhythmias in females. In castrated male dog hearts, I_{Na} amplitudes are similar to those in female hearts.

A study on healthy human transplant donor hearts showed reduced expression of a variety of delayed rectifier K^+ currents (I_K) subunits, including HERG, minK, Kir2.3, Kv1.4, KChIP2, SUR2, and Kir6.2, in women compared with that in men.[2] An isoform switch in Na^+/K^+-ATPase was also found in women. In female mouse hearts, total I_K, transient outward K^+ current (I_{to}), and slow delayed rectifier K^+ current (I_{Ks}) densities are lower in a higher estrogen state, reflecting a direct effect of estrogen on K^+ currents.[3] This lower current density is associated with downregulation of Kv4.3 and Kv1.5 transcript levels. In female canine ventricles, total densities of I_{to}, I_{Ks}, and L-type Ca^{2+} currents are different and lead to transmural variation in cardiac repolarization.[4] Transmural differences in I_K provide a molecular link for the increased susceptibility to ventricular arrhythmias in women. However, this is species-dependent. In male and female guinea pig hearts, expression levels of the different K^+ channels, such as ERG, KvLQT1, minK, and Kir2.1, and the densities of the K^+ currents (rapid delayed rectifier K^+ current [I_{Kr}], I_{Ks}, and inward rectifier K^+ current [I_{K1}]) are similar.[5]

Gender effects on Ca^{2+} channel current (I_{Ca}) function and cardiomyocyte Ca^{2+} content have also been documented. Larger L-type Ca^{2+} (I_{CaL}) currents are present in all layers of female canine ventricles compared with those in males.[4] The I_{CaL} channel plays a significant role in sex-based differences in myocardial excitation–contraction coupling. The required Ca^{2+} for maximum contractile force is significantly lower in males. However, no sex difference in myofilament Ca^{2+} sensitivity has been found in the cat ventricle.

Sarcoplasmic reticulum Ca^{2+} concentration also has an effect on sex-specific cellular Ca^{2+} regulation. Cellular Ca^{2+} transients have been measured in rat epicardial myocytes.[6] Ca^{2+} reuptake was smaller in magnitude and longer in duration, with greater local variability, in females. The rate sensitivity of Ca^{2+} alternans was higher in females without significant heterogeneity in cellular responses. An increase in the Ni^{2+}-sensitive Na^+/Ca^{2+} exchanger and reduced β-adrenergic responsiveness have been noted in male swine LV cardiomyocytes.

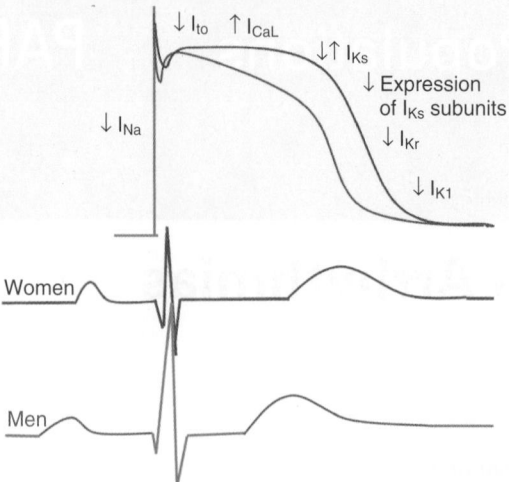

FIGURE 107.1 Sex differences in the basic electrical properties of the heart including ion channel function and action potential morphology are summarized. Action potential duration is longer in women (*red*) than in men (*blue*). Women have slower restitution property, while men have more prominent phase 1 repolarization. This is regulated by altered ionic currents in different phases of the action potential. In parallel, there are significant sex-based differences in electrocardiographic intervals. Women (*red*) have shorter PR intervals, QRS, and P wave durations than men (*blue*). However, rate-corrected QT interval is longer in women. While P wave amplitude is greater in women, R wave amplitude is lower. I_{CaL}, L-type calcium current; I_{K1}, inward rectifier potassium current; I_{Kr}, rapid delayed rectifier potassium current; I_{Ks}, slow delayed rectifier potassium current; I_{Na}, sodium channel current; I_{to}, transient outward potassium current.

Action Potentials

The morphology of the cardiac AP plays an important role in the genesis of arrhythmias. The depolarizing inward and repolarizing outward ionic currents, intracellular ion concentrations, transmembrane potentials, and expression of ion channels determine AP morphology and the electrophysiological properties of cardiomyocytes. Thus AP characteristics including AP duration, repolarization alternans, restitution slope, and adaptation to HR are expected to be different in women from those in men (see Fig. 107.1) based on previously outlined cellular ionic processes. Regional factors, such as transmural dispersion, could also alter AP morphology in women.

AP duration is longer in female ventricles than in male ventricles in various species, including humans (see Fig. 107.1).[4,7,8] Ventricular cardiomyocytes in women have a longer AP duration, larger transmural heterogeneity of AP duration, and greater susceptibility to proarrhythmic early afterdepolarizations (EADs) than men. On the other hand, male cells have more prominent phase 1 repolarization and greater susceptibility to all-or-none repolarization. These differences are associated with altered I_{CaL}, I_{to}, and I_{Kr} densities. Female sex hormones cause prolongation of AP duration.[3] However, in one study, elevated estradiol levels were associated with enhanced KCNH2 membrane trafficking and shorter QTc intervals in healthy women.[9] Slower restitution properties and repolarization alternans have been noted in female rat cardiomyocytes at slower HRs.[6] Underlying ionic mechanisms of rate-dependent changes in AP morphology include variation in transient outward current (I_{to}) and I_{Ks} in AP restitution as well as I_{CaL} and Na$^+$-K$^+$ pump current (I_{NaK}) in AP accommodation.[7] The sex-based difference in AP restitution is thought to be related to heterogeneity in the density and recovery kinetics of I_{to}. Transmural dispersion of cardiac repolarization is associated with I_{to}, I_{Ks}, and I_{CaL} currents. Female M cells have longer AP durations with increasing transmural heterogeneity.[4] The ionic bases of these sex-specific differences are associated

TABLE 107.1 Sex differences in basic electrocardiographic and electrophysiological parameters

PARAMETERS	WOMEN	MEN	REFERENCE
PR interval, ms	155 ± 24	163 ± 27	10
P wave duration, ms	108 ± 12	111 ± 12	10
P wave amplitude, µV	140 ± 45	131 ± 41	11
QRS duration, ms	91 ± 13	98 ± 15	10
QRS axis	31 ± 35	26 ± 40	10
R wave amplitude, µV	450 ± 334	480 ± 365	12
QTc, ms	418 ± 24	406 ± 26	10
QT-dispersion, ms	30 ± 11	37 ± 13	10
Heart rate, beats/min	69 ± 12	67 ± 13	10
Heart rate variability	Lower	Higher	18
Sinus node recovery time	Shorter	Longer	19
Atrial-His (AH) interval	Shorter	Longer	20
His-ventricular (HV) interval	Shorter	Longer	20
Atrioventricular (AV) block CL	Shorter	Longer	21
Slow pathway ERP	Shorter	Longer	21
AV nodal reentrant tachycardia CL	Shorter	Longer	21
Fast pathway ERP	Similar	Similar	21
Anterograde fast pathway ERP	Shorter	Longer	22
AV block CL	Shorter	Longer	22
Retrograde ventriculoatrial (VA) conduction	Longer	Shorter	22
Atrial ERP	Shorter	Longer	19
Ventricular ERP	Longer	Shorter	2

CL, Cycle length; *ERP*, effective refractory period.

with variations in I_{to}, sustained outward K$^+$ current (I_{sus}), ultra-rapid delayed rectifier K$^+$ current (I_{Kur}), I_{K1}, I_K, I_{Kr}, and I_{CaL} in different studies.

Electrocardiography

Baseline Intervals

Sex-based differences in baseline electrocardiographic intervals and HR are summarized in Table 107.1. Substantial sex differences in conduction intervals, as well as in P wave and QRS morphology, have been noted (see Fig. 107.1 and Table 107.1). Women have shorter PR intervals, QRS and P wave durations, and RR intervals than men, while QTc intervals are longer in women.[8,10] P wave amplitude is greater in women than in men of all ages.[11] The differences in PR interval and P wave duration progressively increase with aging, whereas P wave amplitude progressively decreases in both sexes with aging.[11] The QRS complex is shorter in duration and lower in amplitude in women after adjustment for LV mass and body weight.[12] R wave amplitude is also lower in women. Thus the diagnostic accuracy of QRS morphology-based electrocardiographic criteria for LV hypertrophy is significantly lower in women than in men.

Adult women have longer QTc intervals than men (see Fig. 107.1 and Table 107.1). This QT prolongation is associated with a greater risk of ventricular arrhythmias such as polymorphic ventricular tachycardia (VT) or torsades de pointes (TdP). The difference in QT prolongation is associated with sex hormones.[8,10,13] During childhood, QTc intervals are similar in boys and girls, but they shorten in boys at puberty. Among adults, men with higher testosterone levels continue to have shorter QTc intervals than women. Athletes who take large doses of anabolic steroids have shorter QTc intervals too. In parallel, women with virilization syndromes have shorter QTc intervals than castrated men and healthy women. After the age of 65 years, QTc gradually increases in men and becomes comparable with that in women. However, hormone replacement therapy does not have an effect on the QTc intervals of postmenopausal women. Thus compared with estrogen, testosterone modulates QTc more effectively. Significant seasonal variation in QTc intervals has been found among adult men but not in women. Monthly mean QTc intervals were consistently greater in women by 5.2 ± 2.3 ms.[14]

Another important sex difference in the electrocardiogram (ECG) is QT dispersion. Increased QT dispersion has a significant role in the genesis of reentrant arrhythmias and sudden cardiac death (SCD). QT dispersion is greater in men than in women and demonstrates prominent circadian variation.[15] Nevertheless, QT variability is a significant predictor of arrhythmic events following myocardial infarction in women who have a depressed LV ejection fraction (LVEF).[16] Data derived from the Women's Health Initiative Study show that nonspecific repolarization changes are more frequent in women and predict cardiovascular events. Repolarization inhomogeneity, as reflected in variation in mean RR intervals and beat-to-beat QT intervals in an established time domain, is higher in women. Women adapt the QT interval to changes in RR interval faster than men. The QT/RR relationship is steeper and more curved in women.[17]

Heart Rate and Heart Rate Variability

Mean HR at rest is higher in women than in men by 2–6 beats/min.[8,10] This difference persists even with sympathetic and parasympathetic blockade; therefore it is thought to be associated with dissimilarity in intrinsic sinus node properties. Sex differences in HR and HR variability fluctuate on the basis of age, race, physical conditioning, and comorbidities. HR variability is a known sensitive index of cardiac autonomic regulation. One study showed that HR variability is greater in men than in women in the age range of 33–47 years.[18] It is also lower in women with newly diagnosed hypertension and younger women with depressive symptoms after an acute coronary event. Cardiac autonomic modulation is significantly different between men and women during change of posture. Men have higher values of frequency-domain parameters of HR variability (low-frequency power and total power) in the supine and standing positions. However, high-frequency power is similar in both sexes.

Electrophysiological Study

Intracardiac electrophysiological measurements in men and women have demonstrated fundamental differences in the electrical properties of the heart, including sinus node function, atrioventricular (AV) conduction, and atrial and ventricular myocardium (see Table 107.1).

Sinus Node Function

Sinus node function is different in women starting from childhood. Sinus node recovery time is significantly shorter in women than in age-matched men with structurally normal hearts.[19] Similarly, corrected sinus node recovery time remains shorter in young and adult women than in men.

Atrioventricular Conduction Intervals

AV conduction properties are also different in women, as reflected by shorter PR, atrial-His (AH), and His-ventricular (HV) intervals as well as shorter AV block cycle lengths.[20] Overall, men develop AV block more often than women. The incidence of dual AV nodal pathways is similar in both sexes. However, women with symptomatic AV nodal reentrant tachycardia (AVNRT) have shorter slow pathway effective refractory periods (ERPs) and tachycardia cycle lengths than men.[20,21] The anterograde fast

pathway ERP has been found to be similar to or shorter in women than that in men.[22] During ventricular pacing in the absence of pharmacological stimulation, women more often have retrograde ventriculoatrial conduction; men are more likely to exhibit VA dissociation.

Electrophysiological Properties of the Atria and Ventricles

It has been shown that women have shorter atrial ERPs but longer ventricular ERPs than men. The atrial ERP is similarly shorter in girls without structural heart disease than in age-matched boys.[19]

Presentation and Management of Specific Arrhythmias

A sex-specific approach to the diagnosis and treatment of patients is essential to provide optimal care. The clinical presentation and prognosis of cardiovascular diseases, including heart rhythm disorders, are different in women from those in men. This section reviews sex differences in specific arrhythmias, including supraventricular tachyarrhythmias (SVTs), ventricular arrhythmias, SCD, inherited arrhythmias, and syncope (Table 107.2).

Sinus Node Dysfunction/Tachycardia

Sinus node–related disorders are different between the sexes. Women are more frequently affected by sick sinus syndrome, sinus tachycardia, inappropriate sinus tachycardia, postural orthostatic tachycardia syndrome, and sinus node reentry tachycardia than men.[21] On the other hand, carotid sinus syndrome occurs more often in men (see Table 107.2). Inappropriate sinus tachycardia is diagnosed much more commonly in women younger than 40 years. Abnormal autonomic regulation of the sinus node or a related immunological disorder involving cardiac β-adrenergic receptors has been speculated to be the cause of this condition in women.

Supraventricular Tachyarrhythmias

There are significant sex-based differences in the incidence and prevalence of SVT. Symptomatic paroxysmal SVT is more common in women, although SVT is more likely to be misdiagnosed as panic, anxiety, or stress in women than in men.[23] One study showed that the incidence of various arrhythmias in women was 63% AVNRT, 20% AV reentrant tachycardia (AVRT), and 17% atrial tachycardia (AT), while in men it was 45% AVNRT, 39% AVRT, and 17% AT.[21] SVT commonly coexists with atrial fibrillation (AF), with a higher incidence of AF in men than in women.[24]

A clear hormonal effect on triggering of SVT episodes has been noted in women. The frequency of symptomatic SVT episodes is more pronounced during the luteal phase of the menstrual cycle in premenopausal women. SVT is more inducible in a perimenstrual phase during an electrophysiological study (EPS). SVT episodes often cluster during this period; therefore it is important to consider the scheduling of EPS and ablation procedures in women to maximize the chances for successful induction and ablation of arrhythmia.

Atrial Fibrillation

The incidence of AF is lower in women than in men.[8,25] Men have a 1.5-fold higher risk of developing AF than women. The prevalence of AF remains unchanged in women with aging, while it increases in men. However, because of the greater longevity in women, there are more women with AF in the elderly population. Men are more prone to develop postoperative AF and lone AF, particularly the nonfamilial form. A possible relationship between testosterone levels and lone AF has been suggested. Underlying

TABLE 107.2 Sex differences in the incidence and prevalence of heart rhythm disorders

DISEASE	WOMEN	MEN
Sinus node dysfunction	↑	↓
Carotid sinus syndrome	↓	↑
Inappropriate sinus tachycardia	↑	↓
Atrioventricular block	↓	↑
Atrial fibrillation	↓	↑
Atrial flutter	↓	↑
Atrioventricular nodal reentrant tachycardia	↑	↓
Atrioventricular reentrant tachycardia	↓	↑
Atrial tachycardia	↔	↔
Paroxysmal atrial tachycardia	↑	↓
Incessant atrial tachycardia	↓	↑
Tachycardia-mediated cardiomyopathy secondary to focal atrial tachycardia	↓	↑
Left ventricular outflow tract ventricular arrhythmia	↓	↑
Verapamil-sensitive fascicular ventricular tachycardia	↓	↑
Right ventricular outflow tract ventricular arrhythmia	↑	↓
Inducibility of ventricular arrhythmia via programmed stimulation	↓	↑
Sudden cardiac death	↓	↑
Acquired long QT syndrome	↑	↓
Congenital long QT syndrome	↑	↓
Brugada syndrome	↓	↑
Arrhythmogenic right ventricular cardiomyopathy	↓	↑
Catecholaminergic polymorphic ventricular tachycardia	↓	↑
Short QT syndrome	↓	↑
Early repolarization and idiopathic ventricular fibrillation	↓	↑
Syncope	↔	↔
Cardiogenic syncope	↓	↑

valvular heart disease or heart failure is common in women with AF; men more often have AF with coronary artery disease (CAD). Overall, women with AF are older and have a lower quality of life, more significant comorbidities, and more symptoms compared with men. Paroxysmal AF presents with longer episodes and faster ventricular rates in women. AF diminishes the survival advantage in women by increasing the risk of death.

Cardioembolic complications with AF are also more prevalent in women, although men and women receive anticoagulation at similar rates.[25,26] The CHA$_2$DS$_2$-VASc risk score assigns 1 point to each of the following except as noted: Congestive heart failure, Hypertension, Age 65–74 years, Age >75 years (2 points), Diabetes, history of Stroke or transient ischemic attack (2 points), VAscular disease, and Sex category (female). The assignment of 1 point to female sex recognizes the elevated risk of thromboembolism in women compared with men. Women with AF are more likely to present with hypertensive heart failure but less likely to present with dilated cardiomyopathy or CAD.[27]

In general, women with AF are treated less aggressively, with fewer cardioversions and catheter ablations for AF. Consequently, women are not well represented in clinical trials of AF ablation.[25,28,29] Although female sex has been shown to be a predictor of major adverse events during pulmonary vein isolation, particularly a two-fold higher risk of cardiac tamponade, no significant sex difference has been reported for procedural success rate, rate of recurrence, or long-term outcome.[28,29]

Atrial Flutter

The incidence of atrial flutter (AFL) is significantly lower in women than in men.[23–25] AFL is about 2.5 times more common in men after adjustment for age. No sex difference has been documented in the outcome of catheter ablation for AFL. Although the efficacy of cardioversion is similar in men and women, there is a sex-based disparity in the use of cardioversion for the in-hospital management of patients with AFL, with less frequent use of cardioversion in women.[30]

Atrial Tachycardia

Paroxysmal AT is more common in women than in men, while incessant AT has a relatively higher incidence in men.[8,23,24] Women with focal AT are younger and often have other coexisting arrhythmias, with a noted increased incidence of AVNRT in women.[31] The mechanism of AT is typically abnormal automaticity in premenopausal women, and cardiovascular comorbidity is less common. However, no significant sex differences in other electrophysiological characteristics of AT have been found, including number of foci, left atrial involvement, tachycardia cycle length, the rate of success for catheter ablation, or the rate of recurrence of AT. Tachycardia-mediated cardiomyopathy secondary to focal AT is less common in women.

Atrioventricular Nodal Reentrant Tachycardia

A sex-based difference in AVNRT is well known.[8,21–24] AVNRT is twice as common in women as in men, and it starts at a younger age in women. Both typical and atypical types of AVNRT are more common in women. This increased incidence is likely associated with sex differences in AV conduction properties as were described earlier. Anterograde and retrograde AV nodal physiology is different in women.[22] During EPS, women have a higher incidence of multiple jumps, as well as shorter AH intervals, atrial ERPs, anterograde fast pathway ERPs, anterograde slow pathway ERPs, and retrograde slow pathway ERPs, and longer ventricular ERPs. Induction of AVNRT requires less pharmacological intervention in women. No significant sex differences in procedure times, complication rates, or acute success rates have been reported. Younger women (≤50 years old) have been noted to have a higher incidence of anterograde multiple jumps and a retrograde jump phenomenon, as well as shorter anterograde slow pathway ERPs and retrograde slow pathway ERPs, than women over the age of 50. Procedure times, complication rates, and acute success rates are similar in men and women, although recent studies indicate the possibility of a higher recurrence rate in young women.

Atrioventricular Reentrant Tachycardia

The incidence of AVRT is higher in men than in women.[8,23,24,32] AVRT and the Wolff-Parkinson-White (WPW) syndrome are less common in women compared with men by a ratio of 1:2. Concealed AVRT is almost equally distributed in both sexes. The diagnosis of WPW syndrome usually peaks in the fourth decade for women and in the third decade for men. Electrophysiological characteristics of accessory AV pathways in 1821 consecutive patients were evaluated with respect to sex differences.[32] Women comprised 39% of this patient population. The anterograde accessory pathway ERP was shorter in men (<250 ms), and they more often had antidromic AVRT. Women had a higher incidence of right free wall and multiple accessory pathways than men, while anteroseptal pathways were more common in men. Posteroseptal pathways were equally common in men and women. The rates of success of catheter ablation as well as complications and recurrence of accessory pathway conduction after ablation were similar in both sexes. Men with WPW syndrome have a higher incidence of AF and ventricular fibrillation (VF) events.

Ventricular Arrhythmias

Sex-based differences in ventricular arrhythmias, including sustained or nonsustained VT and premature ventricular complexes (PVCs), are well recognized in structurally normal hearts and in structural heart disease.[8,33,34] The incidence of ventricular arrhythmias varies in men and women on the basis of origin and mechanism (see Table 107.2).

Structurally Normal Hearts
A sex difference has been observed in the epidemiology of idiopathic ventricular arrhythmias.[33–35] Right ventricular (RV) outflow tract ventricular arrhythmias are more common in women compared with men, with a ratio of 2:1.[29] On the other hand, most cases of verapamil-sensitive fascicular VT occur in men, with a 3:1 male predominance. This finding is likely related to the shorter AP duration in Purkinje cells and slower distal conduction in men that increase the risk of reentry. LV outflow tract ventricular arrhythmias are more common in men. The success rate with catheter ablation is similar in both sexes for either right or LV outflow tract VT.

Structural Heart Disease
Sustained monomorphic VT often occurs in the presence of scar secondary to myocardial infarction and is more common in men than in women.[33,34,36] However, no significant sex difference has been found in the incidence of VT or electrical storm in patients with nonischemic cardiomyopathy.[30] Myocardial scar burden is a more important predictor of mortality in men than in women. Although the mechanism of sex-based differences in the risk of arrhythmias in structural heart disease is not well understood, women with LV dysfunction have lower arrhythmia-related mortality than men. The outcomes of catheter ablation with respect to success, complications, and recurrence rates are similar in both sexes regardless of age.[36]

Inducibility at Electrophysiological Study
Ventricular arrhythmias are less inducible by programmed stimulation during EPS in women. As shown in the Multicenter UnSustained Tachycardia Trial (MUSTT), inducible sustained ventricular arrhythmias occurred less frequently in women compared with those in men (24% vs. 36%). In some studies, ventricular arrhythmias are induced in men almost three times more often than in women. Among survivors of cardiac arrest, a lower rate of inducibility of sustained monomorphic VT has been reported in women. Male sex and myocardial infarction are independent predictors of arrhythmia inducibility in this population.

Sudden Cardiac Death

The overall incidence of SCD is lower in women that in men.[8,33,34,37] The annual rate of SCD in women is about half of that in men at all ages combined. In patients with out-of-hospital cardiac arrest, women more often present with asystole and pulseless electrical activity, and men usually have VT and VF. Women may have better survival following resuscitation for sudden cardiac arrest.[38] SCD more commonly occurs in women with structurally normal hearts.[37] CAD is less commonly associated with SCD in women (37%) compared with men (56%). Unrecognized myocardial infarction is more common in women. Although CAD markedly elevates the risk of SCD in both sexes, women have a four-fold increased risk of SCD after myocardial infarction compared with a 10-fold increased risk in men.[37] The presence of CAD is an independent predictor of cardiac and total mortality in women.

Heart failure is associated with a higher risk of SCD in both sexes, but the absolute risk of SCD in women is one-third of that in men. Low LVEF (<40%) has no prognostic significance in

female survivors of out-of-hospital cardiac arrest, although it is the strongest independent predictor of mortality in men. Nonsustained VT and PVCs increase the risk of SCD in men but not in women. The fact that women less often have recognized heart disease prior to a cardiac arrest makes risk stratification and institution of appropriate treatment to prevent SCD more challenging than in men.

Inherited Arrhythmia Syndromes

Inherited arrhythmia syndromes such as long QT syndrome (LQTS), Brugada syndrome, arrhythmogenic RV cardiomyopathy (ARVC), catecholaminergic polymorphic VT (CPVT), short QT syndrome (SQTS), early repolarization (ER), and idiopathic VF have recognized sex differences (see Table 107.2).[33,34,37,39] The mechanisms of sex-specific genetic predisposition to inherited arrhythmia syndromes are not well understood.

Long QT Syndrome
Sex differences in the incidence, prevalence, and risk of cardiac events in patients with congenital or acquired LQTS are well recognized.[8,33,34,37,39,40] The LQTS International Registry shows a female predominance in congenital LQTS. The risk of cardiac events in adult women with LQTS is three times higher than that in men. In particular, women with LQTS2 experience the highest rate of events. However, boys have a higher risk of SCD before the age of 15 years. Among family members of patients with LQTS, the cardiac event rate is higher in male than female LQT1 carriers, but no age-sex difference was detected in LQT2 and LQT3 carriers. As has been discussed, women have a longer QTc at baseline, and sex hormones have direct effects on QT prolongation and cardiac events. The result is that women are at a greater risk of developing TdP with drug-induced acquired LQTS.[33,34,37,39,40] The majority of reported cases of drug-induced TdP occur in women.

Brugada Syndrome
Brugada syndrome is more prevalent in men.[33,34,37,39,41] Cardiac events, including VF and SCD, occur more commonly in men with Brugada syndrome compared with women. Men with previous symptoms, type 1 ECGs, and inducible ventricular arrhythmias during EPS have a higher risk of cardiac events. In contrast, a longer PR interval is the only predictor for cardiac events in women.[41] Compared with men, women with Brugada syndrome have been found to have more conduction disturbances and longer QTc intervals in response to Na+ channel blockers.

Arrhythmogenic Right Ventricular Cardiomyopathy
Women are less likely to have ARVC compared with men (29% vs. 71% among 171 consecutive patients).[33,34,37,39,42] At clinical presentation, the male-to-female ratio is 3:1, but no gender difference is noted in genotyped cohorts. ECG abnormalities, including the presence of late potentials, are more often present in men. Half of the female patients with ARVC have normal ECGs. The age at the time of diagnosis and the prevalence of index cases and family members are similar in both sexes. Men have larger RV dimensions than women. However, the incidence of life-threatening ventricular arrhythmias is comparable in men and women.

Other Inherited Syndromes
CPVT is a heterogeneous disease with significant sex-based differences.[33,34,39] Patients with nongenotyped CPVT are predominantly women and become symptomatic at an older age. CPVT patients carrying a cardiac ryanodine receptor gene mutation become symptomatic earlier in life. These patients are more often males and have a high risk of cardiac events and syncope.

Male sex is strongly associated with the ER ECG pattern. It is common in young athletes and adults until middle age. The prevalence of a short QT interval is higher in men and is associated with an increased risk of SCD and AF.[33,34,39] Idiopathic VF is predominantly found in men, who comprise two-thirds of identified cases.

Syncope

The Framingham Heart Study showed that the overall incidence of syncope is similar in men and women. Syncope rates increase in older men and women, particularly beyond 70 years of age. Women with syncope are younger than men. While cardiac causes of syncope and seizure disorders are less common in women, syncope of unknown cause is more frequently found in women and increases the risk of death from any cause. The incidence of stroke or transient ischemic attack, vasovagal syncope, orthostatic hypotension, and syncope due to medications and other causes is similar in both sexes.[43,44] Elderly women are more prone to severe trauma during syncope. Syncope while driving occurs more commonly in men and is mostly neurally mediated.

Evaluation and Diagnostic Testing

The diagnostic yield of clinical evaluation, including the history and physical examination, in patients with syncope is similar in both sexes. No sex-specific difference has been reported regarding the diagnostic utility of initial testing for syncope, including ECG, chest x-ray, brain computed tomography scan, orthostatic test, tilt test, Holter monitoring, implantable loop recorder, and others.[43,44] However, carotid sinus pressure, exercise testing, coronary angiography, and magnetic resonance imaging/computed tomography scans are more commonly performed in men, whereas no type of testing is more common in women.[44] Women have more prominent orthostatic intolerance regardless of their menstrual phase.[43] During tilt-table testing, healthy women have a significantly lower blood pressure and greater orthostatic drop in posterior cerebral artery flow velocity. Women may tolerate tilt-table testing poorly because of a blunted vasoconstrictor response. Mean arterial pressure is lower in women, but HR and cardiac index are similar in both sexes.

Treatment and Outcome

No clear sex distinction has been made regarding the management of patients with syncope or response to conservative treatment of patients with vasovagal syncope. Hospitalization is more common regardless of sex in patients aged ≥65 years. Overall, men are more likely to have cardiac syncope and worse cardiac event–free survival. However, syncope in women is associated with poorer quality of life. New-onset syncope of unknown etiology in the elderly is not an independent predictor of mortality in either sex.

Pharmacotherapy

Overall, women have a greater risk of developing adverse drug reactions as a result of differences in physiology, pharmacokinetics, and pharmacodynamics.[45,46] Many factors cause sex-specific differences in pharmacotherapy in women, such as a lower body mass index, a higher proportion of body fat, a lower creatinine clearance, and smaller organ size.[44] In general, drug absorption may be slower in women. Different pharmacokinetics of drugs in women are important for drugs with narrow therapeutic margins, such as antiarrhythmic drugs. Sex differences are mainly modulated by the activity of drug-metabolizing enzymes, particularly the cytochrome P450 (CYP) system.[45,46] For example, CYP3A4 contributes to first-pass metabolism of most cardiovascular drugs, including diltiazem, quinidine, verapamil, and statins. Higher expression of *CYP3A4* messenger RNA and two-fold higher CYP3A4 levels are found in women on liver biopsy.

A sex-specific difference is controversial for CYP2D6, which has a role in the metabolism of flecainide, mexiletine, propafenone, metoprolol, and, in part, propranolol. Sex hormones affect the pharmacokinetics of drugs. Oral contraceptives are known to increase or decrease drug concentrations of coadministered medications.

Antiarrhythmic Drugs

Women develop proarrhythmia with antiarrhythmic drugs more often than men.[28,33,34,39,45,46] Class I and III antiarrhythmics more often cause TdP in association with QT prolongation in women. As has been discussed, differences in the activity and density of ion channels, particularly K+ channels, in female cardiomyocytes may increase vulnerability to QT prolongation in women. Longer QT intervals have been shown with ibutilide treatment in healthy women. Women have a higher risk than men for mortality and TdP with d,l-sotalol treatment. Female sex is a significant risk factor for the development of TdP with dofetilide treatment. Also, women develop TdP twice as frequently as men with amiodarone. Women have a higher mortality rate with digoxin treatment in association with higher serum levels of digoxin despite lower administered digoxin doses. Also, there are gender-specific differences in cellular Na+ and Ca2+ handling. However, post hoc analysis of the ROCKET AF trial showed a significant digoxin–sex interaction, with an increased risk of all-cause mortality and vascular death in male patients with AF compared with women.[47] Serum levels of β-blockers and procainamide are higher in women than in men. Ca2+ channel blockers demonstrate no sex-specific differences in mortality and morbidity. Both β-blockers and Ca2+ channel blockers provide more prominent blood pressure reduction in women than in men. Despite a greater incidence of side effects, the efficacy of antiarrhythmic drugs in women is relatively comparable with that in men. In general, women are prescribed antiarrhythmic drugs less often than men.

Acquired Long QT Syndrome

Women are more commonly affected by acquired LQTS in association with medications or electrolyte abnormalities compared with men.[33,34,39,45,46] The incidence of antiarrhythmic drug-induced TdP is higher in women, although women receive less antiarrhythmic drug treatment than men. As previously discussed, class IA and class III antiarrhythmic medications, including amiodarone, dofetilide, ibutilide, sotalol, quinidine, disopyramide, and azimilide, cause TdP more often in women than in men. Other medications, such as psychotropic drugs, antibiotics, and antihistamines, including erythromycin, pentamidine, methadone, and bepridil, have been reported to cause acquired LQTS and TdP in women. The mechanism of this vulnerability to acquired LQTS in women is not well understood. Underlying sex-specific changes in ventricular repolarization, cellular electrical properties, genetics, and sex hormones contribute to sex-based susceptibility to acquired LQTS. Thus special precaution is required to prevent acquired LQTS when these medications are initiated in women.

Anticoagulation

Anticoagulation with warfarin is known to be more challenging in women, with a lower probability for optimal anticoagulation and a higher risk of complications. Maintaining anticoagulation levels within the therapeutic range is more difficult in women than in men.[48] Male sex is an independent predictor of stable international normalized ratio (INR) control and of a lower risk of side effects from anticoagulation. Despite similar INRs, women with AF are at a higher risk of stroke than men. As shown in the IMPROVE HF study, women received anticoagulation therapy for AF significantly less often than men.[49] Dabigatran has a 3%–19% higher mean plasma concentration–time curve at steady state in elderly women than in elderly men, although no sex-based side effects have been reported. A meta-analysis showed that women suffer more bleeding complications than men when treated with the novel oral anticoagulants dabigatran, rivaroxaban, and apixaban for venous thromboembolism.[50] However, treatment with apixaban was associated with a similar rate of stroke or systemic embolism but a lower risk of mortality and less clinically relevant bleeding in women than in men.[51]

Implantable Device Therapy

Implantable cardioverter defibrillators (ICDs) and cardiac resynchronization therapy (CRT) are commonly used in both men and women. The smaller number of women in clinical trials and the lower risk of SCD in women have made it difficult to detect differences in outcomes in them with implantable device therapy. However, sex differences in the utilization of these devices and the response to device therapy have been reported.

Implantable Cardioverter Defibrillators

The efficacy of ICDs in the primary or secondary prevention of SCD has been shown in many prospective, randomized trials. ICD therapy significantly reduces mortality in men and women with prior SCD or sustained ventricular arrhythmias and in patients with heart failure and low LVEF compared with antiarrhythmic therapy or placebo.

Utilization

There is significant sex-based disparity regarding the utilization of ICDs. Data from a sample of Medicare beneficiaries who met the criteria for ICD implantation for the primary prevention of SCD revealed that a significantly lower number of women than men received ICDs in the first year of their diagnosis.[52–54] In an observational study including over 13,000 patients with LVEF <30% who were eligible for ICD therapy, the odds of ICD use were 0.62 for Caucasian women and 0.56 for African-American women compared with Caucasian men after adjustment for patient characteristics and hospital factors.[54] In the IMPROVE HF study, the use of ICDs was significantly less frequent in women than in men.[49] Procedural complications are more common in women with ICD implantation.

Response

Several major primary and secondary prevention SCD trials have shown that the overall mortality rate was comparable in men and women despite sex differences in baseline characteristics and clinical arrhythmia at the time of presentation. In a post hoc analysis of the Sudden Cardiac Death in Heart Failure Trial (SCD-HeFT), a significant reduction in mortality was noted in men but not in women with ICD therapy compared with amiodarone or placebo for the primary prevention of SCD in patients with heart failure and LVEF ≤35%. This finding may have been the result of the lower risk of SCD in women and the smaller number of women enrolled in this study. No sex difference in mortality rate was observed in the MADIT II trial. In contrast, the incidence of VT/VF or death was significantly lower in men than in men in both the ICD and the CRT-defibrillator (CRT-D) arms of the recent MADIT-CRT trial.[55] Thus ICD therapy is effective in reducing mortality in women at risk for SCD.

Cardiac Resynchronization Therapy

Several large clinical trials have demonstrated the benefits of CRT in men and women with heart failure refractory to optimal medical therapy, reduced LVEF, and evidence of electromechanical

delay. Recent studies have specifically addressed sex differences in use and response to CRT in this population.

Utilization

A significant gap in the use of CRT has been noted among indicated women. Underutilization of CRT in women is related in part to education among physicians, as the IMPROVE HF trial showed that only 35% of indicated female patients initially had a CRT device; this improved to 65% at 24 months with increased physician education.

Response

CRT is an effective therapy for women with heart failure. In the Multicenter InSync Randomized Clinical Evaluation (MIRACLE) trial, women who received CRT therapy experienced significant improvement in time to first heart failure hospitalization or death compared with women not treated with CRT. In addition, women derived greater benefit than men in this population. This sex difference persisted after adjustments were made for the cause of heart failure, which more often is due to nonischemic cardiomyopathy in women. CRT equally improves clinical and echocardiographic parameters in both sexes. However, female sex is independently associated with a better response to CRT with respect to survival and functional status.[56] Women with CRT-D had a lower risk of VT/VF or death than men.[55] The SMART-AV trial showed that greater reduction of LV end-systolic volume index and a higher rate of biventricular pacing with AV optimization are potential reasons for a better response to CRT in women.[56]

Pregnancy and the Postpartum Period

Arrhythmic events during pregnancy are associated with an increased risk of adverse events in the fetus and the mother. Pregnancy may increase susceptibility to arrhythmias even in the absence of underlying heart disease.[8,23,33,34,39,57–59] Although ECG parameters remain unchanged in pregnancy, resting HR increases by approximately 10 beats/min as a response to hemodynamic changes.[7] A leftward shift of the electrical axis may be seen secondary to enlargement of the gravid uterus. Hemodynamic and neurohormonal changes in the pre- and postpartum periods of pregnancy make women more vulnerable to arrhythmias. Women with SVT or ventricular arrhythmias may have exacerbation of their arrhythmias during pregnancy. Characteristics of arrhythmias in pregnancy are summarized in Table 107.3.

Supraventricular Arrhythmias

The incidence of new onset SVT and the recurrence of SVT episodes increases during pregnancy.[23] Multiple potential mechanisms are associated with these events, including changes in hormonal condition, autonomic tone, or hemodynamics. The first onset of SVT occurred in 3.9% of women during pregnancy. Among women with a history of SVT, 22% reported that pregnancy exacerbated their symptoms.[23] All women with known SVT require close follow-up during pregnancy, and symptomatic patients may require antiarrhythmic drugs to block accessory pathways or suppress tachycardia during pregnancy.

Ventricular Arrhythmias and Sudden Cardiac Arrest

During pregnancy, VT may recur in women who are known to have ventricular arrhythmias.[33,34,39,57–59] The onset of new ventricular arrhythmias during pregnancy has been found to be distributed equally over all three trimesters and exhibits similar characteristics to idiopathic VT.[58] The majority of VT is

TABLE 107.3 Arrhythmias during pregnancy and the postpartum period

CONDITIONS	CHARACTERISTICS	MANAGEMENT
Normal pregnancy	↑ resting HR (~10 beats/min) Leftward shift of the axis ↑ complaints of palpitations ↓ QTc interval with ↑ HR	Monitoring and supportive care

SVA	Recurrences of arrhythmias
	↑ episodes
	↑ symptoms
	↑ incidence of new onset SVA
		Treatment of triggers/underlying conditions
		Terminate tachycardia with following steps:
		    Vagal maneuvers → Adenosine →
		    Metoprolol or verapamil → Cardioversion

VTA	↑ risk of recurrent VTA episodes ↑ incidence of new onset VTA Mostly monomorphic Similar characteristics of idiopathic VTA Frequently originates from RVOT	Cardioversion or defibrillation if hemodynamically unstable Lidocaine if hemodynamically stable Procainamide for long-term therapy Cardioselective β-blocker for prophylaxis
LQTS	↑ risk of cardiac arrest in postpartum period ↑ incidence of torsades de pointes	Cardioselective β-blockers to prevent cardiac events

HR, Heart rate; *LQTS*, long QT syndrome; *RVOT*, right ventricular outflow tract; *SVA*, supraventricular arrhythmia; *VTA*, ventricular tachyarrhythmia.

monomorphic and originates from the RV outflow tract. VT disappeared completely in all patients during the postpartum period. HR variability was lower during pregnancy, and QTc intervals were normal in all patients. In another study, women with LQTS showed a reduced risk of cardiac events during pregnancy.[33,34,39,59] However, cardiac events during the 9-month postpartum period were significantly higher in women with LQTS, particularly with the LQT2 genotype. It is thought that an increased HR during pregnancy infers a protective effect to the QT interval. Women with Brugada syndrome have been shown to have a safe pregnancy and peripartum period.[34]

Management of Arrhythmias During Pregnancy and the Postpartum Period

Although evaluation of arrhythmias in pregnancy is the same as that in the general population, their management requires different approaches.[28] Almost all cardiac medications, including antiarrhythmics, cross the placenta and are secreted in breast milk. The majority of antiarrhythmic drugs and β-blockers are classified as category C for pregnancy. Amiodarone and atenolol are category D, while sotalol and lidocaine are category B.

If paroxysmal SVT episodes occur in pregnant women and vagal maneuvers fail to terminate tachycardia, adenosine, metoprolol, or verapamil can be used in an acute setting. β1-Selective blockers, such as metoprolol, are considered relatively safe in late pregnancy. However, atenolol is reported to be unsafe for pregnant or breastfeeding women since it may cause fetal hypoglycemia and bradycardia. Digoxin, quinidine, adenosine, and verapamil have been used in pregnant women, with no reported adverse fetal effects. Amiodarone causes fetal hypothyroidism and is not recommended for pregnant or breastfeeding women. Dronedarone is contraindicated during pregnancy. To prevent postpartum hemorrhage, verapamil must be discontinued when labor starts.

Management of AF is more challenging in pregnancy. Direct current cardioversion can be used cautiously. Class IC and class III antiarrhythmics for rhythm control are not safe during pregnancy or lactation. Metoprolol or digoxin may be used for rate control. If ventricular arrhythmias occur, lidocaine, procainamide, or cardioversion can be used to terminate them. β-Blockers are effective in reducing cardiac events during the postpartum period in women with LQTS. Thus β-blocker therapy should be continued during pregnancy and the postpartum period in women with LQTS and TdP. An anticoagulation strategy needs to be determined carefully. Warfarin is considered to be contraindicated during pregnancy as it has been associated with fetal defects, spontaneous abortion, stillbirth, and other problems. The novel oral anticoagulants have not been studied in pregnant and lactating women.

REFERENCES

1. Barajas-Martinez H, Haufe V, Chamberland C, et al. Larger dispersion of INa in female dog ventricle as a mechanism for gender-specific incidence of cardiac arrhythmias. *Cardiovasc Res.* 2009;81:82–89.
2. Gaborit N, Varro A, Le Bouter S, et al. Gender-related differences in ion-channel and transporter subunit expression in non-diseased human hearts. *J Mol Cell Cardiol.* 2010;49:639–646.
3. Saito T, Ciobotaru A, Bopassa JC, et al. Estrogen contributes to gender differences in mouse ventricular repolarization. *Circ Res.* 2009;105:343–352.
4. Xiao L, Zhang L, Han W, et al. Sex-based transmural differences in cardiac repolarization and ionic-current properties in canine left ventricles. *Am J Physiol Heart Circ Physiol.* 2006;291:H570–H580.
5. Brouillette J, Lupien MA, St-Michel C, et al. Characterization of ventricular repolarization in male and female guinea pigs. *J Mol Cell Cardiol.* 2007;42:357–366.
6. Wasserstrom JA, Kapur S, Jones S, et al. Characteristics of intracellular Ca²⁺ cycling in intact rat heart: a comparison of sex differences. *Am J Physiol Heart Circ Physiol.* 2008;295:H1895–H1904.

7. Decker KF, Heijman J, Silva JR, et al. Properties and ionic mechanisms of action potential adaptation, restitution, and accommodation in canine epicardium. *Am J Physiol Heart Circ Physiol.* 2009;296:H1017–H1026.
8. Curtis AB, Narasimha D. Arrhythmias in women. *Clin Cardiol.* 2012;35:166–171.
9. Anneken L, Baumann S, Vigneault P, et al. Estradiol regulates human QT-interval: acceleration of cardiac repolarization by enhanced KCNH2 membrane trafficking. *Eur Heart J.* 2016;37:640–650.
10. Mason JW, Ramseth DJ, Chanter DO, et al. Electrocardiographic reference ranges derived from 79,743 ambulatory subjects. *J Electrocardiol.* 2007;40:228–234.
11. Magnani JW, Gorodeski EZ, Johnson VM, et al. P wave duration is associated with cardiovascular and all-cause mortality outcomes: the National Health and Nutrition Examination Survey. *Heart Rhythm.* 2011;8:93–100.
12. Okin PM, Roman MJ, Devereux RB, et al. Gender differences and the electrocardiogram in left ventricular hypertrophy. *Hypertension.* 1995;25:242–249.

13. Zhang Y, Ouyang P, Post WS, et al. Sex-steroid hormones and electrocardiographic QT-interval duration: findings from the third National Health and Nutrition Examination Survey and the Multi-Ethnic Study of Atherosclerosis. *Am J Epidemiol.* 2011;174:403–411.
14. Beyerbach DM, Kovacs RJ, Dmitrienko AA, et al. Heart rate-corrected QT interval in men increases during winter months. *Heart Rhythm.* 2007;4:277–281.
15. Mayuga KA, Thattassery E, Taneja T, et al. Circadian and gender effects on repolarization in healthy adults: a study using harmonic regression analysis. *Ann Noninvasive Electrocardiol.* 2010;15:3–10.
16. Haigney MC, Zareba W, Nasir JM, et al. Gender differences and risk of ventricular tachycardia or ventricular fibrillation. *Heart Rhythm.* 2009;6:180–186.
17. Malik M, Hnatkova K, Kowalski D, et al. QT/RR curvatures in healthy subjects: sex differences and covariates. *Am J Physiol Heart Circ Physiol.* 2013;305:H1798–H1806.
18. Sloan RP, Huang MH, McCreath H, et al. Cardiac autonomic control and the effects of age, race, and sex: the CARDIA study. *Auton Neurosci.* 2008;139:78–85.

19. Sanjeev S, Karpawich PP. Developmental changes in sinus node function in growing children: an updated analysis. *Pediatr Cardiol.* 2005;26:585–588.

20. Liu S, Yuan S, Kongstad O, et al. Gender differences in the electrophysiological characteristics of atrioventricular conduction system and their clinical implications. *Scand Cardiovasc J.* 2001;35:313–317.

21. Liuba I, Jonsson A, Safstrom K, et al. Gender-related differences in patients with atrioventricular nodal reentry tachycardia. *Am J Cardiol.* 2006;97:384–388.

22. Suenari K, Hu YF, Tsao HM, et al. Gender differences in the clinical characteristics and atrioventricular nodal conduction properties in patients with atrioventricular nodal reentrant tachycardia. *J Cardiovasc Electrophysiol.* 2010;21:1114–1119.

23. Page RL, Joglar JA, Caldwell MA, et al. 2015 ACC/AHA/HRS guideline for the management of adult patients with supraventricular tachycardia: A Report of the American College of Cardiology/American Heart Association Task Force on Clinical Practice Guidelines and the Heart Rhythm Society. *J Am Coll Cardiol.* 2016;67:e27–e115.

24. Ozcan C, Strom J, Newell J, et al. Incidence and predictors of atrial fibrillation and its impact on long-term survival in patients with supraventricular arrhythmias. *Europace.* 2014;16:1508–1514.

25. January CT, Wann LS, Alpert JS, et al. 2014 AHA/ACC/HRS guideline for the management of patients with atrial fibrillation: executive summary: a report of the American College of Cardiology/American Heart Association Task Force on practice guidelines and the Heart Rhythm Society. *Circulation.* 2014;130:2071–2104.

26. Avgil Tsadok M, Jackevicius CA, Rahme E, et al. Sex differences in stroke risk among older patients with recently diagnosed atrial fibrillation. *JAMA.* 2012;307:1952–1958.

27. Stewart S, Carrington M, Pretorius S, et al. Standing at the crossroads between new and historically prevalent heart disease: effects of migration and socio-economic factors in the Heart of Soweto cohort study. *Eur Heart J.* 2011;32:492–499.

28. Michowitz Y, Rahkovich M, Oral H, et al. Effects of sex on the incidence of cardiac tamponade after catheter ablation of atrial fibrillation: results from a worldwide survey in 34 943 atrial fibrillation ablation procedures. *Circ Arrhythm Electrophysiol.* 2014;7:274–280.

29. Calkins H, Kuck KH, Cappato R, et al. 2012 HRS/EHRA/ECAS expert consensus statement on catheter and surgical ablation of atrial fibrillation: Recommendations for patient selection, procedural techniques, patient management and follow-up, definitions, endpoints, and research trial design. *Heart Rhythm.* 2012;9:632–696.

30. LaPointe NM, Sun JL, Kaplan S. In-hospital management of patients with atrial flutter. *Am Heart J.* 2010;159:370–376.

31. Hu YF, Huang JL, Wu TJ, et al. Gender differences of electrophysiological characteristics in focal atrial tachycardia. *Am J Cardiol.* 2009;104:97–100.

32. Huang SY, Hu YF, Chang SL, et al. Gender differences of electrophysiologic characteristics in patients with accessory atrioventricular pathways. *Heart Rhythm.* 2011;8:571–574.

33. Zipes DP, Camm AJ, Borggrefe M, et al. ACC/AHA/ESC 2006 guidelines for management of patients with ventricular arrhythmias and the prevention of sudden cardiac death: a report of the American College of Cardiology/American Heart Association Task Force and the European Society of Cardiology Committee for Practice Guidelines (Writing Committee to Develop Guidelines for Management of Patients With Ventricular Arrhythmias and the Prevention of Sudden Cardiac Death). *Circulation.* 2006;114:e385–e484.

34. Priori SG, Blomström-Lundqvist C, Mazzanti A, et al. 2015 ESC Guidelines for the management of patients with ventricular arrhythmias and the prevention of sudden cardiac death: The Task Force for the Management of Patients with Ventricular Arrhythmias and the Prevention of Sudden Cardiac Death of the European Society of Cardiology (ESC). Endorsed by: Association for European Paediatric and Congenital Cardiology (AEPC). *Eur Heart J.* 2015;36:2793–2867.

35. Tanaka Y, Tada H, Ito S, et al. Gender and age differences in candidates for radiofrequency catheter ablation of idiopathic ventricular arrhythmias. *Circ J.* 2011;75:1585–1591.

36. Inada K, Roberts-Thomson KC, Seiler J, et al. Mortality and safety of catheter ablation for antiarrhythmic drug-refractory ventricular tachycardia in elderly patients with coronary artery disease. *Heart Rhythm.* 2010;7:740–744.

37. Deo R, Albert CM. Epidemiology and genetics of sudden cardiac death. *Circulation.* 2012;125:620–637.

38. Teodorescu C, Reinier K, Uy-Evanado A, et al. Survival advantage from ventricular fibrillation and pulseless electrical activity in women compared to men: the Oregon Sudden Unexpected Death Study. *J Interv Card Electrophysiol.* 2012;34:219–225.

39. Priori SG, Wilde AA, Horie M, et al. HRS/EHRA/APHRS expert consensus statement on the diagnosis and management of patients with inherited primary arrhythmia syndromes: document endorsed by HRS, EHRA, and APHRS in May 2013 and by ACCF, AHA, PACES, and AEPC in June 2013. *Heart Rhythm.* 2013;10:1932–1963.

40. Liu JF, Jons C, Moss AJ, et al. Risk factors for recurrent syncope and subsequent fatal or near-fatal events in children and adolescents with long QT syndrome. *J Am Coll Cardiol.* 2011;57:941–950.

41. Benito B, Sarkozy A, Mont L, et al. Gender differences in clinical manifestations of Brugada syndrome. *J Am Coll Cardiol.* 2008;52:1567–1573.

42. Bauce B, Frigo G, Marcus FI, et al. Comparison of clinical features of arrhythmogenic right ventricular cardiomyopathy in men versus women. *Am J Cardiol.* 2008;102:1252–1257.

43. Baron-Esquivias G, Martinez-Alday J, Martin A, et al. Epidemiological characteristics and diagnostic approach in patients admitted to the emergency room for transient loss of consciousness: Group for Syncope Study in the Emergency Room (GESINUR) study. *Europace.* 2010;12:869–876.

44. Edvardsson N, Garutti C, Rieger G, et al. Unexplained syncope: implications of age and gender on patient characteristics and evaluation, the diagnostic yield of an implantable loop recorder, and the subsequent treatment. *Clin Cardiol.* 2014;37:618–625.

45. Nicolson TJ, Mellor HR, Roberts RR. Gender differences in drug toxicity. *Trends Pharmacol Sci.* 2010;31:108–114.

46. Kaiser J. Gender in the pharmacy: does it matter? *Science.* 2005;308:1572.

47. Washam JB, Stevens SR, Lokhnygina Y, et al. Digoxin use in patients with atrial fibrillation and adverse cardiovascular outcomes: a retrospective analysis of the Rivaroxaban Once Daily Oral Direct Factor Xa Inhibition Compared with Vitamin K Antagonism for Prevention of Stroke and Embolism Trial in Atrial Fibrillation (ROCKET AF). *Lancet.* 2015;385:2363–2370.

48. Rose AJ, Hylek EM, Ozonoff A, et al. Patient characteristics associated with oral anticoagulation control: results of the Veterans Affairs Study to Improve Anticoagulation (VARIA). *J Thromb Haemost.* 2010;8:2182–2191.

49. Yancy CW, Fonarow GC, Albert NM, et al. Influence of patient age and sex on delivery of guideline-recommended heart failure care in the outpatient cardiology practice setting: Findings from IMPROVE HF. *Am Heart J.* 2009;157:754–762.

50. Alotaibi GS, Almodaimegh H, McMurtry MS, Wu C. Do women bleed more than men when prescribed novel oral anticoagulants for venous thromboembolism? A sex-based meta-analysis. *Thromb Res.* 2013;132:185–189.

51. Vinereanu D, Stevens SR, Alexander JH, et al. Clinical outcomes in patients with atrial fibrillation according to sex during anticoagulation with apixaban or warfarin: a secondary analysis of a randomized controlled trial. *Eur Heart J.* 2015;36:3268–3275.

52. Ghanbari H, Dalloul G, Hasan R, et al. Effectiveness of implantable cardioverter-defibrillators for the primary prevention of sudden cardiac death in women with advanced heart failure: a meta-analysis of randomized controlled trials. *Arch Intern Med.* 2009;169:1500–1506.

53. Hernandez AF, Fonarow GC, Liang L, et al. Sex and racial differences in the use of implantable cardioverter-defibrillators among patients hospitalized with heart failure. *JAMA.* 2007;298:1525–1532.

54. Mooyaart EA, Marsan NA, van Bommel RJ, et al. Comparison of long-term survival of men versus women with heart failure treated with cardiac resynchronization therapy. *Am J Cardiol.* 2011;108:63–68.

55. Tompkins CM, Kutyifa V, Arshad A, et al. Sex differences in device therapies for ventricular arrhythmias or death in the Multicenter Automatic Defibrillator Implantation Trial with Cardiac Resynchronization Therapy (MADIT-CRT) trial. *J Cardiovasc Electrophysiol.* 2015;26:862–871.

56. Cheng A, Gold MR, Waggoner AD, et al. Potential mechanisms underlying the effect of gender on response to cardiac resynchronization therapy: insights from the SMART-AV multicenter trial. *Heart Rhythm.* 2012;9:736–741.

57. Silversides CK, Harris L, Haberer K, et al. Recurrence rates of arrhythmias during pregnancy in women with previous tachyarrhythmia and impact on fetal and neonatal outcomes. *Am J Cardiol.* 2006;97:1206–1212.

58. Nakagawa M, Katou S, Ichinose M, et al. Characteristics of new-onset ventricular arrhythmias in pregnancy. *J Electrocardiol.* 2004;37:47–53.

59. Seth R, Moss AJ, McNitt S, et al. Long QT syndrome and pregnancy. *J Am Coll Cardiol.* 2007;49:1092–1098.

108 Sudden Cardiac Deaths in Athletes, Including Commotio Cordis

Mark S. Link and N.A. Mark Estes III

Sudden cardiac death (SCD) in athletes continues to draw nearly daily media attention. While the number of these deaths is small, the emotional magnitude is great. Underlying cardiac disease is generally found in these athletes dying young. More data are accumulating on the potentially adverse cardiac remodeling of exercise, especially in certain conditions. The issue of electrocardiogram (ECG) screening has not been resolved. Despite conflicting data on the issue, strong opinions have been formed and continue to be meted out in medical journals and the popular media. Resuscitation has improved likely secondary to the penetration of automated external defibrillators (AEDs) and cardiopulmonary resuscitation (CPR) training.

Epidemiology of Sudden Cardiac Death in Athletes

Each year in the United States, approximately 150 young athletes die suddenly during sporting activities, for an incidence of 0.5/100,000 athletes per year.[1,2] Similar incidences are being observed in Italy.[3] Due to the often intense media attention that SCD in the athlete generates, SCD deaths in athletes appear to be much more common than in nonathletes. However, that impression is not verified by the available data (Table 108.1). While there are observational data that basketball players may be at higher risk of SCD (incidence of 3.6 per 100,000 person-years in male basketball players)[2] and that National Collegiate Athletic Association (NCAA) Division I male basketball players may be at even higher risk (1 in 3100 person-years),[4] most data do not support an increased risk of SCD in athletes.[2,3,5–10]

In most series of SCD in the young, deaths outside of sports far exceed deaths in sports. Indeed in NCAA athletes, deaths unassociated with sports far exceeded the deaths associated with exertion (Fig. 108.1). In the Resuscitation Outcomes Consortium (ROC), the incidence of sudden cardiac arrests in all children was 3.73 in 100,000 person-years in those aged between 1 and 11 years and 6.37 per 100,000 person-years in those aged between 12 and 19 years.[10] In the US pediatric population of over 74 million,[10a] there are between 3000 and 5000 sudden cardiac arrests per year between the ages of 1 and 18 years. There are reasonably good data that there are 100–150 SCDs per year in sports.[1] Thus it appears that most SCDs in the young occur outside of athletics.

This lower incidence of SCD in sports has also been seen in Germany and Denmark. In 48,335 fatalities in Hamburg, Germany, only 176 were involved in sporting activities.[11] In Denmark, among deaths of 5662 individuals aged between 12 and 35 years, only 15 were sport related.[7] The incidence of SCD in athletes (1.21/100,000 person-years) was lower than that in the general population (3.76/100,000 person-years). In a general pediatric population in Japan, the incidence of SCD was 1.32 per 100,000 person-years.[8] In US military recruits the incidence of SCD was 1.32 per 100,000 person-years, with a sudden death rate of 13 per 100,000 person-years.[9] In a Dutch study, the incidence of cardiac arrest in the population aged <21 years was 3.2/100,000 person-years.[12] Thus most of the available data indicate a similar or lower incidence of SCD in athletes compared with nonathletes. Yet these data may be skewed because deaths of athletes are generally only counted as athletic deaths if they occur on the playing field. Deaths in athletes that occur outside of sports are generally not noted by the media and thus are not counted as athletic deaths.

Underlying Structural Heart Disease in the Athlete With Sudden Cardiac Death

As in nonathletes, the majority of athletes with SCD have an underlying cardiac abnormality (Fig. 108.2). In the United States the most common underlying cardiac condition is hypertrophic cardiomyopathy (HCM).[1] Coronary artery anomalies, myocarditis, Marfan syndrome, arrhythmogenic right ventricular cardiomyopathy (ARVC), valvular disease, and dilated cardiomyopathies comprise most of the remaining underlying heart disease. Commotio cordis, one of the few causes of SCD in individuals with a normal heart, accounts for nearly 20% of SCD in athletes, the second most common etiology in the United States.[1] In Italian series of SCD in athletes, ARVC is found in 22%, while HCM is present in 2%.[3] These differences in etiology could be related to the Italian screening process for athletes but also could reflect different genetic penetrations of ARVC and HCM. Anomalous coronary arteries account for a significant percentage of SCD, as does coronary artery disease (CAD).

More recently, in the general population, early repolarization has been reported to be associated with SCD.[13,14] These reports are of potential concern for the athletic community because early repolarization is seen in up to 76% of athletes.[15,16] However, it is apparent that in these studies reporting an association with SCD, early repolarization is defined differently from that previously.[17] In the studies linking early repolarization to SCD, the abnormalities were defined as terminal slurring of the QRS or early notching of the J wave, unlike previous definitions, which primarily were that of J-point elevation with accompanying ST-segment elevation.[17] Early repolarization that is described by the latter definition is very common in trained athletes; however, there have been no data that this early repolarization is a cause of SCD in athletes.[18] In fact, the available data argue that the early repolarization pattern observed in athletes is not a marker of increased arrhythmic risk.[19]

In nonathletic populations, such as the military and general public, the causes of sudden death in the young differ from those

TABLE 108.1 Incidence of sudden death stratified by athletic or general population and the years of the study

COUNTRY	REFERENCE	POPULATION	YEARS	INCIDENCE PER 100,000 PERSON-YEARS
Italy	Corrado[3]	Athletes	1980–81	3.6
Italy	Corrado[3]	Athletes	2007–08	0.4
Israel	Steinvil[5]	Athletes	1985–97	2.54
Israel	Steinvil[5]	Athletes	1998–2009	2.66
United States	VanCamp[2]	Athletes	1983–93	0.33
United States	Maron[6]	Athletes	1985–2006	0.44
Denmark	Holst[7]	Athletes	2000–06	1.21
Denmark	Holst[7]	All children	2000–06	3.76
Japan	Tanaka[8]	All children	1989–97	1.32
United States	Eckart[9]	Military recruits	1997–2001	13
United States and Canada	Atkins[10]	All children aged 1–11 years	2005–07	3.73
United States and Canada	Atkins[10]	All children aged 12–19 years	2005–07	6.37

There is a wide range of incidences of sudden death in both athletes and the general population.
From Link MS, Estes NA. Athletes and arrhythmias. *J Cardiovasc Electrophysiol.* 2010;21:1184-1189.

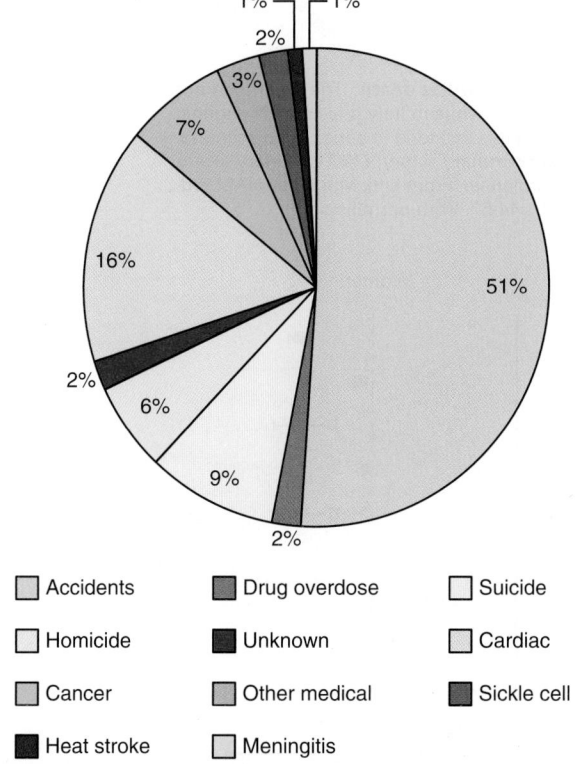

Accidents Drug overdose Suicide
Homicide Unknown Cardiac
Cancer Other medical Sickle cell
Heat stroke Meningitis

FIGURE 108.1 Etiology of deaths in National Collegiate Athletic Association athletes. Note the majority of deaths are not sudden cardiac deaths. (From Harmon KG, Asif IM, Klossner D, Drezner JA. Incidence of sudden cardiac death in National Collegiate Athletic Association athletes. *Circulation.* 2011;123:1594-1600.)

in athletic SCD. Genetic cardiomyopathies are much less common, whereas myocarditis, anomalous coronary arteries, CAD, and normal hearts are more frequent.[9,20,21] In nonpediatric populations, underlying CAD is often found.

Benefits of Exercise

Epidemiological data show the benefit of regular exercise in the prevention of CAD and reduction of mortality (Fig. 108.3).[22–24] The reduction in cardiovascular events is likely brought about by a number of beneficial effects of exercise, including decreased

weight and blood pressure, improved lipids and glucose tolerance, and increased adherence to a healthy lifestyle, which includes an increased attention to diet and reduction in tobacco product consumption. This reduced risk of cardiac events is seen with chronic energy expenditure as minimal as walking and appears to increase with both the time and intensity of exercise.[24–26] In general, the more vigorous the exercise, the greater the long-term benefits. It has been argued that low cardiovascular fitness constitutes the largest attributable risk for all-cause mortality.[27,28] American Heart Association (AHA) physical activity guidelines call for 30 minutes of moderate intensity aerobic activity 5 days a week or vigorous intensity aerobic activity 3 days a week.[29] In addition to a reduction in physical disease, there is also evidence that sport participation, including but not restricted to competitive sports, reduces the risk of suicide, a particularly important consideration for the young in whom suicide is the third leading cause of death.[30,31]

However, for individuals with congenital heart diseases, there has never been any documentation of reduced mortality with exercise.[32] It may even be that the opposite is the case; habitual exercise and especially competitive exercise may increase the risk of SCD.[33] This potentially harmful effect is suggested by epidemiological studies in which diseases such as HCM and arrhythmogenic right ventricular dysplasia (ARVD) are overrepresented in athletic populations with SCD compared with the general population.

Acute Triggering of Sudden Cardiac Death With Athletic Activity

Athletic activity may trigger SCD. In large, well-studied populations, vigorous activity temporarily increases the risk of SCD during vigorous exertion and for 30–60 minutes afterwards.[22,23,34,35] In the Physicians Health Study, acute exercise temporally increased the risk of SCD 11-fold in individuals who were habitual exercisers and 74-fold in those who did not regularly exercise.[23] Yet, even with the association of SCD with exertion, habitual exercise lowered all-cause mortality, likely by affecting the risk factors for CAD.

There is little doubt that intense exercise increases sympathetic tone, intracardiac pressures, and cardiac output. These acute changes likely contribute to the increased risk of triggering SCD.[23] In a registry of athletes with implantable cardioverter defibrillators (ICDs), 47 of 68 (69%) ventricular arrhythmias were associated with exercise (Table 108.2).[36]

How exercise triggers SCD is multifactorial and related to hemodynamic and adrenergic stimulation (Fig. 108.4).[35] The triggering

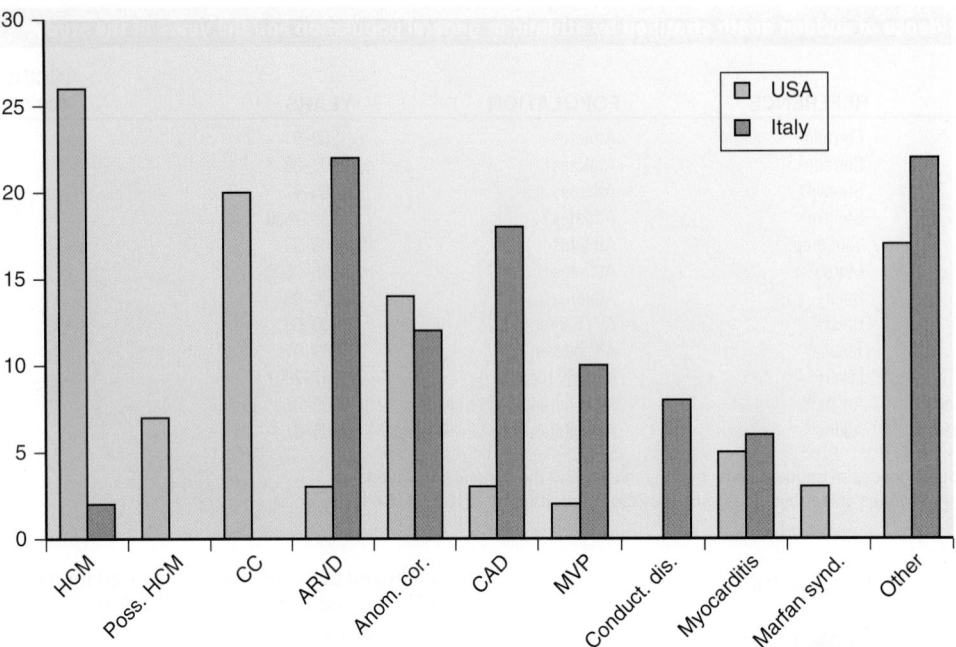

FIGURE 108.2 Underlying heart disease in athletes with sudden cardiac death. The most common abnormality in US athletes is hypertrophic cardiomyopathy (*HCM*), while in Italy it is arrhythmogenic right ventricular dysplasia (*ARVD*). Commotio cordis (*CC*), when it is included in series, also accounts for a significant percentage of deaths. *Anom. cor.,* Anomalous coronary artery; *CAD,* coronary artery disease; *Conduct. dis.,* conduction disease; *MVP,* mitral valve prolapse. (From Link MS, Estes NAM 3rd. Sudden cardiac death in athletes. *Prog Cardiovasc Dis.* 2008;51:44-57. With permission.)

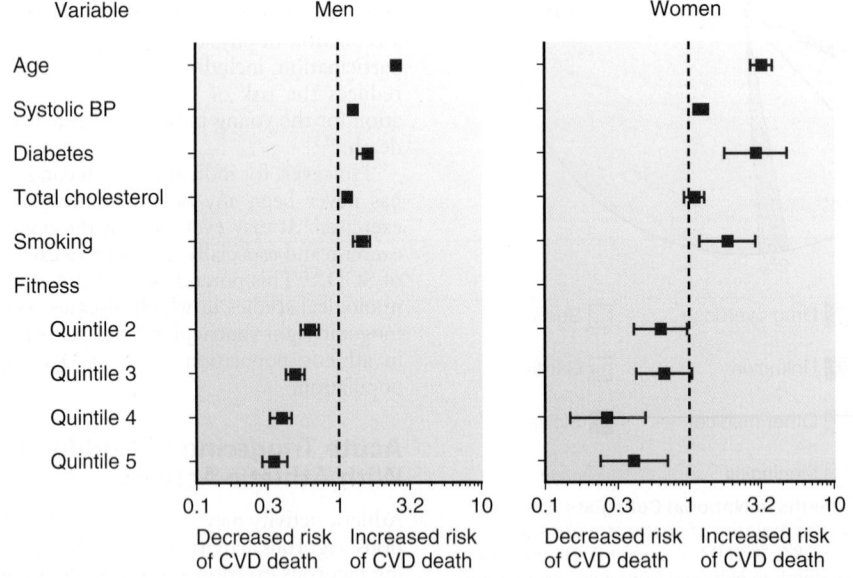

FIGURE 108.3 The benefits of exercise are dose related. In most studies, the more intense the exercise, the greater the health benefits. *BP,* Blood pressure; *CVD,* cardiovascular disease. (From Gupta S, Rohatgi A, Ayers CR, et al. Cardiorespiratory fitness and classification of risk of cardiovascular disease mortality. *Circulation.* 2011;123:1377-1383.)

of SCD with exercise is best documented, but still incompletely understood, in the long QT syndrome (LQTS).[37–39] In LQT1, the most common trigger of syncope and SCD is a state of high sympathetic activation, such as exercise or fright. LQT1 patients, in particular, can experience SCD during swimming. However, individuals with LQT2 and LQT3 have an increased risk of cardiac events not with exercise, but rather with sleep. β-Blocking agents, which block the sympathetic surge with exercise, reduce the risk of arrhythmias in LQT1, but not in LQT3.[37–39]

Patients with catecholaminergic polymorphic ventricular tachycardia (CPVT) also are at an increased risk of arrhythmias with exertion.[40] Arrhythmias are typically provoked at the same level of exertion, and SCD during exertion is typical; β-blockade is particularly effective in this condition. In patients with ARVC, arrhythmias may also be provoked by exercise, and β-blockade may also be effective in decreasing arrhythmias.

Exercise-induced triggering of sudden death is not as well documented in HCM.[41] While there are some data that competitive

TABLE 108.2 Implantable cardioverter defibrillator shocks in an athletic registry of individuals with implantable cardioverter defibrillators[a]

RHYTHM	COMPETITION RELATED[b]	PHYSICAL ACTIVITY RELATED[c]	OTHER	TOTAL (%)
Ventricular tachycardia	22/16	14/11	11/8	47/35 (9)
Ventricular fibrillation	8/6	3/3	10/5	21/14 (4)
Sinus tachycardia	7/6	6/3	1/1	14/10 (3)
Atrial fibrillation	5/3	10/6	3/3	18/12 (3)
Other supraventricular tachycardia	2/2	2/2	0/0	4/4 (1)
Noise	0/0	2/2	6/5	8/7 (2)
T wave oversensing	2/2	1/1	1/1	4/4 (1)
Other	3/2	1/1	1/1	5/4 (1)
TOTAL	49/37 (10)	39/29 (8)	33/24 (6)	121/90 (21)

[a]Note that the majority of shocks are during competition or other physical activity.
[b]Values refer to number of events/number of unique individuals. Percents refer to percent of the study population. Eighteen shocks did not have available implantable cardioverter defibrillator–stored data, so the diagnosis is based on that of the treating physician. Of these, four were ventricular arrhythmia, two were supraventricular, seven were noise, and five were other. Includes competition, postcompetition, and a practice for competition.
[c]Includes physical and postphysical activities.
From Lampert R, Olshansky B, Heidbuchel H, et al. Safety of sports for athletes with implantable cardioverter-defibrillators: results of a prospective, multinational registry. *Circulation.* 2013;127:2021-2030.

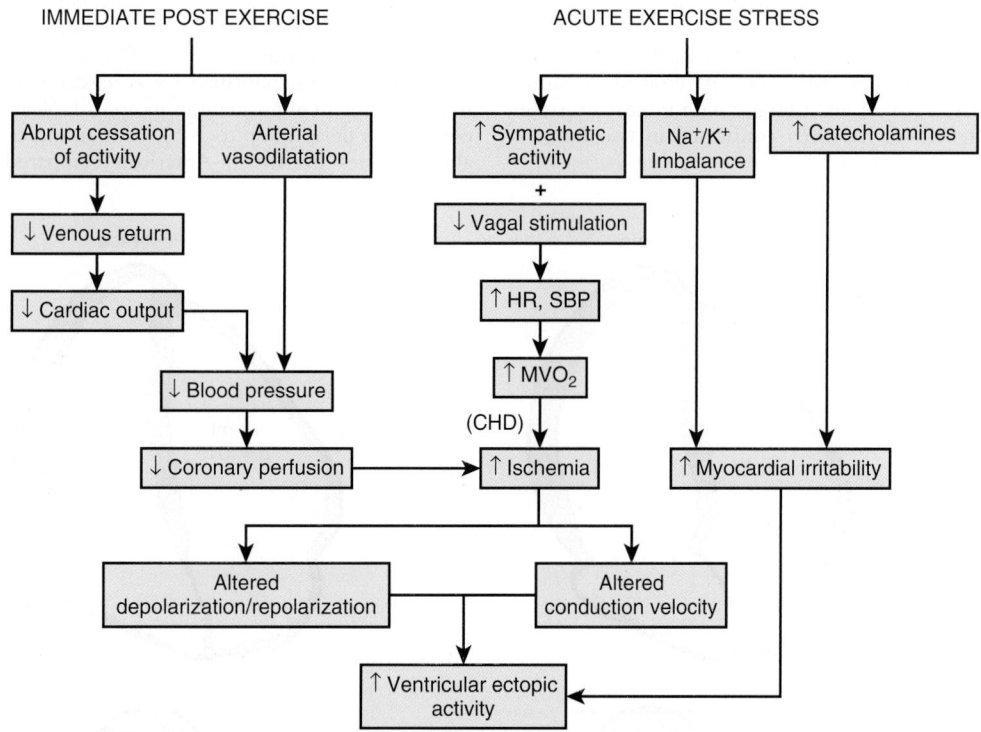

FIGURE 108.4 Exertion- and postexertion-related physiological changes that increase the risk of arrhythmias. *CHD*, Coronary heart disease; *HR*, heart rate; *MVO₂*, myocardial oxygen consumption; *SBP*, systolic blood pressure. (From Thompson PD, Franklin BA, Balady GJ, et al. Exercise and acute cardiovascular events placing the risks into perspective: a scientific statement from the American Heart Association Council on Nutrition, Physical Activity, and Metabolism and the Council on Clinical Cardiology. *Circulation.* 2007;115:2358-2368.)

athletes with HCM are at increased risk for SCD, it is not clear whether this increased risk is due to increased triggering of arrhythmias or remodeling of the substrate, which increases the risk of SCD. Epidemiological data demonstrate that SCD in athletes with HCM occurs most commonly in the afternoon, a time when training and competitive events are held.[42] There are also multiple case reports and descriptions of athletes experiencing SCD during exercise.

Patients with anomalous coronary arteries nearly exclusively die secondary to exercise-induced triggering of arrhythmias,

quite likely mediated via acute coronary ischemia and resultant ventricular arrhythmias. Similarly, acute myocardial ischemia in patients with CAD may trigger arrhythmias. Marfan syndrome is another disease in which exercise can provoke an acute trigger of dissection and sudden death.

Whether sympathetic drive affects the risk of commotio cordis is not entirely clear. In the commotio cordis registry, nearly 60% of the events are during competitive sports. It is extremely unlikely that competitive sports account for 60% of the incidences of being struck in the chest by balls or other objects.

Thus it is possible that the high adrenergic drive associated with competition in commotio cordis also increases the risk of SCD.[43] Regarding Brugada syndrome, myocarditis, and dilated cardiomyopathies, there is currently no evidence that exertion triggers arrhythmias.[38,39]

Potential Adverse Remodeling

Interestingly, there is some evidence that overtraining potentially has adverse cardiovascular effects.[44] Over time, the athlete's heart undergoes physiological adaptation, including ventricular and atrial dilatation, slight increases in wall thickness, and changes in autonomic tone. While these changes are generally thought to be adaptive and reversible, there are accumulating data that these changes may become permanent and maladaptive. There are data that right ventricular (RV) pressures and volumes increase acutely with intense exertion, and these changes may be translated into fibrosis. This RV maladaptation may be particularly relevant in an individual with a genetic predisposition to ARVC. There is increasing evidence that intense exercise increases the likelihood of developing the phenotype of ARVC. RV pressure and volumes increase acutely with intense exertion (Fig. 108.5).[45,46] Repeated and intense exercise and the secondary increases in RV pressures over time, in all likelihood, worsen the phenotype of ARVC, a disease of the adhesive proteins that connect cardiac cells. A mouse ARVC model has shown decreased RV function with intense exercise compared with sedentary controls.[47] More recently, the increased risk of heart failure with intense exercise in individuals with ARVC has been confirmed in two human observational series (Fig. 108.6).[48,49]

With regard to atrial fibrillation (AF), accumulating evidence shows a higher incidence of AF in athletes.[50,51] It is believed that this increased risk is, at least partly, due to the high vagal tone of the athlete, and AF typically initiates during sleep. With deconditioning, episodes of AF may be diminished. Increased left atrial dimensions seen in athletes[52] and subsequent increase in atrial wall strain/stretch may also play a role in the mechanism of AF.[53]

Electrocardiograms in Athletes

Abnormalities in ECGs of athletes are common (Box 108.1).[54] Whether these alterations are due to conditioning effects of sports or underlying cardiac pathology is of critical importance. In the Padua screening series, nearly 10% of the screened individuals had abnormal ECGs.[55] Sinus bradycardias, first-degree heart block, and Mobitz type II Wenckebach are common, as are early repolarization and isolated voltage criteria for left ventricular hypertrophy (LVH).[56] These minor abnormalities are unlikely to be associated with heart disease. However, it is clear that marked abnormalities are far less common.[57] These abnormalities include repolarization abnormalities, pathological Q waves, conduction defects, and ventricular arrhythmias. In another series of 32,652 Italian athletes, the prevalence of ECG abnormalities was 11.8%, which included 2.3% with T wave inversion.[58]

Abnormal ECGs in other populations are increased compared with the series in Italians. In one US series of professional football players, ECG abnormalities were seen in up to 55%, including ST-segment abnormalities in up to 15% and interventricular conduction delay in up to 20%, with an increased prevalence of abnormalities in African-American compared with Caucasian

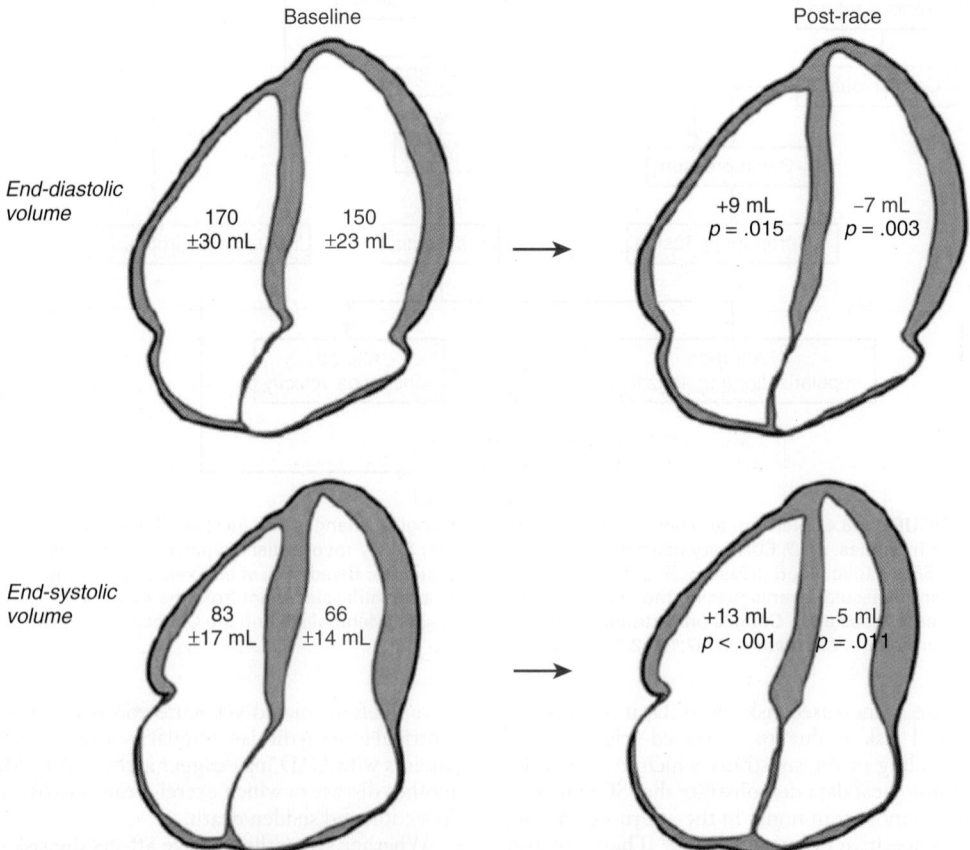

FIGURE 108.5 Acute right ventricular dilatation is observed in athletes. Over time this acute dilatation may be a cause of fibrosis and permanent right ventricular dilatation. (From La Gerche A, Burns AT, Mooney DJ, et al. Exercise-induced right ventricular dysfunction and structural remodeling in endurance athletes. *Eur Heart J.* 2012;33:998-1006.)

players.[59,60] Another US series of professional football players showed that black athletes were more likely than white athletes to have an abnormal ECG (30% vs. 13%, $p < .0001$).[61] In a Dutch series of 428 athletes, 22% had T wave inversion or ST-segment depression, and 7% had right bundle branch block (RBBB) or left bundle branch block (LBBB).[62] In African athletes the incidence of severe ECG abnormalities is markedly increased and includes up to 23% with T wave inversions and up to 13% with RV hypertrophy.[15,16] The reason for the increase in ECG abnormalities

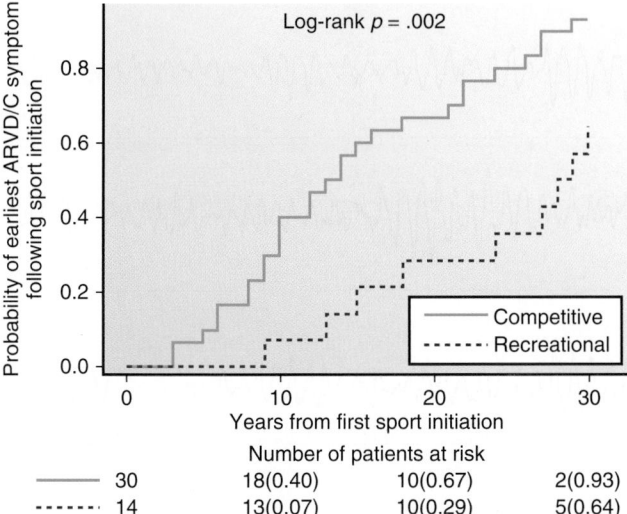

FIGURE 108.6 Among individuals who develop arrhythmogenic right ventricular cardiomyopathy, those who undertake competitive sports develop symptoms at an earlier age. *ARVD/C,* Arrhythmogenic right ventricular dysplasia/cardiomyopathy. (From Ruwald AC, Marcus F, Estes NA 3rd, et al. Association of competitive and recreational sport participation with cardiac events in patients with arrhythmogenic right ventricular cardiomyopathy: results from the North American multidisciplinary study of arrhythmogenic right ventricular cardiomyopathy. *Eur Heart J.* 2015;36:1735-1743.)

BOX 108.1   Classification of abnormalities in athletes' electrocardiograms

Group 1: Common and Training-Related Electrocardiographic Changes
Sinus bradycardia
First-degree atrioventricular block
Incomplete RBBB
Early repolarization
Isolated QRS voltage criteria for left ventricular hypertrophy

Group 2: Uncommon and Training-Unrelated Electrocardiographic Changes
T wave inversion
ST-segment depression
Pathological Q waves
Left atrial enlargement
Left-axis deviation/left anterior hemiblock
Right ventricular hypertrophy
Ventricular preexcitation
Complete LBBB or RBBB
Long or short QT interval
Brugada-like early repolarization

LBBB, Left bundle branch block; *RBBB,* right bundle branch block.
From Corrado D, Pelliccia A, Heidbuchel H, et al. Recommendations for interpretation of 12-lead electrocardiogram in the athlete. *Eur Heart J.* 2010;31:243-259.

---

in other cohorts compared with Italian cohorts is not clear, but clearly has implications for screening athletes with ECGs.

Echocardiographic Changes in Athletes

Adaptive myocardial remodeling is frequent in athletes. These reversible changes include LV dilation and hypertrophy. LV wall dimensions have been shown to increase to up to 14 mm in Italian and British athletes.[63,64] American football players have been demonstrated to have even more marked myocardial hypertrophy of up to 16 mm.[65] In a cohort of 156 asymptomatic National Football League individuals, 23% had evidence of LVH, including 6% with wall thicknesses >14 mm. There was a significant correlation between body weight and LV wall thickness. In a series of British black athletes the incidence of LVH was very similar to that in American football players.[66] While it would be intuitive that larger athletes have thicker hearts, currently there are insufficient data that allow for correlation of weight-based normative LV wall thickness. Differentiation of physiological hypertrophy from HCM can be difficult. In general, physiological hypertrophy is marked by LV dilatation and excellent exercise tolerance, while patients with HCM more commonly demonstrate markedly abnormal ECGs, bizarre patterns of hypertrophy, and left atrial enlargement. Occasionally, deconditioning is necessary to differentiate physiological hypertrophy from HCM.[67,68]

Commotio Cordis

Commotio cordis, sudden death with relatively innocent chest wall impact, was described in the 19th century,[69] but only since 1995 has it become more widely known. Current estimates of incidence range from 10 to 20 events a year.[70,71] Commotio cordis is the second leading cause of sudden death in young athletes in the United States.[1] Commotio cordis is also increasingly being reported in European nations.[72,73]

Based on human and experimental data, commotio cordis is due to immediate ventricular fibrillation (VF) triggered by chest wall impact (Fig. 108.7). A necessary confluence of patient and impact object variables is what underlies the relative rarity of commotio cordis (Fig. 108.8).[74,75] Susceptible patients are young and, typically, male. In the commotio cordis registry the mean age is 15 years and males account for 95% of victims. More compliant chest walls likely explain the predilection for the young age, although the incidence of chest wall impact is also greatly increased in the young compared with individuals aged more than 20 years. There may also be a genetic predisposition or protection from commotio cordis. In an experimental model, approximately 2% of animals were uniquely susceptible to chest impact–induced VF.[76]

The timing of impact is a critical variable in the generation of VF. In an experimental model, only impacts which occurred in a narrow 20-ms time window on the upslope of the T wave caused VF.[77] This time window is similar to but narrower than that of defibrillator shock–induced VF. Impacts outside of this window, but still on the upslope of the T wave, rarely produced sustained VF but did cause nonsustained VF; furthermore, impacts at all other time periods of the cardiac cycle did not produce VF, although they may cause transient heart block, ST-segment elevation, or LBBB. Impact must occur directly over the cardiac silhouette. In humans, minor bruising was found in 22 of 25 and always occurred in the left chest.[78] In an experimental model, only impacts that were directly over the heart caused VF.[79] Glancing blows in this experimental model never caused VF. Impacts with hard spherical objects such as baseballs, softballs, lacrosse balls, and hockey pucks are most commonly reported in commotio cordis. In an experimental model, the smaller the diameter, the more likely the occurrence of VF.[80] Furthermore, in this model, the harder the impact object, the more likely the occurrence of

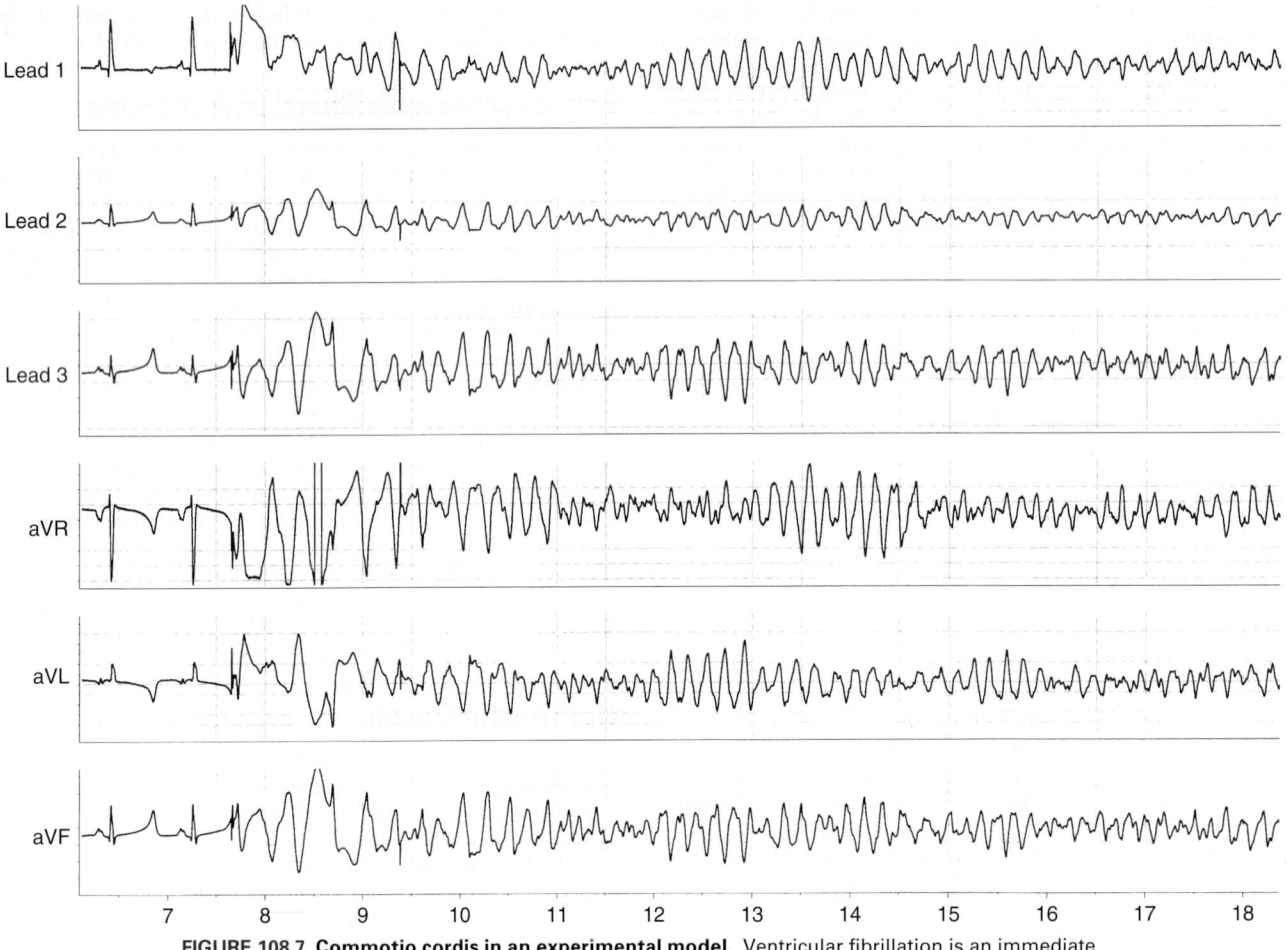

FIGURE 108.7 Commotio cordis in an experimental model. Ventricular fibrillation is an immediate result of an appropriately timed chest wall impact. (From Link MS, Wang PJ, Pandian NG, et al. An experimental model of sudden death due to low-energy chest-wall impact (commotio cordis). *N Engl J Med.* 1998;338:1805-1811.)

VF.[77,81] Commotio cordis has also been reported in nearly every sport and even in nonsport activities due to collision with body parts, such as elbows, fists, and knees.

Impact velocity has been estimated at 40–60 mph with baseballs and well above that with lacrosse balls. In an experimental model, the most deadly velocity was 40 mph.[82] When the baseball impact velocity was 20 mph, VF was never produced. At 30 mph, approximately 30% of impacts caused VF, and at 40 mph nearly 70% of impacts caused it.[82] At impact velocities ≥50 mph, animals less commonly had VF, but now for the first time, structural cardiac damage was seen, including valve rupture, cardiac rupture, and tamponade, suggesting that at these higher velocities, the model was one of cardiac contusion and not commotio cordis.

Resuscitation, originally thought to be rare in commotio, is now routinely being reported, likely due to the increased recognition that VF is the cause of sudden collapse after chest wall impact and the increased penetration of AED as well as knowledge of CPR in the community (Fig. 108.9).[43,83,84]

The risk of commotio cordis can likely be decreased. Coaching and rules should be amended to not allow blocking the ball with the chest in sports. Age-appropriate safety baseballs will decrease the risk of VF due to chest wall impact. Chest protectors have not yet been shown to reduce risk in an experimental model, and in the commotio cordis registry, chest protection was present in one-third of the individuals who suffered commotio during competitive sports.[85,86] In some sports, such as hockey, the arms were lifted, pulling the chest protector upward and thus exposing

the chest.[86] However, in other sports such as lacrosse and baseball, the ball struck the chest protector, which was directly over the heart, still resulting in commotio cordis.

The experimental swine model and a more recently described Langendorff model offer insights into the mechanism of commotio cordis.[87] Commotio cordis is a primary electrical event in which VF is produced directly by a chest wall blow and is not mediated by ischemia, heart block, or cardiac contusion. Similar to other conditions of VF, it is likely that VF requires both a trigger (premature ventricular complex [PVC]) and an abnormal underlying substrate. Both of these requirements are produced by the chest blow, including a premature ventricular contraction caused by direct contact of the ventricular wall and a dispersion of repolarization induced by a marked increase in LV pressure.[87]

LV pressure produced by the chest blow is related to velocity and location of impact, as well as the object hardness and shape. The threshold peak pressure necessary to produce VF is 250–300 mm Hg, and the probability of VF increases with pressure increases up to 600 mm Hg.[79,81,82] Pressure increases beyond that are associated with less VF, but increasing contusions, myocardial rupture, and pericardial tamponade. These pressure thresholds are remarkably conserved across many different experimental protocols including sites of impact,[79] energy of impact,[82] stretch-activated channels,[88] role of autonomic nervous system,[89] and chest wall protectors.[86] The Langendorff model also demonstrated the importance of a critical pressure rise.[87] Pressure rise will increase wall stretch and strain and lead to the activation of

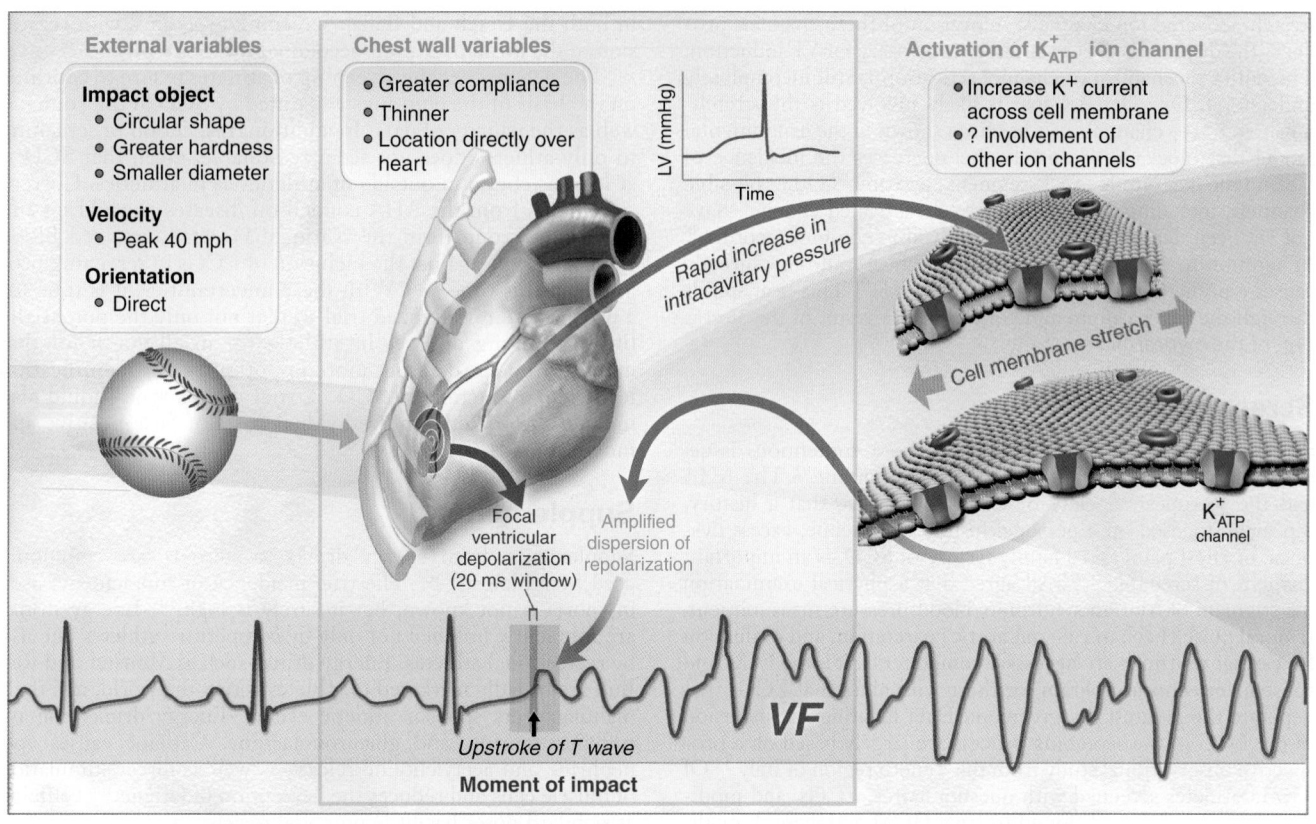

FIGURE 108.8 A necessary confluence of patient and impact object variables is what underlies the relative rarity of commotio cordis. *K⁺_ATP ion channel*, Adenosine triphosphate-sensitive potassium channel; *LV*, left ventricle. (From Link MS, Estes NA. Athletes and arrhythmias. *J Cardiovasc Electrophysiol*. 2010;21:1184-1189.)

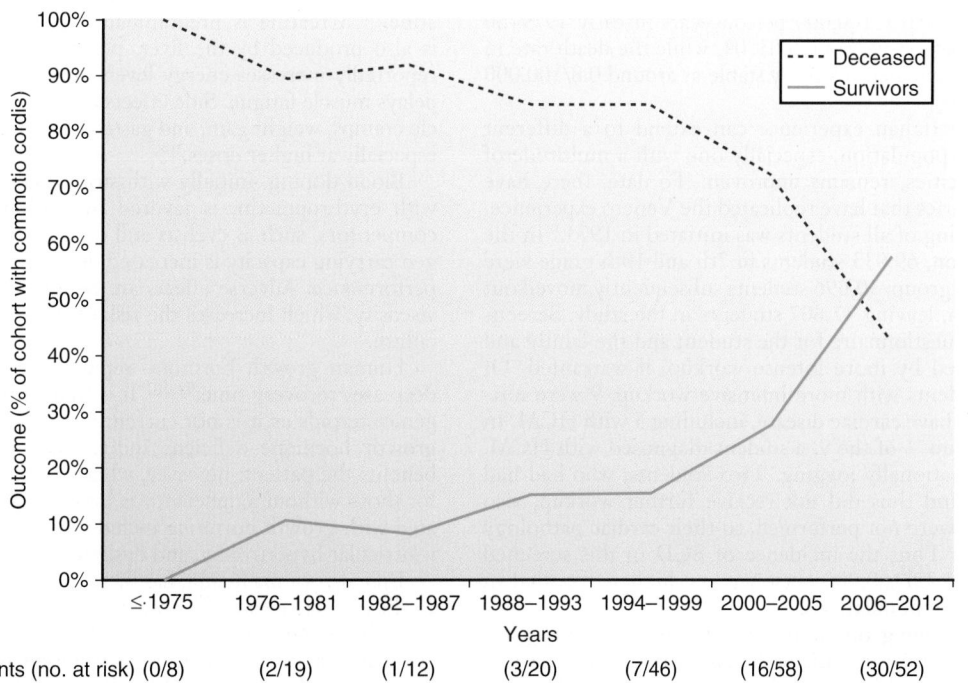

FIGURE 108.9 Resuscitation, originally thought to be rare in commotio, is now routinely reported, likely due to increased recognition that ventricular fibrillation is the cause of sudden collapse after chest wall impact as well as the increased penetration of automated external defibrillator and knowledge of cardiopulmonary resuscitation in the community. (From Maron BJ, Haas TS, Ahluwalia A, Garberich RF, Mark Estes NA 3rd, Link MS. Increasing survival rate from commotio cordis. *Heart Rhythm*. 2013;10:219-223.)

stretch-activated ion channels. Activation of these channels produces the dispersion of repolarization necessary for VF induction. The entire mechanism of channel activation is still incompletely understood. One channel that is likely involved is the stretch-sensitive K^+_{ATP} channel, as it has been shown in the experimental model that blockade of this channel decreases the incidence of VF and the magnitude of ST-segment elevation.[90] Other possible channels, including the calcium stretch–activated channel, have not yet been demonstrated to be involved in commotio cordis.[88] In addition to the altered substrate, the chest wall blow directly causes a premature beat, the first beat of VF.[91] This beat spirals through the myocardium and continues as a result of the alteration of the myocardial substrate.

Screening

Screening young athletes continues to be a contentious issue, even though all agree that screening is important.[92] The AHA and the European Society of Cardiology agree that a history, especially focused on a personal history of syncope, excess dyspnea, or chest pain, and a family history of SCD, is an important element of screening.[93,94] All agree that a physical examination for stigmata of Marfan syndrome, blood pressure measurement, femoral pulse check to rule out aortic coarctation, and evaluation for cardiac murmurs are necessary components. It is the ECG and subsequent echocardiogram for those with abnormal ECGs that generate the greatest disagreement. Data favoring the inclusion of the ECG in the screening process are largely based on a prospective observational study from the Veneto region of Italy.[55] Of 33,735 athletes screened with questionnaires, ECGs, and modified stress test, 22 were found to have HCM and were disqualified from athletics. But these HCM patients only accounted for a small proportion of athletes prohibited from sports. In addition, 238 were disqualified for rhythm and conduction abnormalities, 168 for systemic hypertension, 133 for valvular disease, and 60 for various other diseases. Continued follow-up of this population demonstrated that the incidence of sudden death in athletes decreased from 3.5 per 100,000 person-years in early 1979–80 to 0.4/100,000 person-years in 2003–04, while the death rate in nonathletes has remained relatively stable at around 0.8/100,000 person-years.[3]

Whether the Italian experience can extend to a different or more diverse population, especially one with a multitude of races and ethnicities, remains unproven. To date, there have been no other series that have replicated the Veneto experience. In Japan, screening of all students was initiated in 1973.[8] In the Kagoshima region, 69,033 students in 7th and 10th grade were screened; of this group, 30,696 students subsequently moved out of the study area, leaving 37,807 students in the study. Screening included a questionnaire for the student and the family and an ECG followed by more intense workup, if warranted. Of 1876(2.7%) students with more intensive workup, 9 were ultimately found to have cardiac disease, including 5 with HCM. In a 6-year follow-up, 1 of the 9, a student diagnosed with HCM, died while recreationally jogging. Two students, who had had normal ECGs and thus did not receive further workup, also died. Autopsies were not performed, so their cardiac pathology was not known. Thus the incidence of SCD in this screened population was 1.32/100,000 person-years, higher than that in other nonscreened populations.

An Israeli screening program including an ECG was mandated after an increase in athletic deaths.[5] In a 24-year period, the respective averaged yearly incidence during the decades prior to and after the mandated screening was 2.54 and 2.66 events per 100,000 person-years, respectively (p = .88). Had the 2-year period in which the high number of athletic deaths drove the screening been used as the baseline, the results would have been similar to the Italian series. Thus it is possible that these high baseline rates

in both the Israeli and Italian screening programs, with regression to the mean over time, accounted for the results.[5,95,96]

The debate over the screening of athletes is sure to continue on the basis of the emotions generated by SCD in the young as well as the paucity of data. In addition, restriction of screening to only athletes does not seem reasonable, given that SCD is at least as common outside of athletics as in athletics. Current statements from the AHA council on diseases in children and a working group from the National Heart, Lung, and Blood Institute argue against the inclusion of ECGs in screening programs at this time.[97,98] With these uncertainties, it is time for a prospective randomized trial so that not only the potentially life-threatening diseases in athletes (or in all youth for that matter) are identified but more importantly this identification leads to a reduction of SCD. A trial of this type should also include the societal and individual costs of false positive and indeterminate diagnoses.

Supplements

Supplements, from energy drinks to steroids, are commonly used by athletes.[99–104] The true incidence of supplements used in sports is not known, but it surely is high.[105] Energy drinks are frequently imbibed not only by competitive athletes but also by recreational athletes. Energy drinks such as Monster and Red Bull are broadly marketed to athletes across the world, and their manufacturers sponsor athletic events. Energy drinks contain caffeine, taurine, and glucuronolactone. Caffeine causes epinephrine and acetylcholine release as well as direct stimulation of muscle cells and reduces the perception of fatigue.[106] Caffeine at standard doses has little potential toxicity; however, at higher doses, agitation, tremors, and arrhythmias may result. The benefits of taurine and glucuronolactone are much less clear, as is the potential toxicity. There have been several deaths reputably linked to these energy drinks, and thus several European countries have banned them.[99]

Up to 41% of intercollegiate athletes admit to taking creatine.[107] Creatine is predominantly found in muscle cells but is also produced by the liver, pancreas, and kidneys. Creatine reportedly increases energy levels during anaerobic activity and delays muscle fatigue. Side effects are rare at low doses, but muscle cramps, weight gain, and gastrointestinal distress can be seen, especially at higher doses.[108]

Blood doping, initially with stored blood and more recently with erythropoietin, is favored by prolonged aerobic activity competitors, such as cyclists and cross country skiers.[99–101] Oxygen carrying capacity is increased, leading to improved muscular performance. Adverse effects are related to the increased blood viscosity, which increases the risk of stroke and congestive heart failure.

Human growth hormone reputably increases strength and decreases recovery time.[99–101] It is frequently cycled with androgenic steroids as it is not currently detectable by any means. In growth hormone–deficient individuals, administration clearly benefits the patient; however, whether there is truly any benefit for those without a deficiency is by no means clear. Risks associated with growth hormone include hypertension, cardiomegaly, ventricular hypertrophy, and dyslipidemia.[109]

Ephedra, or ma huang, has increasingly been linked to adverse cardiovascular events.[110] Ephedra is a combination of alkaloids, including ephedrine, pseudoephedrine, norephedrine, and others. Ephedra increases heart rate, blood pressure, and cardiac output.[111] It has been used for the treatment of asthma as well as in weight loss and energy supplements. Multiple cardiovascular toxicities have been associated with ephedra use, including SCD, myocardial infarction, and stroke.[110,112,113] Ephedra has been shown to increase the corrected QT interval (QTc) with a single dose.[114] Although initially protected as a food supplement under the US Dietary Supplemental Health and Education Act of 1994 ruling, the US Congress in 2004 took the extremely unusual course of banning the production and sale of ephedra in the United States.

Androgens have anabolic effects increasing muscle, heart, liver, and kidney mass; decreasing body fat; and stimulating erythropoiesis.[115] They also possess anticatabolic effects, which allow for faster recovery and central nervous system (CNS) effects including increased aggression.[115] With these actions, they are ideal supplements for athletes. They were thus widely utilized by power lifters, track and field athletes, and athletes in any sport in which power and strength were a premium. Androgens have been linked to cardiac toxicity, including myocardial infarction, hypertrophy, and SCD, and to hepatocellular carcinoma, lipid abnormalities, premature closure of growth plates, infertility, and depression.[101] The International Olympic Committee banned the use of androgens in 1975, and most sporting organizations quickly followed, based on not only the toxicity of these agents but also the unfairness they brought to the playing field. Androstenedione was widely used in place of androgens and is believed to be metabolized to androgens. However, a randomized trial and meta-analysis did not show evidence of benefit in athletic performance but did demonstrate that androstenedione lowered high-density lipoproteins (HDLs).[116] It is banned by most sporting organizations. Tetrahydrogestrinone (THG) is a designer steroid solely manufactured for use by athletes. By modification from banned androgens, THG was not detectable by gas chromatography until 2003. It likely has all the beneficial effects of androgens along with the risks.

Resuscitation

Emergency action programs that include ready access to an AED and CPR are critical components of sports programs.[117,118] Emergency action programs encompass not only cardiac events but also trauma, asthma, and any other kind of medical emergency. Data supporting AEDs and early action programs derive from casinos,[119] airlines,[120] and cities.[121] In the much smaller population of athletes, early data showed a dismal survival from cardiac arrest,[122] which appears to be improving, both in athletes[123] and nonathletes.[124] Emergency action plans should include training and certification of athletic trainers and sports participants (a minimum of basic life support and AEDs). Other essential components include prompt access to AEDs, an institutional plan of how to quickly activate the emergency medical service (EMS)

system, integration of the on-site responders and EMS system, and, finally, practice and review of the response plan.[117] All individuals, especially those involved in competitive athletics, should know the basics of resuscitation.[125] It is likely that recognition of SCD and prompt activation of the emergency medical response by all students and athletes would increase the survival rate in SCD.

Sports Participation in Athletes With Heart Disease

Recently the American College of Cardiology (ACC)/AHA updated its Scientific Statement regarding sports participation for athletes with heart disease.[126,127] This comprehensive document included 15 sections on a multitude of topics. While there was little change from the 36th Bethesda document, some important deviations were present. Athletes with congenital LQTS are given the option to participate in competitive sports as long as they are free from symptoms for 3 months and understand and accept some risk.[39] Athletes with definite, probable, or possible ARVC are advised to avoid all competitive and vigorous sports as evidence continues to build regarding the adverse effects of vigorous activity on the expression of this disease.[128] Finally, the restrictions on athletic play with an ICD were loosened. With a frank discussion and understanding of the risks (which include an increased risk of ICD shocks and possibly lead malfunction) and benefits, athletes are permitted to partake in sports.[129]

Conclusion

Athletes with sudden or aborted SCD frequently have an underlying structural heart disease, with the exception of death due to commotio cordis. Exercise, temporally, increases the risk of SCD in an individual with a normal heart and, by implication, also in those with abnormal hearts. Remodeling of the heart by athletics is likely beneficial in individuals with normal hearts and coronary disease, but possibly adverse in individuals with HCM, ARVC, and various other genetic conditions. Screening may be important; however, whether ECGs and modified stress tests are a critical part of the screening and whether all individuals or just athletes should be screened is still unclear. Finally, performance-enhancing agents are widely used, and while randomized-controlled studies will never be performed, it is widely believed that these substances increase the risk of sudden death.

REFERENCES

1. Maron BJ. Sudden death in young athletes. *N Engl J Med.* 2003;349:1064–1075.
2. Van Camp SP, Bloor CM, Mueller FO, Cantu RC, Olsen HG. Nontraumatic sports death in high school and college athletes. *Med Sci Sports Exerc.* 1995;27:641–647.
3. Corrado D, Basso C, Pavei A, Michieli P, Schiavon M, Thiene G. Trends in sudden cardiovascular death in young competitive athletes after implementation of a preparticipation screening program. *JAMA.* 2006;296:1593–1601.
4. Harmon KG, Asif IM, Klossner D, Drezner JA. Incidence of sudden cardiac death in National Collegiate Athletic Association athletes. *Circulation.* 2011;123:1594–1600.
5. Steinvil A, Chundadze T, Zeltser D, et al. Mandatory electrocardiographic screening of athletes to reduce their risk for sudden death: proven fact or wishful thinking? *J Am Coll Cardiol.* 2011;57:1291–1296.
6. Maron BJ, Haas TS, Doerer JJ, Thompson PD, Hodges JS. Comparison of U.S. and Italian experiences with sudden cardiac deaths in young competitive athletes and implications for preparticipation screening strategies. *Am J Cardiol.* 2009;104:276–280.
7. Holst AG, Winkel BG, Theilade J, et al. Incidence and etiology of sports-related sudden cardiac death in Denmark—implications for preparticipation screening. *Heart Rhythm.* 2010;7:1365–1371.

8. Tanaka Y, Yoshinaga M, Anan R, et al. Usefulness and cost effectiveness of cardiovascular screening of young adolescents. *Med Sci Sports Exerc.* 2006;38:2–6.
9. Eckart RE, Scoville SL, Campbell CL, et al. Sudden death in young adults: a 25-year review of autopsies in military recruits. *Ann Intern Med.* 2004;141:829–834.
10. Atkins DL, Everson-Stewart S, Sears GK, et al. Epidemiology and outcomes from out-of-hospital cardiac arrest in children: the Resuscitation Outcomes Consortium Epistry-Cardiac Arrest. *Circulation.* 2009;119:1484–1491.
10a. Howden LM, Meyer JA. Age and sex composition: 2010. <http://www.census.gov/prod/cen2010/briefs/c2010br-03.pdf>; 2010. Accessed 18.08.16.
11. Turk EE, Riedel A, Pueschel K. Natural and traumatic sports-related fatalities: a 10-year retrospective study. *Br J Sports Med.* 2008;42:604–608; discussion 608.
12. Bardai A, Berdowski J, van der Werf C, et al. Incidence, causes, and outcomes of out-of-hospital cardiac arrest in children. A comprehensive, prospective, population-based study in the Netherlands. *J Am Coll Cardiol.* 2011;57:1822–1828.
13. Haissaguerre M, Derval N, Sacher F, et al. Sudden cardiac arrest associated with early repolarization. *N Engl J Med.* 2008;358:2016–2023.
14. Tikkanen JT, Anttonen O, Junttila MJ, et al. Long-term outcome associated with early repolarization on electrocardiography. *N Engl J Med.* 2009;361:2529–2537.

15. Papadakis M, Carre F, Kervio G, et al. The prevalence, distribution, and clinical outcomes of electrocardiographic repolarization patterns in male athletes of African/Afro-Caribbean origin. *Eur Heart J.* 2011;32:2304–2313.
16. Wilson MG, Chatard JC, Carre F, et al. Prevalence of electrocardiographic abnormalities in West-Asian and African male athletes. *Br J Sports Med.* 2012;46:341–347.
17. Derval N, Shah A, Jais P. Definition of early repolarization: a tug of war. *Circulation.* 2011;124:2185–2186.
18. Noseworthy PA, Weiner R, Kim J, et al. Early repolarization pattern in competitive athletes: clinical correlates and the effects of exercise training. *Circ Arrhythm Electrophysiol.* 2011;4:432–440.
19. Tikkanen JT, Junttila MJ, Anttonen O, et al. Early repolarization: electrocardiographic phenotypes associated with favorable long-term outcome. *Circulation.* 2011;123:2666–2673.
20. Puranik R, Chow CK, Duflou JA, Kilborn MJ, McGuire MA. Sudden death in the young. *Heart Rhythm.* 2005;2:1277–1282.
21. Eckart RE, Shry EA, Burke AP, et al. Sudden death in young adults: an autopsy-based series of a population undergoing active surveillance. *J Am Coll Cardiol.* 2011;58:1254–1261.
22. Siscovick DS, Weiss NS, Fletcher RH, Lasky T. The incidence of primary cardiac arrest during vigorous exercise. *N Engl J Med.* 1994;311:874–877.

23. Albert CM, Mittleman MA, Chae CU, Lee IM, Hennekens CH, Manson JE. Triggering of sudden death from cardiac causes by vigorous exertion. *N Engl J Med.* 2000;343:1355–1361.

24. Shiroma EJ, Lee IM. Physical activity and cardiovascular health: lessons learned from epidemiological studies across age, gender, and race/ethnicity. *Circulation.* 2010;122:743–752.

25. Gupta S, Rohatgi A, Ayers CR, et al. Cardiorespiratory fitness and classification of risk of cardiovascular disease mortality. *Circulation.* 2011;123:1377–1383.

26. Sattelmair J, Pertman J, Ding EL, Kohl 3rd HW, Haskell W, Lee IM. Dose response between physical activity and risk of coronary heart disease: a meta-analysis. *Circulation.* 2011;124:789–795.

27. Blair SN. Physical inactivity: the biggest public health problem of the 21st century. *Br J Sports Med.* 2009;43:1–2.

28. Kettunen JA, Kujala UM, Kaprio J, Sarna S. Health of master track and field athletes: a 16-year follow-up study. *Clin J Sport Med.* 2006;16:142–148.

29. Haskell WL, Lee IM, Pate RR, et al. Physical activity and public health: updated recommendation for adults from the American College of Sports Medicine and the American Heart Association. *Med Sci Sports Exerc.* 2007;39:1423–1434.

30. Brown DR, Blanton CJ. Physical activity, sports participation, and suicidal behavior among college students. *Med Sci Sports Exerc.* 2002;34:1087–1096.

31. Taliaferro LA, Rienzo BA, Miller MD, Pigg Jr RM, Dodd VJ. High school youth and suicide risk: exploring protection afforded through physical activity and sport participation. *J Sch Health.* 2008;78:545–553.

32. Maron BJ, Pelliccia A. The heart of trained athletes: cardiac remodeling and the risks of sports, including sudden death. *Circulation.* 2006;114:1633–1644.

33. Corrado D, Basso C, Rizzoli G, Schiavon M, Thiene G. Does sports activity enhance the risk of sudden death in adolescents and young adults? *J Am Coll Cardiol.* 2003;42:1959–1963.

34. Whang W, Manson JE, Hu FB, et al. Physical exertion, exercise, and sudden cardiac death in women. *JAMA.* 2006;295:1399–1403.

35. Thompson PD, Franklin BA, Balady GJ, et al. Exercise and acute cardiovascular events placing the risks into perspective: a scientific statement from the American Heart Association Council on Nutrition, Physical Activity, and Metabolism and the Council on Clinical Cardiology. *Circulation.* 2007;115:2358–2368.

36. Lampert R, Olshansky B, Heidbuchel H, et al. Safety of sports for athletes with implantable cardioverter-defibrillators: results of a prospective, multinational registry. *Circulation.* 2013;127:2021–2030.

37. Kapetanopoulos A, Kluger J, Maron BJ, Thompson PD. The congenital long QT syndrome and implications for young athletes. *Med Sci Sports Exerc.* 2006;38:816–825.

38. Zipes DP, Ackerman MJ, Estes 3rd NA, Grant AO, Myerburg RJ, Van Hare G. Task Force 7: Arrhythmias. 36th Bethesda Conference: Eligibility recommendations for competitive athletes with cardiovascular abnormalities. *J Am Coll Cardiol.* 2005;45:43–52.

39. Ackerman MJ, Zipes DP, Kovacs RJ, Maron BJ. Eligibility and Disqualification Recommendations for Competitive Athletes With Cardiovascular Abnormalities: Task Force 10: The Cardiac Channelopathies: A Scientific Statement From the American Heart Association and American College of Cardiology. *Circulation.* 2015;132:e326–e329.

40. Napolitano C, Priori SG. Diagnosis and treatment of catecholaminergic polymorphic ventricular tachycardia. *Heart Rhythm.* 2007;4:675–678.

41. Maron BJ, Udelson JE, Bonow RO, et al. Eligibility and Disqualification Recommendations for Competitive Athletes With Cardiovascular Abnormalities: Task Force 3: Hypertrophic Cardiomyopathy, Arrhythmogenic Right Ventricular Cardiomyopathy and Other Cardiomyopathies, and Myocarditis: A Scientific Statement From the American Heart Association and American College of Cardiology. *Circulation.* 2015;132:e273–e280.

42. Maron BJ, Semsarian C, Shen WK, et al. Circadian patterns in the occurrence of malignant ventricular tachyarrhythmias triggering defibrillator interventions in patients with hypertrophic cardiomyopathy. *Heart Rhythm.* 2009;6:599–602.

43. Maron BJ, Gohman TE, Kyle SB, Estes 3rd NA, Link MS. Clinical profile and spectrum of commotio cordis. *JAMA.* 2002;287:1142–1146.

44. O'Keefe JH, Patil HR, Lavie CJ, Magalski A, Vogel RA, McCullough PA. Potential adverse cardiovascular effects from excessive endurance exercise. *Mayo Clin Proc.* 2012;87:587–595.

45. La Gerche A, Heidbuchel H. Can intensive exercise harm the heart? You can get too much of a good thing. *Circulation.* 2014;130:992–1002.

46. La Gerche A, Burns AT, Mooney DJ, et al. Exercise-induced right ventricular dysfunction and structural remodelling in endurance athletes. *Eur Heart J.* 2012;33:998–1006.

47. Kirchhof P, Fabritz L, Zwiener M, et al. Age- and training-dependent development of arrhythmogenic right ventricular cardiomyopathy in heterozygous plakoglobin-deficient mice. *Circulation.* 2006;114:1799–1806.

48. Ruwald AC, Marcus F, Estes 3rd NA, et al. Association of competitive and recreational sport participation with cardiac events in patients with arrhythmogenic right ventricular cardiomyopathy: results from the North American multidisciplinary study of arrhythmogenic right ventricular cardiomyopathy. *Eur Heart J.* 2015;36:1735–1743.

49. James CA, Bhonsale A, Tichnell C, et al. Exercise increases age-related penetrance and arrhythmic risk in arrhythmogenic right ventricular dysplasia/cardiomyopathy-associated desmosomal mutation carriers. *J Am Coll Cardiol.* 2013;62:1290–1297.

50. Furlanello F, Bertoldi A, Dallago M, et al. Atrial fibrillation in elite athletes. *J Cardiovasc Electrophysiol.* 1998;9:S63–S68.

51. Grimsmo J, Grundvold I, Maehlum S, Arnesen H. High prevalence of atrial fibrillation in long-term endurance cross-country skiers: echocardiographic findings and possible predictors—a 28-30 years follow-up study. *Eur J Cardiovasc Prev Rehabil.* 2010;17:100–105.

52. Pelliccia A, Culasso F, Di Paolo FM, Maron BJ. Physiologic left ventricular cavity dilatation in elite athletes. *Ann Intern Med.* 1999;130:23–31.

53. Bode F, Sachs F, Franz MR. Tarantula peptide inhibits atrial fibrillation. *Nature.* 2001;409:35–36.

54. Corrado D, Pelliccia A, Heidbuchel H, et al. Recommendations for interpretation of 12-lead electrocardiogram in the athlete. *Eur Heart J.* 2010;31:243–259.

55. Corrado D, Basso C, Schiavon M, Thiene G. Screening for hypertrophic cardiomyopathy in young athletes. *N Engl J Med.* 1998;339:364–369.

56. Corrado D, McKenna WJ. Appropriate interpretation of the athlete's electrocardiogram saves lives as well as money. *Eur Heart J.* 2007;28:1920–1922.

57. Pelliccia A, Zipes DP, Maron BJ. Bethesda Conference #36 and the European Society of Cardiology Consensus Recommendations revisited a comparison of U.S. and European criteria for eligibility and disqualification of competitive athletes with cardiovascular abnormalities. *J Am Coll Cardiol.* 2008;52:1990–1996.

58. Pelliccia A, Culasso F, Di Paolo FM, et al. Prevalence of abnormal electrocardiograms in a large, unselected population undergoing pre-participation cardiovascular screening. *Eur Heart J.* 2007;28:2006–2010.

59. Balady GJ, Cadigan JB, Ryan TJ. Electrocardiogram of the athlete: an analysis of 289 professional football players. *Am J Cardiol.* 1984;53:1339–1343.

60. Choo JK, Abernethy 3rd WB, Hutter Jr AM. Electrocardiographic observations in professional football players. *Am J Cardiol.* 2002;90:198–200.

61. Magalski A, Maron BJ, Main ML, et al. Relation of race to electrocardiographic patterns in elite American football players. *J Am Coll Cardiol.* 2008;51:2250–2255.

62. Bessem B, Groot FP, Nieuwland W. The Lausanne recommendations: a Dutch experience. *Br J Sports Med.* 2009;43:708–715.

63. Whyte GP, George K, Sharma S, et al. The upper limit of physiological cardiac hypertrophy in elite male and female athletes: the British experience. *Eur J Appl Physiol.* 2004;92:592–597.

64. Pelliccia A, Maron BJ, Spataro A, Proschan MA, Spirito P. The upper limit of physiologic cardiac hypertrophy in highly trained elite athletes. *N Engl J Med.* 1991;324:295–301.

65. Abernethy WB, Choo JK, Hutter Jr AM. Echocardiographic characteristics of professional football players. *J Am Coll Cardiol.* 2003;41:280–284.

66. Basavarajaiah S, Boraita A, Whyte G, et al. Ethnic differences in left ventricular remodeling in highly-trained athletes relevance to differentiating physiologic left ventricular hypertrophy from hypertrophic cardiomyopathy. *J Am Coll Cardiol.* 2008;51:2256–2262.

67. Maron BJ. Distinguishing hypertrophic cardiomyopathy from athlete's heart: a clinical problem of increasing magnitude and significance. *Heart.* 2005;91:1380–1382.

68. Maron BJ, Douglas PS, Graham TP, Nishimura RA, Thompson PD. Task Force 1: preparticipation screening and diagnosis of cardiovascular disease in athletes. *J Am Coll Cardiol.* 2005;45:1322–1326.

69. Maron BJ, Doerer JJ, Haas TS, Estes 3rd NA, Link MS. Historical observation on commotio cordis. *Heart Rhythm.* 2006;3:605–606.

70. Maron BJ, Estes 3rd NA. Commotio cordis. *N Engl J Med.* 2010;362:917–927.

71. Link MS, Estes 3rd NA, Maron BJ. Eligibility and Disqualification Recommendations for Competitive Athletes With Cardiovascular Abnormalities: Task Force 13: Commotio Cordis: A Scientific Statement From the American Heart Association and American College of Cardiology. *Circulation.* 2015;132:e339–e342.

72. Solberg E, Embra B, Borjesson M, Herlitz J, Corrado D. Commotio cordis—under-recognized in Europe? a case report and review. *Eur J Cardiovasc Prev Rehabil.* 2011;18:378–383.

73. Maron BJ, Ahluwalia A, Haas TS, Semsarian C, Link MS, Estes 3rd NA. Global epidemiology and demographics of commotio cordis. *Heart Rhythm.* 2011;8:1969–1971.

74. Link MS, Estes NA. Athletes and arrhythmias. *J Cardiovasc Electrophysiol.* 2010;21:1184–1189.

75. Link MS. Commotio cordis: ventricular fibrillation triggered by chest impact-induced abnormalities in repolarization. *Circ Arrhythm Electrophysiol.* 2012;5:425–432.

76. Alsheikh-Ali AA, Madias C, Supran S, Link MS. Marked variability in susceptibility to ventricular fibrillation in an experimental commotio cordis model. *Circulation.* 2010;122:2499–2504.

77. Link MS, Wang PJ, Pandian NG, et al. An experimental model of sudden death due to low-energy chest-wall impact (commotio cordis). *N Engl J Med.* 1998;338:1805–1811.

78. Maron BJ, Poliac LC, Kaplan JA, Mueller FO. Blunt impact to the chest leading to sudden death from cardiac arrest during sports activities. *N Engl J Med.* 1995;333:337–342.

79. Link MS, Maron BJ, VanderBrink BA, et al. Impact directly over the cardiac silhouette is necessary to produce ventricular fibrillation in an experimental model of commotio cordis. *J Am Coll Cardiol.* 2001;37:649–654.

80. Kalin J, Madias C, Alsheikh-Ali AA, Link MS. Reduced diameter spheres increases the risk of chest blow-induced ventricular fibrillation (commotio cordis). *Heart Rhythm.* 2011;8:1578–1581.

81. Link MS, Maron BJ, Wang PJ, Pandian NG, VanderBrink BA, Estes 3rd NA. Reduced risk of sudden death from chest wall blows (commotio cordis) with safety baseballs. *Pediatrics.* 2002;109:873–877.

82. Link MS, Maron BJ, Wang PJ, VanderBrink BA, Zhu W, Estes 3rd NA. Upper and lower limits of vulnerability to sudden arrhythmic death with chest-wall impact (commotio cordis). *J Am Coll Cardiol.* 2003;41:99–104.

83. Link MS, Maron BJ, Stickney RE, et al. Automated external defibrillator arrhythmia detection in a model of cardiac arrest due to commotio cordis. *J Cardiovasc Electrophysiol.* 2003;14:83–87.

84. Maron BJ, Haas TS, Ahluwalia A, Garberich RF. Mark Estes NA 3rd, Link MS. Increasing survival rate from commotio cordis. *Heart Rhythm.* 2013;10:219–223.

85. Doerer JJ, Haas TS, Estes 3rd NA, Link MS, Maron BJ. Evaluation of chest barriers for protection against sudden death due to commotio cordis. *Am J Cardiol.* 2007;99:857–859.

86. Weinstock J, Maron BJ, Song C, Mane PP, Estes 3rd NA, Link MS. Failure of commercially available chest wall protectors to prevent sudden cardiac death induced by chest wall blows in an experimental model of commotio cordis. *Pediatrics.* 2006;117:e656–e662.

87. Bode F, Franz MR, Wilke I, Bonnemeier H, Schunkert H, Wiegand UK. Ventricular fibrillation induced by stretch pulse: implications for sudden death due to commotio cordis. *J Cardiovasc Electrophysiol.* 2006;17:1011–1017.

88. Garan AR, Maron BJ, Wang PJ, Estes 3rd NA, Link MS. Role of streptomycin-sensitive stretch-activated channel in chest wall impact induced sudden death (commotio cordis). *J Cardiovasc Electrophysiol.* 2005;16:433–438.

89. Stout CW, Maron BJ, Vanderbrink BA, Estes 3rd NA, Link MS. Importance of the autonomic nervous system in an experimental model of commotio cordis. *Med Sci Monit.* 2007;13:BR11–15.

90. Link MS, Wang PJ, VanderBrink BA, et al. Selective activation of the K(+)(ATP) channel is a mechanism by which sudden death is produced by low-energy chest-wall impact (commotio cordis). *Circulation.* 1999;100:413–418.

91. Alsheikh-Ali AA, Akelman C, Madias C, Link MS. Endocardial mapping of ventricular fibrillation in commotio cordis. *Heart Rhythm.* 2008;5:1355–1356.

92. Maron BJ, Levine BD, Washington RL, Baggish AL, Kovacs RJ, Maron MS. Eligibility and Disqualification Recommendations for Competitive Athletes With Cardiovascular Abnormalities: Task Force 2: Preparticipation Screening for Cardiovascular Disease in Competitive Athletes: A Scientific Statement From the American Heart Association and American College of Cardiology. *Circulation.* 2015;132:e267–e272.

93. Maron BJ, Thompson PD, Ackerman MJ, et al. Recommendations and considerations related to preparticipation screening for cardiovascular abnormalities in competitive athletes: 2007 update: a scientific statement from the American Heart Association Council on Nutrition, Physical Activity, and Metabolism: endorsed by the American College of Cardiology Foundation. *Circulation.* 2007;115:1643–1455.

94. Pelliccia A, Fagard R, Bjørnstad HH, et al. Recommendations for competitive sports participation in athletes with cardiovascular disease: a consensus document from the Study Group of Sports Cardiology of the Working Group of Cardiac Rehabilitation and Exercise Physiology and the Working Group of Myocardial and Pericardial Diseases of the European Society of Cardiology. *Eur Heart J.* 2005;26:1422–1445.

108

95. Suissa S. Immortal time bias in pharmaco-epidemiology. *Am J Epidemiol.* 2008;167:492–499.

96. van Walraven C, Davis D, Forster AJ, Wells GA. Time-dependent bias was common in survival analyses published in leading clinical journals. *J Clin Epidemiol.* 2004;57:672–682.

97. Mahle WT, Sable CA, Matherne PG, Gaynor JW, Gewitz MH. Key concepts in the evaluation of screening approaches for heart disease in children and adolescents: a science advisory from the American Heart Association. *Circulation.* 2012;125:2796–2801.

98. Kaltman JR, Thompson PD, Lantos J, et al. Screening for sudden cardiac death in the young: report from a National Heart, Lung, and Blood Institute working group. *Circulation.* 2011;123:1911–1918.

99. Dhar R, Stout CW, Link MS, Homoud MK, Weinstock J, Estes 3rd NA. Cardiovascular toxicities of performance-enhancing substances in sports. *Mayo Clin Proc.* 2005;80:1307–1315.

100. Bowers LD. Abuse of performance-enhancing drugs in sport. *Ther Drug Monit.* 2002;24:178–181.

101. Calfee R, Fadale P. Popular ergogenic drugs and supplements in young athletes. *Pediatrics.* 2006;117:e577–e589.

102. Duchan E, Patel ND, Feucht C. Energy drinks: a review of use and safety for athletes. *Phys Sportsmed.* 2010;38:171–179.

103. Estes 3rd NA, Kovacs RJ, Baggish AL, Myerburg RJ. Eligibility and Disqualification Recommendations for Competitive Athletes With Cardiovascular Abnormalities: Task Force 11: Drugs and Performance-Enhancing Substances: A Scientific Statement From the American Heart Association and American College of Cardiology. *J Am Coll Cardiol.* 2015;66:2429–2433.

104. Estes 3rd NA, Kovacs RJ, Baggish AL, Myerburg RJ. Eligibility and Disqualification Recommendations for Competitive Athletes With Cardiovascular Abnormalities: Task Force 11: Drugs and Performance-Enhancing Substances: A Scientific Statement From the American Heart Association and American College of Cardiology. *Circulation.* 2015;132:e330–e333.

105. Alaranta A, Alaranta H, Holmila J, Palmu P, Pietila K, Helenius I. Self-reported attitudes of elite athletes towards doping: differences between type of sport. *Int J Sports Med.* 2006;27:842–846.

106. Bell DG, McLellan TM. Exercise endurance 1, 3, and 6 h after caffeine ingestion in caffeine users and nonusers. *J Appl Physiol.* 2002;93:1227–1234.

107. Metzl JD, Small E, Levine SR, Gershel JC. Creatine use among young athletes. *Pediatrics.* 2001;108:421–425.

108. Bohn AM, Betts S, Schwenk TL. Creatine and other nonsteroidal strength-enhancing aids. *Curr Sports Med Rep.* 2002;1:239–245.

109. Meyers DE, Cuneo RC. Controversies regarding the effects of growth hormone on the heart. *Mayo Clin Proc.* 2003;78:1521–1526.

110. Samenuk D, Link MS, Homoud MK, et al. Adverse cardiovascular events temporally associated with ma huang, an herbal source of ephedrine. *Mayo Clin Proc.* 2002;77:12–16.

111. Jacobs I, Pasternak H, Bell DG. Effects of ephedrine, caffeine, and their combination on muscular endurance. *Med Sci Sports Exerc.* 2003;35:987–994.

112. Shekelle PG, Hardy ML, Morton SC, et al. Efficacy and safety of ephedra and ephedrine for weight loss and athletic performance: a meta-analysis. *JAMA.* 2003;289:1537–1545.

113. Haller CA, Benowitz NL. Adverse cardiovascular and central nervous system events associated with dietary supplements containing ephedra alkaloids. *N Engl J Med.* 2000;343:1833–1838.

114. McBride BF, Karapanos AK, Krudysz A, Kluger J, Coleman CI, White CM. Electrocardiographic and hemodynamic effects of a multicomponent dietary supplement containing ephedra and caffeine: a randomized controlled trial. *JAMA.* 2004;291:216–221.

115. Kutscher EC, Lund BC, Perry PJ. Anabolic steroids: a review for the clinician. *Sports Med.* 2002;32:285–296.

116. King DS, Sharp RL, Vukovich MD, et al. Effect of oral androstenedione on serum testosterone and adaptations to resistance training in young men: a randomized controlled trial. *JAMA.* 1999;281:2020–2028.

117. Drezner JA, Courson RW, Roberts WO, Mosesso Jr VN, Link MS, Maron BJ. Inter-association task force recommendations on emergency preparedness and management of sudden cardiac arrest in high school and college athletic programs: a consensus statement. *Heart Rhythm.* 2007;4:549–565.

118. Link MS, Berkow LC, Kudenchuk PJ, et al. Part 7: Adult Advanced Cardiovascular Life Support: 2015 American Heart Association Guidelines Update for Cardiopulmonary Resuscitation and Emergency Cardiovascular Care. *Circulation.* 2015;132:S444–S464.

119. Valenzuela TD, Roe DJ, Nichol G, Clark LL, Spaite DW, Hardman RG. Outcomes of rapid defibrillation by security officers after cardiac arrest in casinos. *N Engl J Med.* 2000;343:1206–1209.

120. Page RL, Joglar JA, Kowal RC, et al. Use of automated external defibrillators by a U.S. airline. *N Engl J Med.* 2000;343:1210–1216.

121. Link MS, Atkins DL, Passman RS, et al. Part 6: electrical therapies: automated external defibrillators, defibrillation, cardioversion, and pacing: 2010 American Heart Association Guidelines for Cardiopulmonary Resuscitation and Emergency Cardiovascular Care. *Circulation.* 2010;122:S706–S719.

122. Drezner JA, Rogers KJ. Sudden cardiac arrest in intercollegiate athletes: detailed analysis and outcomes of resuscitation in nine cases. *Heart Rhythm.* 2006;3:755–759.

123. Drezner JA, Chun JS, Harmon KG, Derminer L. Survival trends in the United States following exercise-related sudden cardiac arrest in the youth: 2000-2006. *Heart Rhythm.* 2008;5:794–799.

124. Aufderheide TP, Yannopoulos D, Lick CJ, et al. Implementing the 2005 American Heart Association Guidelines improves outcomes after out-of-hospital cardiac arrest. *Heart Rhythm.* 2010;7:1357–1362.

125. Berger S, Utech L, Hazinski MF. Lay rescuer automated external defibrillator programs for children and adolescents. *Pediatr Clin North Am.* 2004;51:1463–1478.

126. Maron BJ, Zipes DP, Kovacs RJ. Eligibility and Disqualification Recommendations for Competitive Athletes With Cardiovascular Abnormalities: Preamble, Principles, and General Considerations: A Scientific Statement From the American Heart Association and American College of Cardiology. *Circulation.* 2015;132:e256–e261.

127. Levine BD, Baggish AL, Kovacs RJ, Link MS, Maron MS, Mitchell JH. Eligibility and Disqualification Recommendations for Competitive Athletes With Cardiovascular Abnormalities: Task Force 1: Classification of Sports: Dynamic, Static, and Impact: A Scientific Statement From the American Heart Association and American College of Cardiology. *J Am Coll Cardiol.* 2015;66:2350–2355.

128. Maron BJ, Udelson JE, Bonow RO, et al. Eligibility and Disqualification Recommendations for Competitive Athletes With Cardiovascular Abnormalities: Task Force 3: Hypertrophic Cardiomyopathy, Arrhythmogenic Right Ventricular Cardiomyopathy and Other Cardiomyopathies, and Myocarditis: A Scientific Statement From the American Heart Association and American College of Cardiology. *J Am Coll Cardiol.* 2015;66:2362–2371.

129. Zipes DP, Link MS, Ackerman MJ, Kovacs RJ, Myerburg RJ, Estes 3rd NA. Eligibility and Disqualification Recommendations for Competitive Athletes With Cardiovascular Abnormalities: Task Force 9: Arrhythmias and Conduction Defects: A Scientific Statement From the American Heart Association and American College of Cardiology. *J Am Coll Cardiol.* 2015;66:2412–2423.

109 Arrhythmias in the Pediatric Population

Edward P. Walsh

Unique Aspects of Pediatric Electrophysiology

Although the basic principles of cardiac electrophysiology (EP) apply broadly across the age spectrum, there are several distinctive characteristics of the pediatric population that deserve emphasis. These begin at the cellular level, with differences in the action potential and calcium handling by immature myocytes, and extend to the gross clinical level, with technical challenges during therapeutic interventions in small hearts. All aspects of pediatric arrhythmia management can be further complicated by the presence of congenital heart defects.

Electrophysiology of the Developing Heart

Our understanding of developmental EP is evolving rapidly but is still far from complete.[1,2] It is generally agreed that the primitive heart tube begins to contract in a peristaltic fashion from its atrial to ventricular poles by about 20–25 days of gestational age and that the cells generating this activity are distributed as several discrete rings along the length of the tube, where action potentials can be recorded with a slow initial upstroke. As the heart tube changes configuration during the process of ventricular looping, a portion of the ring at the atrial pole is retained to form the sinoatrial node, and portions of the other rings combine in a complex fashion to form the specialized atrioventricular (AV) conduction tissues. By about 5 weeks of gestational age, an intact AV conduction axis is established in the normal fetal heart. It is tempting to speculate that failure of apoptosis or failure of insulation for some of the electrically active cells from these various rings may contribute to focal automatic tachycardias[3] later in life (e.g., ectopic atrial tachycardia [EAT] or outflow tract ventricular tachycardia [VT]), although this link has not been established with certainty.

Electrical behavior of young heart cells differs somewhat from that of fully mature myocytes. The most obvious features are enhanced spontaneous depolarization of natural pacemaker cells to account for faster sinus rates and shorter refractory periods to accommodate these rates. Maximum diastolic potentials are also slightly reduced, as are transient outward rectifier potassium currents.[4] These subtle differences are usually not of practical importance during clinical evaluation and treatment, but they do confirm that cellular properties change with age, which may explain why certain tachyarrhythmias presenting in the fetus and newborn (e.g., chaotic atrial rhythm and accelerated ventricular rhythm) will frequently resolve spontaneously over the first year or so of life, while other arrhythmias (e.g., VT in Brugada syndrome) often do not fully manifest until older ages. Perhaps the most therapeutically relevant difference between infant and mature myocytes relates to cell infrastructure, specifically the sarcoplasmic reticulum, which is relatively underdeveloped in the fetus and newborn.[5] This can make infants more reliant on extracellular calcium for myocyte contraction, and this is the likely explanation for past reports of hemodynamic collapse[6] when some young patients received intravenous verapamil (now contraindicated in children under the age of 1 year).

Maturational changes also occur at the gross level of the specialized conduction tissues. It is known from a histopathological study that the posterior extensions off the compact AV node start out very stubby but elongate progressively between birth and teenage years,[7] which may clarify why AV nodal reentrant tachycardia (AVNRT) is relatively uncommon during infancy and early childhood. Similarly, atrioventricular accessory pathways (APs), or the tissues surrounding these pathways, can change during the early years of life. More than 30% of newborns with manifested preexcitation and episodes of AV reentrant tachycardia will have a spontaneous resolution of the delta wave and will be completely noninducible with aggressive transesophageal atrial stimulation by their first birthday.[8] This may relate to ingrowth of fibrous tissue along the AV valve ring or intrinsic changes in the pathway itself, but in either event, the chance for spontaneous resolution has a strong influence on how pathway-mediated tachycardias are managed in very young patients.

Influence of Congenital Heart Disease

The embryological accidents causing congenital heart disease (CHD) can interfere with development of the sinus node and AV conduction tissues. The most extreme examples involve abnormalities of atrial situs with discordant connections of the atria and ventricles (so-called heterotaxy syndromes). Heterotaxy can be divided into the subcategories of polysplenia (sometimes referred to as "bilateral left-sidedness") and asplenia (sometimes referred to as "bilateral right-sidedness"). In the former condition, a true sinus node may be absent and complete heart block is common. In the latter condition, there may actually be two separate sinus nodes,[9] and occasionally the AV conduction system will be duplicated in an arrangement referred to as "twin AV nodes" that can support a variety of reentrant tachycardias.[10]

Even some of the less severe forms of CHD can have associated abnormalities of the AV conduction tissues. One such condition is "congenitally corrected" transposition of the great arteries (L-TGA), where the compact node develops outside of Koch's triangle in an unusual anterior location near the base of the right atrial appendage. This displaced node is often feeble[11] and can deteriorate over time, so that complete heart block is seen in as many as 5% of these patients at birth and in more than 25% by adulthood. Displacement of the AV node also occurs in patients with endocardial cushion defects (i.e., primum atrial septal defects or complete AV canal defects). These hearts do not have a triangle of Koch, and the compact node is consequently displaced in a posterior direction beneath the mouth of the coronary sinus.[12] Similar to L-TGA, AV nodal function can be suboptimal in endocardial cushion defects, with complete heart block at birth in some individuals and a significant risk of surgically induced block following repairs. Congenitally impaired AV nodal function can also be observed in some simple cases of atrial septal defect among patients with Holt-Oram syndrome,[13] an autosomal dominant disorder causing cardiac and upper-limb abnormalities that involves a mutation on the *TBX5* gene.

The incidence of APs in most forms of CHD is not substantially higher than that in the general population, with the notable exceptions of Ebstein anomaly and L-TGA (which can have an Ebstein-like malformation of the left-sided tricuspid valve). Patients with Ebstein anomaly have a greatly elevated risk of APs,[14] in the range of 20%–30%. These can include both AV and atriofascicular connections, which tend to be localized to the region where the tricuspid valve is most abnormal. When preexcitation is present in a patient with Ebstein anomaly, the chances of that patient having multiple pathways may be as high as 50%.[15] Management of these abnormal connections can become a significant challenge in the care of Ebstein patients.[16]

Apart from congenital conduction abnormalities, the hemodynamic stress of CHD and the tissue injury resulting from surgical repairs can have a negative long-term impact on rhythm status. Fibrosis and hypertrophy, in combination with conduction barriers along incisional scars and patches, combine to create a substrate that is conducive to the development of macroreentrant tachycardias.[17] These occur most commonly at the atrial level, especially after surgery that involves extensive atrial baffling, such as the Mustard or Senning procedures for transposition of the great arteries or the Fontan operation for single ventricle. Macroreentrant VTs can also develop in certain CHD lesions, most notably tetralogy of Fallot. Bradyarrhythmias may occur as a consequence of direct surgical trauma to the sinus node and/or the AV conduction tissues.

Autonomic Influences

The intrinsic rate of sinus node discharge in children is naturally faster than that in adults, but it is also noteworthy that autonomic modulation of sinus node activity can result in rather dramatic extremes of rate among young patients that must be differentiated from pathological conditions. Sinus tachycardia can exceed 220 beats/min in a stressed infant, whereas abrupt surges in vagal tone can result in prolonged asystolic pauses lasting more than 30 seconds in some children with an otherwise normal heart.[18] This relative hypersensitivity to autonomic influence is reflected in a high degree of sinus arrhythmia at normal resting rates as well as a strong predisposition to neutrally medicated syncope,[19] both of which become attenuated by adulthood.

Tachycardia-Induced Cardiomyopathy in Children

Some incessant forms of tachycardia can result in severe degrees of ventricular dysfunction. Animal models of this phenomenon[20] have demonstrated that rapid pacing for extended periods will reliably depress left ventricular (LV) performance and that this depression will reverse upon cessation of pacing, although the cellular mechanism underlying the process is still not entirely clear. Tachycardia-induced cardiomyopathy is well described in all age groups and can be caused by a variety of arrhythmia mechanisms,[21] but among pediatric patients, the most common culprits are EAT, the permanent form of junctional reciprocating tachycardia (PJRT), and focal automatic VT.[22] Because the heart rate associated with these disorders is only modestly elevated above expected sinus rates for a child and because young patients can remain relatively asymptomatic until late into the course of ventricular dysfunction, tachycardia may go unrecognized for some time. Consequently, many of these children are

ill with congestive heart failure at presentation. It is imperative that incessant tachycardia always be considered in the differential diagnosis of any young patient with new onset cardiomyopathy and that the electrocardiogram (ECG) is always scrutinized for these curable rhythm disorders.

Hereditary Arrhythmias

Inherited channelopathies and myopathies are discussed in detail elsewhere in this textbook, and their major pediatric features will be reviewed briefly later within this chapter, but it should be stressed here that many of these conditions can cause life-threatening arrhythmias during infancy and childhood and that family screening of young relatives is a required exercise whenever an index case is identified. Box 109.1 provides a partial list of the hereditary disorders that are most relevant to the pediatric population. Most of these are capable of causing serious symptoms at young ages, and in fact, channelopathies have been implicated[23] as the cause for some cases of sudden infant death syndrome (SIDS). Brugada syndrome and arrhythmogenic right ventricular (RV) cardiomyopathy (ARVC) may not be expressed phenotypically until adulthood, although there are well-documented anecdotes of malignant presentations earlier in life.

Size/Age/Anatomical Considerations

Small size is the most distinguishing feature of a pediatric patient, and it greatly impacts all aspects of arrhythmia treatment. Antiarrhythmic medication doses must be titrated carefully on the basis of body weight or surface area (Table 109.1), and oral agents that are not commercially available in the solution form must be compounded to exacting specifications when prescribed for young children who cannot swallow standard pills or capsules.

BOX 109.1 Hereditary conditions causing arrhythmias in pediatric patients

Long QT (LQT) syndromes
- LQT 1
- LQT 2
- LQT 3
- LQT 7 (Andersen-Tawil syndrome)
- LQT 8 (Timothy syndrome)
- Other rare LQT forms

Catecholaminergic polymorphic ventricular tachycardia
Brugada syndrome
Arrhythmogenic right ventricular cardiomyopathy
Short QT syndrome
Hypertrophic cardiomyopathy (errors of metabolism)
- Pompe disease
- Danon disease
- Hurler syndrome
- Hunter syndrome
- Glycogen storage disease
- Barth syndrome

Hypertrophic cardiomyopathy (isolated familial forms)
- β-Myosin heavy chain
- PRKAG2 with Wolff-Parkinson-White syndrome
- Other sarcomeric genes

Hypertrophic cardiomyopathy (other)
- Noonan syndrome
- Friedreich ataxia

Familial dilated cardiomyopathy
Left ventricular noncompaction
Muscular dystrophy
Holt-Oram syndrome

TABLE 109.1 Recommended dosages for commonly used antiarrhythmic drugs in children

CLASS	DRUG	ACUTE INTRAVENOUS DOSAGE	CHRONIC ORAL DOSAGE
IA	Procainamide	5–12 mg/kg load over 30 min, then infuse 20–50 **micro**grams/kg/min	
IB	Lidocaine	1 mg/kg rapid bolus, then infuse 20–50 **micro**grams/kg/min	
IB	Mexiletine		5–15 mg/kg/d (three divided doses)
IC	Flecainide		<6 mo: 50 mg/**m²**/d (three divided doses)
			>6 mo: 80 mg/**m²**/d (three divided doses)
II	Propranolol		1–3 mg/kg/d (three divided doses)
II	Nadolol		0.5–1.0 mg/kg/d (once daily dose)
II	Esmolol	100–500 **micro**grams/kg load over 1 min, then infuse 50–200 **micro**grams/kg/min	
III	Sotalol		80 mg/**m²**/d (two or three divided doses) (consult nomogram if age < 2 years)
III	Amiodarone	5 mg/kg load over 60 min, then infuse 5–10 **micro**grams/kg/min	10 mg/kg/d (two divided doses) × 10 days, then 5 mg/kg/d maintenance
IV	Verapamil	0.1 mg/kg rapid bolus. Do not use in patients under the age of 1 year.	4–8 mg/kg/d (three divided doses)
---	Adenosine	0.1 mg/kg rapid bolus. May repeat with 0.2 mg/kg rapid bolus.	
---	Magnesium	10–25 mg/kg magnesium sulfate slow infusion over 30 min	
---	Atropine	0.01–0.02 mg/kg rapid bolus. Maximum dose 0.4 mg, minimum dose 0.1 mg.	
---	Isoproterenol	0.01–0.10 **micro**grams/kg/min infusion	

Notes:
1. Size-adjusted dosages in older children should never exceed recommended adult dosage.
2. Be alert for milligram (mg) vs. microgram (μg) dosing (micrograms are noted in **bold**).
3. Be alert for body weight (kg) vs. body surface area (m²) dosing (m² is noted in **bold**).
4. Sotalol dosing for patients under the age of 2 years requires adjustment according to a US Food and Drug Administration nomogram.

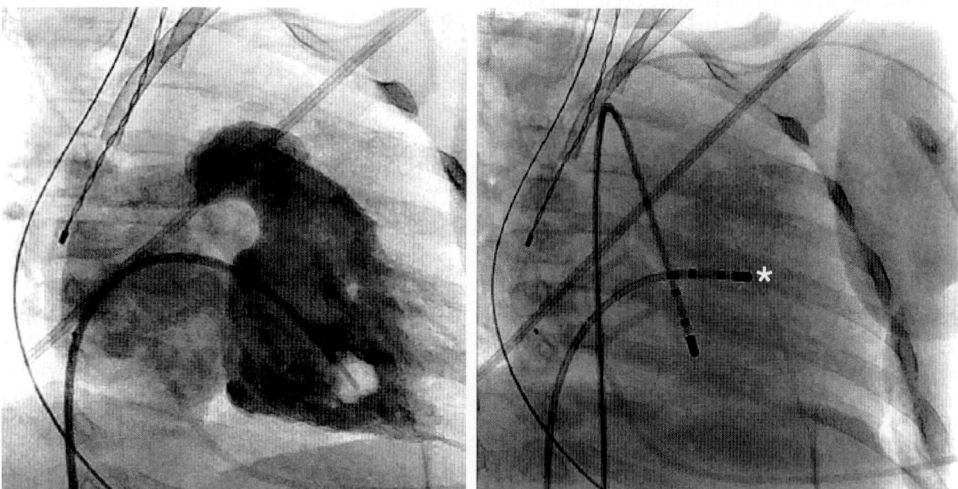

FIGURE 109.1 Ablation in a 6-month-old with incessant ventricular tachycardia (VT) arising near the proximal right bundle branch, leading to cardiomyopathy. *Left panel:* right ventricular angiogram for orientation. *Right panel:* mapping involved two 5-Fr catheters; one, retrograde along the left side of the septum and the other, transvenous into the right ventricle, with an *asterisk* marking the site of successful VT elimination. Ventricular function recovered within 2 weeks of VT elimination.

Techniques used during catheterization for diagnostic testing and ablation must also be tailored to patient age/size (Fig. 109.1). Sedation must be sufficient to quiet a child's anxiety while insuring comfort and immobility during critical step of a procedure, oftentimes necessitating a general anesthetic. Vascular access must be planned carefully within the constraints of a small vessel caliber, downsizing to 4–5-French catheters when necessary and economizing on catheter number[24] by combining functions. During ablation procedures, compulsive mapping is required to minimize unproductive lesions, and extreme caution is naturally required when ablating within or near the reduced dimensions of Koch's triangle in a small heart. Cryoablation has been adopted at many pediatric centers for targets very near the

normal conduction tissues,[25] tolerating the trade-off of higher recurrence rate for improved safety in such cases. Finally, radiation exposure must be minimized in young patients who remain at risk for stochastic tissue injury over many decades following an invasive procedure. Electroanatomical mapping has largely eliminated the need for fluoroscopy[26] and has now been adopted by nearly all pediatric laboratories for ablation of even simple arrhythmia substrates.[27] More detailed discussion of ablation in pediatric patients can be found in Chapter 130.

Pacemaker and implantable cardioverter defibrillator (ICD) procedures are likewise influenced by patient size. Very young children may not be candidates for transvenous hardware and often require epicardial systems until they have grown sufficiently

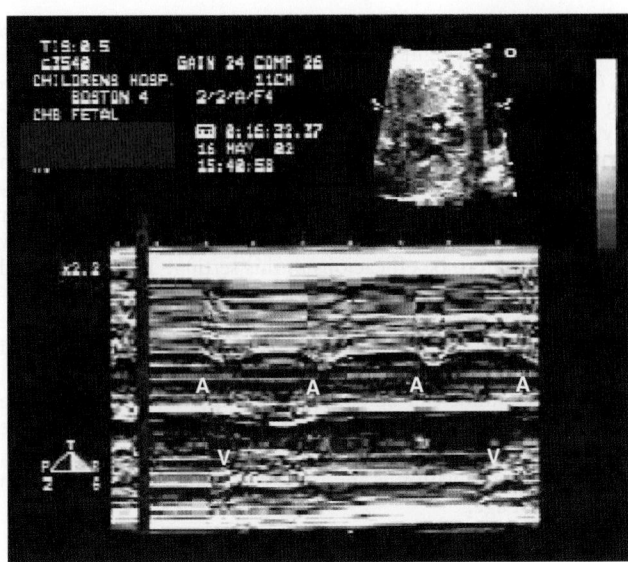

FIGURE 109.2 Fetal M-mode echocardiogram showing dissociated atrial (*A*) and ventricular (*V*) wall motion in a fetus with in utero heart block due to maternal lupus antibodies.

to accommodate conventional leads. Device implantation in children is further complicated by lead attrition during lifelong therapy,[28] which often entails extractions and replacements that can eventually narrow or occlude important vessels. Maintenance of a well-functioning system over many decades can be challenging.

The distorted anatomy that accompanies complex CHD can also confound invasive procedures in both children and adults. It is important that the operator has a clear understanding of the specific defect as well as the surgical patching and vascular redirection involved with its repair. High-resolution registration of anatomy using echocardiography, cardiac magnetic resonance imaging (MRI), angiography, and/or intracardiac echo is essential for ablation procedures as well as device implantation in CHD patients.[29]

Arrhythmias in the Fetus

An interesting branch of pediatric EP is the management of fetal arrhythmias. Because a direct fetal ECG cannot be recorded, alternate methods must be used to decipher abnormal rhythms. Magnetocardiography is one such technique,[30] but the equipment for this procedure is not widely available. A more practical approach is fetal echocardiography, where M-mode recordings of atrial and ventricular wall motion are used in conjunction with Doppler flow analysis (Fig. 109.2) to provide a functional construct of rhythm status.[31] The data obtained by this method are remarkably reliable.

The most commonly detected fetal rhythm disturbance involves frequent atrial premature beats, which are generally benign and resolve before delivery; however, when these ectopic beats occur in a bigeminal pattern (as they often do) and are sufficiently early to be blocked at the AV node (which they often are), they effectively reduce the fetal heart rate and can raise concerns about a true AV conduction disturbance or fetal distress. Echocardiography will clarify the mechanism for the altered rate.

Fetal supraventricular tachycardia (SVT) is a more serious issue.[32] The most common mechanisms are AP reentry and atrial flutter (AFL), either of which can become incessant in utero and result in cardiac decompensation with fetal hydrops, culminating in some unfortunate cases with fetal demise. Treatment can be difficult, but effective control can be achieved in many instances by passive transplacental transfer of antiarrhythmic drugs administered to the mother. Digoxin, flecainide, and sotalol are the

most commonly used agents for this purpose. If the SVT cannot be controlled and the fetus remains compromised, early delivery is the best remaining option if the fetal lungs have matured sufficiently to tolerate extrauterine life.

Complete heart block in the fetus is another complex problem. As will be discussed later in this chapter, exposure of the developing heart to autoantibodies from mothers with systemic lupus erythematosus or Sjögren syndrome can result in permanent heart block, beginning at about 20 weeks of gestation.[33] Escape rhythms at rates of 50–80 beats/min typically ensue and are usually sufficient to support the fetus as well as allow a carefully monitored pregnancy to come to term, but there are exceptions when decompensation may occur. Fetal heart block associated with CHD (heterotaxy, L-TGA, and AV canal defects, as mentioned earlier) tends to be even less well tolerated. Whenever a fetus becomes compromised due to heart block of any etiology, the most expeditious response is early delivery and pacemaker implantation, but this again assumes that the fetal lungs have reached a viable state of maturity. Successful in utero pacing of a human fetus has yet to be perfected, although promising prototype devices are now being developed.[34]

Supraventricular Tachycardia

Some form of SVT accounts for the majority of pediatric arrhythmias. Among patients with structurally normal hearts, the SVT mechanism in more than 50% of the cases involves an AP, while roughly 20% of cases are due to AV nodal reentry; 15% due to automatic ectopic atrial foci; and the remainder an assortment of chaotic atrial rhythm, automatic junctional tachycardia, AFL, and atrial fibrillation (AF).[35] The profile is somewhat different for patients with CHD, in whom AFL and other macroreentrant atrial circuits predominate. This section will not reiterate the detailed EP of these disorders, which is addressed elsewhere in this text, but will instead focus on the clinical presentation, natural history, and treatment approach specific to the pediatric population.

Accessory Pathways

Tachycardias involving an AP are the most common arrhythmias seen in young patients and account for the largest percentage of ablation procedures performed at pediatric centers.[36] Tachycardia events may begin as early as fetal life or any time thereafter, but the frequency peaks during the first year of life and again during early adolescence. The functional properties of AP determine the natural history and the management approach. A large multicenter series of young patients undergoing ablation[37] indicated that pathways with bidirectional conduction (manifest Wolff-Parkinson-White syndrome [WPW]) are present in 59% of pediatric patients undergoing ablation, while APs with unidirectional retrograde conduction (concealed APs) are identified in 37% and the remaining 4% have slowly conducting concealed APs with nearly incessant tachycardia (i.e., PJRT). Pathways with unidirectional anterograde conduction (conventional AV connections as well as atriofascicular fibers) can also be seen in pediatric patients, although their incidence is low. Approximately 10% of all pediatric patients undergoing ablation will be found to have multiple APs. This occurs more commonly among those with underlying heart disease (e.g., Ebstein anomaly or cardiomyopathy) compared with among those with structurally normal hearts.[38]

The initial presentation for pediatric patients with manifest WPW typically involves sustained orthodromic reciprocating tachycardia (ORT). Those who are old enough to verbalize symptoms will usually be brought to medical attention promptly for conversion according to standard pediatric guidelines using an agent such as adenosine.[39] Unfortunately, infants and young children who are preverbal may escape early detection and remain in ORT for hours or perhaps days, resulting in a low cardiac output at presentation that may necessitate emergent electrical cardioversion or transesophageal overdrive pacing to restore sinus rhythm. Apart from the occasional case involving an atriofascicular fiber, antidromic reciprocating tachycardia is unusual as a presenting arrhythmia in pediatric patients with true WPW, but can be encountered as an induced rhythm during EP study in those with multiple APs. Preexcited AF with rapid anterograde conduction over the AP is clearly the most concerning presentation for WPW at any age. AF is exceedingly rare in infants and toddlers with WPW but is certainly well documented in school-age children and adolescents. Acute treatment options for preexcited AF in young patients include electrical cardioversion or intravenous procainamide.

Recommended management for young patients with WPW after acute stabilization varies according to age. The infant age group is always managed medically unless there are extenuating circumstances (e.g., impending surgery for CHD or drug-refractory tachycardia) that justify a higher-than-average-risk ablation attempt.[40] Oral maintenance drugs may include flecainide, sotalol, amiodarone, and sometimes β-blockers. β-Blockers are avoided in older patients with WPW for the fear that they might enhance AP conduction during AF, but the rarity of AF in infants, coupled with the potential toxicity of more potent antiarrhythmic agents in this age group, is reasonable justification for considering the exception. Older children with symptomatic WPW are recommended to undergo catheter ablation as soon as the clinician judges the risk of an invasive procedure to be lower than the risks of continued medical therapy and/or risk of potential break-through episodes of SVT. This calculation is patient- and institution-specific, taking into account age/size, severity of symptoms, efficacy and potential side effects of drugs in use, likely AP location based on the delta wave pattern on ECG, and center experience. All these considerations were reviewed as part of an expert consensus document addressing ablation in children from the Heart Rhythm Society (HRS) in 2002.[41] Multicenter analysis of acute outcome data for WPW ablation in young patients indicates an encouraging acute success rate of over 95%.[37]

Although the risk for sudden cardiac death (SCD) in all large series examining children and young adults with WPW is numerically low, it is clear that SCD can be a sentinel event in the younger age group. For this reason, when a WPW pattern is incidentally detected on ECG in an asymptomatic child and the risk for rapid conduction of preexcited AF is uncertain, it is recommended that some attempt be made to evaluate the anterograde conduction potential of the AP using exercise testing, Holter monitoring, transesophageal pacing, or invasive EP study. A consensus document endorsed by HRS considered persistence of the delta wave at maximum exercise heart rates, measurements of short refractory periods (<220–250 ms), induction of ORT, presence of multiple pathways, and short preexcited RR intervals during AF (<220–250 ms) to be reasonable indications for elective AP ablation in asymptomatic children with a WPW pattern after careful discussion with the family. Asymptomatic patients with only intermittent preexcitation and/or abrupt loss of the delta wave in response to sinus tachycardia during exercise testing are usually followed conservatively.[42]

Management of concealed APs in pediatric patients is more straightforward because the risk of preexcited AF is absent. Acute stabilization of ORT due to a concealed AP is similar to that described for WPW syndrome, but there are more options for long-term management, including periodic use of vagal maneuvers (if episodes are infrequent and well tolerated) and additional drugs such as calcium-channel blockers (assuming age > 1 year). The majority of patients with significant symptoms will usually undergo elective ablation at some point, but as long as episodes can be managed using simple vagal maneuvers or relatively benign

medications, this is deferred at most centers until the patient has grown to a body weight of 25 kg or more.

An important subclass of concealed AP is the slowly conducting variety that can result in PJRT. These pathways are usually located in the posteroseptal area and have remarkably long conduction times with decremental properties that can result in nearly incessant ORT (Fig. 109.3A). Acute therapy with adenosine will terminate reentry, but ORT will promptly resume after only a beat or two of sinus rhythm. Flecainide is one of the few drugs that seem to be efficacious in this setting. The pattern and age of presentation for PJRT is variable because rates are relatively slow compared with conventional ORT and may not cause symptoms until tachycardia-induced myopathy develops.[22,43] If detected early while ventricular function is still well preserved, a trial of flecainide can be considered as a temporizing measure until the patient is judged to be old enough to undergo elective catheter ablation. However, once cardiomyopathy has developed, urgent catheter ablation is the most reasonable course of action regardless of age.

Atrioventricular Nodal Reentry

In children with structurally normal hearts, the EP underlying AVNRT is similar to that seen in adults with the disorder.[44,45] Most cases thus involve typical slow-fast reentry, with sites for successful slow pathway (SP) ablation in the inferior third of Koch's triangle, suggesting involvement of the rightward extension off the compact AV node. It is rare to see AVNRT in infants or toddlers, although it may occur. Most children do not begin to experience symptomatic tachycardia episodes until after the age of 8 years. Vagal maneuvers and adenosine are effective as acute therapy, and chronic therapy with β-blockers or calcium-channel blockers does a reasonable job at preventing recurrences. Even if medical control is successful, most patients and parents will ultimately opt for elective catheter ablation at some point in preference to chronic daily medications. Whenever AV node modification is attempted before the patient has grown to full adult size, the operator must remain mindful of the reduced dimensions of Koch's triangle, and if it ever appears that ablation energy has to be delivered uncomfortably close to the presumptive site of the compact AV node, it is reasonable to consider the use of cryoablation rather than radiofrequency (RF) energy and to accept a higher recurrence rate.[46] However, RF ablation is still a perfectly acceptable option for AVNRT in most pediatric cases. The acute success rate for SP modification in children with normal hearts was reported as 99% in one large multicenter series.[37]

Ablation for AVNRT in the setting of CHD is far more challenging owing to distorted landmarks and displacement of the conduction tissues.[47] This is especially true for patients with heterotaxy syndrome (in whom AV node location can be ambiguous) or those with defects of the AV canal septum (who do not have a triangle of Koch). Successful SP ablation can still be accomplished safely in most cases if proper techniques and precautions are employed.

Ectopic Atrial Tachycardia

Focal atrial tachycardia of nonsinus origin, commonly referred to as ectopic atrial tachycardia (EAT), is an uncommon but difficult disorder in children that can lead to a tachycardia-induced cardiomyopathy if sufficiently rapid and incessant.[48] Its cause remains uncertain, and its precise mechanism is not entirely understood. In most pediatric cases, the ectopic focus behaves like a site of abnormal automaticity because it cannot be interrupted or induced with pacing maneuvers and does not respond to electrical cardioversion, while a smaller percentage of cases display features more consistent with triggered automaticity or microreentry. Despite the uncertainty surrounding etiology, it is clear there is a strong predilection

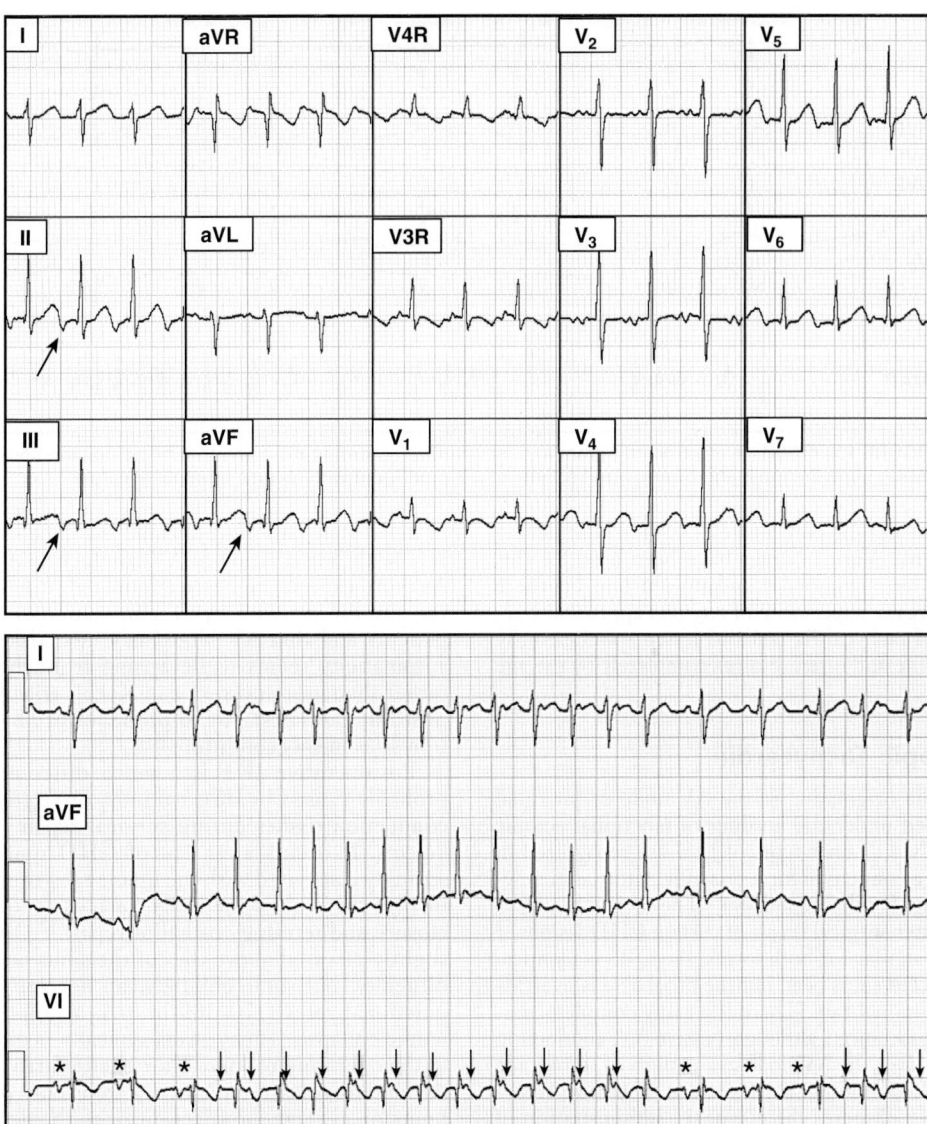

FIGURE 109.3 Two of the common causes of tachycardia-induced myopathy in children. *Upper panel:* Classical electrocardiogram pattern for the permanent form of junctional reciprocating tachycardia with very long RP interval and negative P waves (*arrows*) in the inferior leads. *Lower panel:* Rhythm strip from a patient with ectopic atrial tachycardia showing occasional sinus beats (*asterisks*) interrupted by salvos of atrial tachycardia with a different P wave appearance (*arrows*) and variable atrioventricular relationship.

for EAT to arise from certain specific atrial sites, including the right or left appendage, an orifice of a pulmonary vein, along the crista terminalis, or along the coronary sinus (see Fig. 109.3). Most cases are identified in school-age children and teenagers, but average age of onset is difficult to determine because EAT often does not cause noticeable symptoms unless and until ventricular function begins to suffer. There seems to be a threshold value of roughly 120–130 beats/min for the mean daily ventricular rate on Holter monitor that predicts ventricular dysfunction in otherwise healthy children.[22] Pharmacological treatment for EAT is difficult, and no single agent has proved to be universally effective. Anecdotal success has been reported in children using β-blockers, phenytoin, flecainide, sotalol, and amiodarone; however, choosing a drug still remains a trial-and-error process. Most cases of EAT are managed nowadays with catheter ablation, which has a reported success rate of 92%.[37] If the EAT focus is successfully eliminated, patients who had depressed ventricular function can be expected to recover within 3 months or so.

Chaotic Atrial Tachycardia

Chaotic atrial tachycardia (CAT) is a label given to a rare and poorly understood arrhythmia of infancy that can be fatal if undetected or untreated.[49] The ECG picture is one of very rapid atrial activation with variable P wave morphologies, sometimes degenerating to a pattern that mimics AF (Fig. 109.4). The ventricular response to this rhythm in an infant tends to be quite rapid and is frequently interspersed with periods of a wide QRS due to aberration. The exact mechanism is not known. It seems logical to assume that this is a multifocal atrial disorder, but it might just as well be a single ultra-rapid focus that conducts in a fibrillatory pattern. The latter speculation is supported by a case report of successful restoration of sinus rhythm by catheter ablation at a single site near the orifice of a pulmonary vein.[50]

Tachycardia is usually first detected during the newborn period. Antiarrhythmic medications, even in high-dose combinations, rarely suppress CAT completely. A more realistic

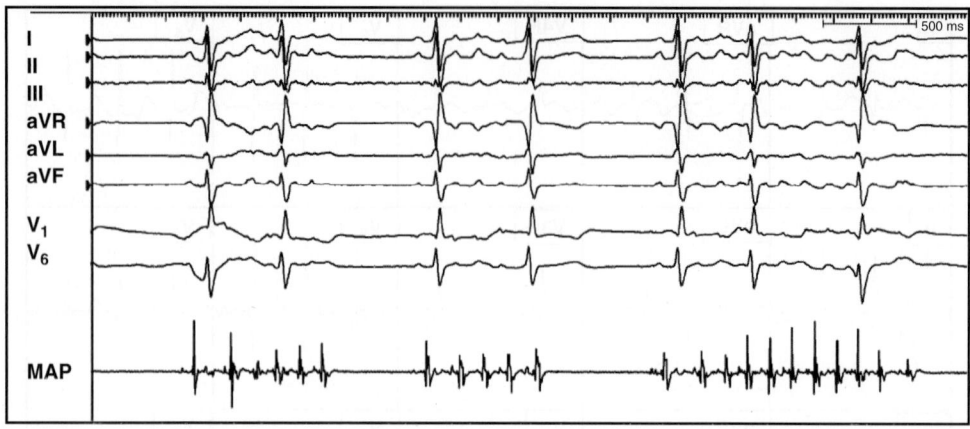

FIGURE 109.4 Surface electrocardiogram and intracardiac recording from an atrial mapping catheter (*MAP*) showing rapid and bizarre atrial activity in a 7-month-old with chaotic atrial tachycardia.

treatment goal is reducing the percentage of CAT and achieving ventricular rate-control. Various drugs have been used for this purpose, including β-blockers, sotalol, and amiodarone, but there are no data to support the superiority of any one approach. Fortunately, this form of tachycardia tends to lessen spontaneously over the first year of life and often resolves completely by the age of 4 years.

Junctional Ectopic Tachycardia

Automatic tachycardia originating in the AV node or proximal His bundle is grouped under the heading of junctional ectopic tachycardia (JET). Two distinct types of JET are recognized in children. The first is a congenital form typically detected in newborns that has a strong familial tendency.[51] The second is a transient disorder seen after surgical repair of certain CHD lesions.[52] The ECG picture is similar for both forms; the QRS is identical to a normally conducted sinus beat, but the atrial rate is overridden by the rapid junctional rate. There is usually complete ventriculoatrial (VA) dissociation, although passive VA conduction can sometimes occur over the AV node in a pattern of retrograde Wenckebach or, less commonly, a 1:1 pattern. If passive retrograde conduction ever obscures the diagnosis, administration of adenosine will result in complete VA dissociation without altering the rapid junctional rate. Rates for JET can vary over time in response to adrenergic state, and occasional irregularity may be seen owing to capture beats from dissociated sinus rhythm.

Congenital JET is a rare but potentially lethal arrhythmia. Only 26 cases were included in the first large published series,[53] but it is notable that 35% of these patients died and that half had a first-degree relative with the same condition. No specific gene defect has yet been identified, nor has a unifying lesion been found in autopsy material. Heart rates in infants with congenital JET can exceed 200 beats/min and, if uncontrolled, can put them at risk for tachycardia-induced myopathy. Medical treatment is difficult, but most published experience indicates that amiodarone is a reasonably effective agent for slowing the rate to a more tolerable range. Nearly one-third of infants with congenital JET surviving till the age of 1 year will have spontaneous resolution of this arrhythmia, and for the remainder, junctional rates tend to become slower and easier to manage with increasing age, which encourages a strong preference for medical therapy over catheter ablation in early years of life. If JET rates cannot be controlled or if the patient remains dependent upon long-term amiodarone use much beyond infancy, catheter ablation can be considered as alternate therapy. Case reports describing successful ablation for congenital JET date back as far as the era of direct current (DC) ablation[54]; in 1990, the first reported RF catheter ablation

in a pediatric patient replicated this by eliminating congenital JET with preservation of AV conduction in a 10-month-old.[55] As more experience has accumulated, it has become clear that the site for successful JET elimination is not the same in all patients and that AV block may be a risk when the focus of automaticity seems to be arising from the anteroseptal area rather than more posterior in Koch's triangle. Cryoablation is probably the safest way to probe for productive and safe ablation sites in this condition.

Postoperative JET is a much different condition that is probably caused by direct trauma or stretch injury to the AV conduction tissues during surgical repair of congenital heart defects. It occurs after 1% of CHD repair surgeries and is strongly associated with the infant age group and surgeries that involve the crux of the heart, such as ventricular septal defect closure and tetralogy of Fallot repair.[52] Often the rate is only slightly elevated above that of the sinus node and causes little difficulty, but some children can develop greatly accelerated junctional rates (170–300 beats/min) that result in hemodynamic collapse. Tachycardia typically begins upon rewarming in the operating room or shortly after arrival in the postoperative intensive care unit. It is a transient condition, lasting 36 hours on average; however, prior to the development of effective management strategies, the mortality during this time was as high as 50% if rates were rapid.[56] Fortunately, diverse treatment options have evolved that now permit nearly all patients to be adequately supported until JET resolves. There are two primary derangements that need to be addressed with treatment. First is loss of AV synchrony, which can be corrected simply by pacing the atria at rates just slightly faster than JET, using postoperative atrial wires or an esophageal lead.[57] However, when JET is extremely rapid, synchrony alone is insufficient, and the second challenge then becomes slowing the rate of junctional automaticity. General supportive measures and cautious weaning of catecholamine infusions will slow JET in about 25% of cases and allow atrial pacing to be carried out at reasonable rates with improved hemodynamics. If rapid JET persists, induction of hypothermia to a core body temperature of 34°C with a cooling blanket can be helpful, and the addition of intravenous procainamide on top of hypothermia in refractory cases will increase efficacy to better than 90%.[52] Intravenous amiodarone has been adopted at some centers as the preferred therapy for postoperative JET because it has the advantage of working under normothermic conditions,[58] but the intravenous formulation of this agent is poorly tolerable in some infants and must be used cautiously.[59] The self-resolving nature of this arrhythmia mandates that every alternative be explored before resorting to a catheter ablation procedure that might permanently damage AV conduction.

Atrial Flutter and Fibrillation in Pediatric Patients With Ostensibly Normal Hearts

In sharp contrast to adult patients, AFL and AF are quite uncommon in pediatric patients with normal hearts, but either may arise under special circumstances. AFL is sometimes seen as an idiopathic disorder in the fetus and neonate.[60] The flutter waves resemble the sawtooth pattern seen with conventional circuits around the tricuspid annulus, but the cycle length is extremely short in this age group (≤150 ms), and AV conduction can be quite rapid. Sustained AFL in the fetus can cause decompensation with hydrops or fetal demise in some cases. If trials of a transplacental drug, such as sotalol or flecainide, administered to the mother do not convert AFL,[61] early delivery needs to be considered as soon as the fetus is sufficiently mature to tolerate extrauterine life. Conversion to sinus rhythm following delivery can then be achieved through a variety of techniques, including synchronized DC cardioversion, transesophageal overdrive pacing, or antiarrhythmic drugs. It is surprisingly rare for fetal AFL to recur after conversion, although most patients are maintained for a few months on a benign agent, such as β-blockers, as a precaution.

AF can be seen occasionally in adolescents with otherwise normal hearts, a completely normal ECG in sinus rhythm, normal thyroid status, and a negative family history of AF. The label "lone AF" is often assigned to such cases, and it is probably sufficient to stick with that diagnosis in patients who do not experience recurrences. However, when AF recurs with any regularity in a young patient, there are often hidden triggers in the form of concealed APs, AVNRT, or intermittent EAT that need to be considered.[62] It is not unreasonable to recommend Holter monitoring, a long-term event recorder, or even intracardiac EP testing to eliminate these concerns. A familial predisposition to AF is also known to exist,[63] sometimes with associated sinus node dysfunction (SND); however, the genetic basis is very heterogeneous, and the penetrance is low for all known genetic variants.

Atrial Tachycardias in Young Patients With Congenital Heart Disease

The most difficult form of SVT encountered in pediatric practice is atrial tachycardia following surgery for CHD. This topic was covered in some detail in Chapter 74, but several highlights are worth mention here.

Macroreentry circuits around atrial scars and other fixed obstacles are the most common form of atrial tachycardia encountered in CHD patients.[64] In many cases the circuit rotates around the tricuspid valve through the cavotricuspid isthmus, similar to conventional AFL, but alternate circuits around atriotomy scars and patches are also seen. The label intraatrial reentrant tachycardia (IART) is generally preferred as a collective term to describe all the possible varieties of atrial circuits in CHD patients.

It is rare to encounter IART in the early postoperative period. Usually it does not surface until a decade or more after repair, suggesting that a period of degenerative atrial remodeling is needed until conduction velocity slows sufficiently for reentry to sustain. Cycle lengths for IART circuits (even those involving the cavotricuspid isthmus) tend to be longer than those for conventional AFL (on the order of 250–320 ms), which allows for a rapid ventricular response that is poorly tolerated in most CHD patients.[65] Acute stabilization is usually accomplished with DC cardioversion or by overdrive atrial pacing if the patient has a device in place. Chronic medical therapy can then be instituted using some combination of AV nodal blocking agents, class Ic and class III drugs intended to prevent reentry, and anticoagulation. Unfortunately, IART is notoriously resistant to pharmacological control, and more than 60% of patients will experience

a recurrence within 1–2 years regardless of the agent chosen.[66] Catheter ablation[67] has now become a common approach to IART at most centers caring for CHD patients (see Chapters 74 and 131).

AF is also being encountered with increasing regularity in CHD patients, particularly those with left heart obstructive lesions, palliated single ventricles, and mitral valve disease. The onset of AF is usually delayed until patients have grown to be young adults, but as the longevity of CHD patients increases, thanks to improvements in surgical techniques, the number of cases is growing rapidly. Medical management is in accordance with the American College of Cardiology/American Heart Association/Heart Rhythm Society (ACC/AHA/HRS) guidelines.[68] The published experience regarding ablation for AF in the CHD population remains limited, but early results show some promise.[69]

Ventricular Arrhythmias

Ventricular arrhythmias in the pediatric age group are variable in their presentation and natural history, ranging from conditions that are self-limited and benign to those that can be abruptly lethal. The challenge is to recognize the clinical pattern and perform the necessary diagnostic testing that assigns the condition to its proper category so that appropriate treatment and surveillance can be instituted. Equally important, compulsive family screening needs to be performed to identify other individuals at potential risk whenever a serious ventricular arrhythmia with a genetic foundation is identified. This section will once again refrain from repetitious discussion of the detailed EP for these arrhythmias, which is addressed elsewhere in this text, and will focus primarily on pediatric presentations and treatment.

Accelerated Ventricular Rhythm of Infancy

Accelerated ventricular rhythm at rates just slightly faster than the underlying sinus rate can be seen occasionally in the fetus and newborn with an otherwise normal heart. The typical ECG pattern supports an origin in the RV outflow region, suggesting that this may in fact be a variant of outflow tract VT that occurs at older ages. Treatment is rarely indicated, and the condition tends to resolve spontaneously within the first 6 months of life.[70]

Focal Ventricular Tachycardias

Idiopathic focal VT with behavior consistent with abnormal automaticity is well recognized in young patients. Detection is most common during early teenage years. Depending upon rate and percentage of the day spent in VT, symptoms can range from nonexistent to congestive heart failure from tachycardia-induced myopathy. The RV or LV outflow tract is the most common location identified in children who have undergone formal mapping for this disorder, but foci can also be found along the superior aspects of the mitral or tricuspid annulus, adjacent to the His bundle on the right side of the intraventricular septum (see Fig. 109.1), or related to a papillary muscle.[71] Although a mechanism of triggered activity has been implicated for some outflow tract VTs, it is rare to see pacing maneuvers successfully induce this sort of VT in a young patient, making an automatic focus the more likely mechanism.[72]

Therapy may not be needed for asymptomatic children with a well-preserved ventricular function and slow VT rates. Over time, some of these VTs may actually undergo spontaneous regression. When the patient is symptomatic and/or ventricular function becomes compromised, medical trials with β-blockers or calcium-channel blockers can be considered, but catheter ablation is the preferred option if the VT burden is high. Having active VT in the laboratory allows high-quality mapping with a success rate for ablation exceeding 90%; however, not infrequently, the VT becomes quiescent when a young patient is inactive and supine on a procedure table, even without sedation. Infusion of isoproterenol or epinephrine may reactivate the focus in some (but not all) patients. If formal activation mapping of spontaneous VT is not possible, pace mapping may be considered, although the long-term success rate of the latter is inferior to that of the former.[71]

Left-Ventricular Septal Fascicular Tachycardia

This tachycardia has been well described in Chapter 82 and is a relatively common form of VT in otherwise healthy school-age children.[71,73] On ECG, the QRS upstroke is sharp with a pattern of right bundle branch block and left anterior hemiblock, all consistent with mapping studies that suggest involvement of the left posterior fascicle. Sensitivity to calcium-channel blockers is a hallmark of this disorder,[74] so verapamil can be considered as long-term suppressive therapy until the patient is of proper size to undergo elective catheter ablation. The success rate for catheter ablation of this disorder (about 90%) is among the highest for any form of childhood VT.[71]

Ventricular Tachycardia in Congenital Heart Disease

It is useful to recognize two varieties of VT in CHD patients. First is the monomorphic reentrant type seen in conditions where underlying anatomy, surgical scarring, and myocardial degeneration result in isolated conduction corridors and central obstacles capable of supporting sustained macroreentry. The classical example is tetralogy of Fallot,[75] where the position of the ventricular septal defect relative to the traditional ventriculotomy incision produces multiple potential circuits in the RV outflow region. Monomorphic VT can also be occasionally seen in patients with Ebstein anomaly related to the thin and fibrotic tissue of the atrialized portion of the RV[76,77] and in a few other rare conditions. The second variety of VT is a less organized type (frequently polymorphic) that may develop in any CHD lesion that causes advanced degrees of hypertrophy and/or dilated cardiomyopathy. Examples include congenital aortic stenosis, transposition of the great arteries following the Mustard or Senning procedures (where the RV is recruited as the systemic ventricle), congenitally corrected transposition, and single ventricle.[78,79]

The most extensive data in this area has been generated from the follow-up of the tetralogy population. Similar to the natural history of IART, VT is quite rare in younger children with tetralogy and usually does not surface until a decade or two after repair, which implies that degenerative remodeling is required before the circuit tissue conducts slowly enough to permit a sustained reentry. Numerous risk-factors for VT and SCD in tetralogy have been identified; these include the following: (1) older age at repair, (2) older chronological age, (3) nonsustained VT on Holter monitoring, (4) dilated and dysfunctional RV, (5) severe pulmonary regurgitation, (6) depressed LV function, (7) very prolonged QRS duration, and (8) symptoms such as syncope or rapid palpitations with dizziness.[80] Unfortunately, none of these have proven to be perfect predictors of high risk and lack the quantitation necessary to direct aggressive therapy. Invasive EP testing with programmed ventricular stimulation can refine risk assessment[81] but still has a high false-positive rate that limits its applicability as a screening tool. The general approach to tetralogy patients nowadays is to repair the lesion early in life and optimize hemodynamics in a fashion that might minimize later deterioration of ventricular function and prevent development of VT. Then, as patients are followed into teenage

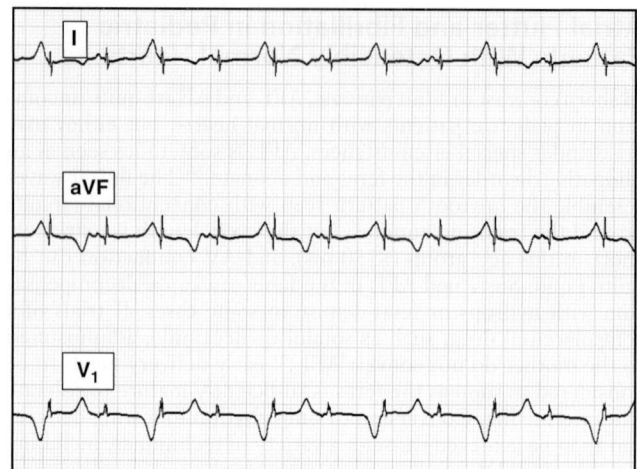

FIGURE 109.5 Dramatic T wave alternans in an infant with LQT8 (Timothy syndrome).

years and early adulthood, routine surveillance is carried out with periodic Holter monitoring and assessment of hemodynamic status, and if the patient appears to accumulate multiple risk factors, invasive EP testing might be recommended. Contemporary treatment[82,83] for either primary or secondary VT prevention in tetralogy is now centered on ICD placement and catheter ablation (see Chapter 131). Medications such as β-blockers or mexiletine are still used occasionally, but solely for primary prevention when risk for sustained VT is judged to be relatively low.

The approach to nonspecific varieties of VT seen in young CHD patients with failing systemic ventricles and/or severe hypertrophy must be tailored to the individual patient. An ICD can be considered as a temporizing measure,[84] although formal selection criteria are not well established, and the implantation risk is elevated by the fact that modified epicardial systems are often needed in CHD patients with complex venous connections or residual intracardiac shunting.[17,29] These tend to be patients with end-stage disease who eventually might have to be considered for cardiac transplant.

Long QT Syndrome

Long QT syndrome (LQTS) is the most common channelopathy seen in children, with an estimated prevalence as high as 1:2000 in some reports. In-depth discussion of the genetic and molecular basis of these disorders was presented in Chapter 93, highlighting both tremendous progress in our scientific understanding and improved options for therapy.

The most malignant forms of LQTS strike early in life.[85] Some neonates with extreme QT prolongation can present with recurrent torsades de pointes, T wave alternans, and even a 2:1 AV conduction pattern due to the very prolonged repolarization times beyond the AV node (Fig. 109.5). This dramatic newborn presentation has been described in conjunction with several disorders within the LQTS family, including LQT2, LQT3, and LQT8. In past, 2:1 block was considered an ominous sign that portended early demise, but the prognosis has improved greatly with early pacing and aggressive β-blocker therapy for many of these cases. The notable exception is LTQ8 (Timothy syndrome, see Chapter 95), which still remains a major management challenge.[86] Undetected LQTS has been implicated as the cause of roughly 10% of SIDS cases on the basis of positive genotype at molecular autopsy.[23]

Beyond the neonatal period, LQTS has a variable presentation depending on genotype, penetrance, and other factors. The rare child with congenital sensorineural deafness and LQTS

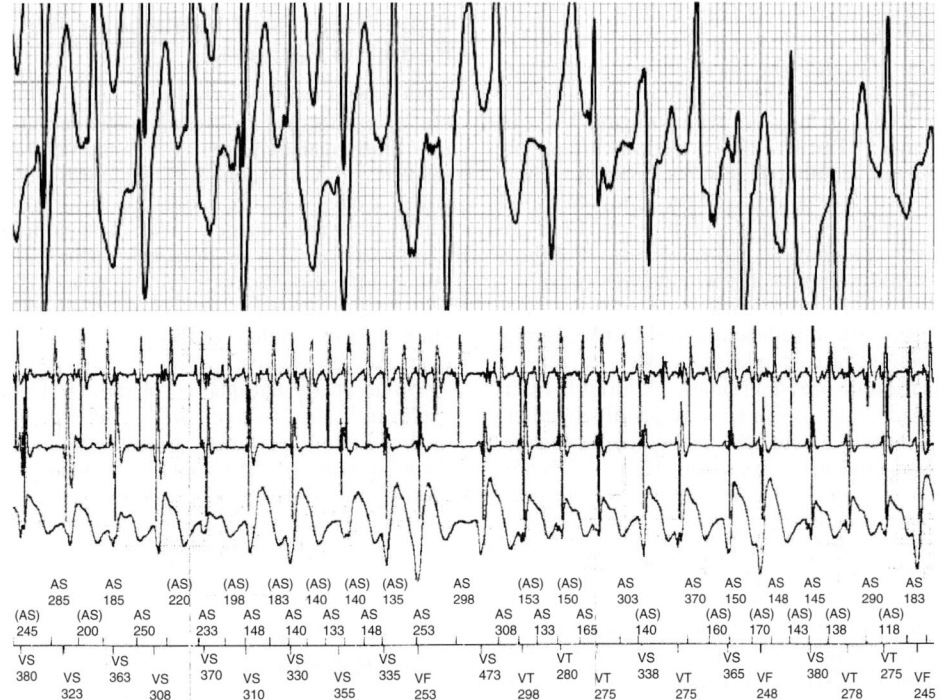

FIGURE 109.6 The variety of tachycardias in young patients with catecholaminergic polymorphic ventricular tachycardia. *Upper panel:* the classical bidirectional ventricular tachycardia (*VT*) that occurred during exercise testing in a 12-year-old. *Lower panel:* Recording from a dual chamber implantable cardioverter defibrillator (ICD) in a 15-year-old who underwent device placement for VT but who also exhibited episodes of rapid irregular atrial tachycardia that triggered multiple inappropriate ICD shocks. *AS,* Atrial sense; *VF,* ventricular fibrillation; *VS,* ventricular sense.

(Jervell and Lange-Nielsen syndrome) tends to have early onset of VT episodes and markedly prolonged QT intervals because this condition is caused by a homozygous state or a compound heterozygous state for mutant genes (usually *KCNQ1*). Patients who are heterozygous for a single abnormal gene (Romano-Ward syndrome) are more likely to develop their first symptoms roughly after the age of 8 years, with escalating frequency into adolescence. An early registry examining childhood LQTS documented initial presentations as cardiac arrest (9%), syncope (26%), "seizures" (10%), and palpitations (6%). The remaining 49% were asymptomatic, with their diagnosis based on family history and ECG findings.[87] This profile has likely changed to a higher percentage of asymptomatic cases in recent years due to improved awareness and more thorough family screening. The diagnosis of LQTS in a symptomatic child or in a child born into a family with known LQTS is usually not difficult, particularly now that family-specific genotyping is possible. More challenging are patients at first presentation without a family history and an abnormal or borderline ECG. The scoring system introduced by Schwartz[88] is the most helpful clinical tool in this situation, using Bazett's formula to correct the QT interval across the wide range of pediatric heart rates. Exercise testing, epinephrine challenge, and genotype screening are sometimes added to the diagnostic evaluation, as necessary.[89]

Emergent treatment for torsades de pointes in children is similar to that for adults and includes lidocaine, magnesium, and esmolol. Electrical cardioversion is reserved for prolonged unremitting episodes of VT, and pacing may occasionally be added if it appears that VT is bradycardia conditioned. The mainstay of chronic therapy for LQTS is β-blockade with propranolol or nadolol. Mexiletine is also used in some cases, especially in those with LQT3, although its efficacy has not been tested systematically. If symptoms continue and/or the patient is considered to be at especially high risk, placement of an ICD and/or left cardiac sympathetic denervation need to be considered.[90,91]

Catecholaminergic Polymorphic Ventricular Tachycardia

Catecholaminergic polymorphic VT (CPVT) is a rare but difficult condition with an estimated prevalence of 1:10,000; it is characterized by stress-induced bidirectional VT that can degenerate into more disorganized rhythms and results in sudden death at young ages.[92] Chapter 88 provided a detailed description of the genetic and molecular basis for this disorder. In children, the bidirectional VT seen in CPVT must be differentiated from that seen in LQT7 (Andersen-Tawil syndrome) that has a much different etiology and treatment approach.[93] The average age of onset of CPVT symptoms is roughly 8 years, and the pediatric phenotype sometimes includes disorganized atrial and junctional tachycardias in addition to VT. The ECG at rest is entirely normal, but exercise testing or Holter monitoring will usually demonstrate the characteristic VT pattern when intrinsic catecholamines are high (Fig. 109.6).

High-dose β-blockers are the first line of treatment in children, usually combined with implantation of a permanent loop recorder for enhanced rhythm surveillance.[94] If VT control is suboptimal, left cardiac sympathetic denervation can be considered. Implantation of an ICD is becoming a less attractive option for young CPVT patients due to the observation that shocks may occur frequently, despite programming long detection times, and often will not terminate these tachycardias. Instead, the shock can precipitate an electrical storm with multiple discharges that are emotionally devastating. Use of an ICD in CPVT is increasingly reserved as a secondary preventive measure in those who have survived cardiac arrest. Flecainide may become a promising option for this disorder, but pediatric experience remains limited.[95]

Brugada Syndrome

The phenotype of Brugada syndrome is usually not fully manifested until late teenage or early adult years, but there are exceptions where classical ECG findings and symptomatic VT can appear as early as infancy.[96] Fever is known to be a very potent trigger for VT in these rare childhood cases, prompting a recommendation that aggressive fever control and even hospitalization for monitoring be considered during febrile illnesses. Data are too limited in children to recommend any specific form of therapy. Anecdotal success has been reported with β-blockers, mexiletine, and quinidine. An ICD can be considered in severe cases once the patient has grown to a sufficient age/size that permits implantation without undue procedural risk.

Referral for evaluation of presymptomatic children is often based on a recently made diagnosis in an older family member, at which point only subtle ECG changes may be present in the child (e.g., mild nonspecific RV conduction delay and 1-mm ST-segment elevation in lead V_1) that are difficult to interpret. Provocative testing with a class I drug may expose more dramatic abnormalities,[97] but the sensitivity of this maneuver in pediatric patients is still uncertain. Genetic screening of young individuals can be considered in a family with a documented abnormal genotype, with the knowledge that a positive screen supports more intense follow-up, but not necessarily active treatment, and that genetic screening is negative in many families with this disorder.

Hypertrophic Cardiomyopathy

As detailed in Chapter 86, hypertrophic cardiomyopathy (HCM) is the most common cause of SCD in young competitive athletes, with a prevalence estimated at 1:500 in the United States.[98] The annual rate of sudden death in children diagnosed with HCM is estimated in some studies to be 2% or higher, placing it among the most lethal cardiac disorders in the pediatric population.[99] Survival is highly dependent upon etiology of the hypertrophic condition. Infants diagnosed with HCM during the first year of life are more likely to suffer from an inborn error of metabolism, resulting in early demise for nearly half this group before the age of 2 years.[100] Children diagnosed with more conventional forms of familial HCM rarely develop symptoms before the age of 8 years, but sudden death can be the first manifestation of the disease.

No form of pharmacological therapy has been identified that reliably alters the sudden death risk in children with HCM. Implantation of an ICD has proved to be the only lifesaving measure to date. In a large study of ICD use in pediatric HCM, 45% of children who received the device for secondary prevention received appropriate shocks within 5 years of implantation, as did 10% of those who received a primary prevention device.[101] There can be no debate regarding the utility of an ICD for secondary prevention in HCM regardless of patient age/size. The real challenge is deciding when the risk of sudden death justifies the risk of a primary prevention implant, particularly during preteen years when narrow vascular caliber and expected thoracic growth complicate lead positioning and long-term maintenance. A number of risk factors for sudden death have been examined in children; these include the following: (1) extreme septal thickness > 30 mm, (2) a history of syncope, (3) family history of HCM with sudden death, (4) nonsustained VT on Holter monitor, and (5) hypotension during exercise. While none of these provide perfect predictive accuracy, many clinicians now consider the presence of two or more risk factors to be an indication for considering primary prevention ICD implantation. The final judgment is still influenced by patient age to some degree, resulting in more liberal adoption of ICD therapy in teenagers with HCM compared with that in children under the age of 10 years.

Other Causes of Ventricular Arrhythmias in Pediatric Patients

There are a number of other rare, but nonetheless important, etiologies that must be considered whenever a child presents with new ventricular arrhythmias or resuscitated cardiac arrest. One of these is ARVC. Although usually not phenotypically manifested at young ages, ARVC can occasionally present with serious symptoms during the teenage years.[102] The pathology of this condition is progressive, so cases detected in this early phase may display only subtle abnormalities on ECG, and RV status may not be dramatically abnormal on echocardiogram or MRI. A positive family history would certainly help raise awareness of ARVC as a diagnostic possibility.

Some unconventional coronary artery abnormalities in children can lead to ischemic VT. These include anomalous origin of the left coronary artery from the pulmonary artery, origin of the left coronary artery from the right sinus of Valsalva (less commonly, origin of the right coronary artery from the left sinus), and acquired coronary occlusion from Kawasaki disease.[103–105] Other causes of VT in children can include cardiac tumors,[106] myocarditis,[107] idiopathic dilated cardiomyopathy,[108] and LV noncompaction.[109]

Bradycardia

Direct trauma to the sinus node or AV node during surgical correction of CHD accounts for most cases of significant bradycardia in the pediatric population. Improvements in the surgical approach to certain CHD lesions (e.g., arterial switch rather than Mustard operation for transposition) have lessened this problem to some degree but have not eliminated it entirely.[110] Indications for permanent pacemakers in children and adolescents (with and without CHD) were included as a subsection within the ACC/AHA/HRS guidelines for device-based therapy of cardiac rhythm and should be consulted when difficult decisions related to implants arise.[111]

Sinus Node Dysfunction

Most cases of symptomatic SND in pediatric patients occur in the setting of CHD, due either to the developmental absence of the node in patients with heterotaxy or to the surgical damage to the nodal tissues or the sinus node artery during the Mustard, Senning, Glenn, or Fontan operations.[112] In the absence of structural heart disease, isolated SND is exceedingly rare in children. There have been sporadic reports of congenital SND with detection of a recessive mutation of the *SCN5A* gene, but such cases are rare.[113] Anorexia nervosa is probably the most common cause of dramatic sinus bradycardia in adolescents, but it is reversible with restoration of adequate nutritional status.[114]

Atrioventricular Block

The most common cause of congenital complete heart block (CCHB) is in utero exposure of the fetus to maternal autoantibodies directed against intracellular ribonucleoproteins Ro (SS-A) and La (SS-B), as occurs in systemic lupus erythematosus or Sjögren syndrome.[33,115] These autoantibodies begin to cross the placenta at about 16 weeks of gestation and have a predilection to injure conduction tissues of a previously normal fetal heart; the injury is irreversible. Infants born to mothers with positive serology have about a 3%–5% risk of CCHB, but this risk rises to 18%–20% if the mother had a previous pregnancy complicated by CCHB. Curiously, more than half of these mothers have no clinical manifestation of connective tissue disease during their pregnancy despite their positive serology. Several trials are ongoing to test whether injury to the fetal conduction tissues can be halted or tempered using maternal steroids or other therapies, but the results have thus far been inconsistent.[116] In most cases the fetus tolerates heart block very well with adequate in utero escape rates and many can be followed for years after delivery without the need for pacing.[117]

The most common cause of acquired heart block in pediatric patients is intraoperative trauma to the specialized conduction tissues during CHD repair. In roughly two-thirds of cases, AV block is a transient issue related to stretch injury or edema that recovers within a few days without any sequelae.[118] Postoperative patients are safely maintained with pacing via temporary epicardial leads until it is clear whether the recovery will occur. If complete or high-grade block persists beyond the tenth postoperative day, it is considered a class I indication for permanent pacemaker implantation. Other causes of acquired heart block in children include viral myocarditis[119] and Lyme disease.[120]

Summary

Pediatric arrhythmia management demands strict attention to unique physiological and anatomical features of the fetus and child. Even though the underlying arrhythmia mechanisms are often similar to those seen in adult patients, smaller patient size and the presence of CHD can greatly alter the natural history and preferred treatment approach.

REFERENCES

1. van Weerd JH, Christoffels VM. The formation and function of the cardiac conduction system. *Development.* 2016;143:197–210.
2. Rothenberg F, Efimov IR, Watanabe M. Functional imaging of the embryonic pacemaking and cardiac conduction system over the past 150 years: technologies to overcome the challenges. *Anat Rec A Discov Mol Cell Evol Biol.* 2004;280:980–989.
3. Blom NA, Gittenberger-de Groot AC, DeRuiter MC, et al. Development of the cardiac conduction tissue in human embryos using HNK-1 antigen expression: possible relevance for understanding of abnormal atrial automaticity. *Circulation.* 1999;99:800–806.
4. Racca AW, Klaiman JM, Pioner JM, et al. Contractile properties of developing human fetal cardiac muscle. *J Physiol.* 2016;594:437–452.
5. Smolich JJ. Ultrastructural and functional features of the developing mammalian heart: a brief overview. *Reprod Fertil Dev.* 1995;7:451–461.
6. Epstein ML, Kiel EA, Victorica BE. Cardiac decompensation following verapamil therapy in infants with supraventricular tachycardia. *Pediatrics.* 1985;75:737–740.
7. Waki K, Kim JS, Becker AE. Morphology of the human atrioventricular node is age dependent: a feature of potential clinical significance. *J Cardiovasc Electrophysiol.* 2000;11:1144–1151.
8. Benson Jr DW, Dunnigan A, Benditt DG. Follow-up evaluation of infant paroxysmal atrial tachycardia: transesophageal study. *Circulation.* 1987;75:542–549.
9. Anderson RH, Brown NA, Moorman AF. The sinus node, isomerism, and heterotaxy. *Cardiovasc Pathol.* 2013;22:243–244.
10. Epstein MR, Saul JP, Weindling SN, et al. Atrioventricular reciprocating tachycardia involving twin atrioventricular nodes in patients with complex congenital heart disease. *J Cardiovasc Electrophysiol.* 2001;12:671–679.
11. Connelly MS, Liu PP, Williams WG, et al. Congenitally corrected transposition of the great arteries in the adult: functional status and complications. *J Am Coll Cardiol.* 1996;27:1238–1243.
12. Ih S, Fukuda K, Okada R, et al. Histopathological correlation between the QRS axis and disposition of the atrioventricular conduction system in common atrioventricular orifice and in its related anomalies. *Jpn Circ J.* 1983;47:1368–1376.
13. Mori AD, Bruneau BG. TBX5 mutations and congenital heart disease: Holt-Oram syndrome revealed. *Curr Opin Cardiol.* 2004;19:211–215.
14. Attenhofer Jost CH, Connolly HM, Edwards WD, et al. Ebstein's anomaly—review of a multifaceted congenital cardiac condition. *Swiss Med Wkly.* 2005;135:269–281.
15. Reich JD, Auld D, Hulse E, et al. The Pediatric Radiofrequency Ablation Registry's experience with Ebstein's anomaly. Pediatric Electrophysiology Society. *Cardiovasc Electrophysiol.* 1998;9:1370–1377.
16. Carmichael TB, Walsh EP, Roth SJ. Anticipatory use of venoarterial extracorporeal membrane oxygenation for a high-risk cardiac procedure. *Respir Care.* 2002;47:1002–1006.
17. Walsh EP. Interventional electrophysiology in patients with congenital heart disease. *Circulation.* 2007;115:3224–3234.
18. Kolterer B, Gebauer RA, Janousek J, et al. Improved quality of life after treatment of prolonged asystole during breath holding spells with a cardiac pacemaker. *Ann Pediatr Cardiol.* 2015;8:113–117.
19. Moodley M. The clinical approach to syncope in children. *Semin Pediatr Neurol.* 2013;20:12–17.
20. Kajstura J, Zhang X, Liu Y, et al. The cellular basis of pacing-induced dilated cardiomyopathy. Myocyte cell loss and myocyte cellular reactive hypertrophy. *Circulation.* 1995;92:2306–2317.

21. Shinbane JS, Wood MA, Jensen DN, et al. Tachycardia-induced cardiomyopathy: a review of animal models and clinical studies. *J Am Coll Cardiol.* 1997;29:709–715.
22. Fishberger SB, Colan SD, Saul JP, et al. Myocardial mechanics before and after ablation of chronic tachycardia. *Pacing Clin Electrophysiol.* 1996;19:42–49.
23. Tester DJ, Ackerman MJ. Postmortem long QT syndrome genetic testing for sudden unexplained death in the young. *J Am Coll Cardiol.* 2007;49:240–246.
24. Dick 2nd M, Law IH, Dorostkar PC, et al. Use of the His/RVA electrode catheter in children. *J Electrocardiol.* 1996;29(suppl):227–233.
25. La MJ, Saul JP, Reed JH. Long-term outcomes for cryoablation of pediatric patients with atrioventricular nodal reentrant tachycardia. *Am J Cardiol.* 2010;105:1118–1121.
26. Smith G, Clark JM. Elimination of fluoroscopy use in a pediatric electrophysiology laboratory utilizing three-dimensional mapping. *Pacing Clin Electrophysiol.* 2007;30:510–518.
27. Mah DY, Miyake CY, Sherwin ED, et al. The use of an integrated electroanatomic mapping system and intracardiac echocardiography to reduce radiation exposure in children and young adults undergoing ablation of supraventricular tachycardia. *Europace.* 2014;16:277–283.
28. Silvetti MS, Drago F, Grutter G, et al. Twenty years of paediatric cardiac pacing: 515 pacemakers and 480 leads implanted in 292 patients. *Europace.* 2006;8:530–536.
29. Walsh EP, Cecchin F. Recent advances in pacemaker and implantable defibrillator therapy for young patients. *Curr Opin Cardiol.* 2004;19:91–96.
30. Strasburger JF, Cheulkar B, Wakai RT. Magnetocardiography for fetal arrhythmias. *Heart Rhythm.* 2008;5:1073–1076.
31. Jaeggi ET, Nii M. Fetal brady- and tachyarrhythmias: new and accepted diagnostic and treatment methods. *Semin Fetal Neonatal Med.* 2005;10:504–514.
32. Wacker-Gussmann A, Strasburger JF, Cuneo BF, et al. Diagnosis and treatment of fetal arrhythmia. *Am J Perinatol.* 2014;31:617–628.
33. Brito-Zerón P, Izmirly PM, Ramos-Casals M, et al. The clinical spectrum of autoimmune congenital heart block. *Nat Rev Rheumatol.* 2015;11:301–312.
34. Bar-Cohen Y, Loeb GE, Pruetz JD, et al. Preclinical testing and optimization of a novel fetal micropacemaker. *Heart Rhythm.* 2015;12:1683–1690.
35. Ko JK, Deal BJ, Strasburger JF, et al. Supraventricular tachycardia mechanisms and their age distribution in pediatric patients. *Am J Cardiol.* 1992;69:1028–1032.
36. Tanel RE, Walsh EP, Triedman JK, et al. Five-year experience with radiofrequency catheter ablation: implications for management of arrhythmias in pediatric and young adult patients. *J Pediatr.* 1997;131:878–887.
37. Van Hare GF, Javitz H, Carmelli D, et al. Prospective assessment after pediatric cardiac ablation: demographics, medical profiles, and initial outcomes. *J Cardiovasc Electrophysiol.* 2004;15:759–770.
38. Zachariah JP, Walsh EP, Triedman JK, et al. Multiple accessory pathways in the young: the impact of structural heart disease. *Am Heart J.* 2013;165:87–92.
39. de Caen AR, Maconochie IK, Aickin R, et al. Pediatric basic life support and pediatric advanced life support: 2015 International Consensus on Cardiopulmonary Resuscitation and Emergency Cardiovascular Care Science With Treatment Recommendations. *Circulation.* 2015;132:S177–S203.
40. Kugler JD, Danford DA, Deal BJ, et al. Radiofrequency catheter ablation for tachyarrhythmias in children and adolescents. *N Engl J Med.* 1994;330:1481–1487.
41. Friedman RA, Walsh EP, Silka MJ, et al. NASPE Expert Consensus Conference: radiofrequency catheter ablation in children with and without congenital heart disease. Report of the writing committee. North American Society of Pacing and Electrophysiology. *Pacing Clin Electrophysiol.* 2002;25:1000–1017.

42. Cohen MI, Triedman JK, Cannon BC, et al. PACES/HRS expert consensus statement on the management of the asymptomatic young patient with a Wolff-Parkinson-White pattern. *Heart Rhythm.* 2012;9:1006–1024.
43. Kang KT, Potts JE, Radbill AE, et al. Permanent junctional reciprocating tachycardia in children: a multicenter experience. *Heart Rhythm.* 2014;11:1426–1432.
44. Van Hare GF, Chiesa NA, Campbell RM, et al. Atrioventricular nodal reentrant tachycardia in children: effect of slow pathway ablation on fast pathway function. *J Cardiovasc Electrophysiol.* 2002;13:203–209.
45. Mahajan T, Berul CI, Cecchin F, et al. Atrioventricular nodal reentrant tachycardia with 2:1 block in pediatric patients. *Heart Rhythm.* 2008;5:1391–1395.
46. Collins KK, Schaffer MS. Use of cryoablation for treatment of tachyarrhythmias in 2010: survey of current practices of pediatric electrophysiologists. *Pacing Clin Electrophysiol.* 2011;34:304–308.
47. Khairy P, Seslar SP, Triedman JK, et al. Ablation of atrioventricular nodal reentrant tachycardia in tricuspid atresia. *J Cardiovasc Electrophysiol.* 2004;15:719–722.
48. Toyohara K, Fukuhara H, Yoshimoto J, et al. Electrophysiologic studies and radiofrequency catheter ablation of ectopic atrial tachycardia in children. *Pediatr Cardiol.* 2011;32:40–46.
49. Yeager SB, Hougen TJ, Levy AM. Sudden death in infants with chaotic atrial rhythm. *Am J Dis Child.* 1984;138:689–692.
50. Bevilacqua LM, Rhee EK, Epstein MR, et al. Focal ablation of chaotic atrial rhythm in an infant with cardiomyopathy. *J Cardiovasc Electrophysiol.* 2000;11:577–581.
51. Collins KK, Van Hare GF, Kertesz NJ, et al. Pediatric non-postoperative junctional ectopic tachycardia. *J Am Coll Cardiol.* 2009;53:690–697.
52. Walsh EP, Saul JP, Sholler GF, et al. Evaluation of a staged treatment protocol for rapid automatic junctional tachycardia after operation for congenital heart disease. *J Am Coll Cardiol.* 1997;29:1046–1053.
53. Villain E, Vetter VL, Garcia JM, et al. Evolving concepts in the management of congenital junctional ectopic tachycardia. A multicenter study. *Circulation.* 1990;81:1544–1549.
54. Gillette PC, Garson Jr A, Porter CJ, et al. Junctional automatic ectopic tachycardia: new proposed treatment by transcatheter His bundle ablation. *Am Heart J.* 1983;106:619–623.
55. Van Hare GF, Velvis H, Langberg JJ. Successful transcatheter ablation of congenital junctional ectopic tachycardia in a ten-month-old infant using radiofrequency energy. *Pacing Clin Electrophysiol.* 1990;13:730–735.
56. Grant JW, Serwer GA, Armstrong BE, et al. Junctional tachycardia in infants and children after open heart surgery for congenital heart disease. *Am J Cardiol.* 1987;59:1216–1218.
57. Till JA, Rowland E. Atrial pacing as an adjunct to the management of post-surgical His bundle tachycardia. *Br Heart J.* 1991;66:225–229.
58. Raja P, Hawker RE, Chaikitpinyo A, et al. Amiodarone management of junctional ectopic tachycardia after cardiac surgery in children. *Br Heart J.* 1994;72:261–265.
59. Saul JP, Scott WA, Brown S, et al. Intravenous amiodarone for incessant tachyarrhythmias in children: a randomized, double-blind, antiarrhythmic drug trial. *Circulation.* 2005;112:3470–3477.
60. Texter KM, Kertesz NJ, Friedman RA, et al. Atrial flutter in infants. *J Am Coll Cardiol.* 2006;48:1040–1046.
61. Jaeggi ET, Carvalho JS, De Groot E, et al. Comparison of transplacental treatment of fetal supraventricular tachyarrhythmias with digoxin, flecainide, and sotalol: results of a nonrandomized multicenter study. *Circulation.* 2011;124:1747–1754.

62. Ceresnak SR, Liberman L, Silver ES, et al. Lone atrial fibrillation in the young—perhaps not so "lone"? *J Pediatr.* 2013;162:827–831.

63. Lai LP, Lin JL, Huang SK. Molecular genetic studies in atrial fibrillation. *Cardiology.* 2003;100:109–113.

64. Sherwin ED, Triedman JK, Walsh EP. Update on interventional electrophysiology in congenital heart disease: evolving solutions for complex hearts. *Circ Arrhythm Electrophysiol.* 2013;6:1032–1040.

65. Triedman JK, Bergau DM, Saul JP, et al. Efficacy of radiofrequency ablation for control of intraatrial reentrant tachycardia in patients with congenital heart disease. *J Am Coll Cardiol.* 1997;30:1032–1038.

66. Triedman JK. Atrial reentrant tachycardias. In: Walsh EP, Saul JP, Triedman JK, eds. *Cardiac Arrhythmias in Children and Young Adults with Congenital Heart Disease.* Philadelphia: Lippincott Williams & Wilkins; 2001:137–159.

67. Saul JP, Triedman JK. Radiofrequency ablation of intraatrial reentrant tachycardia after surgery for congenital heart disease. *Pacing Clin Electrophysiol.* 1997;20:2112–2117.

68. January CT, Wann LS, Alpert JS, et al. 2014 AHA/ACC/HRS guideline for the management of patients with atrial fibrillation: a report of the American College of Cardiology/American Heart Association Task Force on practice guidelines and the Heart Rhythm Society. *Circulation.* 2014;130:e199–e267.

69. Lakkireddy D, Rangisetty U, Prasad S, et al. Intracardiac echo-guided radiofrequency catheter ablation of atrial fibrillation in patients with atrial septal defect or patent foramen ovale repair: a feasibility, safety, and efficacy study. *J Cardiovasc Electrophysiol.* 2008;19:1137–1142.

70. Freire G, Dubrow I. Accelerated idioventricular rhythm in newborns: a worrisome but benign entity with or without congenital heart disease. *Pediatr Cardiol.* 2008;29:457–462.

71. Morwood JG, Triedman JK, Berul CI, et al. Radiofrequency catheter ablation of ventricular tachycardia in children and young adults with congenital heart disease. *Heart Rhythm.* 2004;1:301–308.

72. Fukuhara J, Sumitomo N, Nakamura T, et al. Electrophysiological characteristics of idiopathic ventricular tachycardia in children. *Circ J.* 2011;75:672–676.

73. Collins KK, Schaffer MS, Liberman L, et al. Fascicular and nonfascicular left ventricular tachycardias in the young: an international multicenter study. *J Cardiovasc Electrophysiol.* 2013;24:640–648.

74. Aiba T, Suyama K, Aihara N, et al. The role of Purkinje and pre-Purkinje potentials in the reentrant circuit of verapamil-sensitive idiopathic LV tachycardia. *Pacing Clin Electrophysiol.* 2001;24:333–344.

75. Horowitz LN, Vetter VL, Harken AH. Electrophysiologic characteristics of sustained ventricular tachycardia occurring after repair of tetralogy of Fallot. *Am J Cardiol.* 1980;46:446–452.

76. Shivapour JK, Sherwin ED, Alexander ME, et al. Utility of preoperative electrophysiologic studies in patients with Ebstein's anomaly undergoing the Cone procedure. *Heart Rhythm.* 2014;11:182–186.

77. Obioha-Ngwu O, Milliez P, Richardson A, et al. Ventricular tachycardia in Ebstein's anomaly. *Circulation.* 2001;104:E92–E94.

78. Silka MJ, Hardy BG, Menashe VD, et al. A population-based prospective evaluation of risk of sudden cardiac death after operation for common congenital heart defects. *J Am Coll Cardiol.* 1998;32:245–251.

79. Walsh EP. Sudden death in adult congenital heart disease: risk stratification in 2014. *Heart Rhythm.* 2014;11:1735–1742.

80. Villafañe J, Feinstein JA, Jenkins KJ, et al. Hot topics in tetralogy of Fallot. *J Am Coll Cardiol.* 2013;62:2155–2166.

81. Khairy P, Landzberg MJ, Gatzoulis MA, et al. Value of programmed ventricular stimulation after tetralogy of Fallot repair: a multicenter study. *Circulation.* 2004;109:1994–2000.

82. Khairy P, Harris L, Landzberg MJ, et al. Implantable cardioverter-defibrillators in tetralogy of Fallot. *Circulation.* 2008;117:363–370.

83. Zeppenfeld K, Schalij MJ, Bartelings MM, et al. Catheter ablation of ventricular tachycardia after repair of congenital heart disease: electroanatomic identification of the critical right ventricular isthmus. *Circulation.* 2007;116:2241–2252.

84. Dubin AM, Berul CI, Bevilacqua LM, et al. The use of implantable cardioverter-defibrillators in pediatric patients awaiting heart transplantation. *J Card Fail.* 2003;9:375–379.

85. Lupoglazoff JM, Cheav T, Baroudi G, et al. Homozygous SCN5A mutation in long-QT syndrome with functional two-to-one atrioventricular block. *Circ Res.* 2001;89:E16–E21.

86. Venetucci L, Denegri M, Napolitano C, et al. Inherited calcium channelopathies in the pathophysiology of arrhythmias. *Nat Rev Cardiol.* 2012;9:561–575.

87. Garson Jr A, Dick M, Fournier A, et al. The long QT syndrome in children. An international study of 287 patients. *Circulation.* 1993;87:1866–1872.

88. Schwartz PJ, Moss AJ, Vincent GM, et al. Diagnostic criteria for the long QT syndrome. An update. *Circulation.* 1993;88:782–784.

89. Aziz PF, Wieand TS, Ganley J, et al. Genotype- and mutation site-specific QT adaptation during exercise, recovery, and postural changes in children with long-QT syndrome. *Circ Arrhythm Electrophysiol.* 2011;4:867–873.

90. Daubert JP, Zareba W, Rosero SZ, et al. Role of implantable cardioverter defibrillator therapy in patients with long QT syndrome. *Am Heart J.* 2007;153:53–58.

91. Collura CA, Johnson JN, Moir C, et al. Left cardiac sympathetic denervation for the treatment of long QT syndrome and catecholaminergic polymorphic ventricular tachycardia using video-assisted thoracic surgery. *Heart Rhythm.* 2009;6:752–759.

92. Liu N, Ruan Y, Priori SG. Catecholaminergic polymorphic ventricular tachycardia. *Prog Cardiovasc Dis.* 2008;51:23–30.

93. Nguyen HL, Pieper GH, Wilders R. Andersen-Tawil syndrome: clinical and molecular aspects. *Int J Cardiol.* 2013;170:1–16.

94. Frangini PA, Cecchin F, Jordao L, et al. How revealing are insertable loop recorders in pediatrics? *Pacing Clin Electrophysiol.* 2008;31:338–343.

95. Roston TM, Vinocur JM, Maginot KR, et al. Catecholaminergic polymorphic ventricular tachycardia in children: analysis of therapeutic strategies and outcomes from an international multicenter registry. *Circ Arrhythm Electrophysiol.* 2015;8:633–642.

96. Suzuki H, Torigoe K, Numata O, et al. Infant case with a malignant form of Brugada syndrome. *J Cardiovasc Electrophysiol.* 2000;11:1277–1280.

97. Gehi AK, Duong TD, Metz LD, et al. Risk stratification of individuals with the Brugada electrocardiogram: a meta-analysis. *J Cardiovasc Electrophysiol.* 2006;17:577–583.

98. Maron BJ, Roberts WC, McAllister HA, et al. Sudden death in young athletes. *Circulation.* 1980;62:218–229.

99. Maron BJ. Hypertrophic cardiomyopathy: a systematic review. *JAMA.* 2002;287:1308–1320.

100. Colan SD, Lipshultz SE, Lowe AM, et al. Epidemiology and cause-specific outcome of hypertrophic cardiomyopathy in children: findings from the Pediatric Cardiomyopathy Registry. *Circulation.* 2007;115:773–781.

101. Maron BJ, Spirito P, Ackerman MJ, et al. Prevention of sudden cardiac death with implantable cardioverter-defibrillators in children and adolescents with hypertrophic cardiomyopathy. *J Am Coll Cardiol.* 2013;61:1527–1535.

102. Hamilton RM, Fidler L. Right ventricular cardiomyopathy in the young: an emerging challenge. *Heart Rhythm.* 2009;6:571–575.

103. Lee AC, Foster E, Yeghiazarians Y. Anomalous origin of the left coronary artery from the pulmonary artery: a case series and brief review. *Congenit Heart Dis.* 2006;1:111–115.

104. Hoffman JI. Abnormal origins of the coronary arteries from the aortic root. *Cardiol Young.* 2014;24:774–791.

105. Daniels LB, Gordon JB, Burns JC. Kawasaki disease: late cardiovascular sequelae. *Curr Opin Cardiol.* 2012;27:572–577.

106. Miyake CY, Del Nido PJ, Alexander ME, et al. Cardiac tumors and associated arrhythmias in pediatric patients, with observations on surgical therapy for ventricular tachycardia. *J Am Coll Cardiol.* 2011;58:1903–1909.

107. Miyake CY, Teele SA, Chen L, et al. In-hospital arrhythmia development and outcomes in pediatric patients with acute myocarditis. *Am J Cardiol.* 2014;113:535–540.

108. Nogueira G, Pinto FF, Paixao A, et al. Idiopathic dilated cardiomyopathy in children: clinical profile and prognostic determinants. *Rev Port Cardiol.* 2000;19:191–200.

109. Weisz SH, Limongelli G, Pacileo G, et al. Left ventricular non compaction in children. *Congenit Heart Dis.* 2010;5:384–397.

110. Payne L, Zeigler VL, Gillette PC. Acute cardiac arrhythmias following surgery for congenital heart disease: mechanisms, diagnostic tools, and management. *Crit Care Nurs Clin North Am.* 2011;23:255–272.

111. Epstein AE, Dimarco JP, Ellenbogen KA, et al. ACC/AHA/HRS 2008 guidelines for Device-Based Therapy of Cardiac Rhythm Abnormalities: executive summary. *Heart Rhythm.* 2008;5:934–955.

112. Manning PB, Mayer Jr JE, Wernovsky G, et al. Staged operation to Fontan increases the incidence of sinoatrial node dysfunction. *J Thorac Cardiovasc Surg.* 1996;111:833–839.

113. Benson DW, Wang DW, Dyment M, et al. Congenital sick sinus syndrome caused by recessive mutations in the cardiac sodium channel gene (SCN5A). *J Clin Invest.* 2003;112:1019–1028.

114. Casiero D, Frishman WH. Cardiovascular complications of eating disorders. *Cardiol Rev.* 2006;14:227–231.

115. Michaelsson M, Engle MA. Congenital complete heart block: an international study of the natural history. *Cardiovasc Clin.* 1972;4:85–101.

116. Hutter D, Silverman ED, Jaeggi ET. The benefits of transplacental treatment of isolated congenital complete heart block associated with maternal anti-Ro/SSA antibodies: a review. *Scand J Immunol.* 2010;72:235–241.

117. Friedman RA. Congenital complete AV block. Pace me now or pace me later? *Circulation.* 1995;92:283–285.

118. Weindling SN, Saul JP, Gamble WJ, et al. Duration of complete atrioventricular block after congenital heart disease surgery. *Am J Cardiol.* 1998;82:525–527.

119. Guglin M, Nallamshetty L. Myocarditis: diagnosis and treatment. *Curr Treat Options Cardiovasc Med.* 2012;14:637–651.

120. Costello JM, Alexander ME, Greco KM, et al. Lyme carditis in children: presentation, predictive factors, and clinical course. *Pediatrics.* 2009;123:e835–e841.

110 Sleep-Disordered Breathing and Arrhythmias

Apoor S. Gami, Sean M. Caples, and Virend K. Somers

Obstructive sleep apnea (OSA) and central sleep apnea (CSA), the most common sleep-related breathing disorders, are associated with cardiac arrhythmias. While this had long been recognized anecdotally, only in recent decades have controlled studies confirmed clinicians' suspicions of a strong relationship between these conditions. This chapter will first provide a brief introduction of the pathophysiology and epidemiology of OSA and CSA to cardiologists. Second, it will describe the epidemiological data supporting associations of sleep apnea with bradyarrhythmias, atrial fibrillation (AF), ventricular arrhythmias, and sudden cardiac death (SCD). Next, it will describe the intriguing pathophysiological mechanisms by which OSA and CSA may promote the initiation or maintenance of these arrhythmias. Last, it explores the growing data that identify potential beneficial effects, or otherwise, of sleep apnea therapy on these relationships.

Obstructive Sleep Apnea

Pathophysiology
OSA is characterized by the failure of neuromuscular mechanisms governing upper airway patency during sleep, resulting in airway narrowing or collapse. While apnea can occur in any position, the upper airway is more vulnerable to obstruction in the supine position due to dorsal displacement of the tongue and soft tissues. Upper airway collapse can occur during any stage of sleep, but susceptibility is greatest during rapid eye movement (REM). Heralded by atonia of skeletal muscles, including that of the pharynx and upper airway but excluding the respiratory diaphragm and extraocular muscles, REM occurs cyclically (four to six times) throughout sleep and accounts for about 25% of total sleep time. Of potential pathophysiological importance in arrhythmogenesis, REM is a state of autonomic instability marked by surges in both sympathetic and vagal activity, with attendant variations in heart rate, blood pressure, and peripheral vascular resistance.[1]

Obstructive disordered breathing events are repetitive, numbering in the hundreds per night in extreme cases. Each is associated with oxyhemoglobin desaturation followed by a central nervous system arousal, thereby reestablishing upper airway patency with resumption of ventilation and subsequent reoxygenation. Associated with each repetitive cycle is a cascade of acute stressors, including, among others, hypoxemia, surges in sympathetic neural output, production of reactive oxygen species, and fluctuations of intrathoracic and cardiac transmural pressures. The relevance of these acute pathophysiological changes to specific arrhythmia syndromes will be discussed later.

Diagnosis of OSA is made using attended in-lab multichannel polysomnography. These data generate the apnea–hypopnea index (AHI), which is the average number of apneas and hypopneas per hour of sleep. The AHI is the traditional composite measurement of OSA severity, but it does not directly quantify other processes that are operative in the pathophysiology of cardiovascular disease, which correlate better with the burden of oxygen desaturation. Measurements such as the lowest oxygen saturation that occurs during sleep and the oxygen desaturation index (ODI), which is the average number of times per hour of sleep that the oxygen saturation falls by 3% or more from baseline, are indices that may be more relevant to the cardiologist and are usually available in the polysomnography report.

The diagnosis of OSA is increasingly made using home sleep testing, which is appropriate for patients with a high pretest probability of the disorder but without underlying cardiopulmonary disease. In those with heart failure, COPD, or suspicion for an underlying hypoventilation syndrome (such as neuromuscular disease), in-lab polysomnography remains the standard test.

Epidemiology and Clinical Features

The best available data from population-based studies that utilized polysomnographic monitoring in adults provide estimates of the prevalence of OSA to be between 3% and 28%.[2] Men, in part due to truncal distribution of adipose tissue and muscle, have a higher risk of OSA than women, but the sex prevalence gap narrows after menopause. Age, obesity, and increased neck circumference are additional strong risk factors for OSA.[3] Updated data from the Wisconsin Sleep Cohort show that rates of moderate to severe OSA have increased by as much as 50% over the past two decades.

Excessive daytime sleepiness, a result of frequent nocturnal central nervous system arousals, is the most important symptom of OSA and a potential contributor to motor vehicle accidents. Yet less than 25% of individuals with OSA actually report excessive sleepiness, although it is likely that subjective reporting underrepresents the true symptomatic burden of OSA.[4] Other typical signs and symptoms of OSA include loud snoring, interrupted and unrefreshing sleep, and headache and dry mouth upon awakening. A most helpful and specific sign is provided by a bed partner who witnesses pauses in breathing.

Central Sleep Apnea

Pathophysiology
CSA is characterized by the loss of ventilatory output from the central respiratory generator in the brainstem, resulting in interruptions of respiratory muscle output that lead to apneas and hypopneas. Generally, the maintenance of upper airway patency distinguishes CSA from OSA. However, the conditions may coexist. CSA is broadly composed of a few heterogeneous disorders, such as high-altitude periodic breathing, idiopathic CSA, and some hypoventilation syndromes. The most common and studied form of CSA is Cheyne-Stokes respiration (CSA-CSR), which is most often encountered in the setting of heart failure and manifests as a characteristic waxing and waning periodicity of ventilation.

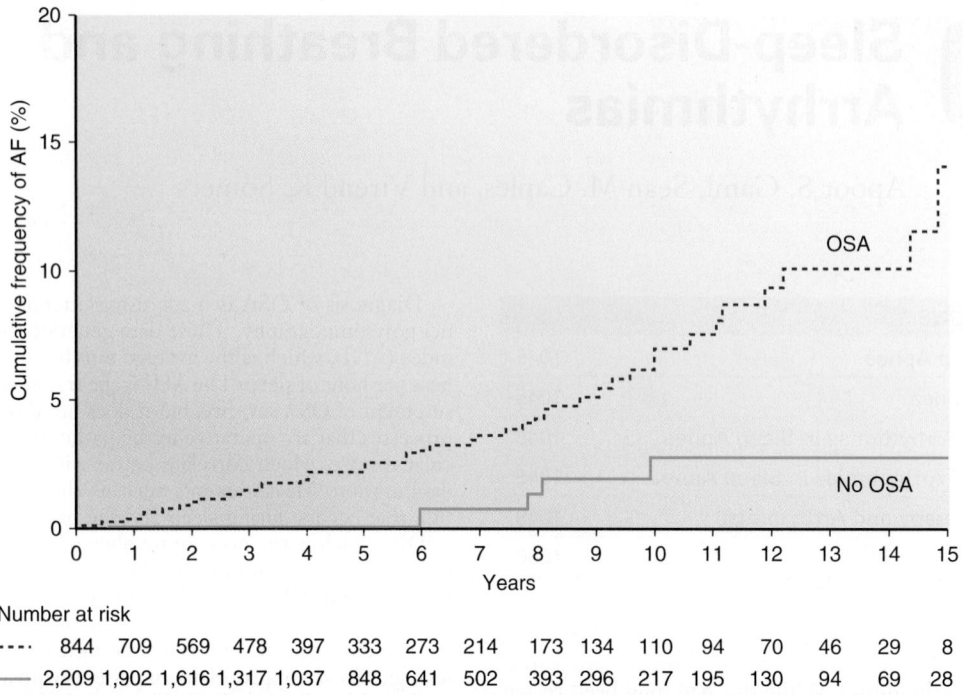

FIGURE 110.1 Obstructive sleep apnea (*OSA*) predicts incident atrial fibrillation (*AF*). Cumulative frequency curves for incident AF for subjects <65 years of age with and without OSA during an average 4.7 years of follow-up. *p* = .002. (From Gami AS, Hodge DO, Herges RM, et al. Obstructive sleep apnea, obesity, and the risk of incident atrial fibrillation. *J Am Coll Cardiol.* 2007;49: 565-571.)

CSA-CSR reflects derangements in ventilatory control mechanisms caused by the hemodynamic consequences of left atrial hypertension and decreased cardiac output (usually due to left ventricular [LV] dysfunction). Partly because of irritant receptor stimulation by pulmonary microvascular congestion, heart failure patients chronically hyperventilate, resulting in low blood carbon dioxide tensions during wakefulness.[5] The relative hypocapnia, together with a heightened chemoreflex response to carbon dioxide and prolonged circulation time, destabilize the ventilatory control system during sleep and result in CSA-CSR. As would be expected by these mechanisms, inhalation of a carbon dioxide–enriched gas abolishes CSA.

CSA-CSR, like OSA, is diagnosed by multichannel polysomnography and is quantified by the central AHI. The characteristic waxing and waning pattern of ventilation, which may also be seen during wakefulness, is most prominent during non-REM sleep and is characteristically absent during REM, where cortical influences on ventilation often override the chemoreflex. Similar to OSA, CSA-CSR is associated with repetitive cycles of acute stressors, including hypoxemia, sympathetic activation, and fluctuations in heart rate and blood pressure.[6] In contrast to OSA, the influence of these processes on cardiovascular outcomes, including arrhythmias, has been relatively unexplored. Some data suggest that CSA-CSR contributes to worse cardiovascular outcomes beyond what is attributable to the accompanying heart failure. However, recent data showing increased mortality in heart failure patients who received state-of-the-art CSA-CSR therapy lend pause to any certainty regarding these complex relationships.[7] What is known regarding the effect of CSA-CSR on specific arrhythmia syndromes is described in subsequent sections.

Epidemiology and Clinical Features

The prevalence of CSA-CSR in the general population or in unselected individuals with LV dysfunction is unknown. In two studies of more than 500 patients with predominantly New York Heart Association class II heart failure and an average LV ejection fraction of about 25%, the prevalence of sleep apnea identified using polysomnography was between 33% and 40%.[8,9] The prevalence of CSA-CSR increases directly with the severity of heart failure. Like OSA, age and male sex increase the risk for CSA-CSR, with narrowing of the gender gap after menopause.

It is unclear if CSA-CSR results in symptoms independent of those related to the underlying cardiac condition. Nocturnal dyspnea attributable to cardiac dysfunction may also be explained by the hyperpneas of CSA-CSR. Despite the fact that CSA may coexist with OSA, symptoms of sleepiness referable to OSA are notably absent in individuals with heart failure.

Mechanisms of Arrhythmias in Sleep Apnea

Obesity, diabetes, dyslipidemia, hypertension, ischemic heart disease, and systolic and diastolic heart failure all cluster with sleep apnea (Fig. 110.1).[10] Simply by association with these conditions, the risk of arrhythmias is increased in patients with OSA and CSA. Intriguingly, sleep apnea itself has several unique pathophysiological mechanisms that may directly promote the initiation or maintenance of specific clinical arrhythmias, as discussed in subsequent sections.

Bradyarrhythmias

Bradycardias during sleep are not uncommon in healthy individuals, and it is helpful to compare the mechanisms of bradycardia between healthy individuals and those with sleep apnea. Although sympathetic neural output and average heart rate are higher during REM sleep than during non-REM sleep, there is evidence for paroxysmal parasympathetic discharges during REM that manifest as abrupt heart rate decelerations. Healthy young adults, often athletes, have periods of exaggerated vagal tone during REM sleep. This results in many benign, albeit sometimes pronounced, bradycardias that are discussed later.

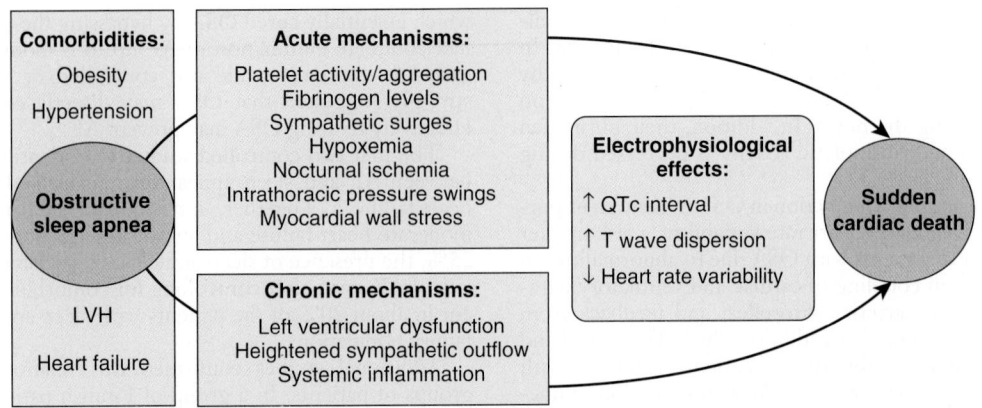

FIGURE 110.2 Obstructive sleep apnea and sudden cardiac death. Obstructive sleep apnea increases the risk of ventricular arrhythmias and sudden cardiac death through associations with comorbidities and its unique pathophysiological mechanisms, both acute and chronic, that may lead to arterial thrombosis and cardiac structural and electrophysiological changes. *LVH*, Left ventricular hypertrophy.

In individuals with OSA, apnea and hypoxemia activate the physiological "diving reflex," so named from observations of oxygen conservation during prolonged water submersion by marine mammals. Hypoxemia, via stimulation of the carotid bodies, normally not only induces hyperventilation but also results in bradycardia. With normal breathing and hyperventilation, this heart rate slowing is attenuated by the vagolytic effects of lung inflation. This latter buffer is lost during apnea and when coupled with the effects of oxyhemoglobin desaturation, results in marked bradycardias.[11] Electrophysiological studies in individuals with OSA and bradycardias who were referred for permanent pacemaker implantation showed no evidence of significant sinus, atrioventricular (AV) node, or His–Purkinje system disease, reflecting the influence of autonomic changes that occur in OSA.

Atrial Fibrillation

Multiple pathophysiological mechanisms may directly link OSA and AF. The marked fluctuations in autonomic tone that occur in OSA have important implications for the initiation and propagation of AF. Cessation of breathing is associated with increases in sympathetic neural output, as measured by peripheral microneurography.[12] Via the aforementioned diving reflex, there may also be a concomitant rise in cardiac vagal activity.[11] Furthermore, surges in sympathetic neural activity occur with each central nervous system arousal that terminates an apnea. While sleep stage–dependent mechanisms have yet to be proved in arrhythmogenesis, the influence of sleep stage on autonomic tone is well recognized. Stage II sleep is punctuated by characteristic "K-complexes," high-amplitude electroencephalogram (EEG) discharges associated with transient increases in peripheral sympathetic neural activity, and a rise in blood pressure.[1] Slow-wave sleep, underrepresented in severe OSA, is a state of parasympathetic predominance. REM sleep is associated with abrupt fluctuations in both sympathetic and parasympathetic activity. While it is clear that the autonomic system plays a major role in the pathophysiology of AF, its specific effects are still being determined.[13] These processes may lead to activation of atrial catecholamine-sensitive ion channels, which could result in ectopy that initiates AF, and also to vagally mediated changes in atrial conduction properties that promote and maintain AF. Additionally, individuals with OSA have chronically elevated sympathetic activity even during the waking period, which may have a deleterious effect on rate-control strategies for AF management.[12]

Increased left atrial size is associated with OSA, independently of other medical conditions.[14] Even among completely healthy, middle-aged men and women with normal left atrial volume indices, those with OSA had a significantly larger left atrium. Left atrial size may be increased in individuals with OSA due to its association with hypertension and diastolic dysfunction.[15] Again, among otherwise healthy individuals, subtle changes in diastolic dysfunction are present in those with OSA, and the severity of diastolic dysfunction correlates directly with the severity of oxygen desaturations. Concomitant obesity likely contributes to an enlarged left atrium due to larger body mass and increased total blood volume.

Wide fluctuations in intrathoracic pressure due to repetitive inspiratory efforts against an obstructed upper airway increase cardiac wall stress.[16] This process may also cause chronic stretching of the atrium, particularly at anchoring regions such as the pulmonary vein ostia, leading to electrical and structural remodeling. Activation of stretch-sensitive ion channels in the atrium may lead to focal impulses that initiate and propagate AF, as an interventional study found a 46% higher frequency of atrial premature depolarizations during simulated obstructive apneas (Muller maneuvers) than during normal breathing.[17]

OSA is associated with systemic inflammation, evidenced by increased levels of C-reactive protein, serum amyloid A, and interleukins, which may contribute to atrial fibrosis and remodeling.[18]

Several measurable electrophysiological abnormalities that promote AF have been demonstrated in patients with OSA. The presence and severity of OSA correlate with interatrial and left atrial electromechanical delay as measured by tissue Doppler imaging and P wave dispersion.[19] Furthermore, atria in patients with OSA demonstrate lower voltage, slower conduction, and more widespread complex fractionated electrograms.[20]

Ventricular Arrhythmias and Sudden Cardiac Death

Numerous pathophysiological mechanisms may directly and indirectly link OSA to ventricular arrhythmias and SCD (Fig. 110.2). The repetitive oxygen desaturations during apneic sleep are temporally associated with ventricular ectopy. This hypoxemia and the simultaneous hypercapnia activate the chemoreflex, which increases peripheral vascular sympathetic nerve activity and circulating catecholamines.[12] Tachycardia and surges in blood pressure at the end of apneas increase myocardial oxygen demand at the same time that hypoxemia decreases myocardial oxygen supply. The resultant nocturnal ischemia, whether manifesting as silent ST-segment changes or nocturnal angina, has been demonstrated in individuals with OSA and may be responsible for ventricular dysrhythmias during sleep.[21]

The risk of myocardial infarction and stroke, which may cause SCD or lead to SCD through dysrhythmias or other complications, is increased in individuals with OSA due to multiple mechanisms that promote nocturnal arterial thrombosis. In contrast to the usual diurnal variation of coagulation in healthy individuals, patients with OSA have increased platelet activation and aggregation during the night. In addition, their fibrinogen levels are increased and fibrinolytic activity is decreased during sleep.

The marked autonomic dysfunction in OSA is likely an important link to SCD. Decreased heart rate variability, a risk marker for SCD, is present in patients with OSA due to abnormalities in central nervous system coupling of cardiac and ventilatory parasympathetic inputs, the arterial baroreflex, and feedback from pulmonary stretch receptors.[22] In addition, the QTc interval and QTc interval dispersion are abnormal in patients with OSA, with the latter correlating directly with the AHI and duration of nocturnal hypoxemia.[23,24] In the special population of patients with congenital long QT syndrome (LQTS), for whom the magnitude of QTc prolongation is a strong marker of SCD risk, a study of 121 patients found that the presence and severity of OSA is associated with an increased QTc interval not only during sleep but also when awake.[25] Importantly, individuals with OSA have increased sympathetic activity that also persists during the awake period, which is associated with an increased risk of SCD.[12,26]

Finally, OSA is present in a large proportion of patients with heart failure, and it is implicated in chronic LV dysfunction through which it may be an important contributor to the neurohumoral response and myocardial remodeling that produce the electrophysiological substrate for SCD.[27]

Epidemiology of Arrhythmias in Sleep Apnea

Bradyarrhythmias

Due to the autonomic changes during normal sleep described earlier, healthy individuals across all age groups commonly have nocturnal sinus bradycardia, marked sinus arrhythmia, sinus pauses or arrest, or first-degree and type I second-degree AV block. This is more prominent in the young and in older athletes.[28] As a result, the American Academy of Sleep Medicine lowered the threshold heart rate for the diagnosis of bradycardia during sleep from the previous 60 to 40 beats/min.[29]

The risk factors for significant bradycardias in OSA include the magnitude of oxygen desaturation, higher AHI, and REM sleep.[30] The prevalence of bradycardias in OSA patients varies widely depending upon the diagnostic strategy. Two months of recordings from an implanted loop recorder identified a prevalence of 47%, while 48 hours of ambulatory electrocardiogram (ECG) monitoring found only a 13% prevalence in the same population.[31] In contrast to the majority of other data, the largest controlled study to assess nocturnal arrhythmias found no increase in bradyarrhythmias among patients with severe sleep apnea compared with individuals without sleep apnea.[32] These similar findings were observed in spite of the fact that the group with sleep apnea comprised individuals who were older and more obese and had more cardiac risk factors. The reason for the discrepant finding is unclear, but it may be due to the lack of distinguishing OSA from CSA in this report.

Atrial Fibrillation

Historically, a 1983 study by Guilleminault and colleagues provided the initial clues to a significant relationship between OSA and AF. Ambulatory ECG monitoring in 400 middle-aged patients with moderate or severe OSA (AHI ≥ 25) revealed that the prevalence of nocturnal paroxysms of AF was more than 3%,[31] which is more than five times the estimated prevalence of AF in middle-aged individuals in the community. Also noteworthy was that all 12 of the study patients who underwent tracheostomy,

which essentially cured OSA by bypassing the obstructed airway, had complete elimination of AF up to 6 months later.[31] These early observations, while not controlled or randomized data, strongly suggested that OSA may directly cause AF and that effectively treating OSA may prevent AF.

The first two controlled studies that identified a relationship between AF and sleep apnea were performed in patients with heart failure.[5,9] Together, in more than 500 patients with mostly moderate heart failure and an average ejection fraction of about 25%, the presence of sleep apnea was associated with a four-fold risk of AF, even after controlling for comorbidities. AF was present in about 20% of the patients with sleep apnea in these heart failure populations.

Additional studies confirmed this relationship in broader groups of patients. In a group of Finnish patients with lone AF (no ischemic or valvular heart disease, heart failure, sick sinus syndrome, pacemaker, hypertension, diabetes mellitus, hyperthyroidism, or acute causes of AF), 32% were found to have sleep apnea (an AHI of 15 or more, without differentiation between OSA and CSA).[33] This was an underestimate of the true prevalence of sleep apnea in lone AF patients because the standard criterion (an AHI of 5 or more) was not used. In an American study, the prevalence of OSA was compared between 151 consecutive patients undergoing electrical cardioversion of AF and 463 consecutive patients without AF being evaluated in a general cardiology practice.[34] The groups had similar age, sex, body mass index, and prevalence of hypertension and heart failure; however, the patients with AF had a significantly higher risk of OSA (49% vs. 33%), and a multivariate analysis demonstrated a strong independent association between OSA and AF (odds ratio 2.2). An analysis of nocturnal arrhythmias in 566 individuals undergoing polysomnography found AF in 5% of patients with severe sleep apnea and only 1% of patients without sleep apnea.[32]

An additional study found that the prevalence of AF was relatively high in patients with idiopathic CSA (no heart failure) compared with patients with OSA or no sleep apnea.[35] While it is possible that CSA in the absence of other cardiopulmonary conditions may increase the risk of AF, it also has been hypothesized that the opposite cause–effect relationship exists, namely that AF and its hemodynamic sequelae may lead to CSA.[36]

Most convincingly, a number of longitudinal studies have identified OSA as a risk factor in the incidence or recurrence of AF. In a prospective study of patients who underwent sleep studies prior to coronary artery bypass graft surgery, an AHI of 5 or more predicted a 32% incidence of postoperative AF requiring intervention, and an ODI of 5 or more predicted a 39% incidence of the same (both compared with 18% in the control groups).[37] A prospective assessment of AF recurrence in 106 patients 1 year after electrical cardioversion found that patients with untreated OSA had a significantly higher recurrence of AF than those for whom OSA status was unknown (82% vs. 53%).[38] Recurrent AF was predicted independently by the severity of nocturnal oxygen desaturation and the proportion of sleep time with oxygen saturation less than 90%. The largest study to date identified the incidence of new-onset AF up to 15 years after diagnostic polysomnography in 3542 patients referred to a sleep center.[39] OSA and multiple measures of its severity, in addition to the usual clinical predictors, were significantly associated with incident AF (Fig. 110.3). In individuals less than 65 years old, independent predictors of incident AF were age, male sex, coronary artery disease, body mass index (hazard ratio [HR] 1.07), and the decrease in nocturnal oxygen saturation (HR 3.29). This study clarified that obesity and OSA, independently of each other, additively increase the risk for AF. Again, the finding that nocturnal oxygen desaturation independently predicted incident AF likely reflects the underlying pathophysiological mechanisms of this relationship. In fact, the previously described three longitudinal studies that were designed to assess AF occurrence based on OSA status

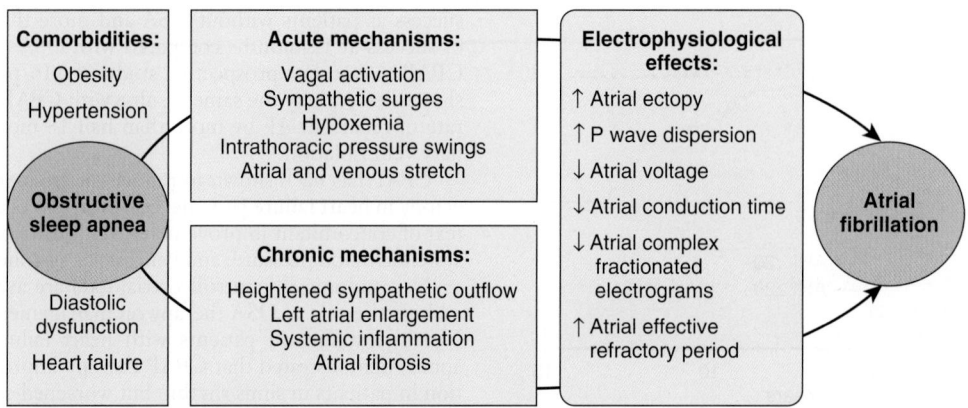

FIGURE 110.3 Obstructive sleep apnea and atrial fibrillation. Obstructive sleep apnea increases the risk of atrial fibrillation through associations with comorbidities and its unique pathophysiological mechanisms, both acute and chronic, that lead to atrial structural and electrophysiological changes.

found that measures of nocturnal oxygen desaturation were the most powerful predictors of AF.

Another important discovery was the independent association of OSA and AF in patients with hypertrophic cardiomyopathy, a condition in which AF is a marker for poorer survival.[40]

Several studies have identified OSA as a risk factor for the inefficacy of AF interventions, such as antiarrhythmic drugs and catheter ablation. One study of 61 patients found that severe sleep apnea nearly halved the response rate to antiarrhythmic drugs compared with less severe sleep apnea.[41] In 424 patients undergoing radiofrequency ablation of AF, OSA was an independent risk factor for acute failure of the procedure (relative risk 2.16).[42] A meta-analysis of six studies including nearly 4000 patients concluded that polysomnogram-diagnosed OSA increased recurrence after AF ablation by 40%, making it a very strong and important predictor of long-term failure.[43]

When attempting to predict the presence of OSA in patients with AF, it is important to recognize that symptoms usually associated with OSA may not be present, as they are in other patients. A prospective study in patients with AF undergoing cardioversion found that excessive daytime sleepiness, which is the hallmark of OSA, was present in only about one-third of them and that it did not correlate with sleep-disordered breathing or its severity.[44] This is important for the clinician who is making a decision to prescribe a sleep study, as a lack of sleepiness should not dissuade one from ordering the test if other predictors exist. It also has implications for a patient's response to OSA therapy. Evidence from randomized controlled trials show muted blood pressure reductions associated with continuous positive airway pressure (CPAP) therapy in nonsleepy OSA patients, suggesting that such symptoms could be a mediator of the cardiovascular system's response to treatment. Additionally, adherence to a treatment such as CPAP may be challenging in the asymptomatic patient.

Ventricular Arrhythmias and Sudden Cardiac Death

Historically, clinical experience and limited observations had suggested an increased frequency of nocturnal ventricular arrhythmias and nocturnal SCD in patients with sleep apnea, particularly in those with severe OSA. A controlled, multicenter study showed that nocturnal nonsustained ventricular tachycardia occurred in 5.3% and complex ventricular ectopy occurred in 25% of patients with severe sleep apnea.[32] After adjustment for comorbidities, patients with sleep apnea had a 3.4-fold risk of nonsustained ventricular tachycardia compared with patients without sleep apnea.

An important observation that demonstrates the acute impact of OSA on SCD is the apparent increase in nocturnal SCD in these patients.[45] The time of SCD was confirmed in 112 patients who had previously undergone polysomnography, and it was discovered that individuals with OSA had a significantly increased risk of SCD from 12 a.m. to 6 a.m. (relative risk 2.57), while individuals without OSA had a diurnal pattern of SCD similar to that expected in the general population (i.e., a peak between 6 a.m. and 12 p.m.). Nearly 50% of SCD in patients with OSA occurred during the sleeping hours, and the severity of OSA correlated directly with the risk of nocturnal SCD.[45] Similarly, in a study of patients with implantable cardioverter defibrillators, individuals with OSA had a significantly higher rate of treated ventricular arrhythmias, which was based on their high proportion of nocturnal events.[46]

In a longitudinal study that examined the risk of SCD in patients with OSA, the rates of SCD were assessed during an average of 7.5 years in 107 OSA patients who were compliant with CPAP therapy and 61 OSA patients who had discontinued CPAP therapy. SCD occurred in four patients (7%) with untreated OSA and in no patients with treated OSA (there was one arrhythmic death in a treated patient during coronary bypass surgery).[47] In the largest observational study of 10,701 adults referred for sleep study, OSA and several measures of its severity predicted incident SCD over an average 5.3 years' follow-up.[47a] Correlating directly with SCA were an AHI greater than 20 (HR 1.60), mean nocturnal oxygen saturation less than 93% (HR 2.93), and lowest nocturnal oxygen saturation less than 78% (HR 2.60). Nocturnal hypoxemia predicted SCD independently of all established clinical risk factors (Fig. 110.4).

Sleep Apnea Therapy and Arrhythmias

Obstructive Sleep Apnea

The most immediately effective and widespread therapy for OSA is CPAP. With regular use, it relieves daytime sleepiness and improves cognitive function. While many patients with highly symptomatic OSA adhere to CPAP therapy, those with limited symptoms may be less compliant. This poses a challenge in managing a growing population of patients with minimally symptomatic OSA and comorbid cardiovascular disease. Tracheostomy eliminates the consequences of upper airway collapse by entirely bypassing the upper airway, but it is typically regarded as a last resort therapy in patients with debilitating or life-threatening OSA. Weight loss is also an exceedingly effective treatment for OSA, as studies of bariatric surgery have suggested, but the long-term durability of this treatment remains to be proved. There are very few controlled studies of other surgical therapies (e.g., uvulopalatopharyngoplasty) for OSA.

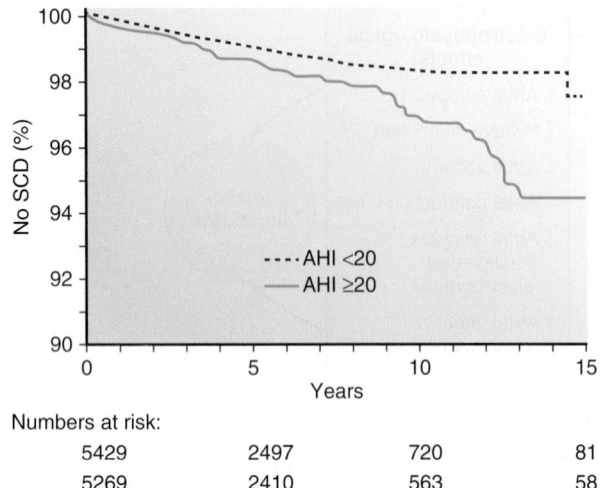

FIGURE 110.4 Obstructive sleep apnea predicts sudden cardiac death (SCD). Survival free of fatal or resuscitated SCD in 10,701 patients during an average 5.3 years of follow-up based on the apnea–hypopnea index (AHI). Hazard ratio: 1.60, 95% confidence interval: 1.14–2.24; p = .007. (From Gami AS, Olson EJ, Shen WK, et al. Obstructive sleep apnea and the risk of sudden cardiac death: a longitudinal study of 10,701 adults. *J Am Coll Cardiol.* 2013;62: 610-616.)

Given the long-standing role of CPAP as the first-line therapy for OSA, it has been most extensively studied in regard to cardiovascular outcomes. Treatment with CPAP has been shown to reduce or abolish many of the putative mechanisms that may link OSA to arrhythmias, including hypoxemia, inflammation, sympathetic overactivity, hypertension, myocardial ischemia, and ventricular systolic dysfunction. Recent studies have also shown specific favorable electrophysiological effects of CPAP therapy. In a study of 42 patients, CPAP therapy for 6 months significantly improved electrocardiographic P wave dispersion and echocardiographic interatrial as well as both left and right intraatrial electromechanical delay, all factors that have been associated with AF risk.[48]

A number of small, observational studies of selected populations demonstrated a reduction in bradyarrhythmias and AV block in individuals with OSA who were treated using CPAP.[30,49] While the usual cautions apply to generalizing these results to the clinical realm, they should encourage clinicians to consider OSA treatment prior to proceeding to more invasive therapies, such as pacemaker implantation, particularly if bradycardias are asymptomatic and limited to sleep.

There are increasing data demonstrating the beneficial effects of OSA therapy on AF. In the Outcomes Registry for Better Informed Treatment of Atrial Fibrillation (ORBIT-AF) registry, 1841 patients with OSA were followed up for 2 years, and those who used CPAP had one-third the rate of progression to more permanent forms of AF compared with those without CPAP.[50] In a prospective study of 118 patients with AF undergoing electrical cardioversion, recurrence was assessed at 1 year.[38] AF recurred in only 42% of OSA patients who were effectively treated with CPAP compared with recurrence in 82% of untreated OSA patients. The recurrence in treated OSA patients was even lower than that in the control group (53%), in whom OSA status was unknown. OSA patients without AF recurrence were three times more likely to have used effective CPAP therapy compared with those with recurrence, and no differences existed between those with and without recurrence with regard to age, gender, body mass index, or hypertension. Several studies have identified benefits of CPAP therapy in improving outcomes after catheter ablation of AF. In an observational study of 62 patients undergoing pulmonary vein isolation, OSA patients using CPAP had similar success as patients without OSA and more than twice the odds of success at 12 months compared with OSA patients not using CPAP.[51] Another prospective study of 116 patients with OSA showed essentially the same results, with CPAP use reducing the rate of recurrent AF by more than half 18 months after pulmonary vein isolation.[52]

CPAP has been shown to reduce the frequency of ventricular ectopy in heart failure patients; however, this occurred in the context of concomitant improvements in global sympathetic activity, systemic blood pressure, and ventricular systolic function.[53]

No randomized controlled trial data are available to directly address the role of OSA therapy on management of arrhythmias. Notably, studies in patients with heart failure (but not sleep apnea) demonstrated that CPAP therapy improved cardiac function in patients in sinus rhythm but worsened cardiac function in patients with AF.[54,55] Thus assumptions cannot be made about the benefit, let alone the safety, of OSA therapy on arrhythmias or other cardiovascular conditions, and this research needs to be designed cautiously. That notwithstanding, the prospect of a noninvasive, safe therapy to decrease the risk of significant clinical arrhythmias, like AF or SCD, is enticing. The recent SAVE study showed no cardiovascular benefit of treating OSA patients with cardiovascular disease with CPAP versus no CPAP, based on intention-to-treat analysis. However, this study was limited to nonsleepy OSA patients who may be at lower risk, and adherence to CPAP was less than optimal. Post hoc analysis suggested that better adherence to CPAP may have been associated with better outcomes.[55a]

Central Sleep Apnea

In contrast to the experience with OSA, there are few established therapies for CSA. Although CPAP was designed to treat OSA, it has been applied to CSA patients in hopes of improving their symptoms, objective heart failure status, and survival. A randomized controlled trial of CPAP in heart failure patients showed improvements in cardiac function but no survival benefit, perhaps because of limited efficacy of CPAP in treating CSA in this patient cohort.[56] CPAP has not been shown to decrease the occurrence or burden of arrhythmias in these patients. Adaptive servo-ventilation is another mode of ventilatory support that has been shown to ameliorate CSA and improve sleep quality. A much anticipated randomized controlled trial published in 2015 showed that adaptive servo-ventilation provided no benefits for cardiac or arrhythmic outcomes while paradoxically *increasing* all-cause and cardiovascular mortality in patients with heart failure and predominantly CSA.[7] The pathophysiological mechanisms of these findings and their reproducibility remain to be clarified. Currently, no data exist regarding potential antiarrhythmic effects of other suggested treatments for CSA-CSR, such as supplemental oxygen, theophylline, and acetazolamide. While it is clear that heart failure treatments (including medical therapy, mitral valve surgery, and biventricular pacing) improve CSA, it is not clear whether improvements in CSA itself are responsible for any potential improvements in arrhythmias.[57]

Approach to the Patient

Identifying and treating sleep apnea, particularly OSA, in patients with AF or at risk or resuscitated from SCD is an important adjunct to the overall care of these patients. Treating OSA favorably modifies the cardiovascular pathophysiological processes that lead to these significant arrhythmias. It should be recognized, however, that currently there are only small observational studies identifying benefits of OSA therapy for managing arrhythmias, and large randomized controlled trials will be challenging to conduct for reasons described earlier.

Generally, patients with benign, vagally mediated sinus node dysfunction or AV block who remain asymptomatic during sleep do not require a pacemaker; however, treatment of OSA should be strongly encouraged. For clinically significant bradyarrhythmias, especially if there is associated hypoperfusion, ventricular dysfunction, or proarrhythmia, OSA therapy alone has not been validated and the usual treatment with a permanent pacemaker should be provided. Based on observational data, treating OSA is likely an important step in improving success for OSA patients undergoing antiarrhythmic drug therapy, cardioversion, or ablation for AF. Certainly, patients under evaluation for an arrhythmia, particularly those who are obese or have hypertension or heart failure, should be questioned about symptoms of sleep apnea so that appropriate treatment may be offered in the hopes of improving quality of life and potentially reducing cardiovascular risk.

REFERENCES

1. Somers V, Dyken M, Mark A, Abboud F. Sympathetic-nerve activity during sleep in normal subjects. *N Engl J Med.* 1993;328:303–307.
2. Young T, Peppard PE, Gottlieb DJ. Epidemiology of obstructive sleep apnea: a population health perspective. *Am J Respir Crit Care Med.* 2002;165:1217–1239.
3. Gami AS, Caples SM, Somers VK. Obesity and obstructive sleep apnea. *Endocrinol Metab Clin North Am.* 2003;32:869–894.
4. Young T, Palta M, Dempsey J, et al. The occurrence of sleep-disordered breathing among middle-aged adults. *N Engl J Med.* 1993;328:1230–1235.
5. Javaheri S. A mechanism of central sleep apnea in patients with heart failure. *N Engl J Med.* 1999;341:949–954.
6. Trinder J, Merson R, Rosenberg JI, et al. Pathophysiological interactions of ventilation, arousals, and blood pressure oscillations during Cheyne-Stokes respiration in patients with heart failure. *Am J Respir Crit Care Med.* 2000;162:808–813.
7. Cowie MR, Woehrle H, Wegscheider K, et al. Adaptive servo-ventilation for central sleep apnea in systolic heart failure. *N Engl J Med.* 2015;373:1095–1105.
8. Javaheri S, Parker TJ, Liming JD, et al. Sleep apnea in 81 ambulatory male patients with stable heart failure. Types and their prevalences, consequences, and presentations. *Circulation.* 1998;97:2154–2159.
9. Sin DD, Fitzgerald F, Parker JD, et al. Risk factors for central and obstructive sleep apnea in 450 men and women with congestive heart failure. *Am J Respir Crit Care Med.* 1999;160:1101–1106.
10. Gami AS, Somers VK. In: Zipes DP, ed. *Braunwald's Heart Disease: A Textbook of Cardiovascular Medicine.* Philadelphia: Saunders; 2007.
11. Somers V, Dyken M, Mark A, Abboud F. Parasympathetic hyperresponsiveness and bradyarrhythmias during apnoea in hypertension. *Clin Auton Res.* 1992;2:171–176.
12. Somers VK, Dyken ME, Clary MP, Abboud FM. Sympathetic neural mechanisms in obstructive sleep apnea. *J Clin Invest.* 1995;96:1897–1904.
13. Chen PS. Douglas P. Zipes lecture. Neural mechanisms of atrial fibrillation. *Heart Rhythm.* 2006;3:1373–1377.
14. Otto ME, Belohlavek M, Romero-Corral A, et al. Comparison of cardiac structural and functional changes in obese otherwise healthy adults with versus without obstructive sleep apnea. *Am J Cardiol.* 2007;99:1298–1302.
15. Chobanian AV, Bakris GL, Black HR, et al. The Seventh Report of the Joint National Committee on Prevention, Detection, Evaluation, and Treatment of High Blood Pressure: the JNC 7 report. *JAMA.* 2003;289:2560–2572.
16. Virolainen J, Ventila M, Turto H, Kupari M. Effect of negative intrathoracic pressure on left ventricular pressure dynamics and relaxation. *J Appl Physiol.* 1995;79:455–460.
17. Schlatzer C, Schwarz EI, Sievi NA, et al. Intrathoracic pressure swings induced by simulated obstructive sleep apnoea promote arrhythmias in paroxysmal atrial fibrillation. *Europace.* 2016;18:64–70.
18. Liu T, Li G, Li L, Korantzopoulos P. Association between C-reactive protein and recurrence of atrial fibrillation after successful electrical cardioversion: a meta-analysis. *J Am Coll Cardiol.* 2007;49:1642–1648.
19. Cagirci G, Cay S, Gulsoy KG, et al. Tissue Doppler atrial conduction times and electrocardiogram interlead P-wave durations with varying severity of obstructive sleep apnea. *J Electrocardiol.* 2011;44:478–482.
20. Dimitri H, Ng M, Brooks AG, et al. Atrial remodeling in obstructive sleep apnea: implications for atrial fibrillation. *Heart Rhythm.* 2012;9:321–327.
21. Alonso-Fernandez A, García-Rio F, Racionero MA, et al. Cardiac rhythm disturbances and ST-segment depression episodes in patients with obstructive sleep apnea-hypopnea syndrome and its mechanisms. *Chest.* 2005;127:15–22.
22. Jo JA, Blasi A, Valladares E, et al. Determinants of heart rate variability in obstructive sleep apnea syndrome during wakefulness and sleep. *Am J Physiol Heart Circ Physiol.* 2005;288:H1103–H1112.

23. Roche F, Gaspoz JM, Court-Fortune I, et al. Alteration of QT rate dependence reflects cardiac autonomic imbalance in patients with obstructive sleep apnea syndrome. *Pacing Clin Electrophysiol.* 2003;26:1446–1453.
24. Nakamura T, Chin K, Hosokawa R, et al. Corrected QT dispersion and cardiac sympathetic function in patients with obstructive sleep apnea-hypopnea syndrome. *Chest.* 2004;125:2107–2114.
25. Shamsuzzaman AS, Somers VK, Knilans TK, et al. Obstructive sleep apnea in patients with congenital long QT syndrome: implications for increased risk of sudden cardiac death. *Sleep.* 2015;38:1113–1119.
26. Zipes DP, Rubart M. Neural modulation of cardiac arrhythmias and sudden cardiac death. *Heart Rhythm.* 2006;3:108–113.
27. Kaneko Y, Floras JS, Usui K, et al. Cardiovascular effects of continuous positive airway pressure in patients with heart failure and obstructive sleep apnea. *N Engl J Med.* 2003;348:1233–1241.
28. Brodsky M, Wu D, Denes P, Kanakis C, Rosen KM. Arrhythmias documented by 24 hour continuous electrocardiographic monitoring in 50 male medical students without apparent heart disease. *Am J Cardiol.* 1977;39:390–395.
29. Caples SM, Rosen CL, Shen WK, et al. The scoring of cardiac events during sleep. *J Clin Sleep Med.* 2007;3:147–154.
30. Becker H, Brandenburg U, Peter JH, Von Wichert P. Reversal of sinus arrest and atrioventricular conduction block in patients with sleep apnea during nasal continuous positive airway pressure. *Am J Respir Crit Care Med.* 1995;151:215–218.
31. Guilleminault C, Conolly SJ, Winkle RA. Cardiac arrhythmia and conduction disturbances during sleep in 400 patients with sleep apnea syndrome. *Am J Card.* 1983;52:490–494.
32. Mehra R, Benjamin EJ, Shahar E, et al. Association of nocturnal arrhythmias with sleep-disordered breathing: The Sleep Heart Health Study. *Am J Respir Crit Care Med.* 2006;173:910–916.
33. Porthan KM, Melin JH, Kupila JT, Venho KK, Partinen MM. Prevalence of sleep apnea syndrome in lone atrial fibrillation: a case-control study. *Chest.* 2004;125:879–885.
34. Gami AS, Pressman G, Caples SM, et al. Association of atrial fibrillation and obstructive sleep apnea. *Circulation.* 2004;110:364–367.
35. Leung RS, Huber MA, Rogge T, et al. Association between atrial fibrillation and central sleep apnea. *Sleep.* 2005;28:1543–1546.
36. Caples SM, Wolk R, Somers VK. Influence of cardiac function and failure on sleep-disordered breathing: evidence for a causative role. *J Appl Physiol.* 2005;99:2433–2439.
37. Mooe T, Gullsby S, Rabben T, Eriksson P. Sleep-disordered breathing: a novel predictor of atrial fibrillation after coronary artery bypass surgery. *Coron Artery Dis.* 1996;7:475–478.
38. Kanagala R, Murali NS, Friedman PA, et al. Obstructive sleep apnea and the recurrence of atrial fibrillation. *Circulation.* 2003;107:2589–2594.
39. Gami AS, Hodge DO, Herges RM, et al. Obstructive sleep apnea, obesity, and the risk of incident atrial fibrillation. *J Am Coll Cardiol.* 2007;49:565–571.
40. Pedrosa RP, Drager LF, Genta PR, et al. Obstructive sleep apnea is common and independently associated with atrial fibrillation in patients with hypertrophic cardiomyopathy. *Chest.* 2010;137:1078–1084.
41. Monahan K, Brewster J, Wang L, et al. Relation of the severity of obstructive sleep apnea in response to antiarrhythmic drugs in patients with atrial fibrillation or atrial flutter. *Am J Cardiol.* 2012;110:369–372.
42. Sauer WH, McKernan ML, Lin D, et al. Clinical predictors and outcomes associated with acute return of pulmonary vein conduction during pulmonary vein isolation for treatment of atrial fibrillation. *Heart Rhythm.* 2006;3:1024–1028.

43. Ng CY, Liu T, Shehata M, et al. Meta-analysis of obstructive sleep apnea as predictor of atrial fibrillation recurrence after catheter ablation. *Am J Cardiol.* 2011;108:47–51.
44. Albuquerque FN, Calvin AD, Sert Kuniyoshi FH, et al. Sleep-disordered breathing and excessive daytime sleepiness in patients with atrial fibrillation. *Chest.* 2012;141:967–973.
45. Gami AS, Howard DE, Olson EJ, Somers VK. Day-night pattern of sudden death in obstructive sleep apnea. *N Engl J Med.* 2005;352:1206–1214.
46. Zeidan-Shwiri T, Aronson D, Atalla K, et al. Circadian pattern of life-threatening ventricular arrhythmia in patients with sleep-disordered breathing and implantable cardioverter-defibrillators. *Heart Rhythm.* 2011;8:657–662.
47. Doherty LS, Kiely JL, Swan V, McNicholas WT. Long-term effects of nasal continuous positive airway pressure therapy on cardiovascular outcomes in sleep apnea syndrome. *Chest.* 2005;127:2076–2084.
47a. Gami AS, Olson EJ, Shen WK, et al. Obstructive sleep apnea and the risk of sudden cardiac death: a longitudinal study of 10,701 adults. *J Am Coll Cardiol.* 2013;62:610–616.
48. Bayir PT, Demirkan B, Bayir O, et al. Impact of continuous positive airway pressure therapy on atrial electromechanical delay and P-wave dispersion in patients with obstructive sleep apnea. *Ann Noninvasive Electrocardiol.* 2014;19:226–233.
49. Grimm W, Koehler U, Fus E, et al. Outcome of patients with sleep apnea-associated severe bradyarrhythmias after continuous positive airway pressure therapy. *Am J Cardiol.* 2000;86:688–692. A9.
50. Holmqvist F, Guan N, Zhu Z, et al. Impact of obstructive sleep apnea and continuous positive airway pressure therapy on outcomes in patients with atrial fibrillation-Results from the Outcomes Registry for Better Informed Treatment of Atrial Fibrillation (ORBIT-AF). *Am Heart J.* 2015;169:647–654.e2.
51. Fein AS, Shvilkin A, Shah D, et al. Treatment of obstructive sleep apnea reduces the risk of atrial fibrillation recurrence after catheter ablation. *J Am Coll Cardiol.* 2013;62:300–305.
52. Naruse Y, Tada H, Satoh M, et al. Concomitant obstructive sleep apnea increases the recurrence of atrial fibrillation following radiofrequency catheter ablation of atrial fibrillation: clinical impact of continuous positive airway pressure therapy. *Heart Rhythm.* 2013;10:331–337.
53. Ryan CM, Usui K, Floras JS, Bradley TD. Effect of continuous positive airway pressure on ventricular ectopy in heart failure patients with obstructive sleep apnoea. *Thorax.* 2005;60:781–785.
54. Liston R, Deegan PC, McCreery C, et al. Haemodynamic effects of nasal continuous positive airway pressure in severe congestive heart failure. *Eur Respir J.* 1995;8:430–435.
55. Kiely JL, Deegan P, Buckley A, et al. Efficacy of nasal continuous positive airway pressure therapy in chronic heart failure: importance of underlying cardiac rhythm. *Thorax.* 1998;53:957–962.
55a. McEvoy RD, Antic NA, Heeley E, et al. CPAP for prevention of cardiovascular events in obstructive sleep apnea. *N Engl J Med.* 2016;375:919–931.
56. Bradley TD, Logan AG, Kimoff RJ, et al. Continuous positive airway pressure for central sleep apnea and heart failure. *N Engl J Med.* 2005;353:2025–2033.
57. Sinha AM, Skobel EC, Breithardt OA, et al. Cardiac resynchronization therapy improves central sleep apnea and Cheyne-Stokes respiration in patients with chronic heart failure. *J Am Coll Cardiol.* 2004;44:68–71.

111 Ventricular Assist Devices and Cardiac Transplantation Recipients

Elvis Teijeira Fernández, Karine Nubret Le Coniat, Pierre Jaïs, and Frederic Sacher

Arrhythmias in Patients With Ventricular Assist Devices

The prevalence of heart failure (HF) is increasing, and it currently reaches 1%–2% of the adult population in developed countries and up to 10% in people above 70 years of age.[1,2] Optimal medical treatment has improved survival dramatically. However, some patients with advanced HF may be refractory to pharmacological therapy. Ventricular assist devices (VADs) are increasingly being used for the treatment of end-stage HF. They may be helpful as bridge-to-recovery (BTR) therapy in acute settings where cardiac support is critical and recovery of heart function is more likely or as bridge-to-decision (BTD) or bridge-to-bridge (BTB) therapy if recovery does not eventually occur. VADs have been shown to improve survival as bridge-to-transplantation (BTT)[3] therapy and even as destination therapy (DT),[4] which has become feasible with the smallest implantable devices and provides long-term support for patients ineligible for heart transplantation. Current survival rates of patients with left ventricular assist devices (LVADs) reported by the Interagency Registry for Mechanically Assisted Circulatory Support (INTERMACS) registry are as high as 80% at 1 year and 70% at 2 years.[5]

Nevertheless, despite the advantages of VADs, adverse events associated with these devices may occur in over one-third of patients. The most common complications of VADs are bleeding (7.79 per 100 patient-months), infection (7.78%), cardiac arrhythmias (4.06%), respiratory failure (2.73%), stroke (1.61%), and renal dysfunction (1.54%). Ventricular arrhythmias (VAs) occur in the range of 20%–50% of patients with VADs (Table 111.1[6–16]), most often within the 4 weeks after surgery.[17] The strongest predictive factor for VAs is the presence of VAs before implantation, but some may develop de novo.[18] Although VAs are usually well tolerated because of the mechanical support of the VAD, they increase morbidity, and there is still controversy about their potential impact on mortality in patients with VADs.[17,19]

Types of Ventricular Assist Devices

VADs can be used for short-term support (days to weeks) or for long-term support (months to years). Short-term VADs are mainly extracorporeal, whereas long-term VADs are intracorporeal or paracorporeal. Long-term VADs require major heart surgery often with the need of extracorporeal circulation, and they are normally implanted in patients with advanced HF but not with acute hemodynamic instability or significant organ damage. VADs can provide support to the left ventricle (LV), right ventricle (RV), or both (biventricular assist devices [BIVADs]), but LVADs are the most widely used. The first generation of VADs developed were large-size pulsatile pumps having low resistance to mechanical wear, but modern small-size continuous-flow devices (either axial or centrifugal) have proved to be more durable and efficient. Besides, the technology of VADs is rapidly evolving, and new devices are under development. A summary of the most common currently available VADs is shown in Table 111.2.

Short-Term Ventricular Assist Devices

Intraaortic Balloon Pump
An intraaortic balloon pump (IABP) (Fig. 111.1A) is the simplest device available for temporary circulatory support. However, it only provides a very modest increase in cardiac output, and in a recent randomized prospective study in patients undergoing early revascularization for myocardial infarction complicated by cardiogenic shock (IABP-SHOCK II), IABP had no impact on all-cause mortality or secondary endpoints at 30 days and 12 months.[20]

Percutaneous Ventricular Assist Devices
Percutaneous devices, such as Impella (Abiomed, Danvers, MA) (Fig. 111.1B) and TandemHeart pVAD (CardiacAssist, Pittsburgh, PA) (Fig. 111.1C), are used for short-term ventricular support. Different Impella devices were developed, but only Impella 5.0 (which delivers 5 L of blood output per minute) can provide sufficient LV support for the treatment of cardiogenic shock. The device is inserted into the LV through the aortic valve. Impella RP is a percutaneous device designed for RV support, and it pumps blood from the inferior vena cava to the pulmonary artery. TandemHeart pVAD consists of an extracorporeal pump connected to a cannula that is inserted in the left atrium via transseptal access and another one placed in the femoral vein. Both Impella and TandemHeart pVAD have been shown to increase cardiac index significantly as compared to IABP in patients with cardiogenic shock after acute myocardial infarction.[21,22]

TABLE 111.1 Prevalence of ventricular arrhythmias in patients with ventricular assist devices

STUDY	YEAR PUBLISHED	% VENTRICULAR ARRHYTHMIAS AFTER IMPLANTATION	N	FOLLOW-UP[a] (DAYS)	CONTINUOUS-FLOW DEVICE (%)
Harding et al.[6]	2005	59	17	14	0
Ziv et al.[18]	2005	35	91	NS[b]	0
Bedi et al.[7]	2007	22	111	98	0
Miller et al.[3]	2007	24	133	126	100
Andersen et al.[8]	2009	52	23	341	100
Ambardekar et al.[9]	2010	24	33	238	53
Cantillon et al.[10]	2010	29	478	84	8
Kuhne et al.[11]	2010	29	76	156	30
Brenyo et al.[12]	2012	31	61	662	100
Raasch et al.[13]	2012	43	61	NS	100
Refaat et al.[14]	2012	20	144	119	51
Enriquez et al.[15]	2013	35	106	217	100
Garan et al.[16]	2015	23	162	30	100

[a]Median or mean follow-up.
[b]Maximum 1 year.
NS, Not specified.

TABLE 111.2 Main currently available ventricular assist devices[a]

DEVICE	INDICATION	VENTRICLE SUPPORTED	MAXIMUM SUPPORT PROVIDED (L/min)	PLACEMENT
IABP	Temporary	L	~0.5	Percutaneous
Impella 5.0	Temporary	L	5	Percutaneous/operative
TandemHeart	Temporary	L	5	Percutaneous
CentriMag	Temporary	R, L, or both	9.9	Percutaneous/operative
ECLS	Temporary	Both[b]	Variable	Percutaneous/operative
Thoratec PVAD/IVAD	BTT, BTR	R, L, or both	7.2	Operative
Berlin Heart EXCOR pumps	BTT, BTR	R, L, or both	Variable (up to 6)	Operative
Jarvik 2000	BTT[c], DT[c]	L	7	Operative
HeartWare HVAD	BTT, DT[c]	L	10	Operative
HeartMate II	BTT, DT	L	10	Operative
HeartMate 3	BTT,[c] DT[c]	L	10	Operative
CardioWest TAH-t	BTT	Both replaced	9.5	Operative

[a]This list is not exhaustive.
[b]And respiratory support.
[c]Currently not approved by the US Food and Drug Administration. CE (*Conformité Européenne*) Mark certification obtained.
ECLS, Extracorporeal life support; *IABP,* intraaortic balloon pump.

Extracorporeal Life Support

Extracorporeal life support (ECLS) (also known as "extracorporeal membrane oxygenation" or ECMO) provides temporary respiratory and mechanical circulatory support (Fig. 111.1D). Different venoarterial and venovenous modes are available. The Extracorporeal Life Support Organization (ELSO) registry reports a survival rate of 39% for cardiac patients treated with ECLS.[23] If myocardial function recovery does not occur, bridging to long-term VADs may be considered in some cases.

Long-Term Ventricular Assist Devices

Most modern long-term VADs are implantable continuous-flow pumps, such as the US Food and Drug Administration (FDA)-approved HeartMate II (Thoratec, Pleasanton, CA) or HeartWare HVAD (HeartWare, Framingham, MA). HeartMate II received approval for use as either BTT therapy or DT,[4,24] and over 20,000 HeartMate II devices have been implanted worldwide. HeartWare HVAD was approved for BTT in 2012 and is currently awaiting approval as DT. However, whereas HeartMate II contains an axial flow pump with a magnetic rotor (Fig. 111.2A), HeartWare

HVAD features a centrifugal pump (Fig. 111.2B). All continuous-flow pumps have external power and control systems, are relatively small, and can provide blood flows of up to 10 L per minute.

Other devices have not been approved by the FDA yet but have received CE (*Conformité Européenne*) Mark certification. Jarvik 2000 (Jarvik Heart, New York, NY) is a small pump that can provide a connection behind the ear, offering the patient the opportunity to have a bath without protection. HeartMate 3 uses a magnetically levitated rotor to minimize shear stress and to provide an artificial pulsatile flow that allows pump washing.

Finally, pneumatic VADs that provide pulsatile flows, such as Thoratec PVAD (paracorporeal) and Thoratec IVAD (intracorporeal), are still in use as BTT or BTR therapies. Berlin Heart EXCOR (Berlin Heart GmbH, Berlin, Germany) pediatric pumps are also pneumatically driven. They are extracorporeal VADs with pumps available in different sizes, thus covering the needs of all pediatric ages.

Total Artificial Heart

Total artificial hearts are not true VADs as they replace the ventricles completely. CardioWest TAH-t (SynCardia Systems,

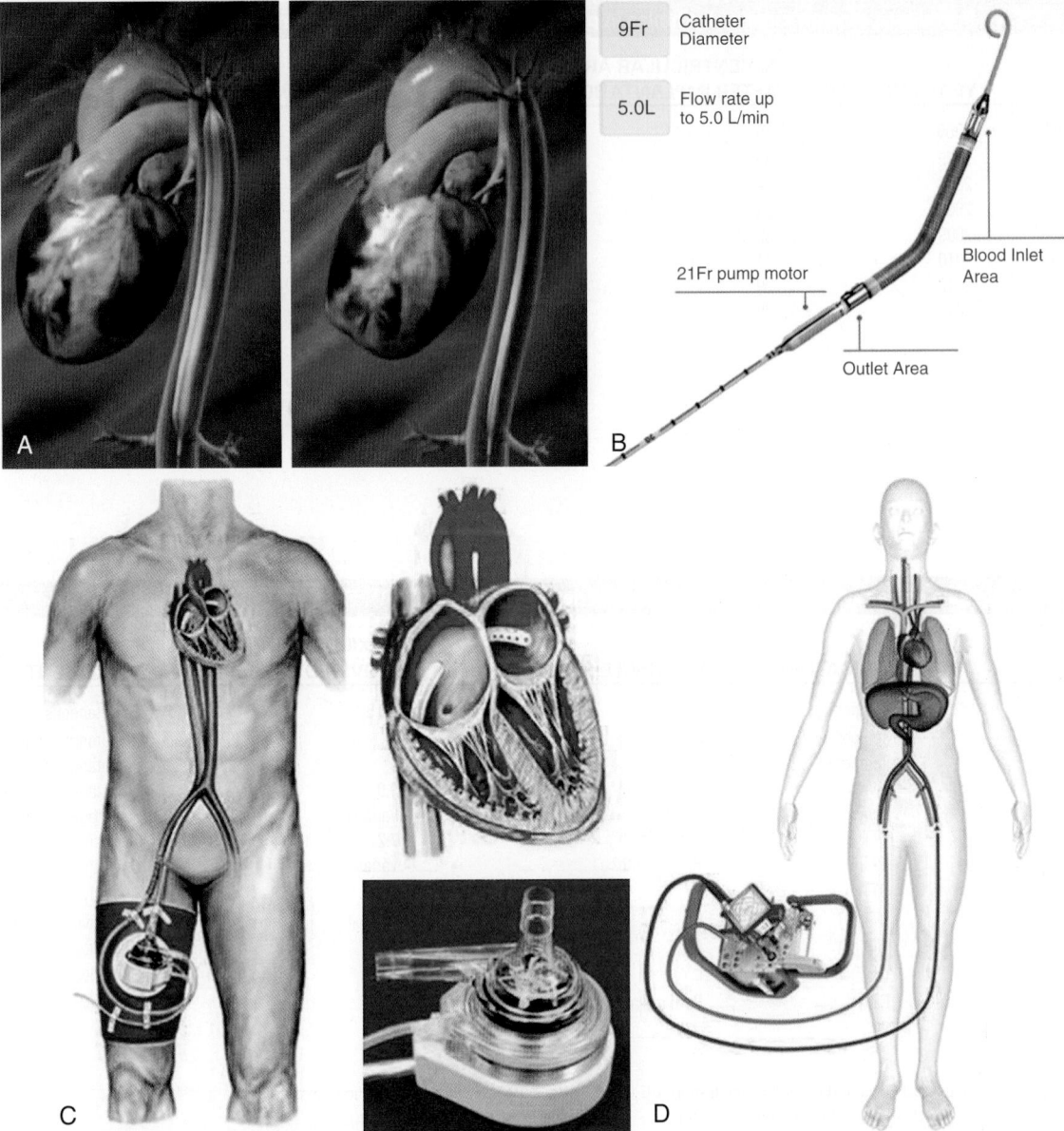

9Fr Catheter Diameter

5.0L Flow rate up to 5.0 L/min

Blood Inlet Area

21Fr pump motor

Outlet Area

FIGURE 111.1 Temporary devices. (A) Intraaortic balloon pump. (B) Impella. (C) TandemHeart. (D) Extracorporeal life support. ([B] with permission from Abiomed, Danvers, MA, copyright 2016. [C] with permission from CardiacAssist, Pittsburgh, PA, copyright 2016.)

Tucson, AZ) provides improved survival compared to heart transplantation[25] and has been approved for BTT by the FDA. It consists of a pneumatic pulsatile pump with an external portable drive unit. Other models of artificial hearts, such as CARMAT and AbioCor (Abiomed, Danvers, MA), have also been developed.

Mechanisms of Arrhythmias in Patients With Ventricular Assist Devices

In certain patients, VADs can reduce the incidence of VAs by mechanical unloading of the ventricles, possibly related to inverse electrical remodeling. However, patients with VADs tend to have a higher incidence of VAs, which suggests that there may be mechanisms of arrhythmogenesis related to these devices. Several risk factors for the development of VAs in these patients have been identified in different studies, but there is considerable discrepancy about these findings. However, previous history of VAs seems to be the most consistent predictive factor.[26]

Acknowledgment of the mechanisms of arrhythmogenesis in patients with VADs could be relevant for the proper management of VAs.

Scar Reentry

Preexisting scar is likely the most frequent cause of VAs in patients with VADs, whereas reentry involving apical scar at the site of insertion of the VAD inflow cannula is much less common.[27,28]

Mechanical Dysfunction

Suction events, especially at the septal wall, occur typically with continuous-flow devices because they provide cardiac output regardless of ventricular preload. They are more frequent in patients with no ventricle dilatation or after bleeding, dehydration, or excessive diuretic treatment. Adequate positioning of the turbine during surgery is critical to avoid suction events.

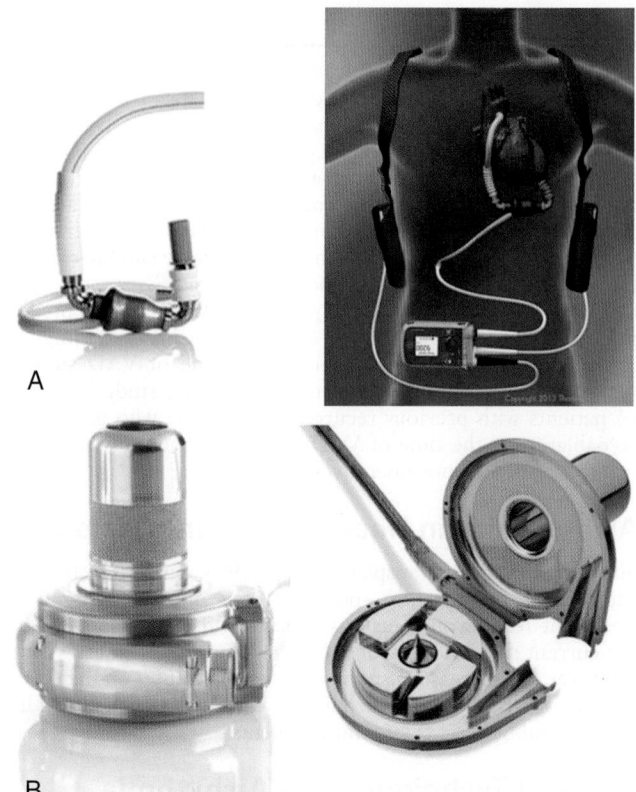

FIGURE 111.2 Long-term ventricular assist devices. (A) Heart-Mate II. (B) HeartWare HVAD. ([A] with permission from Thoratec, Pleasanton, CA, copyright 2016. [B] with permission from HeartWare, Framingham, MA, copyright 2016.)

Myocardial Ischemia

Myocardial ischemia is sometimes overlooked in patients with VADs, but it can be a cause of VAs and should be actively searched for, especially in patients with known ischemic heart disease, as it requires a specific treatment (mainly β-blocker uptitration or revascularization if needed).

Changes in Channel Regulation

Upregulation of the Na^+/Ca^{2+} exchange and downregulation of the voltage-gated K^+ channel, the Na^+/K^+ adenosine triphosphate (ATP) pump, and connexin 43 were observed in patients with VAs after VAD implantation.[29] These changes in channel regulation could lead to the development of delayed afterdepolarizations and to the increase of action potential duration. In addition, upregulation of Ca^{2+} ATPase, ryanodine receptor 2, and fibroblast genes has also been found in patients with VADs.[30]

QTc Prolongation

Although reverse electrical remodeling has been observed in patients with VADs, QTc prolongation may occur within the first weeks postoperatively, and it could be related to the risk for developing VAs.[6]

Metabolites and Drugs

Patients with VADs are usually comorbid and on multiple medications. Therefore it is important that metabolic disturbances and drug toxicity be excluded as the causes of the episodes of VA during initial assessment.[31]

Clinical Implications of Arrhythmias in Patients With Implantable Ventricular Assist Devices

Atrial Arrhythmias

Atrial arrhythmias are common in patients with HF with or without VADs. A recent report found an incidence of 21% (231/1125) over 2 years of follow-up after HeartMate II implantation, with most of the episodes occurring within the first 2 months.[32] Although atrial arrhythmias did not impact survival in this study, the quality of life and the improvement in the 6-minute walk test were lower in patients with atrial arrhythmias as compared with patients with VADs who had not developed them. The lack of atrial contribution to ventricular filling during atrial arrhythmias may have a negative impact and prompt invasive treatment.[33]

Ventricular Arrhythmias

In the acute setting, VAs can be relatively well tolerated due to the mechanical support provided by the VAD. Extreme cases of patients surviving in VF for days or even months have been reported.[34] However, the clinical presentation of VAs can vary enormously from an asymptomatic or mildly symptomatic patient to a scenario of hemodynamic instability warranting immediate intervention, especially in patients with fast ventricular tachycardia (VT) or VF. With LVAD alone, most of the symptoms are due to the lack of RV support. RV function impairment can lead to a decrease in LV preload and in LVAD flow. Patients with VAs can experience palpitations, syncope, or even sudden cardiac death (SCD) depending on the underlying RV function, the degree of pulmonary hypertension, and the tachycardia cycle length. Even in patients with initial tolerance to the VA, long-term complications may develop if the arrhythmia is not treated, including RV failure and thromboembolism. On the other hand, patients with implantable cardioverter defibrillators (ICDs) are likely to experience shocks, which may be painful and increase morbidity. VAs increase the rate of hospitalization,[13] but there is controversy about whether they exert any impact on mortality.[17,19]

Management of Ventricular Arrhythmias

Conservative

Slow VT does not always require treatment if it is well tolerated, especially in BTT patients where preserving RV function may not be a priority. Contrarily, fast VT and VF should normally be treated. Some causes of VAs can successfully be managed conservatively, so they must be searched for actively during initial evaluation of the patient.

Suction events may be corrected by decreasing the VAD flow, which can result in the suppression of nonsustained or even sustained VAs. Avoiding or treating volume depletion caused by dehydration and bleeding are also useful strategies for prevention and management of VAs. However, it is often challenging to find the adequate balance between VAD speed and diuretic treatment, particularly in the early postoperative period. An echocardiogram, chest x-ray, or computed tomography scan may be helpful to assess the VAD inflow cannula position. Ideally, LV end-diastolic pressure should be improved by the VAD without causing suction events. Electrolyte disturbances should be diagnosed and corrected, and potential drug toxicity must also be searched for. Proarrhythmic inotropic drugs are to be limited if possible, and any QT-prolonging drug should also be avoided. Myocardial ischemia may be the etiology of recurrent VAs, especially in patients with known ischemic cardiomyopathy. Revascularization might be required in some cases, whereas simply uptitrating β-blocker therapy might be sufficient for others. β-Blockers may also be a reasonable option for the pharmacological treatment of

VAs themselves. If they are not effective, amiodarone or other antiarrhythmic drugs may be used with caution, as their benefit in patients with VADs has not been demonstrated. Besides, given that the highest risk for VAs is within the first month after VAD surgery, it seems justified to decrease or discontinue antiarrhythmic drugs in stable patients over time.[31]

Implantable Cardioverter Defibrillator and Cardiac Resynchronization Therapy

Even in well-tolerated VAs, RV function deterioration and SCD can still ensue. ICDs could theoretically be beneficial in this setting, but their implantation also carries a significant risk for devastating complications in patients with VADs, including VAD colonization following intravascular infection. ICD therapy was shown to increase survival in patients with pulsatile VADs, in which the native heart contributes to device filling and VAs are poorly tolerated. Nonetheless, in patients with contemporary continuous-flow LVADs, recent studies failed to demonstrate a beneficial effect of ICDs in terms of survival.[19,35] These findings are particularly relevant for patients under consideration for VAD implantation who do not have an ICD, and for those with VADs who require an ICD change. Besides, ICD shocks may be painful and unnecessary in some patients with VAD, and are associated with increased morbidity. Therefore it is of major importance to give priority to the use of ATP rather than shocks and to extend the detection intervals to allow spontaneous termination of nonsustained VTs. Another concern in patients with previous ICDs is the need to review lead parameters, as the sensing amplitude may have decreased and the threshold increased following VAD implantation.[9]

Regarding cardiac resynchronization therapy (CRT), its benefits have not been demonstrated in patients with VADs and no hemodynamic advantage is anticipated. Although CRT could potentially decrease VAs, the contrary has also been reported. Given the lack of evidence supporting the use of CRT in VAD patients, CRT may be turned off in patients developing VAs.[31]

Biventricular Assist Devices vs. Left Ventricular Assist Devices

Although BIVADs remove the risk for RV dysfunction, outcomes with BIVADs may be worse than with LVADs. The INTER-MACS registry showed that patients with BIVADs had lower survival rates and higher rates of complications. However, a selection bias probably influenced these results, as patients selected for BIVAD are more likely to be critically ill.[5]

Catheter Ablation

Catheter ablation is overall a feasible and safe procedure in patients with VADs, provided it is performed in centers with adequate expertise. In the largest multicenter study published so far, 34 patients with HeartMate II underwent 39 ablation procedures. Of 110 VTs targeted, only 9% were related to the apical scar surrounding the cannula. Transseptal approach was used more often than retrograde aortic approach (25 vs. 14). Thirteen of 17 patients who survived and were not transplanted did not experience arrhythmia recurrence during 25 ± 15 months of follow-up.[27] Another series of 28 mapped VTs in 20 patients with VADs also showed that the majority of them originated at intrinsic scar (75%), whereas only 14% came from the area of the inflow cannula, and just a few were focal or due to bundle-branch reentry. Acute success rate was as high as 86%.[28]

Although significant complications of VT ablation associated with VADs are rare, some technical particularities of these procedures should be taken into account. Monitoring invasive arterial pressure is even more important for patients undergoing VT

ablation because of the absence of peripheral pulse. In the case of a transseptal approach, the use of a steerable sheath is strongly recommended as the maneuverability of the catheters is normally very poor without it. A retrograde approach may be challenging because of the lack of flow through the aortic valve. Decreasing the VAD flow may allow certain valves to open, but the presence of a thrombus at the aortic root should be ruled out first. On the other hand, although the catheter will not be aspirated by the inflow cannula, care must be taken to avoid introducing the catheter inside. Interference with ICD telemetry and the electro-anatomical mapping systems is possible but rare.[27]

Given that the occurrence of previous VAs is the main predictive factor for the development of VAs following VAD implantation, prophylactic cryoablation at the time of VAD surgery has been proposed. In a small nonrandomized study including 14 patients with previous recurrent VAs, those who underwent cryoablation at the time of VAD placement had a lower rate of recurrence of VAs postoperatively.[36]

Arrhythmias in Heart Transplant Recipients

Since the first heart transplantation in 1967, surgical techniques and—most importantly—postoperative immunosuppression treatment have evolved extraordinarily and are responsible for the current survival rates of 90% at 1 year and 70% at 5 years. However, the increase in survival has had an impact on the development of arrhythmias, which in turn can affect the quality of life and survival of heart transplant recipients.

Surgical Techniques and Arrhythmia Substrates

Each surgical technique has particular electrical consequences for the heart, and creates different substrates for arrhythmias.

Heterotopic heart transplantation (Fig. 111.3A), in which the donor heart is anastomosed to the recipient heart, permits the recovery of the recipient heart in some cases and was more useful before the current era of advanced immunosuppression therapy and VADs. It was also an option if pulmonary resistances were very high and heart and lung transplantation was not possible. The electrocardiograms (ECGs) of these patients show the electrical activity of both hearts with different axes.

Orthotopic heart transplantation, with removal of the recipient heart, has been by far the most widely used technique. Initially, *biatrial surgery* (Fig. 111.3B) as described by Lower and Shumway was the most popular, but its use has steadily declined since the mid-2000s. With this technique, part of the recipient's right and left atria are left in place and sutured to the atria of the donor heart. The recipient sinus node is preserved, but it is no longer functional. Activation of both donor and recipient atrial tissues may occur, but there is normally complete conduction block at the suture line. Thus a phenomenon of parasystole can be observed and this should not be misinterpreted as atrial flutter. However, if conduction across the anastomosis appears, tachycardias may develop. In addition, atrial scars can also facilitate the development of macroreentry circuits.

The *bicaval technique* (Fig. 111.3C) is the most commonly used technique nowadays. It is slightly less simple and it requires anastomoses at the two venae cavae, the great vessels, and around the pulmonary veins. With this technique, there is less tricuspid regurgitation, less atrial dilatation, less sinus node dysfunction, and less need for pacemaker implantation.[37]

Total orthotopic heart transplantation is seldom performed as it is technically more challenging and it does not convey particular advantages. The recipient's pulmonary veins are anastomosed independently, which requires additional time and increases the risk for pulmonary vein stenosis or bleeding from inaccessible suture lines.

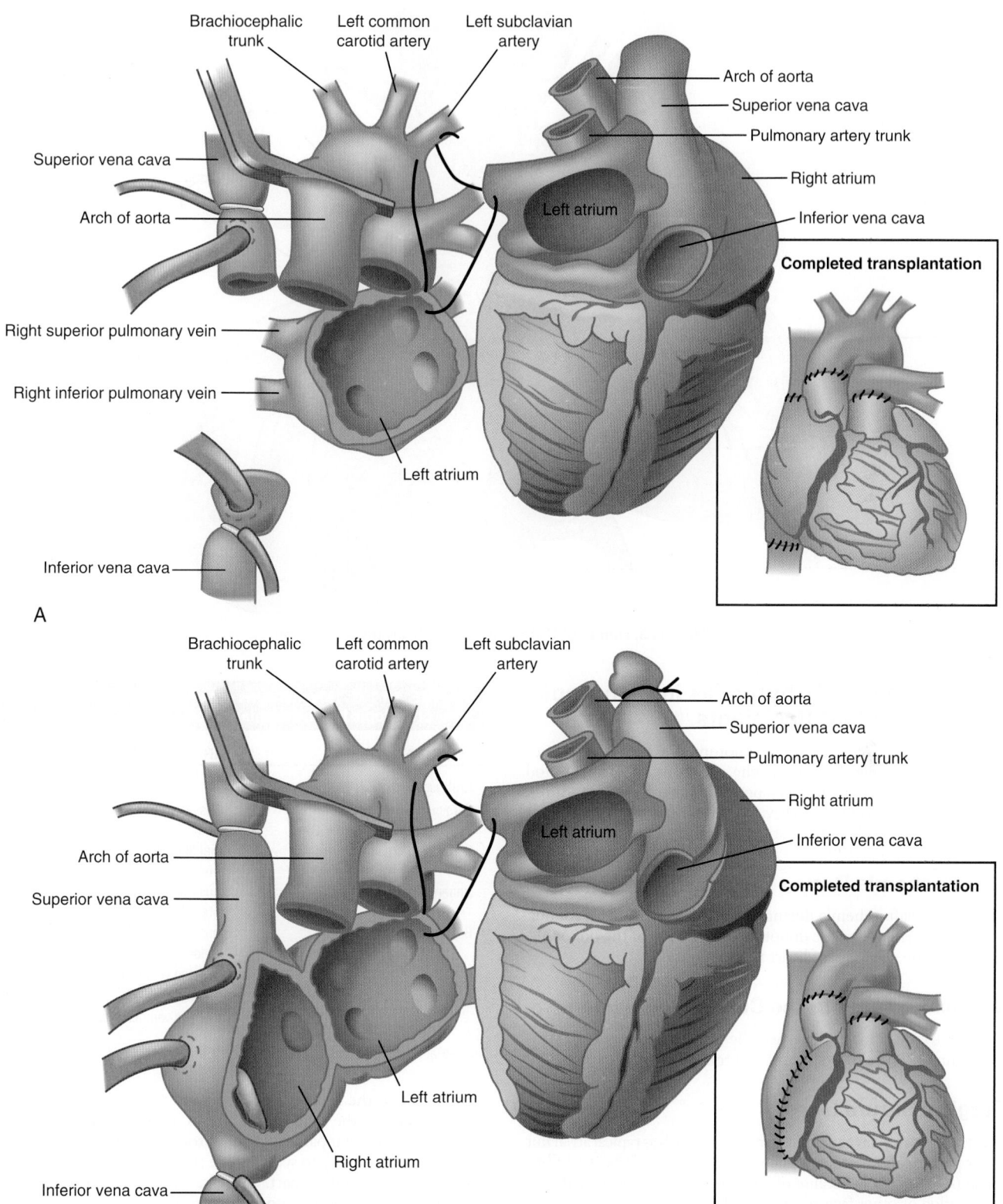

FIGURE 111.3 Heart transplantation techniques. (A) Heterotopic heart transplantation. (B) Orthotopic biatrial heart transplantation.

Continued

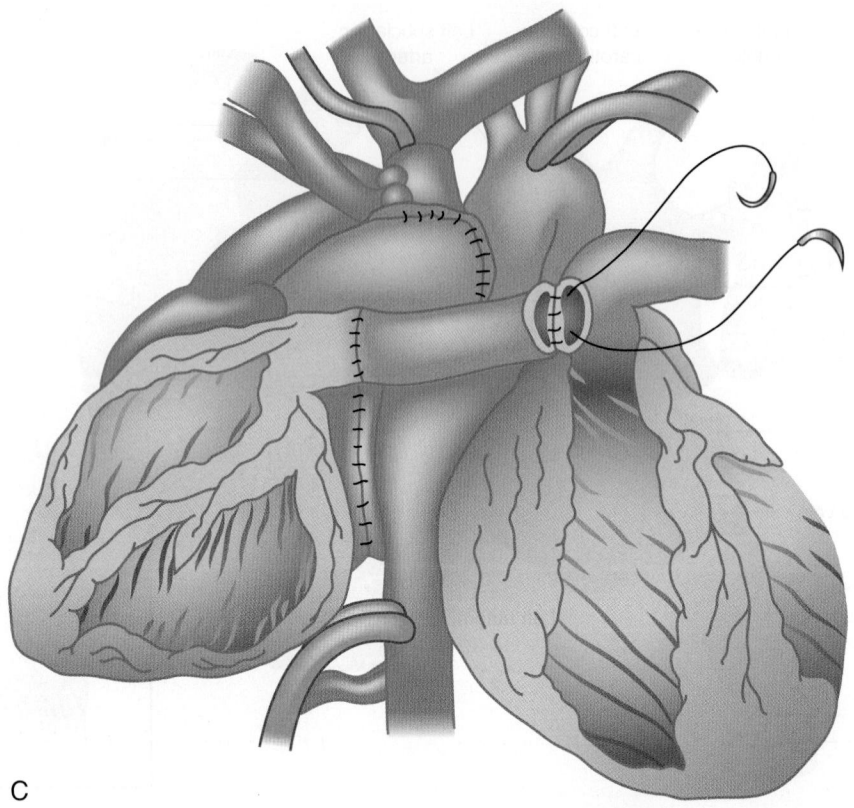

C

FIGURE 111.3, cont'd (C) Orthotopic bicaval heart transplantation.

Mechanisms of Arrhythmias in Orthotopic Heart Transplant Recipients

Arrhythmias are frequent after orthotopic heart transplantation (Table 111.3), especially during the early postoperative period. Different mechanisms can be responsible for cardiac arrhythmias in transplanted patients. However, they should prompt immediate evaluation to rule out rejection or graft vasculopathy.

Graft Ischemia During Preservation

Prolonged graft ischemia during preservation may cause conduction system damage to the donor heart. The age of the donor also influences the outcome of heart transplantation.

Surgical Trauma to the Conduction System

Trauma to the sinus node, especially with the biatrial technique, is a common cause of bradycardia in transplanted patients.

Surgical Suture Lines

Surgical scars may favor certain arrhythmias, such as typical atrial flutter or periscar macroreentry, and prevent others such as atrial fibrillation (AF), probably because of pulmonary vein isolation (although denervation or other factors may also play a protective role).[38]

Denervation and Reinnervation

Denervation occurs after surgery, resulting in chronotropic incompetence after heart transplantation. Reinnervation may occur in around one-third of transplanted hearts after 1 year and continues afterward, although the process is quite heterogeneous. Sympathetic reinnervation is more likely to occur than parasympathetic reinnervation, especially after biatrial surgery. The reason for this

TABLE 111.3 Mechanisms of ventricular arrhythmias after orthotopic heart transplantation

MECHANISMS	ARRHYTHMIAS
Graft ischemia	Sinus node dysfunction
Surgical trauma	Sinus node dysfunction
	AV block
Surgical suture lines	Atrial flutters
	Protect against AF
Denervation and reinnervation	Sinus node dysfunction
	Protect against AF and VF
Rejection	Sinus node dysfunction
	AV block
	Atrial and ventricular arrhythmias
Cardiac allograft vasculopathy	AV block
	Atrial and ventricular arrhythmias

AF, Atrial fibrillation; *AV,* atrioventricular; *VF,* ventricular fibrillation.

is that half of the sympathetic fibers are resected during biatrial surgery, but not the vagus nerve trunks, which results in a lack of stimulus for parasympathetic fiber sprouting. Subsequently, there is increased sensitivity to sympathetic stimuli, due to the lack of the parasympathetic counterpart. The bicaval technique is more likely to stimulate the regeneration of both systems, as both parasympathetic and sympathetic fibers are resected.[39]

Allograft Rejection

Rejection can affect the conduction system, as well as the rest of the myocardium, and cases have been reported where the conduction system was particularly damaged.[40] Rejection phenomena underlie most arrhythmias occurring late after heart transplantation surgery.

TABLE 111.4 Atrial arrhythmias after orthotopic heart transplantation

STUDY	YEAR PUBLISHED	N	MEAN FOLLOW-UP (YEARS)	ATRIAL FLUTTER	ATRIAL FIBRILLATION
Cui et al.[46]	2001	892	1.6	12.7%	13.1%
Ahmari et al.[47]	2006	167	6.5	15%	9.5%
Khan et al.[48]	2006	857	7.5	2.3%	0.3%
Vaseghi et al.[49]	2008	657	6.6	9.1%	7%
Chang et al.[50]	2013	217	6.9	18.4%[a]	11.1%

[a]Atrial flutter or atrial tachycardia.

Allograft Vasculopathy

Accelerated atherosclerosis may cause ischemia and myocardial infarction leading to LV dysfunction and predisposing to VAs and SCD. It may also be the cause of atrial arrhythmias.

Bradycardia

Sinus node dysfunction is very frequent after heart transplantation, but it usually recovers within a few weeks, so observation is recommended during the early postoperative period.[41] Its main causes are sympathetic denervation, surgical trauma to the sinoatrial artery or the sinus node, drug effects, and allograft rejection. The bicaval technique avoids trauma to the sinoatrial artery, and this may explain why permanent pacemaker implantation is less often required.[42] Atrioventricular (AV) conduction usually remains intact despite denervation, with a normal AV node response to circulating catecholamines.[43] Complete AV block is uncommon in transplanted patients, and in some cases, it is caused by surgical trauma or endomyocardial biopsy. First AV block is usually related to allograft rejection or vasculopathy.[44]

American College of Cardiology/American Heart Association/Heart Rhythm Society class I recommendations for pacing in transplanted patients include persistent inappropriate or symptomatic bradycardia that is not expected to resolve, and all other class I indications for permanent pacing. Class IIb indications are prolonged or recurrent bradycardia that limits rehabilitation or discharge, as well as syncope after cardiac transplantation.[45] Noticeably, transplanted patients requiring pacemakers have an excellent long-term prognosis.[10]

Atrial Arrhythmias

Among atrial arrhythmias (Table 111.4[46–50]), typical atrial flutter is the tachycardia most often encountered in heart transplantation patients. Although it was considered to be related to the biatrial technique, it is also found after bicaval surgery. In a series of 657 transplanted patients reported by Vaseghi and colleagues, 9.1% developed typical atrial flutter over a mean follow-up period of 6.6 years. The majority of the episodes occurred postoperatively or were related to graft rejection, severe vasculopathy, or other complications, and only 3.5% occurred in stable patients. Atypical atrial flutter is another common arrhythmia found in stable patients after orthotopic heart transplantation. The underlying mechanism is usually macroreentry involving isthmuses created by surgical scars.[49] Catheter ablation is an excellent treatment option for stable patients, although the procedure may be slightly more challenging in some cases because of anatomical particularities. Preexisting substrates not previously recognized in the donor heart can lead to other types of supraventricular tachycardias, such as atrioventricular nodal reentry tachycardia (AVNRT) or atrioventricular reentrant tachycardia (AVRT), which are also amenable to catheter ablation.

Unlike after other types of heart surgery, AF is very rare in transplanted patients.[48,49] In fact, it is almost exclusively observed in the immediate postoperative period or associated with acute graft rejection or severe vasculopathy. Pulmonary vein isolation due to the suture line created around the recipient pulmonary vein cuff and denervation of the donor heart are the most likely mechanisms protecting transplanted patients against AF. When an episode of AF does occur, prompt diagnosis and eventual treatment of complications of heart transplantation are warranted.

Ventricular Arrhythmias and Sudden Cardiac Death

Ventricular premature beats and nonsustained VTs are common in the early postoperative period, whereas sustained VAs are very rare in transplanted patients, and they are normally associated with allograft vasculopathy or rejection. In an analysis of 37,492 patients from the United Network for Organ Sharing (UNOS) registry, 46% died during 6.5 ± 5.7 years of follow-up, 9.6% of them due to SCD. Reduced left ventricular ejection fraction (LVEF), allograft rejection, and donor age were the main predictive factors for SCD.[51] Another study showed that asystole was the last rhythm documented in most sudden deaths in orthotopic heart transplant patients (14 of 26 patients), followed by pulseless electrical activity (8 patients), and VF (4 patients). The low incidence of VF in transplanted patients may be due to cardiac denervation, and leads to questioning the usefulness of ICD implantation in these patients.[52] A multicenter retrospective study including 36 transplanted patients with an ICD showed that 8 patients received appropriate ICD therapy during an average follow-up of 51 months. Interestingly, all of them had allograft vasculopathy vs. 18/26 in the group without appropriate ICD therapy. The indications for ICD implantation in this study had been severe allograft vasculopathy, unexplained syncope, history of cardiac arrest (n = 8), and severe LV dysfunction. Of note, 17% of patients experienced complications from ICD placement.[53]

Percutaneous Left Ventricular Assist Device Support for Ventricular Tachycardia Ablation

The traditional approach for VT ablation relied on activation and entrainment mapping to find the critical isthmuses of the reentry circuits. However, many VTs are not hemodynamically tolerated, and classical mapping is not possible. Substrate mapping techniques in sinus rhythm have helped to overcome this limitation in the vast majority of cases and are the preferred approach to VT ablation nowadays. However, a clear target may not be found in some patients, and mapping during VT might be a better option for them. Temporary LVADs are currently used in some very high-volume centers to support the LV during VT and allow for extensive mapping of the VT circuit. Experiences with Impella 2.5, TandemHeart, and ECLS have been published so far, but they are mainly limited to small nonrandomized series. Moreover, there are several specific contraindications for these systems, and most of them do not provide adequate support in the case of severe RV dysfunction.

Impella is the easiest system to use, and it requires only 15 minutes for placement with a single femoral arterial approach. However, it may provide insufficient hemodynamic support for VT ablation in some patients,[54] and it is not exempt from potential complications. The device is contraindicated in patients with significant aortic disease or peripheral vascular disease. Besides, it may limit the movement of the catheter or add electromagnetic interference. TandemHeart can provide better hemodynamic support than Impella, but it requires a large cannula to be placed transseptally, apart from a larger arterial sheath to achieve maximal output. Its use virtually impedes the transseptal approach for catheter ablation. The device is also contraindicated in the presence of aortic regurgitation or peripheral vascular disease. ECLS provides the best hemodynamic support, but there are considerable risks related to it, and its placement and manipulation usually require the expertise of a larger multidisciplinary team. Importantly, the sites of cannula insertion should be decided together with the electrophysiologist so that they cause the least impact on the approach selected for the ablation procedure.

In a multicenter observational study, 44 patients supported with Impella or TandemHeart during VT ablation were compared with 22 patients with IABP support. More patients with Impella or TandemHeart could undergo VT mapping, more unstable VTs could be mapped and ablated per patient, more VTs were terminated by ablation, and fewer rescue shocks were required. However, mortality and VT recurrence during 12 ± 5 months of follow-up did not differ between the groups.[55] Another single-center series comparing 34 patients supported with Impella and 34 control patients also failed to demonstrate a decrease in VT recurrence during 19 ± 12 months of follow-up by using LVAD support, despite better mapping during VT.[56] Della Bella and colleagues reported greater use of these devices before the current era of substrate modification, whereas only 3 of 643 patients required support in their high-volume center in more recent years. These patients presented with almost incessant, untolerated fast VT.[57] The net benefit of the use of LVAD support taking into account both the risk for complications and the potential advantages of VT mapping has not been evaluated so far. Its use is limited to patients with untolerated incessant VT and to selected patients with very frequent episodes of VT.

REFERENCES

1. Yancy CW, Jessup M, Bozkurt B, et al. 2013 ACCF/AHA guideline for the management of heart failure: a report of the American College of Cardiology Foundation/American Heart Association Task Force on Practice Guidelines. *J Am Coll Cardiol.* 2013;62:e147–e239.
2. McMurray JJ, Adamopoulos S, Anker SD, et al. ESC guidelines for the diagnosis and treatment of acute and chronic heart failure 2012: The task force for the diagnosis and treatment of acute and chronic heart failure 2012 of the European Society of Cardiology. Developed in collaboration with the Heart Failure Association (HFA) of the ESC. *Eur J Heart Fail.* 2012;14:803–869.
3. Miller LW, Pagani FD, Russell SD, et al. Use of a continuous-flow device in patients awaiting heart transplantation. *N Engl J Med.* 2007;357:885–896.
4. Slaughter MS, Rogers JG, Milano CA, et al. Advanced heart failure treated with continuous-flow left ventricular assist device. *N Engl J Med.* 2009;361:2241–2251.
5. Kirklin JK, Naftel DC, Pagani FD, et al. Seventh INTERMACS annual report: 15,000 patients and counting. *J Heart Lung Transplant.* 2015;34:1495–1504.
6. Harding JD, Piacentino 3rd V, Rothman S, et al. Prolonged repolarization after ventricular assist device support is associated with arrhythmias in humans with congestive heart failure. *J Card Fail.* 2005;11:227–232.
7. Bedi M, Kormos R, Winowich S, et al. Ventricular arrhythmias during left ventricular assist device support. *Am J Cardiol.* 2007;99:1151–1153.
8. Andersen M, Videbaek R, Boesgaard S, et al. Incidence of ventricular arrhythmias in patients on long-term support with a continuous-flow assist device (HeartMate II). *J Heart Lung Transplant.* 2009;28:733–735.
9. Ambardekar AV, Lowery CM, Allen LA, et al. Effect of left ventricular assist device placement on preexisting implantable cardioverter-defibrillator leads. *J Card Fail.* 2010;16:327–331.
10. Cantillon DJ, Tarakji KG, Hu T, et al. Long-term outcomes and clinical predictors for pacemaker-requiring bradyarrhythmias after cardiac transplantation: analysis of the UNOS/OPTN cardiac transplant database. *Heart Rhythm.* 2010;7:1567–1571.
11. Kuhne M, Sakumura M, Reich SS, et al. Simultaneous use of implantable cardioverter-defibrillators and left ventricular assist devices in patients with severe heart failure. *Am J Cardiol.* 2010;105:378–382.
12. Brenyo A, Rao M, Koneru S, et al. Risk of mortality for ventricular arrhythmia in ambulatory LVAD patients. *J Cardiovasc Electrophysiol.* 2012;23:515–520.
13. Raasch H, Jensen BC, Chang PP, et al. Epidemiology, management, and outcomes of sustained ventricular arrhythmias after continuous-flow left ventricular assist device implantation. *Am Heart J.* 2012;164:373–378.
14. Refaat MM, Tanaka T, Kormos RL, et al. Survival benefit of implantable cardioverter-defibrillators in left ventricular assist device-supported heart failure patients. *J Card Fail.* 2012;18:140–145.
15. Enriquez AD, Calenda B, Miller MA, et al. The role of implantable cardioverter-defibrillators in patients with continuous flow left ventricular assist devices. *Circ Arrhythm Electrophysiol.* 2013;6:668–674.
16. Garan AR, Levin AP, Topkara V, et al. Early post-operative ventricular arrhythmias in patients with continuous-flow left ventricular assist devices. *J Heart Lung Transplant.* 2015;34:1611–1616.
17. Makki N, Mesubi O, Steyers C, et al. Meta-analysis of the relation of ventricular arrhythmias to all-cause mortality after implantation of a left ventricular assist device. *Am J Cardiol.* 2015;116:1385–1390.
18. Ziv O, Dizon J, Thosani A, et al. Effects of left ventricular assist device therapy on ventricular arrhythmias. *J Am Coll Cardiol.* 2005;45:1428–1434.
19. Enriquez AD, Calenda B, Miller MA, et al. The role of implantable cardioverter-defibrillators in patients with continuous flow left ventricular assist devices. *Circ Arrhythm Electrophysiol.* 2013;6:668–674.
20. Thiele H, Zeymer U, Neumann FJ, et al. Intra-aortic balloon counterpulsation in acute myocardial infarction complicated by cardiogenic shock (IABP-SHOCK II): final 12 month results of a randomised, open-label trial. *Lancet.* 2013;382:1638–1645.
21. Thiele H, Sick P, Boudriot E, et al. Randomized comparison of intra-aortic balloon support with a percutaneous left ventricular assist device in patients with revascularized acute myocardial infarction complicated by cardiogenic shock. *Eur Heart J.* 2005;26:1276–1283.
22. Seyfarth M, Sibbing D, Bauer I, et al. A randomized clinical trial to evaluate the safety and efficacy of a percutaneous left ventricular assist device versus intra-aortic balloon pumping for treatment of cardiogenic shock caused by myocardial infarction. *J Am Coll Cardiol.* 2008;52:1584–1588.
23. Paden ML, Conrad SA, Rycus PT, et al. Extracorporeal life support organization registry report 2012. *ASAIO J.* 2013;59:202–210.
24. Starling RC, Naka Y, Boyle AJ, et al. Results of the post-U.S. Food and Drug Administration–approval study with a continuous flow left ventricular assist device as a bridge to heart transplantation: a prospective study using the INTERMACS (Interagency Registry for Mechanically Assisted Circulatory Support). *J Am Coll Cardiol.* 2011;57:1890–1898.
25. Copeland JG, Smith RG, Arabia FA, et al. Cardiac replacement with a total artificial heart as a bridge to transplantation. *N Engl J Med.* 2004;351:859–867.
26. Garan AR, Yuzefpolskaya M, Colombo PC, et al. Ventricular arrhythmias and implantable cardioverter-defibrillator therapy in patients with continuous-flow left ventricular assist devices: need for primary prevention? *J Am Coll Cardiol.* 2013;61:2542–2550.
27. Sacher F, Reichlin T, Zado ES, et al. Characteristics of ventricular tachycardia ablation in patients with continuous flow left ventricular assist devices. *Circ Arrhythm Electrophysiol.* 2015;8:592–597.
28. Cantillon DJ, Bianco C, Wazni OM, et al. Electrophysiologic characteristics and catheter ablation of ventricular tachyarrhythmias among patients with heart failure on ventricular assist device support. *Heart Rhythm.* 2012;9:859–864.
29. Refaat M, Chemaly E, Lebeche D, et al. Ventricular arrhythmias after left ventricular assist device implantation. *Pacing Clin Electrophysiol.* 2008;31:1246–1252.
30. Rodrigue-Way A, Burkhoff D, Geesaman BJ, et al. Sarcomeric genes involved in reverse remodeling of the heart during left ventricular assist device support. *J Heart Lung Transplant.* 2005;24:73–80.
31. Healy C, Viles-Gonzalez JF, Sacher F, et al. Management of ventricular arrhythmias in patients with mechanical ventricular support devices. *Curr Cardiol Rep.* 2015;17:59.
32. Brisco MA, Sundareswaran KS, Milano CA, et al. The incidence, risk, and consequences of atrial arrhythmias in patients with continuous-flow left ventricular assist devices. *J Card Surg.* 2014;29:572–580.
33. Maury P, Delmas C, Trouillet C, et al. First experience of percutaneous radio-frequency ablation for atrial flutter and atrial fibrillation in a patient with HeartMate II left ventricular assist device. *J Interv Card Electrophysiol.* 2010;29:63–67.
34. Nishimura M, Ogiwara M, Ishikawa M, et al. Fifteen-month circulatory support for sustained ventricular fibrillation by left ventricular assist device. *J Thorac Cardiovasc Surg.* 2003;126:1190–1192.
35. Lee W, Tay A, Subbiah RN, et al. Impact of implantable cardioverter defibrillators on survival of patients with centrifugal left ventricular assist devices. *Pacing Clin Electrophysiol.* 2015;38:925–933.
36. Mulloy DP, Bhamidipati CM, Stone ML, et al. Cryoablation during left ventricular assist device implantation reduces postoperative ventricular tachyarrhythmias. *J Thorac Cardiovasc Surg.* 2013;145:1207–1213.
37. Weiss ES, Nwakanma LU, Russell SB, et al. Outcomes in bicaval versus biatrial techniques in heart transplantation: an analysis of the UNOS database. *J Heart Lung Transplant.* 2008;27:178–183.
38. Nof E, Stevenson WG, Epstein LM, et al. Catheter ablation of atrial arrhythmias after cardiac transplantation: findings at EP study utility of 3-D mapping and outcomes. *J Cardiovasc Electrophysiol.* 2013;24:498–502.
39. Gallego-Page JC, Segovia J, Alonso-Pulpon L, et al. Reinnervation after heart transplantation: a multidisciplinary study. *J Heart Lung Transplant.* 2004;23:674–682.
40. Knight CS, Tallaj JA, Rayburn BK, et al. Bradycardia and syncope as a presentation of cardiac allograft rejection involving the conducting system. *Cardiovasc Pathol.* 2010;19:117–120.
41. Melton IC, Gilligan DM, Wood MA, Ellenbogen KA. Optimal cardiac pacing after heart transplantation. *Pacing Clin Electrophysiol.* 1999;22:1510–1527.
42. Davies RR, Russo MJ, Morgan JA, et al. Standard versus bicaval techniques for orthotopic heart transplantation: an analysis of the United Network for Organ Sharing database. *J Thorac Cardiovasc Surg.* 2010;140:700–708.
43. Koller-Strametz J, Kratochwill C, Grabenwoger M, et al. PR interval adaptation in the denervated transplanted heart. *Pacing Clin Electrophysiol.* 1997;20:1247–1251.
44. Cui G, Kobashigawa J, Margarian A, Sen L. Cause of atrioventricular block in patients after heart transplantation. *Transplantation.* 2003;76:137–142.
45. Epstein AE, DiMarco JP, Ellenbogen KA, et al. ACC/AHA/HRS 2008 guidelines for device-based therapy of cardiac rhythm abnormalities: a report of the American College of Cardiology/American Heart Association task force on practice guidelines (writing committee to revise the ACC/AHA/NASPE 2002 guideline update for implantation of cardiac pacemakers and antiarrhythmia devices): Developed in collaboration with the American Association for Thoracic Surgery and Society of Thoracic Surgeons. *Circulation.* 2008;117:e350–e408.
46. Cui G, Tung T, Kobashigawa J, et al. Increased incidence of atrial flutter associated with the rejection of heart transplantation. *Am J Cardiol.* 2001;88:280–284.

47. Ahmari SA, Bunch TJ, Chandra A, et al. Prevalence, pathophysiology, and clinical significance of post-heart transplant atrial fibrillation and atrial flutter. *J Heart Lung Transplant.* 2006;25:53–60.

48. Khan M, Kalahasti V, Rajagopal V, et al. Incidence of atrial fibrillation in heart transplant patients: long-term follow-up. *J Cardiovasc Electrophysiol.* 2006;17: 827–831.

49. Vaseghi M, Boyle NG, Kedia R, et al. Supraventricular tachycardia after orthotopic cardiac transplantation. *J Am Coll Cardiol.* 2008;51:2241–2249.

50. Chang H, Lo L, Feng A, et al. Long-term follow-up of arrhythmia characteristics and clinical outcomes in heart transplant patients. *Transplant Proc.* 2013;45:369–375.

51. Vakil K, Taimeh Z, Sharma A, et al. Incidence, predictors, and temporal trends of sudden cardiac death after heart transplantation. *Heart Rhythm.* 2014;11:1684–1690.

52. Vaseghi M, Lellouche N, Ritter H, et al. Mode and mechanisms of death after orthotopic heart transplantation. *Heart Rhythm.* 2009;6:503–509.

53. Tsai VW, Cooper J, Garan H, et al. The efficacy of implantable cardioverter-defibrillators in heart transplant recipients: results from a multicenter registry. *Circ Heart Fail.* 2009;2:197–201.

54. Lu F, Eckman PM, Liao KK, et al. Catheter ablation of hemodynamically unstable ventricular tachycardia with mechanical circulatory support. *Int J Cardiol.* 2013;168:3859–3865.

55. Reddy YM, Chinitz L, Mansour M, et al. Percutaneous left ventricular assist devices in ventricular tachycardia ablation: multicenter experience. *Circ Arrhythm Electrophysiol.* 2014;7:244–250.

56. Aryana A, Gearoid O'Neill P, Gregory D, et al. Procedural and clinical outcomes after catheter ablation of unstable ventricular tachycardia supported by a percutaneous left ventricular assist device. *Heart Rhythm.* 2014;11:1122–1130.

57. Bella PD, Maccabelli G. Temporary percutaneous left ventricular support for ablation of untolerated ventricular tachycardias: is it worth the trouble? *Circ Arrhythm Electrophysiol.* 2012;5:1056–1058.

112 Standard Antiarrhythmic Drugs

Dawood Darbar

Mechanism-Based Approach to Treatment of Arrhythmias

Urgent Need to Define Underlying Mechanisms of Arrhythmias

Cardiac arrhythmias continue to remain a major source of morbidity and mortality and increased healthcare expenditure in developed countries. Despite advances in catheter-based and surgical procedure–based therapies, antiarrhythmic drugs (AADs) remain an important therapeutic option for the acute and chronic treatment of many arrhythmias. However, membrane-active drugs have limited efficacy in suppressing and preventing both atrial and ventricular arrhythmias, and many AADs are associated with significant toxicity. The efficacy in suppressing the most common sustained arrhythmia in clinical practice, atrial fibrillation (AF), is approximately 40%–60% with the possible exception of amiodarone. Sudden cardiac death (SCD), which annually causes over one million deaths in the United States and Europe, is most commonly caused by ventricular fibrillation (VF). Currently, there are no AADs available that can reliably reduce mortality associated with SCD. While implantable cardioverter defibrillators (ICDs) reduce mortality, they do not prevent SCD.

The lack of effective pharmacological therapies for AF and SCD relates not only to the poor understanding of the underlying pathophysiology of the syndromes and heterogeneity of both phenotypes but also a failure to target therapy to the underlying mechanisms. Recent advances in next-generation sequencing have identified rare genetic variants or mutations in genes encoding cardiac ion channels, gap junction proteins and signaling molecules, and single nucleotide polymorphisms (SNPs) associated with AF and SCD. Furthermore, genetic approaches to inherited arrhythmia syndromes have provided important insights into underlying mechanisms.

One universal principle of pharmacological therapy is that the best treatment is that targeted specifically to disease mechanisms.

As our understanding of the molecular and cellular basis of arrhythmias has evolved, so too has the list of arrhythmias for which specific mechanisms have been defined, and therefore specific AAD therapies may be indicated (Table 112.1). However, it is the recent advances in our understanding of molecular mechanisms in specific rare inherited monogenic arrhythmia syndromes (e.g., AF) that has provided important insights into common arrhythmias that may also prompt consideration of specific mechanism-based therapies.

The inherited arrhythmia syndrome catecholaminergic polymorphic ventricular tachycardia (CPVT) provides a good contemporary example of how a mechanism-based approach for drug therapy can be utilized. This syndrome is characterized by VT induced by adrenergic stress in the absence of structural heart disease and a high incidence of SCD. Mutations in two causative genes, i.e., *RYR2*, encoding the cardiac ryanodine receptor (RyR2) Ca^{2+} release channel, and *CASQ2*, encoding cardiac calsequestrin, have been associated with CPVT. Mutations in these two genes destabilize the RyR2 Ca^{2+} release channel complex in sarcoplasmic reticulum and result in spontaneous Ca^{2+} release through RyR2 channels, leading to delayed afterdepolarizations (DADs), triggered activity, and bidirectional/polymorphic VT.[1] While ICDs are recommended for the prevention of SCD in patients with CPVT, painful shocks can trigger further adrenergic stress and arrhythmias, and deaths have occurred despite appropriate ICD shocks. β-Adrenergic blockers have been shown to reduce arrhythmia burden and prevent SCD but are not completely effective. However, because Ca^{2+} leakage through the ryanodine channel is a common mechanism of CPVT, blockade of this channel may have a therapeutic effect. This led Watanabe and colleagues to assess whether direct inhibition of RyR2 channels by flecainide could be used to treat CPVT.[2] They showed that flecainide directly inhibits RyR2 channels and suppresses DADs and triggered activity in *Casq2* null cardiomyocytes.[2,3] Na^+ channel block with flecainide may also prevent CPVT. Flecainide prevents spontaneous VT and inducible VT by exercise or isoproterenol in vivo. Based on these experimental findings, the effects of flecainide in two patients carrying a CPVT-linked mutation in either *RYR2* or *CASQ2* were examined, and it was found that flecainide suppressed exercise-induced arrhythmias and recurrences of VT/VF.[4]

Unfortunately, for most common arrhythmias, such as VT associated with myocardial disease or AF, arrhythmia mechanisms have been difficult to define, and so the choice of drug therapy continues to remain largely empiric. In such settings, drugs shown by clinical experience or controlled trials to be effective often target multiple mechanisms, including modifying the arrhythmia-prone substrate or inhibiting known or putative triggers of arrhythmias. As specific mechanisms for many arrhythmias have not been defined, the expectation that all patients with AF or VT will respond to therapy in a similar fashion makes the assumption that underlying mechanisms are homogeneous across patients.

TABLE 112.1 A mechanism-based approach to antiarrhythmic drug therapy

ARRHYTHMIA	MECHANISM-BASED THERAPY	MECHANISM TARGETED
AF	R-Propafenone	Leaky ryanodine receptor type 2 Ca^{2+} release channels
AV nodal reentry, AV reentry	Adenosine Verapamil	Macroreentry utilizing the AV node
Outflow tract VT	β-Blockers Verapamil, Diltiazem	Adrenergic stimulation
Fascicular VT	β-Blockers, Verapamil, Diltiazem	Reentry within the His-Purkinje system
Torsades de pointes due to drugs	Pacing Isoproterenol K^+ supplementation (to 4.5–5 mEq/L)	I_{Kr} block leading to bradycardia-dependent EADs and unstable intraventricular reentry due to heterogeneity of repolarization
Congenital long QT syndrome, type 1	β-Blockers	Failure of the adrenergically activated K^+ current I_{Ks} to maintain short action potentials during adrenergic stimulation
Congenital long QT syndrome, type 2	K^+ supplementation to 4.5–5 mEq/L	Abnormal action potential prolongation and heterogeneity due to loss of I_{Kr} function
Congenital long QT syndrome, type 3	Na^+ channel block: mexiletine; flecainide	Abnormal action potential prolongation and heterogeneity due to increased inward Na^+ current during the action potential plateau
Brugada syndrome	I_{TO} block: quinidine, sotalol	Increased heterogeneity of action repolarization due to loss of Na^+ channel function and maintained I_{TO}
AF, VF, or T-wave oversensing in short QT syndrome	Quinidine, sotalol	Increased outward current leading to shortened action potentials due to abnormally increased I_{Ks}, I_{Kr}, or I_{K1}.
CPVT	Flecainide	Directly inhibits RyR2 channels and suppresses DADs and triggered activity; prevents CPVT

AF, Atrial fibrillation; *AV,* atrioventricular; *CPVT,* catecholaminergic polymorphic ventricular tachycardia; *DADs,* delayed afterdepolarizations; *EADs,* early afterdepolarizations; *VF,* ventricular fibrillation; *VT,* ventricular tachycardia.

However, as genetic, molecular, and cellular studies continue to demonstrate, this assumption is largely unfounded. Therefore the incomplete efficacy of drugs in treating these arrhythmias, which appear to represent a spectrum of arrhythmia mechanisms, is perhaps not unexpected. Large clinical trials provide the best evidence for choosing among drug therapies and dosages in settings such as AF and VT. The use of evidence-based principles should be complemented by considering patient-specific characteristics that might make one drug more or less desirable than others.

Genetic Approaches to Defining Underlying Mechanisms of Arrhythmias

As AF is the most common sustained arrhythmia for which AADs are currently prescribed, and advances in our understanding of the molecular mechanisms of AF have in part been elucidated by exploring the genetic basis of AF, the discussion here will primarily focus on this common and morbid condition. Some of the genetic approaches that have been pursued in order to better understand the pathophysiology of AF, and how these studies have not only provided important insights into the underlying pathophysiology and enabled subtyping of AF but also allowed us to contemplate a more mechanism-based targeted approach for the treatment of the arrhythmia, will be reviewed (Fig. 112.1).

Over the last 5 years, unraveling the molecular pathogenesis of AF by applying genetic approaches has gained some traction. Familial AF was first described by Wolff in 1943, with subsequent epidemiological studies confirming heritability of the arrhythmia, estimated to be 62%, especially if it occurs in the absence of underlying heart or systemic disease, traditionally called "lone" AF. While recent studies suggest that the number of patients with true lone AF is likely to be much less than we originally assumed, and recent consensus statements recommend not using this term, not all patients with lone AF have a Mendelian form of the arrhythmia, as only 35% have a positive family history.[5] A better term to use is *early onset AF* for those patients who are more likely to have a genetic basis for their arrhythmia.

Linkage Analysis

One approach that has successfully identified novel genes for arrhythmias including AF is linkage analysis and a positional cloning approach. This approach has identified several genes and loci linked with Mendelian forms of early onset AF (Table 112.2). In 2003, the first gene (*KCNQ1*) encoding the delayed rectifier cardiac K^+ channel (I_{Ks}) was linked with familial AF.[6] In collaboration with Mayo investigators, we linked the first non-ion channel atrial gene, natriuretic peptide precursor A (*NPPA*), encoding atrial natriuretic peptide (ANP), with AF.[7]

Candidate Gene Studies

Investigators screened other K^+ and cardiac ion channels as candidate genes for AF upon the discovery that *KCNQ1* was causative for AF. Otway and colleagues[8] identified a *KCNQ1* mutation (R14C) that had no effect on the *KCNQ1/KCNE1* current amplitudes at baseline but the mutant channels demonstrated marked increases in current compared with wild-type (WT) channels upon exposure to hypotonic solution. Importantly, only those patients with left atrial dilatation developed AF. These findings and our data showing that the risk for developing AF is markedly increased when common and rare AF risk alleles combine support a "two-hit" hypothesis (Fig. 112.2). Mutations in genes encoding gap junction proteins (connexins) and signaling molecules (nucleoporin [*NUP155*]) have also been linked with AF. Importantly, an autosomal recessive mutation in *NUP155* was also associated with early SCD.[9]

Association Studies

While most patients with AF have risk factors such as hypertension, the majority of individuals do not develop the arrhythmia. Thus our working *hypothesis* is that common genetic variants increase AF susceptibility in some individuals with other identifiable risk factors (genetic or acquired)—a

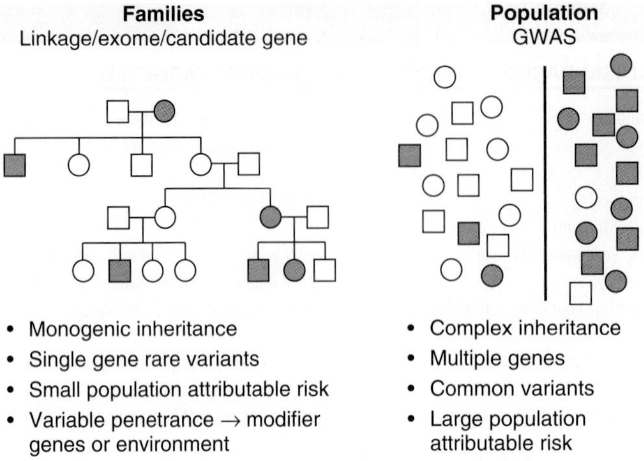

Families
Linkage/exome/candidate gene

Population
GWAS

- Monogenic inheritance
- Single gene rare variants
- Small population attributable risk
- Variable penetrance → modifier genes or environment

- Complex inheritance
- Multiple genes
- Common variants
- Large population attributable risk

FIGURE 112.1 Genetic approaches to defining the underlying genetic mechanisms of arrhythmias. Traditional linkage analysis, whole-exome sequencing, and candidate gene approaches have identified rare genetic variants in single genes in moderate- to large-sized familial kindreds. These mutations are associated with a small population-attributable risk. In contrast, genome-wide association studies (*GWAS*) have identified common genetic variants associated with susceptibility to arrhythmias in multiple genes that are associated with a large population-attributable risk. (Filled-in symbols indicate individuals with the phenotype.)

TABLE 112.2 Rare genetic variants linked with atrial fibrillation (AF)

GENE	MODE OF INHERITANCE	EFFECT ON FUNCTION	PHYSIOLOGICAL EFFECT	ASSOCIATED PHENOTYPES
KCNQ1	AD	Gain-of-function Loss-of-function	↓ Atrial APD	Prolonged QT
KCNE1	AD	Loss-of-function Gain-of-function	↓ Atrial APD	Frequent PACs
KCNE2	AD	Loss-of-function Gain-of-function	↓ Atrial APD	
KCNE5	AD	Gain-of-function	↓ Atrial APD	
KCND3	AD	Gain-of-function	↓ Atrial APD	
KCNJ2	AD	Loss-of-function Gain-of-function	↓ Atrial APD	
GJA5	Somatic mutations Isolated early onset AF cases	↓ Electrical cell-to-cell coupling	Regions of heterogeneous conduction	
KCNA5	AD	Loss-of-function Gain-of-function	↑ Atrial APD, EADs, and TA	
SCN5A	AD	Gain-of-function	↑↓ Atrial APD	HCM, DCM
SCN1B/2B/3B	AD	Loss-of-function	EADs, TA	
SCN10A	AD	Gain-of-function Loss-of-function	↑APD, EADs, TA	Slow ventricular rates
CACNA1C	AD	Gain-of-function	↑APD, EADs, TA	
CACNB2	AD	Loss-of-function	↑APD, EADs, TA	
NPPA	AD	Loss-of-function	↓ Atrial APD	Atrial myopathy
NUP155	AR	Nuclear protein transport (hsp70)		Sudden cardiac death
HSP-1	AD	Modulation of HSP		
EVC2	AD	Associated with long QT and Brugada syndromes		
SCNN1D	AD	Na⁺ channel gene expressed in the heart		
CACNA2D4	AD	Linked with cardiac conduction disease, long QT, and Brugada syndromes		

AD, Autosomal dominant; *APD*, action potential duration; *AR*, autosomal recessive; *EADs*, early afterdepolarizations; *DCM*, dilated cardiomyopathy; *HCM*, hypertrophic cardiomyopathy; *HSP*, heat shock protein; *PACs*, premature atrial contractions; *TA*, triggered activity.
Modified and revised from Darbar D, Roden DM. Genetic mechanisms of atrial fibrillation: impact on response to treatment. *Nat Rev Cardiol*. 2013;10:317-329.

basis for the "two-hit" hypothesis (see Fig. 112.2).[9] Recent advances in next-generation sequencing have resulted in the successful application of the genome-wide association paradigm to AF. In 2007, a chromosome 4q25 locus was highly significantly associated with AF.[10] Although the mechanism for this observed association still remains unclear, the locus is adjacent to the paired-like homeodomain transcription factor 2 (*PITX2*) gene, which is critical for cardiac development.

We replicated this association in the Vanderbilt AF Registry along with other large populations. Two additional AF loci on chromosomes 16q22 and 1q21 have been identified, and a meta-analysis of AF genome-wide association studies (GWAS) performed in 2012 not only validated these three SNPs but also identified and replicated six additional novel AF susceptibility loci. More recently, the AFGen Consortium has identified five more novel AF genes.[9]

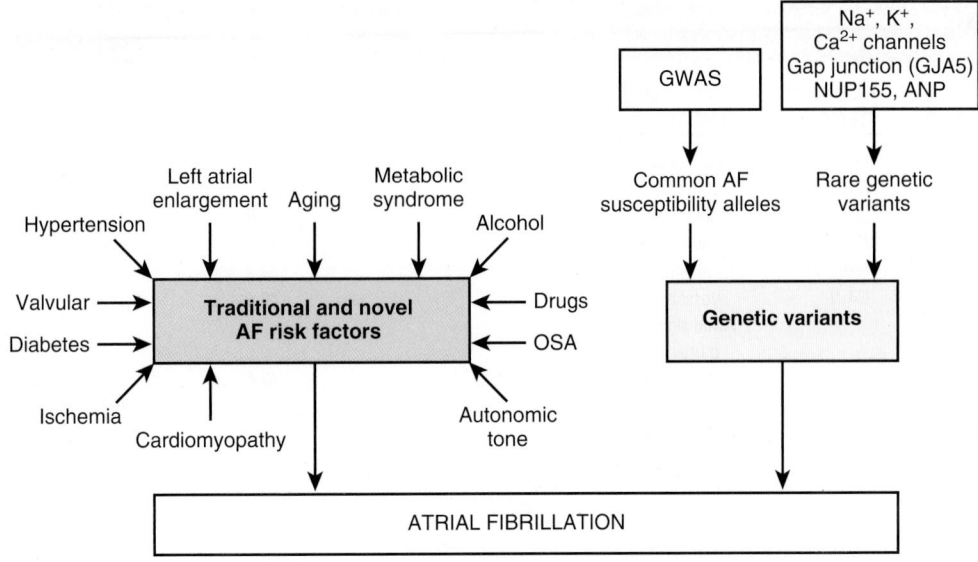

FIGURE 112.2 The two-hit hypothesis states that genetic and acquired risk factors are necessary for the development of atrial fibrillation *(AF)*. *ANP,* Atrial natriuretic peptide; *GWAS,* genome-wide association studies; *OSA,* obstructive sleep apnea.

Impact of Genetic Studies on Pharmacotherapy of Arrhythmias

Positional cloning and candidate gene approaches and GWAS have identified rare genetic variants and SNPs encoding cardiac ion channels, gap junction proteins, and signaling molecules associated with AF. Furthermore, these studies have provided important insights into the underlying pathophysiology of AF, identified novel therapeutic pathways, and formed the basis for a mechanism-based pharmacotherapeutic approach for AF.

Genetic Insights Into Atrial Fibrillation Mechanisms

Linkage studies and candidate gene approaches have demonstrated that genes linked with AF increase susceptibility to the arrhythmia by modulating the atrial action potential duration (APD).[9] While the first cardiac ion channel gene linked with familial AF was associated with a gain-of-function mutation in *KCNQ1*, encoding I_{Ks}, subsequent studies have identified both gain- and loss-of-function mutations in cardiac K+, Na+, and Ca2+ channels (see Table 112.2). We explored whether the WT-*KCNQ1* or the familial AF *KCNQ1*-S140G mutation has distinct pharmacological properties that may enable targeted inhibition by the I_{Ks}-selective blocker HMR-1556.[11] While a low concentration of the blocker had little effect on WT-I_{Ks}, HMR-1556 was capable of inhibiting the mutant channel. In cultured adult rabbit left atrial myocytes, expression of S140G-I_{Ks} shortened APD but cells expressing WT-I_{Ks} did not. The familial *KCNQ1* gain-of-function demonstrated increased sensitivity for the I_{Ks} blocker, which points to the possibility of selective therapeutic targeting. Furthermore, this study illustrates the potential for genotype-specific treatment of familial AF.

To better understand the molecular pathophysiology of AF, it is important to place it in the context of common arrhythmia mechanisms such as focal ectopic activity and reentry. Ectopic activity can be triggered by early afterdepolarizations (EADs), DADs, or enhanced automaticity. Rapid focal activity in the pulmonary veins not only initiates AF but also sustains it. High-frequency firing drivers or rotors or a single localized

reentrant circuit can also give rise to the irregular atrial discharge that is typical of AF. Atrial fibrillatory activity may also be caused by multiple fixed and functional circuits that are time and space dependent. While the cellular mechanisms causing paroxysmal AF in humans are clearly multifactorial, experimental evidence suggests that in mouse models, Ca leak mediated by RyR2 Ca release channels is one important mechanism responsible for triggering this form of the arrhythmia.[12] Ca leak has been demonstrated in atrial tissue from patients with persistent and paroxysmal AF, but the causal relationship to human AF remains controversial. However, recent insights into underlying AF mechanisms have been advanced by genetic studies of AF. GWAS have identified and validated 13 common AF susceptibility alleles, with several loci on chromosome 4q25 having the strongest associations with AF. Mouse studies have shown that reduced *Pitx2* expression generates AF risk in mice. Given how commonly leaky RyR2 channels are found in studies of human AF, and that individuals carrying 4q25 risk alleles respond better to the class IC drugs flecainide and propafenone, both of which also inhibit RyR2 channels, this raises the hypothesis that *PITX2* variants and possibly other rare AF-linked variants may initiate a cascade of cellular signaling events that ultimately leads to deranged RyR2 gating, which then contributes to AF by increasing Ca leak, generation of DADs, and triggered activity. Hence, such derangement of Ca handling may constitute a common electrophysiological mechanism by which both common and rare genetic variants increase susceptibility to paroxysmal AF.[12]

Using a positional cloning approach, a frameshift mutation in *NPPA* was identified in a large kindred with a variable phenotype of AF and atrial myopathy.[7] Infusion of the mutant ANP encoded by the *NPPA* mutation shortened the monophasic APD and effective refractory period in a rat whole-heart Langendorff preparation. While the precise mechanism(s) by which the circulating mutant ANP leads to an atrial myopathy and AF remains unclear, novel insights into underlying mechanisms will be provided by the generation of a transgenic mouse model that overexpresses the frameshift mutation. Both germline and somatic mutations and common SNPs encoding gap junction proteins such as connexin 40 have also been associated with early onset AF. These genetic variants likely mediate increased

TABLE 112.3 Common atrial fibrillation risk loci identified by a meta-analysis of genome-wide association studies and the closest genes that are likely to be modulated by the single nucleotide polymorphisms (SNP)

SNP	LOCUS	CLOSEST GENE	FUNCTIONAL EFFECT	MINOR/MAJOR ALLELE	MAF (%)	RR (95% CI)	P VALUE
rs2200733	4q25	PITX2	Development of pulmonary vein myocardial sleeve	T/C	25.8	1.71 (1.54–2.21)	6.1×10^{-41}
rs10033464	4q25	PITX2		G/C	13.1	1.42 (1.13–1.77)	3.1×10^{-11}
rs7193343	16q22	ZFHX3	unknown	T/C	17.6	1.25 (1.17–1.3)	1.8×10^{-15}
rs13376333	1q21	KCNN3	Ca activated K+ channel	T/C	29.5	1.56 (1.38–1.77)	6.3×10^{-12}
rs3903239	1q24	PRRX1	Development of great vessels	G/A	44.7	1.14 (1.10–1.18)	9.1×10^{-11}
rs3807989	7q31	CAV1	Atrial signal transduction protein	A/G	40.4	0.88 (0.84–0.91)	9.6×10^{-11}
rs10821415	9q22	C9orf3	Modulates TGF-β	A/C	42.4	1.13 (1.08–1.18)	7.9×10^{-9}
rs10821415	10q22	SYNPO2L	Localizes Z-protein	G/A	15.8	0.85 (0.81–0.9)	1.7×10^{-8}
rs1152591	14q23	SYNE2	Cardiac sarcomeric protein	A/G	47.6	1.13 (1.09–1.18)	6.2×10^{-10}
rs7164883	15q24	HCN4	Cardiac pacemaking I_f (funny)	G/A	16.0	1.16 (1.10–1.22)	1.3×10^{-8}

risk for AF by modulating expression of the gap junction proteins and impairing electrical communication and creating heterogeneity between cells.

Another major mechanism by which genetic variants increase susceptibility to AF is by modulating cardiac developmental genes. While the strongest signal associated with AF in GWAS is located at chromosome 4q25, the underlying mechanism(s) by which common SNPs at this locus regulate AF susceptibility remain poorly understood. However, *PITX2*, which encodes a homeobox transcription factor that is critical for development of the pulmonary vein myocardium and modulates signaling pathways important for regulating the electrophysiological substrate for atrial arrhythmias, is a postulated target for AF-associated SNPs at this locus. The identification of *PITX2* as a potential AF developmental gene has resulted in the screening of other cardiac developmental genes such as *GREMLIN2*. A rare genetic variant (Q76E) in this gene was associated with AF. Furthermore, in vivo experiments in zebrafish revealed that this mutation mediated its effects through bone morphogenetic protein (BMP) signaling resulting in *GREMLIN2* overactivity leading to slower cardiac contraction rates and modulation of identified AF candidate genes including *GJA5*, *Sarcolipin*, *Cacna1c*, *Kcne2*, and *Nppa*.[9] This is the first study that has identified the association between BMP signaling and AF and provides important insights into AF mechanisms and potentially a novel therapeutic target.

Genetic approaches to defining the underlying mechanisms of AF have also identified common genetic variants that encode genes that modulate fibrosis pathways and inflammation. Studies in the 1990s suggested that inflammation and atrial fibrosis may play important roles in the pathogenesis of AF when patients with early onset AF were found to have histological evidence of myocarditis. This concept is supported by the suppression of postoperative AF after cardiac surgery by antiinflammatory drugs. Furthermore, animal studies have shown that susceptibility to atrial arrhythmias appears to be mediated by the generation of atrial fibrosis, and the extent of atrial fibrosis was correlated with the success of ablation therapy.

Aside from its role in the development of the pulmonary vein myocardium, *PITX2* may also be involved in structural and electrical remodeling of the atria. Studies in *Pitxc2⁻/⁻* knock-out mice have shown four-chamber enlargement, atrial fibrosis, and upregulation of precursor genes. Conversely, *Pitxc2⁺/⁻* heterozygous mice have normal-sized chambers but increased expression of genes regulating Wnt signaling, a key fibrosis pathway. Additional evidence supporting the association between common

AF-associated SNPs encoding genes important for structural remodeling of the atria and creating a proarrhythmic substrate comes from findings of GWAS that have identified loci at the chromosome 7q31 encoding *caveolin-1*; the 16q22 locus encoding a zinc finger homeobox 3 transcription factor (*ZFHX3*); the 10q22 locus encoding *SYNPO2L*; 14q23 encoding *SYNE2*; and 1q24 encoding a *PRRX1* SNP (Table 112.3). Another possible mechanism by which *NPPA* variants may mediate increased risk for AF is by causing both electrical and structural remodeling of the atria with the development of atrial fibrosis. While overexpression of the humanized *NPPA* variant in mice does not appear to cause atrial enlargement,[13] another *NPPA* mutation identified in four Italian families was associated with an atrial myopathy, massive bi-atrial enlargement, and atrial standstill.[14]

Identification of Novel Therapeutic Targets

Genetic approaches to AF have also identified novel therapeutic targets. A rare variant in *KCNA5* encoding the Kv1.5 cardiac K+ channel and I_{Kur} was linked with AF, identifying the tyrosine signaling pathway as a novel therapeutic target for AF.[15] More recently, rare variants in *SCN10A*, encoding the Nav1.8 Na+ channel, have not only been associated with AF but also were shown to modulate both the peak and late Na+ current (I_{Na-L}).[16,17] Vanderbilt investigators showed that EADs could be blocked by a specific Nav1.8 blocker, supporting I_{Na-L} block as a novel therapeutic target for the treatment of AF.[18]

Novel AAD targets have been identified with the discovery that signaling pathways are important in cardiac protein expression, function, and turnover of cardiomyocytes, a process termed "proteostasis."[19] A novel variant of heat shock factor (HSF-1) was recently identified by whole-exome sequencing of a large AF kindred.[20] Since heat shock proteins (HSPs) play an important role in proteostasis, targeting this pathway with drugs such as geranylgeranylacetone that enhance HSP expression may protect against AF and represents a novel mechanism-based target for the treatment of AF.[19] Importantly, an autosomal recessive mutation in *NUP155* linked with early onset AF regulates transport of *Hsp70* mRNA and protein in and out of the nuclear membrane.[21] While the precise mechanism by which this mutation increases the risk for AF is not clear, upregulation of genes important in the pathogenesis of AF is one potential mechanism. The histone acetyl deacetylases (HDAC) also play an important role in proteostasis. Studies have shown that suppression of HDAC6 with tubastatin A prevented the progression of AF in a tachycardia-induced dog model, suggesting that targeting this pathway may be another novel approach for the treatment of AF.[19]

Identification of Mechanism-Based Genetic Subtypes of Atrial Fibrillation

Genetic studies have not only uncovered AF-associated common and rare genetic variants but also enabled mechanism-based subtyping of AF with differential response to therapy. An early pharmacogenomics study of AF explored the role of the angiotensin-converting enzyme (*ACE*) *I/D* polymorphism in modulating response to AADs for symptomatic AF.[9] Surprisingly, the only significant predictors of failure of AAD therapy were early onset AF and *ACE DD/ID* genotypes. Furthermore, a graded response was observed in patients with the *II* genotype experiencing the greatest suppression of symptomatic AF and those with the *DD* genotype responding the least well to AADs. While the underlying mechanism for this differential effect has not completely been worked out, it has been postulated that patients carrying the *DD* genotype have greater atrial structural remodeling.

More recent studies have assessed whether common AF SNPs at the chromosome 4q25 locus (near *PITX2*), 16q22 (in *ZFHX3*), and 1q21 (in *KCNN3*) modulated symptomatic responses to AADs in patients with symptomatic AF.[22] While multiple clinical variables including age, hypertension, and early onset AF failed to predict response to AAD therapy, an SNP at the chromosome 4q25 locus (rs10033464) was significantly associated with successful symptom control in both the discovery and validation cohorts (odds ratio [OR], 2.97; 95% confidence interval [CI], 1.42–6.21; p = .003). Perhaps the most surprising finding was that individuals who carried the 4q25 SNP responded better to class I versus class III AADs. More recently, our group showed that the same chr4q25 AF locus predicted a 24% shorter recurrence-free time from AF than did the presence of the WT SNP after AF ablation,[23] confirming an earlier study.[24] These variants were also independent predictors of AF recurrence after restoration of sinus rhythm after electrical cardioversion.[25] Collectively, these studies provide strong support for the role of common AF-associated SNPs at the chromosome 4q25 locus (as this is by far the strongest association with the arrhythmia) in modulating response to AADs and cardioversion and ablation therapy for AF. Furthermore, these data provide a basis for potential subtyping of AF that is mechanism-based and selecting AF therapies based on genotype.

Principles of Antiarrhythmic Therapy
Evaluating Risk Versus Benefit of Antiarrhythmic Therapy

The benefits of AAD therapy in the acute setting are clearly evident when a patient presents with a highly symptomatic, sustained arrhythmia that drug therapy terminates rapidly. In this setting, symptomatic benefits are obvious, and the risk is minimized because patients are monitored and exposed to the drug only for a very brief period. By contrast, with chronic therapy, the balance between benefit and risk is more difficult to evaluate. While chronic therapy in a patient with heart disease may be beneficial initially, efficacy may be lost with time because of a changing electrophysiological milieu. Indeed, in virtually all clinical trials to date, chronic antiarrhythmic therapy has been incompletely effective. Furthermore, the consequences of arrhythmia recurrence are clinically important and can vary from recurrent hospitalization to SCD, and the risk for serious adverse effects appears to increase over time. Therefore AADs retain a primary role in the acute termination of arrhythmias and in selected chronic arrhythmia settings, such as AF, in which arrhythmia recurrence might not be catastrophic. By contrast, device-based and ablative therapies are more desirable from a risk-to-benefit point of view in such settings as VT/VF, where AADs have mainly assumed a secondary role. However, as ablative therapies for AF continue to evolve, it is possible that drugs might assume a secondary role

here as well. Nevertheless, the development of new drug therapies for AF (discussed earlier) that are highly effective, and more importantly, safe during chronic therapy is still highly desirable, as ablative therapies are likely limited to a very small section of patients with the arrhythmia.

Historical Perspective on Current Antiarrhythmic Drugs and Their Limitations

Drugs that are currently marketed as antiarrhythmics were initially developed in whole-animal models by screening for their effects on normal cardiac electrophysiology. However, decades elapsed before the initial use of older AADs in humans, and more importantly, the definition of their molecular mechanisms of action. AADs are only partly effective and have many adverse effects. The most important of these is the potential to generate new life-threatening arrhythmias (proarrhythmia). The increasing appreciation of ventricular arrhythmias as a marker of underlying heart disease, and therefore a potential drug target, led to the development of multiple new AADs in the late 1970s and early 1980s. An early animal model that was used to screen for antiarrhythmic activity was the "Harris dog," which demonstrates extremely high-frequency ventricular ectopic activity after two-stage coronary artery ligation. As ventricular arrhythmias are especially sensitive to Na+ channel blockers, the first wave of new antiarrhythmics were drugs that were derived from existing structures and demonstrated activity in this and other models, i.e., primarily Na+ channel blockers.

The Cardiac Arrhythmia Suppression Trial (CAST) represents a landmark trial result, not only for AAD development but for drug development in general.[26] CAST tested the then-prevalent hypothesis that because ventricular ectopy following myocardial infarction (MI) is a risk factor for SCD, suppression of ventricular ectopy would reduce the incidence of SCD. As is now well appreciated, mortality among patients randomized to ventricular ectopic suppression with encainide or flecainide in CAST was approximately threefold higher than that of patients randomized to receive the placebo. It also emphasized the importance of a randomized, placebo-controlled trial with a primary "hard" endpoint, such as death, as opposed to a surrogate endpoint, such as ectopic-beat suppression, in order to sort out if a drug is beneficial or not. The drugs tested in CAST turned out to be potent Na+ channel blocking agents.

For basic and clinical scientists interested in arrhythmia mechanisms, the CAST result provided a strong impetus for further work that defined the way in which loss of Na+ channel function was arrhythmogenic. It is thought that blocking Na+ channels increases the risk for SCD by slowing conduction and/or increasing the heterogeneity of repolarization, both of which can be arrhythmogenic, especially in diseased hearts. Multiple lines of evidence now support the hypothesis that loss of Na+ current (I_{Na}) slows cardiac conduction and may be arrhythmogenic. Such loss may be structural (e.g., mutations in the cardiac Na+ channel gene *SCN5A* leading to loss of peak I_{Na}), pharmacologic, or reflect activation of second messenger systems: e.g., protein kinase A (PKA) activation has been reported to increase peak I_{Na}, at least in part due to altered trafficking, while protein kinase C activation decreases it.[27]

Another consequence of CAST was that development of Na+ channel-blocking drugs came to a rapid halt and QT-prolonging agents then assumed the limelight. Just as procainamide and lidocaine provided the structural starting point for a range of Na+ channel-blocking molecules, two compounds with prominent action potential–prolonging properties formed the framework here: *N*-acetyl procainamide (NAPA) and sotalol. Both compounds also do not block the Na+ channel and gave rise to a generation of QT-prolonging drugs: d-sotalol, dofetilide, almokalant, sematilide, and others. The screening assay to develop these agents usually was

APD in a guinea pig papillary muscle, and as with newer Na+ channel blockers, these compounds were not synthesized to interact with a specific predefined molecular target. Nevertheless, subsequent studies identified block of one specific K+ current, termed I_{Kr} (the rapid component of the cardiac delayed rectifier K+ current), as the major mechanism underlying QT prolongation by AADs. I_{Kr} is encoded by *KCNH2* (also known as HERG). However, blocking I_{Kr} carries the risk for marked QT-interval prolongation and a distinctive form of polymorphic VT, termed torsades de pointes. Indeed, K+ channel-blocking AADs have been tested in CAST-like trials and did not prevent more deaths than placebo. Moreover, the same mechanism underlies the development of torsades de pointes in response to "noncardiovascular" drugs such as certain antihistamines, antibiotics, and antipsychotics.[28]

Classification of Antiarrhythmic Drugs

The earliest schemes classified drugs based on shared efficacies and toxicities. Some AADs share important electrophysiological properties, notably block of Na+ channels or of the K+ current I_{Kr}, and these can provide the basis for predicting shared or "class" actions and toxicities. Block or enhancement of other ionic currents, such as I_{Ks}, the transient outward current (I_{TO}), or acetylcholine-activated current (I_{K-Ach}) may also contribute to clinical drug actions in some cases, and are not usually considered in broad classification schemes. A more modern approach and one that was presciently adopted by the "Sicilian Gambit" investigators is to classify drugs based on key electrophysiological mechanisms involved in arrhythmogenesis, thereby allowing specific drugs to be chosen to target these. This approach is nicely exemplified by the definition of new molecular mechanisms in congenital arrhythmia syndromes, such as AF and the congenital long QT syndrome (LQTS), and the way in which these then lead naturally to mechanism-based therapies, as discussed earlier. As our understanding of the molecular and cellular basis of arrhythmias evolves, a more rational choice of key molecules(s) whose targeting is likely to be safe and effective in the therapy of a particular arrhythmia holds much promise.

The term "antiarrhythmic drugs" has traditionally been used to include drugs targeting ion channels in cardiac myocytes (Na+ channel blockers, Ca2+ channel blockers, and QT-prolonging drugs, generally K+ channel blockers), β-adrenergic receptor blockers, and a series of drugs with diverse mechanisms used primarily for the therapy of arrhythmias, such as digoxin, amiodarone, magnesium, and adenosine. However, recent studies have demonstrated that other widely used cardiovascular therapies, such as ACE and HMG Co-A reductase inhibitors may also exert important antiarrhythmic effects. Such effects may include not only reduction in SCD, an arrhythmic event that represents the final common pathway for many potential disease pathways, but also prevention of AF. These studies not only provide novel potential therapies but also implicate new signaling pathways in the pathogenesis of arrhythmias and therefore as potential targets for the development of effective antiarrhythmic interventions.

Pharmacokinetic Principles

One important mechanism underlying variability in response to AADs is variability in pharmacokinetics, the result of the processes of drug absorption, distribution, metabolism, and elimination. Variability in pharmacokinetics contributes substantially to variability in efficacy or toxicity when there is a narrow therapeutic window (the margin between dosages and plasma concentrations that are associated with efficacy and those associated with toxicity) and when the drug is metabolized or excreted by a single pathway; these criteria apply to many AADs. Sotalol and dofetilide are examples of drugs with narrow therapeutic windows and the risk for toxicity, namely torsades de pointes, increases for both with

increasing dosages. In addition, both drugs are largely excreted by a single pathway, renal excretion. As a result, drug dosages need to be adjusted in renal failure to avoid increased risk for torsades de pointes. By contrast, while the toxicity of flecainide is also concentration-dependent, the drug is eliminated by hepatic metabolism and renal excretion. Thus impaired metabolism or renal dysfunction alone does not generally alter response to the drug, although rare cases of flecainide toxicity due to inhibited drug metabolism in patients with renal dysfunction have been reported.

Cytochrome P450s and Other Drug Elimination Molecules

Drug metabolism, elimination, and disposition are accomplished by specific gene products, most commonly drug-metabolizing enzymes (primarily members of the cytochrome P450 superfamily, or CYPs) and drug transport molecules. DNA variants that alter the activity of these proteins are increasingly well recognized; although some exert only subtle effects on protein function, in other cases, an individual may totally lack enzymatic activity. This is especially important if the affected pathway is critical for elimination of a drug with a narrow therapeutic margin. Furthermore, concomitant drug therapy can modulate the activity of the drug metabolizing and transporting molecules. In most cases, such drug interactions result in inhibition of the elimination pathway. Occasionally, however, concomitant drug therapy can induce expression of drug metabolism and thus accelerate elimination. Under this circumstance, an increase in the drug dosage may be required to maintain a therapeutic effect.

The major drug metabolizing enzymes for AADs are CYP2D6, CYP2C9, and CYP3A4/5. Approximately 5%–10% of Caucasians and African-Americans are homozygous for loss-of-function alleles in CYP2D6; these individuals totally lack enzymatic activity and are designated "poor metabolizers" (PMs). CYP2D6 PMs have markedly decreased propafenone clearance, and accumulate the parent drug to plasma concentrations high enough to produce clinically significant β-blockade; as a result, asthma can be a risk in these subjects. Similarly, CYP2D6 PMs also have higher concentrations of timolol and metoprolol. Propafenone and quinidine are CYP2D6 inhibitors, and may therefore alter the effects of these CYP2D6 substrates. Amiodarone is a potent CYP2C9 inhibitor, and dosages of warfarin must therefore be adjusted downward with amiodarone therapy.

CYP3A4/5 are two closely related enzymes that are the most abundant cytochromes in the liver (and in other sites, like enterocytes) and are responsible for the metabolism of the majority of currently used AADs including quinidine, disopyramide, propafenone, and dofetilide. While individuals totally lacking CYP3A activity have not been described, there is substantial interindividual variability in the activity. However, CYP3A activity can be near-totally inhibited by concomitant drug therapy, notably with certain azole antifungals (ketoconazole), macrolide antibiotics (erythromycin), HIV protease inhibitors (ritonavir), amiodarone, diltiazem, verapamil, and large doses of grapefruit juice. CYP3A activity can also be induced by rifampin, phenytoin, and St. John's wort; reduction in plasma concentrations and loss of drug effects can occur under these conditions. Inhibition of CYP3A-mediated elimination by these drug interactions was the major cause of terfenadine accumulation in plasma, leading to cases of torsades de pointes that eventually prompted the drug's withdrawal from the market.

N-acetyltransferase (NAT) activity is responsible for the elimination of procainamide. There are two NAT genes, *NAT1* and *NAT2*. *NAT1* is expressed in all individuals, but the loss of functional alleles has been reported in *NAT2*. As a result, patients can be divided into rapid and slow acetylators. Slow acetylators have a higher incidence of procainamide-induced lupus syndrome during chronic therapy.

In addition to metabolizing enzymes, transport across biological membranes is another crucial determinant of drug disposition that has received increasing attention over the last few years. The multisubstrate efflux carrier P-glycoprotein is the most well studied to date in terms of cardiovascular drugs. P-glycoprotein is the product of the multidrug resistance 1 (*MDR1; ABCB1*) gene and is a member of the ABCB subfamily of ATP-binding cassette (ABC) transmembrane proteins, which have been implicated in drug resistance in cancer. P-glycoprotein is expressed not only in drug-resistant cancer cells but also in many organs such as the gut and kidney, where it plays important roles in distribution and elimination. It acts as an efflux pump, and in the gut prevents the entry of toxic compounds, while in the liver and kidney it serves to remove xenobiotics from the circulation. Although P-glycoprotein substrates are diverse, there is considerable overlap between the substrates that are transported by P-glycoprotein and those metabolized by CYP3A4/5. One important role for P-glycoprotein in cardiovascular medicine is that it transports cardiac glycosides. A synonymous SNP in exon 26 (C3435T) in the *MDR1* gene has been associated with expression of the transporter and variable digoxin concentration. Furthermore, correlation between the *MDR1* genotype and digoxin uptake in vivo has been described. Many drugs inhibit P-glycoprotein activity and their use with digoxin can lead to increased digoxin plasma concentrations and toxicity: amiodarone, quinidine, verapamil, itraconazole, cyclosporine, and erythromycin are examples.

Pharmacodynamic Principles

Experimental studies even prior to the cloning era indicated that ion channels, the targets of AADs, have specific drug binding sites. Further, a drug binding to these "receptor" sites on the channels to modify their function was found to be modulated by the "state" of the channel (open, closed, or inactivated); these observations led to the formulation of the modulated receptor hypothesis to analyze drug-channel interactions. More contemporary studies have demonstrated the existence of specific drug binding sites on ion channel proteins, and the interaction of drugs with these sites can be modulated by channel protein conformation (or "state"). In some cases, ion channels are blocked by direct binding in the pore region (a common mechanism for most I_{Kr} blockers), whereas in others, drug binding to other regions of the protein alters its function, an "allosteric" effect.

Most Na$^+$ channel blocking drugs inhibit open or inactivated states of the channel; hence, during each cardiac cycle, they associate with and block channels, and then dissociate during diastole, ultimately reaching a steady-state level of block. If the heart rate is increased, there is less time for dissociation, so channel block is enhanced. Furthermore, the rate of dissociation from the channel varies among drugs. For drugs like lidocaine with "fast-off" kinetics, very little block occurs even at fast rates. In contrast, with "slow-off" drugs like flecainide, block accumulates even at physiological rates. As Na$^+$ channel block slows intraventricular conduction, it prolongs QRS duration on the surface electrocardiogram. This explains why QRS widening is apparent at normal heart rates during flecainide (but not lidocaine) therapy and widens further if the heart rate is increased. In addition, since conduction slowing promotes reentry, slowing conduction by the drug at faster rates may explain cases of flecainide-induced VT during exercise.

Class I Antiarrhythmic Drugs

While all class I AADs block the cardiac Na$^+$ channel, the extent of block is dependent not only on the heart rate and membrane potential but also the physicochemical characteristics of each drug that determine the rate of onset and recovery from block. This has given rise to a subclassification of class I AADs based on the magnitude of their effects on cardiac conduction. Class IA drugs such as quinidine, procainamide, and disopyramide have intermediate effects on Na$^+$ channel block and only cause significant prolongation of conduction in cardiac tissue at rapid heart rates. The class IB drugs, lidocaine and mexiletine, have minimal or no effects on the cardiac Na$^+$ channel in normal tissue but cause significant conduction slowing in depolarized tissue. In contrast, class IC drugs, flecainide and propafenone, cause significant prolongation of conduction in cardiac tissue at normal heart rates with an increase in the QRS duration on the electrocardiogram. Many class I AADs have effects on other ion channels and membrane receptors through which some of their electrophysiological effects are mediated.

Class IA Antiarrhythmic Drugs

Quinidine

Pharmacodynamics. Quinidine not only blocks INa but also multiple K+ currents (IKr, IKs, and I_{to}[29]) and has intermediate kinetics of interaction with the channel. While I_{Kr} block can occur at very low concentrations, action potential prolongation in vitro by quinidine is blunted at higher concentrations, likely reflecting an additional effect of Na$^+$ channel blockade.[30] Quinidine's α-blocking properties can produce hypotension when administered intravenously and its vagolytic actions occasionally make it a useful drug for the treatment of vasovagal syncope. Quinidine can also enhance atrioventricular (AV) nodal conduction during atrial flutter. It is a very potent inhibitor of CYP2D6, exerting this pharmacological action at doses as low as 5 mg; indeed low-dose quinidine has actually been used in combination with CYP2D6 substrates to increase the plasma concentrations and make them more uniform. Quinidine is also a potent inhibitor of P-glycoprotein, and as discussed earlier it decreases digoxin clearance and increases its serum concentrations and risk for toxicity.

Pharmacokinetics. Quinidine is well absorbed and is 80% bound to plasma proteins. In high-stress states such as acute MI, greater-than-usual doses may be required to maintain therapeutic concentrations of free quinidine. Quinidine undergoes extensive hepatic oxidative metabolism, with only about 20% excreted unchanged by the kidneys. While the 3-hydroxyquinidine metabolite is nearly as potent as quinidine in blocking I_{Na} or prolonging the action potential,[31] most other metabolites do not contribute significantly to the clinical effects of quinidine. There is substantial interindividual variability in the range of dosages required to achieve therapeutic plasma concentrations of 2–5 μg/mL. In patients with advanced renal disease or heart failure, quinidine clearance is modestly reduced and thus dosage requirements in these patients are similar to those in other patients. Quinidine is eliminated by CYP3A4-mediated hepatic metabolism, with a half-life of 6–12 hours. Drugs such as phenobarbital and phenytoin can induce its metabolism, and in patients receiving these agents, very high doses of quinidine may be required to achieve therapeutic concentrations. If therapy with the inducing agent is then stopped, quinidine concentrations can rise to very high levels, and its dosage must be adjusted downward. Cimetidine and verapamil elevate plasma quinidine concentrations, but these usually are modest.

Adverse Effects. Quinidine is poorly tolerated and diarrhea is the most common adverse effect, occurring in up to 50% of patients. Diarrhea-induced hypokalemia can potentiate the risk for torsades de pointes. While a number of immunological reactions can occur during quinidine therapy including thrombocytopenia, hepatitis, bone marrow suppression, and a lupus-like syndrome, these resolve rapidly with discontinuation of the drug. Quinidine also can produce cinchonism, a symptom complex that includes headache and tinnitus. In contrast to other adverse effects during quinidine therapy, cinchonism usually is related to elevated plasma quinidine concentrations and can be managed by reducing the dose.

It is estimated that 2%–5% of patients who receive quinidine therapy will develop marked QT interval prolongation and torsades de pointes. In contrast to the effects of sotalol, NAPA, and many other drugs, quinidine-associated torsades de pointes generally occurs at therapeutic, or even subtherapeutic, plasma concentrations. The reasons for individual susceptibility to this adverse effect are not known. At high plasma concentrations of quinidine, marked Na+ channel block can occur, with resultant VT. This adverse effect formerly occurred when very high doses of quinidine were used to try to convert AF to normal sinus rhythm, but this aggressive approach to quinidine dosing has now been abandoned, and quinidine-induced VT due to excess Na+ channel block is unusual. Quinidine can exacerbate heart failure or conduction system disease. However, in most patients with congestive heart failure, quinidine is well tolerated, perhaps because of its vasodilating actions.

Clinical Efficacy. While the class IA AADs all have documented efficacy for the treatment of atrial and ventricular tachyarrhythmias, they are less efficacious and more poorly tolerated than other drugs such as amiodarone for the treatment of AF.[32] The combination of quinidine and mexiletine has been shown to have synergistic AAD efficacy for ventricular arrhythmias and is often used in clinical practice for recurrent ventricular arrhythmias. However, the benefits of therapy are often offset by intolerable adverse effects and the risk for ventricular proarrhythmia. All class IA drugs are contraindicated in patients with structural heart disease, including left ventricular hypertrophy, because of the increased risk for death from proarrhythmia, and they can only be considered relatively safe in patients without structural heart disease or in patients with an ICD. Consequently, these drugs are considered second- or third-line therapy for the long-term treatment of AF and other atrial tachyarrhythmias.[32]

Quinidine is now gaining resurgence as an antiarrhythmic for the treatment of ventricular arrhythmias in patients with no demonstrable heart disease. For many years, there was general skepticism toward the use of class I antiarrhythmics and especially quinidine in the treatment of malignant arrhythmias occurring in patients with structurally normal hearts. However, there is increasing evidence for the efficacy of quinidine not only for the treatment of idiopathic VF but also for Brugada syndrome. Belhassen and colleagues[33] reported first the largest series of patients with idiopathic VF or Brugada syndrome in whom quinidine was found to be very effective (96%) in preventing VF reinducibility during an electrophysiology study and this was confirmed by other groups and with long-term follow-up. In addition, quinidine is being successfully used as a first-line therapy for abolishing arrhythmic storms in patients with Brugada syndrome. In these patients, the efficacy of quinidine has been attributed to strong inhibition of the I_{To} current that restores electrical homogeneity and abolishes phase 2 reentry and anticholinergic effects. The mechanism of the efficacy of quinidine is more obscure.

Another syndrome in which quinidine has recently been shown to be efficacious is that associated with arrhythmic SCD and early repolarization anomalies in the inferior and left precordial leads.[34] Many of these patients are prone to electrical storms, and in the acute setting, a continuous infusion of isoproterenol has successfully treated electrical storms associated not only with early repolarization abnormalities but also Brugada syndrome or torsades de pointes associated with bradycardia.[35] Isoproterenol is thought to be effective probably by increasing I_{Ca-L} current and thus decreasing the electrical gradient and possibly by increasing heart rate and reducing inactivation of I_{To}. With chronic therapy, quinidine is highly effective in the prevention of recurrence of VF associated with early repolarization abnormalities.

Procainamide

Pharmacodynamics. Procainamide is a blocker of open Na+ channels, with an intermediate time constant of recovery from block. It also prolongs cardiac action potentials in most tissues, probably by blocking I_{Kr}. Procainamide decreases automaticity, increases refractory periods, and slows conduction. The major metabolite, NAPA, lacks the Na+ channel blocking activity of the parent drug but is equipotent in prolonging action potentials.[31] Because the plasma concentrations of NAPA often exceed those of procainamide, increased refractoriness and QT prolongation during chronic procainamide therapy can be attributed at least in part to the metabolite. However, it is the parent drug that slows conduction and produces QRS interval prolongation. Although hypotension can occur at high plasma concentrations, this effect usually is attributable to ganglionic blockade rather than to any negative inotropic effect, which is minimal.

Pharmacokinetics. Procainamide is rapidly eliminated ($t_{1/2}$, 3–4 hours) by hepatic metabolism and renal excretion of the unchanged drug. The major pathway for hepatic metabolism is conjugation by N-acetyl transferase to form NAPA. NAPA is eliminated by renal excretion ($t_{1/2}$, 6–10 hours) and is not significantly converted back to procainamide. Because of the relatively rapid elimination rates of both the parent drug and its major metabolite, procainamide usually is administered in a slow-release formulation. In patients with renal failure, procainamide and NAPA can accumulate to potentially toxic plasma concentrations. Reduction of procainamide dose and dosing frequency and monitoring of plasma concentrations of both compounds are required in this situation. Because the parent drug and metabolite exert different pharmacological effects, the practice of using the sum of their concentrations to guide therapy is inappropriate. In patients who are slow acetylators, the procainamide-induced lupus syndrome develops more often and earlier during treatment than among rapid acetylators. In addition, the symptoms of procainamide-induced lupus resolve during treatment with NAPA. Procainamide plasma concentrations should be monitored to ensure that concentrations of the parent drug remain in the range of 4–8 µg/mL. NAPA concentrations greater than 20 µg/mL carry a higher risk for torsades de pointes. Procainamide concentrations > 10 µg/mL appear to carry a risk for marked QRS widening and potential arrhythmia exacerbation.

Adverse Effects. Hypotension and marked slowing of conduction are major adverse effects of high concentrations (>10 µg/mL) of procainamide, especially during intravenous use. Dose-related nausea is common during oral therapy and may be attributable in part to a high plasma concentration of NAPA. Torsades de pointes can occur, particularly when the plasma concentration of NAPA rises to greater than 30 µg/mL. Procainamide produces potentially fatal bone marrow aplasia in 0.2% of patients. The mechanism is not known, but high plasma drug concentrations are not suspected. During long-term therapy, most patients develop biochemical evidence of the drug-induced lupus syndrome, such as circulating antinuclear antibodies.[36] Therapy need not be interrupted merely because of the presence of antinuclear antibodies. However, many patients eventually develop symptoms (rash, small-joint arthralgias) of the lupus syndrome. Other symptoms of lupus including pericarditis with tamponade can occur, although renal involvement is unusual.

Clinical Efficacy. While amiodarone gained slow acceptance outside the specialized field of cardiac antiarrhythmic surgery because the side effects are significant, the adoption of amiodarone in the Advanced Cardiac Life Support (ACLS) protocol has popularized this AAD. Procainamide can be effective in converting AF to sinus rhythm and can slow ventricular rate in patients presenting with preexcited AF and rapid ventricular responses. Quinidine has been shown to be effective in preventing VF induction in patients with Brugada syndrome.[37] It also suppresses spontaneous arrhythmias and could prove to be a safe alternative to ICD therapy for a substantial proportion of patients with Brugada syndrome.[33] Intravenous procainamide has been used to unmask the electrocardiographic features of Brugada syndrome.[38]

Disopyramide

Pharmacodynamics. Disopyramide is a Na$^+$ channel blocker with onset and offset kinetics similar to those of quinidine. It also prolongs the QT interval and exerts prominent antiinotropic and anticholinergic effects at clinical dosages.

Pharmacokinetics. Disopyramide is eliminated by hepatic metabolism and renal excretion. The pathways are induced by phenytoin, suggesting participation by CYP3A4 or P-glycoprotein. The drug is administered as a racemate; the enantiomers are equally potent as Na$^+$ channel blockers, but only one, S-disopyramide, prolongs action potentials in vitro. The drug is variably bound to plasma proteins within the therapeutic range, but as its binding is saturable, monitoring plasma concentrations of the total drug is not useful.

Adverse Effects. Torsades de pointes, exacerbation of heart failure, and anticholinergic effects (constipation, urinary retention, glaucoma, dry eyes and mouth) are all adverse effects of disopyramide.

Clinical Efficacy. The anticholinergic actions of disopyramide make it suitable for patients with vagally mediated AF; its negative inotropic effects may also be useful in managing patients with hypertrophic cardiomyopathy and outflow tract obstruction.

Class IB Antiarrhythmic Drugs

Lidocaine

Pharmacodynamics. Lidocaine blocks both open and inactivated cardiac Na$^+$ channels. Recovery from block is very rapid, so lidocaine exerts greater effects in depolarized (e.g., ischemic) or rapidly driven tissues. Lidocaine decreases automaticity by reducing the slope of phase 4 and altering the threshold for excitability. APD usually is unaffected or is shortened; such shortening may be due to block of the few Na$^+$ channels that inactivate late during the cardiac action potential. Lidocaine usually exerts no significant effect on the PR interval, QRS duration, or QT interval. The drug exerts little effect on hemodynamic function, although rare cases of lidocaine-associated exacerbations of heart failure have been reported, especially in patients with very poor left ventricular function.

Pharmacokinetics

While lidocaine is well absorbed, it undergoes extensive first-pass hepatic metabolism, making it inappropriate for oral use. Intravenous lidocaine is the preferred route of administration but it can be given by intermittent intramuscular administration. It is cleared by CYP3A4-mediated metabolism, and two of its metabolites, glycine xylidide (GX) and monoethyl GX (MEGX), both exert modest Na$^+$ channel blockade. GX and lidocaine appear to compete for access to the Na$^+$ channel, suggesting that with infusions during which GX accumulates, lidocaine efficacy may be diminished. After intravenous administration of a bolus of lidocaine, plasma concentrations decline biexponentially. The first phase is rapid, with a half-life of 8 minutes, and is attributed to rapid distribution of the drug from the plasma to the periphery. The drug is then eliminated by hepatic metabolism, with a half-life of approximately 2 hours. Thus after initiation of a lidocaine maintenance infusion, steady-state plasma concentrations are reached in 8–10 hours.

Measuring the drug concentration in plasma is a reasonable guide to the clinical efficacy of lidocaine. To rapidly achieve therapeutic plasma concentrations, a loading regimen of 3–4 mg/kg is generally required to achieve rapid therapeutic plasma concentrations. Central nervous toxicity usually manifests as seizures and is most likely with a single large bolus, so the loading regimen should be administered as a rapid infusion or a series of smaller intravenous boluses, such as 100 mg followed by 50 mg 5–10 minutes later, followed by a further 50 mg 5–10 minutes later. A maintenance infusion is appropriate if the target arrhythmia is suppressed, whereas if the target arrhythmia persists after lidocaine loading, a maintenance infusion is unlikely to add any efficacy. In heart failure, both the loading regimen and the maintenance infusion should be reduced as the central volume of distribution is contracted and clearance is reduced. Similarly, in liver disease, clearance is reduced, so a lower maintenance infusion rate is required.

Adverse Effects. Lidocaine can cause bradyarrhythmias. While prophylactic lidocaine was shown to prevent VF in acute MI in the 1970s, the overall mortality was unaffected, or in fact, increased.[39] Consequently, the drug is no longer used for this indication. Lidocaine is cleared by CYP3A4-mediated hepatic metabolism to metabolites that exert modest antiarrhythmic effects and can mediate some of the central nervous system toxicity. Propranolol and cimetidine reduce lidocaine clearance, and thus lower infusion rates may be required.

Clinical Efficacy. The revised ACLS guidelines recommend amiodarone or procainamide before lidocaine as the initial drug of choice for hemodynamically stable wide-complex tachycardia.[40] Although the revised guidelines state that lidocaine remains an acceptable AAD for the treatment of shock-refractory VF and pulseless VT, the evidence supporting its efficacy is limited, and lidocaine is not recommended as the first drug of choice in this setting.

Mexiletine

Pharmacodynamics. Originally developed as an anticonvulsant, mexiletine is an oral congener of lidocaine used in the treatment of ventricular arrhythmias. The electrophysiological effects of mexiletine are very similar to those of lidocaine.

Pharmacokinetics. Mexiletine is nearly completely absorbed after oral administration, and first-pass metabolism is less than 10%. It is eliminated by hepatic metabolism to inactive metabolites by the genetically variable CYP2D6 enzyme. Slow metabolizers tend to have more adverse effects. Renal excretion of mexiletine is pH sensitive; up to 35% of total clearance can be through the kidneys when the urine is acidic. Clearance is delayed markedly in cirrhosis, but little is seen in renal disease or congestive heart failure.

Side Effects. Gastrointestinal and central nervous system side effects are the most prominent and are dose- and concentration-dependent. Tremor is usually the first sign of central nervous system toxicity, but blurred vision, dysarthria, ataxia, and confusion can also occur. Some of the gastrointestinal effects may be reduced by administering the drug with food, which decreases the peak plasma concentrations without affecting overall absorption.

Clinical Efficacy. Mexiletine is effective in suppressing ventricular ectopy and VT. It is occasionally useful when added to other drugs (amiodarone, quinidine, sotalol) in patients with symptomatic VT. Mexiletine tended to increase mortality in a post-MI trial.[41] However, mexiletine has been used in the congenital LQT type 3 (Na$^+$ channel-linked) subtype, where it can directly block the plateau Na$^+$ current that causes QT prolongation.[42]

Class IC Antiarrhythmic Drugs

Flecainide

Pharmacology. Flecainide is a potent Na$^+$ channel blocker with slow onset and offset kinetics. While it does block I$_{Kr}$, reports of torsades de pointes are exceedingly rare. APD is shortened in Purkinje cells (probably due to block of late-opening Na$^+$ channels) but prolonged in ventricular cells, due to block of I$_{Kr}$. In atrial tissue, flecainide prolongs action potentials disproportionately at fast rates, an especially desirable AAD effect and one that probably contributes to its efficacy for AF. Flecainide prolongs the duration of PR, QRS, and QT intervals, even at normal heart rates.

Pharmacokinetics. Flecainide is well absorbed. The elimination half-life is shorter with urinary acidification (10 hours) than with urinary alkalinization (17 hours), but it is nevertheless sufficiently long to allow dosing twice daily. Elimination occurs by both renal excretion of the unchanged drug and hepatic metabolism to inactive metabolites. The latter is mediated by the polymorphically distributed enzyme CYP2D6. However, even in patients in whom this pathway is absent because of genetic polymorphism or inhibition by other drugs (quinidine, fluoxetine), renal excretion ordinarily is sufficient to prevent drug accumulation. In the rare patient with renal dysfunction and lack of active CYP2D6, flecainide can accumulate to toxic plasma concentrations. Flecainide is a racemate, but there are no differences in the electrophysiological effects or disposition kinetics of its enantiomers.

Adverse Effects. Flecainide produces few subjective complaints in most patients; dose-related blurred vision is the most common noncardiac adverse effect. It can exacerbate congestive heart failure in patients with depressed left ventricular performance. The most serious adverse effects are provocation or exacerbation of potentially lethal arrhythmias. CAST,[26,43] the Cardiac Arrhythmia Suppression Trial Hamburg (CASH),[44] and the Multicentre Unsustained Tachycardia Trial (MUSTT)[45] demonstrated that class IC drugs increase the risk for lethal sudden cardiovascular events in patients with ventricular arrhythmias. Therefore class IC drugs are generally contraindicated in patients with coronary artery disease, and by extension, in patients with advanced structural heart disease.[32] Flecainide can produce atrial flutter with 1:1 AV conduction, increased pacing and defibrillating thresholds, and exacerbation of VT.

Clinical Efficacy. Flecainide is effective for managing supraventricular tachyarrhythmias including atrial tachycardia, reciprocating tachycardia involving an accessory AV bypass tract, atrial flutter, and AF.[32] Flecainide has also been used to unmask right ventricular conduction abnormalities in patients suspected of having Brugada syndrome.[46] Most recently, it is indicated in patients with CPVT who are refractory to β-blockers (mentioned previously).

Propafenone

Pharmacodynamics. Propafenone is a potent Na^+ channel blocker with slow onset and offset kinetics. Like flecainide, propafenone may also block K^+ channels. Its major electrophysiological effect is to slow conduction in fast-response tissues. The drug is prescribed as a racemate. Although the enantiomers do not differ in their Na^+ channel-blocking properties, S-propafenone is a β-adrenergic receptor antagonist in vitro and in some patients. Propafenone prolongs the PR and QRS interval durations.

Pharmacokinetics. Propafenone is well absorbed and is eliminated by both hepatic and renal routes. The activity of CYP2D6, an enzyme that is functionally absent in about 7% of whites and persons of African descent, is a major determinant of plasma propafenone concentrations and thus the clinical action of the drug. In most subjects (extensive metabolizers), propafenone undergoes extensive first-pass hepatic metabolism to 5-hydroxy propafenone, a metabolite equipotent to propafenone as a Na^+ channel blocker but much less potent as a β-adrenergic receptor antagonist. A second metabolite, N-desalkyl propafenone, is formed by non-CYP2D6-mediated metabolism of propafenone and is a less potent blocker of Na^+ channels and β-adrenergic receptors. CYP2D6-mediated metabolism of propafenone is saturable, so small increases in dose can lead to disproportionate increases in plasma propafenone concentration. In poor-metabolizer subjects, in whom functional CYP2D6 is absent, the extent of first-pass hepatic metabolism is much less than in extensive metabolizers, and plasma propafenone concentrations are much higher. The incidence of adverse effects during propafenone therapy is significantly higher in poor than in extensive metabolizers. CYP2D6 activity can be markedly inhibited by a number of drugs, including quinidine and fluoxetine. In extensive-metabolizer subjects receiving such inhibitors or in poor-metabolizer

subjects, plasma propafenone concentrations greater than 1 μg/mL are associated with clinical effects of β-adrenergic receptor blockade, such as a reduction in exercise heart rate.[47] It is recommended that dosages in patients with moderate-to-severe liver disease should be reduced to approximately 20%–30% of the usual dose, with careful monitoring.

Adverse Effects

Propafenone has not been formally tested in patients following MI, but it seems reasonable to assume that it might exert adverse effects in this population, as other Na^+ channel-blocking drugs do. Therefore it is generally contraindicated in patients with coronary disease and those with advanced structural heart disease. Other adverse effects include depressed left ventricular performance, exacerbation of heart failure, atrial flutter with 1:1 AV conduction, and increased pacing and defibrillation thresholds.

Clinical Efficacy. Propafenone is effective for managing supraventricular tachyarrhythmias including atrial tachycardia, reciprocating tachycardias involving an accessory AV bypass tract, atrial flutter, and AF. Flecainide and propafenone are contraindicated for treating atrial tachyarrhythmias or ventricular tachyarrhythmias in patients with structural heart disease.

Class III Antiarrhythmic Drugs

Reentry, one of the most important mechanisms underlying clinical atrial and ventricular arrhythmias, depends on a critical balance between the conduction and refractoriness properties of a potential reentry circuit. Short refractory periods favor reentry, and longer refractory periods make reentry less likely. Because the APD is the principal determinant of refractory periods in normal working atrial and ventricular muscle and the His-Purkinje tissue, the possibility that drugs that selectively prolong the APD of cardiac tissue might prevent and terminate reentrant circuits was first suggested by Kaumann and Olson[48] in 1968. The importance of this drug action and the resultant increase in refractoriness prompted Singh and Vaughan Williams[49] in 1970 to add a new class (III) to their AAD classification scheme. Since the 1990s, there has been increased attention focused on the class III AADs because the class I antiarrhythmics have consistently been shown to increase mortality when used to treat atrial and ventricular arrhythmias.

Amiodarone

Pharmacodynamics. Amiodarone is certainly the "dirtiest" antiarrhythmic, interacting with multiple ion channels, cell surface receptors, and other molecules to block their functions. Because the drug is unusually lipophilic, pharmacological actions including uptake and elimination can be very slow. However, antiadrenergic actions tend to be prominent early, and changes in refractoriness can take longer to be apparent. Thus the drug likely produces both acute and chronic effects by interacting with ion channels and other molecular targets. Amiodarone prolongs myocardial repolarization homogeneously via K^+ channel blockade (I_{Kr} and I_{Ks}) and decreases conduction velocity by blocking cardiac Na^+ channels. It produces noncompetitive β-adrenergic blockade that can cause substantial sinus bradycardia within several days with the peak effect at 3 months, and reduces inward L-type (slow) Ca channel activity in a use-dependent manner. Inhibition of thyroxine (T_4) deiodination to triiodothyronine (T_3) can contribute to antiarrhythmic efficacy. While amiodarone prolongs the QT interval, torsades de pointes is uncommon (incidence, <1%).[50] Amiodarone is a potent inhibitor of CYP3A4, CYP2C9, and P-glycoprotein. The multifaceted electrophysiological effects of amiodarone likely contribute to both its safety and efficacy as an AAD.

Pharmacokinetics. Amiodarone is 30%–50% bioavailable, so intravenous doses are smaller than oral ones. The drug undergoes CYP3A4-mediated metabolism to desethylamiodarone, an active metabolite. As amiodarone has a large volume of distribution (66 L/kg), onset of action is delayed (2 days to 3 weeks for oral therapy) and it has a long elimination half-life. For this reason, loading regimens are required when amiodarone is initiated, and dosages can often be reduced progressively during long-term therapy. While the therapeutic plasma range for amiodarone and desethylamiodarone is 0.5–2.5 µg/mL, measured levels do not correlate well with efficacy or adverse effects.

Adverse Effects. Severe cellulitis and phlebitis can occur with intravenous amiodarone and hence it is advisable to administer the drug through a large bore or central line. Hypotension is common. During chronic therapy, PR, QRS, and QT intervals are all prolonged. Despite QT prolongation, torsades de pointes is exceedingly unusual during amiodarone therapy[50]; the likely explanation is that the drug includes, among its many pharmacological actions, block of inward currents that prevent initiation of torsades de pointes. Amiodarone does not generally produce major depression of left ventricular performance, an advantage when compared with class IA AADs. The major forms of amiodarone toxicity during chronic therapy are extracardiac. The most feared toxicity is pulmonary fibrosis, which can occur in 1%–17% of patients. A reduced diffusion capacity for carbon monoxide (DL_{CO}) is the cardinal laboratory manifestation of amiodarone toxicity. While pulmonary toxicity appears to be dose-related, it can occur during chronic therapy with doses at or below 200 mg daily. Routine annual surveillance with chest X-rays and pulmonary function studies have been advocated as methods to detect early amiodarone toxicity, but the efficacy of these maneuvers is not clearly established. Once pulmonary toxicity is suspected, further diagnostic workups may include transbronchial biopsy, right heart catheterization (to eliminate a role for concomitant heart failure), and gallium scanning. None of these are specific, and biopsy often reveals foam cells but cannot make a definitive diagnosis of toxicity. The drug should be withdrawn if amiodarone toxicity is strongly suspected. Corticosteroids have been used, but their efficacy is not certain. Death from pulmonary insufficiency can occur. Risk factors for the development of pulmonary fibrosis include underlying lung disease, amiodarone dosages greater than 400 mg/day, cumulative dosage, and recent pulmonary insults such as heart failure exacerbation, pneumonia, or general anesthesia. While corneal microdeposits are ubiquitous during chronic amiodarone therapy, they rarely interfere with vision; halos around lights at night may be one complaint. Much more rarely, amiodarone has been associated with optic neuritis.

Another potential toxicity associated with amiodarone is liver dysfunction, although it rarely progresses to cirrhosis. Photosensitivity is very common, and patients should be warned to use sunscreen and broad-brimmed hats. Both hypothyroidism (6%) and hyperthyroidism (0.9%–2%) can occur; hypothyroidism requires thyroid supplementation and hyperthyroidism—which can manifest as worsened arrhythmias, especially AF—can require thyroid ablation or withdrawal of amiodarone. Because of the potential for toxicity, thyroid function studies and liver function tests have been recommended every 6 months, and annual chest X-rays are recommended even in the absence of symptoms.[51] A range of neuropsychiatric adverse effects also can occur including tremor and ataxia, and peripheral neuropathy is uncommon (0.3% annually) but may be severe, requiring dose reduction or discontinuation of therapy. Insomnia, memory disturbances, and delirium also have been reported.

Clinical Efficacy. Although amiodarone is approved by the US Food and Drug Administration only for refractory ventricular arrhythmias, it is also effective in the treatment of symptomatic supraventricular arrhythmias, including AF. A few randomized clinical trials have found amiodarone to be more effective than other AADs for the maintenance of sinus rhythm in patients with AF[52,53] and especially effective at maintaining sinus rhythm in patients with congestive heart failure.[54] Because of adverse effects, however, amiodarone is recommended as a second- or third-line therapy for patients with symptomatic AF. Intravenous amiodarone is also often used to slow the ventricular response rate in AF, and it has been used successfully for rate control in postoperative junctional ectopic tachycardia in children.[55] SCD in patients with ischemic and nonischemic cardiomyopathy remains a substantial problem despite improved medical therapies. Several studies have demonstrated that ICD therapy is superior to medical therapy for the primary and secondary prevention of SCD in patients with ischemic and nonischemic heart disease and congestive heart failure. Many patients, however, require antiarrhythmic therapy to prevent recurrent arrhythmias and ICD shocks. Amiodarone with a β-blocker proved more effective than sotalol or β-blockers alone in preventing shocks, although there was an increase in drug-related adverse effects.[56] Amiodarone might also slow rates of VT, making it more amenable to antitachycardia pacing. However, amiodarone can increase the defibrillation threshold, necessitating repeat ICD testing after initiation of therapy. Intravenous amiodarone has been approved by the FDA for treatment and prevention of VF and hemodynamically unstable VT and for use in patients who require amiodarone therapy but are unable to take it orally.

Dofetilide

Pharmacodynamics. Dofetilide is a potent and specific blocker of I_{Kr} with no other significant pharmacological action. Because of this specificity, it has virtually no extracardiac pharmacological effect. Its only significant toxicity relates to QT prolongation and torsades de pointes. Dofetilide preferentially increases the effective refractory period of the atrium compared with the ventricle. Nonetheless, dofetilide's relative selectivity for the atrium likely contributes to its effectiveness in the pharmacological conversion of atrial arrhythmias. As with many other class III antiarrhythmic agents, dofetilide's I_{Kr} block is reverse use dependent. A potential hazard of reverse use dependence in the ventricle is the development of excessive QT prolongation and risk for torsades de pointes after cardioversion.[57] This is accentuated at slower heart rates, and the increased incidence of torsades de pointes after the restoration of sinus rhythm in part may be related to the relative bradycardia.

Pharmacokinetics. Dofetilide's absolute bioavailability exceeds 90%. Within the therapeutic range, plasma concentrations follow a dose-related linear relation, with peak plasma concentrations achieved within 2–3 hours in a fasting state and 3–4 hours when taken with food. Dofetilide is eliminated largely by renal excretion and to a small extent by CYP3A4-mediated metabolism. Its 10-hour elimination half-life allows twice-daily dosing. Certain drugs inhibit dofetilide elimination and are contraindicated because they can thereby increase the extent of QT prolongation and risk for torsades de pointes. These include cimetidine, verapamil, ketoconazole, trimethoprim-sulfamethoxazole, prochlorperazine, and hydrochlorothiazide.

Adverse Effects. Data on the incidence of torsades de pointes are available from large trials in which the drug was initiated with in-hospital monitoring. In the DIAMOND studies, dofetilide was compared with placebo in patients convalescing from MI and in patients with recent hospitalization for heart failure.[58,59] In the heart failure arm, the incidence of torsades de pointes was 3%, and in the post-MI group, the incidence was lower, 1%. Because of the risk for torsades de pointes, the drug can only be prescribed in the United States by practitioners who have been certified in its use and the drug must be initiated in the hospital. It is unique among antiarrhythmics in that the starting dose, 0.5 mg twice daily, is the highest allowable dose; downward dose adjustments are made if the QT interval is excessively long or if renal function is impaired. The drug is contraindicated in patients with advanced renal failure (creatinine clearance <20 mL/min).

Clinical Efficacy. Dofetilide is about 30% effective at the pharmacological conversion of AF at 0.5 mg twice daily by oral administration. The drug also reduces recurrence of AF following restoration of sinus rhythm.[60] Dofetilide reduces rehospitalization for heart failure, an effect that may be attributable to maintenance of sinus rhythm in patients with AF.[61] While placebo-controlled trials have failed to demonstrate efficacy of the drug in reducing the frequency of episodes of paroxysmal AF or in reducing episodes of VT or ICD discharges, it is often clinically used for these indications.

Ibutilide

Pharmacodynamics. Ibutilide is a methanesulfonamide derivative with structural similarities to sotalol. This drug increases APD as its primary mechanism of action, largely by blocking I_{Kr}.[62] Over a limited range of stimulation rates, ibutilide can increase APD without significant reverse use dependence or loss of effect at rapid pacing rates. In humans, ibutilide causes a dose- and concentration-dependent increase in the QT interval in healthy volunteers and in patients with AF and atrial flutter. Ibutilide can lower the energy threshold required for VF.[63] Although administration of ibutilide can cause mild slowing of sinus rate and AV nodal conduction, there is no significant effect on heart rate, PR interval, or QRS duration.

Pharmacokinetics. Ibutilide is not available for long-term oral use because of extensive first-pass metabolism. After intravenous administration, the plasma concentration declines in a multiexponential manner, with a high systemic plasma clearance that approximates liver blood flow. The elimination half-life of ibutilide is variable, between 2 and 12 hours with a mean of 6 hours, and the drug is extensively metabolized. The parent and most of the inactive metabolites are excreted largely in the urine.[64] Although the metabolic pathways for ibutilide have not been completely determined, they do not appear to involve the CYP3A4 or CYP2D6 pathways, suggesting that previously described drug interactions with other agents are unlikely. Clearance is unaltered by either a reduction in creatinine clearance or left ventricular dysfunction. In patients with liver disease, there is likely reduced clearance and a prolonged pharmacological effect, necessitating longer periods of monitoring after ibutilide administration.

Adverse Effects. The initial dose is 1 mg over 10 minutes. If AF or atrial flutter persists 10 minutes after completion of the first dose, a second 1-mg dose may be given over 10 minutes. If the patient's weight is less than 60 kg, each dose is reduced by 0.01 mg/kg. The infusion is stopped when sinus rhythm is restored, marked QT prolongation occurs, or torsades de pointes develops. Peak pharmacological effects coincide roughly with the end of the infusion. Because the elimination half-life is 6 hours, patients should be observed for at least 4 hours after administration of the drug. The major adverse effect is torsades de pointes, which has been observed in 3.6%–8.3% of patients.[65] The risk for proarrhythmia requires that ibutilide be administered in the hospital, with the necessary monitoring and resuscitation equipment. Administration of ibutilide with other drugs that prolong the APD is not recommended.

Clinical Efficacy. While intravenous ibutilide is effective in converting both AF or atrial flutter to sinus rhythm,[65,66] it is more effective in flutter than in fibrillation. It is also more effective in recent-onset arrhythmias. Cardioversion after ibutilide administration can help maintain sinus rhythm in those in whom cardioversion alone is ineffective.[67] Ibutilide can be safely used in patients receiving chronic amiodarone therapy. Ibutilide is also effective in patients with preexcited AF and rapid ventricular responses due to antegrade accessory pathway conduction; in this setting, it not only can convert AF but also slows conduction down the bypass tract.[68]

Sotalol

Pharmacodynamics. Sotalol is a class III antiarrhythmic that also has nonselective β-blocking effects. This drug is a racemic mixture of its D- (class III effects) and L-stereoisomers (β-blocking effects). In contrast to amiodarone, L-sotalol is a competitive β-blocker and this effect is detectable at relatively low doses. The intrinsic negative inotropic effect of β-blockade is counterbalanced in vivo by a positive inotropic effect related to prolongation of the APD, which allows more time for the rise in intracellular Ca^{2+} that mediates the force of contraction. Clinically, sotalol produces a modest negative inotropic effect. Both enantiomers have class III effects mediated primarily by antagonism of I_{Kr}. The antiarrhythmic does, however, display reverse use dependence, increasing APD at slower heart rates and diminishing effectiveness at faster heart rates. Sotalol slows the sinus rate and prolongs the PR interval, the atrio-His (AH) interval, the AV node refractory period, and the QT interval; it does not change the His-ventricle (HV) interval or QRS duration.

Pharmacokinetics. With a bioavailability of almost 100%, peak sotalol plasma concentrations occur 2–4 hours after oral administration. Sotalol is eliminated exclusively by renal excretion of the unchanged drug, with a half-life of 6–12 hours. In patients with renal dysfunction, the plasma concentrations increase and there is a greater risk for toxicity. Therefore administration and dosing of sotalol need to be tailored to the creatinine clearance. Patients with a creatinine clearance < 40 mL/min should avoid sotalol. The typical oral dosing is 80–320 mg twice a day. Doses less than 120 mg twice a day appear to have primarily a β-blocking effect and little class III action. The benefit of higher doses must be weighed against the risk for QT prolongation and torsades de pointes.

Adverse Effects. Adverse effects of sotalol are related to β-blockade and class III effects. Bradycardia, fatigue, bronchospasm, and dyspnea are related to the β-blockade. The incidence of heart failure or pulmonary edema with sotalol is 3.3%.[69] The incidence of torsades de pointes is estimated to be 2.4% with most events occurring within the first week after initiation of treatment or after a change in dosage. Predisposing factors for torsades de pointes include the female sex, doses greater than 320 mg/day, heart failure, recent cardioversion, hypokalemia, bradycardia, and elevated baseline serum creatinine level.[28]

Clinical Efficacy. Sotalol is effective in preventing the recurrence of a wide range of supraventricular tachycardias including AV nodal reentry, AV reentry, and atrial tachycardia, but its main clinical use lies in the treatment of AF and atrial flutter. In the AFFIRM trial, more than two-thirds of patients in the rhythm control arm were started on either amiodarone or sotalol.[70] While both drugs had a relatively low incidence of adverse effects severe enough to cause discontinuation at 1 year (11.1% [sotalol] vs. 12.3% [amiodarone]), therapy with class I antiarrhythmics had to be stopped more often (28.1% at 1 year) due to frequent adverse effects. However, amiodarone is clearly superior to sotalol and propafenone in maintaining sinus rhythm.[52] Although the impact of sotalol on primary prevention of SCD in patients recovering from MI has been disappointing, it does appear to decrease first defibrillation shock and death in some patients with ICDs.[71] Sotalol also reduced the number of inappropriate ICD shocks, most likely due to its suppression of atrial arrhythmias, and unlike amiodarone, consistently decreases the defibrillation threshold in patients with ICDs. The lowering of the defibrillation threshold, along with the relative lack of noncardiac adverse effects with sotalol, makes it the first-line AAD for patients with ICDs.

Acknowledgment

This work was in part supported by the National Institutes of Health grants R01HL092217, R01HL124935, and R01HL085690.

REFERENCES

1. Watanabe H, Steele DS, Knollmann BC. Mechanism of antiarrhythmic effects of flecainide in catecholaminergic polymorphic ventricular tachycardia. *Circ Res.* 2011;109:712–713.
2. Watanabe H, Chopra N, Laver D, et al. Flecainide prevents catecholaminergic polymorphic ventricular tachycardia in mice and humans. *Nat Med.* 2009;15:380–383.
3. Kang G, Giovannone SF, Liu N, et al. Purkinje cells from RyR2 mutant mice are highly arrhythmogenic but responsive to targeted therapy. *Circ Res.* 2010;107:512–519.
4. Wilde AA, Bhuiyan ZA, Crotti L, et al. Left cardiac sympathetic denervation for catecholaminergic polymorphic ventricular tachycardia. *N Engl J Med.* 2008;358:2024–2029.
5. Darbar D, Herron KJ, Ballew JD, et al. Familial atrial fibrillation is a genetically heterogeneous disorder. *J Am Coll Cardiol.* 2003;41:2185–2192.
6. Chen YH, Xu SJ, Bendahhou S, et al. KCNQ1 gain-of-function mutation in familial atrial fibrillation. *Science.* 2003;299:251–254.
7. Hodgson-Zingman DM, Karst ML, Zingman LV, et al. Atrial natriuretic peptide frameshift mutation in familial atrial fibrillation. *N Engl J Med.* 2008;359:158–165.
8. Otway R, Vandenberg JI, Guo G, et al. Stretch-sensitive KCNQ1 mutation. A link between genetic and environmental factors in the pathogenesis of atrial fibrillation? *J Am Coll Cardiol.* 2007;49:578–586.
9. Darbar D, Roden DM. Genetic mechanisms of atrial fibrillation: impact on response to treatment. *Nat Rev Cardiol.* 2013;10:317–329.
10. Gudbjartsson DF, Arnar DO, Helgadottir A, et al. Variants conferring risk of atrial fibrillation on chromosome 4q25. *Nature.* 2007;488:353–357.
11. Campbell CM, Campbell JD, Thompson CH, et al. Selective targeting of gain-of-function KCNQ1 mutations predisposing to atrial fibrillation. *Circ Arrhythm Electrophysiol.* 2013;6:960–966.
12. Faggioni M, Savio-Galimberti E, Venkataraman R, et al. Suppression of spontaneous Ca elevations prevents atrial fibrillation in calsequestrin 2-null hearts. *Circ Arrhythm Electrophysiol.* 2014;7:313–320.
13. Savio-Galimberti E, Muhammad R, Kannankeril P, et al. NPPA overexpression in mice increases susceptibility to atrial fibrillation. *Circulation.* 2012;126:A19074.
14. Disertori M, Quintarelli S, Grasso M, et al. Autosomal recessive atrial dilated cardiomyopathy with standstill evolution associated with mutation of natriuretic peptide precursor A. *Circ Cardiovasc Genet.* 2013;6:27–36.
15. Yang T, Yang P, Roden DM, Darbar D. Novel KCNA5 mutation implicates tyrosine kinase signaling in human atrial fibrillation. *Heart Rhythm.* 2010;7:1246–1252.
16. Savio-Galimberti E, Weeke P, Muhammad R, et al. SCN10A/Nav1.8 modulation of peak and late sodium currents in patients with early onset atrial fibrillation. *Cardiovasc Res.* 2014;104:355–363.
17. Jabbari J, Olesen MS, Yuan L, et al. Common and rare variants in SCN10A modulate the risk of atrial fibrillation. *Circ Cardiovasc Genet.* 2015;8:64–73.
18. Yang T, Atack TC, Stroud DM, et al. Blocking SCN10A channels in heart reduces late sodium current and is antiarrhythmic. *Circ Res.* 2012;111:322–332.
19. Van Wagoner DR, Piccini JP, Albert CM, et al. Progress towards the prevention and treatment of atrial fibrillation: a summary of the Heart Rhythm Society Research Forum on the Treatment and Prevention of Atrial Fibrillation, Washington, DC, December 9-10, 2013. *Heart Rhythm.* 2014;12:e5–e29.
20. Weeke P, Muhammad R, Delaney JT, et al. Whole-exome sequencing in familial atrial fibrillation. *Eur Heart J.* 2014;35:2477–2483.
21. Zhang X, Chen S, Yoo S, et al. Mutation in nuclear pore component NUP155 leads to atrial fibrillation and early sudden cardiac death. *Cell.* 2008;135:1017–1027.
22. Parvez B, Vaglio J, Rowan S, et al. Symptomatic response to antiarrhythmic drug therapy is modulated by a common single nucleotide polymorphism in atrial fibrillation. *J Am Coll Cardiol.* 2012;60:539–545.
23. Shoemaker MB, Muhammad R, Parvez B, et al. Common atrial fibrillation risk alleles at 4q25 predict recurrence after catheter-based atrial fibrillation ablation. *Heart Rhythm.* 2013;10:394–400.
24. Husser D, Adams V, Piorkowski C, et al. Chromosome 4q25 variants and atrial fibrillation recurrence after catheter ablation. *J Am Coll Cardiol.* 2010;55:747–753.
25. Parvez B, Shoemaker MB, Muhammad R, et al. Common genetic polymorphism at 4q25 locus predicts atrial fibrillation recurrence after successful cardioversion. *Heart Rhythm.* 2013;10:849–855.
26. Preliminary report. effect of encainide and flecainide on mortality in a randomized trial of arrhythmia suppression after myocardial infarction. The Cardiac Arrhythmia Suppression Trial (CAST) Investigators. *N Engl J Med.* 1989;321:406–412.
27. Murray KT, Hu NN, Daw JR, et al. Functional effects of protein kinase C activation on the human cardiac Na^+ channel. *Circ Res.* 1997;80:370–376.
28. Kannankeril P, Roden DM, Darbar D. Drug-induced long QT syndrome. *Pharmacol Rev.* 2010;62:760–781.
29. Paul AA, Witchel HJ, Hancox JC. Inhibition of the current of heterologously expressed HERG potassium channels by flecainide and comparison with quinidine, propafenone and lignocaine. *Br J Pharmacol.* 2002;136:717–729.
30. Antzelevitch C, Shimizu W, Yan GX, et al. The M cell: its contribution to the ECG and to normal and abnormal electrical function of the heart. *J Cardiovasc Electrophysiol.* 1999;10:1124–1152.
31. Thompson KA, Murray JJ, Blair IA, et al. Plasma concentrations of quinidine, its major metabolites, and dihydroquinidine in patients with torsades de pointes. *Clin Pharmacol Ther.* 1988;43:636–642.
32. Fuster V, Ryden LE, Cannom DS, et al. ACC/AHA/ESC 2006 Guidelines for the Management of Patients with Atrial Fibrillation: a report of the American College of Cardiology/American Heart Association Task Force on Practice Guidelines and the European Society of Cardiology Committee for Practice Guidelines (Writing Committee to Revise the 2001 Guidelines for the Management of Patients With Atrial Fibrillation): developed in collaboration with the European Heart Rhythm Association and the Heart Rhythm Society. *Circulation.* 2006;114:e257–e354.
33. Belhassen B, Glick A, Viskin S. Excellent long-term reproducibility of the electrophysiologic efficacy of quinidine in patients with idiopathic ventricular fibrillation and Brugada syndrome. *Pacing Clin Electrophysiol.* 2009;32:294–301.
34. Haissaguerre M, Derval N, Sacher F, et al. Sudden cardiac arrest associated with early repolarization. *N Engl J Med.* 2008;358:2016–2023.
35. Maury P, Couderc P, Delay M, et al. Electrical storm in Brugada syndrome successfully treated using isoprenaline. *Europace.* 2004;6:130–133.
36. Woosley RL, Drayer DE, Reidenberg MM, et al. Effect of acetylator phenotype on the rate at which procainamide induces antinuclear antibodies and the lupus syndrome. *N Engl J Med.* 1978;298:1157–1159.
37. Belhassen B, Glick A, Viskin S. Efficacy of quinidine in high-risk patients with Brugada syndrome. *Circulation.* 2004;110:1731–1737.
38. Brugada R, Brugada J, Antzelevitch C, et al. Sodium channel blockers identify risk for sudden death in patients with ST-segment elevation and right bundle branch block but structurally normal hearts. *Circulation.* 2000;101:510–515.
39. MacMahon S, Collins R, Peto R, et al. Effects of prophylactic lidocaine in suspected acute myocardial infarction. An overview of results from the randomized, controlled trials. *JAMA.* 1988;260:1910–1916.
40. Guidelines 2000 for Cardiopulmonary Resuscitation and Emergency Cardiovascular Care. Part 6: advanced cardiovascular life support: 7B: understanding the algorithm approach to ACLS. The American Heart Association in collaboration with the International Liaison Committee on Resuscitation. *Circulation.* 2000;102:I140–I141.
41. International mexiletine and placebo antiarrhythmic coronary trial: I. Report on arrhythmia and other findings. Impact Research Group. *J Am Coll Cardiol.* 1984;4:1148–1163.
42. Wang DW, Yazawa K, Makita N, et al. Pharmacological targeting of long QT mutant sodium channels. *J Clin Invest.* 1997;99:1714–1720.
43. Echt DS, Liebson PR, Mitchell LB, et al. Mortality and morbidity in patients receiving encainide, flecainide, or placebo. The Cardiac Arrhythmia Suppression Trial. *N Engl J Med.* 1991;324:781–788.
44. Kuck KH, Cappato R, Siebels J, et al. Randomized comparison of antiarrhythmic drug therapy with implantable defibrillators in patients resuscitated from cardiac arrest: the Cardiac Arrest Study Hamburg (CASH). *Circulation.* 2000;102:748–754.
45. Wyse DG, Friedman PL, Brodsky MA, et al. Life-threatening ventricular arrhythmias due to transient or correctable causes: high risk for death in follow-up. *J Am Coll Cardiol.* 2001;38:1718–1724.
46. Rossenbacker T, Priori SG. The Brugada syndrome. *Curr Opin Cardiol.* 2007;22:163–170.
47. Lee JT, Kroemer HK, Silberstein DJ, et al. The role of genetically determined polymorphic drug metabolism in the beta-blockade produced by propafenone. *N Engl J Med.* 1990;322:1764–1768.
48. Kaumann AJ, Olson CB. Temporal relation between long-lasting aftercontractions and action potentials in cat papillary muscles. *Science.* 1968;161:293–295.
49. Singh BN, Vaughan Williams EM. A third class of anti-arrhythmic action. Effects on atrial and ventricular intracellular potentials, and other pharmacological actions on cardiac muscle, of MJ 1999 and AH 3474. *Br J Pharmacol.* 1970;39:675–687.
50. Vorperian VR, Havighurst TC, Miller S, et al. Adverse effects of low dose amiodarone: a meta-analysis. *J Am Coll Cardiol.* 1997;30:791–798.
51. Vassallo P, Trohman RG. Prescribing amiodarone: an evidence-based review of clinical indications. *JAMA.* 2007;298:1312–1322.
52. Roy D, Talajic M, Dorian P, et al. Amiodarone to prevent recurrence of atrial fibrillation. Canadian Trial of Atrial Fibrillation Investigators. *N Engl J Med.* 2000;342:913–920.
53. AFFIRM First Antiarrhythmic Drug Substudy Investigators. Maintenance of sinus rhythm in patients with atrial fibrillation: an AFFIRM substudy of the first antiarrhythmic drug. *J Am Coll Cardiol.* 2003;42:20–29.
54. Deedwania PC, Singh BN, Ellenbogen K, et al. Spontaneous conversion and maintenance of sinus rhythm by amiodarone in patients with heart failure and atrial fibrillation: observations from the veterans affairs congestive heart failure survival trial of antiarrhythmic therapy (CHF-STAT). The Department of Veterans Affairs CHF-STAT Investigators. *Circulation.* 1998;98:2574–2579.
55. Laird WP, Snyder CS, Kertesz NJ, et al. Use of intravenous amiodarone for postoperative junctional ectopic tachycardia in children. *Pediatr Cardiol.* 2003;24:133–137.
56. Connolly SJ, Dorian P, Roberts RS, et al. Comparison of beta-blockers, amiodarone plus beta-blockers, or sotalol for prevention of shocks from implantable cardioverter defibrillators: the OPTIC Study: a randomized trial. *JAMA.* 2006;295:165–171.
57. Choy AM, Darbar D, Dell'Orto S, et al. Exaggerated QT prolongation after cardioversion of atrial fibrillation. *J Am Coll Cardiol.* 1999;34:396–401.
58. Kober L, Bloch Thomsen PE, Moller M, et al. Effect of dofetilide in patients with recent myocardial infarction and left-ventricular dysfunction: a randomised trial. *Lancet.* 2000;356:2052–2058.
59. Pedersen OD, Bagger H, Keller N, et al. Efficacy of dofetilide in the treatment of atrial fibrillation-flutter in patients with reduced left ventricular function: a Danish investigations of arrhythmia and mortality on dofetilide (diamond) substudy. *Circulation.* 2001;104:292–296.
60. Lenz TL, Hilleman DE. Dofetilide: a new antiarrhythmic agent approved for conversion and/or maintenance of atrial fibrillation/atrial flutter. *Drugs Today (Barc).* 2000;36:759–771.
61. Torp-Pedersen C, Moller M, Bloch-Thomsen PE, et al. Dofetilide in patients with congestive heart failure and left ventricular dysfunction. Danish Investigations of Arrhythmia and Mortality on Dofetilide Study Group. *N Engl J Med.* 1999;341:857–865.
62. Yang T, Snyders DJ, Roden DM. Ibutilide, a methanesulfonanilide antiarrhythmic, is a potent blocker of the rapidly activating delayed rectifier K+ current (IKr) in AT-1 cells. Concentration-, time-, voltage-, and use-dependent effects. *Circulation.* 1995;91:1799–1806.
63. Wesley Jr RC, Farkhani F, Morgan D, et al. Ibutilide: enhanced defibrillation via plateau sodium current activation. *Am J Physiol.* 1993;264:H1269–H1274.
64. Naccarelli GV, Lee KS, Gibson JK, et al. Electrophysiology and pharmacology of ibutilide. *Am J Cardiol.* 1996;78:12–16.
65. Stambler BS, Wood MA, Ellenbogen KA, et al. Efficacy and safety of repeated intravenous doses of ibutilide for rapid conversion of atrial flutter or fibrillation. Ibutilide Repeat Dose Study Investigators. *Circulation.* 1996;94:1613–1621.
66. Ellenbogen KA, Stambler BS, Wood MA, et al. Efficacy of intravenous ibutilide for rapid termination of atrial fibrillation and atrial flutter: a dose-response study. *J Am Coll Cardiol.* 1996;28:130–136.
67. Oral H, Souza JJ, Michaud GF, et al. Facilitating transthoracic cardioversion of atrial fibrillation with ibutilide pretreatment. *N Engl J Med.* 1999;340:1849–1854.
68. Glatter KA, Dorostkar PC, Yang Y, et al. Electrophysiological effects of ibutilide in patients with accessory pathways. *Circulation.* 2001;104:1933–1939.
69. MacNeil DJ. The side effect profile of class III antiarrhythmic drugs: focus on d,l-sotalol. *Am J Cardiol.* 1997;80:90G–98G.
70. Wyse DG, Waldo AL, DiMarco JP, et al. A comparison of rate control and rhythm control in patients with atrial fibrillation. *N Engl J Med.* 2002;347:1825–1833.
71. Pacifico A, Hohnloser SH, Williams JH, et al. Prevention of implantable-defibrillator shocks by treatment with sotalol. d,l-Sotalol Implantable Cardioverter-Defibrillator Study Group. *N Engl J Med.* 1999;340:1855–1862.

113 Innovations in Antiarrhythmic Drug Therapy

Paulus Kirchhof and Larissa Fabritz

Background and Current Clinical Context

The past few years have seen several innovations in antiarrhythmic drug therapy. Antiarrhythmic drugs are now commonly used as a part of a multimodal, "hybrid" approach to patients with arrhythmias, new targets for antiarrhythmic drugs have been defined, new compounds are in clinical development, and personalized therapeutic approaches are moving from patients with inherited cardiomyopathies to larger populations. Here, we provide an overview of these developments.

Main Effects of Antiarrhythmic Drugs

Antiarrhythmic drugs counter proarrhythmic mechanisms. These are discussed throughout this book. Antiarrhythmic drugs, such as digitalis and quinidine, were among the first medications subjected to controlled clinical trials. They have a few common electrophysiological effects. Many antiarrhythmic drugs *prolong the cardiac action potential* by inhibiting repolarizing currents (Fig. 113.1). Unfortunately, this potent antiarrhythmic effect also appears to be one of the main mechanisms of drug-induced proarrhythmia by provoking torsades de pointes. Many new antiarrhythmic drugs modify cardiac repolarization using novel ion channel targets in an attempt to improve safety. Sodium channel inhibitors and substances inhibiting intracellular calcium release exert additional antiarrhythmic effects by slowing electrical impulse propagation ("conduction slowing") and by suppressing abnormal, untimely electrical activity. The conduction slowing itself has proarrhythmic risks to be considered. An important beneficial, at times underrecognized, effect of such compounds is the induction of refractoriness beyond the end of the action potential. *Postrepolarization refractoriness* induced by sodium channel blockers prevents ventricular and atrial fibrillation[1-4] and is one of the effects of amiodarone and dronedarone.[1,3,5,6] Recent data suggest that a slightly depolarized resting membrane potential, as found in atria with reduced PITX2 levels, markedly enhances postrepolarization refractoriness induced by sodium channel blockers.[4] It remains to be studied whether a specific cocktail of ion channel inhibitions, time constants of drug binding to the sodium channel, or other factors, such as the resting membrane potential, modify this intriguing effect.[4]

Hybrid Rhythm Control Therapy

As treatment patterns have evolved, most antiarrhythmic drugs are currently used in indications beyond their initially approved use. Recently, antiarrhythmic drugs are increasingly used as part of a "hybrid" therapy, e.g., in patients with defibrillators to reduce shocks or to reduce recurrences of atrial fibrillation in addition to catheter ablation of atrial fibrillation.

The clinical development of new antiarrhythmic drugs is starting to reflect these practice patterns, for example, by detecting recurrent arrhythmias in patients with implanted devices[8] or by studying new atrial fibrillation compounds after catheter ablation. Importantly, this has led to a paradigm shift in the requirements for antiarrhythmic drugs[9]: Complete prevention of arrhythmic events is less aimed for than it was when the current drugs were initially developed. On the other hand, there is a growing appreciation that interventional therapy alone will not be sufficient to suppress arrhythmias.[9a,10] Clinical success is defined as symptom reduction, while the assessment of arrhythmia recurrences is still required in controlled trials,[11] and even for that purpose, hybrid therapy is often needed.[9]

Inhibition of Multiple Ion Channels

Amiodarone is more effective than other clinically available antiarrhythmic drugs, and its proarrhythmic potential is acceptable in many clinical conditions.[12] A prominent feature of amiodarone is its multichannel inhibition, lending support to the assumption that inhibition of multiple ion channels may be more beneficial than single ion channel inhibitors. This has resulted in the preclinical and clinical development of multichannel blockers such as SSR149744C (celivarone), ATI-2042, and dronedarone. Some of these are now used in clinical practice (see later), while others failed because of the lack of efficacy, possibly due to a suboptimal balance of ion channel inhibition.[13] Other compounds, such as azimilide[14] or HMR 1556,[15] often with predominant inhibition of I_{Kr} or I_{Ks}, were abandoned because of ventricular proarrhythmia.

Dronedarone is an amiodarone analog devoid of iodine that prevents atrial fibrillation. It has a favorable safety profile in two large controlled trials that enrolled patients with nonpermanent, often recent-onset atrial fibrillation.[16,17] It even reduced cardiovascular death in a secondary analysis.[17] The fact that dronedarone may be less effective in the prevention of atrial fibrillation than amiodarone in both indirect comparisons (see Singh et al. 2007[16] compared with Singh et al. 2005[18]) and in a direct "head-to-head" comparison[19] suggests that other factors favor amiodarone's effectiveness (see later). Dronedarone also slows the ventricular rate by approximately 8 beats/min[20,21] but should not be used as a rate-controlling agent in patients with permanent atrial fibrillation. Furthermore, dronedarone is unsafe in patients with advanced heart failure.[22,23]

Vernakalant is in clinical use for cardioversion of atrial fibrillation in Europe.[24] Vernakalant is a multichannel blocker that also inhibits I_{Kur} inhibition. The compound terminates recent-onset atrial fibrillation within a few hours. It is not available in oral formulation or in the United States.

Fixed Combinations of Existing Antiarrhythmic Drugs

A fixed combination of *verapamil and quinidine*, another form of a "multichannel blocker" that has been available for many years in Germany, is as effective as sotalol for the prevention of atrial fibrillation but appears to provoke less proarrhythmia than quinidine alone. In the PAFAC and SOPAT trials, telemetric electrocardiogram (ECG) monitoring detected one ventricular tachycardia event in 895 patients treated with the quinidine-verapamil combination over 1 year compared to eight torsade de pointes events in 645 patients treated with sotalol over 1 year.[25,26] More recently, *ranolazine*, which preferentially blocks the late sodium channel and has weak fast sodium channel and I_{Kr} channel blocking, was combined with a low dose of *dronedarone* to suppress atrial fibrillation.[8]

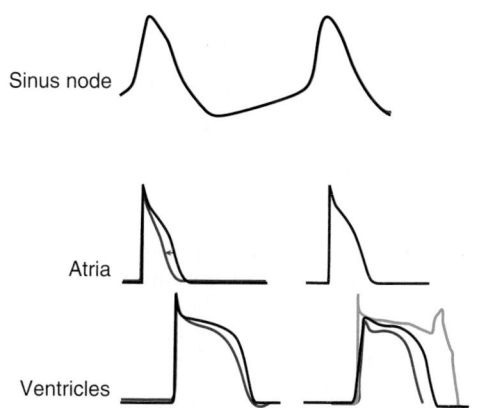

FIGURE 113.1 Modifications of the cardiac action potential of the sinus node *(top tracings)*, atrial *(middle tracings)*, and ventricles *(bottom tracings)* that have been associated with major arrhythmias: *Left:* Electrical changes associated with atrial fibrillation: shortened action potential, depolarized resting membrane potential. *Right:* Electrical changes associated with sudden death due to ventricular arrhythmias in inherited and acquired cardiomyopathies: prolonged action potential leading to afterdepolarziarions, shortened action potential, slow electrical activation.

New Ion Channel Targets for Antiarrhythmic Drugs

Several potassium currents, including the ultra-rapid delayed rectifier I_{Kur}, the background current I_{K1}, and the acetylcholine-activated current $I_{K,ACh}$, are altered in atrial fibrillation, with I_{K1} being increased and $I_{K,ACh}$ becoming in part constitutively active.[27,28] As a consequence, the atrial refractory period is shortened. This creates a condition that supports multiple wavelet reentry and periodic activity of sustained, high-frequency functional reentry sources. In addition, a shift of the resting membrane potential toward more positive potentials via atypical potassium channels (e.g., K2P channels[29,30]) or other background channels[4] may increase the chance of spontaneous depolarizations (e.g., afterdepolarizations) or could activate sodium channels and thereby initiate a premature response. Similarly, a more depolarized resting membrane potential will alter the binding of antiarrhythmic drugs, thus enhancing postrepolarization refractoriness.[4] Modulation of these currents appears to be an attractive target for antiarrhythmic drug therapy (Fig. 113.2).

Abnormal Calcium Release and Arrhythmia Initiation

Abnormal regulation of intracellular calcium is found in fibrillating human atria.[31,32] There is a growing body of evidence to suggest that both atrial ectopy and electrical remodeling are highly calcium-dependent phenomena. Stabilization of abnormal calcium release from the sarcoplasmic reticulum can prevent ventricular tachyarrhythmias in genetically modified models of altered calcium release.[33–36] Prolonged calcium release from the contractile apparatus of cardiomyocytes may have similar effects in cardiac hypertrophy.[37,38] Recent data suggest that altered calcium handling, including modified function of the sodium-calcium exchanger and ryanodine receptor, is also relevant for atrial fibrillation.[39–41] Inhibitors of intracellular kinases (e.g., *CaMKII inhibitors* and *protein phosphatase inhibitors*) can acutely suppress ventricular arrhythmias in a variety of experimental models (hypertrophy, infarction, electrical storm) by modifying sodium influx into cells, sarcoplasmic reticulum calcium release, and cellular function in general.[42–48] Inhibitors of the *sodium-calcium exchanger* and substances targeting the *sodium pump* may suppress ectopic activity.[49–51] Possibly, store-operated calcium also contributes to calcium release-dependent arrhythmogenesis.[52] Atrial fibrillation, however, importantly also causes a silencing of calcium signaling.[53] A thorough understanding

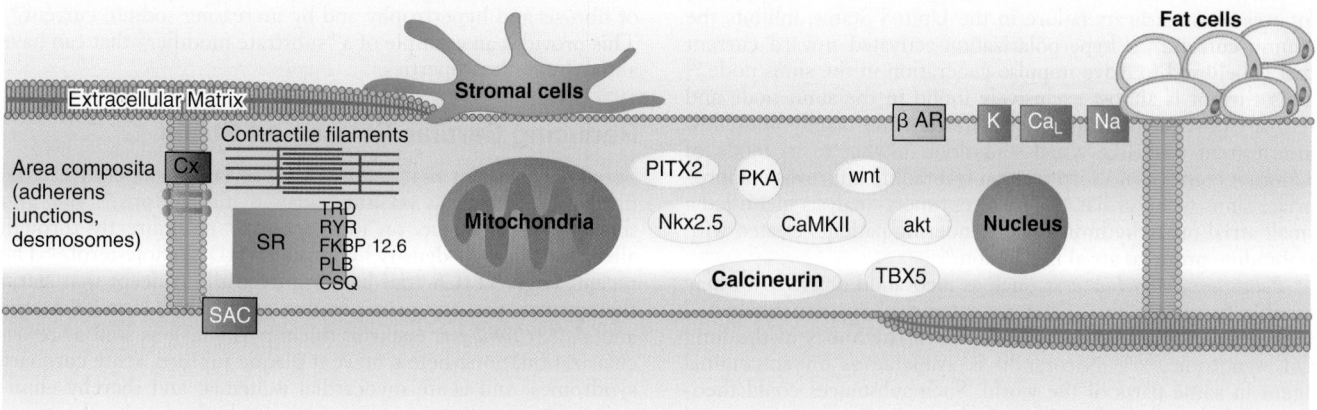

FIGURE 113.2 Targets for antiarrhythmic drug treatment for the prevention of atrial fibrillation and sudden death. Shown is a histological scheme of a cardiomyocyte with some "key" proteins that might represent targets for antiarrhythmic drug therapy. Antiarrhythmic drug classes are indicated within the scheme to illustrate potential sites of action. *Ca_L*, L-type calcium channel; *CaMKII/akt/calcineurin*, examples for relevant protein kinases; *CSQ*, calsequestrin; *Cx*, connexin; *FKBP 12.6*, an accessory protein to the ryanodine receptor; *K*, potassium channel; *Na*, sodium channel; *PLB*, phospholamban; *RYR*, ryanodine receptor; *SAC*, stretch-activated channel; *SR*, sarcoplasmic reticulum; *TRD*, triadin.

of the subcellular calcium compartments that undergo independent calcium regulation will possibly help to devise new compounds that inhibit arrhythmogenesis while maintaining the essential effects of calcium on contractile function, regulation of protein function, and cell function in general.

Targeting Channels Specific to Atrial Tissue and Atrial Fibrillation

The outward currents that determine repolarization in the atria are slightly different than in the ventricle. In theory, inhibition of "atrial-specific" ion currents, especially agents targeting the ultra-rapid rectifying current I_{Kur} encoded by the Kv1.5 channel, could be safer because such compounds would selectively prolong atrial action repolarization without affecting ventricular action potentials or the QT interval (see Fig. 113.1). Importantly, Kv1.5 channels are recycled from endosomes and their atrial expression and function are variable.[54] A model I_{Kur} blocker, *AVE0118*, prevents atrial fibrillation in goats and restores atrial contractility after cardioversion but has never been shown to be clinically effective in patients. Several potassium channel blockers with preferential I_{Kur} inhibition such as XEN-D0101,[55] XEN-D0103/S66913,[56] and others are currently in clinical development. These ongoing studies will provide further information on the validity of atrial-specific ion channel blockade for the treatment of atrial fibrillation.

Clinical Innovation by Off-Label Use

Several drugs with potential antiarrhythmic effects are registered as antianginal medications and thus available in clinical practice. *Ranolazine*, a preferential blocker of the late inward sodium current approved for treatment of angina,[57] inhibits the late sodium current. Ranolazine reduced asymptomatic, nonsustained ventricular arrhythmias in a large study in postinfarction patients, albeit as a secondary outcome parameter.[58] Preclinical data also suggest that ranolazine could prevent torsades de pointes in models of long QT syndrome 3.[59,60] One smaller clinical trial suggested that a combination of ranolazine and dronedarone inhibits atrial high rate episodes detected by pacemakers.[8] Several medium-sized clinical trials are underway to assess the clinical efficacy of ranolazine alone or in combination with dronedarone.[8] In addition to antianginal effects, late sodium channel blockers may have antihypertrophic effects, which could contribute to prevention of arrhythmias. Trials with ranolazine and the compound GS-6615 are ongoing.

Ivabradine, an antianginal medication[61] recently approved for treatment of heart failure in the United States, inhibits the "funny current," a hyperpolarization-activated inward current that is believed to drive impulse generation in the sinus node.[62] This current is almost exclusively found in the sinus node and retina. Consequently, side effects are rare and mainly limited to intermittent flash-like visual sensations. Owing to its mode of action, it comes as no surprise that ivabradine improves inappropriate sinus tachycardias.[63–65] A recent meta-analysis identified a small atrial proarrhythmic effect rendering patients treated with ivabradine prone to atrial fibrillation.[66]

Potassium channel openers, such as nicorandil or NS1643, may be able to reverse the action potential prolongation associated with drug-induced proarrhythmia and arrhythmias in the long QT syndromes.[67,68] Nicorandil is available as an antianginal agent in some parts of the world. Such substances could theoretically help to acutely treat proarrhythmic situations associated with prolongation of the ventricular action potential.[69]

There is a clear need to evaluate such therapies, which are often initial steps toward personalized therapy of arrhythmias, in controlled trials. Funding by the research arms of healthcare systems, public funding bodies, or charities will usually be needed to evaluate these "off-label" antiarrhythmic properties of registered substances, unless specific uses or combinations remain patentable.

Modification of the Arrhythmogenic Substrate

Slowing of atrial impulse propagation[70,71] is an important contributor to the maintenance of atrial fibrillation and to sudden death. Cardiac fibrosis as well as fatty infiltration can enhance conduction defects, while prevention of fibrotic or fatty infiltration will prevent arrhythmias. Modern imaging, especially magnetic resonance imaging of the heart, can visualize likely areas of cardiac fibrosis,[72] and this has been proposed as a risk stratification tool for sudden death and atrial fibrillation, although in atrial fibrillation this needs further validation.[73,74] The "antifibrotic" effect of *angiotensin receptor blockers* and *angiotensin-converting enzyme (ACE) inhibitors* probably explains why these substances prevent new-onset atrial fibrillation in patients with heart failure[75] and in patients with left ventricular hypertrophy,[76] as well as protecting to some extent against sudden death. In several controlled trials enrolling patients without structural heart disease, in contrast, angiotensin receptor blockers and ACE inhibitors did not prevent recurrent atrial fibrillation,[77,78] and their use as antiarrhythmic agents is not recommended in patients without structural heart disease.[24] Furthermore, fibroblasts modify the electrical function of cardiomyocytes,[79–82] making them targets for future antiarrhythmic drugs.

Treatment of Heart Failure

Although treating the underlying heart disease can prevent arrhythmias, treatment of heart failure, unfortunately, is often symptomatic only and can facilitate proarrhythmia, for example, by potassium depletion with use of diuretics. Avoiding proarrhythmic effects of medications is an important part of preventing arrhythmias. Proarrhythmia induced by inotropic substances is an important clinical problem and the use of inotropes, especially in heart failure, faces the dilemma that increased contractility often augments arrhythmic activity as well. Fortunately, there are several recent examples of "heart failure" medications with potential antiarrhythmic effects. A randomized, placebo-controlled clinical trial of human recombinant relaxin-2 for treatment of acute heart failure showed relaxin-2 to be safe and effective.[83] Of note in this context, the positive effect on mortality was primarily driven by prevention of stroke (possibly related to atrial fibrillation) and sudden death,[84] suggesting that this substance may have antiarrhythmic effects. The antifibrotic hormone relaxin has been shown to suppress experimental atrial fibrillation, improving conduction from a combination of reversal of fibrosis and hypertrophy and by increasing sodium current.[85] This provides an example of a "substrate modifier" that can have antiarrhythmic properties.

Reducing Cardiac Stress and Strain

Some data suggest that statins may prevent postoperative atrial fibrillation,[86] mainly via antioxidative mechanisms,[86] but also through direct effects on ion currents[87] or indirectly through alterations in high-density lipoprotein (HDL) cholesterol.[88] The recent, large STICS trial has disproved the concept that statin therapy can prevent postoperative atrial fibrillation.[88a] *Statins* and *platelet inhibitors* (aspirin, thienopyridines), as well as revascularization, nonetheless prevent plaque rupture, acute coronary syndromes, and acute myocardial ischemia, and thereby eliminate relevant triggers for ventricular arrhythmias. Furthermore, prevention of myocardial infarctions will reduce myocardial scar formation. This, in turn, reduces the "substrate" for ventricular arrhythmias. Aldosterone antagonists such as *spironolactone* or *eplerenone*[89] may have similar effects by modulating the activity of the renin-angiotensin-aldosterone system[90] and by direct effects on cardiac gene expression patterns, in addition to balancing cardiac electrolytes.

Fatty Infiltration, Activation of Fat Cells, and Prevention of Atrial Fibrillation

Systematic weight loss can markedly improve rhythm control in atrial fibrillation and may even be sufficient to maintain sinus rhythm in extremely obese patients.[91,92] Obesity increases epicardial fat and leads to atrial infiltration with fat tissue streaks, thus providing a substrate for atrial fibrillation.[93–96] Targeting these processes may provide useful adjuncts to antiarrhythmic therapy in the future.

Intelligent Timing of Antiarrhythmic Drug Therapy

Intelligent timing of antiarrhythmic drug therapy may provide a simple way to enhance the safety of antiarrhythmic drugs while maintaining the bulk of their antiarrhythmic efficacy. Traditionally, antiarrhythmic drug therapy has been long-term therapy. Reducing the duration of antiarrhythmic drug treatment should reduce the risk for proarrhythmia. In patients with atrial fibrillation, two pathophysiological concepts of short-term antiarrhythmic drug therapy have been evaluated in patients.

Pill-in-the-Pocket Treatment of Paroxysmal Atrial Fibrillation

Patients with infrequent (<1 episode per month) symptomatic episodes of paroxysmal atrial fibrillation without overt structural heart disease who respond without side effects to pharmacological conversion of atrial fibrillation by sodium channel blocker administration under close in-hospital monitoring can be advised to take a single dose of a sodium channel-blocking agent (*a single dose of 200–300 mg flecainide or 450–600 mg propafenone*) *at home* as soon as atrial fibrillation recurs. This patient-initiated treatment converts over 90% of atrial fibrillation recurrences.[97] The duration of antiarrhythmic drug treatment was reduced by 99.2% with this type of targeted drug treatment compared to standard long-term treatment.[98]

Targeted Reversal of Electrical Remodeling After Cardioversion

Atrial fibrillation recurrences are "clustered" within the first few weeks after cardioversion of persistent atrial fibrillation. Interestingly, the atrial fibrillation-induced shortening of the atrial action potential and refractory period known as "electrical remodeling"[99] is only reversed after approximately 4 weeks of sinus rhythm.[100] Action potential-prolonging antiarrhythmic drugs may have reduced, if any, antiarrhythmic effects after this period. These considerations have prompted the design of the so-called Flec-SL trial.[101] This trial systematically tested whether *short-term 4-week antiarrhythmic drug therapy after cardioversion* was noninferior to standard long-term therapy. Indeed, short-term antiarrhythmic drug therapy limited to 4 weeks after cardioversion conveyed approximately 80% of the antiarrhythmic effect of standard, long-term therapy over the observation period of 6 months. Nonetheless, short-term therapy was not noninferior to standard long-term therapy.[102] Because of its long half-life, amiodarone does not appear to be suitable for short-term antiarrhythmic drug therapy after cardioversion,[103] although a few weeks of amiodarone therapy can prevent early recurrences of AF after catheter ablation.[10] For other antiarrhythmic drugs, in contrast, short-term therapy after cardioversion may be a suitable treatment option when either a slightly lower effectiveness appears acceptable, or when the risk associated with therapy (e.g., the proarrhythmic risk) appears high.[24]

The Longer, the Better? Half-Life of Antiarrhythmic Drugs

The effectiveness of amiodarone compared to other ion channel-blocking antiarrhythmic drugs remains a puzzling yet consistent clinical finding. The puzzlement is further increased by the only moderate effectiveness of dronedarone compared to amiodarone.[16,17] Compared to all other antiarrhythmic drugs, amiodarone has a uniquely long biological half-life of several months,[104] and its lipophilic properties result in amiodarone accumulation in cell membranes. This may provide a safety net for antiarrhythmic drug therapy: When amiodarone is not taken or not absorbed, even for several days, this will not affect the myocardial drug levels. As most of the other available ion channel-blocking drugs have half-lives in the range of a few hours and are therefore taken twice or thrice a day, omission or reduced absorption of only a few tablets will result in subtherapeutic drug plasma levels.

The Need for Personalized Arrhythmia Management

Cardiovascular medicine has made impressive progress in the last decades, resulting in prolonged survival of entire populations and markedly improved quality of life. This progress has been based on two simple yet important concepts:
1. A choice of therapies based on a thorough understanding of the underlying disease processes
2. Rigorous evaluation of interventions in controlled outcome trials
   The latter and the need for ever-larger trials have created an unwanted intellectual collateral effect, i.e., the broad labeling of patients with different cardiovascular diseases, or at least different and often competing causes of a given disease, into one patient category. "Heart failure," "atrial fibrillation," and "sudden death" are illustrative examples of syndromes rather than diseases.[105] Although we understand arrhythmia mechanisms much better today than in previous generations, this "one size fits all" approach to arrhythmias has hindered the translation of our understanding of arrhythmias into better, stratified clinical management. There is a growing need to bridge this dangerous disconnect between clinical management of arrhythmias and our impressive knowledge of arrhythmia mechanisms.[133]

Personalized Therapy of Patients With Inherited Cardiac Conditions

A notable exception to this observation is the growing number of specialized inherited arrhythmia services that provide access to personalized treatment of inherited conditions such as long QT syndrome or hypertrophic cardiomyopathy. In addition to developing new compounds, clinician-researchers have identified "genotype-" or "patient-specific" approaches to prevent ventricular arrhythmias in patients with inherited cardiomyopathies. In 2001, a small paper appeared suggesting that inhibitors of the late sodium current were able to shorten the QT interval on the ECGs of patients carrying a sodium channel mutation leading to long QT syndrome type 3.[106] This "genotype-specific" therapy would reverse the abnormal sodium channel function induced by the genetic defect and appears pathophysiologically very plausible. Long QT patients with different gene defects seem to benefit from different antiarrhythmic drug therapies. Patients with mutations in the *KVLQT2* (LQTS2) gene may require β-adrenoceptor blockade,[107] while patients with mutations in the *SCN5A* gene (LQTS3) benefit more from prevention of bradycardia.[108] Furthermore, patients with LQTS3 may benefit from sodium channel inhibition, where this "reversal" of the gene defect by antiarrhythmic drugs may prevent both atrial fibrillation and ventricular torsades de pointes.[109–112]

Flecainide, through its direct or indirect modification of ryanodine receptor function, can prevent arrhythmias in patients with catecholaminergic ventricular tachycardias.[113–116] A controlled trial of flecainide in these patients is registered on clinicaltrials.gov (NCT01117454).

Quinidine, a sodium channel-blocking drug that has initially been used in patients with atrial fibrillation, is recommended as

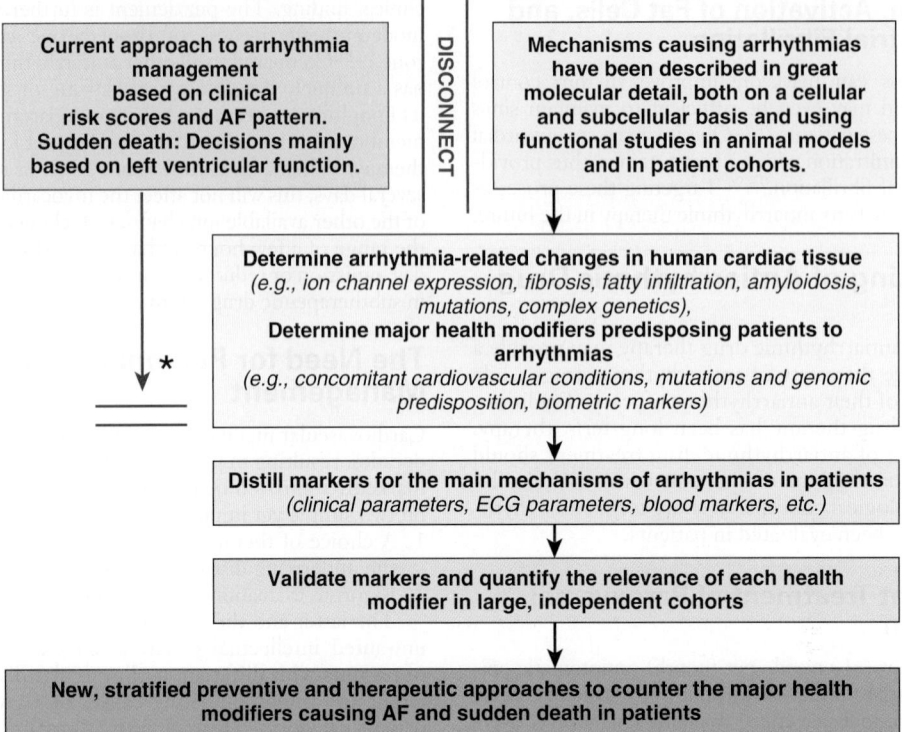

*A notable area that has bridged the disconnect between arrhythmia mechanisms and patient management are patients with inherited arrhythmogenic conditions (e.g., long QT syndrome, hypertrophic cardiomyopathy, ARVC, and others): Specialized inherited arrhythmia clinics offer mechanism-based therapy based on the type of mutation identified for these patients in many parts of the world.

FIGURE 113.3 The current disconnect between clinical management of patients suffering from, or at risk of, sudden death and atrial fibrillation (AF) on one hand (left) and our impressive understanding of arrhythmia mechanisms (right). The current management of patients with inherited arrhythmogenic diseases in specialized clinics and the success of catheter ablation as a cure for many supraventricular tachycardias and Wolff-Parkinson-White syndrome illustrate the strength of a mechanism-based approach to arrhythmias. There is a clear need to bridge this disconnect to improve the prevention and management of sudden death and AF. *ARVC,* Arrhythmogenic right ventricular cardiomyopathy; *ECG,* electrocardiogram. (Modified from Fabritz L, Guasch E, Antoniades C, et al. Defining the major health modifiers causing atrial fibrillation: a roadmap to underpin personalized prevention and treatment. *Nat Rev Cardiol.* 2016;13:230-237.)

a treatment to reduce defibrillator shocks in patients with Brugada syndrome[112] based on observational reports in Brugada syndrome[117-119] and in short QT syndrome.[118,120] Quinidine is known to alleviate some of the electrical inhomogeneities associated with the disease,[121] but so far there has been no controlled trial to assess the antiarrhythmic effects seen in anecdotal reports in a more systematic way.[119] Another recent study suggests that preload-reducing therapy can prevent ventricular arrhythmias in a mouse model of arrhythmogenic right ventricular cardiomyopathy[122,123] that mimics the pathological defect seen in these patients.[124] Based on these experimental findings, an early clinical trial of preload reduction in patients with arrhythmogenic right ventricular cardiomyopathy (ARVC) seems conceivable.[125]

The Electrocardiogram as a Proarrhythmia Predictor

Torsades de pointes and other proarrhythmias only occur in a few patients. A supernormal prolongation of the QT interval on the ECG during initiation of therapy with potassium channel blockers such as sotalol—often estimated as a QT prolongation of more than 0.06 s compared to baseline—is associated with a markedly increased risk for torsades de pointes tachycardias.[126] When therapy with a sodium channel blocker such as flecainide or propafenone is initiated, prolongation of the QRS complex by more than 25% of

the baseline duration is a sign of unexpected conduction slowing and again associated with an increased risk for ventricular proarrhythmia.[127] The ECG, by showing transient large T-U waves, can also identify an imminent risk of proarrhythmia.[128] Hence, the ECG is a valuable tool to identify individual patients who are not suitable for therapy with an existing antiarrhythmic agent.[128a]

Personalized Management of Common Cardiac Arrhythmias

In many patients suffering from atrial fibrillation or sudden death, several competing drivers of the arrhythmia will contribute to the arrhythmic risk. A personalized approach to antiarrhythmic therapy would target these causes. Such a personalized approach to antiarrhythmic drug therapy carries much promise for the future, especially as we are starting to understand the genetic contribution to more common arrhythmias such as atrial fibrillation.[4,129-132] Validation of these concepts requires cooperation between basic scientists and clinicians, most likely in "translational centers" and international consortia. As a basis to evaluate personalized approaches to cardiovascular therapy, the community may have to develop skills to differentiate among causes of these diseases in patients to allow the development of effective, new, personalized therapies (Fig. 113.3[105,133]). Among other fields, arrhythmia management can lead the way toward such a personalized approach to cardiovascular therapy based on the existing knowledge, for example, stemming from inherited cardiac conditions and from the sobering observation of ventricular proarrhythmia.

Outlook

Antiarrhythmic drugs remain an important therapeutic modality for arrhythmias. Ongoing outcome trials such as CABANA (NCT, www.cabanatrial.org) and EAST (NCT, www.easttrial.org[134]) will address whether modern, hybrid rhythm control therapy has a *prognostic* impact on the management of atrial fibrillation. Personalized and intelligently timed antiarrhythmic drug therapy may offer a way to improve safety without compromising efficacy. The preclinical identification of drug targets and development of antiarrhythmic drugs requires blinding and double blinding in experimental studies and predefined hard outcomes in cellular and animal studies to generate more reliable information prior to venturing into clinical trials. The complex environment that makes the clinical use of new medications dependent on regulatory approval, clinical effectiveness, and assessment for reimbursement renders the clinical development of new antiarrhythmic drugs challenging, despite the clear-cut clinical need for new antiarrhythmic drugs. Personalized antiarrhythmic drug therapy appears promising but will require a new taxonomy of patients with common cardiovascular conditions such as heart failure or atrial fibrillation.

Acknowledgments

This work was supported by the British Heart Foundation (FS/13/43/30324), European Union (EUTRAF 25105, grant agreement No. 633196 [CATCH ME]), and Lerucq Foundation.

REFERENCES

1. Kirchhof P, Fabritz L, Franz MR. Post-repolarization refractoriness versus conduction slowing caused by class I antiarrhythmic drugs—antiarrhythmic and proarrhythmic effects. *Circulation.* 1998;97:2567–2574.
2. Burashnikov A, Di Diego JM, Barajas-Martinez H, et al. Ranolazine effectively suppresses atrial fibrillation in the setting of heart failure. *Circ Heart Fail.* 2014;7:627–633.
3. Milberg P, Frommeyer G, Uphaus T, et al. Electrophysiologic profile of dronedarone on the ventricular level: beneficial effect on postrepolarization refractoriness in the presence of rapid phase 3 repolarization. *J Cardiovasc Pharmacol.* 2012;59:92–100.
4. Syeda F, Holmes AP, Yu TY, et al. PITX2 modulates atrial membrane potential and the antiarrhythmic effects of sodium-channel blockers. *J Am Coll Cardiol.* 2016;68:1881–1894.
5. Kirchhof P, Degen H, Franz M, et al. Amiodarone-induced post-repolarization refractoriness suppresses induction of ventricular fibrillation. *J Pharmacol Exp Ther.* 2003;305:257–263.
6. Burashnikov A, Sicouri S, Di Diego JM, et al. Synergistic effect of the combination of ranolazine and dronedarone to suppress atrial fibrillation. *J Am Coll Cardiol.* 2010;56:1216–1224.
7. Deleted in review.
8. Reiffel JA, Camm AJ, Belardinelli L, et al. The HARMONY trial: combined ranolazine and dronedarone in the management of paroxysmal atrial fibrillation: mechanistic and therapeutic synergism. *Circ Arrhythm Electrophysiol.* 2015;8:1048–1056.
9. Kirchhof P, Breithardt G, Bax J, et al. A roadmap to improve the quality of atrial fibrillation management: proceedings from the fifth Atrial Fibrillation Network/ European Heart Rhythm Association consensus conference. *Europace.* 2016;18:37–50.
9a. Kuck KH, Hoffmann BA, Ernst S, et al. Impact of complete versus incomplete circumferential lines around the pulmonary veins during catheter ablation of paroxysmal atrial fibrillation: results from the Gap-Atrial Fibrillation-German Atrial Fibrillation Competence Network 1 Trial. *Circ Arrhythm Electrophysiol.* 2016;9:e003337.
10. Darkner S, Chen X, Hansen J, et al. Recurrence of arrhythmia following short-term oral AMIOdarone after CATheter ablation for atrial fibrillation: a double-blind, randomized, placebo-controlled study (AMIO-CAT trial). *Eur Heart J.* 2014;35:3356–3364.
11. Calkins H, Kuck KH, Cappato R, et al. 2012 HRS/ EHRA/ECAS expert consensus statement on catheter and surgical ablation of atrial fibrillation: recommendations for patient selection, procedural techniques, patient management and follow-up, definitions, endpoints, and research trial design: a report of the Heart Rhythm Society (HRS) Task Force on Catheter and Surgical Ablation of Atrial Fibrillation. Developed in partnership with the European Heart Rhythm Association (EHRA), a registered branch of the European Society of Cardiology (ESC) and the European Cardiac Arrhythmia Society (ECAS); and in collaboration with the American College of Cardiology (ACC), American Heart Association (AHA), the Asia Pacific Heart Rhythm Society (APHRS), and the Society of Thoracic Surgeons (STS). Endorsed by the governing bodies of the American College of Cardiology Foundation, the American Heart Association, the European Cardiac Arrhythmia Society, the European Heart Rhythm Association, the Society of Thoracic Surgeons, the Asia Pacific Heart Rhythm Society, and the Heart Rhythm Society. *Heart Rhythm.* 2012;9: 632.e21–696.e21.
12. Singh SN, Fletcher RD, Fisher SG, et al. Amiodarone in patients with congestive heart failure and asymptomatic ventricular arrhythmia. Survival trial of antiarrhythmic therapy in congestive heart failure. *N Engl J Med.* 1995;333:77–82.
13. Aguilar M, Xiong F, Yan Qi X, et al. Potassium channel blockade enhances atrial fibrillation-selective antiarrhythmic effects of optimized state-dependent sodium channel blockade. *Circulation.* 2015;132:2203–2211.
14. Page RL, Pritchett EL, Connolly S, et al. Azimilide for the treatment of atrial fibrillation, atrial flutter, and paroxysmal supraventricular tachycardia: results of a randomized trial and insights on the concordance of symptoms and recurrent arrhythmias. *J Cardiovasc Electrophysiol.* 2008;19:172–177.
15. Bauer A, Koch M, Kraft P, et al. The new selective I(Ks)-blocking agent HMR 1556 restores sinus rhythm and prevents heart failure in pigs with persistent atrial fibrillation. *Basic Res Cardiol.* 2005;100:270–278.
16. Singh BN, Connolly SJ, Crijns HJ, et al. Dronedarone for maintenance of sinus rhythm in atrial fibrillation or flutter. *N Engl J Med.* 2007;357:987–999.
17. Hohnloser SH, Crijns HJ, van Eickels M, et al. Effect of dronedarone on cardiovascular events in atrial fibrillation. *N Engl J Med.* 2009;360:668–678.
18. Singh BN, Singh SN, Reda DJ, et al. Amiodarone versus sotalol for atrial fibrillation. *N Engl J Med.* 2005;352:1861–1872.
19. Le Heuzey J, De Ferrari GM, Radzik D, et al. A short-term, randomized, double-blind, parallel-group study to evaluate the efficacy and safety of dronedarone versus amiodarone in patients with persistent atrial fibrillation: the DIONYSOS study. *J Cardiovasc Electrophysiol.* 2010;21:597–605.
20. Page RL, Connolly SJ, Crijns HJ, et al. Rhythm- and rate-controlling effects of dronedarone in patients with atrial fibrillation (from the ATHENA trial). *Am J Cardiol.* 2011;107:1019–1022.
21. Davy JM, Herold M, Hoglund C, et al. Dronedarone for the control of ventricular rate in permanent atrial fibrillation: the Efficacy and safety of dRonedArone for the cOntrol of ventricular rate during atrial fibrillation (ERATO) study. *Am Heart J.* 2008;156:527.e1-e9.
22. Kober L, Torp-Pedersen C, McMurray JJ, et al. Increased mortality after dronedarone therapy for severe heart failure. *N Engl J Med.* 2008;358:2678–2687.
23. Connolly SJ, Camm AJ, Halperin JL, et al. Dronedarone in high-risk permanent atrial fibrillation. *N Engl J Med.* 2011;365:2268–2276.
24. Camm AJ, Lip GY, De Caterina R, et al. 2012 focused update of the ESC Guidelines for the management of atrial fibrillation: an update of the 2010 ESC Guidelines for the management of atrial fibrillation. Developed with the special contribution of the European Heart Rhythm Association. *Eur Heart J.* 2012;33:2719–2747.
25. Fetsch T, Bauer P, Engberding R, et al. Prevention of atrial fibrillation after cardioversion: results of the PAFAC trial. *Eur Heart J.* 2004;25:1385–1394.
26. Patten M, Maas R, Bauer P, et al. Suppression of paroxysmal atrial tachyarrhythmias—results of the SOPAT trial. *Eur Heart J.* 2004;25:1395–1404.
27. Voigt N, Trausch A, Knaut M, et al. Left-to-right atrial inward rectifier potassium current gradients in patients with paroxysmal versus chronic atrial fibrillation. *Circ Arrhythm Electrophysiol.* 2010;3:472–480.
28. Voigt N, Heijman J, Trausch A, et al. Impaired Na(+)-dependent regulation of acetylcholine-activated inward-rectifier K(+) current modulates action potential rate dependence in patients with chronic atrial fibrillation. *J Mol Cell Cardiol.* 2013;61:142–152.
29. Glasscock E, Voigt N, McCauley MD, et al. Expression and function of Kv1.1 potassium channels in human atria from patients with atrial fibrillation. *Basic Res Cardiol.* 2015;110:505.
30. Schmidt C, Wiedmann F, Voigt N, et al. Upregulation of K(2P)3.1 K+ current causes action potential shortening in patients with chronic atrial fibrillation. *Circulation.* 2015;132:82–92.
31. Vest JA, Wehrens XH, Reiken SR, et al. Defective cardiac ryanodine receptor regulation during atrial fibrillation. *Circulation.* 2005;111:2025–2032.
32. El-Armouche A, Boknik P, Eschenhagen T, et al. Molecular determinants of altered Ca2+ handling in human chronic atrial fibrillation. *Circulation.* 2006;114:670–680.
33. Wehrens XH, Lehnart SE, Huang F, et al. FKBP12.6 deficiency and defective calcium release channel (ryanodine receptor) function linked to exercise-induced sudden cardiac death. *Cell.* 2003;113:829–840.
34. Wehrens XH, Lehnart SE, Reiken SR, et al. Protection from cardiac arrhythmia through ryanodine receptor-stabilizing protein calstabin2. *Science.* 2004;304:292–296.
35. Lehnart SE, Terrenoire C, Reiken S, et al. Stabilization of cardiac ryanodine receptor prevents intracellular calcium leak and arrhythmias. *Proc Natl Acad Sci U S A.* 2006;103:7906–7910.
36. Lehnart SE, Mongillo M, Bellinger A, et al. Leaky Ca2+ release channel/ryanodine receptor 2 causes seizures and sudden cardiac death in mice. *J Clin Invest.* 2008;118:2230–2245.
37. Knollmann BC, Kirchhof P, Sirenko SG, et al. Familial hypertrophic cardiomyopathy-linked mutant troponin T causes stress-induced ventricular tachycardia and Ca2+-dependent action potential remodeling. *Circ Res.* 2003;92:428–436.
38. Baudenbacher F, Schober T, Pinto JR, et al. Myofilament Ca2+ sensitization causes susceptibility to cardiac arrhythmia in mice. *J Clin Invest.* 2008;118:3893–3903.
39. Voigt N, Heijman J, Wang Q, et al. Cellular and molecular mechanisms of atrial arrhythmogenesis in patients with paroxysmal atrial fibrillation. *Circulation.* 2014;129:145–156.
40. Li N, Chiang DY, Wang S, et al. Ryanodine receptor-mediated calcium leak drives progressive development of an atrial fibrillation substrate in a transgenic mouse model. *Circulation.* 2014;129:1276–1285.
41. Voigt N, Li N, Wang Q, et al. Enhanced sarcoplasmic reticulum Ca2+ leak and increased Na+-Ca2+ exchanger function underlie delayed afterdepolarizations in patients with chronic atrial fibrillation. *Circulation.* 2012;125:2059–2070.
42. Knollmann BC, Chopra N, Hlaing T, et al. Casq2 deletion causes sarcoplasmic reticulum volume increase, premature Ca2+ release, and catecholaminergic polymorphic ventricular tachycardia. *J Clin Invest.* 2006;116:2510–2520.
43. Tsuji Y, Hojo M, Voigt N, et al. Ca(2+)-related signaling and protein phosphorylation abnormalities play central roles in a new experimental model of electrical storm. *Circulation.* 2011;123:2192–2203.
44. El-Armouche A, Wittkopper K, Fuller W, et al. Phospholemman-dependent regulation of the cardiac Na/K-ATPase activity is modulated by inhibitor-1 sensitive type-1 phosphatase. *FASEB J.* 2011;25:4467–4475.

45. Wittkopper K, Fabritz L, Neef S, et al. Constitutively active phosphatase inhibitor-1 improves cardiac contractility in young mice but is deleterious after catecholaminergic stress and with aging. *J Clin Invest*. 2010;120:617–626.
46. Westenbrink BD, Ling H, Miyamoto S, et al. Mitochondrial reprogramming induced by CaMKIIdelta mediates hypertrophy decompensation. *Circ Res*. 2015;116:e28–e39.
47. Li N, Wang T, Wang W, et al. Inhibition of CaMKII phosphorylation of RyR2 prevents induction of atrial fibrillation in FKBP12.6 knockout mice. *Circ Res*. 2012;110:465–470.
48. Yao L, Fan P, Jiang Z, et al. Nav1.5-dependent persistent Na+ influx activates CaMKII in rat ventricular myocytes and N1325S mice. *Am J Physiol Cell Physiol*. 2011;301:C577–C586.
49. Pott C, Muszynski A, Ruhe A, et al. Proarrhythmia in a non-failing murine model of cardiac specific Na+/Ca2+ 2 exchanger overexpression: whole heart and cellular mechanisms. *Bas Res Cardiol*. 2012;107:247.
50. Shpak B, Gofman Y, Shpak C, et al. Effects of purified endogenous inhibitor of the Na+/Ca2+ exchanger on ouabain-induced arrhythmias in the atria and ventricle strips of guinea pig. *Eur J Pharmacol*. 2006;553:196–204.
51. Nagy ZA, Virag L, Toth A, et al. Selective inhibition of sodium-calcium exchanger by SEA-0400 decreases early and delayed after depolarization in canine heart. *Br J Pharmacol*. 2004;143:827–831.
52. Kuwahara K, Wang Y, McAnally J, et al. TRPC6 fulfills a calcineurin signaling circuit during pathologic cardiac remodeling. *J Clin Invest*. 2006;116:3114–3126.
53. Greiser M, Kerfant BG, Williams GS, et al. Tachycardia-induced silencing of subcellular Ca2+ signaling in atrial myocytes. *J Clin Invest*. 2014;124:4759–4772.
54. Boycott HE, Barbier CS, Eichel CA, et al. Shear stress triggers insertion of voltage-gated potassium channels from intracellular compartments in atrial myocytes. *Proc Natl Acad Sci U S A*. 2013;110:E3955–E3964.
55. Ford J, Milnes J, Wettwer E, et al. Human electrophysiological and pharmacological properties of XEN-D0101: a novel atrial-selective Kv1.5/IKur inhibitor. *J Cardiovasc Pharmacol*. 2013;61:408–415.
56. Ford J, Milnes J, El Haou S, et al. The positive frequency-dependent electrophysiological effects of the IKur inhibitor XEN-D0103 are desirable for the treatment of atrial fibrillation. *Heart Rhythm*. 2016;13:555–564.
57. Chaitman BR, Pepine CJ, Parker JO, et al. Effects of ranolazine with atenolol, amlodipine, or diltiazem on exercise tolerance and angina frequency in patients with severe chronic angina: a randomized controlled trial. *JAMA*. 2004;291:309–316.
58. Scirica BM, Morrow DA, Hod H, et al. Effect of ranolazine, an antianginal agent with novel electrophysiological properties, on the incidence of arrhythmias in patients with non ST-segment elevation acute coronary syndrome: results from the Metabolic Efficiency With Ranolazine for Less Ischemia in Non ST-Elevation Acute Coronary Syndrome Thrombolysis in Myocardial Infarction 36 (MERLIN-TIMI 36) randomized controlled trial. *Circulation*. 2007;116:1647–1652.
59. Antoons G, Oros A, Beekman JD, et al. Late Na(+) current inhibition by ranolazine reduces torsades de pointes in the chronic atrioventricular block dog model. *J Am Coll Cardiol*. 2010;55:801–809.
60. Lemoine MD, Duverger JE, Naud P, et al. Arrhythmogenic left atrial cellular electrophysiology in a murine genetic long QT syndrome model. *Cardiovasc Res*. 2011;92:67–74.
61. Fox K, Ford I, Steg PG, et al. Ivabradine for patients with stable coronary artery disease and left-ventricular systolic dysfunction (BEAUTIFUL): a randomised, double-blind, placebo-controlled trial. *Lancet*. 2008;372:807–816.
62. Bucchi A, Baruscotti M, DiFrancesco D. Current-dependent block of rabbit sino-atrial node I(f) channels by ivabradine. *J Gen Physiol*. 2002;120:1–13.
63. Zellerhoff S, Hinterseer M, Krull BF, et al. Ivabradine in patients with inappropriate sinus tachycardia. *Naunyn Schmiedebergs Arch Pharmacol*. 2010;382:483–486.
64. Calo L, Rebecchi M, Sette A, et al. Efficacy of ivabradine administration in patients affected by inappropriate sinus tachycardia. *Heart Rhythm*. 2010;7:1318–1323.
65. Ptaszynski P, Kaczmarek K, Ruta J, et al. Metoprolol succinate vs. ivabradine in the treatment of inappropriate sinus tachycardia in patients unresponsive to previous pharmacological therapy. *Europace*. 2013;15:116–121.
66. Martin RI, Pogoryelova O, Koref MS, et al. Atrial fibrillation associated with ivabradine treatment: meta-analysis of randomised controlled trials. *Heart*. 2014;100:1506–1510.
67. Hansen RS, Diness TG, Christ T, et al. Activation of human ether-a-go-go-related gene potassium channels by the diphenylurea 1,3-bis-(2-hydroxy-5-trifluoromethyl-phenyl)-urea (NS1643). *Mol Pharmacol*. 2006;69:266–277.
68. Shimizu W, Kurita T, Matsuo K, et al. Improvement of repolarization abnormalities by a K+ channel opener in the LQT1 form of congenital long-QT syndrome. *Circulation*. 1998;97:1581–1588.
69. Kirchhof P, Franz MR, Bardai A, Wilde AM. Giant T-U waves precede torsades de pointes in long QT syndrome: a systematic electrocardiographic analysis in patients with acquired and congenital QT prolongation. *J Am Coll Cardiol*. 2009;54:143–149.
70. Kistler PM, Sanders P, Dodic M, et al. Atrial electrical and structural abnormalities in an ovine model of chronic blood pressure elevation after prenatal corticosteroid exposure: implications for development of atrial fibrillation. *Eur Heart J*. 2006;27:3045–3056.
71. Gollob MH, Jones DL, Krahn AD, et al. Somatic mutations in the connexin 40 gene (GJA5) in atrial fibrillation. *N Engl J Med*. 2006;354:2677–2688.
72. Bax JJ, Marsan NA, Delgado V. Non-invasive imaging in atrial fibrillation: focus on prognosis and catheter ablation. *Heart*. 2015;101:94–100.
73. Chan RH, Maron BJ, Olivotto I, et al. Prognostic value of quantitative contrast-enhanced cardiovascular magnetic resonance for the evaluation of sudden death risk in patients with hypertrophic cardiomyopathy. *Circulation*. 2014;130:484–495.
74. Marrouche NF, Wilber D, Hindricks G, et al. Association of atrial tissue fibrosis identified by delayed enhancement MRI and atrial fibrillation catheter ablation: the DECAAF study. *JAMA*. 2014;311:498–506.
75. Pedersen OD, Bagger H, Kober L, Torp-Pedersen C. Trandolapril reduces the incidence of atrial fibrillation after acute myocardial infarction in patients with left ventricular dysfunction. *Circulation*. 1999;100:376–380.
76. Wachtell K, Lehto M, Gerdts E, et al. Angiotensin II receptor blockade reduces new-onset atrial fibrillation and subsequent stroke compared to atenolol: the Losartan Intervention For End Point Reduction in Hypertension (LIFE) study. *J Am Coll Cardiol*. 2005;45:712–719.
77. Disertori M, Latini R, Barlera S, et al. Valsartan for prevention of recurrent atrial fibrillation. *N Engl J Med*. 2009;360:1606–1617.
78. Goette A, Schon N, Kirchhof P, et al. Angiotensin II-antagonist in paroxysmal atrial fibrillation (ANTIPAF) trial. *Circ Arrhythm Electrophysiol*. 2012;5:43–51.
79. Rosker C, Salvarani N, Schmutz S, et al. Abolishing myofibroblast arrhythmogeneicity by pharmacological ablation of alpha-smooth muscle actin containing stress fibers. *Circ Res*. 2011;109:1120–1131.
80. Grand T, Salvarani N, Jousset F, et al. Aggravation of cardiac myofibroblast arrhythmogenicity by mechanical stress. *Cardiovasc Res*. 2014;104:489–500.
81. Qi XY, Huang H, Ordog B, et al. Fibroblast inward-rectifier potassium current upregulation in profibrillatory atrial remodeling. *Circ Res*. 2015;116:836–845.
82. Harada M, Luo X, Qi XY, et al. Transient receptor potential canonical-3 channel-dependent fibroblast regulation in atrial fibrillation. *Circulation*. 2012;126:2051–2064.
83. Teerlink JR, Cotter G, Davison BA, et al. Serelaxin, recombinant human relaxin-2, for treatment of acute heart failure (RELAX-AHF): a randomised, placebo-controlled trial. *Lancet*. 2013;381:29–39.
84. Felker GM, Teerlink JR, Butler J, et al. Effect of serelaxin on mode of death in acute heart failure: results from the RELAX-AHF study. *J Am Coll Cardiol*. 2014;64:1591–1598.
85. Parikh A, Patel D, McTiernan CF, et al. Relaxin suppresses atrial fibrillation by reversing fibrosis and myocyte hypertrophy and increasing conduction velocity and sodium current in spontaneously hypertensive rat hearts. *Circ Res*. 2013;113:313–321.
86. Reilly SN, Jayaram R, Nahar K, et al. Atrial sources of reactive oxygen species vary with the duration and substrate of atrial fibrillation: implications for the antiarrhythmic effect of statins. *Circulation*. 2011;124:1107–1117.
87. Li GR, Sun HY, Zhang XH, et al. Omega-3 polyunsaturated fatty acids inhibit transient outward and ultra-rapid delayed rectifier K+currents and Na+current in human atrial myocytes. *Cardiovasc Res*. 2009;81:286–293.
88. Den Ruijter HM, Franssen R, Verkerk AO, et al. Reconstituted high-density lipoprotein shortens cardiac repolarization. *J Am Coll Cardiol*. 2011;58:40–44.
88a. Zheng Z, Jayaram R, Jiang L, et al. Perioperative rosuvastatin in cardiac surgery. *N Engl J Med*. 2016;374:1744–1753.
89. Swedberg K, Zannad F, McMurray JJ, et al. Eplerenone and atrial fibrillation in mild systolic heart failure: results from the EMPHASIS-HF (Eplerenone in Mild Patients Hospitalization And SurvIval Study in Heart Failure) study. *J Am Coll Cardiol*. 2012;59:1598–1603.
90. Lavall D, Selzer C, Schuster P, et al. The mineralocorticoid receptor promotes fibrotic remodeling in atrial fibrillation. *J Biol Chem*. 2014;289:6656–6668.
91. Abed HS, Wittert GA, Leong DP, et al. Effect of weight reduction and cardiometabolic risk factor management on symptom burden and severity in patients with atrial fibrillation: a randomized clinical trial. *JAMA*. 2013;310:2050–2060.
92. Pathak RK, Middeldorp ME, Meredith M, et al. Long-term effect of goal-directed weight management in an atrial fibrillation cohort: a long-term follow-up study (LEGACY). *J Am Coll Cardiol*. 2015;65:2159–2169.
93. Thanassoulis G, Massaro JM, O'Donnell CJ, et al. Pericardial fat is associated with prevalent atrial fibrillation: the Framingham Heart Study. *Circ Arrhythm Electrophysiol*. 2010;3:345–350.
94. Mahajan R, Lau DH, Brooks AG, et al. Electrophysiological, electroanatomical, and structural remodeling of the atria as consequences of sustained obesity. *J Am Coll Cardiol*. 2015;66:1–11.
95. Venteclef N, Guglielmi V, Balse E, et al. Human epicardial adipose tissue induces fibrosis of the atrial myocardium through the secretion of adipo-fibrokines. *Eur Heart J*. 2015;36:795–805a.
96. Chilukoti RK, Giese A, Malenke W, et al. Atrial fibrillation and rapid acute pacing regulate adipocyte/adipositas-related gene expression in the atria. *Int J Cardiol*. 2015;187:604–613.
97. Alboni P, Botto GL, Baldi N, et al. Outpatient treatment of recent-onset atrial fibrillation with the "pill-in-the-pocket" approach. *N Engl J Med*. 2004;351:2384–2391.
98. Kirchhof P, Breithardt G. New concepts for old drugs to maintain sinus rhythm in patients with atrial fibrillation. *Heart Rhythm*. 2007;4:790–793.
99. Wijffels MC, Kirchhof CJ, Dorland R, Allessie MA. Atrial fibrillation begets atrial fibrillation. A study in awake chronically instrumented goats. *Circulation*. 1995;92:1954–1968.
100. Schotten U, Verheule S, Kirchhof P, et al. Pathophysiological mechanisms of atrial fibrillation: a translational appraisal. *Physiol Rev*. 2011;91:265–325.
101. Kirchhof P, Fetsch T, Hanrath P, et al. Targeted pharmacological reversal of electrical remodeling after cardioversion—rationale and design of the Flecainide Short-Long (Flec-SL) trial. *Am Heart J*. 2005;150:899.
102. Kirchhof P, Andresen D, Bosch R, et al. Short-term versus long-term antiarrhythmic drug treatment after cardioversion of atrial fibrillation (Flec-SL): a prospective, randomised, open-label, blinded endpoint assessment trial. *Lancet*. 2012;380:238–246.
103. Ahmed S, Rienstra M, Crijns HJ, et al. Continuous vs episodic prophylactic treatment with amiodarone for the prevention of atrial fibrillation: a randomized trial. *JAMA*. 2008;300:1784–1792.
104. Connolly SJ. Evidence-based analysis of amiodarone efficacy and safety. *Circulation*. 1999;100:2025–2034.
105. Kirchhof P, Sipido KR, Cowie MR, et al. The continuum of personalized cardiovascular medicine: a position paper of the European Society of Cardiology. *Eur Heart J*. 2014;35:3250–3257.
106. Windle JR, Geletka RC, Moss AJ, et al. Normalization of ventricular repolarization with flecainide in long QT syndrome patients with SCN5A: DeltaKPQ mutation. *Ann Noninvasive Electrocardiol*. 2001;6:153–158.
107. Priori SG, Schwartz PJ, Napolitano C, et al. Risk stratification in the long-QT syndrome. *N Engl J Med*. 2003;348:1866–1874.
108. Fabritz L, Kirchhof P, Franz MR, et al. Effect of pacing and mexiletine on dispersion of repolarisation and arrhythmias in hearts of SCN5A ð-KPQ (LQT3) mice. *Cardiovasc Res*. 2003;57:1085–1093.
109. Fabritz L, Damke D, Emmerich M, et al. Autonomic modulation and antiarrhythmic therapy in a model of long QT syndrome type 3. *Cardiovasc Res*. 2010;87:60–72.
110. Stokoe KS, Thomas G, Goddard CA, et al. Effects of flecainide and quinidine on arrhythmogenic properties of Scn5a+/Delta murine hearts modeling long QT syndrome 3. *J Physiol*. 2007;578:69–84.
111. Fredj S, Lindegger N, Sampson KJ, et al. Altered Na+ channels promote pause-induced spontaneous diastolic activity in long QT syndrome type 3 myocytes. *Circ Res*. 2006;99:1225–1232.
112. Priori SG, Blomström-Lundqvist C, Mazzanti A, et al. 2015 ESC Guidelines for the management of patients with ventricular arrhythmias and the prevention of sudden cardiac death: The Task Force for the Management of Patients with Ventricular Arrhythmias and the Prevention of Sudden Cardiac Death of the European Society of Cardiology (ESC). Endorsed by: Association for European Paediatric and Congenital Cardiology (AEPC). *Eur Heart J*. 2015;36:2793–2867.
113. Bannister ML, Thomas NL, Sikkel MB, et al. The mechanism of flecainide action in CPVT does not involve a direct effect on RyR2. *Circ Res*. 2015;116:1324–1335.
114. Johnson DM, Heijman J, Bode EF, et al. Diastolic spontaneous calcium release from the sarcoplasmic reticulum increases beat-to-beat variability of repolarization in canine ventricular myocytes after beta-adrenergic stimulation. *Circ Res*. 2013;112:246–256.
115. Watanabe H, Chopra N, Laver D, et al. Flecainide prevents catecholaminergic polymorphic ventricular tachycardia in mice and humans. *Nat Med*. 2009;15:380–383.
116. Liu N, Denegri M, Ruan Y, et al. Short communication: flecainide exerts an antiarrhythmic effect in a mouse model of catecholaminergic polymorphic ventricular tachycardia by increasing the threshold for triggered activity. *Circ Res*. 2011;109:291–295.
117. Hermida JS, Denjoy I, Clerc J, et al. Hydroquinidine therapy in Brugada syndrome. *J Am Coll Cardiol*. 2004;43:1853–1860.
118. Schweizer PA, Becker R, Katus HA, et al. Successful acute and long-term management of electrical storm in Brugada syndrome using orciprenaline and quinine/quinidine. *Clin Res Cardiol*. 2010;99:467–470.

119. Viskin S, Wilde AA, Tan HL, et al. Empiric quinidine therapy for asymptomatic Brugada syndrome: time for a prospective registry. *Heart Rhythm*. 2009;6:401–404.

120. Gaita F, Giustetto C, Bianchi F, et al. Short QT syndrome: pharmacological treatment. *J Am Coll Cardiol*. 2004;43:1494–1499.

121. Martin CA, Zhang Y, Grace AA, Huang CL. Increased right ventricular repolarization gradients promote arrhythmogenesis in a murine model of Brugada syndrome. *J Cardiovasc Electrophysiol*. 2010;21:1153–1159.

122. Kirchhof P, Fabritz L, Zwiener M, et al. Age- and training-dependent development of arrhythmogenic right ventricular cardiomyopathy in heterozygous plako-globin-deficient mice. *Circulation*. 2006;114:1799–1806.

123. Fabritz L, Hoogendijk MG, Scicluna BP, et al. Load-reducing therapy prevents development of arrhythmogenic right ventricular cardiomyopathy in plakoglobin-deficient mice. *J Am Coll Cardiol*. 2011;57:740–750.

124. Asimaki A, Tandri H, Huang H, et al. A new diagnostic test for arrhythmogenic right ventricular cardiomyopathy. *N Engl J Med*. 2009;360:1075–1084.

125. Fabritz L, Fortmueller L, Yu TY, et al. Can preload-reducing therapy prevent disease progression in arrhythmogenic right ventricular cardiomyopathy? Experimental evidence and concept for a clinical trial. *Prog Biophys Mol Biol*. 2012;110:340–346.

126. Kääb S, Hinterseer M, Näbauer M, et al. Sotalol testing unmasks altered repolarization in patients with suspected acquired long-QT-syndrome—a case-control pilot study using i.v. sotalol. *Eur Heart J*. 2003;24:649–657.

127. Fabritz L, Kirchhof P. Predictable and less predictable unwanted cardiac drug effects: individual pre-disposition and transient precipitating factors. *Bas Clin Pharm Toxicol*. 2010;106:263–268.

128. Kirchhof P, Franz MR, Bardai A, et al. Giant T-U waves precede torsades de pointes in long QT syndrome. A systematic electrocardiographic analysis in patients with acquired and congenital QT prolongation. *J Am Coll Cardiol*. 2009;54:143–149.

128a. Kirchhof P, Benussi S, Kotecha D, et al. 2016 ESC guidelines for the management of atrial fibrillation developed in collaboration with EACTS. *Eur Heart J*. 2016;37:2893–2962.

129. Kirchhof P, Kahr PC, Kaese S, et al. PITX2c is expressed in the adult left atrium, and reducing Pitx2c expression promotes atrial fibrillation inducibility and complex changes in gene expression. *Circ Cardiovasc Genet*. 2011;4:123–133.

130. Wang J, Klysik E, Sood S, et al. Pitx2 prevents susceptibility to atrial arrhythmias by inhibiting left-sided pacemaker specification. *Proc Natl Acad Sci U S A*. 2010;107:9753–9758.

131. Gudbjartsson DF, Arnar DO, Helgadottir A, et al. Variants conferring risk of atrial fibrillation on chromosome 4q25. *Nature*. 2007;448:353–357.

132. Tucker NR, Ellinor PT. Emerging directions in the genetics of atrial fibrillation. *Circ Res*. 2014;114:1469–1482.

133. Fabritz L, Guasch E, Antoniades C, et al. Defining the major health modifiers causing atrial fibrlilation: a roadmap to underpin personalized prevention and treatment. *Nat Rev Cardiol*. 2016;13:230–237.

134. Kirchhof P, Breithardt G, Camm AJ, et al. Improving outcomes in patients with atrial fibrillation: rationale and design of the Early treatment of Atrial fibrillation for Stroke prevention Trial. *Am Heart J*. 2013;166:442–448.

114 Impact of Nontraditional Antiarrhythmic Drugs on Sudden Cardiac Death

Raul D. Mitrani, Leonard Ilkhanoff, and Jeffrey J. Goldberger

Although mortality from coronary artery disease has declined in the United States, sudden cardiac death (SCD) remains a major clinical problem, with a reported range of 184,000–462,000 deaths occurring annually.[1] Strategies to decrease the incidence of sudden death include preventing underlying structural heart disease, screening for hereditary syndromes and cardiac conditions that predispose persons to sudden death, improving efforts in resuscitation medicine for patients who experience a cardiac arrest (secondary prevention), and identifying patients at high risk for sudden death to provide appropriate intervention.[2,3]

Potential interventions to prevent sudden death include risk factor and lifestyle modification, dietary changes, therapy with antiarrhythmic drugs, therapy with other cardiovascular drugs, catheter ablation, and/or implantation of implantable cardioverter defibrillators (ICDs). Results of therapy with antiarrhythmic drugs that block sodium or potassium channels for the prevention of sudden death have been largely disappointing.[4]

Antiarrhythmic drugs have been classified using several different systems. The Vaughn-Williams classification is the oldest and most commonly used system for antiarrhythmic drugs. In this system, drugs that block sodium channels are considered class I drugs, those that block β-adrenergic receptors are considered class II drugs, those that block potassium channels are considered class III drugs, and those that block calcium channels are considered class IV drugs. Antiarrhythmic drugs that block specific ion channels have been used to treat and prevent ventricular tachycardia (VT) and ventricular fibrillation (VF). However, human studies have been disappointing because drugs that block sodium or potassium channels were either ineffective in preventing SCD or paradoxically increased the risk for life-threatening arrhythmias.[5] In contrast, β-blockers, angiotensin-converting enzyme (ACE) inhibitors, and angiotensin receptor blockers, which are not considered traditional antiarrhythmic drugs, have been shown to reduce overall mortality and sudden death mortality in patients with underlying structural heart disease. Class IV agents—those that block calcium channels—do not reduce the incidence of SCD. This chapter focuses on the prevention of sudden death using pharmacological agents whose primary mode of action is not to block specific ion channels. These drugs, termed "nontraditional antiarrhythmic drugs," and their mechanisms and roles in mortality and sudden death reduction will highlight this chapter.

Assessing the Impact of Nontraditional Antiarrhythmic Drugs on Sudden Cardiac Death

One difficulty in interpreting the results of clinical studies on SCD is the diversity of potential underlying mechanisms of death, with arrhythmic SCD representing a large fraction of underlying etiologies. This is further complicated by variable definitions of SCD[2] and the fact that this is not synonymous with sudden arrhythmic death (i.e., death from myocardial infarction [MI] within the first 24 hours of symptom onset may be unrelated to a primary arrhythmia). Thus in evaluating the effect of nontraditional antiarrhythmic drugs on the incidence of sudden death, we will also consider the effects on total mortality, with the understanding that it is possible that some of the mortality reduction is due to a decreased incidence of sudden death. Studies have suggested that the major mechanisms responsible for sudden arrhythmic death are VT and VF. However, there has been a declining incidence of VT/VF as the cause of cardiac arrest and a concomitant increase in non-VF causes.[2] Therefore evaluating how therapies alter the occurrence of VT and VF provides more specific insight into the pathophysiological action of these agents to reduce SCD.

Broadly, the risk for sudden death stems from several key pathophysiological components, including (1) left ventricular (LV) dysfunction; (2) myocardial scar or substrate; (3) autonomic nervous system modulation; and (4) triggers, such as premature ventricular complexes. In theory, therapies that directly ameliorate these components can indirectly reduce the incidence of SCD. For example, one of the strongest predictors of arrhythmic sudden death is LV dysfunction. The risk of VT and VF varies inversely with LV function. Therefore therapies that may improve myocardial structure and function and decrease disease progression may also reduce the risk of VT and VF and the risk of SCD. In addition, LV dilatation may contribute to arrhythmogenesis by altering cardiac electrophysiological properties through contraction-excitation feedback. Thus pharmacological agents that modulate cardiac hemodynamics may be antiarrhythmic by altering ventricular function and size, even if direct antiarrhythmic activities are not present.

Despite extensive research in the field of sudden death, a coherent pathophysiological framework to identify the series of events or conditions necessary and sufficient to trigger sudden death has not been fully delineated. Although the majority of patients who experience SCD have coronary artery disease, patients with nonischemic cardiomyopathy also have a substantial risk for SCD. While acute MI may be the immediate cause of SCD, this accounts for the minority of cases. Transient autonomic and metabolic factors may also contribute to sudden death. Thus a pathophysiological framework underlying even arrhythmic SCD needs to broadly include many contributing factors, specifically transient factors or triggers that interact with spontaneous arrhythmias on an abnormal,

TABLE 114.1   Pharmacological agents shown to decrease mortality in patients with chronic heart disease

AGENT		POSSIBLE MECHANISMS		
ANTIARRHYTHMIC	ANTIATHEROSCLEROTIC	ANTIINFLAMMATORY/ ANTIFIBROTIC	ANTIISCHEMIC	HEMODYNAMIC
β-Blockers			X	X
ACE inhibitors		X		X
Angiotensin-receptor blockers		X		X
Fish oil	?	X		
Spironolactone		X		X
Aspirin			X	
3-Hydroxy-3-methylglutaryl Coenzyme A–reductase inhibitors	X	X		
Vasodilators (hydralazine, nitrates)				X

ACE, Angiotensin-converting enzyme; *?,* possible effect.

underlying anatomical substrate that contributes to electrophysiological conditions leading to SCD. This model recognizes that the triggering beats may be due to reentry, abnormal automaticity, or triggered activity and that the electrophysiological substrate could consist of either functional or anatomical reentry. Thus transient metabolic and autonomic factors that alter electrophysiological properties can modulate the anatomical substrate to heighten the occurrence of sudden death.

To specifically target the electrophysiological substrate, it is necessary to identify a specific electrophysiological mechanism and to identify specific ion channels or other targets that are present in the region of the myocardium that predispose to sudden death. Drugs, such as β-blockers, also operate on global regions of the myocardium, but their lack of specificity does not appear to be harmful but rather is protective. Given their overall safety profile compared with traditional antiarrhythmic drugs, it should not be surprising that nontraditional drugs that act on more global mechanisms of arrhythmogenesis are more effective in preventing sudden death than drugs that indiscriminately block ion channels throughout the myocardium. Table 114.1 shows treatments that might reduce mortality in patients with heart disease and the potential mechanisms by which they might reduce the incidence of sudden death.

β-Adrenergic Blockers

β-Adrenergic blockers (β-blockers) have emerged as important pharmacological agents for both primary and secondary prevention of SCD (Table 114.2). The mechanism of this class of drugs involves competitive β-adrenergic receptor blockade of sympathetically mediated triggering mechanisms, slowing of the sinus rate, and possibly inhibition of excess calcium release by the ryanodine receptor.[6] Cardiac disease contributes to pathophysiological changes in cardiac sympathetic innervation and regional cardiac denervation that may alter cardiac responsiveness to sympathetic stimulation and circulating catecholamines.

While β-blockers clearly play a beneficial role in reducing mortality in patients with heart failure or after MI, there is some concern that the increasing use of β-blockers may be leading to a higher percentage of out-of-hospital cardiac arrest presenting with nonshockable rhythms (asystole, pulseless electrical activity).[7] However, a recent study from the Toronto Rescu Epistry database did not confirm these findings. In particular, in patients with out-of-hospital cardiac arrest, 18.4% and 17.5% of patients taking or not taking β-blockers at the time of arrest, respectively, had shockable rhythms (*p* = not significant [NS]).[8] Thus there is

no clear evidence that β-blockers influence the presenting rhythm associated with out-of-hospital cardiac arrest.

Efficacy of β-Blockers After Myocardial Infarction

β-Blockers first were recognized as prophylactic agents for preventing sudden death in patients after MI through trials that were designed to address total mortality reduction. Analysis by Freemantle and colleagues[9] of more than 50,000 patients evaluated in numerous randomized clinical trials demonstrated a substantial reduction in total mortality due to β-blocker treatment (relative risk [RR], 0.77; 95% confidence interval [CI], 0.69–0.85). Their effect on reducing SCD is well appreciated, accounting for more than one-half the reduction in total mortality.

As the initial β-blocker trials were performed several decades ago, there have been questions about the current efficacy of β-blockers in patients who receive modern therapy including reperfusion, statins, aspirin, and ACE inhibitors. The benefits of β-blocker therapy were shown to persist in the modern era in the CAPRICORN study.[10] In patients post-MI with an ejection fraction (EF) of ≤40%, carvedilol-treated patients showed a 23% lower total mortality and a 77% reduction in malignant ventricular arrhythmias (0.9% carvedilol treated vs. 3.9% placebo; *p* < .0001) as compared with placebo at 15 months of follow-up.[11]

There is concern about the early use of a β-blocker in the acute phase of MI, particularly an intravenous β-blocker. The COMMIT trial demonstrated that in 45,852 patients, early intravenous β-blocker use was associated with a small benefit in the prevention of VF and reinfarction; however, this early benefit was mitigated by an increase in cardiogenic shock.[11] In data from the GRACE trial, intravenous β-blocker use was associated with higher rates of sustained VT/VF and acute heart failure compared with an oral β-blocker.[12] Furthermore, the administration of any form of β-blocker within 24 hours was associated with higher mortality compared with delayed (>24 hours) β-blocker administration. The Early β-Blocker Administration before Primary PCI in STEMI study showed no effect of early intravenous metoprolol on infarct size, but a significant reduction in malignant arrhythmias during hospitalization from 6.9%–3.6% (*p* = .050).[13] In contrast, data from the VALIANT study showed decreased mortality with early administration of β-blockers, particularly in those patients who had VT/VF or Killip classification I/II.[14] Moreover, a recent

TABLE 114.2 Efficacy of drugs in reducing mortality and preventing sudden death

DRUG	CONTROL	STUDY	PATIENTS	TOTAL N	FOLLOW-UP	TOTAL MORTALITY (95% CI)	SCD (95% CI)
ACE Inhibitors							
Ramipril	Placebo	AIRE[a]	Post-MI + CHF	2006	15 months	RR, 0.73 (0.60–0.89)	RR, 0.70 (0.53–0.92)
Ramipril	Placebo	HOPE	CV disease or DM + CRF	9297	5 years	RR, 0.84 (0.75–0.95)	RR, 0.62 (0.41–0.94)[b]
Captopril	Placebo	SAVE	Post MI + low EF	2231	42 months	RR, 0.81 (0.68–0.97)	NS
Enalapril	Placebo	CONSENSUS I	AMI	6090	6 months	RR, 1.10 (0.93–1.29)	NS
Enalapril	Placebo	SOLVD-P Prevention	EF	4228	37 months	RR, 0.92 (0.79–1.08)	RR, 0.93 (0.70–1.22)
Enalapril	Hydral/isosorbide	V-Heft II	CHF	804	2.5 years	RR, 0.72	RR, 0.65
Zofenopril	Placebo	SMILE	AMI	1556	6 weeks	RR, 0.78 (0.52–1.12)	RR, 0.37 (0.11–1.02)
Trandolapril	Placebo	TRACE	Post MI + low EF	1749	24–50 months	RR, 0.78 (0.67–0.91)	RR, 0.76 (0.59–0.98)
Angiotensin II–Receptor Blockers							
Valsartan	Placebo	Val-Heft	CHF	5010	23 months	RR, 1.02 (0.88–1.18), 98% CI	NS
Losartan	Captopril	ELITE	CHF	722	48 weeks	RR, 0.54 (0.31–0.95)	RR, 0.36 (0.14–0.97)
Losartan	Captopril	ELITE II	CHF	3152	1.5 years	HR, 1.13; 95.7% CI, 0.95–1.35	HR, 1.30 (1.00–1.69)
Losartan	Atenolol	LIFE	HTN + LVH	9193	4.8 years	HR, 0.90 (0.78–1.03)	HR, 1.91 (0.64–5.72)[c]
Losartan	Captopril	OPTIMAAL	Post MI + CHF	5477	2.7 years	RR, 1.13 (0.99–1.28)	RR, 1.19 (0.99–1.43)[d]
Angiotensin-Neprilysin Inhibitors							
LCZ696	Enalapril	PARADIGM-HF	CHF	8399	2.3 years	RR, 0.84 (0.76–0.93)	HR, 0.8 (0.72–0.89)
β-Blockers							
Class	Placebo	1999 meta-analysis[9]	Post-MI	24,974		RR, 0.77 (0.69–0.85)	
Class	Placebo	Medicare database[5]	Post-MI	201,752	2 years	RR, 0.60 (0.57–0.63)	
Carvedilol	Placebo	CAPRICORN	Post-MI + low EF	1959	1.3 years	HR, 0.77 (0.60–0.98)	HR, 0.74 (0.51–1.06)
Metoprolol	Placebo	MERIT-HF	CHF	3991	1 year	RR, 0.66 (0.53–0.81)	RR, 0.59 (0.45–0.78)
Bisoprolol	Placebo	CIBIS-II	CHF	2657	1.3 years	HR, 0.66 (0.54–0.81)	HR, 0.56 (0.39–0.80)

[a]See text for study abbreviations.
[b]Cardiac arrest.
[c]Resuscitated cardiac arrest.
[d]Sudden cardiac death plus resuscitated cardiac arrest.
ACE, Angiotensin-converting enzyme; *AMI*, acute myocardial infarction; *ARB*, angiotensin receptor blockers; *CHF*, congestive heart failure; *CI*, confidence interval; *CRF*, cardiac risk factor; *CV*, cardiovascular; *DM*, diabetes mellitus; *EF*, ejection fraction; *HR*, hazard ratio; *HTN*, hypertension; *Hydral*, hydralazine; *LVH*, left ventricular hypertrophy; *MI*, myocardial infarction; *NS*, not significant; *RR*, relative risk; *SCD*, sudden cardiac death.

meta-analysis of β-blocker trials in over 100,000 patients (including the COMMIT trial) showed no mortality benefit from the use of β-blockers in acute MI in the reperfusion era.[15]

β-Blockers may also mitigate proarrhythmic effects from antiarrhythmic drugs and extend antiarrhythmic effects from one drug in particular, amiodarone.[16,17] A retrospective analysis from the CAST trial showed that concomitant use of a β-blocker with flecainide or encainide substantially mitigated the proarrhythmic effects of these drugs. Furthermore, analyses from the EMIAT and CAMIAT trials showed a favorable interaction between amiodarone and β-blocker usage. In CAMIAT, there was a 29% reduction in RR related to amiodarone therapy versus placebo in patients receiving concomitant therapy with β-blockers.[16]

The majority of post-MI patients are treated with β-blocker doses that are substantially lower than the doses used in clinical trials.[18] The effect of dose on survival benefit has not been definitively demonstrated, though there are reports that suggest low-dose β-blocker therapy does improve survival.[19] Furthermore, one pharmacogenetic study on metoprolol CR/XL in the MERIT–HF study showed that poor metabolizers had substantially higher plasma metoprolol concentrations during dose titration.[20] This validates strategies to uptitrate β-blockers to effect rather than to a specific dose, though the target effect still needs to be elucidated.

Efficacy of β-Blockers in Patients With Congestive Heart Failure

β-Blockers also are important agents in the prevention of SCD in patients with congestive heart failure (CHF).[21] The original β-blocker trials in patients with heart failure demonstrated that carvedilol reduced SCD by 55% (carvedilol, 3.8% vs. placebo, 1.7%), bisoprolol reduced SCD by 44% (bisoprolol, 3.6% vs. placebo, 6.3%) and metoprolol CR/XL reduced SCD by 41% (metoprolol CR/XL, 4.0% vs. placebo, 6.6%). A recent meta-analysis of 30 randomized controlled β-blocker trials[21] for the prevention of SCD in patients with CHF showed an overall reduction in SCD by 31% and in total mortality by 33%, thus confirming the critical therapeutic role of β-blockers in patients with heart failure from either ischemic or nonischemic cardiomyopathy.

Efficacy of β-Blockers in Secondary Prevention of Sudden Death

β-Blockers also demonstrate efficacy in patients known to have significant ventricular tachyarrhythmias. A study from the Antiarrhythmics Versus Implantable Defibrillator (AVID) trial registry provides support for the role of β-blocker therapy in patients with sustained ventricular tachyarrhythmias,[22] where there was an approximately

50% reduction in adjusted RR for mortality due to β-blocker therapy in those patients not treated with an antiarrhythmic drug or ICD. Interestingly, as opposed to primary prevention of SCD where there was a favorable interaction between amiodarone and β-blockers,[16] in the AVID trial and registry there was no protective effect observed from β-blockers in patients treated with amiodarone or an ICD.[22]

In patients with nonischemic dilated cardiomyopathy and ICDs implanted for primary and secondary indications, a multivariate analysis showed that β-blocker therapy was associated with a 0.15 RR (95% CI, 0.05–0.45; $p < .0007$) of appropriate ICD therapy.[23]

Thus β-blockers are indicated in a wide variety of patient populations who also have indications for ICD therapy. The extent to which β-blocker therapy may reduce the recurrence rates of VT/VF in patients who already had a VT/VF event is unclear. However, it is clear that for those patients with VT/VF without reversible causes, a β-blocker would be insufficient as a sole antiarrhythmic therapy but would be indicated as adjuvant therapy based on patient factors.

Renin–Angiotensin–Aldosterone System

Angiotensin-Converting Enzyme Inhibitors

ACE inhibitors have been extensively studied in certain patient populations at risk for SCD. Although studies involving ACE inhibitors have shown substantial reductions in total mortality (with risk reductions ranging from 8% to 40%) and/or cardiovascular mortality, there have been inconsistent effects with respect to arrhythmic death (see Table 114.2).

There are several possible antiarrhythmic actions of ACE inhibitors. ACE inhibitors may mitigate hypokalemia, which may be arrhythmogenic in patients with CHF on diuretic therapy. Moreover, improvement in hemodynamic function is associated with improvements in sympathetic-parasympathetic tone as reflected by heart rate variability and baroreflex sensitivity. Adverse ventricular remodeling, a complex process involving fibrosis and dilatation of the failing heart, has been shown to have adverse effects on the conduction system, including increasing risk for ventricular arrhythmias. ACE inhibitor treatment may limit adverse remodeling, including reductions in LV mass, and this, secondarily, may lead to reductions in ventricular arrhythmias and a lower incidence of sudden death. It is also possible that SCD risk is contributed to by ACE pathways that are, in part, genetically determined.[24]

As shown in Table 114.2, many but not all randomized controlled trials of ACE inhibitors demonstrated reductions in SCD. Among patients studied post-MI, the Acute Infarction Ramipril Efficacy Study (AIRE)[25] and the Trandolapril Cardiac Evaluation (TRACE) study[26] are two placebo-controlled trials that demonstrated significant reductions in SCD. In the AIRE study of patients with recent MI and heart failure, treatment with ramipril (5 mg twice daily) demonstrated a 27% reduction in total mortality and 30% reduction in SCD (12.3%–8.9%) at 15 months compared with placebo. In the TRACE study of patients with postacute MI and with an EF of ≤35%, trandolapril showed a 25% decrease in cardiovascular deaths and a 24% reduction in SCD (RR, 0.76; 95% CI 0.59–0.98; $p = .03$) at 24 months compared with placebo. A meta-analysis of intermediate- or long-term post-MI ACE inhibitor trials involving a total of 15,104 patients[27] showed an overall reduction in SCD with an odds ratio of 0.80 (95% CI, 0.70–0.92).

In the Heart Outcomes Prevention Evaluation (HOPE) study of patients with vascular disease or diabetes mellitus and cardiac risk factors, treatment with ramipril demonstrated a 26% reduction in cardiovascular mortality and a 37% reduction in cardiac arrest compared with placebo at the 5-year follow-up.[28] In a substudy of HOPE examining clinical heart failure or overt LV systolic dysfunction, ramipril reduced the composite outcome of unexpected death, documented arrhythmic death, or resuscitated cardiac arrest by 21% compared with placebo at 4.5 years.[28]

ACE inhibitors appear to reduce SCD if given early after MI[25–27] or to high-risk patients without overt heart failure or LV dysfunction.[28] However, the role of ACE inhibitors in the reduction of SCD in patients with established heart failure or LV dysfunction is less clear. Several major trials including the Cooperative New Scandinavian Enalapril Survival Study (CONSENSUS), the Studies of Left Ventricular Dysfunction (SOLVD)-Treatment, and SOLVD-Prevention did not show a significant reduction in SCD.[5]

Perhaps ACE inhibitors may be more effective early in the disease process (early after MI or in patients with risk factors) where prevention of fibrosis and LV dilatation may decrease the likelihood of future SCD. In patients with established CHF and LV dilatation, ACE inhibitors, although useful at lowering overall mortality, may play less of a role in the prevention of SCD because of the established LV dilatation and fibrosis. Of course, differing definitions of SCD and differing methods of adjudicating events in the different trials make it difficult to draw firm conclusions.

Angiotensin Receptor Blockers

Physiologically active levels of angiotensin II, a potent vasoconstrictor, persist despite long-term therapy with ACE inhibitors and may also be formed by non-ACE-dependent pathways. Possible arrhythmogenic mechanisms of angiotensin II include release of neurohormonal agents (including norepinephrine, aldosterone, and endothelin) as well as increased conduction velocity and shorter refractory periods in cardiac myocytes.[5] Furthermore, unlike ACE inhibitors, angiotensin II receptor blockers (ARBs) do not increase bradykinin levels, which also can increase norepinephrine levels.[5] Therefore these considerations favor direct blockade of angiotensin II receptors that might further reduce morbidity and mortality in patients requiring blockade of the renin–angiotensin–aldosterone system. Similar to ACE inhibitors, ARBs increase serum potassium levels, which may provide a potential protective mechanism against ventricular arrhythmias.

In the Val-HEFT study,[29] a placebo-controlled study of ARBs in patients with established symptomatic CHF and an EF of <40%, there was no difference in overall mortality or SCD. However, the majority of patients (93%) in this trial were on ACE inhibitors and many (35%) were on β-blockers. In fact, this trial raised caution about combining ARBs with ACE inhibitors and β-blockers.

ARBs have mostly been compared with ACE inhibitors in several heart failure or hypertension trials. Although early studies raised the question of the superiority of ARBs over ACE inhibitors, the ELITE II study (3152 patients with heart failure and EF ≤40%) demonstrated no statistically significant differences in all-cause mortality or sudden death or resuscitated arrests between captopril and losartan.[30] In the Optimal Trial in Myocardial Infarction with the Angiotensin II Antagonist Losartan (OPTIMAAL), losartan and captopril were also studied in patients after MI with heart failure.[31] Though not a primary endpoint of the study, the results for the secondary endpoint of SCD or resuscitated cardiac arrest were 9% versus 7% for the losartan group compared with the captopril group (RR, 1.19; 95% CI, 0.98–1.43, $p = .07$). In the CHARM Program, candesartan was compared with placebo in three groups of patients with heart failure (ACE inhibitor intolerant, as adjuvant therapy to ACE inhibitors, or in patients with a preserved EF).[32] The sudden death rate was reduced by candesartan with a hazard ratio (HR) of 0.85 (95% CI, 0.73–0.99; $p = .036$). This drop in SCD rate was seen only in the low-EF group and particularly in the ACE inhibitor intolerant group.

Thus ARBs appear to reduce mortality and may reduce the risk of SCD when given in accordance with standard guidelines. There is no firm evidence that ARBs are superior to ACE inhibitors in reducing SCD, and there is no evidence that combination of ARB and ACE inhibitors confers a lower SCD risk.

Aldosterone Receptor Antagonists

Aldosterone exerts harmful effects on the cardiovascular system in patients with heart failure. Aldosterone promotes sodium retention, magnesium and potassium wasting, sympathetic activation, parasympathetic inhibition, myocardial and vascular fibrosis, baroreceptor dysfunction, vascular damage, and impairment of arterial compliance. Animal models have provided insight into the potential mechanism of arrhythmogenesis in both murine models of mineralocorticoid overexpression, leading to lethal ventricular arrhythmias[33] and canine models of heart failure, in which eplerenone administration reduced susceptibility to life-threatening arrhythmias.[34]

Spironolactone, an aldosterone receptor antagonist and potassium-sparing diuretic, has gained acceptance for the treatment of severe CHF. A meta-analysis of aldosterone antagonists on SCD prevention has demonstrated an overall 19% reduction in SCD in aldosterone-treated patients versus placebo-treated patients[35] with CHF and/or who were post-MI. The Randomized Aldactone Evaluation Study (RALES), showed that in patients with New York Heart Association class III or IV heart failure and an ejection fraction of ≤35%, spironolactone (25 mg daily) reduced cardiac death by 31% and SCD by 29% compared with placebo.[36] The EPHESUS study showed that in postacute MI patients with symptomatic heart failure and an EF of <40%, eplerenone reduced all-cause mortality by 15% ($p < .008$) and SCD by 21% (RR, 0.79; 95% CI, 0.64–0.97; $p < .03$).[37] In the subgroup of patients with an EF ≤ 30%, SCD was reduced by 33% compared with placebo.[38] However, patients with class II CHF did not show a significant reduction in SCD (4.4% in the eplerenone-treated group versus 5.5% in the placebo group, $p = .12$) despite showing a significant reduction in total mortality by 22% ($p = .01$).[39]

There are several possible mechanisms for a therapeutic effect of aldosterone receptor antagonists. Aldosterone enhances positive cardiac remodeling. Fibroblasts and inflammatory cells invade the perivascular space of damaged vessels, leading to fibrosis. These changes can have adverse effects on the mechanical function, vasodilatory reserve, and electrical system of the heart. A substudy of the RALES trial demonstrated that spironolactone decreased the levels of markers of fibrosis at 6 months, in contrast with placebo where these markers remained constant.[40] Several studies have shown that nonpotassium-sparing diuretics were associated with a dose-dependent increase in SCD. Modification of the electrophysiological substrate is another potential mechanism of aldosterone blockade. In a canine model of heart failure induced by rapid ventricular pacing, eplerenone attenuated increases in refractory periods and dispersion of refractoriness, as well as ventricular tachyarrhythmia induction.[34] Thus aldosterone receptor blockers also seem to provide mortality reduction and possibly sudden death reduction in susceptible heart failure and post-MI groups through a variety of pathways.

Combined Angiotensin-Neprilysin Inhibition

Endogenous vasoactive peptides including natriuretic peptides, bradykinins, and adrenomedullin are degraded by neprilysin, a neutral endopeptidase. These vasoactive peptides counter some of the deleterious effects from neurohormonal activation seen in patients with heart failure; therefore inhibition of neprilysin may be beneficial in patients with CHF. In the PARADIGM-HF trial,[41] LCZ696, a combination of the neprilysin inhibitor sacubitril and valsartan, was superior to valsartan in reducing total mortality (HR, 0.84; 95% CI, 0.76–0.93; $p < .001$). SCD was also reduced by LCZ696 (6.0% of patients) compared with standard therapy (7.4% of patients) with an HR of 0.8 (95% CI, 0.68–0.94; $p = .008$).[42]

Modulators of Cholesterol and Inflammation

3-Hydroxy-3-Methylglutaryl-Coenzyme A Reductase Inhibitors

The benefit of statin therapy in patients with coronary artery disease has been well established in multiple large-scale randomized clinical trials. The studies reporting on the effect of statins on ventricular tachyarrhythmias and sudden death risk reduction have been limited. Statins are a group of lipid-lowering drugs that are 3-hydroxy-3-methylglutaryl-coenzyme A reductase inhibitors. As a class, they may indirectly exert an antiarrhythmic benefit by reducing the overall ischemic burden by prevention of plaque progression and reducing ischemia and infarction. However, statins have been shown to have beneficial effects beyond prevention of plaque progression. They can modulate endothelial function, signaling pathways for inflammation, endothelial nitric oxide synthesis, plasminogen, endothelin-1, platelet activation, angiotensin II receptor regulation, oxidative stress, sympathetic nerve activity, LV mass regression, and LV reverse remodeling. Statins may also have a direct antiarrhythmic property by modulating sarcolemmal ion channel function. Reconstituted HDL-C infusion has been shown to shorten cardiac repolarization and thereby provides an alternative plausible mechanism for a reduction in SCD.[43]

The Scandinavian Simvastatin Survival Study (4S) in 4444 patients with coronary artery disease showed a 30% decrease in total mortality and 40% reduction in SCDs (statistical analysis not supplied).[44] Not all statin versus placebo trials were associated with lower rates of SCD.[44] One meta-analysis of 22,275 patients with coronary artery disease showed a 19% reduction in SCD in patients treated with statins after 4.4 years.[45] However, a more recent meta-analysis showed that statins did not significantly reduce the risk for ventricular tachyarrhythmias but did significantly reduce the rate of SCD by 10%.[44] In this analysis, there was a reduction of non-SCD by 20%. Although these meta-analyses do not rule out a direct antiarrhythmic effect from statins, it appears that reduction in sudden death could be due to limitation of progression of atherosclerosis and reduction of acute coronary events, which could trigger a lethal SCD event.[44]

Patients with nonischemic dilated cardiomyopathy have also been shown to derive benefit from statin use, suggesting a pleiotropic effect unrelated to the limitation of atherogenesis. In a post hoc analysis of the DEFINITE study,[46] of 458 patients with nonischemic dilated cardiomyopathy, use of statins was associated with a significant reduction in total mortality (adjusted HR, 0.23; 95% CI, 0.09–0.58; $p = .002$), although there was no difference in the incidence of appropriate shocks. Among 821 patients with nonischemic cardiomyopathy in the MADIT-CRT trial, multivariate analysis showed that time-dependent statin therapy was independently associated with a significant 77% reduction in the risk for fast VT/VF or death ($p < .001$) and with a significant 46% reduction in the risk for appropriate ICD shocks ($p = .01$).[47] Consistent with these findings, the cumulative probability of fast VT/VF or death during 4 years of follow-up was significantly lower among patients who were treated with statins (11%) as compared with study patients who were not treated with statins (19%; $p = .006$ for the overall difference during follow-up). An analysis of the SCD-HeFT study[48] showed that the mortality reduction related to statin use was identical in those with ischemic heart disease and those with nonischemic dilated cardiomyopathy (HRs, 0.69 and 0.67, respectively), supporting the notion that statins may exert a pleiotropic rather than antiatherosclerotic effect. Furthermore, there was no mitigation of the statin effect among patients with ICDs, suggesting that statins improve survival by mechanisms other than, or in addition to, ventricular antiarrhythmic effects.

Several post hoc analyses have suggested that statin therapy is associated with a reduction in ventricular tachyarrhythmias or appropriate ICD therapy in patients with coronary artery disease[49,50] or nonischemic cardiomyopathy.[46,47] Post hoc analyses of the AVID[51] and MADIT-II[50] patients with coronary artery disease treated with an implantable defibrillator demonstrated 40% and 28% reductions, respectively, in VT and VF episodes in patients treated with statins. The cumulative rate of ICD therapy for VT/VF or cardiac death was significantly reduced among those with ≥90% statin usage compared with those with lower statin usage ($p = .01$).[50]

In patients with coronary artery disease, statins have been reported to improve regulation of coronary arterial tone and nitric oxide–mediated endothelial function, inhibit cell proliferation, stabilize atherosclerotic plaques, exert antiinflammatory properties, and provide antioxidant effects. The mechanism by which statins reduce ventricular tachyarrhythmias may relate indirectly to one or more of these effects. For example, the antioxidant and anticell-proliferative effects of statins may play a role in plaque stabilization and thus contribute to an antiarrhythmic effect by reducing ischemia-related ventricular tachyarrhythmias. An antiischemic effect also is plausible in those with nonischemic cardiomyopathy, as a substantial proportion of patients with nonischemic cardiomyopathy may also have underlying coronary artery disease. Finally, small studies that have identified improvements in EF and exercise capacity related to statin therapy support the notion that statins may have beneficial effects on LV remodeling. Thus it is most likely that statin therapy exerts multiple beneficial effects in patients with nonischemic cardiomyopathy through not only its lipid-lowering effects but also its antiinflammatory, antioxidant, and autonomic effects.

Polyunsaturated Fatty Acids

Clues to the cardioprotective benefits of ω-3 polyunsaturated fatty acids (PUFAs) were originally discovered in epidemiological studies in Inuit and Mediterranean populations. Common to those populations' diets were high intakes of fatty fish, which have high levels of these molecules, named for their double-bonded three carbons from the N-terminus. Important ω-3 PUFAs include eicosapentaenoic acid, docosahexaenoic acid, and α-linolenic acid. The cardioprotective mechanisms of ω-3 PUFAs are still being elucidated.[37] Experimental evidence in isolated myocytes and animals points to a possible direct antiarrhythmic effect of PUFAs with an increase in arrhythmogenic threshold. In a canine VF model, ω-3 fatty acid concentrate prevented VF. In an experimental model of long QT 2 and long QT 3, PUFAs were effective in preventing torsades de pointes by mitigating action potential prolongation and reducing spatial and temporal dispersion of repolarization.[52]

Initial studies in the prestatin era generated excitement that PUFAs may reduce cardiac events, ventricular arrhythmias, and SCD. In the DART trial of postinfarct men, subjects randomly assigned to receive a dietary increase in fatty fish consumption demonstrated a 33% relative decrease in deaths due to coronary heart disease.[53] The mortality benefit was mostly seen in the first 6 months. However, a subsequent study by the same author in men with angina showed that a diet with increased fish or fish oil intake resulted in *increased* cardiac and SCD rates.[54]

In the Nurses' Health Study,[55] α-linolenic acid intake was inversely related to the risk for SCD but not nonfatal MI. The GISSI-Prevenzione study, a multicenter, open-label, randomized trial, tested 11,324 patients with recent infarction.[56] At an average of 42 months of follow-up, sudden death was reduced in the group receiving ω-3 PUFA (1 g/day) by 45% compared with the control group ($p < .001$). Total mortality was reduced by 3 months and SCD after only 4 months (RR, 0.47) of therapy with no change in plasma lipid levels. Further substudies found that the reduction in sudden death related to ω-3 PUFAs was greater in patients with LV dysfunction following MI.[57] However, in a randomized

double-blind placebo-controlled trial of patients with heart failure regardless of EF, the use of ω-3 PUFA was associated with a modest reduction in total mortality and no significant change in SCD rate (ω-3 PUFA, 8.8% vs. placebo, 9.3%; $p = .33$).[58] A recent meta-analysis (2012) showed no benefit in mortality, cardiac death, or SCD by ω-3 PUFA supplementation.[59]

Trials using PUFAs in patients with ICDs have shown mixed results[59] with no overall benefit in meta-analysis. In one trial, subjects with recent ICD episodes of sustained VT or VF were randomized to 1.8 g/d of ω-3 PUFAs or placebo. Fish oil supplementation did not prevent recurrent VT/VF and there was a trend toward increases in VT/VF suggesting a potential proarrhythmic effect in certain subgroups.[60] In another trial, Leaf and colleagues found a trend for lower risk for the combined endpoint of ICD discharge and death from any cause (28%; $p = .057$) in the group randomized to PUFAs, with a risk reduction of close to 40% ($p = .03$) when adjusting for probable episodes of malignant arrhythmias and compliance.[61] A third trial showed no significant differences between PUFAs and placebo in patients with ICDs, but in a subgroup with prior MI, the PUFA group had a trend toward benefit ($p = .09$).[62]

Overall, although evidence from in vitro studies, animal experiments, and some human studies remains compelling, confirmation of clinically relevant antiarrhythmic effects of ω-3 PUFA has remained elusive. It is also unclear whether such benefits, if present, are due to direct effects on myocyte electrophysiology or more indirect effects such as improvements in myocardial energetics, autonomic tone, reduction in local inflammatory processes, or other pathways.[63] Further studies have also challenged the notion that PUFAs exert antiarrhythmic effects and suggest potential proarrhythmic effects, possibly increasing the susceptibility to VF in both noninfarcted dogs and low-risk postinfarction dogs.[64] While consumption of fatty fish remains part of a heart-healthy diet, much work remains to be done to elucidate the role of ω-3 PUFA supplementation. In particular, the dose, purity, ratio of different PUFA components, and the target population will remain areas of active scrutiny.[37]

Other
Treatment of Diabetes

Type 2 diabetes is a risk factor for cardiovascular disease; however, there has not been convincing evidence that standard diabetes therapy reduces cardiovascular death, much less SCD.[65,66] Recently, a randomized control study of 7020 patients with type 2 diabetes demonstrated a lower total mortality (32% risk reduction) and cardiovascular mortality (38% risk reduction) using empagliflozin, an inhibitor of sodium-glucose cotransporter 2.[67] There was a 31% decrease in SCD among the pooled empagliflozin group (1.1% SCD rate) versus the placebo group (1.6% SCD rate, statistical analysis not provided) suggesting that this may be the first drug treatment for diabetes that has a clinically significant ventricular antiarrhythmic effect.

Magnesium

Magnesium is an intracellular cation that plays a crucial role in cardiovascular physiology and cardiac electrophysiology.[68] Magnesium is ubiquitous and involved in numerous intracellular enzymatic reactions. Hypomagnesemia is a well-known cause of ventricular arrhythmias. Magnesium deficiency is associated with an increase in intracellular calcium, which may be responsible for some of the cardiovascular effects from low magnesium levels. Hypomagnesemia has also been linked to hypertension, ischemic heart disease, vasospasm, and cardiomyopathies.

Hypomagnesemia has also been linked to ventricular arrhythmias. Animal models have suggested that magnesium has a direct antiarrhythmic effect.[69,70] There are various reports touting its usefulness in various arrhythmic states.[71] Intravenous magnesium therapy is one of the standard therapies for torsades de pointes associated with congenital or acquired long QT syndrome. Its utility to treat other dysrhythmias in the absence of hypomagnesemia is less certain.

In the Nurses' Health Study, magnesium intake was inversely associated with SCD.[72] The RR for the women in the highest quartile of magnesium intake was 0.62 (95% CI, 0.48–0.79) compared with the women in the lowest quartile of magnesium intake. Interestingly, plasma magnesium was not significantly associated with dietary intake. Nevertheless, higher plasma magnesium was also significantly inversely correlated with SCD with an RR of 0.39 (95% CI, 0.20–0.78) between women in the highest and lowest quartiles of plasma magnesium level. After correction for other cardiac risk factors and use of thiazide diuretics, the association with plasma magnesium level remained significant with an RR of 0.23 (95% CI, 0.08–0.87) between women in the highest and lowest quartiles of plasma magnesium level.

Low magnesium levels have also been linked with cardiovascular events, MI, and cardiomyopathy, which are risk factors for SCD. There were some early reports suggesting the benefit of early magnesium therapy in acute MI; however, the MAGIC trial showed no benefit of routine use of intravenous magnesium in patients with acute ST-segment elevation MI.[73]

There is no evidence that routine administration of magnesium supplements can reduce SCD. However, it seems reasonable to prevent hypomagnesemia, given its known effects on the cardiovascular system and role in arrhythmogenesis. Common drugs such as proton pump inhibitors can lead to chronic hypomagnesemia. Chronic alcohol use is also associated with low magnesium levels. Therefore it would appear prudent to monitor magnesium levels in patients with coronary artery disease, cardiomyopathy, or other conditions that predispose to SCD. Magnesium replacement in those patients with hypomagnesemia would be indicated.

Conclusion

In contrast to traditional antiarrhythmic drugs that block sodium or potassium channels, drugs with antiadrenergic effects and neurohormonal effects have been shown to decrease both total and sudden death mortality in patients with underlying structural heart disease. There are important lessons to be learned from the results of drug trials that show decreased sudden death mortality. Life-threatening cardiac arrhythmias are by nature highly sporadic, or at least in part dependent on a complex series of cardiac and extracardiac influences, and can be modulated by drugs that modify the adrenergic and the renin-angiotensin-aldosterone systems. In contrast, drugs whose primary mode of action is on cardiac ion channels are not effective at reducing sudden death. This observation suggests that despite advances in our knowledge of the basic mechanisms of cardiac arrhythmias, our current understanding of the mechanisms of sudden death are not adequate to justify targeting specific ion channels to prevent sudden death. Further studies on regional variations in ion channel properties and myocardial substrate and on genetic interactions will probably be required before it is possible to develop an antiarrhythmic drug that significantly reduces SCD. Integrated strategies spanning a broad range of scales from molecular through organism and population studies will be required to make continued progress in the area of SCD prevention.

In the meantime, clinicians are encouraged to follow guidelines to optimize therapy. Medical therapy with β-blockers, renin-angiotensin inhibitors, and aldosterone blockers may lower the risk of SCD. New and emerging therapies for heart failure and/or diabetes have shown promise in further reducing rates of SCD. However, in some patient groups, even optimal pharmacological therapy is insufficient for prevention of SCD, necessitating nonpharmacological therapy such as the ICD.

REFERENCES

1. Goldberger JJ, Buxton AE, Cain M, et al. Risk stratification for arrhythmic sudden cardiac death: identifying the roadblocks. *Circulation.* 2011;123:2423–2430.
2. Mitrani RD, Myerburg RJ. Ten advances defining sudden cardiac death. *Trends Cardiovasc Med.* 2016;26:23–33.
3. Goldberger JJ, Basu A, Boineau R, et al. Risk stratification for sudden cardiac death: a plan for the future. *Circulation.* 2014;129:516–526.
4. Piccini JP, Berger JS, O'Connor CM. Amiodarone for the prevention of sudden cardiac death: a meta-analysis of randomized controlled trials. *Eur Heart J.* 2009;30:1245–1253.
5. Ilkhanoff L, Goldberger JJ. Impact of nontraditional antiarrhythmic drugs on sudden cardiac death. In: Zipes DP, Jalife J, eds. *Cardiac Electrophysiology: From Cell to Bedside.* Philadelphia: Saunders; 2014:1121–1128.
6. Reiken S, Wehrens XH, Vest JA, et al. Beta-blockers restore calcium release channel function and improve cardiac muscle performance in human heart failure. *Circulation.* 2003;107:2459–2466.
7. Youngquist ST, Kaji AH, Niemann JT. Beta-blocker use and the changing epidemiology of out-of-hospital cardiac arrest rhythms. *Resuscitation.* 2008;76:376–380.
8. Czarnecki A, Morrison LJ, Qiu F, et al. Association of prior beta-blocker use and the outcomes of patients with out-of-hospital cardiac arrest. *Am Heart J.* 2015;170:1018.e2–1024.e2.
9. Freemantle N, Cleland J, Young P, et al. Beta blockade after myocardial infarction: systematic review and meta regression analysis. *BMJ.* 1999;318:1730–1737.
10. McMurray J, Kober L, Robertson M, et al. Antiarrhythmic effect of carvedilol after acute myocardial infarction: results of the Carvedilol Post-Infarct Survival Control in Left Ventricular Dysfunction (CAPRICORN) trial. *J Am Coll Cardiol.* 2005;45:525–530.
11. Chen ZM, Pan HC, Chen YP, et al. Early intravenous then oral metoprolol in 45,852 patients with acute myocardial infarction: randomised placebo-controlled trial. *Lancet.* 2005;366:1622–1632.
12. Park KL, Goldberg RJ, Anderson FA, et al. Beta-blocker use in ST-segment elevation myocardial infarction in the reperfusion era (GRACE). *Am J Med.* 2014;127:503–511.
13. Roolvink V, Ibanez B, Ottervanger JP, et al. Early administration of intravenous beta blockers in patients with ST-elevation myocardial infarction before primary PCI. *J Am Coll Cardiol.* 2016;67:2705–2715.
14. Piccini JP, Hranitzky PM, Kilaru R, et al. Relation of mortality to failure to prescribe beta blockers acutely in patients with sustained ventricular tachycardia and ventricular fibrillation following acute myocardial infarction (from the VALsartan In Acute myocardial iNfarcTion trial [VALIANT] Registry). *Am J Cardiol.* 2008;102:1427–1432.
15. Bangalore S, Makani H, Radford M, et al. Clinical outcomes with beta-blockers for myocardial infarction: a meta-analysis of randomized trials. *Am J Med.* 2014;127:939–953.
16. Kennedy HL. Beta-blocker prevention of proarrhythmia and proischemia: clues from CAST, CAMIAT, and EMIAT. Cardiac Arrhythmia Suppression Trial. Canadian Amiodarone Myocardial Infarction Arrhythmia Trial. European Myocardial Infarct Amiodarone Trial. *Am J Cardiol.* 1997;80:1208–1211.
17. Kennedy HL, Brooks MM, Barker AH, et al. Beta-blocker therapy in the Cardiac Arrhythmia Suppression Trial. CAST Investigators. *Am J Cardiol.* 1994;74:674–680.
18. Goldberger JJ, Bonow RO, Cuffe M, et al. Beta-blocker use following myocardial infarction: low prevalence of evidence-based dosing. *Am Heart J.* 2010;160:435.e1–442.e1.
19. Goldberger JJ, Bonow RO, Cuffe M, et al. Effect of beta-blocker dose on survival after acute myocardial infarction. *J Am Coll Cardiol.* 2015;66:1431–1441.
20. Batty JA, Hall AS, White HL, et al. An investigation of CYP2D6 genotype and response to metoprolol CR/XL during dose titration in patients with heart failure: a MERIT-HF substudy. *Clin Pharmacol Ther.* 2014;95:321–330.
21. Al-Gobari M, El Khatib C, Pillon F, et al. Beta-blockers for the prevention of sudden cardiac death in heart failure patients: a meta-analysis of randomized controlled trials. *BMC Cardiovasc Disord.* 2013;13:52.
22. Exner DV, Reiffel JA, Epstein AE, et al. Beta-blocker use and survival in patients with ventricular fibrillation or symptomatic ventricular tachycardia: the Antiarrhythmics Versus Implantable Defibrillators (AVID) trial. *J Am Coll Cardiol.* 1999;34:325–333.
23. Rankovic V, Karha J, Passman R, et al. Predictors of appropriate implantable cardioverter-defibrillator therapy in patients with idiopathic dilated cardiomyopathy. *Am J Cardiol.* 2002;89:1072–1076.
24. Jong P, Demers C, McKelvie RS, et al. Angiotensin receptor blockers in heart failure: meta-analysis of randomized controlled trials. *J Am Coll Cardiol.* 2002;39:463–470.
25. Cleland JG, Erhardt L, Murray G, et al. Effect of ramipril on morbidity and mode of death among survivors of acute myocardial infarction with clinical evidence of heart failure. A report from the AIRE Study Investigators. *Eur Heart J.* 1997;18:41–51.
26. Kober L, Torp-Pedersen C, Carlsen JE, et al. A clinical trial of the angiotensin-converting-enzyme inhibitor trandolapril in patients with left ventricular dysfunction after myocardial infarction. Trandolapril Cardiac Evaluation (TRACE) Study Group. *N Engl J Med.* 1995;333:1670–1676.
27. Domanski MJ, Exner DV, Borkowf CB, et al. Effect of angiotensin converting enzyme inhibition on sudden cardiac death in patients following acute myocardial infarction. A meta-analysis of randomized clinical trials. *J Am Coll Cardiol.* 1999;33:598–604.
28. Teo KK, Mitchell LB, Pogue J, et al. Effect of ramipril in reducing sudden deaths and nonfatal cardiac arrests in high-risk individuals without heart failure or left ventricular dysfunction. *Circulation.* 2004;110:1413–1417.
29. Cohn JN, Tognoni G. Valsartan Heart Failure Trial Investigators. A randomized trial of the angiotensin-receptor blocker Valsartan in Chronic Heart Failure. *N Engl J Med.* 2001;345:1667–1675.
30. Pitt B, Poole-Wilson PA, Segal R, et al. Effect of losartan compared with captopril on mortality in patients with symptomatic heart failure: randomised trial—the Losartan Heart Failure Survival Study ELITE II. *Lancet.* 2000;355:1582–1587.
31. Dickstein K, Kjekshus J. Effects of losartan and captopril on mortality and morbidity in high-risk patients after acute myocardial infarction: the OPTIMAAL randomised trial. Optimal Trial in Myocardial Infarction with Angiotensin II Antagonist Losartan. *Lancet.* 2002;360:752–760.

32. Solomon SD, Wang D, Finn P, et al. Effect of candesartan on cause-specific mortality in heart failure patients: the Candesartan in Heart failure Assessment of Reduction in Mortality and morbidity (CHARM) program. *Circulation*. 2004;110:2180–2183.

33. Ouvrard-Pascaud A, Sainte-Marie Y, Benitah JP, et al. Conditional mineralocorticoid receptor expression in the heart leads to life-threatening arrhythmias. *Circulation*. 2005;111:3025–3033.

34. Stambler BS, Laurita KR, Shroff SC, et al. Aldosterone blockade attenuates development of an electrophysiological substrate associated with ventricular tachyarrhythmias in heart failure. *Heart Rhythm*. 2009;6:776–783.

35. Le HH, El-Khatib C, Mombled M, et al. Impact of aldosterone antagonists on sudden cardiac death prevention in heart failure and post-myocardial infarction patients: A systematic review and meta-analysis of randomized controlled trials. *PLoS One*. 2016;11:e0145958.

36. Pitt B, Zannad F, Remme WJ, et al. The effect of spironolactone on morbidity and mortality in patients with severe heart failure. Randomized Aldactone Evaluation Study Investigators. *N Engl J Med*. 1999;341:709–717.

37. De Caterina R. n-3 fatty acids in cardiovascular disease. *N Engl J Med*. 2011;364:2439–2450.

38. Pitt B, Gheorghiade M, Zannad F, et al. Evaluation of eplerenone in the subgroup of EPHESUS patients with baseline left ventricular ejection fraction ≤30%. *Eur J Heart Fail*. 2006;8:295–301.

39. Zannad F, McMurray JJ, Krum H, et al. Eplerenone in patients with systolic heart failure and mild symptoms. *N Engl J Med*. 2011;364:11–21.

40. Zannad F, Alla F, Dousset B, et al. Limitation of excessive extracellular matrix turnover may contribute to survival benefit of spironolactone therapy in patients with congestive heart failure: insights from the randomized aldactone evaluation study (RALES). Rales Investigators. *Circulation*. 2000;102:2700–2706.

41. McMurray JJ, Packer M, Desai AS, et al. Angiotensin-neprilysin inhibition versus enalapril in heart failure. *N Engl J Med*. 2014;371:993–1004.

42. Desai AS, McMurray JJ, Packer M, et al. Effect of the angiotensin-receptor-neprilysin inhibitor LCZ696 compared with enalapril on mode of death in heart failure patients. *Eur Heart J*. 2015;36:1990–1997.

43. Den Ruijter HM, Franssen M, Verkerk AO, et al. Reconstituted high-density lipoprotein shortens cardiac repolarization. *J Am Coll Cardiol*. 2011;58:40–44.

44. Rahimi K, Majoni W, Merhi A, Emberson J. Effect of statins on ventricular tachyarrhythmia, cardiac arrest, and sudden cardiac death: a meta-analysis of published and unpublished evidence from randomized trials. *Eur Heart J*. 2012;33:1571–1581.

45. Levantesi G, Scarano M, Marfisi R, et al. Meta-analysis of effect of statin treatment on risk of sudden death. *J Am Coll Cardiol*. 2007;100:1644–1650.

46. Goldberger JJ, Subacius H, Schaechter A, et al. Effects of statin therapy on arrhythmic events and survival in patients with nonischemic dilated cardiomyopathy. *J Am Coll Cardiol*. 2006;48:1228–1233.

47. Buber J, Goldenberg I, Moss AJ, et al. Reduction in life-threatening ventricular tachyarrhythmias in statin-treated patients with nonischemic cardiomyopathy enrolled in the MADIT-CRT (Multicenter Automatic Defibrillator Implantation Trial with Cardiac Resynchronization Therapy). *J Am Coll Cardiol*. 2012;60:749–755.

48. Dickinson MG, Ip JH, Olshansky B, et al. Statin use was associated with reduced mortality in both ischemic and nonischemic cardiomyopathy and in patients with implantable defibrillators: mortality data and mechanistic insights from the Sudden Cardiac Death in Heart Failure Trial (SCD-HeFT). *Am Heart J*. 2007;153:573–578.

49. Chiu JH, Abdelhadi RH, Chung MK, et al. Effect of statin therapy on risk of ventricular arrhythmia among patients with coronary artery disease and an implantable cardioverter-defibrillator. *Am J Cardiol*. 2005;95:490–491.

50. Vyas AK, Guo H, Moss AJ, et al. Reduction in ventricular tachyarrhythmias with statins in the Multicenter Automatic Defibrillator Implantation Trial (MADIT)-II. *J Am Coll Cardiol*. 2006;47:769–773.

51. Mitchell LB, Powell JL, Gillis AM, et al. Are lipid-lowering drugs also antiarrhythmic drugs? An analysis of the Antiarrhythmics versus Implantable Defibrillators (AVID) trial. *J Am Coll Cardiol*. 2003;42:81–87.

52. Milberg P, Frommeyer G, Kleideiter A, et al. Antiarrhythmic effects of free polyunsaturated fatty acids in an experimental model of LQT2 and LQT3 due to suppression of early afterdepolarizations and reduction of spatial and temporal dispersion of repolarization. *Heart Rhythm*. 2011;8:1492–1500.

53. Burr ML, Gilbert JF, Holliday RM, et al. Effects of changes in fat, fish, and fiber intakes on death and myocardial reinfarction: diet and reinfarction trial (DART). *Lancet*. 1989;344:757–761.

54. Burr ML, Ashfield-Watt PA, Dunstan FD, et al. Lack of benefit of dietary advice to men with angina: results of a controlled trial. *Eur J Clin Nutr*. 2003;57:193–200.

55. Albert CM, Oh K, Whang W, et al. Dietary alpha-linolenic acid intake and risk of sudden cardiac death and coronary heart disease. *Circulation*. 2005;112:3232–3238.

56. Marchioli R, Barzi F, Bomba E, et al. Early protection against sudden death by n-3 polyunsaturated fatty acids after myocardial infarction: time-course analysis of the results of the Gruppo Italiano per lo Studio della Sopravvivenza nell'Infarto Miocardico (GISSI)-Prevenzione. *Circulation*. 2002;105:1897–1903.

57. Macchia A, Levantesi G, Franzosi MG, et al. Left ventricular systolic dysfunction, total mortality, and sudden death in patients with myocardial infarction treated with n-3 polyunsaturated fatty acids. *Eur J Heart Fail*. 2005;7:904–909.

58. Tavazzi L, Maggioni AP, Marchioli R, et al. Effect of n-3 polyunsaturated fatty acids in patients with chronic heart failure (the GISSI-HF trial): a randomised, double-blind, placebo-controlled trial. *Lancet*. 2008;372:1223–1230.

59. Rizos EC, Ntzani EE, Bika E, et al. Association between omega-3 fatty acid supplementation and risk of major cardiovascular disease events: a systematic review and meta-analysis. *JAMA*. 2012;308:1024–1033.

60. Raitt MH, Connor WE, Morris C, et al. Fish oil supplementation and risk of ventricular tachycardia and ventricular fibrillation in patients with implantable defibrillators: a randomized controlled trial. *JAMA*. 2005;293:2884–2891.

61. Leaf A, Albert CM, Josephson M, et al. Prevention of fatal arrhythmias in high-risk subjects by fish oil n-3 fatty acid intake. *Circulation*. 2005;112:2762–2768.

62. Brouwer IA, Zock PL, Camm AJ, et al. Effect of fish oil on ventricular tachyarrhythmia and death in patients with implantable cardioverter defibrillators: the Study on Omega-3 Fatty Acids and Ventricular Arrhythmia (SOFA) randomized trial. *JAMA*. 2006;295:2613–2619.

63. Mozaffarian D, Wu JH. Omega-3 fatty acids and cardiovascular disease: effects on risk factors, molecular pathways, and clinical events. *J Am Coll Cardiol*. 2011;58:2047–2067.

64. Billman GE, Carnes CA, Adamson PB, et al. Dietary omega-3 fatty acids and susceptibility to ventricular fibrillation: lack of protection and a proarrhythmic effect. *Circ Arrhythm Electrophysiol*. 2012;5:553–560.

65. Green JB, Bethel MA, Armstrong PW, et al. Effect of sitagliptin on cardiovascular outcomes in type 2 diabetes. *N Engl J Med*. 2015;373:232–242.

66. Holman RR, Sourij H, Califf RM. Cardiovascular outcome trials of glucose-lowering drugs or strategies in type 2 diabetes. *Lancet*. 2014;383:2008–2017.

67. Zinman B, Wanner C, Lachin JM, et al. Empagliflozin, cardiovascular outcomes, and mortality in type 2 diabetes. *N Engl J Med*. 2015;373:2117–2128.

68. Chakraborti S, Chakraborti T, Mandal M, et al. Protective role of magnesium in cardiovascular diseases: a review. *Mol Cell Biochem*. 2002;238:163–179.

69. Fiset C, Kargacin ME, Kondo CS, et al. Hypomagnesemia: characterization of a model of sudden cardiac death. *J Am Coll Cardiol*. 1996;27:1771–1776.

70. Davidenko JM, Cohen L, Goodrow R, et al. Quinidine-induced action potential prolongation, early afterdepolarizations, and triggered activity in canine Purkinje fibers. Effects of stimulation rate, potassium, and magnesium. *Circulation*. 1989;79:674–686.

71. Ho KM. Intravenous magnesium for cardiac arrhythmias: jack of all trades. *Magnes Res*. 2008;21:65–68.

72. Chiuve SE, Korngold EC, Januzzi JL, et al. Plasma and dietary magnesium and risk of sudden cardiac death in women. *Am J Clin Nutr*. 2011;93:253–260.

73. Magnesium in Coronaries (MAGIC) Trial Investigators. Early administration of intravenous magnesium to high-risk patients with acute myocardial infarction in the Magnesium in Coronaries (MAGIC) Trial: a randomised controlled trial. *Lancet*. 2002;360:1189–1196.

115 Prevention of Stroke in Atrial Fibrillation: Warfarin and New Oral Anticoagulants

Luciana Armaganijan and Stuart J. Connolly

Atrial fibrillation (AF) is a very common cardiac rhythm disorder worldwide. Stroke is its most serious complication, causing considerable mortality and morbidity. Therefore stroke prevention is the cornerstone of management of AF. Since the mid-2000s, advances in scientific and therapeutic approaches for stroke prevention in AF have emerged, such as new oral anticoagulants (NOACs) and occlusion of the left atrial appendage (LAA), which have had a major impact on practice and on outcomes. The aim of this chapter is to review the current treatment strategies for stroke prevention in AF.

Risk Stratification in Atrial Fibrillation
Stroke Risk Scores

Patients with AF have a fivefold increased risk for stroke, and one-sixth of all ischemic strokes are attributable to AF.[1] Moreover, strokes complicating AF are often large and clinically disabling.[2] The rate of systemic embolism or stroke in patients with AF varies greatly between patients, ranging from less than 1% to over 10% per year, depending on the presence of additional risk factors. Therefore clinical decision-making regarding stroke prevention in patients with AF must incorporate risk stratification. Many clinical risk factor systems have been developed to facilitate the evaluation of patients with AF. The $CHADS_2$ score is the most widely used and validated. It is based on a point system in which two points are assigned for a history of stroke or transient ischemic attack, and one point is assigned for each of the following risk factors: congestive heart failure, systemic hypertension, age 75 years or older, and diabetes mellitus (Table 115.1). The annual risk for stroke increases with increasing score (see Table 115.1). The CHA_2DS_2-VASc score gives one additional point for the following risk factors: age between 65 and 75 years, female sex, and presence of vascular disease (defined as myocardial infarction, complex aortic plaque, or peripheral artery disease). This risk stratification scheme has been recommended by some international guidelines and is useful for patients with a $CHADS_2$ score of 1 where there is often uncertainty about whether or not the risk for stroke is sufficiently high to justify the use of anticoagulants.[3] The CHA_2DS_2-VASc score of patient with a $CHADS_2$ score of 1 can vary from 1 to 4, with ischemic stroke risk increasing significantly throughout this range of scores.[4] Current guidelines recommend the routine use of $CHADS_2$ or CHA_2DS_2-VASc score in patients with AF.

Bleeding Risk

Bleeding is the major adverse effect of oral anticoagulant (OAC) therapy. Bleeding risk varies by patient, and it should be assessed carefully before starting anticoagulant therapy. Several validated bleeding risk scores have been developed to quantitate this risk, of which the HAS-BLED is currently the most popular. The score is based on a point system in which one point is assigned for any of the following: hypertension, abnormal renal or liver function, stroke, bleeding history or predisposition, labile international normalized ratio (INR), old age, and concomitant use of drugs or alcohol. The annual risk for bleeding increases as the risk score becomes higher. Scores of 3 or greater indicate high risk, requiring caution and regular review following the initiation of antithrombotic therapy[5] (Table 115.2).

Stroke Prevention

Stroke prevention is a key goal in the management of AF. The most successful approach has been the use of antithrombotic agents. However, occlusion of the LAA has been introduced as an alternate approach. Eradication of AF itself has also been proposed, but currently there is still no compelling evidence that it is effective, possibly because there are no treatments that are highly effective and reliable for eradication of all AF episodes.

Antithrombotic Therapy
Aspirin

Several trials have evaluated aspirin and other antiplatelet drugs for stroke prevention in AF. A meta-analysis of these trials suggests that aspirin reduces the risk for stroke by 22% (95% confidence interval [CI], 0.02–0.38).[6] Recently, some authors have questioned whether aspirin is truly effective against stroke in AF, based on an apparent lack of efficacy in at least one large cohort study.[7] However, the trial evidence is more compelling than a potentially confounded cohort study. Nonetheless, because of the greater relative efficacy of warfarin and other OACs, the role of aspirin in stroke prevention in AF is greatly diminishing.

Combination of Aspirin and Clopidogrel

Two trials have evaluated the effectiveness and safety of the combination of aspirin and clopidogrel for the prevention of stroke in patients with AF. The ACTIVE-W study was designed to compare the effects of clopidogrel (75 mg/day) in addition to aspirin (75–100 mg/day) with warfarin (target INR, 2.0–3.0) in patients with AF with at least one additional risk factor for stroke.

TABLE 115.1   CHADS$_2$ score, CHA$_2$DS$_2$-VASc score, and annual adjusted stroke rates

CHADS$_2$ SCORE	ADJUSTED STROKE RATE, %/YEAR (95% CI)	CHA$_2$DS$_2$-VASc SCORE	ADJUSTED STROKE RATE (%/YEAR)
0	1.9 (1.2–3.0)	0	0
1	2.8 (2.0–3.8)	1	1.3
2	4.0 (3.1–5.1)	2	2.2
3	5.9 (4.6–7.3)	3	3.2
4	8.5 (6.3–11.1)	4	4.0
5	12.5 (8.2–17.5)	5	6.7
6	18.2 (10.5–27.4)	6	9.8
		7	9.6
		8	6.7
		9	15.2

CHADS$_2$ score calculation: one point is given for congestive heart failure, an ejection fraction less than 40%, systemic hypertension, age >75 years, and diabetes mellitus; two points are given for a history of stroke or transient ischemic attack. CHA$_2$DS$_2$-VASc score calculation: one point is given for congestive heart failure, an ejection fraction <40%, systemic hypertension, diabetes mellitus, vascular disease (myocardial infarction, complex aortic plaque, and peripheral artery disease [PAD], including prior revascularization, amputation due to PAD, or angiographic evidence of PAD), age between 65 and 75 years, and the female sex; two points are given for a history of stroke, thromboembolism, or transient ischemic attack, and age ≥75 years.

TABLE 115.2   HAS-BLED scoring system

LETTER	CHARACTERISTICS	POINTS
H	Hypertension[a]	1
A	Abnormal renal[b] and liver[c] function (1 point each)	1 or 2
S	Stroke	1
B	Bleeding	1
L	Labile international normalized ratio	1
E	Elderly (>65 years old)	1
D	Drugs[d] or alcohol (1 point each)	1 or 2

[a]Systolic blood pressure >160 mm Hg.
[b]Chronic dialysis, renal transplantation, serum creatinine ≥200 µmol/L.
[c]Chronic hepatic disease (e.g., cirrhosis) or biochemical evidence of significant hepatic derangement (bilirubin >2 × the upper limit of normal in association with AST/ALT >3 × the upper limit of normal).
[d]Concomitant use of drugs such as antiplatelet agents, nonsteroidal antiinflammatory drugs.

The study was terminated early because of the clear superiority of warfarin. Patients who received warfarin had lower rates of primary outcomes (stroke, systemic embolism, myocardial infarction, or vascular death; annual risk of 3.9% and 5.6%, respectively; relative risk [RR], 1.44; 95% CI, 1.18–1.76; p = .0003). The main effect was derived from significant reductions in stroke (RR, 1.72; 95% CI, 1.24–2.37; p = .001) and systemic embolism (RR, 4.66; 95% CI, 1.58–13.8; p = .005) related to warfarin use. Furthermore, there was no difference in major bleeding between the groups (2.42%/year with clopidogrel plus aspirin vs. 2.21%/year with warfarin; RR, 1.1; 95% CI, 0.83–1.45; p = .53).[8]

ACTIVE-A, a double-blind randomized trial, compared clopidogrel (75 mg/day) plus aspirin (75–100 mg/day) with aspirin alone in patients with AF at risk for stroke but who were unsuitable for therapy with vitamin K antagonists (VKAs). The combined antiplatelet therapy was demonstrated to be superior to aspirin alone, with a 28% reduction in stroke (RR, 0.72; 95% CI, 0.62–0.83; p < .001). Dual antiplatelet therapy, however, was associated with a higher risk for major bleeding (RR, 1.57; 95% CI, 1.29–1.92; p < .001).[9]

The results of the two ACTIVE trials indicate clearly that antiplatelet therapy is effective against stroke in AF and that dual antiplatelet therapy is more effective than aspirin alone but at the cost of increased bleeding. The efficacy of dual antiplatelet therapy lies somewhere between that of aspirin alone and VKA therapy. The role of dual antiplatelet therapy for stroke prevention in AF is small because the benefit against stroke is offset by increased bleeding and because other alternatives to warfarin are available.

Vitamin K Antagonist Therapy for Stroke Prevention in Atrial Fibrillation

Oral anticoagulation therapy with VKAs has been the gold standard for stroke reduction in AF since the early 1990s. At that time, several randomized controlled trials demonstrated that warfarin and other VKAs reduce the risk for stroke in AF. In a meta-analysis of the trials of VKAs compared with placebo or usual care, the RR reduction was 62% (95% CI, 0.48–0.72).[6] Some trials have compared warfarin with aspirin, and the meta-analysis of these shows that warfarin reduces the risk for stroke (RR reduction, 36%; 95% CI, 0.14–0.52).[6] The benefit of warfarin comes with an increased risk for hemorrhage. In a comparison with aspirin, the meta-analysis showed that warfarin doubled the risk for major extracranial hemorrhage (RR, 2.0; 95% CI, 1.2–3.4; absolute risk increase, 0.2% per year) and intracranial hemorrhage (RR, 2.1; 95% CI, 1.0–4.6).[6]

Warfarin has been widely recognized as effective and relatively safe for stroke prevention in AF. Despite these clearly demonstrated effects and strong recommendations by international guidelines, one can estimate that approximately 50%–60% of patients at risk for stroke and without major contraindications receive long-term VKA therapy. Rates of use vary greatly globally, with even lower rates of use in many countries. Rates of discontinuation of VKA therapy are high, with approximately one-half of patients discontinuing therapy within 3–5 years. Even for those receiving therapy, in many settings poor control of the INR reduces the effectiveness of therapy.[10–14]

The underprescription of warfarin is in large part related to the many limitations of VKA therapy, which include the narrow therapeutic window, the need for rigorous and inconvenient INR monitoring, the many interactions with food and other drugs, the need for discontinuation and periprocedural bridging with heparin, and the genetic variability in metabolism. These limitations have prompted the development of more convenient alternatives to VKAs.

New Oral Anticoagulants

Several oral drugs directly inhibiting either coagulation factor II (thrombin) or factor Xa have been developed as alternatives to warfarin for stroke prevention in AF (see Table 115.2).

Thrombin Inhibitors: Dabigatran

Dabigatran etexilate is orally administered and rapidly converted to dabigatran by esterases. The bioavailability is 6%–7%, and it has an onset of action within 2 hours of administration. The elimination half-life is 12–14 hours with normal renal function, and approximately 80% of the drug is excreted unchanged by the kidneys.[15] Dabigatran is approved worldwide for prevention of stroke in AF.[15]

The safety and efficacy of dabigatran was assessed in the RE-LY trial, an 18,000-patient noninferiority multicenter randomized clinical trial that compared two different blinded doses of dabigatran to unblinded dose-adjusted warfarin (INR target of 2.0–3.0, achieved 64% of the time). Eligible patients had at least one risk factor for stroke in addition to AF and had an estimated creatinine clearance of 30 mL/min or greater. Dabigatran (150

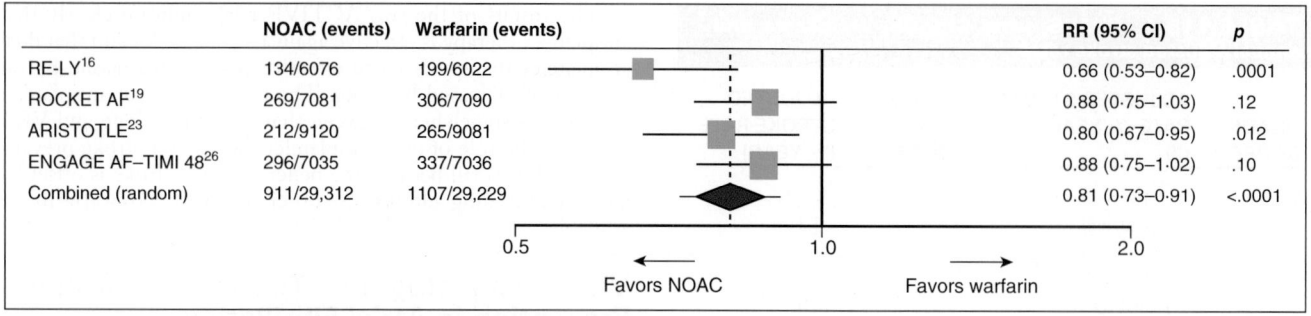

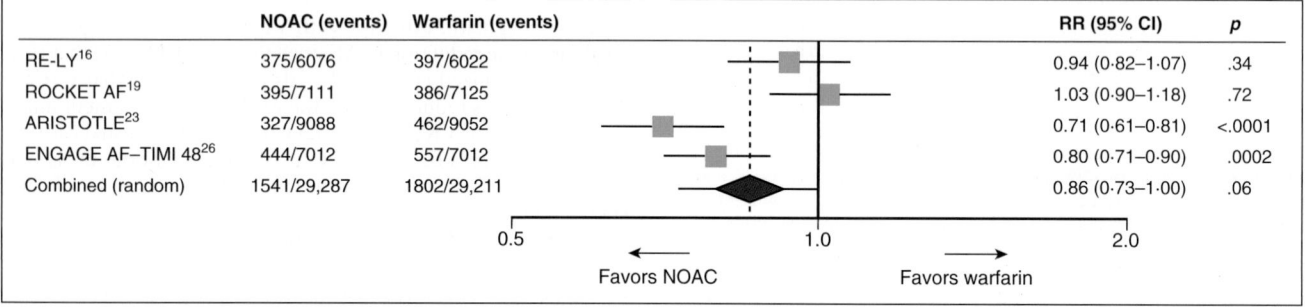

FIGURE 115.1 Cumulative hazard rates for the primary outcome of stroke or systemic embolism according to treatment group. *CI,* Confidence interval; *NOAC,* new oral anticoagulant; *RR,* relative risk.

mg) was shown to be superior to warfarin in reducing the primary outcome, which was stroke (including hemorrhagic) and systemic embolism by 34% (*p* < .001) with no significant difference in major bleeding. Compared with warfarin, dabigatran (110 mg) was noninferior to warfarin in preventing stroke and systemic embolism and was associated with a 20% RR reduction in major bleeding (*p* = .003) (Fig. 115.1).[16]

Both dosages of dabigatran lowered the risk for hemorrhagic stroke and subdural hemorrhage, with highly significant reductions of greater than 50%. Major gastrointestinal bleeding was more common with higher-dose dabigatran than with warfarin, and there was a trend for higher rates of myocardial infarction with dabigatran than with warfarin.[16]

Dabigatran has important advantages over warfarin, including large reductions in intracranial bleeding for both doses, reduction in ischemic stroke with the higher dose, and reduction in major bleeding with the lower dose. The major international guidelines now recommend dabigatran for stroke reduction in AF. The higher dose of dabigatran is recommended for many patients in view of its superior efficacy in the prevention of stroke and systemic embolism. However, the lower dose of dabigatran is recommended in some countries where there is a higher risk for bleeding (HAS-BLED score ≥3), moderate renal impairment (creatinine clearance, 30–49 mL/min), and in most countries, the elderly (age ≥80 years), because of an increase in extracranial bleeding with age on both doses of dabigatran.[17] There was a nonsignificant trend toward lower mortality for both doses of dabigatran compared with warfarin.

Idarucizumab, a specific antidote for dabigatran, has been recently approved for patients who need to undergo emergency surgery or when life-threatening or uncontrolled bleeding occurs. Real-world testing of idarucizumab has shown the agent safely and effectively reverses the anticoagulant effects of dabigatran.[18]

Xa Inhibitors

Rivaroxaban

Rivaroxaban has high bioavailability (90%–100%), rapid onset of action (peak plasma concentration at 2.5–4 hours after dosing), and a half-life of 7–13 hours. Approximately two-thirds of active drug is metabolized by the liver, being 35% renally excreted and 50% excreted via the feces.

The noninferiority of rivaroxaban compared with warfarin was demonstrated in the ROCKET-AF study, which was a randomized, double-blind, double-dummy, event-driven trial in which 14,264 patients with AF and a CHADS$_2$ score of 2 or greater were randomly assigned to receive 20 mg rivaroxaban once daily (15 mg in cases of creatinine clearance between 30 and 49 mL/min) or dose-adjusted warfarin (INR target of 2.0–3.0, achieved 58% of the time). Noninferiority in efficacy was achieved with similar rates of major and nonmajor clinically relevant bleeding events compared with warfarin. There was a large reduction in intracranial hemorrhage, and there was a reduction in fatal bleeding.[19] Several guidelines currently recommend rivaroxaban as an alternative to warfarin. A dose of 20 mg is used for most patients, with a 15-mg dose used for patients with moderate renal impairment (creatinine clearance, 30–49 mL/min). There was a trend toward lower mortality with rivaroxaban.

In a subanalysis of patients with moderate renal impairment, the benefits of lower-dose rivaroxaban were consistent with the effects of usual dose rivaroxaban in those with normal renal function.[20]

Apixaban

Apixaban has a half-life of approximately 12 hours and is administered twice daily. The excretion is approximately 25% renal, and bioavailability is high. Similar to rivaroxaban, cytochrome P450 is involved in metabolism so that strong inhibitors substantially increase drug levels.[21] Two large, randomized, double-blind trials have been conducted on apixaban for stroke prevention in AF. The AVERROES trial compared the efficacy of apixaban (5 mg twice daily) with aspirin (81–324 mg once daily) for prevention of stroke and systemic embolism in 5599 patients with AF who were considered unsuitable for VKA treatment. There was a greater than 50% reduction in stroke or systemic embolism with apixaban (RR, 0.46; 95% CI, 0.33–0.64; *p* < .001). Although minor bleeding was more common in the apixaban group, the rates of major, fatal, and intracranial bleeding did not differ significantly between the groups. Apixaban was better tolerated than aspirin, with significantly fewer study drug discontinuations.[22]

TABLE 115.3 Comparison of pharmacological characteristics of warfarin and the new oral anticoagulants for atrial fibrillation

	WARFARIN	DABIGATRAN	RIVAROXABAN	APIXABAN	EDOXABAN
Administration	Once daily	Twice daily	Once daily	Twice daily	Once daily
Target	Vitamin K–dependent factors	Factor II	Factor Xa	Factor Xa	Factor Xa
Time to peak effect	3–5 days	1 h	2.5–4 h	3 h	1–2 h
Dose	Variable	110 or 150 mg bid	20 mg qd (15 mg qd for renal impairment)	5 mg bid (2.5 mg bid for high risk)	30 or 60 mg qd (with adjustment for high exposure)
Half-life	40 h	12–14 h	7–13 h	12 h	9–11 h
Interactions	Multiple	Inhibitors of the PG transporter[a]	Inhibitors of CYP3A4 and the PG transporter[b]	Inhibitors of CYP3A4[c]	Inhibitors of CYP3A4 and the PG transporter[b]
Renal clearance (%)	0	80	35	25	40
Anticoagulation monitoring	Required	Not required	Not required	Not required	Not required
Antidote	Vitamin K, prothrombin complex, activated factor 7	None	None	None	None

[a]Inhibitors of the PG transporter include amiodarone (cautions with interaction) and verapamil.
[b]Inhibitors of CYP3A4 and the PG transporter include antifungals and protease inhibitors.
[c]Inhibitors of CYP3A4 include antifungals, macrolides, and protease inhibitors.
PG, P-glycoprotein.

Apixaban was also compared with warfarin in the ARIS-TOTLE trial, a randomized, double-blind trial on the prevention of stroke and systemic embolism in 18,201 subjects with nonvalvular AF and at least one additional risk factor for stroke. Compared with warfarin, apixaban reduced stroke and systemic embolism by 21% (p = .01), bleeding by 31% (p < .001), and mortality by 11% (p = .047). Apixaban was well tolerated and resulted in less drug discontinuation.[23] Guidelines recommend apixaban as an alternative to warfarin.

Edoxaban

Edoxaban also has a rapid onset of action, approximately 62% oral bioavailability, and a half-life of 10–14 hours. About 35% of the given substance and 50% of the absorbed substance is excreted renally; cytochrome P450 (CYP) metabolism is less than 4%.[24,25]

The ENGAGE AF-TIMI study was a randomized, double-blind, double-dummy trial that compared two once-daily regimens of edoxaban with warfarin in 21,105 patients with a moderate-to-high risk for AF. For the primary outcome of stroke or systemic embolism, both dose strategies (30 mg and 60 mg daily) showed noninferiority compared with warfarin and neither showed superiority. The annualized rate of the stroke/systemic embolism during treatment was 1.50% for warfarin compared with 1.18% for high-dose edoxaban (p < .001 for noninferiority) and 1.61% for low-dose edoxaban (p = .005 for noninferiority). Both doses markedly reduced hemorrhagic stroke compared with warfarin and neither reduced ischemic stroke. Indeed, there was a nominally significant increase in ischemic stroke with low-dose edoxaban compared with warfarin. Both regimens of edoxaban were associated with significantly lower rates of major bleeding (3.43% for warfarin compared with 2.75% for high-dose edoxaban [p < .001] and 1.61% for low-dose edoxaban [p < .001]) and death from cardiovascular causes. Compared with warfarin, total mortality was reduced with the lower dose of edoxaban; there was a trend toward lower mortality with the higher dose.[26]

A meta-analysis of randomized trials including 42,411 patients on OACs and 29,272 on warfarin showed a favorable risk-benefit profile with NOACs with significant reductions in stroke or systemic embolic events, intracranial hemorrhage, and all-cause mortality, and similar major bleeding as warfarin, but increased gastrointestinal bleeding. The efficacy and safety of NOACs were consistent across a wide range of patients.[27]

Table 115.3 shows a comparison of the pharmacological characteristics of warfarin and the NOACs for AF. Fig. 115.2 summarizes the results of the main randomized clinical trials of new anticoagulants on stroke prevention in patients with AF.

Guidelines Summary

The American Heart Association (AHA)/American College of Cardiology (ACC)/Heart Rhythm Society (HRS) guidelines recommend the use of chronic OACs for patients with nonvalvular AF and prior stroke, transient ischemic attack (TIA), or a CHA2DS2-VASc score of 2 or greater. Options include warfarin with a target INR of 2.0–3.0 (class of recommendation I; level of evidence: A), dabigatran, rivaroxaban, or apixaban (class of recommendation I; level of evidence: B). For patients with CHA2DS2-VASc scores of 0, it is reasonable to omit antithrombotic therapy. For patients with CHA2DS2-VASc scores of 1, no antithrombotic therapy or treatment with an OAC or aspirin is suggested. For those with a creatinine clearance <15 mL/min or on hemodialysis, warfarin is recommended.[28]

The European Society of Cardiology (ESC) guidelines recommend antithrombotic therapy for all patients with AF (male and female), except for those who are at low risk (<65 years old and with lone AF) or have contraindications. In patients with a CHA2DS2-VASc score of 1, either adjusted-dose VKA (targeting an INR between 2.0 and 3.0) or dabigatran or an oral factor Xa inhibitor (rivaroxaban or apixaban) should be considered, based on an assessment of the risk for bleeding complications and patient preference. In patients with a CHA2DS2-VASc score of 2 or greater, therapy with an adjusted-dose VKA or a new anticoagulant (dabigatran, rivaroxaban, or apixaban) is recommended, unless contraindicated. In the absence of stroke risk factors (e.g., CHA2DS2-VASc of 0) no antithrombotic therapy is recommended. NOACs are not recommended in patients with severe renal impairment (creatinine clearance ≤30 mL/min).[17]

The Canadian Cardiovascular Society (CCS) AF guidelines suggest that all patients with AF or atrial flutter (paroxysmal, persistent, or permanent) should be stratified using the CCS algorithm based on the CHADS2 model and that most patients should receive antithrombotic therapy. Patients at low risk of stroke (no CHADS2 risk factors, age <65 years, and free of arterial vascular disease [coronary, aortic, peripheral]) are recommended to receive no antithrombotic therapy. Aspirin (81 mg/day) is recommended for patients aged <65 with no CHADS2 risk factors who have arterial disease (coronary, aortic, or peripheral).

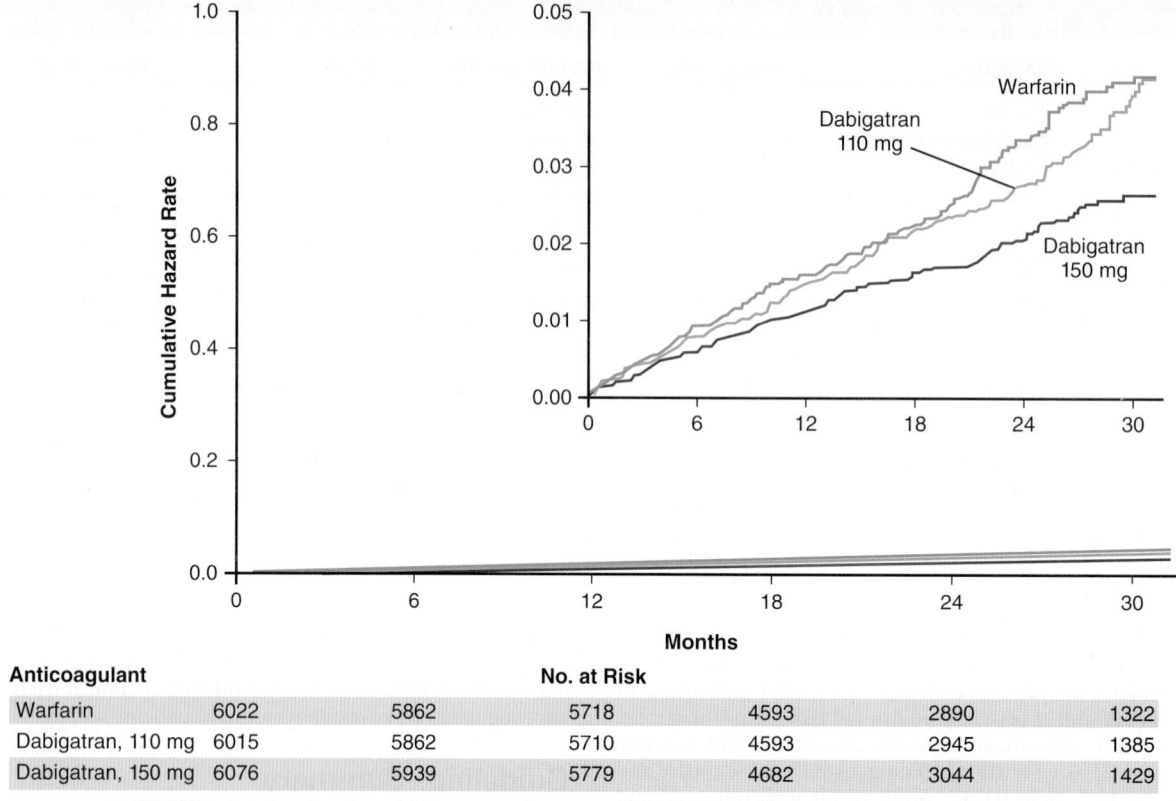

FIGURE 115.2 Results of the RE-LY trial for stroke prevention in atrial fibrillation patients, comparing dabigatran to warfarin.

For patients with a moderate-to-high risk for stroke (CHADS$_2$ ≥1 or ≥65 years), OAC therapy is indicated with a preference for NOACs (dabigatran, apixaban, rivaroxaban, or edoxaban) over warfarin.[29]

It is likely that with the advent and further familiarization with NOACs that have a better safety profile than VKAs, more patients with a low-intermediate risk will be given these newer agents.

Special Groups

Antithrombotic Therapy for Patients With Atrial Fibrillation and Valvular Disease

For the purpose of discussion about patients with AF, nonvalvular AF is usually defined as AF not associated with rheumatic valvular heart disease (VHD; mainly moderate/severe mitral stenosis) or with mechanical heart valves. Patients with nonrheumatic valvular disease including those without prosthetic valves were included in the main clinical trials assessing the efficacy and safety of OAC therapy and the NOACs as long as they were considered unlikely to undergo valve surgery before study completion. Patients with rheumatic VHD and mechanical heart valves were excluded. Ezekowitz and colleagues reported that compared with patients without VHD, patients with VHD derived similar benefits from dabigatran compared with warfarin. Of the 18,113 patients enrolled in the RE-LY trial, 3950 patients (21.8%) had some degree of VHD. Patients with VHD had similar rates of stroke and systemic embolism but were at higher risk for death and major bleeding compared with patients without VHD. The efficacy and safety of dabigatran was not significantly influenced by the presence of valvular disease.[30]

The question of whether dabigatran could be used in patients with mechanical valves was addressed in the RE-ALIGN study, a randomized, open-label, prospective controlled phase II clinical trial of patients with mechanical bileaflet heart valves from 39 centers in 10 countries. Both patients in the immediate postoperative period and those who had undergone valve replacement (aortic or mitral or both) at least 3 months earlier were randomized to receive either dabigatran or warfarin for 12 weeks. The trial was terminated early because of concerns regarding excess rates of thromboembolic and bleeding events in the dabigatran group. Although not statistically significant but trending toward harm, the rate of the composite of stroke, transient ischemic attack, systemic embolism, myocardial infarction, and death was higher in the dabigatran group (8% vs. 2%, p = .11).[31] All health authorities have issued warnings about using dabigatran in patients with mechanical heart valves.

Recently, Avezum and colleagues published the effects of apixaban on the occurrence of thromboembolic events and major bleeding in patients with AF and nonrheumatic VHD (not including mechanical valves) compared with those of warfarin. Data from patients with AF enrolled in the ARISTOTLE trial were analyzed. Those with VHD had a greater risk for thromboembolic and bleeding events compared with non-VHD AF patients. The benefits of apixaban compared with warfarin regarding stroke and status epilepticus (SE), major bleeding, and death were similar in patients with VHD compared with those without it.[32]

Patients with mitral stenosis and mechanical heart valves were excluded from the ROCKET-AF trial. However, 14% of patients had significant VHD. A post hoc analysis of the ROCKET-AF trial reported similar rates of stroke and SE with rivaroxaban compared with warfarin irrespective of the presence of VHD. However, rates of major and nonmajor clinically relevant bleeding with rivaroxaban versus warfarin were higher in patients with VHD versus those without. In intracranial hemorrhage, there was no interaction between patients with and without VHD where the overall rate was lower among those randomized to rivaroxaban.[33]

TABLE 115.4   New oral anticoagulants for patients with valvular heart disease: indications and contraindications

	ELIGIBLE	CONTRAINDICATED
Mechanical prosthetic valve		X
Moderate-to-severe mitral stenosis (usually of rheumatic origin)		X
Mild-to-moderate other native valvular disease	X	
Severe aortic stenosis	Limited data Most will undergo intervention	
Bioprosthetic valve[a]	Except for the first 3 months postoperatively	
Mitral valve repair[a]	Except for the first 3–6 months postoperatively	
PTAV and TAVI	No prospective data May require combination with single or double antiplatelet therapy Consider bleeding risk	

PTAV, Percutaneous transluminal aortic valvuloplasty; TAVI, transcatheter aortic valve implantation.
[a]Current guidelines do not recommend the use of new oral anticoagulants in patients with bioprothesis and valve repair.
From Heidbuchel H, Verhamme P, Alings M, et al. Updated European Heart Rhythm Association practical guide on the use of non-vitamin K antagonist anticoagulants in patients with non-valvular atrial fibrillation. *Europace.* 2015;17:1467-1507.

In conclusion, in patients with AF associated with VHD excluding moderate/severe mitral stenosis and mechanical prosthetic heart valves at risk for stroke or systemic embolism, NOACs have been shown to be effective, safe, and convenient therapies for prevention of stroke and systemic embolism. No data are available on the efficacy and safety of any NOAC in patients with clinically significant mitral stenosis and mechanical prosthetic valves, and therefore they are not approved for use in these patients. VKAs remain the only proven strategy for the prevention of thromboembolic events in patients with mechanical heart valves.

Table 115.4[34] summarizes the indications and contraindications for the use of NOACs in patients with VHD.

Antithrombotic Therapy in Patients With Coronary Artery Disease and Atrial Fibrillation

The combination of aspirin plus clopidogrel is usually recommended for patients with acute coronary syndrome (ACS), particularly in the context of percutaneous coronary intervention (PCI; for both elective and urgent procedures).[35] However, an OAC continues to be the optimal antithrombotic therapy for patients with chronic AF and a moderate-to-high risk for thromboembolic events.[8] In patients with both AF and ACS, concerns have arisen about the safety of triple therapy, currently defined as aspirin plus clopidogrel and warfarin, and the optimal antithrombotic strategy for patients with ACS and AF is still uncertain.

In 40,812 patients with myocardial infarction, Sorensen and colleagues[36] showed that hospital admission for bleeding increased with the number of antithrombotic drugs used. The authors reported annual incidences of bleeding of 2.6% among those receiving aspirin, 4.6% for clopidogrel, 4.3% for a VKA,

3.7% for aspirin plus clopidogrel, 5.1% for aspirin plus a VKA, 12.3% for clopidogrel plus a VKA, and 12% for triple therapy. Using aspirin alone as a reference, the adjusted hazard ratios for bleeding were 1.33, 1.23, 1.47, 1.84, 3.52, and 4.05, respectively.[37]

Strategies that can reduce the risk for bleeding in patients who receive triple therapy include the use of low doses of aspirin, the coadministration of acid-suppressive therapy to prevent gastrointestinal bleeding (a proton pump inhibitor), and INR targets of 2.0–2.5.

The WOEST trial was designed to address the question of the optimal antithrombotic treatment for patients taking an OAC who undergo coronary stenting. The study included 573 patients receiving a VKA and requiring coronary stent procedures, prospectively randomized to either additional clopidogrel only (double therapy) or clopidogrel plus aspirin (triple therapy). The strategy of adding clopidogrel only to anticoagulants (and omitting aspirin) was associated with less bleeding and lower overall mortality rates compared with triple therapy. Furthermore, there was no increase in the occurrence of myocardial infarction or stent thrombosis compared with the triple-therapy group.[38] Despite the limited number of patients in this study, this is an important finding with implications for future treatment and guidelines.

Two trials with NOACs are ongoing to define the optimal strategy related to ACS/PCI and the use of dual or triple antiplatelet therapy in patients with AF. The PIONEER AF-PCI study is comparing rivaroxaban at two different doses versus VKA along with single-agent antiplatelet therapy, while the RE-DUAL PCI study is comparing dabigatran in addition to a single nonaspirin antiplatelet versus warfarin plus dual antiplatelet therapy in patients with AF undergoing PCI. A 2 × 2 factorial trial of apixaban versus a VKA and dual antiplatelet versus single antiplatelet therapy is ongoing in patients with ACS or PCI primarily evaluating safety (clinicaltrials.gov; NCT02415400).

For patients at low or intermediate risk for bleeding undergoing elective bare metal stent implantation, the ESC, European Heart Rhythm Association, and European Association of Percutaneous Cardiovascular Interventions guidelines recommend 1 month of triple therapy followed by long-term oral anticoagulation with warfarin. For patients at high risk for bleeding, triple therapy is recommended for 2–4 weeks followed by long-term oral anticoagulation with warfarin. In those with an implanted drug-eluting stent (DES) and at a low or intermediate risk for bleeding, triple therapy is suggested for 3 months (for those with an olimus group DES) to 6 months (for those with a paclitaxel DES), followed by dual therapy with warfarin plus clopidogrel for up to 12 months, and then long-term anticoagulation with warfarin. In the setting of ACS, triple therapy is indicated for 6 months regardless of the type of stent for patients with a low or intermediate bleeding risk, and for 4 weeks for those at a high bleeding risk, followed by dual therapy with clopidogrel plus warfarin for a period of up to 12 months, and then long-term therapy with warfarin.[39,40] On the other hand, the ACC/AHA/ESC AF guidelines recommend that after clopidogrel is discontinued, warfarin should be continued as monotherapy.[41]

The Elderly

Age is one of the strongest and best-documented risk factors for stroke in patients with AF. However, OACs tend to be underprescribed in the elderly for several reasons such as the high prevalence of comorbidities, cognitive deficits, and high rates of falls, which raise concerns about the potential risk for intracranial bleeding. The discontinuation of anticoagulation therapy is particularly high in patients older than 80 years because of worries about safety and inadequate use. A cohort of elderly patients given warfarin found that 26% of patients 80 years or older had discontinued warfarin by 1 year. Rates of major bleeding were very high: 7.2%/100 person-years (95% CI, 4.9–10.6), and the rate of intracranial hemorrhage was 2.5% (95% CI, 1.1–4.7). Patients older than 80 years experienced higher rates of major bleeding compared with younger patients (13.08/100 person-years vs. 4.75/100 person-years; $p = .01$). The rates of bleeding were higher during the first 90 days, illustrating the vulnerability of warfarin during initiation. In addition, INRs were in the target range of 2.0–3.0 only 58% of the time.[42]

Should Lower International Normalized Ratio Values Be Considered in the Elderly?

Advanced age (>74 years) is an independent risk factor for anticoagulation-related bleeding events. Some authors defend that a lower INR (1.8–2.5) is a reasonable strategy in this population.[43]

However, the BAFTA[44] and WAPSO[45] studies have demonstrated the clear superiority of dose-adjusted warfarin (INR target, 2.0–3.0) over low doses of aspirin (75 mg daily) for stroke prevention. In the BAFTA study (mean age, 81.5 years), the rates of stroke in patients older than 75 years were 5% in the aspirin group compared with 2.7% in the warfarin group (RR reduction, 46%; 95% CI, 0.33–0.80; $p = .002$). The rates of major bleeding were low and did not differ between the groups (1.9% vs. 2.0% for the warfarin and aspirin arms, respectively; $p = .9$). The WAPSO study enrolled 75 patients between 80 and 90 years of age, and although this was not statistically significant, it showed higher rates of adverse events in the group treated with 300 mg of aspirin daily compared with dose-adjusted warfarin (33% vs. 6%; $p < .05$), which resulted in higher rates of discontinuation of the treatment in the aspirin group.

A subanalysis of the RE-LY trial showed an evident interaction with age for extracranial bleeding, but not for intracranial bleeding, with the risk for the latter being consistently reduced with dabigatran compared with warfarin regardless of age. Dabigatran (110 mg) compared with warfarin was associated with a similar risk for extracranial bleeding (4.43% vs. 4.37%; $p = .89$; p for interaction < .001), whereas 150 mg of dabigatran twice per day was associated with a trend toward a higher risk for major bleeding in patients aged 75 years or older (5.10% vs. 4.37%; $p = .07$; p for interaction < .001).[46] This interaction is the main reason that most regulatory agencies have recommended that the lower dose of dabigatran be used in older patients.

Left Atrial Appendage Closure

Approximately 86%–90% of LA thrombi are located in the LAA.[47,48] This observation has led to testing of both surgical removal and percutaneous device occlusion of the LAA. Surgical removal or occlusion of the LAA can be done either at the time of other cardiac surgery or in a dedicated thoracoscopic procedure.[49,50] For the percutaneous approach, three devices have been developed: the PLAATO, the Watchman, and the Amplatzer cardiac plug. The Watchman device fills the LAA, and the Amplatzer device seals the ostium.

The effectiveness and safety of the Watchman device were assessed in the randomized, multicenter, prospective PROTECT-AF trial that included 707 patients with nonvalvular AF and at least one additional risk factor for thromboembolic events; these patients were randomized to Watchman device implantation or standard care with warfarin. Patients randomized to LAA occlusion were treated with an OAC for 45 days after the procedure, followed by dual platelet inhibition for 6 months and aspirin alone as chronic therapy. The initial procedural success rate was high (91%) with effective sealing of the LAA. The trial met its predefined noninferiority endpoint (composite endpoint of stroke, cardiovascular death, and systemic embolism), but ischemic strokes were more frequent in the device group (RR, 1.53; 95% CI, 0.654–5.43). Adverse events in the intervention

group were common, including device migration, tamponade, and stroke.[51] Over time, the risk for procedure-related adverse events, including device embolization, was reduced, demonstrating the "learning curve effect."[52]

The PREVAIL trial was a multicenter, prospective, randomized clinical trial designed to confirm the results of the PROTECT AF trial and validate the safety of the implant procedure. High rates of implant success were observed for both new and experienced operators. Although no difference was reported between the two strategies for the composite of stroke, systemic embolism, and cardiovascular/unexplained death (0.064 in the device group vs. 0.063 in the control group), LAA occlusion was noninferior to warfarin for ischemic stroke or systemic embolism >7 days postprocedure and procedural safety has significantly improved. Early safety events were significantly lower than in the PROTECT AF trial. Pericardial effusions requiring surgical repair decreased from 1.6% to 0.4% ($p = .027$), and those requiring pericardiocentesis decreased from 2.9% to 1.5% ($p = .36$).[53]

A recent meta-analysis of the two randomized trials including 2406 patients with 5931 patient-years and their respective registries demonstrated significantly fewer hemorrhagic strokes (0.15 vs. 0.96 events/100 patient-years; $p = .004$), cardiovascular/unexplained death (1.1 vs. 2.3 events/100 patient-years; $p = .006$), and nonprocedural bleeding (6.0% vs. 11.3%; $p = .006$) with LAA closure compared with warfarin. No differences in all-cause stroke or systemic embolism were seen between the strategies (1.75 vs. 1.87 events/100 patient-years; $p = .94$). More ischemic strokes were observed in the device group.[54]

The Watchman device is now approved in both Europe (since 2005) and the United States (2015). Interventional LAA closure might be considered in AF patients at high risk for stroke for whom a long-term OAC is contraindicated; however, long-term data following device implantation are few; and medical therapy is evolving rapidly with the introduction of several alternatives to OACs that are more effective and safer.[17,29]

Cardioversion

The prevalence of thromboemboli in patients with AF undergoing cardioversion without anticoagulation has been reported to be between 1% and 6% in the weeks following cardioversion.[55–57] This prevalence is derived from old retrospective studies, and the risk could possibly be lower in a contemporary population with a much lower prevalence of rheumatic heart disease (RHD) and better control of risk factors such as hypertension and diabetes.

Theoretically, thromboembolism is thought to be due to dislodgment of preformed LA thrombi at the time of cardioversion when restoration of atrial contraction occurs. Thrombi can also form during the period of "mechanical stunning or dysfunction" that usually lasts a few weeks following cardioversion.[58] Pharmacological cardioversion can have an equivalent thromboembolic risk to direct current cardioversion.[59] Pericardioversion oral anticoagulation aims to reduce the formation of potential atrial thrombi, assist in the resolution of preformed thrombi, and prevent thrombi formation during the period of transient myocardial stunning. It is interesting to note that spontaneous conversion of paroxysmal AF to sinus rhythm has only an equivalent or slightly lower stroke risk compared with patients with persistent AF not undergoing cardioversion.[60] This observation suggests that the risk for thromboemboli could be related less to the cardioversion itself and could be influenced more by the patient's stroke risk factors.

Routine precardioversion anticoagulation was first proposed by Lown in 1967 and has been accepted without there ever being a randomized trial evaluating this approach.[55] All the following recommendations are based on indirect observational studies. For AF lasting 48 hours or more or of unknown duration, major society guidelines recommend a minimum period of 3 weeks of an OAC before cardioversion and a minimum period of 4 weeks after cardioversion.[61,62] The short-term risk for thromboembolism using this OAC regimen in a contemporary population appears to be low (0.5%–0.6%).[48]

For AF lasting less than 48 hours, major society guidelines recommend no OAC before cardioversion. Observational data suggest the stroke risk to be low for AF less than 48 hours (0.8%) when cardioversion is performed without an OAC.[63] Guidelines recommend intravenous (IV) unfractionated heparin (UFH) or low-molecular-weight heparin (LMWH) in patients undergoing pericardioversion without any evidence from clinical trials.[61] An OAC is recommended for a minimum of 4 weeks after cardioversion regardless of stroke risk. For hemodynamically unstable AF, immediate cardioversion with IV UFH or LMWH pericardioversion should be followed by a minimum of 4 weeks of an OAC, but there are no data to support this recommendation.

VKAs are the most widely used OACs in the pericardioversion period. Although no studies have strictly determined the optimal INR control in the pericardioversion period, a target INR of 2.0–3.0 is reasonable, similar to chronic AF. This recommendation is supported by a warfarin study that suggested that an INR of 2.5 or greater at the time of cardioversion was associated with a significant reduction in the incidence of systemic embolism compared with patients with an INR of 1.5–2.5 (0% vs. 1.2% of patients, respectively).[64] LMWH can be a reasonable alternative to an OAC in the pericardioversion setting. A randomized study of enoxaparin given subcutaneously for 3 weeks before and 4 weeks after cardioversion was shown to be noninferior for the primary endpoint of stroke, thromboembolism, and bleeding compared with IV UFH for at least 72 hours and phenprocoumon for 3 weeks before cardioversion and then 4 weeks after cardioversion (3.2% vs. 5.7% of patients, respectively).[65]

A comparison of dabigatran and warfarin in the RE-LY trial reported that the incidence of thromboembolism at 30 days was similar in the warfarin group (0.6%) compared with the dabigatran groups (110 mg twice daily [0.8%] and 150 mg twice daily [0.3%]). This trial was underpowered to detect a true difference between the groups, but it suggests that dabigatran is a reasonable alternative to warfarin in the pericardioversion setting.[66] Post hoc analyses of the ROCKET and ARISTOTLE trials have shown similar rates of bleeding and thromboembolic events when warfarin was compared with rivaroxaban[67] and apixaban,[68] respectively, in patients undergoing cardioversion.

The X-VeRT study was the first prospective randomized trial to investigate the efficacy and safety of NOACs in patients undergoing elective cardioversion. Patients were randomly assigned to receive rivaroxaban 20 mg once daily (or an adjusted dose in cases of renal dysfunction) or VKA and were selected for either an early (1–5 days after randomization) or delayed (3–8 weeks) cardioversion strategy. Low rates of the primary efficacy endpoint (a composite of stroke, TIA, peripheral embolism, myocardial infarction, and cardiovascular death) were seen in both groups (0.51% in the rivaroxaban arm and 1.02% in the VKA group). Similarly, major bleeding rates were low in both treatment groups (0.6% and 0.8% in the rivaroxaban and warfarin arms, respectively). No differences were seen between early and delayed cardioversion for the primary efficacy and safety endpoints. Rivaroxaban was associated with a shorter time to cardioversion compared with VKA (p < .001).[69]

An alternative to the conventional 3 weeks of an OAC for AF lasting 48 hours or longer or of unknown duration before cardioversion is the transesophageal echocardiography (TEE)-guided strategy. With the TEE-guided strategy, a TEE is performed to exclude LA thrombi before cardioversion, preventing the need for an OAC before cardioversion. If LA thrombi are present, then the cardioversion is postponed for an additional 3 weeks on an OAC before the TEE is repeated. Patients should be given an anticoagulant at the time of cardioversion (usually a therapeutic OAC for a few days or IV bolus of UFH or LMWH before cardioversion). This TEE-guided strategy is supported by a randomized trial (ACUTE) of 1222 patients randomized to a TEE-guided approach followed by 4 weeks of warfarin after cardioversion compared with a conventional group of 3 weeks of warfarin before and 4 weeks after cardioversion.[48] There was no significant difference in embolic events between the two groups (0.8% in the TEE group vs. 0.5% of patients in the conventional group). The TEE-guided strategy had significantly fewer bleeding events and a shorter time to cardioversion, but a trend toward an unexplained increase in all-cause mortality. This approach may be suitable for patients who are symptomatic and require hospitalization or who have an increased bleeding risk. There appears to be no compelling evidence to use a TEE-guided approach routinely for cardioversion.

Future Directions

For decades, warfarin was the only available OAC for stroke prevention in patients with AF. Although it is highly effective under optimal conditions, its limitations hamper its long-term use. Several large-scale, randomized clinical trials have shown important advantages of the NOACs on clinical outcomes, including stroke reduction, a large reduction in intracranial hemorrhage, and lower mortality. As a result, VKAs will most likely be replaced in a majority of patients for these indications. Interventional LAA closure might be considered in AF patients at high risk for stroke for whom a long-term OAC is contraindicated; however, long-term data following device implantation are few. Advances in risk stratification are expected, especially related to silent AF and biomarkers that predict development of AF and development of stroke in those with AF. A key area for discovery will be to learn whether ablation for AF can ultimately reduce stroke and in which situations.

REFERENCES

1. Wolf PA, Abbott RD, Kannel WB. Atrial fibrillation as an independent risk factor for stroke: the Framingham Study. *Stroke.* 1991;22:983–988.
2. Lin HJ, Wolf PA, Kelly-Hayes M, et al. Stroke severity in atrial fibrillation. The Framingham Study. *Stroke.* 1996;27:1760–1764.
3. Coppens M, Eikelboom JW, Hart RG, et al. The CHA2DS2-VASc score identifies those patients with atrial fibrillation and a CHADS2 score of 1 who are unlikely to benefit from oral anticoagulant therapy. *Eur Heart J.* 2013;34:170–176.
4. Olesen JB, Torp-Pedersen C, Hansen ML, et al. The value of the CHA2DS2-VASc score for refining stroke risk stratification in patients with atrial fibrillation with a CHADS2 score 0-1: a nationwide cohort study. *Thromb Haemost.* 2012;107:1172–1179.
5. Pisters R, Lane DA, Nieuwlaat R, et al. A novel user-friendly score (HAS-BLED) to assess 1-year risk of major bleeding in patients with atrial fibrillation: the Euro Heart Survey. *Chest.* 2010;138:1093–1100.

6. Hart RG, Benavente O, McBride R, et al. Antithrombotic therapy to prevent stroke in patients with atrial fibrillation: a meta-analysis. *Ann Intern Med.* 1999;131:492–501.
7. Olesen JB, Lip GY, Lindhardsen J, et al. Risks of thromboembolism and bleeding with thromboprophylaxis in patients with atrial fibrillation: a net clinical benefit analysis using a 'real world' nationwide cohort study. *Thromb Haemost.* 2011;106:739–749.
8. ACTIVE Writing Group of the ACTIVE Investigators, Connolly S, Pogue J, et al. Clopidogrel plus aspirin versus oral anticoagulation for atrial fibrillation in the Atrial fibrillation Clopidogrel Trial with Irbesartan for prevention of Vascular Events (ACTIVE W): a randomised controlled trial. *Lancet.* 2006;367:1903–1912.
9. ACTIVE Investigators, Connolly SJ, Pogue J, et al. Effect of clopidogrel added to aspirin in patients with atrial fibrillation. *N Engl J Med.* 2009;360:2066–2078.
10. Nieuwlaat R, Capucci A, Lip GY, et al. Antithrombotic treatment in real-life atrial fibrillation patients: a report

from the Euro Heart Survey on Atrial Fibrillation. *Eur Heart J.* 2006;27:3018–3026.
11. Hylek EM, D'Antonio J, Evans-Molina C, et al. Translating the results of randomized trials into clinical practice: the challenge of warfarin candidacy among hospitalized elderly patients with atrial fibrillation. *Stroke.* 2006;37:1075–1080.
12. Waldo AL, Becker RC, Tapson VF, et al. Hospitalized patients with atrial fibrillation and a high risk of stroke are not being provided with adequate anticoagulation. *J Am Coll Cardiol.* 2005;46:1729–1736.
13. Go AS, Hylek EM, Borowsky LH, et al. Warfarin use among ambulatory patients with nonvalvular atrial fibrillation: the anticoagulation and risk factors in atrial fibrillation (ATRIA) study. *Ann Intern Med.* 1999;131:927–934.
14. Baker WL, Cios DA, Sander SD, et al. Meta-analysis to assess the quality of warfarin control in atrial fibrillation patients in the United States. *J Manag Care Pharm.* 2009;15:244–252.

15. Eriksson BI, Quinlan DJ, Weitz JI. Comparative pharmacodynamics and pharmacokinetics of oral direct thrombin and factor Xa inhibitors in development. *Clin Pharmacokinet*. 2009;48:1–22.
16. Connolly SJ, Ezekowitz MD, Yusuf S, et al. Dabigatran versus warfarin in patients with atrial fibrillation. *N Engl J Med*. 2009;361:1139–1151.
17. Camm AJ, Lip GY, De Caterina R, et al. 2012 focused update of the ESC Guidelines for the management of atrial fibrillation: an update of the 2010 ESC Guidelines for the management of atrial fibrillation–developed with the special contribution of the European Heart Rhythm Association. *Europace*. 2012;14:1385–1413.
18. Pollack Jr CV, Reilly PA, Eikelboom J, et al. Idarucizumab for dabigatran reversal. *N Engl J Med*. 2015;373:511–520.
19. Patel MR, Mahaffey KW, Garg J, et al. Rivaroxaban versus warfarin in nonvalvular atrial fibrillation. *N Engl J Med*. 2011;365:883–891.
20. Fox KA, Piccini JP, Wojdyla D, et al. Prevention of stroke and systemic embolism with rivaroxaban compared with warfarin in patients with non-valvular atrial fibrillation and moderate renal impairment. *Eur Heart J*. 2011;32:2387–2394.
21. Eikelboom JW, Weitz JI. New anticoagulants. *Circulation*. 2010;121:1523–1532.
22. Connolly SJ, Eikelboom J, Joyner C, et al. Apixaban in patients with atrial fibrillation. *N Engl J Med*. 2011;364:806–817.
23. Granger CB, Alexander JH, McMurray JJ, et al. Apixaban versus warfarin in patients with atrial fibrillation. *N Engl J Med*. 2011;365:981–992.
24. Ogata K, Mendell-Harary J, Tachibana M, et al. Clinical safety, tolerability, pharmacokinetics, and pharmacodynamics of the novel factor Xa inhibitor edoxaban in healthy volunteers. *J Clin Pharmacol*. 2010;50:743–753.
25. Ansell J. Will the new target-specific oral anticoagulants improve the treatment of venous thromboembolism? *Thromb Haemost*. 2012;107:1009–1011.
26. Giugliano RP, Ruff CT, Braunwald E, et al. Edoxaban versus warfarin in patients with atrial fibrillation. *N Engl J Med*. 2013;369:2093–2104.
27. Ruff CT, Giugliano RP, Braunwald E, et al. Comparison of the efficacy and safety of new oral anticoagulants with warfarin in patients with atrial fibrillation: a meta-analysis of randomised trials. *Lancet*. 2014;383:955–962.
28. January CT, Wann LS, Alpert JS, et al. 2014 AHA/ACC/HRS guideline for the management of patients with atrial fibrillation: executive summary. A report of the American College of Cardiology/American Heart Association Task Force on practice guidelines and the Heart Rhythm Society. *J Am Coll Cardiol*. 2014;64:2246–2280.
29. Verma A, Cairns JA, Mitchell LB, et al. 2014 focused update of the Canadian Cardiovascular Society Guidelines for the management of atrial fibrillation. *Can J Cardiol*. 2014;30:1114–1130.
30. Ezekowitz MD, Parise H, Nagarakanti R, et al. Comparison of dabigatran versus warfarin in patients with atrial fibrillation and valvular heart disease: the RE-LY® trial. *J Am Coll Cardiol*. 2014;63. http://dx.doi.org/10.1016/S0735-1097(14)60325-9.
31. Eikelboom JW, Connolly SJ, Brueckmann M, et al. Dabigatran versus warfarin in patients with mechanical heart valves. *N Engl J Med*. 2013;369:1206–1214.
32. Avezum A, Lopes RD, Schulte PJ, et al. Apixaban in comparison with warfarin in patients with atrial fibrillation and valvular heart disease: findings from the Apixaban for Reduction in Stroke and Other Thromboembolic Events in Atrial Fibrillation (ARISTOTLE) trial. *Circulation*. 2015;132:624–632.
33. Breithardt G, Baumgartner H, Berkowitz SD, et al. Clinical characteristics and outcomes with rivaroxaban vs. warfarin in patients with non-valvular atrial fibrillation but underlying native mitral and aortic valve disease participating in the ROCKET AF trial. *Eur Heart J*. 2014;35:3377–3385.
34. Heidbuchel H, Verhamme P, Alings M, et al. Updated European Heart Rhythm Association practical guide on the use of non-vitamin K antagonist anticoagulants in patients with non-valvular atrial fibrillation. *Europace*. 2015;17:1467–1507.
35. Steinhubl SR, Berger PB, Mann 3rd JT, et al. Early and sustained dual oral antiplatelet therapy following percutaneous coronary intervention: a randomized controlled trial. *JAMA*. 2002;288:2411–2420.
36. Sorensen R, Hansen ML, Abildstrom SZ, et al. Risk of bleeding in patients with acute myocardial infarction treated with different combinations of aspirin, clopidogrel, and vitamin K antagonists in Denmark: a retrospective analysis of nationwide registry data. *Lancet*. 2009;374:1967–1974.
37. Dans AL, Connolly SJ, Wallentin L, et al. Concomitant use of antiplatelet therapy with dabigatran or warfarin in the Randomized Evaluation of Long-Term Anticoagulation Therapy (RE-LY) trial. *Circulation*. 2013;127:634–640.
38. Dewilde WJ, Oirbans T, Verheugt FW, et al. Use of clopidogrel with or without aspirin in patients taking oral anticoagulant therapy and undergoing percutaneous coronary intervention: an open-label, randomised, controlled trial. *Lancet*. 2013;381:1107–1115.
39. King 3rd SB, Smith Jr SC, Hirshfeld Jr JW, et al. 2007 focused update of the ACC/AHA/SCAI 2005 guideline update for percutaneous coronary intervention: a report of the American College of Cardiology/American Heart Association Task Force on practice guidelines. *J Am Coll Cardiol*. 2008;51:172–209.
40. Lip GY, Huber K, Andreotti F, et al. Antithrombotic management of atrial fibrillation patients presenting with acute coronary syndrome and/or undergoing coronary stenting: executive summary–a Consensus Document of the European Society of Cardiology Working Group on Thrombosis, endorsed by the European Heart Rhythm Association (EHRA) and the European Association of Percutaneous Cardiovascular Interventions (EAPCI). *Eur Heart J*. 2010;31:1311–1318.
41. Fuster V, Rydén LE, Cannom DS, et al. ACC/AHA/ESC 2006 guidelines for the management of patients with atrial fibrillation–executive summary: a report of the American College of Cardiology/American Heart Association Task Force on Practice Guidelines and the European Society of Cardiology Committee for Practice Guidelines (Writing Committee to Revise the 2001 Guidelines for the Management of Patients With Atrial Fibrillation). *J Am Coll Cardiol*. 2006;48:854–906.
42. Hylek EM, Evans-Molina C, Shea C, et al. Major hemorrhage and tolerability of warfarin in the first year of therapy among elderly patients with atrial fibrillation. *Circulation*. 2007;115:2689–2696.
43. Pengo V, Cucchini U, Denas G, et al. Lower versus standard intensity oral anticoagulant therapy (OAT) in elderly warfarin-experienced patients with non-valvular atrial fibrillation. *Thromb Haemost*. 2010;103:442–449.
44. Mant J, Hobbs FD, Fletcher K, et al. Warfarin versus aspirin for stroke prevention in an elderly community population with atrial fibrillation (the Birmingham Atrial Fibrillation Treatment of the Aged Study, BAFTA): a randomised controlled trial. *Lancet*. 2007;370:493–503.
45. Rash A, Downes T, Portner R, et al. A randomised controlled trial of warfarin versus aspirin for stroke prevention in octogenarians with atrial fibrillation (WASPO). *Age Ageing*. 2007;36:151–156.
46. Eikelboom JW, Wallentin L, Connolly SJ, et al. Risk of bleeding with 2 doses of dabigatran compared with warfarin in older and younger patients with atrial fibrillation: an analysis of the randomized evaluation of long-term anticoagulant therapy (RE-LY) trial. *Circulation*. 2011;123:2363–2372.
47. Nakai T, Lesh MD, Gerstenfeld EP, et al. Percutaneous left atrial appendage occlusion (PLAATO) for preventing cardioembolism: first experience in canine model. *Circulation*. 2002;105:2217–2222.
48. Klein AL, Grimm RA, Murray RD, et al. Use of transesophageal echocardiography to guide cardioversion in patients with atrial fibrillation. *N Engl J Med*. 2001;344:1411–1420.
49. Gillinov AM. Advances in surgical treatment of atrial fibrillation. *Stroke*. 2007;38:618–623.
50. Salzberg SP, Plass A, Emmert MY, et al. Left atrial appendage clip occlusion: early clinical results. *J Thorac Cardiovasc Surg*. 2010;139:1269–1274.
51. Holmes DR, Reddy VY, Turi ZG, et al. Percutaneous closure of the left atrial appendage versus warfarin therapy for prevention of stroke in patients with atrial fibrillation: a randomised non-inferiority trial. *Lancet*. 2009;374:534–542.
52. Reddy VY, Holmes D, Doshi SK, et al. Safety of percutaneous left atrial appendage closure: results from the Watchman Left Atrial Appendage System for Embolic Protection in Patients with AF (PROTECT AF) clinical trial and the Continued Access Registry. *Circulation*. 2011;123:417–424.
53. Holmes Jr DR, Kar S, Price MJ, et al. Prospective randomized evaluation of the Watchman Left Atrial Appendage Closure device in patients with atrial fibrillation versus long-term warfarin therapy: the PREVAIL trial. *J Am Coll Cardiol*. 2014;64:1–12.
54. Holmes Jr DR, Doshi SK, Kar S, et al. Left atrial appendage closure as an alternative to warfarin for stroke prevention in atrial fibrillation: a patient-level meta-analysis. *J Am Coll Cardiol*. 2015;65:2614–2623.
55. Lown B. Electrical reversion of cardiac arrhythmias. *Br Heart J*. 1967;29:469–489.
56. Bjerkelund CJ, Orning OM. The efficacy of anticoagulant therapy in preventing embolism related to D.C. electrical conversion of atrial fibrillation. *Am J Cardiol*. 1969;23:208–216.
57. Arnold AZ, Mick MJ, Mazurek RP, et al. Role of prophylactic anticoagulation for direct current cardioversion in patients with atrial fibrillation or atrial flutter. *J Am Coll Cardiol*. 1992;19:851–855.
58. Fatkin D, Kuchar DL, Thorburn CW, et al. Transesophageal echocardiography before and during direct current cardioversion of atrial fibrillation: evidence for "atrial stunning" as a mechanism of thromboembolic complications. *J Am Coll Cardiol*. 1994;23:307–316.
59. Antonielli E, Pizzuti A, Bassignana A, et al. Transesophageal echocardiographic evidence of more pronounced left atrial stunning after chemical (propafenone) rather than electrical attempts at cardioversion from atrial fibrillation. *Am J Cardiol*. 1999;84:1092–1096. A9-A10.
60. Falcone RA, Morady F, Armstrong WF. Transesophageal echocardiographic evaluation of left atrial appendage function and spontaneous contrast formation after chemical or electrical cardioversion of atrial fibrillation. *Am J Cardiol*. 1996;78:435–439.
61. European Heart Rhythm Association; European Association for Cardio-Thoracic Surgery, Camm AJ, et al. Guidelines for the management of atrial fibrillation: the Task Force for the Management of Atrial Fibrillation of the European Society of Cardiology (ESC). *Europace*. 2010;12:1360–1420.
62. Fuster V, Ryden LE, Cannom DS, et al. ACC/AHA/ESC 2006 Guidelines for the Management of Patients with Atrial Fibrillation: a report of the American College of Cardiology/American Heart Association Task Force on Practice Guidelines and the European Society of Cardiology Committee for Practice Guidelines (Writing Committee to Revise the 2001 Guidelines for the Management of Patients With Atrial Fibrillation): developed in collaboration with the European Heart Rhythm Association and the Heart Rhythm Society. *Circulation*. 2006;114:e257–e354.
63. Weigner MJ, Caulfield TA, Danias PG, et al. Risk for clinical thromboembolism associated with conversion to sinus rhythm in patients with atrial fibrillation lasting less than 48 hours. *Ann Intern Med*. 1997;126:615–620.
64. Gallagher MM, Hennessy BJ, Edvardsson N, et al. Embolic complications of direct current cardioversion of atrial arrhythmias: association with low intensity of anticoagulation at the time of cardioversion. *J Am Coll Cardiol*. 2002;40:926–933.
65. Stellbrink C, Nixdorff U, Hofmann T, et al. Safety and efficacy of enoxaparin compared with unfractionated heparin and oral anticoagulants for prevention of thromboembolic complications in cardioversion of nonvalvular atrial fibrillation: the Anticoagulation in Cardioversion using Enoxaparin (ACE) trial. *Circulation*. 2004;109:997–1003.
66. Nagarakanti R, Ezekowitz MD, Oldgren J, et al. Dabigatran versus warfarin in patients with atrial fibrillation: an analysis of patients undergoing cardioversion. *Circulation*. 2011;123:131–136.
67. Piccini JP, Stevens SR, Lokhnygina Y, et al. Outcomes after cardioversion and atrial fibrillation ablation in patients treated with rivaroxaban and warfarin in the ROCKET AF trial. *J Am Coll Cardiol*. 2013;61:1998–2006.
68. Flaker G, Lopes RD, Al-Khatib SM, et al. Efficacy and safety of apixaban in patients after cardioversion for atrial fibrillation: insights from the ARISTOTLE Trial (Apixaban for Reduction in Stroke and Other Thromboembolic Events in Atrial Fibrillation). *J Am Coll Cardiol*. 2014;63:1082–1087.
69. Cappato R, Ezekowitz MD, Klein AL, et al. Rivaroxaban vs. vitamin K antagonists for cardioversion in atrial fibrillation. *Eur Heart J*. 2014;35:3346–3355.

116 Implantable Cardioverter Defibrillators: Technical Aspects

Mohamed H. Kanj and Bruce L. Wilkoff

Implantable cardioverter defibrillators (ICDs) have revolutionized the treatment of malignant ventricular arrhythmias. The basic functions include tachycardia detection and tachycardia termination. The ICD relies on a very complex series of steps, including sensing of myocardial potentials, delivering these signals to the ICD circuit board to be filtered and analyzed, and then delivering life-saving therapies back to the heart. This chapter outlines the technical aspects of these life-saving devices, including those of the ICD's programmer, diagnostic information, and radiofrequency telemetry.

System Elements

The physical components of an implanted system consist of the ICD generator, the pacing and sensing electrodes, and one or more high-energy electrodes. The titanium casing of the ICD generator usually constitutes one of the high-energy electrodes. The electrodes or leads attach to the generator header through sealed connectors. Until recently the ICD leads were all divided into two or three 3.2-mm diameter terminal connectors, one bipolar IS-1 (bradycardia) and one or two DF-1 (high energy) connectors that are inserted into the ICD generator header. Now a fully approved (March 15, 2010) International Organization for Standardization (ISO) standard (ISO 27186) implemented by several manufacturers is the DF-4 connector standard that is also 3.2 mm in diameter but integrates the three functions into a single connector for both low-energy (pacing and sensing) and high-energy (shocking) electrode functions. The older IS-1/DF-1 lead design is bulky in the device pocket and adds to the length of the lead. In addition, the trifurcation/bifurcation of the lead also creates the potential for errors in making connections to the header. A similarly constructed (IS-4) connection standard is also implemented for quadrupolar low-voltage leads. Currently this is implemented only for left ventricular (LV) cardiac venous leads and permits noninvasive programming of the pacing vectors after the incision is closed. The IS-4 for LV leads and DF-4 for ICD leads are similar but distinct enough to not allow connection errors to the header (Fig. 116.1).

The DF-4 connector design provides a single set screw that secures on the terminal pin of the lead with spring contacts for the ring and defibrillation electrodes. Inside the DF-4 connector, there are double sealing rings between the electrodes to secure good isolation between the high- and low-voltage electrode contacts. These sealing rings have been moved from the lead to the connector block to prevent any damage that may occur during lead implantation.

The advantages of the DF-4 design include quicker connections to the ICD because of the single terminal pin, improved patient comfort/satisfaction, and easier reoperations with decreased debridement due to a shorter and less complex lead body in the pocket. The risk for procedural errors, including loose or stripped set screws and port mismatch (switching RV DF-1 and SVC DF-1 pins in the header) should decrease. Subcutaneous tunneling (submammary implant) may be easier as well.

The potential limitations of this lead design are initially the lack of adapters to modify the lead system to include additional high- or low-voltage leads. These are sometimes required for high defibrillation threshold (DFT) patients and include the subclavian, subcutaneous, and azygos veins or coronary sinus coils. As with any change there are potential unidentified reliability risks, but this development was carefully designed and tested over a decade of research and now has been in the market for over 5 years.

Implantable Cardioverter Defibrillator Generator

ICD generators have decreased significantly in size because of the significant advancements in battery and microprocessor technologies. Most of the volume of current ICDs is occupied by its battery and capacitors. The newest generations of devices have added device-initiated long-range telemetry device interrogation, automatic alert notifications, and bioimpedance measurement capability along with other advanced features.

Current devices provide all these options with a generator size of about 30 cm^3 in volume. The ICD generator casing is made of electrically active titanium, considered to be the preferred material because of its conductivity, strength, biocompatibility, corrosion resistance, and light weight. The casing not only serves mainly to protect the circuitry from the corrosive effects of body fluids but also serves as an active high-voltage electrode in many current ICD models. Some devices have a Parylene coating as a protective barrier to reduce friction between the lead and ICD can. Bench studies reported a six-fold reduction in friction with the use of this coating, but clinical human data are lacking on whether this will decrease the incidence of ICD lead failures, which is relevant particularly in Silastic insulated leads.

The header is generally made of a clear material, polymethylmethacrylate, so that the connections with the leads can be visually confirmed during implantation and can be inspected if ICD

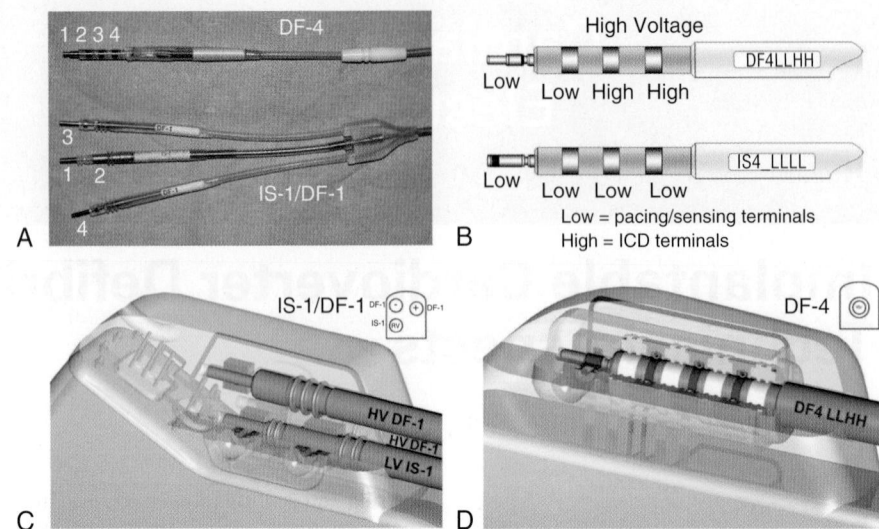

FIGURE 116.1 DF-4/IS-4 lead design. (A) The DF-4 lead design eliminates the yoke and the redundant lead furcation seen in the IS-1/DF-1 design. 1, Distal pace/sense electrode contact; 2, proximal pace/sense electrode contact; 3, distal DF-1 coil electrode contact; and 4, proximal DF-1 coil electrode contact. (B) The IS-4 lead design is similar to the DF-4 lead design except that all electrodes are pace/sense low-voltage electrodes. (C) The IS-1/DF-1 lead connector has three set screws with the sealing rings built on the lead. (D) The DF-4/IS-4 connector has a single set screw that secures on the tip of the lead with spring contacts for the ring and DF electrodes. Inside the DF-4 connector, there are double sealing rings (*blue*) between the electrodes to secure good isolation between the high- and low-voltage electrode insulation. *ICD,* Implantable cardioverter defibrillator.

system troubleshooting is required for component malfunction or suspicion of failure. The lead connections gain access to the ICD circuitry through feedthrough wires, which penetrate the casing through sealed openings.

The interior of the ICD consists of one or more batteries, capacitors, a DC-DC converter, hybrid with a microprocessor, telemetry communication coil, and their connections. The sensed ventricular signals, generally 5–25 mV in amplitude, enter the generator through the leads, are filtered, and then are analyzed by the algorithms programmed into the hybrid. The hybrid consists of electronic circuitry embedded in a silicon wafer, specifically designed for the analysis of these signals and identification of either tachycardia or fibrillation. Once the detection criteria are met, the specifically programmed pacing and high-energy shock therapies are then delivered to the patient.

Battery

Unlike other batteries, ICD batteries have many performance requirements. Besides its compact size, the battery must be capable of charging the capacitors by delivering high-energy currents of approximately 75 amperes to charge the capacitors within seconds and must have a low current drain in the order of milliamperes. Factors affecting the current drain include pacing and defibrillation needs and the quiescent current needed for ongoing tasks such as powering the hybrid, monitoring intrinsic rhythm, and logging the data in the memory. Additionally, the battery performance over time must be predictable to allow for adequate warnings before it is depleted.

The battery used by many current ICD generators is a lithium silver vanadium oxide (Li/SVO) cell. There are two kinds of Li/SVO batteries, anode-limited (Li) and cathode-limited (SVO) batteries. Anode-limited (Li) batteries have two voltage plateaus: a very early short-lived one followed by a later long-lived one. Current ICD batteries are often cathode-limited (SVO) batteries and carry a charge between 1000 and 2000 mA·h at their beginning of life (BOL). This generates approximately 3.2 V at full charge. At middle of life (MOL), these batteries suffer from

inherent internal impedance buildup, resulting from the accumulation of a film on the Li electrode. Although this may result in a prolonged charge time, pulsing the battery frequently by charging the capacitors is usually sufficient to prevent this phenomenon.

The battery status is generally estimated by its measured output voltage. With a significant decline in open-circuit voltage and a rise in internal resistance, the ability to deliver adequate current to charge the capacitors becomes impaired, causing a significant prolongation in charge time. This is called the elective replacement indicator (ERI) or recommended replacement time (RRT). Once the ERI is reached, generator replacement can be electively scheduled, usually within 3 months, depending on the frequency of therapy (which determines the depletion rate). A later indicator, end of life (EOL), reflects a significantly lower voltage and indicates a more urgent need for generator replacement because of the associated long capacitor charge times required to achieve an appropriate shock energy. In addition to voltage criteria, the time required to charge the capacitors to full energy is also used as a measurement of the battery status and may activate the ERI. In certain devices, charging the capacitors stops after 20 seconds and delivers the stored energy as shock therapy. When these devices reach the ERI, the stored energy may be significantly less than the programmed energy.

Newer ICDs have incorporated newer battery technologies to improve battery performance and longevity. Balancing the cell to an appropriate electron reduction slows the progression of internal battery impedance over time. Additionally, the development of hybrid cathode batteries (Li/SVO blended with carbon monofluoride: Li/CFx-SVO) as well as lithium manganese dioxide (LiMnO2) have improved service life and resulted in a stable charge time throughout the lifetime of the battery. In addition, LiMnO2 batteries have no midlife impedance rise and stable voltage during the lifetime of the device, with a slow gradual decay toward the ERI independent of the rate of energy use. Significant work has been done to optimize device efficiency in an effort to decrease the current drain needed for daily operation of the device, memory management telemetry, and remote monitoring.

Capacitors

The rate of energy delivery for cardiac defibrillation is much greater than can be delivered directly from ICD batteries. Hence, capacitors are used to store the energy over a longer period of time (seconds) and deliver it over a shorter period of time (milliseconds). Capacitors are measured by their capacitance (C) which is a measure of the amount of electrical charge that the capacitor can store for a given voltage. Multiple capacitors are charged in a parallel configuration by the battery through a DC-DC converter, and then are connected in series to be able to deliver the stored energy (30–80 J) but at high voltages (up to 890 V) within 10–20 milliseconds. The rate with which the capacitor is being charged depends on its capacitance (C) and the internal impedances of the battery and the circuitry. However, the rate with which the capacitor delivers its charge to the patient depends on its capacitance and the lead/body impedance.

To achieve a high stored charge, current ICDs incorporate new designs such as the use of multiple capacitors in series and the use of capacitors with convoluted surfaces to increase surface area. Most capacitors used in the ICD industry are aluminum and tantalum electrolytic capacitors because of their ability to charge within the prescribed time limitations. With time, the dielectric layers in these capacitors become deformed, causing current to flow through them ("capacitor leak"). This will result in a suboptimal charge and prolonged charge time. Capacitor reformation, where the capacitors are discharged through high-impedance circuitry to allow for a longer discharge time, will usually regenerate the dielectric layer and fix the leak.

Electrodes

There are three essential functions of defibrillator systems: (1) detection of the tachycardia, (2) pacing stimulation of the heart, and (3) shock stimulation of the heart. The electrodes are the noninsulated segments of the leads that deliver these functions. The technology used for detection (sensing) and pacing is similar to that used by pacemakers. However, the bipole for sensing and pacing is sometimes from the tip of the ventricular lead to the distal shocking electrode instead of from the tip to the ring electrode. This is called an integrated bipolar system instead of a true bipolar system.

High-voltage coil electrodes are ideal for high-energy shocks. The lower impedance of the coils and the conductor cables to the coils permit a high-current charge discharge from the capacitors. In addition, their wide surface area creates a broader electrical field that may enable the defibrillation of more myocardial mass and reduce the current density near the coil. To better distribute the current drain along the length of the coil, the proximal and distal ends of each coil are sometimes connected via a shunt wire.

Nonthoracotomy or Transvenous Leads

Nonthoracotomy ICD leads (NTLs) were designed to carry high defibrillation energy to the inside of the heart. They can have a dedicated proximal sensing/pacing ring electrode (true bipolar) or utilize the distal high-voltage shocking coil as the proximal sensing/pacing electrode (integrated bipolar). True bipolar leads often offer better discrimination for sensing, being less susceptible to far-field oversensing and postshock undersensing. The latter is due to the remoteness of the distal coil from the distal electrode. They often have better pacing performance as well, due to lower current drain and being less susceptible to postshock loss-of-capture. On the other hand, integrated bipolar leads may offer better defibrillation performance due to the shorter tip to distal coil distance. In an individual patient, programming from one to the other configuration may avoid the need for a new lead system surgery.

NTLs can have one right ventricular (single-coil) or two (dual-coil) high-voltage shocking electrode(s). The distal coil is usually placed in the right ventricular apex or along the RV septum and the proximal coil in the superior vena cava. The effect of a dual-coil ICD lead on the DFT is multifactorial. It changes the shock vector; it lowers high-voltage shock impedance and therefore results in shortening the shock waveform duration. Although dual-coil ICD lead systems have predominated in the United States and Europe, their clinical superiority over the single-coil lead system is not well established. Defibrillation efficiency is slightly improved, usually by 1–3 joules.[1] This may be justified in patients with anticipated high DFTs. However, this potential benefit needs to be weighed against the added complexity of the lead construction and its potential effect on lead reliability as well as the potential for more complex extraction when needed. Additionally, a low right atrial position of the proximal coil, in the case of a severely enlarged right ventricle, may in fact increase the DFT by the negative current vector effect. In other patients, there may be a need to implant other coils (a coronary sinus, middle cardiac vein, subcutaneous, or azygos coil) when maximal shocks are ineffective and are almost always more effective in reducing the required defibrillation energy by 5–15 joules.[2]

ICD leads are designed with either coaxial or multilumen constructions. A coaxial design, where layered conductors are separated by layers of polyurethane insulation material, was formerly used in some of the original designs. This was associated with insulation failure due to metal ion oxidation of the middle polyurethane insulation layer, identical to that seen in coaxial polyurethane pacemaker leads in the Medtronic Transvene family of leads. Clinically, this manifested as low stimulation impedance and under- and oversensing. Current ICD leads employ multilumen construction designs, where conductors run in parallel through a single insulating body. This design has allowed these leads to be more resistant to this mode of failure and thinner. However, some variations of this design have been the subject of other failure mechanisms, such as in the cases of Sprint Fidelis (Medtronic) and Riata leads (St. Jude Medical). In this multiluminal configuration, the conductor of the distal pace/sense electrode is a coil conductor, while the rest are cable conductors. Although the latter are more resistant to mechanical stress, coil conductors are still needed to allow the stylet to go through the lead.

To insulate these conductors, manufacturers use a combination of insulators: silicone, polyurethane, fluoropolymers, and silicone-polyurethane copolymers. Silicone has the best biostability characteristics but it lacks tensile strength and tear resistance, making it flimsy and prone to abrasions, and has a high coefficient of friction, complicating implantation. Polyurethane, on the other hand, has excellent tensile strength and a lower coefficient of friction; however, it has poor biostability and is prone to degradation, including environmental stress cracking and metal ion oxidation. Instead, a thin layer of Teflon-like fluoropolymer (ethylene tetrafluoroethylene [ETFE] or polytetrafluoroethylene [PTFE]) is often used to coat the conductors to prevent corrosion. However, this increases the stiffness of the lead and does not have strong physical characteristics. Recently, a silicone-polyurethane copolymer (Optim, St. Jude Medical) has been used as a component of the insulation. Bench studies of this copolymer showed that it exhibits the biostability and flexibility of silicone and the durability and abrasion resistance and low friction coefficient of polyurethane.[3]

Currently available leads either have silicone insulation backfilling in between and behind the metal defibrillation coils or have a flat wire coil technology to decrease tissue ingrowth. Alternatively, the coils have been covered with expanded PTFE (Gore ePTFE). This ePTFE coating is slippery, permits the defibrillation current to be transmitted, and prevents tissue ingrowth and an inflammatory fibrous reaction. These techniques may result in easier lead extraction.

TABLE 116.1 Summary of the characteristics of currently available nonthoracotomy leads

MANUFACTURER	MODEL	CONDUCTORS PACE:SENSE/COIL	ELECTRODES PACE:SENSE/COIL	NO. OF COILS	SENSING CONFIGURATION
Boston Scientific/Guidant, St. Paul, MN	All	MP35N/DBS	Pt-Ir/Pt-coated titanium	1 or 2	Integrated bipolar
Medtronic, St. Paul, MN	Sprint Fidelis	MP35N/MP35N	TN-Pt-Ir/Pt-clad tantalum	1 or 2	True bipolar
Medtronic	Quattro	MP35N/MP35N-Ag	Pt-Ir/Pt-Ir-clad tantalum	2	True bipolar
Medtronic	All others	MP35N/MP35N-Ag	Pr-Ir/Pt-Ir	1 or 2	True or integrated bipolar
St. Jude Medical, Sylmar, CA	Riata/TVL-ADX	MP35N/MP35N	TN-Pt-Ir/Pt-Ir	1 or 2	True bipolar
St. Jude Medical	Optisure/Durata	MP35N/MP35N	TN-Pt-Ir/Pt-Ir	1 or 2	True bipolar
St. Jude Medical	All others	MP35N/MP35N	Pt-Ir/Pt-Ir	1 or 2	Integrated bipolar
Biotronik, Portland, OR	Linox	MP35N/MP35N	Pt-Ir-Fr/Pt-Ir-Fr	1 or 2	True bipolar
Biotronik	Kentrox	MP35N/MP35N	Pt-Ir-Fr/Pt-Ir-Fr	1 or 2	Integrated bipolar
Sorin, Plymouth, MN	Swift	MP35N/MP35N-Ag	Pr-Ir/Pt-Ir	1	Integrated bipolar

DBS, Drawn brazed strand cable; *MP35N,* cobalt-chrome-nickel alloy; *MP35N-Ag,* cobalt-chrome-nickel alloy with a silver core; *Pt-Ir,* platinum-iridium alloy; *Pt-Ir-Fr,* platinum-iridium fractal-coated; *TN-Pt-Ir,* titanium nitride-coated iridium alloy.

Invariably, NTLs have a high-energy coil located near the distal end and lying within the right ventricular cavity. Manufacturers have released NTLs with similar constructions, although some details differ (Table 116.1). The physics of DC current flow, however, requires at least one other electrode to complete the shocking circuit. The development of smaller ICD generators has allowed for pectoral implantation, which has enabled the use of the generator casing as the second electrode (i.e., a "hot can"). An animal study compared the defibrillation efficacy of a hot can ICD system placed in a left pectoral or subaxillary location with right pectoral and left or right abdominal locations. The left pectoral and axillary subcutaneous positions were superior to all other locations. The right pectoral location was superior to both abdominal locations. These results imply that alternative ICD implantation sites are feasible in the event of inability to implant a left prepectoral device because of left subclavian venous occlusion, history of left mastectomy/radiation, left-sided arteriovenous fistula, or other reasons to avoid the left prepectoral area.

Tachyarrhythmia Detection

The recognition of tachyarrhythmias by an ICD is a complex interaction of several dependent variables. However, the task of the ICD is more complicated because it must also recognize the lack of tachyarrhythmias. This central insight is crucial because the patient will spend all but a small fraction of his or her life in a nontachycardic rhythm. Therefore assuming the efficacy of the pacing and shock therapies, rhythm recognition arbitrates between the quality and length of life.

Not all of the factors required for accurate rhythm recognition are potentially affected by ICD technology. Most notably, the rate and mechanism of the arrhythmia and the programming of the ICD are major determinants of rhythm recognition and are factors that are almost completely independent of the technological solution. However, by understanding the nature of the signals presented to the ICD, allowing the ICD to adapt to these signals, and limiting programming options, appropriate ICD function is frequently achieved.

Sensing

All current ICDs use ventricular heart rate as the cornerstone variable in tachycardia recognition. However, to determine heart rate, the interval between each depolarization of the ventricle must be measured. It is not interval recognition but the detection of individual electrogram events that becomes the basic building block in this process. The process begins with the placement of the sensing lead. The sensed electrogram depends on the health of the myocardium in close proximity to the lead, the far-field structures of the diaphragm, anterior chest wall, and right atrium, and other electrical devices such as pacemakers, cellular phones, and other sources of electromagnetic interference. Detection of the electrogram events is completely dependent on the quality of the signal, and the quality of the signal is determined primarily at the time of the lead placement. Additional aspects potentially dependent on the position of the lead are measures of electrogram morphology such as electrogram event width.

In dual-chamber devices, the accurate recognition of arrhythmias adds another layer of complexity and hopefully specificity with the inclusion of atrial lead data input into the generator. The intracardiac location of the atrial lead (far away from the annulus to minimize the far-field right ventricular signal) and a short interelectrode distance between the distal and proximal electrodes improve the signal-to-noise ratio of the sensed atrial signal and may thus improve the accuracy of the data used for tachycardia discrimination.

Band-Pass Filtering

The sense amplifier processes signals presented to the pulse generator by the sensing electrodes and allows signals of certain frequencies to be presented to the detection logic, whereas others are filtered out. This band-pass filter consists of a high-frequency cutoff to filter out myopotential signals and a low-frequency cutoff to filter out repolarization T wave signals. The midrange is intended to represent a band of frequency containing true signal events. The intent is to prevent extraneous signals from fooling the device into falsely detecting tachyarrhythmias. Unfortunately, there is some frequency overlap between repolarization and depolarization waves, atrial and ventricular events, postpacing polarization and depolarization of the ventricles, myopotentials, cardiac depolarizations, and environmental signals and cardiac events.

Frequency and Amplitude

Both a large signal amplitude and high-frequency content improve the chances of the signal being detected. In addition, there is a strong relation between the amplitude of the signal presented to the band-pass filter and the frequencies contained within that signal. Larger signals usually improve the specificity of electrogram event detection by placing the frequency content into the center frequencies of the band-pass filter. However, a signal that is relatively small, such as 4–6 mV, but has good frequency content as represented by the slow rate measured on the pacing system analyzer of more than 1 V/s will probably do better than a larger signal such as 8–10 mV with a much poorer frequency content of less than 0.1 V/s.

Autogain and Autothreshold

One of the larger challenges present in ICD detection algorithms is the marked variability in the amplitudes of the signals presented to the ventricular lead: naturally conducted beats through the His-Purkinje system are 5–25 mV, paced amplitudes are 5000 mV with a polarization voltage after each pacer spike, premature ventricular contractions and ventricular tachycardia (VT) amplitudes range from 2 to 25 mV, asystolic electrogram amplitudes are 0–0.15 mV, and ventricular fibrillation (VF) amplitudes range from 0.2 to 20 mV. The transitions between each of the rhythms must be accurately identified.

The most difficult problems are distinguishing frequent excursions from low to high and back to low amplitude electrogram events. The two approaches are the use of autogain and autothreshold. The autogain technique uses fixed-amplitude voltage thresholds and amplifies the signal at continually varying gains according to various algorithms to single-count both small and large signals. The autothreshold technique uses one amplifier gain and a continuously varying threshold to accomplish the same end. Usually, the threshold will vary within a single cycle, decaying after each sensed event after an adjustment proportional to the amplitude of the signal. Sometimes the floor or minimum voltage limit can be programmed to distinguish between noise in the signal and low-amplitude VF signals. After a paced beat, the autogain is set to the maximum, and the autothreshold is set to the minimum. In some devices, a time delay for the threshold to initiate its decay can be programmed to reduce the detection of a large T wave from being misidentified as a second R wave.

Estimation of Adequate Amplitude

The ventricular sensing electrode is placed during a nontachycardic rhythm. Therefore the adequacy of that placement must be determined before the VF is induced for defibrillation adequacy testing. Although there is marked variability in the average electrogram event amplitude between VF episodes and within a single VF episode, there are relations between the amplitude of the sinus rhythm electrogram amplitude and the average, minimum, and maximum VF electrogram events of subsequently induced arrhythmias. As an estimate of adequacy, sinus rhythm electrograms of at least 5 mV reliably predict that less than 10% of the electrogram events will be undersensed and that failure of tachyarrhythmia detection is eliminated.

Detection Algorithms

Once an electrogram event is marked or detected, the detection algorithm interprets the pattern of the intervals between the events. The algorithms attempt to develop a hierarchy of detected rhythms that require different therapies such as bradycardia, VT requiring antitachycardia pacing (ATP), VT requiring low-energy shocks, and VF requiring higher-energy shocks. The exclusion of sinus tachycardia and atrial fibrillation with overlapping rates from ventricular arrhythmias is particularly difficult. Added to the ventricular rate criterion is the duration of the arrhythmia, the acuteness of the increase in rate, and the beat-to-beat variation in the cycle length to distinguish these rhythms. Derivatives of the electrogram morphology include templates, duration, and vector correlations, and with the addition of an atrial electrode, the pattern of the relation between the atrial and ventricular events has more recently improved the specificity of arrhythmia detection.

Sensitivity Versus Specificity (Discriminating Supraventricular From Ventricular Arrhythmias)

Life-threatening arrhythmias must always be detected and terminated. However, an arrhythmia's mechanism, rate, or both do not always correlate with its hemodynamic significance. Atrial flutter with 1:1 atrioventricular (AV) conduction or monomorphic VT at 110 beats/min could result in hemodynamic collapse. The lower the rate cutoff, the greater the sensitivity, but the poorer the specificity for truly life-threatening situations. The challenge is to use the algorithms to avoid the delivery of inappropriate therapy so that the ICD is better tolerated and contributes to an improved quality of life.

Rate and Duration

The primary characteristics of ventricular arrhythmias requiring treatment are the rate and duration of the arrhythmia. Slow or nonsustained arrhythmias do not require therapy. However, the negative consequence of waiting to see if an arrhythmia is going to end without an intervention from the ICD increases with rapid rates. The possibility that failure to detect low-amplitude electrogram events will cause a delay or prevent detection is also a serious issue. Consequently, the faster the rhythm, the shorter the duration that should be required for detection. Arrhythmia rates are measured by measuring the beat-to-beat interval and then classified as VT or VF. The duration of the arrhythmia is then measured by the number of intervals to detect (NID) or the length of time to detect (seconds). For VT detection, consecutive intervals faster than the programmed rate provide an effective algorithm. However, for VF, a probabilistic NID counter where X short cycle length intervals out of a larger number of Y consecutive intervals is more sensitive because of the marked variability of electrogram amplitudes and intervals during VF.

Sudden Onset

Reentrant VT and some not clearly reentrant arrhythmias start at a rapid rate, which is usually distinct from the preceding nontachycardic rhythm. The sudden shortening of the cycle length is a factor that is somewhat useful in differentiating sinus tachycardia from slow VT. The best criterion for preventing VT detection during sinus tachycardia is programming a more rapid VT detection rate; however, when that is not possible there is some, but limited, value in using sudden onset. Unfortunately, using this approach increases the risk that the arrhythmia will not be treated if the VT arises in the setting of sinus tachycardia or exercise. In addition, this discriminator might inhibit therapies for VT that started below the programmed detection rate even when it accelerates beyond the programmed detection rate.

Cycle Length Stability

Most VTs, in distinction from the ventricular response in atrial fibrillation, have a stable cycle length with little beat-to-beat variation (<40 msec) in the interval. Unfortunately, this is not always the case, but when the ventricular response is rapid during relatively infrequent episodes of atrial fibrillation, this can be an effective tool. If there is continuous atrial fibrillation or frequent paroxysmal episodes, especially in the setting of a slow VT that also needs treatment, then AV junctional ablation with a rate-responsive pacemaker mode is a better choice.

Morphology and QRS Width

Electrogram width measurements, morphology criteria, and most recently, morphology template matching and vector correlation techniques have been used to enhance the quickness and specificity of tachycardia detection with some success. The digital image of every tachycardia electrogram is compared to a presaved template of the baseline rhythm. Although very helpful, this discriminator is limited by multiple scenarios including physiological rate-dependent changes in electrogram morphology and truncation and alignment errors in the digitalization process.

Atrial Lead Criteria

With placement of an atrial lead, the relation of atrial activity to ventricular activity is available for analysis. If the data are accurate, with the caveats mentioned earlier concerning far-field signals, then AV dissociation during a rapid ventricular rhythm makes the diagnosis of VT certain. The same is true when the ventricular rate is faster than the atrial rate.

However, if there is a 1:1 relation, the chance that the rhythm is VT or supraventricular tachycardia (SVT) is dependent on the ratio of the durations of the AV to the ventriculoatrial (VA) interval. Unfortunately, it is still possible to have atrial tachyarrhythmia and ventricular tachycardia at the same time. Newer device algorithms track the position and sequence of the sensed atrial signal (P wave) among consecutive sensed ventricular signals (R waves). Atrial tachycardias are usually long RP tachycardias and thus are diagnosed when the P wave falls in the distal half of the RR interval. Junctional and AV nodal atrial tachycardias are very short RP tachycardias and thus are diagnosed when the P wave falls immediately before or after an R wave. P waves falling in the proximal half of the RR interval are considered retrograde and thus support the diagnosis of VT.

Other devices continuously monitor the average PP, RR, and PR intervals and use this information for analysis of the tachycardia rhythm. For example, a stable PR (PR association) interval when the RR interval is unstable suggests that the ventricle is being driven by the atrium and thus the arrhythmia is SVT. Monotonous change in the PR interval (progressive increase or decrease in the PR interval) suggests AV dissociation and thus VT.

The origin of acceleration (comparing consecutive PP and RR intervals) is also used in differentiating SVT from VT. In the end, the ICD uses all the input from all of the above criteria as well as others in a multistep algorithm to help differentiate SVT from VT.

Atrial leads reduce the incidence, but will not prevent inappropriate therapy because all algorithms are biased so that VF is rarely, if ever, missed. In one study, the addition of an atrial lead significantly decreased the rate of inappropriate SVT detection (as VT) and the rate of inappropriate therapy delivery but it did not decrease the rate of ICD shock, but this is not a consistent finding.[4]

Some devices would allow delivery of therapy after a programmed duration even if the discriminators suggest a SVT. This provides treatment of potentially hemodynamically significant SVTs and improves the chances that misdiagnosed life-threatening ventricular arrhythmias will receive therapy ("sustained rate duration," "high rate timeout"). Newer devices will allow different programmability settings for the different VT and VF zones.

Confirmation and Redetection and Reconfirmation

Detection of tachycardia, like any other test, follows Bayesian statistics. The probability of a truly positive result is directly proportional to the prevalence of the condition in the population being treated. Once a rhythm has been detected with rigorous criteria and treated, it is likely that a rhythm that meets the rate criteria will need to be treated again, and quickly, to prevent syncope.

Confirmation is the process whereby the ICD confirms that the ventricular arrhythmia is present after the delivery of ATP or before the first high-voltage shock. After ventricular arrhythmia detection is met, it takes time to charge the ICD capacitors, during which time the arrhythmia may have terminated. For this reason, before the delivery of therapy, confirmation of the tachycardia is required to prevent shocks when treating patients with nonsustained tachycardia during sinus rhythm. The danger is that the autogain or autothreshold algorithm has failed to pick up very low amplitude VF during progressive hemodynamic collapse. Thus confirmation of rhythms in the VF zone should be used with care. Some devices permit the allocation of committed and noncommitted shocks in VF or VT and VF rate zones. In most devices, confirmation applies only to the first therapy; the rest of the therapies are committed therapies and no reconfirmation is needed.

Redetection is the process in which the ICD examines whether the programmed therapy was effective in terminating the presenting arrhythmia. In most ICDs, the SVT-VT discriminators are not applied during this process and redetection is based solely on the programmed rate cutoff. The quickness and sensitivity of arrhythmia algorithms are enhanced during "redetection" by reducing the number of intervals required and by eliminating additional criteria.

Tachyarrhythmia Therapy

Pacing Therapy

All transvenous ICDs provide for bradycardia support with single-, dual-, or triple-chamber stimulation; however, the subcutaneous defibrillator only provides temporary postshock cardiac stimulation. The pacing mode, rate, and stimulation output are often separately programmable after a high-energy shock for a period to provide overdrive suppression of arrhythmias. Although many patients with ICDs receive dual-chambered rate-adaptive pacemakers, a small minority of these patients has an indication or need for pacing. The Dual Chamber and VVI Implantable Defibrillator (DAVID) trial examined the effect of pacing in the DDDR mode compared with ventricular backup pacing in patients who had an ICD but no pacing indications. In these patients, DDDR pacing increased the combined end point of hospitalization for congestive heart failure (CHF) or death.[5] In the DAVID-II trial, atrial support pacing at AAI-70 was tested and showed no significant improvement in quality-of-life outcomes compared with VVI-40.[6] Thus patients without clear indications for antibradycardia pacing should be set to ventricular backup pacing. In patients with wide QRS durations and New York Heart Association functional class III or IV CHF, biventricular stimulation is appropriate. This therapy may also be applied in patients with less severe CHF or the need for antibradycardia pacing.[7]

In addition, ATP is available in all of the current transvenous ICDs, but not in a subcutaneous defibrillator. This therapy consists of the delivery of a short burst of ventricular pacing at a (programmable) rate faster than the detected VT rate. A variety of ATP techniques are available, and their effectiveness has been demonstrated to be 90% and 72% in terminating slower and fast VTs, respectively. Its effectiveness was 95% when the testing of the ATP modality was performed prior to discharge. ATP was also effective in terminating SVTs for which patients would have received a shock.

A drawback to ATP in some patients is the potential for acceleration of the tachycardia to greater rates or to VF so that high-energy shocks are required. Although 4% of patients experience acceleration of the tachycardia from ATP, this was not associated with any increase in mortality or the incidence of syncopal events.[7,8] Compared with shock therapy, ATP can be delivered with no delay

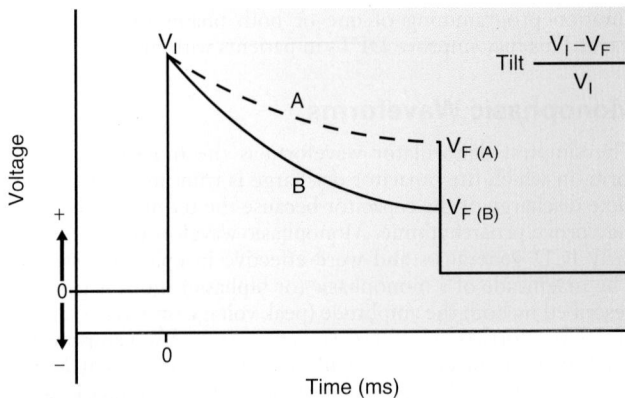

FIGURE 116.2 The monophasic waveform is created by truncation of the capacitor discharge and is the simplest implantable cardioverter defibrillator waveform. The initial voltage (V_I) is dependent on the charge placed on the capacitor. The waveform is truncated after a variable duration (depending on the manufacturer) when a certain final voltage (V_F) is reached. The rate of voltage decay (tilt) is inversely proportional to both the impedance of the lead system and the total capacitance of the implantable cardioverter defibrillator. Tilt is calculated according to the formula given such that waveform A demonstrates a lower tilt than waveform B.

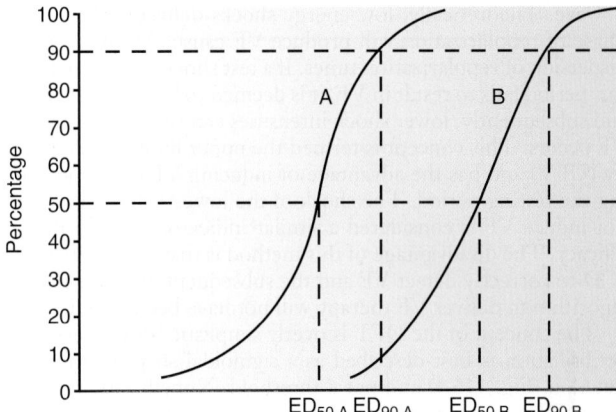

FIGURE 116.3 The graph shows the relation between the probability of successful defibrillation and the intensity of the shock—that is, the greater the shock intensity, the higher the probability of success. The ED_{50} and ED_{90} refer to the shock intensities that result in successful defibrillation 50% and 90% of the time, respectively. In the examples given, curves A and B represent waveforms A and B with different defibrillation efficacies. Waveform A shows a greater efficacy (lower ED_{50} and ED_{90}) than waveform B.

from the detection of the tachycardia (no capacitor to charge), with less morbidity (pain and ventricular stunning), and less battery usage. Once ATP therapy fails to terminate the tachyarrhythmia, shock therapy is delivered. In fact, in the EMPIRIC trial, standardized prespecified ICD programming with ATP during slow and fast VT was at least as effective as physician-tailored programming without an increase in mortality or shock-related morbidity.[8]

ATP therapy could be delivered before or while the capacitors are changing. The main advantage of attempting ATP therapy before charging is to reduce unnecessary capacitor charging and thus increasing battery life since most ATP therapies work. However, the disadvantage is the slight delay in shock delivery in case this therapy is not effective. ATP therapy while the capacitors are charging addresses the last concern. Some devices allow the programmability of these features depending on the response of past ATP therapies (*Smart Mode* disables ATP therapies if prior ATP therapies failed, *Charge Saver* switches from ATP during charging to ATP before charging if prior ATP therapies were successful, and the *Switchback* feature switches back to ATP during charging if prior ATP therapies failed). ATP therapy programming is mainly done in the VT zones but a one-shot ATP therapy during charging could be given in the VF zone.

Each ATP therapy *sequence* (or *salvo*) is defined by the *number* and the *cycle length* of its paced *pulses* (Fig. 116.2). The programmed *cycle length* is set as a percentage of the tachycardia cycle length. The cycle length is fixed in a *burst* sequence but will decrement by a programmable duration in a *ramp* sequence. In *burst+* or *ramp+*, a pulse is added to each sequence. A *scan decrement* (or a *sweep*) feature could be applied when more than one sequence of the same ATP therapy is to be delivered. This feature will decrement the cycle length of the consecutive sequence by a programmed duration.

Shock Therapy

The electrical shocks delivered by ICDs arise from the discharge of the capacitors through the heart via the high-voltage electrodes. Capacitor discharge follows an exponential decay (Fig. 116.3) dependent on two variables: the capacitance and the impedance of the electrode/patient body system. As either of these variables is increased, the voltage and current discharge decay more slowly, producing a flatter waveform. One to three capacitors are commonly used in each generator, each rated for about 106–480 μF of capacitance and capable of a maximal voltage of about 350–890 V. These

capacitors are usually charged in parallel to a programmable voltage up to the maximum. When discharged, however, these capacitors are configured in series, so that the total voltage is doubled or tripled depending on the number of capacitors. Although the voltage is multiplied in the series configuration, the capacitance is reduced by the number of capacitors used. Hence, the resultant system capacitance is 120–150 μF for most currently available clinical devices. Lowering the capacitance of the system will have a favorable clinical outcome by decreasing the discharge time. Because most lead impedance values are between 30 and 70 ohms, these result in a voltage that decreases by about 60%–90% in 20 msec. The shock waveform (see later) is generated by the discharge of the capacitors through the electrode system to the patient. Unlike with ATP, ICD shocks may be associated with increased mortality and morbidity. In the PREPARE and MADIT-RIT studies, programming strategies to decrease ICD shocks by avoiding therapy for slow and nonsustained VT and applying antitachycardia even to faster VT were associated with less morbidity as well as mortality.[9,10]

Defibrillation Threshold and Safety Margin

The main determinant of the success of defibrillation is the magnitude of the electrical field generated across the heart, which is proportional to the spatial derivative of the stored voltage. However, since device companies report their device outputs in energy units (joules), there has been a trend to refer to the effective defibrillation energy in joule units. The simplest measure of defibrillation effectiveness is usually simplistically termed the DFT, defined as the lowest delivered shock strength required to defibrillate. However, the clinical predictive value of defibrillation testing is limited by the probabilistic nature of defibrillation. The DFT is often estimated in a step-down manner, in which progressively lower intensity shocks are delivered after VF is induced, and the lowest successful shock strength is labeled as the DFT. Alternatively, shocks can be delivered in a step-up fashion, beginning at low energies. However, the step-up method will have more failed shocks for patients with high energy requirements. Actually, the duration of circulatory arrest is shorter for most patients with the step-up method because the charge times are much shorter with lower energies, but longer for the few patients with high energy requirements. A third method of estimating defibrillation efficacy has been validated, in which test shocks are delivered during the vulnerable period of the cardiac cycle, near the peak of the surface

T wave. Theoretically, low-energy shocks delivered during this phase of repolarization will produce VF caused by the resultant dispersion of repolarization times. If a test shock delivered during this period fails to result in VF, it is deemed to be above the DFT, and subsequently, lower shock intensities can then be tested until VF occurs. This concept is termed the upper limit of vulnerability (ULV) and has the advantage of inducing VF only once during the testing period. The shock of the lowest energy that does not induce VF is considered a similar indicator of defibrillation efficacy. The disadvantage of this method is that the ability of the ICD to correctly detect VF and the subsequent decision-making algorithm to deliver VF therapy will not have been tested.

The concept of the DFT is overly simplistic because electrical defibrillation is best described as a sigmoidal-shaped probability function (Fig. 116.4) and not a threshold. Nonetheless, the step-down DFT estimation is a convenient clinical measurement to obtain during implantation and generally correlates with an 80% probability of success for the initial clinical shock. The probability of success approach has significant clinical relevance because appropriate implantation of ICDs requires a high confidence that the first shock will be successful. Historically, using epicardial leads and monophasic waveforms, a safety margin (a margin between the estimated DFT and the maximum output of the ICD) of 10 J was considered minimal implantation criteria. More recent studies have suggested that with biphasic shocks and NTLs, a margin of 1.9 times the DFT energy provides a 95% probability of success. One thing to keep in mind is that DFT testing is device- and lead-specific since the delivered energy is not the only parameter to ensure successful defibrillation. Other parameters include lead/body impedance, waveform tilt, truncation, pulse duration, and positive- and negative-phase peak voltage, and may all affect defibrillation success and are usually device/lead specific.[11,12]

To maximize the success of defibrillation, ICD devices will allow the programming of the shock polarity, shock vector, shock energy, shock waveforms, and the number of shocks. The latter is usually limited to six to decrease the risk for endless shock therapies in patients with inappropriate detection and because there is no proven data that more shocks are beneficial when prior shocks have failed to restore a perfusing rhythm. Shock polarity can be programmed to be normal (where the RV coil is the anode), reversed (the RV coil is the cathode), or alternating to improve the success rate of defibrillation. The shock vector could be altered depending on the inclusion of the SVC or another coil in the defibrillation wavefront. Some devices will allow pulse

duration programming of one or both phases of the biphasic wave. This may improve DFTs in patients with high DFTs.

Monophasic Waveforms

The simplest defibrillator waveform is the monophasic waveform, in which the capacitor discharge is truncated before complete discharge of the capacitor because the terminal voltage tail may prove proarrhythmic. Monophasic waveforms were used in early ICD generators and were effective in epicardial systems. The magnitude of a monophasic (or biphasic) shock is generally described by both the amplitude (peak voltage or current) and tilt of the waveform (see Fig. 116.3). For example, a waveform whose amplitude is reduced to one-half the initial value has a 50% tilt.

When the NTL was first developed and monophasic waveforms were used, the right ventricular coil electrode was configured as the cathode (negative), whereas the superior vena cava coil or subcutaneous patch electrode was configured as the anode (positive). When subsequent animal and clinical studies were performed comparing the right ventricular cathodal configuration with the right ventricular anodal configuration, the anodal right ventricular electrode resulted in a significantly lower DFT in patients and a lower need for supplementary electrodes.

Biphasic Waveforms

The most beneficial ICD innovation from the viewpoint of defibrillation efficacy was the development of the biphasic defibrillation waveform (Fig. 116.5). This waveform consists of the capacitor discharge divided into two phases of opposite polarity. The first phase is identical to a monophasic waveform (although usually of a shorter duration) before the capacitor discharge is truncated. The duration of the first phase is either programmable or continues until the voltage across the capacitor drops by a certain percentage of the original voltage (Tilt #1). The electrical connection within the generator is then quickly reversed

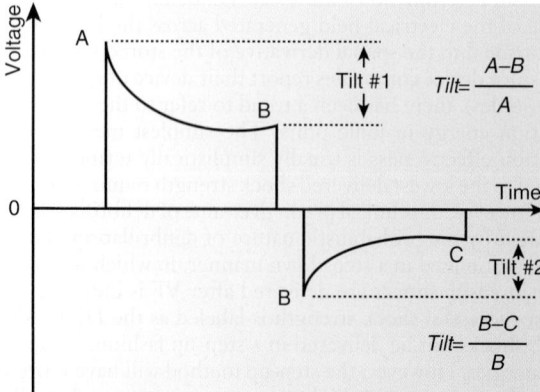

FIGURE 116.4 The biphasic waveform now used in all current implantable defibrillators. It is composed of a capacitor discharge divided into two phases of opposite polarity. The duration of each phase is dependent on the manufacturer and may be programmable in some devices. The initial voltage of the second phase is equivalent to the remaining voltage from the capacitor after truncation of phase 1 in most cases.

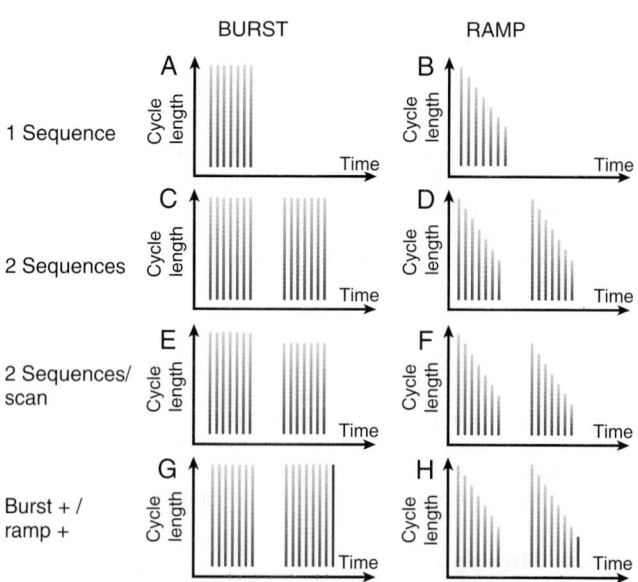

FIGURE 116.5 An antitachycardia pacing modality. (A) One sequence of burst, which is a salvo of pacing pulses at a fixed cycle length; (B) one sequence of ramp, which is a salvo of pacing pulses at a decremental cycle length; (C) two sequences of burst, both identical; (D) two sequences of ramp, both identical; (E) a burst with scan or sweep where the second burst sequence has a shorter cycle length; (F) a ramp with scan or sweep where the second ramp sequence starts with a shorter cycle length; (G) burst+ where the second burst sequence exhibits an extra pulse; and (H) ramp+ where the second ramp sequence exhibits another pulse.

(usually within 2–3 μsec) and the second phase is discharged in the opposite polarity for an additional set period or until the voltage across the capacitor(s) drop by another percentage (Tilt #2). Table 116.2 lists the biphasic waveform characteristics currently available in clinical ICDs.

The basic physiology of defibrillation and its relationship to the best or optimized biphasic waveform is well studied. Biphasic waveform characteristics in animals identified two factors that appear to maximize defibrillation efficacy as follows: (1) the first phase should be longer than the second phase; and (2) the polarity of the first phase appears to be important only for phase 1 durations greater than 10 msec or when the second phase duration is greater than that of the first phase.

Additional studies have examined the effectiveness of other phase characteristics. One interesting modification involves doubling the second phase initial voltage by switching the capacitance from series to parallel between the first and second phases. This also reduces the capacitance of the second phase by half, resulting in an increased tilt and a more rapid decay of voltage. Animal studies have suggested that this improves the defibrillation efficacy. Multiple recent studies have reported improved DFTs with modification of the tilt percentages. The results of these studies were then used to modify the preset tilts in the currently available devices. Some devices also have the capacity to specify the durations of the first and second phases of the biphasic shock, which determines the tilt. Although this can make a difference in a few patients, in general, this is not required.

System Malfunction

ICDs and their lead systems are very complex medical device systems. Their system integrity is challenged by several factors including a high-temperature, high-osmolar, high-salt environment and continuous mechanical stress from the beating heart and body movement. Despite all of these challenges, the "failure prediction" is very small: less than 1% over 5 years. ICD safety alerts or recalls are usually generated in response to a higher than normal projected risk for failure or if the failure would subject the patient to a serious adverse consequence. System failure could occur in the device battery, device electronics, or in the lead design and interact with the implantation techniques and patient characteristics.

Fortunately, primary battery failure is extremely rare. More often, battery depletion is caused by excessive power drain from pacing, capacitor charge, and electrogram storage. High pacing thresholds and lead insulation failure are additional causes of excessive current drain. On the other hand, repetitive capacitor charges due to nonsustained VT or temporary ventricular oversensing can cause important reductions in battery longevity. In 2012, Medtronic identified a rare (0.04%–0.15%) dysfunction resulting in a greater than expected drop in the Entrust ICD battery voltage. This resulted in this ICD having a shortened predicted longevity and quicker transition from the ERI to EOL. Usually, these high current drain issues can be managed with increased frequency of battery assessments.

In 2005, the US Food and Drug Administration (FDA) issued a class I recall (reasonable probability that the use of these devices will cause serious adverse health consequences or death with failure) regarding the use of Guidant PRIZM 2 DR CONTAK Renewal and CONTAK Renewal 2 devices due to failure to deliver a life-saving therapy due to short circuiting that occurs across the space between the anode (+) backfill tube and the cathode (-) defibrillation (DF) feedthrough wire. In 2005, there was also a voluntary class II recall (risk for adverse health consequences or death is remote) for the Medtronic Marquis with regard to a battery short.

TABLE 116.2 Summary of biphasic waveform characteristics in currently available commercial implantable cardioverter defibrillators

MANUFACTURER	MODEL	CAPACITANCE	PHASE 1 CHARACTERISTIC	PHASE 2 CHARACTERISTIC	MONOPHASIC
Boston Scientific, St. Paul, MN	Dynagen/Teligen	140 μF	60% tilt (nonprogrammable)	50% tilt (nonprogrammable)	80%
	Vitality HE	130–150 μF	60% tilt (nonprogrammable)	50% tilt (nonprogrammable)	80%
	Prizm II	158 μF	60% tilt (nonprogrammable)	50% tilt (nonprogrammable)	67%
Medtronic, St. Paul, MN	Evera/Protecta (XT)/ Secura/Virtuoso (II)/ Entrust	128 μF	50% tilt (programmable)[a]	50% tilt (programmable)[a]	None
	GEM III AT	118 μF	50% tilt (programmable)[a]	50% tilt (programmable)[a]	None
St. Jude Medical, Sylmar, CA	Assura/Fortify	80–120 μF	65% tilt (programmable) or 5.5 msec PW (programmable)	65% tilt (programmable) or 5.5 msec PW (programmable)	65% (programmable)
	Photon/Atlas	106–126 μF	65% tilt (programmable) or 5.5 msec PW (programmable)	65% tilt (programmable) or 5.5 msec PW (programmable)	65% (programmable)
	Epic/Photon	99–102 μF	65% tilt (programmable) or 5.5 msec PW (programmable)	65% tilt (programmable) or 5.5 msec PW (programmable)	65% (programmable)
Sorin, Plymouth, MN	Ovatio/Alto/Paradym	105–120 μF	50% tilt (nonprogrammable)	50% tilt (nonprogrammable)	None
Biotronik, Portland, OR	Ilesto/Lumax	160 μF	60% tilt, 16 msec maximum PW	50% tilt, 10 msec maximum PW	None
	Lumos	145 μF	60% tilt, 16 msec maximum PW	50% tilt, 10 msec maximum PW	None

[a]Applies only to the atrial shock tilt; the ventricular shocks are not tilt-programmable.

Capacitance values may vary between models within a given manufacturer and older models may vary from these specifications. In models in which phase parameters are programmable, the value given is the default value programmed at the factory. When a range of values is given, it refers to different models offered by the same manufacturer.

PW, Pulse width.

Failure of transvenous high-voltage ICD leads may be the result of a combination of multiple factors: patient-related, operator-related, and engineering-design-related factors. Patient-related factors include thoracic inlet syndrome, twiddler's syndrome, and certain activities like bench pressing. Operator methods that have contributed to lead failure include subclavian or second rib approach venous access, poorly applied suture sleeves, excessively tight lead coiling within the pocket, overtorquing of the lead, and iatrogenic damage to the leads during implantation. Lead-related factors that may contribute to lead failure include lead engineering and suture design flaws.

Sprint Fidelis ICD leads (Medtronic) were the subject of class I recall due to a higher than expected conductor fracture rate. There was also evidence of an increased risk for high-voltage conductor fracture if a pace/sense conductor fracture had previously occurred; thus it is recommended that one implant a new high-voltage lead instead of a pace/sense lead if a lead fracture of any type has occurred. It is recommended to use the lead integrity alert (LIA) algorithm extending arrhythmia detection, activating audible alarms and quick alert notification to monitor fully functional leads. The LIA algorithm could provide most patients with a 3-day warning prior to inappropriate shocks.

St. Jude Medical Riata and Riata ST leads were the subjects of class I recalls due to higher than expected erosion in the silicone coating around their conductors. Insulation breaks seen in these leads could be caused by either an "inside out" or by an "outside in" abrasion. The latter often occurs close to the pocket and is often due to lead contact with another part of the lead or the pulse generator. While "inside out" externalizations of the inner cables are not uncommon and can easily be visualized using fluoroscopy, they do not seem to place patients at a significant risk for electrical dysfunction (Fig. 116.6). However, "outside in" abrasions are difficult to identify using fluoroscopy and can result in shorting of the high voltage. This is neither unique to the Riata lead family nor is it a new failure mechanism.

Optisure is the newer generation of Optim leads from St. Jude Medical. They incorporated a few changes into the lead design to help address lead failure seen with the Riata lead. These changes include a larger lead body (8 Fr), redundant conductors that may serve as a backup system in the event of conductor failure, symmetrically aligned cables to provide better protection for the centrally located inner coil, and additional Optim insulation at the proximal end of the lead and under the SVC coil.

Currently, the FDA does not support routine replacement of leads that do not show evidence of electrical dysfunction, although clinical management of patients should be individualized. Multiple issues should be addressed prior to replacement including the risk for keeping the recalled unit, risk for replacement (infection and extraction), risk for failure of the new element to be placed, and the age of the unit that needs to be replaced.

Some devices have embedded algorithms to detect early lead failure, with the aim of decreasing inappropriate shocks in response to nonphysiological sensing. These algorithms monitor for an abrupt change in pace/sense impedance (increase or decrease), the presence of nonphysiological and extremely short R-R intervals, and the presence of frequent rapid nonsustained VT episodes. If present, this will automatically generate an alert to the patient and/or physician.

Newer algorithms (SecureSense from St. Jude Medical and SmartShock from Medtronic) utilize far-field channel signals during arrhythmia (RV coil to can or RV tip to can or RV coil to SVC coil) and withhold therapy if no arrhythmia is detected on the far-field channel even if fast events are detected on the near-field channel.

To protect from compromised shock therapy delivery as a result of lead insulation failure, St. Jude Medical uses a proprietary algorithm called DynamicTx. It effectively switches the defibrillation vector to one capable of delivering a defibrillation shock in case one coil is compromised. This algorithm may prove valuable for improving patient safety.

Recent and Future Directions

Remote Monitoring

The development of device monitoring systems with or without wandless communication has permitted the early diagnosis of arrhythmias and system malfunction from the patient's home and with few limits in geographic location or distance from the monitoring physician. Some devices could offer 24/7 remote monitoring via cellular phone communications. It has the potential to safely decrease clinic visits by 40%, as seen in

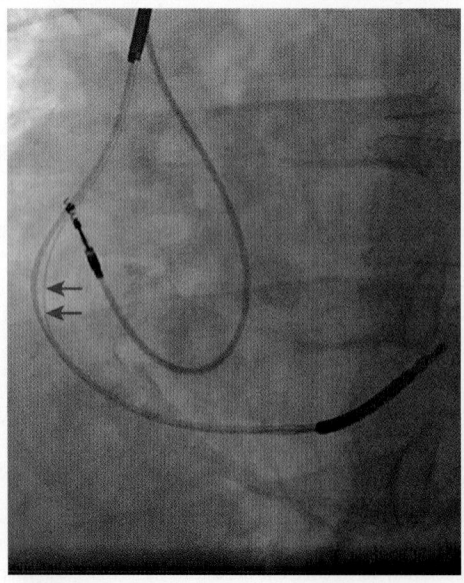
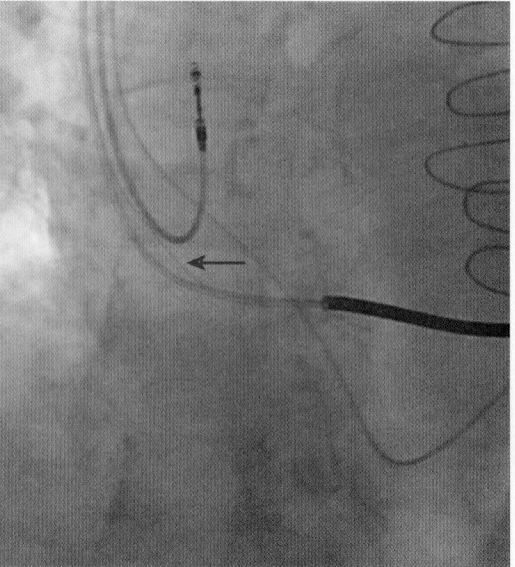

FIGURE 116.6 "Inside out" externalizations of the inner cables of Riata leads visualized using fluoroscopy (*arrows*).

the TRUST trial. The CONNECT trial showed that remote monitoring with automatic clinician alerts can reduce the time between clinical events and clinical decisions as well as the length of hospitalization stay. The ECOST trial showed that remote monitoring allowed for early and reliable detection of ICD lead failure and can reduce inappropriate ICD shocks and save battery life. However, other trials such as the Tele-HF and EVATEL did not show any significant benefit from remote monitoring on hospital readmission, all-cause mortality, or major clinical events. However, in patients with symptomatic heart failure, the IN-TIME trial demonstrated improved clinical benefits for patients with daily remote monitoring; this improvement was mainly driven by declines in cardiovascular and all-cause mortality.[13] Patients whose devices were remotely monitored showed better compliance with medical therapy. In addition to compliance, it was believed that the early detection and management of atrial and ventricular arrhythmias and the early recognition of suboptimal device programming might be responsible for the improved clinical outcomes.

Remote Device Programming

Remote device programming may have a significant impact on device management. Potential benefits include economical savings, patient convenience, and the ability to provide care to patients in remote areas. Although the technology is currently available, it is not accessible due to the lack of widespread acceptance from the medical community and regulatory bodies. Issues with this technology include the safety of communication and the scope of programming parameters allowable via this method. The impact of these issues could be mitigated if remote programming is allowed in the presence of medical personnel.

Long-Distance Telemetric Communication

Long-distance telemetric communication (wandless telemetry) in these devices is sometimes accomplished through the Medical Implant Communications Service (MICS). MICS is an ultra-low power, mobile radiofrequency service designed for transmitting diagnostic and therapeutic information from implanted medical devices. Its band operates between 402 and 405 MHz. This bandwidth does not need any licensing and is shared by different manufacturers (currently Medtronic, St. Jude Medical, and Biotronik). Each manufacturer has applied mechanisms to avoid interference and cross-communication with other devices. There is another frequency spectrum: the Industrial, Scientific, and Medical (ISM) band (902–928 MHz) is in use for long-range telemetry by Boston Scientific. They use precisely 914 MHz for communication from the ICD to the home monitor, which is also coupled with Bluetooth communication with a weight scale and blood pressure cuff.

Investigational Shock Waveforms

Multiple triphasic waveform patterns were tested in animals and failed to improve shock efficacy in terminating VF over biphasic waves.[14] However, multiple serial monophasic shocks were shown to terminate monomorphic VT with a lesser total energy requirement and peak voltage compared with a single monophasic or biphasic shock in a canine myocardial infarction model.[15] If these findings could be replicated in humans, this may translate into prolonged battery life, less pain, and less myocardial stunning and necrosis from the ICD shocks.

Magnetic Resonance Imaging–Conditional Implantable Cardioverter Defibrillators

Several interactions can be seen during magnetic resonance imaging (MRI) scanning of patients with ICDs: displacement of ferromagnetic material, reed switch interaction, magnetic saturation of the ICD transformer, heating-induced myocardial

necrosis, myocardial stimulation, device reset, and over- and undersensing of ventricular arrhythmias. As of early October 2015, there are two available MRI-conditional ICD devices (FDA designation) approved for full-body scans in the United States: the Evera MRI (up to 1.5 T) ICD from Medtronic and the Lumax, Iforia, and Ilesto (up to 1.5 T for the Lumax and 3 T for the Iforia and Ilesto) ICDs and CRT-Ds from Biotronik. Boston Scientific and St. Jude Medical have the CE Mark for European Union use for their MRI-conditional ICD systems.

Displacement was addressed by reducing the ferromagnetic components of the ICD. The undesirable interactions seen with the reed switch were avoided by replacing it with a Hall sensor. The internal circuitry was isolated to prevent unintentional ICD reset or reprogramming. Finally, the lead design was modified to decrease polarization, improve evoked response sensing, and improve heat dispersion, thus preventing lead tip heating.

Adjunctive Sensor Technology

Newer devices have incorporated special adjunctive features like intrathoracic impedance monitoring and left atrial/right ventricular pressure monitoring. Variations in intrathoracic impedance, measured by the subthreshold electrical impulse between the can and the RV coil +/– LV lead, correlate with changes in pulmonary fluid accumulation. Since fluid is a good conductor, decompensated heart failure often leads to a decrease in intrathoracic impedance. However, decreases in impedance are also seen in other clinical scenarios like pleural/pericardial effusion, pneumonia, an increase in intraabdominal pressure, and shortly after device implantation. Studies are currently under way to evaluate its impact on heart failure mortality and hospitalization.

Implantable right ventricular or left atrial pressure sensors, which allow for continuous hemodynamic monitoring, have also been used in ICDs. These pressure measurements can then be used to adjust medical therapy. The hope is to prevent acute heart failure decompensation with pulmonary edema or complications related to overtreatment.

Monitoring of ST-segment changes derived from a far-field intracardiac electrogram was recently evaluated in the management of patients with coronary artery disease. However, this limited study showed low sensitivity and specificity in detecting coronary events.

Battery Technologies

Because of the increased risk for infection with device changes, there has been significant work to produce batteries with longer longevity, including biothermal and biodegradable batteries. If proven to be effective, these batteries could extend the life of the device by more than 15–20 years. There has also been significant recent interest in rechargeable devices. If successful, it may allow the implantation of cardiac devices deep inside the body. These devices will be charged via a mid-field wireless transfer, which has the power delivery of near-field waves with the reach of far-field waves. This will essentially transfer electromagnetic waves safely into the body to power as well as to alter the function of a biomedical device if needed. Another promising method is the ability to charge pacemaker and ICD batteries via the physiological movement of the body organs. This is achieved by the transduction of mechanical energy into electrical energy via a specialized piezoelectric crystal on a nanoribbon. When attached to an animal heart, it was able to generate up to 7–8 volts. Although these options are very promising, there is still a significant amount of work that needs to be done to establish the safety and reliability of these battery technologies in a lifesaving device like an ICD.

REFERENCES

1. Gold M, Val-Mejias J, Lennan RB, et al. Optimization of superior vena cava coil position and usage for transvenous defibrillation. *Heart Rhythm.* 2008;5:394–399.

2. Cesario D, Bhargava M, Valderrábano M, et al. Azygos vein lead implantation: a novel adjunctive technique for implantable cardioverter defibrillator placement. *J Cardiovasc Electrophysiol.* 2004;15:780–783.

3. Wilkoff BL, Rickard J, Tkatchouk E, et al. The biostability of cardiac lead insulation materials as assessed from long-term human implants. *J Biomed Mater Res B Appl Biomater.* 2016;104:411–421.

4. Friedman PA, McClelland RL, Bamlet WR, et al. Dual-chamber versus single-chamber detection enhancements for implantable defibrillator rhythm diagnosis. The detect supraventricular tachycardia study. *Circulation.* 2006;113:2871–2879.

5. Wilkoff BL, Cook JR, Epstein AE, et al. Dual-chamber pacing or ventricular backup pacing in patients with an implantable defibrillator: the Dual Chamber and VVI Implantable Defibrillator (DAVID) Trial. *JAMA.* 2002;288:3115–3123.

6. Cook JR, et al. Impact of atrial pacing on quality of life in the dual chamber and VVI implantable defibrillator (DAVID) II trial. Presented at: *Heart Failure Society of America 2006 Scientific Meeting.* Washington, DC: Recent and Late-Breaking Trials; September 19, 2007.

7. Moss AJ, Hall WJ, Cannom DS, et al. Cardiac-resynchronization therapy for the prevention of heart-failure events. *N Engl J Med.* 2009;361:1329–1338.

8. Wilkoff BL, Ousdigian KT, Sterns LD, et al. A comparison of empiric to physician-tailored programming of implantable cardioverter-defibrillators: results from the prospective randomized multicenter EMPIRIC trial. *J Am Coll Cardiol.* 2006;48:330–339.

9. Wilkoff BL, Williamson BD, Stern RS, et al. Strategic programming of detection and therapy parameters in implantable cardioverter-defibrillators reduces shocks in primary prevention patients: results from the PREPARE (Primary Prevention Parameters Evaluation) Study. *J Am Coll Cardiol.* 2008;52:541–550.

10. Moss AJ, Schuger C, Beck CA, et al. Reduction in inappropriate therapy and mortality through ICD programming. *N Engl J Med.* 2012;367:2275–2283.

11. Sweeney MO, Natale A, Volosin KJ, et al. Prospective randomized comparison of 50/50% versus 65/65% tilt biphasic waveform on defibrillation in humans. *Pacing Clin Electrophysiol.* 2001;24:60–65.

12. Schauerte PN, Ziegert K, Waldmann M, et al. Effect of biphasic shock duration on defibrillation threshold with different electrode configurations and phase 2 capacitances: prediction by upper-limit-of-vulnerability determination. *Circulation.* 1999;99:1516–1522.

13. Hindricks G, Taborsky M, Glikson M, et al. Implant-based multiparameter telemonitoring of patients with heart failure (IN-TIME): a randomised controlled trial. *Lancet.* 2014;384:583–590.

14. Davis R, Malkin R. Simultaneous comparison of many triphasic defibrillation waveforms. *Open Biomed Eng J.* 2012;6:1–4.

15. Janardhan A, Li W, Gutbrod S, et al. Low-energy three-stage electrotherapy delivered through implantable leads significantly reduces the cardioversion threshold in a canine model of persistent atrial fibrillation. *Circulation.* 2011;124:A15917.

117 Implantable Cardioverter Defibrillator: Clinical Aspects

Charles Swerdlow and Paul Friedman

Implantable cardioverter defibrillators (ICDs) are the preferred treatment for most patients who are at a high risk for ventricular fibrillation (VF) or life-threatening ventricular tachycardia (VT). This chapter complements Chapter 116 with the technical aspects.

Indications and Use

For many years, ICDs have been the treatment of choice for secondary prevention of VT/VF. The MADIT II and SCD-HeFT clinical trials demonstrated 5%–7% absolute mortality reductions over 2–4 years and established ICDs as a standard of care for primary prevention in high-risk patients. Presently, more than 80% of ICDs are implanted for primary prevention. Guidelines based on these trials identify patients with ischemic or nonischemic cardiomyopathy primarily by heart failure class and left-ventricular ejection fraction ≤30%–40%.[1] Guidelines based on more limited evidence identify subgroups of high-risk patients with less common diseases, including hypertrophic cardiomyopathy and ion channelopathies.[1] Some patient groups at a high risk for VT/VF have not been studied in clinical trials. Expert consensus documents provide recommendations for ICD implantation in these patients (Table 117.1).[2,3]

An overwhelming consensus supports secondary prevention guidelines, but primary prevention guidelines are applied inconsistently. Experts vary in their level of concern about comorbidities as contraindications, complications, and the number of patients who need to receive ICDs to save one life (15–20). Patients vary in their acceptance of ICDs to treat a statistical risk. Retrospective analyses provide cautionary evidence that ICDs (excluding cardiac resynchronization devices) do not prolong life in identifiable subgroups of MADIT II and SCD-HeFT patients with extensive comorbidities, including advanced heart failure and renal failure.[4,5]

Implantable Cardioverter Defibrillator System Selection

ICD systems first used epicardial leads and evolved to using transvenous leads that permit single- and dual-chamber antibradycardia pacing as well as cardiac resynchronization pacing (see Chapter 120). Recently, a totally subcutaneous (S)-ICD system has been introduced. Fig. 117.1 provides an overview of ICD system selection. Fig. 117.2 compares the advantages and limitations of transvenous versus S-ICD systems.

Transvenous Versus Subcutaneous Implantable Cardioverter Defibrillators

The S-ICD[6] eliminates morbidity associated with transvenous leads, lead-related complications during magnetic resonance imaging (MRI) scanning, and the costs and hazards of transvenous extraction when lead removal is required. In comparison with closely spaced, endocardial sensing electrograms (EGMs), widely spaced, far-field, subcutaneous EGMs have lower amplitudes (0.3–4.0 mV vs. 3–30 mV), longer durations, lower frequency contents, greater postural variations, and lower signal-to-noise ratios (Fig. 117.3). Thus they are more likely to double-count R waves or oversense T waves and noncardiac signals. Candidates for S-ICD undergo screening utilizing surface electrocardiogram (ECG) electrodes to assess the risks for T wave oversensing or R wave double-counting; 7%–10% of S-ICD candidates fail screening.[7]

The S-ICD's extrathoracic electrodes cannot perform painless antitachycardia, resynchronization, or antibradycardia pacing. If bradycardia pacing is not required at implantation, the risk for subsequent clinical bradycardia is low over a few years in most patient populations. As discussed later, antitachycardia pacing (ATP) is an important tool for secondary prevention patients with clinical monomorphic VT, but experts differ on its role for primary prevention patients.

Since most primary prevention patients do not receive ICD therapy for VT/VF, they may benefit most from the S-ICD's reduction of transvenous lead-related risks. S-ICDs may also be preferred in niche groups (see Fig. 117.2).

Dual-Chamber Versus Single-Chamber Transvenous Implantable Cardioverter Defibrillators

Dual-chamber ICDs provide dual-chamber pacing, diagnostics for atrial fibrillation (AF), and supraventricular tachycardia (SVT)-VT discriminators that are not available in single-chamber ICDs. Dual-chamber stored EGMs provide higher diagnostic accuracy than single-chamber EGMs.[8] Disadvantages of dual-chamber ICDs include higher cost, atrial lead complication, and decreased longevity. Dual-chamber pacing modes that minimize ventricular pacing reduce the risk for heart failure due to obligatory right ventricular (RV) pacing. In secondary prevention patients who have SVT and monomorphic VT at overlapping ventricular rates, dual-chamber SVT-VT discrimination is superior to single-chamber discrimination.[9] Primary prevention patients are less likely to benefit because their monomorphic VT tends to be sufficiently fast that rate overlap with SVT is infrequent.[10]

TABLE 117.1	Indications for primary prevention implantable cardioverter defibrillators	
	GUIDELINES	**EXPERT CONSENSUS**
CLASS I		**>40 DAYS POST MI**
EF ≤35%	Ischemic[a]: NYHA 2, 3 DCM, NYHA 1, 2, 3	• Needs nonelective pacing, meets primary prevention for ICD • >48 h post MI, sustained VT/VF, without treatable ischemia[b]
EF ≤30%	Ischemic[a]: NYHA 1	• >48 h post MI, syncope thought to be due to VT[b]
EF ≤40%	Ischemic: nsVT, inducible sustained VT	• Post MI, ICD at ERI, generator change indicated
		>90 DAYS POST PCI/CABG
		• Previous primary prevention indication; EF unlikely to improve >35% • Previous secondary prevention indication,[b] ICD considered if either abnormal EF postrevascularization or previous VT/VF arrest unlikely related to ischemia • Needs nonelective pacing, meeting primary prevention for ICD • Syncope thought to be due to VT • PCI/CABG, ICD at ERI, generator change recommended
CLASS II: SPECIAL CONDITIONS AND RISK FACTORS		**DCM >9 MONTHS**
HCM LQTS Brugada syndrome Awaiting transplant Myocarditis Sarcoid Chagas disease		• >3 months since diagnosis, improvement in EF unlikely • Spontaneous sustained VT/VF[b] • Syncope thought to be due to VT/VF ·

[a]>40 days post MI, >90 days PCI/CABG.
[b]Secondary prevention indication, included for clarity.
CABG, Coronary artery bypass surgery; *DCM*, dilated cardiomyopathy; *EF*, left-ventricular ejection fraction; *ERI*, elective replacement indicator; *HCM*, hypertrophic cardiomyopathy; *ICD*, implantable cardioverter defibrillator; *LQTS*, long QT syndrome; *MI*, myocardial infarction; *NYHA*, New York Heart Association functional class; *PCI*, percutaneous coronary intervention; *VF*, ventricular fibrillation; *VT*, ventricular tachycardia.

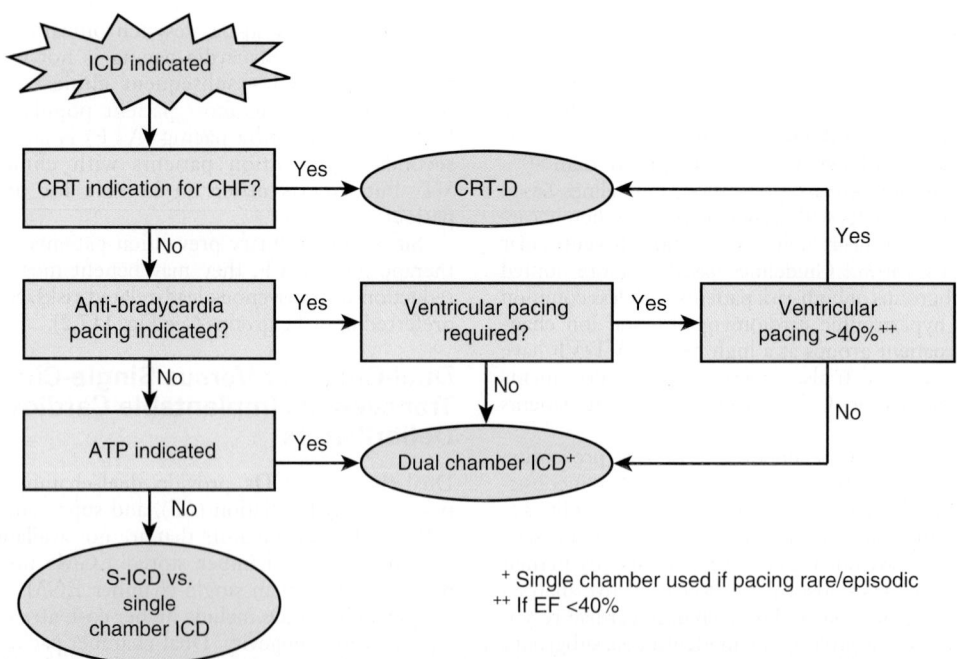

FIGURE 117.1 Selection of an appropriate implantable cardioverter defibrillator (*ICD*) system. A transvenous resynchronization system is indicated if patients have (1) heart failure, (2) left-ventricular ejection fraction (*EF*) ≤35%, and (3) left bundle branch block, QRS >150 msec, or ≥40% ventricular pacing. Patients who need atrial pacing receive a dual-chamber ICD. Patients with ventricular tachycardia (VT) with rates that overlap supraventricular tachycardia (SVT) rates (most commonly secondary prevention patients) may also benefit from dual-chamber ICDs for SVT-VT discrimination. Otherwise, subcutaneous (S)-ICD or single-chamber ICD is used. See also Fig. 117.3. *ATP,* Antitachycardia pacing; *CHF,* congestive heart failure; *CRT-D,* cardiac resynchronization therapy defibrillator.

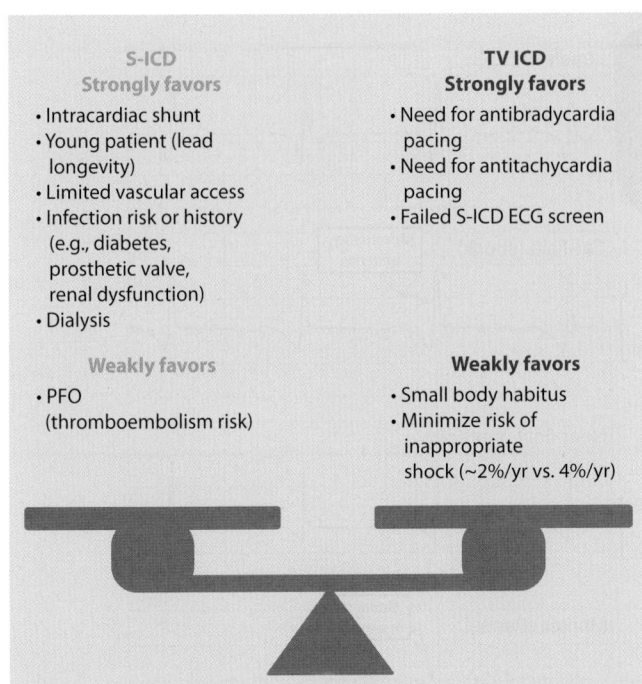

FIGURE 117.2 Choosing a subcutaneous (*S*) or transvenous (*TV*) single-chamber implantable cardioverter defibrillator (*ICD*). *ECG*, Electrocardiogram; *PFO*, patent foramen ovale.

Transvenous Defibrillation Leads

Dual Coil Versus Single Coil

Dual-coil leads (see Chapter 116) defibrillate with slightly lower mean shock strengths than single-coil leads, but there is no difference in first-shock efficacy, the risk for atrial tachyarrhythmias, or all-cause mortality.[11] Atrial cardioversion is more effective with dual-coil than with single-coil leads. EGMs recorded between the proximal coil and ICD housing record atrial signals that are useful for physician interpretation of single-chamber stored EGMs and may replace surface ECG electrodes during follow-up. However, in practice, single-coil leads are often preferred because dual-coil leads increase the difficulty and risk for extraction.

Integrated Versus Dedicated Sensing Bipoles

Integrated bipolar leads require one less conductor than dedicated bipolar leads (see Chapter 116) and thus might be more reliable. In practice, highly reliable leads have been developed with both designs. Oversensing of extracardiac signals is more common with integrated bipolar sensing.[11] Presently, T wave oversensing is more common with dedicated bipoles.[12]

Implant Procedure and Testing

Test sensing and defibrillation at implantation was mandatory for early ICDs to ensure adequate sensing of VF EGMs and reliable defibrillation. Improved ICD performance and inherent risks for defibrillation testing led to a reappraisal of the need for such testing and then to evidence-based omission of defibrillation testing in many primary prevention patients.

Testing Sensing in Ventricular Fibrillation

Sensing is the process of identifying the electrical signals (EGMs) that correspond to individual cardiac depolarization. In modern ICDs, the combination of dynamic adjustment of sensitivity and short blanking periods produce reliable sensing during VF if the R wave during native rhythm is at least 5–7

mV[13] and perhaps as low as 3 mV with dedicated bipolar sensing.[14] Presently, undersensing of VF is caused primarily by variations in VF EGM amplitude that occur faster than dynamically adjusting sensitivity can track them (Fig. 117.4A).[12] Thus induction of VF is not required to test sensing for the vast majority of implants. However, confirmation of sensing during VF is important in specific circumstances (e.g., when nominal sensing parameters have been reprogrammed to minimize oversensing of T waves or other signals, possible device-device interactions, and potentially when using features that withhold shocks for rapid oversensing).[12]

Testing Defibrillation Efficacy

Methods

Defibrillation efficacy is usually assessed directly by fibrillation-defibrillation ("defibrillation") testing, but it also can be assessed indirectly by vulnerability testing (see Chapter 116). Either method can determine the minimum shock strength that defibrillates reliably (patient-specific strategy) or estimate if the maximum output of the ICD will defibrillate reliably (safety margin strategy). Most clinical testing determines the safety margin between the ICD's maximum shock strength and an estimated high point on the defibrillation probability of success curve. Vulnerability testing is based on the close relationship between the highly reproducible upper limit of vulnerability (ULV) and the minimum shock strength that defibrillates approximately 90% of the time.[15] The principal advantage of vulnerability testing is that it can confirm reliable defibrillation without inducing VF in 80%–95% of patients.[16]

Clinical Utility, Necessity, and Recommendations

Identifying ICD systems with insufficient defibrillation safety margins is challenging because of their low prevalence (about 5% of new left-pectoral implants) and the probabilistic nature of defibrillation (see Chapter 116). Statistical modeling of clinical data shows that safety margin testing is superior to clinical estimates of defibrillation threshold for implant testing.[17] However, there is substantial uncertainty regarding defibrillation efficacy in patients who fail conventional testing; almost half of these patients pass repeat testing without system revision because of regression to the mean.[17] Defibrillation testing has two additional limitations. First, clinical defibrillation failures may be caused by factors that cannot be measured at implantation, such as ischemia. Second, the low incidence of VT/VF requiring shocks in primary prevention patients limits the impact of differences in defibrillation efficacy on total mortality.

Recent prospective data from registries and randomized controlled trials have established that clinically used safety margin defibrillation testing does not improve either overall mortality or first-shock defibrillation efficacy for large populations of patients with new left-sided implants with well-positioned defibrillation leads that have satisfactory sensing and pacing thresholds and the RV defibrillation coil programmed as the anode.[18–20] They also found that testing had no significant effect on adverse events, which are dominated by mechanical complications, infections, and—in cardiac resynchronization patients—decompensated heart failure.

The earlier considerations and data do not favor routine testing in all new left-sided pectoral implants of transvenous ICDs. However, assessment of defibrillation efficacy or shock testing is recommended under different clinical conditions (Table 117.2).

Implant Complications

ICD implantation has well-known surgical risks. Additionally, defibrillation testing has risks related to VF (e.g., circulatory arrest and hypoperfusion) and shocks (pulseless electrical activity).[21] With experienced operators, overall combined complications

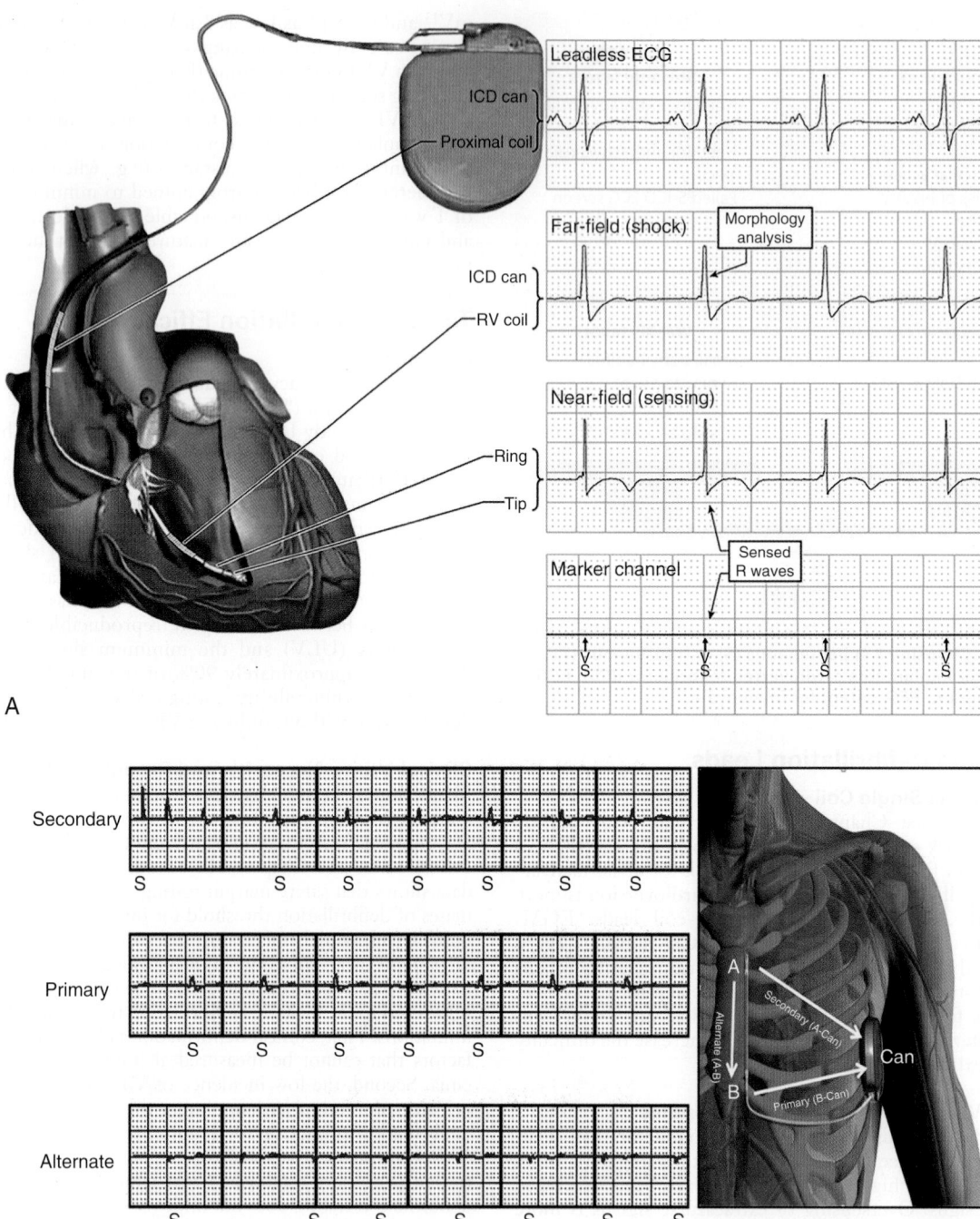

FIGURE 117.3 Implantable cardioverter defibrillator (*ICD*) leads and electrograms (EGMs). (A) A single-chamber ICD system including a left pectoral active can and right ventricular (*RV*) lead is shown on the left; a telemetered EGM recorded between the proximal coil and can ("leadless electro-cardiogram [*ECG*]"), high-voltage (shock) far-field EGM, and sensing near-field EGM are shown with annotated markers on the right. The dual-coil lead uses true bipolar sensing between the tip and ring electrodes. The marker channel denotes timing of sensed R waves from the near-field EGM (*arrows*) and the ICD's classification of each ventricular event by letter symbols. Numbers indicate RR intervals in milliseconds. *S* denotes sensed ventricular events in the sinus rate zone. Sensing is accurate because there is a 1:1 correspondence between ventricular EGMs and markers. The morphology of shock EGMs stored during detected tachycardias is useful for distinguishing ventricular tachycardia from supraventricular tachycardia. Leadless ECGs provide a signal with an identifiable atrial EGM with a single-chamber ICD if a dual-coil lead is used. (B) A subcutaneous (S)-ICD records subcutaneous EGMs from one of three vectors. The amplitude of the alternate vector is smallest (as in this tracing) because it often overlies atrial tissue and the sternum. The secondary vector is prone to myopotential artifacts because it usually overlies the pectoralis muscles. EGMs are displayed at 1× gain. Displaying them at 2× gain may facilitate clinician review but does not affect rhythm determination.

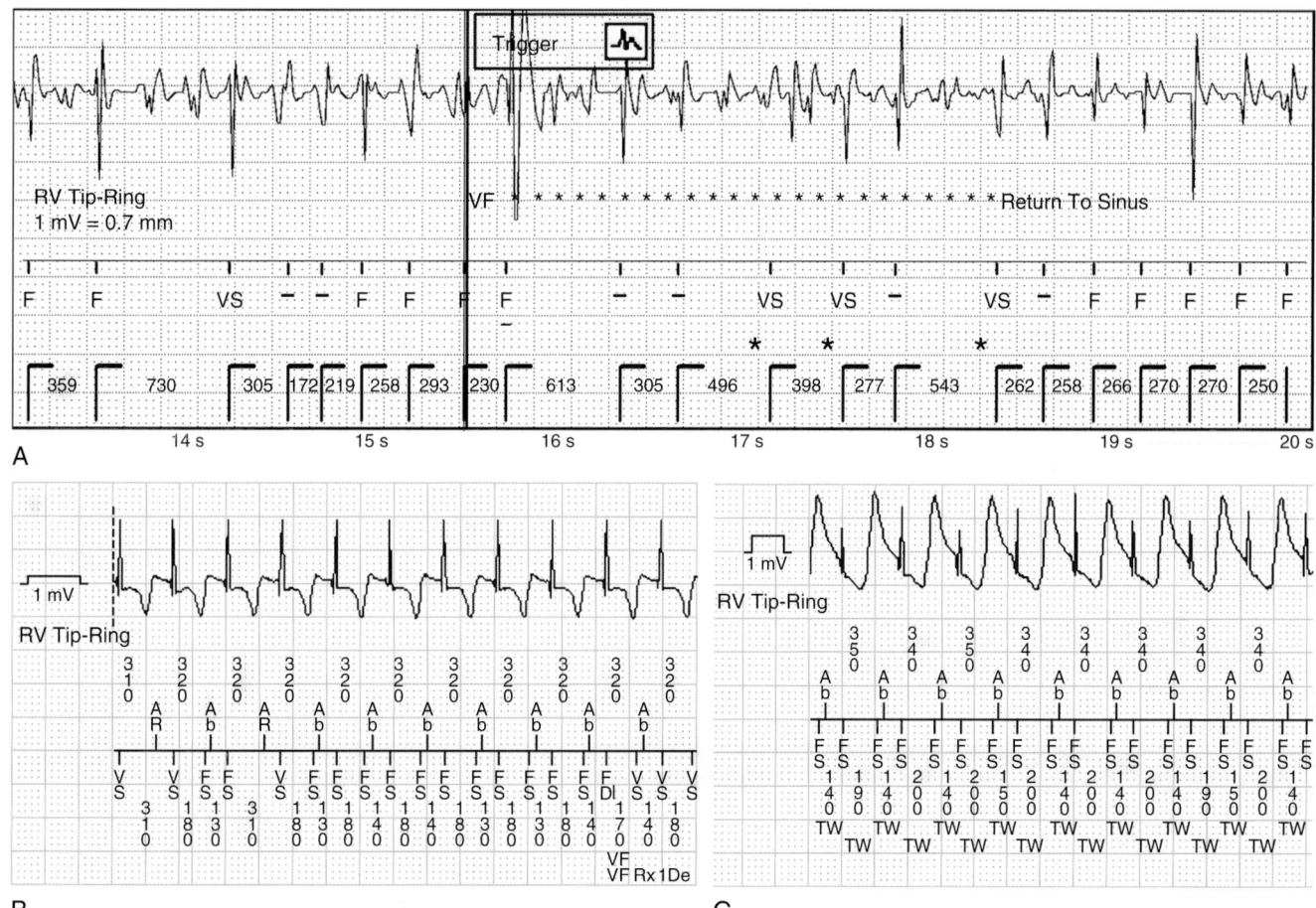

FIGURE 117.4 Undersensing and oversensing. (A) Undersensing. A dedicated bipolar filtered electrogram (EGM) is shown during ongoing ventricular fibrillation (*VF*). Between the first 5 seconds and before the 18-second marker, there are fewer markers than true EGMs indicating undersensing, The single-zone VF detection interval is 360 msec, and programmed minimum sensitivity is 0.3 mV. Undersensing occurs primarily because of the amplitude of EGMs changing faster than dynamic sensitivity can adjust despite EGM amplitudes that exceed the programmed sensitivity. Shortly after detection of VF at a vertical line (*Trigger, VF*), three consecutive binned intervals (*asterisks*) separated by one unbinned interval result in clinically incorrect termination of the device-defined VF episode (Return to Sinus) despite ongoing VF. The implantable cardioverter defibrillator subsequently performed a second initial detection of VF and delivered a successful shock. (B and C) Oversensing of T waves. Wide-band dedicated bipolar right ventricular (*RV*) EGMs during sinus tachycardia with dual-chamber markers are shown. Each EGM shows the characteristic pattern of alternating high- and low-frequency sensed events with two ventricular events for each atrial event. One of the mV calibration markers is shown on the left. (B) Oversensing causes inappropriate detection of VF. High-amplitude T waves cause intermittent oversensing despite adequate (10 mV base to peak) R waves. *VF Therapy 1 Defib* at the lower right denotes inappropriate detection of VF. (C) An enhanced sensing algorithm identifies the pattern of T wave oversensing therapy (TW markers) and prevents inappropriate detection of VF despite consistent T wave oversensing. (B) Low-amplitude (1.5–4 .0 mV) R waves are the root cause of this T wave oversensing.

total 3%–5% for single- or dual-chamber ICDs.[22] The NCDR registry[23] reported a total mortality of 0.3%. However, these data were neither collected nor adjudicated uniformly. When a new transvenous lead is added at the time of replacement or upgrade, the complication rate increases to 15%.[24]

Programming Sensing, Detection, and Therapies for Shock Reduction

When delivered for hypotensive VT/VF, ICD therapies reduce mortality and prevent hospitalizations. However, shocks are painful and cause adverse psychosocial effects; they also cause acute adverse physiological effects of uncertain clinical significance.[25] Further, both shocks and ATP may be proarrhythmic.

Programming to minimize therapies is the focus of a recent expert consensus statement[13] that classifies them as *appropriate* if delivered for sustained VT/VF and *inappropriate* if delivered during a rhythm other that VT/VF. In addition, it classifies appropriate therapy as *avoidable* if it could have been withheld without adverse clinical consequences; avoidable shocks are also referred to as *unnecessary*. Examples include shocks for self-terminating VT or VT that could be terminated by ATP. Strategic programming of sensing, VT/VF detection, and VT/VF therapy reduce inappropriate and avoidable therapies[26] and may reduce overall mortality.[27] See Chapter 119 for strategic programming of bradycardia pacing mode and rate in ICD patients.[13] Table 117.3 summarizes key recommendations regarding programming of tachycardia parameters.[13]

TABLE 117.2 Consensus recommendations: implant testing of defibrillation efficacy

RECOMMENDATION	CLASS	LEVEL OF EVIDENCE[13]	COMMENT
Reasonable to omit testing in patients undergoing *initial left-pectoral transvenous ICD implantation* procedures where appropriate sensing, pacing, and impedance values are obtained with fluoroscopically well-positioned RV leads	IIa	B-R	
Testing recommended in patients undergoing a *subcutaneous ICD* implantation	I	C-LD	Limited data; subcutaneous ICDs use shocks to terminate all VT/VF, but transvenous ICDs terminate most VTs using ATP
Testing reasonable in patients undergoing a right-pectoral transvenous ICD implantation	IIa	B-NR	Right-pectoral ICDs have suboptimal shock vectors and defibrillation thresholds compared with left-pectoral ICDs
Testing reasonable in patients undergoing ICD pulse generator changes	IIa	B-NR	At generator change, the impedance of a high-voltage shock may be the only way to identify an insulation breach of a high-voltage conductor
Testing should not be performed in patients with specific contraindications[a]	III (Harm)	C-LD	

[a]Documented nonchronic cardiac thrombus, atrial fibrillation, or atrial flutter without adequate systemic anticoagulation, critical aortic stenosis, unstable coronary artery disease, recent stroke or transient ischemic attack, hemodynamic instability, or other known morbidities associated with poor outcomes.
ATP, Antitachycardia pacing; *ICD,* implantable cardioverter defibrillator; *RV,* right ventricular; *VF,* ventricular fibrillation; *VT,* ventricular tachycardia.
Modified from Wilkoff B, Fauchier L, Stiles M, et al. 2015 HRS/EHRA/APHRS/SOLAECE expert consensus statement on optimal implantable cardioverter-defibrillator programming and testing. *Heart Rhythm.* 2016;13:e50–86.

TABLE 117.3 Selected consensus recommendations for strategic implantable cardioverter defibrillator programming

TACHYCARDIA DETECTION PROGRAMMING RECOMMENDATIONS	CLASS	LEVEL OF EVIDENCE[13]	COMMENT
Detection duration should be programmed to at least 6–12 s or 30 intervals	I	A/B-R[a]	Reduce total therapies
For primary prevention adult patients, the slowest detection rate should be programmed to 185–200 beats/min	I	A	Reduce total therapies
For secondary prevention patients, it is reasonable to program the slowest detection rate to at least 10 beats/min < documented VT rate but not >200 beats/min	IIa	C-EO	Reduce total therapies
SVT-VT discrimination algorithms should be programmed ON up to 200–230 beats/min	I	B-R	Reduce inappropriate therapies
ATP should be programmed for all VT/VF zones up to 230 beats/min in all patients with structural heart disease	I	A	Reduce shocks

[a]Primary prevention, A; secondary prevention, B-R.
ATP, Antitachycardia pacing; *SVT,* supraventricular tachycardia; *VF,* ventricular fibrillation; *VT,* ventricular tachycardia.
Modified from Wilkoff B, Fauchier L, Stiles M, et al. 2015 HRS/EHRA/APHRS/SOLAECE expert consensus statement on optimal implantable cardioverter-defibrillator programming and testing. *Heart Rhythm.* 2016;13:e50–86.

Sensing

Basic sensing occurs when the filtered signal crosses an amplitude threshold. *Oversensing* occurs when signals that do not correspond to local myocardial depolarization are sensed. Conversely, *undersensing* occurs when signals that correspond to local myocardial depolarization are not sensed. *Markers* telemetered from the ICD to the programmer indicate the timing of sensed events. The marker channel plays a critical role in identifying both oversensing and undersensing (see Fig. 117.4). *Enhanced* sensing features minimize oversensing by rejecting signals that satisfy amplitude and frequency content for basic sensing but do not represent cardiac depolarizations. In S-ICDs and some newer ICDs, these features reduce inappropriate therapies due to oversensing (see Fig. 117.4C).

Detection

Detection is the process by which ICD algorithms count and classify a sequence of sensed signals to determine the cardiac rhythm.

Detection Rate and Duration

A device-defined tachycardia episode begins when rate and duration criteria are fulfilled (see Chapter 116). Rate thresholds of 185–200 beats/min and durations of at least 6–12 seconds or 30 intervals reduce avoidable shocks in primary prevention patients and have at most a minimal impact on syncope (Fig. 117.5A).[13] This programming strategy is based on three premises: (1) Primary prevention patients usually have fast VTs, (2) slower VT often terminates spontaneously and rarely leads to cardiac collapse, and (3) rapid ventricular rates during conducted AF often are transient, so longer duration reduces inappropriate detection. For secondary prevention patients, data support the same 6–12 seconds or 30-interval detection duration[28,29] and, if the clinical VT rate exceeds 200 beats/min, the same rate threshold.

Zones for Detection and Therapy

ICDs have up to three ventricular rate zones for detection duration and therapy (VT, fast VT, and VF) (Fig. 117.6). These permit programming of zone-specific detection durations and

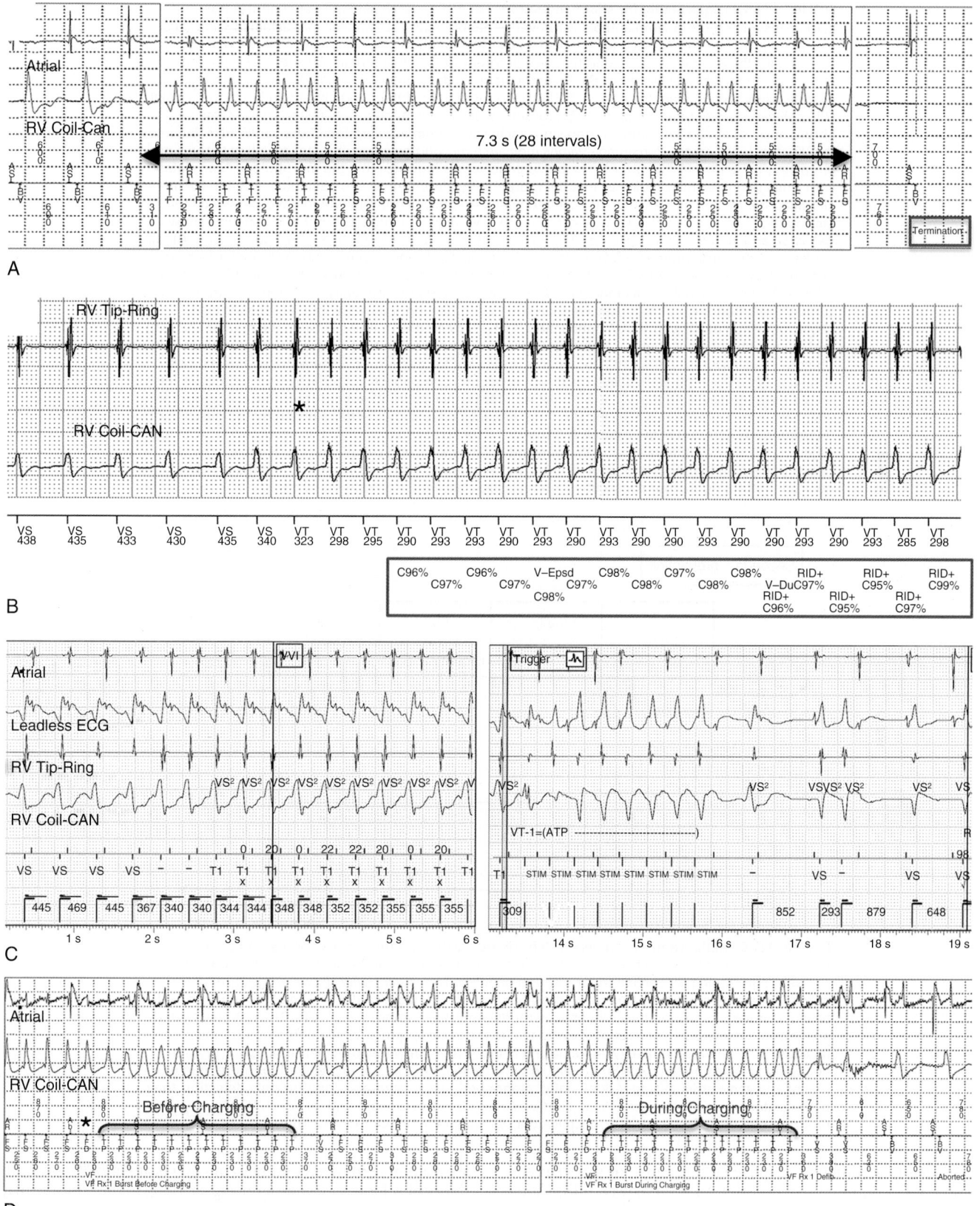

FIGURE 117.5 For legend, see next page.

FIGURE 117.5 Programming for shock reduction. (A) Atrial, shock, and marker channels from a cardiac resynchronization implantable cardioverter defibrillator (ICD) shows nonsustained ventricular tachycardia (*VT*) lasting 7.3 seconds (28 beats) at a cycle length of 250–290 msec. This VT was not detected for therapy because the duration was programmed to 30 intervals. Episode "Termination" is denoted in the red box at the right. *BV*, Biventricular paced; *TF*, intervals in fast VT zone. (B) Single-chamber supraventricular tachycardia (SVT)-VT discrimination. Integrated bipolar and right ventricular (*RV*) coil-can electrograms are shown. An abrupt increase in ventricular rate (*asterisk*) indicates the abrupt onset of atrial tachycardia during sinus tachycardia with acceleration of the ventricular rate into the VT zone (<340 msec). Percentage values indicate a morphology discriminator match with the sinus template (SVT ≥94%). A "C" prior to the percentage values indicates that the morphology "correlates" with sinus template. RID+ indicates that the morphology algorithm (Boston Scientific Rhythm ID) has classified the rhythm as SVT after 10 analyzed beats. An onset algorithm would have classified this tachycardia incorrectly as VT. (C) Dual-chamber SVT-VT discrimination. Discontinuous panels show detection and antitachycardia pacing (*ATP*) therapy of monomorphic VT with 1:1 VT conduction. Atrial, leadless electrocardiogram (*ECG*) (see Fig. 117.3), dedicated bipolar, shock, and marker channels are shown. The clinical onset of VT is not shown because it begins at a rate slower than the VT detection interval. In the left panel, VT is detected as the rhythm accelerates gradually across the programmed sinus-VT rate boundary of 350 msec (vertical line "VVI"). The right panel (about 10 seconds later) shows detection of VT with 1:1 VA conduction ("VT-1") treated with ATP (*STIM* on the marker channel) and resumption of sinus rhythm. Numeric values on the upper side of the marker channel denote morphology match scores (≥90% = match). Scores in VT vary from 0% to 22%; the score on the last best (sinus) is 98%. Discriminators based on abrupt onset and comparisons of atrial versus ventricular rates would have misclassified this VT as SVT. (D) ATP for fast VT in the VF zone. Atrial, shock, and marker channels from a cardiac resynchronization therapy device are shown. After a programmed duration of 30 beats, VF is detected at the asterisk (*FD* marker). The first sequence of ATP is unsuccessful. The ICD redetects VF after 12 intervals in the VF zone and delivers a second sequence of ATP while simultaneously charging the shock capacitor. The second sequence of ATP is successful, and the shock is aborted (bottom right); four consecutive intervals are classified in a nontherapy zone.

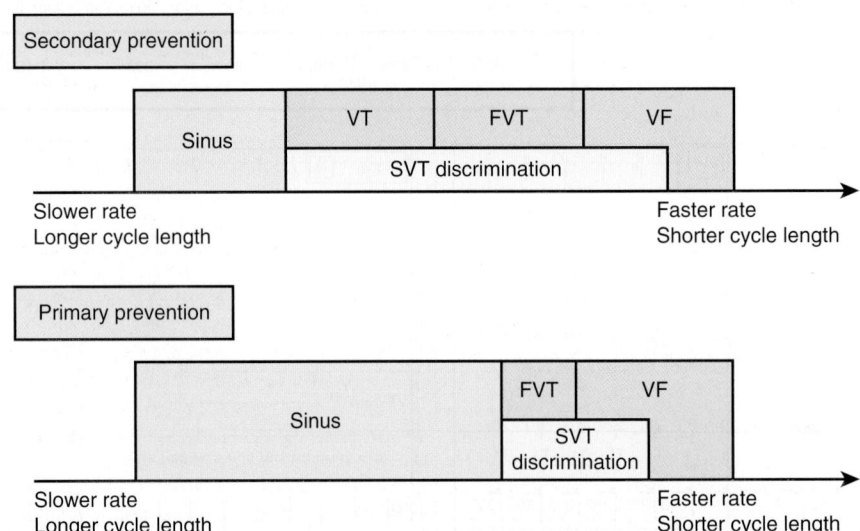

FIGURE 117.6 Implantable cardioverter defibrillator rate detection zones. Some implantable cardioverter defibrillators permit programming of an additional monitor-only zone. The *upper panel* shows programming for secondary prevention patients. The *lower panel* shows programming for primary prevention patients. Generally, the sinus–ventricular tachycardia (*VT*) rate boundary should be slow enough to ensure detection of all hemodynamically compromising VTs. The optional boundary between the two VT zones should be based on the cycle length at which different durations for detection or a different antitachycardia pacing is preferred. The VT–ventricular fibrillation (*VF*) rate boundary is based on the cycle length below which shocks should not be delayed for more than one trial of antitachycardia pacing. Additionally, programming a nontherapy, monitor-only detection zone permits storing electrograms for tachycardias slower than the slowest zone at which VT therapy is programmed. *FVT,* Fast ventricular tachycardia; *SVT,* supraventricular tachycardia.

therapies (e.g., different adaptive cycle lengths for slower versus faster VTs and more sequences of ATP for slower VTs). Additionally, because most manufacturers link SVT discriminators to specific therapy zones, multizone programming may facilitate SVT-VT discrimination. Multizone programming increases flexibility in relation to detection duration, SVT-VT discrimination, and therapy, but the supporting evidence base is limited. Observational data from a large remote monitoring database based reported fewer shocks with dual-zone versus single-zone

programming for detection rates of <200 beats/min.[30] The availability of ATP before and/or during charging in the VF zone may reduce the ATP-related benefits of multizone programming.

Supraventricular Tachycardia Versus Ventricular Tachycardia Discriminators
Ventricular rate and duration serve as implicit SVT-VT discriminators and suffice in many patients,[31] but patients with overlapping SVT and VT rates require an explicit SVT-VT discrimination

process. *Discriminators* are individual algorithm components that provide a partial or complete rhythm classification for a subset of rhythms. *Discrimination algorithms* integrate complementary component discriminators to classify tachycardias as VT/VF or SVT.

Chapter 116 describes individual discriminators, which may be considered in relation to the EGMs analyzed (ventricular only or both atrial and ventricular), the rhythm that they identify (e.g., AF, sinus tachycardia, VT), or the type of EGM information analyzed (intervals vs. morphology).[9,13] Morphology of the ventricular far-field (shock) EGM is the most versatile single-chamber discriminator and the only one that does not rely on inter-EGM intervals (see Fig. 117.5B and C). Dual-chamber algorithms combine single-chamber discriminators with an absolute measure of atrial rate, comparisons of atrial and ventricular rates, and measures of AV association.[9,13] Dual-chamber discrimination should not be used if the atrial lead is unstable or atrial sensing is unreliable.

SVT-VT discriminators apply in a range of cycle lengths bounded on the slower end by the VT detection interval and on the faster end by a minimum cycle length. Programming a sufficiently short minimum cycle length for SVT-VT discrimination is critical. In clinical trials, about 25% of inappropriate therapies have been caused by SVT faster than the programmed minimum value.

The value of SVT-VT discrimination was demonstrated in the 1990s and has not been restudied systematically. Patients benefit most if the rates of their VTs and SVTs overlap.[30] This includes patients with slower monomorphic VT, those at risk for AF with rapid ventricular rates, or those capable of exercising to sinus rates in the VT zone.[32] The benefit is less in primary prevention patients, secondary prevention patients at risk only for VF, and those who cannot sustain rapid atrioventricular (AV) conduction. The risk is misclassification of VT as SVT, delaying therapy, or preventing VT detection (underdetection). When modern algorithms are programmed to recommended parameters, clinically significant underdetection is vanishingly rare.

Programming Ventricular Antitachycardia Pacing

ATP is preferable to shocks for patients at risk for monomorphic VT:[33] (1) Shocks reduce quality of life, but ATP does not. (2) ATP delivered inappropriately for SVT either terminates SVT or slows the ventricular rate below the VT detection rate in about 50% of episodes; thus inappropriate ATP may prevent inappropriate shocks. (3) The response to ATP that does not terminate tachycardia can be used to differentiate VT from sinus or atrial tachycardia with 1:1 AV conduction and thus to optimized ICD programming.[34] (4) Frequent delivered or aborted shocks deplete the ICD's battery, but ATP does not. (5) Shocks depress myocardial contractility acutely, but ATP does not.

However, ATP may fail for reasons that do not affect shocks, such as pacing-induced T wave oversensing, a rise in pacing threshold, or conduction block between the pacing site and the reentry circuit. Multiple ineffective ATP sequences may delay an effective shock, permitting syncope. Rarely, ATP may be proarrhythmic or accelerate hemodynamically stable VT into unstable VT/VF.

Early studies reported that ATP terminated 80%–95% of slower VT (cycle length >320 msec) and ≥70% of fast VT (cycle length, 240–320 msec). However, these studies were performed with short detection durations of 12–16 beats, and many of these VTs probably would have terminated spontaneously if the duration had been longer,[35] emphasizing the concept of avoidable therapy. The PREPARE[26] and ADVANCE III[36] trials programmed detection to 30–40 beats for fast VT; these studies report ATP success rates of 49% and 44%, respectively (see Fig. 117.5D).

Usually, adaptive burst cycle lengths should be programmed to 85%–90% of the VT cycle length for faster VTs and 70%–80% for slower VTs.[33]

Strategic Programming and Clinical Outcomes

The EMPIRIC[37] trial found that standardized strategic programming reduced shocks compared with physician-guided individualized programming. Although this study was performed with older ICDs, no study has demonstrated the superior performance of individualized programming. In a contemporary observational study of 2770 closely followed patients with both initial and replacement implants, strategic programming resulted in an inappropriate shock rate at 1 year of 1.5% in dual/triple-chamber ICDs and 2.5% in single-chamber ICDs.[28]

Patient Alerts, Clinical Follow-up, and Remote Monitoring

Patient Alerts

ICDs provide alerts related to ICD system malfunction (e.g., suspected lead failure), potential programming errors (e.g., VF detection or therapy OFF), and spontaneous arrhythmias. Alerts for AF facilitate early anticoagulation and adjustment of rate and rhythm control medications. Alerts include audible tones, pulse generator vibration, and wireless internet transmissions. A lead integrity alert (see later) reduces inappropriate shocks caused by lead failure.[38]

Remote Monitoring

Technically, remote interrogation refers to scheduled, routine device interrogation at a distance corresponding to in-clinic interrogation; remote monitoring refers to automatic data transmission based on device-generated alerts.[39] Colloquially, "remote monitoring" includes both. All ICD manufacturers sell ICDs with "wireless telemetry" that automatically transmits data stored in the ICD to a home monitor, which then relays the data to a server via an internet connection. This enables immediate or daily transmission of alerts. Additionally, patients may initiate transmissions in response to symptoms. Healthcare providers log into a web server to review alerts and transmitted data.

Remote monitoring is recommended for all ICD patients.[39] It reduces the time for diagnosis of both new arrhythmias (primarily AF) and ICD system problems identified by alerts. It reduces patient expense, reduces the burden on the healthcare system by reducing in-office visits, improves adherence to follow-up, shortens the time for decision-making following clinical events, and reduces the length of cardiovascular hospitalizations. It also correlates with fewer appropriate and inappropriate shocks and lower mortality.[39,40]

Troubleshooting

Ventricular Oversensing: Diagnosis and Management

Ventricular oversensing of rapid signals presents as oversensing alerts, inappropriate detection of nonsustained VT/VF, inappropriate detection of sustained VT/VF with delivered therapy or aborted shocks, or inhibition of bradycardia pacing. Excluding recalled leads, ventricular oversensing accounts for <10% of inappropriate shocks, but it often results in repetitive shocks and severe symptoms.[12]

Oversensing may be classified by EGM morphology, temporal pattern (cyclic vs. noncyclic), source type (physiological vs. nonphysiological), and source location (intracardiac vs. extracardiac). Specific sources may generate oversensed signals with

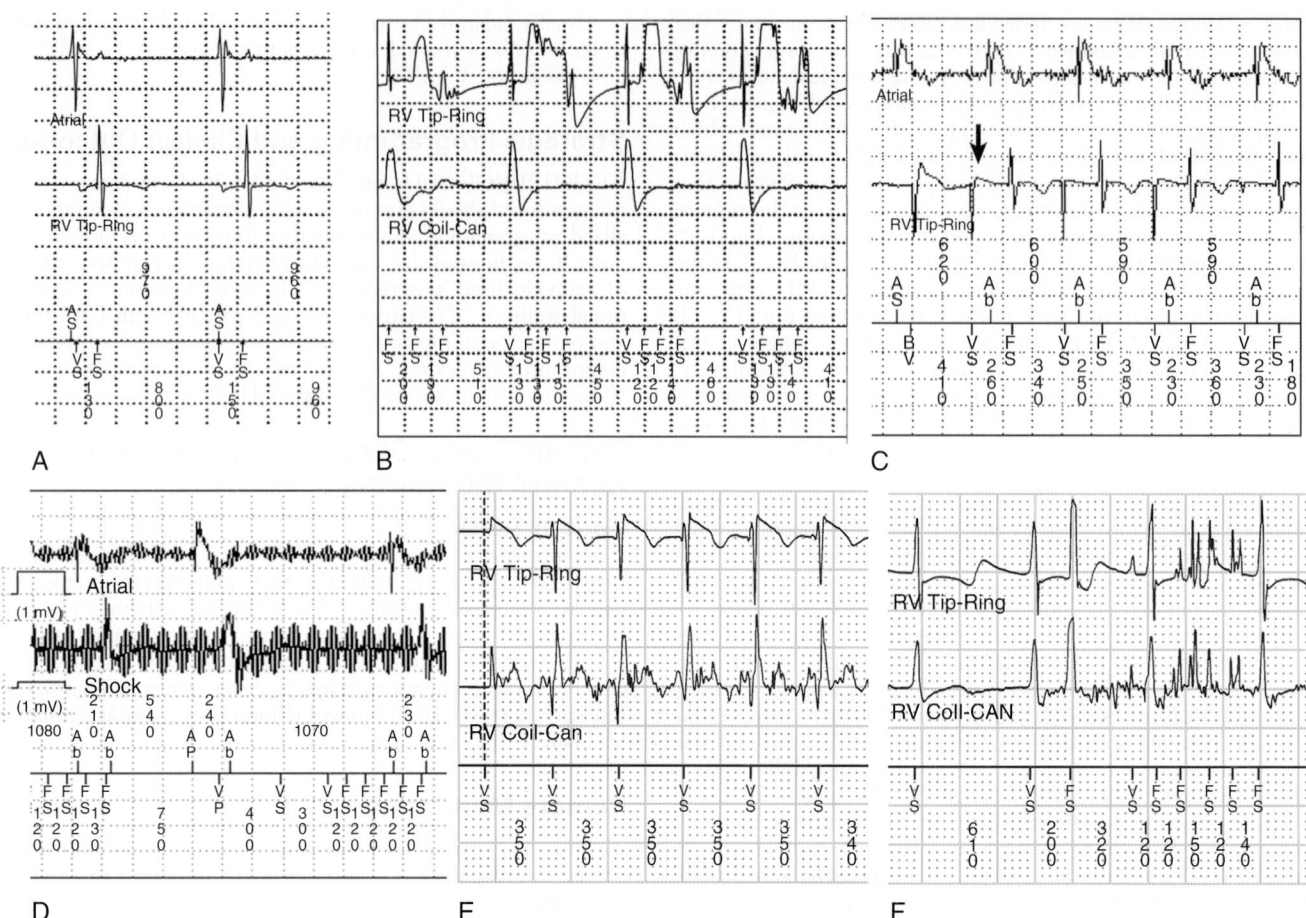

FIGURE 117.7 Electrogram (EGM) patterns of ventricular oversensing. Each panel shows labeled EGMs and the marker channel. *Upper panel,* cyclic oversensing patterns of intracardiac signals. (A) Atrial and ventricular sensing EGMs in P wave oversensing. Cyclic oversensing of physiological T waves (see Fig. 117.4) and P waves or R wave double-counting results in a pattern of one oversensed signal per true cardiac cycle that corresponds consistently to P waves, T waves, or a second component of R waves. In contrast, oversensing of cyclic, nonphysiological signals from intracardiac lead failure is diagnosed by the superimposition of nonphysiological signals on true ventricular EGMs at a fixed time in the ventricular cycle. (B) A multiphasic signal superimposed on the ST segment and T wave in a Fidelis lead (Medtronic Inc.) ring-cable fracture results in multiple oversensed events per cardiac cycle. (C) Cyclic spikes caused by an inside-out insulation breach of Riata lead (St. Jude Medical). *Lower panel,* noncyclic oversensing patterns of extracardiac signals. (D) External electromagnetic interference (EMI) typically appears on multiple channels. The 60-Hz signal from the line current appears with an 8-Hz modulation due to telemetry sampling at 128 Hz, just above the Nyquist limit. (E) High-frequency pectoral myopotentials are a *normal* finding on EGMs that include the can as one electrode. No oversensing occurs on the marker channel. (F) An in-pocket lead insulation breach results in oversensing of pectoral myopotentials on a dedicated bipole in the right ventricular (*RV*) apex (upper EGM). The myopotential on the lower (shock) EGM is a normal finding (see E) and does not indicate a breach of the conductor to the RV coil.

characteristic features that differ from true cardiac EGMs in frequency content and amplitude (Fig. 117.7).[12]

Temporally, oversensing may vary consistently with the ventricular cycle (*cyclic*) or independently of the ventricular cycle (*noncyclic*). Cyclic oversensing indicates an intracardiac signal, usually physiological—R wave double-counting or P/T wave oversensing. These produce a characteristic pattern of one oversensed event and corresponding marker for each true ventricular cycle. Nonphysiological, intracardiac signals—most commonly caused by lead problems—may be both noncyclic and cyclic; the latter may cause multiple oversensed events for each true ventricular cycle. In contrast, extracardiac signals (physiological or nonphysiological) always produce noncyclic oversensing.

Oversensing in the Diagnosis of Implantable Cardioverter Defibrillator Lead Failure

Of all the causes of oversensing, early diagnosis may be most important in lead failure.

Oversensing Nonphysiological Signals from Lead Problems

The mechanism(s) by which conductor fractures cause nonphysiological signals are not understood completely, but the signals are well characterized (Fig. 117.8).[41] Pacing, especially high-output pacing, may precipitate these signals and oversensing. Importantly, connection problems between the lead and header may cause identical EGM patterns.[42]

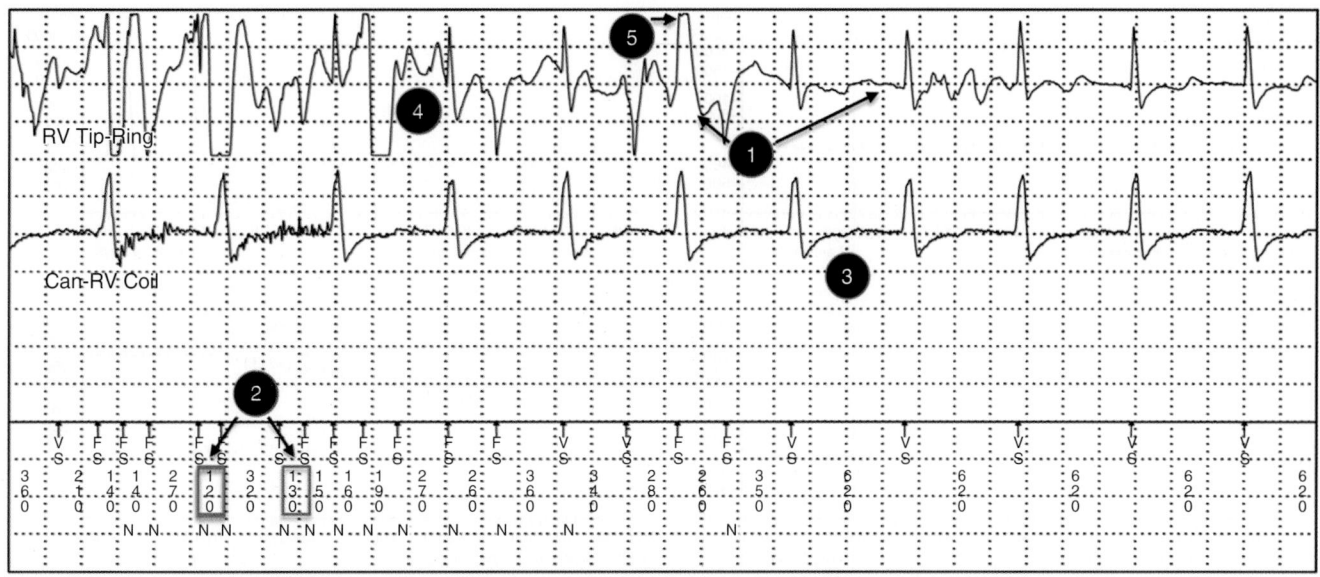

FIGURE 117.8 Characteristic features of electrogram (EGM) in conductor fracture or a connection problem between the DF-1 lead and header. (1) Intermittent nonphysiological signals; (2) "nonphysiological" intervals too short to correspond to successive ventricular depolarizations; (3) no abnormal signal on the shock channel of a dedicated sensing bipole; (4) variable amplitude, morphology, and frequency; may saturate the sensing amplifier. An enhanced sensing feature (lead noise algorithm) prevents inappropriate detection of VF, classifying intervals as "N" (noise) on the marker channel. A high-frequency signal superimposed onto the shock channel is probably caused by pectoral myopotentials, which are a normal finding on EGMs including the can (see Fig. 117.7E and F). *RV,* Right ventricular.

Unlike conductor fractures, insulation breaches themselves do not generate abnormal signals. Instead, oversensing occurs because external signals enter the conductor at the insulation breach; EGM patterns vary, reflecting the source signal. Nonphysiological signals may be recorded from multiple conductors (e.g., inside-out abrasion) or multiple leads (lead-lead abrasion). Similar to fracture-related oversensing, oversensing related to insulation breaches usually is intermittent and transient (see Fig. 117.7F).

Lead Integrity Diagnostics That Incorporate Oversensing

Lead integrity diagnostics incorporate specific features of lead-related oversensing. Recurrent, transient oversensing is often detected as rapid nonsustained VT. Short "nonphysiological" R-R intervals near the ventricular blanking period are common in lead-related oversensing and cannot represent successive cardiac depolarizations, except occasionally during VF.

The occurrence of an abrupt change in pace-sense impedance with either nonphysiological intervals or repetitive, rapid nonsustained "VT" is highly specific for pace-sense lead failure; the combination of both with normal impedance is relatively specific in dedicated bipolar leads.[11] A lead integrity alert incorporating these features improves early detection of both conductor fracture[38] and insulation breaches,[11] reducing shocks caused by lead-related oversensing.

A different type of lead failure algorithm operates on the principle that true ventricular EGMs occur simultaneously on the sensing and shock channels, so the occurrence of more signals on the sensing channel than on the shock channel indicates oversensing (see Fig. 117.8).[12] These algorithms withhold therapy from device-detected VT/VF if a sufficient fraction of sensed EGMs do not have corresponding EGMs on the shock channel. While designed for oversensing related to pace-sense lead failures, these algorithms will withhold shocks from oversensing of any cause limited to the sensing channel (e.g., T wave oversensing). Two such algorithms have been introduced.[12,28]

Impedance and Impedance Trends in the Diagnosis of Lead Failure

ICDs measure direct current electrical resistance ("impedance") periodically for both pace-sense and high-voltage conductors. Conductor fractures may cause high impedance; conversely, insulation breaches may cause low impedance, but oversensing usually precedes impedance changes in both conductor fractures and insulation breaches. Fig. 117.9 shows examples of impedance trends in various conditions.

Pace-Sense Impedance

An *abrupt* 50%–75% relative increase in impedance is a highly specific indicator of an ICD system problem, either conductor fracture or a connection problem between the lead and header.[38,42] Conversely, a gradual impedance increase without oversensing usually occurs at the electrode-myocardial interface,[42] caused—at least in some cases—by calcium deposition in the form of hydroxyapatite; lead replacement is not indicated unless pacing or sensing is compromised. Occasionally, silicone insulation breaches present with low or decreasing pacing impedance; impedance decreases have also been reported in RV lead perforations.[12]

High-Voltage Impedance

Fractures of high-voltage conductors may present as abrupt increases in shock impedance.[43] High shock impedance may also be caused by high-voltage connection issues or improper calibration of low-voltage measurements. Low shock impedance has been reported in some high-voltage insulation breaches. However, diagnosing high-voltage insulation breaches by painless measurements of shock impedance is challenging because high-voltage shocks above the insulating material's dielectric breakdown voltage can cause catastrophic short circuits even if low-voltage test pulses encounter intact insulation.

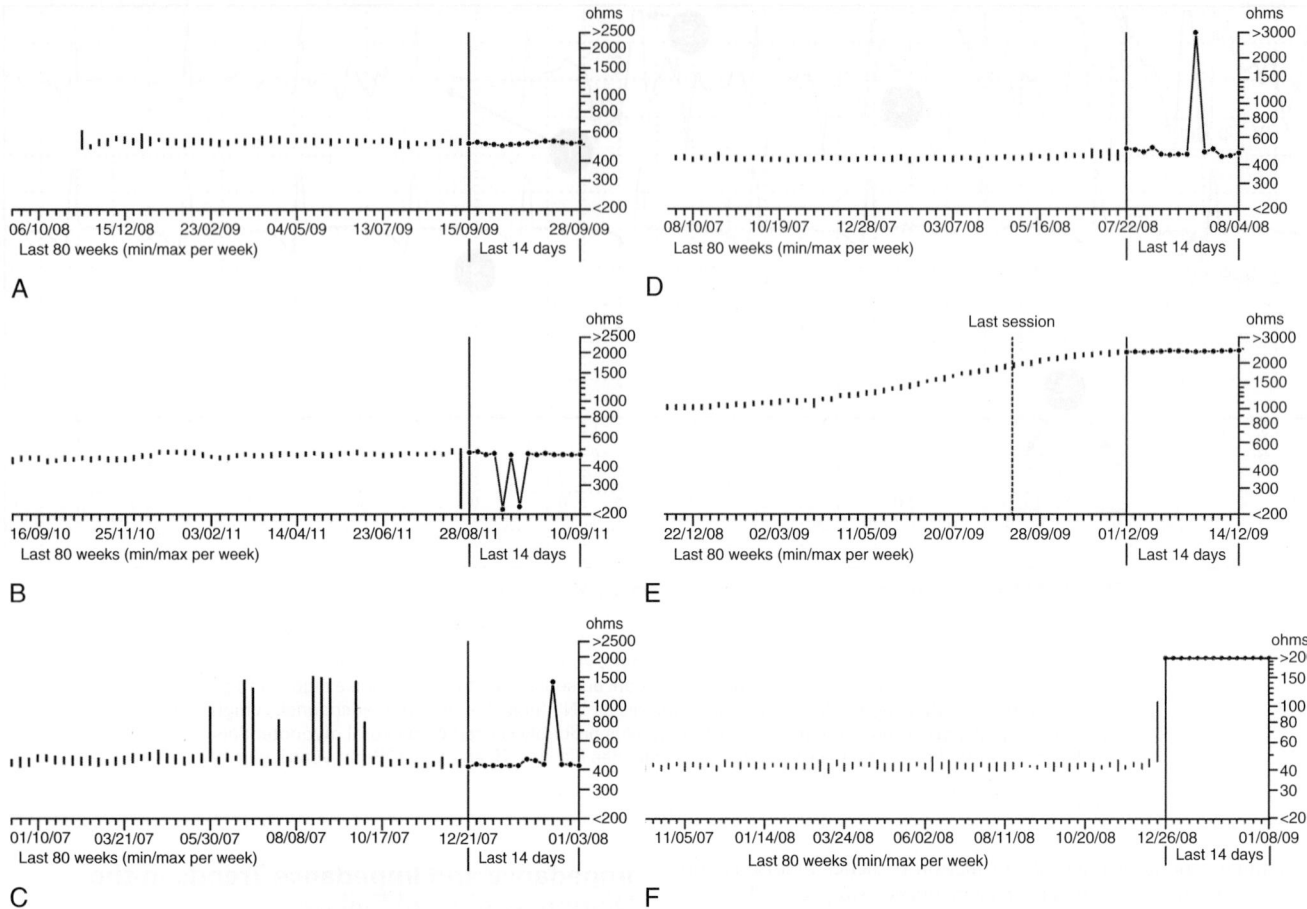

FIGURE 117.9 Impedance trends. (A–E) show pace-sense impedance trends; (F) shows a high-voltage impedance trend. To the left of the longest vertical line, impedance measurements are displayed as vertical bars connecting weekly maximum and minimum impedance values. To the right, black points indicate daily values. (A) A normal impedance trend. Normal trends commonly occur in conductor fractures and insulation failures. (B) Lead insulation failure shows a late abrupt fall in impedance. (C) A connection problem between the header and lead due to incomplete pin insertion shows highly variable impedances beginning about 4 months after implantation followed by a return to baseline for about 2 months between early October and December 2007. (D) A lead conductor fracture with a late, abrupt increase in impedance to the highest reported value (>3000 Ω). (E) A gradual increase in impedance in a normally functioning lead thought to be due to changes at the electrode-myocardial interface. (F) A high-voltage conductor fracture. Note the lower impedance range (0–200 Ω vs. 200–2500/3000 Ω). (Modified from Swerdlow CD, Asirvatham SJ, Ellenbogen KA, et al. Troubleshooting implanted cardioverter defibrillator sensing problems I. *Circ Arrhythm Electrophysiol.* 2014;7:1237-1261.)

Lead Failure and Lead Alerts: Presentation and Management

Excluding leads with known high failure rates, the overall incidence of clinical failure of defibrillation leads is about 1.3 per 100 lead-years.[44]

Clinical Presentations of Lead Failure

Pace-sense malfunctions account for most clinically diagnosed lead failures. Oversensing with normal pacing impedance is the most common initial electrical abnormality with either conductor fracture or insulation breach.[11,38,45] Pace-sense malfunctions may also present with pacing impedance changes, loss of capture, or an abrupt decrease in R wave amplitude. Shock component malfunction presents with shock impedance changes, abnormal signals on shock EGMs, or failed defibrillation shocks. Insulation breaches that cause high-voltage short circuits may also cause ICD generator failure.

Imaging

The chest x-ray is unrevealing in most cases of lead failure, but it should be inspected for lead conductor discontinuity, kinks or acute angles that indicate stress points, twisting suggesting "twiddler's syndrome," or cables that protrude outside the outer insulation (externalized cables).[41] It is important for excluding alternative causes of oversensing such as lead dislodgement, abandoned leads or lead fragments that cause a lead-lead interaction, and incomplete insertion of DF-1 pins into the header. [42] Cinefluoroscopy in multiple views is more sensitive for identifying externalized conductors in Riata leads[46] (see Fig. 117.7).

Approach to the Patient

Clinical Lead Failure. Fig. 117.10 summarizes the approach to the diagnosis of patients with electrical findings suggestive of lead failure. All lead failure diagnostics have false-positives, and the diagnosis of lead failure must be confirmed before surgical intervention to remove the failed lead from the ICD system. Table 117.4 summarizes the major alternate causes of rapid oversensing that may be confused with lead failure. System revision may be accomplished by adding a new lead, extracting the failed lead and inserting a replacement lead, or abandoning the transvenous system and implanting an S-ICD. The most common decision is between the addition of a new lead or extraction and

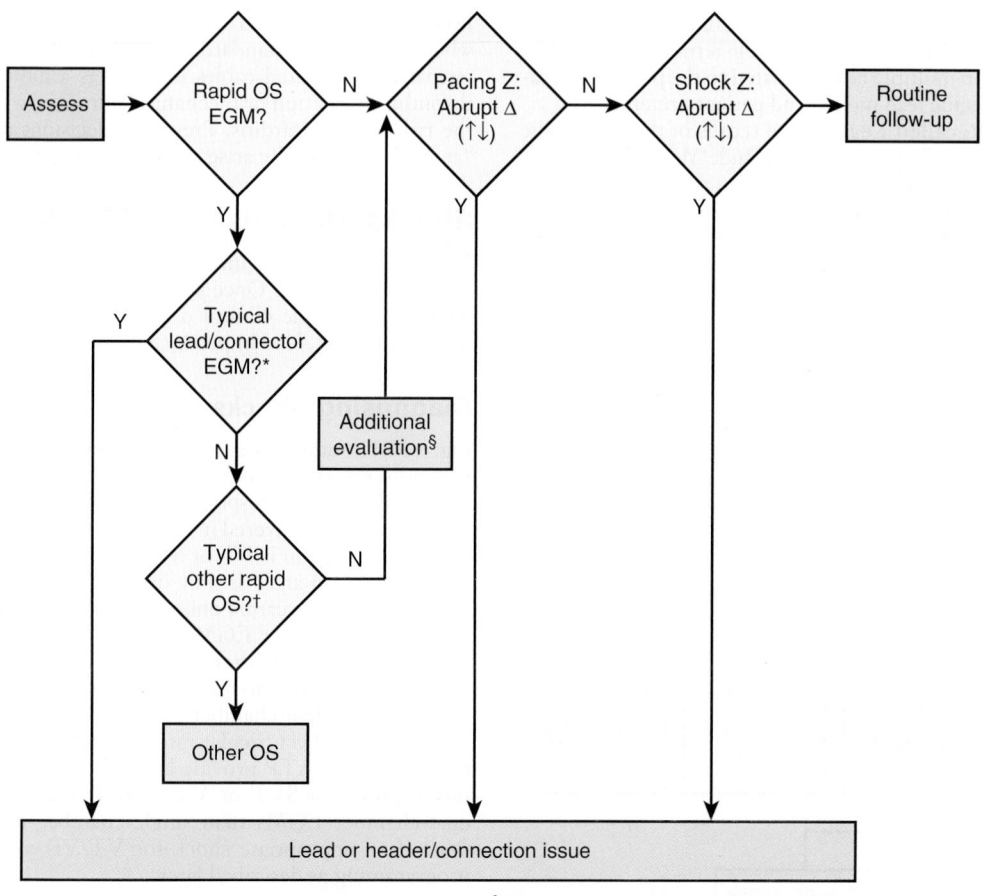

*See Figs. 117-7B,C,F and 117-8
†See Box 117-1

§Additional evaluation
• Real-time EGMs with muscle
  exercise and pocket manipulation
• Shock EGMs
• Differential EGMs
• Pacing threshold
• R-wave amplitude

FIGURE 117.10 Approach to the patient with suspected lead failure. See text for details. *EGM,* Electrogram; *OS,* oversensing; *Z,* impedance.

TABLE 117.4	Rapid oversensing with normal pacing impedance: differential diagnosis of lead failure	
	SENSING EGM CHARACTERISTICS	**CLUES TO DIAGNOSIS**
Early or Late Postimplantation		
Conductor fracture	Typical nonphysiological signals (see Fig. 117.8)	Postpacing oversensing
Insulation breach – in pocket	Pectoral myopotentials on dedicated bipolar EGM (see Fig. 117.4F)	Pectoral muscle exercise reproduces oversensing
Insulation breach – inside out	Spikes (see Fig. 117.4C)	Simultaneous spikes on multiple EGM channels
Electromagnetic interference	Reflects characteristics of source	More common in integrated bipolar than dedicated bipolar leads; history may suggest source; in dedicated bipolar leads, amplitude is usually greater on the shock channel than the sensing channel
Diaphragmatic myopotentials	Uniformly low-amplitude and relatively uniform morphology vs. lead failure signals, which vary in morphology, amplitude, or both[a]	Usually occur in paced rhythm or bradycardia with integrated bipolar leads at the right ventricular apex; may be reproduced by a deep breath or Valsalva maneuver
Ventricular fibrillation	Variable	Present on both shock and sensing channels
Lead-lead mechanical interactions	Spikes on both leads	Presence of other leads; cinefluoroscopy with real-time EGM recordings confirms diagnosis
Connection problems	Indistinguishable from lead fracture	Radiography, pocket manipulation, repeat measurement of impedance; most common in the first year after surgery
Perioperative Period Only		
Air trapped in header	Uniform, medium-frequency signals	Postoperatively it is a diagnosis of exclusion

EGM, Electrogram.

replacement. Usually, the former is associated with lower procedural risk and the latter with fewer long-term problems. The tradeoffs depend on multiple factors related to the patient, operator/institution, specific lead model, and patient preference.[41]

Functioning Recalled Leads. The recalls of the Medtronic Sprint Fidelis ("Fidelis") lead and the St. Jude Medical Riata lead family presented the challenge of managing patients with functioning leads that have a higher than anticipated risk for conductor fracture and inside-out insulation breach, respectively. Management begins with a baseline assessment. To minimize patient morbidity in the event of a lead failure, utilize both lead-specific programming[41] and lead alerts/shock-withholding algorithms in combination with remote monitoring. Most Riata

leads with externalized cables have normal electrical function when evaluated by standard, low-voltage ICD diagnostics. Infrequently, externalized cables may act as a nidus for intracardiac thrombus formation or mechanical abrasion, which may increase the risk for endocarditis. Presently, decisions about functioning "at-risk" leads usually arise at the time of generator change.[47]

Shocks: Diagnosis and Management

Minimizing shocks requires proper programming, use alerts, and remote monitoring. Once shocks occur, diagnosis and management tools include clinical data (history, chest x-ray) and ICD diagnostics (e.g., lead impedance trends) and stored EGMs.

Diagnosing Shocks

Fig. 117.11 summarizes our three-step approach to the patient who presents with a shock: (1) Analyze stored EGMs to determine if it was delivered in response to a tachycardia or oversensing. (2) If the shock was delivered in response to a true tachycardia, determine if the rhythm is VT or SVT using established principles of ECG and EGM analysis. For single-chamber ICDs, diagnosis is based on the tachycardia onset and the morphology and regularity of the ventricular EGM. A real-time, reference sinus EGM should be recorded with the patient in the same position in which the episode occurred to minimize postural changes in EGM morphology. For dual-chamber ICDs, analyses of the chamber of onset, atrial and ventricular rates, AV relationships, and response to unsuccessful ATP provide key information. Experts agree on the diagnosis of SVT or VT more frequently when reviewing dual-chamber EGMs than single-chamber EGMs.[8] (3) Determine if an appropriate shock for VT/VF could be avoided by programming as described later.

Approach to the Patient With Shocks

Fig. 117.12 summarizes the clinical response to a patient with shocks. Shocks for VT/VF or rapidly conducted AF are associated with increased mortality over weeks to months, primarily due to heart failure.[48] Although the primary cause of this excess

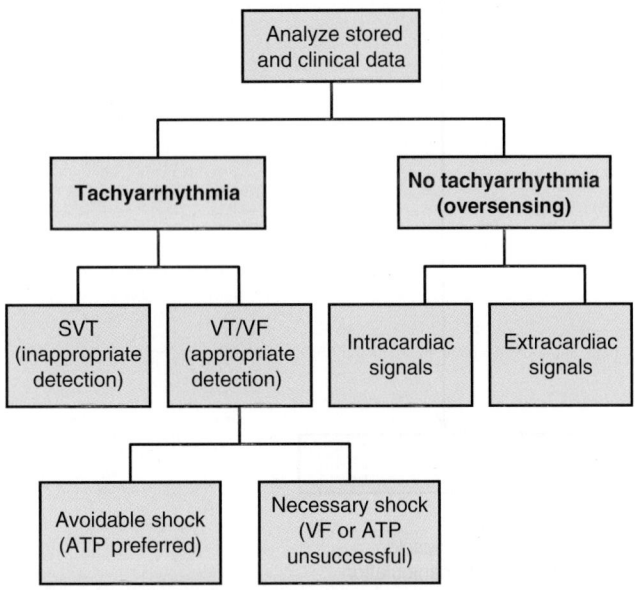

FIGURE 117.11 Differential diagnosis of implantable cardioverter defibrillator shocks. See text for details. *ATP,* Antitachycardia pacing; *SVT,* supraventricular tachycardia; *VF,* ventricular fibrillation; *VT,* ventricular tachycardia.

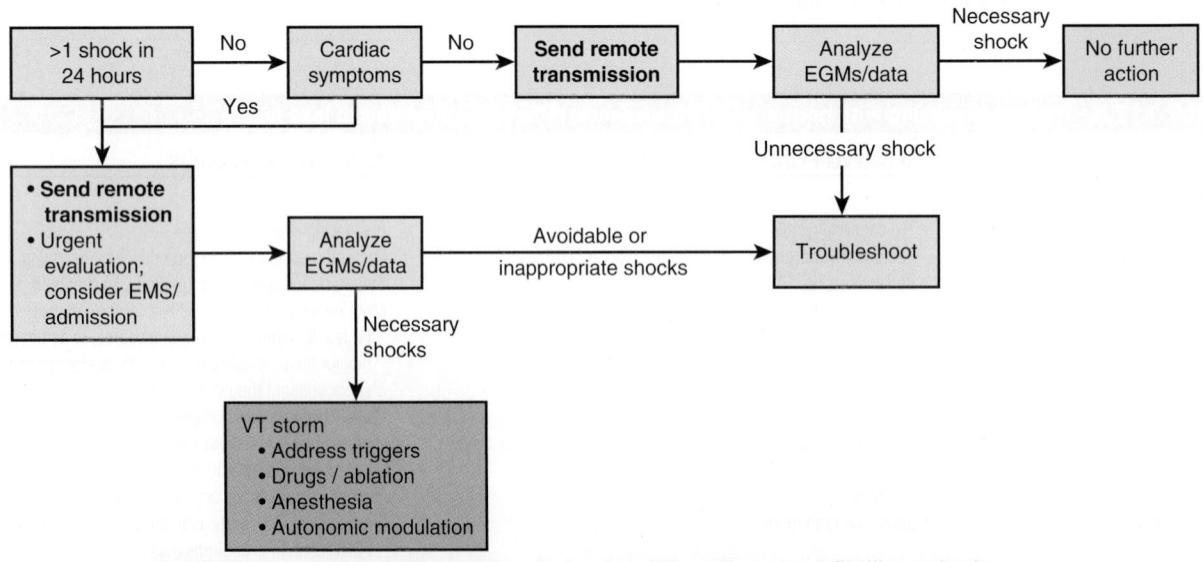

FIGURE 117.12 Approach to the patient with implantable cardioverter defibrillator shocks at home. Remote monitoring facilitates care of patients who receive shocks. In the absence of ongoing cardiac symptoms, a single appropriate shock (reviewed remotely) does not require further intervention. Multiple shocks or ongoing symptoms require urgent action to treat ventricular tachycardia (*VT*) storm, treat supraventricular tachycardia, or troubleshoot to prevent oversensing. *EGM,* Electrogram; *EMS,* emergency medical service.

mortality is likely underlying disease rather than the shocks themselves,[25] the approach to the patient requires not only diagnosis and treatment of the immediate cause of shocks but also the consideration of treatments to reduce delayed mortality. Heart failure and ischemia status should be reassessed if a patient presents with a change in shock pattern.

The approach to the treatment of shocks delivered for oversensing is guided by the cause of oversensing as discussed previously. Shocks for SVT may be corrected by reprogramming (rate zones or SVT-VT discriminators), treatment with β-blockers, antiarrhythmic drugs, or ablation.

Avoidable shocks for self-terminating VT may be prevented by reprogramming shock confirmation or episode termination in addition to the duration for detection. Shocks for sustained VT may be reduced by programming ATP, antiarrhythmic drugs, β-blockers, and VT ablation. Box 117.1 summarizes interactions between antiarrhythmic drugs and ICDs. Drugs such as amiodarone that slow VT may result in failure to detect VT if the detection rate is not decreased when treatment is initiated.

Patients who have *single or infrequent* shocks should send an immediate remote-monitoring transmission to permit prompt diagnosis. If this is not possible, the ICD should be interrogated within 24–48 hours. In contrast, *repetitive shocks* constitute an emergency (see Fig. 117.12); detection may be disabled using a programmer or magnet. Repetitive shocks for VT may be caused by recurring episodes of VT after successful shock termination of VT (VT storm) or by multiple unsuccessful shocks for a single episode. Therapeutic approaches differ. Treatment of VT storm requires reversal of the precipitating events and/or antiarrhythmic

---

BOX 117.1 Interactions between drugs and implantable cardioverter defibrillators

Frequency of Ventricular Tachycardia or Fibrillation
Increased
- Drugs with proarrhythmic side effects (all except β-blockers)
- Drugs that interact with proarrhythmic drugs

Decreased
- β-Blockers
- Antiarrhythmic drugs

Consideration for Detection of Ventricular Tachycardia or Fibrillation
VT Rate
- Decrease (class IC, amiodarone)

SVT Ventricular Rate
- Decrease (β-blockers, amiodarone, sotalol)
- Increase (class IC drugs, 1:1 conduction of atrial flutter)

ICD SVT-VT Discrimination Algorithms
- VT interval stability (IC, amiodarone—more irregular)
- Altered electrogram morphology

Therapy for Ventricular Tachycardia or Fibrillation
Defibrillation Energy Requirement
- Increase (class IB, class IC, chronic amiodarone, verapamil)
- Decrease (sotalol, dofetilide)

Effect on Pacing
- Elevated pacing threshold and use-dependent effect during antitachycardia pacing (class 1C)
- Bradycardia pacing-induced battery drain if drug-induced sinus bradycardia or atrioventricular delay

ICD, Implantable cardioverter defibrillator; *SVT,* supraventricular tachycardia; *VT,* ventricular tachycardia.

---

therapy. Causes include acute ischemia, exacerbation of heart failure, metabolic abnormalities (e.g., hypokalemia, amiodarone-induced hyperthyroidism), and drug effects (e.g., proarrhythmia or noncompliance). Diagnosis of acute coronary syndromes during a VT storm is difficult because shocks can cause changes in repolarization and elevations of troponin I. In addition to previously mentioned therapies, neuraxial interventions may also be useful.[49]

Unsuccessful Shocks

If an ICD classifies a shock delivered for true VT/VF as unsuccessful, stored EGMs should be reviewed to determine if the shock truly failed to terminate VT/VF or if the ICD misclassified effective therapy as ineffective, possibly due to immediate arrhythmia recurrence.

Because defibrillation success is probabilistic, occasional shocks fail; but the failure of two maximum-output shocks is rare if the safety margin is adequate. Shocks from chronic ICD systems fail to terminate true VT/VF for both patient-related or ICD system-related causes. Most patient-related causes can be reversed (e.g., hyperkalemia, hypoxemia, hypercapnia, acidemia, ischemia), but system-related causes usually require operative intervention. ICD data should be reviewed for clues to system-related causes including excessive detection or charge times, evidence of lead or connection failure, a mismatch between programmed and delivered shock strength suggesting a short circuit, or out-of-range high-voltage impedance. In the absence of such findings, defibrillation testing should be performed, especially if it was not performed at implantation.

Failure to Deliver Therapy or Delayed Therapy

Delayed therapy and failure to deliver therapy may be caused by sensing problems, programmed detection parameters, or ICD system malfunction. VF may be undersensed because of low-amplitude EGMs, rapidly varying EGM amplitudes, drug effects, postshock tissue changes, device-device interactions, or intradevice interactions.[12] VF may be underdetected because of device inactivation or programming (sensitivity, rate, duration, SVT-VT discriminators). Lead, connector, or generator malfunction can also prevent delivery of therapy.

Other Common Clinical Issues

Psychosocial, Lifestyle, and End-of-Life Issues

ICD patients may experience anxiety about shocks, but they may also feel protected from sudden death.[50] Patients who receive shocks have reduced quality of life. ICD recipients may benefit from counseling, education, and support groups.[50,51]

Decisions regarding sports participation should be based on the patient's underlying disease, indication for ICD therapy (e.g., primary vs. secondary prevention), and risks for specific sports (e.g., ICD system damage in contact sports, risk for trauma with transient loss of consciousness). Athletes with ICDs experience shocks for both VT/VF and SVT more frequently during sports than at rest, but the risk for injury or failure to terminate VT/VF is low.[52] A recently updated consensus statement provides extensive guidance.[53]

Guidelines for driving and flying are based on arrhythmia symptoms and frequency.[54] Patients in whom ICDs are implanted for primary prevention are not restricted from driving personal cars (as opposed to commercial vehicles). Guidelines recommend that patients refrain from all driving for 6 months both after ICD implantation for secondary prevention and each shock. Although most patients resume driving earlier, accidents in ICD recipients occur less often than in the general driving population.[51]

A consensus statement addresses legal and ethical issues related to withdrawal of ICD therapy to reduce suffering at the end of life.[55] This is important because 20% of ICD patients receive painful shocks in their last weeks of life. A patient (or legally defined surrogate decision-maker) has the right to request withdrawal of any medical therapy, including ICD therapy, even if such withdrawal allows the patient to die naturally from an underlying disease.

Electromagnetic Interference with Implantable Cardioverter Defibrillators

Electromagnetic interference (EMI) has been reviewed extensively.[56] It may cause temporary or permanent inactivation, inappropriate detection of VT/VF, or inappropriate pacing or inhibition of pacing.[57]

Nonmedical Sources

Routine use of household articles should not interfere with ICD function. Although the risk for clinical interference is extremely low, patients should hold activated digital cellular phones to the contralateral ear and avoid carrying them in the ipsilateral breast pocket. ICD patients may walk through airport metal detectors and electronic article surveillance devices at a normal pace. Prolonged exposure can inhibit pacing and detection of VT/VF, cause inappropriate detection of VT/VF, or (in some ICDs) program VT/VF detection OFF.

Medical Sources

Medical sources of EMI are most frequently associated with surgical procedures or MRI.

Surgical Procedures. A consensus statement[58] provides recommendations for intraoperative management of ICD patients, which may include magnet application or perioperative reprogramming. A magnet placed over an ICD disables detection of VT/VF but does not alter the pacing mode. If the surgical site and dispersive ground pad are both below the umbilicus, the risk for EMI is low, and additional ICD-related care typically is not needed.[58]

Magnetic Resonance Imaging. MRI exposes ICD patients to risks due to mechanical forces generated by the static magnetic field, heat and current flow in the leads induced by the radiofrequency fields, and current induced by gradient magnetic fields. New MRI-conditional ICD systems employ pulse generators and leads designed to permit safe imaging under specific MRI conditions.[59] MRI imaging of patients with standard ICDs may be achieved safely by implementing rigorous risk mitigation strategies including pre- and postimaging ICD interrogation; disabling VT/VF detection during scanning; monitoring blood pressure, ECG, and oximetry; and limiting the tissue-specific absorption rate (SAR) during imaging to <2 W/kg.[60]

Other Medical Procedures and Devices. If possible, cardioversion of AF should be performed through the ICD. When external cardioversion is required, defibrillation pads should be placed at least 8 inches from the pulse generator. Because radiation therapy can damage ICD circuitry, ICDs should be shielded or moved to the contralateral side. VT/VF detection should be disabled, and oversensing should be anticipated. Left-ventricular assist devices (LVADs) cause specific forms of EMI.[56]

REFERENCES

1. Epstein AE, DiMarco JP, Ellenbogen KA, et al. 2012 ACCF/AHA/HRS focused update incorporated into the ACCF/AHA/HRS 2008 guidelines for device-based therapy of cardiac rhythm abnormalities: a report of the American College of Cardiology Foundation/American Heart Association Task Force on Practice Guidelines and the Heart Rhythm Society. *Circulation.* 2013;127:e283–e352.
2. Russo AM, Stainback RF, Bailey SR, et al. CCF/HRS/AHA/ASE/HFSA/SCAI/SCCT/SCMR 2013 appropriate use criteria for implantable cardioverter-defibrillators and cardiac resynchronization therapy: a report of the American College of Cardiology Foundation appropriate use criteria task force, Heart Rhythm Society, American Heart Association, American Society of Echocardiography, Heart Failure Society of America, Society for Cardiovascular Angiography and Interventions, Society of Cardiovascular Computed Tomography, and Society for Cardiovascular Magnetic Resonance. *Heart Rhythm.* 2013;10:e11–e58.
3. Kusumoto FM, Calkins H, Boehmer J, et al. HRS/ACC/AHA expert consensus statement on the use of implantable cardioverter-defibrillator therapy in patients who are not included or not well represented in clinical trials. *J Am Coll Cardiol.* 2014;130:94–125.
4. Levy WC, Lee KL, Hellkamp AS, et al. Maximizing survival benefit with primary prevention implantable cardioverter-defibrillator therapy in a heart failure population. *Circulation.* 2009;120:835–842.
5. Goldenberg I, Vyas AK, Hall WJ, et al. Risk stratification for primary implantation of a cardioverter-defibrillator in patients with ischemic left ventricular dysfunction. *J Am Coll Cardiol.* 2008;51:288–296.
6. Burke MC, Gold MR, Knight BP, et al. Safety and efficacy of the totally subcutaneous implantable defibrillator: 2-year results from a pooled analysis of the IDE study and EFFORTLESS registry. *J Am Coll Cardiol.* 2015;65:1605–1615.
7. Groh CA, Sharma S, Pelchovitz DJ, et al. Use of an electrocardiographic screening tool to determine candidacy for a subcutaneous implantable cardioverter-defibrillator. *Heart Rhythm.* 2014;11:1361–1366.
8. Powell BD, Cha YM, Asirvatham SJ, et al. Implantable cardioverter defibrillator electrogram adjudication for device registries: methodology and observations from ALTITUDE. *Pacing Clin Electrophysiol.* 2011;34:1003–1012.
9. Madhavan M, Friedman PA. Optimal programming of implantable cardiac-defibrillators. *Circulation.* 2013;128:659–672.

10. Wilkoff BL, Hess M, Young J, Abraham WT. Differences in tachyarrhythmia detection and implantable cardioverter defibrillator therapy by primary or secondary prevention indication in cardiac resynchronization therapy patients. *J Cardiovasc Electrophysiol.* 2004;15:1002–1009.
11. Ellenbogen KA, Gunderson BD, Stromberg KD, Swerdlow CD. Performance of lead integrity alert to assist in the clinical diagnosis of implantable cardioverter defibrillator lead failures: analysis of different implantable cardioverter defibrillator leads. *Circ Arrhythm Electrophysiol.* 2013;6:1169–1177.
12. Swerdlow CD, Asirvatham SJ, Ellenbogen KA, Friedman PA. Troubleshooting implanted cardioverter defibrillator sensing problems I. *Circ Arrhythm Electrophysiol.* 2014;7:1237–1261.
13. Wilkoff B, Fauchier L, Stiles M, et al. 2015 HRS/EHRA/APHRS/SOLAECE expert consensus statement on optimal implantable cardioverter-defibrillator programming and testing. *Heart Rhythm.* 2016;13:e50–86.
14. Ruetz LL, Koehler JL, Brown ML, et al. Sinus R-wave amplitude as a predictor of ventricular fibrillation undersensing in implantable cardioverter defibrillator patients. *Heart Rhythm.* 2015;12:2411–2418.
15. Swerdlow CD, Shehata M, Chen PS. Using the upper limit of vulnerability to assess defibrillation efficacy at implantation of ICDs. *Pacing Clin Electrophysiol.* 2007;30:258–270.
16. Birgersdotter-Green U, Ruetz LL, Anand K, et al. Automated vulnerability testing identifies patients with inadequate defibrillation safety margin. *Circ Arrhythm Electrophysiol.* 2012;5:1073–1080.
17. Smits K, Virag N, Swerdlow CD. Impact of defibrillation testing on predicted ICD shock efficacy: implications for clinical practice. *Heart Rhythm.* 2013;10:709–717.
18. Baccillieri MS, Gasparini G, Benacchio L, et al. Multicentre comparison Of shock efficacy using single-vs. Dual-coil lead systems and Anodal vs. cathodaL polarITY defibrillation in patients undergoing transvenous cardioverter-defibrillator implantation. The MODALITY study. *J Interv Card Electrophysiol.* 2015;43:45–54.
19. Healey JS, Hohnloser SH, Glikson M, et al. Cardioverter defibrillator implantation without induction of ventricular fibrillation: a single-blind, non-inferiority, randomised controlled trial (SIMPLE). *Lancet.* 2015;385:785–791.
20. Bänsch D, Bonnemeier H, Brandt J, et al. Intra-operative defibrillation testing and clinical shock efficacy in patients with implantable cardioverter-defibrillators: the NORDIC ICD randomized clinical trial. *Eur Heart J.* 2015;36:2500–2507.

21. Birnie D, Tung S, Simpson C, et al. Complications associated with defibrillation threshold testing: The Canadian experience. *Heart Rhythm.* 2008;5:387–390.
22. Lee DS, Krahn AD, Healey JS, et al. Evaluation of early complications related to De Novo cardioverter defibrillator implantation insights from the Ontario ICD database. *J Am Coll Cardiol.* 2010;55:774–782.
23. Kremers MS, Hammill SC, Berul CI, et al. The National ICD Registry Report: version 2.1 including leads and pediatrics for years 2010 and 2011. *Heart Rhythm.* 2013;10:e59–e65.
24. Poole JE, Gleva MJ, Mela T, et al. Complication rates associated with pacemaker or implantable cardioverter-defibrillator generator replacements and upgrade procedures: results from the REPLACE registry. *Circulation.* 2010;122:1553–1561.
25. Swerdlow C, Ellenbogen KA, Klein GJ. Resolving the conflict: implantable cardioverter-defibrillator shocks for ventricular tachyarrhythmias increase mortality. *Heart Rhythm.* 2012;9:1328–1330.
26. Wilkoff BL, Williamson BD, Stern RS, et al. Strategic programming of detection and therapy parameters in implantable cardioverter-defibrillators reduces shocks in primary prevention patients: results from the PREPARE (Primary Prevention Parameters Evaluation) study. *J Am Coll Cardiol.* 2008;52:541–550.
27. Tan VH, Wilton SB, Kuriachan V, et al. Impact of programming strategies aimed at reducing nonessential implantable cardioverter defibrillator therapies on mortality: a systematic review and meta-analysis. *Circ Arrhythm Electrophysiol.* 2014;7:164–170.
28. Auricchio A, Schloss EJ, Kurita T, et al. Low inappropriate shock rates in patients with single- and dual/triple-chamber implantable cardioverter-defibrillators using a novel suite of detection algorithms: painFree SST trial primary results. *Heart Rhythm.* 2015;12:926–936.
29. Kloppe A, Proclemer A, Arenal A, et al. Efficacy of long detection interval implantable cardioverter-defibrillator settings in secondary prevention population: data from the Avoid Delivering Therapies for Nonsustained Arrhythmias in ICD Patients III (ADVANCE III) trial. *Circulation.* 2014;130:308–314.
30. Gilliam FR, Hayes DL, Boehmer JP, et al. Real world evaluation of dual-zone ICD and CRT-D programming compared to single-zone programming: the ALTITUDE REDUCES study. *J Cardiovasc Electrophysiol.* 2011;22:1023–1029.
31. Moss AJ, Schuger C, Beck CA, et al. Reduction in inappropriate therapy and mortality through ICD programming. *N Engl J Med.* 2012;367:2275–2283.

32. Fischer A, Ousdigian KT, Johnson JW, et al. The impact of atrial fibrillation with rapid ventricular rates and device programming on shocks in 106,513 ICD and CRT-D patients. *Heart Rhythm.* 2012;9:24–31.

33. Cantillon DJ, Wilkoff BL. Antitachycardia pacing for reduction of implantable cardioverter-defibrillator shocks. *Heart Rhythm.* 2015;12:1370–1375.

34. Michael KA, Enriquez A, Baranchuk A, et al. Failed anti-tachycardia pacing can be used to differentiate atrial arrhythmias from ventricular tachycardia in implantable cardioverter-defibrillators. *Europace.* 2015;17:78–83.

35. Gasparini M, Menozzi C, Proclemer A, et al. A simplified biventricular defibrillator with fixed long detection intervals reduces implantable cardioverter defibrillator (ICD) interventions and heart failure hospitalizations in patients with non-ischaemic cardiomyopathy implanted for primary prevention: the RELEVANT [Role of long dEtection window programming in patients with LEft VentriculAr dysfunction, Non-ischemic eTiology in primary prevention treated with a biventricular ICD] study. *Eur Heart J.* 2009;30:2758–2767.

36. Gasparini M, Proclemer A, Klersy C, et al. Effect of long-detection interval vs standard-detection interval for implantable cardioverter-defibrillators on antitachycardia pacing and shock delivery: the ADVANCE III randomized clinical trial. *JAMA.* 2013;309:1903–1911.

37. Wilkoff BL, Ousdigian KT, Sterns LD, et al. A comparison of empiric to physician-tailored programming of implantable cardioverter-defibrillators: results from the prospective randomized multicenter EMPIRIC trial. *J Am Coll Cardiol.* 2006;48:330–339.

38. Swerdlow CD, Gunderson BD, Ousdigian KT, et al. Downloadable software algorithm reduces inappropriate shocks caused by implantable cardioverter-defibrillator lead fractures: a prospective study. *Circulation.* 2010;122:1449–1455.

39. Slotwiner D, Varma N, Akar JG, et al. HRS Expert Consensus Statement on remote interrogation and monitoring for cardiovascular implantable electronic devices. *Heart Rhythm.* 2015;12:e69–e100.

40. Akar JG, Bao H, Jones PW, et al. Use of remote monitoring is associated with lower risk of adverse outcomes among patients with implanted cardiac defibrillators. *Circ Arrhythm Electrophysiol.* 2015;8:1173–1180.

41. Swerdlow CD, Ellenbogen KA. Implantable cardioverter-defibrillator leads: design, diagnostics, and management. *Circulation.* 2013;128:2062–2071, 1-9.

42. Swerdlow CD, Sachanandani H, Gunderson BD, et al. Preventing overdiagnosis of implantable cardioverter-defibrillator lead fractures using device diagnostics. *J Am Coll Cardiol.* 2011;57:2330–2339.

43. Koneru JN, Gunderson BD, Sachanandani H, et al. Diagnosis of high-voltage conductor fractures in Sprint Fidelis leads. *Heart Rhythm.* 2013;10:813–818.

44. Borleffs CJ, van Erven L, van Bommel RJ, et al. Risk of failure of transvenous implantable cardioverter-defibrillator leads. *Circ Arrhythm Electrophysiol.* 2009;2:411–416.

45. Sung RK, Massie BM, Varosy PD, et al. Long-term electrical survival analysis of Riata and Riata ST silicone leads: National Veterans Affairs experience. *Heart Rhythm.* 2012;9:1954–1961.

46. Abdelhadi RH, Saba SF, Ellis CR, et al. Independent multicenter study of Riata and Riata ST implantable cardioverter-defibrillator leads. *Heart Rhythm.* 2013;10:361–365.

47. U.S. Food and Drug Administration. FDA safety communication: premature insulation failure in recalled riata implantable cardioverter defibrillator leads manufactured by St. Jude Medical, Inc. 2012; http://www.fda.gov/MedicalDevices/Safety/AlertsandNotices/ucm314930.htm. Accessed April 7, 2013.

48. Poole JE, Johnson GW, Hellkamp AS, et al. Prognostic importance of defibrillator shocks in patients with heart failure. *N Engl J Med.* 2008;359:1009–1017.

49. Bourke T, Vaseghi M, Michowitz Y, et al. Neuraxial modulation for refractory ventricular arrhythmias: value of thoracic epidural anesthesia and surgical left cardiac sympathetic denervation. *Circulation.* 2010;121:2255–2262.

50. Dunbar SB, Dougherty CM, Sears SF, et al. Educational and psychological interventions to improve outcomes for recipients of implantable cardioverter defibrillators and their families: a scientific statement from the American Heart Association. *Circulation.* 2012;126:2146–2172.

51. Lampert R. Managing with pacemakers and implantable cardioverter defibrillators. *Circulation.* 2013;128:1576–1585.

52. Lampert R, Olshansky B, Heidbuchel H, et al. Safety of sports for athletes with implantable cardioverter-defibrillators: results of a prospective, multinational registry. *Circulation.* 2013;127:2021–2030.

53. Zipes DP, Link MS, Ackerman MJ, et al. Eligibility and disqualification recommendations for competitive athletes with cardiovascular abnormalities: Task Force 9: arrhythmias and conduction defects: a scientific statement from the American Heart Association and American College of Cardiology. *J Am Coll Cardiol.* 2015;66:2412–2423.

54. Epstein AE, Baessler CA, Curtis AB, et al. Addendum to "Personal and public safety issues related to arrhythmias that may affect consciousness: implications for regulation and physician recommendations: a medical/scientific statement from the American Heart Association and the North American Society of Pacing and Electrophysiology": public safety issues in patients with implantable defibrillators: a scientific statement from the American Heart Association and the Heart Rhythm Society. *Circulation.* 2007;115:1170–1176.

55. Lampert R, Hayes DL, Annas GJ, et al. HRS Expert Consensus Statement on the Management of Cardiovascular Implantable Electronic Devices (CIEDs) in patients nearing end of life or requesting withdrawal of therapy. *Heart Rhythm.* 2010;7:1008–1026.

56. Beinart R, Nazarian S. Effects of external electrical and magnetic fields on pacemakers and defibrillators: from engineering principles to clinical practice. *Circulation.* 2013;128:2799–2809.

57. Napp A, Joosten S, Stunder D, et al. Electromagnetic interference with implantable cardioverter-defibrillators at power frequency: an in vivo study. *Circulation.* 2014;129:441–450.

58. Crossley GH, Poole JE, Rozner MA, et al. The Heart Rhythm Society (HRS)/American Society of Anesthesiologists (ASA) Expert Consensus Statement on the perioperative management of patients with implantable defibrillators, pacemakers and arrhythmia monitors: facilities and patient management. This document was developed as a joint project with the American Society of Anesthesiologists (ASA), and in collaboration with the American Heart Association (AHA), and the Society of Thoracic Surgeons (STS). *Heart Rhythm.* 2011;8:1114–1154.

59. Gold MR, Sommer T, Schwitter J, et al. Full-body MRI in patients with an implantable cardioverter-defibrillator: primary results of a randomized study. *J Am Coll Cardiol.* 2015;65:2581–2588.

60. Nazarian S, Hansford R, Roguin A, et al. A prospective evaluation of a protocol for magnetic resonance imaging of patients with implanted cardiac devices. *Ann Intern Med.* 2011;155:415–424.

118 Subcutaneous Implantable Cardioverter Defibrillators

Andrew Grace and Gust H. Bardy

Evidence supporting the use of implantable cardioverter defibrillators (ICDs) for protection against the consequences of ventricular fibrillation (VF) is extensive and secure.[1,2] Standard ICDs have evolved considerably, being initially somewhat cumbersome and requiring surgical placement of epicardial patches.[1] Abdominally placed generators with long, subcutaneously tracked, transvenous leads followed. A major technical step was the simplified unipolar approach allowing devices to be placed in deep and then prepectoral locations.[3] Subsequent extensive use for core-task defibrillation set the stage for increasingly complex pacing applications, and later, cardiac resynchronization.[4] Each of these later advances depended on intravascular leads (Fig. 118.1[5–8]).

Landmark studies supporting primary prevention indications[1,5,6] led to predictions of several hundred thousand extra ICD implants each year.[9] Evidence of potential efficacy was not, however, followed by the anticipated sustained expansion in demand with a grumbling, persistent disinclination from referrers, especially for primary prevention indications.[10,11] Patients had also become aware of adverse events mostly related to the leads,[12] blunting their own enthusiasm even with the knowledge of proven lifesaving potential. The usual problems arising with transvenous pacemaker leads (e.g., vascular obstruction, thrombosis, and systemic infection) were joined by a veritable flood of other concerns, many related to design and manufacture (Fig. 118.2).[7,13,14] It also became apparent that lead performance deteriorated over time,[14] with some leads, especially those with a low-profile construction, showing accelerated aging with several consequences including breakdown, the possibility of inappropriate shocks, and a need for premature replacement.[12] Transvenous leads became viewed as the "weakest link"[14] and the "most vulnerable component"[12] in the effective delivery of ICD therapy. The fact that leads in response to advisories on occasion needed extrication from the heart and vascular system further blunted the community view of singular benefit.[15,16]

It was against this background that the concept of the subcutaneous ICD (S-ICD) developed, with a key objective being a return to pure goal-directed functionality providing simple, effective defibrillation not confounded by the safety issues necessarily attached to intravascular leads.[8,17–19] In fact, it was from the problem of lead failure leading to the death of a patient in 1994 that the concept of the S-ICD was born. During the protracted program of development of the S-ICD, transvenous devices were also transformed both technically—with much more reliable leads,[12,20] improved sensing algorithms, and longer battery life—and clinically, mainly through more rational programming.[21,22] The S-ICD tended to gain also through these advances to become a critical option in the therapeutic toolbox of the electrophysiologist.

Early Development

The first question to be addressed was the energy requirement for defibrillation with an electrode and device in subcutaneous locations.[8,17,23] Conceptually, this followed from early efforts at reducing transthoracic defibrillation energy requirements, which had provided the energy upper limits that an ICD would require.[24] Then followed exploratory studies that demonstrated the capability for clinical defibrillation employing subcutaneous electrodes and an active can emulator,[8,25] at which point it also was shown that if a device were to be placed in a lateral location, patients would tolerate it.[8] Subsequently, in dogs paced into VF electrode configurations for defibrillation, it was identified that it would then also be open to implementation in humans.[23] Parallel clinical research established the optimal device/lead locations for defibrillation in humans.[8,26] The protocols required that patients undergoing routine ICD implantation under general anesthesia (GA) were paced into VF with defibrillation thresholds (DFTs) obtained from a range of device/lead configurations.[8] It was found that with a laterally placed emulator and an 8-cm coil running parallel and 1–2 cm away from the left sternal border (parasternal), the DFT was at its lowest, but also that other configurations could achieve effective, clinically useful defibrillation.[8]

In order to assess more formally the comparative efficacy of the planned clinical device configuration, a randomized evaluation was conducted.[8,27] Patients under GA underwent temporary placement of subcutaneous electrodes and a step-down/skip-up protocol either through a transvenous lead placed as part of the routine clinically required procedure or a subcutaneous electrode. The headline finding was that the DFT (35 J with reasonably tight confidence intervals) strongly suggested than an 80-J device would likely provide a clinically acceptable margin of safety.[17] In the study required for European CE mark approval during implant testing, all 137 episodes of induced VF were cardioverted reliably at 65 J,[8] with this observation of high efficacy then reproduced in the pivotal IDE trial.[28]

Characteristics of the Subcutaneous Implantable Cardioverter Defibrillator System

The first generation S-ICD (SQ-RX 1010, Boston Scientific Inc.) had a significantly larger volume (70 cm³) and was heavier (165 g) than contemporary conventional devices in order to accommodate the capacitors that provided the higher energy outputs required.[17] The necessarily large size was then employed as an

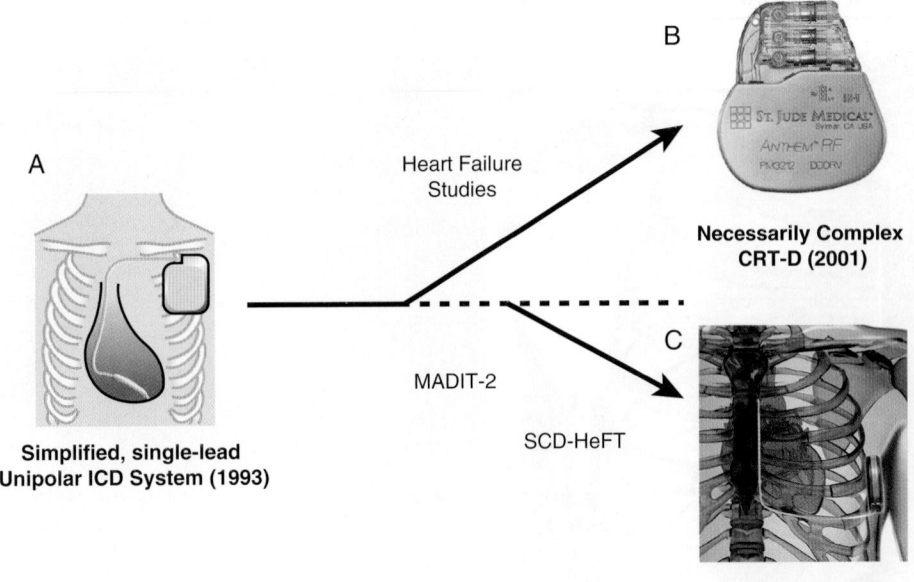

FIGURE 118.1 Development of key ideas in high-energy implantable cardioverter defibrillator (*ICD*) arrhythmia device therapy. (A) Complex transvenous ICDs have represented the standard of care since the mid-1990s with demonstrable efficacy against ventricular arrhythmia and positive effects on mortality.[5,6] However, the leads of these devices remain their "weakest link," being prone to acute complications and time-dependent failure.[7] (B) Cardiac resynchronization therapy with high-energy (ICD) capability (*CRT-D*) is appropriate for patients with impaired ventricular function according to current guidelines.[4] (C) Subcutaneous devices (e.g., subcutaneous ICDs [*S-ICD*]) have been introduced more recently[8] and essentially provide protection against ventricular fibrillation, and other than for a short period of time after defibrillation, are unable to pace. Accordingly, these devices are not suitable for patients with a "pacing" indication whether due to bradycardia, conduction system disease, or the relatively modest number of patients with primary prevention indications who need antitachycardia pacing capabilities. ([B] Courtesy St. Jude Medical, St. Paul, MN. Anthem and St. Jude Medical are trademarks of St. Jude Medical, LLC or its related companies. Reproduced with permission of St. Jude Medical, ©2017. All rights reserved. [C] Courtesy Boston Scientific, Marlborough, MA.)

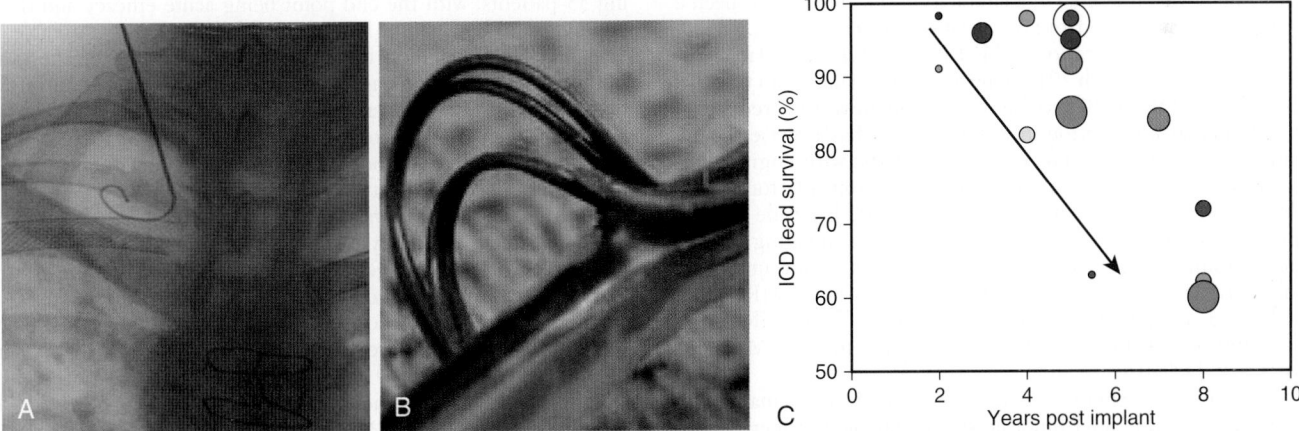

FIGURE 118.2 Key drivers in the development of the subcutaneous implantable cardioverter defibrillator (*ICD*) system. (A) An x-ray obtained from a patient suffering extreme consequences (including infective endocarditis) of conventional transvenous ICD therapy with bilateral venous occlusion requiring stent placements and tricuspid valve avulsion requiring surgical repair. (B) Externalization of cables from a low-profile lead (Riata) with the potential consequences of inappropriate shocks and need for extraction and replacement. (C) Deterioration of lead functionality over time. The plot refers to a series of papers that included over 4000 patients showing a consistent trend of a time-dependent drop-off in functional lead survival.[7] The most striking example seemingly (which was subsequently challenged)[7] is that of Kleemann (n = 990, *blue circle, bottom right*) with a 20% annual failure rate at 10 years.[14] ([C] Modified from Maisel WH. Transvenous implantable cardioverter-defibrillator leads: the weakest link. *Circulation.* 2007;115:2461–2463.)

argument against it by detractors when considering the possibilities for broad deployment, then further supported by limited but ill-advised, premature use of first-generation S-ICDs in children, which resulted in some predictable size-/programming-related problems.[29] The main design advantage of the S-ICD was that the electrode was unconstrained by the conditions implied by the prior requirements for intravascular placement.[17] The lead, for example, needed neither a hollow core nor inner coils and could therefore be manufactured primarily to have long-term durability with multistrand core cables and polyurethane insulation.[17] The

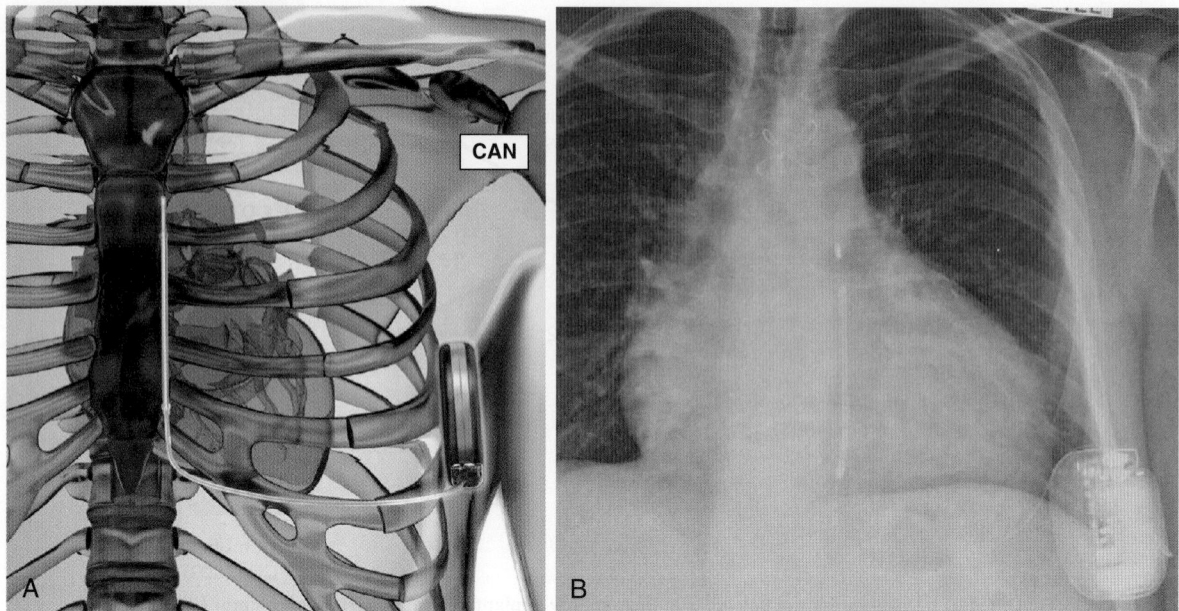

FIGURE 118.3 General setup of the subcutaneous implantable cardioverter defibrillator (S-ICD) system. (A) The pulse generator is placed in a left lateral location. The lead is tunneled to the left parasternal location with the proximal, mid-coil, and distal tips highlighted.[17] (B) A posteroanterior chest x-ray (CXR) shows the ideal device location. It is important that the device be placed sufficiently posteriorly so as to capture as much myocardial tissue in the field of activity as possible. This CXR image is from the first patient who received an S-ICD in July 2008. ([A] Courtesy Boston Scientific, Marlborough, MA. [B] Courtesy Dr. Warren Smith, Auckland, New Zealand.)

overall design of the device and the dimensions and characteristics of the lead have changed little from the initial vision (Fig. 118.3) with the main structural change being downsizing of the can in the most recent design (EMBLEM, Boston Scientific Inc., 2015). It was clear that even the first iteration of the device was surprisingly well tolerated in a lateral location, and this has been a consistent observation from physicians and their patients.[8,30]

The second-generation EMBLEM S-ICD was launched commercially in March 2015. The device is smaller than those of the first generation (20% reduction in thickness, 15% reduction in volume, 10% reduction in weight), and it has a revised shape and increased battery longevity (to 7.3 years) with engineering based on principles common to the transvenous platform. It is also enabled for use on the Boston Scientific Latitude remote monitoring platform.[31] Magnetic resonance imaging (MRI) compatibility has been assessed with first-generation units in a cohort of 15 patients who underwent a total of 22 MRI scans with a 1.5-T magnet without adverse effects,[32] and MRI compatibility is now an embedded characteristic in the EMBLEM MRI S-ICD (2016).

The delivered energy of the EMBLEM device remains at a nonprogrammable 80-J biphasic shock, having a longer charge time than conventional devices with their lower outputs. The charge time was seen initially by some to be a hazard,[33] but more conservative programming of conventional systems supported by numerous studies[21,22] quelled much of that concern and has actually proved to be a benefit in limiting inappropriate shocks. The time to therapy remains in the range of 15–20 seconds. If the initial shock is unsuccessful, then the shock polarity of the S-ICD is automatically inverted. The device is also capable of transcutaneous postshock pacing for 30 seconds. The engineering needed to provide a device for effective defibrillation and postshock pacing was provided relatively early, and the major hurdle in the implementation project was in fact development of the hardware and software algorithms needed to achieve effective sensing and discrimination of the cardiac rhythm—see later[17] (Fig. 118.4[8,34]).

Initial Observational Studies/IDE Submission Trial

The first fully implanted system was placed on July 28, 2008.[8] Studies that led to European CE mark approval then followed, involving 55 patients, with the end point being acute efficacy and then short-term safety[8] with a longer-term follow-up now available.[35] The S-ICD IDE clinical investigation was required for approval in the United States through the US Food and Drug Administration (FDA) and began recruitment in January 2010.[28] This was a prospective, single-arm comparison to an objective performance criterion (OPC) that had been carefully developed with the regulators and was based on that used in prior transvenous ICD trials.[36] The efficacy end point was acute VF conversion and the safety end point was the 180-day system complication-free rate. Three-hundred thirty patients were enrolled, with a distribution of primary and second prevention indications similar to those recorded in the National Cardiovascular Data Registry (NCDR)[37] with low ejection fractions (EFs) well represented (70% of patients had an EF <35%).[28] The primary effectiveness end point was met. In 304 relevant patients, conversion was achieved in 100% of cases. All analyses exceeded the OPC. In addition to these acute conversions, there were 22 episodes of monomorphic ventricular tachycardia (VT) and 16 episodes of VF with first (92%) and second (97%) shock success also in the context of four VT/VF storms. The results were again similar to those seen earlier for transvenous systems. The primary safety end point was met with a 180-day type 1 complication-free rate of 99%. Among the patients, 92.1% were free of type 1–3 complications (those related respectively to the device, to labeling, or to the procedure). The performance goal was 79% and was therefore readily exceeded.[28] The overall conclusions of this purpose-driven pivotal (IDE) study were that the effectiveness end point was met, and the safety end point was met, leading to an almost unanimous FDA advisory panel approval when presented in Washington, DC on April 26, 2012. The thoughtful, reasonable points of concern offered by the dissenting panel member were subsequently presented in detail.[33]

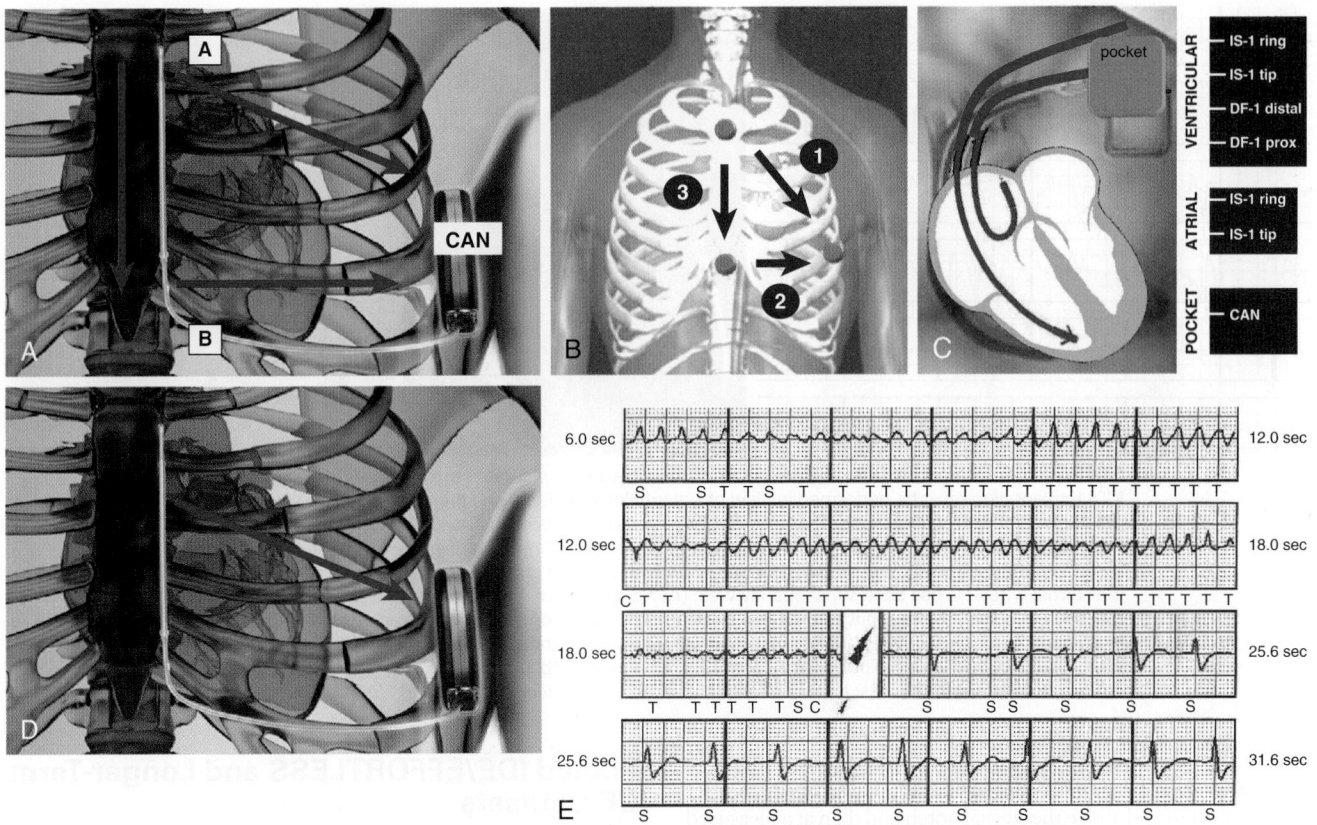

FIGURE 118.4 Key functions of the subcutaneous implantable cardioverter defibrillator (ICD) for sensing and defibrillation. (A) Sensing vectors. The device has three possible sensing vectors with the optimal vector automatically selected by the device. The first iteration device was ~70 cm³ in volume, weighed 145 g, delivered 80 J in a biphasic shock, had postshock pacing for 30 seconds, two zones for shock programming, episode storage, and was simple to program.[8] (B) and (C) The Subcutaneous versus Transvenous Arrhythmia Recognition Testing (START) study[34] evaluated the specificity and sensitivity of the subcutaneous ICD when compared with conventional transvenous ICDs obtained from various manufacturers. In this multicenter study, patients being evaluated for ICD implantation were paced into arrhythmia and the capacities of the different systems to discriminate *shockable* and *nonshockable* rhythms were examined.[34] The results showed that both subcutaneous and transvenous ICDs could identify the presence of a rapid rhythm (high sensitivity) but the performance of the subcutaneous ICD detection arrangement was much higher in terms of discrimination of *shockable* versus *nonshockable* rhythms (high specificity) when compared with transvenous ICDs that in this experimental setting generally had relatively low specificity. (D) The essential effector function of the device is to give an 80-J defibrillation biphasic shock in response to the observation of fully observed ventricular fibrillation. This can be achieved between the *active can* and the parasternal lead in either a lead-to-can (as here) or a can-to-lead vector and this is programmable.[8] (E) In response to the observation of ventricular fibrillation, the capacitor in the device charges up and then discharges with a programmed 80 J of delivered energy. This example from the device memory function taken from the first patient who received a subcutaneous ICD (July 2009; also see Fig. 118.3) shows a charge time of around 20 seconds with effective correction of ventricular fibrillation. ([A and D] Courtesy Boston Scientific, Marlborough, MA. [B and C] Modified from Gold MR, Theuns DA, Knight BP, et al. Head-to-head comparison of arrhythmia discrimination performance of subcutaneous and transvenous ICD arrhythmia detection algorithms: the START study. *J Cardiovasc Electrophysiol.* 2012;23:359–366.)

Practical Clinical Aspects

The techniques for implantation of the S-ICD resemble in many respects those developed for abdominal transvenous systems with tunneled leads. The procedure for implantation of the S-ICD became established with the first few experimental cases.[8] Movies made several years ago provided the basis for later animations with a consistency of approach over time that is striking. It was clear from the outset that following a simple set of rules resulted in good outcomes. The learning curve for implantation is therefore steep,[8] as further evidenced by an analysis of implant duration and inappropriate shocks at 180 days as reasonable indices.[38] Anatomical deterrents are few and implantation is predictable in terms of duration (65–75 minutes[38]) with few unforeseen consequences,

although the current short implantation times for single-lead transvenous systems are unlikely to be exceeded.

DFT testing is still generally recommended, although in the IDE trial, 16 patients did not undergo DFT testing in view of physician concern.[28] In 17% of patients in the IDE trial, reversal of shocking polarity followed DFT failure.[28] In addition, there are a few reports of high DFTs on occasion needing novel methods of resolution (e.g., with substernal lead positioning),[39] although there is no evidence that such patients would fare any better with transvenous systems.

Skin care should be meticulous with diligent skin preparation, removal of all excess hair (including careful attention to the axilla), and antibiotic prophylaxis according to local guidance reliably administered[40] with the physician involved at all stages.[38] The incision needed to accommodate the main body of the device is made

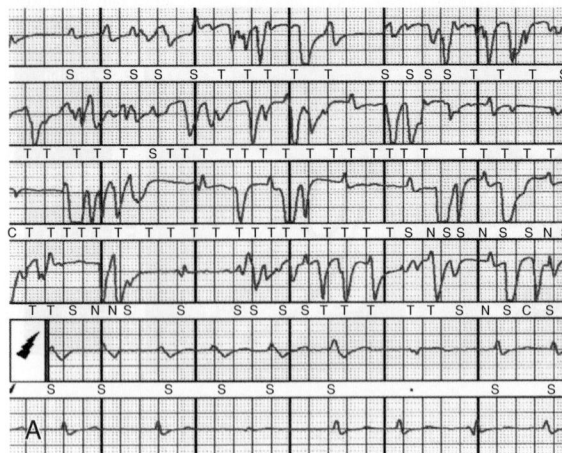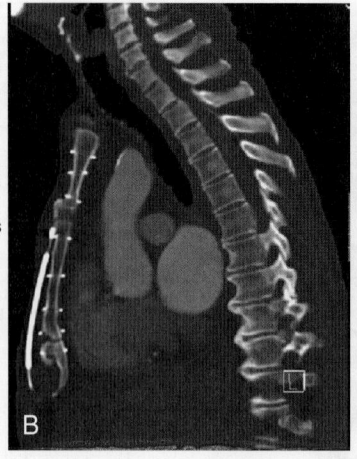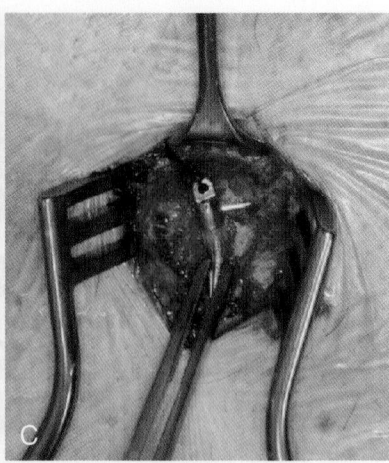

FIGURE 118.5 Interaction with sternal wires. Subcutaneous implantable cardioverter defibrillator (S-ICD) implantation must be performed in view of potential interactions, and there are at least two reports of interactions with sternal wires. This case is a 71-year-old man receiving an ICD for primary prevention. Procedural checks were fine, but he then received inappropriate shocks on days 2 and 3. Distal tip manipulation reproduced noise, and he was reoperated on with the lead distal electrode then relocated between the sternal wires. He has been subsequently well. (A) An episode of inappropriate therapy delivered in response to noise/baseline shift with bizarre electrograms. (B) A computed tomography scan with distal impingement on sternal wires. (C) At reoperation, the distal electrode tip was observed lying on a sternal wire. ([A–C] From Winter J, Kohlmeier A, Shin DI, O'Connor S. Subcutaneous implantable cardioverter-defibrillators and sternal wires: a cautionary tale. *Circ Arrhythm Electrophysiol.* 2014;7:986–987.)

in the left inframammary crease and in the mid-thoracic line with usually two other small incisions made at the lower sternal border just to the left of and above the sternal notch and then at a measured distance upwards (determined by the 8-cm length of the electrode, taking into account the characteristics of the individual patient) to accommodate the electrode also at the left sternal border. The lead is then placed absolutely parallel to the sternum using a proprietary tunneling tool.[41] The tip at the superior (distal) end needs to be fastened securely to the fascia to avoid lead drift. Downward drift was observed in the initial CE study but was solved by the use of a suture sleeve and should no longer happen.[8] Similarly, anterior drift to the skin surface leads to skin irritation, an eczematous reaction, and the potential for erosion, and again is a problem that can be easily avoided. A different approach to lead placement with the use of just two incisions has been proposed, offering the advantage of simplicity,[42] but comparative studies are needed and most implanters still use three incisions, and as such, the greatest experience was acquired with this technique.[41] In patients with prior sternotomy, careful attention needs to be paid to issues of proximity to sternal wires[43] (Fig. 118.5).

The device is placed without the need for routine radiography, although in early postapproval cases, some still advocated screening to verify position.[41] Accordingly, the implanter does not usually require protection against x-rays. In many labs, the procedures are still conducted under GA. It is possible to use conscious sedation but this needs to be efficient and effective. The importance of using sufficient local anesthetic to make conscious sedation cases tolerable and the early period of recovery from the procedure comfortable needs emphasis. Effective use of local anesthetic requires infiltration around the pocket, into the deep fascia, and along the route taken by the lead.[8] Care should be taken with hemostasis; although there are only a few reports of hematoma,[29] the area where the device will reside has many small vessels and it is possible that published reports understate the potential for hematoma as a clinically relevant problem. Erosion has been strikingly rare,[41] although again in one early report 3/16 (18.8%) of children/teenagers suffered erosion,[29] although this reflected inexperience in both case selection and technique.[44] Location within an intermuscular pocket can be considered and may be a helpful approach to improving both comfort and security.[45]

Pooled IDE/EFFORTLESS and Longer-Term CE Datasets

The best current data to support the safety/efficacy of the S-ICD are from the combined data of the IDE trial and the EFFORTLESS (Evaluation of the Factors Impacting Clinical Outcome and Cost Effectiveness of the SICD) European/New Zealand registry.[30] The pooled analysis is based on observations made from 882 patients (mean age, 50.3 ± 16.9 years) with 70% with a primary prevention indication and a mean EF of 40%.[30] In the initial report, patients were followed for 651 ± 345 days (1571.5 patient-years). Device-treated arrhythmias were seen in 11.1% at 3 years, the success of defibrillation after up to five shocks was 98.2%, and the 3-year inappropriate shock rate was 13.1%.[46] Clinical studies continue with longer-term observational data already available from the initial CE patient cohort.[35] Fifty-five patients were followed for 5.8 years during which period 47% had device replacement and 9% had device explantation. The mean time to replacement was 5 years.

Sensing and Discrimination

The issue of greatest initial concern for engineers was the capacity of the device to discriminate between noise and clinically relevant rhythms. This took longer than anticipated to resolve.[17] The algorithms that resulted, however, were refined, sophisticated, and effective. The early experience with the S-ICD was a 13.1% inappropriate shock rate over 11 months[28]; nevertheless, this compared somewhat unfavorably to that seen, for example, in MADIT II (11.5% at 20 months).[46] The main reason for inappropriate shocks from the S-ICD is T wave oversensing (TWOS) and unlike transvenous devices, the device is good at appropriately recognizing and correctly classifying supraventricular arrhythmias.[34,41] Of course, inappropriate shock rates with transvenous devices are now often <5% because of the availability of newer algorithms, longer detection times, and higher cutoff rates,[21] so the bar has moved considerably higher regarding views of its competitive advantage.[41]

Three possible sensing vectors (primary [ring-to-can], secondary [tip-to-can], alternate [tip-to-ring]) are intrinsic and the device automatically selects the optimal sense vector. The system sees a signal not dissimilar to the surface electrocardiogram with a far-field electrogram. The algorithm must therefore integrate the signals obtained from the whole heart.[17] When the R wave amplitude is reduced, the R/T wave ratio may diminish dependent on body habitus, posture, activity, and heart rate, thus providing the setting for TWOS. This problem may be foreseen in certain patients during postimplant alternative posture and activity testing allowing the detection vector to be reprogrammed. The S-ICD has two possible detection zones—shock only (based on rate alone) and a conditional zone based also on a morphology analysis algorithm.[17] Ventricular rate detection relies on a large surface R wave, rejection of mid-sized T waves, and dynamic adjustment to detect smaller signals occurring during VF—these are substantially different from endocardial signals and endocardial detection methods.[17]

The advanced discriminant algorithm of the S-ICD moves through three phases: detection, certification, and decision.[17] The conditional zone discriminant algorithm relies on sequential analysis: (1) Correlation waveform analysis of each beat with a stored baseline template; (2) beat-to-beat analysis; and (3) QRS width analysis. It underwent its first formal comparison in the Subcutaneous versus Transvenous Arrhythmia Recognition Testing (START) study.[34] This investigation compared the sensitivity and specificity of the transvenous lead setup and subcutaneous lead placements in response to a variety of induced arrhythmias in an acute setting. The key findings were that the sensitivity of VF detection by the S-ICD equivalent system was comparable to transvenous systems with essentially 100% capability across the board. However, the specificity of arrhythmia discrimination by the S-ICD system at 98% was superior to both contemporary single- and dual-chamber transvenous systems.[34]

The introduction of the discriminant algorithm during the course of the IDE had a striking impact.[28,47] Eighty-eight patients had a single shock zone programmed and 226 later recruited patients had two shock zones with the discriminant algorithm programmed in the lower rate zone. At follow-up at 661 ± 174 days, inappropriate shocks occurred in 26.1% of the single-zone programmed devices but in only 10.2% of the dual-zone programmed devices.[47] These findings were not associated with prolonged detection times or an increased risk of syncope and the discriminant algorithm is now routinely programmed "on." Newer algorithms continue to be developed that further compare observed complexes with those developed through a database of stored episodes.[48] The possibility of a decrease in inappropriate episodes of 30.7% has been suggested through the use of this refinement alone.

A preimplant surface electrocardiogram (ECG) screening template was developed early to help physicians make rational decisions regarding patient suitability, with the intention that this be used in various postures and configurations. In order to further refine programming and detection of appropriate vectors, different postures are recommended once the device has been implanted.[49] The eligibility of patients has varied with 8% disqualified in an early study,[50] rising to 14.8%[51] and higher (16%) in those with hypertrophic cardiomyopathy (HCM)[52] due to high T wave voltage. Certainly in selected cases, such as younger patients with channelopathies/cardiomyopathies, exercise testing may enhance device setups.[53] In HCM with T wave inversion and prior myectomy, the ECG screening tool may in fact not be usefully applicable.[52] However, in general, the S-ICD has proved useful and effective in HCM. In a pooled data analysis, 99 HCM patients (out of 872 total)[54] with a median follow-up of 637 days suffered three episodes of VT in three patients. The conclusion was that in HCM, the S-ICD was also safe and effective.[54]

Bradycardia Support and Antitachycardia Pacing

One consistent initial objection to the S-ICD was its inability in the absence of transvenous leads to pace, and most particularly, to provide antitachycardia pacing (ATP).[8] The attitude to ATP has, however, evolved considerably over the 5–10 years during which the S-ICD concept developed.[8,21,55] MADIT-RIT showed that ignoring slower rhythms and being more conservative with ATP reduced inappropriate therapy and improved patient survival.[21] In fact, it looks like conventional "aggressive" ICD programming overestimates the real incidence of appropriate discharges, and in the S-ICD pooled data, 36% of detected VT/VF episodes self-terminated without the need for therapy.[30] The Sudden Cardiac Death in Heart Failure Trial (SCD-HeFT) was designed specifically to avoid ATP,[6] and also showed improved survival with shock-only therapy as well as a very low incidence of monomorphic VT with most, if not all, lethal arrhythmias being VF or very rapid VT/ventricular flutter.[6]

Of course, the indications for the S-ICD were neither bradycardia nor cardiac resynchronization.[56] Although the device has the capability for postshock pacing, the number of patients with a primary prevention indication for an ICD who require long-term pacing is modest and so the device should not be considered in those who also need a pacemaker.[41] In the European CE trial over longer-term follow-up, 1/55 (1.8%) patients developed a bradycardia indication and 2/55 developed heart failure leading to the institution of cardiac resynchronization therapy (CRT).[35] In a retrospective cohort study of patients receiving ICDs without pacing indications (2002–2011), <50% went on to a pacing indication at 5 years, indicating the high potential suitability of patients for consideration of the S-ICD.[57] Furthermore, SCD-HeFT also showed an extremely low need for pacing in primary prevention pacing if no clear need had been identified prior to implantation.

The substantial potential for complications with transvenous device upgrades[58] may make one consider an S-ICD in those with a CRT-P who now need ICD support and are being considered for an upgrade to a CRT-D.[41] Although there are no trial data, one could surmise that the approach of an S-ICD added to a CRT-P would carry less risk and be less costly than the insertion of a shocking lead and replacement of a preexisting CRT-P generator.[58] The addition of an S-ICD to patients who already have an implanted pacemaker (simple or CRT-P) needs only careful checks to avoid potential interactions due to cross-talk.[59] There is a current trend for the consideration of the use of the S-ICD in conjunction with "leadless" pacemakers, and in that context, consideration of potential interactions also apply.[60]

Shock Size

Another issue of concern was that of shock size. Again, during development of the S-ICD, the possibility that transvenous shocks themselves could damage the myocardium was being highlighted.[61–63] This question remains unresolved despite some tangential clinical evidence to support the possibility.[61,64,65] The concern was therefore that with the larger 80-J shock, more damage to the myocardium may be sustained.

In fact, this seems not to be the case.[66] Important work has shown the diffusibility of external shocks.[67] Direct comparison of the consequences of shocks using transvenous and subcutaneous systems in swine indicated that the elevations in serum biomarkers reflective of myocardial damage were actually less with a subcutaneous system compared with a transvenous system[66] (Fig. 118.6). Clinically observed acute necrosis and cell injury seen with transvenous shocks presumably contribute to such elevations due to intense field strengths near the right ventricle (RV) coil[61] (see Fig. 118.6).

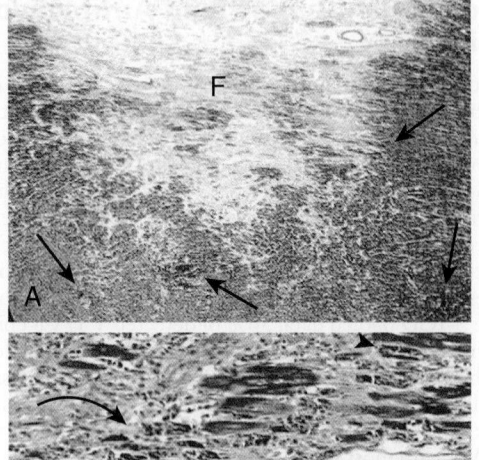

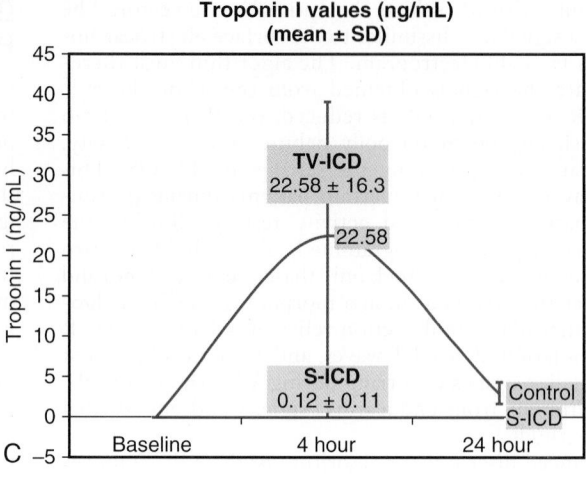

FIGURE 118.6 Myocardial consequences of defibrillation. (A) Acute necrosis (*arrows*) and chronic fibrosis (*F*) in response to transvenous shocks.[61] (B) At higher power, acute cell injury is seen mixed in with fibrosis and other viable myocytes.[61] (C) Evidence of myocellular injury observed with transvenous but not subcutaneous shocks.[66] In this experiment, four swine received five deliveries each of 35 J transvenously and a second group of four swine received five deliveries each of 80 J subcutaneously to model clinical situations. There was a significant rise in troponin I of cardiac origin from the transvenous shocks along with observed arrhythmia. The subcutaneous shocks had no apparent adverse impact on the heart but they did give rise to an increase in skeletal muscle enzymes and histology, indicating local inflammation that was, however, thought unlikely to have any significant clinical consequence.[66] *S-ICD,* Subcutaneous implantable cardioverter defibrillator; *SD,* standard deviation; *TV-ICD,* transvenous implantable cardioverter defibrillator. ([A] From Epstein AE, Kay GN, Plumb VJ, Dailey SM, Anderson PG. Gross and microscopic pathological changes associated with nonthoracotomy implantable defibrillator leads. *Circulation.* 1998;98:1517–1524. [B] From Killingsworth CR, Melnick SB, Litovsky SH, Ideker RE, Walcott GP. Evaluation of acute cardiac and chest wall damage after shocks with a subcutaneous implantable cardioverter defibrillator in swine. Pacing *Clin Electrophysiol.* 2013;36:1265–1272.)

Infection

One of the main issues with all cardiac implanted electronic devices (CIEDs) is that of systemic infection and is possibly of greater impact than previously thought.[40,68] The S-ICD was anticipated to have a low risk of systemic infection, and this has now been seen in practice in all relevant studies.[41] For example, only 1.7% of patients needed extraction in the IDE trial,[30] and in the initial 5.8-year follow-up from the CE study, only one device was removed in view of infection.[35] In regard to other findings, one striking observation was the resolution of infection in the patients later recruited through simple antibiotic administration rather than through explantation.[28] It should be pointed out that many implanting those devices were new to the use of this technology and yet still demonstrated good outcomes. A compelling explanation for infections reported in early studies[28,29] is that most implanters were most used to a pectoral insertion site and once field preparation was mastered, infection rates appeared to fall.[28,38]

Future Developments

The current S-ICD design is a second-generation device that is downsized with improved longevity, further improved detection algorithms, remote monitoring capability, and MRI compatibility. It is anticipated that there will be further improvements in the algorithms for sense amplification, patient-specific morphology detection, and also further size reductions. In addition, alternative shock pathways such as the various configurations tested in early studies,[8] the anteroposterior subcutaneous shock pathways,[69] and the right parasternal location as described in case reports[70] and supported also by modeling studies may be tried, but these vectors require substantial testing before leaving the reliable vector currently employed. Together, the application of such approaches may result in the development of specifically targeted devices, for example, for pediatric applications in which possibly lower energy output is needed based on both lower cardiac mass and transthoracic impedances.[71] The main technical thrust beyond the core S-ICD device itself may relate to the incorporation of other features with combined or independent pacing capability and the inclusion of monitor zones from atrial and ventricular arrhythmias in an attempt to capture more widely relevant events including, for example, episodes of atrial fibrillation to guide decisions on thromboprophylaxis. However, the adverse consequences arising in the pursuit of perfection (unneeded enhancements/undue complexity) with transvenous systems should not be forgotten.

There is also a need for a more conventional prospective evaluation and long-term data-gathering. The much anticipated PRAETORIAN trial[72] is a randomized (1:1), controlled, multicenter, prospective, double-arm comparison of S-ICDs and transvenous ICDs in 700 patients and is due for completion in

2018.[72] The FDA required observation of the performance of the device over time, and the S-ICD postapproval study is a nonrandomized registry of 1600 patients at 150 sites looking at 5-year outcomes.

Conclusions

Leads have always proved problematic in ICD therapy, and there is little reason to believe that the well-documented issues of the transvenous approach (due to entry into a relatively unwelcoming intravascular environment) will abate. The S-ICD had an almost 15-year gestation from concept to delivery, but now with wider implementation there is a general enthusiasm to an extent that for many indications it may prove to be the approach of choice.[41] Many commentators now see it as an option that should be considered in all patients for both primary and secondary prevention of sudden arrhythmic death who do not have an additional pacing indication.[41] A particular focus has been on those who are younger and needing longer periods of protection[41] and those with vascular access issues, including renal patients.[73] In addition, those with an apparent predisposition to infection, including the immunosuppressed and those with prior infected CIEDs, can clearly do well.[74]

Of course, there are things we know and things we do not. What is absolutely clear is that the S-ICD is effective in protection essentially at a level seen with transvenous systems.[41] S-ICDs also demonstrate reliable detection and discrimination[41] generally comparable to those seen with conventional systems. We are fortunate that improved algorithms and revised conservative programming have had such a positive impact on inappropriate shock rates in general, supporting the technical position of longer detection also adopted by the S-ICD.

Further studies will provide data regarding long-term performance and further insights into the prognostic impact of subcutaneous versus transvenous shocks. This along with overall physician and patient perceptions of a device that has clear intuitive advantages are likely to influence strongly how we see targeted protection against the risk of sudden arrhythmic death over the next few years.

Commercial and Funding Relationships

Dr. Grace received stock options from Cameron Health Inc., the company responsible for the development of the subcutaneous ICD; he is now a member of the Patient Safety Advisory Board of Boston Scientific Inc. Dr. Bardy was an inventor, founder, and a stockholder of Cameron Health, acquired in 2012 by Boston Scientific Inc.

Acknowledgments

The authors are grateful for all the members of the Clinical Field Team from Cameron Health who played a critical role in making the S-ICD a reality. Among many others, team leader Jon Hunt along with Stephen O'Connor, Rick Sanghera, Don Scheck, Perry Seltz, and Linda Smith deserve our thanks and particular recognition.

REFERENCES

1. Yousuf O, Chrispin J, Tomaselli GF, Berger RD. Clinical management and prevention of sudden cardiac death. *Circ Res.* 2015;116:2020–2040.
2. Hohnloser SH, Israel CW. Current evidence base for use of the implantable cardioverter-defibrillator. *Circulation.* 2013;128:172–183.
3. Bardy GH, Johnson G, Poole JE, et al. A simplified, single-lead unipolar transvenous cardioversion-defibrillation system. *Circulation.* 1993;88:543–547.
4. Abraham WT, Smith SA. Devices in the management of advanced, chronic heart failure. *Nat Rev Cardiol.* 2013;10:98–110.
5. Moss AJ, Zareba W, Hall WJ, et al. Prophylactic implantation of a defibrillator in patients with myocardial infarction and reduced ejection fraction. *N Engl J Med.* 2002;346:877–883.
6. Bardy GH, Lee KL, Mark DB, et al. Amiodarone or an implantable cardioverter-defibrillator for congestive heart failure. *N Engl J Med.* 2005;352:225–237.
7. Maisel WH. Transvenous implantable cardioverter-defibrillator leads: the weakest link. *Circulation.* 2007;115:2461–2463.
8. Bardy GH, Smith WM, Hood MA, et al. An entirely subcutaneous implantable cardioverter-defibrillator. *N Engl J Med.* 2010;363:36–44.
9. McClellan MB, Tunis SR. Medicare coverage of ICDs. *N Engl J Med.* 2005;352:222–224.
10. Narayanan K, Reinier K, Uy-Evanado A, et al. Frequency and determinants of ICD deployment among primary prevention candidates with subsequent sudden cardiac arrest in the community. *Circulation.* 2013;128:1733–1738.
11. LaPointe NM, Al-Khatib SM, Piccini JP, et al. Extent of and reasons for nonuse of implantable cardioverter defibrillator devices in clinical practice among eligible patients with left ventricular systolic dysfunction. *Circ Cardiovasc Qual Outcomes.* 2011;4:146–151.
12. Swerdlow CD, Ellenbogen KA. Implantable cardioverter-defibrillator leads: design, diagnostics, and management. *Circulation.* 2013;128:2062–2071. 1-9.
13. Cheung JW, Al-Kazaz M, Thomas G, et al. Mechanisms, predictors, and trends of electrical failure of riata leads. *Heart Rhythm.* 2013;10:1453–1459.
14. Kleemann T, Becker T, Doenges K, et al. Annual rate of transvenous defibrillation lead defects in implantable cardioverter-defibrillators over a period of >10 years. *Circulation.* 2007;115:2474–2480.
15. Tung R, Zimetbaum P, Josephson ME. A critical appraisal of implantable cardioverter-defibrillator therapy for the prevention of sudden cardiac death. *J Am Coll Cardiol.* 2008;52:1111–1121.

16. Mulpuru SK, Pretorius VG, Birgersdotter-Green UM. Device infections: management and indications for lead extraction. *Circulation.* 2013;128:1031–1038.
17. Sanghera R, Sanders R, Husby M, Bentsen JG. Development of the subcutaneous implantable cardioverter-defibrillator for reducing sudden cardiac death. *Ann N Y Acad Sci.* 2014;1329:1–17.
18. Burke MC, Coman JA, Cates AW, et al. Defibrillation energy requirements using a left anterior chest cutaneous to subcutaneous shocking vector: implications for a total subcutaneous implantable defibrillator. *Heart Rhythm.* 2005;2:1332–1338.
19. Lieberman R, Havel WJ, Rashba E, et al. Acute defibrillation performance of a novel, non-transvenous shock pathway in adult ICD indicated patients. *Heart Rhythm.* 2008;5:28–34.
20. Kramer DB, Hatfield LA, McGriff D, et al. Transvenous implantable cardioverter-defibrillator lead reliability: implications for postmarket surveillance. *J Am Heart Assoc.* 2015;4:e001672.
21. Moss AJ, Schuger C, Beck CA, et al. Reduction in inappropriate therapy and mortality through ICD programming. *N Engl J Med.* 2012;367:2275–2283.
22. Gasparini M, Proclemer A, Klersy C, et al. Effect of long-detection interval vs standard-detection interval for implantable cardioverter-defibrillators on antitachycardia pacing and shock delivery: the ADVANCE III randomized clinical trial. *JAMA.* 2013;309:1903–1911.
23. Cappato R, Castelvecchio S, Erlinger P, et al. Feasibility of defibrillation and automatic arrhythmia detection using an exclusively subcutaneous defibrillator system in canines. *J Cardiovasc Electrophysiol.* 2013;24:77–82.
24. Bardy GH, Gliner BE, Kudenchuk PJ, et al. Truncated biphasic pulses for transthoracic defibrillation. *Circulation.* 1995;91:1768–1774.
25. Bardy GH, Cappato R, Smith WM, et al. The totally subcutaneous ICD system (the S-ICD). *Pacing Clin Electrophysiol.* 2002;25:578.
26. Grace AA, Hood MA, Smith WM, et al. Evaluation of four distinct subcutaneous implantable defibrillator (S-ICD) lead systems in humans. *Heart Rhythm.* 2006;3:S128–S129.
27. Grace AA, Smith WM, Hood MA, et al. A prospective, randomised comparison in humans of defibrillation efficacy of a standard transvenous ICD system with a totally subcutaneous ICD system (The S-ICD® System). Heart Rhythm, Vol 2, No 9, p 1036. Heart Rhythm Society Meetings, New Orleans, May 7, 2005.
28. Weiss R, Knight BP, Gold MR, et al. Safety and efficacy of a totally subcutaneous implantable-cardioverter defibrillator. *Circulation.* 2013;128:944–953.

29. Jarman JW, Lascelles K, Wong T, et al. Clinical experience of entirely subcutaneous implantable cardioverter-defibrillators in children and adults: cause for caution. *Eur Heart J.* 2012;33:1351–1359.
30. Burke MC, Gold MR, Knight BP, et al. Safety and efficacy of the totally subcutaneous implantable defibrillator: 2-year results from a pooled analysis of the IDE study and EFFORTLESS registry. *J Am Coll Cardiol.* 2015;65:1605–1615.
31. Boriani G, Ritter P, Biffi M, et al. Battery drain in daily practice and medium-term projections on longevity of cardioverter-defibrillators: an analysis from a remote monitoring database. *Europace.* 2016;18:1366–1373.
32. Keller J, Neuzil P, Vymazal J, et al. Magnetic resonance imaging in patients with a subcutaneous implantable cardioverter-defibrillator. *Europace.* 2015;17:761–766.
33. Rav Acha M, Milan D. Who should receive the subcutaneous implantable cardioverter defibrillator? Timing is not right to replace the transvenous implantable cardioverter defibrillator. *Circ Arrhythm Electrophysiol.* 2013;6:1246–1251. discussion 1251.
34. Gold MR, Theuns DA, Knight BP, et al. Head-to-head comparison of arrhythmia discrimination performance of subcutaneous and transvenous ICD arrhythmia detection algorithms: the START study. *J Cardiovasc Electrophysiol.* 2012;23:359–366.
35. Theuns DA, Crozier IG, Barr CS, et al. Longevity of the subcutaneous implantable defibrillator: long-term follow-up of the European Regulatory Trial cohort. *Circ Arrhythm Electrophysiol.* 2015;8:1159–1163.
36. Nisam S, Reddy S. The story of... a lead. *Europace.* 2015;17:677–688.
37. Kramer DB, Kennedy KF, Noseworthy PA, et al. Characteristics and outcomes of patients receiving new and replacement implantable-cardioverter defibrillators: results from the NCDR. *Circ Cardiovasc Qual Outcomes.* 2013;6:488–497.
38. Knops RE, Brouwer TF, Barr CS, et al. The learning curve associated with the introduction of the subcutaneous implantable defibrillator. *Europace.* 2016;18:1010–1015.
39. Guenther M, Kolschmann S, Knaut M. Substernal lead implantation: a novel option to manage DFT failure in S-ICD patients. *Clin Res Cardiol.* 2015;104:189–191.
40. Padfield GJ, Steinberg C, Bennett MT, et al. Preventing cardiac implantable electronic device infections. *Heart Rhythm.* 2015;12:2344–2356.
41. Lewis GF, Gold MR. Safety and efficacy of the subcutaneous implantable defibrillator. *J Am Coll Cardiol.* 2016;67:445–454.
42. Knops RE, Olde Nordkamp LR, de Groot JR, Wilde AA. Two-incision technique for implantation of the subcutaneous implantable cardioverter-defibrillator. *Heart Rhythm.* 2013;10:1240–1243.

43. Winter J, Kohlmeier A, Shin DI, O'Connor S. Subcutaneous implantable cardioverter-defibrillators and sternal wires: a cautionary tale. *Circ Arrhythm Electrophysiol.* 2014;7:986–987.

44. Pettit SJ, McLean A, Colquhoun I, et al. Clinical experience of subcutaneous and transvenous implantable cardioverter defibrillators in children and teenagers. *Pacing Clin Electrophysiol.* 2013;36:1532–1538.

45. Winter J, Siekiera M, Shin DI, et al. Intermuscular technique for implantation of the SICD. *Europace.* 2016. in press.

46. Daubert JP, Zareba W, Cannom DS, et al. Inappropriate implantable cardioverter-defibrillator shocks in MADIT II: frequency, mechanisms, predictors, and survival impact. *J Am Coll Cardiol.* 2008;51:1357–1365.

47. Gold MR, Weiss R, Theuns DA, et al. Use of a discrimination algorithm to reduce inappropriate shocks with a subcutaneous implantable cardioverter-defibrillator. *Heart Rhythm.* 2014;11:1352–1358.

48. Brisben AJ, Burke MC, Knight BP, et al. A new algorithm to reduce inappropriate therapy in the S-ICD system. *J Cardiovasc Electrophysiol.* 2015;26:417–423.

49. Zeb M, Curzen N, Allavatam V, et al. Sensitivity and specificity of the subcutaneous implantable cardioverter defibrillator pre-implant screening tool. *Int J Cardiol.* 2015;195:205–209.

50. Groh CA, Sharma S, Pelchovitz DJ, et al. Use of an electrocardiographic screening tool to determine candidacy for a subcutaneous implantable cardioverter-defibrillator. *Heart Rhythm.* 2014;11:1361–1366.

51. Randles DA, Hawkins NM, Shaw M, et al. How many patients fulfill the surface electrocardiogram criteria for subcutaneous implantable cardioverter-defibrillator implantation? *Europace.* 2014;16:1015–1021.

52. Maurizi N, Olivotto I, Olde Nordkamp LR, et al. Prevalence of subcutaneous implantable cardioverter-defibrillator candidacy based on template ECG screening in patients with hypertrophic cardiomyopathy. *Heart Rhythm.* 2016;13:457–463.

53. Kooiman KM, Knops RE, Olde Nordkamp L, et al. Inappropriate subcutaneous implantable cardioverter-defibrillator shocks due to T-wave oversensing can be prevented: implications for management. *Heart Rhythm.* 2014;11:426–434.

54. Lambiase PD, Gold MR, Hood M, et al. Evaluation of subcutaneous ICD early performance in hypertrophic cardiomyopathy from the pooled EFFORTLESS and IDE cohorts. *Heart Rhythm.* 2016;13:1066–1074.

55. Wilkoff BL. Improved programming of ICDs. *N Engl J Med.* 2012;367:2348–2349.

56. Bardy GH, Smith WM, Grace AA. An entirely subcutaneous implantable cardioverter-defibrillator. *N Engl J Med.* 2010;363:1577–1578.

57. de Bie MK, Thijssen J, van Rees JB, et al. Suitability for subcutaneous defibrillator implantation: results based on data from routine clinical practice. *Heart.* 2013;99:1018–1023.

58. Poole JE, Gleva MJ, Mela T, et al. Complication rates associated with pacemaker or implantable cardioverter-defibrillator generator replacements and upgrade procedures: results from the REPLACE registry. *Circulation.* 2010;122:1553–1561.

59. Kuschyk J, Stach K, Tulumen E, et al. Subcutaneous implantable cardioverter-defibrillator: first single-center experience with other cardiac implantable electronic devices. *Heart Rhythm.* 2015;12:2230–2238.

60. Miller MA, Neuzil P, Dukkipati SR, et al. Leadless cardiac pacemakers: back to the future. *J Am Coll Cardiol.* 2015;66:1179–1189.

61. Epstein AE, Kay GN, Plumb VJ, et al. Gross and microscopic pathological changes associated with nonthoracotomy implantable defibrillator leads. *Circulation.* 1998;98:1517–1524.

62. Poole JE. Shocks: The whole truth, the partial truth, or nowhere near the truth. *Circ Arrhythm Electrophysiol.* 2011;4:424–425.

63. Sweeney MO. The contradiction of appropriate shocks in primary prevention ICDs: increasing and decreasing the risk of death. *Circulation.* 2010;122:2638–2641.

64. Deyell MW, Qi A, Chakrabarti S, et al. Prognostic impact of inappropriate defibrillator shocks in a population cohort. *Heart.* 2013;99:1250–1255.

65. Ha AH, Ham I, Nair GM, et al. Implantable cardioverter-defibrillator shock prevention does not reduce mortality: a systemic review. *Heart Rhythm.* 2012;9:2068–2074.

66. Killingsworth CR, Melnick SB, Litovsky SH, et al. Evaluation of acute cardiac and chest wall damage after shocks with a subcutaneous implantable cardioverter defibrillator in swine. *Pacing Clin Electrophysiol.* 2013;36:1265–1272.

67. Allred JD, Killingsworth CR, Allison JS, et al. Transmural recording of shock potential gradient fields, early postshock activations, and refibrillation episodes associated with external defibrillation of long-duration ventricular fibrillation in swine. *Heart Rhythm.* 2008;5:1599–1606.

68. Kirkfeldt RE, Johansen JB, Nohr EA, et al. Complications after cardiac implantable electronic device implantations: an analysis of a complete, nationwide cohort in Denmark. *Eur Heart J.* 2014;35:1186–1194.

69. Kuschyk J, Milasinovic G, Kuhlkamp V, et al. A multicenter study of shock pathways for subcutaneous implantable defibrillators. *J Cardiovasc Electrophysiol.* 2014;25:29–35.

70. Zumhagen S, Grace AA, O'Connor S, et al. Totally subcutaneous implantable cardioverter defibrillator with an alternative, right parasternal, electrode placement. *Pacing Clin Electrophysiol.* 2012;35:e254–e257.

71. Jolley M, Stinstra J, Tate J, et al. Finite element modeling of subcutaneous implantable electrodes in an adult torso. *Heart Rhythm.* 2010;7:692–698.

72. Olde Nordkamp LR, Knops RE, Bardy GH, et al. Rationale and design of the PRAETORIAN trial: a prospective, randomized comparison of subcutaneous and transvenous implantable cardioverter-defibrillator therapy. *Am Heart J.* 2012;163:753.e2–760.e2.

73. Dhamija RK, Tan H, Philbin E, et al. Subcutaneous implantable cardioverter defibrillator for dialysis patients: a strategy to reduce central stenoses and infections. *Am J Kidney Dis.* 2015;66:154–158.

74. Boersma L, Burke MC, Neuzil P, et al. Infection and mortality after implantation of a subcutaneous ICD after transvenous ICD extraction. *Heart Rhythm.* 2016;13:157–164.

119 Implantable Pacemakers

Paul J. Wang and David L. Hayes

The use and sophistication of permanent pacemakers have increased steadily since the first pacemaker was implanted in 1958. Indications for their use have broadened as the technology has advanced, and pacemakers have become a mainstay of therapy. Those involved in arrhythmia management must have a good understanding of this discipline.

History of Pacing

Since the first epicardial pacing system was implanted in 1958, pacemaker technology has evolved rapidly. The sophistication of sensing circuitry led to the introduction of single-chamber demand pacing systems in 1963. Although atrial-synchronous systems and dual-chamber systems were described in the 1950s, clinical use of such devices did not occur for many years. In the 1970s, lithium batteries and programmability were introduced. Milestones of the 1980s include greater acceptance of dual-chamber pacing systems and the introduction of rate-adaptive pacing systems. The 1990s and the 2000s witnessed the introduction of advanced sensor technology, new pacemaker algorithms, and enhanced automaticity of many programmable features. The utilization of pacing has increased significantly from 46.7/100,000 in 1993 to 61.6/100,000 in 2009, with the percentage of dual-chamber devices increasing from 62% to 82% during this time period.[1]

Pacemaker Nomenclature

Since the first introduction of a three-letter code describing basic pacemaker functions in 1974, the code has been updated periodically by a committee comprising members of the North American Society of Pacing and Electrophysiology and the British Pacing and Electrophysiology Group (NASPE/BPEG). The most recent code consists of a five-letter code (Box 119.1). The first position indicates the chamber or chambers that are *stimulated:* A (atrium), V (ventricle), or D (dual-chamber, both A and V). The second position indicates the chamber or chambers in which *sensing* occurs: A (atrium), V (ventricle), or D (dual-chamber, both A and V). The third position indicates the *function:* I (inhibition), T (triggered), or D (a dual function of atrial tracking and ventricular inhibition). The fourth position of the code indicates that *rate modulation* is present by the letter *R*. Rate modulation is the use of a sensor to meet the patient's metabolic demands, independent of intrinsic cardiac activity. The fifth position indicates whether *multisite pacing* is present: A (atrium), V (ventricle), or D (both A and V). Multisite pacing is defined as more than one stimulation site in any single chamber. In any of the positions, *O* indicates that pacing, sensing, or a function is not present.

Indications for Cardiac Pacing

Criteria established by a joint committee of the American College of Cardiology (ACC), the American Heart Association (AHA), and the Heart Rhythm Society (HRS) have categorized indications for pacing as class I, generally indicated; class II, possibly indicated; and class III, not indicated.[2] Class II has been divided into class IIa for recommendations for which there is general agreement and class IIb for which there is some disagreement. The evidence supporting the recommendations is ranked as follows: The weight of evidence is ranked A if there are multiple randomized trials involving a large number of subjects and B if data were derived from a limited number of trials involving a relatively small number of subjects. The weight of evidence is ranked C if expert consensus is the primary source of the recommendation.[2] Although some indications for permanent pacing are relatively certain or unambiguous, others require considerable expertise and judgment. The clinician prescribing permanent pacing systems should be aware of the indications and controversies regarding indications.

Acquired Atrioventricular Block

Acquired atrioventricular (AV) block is most commonly idiopathic and related to aging, but the potential causes are many.

Class I indications for permanent pacing in patients with acquired AV block include any AV block with associated symptoms, as well as AV block after AV node ablation or persistent AV block after cardiac surgery. For some patients, heart failure may be a manifestation of AV block. In addition, some patients require medications that can cause symptomatic bradycardia and might need pacing. For postoperative AV block, the guidelines do not specify a period to wait postoperatively for recovery of conduction. Class I indications also include acquired AV block below the level of the AV node or associated with marked pauses, such as longer than 3.0 seconds or a ventricular escape rate less than 40 beats/min. Permanent pacemaker implantation is also indicated in awake, symptom-free patients with atrial fibrillation (AF) and bradycardia with pauses of 5 seconds or more.[2] Because the cardiovascular risk is felt to be particularly high in patients with second- or third-degree block and specific underlying conditions, permanent pacing is felt to be indicated in these patients even in the absence of symptoms. These conditions include neuromuscular diseases such as myotonic dystrophy, Kearns-Sayre syndrome, peroneal muscular atrophy, and Erb limb-girdle dystrophy. Myotonic dystrophy has been associated with an increased risk of sudden death thought to be due to progressive conduction system disease.[3]

BOX 119.1   The revised NASPE/BPEG generic code for antibradycardia pacing

Chamber(s) Paced
0 = None
A = Atrium
V = Ventricle
D = Dual (A + V)
S = Single (A or V) (manufacturers' designation only)

Chamber(s) Sensed
0 = None
A = Atrium
V = Ventricle
D = Dual (A + V)
S = Single (A or V) (manufacturers' designation only)

Response to Sensing
0 = None
T = Triggered
I = Inhibited
D = Dual (T + I)

Rate Modulation
0 = None
R = Rate modulation

Multisite Pacing
0 = None
A = Atrium
V = Ventricle
D = Dual (A + V)

BPEG, British Pacing and Electrophysiology Group; *NASPE,* North American Society of Pacing and Electrophysiology.

Exercise-related AV block is also felt to be an indication for pacing. Advanced second-degree AV block or alternating bundle branch block in the setting of bifascicular block is considered a class I indication. Asymptomatic type II second-degree AV block with a wide QRS is a class I indication. Transient, infranodal, high-grade AV block and associated bundle branch block is a class I indication.[2]

Class IIa indications include asymptomatic type II second-degree AV block with a narrow QRS complex, and asymptomatic second-degree AV block at intra-His or infra-His levels based on electrophysiological testing.[2] First-degree or second-degree AV block with hemodynamic compromise is also considered a class IIa indication because some patients develop pacemaker-like syndrome due to conduction delay. In patients with bifascicular block, asymptomatic severe prolongation of the His-ventricle interval (>100 ms), asymptomatic pacing-induced infra-His block that is not felt to be physiological, or syncope when other causes such as ventricular tachycardia have been excluded are considered class IIa indications for pacing.

First-degree AV block in patients with neuromuscular disorders is considered a class IIb indication because the risk of progression to AV block is felt to be high. Another class IIb indication includes AV block that might have occurred because of drug use or toxicity, but there is a risk of recurrence of AV block. First-degree AV block in a patient with left ventricular dysfunction and congestive heart failure in whom hemodynamic improvement with AV interval optimization can be demonstrated is a class IIb indication.[2] Asymptomatic persistent second-degree or third-degree block at the AV node level is classified as a class IIb indication.[2]

Class III indications include asymptomatic first-degree AV block, asymptomatic second-degree AV block at the supra-His level or not known to be intra-His or infra-His, and AV block occurring in the setting of reversible conditions such as drug toxicity that is unlikely to recur, Lyme disease, transient increases in vagal tone, or during sleep apnea.

After a myocardial infarction, a pacemaker is generally considered to be indicated for persistent second-degree bilateral bundle branch block, third-degree AV block within or below the His bundle, or persistent symptomatic second-degree or third-degree AV block.

Congenital Complete Heart Block

Symptomatic congenital complete AV block remains a class I indication for pacing in pediatric patients.[2] In addition, in pediatric patients with congenital complete AV block, the presence of a wide QRS escape rhythm, ventricular dysfunction, or complex ventricular ectopy is also a class I indication. In pediatric patients, an average heart rate less than 50 beats/min, pauses two to three times the basic cycle length, or symptoms associated with chronotropic incompetence are considered class IIa indications. In pediatric and adult patients with an adequate rate, narrow QRS complex, and normal ventricular function, pacing is a class IIb indication.

For adult patients with congenital complete AV block, the timing and indications for permanent pacing are more controversial and continue to evolve.[4] As a result of data regarding the high incidence of unexpected syncope in adult patients with congenital complete AV block, prophylactic pacemaker implantation is often considered.[2,4]

Sinus Node Dysfunction

Sinus node dysfunction may be manifested by abrupt sinus pauses or gradual sinus slowing. Symptomatic chronotropic incompetence and symptomatic sinus bradycardia occurring spontaneously or as the result of drug therapy are considered class I indications for pacing. In patients with minimal or no symptoms and chronic heart rates less than 40 beats/min, pacing is a class IIb indication.[2]

Class III indications for pacing include asymptomatic sinus node dysfunction. Sinus pauses occurring during sleep are generally not considered indications for pacing. Many patients, particularly trained athletes, have high levels of vagal tone and have significant pauses greater than 3 seconds and periods of sinus bradycardia. These patients do not require permanent pacing.

Neurocardiogenic Syncope

Neurocardiogenic syncope typically has both cardioinhibitory and vasodepressor components. Pacing during most episodes of neurocardiogenic syncope is still associated with a significant fall in blood pressure and symptoms because of the continued vasodepressor response. Therefore, even in the presence of significant bradycardia, pacing is usually not considered first-line therapy. A number of randomized trials have failed to show a substantial benefit in increasing the freedom from recurrent syncope.[5,6] As a result, neurocardiogenic syncope with documented bradycardia is considered a class IIb indication for pacing. However, there are some recent studies that may indicate the selective use of pacing. In the Third International Study on Syncope of Uncertain Etiology (ISSUE-3) trial, in patients 40 years of age or older with at least three syncopal episodes in 2 years, and with documentation of syncope with 3 or more seconds of asystole or 6 or more seconds of asystole without syncope, 77 patients were randomized to dual-chamber pacing on or off with an algorithm to increase the pacing rate with a sudden decrease in heart rate. The syncope recurrence rate was 57% in the pacing off group and 25% in the pacing on group (*p* = .039).[7]

When pacing is performed in this setting, dual-chamber pacing is necessary to preserve the atrial contribution to cardiac output. Modifications to the pacing strategy are being studied to make dual-chamber pacing more effective in ameliorating neurocardiogenic syncope. The heart rate may be adjusted according to measured changes in impedance to estimate myocardial contractility, using so-called closed-loop stimulation (CLS). While retrospective data suggest that this approach may reduce the frequency of recurrence of syncope, further prospective studies are needed.[8]

In patients with syncope of unknown origin, a randomized, multicenter study examined patients exhibiting a pause of 10 seconds or more when given an intravenous bolus of 20 mg adenosine triphosphate (ATP). These patients were randomized to AAI at 30 beats/min versus DDD pacing at 70 beats/min. In the DDD pacing group, 21% of patients had recurrence of syncope compared to 66% of patients in the AAI group. Of note, the mean age in these studies was 76 years of age.[9]

Carotid Sinus Hypersensitivity

Carotid sinus hypersensitivity has been shown to be a cause of syncope, particularly in the elderly. However, because an abnormal response can occur even in asymptomatic persons, caution must be used when spontaneous bradycardia has not been demonstrated. In cases in which syncope has occurred during carotid sinus stimulation and carotid sinus pressure has resulted in pauses of 3 seconds or more, a class I indication is felt to be present. If such an abnormal carotid sinus pressure response is obtained but syncope did not occur in circumstances suggesting carotid sinus stimulation, a class IIa indication is present. In addition, there may be a role for pacing in patients with unexplained falls and evidence of carotid sinus hypersensitivity. Recent studies did not show a difference in the recurrence of events in patients pacing on treatment using ventricular-inhibited (VVI) pacing, dual-chamber rate adaptive pacemaker (DDDR), or DDDR with a sudden bradycardia response.[10]

Nonbradycardic Indications for Pacing

An increasing number of patients are receiving pacemakers for nonbradycardic indications. Cardiac resynchronization therapy for refractory congestive heart failure is the major indication in this category. Dual-chamber pacing for medically refractory symptoms of hypertrophic obstructive cardiomyopathy and pacing therapy for prevention of AF are no longer considered major nonbradycardic indications for pacing.

Pacing for Atrial Fibrillation

There are numerous studies that examined various pacing algorithms to prevent AF. Most such algorithms involve increasing the pacing rate to suppress atrial ectopy felt to trigger AF. Although most randomized studies have not demonstrated a beneficial effect, selected studies have suggested a modest decrease in the occurrence of AF. In the SAFARI trial, patients with AF recorded were randomized to AF pacing prevention strategies. Overall, there was a small reduction in the occurrence of AF. In patients with a high burden of AF, the reduction in AF was greater.[11] At present, pacing for AF reduction is a class III indication.

Resynchronization Therapy

Numerous randomized, controlled trials have demonstrated the benefit of cardiac resynchronization therapy in improving symptoms and outcomes in patients with drug-refractory heart failure. Cardiac resynchronization therapy is the pacing of the left and right ventricles to improve the hemodynamics that are impaired due to bundle branch block. These randomized studies have shown improvement in New York Heart Association (NYHA) classes, 6-minute walk time, oxygen consumption, brain natriuretic peptide levels, neurohormonal levels, ejection fraction, end-diastolic and end-systolic dimensions, heart failure hospitalizations, and all-cause mortality.[12] The current indications for resynchronization therapy (class I) include left bundle branch block, QRS duration of 150 ms or greater, left ventricular ejection fraction of 35% or less, sinus rhythm, and class II, III, or ambulatory class IV heart failure symptoms on optimal medical therapy. Class IIa indications include a left ventricular ejection fraction of 35% or less and NYHA class II, III, and ambulatory IV symptoms on optimal medical therapy with (1) left bundle branch block, QRS duration of 120–149 ms, or (2) non–left bundle branch block and a QRS duration of 150 ms or greater. Class IIa indications also include patients with a left ventricular ejection fraction of 35% or less on optimal medical therapy and (1) who are undergoing new or replacement device implantation with anticipated 40% or more ventricular pacing or (2) have AF that requires ventricular pacing or meets other criteria and near 100% ventricular pacing.[2,12]

Hypertrophic Cardiomyopathy

Early studies suggested that right ventricular apical pacing resulted in a significant reduction in the outflow tract gradient and ameliorated symptoms. However, a subsequent randomized multicenter trial failed to demonstrate a benefit in patients with pacing. A subset of elderly patients might have exhibited some improvement. An analysis from the Cochrane Database concluded that clinical trial data are inconclusive for evidence of an effect of pacing on outcomes in this patient population.[13] Therefore at present, pacing in medically refractory symptomatic patients with a significant resting or provoked gradient due to hypertrophic cardiomyopathy is a class IIb indication.[2] Many such patients should be considered for a dual-chamber implantable cardioverter defibrillator (ICD) because of the risk of sudden death.

Basic Pacemaker Function and Modes
Ventricular Inhibited Pacing

In the VVI pacing mode, pacemaker output is inhibited by a sensed ventricular event (Fig. 119.1). The lower rate interval determines the longest interval between any sensed or paced ventricular events. The interval from the previous sensed or paced ventricular event to the subsequent paced ventricular event is the lower rate interval. If the time interval from the last sensed ventricular event to the first paced ventricular beat is longer than the time interval between ventricular paced beats, ventricular hysteresis is present. Any ventricular event occurring after a paced or sensed ventricular event within the ventricular refractory period is not sensed and does not reset the timing cycle.

Atrial Inhibited Pacing

Atrial inhibited (AAI) pacing incorporates the same timing cycles as VVI pacing, with the obvious difference that pacing and sensing occur in the atrium, and pacemaker output is inhibited by a sensed atrial event (Fig. 119.2). An atrial paced or sensed event initiates a refractory period during which atrial events do not reset the timing cycle. Confusion can arise when multiple ventricular events occur during atrial pacing. For example, when the atrial timing cycle ends, an atrial pacing stimulus is delivered regardless of ventricular events, because an AAI pacemaker does not sense in the ventricle. If the ventricular signal is inappropriately sensed by the atrial lead (far-field sensing), the atrial timing cycle

VVI

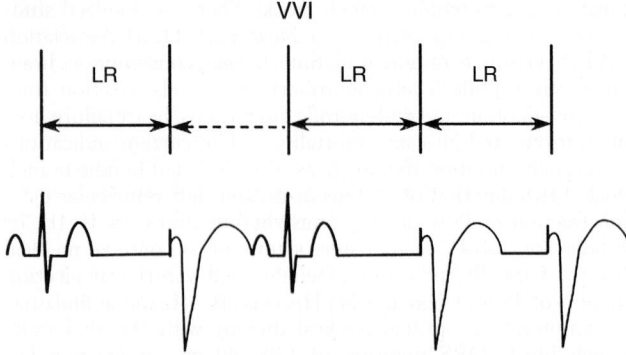

FIGURE 119.1 In ventricular-inhibited (*VVI*) pacing, the lower rate interval (*LR*) is the time from the last intrinsic or paced ventricular event to a ventricular paced event. When the LR interval has been completed, a ventricular paced event will occur. If an intrinsic beat occurs before the LR is completed, the ventricular output will be inhibited. The first QRS complex is intrinsic and after the LR interval is completed, a second intrinsic beat has not occurred, and thus the second QRS complex is a paced ventricular event. The third QRS complex is again intrinsic. Following the third QRS complex, intrinsic QRS complexes do not occur within the LR interval. Thus the fourth and fifth QRS complexes are paced. The *double-headed arrows* indicate that the full LR interval has transpired. The *dotted single-headed arrow* indicates that the full LR interval has not been completed and an intrinsic QRS complex inhibits ventricular pacing.

AAI

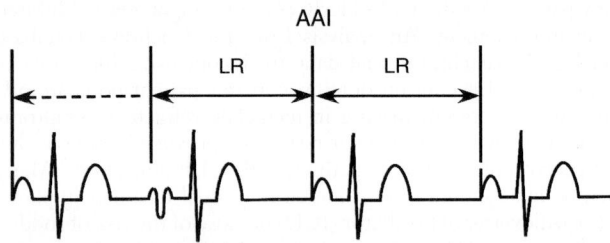

FIGURE 119.2 In atrial inhibited (*AAI*) pacing, the lower rate interval (*LR*) is the time from the last intrinsic or paced atrial event to an atrial paced event. When the LR interval has been completed, an atrial paced event will occur. If an intrinsic beat occurs before the LR interval is completed, the atrial output will be inhibited. The first atrial complex is paced. The second atrial complex occurs before the LR is completed. A third atrial complex does not occur spontaneously, and instead, after the LR interval has been completed, an atrial paced beat occurs. The fourth atrial complex is also paced and occurs after another LR interval. The *double-headed arrows* indicate that a full LR interval has transpired. The *dotted single-headed arrow* indicates that the full LR interval has not been completed and an intrinsic QRS complex inhibits ventricular pacing.

is reset. This abnormality can sometimes be corrected by making the atrial channel less sensitive or by lengthening the atrial refractory period so that a conducted ventricular complex is not sensed.

Single-chamber, rate-adaptive pacing modes (AAIR, VVIR) have timing cycles that are not markedly different from those of their non–rate-adaptive counterparts. The difference lies in the potential variability of the paced rate. Depending on the sensor incorporated and the patient's level of exertion, the basic interval shortens from the programmed lower rate limit. Shortening requires that an upper rate limit be programmed to define the absolute shortest cycle length allowable.

DDD Pacing

Four different rhythms can be seen as a result of normal DDD function: normal sinus rhythm, atrial pacing, AV sequential pacing, and P-synchronous pacing. In the DDD mode, the lower

DDD

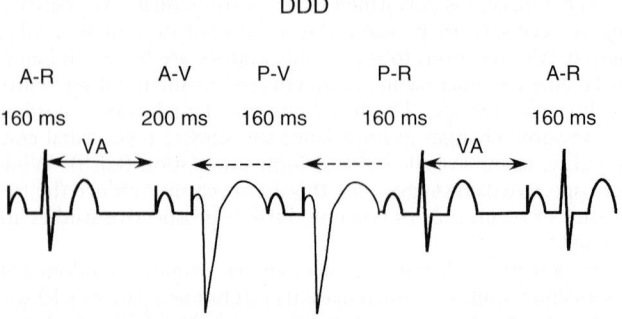

FIGURE 119.3 The DDD timing cycle consists of a lower rate limit interval, an atrioventricular interval (AVI), a postventricular atrial refractory period (PVARP), and an upper rate limit. In the figure, the first complex consists of an atrial paced event and an intrinsic QRS complex. Following the sensed ventricular event, a ventriculoatrial (*VA*) interval is created to indicate the time of the next atrial paced event if no intrinsic atrial event (after the PVARP) and no intrinsic ventricular event occur. The VA interval equals the lower rate interval minus the programmed AV interval. A completed VA interval is indicated by the *double-headed solid arrow*. In the second complex, following the atrial paced event there is no intrinsic QRS complex within the AV interval of 200 ms. Thus a paced ventricular event occurs. If an intrinsic atrial event occurs before the VA interval is completed but after the PVARP, the atrial event will be tracked or followed by a paced ventricular event (the third QRS complex). As long as the V-V interval does not occur before the upper rate limit interval is complete, the AV interval will occur after the tracked atrial event. Following the third QRS complex, an intrinsic atrial event occurs before the VA interval is complete, but an intrinsic QRS complex occurs before the AV interval is finished. Following the fourth QRS complex, the VA interval is completed and another atrial paced event occurs. The *dotted single-headed arrow* indicates that the full LR interval has not been completed and an intrinsic QRS complex inhibits ventricular pacing.

rate limit determines the lowest rate at which the atrial and ventricular events will occur (Fig. 119.3). If the intrinsic atrial rate is too slow, an atrial paced event will occur. After a paced or intrinsic atrial event, if there is no ventricular event, a paced ventricular event occurs at the programmed interval called the *AV delay* or *interval*. If an intrinsic atrial event occurs before the programmed lower rate, the atrial event will be followed by a ventricular paced event, a function called *atrial tracking*. This permits the ventricular pacing to follow the atrial rate as the metabolic demands change. There is a maximum tracking rate to prevent the tracking of atrial arrhythmias and extraneous signals at excessively rapid rates. In addition, if the P wave occurs too early after the previous ventricular event, it will occur in the postventricular atrial refractory period (PVARP) and therefore will not be tracked. The atrial rate at which two atrial sensed events will be followed by one ventricular paced event is equal to the total atrial refractory period (TARP), which is the sum of the programmed AV delay and the PVARP.

The timing from the last ventricular beat to the next atrial paced beat is determined by the ventriculoatrial (VA) interval. This interval is determined by subtracting the AV interval (AVI) from the lower rate interval in milliseconds. Thus the lower rate interval minus the AVI equals the VA interval. The AV interval may be adjusted based on the ventricular rate, a parameter called the *rate-responsive AV interval*. In patients with AV block and rapid sinus rates that might exceed the programmed upper rate limit and 2:1 atrial tracking rate, the rate-responsive AV interval might permit much higher upper rate limit tracking rates and maximum 2:1 atrial tracking rates. The AV interval might also be extended to promote intrinsic AV conduction, a function called *positive AV hysteresis* (see "Intrinsic Conduction Preference"). Negative AV hysteresis refers to a function in which the

AV interval is shortened to promote ventricular pacing, which is desirable in biventricular pacing.

Selecting the Appropriate Pacing Mode

Selection Criteria

In selecting the optimal pacing mode, the patient's overall physical condition, associated medical problems, exercise capacity, and chronotropic response to exercise must be considered, along with the underlying rhythm disturbance.[14]

VVIR pacing is indicated for patients with chronic AF and slow ventricular response. Although VVI pacing protects the patient from lethal bradycardia, its limitations include its inability to restore or to maintain AV synchrony and to provide rate responsiveness in the chronotropically incompetent patient. In addition, some patients with VVI pacing experience symptomatic hemodynamic deterioration with ventricular pacing. Adverse hemodynamics due to pacing are referred to as *pacemaker syndrome* if the normal coordination of atrial filling and ventricular emptying is absent because of VA conduction or long AV conduction times. During ventricular pacing with VA conduction, the systolic blood pressure might decline. The incidence of pacemaker syndrome depends on the definition used, and its incidence has been estimated to be 7%–10% of patients with VVI or VVIR pacing. The most common symptoms reported were shortness of breath, dizziness, fatigue, pulsations in the neck or abdomen, cough, and apprehension.

AAIR pacing is appropriate for patients with sinus node dysfunction. The obvious disadvantage of atrial pacing is the lack of ventricular support if AV block occurs. If the patient with sinus node dysfunction is carefully assessed for the presence of AV node disease at the time of pacemaker implantation, the occurrence of clinically significant AV node disease is very low, less than 2% per year. The concern of progression to AV block when patients are carefully selected for AAI(R) pacing has been dispelled by long-term follow-up of patients. Assessment before AAI pacemaker implantation should include incremental atrial pacing with an adequate response defined as 1:1 AV nodal conduction to atrial pacing rates of 120–140 beats/min. Newer pacing algorithms (discussed later) to avoid the deleterious effects of ventricular pacing allow atrial pacing to occur, and they switch to a mode that supports ventricular pacing only when necessary.

The DDD pacing mode is most appropriate for patients with normal sinus node function and AV block. DDDR pacemakers are capable of all the variations described for DDD pacemakers. In addition to the use of P-synchronous pacing as a method for increasing the heart rate, the sensor incorporated in the pacemaker might also drive the increase in heart rate. The resulting rhythm may be sinus-driven (alternatively called *atrial-driven* or *P-synchronous*) or sensor-driven.

DDDR pacing is indicated in patients with sinus node dysfunction and AV conduction disease. DDDR pacing is also appropriate for patients with pure sinus node dysfunction and when backup ventricular pacing is desired.

Effect of Pacing Mode on Morbidity and Mortality

Several large randomized, controlled trials have demonstrated the benefits of physiological AAI(R) or DDD(R) versus VVI(R). Andersen and associates published prospective data on pacing mode and survival with the random assignment of 225 patients with sinus node dysfunction to AAI or VVI pacing. The study demonstrated a lower incidence of AF and thromboembolism in the AAI group than in the VVI group. The Canadian Trial of Physiologic Pacing (CTOPP) randomly assigned 2568 patients to physiological pacing (dual-chamber or AAIR) or ventricular pacing (VVI). No difference in mortality rate or quality of life was demonstrated. However, there was an 18% relative risk reduction for AF.

Two additional trials have examined the outcomes of physiological pacing: Pacing Mode Selection in the Elderly (PASE) and the Mode Selection Trial (MOST). PASE failed to demonstrate any statistically significant benefit of physiological pacing over ventricular pacing. When the patients were separated by underlying rhythm disturbance—that is, sinus node dysfunction versus AV block—the sinus node dysfunction group had some quality-of-life improvements. In addition, there was a crossover of 26% of the patients assigned to ventricular pacing because they were unable to tolerate ventricular pacing. The MOST study, like CTOPP, did not demonstrate any difference in mortality rates, but it did demonstrate a lower incidence of AF with physiological pacing, reduced signs and symptoms of heart failure, and a slightly improved quality of life. The study concluded that overall, dual-chamber pacing offered a significant improvement compared with ventricular pacing. Most recently, the DANPACE trial randomized 1415 patients to AAIR or DDR pacing. There were no significant differences in stroke, heart failure, death, and chronic AF, but there was a lower incidence of paroxysmal AF of 28.4% in the AAIR group compared to 23.0% in the DDDR group.[15]

Taken together, these studies demonstrate the benefit of physiological pacing with the maintenance of AV synchrony compared with ventricular-only pacing in terms of AF and possibly quality of life.

Selecting the Appropriate Sensor for Rate-Adaptive Pacing

A variety of sensors appropriate for rate-adaptive pacing has been developed and achieves excellent responses in heart rate to exertion and changes in metabolic demand.[16]

Activity and Accelerometer Sensors

Accelerometer sensors have replaced basic vibration-based activity sensors. Both these sensors use a piezoelectric crystal, which produces a minute electrical current in response to motion. The piezoelectric vibration activity sensor senses vibration from up and down motion, and the accelerometer senses anterior and posterior motion. The accelerometer is relatively free from detection of motion leading to inappropriate increases in heart rate and responds rapidly to the onset of exertion. The accelerometer is the most widely used form of rate-adaptation sensor because it is simple, easy to apply clinically, and rapid in the onset of rate response.

Minute-Ventilation Sensor

Minute volume (respiratory rate × tidal volume) has an excellent correlation with metabolic demand. The transthoracic impedance, which varies with respiration, can be used to determine minute volume. Because minute ventilation maintains a predictable relation with metabolic demand, minute-ventilation values can be used to modulate the heart rate during various levels of activity for the patient. Long-term reliability of the minute-volume sensor has been excellent.

Stimulus-T or QT-Sensing Sensor

The interval from the onset of a paced QRS complex to the end of the T wave has been used for rate adaptation for many years. This stimulus-T interval is affected by autonomic activity and heart rate. The relation allows measurement of the stimulus-T interval to be used for rate adaptation. The QT-sensing, rate-adaptive pacing system has been successful clinically and responds well to mental and emotional stress.

BOX 119.2   Implant- and hardware-related complications

Complications Usually Seen Early
Air embolism
Brachial plexus injury
Extracardiac stimulation
Hematoma formation
Intraoperative lead damage
Lead perforation
Pain or ecchymoses
Pneumothorax
Subclavian artery puncture
Subcutaneous emphysema
Thoracic duct injury

Complications Usually Seen Late
Lead fracture or insulation defect
Skin adherence
Skin erosion
Thrombosis

Complications Seen Early or Late
Allergy to pacemaker
Circuit failure
Exit block
Infection
Lead dislodgement
Loose lead or connector block interface
Pacemaker-related arrhythmias
Pacemaker syndrome
Twiddler syndrome

BOX 119.3   Pacemaker troubleshooting

Failure to Capture
Air in the pocket of a unipolar pacemaker
Circuit failure
Functional noncapture
High thresholds with inadequately programmed output
Impending total battery depletion
Insulation defect
Lead dislodgement or perforation
Partial conductor coil fracture
Poor or incompatible connection at the connector block

Failure to Output
Circuit failure
Complete or intermittent conductor coil fracture
Intermittent or permanently loose setscrew
Internal insulation failure (bipolar lead)
Lack of anodal connector contact[a]
Oversensing any noncardiac activity
Total battery depletion

Sensing Abnormalities
Battery depletion
Circuit failure
Electromagnetic interference
Lead dislodgement or poor lead positioning
Lead insulation failure
Magnet application
Malfunction of the reed switch
Structure of the intrinsic event different from that measured at implantation

Altered Pacing Rate
Battery depletion
Circuit failure
Crosstalk
Hysteresis
Magnet application
Malfunction of the electrocardiographic recording equipment (i.e., alteration of paper speed)
Oversensing
Runaway
Undocumented reprogramming of the pacemaker

[a]Examples include a unipolar lead in a bipolar generator, bipolar lead in a pacemaker programmed to be unipolar, air in the pocket of a unipolar device, and a unipolar pacemaker not in the pocket.

Peak Endocardial Acceleration Sensor

Using a miniature accelerometer within a pacing lead, an index called *peak endocardial acceleration* has been introduced. This sensor, placed in the right ventricular lead, provides a surrogate measure of myocardial contractility and sympathetic activation. The sensor is also being tested as a means to optimize the AV interval and right ventricle–left ventricle timing in dual-chamber and biventricular pacing devices.

Right Ventricular Impedance-Based Sensor

CLS measures impedance from the right ventricular unipolar pacing. The impedance measurements are felt to correlate with dP/dt_{max}, which is a surrogate for ventricular contractility, and in turn, is a reflection of autonomic activity. As a reflection of autonomic activity, this sensor has the potential to respond to nonexertional stimuli such as mental stress.[17]

Dual-Sensor Combinations

The perfect sensor would be resistant to all nonphysiological stimuli. A multisensor, rate-adaptive pacing system could improve specificity by having one sensor verify or crosscheck the other. The most widely used sensor combination is the accelerometer–minute ventilation combination or blended sensor. Using this combination, the accelerometer provides a rapid response to exertion and the minute ventilation provides an excellent physiological response, achieving a more normal physiological heart rate response.[18] A dual sensor using a CLS and an accelerometer may have the advantage of being able to result in increased heart rates with mental stress.[19]

Pacemaker Complications

Complications can occur related to the implantation procedure or because of failure of a component of the pacing system. Box 119.2 lists the most commonly encountered complications and whether they are more likely to be seen immediately or over the long term.

Troubleshooting Electrocardiographic Abnormalities

Electrocardiographic abnormalities in patients with pacemakers can be broadly categorized into failure to capture, failure to output, oversensing, undersensing, and inappropriate rate change.[20]

Failure to capture indicates that a pacing artifact is present without subsequent cardiac depolarization (Box 119.3).

True failure to output is caused by failure to output from the pacemaker so that the electrical signal cannot reach the heart (see Box 119.3).

Oversensing is caused by the sensing of signals interpreted as the atria or ventricles deflecting in their respective channels. Sensing of signals originating in the opposite chamber is called *crosstalk*. For example, the ventricular deflection may be sensed on the atrial channel. More seriously, the atrial stimulus may be detected on the ventricular channel, resulting in ventricular inhibition and asystole. Such an occurrence may be prevented by programming

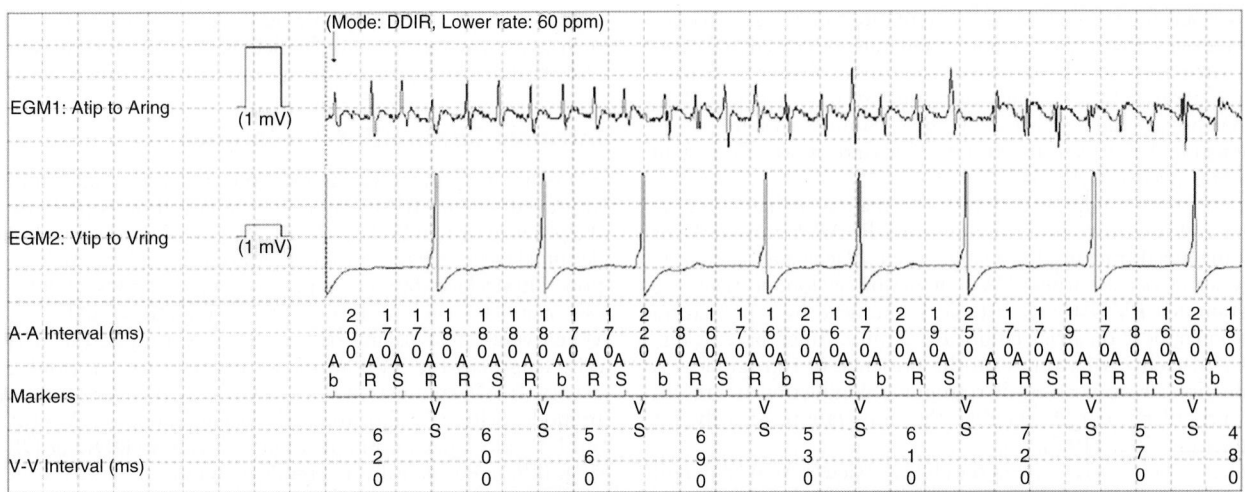

FIGURE 119.4 **Intracardiac electrogram** *(EGM)* **recordings and a marker channel demonstrating mode switching** *Top channel,* bipolar atrial electrogram (tip-ring). *Second channel,* bipolar ventricular electrogram (tip-ring). *Third channel,* atrial intervals in milliseconds. *Fourth channel,* marker channel. *Bottom channel,* ventricular intervals in milliseconds. The pacemaker has detected rapid atrial signals noted by AR and AS, meeting criteria for atrial arrhythmia, and has automatically switched its mode to DDIR, a nontracking mode. AB indicates an atrial event occurring during an atrial blanking period after a ventricular sensed event.

safety pacing so that a ventricular stimulus is given if a ventricular event is sensed shortly after an atrial stimulus is delivered. The electrocardiographic hallmark of safety pacing is the presence of pacing with a shortened AV interval, ranging from 80 to 130 ms. Ventricular oversensing results in a prolonged ventricular interval and atrial oversensing in the DDD mode results in the tracking of atrial signals and rapid ventricular pacing.

The differential diagnoses of the electrocardiographic abnormalities might overlap. For example, a ventricular lead fracture can result in failure to capture and to ventricular oversensing of noise, causing inhibition of pacing. A lead fracture can also result in undersensing.

Insulation defects similarly can manifest with oversensing or with failure to capture, although the most common presentation of insulation failure is a sensing abnormality. Lead impedance measurements are helpful in making the diagnosis, with lead fractures resulting in high impedances (>2500 Ω) and insulation breaks resulting in low impedances (<250 Ω). As pacemaker battery power is depleted, there may be decreased output or no output at all. This degree of battery depletion is avoidable with appropriate pacemaker follow-up. The pacemaker also might revert to VVI or VOO mode from DDD(R) mode when the replacement indicator occurs.

Sensing abnormalities can be divided into true abnormalities and functional sensing abnormalities (see Box 119.3). True abnormalities include undersensing, which is a failure to recognize normal intrinsic cardiac activity, and oversensing, which is unexpected sensing of an intrinsic or extrinsic electrical signal. An artifact might also give the appearance of oversensing. True undersensing is most commonly caused by lead dislodgement or inadequate intrinsic amplitude. Sensing abnormalities are commonly seen secondary to insulation defects and lead fracture.

Functional undersensing is present when an intrinsic cardiac event is not sensed because it falls within a programmed refractory period. For example, if an intrinsic atrial event occurs within the PVARP, the event is not sensed. However, without a thorough understanding of the timing cycle, it might appear as though true undersensing has occurred. Similarly, apparent failure to capture is noted if a pacemaker stimulus occurs during the physiological refractory period of a spontaneous beat. This condition is referred to as *functional noncapture.*

Every pacing mode has a defined lower rate limit, and dual-chamber and rate-adaptive pacemakers also require a defined upper rate limit. One must be familiar with the timing cycle of a particular pacing mode, as well as any idiosyncrasies of the specific pacemaker, to determine whether the paced rate is appropriate. The causes of an altered pacing rate are numerous (see Box 119.3).

Drugs can affect sensing and pacing thresholds and result in electrocardiographic abnormalities. Although many drugs have been reported to affect pacing thresholds, only the class IC agents commonly result in a clinical problem. If these drugs are administered to a patient with a pacemaker, especially a pacemaker-dependent patient, he or she should be monitored for an increase in pacing threshold. Class IC agents can also cause sensing abnormalities.

Electrolyte and metabolic abnormalities can also affect pacing and sensing thresholds. Hyperkalemia is the most common electrolyte abnormality that causes clinically significant problems, but severe acidosis or alkalosis, hypercapnia, severe hyperglycemia, hypoxemia, and myxedema should also be considered.

Automatic Pacemaker Function

Atrial Arrhythmia Detection and Automatic Mode Switching

The onset of atrial arrhythmias in the DDD or DDDR mode results in tracking of the atrial activity and rapid ventricular pacing, typically at the upper rate limit. Modern algorithms detect the rapid atrial rate on the atrial channel and result in automatic switching of the mode to a nontracking mode such as DDI, DDIR, VVI, or VVIR (Fig. 119.4). In all of these modes, tracking of atrial activity ceases. Once the atrial arrhythmia stops, the mode switches back to the DDD or DDDR mode. Atrial mode switching is generally considered to be accurate. Since mode switching detects atrial arrhythmias by rapid rates, it is able to detect both atrial flutter and AF. Pacemakers can display the frequency of atrial arrhythmias over time in a tabular or graphical format (Fig. 119.5). However, since atrial flutter is regular and rapid, atrial signals can fall within postventricular atrial blanking periods, and atrial flutter may be undersensed. Undersensing and oversensing atrial rhythms are limitations of using devices to detect atrial arrhythmias accurately and must be considered carefully when using such data to make clinical decisions. Atrial oversensing of far-field ventricular signals or atrial noise (Fig. 119.6) can be misclassified as atrial arrhythmias. Simulation studies have demonstrated that rate-based algorithms are most effective in detecting atrial arrhythmias.[21]

Algorithms might also detect pacemaker-mediated tachycardia and intervene by prolonging the PVARP transiently or avoiding atrial tracking for a single cycle. Pacemaker-mediated tachycardia occurs when VA conduction is longer than the programmed PVARP and is typically induced by a premature ventricular beat or atrial failure to capture. Since pacemaker-mediated tachycardia relies on the presence of retrograde VA conduction, we can assess if retrograde conduction is present by ventricular pacing faster than the sinus rate to identify VA conduction. (Fig. 119.7).

There is some variability in the ability to detect AF by different atrial tachyarrhythmia detection algorithms. Undersensing may lead to decreased detection of episodes but also may result in an incorrect determination that an episode has terminated. In such a situation, a greater number of shorter episodes might be recorded rather than fewer longer episodes. Longer detection times during onset may decrease inappropriate far-field oversensing. Atrial

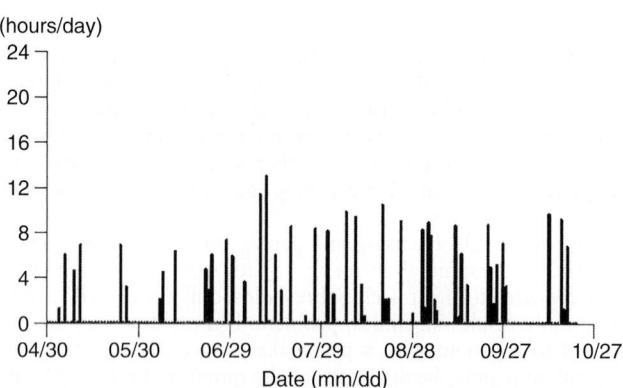

FIGURE 119.5 **Graphical display of atrial arrhythmia events** On the x-axis, the day and month of the atrial arrhythmia event is noted. On the y-axis, the duration of the atrial arrhythmia event in hours per day is shown. Each bar represents an arrhythmia event.

electrodes with shorter tip-to-ring distances, particularly shorter than 10 mm, may also reduce far-field R wave sensing. Postventricular atrial blanking periods may also contribute to undersensing.[22]

Intrinsic Conduction Preference

There has been an increasing recognition that hemodynamics are improved when intrinsic ventricular conduction is permitted in the absence of bundle branch block. New algorithms have been designed to permit the automatic restoration of intrinsic conduction. These algorithms can represent a form of AV search hysteresis or mode switching from DDD or DDDR to AAI or AAIR. When ventricular pacing occurs, AV search hysteresis periodically lengthens the AV interval so that intrinsic AV conduction occurs. If AV conduction does not occur, AV pacing resumes. In mode-switching algorithms, the pacing mode is AAI or AAIR until AV block occurs and the mode switches to DDD or DDDR (Fig. 119.8). Periodically, the mode switches back to AAI or AAIR to check if AV conduction has resumed (Fig. 119.9). These algorithms are extremely successful in decreasing the incidence of ventricular pacing in patients with intact AV conduction and can decrease the incidence of AF.

Automatic Testing and Data Storage

Many pacemakers can perform reliable automatic threshold testing of the leads. These data may be used to automatically adjust the pacing output. Automatic capture verification appears to be reliable in long-term follow-up and provides the benefit of maintaining an adequate safety margin even when the threshold has changed. Data about automatic capture threshold testing are frequently available and provide insight into any changes in pacing threshold (Fig. 119.10). In addition, use of automatic capture verification may prolong pacemaker battery life.[23] Such automatic features may be effectively programmed with a need for reprogramming in 6% of patients in 12 months.[24] Pediatric patients with constant intrinsically high heart rates may not be able to have effective automatic threshold testing.[25] In addition, many pacemakers keep long-term data regarding lead thresholds, lead impedances, and R wave and P wave amplitudes. Such trends are extremely helpful in detecting early abnormalities in lead function and in identifying pacing abnormalities. Many pacemakers can store events that are classified as pacemaker-mediated tachycardia, atrial tachyarrhythmia, or a rapid ventricular rate.

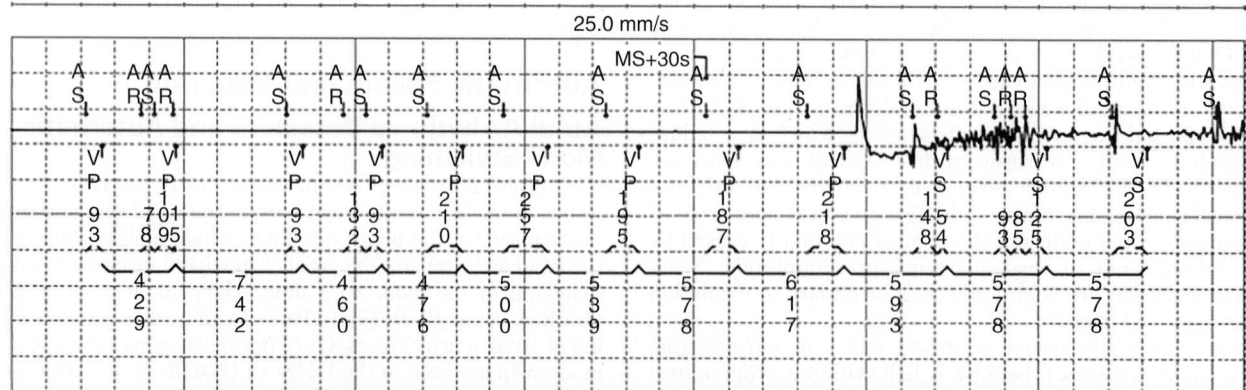

FIGURE 119.6 **Electrograms demonstrating atrial oversensing** The *top channel* is the atrial marker channel. *A* indicates an atrial paced event, *P* indicates intrinsic atrial activity, *V* indicates a ventricular paced event, and *R* indicates a ventricular sensed event. The *second channel* is the bipolar atrial electrogram. The *third channel* is the ventricular marker channel. The *bottom channel* is interval data. On the right-hand part of the panel in the atrial electrogram channel, there is atrial noise consistent with a lead abnormality. The AR events indicate atrial oversensed events due to sensing noise on the atrial channel.

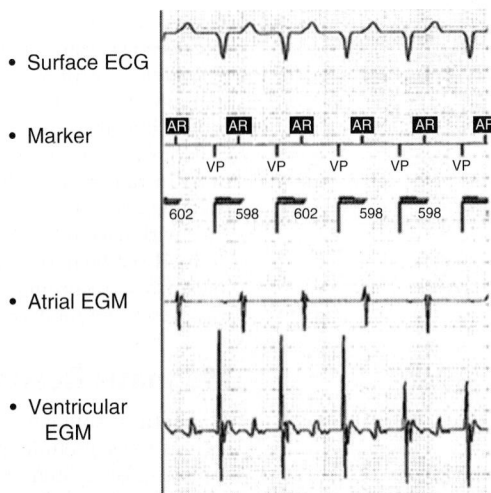

FIGURE 119.7 A surface electrocardiogram (*ECG*) and intracardiac electrogram (*EGM*) during ventricular pacing demonstrating retrograde ventriculoatrial conduction The *top channel* is the surface ECG. The *second channel* is the marker channel. The *third channel* is the bipolar atrial EGM. The *bottom channel* is the bipolar ventricular EGM. VP indicates ventricular pacing. AR indicates an atrial event. Because each VP is followed by an AR, there is likely 1:1 ventriculoatrial conduction. Setting the postventricular refractory period longer than the measured retrograde conduction time will likely prevent pacemaker-mediated tachycardia.

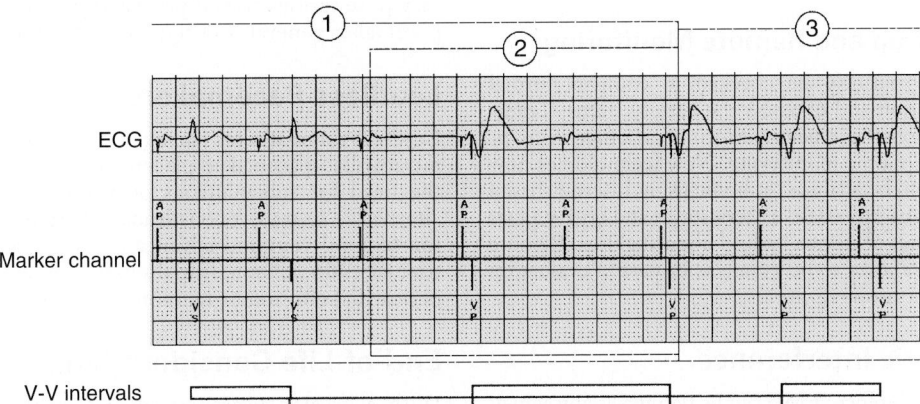

FIGURE 119.8 An electrocardiographic (*ECG*) tracing reveals a mode-switching algorithm from AAI or AAIR to DDD or DDDR. The managed ventricular pacing algorithm significantly decreases the incidence of ventricular pacing in patients with intact AV conduction. If transient AV block occurs in the AAIR mode after an A-A interval without a ventricular sensed event, a ventricular paced event occurs 80 ms after the escape interval. If two of the four most recent A-A intervals are missing a ventricular event, the device will switch from AAIR to DDDR or from AAI to DDD. (From the Medtronic Adapta/Versa/Sensia Device Manual.)

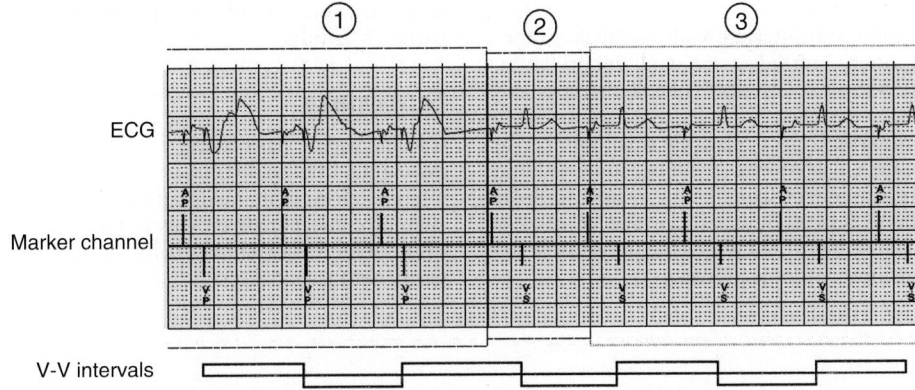

FIGURE 119.9 An electrocardiographic (*ECG*) tracing reveals a mode-switching algorithm from DDD or DDDR to AAI or AAIR. The algorithm checks for AV conduction at progressively longer intervals, initially 1 minute in duration but increasing up to 16 hours. If AV conduction is present, the mode changes to AAIR. (From the Medtronic Adapta/Versa/Sensia Device Manual.)

Max amplitude(V)	Average Threshold(V)	Maximum Threshold(V)
2 - Adapted	0.875	1
2 - Adapted	0.875	0.875
2 - Adapted	0.875	0.875
2 - Adapted	0.875	1
2 - Adapted	0.875	0.875
2 - Adapted	0.875	0.875
2 - Adapted	0.875	0.875
2 - Adapted	0.875	1
2 - Adapted	0.875	0.875
2 - Adapted	0.875	0.875
2 - Adapted	0.875	1
2 - Adapted	0.875	1
2 - Adapted	0.875	0.875
2 - Adapted	0.875	1
2 - Adapted	0.875	1

FIGURE 119.10 A tabular display from the programmer of automatic capture management results The adapted voltage in the first column is selected by the device. The middle and right columns indicate the average threshold and the maximum threshold recorded by the device, respectively.

Routine Follow-up and Remote Monitoring

Pacemakers should routinely be checked to confirm normal device and lead function and to assess the battery status. Traditionally, these functions have been performed at office visits or using home transtelephonic monitoring. New technologies now permit some devices to be analyzed at home using Internet-based services. These systems can assess battery status and create alerts notifying the physician of device or lead abnormalities. Remote monitoring has been shown to be as safe as in-person evaluation and may lead to fewer hospitalizations.

Electromagnetic Interference

Electromagnetic interference (EMI) can be defined as any signal, either biological or nonbiological, that falls within a frequency spectrum that may be detected by the sensing circuitry of the pacemaker. EMI can result in rate alteration, sensing abnormalities, magnet mode response, initiation of pacing algorithms, or reprogramming.[26,27]

Biological signals that may be responsible for oversensing include T waves, myopotential interference, afterpotential delay, and P waves. Isoelectric extrasystoles can give the appearance of oversensing.

Hospital equipment that can interfere with pacemaker function includes electrocautery, cardioversion and defibrillation, lithotripsy, radiofrequency ablation, electroshock therapy, and diathermy.

Potential EMI might arise from a relatively small number of sources in the nonhospital environment, including some welding equipment, degaussing equipment, conduction heaters, cellular telephones, and antitheft devices. Interference due to cellular telephone use is rare, and if the patient places the phone over the pacemaker, an adverse clinical event is unlikely.

Certain antitheft devices have the potential for pacemaker interference, causing pacemaker inhibition, sensing abnormalities, and induction of extrasystoles. However, from a practical standpoint, if the patient walks through antitheft gates at a regular pace, clinically significant abnormalities are unlikely.

Consumer products may also interfere with pacemaker function. In one report, iPods placed within 2 inches of implanted pacemakers may result in telemetry interference but no interference with pacemaker function or programmed parameters.[28]

EMI can be noticed as high-frequency repetitive signals on the intracardiac recordings, and can be particularly easily identified if it is present on both atrial and ventricular channels.

Magnetic Resonance Imaging

Magnetic resonance imaging (MRI) has been shown to pose serious risks, including life-threatening arrhythmias and death. A pacemaker system designed for safe use in MRIs is US Food and Drug Administration (FDA)-approved. Wilkoff and colleagues examined 464 patients randomized to undergo MRI scanning between 9 and 12 weeks postimplantation or not to undergo an MRI scan. During 1.5-T brain and lumbar MRI scans, there were no clinically significant ventricular arrhythmias, pacemaker inhibition, or changes in threshold.[29] Bailey and associates demonstrated the feasibility and safety of thoracic or cardiac MRI in an MRI conditional pacemaker.[30] MRI may pose serious risks if preexisting leads are in place even if a pacemaker generator designed for MRI use is in place.

Leadless Pacemakers

Leadless transcatheter pacing systems have been developed for intracardiac pacemaker placement.[31,32] These systems obviate the need for subcutaneous pocket formation and provide an alternative to transvenous leads. These devices are inserted via the femoral vein and advanced and secured to the right ventricular endocardium. Initial series demonstrate some reports of pericardial effusion or tamponade or dislodgement.

End-of-Life Considerations

With a greater awareness of end-of-life considerations, the field has created guidance regarding the management and ethics of pacemaker therapy at the end of a patient's life placement.[33,34] Clinicians should discuss the overall goals of care, the role of pacemaker therapy, and the option of withdrawal of pacemaker therapy. For the pacemaker-dependent patient, withdrawal of the pacing function may be quickly followed by the patient's death. For a patient that is not dependent on pacing, withdrawal may have little impact. In all cases, the possible outcomes should be discussed with the patient and the patient's family.

Summary

Cardiac pacing has become a sophisticated and critical aspect of managing bradyarrhythmias. Changes in indications represent ongoing changes in the discipline of cardiac pacing and the influence of clinical trials on this practice. The future will certainly result in increasing automaticity, flexibility, and self-regulation of permanent pacemakers.

REFERENCES

1. Greenspon AJ, Patel J, Lau E, et al. Trends in permanent pacemaker implantation in the United States 1993-2009: increasing complexity of patients and procedures. *J Am Coll Cardiol.* 2012;59:1016–1097.

2. Tracy CM, Epstein AE, Darbar D, et al. 2012 ACCF/AHA/HRS focused update incorporated into the ACCF/AHA/HRS 2008 guidelines for device-based therapy of cardiac rhythm abnormalities. *J Am Coll Cardiol.* 2013;61:e6–e75.

3. Nazarian S, Wagner KT, Caffo BS, et al. Clinical predictors of conduction disease progression in type I myotonic muscular dystrophy. *Pacing Clin Electrophysiol.* 2011;34:171–176.

4. Serwer GA, Shetty I. Pediatric pacing and defibrillator use. In: Ellenbogen KA, Kay GN, Lau CP, Wilkoff BL, eds. *Clinical Cardiac Pacing and Defibrillation, and Resynchronization Therapy.* 4th ed. Philadelphia: Saunders; 2011:393–427.

5. Romme JJ, Reitsma JB, Black CN, et al. Drugs and pacemakers for vasovagal, carotid sinus and situational syncope. *Cochrane Database Syst Rev.* 2011;5:CD004194.

6. Solbiati M, Sheldon RS. Implantable rhythm devices in the management of vasovagal syncope. *Autonomic Neurosci.* 2014;184:33–39.

7. Brignole M, Menozzi C, Moya A, et al. Pacemaker therapy in patients with neutrally-mediated syncope and documented asystole: Third International Study on Syncope of Uncertain Etiology (ISSUE-3): A randomized trial. *Circulation.* 2012;125:2566–2571.

8. Palmisano P, Zaccaria M, Luzzi G, et al. Closed-loop cardiac pacing vs. conventional dual-chamber pacing with specialized sensing and pacing algorithms for syncope prevention in patients with refractory vasovagal syncope: results of a long-term follow up. *Europace.* 2012;14:1038–1043.

9. Flammang D, Church TR, De Roy L, et al. Treatment of unexplained syncope: a multicenter, randomized trial of cardiac pacing guided by adenosine 5′-triphosphate testing. *Circulation.* 2012;125:31–36.

10. McLeod CJ, Trusty JM, Jenkins SM, et al. Method of pacing does not affect the recurrence of syncope in carotid sinus syndrome. *Pacing Clin Electrophysiol.* 2012;35:827–833.

11. Gold MR, Adler S, Fauchier L, et al. Impact of atrial prevention pacing on atrial fibrillation burden: primary results of the study of atrial fibrillation (SAFARI) trial. *Heart Rhythm.* 2009;6:295–301.

12. Talwar S, Saxon LA. Clinical trials of cardiac resynchronization therapy: Pacemakers and defibrillators. In: Ellenbogen KA, Kay GN, Lau CP, Wilkoff BL, eds. *Clinical Cardiac Pacing and Defibrillation, and Resynchronization Therapy.* 4th ed. Philadelphia: Saunders; 2011:279–299.

13. Qintar M, Morad A, Alhawasli H, et al. Pacing for drug-refractory or drug-intolerant hypertrophic cardiomyopathy. *Cochrane Database Syst Rev.* 2012;5:CD008523.11.

14. Prinzen F, Strik M, Regoli F, et al. Basic physiology and hemodynamics of cardiac pacing. In: Ellenbogen KA, Kay GN, Lau CP, Wilkoff BL, eds. *Clinical Cardiac Pacing and Defibrillation, and Resynchronization Therapy.* 4th ed. Philadelphia: Saunders; 2011:203–233.

15. Nielsen JC, Thomsen PE, Hojberg S, et al. A comparison of single-lead atrial pacing with dual chamber pacing in sick sinus syndrome. *Eur Heart J.* 2011;32:686–696.

16. Lau CP, Siu CW, Tse HF. Implantable sensors for rate adaption and hemodynamic monitoring. In: Ellenbogen KA, Kay GN, Lau CP, Wilkoff BL, eds. *Clinical Cardiac Pacing and Defibrillation, and Resynchronization Therapy.* 4th ed. Philadelphia: Saunders; 2011:144–174.

17. Proietti R, Manzoni G, DiBiase L. Closed loop stimulation is effective in improving heart rate and blood pressure response to mental stress: report of a single-chamber pacemaker study in patients with chronotropic incompetent atrial fibrillation. *Pacing Clin Electrophysiol.* 2012;35:990–998.

18. Coman J, Freedman R, Koplan BA, et al. A blended sensor restores chronotropic response more favorably than an accelerometer alone in pacemaker patients: the LIFE study results. *Pacing Clin Electrophysiol.* 2008;31:1433–1442.

19. Coenen M, Malinowski K, Spitzer W, et al. Closed loop stimulation and accelerometer-based rate adaptation: results of the PROVIDE study. *Europace.* 2008;10:327–333.

20. Love CJ. Pacemaker troubleshooting and follow-up. In: Ellenbogen KA, Kay GN, Lau CP, Wilkoff BL, eds. *Clinical Cardiac Pacing and Defibrillation, and Resynchronization Therapy.* 3rd ed. Philadelphia: Saunders; 2007:1005–1062.

21. Santamauro M, Ottaviano L, Borreli A, et al. Efficacy of automatic mode switching in DDDR mode parameters: the most 2 study. *J Interv Card Electrophysiol.* 2008;21:13–17.

22. Silberbauer J, Arya A, Veasey R, et al. The effect of bipole tip-to-ring distance in atrial electrodes upon atrial tachyarrhythmia sensing capability in modern dual-chamber pacemakers. *Pacing Clin Electrophysiol.* 2010;33:85–93.

23. Biffi M, Bertini M, Mazzotti A, et al. Long-term RV threshold behavior by automated measurements: safety is the standpoint of pacemaker longevity. *Pacing Clin Electrophysiol.* 2011;34:89–95.

24. Ailings M, Vireca E, Bastian D, et al. Clinical use of automatic pacemaker algorithms: results of AUTOMATICITY registry. *Europace.* 2011;13:976–983.

25. Hiippala A, Serwer G, Clausson E, et al. Automatic atrial threshold measurement and adjustment in pediatric patients. *Pacing Clin Electrophysiol.* 2010;33:309–313.

26. Wang PJ, Chen H, Okamura H, et al. Timing cycles of implantable devices. In: Ellenbogen KA, Kay GN, Lau CP, Wilkoff BL, eds. *Clinical Cardiac Pacing and Defibrillation, and Resynchronization Therapy.* 3rd ed. Philadelphia: Saunders; 2007:969–1004.

27. Misiri J, Kusomoto F, Goldshlager N. Electromagnetic interference and implanted devices: the non-medical environment (part I). *Clin Cardiol.* 2012;35:276–280.

28. Misiri J, Kusomoto F, Goldshlager N. Electromagnetic interference and implanted devices: the medical environment (part II). *Clin Cardiol.* 2012;35:321–328.

29. Thaker JP, Patel MP, Shah AJ. Do media players cause interference with pacemakers? *Clin Cardiol.* 2009;32:653–657.

30. Wilkoff B, Bellow D, Taborsky M, et al. Magnetic resonance imaging in patients with a pacemaker system designed for the magnetic resonance environment. *Heart Rhythm.* 2011;8:65–73.

31. Reddy VY, Exner DV, Cantillon DJ, et al. Percutaneous implantation of an entirely intracardiac leadless pacemaker. *N Engl J Med.* 2015;373:1125–1135.

32. Reynolds D, Duray GZ, Omar R, et al. A leadless intracardiac transcatheter pacing system. *N Engl J Med.* 2016;374:533–541.

33. Pasalic D, Gazelka HM, Topazian RJ, et al. Palliative care consultation and associated end-of-life care after pacemaker or implantable cardioverter-defibrillator deactivation. *Am J Hosp Palliat Care.* 2016;33:966–971.

34. Karches KE, Sulmasy DP. Ethical considerations for turning off pacemakers and defibrillators. *Card Electrophysiol Clin.* 2015;7:547–555.

120 Use of QRS Fusion Complex Analysis in Cardiac Resynchronization Therapy

Michael O. Sweeney

Cardiac resynchronization therapy (CRT) is a term that implies the restoration of the normal, ordered, four-chamber coupling of the heart. This is misleading at multiple levels because neither atrioventricular synchronization nor interventricular (I-V) synchronization is a requisite. The target of CRT is electrical delay in the *left ventricle* (LV) imposed by the *left bundle branch block* (LBBB) or its surrogate in the form of obligatory right ventricular (RV) stimulation.[1] The electrical delay disturbs the normally synchronized muscle contraction sequence generated by the "infinite" electrode of the Purkinje system. Consequently, the normal evenly distributed load-bearing arrangement of the LV is degraded. Over time, adverse biomechanical changes in the LV are induced by asynchronous electrical activation. These changes in function manifest clinically as heart failure with a low ejection fraction and are highlighted by progressive ventricular enlargement, asymmetric hypertrophy, reduced pump function, and functional mitral regurgitation. Therefore while "CRT" is an embedded concept, a better use of the acronym is "conduction replacement therapy" because only the correction of LV conduction delay unloads the overstretched LV for clinical effect.

As an electrical therapy for cardiac disease, CRT has no peer except perhaps high-voltage shocks for ventricular fibrillation. There is no suitable replacement for either. Most patients benefit clinically from CRT, even those with significant comorbidities, such as moderate-to-severe chronic kidney disease,[2] assuming that LBBB is well represented and that LV conduction delay is efficiently remediated. Interestingly, symptomatic improvement is not necessarily accompanied by an improvement in LV size and structure. However, the reduction in LV volume and increased pump function dominates clinical response. Moreover, a small subset of patients experience left ventricular ejection fraction normalization, which is associated with an extraordinarily low rate of ventricular arrhythmia, suggesting that CRT delivery can be uncoupled from defibrillator backup in some instances.[3]

Virtually every available assessment methodology (nuclear medicine, magnetic resonance imaging, echocardiography, invasive hemodynamics, etc.) has been applied to interpret the basis of the improvement in pump function in response to CRT. Many of these methods are technically cumbersome, time consuming, clinically impractical, ultra-expensive, and largely unavailable to the implanting physician. Moreover, while providing insight, there are several degrees of separation removed from the clinical phenomenology of electrically asynchronous heart failure. It is therefore not surprising that none of these methods has reliably improved the remodeling response to CRT for individual patients and is therefore infrequently applied in clinical practice. Consequently, most clinicians approach the CRT candidate as a "black box" response function, reflecting uncertainty of the clinical outcome beyond successful completion of the implantation procedure.

In contrast, the standard 12-lead electrocardiogram (ECG), which is used to identify patients who qualify for therapy, has seen a resurrection of interest as the most readily available, widely applied, least expensive, and easily interpreted means of describing ventricular activation before and after CRT. An additional virtue of the QRS fusion method for CRT is that the standard ECG is the familiar currency of the cardiologist implementing the therapy. The translational mechanism for improvement in ventricular pump function and reverse remodeling during CRT is the activation sequence change induced by pacing. QRS fusion complex analysis has proved remarkably useful for interpreting the linkage between foundational activation sequence changes induced by CRT and the clinical response, specifically LV reverse remodeling. This is important because physical reduction in LV volume is associated with clinical improvement and reduced mortality, similar to or exceeding the effects of neurohormonal antagonists for heart failure.

The study of ventricular fusion using surface ECG has a long and rich history in electrocardiology. The first published study of ventricular fusion by Sir Thomas Lewis in 1913, accompanied by the following mechanistic explanation that could not be improved upon more than 100 years later, is reproduced in Fig. 120.1. "When a premature contraction falls very late in diastole, the disturbance of ventricular rhythm is slight, for it comes at an instant close to that at which a rhythmic beat is expected. The auricle may even contract before the premature beat appears, so that there is an appreciable, though shortened, interval between the auricular beat and the premature one. The origin of the latter is nevertheless clearly shown by the *shape of its electric complex*. But suppose that the premature beat comes so late that an auricular impulse is already well on its way to the ventricle, then two waves of contraction, one from the normal source and one from the source of the irritation in the ventricle, may travel over that chamber and meet somewhere in the walls. Under these circumstances, the *electrical complex of the ventricular contraction will be of transitional form*. The resultant ventricular curve has a distinct form, in which traces of the normal and traces of the abnormal electric curves are seen. Such a contraction is the result of two impulses giving rise to simultaneous contraction curves, which meet in the ventricular walls."[4] Refinements to the ECG method for analysis of LBBB remediation during CRT were acquired from analysis of QRS patterns during spontaneous biventricular (BV) fusion in classical electrocardiology. The principles of fusion resulting from the interaction between two independent ventricular activation wavefronts stipulate a conformational change in the QRS complex, generating a hybrid combined wave complex possessing recognizable features of the patterns produced by each wavefront alone.[4,5] The QRS fusion contour is *most often* intermediate in shape and duration between the QRS contours of the independent wavefronts.

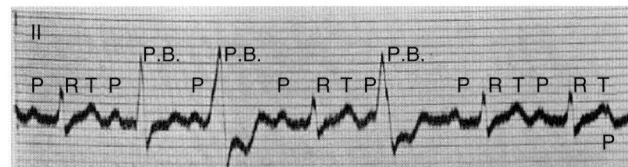

FIGURE 120.1 Electrocardiogram taken from a single-limb lead (II). "Premature ventricular contractions (P-B) are shown that arise in the right ventricle late in diastole. There are three such in the curve; in the second and third instances, the wave has spread throughout the whole ventricle from the point at which the new pulse arose. The first abnormal beat has fallen later in diastole so late that the ventricle responds in part to the natural impulse and in part to the new impulse; the ventricular complex is therefore transitional...in shape it is intermediate between the natural complex and the extrasystolic form...due to *interference between two excitation waves*." (From Lewis T. *Clinical Electrocardiology*. London: Shaws and Sons; 1913.)

The appearance of the combined wave QRS contour reflects the volume of myocardium controlled by each advancing wavefront. The *exception* to this principle occurs when the interacting wavefronts, each generating a uniquely abnormal QRS complex, fuse to create a normal-looking narrow complex that bears no resemblance to one or both component complexes (Fig. 120.2). The fusion QRS contours are explained by interference and the principle of superposition during periodic wave propagation. These examples of spontaneous BV QRS fusion are the wave interference products of independent RV and LV activation. The appearance of the QRS fusion contour is an admixture that necessarily reflects the extent to which each activation wavefront controls the ventricular muscle mass and displays sensitivity to (1) the site of origin of interfering wavefronts (e.g., RV and LV are antiphase) and (2) the relative timing of interfering wavefronts. Consequently, more than one QRS fusion type can occur in a single patient. This phenomenology duplicates the electrical wavefront interactions generated by BV pacing in experimental models.[6] These concepts were transferred to QRS complex analysis for classifying and quantifying BV electrical wave fusion.

Wave Interference for QRS Fusion

When two or more waves arrive at the same point and time they interact, or *interfere*, to create a unique disturbance. The waves superimpose according to the principle of superposition, which states that when two waves interfere, the resulting wave is the sum of their individual effects. Algebraically, the resultant displacement is the sum of the displacements of the individual waves at that same point, irrespective of the individual wave shapes and amplitudes. If the two interfering waves are identical in shape and amplitude and exactly in phase (peaks aligned with peaks, troughs aligned with troughs), the displacements add, yielding a fusion wave that is twice the amplitude of the individual waves but has the same wavelength. This superposition produces pure constructive interference. If the two interfering waves are identical in shape and amplitude but exactly out of phase (peaks aligned with troughs), the displacements completely destroy each other, or *cancel*, and the resulting amplitude is zero. This superposition produces pure destructive interference. Pure constructive and pure destructive interferences require precisely aligned identical waves. Most interacting waves are not identical and are at least partially out of phase. The superposition of nonidentical waves produces a *mosaic* of constructive and destructive interferences, displayed as a conformational hybrid of the two interfering waves, which can vary from place to place and time to time. Therefore the superposition of simple but dissimilar waves generates complex fusion wave patterns due to mixed addition and subtraction of wave forces (Fig. 120.3).

Wave Interference and the QRS During Normal Activation, Left Bundle Branch Block, and Biventricular Fusion

Cardiac electrical activation can be characterized as a volume model of periodic wave propagation. Wave interference is responsible for the expression of the normal QRS complex. Normal synchronous ventricular electrical activation generates a large number of wavefronts propagating simultaneously in many directions. Most of these wavefronts are antiphase and undergo cancelation (destructive interference). The QRS complex is therefore formed by residual in-phase (noncanceled) wavefronts, which add forces (constructive interference) to generate the normal narrow QRS.

During LBBB, RV and LV activation occur sequentially; therefore a large number of wavefronts are in phase, forces add (constructive interference), cancelation (destructive interference) is reduced, and the electrocardiographically recorded potential has greater amplitude and duration as compared with normal synchronous electrical activation.

Similarly, wave interference accounts for the classical examples of QRS fusion exemplified in Fig. 120.2. The naturally occurring spontaneous phenomenon of two independent and opposing pacemakers generating ventricular fusion simulates the objective of BV pacing to correct LV conduction delay. Idioventricular RV activation duplicates RV monochamber pacing (LBBB activation), idioventricular LV activation duplicates LV monochamber pacing (right bundle branch block [RBBB] activation), and the QRS fusion contour is the predictable wave interference product of these opposing wavefronts.

Consequently, a methodological solution for QRS fusion analysis was elaborated using the principles of wave interference.[9] In this model, BV fusion is an example of a stable two-point source interference where electrical wave generation is controlled by timed pacing stimulation. Because the point sources produce waves at the same frequency, they have identical wavelengths but typically different shapes and amplitudes, which influence the interference pattern of the combined wave. The interference pattern is also potentially influenced by the difference in the distance the two waves travel from their respective sources to a common point. This *path difference* is described in terms of the number of full waves that travel from each point source to the interference point. Path difference influences superposition; constructive interference occurs when the path difference between two wavefronts is equal to a whole number of wavelengths, whereas destructive interference occurs when the path difference is equal to a half number of wavelengths. During BV pacing, single waves from each stimulation site interact and complete before the subsequent wave from each site is emitted. However, the path length and conduction velocity from each site to the interference point (e.g., different ECG lead viewpoints) may differ depending on the contribution of muscle path conduction and Purkinje system engagement influencing the superposition pattern. For example, dominantly constructive interference may be observed from one point of view, whereas mixed constructive and destructive interferences may be observed from another.

Brief Summary of QRS Fusion Analysis to Predict Reverse Remodeling During Cardiac Resynchronization Therapy

The principles of wave interference, exemplified by the examples in Figs. 120.1 to 120.3, were applied to QRS fusion pattern recognition. Accordingly, initial attention was focused on the QRS contour before and after BV pacing in leads V1-V2 because they are best positioned to register the interference product of RV and LV pacing, which is typically antiphase in this vector (Fig. 120.4).

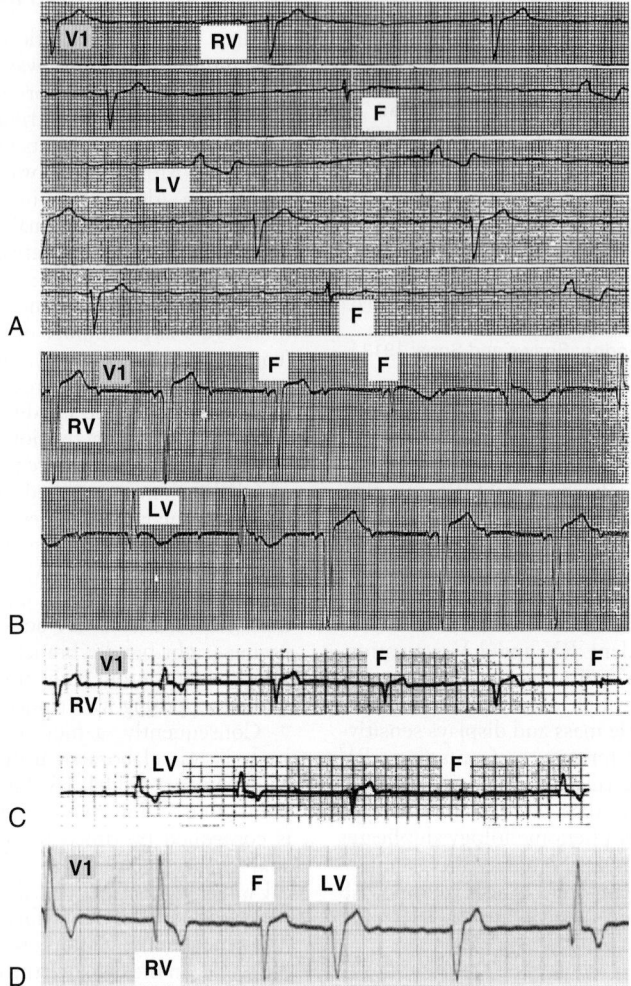

FIGURE 120.2 (A) An electrocardiogram (ECG) taken from a single anterior precordial lead (*V1*) showing complete atrioventricular (AV) block with two competing idioventricular escape rhythms.[5] *First and fourth rows* show right ventricular (*RV*) rhythm generating a left bundle branch block (LBBB) activation. *Third row* shows a left ventricular (*LV*) rhythm generating a right bundle branch block (RBBB) activation. Narrow beats in the *second and fifth rows* are fusion (*F*) QRS complexes generated by simultaneous activation of RV and LV by competing idioventricular rhythms. Note the QRS fusion contour contains recognizable features of both activation wavefronts (R wave component from the LV escape QRS, S wave component from RV escape QRS) but is *normally narrow*. This exemplifies the exception to the rule that the fusion QRS must be intermediate in form *and* width between the fusing complexes. (B) An ECG taken from a single anterior precordial lead (*V1*).[5] The rhythm is a 2:1 AV block. Note LBBB activation (RV) at the *beginning of the top strip* and *second half of the bottom strip*. Last two beats on the *top strip* and first two beats on the *bottom strip* are competitive idioventricular escape pacemakers from LV (RBBB activation). The third and fourth beats on the *top strip* are fusion (*F*) beats; note the large reduction in QRSd and absence of conformational change (R emergence is absent) in the QRS fusion contour. Fourth beat (second fusion complex) is "normally narrow"; note QS regression. (C) An ECG taken from a single anterior precordial lead (V1).[7] The rhythm is a complete AV block with two competing idioventricular pacemakers. QRS complexes 1, 3, 5, and 9 are RV escape pacemakers; QRS complexes 2, 7, 8, and 11 arise in the LV. QRS complexes 4, 6, and 10 are fusion complexes generated by simultaneous activation of RV and LV. Note that QRS fusion complex 4 is similar to the RV escape pacemaker except that QRSd is reduced; fusion QRS complexes 6 and 10 are conformational hybrids of the competing RV and LV idioventricular escape pacemakers. The explanation for the variation in QRS contour is that the timing of the idioventricular escape rhythms differs: for the fusion QRS 4, they are simultaneous; for QRS 6 and 10, they are sequential with the LV first, which accounts for the new R wave emergence. (D) The rhythm is atrial fibrillation (AF) with conducted LBBB (RV), an LV escape rhythm with RBBB, and normalization of the QRS complex as represented by the third beat in V1.[8] This is because of ventricular fusion between RBBB conduction in AF and the LV escape rhythm.

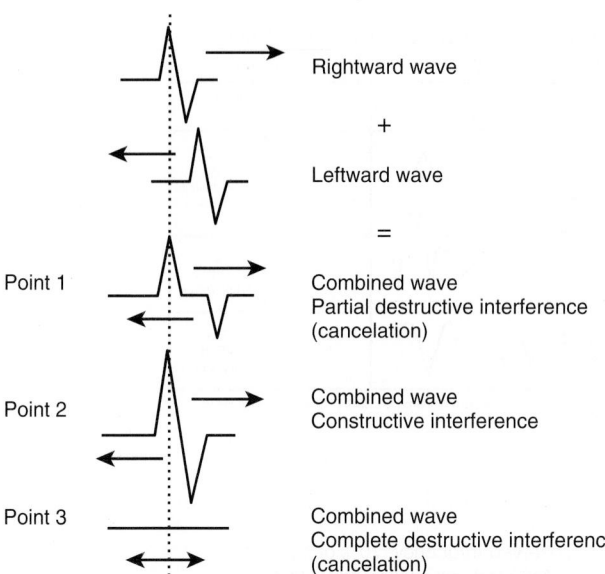

Rightward wave

+

Leftward wave

=

Point 1 — Combined wave
Partial destructive interference (cancelation)

Point 2 — Combined wave
Constructive interference

Point 3 — Combined wave
Complete destructive interference (cancelation)

FIGURE 120.3 Wave interference superposition. *Top,* Two waves having identical shapes and displacement amplitudes are depicted moving along the same line in opposite directions. At the first point of interaction, the negative component (trough or downward displacement) of the rightward wave and the positive component (peak or upward displacement) of the leftward wave are precisely aligned and cancel, yielding a combined fusion wave contour intermediate in shape between the two independent interfering waves, termed a *conformational change.* At the second point of interaction, the positive (peaks) and negative (troughs) displacements of both waves reinforce because of constructive interference; note the wave contour that duplicated independent interfering waves but with increased amplitudes. At the third point of interaction, the reinforced positive (peak) and negative (trough) components are perfectly aligned and completely cancel (zero amplitude). Waves are destroyed.

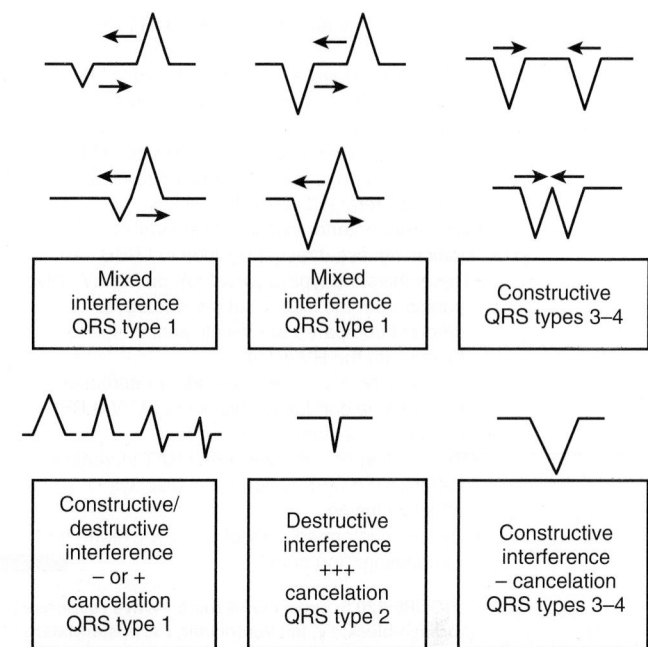

| Mixed interference QRS type 1 | Mixed interference QRS type 1 | Constructive QRS types 3–4 |

| Constructive/ destructive interference – or + cancelation QRS type 1 | Destructive interference +++ cancelation QRS type 2 | Constructive interference – cancelation QRS types 3–4 |

FIGURE 120.4 Waves are depicted to represent typical QRS complex interactions between the right ventricular (RV) monochamber (QS), left ventricular (LV) monochamber (R), and biventricular pacing from the viewpoint of leads V1-V2. Assume the left bundle branch block (LBBB) activation displays a typical QS complex (not shown). Note that the wave shapes, amplitudes, and durations vary and influence the interference product. *Row 1,* RV pacing generates the QS complex (moving right → left and anterior → posterior) and lateral LV pacing generates the R complex (moving left → right and posterior → anterior). *Column 1,* wave shapes are similar but amplitudes differ and forces are opposing. *Column 2,* wave shapes and amplitudes are nearly identical and forces are opposing. *Column 3,* wave shapes and amplitudes are identical and forces are reinforced because LV pacing is conducted from a site that does not oppose LBBB conduction. *Row 2,* The onset of fusion results in a conformational change of the QRS complex showing recognizable elements of the independent interacting waves (e.g., qR in *column 1,* QR in *column 2,* QrS in *column 3*). *Row 3, column 1,* The final fusion QRS complex is R, Rs, rS, etc. (conformational hybrid); note the admixture of constructive and destructive interference. Amplitudes and duration are reduced versus baseline waveforms if destructive interference (cancelation) dominates. These are exemplary forms of QRS Type 1 (a new R wave, with or without a reduction in QRSd) as compared with LBBB. *Column 2,* The final fusion complex is qs (QRS normalization, nonconformational change); note the destruction of both the R wave and QS waves (wave suppression) and marked reduction in wave duration versus baseline waveforms because of a large, dominant cancelation effect. This is an example of QRS Type 2. *Column 3,* The final fusion complex is QS; note that the QS complex is increased in amplitude and duration because of a dominant constructive interference effect. This is an example of QRS Types 3 and 4.

This provides a reproducible pivot point between anterior (right sided) and posterior (left sided) cardiac electrical activation,[6,10–12] suitable for preliminarily characterizing LBBB remediation.

Four distinctive QRS fusion types to represent BV activation wavefronts were identified and ordered by observed frequency. These QRS fusion types recite the principles of BV fusion epitomized in Figs 120.1 to 120.4. *From the viewpoint of leads V1-V2:*

- QRS Type 1 (Fig. 120.5): A conformational change in the QRS contour showing new R wave *and* (QRS_{diff}, in milliseconds = $QRS_{BV} - QRS_{LBBB}$) any value ($QRS_{BV} <, =, > QRS_{LBBB}$) but typically a positive value. The QRS fusion wave is a hybrid, intermediate in shape between the shapes of the interacting wavefronts, and follows the rule that the fusion complex admixture resembles both independent QRS types (i.e., shows features of both).

- QRS Type 2 (Fig. 120.6): A nonconformational change in the QRS contour showing *QRS wave force normalization,* obligatory and generally large (–) QRS_{diff} ($QRS_{BV} < QRS_{LBBB}$), *and* no new R wave.

- QRS Type 3 (Fig. 120.7): A persistent LBBB QRS contour,[11,13,14] no new R wave, *and* neutral or (+) QRS_{diff} ($QRS_{BV} \geq QRS_{LBBB}$); LBBB reinforcement.

- QRS Type 4 (Fig. 120.8): A "pseudopersistent LBBB" QRS contour resembling QRS Type 3. QRS contour duplicating LBBB (or RV pacing), no new R wave, *and* neutral or (+) QRS_{diff} ($QRS_{BV} \geq QRS_{LBBB}$). Concealed QRS fusion is only revealed by manipulation of BV timing. Real-time manipulation of ventricular activation using BV timing parameters identified a fourth QRS type superficially similar to Type 3, but in which timing changes can induce a transformation to Type 1.

Because stimulation from the lateral/posterolateral LV generates a large monophasic R wave in V1-V2,[1–3,6] which opposes the QS in V1-V2 during typical LBBB and RV pacing, QRS Types 1 and 2 must be variations on the interference product of RV and LV paced wavefronts. The QRS Type 1 conformational change is due to a mosaic of constructive and destructive interferences. The resulting QRS contour represents the extent to which elements of the interfering wavefronts reinforce or cancel one another; similarly, QRSd may increase or decrease depending on the balance of constructive and destructive interferences. QRS Type 2 is dominated by destructive interference, generating greater cancelation, wave suppression, and QRSd shortening. The greater contribution of destructive interference accounts for the larger reduction in QRSd observed in

Type 1: R dominant (R, qR, qRs, RsR', Rs)

- QRS fusion wave is a conformational hybrid with recognizable elements of both RV and LV waveforms.
- LV waveform is modestly oppositional to LBBB
- This waveform is observed most often from posterolateral (PL) wall stimulation
- Also from anterior vein, but R is smaller indicating less direct opposition to LBBB
- Resembles the typical waveform during LV-only pacing from the PL LV but morphology is different compared to LV-only pacing due to fusion with the RV wave.
- VAT may be increased, neutral, or decreased. Likely some conduction block out of LV (LBB conduction is completely "out")
- Remodeling occurs even when VAT increases because the QRS fusion wave displays effective fusion.
- This is an intermediately efficient waveform for remodeling; "the norm"

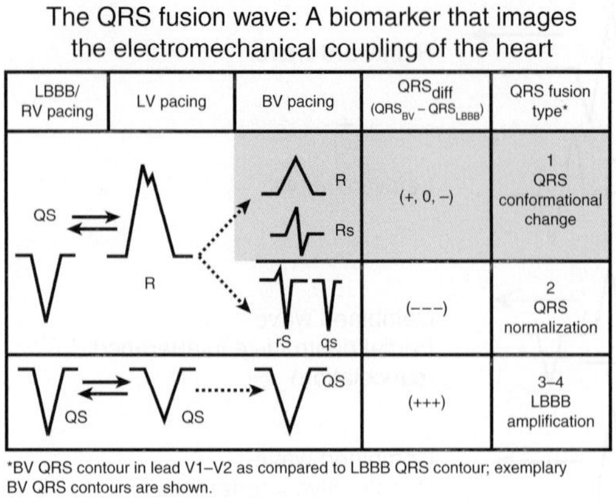

The QRS fusion wave: A biomarker that images the electromechanical coupling of the heart

LBBB/RV pacing	LV pacing	BV pacing	QRS$_{diff}$ (QRS$_{BV}$ − QRS$_{LBBB}$)	QRS fusion type*
		R / Rs	(+, 0, −)	1 QRS conformational change
		rS / qs	(−−−)	2 QRS normalization
		QS	(+++)	3–4 LBBB amplification

*BV QRS contour in lead V1–V2 as compared to LBBB QRS contour; exemplary BV QRS contours are shown.

Observed frequency: 70% of patients
Adjusted remodeling odds: 60%

FIGURE 120.5 Type 1 QRS fusion wave response to biventricular (*BV*) stimulation. *LBBB*, Left bundle branch block; *LV*, left ventricular; *PL*, posterolateral; *RV*, right ventricular; *VAT*, ventricular activation time.

Type 2: S-dominant waveform (QS, rS)

- QRS fusion wave in V1-V2 appears "normally narrow," duplicating the normal QRS
- LV wave is highly oppositional to LBBB
- This waveform is observed most often from PL stimulation
- Rarely generated from anterior wall or inferior wall stimulation unless lucky "wrap-around" wave propagation path
- Visual evidence of highly effective wave cancelation in the form of
  - Wave force normalization in multiple leads
  - Normalization of frontal plane electrical axis
  - Largest decrease in VAT (− value QRS$_{diff}$)
- This is a highly efficient waveform for remodeling; the "super-responder"

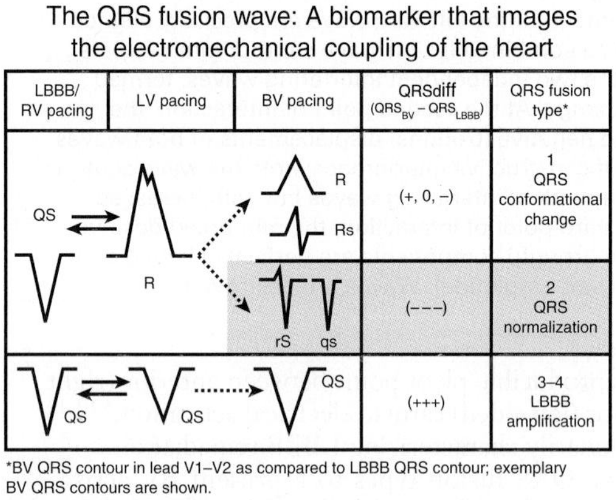

The QRS fusion wave: A biomarker that images the electromechanical coupling of the heart

LBBB/RV pacing	LV pacing	BV pacing	QRSdiff (QRS$_{BV}$ − QRS$_{LBBB}$)	QRS fusion type*
		R / Rs	(+, 0, −)	1 QRS conformational change
		rS / qs	(−−−)	2 QRS normalization
		QS	(+++)	3–4 LBBB amplification

*BV QRS contour in lead V1–V2 as compared to LBBB QRS contour; exemplary BV QRS contours are shown.

Observed frequency: 20% of patients
Adjusted remodeling odds: 90%

FIGURE 120.6 Type 2 QRS fusion wave response to biventricular (*BV*) stimulation. *LBBB*, Left bundle branch block; *LV*, left ventricular; *PL*, posterolateral; *RV*, right ventricular; *VAT*, ventricular activation time.

Type 3: S-dominant (QS, rS)

- QRS wave in V1–V2 duplicates LBBB; fusion absent
- LV wave is non-oppositional to LBBB
  - Stimulation site is MCV or distal AIV
  - Apical LV stimulation site
- Visual evidence of wave summation in the form of
  - Right to left dominant waveform, ↑QRSd
  - Wave amplification across multiple leads
- Obligatory increase in VAT (+value QRS$_{diff}$)
- This is an ineffective waveform for remodeling; the "non-responder"
- Cannot be corrected by wave timing maneuver

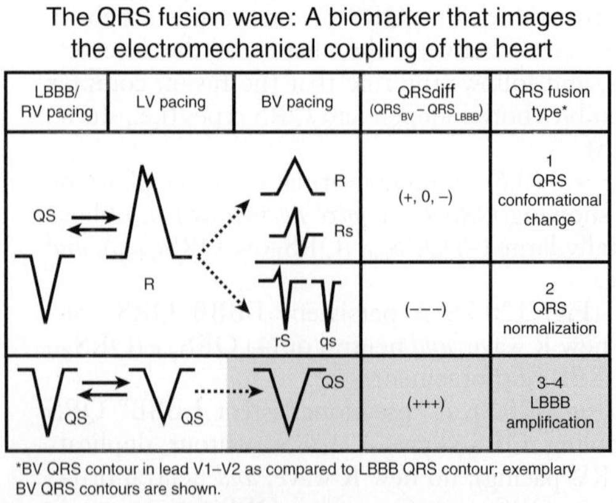

The QRS fusion wave: A biomarker that images the electromechanical coupling of the heart

LBBB/RV pacing	LV pacing	BV pacing	QRSdiff (QRS$_{BV}$ − QRS$_{LBBB}$)	QRS fusion type*
		R / Rs	(+, 0, −)	1 QRS conformational change
		rS / qs	(−−−)	2 QRS normalization
		QS	(+++)	3–4 LBBB amplification

*BV QRS contour in lead V1–V2 as compared to LBBB QRS contour; exemplary BV QRS contours are shown.

Observed frequency: 10% of patients
Adjusted remodeling odds: <40% (nil)

FIGURE 120.7 Type 3 QRS fusion wave response to biventricular (*BV*) stimulation. *LBBB*, Left bundle branch block; *LV*, left ventricular; *MCV*, middle cardiac vein; *RV*, right ventricular; *VAT*, ventricular activation time.

Type 4: S-dominant (QS, rS)

- QRS wave in V1–V2 duplicates LBBB; fusion absent
- LV wave is oppositional to LBBB
- LV wave is "jailed" at or near the stimulation site
- Obligatory increase in VAT (+value QRS$_{diff}$)
- This is an ineffective waveform for remodeling; the "non-responder"
- Cannot be corrected by timing maneuver
- A special case is observed where T3 activation occurs even though the LV lead is confirmed on the PL wall and monochamber activation wave is oppositional to LBBB
- This is a special form of severe conduction block or delay out of the LB which can only be overcome by advancing the LV wave, usually by >40 ms to generate Type 1 QRS fusion
- Even then VAT increases (QRS$_{diff}$ is +++) and remodeling odds are only modest (60%) probably due to prohibitive scar.

Observed frequency: Rare
Remodeling odds: Low

The QRS fusion wave: A biomarker that images the electromechanical coupling of the heart

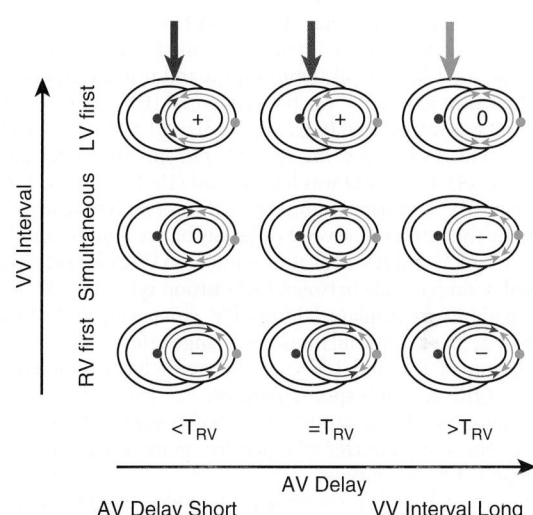

LBBB/ RV pacing	LV pacing	BV pacing	QRSdiff (QRS$_{BV}$ – QRS$_{LBBB}$)	QRS fusion type*
		Sequential LV	(+++)	1 QRS conformational change
		Simultaneous	(+++)	4 LV conduction block
			(+++)	3 LBBB amplification

*BV QRS contour in lead V1–V2 as compared to LBBB QRS contour; exemplary BV QRS contours are shown.

FIGURE 120.8 Type 4 QRS fusion wave response to biventricular (*BV*) stimulation. *LBBB*, Left bundle branch block; *LV*, left ventricular; *RV*, right ventricular; *VAT*, ventricular activation time.

QRS Type 2 versus Type 1. QRS Types 1 and 2 are therefore distinguished primarily by the extent to which wavefront cancelation due to destructive interference contributes to the final QRS contour. QRS Types 3 and 4 are dominated by constructive interference, which reinforces LBBB activation (wave force amplification).

These observations regarding wave interference and the genesis of QRS fusion patterns during spontaneous or pacing-initiated BV activation support the following conceptualization of the electrical mechanism of ventricular resynchronization:

1. Normal synchronous ventricular electrical activation is the interference product of a multitude of simultaneously activating and canceling wavefronts.
2. Sequential ventricular activation during LBBB reduces wavefront cancelation and increases electrical asynchrony (EAS) due to unopposed wavefronts. Wavefronts are reinforcing, wave forces sum, and conduction delay is amplified.
3. BV fusion restores wavefront cancelation and reduces EAS with two large opposing wavefronts that simulate normal ventricular activation. Wavefronts are highly oppositional, wave forces cancel, LBBB conduction delay is reduced, and EAS is reduced. The overall pattern approximates normal ventricular activation.
4. QRS Types 1 and 2 are the interference products of two opposing wavefronts that represent different forms of LBBB remediation. QRS Type 2 generally displays greater restoration of cancelation and reduction of EAS compared with QRS Type 1. QRS Type 3 is the interference product of two nonopposing wavefronts. Wavefronts are reinforcing, wave forces sum, LBBB conduction delay is amplified, and EAS is increased. QRS Type 4 resembles Type 3; however, manipulation of I-V timing reveals the concealed oppositional LV wavefront.

In summary, a foundational principle is formed: LBBB reduces wave cancelation, which results in EAS; BV fusion restores wave cancelation, which results in electrical resynchronization.

BV fusion requires that (1) stimulation must occur from a site capable of reversing LV conduction delay and (2) stimulation must be delivered in a fashion that effectuates reversal of LV conduction delay. Changes in the QRS complex provide evidence for or against effective wavefront opposition to LBBB (LBBB remediation). These include (1) a change in directionality of specific QRS waveform components, (2) a change in amplitude of specific QRS waveform components (emergence of or increased amplitude; regression of or decreased amplitude), and (3) a change in

VV Interval
LV first
Simultaneous
RV first

<T_{RV} =T_{RV} >T_{RV}

AV Delay

AV Delay Short   VV Interval Long

3 types of LV pacing fusion

1. ↓ No RBB fusion
2. ↓ RBB/RV pacing fusion
3. ↓ Pure RBBB fusion

— RV pacing activation
— LV pacing activation
— Intrinsic activation
— RV pacing/intrinsic activation

FIGURE 120.9 Interactions between the PR interval, atrioventricular (*AV*) delay, and interventricular timing during biventricular pacing for the left bundle branch block. *LV*, Left ventricular; *RBBB*, right bundle branch block; *RV*, right ventricular. (Data from Vernooy K, Cornelussen RN, Verbeek XA, et al. Cardiac resynchronization therapy cures dyssynchronopathy in canine left bundle-branch block hearts. *Eur Heart J.* 2007;28:2148-2155; and Verbeek XA, Vernooy K, Peschar M. Intra-ventricular resynchronization for optimal left ventricular function during pacing in experimental left bundle branch block. *J Am Coll Cardiol.* 2003;42:558-567.)

ventricular activation time (VAT) as a surrogate for EAS. QRS waveform changes should demonstrate opposition to LBBB forces.

Effects of Stimulation Timing and Site on QRS Fusion Wave Interference

Interactions between the PR interval, atrioventricular delay (AVD), and I-V timing during BV pacing for LBBB are displayed in Fig. 120.9.[15,16] During LBBB the RV is activated by RBB conduction

(RBBc) before the LV, and the time difference between $RV(T_{RVi})$ and $LV(T_{LV})$ activation is the intrinsic I-V conduction delay.[17] Experimental models show that maximally effective ventricular resynchronization occurs when electrical wavefronts fuse midway between the earliest (RBBc) and latest LV activation sites. The optimum AVD achieves maximally effective ventricular resynchronization by advancing LV activation sufficiently to minimize the I-V interval. When the AVD is substantially shorter than the PR interval, the RV and LV advance, and ventricular conduction is completely controlled by pacing wavefronts (column 1). Intermediate AVDs approaching the PR interval result in three-way fusion between RBBc, RV paced activation, and LV paced activation (column 2).[6,17] Moreover, LV activation can still be advanced when AVD is equal to or exceeds the PR interval because the LV is delayed relative to the RV[17-19] (column 3). Then, BV fusion occurs between RBBc and LV pacing wavefronts; RV pacing is not required to achieve fusion. Consequently, correction of LV conduction delay is possible across a range of AVDs and I-V timing arrangements to time the relative prematurity of LV stimulation.

BV fusion wave interference patterns should display sensitivity to timing manipulations and stimulation site due to their effects on activation wavefront shapes, conduction path, and superposition patterns. Several exemplary QRS fusion type response scenarios are systematically illustrated using this ECG method (Figs. 120.10 to 120.14). (1) The nominal QRS fusion type was established during simultaneous BV (BV_sim) pacing at short AVD = 100 ms (150 ms during obligatory atrial pacing), a typically applied value within the observed range for LV preload optimization and utilized in CRT trials and clinical practice.[20-23] (2) BV sequential (BV_seq) pacing ($R \rightarrow L$, $L \rightarrow R$) was introduced (e.g., 10, 20, 30...80 ms) at an AVD of 100 ms. (3) The AVD was shortened (80, 60, and 40 ms) during BV_sim pacing. (4) The AVD was lengthened (100, 110, 120, 130 ms, etc.) during BV_sim pacing until the PR interval was reached. In this manner the effects of several different but related methods for manipulating LV and RV activation timing on QRS fusion type were assessed. Comparisons between QRS fusion types by LV site for selected patients are displayed during BV_sim pacing at AVD = 100 ms to isolate the LV stimulation site change effect.

Manipulation of RV and LV wave behavior has predictable effects on the QRS fusion response pattern.

These examples demonstrate that BV wavefront timing changes alter the wave interference pattern, generating predictable effects on QRS fusion type.

1. Advancing the LV activation wavefront reinforces QRS Type 1 and transforms QRS Type 2 and QRS Type 4 to Type 1. These conformational changes reflect a phase shift, resulting in a greater contribution of LV wavefront forces to the BV wave interference pattern. During typical activation from a lateral or posterolateral LV site, this change is represented as increasing R wave amplitude in V1-V2 (e.g., QS, rS → RS, Rs, R) and ↑VAT (↓wavefront cancelation). S wave regression may coexist because of diminished contribution of RV wavefront forces to the BV fusion wave. Advancing the LV activation wavefront amplifies QRS Type 3 since RV and LV wavefronts are nonoppositional, wavefronts are reinforcing, and wave forces sum.

2. Withdrawing the LV activation wavefront progressively transforms QRS Type 1 → Type 2 → Type 4 → LBBB conduction. These changes reflect a phase shift, resulting in lesser contribution of LV wavefront forces to the BV wave interference pattern ending in the reemergence of LBBB conduction. For QRS Type 1, this represents a reverse conformational change. For QRS Type 2 the "normalized" QRS complex is transformed to a wide QRS duplicating LBBB conduction. Withdrawing LV activation regresses QRS Type 3 by reducing wavefront reinforcement.

3. Advancing the RV activation wavefront progressively transforms QRS Type 1 and Type 2 → Type 4 → RV monochamber pacing conduction. These changes reflect a phase shift resulting in greater contribution of RV wavefront forces to

the BV wave interference pattern. For QRS Type 1, this represents a "reverse" conformational change. For QRS Type 2, the "normalized" QRS complex is transformed to a wide QRS duplicating RV pacing. Advancing the RV activation wavefront amplifies QRS Type 3 since RV and LV wavefronts are nonoppositional, wavefronts are reinforcing, and wave forces sum.

Advancing RV activation exerts similar effects to withdrawing LV activation on the wave interference pattern. Likewise, advancing LV activation and withdrawing RV activation exert similar, but reciprocal, effects on the wave interference pattern.

These examples of wave behavior confirm that cancelation due to wavefront superposition is the mechanism of QRS shortening during CRT. The combined wave has a shorter VAT than either independent wave, both of which typically exceed LBBB duration during muscle path conduction. Cancelation is reflected in wave suppression (reduced wave amplitude), restoration of normal QRS forces, and ↓VAT. Moreover, complete wavefront destruction occurs when the interfering waves are antiphase and have equivalent amplitudes (see Fig. 120.11B). These examples also demonstrate that two simple waves interact differently at separate points throughout the ventricular muscle. This can generate complex waves with multiple superposition patterns because of the changes in wave shapes and path length as the wavefronts propagate from their sources to the different interference boundaries displayed by the 12-lead ECG. The magnitude of constructive and destructive interference displayed in the QRS fusion wave complex therefore may be the same or vary from point to point, which accounts for concordance or discordance of QRS fusion types (conformational change, QRS normalization) between ECG viewpoints. Wavefront fusion during CRT is a complex process functioning on multiple levels and in multiple dimensions.

These examples support the conceptualization of QRS fusion during BV pacing as a problem of interference during electrical wave propagation. Moreover, the QRS fusion wave interference pattern can be predictably manipulated by electrical timing instructions to achieve certain goals. From this perspective, BV pacing is a two-source generator of electrical wave interference, and the AVD and I-V timing operate as wave interference control parameters. Finally, a change in LV stimulation site influences LV wave constituents (shape, amplitude, and duration), muscle path to the interference boundary, and possibly access to the Purkinje system.

Regression Equations for Predicting Reverse Remodeling During QRS Fusion

Several generations of multivariable prediction models for reverse remodeling in response to CRT have been elaborated. A current model[24] for predicting patient-specific odds of reverse remodeling is defined by the interaction between (1) QRS fusion type, (2) QRS_{diff} induced by the QRS fusion response and indicative of the efficiency in the reduction of EAS, and (3) LV scar (where more scar reduces remodeling odds). The ranking of variables by predictive significance is QRS fusion type (highest), QRS score, and QRS_{diff} (reduction in VAT or EAS due to LBBB). This is important because QRS fusion type is the only variable that can be modulated for clinical effect.

This model also confirms that the method of QRS fusion analysis applies to all qualifying patients with LBBB heart failure (or RV apical stimulation) irrespective of substrate (ischemic, nonischemic), lack of sinus rhythm (e.g., atrial fibrillation [AF]), clinical demographics, or New York Heart Association (NYHA) functional class. In other words, the method applies to all patients qualifying for CRT with LBBB and/or obligatory RV apical stimulation. The c-index for all of these models has consistently been in the range of 0.71–0.75. This is quite striking in that ECG-based quantitative measures are capable of accurately forecasting change in ventricular volumes during CRT. No other method has proven to have this singular capacity.

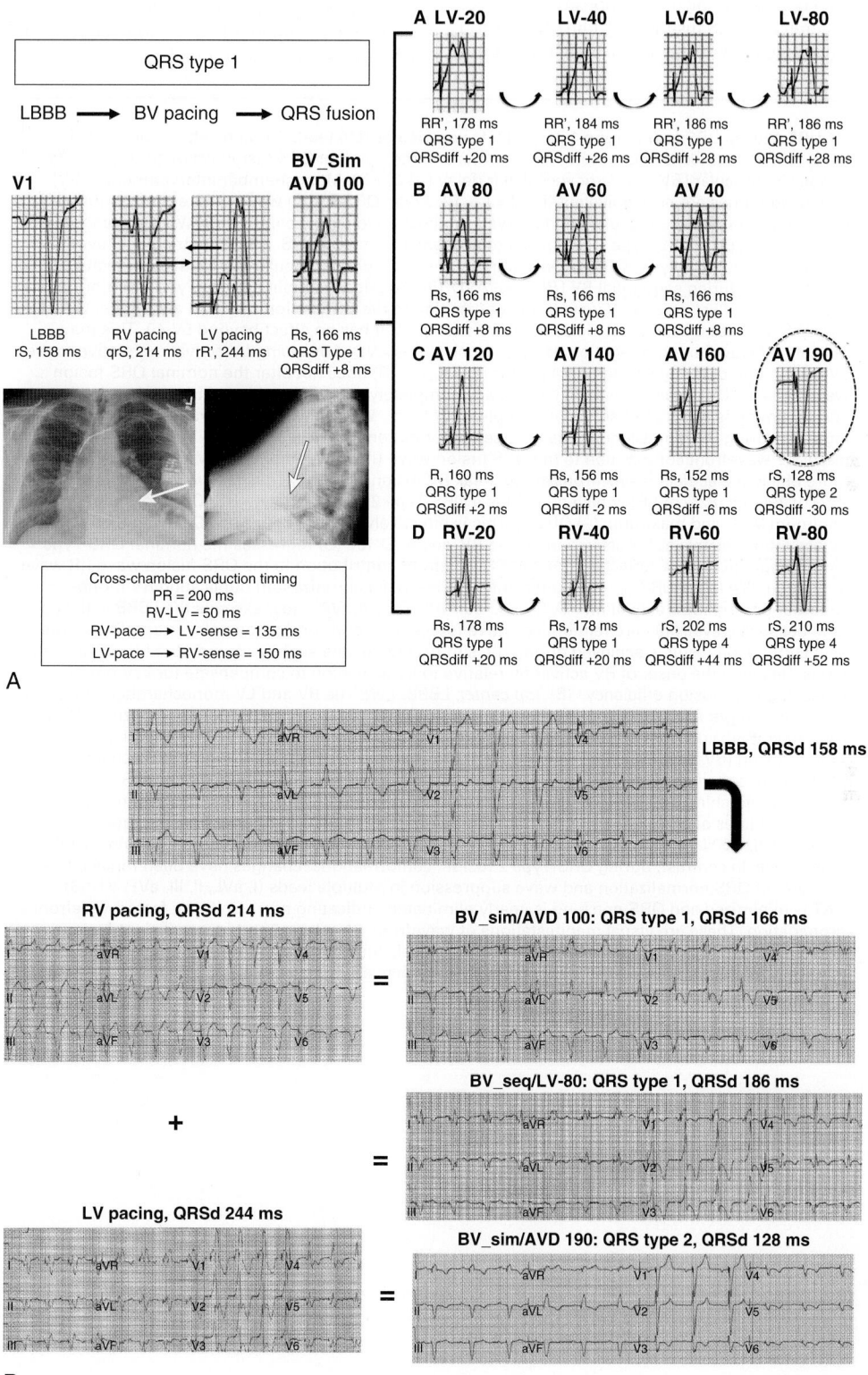

FIGURE 120.10 For legend, see next page.

Clinical Implications

Multiple investigations indicate that clinical response, including reverse remodeling, is driven by the interaction between baseline LV conduction delay and one or more oppositional wavefronts that interact to generate QRS fusion.[25,26] The QRS fusion wave displays anatomical sensitivity to single and multipoint stimulation sites[6,27] and can be rationalized using QRS fusion analysis. The QRS fusion contour displays predictable sensitivity to timing manipulations and stimulation site consistent with the principles of wave interference. These changes are instantaneously expressed on the 12-lead ECG[28] and could guide quantitative assessment of activation sequence titration to improve LV reverse remodeling odds.

FIGURE 120.10 QRS fusion type 1; lateral left ventricular (*LV*) lead. (A) *Left*, left bundle branch block (*LBBB*); monochamber pacing waveforms; and the nominal QRS fusion wave during simultaneous biventricular (*BV_sim*)/atrioventricular delay (*AVD*) 100. Monochamber interventricular (I-V) conduction times are nonequivalent (R → L< L → R). *Right*, QRS fusion wave progressions during I-V timing titration. Selected results are displayed for illustrative purposes. BV_sim/AVD 100 (*left top*) generates a typical QRS Type 1 conformational change from LBBB: rS → Rs, ↑ ventricular activation time (VAT), and slightly (+) QRS$_{diff}$. Delaying the onset of right ventricular (*RV*) activation relative to LV activation during sequential BV (*BV_seq*)/AVD 100 (A) initially amplifies QRS Type 1 conformational change to reflect greater LV wavefront contribution to the QRS fusion wave (↑R amplitude, ↑VAT, ↑[+] QRS$_{diff}$ → less efficient electrical resynchronization) but has no effect beyond LV-40. This may indicate LV wavefront propagation delay or block at this AVD. Advancing LV activation relative to the LV conduction delay by shortening AVD during BV_sim (B) does not alter the nominal QRS fusion wave because BV pacing activation has already completely replaced native ventricular conduction and I-V timing is fixed, as observed in complete AV block. Withdrawing LV activation by lengthening AVD during BV_sim (C) induces a reverse conformational change from QRS Type 1 to reflect the lesser LV wavefront contribution to the QRS fusion wave (↓R wave amplitude, ↓VAT, ↑[–] QRS$_{diff}$ → more efficient electrical resynchronization). Peak BV fusion efficiency (*dashed circle*) is achieved at an AVD of 190 ms (82% of PR), which generates a QRS Type 2 transformation (rS, QRS normalization), minimum VAT, and maximum (–) QRS$_{diff}$. This is effectively "LV-only" pacing. Delaying the onset of LV activation relative to RV activation during BV_seq/AVD 100 (D) regresses the nominal QRS Type 1 conformational change reflecting greater RV wavefront contribution to the QRS fusion wave (↓R wave amplitude, ↑VAT, ↑[+] QRS$_{diff}$ → least efficient electrical resynchronization) duplicating RV monochamber pacing/LBBB activation (rS, RV-60, -80; QRS Type 4). VAT now exceeds the LBBB activation time because wavefronts are reinforcing, wave forces sum, and conduction delay is amplified. The best QRS fusion result is achieved during BV_sim pacing despite slightly asymmetric I-V conduction times. Delaying the onset of RV activation relative to LV activation to compensate for asymmetric I-V times degrades fusion efficiency. (B) *Top center*, LBBB. *Left*, The RV and LV monochamber activation sequences. *Right top*, QRS Type 1 during BV_sim/AVD 100; *right middle*, QRS Type 1 during BV_seq/AVD 100/LV-80; and *right bottom*, QRS Type 2 (best result) during BV_sim/AVD 190. During QRS Type 1 fusion (BV_sim/AVD 100), concordant conformational changes indicating LBBB activation reversal are observed in the frontal (R → QR in I, R → qR in aVL) and horizontal planes (QS → RS in V1-V2).[10] QRS notching persists in multiple leads indicating nonuniform wavefront propagation probably because of lines of block (slow conduction). These conformational changes are exaggerated during BV_seq/AVD 100/LV-80 pacing (↑↑R wave in V1-V5, ↑QRS notching, ↑VAT) because of LV wavefront dominance. In contrast, during QRS Type 2 fusion, conformational changes have been replaced by concordant QRS normalization and wave suppression in multiple leads (I, aVL, II, III, aVF, V1-V3). VAT is minimized and QRS notching is nearly eliminated, indicating more uniform, faster wavefront propagation. These are visual manifestations of wavefront cancelation and more efficient fusion. Wavefronts are highly oppositional, wave forces cancel, and conduction delay is reduced. The overall pattern now closely approximates normal ventricular activation.

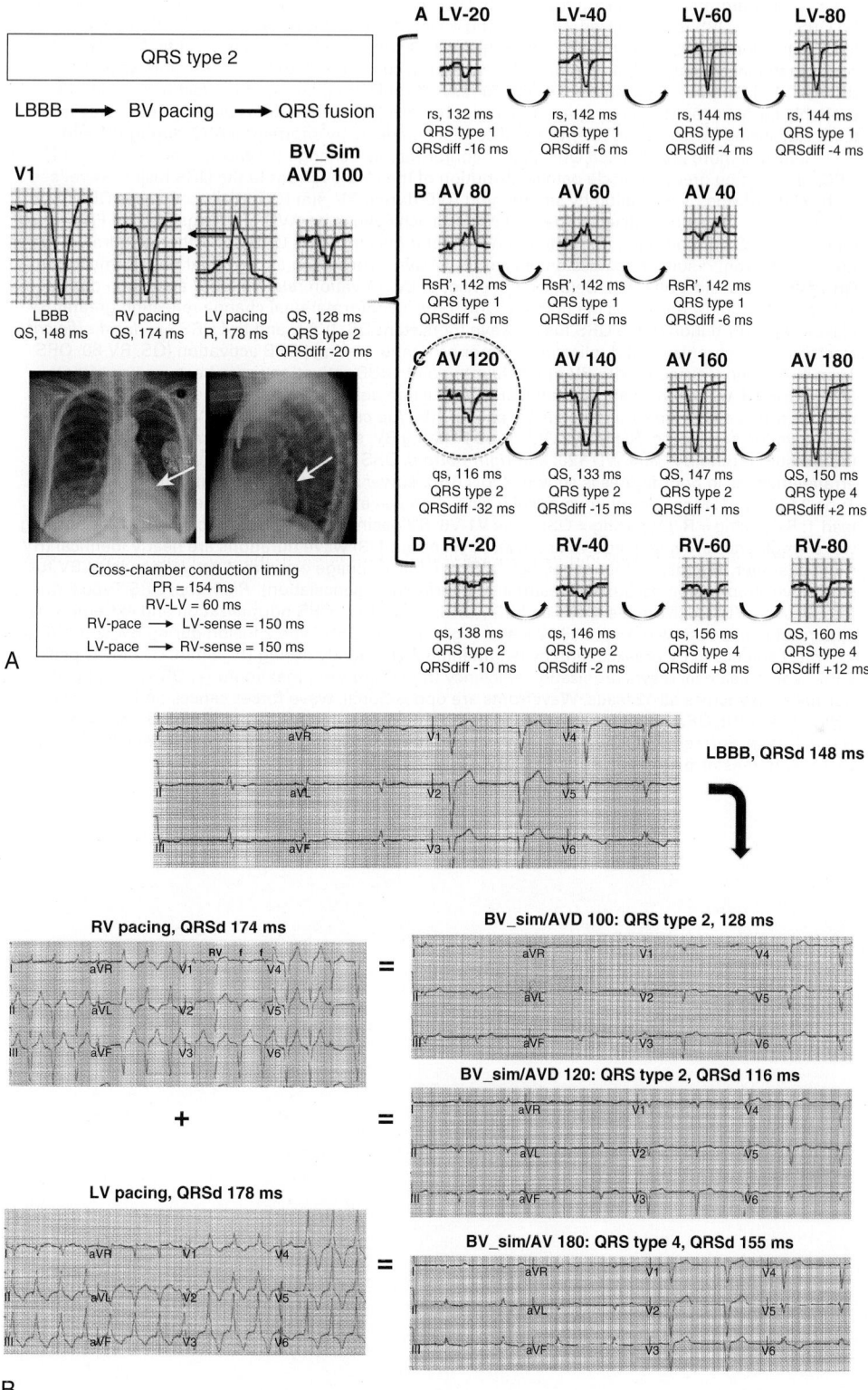

FIGURE 120.11 For legend, see next page.

FIGURE 120.11 QRS fusion Type 2; lateral left ventricular (*LV*) lead. (A) *Left,* left bundle branch block (*LBBB*), monochamber pacing waveforms, and the nominal QRS fusion wave during simultaneous biventricular (*BV_sim*)/atrioventricular delay (*AVD*) 100. Monochamber interventricular (I-V) conduction times are equivalent. *Right,* QRS fusion wave progressions during I-V timing titration. Selected results are displayed for illustrative purposes. BV_sim/AVD 100 (*left top*) generates a QRS Type 2 nonconformational change from LBBB: QS → qs, ⬇⬇⬇ventricular activation time (VAT), and large (−) QRS_diff. The QRS is normalized. Delaying the onset of right ventricular (*RV*) activation relative to LV activation during sequential BV (BV_seq)/AVD 100 (A) initially results in a subtle QRS Type 1 conformational change reflecting greater LV wavefront contribution to the QRS fusion wave (QS → rS, ⬆VAT, ⬇[−] QRSdiff → *less efficient* electrical resynchronization) but has no effect beyond LV-40, probably because rapid wave propagation through Purkinje engagement is already under way (see text). Advancing LV activation relative to LV conduction delay by shortening AVD during BV_sim (B) results in a more pronounced QRS Type 1 conformational change (⬆R wave, ⬇S wave, ⬆VAT, ⬇[−] QRS_diff) reflecting greater muscle path contribution of the LV wavefront to the QRS fusion wave (see text). Withdrawing LV activation by lengthening AVD during BV_sim (C) initially enhances QRS Type 2 fusion; peak BV fusion efficiency (*dashed circle*) is achieved at an AVD of 120 ms (78% of PR), which generates QRS normalization (*qs*), minimum VAT, and maximum (−) QRS_diff. Further withdrawal of the LV wavefront results in regression of electrical resynchronization and gradual transformation to QRS Type 4 (BV_sim/AVD 180). Delaying the onset of LV activation relative to RV activation during BV_sim/AVD 100 (D) regresses the nominal QRS Type 1 conformational change reflecting greater RV wavefront contribution to the QRS fusion wave (persistent QS, ⬆VAT, and ⬆[+] QRS_diff → *least efficient* electrical resynchronization) duplicating RV monochamber pacing/LBBB activation (QS, RV-80, QRS Type 4). VAT now exceeds both RV monochamber and LBBB activation times because wavefronts are reinforced, wave forces are summed, and conduction delay is amplified. The best QRS fusion result is achieved during simultaneous BV pacing. (B) *Top center,* LBBB. *Left,* RV and LV monochamber activation sequences. *Right top,* QRS Type 2 during BV_sim/AVD 100; *right middle,* QRS Type 2 (best result) during BV_sim/AVD 120; and *right bottom,* QRS Type 4 during BV_sim/AVD 180. Same arrangement as in prior figures is shown. *Top,* LBBB. *Lower left,* Ideal wavefront conditions for QRS Type 2 fusion. (1) Monochamber ventricular activation wavefronts are antiphase in all 12 leads (e.g., lead 1: RV pacing = R, LV pacing = QS; leads V1-V6: RV pacing = QS, and LV pacing = R); (2) opposing wave amplitudes are nearly equivalent in all 12 leads; and (3) wave durations are nearly identical (RV monochamber, 174 ms; LV monochamber, 178 ms). Mirror image wavefront activation yields BV fusion wave suppression because of destructive interference (cancelation). *Right top,* QRS Type 2 during BV_sim/AVD 100. Note the ⬇⬇VAT and ⬆⬆(−) QRS_diff (−20 ms). QRS normalization and extreme wave suppression are observed across all 12 leads. *Right middle,* QRS Type 2 fusion during BV_sim/AVD 120 ms. Leniency in LV preexcitation by lengthening AVD slightly during BV_sim (C) achieves peak QRS Type 2 electrical resynchronization efficiency (minimum VAT, maximum [−] QRS_diff) and QRS normalization across all 12 leads. Wavefronts are oppositional, wave forces cancel, and conduction delay is reduced. QRS notching is abolished, indicating more uniform, faster wavefront propagation. *Right bottom,* Further withdrawal of the LV wavefront results in regression of electrical resynchronization and transformation to QRS Type 4 (BV_sim/AVD 180).

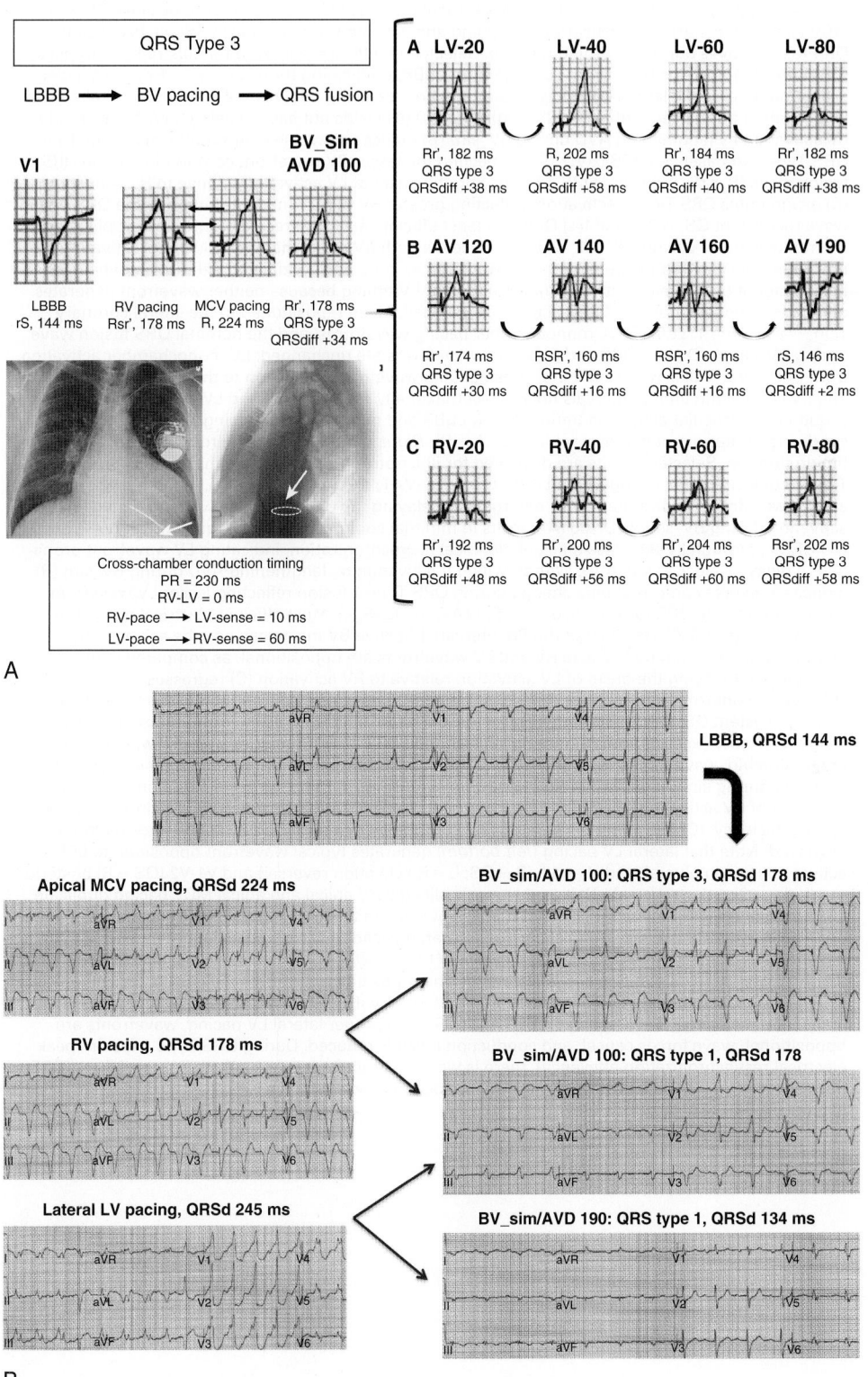

FIGURE 120.12 For legend, see next page.

FIGURE 120.12 QRS fusion Type 3; left ventricular (*LV*) lead in the apical middle cardiac vein (*MCV*). (A) *Left,* left bundle branch block (*LBBB*), monochamber pacing waveforms, and the nominal QRS fusion wave during simultaneous biventricular (*BV_sim*)/atrioventricular delay (*AVD*) 100. The LBBB activation sequence is typical. Right ventricular (*RV*) pacing displays an atypical R complex in V1-V2. The apical MCV ("LV") lead duplicates RV pacing activation except that the QRSd is longer because of the epicardial location. The interventricular (I-V; RV-LV interval) is zero because RV and MCV stimulation sites are physically overlapping and activated simultaneously. *Right,* Pseudo-BV QRS fusion waves during I-V timing titration. Selected results are displayed for illustrative purposes. BV_sim/AVD 100 yields QRS Type 3 change from LBBB, duplicating RV pacing: rS → Rr', ↑ventricular activation time (VAT), large (+) QRS$_{diff}$. In this situation, delaying the onset of RV activation relative to LV activation during sequential BV (BV_seq)/AVD 100 (A) yields but has little effect. Withdrawing the LV activation by lengthening AVD during BV_sim (B) induces a reverse conformational change from QRS Type 3 to baseline LBBB (AVD 190), reflecting the lesser BV wavefront contribution to the QRS fusion wave (R → rS, ↓VAT, ↓[+] QRS$_{diff}$). Delaying the onset of LV activation relative to RV activation (C) exaggerates QRS Type 3 activation, reflecting greater RV wavefront contribution to the QRS fusion wave (persistent QS, ↑VAT, and ↑[+] QRS$_{diff}$ → least efficient electrical resynchronization) duplicating RV monochamber pacing (*RV-80*). VAT now exceeds both RV monochamber and LBBB activation times because wavefronts are reinforcing, wave forces sum, and conduction delay is amplified. BV fusion cannot be achieved with any manipulation of I-V timing because neither wavefront generates opposition to one another or LBBB activation. (B) The LV lead repositioned to the lateral coronary vein → QRS Type 1. *Left,* LBBB, monochamber pacing waveforms, and the nominal QRS fusion wave during BV_sim/AVD 100. LBBB and RV paced waveforms are unchanged; LV monochamber activation from the lateral wall is typical and indicates genuine wavefront opposition to the LBBB activation. The I-V conduction timing intervals now reflect maximally separated RV and LV stimulation sites and sequential ventricular activation timing during LBBB and monochamber pacing. Monochamber I-V conduction times are nonequivalent (R → L < L → R). *Right,* QRS fusion wave progressions during I-V timing titration. Selected results are displayed for illustrative purposes. BV_sim/AVD 100 yields QRS Type 1 conformational change from LBBB: QS → Rs, ↑VAT, and large (+) QRS$_{diff}$. In this situation, RV and LV wavefronts contribute to V1R emergence. Delaying the onset of RV activation relative to LV activation during BV_seq/AVD 100 (A) results in minimal conformational change, modest ↑VAT, and ↑(+) QRS$_{diff}$ through LV-80 → less efficient electrical resynchronization, indicating LV wavefront propagation delay or block at this AVD. Withdrawing LV activation by lengthening AVD during BV_sim (B) induces a reverse conformational change during QRS Type 1 fusion reflecting lesser LV wavefront contribution to the QRS fusion wave (R → rS, ↓VAT, ↑[−] QRS$_{diff}$). Most efficient electrical resynchronization occurs at AVD 190 (73% of the PR interval). Effective BV fusion can now be achieved by manipulation of I-V timing because RV and LV wavefronts are oppositional, as compared with RV + MCV pacing. Delaying the onset of LV activation relative to RV activation (C) regresses the nominal QRS type 1 conformational change reflecting greater RV wavefront contribution to the QRS fusion wave (persistent QS, ↑VAT, and ↑[+] QRS$_{diff}$ → least efficient electrical resynchronization), duplicating RV-80. VAT now exceeds both RV monochamber and LBBB activation times because wavefronts are reinforcing, wave forces sum, and conduction delay is amplified. The best QRS fusion result is achieved during simultaneous BV pacing despite slightly asymmetric I-V conduction times. Delaying the onset of RV activation relative to LV activation to compensate for asymmetric I-V times degrades fusion efficiency. (C) The effect of change in LV stimulation site on BV wave interference patterns is displayed. Note that lateral LV pacing (*left bottom*) generates typical wavefront opposition to LBBB activation (*top*) in pivotal leads I and L (R → QS; L → R activation reversal) and V1-V2 (QS → R; posterior → anterior activation reversal). Ordinarily, uncomplicated RV apical and apical MCV pacing duplicate LBBB activation (QS in V1-V2, dominant R in I). However, in this case, an atypical activation pattern during RV and MCV pacing, presumably due to scar, misleadingly resembles lateral LV pacing. During lateral LV pacing, large dominant R waves in V1-V5 (posterior → anterior forces) and QS in I/aVL (L → R forces) indicate genuine activation wavefront opposition to LBBB. In the case of RV and apical MCV pacing, opposition to LBBB is not demonstrated, wavefronts are reinforcing, wave forces sum, and conduction delay is worsened. In the case of RV and proper lateral LV pacing, wavefronts are oppositional, wave forces cancel, and conduction delay is reduced. During QRS Type 1 fusion (peak electrical resynchronization efficiency), there is wave destruction in leads I, II, III, R, L, and F and QRS normalization in leads V1-V6. Wavefronts are oppositional, wave forces cancel, and conduction delay is reduced.

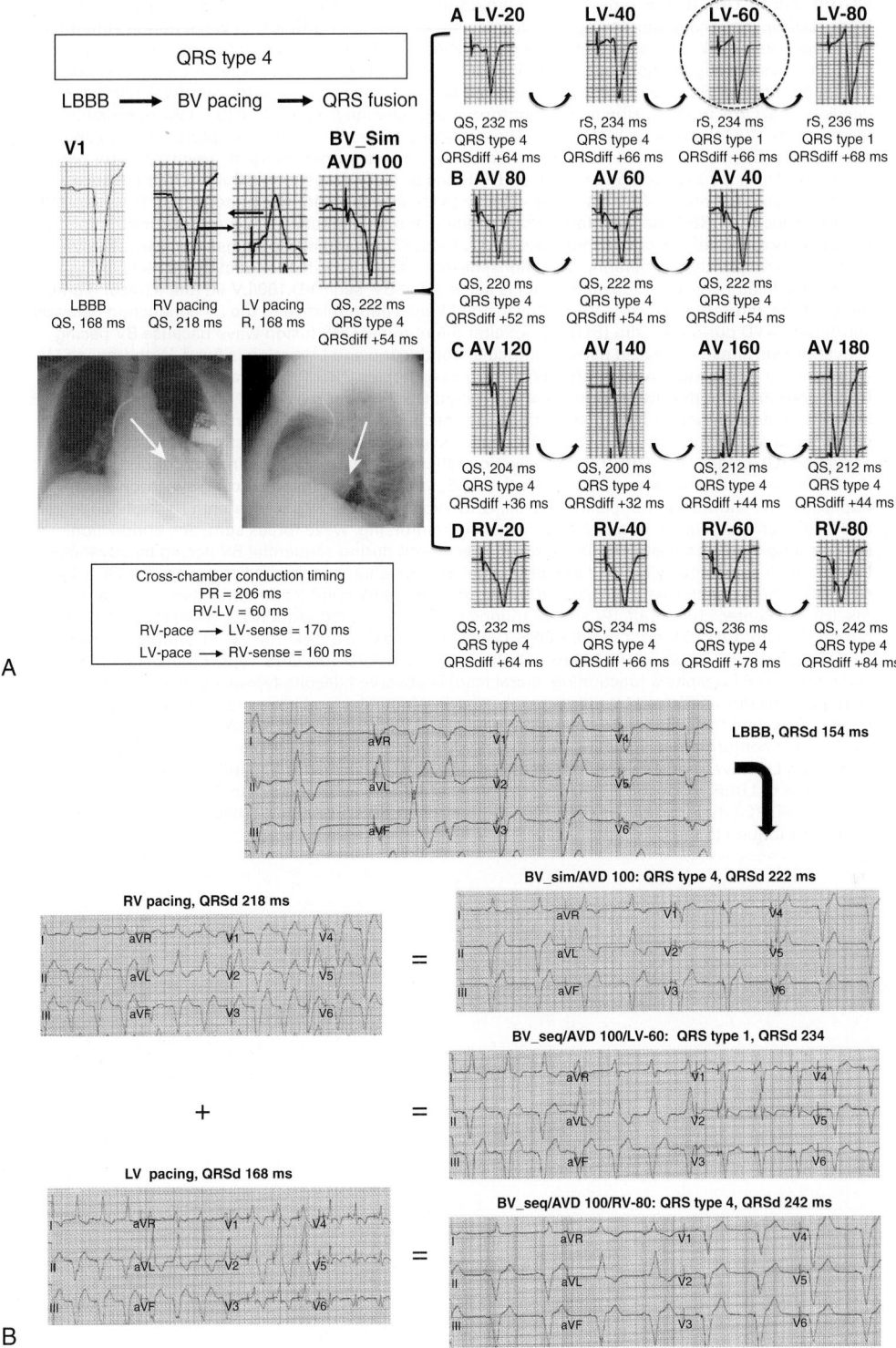

FIGURE 120.13 For legend, see next page.

FIGURE 120.13 QRS fusion Type 4; lateral left ventricular (*LV*) lead. (A) *Left,* left bundle branch block (*LBBB*), monochamber pacing waveforms, and the nominal QRS fusion wave during simultaneous biventricular (*BV_sim*)/atrioventricular delay (*AVD*) 100. Monochamber interventricular (I-V) conduction times are slightly nonequivalent (R → L > L → R). *Right,* QRS fusion wave progressions during I-V timing titration. Selected results are displayed for illustrative purposes. BV_sim/AVD 100 (*left top*) yields typical QRS Type 4 fusion and no conformational change from LBBB (QS → QS, ↑ventricular activation time [VAT], and large [+] QRS_{diff}). The nonlateral LV lead site, LV noncapture, and LV capture latency have been excluded; the LV monochamber pacing wavefront is directly opposed to RV pacing in V1. Therefore the explanation must be an L → R line of block preventing LV wavefront advancement. Delaying the onset of RV activation relative to LV activation during sequential BV (*BV_seq*)/AVD 100 (A) induces a QRS Type 1 conformational change to reflect greater LV wavefront contribution to the QRS fusion wave[13] (↑R wave amplitude, ↑VAT, ↑[+] QRS_{diff}), and best obtainable electrical resynchronization under these operating conditions, despite asymmetric I-V conduction times favoring L → R. Peak BV fusion efficiency (dashed circle) is achieved at BV_seq/AVD 100/LV-60 (the earliest R emergence at the shortest achievable VAT). Advancing LV activation relative to the LV conduction delay by shortening AVD during BV_sim (B) does not alter the nominal QRS fusion wave because BV pacing activation has already replaced native ventricular conduction and I-V timing is fixed. Withdrawing LV activation by lengthening AVD during BV_sim (C) exaggerates QRS Type 4, reflecting lesser LV wavefront contribution to the QRS fusion wave (persistent QS, ↑VAT, and ↑[+] QRS_{diff}). VAT now exceeds both RV monochamber and LBBB activation times because RV pacing reinforces LBBB conduction delay → *less efficient* electrical resynchronization. Delaying the onset of LV activation relative to RV activation (D) exaggerates QRS Type 4 activation reflecting greater RV wavefront contribution to the QRS fusion wave (persistent QS, ↑VAT, ↑[+] QRS_{diff} → least efficient electrical resynchronization) duplicating RV monochamber pacing (RV-80, QRS Type 4). VAT now exceeds both RV monochamber and LBBB activation times because wavefronts are reinforcing, wave forces sum, and conduction delay is amplified. The best QRS fusion result is achieved during sequential BV pacing by advancing LV activation substantially beyond the differential in monochamber conduction times. The QRS Type 4 → QRS Type 1 transformation occurs at LV-60, though the I-V conduction times differ by only 10 ms. (B) *Top center,* LBBB. *Left,* RV and LV monochamber activation sequences. *Right top,* QRS Type 4 during BV_sim/AVD 100; *right middle,* QRS Type 1 during BV_seq/AVD 100/LV-60; and *right bottom,* QRS Type 4 during BV_seq/AVD 100/RV-80. During BV_sim/AVD 100, QRS Type 4 (persistent LBBB activation + ↑VAT despite a functioning lateral lead) is observed despite typical oppositional wavefront patterns during RV and LV monochamber pacing (note the lead I paradox during LV pacing; see earlier). Delaying the onset of RV activation relative to LV activation (BV_seq/AVD 100/LV-60) induces QRS Type 1 conformational change, presumably by overcoming a line of block encountered by the advancing LV wavefront. The emergence of R waves in V1-V2 indicates a manifestation of wavefront opposition to LBBB conduction. Delaying the onset of LV activation relative to RV activation during BV_seq/AVD 100/RV-80 amplifies QRS Type 4 (persistent LBBB) activation reflecting greater RV wavefront contribution to the QRS fusion wave.

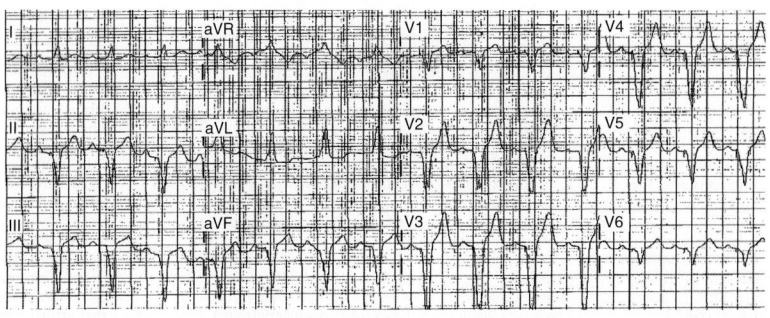

LBBB, QRSd 163 ms

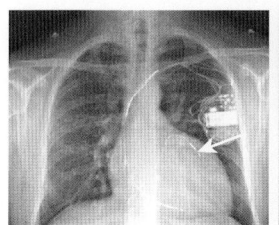

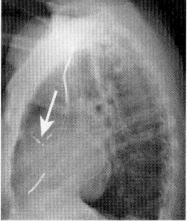

LV Site 1: Mid-anterior vein

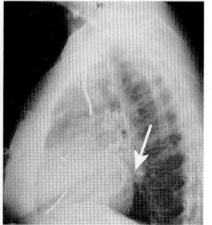

LV Site 2: Mid-lateral vein

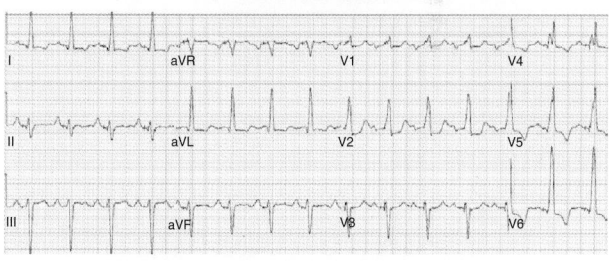

QRS Type 3, QRSd 180 ms, QRSdiff +17 ms   **QRS Type 1, QRSd 118 ms, QRSdiff -45 ms**

FIGURE 120.14 Effect of a change in left ventricular (*LV*) stimulation site on QRS fusion type. The underlying rhythm is sinus + complete atrioventricular block + ventricular asystole; biventricular (BV) wave interference products (*bottom*) are compared with right ventricular (RV) pacing (left bundle branch block [*LBBB*] surrogate, *top*). The RV apical site is fixed during simultaneous BV/atrioventricular delay 100 pacing. BV fusion during LV stimulation from midchamber AIV (site 1) generates QRS Type 3 (RV pacing/LBBB reinforcement). BV fusion during LV stimulation from a mid-chamber lateral vein (site 2) generates QRS Type 1 with ⅢVAT, indicating a large cancelation effect (LBBB remediation). Note in the anteroposterior view, AIV and lateral stimulation sites appear to be anatomically overlapping. However, in the lateral view, the posterior location of the lateral site and anterior location of the AIV site are realized.

REFERENCES

1. Tayal B, Gorcsan 3rd J, Delgado-Montero A, et al. Comparative long-term outcomes after cardiac resynchronization therapy in right ventricular paced patients versus native wide left bundle branch block patients. *Heart Rhythm.* 2016;13:511–518.

2. Friedman DJ, Singh JP, Curtis JP, et al. Comparative effectiveness of CRT-D versus defibrillator alone in HF patients with moderate-to-severe chronic kidney disease. *J Am Coll Cardiol.* 2015;66:2618–2629.

3. Ruwald MH, Solomon SD, Foster E, et al. Left ventricular ejection fraction normalization in cardiac resynchronization therapy and risk of ventricular arrhythmia and clinical outcomes: results from the Multicenter Automatic Defibrillator Implantation Trial with Cardiac Resynchronization Therapy (MADIT-CRT) Trial. *Circulation.* 2014;130:2278–2286.

4. Lewis T. *Clinical Electrocardiology.* London: Shaws and Sons; 1913.

5. Marriott HJL. *Practical Electrocardiology.* Baltimore, MD: Williams & Wilkins; 1988.

6. Ploux S, Strik M, van Hunnik A, et al. Acute electrical and hemodynamic effects of multisite left ventricular pacing for cardiac resynchronization therapy in the dyssynchronous canine heart. *Heart Rhythm.* 2014;11:119–125.

7. Lee YC. Ventricular fusion beats. *JAMA.* 1967;202:991.

8. Schamroth L, Agathangelou N. QRS normalization by ventricular fusion. *Pacing Clin Electrophysiol.* 1981;4:448–451.

9. Sweeney MO, Hellkamp AS, van Bommel RJ, et al. QRS fusion complex analysis using wave interference to predict reverse remodeling during cardiac resynchronization therapy. *Heart Rhythm.* 2014;11:806–813.

10. Sweeney MO, van Bommel RJ, Schalij MJ, et al. Analysis of ventricular activation using surface electrocardiography to predict left ventricular reverse volumetric remodeling during cardiac resynchronization therapy. *Circulation.* 2010;121:626–634.

11. Ammann P, Sticherling C, Kalusche D, et al. An electrocardiogram-based algorithm to detect loss of left ventricular capture during cardiac resynchronization therapy. *Ann Intern Med.* 2005;142:968–973.

12. Giudici MC, Tigrett DW, Carlson JI, et al. Electrocardiographic patterns during pacing the great cardiac and middle cardiac veins. *Pacing Clin Electrophysiol.* 2007;30:1376–1380.

13. Jia P, Ramanathan C, Ghanem RN, et al. Electrocardiographic imaging of cardiac resynchronization therapy in heart failure: observation of variable electrophysiologic responses. *Heart Rhythm.* 2006;3:296–310.

14. Varma N, Jia P, Rudy Y, Placebo CRT. *J Cardiovasc Electrophysiol.* 2008;19:878.

15. Vernooy K, Cornelussen RN, Verbeek XA, et al. Cardiac resynchronization therapy cures dyssynchronopathy in canine left bundle-branch block hearts. *Eur Heart J.* 2007;28:2148–2155.

16. Verbeek XA, Vernooy K, Peschar M. Intra-ventricular resynchronization for optimal left ventricular function during pacing in experimental left bundle branch block. *J Am Coll Cardiol*. 2003;42:558–567.

17. Vernooy K, Verbeek XA, Cornelussen RN, et al. Calculation of effective VV interval facilitates optimization of AV delay and VV interval in cardiac resynchronization therapy. *Heart Rhythm*. 2006;4:75–82.

18. Van Gelder BM, Bracke FA, Meijer A, et al. Morphology of the RV electrogram during LV pacing is related to the hemodynamic effect in cardiac resynchronization therapy. *Pacing Clin Electrophysiol*. 2007;30:1381–1387.

19. Van Gelder BM, Bracke FA, Van Der Voort PH, et al. Optimal sensed atrio-ventricular interval determined by paced QRS morphology. *Pacing Clin Electrophysiol*. 2007;30:476–481.

20. Auricchio A, Stellbrink C, Block M, et al. Effect of pacing chamber and atrioventricular delay on acute systolic function of paced patients with congestive heart failure. The Pacing Therapies for Congestive Heart Failure Study Group. The Guidant Congestive Heart Failure Research Group. *Circulation*. 1999;99:2993–3001.

21. Auricchio A, Klein H. Beyond expectations: A decade of positive results with cardiac resynchronization therapy for heart failure. *Eur Heart J Suppl*. 2002;4:D95–D101.

22. Cazeau S, Leclerlq C, Lavergne T, et al. Effects of multisite biventricular pacing in patients with heart failure and intraventricular conduction delay. *N Engl J Med*. 2001;344:873–880.

23. Abraham WT, Fisher WG, Smith AL, et al. Cardiac resynchronization in chronic heart failure. *N Engl J Med*. 2002;346:1845–1853.

24. Sweeney MO, Hellkamp A, van Bommel RJ, et al. QRS fusion complex analysis using wave interference to predict reverse remodeling during cardiac resynchronization therapy. *Heart Rhythm*. 2014;11:806–813.

25. Bode WD, Bode MF, Gettes L, et al. Prominent R wave in ECG lead V1 predicts improvement of left ventricular ejection fraction after cardiac resynchronization therapy in patients with or without left bundle branch block. *Heart Rhythm*. 2015;12:2141–2147.

26. Birnie D, Lemke B, Aonuma K, et al. Clinical outcomes with synchronized left ventricular pacing: Analysis of the Adaptive CRT trial. *Heart Rhythm*. 2013;10:1368–1374.

27. Zanon F, Baracca E, Pastore G, et al. Multipoint pacing by a left ventricular quadripolar lead improves the acute hemodynamic response to CRT compared with conventional biventricular pacing at any site. *Heart Rhythm*. 2015;12:975–981.

28. Del-Carpio Munoz F, Powell BD, Cha YM, et al. Delayed instrinsicoid deflection onset in surface ECG lateral leads predicts left ventricular reverse remodeling after cardiac resynchronization therapy. *Heart Rhythm*. 2013;10:979–987.

121 Newer Applications of Cardiac Pacemakers and Extracardiac Stimulation

Frank Cuoco and Michael R. Gold

Permanent pacemaker technology has evolved significantly over more than 50 years. From primitive, asynchronous, fixed-rate single-chamber devices (i.e., VOO mode) used initially to treat life-threatening heart block, these devices are currently used more commonly for symptomatic improvement rather than to treat asystole. In this process, pacemakers have undergone a major transformation in both sophistication and complexity. These technological advances and improved understanding of cardiac conduction have led to pacemaker therapy being applied to a variety of additional disorders. Many of these applications are not directly related to treatment of bradycardia but rather use pacing to alter myocardial activation patterns, suppress tachyarrhythmias, or improve hemodynamic function. This chapter focuses on the role of permanent pacing in less common cardiac disorders, the use of pacing after novel procedures, and potential newer applications of permanent pacing technology.

Pacing for Specific Cardiac Conditions

Permanent pacing has been employed to treat a variety of disorders in addition to traditional indications of chronotropic incompetence, sick sinus syndrome, and atrioventricular (AV) block. For example, cardiac resynchronization therapy (CRT), discussed in detail in a separate chapter, has become an important and commonly employed application for the treatment of patients with left ventricular (LV) systolic dysfunction, congestive heart failure, and electrical dyssynchrony. CRT is now also being used to counteract the deleterious effects of chronic right ventricular pacing.[1a] Pacemakers have also played an important role in the treatment of atrial fibrillation, including rate support for slow ventricular response, arrhythmia suppression, and after AV nodal ablation. The applications of pacemakers in the treatment of a variety of less common disorders or special situations are discussed below and are summarized in Table 121.1.

Hypertrophic Cardiomyopathy

Hypertrophic cardiomyopathy (HCM) is a condition characterized by disarray of myocardial fibers and myofibrils, producing excessive and inappropriate hypertrophy of the LV, most frequently the interventricular septum. The hypertrophy interferes with diastolic function and ventricular relaxation, and in up to 25% of patients, hypertrophy causes dynamic obstruction across the LV outflow tract. Early observational studies of right ventricular apical pacing suggested regression of ventricular hypertrophy and dramatic clinical improvement.[1] However, this benefit was not substantiated in subsequent randomized controlled clinical trials,[1] so this strategy has been largely abandoned, except when there is another indication for pacing, such as AV block after alcohol septal ablation (ASA) (discussed later).

Neurocardiogenic Syncope

Neurocardiogenic syncope is a common problem that accounts for approximately 6% of hospital admissions in the United States annually. Despite improved diagnostic techniques, the cause of syncope is undiagnosed in up to 50% of cases. It is likely that many of these are neurally mediated. The term neurocardiogenic syncope (also termed vasovagal syncope or neurally mediated syncope) is used to describe a group of related conditions that include carotid sinus hypersensitivity, posttussive syncope, and postmicturition syncope. Because episodes are often accompanied by bradycardia, it was hypothesized that permanent pacing may be of benefit. Unfortunately, as with HCM, early uncontrolled studies suggested that permanent pacing offered major clinical benefits, which have not been confirmed by subsequent randomized clinical trials.[1,2] Currently, permanent pacing is not considered a standard treatment of neurocardiogenic syncope. However, a subgroup of patients who experience very long pauses (>6 seconds) or marked bradycardia during ambulatory monitoring may benefit from pacing therapy.[3]

Long QT Syndrome

The long QT syndrome is a heterogeneous group of disorders characterized by QT prolongation and a tendency to develop torsades de pointes and sudden cardiac death. Congenital forms of this disorder have been linked to point mutations in specific genes associated with sodium or potassium channel activity. Acquired forms of the long QT syndrome are usually associated with use of QT-prolonging medications (e.g., sotalol, tricyclic antidepressants), the list of which continues to grow. It is also possible that the congenital and acquired forms are actually a continuum with some individuals manifesting the abnormality in the baseline state, with others requiring trigger factors to elicit QT prolongation. The pathogenesis of ventricular arrhythmias in this syndrome has not been completely elucidated but seems related to sympathetic activation and early afterdepolarizations.

Initial therapy of long QT disorders has traditionally been pharmacological (β-blockers), although left stellate ganglion ablation and permanent pacing have also been advocated. Although the exact mechanism by which pacing exerts its beneficial effect is unclear, it is probably related to preventing pauses that characteristically precede episodes of torsades, with elimination of early afterdepolarizations and decrease in dispersion of refractoriness.

TABLE 121.1 Pacing for specific cardiac conditions

CARDIAC CONDITION	INDICATION FOR PERMANENT PACING
Hypertrophic cardiomyopathy	Largely abandoned for symptoms of obstruction Indicated for AV block after ASA or SSM
Neurocardiogenic syncope	Limited benefit, unless very long pauses/asystole
Long QT syndrome	Reserved for symptomatic bradycardia ICD may be indicated for SCD or recurrent syncope
MUSCULAR DYSTROPHIES	**INDICATION FOR PERMANENT PACING**
Duchenne	Second- or third-degree AVB (especially if wide QRS)
Becker	Second- or third-degree AVB (especially if wide QRS)
Myotonic	HV >70 ms or high-degree AVB
Emery-Dreifuss	Second- or third-degree AVB or unexplained syncope
Limb-girdle	High-grade AVB or family history of AVB/SCD
Kearns-Sayre	Marked first-degree or high-grade AVB
INFILTRATIVE DISORDERS	**INDICATION FOR PERMANENT PACING**
Amyloidosis	First-degree or high-grade AVB, WBCL <100 beats/min
Sarcoidosis	Symptomatic bradycardia, ICD may be indicated
Collagen vascular diseases	Symptomatic bradycardia or high-grade AVB only
Lyme carditis	Usually reversible with treatment, rarely required

ASA, Alcohol septal ablation; *AVB,* atrioventricular block; *ICD,* implantable cardioverter defibrillator; *SCD,* sudden cardiac death; *SSM,* surgical septal myectomy; *WBCL,* Wenckebach cycle length.

In addition, overdrive pacing to increase heart rate decreases QT interval. Currently, it is standard to use an implantable cardioverter defibrillator (ICD) in any individual with documented cardiac arrest, sustained ventricular tachycardia, or recurrent syncope refractory to β-blockers, with pacing reserved for symptomatic bradycardia.

Chronic Disorders of the Neuromuscular System

Muscular dystrophies are a diverse group of inherited, chronic degenerative conditions primarily affecting skeletal muscle. It has long been appreciated that these disorders can also affect cardiac muscle, resulting in fibrosis and fatty replacement of the myocardium. There is now a growing awareness that the prevalence of arrhythmias, conduction system disease, and sudden cardiac death in these patients may warrant early intervention.[4] Because these conditions are infrequent, the therapeutic guidelines are necessarily nonspecific. In general, it can be recommended that unexplained syncope, presyncope, and other transient neurological symptoms should be aggressively investigated using ambulatory electrocardiographic recordings, long-term event recorders and loop recorders, and, in more worrisome situations (e.g., unexplained sudden syncope associated with injury), hospitalization with inpatient monitoring. In most cases, the finding of second-degree AV block, particularly Mobitz II, even when asymptomatic, may warrant permanent pacemaker implantation. It should be noted that ventricular tachyarrhythmias are also common in

this population, so, depending on the clinical scenario, an ICD should also be considered.

Duchenne Muscular Dystrophy
Duchenne muscular dystrophy is a progressive neuromuscular disease that clinically manifests in the mid-teens and is usually fatal by the end of the third decade, generally from heart failure. Although cardiac involvement is the rule, the conduction system is not always involved. Permanent pacing is warranted for second- or third-degree AV block, especially in the setting of a widened QRS complex.

Becker Muscular Dystrophy
Becker muscular dystrophy is similar to Duchenne muscular dystrophy but is more slowly progressive and appears with less frequent cardiac involvement. The indications for permanent pacing appear similar to those for Duchenne muscular dystrophy.

Myotonic Muscular Dystrophy
In myotonic muscular dystrophy, cardiac involvement is common and usually affects the conduction system. Published data indicate that permanent pacing is warranted with an HV interval of greater than 70 ms, even in the absence of high-degree AV block.[5] More recently, it was demonstrated that patients with myotonic dystrophy who underwent an invasive approach with electrophysiology study and prophylactic pacing had a longer 9-year survival rate than those treated conservatively.[6]

Emery-Dreifuss Muscular Dystrophy
In Emery-Dreifuss muscular dystrophy, conduction system disease is frequent. Sudden cardiac death due to high-grade AV block has been documented, and permanent pacing should be offered with the development of any unexplained transient neurological symptoms or second- or third-degree AV block.

Limb-Girdle Muscular Dystrophy
Limb-girdle muscular dystrophy is a heterogeneous group of disorders characterized by weakness in the pelvic musculature and upper legs. The familial form has a high incidence of conduction system disease, and permanent pacing should be considered for anyone with a family history of heart block or sudden death.

Kearns-Sayre Syndrome
Kearns-Sayre syndrome is a multisystem disorder of the mitochondria with diverse clinical manifestations. Progressive conduction system disease is common, and permanent pacing is probably warranted for marked first-degree AV block.

Infiltrative Diseases of the Myocardium

These are a diverse variety of disorders in which the myocardium is infiltrated and replaced by nonmyocardial tissue. Although the prognosis is usually determined more by the type and severity of the underlying disease, cardiac and conduction system involvement is not unusual and may be accompanied by potentially life-threatening brady- or tachyarrhythmias. In these situations, permanent pacemakers may be helpful symptomatically, although they may not necessarily prolong life.

Amyloidosis

Amyloidosis is characterized by deposition of an insoluble protein in the myocardium, often involving the conduction system.[7] Restrictive cardiomyopathy may develop with death from congestive heart failure. Sinus node dysfunction, AV block, and intraventricular blocks are not uncommon and may require permanent pacemaker implantation if associated with symptoms. In one large study, a group of 95 patients with familial amyloid polyneuropathy (FAP) was followed after prophylactic pacemaker implantation.[8] In this series, 25% of patients developed high-degree AV block over a mean follow-up of 45 months. Predictors of development of high-grade AV block included existing first-degree AV block and Wenckebach anterograde block at ≤100 beats/min. Therefore prophylactic pacemaker implantation may be warranted in this population to reduce the risk for syncope and sudden death related to the development of significant conduction system disease.

Sarcoidosis

Sarcoidosis is a multisystem, infiltrative disorder characterized by noncaseating granulomas, which often involve the heart and conduction system.[9] The disease tends to be progressive, and the mortality rate of patients with extensive myocardial sarcoid is high. Permanent pacemakers may be implanted for symptomatic bradyarrhythmias, although the frequency of malignant ventricular tachyarrhythmias often warrants an ICD, particularly when noninvasive evaluation shows evidence of ventricular involvment.[10]

Collagen Vascular Diseases

Cardiac involvement is fairly common in collagen vascular diseases, especially polymyositis and systemic lupus erythematosus. Fibrosis of the conduction system may occur, and the resulting AV block may require a permanent pacemaker based on standard criteria for implantation.

Lyme Carditis

Lyme carditis is a Lyme disease spirochetal infection caused by *Borrelia burgdorferi* and carried by the deer tick *Ixodes dammini*. It is a systemic illness characterized by a "target"-shaped rash (erythema chronicum migrans) as well as fever, arthralgia, myalgia, and lymphadenopathy. When untreated, this illness can result in later complications, including neurological and cardiac involvement. Lyme carditis is typically characterized by AV block and is often reversible with antibiotic therapy, obviating the need for permanent pacing.[11] To avoid unnecessary pacemaker implantation, Lyme carditis should be considered by physicians when the clinical scenario occurs in an area where Lyme disease is endemic.

Permanent Pacing Post–Myocardial Infarction

In the setting of acute myocardial infarction, conduction abnormalities can occur immediately or within hours to days after infarction. Conduction abnormalities associated with inferior wall myocardial infarction, including high-degree AV block, are usually secondary to increased vagal tone in the acute phase and secondary to edema and local release of adenosine in the subacute phase (>24 hours after infarction). Both scenarios are often reversible (within several days to up to 2 weeks), and while they may warrant temporary pacing, they rarely require permanent pacemaker implantation. In contrast, conduction abnormalities associated with anterior myocardial infarction are often a result of infarction and necrosis of the intramyocardial conduction system. This almost always occurs in the setting of a proximal occlusion of the left anterior descending (LAD) artery, and complete AV block usually occurs within the first 24 hours post–myocardial infarction. Because the left anterior fascicle and the right bundle branch (RBB) are supplied by septal branches of the proximal LAD, the development of bifascicular block (especially with PR prolongation) after anterior infarction is associated with a high incidence of complete heart block and warrants empiric temporary pacemaker placement. Permanent pacemaker placement, however, is reserved for patients with high-grade AV block,

including those with alternating bundle branch block and transient or persistent second- or third-degree AV block in the His–Purkinje system.[12]

Preventing Remodeling After Myocardial Infarction

After myocardial infarction, there is a redistribution of cardiac workload with an increase in mechanical wall stress in the ischemic and surrounding areas. These pathophysiological responses are associated with LV remodeling and subsequent dysfunction, and the activation of cytokines and neurohormonal factors are often associated with adverse clinical outcome. It has been shown that pacing areas of high wall stress ("electrical preexcitation") alters regional distribution of stroke work in a normal heart, reducing stroke work adjacent to the stimulation site and increasing stroke work in distant regions. Shuros and coworkers used a swine model to demonstrate that pacing from the peri-infarct area improves hemodynamics and attenuates cardiac remodeling.[13] Saba and colleagues used a rabbit infarct model to demonstrate that biventricular pacing prevented mechanical and electrical remodeling, including preventing LV systolic and diastolic function, as well as restoring QRS width and rate-dependent AT intervals. Similar beneficial effects were found in a preliminary study by Chung and associates among patients randomized to biventricular pacing (compared with right ventricular stimulation).[14] However, two subsequent randomized trials of after infarct pacing (MENDMI and PRomPT) showed no effect on LV dimensions or clinical outcomes, including quality of life, 6-minute walk distance, heart failure, hospitalization, or death.[15,16]

Vagal Stimulation for the Treatment of Heart Failure

Chronic heart failure is characterized by autonomic dysfunction involving increased sympathetic tone, downregulation of adrenoreceptors, and decreased parasympathetic outflow and heart rate variability. In addition to neurohormonal activation (i.e., renin-angiotensin-aldosterone system), these changes can result in a positive feedback mechanism that causes worsening vasoconstriction, LV dysfunction, negative remodeling, and ultimately, end organ dysfunction and death. Vagal stimulation and carotid sinus baroreflex (CSB) activation may inhibit these effects but are often blunted in chronic heart failure states. Vagal stimulation also has potentially beneficial pleomorphic actions, including antiinflammatory effects and inhibition of apoptosis. Therefore there has been great interest and hope that stimulation of these reflexes and thereby increasing parasympathetic outflow may halt or even reverse the negative effects of the increased sympathetic tone in heart failure. Similarly, spinal cord stimulation has been effective in the treatment of chronic chest pain and can modulate autonomic activity. It has now been applied in the treatment of heart failure as well and is discussed in detail in a separate chapter.

Initial studies on vagal nerve stimulation demonstrated favorable changes in tissue and plasma biomarkers.[17] More recently, investigators demonstrated that chronic electrical stimulation of the CSB improved LV function and promoted LV remodeling in dogs with chronic heart failure.[18] This study demonstrated that chronic vagal stimulation resulted in changes at the global and cellular/molecular levels, including decreased LV end-diastolic pressure, decreased circulating catecholamines, normalized β-receptor expression, and reduced interstitial fibrosis and myocyte hypertrophy.

The CardioFit Multicenter Trial was a small (n = 32), open-label study of vagal nerve stimulation in patients with severe systolic heart failure.[19] In this study, vagal stimulation was performed using a cuff electrode and implantable generator and regulated according

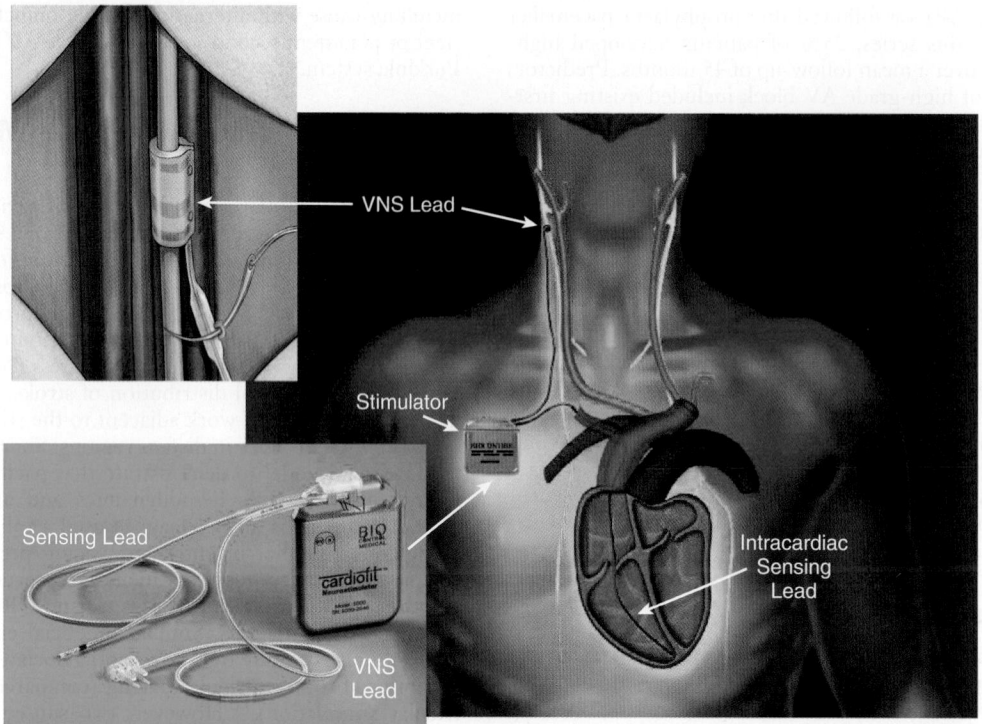

FIGURE 121.1 *Right,* Depiction of an implanted CardioFit vagus nerve stimulation (*VNS*) device showing the position of the VNS lead on the right vagus nerve, the intracardiac pacing lead in the right ventricular apex, and the implantable CardioFit neurostimulator in the right subclavicular region. *Top left,* Positioning of the CardioFit stimulation lead around the right vagus nerve. *Bottom left,* The CardioFit VNS implantable neurostimulator, sensing lead, and VNS lead. (Courtesy BioControl Medical, Ltd., Yehud, Israel.)

to the patient's heart rate using an intracardiac sensor (Fig. 121.1). The results of this study demonstrated significant improvements at 6 months in New York Heart Association (NYHA) class, quality of life, 6-minute walk times, and LV ejection fraction and volumes. Serious adverse events that occurred in this trial were common (40%), but only two (6%, no deaths) were directly attributable to the implantation procedure and device.

More recently, a randomized sham-controlled trial of vagal stimulation in 96 patients with medically refractory heart failure with severe LV dysfunction (NECTAR HF) was completed.[20] Unfortunately, vagal nerve stimulation failed to demonstrate a benefit in measures of cardiac remodeling or functional capacity, although patients with vagal stimulation did report improvements in quality of life scores. In contrast, the ANTHEM-HF trial, which utilized a different vagal stimulation device, showed improved remodeling with either right or left vagal stimulation. These conflicting results[21] may be due to a number of differences among trials, including study design and stimulation current.[22] The first pivotal trial of vagal stimulation for advanced heart failure, INcrease Of Vagal TonE in Heart Failure study (INOVATE-HF), has completed enrollment of over 700 patients. This study should help determine if this novel approach of vagal stimulation in the treatment of chronic heart failure may provide some clinical benefits to the most refractory of cases.

Indication for Pacemakers After Cardiac Procedures

After some cardiac procedures, there is a risk for injury to the sinus node and AV conduction system, resulting in symptomatic bradycardia and the need for permanent pacing. Catheter and surgical ablation of cardiac arrhythmias, including atrial fibrillation, are among the more common procedures associated with

these risks; however, these procedures are discussed elsewhere. Table 121.2 summarizes the incidence of advanced AV block requiring permanent pacing after the procedures discussed later.

Septal Reduction Procedures for Hypertrophic Cardiomyopathy

Symptoms related to LV outflow tract obstruction in HCM may be treated with both surgical septal myectomy (SSM) and ASA. Both of these procedures have been associated with injury to the conduction system, including AV block and the need for permanent pacing. Typically, patients undergoing ASA develop an RBB block (RBBB) after the procedure, whereas post-SSM patients develop a left bundle branch block (LBBB). In one series, the rates of RBBB and complete heart block after ASA were 36% and 12%, respectively, whereas the rates of LBBB and complete heart block after SSM were 40% and 3%, respectively.[23] Predisposing contralateral BBB is an important predictor of complete AV block and the need for permanent pacing after these procedures.[23,24] Other factors predictive of complete heart block after ASA include female sex, multiple or bolus injections of ethanol, preexisting first-degree AV block, and acute AV block during ASA.[24,25] There is likely a significant "learning curve" with these procedures as the need for pacing decreases (<10%) at high-volume centers.[26] Patients who require permanent pacing after these procedures derive similar clinical and hemodynamic benefits to those who do not require pacing.

Percutaneous Aortic Valve Procedures

Indications for percutaneous procedures for aortic valve disease, especially transcatheter aortic valve replacement (TAVR), are growing rapidly, and these procedures are being performed

TABLE 121.2 Pacing indications after cardiac procedures

CARDIAC PROCEDURE	INCIDENCE OF AVB REQUIRING PPM
Septal Reduction for HCM	
Alcohol septal ablation	RBBB is most common (~35%)
	High-grade AVB <10% at experienced centers
Surgical septal myectomy	LBBB is common (~40%)
	High-grade AVB <5%
Percutaneous AV Procedures	
Aortic valvuloplasty	Second- or third-degree AVB (especially if wide QRS)
TAVR	Second- or third-degree AVB (especially if wide QRS)
Cardiac Surgery	
Pooled surgeries (CABG, AVR, MVR)	1.4% overall
	Higher likelihood if LBBB present or AVR
AVR	7% overall, highest incidence if combined MVR

AV, aortic valve; *AVB,* atrioventricular block; *AVR,* aortic valve replacement; *CABG,* coronary artery bypass graft; *HCM,* hypertrophic cardiomyopathy; *LBBB,* left bundle branch block; *MVR,* mitral valve replacement; *PPM,* permanent pacemaker; *RBBB,* right bundle branch block; *TAVR,* transcatheter aortic valve replacement.

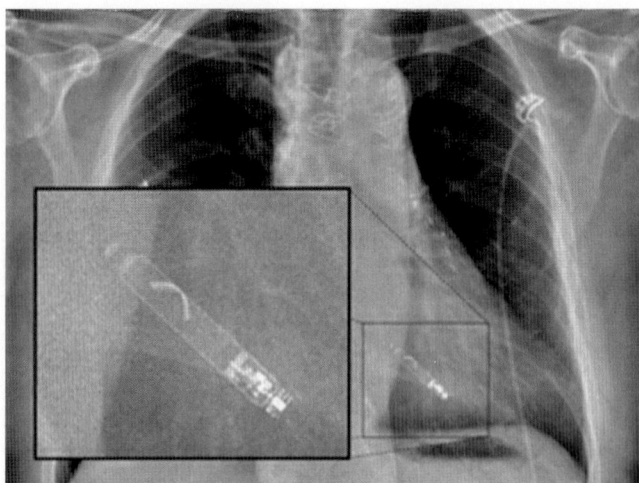

FIGURE 121.2 The Nanostim leadless cardiac pacemaker. (Courtesy St. Jude Medical, St. Paul, MN.)

more commonly today. Because of the proximity of the aortic valve to the AV conduction system, procedures that aim to treat aortic valve disease, particularly senile calcification, can lead to AV block. The incidence of new advanced AV block after balloon valvuloplasty of the aortic valve alone is low (<2%) and may be related to oversizing of the balloon employed during the procedure.[27] TAVR carries a known risk for pacemaker implantation, and a recent systematic literature review demonstrated that the risk is 15% overall but appears to be higher with the CoreValve prosthesis compared with the Edwards-Sapiens valve (odds ratio [OR], 4.91; $p < .0001$).[28] This trend seems to continue with newer devices, suggesting that self-expanding valves have a high risk for heart block. The prevalence of new LBBB is increased following TAVR, and therefore the presence of baseline RBBB is an important predictor of AV block after the procedure. Additionally, >90% of AV block requiring long-term pacing occurs immediately or within 1 week after the procedure, suggesting that this is due to direct mechanical injury to the conduction system during valve implantation.

Cardiac Surgery

The requirement for acute pacing after cardiac surgery is common (10%–15%); however, most of these conditions will recover, and only 1%–3% of patients will require permanent pacing postoperatively. In a review of almost 5000 patients undergoing cardiac surgery (81% coronary bypass surgery, 14% AVR, and 18% mitral valve replacement), the incidence of new permanent pacing postoperatively was 1.4%.[29] The indications for pacing were predominantly high-grade AV block, and approximately two-thirds of patients were pacemaker dependent at 6-year follow-up. The predictors for requiring permanent pacing included baseline LBBB and AVR. In another series, 7% of patients undergoing AVR required permanent pacing postoperatively, 70% of whom were pacemaker dependent at follow-up.[30] Patients who had baseline first-degree AV block with or without left anterior fascicular block or intraventricular

conduction delay, as well as those who underwent combined aortic and mitral valve replacement, had the highest risk for permanent pacing. Surgery for congenital heart disease can be very complex and can damage the conduction system, thereby requiring permanent pacing.

Novel Approaches and Technology for Cardiac Pacing

Leadless Pacemakers

It is well recognized that the "weak link" in a pacemaker system is the leads required for sensing and carrying electrical impulses from the pulse generator to the cardiac tissue. Lead failure occurs in up to 20% of patients within 10 years of implantation.[31] Additionally, the risks for vascular occlusion, pacemaker lead–associated endocarditis, and extraction procedures when leads fail all make the concept of developing leadless pacing technologies attractive.

One approach that is in development employs a miniaturized device that is completely implantable within the heart, thus eliminating the need for a pocket or leads. Such technology was first proposed by Spickler and colleagues in 1970.[32] The initial designs of these pacemakers include a fully self-contained capsule-shaped device with combined battery, electronics, and electrodes (Fig. 121.2).[33] The initial versions of these devices are implanted in the right ventricular apex via a transfemoral approach. Recently, a large, multicenter trial reported outcomes for over 500 implanted leadless pacemakers (Nanostim LP, St. Jude Medical, St. Paul, MN).[33] Stable and acceptable sensing and pacing thresholds were achieved in the vast majority of implants. Adverse events occurred in approximately 6% of implants and included device dislodgement requiring retrieval (1.7%), cardiac perforation (1.3%), and elevated thresholds requiring device reimplantation (1.3%). Another leadless pacemaker design (Micra, Medtronic, Inc.) reported similar highly successful implant rates with relatively low complications, including no device dislodgements.[34] Again, the most common major complication was cardiac injury during implantation (1.6%). Challenges in the development of a miniaturized pacemaker system will include the ability to produce sequential (i.e., AV) pacing between devices implanted in different chambers, integration with ICD systems (particularly subcutaneous ICD systems), ability[35] to extract the device, and approaches for device replacement at battery depletion.

Another area of research and development involves the use of external transmission of an energy source to a stand-alone intracardiac transducer localized in the chamber to be paced. Wienke and associates successfully showed that induction technology can be used for cardiac pacing; they employed alternating magnetic fields to generate voltage pulses in a receiver that was screwed into the right ventricular apex.[31] Ultrasound technology has also been used to generate pacing with consistent capture from a receiver electrode in the right atrium, right ventricle, and LV.[36] Investigators have studied ultrasound stimulation for LV pacing in heart failure patients, demonstrating reliable capture and predictable acoustic windows during positional changes and respiration to guide development of future implantable devices.[37]

Biological Pacemakers

The notion of using a biological pacemaker to replace an electronic pacemaker may be attractive, potentially avoiding the expense and complications associated with device replacement, device or lead failure, and infection; however, despite their limitations, electronic pacemakers are effective, durable, and have withstood the test of time for over five decades. "Niche" applications, such as use in patients with chronic infections, loss of vascular access, or other "bridge-to-device" applications, may be suitable for a biological pacemaker. Several approaches, including gene therapies, gene-cell hybrid approaches, and use of stem cells, have been proposed and tested to convert nonexcitable cells into self-contained biological pacemakers through ion channel expression.[38] Future research will focus on generating the cells necessary to generate action

potentials reliably with automaticity, as well as developing delivery systems and avoiding pitfalls such as the durability of these systems over time and the potential tumorigenicity of stem cells.

Conclusions

As techniques continue to evolve, the indications for permanent pacing will undoubtedly change. This chapter described some of the indications for permanent pacing in less common cardiac conditions, including inherited structural and electrical disorders, as well as systemic illnesses affecting the cardiac conduction system. In addition to these indications for pacing, the risks for conduction system injury, requiring permanent pacing, from other cardiac procedures and the indications for pacing post–myocardial infarction were reviewed. There is potential benefit and hope for using vagal stimulation to improve symptoms and outcomes in patients with chronic heart failure; however, initial randomized trial results have been mixed. The concept of local stimulation adjacent to the site of acute myocardial infarction as a means of preventing ventricular remodeling has also failed to show benefit in multiple clinical trials. Finally, novel technologies for pacing, including leadless pacemakers, employing ultrasound technology, as well as the concept of biological pacemakers, are developing rapidly. In combination, these new applications and developing technology may allow the role of permanent pacing to assume greater applicability, and the number of potential uses may continue to expand.

REFERENCES

1. Gold M, Peters RW. Newer applications of pacemakers. In: Zipes DP, Jalife J, eds. *Cardiac Electrophysiology: From Cell to Bedside*. 5th ed. Philadelphia: Saunders; 2009.
1a. Curtis AB, Worley SJ, Adamson PB, et al; for the Biventricular versus Right Ventricular Pacing in Heart Failure Patients with Atrioventricular Block (BLOCK HF) Trial Investigators. Biventricular pacing for atrioventricular block and systolic dysfunction. *N Engl J Med*. 2013;368:1585–1593.
2. Connolly SJ, Sheldon R, Thorpe KE, et al. Pacemaker therapy for prevention of syncope in patients with recurrent severe vasovagal syncope: Second Vasovagal Pacemaker Study (VPS II): a randomized trial. *JAMA*. 2003;289:2224–2229.
3. Brignole M, Menozzi C, Moya A, et al. Pacemaker therapy in patients with neurally mediated syncope and documented asystole: Third International Study on Syncope of Uncertain Etiology (ISSUE-3): a randomized trial. *Circulation*. 2012;125:2566–2571.
4. Groh WJ. Arrhythmias in the muscular dystrophies. *Heart Rhythm*. 2012;9:1890–1895.
5. Lazarus A, Varin J, Babuty D, et al. Long-term follow-up of arrhythmias in patients with myotonic dystrophy treated by pacing: a multicenter diagnostic pacemaker study. *J Am Coll Cardiol*. 2002;40:1645–1652.
6. Wahbi K, Meune C, Porcher R, et al. Electrophysiological study with prophylactic pacing and survival in adults with myotonic dystrophy and conduction system disease. *JAMA*. 2012;307:1292–1301.
7. Shah KB, Inoue Y, Mehra MR. Amyloidosis and the heart: a comprehensive review. *Arch Intern Med*. 2006;166:1805–1813.
8. Algalarrondo V, Dinanian S, Juin C, et al. Prophylactic pacemaker implantation in familial amyloid polyneuropathy. *Heart Rhythm*. 2012;9:1069–1075.
9. Doughan AR, Williams BR. Cardiac sarcoidosis. *Heart*. 2006;92:282–288.
10. Kim JS, Judson MA, Donnino R, et al. Cardiac sarcoidosis. *Am Heart J*. 2009;157:9–21.
11. McAlister HF, Klementowicz PT, Andrews C, et al. Lyme carditis: an important cause of reversible heart block. *Ann Intern Med*. 1989;110:339–345.
12. Zimetbaum PJ, Josephson ME. Use of the electrocardiogram in acute myocardial infarction. *N Engl J Med*. 2003;348:933–940.
13. Shuros AC, Salo RW, Florea VG, et al. Ventricular preexcitation modulates strain and attenuates cardiac remodeling in a swine model of myocardial infarction. *Circulation*. 2007;116:1162–1169.

14. Chung ES, Menon SG, Weiss R, et al. Feasibility of biventricular pacing in patients with recent myocardial infarction: impact on ventricular remodeling. *Congest Heart Fail*. 2007;13:9–15.
15. Chung ES, Dan D, Solomon SD, et al. Effect of peri-infarct pacing early after myocardial infarction: results of the prevention of myocardial enlargement and dilation post myocardial infarction study. *Circ Heart Fail*. 2010;3:650–658.
16. Stone GW, Chung ES, Stancak B, et al. Peri-infarct zone pacing to prevent adverse left ventricular remodeling in patients with large myocardial infarction. *Eur Heart J*. 2016;37:484–493.
17. Ruble SB, Hamann JJ, Gupta RC, et al. Chronic vagal Nerve Stimulation Impacts Biomarkers of Heart Failure in Canines. *J Am Coll Cardiol*. 2010;55:A16–E153.
18. Sabbah HN, Gupta RC, Imai M, et al. Chronic electrical stimulation of the carotid sinus baroreflex improves left ventricular function and promotes reversal of ventricular remodeling in dogs with advanced heart failure. *Circ Heart Fail*. 2011;4:65–70.
19. Sabbah HN. Electrical vagus nerve stimulation for the treatment of chronic heart failure. *Cleve Clin J Med*. 2011;78:S24–S29.
20. Zannad F, De Ferrari GM, Tuinenburg AE, et al. Chronic vagal stimulation for the treatment of low ejection fraction heart failure: results of the NEural Cardiac TherApy foR Heart Failure (NECTAR-HF) randomized controlled trial. *Eur Heart J*. 2015;36:425–433.
21. Premchand RK, Sharma K, Mittal S, et al. Autonomic regulation therapy via left or right cervical vagus nerve stimulation in patients with chronic heart failure: results of the ANTHEM-HF trial. *J Card Fail*. 2014;20:808–816.
22. Gold MR, van Veldhuisen DJ, Mann DL. Vagal nerve stimulation for heart failure: new pieces to the puzzle? *Eur J Heart Fail*. 2015;17:125–127.
23. Talreja DR, Nishimura RA, Edwards WD, et al. Alcohol septal ablation versus surgical septal myectomy: comparison of effects on atrioventricular conduction tissue. *J Am Coll Cardiol*. 2004;44:2329–2332.
24. Chang SM, Nagueh SF, Spencer 3rd WH, et al. Complete heart block: determinants and clinical impact in patients with hypertrophic obstructive cardiomyopathy undergoing nonsurgical septal reduction therapy. *J Am Coll Cardiol*. 2003;42:296–300.
25. Chen AA, Palacios IF, Mela T, et al. Acute predictors of subacute complete heart block after alcohol septal ablation for obstructive hypertrophic cardiomyopathy. *Am J Cardiol*. 2006;97:264–269.

26. Fernandes VL, Nielsen C, Nagueh SF, et al. Follow-up of alcohol septal ablation for symptomatic hypertrophic obstructive cardiomyopathy: the Baylor and Medical University of South Carolina experience 1996 to 2007. *JACC Cardiovasc Interv*. 2008;1:561–570.
27. Laynez A, Ben-Dor I, Hauville C, et al. Frequency of cardiac conduction disturbances after balloon aortic valvuloplasty. *Am J Cardiol*. 2011;108:1311–1315.
28. Erkapic D, De Rosa S, Kelava A, et al. Risk for permanent pacemaker after transcatheter aortic valve implantation: a comprehensive analysis of the literature. *J Cardiovasc Electrophysiol*. 2012;23:391–397.
29. Merin O, Ilan M, Oren A, et al. Permanent pacemaker implantation following cardiac surgery: indications and long-term follow-up. *Pacing Clin Electrophysiol*. 2009;32:7–12.
30. Huynh H, Dalloul G, Ghanbari H, et al. Permanent pacemaker implantation following aortic valve replacement: current prevalence and clinical predictors. *Pacing Clin Electrophysiol*. 2009;32:1520–1525.
31. Wieneke H, Konorza T, Erbel R, et al. Leadless pacing of the heart using induction technology: a feasibility study. *Pacing Clin Electrophysiol*. 2009;32:177–183.
32. Spickler JW, Rasor NS, Kezdi P, et al. Totally self-contained intracardiac pacemaker. *J Electrocardiol*. 1970;3:325–331.
33. Reddy VY, Exner DV, Cantillon DJ, et al. Percutaneous implantation of an entirely intracardiac leadless pacemaker. *N Engl J Med*. 2015;373:1125–1135.
34. Reynolds D, Duray GZ, Omar R, et al. A leadless intracardiac transcatheter pacing system. *N Engl J Med*. 2016;374:2604–2605.
35. Gold MR. Are leadless pacemakers a niche or the future of device therapy? *J Am Coll Cardiol*. 2015;65:1505–1508.
36. Lee KL, Lau CP, Tse HF, et al. First human demonstration of cardiac stimulation with transcutaneous ultrasound energy delivery: implications for wireless pacing with implantable devices. *J Am Coll Cardiol*. 2007;50:877–883.
37. Lee KL, Tse HF, Echt DS, et al. Temporary leadless pacing in heart failure patients with ultrasound-mediated stimulation energy and effects on the acoustic window. *Heart Rhythm*. 2009;6:742–748.
38. Cho HC, Marban E. Biological therapies for cardiac arrhythmias: can genes and cells replace drugs and devices? *Circ Res*. 2010;106:674–685.

122 Remote Monitoring of Cardiac Implantable Electronic Devices

Emily P. Zeitler, Ruth Ann Greenfield, and Jonathan P. Piccini

Evolution of Remote Monitoring

Utilization of cardiac implantable electronic devices (CIEDs), including pacemakers, implantable cardioverter defibrillators (ICDs), cardiac resynchronization therapy (CRT) devices, and implanted rhythm monitors, has increased globally over the past few decades in light of expanding indications for their use and improved access. These combined forces have led to an increasing prevalence of CIEDs worldwide.[1,2]

Concordant with the increasing prevalence of CIEDs, there has also been a progressive evolution in remote monitoring (RM) technology. Today, RM plays a critical role in the surveillance of device function, and in many centers, RM also plays a role in disease management. A tremendous amount of information recorded and stored by CIEDs has become increasingly available to health care providers without the need for face-to-face interaction. In the earliest days of RM, pacemakers could be followed transtelephonically to provide basic information on device function only (e.g., battery status and rhythm strips with a magnet applied). Transtelephonic monitoring requires patient initiation and uses analog transmission to send sensing and capture data and information about the battery status. Importantly, transtelephonic monitoring cannot transmit recorded data. Some legacy devices are still monitored this way; in other cases, patients without access to and/or familiarity with modern telecommunications opt for this form of remote interrogation (Fig. 122.1).

Following transtelephonic monitoring, the next generation of RM, termed "remote interrogation," incorporated additional portions of a traditional in-person follow-up visit for pacemakers and other devices into transmissions. For example, a remote interrogation transmission might include automated capture threshold testing results. Remote interrogation still required patient interaction to accomplish inductive transmission over phone lines.

As CIEDs, RM platforms, and telecommunication technologies progressed, true RM became possible. In this paradigm, automatic data acquisition occurs wirelessly on a frequent basis (e.g., daily) without patient interaction. Additionally, these systems provide unscheduled transmission of any predefined alerts to the CIED provider (Fig. 122.2). These alerts can include information and warnings about device integrity (e.g., lead impedance), programming issues (e.g., insufficient safety margins for sensing or capture), or medical data (e.g., arrhythmia events, change in thoracic impedance). The frequency and content of these automatic transmissions depend on the capabilities of different CIEDs (Table 122.1) and associated RM platforms as well as the personalized programming of the device by physicians or other providers (Fig. 122.3). RM is now considered the standard of care and is preferred to older methods of home-based follow-up. Some investigators advocate that daily transmission has advantages over other schedules.[3,4] However, RM platforms have not been directly compared for their effectiveness.

Logistics of Remote Monitoring

Globally, five device manufacturers have approved RM systems: Biotronik, Boston Scientific, Medtronic Inc., Sorin, and St. Jude Medical. While the various RM systems are all capable of the same basic functions, each system has special features that may be relevant for an individual patient (see Table 122.1). Therefore for a successful RM relationship between patients and providers, responsibilities should be well delineated. In other words, all involved parties, including patients, physicians, physician extenders, office staff, the health care system, and device manufacturers, have necessary functions.

In addition, the local telecommunications infrastructure can play an important role. For example, while RM systems are moving more and more toward mobile communication–based systems, legacy CIEDs, which require an analog phone line for RM, will remain relevant as long as these devices are in service, and this can represent a significant share of CIED patients, especially in more resource-poor settings. Furthermore, in more rural settings, the availability of mobile technologies versus traditional analog phone line systems must be weighed when choosing an appropriate CIED for a patient.

Patient Participation

Active patient participation in RM is essential—perhaps more so than in other patient-provider relationships. High-quality data have demonstrated RM to be acceptable in patients,[5-8] convenient,[8,9] and associated with good quality of life,[10] but challenges to RM compliance remain. For example, in some RM systems, patient-initiated transmission is required, in which case patients must comply with transmission schedules. In some series, one-fifth of patients demonstrate poor compliance with RM, so there is generally substantial room for improvement in regard to patient adherence with RM programs,[11,12] especially because some of the clinical benefits of RM are dose responsive to the level of adherence.[13]

Reasons for this poor compliance can be divided into several categories. First, some issues are patient related: age older than 80 years has been associated with lower adherence. Second, clinical

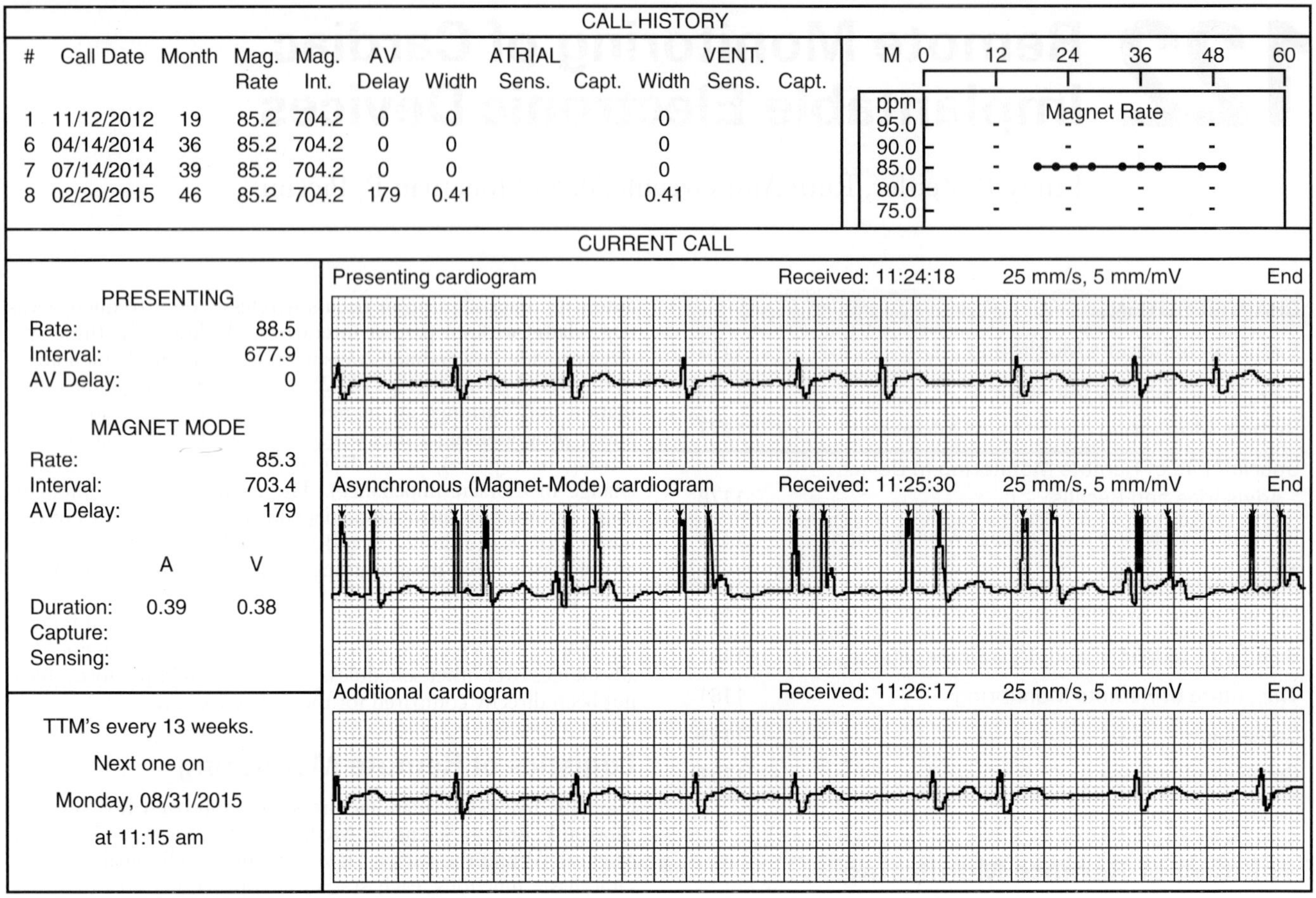

CALL HISTORY

#	Call Date	Month	Mag. Rate	Mag. Int.	AV Delay	ATRIAL Width	ATRIAL Sens.	ATRIAL Capt.	VENT. Width	VENT. Sens.	VENT. Capt.
1	11/12/2012	19	85.2	704.2	0	0			0		
6	04/14/2014	36	85.2	704.2	0	0			0		
7	07/14/2014	39	85.2	704.2	0	0			0		
8	02/20/2015	46	85.2	704.2	179	0.41			0.41		

M   0   12   24   36   48   60

ppm
95.0   Magnet Rate
90.0
85.0 ●●●●● ●●●   ●
80.0
75.0

CURRENT CALL

PRESENTING

Rate:	88.5
Interval:	677.9
AV Delay:	0

MAGNET MODE

Rate:	85.3
Interval:	703.4
AV Delay:	179

	A	V
Duration:	0.39	0.38
Capture:		
Sensing:		

TTM's every 13 weeks.

Next one on

Monday, 08/31/2015

at 11:15 am

Presenting cardiogram　　　Received: 11:24:18　　25 mm/s, 5 mm/mV　　End

Asynchronous (Magnet-Mode) cardiogram　　Received: 11:25:30　　25 mm/s, 5 mm/mV　　End

Additional cardiogram　　　Received: 11:26:17　　25 mm/s, 5 mm/mV　　End

FIGURE 122.1 Transtelephonic device monitoring. An excerpt from a transtelephonic monitoring (*TTM*) session of a 94-year-old male patient with a legacy dual-chamber pacemaker system. In this transmission, a magnet is applied, revealing the asynchronous magnet mode at a rate of 85 beats/min. As battery life declines, the magnet rate will decrease, alerting the physician to consider generator replacement. *AV,* Atrioventricular.

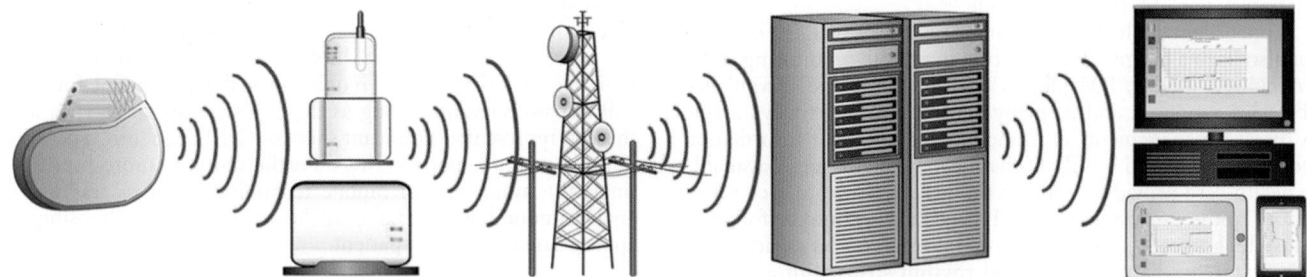

FIGURE 122.2 Transmission of data from patient to provider. In a traditional remote monitoring system, data moves unidirectionally from the implanted device to the responsible provider. First, a very low–power transmitter integrated within the pulse generator transmits stored data on a predetermined basis (typically daily) to a mobile communicator in the patient's home. The data are relayed to a service center, which is monitored at all times by an independent diagnostic testing facility. A report is generated and made available to the physician typically through a web-based platform. (From Varma N, Ricci RP. Telemedicine and cardiac implants: what is the benefit? *Eur Heart J.* 2013;34:1885-1895.)

sites with the greatest proportion of patients enrolled in RM have greater patient adherence, suggesting that site-specific or health care system specific-infrastructure, operations, and behavior can impact compliance. One important step for improving utilization and adherence to RM is the provision of patient education at the time of implantation and enrollment in RM systems before hospital discharge. Lastly, but perhaps most importantly, technical properties of the RM system can play a role in compliance such that patients who used systems that required active inductive transmission with a "wand" had poorer compliance compared with those who used automatic wireless home systems for RM. These considerations underscore the importance of appropriate hardware selection at the time of implantation and detailed counseling prior to the initiation of RM.

Some common sense interventions to improve patient engagement have been explored. For example, the setup of RM equipment for pacemakers during a health care encounter may improve compliance.[11] Another strategy is to establish an RM patient contract to explicitly outline patient responsibilities at the time of RM initiation. This strategy has been endorsed by the

TABLE 122.1 Comparison of available remote monitoring systems by device manufacturer

FEATURE	BIOTRONIK	BOSTON SCIENTIFIC	MEDTRONIC	SORIN	ST. JUDE MEDICAL
Remote monitoring system	Home Monitoring	Latitude	CareLink	SMARTVIEW	Merlin.net
Data transmission	Analog phone line and GSM network	Analog or digital cellular adapter, wired Ethernet adapter, and wireless Internet adapter	Analog phone line, GSM network, Ethernet, mobile cellular network, and Wi-Fi (pacemakers only)	Analog phone line and GSM network	Analog, GSM, or broadband
Transmitter	Mobile or stationary	Stationary	Mobile or stationary	Stationary	Stationary
Provider communication method	SMS, email, fax	Email, SMS, website	SMS, email, voicemail, pager, mobile app	Fax, email, SMS	Fax, email, SMS
FDA clearance	Yes	Yes	Yes	Yes	Yes
CE mark	Yes	Yes	Yes	Yes	Yes
Special features	Automatic RV and LV thresholds, impedance, and sensing measurements; configurable red and yellow alerts; fully configurable online; patient callback feature; electronic health record export compatibility; hands-free automatic transmission	Optional Bluetooth weight scales and BP cuffs; configurable data transmission to associated caregivers; configurable red and yellow alerts; electronic health record data export capability; hands-free automatic data transmissions for newer devices (older devices require a "wand"); iPhone app available	Optivol thoracic impedance alert (CE mark only); configurable red and yellow alerts; RM available for ILR; PDF exports of patient reports; Cardiac Compass HF report; 99% of implanted devices are able to be remotely monitored; electronic health record data export capability; supports IDCO profile; automatic hands-free transmission for some devices (others require a "wand")	7-second real-time IEGM for scheduled follow-ups, alerts, reports, and patient-initiated transmissions (PIT)	Alerts fully configurable online; send phone calls to patients; CorVue fluid status alert; automatic RA, RV, and LV pacing thresholds; integrated HF website showing correlations between pulmonary artery pressures and the device; and diagnostics, such as AF burden, percent pacing, and day/night HR when the patient is implanted with both the CardioMEMS PA sensor and SJM CIED; hands-free automatic transmission
Default alert assessment frequency	Daily	Daily	Immediate (when the device is within the range of the transmitter)	Daily	Daily
Representative picture of the home transmission unit[a]					

[a]Images of these systems appear courtesy of the manufacturers.
AF, Atrial fibrillation; *BP*, blood pressure; *CE*, Conformité Européene; *CIED*, cardiac implantable electronic device; *FDA*, US Food and Drug Administration; *GSM*, global system for mobile communications; *HF*, heart failure; *HR*, heart rate; *IDCO*, implantable device cardiac observation; *ILR*, implantable loop recorder; *IEGM*, intracardiac electrogram; *LV*, left ventricular; *PDF*, portable document format; *RA*, right atrial; *RM*, remote monitoring; *RV*, right ventricular; *SJM*, St. Jude Medical; *SMS*, short message service.

Heart Rhythm Society[14] and can be implemented relatively easily and at low cost.

Responsibilities of Physicians and Other Providers

Physicians are ultimately responsible for managing their CIED patients and any associated RM programs. Therefore frequent adaptation to changes by manufacturers, the health care system, and patient preferences requires modifications to patient management. RM almost always requires dedicated personnel who are responsible for ensuring and facilitating its operational success, including timely review and action on RM information. Increased utilization of RM often shifts the workload in device clinics and necessitates some restructuring of practice infrastructure. Regardless of a particular practice pattern, physicians must provide the final evaluation of any RM transmission.

All available RM platforms allow physicians to tailor alerts based on unique patient characteristics (e.g., heart failure [HF]), indications for the CIED (e.g., sustained ventricular tachycardia

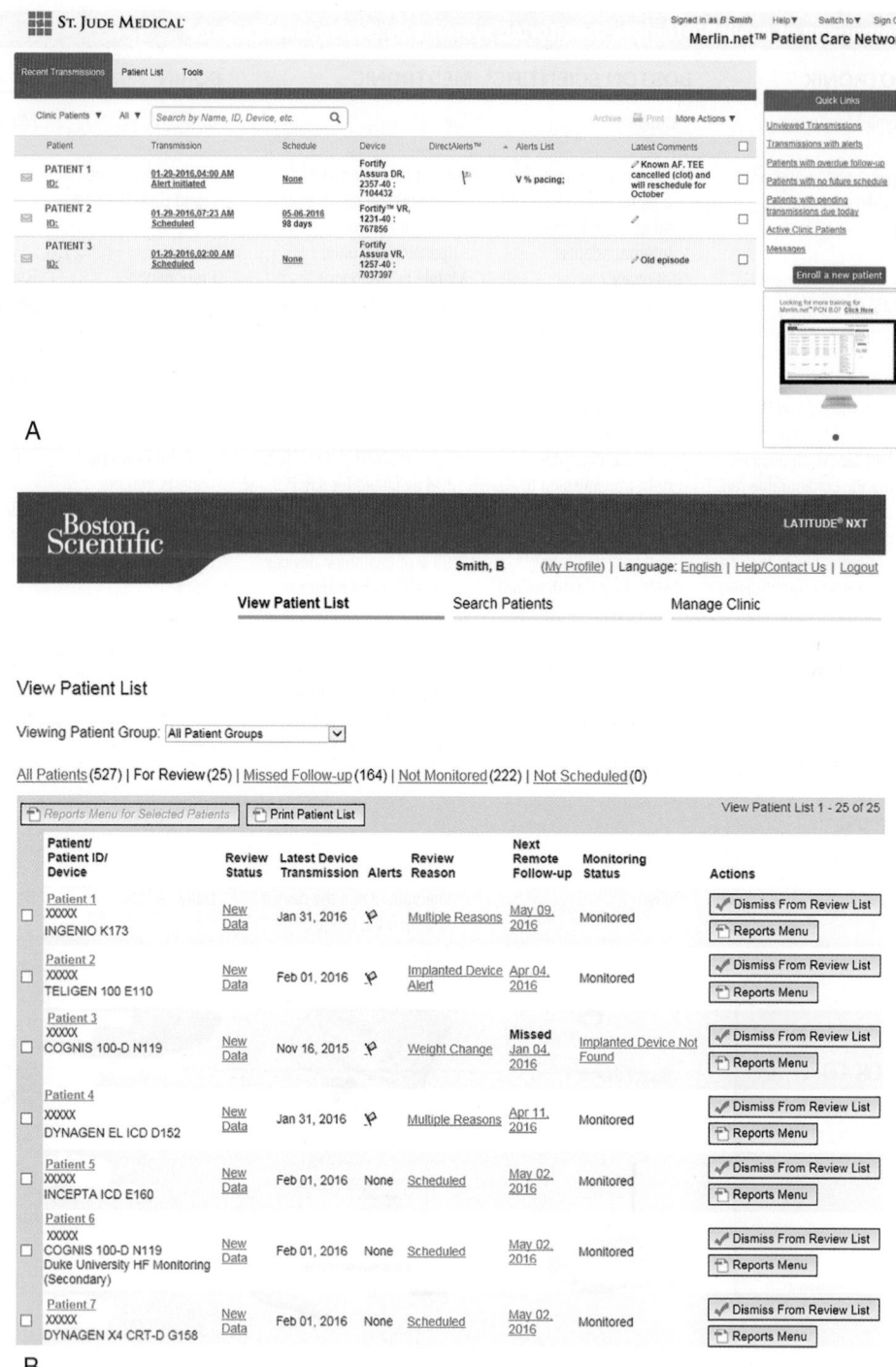

FIGURE 122.3 Provider portal for extraction and interpretation of remote transmission data. Providers can access remote transmissions through web-based portals. (A) The provider portal for Merlin.net. (B) The provider portal for Latitude NXT. ([A] Courtesy St. Jude Medical, St. Paul, MN; [B] courtesy Boston Scientific, Marlborough, MA.)

[VT]), and the presence of lead or device advisories. Therefore the needs of an individual patient should be considered at the time of RM initiation and continually thereafter as the patient's clinical status and preferences change along with the evolution in clinical evidence and device capabilities. While some patients may decline the substitution of RM visits in favor of traditional in-person visits, these patients should still be enrolled in RM networks so that they can take advantage of RM for safety and unexpected needs (e.g., evaluation of sustained palpitations on a weekend).

Mid-level providers and physician extenders (nurse practitioners or physician assistants), as well as allied professionals trained in CIED management, can effectively serve as the "first contact" for CIED patients by reviewing RM transmissions or troubleshooting clinical events in collaboration with the supervising physician. In addition, physicians and other providers collaboratively engaged in a CIED RM program can develop and implement patient education programs for different stages of patient care because educational needs will change from the time of implantation to a revision or upgrade procedure. Changes in technology or clinical status may also necessitate revised or additional patient education. Finally, all health care providers share the responsibility to document patient interactions—remote or otherwise—in medical records. Innovative ways of sharing this documentation with patients through automated messaging to confirm receipt of transmission or to communicate other findings that require follow-up improve transparency and may improve patient adherence and satisfaction.

Role of Health Care Systems and Infrastructure

As described, RM relies on interoperability between various systems, including the implanted CIED itself, the home transmitting device, existing telecommunications technology, and servers that communicate with physician offices typically through web-based platforms. Moreover, these complex system interactions are frequently changing. When one or more of these systems are unavailable, RM may be challenging or impossible for a particular patient. Therefore these logistic considerations also impact hardware selection for an individual patient. Underscoring this point, clinical trials have demonstrated that many transmissions are often unsuccessful.[15]

Sustainability of a CIED RM program relies on adequate coverage and reimbursement for nontraditional services. Without adequate resources or coverage, it is often impractical to conduct RM successfully. Despite similar CIED and RM technologies and RM standards of care, coverage and reimbursement structures vary across international borders, geographic regions, and even within the same health care system.[16,17]

Remote Monitoring and Patient Outcomes

Extensive, rigorous study of RM in regard to a wide range of important outcomes, including mortality, health care utilization, and incidence of inappropriate shocks, has generally demonstrated the value of RM. Because of the centralized nature of RM data storage, RM lends itself well to observational registry-based studies, which, in some cases, include hundreds of thousands of patients. While observational data have limitations, the sheer numbers of patients in these registries provide very important data about the use of RM and its outcomes. It is important to note that the available clinical evidence applies almost exclusively to adult patients in part because the population of CIED patients cared for by pediatric providers is limited. RM in pediatric patients has been demonstrated to be feasible, safe, and useful in some circumstances.[18,19] However, the paucity of evidence and significant variability in practice and outcomes likely contribute to the lack of specific guidelines for the use of RM in pediatric patients.[20]

Mortality

Beginning in the 2000s, several studies have examined the relationship between mortality risk and the use of RM compared with standard follow-up of CIED patients. These early studies were conducted primarily in single centers and were not designed or powered to detect differences in mortality, but there was no indication that patients managed with RM had worse survival compared with patients in the usual care groups.[21–23] These reassuring findings paved the way for larger, randomized, adequately powered investigations of mortality in RM.

In a 2014 study of patients with high-voltage devices (ICD or CRT-defibrillator [CRT-D]), those randomized to RM using the Home Monitoring platform along with traditional in-office visits had reduced mortality compared with those receiving only quarterly in-office visits (1-year Kaplan–Meier estimates of all-cause mortality, 3.4% in the RM group and 8.7% in the control group

[p = .004]).[24] Six other randomized trials have reported the effect of RM on mortality in ICD patients, representing nearly 5000 patients with a variety of devices and RM systems.[15,22,23,25–27] When the findings from these seven studies were meta-analyzed in a 2015 study, the odds ratio (OR) for mortality with RM was not significantly different from in-office follow-up alone (OR, 0.83; 95% confidence interval [CI], 0.58–1.17; p = .285; I² = 34.8%).[4] One of the most striking randomized clinical trials was the implant-based multiparameter telemonitoring of patients with HF (IN-TIME) trial, where RM of ICD and CRT-D recipients led to a 50% reduction in mortality.[24] Observational studies using "big data" from hundreds of thousands of patients have also reported survival comparisons between CIED patients managed with and without RM and have consistently demonstrated a survival benefit associated with RM.[13,28]

Health Care Utilization

At the point of care, RM has been shown to be less resource intensive than in-person visits for both clinic staff and patients[29,30] because of the decreased time required for completing a review of data obtained from a remote transmission compared with that required for completing an in-office visit. Accordingly, RM results in time saved by patients by eliminating travel to and from a physician's office and receiving care (including office wait times). It remains to be seen if these savings in health care utilization at the point of care translate to the wide variety of clinical settings in which CIED patients are managed. Moreover, differences at the point of care are only a part of the total management strategy. As such, a number of studies have evaluated the differences in other aspects of health care utilization between patients managed with RM versus those who are not. In the 2010 Lumos-T Safely Reduces Routine Office Device Follow-Up (TRUST) trial, there was a significant reduction in scheduled and unscheduled office and hospital visits in ICD patients randomized to RM versus usual care (2.1 visits per patient-year compared with 3.8, p < .001).[23] However, when hospitalizations were examined in isolation, six randomized studies failed to show any decrease among RM patients compared with those receiving usual care.[15,21,22,25,27,31]

Because hospitalizations are expected to be relatively infrequent in CIED patients, the impact of RM on unscheduled office visits also has important implications for the efficiency and sustainability of an RM program. This end point has been examined specifically, and results are inconsistent with some demonstrating reductions in ambulatory visits,[21,27] some showing a measurable increase in visits,[23,25,26] and one showing no difference.[15] This variability suggests that differences in findings related to unscheduled visits depend on local standards of care and the characteristics of patients included in these studies. It is notable that two of the largest of those studies (The TRUST trial and The Clinical Evaluation of Remote Notification to Reduce Time to Clinical Decision [CONNECT] trial) demonstrated a decrease in overall office visits of RM patients despite no reduction in unscheduled visits.[15,23]

Time to Clinical Decision Making

One of the greatest promises of RM is the potential to decrease the time between the identification of a clinical event and the therapeutic intervention. RM should not only allow earlier identification of arrhythmias or other problems but also allow a more timely application of a therapy. For example, in theory, RM should decrease the time between the diagnosis of sustained atrial fibrillation (AF) and the initiation of oral anticoagulation in patients at risk for stroke. It appears that the promise of RM to decrease time to clinical intervention has been realized. In the CONNECT study of 1997 patients from

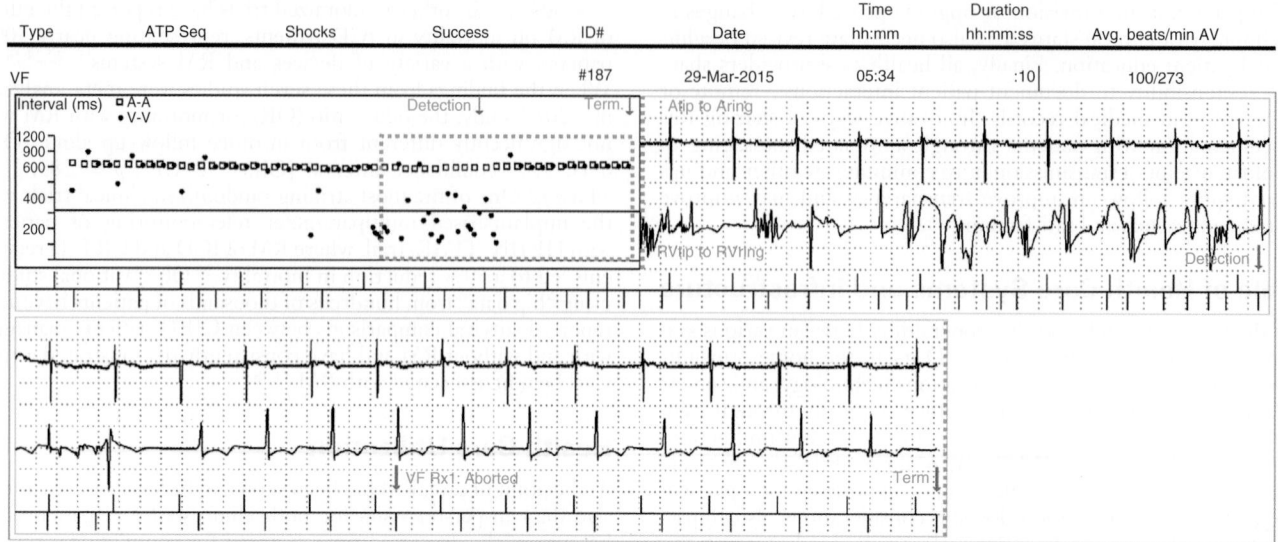

FIGURE 122.4 Malfunctioning implantable cardioverter defibrillator (ICD) leads that may be monitored more closely. The recalled Sprint Fidelis defibrillator lead is prone to fracture. For Fidelis leads still in service, heightened surveillance may help identify patients at risk for serious complications. One event strip from a remote monitoring transmission of a 48-year-old male who had an ICD system implanted for primary prevention including a Sprint Fidelis defibrillator lead is shown. The transmission included 333 ventricular sensing events, suggesting lead fracture. This transmission resulted in immediate referral to the emergency department to urgently disable tachytherapies. The patient ultimately had the problematic lead extracted and replaced. *AV,* Atrioventricular; *RV,* right ventricular; *VF,* ventricular fibrillation.

136 sites with ICD or CRT-D who were randomized to either RM using the Carelink platform or standard care, patients receiving RM had a reduction in the time to a clinical decision, from a median of 22 days to 4.6 days ($p < .001$).[15] Other randomized investigations have shown similar benefits in this regard,[23,25,27] as have large observational studies from the earliest days of widespread RM.[32]

RM may also lead to more frequent CIED programming optimization. Device reprogramming is generally focused on improving patient outcomes (e.g., reducing right ventricular [RV] pacing or increasing biventricular [BiV] pacing) but may have the added benefit of increasing battery longevity.[33]

Inappropriate Shocks

It has become increasingly recognized that inappropriate and unnecessary ICD shocks have important consequences on the quality of life and cardiovascular outcomes. Thus significant investment has been made in developing systems—mainly software algorithms—to avoid inappropriate and all-cause shocks. In some cases, inappropriate shocks may be delivered for ventricular arrhythmias that would have otherwise self-terminated (nonsustained) and been non–life-threatening.[34] In other cases, tailored software algorithms and programming methods can address common sources of inappropriate shocks related to AF or supraventricular tachycardias, electromagnetic interference, and T wave oversensing, to name a few. In still other cases, inappropriate shocks may be caused by device or lead malfunction.[35] In all of these cases, RM offers the potential to identify shock risks earlier and intervene to avoid future inappropriate or unnecessary shocks. Clinical trial data have shown that patients randomized to an RM management program had less than one-half the incidence of inappropriate shocks compared with those randomized to a standard in-office follow-up. This reduction in inappropriate shocks was because of the timely diagnosis of supraventricular tachycardia, oversensing secondary to noise, lead dysfunction, and T wave oversensing.[26]

Special Role of Remote Monitoring in Device Advisories and Recalls

As CIEDs have become more advanced and complex, advisories and recalls have increased over the past several decades with respect to frequency and impact. When an advisory or recall is announced, RM has a particularly important role to play. For example, some parameters available through RM can identify lead defects (e.g., rapid change in lead impedance) that may place patients at risk for inappropriate shocks (Fig. 122.4). Data from clinical practice in the wake of high-profile device advisories have demonstrated that RM may be a much more effective way of monitoring patients compared with routine in-office follow-up.[36] Heightened surveillance of lead parameters and device alerts may avoid catastrophic outcomes[37] in patients awaiting device revision[38,39] and provide a reasonable alternative to device replacement for patients in whom a replacement procedure is undesirable or unreasonable. Indeed, device manufacturers have incorporated special surveillance algorithms to respond to device advisories and recalls, which may improve sensitivity to detect a malfunction and reduce associated risks (e.g., inappropriate shocks).[39,40] Based on the aggregate evidence, the Heart Rhythm Society issued a specific class I recommendation that patients with a CIED component under advisory or recall should be enrolled in RM in addition to the general recommendation to use RM in all patients in whom it is technically feasible.[14] Device clinics should flag patients with devices under advisory, and advisory status should be known to the health care professional who is reviewing the RM data, as this knowledge may impact interpretation and management.

Remote Monitoring and Disease Management
Heart Failure

As the population of CIED patients overlaps more and more with the general HF population, there has been increasing interest and investment in CIED-based technologies to monitor HF events.

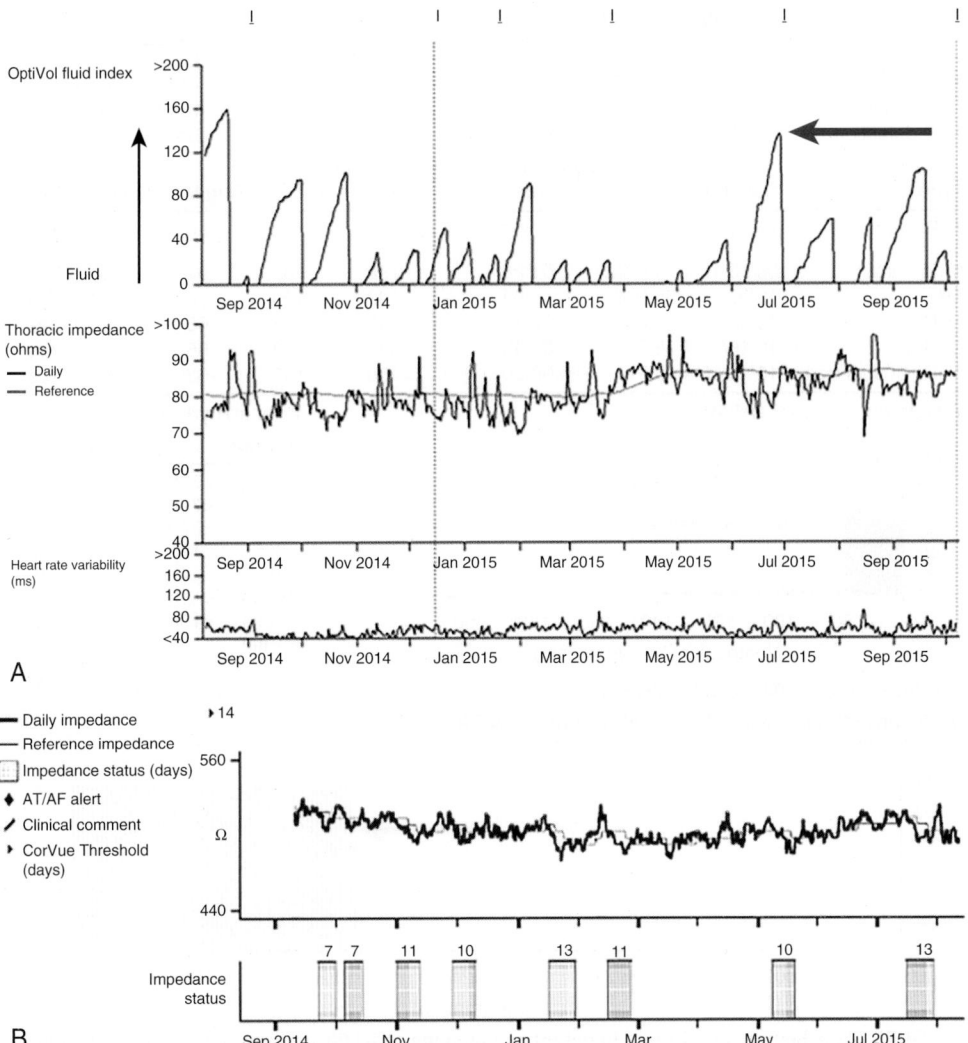

FIGURE 122.5 Heart failure management systems. (A) This is an excerpt from the Cardiac Compass report (Medtronic, Minneapolis, MN) from a remote transmission of a biventricular implantable cardioverter defibrillator in a 49-year-old patient with heart failure secondary to peripartum cardiomyopathy. At the *red arrow*, the patient had an exacerbation of heart failure symptoms, resulting in an increase in oral diuretic therapy, and was able to avoid hospitalization. (B) The CorVue monitoring system (St. Jude Medical, St. Paul, MN) measures thoracic impedance based on a regularly updated reference measure. The line graph depicts daily impedance trends compared with a continuously updated reference value. In the bar graph below, the number of days the impedance decreases below the reference value, suggesting volume overload, is depicted, with seven being the lowest reportable number. *AT/AF*, Atrial tachycardia/atrial fibrillation.

HF hospitalization is a major source of health care utilization and patient morbidity and mortality, so device-based monitoring that can anticipate HF exacerbations for outpatient intervention is particularly attractive.

One of the most well-known RM technologies for HF monitoring is the thoracic impedance measure, which can be calculated by many CIEDs and reported through device interrogation and RM. Some evidence suggests that monitoring thoracic impedance trends can alert providers to an impending or active HF exacerbation, which may reduce hospitalizations and improve other clinical outcomes.[41] Like many diagnostic tests, this function in isolation has a limited value[14,42] but may be an important component in the comprehensive assessment of a given HF patient.

Some device manufacturers have therefore developed a suite of HF diagnostic data, including thoracic impedance along with heart rate variability, patient activity, and other measures to provide a more complete picture of HF disease status (Fig. 122.5). When used in combination, these measures can be a powerful tool for predicting (and avoiding) HF hospitalizations.[43] The maximum value from these features may best be realized when HF specialists work closely with electrophysiologists. There is no consensus regarding the best models for this type of cooperation as this emerging field continues to develop.

Atrial Fibrillation

As mentioned previously, RM is also useful for the earlier detection of AF[44,45] over standard follow-up. An important example is the use of RM in patients with cryptogenic stroke wherein an implantable monitor identified significantly more patients with AF within 6 months than those who underwent standard follow-up.[46] In addition to improving the sensitivity of AF detection, RM can reduce the time for making a clinical decision by more than 20% (Fig. 122.6). An earlier and more sensitive detection of AF can facilitate important CIED programming changes to avoid inappropriate shocks or to improve the percentage of BiV

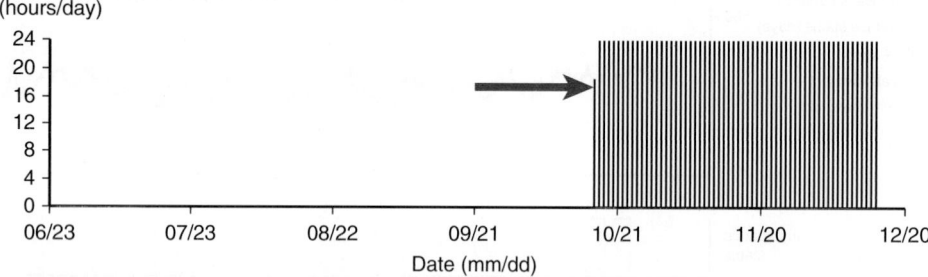

Arrhythmia summary: 06/02/15 to 12/15/15

Mode switch count	25 (7.3 hrs/day – 30.5%)	VHR episodes	1
AHR episode trigger	Mode switch >30 s	VHR detection	180 ppm for 5 beats
AHR episodes	9	VHR termination	180 ppm for 5 beats
AHR detection	175 beats/min - No delay	SVT filter	On

			Duration	Rates (beats/min):				
Type		Date/time	hh:mm:ss	Max A	Max V	Avg V	Sensor	EGM
VHR	Longest...	08/07/15 7:33 AM	:04	62	183	180	62	Yes
AHR	First	06/03/15 11:54 AM	:01:28	182	85	61	60	No
AHR		10/09/15 8:55 PM	:44	182	100	94	93	Yes
AHR		10/16/15 3:44 PM	:50:33	346	98	65	95	Yes
AHR		10/16/15 4:35 PM	:09:40	331	93	66	61	Yes
AHR	Suspended...	10/16/15 4:45 PM	>96:00:00	>400	187	63	83	Yes

V. Rate during atrial arrhythmias

% of V. Beats
□ VS ■ VP

Ventricular rate (beats/min)

Atrial arrhythmias

Duration		Count
	≥72hr	1
24hr	- <72hr	0
12hr	- <24hr	0
4hr	- <12hr	0
1hr	- < 4hr	0
10min	- < 1hr	1
1min	- <10min	5
<1min		18
		25

Cardiac compass: 06/23/15 to 12/15/15

Atrial arrhythmia trend: 60 days with >4 hours AT/AF

(hours/day)

Date (mm/dd)

FIGURE 122.6 Remote monitoring to detect and manage atrial fibrillation. Remote interrogation from an 82-year-old man with a dual-chamber pacemaker indicated for complete heart block demonstrates the abrupt onset of persistent atrial fibrillation in October (*red arrow*). The patient was entirely asymptomatic, caused at least in part from experiencing no change in paced rate (*green arrow*). *AHR,* Atrial high rate; *AT/AF,* atrial tachycardia/atrial fibrillation; *EGM,* electromyogram; *SVT,* supraventricular tachycardia; *VHR,* ventricular high rate.

pacing. Moreover, because even relatively brief episodes of AF can appreciably increase the risk for stroke,[47] better detection can help guide physicians in discussions with patients about anticoagulation for stroke prevention. While early clinical trials have been challenging with negative results, ongoing clinical trials will help clarify how much AF is actionable.[48,49] These trials will also help identify the optimal pharmacological management of these patients.

Cost Effectiveness

Cost effectiveness is an important consideration for any health care technology, and RM is no exception. Several cost-effectiveness studies of RM have been conducted as stand-alone investigations or as embedded studies in larger clinical trials. These studies have generally demonstrated cost savings.

When RM is integrated in the routine care of CIED patients, cost savings accrue for both the health care system at large and the patients directly, but the magnitude of these savings vary. Consistently, however, cost savings result from decreased in-clinic visits and hospitalizations.[30,50–55] As health care systems and technologies evolve, the magnitude of the cost effectiveness of RM is likely to change. An ongoing study is needed to update

the understanding of RM to inform policies for coverage and reimbursement.[56,57]

Mega-Cohorts and "Big Data"

Not coincidentally, the rise of RM programs has occurred in parallel with the improvement in the availability to store, handle, and analyze "big data," giving rise to the development of "mega-cohorts." CIED manufacturers have developed separate RM systems specific to their devices (see Table 122.1), and these systems can act as a repository for all CIED data that are collected, stored, and transmitted by CIEDs. In turn, these data collection and transmission systems can be leveraged to provide important longitudinal information, including device integrity data, and clinical information about CIED patients across health care systems and vast geographic regions. These capabilities have enabled some of the largest studies of CIED patients.

While analyses of these data have limitations, including limited patient characteristics and the usual limitations inherent in retrospective observational analysis, these studies are not limited by power, as they include enormous numbers of patients. For example, in an analysis of nearly 270,000 patients in a clinical practice with CIEDs monitored through Merlin.net, an association was found between the use of RM and improved survival rate across all device types. Furthermore, the survival advantage appeared to correlate with the degree of RM adherence, suggestive of a dose response.[13] Another strikingly large cohort study of >185,000 patients with defibrillators (ICDs and CRT-Ds) engaged in RM with the Latitude system also demonstrated that the use of RM was associated with improved survival rate compared with patients followed up with traditional in-office visits only.[28]

Relevant Guidelines and Recommendations

Several heart rhythm professional societies have produced guidelines and recommendations for the integration of RM into the care of CIED patients.[14,16,58,59] As the clinical evidence has grown, it has become clear that in summation, the clinical evidence strongly favors the use of RM as part of the management of all CIED patients in whom the use of RM is technically feasible (Table 122.2). The special benefits of RM in the context of disease management (e.g., HF and AF) and surveillance of recalled or advisory devices or lead components are specifically recognized in the most recent iterations of these guidelines.

The Future of Remote Monitoring

RM technologies will continue to evolve. In the current paradigm, information flows primarily in one direction: from patients' CIEDs to a provider. However, one may imagine clear benefits to a bidirectional flow of data. For example, if technological barriers and privacy concerns can be adequately addressed, there may be the opportunity to program CIEDs remotely. This may be particularly valuable for patients in remote geographic locations, those with an urgent/emergent need based on a clinical event, and for the administration of software upgrades or execution of advisories and recalls amenable to reprogramming.

Wearable technologies are gaining popularity and usefulness such that patients can now detect and monitor a variety of biometric data, including peripheral oxygen saturation, serum glucose, and heart rate, using a smartphone. A similar potential exists for CIED patients to interact with their CIEDs. Currently, some device manufacturers have made progress by moving toward RM systems that leverage the power and ubiquity of smartphones and mobile communications technology (Fig. 122.7). More fully engaging patients in their health care through sharing CIED-generated and CIED-stored information could enhance patient satisfaction, patient–provider interactions, and clinical outcomes.

Finally, as previously described, the sheer quantity of data involved in RM has facilitated tremendous data collection and produced compelling evidence through mega-cohorts. However, high-quality randomized data remain the standard. As such, developing RM platforms that could facilitate the conduct of randomized clinical trials that may include remote programming or other interventions would be a transformative innovation.

Conclusion

The central role that RM plays in the management of many CIED patients worldwide is supported by abundant high-quality clinical evidence and endorsed by authoritative guidelines and recommendations from professional societies. This role is expanding to include more than routine parameters of CIED function. Enhanced disease management of HF and AF and heightened surveillance of advisory or recalled CIEDs or components are all now part of the standard of care in most practice environments. These capabilities have been shown to be cost effective for both patients and health care systems. Technical capabilities continue to expand, resulting in increasing possibilities for improved patient management, satisfaction, and outcomes.

Conflicts of Interest

Dr. Zeitler was funded by National Institutes of Health (NIH) T-32 training grant #2 T32 HL 69749-11 A1; however, no relationships exist related to the content presented. Dr. Greenfield reports no conflict of interest. Dr. Piccini receives grants for clinical research from Boston Scientific and St. Jude Medical and serves as a consultant to Medtronic.

TABLE 122.2 Comparison of recent professional society guidelines and recommendations

DOMAIN	HEART RHYTHM SOCIETY[14]		CANADIAN CARDIOVASCULAR SOCIETY[58]		INTERNATIONAL SOCIETY FOR HOLTER AND NONINVASIVE ELECTROCARDIOLOGY (ISHNE) AND EUROPEAN HEART RHYTHM ASSOCIATION (EHRA)[16]
	RECOMMENDATION	STRENGTH	RECOMMENDATION	STRENGTH	CONSENSUS[a]
Eligibility and application of RM for CIED patients	All CIED patients should be offered RM as part of standard management	Class I, LOE A	Integrate RM into routine care functions of CIED patients	Strong recommendation, moderate-quality evidence	RM transmissions between scheduled in-office visits can detect important events more quickly than traditional follow-up
	RM combined with ≥ annual follow-up is favorable over in-person evaluation alone	Class I, LOE A	Routine follow-up of CIED patients (after 3 months postimplantation) should include alternating RM and in-clinic visits in a 1:1 ratio	Conditional recommendation, low-quality evidence	Continuous patient and device RM as a replacement for some in-office follow-up visits would improve prevention, detection, and management of medical or technical events
			RM should be used to supplement in-person monitoring in clinical circumstances warranting more intensive surveillance	Strong recommendation, low-quality evidence	
Patient education	Before implementing RM, patients should be educated regarding their responsibilities and expectations; this should be documented in medical records	Class I, LOE E	RM should only be implemented after explicit consent and proper patient education including medico-legal implications and effects on patient privacy and confidentiality	Strong recommendation, very low-quality evidence	Patients need to be informed of the purposes and limitations of RM
					Before RM initiation, patients may be asked to sign an informed consent document, authorizing transmission of personal data to third parties
Frequency and initiation of RM	All CIEDs should be checked in a person 2–12 weeks postimplantation	Class I, LOE E	Follow-up of CIED patients should be done in person until 3 months postimplantation	Conditional recommendation, low-quality evidence	Automatic testing and data transmission may be especially important for potentially dangerous silent clinical or device events
	It may be beneficial to initiate RM within 2 weeks of implantation	Class IIa, LOE C			
Role of allied health care professionals	Allied health care providers responsible for interpreting RM should have the same qualifications as those performing in-clinic assessments	Class I, LOE E	Health care professionals responsible for RM interpretation and subsequent patient management decisions should have the same qualifications, training, and experience as those performing in-clinic assessments	Strong recommendation, low-quality evidence	N/A
RM program management	Develop and document appropriate policies and procedures to govern program operations, roles, and responsibilities of those involved and expected timelines for providing service	Class I, LOE E	Develop infrastructure, resources, policies, and procedures to optimally support an RM program analogous to in-clinic assessment	Strong recommendation, very low-quality evidence	Reimbursement policies for RM need to be enforced in a timely manner to remove barriers to more widespread use of RM; RM should not be limited by discriminative reimbursement policies
Recalls and advisories	Patients with a CIED component under advisory or recall should be enrolled in RM	Class I, LOE E	N/A		RM strongly benefits patients' safety specifically following an advisory
Role of industry representatives	Industry should refrain from direct patient care, either within the clinic or at home	Noted in the text only	Representatives of private industry involved in RM can provide support but should not be involved in RM-related patient care	Strong recommendation, very low-quality evidence	N/A

aThe document in this column is an expert consensus document without traditional recommendations for management.
CIED, Cardiac implantable electronic device; LOE, level of evidence; N/A, not addressed; RM, remote monitoring.

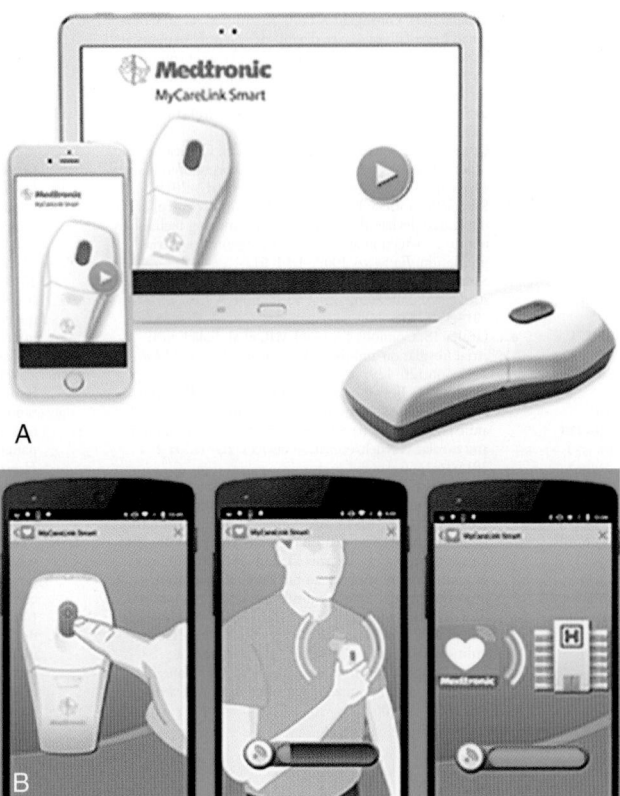

FIGURE 122.7 Use of Bluetooth technology that leverages patients' smartphones for remote transmissions. For some Medtronic devices, data are captured by the patient wand and transmitted wirelessly via Bluetooth to a software application running on a paired device. The data are then automatically forwarded via Internet connectivity to the manufacturer's server. (A) Representative image of the patient wand and potential paired devices (smartphone or tablet). (B) Excerpts from the patient-facing instructions for setup and transmission. (Images courtesy Medtronic, Minneapolis, MN.)

REFERENCES

1. Zhan C, Baine WB, Sedrakyan A, et al. Cardiac device implantation in the United States from 1997 through 2004: a population-based analysis. *J Gen Intern Med.* 2008;23:13–19.
2. Mond HG, Proclemer A. The 11th world survey of cardiac pacing and implantable cardioverter-defibrillators: calendar year 2009—a World Society of Arrhythmia's project. *Pacing Clin Electrophysiol.* 2011;34:1013–1027.
3. Varma N, Ricci RP. Telemedicine and cardiac implants: what is the benefit? *Eur Heart J.* 2013;34:1885–1895.
4. Parthiban N, Esterman A, Mahajan R, et al. Remote monitoring of implantable cardioverter-defibrillators: a systematic review and meta-analysis of clinical outcomes. *J Am Coll Cardiol.* 2015;65:2591–2600.
5. Morichelli L, Porfili A, Quarta L, et al. Implantable cardioverter defibrillator remote monitoring is well accepted and easy to use during long-term follow-up. *J Interv Card Electrophysiol.* 2014;41:203–209.
6. Petersen HH, Larsen MC, Nielsen OW, et al. Patient satisfaction and suggestions for improvement of remote ICD monitoring. *J Interv Card Electrophysiol.* 2012;34:317–324.
7. Ricci RP, Morichelli L, Quarta L, et al. Long-term patient acceptance of and satisfaction with implanted device remote monitoring. *Europace.* 2010;12:674–679.
8. Schoenfeld MH, Compton SJ, Mead RH, et al. Remote monitoring of implantable cardioverter defibrillators: a prospective analysis. *Pacing Clin Electrophysiol.* 2004;27:757–763.
9. Marzegalli M, Lunati M, Landolina M, et al. Remote monitoring of CRT-ICD: the multicenter Italian CareLink evaluation–ease of use, acceptance, and organizational implications. *Pacing Clin Electrophysiol.* 2008;31:1259–1264.
10. Hindricks G, Elsner C, Piorkowski C, et al. Quarterly vs. yearly clinical follow-up of remotely monitored recipients of prophylactic implantable cardioverter-defibrillators: results of the REFORM trial. *Eur Heart J.* 2014;35:98–105.
11. Ren X, Apostolakos C, Vo TH, et al. Remote monitoring of implantable pacemakers: in-office setup significantly improves successful data transmission. *Clin Cardiol.* 2013;36:634–637.
12. Rosenfeld LE, Patel AS, Ajmani VB, et al. Compliance with remote monitoring of ICDS/CRTDS in a real-world population. *Pacing Clin Electrophysiol.* 2014;37:820–827.
13. Varma N, Piccini JP, Snell J, et al. The relationship between level of adherence to automatic wireless remote monitoring and survival in pacemaker and defibrillator patients. *J Am Coll Cardiol.* 2015;65:2601–2610.
14. Slotwiner D, Varma N, Akar JG, et al. HRS Expert Consensus Statement on remote interrogation and monitoring for cardiovascular implantable electronic devices. *Heart Rhythm.* 2015;12:e69–e100.
15. Crossley GH, Boyle A, Vitense H, et al. The CONNECT (Clinical Evaluation of Remote Notification to Reduce Time to Clinical Decision) trial: the value of wireless remote monitoring with automatic clinician alerts. *J Am Coll Cardiol.* 2011;57:1181–1189.
16. Dubner S, Auricchio A, Steinberg JS, et al. ISHNE/EHRA expert consensus on remote monitoring of cardiovascular implantable electronic devices (CIEDs). *Europace.* 2012;14:278–293.
17. Slotwiner D, Wilkoff B. Cost efficiency and reimbursement of remote monitoring: a US perspective. *Europace.* 2013;15:i54–i58.
18. Dechert BE, Serwer GA, Bradley DJ, et al. Cardiac implantable electronic device remote monitoring surveillance in pediatric and congenital heart disease: utility relative to frequency. *Heart Rhythm.* 2015;12:117–122.
19. Leoni L, Padalino M, Biffanti R, et al. Pacemaker remote monitoring in the pediatric population: is it a real solution? *Pacing Clin Electrophysiol.* 2015;38:565–571.
20. Boyer SL, Silka MJ, Bar-Cohen Y. Current practices in the monitoring of cardiac rhythm devices in pediatrics and congenital heart disease. *Pediatr Cardiol.* 2015;36:821–826.
21. Mabo P, Victor F, Bazin P, et al. A randomized trial of long-term remote monitoring of pacemaker recipients (the COMPAS trial). *Eur Heart J.* 2012;33:1105–1111.
22. Al-Khatib SM, Piccini JP, Knight D, et al. Remote monitoring of implantable cardioverter defibrillators versus quarterly device interrogations in clinic: results from a randomized pilot clinical trial. *J Cardiovasc Electrophysiol.* 2010;21:545–550.
23. Varma N, Epstein AE, Irimpen A, et al. Efficacy and safety of automatic remote monitoring for implantable cardioverter-defibrillator follow-up: the Lumos-T Safely Reduces Routine Office Device Follow-up (TRUST) trial. *Circulation.* 2010;122:325–332.
24. Hindricks G, Taborsky M, Glikson M, et al. Implant-based multiparameter telemonitoring of patients with heart failure (IN-TIME): a randomised controlled trial. *Lancet.* 2014;384:583–590.
25. Boriani G, Da Costa A, Ricci RP, et al. The MOnitoring Resynchronization dEvices and CARdiac patiEnts (MORE-CARE) randomized controlled trial: phase 1 results on dynamics of early intervention with remote monitoring. *J Med Internet Res.* 2013;15:e167.
26. Guedon-Moreau L, Lacroix D, Sadoul N, et al. A randomized study of remote follow-up of implantable cardioverter defibrillators: safety and efficacy report of the ECOST trial. *Eur Heart J.* 2013;34:605–614.
27. Landolina M, Perego GB, Lunati M, et al. Remote monitoring reduces healthcare use and improves quality of care in heart failure patients with implantable defibrillators: the evolution of management strategies of heart failure patients with implantable defibrillators (EVOLVO) study. *Circulation.* 2012;125:2985–2992.
28. Saxon LA, Hayes DL, Gilliam FR, et al. Long-term outcome after ICD and CRT implantation and influence of remote device follow-up: the ALTITUDE survival study. *Circulation.* 2010;122:2359–2367.
29. Cronin EM, Ching EA, Varma N, et al. Remote monitoring of cardiovascular devices: a time and activity analysis. *Heart Rhythm.* 2012;9:1947–1951.
30. Raatikainen MJ, Uusimaa P, van Ginneken MM, et al. Remote monitoring of implantable cardioverter defibrillator patients: a safe, time-saving, and cost-effective means for follow-up. *Europace.* 2008;10:1145–1151.
31. Perl S, Stiegler P, Rotman B, et al. Socio-economic effects and cost saving potential of remote patient monitoring (SAVE-HM trial). *Int J Cardiol.* 2013;169:402–407.
32. Lazarus A. Remote, wireless, ambulatory monitoring of implantable pacemakers, cardioverter defibrillators, and cardiac resynchronization therapy systems: analysis of a worldwide database. *Pacing Clin Electrophysiol.* 2007;30:S2–S12.

33. Ricci RP, Morichelli L, Quarta L, et al. Effect of daily remote monitoring on pacemaker longevity: a retrospective analysis. *Heart Rhythm.* 2015;12:330–337.

34. Moss AJ, Schuger C, Beck CA, et al. Reduction in inappropriate therapy and mortality through ICD programming. *N Engl J Med.* 2012;367:2275–2283.

35. Hauser RG, Kallinen LM, Almquist AK, et al. Early failure of a small-diameter high-voltage implantable cardioverter-defibrillator lead. *Heart Rhythm.* 2007;4:892–896.

36. Guedon-Moreau L, Chevalier P, Marquie C, et al. Contributions of remote monitoring to the follow-up of implantable cardioverter-defibrillator leads under advisory. *Eur Heart J.* 2010;31:2246–2252.

37. Hauser RG, Abdelhadi R, McGriff D, et al. Deaths caused by the failure of Riata and Riata ST implantable cardioverter-defibrillator leads. *Heart Rhythm.* 2012;9:1227–1235.

38. Spencker S, Coban N, Koch L, et al. Potential role of home monitoring to reduce inappropriate shocks in implantable cardioverter-defibrillator patients due to lead failure. *Europace.* 2009;11:483–488.

39. Blanck Z, Axtell K, Brodhagen K, et al. Inappropriate shocks in patients with Fidelis(R) lead fractures: impact of remote monitoring and the lead integrity algorithm. *J Cardiovasc Electrophysiol.* 2011;22:1107–1114.

40. Ellenbogen KA, Gunderson BD, Stromberg KD, et al. Performance of Lead Integrity Alert to assist in the clinical diagnosis of implantable cardioverter defibrillator lead failures: analysis of different implantable cardioverter defibrillator leads. *Circ Arrhythm Electrophysiol.* 2013;6:1169–1177.

41. Catanzariti D, Lunati M, Landolina M, et al. Monitoring intrathoracic impedance with an implantable defibrillator reduces hospitalizations in patients with heart failure. *Pacing Clin Electrophysiol.* 2009;32:363–370.

42. van Veldhuisen DJ, Braunschweig F, Conraads V, et al. Intrathoracic impedance monitoring, audible patient alerts, and outcome in patients with heart failure. *Circulation.* 2011;124:1719–1726.

43. Whellan DJ, Ousdigian KT, Al-Khatib SM, et al. Combined heart failure device diagnostics identify patients at higher risk of subsequent heart failure hospitalizations: results from PARTNERS HF (Program to Access and Review Trending Information and Evaluate Correlation to Symptoms in Patients With Heart Failure) study. *J Am Coll Cardiol.* 2010;55:1803–1810.

44. Crossley GH, Chen J, Choucair W, et al. Clinical benefits of remote versus transtelephonic monitoring of implanted pacemakers. *J Am Coll Cardiol.* 2009;54:2012–2019.

45. Ricci RP, Morichelli L, Santini M. Remote control of implanted devices through Home Monitoring technology improves detection and clinical management of atrial fibrillation. *Europace.* 2009;11:54–61.

46. Sanna T, Diener HC, Passman RS, et al. Cryptogenic stroke and underlying atrial fibrillation. *N Engl J Med.* 2014;370:2478–2486.

47. Healey JS, Connolly SJ, Gold MR, et al. Subclinical atrial fibrillation and the risk of stroke. *N Engl J Med.* 2012;366:120–129.

48. Martin DT, Bersohn MM, Waldo AL, et al. Randomized trial of atrial arrhythmia monitoring to guide anticoagulation in patients with implanted defibrillator and cardiac resynchronization devices. *Eur Heart J.* 2015;36:1660–1668.

49. Institute PHR. Apixaban for the reduction of thromboembolism in patients with device-detected sub-clinical atrial fibrillation (ARTESiA). ClinicalTrials.gov [Internet]. Bethesda (MD): National Library of Medicine (US). 2015.

50. Guedon-Moreau L, Lacroix D, Sadoul N, et al. Costs of remote monitoring vs. ambulatory follow-ups of implanted cardioverter defibrillators in the randomized ECOST study. *Europace.* 2014;16:1181–1188.

51. Zanaboni P, Landolina M, Marzegalli M, et al. Cost-utility analysis of the EVOLVO study on remote monitoring for heart failure patients with implantable defibrillators: randomized controlled trial. *J Med Internet Res.* 2013;15:e106.

52. Klersy C, De Silvestri A, Gabutti G, et al. Economic impact of remote patient monitoring: an integrated economic model derived from a meta-analysis of randomized controlled trials in heart failure. *Eur J Heart Fail.* 2011;13:450–459.

53. Fauchier L, Sadoul N, Kouakam C, et al. Potential cost savings by telemedicine-assisted long-term care of implantable cardioverter defibrillator recipients. *Pacing Clin Electrophysiol.* 2005;28:S255–S259.

54. Calo L, Gargaro A, De Ruvo E, et al. Economic impact of remote monitoring on ordinary follow-up of implantable cardioverter defibrillators as compared with conventional in-hospital visits. A single-center prospective and randomized study. *J Interv Card Electrophysiol.* 2013;37:69–78.

55. Burri H, Sticherling C, Wright D, et al. Cost-consequence analysis of daily continuous remote monitoring of implantable cardiac defibrillator and resynchronization devices in the UK. *Europace.* 2013;15:1601–1608.

56. Zabel M, Muller-Riemenschneider F, Geller JC, et al. Rationale and design of the MONITOR-ICD study: a randomized comparison of economic and clinical effects of automatic remote MONITORing versus control in patients with Implantable Cardioverter Defibrillators. *Am Heart J.* 2014;168:430–437.

57. Ricci RP, D'Onofrio A, Padeletti L, et al. Rationale and design of the health economics evaluation registry for remote follow-up: TARIFF. *Europace.* 2012;14:1661–1665.

58. Yee R, Verma A, Beardsall M, et al. Canadian Cardiovascular Society/Canadian Heart Rhythm Society joint position statement on the use of remote monitoring for cardiovascular implantable electronic device follow-up. *Can J Cardiol.* 2013;29:644–651.

59. de Cock CC, Elders J, van Hemel NM, et al. Remote monitoring and follow-up of cardiovascular implantable electronic devices in the Netherlands: an expert consensus report of the Netherlands Society of Cardiology. *Neth Heart J.* 2012;20:53–65.

123　Catheter Ablation: Technical Aspects

Eric Buch, Noel G. Boyle, and Kalyanam Shivkumar

Interventional cardiac electrophysiology requires energy delivery to myocardial tissue to render it nonexcitable, thereby preventing initiation or maintenance of cardiac arrhythmias. The goal of catheter-based ablation technologies is to create precise and permanent myocardial lesions and to minimize collateral damage. This chapter describes biophysical principles of lesion formation, reviews available energy sources for catheter ablation, and surveys evolving technologies for lesion formation (Table 123.1).

Historical Context of Catheter Ablation

The first catheter-based method of ablating cardiac tissue—high-energy direct current (DC) shock—was reported in 1982. To ablate the atrioventricular (AV) node, DC shocks from an external defibrillator were delivered to the heart via a transvenous electrode catheter positioned adjacent to the His bundle.[1] This procedure was effective but caused significant complications, including cardiac perforation and tamponade, with in-hospital mortality rates approaching 6%. Safer methods of creating ablative lesions were needed for catheter-based ablation to gain widespread acceptance. The application of radiofrequency (RF) ablation in the treatment of cardiac arrhythmias was first reported by Huang and colleagues in 1985[2] and quickly became recognized as both safer and more effective. RF ablation was rapidly incorporated in the treatment of multiple arrhythmias, including Wolff-Parkinson-White (WPW) syndrome,[3] supraventricular tachycardia (SVT),[4] atrial flutter,[5] and ventricular tachycardia (VT).[6]

Radiofrequency Ablation

Since the 1980s, RF catheter ablation has revolutionized the treatment of cardiac arrhythmias, providing long-term curative therapy for many arrhythmias without the need for medications. This section discusses the biophysics of RF catheter ablation.

Radiofrequency Energy Sources

Most cardiac ablation systems deliver RF energy between a unipolar platinum-iridium electrode at the tip of the ablation catheter and a large dispersive grounding patch on the patient's skin, typically on the abdomen or thigh. As RF current passes from the tip of the ablation catheter to the grounding patch, resistive heating occurs in the intervening tissue at a rate proportional to the square of current density. Current density is highest in the immediate vicinity of the ablation catheter tip, which has a small surface area. As a result, significant resistive heating occurs only at the catheter tip–tissue interface and in a small volume of surrounding tissue. Deeper lesions result from conductive heating of myocardium adjacent to the site of resistive heating. Significant tissue heating during RF delivery causes changes in tissue electrical properties that are usually associated with impedance drops of 5–10 ohms.

Electromagnetic energy is delivered via a catheter to the targeted tissue until it is adequately heated to cause irreversible thermal damage. The RF spectrum refers to the oscillating electrical current in the range of frequencies from 3 kHz to 300 GHz. RF generators typically deliver unmodulated sine wave alternating current at frequencies between 500 and 1000 kHz, which oscillates too rapidly to depolarize myocardium and induce arrhythmias or to depolarize neurons and create the sensation of electrical current.

Heat Transfer to Tissue in Radiofrequency Ablation

In *resistive heating*, energy dissipated per unit time (W) is directly proportional to current and voltage, as described by the power equation:

$$W = VI = (IR)\,I = I^2 R \text{ (watts)}$$

(V is voltage, I is current, R is resistance, and V = IR by Ohm's law.)

Because current disperses radially from the electrode tip, current density is inversely proportional to the square of the distance from the catheter tip. Therefore, at double the distance from the catheter tip, current density is 75% lower. This is specified by the current density (Q) equation for a spherical electrode:

$$Q = 1/4\pi r^2 \,\left(\text{amp/cm}^2\right)$$

Resistive heating is proportional to the square of current density, which means that heat generated directly by RF energy is inversely related to the fourth power of the distance from the catheter tip. Therefore, at double the distance from the catheter tip, resistive heating is 94% lower. Because of this rapid reduction in heating with distance, lesions created by RF energy are

TABLE 123.1 Comparison of energy sources for catheter ablation

SOURCE	ENERGY SPECTRUM	MECHANISM OF INJURY	CONTACT
Radiofrequency	500–1000 kHz	Resistive heating	Critical
Cryotherapy	Cooling to –75°C	Direct cell injury	Critical
HIFU	20 kHz–200 MHz	Dielectric heating	Not critical
Laser	980-nm near-infrared light	Photonic heating	Not critical
Microwave	915 MHz or 2420 MHz	Dielectric heating	Not critical

HIFU, High-intensity focused ultrasound.

BOX 123.1 Signs of effective lesion formation with radiofrequency ablation

Sustained increase in catheter tip temperature (nonirrigated catheters)
Reduction in local electrogram amplitude
Decrease in impedance, usually 5–10 ohms
Appearance of split potentials reflecting local conduction block
Increase in the local capture threshold or rendering tissue nonexcitable
Adequate tissue contact force during ablation

BOX 123.2 Factors affecting lesion formation with radiofrequency ablation

Catheter tip–tissue contact force
Tip temperature achieved
Power delivered
Duration of energy delivery
Blood flow cooling
Active catheter tip cooling (irrigation)
Catheter tip orientation

---

typically small and well circumscribed. Only a 1- to 2-mm rim of tissue directly adjacent to the catheter tip is heated resistively; deeper tissues are heated by passive thermal conduction. This *conductive heating* is responsible for most of the lesion volume from RF ablation catheters.

Experimental studies have shown that irreversible loss of conduction occurs when tissue temperature exceeds 50°C for a sufficient duration.[7] The radius of the 50°C isotherm in the tissue, representing the lesion boundary, increases proportionally with the temperature of the catheter tip, up to the catheter tip–tissue interface temperatures of around 100°C. Plasma boils at higher temperatures, resulting in increased abrupt impedance, reduced current delivery, and ineffective tissue heating.[8] Such temperatures can also result in coagulum or char at the catheter tip and potential embolization.

To avoid excessive heating, RF ablation catheters incorporate thermocouples or thermistors for real-time monitoring of catheter tip temperature during ablation, allowing RF generators to titrate power based on a maximum preset catheter temperature. This is called *temperature-guided* mode, which is in contrast to *power-guided* mode wherein the operator manually sets the power. Although current technology does not allow direct measurement of myocardial tissue temperature, surrogate markers of tissue temperature and tissue destruction during RF ablation include impedance drop, electrogram amplitude reduction, and excitability loss with pacing (Box 123.1). With standard nonirrigated ablation catheters, the power output of the RF generator is usually adjusted manually or automatically to achieve a temperature of 50°C–60°C at the electrode–tissue interface.

The catheter tip–tissue contact is a key determinant of lesion formation with RF catheter ablation (Box 123.2). If the catheter does not directly contact myocardial tissue, a large proportion of energy delivered will dissipate in the blood pool without effective tissue heating. Operators rely on multiple sources of information to assess the catheter tip–tissue contact, including tactile feedback, fluoroscopic catheter movement, intracardiac echocardiography, catheter tip impedance, unipolar injury current, and electrogram variability from beat to beat. However, even with all of these data, significant discrepancies are seen between estimated and actual tissue contact force.[9] The most recent generation of RF ablation catheters incorporates sensors into the ablation catheter tip to estimate contact force and catheter orientation (Fig. 123.1). One technology incorporates three fiberoptic sensors in the catheter tip to measure deformation of the catheter tip, which is tightly correlated with the magnitude and vector of axial and lateral forces on the catheter tip (TactiCath, St. Jude Medical, Minneapolis, MN).[10] Another method relies on three magnetic sensors near the catheter tip to measure forces acting on a spring coil (SmartTouch, Biosense Webster, Diamond Bar, CA).[11] As expected, greater contact force results in larger lesions but more steam pops.[12] Higher contact force, especially during RF delivery, increases the odds of cardiac chamber perforation.[13] Clinical studies generally support the expectation that such catheters can improve both efficacy and safety of RF catheter ablation by helping the operator achieve sufficient but not excessive catheter tip–tissue contact and that clinical outcomes are improved when contact force is optimal—that is, 10–30 g in the left atrium.[14–16]

A major consideration for RF ablation is that catheter tip temperature can differ substantially from underlying tissue temperature because of the complex relationship between RF heating of adjacent tissue and convective cooling from intracavitary blood flow. This can result in a measured catheter tip temperature that is significantly lower than true tissue temperature, especially with larger-tip catheters, which are exposed to more convective cooling due to larger surface area. In fact, tissue temperatures can exceed 100°C, even while a much lower temperature is recorded from the catheter tip. This can boil fluid within the tissue, resulting in an explosive steam pop, damage to adjacent structures, crater formation, cardiac perforation, and tamponade.

A typical 7-French diameter RF ablation catheter with a 4-mm–long ablation electrode tip creates a lesion with 5- to 6-mm diameter and 2- to 3-mm depth. RF ablation catheters with 8- to 10-mm tips expose a greater surface area of the ablation electrode to the blood pool, increasing convective cooling at any given level of blood flow and creating a larger tissue–catheter tip interface, which results in larger lesions. As described in detail later, irrigated RF ablation catheters allow delivery of more power without excessive heating at the catheter tip, resulting in larger lesions (Fig. 123.2).

An alternative to the conventional platinum-iridium RF ablation catheter tip is the gold-tip ablation catheter, which provides much higher thermal conductivity and allows greater power delivery without excessive heating of the catheter tip–tissue interface in vitro.[17] Theoretically, this should result in more effective lesion formation, but clinical studies have not demonstrated increased efficacy in the treatment of common arrhythmias.[18,19] In the future, other elements, compounds, or alloys may prove superior to platinum-iridium for catheter tip construction.

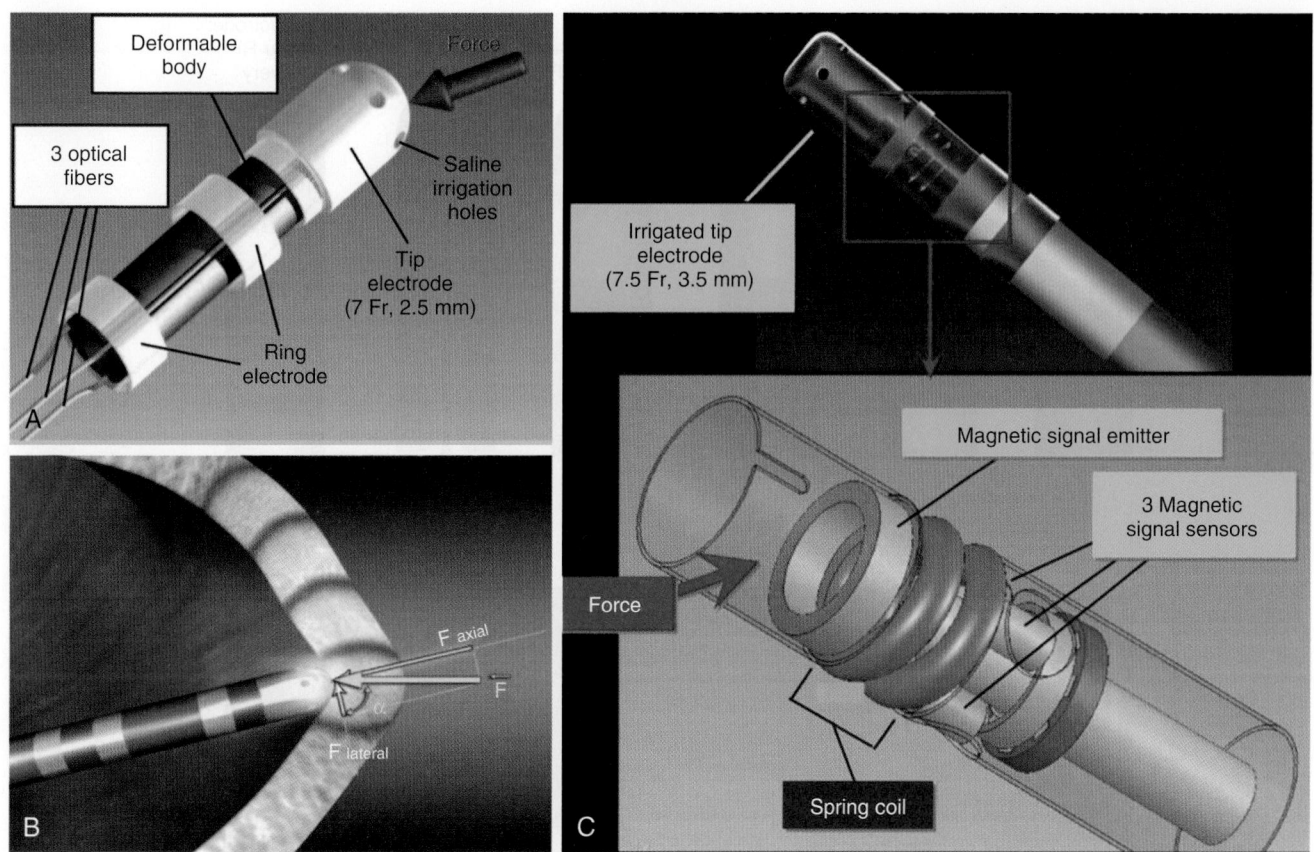

FIGURE 123.1 Design of contact force-sensing catheters. (A) Force on the deformable body of the catheter tip changes the reflected wavelength of light in three optic fibers (Fabry-Perot interferometer), allowing the calculation of the contact force (TactiCath, St. Jude Medical, St. Paul, MN). (B) Current systems can display total force magnitude and orientation, as well as axial and lateral constituents of the contact force. (C) Magnetic sensors near the catheter tip determine the proximity of a magnetic spring coil, which varies based on the magnitude and direction of the contact force (SmartTouch, Biosense Webster, Diamond Bar, CA). ([A] and [B] from Yokoyama K, Nakagawa H, Shah DC, et al. Novel contact force sensor incorporated in irrigated radiofrequency ablation catheter predicts lesion size and incidence of steam pop and thrombus. *Circ Arrhythm Electrophysiol.* 2008;1:354-362; [C] from Nakagawa H, Kautzner J, Natale A, et al. Locations of high contact force during left atrial mapping in atrial fibrillation patients: electrogram amplitude and impedance are poor predictors of electrode-tissue contact force for ablation of atrial fibrillation. *Circ Arrhythm Electrophysiol.* 2013;6:746-753.)

Limitations of Standard Catheter-Based Radiofrequency Ablation

One challenge of RF ablation is the lack of information about true tissue temperature. Another issue is delayed tissue injury after RF application; because most tissue heating is conductive, the temperature can continue to increase after the termination of RF delivery, with the potential for late lesion growth and collateral damage. Challenges have also arisen during RF energy delivery in the pericardial space. Uncooled RF catheters reach high temperatures quickly in this confined space without cooling blood flow, limiting energy delivery. Therefore internally or externally cooled catheters are usually chosen.

A challenge for all ablation technologies is creating permanent transmural lesions. Nontransmural lesions may be associated with temporary conduction block due to edema or transient tissue injury, then subsequent recovery of conduction and recurrence of arrhythmia. Because most RF ablation catheters deliver energy to a single point, creating a line of contiguous lesions can be difficult; this becomes more significant for longer lines of ablation. Gaps in lesion lines can be proarrhythmic, thereby acting as a zone of slow conduction and facilitating reentrant arrhythmias.

Advances in Radiofrequency Ablation

Newer catheters have been designed to address some of the special challenges encountered during RF ablation. Linear catheters with multiple electrodes, which can ablate sequentially or simultaneously, have been developed with the goal of creating more continuous linear lesions without gaps.[20,21] Bipolar RF catheters deliver current between two adjacent electrodes, rather than between one electrode and a grounding patch on the body surface. Duty-cycled phased RF systems alternate between uni- and bipolar energy delivery. These catheters were designed to facilitate pulmonary vein (PV) isolation and left atrial substrate modification, which can be technically demanding procedures requiring long contiguous lesion sets.[22] Acute and medium-term success rates for multielectrode catheters in the treatment of atrial flutter and atrial fibrillation (AF) are similar to those seen for conventional point-by-point ablation, with lower procedure and fluoroscopy times.[23,24] Controversy remains about whether nonirrigated multielectrode ablation catheters are associated with a greater risk for asymptomatic cerebral emboli, and effective strategies for minimizing these events have been demonstrated.[25,26]

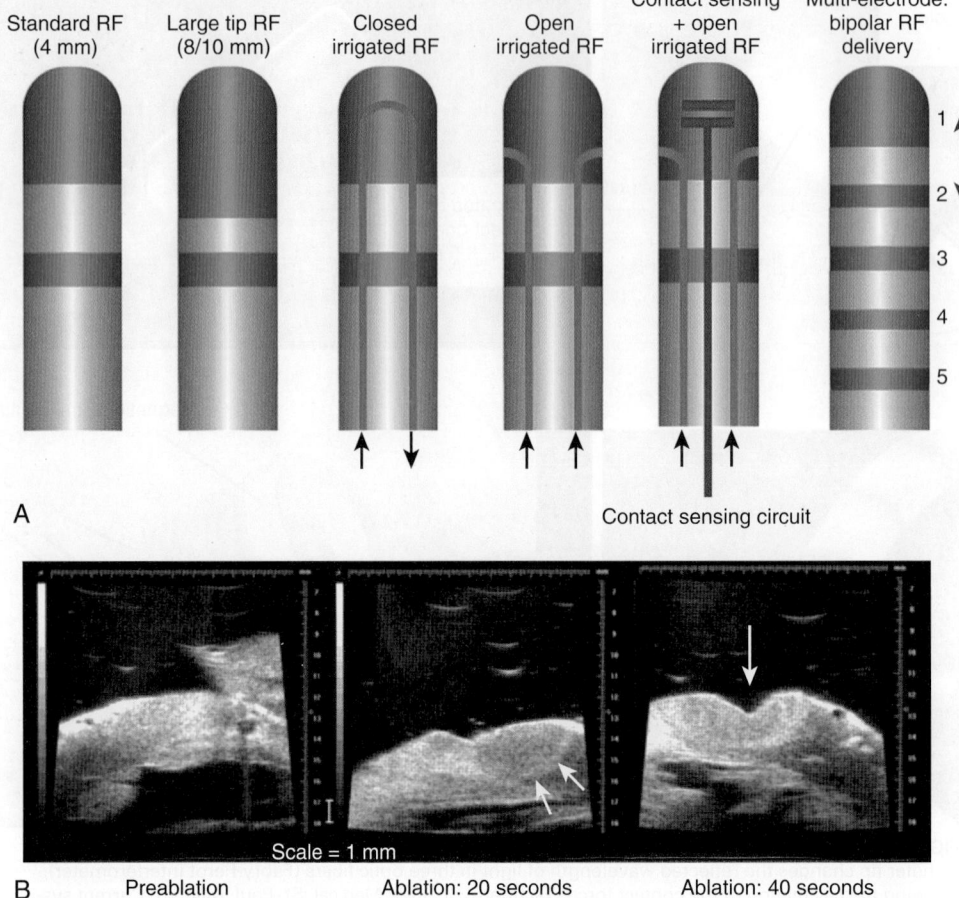

FIGURE 123.2 (A) Currently available radiofrequency (*RF*) ablation catheter designs. For irrigated catheters, *black arrows* represent flow of saline irrigation. For bipolar RF catheter, *red arrows* represent examples of bipoles between which RF energy can be delivered. (B) Lesion formation during RF delivery on the epicardial (*arrow*) surface of a Langendorff-perfused rabbit heart. This heart was imaged using a 30-MHz ultrasound system (VisualSonics, Toronto, Canada). (Courtesy Aman Mahajan, MD, PhD, UCLA.)

Radiofrequency Ablation With Irrigated Catheters

The development of irrigated or cooled-tip RF catheters was a major advance in RF ablation technology. With this approach the ablation catheter is irrigated with saline internally or externally during ablation, allowing greater power delivery with less catheter tip heating. This shifts the zone of maximal heating deeper into the tissue and increases the radius of resistive heating, resulting in larger and deeper lesions.[27] Because irrigation lowers the electrode–tissue interface temperature to well below 100°C, coagulum and impedance increases are rare. However, it is important to remember that with irrigated RF ablation, the temperature recorded at the catheter tip substantially underestimates the deeper tissue temperature,[28] potentially increasing the risk for steam pops and mechanical complications.[29,30]

The most common types of cooled-tip RF ablation catheters are closed-loop irrigated catheters, which circulate saline within the electrode tip to cool it internally, and open irrigation catheters, which flush saline through ports near the catheter tip to provide both internal and external cooling (see Fig. 123.2). Yokoyama and associates found that open-irrigated catheters resulted in greater interface cooling, lower tip temperature, and lower incidence of thrombus formation and steam pops than closed-loop irrigated catheters.[31] One disadvantage is that open irrigation can result in substantial intravenous saline infusion, occasionally leading to volume overload in patients with heart failure or renal insufficiency.

Irrigated ablation catheters are useful in epicardial ablation because in this space there is no convective cooling from circulating blood, resulting in high electrode temperatures and limited power delivery with standard nonirrigated catheters. D'Avila and coworkers compared the efficacy of standard versus cooled-tip RF catheters for epicardial ablation in animal models and found significantly larger lesions with irrigated catheters.[32] Externally irrigated catheters may infuse a substantial volume into the epicardial space, which must be periodically aspirated to avoid cardiac compression and tamponade physiology.

Cryoablation

Cryoablation employs extreme cooling to damage myocardial tissues and create nonconductive ablation lesions. The first application of cryoablation in the treatment of arrhythmia was described by Klein and colleagues for the epicardial ablation of accessory pathways using a surgical approach.[33] After intraoperative mapping localized the accessory pathway, a cryoprobe cooled to –60°C was applied to the target site to ablate the pathway.

Endovascular cryoablation systems use a steerable ablation catheter that can be cooled to –70°C or lower, resulting in tissue necrosis with a similar lesion size to that attained with irrigated RF ablation catheters.[34] Commercially available systems cool the catheter tip by delivering nitrous oxide under pressure via a hollow injection tube that spans the length of the ablation catheter into a widened lumen at the catheter tip. Nitrous oxide expands and decompresses within a small chamber at the catheter tip, resulting in cooling based on the Joule-Thomson effect. The cooled catheter then extracts heat from the tissue in contact with the distal electrode.[35] Similar to RF catheters, cryoablation systems can monitor tip temperature and adjust refrigerant flow to maintain a specified temperature.

Lesion formation in cryoablation occurs through direct cellular injury and vascular-mediated tissue injury. Direct injury results from ice formation, resulting in a hyperosmotic environment that causes cells to shrink and damages the plasma membrane. Irreversible cellular injury can also occur in the rewarming phase. Cooling myocardial tissue to temperatures low enough to result in extracellular ice formation causes cellular death when applied for prolonged periods. However, when only briefly cooled to this temperature, most cell damage is reversible, and cellular function usually recovers without permanent damage. This makes it possible to deliver a functionally reversible lesion in many cases. A technique referred to as *cryomapping* is accomplished by cooling tissue to −30°C for 30–60 seconds to identify transient physiological changes, such as abolition of accessory pathway conduction or prolongation of the A-H interval.[36] If cryomapping achieves the desired result without signs of collateral damage, a cryoablation lesion is delivered at the same location by maintaining a tissue–catheter tip interface temperature below −50°C for 4 minutes, resulting in irreversible tissue destruction. Another useful feature of cryoablation is catheter stability during ablation, resulting from *cryoadhesion* of catheter to tissue resulting from ice formation.

In addition to direct tissue injury, cryoablation also results in lesion formation via vascular-mediated tissue necrosis. Initially, the application of cryothermal energy results in decreased perfusion from vasoconstriction. When tissue temperature drops to below freezing, circulation ceases, resulting in tissue damage via ischemic necrosis, as well as endothelial damage, platelet aggregation, and microthrombus formation. Subsequently, rewarming of frozen tissue causes hyperemia, with increased vascular permeability and edema.

In catheter-based focal cryoablation systems, the coldest area is adjacent to the catheter tip, and the effects are first observed at these sites. Farther away, at the periphery of the cryoablation lesion, cooling is delayed and of a lower magnitude, often resulting in reversible tissue damage. Thus effects noted late during the application of cryoenergy are less likely to be permanent and may reverse upon rewarming. In general, ablation success is correlated with early functional modification, usually within 30–60 seconds of cryoenergy application.

Cryoenergy has been used in several different forms for myocardial lesion formation to treat cardiac arrhythmias. In surgical AF ablation, epicardial cryoenergy can be applied to isolate PVs.[37] Ventricular arrhythmias have also been treated with epicardial cryoablation.[38] Percutaneous endocardial catheter cryoablation is also used in the treatment of arrhythmia. An early application of focal cryoenergy catheter ablation was slow pathway ablation in the treatment of AV node reentrant tachycardia (AVNRT). Cryoablation is useful in this setting because of the proximity of the compact AV node and concerns about iatrogenic AV block. In this or other high-risk areas (e.g., near the phrenic nerve, His bundle, or coronary artery), cryomapping allows assessment of the safety of a potential ablation site before ablation causes permanent irreversible tissue damage. A randomized comparison between cryoablation and conventional RF ablation for AVNRT showed equivalent acute success and no AV block in the cryoablation group but with a higher risk for recurrence (9.4% vs. 4.4%).[39] The potential benefits of cryoablation over RF ablation must be weighed against the possibility of higher risk for recurrence and reoperation.

Another promising application of cryoablation is ablation of accessory pathways in high-risk anatomical locations, such as near the native conduction system or within the coronary sinus, in which application of RF energy carries a higher risk for complications. Concerns about durable efficacy persist; for accessory pathways located within the coronary sinus, Collins and colleagues

reported only 71% acute success and 40% risk for recurrence.[40] Cryoablation has also been used in the treatment of typical right atrial flutter, resulting in longer procedural times, similar acute outcomes, and improved patient tolerability.[41]

Endocardial cryoablation is an increasingly common modality for PV isolation in the treatment of AF (Fig. 123.3). In this system, a catheter delivers nitrous oxide to an inner balloon, where it undergoes a phase change resulting in a temperature drop to near −80°C. The balloon catheter has a central lumen for a spiral mapping catheter to guide balloon position, reduce perforation risk, and record PV potentials during ablation. Kinetics of tissue destruction are similar to RF ablation, related both to proximity of targeted tissue to cryoballoon surface, and duration of energy application (Fig. 123.4). In a multicenter study, 97% of 1403 PVs were acutely isolated using cryothermal energy delivered via a balloon catheter, and 1-year outcomes were similar to those observed with RF ablation.[42] The randomized STOP-AF trial found that cryoballoon ablation was more effective than antiarrhythmic drugs for rhythm control (70% vs. 7% success at 1 year) but with 11% risk for transient or persistent phrenic nerve injury.[43] Besides phrenic nerve injury, other complications have been observed, including PV stenosis[44] and esophageal injury.[45] The second-generation cryoballoon, which uses multiple nitrous oxide jets to cool the entire distal hemisphere of the balloon, is likely to be more effective but with greater potential for damage to adjacent anatomical structures.[46,47] Current evidence suggests that cryoballoon and RF ablation have similar efficacy and safety for PV isolation with shorter procedure time,[48–50] recently confirmed in a large randomized study comparing the two approaches.[51]

Laser Catheter Ablation

In laser ablation, a high-intensity coherent beam at a precise frequency of the electromagnetic spectrum is used to deliver energy. Absorbed laser energy causes tissue ablation by heating and evaporation. Balloon-based laser ablation technologies are under development for PV isolation (see Fig. 123.3). A catheter combining a variable-diameter compliant balloon with an endoscope for tissue visualization and a 980-nm near-infrared diode laser for lesion formation received premarket approval for clinical use by the US Food and Drug Administration in 2016 (CardioFocus, Marlborough, MA). In a feasibility study, 91% of 116 PVs were successfully isolated using this technology, although adverse events of phrenic nerve palsy, stroke, and cardiac tamponade were observed.[52] This technology does not deliver circumferential energy as does the cryoballoon, potentially avoiding critical structures. PV isolation appears to be durable with laser balloon technology; in one study, 86% of PVs remained isolated at an average of 3 months later.[53] The first randomized controlled trial of laser balloon versus RF ablation for AF showed similar safety and efficacy in the two treatment arms.[54]

High-Intensity Focused Ultrasound Catheter Ablation

High-intensity focused ultrasound (HIFU) uses ultrasonic energy in the frequency range of 20 kHz–200 MHz to create focused thermal ablation lesions by molecular vibration and friction, without affecting intervening structures (Fig. 123.5). HIFU energy delivered circumferentially via a balloon at the PV ostium was developed for PV isolation. Although early studies showed promise, significant complications, including phrenic nerve palsy and fatal atrioesophageal fistula, were observed.[55] Human trials of this technology (ProRhythm, Ronkonkoma, NY) were suspended because of safety concerns. Another possible application of HIFU is for surgical epicardial ablation, although preliminary results have not shown a high rate of PV isolation.[56]

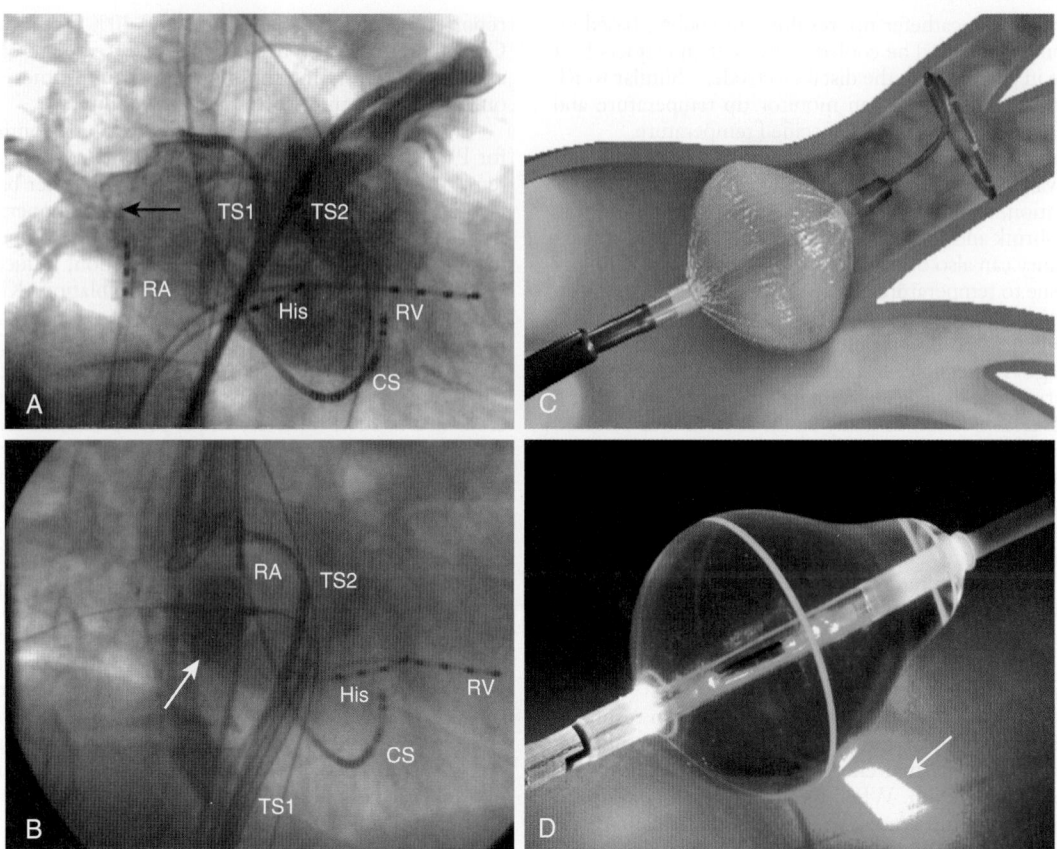

FIGURE 123.3 Balloon-based catheter ablation. (A) A right anterior oblique (RAO) fluoroscopic image showing left atrial and pulmonary vein (PV) angiography via a transseptal sheath (*arrow* shows the right PV antrum). A second transseptal sheath has selectively engaged the left superior PV. (B) An RAO fluoroscopic image of a balloon ablation catheter engaging the right inferior PV ostium (*white arrow*). A circular mapping catheter is positioned at the right superior PV ostium. (C) A schematic of the Arctic Front Advance cryoballoon engaged in the PV–left atrial junction (Medtronic, Minneapolis, MN). (D) A visually guided laser balloon catheter (HeartLight, CardioFocus, Marlborough, MA), a variable-diameter compliant balloon delivered through a 12-F deflectable sheath. *CS,* Coronary sinus catheter; *His,* His bundle catheter; *RA,* right atrial catheter; *RV,* right ventricular catheter; *TS1* and *TS2,* transseptal sheaths. ([D] From Dukkipati SR, Cuoco F, Kutinsky I, et al. Pulmonary vein isolation using the visually guided laser balloon: a prospective, multicenter, and randomized comparison to standard radiofrequency ablation. *J Am Coll Cardiol.* 2015;66:1350-1360.)

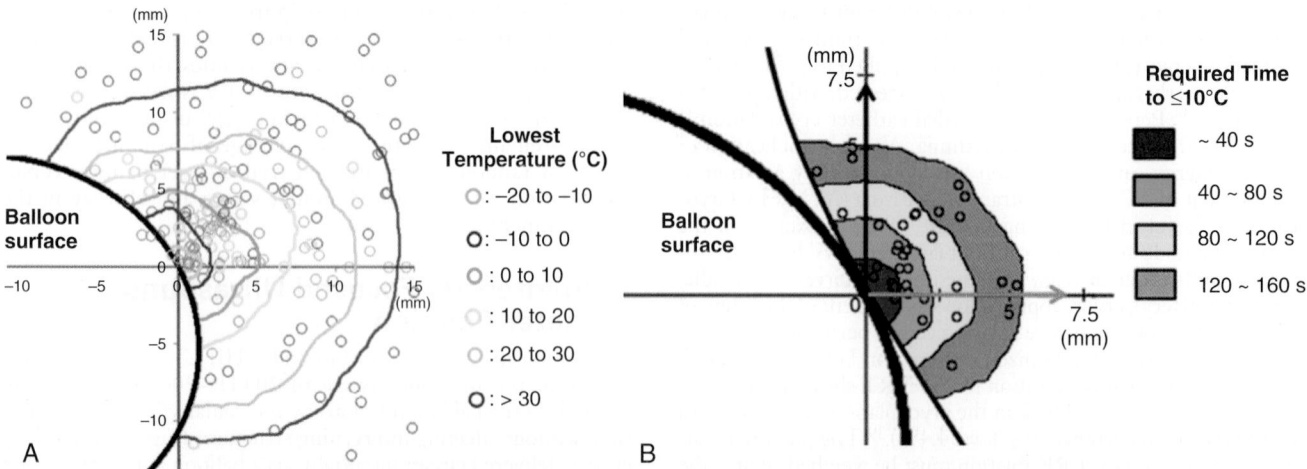

FIGURE 123.4 Biophysics of cryoballoon ablation. (A) The lowest temperature distribution of thermocouples during a second-generation cryoballoon ablation in an animal model. Each point represents the location and tissue temperature achieved in relation to the balloon surface. (B) The time needed to cool the tissue to 10°C based on the proximity to the cryoballoon surface. During energy application, freezing of the tissue proceeds radially over time. (Modified from Takami M, Misiri J, Lehmann HI, et al. Spatial and time-course thermodynamics during pulmonary vein isolation using the second-generation cryoballoon in a canine in vivo model. *Circ Arrhythm Electrophysiol.* 2015;8:186-192.)

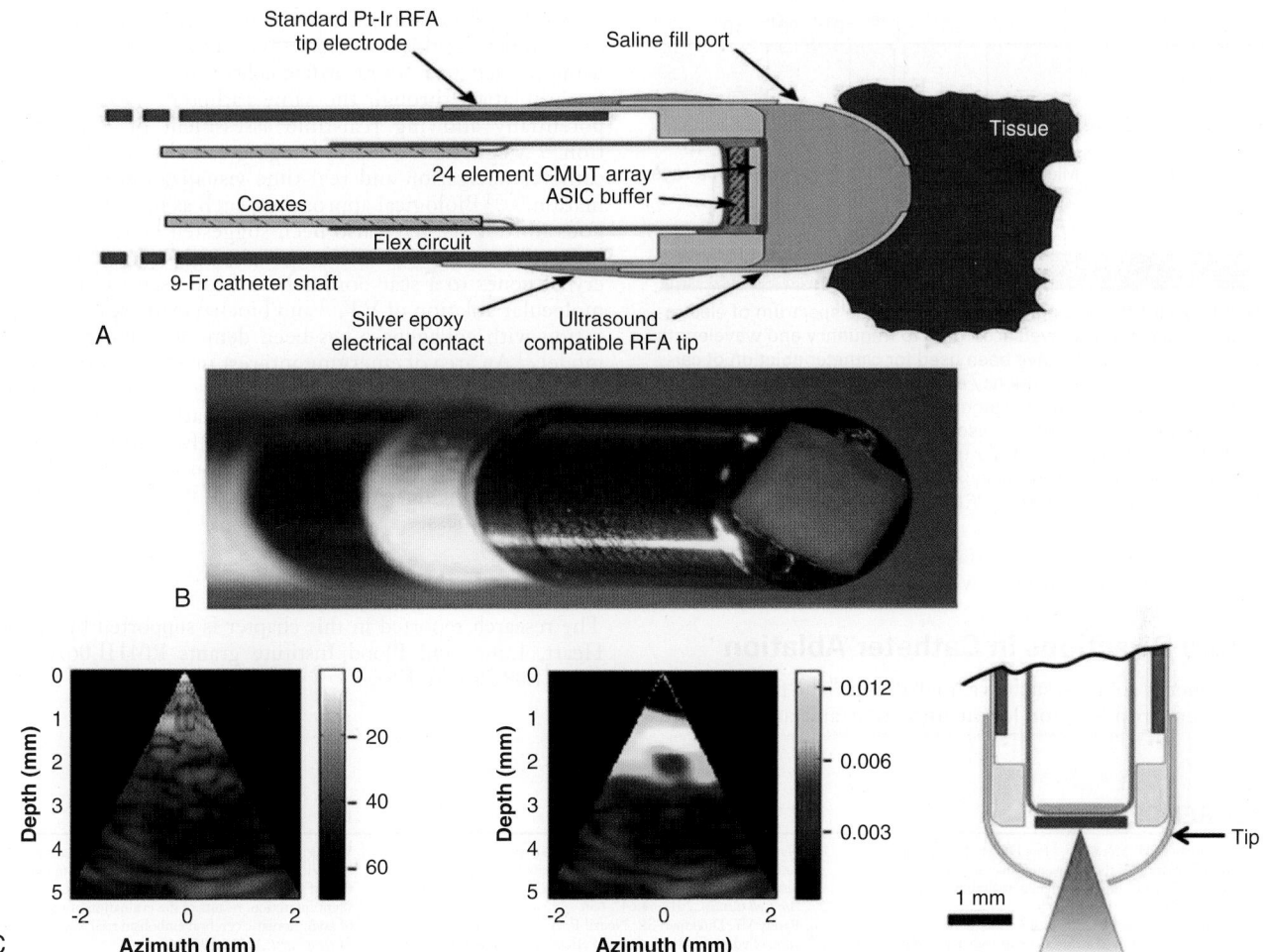

FIGURE 123.5 Multifunctional catheter: radiofrequency ablation (*RFA*), imaging, and tissue thermometry. (A) A graphical depiction of a microlinear capacitive micromachined ultrasound transducer (*CMUT*) catheter with a special ultrasound-transparent ablation tip, which contacts the endocardial wall for RFA and simultaneous thermal strain echo collection. *ASIC*, Application-specific integrated circuit; *Pt-Ir*, platinum-iridium. (B) An image of the catheter with the tip removed. (C) Thermal strain imaging based on in vivo real-time echo from porcine endocardium during ablation. The *left panel* is the unprocessed B-mode sector image in grayscale gradients on a decibel scale. The *middle panel* shows the ultrasound-based "strain" image of the tissue at 12 seconds after the start of ablation. The *color bar* depicts thermal strain, which can be converted to temperature. A schematic of the ultrasound-compatible RFA tip and the approximate ultrasound image sector is shown at the *right* (the tip is attached to the catheter shown in [B]). (From Stephens DN, Truong UT, Nikoozadeh A, et al. First in vivo use of a capacitive micromachined ultrasound transducer array-based imaging and ablation catheter. *J Ultrasound Med.* 2012;31:247-256.)

Microwave Catheter Ablation

Microwave energy (frequency range, 300 MHz–300 GHz) can produce an electrical field that results in oscillation of water molecules in tissue, causing *dielectrical heating*. Most commercially available generators operate at 915 or 2420 MHz (Fig. 123.6). The amount of energy absorbed depends on dielectric permittivity, which varies with water content. Microwave energy penetrates up to four times deeper in fat compared with blood or muscle, propagating through tissue with low water content and delivering energy to tissue with higher water content, such as myocardium.[57] As with other energy sources, conductive heating affects myocardium adjacent to directly heated tissue. Unlike RF energy, however, microwave ablation does not require tissue contact or a dispersive electrode and can penetrate more deeply than RF.

Microwave catheter ablation has been used to achieve bidirectional cavotricuspid isthmus block in seven consecutive patients with isthmus-dependent atrial flutter.[58] In preclinical studies, microwave noncontact catheters have been used to create a line of conduction block in the right atrium and deliver energy circumferentially to model PV antra.[59,60] Eventually, this technology may improve our ability to quickly create contiguous linear lesions without conduction gaps.

Robotic Catheter Ablation

Currently two systems—the magnetically guided Niobe system[61] (Stereotaxis Inc., St. Louis, MO) and the robotically driven Sensei system[62] (Hansen Medical, Mountain View, CA)—are widely used, and additional technologies are in development. These systems aim to provide ease of navigation and increased catheter stability, potentially with reduced radiation exposure. Availability of an irrigated tip catheter for the magnetically guided system has increased the utility of this system for AF and VT ablation procedures.[61]

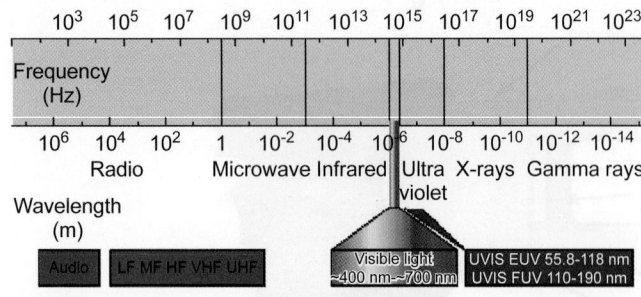

FIGURE 123.6 Electromagnetic spectrum. The spectrum of electromagnetic waves is displayed according to frequency and wavelength. Various energy sources have been used for catheter ablation of cardiac arrhythmias. Radiofrequency energy is currently the most commonly used energy source in catheter ablation of cardiac arrhythmias. Microwave, laser, and ultrasound energy have also been used. *EUV,* Extreme ultraviolet; *FUV,* far ultraviolet; *HF,* high frequency; *LF,* low frequency; *MF,* mid frequency; *UHF,* ultrahigh frequency; *UVIS,* ultraviolet imaging spectrum; *VHF,* very high frequency.

Both systems have significant startup costs, and it remains to be assessed whether these benefits will outweigh the costs.

Future Directions in Catheter Ablation

Other energy sources, such as a hot balloon[63] and β-radiation,[64] have been proposed for lesion formation and are in various stages of development. Experimental catheters currently in development could allow electrophysiologists to collect images using phased array intracardiac echocardiography and to perform ablation through the same catheter[65] (see Fig. 123.5), potentially allowing real-time assessment of lesion formation.[66] Magnetic resonance imaging can also be used for both catheter navigation and real-time visualization of lesion formation.[67,68] Biological approaches, such as injection of autologous fibroblasts, have also been suggested as an approach for lesion formation.[69] Gene-based strategies that target delivery of genes to a scar border have been used successfully for molecular ablation of VT,[70] and bioenzymatic scar homogenization with collagenase has been demonstrated in an animal model.[71] An area of emerging interest involves optimizing epicardial ablation and delivery of energy; RF and cryoablation have been used in this location with catheters developed for endocardial use.[72] However, unipolar RF ablation remains the primary technology for lesion formation today and is likely to remain so in the near future because of its efficacy, safety, and cost effectiveness.

Acknowledgment

The research reported in this chapter is supported by National Heart, Lung, and Blood Institute grants R01HL067647 and R01HL084261 (to KS).

REFERENCES

1. Scheinman MM, Morady F, Hess DS, et al. Catheter-induced ablation of the atrioventricular junction to control refractory supraventricular arrhythmias. *JAMA.* 1982;248:851–855.
2. Huang SK, Jordan N, Graham AR. Closed-chest catheter desiccation of atrioventricular junction using radiofrequency energy: a new method of catheter ablation. *Circulation.* 1985;72:389.
3. Jackman WM, Wang XZ, Friday KJ, et al. Catheter ablation of accessory atrioventricular pathways (Wolff-Parkinson-White syndrome) by radiofrequency current. *N Engl J Med.* 1991;324:1605–1611.
4. Calkins H, Sousa J, el-Atassi R, et al. Diagnosis and cure of the Wolff-Parkinson-White syndrome or paroxysmal supraventricular tachycardias during a single electrophysiologic test. *N Engl J Med.* 1991;324:1612–1618.
5. Feld GK, Fleck RP, Chen PS, et al. Radiofrequency catheter ablation for the treatment of human type 1 atrial flutter. Identification of a critical zone in the reentrant circuit by endocardial mapping techniques. *Circulation.* 1992;86:1233–1240.
6. Stevenson WG, Khan H, Sager P, et al. Identification of reentry circuit sites during catheter mapping and radiofrequency ablation of ventricular tachycardia late after myocardial infarction. *Circulation.* 1993;88:1647–1670.
7. Haines DE. The biophysics of radiofrequency catheter ablation in the heart: the importance of temperature monitoring. *Pacing Clin Electrophysiol.* 1993;16:586–591.
8. Haemmerich D. Biophysics of radiofrequency ablation. *Crit Rev Biomed Eng.* 2010;38:53–63.
9. Burkhardt JD, Natale A. New technologies in atrial fibrillation ablation. *Circulation.* 2009;120:1533–1541.
10. Yokoyama K, Nakagawa H, Shah DC, et al. Novel contact force sensor incorporated in irrigated radiofrequency ablation catheter predicts lesion size and incidence of steam pop and thrombus. *Circ Arrhythm Electrophysiol.* 2008;1:354–362.
11. Nakagawa H, Kautzner J, Natale A, et al. Locations of high contact force during left atrial mapping in atrial fibrillation patients: electrogram amplitude and impedance are poor predictors of electrode-tissue contact force for ablation of atrial fibrillation. *Circ Arrhythm Electrophysiol.* 2013;6:746–753.
12. Thiagalingam A, D'Avila A, Foley L, et al. Importance of catheter contact force during irrigated radiofrequency ablation: evaluation in a porcine ex vivo model using a force-sensing catheter. *J Cardiovasc Electrophysiol.* 2010;21:806–811.
13. Perna F, Heist EK, Danik SB, et al. Assessment of catheter tip contact force resulting in cardiac perforation in swine atria using force sensing technology. *Circ Arrhythm Electrophysiol.* 2011;4:218–224.

14. Natale A, Reddy VY, Monir G, et al. Paroxysmal AF catheter ablation with a contact force sensing catheter: results of the prospective, multicenter SMART-AF trial. *J Am Coll Cardiol.* 2014;64:647–656.
15. Reddy VY, Dukkipati SR, Neuzil P, et al. Randomized, controlled trial of the safety and effectiveness of a contact force-sensing irrigated catheter for ablation of paroxysmal atrial fibrillation: results of the TactiCath Contact Force Ablation Catheter Study for Atrial Fibrillation (TOCCASTAR) study. *Circulation.* 2015;132:907–915.
16. Kautzner J, Neuzil P, Lambert H, et al. EFFICAS II: optimization of catheter contact force improves outcome of pulmonary vein isolation for paroxysmal atrial fibrillation. *Europace.* 2015;17:1229–1235.
17. Lewalter T, Bitzen A, Wurtz S, et al. Gold-tip electrodes–a new "deep lesion" technology for catheter ablation? In vitro comparison of a gold alloy versus platinum-iridium tip electrode ablation catheter. *J Cardiovasc Electrophysiol.* 2005;16:770–772.
18. Sacher F, O'Neill MD, Jais P, et al. Prospective randomized comparison of 8-mm gold-tip and 8-mm platinum-iridium tip catheters for cavotricuspid isthmus ablation. *J Cardiovasc Electrophysiol.* 2007;18:709–713.
19. Stuhlinger M, Steinwender C, Schnoll F, et al. GOLD-ART—Gold Alloy Versus Platinum-Iridium Electrode for Ablation of AVNRT. *J Cardiovasc Electrophysiol.* 2008;19:242–246.
20. Boll S, Dang L, Scharf C. Linear ablation with duty-cycled radiofrequency energy at the cavotricuspid isthmus. *Pacing Clin Electrophysiol.* 2010;33:444–450.
21. Fredersdorf S, Weber S, Jilek C, et al. Safe and rapid isolation of pulmonary veins using a novel circular ablation catheter and duty-cycled RF generator. *J Cardiovasc Electrophysiol.* 2009;20:1097–1101.
22. Scharf C, Boersma L, Davies W, et al. Ablation of persistent atrial fibrillation using multielectrode catheters and duty-cycled radiofrequency energy. *J Am Coll Cardiol.* 2009;54:1450–1456.
23. Erdogan A, Guettler N, Doerr O, et al. Randomized comparison of multipolar, duty-cycled, bipolar-unipolar radiofrequency versus conventional catheter ablation for treatment of common atrial flutter. *J Cardiovasc Electrophysiol.* 2010;21:1109–1113.
24. Tivig C, Dang L, Brunner-La Rocca HP, et al. Duty-cycled unipolar/bipolar versus conventional radiofrequency ablation in paroxysmal and persistent atrial fibrillation. *Int J Cardiol.* 2012;157:185–191.
25. Herrera Siklody C, Deneke T, Hocini M, et al. Incidence of asymptomatic intracranial embolic events after pulmonary vein isolation: comparison of different atrial fibrillation ablation technologies in a multicenter study. *J Am Coll Cardiol.* 2011;58:681–688.

26. Verma A, Debruyne P, Nardi S, et al. Evaluation and reduction of asymptomatic cerebral embolism in ablation of atrial fibrillation, but high prevalence of chronic silent infarction: results of the evaluation of reduction of asymptomatic cerebral embolism trial. *Circ Arrhythm Electrophysiol.* 2013;6:835–842.
27. Wittkampf FH, Nakagawa H. RF catheter ablation: Lessons on lesions. *Pacing Clin Electrophysiol.* 2006;29:1285–1297.
28. Bruce GK, Bunch TJ, Milton MA, et al. Discrepancies between catheter tip and tissue temperature in cooled-tip ablation: relevance to guiding left atrial ablation. *Circulation.* 2005;112:954–960.
29. Seiler J, Roberts-Thomson KC, Raymond JM, et al. Steam pops during irrigated radiofrequency ablation: feasibility of impedance monitoring for prevention. *Heart Rhythm.* 2008;5:1411–1416.
30. Everett 4th TH, Lee KW, Wilson EE, et al. Safety profiles and lesion size of different radiofrequency ablation technologies: a comparison of large tip, open and closed irrigation catheters. *J Cardiovasc Electrophysiol.* 2009;20:325–335.
31. Yokoyama K, Nakagawa H, Wittkampf FH, et al. Comparison of electrode cooling between internal and open irrigation in radiofrequency ablation lesion depth and incidence of thrombus and steam pop. *Circulation.* 2006;113:11–19.
32. d'Avila A, Houghtaling C, Gutierrez P, et al. Catheter ablation of ventricular epicardial tissue: a comparison of standard and cooled-tip radiofrequency energy. *Circulation.* 2004;109:2363–2369.
33. Klein GJ, Guiraudon GM, Perkins DG, et al. Surgical correction of the Wolff-Parkinson-White syndrome in the closed heart using cryosurgery: a simplified approach. *J Am Coll Cardiol.* 1984;3:405–409.
34. Parvez B, Pathak V, Schubert CM, et al. Comparison of lesion sizes produced by cryoablation and open irrigation radiofrequency ablation catheters. *J Cardiovasc Electrophysiol.* 2008;19:528–534.
35. Cummings JE, Pacifico A, Drago JL, et al. Alternative energy sources for the ablation of arrhythmias. *Pacing Clin Electrophysiol.* 2005;28:434–443.
36. Wong T, Markides V, Peters NS, et al. Clinical usefulness of cryomapping for ablation of tachycardias involving perinodal tissue. *J Interv Card Electrophysiol.* 2004;10:153–158.
37. Christiansen S, Klocke A, Schmid M, et al. Short and midterm results of epi and endocardial cryoablation. *Ann Thorac Cardiovasc Surg.* 2010;16:340–344.
38. Choi EK, Nagashima K, Lin KY, et al. Surgical cryoablation for ventricular tachyarrhythmia arising from the left ventricular outflow tract region. *Heart Rhythm.* 2015;12:1128–1136.

39. Deisenhofer I, Zrenner B, Yin YH, et al. Cryoablation versus radiofrequency energy for the ablation of atrioventricular nodal reentrant tachycardia (the CYRANO study): results from a large multicenter prospective randomized trial. *Circulation*. 2010;122:2239–2245.

40. Collins KK, Rhee EK, Kirsh JA, et al. Cryoablation of accessory pathways in the coronary sinus in young patients: a multicenter study from the Pediatric and Congenital Electrophysiology Society's Working Group on Cryoablation. *J Cardiovasc Electrophysiol*. 2007;18:592–597.

41. Collins NJ, Barlow M, Varghese P, et al. Cryoablation versus radiofrequency ablation in the treatment of atrial flutter trial (CRAAFT). *J Interv Card Electrophysiol*. 2006;16:1–5.

42. Neumann T, Vogt J, Schumacher B, et al. Circumferential pulmonary vein isolation with the cryoballoon technique results from a prospective 3-center study. *J Am Coll Cardiol*. 2008;52:273–278.

43. Packer DL, Kowal RC, Wheelan KR, et al. Cryoballoon ablation of pulmonary veins for paroxysmal atrial fibrillation: first results of the North American Arctic Front (STOP AF) pivotal trial. *J Am Coll Cardiol*. 2013;61:1713–1723.

44. Thomas D, Katus HA, Voss F. Asymptomatic pulmonary vein stenosis after cryoballoon catheter ablation of paroxysmal atrial fibrillation. *J Electrocardiol*. 2011;44:473–476.

45. Stockigt F, Schrickel JW, Andrie R, et al. Atrioesophageal fistula after cryoballoon pulmonary vein isolation. *J Cardiovasc Electrophysiol*. 2012;23:1254–1257.

46. Kaszala K, Ellenbogen KA. Biophysics of the second-generation cryoballoon: cryobiology of the big freeze. *Circ Arrhythm Electrophysiol*. 2015;8:15–17.

47. Takami M, Misiri J, Lehmann HI, et al. Spatial and time-course thermodynamics during pulmonary vein isolation using the second-generation cryoballoon in a canine in vivo model. *Circ Arrhythm Electrophysiol*. 2015;8:186–192.

48. Luik A, Radzewitz A, Kieser M, et al. Cryoballoon versus open irrigated radiofrequency ablation in patients with paroxysmal atrial fibrillation: the prospective, randomized, controlled, noninferiority FreezeAF study. *Circulation*. 2015;132:1311–1319.

49. Hunter RJ, Baker V, Finlay MC, et al. Point-by-point radiofrequency ablation versus the cryoballoon or a novel combined approach: a randomized trial comparing 3 methods of pulmonary vein isolation for paroxysmal atrial fibrillation (the Cryo Versus RF Trial). *J Cardiovasc Electrophysiol*. 2015;26:1307–1314.

50. Kojodjojo P, O'Neill MD, Lim PB, et al. Pulmonary venous isolation by antral ablation with a large cryoballoon for treatment of paroxysmal and persistent atrial fibrillation: medium-term outcomes and non-randomised comparison with pulmonary venous isolation by radiofrequency ablation. *Heart*. 2010;96:1379–1384.

51. Kuck KH, Brugada J, Furnkranz A, et al. Cryoballoon or radiofrequency ablation for paroxysmal atrial fibrillation. *N Engl J Med*. 2016;374:2235–2245.

52. Reddy VY, Neuzil P, Themistoclakis S, et al. Visually-guided balloon catheter ablation of atrial fibrillation: experimental feasibility and first-in-human multicenter clinical outcome. *Circulation*. 2009;120:12–20.

53. Dukkipati SR, Neuzil P, Kautzner J, et al. The durability of pulmonary vein isolation using the visually guided laser balloon catheter: multicenter results of pulmonary vein remapping studies. *Heart Rhythm*. 2012;9:919–925.

54. Dukkipati SR, Cuoco F, Kutinsky I, et al. Pulmonary vein isolation using the visually guided laser balloon: a prospective, multicenter, and randomized comparison to standard radiofrequency ablation. *J Am Coll Cardiol*. 2015;66:1350–1360.

55. Neven K, Schmidt B, Metzner A, et al. Fatal end of a safety algorithm for pulmonary vein isolation with use of high-intensity focused ultrasound. *Circ Arrhythm Electrophysiol*. 2010;3:260–265.

56. Pozzoli A, Benussi S, Anzil F, et al. Electrophysiological efficacy of Epicor high-intensity focused ultrasound. *Eur J Cardiothorac Surg*. 2012;42:129–134.

57. Lin JC. Studies on microwaves in medicine and biology: from snails to humans. *Bioelectromagnetics*. 2004;25:146–159.

58. Chan JY, Fung JW, Yu CM, et al. Preliminary results with percutaneous transcatheter microwave ablation of typical atrial flutter. *J Cardiovasc Electrophysiol*. 2007;18:286–289.

59. Lim TW, Clout R, Barry MA, et al. Percutaneous microwave ablation with a long side-firing antenna array can successfully treat a nonsurgical chronic ovine atrial flutter model. *J Cardiovasc Electrophysiol*. 2009;20:1255–1261.

60. Qian P, Barry MA, Nguyen T, et al. A novel microwave catheter can perform noncontact circumferential endocardial ablation in a model of pulmonary vein isolation. *J Cardiovasc Electrophysiol*. 2015;26:799–804.

61. Bradfield J, Tung R, Mandapati R, et al. Catheter ablation utilizing remote magnetic navigation: a review of applications and outcomes. *Pacing Clin Electrophysiol*. 2012;35:1021–1034.

62. Aagaard P, Natale A, Di Biase L. Robotic navigation for catheter ablation: benefits and challenges. *Expert Rev Med Devices*. 2015;12:457–469.

63. Yamaguchi Y, Sohara H, Takeda H, et al. Long-term results of radiofrequency hot balloon ablation in patients with paroxysmal atrial fibrillation: safety and rhythm outcomes. *J Cardiovasc Electrophysiol*. 2015;26:1298–1306.

64. Guerra PG, Talajic M, Thibault B, et al. Beta-radiation for the creation of linear lesions in the canine atrium. *Circulation*. 2004;110:911–914.

65. Stephens DN, Truong UT, Nikoozadeh A, et al. First in vivo use of a capacitive micromachined ultrasound transducer array-based imaging and ablation catheter. *J Ultrasound Med*. 2012;31:247–256.

66. Wright M, Harks E, Deladi S, et al. Real-time lesion assessment using a novel combined ultrasound and radiofrequency ablation catheter. *Heart Rhythm*. 2011;8:304–312.

67. Ranjan R, Kholmovski EG, Blauer J, et al. Identification and acute targeting of gaps in atrial ablation lesion sets using a real-time magnetic resonance imaging system. *Circ Arrhythm Electrophysiol*. 2012;5:1130–1135.

68. Vergara GR, Vijayakumar S, Kholmovski EG, et al. Real-time magnetic resonance imaging-guided radiofrequency atrial ablation and visualization of lesion formation at 3 Tesla. *Heart Rhythm*. 2011;8:295–303.

69. Bunch TJ, Mahapatra S, Bruce GK, et al. Impact of transforming growth factor-beta1 on atrioventricular node conduction modification by injected autologous fibroblasts in the canine heart. *Circulation*. 2006;113:2485–2494.

70. Sasano T, McDonald AD, Kikuchi K, et al. Molecular ablation of ventricular tachycardia after myocardial infarction. *Nat Med*. 2006;12:1256–1258.

71. Yagishita D, Ajijola OA, Vaseghi M, et al. Electrical homogenization of ventricular scar by application of collagenase: a novel strategy for arrhythmia therapy. *Circ Arrhythm Electrophysiol*. 2013;6:776–783.

72. Boyle N, Shivkumar K. Epicardial interventions in electrophysiology. *Circulation*. 2012;126:1752–1769.

124 Catheter Ablation: Clinical Aspects

Luigi Di Biase, Philip Aagaard, Pasquale Santangeli, and Andrea Natale

The last decades have witnessed intense research directed toward the discovery and validation of electrophysiological and anatomical targets responsible for triggering and maintaining cardiac arrhythmias. Because it has curative potential, catheter ablation may, in many cases, be superior to other therapies, such as antiarrhythmic drugs (AADs). Several randomized clinical trials have demonstrated the benefits of catheter ablation, and today, catheter ablation has become an established treatment for a substantial proportion of patients with cardiac arrhythmias. Patient selection and peri- and postprocedural management are important clinical aspects that play key roles in appropriately planning the best ablation strategy, as well as predicting procedural outcomes. This chapter focuses on clinical aspects relevant to catheter ablation of cardiac arrhythmias, with an emphasis on the selection and clinical management of patients undergoing catheter ablation procedures. More detailed descriptions of clinical diagnoses, electrophysiological characteristics, and arrhythmia treatments are provided in other chapters of this book.

Preprocedural Management

Clinical Indications and Patient Selection

Supraventricular Arrhythmias

Supraventricular arrhythmias (SVAs) encompass a wide group of relatively common cardiac rhythm disturbances. They typically occur in repetitive bouts and are rarely life threatening.[1] In current guidelines, catheter ablation is a class I indication for patients with symptomatic SVAs who are drug resistant, drug intolerant, or do not want to undergo long-term drug therapy (Table 124.1).[1] Of note, the clinical effectiveness of AAD therapy in patients with SVAs is typically suboptimal, and patients often experience arrhythmia recurrence despite drug compliance. Furthermore, the risks associated with long-term AAD therapy are not negligible. Therefore most clinicians support the appropriateness of considering catheter ablation as first-line therapy for the majority of patients with symptomatic SVAs. Asymptomatic SVAs, on the other hand, have an overall benign prognosis, and invasive electrophysiological study and catheter ablation are rarely indicated.

Age and gender are important factors influencing both the prevalence and mechanisms of SVA. Age at tachycardia onset is typically higher (average of 30 years), and female gender is more prevalent in patients with atrioventricular node reentrant tachycardia (AVNRT) than in those with atrioventricular reentrant tachycardia (AVRT).[2] Female gender is also associated with a higher incidence of focal automatic atrial tachycardia (AT), especially during premenopause. On the other hand, females have a lower risk for sudden cardiac death in the presence of AV bypass tracts, related to the lower incidence of concomitant atrial fibrillation (AF).[2]

Although most patients with a history of SVAs are asymptomatic at the time of initial evaluation, careful history-taking might provide important clues regarding the SVA mechanism. This is relevant for planning the ablation procedure and also for predicting outcomes. Irregular palpitations may be caused by premature atrial contractions (PACs), AT, atrial flutter (AFL), or AF. Regular palpitations with abrupt onset and termination, on the other hand, are hallmarks of reentrant SVAs, such as AVNRT or AVRT. Termination of SVAs with vagal maneuvers or AV node–blocking agents supports the participation of the AV node in the SVA and suggests either AVNRT or AVRT. More severe symptoms, such as syncope or sudden cardiac arrest, suggest AF with a concomitant rapidly conducting AV bypass tract, an underlying cardiomyopathic substrate, and/or sinus node dysfunction leading to prolonged sinus arrest after SVA termination. Such symptoms warrant prompt intervention with invasive electrophysiological study and often require catheter ablation.

Importantly, in patients with persistent SVAs, such as focal AT, the main signs and symptoms may be related to heart failure (HF) secondary to tachycardia-induced cardiomyopathy, rather than palpitations. In a study of 345 patients undergoing radiofrequency (RF) catheter ablation of focal AT, 10% of patients had tachycardia-mediated cardiomyopathy.[3] Younger males (mean age, 39 ± 22 years vs. 51 ± 17 years; p = .006) and a relatively long tachycardia cycle length (502 ± 131 ms vs. 402 ± 105 ms; p < .001) were important predictors of cardiomyopathy development. Importantly, catheter ablation restored normal left ventricular function in almost all (97%) patients after a mean follow-up of 3 months.

With regard to patients with AV accessory connections, the clinical presentation may be highly variable, ranging from no symptoms to sudden cardiac arrest. Because of the unpredictable risk for sudden cardiac death, some clinicians also advocate early invasive risk stratification with an electrophysiological study in asymptomatic patients with manifest preexcitation. However, data have consistently shown that the actual risk for major cardiac events in patients with asymptomatic preexcitation is exceedingly low, which calls into question the appropriateness of such routine invasive management.[4]

When planning an ablation procedure for patients with accessory pathways, several clinical and electrocardiographic (ECG) characteristics are useful to determine the best ablation approach, as well as to predict procedural success and complication risk. From a clinical standpoint, it is important to emphasize that preexcitation syndromes can be associated with underlying structural heart disease, which might pose unique challenges during catheter ablation. Ebstein anomaly of the tricuspid valve is the most common form of congenital heart disease associated with accessory pathways (up to 10%–30% of cases), which are typically right sided and often multiple.[5] In these patients, catheter ablation of accessory pathways has been reported to have a slightly lower success rate, likely as a result of impaired catheter stability in the presence of an anatomically abnormal right AV groove.[5] Univentricular heart syndromes, atrial septal defects, and congenitally corrected transpositions of the great vessels are other examples of congenital heart diseases associated with the presence of accessory pathways. Recent data support the usefulness of remote magnetic navigation (RMN) for ablation in patients with corrected congenital heart disease.[6] Rarely, accessory AV

TABLE 124.1   Guideline indications for catheter ablation of cardiac arrhythmias

	CLASS I	CLASS II (IIa/IIb)	CLASS III
Supraventricular Arrhythmia			
AVNRT	• Hemodynamically unstable • Recurrent, symptomatic • Patients refractory, intolerant, or not willing to take AADs	—	—
AVRT	• Symptomatic arrhythmia • Preexcitation with AF and rapid conduction or poorly tolerated AVRT	• Asymptomatic preexcitation (IIa)	—
AT	• Recurrent symptomatic • Incessant AT	—	• Nonsustained and asymptomatic
Atrial Fibrillation			
PAF	• Symptomatic drug-refractory AF	• Symptomatic as first-line therapy (IIa)	—
NPAF	—	• Symptomatic drug-refractory persistent AF (IIa) • Symptomatic drug-refractory long-standing persistent AF (IIb) • Symptomatic as first-line therapy (IIb)	—
Ventricular Tachycardia			
Structural heart disease	• Symptomatic drug-refractory VT • Incessant sustained monomorphic VT • VT storm not because of a transient or reversible cause • Frequent PVCs, NSVTs, or VT that is presumed to cause ventricular dysfunction • Bundle branch reentrant or interfascicular VTs • Trigger-dependent sustained polymorphic VT or drug refractory VF	• ≥1 episode of sustained monomorphic drug-refractory VT • Recurrent sustained monomorphic VT, LVEF ≤ 30%, life expectancy ≥ 1 year • First-line therapy in hemodynamically stable VT and LVEF ≥ 35%	—
No structural heart disease	• Monomorphic VT, severely symptomatic • Monomorphic drug-refractory VT • Patients intolerant to AADs or not willing to take drugs • Recurrent trigger-dependent sustained polymorphic VT and VF (electrical storm) refractory to AADs	• Asymptomatic drug-refractory sustained VT or RV origin (IIa) • Symptomatic drug-refractory VT/PVCs originating from uncommon left ventricular sites (aortic SOV, epicardium) (IIb) • Asymptomatic drug-refractory sustained VT of LV origin (IIb)	• Asymptomatic and infrequent PVCs not causing cardiomyopathy

AADs, Antiarrhythmic drugs; *AF,* atrial fibrillation; *AVNRT,* atrioventricular node reentrant tachycardia; *AVRT,* atrioventricular reentrant tachycardia; *AT,* atrial tachycardia; *LV,* left ventricle; *LVEF,* left ventricular ejection fraction; *NPAF,* nonparoxysmal atrial fibrillation; *NSVT,* nonsustained ventricular tachycardia; *PAF,* paroxysmal atrial fibrillation; *PVCs,* premature ventricular contractions; *RV,* right ventricle; *SOV,* sinus of Valsalva; *VF,* ventricular fibrillation; *VT,* ventricular tachycardia.
From references 1, 12, 19, and 110.

connections could be iatrogenically provoked through surgical anastomosis of atrial tissue to the underlying ventricular myocardium when the Bjork variant of the Fontan operation is performed.[7] In these cases, an endocardial-only approach might be insufficient, given the possibility of epicardial connections at the level of the surgical anastomosis.

A careful family history is important in patients with Wolff-Parkinson-White syndrome to disclose rare forms of familial syndromes that are often associated with glycogen storage cardiomyopathy caused by a mutation in the *PRKAG2* gene.[8] Clinically, such patients typically display evidence of accessory AV connections (often fasciculoventricular pathways) and signs of left ventricular hypertrophy and are characterized by a high incidence of other cardiac rhythm disturbances such as sick sinus syndrome and complete AV block.[8]

When planning the ablation procedure in patients with an accessory pathway, proper recognition of pathways with high risk for iatrogenic AV block during ablation (i.e., antero- or midseptal pathways) or of those requiring special approaches, such as epicardial access for mapping and ablation, is of utmost importance. Antero- and midseptal pathways are typically characterized by a negative delta wave in lead V_1 with transition before lead V_3 and a frankly positive polarity in the inferior leads (i.e., DII, DIII, and aVF).[9] Some of these pathways are classified as para-Hisian; according to their initial description, a clear His bundle deflection (usually >0.1 mV) should be recorded on the ablation catheter in such cases, and the tip of the ablation catheter should overlap with the tip of a diagnostic His bundle catheter on any fluoroscopic view.[10] Therefore, by definition, para-Hisian pathways cannot be diagnosed on the basis of ECG criteria alone. Nonetheless, antero- or midseptal pathways are usually easily detected by means of ECG criteria. This is important for correctly informing patients about the estimated success and possible complications of the procedure and for advance planning of ablation with alternative sources of energy, such as cryoenergy (see Chapter 123).

Few clinical and ECG criteria have been proposed for selection of patients who are likely to require epicardial access for mapping and ablation of accessory pathways. Usually, these patients present after multiple failed endocardial procedures or have some peculiar clinical clues suggestive of epicardial AV connections, such as surgical anastomosis after the Fontan

TABLE 124.2 Baseline characteristics and main outcomes of randomized clinical trials evaluating catheter ablation as first-line therapy for paroxysmal atrial fibrillation (AF)

STUDY	YEAR	NO. OF PATIENTS	DESIGN	CA APPROACH	PRIMARY ENDPOINT	NO. OF INSTITUTIONS	FOLLOW-UP (MONTHS)	AF RECURRENCE AT FU (%)	COMPLICATIONS (%)
RAAFT[13]	2005	70	RFCA vs. AADs in patients with AF	PVAI with 8-mm NIC	AF recurrence	4	12	AADs 63[a] RFCA 13[a]	AADs 11.5 RFCA 12.5
MANTRA-PAF[14]	2011	294	RFCA vs. AADs in patients with paroxysmal AF	CPVA or PVAI, OIC, or 8-mm NIC	AF burden	10	24	AADs 29[a] RFCA 15[a]	AADs 19 RFCA 19
RAAFT-2[15]	2012	127	RFCA vs. AADs in patients with paroxysmal AF	PVAI with OIC	AF recurrences	16	25	AADs 72[a] RFCA 55[a]	AADs 19.5 RFCA 7.7

[a]$p < .05$.
AADs, Antiarrhythmic drugs; *CPVA,* circumferential pulmonary vein ablation; *FU,* follow-up; *NIC,* nonirrigated ablation catheter; *OIC,* open irrigated ablation catheter; *PVAI,* pulmonary vein antrum isolation; *RFCA,* radiofrequency catheter ablation.

operation, as was previously discussed. With regard to ECG criteria, some authors have suggested that a steeply negative delta wave in lead DII in the setting of a posteroseptal accessory pathway predicts the need for epicardial mapping and ablation,[10] although this criterion has not been adequately validated in large cohorts of patients. Focal ATs might also originate from the atrial subepicardial tissue, although no clinical criteria have been demonstrated that can predict the need for epicardial access in these patients.

Atrial Fibrillation
The 2014 edition of the American College of Cardiology (ACC)/American Heart Association (AHA)/Heart Rhythm Society (HRS) guidelines for the management of AF gives a class I indication, with the highest level of evidence, to catheter ablation in patients with symptomatic paroxysmal AF who have failed treatment with an AAD (see Table 124.1).[11] Such a position has also been endorsed by the HRS/European Heart Rhythm Association (EHRA)/European Cardiac Arrhythmia Society (ECAS) expert consensus statement on catheter and surgical ablation of AF.[12] An initial strategy of catheter ablation is considered reasonable (class IIa; level of evidence, B) for patients with recurrent symptomatic AF, even before a trial of AADs. This recommendation is based on data from randomized trials comparing catheter ablation with AADs as first-line therapy for paroxysmal AF (Table 124.2).[13–15] The most recent guidelines have also introduced new recommendations for catheter ablation in patients with nonparoxysmal AF (see Table 124.1).

While not mentioned in their US counterpart, European guidelines give a class IIb recommendation for catheter ablation to prevent recurrent AF in athletes, hypertrophic cardiomyopathy (HCM) patients with symptomatic AF refractory to pharmacological control, and patients with HF when antiarrhythmic medication, including amiodarone, fails to control symptoms.[16] Emerging data suggest that catheter ablation is also useful in certain patients who are not yet specifically included in guideline recommendations, such as those with previous cardiac surgery history or valvular heart disease,[17] and subgroups such as the elderly.[18] In brief, we believe that catheter ablation should be offered to virtually all patients with symptomatic drug-refractory AF.

As will be highlighted later in the chapter, the type of AF, namely paroxysmal versus nonparoxysmal, is the major clinical determinant of the procedural approach. However, other clinical features might also predict the need for a more extensive ablation beyond pulmonary vein isolation (PVI) due to a high prevalence of non-PV triggers. These include, but are not limited to, female gender, the elderly, presence of mechanical cardiac valves, metabolic syndromes, obstructive sleep apnea, and HF.[11,16]

Before the procedure, we believe that it is crucial to have a frank discussion with the patient to manage expectations. For example, patients with severely dilated left atrium (LA; >60 mm) should, if not excluded, at the very least be informed that multiple procedures will likely be needed and that their chances of maintaining sinus rhythm (SR) are very limited, particularly if the ablation procedure is limited to PVI. This concept is recognized in the current US guidelines, which downgrade their recommendation to class IIb in patients with significant LA dilatation (European guidelines currently do not factor in LA size).[11,16] Furthermore, many patients are motivated to undergo ablation to enable discontinuation of anticoagulation. However, because of the relatively high recurrence rate, it should be emphasized that ablation is performed primarily to ameliorate symptoms. Other issues that should be discussed with the patient include the need to aggressively treat comorbidities that favor AF recurrence, including obesity, sleep apnea, hypertension, and HF.

Ventricular Arrhythmias
According to the EHRA/HRS expert consensus, catheter ablation of ventricular arrhythmias (VAs) is recommended for patients with symptomatic sustained monomorphic ventricular tachycardia (VT) refractory to AAD therapy, for those with bundle branch reentrant or fascicular reentrant VT, and for those with drug refractory VT storm not due to a transient cause (see Table 124.1).[19] Data also support the benefit of early adoption of catheter ablation in patients with postinfarct VT, although no evidence indicates that such a strategy improves long-term freedom from recurrent arrhythmia compared with conventional ablation of drug refractory VT (Fig. 124.1).[20]

From a clinical perspective, a correct diagnosis of the substrate underlying VAs is crucial, as it bears relevant prognostic information. Unfortunately, current noninvasive techniques, including

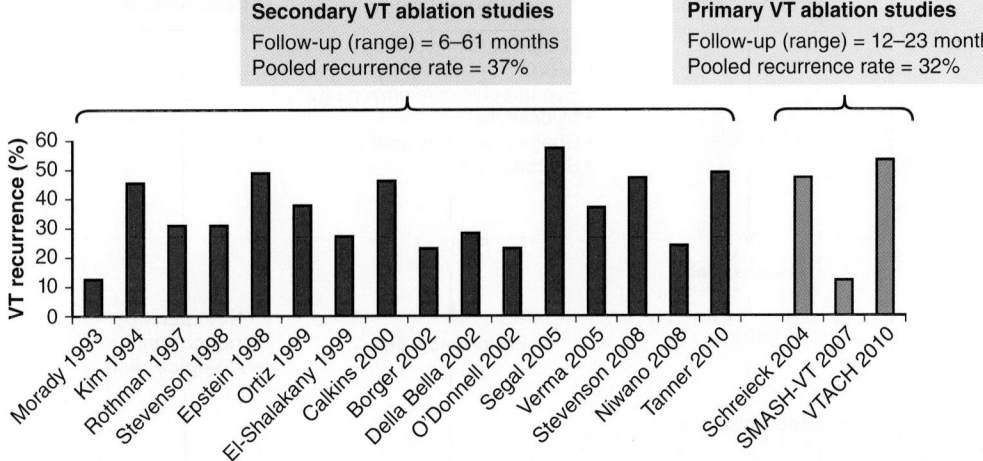

FIGURE 124.1 Individual and pooled ventricular tachycardia (*VT*) recurrence rates after catheter ablation of postinfarct VT. Secondary VT ablation indicates conventional ablation of drug refractory VT. Primary VT ablation indicates the early adoption of catheter ablation before the failure of multiple antiarrhythmic drugs.

cardiac magnetic resonance (MR), can miss subtle cardiomyopathic substrates underlying VAs, and more sophisticated invasive tests, such as electroanatomical mapping with biopsy, might be necessary when the clinical suspicion of underlying structural heart disease is high.[21] The substrate underlying VAs has been demonstrated to be a powerful predictor of the most appropriate procedural approach. Patients with nonischemic cardiomyopathies have a high rate of epicardial VT substrates. Therefore it is advisable to program an epicardial access for mapping and ablation from the beginning of the procedure in these patients (Fig. 124.2). Such an approach is supported by adequate evidence. For instance, several studies have compared endoepicardial ablation with an endocardial-only approach in patients with arrhythmogenic right ventricular cardiomyopathy (ARVC).[22] Overall, 160 ARVC patients with drug refractory VT have been included in such studies, of whom 87 (54%) underwent catheter ablation with an endocardial-only approach and 73 (46%) underwent endoepicardial mapping and ablation. After a mean follow-up of 32 ± 22 months, VT-free survival was achieved in 24 of 87 (28%) patients treated with an endocardial-only approach compared with 52 of 73 (71%) patients treated with an endoepicardial approach. Similar results have been obtained for other nonischemic substrates, such as idiopathic dilated cardiomyopathy and HCM.[23,24]

Most patients with ischemic substrates, on the other hand, may be successfully ablated through an endocardial-only approach. However, emerging data suggest that epicardial mapping and ablation are also beneficial in these patients (see Fig. 124.2). We reported our experience that evidence of epicardial scar with late and fragmented electrograms was seen in up to one-third of patients who were referred to our center for catheter ablation of postinfarct VT.[25] Other groups have confirmed the importance of epicardial mapping and ablation in current populations of patients with postinfarct VT, especially in those with inferior–posterior scars.[26]

Several ECG criteria have been proposed to detect the origin of VAs and to plan the most appropriate ablation strategy. A detailed discussion on ECG criteria to guide VA ablation is provided in Chapters 80–82, 85, and 128.

Preprocedural Drug Therapy

Pre- and Periprocedural Anticoagulation

No specific preprocedural anticoagulation protocol is required for patients undergoing catheter ablation of SVAs (other than AF) and VAs. As a general rule, patients under long-term treatment with oral anticoagulant agents should discontinue oral anticoagulants during the periprocedural period and should bridge with low molecular weight heparin (LMWH) for procedures requiring an arterial or a percutaneous epicardial access. On the other hand, catheter ablation procedures requiring only a transvenous approach can be safely performed under therapeutic anticoagulation.[27,28]

The optimal anticoagulation strategy during AF ablation to reduce the incidence of neurological sequelae (e.g., stroke and transient ischemic attacks [TIAs]), while minimizing bleeding complications, remains an area of active investigation. Current guidelines recommend at least 3 weeks of effective anticoagulation prior to ablation.[12] If these criteria are not met, transesophageal echocardiography (TEE) is recommended to rule out LA thrombus, although many centers routinely perform TEE prior to ablation regardless of anticoagulation status.

Previously, it was common practice to discontinue oral anticoagulation and bridge patients with LMWH a few days before the procedure.[29] However, the COMPARE trial definitively showed that uninterrupted anticoagulation was superior to bridging, both in terms of preventing periprocedural neurological sequelae and reducing bleeding events (Fig. 124.3).[30] Stroke or TIA occurred in 4.9% (n = 39) of patients when anticoagulation (warfarin [Coumadin]) was discontinued but only in 0.25% (n = 2) when full anticoagulation was continued (international normalized ratio [INR] goal, 2–3.5). Furthermore, few bleeding events occurred in the group in which full anticoagulation was continued. Therefore uninterrupted anticoagulation is considered the current best clinical practice.

If preprocedural INR is above 3.5, we partially reverse the anticoagulant effect with 1–2 units of fresh frozen plasma. Furthermore, we type- and crossmatch all patients on warfarin prior to ablation, which allows us to keep packed red blood cells and fresh frozen plasma available for infusion in case of periprocedural hemorrhagic complications.

While vitamin K antagonists (VKAs) (e.g., warfarin) have been the standard of care for stroke prevention in AF patients for decades, new oral anticoagulants (NOACs) have emerged as an alternative treatment. Although NOACs have demonstrated noninferiority to warfarin for stroke prevention in AF patients, the feasibility and safety of NOACs in preventing AF ablation periprocedural thromboembolic events remain controversial.[31] Recently, the VENTURE-AF trial demonstrated that the use of uninterrupted oral rivaroxaban was feasible in patients undergoing AF ablation and that complication rates were similar to those undergoing uninterrupted VKA therapy.[32] Similar results have been demonstrated with periprocedural anticoagulation using

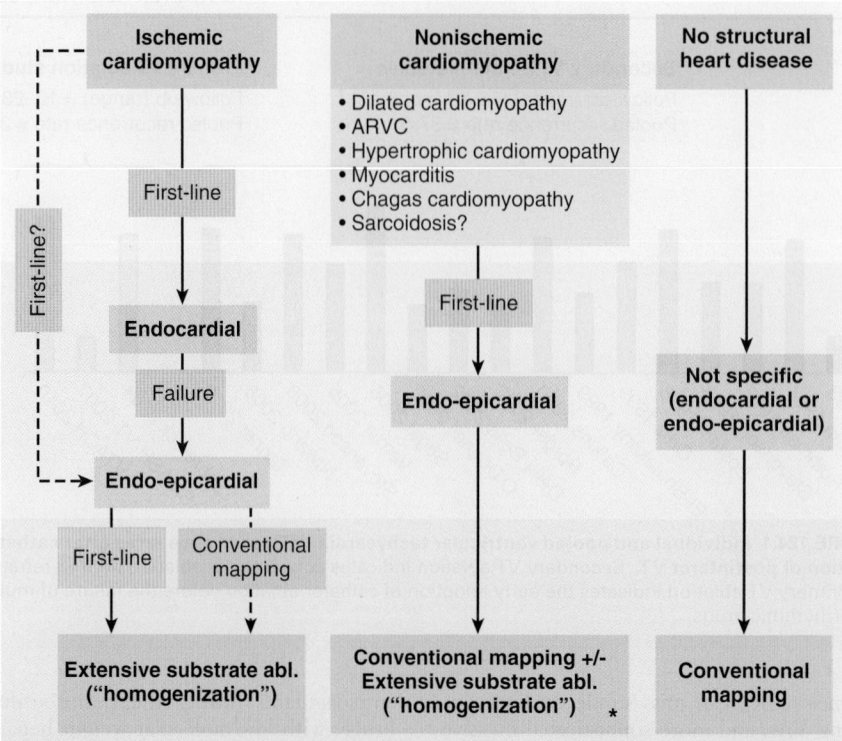

FIGURE 124.2 Preprocedural planning of the ablation approach based on the myocardial substrate that underlies ventricular tachycardia. *Asterisk* indicates that scarring is present, and ventricular tachycardia is demonstrated to originate from the scar. Conventional mapping indicates conventional entrainment/activation mapping and pace mapping techniques. Extensive substrate ablation (*abl.*) indicates ablation of all abnormal electrograms within the scar (fragmented and late electrograms) (see text for details). *ARVC,* Arrhythmogenic right ventricular cardiomyopathy.

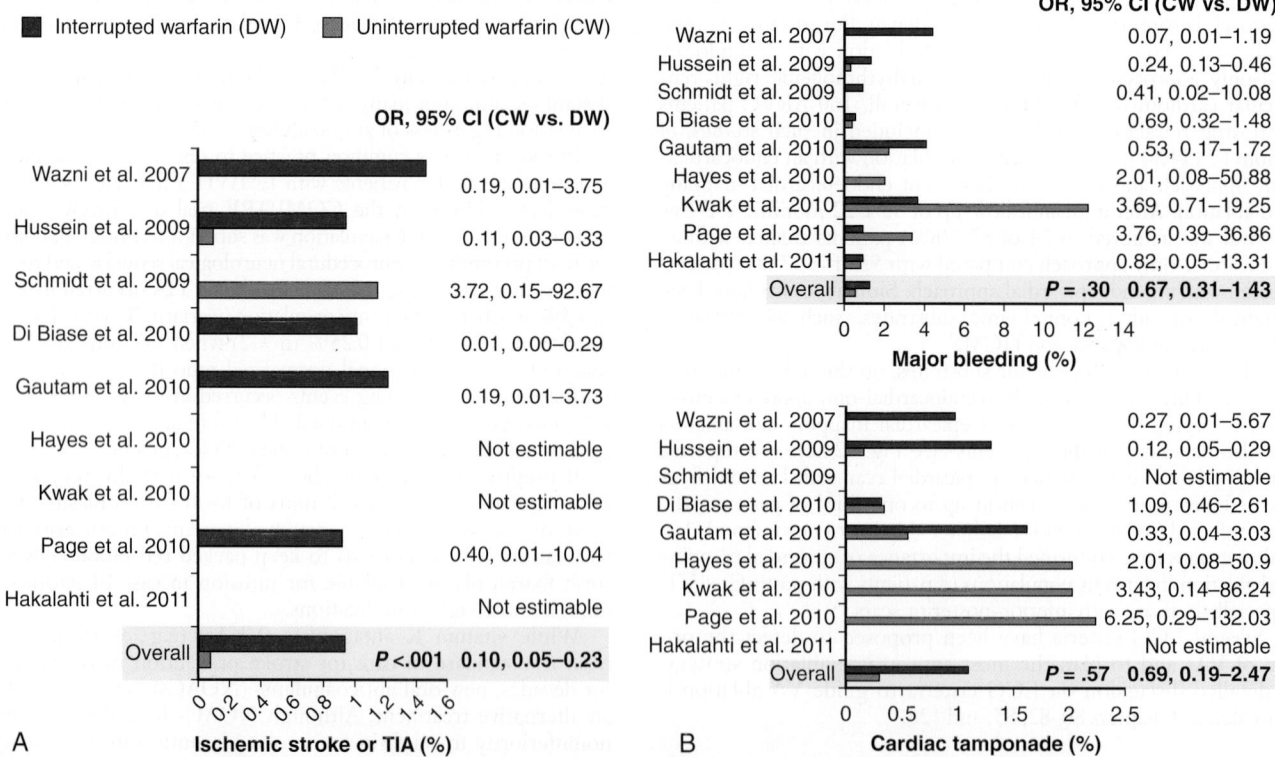

FIGURE 124.3 (A) A plot showing individual and pooled event rates and odds ratios (*OR*) with 95% confidence intervals (*CI*) of periprocedural ischemic stroke/transient ischemic attack (*TIA*) comparing periprocedural warfarin continuation (*CW*) with warfarin discontinuation plus heparin bridging (*DW*). (B) Plots showing individual and pooled event rates and ORs with 95% CIs for major bleeding (*upper panel*) and separately for cardiac tamponade (*lower panel*) with a comparison of CW versus DW. (Modified from Santangeli P, Di Biase L, Horton R, et al. Ablation of atrial fibrillation under therapeutic warfarin reduces periprocedural complications: evidence from a meta-analysis. *Circ Arrhythm Electrophysiol.* 2012;5:302-311.)

apixaban.[33] However, there is concern regarding the use of dabigatran for periprocedural anticoagulation. A multicenter prospective registry showed a significantly higher rate of major bleeding, as well as a higher rate of the composite endpoint of bleeding and thromboembolic complications (6% and 16%, respectively) with dabigatran compared with warfarin (1% and 6%, respectively).[34] On the other hand, one study found no difference in the incidence of symptomatic and asymptomatic cerebral thromboembolism after AF ablation in patients treated with dabigatran and warfarin, respectively.[35] However, a higher risk for thromboembolic complications using dabigatran was reported in a meta-analysis.[36] Therefore, although NOACs show great promise as an alternative agent to warfarin for uninterrupted periprocedural anticoagulation, more data are needed. Currently, periprocedural anticoagulation with dabigatran cannot be recommended.

Antiarrhythmic Drug Therapy

AAD therapy should be discontinued in all patients at least four half-lives before they undergo catheter ablation of cardiac arrhythmias. AADs significantly interfere with arrhythmia inducibility, might conceal underlying arrhythmogenic areas during substrate mapping, and may reduce the effectiveness of catheter ablation. Although adequate drug washout can be achieved in a reasonable time before the procedure (i.e., 4–7 days) in most patients treated with conventional antiarrhythmic agents, subjects who undergo long-term treatment with amiodarone represent a particular challenge because of the long elimination half-life of the drug (58 days on average). Recent evidence, however, strongly supports an incremental benefit of preprocedural amiodarone washout.[37] The success rate was significantly lower in patients with long-standing AF who were maintained on amiodarone than in whom amiodarone was discontinued. Given these data, we discontinue amiodarone 4–6 months prior to ablation and all other AADs 3–5 days prior to ablation to avoid suppression of AF triggers during the procedure. Patients on amiodarone are sometimes bridged with dofetilide (Tikosyn) until 5 days before the procedure if rhythm control is also strongly desired in the months that lead up to the procedure. It is our opinion that AAD discontinuation is particularly important in patients with long-standing persistent AF, in whom the search for non-PV triggers plays a larger role than in patients with paroxysmal AF. Whether the benefits of amiodarone discontinuation in patients undergoing catheter ablation of AF might be generalizable to those undergoing VA ablation requires further investigation.

β-Blockers

Although no data are available from clinical studies, a strong rationale supports the benefit of β-blocker discontinuation before catheter ablation. β-Blockers might interfere with arrhythmia inducibility, negatively affect blood pressure response during sustained arrhythmias, and can significantly blunt the effects of drugs commonly used to induce arrhythmias such as isoproterenol (ISP). In particular, ISP testing in patients who are undergoing long-term therapy with cardioselective β-blockers might induce significant hypotension because of the need to increase dosages to overcome the β1 blockade, coupled with the unrestricted stimulation of $β_2$-adrenergic receptors in vascular smooth muscle cells, leading to systemic vasodilatation.

Patients with HF are an exception to this; however, periprocedural β-blocker discontinuation has been associated with increased risk for worsening HF and mortality.[38] Therefore it is recommended to continue β-blocker therapy in the presence of HF. Similarly, patients with risk factors for ischemic heart disease and those with established ischemic heart disease benefit from periprocedural continuation of β-blockers.[39] As will be highlighted later in the chapter, ISP testing should be avoided in these patients.

Other appropriate drug treatments for an underlying concomitant cardiac condition, such as antihypertensive medications, HF therapies (e.g., renin-angiotensin system blockers), and lipid-lowering drugs, should also be maintained during the periprocedural period.[40]

Preprocedural Imaging

We do not routinely perform preprocedural imaging of PVs or the LA with computed tomography (CT) or MR imaging (MRI) prior to AF ablation. It is our opinion that modern three-dimensional (3D) mapping systems used during the procedure are sufficient for accurate chamber reconstruction. However, we commonly perform such preprocedural imaging in patients undergoing repeat procedures, primarily to rule out PV stenosis. Preprocedural imaging is also routinely performed if the anatomy is complex, for example, in patients with congenital heart disease. We do, however, routinely perform CT or MRI 3 months postprocedure to assess for PV stenosis.

Intraprocedural Management
Sedation and Anesthesia

The main goals of intraprocedural sedation and anesthesia are to minimize or abolish pain, control the patient's ventilation and movements, avoid abnormal autonomic responses, and reduce intraoperative patient awareness and recall. For many years, conscious sedation has been the most commonly adopted anesthesia protocol during electrophysiological procedures. Using this protocol, a short-acting benzodiazepine (e.g., midazolam) usually in combination with an opioid analgesic (e.g., fentanyl) is administered to patients shortly before the procedure.

In recent years, general anesthesia has gained increasing interest, given the increasing numbers of complex and long procedures such as catheter ablation of AF or VA. The main advantages of general anesthesia are the almost complete abolition of pain and patient awareness, the abolition of patient movement for prolonged periods, and complete control of ventilation. On the other hand, general anesthesia is associated with autonomic lability, which can manifest as decreases in blood pressure and/or reflex tachycardia, which might require active intervention. Thus far, only one randomized trial of 257 consecutive patients has formally evaluated the outcomes of conscious sedation compared with those of general anesthesia in patients undergoing catheter ablation of AF.[41] General anesthesia was initiated with propofol (2 mg/kg) and fentanyl (1–2 µg/kg), followed by a neuromuscular blocking agent (usually rocuronium 0.6–1 mg/kg) and by endotracheal intubation with intermittent positive-pressure ventilation. Conscious sedation was attained with fentanyl or midazolam. After a mean follow-up of 17 ± 8 months, 88 (69%) patients assigned to conscious sedation were free of atrial arrhythmias when off AADs compared with 114 (88%) patients randomly assigned to general anesthesia (p < .001). All patients with recurrence underwent a second procedure. Notably, at the time of the repeat procedure, 42% of PVs in the conscious sedation arm had recovered PV conduction compared with 19% of PVs in the general anesthesia group (p = .003).[41] Therefore current evidence supports an incremental benefit of general anesthesia compared with conscious sedation in patients undergoing catheter ablation of AF. Because the procedure requires more extensive lesion sets and a longer total procedure time, we perform all ablations of patients with long-standing persistent AF under general anesthesia. We typically induce anesthesia with propofol (2 mg/kg) and fentanyl (1–2 µg) followed by neuromuscular blockade, typically rocuronium (0.6–1 mg/kg). We avoid muscle paralysis to better enable the detection of diaphragmatic complications. The airway is managed by endotracheal intubation and with intermittent positive-pressure ventilation. While we recognize that this is contrary to the practice at some other centers, it is our opinion that general anesthesia conditions are superior to other forms of sedation during the longer and more complex ablations performed in patients with long-standing persistent AF. This is based in part on data showing a higher success rate, as well as reduced fluoroscopy and procedural times under such conditions, possibly due to better mapping and improved catheter stability, enabling superior lesion formation.[41] Furthermore, general anesthesia is generally preferred by patients and may increase their willingness to undergo repeat procedures.[42] The latter is particularly important in patients with long-standing persistent AF, in whom multiple procedures are often required to achieve long-term freedom from AF.

Other strategies to achieve better catheter stability, such as high-frequency jet ventilation, have been proposed as a valuable alternative to conscious sedation. However, high-frequency jet ventilation has been associated with several complications, including problems with humidification and warming, high gas flow rates, and rapid increases in lung volume that might cause lung injury through the generation of shear forces at the interface of compliant and atelectatic airways.[43] Furthermore, an extensive learning curve is needed for one to become proficient at using this technique safely, and few anesthesia providers have sufficient experience for the technique to be considered the standard of care.

No data are available to compare conscious sedation with general anesthesia in patients undergoing catheter ablation of VAs. At our institution, we routinely implement conscious sedation in patients undergoing catheter ablation of VAs, given the putative higher risk for hemodynamic decompensation with general anesthesia. Data also suggest an antiarrhythmic effect of general anesthesia, which might limit VA inducibility. However, in the absence of comparative data, both anesthesia protocols are reasonable choices based on the preference of operators and/or patients.

Venous Access

The modified Seldinger technique is the preferred method for obtaining vascular access during electrophysiological procedures. Typically, femoral venous accesses in the right and left groin are used to position most diagnostic catheters, the intracardiac echocardiography (ICE) catheter, and the ablation catheter when procedures are performed through a transvenous approach. The major contraindication to femoral vein catheterization is the presence of acute or recurrent iliofemoral deep vein thrombosis. In some patients, such as those with a history of recurrent femoral vein catheterization or those with a history of radiotherapy, the femoral vein might be partially or totally occluded. Sporadic reports of inferior vena cava interruption have been described. In these cases, a superior approach from the right internal jugular vein might be implemented, also for complex ablation procedures (e.g., catheter ablation of AF).[44]

A coronary sinus diagnostic catheter might be introduced through a variety of venous accesses at the discretion of the operator, including the femoral vein, internal jugular vein, subclavian vein, or median basilic vein. Although the adoption of special precautions for obtaining venous access, such as the use of ultrasound, appears justifiable in patients undergoing electrophysiological procedures without interruption of therapeutic anticoagulation, the risk for vascular-related bleeding with such an anticoagulation protocol has been consistently demonstrated as smaller than that with warfarin discontinuation and heparin bridging.[27] No evidence has been found of an incremental benefit of ultrasound-guided femoral venous access compared with the standard manual approach. At our institution, over the past 7188 AF ablations performed, ultrasound-assisted femoral venous access was attained in 1079 (15%) cases. No difference in the rate of vascular-related complications was observed between patients who received ultrasound-assisted vascular access and those who received conventional manual access (3.2% vs. 3.8%; $p = .44$).

With regard to nonfemoral venous access, such as access to the internal jugular vein, published data suggest an incremental benefit of ultrasound guidance compared with a blind technique.[45] In patients undergoing venous access without interruption of therapeutic anticoagulation, the risks associated with a blind puncture of the internal jugular vein represent a major concern, and conventional blind puncture should be discouraged. At our institution, we systematically avoid a blind puncture of the internal jugular vein and perform access under fluoroscopic guidance after advancing a catheter from the femoral vein into the internal jugular vein. This approach can also be helpful in eliminating the risk for pneumothorax by allowing access in the neck at a higher level.

Transseptal Access

At our institution, transseptal access is attained under ICE guidance. Although no formal comparison between ICE-assisted and conventional fluoroscopy-assisted transseptal access has been performed, our experience with ICE strongly suggests a high degree of safety when transseptal access is performed under ICE guidance, with no complications over the past 12,000 transseptal punctures. TEE is another imaging method available for facilitating transseptal puncture.

The technique of ICE-assisted transseptal access is described in detail elsewhere.[46] In brief, once the ICE catheter is positioned in the right atrium in the "home" position (view of the right atrium, tricuspid valve, and RV), a clockwise torque brings into sequential view the aortic arch (more anterior), followed by the anterior LA, mitral valve and LA appendage (LAA), left PVs, posterior wall, and right PVs. The interatrial septum is visualized in the near field. If the septum is too close to the probe, gentle bending of the transducer toward the right atrial free wall moves the imaging plane of the septum toward the midfield of the view. The site of the septum suitable for transseptal puncture typically intersects an ICE section plane between the left PVs. Under ICE assistance, physicians are able to direct the transseptal puncture toward specific areas of the fossa ovalis; a posterior puncture is warranted for procedures involving posterior structures, such as PVs in case of AF ablation, whereas a more anterior puncture is helpful for VA ablation, given the anterior position of the mitral valve with respect to the fossa ovalis. Furthermore, ICE monitoring could be of significant value for challenging transseptal accesses, as in patients with interatrial septum aneurysm and those with atrial septal defect closure devices.[47]

RF application through a surgical electrocautery pen (usually 30–35 W in the cut mode) applied to the proximal hub of a standard Brockenbrough needle or a special RF needle (Baylis, Montreal, QC, Canada) might be necessary in cases of increased resistance to transseptal puncture (e.g., lipomatous hypertrophy of the interatrial septum, postcardiac surgery). Recent data on animal models have raised concerns about the safety of RF-assisted transseptal puncture because of a relatively high incidence of tissue coring.[48] Notably, in this study, periprocedural maintenance of therapeutic INR was not required, and heparin was not administered before the transseptal puncture was performed. Therefore the extent to which these results might be extended to humans is unclear; in this regard, we have found no evidence of clinical or silent cerebral thromboembolism in a large series of patients undergoing RF-assisted double transseptal access under fully therapeutic anticoagulation (with an intravenous [IV] heparin bolus before transseptal puncture).[49]

Arterial Access

Arterial femoral access is usually obtained when performing retrograde aortic approaches. In some laboratories, an arterial line

Table 124.3 Complications of subxiphoid percutaneous epicardial access for mapping and ablation of ventricular tachycardia

MAJOR COMPLICATIONS	N (%)
Intrapericardial bleeding	11[3]
Coronary artery stenosis	1 (0.3)
Significant pericarditis	1 (0.3)
Delayed cardiac tamponade	5 (1.4)
Myocardial infarction	1 (0.3)
Peridiaphragmatic hematoma	1 (0.3)
MINOR COMPLICATIONS	**N (%)**
RV puncture without consequence	24 (6.8)
Pleural catheterization with guidewire	2 (0.6)
Chest pain	182[51]

N, Number of patients; *RV,* right ventricle.
Data from Sacher F, Roberts-Thomson K, Maury P, et al. Epicardial ventricular tachycardia ablation: a multicenter safety study. *J Am Coll Cardiol.* 2010;55:2366-2372; Della Bella P, Brugada J, Zeppenfeld K, et al. Epicardial ablation for ventricular tachycardia: a European multicenter study. *Circ Arrhythm Electrophysiol.* 2011;4:653-659.

TABLE 124.4 Relative merits and limitations of standard fluoroscopy versus three-dimensional nonfluoroscopic mapping systems for intraprocedural catheter manipulation

	FLUOROSCOPY	THREE-DIMENSIONAL NONFLUOROSCOPIC MAPPING SYSTEMS
Pros	• Reliable tracking of catheter motion • Allows imaging of the entire catheter and sheath(s) • Reliable imaging of beat-to-beat cardiac motion • Imaging of respiratory excursions • Real-time imaging of multiple structures	• No radiation exposure • Faster tracking of catheter tip motion • Three-dimensional reconstruction of cardiac anatomy
Cons	• Radiation exposure • Only two-dimensional images	• Not reliable for imaging of beat-to-beat variability in cardiac motion and respiratory excursions • Allows visualization of only the catheter tip

is placed in the radial or femoral artery for invasive monitoring of blood pressure. However, there are no data to support that procedural safety is increased with invasive blood pressure monitoring, especially when more advanced technologies for complication monitoring, such as ICE, are implemented. Arterial access is attained with the modified Seldinger technique, and no evidence supports the use of ultrasound-assisted arterial puncture. Although it is generally recommended to interrupt long-term warfarin therapy in patients in whom an arterial puncture is planned, observational data from our institution suggest that performing arterial femoral access for invasive monitoring of blood pressure (5-Fr sheath) is feasible and safe, even in patients who are therapeutically anticoagulated.

Pericardial Access

A detailed description of the percutaneous pericardial access technique will be provided in Chapter 128. In brief, the subxiphoid approach involves the fluoroscopically guided passage of an 18-gauge needle from the skin through the subcutaneous fat, rectus abdominis muscle, and usually through the diaphragm inside the virtual pericardial space. Physicians should be aware of the possible risks associated with subxiphoid pericardial access, which involve both noncardiac and cardiac structures. Among noncardiac structures, the left lobe of the liver might be injured in patients with an enlarged liver, such as those with congestive HF[50]; inadvertent puncture of arterial branches providing blood supply to the diaphragm might cause hemoperitoneum, and the transverse colon might be injured in patients with megacolon due to Chagas disease. Among cardiac structures, inadvertent puncture of the RV is most common, and injury of the coronary arteries or of the coronary sinus has been reported in sporadic cases.[50] Notwithstanding these possible risks, the total rate of complications related to percutaneous epicardial access has been consistently reported as very low, ranging from 4% to 5% in large multicenter series (Table 124.3[3,51]).[24]

Catheter Manipulation and the Role of Intraoperative Imaging Techniques

The order in which specific catheters are inserted into the cardiac chambers is generally not important. One notable exception is in patients with preexisting left bundle branch block, in whom it is recommended that the first catheter inserted should be advanced into the RV for rescue pacing in case of traumatic right bundle branch block leading to complete heart block when catheters are manipulated in the region of the AV junction (e.g., during positioning of the coronary sinus or the His bundle catheters). Intraprocedural catheter manipulation might be assisted by conventional fluoroscopy or by a 3D nonfluoroscopic mapping system, with diverse relative merits and limitations (Table 124.4). Intraprocedural ICE monitoring is also used as an adjuvant strategy to assist catheter positioning and complication monitoring. In the near future, 3D echocardiographic imaging and MRI will become additional methods of intraoperative monitoring of catheter manipulation. In the absence of comparative data between different imaging modalities to assist catheter manipulation and complication monitoring, surgeons might choose an intraprocedural imaging modality to guide catheter manipulation based on their own preference.

Management of Intraprocedural Thromboembolic Risk

During the procedure, important steps to reduce the risk for thromboembolic events include administering unfractionated heparin (UFH) and monitoring for thrombus formation on sheaths and catheters using ICE. UFH should be administered as an IV bolus, followed by a continuous infusion to maintain target-activated clotting time (ACT). To prevent thrombus formation on the transseptal sheath, the bolus is usually administered before or immediately after the transseptal puncture. The currently recommended target ACT is 300–400 seconds, with some centers aiming for a level of >350 seconds. The target ACT should be achieved prior to the first energy delivery and rechecked every 20–30 minutes to ensure that an adequate level is maintained throughout the procedure. Additional UFH boluses can be administered as needed. Importantly, when performing ablations on patients administered NOACs, it is often necessary to use larger doses of UFH to maintain an adequate ACT level.[35] UFH is discontinued once all catheters and sheaths have exited the LA. Some centers use protamine at the end of the procedure to reverse the effects of UFH.

Because all sheaths and catheters are potential sources of thrombus formation, particularly in the absence of appropriate and timely anticoagulation, ICE can play an important role during the ablation procedure to detect catheter-related sources of emboli. At many centers, sheaths are retracted to the right atrium once the diagnostic and ablation catheters have been placed in the LA to reduce further

COMPARATIVE EFFECTIVENESS OF WIDE ANTRAL VERSUS OSTIAL PULMONARY VEIN ISOLATION

Study or subgroup	Wide antral PVI Events	Wide antral PVI Total	Ostial PVI Events	Ostial PVI Total	Weight	Odds ratio M-H, fixed, 95% CI
Arentz T	18	55	28	55	12.2%	0.47 [0.22, 1.02]
Fiala M	5	56	6	54	3.6%	0.78 [0.22, 2.74]
Hwang HJ	12	45	18	36	9.5%	0.36 [0.14, 0.92]
Li-Wei Lo	3	27	4	46	1.7%	1.31 [0.27, 6.36]
Liu X	9	55	12	55	6.5%	0.70 [0.27, 1.83]
Mansour M	10	40	16	40	7.8%	0.50 [0.19, 1.30]
Nilsson B	20	46	38	54	12.9%	0.32 [0.14, 0.74]
Oral H	4	40	13	40	7.6%	0.23 [0.07, 0.79]
Sawhney	5	33	5	33	2.8%	1.00 [0.26, 3.84]
Tan HB	7	45	12	40	7.0%	0.43 [0.15, 1.23]
Yamada	11	51	22	50	11.3%	0.35 [0.15, 0.84]
Yamane T*	6	79	11	44	8.5%	0.25 [0.08, 0.72]
Yamane T†	8	38	14	26	8.5%	0.23 [0.08, 0.68]
Total (95% CI)		**610**		**573**	**100.0%**	**0.42 [0.32, 0.56]**
Total events	118		199			

Heterogeneity: Chi^2 = 9.54, df = 12 (P = .66); I^2 = 0%
Test for overall effect: Z = 6.03 (P <.00001)

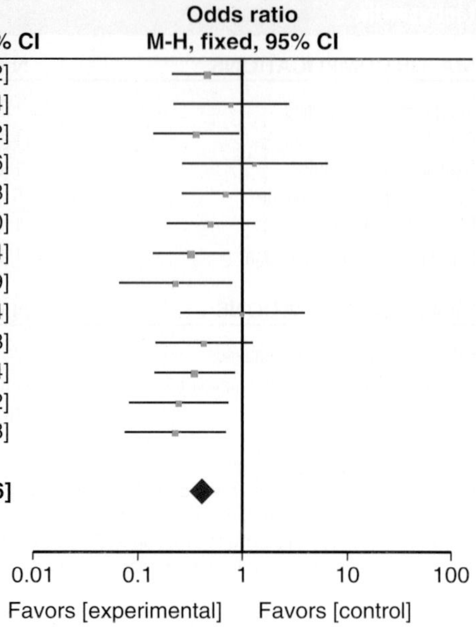

Odds ratio M-H, fixed, 95% CI (scale: 0.01, 0.1, 1, 10, 100)
Favors [experimental]   Favors [control]

FIGURE 124.4 Impact of wide antral versus ostial pulmonary vein isolation in patients undergoing atrial fibrillation ablation. Wide antral pulmonary vein isolation (*PVI*) is more effective than ostial PVI with a striking reduction in overall atrial arrhythmia recurrences (mainly driven by a reduction in atrial fibrillation recurrences) and a comparable rate of complications. Yamane reported separately for paroxysmal atrial fibrillation (*asterisk*) and persistent atrial fibrillation (*dagger*). *CI*, Confidence interval. (Modified from Proietti R, Santangeli P, Di Biase L, et al. Comparative effectiveness of wide antral versus ostial pulmonary vein isolation: a systematic review and meta-analysis. *Circ Arrhythm Electrophysiol.* 2014;7:39-45.)

systemic embolic risk. Removal of sheaths from the groin can be safely performed when the ACT is <200 seconds. Other factors that can potentially affect embolic risk include more extensive ablation protocols, total time spent in the LA, and periprocedural cardioversion. However, data in these areas are conflicting.[52,53]

Temperature Monitoring

We use esophageal probes in all patients to monitor esophageal temperature when ablating in proximity to the esophagus, e.g., the posterior LA wall. While we use up to 45 W of energy and allow temperatures up to 41°C during some ablation steps, we limit the power to 35 W during ablation of the posterior atrial wall. Furthermore, we limit each RF application to 20 seconds and discontinue energy delivery when the esophageal temperature probe detects a rapid temperature increase and/or when the temperature reaches 39°C. However, even with these safety features in place, it is prudent to still use caution during ablation in these areas as esophageal fistula formation has been demonstrated even with the use of esophageal probes.[51] Although positive esophageal findings (but not severe esophageal complications) during postprocedural upper endoscopy are more common in patients ablated under general anesthesia, we are of the opinion that the benefits clearly outweigh the risks. We do not routinely use a prophylactic proton pump inhibitor therapy after the procedure.

Ablation Targets During Atrial Fibrillation Ablation

As mentioned, AF type is the major factor that determines which structures to target during catheter ablation. In most patients with paroxysmal AF, PVs represent the most important structure to be targeted to achieve a cure. Importantly, wide antral PVI has been recently shown to be more effective than ostial PVI, with a striking reduction in overall atrial arrhythmia recurrences (mainly driven by reduction of AF recurrences) and a comparable rate of complications (Fig. 124.4).[54]

However, several studies have demonstrated that non-PV foci also play an important role in the initiation, maintenance, and recurrence of AF.[55] The prevalence of non-PVI triggers significantly increases in nonparoxysmal AF, although recent data have highlighted their importance in specific subsets of patients with paroxysmal AF, particularly those with enlarged LA and those with underlying heart disease, including HF. Therefore, although we agree that PVI remains the cornerstone of AF ablation, we routinely target non-PVI triggers, particularly in patients with long-standing persistent AF. Common non-PVI foci include the posterior wall of the LA, coronary sinus, LAA, superior vena cava (SVC), crista terminalis, interatrial septum, ligament of Marshall, and areas adjacent to the AV valve annuli. This practice is based on data from several studies and meta-analyses showing better overall results in long-standing persistent AF ablation using more extensive lesion sets.[56]

It has been speculated that AF recurrence can occur either through activation of non-PV foci that were dormant during the initial procedure or through progressive worsening of the atrial substrate, causing new non-PVI foci to emerge. The latter explanation is supported by evidence of progressive structural atrial remodeling in patients with AF recurrence, in contrast to the reverse atrial remodeling often seen in patients who remain free from AF.[57] Because HF is generally a progressive disease, atrial remodeling and non-PV triggers may well account for the higher risk for AF recurrence after ablation in patients with HF compared with those that do not have this diagnosis.

High-dose ISP (up to 30 μg/min for 15 minutes) infusion is the most commonly used method for disclosing latent non-PV triggers and has been shown to reveal more non-PV triggers than adenosine or rapid atrial pacing.[58] High-dose ISP may reveal non-PVI foci by increasing arrhythmogenicity through vagally mediated bradycardia, and by reducing the atrial refractory period, thereby inducing early afterdepolarizations and delayed afterdepolarizations.[59] We therefore perform mapping during

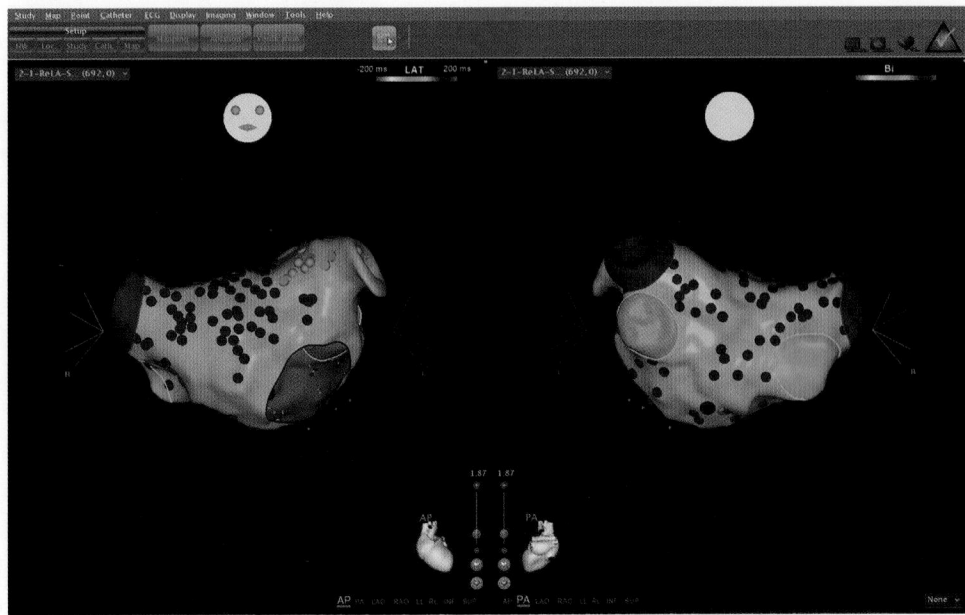

FIGURE 124.5 An example of pulmonary vein isolation plus non–pulmonary vein trigger ablation in a patient with long-standing persistent atrial fibrillation.

ISP positioning with a circular mapping catheter at the ostium of the left superior PV, registering the far field from the LAA and the ablation catheter in the right superior PV. Differential activation between the distal coronary sinus and the circular mapping catheter can distinguish LAA from left PV firing. In the presence of rapid conduction through the Bachmann bundle, the circular mapping catheter registering the LAA far-field electrogram is an invaluable aid for correctly detecting LAA firing, which in this case is usually associated with a rapid septal–right atrial activation. In cases of right-sided atrial ectopy, the site of origin can be detected by analyzing the activation sequence of the duodecapolar catheter, which is similar to SR. In this way, the site of origin of any significant ectopic atrial activity can be mapped and targeted for ablation (Fig. 124.5).

As mentioned, the major drawback of ISP infusion is its relatively unpredictable hypotensive response, caused by the stimulation of vascular β_2-adrenergic receptors. As mentioned earlier, this is more likely to occur in patients under long-term cardioselective β-blocker therapy and should therefore be avoided in this patient subset. Furthermore, ISP testing is contraindicated in patients with obstructive coronary artery disease due to the risk for precipitating acute myocardial ischemia.

The benefit of targeting specific types of atrial electrograms, such as complex fractionated atrial electrograms (CFAEs), has been reported in multiple randomized trials and meta-analyses.[60] In brief, such benefit is confined to patients with nonparoxysmal AF. Whether this is the result of elimination of CFAE or merely reflects a more extensive ablation of arrhythmogenic anatomical structures, such as the posterior LA wall or the coronary sinus, remains incompletely clear. In this regard, the pathophysiological significance of CFAEs has been challenged. In particular, CFAEs appear to represent areas of wavefront collision rather than the electrical expression of underlying atrial structural abnormalities.[61]

Other evolving techniques in AF ablation include linear ablation and focal ablation of areas with scar or areas that demonstrate fractionation or perpetuation of rotors. Several small studies have shown that such techniques, in addition to PVI, improve arrhythmia-free outcomes.[62–64] Other emerging technologies include algorithms based on catheter stability and impedance drops, as well as contact force sensing.

Ablation Endpoints During Atrial Fibrillation Ablation

Although the targets of current AF ablation approaches are represented by different anatomical structures (e.g., PVs, LA posterior wall, coronary sinus, LAA), the endpoint is to achieve electrical isolation. This concept, extensively validated for PVs, has also been confirmed for other non-PV structures such as the coronary sinus and LAA.[65] Currently, the only reliable method for assessing electrical isolation involves positioning a circular mapping catheter within the area targeted and verifying the presence of electrical disconnection from the rest of the atrium. Other methods used to verify isolation, such as 3D mapping systems, have proved unreliable for detecting electrical isolation.[66] For the coronary sinus, electrical isolation is verified through the absence of atrial electrogram recordings and the failure to capture the atrium when pacing from within the coronary sinus.

Procedural endpoints beyond PVI itself are a contested topic. There is ongoing debate whether procedural AF termination improves long-term freedom from AF or not, with some investigators preferring empirical lesion sets.[67] The benefit of procedural cardioversion is also controversial, and, as previously mentioned, there is concern over an increased risk for thromboembolic events when cardioversion is performed. It has therefore been suggested that cardioversion should be deferred until after the procedure to allow healing of atrial lesions.[52]

However, based on results from a prospective study of 306 patients with long-standing persistent AF, we do not consider procedural AF termination as an endpoint in and of itself.[68] In this study, there was no difference in long-term freedom from AF between patients in whom procedural AF termination was or was not achieved, and there is some concern that pursuing procedural AF termination prolongs procedure times and increases the risk for complications. If AF termination has not been achieved after extensive ablation of all potential AF trigger structures, we perform cardioversion.

After achieving stable SR (either procedurally or by cardioversion), we administer ISP of up to 30 μg/min for 15–20 minutes to reveal additional non-PV triggers and/or acute PV reconnections. Mapping during ISP is performed with the circular mapping catheter at the ostium of the LAA and the ablation catheter in the right superior PV. This way, any significant ectopic atrial activity can be identified by comparing the activation sequences

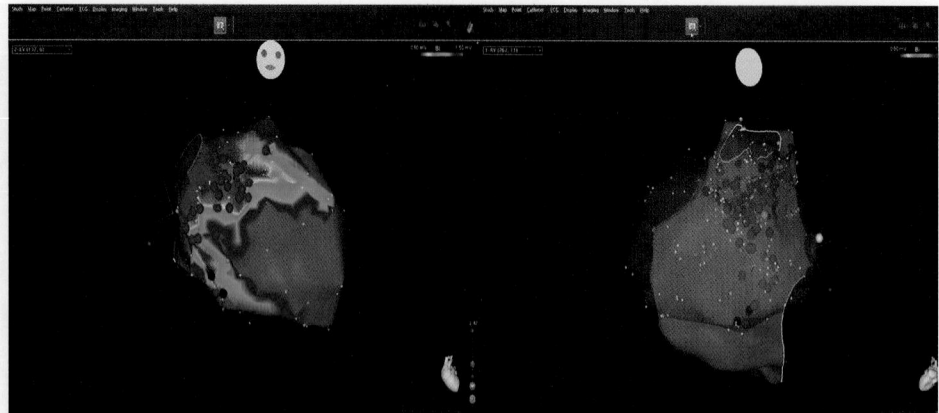

FIGURE 124.6 Lesion sets in a septal ventricular tachycardia successfully ablated targeting both sides of the septum in a patient with nonischemic cardiomyopathy.

of the sinus and the ectopic beats. If triggers are seen from the coronary sinus or the LAA, these sites become targets for electrical isolation. Finally, after completing the abovementioned steps, the catheters and sheaths are pulled back into the right atrium. Under ICE guidance, the circular mapping catheter is positioned at the SVC and high right atrial junction, after which ablation to achieve isolation of the SVC is performed, beginning with targets at the septal aspects. When ablating the lateral aspect of the SVC, we use high-voltage pacing (at least 30 mA) to identify the phrenic nerve to avoid diaphragmatic complications.

Intraprocedural Radiofrequency Power Titration

A detailed description of different energy sources already available and under development for catheter ablation of AF and other arrhythmias is provided in Chapter 123. The main endpoint of catheter ablation is producing irreversible damage to the target tissue, resulting in permanent loss of conduction. The most important factors influencing the size and depth of an ablation lesion include the current density at the catheter tip, which might be approximated to the power setting at the equality of ablation catheter tip diameters; the electrode–myocardium contact; the orientation of the catheter tip; and the efficiency of heat dissipation from the catheter tip, cooling, intracavitary blood, and cardiac vessels close to the targeted structure. With current ablation catheters incorporating open irrigation technologies, we safely deliver RF ablation lesions at a power of 40–45 W, slightly reducing the ablation power (35 W) when delivering lesions in the posterior wall close to the esophagus or in the coronary sinus. In the clinical setting, power titration is dynamically modulated by impedance and temperature monitoring and by other intraoperative tools, such as esophageal temperature monitoring. RF delivery should be interrupted if the esophageal temperature rises to above 39°C; close monitoring of the esophageal temperature during RF delivery is particularly important in patients undergoing AF ablation under general anesthesia because of the reduced esophageal motility and the lack of patient swallowing.[69] Other tools of intraoperative RF energy delivery monitoring, such as ICE, lost their clinical significance after the advent and widespread adoption of open irrigated ablation catheters.

On the other hand, with open irrigated ablation catheters, fluid overload may become an issue, particularly in patients with significant left ventricular dysfunction (both systolic and diastolic). Careful monitoring of fluid balance is required in such cases, and diuretic administration during the procedure may be needed. Recently, an open irrigated catheter with a porous tip technology has been released (ThermoCool SF, Biosense Webster, Diamond Bar, CA). The porous tip technology allows halving of the amount of fluid necessary to effectively cool the catheter tip (from 30 to 15 mL/min). Whether such fluid reduction translates into clinical benefit warrants further investigation.

Contact force is another key contributor to lesion size and depth, and it can predict major procedure-related complications such as steam pop, perforation, and coagulum formation.[70] Open irrigated catheters with contact force sensors (TactiCath, EndoSense, Geneva, Switzerland; ThermoCool SmartTouch, Biosense Webster) have been made available. These catheters allow the operator to apply appropriate force and deliver optimal lesions without risk of pressure-related complications.[71]

Other technologies aimed at assessing the degree of tissue–catheter contact are being actively investigated. Among these, novel open irrigated ablation catheters with incorporated temperature-sensing chips are capable of measuring and interpreting microwaves emitted from heated tissue during ablation (i.e., microwave radiometry technology; Tempasure, Advanced Cardiac Therapeutics, Laguna Beach, CA), which provide indirect assessment of tissue–catheter contact. In addition, microwave radiometry has the capacity of providing real-time feedback on tissue temperature and lesion growth. This novel technology has just entered clinical investigation.

Ablation Targets During Ventricular Tachycardia Ablation

In general terms, the ablation targets for VT largely depend on the mechanism underlying the arrhythmia, namely whether the arrhythmia has a focal as opposed to a reentrant mechanism. With focal VTs, the target is the localized arrhythmia focus, typically identified as the earliest intracardiac activation site, together with pace mapping techniques, whereas in reentrant arrhythmias, resection of a larger area of slow conduction (e.g., VT isthmus) is necessary to render the arrhythmia noninducible. As has been mentioned, simple baseline clinical characteristics together with ECG criteria are helpful for predicting both the arrhythmia mechanism and optimal sites for mapping and ablation (see Chapters 80–82, 85, and 128). VAs associated with cardiomyopathic substrates leading to scar tissue more likely have a scar-related reentrant mechanism, and slow conduction areas within the scar tissue represent the ablation targets (see Chapter 127). On the other hand, patients without structural heart disease typically have a focal mechanism of VT, with outflow tract VTs (right or left ventricular) constituting the most prevalent type of focal VTs (Fig. 124.6). Although most of these arrhythmias can be successfully ablated with focal applications of RF energy at specific sites identified during intracardiac mapping, a small but definite subset of patients might require RF energy application at multiple sites. We have described a series of patients with left ventricular outflow tract VTs in whom intracardiac mapping disclosed multiple sites of equally early activation (i.e., anterior

TABLE 124.5 Ventricular arrhythmia recurrence rates after catheter ablation of infarct-related ventricular tachycardia (VT)

	YEAR	NO. OF PATIENTS	LVEF (%)	FOLLOW-UP (MONTHS)	VT RECURRENCE (%)
Morady et al.[74]	1993	15	27	9	13
Kim et al.[75]	1994	21	32	13	45
Rothman et al.[76]	1997	35	24	14	31
Stevenson et al.[77]	1998	52	33	18	31
Epstein et al.[78]	1998	73	30	6	49
Ortiz et al.[79]	1999	34	31	26	38
El-Shalakany et al.[80]	1999	15	26	15	27
Calkins et al.[81]	2000	119	31	8	46
O'Callaghan et al.[82]	2001	55	32	39	—[a]
Borger et al.[83]	2002	89	29	34	23
Della Bella et al.[84]	2002	124	34	41	28
O'Donnell et al.[85]	2002	109	—	61	23
Segal et al.[86]	2005	40	36	36	57
Verma et al.[87]	2005	46	—	16	37
Stevenson et al.[88]	2008	231	25	6	47
Niwano et al.[89]	2008	58	35	31	24
Tanner et al.[90]	2010	63	30	12	49
Schreieck et al.[91]	2004	39	33	12	47
SMASH-VT[92]	2007	128	32	23	12
VTACH[93]	2010	107	34	23	53
Summary	—	1453	—	—	36

[a]Not included in the summary estimate because of lack of data on VT recurrence rate.
LVEF, Left ventricular ejection fraction.

interventricular vein, mitro–aortic continuity, left coronary cusp, and epicardial left ventricular outflow tract). In these patients, RF applications were necessary at multiple sites to achieve acute VT suppression and long-term success.[72] It bears emphasis that no specific clinical or ECG characteristic could be used to accurately identify this population of patients, and invasive electrophysiological study with detailed mapping was always necessary.

Ablation of VT arising close to coronary vessels, such as coronary cusp VTs or epicardial VTs, carries the potential risk for coronary artery damage. Traditionally, coronary artery angiography has been performed in these cases to assess the distance between the ablation catheter tip and coronary artery vessels. For coronary cusp ablation, ICE monitoring might replace the need for coronary artery angiography, especially for ablation in the left coronary cusp. In a large multicenter series, we assessed the feasibility of ICE-guided coronary cusp ablation in a consecutive series of 122 patients with coronary cusp VT. A total of 151 ablation procedures were performed, 105 (70%) from within the left coronary cusp and 46 (30%) from within the right coronary cusp. ICE was the only imaging modality used in all 151 cases of left coronary cusp ablation and in 44 of 46 (96%) cases of right coronary cusp ablation. In this group, coronary angiography was required in two (4%) cases because of failure to image the right coronary artery ostium. Of note, no periprocedural complication was observed. Therefore, in experienced hands, ICE monitoring is able to abolish the need for intraprocedural coronary angiography in all cases of left coronary cusp ablation and in most cases of right coronary cusp ablation.

With regard to ablation of epicardial VTs, we routinely do not perform angiography when the mechanism of VT is scar-related reentry. In these cases, the small risk for coronary artery damage is very unlikely to produce clinically significant manifestations, given the selective delivery of RF energy within areas of myocardial scarring. In a consecutive series of 153 patients undergoing catheter ablation of scar-related epicardial VT, intraprocedural coronary angiography was performed in 34 (22%) patients, while the remaining 119 (78%) underwent epicardial ablation without intraprocedural angiography.[73] The distribution of successful

ablation sites was not different between the two groups. Periprocedural complications occurred in 13 (8.4%) patients (3 [8.8%] in the coronary angiography group and 10 [8.4%] in the no coronary angiography group; $p = .94$) and consisted of minor intrapericardial bleeding without consequence in 11 (7.2%) cases, mild abdominal discomfort that did not require further intervention in 1 case, and acute HF in 1 case. No other complications occurred; in particular, no case of coronary artery damage was observed both acutely and at follow-up, as assessed by nuclear imaging stress testing. The results of this large observational study suggest that epicardial scar–related VT ablation can be safely performed without intraprocedural coronary angiography and without acute and follow-up risks for coronary artery damage. The latter is an extremely rare complication in these patients, probably reflecting exclusive ablation within the scar area, together with the insulating properties of pericoronary epicardial adipose tissue and the convective cooling effect of the coronary blood flow.

Ablation Endpoints During Ventricular Tachycardia Ablation

Acute arrhythmia termination and noninducibility of any sustained arrhythmia are the most widely adopted endpoints during catheter ablation of VT. For focal VTs, mapping and ablation during VT are associated with the greatest likelihood of acute termination, postprocedural noninducibility, and long-term success. On the other hand, for scar-related VTs, the abolition of only clinical or inducible VT(s) has been reported to result in long-term arrhythmia–free survival in no more than 70% of patients (Table 124.5[74–93]). In this regard, targeting only the clinical or inducible VT(s) does not necessarily abolish all of the potential reentrant circuits within the scar.

We have described a pure substrate-based ablation approach in scar-related VT, namely, the endoepicardial scar homogenization approach.[25] With such an approach, all potential arrhythmogenic areas within the scar, defined as abnormal late and fragmented electrograms, are targeted during ablation, irrespective of their participation in clinical/inducible VT(s). We have evaluated the benefit of the scar homogenization approach in a consecutive case series of 92 patients with postinfarction scar–related VT storm.[25] Patients were treated by confining RF lesions to the putative isthmus sites of clinical/inducible VT(s), as assessed using conventional mapping techniques such as entrainment, activation, and pace mapping (conventional VT ablation; n = 49), or they underwent endo- and epicardial ablation of all abnormal potentials within the scar (homogenization of the scar; n = 43). During a mean follow-up of 25 ± 10 months, the VT recurrence rate was 47% in the conventional ablation group and 19% in the endo-epicardial scar homogenization group (log rank p = .006). The results of this study provide the first demonstration in a large series of patients that extensive substrate modification with catheter ablation improves long-term arrhythmia–free survival in patients undergoing catheter ablation of scar-related VT. Other groups have reported results comparable with ours with similarly extensive substrate-based ablation approaches in patients with ischemic cardiomyopathy.[94]

Importantly, we recently published findings from the Ablation of Clinical Ventricular Tachycardia Versus Addition of Substrate Ablation on the Long Term Success Rate of VT Ablation (VISTA) trial.[95] This was a randomized multicenter trial comparing substrate-based ablation (scar homogenization, n = 58) and conventional VT ablation (n = 60), which showed that substrate-based ablation was superior in terms of preventing VT recurrence, less requirement for AADs, and fewer rehospitalizations. This was achieved with a similar complication rate between groups. However, there was no difference in terms of mortality. This trial lends further support to using the substrate-based ablation approach.

Postprocedural Management

Atrial Fibrillation

Monitoring for Recurrences: Methods and Relative Merits

All patients are monitored overnight with respect to frequent symptoms, access sites, and neurological assessments. Following discharge, the optimal method for long-term monitoring of atrial arrhythmia recurrence after AF ablation is a crucial yet unsolved issue. Clinical assessment based on patients' symptoms has been demonstrated to be largely unreliable for predicting postablation recurrences, and a substantial number of patients experience asymptomatic AF recurrences.[12] From a clinical standpoint, accurate detection of postablation recurrences bears important implications, including the selection of patients who might benefit from AAD continuation or a repeat ablation procedure and for clinical decision making with regard to oral anticoagulation discontinuation. Several noncontinuous and continuous ECG monitoring techniques have been employed in clinical studies on AF ablation; in general, more intensive monitoring is associated with a greater likelihood of detecting both symptomatic and asymptomatic AF episodes.[12] Serial or symptom-initiated standard ECGs, Holter monitoring (24 hours to 7 days) and transtelephonic recordings, patient-activated and automatically activated devices, and external loop recorders are among the commonly used noncontinuous monitoring tools.

At our institution, we routinely adopt scheduled 7-day Holter ECG recordings with random and symptom-activated external event recordings. By adopting a similar protocol, other groups have reported a sensitivity of 70% for detecting recurrent arrhythmia, with a negative predictive value for the absence of AF, ranging between 25% and 40%.[96] In recent years, the value of continuous ECG monitoring with implantable devices (e.g., pacemakers/defibrillators with atrial leads, long-term subcutaneous monitors) has been increasingly reported.[71] In the recently terminated Discerning the Incidence of Symptomatic and Asymptomatic Episodes of Atrial Fibrillation Pre- and Post-Radiofrequency Ablation (DISCERN AF) trial, Verma and colleagues equipped 50 patients with an implantable loop recorder at least 3 months before the scheduled ablation procedure and for up to 18 months after ablation. Notably, after ablation, the ratio of asymptomatic to symptomatic AF episodes increased from 1.1 to 3.7, with patients' symptoms markedly underestimating AF burden after ablation (12% of patients had only asymptomatic AF recurrences).[97] Although implantable loop recorders appear promising for the long-term assessment of AF burden, important limitations include less than 100% specificity due to myopotentials and atrial and ventricular premature beats, as well as limited memory, resulting in unretrievable electrograms that cannot be used to verify the correct rhythm diagnosis. We consider any episode of AF/AFL or AT that occurs after the blanking period and that lasts for more than 30 seconds to be a recurrence. If AF recurrence occurs after the blanking period, patients are initially restarted on their previous AAD regimen and are considered for a redo procedure.

Both US and European guidelines recognize the significant rate of postprocedural AF recurrence, but no specific recommendations regarding postprocedural surveillance (e.g., Holter monitoring) are made, which appears reasonable given that current treatment strategies are largely driven by patient symptoms. However, the European guidelines do suggest (class IIa recommendation) that when AF recurs within the first 6 weeks after catheter ablation, a watch-and-wait rhythm control therapy should be considered.[11,16]

Postablation Use of Antiarrhythmic Drugs

It is common practice to continue previously ineffective AADs during the blanking period after ablation. However, this practice is not supported by adequate evidence. In a randomized study of 110 patients undergoing catheter ablation of AF, Leong-Sit and colleagues showed that empirical use of AADs (e.g., flecainide, propafenone, sotalol, dofetilide, dronedarone, amiodarone) during the first 6 weeks after AF ablation was associated with a reduced incidence of early (within 6 weeks) clinically significant atrial arrhythmias and the need for cardioversion or hospitalization for arrhythmia management, although it had no effect on prediction or prevention of arrhythmia recurrence at 6 months.[98]

The role of antiinflammatory drugs, such as steroids, in preventing early postablation recurrences has been recently assessed in a randomized study.[99] In this trial, a total of 125 patients with paroxysmal AF were randomly assigned to receive either corticosteroids (IV hydrocortisone [2 mg/kg] on the day of the procedure and oral prednisolone [0.5 mg/kg/day] for 3 days after ablation) or placebo. The prevalence of immediate AF recurrences (within 3 days after ablation) was significantly lower in the corticosteroid group than in the placebo group (7% vs. 31%), and the AF-free rate at 14 months postablation was better in the corticosteroid group than in the placebo group (85% vs. 71%; p = .032).[100]

Other drugs, such as upstream therapies for AF (e.g., renin-angiotensin system blockers, statins), have not been shown to affect SR maintenance after catheter ablation of AF.[101]

Postablation Anticoagulation

Immediately after concluding the procedure, heparin is partially reversed with IV protamine (30–50 mg) and sheaths are removed when ACT is ≤250 seconds. All patients are administered 325 mg of aspirin and continue their warfarin therapy to maintain target INR; an echocardiogram is performed 6 hours postprocedure to rule out pericardial effusion. Observational data suggest that the majority of cerebral insults occur within 2 weeks after the procedure,[102] and postablation anticoagulation is recommended in all patients for at least 2 months.[12] There is a variable degree of atrial stunning following AF ablation, which may promote thrombus formation. Furthermore, there is concern that the endothelial damage incurred during the energy application to the LA is thrombogenic.

There is currently no evidence from large randomized trials to guide long-term anticoagulation strategies following AF ablation. Therefore, at present, patients should be risk stratified according to the same principles (CHADS2 or CHADS2-VASc score) used in patients who did not undergo ablation, even if SR is initially restored.[16,103,104] These scores have been recently shown to provide prognostic value in patients after ablation.[105] However, emerging data suggest that successful AF ablation does reduce the risk for stroke and that long-term anticoagulation may not be necessary in all patients. A nonrandomized study followed 755 patients for 25 months after ablation.[102] In a subgroup of 180 patients with ≥1 stroke risk factor who remained in SR, anticoagulation was discontinued at a median of 5 months postablation without any cardioembolic events. Furthermore, in a recent observational study including 3344 AF ablation patients, anticoagulation was discontinued in patients without significant LA mechanical dysfunction who remained in SR, regardless of the CHADS2 score.[106] All patients were transitioned to aspirin, and in patients with a CHADS2 score of ≥1, anticoagulation was restarted only in the event of AF recurrence. Using this strategy, no cardioembolic events occurred during a mean follow-up of 28 months in 347 patients with a mean CHADS2 score of ≥2. Such results were recently confirmed in a large single-center series.[107] While these data are promising, large randomized trials to evaluate the best postprocedural long-term anticoagulation strategy are needed to help guide the best postablation anticoagulation approach.

In patients where LAA isolation was performed as part of the AF ablation procedure, it is important to consider the mechanical function of the LAA postablation. For patients with impaired LAA contractility at 6 months follow-up, we continue anticoagulation indefinitely, unless an LAA closure device is placed. However, in our experience, 40%–45% of patients have preserved LAA contraction on TEE 6 months postprocedure, which may be due to LAA reconnection and/or passive LAA contraction following ventricular contraction.

We discontinue long-term anticoagulant therapy 6 months after the procedure if (1) the patient maintains stable SR, (2) LAA velocity is normal (i.e., >0.3 m/s) on TEE, and (3) evidence suggests a consistent A wave on the transmitral Doppler flow study. In the future, the widespread availability of percutaneous LAA closure devices (e.g., WATCHMAN, Atritech, Plymouth, MN; LARIAT, SentreHEART, Inc., Palo Alto, CA) might allow more patients undergoing LAA isolation to safely discontinue long-term oral anticoagulation therapy. In this context, it should be noted that the PROTECT-AF trial recently reported more long-term follow-up data in patients with nonvalvular AF undergoing LAA closure.[108] Compared with warfarin, percutaneous LAA closure met criteria for both noninferiority and superiority and for the prevention of the combined outcome of stroke, systemic embolism, and cardiovascular death, as well as superiority for cardiovascular and all-cause mortality after 3.8 years of follow-up.[108]

Other Postprocedural Management Considerations

With the use of tip-irrigated catheters, fluid overload can become an issue, as several liters of saline may be administered. This is particularly important to consider in patients with long-standing persistent AF as a more extensive ablation protocol is often used in these patients. Therefore we routinely administer 40–60 mg of IV furosemide immediately after the procedure, followed by additional IV and/or per os (PO) furosemide as needed for 2–3 days postprocedure. Patients are counseled to monitor their weight and contact their assigned AF nurse if body weight does not approach the preprocedural value or if complications or new symptoms emerge. We consider these dedicated AF nurses, who are in charge of preprocedural education and postprocedural follow-up, to be an integral part of a state-of-the-art ablation center.

Role of Repeat Ablation Procedures

Patients experiencing recurrent drug refractory arrhythmia after catheter ablation of AF are usually managed with a repeat ablation procedure. In general, reconnection of previously ablated areas (mostly PVs) represents the most common finding in these patients and the achievement of permanent reisolation often results in a lasting cure. On the other hand, a relatively small but definitive subset of patients experience recurrent arrhythmia in the absence of reconnection of previously targeted areas. The exact prevalence of this phenomenon is yet undefined and depends largely on how many structures have been targeted for isolation during the index procedure (e.g., only PVs as opposed to wider areas of isolation, including the entire posterior wall). For instance, in a recent observational case series of 52 patients with paroxysmal AF undergoing ostial PVI with a laser balloon catheter, arrhythmia-free survival after a mean follow-up of 12 ± 1.8 months was 71.2% despite proven permanent PVI.[109] More proximal triggers (e.g., posterior wall between the veins) or other non-PV triggers (e.g., coronary sinus, interatrial septum, LAA, crista terminalis/SVC) constitute likely explanations for the results by Dukkipati and coworkers.[109] In this regard, we have already reported in a large multicenter prospective study the relevance of the LAA as a trigger site for AF.[65] In this study, we included a consecutive series of 987 patients (29% paroxysmal AF, 71% nonparoxysmal AF) referred to our institution for redo catheter ablation. LAA firing was assessed only after all potential sites of reconnection, including the PV antra, posterior wall, and septum, were checked and targeted if reconnected. Overall, 266 (27%) patients showed firing from the LAA at baseline or after administration of ISP, and in 8.7% of patients, the LAA was found to be the only source of arrhythmia. LAA firing was defined as consistent PACs with earliest activation in the LAA or as AF/atrial tachyarrhythmia originating from the LAA. In these cases, complete isolation of the LAA is the ablation strategy that provides the best long-term outcome. Of 266 patients presenting with LAA firing, 43 were not ablated (group 1), 56 received a focal ablation (group 2), and 167 underwent LAA isolation guided by a circular mapping catheter and ICE (group 3). After a mean follow-up of 1 year, AF recurred in 74% of group 1 patients compared with 68% of group 2 and 15% of group 3 patients ($p <$ .001 for multiple comparison).[65]

Ventricular Tachycardia

Monitoring for Recurrences: Methods and Relative Merits

Few clinical data are available to compare different methods of monitoring for VT recurrence after catheter ablation.[110] However, most patients undergoing VT ablation either already have an implantable cardioverter defibrillator (ICD) or will have an ICD implanted after the procedure, and recurrent arrhythmia could be easily monitored by analyzing the ventricular events stored in the ICD (i.e., device telemetry or ventricular events leading to appropriate ICD intervention). In 1999, the US Food and Drug Administration (FDA) suggested that any VT requiring ICD therapy or nonsustained VT episodes lasting more than 20 seconds should be documented, and proposed a minimum follow-up of 6 months.[111] The last consensus document on VT ablation has proposed that the minimum follow-up should be extended to 1 year.[110]

For patients without an ICD, no consensus has been reached regarding the best method for monitoring recurrent arrhythmia. Typically, patients have no evidence of structural heart disease and present with symptomatic but hemodynamically tolerated VAs; in these cases, absence of symptomatic recurrence is considered a valid endpoint. For patients with few or no symptoms and for those with infrequent arrhythmia episodes before ablation, prolonged monitoring with loop recorders or transtelephonic monitoring is justifiable. Exercise stress testing could be indicated to monitor the ablation outcomes of patients with exercise-induced VTs, and follow-up echo monitoring is advisable for patients with VA-induced cardiomyopathy.

Postablation Use of Antiarrhythmic Drugs

With regard to catheter ablation of AF, long-term freedom from recurrent VT without AAD therapy is the main goal of catheter ablation of VT. In patients without structural heart disease, all AADs are usually discontinued postablation; such an approach allows more reliable monitoring for recurrences. In patients with structural heart disease, AADs are usually continued after ablation, given the greater complexity of arrhythmia substrates in these cases. Amiodarone is the drug used most commonly in these patients. Current guidelines suggest that amiodarone should be discontinued after catheter ablation of VT and that attempts should be made to reduce its dosage when complete discontinuation is not possible,[110] given the dose-dependent risk for side effects related to amiodarone use.

Role of Repeat Ablation Procedures

Recurrent arrhythmia after failed VT ablation might be due to recovery of conduction in a previously ablated area or to a deeper substrate (midmyocardial or epicardial) that was incompletely targeted during the previous ablation, or it might merely reflect the development of a new VT circuit.[112]

The decision of whether to perform a repeat VT ablation and its timing are highly dependent on the clinical context and on the suspected mechanism of arrhythmia recurrence. For instance, a recurrent VT displaying exactly the same ECG morphology and cycle length as the previously ablated one suggests recovery or conduction in the previously ablated area or a deeper myocardial substrate. On the other hand, when the recurrent VT has different ECG morphology and cycle length, the clinician should suspect the development of a new VT circuit.[112]

Thus far, no data are available for evaluation of the optimal timing of repeat VT ablation. According to FDA guidelines, clinicians should wait at least 1 week after ablation.[111] However, in the case of frequent recurrences or even an electrical storm, the repeat procedure should be scheduled as soon as possible.[110]

Conclusions

When a catheter ablation procedure is planned, clinical aspects related to patient history, symptoms, mode of presentation, and arrhythmia characteristics are crucial for anticipating the optimal ablation approach and predicting outcomes. For instance, in the case of catheter ablation of complex arrhythmias, such as AF and VT, simple baseline clinical characteristics provide key information. The type of AF, namely, paroxysmal versus nonparoxysmal AF, can help clinicians to predict the need for more extensive ablation beyond PVI. Other clinical characteristics, including gender, comorbidities, and duration of arrhythmia episodes, are also useful for this purpose. After AF ablation, optimizing arrhythmia recurrence monitoring and developing criteria for selecting patients in whom discontinuation of anticoagulation may be appropriate are areas of active investigation.

In patients with VT, the presence of nonischemic structural heart disease predicts the need for an endo-epicardial procedure as a first-line approach, whereas most patients with ischemic substrates can be effectively managed with an endocardial procedure. After ablation, the mode and intensity of arrhythmia monitoring are important for timely detection of recurrent arrhythmia and for planning of a repeat ablation procedure.

REFERENCES

1. Blomström-Lundqvist C, Scheinman MM, Aliot EM, et al. ACC/AHA/ESC guidelines for the management of patients with supraventricular arrhythmias—executive summary. A report of the American College of Cardiology/American Heart Association task force on practice guidelines and the European Society of Cardiology committee for practice guidelines (writing committee to develop guidelines for the management of patients with supraventricular arrhythmias) developed in collaboration with NASPE-Heart Rhythm Society. *J Am Coll Cardiol.* 2003;42:1493–1531.
2. Santangeli P, di Biase L, Pelargonio G, et al. Outcome of invasive electrophysiological procedures and gender: are males and females the same? *J Cardiovasc Electrophysiol.* 2011;22:605–612.
3. Medi C, Kalman JM, Haqqani H, et al. Tachycardia-mediated cardiomyopathy secondary to focal atrial tachycardia: long-term outcome after catheter ablation. *J Am Coll Cardiol.* 2009;53:1791–1797.
4. Pediatric and Congenital Electrophysiology Society (PACES), Heart Rhythm Society (HRS), American College of Cardiology Foundation (ACCF), et al. PACES/HRS expert consensus statement on the management of the asymptomatic young patient with a Wolff-Parkinson-White (WPW, ventricular preexcitation) electrocardiographic pattern: developed in partnership between the Pediatric and Congenital Electrophysiology Society (PACES) and the Heart Rhythm Society (HRS). Endorsed by the governing bodies of PACES, HRS, the American College of Cardiology Foundation (ACCF), the American Heart Association (AHA), the American Academy of Pediatrics (AAP), and the Canadian Heart Rhythm Society (CHRS). *Heart Rhythm.* 2012;9:1006–1024.
5. Roten L, Lukac P, De Groot N, et al. Catheter ablation of arrhythmias in Ebstein's anomaly: a multicenter study. *J Cardiovasc Electrophysiol.* 2011;22:1391–1396.
6. Ernst S, Babu-Narayan SV, Keegan J, et al. Remote-controlled magnetic navigation and ablation with 3D image integration as an alternative approach in patients with intra-atrial baffle anatomy. *Circ Arrhythm Electrophysiol.* 2012;5:131–139.
7. Razzouk AJ, Gow R, Finley J, et al. Surgically created Wolff-Parkinson-White syndrome after Fontan operation. *Ann Thorac Surg.* 1992;54:974–977.

8. Sternick EB, Oliva A, Gerken LM, et al. Clinical, electrocardiographic, and electrophysiologic characteristics of patients with a fasciculoventricular pathway: the role of PRKAG2 mutation. *Heart Rhythm.* 2011;8:58–64.
9. Arruda MS, McClelland JH, Wang X, et al. Development and validation of an ECG algorithm for identifying accessory pathway ablation site in Wolff-Parkinson-White syndrome. *J Cardiovasc Electrophysiol.* 1998;9:2–12.
10. Haissaguerre M, Marcus F, Poquet F, et al. Electrocardiographic characteristics and catheter ablation of parahisian accessory pathways. *Circulation.* 1994;90:1124–1128.
11. January CT, Wann LS, Alpert JS, et al. 2014 AHA/ACC/HRS guideline for the management of patients with atrial fibrillation: executive summary: a report of the American College of Cardiology/American Heart Association Task Force on practice guidelines and the Heart Rhythm Society. *Circulation.* 2014;130:2071–2104.
12. Calkins H, Kuck KH, Cappato R, et al. 2012 HRS/EHRA/ECAS expert consensus statement on catheter and surgical ablation of atrial fibrillation: recommendations for patient selection, procedural techniques, patient management and follow-up, definitions, endpoints, and research trial design: a report of the Heart Rhythm Society (HRS) Task Force on Catheter and Surgical Ablation of Atrial Fibrillation. Developed in partnership with the European Heart Rhythm Association (EHRA), a registered branch of the European Society of Cardiology (ESC) and the European Cardiac Arrhythmia Society (ECAS); and in collaboration with the American College of Cardiology (ACC), American Heart Association (AHA), the Asia Pacific Heart Rhythm Society (APHRS), and the Society of Thoracic Surgeons (STS). Endorsed by the governing bodies of the American College of Cardiology Foundation, the American Heart Association, the European Cardiac Arrhythmia Society, the European Heart Rhythm Association, the Society of Thoracic Surgeons, the Asia Pacific Heart Rhythm Society, and the Heart Rhythm Society. *Heart Rhythm.* 2012;9:632–696.e21.
13. Wazni OM, Marrouche NF, Martin DO, et al. Radiofrequency ablation vs antiarrhythmic drugs as first-line treatment of symptomatic atrial fibrillation: a randomized trial. *JAMA.* 2005;293:2634–2640.

14. Cosedis Nielsen J, Johannessen A, Raatikainen P, et al. Radiofrequency ablation as initial therapy in paroxysmal atrial fibrillation. *N Engl J Med.* 2012;367:1587–1595.
15. Morillo CA, Verma A, Connolly SJ, et al. Radiofrequency ablation vs antiarrhythmic drugs as first-line treatment of paroxysmal atrial fibrillation (RAAFT-2): a randomized trial. *JAMA.* 2014;311:692–700.
16. Camm AJ, Lip GY, De Caterina R, et al. 2012 focused update of the ESC Guidelines for the management of atrial fibrillation: an update of the 2010 ESC Guidelines for the management of atrial fibrillation. Developed with the special contribution of the European Heart Rhythm Association. *Eur Heart J.* 2012;33:2719–2747.
17. Lakkireddy D, Nagarajan D, Di Biase L, et al. Radiofrequency ablation of atrial fibrillation in patients with mitral or aortic mechanical prosthetic valves: a feasibility, safety, and efficacy study. *Heart Rhythm.* 2011;8:975–980.
18. Santangeli P, Di Biase L, Mohanty P, et al. Catheter ablation of atrial fibrillation in octogenarians: safety and outcomes. *J Cardiovasc Electrophysiol.* 2012;23:687–693.
19. Aliot EM, Stevenson WG, Almendral-Garrote JM, et al. EHRA/HRS Expert Consensus on Catheter Ablation of Ventricular Arrhythmias: developed in a partnership with the European Heart Rhythm Association (EHRA), a Registered Branch of the European Society of Cardiology (ESC), and the Heart Rhythm Society (HRS); in collaboration with the American College of Cardiology (ACC) and the American Heart Association (AHA). *Heart Rhythm.* 2009;6:886–933.
20. Tanawuttiwat T, Nazarian S, Calkins H. The role of catheter ablation in the management of ventricular tachycardia. *Eur Heart J.* 2016;37:594–609.
21. Santangeli P, Pieroni M, Dello Russo A, et al. Correlation between signal-averaged ECG and the histologic evaluation of the myocardial substrate in right ventricular outflow tract arrhythmias. *Circ Arrhythm Electrophysiol.* 2012;5:475–483.
22. Bai R, Di Biase L, Shivkumar K, et al. Ablation of ventricular arrhythmias in arrhythmogenic right ventricular dysplasia/cardiomyopathy: arrhythmia-free survival after endo-epicardial substrate based mapping and ablation. *Circ Arrhythm Electrophysiol.* 2011;4:478–485.
23. Santangeli P, Di Biase L, Lakkireddy D, et al. Radiofrequency catheter ablation of ventricular arrhythmias in patients with hypertrophic cardiomyopathy: safety and feasibility. *Heart Rhythm.* 2010;7:1036–1042.

24. Della Bella P, Brugada J, Zeppenfeld K, et al. Epicardial ablation for ventricular tachycardia: a European multicenter study. *Circ Arrhythm Electrophysiol.* 2011;4:653–659.

25. Di Biase L, Santangeli P, Burkhardt DJ, et al. Endo-epicardial homogenization of the scar versus limited substrate ablation for the treatment of electrical storms in patients with ischemic cardiomyopathy. *J Am Coll Cardiol.* 2012;60:132–141.

26. Yoshiga Y, Mathew S, Wissner E, et al. Correlation between substrate location and ablation strategy in patients with ventricular tachycardia late after myocardial infarction. *Heart Rhythm.* 2012;9:1192–1199.

27. Santangeli P, Di Biase L, Horton R, et al. Ablation of atrial fibrillation under therapeutic warfarin reduces peri-procedural complications: evidence from a meta-analysis. *Circ Arrhythm Electrophysiol.* 2012;5:302–311.

28. Di Biase L, Burkhardt JD, Mohanty P, et al. Periprocedural stroke and management of major bleeding complications in patients undergoing catheter ablation of atrial fibrillation: the impact of periprocedural therapeutic international normalized ratio. *Circulation.* 2010;121:2550–2556.

29. Briceno DF, Natale A, Di Biase L. Heparin kinetics: the "holy grail" of periprocedural anticoagulation for ablation of atrial fibrillation. *Pacing Clin Electrophysiol.* 2015;38:1137–1141.

30. Di Biase L, Burkhardt JD, Santangeli P, et al. Periprocedural stroke and bleeding complications in patients undergoing catheter ablation of atrial fibrillation with different anticoagulation management: results from the Role of Coumadin in Preventing Thromboembolism in Atrial Fibrillation (AF) Patients Undergoing Catheter Ablation (COMPARE) randomized trial. *Circulation.* 2014;129:2638–2644.

31. Di Biase L, Natale A. Apixaban is dear to me, but dearer still is warfarin. *Pace Clin Electrophysiol.* 2015;38:153–154.

32. Cappato R, Marchlinski FE, Hohnloser SH, et al. Uninterrupted rivaroxaban vs. uninterrupted vitamin K antagonists for catheter ablation in non-valvular atrial fibrillation. *Eur Heart J.* 2015;36:1805–1811.

33. Di Biase L, Lakkireddy D, Trivedi C, et al. Feasibility and safety of uninterrupted periprocedural apixaban administration in patients undergoing radiofrequency catheter ablation for atrial fibrillation: results from a multicenter study. *Heart Rhythm.* 2015;12:1162–1168.

34. Lakkireddy D, Reddy YM, Di Biase L, et al. Feasibility and safety of dabigatran versus warfarin for periprocedural anticoagulation in patients undergoing radiofrequency ablation for atrial fibrillation: results from a multicenter prospective registry. *J Am Coll Cardiol.* 2012;59:1168–1174.

35. Kaseno K, Naito S, Nakamura K, et al. Efficacy and safety of periprocedural dabigatran in patients undergoing catheter ablation of atrial fibrillation. *Circ J.* 2012;76:2337–2342.

36. Dentali F, Riva N, Crowther M, et al. Efficacy and safety of the novel oral anticoagulants in atrial fibrillation: a systematic review and meta-analysis of the literature. *Circulation.* 2012;126:2381–2391.

37. Mohanty S, Di Biase L, Mohanty P, et al. Effect of periprocedural amiodarone on procedure outcome in patients with longstanding persistent atrial fibrillation undergoing extended pulmonary vein antrum isolation: results from a randomized study (SPECULATE). *Heart Rhythm.* 2015;12:477–483.

38. Fonarow GC, Abraham WT, Albert NM, et al. Influence of beta-blocker continuation or withdrawal on outcomes in patients hospitalized with heart failure: findings from the OPTIMIZE-HF program. *J Am Coll Cardiol.* 2008;52:190–199.

39. Bangalore S, Wetterslev J, Pranesh S, et al. Perioperative beta blockers in patients having non-cardiac surgery: a meta-analysis. *Lancet.* 2008;372:1962–1976.

40. Kristensen SD, Knuuti J, Saraste A, et al. 2014 ESC/ESA Guidelines on non-cardiac surgery: cardiovascular assessment and management: The Joint Task Force on non-cardiac surgery: cardiovascular assessment and management of the European Society of Cardiology (ESC) and the European Society of Anaesthesiology (ESA). *Eur Heart J.* 2014;35:2383–2431.

41. Di Biase L, Conti S, Mohanty P, et al. General anesthesia reduces the prevalence of pulmonary vein reconnection during repeat ablation when compared with conscious sedation: results from a randomized study. *Heart Rhythm.* 2011;8:368–372.

42. Ezzat VA, Chew A, McCready JW, et al. Catheter ablation of atrial fibrillation-patient satisfaction from a single-center UK experience. *J Interv Card Electrophysiol.* 2013;37:291–303.

43. Fernandez-Bustamante A, Ibanez V, Alfaro JJ, et al. High-frequency jet ventilation in interventional bronchoscopy: factors with predictive value on high-frequency jet ventilation complications. *J Clin Anesth.* 2006;18:349–356.

44. Lim HE, Pak HN, Tse HF, et al. Catheter ablation of atrial fibrillation via superior approach in patients with interruption of the inferior vena cava. *Heart Rhythm.* 2009;6:174–179.

45. Hind D, Calvert N, McWilliams R, et al. Ultrasonic locating devices for central venous cannulation: meta-analysis. *BMJ.* 2003;327:361.

46. Natale A, Thakur R. *Transseptal Catheterization and Interventions.* Minneapolis: Cardiotext; 2010.

47. Santangeli P, Di Biase L, Burkhardt JD, et al. Transseptal access and atrial fibrillation ablation guided by intracardiac echocardiography in patients with atrial septal closure devices. *Heart Rhythm.* 2011;8:1669–1675.

48. Greenstein E, Passman R, Lin AC, et al. Incidence of tissue coring during transseptal catheterization when using electrocautery and a standard transseptal needle. *Circ Arrhythm Electrophysiol.* 2012;5:341–344.

49. Di Biase L, Natale A, Blandino A, et al. Diffusion magnetic cerebral imaging (dMRI) pre and 24 hours post ablation of atrial fibrillation: results on therapeutic anticoagulation with Coumadin. *Circulation.* 2011;124. A10868.

50. Koruth JS, Aryana A, Dukkipati SR, et al. Unusual complications of percutaneous epicardial access and epicardial mapping and ablation of cardiac arrhythmias. *Circ Arrhythm Electrophysiol.* 2011;4:882–888.

51. Singh SM, d'Avila A, Doshi SK, et al. Esophageal injury and temperature monitoring during atrial fibrillation ablation. *Circ Arrhythm Electrophysiol.* 2008;1:162–168.

52. Gaita F, Caponi D, Pianelli M, et al. Radiofrequency catheter ablation of atrial fibrillation: a cause of silent thromboembolism? Magnetic resonance imaging assessment of cerebral thromboembolism in patients undergoing ablation of atrial fibrillation. *Circulation.* 2010;122:1667–1673.

53. Di Biase L, Gaita F, Toso E, et al. Does periprocedural anticoagulation management of atrial fibrillation affect the prevalence of silent thromboembolic lesion detected by diffusion cerebral magnetic resonance imaging in patients undergoing radiofrequency atrial fibrillation ablation with open irrigated catheters? Results from a prospective multicenter study. *Heart Rhythm.* 2014;11:791–798.

54. Proietti R, Santangeli P, Di Biase L, et al. Comparative effectiveness of wide antral versus ostial pulmonary vein isolation: a systematic review and meta-analysis. *Circ Arrhythm Electrophysiol.* 2014;7:39–45.

55. Trulock KM, Narayan SM, Piccini JP. Rhythm control in heart failure patients with atrial fibrillation: contemporary challenges including the role of ablation. *J Am Coll Cardiol.* 2014;64:710–721.

56. Tilz RR, Rillig A, Thum AM, et al. Catheter ablation of long-standing persistent atrial fibrillation: 5-year outcomes of the Hamburg Sequential Ablation Strategy. *J Am Coll Cardiol.* 2012;60:1921–1929.

57. Tsao HM, Wu MH, Huang BH, et al. Morphologic remodeling of pulmonary veins and left atrium after catheter ablation of atrial fibrillation: insight from long-term follow-up of three-dimensional magnetic resonance imaging. *J Cardiovasc Electrophysiol.* 2005;16:7–12.

58. Crawford T, Chugh A, Good E, et al. Clinical value of noninducibility by high-dose isoproterenol versus rapid atrial pacing after catheter ablation of paroxysmal atrial fibrillation. *J Cardiovasc Electrophysiol.* 2010;21:13–20.

59. Chen PS, Maruyama M, Lin SF. Arrhythmogenic foci and the mechanisms of atrial fibrillation. *Circ Arrhythm Electrophysiol.* 2010;3:7–9.

60. Li WJ, Bai YY, Zhang HY, et al. Additional ablation of complex fractionated atrial electrograms after pulmonary vein isolation in patients with atrial fibrillation: a meta-analysis. *Circ Arrhythm Electrophysiol.* 2011;4:143–148.

61. Jadidi AS, Duncan E, Miyazaki S, et al. Functional nature of electrogram fractionation demonstrated by left atrial high-density mapping. *Circ Arrhythm Electrophysiol.* 2012;5:32–42.

62. Shivkumar K, Ellenbogen KA, Hummel JD, et al. Acute termination of human atrial fibrillation by identification and catheter ablation of localized rotors and sources: first multicenter experience of focal impulse and rotor modulation (FIRM) ablation. *J Cardiovasc Electrophysiol.* 2012;23:1277–1285.

63. Calkins H. Catheter ablation to maintain sinus rhythm. *Circulation.* 2012;125:1439–1445.

64. Narayan SM, Krummen DE, Shivkumar K, et al. Treatment of atrial fibrillation by the ablation of localized sources: CONFIRM (Conventional Ablation for Atrial Fibrillation With or Without Focal Impulse and Rotor Modulation) trial. *J Am Coll Cardiol.* 2012;60:628–636.

65. Di Biase L, Burkhardt JD, Mohanty P, et al. Left atrial appendage: an underrecognized trigger site of atrial fibrillation. *Circulation.* 2010;122:109–118.

66. Santangeli P, Di Biase L, Pelargonio G, et al. Catheter ablation of atrial fibrillation: randomized controlled trials and registries, a look back and the view forward. *J Interv Card Electrophysiol.* 2011;31:69–80.

67. Gaita F, Caponi D, Scaglione M, et al. Long-term clinical results of 2 different ablation strategies in patients with paroxysmal and persistent atrial fibrillation. *Circ Arrhythm Electrophysiol.* 2008;1:269–275.

68. Elayi CS, Di Biase L, Barrett C, et al. Atrial fibrillation termination as a procedural endpoint during ablation in long-standing persistent atrial fibrillation. *Heart Rhythm.* 2010;7:1216–1223.

69. Di Biase L, Saenz LC, Burkhardt DJ, et al. Esophageal capsule endoscopy after radiofrequency catheter ablation for atrial fibrillation: documented higher risk of luminal esophageal damage with general anesthesia as compared with conscious sedation. *Circ Arrhythm Electrophysiol.* 2009;2:108–112.

70. Di Biase L, Natale A, Barrett C, et al. Relationship between catheter forces, lesion characteristics, "popping," and char formation: experience with robotic navigation system. *J Cardiovasc Electrophysiol.* 2009;20:436–440.

71. Reddy VY, Shah D, Kautzner J, et al. The relationship between contact force and clinical outcome during radiofrequency catheter ablation of atrial fibrillation in the TOCCATA study. *Heart Rhythm.* 2012;9:1789–1795.

72. Di Biase L, Burkhardt D, Sanchez J, et al. Variant of left ventricular outflow tract tachycardia requiring ablation from multiple sites. *Eur Heart J.* 2011;32:178. Abstract 1253.

73. Santangeli P, Di Biase L, Burkhardt D, et al. Safety of epicardial scar-related ventricular tachycardia ablation without performing coronary angiography: results from a multicenter study. *Heart Rhythm.* 2012;9:S355.

74. Morady F, Harvey M, Kalbfleisch SJ, et al. Radiofrequency catheter ablation of ventricular tachycardia in patients with coronary artery disease. *Circulation.* 1993;87:363–372.

75. Kim YH, Sosa-Suarez G, Trouton TG, et al. Treatment of ventricular tachycardia by transcatheter radiofrequency ablation in patients with ischemic heart disease. *Circulation.* 1994;89:1094–1102.

76. Rothman SA, Hsia HH, Cossu SF, et al. Radiofrequency catheter ablation of postinfarction ventricular tachycardia: long-term success and the significance of inducible nonclinical arrhythmias. *Circulation.* 1997;96:3499–3508.

77. Stevenson WG, Wilber DJ, Natale A, et al. Irrigated radiofrequency catheter ablation guided by electroanatomic mapping for recurrent ventricular tachycardia after myocardial infarction: the multicenter thermocool ventricular tachycardia ablation trial. *Circulation.* 2008;118:2773–2782.

78. Epstein AE, Wilber D, Calkins H, et al. Randomized controlled trial of ventricular tachycardia treatment by cooled tip catheter ablation vs drug therapy. *J Am Coll Cardiol.* 1998;31:118A.

79. Ortiz M, Almendral J, Villacastin J, et al. [Radiofrequency ablation of ventricular tachycardia in patients with ischemic cardiopathy]. *Rev Esp Cardiol.* 1999;52:159–168.

80. El-Shalakany A, Hadjis T, Papageorgiou P, et al. Entrainment/mapping criteria for the prediction of termination of ventricular tachycardia by single radiofrequency lesion in patients with coronary artery disease. *Circulation.* 1999;99:2283–2289.

81. Calkins H, Epstein A, Packer D, et al. Catheter ablation of ventricular tachycardia in patients with structural heart disease using cooled radiofrequency energy: results of a prospective multicenter study. Cooled RF Multi Center Investigators Group. *J Am Coll Cardiol.* 2000;35:1905–1914.

82. O'Callaghan PA, Poloniecki J, Sosa-Suarez G, et al. Long-term clinical outcome of patients with prior myocardial infarction after palliative radiofrequency catheter ablation for frequent ventricular tachycardia. *Am J Cardiol.* 2011;87:975–979.

83. Borger van der Burg AE, de Groot NM, van Erven L, et al. Long-term follow-up after radiofrequency catheter ablation of ventricular tachycardia: a successful approach? *J Cardiovasc Electrophysiol.* 2002;13:417–423.

84. Della Bella P, De Ponti R, Uriarte JA, et al. Catheter ablation and antiarrhythmic drugs for haemodynamically tolerated post-infarction ventricular tachycardia: long-term outcome in relation to acute electrophysiological findings. *Eur Heart J.* 2002;23:414–424.

85. O'Donnell D, Bourke JP, Anilkumar R, et al. Radiofrequency ablation for post infarction ventricular tachycardia: report of a single centre experience of 112 cases. *Eur Heart J.* 2002;23:1699–1705.

86. Segal OR, Chow AW, Markides V, et al. Long-term results after ablation of infarct-related ventricular tachycardia. *Heart Rhythm.* 2005;2:474–482.

87. Verma A, Marrouche NF, Schweikert RA, et al. Relationship between successful ablation sites and the scar border zone defined by substrate mapping for ventricular tachycardia post-myocardial infarction. *J Cardiovasc Electrophysiol.* 2005;16:465–471.

88. Stevenson WG, Wilber DJ, Natale A, et al. Irrigated radiofrequency catheter ablation guided by electroanatomic mapping for recurrent ventricular tachycardia after myocardial infarction: The multicenter thermocool ventricular tachycardia ablation trial. *Circulation.* 2008;118:2773–2782.

89. Niwano S, Fukaya H, Yuge M, et al. Role of electrophysiologic study (EPS)-guided preventive therapy for the management of ventricular tachyarrhythmias in patients with heart failure. *Circ J*. 2008;72:268–273.

90. Tanner H, Hindricks G, Volkmer M, et al. Catheter ablation of recurrent scar-related ventricular tachycardia using electroanatomical mapping and irrigated ablation technology: results of the prospective multicenter Euro-VT-study. *J Cardiovasc Electrophysiol*. 2010;21:47–53.

91. Schreieck J, Schneider MAE, Röhling M, et al. Preventive ablation of post infarction ventricular tachycardias: results of a prospective randomized study. *Heart Rhythm*. 2004;1:S35–S37.

92. Reddy VY, Reynolds MR, Neuzil P, et al. Prophylactic catheter ablation for the prevention of defibrillator therapy. *N Engl J Med*. 2007;357:2657–2665.

93. Kuck KH, Schaumann A, Eckardt L, et al. Catheter ablation of stable ventricular tachycardia before defibrillator implantation in patients with coronary heart disease (VTACH): a multicenter randomised controlled trial. *Lancet*. 2010;375:31–40.

94. Jais P, Maury P, Khairy P, et al. Elimination of local abnormal ventricular activities: a new end point for substrate modification in patients with scar-related ventricular tachycardia. *Circulation*. 2012;125:2184–2196.

95. Di Biase L, Burkhardt JD, Lakkireddy D, et al. Ablation of stable VTs versus substrate ablation in ischemic cardiomyopathy: the VISTA randomized multicenter trial. *J Am Coll Cardiol*. 2015;66:2872–2882.

96. Edgerton JR, Mahoney C, Mack MJ, et al. Long-term monitoring after surgical ablation for atrial fibrillation: how much is enough? *J Thorac Cardiovasc Surg*. 2011;142:162–165.

97. Verma A, Champagne J, Sapp J, et al. Discerning the incidence of symptomatic and asymptomatic episodes of atrial fibrillation before and after catheter ablation (DISCERN AF): a prospective, multicenter study. *JAMA Intern Med*. 2013;173:149–156.

98. Leong-Sit P, Roux JF, Zado E, et al. Antiarrhythmics after ablation of atrial fibrillation (5A Study): six-month follow-up study. *Circ Arrhythm Electrophysiol*. 2011;4:11–14.

99. Koyama T, Tada H, Sekiguchi Y, et al. Prevention of atrial fibrillation recurrence with corticosteroids after radiofrequency catheter ablation: a randomized controlled trial. *J Am Coll Cardiol*. 2010;56:1463–1472.

100. Patel D, Mohanty P, Di Biase L, et al. The impact of statins and renin-angiotensin-aldosterone system blockers on pulmonary vein antrum isolation outcomes in post-menopausal females. *Europace*. 2010;12:322–330.

101. Suleiman M, Koestler C, Lerman A, et al. Atorvastatin for prevention of atrial fibrillation recurrence following pulmonary vein isolation: a double-blind, placebo-controlled, randomized trial. *Heart Rhythm*. 2012;9:172–178.

102. Oral H, Chugh A, Ozaydin M, et al. Risk of thromboembolic events after percutaneous left atrial radiofrequency ablation of atrial fibrillation. *Circulation*. 2006;114:759–765.

103. Anderson JL, Halperin JL, Albert NM, et al. Management of patients with atrial fibrillation (compilation of 2006 ACCF/AHA/ESC and 2011 ACCF/AHA/HRS recommendations): a report of the American College of Cardiology/American Heart Association Task Force on practice guidelines. *Circulation*. 2013;127:1916–1926.

104. European Heart Rhythm Association, European Association for Cardio-Thoracic Surgery, Camm AJ, et al. Guidelines for the management of atrial fibrillation: the Task Force for the Management of Atrial Fibrillation of the European Society of Cardiology (ESC). *Eur Heart J*. 2010;31:2369–2429.

105. Chao TF, Lin YJ, Tsao HM, et al. CHADS(2) and CHA(2)DS(2)-VASc scores in the prediction of clinical outcomes in patients with atrial fibrillation after catheter ablation. *J Am Coll Cardiol*. 2011;58:2380–2385.

106. Themistoclakis S, Corrado A, Marchlinski FE, et al. The risk of thromboembolism and need for oral anticoagulation after successful atrial fibrillation ablation. *J Am Coll Cardiol*. 2010;55:735–743.

107. Saad EB, d'Avila A, Costa IP, et al. Very low risk of thromboembolic events in patients undergoing successful catheter ablation of atrial fibrillation with a CHADS2 score ≤3: a long-term outcome study. *Circ Arrhythm Electrophysiol*. 2011;4:615–621.

108. Reddy VY, Sievert H, Halperin J, et al. Percutaneous left atrial appendage closure vs warfarin for atrial fibrillation: a randomized clinical trial. *JAMA*. 2014;312:1988–1998.

109. Dukkipati SR, Neuzil P, Kautzner J, et al. The durability of pulmonary vein isolation using the visually guided laser balloon catheter: multicenter results of pulmonary vein remapping studies. *Heart Rhythm*. 2012;9:919–925.

110. Natale A, Raviele A, Al-Ahmad A, et al. Venice Chart International Consensus document on ventricular tachycardia/ventricular fibrillation ablation. *J Cardiovasc Electrophysiol*. 2010;21:339–379.

111. U.S. Food and Drug Administration Center for Devices and Radiological Health. Recommended clinical study design for ventricular tachycardia ablation; 1999. http://wwwfdagov/cdrh/ode/tachyablpdf

112. Santangeli P, Di Biase L, Burkhardt JD, et al. Lesion recovery, epicardial substrate, or new circuit? Exploring the dark side of recurrent ventricular tachycardia after endocardial ablation. *Heart Rhythm*. 2011;8:1523–1524.

125 Ablation for Atrial Fibrillation

Nathaniel Thompson, Antonio Frontera, Masateru Takigawa, Arnaud Denis, Nicolas Derval, Mélèze Hocini, Pierre Jaïs, and Michel Haïssaguerre

Historical Context

Since the initial description of pulmonary vein (PV) triggers,[1] catheter ablation of atrial fibrillation (AF) has become a frequently performed ablation procedure. It is possible to trace the first attempts at catheter ablation of AF to prior experience with surgical techniques. Cox and colleagues[2] pioneered a surgical procedure based on the multiple wavelet reentry theory of AF as described by Moe. Segmentation of both atria using linear lesions aimed to reduce the surface area of electrically contiguous atrial tissue below the critical threshold required for AF maintenance. Electrical isolation of each PV and the posterior left atrium (LA) has been consistently retained in each modification of the procedure (Maze I–III).[3] Although the long-term success rate stands at 80% and up to 99% with antiarrhythmic drugs, these surgical techniques remain complex and are associated with significant morbidity and mortality.[3]

Initial catheter ablation approaches attempted to reproduce the linear lesions of the Maze procedure.[4] For safety reasons, lesions were initially limited to the right atrium (RA); however, the success of this approach was <20% in patients with paroxysmal AF.[5,6] Extension of linear lesions to the LA was more effective in patients with paroxysmal and particularly persistent AF.[7] However, most published series reported significant complications as well as long procedural times.[4]

The subsequent demonstration of triggers initiating AF, most often in or near the PVs, prompted a shift toward a "focal" ablation strategy.[1] This approach comprised mapping the earliest electrical activity responsible for AF initiation followed by discrete ablation at that site. Fig. 125.1 demonstrates the characteristic features of AF triggered by a PV focus. However, the limitations of this strategy were rapidly identified. First, this approach relies on focal firing and AF initiation at the time of the electrophysiological (EP) study (which is unreliable). In addition, if focal firing was identified in a PV, the elimination of one focus in a particular PV did not prevent another focus from firing at a later time. Maneuvers were used to improve foci identification, but they frequently resulted in initiation of AF that required electrical cardioversion.

The limited success and long procedural times of the focal ablation technique led to circumferential, electrical isolation of PVs.[8] This can be considered a pragmatic approach to AF ablation as it assumes that all PVs can potentially harbor AF triggers. Circumferential, en bloc isolation of PVs is now common; results suggest this approach may be superior to segmental PV isolation (PVI), notably in persistent AF.[9–11]

Since first adopted in the 2000s, catheter ablation techniques, technology, and operator expertise have steadily improved. In particular, new technological advances have given us insight into the substrate that is likely critical in the perpetuation of AF. Catheter ablation has been successively offered to a greater proportion of the global AF population, and this can be expected to continue.

Indications and Preprocedure Assessment

The rationale behind catheter ablation of AF is to mitigate symptoms and improve the quality of life of the patient. Current guidelines recommend that ablation can be considered in symptomatic patients who have failed treatment with antiarrhythmic drugs or those who present with significant consequences of arrhythmia such as a tachycardia-mediated cardiomyopathy.[12] There are randomized data to support the superiority of catheter ablation over antiarrhythmic drugs in symptomatic patients with drug-refractory paroxysmal AF and a relatively normal LA size.[13,14] Catheter ablation of AF has not yet been demonstrated to reduce the risk for AF mortality or stroke and is generally not considered a first-line treatment for AF.[12] However, there are currently ongoing multicenter trials to assess radiofrequency (RF) ablation as a first-line therapy.

Prior to ablation, patients must be carefully assessed for the management of comorbidities, including hypertension, sleep apnea, obesity, cardiac ischemia, and heart failure. It is also important to characterize the arrhythmia, as a greater degree of atrial remodeling accompanies the progression from paroxysmal to persistent AF and generally dictates ablation strategy. PVI is an accepted cornerstone of AF ablation.[12] In patients with persistent AF, additional modification of the atrial substrate is recommended, although an ideal ablation strategy in this group of patients has not yet been determined.

The approach to periprocedural anticoagulation varies. The safest way to manage patients is similar to how patients considered for electrical cardioversion are managed. Thus patients with a high CHADS$_2$ or CHA$_2$DS$_2$-VASc score, hypertrophic cardiomyopathy, or valvular heart disease should be fully anticoagulated. A majority of operators advocate systemic anticoagulation for 1 month before AF ablation.[12] More recently, new oral anticoagulants (NOACs) have been available on the market. A higher stroke risk was initially reported with their use.[15] The use of oral apixaban, dabigatran, and rivaroxaban has since been demonstrated as feasible, with complication rates that were noninferior to uninterrupted warfarin therapy.[16]

Transthoracic echocardiography should be performed prior to ablation to assess the LA size and exclude significant structural abnormalities. Transesophageal echocardiography (TEE) can be used to screen for LA thrombus and define the anatomy of the

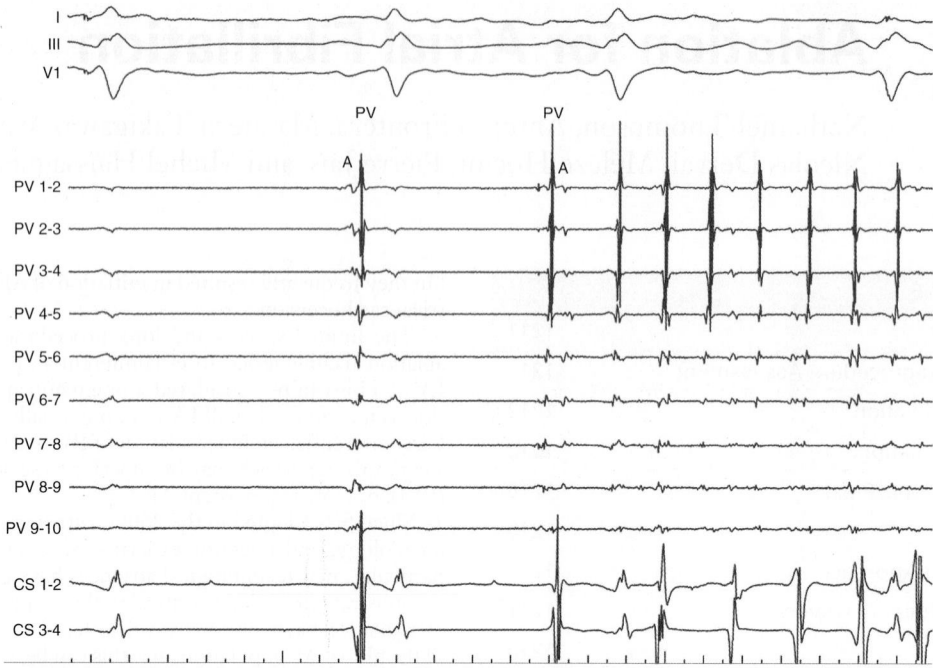

FIGURE 125.1 Characteristic features of atrial fibrillation (AF) triggered by pulmonary vein (*PV*) focus. The *top panel* demonstrates "P on T" monomorphic atrial ectopy on the surface electrocardiogram, with the second ectopic beat initiating AF (*arrow*). The *bottom panel* shows the simultaneous intracardiac recordings, with the middle tracing taken from the distal bipole of a quadripolar mapping catheter placed at the PV ostium. During ectopy, the PV potential is seen preceding the far-field atrial signal, whereas during AF, repetitive PV firing (*asterisk*) is demonstrated. *CS*, Coronary sinus.

septum, including the presence of a patent foramen ovale. TEE may detect LA thrombus in patients taking therapeutic anticoagulants; predictors of this occurrence include a high $CHADS_2$ score, LA size, and persistent AF.[17] Although TEE is recommended in all persistent AF cases, this practice is variable in paroxysmal AF.

Cardiac computed tomography (CT) scanning with three-dimensional reconstruction of the LA and PVs offers a powerful tool for ablation planning and guidance,[18] including assessment for LA thrombus. CT imaging is able to demonstrate the highly variable anatomy of PVs (Fig. 125.2). The veins may demonstrate early branching or a relatively long common trunk before the first branch.[18] A common trunk is seen on the left side in approximately 30% of cases, whereas a right middle PV is seen in 18%–29% of cases.[12] Rare variants may be seen, including roof veins.[19] PV pseudostenosis, caused by external compression from the descending aorta, is most commonly seen in the left inferior PV.[20] The anatomy and location of the LA appendage (LAA) are variable, and the ostium may be located high or low relative to the mitral annulus; the ridge of tissue between the left-sided veins and LAA is variable in its location, extent, and thickness.[21] The location and presence of a fat pad between the esophagus and LA are relevant for risk management due to thermal injury with RF ablation.[22]

Cardiac magnetic resonance imaging (MRI) with delayed enhancement has been described as a technique to visualize and quantify the amount of preexisting atrial fibrosis.[23] This type of imaging currently has some limitations but can provide insights into the atrial substrate; studies have demonstrated that the quantum of preexisting LA fibrosis can predict the outcomes of catheter ablation of AF, with a lower likelihood of success as the area of delayed enhancement increases.[24] The use of stronger magnets with improving image resolution, as well as the absence of ionizing radiation and the provision of additional information, may make MRI an imaging modality of higher preference than CT.

The data obtained from the CT scan can be directly imported into three-dimensional mapping systems or presented as an overlaid and linked image on fluoroscopic imaging to assist the operator during the procedure. A variety of three-dimensional navigation tools, such as Ensite Velocity (St. Jude Medical, St. Paul, MN), CARTO (Biosense-Webster, Diamond Bar, CA), and Rhythmia (Boston Scientific, Marlborough, MA), can integrate images from cardiac CT or MRI and may be used to assist with the ablation of AF or secondary atrial tachycardia (AT) (Fig. 125.3).

Pulmonary Vein Isolation

PVI is an accepted cornerstone for all AF ablation. In patients with persistent AF, unlike those with paroxysmal AF, the LA antra often contain sites with high-frequency electrograms and are likely drivers of this rhythm as opposed to the veins themselves. Therefore PVI is generally preferred with a wide antral approach, with a universal endpoint of achieving electrical isolation.

Mapping of PVs is facilitated by the use of multielectrode circular mapping catheters.[8] The recorded electrograms representing electrical activation of PV sleeves are referred to as *PV potentials* (PVPs). The electrograms recorded by the circumferential mapping catheter are often a fusion of far- and near-field signals, i.e., LAA (with the left superior PV) or RA (with the right PVs). Higher spatial resolution of the recording catheter reduces the relative inclusion of far-field signals. Even so, an understanding of far-field signals is critical to avoid misinterpretation and unnecessary ablation. Pacing the distal coronary sinus (CS) or directly pacing the LAA alters the activation sequence and is a practical and effective way to separate far-field signals from the PVP (Fig. 125.4).

At the end of the procedure, electrical entrance block (into the PV from the LA) is easier to demonstrate than exit block (from the PV to the LA). PV entrance block without exit block is rare, and thus it is reasonable to only demonstrate entrance block as the

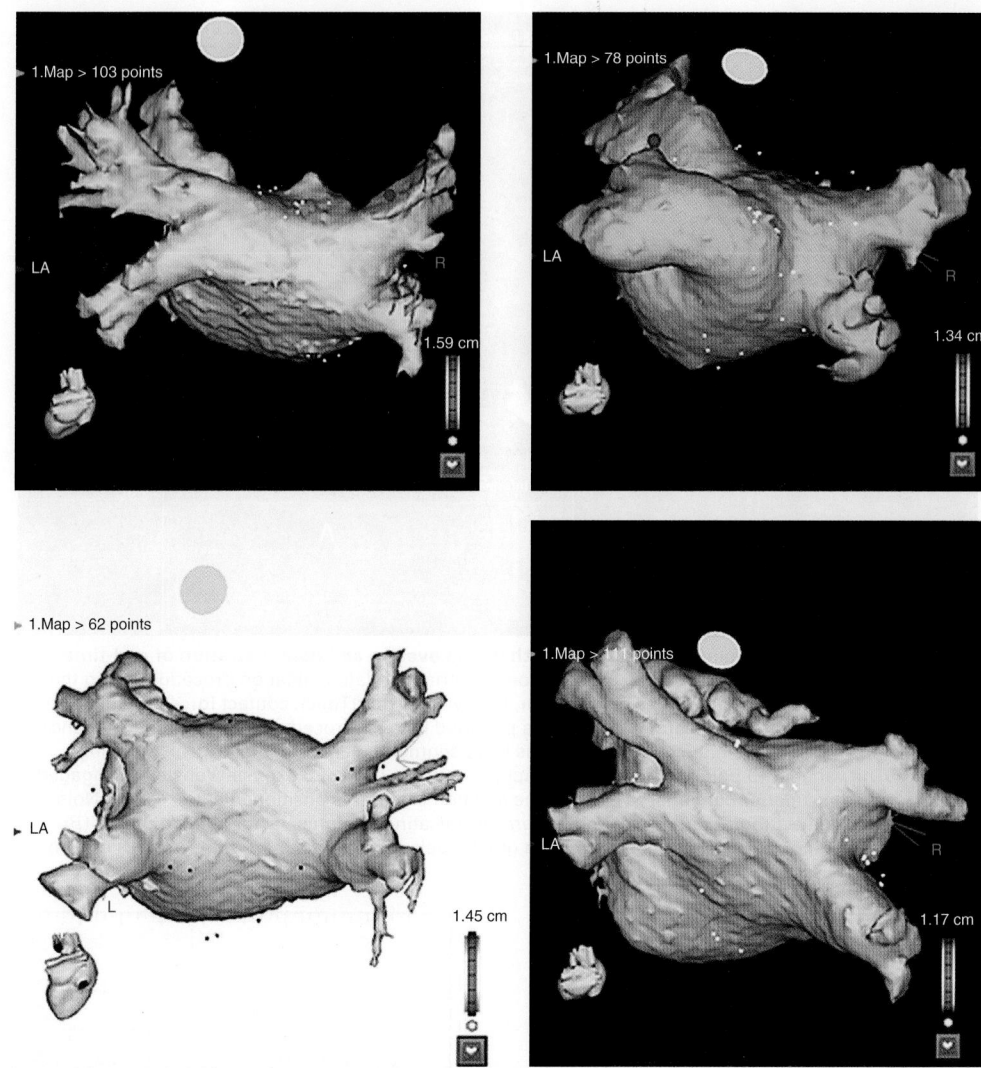

FIGURE 125.2 Highly variable pulmonary vein (PV) anatomy. Three-dimensional reconstruction from 64-slice computed tomographic PV angiography demonstrates the highly variable anatomy of the PV–left atrial junction. The *upper panels* show a left common pulmonary trunk, and the *lower panels* demonstrate the right middle vein variant. Different PV calibers and branching patterns can also be appreciated from these images. *LA,* Left atrium.

endpoint of PVI. Correct demonstration of exit block requires capture of the PV myocardium, which may be difficult owing to pacing artifact and the reduction in amplitude of these signals after ablation. In cases in which dissociated PV activity is seen after isolation, both entrance and exit block are easily demonstrated. Preliminary results suggest that contact force technology will also improve the durability of PVI as better quality lesions can be delivered.[25]

Atrial Substrate Ablation

HRS/EHRA/ESC guidelines recommend that atrial substrate ablation be considered in patients with persistent AF.[12] Unfortunately, these patients often have complex atrial electrograms that do not allow for accurate analysis of the electrogram cycle length, morphology, or activation sequence. Distinguishing passive from active sites harboring critical atrial drivers remains the most challenging part of AF mapping.

Electrogram-guided ablation aims to modify specific atrial substrate. These include targeting complex fractionated atrial electrograms (CFAEs),[26] high-frequency electrograms,[27] and localized drivers.[28] Linear ablation techniques modeled after the

surgical Maze procedure take a more probabilistic approach to ablation, with the aim to transect the electrical circuits of meandering reentrant wavelets (or rotors).[29] Although the autonomic nervous system is not specifically targeted using these strategies, the ganglionic plexi are often ablated along the trajectory of ablation lesions.

In a randomized trial (STAR AF II), the addition of nonspecific atrial ablation techniques, CFAE, and linear ablation to PVI did not improve outcomes in patients with persistent AF versus those who received PVI alone.[30] This and other studies suggest that antral PV ablation is at least necessary to achieve a success rate between 24%[31] and 59%.[30] In a prior meta-analysis of published literature,[32,33] persistent AF has been effectively treated with substrate ablation (although with variation of success). These variable results highlight our lack of clear understanding of what occurs in the atrial substrate to thereby create a specific and effective ablation strategy. Recently, the reports of direct mapping of sources, including foci and rotating waves, provide a potential insight into the mechanisms underlying human AF.[34,35] Similarly, although with a different method, noncontact mapping offers as well an opportunity to individually map and guide RF ablation.[36]

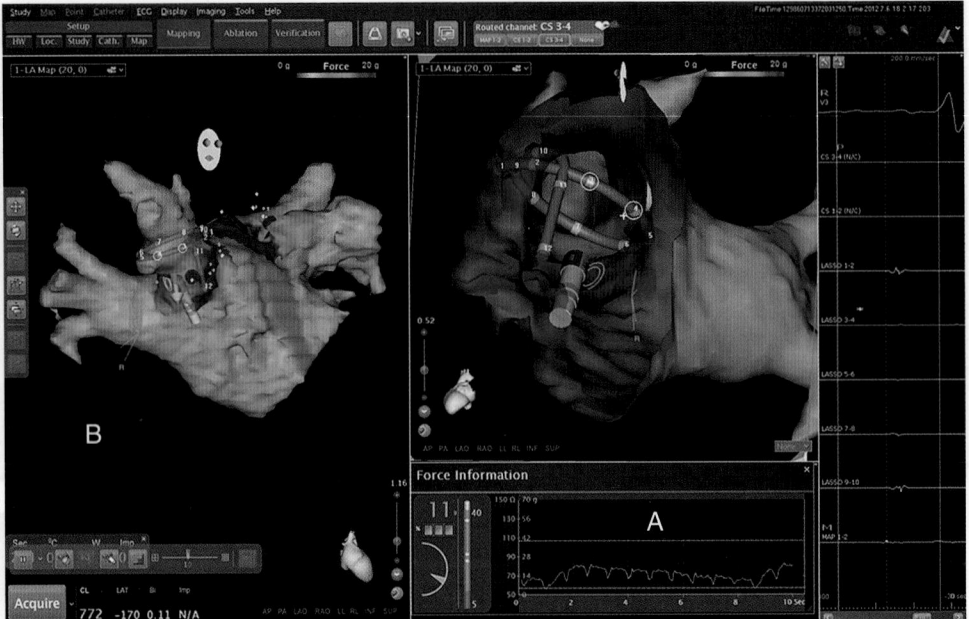

FIGURE 125.3 Three-dimensional mapping with image overlap and demonstration of real-time contact force. This figure is a screen capture from an atrial fibrillation ablation procedure using the Carto 3 system (Biosense-Webster, Diamond Bar, CA) with a SmartTouch contact force–sensing catheter (Biosense-Webster). The cardiac anatomy is provided by a preprocedure 3T magnetic resonance imaging scan (with gadolinium contrast) that has been segmented and rendered by the mapping system. The variable 10-pole circumferential mapping catheter (Lasso, Biosense-Webster) is engaged within the right superior pulmonary vein, and the ablation catheter is positioned at the carina. Note the real-time contact force window (*A*) and the *arrow* indicating the force vector and amplitude (*B*). The *color scale* indicates the amount of force (in grams) delivered to each part of the venous ostium.

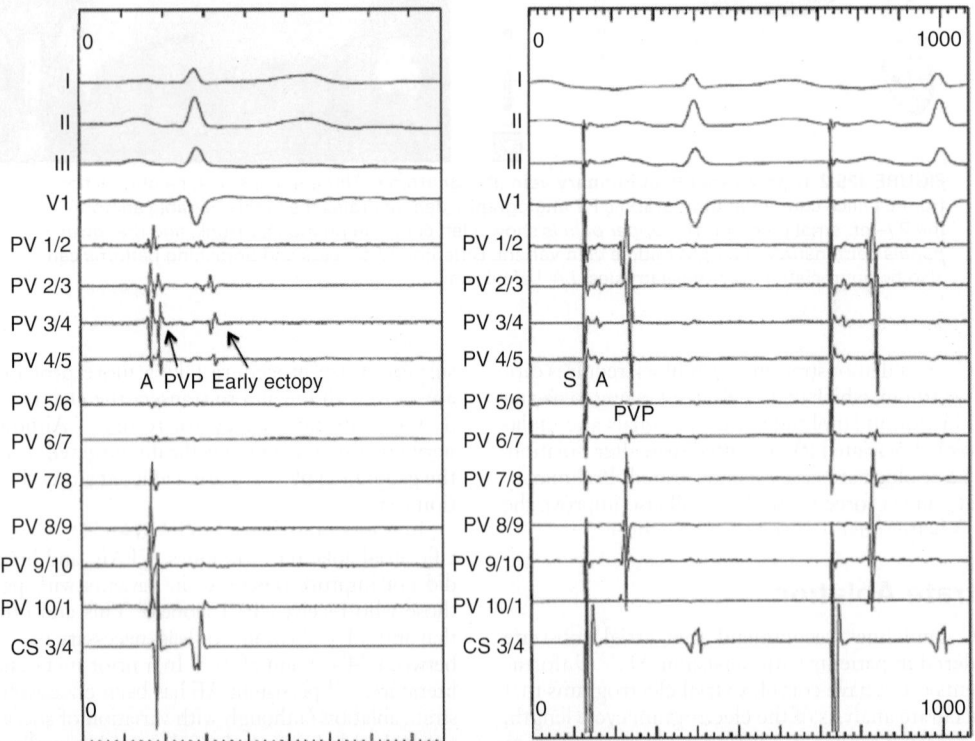

FIGURE 125.4 Use of coronary sinus (*CS*) pacing during mapping of left-sided veins. The left superior pulmonary vein (*PV*) tracing during sinus rhythm demonstrates concealed PV ectopy synchronous with QRS on surface electrocardiogram, which disappears during CS pacing (*right panel*). During CS pacing (*right panel*), atrial far-field signals (*A*) are revealed, and the PV potentials (*PVP*) are more easily seen.

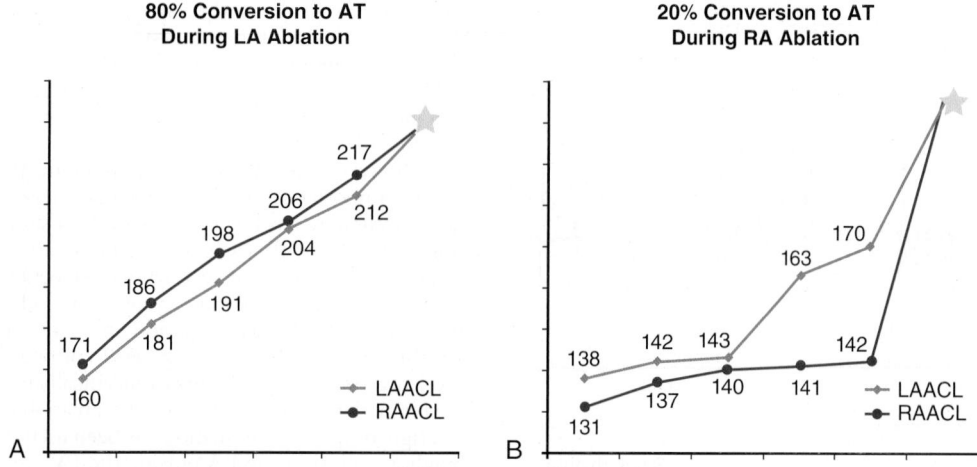

FIGURE 125.5 Disparate evolution of right and left atrial cycle length during stepwise abla-tion. (A) Stepwise ablation in the left atrium (*LA*) results in progressive prolongation of the atrial fibrillatory (cycle length) in both the left and right atria (*RA*) until the eventual termination of the arrhythmia (*star*). This pattern is observed in 80% of cases of persistent atrial fibrillation. (B) Progres-sive cycle length prolongation is only seen in the LA, indicating that the ablation target is in the RA. When the RA is targeted, cycle length prolongation and termination occur (*star*). This pattern is seen in 20% of cases of persistent atrial fibrillation. *AT*, Atrial tachycardia; *LAACL*, left atrial appendage cycle length; *RAACL*, right atrial appendage cycle length.

Fractionated Electrograms and Complex Fractionated Atrial Electrograms

Fractionated atrial electrograms were first described as continu-ous activity or electrograms with a fibrillatory interval of <100 ms and were irregularly distributed across the RA and LA.[27] CFAEs were subsequently described by Nademanee and colleagues[26] as low-voltage electrograms (0.05–0.25 mV) with a cycle length shorter than 120 ms, displaying two or more deflections or hav-ing a continuous deflection from baseline. Regional differences in electrogram characteristics are often observed; the septum or structures adjacent to the LA such as the CS and appendage often display the most complex fractionation and rapid atrial activity.[37]

Different tissue activation patterns have been shown to result in electrogram fractionation, including meandering rotors, wave collision, and slow conduction.[26,38] Given the nonsingular relationship of electrogram fractionation and tissue activity, it is difficult to characterize CFAEs as either active or passive phenomena. Shortening of the AF cycle length (AFCL) by at least 10 ms has been shown to precede complex fractionation in 91% and 88% of the regions sampled in the atria and CS, respectively, implying that fractionation is a passive follower of a high-frequency driver.[39] These passive CFAEs displayed nearly simultaneous activation over a limited part of AFCL, whereas active CFAEs displayed nonsimulta-neous activation spanning the majority of AFCL, potentially indicating a rotating wave.[39]

In two studies, electrogram characteristics were investigated to determine their impact on AFCL and AF termination. A sig-nificant predictor of the prolongation of AFCL was targeting sites displaying continuous electrical activity (>70% of the local cycle interval), with positive and negative predictive values of 52% and 67%, respectively.[40] Other variables, such as fractionation index (number of deflections of fractionated activity in a 4-second win-dow), electrogram voltage, and local mean cycle length, were not significant predictors. The degree of CFAE fractionation has been quantified with a grading system, with ablation of certain grades having an appreciable impact on AFCL.[41] The spatial resolution of the recording electrodes can also impact the degree of fractionated electrograms; mapping catheters with lower-reso-lution electrodes will have more fractionated signals.[42,43]

Monitoring the Progress of Ablation Using Atrial Fibrillation Cycle Length

AFCL is generally considered a surrogate for local tissue refrac-toriness. Earlier studies have shown that AFCL accurately tracks the shortening in local refractory periods seen with prolonged AF duration or lengthening in local refractory periods during antiar-rhythmic drug therapy. The gradual prolongation in AFCL before AF termination during catheter ablation supports the use of AFCL to monitor substrate modification during AF ablation.[37,44] The impact of ablation on AFCL at sites remote from ablation, such as the appendages, indicates changes in the substrate maintaining AF.

Measurements of AFCL can be determined reliably by averag-ing 30 consecutive cycles taken from the LAA and the RA append-age, where unambiguous high-voltage, discrete, and reproducible electrograms are observed. Baseline AFCL measurement has been shown to be the strongest predictor of success for persis-tent AF ablation of fewer than 5 years' duration. A longer initial AFCL is observed among patients in whom AF terminates dur-ing ablation (156 ± 23 ms vs. 130 ± 14 ms).[37] AFCL of <140 ms is associated with AF termination in fewer than 69% of patients, and a longer AFCL is associated with >89% AF termination.

Changes in AFCL can be used to monitor the progress of sub-strate modification. Based on previous experience, after stepwise ablation, including PVI, ablation of complex fractionated elec-trograms, and linear lesions, a gradual prolongation of AFCL was found, culminating in conversion to sinus rhythm or AT. The lat-ter is observed when AFCL reaches 180–200 ms. In other words, more ablation is required to terminate AF with a lower baseline AFCL of <140 ms compared with AFCL of 200 ms. A simultane-ous increase in LAA and RA appendage AFCL during ablation is observed in a majority of patients. An increase in LAA AFCL while the right remains short is seen in a subset of patients (20%–30%) in whom AF may eventually terminate during ablation in the RA (Fig. 125.5).[45] This finding highlights the role of AFCL in further defining the atrial chamber that drives AF.

Dominant Frequency

An alternative method for assessing complex electrograms is to analyze them according to their frequency spectra. This approach

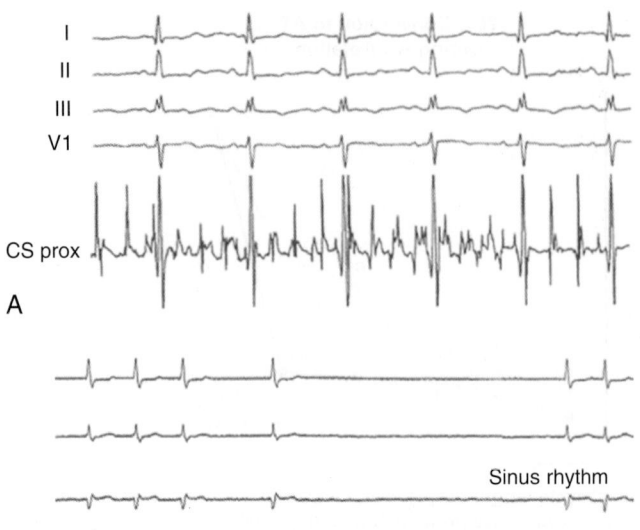

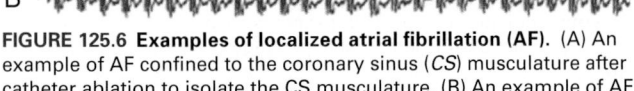

FIGURE 125.6 Examples of localized atrial fibrillation (AF). (A) An example of AF confined to the coronary sinus (*CS*) musculature after catheter ablation to isolate the CS musculature. (B) An example of AF confined to an isolated segment of the right atrium. When isolation occurs, sinus rhythm is restored in this case.

is based on experimental and clinical studies demonstrating that AF can be maintained by high-frequency sources displaying spatially distributed frequency gradients.[46–51] Using fast Fourier transform, signals can be deconstructed into sine waves and quantified according to the most prevalent sine wave frequency, known as the *dominant frequency* (DF). Analysis of DF can be used to assess changes in activation rates and organization of AF after ablation in an attempt to understand the pathophysiology of AF.[50,52]

Catheter ablation studies incorporating DF mapping have shown that PVs harbor important DF sites in patients with paroxysmal AF but not in those with persistent AF.[48,53] Targeting the sites of DF in persistent AF is much less effective, possibly due to the spatiotemporal complexity of the atrial substrate. Inaccuracies of DF analysis may be related to complex fractionation, double potentials, effects of far-field electrograms, or multiple sources averaging in multiple frequency peaks with very similar power rather than one clear DF as seen in paroxysmal AF.[54]

Stable Sources Maintaining Atrial Fibrillation

After extensive ablation, localized sources perpetuating AF can be identified and ablated by converging on an area displaying centrifugal activation.[28] Using a 20-pole catheter (Pentaray, Biosense-Webster) for high-density mapping, Haïssaguerre and associates[28] reported that the localized source driving AF may originate not only from a discrete focal point but also from a region harboring a small, discrete reentrant circuit with local electrical activity covering 75%–100% of the cycle length, indicating localized reentry. Human studies have also confirmed persistent fibrillatory activity confined within small isolated portions of the atria (Fig. 125.6).[55] Similarly, animal studies during pacing and acetylcholine-induced AF,[56] as well as computational models of AF,[57] have supported the perpetuation of AF from localized sources. These are specific conditions of stable reentry whereby the spatiotemporal complexity of the rhythm was reduced by ablation.

Autonomic Ganglionic Plexi

Autonomic innervation of the heart consists of both the extrinsic and intrinsic autonomic systems. The extrinsic autonomic system

innervates the heart via the vagosympathetic trunk. Innervation from the intrinsic autonomic system is via the ganglionated plexi and interganglionic axons distributed in the cardiac epicardial fat pads found predominantly at the PV antrum and superior vena cava junction.[58] Modulation of either extrinsic autonomic system by stimulation of vagosympathetic trunk or the ganglia have both been shown to affect the heart rate and inducibility of AF.[59]

The importance of the autonomic nervous system in PV pathophysiology has been underscored in studies demonstrating rapid firing from PVs when the ganglia are activated by high-frequency stimulation or acetylcholine injection.[60–62] In addition, acceleration of the fibrillatory cycle length in PVs due to shortening of the atrial refractory period and action potential duration has also been described during vagal episodes.[63] These findings have encouraged investigators to specifically target the ganglionic plexi in patients undergoing catheter ablation of AF.

High-frequency stimulation has been used to locate clusters of ganglionic plexi in the LA outside the PV antrum and to determine the efficacy of ganglia ablation.[64–66] Stimulation of the ganglia resulted in a vagal reflex that manifested as atrioventricular (AV) block, bradycardia (with an increase in the RR interval of at least 50%), or hypotension. Putative ganglionated plexi ablation, as evidenced by the abolition of vagal response, has been associated with reduction in AF recurrence compared with circumferential PV ablation alone in patients with paroxysmal AF.[64,67] However, there is considerable overlap among the anatomical locations of the ganglionic plexi, CFAE, and lesions of wide circumferential PV ablation, which impedes the ability to differentiate the role of each component individually.[66,67]

Linear Ablation

Although technically challenging, the primary purpose of linear ablation is to interrupt the reentrant wavefronts of AF (and macroreentrant circuits). Verification of linear block is necessary to prevent macroreentrant AT from occurring around areas of scar.[68,69] However, some patients with persistent AF may not respond to linear ablation, either because mechanisms are too diffuse or they are localized but not appropriately targeted. Therefore these are specific cases of ablation, most often limited to ATs that occur after ablation.

Technique for Ablation of the Mitral Isthmus

The mitral line consists of lesions joining the posterior mitral annulus to the left inferior PV. Because of the difficulty and risk associated with ablation at this location,[68] a more anterior mitral line has been recommended.[70] To perform the standard mitral line, an irrigated ablation catheter is positioned at the lateral mitral annulus, where the ratio of amplitude of ventricular to atrial electrogram is 2:1. The ablation line is started at the 3- or 4-o'clock position on the mitral annulus, reaching up to the 2- to 3-o'clock position at the top of the line. RF energy is typically delivered for 60–120 seconds at each site using a power of 30–35 W with an irrigated catheter. Care must be taken to ensure catheter stability and to avoid its inadvertent movement, which can result in high-energy delivery within the left inferior PV or LAA. If conduction block is not achieved, potential conduction gaps along the line should be explored and ablated. Failing this, ablation can be performed on the anterior wall.

Approximately two-thirds of patients require ablation from within the CS to achieve mitral isthmus block. Ablation within the CS is performed using an irrigated-tip catheter, with power delivery of 20–25 W and increased flow rates to reduce the risk for circumflex artery injury and cardiac tamponade. The epi- and endocardial lesions effectively oppose the lateral mitral isthmus to obtain a transmural lesion set.

The endpoint of linear ablation is the confirmation of bidirectional block using criteria similar to those described for

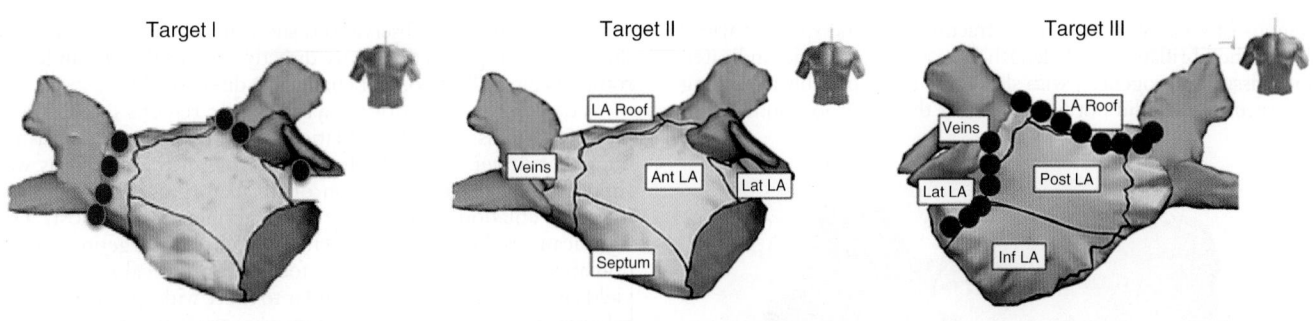

Target I

Target II

Target III

Antral pulmonary vein isolation · *Electrogram-based ablation* · *Linear lesions*

FIGURE 125.7 Stepwise ablation of persistent atrial fibrillation. The first target is the pulmonary veins, which are encircled en bloc two at a time. The second ablation target is complex, fractionated atrial electrograms. Finally, linear ablation is performed at the roof and mitral isthmus. *LA,* Left atrium.

cavotricuspid isthmus (CTI) block. Along the line, there is a corridor of double potentials, proximal to distal CS activation during pacing from the LAA, and delayed LAA activation with distal compared with proximal CS pacing.

Technique for Ablation of the Left Atrial Roof

The LA roofline is a line of lesions joining the left and right superior PVs. An irrigated ablation catheter is introduced with its tip oriented toward the LA roof. Starting at the left superior PV, the ablation catheter is gradually dragged toward the right superior PV by rotating the sheath and catheter assembly clockwise and posteriorly.

RF energy is typically delivered for 60–120 seconds at each site with power delivery guided by the catheter orientation. When the catheter tip is perpendicular to the tissue interface, power is reduced to 25 W; a power of 30 W is safe with a more parallel catheter tip position. The ablation endpoint is the demonstration of a line of conduction block. Conduction block is suggested by a line of double potential along the ablation line (not always observed) or by caudocranial activation of the posterior LA in sinus rhythm or LAA pacing.

Stepwise Ablation Approach

The stepwise ablation approach incorporates the previously described techniques, targeting sites contributing to the initiation and maintenance of AF (Fig. 125.7). Using this strategy, PVI, electrogram-based ablation of atrial substrate, and linear ablation were performed in patients with persistent AF.[37,71] Each region of the LA was targeted in sequence, and the impact of each step of ablation was assessed by the measurements of AFCL at the RA appendage and LAA. Structures outside the LA (CS, superior vena cava, and RA) were targeted based on electrogram morphology and frequency. Linear ablation of the roof and mitral isthmus was performed for cases in which AF persisted. In the initial study, stepwise ablation was associated with acute AF termination (sinus rhythm or AT) in 87% of patients during catheter ablation and was preceded by a 40-ms increase in both the LAA and RA appendage AFCL.[37] In roughly 20% of patients, a disparate increase in left-to-right AFCL was observed.[45] In these patients, ablation within the RA was successful.

Patients may present with AT or AF recurrence, and multiple procedures may be required for AF maintenance.[72] Disease-free survival was 87% at 5 years. Meta-analysis has reported long-term success rates of 80%, with significant heterogeneity in the success of single-procedure outcomes.[73] Strong predictors of success include longer AFCL and procedural AF termination.[74]

A concern with extensive ablation for substrate modification is the effect on atrial mechanical function caused by the replacement of healthy myocardium with scar tissue. Areas of scar tissue and low-voltage atrial tissue, as assessed by electroanatomical mapping, accounted for 31% ± 12% and 32% ± 17% of the total LA surface area, respectively (the majority of the scar burden related to PVI: 20% ± 4% of the LA surface). However, recovery of atrial mechanical function was observed at 3 months in almost all patients.[75]

The possibility of mapping AF sources more directly may offer a safer and more efficient strategy for persistent AF, potentially reducing the total ablation burden.

New Methods to Identify Drivers

Experimental models in which rapidly activating transient reentrant waves are a mechanism of AF have been pioneered by Jalife and colleagues.[51] Narayan and associates have provided putative evidence of these mechanisms in human AF using biatrial basket catheter mapping and a computational approach based on tissue conduction and repolarization to create individualized spatiotemporal maps.[34,35,76] This method identified both rotors and focal sources in all AF patients (paroxysmal and persistent). The rotors have the main characteristics of being stable at a single site (over hours and days) independent of AF type. The ablation strategy has been subsequently developed with brief 3–5-minute applications of RF energy at each site, with the endpoint of AF slowing or termination. The main advantage is a reduction in the amount of atrial ablation. The authors reported an impressive 84% success rate at 600 days for persistent AF after a single procedure. Since then, reports have indicated less favorable success rates.[77]

Noninvasive (surface) mapping offers an alternative means of understanding the substrate of AF and creating an individualized ablation strategy. Rudy and Messinger-Rapport[78] and Cuculich and coworkers[79] reported the feasibility of this external mapping technique incorporating a 252-electrode vest worn by the patient. After developing a signal-processing technique, it has been possible to identify drivers in both atria (excluding the septum, which is indirectly mapped) of both foci and reentrant wavefronts. Their interplay with PV and atrial foci and macroreentrant loops can be directly visualized (Fig. 125.8).

In a recent study, noninvasive mapping was applied to identify drivers in 103 patients with persistent AF.[80] The driver domains were targeted with AF termination as the procedural endpoint compared with the stepwise ablation control group. The maps showed changing beat-to-beat wavefronts and varying spatiotemporal complexity. Reentries were not sustained and meandered substantially but recurred repeatedly in clustered regions. Driver ablation alone terminated 75% and 15% of persistent and long-lasting AF, respectively. The number of driver regions increased with the duration of continuous AF. The mean RF delivery for AF termination was 28 ± 17 minutes versus 65 ± 33 minutes in the control group. At 12 months, 85% of patients with AF termination were free from AF, similar to the control population (87%). In keeping with previous reports, the endocardial electrograms from regions of reentry showed more fractionation and spanned wider across the fibrillatory cycle length. These characteristics indicated local tissue heterogeneity with slow conduction possibly anchoring the reentries but did not firmly predict the driver locations. They

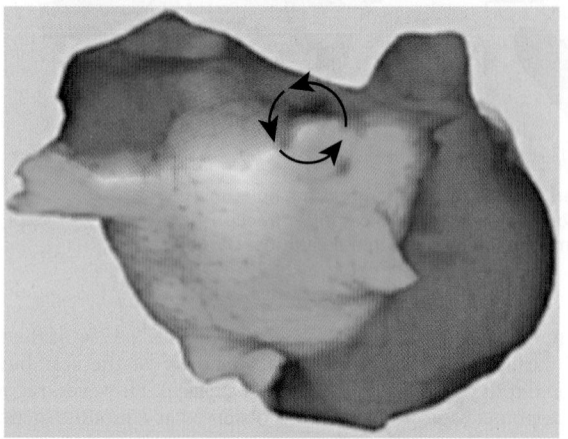

FIGURE 125.8 Surface mapping of atrial fibrillation. An example of a panoramic map obtained by surface mapping techniques utilizing a 252-electrode wearable vest. The posterior surface of the left atrium is shown with a snapshot of a wandering rotor. *Arrows* indicate counterclockwise rotation.

corroborate previous observations showing fractionated activity at the wave pivot points or activity directly produced by meandering rotors owing to beat-to-beat changes in directionality.

We utilize the term of arrhythmogenic regions to substitute discrete sites as targets of ablation to address the spatial distribution of driver sites. The functional role of these regions was supported by the prolongation of fibrillatory cycle length during their ablation, culminating in AF termination in most. The significant reduction in RF energy delivery targeting driver domains indicated that ablation focused on critical regions may yield an AF termination rate similar to more widespread anatomical energy delivery. A critical point appeared after a few months where a decrease in the acute efficacy of driver ablation was observed (although it did not impact the final clinical outcome, because patients in whom AF was not terminated by driver ablation received ablation lines to achieve AF termination).

In some cases, remapping of persistent AF after ablation of driver regions has shown the emergence of a second set of drivers that may be new or possibly preexisting but unveiled after the first set of drivers has been eliminated (Fig. 125.9). The characteristics of a second set of drivers and how this added information may help guide ablation are being investigated.

In the current AFACART trial[81] involving eight European centers, a high rate of acute termination (65%) by driver-only ablation has been reported despite the fact that these centers had no practical experience with the noninvasive mapping system. The mean atrial surface covered by CFAEs was 49% of the total

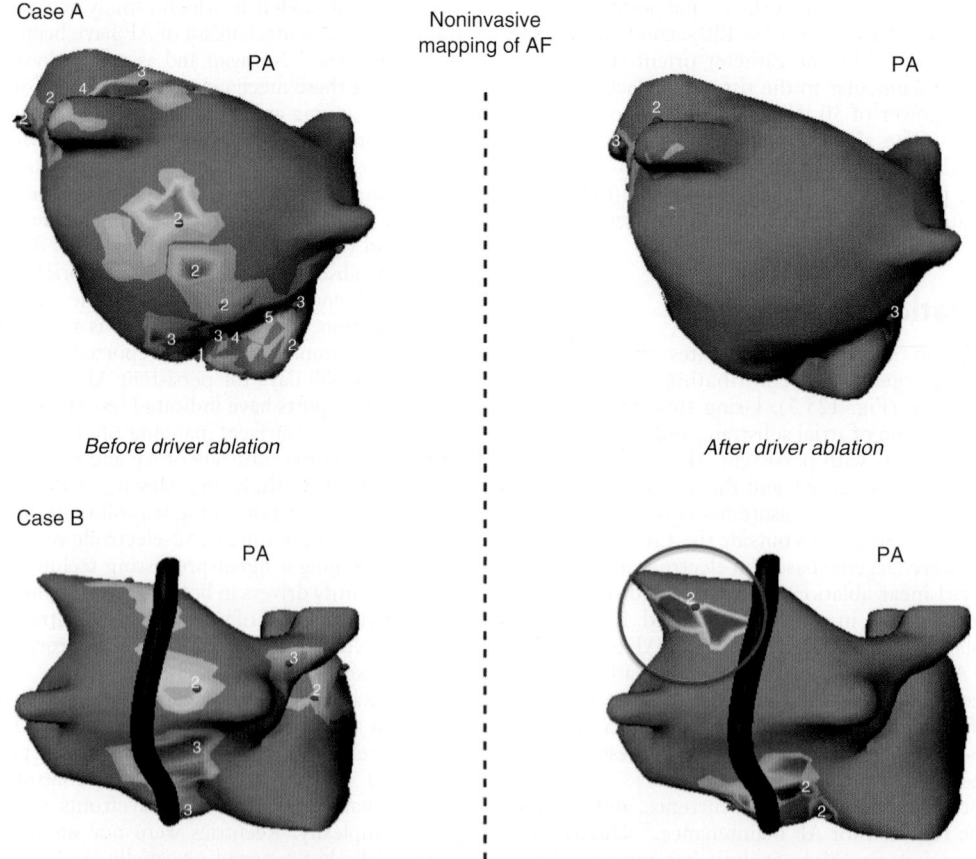

FIGURE 125.9 Arrhythmogenic driver-density maps of two patients before and after driver ablation. Areas of *red* are regions and numbers of focal drivers/rotor cores superimposed on a computed tomography shell of the right and left atria. In patient A, there is a reduction in driver sites; in patient B, there are new driver sites that are unmasked (adjacent to the left veins on the posterior wall on the posteroanterior [*PA*] view; circled in red) with persistence of driver sites on the floor of the left atrium. *AF,* Atrial fibrillation.

atrial surface, while the one occupied by driver domains was 19%, indicating a better specificity of targets using a focal/reentrant driver mapping strategy.

In a modification of the stepwise approach (Table 125.1), we currently perform wide antral PVI for all patients with persistent AF (with ~10% termination of AF during ablation), and subsequent targeting of drivers. The impact of ablation is assessed by calculating AFCL after each targeted region. Instead of the complete elimination of local signals on the ablation catheter, we instead try to achieve a local increase in cycle length and organization of the local recordings (Fig. 125.10). We reserve linear lesions for recalcitrant and specific cases of AF (and macroreentrant tachycardias).

Complications

Catheter ablation of AF is a complex procedure with the potential for significant complications.[12] The rate of serious

TABLE 125.1 **Approach to ablation of paroxysmal and persistent atrial fibrillation (AF)**

AF TYPE		TARGET	ASSESSMENT
Paroxysmal		Antral PVI	PV block confirmation
Persistent	Stepwise approach	Antral PVI	PV block confirmation
		Substrate driver sites with mapping during AF	AFCL calculated after each region
Secondary atrial tachycardias		Sites of centrifugal activation	Block is confirmed for all lines
Localized and macroreentry		Linear lesions (including mitral and roof lines)	

Ablation of persistent AF is a modification of the stepwise approach with sequential driver regions targeted.
AFCL, Atrial fibrillation cycle length; *PV,* pulmonary vein; *PVI,* pulmonary vein isolation.

complications is <2% with an experienced team. Good risk management dictates that the primary operator and other members of the team (assistant physicians, cardiac technicians, nurses, and anesthesiologists) have a sound understanding of the risks involved and how to mitigate them. The most commonly described complications involve vascular access (false aneurysm, arteriovenous fistula, retroperitoneal hematoma).[82] Serious complications include cardiac tamponade, stroke, PV stenosis, esophageal injury (including atrioesophageal fistula), phrenic nerve palsy, gastroparesis, mitral valve damage caused by catheter entrapment, endocarditis, and aortic root injury during transseptal puncture.[82]

Clinical Results

There is a significant amount of published data concerning the success rates of catheter ablation of AF. A meta-analysis of randomized clinical trials (largely paroxysmal AF patients) described an overall success rate of 78% in the ablation arm compared with 23% in the control group at 12 months.[83] Fig. 125.11 is a summary of the different strategies and results for persistent AF ablation.[32] The results are variable; however, what is consistent is more than a single procedure typically required for ablation success. Long-term follow-up studies have demonstrated a slow but steady decline in arrhythmia-free survival over time.[72,73,84]

Conclusion

Catheter-based ablation therapy for AF is an accepted strategy by scientific committees. Although the strategy for paroxysmal AF is standard, largely comprising PVI, there is a need for improving single procedure and long-term outcomes, potentially with new and safer technologies. Concerning catheter ablation for persistent AF, ongoing research will help in better understanding the atrial substrate maintaining AF, including both imaging and mapping systems. Targeted ablation of drivers appears to be capable of terminating most persistent AF using an ablation time similar to that for nonspecific AF ablation. Earlier intervention for persistent AF is a suggested strategy.

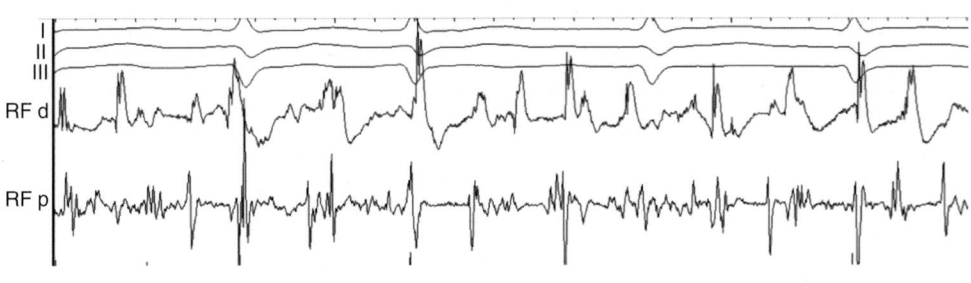

A   Local electrogram recording before ablation

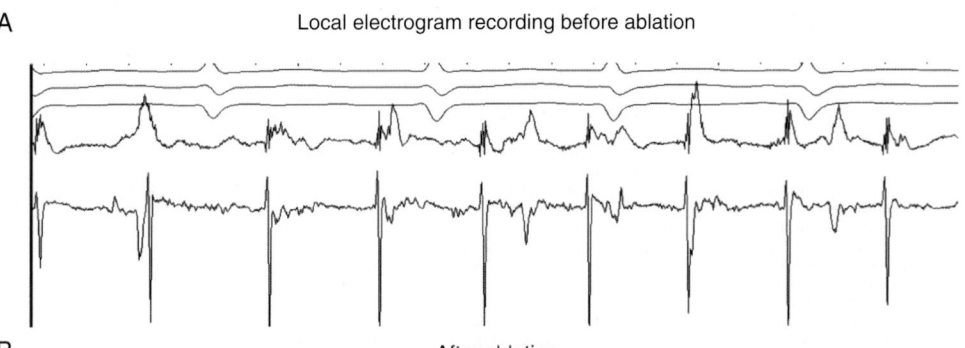

B   After ablation

FIGURE 125.10 An example of electrogram organization with an increase in local atrial fibrillation cycle length after the initiation of radiofrequency *(RF)* ablation.

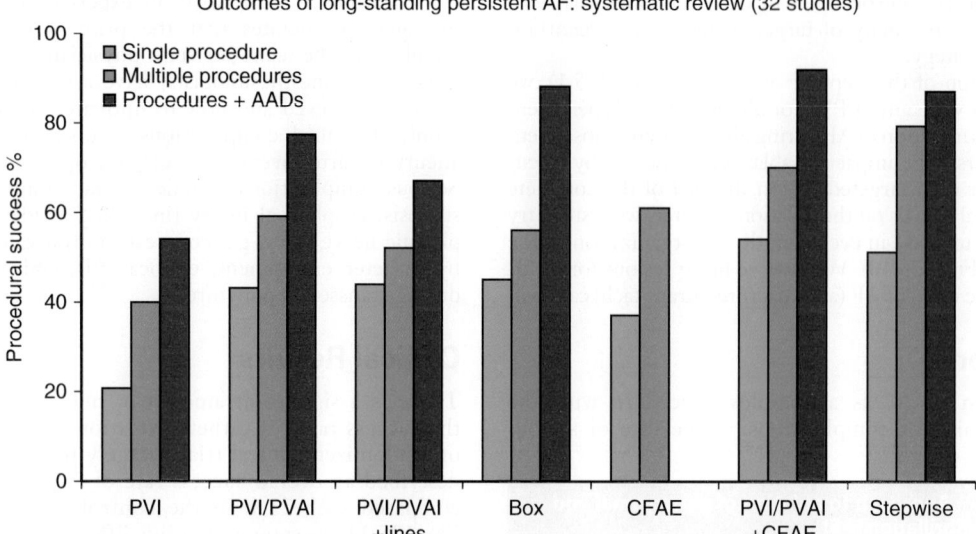

Outcomes of long-standing persistent AF: systematic review (32 studies)

FIGURE 125.11 Summary of the results of catheter ablation of persistent atrial fibrillation (AF). Multiple procedures with the addition of antiarrhythmic drugs (*AADs*) are most commonly required for success. *CFAE*, Complex fractionated atrial electrogram, *PVAI*, pulmonary vein antrum isolation; *PVI*, pulmonary vein isolation.

REFERENCES

1. Haïssaguerre M, Jaïs P, Shah DC, et al. Spontaneous initiation of atrial fibrillation by ectopic beats originating in the pulmonary veins. *N Engl J Med.* 1998;339:659–666.
2. Cox JL, Schuessler RB, D'Agostino Jr HJ, et al. The surgical treatment of atrial fibrillation. III. Development of a definitive surgical procedure. *J Thorac Cardiovasc Surg.* 1991;101:569–583.
3. Saint LL, Bailey MS, Prasad S, et al. Cox-Maze IV results for patients with lone atrial fibrillation versus concomitant mitral disease. *Ann Thorac Surg.* 2012;93:789–794. discussion 794–795.
4. Jaïs P, Weerasooriya R, Shah DC, et al. Ablation therapy for atrial fibrillation (AF): past, present and future. *Cardiovasc Res.* 2002;54:337–346.
5. Haïssaguerre M, Gencel L, Fischer B, et al. Successful catheter ablation of atrial fibrillation. *J Cardiovasc Electrophysiol.* 1994;5:1045–1052.
6. Gaita F, Riccardi R, Calo L, et al. Atrial mapping and radiofrequency catheter ablation in patients with idiopathic atrial fibrillation: electrophysiological findings and ablation results. *Circulation.* 1998;97:2136–2145.
7. Swartz J. A catheter-based curative approach to atrial fibrillation in humans. *Circulation.* 1994;90:I-335.
8. Haïssaguerre M, Jaïs P, Shah DC, et al. Electrophysiological end point for catheter ablation of atrial fibrillation initiated from multiple pulmonary venous foci. *Circulation.* 2000;101:1409–1417.
9. Arentz T, Weber R, Burkle G, et al. Small or large isolation areas around the pulmonary veins for the treatment of atrial fibrillation? Results from a prospective randomized study. *Circulation.* 2007;115:3057–3063.
10. Oral H, Scharf C, Chugh C, et al. Catheter ablation for paroxysmal atrial fibrillation segmental pulmonary vein ostial ablation versus left atrial ablation. *Circulation.* 2003;108:2355–2360.
11. Karch MR, Zrenner B, Deisenhofer I, et al. Freedom from atrial tachyarrhythmias after catheter ablation of atrial fibrillation: a randomized comparison between 2 current ablation strategies. *Circulation.* 2005;111:2875–2880.
12. Calkins H, Kuck KH, Cappato R, et al. 2012 HRS/EHRA/ECAS expert consensus statement on catheter and surgical ablation of atrial fibrillation: recommendations for patient selection, procedural techniques, patient management and follow-up, definitions, endpoints, and research trial design: a report of the Heart Rhythm Society (HRS) Task Force on Catheter and Surgical Ablation of Atrial Fibrillation. Developed in partnership with the European Heart Rhythm Association (EHRA), a registered branch of the European Society of Cardiology (ESC) and the European Cardiac Arrhythmia Society (ECAS); and in collaboration with the American College of Cardiology (ACC), American Heart Association (AHA), the Asia Pacific Heart Rhythm Society (APHRS), and the Society of Thoracic Surgeons (STS). Endorsed by the governing bodies of the American College of Cardiology Foundation, the American Heart Association, the European

Cardiac Arrhythmia Society, the European Heart Rhythm Association, the Society of Thoracic Surgeons, the Asia Pacific Heart Rhythm Society, and the Heart Rhythm Society. *Heart Rhythm.* 2012;9:632–696.e21.
13. Jaïs P, Cauchemez B, Macle L, et al. Catheter ablation versus antiarrhythmic drugs for atrial fibrillation: the A4 study. *Circulation.* 2008;118:2498–2505.
14. Wilber DJ, Pappone C, Neuzil P, et al. Comparison of antiarrhythmic drug therapy and radiofrequency catheter ablation in patients with paroxysmal atrial fibrillation: a randomized controlled trial. *JAMA.* 2010;303:333–340.
15. Lakkireddy D, Reddy YM, Di Biase L, et al. Feasibility and safety of dabigatran versus warfarin for periprocedural anticoagulation in patients undergoing radiofrequency ablation for atrial fibrillation: results from a multicenter prospective registry. *J Am Coll Cardiol.* 2012;59:1168–1174.
16. January CT, Wann LS, Alpert JS, et al. 2014 AHA/ACC/HRS guideline for the management of patients with atrial fibrillation: a report of the American College of Cardiology/American Heart Association Task Force on practice guidelines and the Heart Rhythm Society. *Circulation.* 2014;130:e199–e267.
17. Scherr D, Dalal D, Chilukuri K, et al. Incidence and predictors of left atrial thrombus prior to catheter ablation of atrial fibrillation. *J Cardiovasc Electrophysiol.* 2009;20:379–384.
18. Schwartzman D, Lacomis J, Wigginton WG. Characterization of left atrium and distal pulmonary vein morphology using multidimensional computed tomography. *J Am Coll Cardiol.* 2003;41:1349–1357.
19. Lickfett L, Kato R, Tandri H, et al. Characterization of a new pulmonary vein variant using magnetic resonance angiography: incidence, imaging, and interventional implications of the "right top pulmonary vein". *J Cardiovasc Electrophysiol.* 2004;15:538–543.
20. Wongcharoen W, Tsao HM, Wu MH, et al. Preexisting pulmonary vein stenosis in patients undergoing atrial fibrillation ablation: a report of five cases. *J Cardiovasc Electrophysiol.* 2006;17:423–425.
21. Wongcharoen W, Tsao HM, Wu MH, et al. Morphologic characteristics of the left atrial appendage, roof, and septum: implications for the ablation of atrial fibrillation. *J Cardiovasc Electrophysiol.* 2006;17:951–956.
22. Tsao HM, Wu MH, Churn MS, et al. Anatomic proximity of the esophagus to the coronary sinus: implication for catheter ablation within the coronary sinus. *J Cardiovasc Electrophysiol.* 2006;17:266–269.
23. McGann CJ, Kholmovski EG, Oakes RS, et al. New magnetic resonance imaging-based method for defining the extent of left atrial wall injury after the ablation of atrial fibrillation. *J Am Coll Cardiol.* 2008;52:1263–1271.
24. Mahnkopf C, Badger TJ, Burgon NS, et al. Evaluation of the left atrial substrate in patients with lone atrial fibrillation using delayed-enhanced MRI: implications for disease progression and response to catheter ablation. *Heart Rhythm.* 2010;7:1475–1481.

25. Kuck KH, Reddy VY, Schmidt B, et al. A novel radiofrequency ablation catheter using contact force sensing: Toccata study. *Heart Rhythm.* 2012;9:18–23.
26. Nademanee K, McKenzie J, Kosar E, et al. A new approach for catheter ablation of atrial fibrillation: mapping of the electrophysiologic substrate. *J Am Coll Cardiol.* 2004;43:2044–2053.
27. Jaïs P, Haïssaguerre M, Shah DC, et al. Regional disparities of endocardial atrial activation in paroxysmal atrial fibrillation. *Pacing Clin Electrophysiol.* 1996;19:1998–2003.
28. Haïssaguerre M, Hocini M, Sanders P, et al. Localized sources maintaining atrial fibrillation organized by prior ablation. *Circulation.* 2006;113:616–625.
29. Spector PS, de Sa DD, Tischler ES, et al. Ablation of multi-wavelet re-entry: general principles and in silico analyses. *Europace.* 2012;14:v106–v111.
30. Verma A, Jiang CY, Betts TR, et al. Approaches to catheter ablation for persistent atrial fibrillation. *N Engl J Med.* 2015;372:1812–1822.
31. Tilz RR, Rillig A, Thum AM, et al. Catheter ablation of long-standing persistent atrial fibrillation: 5-year outcomes of the Hamburg Sequential Ablation Strategy. *J Am Coll Cardiol.* 2012;60:1921–1929.
32. Brooks AG, Stiles MK, Laborderie J, et al. Outcomes of long-standing persistent atrial fibrillation ablation: a systematic review. *Heart Rhythm.* 2010;7:835–846.
33. Hayward RM, Upadhyay GA, Mela T, et al. Pulmonary vein isolation with complex fractionated atrial electrogram ablation for paroxysmal and nonparoxysmal atrial fibrillation: a meta-analysis. *Heart Rhythm.* 2011;8:994–1000.
34. Narayan SM, Krummen DE, Rappel WJ. Clinical mapping approach to diagnose electrical rotors and focal impulse sources for human atrial fibrillation. *J Cardiovasc Electrophysiol.* 2012;23:447–454.
35. Narayan SM, Patel J, Mulpuru S, et al. Focal impulse and rotor modulation ablation of sustaining rotors abruptly terminates persistent atrial fibrillation to sinus rhythm with elimination on follow-up: a video case study. *Heart Rhythm.* 2012;9:1436–1439.
36. Haïssaguerre M, Hocini M, Sha AJ, et al. Noninvasive panoramic mapping of human atrial fibrillation mechanisms: a feasibility report. *J Cardiovasc Electrophysiol.* 2013;24:711–717.
37. Haïssaguerre M, Hocini M, Sanders P, et al. Catheter ablation of long-lasting persistent atrial fibrillation: clinical outcome and mechanisms of subsequent arrhythmias. *J Cardiovasc Electrophysiol.* 2005;16:1138–1147.
38. Kalifa J, Tanaka K, Zaitsev AV, et al. Mechanisms of wave fractionation at boundaries of high-frequency excitation in the posterior left atrium of the isolated sheep heart during atrial fibrillation. *Circulation.* 2006;113:626–633.
39. Rostock T, Rotter M, Sanders P, et al. High-density activation mapping of fractionated electrograms in the atria of patients with paroxysmal atrial fibrillation. *Heart Rhythm.* 2006;3:27–34.

40. Takahashi Y, O'Neill MD, Hocini M, et al. Characterization of electrograms associated with termination of chronic atrial fibrillation by catheter ablation. *J Am Coll Cardiol.* 2008;51:1003–1010.

41. Hunter RJ, Diab I, Tayebjee M, et al. Characterization of fractionated atrial electrograms critical for maintenance of atrial fibrillation: a randomized, controlled trial of ablation strategies (the CFAE AF trial). *Circ Arrhythm Electrophysiol.* 2011;4:622–629.

42. de Sa DD, Thompson N, Stinnet-Donnelly J, et al. Electrogram fractionation: the relationship between spatiotemporal variation of tissue excitation and electrode spatial resolution. *Circ Arrhythm Electrophysiol.* 2011;4:909–916.

43. Jadidi AS, Duncan E, Miyazaki S, et al. Functional nature of electrogram fractionation demonstrated by left atrial high-density mapping. *Circ Arrhythm Electrophysiol.* 2012;5:32–42.

44. Haïssaguerre M, Sanders P, Hocini M, et al. Changes in atrial fibrillation cycle length and inducibility during catheter ablation and their relation to outcome. *Circulation.* 2004;109:3007–3013.

45. Hocini M, Nault I, Wright M, et al. Disparate evolution of right and left atrial rate during ablation of long-lasting persistent atrial fibrillation. *J Am Coll Cardiol.* 2010;55:1007–1016.

46. Sahadevan J, Ryu K, Peltz L, et al. Epicardial mapping of chronic atrial fibrillation in patients: preliminary observations. *Circulation.* 2004;110:3293–3299.

47. Lazar S, Dixit S, Marchlinski FE, et al. Presence of left-to-right atrial frequency gradient in paroxysmal but not persistent atrial fibrillation in humans. *Circulation.* 2004;110:3181–3186.

48. Sanders P, Barenfeld O, Hocini M, et al. Spectral analysis identifies sites of high-frequency activity maintaining atrial fibrillation in humans. *Circulation.* 2005;112:789–797.

49. Lin YJ, Tai CT, Kao T, et al. Frequency analysis in different types of paroxysmal atrial fibrillation. *J Am Coll Cardiol.* 2006;47:1401–1407.

50. Huang JL, Tai CT, Lin YJ, et al. The mechanisms of an increased dominant frequency in the left atrial posterior wall during atrial fibrillation in acute atrial dilatation. *J Cardiovasc Electrophysiol.* 2006;17:178–188.

51. Berenfeld O, Zaitsev AV, Mironov SF, et al. Frequency-dependent breakdown of wave propagation into fibrillatory conduction across the pectinate muscle network in the isolated sheep right atrium. *Circ Res.* 2002;90:1173–1180.

52. Ryu K, Sahadevan J, Khrestian CM, et al. Use of fast Fourier transform analysis of atrial electrograms for rapid characterization of atrial activation—implications for delineating possible mechanisms of atrial tachyarrhythmias. *J Cardiovasc Electrophysiol.* 2006;17:198–206.

53. Sanders P, Nalliah CJ, Dubois R, et al. Frequency mapping of the pulmonary veins in paroxysmal versus permanent atrial fibrillation. *J Cardiovasc Electrophysiol.* 2006;17:965–972.

54. Ng J, Kadish AH, Goldberger JJ. Effect of electrogram characteristics on the relationship of dominant frequency to atrial activation rate in atrial fibrillation. *Heart Rhythm.* 2006;3:1295–1305.

55. Rostock T, Rotter M, Sanders P, et al. Fibrillating areas isolated within the left atrium after radiofrequency linear catheter ablation. *J Cardiovasc Electrophysiol.* 2006;17:807–812.

56. Schuessler RB, Kawamoto T, Hand DE, et al. Simultaneous epicardial and endocardial activation sequence mapping in the isolated canine right atrium. *Circulation.* 1993;88:250–263.

57. Kneller J, Zou R, Vigmond EJ, et al. Cholinergic atrial fibrillation in a computer model of a two-dimensional sheet of canine atrial cells with realistic ionic properties. *Circ Res.* 2002;90:E73–E87.

58. Chevalier P, Tabib A, Meyronnet D, et al. Quantitative study of nerves of the human left atrium. *Heart Rhythm.* 2005;2:518–522.

59. Hou Y, Scherlag BJ, Lin J, et al. Ganglionated plexi modulate extrinsic cardiac autonomic nerve input: effects on sinus rate, atrioventricular conduction, refractoriness, and inducibility of atrial fibrillation. *J Am Coll Cardiol.* 2007;50:61–68.

60. Patterson E, Po SS, Scherlag BJ, et al. Triggered firing in pulmonary veins initiated by in vitro autonomic nerve stimulation. *Heart Rhythm.* 2005;2:624–631.

61. Zhou J, Scherlag BJ, Edwards BJ, et al. Gradients of atrial refractoriness and inducibility of atrial fibrillation due to stimulation of ganglionated plexi. *J Cardiovasc Electrophysiol.* 2007;18:83–90.

62. Po SS, Scherlag BJ, Yamanashi WS, et al. Experimental model for paroxysmal atrial fibrillation arising at the pulmonary vein-atrial junctions. *Heart Rhythm.* 2006;3:201–208.

63. Takahashi Y, Jaïs P, Hocini M, et al. Shortening of fibrillatory cycle length in the pulmonary vein during vagal excitation. *J Am Coll Cardiol.* 2006;47:774–780.

64. Scherlag BJ, Nakagawa H, Jackman WM, et al. Electrical stimulation to identify neural elements on the heart: their role in atrial fibrillation. *J Interv Card Electrophysiol.* 2005;13(suppl 1):37–42.

65. Verma A, Saliba WI, Lakkireddy D, et al. Vagal responses induced by endocardial left atrial autonomic ganglion stimulation before and after pulmonary vein antrum isolation for atrial fibrillation. *Heart Rhythm.* 2007;4:1177–1182.

66. Lemery R, Birnie D, Tang AS, et al. Feasibility study of endocardial mapping of ganglionated plexuses during catheter ablation of atrial fibrillation. *Heart Rhythm.* 2006;3:387–396.

67. Pappone C, Santinelli V, Manguso F, et al. Pulmonary vein denervation enhances long-term benefit after circumferential ablation for paroxysmal atrial fibrillation. *Circulation.* 2004;109:327–334.

68. Jaïs P, Hocini M, Hsu LF, et al. Technique and results of linear ablation at the mitral isthmus. *Circulation.* 2004;110:2996–3002.

69. Hocini M, Jaïs P, Sanders P, et al. Techniques, evaluation, and consequences of linear block at the left atrial roof in paroxysmal atrial fibrillation: a prospective randomized study. *Circulation.* 2005;112:3688–3696.

70. Tzeis S, Luik A, Jilek C, et al. The modified anterior line: an alternative linear lesion in perimitral flutter. *J Cardiovasc Electrophysiol.* 2010;21:665–670.

71. O'Neill MD, Jaïs P, Takahashi Y, et al. The stepwise ablation approach for chronic atrial fibrillation—evidence for a cumulative effect. *J Interv Card Electrophysiol.* 2006;16:153–167.

72. Weerasooriya R, Khairy P, Litalien J, et al. Catheter ablation for atrial fibrillation: are results maintained at 5 years of follow-up? *J Am Coll Cardiol.* 2011;57:160–166.

73. Ganesan AN, Shipp NJ, Brooks AG, et al. Long-term outcomes of catheter ablation of atrial fibrillation: a systematic review and meta-analysis. *J Am Heart Assoc.* 2013;2:e004549.

74. Rostock T, Salukhe TV, Steven D, et al. Long-term single- and multiple-procedure outcome and predictors of success after catheter ablation for persistent atrial fibrillation. *Heart Rhythm.* 2011;8:1391–1397.

75. Takahashi Y, O'Neill MD, Hocini M, et al. Effects of stepwise ablation of chronic atrial fibrillation on atrial electrical and mechanical properties. *J Am Coll Cardiol.* 2007;49:1306–1314.

76. Narayan SM, Wright M, Derval N, et al. Classifying fractionated electrograms in human atrial fibrillation using monophasic action potentials and activation mapping: evidence for localized drivers, rate acceleration, and nonlocal signal etiologies. *Heart Rhythm.* 2011;8:244–253.

77. Benharash P, Buch E, Frank P, et al. Quantitative analysis of localized sources identified by focal impulse and rotor modulation mapping in atrial fibrillation. *Circ Arrhythm Electrophysiol.* 2015;8:554–561.

78. Rudy Y, Messinger-Rapport BJ. The inverse problem in electrocardiography: solutions in terms of epicardial potentials. *Crit Rev Biomed Eng.* 1987;16:215–268.

79. Cuculich PS, Wang Y, Lindsay BD, et al. Noninvasive characterization of epicardial activation in humans with diverse atrial fibrillation patterns. *Circulation.* 2010;122:1364–1372.

80. Haïssaguerre M, Hocini M, Denis A, et al. Driver domains in persistent atrial fibrillation. *Circulation.* 2014;130:530–538.

81. Non invasive mapping before ablation for atrial fibrillation: the AFACART study. Available from: https://clinicaltrials.gov/ct2/show/NCT02113761; January 2015.

82. Cappato R, Calkins H, Chen SA, et al. Updated worldwide survey on the methods, efficacy, and safety of catheter ablation for human atrial fibrillation. *Circ Arrhythm Electrophysiol.* 2010;3:32–38.

83. Bonanno C, Paccanaro M, La Vecchia L, et al. Efficacy and safety of catheter ablation versus antiarrhythmic drugs for atrial fibrillation: a meta-analysis of randomized trials. *J Cardiovasc Med (Hagerstown).* 2010;11:408–418.

84. Ouyang F, Tilz R, Chun J, et al. Long-term results of catheter ablation in paroxysmal atrial fibrillation: lessons from a 5-year follow-up. *Circulation.* 2010;122:2368–2377.

126 Ablation of Supraventricular Tachyarrhythmias

Feifan Ouyang, Ardan M. Saguner, Andreas Metzner, and Karl Heinz Kuck

Current international guidelines firmly establish catheter ablation of supraventricular tachycardia (SVT) as first-line therapy in patients with recurrent episodes.[1] Historically, lessons from the surgical resection of arrhythmic tissue paved the way for percutaneous catheter ablation. Today, catheter ablation is typically performed as a combined procedure following a diagnostic electrophysiology study. This chapter will discuss the role of catheter ablation for the treatment of paroxysmal and persistent SVT/flutter, while ablation of atrial fibrillation (AF) is covered elsewhere.

Ablation of Atrioventricular Nodal Reentrant Tachycardia

Indications

The 2015 ACC/AHA/HRS guidelines for the management of adult patients with supraventricular arrhythmias list catheter ablation as a class I indication in patients with recurrent atrioventricular nodal reentrant tachycardia (AVNRT).[1] Catheter ablation, the preferred choice of most patients, prevents recurrent episodes and the need for drug therapy.

General Principles

Catheter ablation of AVNRT is based on the concept of dual AVN pathways with distinct anatomical and functional entities.[2] The triangle of Koch describes the anatomical region incorporating the slow and fast AVN pathways. The His bundle marks the apex of the triangle of Koch, while the fast AVN pathway borders just posteriorly, extending into the compact AVN. The tendon of Todaro forms a band-like structure extending posteriorly and inferiorly from the AVN to the eustachian ridge, marking the posterior border of the triangle of Koch, while the ostium of the coronary sinus (CS) marks its base and the tricuspid valve marks its anterior boundary. The slow pathway extends between the CS ostium and the tricuspid valve annulus toward the compact AVN. It has been demonstrated that AVNRT patients have a larger CS ostium than control patients, a fact that needs to be appreciated when positioning the ablation catheter in the region of the slow pathway.[3]

During sinus rhythm, conduction typically spreads rapidly via the fast pathway that exhibits a relatively long refractory period, while conduction generally spreads less rapidly via the slow pathway that demonstrates a shorter refractory period.

Retrograde conduction over the fast AVN pathway results in the recording of concentric earliest atrial activation at the interatrial septum superoposterior to the tendon of Todaro, while retrograde conduction over the slow AVN pathway demonstrates earliest atrial activation in the vicinity of the CS ostium.[2]

Slow Pathway Ablation

In the pioneering days of radiofrequency (RF) ablation, the fast pathway was targeted for ablation, resulting in a prolonged PR interval during sinus rhythm and a high rate of complete AV block due to close proximity to the compact AVN.[2] Today, the standard approach is to target the slow pathway for ablation. Two techniques for successful slow AVN pathway ablation, slow pathway potential mapping and an anatomical approach, have been described.

Using a detailed mapping approach, Jackman et al. recorded large, sharp, slow pathway potentials along the inferior septum between the tricuspid annulus and CS ostium, which if targeted during catheter ablation, resulted in the modification or ablation of the slow pathway with a high rate of success.[4] Haïssaguerre and colleagues reported a high success rate following catheter ablation of typical slow/fast AVNRT targeting discrete low-frequency, low-amplitude potentials posteroinferior to the AVN and anterior to the CS ostium.[5] While the electrophysiological characterization of slow pathway potentials has been variable, targeting these potentials during ablation has been proved highly effective.

Alternatively, an anatomical approach for slow pathway ablation may be utilized. For this purpose, the triangle of Koch is divided into three sections, as seen during fluoroscopic imaging. The superior third harbors the AVN and fast pathway and correlates fluoroscopically with the position of the His bundle recording catheter. The middle third extends inferiorly to the CS roof. The inferior third incorporates the CS ostium and is inferred fluoroscopically by the catheter positioned in the proximal CS. The inferior third of the triangle of Koch represents the typical site for slow pathway ablation. At this location, the ablation catheter will record a large ventricular signal and a single or multicomponent atrial potential with an atrial-to-ventricular ratio of 0.1:0.5. A conventional nonirrigated 4-mm-tip ablation catheter in temperature mode is generally used with a target temperature of 55°C and an initial power of 20 W that is gradually titrated to 30–40 W if junctional ectopy ensues. If initial attempts are unsuccessful, the catheter is gradually advanced superiorly until energy application results in successful slow pathway ablation. It is important to note that ablation at a more superior position may increase the risk for inadvertent AV block due to closer proximity to the AVN. Ablation between the tricuspid annulus and CS ostium (slow pathway recording site) produces junctional ectopy but fails to abolish AVNRT in <2% of patients with typical slow/fast AVNRT. In these patients, a leftward inferior extension of the AVN may form the antegrade slow pathway. Instead of delivering RF energy at higher sites in the triangle of Koch, the atrial end of the leftward inferior extension along the proximal CS roof can be targeted for ablation. CS venography can be used to localize the CS ostium and CS roof to facilitate ablation.[3] Rarely, if repeat attempts at common right atrial sites prove unsuccessful, after transseptal puncture, RF application to the inferior

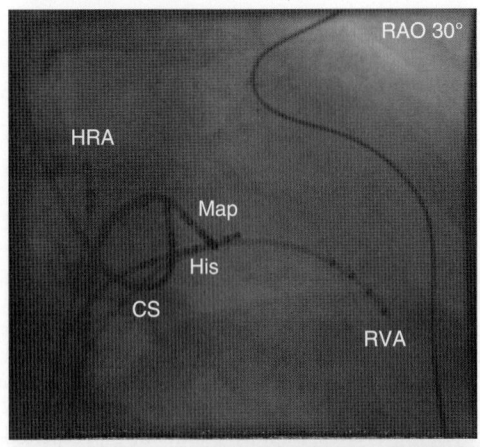

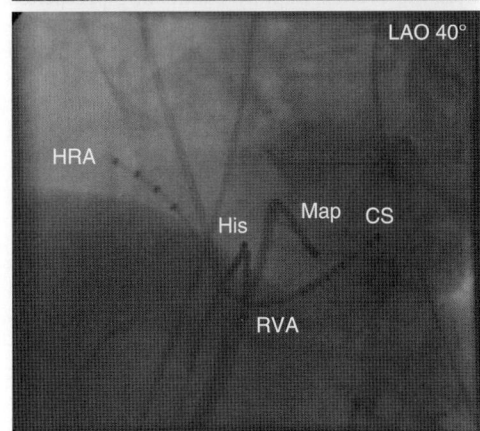

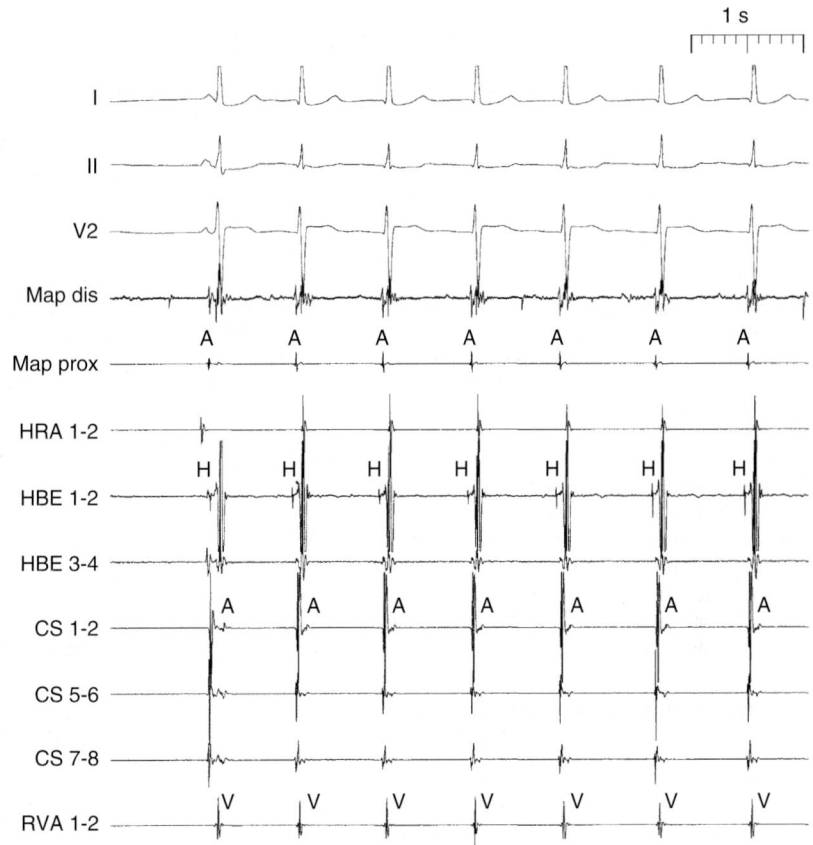

FIGURE 126.1 Successful ablation of the left slow pathway via a transseptal approach in a 45-year-old female patient with typical (slow–fast) atrioventricular nodal reentry tachycardia and two failed ablation attempts in the right atrium and within the coronary sinus. *Left,* Fluoroscopic catheter position (in the right anterior oblique *[RAO]* view, 30–degree projections and in the left anterior oblique *[LAO]* view, 40-degree projections) during ablation. *CS,* Catheter in the coronary sinus; *His,* catheter at the His bundle region; *HRA,* catheter in the high right atrium; *Map,* ablation catheter at the left atrial midseptum; *RVA,* catheter in the right ventricular apex. *Right,* Tracings are electrocardiogram leads I, II, and V$_2$, and an intracardiac electrogram recorded from a mapping catheter (Map dis and Map prox) positioned at the left atrial midseptum, a catheter at the high right atrium (HRA 1-2), a catheter at the His bundle region (*HBE 1-2, HBE 3-4*), a catheter within the coronary sinus (CS 1-2 to CS 7-8), and a catheter at the right ventricular apex during ablation of the left slow pathway. Note that continuous junctional beats with variable cycle length and retrograde one-to-one conduction are present during ablation.

left atrial (LA) septum is required for successful slow pathway ablation (Fig. 126.1).[3] Comparing the technique of detailed slow pathway potential mapping with an anatomical approach, a prospective randomized study found both methods comparable in efficacy, procedure duration, fluoroscopy time, and mean number of RF applications.[3] Frequently, both techniques are combined to scan the inferior septum in the proximity of the CS ostium for a multicomponent atrial potential and a larger ventricular signal.

As an alternative energy source, the use of cryoenergy for ablation of AVNRT was first reported by Skanes and colleagues.[3] Applying cryoenergy allows for testing of the functional impact of each freeze application at specific sites (cryomapping) before delivery of an irreversible lesion. Ice formation at the catheter tip will prevent catheter dislodgement, while cryoablation is less painful to the patient.[6,7] Cryoenergy application at the site of the slow pathway will not induce junctional rhythm and thus cannot be used to guide lesion delivery.[3]

Endpoints for Slow Pathway Ablation

During successful RF ablation of the slow pathway, an accelerated, irregular junctional rhythm is commonly seen. Albeit sensitive, development of a junctional rhythm is a nonspecific finding also noted in 65% of ineffective RF applications.[8] Rarely, successful slow pathway ablation can be achieved with RF current in the absence of a junctional rhythm.[3] Complete elimination of slow pathway conduction serves as the optimal endpoint for ablation. However, modulation of the slow pathway, that is, presence of residual slow pathway conduction limited to single echo beats without inducibility of tachycardia after isoproterenol infusion, is an acceptable endpoint, especially in pediatric patients if AVNRT was inducible prior to ablation. In this scenario, slow pathway modulation demonstrates comparable long-term success rates to complete elimination of slow pathway conduction.[3]

In patients with baseline prolongation of the PR interval and AVNRT, the procedural endpoint should aim at modulating slow pathway conduction because the complete slow pathway ablation will lead to a higher rate of late complete AV block.[9] In contrast, AV conduction may improve once slow pathway conduction has been eliminated, likely due to reversal of electrotonic inhibition by the slow pathway imposed on the fast pathway.[3] In about 10% of patients, AVNRT remains noninducible during the electrophysiology study despite the use of intravenous isoproterenol.[3] Most commonly, this is due to block in the fast pathway. If

AVNRT cannot be induced in the presence of dual AVN physiology and the documented SVT suggests AVNRT, slow pathway ablation should be performed, demonstrating excellent long-term results.[3] A recent large observational study indicated that this recommendation is also applicable to patients with typical electrocardiogram (ECG) documentation but with the absence of dual AVN physiology.[10]

In the atypical forms of AVNRT, the slow pathway (rightward inferior extension) is also targeted for ablation.[2] Alternatively, for ablation of slow/slow AVNRT, retrograde slow pathway (leftward inferior extension) conduction can be targeted. Therefore RF energy is delivered to the site of earliest retrograde atrial activation, which is usually at the proximal CS roof. During ablation of slow/slow AVNRT, accelerated junctional rhythm is frequently associated with a ventriculoatrial (VA) block because retrograde fast pathway conduction is either absent or poor in these patients. In this situation, a safe ablation strategy can be pursued by fast atrial pacing with one-to-one AV conduction to monitor PR interval and minimize potential injury to the AVN. In elderly patients with atypical fast/slow AVNRT, rarely successful ablation can be achieved from the noncoronary cusp of Valsalva.[11]

The procedural endpoint for fast/slow or slow/slow AVNRT is complete elimination of VA conduction over the retrograde slow pathway as mere slow pathway modulation results in a higher rate of recurrence.

Risk for Atrioventricular Block

The risk for AV block during ablation of the slow pathway has been estimated to be <1% at experienced centers.[4,5] Unstable catheter tip-to-tissue contact due to deep inspiration or anatomical features, such as a large CS ostium or a narrow triangle of Koch, are often overcome by intensifying sedation and the use of a long sheath facilitating catheter stability. Anterograde AV conduction is carefully monitored during RF application and energy delivery is aborted if prolongation of the AV interval is noted. Induction of a fast junctional rhythm with a cycle length <350 ms was predictive for the development of AV conduction block.[2] The VA interval should be continuously monitored and stable catheter position verified to minimize the risk for AV block during energy delivery. Prolonging or blocking VA conduction suggests imminent high-grade anterograde AV block, and immediate termination of RF delivery is warranted.[2] Alternatively, ablation can be performed during atrial pacing at a rate sufficient to override the junctional rhythm, while closely monitoring anterograde AV conduction. Results from a large multicenter prospective randomized trial (the CYRANO study) show that the risk for permanent AV block did not significantly differ between cryoablation and RF ablation.[7]

Outcome

RF ablation of the slow pathway has been proved to be highly effective, with a reported acute success rate of 96%–100%.[1,4,5] During long-term follow-up, 1.3%–6.9% of patients develop recurrent AVNRT. Acute success rates of cryoablation are similar to those of RF ablation.[7] However, in the CYRANO study enrolling 509 patients, long-term results demonstrated a significantly higher rate of recurrence in patients undergoing cryoablation compared with those undergoing RF ablation (9.4% vs. 4.4%) without differences in risk for permanent AV block. The reduced long-term efficacy of cryoablation was confirmed in a recent meta-analysis and systematic review.[12] In light of these findings, RF ablation should be the first choice for patients undergoing slow pathway ablation. Electroanatomical mapping has been shown to guide slow pathway ablation with no or minimal fluoroscopy, with success and complication rates similar to those obtained with standard techniques, which may be particularly important in pregnant women and children.[13]

Ablation of Atrioventricular Reentrant Tachycardia

Indications

Catheter ablation, the mainstay of treatment for patients with AV reentrant tachycardia (AVRT), demonstrates excellent long-term outcomes and a low rate of complications.[1,14,15] Although low in prevalence (10-year risk ranges from 0.15% to 0.24%),[16,17] rapid anterograde conduction over an accessory pathway (AP) in the setting of AF may result in ventricular fibrillation and sudden cardiac death. The most recent 2015 ACC/AHA/HRS guidelines give catheter ablation a class I indication in patients with orthodromic/antidromic AVRT and preexcited AF and a class IIa indication in asymptomatic patients with preexcitation (without documented AVRT) if electrophysiological study identifies a high risk for arrhythmic events. Rapidly conducting preexcited AF (<250 ms between two preexcited complexes during spontaneous or induced AF), the finding of AVRT precipitating preexcited AF, an AP refractory period <240 ms, and the presence of multiple APs are indicative of high-risk patients. Of note, malignant arrhythmias seem to correlate more with the electrophysiological properties of the AP rather than the presence of symptoms.[1]

Accessory Pathway Localization

APs are commonly located along the tricuspid or mitral annulus or within the subepicardial pyramidal space in the inferoseptal region (Fig. 126.2), forming connections between atrial and ventricular tissue. Rarely, an AP spans from the atrium (atriofascicular), AVN (nodofascicular or nodoventricular), or His-Purkinje system (fasciculoventricular) to a more distal branch of the His-Purkinje system or ventricular musculature. The 12-lead surface ECG will aid in pathway localization and preparation for the best ablation strategy. Arruda and colleagues developed an algorithm for AP localization by correlating the surface 12-lead ECG pattern with the successful ablation site in 135 patients with manifest anterogradely conducting pathways.[18] In a prospective evaluation of 121 patients, the authors could demonstrate that the vector of the initial portion of the surface delta wave in leads I, II, aVF, and V_1, as well as the R-to-S ratios in leads III and V1, accurately predicted 1 of 10 sites around the AV annuli or subepicardial region with a sensitivity of 90% and a specificity of 99%.[18]

Following successful catheter ablation, the 12-lead surface ECG commonly demonstrates repolarization changes in the direction of the delta wave, dominating in patients with right-sided APs. These alterations in repolarization are caused by cardiac memory and require no further treatment, resolving spontaneously over time.[3]

Multiple APs may occur in up to 13% of patients with Wolff-Parkinson-White (WPW) syndrome, and its prevalence is as high as 52% (range, 35%–52%) in patients with Ebstein anomaly.[19] The presence of additional APs may only be evident after ablation of the first or may be suggested during intracardiac mapping by variations in the activation sequence due to simultaneous or alternating conduction across multiple pathways.

Accurate localization of an AP will require careful intracardiac mapping during the electrophysiology study. At the AV groove, ventricular myocardium is relatively thick, resulting in an atrial-to-ventricular signal amplitude ratio <1, while a position at the atrial insertion site has a ratio of about 1, and a position at the ventricular insertion site has a ratio of 1/2–1/6. Catheter stability is verified by <20% variation in the atrial potential amplitude.[3]

The most reliable mapping criterion is the recording of an AP potential.[2] In manifest pathways, the distal bipolar recording at the successful ablation site will demonstrate a discrete, low-amplitude AP potential between the local atrial and ventricular electrogram that precedes the onset of the delta wave on the surface ECG (Fig. 126.3). Generally, pacing maneuvers at atrial and ventricular sites are used to dissociate the pathway potential from

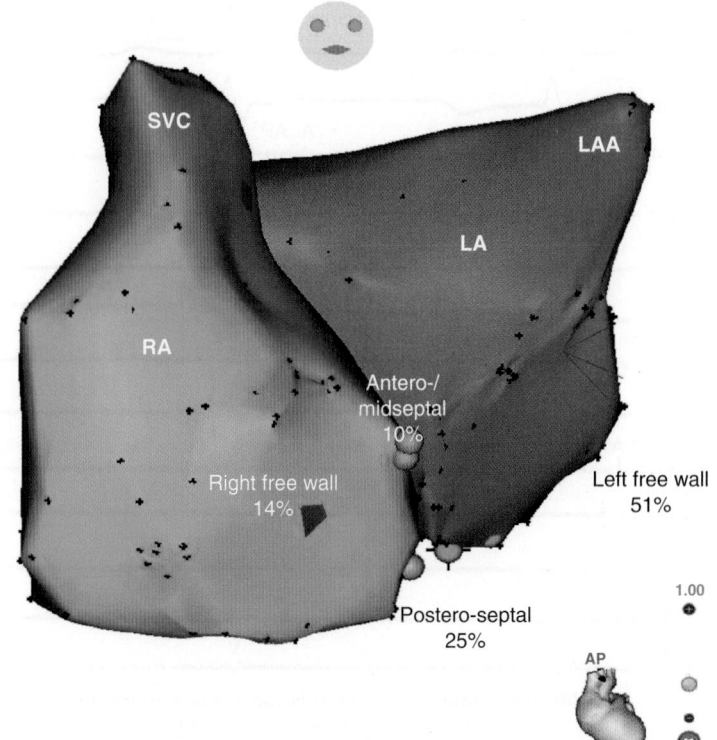

FIGURE 126.2 Distribution of the accessory pathway *(AP)* location. A three-dimensional schematic of tricuspid and mitral atrioventricular rings in an anterior-posterior projection, showing the locations of APs including Ebstein anomaly from 1969 consecutive patients receiving catheter ablation of APs at the Asklepios Clinic, St. Georg, Hamburg, Germany between 1994 and 2001. The anatomically correct terminology is used. The table shows the number of APs per patient for the total cohort and in those with Ebstein anomaly. *LA,* Left atrium; *LAA,* left atrial appendage; *RA,* right atrium; *SVC,* superior vena cava.

N = 1969 (1146 males)
Mean age 36 ± 18 years

	Patients	Ebstein
	1969	40/1969
	2325 APs	86 APs
1 AP	1705	12
2 APs	193	15
3 APs	57	10
4 APs	8	1
5 APs	5	2
6 APs	1	0

the atrial and ventricular electrogram. Importantly, the number of RF energy applications necessary for successful pathway ablation is lower if an AP potential can be identified.[2]

In clinical practice, the earliest local ventricular or atrial activation will identify the AP insertion site. In antegradely conducting APs, the timing of the preexcited local ventricular electrogram on the bipolar recording during sinus rhythm, atrial pacing, or antidromic AVRT in reference to the earliest onset of the delta wave on the surface ECG is used to accurately localize the ventricular insertion site of the AP.[3] At this site, the unipolar electrogram will demonstrate a QS pattern indicating spread of activation from the insertion of the AP toward local ventricular tissue (see Fig. 126.3).

In concealed APs or retrogradely conducting manifest pathways, the site of earliest atrial activation during orthodromic AVRT or ventricular pacing identifies the atrial insertion site. Clinically, it is difficult to identify the onset of local atrial and ventricular activation if the local atrial activation is superimposed on the ventricular activation during atrial and ventricular pacing. Programmed stimulation with extrastimuli at AP refractoriness can differentiate them (Fig. 126.4). The local AV or VA intervals are insufficient parameters to predict the successful ablation site because pathway conduction in most patients will follow an oblique course or the local activation wavefront recorded on the distal mapping electrode may vary in direction.[2,20]

Free Wall Accessory Pathways

In the presence of a left AP, access is gained through a transseptal or retrograde transaortic approach. Lesh and associates compared a transseptal with a retrograde transaortic approach and concluded that both complement each other, resulting in nearly 100% success if used in combination.[3] In most cases, the primary determinant of which approach to choose is one of operator preference. Transseptal access carries the risk of systemic air embolism and cardiac tamponade due to perforation but avoids aortic valve injury or coronary artery dissection reported using a retrograde transaortic approach.[3] Transseptal access is preferred in children or elderly patients or in the presence of aortic valve stenosis, mechanical aortic valve prosthesis, or significant arterial disease.

While reported success rates for ablation of left free wall APs range from 95% to 97%, those for ablation of right free wall APs are lower (90%) because of a lack of any marker along the tricuspid annulus and thick trabeculated myocardium near the tricuspid annulus. A high-density multielectrode mapping catheter positioned around the tricuspid annulus will facilitate localization of a right free wall AP. Catheter stability is improved by using a long sheath placed via the femoral vein and/or targeting the ventricular insertion site by making a reverse loop in the right ventricle (RV) (Fig. 126.5). Ebstein anomaly is associated with a higher incidence of right APs, and multiple right-sided pathways are present in up to 52% of patients.[3] In the region of the "atrialized" RV, the presence of extensive fractionated endocardial electrograms may confound proper identification of local preexcited potentials and discrete pathway potentials.[3] Importantly, APs are always located at the true annulus in these patients. A right atrial/RV angiogram with or without three-dimensional (3D) electroanatomical mapping can facilitate identification of the AV groove, enabling a high procedural success rate.[21]

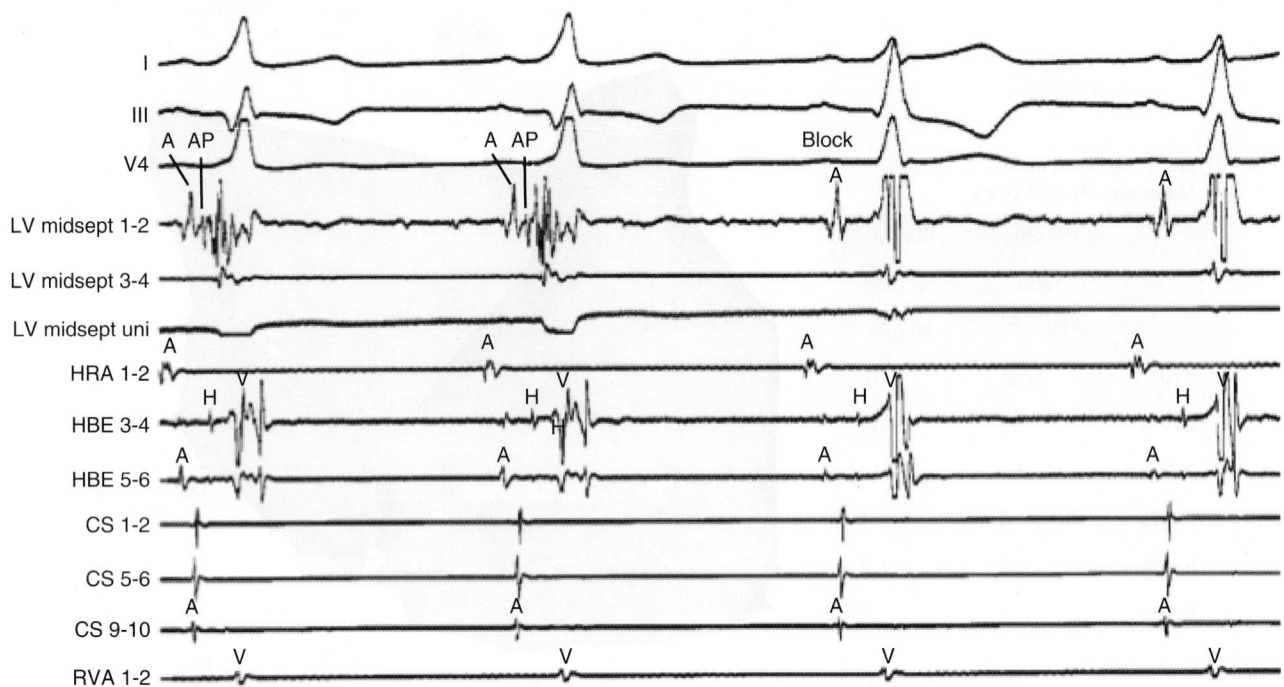

FIGURE 126.3 Radiofrequency ablation of a left midseptal (paraseptal) accessory pathway (*AP*). The *top tracings* show surface electrocardiogram leads I, III, and V$_4$ with a prominent delta wave in the first two beats followed by the disappearance of preexcitation in beats 3 and 4 once AP is blocked (*Block*). Intracardiac tracings were recorded from the ablation catheter (left ventricular *[LV]* midsept 1-2, 3-4, and LV midsept uni) positioned at the insertion site of the midseptal (paraseptal) AP. The distal bipolar electrode (LV midsept 1-2) records an atrial signal (*A*), followed by an AP potential and a ventricular signal (*V*) in beats 1 and 2. Note the prolongation of the local atrial-to-ventricular interval once a conduction block in AP occurs (beats 3 and 4). The unipolar electrode (midsept uni) located at the AP insertion site records a QS complex, indicating activation away from the unipolar electrode. *CS 1-2, 5-6, and 9-10,* Recordings from the coronary sinus; *HBE 3-4 and 5-6,* His bundle recordings; *HRA 1-2,* recording from the high right atrium; *RVA 1-2,* recording from the right ventricular apex.

Septal Accessory Pathways

Septal APs are subdivided into anteroseptal (superoparaseptal), midseptal (paraseptal), and posteroseptal (inferoparaseptal) locations.[22] An anteroseptal or para-Hisian (superoparaseptal) pathway is present if the site recording a pathway potential simultaneously displays a His bundle potential. A superior approach targeting the ventricular insertion site through a long sheath placed via the right jugular vein will facilitate catheter stability during energy delivery, minimizing the potential risk for AV block. Judicious titration of RF energy will result in blocking the superficially situated anteroseptal (superoparaseptal) pathway without damaging the His bundle, which is protected by layers of fibrous tissue. Alternatively, cryoenergy can be used for pathway ablation. A single tip cryoablation catheter allows reversible cryomapping at a temperature of –30°C, before definitive energy delivery at lower temperatures causes an irreversible loss of myocardial cell function, thus reducing the risk for inadvertent AV block.[23] However, compared with RF ablation, long-term success rates of 80% are less favorable with cryoablation.[3] Epicardial anteroseptal (superoparaseptal) pathways may rarely require irrigated RF ablation from the noncoronary aortic valve cusp.[3]

Compared with anteroseptal (superoparaseptal) pathways, the risk for accidental AV block is higher during ablation of midseptal pathways due to the close proximity to the compact AVN. Targeting a right-sided midseptal (paraseptal) pathway, the local recording site should demonstrate a small atrial and a large ventricular signal, indicating a catheter position closer to the ventricular aspect of the tricuspid annulus (see Fig. 126.3). Left midseptal (paraseptal) pathways are targeted using a left-sided retrograde or antegrade approach.

Posteroseptal (inferoparaseptal) APs traverse the pyramidal space posterior to the septum and are subdivided into right and left posteroseptal (inferoparaseptal) pathways. Right posteroseptal (inferoparaseptal) pathways are located in the vicinity of the ostium of the CS. If careful mapping fails to identify an AP potential along the endocardial right posteroseptal (inferoparaseptal) region or within the CS ostium and its trajectories, retrograde transaortic or transseptal access is obtained to search for a suitable ablation site along the left posteroseptal (inferoparaseptal) region at the medial aspect of the mitral annulus. Occasionally, successful ablation of left posteroseptal APs can only be achieved via the transaortic approach due to the mismatch of the atrial and ventricular septa.

Epicardial Accessory Pathways

Epicardial APs most commonly utilize muscular sleeves extending into the CS and its tributaries, acting as a bridge between atrial and ventricular myocardium. Because of low blood flow within the CS or its branches, ablation requires the use of an irrigated-tip catheter targeting the ostium of the middle cardiac vein or the posterior coronary vein. In 21% of patients with previously failed ablation of a posteroseptal (inferoparaseptal) AP, CS angiography will demonstrate a diverticulum emanating from the CS or middle cardiac vein.[2] In these patients, the successful ablation site is commonly located within the neck of the diverticulum. Coronary angiography should be performed to identify the relationship between the targeted site and the coronary artery before ablation. Rarely, APs are confined to the epicardial space along the right free wall or utilize an LA appendage (LAA)- or

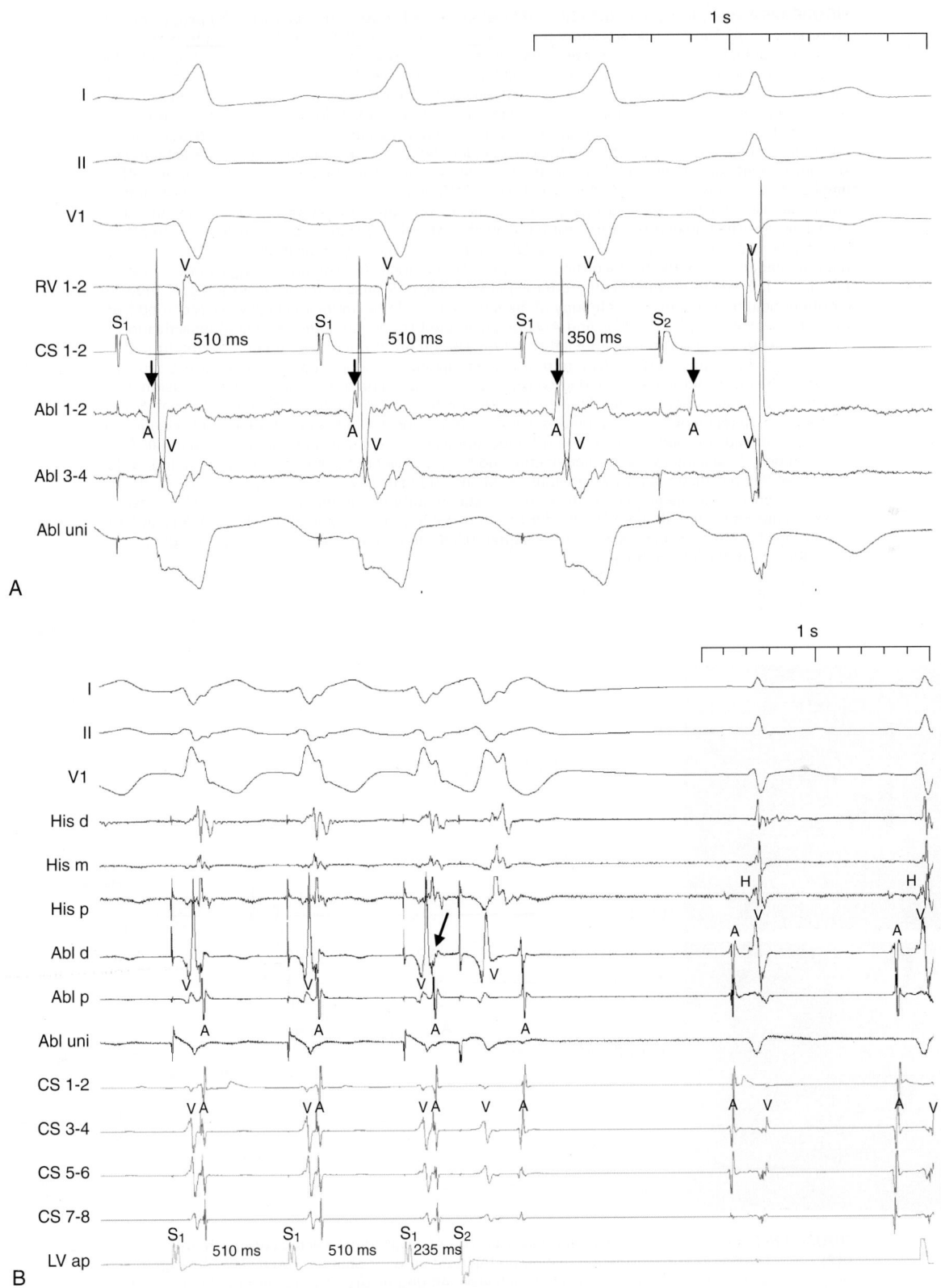

FIGURE 126.4 For legend, see next page.

FIGURE 126.4 Identification of the onset of local atrial and ventricular activation by programmed stimulation. (A) The *top tracings* show surface electrocardiogram (ECG) leads I, II, and V₁ with a prominent delta wave in the first three beats followed by the disappearance of preexcitation in beat 4. Intracardiac tracings were recorded from the ablation catheter (*Abl 1-2, 3-4,* and *Abl uni*) positioned at the insertion site of a right-sided accessory pathway (AP). During programmed atrial pacing from the distal coronary sinus (*CS* 1-2) at a basic cycle length of 510 ms (S₁), atrioventricular conduction occurs over the AP causing a fusion of the local atrial (*A, red arrow*) and ventricular (*V*) activation on the ablation catheter. Fusion may obscure the correct identification of the earliest ventricular activation. A programmed stimulation with a single atrial extrabeat (S₂) causes the loss of conduction over AP, and conduction now occurs via the atrioventricular (AV) node that unmasks the local atrial (A) and ventricular (V) signal in beat 4, facilitating the correct identification of the onset of earliest ventricular activation. The unipolar recording from the ablation distal electrode (*Abl uni*) located at the AP ventricular insertion site records a classical QS complex morphology, indicating activation away from the unipolar electrode. *RV 1-2,* recording from the right ventricle. (B) The *top tracings* show surface ECG leads I, II, and V₁ during pacing from the left ventricle (*LV*) close to the AP insertion site, showing a right bundle branch block morphology of the surface ECG. Intracardiac tracings were recorded from the ablation catheter (*Abl d, Abl p,* and *Abl uni*) positioned at the site of the earliest atrial activation, which indicates the insertion site of a left-sided AP. During programmed ventricular pacing from LV at a basic cycle length of 510 ms (S₁), retrograde ventriculoatrial conduction occurs over AP, causing fusion of the local ventricular (V) and atrial (*A, arrow*) activation on the ablation catheter. Fusion may obscure the correct identification of the earliest atrial activation. A single ventricular extrabeat (S₂) with an S₁-S₂ interval of 235 ms is delivered at AP refractoriness and results in the loss of conduction over AP and leads to conduction via the AV node, unmasking the local ventricular (V) and atrial (A) signal in beat 4, facilitating the correct identification of the onset of the earliest atrial activation. Note that the ablation catheter is positioned at the atrial insertion site of AP via a transseptal approach (A>V); the position of the ablation catheter is very stable during mapping of AP, reflected by a stable V-A ratio during beats 1–4 and A-V ratio during sinus rhythm (beats 5 and 6). *CS 1-2, 3-4, 5-6,* and *7-8,* Recordings from the coronary sinus; *H,* His signal; *His d, His m,* and *His p,* His bundle recordings; *LV,* recordings from the left ventricle.

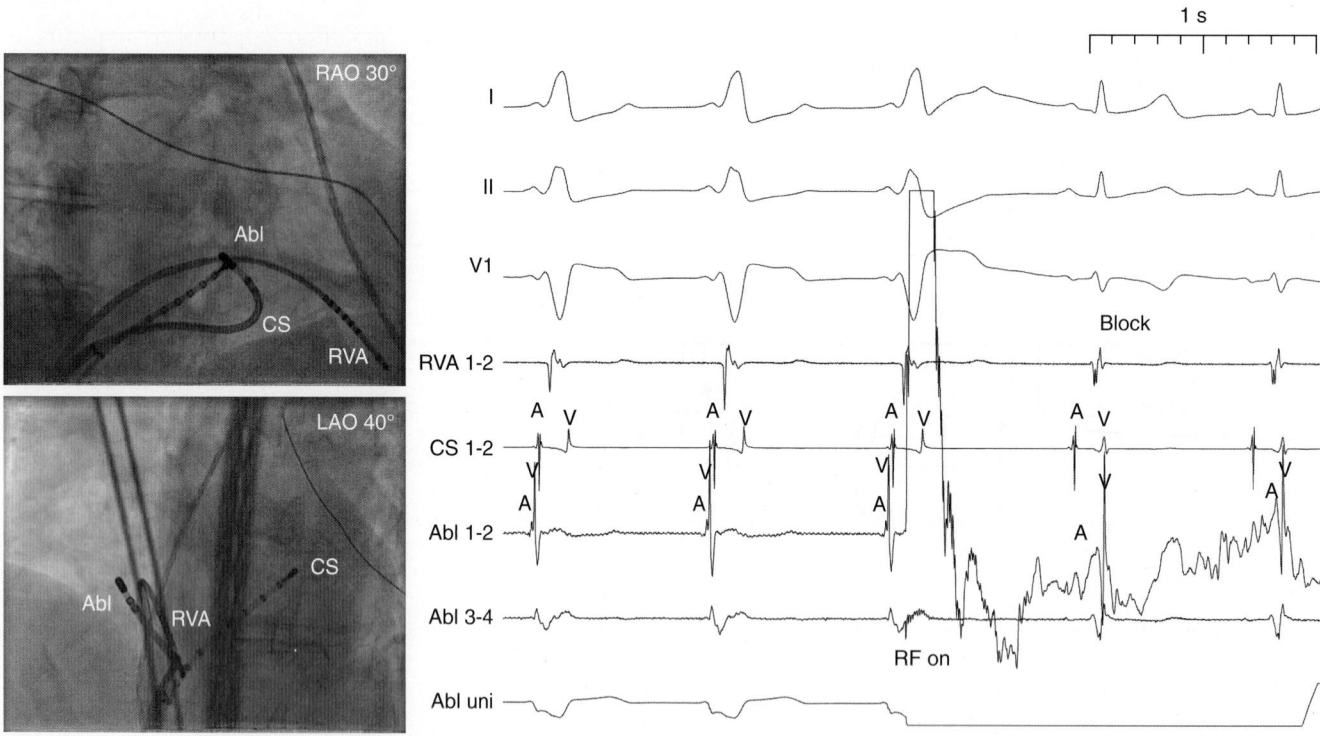

FIGURE 126.5 Targeting the ventricular insertion site of a right-sided accessory pathway (AP). *Left,* The fluoroscopic catheter position (in the right anterior oblique *[RAO]* view, 30-degree projections and in the left anterior oblique *[LAO]* view, 40-degree projections) during ablation of a right-sided AP. Note that ablation catheter stability (LAO, 40 degrees, 11-o'clock position) is improved by using a long sheath placed via the femoral vein and targeting the ventricular insertion site by making a reverse loop (reverse C curve) in the right ventricle. *Abl,* Ablation catheter; *CS,* catheter in the coronary sinus; *RVA,* catheter in the right ventricular apex. *Right,* Tracings show surface ECG leads I, II, and V₁ and intracardiac recordings from the wave in the first three beats followed by the disappearance of preexcitation in beats 4 and 5 once AP is blocked *(Block).* Intracardiac tracings were recorded from the ablation catheter (*Abl 1-2, Abl 3-4,* and *Abl uni*) positioned at the ventricular insertion site of the right-sided AP. The distal bipolar electrode (*Abl 1-2*) records fusion of the atrial (A) and ventricular signal (V) in beats 1–3. Radiofrequency delivery (*RF on*) at this site immediately eliminates AP conduction with the normalization of the surface QRS complex (beats 4 and 5). The unipolar electrode (*Abl uni*) located at the AP insertion site records a QS complex, indicating activation away from the unipolar electrode. *CS 1-2,* Recording from the coronary sinus; *RVA,* recording from the right ventricular apex.

right atrial appendage-to-ventricular connection. In the latter, an AP potential is not recorded endocardially because these pathways result from a direct connection between the atrial appendages and the ventricular myocardium. It may require cautious endocardial ablation within the atrial appendage base far from the tricuspid annulus and generally requires multiple irrigated RF ablation lesions at the right atrial appendage base. Finally, a percutaneous pericardial or surgical approach may be considered after multiple failed attempts at endocardial ablation.[2,24,25]

Accessory Pathways With Decremental Conduction

An atriofascicular pathway (Mahaim fiber) is characterized by decremental antegrade conduction properties in the absence of retrograde conduction. During antidromic AVRT, the surface

ECG demonstrates left bundle branch block morphology (sharp QS pattern in V_1) with late precordial transition. Essentially, right atriofascicular pathways consist of a duplicate His bundle located along the lateral tricuspid annulus that produces a characteristic M potential and an accessory right bundle branch that inserts into the apical RV free wall or the original distal right bundle branch.[2] Catheter ablation generally targets the atrial insertion site at the lateral tricuspid annulus where a discrete low-amplitude, high-frequency pathway potential (M potential) is recorded, the distal ventricular insertion site or, alternatively, the earliest site of ventricular activation. Mapping at the ventricular aspect of the tricuspid annulus is sometimes required to achieve a stable catheter position using 3D mapping where a clear M potential is also recorded during sinus rhythm or orthodromic AVRT (Fig. 126.6). Ablation close to the RV apex should be avoided to prevent ablation of the distal right bundle branch,

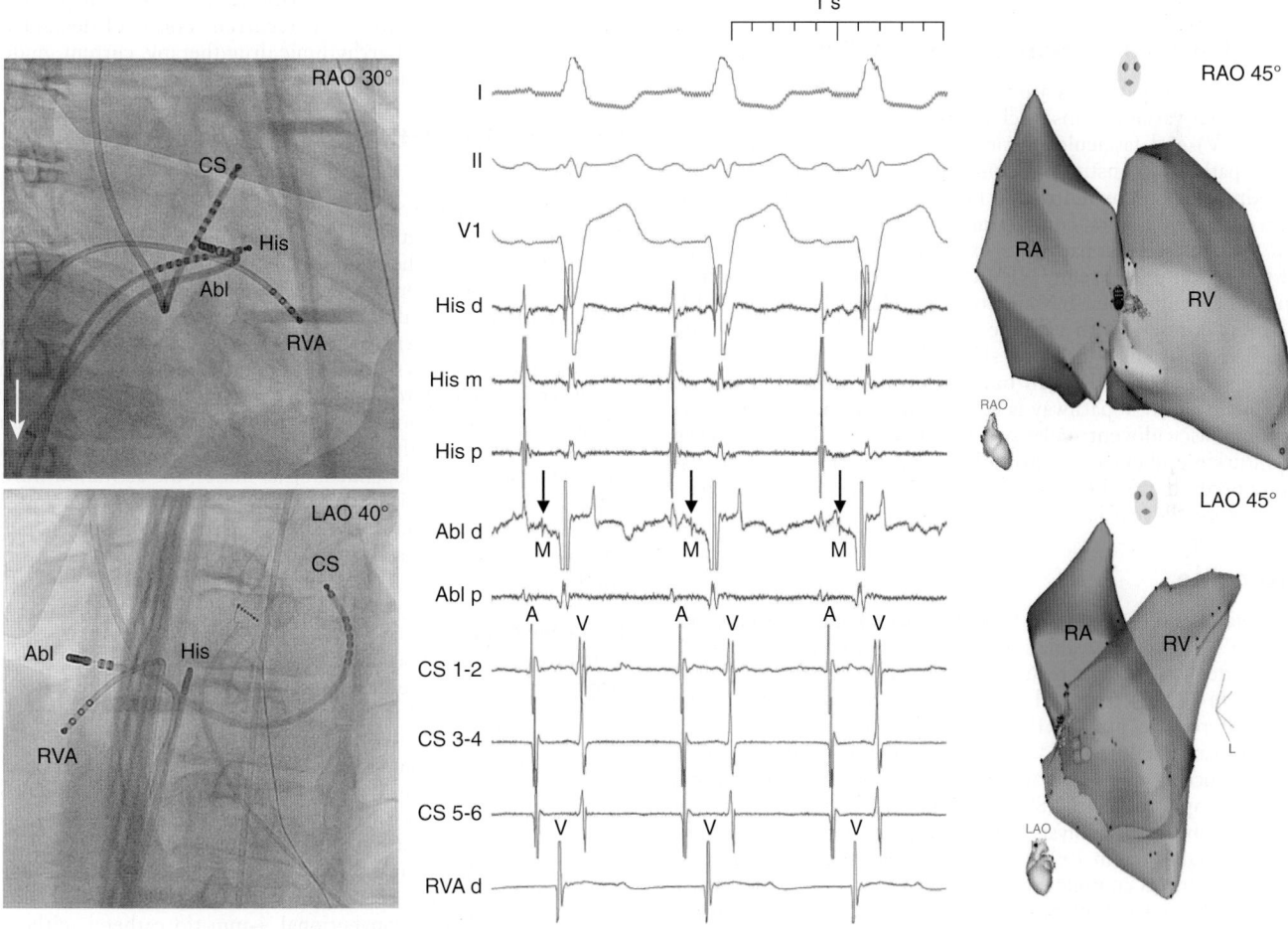

FIGURE 126.6 Ablation of a right-sided decremental atriofascicular pathway (Mahaim). *Left,* The fluoroscopic catheter position (in the right anterior oblique *[RAO]* view, 30-degree projections and in the left anterior oblique *[LAO]* view, 40-degree projections) during ablation of a right-sided decremental atriofascicular pathway (Mahaim). Note that ablation catheter stability (LAO, 40 degrees; 10-o'clock position) is improved by using a long sheath (*white arrow*) placed via the femoral vein and by making a reverse loop (reverse C curve) in the right ventricle. *Abl,* ablation catheter; *CS,* catheter in the coronary sinus; *His:* catheter in the His bundle region; *RVA,* catheter in the right ventricular apex. *Middle, The top tracings* show surface ECG leads I, II, and V_1 with preexcitation (typical left bundle branch block morphology and a superior axis). Intracardiac tracings recorded from the ablation catheter (*Abl* d and Abl p) positioned at the tricuspid annulus show a characteristic Mahaim (*M, arrows*) potential. *A,* Atrial signal; *CS 1-2, 3-4, 5-6,* recordings from the coronary sinus; *His d, His m, His p,* His bundle recordings; *RV d,* recording from the right ventricular apex; *V,* ventricular signal. *Right,* The RAO (45 degrees) and LAO (45 degrees) projections show a 3D electroanatomical reconstruction of the right atrium (*blue*) and the right ventricle (*gray*) during sinus rhythm with point-by-point mapping technology. Note that (1) a Mahaim potential (M) is found in a small area (marked with *red color*) on the free wall of the tricuspid annulus, and (2) *pink points* indicate the site of successful ablation with irrigated radiofrequency energy. *RA,* Right atrium; *RV,* right ventricle.

which may increase antidromic AVRT cycle length, occasionally producing incessant tachycardia. Because the atriofascicular fibers are located superficially endocardially in contrast to common APs, due to a different embryological origin, they can be easily bumped during mapping along the tricuspid annulus.

More common in infants, children, or young adults, permanent junctional reciprocating tachycardia (PJRT) is defined as orthodromic AVRT utilizing a mostly posteroseptal (inferoparaseptal) pathway with slow decremental retrograde conduction properties that may result in tachycardia-mediated cardiomyopathy.[3] This tachycardia has deeply inverted retrograde P waves in leads II, III, and aVF, with a long RP interval due to the location and decremental conduction properties of the AP. During tachycardia or ventricular pacing, an AP potential is most often found at the right posteroseptal (inferoparaseptal) region or within the proximal CS, and successful ablation will usually result in normalization of left ventricular function if successful ablation is performed not too late.

Rare Forms of Variant Accessory Pathways

Atriofascicular pathways are the most common form of variant APs. Other variant forms, such as nodofascicular/nodoventricular (NFV) and fasciculoventricular pathways, are rather rare. NFV pathways constitute a connection between the AVN and Purkinje fascicles or ventricular myocardium, causing preexcitation with decremental conduction. The pathophysiology is similar to atriofascicular pathways, except that the atrium is not part of the arrhythmia circuit. NFV can constitute a critical part of an SVT circuit or be a bystander. Studies have shown that NFV pathways present with variable QRS morphologies depending on their ventricular insertion site and often coexist with other SVTs such as AVNRT. In most cases, the atrial insertion of the manifest NFV pathway is located close to the slow pathway region. Fasciculoventricular pathways (short-circuiting between the Purkinje fibers and ventricular myocardium) can cause discrete preexcitation but have not been described to actively participate in tachycardia.

Outcome

Nakagawa and colleagues reported an overall acute success rate of 98.8% for catheter ablation of APs with a recurrence rate of 5.4% after 1 year.[2] The recurrence rate was lowest for left (2.2%) and right (2.8%) free wall APs, intermediate for posteroseptal APs (inferoparaseptal, 10.1%), and highest for anteroseptal APs (superoparaseptal, 14.7%). Current guidelines[1] state a lower overall success rate of 93% with a recurrence rate of 8%, and major complications in 2.8% (death in 0.1%) based on a recent observational meta-analysis[26] and a prospective, multicenter clinical trial published in 1999.[1] In another pooled analysis, Morady reported serious complications in 0.6% of patients, with cardiac tamponade and complete AV block being the most common adverse events.[3] Death occurred in 0.02% of patients undergoing catheter ablation of an AP, while the risk for malignant arrhythmias causing hemodynamic collapse or ventricular fibrillation was 1.1% over 5 years in patients with untreated symptomatic WPW syndrome.[3] Recent studies have demonstrated that catheter ablation with 3D mapping can not only maintain high success rates but also reduces the amount of radiation exposure to physicians and patients during ablation of APs. In this regard, it is especially used in children or pregnant women with incessant drug-refractory tachycardia.[27,28] In patients with previously failed AP ablation, a repeat ablation procedure yields a success rate of 91%.[29] Causes for ablation failure during the initial procedure include inappropriate identification of the atrial or ventricular AP insertion site due to an oblique course, a difficult or unexpected anatomical location of the AP, technical issues of limiting RF energy delivery, or lack of operator experience.[3]

Ablation of Typical Atrial Flutter and Non–Isthmus-Dependent Macroreentrant Atrial Tachycardia

Indications

Cavotricuspid isthmus (CTI)-dependent atrial flutter is the most common type of macroreentrant atrial tachycardia (AT), while the remaining 10% are termed non-CTI-dependent macroreentrant AT or atypical atrial flutter. Macroreentrant AT presenting after corrective cardiac surgery or following catheter ablation of AF will be discussed elsewhere.

Because catheter ablation for typical atrial flutter has been proven superior to antiarrhythmic drug therapy in two randomized trials[1,3] and further studies, the 2015 ACC/AHA/HRS guidelines give catheter ablation a class I indication in patients with CTI-dependent atrial flutter that is either symptomatic or refractory to pharmacological rate control and a class IIb indication in patients with asymptomatic recurrent CTI-dependent atrial flutter.[1] For patients with recurrent non-CTI-dependent atrial flutter despite antiarrhythmic drug therapy, current guidelines list catheter ablation as a class I indication.

Cavotricuspid Isthmus–Dependent Atrial Flutter

CTI-dependent atrial flutter comprises 90% of macroreentrant ATs in patients without prior ablation of AF. The preferential path of activation involves the region posterior to the tricuspid valve and anterior to the crista terminalis and eustachian ridge, while its narrowest portion (mean distance, 2–3 cm), situated between the tricuspid annulus and inferior vena cava, is termed CTI.[3] Conduction traverses the interatrial septum in an inferior-to-superior direction, resulting in a counterclockwise activation (typical atrial flutter) around the tricuspid annulus in a left anterior oblique projection with late activation of the inferolateral right atrial free wall. In 10% of patients with CTI-dependent atrial flutter, the activation wavefront proceeds in a clockwise direction (reverse typical atrial flutter) around the tricuspid annulus.[30] The 3D electroanatomical mapping studies confirmed that activation across the CTI is constant, while conduction varies along other parts of the tachycardia circuit.[3]

Catheter Ablation

If CTI-dependent atrial flutter is present at the time of electrophysiology study, entrainment and activation mapping will confirm that the CTI is an integral part of the macroreentrant circuit. At times, local conduction delay at the site of entrainment pacing may result in a falsely long postpacing interval.[31] Catheter ablation is performed during ongoing tachycardia or if the patient is in sinus rhythm while pacing from the proximal CS to identify block of the CTI. Variable length, muscle thickness, and pouch-like recesses are frequent anatomical features of the CTI.[32] Therefore ablation catheters capable of creating larger lesions than a conventional 4-mm-tip catheter, either a nonirrigated 8-mm tip or an irrigated-tip catheter, are used for CTI ablation. In one randomized trial, the open-irrigated catheter demonstrated superiority over a conventional 8-mm tip or an internally irrigated tip ablation catheter,[3] whereas in another more recent randomized trial, complete CTI block was achieved more rapidly using a large-tip (10 mm) catheter than an externally irrigated catheter, providing similar clinical efficacy.[33]

For RF energy delivery, the ablation catheter is positioned on the CTI at a 6:00- to 6:30-o'clock position where the distal bipole records a large ventricular and a small atrial electrogram. Gradual withdrawal of the catheter during energy delivery will result in a continuous linear lesion set. Alternatively, individual lesions are placed contiguously in a point-by-point fashion until the catheter reaches the eustachian ridge along the anterior margin of the inferior vena cava. In an electrogram-based approach, single or narrowly split atrial electrograms are targeted along the CTI (Fig. 126.7), especially in patients with recurrent typical atrial flutter, despite an initially successful ablation. In a randomized comparison, an electrogram mapping technique was superior to an anatomical approach when deployment of an initial ablation line failed to achieve complete isthmus block.[3] In addition, a long or steerable sheath may provide greater catheter stability, allowing proper energy delivery to regions difficult to reach.[34] Although ablation of the CTI is readily accomplished in most instances, a 3D mapping system may provide the necessary support if conventional methods fail.[3] Furthermore, 3D mapping has been shown to reduce fluoroscopic exposure time by almost 50% compared with a conventional approach but at the expense of increased cost of the procedure.[35] Cryoenergy has demonstrated similar acute and long-term success rates to RF ablation and may offer the advantage of decreased pain perception during energy delivery.[6]

Procedural Endpoints

Termination into sinus rhythm during ablation and subsequent inability to reinduce tachycardia was once considered to be an acceptable procedural endpoint but is flawed by a significant rate of arrhythmia recurrence as high as 40% (see Fig. 126.7).[3] In current clinical practice, the accepted procedural endpoint has become a bidirectional conduction block across the CTI, decreasing the long-term recurrence rate to <10%.[3] Several diagnostic techniques have been published to verify that bidirectional block is present. Differential pacing from the low lateral right atrium, which is of greater distance from the medial aspect of the CTI line, will demonstrate a longer conduction interval to the proximal CS than pacing from the mid-lateral right atrial wall. During ablation, the local atrial signal should decrease in amplitude until double potentials are seen (see Fig. 126.7). Widely split double potentials separated by an isoelectric interval of ≥110 ms with little variation along the ablation line indicate local conduction block.[3] Scanning the CTI line for convergence of double potentials will identify gaps capable of continued slow conduction, requiring additional ablation lesions. Polarity reversal in the second component of the double potential during CS pacing or a transisthmus conduction interval increase of ≥50% compared with baseline are other methods to ensure bidirectional isthmus block.[3] Incremental atrial pacing maneuvers from the CS and low lateral right atrium can be valuable to distinguish complete CTI block from persistent slow conduction because a >20-ms increase in the double potential distance during incremental pacing has been reported to indicate incomplete CTI block.[36]

Lower Loop Reentry

In some patients, the macroreentrant circuit may cross the crista terminalis with activation proceeding around the inferior vena cava, resulting in lower loop reentry, which generally has a shorter cycle length than typical atrial flutter.[3] Lower loop reentry is amenable to CTI ablation because CTI is a critical part of the macroreentrant circuit.

Outcome

In a randomized trial, RF ablation of typical atrial flutter resulted in 80% of patients maintaining sinus rhythm, while only 36% of patients on antiarrhythmic drug therapy were free of arrhythmia recurrence during a mean follow-up period of 22 ± 11 months.[3] In a survey of electrophysiology laboratories published in 2004, Morady reported a 97% long-term success rate, with 4% of patients necessitating a repeat ablation procedure.[3] The rate of complications was 0.4% with AV block, accounting for half of reported complications. Two meta-analyses comprising 176 studies published between 1988 and 2008 on the outcome of catheter ablation of typical atrial flutter reported a single-procedure success rate of 91%, a

multiprocedure success rate of 97.0%, an arrhythmia recurrence rate of ~5% with an 8-mm tip or irrigated RF ablation catheter, and an acute complication rate of up to 2.6%.[26,37] One study demonstrated that 50% of patients undergoing CTI ablation of typical atrial flutter subsequently developed AF.[38] Importantly, studies have shown that early AF after the first typical atrial flutter ablation in patients without a previous history of AF occurred in up to 8%,[38] reaching similar incidences after 5 years in those with and without AF before atrial flutter ablation.[37] According to a recent position paper by the European Heart Rhythm Association (EHRA) on antithrombotic management in patients undergoing catheter ablation, after ablation of isolated CTI-dependent atrial flutter, an oral anticoagulant may be continued in patients with a CHA_2DS_2-VASc score of ≥2 because a very high incidence of subsequent AF has been reported in these patients.[39] At least, these data highlight the need for careful long-term follow-up to detect AF in this patient population.

Ablation of Non–IsthmusI-Dependent Macroreentrant Atrial Tachycardia and Atypical Atrial Flutter

Nonisthmus-dependent atrial macroreentry originates in the right atrium or LA or may involve the interatrial septum or traverse both atria. Atypical atrial flutter is a descriptive term for a non-CTI–dependent atrial macroreentrant tachycardia, fulfilling the classic ECG definition of a continuous undulating pattern without satisfying the 12-lead surface ECG criteria of typical clockwise or counterclockwise CTI-dependent atrial flutter.[30] Of note, flutter wave morphology of atypical atrial flutter is highly variable and infrequently gives a clue to precise anatomical location. If severe atrial fibrosis is present, sawtooth flutter waves may even be absent, and P waves can be separated by an isoelectric line. The reentrant circuit commonly evolves around anatomical boundaries, such as atrial fibrosis, mitral isthmus, or surgical scar following repair of congenital or valvular heart disease.[3] These circuits, as well as non-CTI–dependent atrial macroreentrant tachycardia or atypical atrial flutter following catheter ablation of AF, will be covered elsewhere.

In patients without prior cardiac surgery, the macroreentrant circuit is constrained between islands of acquired scar tissue and a fixed anatomical structure.[40] These patients often demonstrate underlying structural heart disease, and during electrophysiology study, multiple reentrant circuits may be inducible.[40,41] Within the right atrium, spontaneous scarring most commonly occurs along the right atrial free wall.[40] LA scarring is predominantly found along the anterior and posterior atrial wall, particularly in elderly patients with enlarged LA.[41,42]

Mapping Techniques

Activation, voltage, and entrainment mapping are common techniques used to further delineate the macroreentrant circuit (Fig. 126.8). Entrainment mapping from the CTI, CS, and lateral right atrial wall readily distinguishes between a right or left site of origin, precluding the need for unnecessary transseptal puncture.[3] Entrainment mapping from a critical isthmus within the reentrant circuit will demonstrate concealed entrainment without evident fusion of intracardiac activation, and on the surface it will demonstrate P-wave morphology during the pacing cycle, a postpacing interval within 30 ms of the tachycardia cycle length, and a stimulus time-to-activation time interval <30 ms. Local recordings from a critical isthmus site frequently demonstrate slowing of conduction and a low-amplitude, fractionated, broad bipolar signal in the majority of patients. Pacing with multielectrode catheters from downstream activation sites during tachycardia with a paced cycle length of 10–30 ms below

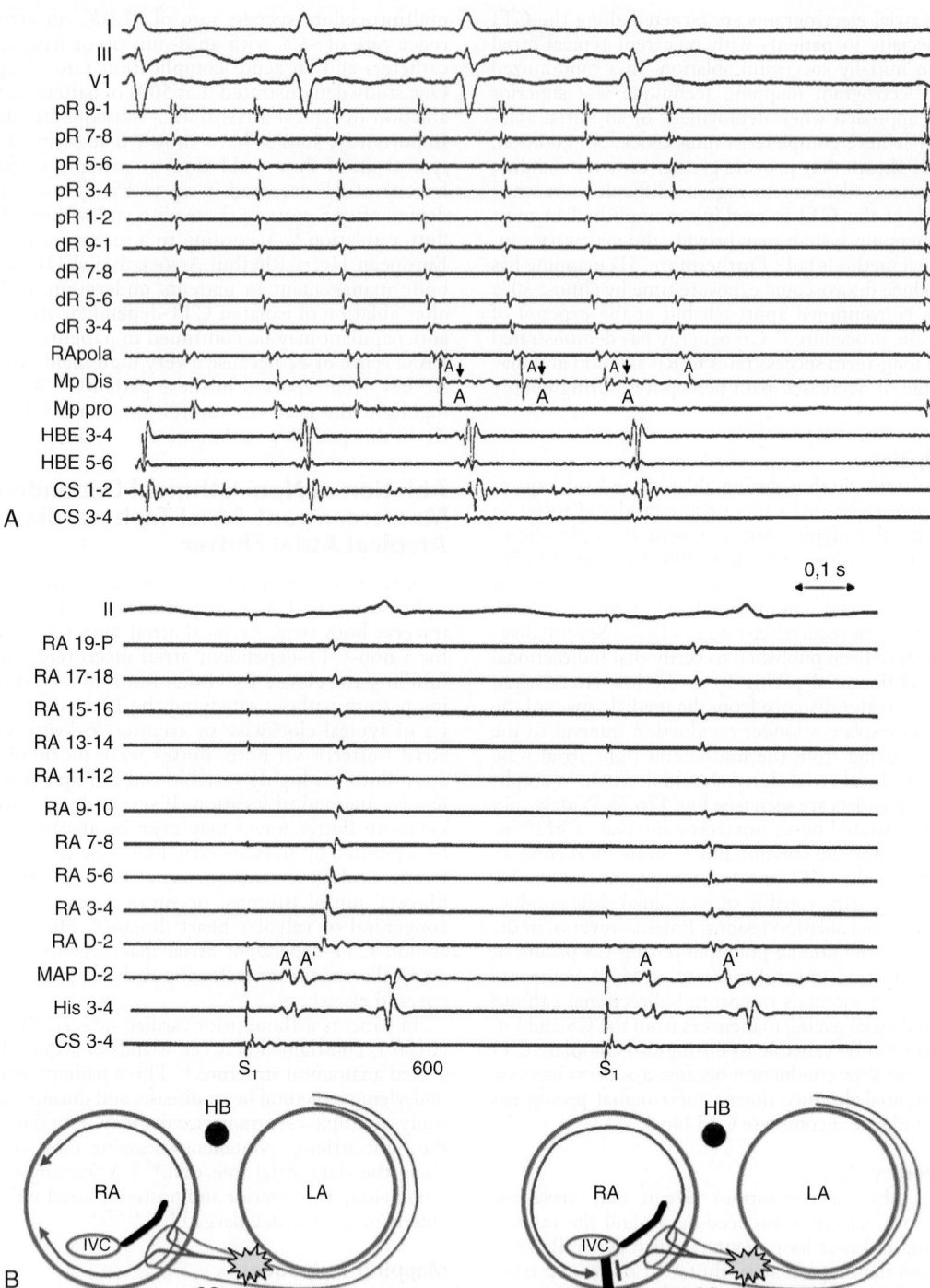

FIGURE 126.7 Termination of typical (counterclockwise) isthmus-dependent right atrial flutter during radiofrequency energy delivery. (A) The top three tracings are surface ECG leads I, III, and V₁ that demonstrate negative flutter waves in the inferior lead III and positive flutter waves in precordial lead V₁. Intracardiac tracings from a multipolar catheter are positioned around the tricuspid valve annulus (proximal pR 9-1 to distal dR 3-4 and RA pola). The activation spreads in a counterclockwise pattern around the tricuspid annulus. The mapping catheter (*Mp Dis* and *Mp pro*) records a local double potential (*arrow*) before the termination of tachycardia. (B) Radiofrequency ablation of the cavotricuspid isthmus with the development of an isthmus block during coronary sinus pacing. *Top,* During pacing from the coronary sinus (*CS* 3-4), a narrowly split atrial signal (AA') is recorded on the distal electrode (*MAP D-2*) of the ablation catheter. Following the second paced beat, a widely split double potential is recorded on the distal electrode, indicating a local conduction block. Note that at the time of a local conduction block, the activation sequence recorded on the multipolar mapping catheter (*RA 19-P* to *RA D-2*) changes, indicating a cavotricuspid isthmus block. *His 3-4,* recording from the His bundle catheter; *S₁,* pacing stimulus. *Bottom,* A schematic of the ensuing cavotricuspid isthmus block. *Left,* Pacing from the coronary sinus (*yellow*) results in two wavefronts (*red double arrow*) traveling simultaneously from the inferior and superior directions with the late activation of the mid-lateral right atrial wall (*RA 13-14* in the *top tracing*). *Right,* Once a cavotricuspid isthmus block is achieved, direct activation of the lateral right atrial wall from an inferior direction is interrupted (*black vertical line*), resulting in a superior-to-inferior activation (*red arrow*) and late activation of the infero-lateral right atrial wall (*RA D-2* in the *top tracing*). *HB,* His bundle. *LA,* left atrium; *RA,* right atrium.

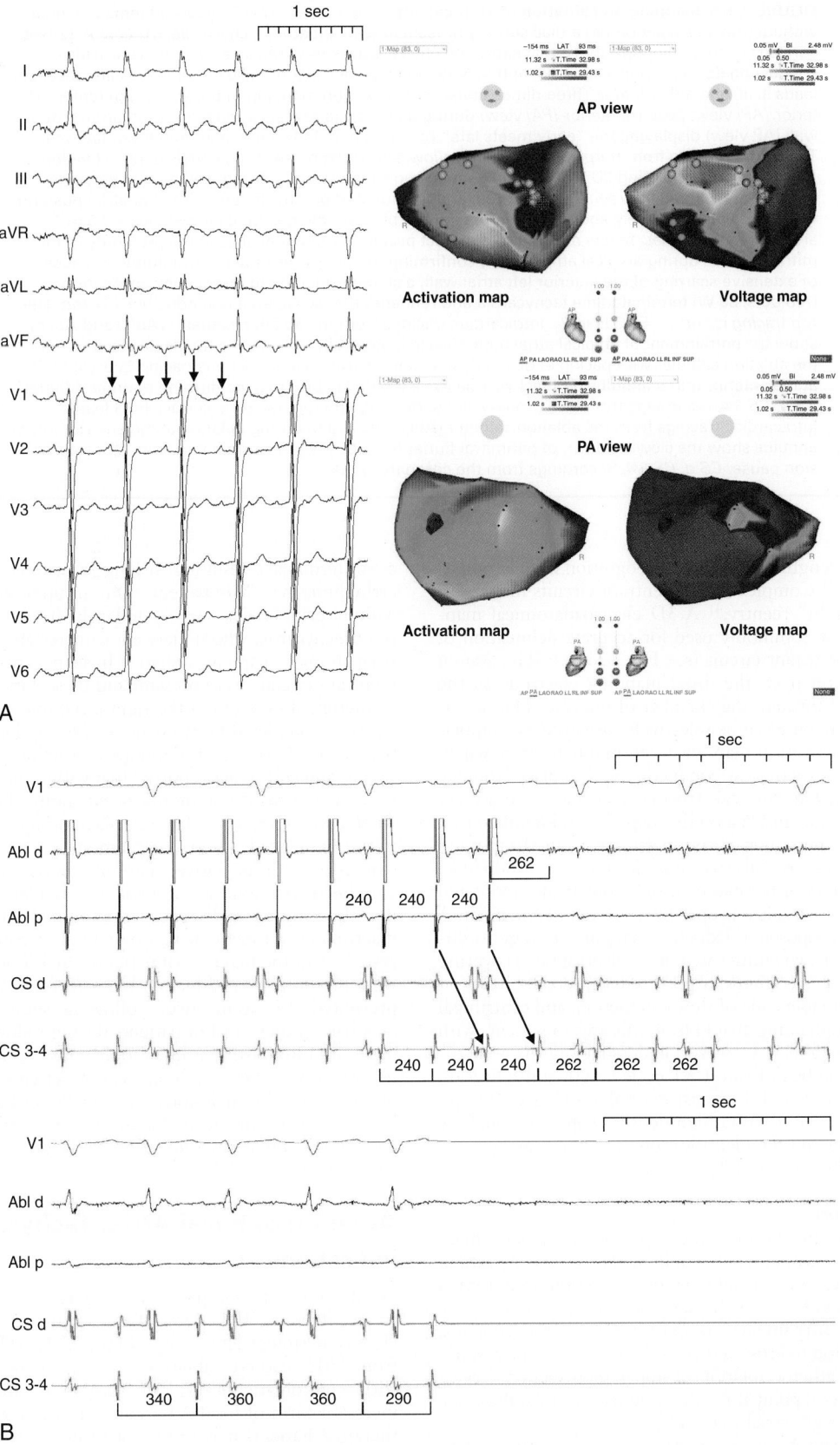

FIGURE 126.8 For legend, see next page.

FIGURE 126.8 Mapping and ablation of atypical left atrial flutter. This 82-year-old female patient without previous ablation or cardiac surgery presented with left atrial tachycardia. (A) *Left*, A 12-lead surface electrocardiogram (ECG) that shows positive P waves in V_1 (*arrows*) with 2:1 ventricular conduction during atypical left atrial flutter. Note that typical sawtooth-like flutter waves are absent in leads II, III, and aVF. *Middle*, Three-dimensional (3D) activation mapping of the left atrium (anteroposterior *[AP]* view; posteroanterior *[PA]* view) during tachycardia reveals a zone in the left atrial anterior wall (AP view) displaying the "early meets late" phenomenon, indicating macroreentrant tachycardia. The colors ranging from *purple, blue, green, yellow*, and *red* represent late versus early activation. *Right*, The corresponding 3D bipolar voltage map shows low-amplitude signals (bipolar voltages <0.5 mV are colored in *green, blue*, and *red*) and fractionated potentials (*pink*). The left atrial posterior wall is activated passively and shows almost normal bipolar voltages (bipolar voltages > 0.5 mV are colored in *purple*). *Yellow dots* indicate perfect pacing entrainment sites in the proximity of the mitral annulus during atypical atrial flutter, confirming the diagnosis of perimitral flutter. Because of extensive scarring of the anterior left atrial wall, a single irrigated radiofrequency application (*red dots*, 30 W) terminated the tachycardia and rendered the tachycardia noninducible. (B) *Top*, The *top tracing* is surface ECG lead V_1. Intracardiac tracings from the ablation catheter (*Abl d* and *Abl p*) show the entrainment of atypical atrial flutter (cycle length [CL], 262 ms) via the distal electrode of the ablation catheter with pacing at CL of 240 ms, demonstrating a perfect postpacing interval (PPI) at the anterior mitral annulus (PPI-tachycardia cycle length [TCL], 0 ms), confirming perimitral flutter. *CS d, CS 3/4*, recordings from the coronary sinus. *Bottom*, The *top tracing* is surface ECG lead V_1. Intracardiac tracings from the ablation catheter (Abl d and Abl p) during ablation at the anterior mitral annulus show the slowing down of perimitral flutter (CL, 360 ms) and termination with a postconversion pause. *CS d, CS 3/4*, Recordings from the coronary sinus.

tachycardia cycle length can facilitate recognition of macroreentrant tachycardia.[43] Complex macroreentrant circuits may result in a "figure-of-eight" reentry.[41] A 3D electroanatomical mapping system is now commonly used for accurate delineation of the atrial macroreentrant circuit (see Fig. 126.8).[42] The system collects information from the distal mapping electrode as the catheter is steered through the chamber of interest. The reconstructed virtual anatomy can be selectively displayed as a bipolar voltage map, an activation map, or an entrainment map, which helps to identify zones of slow conduction and to place strategic linear lesions. Fixed anatomical structures, such as valve orifices or venous ostia, can be marked on the map. Scar is identified by a low-voltage area where high-output pacing (e.g., at ≥10 mA and a pulse duration of 2 ms) fails to capture local tissue.[44] Individual ablation points can be either manually or automatically annotated on a virtual map to visualize proper linear lesion deployment. A recent study has proposed a deductive mapping strategy to differentiate the latter two entities with local electrograms covering ≥75% of the AT cycle length, a postpacing interval <30 ms at that site, an identifiable zone of slow conduction, and centrifugal activation of the remaining atrium from this area in patients with stable AT cycle lenghts.[45] However, understanding the arrhythmia mechanism can be difficult if AT cycle length and activation sequence are variable and if extensive atrial scarring is present. With the recent advent of ultra high-density mapping, hopefully our understanding and the identification of complex arrhythmia mechanisms can be improved.[46]

Catheter Ablation

Catheter ablation aims at transecting a critical portion of the macroreentrant circuit, resulting in noninducibility of tachycardia. Typically, two inert anatomical structures are connected using a linear lesion set that traverses through the critical isthmus.

Upper loop reentry involves a gap within the crista terminalis, allowing conduction to cross and encircle the orifice of the superior vena cava. Catheter ablation of upper loop reentry targets the lower turnaround point along the conduction gap of the crista terminalis on the right atrial free wall.[3]

In a study by Stevenson and colleagues on eight patients with right atrial macroreentrant tachycardia, spontaneous regions of scar were predominantly located along the posterolateral right atrial free wall, forming the central obstacle around which macroreentry would circulate.[3] RF ablation targeted the critical isthmus between scar tissue and the superior or inferior vena cava or the

crista terminalis, resulting in long-term freedom from recurrent arrhythmia in 75% of patients. Our group reported on 17 patients without prior cardiac surgery and right atrial free wall macroreentrant tachycardia who underwent catheter ablation using an electroanatomical mapping system.[40] In six patients, multiple unstable reentrant circuits were present, and these patients underwent circumferential isolation of the right atrial free wall, which was successfully completed in five patients. During long-term follow-up, two of six (33%) patients developed arrhythmia recurrence.

Jaïs and colleagues reported that within the LA, areas of fibrosis and scar most commonly occur along the posterior wall.[41] Regions of scar act as barriers, facilitating reentry around the mitral annulus, LA roof, or pulmonary vein ostia. Connecting scar tissue with the native anatomical barriers, such as the mitral annulus or pulmonary vein ostia, can render tachycardia noninducible. Ouyang and associates examined 28 patients with LA macroreentrant tachycardia using an electroanatomical mapping system.[42] In the majority of patients, dual-loop reentrant circuits were present, and conduction block through the critical isthmus prevented AT recurrence. Following successful ablation, AF occurred in one-third of patients during follow-up. The deployment of a mitral isthmus line should consider the location of atrial fibrosis, LA diameter, and operator experience. We strongly recommend that linear lesions crossing the critical isthmus should be performed individually based on the presumed reentrant circuit, slow conduction zone, global voltage on 3D mapping, and LAA activation.

Ablation of Focal Atrial Tachycardia

Indications

Focal AT due to automaticity, triggered activity, or microreentry accounts for 10%–15% of cases referred for ablation to the electrophysiology laboratory.[3] In the ACC/AHA/HRS guidelines from 2015, catheter ablation is a class I indication in patients with symptomatic focal AT or in asymptomatic patients with the incessant form of focal AT as an alternative to pharmacological therapy.[1] Patients may present with nonsustained or paroxysmal AT or with incessant AT, with 10% of patients developing tachycardia-mediated cardiomyopathy.[3] Most patients have no underlying structural heart disease even in the presence of more than one inducible focal AT, although localized abnormalities including fibrosis, at the tachycardia origin may be present.

Correlating Site of Origin With Surface P-Wave Morphology

The majority of focal ATs (75%) originate from the right atrium, most frequently along the crista terminalis. ATs from this site have also been referred to as sinus node reentry.[3] Other common right atrial sites are the tricuspid annulus or the vicinity of the CS ostium. In the LA, the pulmonary vein ostia and mitral annulus constitute common focal sites of origin (Fig. 126.9).[47] Focal ATs may also emanate from the noncoronary aortic cusp, peri-AVN region, right atrial appendage/LAA, superior vena cava, or vein of Marshall.[48]

During AT, centrifugal spread from a point source within the atrial myocardium will result in a characteristic P-wave configuration on 12-lead surface ECG.[30,49] A right atrial focus is suggested by a negative monophasic or initially positive than negative biphasic P wave in V_1.[3] A monophasic positive P wave in lead V_1 or a monophasic negative P wave in lead aVL implies an LA origin. Focal ATs originating from the atrial septum display a narrower P wave compared with sinus rhythm, while an inferior site of origin will result in negative P waves, and a superior site in positive P waves in leads II, III, and aVF. An algorithm developed by Kistler and colleagues predicted the correct location of focal AT in the majority of patients.[49]

Mapping Techniques

During ongoing tachycardia or frequent atrial extrasystoles with identical P-wave morphology as the clinical AT, activation mapping can be performed to accurately locate the site of origin.[3] Atrial pacing and intravenous isoprenaline infusion will aid in induction of tachycardia, which may be suppressed by sedatives. A multielectrode mapping catheter positioned around the tricuspid annulus, a His bundle catheter, and a CS catheter facilitate sequential point-by-point activation mapping within the atria during AT. Overdrive pacing at a rate slightly faster than the tachycardia cycle length can be used to accurately localize the focal site of origin. A difference in the postpacing interval to tachycardia cycle length of <20 ms is indicative of the site of origin and predicted successful ablation.[3] If AT is noninducible or spontaneous atrial extrasystoles are infrequent, pace mapping with comparison of the paced P-wave and clinical P-wave morphology, as well as intraatrial activation, can be attempted.[50] Pacing from the distal bipole of the ablation catheter at different locations within the atrium will generate a characteristic P-wave configuration and intraatrial activation sequence for each site. A perfect match to the P-wave morphology and intraatrial activation sequence of the documented clinical AT or atrial extrasystole will indicate the focal site of origin where ablation will likely be successful. At the focal site of origin, the local atrial electrogram is often prolonged and fractionated, preceding the onset of the surface P wave by ≥30 ms.[3] If the P-wave onset is obscured by the preceding T wave, an alternate reference, such as the CS atrial electrogram with a known constant relationship to the P-wave onset, should be selected. In addition, introducing paced premature ventricular extrastimuli can facilitate proper P wave analysis.

A QS complex recorded on the unipolar electrogram indicates spread of activation away from the focal source, while remote sites will demonstrate an RS complex. During catheter mapping, "bumping" the focal site of origin may rarely cause inadvertent mechanical termination of AT. Ablation should be attempted if the local atrial electrogram at the site of inadvertent termination precedes the surface P wave by ≥30 ms or pace mapping at this site demonstrates a perfect match.

An electroanatomical mapping system can aid in localizing the site of origin (see Fig. 126.9).[3] During activation mapping, each point is tagged and color coded on a virtual 3D atrial map. Precise localization of the earliest activation site within the reconstructed anatomy facilitates successful catheter ablation. However, frequent atrial ectopics or inducible AT is a prerequisite for detailed point-by-point electroanatomical mapping with conventional 3D mapping systems. In patients with only difficult-to-induce and nonsustained focal AT, pace mapping of P wave and atrial activation sequence can guide successful ablation (Fig. 126.10). Ultra high-density contact mapping using a multipolar basket catheter will hopefully facilitate ablation in this scenario.

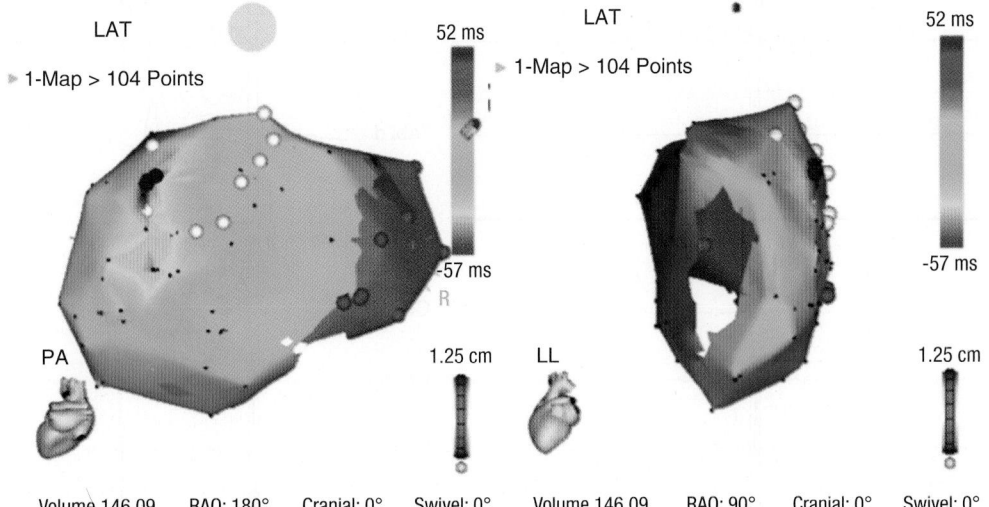

FIGURE 126.9 A three-dimensional electroanatomical activation map of a focal left atrial tachycardia (*LAT*) with a cycle length of 260 ms. Note that the activation map covers <50% of the tachycardia cycle length (109 ms vs. 260 ms), indicating focal spread from a point source. The colors ranging from *purple, blue, green, yellow,* and *red* represent late versus early activation. Left map in posterior-anterior *(PA)* projection and right map in left lateral *(LL)* projection. The *gray area* represents regions of scarring. *Gray dots* indicate sites where pacing with maximal output from the distal mapping electrode failed to capture local tissue. *White dots* are location points that encircle the ipsilateral left pulmonary veins. The focal (earliest) site of activation is located at the ostium (anterior ridge) of the left inferior pulmonary vein. Ablation at this site *(red dots)* eliminated focal atrial tachycardia.

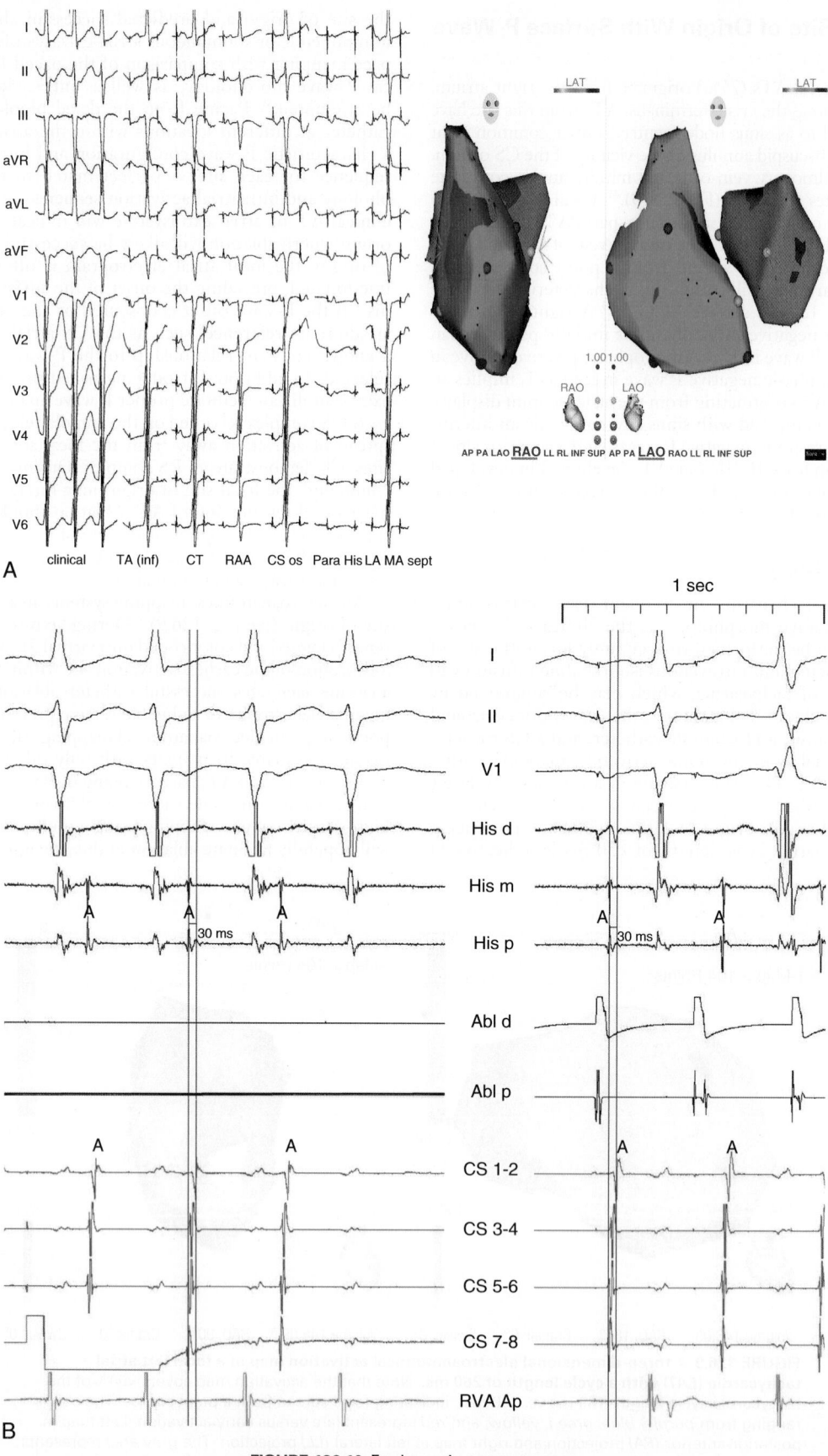

FIGURE 126.10 For legend, see next page.

FIGURE 126.10 Ablation of noninducible focal atrial tachycardia. (A) *Left,* A 12-lead surface electrocardiogram (ECG) that shows the clinical nonsustained and difficult-to-induce focal atrial tachycardia (clinical) and pace mapping from different atrial sites. *CS os,* coronary sinus ostium; *CT,* crista terminalis; *LA MA septal,* septal mitral annulus; *Para His,* para-Hisian region; *RAA,* right atrial appendage; *TA inf,* inferior tricuspid annulus. Note that pacing from the distal bipole of the ablation catheter at different locations within the atria will generate a characteristic P-wave configuration that is compared with the clinical P-wave morphology during atrial tachycardia. Pacing should be performed at the cycle length of the clinical tachycardia with the lowest output that captures the atrium. *Right,* Pace mapping is performed with the annotation of pacing sites on a three-dimensional mapping system (*green:* right atrium; *purple:* left atrium). Pacing is shown from the inferior tricuspid annulus (TA, *blue dot*), crista terminalis (CT, *light blue dot*), right atrial appendage (RAA, *brown dot*), right atrial free wall (*gray dot*), coronary sinus ostium (CS os, *light brown dot*), para-Hisian region (Para His, *yellow dot*), and septal mitral annulus (LA MA septal, *pink dot*). The best P-wave pace map was obtained during pacing from the inferior tricuspid annulus (*blue dot*). Radiofrequency (RF) ablation at this site eliminated the tachycardia. *LAO,* left anterior oblique; *RAO,* right anterior oblique. (B) *Left,* The *top tracings* show surface ECG leads I, II, and V₁ during nonsustained clinical atrial tachycardia. The *bottom intracardiac tracings* were recorded from the His bundle region (His d, His m, and His p), coronary sinus (CS 1-2, 3-4, 5-6, 7-8), and right ventricular apex (RVAp). A match of the intraatrial activation sequence during clinical tachycardia and atrial pace mapping (atrial signal *[A]* on the proximal His [His p; positive peak] to the A in the distal coronary sinus [CS 1-2; positive peak] during tachycardia and pacing from the inferior tricuspid annulus both measure 30 ms) with the distal electrode of the ablation catheter (Abl d) reveals the origin of the clinical tachycardia. In comparison, during pacing from RAA, this measurement yielded 65 ms; from the CS ostium, −5 ms; and from the crista terminalis, 15 ms. Ablation at the inferior tricuspid annulus eliminated the clinical tachycardia. *Abl d and Abl p,* Recordings from the distal and proximal ablation catheter; *CS 1-2, 3-4, 5-6, 7-8,* recordings from the coronary sinus; *His d, His m, His p,* recordings from the His bundle region; *LAT,* left atrial tachycardia; *RVAp,* recording from the right ventricular apex.

Catheter Ablation

Most commonly, RF energy is used for catheter ablation of focal AT. In regions of low blood flow, e.g., CS or atrial appendage, or in the noncoronary aortic cusps, an irrigated-tip catheter will allow sufficient energy delivery to achieve successful lesion formation. ATs from the atrial appendages can be particularly challenging to ablate. In these cases, successful ablation with a cryoballoon, epicardial RF ablation, or surgical techniques have been reported in some studies.[51–53] However, these need further investigation in larger patient cohorts. Successful RF ablation is suggested by acceleration of the tachycardia prior to termination and/or termination within 10 seconds of energy delivery. Following ablation, acute procedural success is defined as noninducibility of AT after repeating the arrhythmia induction protocol with or without isoprenaline and completing a 30-minute waiting period.

Outcome

Reported acute success rates from nonrandomized studies range from 69% to 100% and are dependent on tachycardia inducibility during the procedure, mapping technique, anatomical location, and operator's experience.[1] The recurrence rate varied between 0% and 33%, and 3D mapping systems have improved success rates. In a multivariable analysis, a right atrial focus was the only independent predictor of successful ablation, while underlying heart disease, older age, and multiple tachycardia foci predicted AT recurrence.[3] Yet, a recent study with 10 patients has reported that catheter ablation for focal AT with ≤3 foci is feasible and yields excellent long-term outcome.[54] In patients with focal AT, originating from within the pulmonary veins and no prior history of AF, catheter ablation with pulmonary vein isolation or focal ablation resulted in freedom from new-onset AF in all patients over a mean follow-up of 7.2 years.[55] The overall major complication rate of focal AT ablation is <2%. Yet, because spontaneous resolution of focal AT is common in young children, delayed ablation in this particular patient population is warranted.[56]

Conclusions

In patients suffering from regular SVT, catheter ablation demonstrates excellent acute and long-term success rates with a low rate of complications. An ablative strategy should be considered in all patients with symptomatic SVT and as first-line therapy in those patients who desire a definitive cure.

REFERENCES

1. Page RL, Joglar JA, Caldwell MA, et al. 2015 ACC/AHA/HRS guideline for the management of adult patients with supraventricular tachycardia: a report of the American College of Cardiology/American Heart Association Task Force on Clinical Practice Guidelines and the Heart Rhythm Society. *J Am Coll Cardiol.* 2016;67:e27–e115.
2. Nakagawa H, Jackman WM. Catheter ablation of paroxysmal supraventricular tachycardia. *Circulation.* 2007;116:2465–2478.
3. Wissner E, Ouyang F, Metzner A, et al. Ablation of supraventricular tachyarrhythmias. In: Zipes DP, Jalife J, eds. *Cardiac Electrophysiology from Cell to Bedside.* 6th ed. Philadelphia: WB Saunders; 2014:1239–1248.
4. Jackman WM, Beckman KJ, McClelland JH, et al. Treatment of supraventricular tachycardia due to atrioventricular nodal reentry, by radiofrequency catheter ablation of slow-pathway conduction. *N Engl J Med.* 1992;327:313–318.
5. Haïssaguerre M, Gaita F, Fischer B, et al. Elimination of atrioventricular nodal reentrant tachycardia using discrete slow potentials to guide application of radiofrequency energy. *Circulation.* 1992;85:2162–2175.
6. Timmermans C, Ayers GM, Crijns HJ, et al. Randomized study comparing radiofrequency ablation with cryoablation for the treatment of atrial flutter with emphasis on pain perception. *Circulation.* 2003;90:1250–1252.
7. Deisenhofer I, Zrenner B, Yin YH, et al. Cryoablation versus radiofrequency energy for the ablation of atrioventricular nodal reentrant tachycardia (the Cyrano study): results from a large multicenter prospective randomized trial. *Circulation.* 2010;122:2239–2245.
8. Jentzer JH, Goyal R, Williamson BD, et al. Analysis of junctional ectopy during radiofrequency ablation of the slow pathway in patients with atrioventricular nodal reentrant tachycardia. *Circulation.* 1994;90:2820–2826.
9. Li YG, Gronefeld G, Bender B, et al. Risk of development of delayed atrioventricular block after slow pathway modification in patients with atrioventricular nodal reentrant tachycardia and a pre-existing prolonged PR interval. *Eur Heart J.* 2001;22:89–95.
10. Pott C, Wegner FK, Bogeholz N, et al. Outcome predictors of empirical slow pathway modulation: clinical and procedural characteristics and long-term follow-up. *Clin Res Cardiol.* 2015;104:946–954.
11. Kaneko Y, Naito S, Okishige K, et al. Atypical fast-slow atrioventricular nodal reentrant tachycardia incorporating a "superior" slow pathway: a distinct supraventricular tachyarrhythmia. *Circulation.* 2015;133:114–123.
12. Hanninen M, Yeung-Lai-Wah N, Massel D, et al. Cryoablation versus RF ablation for AVNRT: a meta-analysis and systematic review. *J Cardiovasc Electrophysiol.* 2013;24:1354–1360.
13. Alvarez M, Tercedor L, Almansa I, et al. Safety and feasibility of catheter ablation for atrioventricular nodal re-entrant tachycardia without fluoroscopic guidance. *Heart Rhythm.* 2009;6:1714–1720.
14. Jackman WM, Wang XZ, Friday KJ, et al. Catheter ablation of accessory atrioventricular pathways (Wolff-Parkinson-White syndrome) by radiofrequency current. *N Engl J Med.* 1991;324:1605–1611.

15. Kuck KH, Schluter M, Geiger M, et al. Radiofrequency current catheter ablation of accessory atrioventricular pathways. *Lancet.* 1991;337:1557–1561.
16. Munger TM, Packer DL, Hammill SC, et al. A population study of the natural history of Wolff-Parkinson-White syndrome in Olmsted County, Minnesota, 1953-1989. *Circulation.* 1993;87:866–873.
17. Pappone C, Vicedomini G, Manguso F, et al. Wolff-Parkinson-White syndrome in the era of catheter ablation: insights from a registry study of 2169 patients. *Circulation.* 2014;130:811–819.
18. Arruda MS, McClelland JH, Wang X, et al. Development and validation of an ECG algorithm for identifying accessory pathway ablation site in Wolff-Parkinson-White syndrome. *J Cardiovasc Electrophysiol.* 1998;9:2–12.
19. Wei W, Zhan X, Xue Y, et al. Features of accessory pathways in adult Ebstein's anomaly. *Europace.* 2014;16:1619–1625.
20. Otomo K, Gonzalez MD, Beckman KJ, et al. Reversing the direction of paced ventricular and atrial wavefronts reveals an oblique course in accessory AV pathways and improves localization for catheter ablation. *Circulation.* 2001;104:550–556.
21. Guo XG, Liu XU, Zhou GB, et al. Frequency of fractionated ventricular activation and atrial/ventricular electrogram amplitude ratio at successful ablation target of accessory pathways in patients with Ebstein's anomaly. *J Cardiovasc Electrophysiol.* 2015;26:404–411.
22. Cosio FG, Anderson RH, Kuck KH, et al. Living anatomy of the atrioventricular junctions. A guide to electrophysiologic mapping. A consensus statement from the Cardiac Nomenclature Study Group, Working Group of Arrhythmias, European Society of Cardiology, and the Task Force on Cardiac Nomenclature from NASPE. *Circulation.* 1999;100:e31–e37.
23. Insulander P, Bastani H, Braunschweig F, et al. Cryoablation of substrates adjacent to the atrioventricular node: acute and long-term safety of 1303 ablation procedures. *Europace.* 2014;16:271–276.
24. Mah D, Miyake C, Clegg R, et al. Epicardial left atrial appendage and biatrial appendage accessory pathways. *Heart Rhythm.* 2010;7:1740–1745.
25. Guo XG, Sun QI, Ma J, et al. Electrophysiological characteristics and radiofrequency catheter ablation of accessory pathway connecting the right atrial appendage and the right ventricle. *J Cardiovasc Electrophysiol.* 2015;26:845–852.
26. Spector P, Reynolds MR, Calkins H, et al. Meta-analysis of ablation of atrial flutter and supraventricular tachycardia. *Am J Cardiol.* 2009;104:671–677.
27. Earley MJ, Showkathali R, Alzetani M, et al. Radiofrequency ablation of arrhythmias guided by non-fluoroscopic catheter location: a prospective randomized trial. *Eur Heart J.* 2006;27:1223–1229.
28. Casella M, Dello Russo A, Pelargonio G, et al. Near zerO fluoroscopic exPosure during catheter ablAtion of supRavenTricular arrhYthmias: the NO-PARTY multicentre randomized trial. *Europace.* 2015;pii: euv344. [Epub ahead of print].

29. Sacher F, Wright M, Tedrow UB, et al. Wolff-Parkinson-White ablation after a prior failure: a 7-year multicentre experience. *Europace.* 2010;12:835–841.
30. Saoudi N, Cosio F, Waldo A, et al. A classification of atrial flutter and regular atrial tachycardia according to electrophysiological mechanisms and anatomical bases; a statement from a joint expert group from the Working Group of Arrhythmias of the European Society of Cardiology and the North American Society of Pacing and Electrophysiology. *Eur Heart J.* 2001;22:1162–1182.
31. Vollmann D, Stevenson WG, Luthje L, et al. Misleading long post-pacing interval after entrainment of typical atrial flutter from the cavotricuspid isthmus. *J Am Coll Cardiol.* 2012;59:819–824.
32. Cabrera JA, Sanchez-Quintana D, Ho SY, et al. The architecture of the atrial musculature between the orifice of the inferior caval vein and the tricuspid valve: the anatomy of the isthmus. *J Cardiovasc Electrophysiol.* 1998;9:1186–1195.
33. Ilg KJ, Kuhne M, Crawford T, et al. Randomized comparison of cavotricuspid isthmus ablation for atrial flutter using an open irrigation-tip versus a large-tip radiofrequency ablation catheter. *J Cardiovasc Electrophysiol.* 2011;22:1007–1012.
34. Matsuo S, Yamane T, Tokuda M, et al. Prospective randomized comparison of a steerable versus a non-steerable sheath for typical atrial flutter ablation. *Europace.* 2010;12:402–409.
35. Hindricks G, Willems S, Kautzner J, et al. Effect of electroanatomically guided versus conventional catheter ablation of typical atrial flutter on the fluoroscopy time and resource use: a prospective randomized multicenter study. *J Cardiovasc Electrophysiol.* 2009;20:734–740.
36. Bazan V, Marti-Almor J, Perez-Rodon J, et al. Incremental pacing for the diagnosis of complete cavotricuspid isthmus block during radiofrequency ablation of atrial flutter. *J Cardiovasc Electrophysiol.* 2010;21:33–39.
37. Perez FJ, Schubert CM, Parvez B, et al. Long-term outcomes after catheter ablation of cavo-tricuspid isthmus dependent atrial flutter: a meta-analysis. *Circ Arrhythm Electrophysiol.* 2009;2:393–401.
38. Chinitz JS, Gerstenfeld EP, Marchlinski FE, et al. Atrial fibrillation is common after ablation of isolated atrial flutter during long-term follow-up. *Heart Rhythm.* 2007;4:1029–1033.
39. Sticherling C, Marin F, Birnie D, et al. Antithrombotic management in patients undergoing electrophysiological procedures: a European Heart Rhythm Association (EHRA) position document endorsed by the ESC Working Group Thrombosis, Heart Rhythm Society (HRS), and Asia Pacific Heart Rhythm Society (APHRS). *Europace.* 2015;17:1197–1214.
40. Satomi K, Chun KR, Tilz R, et al. Catheter ablation of multiple unstable macroreentrant tachycardia within the right atrium free wall in patients without previous cardiac surgery. *Circ Arrhythm Electrophysiol.* 2010;3:24–31.
41. Jaïs P, Shah DC, Haïssaguerre M, et al. Mapping and ablation of left atrial flutters. *Circulation.* 2000;101:2928–2934.
42. Ouyang F, Ernst S, Vogtmann T, et al. Characterization of reentrant circuits in left atrial macroreentrant

tachycardia: critical isthmus block can prevent atrial tachycardia recurrence. *Circulation.* 2002;105:1934–1942.
43. Barbhaiya CR, Kumar S, Ng J, et al. Overdrive pacing from downstream sites on multielectrode catheters to rapidly detect fusion and to diagnose macroreentrant atrial arrhythmias. *Circulation.* 2014;129:2503–2510.
44. Steven D, Sultan A, Reddy V, et al. Benefit of pulmonary vein isolation guided by loss of pace capture on the ablation line: results from a prospective 2-center randomized trial. *J Am Coll Cardiol.* 2013;62:44–50.
45. Jaïs P, Matsuo S, Knecht S, et al. A deductive mapping strategy for atrial tachycardia following atrial fibrillation ablation: importance of localized reentry. *J Cardiovasc Electrophysiol.* 2009;20:480–491.
46. Bollmann A, Hilbert S, John S, et al. Initial experience with ultra high-density mapping of human right atria. *J Cardiovasc Electrophysiol.* 2016;27:154–160.
47. Yamada T, Murakami Y, Yoshida Y, et al. Electrophysiologic and electrocardiographic characteristics and radiofrequency catheter ablation of focal atrial tachycardia originating from the left atrial appendage. *Heart Rhythm.* 2007;4:1284–1291.
48. Ouyang F, Ma J, Ho SY, et al. Focal atrial tachycardia originating from the non-coronary aortic sinus: electrophysiological characteristics and catheter ablation. *J Am Coll Cardiol.* 2006;48:122–131.
49. Kistler PM, Roberts-Thomson KC, Haqqani HM, et al. P-wave morphology in focal atrial tachycardia: development of an algorithm to predict the anatomic site of origin. *J Am Coll Cardiol.* 2006;48:1010–1017.
50. Hayashi K, Heeger CH, Mathew S, et al. Efficacy of P wave pace-mapping to identify the site of ectopic atrial tachycardia origin. *Clin Res Cardiol.* 2015;104.
51. Chun KJ, Ouyang F, Schmidt B, et al. Focal atrial tachycardia originating from the right atrial appendage: first successful cryoballoon isolation. *J Cardiovasc Electrophysiol.* 2009;20:338–341.
52. Guo XG, Zhang JL, Ma J, et al. Management of focal atrial tachycardias originating from the atrial appendage with the combination of radiofrequency catheter ablation and minimally invasive atrial appendectomy. *Heart Rhythm.* 2014;11:17–25.
53. Hanumandla A, Kaur D, Shah M, et al. Epicardial ablation of focal atrial tachycardia arising from left atrial appendage in children. *Indian Pacing Electrophysiol J.* 2014;14:199–202.
54. Hillock RJ, Kalman JM, Roberts-Thomson KC, et al. Multiple focal atrial tachycardias in a healthy adult population: characterization and description of successful radiofrequency ablation. *Heart Rhythm.* 2007;4:435–438.
55. Teh AW, Kalman JM, Medi C, et al. Long-term outcome following successful catheter ablation of atrial tachycardia originating from the pulmonary veins: absence of late atrial fibrillation. *J Cardiovasc Electrophysiol.* 2010;21:747–750.
56. Kang KT, Etheridge SP, Kantoch MJ, et al. Current management of focal atrial tachycardia in children: a multicenter experience. *Circ Arrhythm Electrophysiol.* 2014;7:664–670.

127 Catheter Ablation for Ventricular Tachycardia With or Without Structural Heart Disease

William G. Stevenson and Usha B. Tedrow

Catheter ablation has an important role in reducing or preventing ventricular arrhythmias both in patients with heart disease and in those with idiopathic ventricular tachycardia (VT) that is not associated with structural heart disease (SHD). The approach to ablation and efficacy is determined by the characteristics of the arrhythmia as well as the anatomy and location of the arrhythmia substrate, which can often be anticipated from the electrocardiogram (ECG) of VT and the nature of any underlying heart disease (see Chapter 60). Most VTs that are considered for ablation are monomorphic, with the same QRS complex from beat to beat, indicating repetitive ventricular activation from a structural substrate or focus that can be targeted for ablation. Patients with heart disease often have multiple morphologies of inducible VT. VT that has the same QRS morphology and cycle length as one that has been observed to occur spontaneously is designated a "clinical VT."[1] Often the ECG morphology of VT is not completely defined, as the arrhythmia is promptly terminated by an implantable cardioverter defibrillator (ICD). VTs that are similar in cycle length and morphology to available ECG leads or recordings are designated "presumed clinical VTs."[1] Inducible VTs that have not been documented to occur spontaneously are designated "undocumented VTs." Polymorphic VTs have a continually changing activation sequence but may respond to ablation when triggering foci or a substrate can be identified (see Chapter 129).

Preprocedure Preparation and Consideration of Risks

In patients without SHD, mortality from ablation is rare, but perforation and tamponade, coronary injury, and atrioventricular (AV) block can occur (Table 127.1).[2–9] A review of administrative data from 6635 patients found any adverse event in 6%, a major adverse event in 1.4%, and periprocedural mortality of 0.3%.[4] In patients with SHD, major complications occur in approximately 7% of patients and while periprocedural death is <1%, in-hospital death is 3%–5%.[3,4] Adverse outcomes are associated with SHD, increasing age, anemia, atrial fibrillation (AF), renal disease, emergency admission or hospital transfer, or VT storm.[1,3–5]

Preprocedure planning is important to minimize risks. Underlying heart disease should be defined. The potential for myocardial ischemia should be assessed. Although ischemia is not usually the cause of monomorphic VT, it may contribute to hemodynamic instability and increase the risk of the procedure if not addressed. It is important to consider fluid balance, electrolyte abnormalities, anemia, and metabolic abnormalities, such as hyperthyroidism, that might contribute to hemodynamic deterioration or development of uncontrollable arrhythmias during the procedure. The use of external irrigation catheters administers intravascular volume that requires attention to managing fluid balance.

Echocardiography should be performed before left ventricular (LV) endocardial mapping; a mobile LV thrombus is a contraindication to LV mapping. If laminated thrombus is suspected, a period of chronic anticoagulation using warfarin may be considered with the hope of reducing the chance of a friable thrombus being present, although whether this improves safety is not known. During LV or aortic mapping, systemic anticoagulation is achieved with heparin. After LV or aortic ablation, the anticoagulation is continued with aspirin. Warfarin is often recommended if ablation over large areas was performed.[1] The anticoagulation regimen is often determined by other concerns such as stents or AF.

LV access may be achieved through a retrograde aortic approach. Damage to the aortic valve or coronary artery ostia or the mitral valve is possible, but rare. Significant vascular access complications including bleeding, arterial dissection, and femoral AV fistulas occur in 1%–2% of patients.[9] A transseptal approach to the left atrium allows access to the LV through the mitral valve for patients with peripheral vascular disease, a mechanical aortic valve, or when it is desirable to avoid a large arterial sheath when ablation is performed without interrupting oral anticoagulation.

Discontinuation of antiarrhythmic drug therapy is usually desirable to facilitate induction of VT and assessment of the ablation endpoint, but it is not always feasible or necessary in patients with frequent episodes and may precipitate an electrical storm in some patients.

Approach to Mapping and Ablation

If VT is incessant, mapping proceeds during VT. Otherwise, programmed stimulation is used to induce VT to confirm the diagnosis, establish the absence of inducible VT as a potential procedural endpoint, and to obtain ECG and intracardiac recordings that suggest the type of VT and its likely origin to guide the procedure. Recordings from the His bundle and right ventricular (RV) apex are usually obtained. An associated His bundle potential suggests the possibility of bundle branch reentry (see Chapter 83). Pacing is often performed from the RV apex to entrain or terminate VT. Entrainment from the RV apex with a postpacing interval (PPI) of 30 ms or less suggests bundle branch reentry or a VT circuit close to the apex.[10]

TABLE 127.1   Complications of catheter ablation

	12 EXPERT CENTERS VT WITH HEART DISEASE TUNG ET AL. 2015[5]	VT WITH HEART DISEASE ADMINISTRATIVE DATABASE KATZ ET AL. 2015[4]	VT WITH NO HEART DISEASE ADMINISTRATIVE DATABASE KATZ ET AL. 2015[4]	PROCEDURES WITH EPICARDIAL MAPPING IN EXPERT CENTERS[6–8]
Patients	2061	3064	6635	411
Major complications	6%	6.5%	1.4%	7%
Death	0.1%	3%	0.3%	0.5%
Vascular access	1.6%			<1%
Hemopericardium	1.7%			4%
AV block	0.9%			
Stroke/TIA	0.5%			
Coronary injury	0.2%			0.5%
Phrenic nerve injury				<1%

AV, Atrioventricular; *TIA*, transient ischemic attack; *VT*, ventricular tachycardia.

QRS Morphology During Ventricular Tachycardia and Pace-Mapping

The QRS morphology of VT is an indication of the location of the arrhythmia focus or reentry circuit exit.[11] A left bundle branch block (LBBB)-like configuration in lead V_1 (dominant S wave) suggests an origin in the RV or interventricular septum; dominant R waves in V_1 indicate an LV origin. The frontal plane axis points away from the origin. A superiorly directed axis indicates an inferior wall exit. An inferiorly directed axis indicates an anterior wall exit. The closer an exit is to a precordial lead, the more negative the S wave is in that lead, providing an indication of exit location between the base and apex. Apical exits generate dominant S waves in leads V_3 and V_4. Basal exits generate dominant R waves in these leads.

For idiopathic VTs, the QRS morphology is a particularly important guide to the likely origin (see Chapters 81 and 82). An interval from the QRS onset (determined from a simultaneous recording of all 12 leads) to the earliest initial peak in all precordial leads that is >56% of the total QRS duration ("maximal deflection index," or MDI) suggests an epicardial focus.[11] In nonischemic cardiomyopathy, an epicardial origin is suggested by a VT QRS with a relatively long QRS duration; slow QRS upstroke, producing a pseudodelta waves; or a QS complex in lead I for VTs originating from the basal lateral LV.[11] Exceptions occur, and in patients with prior myocardial infarction, the VT QRS morphology does not reliably identify epicardial VTs.[11]

The QRS morphology during pace-mapping usually suggests the direction in which the catheter should be directed to approach the VT focus or reentry circuit exit. Moving farther from a positive electrode (e.g., the left arm for lead I or a precordial lead) increases the R-wave in that lead during pace-mapping. Moving closer to the lead decreases the R-wave and increases the S-wave.

The QRS morphology only suggests a starting point for mapping. Individual differences in cardiac position, areas of scars, conduction block, and abnormal ventricular anatomy can render the QRS morphology misleading, particularly in scar-related arrhythmias.

Focal Origin Ventricular Arrhythmias

Focal origin arrhythmias should be particularly suspected in patients without SHD who have repetitive monomorphic and nonsustained VTs and PVCs or who have sustained VT from the outflow tract (see Chapter 81). Automaticity or small reentry circuits are possible mechanisms. A focal origin is confirmed by mapping that shows spread of activation away in all directions from the site of earliest activation relative to the QRS onset (see Chapter 61). Unipolar unfiltered (or minimally high-pass filtered at 0.5 Hz) electrograms typically display a QS configuration at the site of origin.[12] Pacing at the origin will replicate the VT/ premature ventricular complexes (PVCs) QRS morphology, but matching pacemaps are often found within 1 cm of the site of earliest activation.[13] Pace-mapping is particularly unreliable for VTs originating from the aortic sinuses (see Chapter 81).

Inability to induce the VT for mapping is a common problem for idiopathic focal arrhythmias. On arrival in the electrophysiology laboratory, attention should be directed to recording a 12-lead ECG of any spontaneous arrhythmia to provide a template for pace-mapping if the arrhythmia is not inducible after the placement of catheters. Minimizing sedation, while avoiding excess administration of local lidocaine anesthesia, which can be absorbed, and achieving therapeutic levels are considerations.[14] Administration of β-agonists, such as isoproterenol, or epinephrine infusions or boluses may be effective; the arrhythmia may emerge as the heart rate slows during the washout.

The most common location of focal idiopathic ventricular arrhythmias is the RV outflow tract near the pulmonary valve annulus. When this arrhythmia is inducible, ablation success rates are high. Origins above the pulmonic valve annulus, in the LV outflow tract near the aortic valve, and in the aortic sinuses of Valsalva are also usually amenable to ablation (see Chapter 81). Ablation at the focus is not always possible for foci deep within the septum or beneath the epicardial fat and coronary arteries at the summit of the LV.[15–17] Ablation attempts from within the great cardiac vein or epicardium in this region should be preceded by the definition of adjacent coronary anatomy with angiography; ablation is often precluded or limited by proximity to a coronary artery with a risk of coronary occlusion.[15,16,18,19] Electroanatomical mapping systems, imaging with intracardiac ultrasound, angiography, and incorporation of preprocedure cardiac computed tomography (CT) or magnetic resonance (MR) images can be helpful in clarifying anatomical complexities (see Chapters 62 and 63).

Focal arrhythmias are also found along the mitral and tricuspid valve annuli, in the LV and RV papillary muscles, and in the Purkinje system.[20–22] Papillary muscle arrhythmias usually cause PVCs or nonsustained VT rather than sustained VT (see Chapter 80). Mapping and ablation are difficult because of the variable anatomy and motion that hinder the maintenance of a stable contact. Intracardiac ultrasound is helpful in assessing appropriate catheter position. Mapping shows activation preceding the QRS by 10–30 ms. Multiple ablation applications are often required.

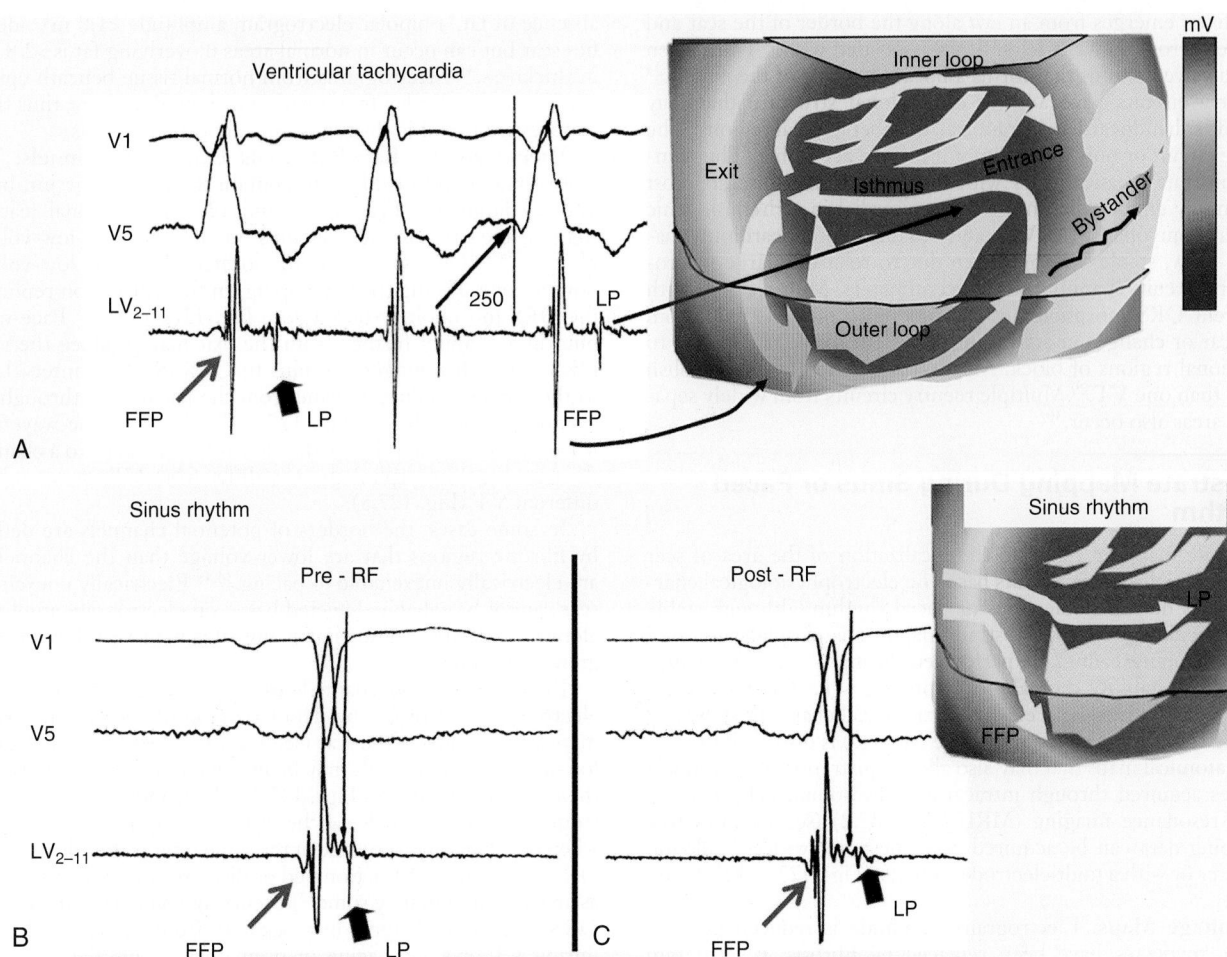

FIGURE 127.1 The schematic at the upper right depicts a theoretical figure-eight reentry circuit. The reentry wavefront propagates through a central isthmus/channel emerging at the exit region to propagate across the ventricles. From the exit, one reentry wave continues clockwise through an inner loop, which is another channel through the scar, and a second wave propagates counterclockwise through an outer loop along the border of the scar to reach the entrance to the isthmus. Colors indicate electrogram amplitude, with *red* being lowest followed by *yellow, green,* and *blue,* typical of a scar region. *Gray* regions are fibrosis without myocytes. Bystander areas are not involved in the reentry circuit. The tracings in each panel are recordings from a patient with ventricular tachycardia (VT) due to a prior infarct. From the top are electrocardiogram (ECG) leads V_1 and V_5 and a bipolar recording from *LV site 2–11.* In the tracing in (A), VT is present. The recording site shows an early diastolic potential (*LP*), the timing of which is consistent with its origin from the proximal isthmus, as was shown by entrainment (not shown). During sinus rhythm (B), the potentials are closer together, and the second potential occurs after the end of the QRS (designated by the *vertical arrow*) and is hence a late potential (*LP*). (C) shows the same site after ablation at this site. Note that the *LP* is markedly diminished in amplitude, consistent with ablation, but the larger initial potential is essentially unchanged, indicating that it is a far-field potential (*FFP*) that originates from the depolarization of myocardium remote from the ablation site. The genesis of the potentials during sinus rhythm is shown in the schematic at the right.

Reentrant Ventricular Tachycardias Related to the Purkinje System

Reentry in or near the fascicles of the LV Purkinje system gives rise to an idiopathic, verapamil-sensitive VT that can be effectively treated with ablation (see Chapter 82). Bundle branch macroreentrant VT is also effectively treated with ablation (see Chapter 83).

Scar-Related Reentry

Scar-related reentry is the most common cause of sustained monomorphic VT in SHD.[1] Scars can be due to prior myocardial infarction, cardiomyopathies, or surgical incisions. Preprocedure imaging is useful to identify the scar location. Areas of delayed gadolinium enhancement on MR images correlate with voltage maps and can suggest the need for an epicardial approach (see Chapter 63).[23–26] Scars may also be evident as areas of absent perfusion on nuclear imaging or thinning and diminished perfusion on CT imaging.[27] Intracardiac ultrasound imaging during the procedure shows some scar areas as akinetic or dyskinetic regions that are sometimes associated with thinning and increased echogenicity.[28] Regions of fibrosis with surviving myocyte bundles create fixed and/or functional conduction block and slow conduction that are the substrate for reentry (see Chapter 48). Stable circuits can be modeled as having an *isthmus* or *channel* comprised of a small mass of tissue that does not contribute to the surface ECG (Fig. 127.1). The QRS onset occurs when the excitation wavefront emerges from an *exit* along the border of the scar and spreads across the ventricles. Scars associated with VT are often near a valve annulus that forms a border for part of the circuit.[23] Reentry circuits have a three-dimensional structure that may include subendocardial, intramural, or subepicardial regions. The entire circuit or only a portion of it may be accessible. The reentry substrate locations vary with the type of heart disease, most commonly endocardial in infarcts, epicardial in arrhythmogenic RV cardiomyopathy (ARVC), and variable in other cardiomyopathies. Slow, stable VTs are often due to relatively large macroreentry circuits spanning several centimeters. Multiple VTs with different QRS morphologies can be due to multiple exits from the scar or changes in activation remote from the circuit due to functional regions of block. Ablation at one region may abolish more than one VT.[29] Multiple reentry circuits from widely separated areas also occur.[30]

Substrate Mapping During Sinus or Paced Rhythm

Substrate mapping refers to the localization of the area of scar and potential reentry circuits based on electrophysiological characteristics during stable sinus or paced rhythm (although stable VT may also be used). Substrate mapping is particularly useful when mapping cannot be performed during VT due to hemodynamic instability or inability to induce VT. The ventricular anatomy combined with electrophysiological characteristics such as electrogram timing or amplitude (voltage) is displayed in electroanatomical maps that may also allow registration of anatomical images acquired through intracardiac ultrasound, CT, or magnetic resonance imaging (MRI) (Fig. 127.2) (see Chapter 61). Mapping data can be acquired point by point with an ablation catheter or with a multielectrode catheter (Figs. 127.2, 127.3, and 127.4).

Voltage Maps. Electrogram amplitude is reduced in areas where myocytes have been replaced by fibrosis. Electrogram amplitude is influenced by the orientation of the recording bipole compared with the direction and speed of propagation, electrode size, spacing and tissue contact, and signal processing (notably filtering).[31,32] Using bipolar recordings between the tip and distal ring of radiofrequency (RF) ablation catheters, more than 95% of sites in the normal LV have a peak-to-peak electrogram amplitude >1.5 mV.[33] MRI shows that fibrosis usually extends through more than 75% of the LV wall in regions with voltage <1.5 mV. Some laboratories consider the infarct border zone as the region of 1- to 1.5-mV amplitude and the areas of <0.5 mV as dense scar. It is important to recognize that "dense scar" based on voltage does not indicate absence of myocardium; pacing often captures in these areas of <0.5 or even <0.1 mV, and they often contain channels.[29,34] An electrogram amplitude >1.5 mV does not necessarily indicate that the region is normal. An endocardial myocardial rim of 2 mm or more can produce a signal of >1.5 mV.[24,35,36] Intramural or epicardial fibrosis overlying endocardial regions of >1.5 mV is common in and can be detected from the analysis of minimally filtered (high-pass filter of 0–0.5 Hz) unipolar recordings, which contain a greater contribution of far-field signals.[37] Endocardial unipolar electrograms exceed 8.3 mV at 95% of nonannular, normal LV sites and are >5.5 mV at 95% of nonannular RV sites.[37–39] An endocardial unipolar electrogram amplitude <5.1 mV had a specificity of 72% for identifying epicardial low-voltage regions.[40] Exceptions occur, and a normal unipolar endocardial map does not exclude the presence of subepicardial arrhythmia substrate.

During epicardial mapping the bipolar electrogram amplitude exceeds 1 mV at 95% of normal sites; however, low-amplitude signals are recorded normally over regions of thick fat along the AV groove and coronary arteries. CT and MRI can be used to detect fat to improve accuracy of epicardial voltage maps. In the absence of fat, a bipolar electrogram amplitude <1.8 mV identifies scar but can occur in normal areas if overlying fat is >2.8 mm in thickness.[41] Electrograms from normal tissue beneath epicardial fat do not display fractionation or long durations; thus these features are useful in distinguishing abnormal regions.

Pace-Mapping, Late Potentials, Exits, and Channels. The low-voltage region is likely to contain the reentry circuit, but it is often large (see Figs. 127.1 and 127.3). Additional features suggest reentry circuit locations in and around low-voltage regions.[29,36,42] Exits are typically located along the low-voltage border zone. Pacing (pace-mapping) in the exit region replicates the QRS morphology of VT (see Fig. 127.3).[29,43–45] Pace-mapping in a channel further from the exit may produce the same QRS but with a longer stimulus to QRS (S-QRS) interval due to the longer conduction time from the pacing site through the channel to the exit (see Fig. 127.3).[29,43,44,46,47] If the wavefront leaves the scar by another path, such as the entrance to a channel, the paced QRS morphology may differ from VT, or resemble a different VT (Fig. 127.5).

In some cases, the borders of potential channels are defined by fibrotic regions that are lower voltage than the channel, or are electrically unexcitable to pacing.[34,48] Electrically unexcitable scar cannot be reliably detected based on electrogram amplitude alone.[29,49] Pacing captures at many sites with very-low-electrogram amplitude.

Electrograms from channels are often smaller than the far-field electrograms produced by depolarization of the larger mass of myocardium outside the scar (see Figs. 127.1 and 127.5).[49] These low-amplitude potentials may be inscribed as late potentials after the end of the QRS (see Figs. 127.1, 127.5, and 127.4).[50–52] Electrograms from channels can be difficult to appreciate, however, when the channel is activated at the same time as the adjacent normal myocardium. A fractionated or discrete potential (referred to as an early potential by some[42]) occurring coincidentally with the QRS and far-field signal may separate from the far-field signal during VT or when pacing or premature stimuli delay conduction into the channel (see Fig. 127.1).[51] Jaïs and coworkers have applied the term "local abnormal ventricular activities" (LAVA) to describe late potentials and other potentials that can be separated in time from the activation of adjacent myocardium, consistent with conduction through a potential channel.[51]

Pace-mapping and analysis of sinus rhythm electrograms are complementary methods, and some channels/isthmuses for conduction may be appreciated by one method and not the other.[29] Nayyar and coworkers performed high-density mapping with both pace-mapping and electrogram analysis in 22 patients with prior infarction and 73 different inducible VTs. Channels were defined by two or more pace-mapping sites with the same QRS, with an S-QRS of >40 ms at least one site. By this definition, 240 possible channels were identified: 57 matching a VT and 183 that appeared to be bystanders. VT channels had a longer average length (53 ± 5 mm) and an average longest S-QRS (130 ± 12 ms) than bystander channels. This method failed to identify a channel for 16 VTs. Fractionated, late (>20 ms after the end of the QRS) and very late (>100 ms after the end of the QRS) potentials were associated with VT channels, but over 70% of the sites where late potentials were recorded were bystanders. Substrate mapping identifies many bystander regions as well as potential VT channels. It is possible, however, that some bystanders could participate in previously undetected VTs.

Mapping During Ventricular Tachycardia

During VT, activation and entrainment mapping are useful for identifying targets.[53–55] When VT is not stable for extensive mapping, mapping during brief episodes may be sufficient to confirm that a region identified during substrate mapping is involved in the tachycardia. Hemodynamic support with percutaneously

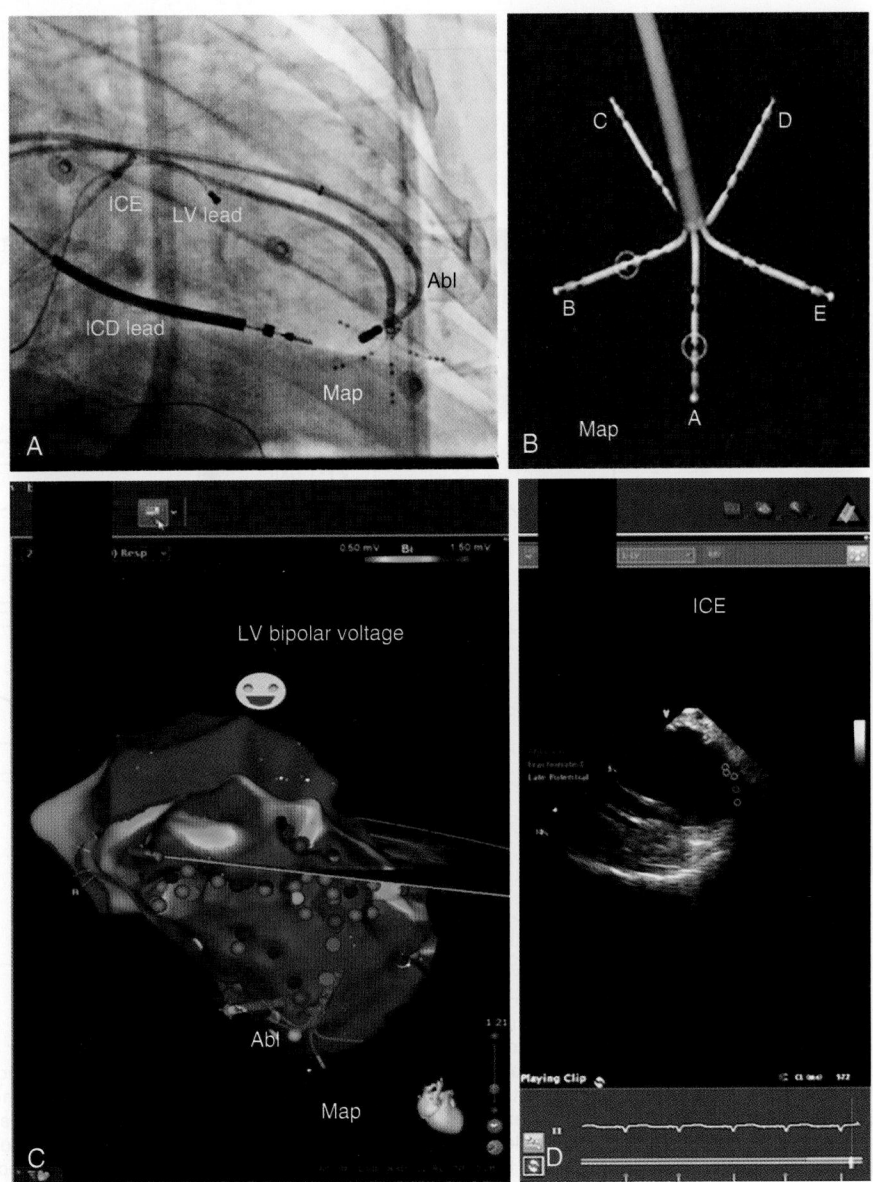

FIGURE 127.2 Images from electroanatomical mapping of ventricular tachycardia in a patient with prior anterior wall infarction are shown. (A) shows a right anterior oblique fluoroscopic image. A right ventricular (RV) implantable cardioverter defibrillator (*ICD*) lead and left ventricular (*LV*) epicardial lead in a lateral LV vein are labeled. An intracardiac phased array ultrasound probe (*ICE*) is present in the RV. An ablation catheter (*Abl*) and a 5-spline mapping catheter (*Map*; also shown in [B]) have been introduced into the LV via a transatrial septal approach and are positioned at the inferoapical LV. (C) shows the voltage map. The anatomy was constructed from a series of intracardiac ultrasound images, one of which is shown in (D). The plane of the ultrasound image is also visible in (C). The mapping and ablation catheters were then moved throughout the chamber to obtain electrogram data for the voltage map (C). The colors are electrogram amplitudes, with *red* representing <0.5 mV and *purple* >1.5 mV. Colored tags are as follows: *red,* ablation site; *blue,* fractionated or late potential site; *green* and *teal,* in-circuit entrainment sites. Recordings from this map are shown in Fig. 127.4.

placed ventricular rotary pumps, left atrial–femoral bypass, or femoral vein to femoral artery cardiopulmonary bypass may be used to allow mapping during VT, but whether this approach improves outcomes is not clear.[56-58] Potential complications related to vascular access, thromboembolism, and interference with electroanatomical mapping systems are concerns.

Activation Mapping and Electrograms. During VT, presystolic activation is recorded at the circuit exit, and earlier, diastolic activation is recorded from more proximal isthmus sites, often in the form of an isolated potential (see Figs. 127.3 and 127.5). Electrogram timing alone is not a reliable indicator of

reentry circuit sites because sites that are proximal in the isthmus can be activated during the end of the QRS complex, without diastolic electrical activity, and presystolic and diastolic electrograms can also occur at bystander sites that are not in the circuit.

Entrainment Mapping. Entrainment is used to assess the relationship of an individual site to the reentry circuit.[59] During entrainment, pacing at a rate faster than the VT continuously resets the reentry circuit (see Figs. 127.3, 127.5, and 127.6). Entrainment is confirmed by evidence of constant fusion between paced orthodromic and antidromic wavefronts and/or progressive fusion due to proportionately greater activation of the

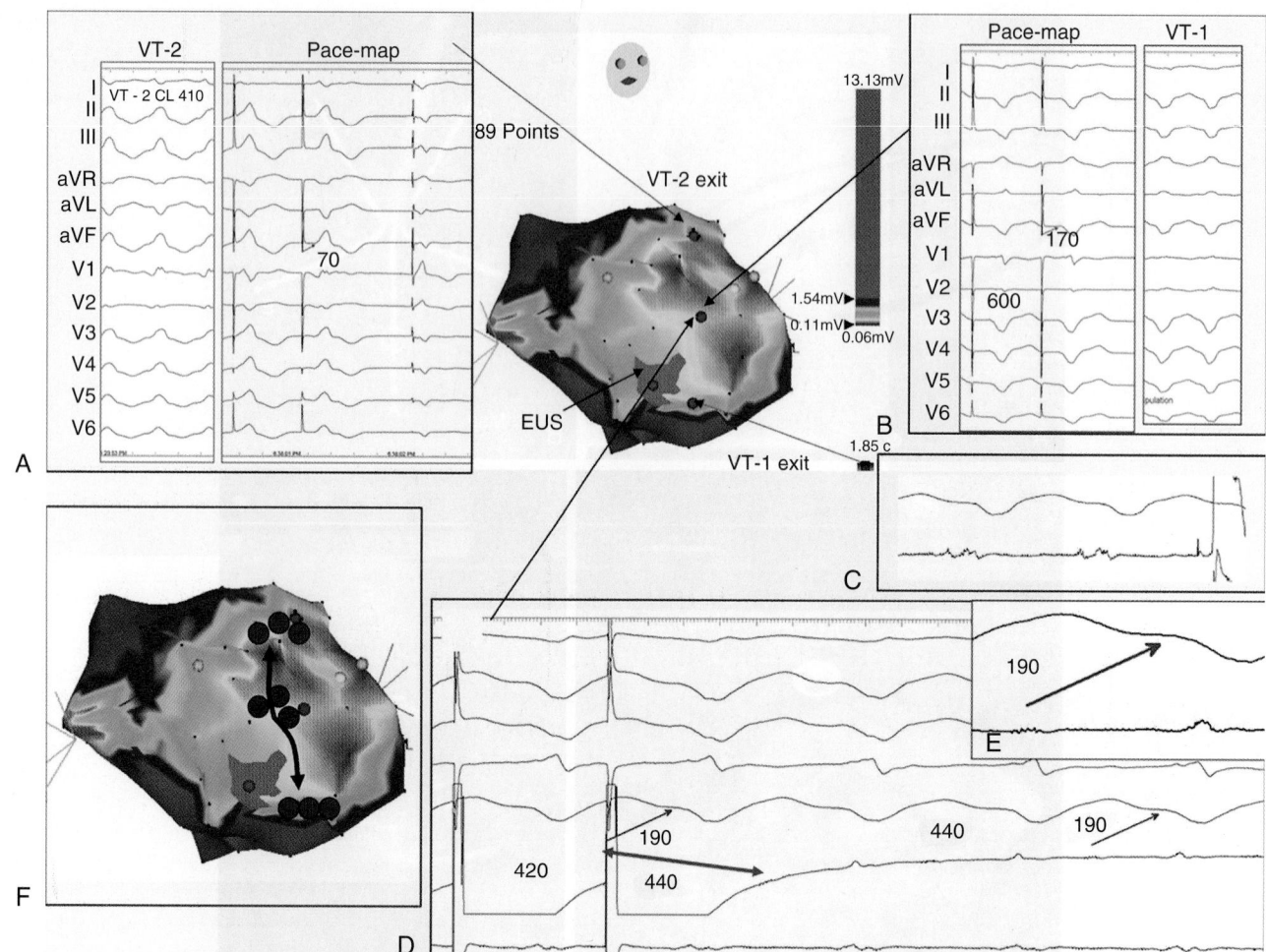

FIGURE 127.3 Findings from mapping in a patient with a prior anterior wall infarction are shown. The center and (F) show a voltage map viewed from the right anterior projection. *Purple* indicates electrogram amplitude of 1.5 mV or greater. A *gray* region of electrically unexcitable scar is present. (A) shows a ventricular tachycardia (*VT*)-2 that has a right bundle branch block configuration and an inferior axis configuration. Pacing at the superior aspect of the infarct (*arrow*) reproduces the *VT-2* QRS morphology, indicating that the exit for *VT-2* is near the pacing site. (B) shows pacing at a site in the middle of the infarct. There is a delay of 170 ms from the pacing stimulus to the QRS, indicating slow conduction through the scar to the margin of the infarct. The paced QRS has a left bundle branch block and superior axis configuration that matched *VT-1*, suggesting that the pacing site was in a channel used by *VT-1* and is confirmed by pacing during *VT-1* (D). (D) shows entrainment with concealed fusion, with a postpacing interval (PPI) that matches the VT cycle length (*CL*). Pacing resets tachycardia with a long stimulus to QRS interval of 190 ms without changing the QRS morphology and with a PPI, measured to the low-amplitude diastolic potential that is enlarged in the inset of (D), which matches the *VT CL*. The S-QRS matches the electrogram to QRS interval (E). (C) shows a recording of presystolic activity during VT from the exit for *VT-1* at the inferior margin of the infarct. (F) shows the potential channel (*black arrow*) with exits at the superior and inferior septal margin of the infarct. Potential ablation targets include the exits (*red circles*) and/or the channel (*blue circles*). EUS, Endoscopic ultrasonography. (Modified from Stevenson WG, Soejima K. Catheter ablation for ventricular tachycardia. *Circulation.* 2007;115:2750-2760.)

ventricles by paced antidromic wavefronts as the pacing rate is increased. The demonstration of entrainment indicates reentry with an excitable gap.

The PPI following entrainment is an indication of the proximity of the pacing site to the reentry circuit.[59] The last stimulus that entrains VT produces a wavefront that propagates to the reentry circuit, orthodromically through the circuit, and returns to the pacing site (see Figs. 127.5 and 127.6). The time from the last pacing stimulus to the next activation at the pacing site is equal to the sum of the conduction times from the pacing site to the circuit, one revolution through the circuit (the tachycardia cycle length) and then back to the pacing site. For sites that are in the circuit, PPI equals the VT cycle length. At sites removed

from the circuit, PPI increases as a function of the conduction time between the site and the circuit.

Use of the PPI requires that three assumptions are satisfied: first, that the pacing stimuli reliably capture; second, that pacing does not alter the conduction through the circuit, as may be suggested by oscillations in VT cycle length; and third, that the time of activation *at the pacing site* following the last stimulus can be determined from the electrograms.[60] Identification of local activation is often complicated by the presence of multicomponent electrograms, some of which are far-field potentials due to depolarization of tissue remote from the pacing site (see Fig. 127.5). Far-field electrograms can often be recognized by their visible presence during pacing, typically distinct from the pacing artifact,

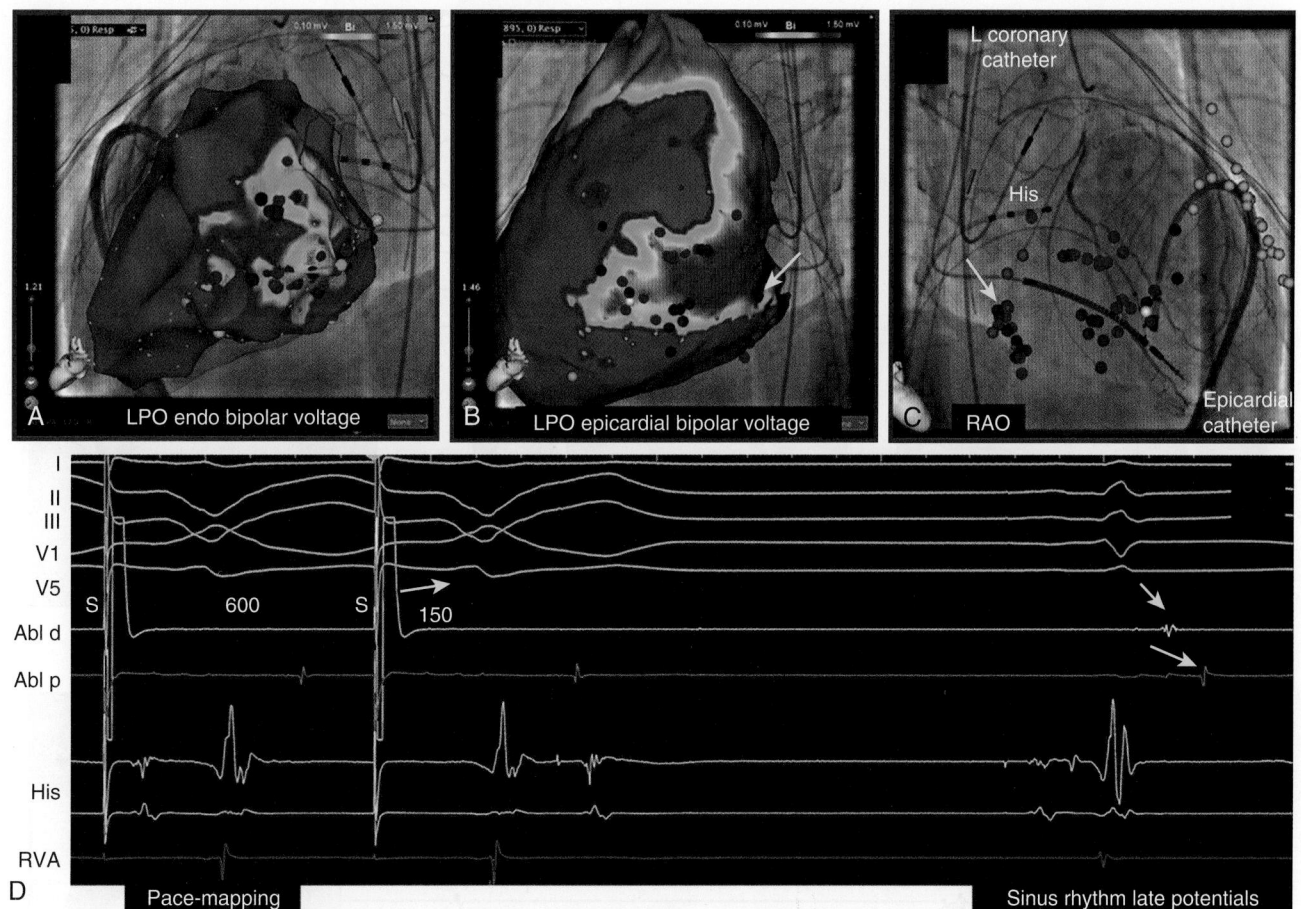

FIGURE 127.4 Data from endocardial and epicardial mapping in a patient with recurrent ventricular tachycardia (VT) due to nonischemic dilated cardiomyopathy. (A)–(C) show the electroanatomical map registered with the fluoroscopic image in the mapping system that was obtained during left coronary angiography. (A) shows the endocardial voltage map, and (B) shows the epicardial voltage map viewed from a left posterior oblique projection. *Red* indicates bipolar voltage <0.1 mV, and *purple* indicates bipolar voltage >1.5 mV. A low-voltage area larger in the epicardium than in the endocardium is present in the inferolateral left ventricle (LV) and extends superiorly along the mitral annulus. *Red* tags indicate ablation sites, and *blue* tags indicate fractionated and late potentials. (C) shows a right anterior oblique projection cine image following left coronary artery injection. The tip of the epicardial ablation catheter is positioned between two marginal coronary artery branches. Radiofrequency (RF) lesions (*red tags*) are clustered between coronary arterial branches. The right ventricle (RV) and atrial leads from the implantable cardioverter defibrillator (ICD) are visible, as are the His catheter (*His*) and RV apical catheter. (D) shows pace-mapping and a sinus rhythm beat recorded at the site indicated by the *yellow arrow* in (B) and (C). The paced QRS has a right bundle branch block superior axis configuration, consistent with the pacing site and resembling one of the inducible VTs (not shown). The S-QRS is 150 ms, consistent with a long conduction time from the pacing site. During sinus rhythm, late potentials are recorded from the distal (*Abl d*) and proximal (*Abl p*) electrodes of the ablation catheter. *His*, His bundle catheter; *RVA*, recording from the RV apical catheter.

indicating that they are not directly depolarized by the pacing stimulus. In contrast, the local potential is obscured by the stimulus artifact during pacing. When the electrograms recorded from the pacing electrode are not visible due to the saturation of the recording amplifier during pacing, measuring the PPI to an electrogram recorded on the adjacent proximal electrodes that is on time with a signal on the distal electrode pair that is not a far-field potential is a good approximation. The S-QRS n+1 measures can also be used to assess the PPI.[61]

Whether the pacing site is in an isthmus is determined through the assessment of QRS fusion. During pacing at an isthmus site, the stimulated orthodromic wavefronts follow the path of the reentry circuit, emerging from the exit. The stimulated antidromic wavefronts are contained in or near the circuit by areas of block that define the isthmus and by collision with returning orthodromic wavefronts. Fusion, due to collision of stimulated

antidromic and orthodromic wavefronts, occurs in or near the pacing site and is not evident as fusion in the surface ECG. VT is accelerated to the pacing rate with a QRS morphology that remains identical to that of the VT (entrainment with concealed fusion). During entrainment with concealed fusion, the stimulus to QRS interval (S-QRS) indicates the conduction time from the pacing site to the reentry circuit exit, is short near the exit, longer at sites proximal to the exit, and matches the electrogram to QRS interval (see Fig. 127.5).

At sites that are in broad portions of the reentry circuit, such as reentry loops along the border of the scar, entrainment occurs with QRS fusion due to propagation of stimulated wavefronts away from the pacing site, but the PPI indicates that the pacing site is in the circuit (see Fig. 127.6F).

Termination of VT by pacing stimuli that capture without producing a propagated response, such that no QRS complex

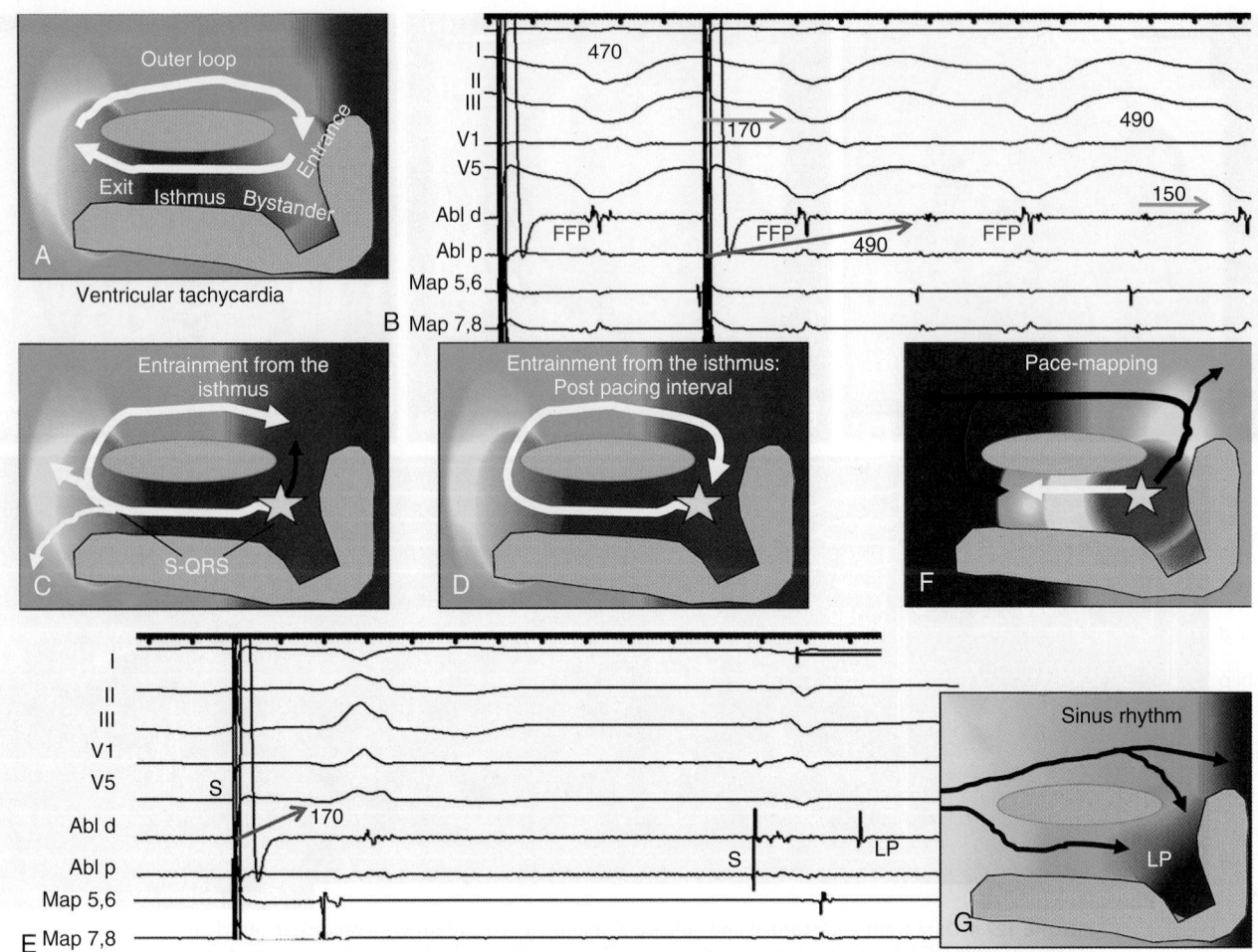

FIGURE 127.5 Tracings from the patient shown in Fig. 127.3 are shown along with schematics of the theoretical reentry substrate. Colors in the schematics indicate the sequence of activation proceeding from *red* to *yellow, green, blue,* and *purple*. (A) shows the theoretical reentry circuit comprising an isthmus/channel and outer loop. (B) and (E) are tracings recorded from the same site with surface electrocardiogram leads I, II, III, V$_1$, and V$_5$ and recordings from the distal (*Abl d*) and proximal (*Abl p*) electrodes of the mapping catheter and from one of the splines of the mapping catheter (*Map 5,6* and *Map 7,8*). In (B), sustained monomorphic ventricular tachycardia (VT) is present, and the last two stimuli of a pacing train at a cycle length of 470 ms are shown. Pacing entrains VT with concealed fusion, a postpacing interval (PPI) (*blue arrow*) of 490 ms, and a S-QRS of 170 ms (approximating the electrogram to QRS of 150 ms [*arrow*]), all consistent with pacing from the isthmus as shown schematically in (C) and (D). During VT, two potentials are recorded from the ablation catheter. The larger potential occurs during the QRS and is not directly depolarized by the pacing stimulus, as it is visible and unperturbed during pacing, indicating it is a far-field potential (*FFP*). The smaller potential is inscribed 150 ms preceding the QRS onset and is obscured by the stimulus artifact during pacing, consistent with capture; hence, it is likely that the local potential should be used for PPI measurement. (E) shows recordings from the site after termination of VT. The first beat is the last of a train of pacing stimuli applied for pace-mapping. Note that although the site is in the VT channel, as seen in (B), the paced QRS morphology is different from that of VT. The mechanism is illustrated in (F); in the absence of VT, the paced wavefront emerges from the entrance region of the isthmus, producing a QRS different from that of VT. In (E), the second beat is produced by the patient's biventricular pacer (*S*). A late potential (*LP*) is present at the site. The mechanism is illustrated in (G).

follows the stimulus, also indicates that the site is likely to be in a narrow isthmus.[62] The mechanism is collision of the stimulated antidromic wavefront with a returning orthodromic wavefront and block of the stimulated orthodromic wavefront before it emerges from the exit. Termination of VT by catheter-induced mechanical pressure or by ablation without eliciting premature beats also indicates that the site is likely in an isthmus.[62,63]

Other Ablation Targets
Approximately 8% of patients with sustained monomorphic VT associated with SHD have bundle branch reentry as the cause of one of their VTs, although scar-related reentry is often also

present (see Chapter 83).[64] Portions of the Purkinje system can also be involved in scar-related reentry circuits.[65] These VTs can have a relatively narrow QRS duration of ≤145 ms, with Purkinje potentials present in the exit region. Rarely, automaticity in the Purkinje system is the cause of VT in patients with SHD.[64,66] Some patients have premature ventricular beats that originate from the VT exit region that can serve as a target for ablation.[67]

Ablation Strategies and Acute Endpoints for Scar-Related Ventricular Tachycardia
Ablation in scar areas seeks to create relatively deep ablation lesions, usually using irrigated ablation electrodes (Chapter 123).

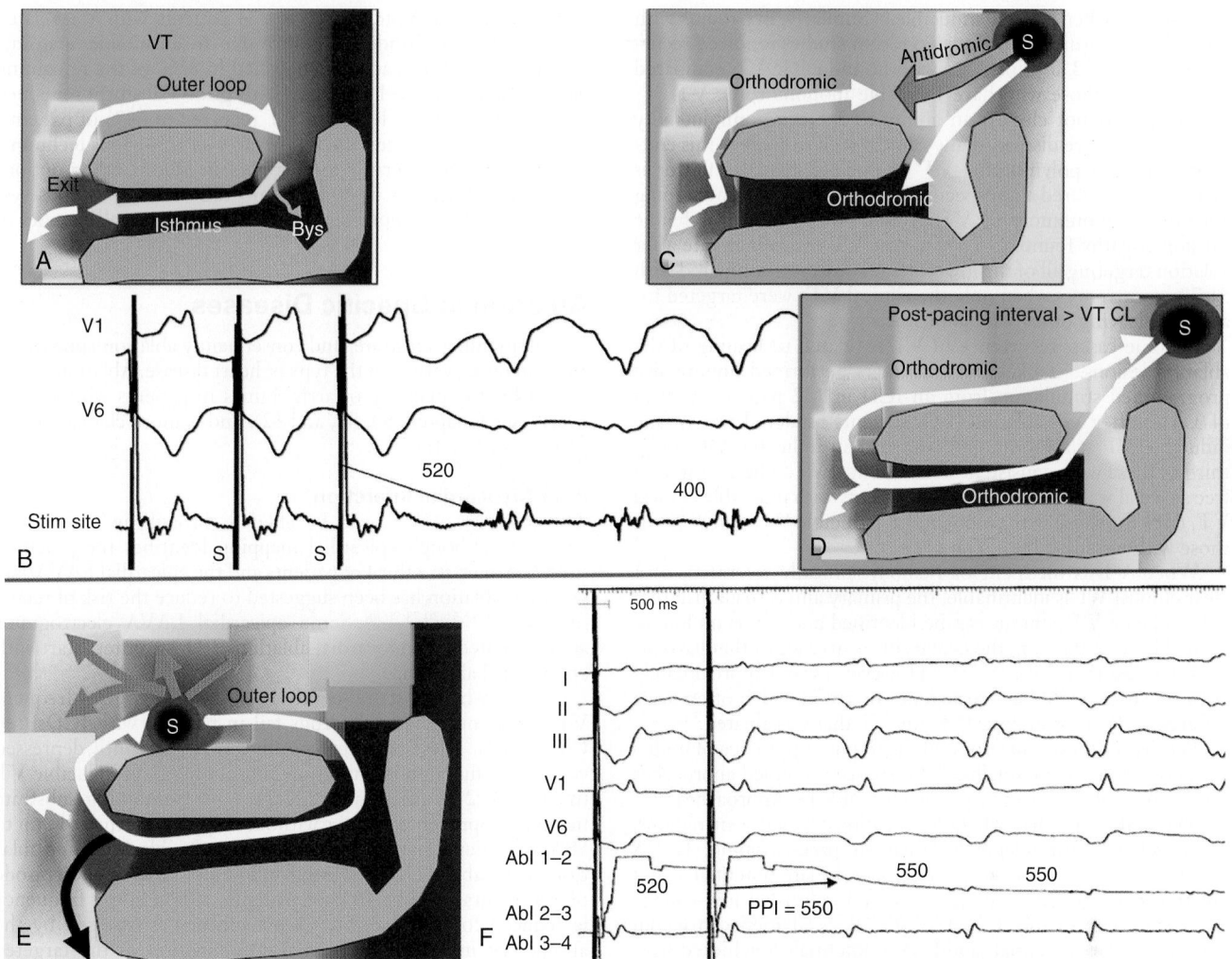

FIGURE 127.6 Entrainment of reentrant ventricular tachycardia (*VT*) from a bystander (*top*) and outer loop (*bottom*) site. (A), (C), (D), and (E) show the schematics of a theoretic reentry circuit with areas of dense scar (*gray*) defining the circuit. The activation sequence is indicated by *arrows* and *colors* proceeding from *red* to *yellow* to *green* to *blue* to *purple*. (A) shows the VT circuit with an isthmus (*yellow arrow*), an outer loop along the border of the scar (*white arrow*), and a bystander region (*Bys, gray arrow*). The QRS onset would occur when the wavefront emerged from the exit region. (B), (C), and (D) show entrainment from a remote bystander. In (B), VT with a cycle length of 400 ms is present. The last three stimuli of a pacing train accelerate the QRS complexes and electrograms to the pacing cycle length with a change in QRS morphology compared to VT. The postpacing interval (PPI) is 520 ms, exceeding the VT cycle length by 120 ms. (C) shows that the stimulated wavefronts divide into antidromic wavefronts (*gray arrow*), which alter the ventricular activation sequence compared to VT. The stimulated orthodromic wavefront resets the tachycardia circuit. Following the last stimulus, the stimulated orthodromic wavefront propagates through the circuit and back to the pacing site, such that the PPI is equal to the tachycardia cycle length (*VT CL*) plus the conduction time from the pacing site to the circuit and from the circuit back to the pacing site (D). (E) and (F) show the effects of pacing at an outer loop site along the border of the scar. In (F), pacing accelerates the QRS complexes and electrograms. The *PPI* of 550 ms matches the VT cycle length, indicating that the site is in the circuit as shown schematically by the *white arrow* in (E). Subtle QRS fusion is evident in the change in QRS morphology in lead I during pacing. Absence of any delay between stimulus and QRS also indicates that the site is not in an isthmus.

We attempt to achieve >10 g of contact force and an impedance fall during ablation approaching 15 ohms. Impedance falls exceeding 18 ohms are associated with an increased risk of steam pops, although perforation in areas of scar is rare.[68] In low-voltage regions, we apply RF to render the targeted area unexcitable to pacing at 10 mA, 2-ms pulse width.[34] Unexcitability may not be achieved in border zone areas, likely due to the adjacent more normal myocardium.

Programmed stimulation is commonly used to assess inducible VT after ablation. Stimulation protocols for this purpose have not been standardized but most include 1, 2, and 3 extrastimuli from two RV sites following two or more different drive cycle lengths. Some centers use up to 4 extrastimuli, additional LV stimulation for VTs arising from the LV and adjunctive isoproterenol.[42,69–71] In approximately 10% of patients in reported series, programmed stimulation is not tested after ablation to avoid additional hemodynamic stress. In a multicenter retrospective analysis of patients with postinfarction VT, the absence of any inducible monomorphic VT after ablation was associated with a lower risk of arrhythmia recurrence (38% vs. 55%)

compared to when any VT inducible.[69] Similarly, in patients with nonischemic cardiomyopathy, two recent studies reported recurrence in 18%–53% of patients with no inducible VT compared with 75% of those who have inducible monomorphic VT.[71,72] Although it is not clear if an ability to achieve noninduciblity reflects less severe disease, many centers seek to achieve this endpoint. Induced polymorphic VT or rapid ventricular flutter is generally considered a nonspecific finding in patients undergoing ablation for monomorphic VT. A randomized trial in ischemic cardiomyopathy found a 15.5% 1-year VT recurrence rate after ablation targeting all of the low-voltage substrates compared with 51.7% recurrences when only the clinical VTs were targeted for ablation, leaving other VTs inducible.[73]

In some cases, recurrence of VT is related to healing of the ablation lesions. Frankel and coworkers performed noninvasive programmed stimulation from an ICD in 132 patients a mean of 3 days after VT ablation.[74] Of patients rendered free of any inducible VT at ablation, half later had an inducible VT, and a third of these were consistent with a clinical VT. The 1-year VT-free survival was less than 30% for patients with inducible clinical VT, 65% for those with a nonclinical inducible VT, and 85% for those without inducible VT.

When VT is incessant or hemodynamically tolerated, or a clear clinical VT is identifiable, the primary aim is to abolish that VT. When a VT isthmus can be identified and VT is no longer inducible after ablation, the chance of recurrence of that particular VT is less than 15%.[53,54,75,76] However, overall approximately 30% of patients will have recurrence of a VT, which often has a different QRS morphology than the VT that was ablated.[54,75–77]

Because of these concerns and the frequent presence of multiple poorly tolerated inducible VTs, substrate-guided approaches are often combined with targeting clinical VTs. Approaches vary among centers and have included ablation through exit regions, identified isthmuses/channels based on pace-mapping, LAVA (local abnormal ventricular activity, such as late potentials), and ablation over the entire endocardial and epicardial low-voltage (<1.5 mV) area (Table 127.2).[29,42,45,50,51,73,78] Patients in whom abolition of late potentials and LAVA potentials is achieved have a lower risk of recurrent VT compared with those in whom these potentials persist, although it is unclear whether the ability to eliminate these potentials is a marker for substrate accessible to ablation or less severe disease.[42,51] Confirmation of channel block by demonstrating a change in conduction away from the pace-mapping site in the scar or isolation of regions of low-voltage scar have also been used as endpoints.[47,79,80] Electrical isolation of the low-voltage region that surrounds areas that contain isthmus, entrance, or exit sites with an endpoint of inability to capture the ventricle by pacing at 20 mA, 2-ms pulse width from within the isolation region, an approach termed "core isolation," was associated with a low risk of recurrence (see Table 127.2).[79] Complete encirclement for isolation of the low-voltage area has also been attempted and can be effective, but it is difficult with present methods and was achievable in only half of the patients.[81]

When endocardial ablation is not successful despite apparently adequate ablation, the reentry circuit may be subepicardial or intramural.[83] An intramural septal origin is suspected when the sites closest to the VT circuit are located on either side of the ventricular septum or at adjacent endocardial and epicardial sides of the ventricular free wall.[38,84] Voltage maps (bipolar and unipolar) usually suggest septal scar. Ablation at the best adjacent sites is usually attempted. Bipolar RF ablation between two catheters positioned on either side of the septum or across the free wall of the ventricle for intramural arrhythmias is feasible.[85]

When endocardial and epicardial ablation attempts fail, transcoronary ethanol ablation can be considered.[83,86] This approach requires identification and cannulation of a target artery that is supplying the VT substrate and injecting absolute ethanol to directly damage the myocardium and close the vessel. This approach was attempted in 27 of 274 patients with VT related to SHD. It was abandoned in five due to unsuitable anatomy; the targeted VT was acutely abolished in 82% of the remaining patients, and 9 of the 11 patients with prior VT storm remained free of VT storm. At least one VT recurred in 64% of patients, and the mortality during the follow-up was 32%. This technique continues to be reserved for patients in whom other options have failed. Injection of ethanol into the coronary venous system has also been reported to be successful in a small number of patients.[87]

Ablation in Specific Diseases

The arrhythmia substrate, and consequently ablation approaches and outcomes, vary with the type of heart disease. Ablation is successful for the majority of arrhythmias in patients with normal hearts (see Chapters 80, 81, and 82), and is more challenging in patients with SHD.

Prior Myocardial Infarction

The majority of VTs can be ablated through an endocardial approach, although epicardial mapping identifies the potential substrate in up to a third of patients and the epicardial LAVA/late potential ablation has been suggested to reduce the risk of recurrent VT.[36,42,51,70,73,78,88] Some epicardial LAVA electrograms are eliminated by endocardial ablation.[89] Most centers start with endocardial ablation.

Ablation has most frequently been used to control frequent VT when antiarrhythmic drugs fail in patients with ICDs (see Chapter 84). These patients typically have significantly depressed ventricular function and multiple morphologies of inducible VT (median of 2–3) (see Table 127.2).[1,5,9,73] Combining substrate mapping approaches with or without mapping during VT, up to 88% of patients have no immediately inducible VT after ablation (see Table 127.2).[5] During follow-up, at least one episode of VT recurs in 15%–50% of patients, although the frequency is reduced for the majority. Acute efficacy as assessed by the absence of inducible VT and the elimination of the targeted substrate is associated with lower risk of recurrence. Multiple morphologies of inducible VT, failure of multiple antiarrhythmic drugs, history of VT storm (three or more episodes of VT within 24 hours), and the severity of heart disease, as indicated by functional class, lower LV ejection fraction, and presence of cardiac resynchronization therapy, are associated with increased risk of recurrence.[5,70]

The annual mortality following catheter ablation for recurrent VT that is failing drug therapy ranges from 9% to 18%. Patients who have recurrent VT after ablation have a substantially increased risk of mortality, particularly when VT recurs early.[5,90] Progressive heart failure is the most common single cause of death and is consistent with the severity of heart disease and the association of VT as a marker for mortality and heart failure. Older age, history of electrical storm, severe ventricular dysfunction, and kidney disease are associated with increased mortality. The potential for ablation to adversely affect LV function is of concern. Assessment of LV ejection fraction after ablation has not shown deterioration, but confining ablation to regions of scar, when feasible, and attention to medical therapy for ventricular dysfunction seems prudent. Because of these concerns, an ICD is usually recommended when not already present.

It has been suggested that outcomes will be better in patients with less severe disease or in those treated earlier in the course of the disease.[70,91] In the VTACH trial, 110 patients were randomized to ablation and ICD implantation versus ICD implantation alone after presenting with hemodynamically stable VT. VT recurrences were reduced from 71% to 53%, the median time to recurrent VT increased from 6 to 19 months and hospitalizations were reduced.[92,93] The total number of VT episodes

TABLE 127.2   Scar-related ventricular tachycardia (VT) ablation guided by substrate mapping with or without mapping during VT

	PATIENTS	DISEASE	LVEF	MAPPING DURING AT LEAST ONE VT	SUBSTRATE GUIDED ABLATION TARGETS	EPICARDIAL	NO INDUCIBLE VT AFTER ABLATION	FOLLOW-UP	RECURRENT VT	TOTAL MORTALITY
Nayyar et al. 2014 [29]	22	CAD 100%	0.32	11 pts	Pace-mapping and Abn EGs	0	64%	16 mos (mean)	23%	14%
De Riva et al. 2015 [70]	91	CAD 100%	0.34	>30%	Pace-mapping and Abn EGs	8%	47%	23 mos (med.)	38%	27%
Tzou et al. 2015 [79]	44	CAD 73%	0.31	14 pts	Core isolation + additional ablation	6 pts	84%	17.5 mos (mean)	14%	NR
Silberbauer et al. 2014 [42]	160	CAD 100%		26% at least one tolerated VT	LP EP where pacing has S-QRS >40 ms	21%	88%	18.7 mos (med.)	32%	17%
	73		0.34		LP/EP abolished	21%	100%	20 mos	16%	8%
	63		0.31		LP/EP not abolished	18%	100%	19 mos	47%	18%
	19		0.28		VT inducible	32%	0	8.5 mos	47%	47%
Di Base et al. 2015 [73]	60	CAD 100%	0.33	Yes	Clinical VT	11%	A mean of two VTs inducible	12 mos	48.3%	15%
Jaïs et al. 2012 [51]	58	CAD 100%	0.32	No	All low-voltage substrate	10%	NA	12 mos	15.5%	8.6%
	70	CAD 80%	0.35	32%	LAVA potentials	30%	30%	22 mos (med.)	46%	19%
	47	CAD 85%	0.34		LAVA eliminated	36%	32%		32%	19%
	20	CAD 70%	0.37		LAVA not eliminated	20%	30%		75%	20%
Oloriz et al. 2014 [82]	87	NICM	0.28–0.53	54%	LP EP where pacing has S-QRS >40 ms	74%	81%	18 mos	51%	15%

CAD, Coronary artery disease; *EP,* early potentials; *LP,* late potentials; *LVEF,* left ventricular ejection fraction; *med.,* median; *NICM,* nonischemic cardiomyopathy; *LAVA,* local abnormal ventricular activities.

was markedly reduced in the ablation group. In the SMASH VT trial, 128 patients with hemodynamically unstable VTs who were receiving an ICD were randomized to ablation of the VT substrate or ICD alone. After 2 years of follow-up, VT had recurred in 12% of the ablation and 33% of the control groups (hazard ratio [HR], 0.35; p = .007). These trials were too small to assess an impact on mortality. Both were conducted between 2002 and 2006, and there have been substantial advances since.

Although patients with sustained VT and SHD usually warrant an ICD, favorable outcomes in selected patient groups with relatively preserved LV function (LV ejection fraction >0.35) who are rendered free of inducible VT after, and in some cases at repeat programmed stimulation 3 months after ablation, has led some to avoid ICD implantation in selected patients.[70,94,95]

Dilated Cardiomyopathy and Valvular Heart Disease

More than 80% of patients with sustained monomorphic VT have scar-related reentry; in the remainder, VT is due to bundle branch reentry (see Chapter 83) or has a focal origin.[45,82,96,97] Scars typically have a noncoronary distribution and are often intramural or epicardial (see Chapter 128).[98] Low-voltage areas tend to be smaller, with less evidence of abnormal delayed potentials, compared with patients with infarct scars.[45,50] With intramural substrate, the best ablation targets can be in regions with bipolar voltage >1.5 mV, often with low-unipolar voltage, but may require mapping during VT for identification.[97]

The most common scar locations in patients with sustained monomorphic VT involve the base of the LV.[23,38,72,82,84] The location of the scar can often be inferred from the QRS morphology of VTs. Scars along the lateral and inferior mitral annulus produce VTs that have a right bundle branch block, right axis configuration; and a QS configuration in lead I and often indicate an epicardial exit.[99] These VTs often require epicardial ablation, where branches of the circumflex coronary artery and the left phrenic nerve are concerns (see Fig. 127.4). A second common scar location involves the basal septum. One or more of the VTs have an LBBB-like configuration. Late potentials are often absent, possibly related to relatively early activation of the septum.[72,82] Epicardial mapping is usually not helpful.[71] For septal VTs, AV block is a risk that is sometimes unavoidable if ablation is to be attempted. With either of these patterns, extension of scar along the aortic valve region including the area beneath the aortic mitral continuity is common. Ablations from the LV endocardium, RVOT, aortic sinuses, and great cardiac vein have been performed for VTs in this area but still fail in some patients. VTs that have dominant S waves in V_3 and V_4 suggest low-voltage scar extending to the apex associated with a worse prognosis, likely reflecting extensive ventricular scar.[100]

In recent series including 234 patients, abolition of inducible VT was achieved in 38%–61% of patients.[71,72,82] Epicardial mapping was performed in 35%–74% of patients. During an average follow-up of 18–25 months, 44%–49% of patients were free of VT. Despite recurrences in about half of the patients, the frequency of VT was reduced by ≥75% in 79% of patients in one study.[72] Procedural complications occurred in 9%–11% of patients.

Incessant idiopathic VT or frequent ventricular ectopy can cause tachycardia-induced cardiomyopathy that improves after ablation (see Chapter 80).[101]

Right Ventricular Cardiomyopathies

Scar-related RV tachycardias occur in idiopathic cardiomyopathy, ARVC (see Chapter 87), cardiac sarcoidosis, and repaired congenital heart disease, notably tetralogy of Fallot (see Chapter 102).[102-104] Scars causing VT are often adjacent to the tricuspid or pulmonic annulus. Focal origin VTs also occur.

Epicardial circuits are usually present in ARVC, and epicardial ablation combined with endocardial ablation improves outcomes.[103,104] In a nonrandomized case series, 85% of patients were free from VT over 3 years following combined endocardial and epicardial ablation compared with 52% of patients treated with endocardial ablation only.[102]

Cardiac sarcoidosis can mimic ARVC, and the two diseases cannot be reliably distinguished on the basis of electrophysiological characteristics alone, although AV conduction disease favors sarcoidosis.[105,106] Endomyocardial biopsy, positron emission tomography (PET), and MRI can help identify sarcoid.[107] Ablation for VT due to sarcoidosis can reduce VT episodes, but recurrence rates were 63% at 1 year in one study.[108]

Other Diseases

Ablation has been successfully used to control scar-related recurrent VT in patients with repaired congenital heart disease (see Chapter 102), a history of myocarditis,[96,109,110] hypertrophic cardiomyopathy,[111,112] valvular heart disease,[113] and LV assist devices (see Chapter 111).[114]

Ablation for Polymorphic Ventricular Tachycardia and Ventricular Fibrillation

Recurrent polymorphic VT causing "electrical storm" that is not due to ongoing acute ischemia is rare, but it occurs in idiopathic ventricular fibrillation, long QT syndrome, Brugada syndrome, and early and late after myocardial infarction. VT is often initiated by premature beats from foci that can be targeted for ablation (see Chapter 129). In Brugada syndrome, epicardial ablation of abnormal areas in the RV outflow region can abolish recurrent VF (see Chapter 92).[115]

Summary

Catheter ablation of VT has an important role in reducing VT episodes in patients with ICDs and controlling incessant VT and electrical storms. Epicardial mapping and ablation have improved outcomes in patients with arrhythmias that are not endocardial in origin, particularly nonischemic cardiomyopathy and ARVC. The approach is determined by the characteristics of the arrhythmia and underlying heart disease. Present techniques enable ablation for multiple and hemodynamically unstable VTs, formerly considered "unmappable." Failures are often due to anatomical obstacles that will continue to be addressed by technological advances.

REFERENCES

1. Aliot EM, Stevenson WG, Almendral-Garrote JM, et al. EHRA/HRS Expert Consensus on Catheter Ablation of Ventricular Arrhythmias: developed in a partnership with the European Heart Rhythm Association (EHRA), a Registered Branch of the European Society of Cardiology (ESC), and the Heart Rhythm Society (HRS); in collaboration with the American College of Cardiology (ACC) and the American Heart Association (AHA). *Heart Rhythm*. 2009;6:886–933.
2. Bohnen M, Stevenson WG, Tedrow UB, et al. Incidence and predictors of major complications from contemporary catheter ablation to treat cardiac arrhythmias. *Heart Rhythm*. 2011;8:1661–1666.
3. Peichl P, Wichterle D, Pavlu L, et al. Complications of catheter ablation of ventricular tachycardia: a single-center experience. *Circ Arrhythm Electrophysiol*. 2014;7:684–690.
4. Katz DF, Turakhia MP, Sauer WH, et al. Safety of ventricular tachycardia ablation in clinical practice: findings from 9699 hospital discharge records. *Circ Arrhythm Electrophysiol*. 2015;8:362–370.
5. Tung R, Vaseghi M, Frankel DS, et al. Freedom from recurrent ventricular tachycardia after catheter ablation is associated with improved survival in patients with structural heart disease: An International VT Ablation Center Collaborative Group study. *Heart Rhythm*. 2015;12:1997–2007.
6. Sacher F, Roberts-Thomson K, Maury P, et al. Epicardial ventricular tachycardia ablation: a multicenter safety study. *J Am Coll Cardiol*. 2010;55:2366–2372.
7. Della Bella P, Brugada J, Zeppenfeld K, et al. Epicardial ablation for ventricular tachycardia: a European multicenter study. *Circ Arrhythm Electrophysiol*. 2011;4:653–659.
8. Schmidt B, Chun KR, Baensch D, et al. Catheter ablation for ventricular tachycardia after failed endocardial ablation: epicardial substrate or inappropriate endocardial ablation? *Heart Rhythm*. 2010;7:1746–1752.
9. Stevenson WG, Wilber DJ, Natale A, et al. Irrigated radiofrequency catheter ablation guided by electroanatomic mapping for recurrent ventricular tachycardia after myocardial infarction: the multicenter thermocool ventricular tachycardia ablation trial. *Circulation*. 2008;118:2773–2782.
10. Merino JL, Peinado R, Fernandez-Lozano I, et al. Bundle-branch reentry and the postpacing interval after entrainment by right ventricular apex stimulation: a new approach to elucidate the mechanism of wide-QRS-complex tachycardia with atrioventricular dissociation. *Circulation*. 2001;103:1102–1108.
11. de Riva M, Watanabe M, Zeppenfeld K. Twelve-lead ECG of ventricular tachycardia in structural heart disease. *Circ Arrhythm Electrophysiol*. 2015;8:951–962.
12. Sorgente A, Epicoco G, Ali H, et al. Negative concordance pattern in bipolar and unipolar recordings: an additional mapping criterion to localize the site of origin of focal ventricular arrhythmias. *Heart Rhythm*. 2016;13:519–526.
13. Bogun F, Taj M, Ting M, et al. Spatial resolution of pace mapping of idiopathic ventricular tachycardia/ectopy originating in the right ventricular outflow tract. *Heart Rhythm*. 2008;5:339–344.
14. Nof E, Reichlin T, Enriquez AD, et al. Impact of general anesthesia on initiation and stability of VT during catheter ablation. *Heart Rhythm*. 2015;12:2213–2220.
15. Santangeli P, Marchlinski FE, Zado ES, et al. Percutaneous epicardial ablation of ventricular arrhythmias arising from the left ventricular summit: outcomes and electrocardiogram correlates of success. *Circ Arrhythm Electrophysiol*. 2015;8:337–343.
16. Nagashima K, Choi EK, Lin KY, et al. Ventricular arrhythmias near the distal great cardiac vein: challenging arrhythmia for ablation. *Circ Arrhythm Electrophysiol*. 2014;7:906–912.
17. Ouyang F, Mathew S, Wu S, et al. Ventricular arrhythmias arising from the left ventricular outflow tract below the aortic sinus cusps: mapping and catheter ablation via transseptal approach and electrocardiographic characteristics. *Circ Arrhythm Electrophysiol*. 2014;7:445–455.
18. Roberts-Thomson KC, Steven D, Seiler J, et al. Coronary artery injury due to catheter ablation in adults: presentations and outcomes. *Circulation*. 2009;120:1465–1473.
19. Baldinger SH, Kumar S, Barbhaiya CR, et al. Epicardial radiofrequency ablation failure during ablation procedures for ventricular arrhythmias—reasons and implications for outcomes. *Circ Arrhythm Electrophysiol*. 2015;CIRCEP-115.
20. Wasmer K, Kobe J, Dechering DG, et al. Ventricular arrhythmias from the mitral annulus: patient characteristics, electrophysiological findings, ablation, and prognosis. *Heart Rhythm*. 2013;10:783–788.
21. Al'Aref SJ, Ip JE, Markowitz SM, et al. Differentiation of papillary muscle from fascicular and mitral annular ventricular arrhythmias in patients with and without structural heart disease. *Circ Arrhythm Electrophysiol*. 2015;8:616–624.
22. Yamada T, Doppalapudi H, McElderry HT, et al. Idiopathic ventricular arrhythmias originating from the papillary muscles in the left ventricle: prevalence, electrocardiographic and electrophysiological characteristics, and results of the radiofrequency catheter ablation. *J Cardiovasc Electrophysiol*. 2010;21:62–69.
23. Piers SR, Tao Q, van Huls van Taxis CF, et al. Contrast-enhanced MRI-derived scar patterns and associated ventricular tachycardias in nonischemic cardiomyopathy: implications for the ablation strategy. *Circ Arrhythm Electrophysiol*. 2013;6:875–883.
24. Dickfeld T, Tian J, Ahmad G, et al. MRI-Guided ventricular tachycardia ablation: integration of late gadolinium-enhanced 3D scar in patients with implantable cardioverter-defibrillators. *Circ Arrhythm Electrophysiol*. 2011;4:172–184.
25. Bala R, Ren JF, Hutchinson MD, et al. Assessing epicardial substrate using intracardiac echocardiography during VT ablation. *Circ Arrhythm Electrophysiol*. 2011;4:667–673.
26. Piers SR, Tao Q, de Riva Silva M, et al. CMR-based identification of critical isthmus sites of ischemic and nonischemic ventricular tachycardia. *JACC Cardiovasc Imaging*. 2014;7:774–784.
27. Tian J, Jeudy J, Smith MF, et al. Three-dimensional contrast-enhanced multidetector CT for anatomic, dynamic, and perfusion characterization of abnormal myocardium to guide ventricular tachycardia ablations. *Circ Arrhythm Electrophysiol*. 2010;3:496–504.
28. Hussein A, Jimenez A, Ahmad G, et al. Assessment of ventricular tachycardia scar substrate by intracardiac echocardiography. *Pacing Clin Electrophysiol*. 2014;37:412–421.
29. Nayyar S, Wilson L, Ganesan AN, et al. High-density mapping of ventricular scar: a comparison of ventricular tachycardia (VT) supporting channels with channels that do not support VT. *Circ Arrhythm Electrophysiol*. 2014;7:90–98.
30. Stevenson WG, Soejima K. Catheter ablation for ventricular tachycardia. *Circulation*. 2007;115:2750–2760.
31. Anter E, Josephson ME. Bipolar voltage amplitude: What does it really mean? *Heart Rhythm*. 2016;13:326–327.
32. Mizuno H, Vergara P, Maccabelli G, et al. Contact force monitoring for cardiac mapping in patients with ventricular tachycardia. *J Cardiovasc Electrophysiol*. 2013;24:519–524.
33. Marchlinski FE, Callans DJ, Gottlieb CD, et al. Linear ablation lesions for control of unmappable ventricular tachycardia in patients with ischemic and nonischemic cardiomyopathy. *Circulation*. 2000;101:1288–1296.
34. Soejima K, Stevenson WG, Maisel WH, et al. Electrically unexcitable scar mapping based on pacing threshold for identification of the reentry circuit isthmus: feasibility for guiding ventricular tachycardia ablation. *Circulation*. 2002;106:1678–1683.
35. Wijnmaalen AP, van der Geest RJ, van Huls van Taxis CF, et al. Head-to-head comparison of contrast-enhanced magnetic resonance imaging and electroanatomical voltage mapping to assess post-infarct scar characteristics in patients with ventricular tachycardias: real-time image integration and reversed registration. *Eur Heart J*. 2011;32:104–114.
36. Tsiachris D, Silberbauer J, Maccabelli G, et al. Electroanatomical voltage and morphology characteristics in postinfarction patients undergoing ventricular tachycardia ablation: pragmatic approach favoring late potentials abolition. *Circ Arrhythm Electrophysiol*. 2015;8:863–873.
37. Hutchinson MD, Gerstenfeld EP, Desjardins B, et al. Endocardial unipolar voltage mapping to detect epicardial ventricular tachycardia substrate in patients with nonischemic left ventricular cardiomyopathy. *Circ Arrhythm Electrophysiol*. 2011;4:49–55.
38. Haqqani HM, Tschabrunn CM, Tzou WS, et al. Isolated septal substrate for ventricular tachycardia in nonischemic dilated cardiomyopathy: incidence, characterization, and implications. *Heart Rhythm*. 2011;8:1169–1176.
39. Polin GM, Haqqani H, Tzou W, et al. Endocardial unipolar voltage mapping to identify epicardial substrate in arrhythmogenic right ventricular cardiomyopathy/dysplasia. *Heart Rhythm*. 2011;8:76–83.
40. Tokuda M, Tedrow UB, Inada K, et al. Direct comparison of adjacent endocardial and epicardial electrograms: implications for substrate mapping. *J Am Heart Assoc*. 2013;2:e000215.
41. Piers SR, van Huls van Taxis CF, Tao Q, et al. Epicardial substrate mapping for ventricular tachycardia ablation in patients with non-ischaemic cardiomyopathy: a new algorithm to differentiate between scar and viable myocardium developed by simultaneous integration of computed tomography and contrast-enhanced magnetic resonance imaging. *Eur Heart J*. 2013;34:586–596.
42. Silberbauer J, Oloriz T, Maccabelli G, et al. Noninducibility and late potential abolition: a novel combined prognostic procedural end point for catheter ablation of postinfarction ventricular tachycardia. *Circ Arrhythm Electrophysiol*. 2014;7:424–435.
43. Sinno MC, Yokokawa M, Good E, et al. Endocardial ablation of postinfarction ventricular tachycardia with nonendocardial exit sites. *Heart Rhythm*. 2013;10:794–799.
44. de Chillou C, Groben L, Magnin-Poull I, et al. Localizing the critical isthmus of postinfarct ventricular tachycardia: the value of pace-mapping during sinus rhythm. *Heart Rhythm*. 2014;11:175–181.
45. Kuhne M, Abrams G, Sarrazin JF, et al. Isolated potentials and pace-mapping as guides for ablation of ventricular tachycardia in various types of nonischemic cardiomyopathy. *J Cardiovasc Electrophysiol*. 2010;21:1017–1023.
46. Yokokawa M, Liu TY, Yoshida K, et al. Automated analysis of the 12-lead electrocardiogram to identify the exit site of postinfarction ventricular tachycardia. *Heart Rhythm*. 2012;9:330–334.
47. Tung R, Mathuria N, Michowitz Y, et al. Functional pace-mapping responses for identification of targets for catheter ablation of scar-mediated ventricular tachycardia. *Circ Arrhythm Electrophysiol*. 2012;5:264–272.
48. Mountantonakis SE, Park RE, Frankel DS, et al. Relationship between voltage map "channels" and the location of critical isthmus sites in patients with post-infarction cardiomyopathy and ventricular tachycardia. *J Am Coll Cardiol*. 2013;61:2088–2095.
49. Baldinger SH, Nagashima K, Kumar S, et al. Electrogram analysis and pacing are complimentary for recognition of abnormal conduction and far-field potentials during substrate mapping of infarct-related ventricular tachycardia. *Circ Arrhythm Electrophysiol*. 2015;8:874–881.
50. Nakahara S, Tung R, Ramirez RJ, et al. Characterization of the arrhythmogenic substrate in ischemic and nonischemic cardiomyopathy implications for catheter ablation of hemodynamically unstable ventricular tachycardia. *J Am Coll Cardiol*. 2010;55:2355–2365.
51. Jaïs P, Maury P, Khairy P, et al. Elimination of local abnormal ventricular activities: a new end point for substrate modification in patients with scar-related ventricular tachycardia. *Circulation*. 2012;125:2184–2196.
52. Irie T, Yu R, Bradfield JS, et al. Relationship between sinus rhythm late activation zones and critical sites for scar-related ventricular tachycardia: systematic analysis of isochronal late activation mapping. *Circ Arrhythm Electrophysiol*. 2015;8:390–399.
53. Bogun F, Kim HM, Han J, et al. Comparison of mapping criteria for hemodynamically tolerated, postinfarction ventricular tachycardia. *Heart Rhythm*. 2006;3:20–26.
54. Soejima K, Suzuki M, Maisel WH, et al. Catheter ablation in patients with multiple and unstable ventricular tachycardias after myocardial infarction: short ablation lines guided by reentry circuit isthmuses and sinus rhythm mapping. *Circulation*. 2001;104:664–669.
55. Verma A, Marrouche NF, Schweikert RA, et al. Relationship between successful ablation sites and the scar border zone defined by substrate mapping for ventricular tachycardia post-myocardial infarction. *J Cardiovasc Electrophysiol*. 2005;16:465–471.
56. Reddy YM, Chinitz L, Mansour M, et al. Percutaneous left ventricular assist devices in ventricular tachycardia ablation: multicenter experience. *Circ Arrhythm Electrophysiol*. 2014;7:244–250.
57. Bunch TJ, Darby A, May HT, et al. Efficacy and safety of ventricular tachycardia ablation with mechanical circulatory support compared with substrate-based ablation techniques. *Europace*. 2012;14:709–714.
58. Aryana A, Gearoid O'Neill P, Gregory D, et al. Procedural and clinical outcomes after catheter ablation of unstable ventricular tachycardia supported by a percutaneous left ventricular assist device. *Heart Rhythm*. 2014;11:1122–1130.
59. Stevenson WG, Khan H, Sager P, et al. Identification of reentry circuit sites during catheter mapping and radiofrequency ablation of ventricular tachycardia late after myocardial infarction. *Circulation*. 1993;88:1647–1670.
60. Tung S, Soejima K, Maisel WH, et al. Recognition of far-field electrograms during entrainment mapping of ventricular tachycardia. *J Am Coll Cardiol*. 2003;42:110–115.
61. Soejima K, Stevenson WG, Maisel WH, et al. The N + 1 difference: a new measure for entrainment mapping. *J Am Coll Cardiol*. 2001;37:1386–1394.
62. Bogun F, Krishnan SC, Marine JE, et al. Catheter ablation guided by termination of postinfarction ventricular tachycardia by pacing with nonglobal capture. *Heart Rhythm*. 2004;1:422–426.
63. Bogun F, Good E, Han J, et al. Mechanical interruption of postinfarction ventricular tachycardia as a guide for catheter ablation. *Heart Rhythm*. 2005;2:687–691.

64. Lopera G, Stevenson WG, Soejima K, et al. Identification and ablation of three types of ventricular tachycardia involving the His-Purkinje system in patients with heart disease. *J Cardiovasc Electrophysiol.* 2004;15:52–58.

65. Bogun F, Good E, Reich S, et al. Role of Purkinje fibers in post-infarction ventricular tachycardia. *J Am Coll Cardiol.* 2006;48:2500–2507.

66. Fiek M, Remp T, Fleckenstein M, et al. Incidence and relevance of nonreentrant monomorphic ventricular tachycardia in patients with frequent implantable cardioverter defibrillator interventions. *J Interv Card Electrophysiol.* 2015;42:151–160.

67. Bogun F, Crawford T, Chalfoun N, et al. Relationship of frequent postinfarction premature ventricular complexes to the reentry circuit of scar-related ventricular tachycardia. *Heart Rhythm.* 2008;5:367–374.

68. Seiler J, Roberts-Thomson KC, Raymond JM, et al. Steam pops during irrigated radiofrequency ablation: feasibility of impedance monitoring for prevention. *Heart Rhythm.* 2008;5:1411–1416.

69. Yokokawa M, Kim HM, Baser K, et al. Predictive value of programmed ventricular stimulation after catheter ablation of post-infarction ventricular tachycardia. *J Am Coll Cardiol.* 2015;65:1954–1959.

70. de Riva M, Piers SR, Kapel GF, et al. Reassessing noninducibility as ablation endpoint of post-infarction ventricular tachycardia: the impact of left ventricular function. *Circ Arrhythm Electrophysiol.* 2015;8:853–862.

71. Dinov B, Arya A, Schratter A, et al. Catheter ablation of ventricular tachycardia in patients with nonischemic dilated cardiomyopathy: can noninducibility after ablation be a predictor for reduced mortality? *Circ Arrhythm Electrophysiol.* 2015;8:598–605.

72. Piers SR, Leong DP, van Huls van Taxis CF, et al. Outcome of ventricular tachycardia ablation in patients with nonischemic cardiomyopathy: the impact of noninducibility. *Circ Arrhythm Electrophysiol.* 2013;6:513–521.

73. DiBiase LB, Burkhardt JD, Lakkireddy D, et al. Ablation of stable VTs versus substrate ablation in ischemic cardiomyopathy. The VISTA randomized multicenter trial. *J Am Coll Cardiol.* 2015;66:2872–2882.

74. Frankel DS, Mountantonakis SE, Zado ES, et al. Non-invasive programmed ventricular stimulation early after ventricular tachycardia ablation to predict risk of late recurrence. *J Am Coll Cardiol.* 2012;59:1529–1535.

75. El-Shalakany A, Hadjis T, Papageorgiou P, et al. Entrainment/mapping criteria for the prediction of termination of ventricular tachycardia by single radiofrequency lesion in patients with coronary artery disease. *Circulation.* 1999;99:2283–2289.

76. Yokokawa M, Desjardins B, Crawford T, et al. Reasons for recurrent ventricular tachycardia after catheter ablation of post-infarction ventricular tachycardia. *J Am Coll Cardiol.* 2013;61:66–73.

77. Tokuda M, Kojodjojo P, Tung S, et al. Characteristics of clinical and induced ventricular tachycardia throughout multiple ablation procedures. *J Cardiovasc Electrophysiol.* 2016;27:88–94.

78. Di Biase L, Santangeli P, Burkhardt DJ, et al. Endo-epicardial homogenization of the scar versus limited substrate ablation for the treatment of electrical storms in patients with ischemic cardiomyopathy. *J Am Coll Cardiol.* 2012;60:132–141.

79. Tzou WS, Frankel DS, Hegeman T, et al. Core isolation of critical arrhythmia elements for treatment of multiple scar-based ventricular tachycardias. *Circ Arrhythm Electrophysiol.* 2015;8:353–361.

80. Kapel GF, Reichlin T, Wijnmaalen AP, et al. Re-entry using anatomically determined isthmuses: a curable ventricular tachycardia in repaired congenital heart disease. *Circ Arrhythm Electrophysiol.* 2015;8:102–109.

81. Tilz RR, Makimoto H, Lin T, et al. Electrical isolation of a substrate after myocardial infarction: a novel ablation strategy for unmappable ventricular tachycardias–feasibility and clinical outcome. *Europace.* 2014;16:1040–1052.

82. Oloriz T, Silberbauer J, Maccabelli G, et al. Catheter ablation of ventricular arrhythmia in nonischemic cardiomyopathy: anteroseptal versus inferolateral scar sub-types. *Circ Arrhythm Electrophysiol.* 2014;7:414–423.

83. Kumar S, Barbhaiya CR, Sobieszczyk P, et al. Role of alternative interventional procedures when endo- and epicardial catheter ablation attempts for ventricular arrhythmias fail. *Circ Arrhythm Electrophysiol.* 2015;8:606–615.

84. Betensky BP, Kapa S, Desjardins B, et al. Characterization of trans-septal activation during septal pacing: criteria for identification of intramural ventricular tachycardia substrate in nonischemic cardiomyopathy. *Circ Arrhythm Electrophysiol.* 2013;6:1123–1130.

85. Koruth JS, Dukkipati S, Miller MA, et al. Bipolar irrigated radiofrequency ablation: a therapeutic option for refractory intramural atrial and ventricular tachycardia circuits. *Heart Rhythm.* 2012;9:1932–1941.

86. Tokuda M, Sobieszczyk P, Eisenhauer AC, et al. Transcoronary ethanol ablation for recurrent ventricular tachycardia after failed catheter ablation: an update. *Circ Arrhythm Electrophysiol.* 2011;4:889–896.

87. Schurmann P, Penalver J, Valderrabano M. Ethanol for the treatment of cardiac arrhythmias. *Curr Opin Cardiol.* 2015;30:333–343.

88. Sarkozy A, Tokuda M, Tedrow UB, et al. Epicardial ablation of ventricular tachycardia in ischemic heart disease. *Circ Arrhythm Electrophysiol.* 2013;6:1115–1122.

89. Komatsu Y, Daly M, Sacher F, et al. Endocardial ablation to eliminate epicardial arrhythmia substrate in scar-related ventricular tachycardia. *J Am Coll Cardiol.* 2014;63:1416–1426.

90. Nagashima K, Choi EK, Tedrow UB, et al. Correlates and prognosis of early recurrence after catheter ablation for ventricular tachycardia due to structural heart disease. *Circ Arrhythm Electrophysiol.* 2014;7:883–888.

91. Dinov B, Arya A, Bertagnolli L, et al. Early referral for ablation of scar-related ventricular tachycardia is associated with improved acute and long-term outcomes: results from the Heart Center of Leipzig ventricular tachycardia registry. *Circ Arrhythm Electrophysiol.* 2014;7:1144–1151.

92. Kuck KH, Schaumann A, Eckardt L, et al. Catheter ablation of stable ventricular tachycardia before defibrillator implantation in patients with coronary heart disease (VTACH): a multicentre randomised controlled trial. *Lancet.* 2010;375:31–40.

93. Delacretaz E, Brenner R, Schaumann A, et al. Catheter ablation of stable ventricular tachycardia before defibrillator implantation in patients with coronary heart disease (VTACH): an on-treatment analysis. *J Cardiovasc Electrophysiol.* 2013;24:525–529.

94. Pauriah M, Cismaru G, Magnin-Poull I, et al. A stepwise approach to the management of postinfarct ventricular tachycardia using catheter ablation as the first-line treatment: a single-center experience. *Circ Arrhythm Electrophysiol.* 2013;6:351–356.

95. Maury P, Baratto F, Zeppenfeld K, et al. Radio-frequency ablation as primary management of well-tolerated sustained monomorphic ventricular tachycardia in patients with structural heart disease and left ventricular ejection fraction over 30%. *Eur Heart J.* 2014;35:1479–1485.

96. Dello Russo A, Casella M, Pieroni M, et al. Drug-refractory ventricular tachycardias following myocarditis: endocardial and epicardial radiofrequency catheter ablation. *Circ Arrhythm Electrophysiol.* 2012;5:492–498.

97. Nazer B, Woods C, Dewland T, et al. Importance of ventricular tachycardia induction and mapping for patients referred for epicardial ablation. *Pacing Clin Electrophysiol.* 2015;38:1333–1342.

98. Piers SR, Everaerts K, van der Geest RJ, et al. Myocardial scar predicts monomorphic ventricular tachycardia but not polymorphic ventricular tachycardia or ventricular fibrillation in nonischemic dilated cardiomyopathy. *Heart Rhythm.* 2015;12:2106–2114.

99. Valles E, Bazan V, Marchlinski FE. ECG criteria to identify epicardial ventricular tachycardia in nonischemic cardiomyopathy. *Circ Arrhythm Electrophysiol.* 2010;3:63–71.

100. Frankel DS, Tschabrunn CM, Cooper JM, et al. Apical ventricular tachycardia morphology in left ventricular nonischemic cardiomyopathy predicts poor transplant-free survival. *Heart Rhythm.* 2013;10:621–626.

101. Sadron Blaye-Felice M, Hamon D, Sacher F, et al. Premature ventricular contraction-induced cardiomyopathy: related clinical and electrophysiologic parameters. *Heart Rhythm.* 2016;13:103–110.

102. Bai R, Di Biase L, Shivkumar K, et al. Ablation of ventricular arrhythmias in arrhythmogenic right ventricular dysplasia/cardiomyopathy: arrhythmia-free survival after endo-epicardial substrate based mapping and ablation. *Circ Arrhythm Electrophysiol.* 2011;4:478–485.

103. Berruezo A, Fernandez-Armenta J, Mont L, et al. Combined endocardial and epicardial catheter ablation in arrhythmogenic right ventricular dysplasia incorporating scar dechanneling technique. *Circ Arrhythm Electrophysiol.* 2012;5:111–121.

104. Philips B, te Riele AS, Sawant A, et al. Outcomes and ventricular tachycardia recurrence characteristics after epicardial ablation of ventricular tachycardia in arrhythmogenic right ventricular dysplasia/cardiomyopathy. *Heart Rhythm.* 2015;12:716–725.

105. Dechering DG, Kochhauser S, Wasmer K, et al. Electrophysiological characteristics of cardiac arrhythmias in cardiac sarcoidosis versus arrhythmogenic right ventricular cardiomyopathy. *Heart Rhythm.* 2013;10:158–164.

106. Birnie DH, Sauer WH, Bogun F, et al. HRS expert consensus statement on the diagnosis and management of arrhythmias associated with cardiac sarcoidosis. *Heart Rhythm.* 2014;11:1305–1323.

107. Blankstein R, Osborne M, Naya M, et al. Cardiac positron emission tomography enhances prognostic assessments of patients with suspected cardiac sarcoidosis. *J Am Coll Cardiol.* 2014;63:329–336.

108. Kumar S, Barbhaiya C, Nagashima K, et al. Ventricular tachycardia in cardiac sarcoidosis: characterization of ventricular substrate and outcomes of catheter ablation. *Circ Arrhythm Electrophysiol.* 2015;8:87–93.

109. Maccabelli G, Tsiachris D, Silberbauer J, et al. Imaging and epicardial substrate ablation of ventricular tachycardia in patients late after myocarditis. *Europace.* 2014;16:1363–1372.

110. Berte B, Sacher F, Cochet H, et al. Postmyocarditis ventricular tachycardia in patients with epicardial-only scar: a specific entity requiring a specific approach. *J Cardiovasc Electrophysiol.* 2015;26:42–50.

111. Inada K, Seiler J, Roberts-Thomson KC, et al. Substrate characterization and catheter ablation for monomorphic ventricular tachycardia in patients with apical hypertrophic cardiomyopathy. *J Cardiovasc Electrophysiol.* 2011;22:41–48.

112. Dukkipati SR, d'Avila A, Soejima K, et al. Long-term outcomes of combined epicardial and endocardial ablation of monomorphic ventricular tachycardia related to hypertrophic cardiomyopathy. *Circ Arrhythm Electrophysiol.* 2011;4:185–194.

113. Eckart RE, Hruczkowski TW, Tedrow UB, et al. Sustained ventricular tachycardia associated with corrective valve surgery. *Circulation.* 2007;116:2005–2011.

114. Sacher F, Reichlin T, Zado ES, et al. Characteristics of ventricular tachycardia ablation in patients with continuous flow left ventricular assist devices. *Circ Arrhythm Electrophysiol.* 2015;8:592–597.

115. Nademanee K, Veerakul G, Chandanamattha P, et al. Prevention of ventricular fibrillation episodes in Brugada syndrome by catheter ablation over the anterior right ventricular outflow tract epicardium. *Circulation.* 2011;123:1270–1279.

128 Epicardial Approach in Electrophysiology

Arnaud Chaumeil, Frederic Sacher, Michel Haïssaguerre, and Pierre Jaïs

The pericardial space was historically the first access used to study cardiac electrophysiology.[1] During its golden age—from the 1970s through the 1980s—the first electrical activation maps were acquired in the operating room by surgeons.[2-4] These studies helped in understanding the main atrial and ventricular arrhythmia mechanisms. These maps also paved the way for the first surgical procedures used to cure the most severe and even lethal electrical disorders.[5-7] Later on, endocardial access progressively replaced surgical mapping because of its superior simplicity and safety and because of the importance of the endocardial substrate, especially in ischemic ventricular or supraventricular tachycardias. The development of diagnostic and ablation catheters as well as energy sources (from fulguration to radiofrequency [RF]) has made the surgical approach anecdotal.[8]

For many years, the use of epicardial access was restricted to cardiac defibrillation or for treating refractory arrhythmias. In 1996, Sosa et al. developed a technique of percutaneous access to the epicardium for treating recurrent electrical storms in a subpopulation of patients with Chagas disease.[9] The spread of this technical knowledge allowed the treatment of refractory arrhythmias, mainly from the ventricles, and provided a better understanding of the epicardial arrhythmogenic substrate of different cardiomyopathies.

Nowadays, this approach is commonly performed in tertiary electrophysiology centers for ventricular tachycardia (VT) ablation in different pathologies such as nonischemic dilated cardiomyopathy or arrhythmogenic right ventricular cardiomyopathy (ARVC).

Anatomy

The pericardial sac is situated posterior to the sternum and at the level of the second to sixth costal cartilages. To help maintain its position, the fibrous pericardium, the outermost layer of the sac, has attachments to the sternum anteriorly and to the central tendon of the diaphragm inferiorly and fuses with the adventitia of the great vessels superiorly. The inner fibrous pericardium is lined by the parietal serous pericardium. The parietal serous pericardium reflects on itself to form the visceral serous pericardium, which is adherent to the epicardium. The pericardial cavity is the potential space between the outer parietal layer and the inner visceral layer of the serous pericardium. In about 1/10,000 patients, the pericardium is congenitally absent. Features suggestive of this rare disorder include electrocardiographic (ECG) changes, cardiac displacement, and a sharp aortopulmonary window on the chest radiograph, which can be confirmed by computed tomography (CT) or magnetic resonance imaging (MRI). Within the pericardial sac, the catheter moves freely over most of the epicardial surface, apart from the specific regions bound by the pericardial reflections, such as the oblique and transverse sinuses, and the pulmonary vein recesses.

The oblique sinus is a cul-de-sac along the posterior left atrial (LA) wall and is bounded by the pericardial reflections of the left and right pulmonary veins and superiorly by the transverse sinus/LA roof. Its inferior opening is bounded by the two inferior pulmonary veins. The ligament of Marshall is situated at the posterolateral aspect of the LA, and the fold of Marshall may be seen to the left of the oblique sinus.

The transverse sinus is a tunnel-shaped anatomical space between the great vessels and the roof of the LA, connecting the left and right sides of the pericardial cavity.

The right pulmonary artery lies superior to the transverse sinus, and the roof of the LA forms its floor. The phrenic nerves lie near the pericardium. The left phrenic nerve passes behind the left brachiocephalic vein, over the aortic arch and pulmonary trunk, over the LA appendage, and in the majority of patients laterally over the obtuse margin of the left ventricle (LV) and in a minority of patients anteriorly close to the left anterior descending artery. The right phrenic nerve descends along the brachiocephalic vein, follows the right anterolateral border of the superior vena cava, passes close to the anterior wall of the right superior pulmonary vein, and then travels along the lateral aspect of the right atrial wall to finally join the lateral inferior vena cava (IVC).[10]

Indications

The indications for epicardial access are not clearly established by scientific societies. The real benefit of this approach will largely remain unknown and probably underestimated until several studies systematically investigate this issue. Because of its potential morbidity, this approach is mainly performed in high-volume expert centers with surgical backup. The majority of epicardial access procedures are considered for VT, but it remains challenging to screen patients in whom this approach will be needed and is beneficial. Presented next are some criteria that have been reported to help making a decision.

Previous Failure of Endocardial Ablation

A prior unsuccessful endocardial ablation is possibly the clearest indication for considering an epicardial access procedure, as an epicardial substrate is commonly found in almost 80% of these cases irrespective of the type of cardiopathy.[11] Schmidt et al. mentioned epicardial participation in three-fourths of patients with a prior unsuccessful endocardial ablation.[12]

Predictive Electrocardiographic Criteria

Many decisional algorithms have been suggested. They seem to be more discriminant for patients with nonischemic cardiomyopathy (NICM).

According to Berrueza et al.,[13] the following criteria are predictive of an epicardial ventricular location:

- A pseudodelta wave of >34 ms has a sensitivity of 83% and a specificity of 95%.
- An intrinsic deflection time of >85 ms has a sensitivity of 87% and a specificity of 90%.
- An RS complex duration of >121 ms has a sensitivity of 76% and a specificity of 85% for identifying an epicardial origin of the VT.

Complementary studies were produced to improve their sensibility according to the origin of the circuit (Fig. 128.1).

The presence of a Q wave in the inferior leads or D1 increases the diagnostic specificity.[14] Marchlinski et al. pooled these criteria in a validated algorithm for patients with an NICM that reaches 96% sensitivity and 93% specificity[15](Fig. 128.2).

Type of Cardiomyopathy Scar Localization on Magnetic Resonance Imaging

The location of the scar varies considerably among patients, but some patterns linking to the disease have to be demonstrated. The likelihood of an epicardial substrate varies with the etiology, as summarized in Table 128.1.[12,16–28]

Chagas Disease

The pathology of patients with acquired Chagas disease initiated the development of nonsurgical epicardium access. Chagas disease, caused by a parasite (*Trypanosoma cruzi*), is mainly found in South and Central America. Myocardium and coronary arteries are the target of chronic extensive infectious and inflammatory injuries that cause refractory incessant VT. The critical isthmus of the VT circuits is typically located in the epicardium.[17,18]

Myocarditis Sequelae

Mainly of viral origin, arrhythmias complicate almost 50% of myocarditis episodes during the acute phase. Then, late tachycardia recurrences occur independently of left ventricular dysfunction. In a series with 20 chronic stage patients scheduled for a refractory VT ablation, epicardial access was needed in 30% of cases.[19]

With use of late gadolinium enhancement, MRI has the capability of showing a relative increase in fibrotic tissue. This allows the detection of a scar with a spatial resolution of approximately 2 mm. The scar and therefore the area critical for VT maintenance can be preoperatively localized to the epicardium or even midwall in some cases. These data are critical for deciding about an epicardial access procedure and refining the ablation targets and strategy[29] (eFig. 128.1).

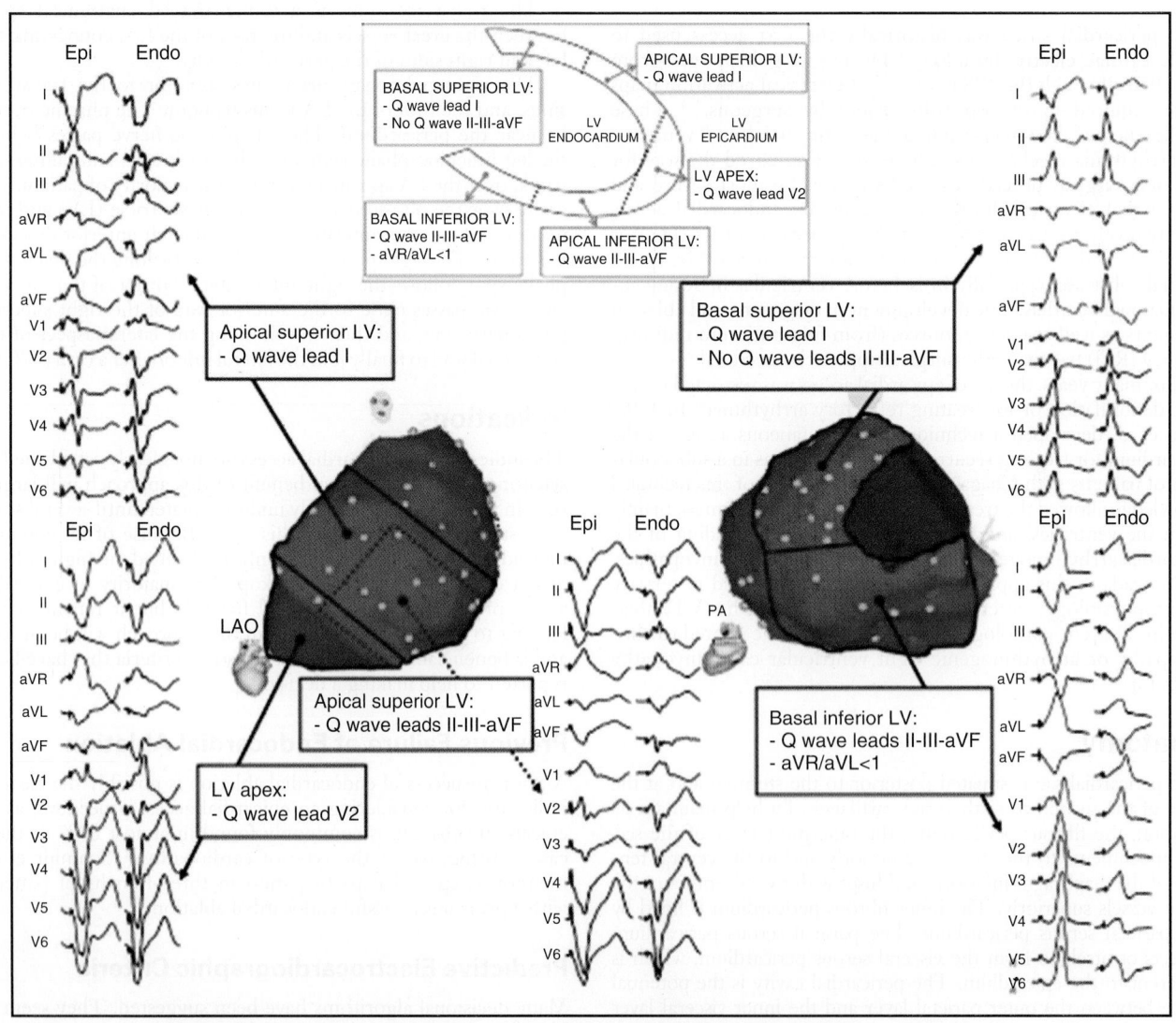

FIGURE 128.1 Epicardial ventricular tachycardia (VT) circuit location according to electrocardiographic criteria.[13] *LV,* Left ventricle.

Arrhythmogenic Right Ventricular Cardiomyopathy

ARVC is an inherited myocardial disease that is characterized by a fibrofatty replacement of the myocardial cells that begins

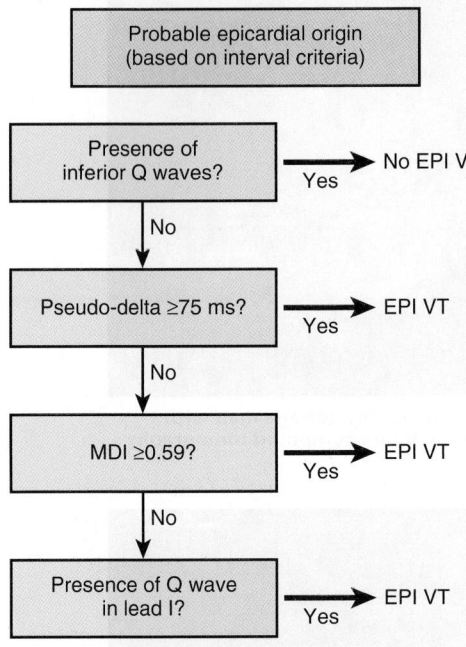

FIGURE 128.2 Four steps identifying an epicardial (*EPI*) origin from the basal superior and lateral left ventricle in the setting of non-ischemic cardiomyopathy. MDI is defined as the interval measured from the earliest ventricular activation (or from the stimulation artifact) to the peak of the largest-amplitude deflection in each precordial lead divided by the QRS duration. *SN*, Sensibility; *SP*, specificity; *VT*, ventricular tachycardia. (From Valles E, Bazan V, Marchlinski FE. ECG criteria to identify epicardial ventricular tachycardia in nonischemic cardiomyopathy. *Circ Arrhythm Electrophysiol.* 2010;3:63-71.)

in the most epicardial layers of the right ventricle (RV). More extensive epicardial substrate has been found histologically in small clinical studies. This anatomical profile can explain the high rate of recurrences after endocardial VT ablation.[30] In some experienced centers, the epicardial approach is used as a first-line strategy in this condition, given the importance of epicardial substrate.

Fernandez-Armanta et al.'s series with 22 patients found up to 90% of patients with a critical isthmus in the epicardium,[25] and Haqqani et al. found all pathological areas to be epicardial in 18 patients.[26] The main location is usually in the sub- and latero-tricuspid annulus zone and also in the RV free wall and outflow tract. A VT critical isthmus was found in almost 69% of cases[31] (Fig. 128.3 and eFig. 128.2).

This point has also largely been confirmed by other groups.[32] Interestingly, CT scan is a powerful imaging modality to describe fibrofatty infiltration in this condition, with the advantage over MRI of a spatial resolution of 0.3 mm and a universal cut that can be set at 0 Hounsfield unit.[33]

Nonischemic Cardiomyopathy

NICM is very heterogeneous, and MRI may establish the diagnosis or allow for scar identification and localization. Scar location is highly predictive of abnormal potentials. In a heterogeneous group of cardiomyopathies, most of the clinical studies targeted the failure of the endocardial approach and found a 100% rate of low-voltage areas or abnormal electrogram (EGM) in the epicardium.[34] Nakahara et al. found a 100% epicardial substrate rate in seven patients with previous ablation failure.[27] The common location of scars in this condition is the basolateral and inferolateral LV (Fig. 128.4).

Ischemic Cardiomyopathy

During myocardial infarction, the endocardium is the first to be injured, and as a consequence, the critical isthmus of the VT circuit is most frequently endocardial. The epicardium substrate is implicated in only 6%–41% of patients, particularly in the inferior territory, but in nearly all patients with arrhythmic recurrences after endocardial ablation.[24] However, in the absence of studies in which an epicardial approach would be routinely used

TABLE 128.1	Importance of epicardial substrate according to the pathology						
REFERENCE	NO. OF PATIENTS	ICM (%)	DCM INCLUDING MYOCARDITIS SEQUELAE (%)	ARVC (%)	HCM (%)	IDIOPATHIC VT (%)	CHAGAS DISEASE (%)
Schmidt et al.[12]	59	NA	80	83	NA	75	NA
Sacher et al.[16]	156	82	92	100	NA	71	NA
Henz et al.[17]	17	NA	NA	NA	NA	NA	82
Sosa et al.[18]	10	NA	NA	NA	NA	NA	100
Dello Russo et al.[19]	218	NA	30	NA	NA	NA	NA
Ueda et al.[20]	5	NA	NA	NA	60	NA	NA
Santangelli et al.[21]	22	NA	NA	NA	59.1	NA	NA
Inada et al.[22]	4	NA	NA	NA	75	NA	NA
Dukkipati et al.[23]	10	NA	NA	NA	80	NA	NA
Sarkozy et al.[24]	444	6	NA	NA	NA	NA	NA
Fernandez-Armenta et al.[25]	22	NA	NA	90	NA	NA	NA
Haqqani et al.[26]	18	NA	NA	100	NA	NA	NA
Nakahara et al.[27]	19	41	83	NA	NA	NA	NA
Cano et al.[28]	22	NA	82	NA	NA	NA	NA

ARVC, Arrhythmogenic right ventricular cardiomyopathy; *DCM*, dilated cardiomyopathy; *HCM*, hypertrophic cardiomyopathy; *ICM*, ischemic cardiomyopathy; *VT*, ventricular tachycardia.

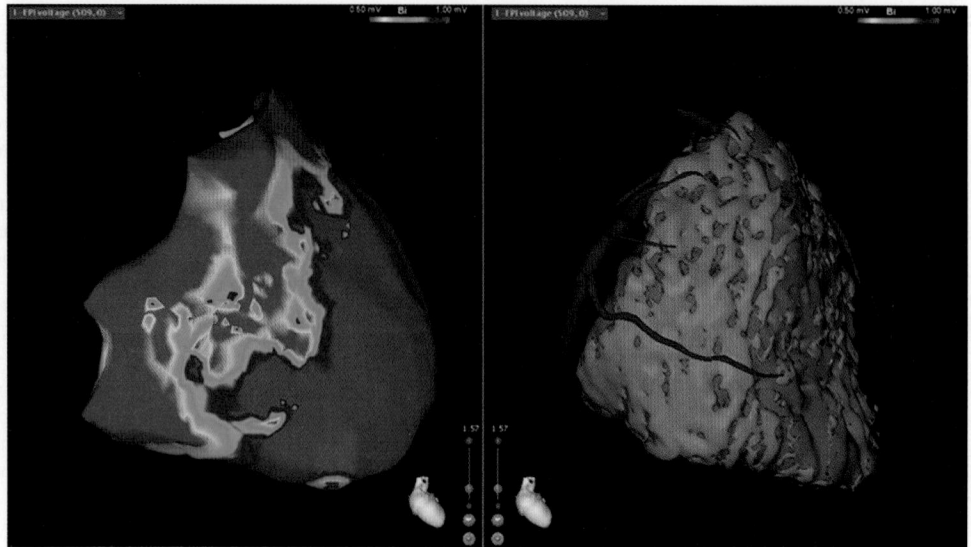

FIGURE 128.3 Typical arrhythmogenic right ventricular cardiomyopathy voltage map with basal- and laterotricuspid annulus scar well correlated with the fat on computed tomography scan imaging.

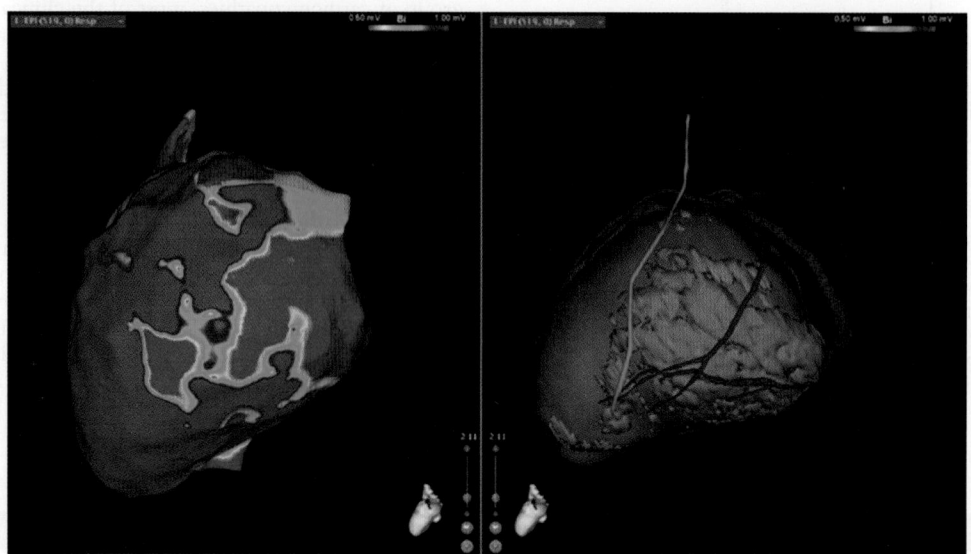

FIGURE 128.4 A patient with nonischemic cardiomyopathy. Normal endocardial voltage with large electrical scar in the epicardium of the posterobasal and lateral left ventricle part (*left*) confirmed by magnetic resonance imaging–related scar integration (*right*).

in the index VT ablation procedure, we have no idea of what the exact numbers are.

Brugada Syndrome

First described by Brugada et al., the Brugada syndrome associates a typical ECG pattern with recurrent malignant arrhythmias and sudden cardiac death. Experimental data have shown the presence of abnormal signals on the RV outflow tract epicardial surface.[35]

A clinical study confirmed these data. Nademanee et al. found an epicardial substrate on the RV outflow tract surface in all nine patients of the series with type 1 Brugada syndrome. Ablation at these sites made ventricular arrhythmia noninducible (in seven of nine patients [78%]) and normalized the Brugada ECG pattern in 89% of patients. The long-term outcomes (at 20 ± 6 months) were excellent, with no recurrent arrhythmia in any patient without medication (except in one patient on amiodarone).[36] In other

cases, this access can increase the efficacy and transmurality of ablation lesions.

Hypertrophic Cardiomyopathy

Hypertrophic cardiomyopathy is defined by a heterogeneous substrate composed of areas with interconnected endocardial, intracardial, and epicardial fibrosis and hypertrophic myocytes. Monomorphic VT is less frequent than polymorphic VT or ventricular fibrillation (VF) in this population. Myocardial thickness and the presence of important trabeculations (especially in the apex of the LV) limit intracardiac mapping. More importantly, transmurality of RF lesions is impossible to achieve because of muscle thickness. The benefit of the epicardial approach was confirmed in a nine-patient series in which an abnormal substrate was documented in 80% of cases (mainly in the apical region: 70%), versus 60% in the endocardium. Interestingly, no substrate was found in a particular case of a probable intramural scar.[21,23]

Left Ventricular Noncompaction

Case reports also have described the use of epicardial ablation in cases of rare inherited diseases (left ventricular noncompaction, and Fabry disease).[37]

Can Electrograms Suggest an Epicardial Origin?

In an NICM group, Tzou et al.[38] noted the following intracardiac electrophysiological criteria during VT as predictive of an epicardial origin:

- Diffusely early activation (>2 cm^2 region of sites with equally earliest activation within 10 ms)
- Sequence of a far-field EGM followed by a near-field EGM in the region of earliest endoactivation
- Inability to capture the far-field component of the earliest EGM (stim-QRS < EGM-QRS time) or reproduce morphological features of the VA complex with stimulation at the earliest endocardial site of activation

Moreover, unipolar endocardial voltage has been shown to be well correlated with epicardial bipolar voltage and scar. In the LV, a value <8.27 mV has been reported to be associated with an epicardial scar in NICM.[39] With right-sided VT, the presence of unipolar peak-negative voltage of <1.66 mV in the endocardium predicts the presence of an epicardial dense scar (<0.5 mV). However, the unipolar endocardial voltage threshold for an epicardial scar in the RV has been identified as ≤5.5 mV in ARVC patients.[40]

Very rarely, nonventricular arrhythmias have been targeted using an epicardial approach. Accessory pathways (specifically between the right appendage and RV) have been targeted as well, as in one case of resistant arrhythmia from the right pulmonary veins (PVs).[41,42]

Situations at Risk

The epicardial approach is associated with an increased risk for complications as reported in multicenter observational registries allowing the clarification of some relative contraindications. In general, all circumstances where a percutaneous pericardial puncture is challenging should be proscribed:

- Previous cardiac surgery increases the risk and limits the feasibility. However, it has been used, as reported by some expert centers. In addition to the challenging pericardial puncture, pericardial adhesions limit mapping and can cause significant bleeding if they are torn. They are more frequently found in the anterior aspect of the LV.[43] It is our opinion that percutaneous epicardial access should probably not be performed in patients with previous cardiac surgery, particularly in cases of previous coronary artery bypass grafting (CABG) and when the operator is less experienced. It is safer to ask a surgeon to perform a subxiphoid/laterothoracic window and eliminate the adhesions.
- The presence of organomegaly (hepatomegaly, splenomegaly, occlusive syndrome) exposes the patient to a major risk for infradiaphragmatic injuries.
- Patients with ventricular assist devices requiring compulsory anticoagulation can be exposed to a fatal hemorrhage risk.
- Morbid obesity can prolong the needle route, change its angle of penetration, and challenge the subcostal approach.

In contrast, repeated procedures using epicardial access have not been associated with increased risk.[44]

Alternatives to be considered when percutaneous access is not possible include the following:

- A classical surgical approach (sternotomy, mini-invasive procedure, subxiphoid access) allows a good exposition of most target sites.[45]
- Some other techniques have been proposed, such as endocardial puncture through the right appendage or a direct intercostal access,[46,47] but this remains anecdotal.

Practical Aspects

Preparation

The procedure is currently performed in the electrophysiology lab, with surgical backup. Prior anticoagulation is stopped or in some circumstances reversed. Epicardial percutaneous puncture is performed best before any anticoagulation. An imaging procedure (MRI or CT scan) can help in case of abnormal anatomical landmarks.

Cardiac CT localizes coronary arteries, veins, nerves (phrenic), and myocardial wall thinning area as a surrogate for a scar when good-quality MRI is precluded by presence of an implantable cardioverter defibrillator (ICD) and influences the ablation strategy.[48–50]

General anesthesia is not mandatory, but epicardial access and mapping are painful, necessitating premedication and powerful analgesics. A long-acting paralytic agent should not be used during general anesthesia.

After careful cutaneous disinfection, an operative field covers the upper part of the patient except the xiphoid process and 5 cm below it. Antibiotic prophylaxis is not done in every patient.

Access

The puncture is commonly performed with a hollow atraumatic, curved-tip Tuohy needle (Tuohy bevel, 18 gauge, 1.3 × 80 or 150 mm; Braun, Kronberg, Germany).

Additional materials needed are as follows:

- An iodine injection, which confirms the good location of the needle once it crosses the pericardial membranes and splits them, making it easy for guidewire progression
- More than 1-m-long guidewire 0.32
- A 10-French (Fr) introducer for predilation
- A deflectable small-curve sheath, which may facilitate mapping and catheter contact on the epicardium
- A pressure sensor or an ECG analyzer, which may be connected to the needle to facilitate the puncture and prevent myocardial injury

The needle direction above the operating field is changed according to the radioscopic anteroposterior view toward the mesocardiac area. Endocardiac leads (diagnostic or defibrillation leads) are good landmarks in the frontal plane.

After local anesthesia, the puncture is made 1 to 2 cm below the xiphoid process on the midline with an angle of 20 to 40 degrees. At the same time, a mild abdominal depression helps move away the hepatic lobe and digestive system.

Afterward, among many techniques, we prefer the use of a left lateral view to visualize the xiphoid process and the upper part of the sternum, the cardiac silhouette and the middle part of the diaphragmatic dome, and the lung lightness in the lower part (Fig. 128.5). This is the only view that really allows one to control the needle depth throughout the entire route, from the skin to the pericardium. This is a major safety aspect, as by maintaining a route that is right below the sternum, the needle will never enter the abdominal space, and all related complications can be avoided.

Transiently increased x-ray penetrance and image rate may improve the definition of different component boundaries.

Starting from the cutaneous plane, the needle crosses the following successively:

- The cutaneous plane
- The superficial fascia
- The anterior rectus sheath/linea alba
- The rectus abdominis muscle
- The posterior rectus sheath
- The diaphragmatic dome
- Parietal and serous fibrous pericardial membranes

For an anterior access, the needle heads to the RV free wall, with a more superficial direction. Subdiaphragmatic organ injuries are avoided this way. A puncture on the median line is necessary to avoid the internal mammal artery. A posterior access approach reaches the left ventricular posterior wall but increases the risk for deep organ injuries.

Heartbeats can be felt when the tip of the needle touches the radioscopic cardiac shadow. To cross the pleura and parietal pericardial layer, the needle may need more pressure. A light iodine injection localizes the needle position (diaphragmatic

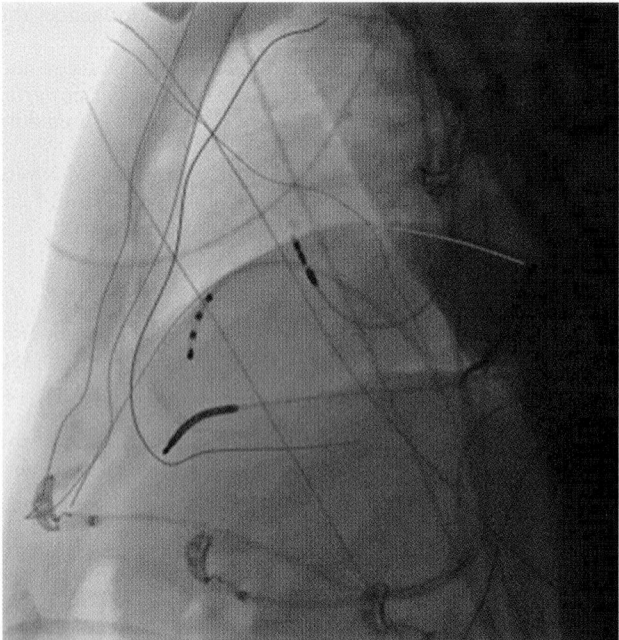

FIGURE 128.5 **X-ray profile view.** The *orange line* tags the sternum and xiphoid process, *blue line* cardiac silhouette (right ventricular free wall, left ventricular inferior wall), and *green line* diaphragmatic dome projection.

or intramyocardial if myography and pericardial space if heart molding iodine border). Importantly, radioscopic landmarks can be hidden by excessive contrast injection (Fig. 128.6A and B).

For safety reasons, a pressure sensor can be used to help identify an accidental intracardiac location, but this is not our current practice.[51]

An RV puncture rarely causes massive hemorrhage if the needle is mobilized in only a forward and backward move (Fig. 128.6C). Significant active bleeding is rather due to a coronary or diaphragmatic artery injury.

Another injection given during slow withdrawal of the needle may then split the pericardial membranes, allowing for pericardial catheterization and thereby avoiding a repeated puncture. The guidewire is then pushed through the needle with limited resistance, if any, and buckled in the pericardial space around the heart silhouette. No overlap is found with the lung lightness in at least two incidences, particularly in the left anterior oblique view (Fig. 128.6D). Importantly, the route of the guidewire should never be compatible with an intracardiac location. A guidewire over the lung frame means a pleural location and has to be withdrawn, but usually without clinical significance. Before introducing the sheath over the wire, a predilatation facilitates the subcutaneous and subcostal path.

The constant presence of a catheter or a guidewire in the sheath is necessary to prevent cardiac tissue laceration.

We use a smooth aspiration between the sheath and a wall outlet for fluid drainage. It also immediately alerts the occurrence of bleeding.

Many different irrigated tip ablation catheters or multipolar diagnostic catheters can be introduced through the sheath. The lack of natural cooling forces the use of irrigated tip ablation catheters to limit the temperature increase and effectively ablate.[52]

Some groups also use the micropuncture or "needle-in-the-needle" technique, described as follows:[53]

1. Subxiphoid insertion of an 18-gauge Cook needle is made through superficial tissue to a point just before the cardiac silhouette.
2. A 21-gauge micropuncture needle is inserted through the 18-gauge Cook needle.
3. The 21-gauge needle alone is used to enter the pericardial space while maintaining the position of the Cook needle steady with the aid of contrast, fluoroscopy, and tactile sensation for entry into the pericardial space.
4. A 0.18-gauge guidewire with a floppy tip (HiTorqueSteel-core 18 guidewire with a microglide coating, 0.018 inch, 190 cm; Abbott Vascular, Santa Clara, CA) is then advanced through the 21-gauge needle into the pericardial space. As with the Sosa technique, confirmation that the wire is in the pericardial

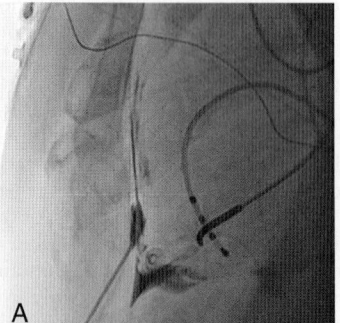
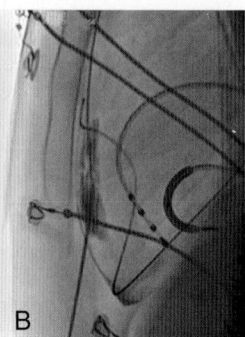
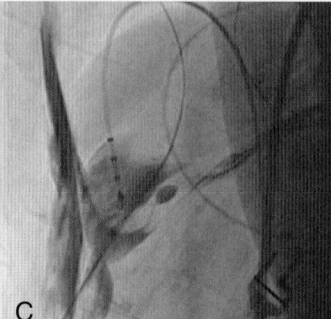
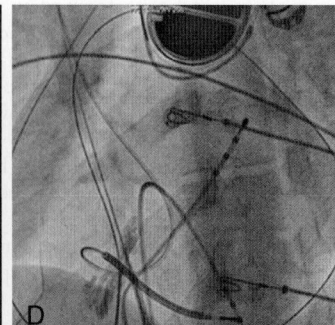

FIGURE 128.6 (A) Intrapericardial puncture with a heart molding contrast injection. (B) Intramyocardial puncture with right ventricular wall myography. (C) Intraventricular puncture confirmed by contrast injection and abnormal guidewire route. (D) Anteroposterior view. Guidewire loops largely circling the heart shadow.

space is obtained by demonstrating using fluoroscopy that the wire crosses multiple cardiac chambers and hugs the border of the lateral left cardiac silhouette in the left anterior oblique projection.

5. Both needles are then removed, and a micropuncture dilator is advanced into the pericardial space over the 0.18-gauge guidewire and exchanged for a 6- or 8-Fr dilator.

6. Confirmation of pericardial entry is again obtained using contrast and/or fluid aspiration.

7. The 0.18-gauge guidewire is exchanged for a 0.35-inch floppy tip Bentsonwire (CookMedical).

8. An 8-Fr sheath with dilator is inserted over the 0.35-inch wire.

Mapping

A three-dimensional mapping system may help reduce x-ray exposure and improve spatial tracking (especially with an imaging merge).

In our experience, the contact force data made available recently on the mapping system are very useful, particularly for epicardial mapping. The contact vector provides crucial information confirming that the ablation catheter is in contact with the cardiac surface (muscle) and not pushing against the fibrous pericardium, compromising both safety and efficacy. When epicardial mapping is considered, the natural tendency of the mapping catheter is to push against the most external structure, i.e., the pericardial sac. Therefore the absolute value of the contact force is not relevant and attention should first be drawn to the vector of the contact force.[54]

The bipolar voltage value range for defining a scar tissue should be modified for epicardial mapping: 1 mV should be the upper value for healthy tissue, and 0.5 mV for dense scar.[28]

Of note, however, insufficient contact or extensive fatty deposit may lead to misidentification of the scar location. Therefore a signal analysis rather than voltage value is the main element to take into account.

Mapping distortion or catheter malpositioning can occur with development of progressive and significant pericardial effusion and the use of an impedance field–based system. Continuous aspiration or mapping without cool flow irrigation may prevent this problem.

Ablation

Ablation and irrigation setup can vary (20–50 W). The amount of contact as well as the interposition of fat may affect lesion depth and size. Moreover, presence of a coronary vessel ≤5 mm to the ablation tip should be considered,[55] especially if the target zone is basal, close to the interventricular groove, or in a periannular region, and should preclude ablation (eFig. 128.3).

The left phrenic nerve route is close to the left appendage and the anterolateral ventricular wall and should be carefully tagged with the help of high-output pacing to avoid postoperative diaphragmatic paralysis. Upper-level phrenic stimulation (left appendage) can be used to monitor diaphragmatic contraction during ablation. The presence of myocardial wall <5 mm thick (identified by CT scan and merged in a three-dimensional electroanatomical system) allows transmural ablation from the endocardium and therefore prevents epicardial structure damage compared with epicardial energy delivery.[56]

As a rule, we always start the ablation with endocardial attempts for safety reasons and to reduce as much as possible epicardial RF delivery, acknowledging a much higher risk for extracardiac damage with this approach.

An additional important point is to ascertain the absence of air in the pericardium before VT/VF induction because it could prevent an effective cardioversion.[57]

Postprocedure

After fluid aspiration, the catheter is usually removed in an attempt to reduce risks for inflammation/infection. In some centers, corticosteroids are infused in the pericardium. It does not affect the postoperative pericarditis rate but reduces pain significantly.[58]

Analgesic/oral nonsteroidal antiinflammatory drugs or colchicine is routinely given after the procedure. Cardiac echography is typically performed at day 1 or in case of symptoms.

Results

Access

The epicardial procedure is restricted to expert centers for safety reasons and also because these procedures are rare and should not be used in low-volume centers. The success rate is usually important.

In a single-center North American series, access was obtained in 89.3% of 149 procedures.[59] In Europe, Della Bella et al. reported a success rate of 97.2% with 218 patients in 6 high-volume centers.[60]

In another observational study, >87.2% success was reached in 156 procedures in three centers.[16] Other smaller, single-center series have reported 93.3%–95% good results.[61] Most failures are due to a prior cardiac surgery or pericarditis (in 80% of cases).

Epicardial Ablation Success

Epicardial ablation is overall effective, with a 70% mean acute success rate. Postprocedure results are summarized in Table 128.2.[12,16,59,60] These results have been categorized by substrate origin, as discussed next.

Ischemic Cardiomyopathy

A systematic epicardial access in case of an ischemic cardiomyopathy does not achieve any evident benefit unless a previous endocardial ablation has failed.[62]

TABLE 128.2 **Epicardial ablation acute results**

REFERENCE	NO. OF PATIENTS	TYPE OF PROCEDURE	SUCCESS (%)	NONINDUCIBILITY (%)	OTHER TACHYCARDIA INDUCIBILITY (%)	NOT TESTED
Schmidt et al.[12]	59	VT	78	46	32	NA
Roberts-Thomson et al.[59]	137	VT and SVT	80	50	30	6.8
Della Bella et al.[60]	218	VT	71.6	71.6	NA	NA
Sacher et al.[16]	156	VT	71	NA	NA	NA

NA, Nonaddressed; *SVT*, supraventricular tachycardia; *VT*, ventricular tachycardia.

TABLE 128.3 Nonischemic cardiomyopathy ventricular tachycardia ablation midterm results

	NO. OF PATIENTS	FOLLOW-UP	RESULTS
Nakahara et al.[27]	12	15 months	50%
Soejima et al.[34]	8	115 ± 49 days	57%
Cano et al.[28]	14	18 months	71%

Nonischemic Cardiomyopathy

The success rate ranges from 50% to 71% (Table 128.3[27,28,34]). An endoepicardial approach gives better results than with endocardial ablation alone (57% recurrence free at 115 ± 49 days vs. 46% at 1 year).[34]

Arrhythmogenic Right Ventricular Dysplasia

Some studies have shown that a combined endoepicardial substrate–guided ablation in patients with ARVC could improve the procedure results and midterm outcomes. Bai et al. compared endocardial with double access in 49 procedures; 26 patients (100%) in the epicardial group had a significant substrate. After a 3-month follow-up, positive results were 84.6% in the second group versus 69.2% in the first one without any antiarrhythmic treatment.[32] In another series,[63] mid- and long-term results showed a better outcome with epicardial ablation in 30 patients (follow-up of 88.3 ± 66.1 months): VT-free survival was 83% at 6 months, 76% at 12 months, and 70% at 24 months. Fernandez-Armanta et al.[25] reported 13.6% VT recurrence after a mean follow-up of 28 ± 18 months.

Hypertrophic Cardiomyopathies

Despite a limited VT-treated population, Dukkipati et al. found positive results. After 37 ± 17 months (median, 37 months), the freedom from recurrent ICD shocks was 78% (7/9 patients) in those who underwent ablation.[23] Santangeli et al. reported similar results with 77% success at 1-year follow-up.[21]

Myocarditis Sequelae

An epicardial ablation procedure in a postmyocarditis population had good results in a report by Berte et al. After a mean follow-up of 28 ± 16 months, recurrence of VT was seen in only 16.7% of cases.[29]

Complications

In addition to the expected complications associated with an endocardial ablation procedure, complications attributable to the epicardial approach are listed in Box 128.1.[10,12,48,61,64,65] The most frequent are detailed next.

Early Complications Related to the Puncture

Pericardial Bleeding

Because of the presence of small superficial vessels, the puncture usually causes a limited bloody-colored effusion but always of small volume (<80 mL). Ventricular puncture may occur in up to 17%, but massive bleeding is not frequent. It may be the result of improper needle handling or an inappropriate sheath introduction.

Coronary vessel laceration is unusual but may cause uncontrollable bleeding requiring surgical repair. Prolonged angioplasty balloon occlusion or placement of a covered stent has resolved some emergency situations.[66] Transient bleeding can also be due to postsurgical or inflammatory adherence trauma. Although extremely rare, fatal hemorrhage can occur.[67] If significant bleeding is observed, anticoagulation should be reversed and

---

BOX 128.1 Summary of main early and late complications occurring during epicardial ablation

Potential Early Complications
Pericardial effusion
    Right or left ventricular puncture
    Epicardial ablation bleb
    Coronary vessel laceration
    Sheath mechanical injury
Abdominal injury
    Hepatic, splenic, biliary tree laceration
    Subdiaphragmatic vessel injury
    Stomach, intestine perforation
Pulmonary injury
    Pleuropericardial fistula
    Pulmonary parenchymal puncture
Nerve injury
    Phrenic nerve lesion with diaphragmatic paralysis
    Vagal nerve lesion
    Recurrent laryngeal nerve lesion
Coronary vasospasm and ventricular fibrillation

Potential Late Complications
Recurrent pericarditis
Late pericardial effusion
Constrictive pericarditis
Coronary stenosis

---

the pericardium continuously aspirated. In most situations, bleeding stops spontaneously, allowing the procedure to continue.

Infradiaphragmatic Injuries

Infradiaphragmatic injuries are probably more frequent with a posterior access. Puncture can cause hematoma in solid organs or pneumoperitoneum and/or peritonitis in case of digestive tract perforation. Subcutaneous or digestive vessels can also be inadvertently punctured, with the potential for significant bleeding. With a silent evolution, such injuries sometimes cause a delayed fall in hemoglobin or hemorrhagic shock. The presence of abdominal pain after such a procedure should trigger an emergency imaging procedure.

Pleuropulmonary Complications

Pleuropulmonary complications are infrequent. The guidewire may enter the pleural space without any consequence. Nevertheless, pleuropericardial fistula has been reported.[68]

Early Complications Related to the Ablation

Adjacent structures (coronary vessels, phrenic nerve, lungs, bronchi, etc.) and all cardiac layers can be affected. The left phrenic nerve can be injured in case of RF/cryoapplications over its course (it crosses the anterolateral ventricular wall). Such injury could result in left phrenic nerve palsy with hemidiaphragmatic paralysis and consequent dyspnea or respiratory insufficiency. When mapping over the epicardial lateral LV wall, it is important to identify the phrenic nerve course and tag it using an electroanatomical mapping system. Cardiac CT scan merge may help identify its course. Pacing in an upper location (left appendage, left subclavian vein) enables continuous safety monitoring.[21]

Different strategies have been proposed to remove it far from the ablation site. A very slow infusion of air–sodium chloride mixture up to the loss of the pacing capture is an effective technique.[69] Nevertheless, care is required, and the inflated air has to be drained to avoid the risk for direct current cardioversion failure in case of VT/VF induction. The main coronary arteries (circumflex and right and left anterior descending arteries) have an epicardial location, necessitating caution in case of a nearby ablation site.[55] Preablation coronary angiography identifies precisely the distance between the ablation catheter and the coronary artery, and this distance for a safe ablation is probably around 5 mm. An accurate merge of CT scan images displaying coronary arteries may facilitate ablation in areas where coronary artery is present. Adjacent organ injuries are not well known because they are often silent. However, some animal experimental data have shown parenchymal lung lesions. Esophagus is almost never of concern because of the lack of ablation needs in this region and the particular anatomy (cul-de-sac of oblique and transverse sinuses).

Postprocedure Complications

Pain can occur in the early postoperative period, and analgesic and antiinflammatory medications are needed. In situ corticosteroid infusions may reduce the pain level.[58] Supplemental oral treatment can be given for a few weeks. In some reported cases, pericardiocentesis was needed for refractory painful chronic pericarditis treatment. A chronic inflammatory mechanism may cause recurrent abundant pericardial effusion. The size of the effusion and the degree of clinical effect will dictate the need for drainage. Some atrial arrhythmia related to inflammation may occur.[70]

Conclusion

Percutaneous epicardial access is a valuable adjunct for catheter ablation of complex arrhythmias. Depending on the underlying substrate, it may be used as a first-line strategy for VT ablation in ARVC and postmyocarditis particularly. However, knowledge of potential complications and pertinent preventive measures is vital to ensure safe implementation of the procedure. Cardiac imaging (MRI and CT scans) is extremely useful for substrate and anatomical structure identification.

REFERENCES

1. Brusca A, Magri G. Direct epicardial electrocardiography from the exposed human heart in cases of right bundle branch block. *Acta Cardiol*. 1956;11:274–281.
2. Durrer D, Roos JP. Epicardial excitation of the ventricles in a patient with Wolff-Parkinson-White syndrome (type B). *Circulation*. 1967;35:15–21.
3. Wellens HJ, Janse MJ, van Dam RT, et al. Epicardial excitation of the atria in a patient with atrial flutter. *Br Heart J*. 1971;33:233–237.
4. Waldo AL, Ross SM, Kaiser GA. The epicardial electrogram in the diagnosis of cardiac arrhythmias following cardiac surgery. *Geriatrics*. 1971;26:108–112.
5. Wellens HJ, Janse MJ, Van Dam RT, et al. Epicardial mapping and surgical treatment in Wolff-Parkinson-White syndrome Type A. *Am Heart J*. 1974;88:69–78.
6. Fontaine G, Guiraudon G, Frank R, et al. Epicardial cartography and surgical treatment by simple ventriculotomy of certain resistant re-entry ventricular tachycardias. *Arch Mal Coeur Vaiss*. 1975;68:113–124.
7. Horowitz LN, Harken AH, Kastor JA, et al. Ventricular resection guided by epicardial and endocardial mapping for treatment of recurrent ventricular tachycardia. *N Engl J Med*. 1980;302:589–593.
8. Kuck KH, Kunze KP, Schluter M, et al. Modification of a left-sided accessory atrioventricular pathway by radiofrequency current using a bipolar epicardial-endocardial electrode configuration. *Eur Heart J*. 1988;9:927–932.
9. Sosa E, Scanavacca M, d'Avila A, et al. A new technique to perform epicardial mapping in the electrophysiology laboratory. *J Cardiovasc Electrophysiol*. 1996;7:531–536.
10. Lim HS, Sacher F, Cochet H, et al. Safety and prevention of complications during percutaneous epicardial access for the ablation of cardiac arrhythmias. *Heart Rhythm*. 2014;11:1658–1665.
11. Schweikert RA, Saliba WI, Tomassoni G, et al. Percutaneous pericardial instrumentation for endo-epicardial mapping of previously failed ablations. *Circulation*. 2003;108:1329–1335.
12. Schmidt B, Chun KR, Baensch D, et al. Catheter ablation for ventricular tachycardia after failed endocardial ablation: epicardial substrate or inappropriate endocardial ablation? *Heart Rhythm*. 2010;7:1746–1752.
13. Berruezo A, Mont L, Nava S, et al. Electrocardiographic recognition of the epicardial origin of ventricular tachycardias. *Circulation*. 2004;109:1842–1847.
14. Bazan V, Gerstenfeld EP, Garcia FC, et al. Site-specific twelve-lead ECG features to identify an epicardial origin for left ventricular tachycardia in the absence of myocardial infarction. *Heart Rhythm*. 2007;4:1403–1410.
15. Valles E, Bazan V, Marchlinski FE. ECG criteria to identify epicardial ventricular tachycardia in nonischemic cardiomyopathy. *Circ Arrhythm Electrophysiol*. 2010;3:63–71.
16. Sacher F, Roberts-Thomson K, Maury P, et al. Epicardial ventricular tachycardia ablation: a multicenter safety study. *J Am Coll Cardiol*. 2010;55:2366–2372.
17. Henz BD, do Nascimento TA, Dietrich Cde O, et al. Simultaneous epicardial and endocardial substrate mapping and radiofrequency catheter ablation as first-line treatment for ventricular tachycardia and frequent ICD shocks in chronic chagasic cardiomyopathy. *J Interv Card Electrophysiol*. 2009;26:195–205.
18. Sosa E, Scanavacca M, D'Avila A, et al. Radiofrequency catheter ablation of ventricular tachycardia guided by nonsurgical epicardial mapping in chronic Chagasic heart disease. *Pacing Clin Electrophysiol*. 1999;22:128–130.
19. Dello Russo A, Casella M, Pieroni M, et al. Drug-refractory ventricular tachycardias after myocarditis: endocardial and epicardial radiofrequency catheter ablation. *Circ Arrhythm Electrophysiol*. 2012;5:492–498.
20. Ueda A, Fukamizu S, Soejima K, et al. Clinical and electrophysiological characteristics in patients with sustained monomorphic reentrant ventricular tachycardia associated with dilated-phase hypertrophic cardiomyopathy. *Europace*. 2012;14:734–740.
21. Santangeli P, Marchlinski FE, Zado ES, et al. Percutaneous epicardial ablation of ventricular arrhythmias arising from the left ventricular summit: outcomes and electrocardiogram correlates of success. *Circ Arrhythm Electrophysiol*. 2015;8:337–343.
22. Inada K, Seiler J, Roberts-Thomson KC, et al. Substrate characterization and catheter ablation for monomorphic ventricular tachycardia in patients with apical hypertrophic cardiomyopathy. *J Cardiovasc Electrophysiol*. 2011;22:41–48.
23. Dukkipati SR, d'Avila A, Soejima K, et al. Long-term outcomes of combined epicardial and endocardial ablation of monomorphic ventricular tachycardia related to hypertrophic cardiomyopathy. *Circ Arrhythm Electrophysiol*. 2011;4:185–194.
24. Sarkozy A, Tokuda M, Tedrow UB, et al. Epicardial ablation of ventricular tachycardia in ischemic heart disease. *Circ Arrhythm Electrophysiol*. 2013;6:1115–1122.
25. Fernandez-Armenta J, Andreu D, Penela D, et al. Sinus rhythm detection of conducting channels and ventricular tachycardia isthmus in arrhythmogenic right ventricular cardiomyopathy. *Heart Rhythm*. 2014;11:747–754.
26. Haqqani HM, Tschabrunn CM, Betensky BP, et al. Layered activation of epicardial scar in arrhythmogenic right ventricular dysplasia: possible substrate for confined epicardial circuits. *Circ Arrhythm Electrophysiol*. 2012;5:796–803.
27. Nakahara S, Tung R, Ramirez RJ, et al. Characterization of the arrhythmogenic substrate in ischemic and nonischemic cardiomyopathy implications for catheter ablation of hemodynamically unstable ventricular tachycardia. *J Am Coll Cardiol*. 2010;55:2355–2365.
28. Cano O, Hutchinson M, Lin D, et al. Electroanatomic substrate and ablation outcome for suspected epicardial ventricular tachycardia in left ventricular nonischemic cardiomyopathy. *J Am Coll Cardiol*. 2009;54:799–808.
29. Berte B, Sacher F, Cochet H, et al. Postmyocarditis ventricular tachycardia in patients with epicardial-only scar: a specific entity requiring a specific approach. *J Cardiovasc Electrophysiol*. 2015;26:42–50.
30. Garcia FC, Bazan V, Zado ES, et al. Epicardial substrate and outcome with epicardial ablation of ventricular tachycardia in arrhythmogenic right ventricular cardiomyopathy/dysplasia. *Circulation*. 2009;120:366–375.
31. Philips B, Madhavan S, James C, et al. Outcomes of catheter ablation of ventricular tachycardia in arrhythmogenic right ventricular dysplasia/cardiomyopathy. *Circ Arrhythm Electrophysiol*. 2012;5:499–505.
32. Bai R, Di Biase L, Shivkumar K, et al. Ablation of ventricular arrhythmias in arrhythmogenic right ventricular dysplasia/cardiomyopathy: arrhythmia-free survival after endo-epicardial substrate based mapping and ablation. *Circ Arrhythm Electrophysiol*. 2011;4:478–485.
33. Komatsu Y, Jadidi A, Sacher F, et al. Relationship between MDCT-imaged myocardial fat and ventricular tachycardia substrate in arrhythmogenic right ventricular cardiomyopathy. *J Am Heart Assoc*. 2014:3.
34. Soejima K, Stevenson WG, Sapp JL, et al. Endocardial and epicardial radiofrequency ablation of ventricular tachycardia associated with dilated cardiomyopathy: the importance of low-voltage scars. *J Am Coll Cardiol*. 2004;43:1834–1842.
35. Morita H, Zipes DP, Morita ST, et al. Epicardial ablation eliminates ventricular arrhythmias in an experimental model of Brugada syndrome. *Heart Rhythm*. 2009;6:665–671.
36. Nademanee K, Veerakul G, Chandanamattha P, et al. Prevention of ventricular fibrillation episodes in Brugada syndrome by catheter ablation over the anterior right ventricular outflow tract epicardium. *Circulation*. 2011;123:1270–1279.
37. Lim HE, Pak HN, Shim WJ, et al. Epicardial ablation of ventricular tachycardia associated with isolated ventricular noncompaction. *Pacing Clin Electrophysiol*. 2006;29:797–799.
38. Tzou WS, Nguyen DT, Aleong RG, et al. Endocardial electrogram characteristics of epicardial ventricular arrhythmias. *J Cardiovasc Electrophysiol*. 2013;24:649–654.
39. Hutchinson MD, Gerstenfeld EP, Desjardins B, et al. Endocardial unipolar voltage mapping to detect epicardial ventricular tachycardia substrate in patients with nonischemic left ventricular cardiomyopathy. *Circ Arrhythm Electrophysiol*. 2011;4:49–55.
40. Polin GM, Haqqani H, Tzou W, et al. Endocardial unipolar voltage mapping to identify epicardial substrate in arrhythmogenic right ventricular cardiomyopathy/dysplasia. *Heart Rhythm*. 2011;8:76–83.
41. Lam C, Schweikert R, Kanagaratnam L, et al. Radiofrequency ablation of a right atrial appendage-ventricular accessory pathway by transcutaneous epicardial instrumentation. *J Cardiovasc Electrophysiol*. 2000;11:1170–1173.
42. Reddy VY, Neuzil P, Ruskin JN. Extra-ostial pulmonary venous isolation: use of epicardial ablation to eliminate a point of conduction breakthrough. *J Cardiovasc Electrophysiol*. 2003;14:663–666.
43. Tschabrunn CM, Haqqani HM, Cooper JM, et al. Percutaneous epicardial ventricular tachycardia ablation after noncoronary cardiac surgery or pericarditis. *Heart Rhythm*. 2013;10:165–169.
44. Tschabrunn CM, Haqqani HM, Zado ES, et al. Repeat percutaneous epicardial mapping and ablation of ventricular tachycardia: safety and outcome. *J Cardiovasc Electrophysiol*. 2012;23:744–749.
45. Soejima K, Couper G, Cooper JM, et al. Subxiphoid surgical approach for epicardial catheter-based mapping and ablation in patients with prior cardiac surgery or difficult pericardial access. *Circulation*. 2004;110:1197–1201.
46. Hsieh CH, Thomas SP, Ross DL. Direct transthoracic access to the left ventricle for catheter ablation of ventricular tachycardia. *Circ Arrhythm Electrophysiol*. 2010;3:178–185.
47. Scanavacca MI, Venancio AC, Pisani CF, et al. Percutaneous transatrial access to the pericardial space for epicardial mapping and ablation. *Circ Arrhythm Electrophysiol*. 2011;4:331–336.
48. Yamashita S, Sacher F, Mahida S, et al. Role of high-resolution image integration to visualize left phrenic nerve and coronary arteries during epicardial ventricular tachycardia ablation. *Circ Arrhythm Electrophysiol*. 2015;8:371–380.
49. Njeim M, Yokokawa M, Frank L, et al. Value of cardiac magnetic resonance imaging in patients with failed ablation procedures for ventricular tachycardia. *J Cardiovasc Electrophysiol*. 2016;27:183–189.

50. Cochet H, Komatsu Y, Sacher F, et al. Integration of merged delayed-enhanced magnetic resonance imaging and multidetector computed tomography for the guidance of ventricular tachycardia ablation: a pilot study. *J Cardiovasc Electrophysiol.* 2013;24:419–426.

51. Mahapatra S, Tucker-Schwartz J, Wiggins D, et al. Pressure frequency characteristics of the pericardial space and thorax during subxiphoid access for epicardial ventricular tachycardia ablation. *Heart Rhythm.* 2010;7:604–609.

52. d'Avila A, Houghtaling C, Gutierrez P, et al. Catheter ablation of ventricular epicardial tissue: a comparison of standard and cooled-tip radiofrequency energy. *Circulation.* 2004;109:2363–2369.

53. Kumar S, Bazaz R, Barbhaiya CR, et al. "Needle-in-needle" epicardial access: Preliminary observations with a modified technique for facilitating epicardial interventional procedures. *Heart Rhythm.* 2015;12:1691–1697.

54. Sacher F, Wright M, Derval N, et al. Endocardial versus epicardial ventricular radiofrequency ablation: utility of in vivo contact force assessment. *Circ Arrhythm Electrophysiol.* 2013;6:144–150.

55. D'Avila A, Gutierrez P, Scanavacca M, et al. Effects of radiofrequency pulses delivered in the vicinity of the coronary arteries: implications for nonsurgical transthoracic epicardial catheter ablation to treat ventricular tachycardia. *Pacing Clin Electrophysiol.* 2002;25:1488–1495.

56. Komatsu Y, Daly M, Sacher F, et al. Endocardial ablation to eliminate epicardial arrhythmia substrate in scar-related ventricular tachycardia. *J Am Coll Cardiol.* 2014;63:1416–1426.

57. Yamada T, McElderry HT, Platonov M, et al. Aspirated air in the pericardial space during epicardial catheterization may elevate the defibrillation threshold. *Int J Cardiol.* 2009;135:e34–e35.

58. Dyrda K, Piers SR, van Huls van Taxis CF, et al. Influence of steroid therapy on the incidence of pericarditis and atrial fibrillation after percutaneous epicardial mapping and ablation for ventricular tachycardia. *Circ Arrhythm Electrophysiol.* 2014;7:671–676.

59. Roberts-Thomson KC, Seiler J, Steven D, et al. Percutaneous access of the epicardial space for mapping ventricular and supraventricular arrhythmias in patients with and without prior cardiac surgery. *J Cardiovasc Electrophysiol.* 2010;21:406–411.

60. Della Bella P, Brugada J, Zeppenfeld K, et al. Epicardial ablation for ventricular tachycardia: a European multicenter study. *Circ Arrhythm Electrophysiol.* 2011;4:653–659.

61. Tung R, Michowitz Y, Yu R, et al. Epicardial ablation of ventricular tachycardia: an institutional experience of safety and efficacy. *Heart Rhythm.* 2013;10:490–498.

62. Izquierdo M, Sanchez-Gomez JM, Ferrero de Loma-Osorio A, et al. Endo-epicardial versus only-endocardial ablation as a first line strategy for the treatment of ventricular tachycardia in patients with ischemic heart disease. *Circ Arrhythm Electrophysiol.* 2015;8:882–889.

63. Philips B, te Riele AS, Sawant A, et al. Outcomes and ventricular tachycardia recurrence characteristics after epicardial ablation of ventricular tachycardia in arrhythmogenic right ventricular dysplasia/cardiomyopathy. *Heart Rhythm.* 2015;12:716–725.

64. Koruth JS, Aryana A, Dukkipati SR, et al. Unusual complications of percutaneous epicardial access and epicardial mapping and ablation of cardiac arrhythmias. *Circ Arrhythm Electrophysiol.* 2011;4:882–888.

65. Killu AM, Friedman PA, Mulpuru SK, et al. Atypical complications encountered with epicardial electrophysiological procedures. *Heart Rhythm.* 2013;10:1613–1621.

66. Roberts-Thomson KC, Steven D, Seiler J, et al. Coronary artery injury due to catheter ablation in adults: presentations and outcomes. *Circulation.* 2009;120:1465–1473.

67. Koruth JS, d'Avila A. Management of hemopericardium related to percutaneous epicardial access, mapping, and ablation. *Heart Rhythm.* 2011;8:1652–1657.

68. Mathuria N, Buch E, Shivkumar K. Pleuropericardial fistula formation after prior epicardial catheter ablation for ventricular tachycardia. *Circ Arrhythm Electrophysiol.* 2012;5:e18–e19.

69. Di Biase L, Burkhardt JD, Pelargonio G, et al. Prevention of phrenic nerve injury during epicardial ablation: comparison of methods for separating the phrenic nerve from the epicardial surface. *Heart Rhythm.* 2009;6:957–961.

70. Mahapatra S, LaPar DJ, Bhamidipati CM, et al. Incidence, risk factors, and consequences of new-onset atrial fibrillation following epicardial ablation for ventricular tachycardia. *Europace.* 2011;13:548–554.

129 Ventricular Fibrillation

Mélèze Hocini, Ashok J. Shah, Pippa McKelvie-Sebileau, and Michel Haïssaguerre

Ventricular fibrillation (VF) is an important cause of morbidity and sudden death (SD), yet it is one of the most difficult arrhythmias to effectively treat. The implantable cardioverter defibrillator (ICD) offers prolonged survival by protecting against death due to arrhythmia and is the gold standard treatment for primary and secondary prevention for at-risk patients. However, device implantation does not affect the underlying substrate. Furthermore, up to 20% of patients with an ICD experience recurrent episodes of VF or electrical storms, resulting in multiple device therapies, which not only deteriorate the quality of life[1] but also increase associated mortality.[2,3] Antiarrhythmic drugs such as amiodarone, β-blockers, and lidocaine have been used for life-threatening arrhythmias, including VF, but their efficacy has not yet been demonstrated on a large scale. Moreover, they are associated with various side effects, which often outweigh the uncertain prognostic benefit.

Catheter ablation of VF has been proposed as a strategy, after both drugs and ICD fail, for a subset of patients in whom the VF-triggering area can be identified. Since the 1980s, while various case reports have been published detailing the technical and clinical aspects of ablation, most of them have focused on ventricular arrhythmias, including VT and VF as a whole. The only international consensus document on ablation of ventricular arrhythmias largely focuses on ventricular tachycardia (VT) and provides limited information specifically for VF. Because of the inherent difficulties of studying the rapidly syncopal and strikingly lethal VF storms and the nonrepetitive nature of VF-initiating triggers, it is not surprising that there is just one literature review[4] and only four studies describing ablation of >10 VF patients[5-8] in the vast corpus of scientific literature. It should be noted that animal models of spontaneous VF are rare.

This chapter provides a comprehensive clinical review of catheter ablation of VF in patients with structural and nonstructural heart disease, offering detailed illustrations of various premature ventricular beat (PVB) origins and particularly focusing on the role of the Purkinje system in triggering and maintaining VF.

Ablation of Purkinje Triggers in Nonstructural Heart Disease

Coronary heart disease is the most frequent cause of clinically documented VF, accounting for around 80% of cases.[9] In approximately 6%–14% of patients, no documented heart disease or surface electrocardiogram (ECG) abnormalities can be identified when the first electrical storm occurs.[10,11] Patients experiencing primary VF with no evidence of structural heart disease can be classified according to five types: idiopathic long QT syndrome (LQTS), short QT syndrome, Brugada syndrome, early repolarization syndrome (ERS), and catecholaminergic polymorphic VT (CPVT), where the triggers are amenable to catheter ablation.

In this context, catheter ablation is offered in the rare cases of patients who, after surviving an out-of-hospital cardiac arrest and receiving an ICD, experience electrical storms or repeated shocks and do not respond to drug therapy. In addition, PVBs, which serve as triggers of VF, need to be identified on electrophysiology mapping to target ablation sites. Idiopathic VF accounts for 8% of victims of sudden cardiac death,[12] representing approximately 24,000 deaths per year in Europe.

Idiopathic Ventricular Fibrillation

The first successful ablation of triggered idiopathic VF reported immediate suppression of electrical storms after ablation of PVBs located in the posterolateral wall of the left ventricle (LV).[13] In one of the largest multicenter studies to date, Haïssaguerre et al.[5] described ablation of idiopathic VF by mapping and ablating PVBs with short coupling intervals initiating VF in 27 patients. The triggering PVBs were mapped and localized to the peripheral Purkinje system of both ventricles in 23 patients and to the right ventricular outflow tract (RVOT) myocardium in the remaining four.

The His-Purkinje system makes up a small fraction of the myocardial mass (<2%), consisting of specialized fibers insulated from the underlying ventricular myocardium until their peripheral arborization into muscle. The complex architecture, the specific transcriptional signatures and functional properties of His-Purkinje cells, including their intracellular calcium dynamics, underlie a disproportionately higher arrhythmogenic role in comparison with their total mass. The His-Purkinje system is specialized for rapid synchronous activation of both ventricles, and, as such, it is the most frequent site of VF initiation, which is usually initiated by a PVB during the vulnerable period of cardiac repolarization.[5,6,14,15] However, its role in the maintenance and triggering of arrhythmia mechanisms has not yet been fully characterized.[16]

Recording the 12-lead ECG of the triggering beat can prove invaluable in localizing the origin of the triggering PVB for more detailed subsequent mapping, and efforts to record such triggers should be routine for all patients. The probable optimal target site can be identified from the 12-lead ECG results. Premature beats that originate from the LV are positive in V_1 and usually have clinically important variations, mainly in limb leads, with a short QRS duration of <120 ms (Fig. 129.1). Premature beats that originate from the RV are negative in V_1, with inferior or

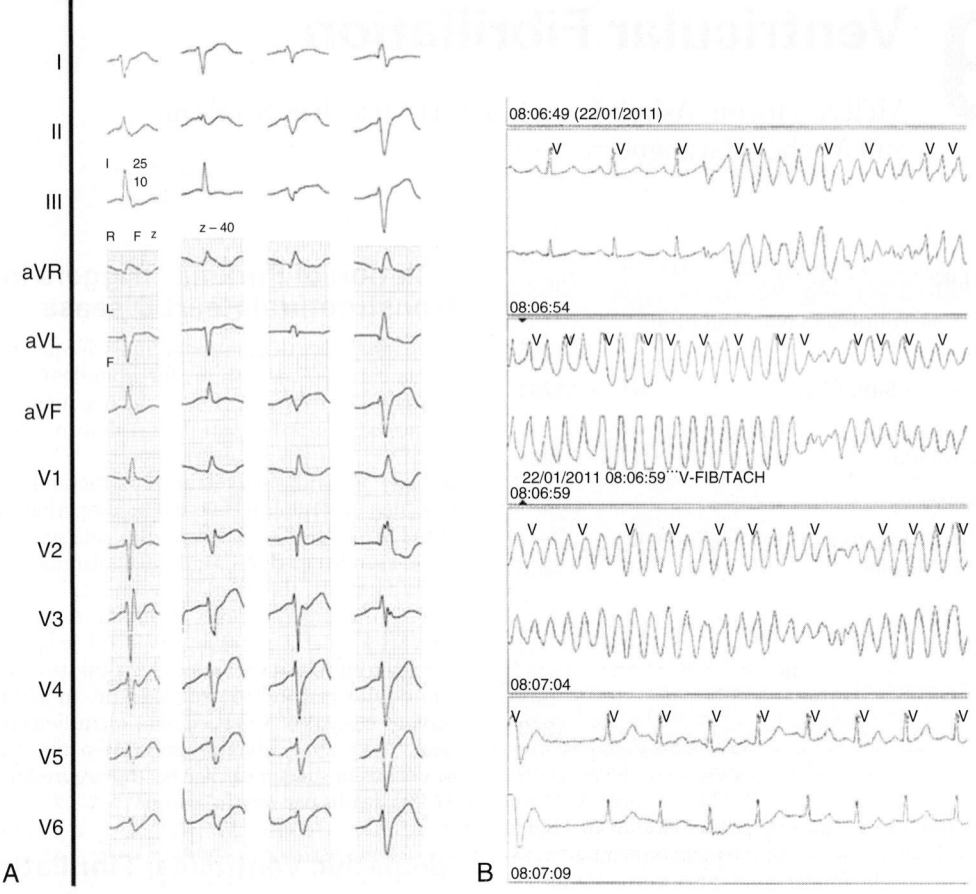

FIGURE 129.1 (A) Various 12-lead electrocardiogram morphologies of premature ventricular beats that originate in the left Purkinje system in the same patient. (B) Holter results showing a self-terminating episode of ventricular fibrillation triggered by short-coupled premature ventricular beat and demonstrating the R-on-T phenomenon.

superior axes, subtle morphological variations, and a longer QRS duration than beats that originated in the LV at ~145 ms.

During intracardiac mapping, the source of PVB triggers is localized by the earliest electrograms relative to the onset of the ectopic QRS complex. An initial sharp potential (<10 ms in duration) preceding the ventricular electrograms during sinus rhythm as well as during PVB indicates that the latter originates from the distal His-Purkinje arborization, whereas its absence at the site of earliest activation indicates an origin from ventricular muscle.[6] During premature beats, conduction delay from the Purkinje network to the myocardium was shorter in the RV than the LV, with variable conduction delays and dissociated Purkinje potentials in some patients.[6] Ectopy arising from the Purkinje system produces a characteristic 12-lead ECG pattern; PVBs originating in the right Purkinje system typically have a left bundle branch block pattern with left superior axis (Fig. 129.2). PVBs originating in the left Purkinje system produce more variable 12-lead ECG patterns, reflecting the more complex and extended Purkinje arborization on the left. During double or triple repetitive beats, each complex is preceded by a Purkinje potential, with variable conduction time. Radiofrequency (RF) current application targeting these Purkinje beats usually produces a spurt of the arrhythmia, including VF with subsequent disappearance of the premature beats and abolition of the local Purkinje potentials. After ablation, patients can develop nonspecific intraventricular conduction defects not meeting formal criteria for a bundle branch block.

In idiopathic polymorphic VF, Purkinje triggers are the primary target for ablation, but other initiating events have been demonstrated distinct from the cardiac conduction system (e.g.,

RVOT),[5] and a recent large series indicates that the LV outflow tract (LVOT) and papillary muscles may also be sites of origin of VF triggers.[17]

Outcome of Purkinje Ablation in Idiopathic Ventricular Fibrillation

Patient outcomes after ablation of idiopathic VF triggers are excellent compared with those after ablation of VT or VF with structural heart disease, and ablation can be curative.[18] Immediate (procedural) success rates range between 73% and 88%.[5–7,19] In a multicenter study with the longest available follow-up (63 months), 18% recurrence was observed, confirming that ablation for idiopathic VF, targeted at its potential ventricular ectopic triggers, may effectively prevent VF recurrence in this high-risk population.[7]

However, other than a handful of case reports[20–24] and the four series cited earlier, no randomized study is available. Follow-up durations are relatively short in all but one[7] of the studies.

Long QT Syndrome

In LQTS, the mechanism of VF appears to be focal ectopy and reentry.[25] Purkinje fibers have also been implicated.[26,27] In preclinical studies, prolonged ventricular repolarization (long QT interval) has been reproduced in anthopleurin-A–treated animals or animal models of inward rectifying K+ current (IKr) block.[28,29] In these models, Purkinje early afterdepolarizations were sources of torsades de pointes arrhythmias, with the twisting

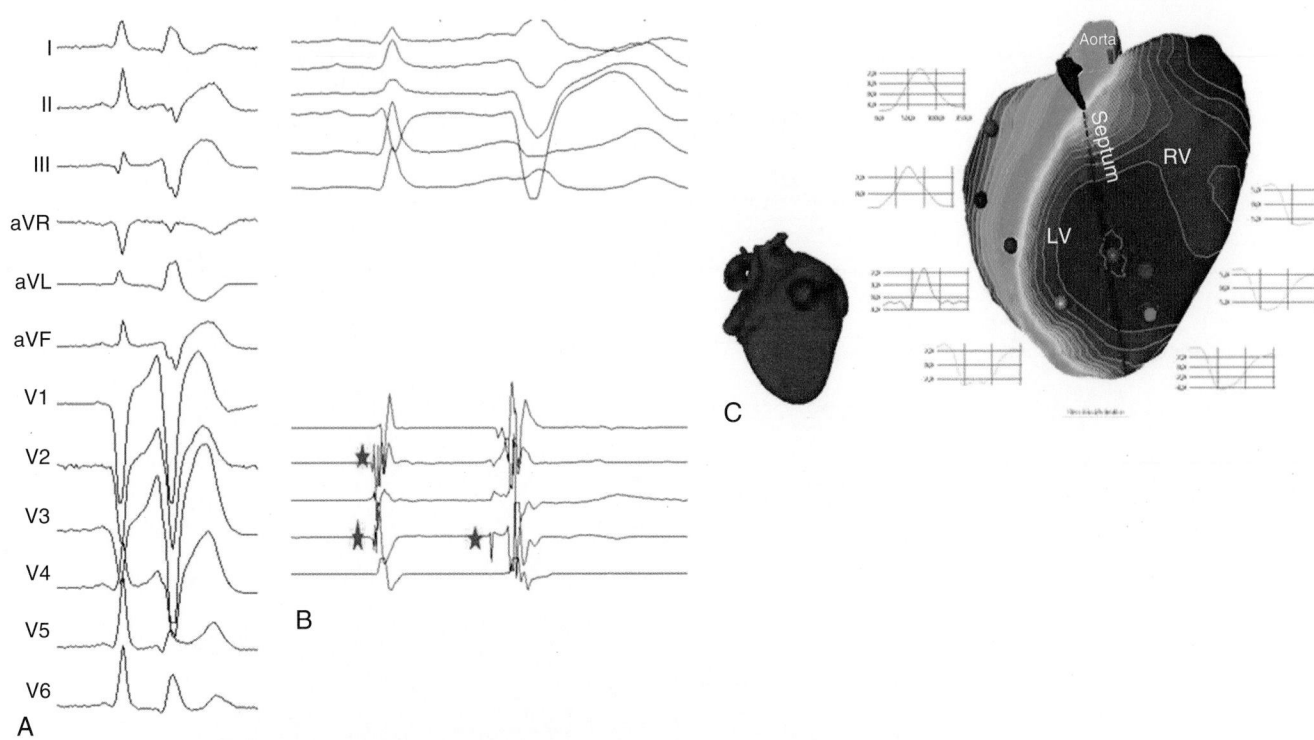

FIGURE 129.2 Idiopathic ventricular fibrillation originating from the right ventricular Purkinje tissue. (A) A 12-lead electrocardiogram showing short-coupled premature ventricular beat (PVB). Note the R-on-T phenomenon. (B) An intracardiac recording shows Purkinje potential (*stars*) in sinus rhythm and during PVB. Note the precocity of the sharp, narrow potential that triggers PVB. (C) ECVUE electrocardiographic mapping (CardioInsight Technologies, Cleveland, OH) of the culprit PVB shows its location in the posteroinferior midseptal region. Reconstructed unipolar local signals from various sites in the right ventricle (*RV*) and left ventricle (*LV*) are shown in *insets*. The QS morphology is noted at the source of PVB (color code: the earliest activation is depicted in *red* and subsequent ones in other sequential colors of the rainbow).

morphology being attributed to varying conduction delays in the myocardium.[28-30] Endocardial ablation suppressed spontaneous arrhythmias; however, new sources could generate arrhythmias, indicating that the Purkinje tissue was an important, but not the sole, trigger of long QT–related arrhythmias.[31]

Catheter ablation of culprit PVB–triggering VF may be necessary in patients with LQTS refractory to conventional treatment. Only three reports of ablation of VF in LQTS are available, all describing patients with congenital LQTS.[4,26,32] In our series,[26] we described VF ablation in four patients with LQTS. The triggering PVB was monomorphic in two patients and polymorphic and repetitive (sometimes bidirectional) with a positive QRS morphology in lead V_1 in the other two. The initiating PVB arose from the distal Purkinje fibers in three of four patients and from the RVOT in the remaining one. The latter was repetitive, lasting for 3–45 beats with varying cycle lengths of 280–420 ms. Ablation of triggers in the distal Purkinje fibers or RVOT and the LVOT resulted in excellent results with no recurrence during follow-up (18–24 months).

Brugada Syndrome

Mechanisms of VF in Brugada syndrome are conflicting, and it is not clear whether it is a re- or depolarization disorder. The repolarization hypothesis is based on transmural inhomogeneity with epicardial action potentials shorter than those in the endocardium. It leads to short-coupled PVBs that may induce VF mediated by phase 2 reentry in a canine RV wedge preparation.[25] The depolarization hypothesis observes conduction slowing with localized conduction delay in the RVOT as the likely mechanism of VF.[33] The ablation targets are generally located in the

RVOT[26,34-37] or more rarely in the Purkinje system.[26] The largest prospective study to date included nine patients with 20 ± 6 months of follow-up.[35] In this study, the depolarization substrate was characterized by abnormal low-voltage fractionated ventricular electrograms that have a markedly delayed conduction and a markedly prolonged duration. These abnormal electrograms were exclusively localized in a cluster over the epicardium of the anterior aspect of the RVOT. Catheter ablation targeting the abnormal arrhythmogenic substrate suppressed any further VT/VF episodes in eight of nine patients. Interestingly, catheter ablation in the RVOT resulted in normalization of the Brugada ECG pattern in five of nine patients. Shah and Hocini[37] also described abolition of the ECG pattern of Brugada syndrome immediately after ablation of the substrate in anteroseptal and lateral RVOT in one patient. The ECG has shown no reappearance of the Brugada pattern after almost 7 years of follow-up, suggestive of a potential role of ablation in curing the primary electrical disorder.

Early Repolarization Syndrome

The pathophysiological basis of the ER pattern is not fully understood. A prevailing theory presumes that J-point elevation arises because of a more pronounced phase that is one notch of the epicardial action potential relative to that of the endocardium, which manifests as J-point elevation.[38] With regard to the mechanism underlying ventricular arrhythmogenesis, it is likely that the dispersion of repolarization associated with ER increases susceptibility to phase 2 reentry.[38] The result is a premature ventricular contraction that interacts with a susceptible ventricular substrate to trigger transmural reentry. To date, the largest report on out-of-hospital cardiac arrests in patients with idiopathic VF involved

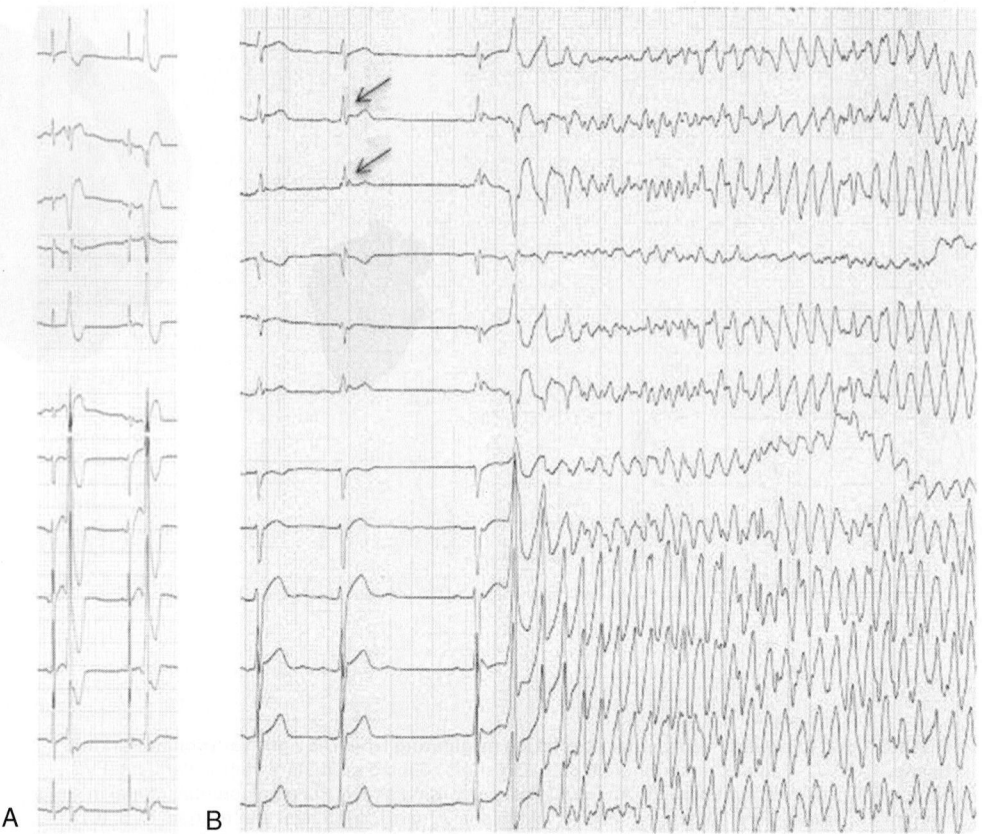

FIGURE 129.3 Early repolarization syndrome. (A) An isolated ventricular premature beat (with a left axis). (B) A similar beat triggered ventricular fibrillation a few hours later. Note that the origin of ventricular ectopy is concordant with the localization of repolarization abnormalities.

a series of 206 patients across 22 centers worldwide.[19] We found that ER, previously considered a benign ECG feature, was significantly more frequent in patients who had been resuscitated from VF compared with a control group (31% vs. 5%). The origin of ectopy that initiated the VF episodes was concordant with the localization of repolarization abnormalities (Fig. 129.3). In total, 26 different PVBs were mapped either to the ventricular myocardium or Purkinje tissue. Catheter ablation was successful in eliminating ventricular ectopy in five of eight patients. Catheter ablation of triggering PVBs therefore does not currently appear to be a cure for VF or a substitute for an ICD, although it has a useful role in controlling electrical storm.

Ablation of Purkinje Triggers in Various Types of Structural Heart Disease

Discrete His-Purkinje sources can also serve as critical VF triggers in a wide spectrum of patients with structural heart disease. The Purkinje arborization along the border zone of scar has an important role in the mechanism of polymorphic VT (PMVT) or VF in patients with structural heart disease, and ablation of the local Purkinje network allows suppression of PMVT or VF.

Ischemic Heart Disease

For patients with recent or anterior myocardial infarction, ablation targets include the VF-initiating PVBs that arise from the His-Purkinje system and/or the border of the scar. Various reports of successful ablation have been published. Marrouche et al.[39] ablated PVBs triggering drug-refractory VF storm in eight patients with myocardial infarction at least 6 months prior. The earliest

activation site was consistently located in the scar border zone and always marked by a Purkinje-like potential. Ablation targeting these potentials eliminated VF storm in all patients over a follow-up of 10 ± 6 months. Isolated episodes of VF occurred in one patient. Monomorphic VT, which may be considered as a mechanistically unrelated arrhythmia, was found in another patient.

Enjoji et al.[40] reported ablation of posterior/posteroseptal LV Purkinje–triggered VF/VT storm in four patients precipitated by an acute coronary event. Acute success was sustained during the follow-up period of 1–4 years in all four patients. Similarly, Bansch et al.[41] mapped and ablated LV Purkinje triggers of refractory VF/VT storm within 1 week of acute myocardial infarction in four patients. No recurrence was observed between 5 and 33 months of follow-up.

Peichl et al. successfully ablated PVBs triggering PMVT/VF storm in eight of nine patients with previous myocardial infarction (3 days to 6 months).[42] PVBs were mapped to the border zone of the septal, inferior, and lateral LV scar. During the follow-up of 13 ± 7 months, electrical storms triggered by PVBs of different morphologies were successfully reablated in one patient.

Szumowski et al.[43] mapped and ablated recurrent episodes of PMVT after anterior wall myocardial infarction triggered by PVBs arising from the Purkinje arborization in the infarct border zone. Ablation at these sites eliminated all PVBs, and during 16 ± 5 months of follow-up, no patient had recurrence of arrhythmia.[44] Finally, Bode et al.[44] mapped and successfully ablated PMVT/VF triggered by PVBs arising from the distal Purkinje arborization in four patients with myocardial infarction and severe LV dysfunction. While two patients died due to refractory heart failure, the other two had no recurrence of PMVT and VF during follow-up at 10 and 27 months, respectively.

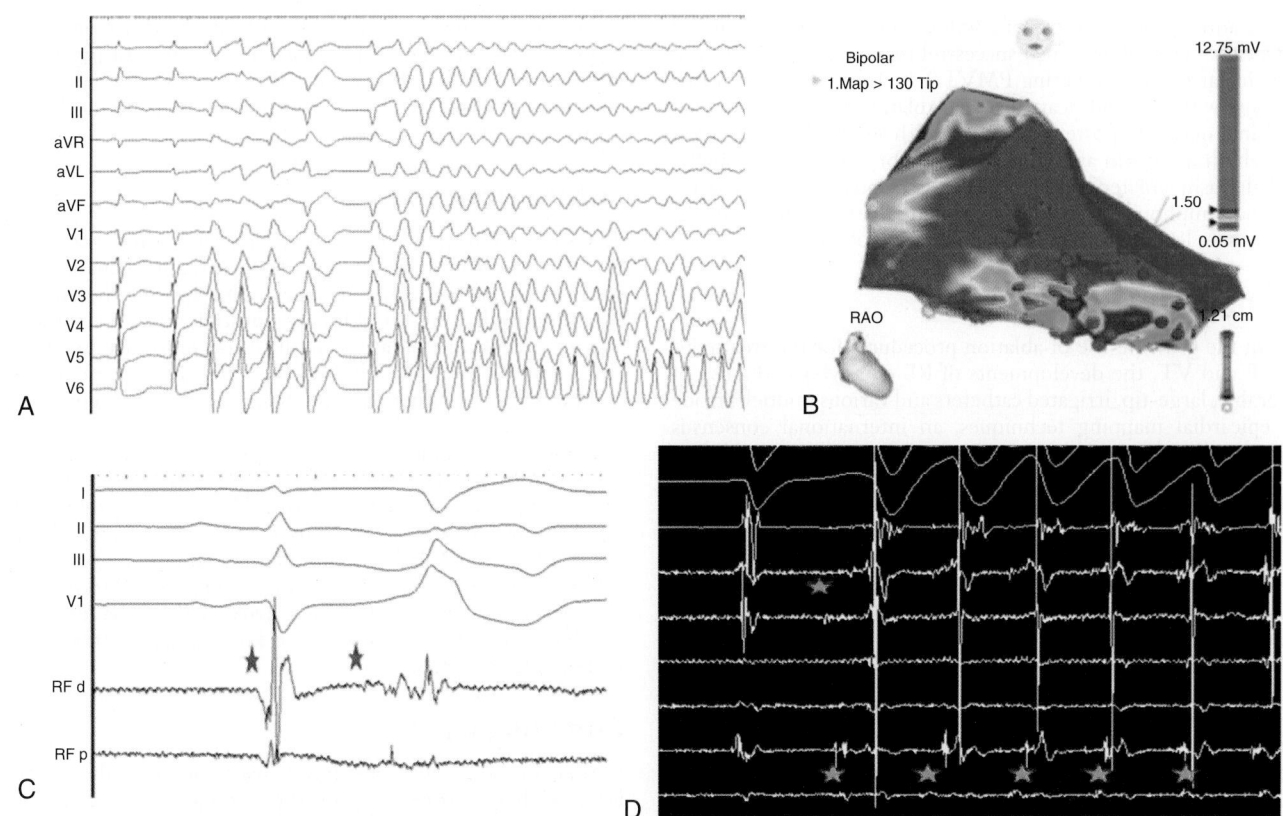

FIGURE 129.4 Spontaneous initiation of ventricular fibrillation (VF) in ischemic heart disease.
(A) A 12-lead electrocardiogram showing spontaneous VF initiation by short-coupled premature ventricular beat (PVB), falling on the descending limb of the T wave of the preceding sinus beat. (B) An electroanatomical map showing surviving Purkinje cells bordering the infarcted tissue (*pink dots*). *RAO*, Right anterior oblique. (C) A multipolar (Pentaray) catheter recording intracardiac Purkinje potentials *(stars)* in sinus rhythm and precocity during the five first beats of VF, indicating that the Purkinje tissue is maintaining VF during the first beats. (D) The ablation catheter records the Purkinje potential *(stars)* in sinus rhythm and with remarkable precocity prior to a Purkinje-triggered PVB.

In our experience in Bordeaux, we have successfully mapped and ablated ischemic VF in 25 patients (aged 63–74 years). VF storms (10–72 shocks) occurred within 2 weeks of myocardial infarction with low ejection fraction. All patients were revascularized. Severe heart failure was present in four patients (intubation, under pump). Pharmacotherapy, deep sedation, and overdrive pacing were unsuccessful. Ablation of the VF-triggering PVBs arising from the Purkinje fibers in the scar area eliminated PMVT/VF in 17 of 25 patients. The PVBs were mapped to the border zone of the ventricular scar (Fig. 129.4).

Dilated Cardiomyopathy

Sinha et al.[45] reported monomorphic PVB–triggered VF storm in five patients. Using voltage criteria to define the scar (<0.5 mV) on the three-dimensional electroanatomical mapping system CARTO (Biosense-Webster Inc., Diamond Bar, CA), basal posterior wall scars near the mitral annulus were found in four of five patients. Purkinje-like potentials were recorded around the scar border in sinus rhythm in these four patients. RF elimination of these potentials was successfully undertaken. One patient without Purkinje-like potentials did not undergo ablation. During follow-up (12 ± 5 months), only the patient without ablation had four VF recurrences.

Santoro et al.[46] ablated VF triggered by PVBs originating from the LV posteromedial papillary muscle in a patient with nonischemic cardiomyopathy. Purkinje potentials were present in the septal endocardial scar, which extended to the medial border of the papillary muscle. The potentials were targeted for ablation with consolidating lesions in the area. No recurrence was reported at the end of 5 years.

Hypertrophic Cardiomyopathy

In contrast to what may be ordinarily assumed, recent results indicate that VF in hypertrophic cardiomyopathy initiates from Purkinje arborization instead of the thickened myocardial tissue. In a series of five patients followed up for over 3 years, focal RF ablation resulted in complete suppression of VF in all but one patient. VF recurred once after ablation in one patient. Ablation therapy can be considered to at least reduce the VF burden substantially in hypertrophic cardiomyopathy.[47] A further case report described successful ablation of pleomorphic VT accompanied by monomorphic VTs arising from the left anterior fascicular Purkinje network in a middle-aged woman.[48]

Other Structural Heart Disease

Smaller series, including patients with various structural heart diseases, have also described successful ablation of Purkinje triggers of PVBs. Bode et al.[44] reported ablation of PMVT/VF storms initiated by monomorphic Purkinje-triggered PVBs in three patients, two with myocarditis and one with aortic valve disease, and no recurrence was observed at 1–15 months of follow-up. Purkinje triggers of electrical storms were successfully ablated in six patients with dilated cardiomyopathy (one), hypertrophic cardiomyopathy (two), noncompaction cardiomyopathy (one), aortic valve replacement (one), and myocarditis (one).[49] Mlcochova et al.[50] described successful mapping and ablation of ventricular ectopy triggering PMVT/VF electrical storm in two patients with amyloid heart disease. Ablation involved proximal Purkinje network (posterior fascicle) with successful elimination of arrhythmic storm and clinical ectopy for one patient. Finally, Nakabayashi ablated refractory VF associated with malignant cardiac lymphoma.[51] A Purkinje potential was targeted at the tumor site, leading to successful elimination of VF.

Technical Aspects

Given the growing use of ablation procedures for the treatment of VF and VT, the developments of RF energy, and the use of steerable, large-tip, irrigated catheters and various multielectrode or epicardial mapping techniques, an international consensus document was issued in 2010 to standardize practices for ablation of VT and VF.[9] When RF energy is used for ablation, the use of irrigated-tip catheters is recommended with power delivery of up to 40 watts.

In VF-trigger ablation, RF is applied at the earliest Purkinje site(s), often producing a flurry of premature beats and PMVT, followed by complete quiescence. Additional applications can be utilized in surrounding Purkinje sites to "prune" the regional arborization and reduce recurrences.[16] An important limitation is that triggers are momentary and might be absent if mapping is programmed later. In contrast to inducible reentrant VT, no technique or agent reproducibly provokes Purkinje firing. Distinct individual precipitating factors and drugs and electrolytes (Ca^{2+}) that can reinitiate VF have been reported, but their range and variety prevent their practical use.[52–54] When feasible, 12-lead ECG documentation of culprit ectopies is essential to permit future ablation of VF sources using pace mapping techniques or potentially using the electrogram morphology or sequence stored in the defibrillator.

Challenges

Although much technical progress has been achieved, such as greatly improved mapping techniques and the introduction of irrigated catheters creating deeper lesions more safely, many technical challenges remain to be solved, such as more precise mapping of VF triggers and better identification of patients eligible for treatment. This is due in part to the limited imaging data available and the scarce reports regarding the mechanisms that trigger VF.[15,55,56]

Future Directions

The role of Purkinje cells in triggering VF storms is confirmed by discrete ablation, reversing life-threatening situations in a wide spectrum of cardiac diseases. This has set the stage for a randomized, long-term follow-up study to understand the impact of Purkinje ablation on all-cause mortality in relevant clinical scenarios. The role of the Purkinje system in more common clinical situations, involving one or a few episodes of VF and possibly in VF ensuing from the degeneration of VT, remains to be deciphered.

Furthermore, besides the Purkinje system, ablation of the underlying substrate may be a useful technique for complex VF, but these strategies are still being developed and preclinical validation still being conducted. Research to understand differential characteristics of arrhythmogenic Purkinje cells in a given clinical scenario, as a part of the broader project involving SD, may improve our knowledge of this incompletely known entity.

Conclusions

Cardiac Purkinje cells, constituting just a fraction of the ventricular mass, harbor sources of life-threatening ventricular arrhythmias. Although clinical data are limited, they support catheter ablation of Purkinje triggers of refractory VF as a rescue therapy with an excellent acute success rate and sustained freedom from recurrence in a wide range of patients with structurally normal and diseased hearts.

Acknowledgment

This work has been supported by IHU LIRYC ANR-10-IAHU-04, European Research Council ERC-2012-ADG 20120314, and Fondation Coeur et Artères.

REFERENCES

1. Tomzik J, Koltermann KC, Zabel M, et al. Quality of life in patients with an implantable cardioverter defibrillator: a systematic review. *Front Cardiovasc Med.* 2015;2:34.
2. Huang DT, Traub D. Recurrent ventricular arrhythmia storms in the age of implantable cardioverter defibrillator therapy: a comprehensive review. *Prog Cardiovasc Dis.* 2008;51:229–236.
3. Villacastin J, Almendral J, Arenal A, et al. Incidence and clinical significance of multiple consecutive, appropriate, high-energy discharges in patients with implanted cardioverter-defibrillators. *Circulation.* 1996;93:753–762.
4. Tan VH, Yap J, Hsu LF, Liew R. Catheter ablation of ventricular fibrillation triggers and electrical storm. *Europace.* 2012;14:1687–1695.
5. Haïssaguerre M, Shoda M, Jais P, et al. Mapping and ablation of idiopathic ventricular fibrillation. *Circulation.* 2002;106:962–967.
6. Haïssaguerre M, Shah DC, Jais P, et al. Role of Purkinje conducting system in triggering of idiopathic ventricular fibrillation. *Lancet.* 2002;359:677–678.
7. Knecht S, Sacher F, Wright M, et al. Long-term follow-up of idiopathic ventricular fibrillation ablation: a multicenter study. *J Am Coll Cardiol.* 2009;54:522–528.
8. Kozeluhova M, Peichl P, Cihak R, et al. Catheter ablation of electrical storm in patients with structural heart disease. *Europace.* 2011;13:109–113.
9. Natale A, Raviele A, Al-Ahmad A, et al. Venice Chart International Consensus document on ventricular tachycardia/ventricular fibrillation ablation. *J Cardiovasc Electrophysiol.* 2010;21:339–379.
10. Priori SG. Survivors of out-of-hospital cardiac arrest with apparently normal heart: need for definition and standardized clinical evaluation: consensus statement of the Joint Steering Committees of the Unexplained Cardiac Registry of Europe and of the Idiopathic Ventricular Fibrillation Registry of the United States. *Circulation.* 1997;95:265–272.
11. Zipes D, Wellens H. Sudden cardiac death. *Circulation.* 1998;98:2334–2351.
12. Myerburg RJ, Kessler KM, Zaman L, et al. Survivors of prehospital cardiac arrest. *JAMA.* 1982;247:1485–1490.
13. Aizawa Y, Tamura M, Chinushi M, et al. An attempt at electrical catheter ablation of the arrhythmogenic area in idiopathic ventricular fibrillation. *Am Heart J.* 1992;123:257–260.
14. Hooks DA, Berte B, Yamashita S, et al. New strategies for ventricular tachycardia and ventricular fibrillation ablation. *Expert Rev Cardiovasc Ther.* 2015;13:263–276.
15. Scheinman MM. Role of the His-Purkinje system in the genesis of cardiac arrhythmia. *Heart Rhythm.* 2009;6:1050–1058.
16. Haïssaguerre M, Vigmond E, Stuyvers B, et al. Ventricular arrhythmias and the His-Purkinje system. *Nat Rev Cardiol.* 2016;13:155–166.
17. Van Herendael H, Zado ES, Haqqani H, et al. Catheter ablation of ventricular fibrillation: importance of left ventricular outflow tract and papillary muscle triggers. *Heart Rhythm.* 2014;11:566–573.
18. Peichl P, Wichterle D, Pavlu L, et al. Complications of catheter ablation of ventricular tachycardia: a single-center experience. *Circ Arrhythm Electrophysiol.* 2014;7:684–690.
19. Haïssaguerre M, Derval N, Sacher F, et al. Sudden cardiac arrest associated with early repolarization. *N Engl J Med.* 2008;358:2016–2023.
20. Kataoka M, Takatsuki S, Tanimoto K, et al. A case of vagally mediated idiopathic ventricular fibrillation. *Nat Clin Pract Cardiovasc Med.* 2008;5:111–115.
21. Kohsaka S, Razavi M, Massumi A. Idiopathic ventricular fibrillation successfully terminated by radiofrequency ablation of the distal Purkinje fibers. *Pacing Clin Electrophysiol.* 2007;30:701–704.
22. Nogami A, Sugiyasu A, Kubota S, et al. Mapping and ablation of idiopathic ventricular fibrillation from the Purkinje system. *Heart Rhythm.* 2005;2:646–649.
23. Saliba W, Abul Karim A, Tchou P, et al. Ventricular fibrillation: ablation of a trigger? *J Cardiovasc Electrophysiol.* 2002;13:1296–1299.
24. Takatsuki S, Mitamura H, Ogawa S. Catheter ablation of a monofocal premature ventricular complex triggering idiopathic ventricular fibrillation. *Heart.* 2001;86:E3.
25. Yan GX, Antzelevitch C. Cellular basis for the Brugada syndrome and other mechanisms of arrhythmogenesis associated with ST-segment elevation. *Circulation.* 1999;100:1660–1666.
26. Haïssaguerre M, Extramiana F, Hocini M, et al. Mapping and ablation of ventricular fibrillation associated with long-QT and Brugada syndromes. *Circulation.* 2003;108:925–928.
27. Li YG, Gronefeld G, Israel C, et al. Catheter ablation of frequently recurring ventricular fibrillation in a patient after aortic valve repair. *J Cardiovasc Electrophysiol.* 2004;15:90–93.
28. el-Sherif N, Caref EB, Yin H, et al. The electrophysiological mechanism of ventricular arrhythmias in the long QT syndrome. Tridimensional mapping of activation and recovery patterns. *Circ Res.* 1996;79:474–492.

29. el-Sherif N, Zeiler RH, Craelius W, et al. QTU prolongation and polymorphic ventricular tachyarrhythmias due to bradycardia-dependent early afterdepolarizations. Afterdepolarizations and ventricular arrhythmias. *Circ Res.* 1988;63:286–305.

30. Asano Y, Davidenko JM, Baxter WT, et al. Optical mapping of drug-induced polymorphic arrhythmias and torsade de pointes in the isolated rabbit heart. *J Am Coll Cardiol.* 1997;29:831–842.

31. Choi BR, Burton F, Salama G. Cytosolic Ca2+ triggers early afterdepolarizations and Torsade de Pointes in rabbit hearts with type 2 long QT syndrome. *J Physiol.* 2002;543:615–631.

32. Srivathsan K, Gami AS, Ackerman MJ, et al. Treatment of ventricular fibrillation in a patient with prior diagnosis of long QT syndrome: importance of precise electrophysiologic diagnosis to successfully ablate the trigger. *Heart Rhythm.* 2007;4:1090–1093.

33. Coronel R, Casini S, Koopmann TT, et al. Right ventricular fibrosis and conduction delay in a patient with clinical signs of Brugada syndrome: a combined electrophysiological, genetic, histopathologic, and computational study. *Circulation.* 2005;112:2769–2777.

34. Darmon JP, Bettouche S, Deswardt P, et al. Radiofrequency ablation of ventricular fibrillation and multiple right and left atrial tachycardia in a patient with Brugada syndrome. *J Interv Card Electrophysiol.* 2004;11:205–209.

35. Nademanee K, Veerakul G, Chandanamattha P, et al. Prevention of ventricular fibrillation episodes in Brugada syndrome by catheter ablation over the anterior right ventricular outflow tract epicardium. *Circulation.* 2011;123:1270–1279.

36. Nakagawa E, Takagi M, Tatsumi H, et al. Successful radiofrequency catheter ablation for electrical storm of ventricular fibrillation in a patient with Brugada syndrome. *Circ J.* 2008;72:1025–1029.

37. Shah AJ, Hocini M, Lamaison D, et al. Regional substrate ablation abolishes Brugada syndrome. *J Cardiovasc Electrophysiol.* 2011;22:1290–1291.

38. Yan GX, Antzelevitch C. Cellular basis for the electrocardiographic J wave. *Circulation.* 1996;93:372–379.

39. Marrouche NF, Verma A, Wazni O, et al. Mode of initiation and ablation of ventricular fibrillation storms in patients with ischemic cardiomyopathy. *J Am Coll Cardiol.* 2004;43:1715–1720.

40. Enjoji Y, Mizobuchi M, Shibata K, et al. Catheter ablation for an incessant form of antiarrhythmic drug-resistant ventricular fibrillation after acute coronary syndrome. *Pacing Clin Electrophysiol.* 2006;29:102–105.

41. Bansch D, Oyang F, Antz M, et al. Successful catheter ablation of electrical storm after myocardial infarction. *Circulation.* 2003;108:3011–3016.

42. Peichl P, Cihak R, Kozeluhova M, et al. Catheter ablation of arrhythmic storm triggered by monomorphic ectopic beats in patients with coronary artery disease. *J Interv Card Electrophysiol.* 2010;27:51–59.

43. Szumowski L, Sanders P, Walczak F, et al. Mapping and ablation of polymorphic ventricular tachycardia after myocardial infarction. *J Am Coll Cardiol.* 2004;44:1700–1706.

44. Bode K, Hindricks G, Piorkowski C, et al. Ablation of polymorphic ventricular tachycardias in patients with structural heart disease. *Pacing Clin Electrophysiol.* 2008;31:1585–1591.

45. Sinha AM, Schmidt M, Marschang H, et al. Role of left ventricular scar and Purkinje-like potentials during mapping and ablation of ventricular fibrillation in dilated cardiomyopathy. *Pacing Clin Electrophysiol.* 2009;32:286–290.

46. Santoro F, Di Biase L, Hranitzky P, et al. Ventricular fibrillation triggered by PVCs from papillary muscles: clinical features and ablation. *J Cardiovasc Electrophysiol.* 2014;25:1158–1164.

47. Hocini M, Denis A, Szumowski L, et al. Ventricular fibrillation in hypertrophic cardiomyopathy is Purkinje-triggered. *Heart Rhythm.* May 4-7, 2016. San Francisco.

48. Yokoshiki H, Mitsuyama H, Watanabe M, et al. Suppression of ventricular fibrillation by electrical modification of the Purkinje system in hypertrophic cardiomyopathy. *Heart Vessels.* 2014;29:709–717.

49. Kozluk E, Gaj S, Kiliszek M, et al. Efficacy of catheter ablation in patients with an electrical storm. *Kardiol Pol.* 2011;69:665–670.

50. Mlcochova H, Saliba WI, Burkhardt DJ, et al. Catheter ablation of ventricular fibrillation storm in patients with infiltrative amyloidosis of the heart. *J Cardiovasc Electrophysiol.* 2006;17:426–430.

51. Nakabayashi K, Sugiura R, Oka T. Catheter ablation targeting Purkinje potentials controlled ventricular fibrillation in a patient with a malignant lymphoma occurring in the ventricular septum. *BMJ Case Rep.* 2015;2015.

52. Kimura T, Takatsuki S, Aizawa Y, et al. Ventricular fibrillation associated with J-wave manifestation following pericarditis after catheter ablation for paroxysmal atrial fibrillation. *Can J Cardiol.* 2013;29:1330.e1–1330.e3.

53. Pasquie JL, Sanders P, Hocini M, et al. Fever as a precipitant of idiopathic ventricular fibrillation in patients with normal hearts. *J Cardiovasc Electrophysiol.* 2004;15:1271–1276.

54. Yagishita A, Yamauchi Y, Obayashi T, et al. Idiopathic ventricular fibrillation associated with early repolarization which was unmasked by a sodium channel blocker after catheter ablation of atrial fibrillation. *J Interv Card Electrophysiol.* 2014;41:145–146.

55. Boyden PA, Hirose M, Dun W. Cardiac Purkinje cells. *Heart Rhythm.* 2010;7:127–135.

56. John RM, Tedrow UB, Koplan BA, et al. Ventricular arrhythmias and sudden cardiac death. *Lancet.* 2012;380:1520–1529.

130 Ablation in Pediatrics

Jennifer N.A. Silva and George F. Van Hare

Indications for Ablation in the Pediatric Age Group

The indications for catheter ablation in the pediatric age group are similar to, but not identical to, those in the adult group. As with any invasive procedure, the indications depend on the natural history of the condition, the success rate of the proposed intervention, and the complication rates. In the pediatric age group, these considerations are largely dependent on the age and size of the child, as growth and development change both incidences and mechanisms of tachycardia, and the potential for a safe, uncomplicated procedure.

Incidence of Heart Rhythm Abnormalities by Age and Congenital Heart Disease

The respective incidences of heart rhythm disorders change throughout childhood, from fetal life, through newborn infants, and up through the teen years to adulthood. In adults, the most common form of supraventricular tachycardia (SVT) other than atrial fibrillation (AF) is atrioventricular nodal reentrant tachycardia (AVNRT). In contrast, in the newborn infant, this diagnosis is unusual, and accessory pathway (AP)–mediated tachycardia is the most common form of SVT observed. Through childhood, AVNRT becomes progressively more likely and is common in teenagers.[1]

Specific arrhythmia mechanisms are much more common in children than in adults. Atrial flutter can be seen in the newborn period, with atrial rates in the range of 400–600 beats/min, but once converted back to normal sinus rhythm, most will never require therapy or ablation.[2] Neonates can exhibit hydrops caused by in utero SVT, but most can be managed with medication once they are born. Furthermore, the natural history of SVT in infants is fairly well characterized, particularly when Wolff-Parkinson-White (WPW) syndrome is present.[3] Most will experience spontaneous resolution by 1 year of age, and this argues strongly for avoiding invasive procedures in infants if possible. Occasionally, incessant SVT, especially persistent junctional reciprocating tachycardia (PJRT), or other mechanisms, such as atrial or junctional ectopic tachycardia, can be difficult to manage and rarely require catheter ablation. It is generally agreed that once the child reaches 3–4 years of age, if SVT is still occurring clinically, it is unlikely that the substrate will spontaneously resolve. The specific situation of congenital heart disease (CHD) should be noted. Certain forms of CHD are highly associated with arrhythmias. Most importantly, patients with Ebstein anomaly of the tricuspid valve have a high incidence of coexisting WPW syndrome, generally because of right-sided

APs.[4] One subtype of hypertrophic cardiomyopathy is associated with WPW syndrome, specifically Danon disease, a form of glycogen storage disease caused by lysosome-associated membrane protein 2 (LAMP2) mutation.[5] In patients who underwent CHD repair, a variety of tachyarrhythmias are seen, generally in the late postoperative period and sometimes decades later. This topic is discussed in Chapter 131. Intraatrial reentrant tachycardia, also known as *postoperative atrial flutter*, is seen commonly after extensive atrial surgery, such as a Senning or Mustard procedure, but can also be seen after any operation that involves an atriotomy, including repair of tetralogy of Fallot, ventricular septal defect, atrial septal defect, or other conditions.[6]

General Procedural Success and Complication Rates That Inform Indications

The first case reports and single-center reports concerning catheter ablation in children appeared in the early 1990s, but organized multicenter research quickly followed. There are now reasonable benchmarks for likely success rates, complication rates, and recurrence risks based on these multicenter studies. The collaborative Prospective Assessment after Pediatric Cardiac Ablation (PAPCA) study began enrolling patients on April 1, 1999 in an effort to better determine success rates, complication rates, and time courses of recurrence following initially successful ablation. The PAPCA study included children up to 16 years of age with either AP tachycardias or AVNRT. The first PAPCA report included 2761 patients and revealed an initial procedural success rate of 95.7%, which was higher for left-sided (97.8%) than for right-sided (90.8%) pathways.[7] Acute complications were uncommon (approximately 4%). The incidence of AV block was 1.2% for all procedures, but 2.1% for AVNRT and 3.0% for septal AP procedures. Success rates were high in younger-aged children and teenagers, and complication rates were similar. The second PAPCA report focused on recurrence.[8] This study involved 517 successfully ablated substrates (540 attempted; 95.7%). The recurrence rate 12 months after ablation was related to substrate type (AP, AVNRT) and AP location. It was highest for right septal pathways (24.6%) and lowest for left septal AP and AVNRT (both 4.8%). Serial echocardiography results after ablation were the subject of the third PAPCA report.[9] Previously, only anecdotal or retrospective nonblinded data had been reported addressing the issue of potential cardiac structural damage (e.g., valvar regurgitation, perforation, coronary occlusion) by ablation.[10] In the small hearts of pediatric patients, this has been an important concern. Of the total 481 patients (follow-up at 2, 6, and 12 months) who were recruited, two-dimensional echocardiography was obtained before and at intervals following the ablation procedure, and these studies were reviewed by a reference laboratory in a blinded fashion. Moderate valve regurgitation was uncommon (0.12%), and severe valve abnormalities were not seen at all. With the exception of the association of mild tricuspid valve regurgitation to right free wall AP and AVNRT, there was no other association of ablation targets to valve proximity. No intracardiac thrombosis or ventricular wall motion or function problems were found.

Since the publication of the PAPCA studies, technology has changed, with the availability of catheter cryoablation and reports of the use of three-dimensional (3D) mapping as a technique for avoiding fluoroscopy exposure. The risk for inadvertent AV block has been lowered substantially with the use of cryoablation.[11,12] Only transient block has been reported. This is comparable with the data for radiofrequency (RF) ablation that have consistently shown a 1% risk for AV block in slow AVN modification for AVNRT, 3% for ablation of anteroseptal AP, and 10% for midseptal AP.[13]

Since the beginning of the catheter ablation era, there has been concern about the fate of the coronary arteries because of the frequent close anatomical proximity of the catheter ablation to the tricuspid and mitral valve annuli. It is considered that high coronary flow dissipates any heat that reaches coronary arteries, and results have shown, with few exceptions, no evidence of gross catheter ablation damage using standard ablation techniques for APs. However, the concern for potential catheter ablation damage to coronary arteries has never completely receded. There has been occasional but persistent case reports of coronary damage, especially in small children.[14] Further animal investigation demonstrated catheter ablation effects by more sensitive tests, such as ultrasound, suggesting that perhaps the absence of gross catheter ablation damage did not negate the potential cellular damage that could lead to clinical problems in the future in the older pediatric population and adults.[15] Although there are essentially no reports of the late development of coronary artery disease following catheter ablation, no prospective studies investigating the status of the coronary arteries have been performed.

Consensus Indications (Class I, II, III) for Catheter Ablation in Children

From the factors and available data detailed earlier, it appears reasonable that indications for catheter ablation in pediatric patients should vary with age and symptoms. The 2002 National Association for Sport and Physical Education (NASPE) Expert Consensus Conference reported guidelines for indications of ablation in children by applying the American Heart Association (AHA) and American College of Cardiology (ACC) definitions used for other published indications: class I, class II, and class III (Box 130.1).[16] No other consensus guidelines for pediatric indications have been developed; however, several reports continue to stimulate opinion and discussion.

A recent joint expert consensus statement from the Pediatric and Congenital Electrophysiology Society and the Heart Rhythm Society addressed the topic regarding management of asymptomatic younger patients with WPW syndrome. Traditionally, the risk for sudden death in asymptomatic individuals has been considered to be low (0.1% per year), but it is clear that these data, accumulated from adults, do not necessarily apply to the pediatric population. There have always been reports of pediatric patients with sudden death as their first sign of WPW, but the actual risk for such an event has been difficult to determine. The availability of electrophysiology study (EPS) and the high success rate and low complication rate of catheter ablation have prompted many clinicians to take an aggressive approach for studying asymptomatic pediatric patients with WPW syndrome and offering catheter ablation when safe and feasible. The recent consensus document supports the use of noninvasive testing for risk stratification, specifically exercise treadmill testing to identify individuals who have had a spontaneous loss of preexcitation indicating low risk.[17] Another approach is the use of Holter monitoring to identify intermittent preexcitation. For individuals who are 8–21 years old and exhibit constant preexcitation but are asymptomatic, transvenous or esophageal EPS is judged to be reasonable, primarily to evaluate the shortest preexcited RR interval during AF, with subsequent catheter ablation depending on the findings. The decision concerning ablation also depends on the proximity of the pathway to critical structures, such as the conduction system or coronary arteries, and the inducibility of AV reciprocating tachycardia.

BOX 130.1   Indications for pediatric catheter ablation

Class I
- WPW syndrome following an episode of aborted sudden cardiac death
- WPW syndrome associated with syncope when there is a short preexcited RR interval during atrial fibrillation (preexcited RR interval <250 ms) or anterograde effective refractory period of the accessory pathway measured during programmed electrical stimulation <250 ms
- Chronic or recurrent SVT associated with ventricular dysfunction
- Recurrent VT that is associated with hemodynamic compromise and is amenable to catheter ablation

Class IIA
- Recurrent or symptomatic SVT refractory to conventional medical therapy and age >4 years
- Impending congenital heart surgery when vascular or chamber access may be restricted following surgery
- Chronic (occurring for >6–12 months following an initial event) or incessant SVT in the presence of normal ventricular function
- Chronic or frequent recurrences of intraatrial reentrant tachycardia
- Palpitations with inducible sustained SVT during electrophysiological testing

Class IIB
- Asymptomatic preexcitation (WPW pattern) on ECG, age >5 years, no recognized tachycardia, and when the risks and benefits of the procedure and arrhythmia have been clearly explained
- SVT, age >5 years, as an alternative to chronic antiarrhythmic therapy that has been effective in controlling arrhythmia
- SVT, age <5 years (including infants), when antiarrhythmic medications, including sotalol and amiodarone, are not effective or are associated with intolerable side effects
- IART, one to three episodes per year, requiring medical intervention
- AV node ablation and pacemaker insertion as an alternative therapy for recurrent or intractable intraatrial reentrant tachycardia
- One episode of VT that is associated with hemodynamic compromise and that is amenable to catheter ablation

Class III
- Asymptomatic WPW syndrome, age <5 years
- SVT controlled with conventional antiarrhythmic medications, age <5 years
- Nonsustained, paroxysmal VT that is not considered incessant (i.e., present on monitoring for hours at a time or on nearly all strips recorded during any 1-hour period) and where no concomitant ventricular dysfunction exists
- Episodes of nonsustained SVT that do not require other therapy or are minimally symptomatic

AV, Atrioventricular; *ECG,* electrocardiogram; *IART,* intraatrial reentry; *SVT,* supraventricular tachycardia; *VT,* ventricular tachycardia; *WPW,* Wolff-Parkinson-White.

Modified from Friedman RA, Walsh EP, Silka MJ, et al. NASPE Expert Consensus Conference: radiofrequency catheter ablation in children with and without congenital heart disease. Report of the Writing Committee. *Pacing Clin Electrophysiol.* 2002;25:1000-1017.

Another frequently discussed issue is ablation in infants and small children. Data from individual centers suggest that younger and smaller patients appear to have a higher risk for complications, although small numbers of patients limit meaningful statistical analysis. Blaufox et al.[18] showed a good success rate in their 14 small-sized patients (18 procedures) weighing <15 kg. They reported a higher incidence of complications that were significantly associated with greater total RF applications. The consensus is that ablation is recommended only in dire circumstances in this population and, when necessary, to limit RF application duration to 20 seconds.

Finally, the role of ablation in high-risk pediatric patients on mechanical support was reported in 2014.[19] In this multicenter cohort of 39 patients (median age, 5.5 months; weight, 6 kg),

33% of pediatric patients on mechanical support for a primary diagnosis of tachycardia underwent EPS +/– transcatheter ablation. The reported complication rate from EPS and ablation in this population was 15%, although successful ablation was performed in all (100%) patients. While ablations can be performed in very young high-risk patients, risks and benefits of the procedure must be carefully considered and discussed with the family.

Preparation for the Procedure

Developmental and Psychosocial Considerations and Procedure Consent

Most children older than 6 years should be involved in some way in the consent process, and the level of involvement depends on age and developmental status. Preparation for the procedure should start well in advance and is particularly important in teenagers who need to be completely cognizant of the issues involved. Often, pediatric patients and families who have previously gone through the experience can be helpful in answering questions and allaying fears.

Preprocedural Studies

The results of all prior cardiovascular testing should be reviewed, paying particular attention to electrocardiographic records of the arrhythmia in question. Most clinicians routinely obtain a complete echocardiogram in children who visit the EP laboratory, even when there is no clinical evidence of structural heart disease. Certain abnormalities are important to detect before insertion of catheters, such as left superior vena cava to coronary sinus (CS) connection, patent foramen ovale, and more rare abnormalities of venous connections. In patients with preexcitation, particularly those with apparent right-sided pathway locations, Ebstein anomaly of the tricuspid valve should be excluded because this defect dramatically changes the expected technical challenges and likely outcomes.

Laboratory Setting

Sedation and Anesthesia

Virtually all pediatric patients require sedation, anesthesia, or both. For younger children, general anesthesia is essentially always used. Although older teenagers can often cooperate with an invasive procedure lasting several hours with conscious sedation, many cannot, and it can be difficult to predict which teenagers will do well. In general, patient and family acceptance is highest when general anesthesia is offered.

Anesthesia techniques vary, and patients can undergo deep sedation and anesthesia without airway instrumentation or with the use of laryngeal mask airway or endotracheal intubation. The anesthetic agent dexmedetomidine should be avoided; it is a vagotonic agent and suppresses sinus and AV node function,[20] and it can interfere with automatic focus tachycardias.[21] However, the use of general anesthesia has implications for the pediatric patient. First, the inducibility of arrhythmias, particularly AVNRT, may be decreased, and it is frequently necessary to use provocative agents, such as isoproterenol, to allow for tachycardia initiation. Recovery from general anesthesia will generally take longer than that from conscious sedation, and postprocedure nausea is sometimes an issue; therefore same-day discharge is not always possible.

Radiation Concerns

Nearly all ablation procedures require some level of radiation exposure, and for years, there has been concern over the effects of such exposure in young patients, particularly before modern

pulsed fluoroscopy systems became available. Bacher et al.,[22] Campbell et al.,[23] and Davies et al.[24] have addressed the issues of various measurements, new technologies of radiation direct measurement, and radiation exposure–reduction strategies. The calculated effective doses in children are as high as those in adult interventional cardiology, resulting in higher radiation risks. It is important to monitor the patient using dose–area product (DAP) instrumentation and to maintain records of cumulative DAP for individual patients for repeat procedures. DAP can be reduced using beam filtration to maintain the effective dose as low as possible. Strategies to reduce radiation exposure have been developed.

The availability of advanced 3D mapping systems has led to much interest in the development of nonfluoroscopic catheter navigation techniques in children. In addition, intracardiac echocardiography particularly contributes to the safe performance of transseptal puncture. Interestingly, a 2011 study evaluated the radiation doses applied to patients undergoing EPS and ablation using an integrated electroanatomical mapping system plus intracardiac echocardiogram versus electroanatomical mapping alone.[25] They found that the integration of intracardiac echocardiogram did not further limit radiation but was helpful for patients who needed transseptal punctures. The performance of catheter ablation in children completely without fluoroscopy is clearly possible, but it is much more likely that these technologies will lead to a dramatic reduction in fluoroscopy exposure rather than its complete elimination[25] (Fig. 130.1).

Recording and Mapping Systems

All modern pediatric EP laboratories incorporate the use of 3D mapping systems. These systems are particularly valuable for mapping complex arrhythmias, such as those seen after repaired CHD. They provide excellent assistance to catheter navigation, even for simple substrates that normally do not require 3D mapping, such as AVNRT and AP. In addition to reducing fluoroscopy exposure, as discussed earlier, they allow for the accurate placement of catheters at previously mapped and ablated locations, such as when a successful lesion is followed by recurrence of AP conduction. These systems can be used in the smallest patients.

Energy Sources

Various technologies available for creating intracardiac lesions are covered extensively elsewhere in this text. Standard RF ablation, irrigated-tip ablation, and ablation with large tips are useful in the pediatric population; however, techniques such as irrigated-tip ablation designed to create larger and deeper lesions are rarely used in children, particularly those with smaller hearts, because of a fear of serious complications.

The development of cryoablation techniques has enhanced the safety of catheter ablation. The avoidance of inadvertent AV block is of paramount concern in children as those with this complication will require a lifetime of pacing. Cryoablation essentially allows for the complete avoidance of this complication. In addition, RF lesions are often ineffective in areas of low flow, such as the CS, and cryoablation offers an advantage here.[26] The details of biophysics and engineering considerations are covered elsewhere. The limitations of this technology in children are partly related to the stiffness of the currently available catheters, as well as the lower reported success rate initially and higher reported recurrence rate with cryoablation compared with RF ablation in pediatric patients.[27] In general, larger-tip cryoablation catheters seem to be more effective in early reports.

New technology, measuring catheter–tissue contact force, is now available for RF ablation catheters (Fig. 130.2). When

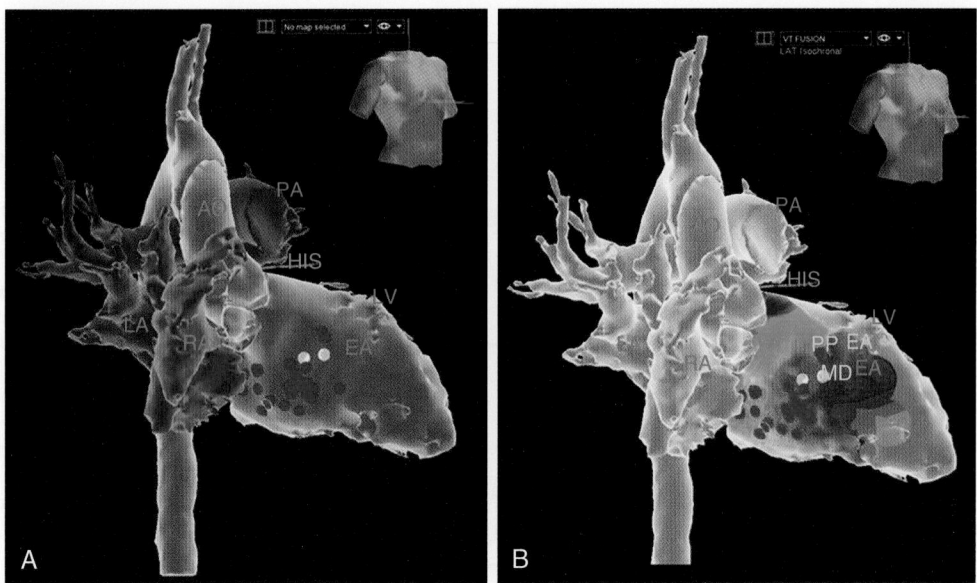

FIGURE 130.1 (A) This example of fusion merges an anatomical shell from cardiac magnetic resonance imaging (MRI) with the electroanatomical mapping from a NavX system. (B) Fusion is an example of new tools being employed to reduce radiation exposure during electrophysiology study (EPS) and ablation. In this instance, a patient with left ventricular tachycardia had cardiac MRI prior to EPS. MRI was then imported into the NavX system and merged with the electroanatomical activation data. *Red lesions* mark ablation sites. *AO,* Aorta; *EA,* early activation; *HIS,* His bundle; *LA,* left atrium; *LV,* left ventricle; *MD,* mid-diastolic potential; *PA,* pulmonary artery; *PP,* prepotential; *RA,* right atrium.

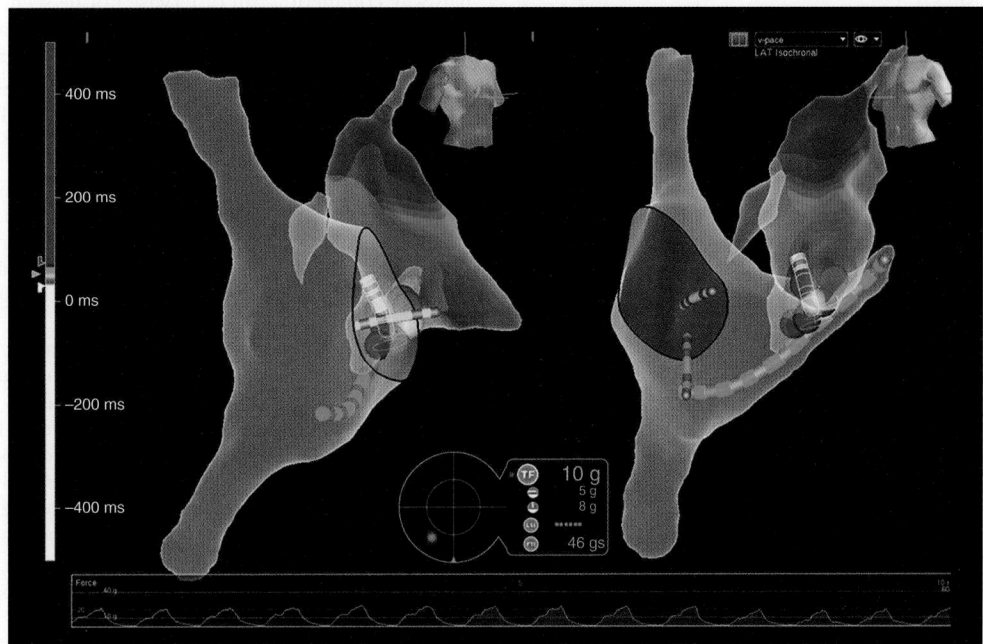

FIGURE 130.2 This image was obtained during an ablation of left posteroseptal accessory pathway using a force sensing catheter. In this case, a St. Jude force sensing ablation catheter is used that delivers real-time data following contact being made during the lesion. Further calculated parameters are included to provide the user a sense of lesion depth.

comparing force sensing catheters with standard RF ablation catheters, data have shown that higher contact force results in a greater impedance decrease.[28] Because monitoring impedance during RF ablations is widely available, a decrease in impedance can be used as an indicator of good catheter contact. Additional data from adult AF patients have generated target force parameters for creation of transmural lesions.[29,30]

Child-Specific Resources

The pediatric EP laboratory is ideally equipped with devices and catheters that allow for the performance of procedures in small hearts. The staff members should be trained in the care of children; this group includes cardiologists, nurses, and anesthesiologists. In addition, the laboratory should exist in an environment that supports all aspects of pediatric care. The availability of a pediatric intensive care unit is essential, as is a recovery area with personnel experienced in caring for children after anesthesia. The institution should have pediatric cardiothoracic surgery services available in the infrequent event of a catastrophic complication. Other features of a children's hospital are also important, such as the availability of child life services.

Clinical and Procedural Considerations Related to Specific Pediatric Ablation Procedures

General Technical Considerations

Few if any of the catheters designed and marketed for ablation procedures are designed for children; therefore a pediatric electrophysiologist must adapt currently available equipment to the situation of smaller anatomy. Size 4- and 5-French diagnostic catheters are available, which minimize the effect on vessels. In small children and in those with limited venous access, the use of an esophageal lead allows a complete study, with fewer intravascular catheters.

In smaller children, the amount of cardiac movement and effect of diaphragm movement can be significant. Long vascular sheaths are available for stabilizing catheter positions, but they are designed for adults and are difficult to deploy in smaller hearts. Catheter stability can often be achieved with nonstandard catheter approaches, such as via the subclavian or jugular vein. In cases of ablation close to the AV junction, the effect of respiratory movement on catheter position can be minimized by a held inspiration in the anesthetized patient, with the cooperation of the anesthesiologist.[31]

Wolff-Parkinson-White Syndrome and Concealed Accessory Pathways

The standard techniques for diagnosis, intracardiac mapping, and catheter ablation, discussed elsewhere in this text, apply to all children. However, pediatric cardiac physiology can present some particular challenges. For example, AVN conduction tends to be naturally robust in children. The PR interval in children is relatively short compared with that in adults, and retrograde conduction via the AV node is common. Thus, in WPW syndrome, preexcitation tends to be less prominent, making prediction of pathway location more difficult. Furthermore, it is possible for a robust anterograde AP to exhibit essentially no preexcitation on the surface electrocardiograms during sinus rhythm if that pathway is located in the left lateral location and AVN conduction is brisk (Fig. 130.3). In the laboratory, excellent retrograde conduction via AVN occasionally makes identification of left lateral pathways challenging when pacing is performed from the right ventricular apex. At times, the only way to show eccentric retrograde atrial activation clearly via a left-sided pathway is by left ventricular pacing or by the administration of adenosine during ventricular pacing.

The approach to left-sided APs can be via a patent foramen ovale, transseptal puncture, or retrograde approach via the femoral artery. Each of these approaches has advantages and disadvantages. In all, full systemic heparinization is considered the standard of care, and most laboratories use a target-activated clotting time of >240 seconds. It should be noted that there is no clinical evidence that any given activated clotting time level is effective for preventing thromboembolic stroke in left-sided catheter ablation of SVT. The transseptal approach has the advantage of avoiding an arterial puncture, and most sites on the mitral annulus can be reached relatively easily. Possible exceptions to this rule include pathways that are located anteriorly, as well as left posteroseptal pathways in which the curve of the sheath may make it difficult to reach these locations. Careful attention must be paid to avoid

blood clot formation between the sheath and the ablation catheter, and particular attention must be paid when ablation catheters are exchanged so that air is not introduced and then delivered to the left atrium. The retrograde approach is highly effective, and all parts of the mitral annulus can be reached, including anterior and left posteroseptal locations. The retrograde approach allows the catheter tip to be positioned under the mitral valve leaflet, where catheter stability is excellent, and tip temperatures are also excellent at moderate power (Fig. 130.4). Alternatively, the catheter can be retroflexed through the mitral valve and positioned in the left atrium and then balanced on the mitral annulus. With this approach, adequate tip temperatures are sometimes difficult to achieve. This latter approach is generally required if the pathway is located adjacent to the commissure between anterior and posterior mitral valve leaflets. Although there initially was concern that the retrograde approach put the aortic valve at risk for aortic insufficiency as a complication, the PAPCA study identified no such risk.[9]

RF energy can be delivered during sinus rhythm in WPW syndrome or during atrial pacing to bring out preexcitation. For concealed and manifest pathways, energy can be delivered during ventricular pacing, observing for a sudden shift in retrograde atrial activation sequence or loss of retrograde conduction entirely. This latter technique is problematic if retrograde nodal conduction is robust and eccentric retrograde atrial activation is difficult to appreciate. One approach to this problem is to pace the ventricle faster, achieving decremental retrograde conduction in the node and bringing out retrograde pathway conduction, but this is sometimes not tolerated in the anesthetized child. Another approach is to pace from the left ventricle if left-sided pathway conduction can otherwise not be seen, but this requires an additional catheter to be placed in most cases. Finally, one helpful technique is to initiate sustained AV reciprocating tachycardia, and then entrain the tachycardia using ventricular pacing at a slightly faster rate, thereby eliminating the problem of retrograde fusion. This technique also avoids the problem of catheter dislodgement, which can result from successful ablation and sudden termination of tachycardia. When pathways are located on the septum, this approach should not be taken, as one needs to observe for the occurrence of junctional rhythm as an indication of impending damage to AVN. In this situation, most clinicians deliver energy in sinus rhythm and test retrograde conduction after each lesion.

The techniques for using cryoablation for AP ablation are similar. However, one advantage of cryoablation is the phenomenon of cryoadhesion, in which the tip of the catheter adheres to the myocardium once the temperature is less than –35°C. Because of this phenomenon, cryoablation can be performed during sustained AV reciprocating tachycardia without entrainment pacing because when tachycardia terminates because of successful ablation, the catheter tip will not dislodge. When using this technique, of course, the clinician must confirm immediately that tachycardia has terminated because of retrograde pathway block rather than anterograde AVN block.

Because results of cryoablation of APs have been somewhat disappointing, both in terms of the initial success rate and the high incidence of recurrence, in most laboratories cryoablation is reserved for pathways that are close to the AVN or located in structures such as the CS, where inadequate tip cooling prevents adequate lesion formation with RF energy.[27,32]

A particular form of AV reciprocating tachycardia that is relatively uncommon and principally seen in the pediatric population is PJRT. Patients with PJRT can present with heart failure caused by tachycardia-induced cardiomyopathy. This form of SVT is mediated by a slowly conducting concealed AP that in almost all cases is found in the posteroseptal region. Most cases of PJRT tend to be incessant, and ablation during tachycardia is the usual approach. It is helpful, but not mandatory, to differentiate PJRT

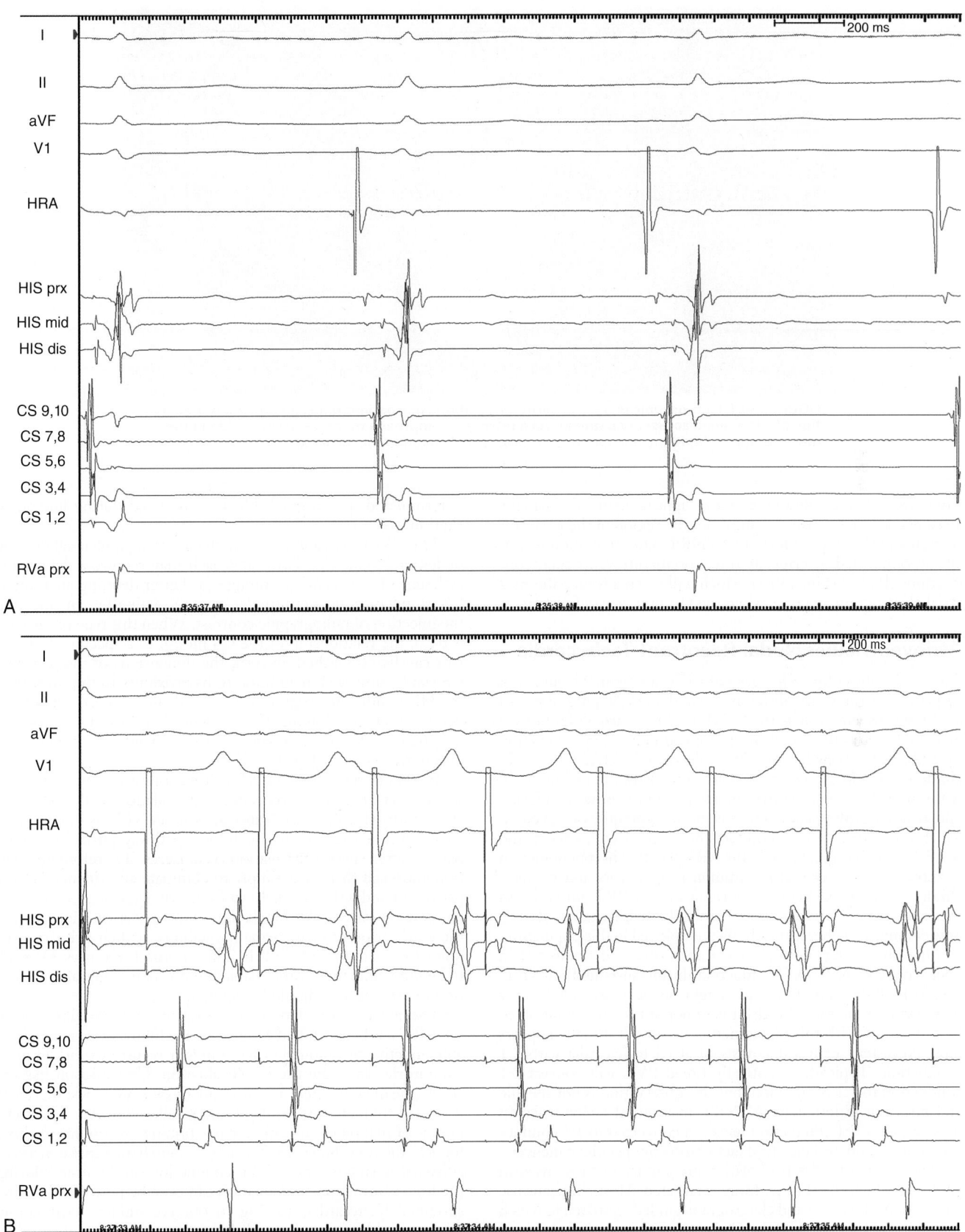

FIGURE 130.3 Surface and intracardiac electrograms in a 12-year-old patient with Wolff-Parkinson-White syndrome. (A) Note that there is essentially no preexcitation on surface ECG in sinus rhythm, (B) but preexcitation is seen easily with high right atrial pacing at a cycle length of 320 ms. *CS,* Coronary sinus; *dis,* distal; *HIS,* His bundle; *HRA,* high right atrium; *mid,* middle; *prx,* proximal; *RVa prx,* proximal right ventricular apex.

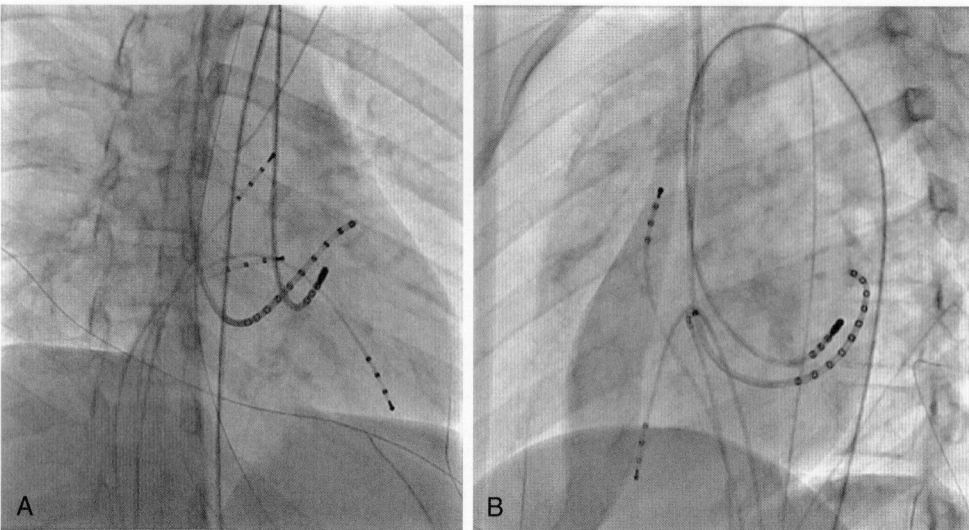

FIGURE 130.4 Fluoroscopic images of catheter positions in a patient undergoing catheter abla-tion of a left-sided accessory pathway via a retrograde approach to the ventricular side of the mitral annulus. (A) Right anterior oblique view. (B) Left anterior oblique view.

from two other conditions that can appear identical—namely, atrial ectopic tachycardia arising from the region of the posterior septum and the atypical form of AVNRT. Differentiation is usu-ally accomplished by critically timed premature ventricular con-tractions (PVCs) (Fig. 130.5), which will often advance the next atrial electrogram at a time when the His bundle is refractory.

Atrioventricular Nodal Reentrant Tachycardia

The AVN physiology changes with development,[33,34] and, not surprisingly, there are differences in the AVN physiology of adults versus children with AVNRT. The usual definition of dual AVN pathways is a 50-ms prolongation in AVN conduction time (A2H2) in response to a 10-ms decrease in A1A2 interval. In children and adolescents, a clear-cut demonstration of dual AVN pathways is less common than in adults. On the other hand, sus-tained slow pathway conduction is more commonly observed, in which rapid atrial pacing conducts down the slow pathway and the PR interval is greater than the RR interval. This phenomenon is known as *crossover* and is common in teenagers and younger children. The need for isoproterenol for AVNRT initiation in the laboratory is also common, probably at least partly due to how commonly general anesthesia is employed in this population.

One interesting phenomenon that is observed frequently in young patients is 2:1 AV conduction during sustained AVNRT, caused by either His-Purkinje system block or so-called lower final common pathway block. It is important for the clinician to be acquainted with this phenomenon because it initially appears most consistent with a diagnosis of atrial tachycardia with 2:1 conduction. Typically, a critically timed PVC will convert 2:1 conduction to 1:1 conduction, but this observation is not specific and does not differentiate AVNRT from atrial tachycardia. In practice, once 2:1 conduction has been converted to 1:1 conduc-tion, one should exclude atrial tachycardia by specific maneuvers.

The techniques for RF ablation are similar to those used in adults, in which the slow pathway is targeted. Most clinicians use an anatomically based and electrogram-guided approach in which the region of the mouth of the CS is explored for typical electrical potentials. Energy is delivered during sinus rhythm, observing for junctional accelerated rhythm as an indicator of correct abla-tion location. In some laboratories, atrial pacing is performed at a rate faster than the junctional rhythm, observing for AV block; in others, junctional rhythm is simply observed and energy delivery

is terminated if retrograde block is observed during junctional rhythm.

The CS can be cannulated via the internal jugular, subclavian, or femoral vein. The latter approach may require a deflectable catheter. One available technique for better defining anatomy is CS cannulation by a multipolar catheter with a lumen, allowing the injection of radiographic contrast. When this type of catheter is used, the relationship of the CS mouth to a specific electrode pair can be established; in turn, the dimensions of the proximal CS can be observed in addition to its proximity to the site where the His bundle electrogram is recorded (Fig. 130.6). The proxi-mal CS is enlarged in many cases. Knowledge of this anatomical information allows the clinician to better avoid delivering energy inside the CS itself (Fig. 130.7).

It is important that AVNRT inducibility in any patient be well established before proceeding with ablation. Unlike the situ-ation with APs, the basic substrate for AVNRT is not particu-larly well understood, and dual AVN pathway physiology often persists after successful ablation procedures. Therefore an abla-tion approach that seeks simply to eliminate all evidence of slow pathway conduction is likely to be overly aggressive and might increase the risk for AV block. Thus most pediatric clinicians use the elimination of tachycardia inducibility as their primary end-point for ablation in AVNRT. This approach requires AVNRT to be inducible; therefore reliable methods for tachycardia initia-tion in each patient should be defined.

The use of cryoablation for posterior AVN modification in AVNRT has been studied extensively in children.[12] It is a reason-ably effective technique but has a higher recurrence risk in most laboratories than the use of RF ablation. Cryoablation has the advantage of completely avoiding any risk for AV block; therefore it is used frequently in younger and smaller children. The tech-niques of mapping and catheter positioning are similar to those for RF ablation; however, because of the characteristic of cryo-adhesion, characteristics of AV conduction can be tested during the lesion formation, and ablation can even be performed during sustained tachycardia, seeking to observe sudden termination. With cryoablation, catheter dislodgement is not a problem dur-ing sudden termination, and lesion formation can be continued for a full 4 minutes. When using this technique, however, the clinician must immediately determine the mechanism of termina-tion to confirm that it is by slow pathway block rather than fast pathway block.

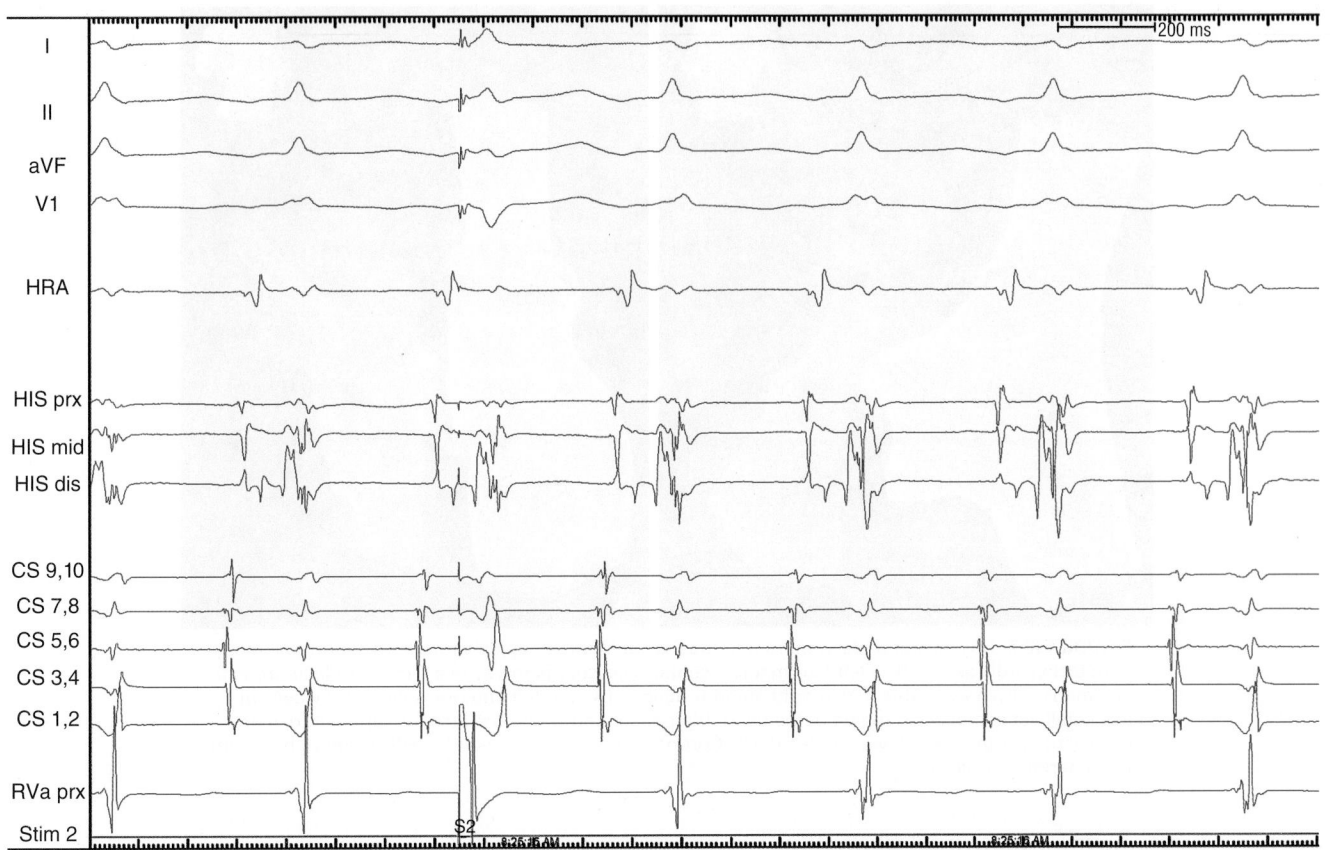

FIGURE 130.5 Incessant persistent junctional reciprocating tachycardia in a 6-year-old boy. Note the long RP tachycardia with inverted P waves in leads II and aVF. Earliest retrograde atrial activation is seen in the coronary sinus (*CS*) pair 5,6, which by fluoroscopy was at the mouth of the CS. A premature contraction is introduced after the inscription of the His bundle (*HIS*) electrogram, which advances the next atrial electrogram without changing the retrograde atrial activation sequence, proving the presence of an extranodal pathway. *dis,* Distal; *HRA,* high right atrium; *mid,* middle; *prx,* proximal; *RVa prx,* proximal right ventricular apex; *Stim 2,* stimulus marker.

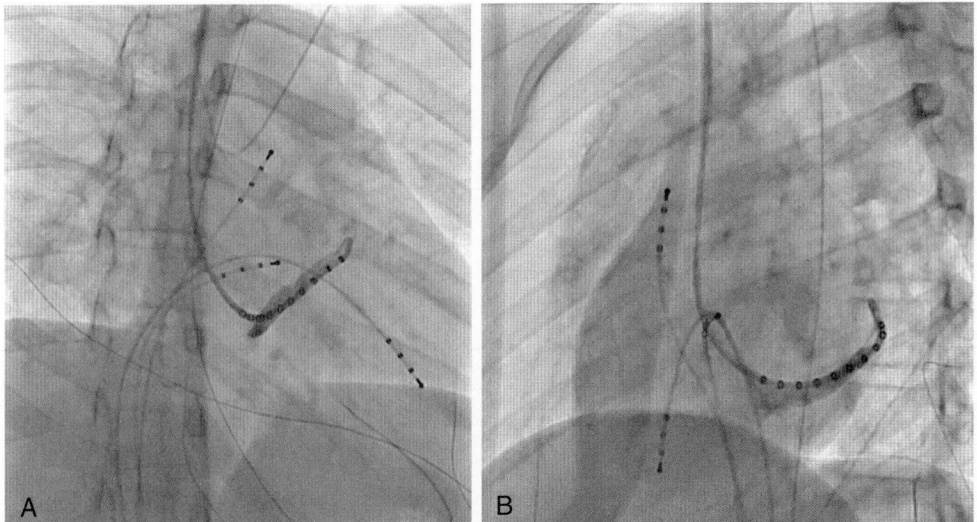

FIGURE 130.6 Fluoroscopic images of catheter positions in a patient with atrioventricular nodal reentrant tachycardia. Note that radiographic contrast is injected via the coronary sinus (CS) catheter, enabling the identification of the relationship between the CS mouth and CS electrodes. (A) Right anterior oblique view. (B) Left anterior oblique view.

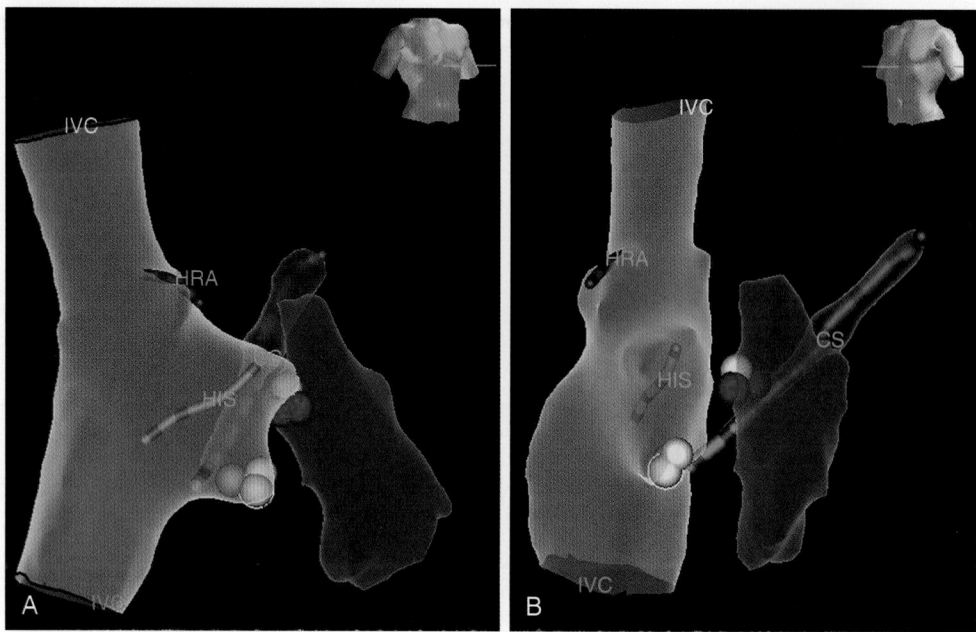

FIGURE 130.7 This patient underwent radiofrequency ablation of typical atrioventricular nodal reentrant tachycardia as well as a left intermediate septal accessory pathway (via a retrograde approach). The maps shown were obtained in right anterior oblique (A) and left anterior oblique (B) views. In this small yet complicated region of the heart, the patient had two substrates for supraventricular tachycardia, both of which were ablated. *CS,* Coronary sinus; *HIS,* His bundle; *HRA,* high right atrium; *IVC,* inferior vena cava.

Automatic Focus Tachycardias, Especially Junctional Ectopic Tachycardia

The approach to most automatic focus tachycardias in children is similar to that used in adults. The 3D mapping has proved itself useful in atrial ectopic tachycardia and various forms of ventricular tachycardia, especially those arising from the right ventricular outflow tract. One problem often presents itself in pediatric cases of automatic tachycardia, i.e., the tendency for the suppression of automatic focus with anesthesia administration.

Congenital junctional ectopic tachycardia is another rare condition that is seen mainly in children. It seems to have a familial occurrence, tends to be incessant, presents as a narrow QRS tachycardia with AV dissociation and capture beats, and can present with tachycardia-induced cardiomyopathy. Catheter ablation is necessarily hazardous because of the proximity of the AV conduction system. A multicenter study published in 2009[35] on the management of pediatric nonpostoperative junctional ectopic tachycardia reported that 47% of patients underwent ablation, with successful RF ablation in 82% (14/17) and successful

cryoablation in 85% (23/27) and with a significant difference between the two groups. Inadvertent AV block was documented in 18% (3/17) of patients undergoing RF ablation with no permanent AV block in those who had cryoablation.[35] In addition, the advantages of cryoablation are obvious in this condition because complete AV block should be completely avoidable using cryoablation.

Follow-up

Patients should be followed up after initial successful catheter ablation procedures, principally to monitor for possible recurrence of the ablated substrate. Clinical studies have shown that most documented recurrences are evident by 6 months after the procedure.[8] Most clinicians perform follow-up evaluations in patients at several intervals out to 1 year.

For patients who have undergone ablation of an incessant tachycardia, follow-up generally involves serial echocardiography to document the resolution of ventricular dysfunction, as well as Holter monitoring to detect episodes of tachycardia.

REFERENCES

1. Blaufox AD, Warsy I, D'Souza M, et al. Transesophageal electrophysiological evaluation of children with a history of supraventricular tachycardia in infancy. *Pediatr Cardiol.* 2011;32:1110–1114.
2. Drago F, Mazza A, Garibaldi S, et al. Isolated neonatal atrial flutter: clinical features, prognosis and therapy. *G Ital Cardiol.* 1998;28:365–368.
3. Perry JC, Garson Jr A. Supraventricular tachycardia due to Wolff-Parkinson-White syndrome in children: early disappearance and late recurrence. *J Am Coll Cardiol.* 1990;16:1215–1220.
4. Delhaas T, Sarvaas GJ, Rijlaarsdam ME, et al. A multicenter, long-term study on arrhythmias in children with Ebstein anomaly. *Pediatr Cardiol.* 2010;31:229–233.
5. Cheng Z, Fang Q. Danon disease: focusing on heart. *J Hum Genet.* 2012;57:407–410.

6. Chan DP, Van Hare GF, Mackall JA, et al. Importance of atrial flutter isthmus in postoperative intra-atrial reentrant tachycardia. *Circulation.* 2000;102:1283–1289.
7. Van Hare GF, Javitz H, Carmelli D, et al. Prospective assessment after pediatric cardiac ablation: demographics, medical profiles, and initial outcomes. *J Cardiovasc Electrophysiol.* 2004;15:759–770.
8. Van Hare GF, Javitz H, Carmelli D, et al. Prospective assessment after pediatric cardiac ablation: recurrence at 1 year after initially successful ablation of supraventricular tachycardia. *Heart Rhythm.* 2004;1:188–196.
9. Van Hare GF, Colan SD, Javitz H, et al. Prospective assessment after pediatric cardiac ablation: fate of intracardiac structure and function, as assessed by serial echocardiography. *Am Heart J.* 2007;153:815–820, 820.e1-820.e6.

10. Minich LL, Snider AR, Dick 2nd M. Doppler detection of valvular regurgitation after radiofrequency ablation of accessory connections. *Am J Cardiol.* 1992;70:116–117.
11. Bar-Cohen Y, Cecchin F, Alexander ME, et al. Cryoablation for accessory pathways located near normal conduction tissues or within the coronary venous system in children and young adults. *Heart Rhythm.* 2006;3:253–258.
12. Collins KK, Dubin AM, Chiesa NA, et al. Cryoablation versus radiofrequency ablation for treatment of pediatric atrioventricular nodal reentrant tachycardia: initial experience with 4-mm cryocatheter. *Heart Rhythm.* 2006;3:564–570.
13. Schaffer MS, Silka MJ, Ross BA, et al. Inadvertent atrioventricular block during radiofrequency catheter ablation. Results of the Pediatric Radiofrequency Ablation Registry. Pediatric Electrophysiology Society. *Circulation.* 1996;94:3214–3220.

14. Schneider HE, Kriebel T, Gravenhorst VD, et al. Incidence of coronary artery injury immediately after catheter ablation for supraventricular tachycardias in infants and children. *Heart Rhythm.* 2009;6:461–467.

15. Aoyama H, Nakagawa H, Pitha JV, et al. Comparison of cryothermia and radiofrequency current in safety and efficacy of catheter ablation within the canine coronary sinus close to the left circumflex coronary artery. *J Cardiovasc Electrophysiol.* 2005;16:1218–1226.

16. Friedman RA, Walsh EP, Silka MJ, et al. NASPE expert consensus conference: radiofrequency catheter ablation in children with and without congenital heart disease. Report of the writing committee. North American Society of Pacing and Electrophysiology. *Pacing Clin Electrophysiol.* 2002;25:1000–1017.

17. Cohen MI, Triedman JK, Cannon BC, et al. PACES/HRS expert consensus statement on the management of the asymptomatic young patient with a Wolff-Parkinson-White (WPW, ventricular preexcitation) electrocardiographic pattern: developed in partnership between the Pediatric and Congenital Electrophysiology Society (PACES) and the Heart Rhythm Society (HRS). Endorsed by the governing bodies of PACES, HRS, the American College of Cardiology Foundation (ACCF), the American Heart Association (AHA), the American Academy of Pediatrics (AAP), and the Canadian Heart Rhythm Society (CHRS). *Heart Rhythm.* 2012;9:1006–1024.

18. Blaufox AD, Paul T, Saul JP. Radiofrequency catheter ablation in small children: relationship of complications to application dose. *Pacing Clin Electrophysiol.* 2004;27:224–229.

19. Silva JN, Erickson CC, Carter CD, et al. Management of pediatric tachyarrhythmias on mechanical support. *Circ Arrhythm Electrophysiol.* 2014;7:658–663.

20. Hammer GB, Drover DR, Cao H, et al. The effects of dexmedetomidine on cardiac electrophysiology in children. *Anesth Analg.* 2008;106:79–83. table of contents.

21. Chrysostomou C, Beerman L, Shiderly D, et al. Dexmedetomidine: a novel drug for the treatment of atrial and junctional tachyarrhythmias during the perioperative period for congenital cardiac surgery: a preliminary study. *Anesth Analg.* 2008;107:1514–1522.

22. Bacher K, Bogaert E, Lapere R, et al. Patient-specific dose and radiation risk estimation in pediatric cardiac catheterization. *Circulation.* 2005;111:83–89.

23. Campbell RM, Strieper MJ, Frias PA, et al. Quantifying and minimizing radiation exposure during pediatric cardiac catheterization. *Pediatr Cardiol.* 2005;26:29–33.

24. Davies AG, Cowen AR, Kengyelics SM, et al. X-ray dose reduction in fluoroscopically guided electrophysiology procedures. *Pacing Clin Electrophysiol.* 2006;29:262–271.

25. Miyake CY, Mah DY, Atallah J, et al. Nonfluoroscopic imaging systems reduce radiation exposure in children undergoing ablation of supraventricular tachycardia. *Heart Rhythm.* 2011;8:519–525.

26. Collins KK, Rhee EK, Kirsh JA, et al. Cryoablation of accessory pathways in the coronary sinus in young patients: a multicenter study from the Pediatric and Congenital Electrophysiology Society's working group on cryoablation. *J Cardiovasc Electrophysiol.* 2007;18:592–597.

27. Kriebel T, Broistedt C, Kroll M, et al. Efficacy and safety of cryoenergy in the ablation of atrioventricular reentrant tachycardia substrates in children and adolescents. *J Cardiovasc Electrophysiol.* 2005;16:960–966.

28. Reichlin T, Knecht S, Lane C, et al. Initial impedance decrease as an indicator of good catheter contact: insights from radiofrequency ablation with force sensing catheters. *Heart Rhythm.* 2014;11:194–201.

29. Neuzil P, Reddy VY, Kautzner J, et al. Electrical reconnection after pulmonary vein isolation is contingent on contact force during initial treatment: results from the EFFICAS I study. *Circ Arrhythm Electrophysiol.* 2013;6:327–333.

30. Reddy VY, Shah D, Kautzner J, et al. The relationship between contact force and clinical outcome during radiofrequency catheter ablation of atrial fibrillation in the TOCCATA study. *Heart Rhythm.* 2012;9:1789–1795.

31. Pecht B, Maginot KR, Boramanand NK, et al. Techniques to avoid atrioventricular block during radiofrequency catheter ablation of septal tachycardia substrates in young patients. *J Interv Card Electrophysiol.* 2002;7:83–88.

32. Collins KK, Schaffer MS. Use of cryoablation for treatment of tachyarrhythmias in 2010: survey of current practices of pediatric electrophysiologists. *Pacing Clin Electrophysiol.* 2011;34:304–308.

33. Blaufox AD, Rhodes JF, Fishberger SB. Age related changes in dual AV nodal physiology. *Pacing Clin Electrophysiol.* 2000;23:477–480.

34. Cohen MI, Wieand TS, Rhodes LA, et al. Electrophysiologic properties of the atrioventricular node in pediatric patients. *J Am Coll Cardiol.* 1997;29:403–407.

35. Collins KK, Van Hare GF, Kertesz NJ, et al. Pediatric nonpost-operative junctional ectopic tachycardia medical management and interventional therapies. *J Am Coll Cardiol.* 2009;53:690–697.

131 Catheter Ablation in Congenital Heart Disease

Edward P. Walsh

Technical Challenges

The presence of congenital heart disease (CHD) can complicate catheter ablation procedures at several levels. First is the simple matter of vascular access and catheter navigation through distorted anatomy. Patients with major defects have frequently undergone multiple prior cardiac catheterizations for hemodynamic purposes, so it is not unusual for femoral vessels to be occluded or narrowed. The jugular vein, retrograde approach, or even more inventive techniques (e.g., transhepatic) may be required to advance catheters into the heart.[1,2] Beyond vessel access, catheter positioning at certain target sites can be impeded by atrial baffles, septal patches, and occlusion devices, which may be difficult to traverse with a standard Brockenbrough needle. Such barriers may require the use of radiofrequency (RF) energy delivered through the needle tip to reach a desired cardiac chamber.[3] Once inside the chamber of interest, the geometry can be dilated and misshapen, in which case a long deflectable sheath is an effective way to ensure thorough electrogram sampling and proper tissue contact for ablation. Institutions equipped with magnetic navigation systems report the technology to be very helpful for positioning the catheter tip in desired locations in difficult CHD patients.[4,5] Obviously, it is essential that these anatomical challenges be anticipated in advance of the procedure. All available imaging studies, operative notes, and prior catheterization reports need to be reviewed. If available, anatomical shells from cardiac magnetic resonance imaging (MRI) or computed tomography (CT) should be merged into electroanatomical mapping systems prior to the procedure, then further structural detail can be gathered with intraprocedural imaging using intracardiac echo and angiography.[6]

A second issue is abnormal development and location of specialized atrioventricular (AV) conduction tissues in certain CHD types.[7] Patients with heterotaxy (abnormal atrial situs and/or discordant alignment of atria and ventricles) exhibit the most dramatic variants,[8] ranging from complete absence of the AV node (AVN) all the way to a duplicated conduction system referred to as "twin AVNs."[9,10] Other important variants include the anteriorly displaced AVN seen in patients with "congenitally corrected" transposition of the great arteries (L-TGA) and the posteriorly displaced node seen in patients with AV canal defects.[7] Even when the node is not actually displaced, abnormal chamber dimensions in conditions such as Ebstein anomaly can distort the customary landmarks for the triangle of Koch and can make node localization challenging. Care must therefore be taken to understand these deviations and localize the AVN and His bundle as precisely as possible before delivering ablation energy that could inadvertently damage normal conduction.

Arrhythmia substrates encountered in CHD patients (as detailed in this chapter as well as in Chapters 74, 102, and 109) must also be well understood. Some of these, such as accessory pathways (APs) and AVN reentry, are quite conventional in their electrophysiology, but distorted anatomy can increase the degree of difficulty during ablation. Other substrates, including atrial macroreentrant circuits in patients with extensive atrial scarring[11,12] or ventricular macroreentry in tetralogy of Fallot[13] involve somewhat unique mechanisms that must be understood fully to facilitate mapping and ensure creation of an effective ablative lesion set.

A final technical challenge during ablation in CHD is the issue of tissue thickness and limitations of ablative lesion depth. Atrial walls can become densely fibrotic and more than twice the normal thickness in response to abnormal pressure and volume loads,[14] and the right ventricle (RV) in a condition such as tetralogy of Fallot can develop a wall thickness that exceeds that of a normal left ventricle. Consequently, creating effective transmural lines of conduction block with endocardial ablation can occasionally be more challenging than anticipated. The adoption of irrigated-tip technology has definitely improved outcomes,[15,16] but frustrations remain in terms of both acute success and recurrence rate. Reinforcing ablative lesions from the epicardial surface via an intrapericardial approach is usually not a reliable option in patients with mediastinal and pericardial adhesions from previous surgery. Therefore occasions still arise when an open chest surgical approach becomes the only effective way to address a difficult tachycardia in select CHD patients.[17]

Ablation of Supraventricular Tachycardia

Supraventricular tachycardia (SVT) is a major source of morbidity among CHD patients, and for those with poor ventricular function, it is also a potential cause of mortality. In a large 2009 cohort study of adult survivors with CHD, the prevalence of some type of SVT was 15%, with a lifetime risk of approximately 50% regardless of the severity of the underlying lesion. These tachycardias were associated with a 50% increase in mortality, a two-fold increased risk for heart failure or stroke, and a three-fold higher risk for requiring some major cardiac intervention.[18] Single-ventricle patients with a Fontan circulation and those with TGA following Mustard or Senning operations have the highest burden of SVT, but even simple atrial septal defect closure can be associated with atrial rhythm disturbances during long-term follow-up. Furthermore, SVT can coexist with ventricular arrhythmias in this population, such that patients who have an implanted cardioverter defibrillator (ICD) not infrequently receive inappropriate shocks from their device in response to rapidly conducted SVT episodes.[19] Although antiarrhythmic medications retain a role under certain circumstances, there is growing reliance on ablation procedures to address SVT in both children and adults with CHD.[20]

Ablation of Atrial Macroreentrant Tachycardia

Atrial macroreentrant tachycardias account for the majority of ablation procedures performed in CHD patients. These can involve a traditional peritricuspid circuit of atrial flutter or more novel circuits related to scars and patches at other atrial sites.

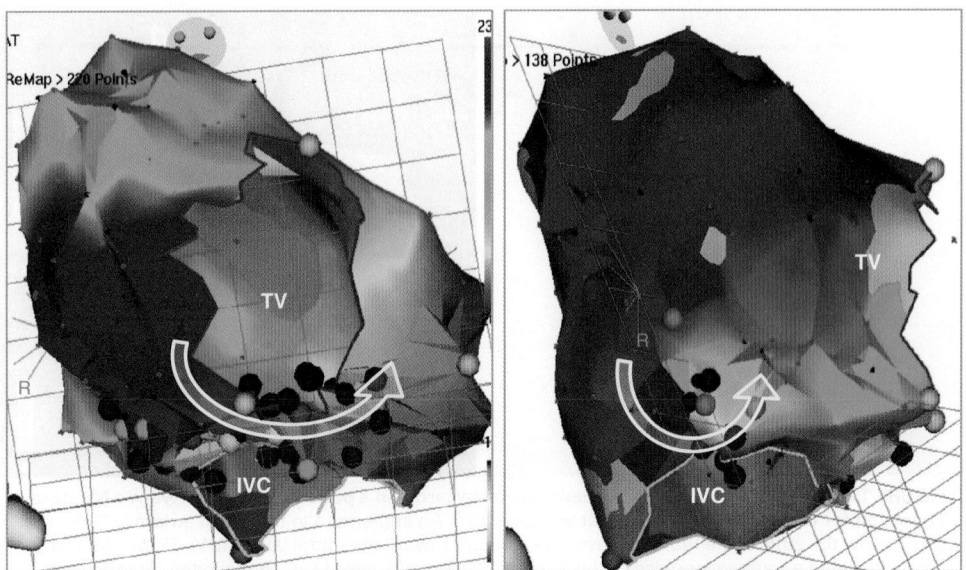

FIGURE 131.1 Electroanatomical maps of the right atrium in an adult patient with intraatrial reentrant tachycardia (IART) who underwent repair of tetralogy of Fallot as a child. *Left,* The first induced IART involved a counterclockwise circuit around the tricuspid valve (*TV*) that was successfully interrupted with ablation (*red dots*) in the cavotricuspid isthmus. *Right,* A second IART was then induced, involving a counterclockwise circuit on the right atrial lateral wall that used an atriotomy scar (*light blue dots*) as the central obstacle. This second circuit was interrupted with a line of ablation (*red dots*) from the lower edge of the atriotomy scar down to the inferior vena cava (*IVC*).

The label "intraatrial reentrant tachycardia" (IART) has been adopted as a general term to describe all possible circuits in CHD patients.[21]

Perhaps the most useful observation generated during the early years of IART ablation was that predictable patterns of circuit location could be linked to the underlying CHD lesion and method used for surgical repair.[11,12,22,23] For example, it is now well established that the culprit circuit for IART in simple four-chamber CHD (e.g., solitary atrial or ventricular septal defect closure, tetralogy of Fallot repair) typically involves the cavotricuspid isthmus but is frequently complicated by a figure-of-eight or dual-loop configuration with an outer loop around an atriotomy scar on the lateral right atrial (RA) wall (Fig. 131.1). Thus effective ablation typically requires interruption of both loops by creating conduction block along the isthmus, as well as at the narrow corridor between the lower edge of the atriotomy scar and inferior vena cava.[24] The atriotomy location can usually be identified by careful mapping of a narrow scar region with split potentials along the lateral RA wall that usually runs parallel but anterior to the crista terminalis. The typical IART circuit found in patients after Mustard or Senning operations for transposition also involves the cavotricuspid isthmus, but in these cases, the true isthmus is located on the pulmonary venous side of the large atrial baffle.[25] Access to the pulmonary venous atrium is almost always necessary for ablation of IART in these hearts (Fig. 131.2). This can be accomplished via a retrograde aortic approach through the tricuspid valve or by transbaffle puncture, which has become the preferred method at many centers.[3,26]

The most difficult IART circuits to map and ablate involve patients with a single ventricle who have undergone some variation of the Fontan operation.[27–29] The surgical design of this operation has evolved over the years, and the different designs vary in terms of both arrhythmogenic potential and IART circuit location. The original Fontan design used a RA–pulmonary artery anastomosis that usually resulted in dramatic atrial dilation, with large areas of low-voltage or fractionated potentials and an IART incidence as high as 40%.[30] The IART circuits in such patients are often multiple and can occur just about anywhere within the dilated

RA chamber (Fig. 131.3). Ablation success and freedom from recurrence tends to be lower in this group than in any other CHD category, prompting some centers to advocate operative intervention for conversion to one of the newer Fontan designs, along with excision of redundant RA tissue and surgical maze.[31,32] Newer Fontan designs bypass RA to a large extent, using either a lateral tunnel or an extracardiac conduit, thereby reducing RA dilation and significantly reducing IART incidence to <10%. However, for the occasional patient who does develop IART with a more modern Fontan design, circuit locations are typically on the pulmonary venous side of the tunnel or conduit, requiring complex techniques for transseptal access.[33]

Mapping of IART circuits in any form of CHD requires accurate registration of the underlying anatomy. Nearly all these procedures are now performed using three-dimensional (3D) electroanatomical mapping systems, augmenting the spatial shell geometry by merging one or more alternate imaging modalities (MRI, CT, intracardiac echocardiography, angiography). After registration of the anatomy, it can be helpful to perform a substrate map in baseline rhythm to locate low-voltage areas corresponding to scars and patches that may serve as central obstacles or the border of a conduction corridor for IART circuits, as well as to locate positions of normal conduction tissues and the course of the phrenic nerve to avoid potential injury.[34,35] Activation mapping and entrainment maneuvers are then performed during IART to localize and confirm the circuit according to the standard methodology for macroreentry. It should be noted that atrial cycle lengths for IART circuits tend to be far longer (250–330 ms) than those in conventional atrial flutter,[36] allowing rapid AV conduction that may be poorly tolerated in CHD patients with depressed ventricular function. Administration of AVN-blocking agents, such as diltiazem, is often required to titrate the ventricular response rate and allow mapping to be completed. Experience suggests that creation of effective ablation lines in CHD patients with potentially increased atrial wall thickness is greatly aided by the use of an irrigated-tip ablation catheter.[15,16,37] Whenever possible, postablation pacing maneuvers should be performed

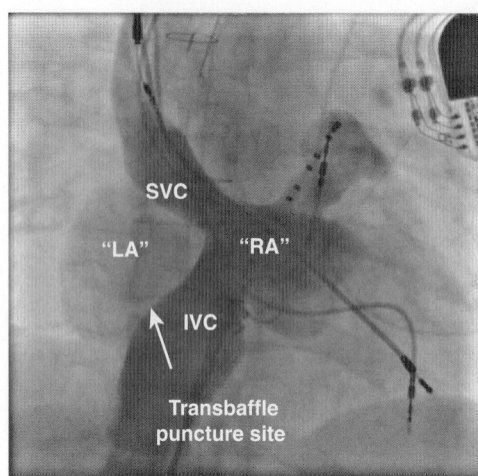
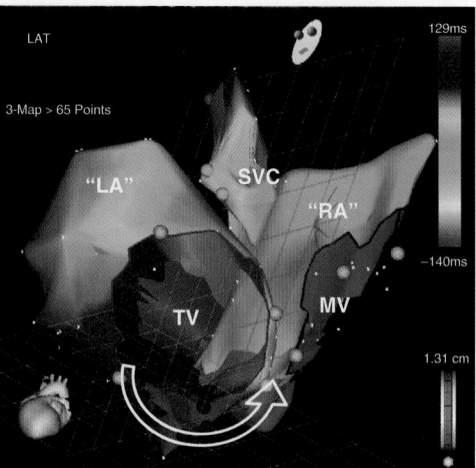

FIGURE 131.2 Ablation for intraatrial reentrant tachycardia in a patient who underwent a Mustard operation for transposition of the great arteries. *Left,* An angiogram in the "right atrium" ("*RA*") that shows how the atrial baffle redirects caval blood return toward the mitral valve (*MV*). *Right,* The tachycardia involved a counterclockwise circuit around the tricuspid valve (*TV*). To reach the cavotricuspid isthmus region for ablation, a transbaffle puncture technique was employed to enter the "left atrium" ("*LA*"). *IVC,* Inferior vena cava; *LAT,* left atrial tachycardia; *SVC,* superior vena cava.

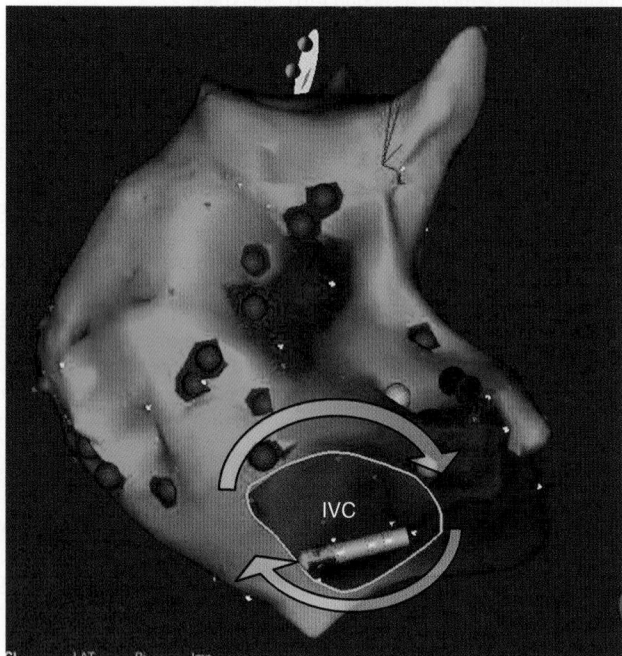

FIGURE 131.3 Electroanatomical map of a dilated right atrium in a patient who underwent an atriopulmonary-style Fontan operation for a single ventricle. The activation pattern represents an unusual circuit of intraatrial reentrant tachycardia rotating around a dilated inferior vena cava (*IVC*).

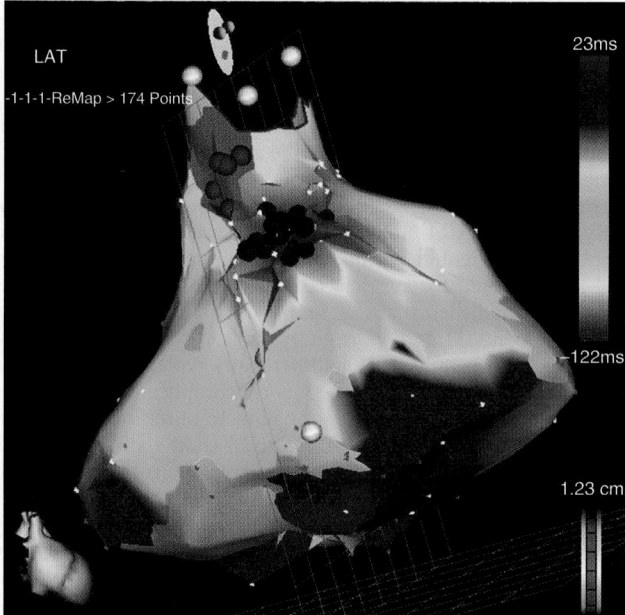

FIGURE 131.4 Electroanatomical map of a dilated right atrium in a patient who underwent an atriopulmonary-style Fontan operation for a single ventricle. The activation pattern is generated by a focal atrial tachycardia that originates near a scar zone (*dark gray area*) in the region of the superior vena cava–right atrium junction, which likely represents a caval cannulation site from prior surgery.

to prove bidirectional conduction block across the ablation site, although the awkward anatomy of some CHD lesions can make it difficult to position the pacing electrode at ideal sites to verify this unequivocally.

As a consequence of more sophisticated mapping, more effective ablation, and expanded procedural experience, the acute success rate for catheter ablation of IART has now improved to approximately 85%.[15,35–42] The recurrence rate after acutely successful procedures remains relatively high (10%–30%), particularly in the Fontan subgroup. However, these outcomes are still far superior to the control achieved with drug therapy and continue to improve along with refinements in technology.

Ablation of Focal Atrial Tachycardia

A subset of atrial tachycardias in CHD patients involves a focal disorder that can be triggered with programmed atrial stimulation and terminated with overdrive pacing and electrical cardioversion, suggesting a mechanism of either triggered activity or a small region of microreentry.[43] It is estimated that 5%–10% of atrial tachycardias mapped and ablated in CHD patients involve such a mechanism. These foci tend to be localized along the edge of a scar zone or suture line[44] and occur most commonly in patients who have undergone the Fontan operation (Fig. 131.4). Mapping reveals a point source for early activation with centrifugal spread of atrial depolarization away from a scar zone. Ablation can be successful in over 90% of these cases.

Ablation of Atrial Fibrillation

Atrial fibrillation (AF) is being reported with increasing frequency in CHD patients, particularly those who have reached adult age with diastolic dysfunction of their systemic ventricle, left heart obstruction, mitral valve disease, or other lesions, contributing to left atrial (LA) dilation.[39,45] There is a small but growing amount of literature that describes transcatheter pulmonary vein isolation for AF in this population. Most cases reported to date have involved straightforward lesions, such as atrial septal defects,[46,47] although the technique is being cautiously expanded to more complex anatomy. One item that may distinguish these cases from more conventional AF ablation in a structurally normal heart is the challenge of achieving LA access across patches and septal occlusion devices, but this can be overcome in nearly all instances.[3,48] A second issue is that CHD patients with cyanotic lesions (e.g., palliated single ventricle, Eisenmenger syndrome) have little or no reserve in terms of pulmonary blood flow so that even small degrees of pulmonary venous narrowing from ablation too near an orifice is likely to be catastrophic. This concern has led many centers to adopt the cryothermal (CRYO) balloon technique in preference to RF ablation in cyanotic CHD patients undergoing AF ablation (Fig. 131.5). Experience is still too limited to define success and recurrence rates for AF ablation in the CHD population, and selection criteria are still being developed.

Ablation of Atrioventricular Nodal Reentry

The high success rate associated with slow pathway modification for AVN reentrant tachycardia (AVNRT) in patients with structurally normal hearts is largely based on a predictable location of compact AVN and its extensions, but as mentioned earlier in this chapter, certain CHD patients can have a displaced node and/or distorted landmarks for the triangle of Koch that add a level of complexity whenever slow pathway modification is attempted. Furthermore, surgical patching can complicate catheter positioning near the nodal region following the Mustard or Senning operations for D-looped TGA or following the Fontan operation for a single ventricle. Although tachycardia behavior and electrophysiology are conventional in every other sense, this anatomical variance could affect both ablation success and risk for inadvertent AVN injury. The experience with ablation of AVNRT in CHD is still somewhat limited, but there are a growing number of case reports[49–52] and clinical series[53,54] that indicate that the procedure can be accomplished safely if proper technical modifications and precautions are employed. Publications now describe successful AVN modification in patients with D-looped TGA, "congenitally corrected" TGA, a single ventricle, and others (Fig. 131.6). Most cases have been performed using RF energy, but CRYO is used for safety reasons whenever the precise location of the compact node is ambiguous. The largest series to date, involving 39 patients[54] with an assortment of CHD lesions, reported acute success in 92%, with no major complications and only one recurrence over approximately 3 years of follow-up.

A rare but fascinating variation on the AVNRT theme in CHD patients is a condition known as twin AVNs.[9,10,55] This phenomenon occurs most commonly in patients with heterotaxy of the asplenia type (bilateral right sidedness), often characterized by single-ventricle physiology due to a malaligned AV canal defect, favoring RV with a discordant relationship between atria and ventricles. The twin node conduction system features two compact nodes and two His bundles that typically fuse at the ventricular level with a connecting sling of specialized conduction tissue. Tachycardia due to node–node reentry across the sling is the most common arrhythmia seen in this condition, but other reentrant circuits may also occur. Ablation of the less robust of the two nodes is a practical approach to this unusual disorder.[9,56] Twin node reentry shares some features in common with

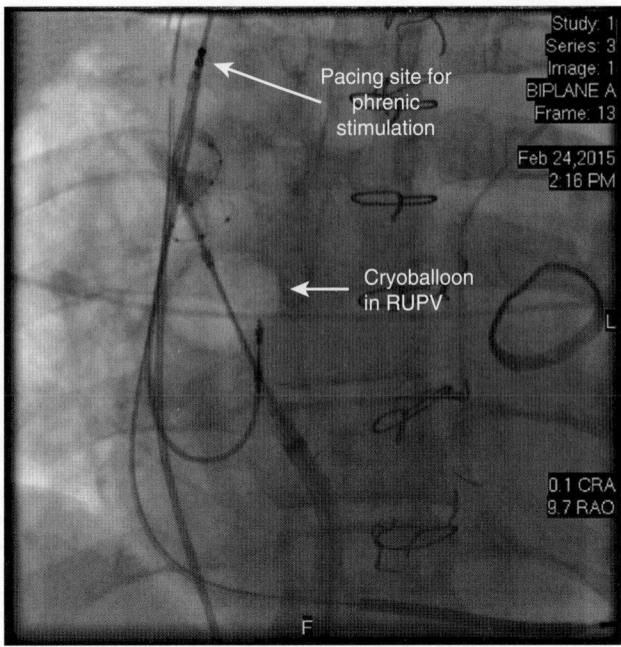

FIGURE 131.5 Pulmonary vein isolation in a 55-year-old with recurrent atrial fibrillation who underwent tetralogy of Fallot repair as a child. The cryoballoon is inflated in the right upper pulmonary vein (*RUPV*), and a quadripolar pacing catheter is used in the superior vena cava to monitor phrenic nerve integrity during the freeze. *CRA,* Cranial; *RAO,* right anterior oblique.

antidromic tachycardia due to an atriofascicular fiber, except that neither of the twin nodes generates a preexcited QRS and both nodes are usually capable of bidirectional conduction. Still, it has to be wondered if there is some embryological overlap between these two disorders.

Ablation of Accessory Pathways in Ebstein Anomaly

Some form of SVT is extremely common in patients with Ebstein anomaly.[57] More than 20% have Wolff-Parkinson-White syndrome,[58] quite often involving multiple APs that tend to localize in the region where the tricuspid valve is most displaced down into the RV body.[59,60] Concealed APs, atriofascicular pathways, and AVNRT are also far more common in the population with Ebstein anomaly than in the general population.[61] Over time, IART and AF often develop due to atrial distension.[62]

Ablation of APs in patients with Ebstein anomaly can be challenging. The technique is similar to that of conventional APs, except that the level of true AV annulus, where ablation is most likely to be productive, can be hard to define owing to the abnormal tricuspid valve. A right coronary artery angiogram can be very helpful for localizing the true AV groove, but a second challenge then becomes interpretation of the electrograms along the groove (Fig. 131.7). Because RV muscle is very thin and "atrialized" in this region of interest, the ventricular component of the electrogram is often of a lower amplitude than expected. Mapping can become surprisingly difficult, with the possibility of multiple APs. Severe RA dilation, which is common in Ebstein anomaly, can further complicate matters by affecting catheter navigation and tip stability. As a result, ablation of AP is less successful in Ebstein anomaly than in normal hearts. Early reports from the 1990s[61] suggested an acute success rate of 88% and a high recurrence rate of 22%, which initially were attributed to lack of experience, but more contemporary reports[63] confirm similar outcomes despite all advances in imaging, mapping, and ablation energy delivery. APs in this condition may be anatomically more complex than

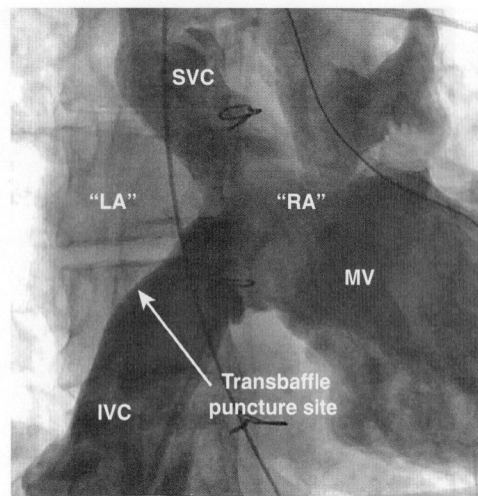 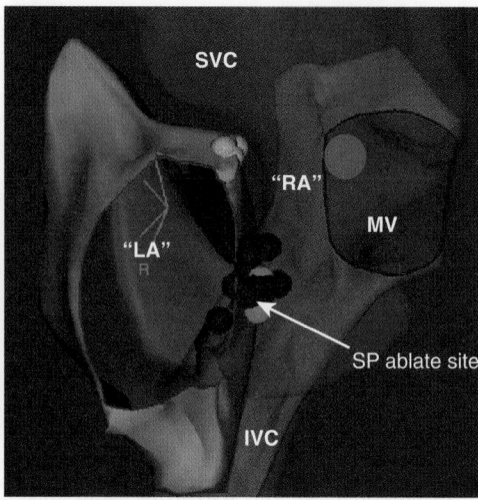

FIGURE 131.6 Slow pathway *(SP)* ablation in a Mustard patient with typical slow–fast atrioventricular nodal reentrant tachycardia. *Left,* An angiogram in the "right atrium" (*"RA"*) that shows how the atrial baffle redirects caval blood return toward the mitral valve (*MV*). *Right,* An anatomical shell focused on the "left atrium" (*"LA"*). The SP was located in the expected area of the triangle of Koch, albeit on the left side of the atrial baffle, which was crossed by a transbaffle puncture technique. Sites of recording for the His bundle are marked with *orange dots.* Cautious radiofrequency applications were made in the lower third of the triangle of Koch. *Red dots* indicate unsuccessful test sites. *Light blue dots* indicate sites that caused junctional acceleration but did not eliminate the SP. The *dark blue dot* marks a site of success. *IVC,* Inferior vena cava; *SVC,* superior vena cava.

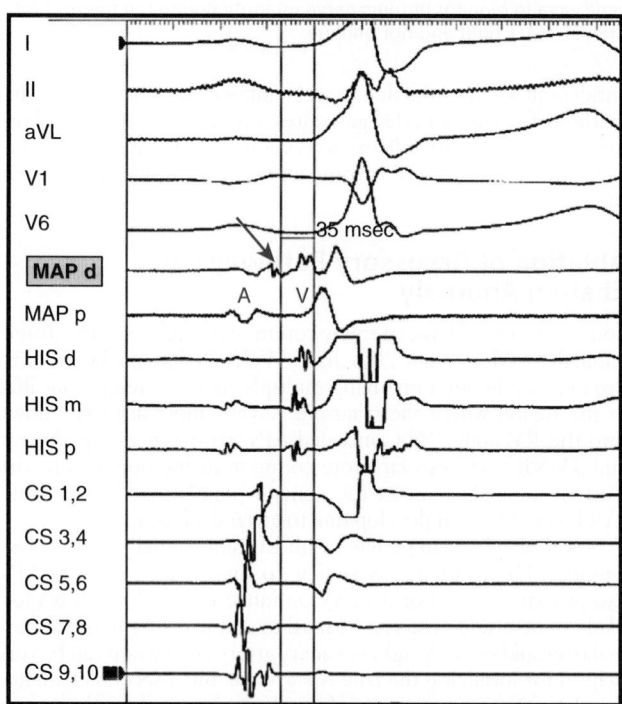

FIGURE 131.7 Mapping of an accessory pathway along the true atrioventricular groove in a patient with Ebstein anomaly. The distal electrode pair of the mapping catheter (*MAP d*) is located at the site of successful ablation. The signal at this site contains a sharp middle component (*arrow*) that likely represents an accessory pathway potential. However, the ventricular (*V*) amplitude is relatively low at this site because the regional myocardium is thin and fibrotic. *CS,* Coronary sinus; *HIS,* His bundle.

standard AV connections. Regardless, strong efforts must be made to eliminate APs in patients with Ebstein anomaly, particularly in advance of surgical tricuspid valve reconstructions, which could make any subsequent catheter tip positioning along the AV groove difficult. If AP proves resistant to preoperative catheter

ablation, it is possible to map the location carefully and resort to cryoablation under direct vision in the operating room.[62]

Ablation of Ventricular Tachycardia

It is useful to distinguish two categories of ventricular tachycardia (VT) in the CHD population.[64] The first involves developmental and surgical features that create discrete conduction corridors capable of supporting one or more monomorphic reentrant VT circuits. Specific CHD lesions that exemplify this anatomical predisposition to macroreentrant VT include (1) tetralogy of Fallot, (2) Ebstein anomaly, and (3) other rare defects repaired through a free wall ventriculotomy. These are patients who are most likely to benefit from catheter ablation and hence are the source of most VT mapping data in the CHD population. The second category involves less organized VT and/or ventricular fibrillation that can develop in diffusely abnormal myocardium, similar to VT seen in other forms of hypertrophic or dilated cardiomyopathy. The myopathic substrate in CHD patients is generated by long-standing pressure and volume loads, often complicated by cyanosis, that ultimately result in advanced degrees of hypertrophy, fibrosis, and ventricular dilation. Lesions and conditions associated with this myopathic type of VT include (1) congenital left-heart outflow obstruction, (2) TGA following Mustard or Senning operations where the RV has been recruited as the systemic ventricle, (3) tetralogy of Fallot with advanced ventricular dilation and dysfunction, (4) unrepaired ventricular septal defect with Eisenmenger physiology, and (5) palliated single ventricle. Generally, these are ill patients with poor hemodynamics in whom treatment with an ICD is the preferred approach, although ablation may still be indicated to reduce the shock burden from the device. Naturally, the potential exists for both VT categories to occur in a given patient whenever there is a combination of underlying anatomical substrate and ventricular dysfunction.

Mapping and ablation techniques for VT in CHD are similar to those employed for any other form of heart disease, with a few important differences related to ventricular geometry, location of surgical scars, and other muscle features that influence reentrant

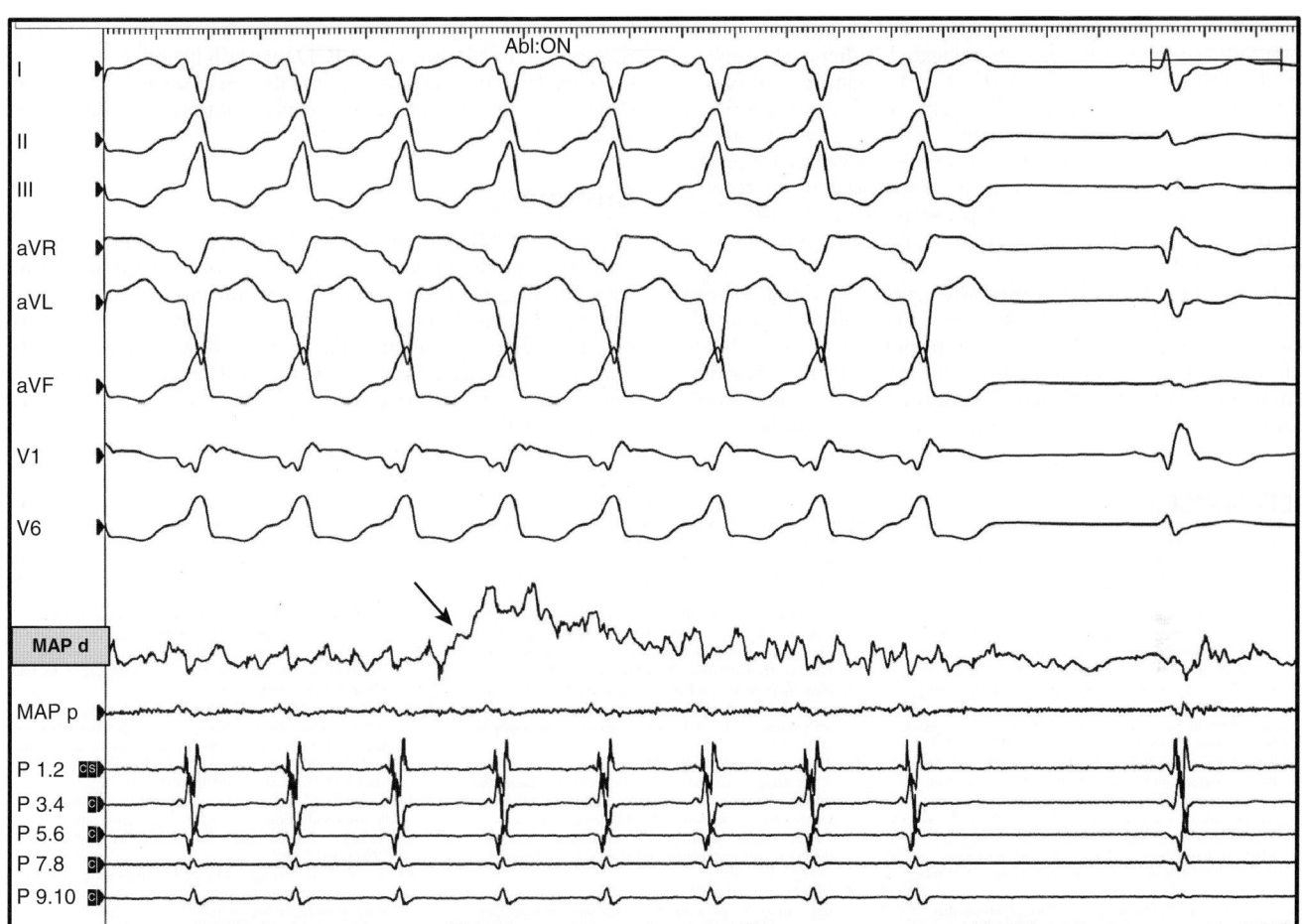

FIGURE 131.8 Ablation of monomorphic ventricular tachycardia (VT) in an adult with repaired tetralogy of Fallot. The tachycardia has left bundle branch block morphology and an inferior axis, consistent with an origin in the right ventricular outflow region. Note the signal on the distal mapping electrode (*MAP d*), which has a nearly continuous low-amplitude electrical activity, including middiastolic activation time. A radiofrequency application was initiated at this site (*arrow*) that terminated VT promptly.

propagation patterns. The anatomical predilection for macroreentrant VT circuits to arise from the RV outflow region in tetralogy of Fallot has been appreciated since the landmark 1980 article from Horowitz et al.[65] that contributed to the first successful surgical ablations of VT in tetralogy of Fallot patients.[66] More recently, a refined understanding of VT circuits in tetralogy of Fallot was provided by Zeppenfeld et al.,[67] who highlighted multiple discrete conduction corridors in the RV outflow region, including (1) the conal septum running between the ventricular septal defect and pulmonary valve, (2) a rim of RV muscle between the anterior ventriculotomy scar and pulmonary valve (when a nontransannular patch technique was used), and (3) RV free wall muscle between the ventriculotomy and tricuspid valve. Importantly, they were able to verify the importance of these corridors by proving that empirical ablation, even in the absence of propagation mapping, could effectively eliminate monomorphic VT in most instances. On rare occasions, VT in tetralogy of Fallot has to be ablated from the left side of the outflow tract within the aortic root.[68]

The substrate for monomorphic VT in Ebstein anomaly is less discrete, but most cases appear to involve the thin and fibrotic RV tissue along the AV groove that is said to be "atrialized." There are isolated case reports and small series describing successful RF ablation of monomorphic VT in this setting.[62,69]

Most reports of successful VT ablation in CHD stress the need for a careful baseline substrate map focused on scar areas that correspond to surgical patches, incision lines, and other regions of low-amplitude and fragmented electrograms. Assuming

successful VT induction, circuit stability, and patient tolerance, detailed activation mapping can then be attempted to outline the propagation pattern. Diastolic potentials with fractionated activity of low amplitude will typically be recorded in relevant conduction corridors (Fig. 131.8), and pacing maneuvers within these corridors should result in a classic pattern of concealed entrainment with a postpacing interval identical to the tachycardia cycle length.[13,70,71] In cases where VT is too rapid for the patient to tolerate, alternate techniques, such as noncontact mapping[72] and pace mapping,[73] have been effectively used to localize macroreentrant circuits in CHD. If it proves difficult to induce and sustain the patient's clinical VT, an empirical lesion set directed at potential narrow conduction corridors, identified on the baseline substrate map, may be a workable strategy even when detailed activation mapping is impossible.[67,72] This is particularly true for tetralogy of Fallot patients in whom candidate paths for reentry are fairly well defined.

Most outcome data for transcatheter VT ablation in CHD involve the tetralogy of Fallot population. Descriptions of successful ablation of VT in this group first appeared in the early 1990s, beginning as isolated case reports[73,74] and gradually growing to small clinical series.[67,71,75] The acute success rate for RF catheter ablation now approaches 90% in this group, although VT recurrence or positive follow-up ventricular stimulation studies are still seen in approximately 18% of patients. Recurrences are not surprising given the dramatic thickness of RV muscle that may be hard to penetrate in some of these cases even when using irrigated-tip catheters. The uneasiness surrounding recurrence has largely relegated catheter ablation to an adjunctive role along with an ICD in the management of VT in tetralogy of Fallot patients.[76] There may be an exceptional case of well-tolerated VT in a patient with preserved ventricular function where ablation might be used as isolated therapy, but if an ICD is ever deferred, it seems prudent to recommend that follow-up testing with programmed stimulation[77] be performed at some later date before the need for an ICD is dismissed entirely.

If catheter ablation is not successful, surgical VT ablation can be considered. The surgical option remains important for tetralogy of Fallot patients because a large number are now being referred back to the operating room for replacement of regurgitant pulmonary valves. When valve replacement is combined with careful pre- or intraoperative mapping, strategic cryoablation can be performed by the surgeon to reduce the likelihood of macroreentrant VT.[78] However, an ICD may still be indicated because most available data suggest that the degree of reverse RV remodeling after valve replacement is insufficient to completely remove all VT risk.[79]

Summary

Ablation in CHD patients demands strict attention to anatomical details of the underlying cardiac lesion and the technique used for surgical repair. Macroreentrant circuits at the atrial and ventricular level account for the majority of the serious arrhythmias requiring ablation in these patients. As the population of adult survivors with CHD continues to grow, the number of cases requiring ablation therapy will increase proportionally.

REFERENCES

1. Emmel M, Brockmeier K, Sreeram N. Combined transhepatic and transjugular approach for radiofrequency ablation of an accessory pathway in a child with complex congenital heart disease. *Z Kardiol*. 2004;93:555–557.
2. Nehgme RA, Carboni MP, Care J, et al. Transthoracic percutaneous access for electroanatomic mapping and catheter ablation of atrial tachycardia in patients with a lateral tunnel Fontan. *Heart Rhythm*. 2006;3:37–43.
3. Esch JJ, Triedman JK, Cecchin F, et al. Radiofrequency-assisted transseptal perforation for electrophysiology procedures in children and adults with repaired congenital heart disease. *Pacing Clin Electrophysiol*. 2013;36:607–611.
4. Akca F, Bauernfeind T, Witsenburg M, et al. Acute and long-term outcomes of catheter ablation using remote magnetic navigation in patients with congenital heart disease. *Am J Cardiol*. 2012;110:409–414.
5. Suman-Horduna I, Babu-Narayan SV, Ueda A, et al. Magnetic navigation in adults with atrial isomerism (heterotaxy syndrome) and supraventricular arrhythmias. *Europace*. 2013;15:877–885.
6. Kedia A, Hsu PY, Holmes J, et al. Use of intracardiac echocardiography in guiding radiofrequency catheter ablation of atrial tachycardia in a patient after the Senning operation. *Pacing Clin Electrophysiol*. 2004;26:2178–2180.
7. Anderson RH, Ho SY. The disposition of the conduction tissues in congenitally malformed hearts with reference to their embryological development. *J Perinat Med*. 1991;19:201–206.
8. Anderson RH, Brown NA, Moorman AF. The sinus node, isomerism, and heterotaxy. *Cardiovasc Pathol*. 2013;22:243–244.
9. Epstein MR, Saul JP, Weindling SN, et al. Atrioventricular reciprocating tachycardia involving twin atrioventricular nodes in patients with complex congenital heart disease. *J Cardiovasc Electrophysiol*. 2001;12:671–679.
10. Bae E-J, Noh C-I, Choi J-Y, et al. Twin AV node and induced supraventricular tachycardia in Fontan palliation patients. *Pacing Clin Electrophysiol*. 2005;28:126–134.
11. Collins KK, Love BA, Walsh EP, et al. Location of acutely successful radiofrequency catheter ablation of intraatrial reentrant tachycardia in patients with congenital heart disease. *Am J Cardiol*. 2000;86:969–974.
12. Lukac P, Pedersen AK, Mortensen PT, et al. Ablation of atrial tachycardia after surgery for congenital and acquired heart disease using an electroanatomic mapping system: which circuits to expect in which substrate? *Heart Rhythm*. 2005;2:64–72.
13. Walsh EP. Interventional electrophysiology in patients with congenital heart disease. *Circulation*. 2007;115:3224–3234.
14. Wolf CM, Seslar SP, den Boer K, et al. Atrial remodeling after the Fontan operation. *Am J Cardiol*. 2009;104:1737–1742.
15. Triedman JK, DeLucca JM, Alexander ME, et al. Prospective trial of electroanatomically guided, irrigated catheter ablation of atrial tachycardia in patients with congenital heart disease. *Heart Rhythm*. 2005;2:700–705.
16. Tanner H, Lukac P, Schwick N, et al. Irrigated-tip catheter ablation of intraatrial reentrant tachycardia in patients late after surgery of congenital heart disease. *Heart Rhythm*. 2004;1:268–275.
17. Mavroudis C, Deal BJ, Backer CL, et al. The J Maxwell Chamberlain Memorial Paper for congenital heart surgery. 111 Fontan conversions with arrhythmia surgery: surgical lessons and outcomes. *Ann Thorac Surg*. 2007;84:1457–1465.
18. Bouchardy J, Therrien J, Pilote L, et al. Atrial arrhythmias in adults with congenital heart disease. *Circulation*. 2009;120:1679–1686.
19. Love BA, Barrett KS, Alexander ME, et al. Supraventricular arrhythmias in children and young adults with implantable cardioverter defibrillators. *J Cardiovasc Electrophysiol*. 2001;12:1097–1101.
20. Khairy P, Van Hare GF, Balaji S, et al. PACES/HRS Expert Consensus Statement on the Recognition and Management of Arrhythmias in Adult Congenital Heart Disease. *Heart Rhythm*. 2014;11:e102–e165.
21. Mandapati R, Walsh EP, Triedman JK. Pericaval and periannular intra-atrial reentrant tachycardias in patients with congenital heart disease. *J Cardiovasc Electrophysiol*. 2003;14:119–125.
22. Triedman JK, Alexander ME, Berul CI, et al. Electroanatomic mapping of entrained and exit zones in patients with repaired congenital heart disease and intra-atrial reentrant tachycardia. *Circulation*. 2001;103:2060–2065.
23. Drago F, Russo MS, Marazzi R, et al. Atrial tachycardia in patients with congenital heart disease. *Europace*. 2011;13:689–695.
24. Mah D, Alexander ME, Cecchin F, et al. The electroanatomic mechanisms of atrial tachycardia in patients with tetralogy of Fallot and double outlet right ventricle. *J Cardiovasc Electrophysiol*. 2011;22:1013–1017.
25. Van Hare GF, Lesh MD, Ross BA, et al. Mapping and radiofrequency ablation of intraatrial reentrant tachycardia after the Senning or Mustard procedure for transposition of the great arteries. *Am J Cardiol*. 1996;77:985–991.
26. Perry JC, Boramanand NK, Ing FF. "Transseptal" technique through atrial baffles for 3-dimensional mapping and ablation of atrial tachycardia in patients with d-transposition of the great arteries. *J Interv Card Electrophysiol*. 2003;9:365–369.
27. Abrams DJ, Earley MJ, Sporton SC, et al. Comparison of noncontact and electroanatomic mapping to identify scar and arrhythmia late after the Fontan procedure. *Circulation*. 2007;115:1738–1746.
28. Yap SC, Harris L, Downar E, et al. Evolving electroanatomic substrate and intra-atrial reentrant tachycardia late after Fontan surgery. *J Cardiovasc Electrophysiol*. 2012;23:339–345.
29. Stephenson EA, Lu M, Berul CI, et al. Arrhythmias in a contemporary Fontan cohort: prevalence and clinical associations in a multicenter cross-sectional study. *J Am Coll Cardiol*. 2010;56:890–896.
30. Fishberger SB, Wernovsky G, Gentles TL, et al. Factors that influence the development of atrial flutter after the Fontan operation. *J Thorac Cardiovasc Surg*. 1997;113:80–86.
31. Deal BJ, Costello JM, Webster G, et al. Intermediate-term outcome of 140 consecutive Fontan conversions with arrhythmia operations. *Ann Thorac Surg*. 2016;101:717–724.
32. Aboulhosn J, Williams R, Shivkumar K, et al. Arrhythmia recurrence in adult patients with single ventricle physiology following surgical Fontan conversion. *Congenit Heart Dis*. 2010;5:430–434.
33. Correa R, Sherwin ED, Kovach J, et al. Mechanism and ablation of arrhythmia following total cavopulmonary connection. *Circ Arrhythm Electrophysiol*. 2015;8:318–325.
34. Love BA, Collins KK, Walsh EP, et al. Electroanatomic characterization of conduction barriers in sinus/atrially paced rhythm and association with intra-atrial reentrant tachycardia circuits following congenital heart surgery. *Cardiovasc Electrophysiol*. 2001;12:17–25.
35. de Groot NM, Schalij MJ, Zeppenfeld K, et al. Voltage and activation mapping: how the recording technique affects the outcome of catheter ablation procedures in patients with congenital heart disease. *Circulation*. 2003;108:2099–2106.
36. Triedman JK, Bergau DM, Saul JP, et al. Efficacy of radiofrequency ablation for control of intraatrial reentrant tachycardia in patients with congenital heart disease. *J Am Coll Cardiol*. 1997;30:1032–1038.
37. Triedman JK, Alexander ME, Love BA, et al. Influence of patient factors and ablative technologies on outcomes of radiofrequency ablation of intra-atrial reentrant tachycardia in patients with congenital heart disease. *J Am Coll Cardiol*. 2002;39:1827–1835.
38. de Groot NM, Atary JZ, Blom NA, et al. Long-term outcome after ablative therapy of postoperative atrial tachyarrhythmia in patients with congenital heart disease and characteristics of atrial tachycardia recurrences. *Circ Arrhythm Electrophysiol*. 2010;3:148–154.
39. Teh AW, Medi C, Lee G, et al. Long-term outcome following ablation of atrial flutter occurring late after atrial septal defect repair. *Pacing Clin Electrophysiol*. 2011;34:431–435.
40. Koyak Z, de Groot JR, Mulder BJ. Interventional and surgical treatment of cardiac arrhythmias in adults with congenital heart disease. *Expert Rev Cardiovasc Ther*. 2010;8:1753–1766.
41. de Groot NM, Lukac P, Schalij MJ, et al. Long-term outcome of ablative therapy of post-operative atrial tachyarrhythmias in patients with tetralogy of Fallot: a European multi-centre study. *Europace*. 2012;14:522–527.
42. Yap SC, Harris L, Silversides CK, et al. Outcome of intra-atrial re-entrant tachycardia catheter ablation in adults with congenital heart disease: negative impact of age and complex atrial surgery. *J Am Coll Cardiol*. 2010;56:1589–1596.
43. Seslar SP, Alexander ME, Berul CI, et al. Ablation of nonautomatic focal atrial tachycardia in children and adults with congenital heart disease. *J Cardiovasc Electrophysiol*. 2006;17:359–365.
44. de Groot N, Zeppenfeld K, Wijffels MC, et al. Ablation of focal atrial arrhythmia in patients with congenital heart defects after surgery: role of circumscribed areas with heterogeneous conduction. *Heart Rhythm*. 2006;3:526–535.
45. Kirsh JA, Walsh EP, Triedman JK. Prevalence of and risk factors for atrial fibrillation and intraatrial reentrant tachycardia among patients with congenital heart disease. *Am J Cardiol*. 2002;90:338–340.
46. Philip F, Muhammad KI, Agarwal S, et al. Pulmonary vein isolation for the treatment of drug-refractory atrial fibrillation in adults with congenital heart disease. *Congenit Heart Dis*. 2012;7:392–399.
47. Lakkireddy D, Rangisetty U, Prasad S, et al. Intracardiac echo-guided radiofrequency catheter ablation of atrial fibrillation in patients with atrial septal defect or patent foramen ovale repair: a feasibility, safety, and efficacy study. *J Cardiovasc Electrophysiol*. 2008;19:1137–1142.
48. Katritsis DG. Transseptal puncture through atrial septal closure devices. *Heart Rhythm*. 2011;8:1676–1677.
49. Kanter RJ, Papagiannis J, Carboni MP, et al. Radiofrequency catheter ablation of supraventricular tachycardia substrates after Mustard and Senning operations for d-transposition of the great arteries. *J Am Coll Cardiol*. 2000;35:428–441.
50. Khairy P, Seslar SP, Triedman JK, et al. Ablation of atrioventricular nodal reentrant tachycardia in tricuspid atresia. *J Cardiovasc Electrophysiol*. 2004;15:719–722.
51. Abrams DJ, Earley MJ, Sporton SC, et al. Successful ablation of atrioventricular nodal reentry tachycardia following the atriopulmonary Fontan procedure. *Europace*. 2006;8:907–910.
52. Ernst S, Ouyang F, Linder C, et al. Modulation of the slow pathway in the presence of a persistent left superior caval vein using the novel magnetic navigation system Niobe. *Europace*. 2004;6:10–14.

53. Liao Z, Chang Y, Ma J, et al. Atrioventricular node reentrant tachycardia in patients with congenitally corrected transposition of the great arteries and results of radiofrequency catheter ablation. *Circ Arrhythm Electrophysiol.* 2012;5:1143–1148.

54. Upadhyay S, Valente AM, Triedman JK, et al. Catheter ablation for atrioventricular nodal reentry tachycardia in patients with congenital heart disease. *Heart Rhythm.* 2016;13:1228–1237.

55. Takahashi K, Kurosawa H, Nakanishi T. Twin atrioventricular nodes connecting to sling of conduction tissue in congenitally corrected transposition associated with straddling tricuspid valve. *World J Pediatr Congenit Heart Surg.* 2011;2:312–315.

56. Czosek RJ, Anderson J, Connor C, et al. Nodoventricular pathway associated with twin AV nodes: complexity of ablation in single ventricle physiology. *Cardiovasc Electrophysiol.* 2010;21:936–939.

57. Paranon S, Acar P. Ebstein's anomaly of the tricuspid valve: from fetus to adult: congenital heart disease. *Heart.* 2008;94:237–243.

58. Attenhofer Jost CH, Connolly HM, Edwards WD, et al. Ebstein's anomaly - review of a multifaceted congenital cardiac condition. *Swiss Med Wkly.* 2005;135:269–281.

59. Chetaille P, Walsh EP, Triedman JK. Outcomes of radiofrequency catheter ablation of atrioventricular reciprocating tachycardia in patients with congenital heart disease. *Heart Rhythm.* 2004;1:168–173.

60. Zachariah JP, Walsh EP, Triedman JK, et al. Multiple accessory pathways in the young: the impact of structural heart disease. *Am Heart J.* 2013;165:87–92.

61. Reich JD, Auld D, Hulse E, et al. The Pediatric Radiofrequency Ablation Registry's experience with Ebstein's anomaly. Pediatric Electrophysiology Society. *J Cardiovasc Electrophysiol.* 1998;9:1370–1377.

62. Shivapour JK, Sherwin ED, Alexander ME, et al. Utility of preoperative electrophysiologic studies in patients with Ebstein's anomaly undergoing the Cone procedure. *Heart Rhythm.* 2014;11:182–186.

63. Roten L, Lukac P, De Groot N, et al. Catheter ablation of arrhythmias in Ebstein's anomaly: a multicenter study. *J Cardiovasc Electrophysiol.* 2011;22:1391–1396.

64. Walsh EP. Sudden death in adult congenital heart disease: risk stratification in 2014. *Heart Rhythm.* 2014;11:1735–1742.

65. Horowitz LN, Vetter VL, Harken AH, et al. Electrophysiologic characteristics of sustained ventricular tachycardia occurring after repair of tetralogy of Fallot. *Am J Cardiol.* 1980;46:446–452.

66. Harken AH, Horowitz LN, Josephson ME. Surgical correction of recurrent sustained ventricular tachycardia following complete repair of tetralogy of Fallot. *J Thorac Cardiovasc Surg.* 1980;80:779–781.

67. Zeppenfeld K, Schalij MJ, Bartelings MM, et al. Catheter ablation of ventricular tachycardia after repair of congenital heart disease: electroanatomic identification of the critical right ventricular isthmus. *Circulation.* 2007;116:2241–2252.

68. Kapel GF, Reichlin T, Wijnmaalen AP, et al. Left-sided ablation of ventricular tachycardia in adults with repaired tetralogy of Fallot: a case series. *Circ Arrhythm Electrophysiol.* 2014;7:889–897.

69. Obioha-Ngwu O, Milliez P, Richardson A, et al. Ventricular tachycardia in Ebstein's anomaly. *Circulation.* 2001;104:E92–E94.

70. Schneider HE, Schill M, Kriebel T, et al. Value of dynamic substrate mapping to identify the critical diastolic pathway in postoperative ventricular reentrant tachycardias after surgical repair of tetralogy of Fallot. *J Cardiovasc Electrophysiol.* 2012;23:930–937.

71. Morwood JG, Triedman JK, Berul CI, et al. Radiofrequency catheter ablation of ventricular tachycardia in children and young adults with congenital heart disease. *Heart Rhythm.* 2004;1:301–308.

72. Kriebel T, Saul JP, Schneider H, et al. Noncontact mapping and radiofrequency catheter ablation of fast and hemodynamically unstable ventricular tachycardia after repair of tetralogy of Fallot. *J Am Coll Cardiol.* 2007;50:2162–2168.

73. Burton ME, Leon AR. Radiofrequency catheter ablation of right ventricular outflow tract tachycardia late after complete repair of tetralogy of Fallot using the pace mapping technique. *Pacing Clin Electrophysiol.* 1993;16:2319–2325.

74. Biblo LA, Carlson MD. Transcatheter radiofrequency ablation of ventricular tachycardia following surgical correction of tetralogy of Fallot. *Pacing Clin Electrophysiol.* 1994;17:1556–1560.

75. Gonska BD, Cao K, Raab J, et al. Radiofrequency catheter ablation of right ventricular tachycardia late after repair of congenital heart defects. *Circulation.* 1996;94:1902–1908.

76. Khairy P, Harris L, Landzberg MJ, et al. Implantable cardioverter-defibrillators in tetralogy of Fallot. *Circulation.* 2008;117:363–370.

77. Khairy P, Landzberg MJ, Gatzoulis MA, et al. Prognostic significance of electrophysiologic testing post tetralogy of Fallot repair: a multicenter study. *Circulation.* 2004;109:1994–2000.

78. Karamlou T, Silber I, Lao R, et al. Outcomes after late reoperation in patients with repaired tetralogy of Fallot: the impact of arrhythmia and arrhythmia surgery. *Ann Thorac Surg.* 2006;81:1786–1793.

79. Harrild DM, Berul CI, Cecchin F, et al. Pulmonary valve replacement in tetralogy of Fallot: impact on survival and ventricular tachycardia. *Circulation.* 2009;119:445–451.

132 Anesthesiology Considerations for the Electrophysiology Laboratory

Wendy L. Gross, Mark S. Weiss, Lebron Cooper, and William G. Stevenson

Setting the Stage for an Effective Partnership

The evolution of clinical electrophysiology (EP) from a diagnostic discipline to a technologically sophisticated therapeutic subspecialty has been accompanied by an increased need for anesthesiology support. While some procedures may be performed using local anesthesia with minimal sedation, many now require general anesthesia (GA) with intensive physiological monitoring. Procedures are longer, demanding more precision and interventional expertise. Technological development has occurred at an unprecedented rate. Simultaneously, an increasingly elderly, high-acuity patient population has emerged. We are witnessing an exponential increase in the number of EP procedures worldwide, and EP is currently the fastest growing subspecialty of cardiology.[1] Anesthesiologists are asked to participate in EP procedures to assure patient comfort during extended procedures, facilitate optimal outcomes by establishing and maintaining a relatively motionless ablation target, and provide additional imaging and guidance via transesophageal echocardiography (TEE) when necessary.

Pharmacological and technical progress in anesthesiology care continues to enhance the development of tailored approaches to sedation and GA. A well-orchestrated interface between electrophysiologists and anesthesiologists that includes preemptive discussion and consensus about procedural processes and goals can decrease procedure and recovery time and enhance laboratory throughput.[2–4] Effective communication between anesthesiologists and electrophysiologists ensures conditions that enhance performance of the intervention, thus increasing the likelihood of achieving desired outcomes. Specialization, however, can make collaborative practice difficult. Technical vocabularies can be forbidding and exclusive. Interdisciplinary knowledge gaps can make planning problematic. The purpose of this chapter is to identify important aspects of anesthesiology practice and care that potentially impact the course of EP procedures to facilitate meaningful dialogue between anesthesiologists and electrophysiologists. The care of patients with advanced disease requires discussion and alignment of goals. Preprocedural identification and assessment of comorbidities and potential complications should be a routine part of multidisciplinary periprocedural planning. This does not have to be time consuming if it is organized and routine. Advance recognition of possible difficulties enables the creation of collaborative practice platforms that serve to optimize patient care, procedural process, and outcome.

Anesthesiologists and Anesthesiology: Who We Are and What We Do

In the United States, anesthesia can be administered by anesthesiologists (physicians), certified registered nurse anesthetists (CRNAs), or certified anesthesia assistants (CAAs). CAAs are unique to the United States. Although many European countries train and utilize CRNAs, their range of practice is quite variable by country. CRNAs are advanced practice nurses who complete a graduate level post-RN program in anesthesiology practice.[5] CAAs are nonphysicians who are qualified by advanced education and clinical training to work cooperatively with an anesthesiologist to develop and implement the anesthesia care plan.[6] CRNAs usually administer anesthesia under the supervision of a physician anesthesiologist, although in 17 states, physician supervision is not mandatory.[7] Physician anesthesiologists complete a minimum of 1-year internship and 3-year anesthesiology residency. Many also complete 1–3 years of postresidency fellowships in critical care and cardiothoracic anesthesiology. Although anesthesiologists historically focused on procedures, their responsibilities now include an individualized assessment of risks, benefits, and likely sequelae of anesthesia and discussion with the electrophysiologist.

Anesthesiology has a long tradition of improving patient safety in the operating room (OR), and although the foray into non-OR areas is relatively new, the goal of any anesthetic administered in the EP laboratory is the same as that in the OR: to enhance and facilitate safe and comfortable performance of the procedure. This includes the maintenance of hemodynamic, respiratory, neurological, and metabolic homeostasis during and immediately following procedures.

The implementation and management of invasive and noninvasive monitoring are standard components of anesthesiology training and practice. Standard anesthesia monitors include five-lead electrocardiogram (ECG), capnography, noninvasive blood pressure (BP) cuff, and ventilator monitors if the ventilator/anesthesia machine is in use. Modified electroencephalogram (EEG) monitors and cerebral oximeters are also often utilized. Cardiac anesthesiologists handle mechanical support options for decompensated patients (ventricular assist devices [VADs], intraaortic balloon counterpulsation [IABP], percutaneous VADs [PVADs], and extracorporeal membrane oxygenation [ECMO]) in the OR, which are sometimes needed in the EP laboratory. Cardiac anesthesiologists are trained echocardiographers and can provide intraprocedural TEE. Anesthesiologists should be involved in the pre- and intraprocedure discussions about how, when, and where to utilize invasive monitoring or mechanical support devices for ill patients. It is also important for the anesthesia team to recognize that precise procedural pathways may not be predictable at the outset and that even arrhythmia diagnosis may not be clear until the diagnostic portion of the EP study is completed. Therefore anesthetic plans must be flexible and are best made via a team approach that considers the goals and constraints of electrophysiologists, anesthesiologists, and postoperative care teams.

Preprocedural Evaluation of Patients

Catheter ablations and device implantations, like all cases, require thorough preoperative preparation, planning, and interdisciplinary discussion. Prior to initiating care, anesthesiologists are required to perform "... an evaluation ... that carefully considers both the patient's current state of health and the planned surgical procedure [in order to develop] the safest anesthesia plan for each individual patient."[8] Regardless of the procedure, a thorough preanesthetic review is needed and is required by regulatory agencies.[9] Coexisting conditions that might have nothing to do with the EP intervention at hand can impact outcomes such that even a simple undertaking can become difficult to manage in the context of significant comorbidities. Tenuous hemodynamic status, respiratory compromise that may render patients unable to maintain adequate oxygenation in the supine position, altered mental status, or extremes of age may reduce the effectiveness and therapeutic index of some sedatives. Any of these situations may set the stage for failure of nurse-administered sedation or even local anesthesia. Comorbidities that impact anesthetic planning must be recognized and communicated among team members. Preemptive discussion among electrophysiologists, nurses, and anesthesiologists can prevent intraprocedural emergencies. Preprocedural planning is always preferable to intraprocedural crisis management. Preprocedural discussion also ensures that specialty-related considerations, which might not be the principal focus of individual team members, are considered as part of the overall plan. For example, the need for and extent to which patients can tolerate a period of minimal sedation to facilitate mapping of arrhythmias that may be suppressed by anesthesia should be considered at the outset of the case. Cardiopulmonary abnormalities, such as pleural effusions, lung disease, and

intracardiac shunt, should be clear to everyone because these conditions may dictate the nature of postprocedure care (intensive care unit [ICU] vs. postoperative recovery unit [PACU]). The approach to vascular and ventricular access (venous, arterial, retrograde aortic, or transseptal approaches) and need for angiography or percutaneous pericardial access should be made clear. Ideally, therapy for heart failure and myocardial ischemia has been optimized, but this is not possible when the arrhythmia requiring treatment is aggravating the condition. The severity of ventricular dysfunction and heart failure should be discussed, with the recognition that poor perfusion may induce vascular, pulmonary, or renal derangements that dictate subsequent management. Preprocedural evaluation, which is context sensitive, creates a platform for appropriate utilization of anesthesiology resources and support. Because advancement of sedation depth from moderate to deep can encompass the need for airway support, it is wise to plan for anesthesia support if this is likely. Interjection of unplanned anesthesiology support when anesthesia providers have not previously evaluated the patient should be reserved only for emergency situations.

Intraprocedural Considerations

Local Anesthetics

Local anesthetics are used to minimize painful stimulation during vascular access. All local anesthetics (except for cocaine) are synthetic. They differ in potency, therapeutic index, duration of action, and plasma half-life. Knowledge of the basic chemical characteristics, mechanism of action, and potential for toxicity of these agents is important. Local anesthetics inhibit depolarization of the nerve membrane by interfering with both Na^+ and K^+ currents. All have the capability of blocking cardiac sodium current (I_{Na}). Bupivacaine can block several cardiac potassium currents (I_{to}, I_{KATP}, and $K_V1.5$) and procaine blocks Ikr.[10,11] Systemic absorption can produce significant electrophysiological effects. Bupivacaine can precipitate polymorphic ventricular tachycardia (VT) in Brugada syndrome.[12]

All local anesthetics have a similar chemical structure that includes three components: aromatic portion, intermediate chain, and amine group (Fig. 132.1). The nature of the intermediate chain divides local anesthetics into two classes: esters and amides (see Fig. 132.1 and Table 132.1). The aromatic portion, usually composed of a benzene ring, is lipophilic; the amine portion is hydrophilic. The lipid solubility of each anesthetic determines its potency because this property enables diffusion through nerve membranes. Local anesthetics are weak bases that require the addition of hydrochloride salt to be water soluble and therefore injectable. The salt equilibrates between an ionized form and a nonionized form in aqueous solution. Equilibration is crucial because although the ionized form is injectable, the nonionized base possesses lipophilic properties responsible for diffusion across the nerve cell membrane. Neutralization of local anesthetics with bicarbonate can minimize injection pain and speed onset

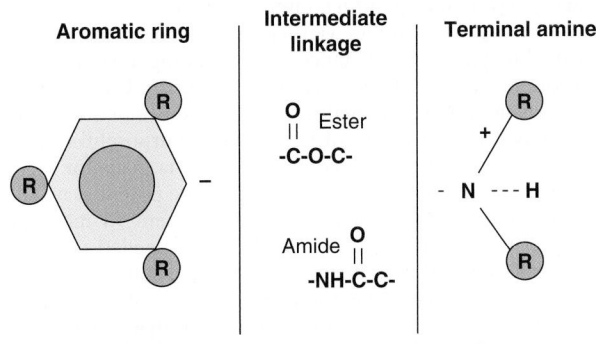

FIGURE 132.1 Structure of local anesthetics.

LOCAL ANESTHETIC	DURATION (min) (WITHOUT EPI)	DURATION (min) (WITH EPI)	MAXIMUM DOSE (mg/kg) (WITHOUT EPI)	MAXIMUM DOSE (mg/kg) (WITH EPI)
TABLE 132.1 Characteristics of local anesthetics				
Esters				
Procaine	15–30	30–90	7	8.5
Amides				
Lidocaine	30–120	60–400	4.5	7
Bupivacaine	120–240	240–480	2.5	3

EPI, Epinephrine.

of action. The duration of action of local anesthesia is determined by its protein-binding activity. This property is expressed as the percentage of circulating drug that is protein bound and correlates with the affinity for protein within sodium channels.

The ester–amide classification identifies the pathway by which local anesthetics are metabolized, and metabolic byproducts determine allergic potential. Ester anesthetics (e.g., procaine) are metabolized by hydrolysis via plasma pseudocholinesterase, which generates the allergen paraaminobenzoic acid (PABA). Patients with a (rare) genetic defect in the structure of this enzyme may be unable to metabolize ester-type anesthetics, increasing the potential for toxicity. Amide-type local anesthetics (e.g., lidocaine and bupivacaine) are metabolized by hepatic microsomal enzymes. Lidocaine is metabolized by cytochrome P450 3A4. Factors predisposing to increased systemic levels of amide-type anesthetics include severe liver disease, inhibitors of cytochrome P450 enzymes, and β-blockers, which can decrease hepatic blood flow. Systemic blood levels may also suppress target arrhythmia.[13] Known allergy to an amide local anesthetic limits the choice of local anesthetic to procaine, which has a relatively short half-life.

Toxicity

All team members should be aware of the signs and symptoms of systemic toxicity from excessive blood levels of local anesthetics, which can occur due to excessive administration or inadvertent intravascular injection. Systemic toxicity manifests clinically as adverse central nervous system (CNS) or cardiovascular reactions. CNS is affected in a predictable and dose-dependent manner. Serum lidocaine levels in the range of 1–5 μg/mL produce tinnitus, lightheadedness, circumoral numbness, diplopia, or a sensation of metallic taste. Nausea and/or vomiting can also occur. As serum lidocaine levels increase to 5–8 μg/mL, nystagmus, slurred speech, localized muscle twitching or fine tremors, and hallucinations may occur. If blood lidocaine levels reach 8–12 μg/mL, focal seizure activity occurs, which can progress to generalized tonic–clonic seizures. Respiratory depression occurs at extremely high blood levels (20–25 μg/mL) and can progress to coma. If signs of CNS toxicity are noted, attention to airway maintenance is critical. Increased partial pressure of carbon dioxide (pCO_2) decreases the protein binding of lidocaine and increases blood levels of free lidocaine. If convulsions occur, the patient's airway should be maintained and supplemental oxygen administered. If seizure activity is sustained, benzodiazepines are indicated. Propofol and thiopental are also useful. Very high plasma levels of local anesthetics can depress cardiac contractility, exacerbating the hemodynamic impact of their direct vasodilatory effects. Atrioventricular (AV) block, bradycardia, and ventricular arrhythmias can occur and are more common in patients known to require antiarrhythmic medications. Lidocaine toxicity produces bradycardia and hypotension prior to cardiac arrest,

while bupivacaine may cause sudden cardiovascular collapse due to ventricular dysrhythmias.[14] Maintenance of perfusion and ventilation through prolonged cardiopulmonary resuscitation (CPR) is critical because dissociation of the local anesthetic from its ion channels is necessary to resolve the problem, and this may take some time. Cardiopulmonary bypass has been discussed as an option, and case reports suggest that the infusion of lipid emulsions can reverse cardiac and neurological effects, but there are no controlled studies in humans.[15]

Anesthesia Options (Sedation, Monitored Anesthesia Care, General Anesthesia, and General Endotracheal Anesthesia): What's What and What's Best

The degree of sedation-analgesia-anesthesia (Table 132.2) provided for patients follows a continuum of depth as described by the American Society of Anesthesiologists (ASA).[16] Support levels are as defined later; however, in practice, there is significant overlap between categories.

Levels of Sedation: What Do They Mean?

According to the ASA, *moderate sedation/analgesia* ("conscious sedation") is a drug-induced depression of consciousness during which an individual responds purposefully to verbal commands, either alone or accompanied by light tactile stimulation. No interventions are required to maintain a patent airway; spontaneous ventilation is adequate. Cardiovascular function is usually maintained. Conscious sedation can be provided with nurse administration of midazolam and fentanyl or by an anesthesiologist using other drugs if a different pharmacological profile is more suitable for the case/patient. If pulmonary status or airway anatomy requires the use of drugs that have fewer respiratory side effects or a shorter half-life, anesthesiologists can provide moderate sedation with infusions of short-acting drugs (propofol/remifentanil), which can be titrated as needed. *Deep sedation/analgesia* is a drug-induced depression of consciousness from which an individual cannot be easily aroused but responds purposefully following repeated or painful stimulation.

The ability to maintain ventilation may be impaired. The individual may require assistance in maintaining a patent airway, and spontaneous ventilation may be inadequate. Cardiovascular function is usually maintained. Each of the abovementioned levels is defined by the extent of the patient's purposeful response to stimuli. Decisions about sedation/anesthesia goals for a given procedure should include consideration of the potential need for uncompromised sympathetic tone, advancement to more profound sedation, and availability of the skills needed to achieve the patient's desired mental and physiological status. Anesthesia support can be provided via the administration of sedative-hypnotics, opiates, or other classes of medications that achieve a state

TABLE 132.2	American Society of Anesthesiologists levels of sedation			
	I: MINIMAL/ ANXIOLYSIS	**II: MODERATE/ CONSCIOUS SEDATION**	**III: DEEP SEDATION**	**IV: GENERAL ANESTHESIA (GA/GETA)**
Response to stimuli	Normal to verbal	Purposeful to verbal or tactile	Purposeful to repeated verbal or to pain	Unresponsive to pain
Airway	Normal	No required intervention	May require intervention	Often requires intervention
Breathing	Normal	Adequate	May require assistance	Often requires intervention
Cardiovascular parameters	Normal	Usually normal	Usually normal	May be impaired

GA/GETA, General anesthesia/general endotracheal anesthesia.

of depressed consciousness, which facilitates the procedure but maintains the patient in a safe and comfortable state. *Deep sedation* and *GA* with or without intubation or a combination of these support levels is purely the province of anesthesiology providers.

GA can be accomplished with a natural airway (without endotracheal intubation) but requires the vigilance of a provider who can manage and control the airway and implement endotracheal intubation if necessary. Monitored anesthesia care (MAC) is a term commonly misused to describe that depth of sedation between conscious and deep sedation but that falls short of general endotracheal anesthesia (GETA). The term "MAC" was originally devised as a billing code, which was coined to denote oversight of surgical "local only" cases by anesthesiologists. MAC does not define any depth of sedation or drug regimen and is actually meaningless when used to describe levels of sedation. Any case that requires a level of sedation beyond conscious sedation or a widely fluctuating level of support, which includes deep sedation and beyond, requires either an anesthesiologist or a clinician credentialed to administer anesthetics under the medical direction of an anesthesiologist (or CRNA or CAA in the United States). Nonanesthesiologists often mistakenly label any anesthetic that does not involve endotracheal intubation as "sedation." However, anesthesiologists are adept at administering GA that does not require respiratory support or intubation. GA with a natural airway is possible if the procedure and patient's anatomy and physiology permit. Patients can be unconscious and unresponsive but have adequate respiratory and hemodynamic stability under some conditions; however, frequent induction of unstable VTs, during which cardiac output is reduced, would not be conducive to such an approach. The level of drug administered during these cases may be equivalent to that administered during GETA, but the absence of positive pressure ventilation can mitigate the need for pharmacological hemodynamic support, although this is not always the case.

The decision to proceed with sedation or GA for a particular case should be the result of a preoperative discussion between the electrophysiologist and anesthesiologist. Some procedures that can usually be performed with little or no sedation may require a more advanced approach due to comorbidities that render the patient unable to maintain the supine position, such as morbid obesity, obstructive sleep apnea, dementia, and extreme anxiety. Lengthy procedures prove challenging for some patients if they are not asleep. It is important to realize that lighter sedation is not necessarily safer or better than general anesthetics, especially when risks for unmanageable behavior, airway obstruction, hypercarbia, and hypoxia are significant.

General Anesthesia and General Endotracheal Anesthesia: Definitions and Risks/Benefits

The ASA defines GA as "a drug-induced loss of consciousness during which an individual is not arousable, even by painful stimulation" (see Table 132.2). The ability to independently maintain ventilatory function is often but not always impaired. The individual often requires assistance in maintaining a patent airway, and positive pressure ventilation may be required because of depressed spontaneous ventilation or drug-induced depression of neuromuscular function. Cardiovascular function may be impaired.[16] GA can be accomplished with or without intubation, with or without spontaneous ventilation, with volatile (gas) or intravenous (IV) agents, and with or without paralysis. It is sometimes mistakenly assumed that GA by definition includes one or more of the abovementioned factors. Conversely, it is assumed that because a patient is receiving anesthetics via IV medications only, they are not receiving GA. These assumptions are not correct; GA is defined by the patient's response to stimulation, not by the drugs he or she receives.

The goal of GA is to induce a state of amnesia, analgesia, and immobility through depression of autonomic reflexes and controlled temporary disruption of CNS function. The precise mechanisms of action of general anesthetics remain unclear, despite their use for >150 years. Ideally, general anesthetics induce loss of consciousness, but vital functions continue to work, although pharmacological augmentation may be required.

Inhalational Agents

The inhaled general anesthetics are liquid at room temperature and are therefore administered through vaporizers via a breathing circuit. Hence, they are often referred to as volatile anesthetics. These agents have narrow therapeutic indices, and none are reversible via pharmacological competitors. They are structurally related to ether. Their primary site of action is in the CNS, where they inhibit excitatory and potentiated nerve transmission via reduction in synaptic transmission. Volatile anesthetics are lipid soluble; they disrupt the function of ion channels and neurotransmitter receptor proteins in the membranes of neurons. $GABA_A$ and NMDA receptors, as well as Na^+ and K_{2P}, are known targets.

Volatile anesthetics bind very weakly to their site(s) of action, so high concentrations are needed to achieve an anesthetic state. This makes isolating key mediators of synaptic inhibition challenging because at high concentrations, the function of many proteins in nerve cell membranes is affected. In addition, because volatile agents are lipid soluble, they affect components of the surrounding membrane, so it is unclear whether anesthetics exert their primary effects via direct interaction with membrane proteins or via interaction with the lipids surrounding them. In any case, we do not have a comprehensive explanation for how these drugs produce CNS depression. The fact that cell membranes and ion channels in the CNS are perturbed by general anesthetics raises the question of how these agents might influence excitable cardiac tissue. Although the general cardiovascular effects of common volatile anesthetics are well known, the precise molecular level effects of volatile anesthetics on cardiac conduction are not well understood.

Commonly used volatile agents include isoflurane, sevoflurane, and desflurane (Fig. 132.2). They are all nonflammable, nonexplosive halogenated ether derivatives. The potency of a volatile anesthetic is indicated by its minimum alveolar concentration, which is essentially its ED_{50}, the alveolar concentration of a gas that renders 50% of subjects unresponsive to painful stimuli.

Inhalational agents produce GA when the necessary partial pressure develops within the brain. For this to occur, inspired gas must pass from the breathing circuit to the alveoli and to the brain. Steady state is achieved when equilibration occurs between brain, alveoli and body tissue stores (particularly vessel-rich organs),

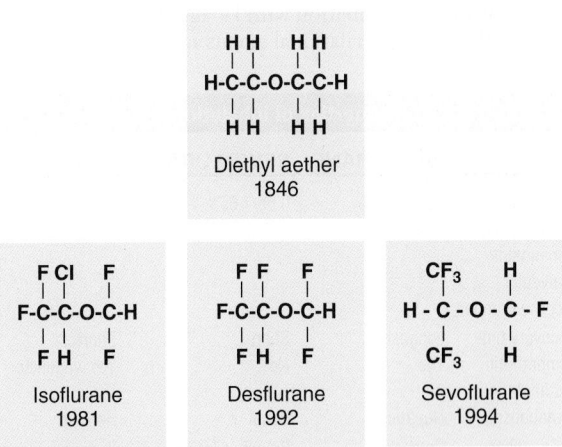

FIGURE 132.2 Structure of inhalational anesthetics.

muscle, and fat stores. The alveolar concentration depends on the balance of variables affecting delivery of anesthetic to the lungs and those affecting removal (uptake to tissues) from the lungs. Delivery is affected by inspired concentration and ventilation. Removal is affected by solubility of the agent in blood, cardiac output, and the difference in concentration of agent between venous blood and alveolar gas. Alveolar partial pressure reflects brain partial pressure. The brain and other tissues equilibrate with the alveoli via the blood as a function of the blood/gas partition coefficient of the agent. This coefficient indicates the concentration of an anesthetic in the blood phase relative to that in the gas phase *when the anesthetic is in equilibrium between the two phases*. A high blood/gas partition coefficient means that equilibration between alveoli and blood requires that a large amount of gas be dissolved in the blood. The blood/gas partition coefficients of commonly used agents range from 0.45 for desflurane to 0.65 for sevoflurane and 1.4 for isoflurane (Table 132.3). Higher blood/gas partition coefficients indicate that increased inspired concentrations are needed to induce anesthesia and that recovery from or elimination of anesthetic gas will be longer. Accordingly, recovery from desflurane is faster than that from sevoflurane or isoflurane (in the absence of other agents). Tissue uptake depends on blood/tissue solubility, tissue blood flow, and concentration gradient between arterial blood and the tissue itself. The tissue:gas partition coefficient is the ratio of the concentration of anesthetic in tissue to that in the gas phase when the anesthetic is in equilibrium between the two phases. A low tissue:gas partition coefficient indicates low tissue solubility. Desflurane tissue solubility is approximately half that of sevoflurane, which is half as soluble as isoflurane. Vessel-rich tissues (brain, heart, kidneys, splanchnic bed) quickly uptake anesthetics. Muscle is less well perfused but still has a moderately good blood supply. Fat has a poor blood supply but large capacity, so it continues to contribute to anesthetic uptake long after vessel-rich tissues attain equilibrium.[17]

Factors affecting recovery from inhalational anesthesia are the same as those affecting its uptake. Solubility, cardiac output, and venous to alveolar anesthetic partial pressure differences govern the time to wake up. Inhalational anesthetics accumulate slowly in fat, but during long procedures, fat stores can become saturated and the time to wake up may be prolonged, and thus obese patients may require a longer time to wake up even from a short-acting inhalational agent. All inhalational agents increase cerebral perfusion, intracranial pressure, and bronchodilation and decrease pulmonary and systemic vascular resistance. All have negative inotropic properties.[18]

For the most part, inhaled anesthetics are used in combination with IV agents. Induction of anesthesia is usually via IV medications; inhalational agents are used to maintain anesthetic depth either alone or in combination with IV agents. An anesthetic that utilizes both IV and inhalational agents may be preferable when gas delivery is impacted by pulmonary compromise or ventilation technique (as with high-frequency jet ventilation [HFJV]; see later) or apneic periods implemented to improve catheter stability. The effects are additive, so when multiple agents are used to maintain anesthetic depth, less of any one agent is needed and estimation of the recovery time is more complex. Other factors that decrease minimum alveolar concentration of volatile agents include increased age, hypothermia, alcohol intoxication, hyponatremia, and the presence of other sedating agents. Factors that increase minimum alveolar concentration include alcoholism, CNS stimulants, and hyperthermia.

All volatile anesthetics can precipitate malignant hyperthermia (MH) in susceptible individuals. MH is a pharmacogenetic disorder caused by a defect in the type I ryanodine receptor in skeletal muscle. More than 30 causative mutations are known. Genetic testing is available, but the caffeine halothane contracture test (CHCT) remains the standard diagnostic test. In susceptible patients, exposure to a triggering agent results in the release of large quantities of calcium from the sarcoplasmic reticulum of skeletal muscle, which induces a hypermetabolic state with excessive stimulation of aerobic and anaerobic glycolytic metabolism, respiratory and metabolic acidosis, altered cell permeability, hyperkalemia, and rigidity. Treatment is dantrolene.[19]

Intravenous General Anesthetics

Common IV anesthetics include propofol, remifentanil, and sufentanil. These compounds are used for induction and maintenance of anesthesia, both as part of total IV anesthesia (TIVA) and as adjuncts to volatile agents. Propofol is a phenol emulsion in Intralipid, which works at GABA receptors. It is highly lipid soluble and crosses the blood–brain barrier very quickly; redistribution occurs within 8 minutes. Biotransformation occurs in the liver by conjugation; excretion is via the kidney, but renal failure patients do not require dose reduction. Decreased systemic vascular resistance, depressed cardiac contractility, and lowered BP are usual effects. Propofol can inhibit barostatic reflexes, cause vagal stimulation, and attenuate reflex heart rate response, creating an exaggerated hypotensive effect. Propofol decreases cerebral blood flow, intracranial pressure, and cerebral metabolic oxygen requirement ($CMRO_2$). Propofol is not an analgesic and therefore is often mixed with an opioid or inhaled anesthetic.

Dexmedetomidine is an α_2 receptor agonist that can be used as a sedative or an adjunct to GA. Hypotension and bradycardia are common with this drug, so it is not likely to be useful in the EP lab. It can be used for device implantations in some patients because it does not depress respiration.[20]

Short-acting opioids can also be used as adjuvants to GA or as sedatives. Sufentanil is highly lipid soluble and is a protein-bound lipid with the ability to decrease minimum alveolar concentration of volatile agents by 50%–70%. It is 10 times more potent than fentanyl and has a shorter half-life of about 160 minutes. Metabolites are excreted in urine and bile. Remifentanil has an extremely rapid onset of effect and is ultra-short acting. It is metabolized by plasma esterases, its skeletal muscle half-life is about 4 minutes, and clearance is unchanged in patients with hepatic or renal impairment. It is ideal for patients who are not expected to have postoperative pain. It can decrease minimum alveolar concentration by up to 90%. Postoperative hyperalgesia is an uncommon side effect of remifentanil.

Impact of Technique on Ablation

Data comparing conscious sedation and anesthetic regimens for EP procedures are limited. GA provides more complete relief of pain and anxiety. Patients undergoing procedures with GA seem more satisfied with their experiences than those receiving sedation; patients undergoing repeat procedures ask for GA more

TABLE 132.3	Properties of inhalational agents		
	ISOFLURANE	**SEVOFLURANE**	**DESFLURANE**
Blood:gas coefficient/ minimum alveolar concentration	1.49/1.15%	0.65/1.85%	0.45/6.0%
Recovery time	Longest	Short	Shortest
Sympathetic stimulation	Yes	No	Yes; vagolytic
Metabolism	Hepatic	Renal	Hepatic
Unique characteristics	Coronary vasodilation	Bronchodilation	Pungency; airway irritant

often.[21] However, the impact on patient motion, autonomic function, and arrhythmia inducibility is an important consideration.

There is evidence that GA rather than conscious sedation can improve the outcomes of radiofrequency (RF) catheter ablation of atrial fibrillation.[3] In a study of 257 patients, randomized to conscious sedation versus GA, pulmonary vein isolation was achieved in all patients, but at 17 months' postprocedure, 88% of GA patients were arrhythmia free compared with 69% of sedation patients. In restudied patients, pulmonary vein reconnection was present in fewer who had GA (19% vs. 42%). Other centers report decreases in procedure time, time to successful transseptal puncture, and recovery time for patients receiving GA.[4] There is speculation that the inability to feel pain during ablation under GA might increase the potential for esophageal or mediastinal injury[22,23]; however, with esophageal temperature monitoring and decreased ablation power in the posterior left atrium, this risk appears to be low.

It is likely that GA facilitates the ability to achieve ablation catheter contact and stability by minimizing patient movement and reducing or allowing control of respiratory movement. Risks and benefits of various ventilation strategies for atrial fibrillation ablation are currently under scrutiny. Cardiopulmonary interactions contribute to mediastinal and cardiac motion. Reduced tidal volumes and more rapid respiratory rates, as well as utilization of pressure-controlled or pressure-support ventilation modes, can enhance conditions for catheter stability and also influence impedance of the ablation system. Two retrospective reviews suggest that HFJV, which reduces thoracic motion by delivering very low tidal volumes at a rapid rate, improves the ease, precision, and stability of catheter placement,[24,25] but there have been no randomized trials of HFJV versus conventional mechanical ventilation. The precise contribution of HFJV in improving outcomes achieved with modern procedures utilizing current mapping systems and catheters remains unclear. HFJV may be problematic in patients with chronic obstructive pulmonary disease (COPD) and other lung pathology. It requires blood gas monitoring of pCO_2 because end-tidal CO_2 monitoring is not possible due to high rates of gas flow. Because monitoring of inhalational agents is not possible in this ventilation mode, TIVA is needed. Vasopressors are also usually required.[26] An alternative to HFJV, which we and others have found helpful to improve catheter positioning, is the use of brief periods of apnea during conventional ventilation. Apnea may also be helpful when catheter stability is critical for avoiding complications, as with ablation of accessory pathways that are in close proximity to the AV node and during pericardial puncture. As previously noted, during repeated or long periods of apnea or HFJV, IV anesthetics must be used to maintain anesthetic depth. Infusions of short-acting narcotics and propofol are acceptable. Infusions of phenylephrine or inotropic agents may be necessary during TIVA to offset drug-induced vasodilation. Use of vasoactive drugs to treat hypotension should always be communicated between anesthesiologists and cardiologists because the need for these agents may indicate something more worrisome than anesthetic-induced vasodilation, i.e., complications such as tamponade or hemorrhage.

Optimal anesthetics for EP procedures are not established. Controversy surrounds the antiarrhythmic potential of volatile agents. Limited studies have compared electrophysiological effects of propofol and isoflurane in children undergoing ablation of tachyarrhythmias.[27,28] No differences were found in one study, and the other found no differences in inducibility but did note that propofol seemed to slow AV nodal conduction whereas isoflurane prolonged ventricular repolarization. More studies utilizing modern techniques in adult populations are needed.

For VT ablation, the question of anesthetic technique is again complex and data are limited. The concern for sympathetic damping reducing the ability to initiate ventricular arrhythmias is under active investigation. Recent reports indicate that propofol and

sevoflurane seem to differ little in their effects on electrophysiological parameters.[29] Often, the need to maintain inducibility of the arrhythmia for mapping requires that minimal medication be administered at the beginning of the case with transition to deep sedation or GA once the ablation target region is identified. Patients with VT and depressed ventricular function can be hemodynamically tenuous, and invasive monitoring with an arterial line is often preferred both for inducing anesthesia and monitoring during the case. Monitoring cerebral oxygenation is helpful during periods when the patient's ventricular tachyarrhythmia is induced and can help direct the need for timing of arrhythmia termination, particularly when ventricular support devices are used to maintain peripheral arterial pressure.[4] Right heart dysfunction can be exacerbated when left ventricular (LV) dysfunction is further exacerbated by arrhythmias. Cardiac anesthesiologists are adept at the management of patients with poor cardiac function and can compensate for hemodynamic perturbations pharmacologically to some degree. Often, vasopressors are required. Hemodynamic and fluid management are more reliably achieved with invasive monitoring of arterial and venous pressures. In severely compromised patients, all team members (anesthesiologists, electrophysiologists, interventional cardiologists, and cardiac surgeons) should be aware of and discuss plans for any mechanical support that may be needed, including intraaortic balloon pumps, PVADs, or ECMO.[30] Planning for therapies that are difficult to implement on an ad hoc basis should occur in advance whenever possible.

Postprocedural Planning and Disposition

Anesthesiologists and electrophysiologists should collaborate in planning postprocedural disposition, including ventilation and extubation parameters. Careful reconciliation of fluid balance, including consideration of fluid administered from irrigated ablation catheters, should take place explicitly and on a regular basis throughout the case, as it is easy for anesthesiologists and cardiologists to be unaware of each other's contributions to fluid balance. For patients who are morbidly obese or whose respiratory limitations require that they be sitting up to breathe adequately, postprocedure ventilation and ICU disposition may be required. Even for postoperative recovery room admission, parameters for patient recovery should be clear so that postprocedure medication and ventilation needs are anticipated. GA with immobility on hard x-ray tables during long procedures can precipitate musculoskeletal pain. Often, larger patients awaken with shoulder and wrist pain because they are not optimally supported by narrow fluoroscopy tables. Administration of ketorolac is usually effective if this occurs. Lorazepam, ondansetron, Decadron, and haloperidol are useful antiemetics for postprocedure nausea. Ondansetron is best avoided in patients who suffer from migraine headache.

Summary

The need for anesthesiology services in the EP laboratory will continue to increase. Patients are increasing in numbers and complexity, and technological advances continue to address the ever-extending medical horizon. These factors and the EP laboratory environment create dynamic and unique challenges for achieving optimal anesthesia. Anesthesiology options for interventional medicine are also expanding in terms of new drugs and equipment. Favorable pharmacological profiles, sophisticated delivery systems, and the possibility of service line approaches to health care make likely the continued integration of anesthesiology support and therapeutic EP. Electrophysiologists and anesthesiologists should take the time to acquire a basic understanding of each other's vocabulary, technical platforms, and available options. Development of robust, collaborative, interdisciplinary interfaces will enable anesthesiologists to facilitate the goals of EP procedures and enhance outcomes.

REFERENCES

1. Heart Rhythm Society. http://www.heartrhythmfoundation.org/facts/electrophysiology.asp.
2. *Anesthesia for electrophysiology procedures in the cardiac catheter laboratory*, Ashley EMC. http://ceaccp.oxfordjournals.org/content/early/2012/05/26/bjaceaccp.mks032.full.
3. DiBiase L, Conti S, Mohanty P, et al. General anesthesia reduces the prevalence of pulmonary vein reconnection during repeat ablation when compared with conscious sedation: results from a randomized study. *Heart Rhythm*. 2011;8:368–372.
4. Gross WL, Roberts JD, Shook DC, et al. *Anesthesiologists in the EP lab: general anesthesia administered by anesthesiologists reduces both procedure length and recovery time for radiofrequency ablations for persistent atrial fibrillation*. Society of Cardiovascular Anesthesia meetings; October 2012.
5. American Association of Nurse Anesthetists. *Certified registered nurse anesthetists fact sheet*. http://www.aana.com/ceandeducation/becomeacrna/Pages/Nurse-Anesthetists-at-a-Glance.aspx.
6. American Academy of Anesthesiologist Assistants. http://www.anesthetist.org.
7. Fields R. *17 states opting out of the physician supervision of anesthesia rule*. http://www.beckersasc.com/anesthesia/17-states-opting-out-of-the-physician-supervision-of-anesthesia-rule.html.
8. American Society of Anesthesiologists. *About the profession*. https://www.asahq.org/For-the-Public-and-Media/About-Profession.aspx.
9. Centers for Medicare & Medicaid Services. *State operations manual*. http://www.cms.gov/Regulations-and-Guidance/Guidance/Manuals/downloads/som107ap_a_hospitals.pdf. Accessed October 31, 2012.
10. Butterworth JF. Models and mechanisms of local anesthetic cardiac toxicity. *Reg Anesth Pain Med*. 2010;35:167–176.
11. Doggrell SA, Bishop BE. Effects of potassium channel blockers on the action potentials and contractility of the rat right ventricle. *Gen Pharmacol*. 1996;27:379–385.
12. Vernooy K, Sicouri S, Dumaine R, et al. Genetic and biophysical basis for bupivacaine-induced ST segment elevation and VT/VF. Anesthesia unmasked Brugada syndrome. *Heart Rhythm*. 2006;3:1074–1078.
13. Nattel S, Rinkenberger RL, Lehrman LL, et al. Therapeutic blood lidocaine concentrations after local anesthesia for cardiac electrophysiologic studies. *N Engl J Med*. 1979;301:418–420.
14. Kapitanyan R. *Local anesthetic toxicity*. http://emedicine.medscape.com/article/1844551-overview.
15. Picard J, Meek T. Lipid emulsion to treat overdose of local anesthetic: the gift of the glob. *Anaesthesia*. 2006;61:107–109.
16. American Society of Anesthesiologists. *Continuum of depth of sedation: definition of general anesthesia and levels of sedation/analgesia*, http://www.asahq.org/publicationsAndServices/standards/20.pdf.
17. McKay RE. Inhaled anesthetics. In: Miller RD, Pardo Jr MC, eds. *Basics of Anesthesia*. 6th ed. Philadelphia: Elsevier; 2011:78–98.
18. Eger 2nd EI. Characteristics of anesthetic agents used for induction and maintenance of general anesthesia. *Am J Health Syst Pharm*. 2004;61:S3–S10.
19. Schneiderbanger D, Johannsen S, Roewer N, et al. Management of malignant hyperthermia: diagnosis and treatment. *Ther Clin Risk Manag*. 2014;10:355–362.
20. Hillier SC, Mazurek MS. Monitored anesthesia care. In: Barash PG, Cullen BF, Stoelting RK, et al., eds. *Clinical Anesthesia*. 6th ed. Philadelphia: Lippincott Williams and Wilkins; 2009:815–832.
21. Ezzat V, Chew A, McCready J, et al. The atrial fibrillation patient journey—patient satisfaction from a single center UK experience. *Europace*. 2010;12:ii9.
22. Di Biase L, Saenz LC, Burkhardt DJ, et al. Esophageal capsule endoscopy after radiofrequency catheter ablation for atrial fibrillation: documented higher risk of luminal esophageal damage with general anesthesia as compared with conscious sedation. *Circ Arrhythm Electrophysiol*. 2009;2:108–112.
23. Zellerhoff S, Ullerich H, Lenze F, et al. Damage to the esophagus after atrial fibrillation ablation: just the tip of the iceberg? High prevalence of mediastinal changes diagnosed by endosonography. *Circ Arrhythm Electrophysiol*. 2010;3:155–159.
24. Hutchinson M, Garcia FC, Mandel JM, et al. Efforts to enhance catheter stability improve atrial fibrillation outcome. *Heart Rhythm*. 2013;10:347–353.
25. Goode JS, Taylor RL, Buffington CW, et al. High-frequency jet ventilation: utility in posterior left atrial catheter ablation. *Heart Rhythm*. 2006;3:13–19.
26. Tanner JW, Moore RA, Weiss MS. Anesthesia for electrophysiology procedures. In: Weiss MS, Fleisher LA, eds. *Non-Operating Room Anesthesia*. Philadelphia: Elsevier; 2014:91–116.
27. Lavoie J, Walsh E, Burrows F, et al. Effects of propofol or isoflurane anesthesia on cardiac conduction in children undergoing radiofrequency ablation for tachydysrhythmias. *Anesthesiology*. 1995;82:884–887.
28. Erb T, Kanter R, Hall J, et al. Comparison of electrophysiological effects of propofol and isoflurane-based anesthetics in children undergoing radiofrequency catheter ablation for SVT. *Anesthesiology*. 2002;96:1386–1394.
29. Nof E, Reichlin T, Enriquez AD, et al. Impact of general anesthesia on initiation and stability of VT during catheter ablation. *Heart Rhythm*. 2015;12:2213–2220.
30. Miller MA, Dukkipati SR, Koruth JS, et al. How to perform ventricular tachycardia ablation with a percutaneous left ventricular assist device. *Heart Rhythm*. 2012;9:1168–1176.

133 Surgery for Atrial Fibrillation and Other Supraventricular Tachycardias

Matthew R. Schill, Spencer J. Melby, Richard B. Schuessler, and Ralph J. Damiano, Jr.

Atrial Fibrillation

The need for interventional therapies to treat atrial fibrillation (AF) has arisen from the shortcomings of pharmacological management. Antiarrhythmic medications have been limited by modest efficacies, significant proarrhythmic side effects, and systemic toxicities.[1] Conversely, rate-control strategies leave patients in AF, do not address the impaired hemodynamics or symptoms associated with this arrhythmia, and may render subsequent attempts at rhythm-control therapies less effective when patients suffer from irreversible atrial remodeling after spending prolonged time in AF. Both rate- and rhythm-control strategies necessitate the use of warfarin or novel oral anticoagulants and as a result, carry a defined risk for major bleeding complications.

Theoretically, restoration of normal sinus rhythm (NSR) has several potential benefits over other strategies. These include improvements in atrial systolic function, which improves cardiac output and prevents the development of worsening symptoms in patients with congestive heart failure; a lower risk for stroke; the possibility for discontinuation of anticoagulation; and the potential benefit of reversing atrial structural and/or electrical remodeling. While the *strategy* of pharmacological rhythm control has never been shown to be superior to that of rate control, largely because of the aforementioned problems, a follow-up analysis of outcomes in the Atrial Fibrillation Follow-Up Investigation of Rhythm Management (AFFIRM) trial did show that the presence of NSR was associated with a significant 47% reduction in mortality.[2] A recent meta-analysis of 10 studies including more than 7000 patients showed a lower rate of readmission using a rate-control strategy, but identified a higher mortality associated with a rate-control strategy in patients younger than 65 years of age, presumably due to the proarrhythmic effects of common antiarrhythmic drugs (RR, 3.03; $p < .0007$).[3] Given the significant prevalence and public health burden of AF, restoration of NSR with surgical or catheter ablation may be of significant benefit to selected patients.

Development of Surgery for Atrial Fibrillation

The first effective interventional procedure for AF was introduced clinically by Dr. James Cox in 1987 after an extensive animal investigation at Washington University in St. Louis. This operation, now known as the Cox-Maze procedure, was developed to provide a standardized anatomic approach that would be applicable to all patients. After initial attempts at both the laboratory and the operating room failed to define the precise mechanisms of AF in the individual patient this operation was designed to prevent AF by interrupting most of the potential macroreentrant circuits that could develop in the atria, thereby precluding the ability of the atrium to flutter or fibrillate (Fig. 133.1). The operation consisted of a myriad of incisions arranged across the left and right atria in such a fashion that the sinoatrial (SA) node could still direct the propagation of the sinus impulse. The pattern of incisions was designed such that the propagation of the impulse into dead-end pathways would allow sufficient atrial myocardial depolarization to ensure contraction while preventing reentry. The Cox-Maze procedure was successful in restoring the sinus rhythm and AV synchrony, thereby significantly reducing the risk for thromboembolism and hemodynamic compromise from the arrhythmia.[4,5] It has also allowed for the preservation of atrial transport function in most patients.[6]

The Cox-Maze procedure has evolved through several iterations as clinical experience has increased and technology has advanced. The early versions of the Cox-Maze procedure were complicated by late chronotropic incompetence and a high incidence of postoperative pacemaker requirement. The Cox-Maze III procedure, the third iteration, became the gold standard for the surgical treatment of AF.[5] However, despite its clinical success, the Cox-Maze III procedure was not widely adopted

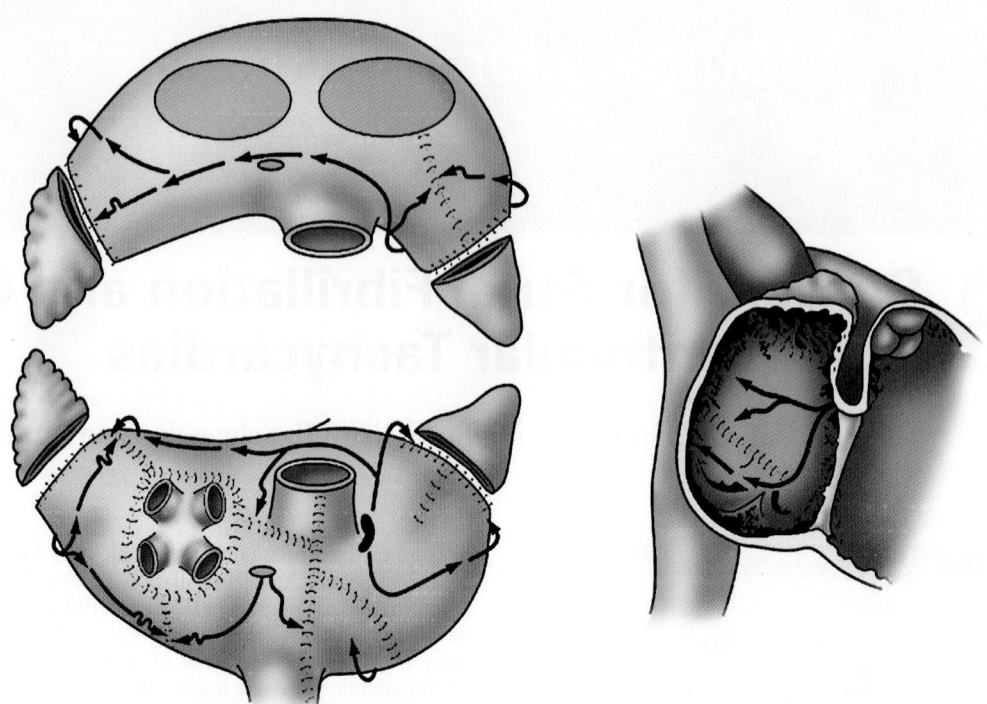

FIGURE 133.1 The lesion set of the traditional cut-and-sew Cox-Maze III operation.

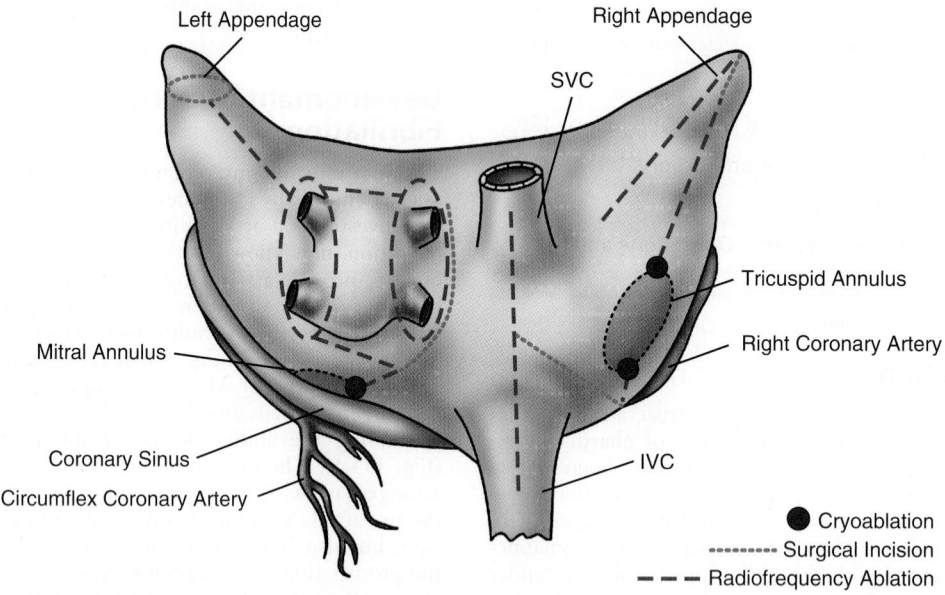

FIGURE 133.2 Diagram illustrating the incisions, lesions, and energy sources that are typically used for the Cox-Maze IV procedure. *IVC,* Inferior vena cava; *SVC,* superior vena cava. (From Weimar T, Bailey MS, Watanabe Y, et al. The Cox-Maze IV procedure for lone atrial fibrillation: a single-center experience in 100 consecutive patients. *J Interv Card Electrophysiol.* 2011;31:47-54.)

because it remained technically demanding with a prolonged cardiopulmonary bypass time. During the last decade, many groups around the world have attempted to make the operation simpler and faster to perform by replacing the traditional "cut-and-sew" lesions with ablation lines created using various energy sources.[7] In 2002, our group introduced the Cox-Maze IV operation, which uses a combination of bipolar radiofrequency (RF) ablation and cryoablation to effectively replace the

majority of incisions that comprise the Cox-Maze III procedure (Fig. 133.2).[8]

These ablation-based procedures have resulted in a continued increase in the number of operations performed annually for AF. In 2005, 12,737 patients were reported in the Society of Thoracic Surgeons (STS) Database as having undergone a surgical procedure for AF, whereas 1 year prior the number was 3987 patients.[9] Before 2004, the volume was so low that the operation was not even reported. An analysis of the STS Adult Cardiac Surgery Database by Ad et al. showed an increase in the volume of concomitant AF ablation from 8461 in 2005 to 11,363 in 2010.[10] The volume of standalone ablation procedures per year also increased from 552 in 2005 to 1014 in 2010.

Surgical Ablation Technology

The development of surgical ablation technology has transformed the field of arrhythmia surgery by reshaping the Cox-Maze procedure into an operation that is technically easier, shorter, and less invasive. Several devices have been used with varying success; therefore it is imperative that the relative advantages and disadvantages of each available ablation modality are understood.[11,12]

Several criteria must be met for an ablation device to be considered suitable for arrhythmia surgery. First, it must reliably produce bidirectional conduction block across the line of ablation. It is important to understand that this requires a transmural lesion, as even small gaps can conduct both sinus and fibrillatory wavefronts.[13] Second, the ablation device must be safe. This requires a precise definition of dose–response curves to limit excessive or inadequate ablation and potential hazards to surrounding vital cardiac structures, such as the coronary sinus, coronary arteries, and valvular structures. Third, the ablation device should facilitate efficient completion of the operation. This would require the device to create lesions rapidly, be intuitive to use, and have adequate length and flexibility. Finally, the device should be adaptable to a minimally invasive approach. This would include the ability to insert the device through minimal access incisions or ports. For the treatment of lone AF, devices that are able to create transmural lesions on the beating heart without the need for cardiopulmonary bypass are desirable. The failure to reliably create linear epicardial lesions on the beating heart is the biggest shortcoming of unipolar energy sources, and has resulted in the development of hybrid procedures to allow for less-invasive surgical options. Currently, no single device has properly met all these criteria.

Microwave, laser, and high-frequency ultrasound (HIFU) technologies have been proved unreliable in the formation of transmural lesions and have been removed from the market. This chapter will focus on cryothermy and RF energy, the two most common ablation technologies now in use.

Cryoablation

Cryoablation devices work by delivering refrigerated fluid through a hollow shaft under a high pressure to a distal closed electrode tip. Rapid expansion induces cooling, and the resultant gas is aspirated via a vacuum tip and returned through a separate circuit.

Cryoablation is unique in that it destroys myocardial tissue by freezing rather than heating. Since this technology preserves the myocardial fibrous skeleton and collagen structure, it is considered safe for use around valvular tissue. The size and depth of the lesion depend on the probe temperature, probe size, duration and number of freeze cycles, gas type, and thermal conductivity and temperature of the tissue.[7]

There are currently two commercially available sources of cryothermal energy being used in cardiac surgery: nitrous oxide and argon. At 1 atm pressure, nitrous oxide is capable of achieving a temperature of −89.5°C, whereas argon has a minimum temperature of −185.7°C. The goal of cryoablation is to cause irreversible cell injury while maintaining the extracellular matrix; a temperature of −40°C is required to be certain of intracellular ice formation.[14,15] The nitrous oxide technology has been extensively used and is generally safe and efficacious, except around the coronary arteries, where studies have

shown late intimal hyperplasia after cryoablation.[16] Disadvantages of cryoablation include the relatively long time required to create lesions (1–3 minutes) and the difficulty encountered when attempting epicardial creation of transmural lesions on the beating heart.[7] The latter shortfall is in part a result of dissipation of thermal energy through convective warming from the circulating endocardial blood, which is known as the "heat-sink" effect. Finally, there is a risk for thromboembolism if blood freezes and coagulates during epicardial ablation on the beating heart. This problem can be overcome by placing the probe endocardially and freezing outward; however, this requires cardiopulmonary bypass. Recent developments in cryoablation include the development of malleable cryoprobes that facilitate minimally invasive application. The ability of one such cryoprobe to reliably produce transmural lesions has been shown to be equivalent to that of a rigid cryoprobe in in vitro and in vivo studies.[15,17]

Radiofrequency Energy

RF was among the earliest energy sources to be reliably applied in the operating room for treating AF. Devices that employ RF emit electromagnetic energy through the delivery of high-density, unmodulated alternating current at a frequency of 350–1000 kHz.[7] This frequency is high enough to prevent rapid myocardial depolarization and induction of ventricular fibrillation yet low enough to prevent tissue vaporization and perforation. Approximately 1 mm of tissue adjacent to the probes is directly heated by a resistive effect, while deeper tissue layers are heated via conduction. Tissue temperatures of approximately 50°C–60°C result in coagulation and permanent destruction of cell structures and collagen. The lesion size depends on the electrode–tissue contact area, interface temperature, current and voltage (power), topical cooling, and tissue resistance. Accordingly, the depth of the lesion can be limited by char formation, epicardial fat, myocardial and endocardial blood flow, and tissue thickness.

Currently available devices are capable of delivering RF energy through either bipolar or unipolar electrodes. Some of these devices are also irrigated, using circulating saline to prevent overheating the thermocouples, avoid insulating char formation, and allow a low-impedance path for energy to penetrate deeper into the tissue. Certain devices intended for epicardial ablation, particularly those intended for use via a minimally invasive approach, employ suction for stabilizing the electrode and promoting better tissue contact.

There have been a number of unipolar RF devices developed for ablation. Although unipolar RF devices have been shown to create transmural lesions on the arrested heart in animals with sufficiently long ablation times, they have not been consistently successful in humans. After 2-minute endocardial ablations during mitral valve surgery, only 20% of the in vivo lesions were transmural.[18] Epicardial ablation on the beating heart has been even more problematic. Animal studies have consistently shown that epicardial application of unipolar RF is incapable of reliably creating transmural lesions on the beating heart,[19] and epicardial RF ablation in humans resulted in only 10% of the lesions being transmural.[20]

Bipolar RF clamps were developed to overcome the shortcomings of unipolar RF ablation by embedding the electrodes in the jaws of a clamp to focus the delivery of energy. An example is shown in Fig. 133.3. This design shields the electrodes from both the circulating blood pool and surrounding tissues, which shortens lesion formation and limits collateral injury. Bipolar ablation has been shown to be capable of creating precise transmural lesions on the beating heart both in animals and humans, with ablation times typically between 10 and 20 seconds.[7,21] Bipolar clamps have also been consistently shown to not damage commonly used polypropylene suture material.[22]

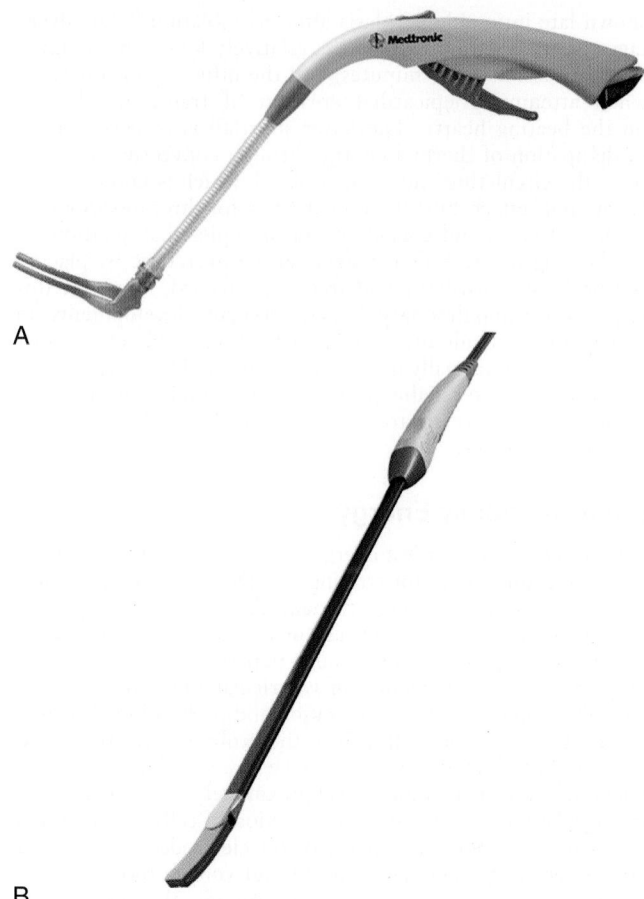

FIGURE 133.3 (A) An example of a bipolar radiofrequency clamp (©Medtronic 2016). (B) An example of a surface bipolar radiofrequency device (©AtriCure 2016).

Bipolar devices have been shown to be safer than unipolar devices. Although relatively infrequent, a number of clinical complications from unipolar RF devices have been reported, including coronary artery injuries, cerebrovascular accidents, and esophageal perforation leading to atrioesophageal fistula.[7] Bipolar RF technology has virtually eliminated this collateral damage by confining the energy within the jaws of the clamp, and no device-related injuries have been reported in the literature with the use of bipolar RF clamps. Presently available devices employ algorithms capable of predicting lesion transmurality either by measuring the tissue conductance between the electrodes or through the use of temperature-based feedback, thereby allowing these devices to tailor the energy delivery to the physiological characteristics of tissue. One drawback of bipolar RF clamps is the requirement for the tissue to be clamped. This has limited potential lesion sets, particularly on the beating heart, and requires the use of adjunctive unipolar or cryothermal technology to create a complete Cox-Maze IV lesion set.

A shortcoming of bipolar clamps is that they are limited in their application on the beating heart to pulmonary vein isolation (PVI). This has led to the development of surface bipolar electrodes that are specially designed to create linear ablation lines from the epicardial surface. These surface bipolar RF devices would ideally be able to perform an off-pump Maze-like lesion set. Several iterations of these devices have been produced, some with features such as suction to aid in affixing the device to the surface being ablated.

Unfortunately, there has been some concern regarding the transmurality of lesions created with surface bipolar RF devices.

Animal studies in our laboratory have shown that despite acute conduction block, none of the lesions produced with one linear device exhibited conduction block at 4 weeks, even though 76% of histological sections were transmural.[23] A suction-assisted device was tested by two independent groups in a porcine model; one study showed a 96% rate of transmural lesions,[24] while the other showed a similar rate of transmurality on a per-section basis but only a 68% rate of transmurality for the entire lesion.[25] In general, the bipolar clamps have been much more effective at creating transmural lesions than the surface bipolar devices.[21,23,26] Careful attention to surgical technique, meticulous testing for entrance and/or exit block when possible, and improvement in device technology are still needed. This technology may improve with future iterations.

In summary, each ablation technology has its own advantages and disadvantages. Although efforts have been made to indirectly compare the merits of different ablation devices, no randomized controlled trial data directly compared them with one another. Situations exist where the use of each of these devices is appropriate, but it is necessary to understand the advantages and disadvantages of each to ensure that the devices are applied correctly. Failure to do so will result in suboptimal clinical outcomes.

Indications for Surgical Ablation of Atrial Fibrillation

The Cox-Maze procedure is indicated for both patients with medically refractory, lone AF and patients undergoing cardiac surgery who have concomitant AF that would benefit from treatment. The latter group is sizable and represents the majority of patients in most clinical experiences. In a review of our experience at Washington University from 1996 to 2005, the incidence of preoperative AF was 22% and 24% in patients referred for valvular or combined valvular/coronary surgery, respectively. However, this remains an undertreated cohort of patients. A review of the STS Adult Cardiac Surgery Database by Ad et al. from 2005 to 2010 showed that only 40.6% patients with preoperative AF received surgical ablation.[10] A higher proportion of patients with preoperative AF referred for mitral valve repair (61.5%) received concomitant surgical ablation compared with 27.5% of patients with preoperative AF undergoing coronary artery bypass grafting (CABG). The role of surgery for AF was clarified and endorsed in a consensus statement released by the Heart Rhythm Society in partnership with the European Heart Rhythm Association, the European Cardiac Arrhythmia Society, the American College of Cardiology, the American Heart Association, and the STS.[27] Surgical ablation for AF is indicated for the following: (1) all symptomatic AF patients undergoing other cardiac surgery; (2) selected asymptomatic AF patients undergoing cardiac surgery in which the ablation can be performed with minimal additional risk; and (3) symptomatic lone AF patients who prefer a surgical approach, have failed one or more attempts at catheter ablation, or are not candidates for catheter ablation. Thus for lone AF, surgery is a complementary approach to catheter ablation.

A relative indication for surgery exists for AF patients at a high risk for cerebrovascular thromboembolic events. This would include patients with persistent AF and a $CHADS_2$ score ≥ 2 who develop a contraindication to long-term anticoagulation.[28] The annual risk for stroke in patients with a CHA_2DS_2-VASc score >2 is between 3% and 15%,[29] whereas the annual risk for stroke after a Cox-Maze procedure in 433 patients followed at our institution for a mean of 6.6 ± 5 years was 0.2%. In the latter study, no association was found between postoperative neurological events and either the $CHADS_2$ score or warfarin use.[28] Although these benefits have not been demonstrated in prospective randomized trials, they are thought to be a result of both successful restoration of sinus rhythm and exclusion of the left atrial appendage (LAA), which is considered a major source of thromboemboli in patients with AF.

Surgical treatment for AF with management of the LAA should also be considered in high-risk patients with persistent AF and cerebrovascular events that have occurred while on therapeutic anticoagulation, as these patients are at high risk for further embolic events. Although warfarin is capable of reducing the risk for ischemic and hemorrhagic strokes by more than 60% in patients with AF, it does not completely eliminate this serious complication.[30] At our institution, 20% of patients who underwent the Cox-Maze III procedure had experienced at least one cerebral thromboembolic event preoperatively.[5] Furthermore, studies have shown that adding the Cox-Maze procedure in patients undergoing concomitant valve surgery can decrease the late risk for cardiac- and stroke-related deaths.[31] A series from Japan demonstrated a 10% increase in the incidence of stroke at an 8-year follow-up for patients with chronic AF who underwent mitral valve replacement alone when compared with similar patients who had mitral valve replacement with a concomitant Cox-Maze procedure.[32] Current European guidelines note no benefit of LAA exclusion in reducing stroke risk.[33] If LAA exclusion is performed, we recommend that the LAA be excised or that a dedicated LAA exclusion device be used.

The Cox-Maze Procedure

Surgical Technique

The Cox-Maze III procedure is rarely performed at the present time, as most centers have replaced the surgical incisions described in the original "cut-and-sew" procedure with lines of ablation created by a variety of different energy sources. At our institution, we have successfully used bipolar RF energy and cryoablation to replace most of the surgical incisions of the Cox-Maze III procedure in an operation termed Cox-Maze IV (see Fig. 133.2).

The Cox-Maze IV procedure is performed using cardiopulmonary bypass with either a median sternotomy, often in combination with other cardiac surgery, or a less-invasive right minithoracotomy. The latter is our procedure of choice in patients referred for a stand-alone Cox-Maze procedure or in conjunction with mitral valve repair. All patients undergo intraoperative transesophageal echocardiography. If a patient has AF at the time of surgery, amiodarone is administered and the patient is electrically cardioverted after excluding the presence of an LAA clot. Both the right and left pulmonary veins (PVs) are bluntly dissected. Pacing thresholds are measured from each PV. The PVs are then isolated using a bipolar RF ablation device, such that a line of ablation surrounds a cuff of atrial tissue encompassing the right and left PVs, respectively (Fig. 133.4). The adequacy of electrical isolation is demonstrated by confirming exit block by pacing from each PV in patients who have undergone a full sternotomy, and from the right PVs in minithoracotomy patients.

The right atrial lesion set is typically performed on the beating heart during cardiopulmonary bypass through a small incision at the base of the right atrial appendage and a single vertical atriotomy (Fig. 133.5). Recently, a three-purse-string approach has been adopted to eliminate the atriotomy in some patients. All ablations are performed using a bipolar RF clamp except for the two endocardial ablation lines to the tricuspid annulus, which are created using a linear cryoprobe. All cryoablations using nitrous oxide devices are performed for 3 minutes at −60°C.

The heart is then arrested by cold cardioplegia. The LAA is amputated or oversewn, and the bipolar RF ablation is performed through the appendage site toward either left PV. The remaining ablation lines are then created using the bipolar clamp through a standard left atriotomy (see Fig. 133.4). Connecting lesions

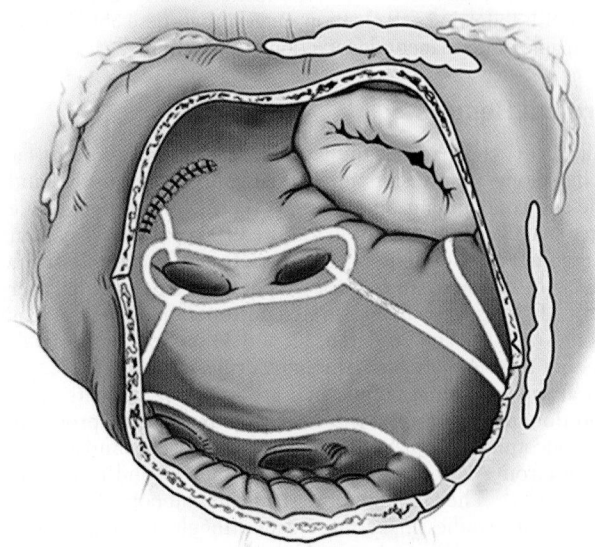

FIGURE 133.4 The left atrial lesion set of the Cox-Maze IV. This comprises right and left pulmonary vein isolation, connecting lesions between the left and right superior and inferior pulmonary veins, a lesion from the left atrial appendage excision site to the pulmonary vein, and a lesion to the mitral valve annulus. (From Weimar T, Bailey MS, Watanabe Y, et al. The Cox-maze IV procedure for lone atrial fibrillation: a single center experience in 100 consecutive patients. *J Interv Card Electrophysiol.* 2011;31:47-54.)

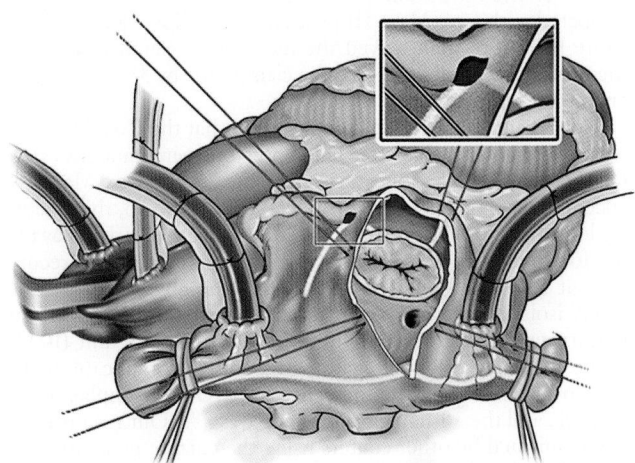

FIGURE 133.5 The right atrial lesion set of the Cox-Maze IV. This consists of lines of ablation along the superior and inferior vena cavae, the free wall of the right atrium, and down to the tricuspid valve annulus. (From Weimar T, Bailey MS, Watanabe Y, et al. The Cox-Maze IV procedure for lone atrial fibrillation: a single center experience in 100 consecutive patients. *J Interv Card Electrophysiol.* 2011; 31:47-54.)

into the left superior and inferior PVs effectively isolate the entire posterior left atrium, and a linear line of ablation is created toward the mitral annulus. Cryoablation is then used to connect the lesion to the mitral annulus and to complete the left atrial isthmus line. In patients undergoing a right minithoracotomy, cryoablation is more extensively used to complete the posterior left atrial isolation.

Some groups have added additional ganglionated plexus (GP) ablation to the Cox-Maze IV procedure; however, definite clinical evidence supporting the use of GP ablation is lacking.[34] Moreover, in animal studies in our laboratory, evidence of early reinnervation at 1 month following GP ablation suggest that these ablations are not capable of permanent denervation of the atrium.[35]

Surgical Results

Similar to Cox-Maze III, the Cox-Maze IV procedure has had excellent long-term results for patients undergoing both stand-alone and concomitant operations. A recent prospective, single-center trial from our institution followed 100 consecutive patients undergoing a stand-alone procedure between January 2002 and May 2010.[36] More than 60% of patients had long-standing persistent AF. This study demonstrated postoperative freedom from AF of 93%, 90%, and 90% at 6, 12, and 24 months, respectively. Freedom from AF off antiarrhythmic drugs was 82%, 82%, and 84% at the same time points. In a group of 282 patients at our institution, the majority of whom had a Cox-Maze IV procedure with concomitant cardiac surgery, the results were similar with a freedom from AF of 89%, 93%, and 89% at 3, 6, and 12 months, respectively.[37] The fact that more stringent end points were used in the recent studies make these data difficult to compare with prior Cox-Maze III results. Instead of relying on symptomatic recurrences, electrocardiogram (ECG) and Holter monitor recordings were performed, and AF recurrence was defined as any episode lasting for over 30 seconds. Despite these variations in the follow-up methodology, a propensity analysis performed by our group has shown no significant difference in the freedom from AF between Cox-Maze III and IV patients.[38] In our consecutive series of stand-alone procedures, no difference was found in outcomes between the Cox-Maze III and IV procedures, the complication rate was significantly lower with the ablation-assisted procedure, and the operative time was shorter. Compared with Cox-Maze III procedure, the Cox-Maze IV procedure had more than halved the mean cross-clamp time for a lone procedure[36] and decreased the clamp time by 30 minutes for concomitant procedures.[8]

Two recent studies have demonstrated that the Cox-Maze IV results were comparable after failed previous percutaneous catheter ablation.[39,40] The long-term outcomes of the Cox-Maze IV procedure have remained good; at a 5-year follow-up, the overall freedom from AF after 5 years in 119 consecutive patients available for follow-up was 78%.[41] Significant predictors of recurrence at 5 years in our cohort included the absence of a "box lesion" isolating the entire left atrial posterior wall, early atrial tachyarrhythmias, extended length of intensive care unit (ICU) and hospital stay, and aggregate perioperative complications. In our 576-patient series, the incidence of pacemaker implantation was 12%, and the 30-day mortality rate was 3%. Our results have been confirmed by other centers using the current generation of bipolar RF clamps and/or cryothermy.[42]

Although electrical and mechanical exclusion of the entire posterior left atrium was expected to compromise atrial function, cardiac magnetic resonance imaging (MRI) demonstrated that this was not the case.[43] In fact, our group has shown that isolating the entire posterior left atrium by creating a "box" is greatly preferable to isolating the left and right PVs separately, with or without a connecting lesion (see Fig. 133.5). Box-lesion patients have been shown to have significantly higher freedom from AF (96% vs. 86%) and from AF off antiarrhythmic drugs (79% vs. 47%) compared with patients who underwent a non-box-lesion set.[36] For this reason, all patients now receive a non-box lesion set at our institution. In a small study, using cardiac MRI to evaluate atrial function, we found that patients with paroxysmal AF had significant left atrial wall motion abnormalities compared with healthy volunteers, and patients who had undergone Cox-Maze IV procedures had wall motion abnormalities similar to those of patients with AF.[44]

Risk factors for recurrence of AF at 1 year include enlarged left atrial diameter, failure to isolate the entire posterior left atrium, and early atrial tachyarrhythmias.[37] Increasing left atrial size has been related to operative failure in several studies, and our group has demonstrated that the probability of recurrence exceeds 50% once the diameter of the left atrium is >8 cm.[37] Early atrial tachyarrhythmias were also associated with recurrence, and it is thought that these might be a marker of more advanced atrial pathology in patients with AF of long duration. Other authors have shown longer AF duration, surgeon inexperience, and greater left atrial diameter to be significant predictors of recurrence.[45] It is clear that surgeon-dependent factors such as hasty or incorrect use of ablation technology or failure to properly perform certain lesions can also affect outcomes.

When compared with other minimally invasive surgical methods for ablation of AF, the Cox-Maze IV procedure remains the most effective. A recent systematic review and meta-analysis including 1877 patients showed rates of freedom from AF of 93%, 80%, and 70%, respectively, for Cox-Maze IV, epicardial procedures including PVI, and hybrid procedures.[46] It also has been shown that the Cox-Maze IV lesion set and minimally invasive approaches are equally effective when cryothermal energy is used in place of bipolar RF ablation.[47]

Retrospective studies have shown the Cox-Maze IV procedure to be effective when performed concomitantly with other cardiac operations, including mitral valve surgery,[48–52] CABG,[53] and aortic valve replacement,[54] and also when the operative risk is high.[55] The addition of a Maze procedure does not appear to add to the operative risk for CABG or aortic valve replacement (AVR).[56] A Cox-Maze procedure has been shown to improve the durability of mitral valve repair in selected patients with preoperative AF.[57]

The Concomitant Utilization of Radiofrequency Energy for Atrial Fibrillation (CURE-AF) trial, a prospective multicenter trial of concomitant biatrial Cox-Maze IV using irrigated unipolar and bipolar RF ablation, showed 66% freedom from atrial tachyarrhythmias at 6–9 months.[58] These results were less encouraging, although issues with the study's methodology and surgeon-to-surgeon variability in technique may explain some of the discrepancies between the results of this study and those reported retrospectively by high-volume centers. The reduced efficacy seen in this study may be related to heterogeneity in ablation technique among centers. Another recent multicenter trial comparing "biatrial procedures" and PVI versus no ablation at the time of mitral valve repair showed no difference in freedom from AF or mortality between patients treated with a biatrial procedure and patients treated with PVI.[59] However, a major shortcoming of this study was the lack of standardization of the biatrial procedure, making it difficult to interpret the results.

Left Atrial Lesion Sets

Surgical Technique

There is a high degree of variability in how surgeons perform left-sided atrial lesion sets. Techniques have utilized all available ablation technologies and vary in whether the energy is applied from the endocardial or epicardial surface. From a procedural standpoint, all these procedures have incorporated a subset of the left atrial lesion set of the Cox-Maze IV procedure. Typically, electrical isolation of the PVs is attempted and may be accompanied by a lesion to the mitral annulus with or without the removal of the LAA. The use of a box lesion isolating all four PV ostia with the left atrial posterior wall has become an increasingly common feature of these lesion sets. One iteration, introduced by Edgerton et al., is the Dallas lesion set, which can be performed epicardially on the beating heart using minimally invasive techniques. This lesion set, which combines PVI with connecting lesions formed on the dome of the left atrium, electrophysiologically mimics most of the left atrial lesions of the Cox-Maze lesion set and has shown promising results at both 6 and 12 months.[60]

Surgical Results

The value of left atrial lesion sets in the surgical management of AF has been proven in the literature, but results have varied. In a randomized trial of patients with persistent AF undergoing mitral valve surgery and radiofrequency ablation (RFA) of the left atrium versus mitral valve surgery alone, sinus rhythm was present in 44.4% of RFA patients at a 1-year follow-up compared with 4.5% in the mitral valve surgery–only group.[61] In this trial, the lines of ablation were created using a monopolar RF device applied from the endocardial surface, which may have had limited efficacy in creating transmural lesions. Although these results were inferior to those of the complete biatrial Cox-Maze lesion set, it is important to note that a more limited lesion set was superior to no intervention for patients with AF in this study, as well as in several other randomized trials of patients undergoing concomitant cardiac surgery in which only a left atrial lesion set was used.[27] In the PRAGUE-12 study, a randomized multicenter study of the left atrial lesion set compared with no ablation performed concomitantly with coronary or valve surgery, 60.2% of ablated patients were in sinus rhythm at 1 year compared with 35.5% of patients who did not undergo ablation (p =.002).[62] Most of this effect seems to have occurred in patients with long-standing persistent AF. The results of left atrial lesion sets have also been shown in randomized trials to have results superior to those of PVI alone.[63]

The importance of the right atrial lesion set is difficult to define, as biatrial versus left atrial surgical ablation has not been compared in an adequately powered randomized controlled trial. Although some evidence suggests that a left atrial lesion set is as effective as a biatrial lesion set in patients with chronic AF undergoing concomitant open heart procedures,[64] other studies have not substantiated this finding. A meta-analysis of a published study including 2225 patients showed significantly higher freedom from AF at 1 year in patients treated with biatrial versus left atrial lesion sets (77% vs. 70%, p = .005), but obtained similar results between the two groups at late follow-up.[65] In another meta-analysis, a greater benefit of biatrial ablation was obtained compared with left atrial ablation (89% vs. 76%, p = .001).[66]

These results were consistent with our intraoperative mapping experience, which showed distinct regions of stable dominant frequencies in the left atrium, indicating stable left atrial origins for AF, only 30% of the time. In 12% of patients, the AF originated from the right atrium, and in almost half of the patients mapped, the origin was unstable and moved around the atria.[67] It must be kept in mind that recurrent right atrial flutter or tachycardia is a well-known complication of performing only left atrial ablations.

Data are available on the importance of several of the lines that comprise the left atrial lesions of the Cox-Maze procedure. Retrospective work from Gillinov et al. has shown the significance of the left atrial isthmus lesion in patients with permanent AF,[68] and patients are at risk for late left atrial flutter if the isthmus line is either incomplete or omitted. In a randomized trial, Gaita and coauthors examined PVI alone versus two alternate lesion sets that both included ablation of the left atrial isthmus. In this study, freedom from AF off antiarrhythmic drugs at a 2-year follow-up using a Holter monitor was only seen in 20% in the PVI group versus 57% in the other groups (p < .006).[69] Moreover, we have demonstrated the importance of a "box" lesion around the PVs and the entire posterior left atrium.[37,41,70] Therefore most of the left atrial Cox-Maze lesion set is likely needed to ensure a high success rate.

With the advent of ablation technology, which has simplified the performance of the operation, it is our opinion that all patients undergoing AF ablation with concomitant cardiac surgery should have at least the full Cox-Maze left atrial lesion set. There is little justification for more limited left atrial lesion sets at the present time.

Pulmonary Vein Isolation

Surgical Technique

The term *pulmonary vein isolation* or PVI is used to describe an amalgamation of techniques that result in the electrical isolation of the PVs from the remainder of the heart. PVI can be performed with lesions encircling the right and left PVs individually, with or without an intervening connecting lesion, or as a box lesion isolating the entire posterior left atrium (Fig. 133.6). Regardless of the lesion set used, PVI can be performed without the need for cardiopulmonary bypass, making it an attractive treatment option, especially for patients with lone AF in whom the procedure can be performed via a minimally invasive approach. Various energy sources have been used for PVI; however, our institution favors bipolar RF clamps for this procedure.

Before attempting a minimally invasive approach, an intraoperative transesophageal echocardiogram is performed to evaluate whether a left atrial thrombus is present. If a left atrial clot is identified, the procedure is either aborted or converted to an open procedure to minimize the risk for systemic thromboembolism. If no clot is identified, external defibrillator pads are placed, and the patient is positioned in the left lateral decubitus position with the right arm extended over the head. A camera port is then placed in the fourth intercostal space, approximately 2 cm anterior to the midaxillary line, and additional working ports are placed in the second and sixth intercostal spaces along the anterior axillary line.

The pericardium is opened anterior and parallel to the phrenic nerve, and blunt dissection is used to identify the space between the right superior PV and the right pulmonary artery. A specialized thoracoscopic dissector and guide sheath are then introduced via a second 10-mm port placed adjacent to the scope port. The device is advanced through the previously dissected space until the tip is between the right superior PV and the right pulmonary artery, at which time the dissector is removed, leaving only the guide sheath in place.

The patient is cardioverted into the sinus rhythm at this time, and pacing thresholds are obtained for each PV to evaluate for conduction block at the end of the procedure. A bipolar RF clamp is introduced into the guide sheath and placed around the right PVs, where two consecutive ablations are performed, the second after advancing the clamp slightly farther onto the surrounding left atrium. Further ablations are performed until electrical isolation is confirmed. Multielectrode catheters have been developed to facilitate minimally invasive epicardial mapping.[71]

The patient is then repositioned into the right lateral decubitus position, with the left arm extended over the head. The procedure is duplicated on the left side, with minimal adjustments based on anatomy: the thoracoscopic port is placed slightly posterior to the midaxillary line, and the pericardotomy is performed parallel and posterior to the phrenic nerve to expose the left PVs. Prior to closing the chest, the LAA is managed with either a stapler or an occluding device.[72] Because of the significant risk for tears and bleeding posed by using an endoscopic stapler in this location, our group prefers to use clip devices to exclude the LAA.[73]

Surgical Results

Although PVI can be performed via a minimally invasive approach without the need for cardiopulmonary bypass, the success of this technique has been variable and highly dependent on patient selection. In one of the first case series on surgical PVI, Wolf

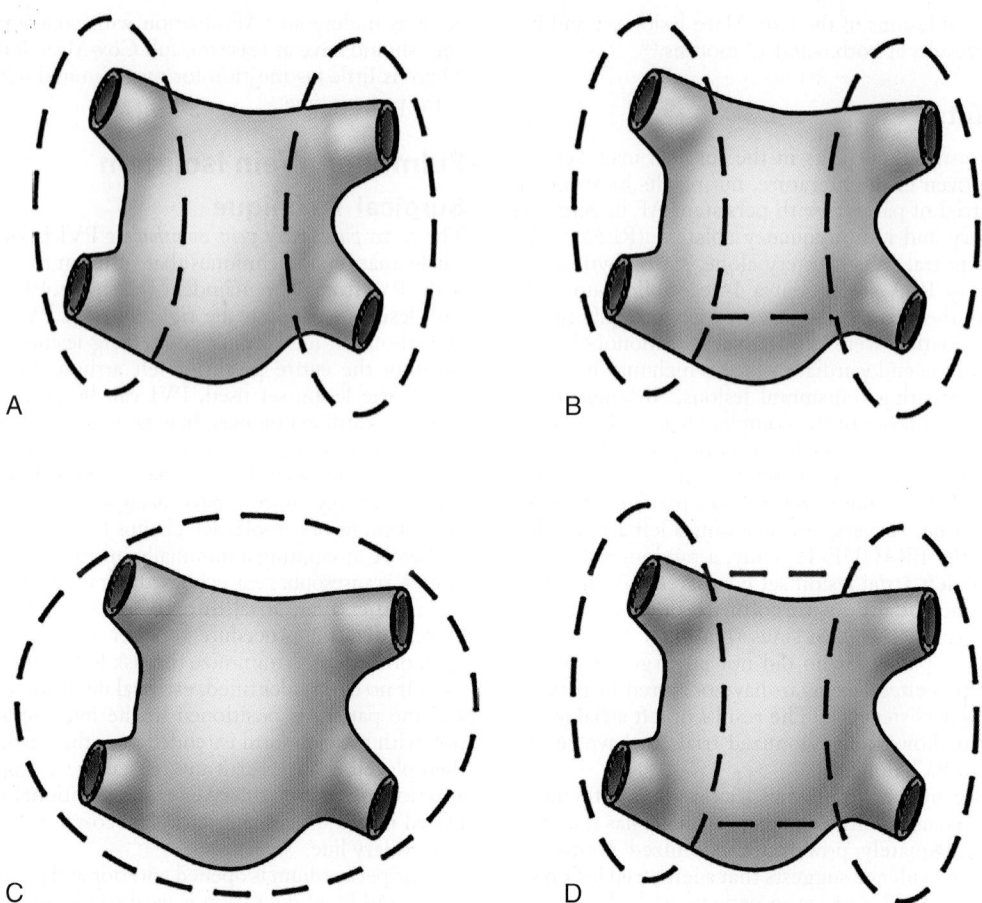

FIGURE 133.6 Schematic illustration of the methods used to isolate the pulmonary veins. Pulmonary vein isolation may be performed (A) separately, (B) with a single connecting lesion, (C) as a complete set, encircling posterior left atrium isolation, or (D) as a "box-lesion" set. Both C and D isolate the entire posterior left atrium, but the lesion pattern in C is typical of minimally invasive ablation devices that snake around the pulmonary veins.

et al. reported 91% freedom from AF and 65% freedom from AF off antiarrhythmic drugs, in patients primarily with paroxysmal AF (66%) who underwent video-assisted, bilateral PVI and LAA exclusion.[74] However, this was a small group of only 27 patients with a very limited follow-up of just 3 months.

A larger study, which focused on 52 paroxysmal AF patients undergoing bilateral PVI, autonomic denervation, and excision of the LAA, demonstrated 81% freedom from AF at 12 months with prolonged monitoring; 89% of those without AF 1-year postoperatively were also free from antiarrhythmic medications.[75] In a larger multicenter trial of 100 patients undergoing minimally invasive bilateral PVI, autonomic denervation, and LAA resection, 87% were found to be in NSR using Holter monitoring at a mean follow-up of 13.6 ± 8.2 months.[76] Although this study included a diverse group of patients, those patients with long-standing persistent AF only had a 71% incidence of NSR at the conclusion of the study period. Moreover, the strongest predictor of AF recurrence in this trial was found to be the presence of long-standing persistent AF (hazard ratio = 9.3, confidence interval [CI] = 2.2–38.5). A study by Edgerton et al. showed even less success in patients with long-standing persistent AF, demonstrating only 56% freedom from AF, with only 35% of patients off antiarrhythmic drugs, at 6 months.[77] Similar results have been reported by Zheng et al. in China; in their series, only 28.2% of patients with persistent AF and 28.6% of patients with long-standing persistent AF were free from AF at 5 years after PVI with GP ablation.[78] These results stress the necessity of appropriate patient selection.

Most recently, the Atrial Fibrillation Catheter Ablation Versus Surgical Ablation Treatment (FAST) trial, which was a two-center, randomized clinical trial, compared catheter-based ablation with thoracoscopic PVI in patients with antiarrhythmic drug–refractory AF with LA dilatation and hypertension or failed prior catheter ablation.[79] This study demonstrated that the 12-month freedom from AF and antiarrhythmic drugs was 37% for the catheter ablation group and 66% for the PVI group (p = .0022). Therefore while results with surgical PVI were not as good as with a biatrial Cox-Maze lesion set, they have been superior to catheter-based ablation in selected patients.

There is some need to balance the higher efficacy of surgical PVI with its higher risk for complications compared with catheter ablation. A recent systematic review and meta-analysis, which analyzed the results of 245 patients who underwent PVI and 204 patients who underwent catheter ablation, showed much higher freedom from AF off antiarrhythmic drugs at 12 months in the surgical ablation group (odds ratio [OR] = 1.54, 95% CI = 1.24–1.91), but also a significantly higher rate of major complications (28.2% vs. 7.8%, p = .0003).[80] Similar results were found in a cohort study of 33 patients who underwent surgical PVI matched with 66 patients who underwent transcatheter PVI; freedom from atrial arrhythmias off antiarrhythmic drugs was 88% in the surgical PVI group compared with 41% in the transcatheter PVI group (p < .001).[81] However, the complication rate was much higher in the surgical PVI group (21% vs. 5%, p = .015), and 77% of the patients had paroxysmal AF.

The success of PVI is even lower in patients undergoing concomitant operations. In the setting of mitral valve replacement ± other concomitant operations (including aortic and tricuspid valve procedures, and atrial septal defect closure), one study showed 61% freedom from AF, and only 17% freedom from antiarrhythmic medications at a follow-up of 31 ± 16 months.[82] These results highlight the need to fully understand the electrophysiological substrate of AF to perform the optimal operation for any given individual patient. As discussed earlier, a recent multicenter trial comparing "biatrial procedures" and PVI versus no ablation at the time of mitral valve repair showed no difference in freedom from AF or mortality between "biatrial procedures" and PVI, although the biatrial procedures were not standardized.[59] Also, the success rates with surgical ablation in this trial were very low, obscuring differences in procedural outcomes. Moreover, the trial was not powered to detect differences between surgical procedures. A retrospective study including 160 patients undergoing PVI concomitant with aortic valve replacement or CABG revealed inferior freedom from AF at 6 months and a higher risk for adverse events in patients with LA diameter >4.5 cm.[83] At present, surgical PVI can only be recommended for patients with lone paroxysmal AF and should be avoided in patients with large left atria (diameter ≥ 4.5 cm).

Ganglionated Plexus Ablation

Some surgeons advocate taking advantage of the surgical exposure afforded by PVI to perform autonomic denervation via ablation of the GP. The GP innervates both the PV myocardial sleeves and adjacent atrial muscle, and the autonomic ganglia within these plexuses have been found to play a role in the initiation and maintenance of AF.[84] In theory, ablating the region of the epicardial fat pads in which the GP reside at the time of PVI should increase procedural efficacy by removing these proarrhythmic influences. However, the efficacy of surgical GP ablation is unknown. No direct comparisons between conventional PVI and PVI plus GP ablation have been made as part of a randomized clinical trial.

There are additional concerns regarding the long-term efficacy of routine GP ablation at the time of PVI. Experimental evidence from our laboratory and other groups has demonstrated recovery of autonomic function in as few as 4 weeks following GP ablation[35] and that GP ablation may be proarrhythmic.[85] It is worrisome that the reinnervation of tissues occurring following GP ablation may not be homogeneous, leading to an even more arrhythmogenic substrate than existed preoperatively.

Given the lack of data concerning the long-term efficacy of GP ablation, our practice is not to perform GP ablation at the time of AF correction surgery. GP ablation should only be performed in experienced centers participating in clinical trials.

Hybrid Procedures

There has been great interest in the development of hybrid procedures utilizing thoracoscopic epicardial ablation performed by a surgeon and transcatheter endocardial ablation performed by an electrophysiologist. This has been because of the inability of surgical epicardial ablation to reliably create transmural linear lesions due to the limitations of present technology. These hybrid procedures have been performed either simultaneously or as a staged operation. Two-stage hybrid procedures that combine PVI, LAA exclusion, and other variable biatrial lesions via a minimally invasive approach with subsequent endocardial catheter-based ablations are being investigated with promising early results.[86] Hybrid procedures using a suction-based unipolar RF device for epicardial ablation have shown encouraging results at some institutions, although questions regarding the reliability with which unipolar technology is able to create transmural linear lesions on the beating heart remain unanswered.[87,88] In particular, Muneretto et al. have had excellent results with a two-stage hybrid approach, with restoration of sinus rhythm in 87.5% of patients at 28 months.[89] However, as described in an excellent recent review by Kumar et al., the hybrid AF ablation literature currently consists of several small case series with variable lesion sets and devices used.[90] As yet, there has been no randomized controlled trial comparing hybrid ablation with catheter ablation for persistent AF. We await the results of the Staged Transthoracic Approach to Persistent Atrial Fibrillation (TOP-AF) trial, proposed in 2014 by Pragliola et al.[91] Further research will be needed to determine whether a simultaneous or a staged procedure is more effective.

Follow-up After Surgical Ablation of Atrial Fibrillation

There has been recent interest in improving methods of follow-up after surgical ablation of AF. Current guidelines recommend performing an ECG at each follow-up visit and at least 24-hour Holter monitoring once every 12 months for paroxysmal AF and every 6 months for persistent AF to document freedom from AF.[27] Numerous small studies have evaluated the use of an implantable loop recorder (ILR) to assess freedom from AF after surgical ablation.[63,92,93] We recently published a multicenter study enrolling 47 patients, each of whom underwent continuous monitoring with an ILR.[94] We found no difference in freedom from atrial tachyarrhythmias at 1 year, assessed using ILR compared with standard ECG or Holter monitoring. We feel that the current iteration of this technology is limited by the high rate of false-positive events and the limited storage space available on the ILR device.

Future Directions in Atrial Fibrillation Surgery

Novel advances in diagnostic techniques are addressing concerns with current ablation strategies. For certain populations, such as those with enlarged atria, even the Cox-Maze procedure has had high postoperative failure rates. Additionally, while most of the triggers for paroxysmal AF originate around the PVs, and are thus amenable to PVI, over 30% of triggers originate elsewhere.[95] It would be a significant advance if the mechanisms of AF could be identified and used to guide the intervention.

Electrocardiographic imaging (ECGI), a relatively new, noninvasive, multipoint mapping modality, may facilitate a patient-specific approach to AF surgery. By combining computed tomography (CT) scanning with body surface potential mapping and 250 electrodes representing over 800 epicardial sites, ECGI is able to obtain patient-specific, heart–torso geometry and create maps of cardiac activation.[96] This technique has been well described in patients with a variety of AF types, and allows activation times to be calculated and displayed as either static or dynamic activation maps on a three-dimensional (3D) surface model of an individual patient's atria.[97] Individual conduction velocities and refractory periods can be surmised from these data and, when combined with information regarding the patient's atrial geometry, used to calculate the critical mass of tissue needed to sustain AF in an individual patient.[98,99] In patients with stable and focal electrophysiological mechanism, ECGI may be used to guide a more targeted surgical or catheter procedure. In patients with multiple or poorly defined nonfocal mechanisms of AF, ECGI may allow a more patient-tailored approach based on critical mass calculations or other metrics. A case series published by Cuculich et al. in 2010 mapped paroxysmal and persistent AF using ECGI, identifying various AF mechanisms and defining a semiquantitative "complexity index."[97] Haissaguerre et al. recently published a series of 102 patients with persistent AF who underwent noninvasive mapping using a novel commercial mapping system based on the ECGI technology (ECVUE [Medtronic; Dublin, Ireland]).[100] They identified "driver domains," using phase mapping. Catheter ablation was subsequently performed, with results comparable with a control sequential linear ablation strategy.

In theory, a surgeon would be able to use ECGI to identify certain patients who would benefit from either atrial reduction surgery or additional ablative lines that further subdivide the atria in order to reduce the size of contiguous atrial tissue below that "critical mass" requisite for AF, making the patients AF proof.

Although the advent of ablation technology has made the Cox-Maze IV procedure technically easier and faster to perform than its initial iterations, it still requires cardiopulmonary bypass. The development of new ablation technologies has spurred the development of novel surgical techniques that can be performed through small incisions without the need for cardiopulmonary bypass.

The limitations of the current ablation devices also have impeded the development of a truly minimally invasive procedure because the creation of reliable transmural lines of ablation from the epicardial surface on the beating heart has been difficult. Future advances may offer devices that overcome this limitation or allow expanded use of hybrid procedures in which surgeons and electrophysiologists work together to complete the lesion sets. Some investigators have already investigated the robot-assisted epicardial application of a dual-energy bipolar–unipolar RF device with promising early results.[101]

Conclusions

Although various strategies exist for the management of AF, the results of the Cox-Maze procedure have been excellent in all patient subgroups. In patients with AF undergoing mitral valve procedures, a concomitant Cox-Maze IV lesion set incurs minimal additional cross-clamp time and overall operative risk and has demonstrated superior freedom from AF compared with mitral valve surgery alone.[52,102] The Cox-Maze lesion set has also been shown to have a high success rate in patients undergoing CABG.[53] It is recommended that a biatrial Cox-Maze procedure be performed in all patients undergoing aortic or mitral valve operations and all on-pump CABG patients. In patients with paroxysmal AF undergoing off-pump CABG, we perform PVI alone due to the reasonably good results demonstrated with this strategy in this patient subgroup. Nonetheless, in patients with long-standing persistent AF, the results of PVI alone have been suboptimal, indicating the need for a more extensive approach. Because of the excellent results obtained with the Cox-Maze lesion set in this patient population, our practice is to either change plans from an off-pump to an on-pump CABG or simply exclude the LAA with a clip device.

In conclusion, the development of ablation technology has dramatically changed the field of AF surgery by transforming a technically demanding procedure into one that is accessible to the majority of surgeons and introducing the possibility of minimally invasive approaches. As we learn more about the mechanisms of AF and develop improved preoperative diagnostic technologies capable of precisely locating the areas responsible for AF, it will become possible to tailor specific lesion sets and ablation modalities to individual patients. This would make the surgical treatment of AF more effective and available to a larger population of patients.

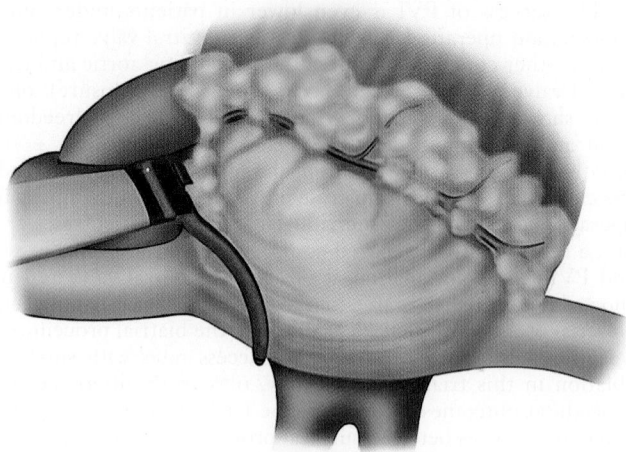

FIGURE 133.7 Surgical isolation of the sinoatrial node using a bipolar radiofrequency clamp. (From Kreisel D, Bailey M, Lindsay BD, et al. A minimally invasive surgical treatment for inappropriate sinus tachycardia. *J Thorac Cardiovasc Surg.* 2005;130:598-599.)

Inappropriate Sinus Tachycardia

Background and Indications

Inappropriate sinus tachycardia (IST) is an uncommon clinical diagnosis characterized by a resting heart rate ≥100 and a rapid rise in heart rate with mild exertion in a structurally normal heart. The tachycardia is deemed an *inappropriate* chronotropic response because both the resting heart rate and the increasing heart rate seen with exercise are generally out of proportion to the physiological need.[103] Although IST is a rare disorder, the prevalence of IST is likely higher than what presents clinically, and may be as high as 1% of the population.[104]

Initial therapy consists of dietary modification and medical management. Until recently, medical management consisted solely of β-blockers and calcium channel blockers. Ivabradine, a specific I_f blocker, has been in use in Europe for 10 years and was approved by the US Food and Drug Administration (FDA) in 2015 for treating stable, symptomatic chronic heart failure with reduced ejection fraction (EF) and a resting heart rate >70 beats/min on maximal doses of β-blockers. Ivabradine has shown promising results in treating IST, completely eliminating symptoms in 47% of patients in a small randomized controlled trial.[105] Adverse reactions to ivabradine include bradycardia and AF. Ivabradine has significant fetal toxicity and cannot be used in pregnant patients. Patients that experience symptoms refractory to conservative measures often undergo catheter ablation therapy. However, this treatment modality remains controversial, and a small reported series demonstrated a high failure rate at a long-term follow-up.[106] This has led some centers to consider a surgical approach.

Surgical Technique: Superior Right Atrial Isolation

Although surgical isolation of the SA node has traditionally been performed through a median sternotomy with intraoperative mapping and cardiopulmonary bypass, our institution has adopted a minimally invasive approach that utilizes epicardial bipolar RF energy to obviate the need for cardiopulmonary bypass.[107]

After positioning the patient in a left lateral decubitus position, a right minithoracotomy is made and a bipolar RF clamp is used to isolate the sinus node along with the entire proximal right atrium (Fig. 133.7). Intraoperative isoproterenol is administered to induce sinus tachycardia to a rate of 150–180 beats/min. Circumferential ablations are then performed around the right atrium until an inversion of the P-wave morphology is seen in the inferior leads, and blunting of the response to isoproterenol is achieved. In our experience of five patients, an average of 8.3 ± 1.5 ablations were needed to fully isolate the SA node, along with a generous cuff of right atrial tissue extending below the junction of the superior vena cava and right atrium. Bipolar pacing is then used to confirm electrical isolation of the SA node and the surrounding atrium from the remainder of the heart in each case. Isoproterenol is used before and after SA node isolation to demonstrate the effectiveness of the procedure.

Surgical Results

The results of superior right atrial isolation have been good. However, both the traditional and minimally invasive techniques have been hampered by symptomatic bradycardia requiring permanent pacemaker implantation, as well as recurrent supraventricular tachycardia from ectopic foci.[107]

In our series of 13 patients, sinus tachycardia was eliminated in all patients in the immediate postoperative period as noted on ECG. Nine patients had an atrial escape rhythm, and only two patients had a junctional rhythm that required postoperative pacemaker implantation immediately following surgery. At the late follow-up of 5.6 ± 5.7 years, four patients had new pacemakers, and three patients developed atrial tachyarrhythmias, with two requiring catheter ablations and one requiring medical therapy for AF. Of the five patients who received the minimally invasive approach, only one required pacemaker implantation

during the follow-up period, and all patients were free from cardiac symptoms at the late follow-up.

Conclusions

Surgical isolation of the SA node should be reserved for highly symptomatic patients with IST that is refractory to medical management. Less-invasive techniques offer a more attractive option for surgical management of refractory IST, with acceptable long-term success in patients for whom medical therapy has failed. Although current clinical practice guidelines do not recommend catheter or surgical ablation for IST,[108] it is our opinion that in selected, highly symptomatic patients, surgical ablation is reasonable.

Other Supraventricular Tachycardia Operations and Conclusions

Although operations developed for treating other supraventricular arrhythmias, such as Wolff-Parkinson-White syndrome, atrial flutter, and atrioventricular nodal reentry, were important precursors in the development of catheter-based procedures, they are currently most notable for their historical significance. Traditional surgical approaches will continue to have a role in patients with atrial arrhythmias refractory to catheter-based procedures as well as in patients with other cardiac or vascular diseases that prohibit a percutaneous approach.

REFERENCES

1. Prystowsky EN, Padanilam BJ, Fogel RI. Treatment of atrial fibrillation. *JAMA*. 2015;314:278–288.
2. Corley SD, Epstein AE, DiMarco JP, et al. Relationships between sinus rhythm, treatment, and survival in the Atrial Fibrillation Follow-Up Investigation of Rhythm Management (AFFIRM) Study. *Circulation*. 2004;109:1509–1513.
3. Chatterjee S, Sardar P, Lichstein E, et al. Pharmacologic rate versus rhythm-control strategies in atrial fibrillation: an updated comprehensive review and meta-analysis. *Pacing Clin Electrophysiol*. 2013;36:122–133.
4. Cox JL, Ad N, Palazzo T. Impact of the maze procedure on the stroke rate in patients with atrial fibrillation. *J Thorac Cardiovasc Surg*. 1999;118:833–840.
5. Prasad SM, Maniar HS, Camillo CJ, et al. The Cox maze III procedure for atrial fibrillation: long-term efficacy in patients undergoing lone versus concomitant procedures. *J Thorac Cardiovasc Surg*. 2003;126:1822–1828.
6. Feinberg MS, Waggoner AD, Kater KM, et al. Restoration of atrial function after the maze procedure for patients with atrial fibrillation. Assessment by Doppler echocardiography. *Circulation*. 1994;90:II285–II292.
7. Lall SC, Damiano Jr RJ. Surgical ablation devices for atrial fibrillation. *J Interv Card Electrophysiol*. 2007;20:73–82.
8. Gaynor SL, Diodato MD, Prasad SM, et al. A prospective, single-center clinical trial of a modified Cox maze procedure with bipolar radiofrequency ablation. *J Thorac Cardiovasc Surg*. 2004;128:535–542.
9. Gammie JS, Haddad M, Milford-Beland S, et al. Atrial fibrillation correction surgery: lessons from the Society of Thoracic Surgeons National Cardiac Database. *Ann Thorac Surg*. 2008;85:909–914.
10. Ad N, Suri RM, Gammie JS, et al. Surgical ablation of atrial fibrillation trends and outcomes in North America. *J Thorac Cardiovasc Surg*. 2012;144:1051–1060.
11. Schuessler RB, Lee AM, Melby SJ, et al. Animal studies of epicardial atrial ablation. *Heart Rhythm*. 2009;6:S41–S45.
12. Melby SJ, Schuessler RB, Damiano Jr RJ. Ablation technology for the surgical treatment of atrial fibrillation. *ASAIO J*. 2013;59:461–468.
13. Melby SJ, Lee AM, Zierer A, et al. Atrial fibrillation propagates through gaps in ablation lines: implications for ablative treatment of atrial fibrillation. *Heart Rhythm*. 2008;5:1296–1301.
14. Gage AA, Baust J. Mechanisms of tissue injury in cryosurgery. *Cryobiology*. 1998;37:171–186.
15. Weimar T, Lee AM, Ray S, et al. Evaluation of a novel cryoablation system: in vivo testing in a chronic porcine model. *Innovations (Phila)*. 2012;7:410–416.
16. Holman WL, Ikeshita M, Ungerleider RM, et al. Cryosurgery for cardiac arrhythmias: acute and chronic effects on coronary arteries. *Am J Cardiol*. 1983;51:149–155.

17. Weimar T, Lee AM, Ray S, et al. Evaluation of a novel cryoablation system: in vitro testing of heat capacity and freezing temperatures. *Innovations (Phila)*. 2012;7:403–409.
18. Santiago T, Melo JQ, Gouveia RH, et al. Intra-atrial temperatures in radiofrequency endocardial ablation: Histologic evaluation of lesions. *Ann Thorac Surg*. 2003;75:1495–1501.
19. Thomas SP, Guy DJ, Boyd AC, et al. Comparison of epicardial and endocardial linear ablation using handheld probes. *Ann Thorac Surg*. 2003;75:543–548.
20. Santiago T, Melo J, Gouveia RH, et al. Epicardial radiofrequency applications: in vitro and in vivo studies on human atrial myocardium. *Eur J Cardiothorac Surg*. 2003;24:481–486. discussion 486.
21. Voeller RK, Zierer A, Schuessler RB, et al. Performance of a novel dual-electrode bipolar radiofrequency ablation device: a chronic porcine study. *Innovations (Phila)*. 2011;6:17–22.
22. Bohn J, Gehron J, Dellmann A, Boening A. Influence of radiofrequency energy on polypropylene sutures in atrial tissue. *Thorac Cardiovasc Surg*. 2012;60:290–292.
23. Lee AM, Aziz A, Clark KL, et al. Chronic performance of a novel radiofrequency ablation device on the beating heart: Limitations of conduction delay to assess transmurality. *J Thorac Cardiovasc Surg*. 2012;144:859–865.
24. Kiser AC, Pappas HR, Garner KC, et al. Evaluation of an integrated bipolar and unipolar ablation device. *Innovations (Phila)*. 2014;9:33–37.
25. Saint LL, Lawrance CP, Okada S, et al. Performance of a novel bipolar/monopolar radiofrequency ablation device on the beating heart in an acute porcine model. *Innovations (Phila)*. 2013;8:276–283.
26. Kasirajan V, Sayeed S, Filler E, et al. Histopathology of bipolar radiofrequency ablation in the human atrium. *Ann Thorac Surg*. 2015;101:638–643.
27. Calkins H, Kuck KH, Cappato R, et al. 2012 HRS/EHRA/ECAS expert consensus statement on catheter and surgical ablation of atrial fibrillation: recommendations for patient selection, procedural techniques, patient management and follow-up, definitions, endpoints, and research trial design: a report of the Heart Rhythm Society (HRS) Task Force on Catheter and Surgical Ablation of Atrial Fibrillation. Developed in partnership with the European Heart Rhythm Association (EHRA), a registered branch of the European Society of Cardiology (ESC) and the European Cardiac Arrhythmia Society (ECAS); and in collaboration with the American College of Cardiology (ACC), American Heart Association (AHA), the Asia Pacific Heart Rhythm Society (APHRS), and the Society of Thoracic Surgeons (STS). Endorsed by the governing bodies of the American College of Cardiology Foundation, the American Heart Association, the European Cardiac Arrhythmia Society, the European Heart Rhythm

Association, the Society of Thoracic Surgeons, the Asia Pacific Heart Rhythm Society, and the Heart Rhythm Society. *Heart Rhythm*. 2012;9:632–696.e21.
28. Pet M, Robertson JO, Bailey M, et al. The impact of CHADS(2) score on late stroke after the Cox maze procedure. *J Thorac Cardiovasc Surg*. 2012;146:85–89.
29. Pieri A, Lopes TO, Gabbai AA. Stratification with CHA2DS2-VASc score is better than CHADS2 score in reducing ischemic stroke risk in patients with atrial fibrillation. *Int J Stroke*. 2011;6:466.
30. Risk factors for stroke and efficacy of antithrombotic therapy in atrial fibrillation. Analysis of pooled data from five randomized controlled trials. *Arch Intern Med*. 1994;154:1449–1457.
31. Bando K, Kobayashi J, Kosakai Y, et al. Impact of Cox maze procedure on outcome in patients with atrial fibrillation and mitral valve disease. *J Thorac Cardiovasc Surg*. 2002;124:575–583.
32. Bando K, Kobayashi J, Hirata M, et al. Early and late stroke after mitral valve replacement with a mechanical prosthesis: risk factor analysis of a 24-year experience. *J Thorac Cardiovasc Surg*. 2003;126:358–364.
33. Dunning J, Nagendran M, Alfieri OR, et al. Guideline for the surgical treatment of atrial fibrillation. *Eur J Cardiothorac Surg*. 2013;44:777–791.
34. Gelsomino S, Lozekoot P, La Meir M, et al. Is ganglionated plexi ablation during Maze IV procedure beneficial for postoperative long-term stable sinus rhythm? *Int J Cardiol*. 2015;192:40–48.
35. Sakamoto S, Schuessler RB, Lee AM, et al. Vagal denervation and reinnervation after ablation of ganglionated plexi. *J Thorac Cardiovasc Surg*. 2010;139:444–452.
36. Weimar T, Bailey MS, Watanabe Y, et al. The Cox-maze IV procedure for lone atrial fibrillation: a single center experience in 100 consecutive patients. *J Interv Card Electrophysiol*. 2011;31:47–54.
37. Damiano Jr RJ, Schwartz FH, Bailey MS, et al. The Cox maze IV procedure: predictors of late recurrence. *J Thorac Cardiovasc Surg*. 2011;141:113–121.
38. Lall SC, Melby SJ, Voeller RK, et al. The effect of ablation technology on surgical outcomes after the Cox-maze procedure: a propensity analysis. *J Thorac Cardiovasc Surg*. 2007;133:389–396.
39. Ad N, Henry L, Hunt S, et al. The outcome of the Cox Maze procedure in patients with previous percutaneous catheter ablation to treat atrial fibrillation. *Ann Thorac Surg*. 2011;91:1371–1377. discussion 1377.
40. Okada S, Weimar T, Moon MR, et al. The impact of previous catheter-based ablation on the efficacy of the Cox-maze IV procedure. *Ann Thorac Surg*. 2013;96:786–791. discussion 791.
41. Henn MC, Lancaster TS, Miller JR, et al. Late outcomes after the Cox maze IV procedure for atrial fibrillation. *J Thorac Cardiovasc Surg*. 2015;150:1168–1178.e2.

42. Philpott JM, Zemlin CW, Cox JL, et al. The ABLATE Trial: safety and efficacy of Cox Maze-IV using a bipolar radiofrequency ablation system. *Ann Thorac Surg*. 2015;100:1541–1548.
43. Voeller RK, Zierer A, Lall SC, et al. The effects of the Cox maze procedure on atrial function. *J Thorac Cardiovasc Surg*. 2008;136:1257–1264. 1264 e1–3.
44. Robertson JO, Lee AM, Voeller RK, et al. Quantification of the functional consequences of atrial fibrillation and surgical ablation on the left atrium using cardiac magnetic resonance imaging. *Eur J Cardiothorac Surg*. 2014;46:720–728.
45. Ad N, Holmes SD. Prediction of sinus rhythm in patients undergoing concomitant Cox maze procedure through a median sternotomy. *J Thorac Cardiovasc Surg*. 2014;148:881–886. discussion 886–887.
46. Je HG, Shuman DJ, Ad N. A systematic review of minimally invasive surgical treatment for atrial fibrillation: a comparison of the Cox-Maze procedure, beating-heart epicardial ablation, and the hybrid procedure on safety and efficacy. *Eur J Cardiothorac Surg*. 2015;48:531–540. discussion 540–541.
47. Ad N, Henry L, Friehling T, et al. Minimally invasive stand-alone Cox-maze procedure for patients with nonparoxysmal atrial fibrillation. *Ann Thorac Surg*. 2013;96:792–798. discussion 798–799.
48. Lawrance CP, Henn MC, Miller JR, et al. Comparison of the stand-alone Cox-Maze IV procedure to the concomitant Cox-Maze IV and mitral valve procedure for atrial fibrillation. *Ann Cardiothorac Surg*. 2014;3:55–61.
49. Bum Kim J, Suk Moon J, Yun SC, et al. Long-term outcomes of mechanical valve replacement in patients with atrial fibrillation: impact of the maze procedure. *Circulation*. 2012;125:2071–2080.
50. Ad N, Holmes SD, Massimiano PS, et al. The effect of the Cox-maze procedure for atrial fibrillation concomitant to mitral and tricuspid valve surgery. *J Thorac Cardiovasc Surg*. 2013;146:1426–1434. discussion 1434–1435.
51. Saint LL, Damiano Jr RJ, Cuculich PS, et al. Incremental risk of the Cox-maze IV procedure for patients with atrial fibrillation undergoing mitral valve surgery. *J Thorac Cardiovasc Surg*. 2013;146:1072–1077.
52. Saint LL, Bailey MS, Prasad S, et al. Cox-Maze IV results for patients with lone atrial fibrillation versus concomitant mitral disease. *Ann Thorac Surg*. 2012;93:789–794. discussion 794–795.
53. Damiano Jr RJ, Gaynor SL, Bailey M, et al. The long-term outcome of patients with coronary disease and atrial fibrillation undergoing the Cox maze procedure. *J Thorac Cardiovasc Surg*. 2003;126:2016–2021.
54. Henn MC, Lawrance CP, Sinn LA, et al. Effectiveness of surgical ablation in patients with atrial fibrillation and aortic valve disease. *Ann Thorac Surg*. 2015;100:1253–1259. discussion 1259–1260.
55. Ad N, Holmes SD, Pritchard G, Shuman DJ. Association of operative risk with the outcome of concomitant Cox Maze procedure: a comparison of results across risk groups. *J Thorac Cardiovasc Surg*. 2014;148:3027–3033.
56. Ad N, Henry L, Hunt S, Holmes SD. Do we increase the operative risk by adding the Cox Maze III procedure to aortic valve replacement and coronary artery bypass surgery? *J Thorac Cardiovasc Surg*. 2012;143:936–944.
57. Kim GS, Lee CH, Kim JB, et al. Echocardiographic evaluation of mitral durability following valve repair in rheumatic mitral valve disease: impact of Maze procedure. *J Thorac Cardiovasc Surg*. 2014;147:247–253.
58. Damiano Jr RJ, Badhwar V, Acker MA, et al. The CURE-AF trial: a prospective, multicenter trial of irrigated radiofrequency ablation for the treatment of persistent atrial fibrillation during concomitant cardiac surgery. *Heart Rhythm*. 2014;11:39–45.
59. Gillinov AM, Gelijns AC, Parides MK, et al. Surgical ablation of atrial fibrillation during mitral-valve surgery. *N Engl J Med*. 2015;372:1399–1409.
60. Edgerton JR, Jackman WM, Mack MJ. A new epicardial lesion set for minimal access left atrial maze: the Dallas lesion set. *Ann Thorac Surg*. 2009;88:1655–1657.
61. Doukas G, Samani NJ, Alexiou C, et al. Left atrial radiofrequency ablation during mitral valve surgery for continuous atrial fibrillation: a randomized controlled trial. *JAMA*. 2005;294:2323–2329.
62. Budera P, Straka Z, Osmancik P, et al. Comparison of cardiac surgery with left atrial surgical ablation vs. cardiac surgery without atrial ablation in patients with coronary and/or valvular heart disease plus atrial fibrillation: final results of the PRAGUE-12 randomized multicentre study. *Eur Heart J*. 2012;33:2644–2652.
63. Bogachev-Prokophiev A, Zheleznev S, Pivkin A, et al. Assessment of concomitant paroxysmal atrial fibrillation ablation in mitral valve surgery patients based on continuous monitoring: does a different lesion set matter?. *Interact Cardiovasc Thorac Surg*. 2014;18:177–181. discussion 182.
64. Deneke T, Khargi K, Grewe PH, et al. Left atrial versus bi-atrial Maze operation using intraoperatively cooled-tip radiofrequency ablation in patients undergoing open-heart surgery: safety and efficacy. *J Am Coll Cardiol*. 2002;39:1644–1650.
65. Phan K, Xie A, Tsai YC, et al. Biatrial ablation vs. left atrial concomitant surgical ablation for treatment of atrial fibrillation: a meta-analysis. *Europace*. 2015;17:38–47.
66. Barnett SD, Ad N. Surgical ablation as treatment for the elimination of atrial fibrillation: a meta-analysis. *J Thorac Cardiovasc Surg*. 2006;131:1029–1035.
67. Schuessler RB, Kay MW, Melby SJ, et al. Spatial and temporal stability of the dominant frequency of activation in human atrial fibrillation. *J Electrocardiol*. 2006;39:S7–S12.
68. Gillinov AM, McCarthy PM, Blackstone EH, et al. Surgical ablation of atrial fibrillation with bipolar radiofrequency as the primary modality. *J Thorac Cardiovasc Surg*. 2005;129:1322–1329.
69. Gaita F, Riccardi R, Caponi D, et al. Linear cryoablation of the left atrium versus pulmonary vein cryoisolation in patients with permanent atrial fibrillation and valvular heart disease: correlation of electroanatomic mapping and long-term clinical results. *Circulation*. 2005;111:136–142.
70. Voeller RK, Bailey MS, Zierer A, et al. Isolating the entire posterior left atrium improves surgical outcomes after the Cox maze procedure. *J Thorac Cardiovasc Surg*. 2008;135:870–877.
71. Sabashnikov A, Weymann A, Haldar S, et al. Position of totally thoracoscopic surgical ablation in the treatment of atrial fibrillation: an alternative method of conduction testing. *Med Sci Monit Basic Res*. 2015;21:76–80.
72. Dawson AG, Asopa S, Dunning J. Should patients undergoing cardiac surgery with atrial fibrillation have left atrial appendage exclusion? *Interact Cardiovasc Thorac Surg*. 2010;10:306–311.
73. Ailawadi G, Gerdisch MW, Harvey RL, et al. Exclusion of the left atrial appendage with a novel device: early results of a multicenter trial. *J Thorac Cardiovasc Surg*. 2011;142:1002–1009 e1.
74. Wolf RK, Schneeberger EW, Osterday R, et al. Video-assisted bilateral pulmonary vein isolation and left atrial appendage exclusion for atrial fibrillation. *J Thorac Cardiovasc Surg*. 2005;130:797–802.
75. Edgerton JR, Brinkman WT, Weaver T, et al. Pulmonary vein isolation and autonomic denervation for the management of paroxysmal atrial fibrillation by a minimally invasive surgical approach. *J Thorac Cardiovasc Surg*. 2010;140:823–828.
76. Beyer E, Lee R, Lam BK. Point: Minimally invasive bipolar radiofrequency ablation of lone atrial fibrillation: early multicenter results. *J Thorac Cardiovasc Surg*. 2009;137:521–526.
77. Edgerton JR, Edgerton ZJ, Weaver T, et al. Minimally invasive pulmonary vein isolation and partial autonomic denervation for surgical treatment of atrial fibrillation. *Ann Thorac Surg*. 2008;86:35–38. discussion 39.
78. Zheng S, Li Y, Han J, et al. Long-term results of a minimally invasive surgical pulmonary vein isolation and ganglionic plexi ablation for atrial fibrillation. *PloS One*. 2013;8. e79755.
79. Boersma LV, Castella M, van Boven W, et al. Atrial fibrillation catheter ablation versus surgical ablation treatment (FAST): a 2-center randomized clinical trial. *Circulation*. 2012;125:23–30.
80. Phan K, Phan S, Thiagalingam A, et al. Thoracoscopic surgical ablation versus catheter ablation for atrial fibrillation. *Eur J Cardiothorac Surg*. 2015;49:1044–1051.
81. De Maat GE, Van Gelder IC, Rienstra M, et al. Surgical vs. transcatheter pulmonary vein isolation as first invasive treatment in patients with atrial fibrillation: a matched group comparison. *Europace*. 2014;16:33–39.
82. Tada H, Ito S, Naito S, et al. Long-term results of cryoablation with a new cryoprobe to eliminate chronic atrial fibrillation associated with mitral valve disease. *Pacing Clin Electrophysiol*. 2005;28:S73–S77.
83. Kainuma S, Mitsuno M, Toda K, et al. Dilated left atrium as a predictor of late outcome after pulmonary vein isolation concomitant with aortic valve replacement and/or coronary artery bypass grafting dagger. *Eur J Cardiothorac Surg*. 2015;48:765–777.
84. Scherlag BJ, Nakagawa H, Jackman WM, et al. Electrical stimulation to identify neural elements on the heart: their role in atrial fibrillation. *J Interv Card Electrophysiol*. 2005;13:37–42.
85. Mao J, Yin X, Zhang Y, et al. Ablation of epicardial ganglionated plexi increases atrial vulnerability to arrhythmias in dogs. *Circ Arrhythm Electrophysiol*. 2014;7:711–717.
86. Mahapatra S, LaPar DJ, Kamath S, et al. Initial experience of sequential surgical epicardial-catheter endocardial ablation for persistent and long-standing persistent atrial fibrillation with long-term follow-up. *Ann Thorac Surg*. 2011;91:1890–1898.
87. La Meir M, Gelsomino S, Lorusso R, et al. The hybrid approach for the surgical treatment of lone atrial fibrillation: one-year results employing a monopolar radiofrequency source. *J Cardiothorac Surg*. 2012;7:71.
88. Zembala M, Filipiak K, Kowalski O, et al. Minimally invasive hybrid ablation procedure for the treatment of persistent atrial fibrillation: one year results. *Kardiol Pol*. 2012;70:819–828.
89. Muneretto C, Bisleri G, Bontempi L, et al. Successful treatment of lone persistent atrial fibrillation by means of a hybrid thoracoscopic-transcatheter approach. *Innovations (Phila)*. 2012;7:254–258.
90. Kumar P, Kiser AC, Gehi AK. Hybrid treatment of atrial fibrillation. *Prog Cardiovasc Dis*. 2015;58:213–220.
91. Pragliola C, Mastroroberto P, Gaudino M, et al. Staged transthoracic approach to persistent atrial fibrillation (TOP-AF): study protocol for a randomized trial. *Trials*. 2014;15:190.
92. Pecha S, Aydin MA, Ahmadzade T, et al. Implantable loop recorder monitoring after concomitant surgical ablation for atrial fibrillation (AF): insights from more than 200 continuously monitored patients. *Heart Vessels*. 2016;31:1347–1353.
93. Pokushalov E, Romanov A, Cherniavsky A, et al. Ablation of paroxysmal atrial fibrillation during coronary artery bypass grafting: 12 months' follow-up through implantable loop recorder. *Eur J Cardiothorac Surg*. 2011;40:405–411.
94. Damiano Jr RJ, Lawrance CP, Saint LL, et al. Detection of atrial fibrillation after surgical ablation: conventional versus continuous monitoring. *Ann Thorac Surg*. 2016;101:42–48.
95. Lee SH, Tai CT, Hsieh MH, et al. Predictors of non-pulmonary vein ectopic beats initiating paroxysmal atrial fibrillation: implication for catheter ablation. *J Am Coll Cardiol*. 2005;46:1054–1059.
96. Ramanathan C, Ghanem RN, Jia P, et al. Noninvasive electrocardiographic imaging for cardiac electrophysiology and arrhythmia. *Nat Med*. 2004;10:422–428.
97. Cuculich PS, Wang Y, Lindsay BD, et al. Noninvasive characterization of epicardial activation in humans with diverse atrial fibrillation patterns. *Circulation*. 2010;122:1364–1372.
98. Byrd GD, Prasad SM, Ripplinger CM, et al. Importance of geometry and refractory period in sustaining atrial fibrillation: testing the critical mass hypothesis. *Circulation*. 2005;112:I7–I13.
99. Lee AM, Aziz A, Didesch J, et al. Importance of atrial surface area and refractory period in sustaining atrial fibrillation: testing the critical mass hypothesis. *J Thorac Cardiovasc Surg*. 2012;146:593–598.
100. Haissaguerre M, Hocini M, Denis A, et al. Driver domains in persistent atrial fibrillation. *Circulation*. 2014;130:530–538.
101. Balkhy HH, Vloka ME, Chapman PD, et al. Robotic application of a novel dual-energy device for left atrial ablation: intraoperative and early postoperative results. *Innovations (Phila)*. 2014;9:439–444.
102. Saint LL, Damiano Jr RJ, Cuculich PS, et al. Incremental risk of the Cox-Maze IV procedure for patients with atrial fibrillation undergoing mitral valve surgery. *J Thorac Cardiovasc Surg*. 2013;146:1072–1077.
103. Shen WK. How to manage patients with inappropriate sinus tachycardia. *Heart Rhythm*. 2005;2:1015–1019.
104. Still AM, Raatikainen P, Ylitalo A, et al. Prevalence, characteristics and natural course of inappropriate sinus tachycardia. *Europace*. 2005;7:104–112.
105. Cappato R, Castelvecchio S, Ricci C, et al. Clinical efficacy of ivabradine in patients with inappropriate sinus tachycardia: a prospective, randomized, placebo-controlled, double-blind, crossover evaluation. *J Am Coll Cardiol*. 2012;60:1323–1329.
106. Man KC, Knight B, Tse HF, et al. Radiofrequency catheter ablation of inappropriate sinus tachycardia guided by activation mapping. *J Am Coll Cardiol*. 2000;35:451–457.
107. Kreisel D, Bailey M, Lindsay BD, et al. A minimally invasive surgical treatment for inappropriate sinus tachycardia. *J Thorac Cardiovasc Surg*. 2005;130:598–599.
108. Sheldon RS, Grubb 2nd BP, Olshansky B, et al. 2015 Heart Rhythm Society expert consensus statement on the diagnosis and treatment of postural tachycardia syndrome, inappropriate sinus tachycardia, and vasovagal syncope. *Heart Rhythm*. 2015;12:e41–e63.

134 Surgery for Ventricular Arrhythmias

Sanjay Dixit and Y. Joseph Woo

Historical Perspective

Open-heart surgery was commonly used in the past to treat refractory ventricular arrhythmias.[1] The predominant population subjected to this management strategy comprised patients with healed myocardial infarcts who experienced sustained ventricular tachycardia (VT). The original technique used resection of the dyskinetic/akinetic scarred myocardial tissue (aneurysmectomy) with only modest success (~40%) for long-term arrhythmia control.[2] Subsequent mapping studies revealed that critical components of the VT reentrant circuit used the border zone between the dense scar and healthy myocardium. This resulted in the development of subendocardial resection (removing tissue up to a depth of 2–4 mm in the area surrounding the dense aneurysm),[3] which improved the overall success rate of long-term arrhythmia control to 90%.[4] Subsequent innovations in mapping tools (multielectrode epicardial shock and endocardial basket) allowed operators to better characterize VT circuits for more effective surgical ablation.[5] Nevertheless, a major limitation of the technique remained its highly invasive nature (median sternotomy with cardiopulmonary bypass and ventriculotomy).[6] Furthermore, because the technique was typically performed on sick patients with impaired cardiac function (who experienced recurrent ventricular arrhythmias refractory to multiple antiarrhythmic drugs [AADs]), the periprocedural mortality rate was high.[1,4,5,7] For these reasons, the technique was never widely adopted. Furthermore, with the invention of implantable cardioverter defibrillators (ICDs) and advances in percutaneous catheter mapping and ablation techniques, there was steady decline of surgical VT ablation. Nowadays, it is used only rarely in a select group of patients for treating refractory ventricular arrhythmias.

Indications

Surgical VT ablation is generally the treatment of last resort reserved primarily for patients who have failed a combination of AADs and percutaneous catheter ablation attempts.[8,9] The more contemporary experience at the Hospital of The University of Pennsylvania is consistent with this.[10] Over an 8-year period (2007–2015), 2353 patients underwent VT ablations at our center. Of these, 608 patients (25.8%) had heart disease categorized as nonischemic based on the lack of a prior infarct and absence of coronary disease. In 21 of these patients (3.5%, 18 males), all with a nonischemic substrate (median left ventricular ejection fraction of 41% ± 20%), the arrhythmia remained refractory to medications and endocardial/epicardial percutaneous radiofrequency (RF) ablation attempts. These patients eventually underwent surgical VT ablation for arrhythmia control. Eleven patients had idiopathic dilated cardiomyopathy, four had valvular cardiomyopathy, two had long-standing hypertrophic cardiomyopathy, and three had arrhythmogenic right ventricular dysplasia/cardiomyopathy.[11] Cardiac magnetic resonance imaging (MRI) was performed in 13 patients, and late gadolinium enhancement was identified in the midmyocardium in four patients, subepicardium in three, and interventricular septum (IVS) in six. The latter group was particularly interesting because in the majority, the basal septum was markedly thickened (>20 mm). Consistent with these observations, case reports from other investigators also suggest that ventricular arrhythmias arising from the basal IVS are challenging to ablate percutaneously.[12] Thus in patients with VT, which manifests electrocardiogram (ECG) characteristics suggestive of origin from the IVS region, attempts should be made a priori to identify septal scar using MRI, positron emission tomography scan, and transthoracic or intracardiac echocardiography (Fig. 134.1). Typical ECG features suggesting VT origin from the IVS region include (1) left bundle branch block morphology with superior or inferior axis and early precordial transition (before lead V_3) or (2) right bundle branch block morphology with inferior or superior axis and an unusual precordial transition pattern with lead V_2 manifesting predominantly negative complexes (rS or QS) compared with leads V_1 and V_2 (Fig. 134.2).[13,14] In these cases, especially if a scar is identified in the IVS, it is prudent to make the patient aware of the possibility that percutaneous catheter ablation may not be successful. Similarly, in patients with left ventricular (LV) hypertrophy who have ventricular arrhythmias in the setting of midmyocardial scar, consideration should be given to a surgical option if an attempt at percutaneous catheter ablation fails.[10,11] In addition to this, surgical ablation of ventricular arrhythmias should be considered in patients who are undergoing open-heart surgery for other cardiac conditions, such as valve surgery or coronary artery bypass grafting, and have manifested recurrent VT despite AAD therapy and/or percutaneous catheter ablation attempts. For patients undergoing surgical placement of ventricular assist devices (VADs) who have clinically experienced VT, surgical VT ablation may be considered. We have recently reported our experience on this scenario in six patients at the time of left VAD placement.[15] Patel and colleagues have also reported a series of five patients in whom they performed VT ablation during the VAD placement.[16] Unlike our approach where the VT substrate was targeted through the "cored-out" LV apex prior to left VAD placement, Patel and colleagues allowed the patients to recover from the left VAD surgery for 24–48 hours and then performed open-chest electrophysiological and electroanatomical mapping (EAM) on exposed heart in the hybrid operation room.

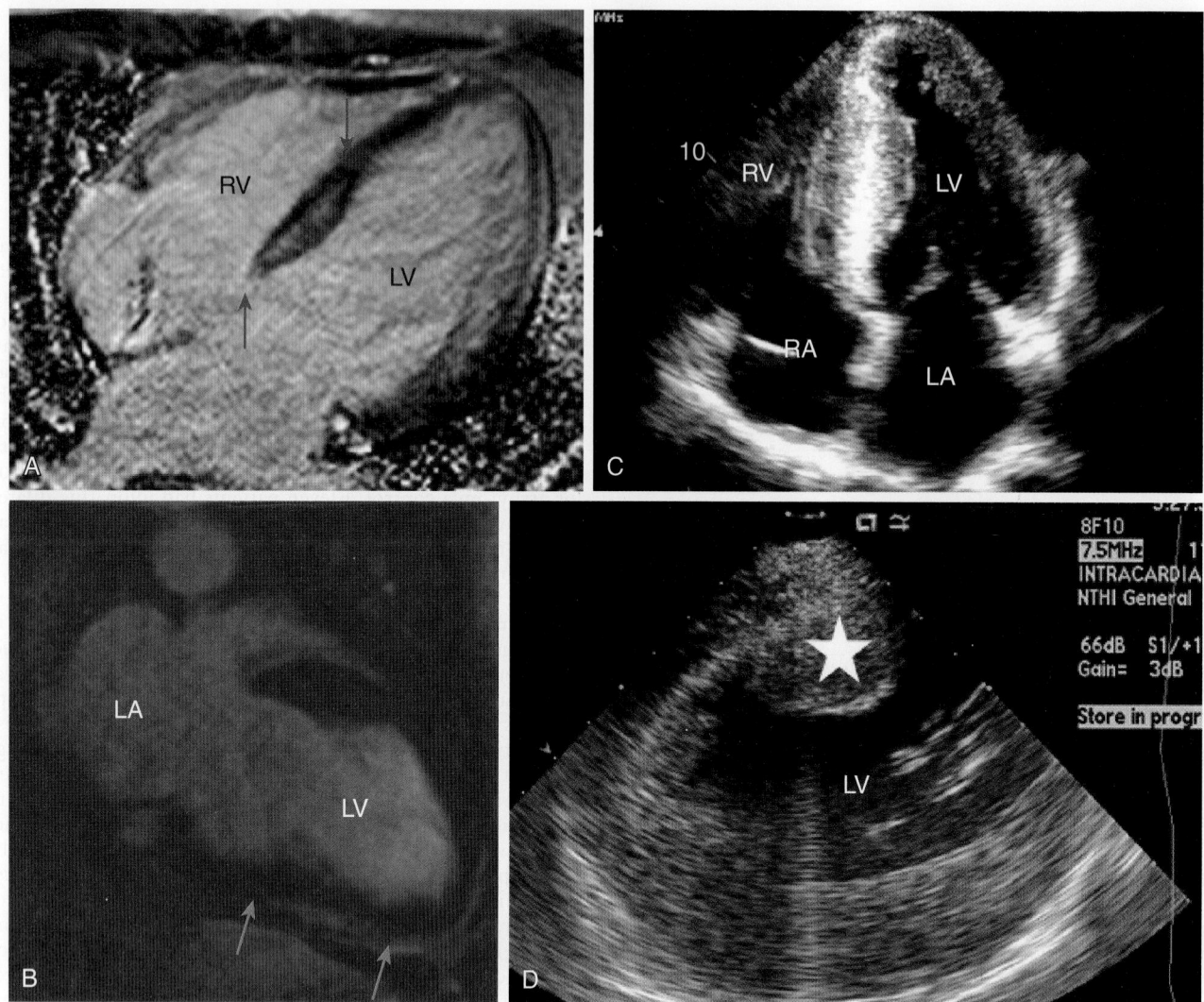

FIGURE 134.1 Septal scar identified by magnetic resonance imaging (MRI) and echocardiographic imaging. (A) Proximal interventricular scar (*red arrows*). (B) Scar in the distal interventricular distribution extending to the apex (*blue arrows*) identified by MRI. (C) Apical four-chamber transthoracic echocardiographic view showing thickened septum with marked echogenicity representing infiltrative disease process. (D) Thickened proximal interventricular septum (*star*) identified using intracardiac echocardiography in a patient with hypertrophic cardiomyopathy. In all these patients, refractory ventricular arrhythmias originated from the septal substrate, which was targeted during surgical ablation. *LA,* Left atrium; *LV,* left ventricle; *RA,* right atrium; *RV,* right ventricle.

Different Approaches for Accessing the Ventricle

Adequate access to all cardiac surfaces is critical to the success of surgical VT ablation. Median sternotomy typically provides the best visualization of the entire heart.[1,4,10,11] The epicardial aspect of the right ventricle (RV), superior IVS, and anterior LV wall are well visualized through median sternotomy without additional cardiac manipulation (Fig. 134.3). However, to adequately inspect the posterolateral LV wall, the heart has to be physically lifted. Although this can cause a drop in cardiac output and blood pressure, proper pericardial and cardiac manipulation as conducted during off-pump coronary artery bypass grafting can facilitate good exposure of the posterolateral LV for inspection and mapping if necessary.[17] Actual ablation, particularly cryoablation, is typically best performed in our experience with cardiopulmonary bypass on an arrested heart to avoid the energy sink of warm blood within the heart. To access the LV endocardium, several options are available. The transaortic approach offers the best

visualization of the basal LV, including the IVS region as well as the anterior and lateral LV walls.[17,18] To achieve this, a standard aortotomy for aortic valve (AV) replacement is performed above the sinotubular junction.[10] The AV leaflets are carefully retracted against the sinus of Valsalva, and the LV outflow tract is exposed (see Fig. 134.3). The IVS is seen immediately under the right coronary AV cusp. The basal anterior and lateral LV endocardium is visualized under the junction of right–left commissures and the left coronary cusp, respectively (see Fig. 134.3). A transatrial trans-mitral valve (MV) approach offers the best visualization of both papillary muscles, the posterior LV endocardium, and the LV apex.[17,19,20] These structures are frequently involved in VT circuits in patients with healed inferior infarcts and can also be the source of VT in patients with nonischemic cardiomyopathy. In patients with mechanical AV and MV, apical ventriculotomy has been used to access the LV endocardium.[18] In patients undergoing surgical ventricular aneurysm repair, the site of aneurysmectomy can also be used to access the LV endocardium before aneurysm resection and closure. More recently

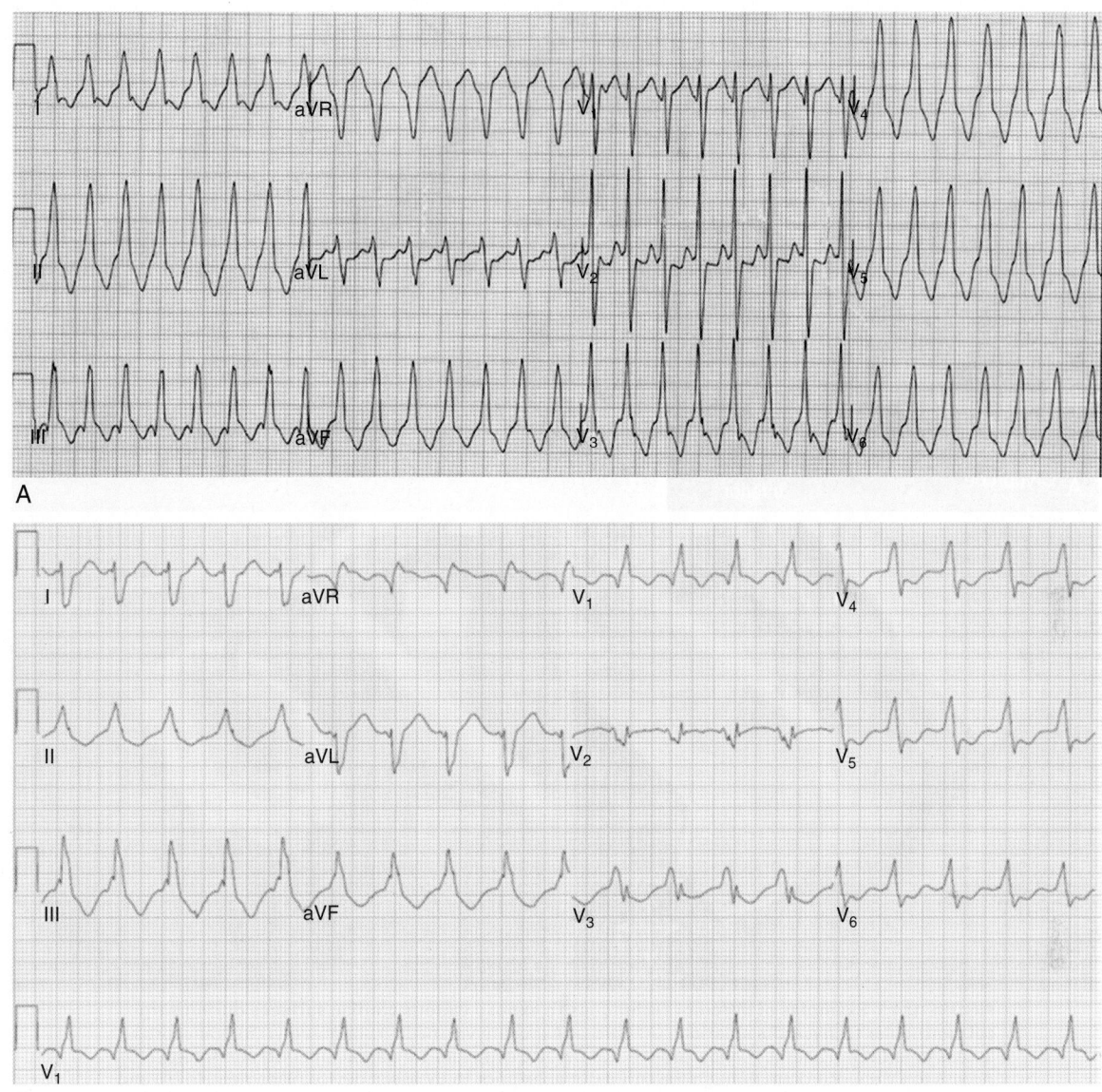

FIGURE 134.2 (A) A 12-lead electrocardiogram (ECG) of ventricular tachycardia (VT) manifesting a left bundle branch block morphology and inferior axis with early transition ($\leq V_3$). (B) A 12-lead ECG of VT manifesting a right bundle branch block morphology, inferior axis, and unusual transition pattern (predominantly positive forces in leads V_1 and V_3–V_6 but negative forces in lead V_2). These features are characteristic of VT originating from the interventricular septal region. *aVF,* Augmented vector foot; *aVL,* augmented vector left; *aVR,* augmented vector right.

in patients undergoing left VAD placement, the "cored-out" LV apex (see Fig. 134.3) can provide access to the LV endocardium.[15] The RV too can be accessed either via a transatrial trans-tricuspid valve approach or directly through the RV free wall.[17,21] An important difference between epicardial alone versus additional endocardial cardiac access pertains to cardiopulmonary bypass use.[22] When the arrhythmia originates from the RV free wall or the inferior IVS region, access to these locations can be obtained by partial sternotomy, sparing the upper half of the sternum (see Fig. 134.3).[23] The advantages of this approach are shorter postprocedure recovery and more stable sternal healing. We have used this approach successfully in a patient undergoing ablation for refractory VT originating from the inferior IVS region and the anterior epicardial LV surface. There are also case series and larger patient experiences describing access to the epicardium using a surgical window via an epigastric incision with

or without removal of the xyphoid process,[21,24] or a left anterior thoracotomy using a limited left anterior incision extending from the third to fifth intercostal spaces. Both these techniques have been successfully accomplished in the cardiac electrophysiology (EP) laboratory. However, using this approach in the EP laboratory, only the epicardial aspect of the inferior, anterior, and parts of the lateral cardiac surfaces were accessed[25] (Video 134.1).

Tools and Techniques for Mapping

Early attempts at mapping ventricular arrhythmias in the operating room (OR) used finger-mounted bipolar electrodes that were sequentially manipulated to various locations in the chamber of interest.[3,4] Subsequently, multipolar meshes and basket catheters were developed that had the ability to record simultaneous electrical activity at a higher resolution.[26,27] However, interpretation

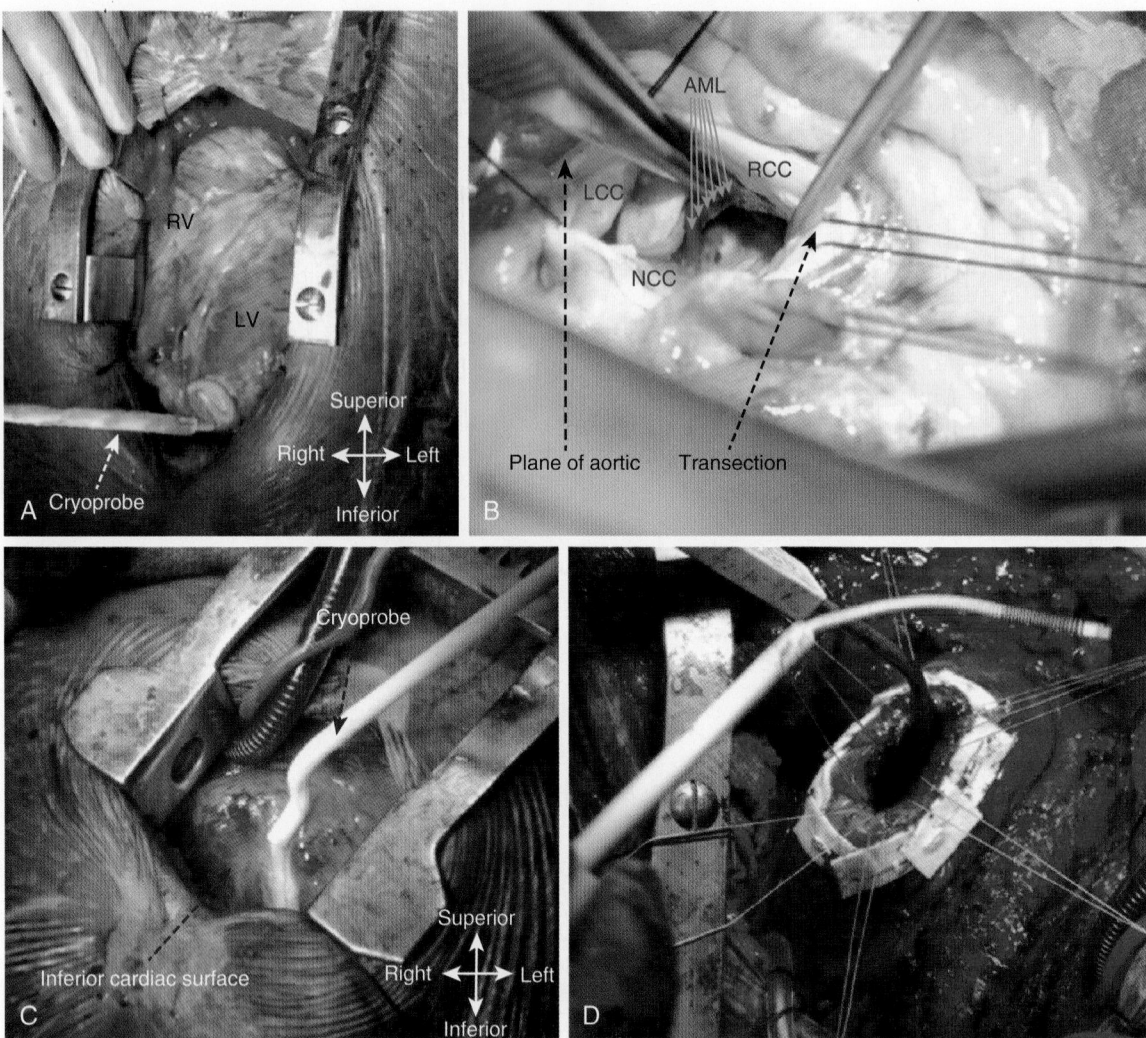

FIGURE 134.3 Examples of different techniques to expose various cardiac surfaces during surgical ventricular tachycardia ablation. (A) Cardiac exposure via median sternotomy. (B) Transaortic access to left ventricular (LV) endocardium. (C) Cardiac exposure via partial (inferior) sternotomy. (D) Access to LV endocardium through the cored-out apex prior to LV assist device placement. In (A) and (C), the cryoprobe can be seen deployed at the LV apex and the inferior interventricular septal region, respectively. *AML,* Anterior mitral leaflet; *LCC,* left coronary cusp; *LV,* left ventricle; *NCC,* noncoronary cusp; *RCC,* right coronary cusp; *RV,* right ventricle.

of data required special signal processing that made these tools cumbersome to use in the OR. With the development of EAM techniques, electrophysiologists are now able to create a three-dimensional shell of the chamber of interest during ongoing arrhythmia.[28] This tool provides more intuitive visualization of the tachycardia circuit vis-à-vis the underlying anatomy and substrate. EAM requires a low-intensity magnetic field around the patient, which requires a special setup. In hybrid ORs that are specifically designed for both percutaneous catheter and open-heart surgical interventions, use of advanced cardiac EP mapping tools including EAM is possible.[16,21,29] To accomplish this, typically the magnet is set up under the operating table, reference electrodes are sutured to the epicardial surface of either ventricle (exposed via sternotomy), and the mapping catheter is manipulated on or within the chamber of interest (Fig. 134.4 and Video 134.2). However, to sustain and map ventricular arrhythmias in the OR, the heart usually has to be actively "beating." In some cases, ventricular arrhythmias can be induced and sustained with the heart connected to cardiopulmonary bypass, but without aortic cross-clamping. However, in these instances, the

cardiac temperatures on bypass need to be maintained in the normothermic range. Furthermore, if cryothermy is used for ablation, then the most effective lesions are created on a cooled, cardioplegia-arrested heart. The downside of cold cardioplegia is that it is impossible to sustain ventricular arrhythmias.[10,12,26] Even without using cold cardioplegia, reproducible induction and maintenance of the clinical arrhythmia(s) during open-heart surgery (in patients under deep anesthesia) can be challenging. The loss of autonomic tone as well as the effects of various anesthetic agents coupled with underfilled hearts can make this hard. An alternative to mapping ventricular arrhythmias in the OR is to perform detailed mapping of these a priori in the cardiac EP laboratory. We have used this strategy in the majority of patients who have undergone surgical VT ablation at our institution.[10,11] In each case, detailed endocardial and, when indicated, epicardial mapping of the arrhythmia was performed in the EP laboratory. Using activation, entrainment, and EAM, the critical components of the reentrant circuit and/or the site of origin of VT (vis-à-vis the underlying substrate) were characterized. These locations were then targeted by conventional RF energy.

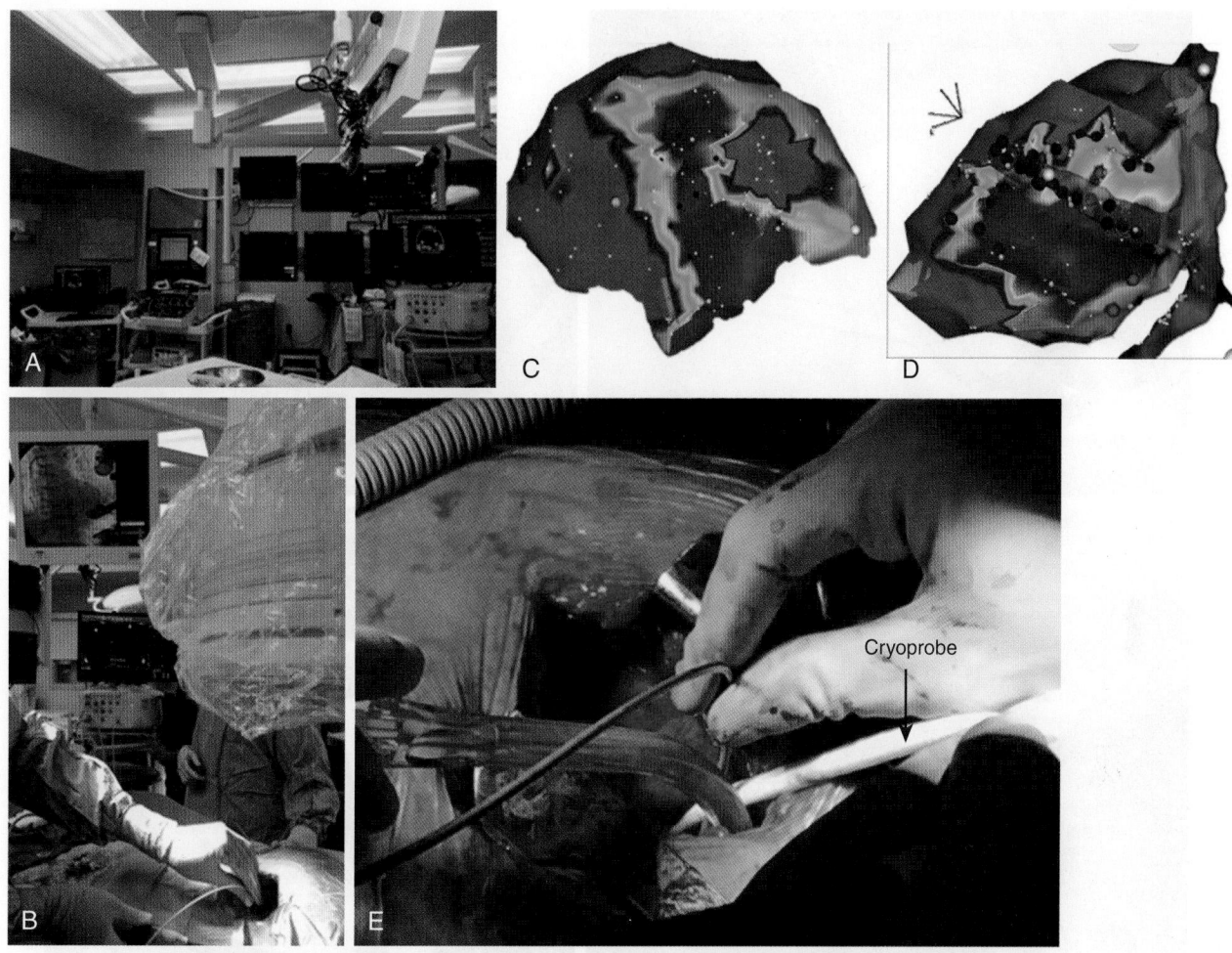

FIGURE 134.4 Example of electroanatomical mapping (EAM)-guided surgical ventricular tachycardia (VT) ablation. (A) The typical setup for EAM in the hybrid operating room (OR) at our institution. (B) Access to the epicardial surface of the heart was obtained via partial sternotomy, and epicardial EAM was performed via a standard mapping catheter under fluoroscopic guidance. (C and D) The scar distribution on the EAM of epicardial surface in the OR (C, *red color*) closely approximated the scar distribution seen on the EAM obtained in the electrophysiology lab (D). (E) Successful surgical VT ablation was achieved by positioning the cryoprobe in close approximation to the mapping catheter (under fluoroscopic guidance) through the partial sternotomy.

Although percutaneous RF ablation in these cases was not effective in suppressing the arrhythmias, in the OR the RF lesions were identifiable and served as targets for cryothermy application (Fig. 134.5). This precluded the need for additional arrhythmia induction or mapping during open-heart surgical ablation. In the OR (under cold cardioplegia), the cryoprobe was positioned over the RF lesion site and full-duration (3 minutes) cryothermy application was made. This procedure typically resulted in a large lesion, the induration from which could be palpated on the opposing surface (see Fig. 134.5). Thus cryolesions delivered on the endocardial surface could be palpated from the epicardial aspect and vice versa. As a result, it was possible to make an additional cryothermy application on the opposing cardiac surface to ensure a transmural lesion that would extend through the entire thickness of the targeted LV myocardium (Video 134.3).

Energy Sources for Surgical Ablation

Several energy sources have been used to create effective lesions during surgical ablation of ventricular arrhythmias. These include RF energy, cryothermy, microwave, and laser energy. Among these, the largest experience has been with cryothermy.

The cryoablation technology used earlier during surgical VT ablation utilized a stiff handheld probe that was able to achieve tissue temperatures of −60° C.[26] Although this was found to be adequate for targeting VT circuits around the aneurysm of healed infarcts, it likely created lesions no larger than 5 mm. Thus for deeper intramural VT circuits/sources, this may not be an effective energy source.[12] In comparison, for our current surgical VT ablation cases, we have utilized the Surgifrost Surgical Cryoablation System (Medtronic CryoCath LP, Quebec, Canada).[10,11] This system uses a flexible metal probe with an adjustable insulation sheath and can be molded to conform to cardiac contours. It uses argon gas to achieve rapid cooling to a temperature of −150° C and is capable of creating lesions up to 60 mm in size. The standard duration of cryoapplication with this unit is for a maximum of 3 minutes and comprises both the cooling and thawing phases. The best results are achieved under cold cardioplegia, which allows the probe to achieve the lowest tissue temperatures. The malleable probe can be configured into various shapes, which is helpful for ablating at different cardiac locations and surfaces. The entire length of the probe is positioned to create linear lesions when targeting large epicardial scars in the IVS region (Fig. 134.6). In instances where the epicardial source of

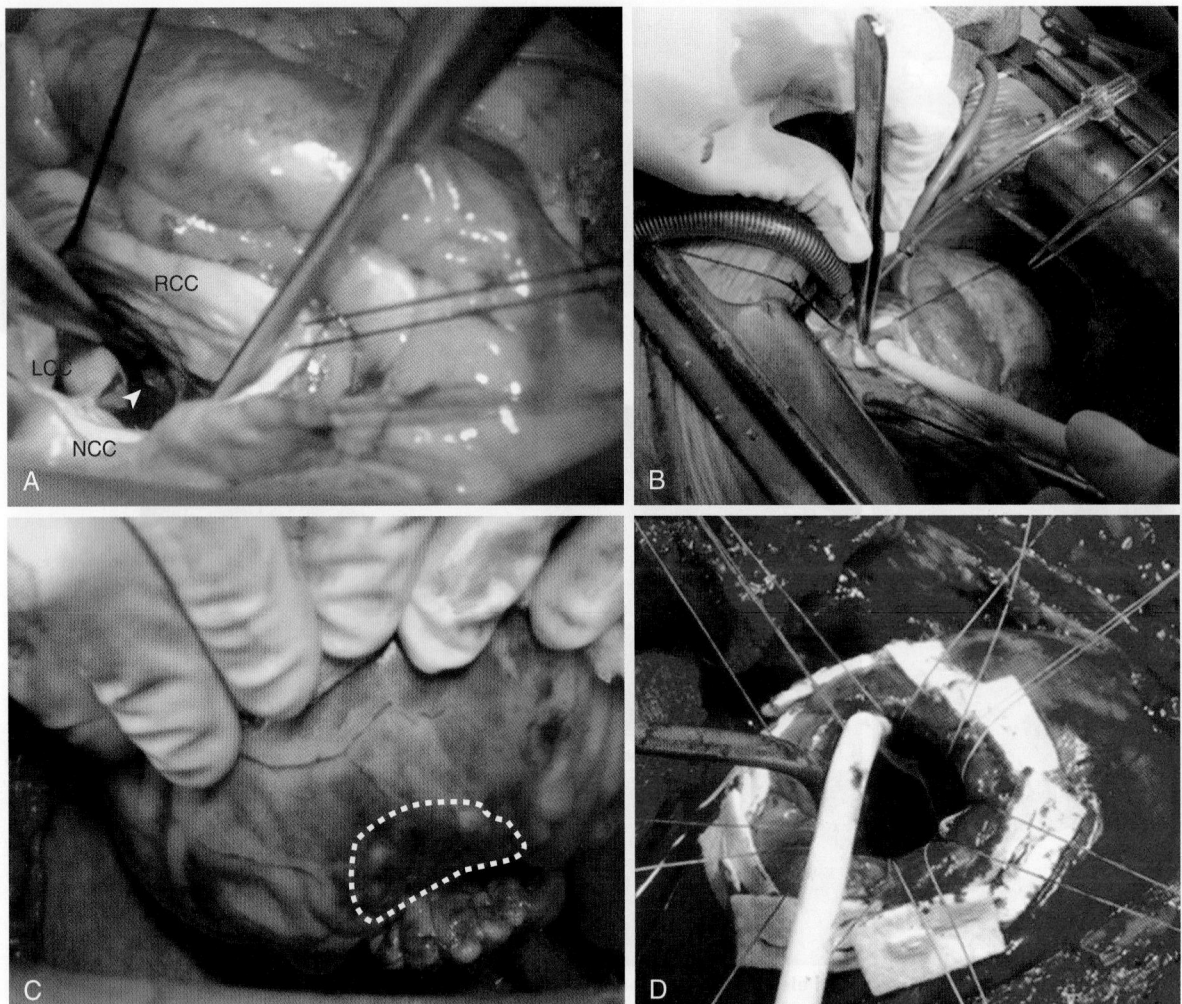

FIGURE 134.5 Our approach to surgical ventricular tachycardia ablation by cryothermy. (A) Example in which radiofrequency lesions delivered during percutaneous mapping and ablation in the cardiac electrophysiology laboratory on the posterolateral left ventricular (LV) endocardial surface were identifiable at the time of surgical ablation (7 days later; *arrowhead*). (B and C) This location is targeted by cryothermy (transaortic deployment of cryoprobe tip). The induration created by cryothermal application (3-minute lesion) at this endocardial location was easily palpable on the corresponding epicardial surface (C, *dotted enclosed area*). (D) Deployment of cryoprobe through the cored-out LV apex for placing an LV assist device. *LCC,* Left coronary cusp; *NCC,* noncoronary cusp; *RCC,* right coronary cusp.

VT is more focal, the probe can be coiled to create large circular lesions (see Fig. 134.6). For targeting VT circuits and sources endocardially, the probe can be deployed at the ablation site without modifying the tip (see Fig. 134.5). Because the entire length of the probe cools during energy application, care has to be taken to avoid making contact of the proximal end of the probe with critical cardiac structures (e.g., valve leaflets, conduction system), which can sometimes be frozen inadvertently. This is particularly important when the probe is deployed across the aortic or MVs (see Fig. 134.5).

Conventional RF energy has been infrequently used to create lesions during surgical VT ablation. Typically, RF ablation requires a generator, delivery platform, and impedance pads. These may be cumbersome to deploy in the OR setting. Furthermore, creating lesions using resistive heating may not be as effective in cooled hearts. In the recent literature, there are only limited case series describing successful targeting of VT originating from the posteromedial papillary muscle in two patients with healed infarcts and in five patients acutely after left VAD

placement. In both these series, monopolar RF energy was used through a cool-tip ablation catheter platform.[16,20] Laser energy (Nd-YAG, pulsed argon) has also been used for surgical VT ablation in patients with healed infarcts.[30,31] In a single-center experience that used pulsed argon laser energy source, this technique was found to be helpful in targeting VT originating from all LV locations, with excellent long-term arrhythmia-free survival (90% freedom from VT or death at 1 year).[31] However, it remains unclear why this technology is no longer used for surgical VT ablation. Microwave has also been infrequently used to create cardiac lesions.[32] This technology has been utilized for isolating pulmonary veins and creating linear lesions in patients undergoing surgical atrial fibrillation (AF) ablation. A case report has also described the efficacy of this technology during surgical VT ablation.[33]

Although cryothermy seems to be the most popular energy source in patients undergoing surgical ablation of ventricular arrhythmias, no studies have yet compared the efficacy of this source with other ablation platforms in this patient population.

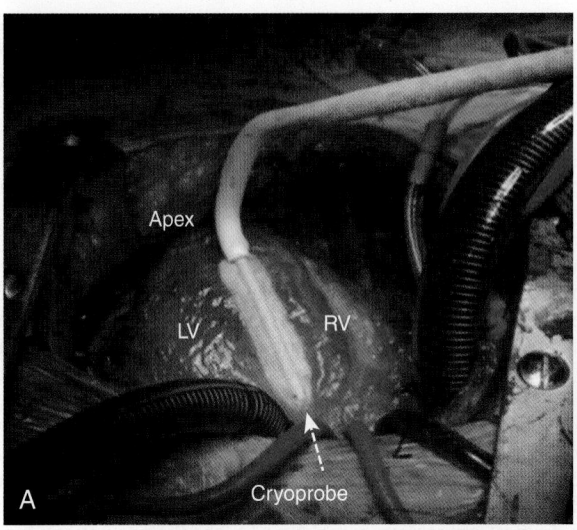
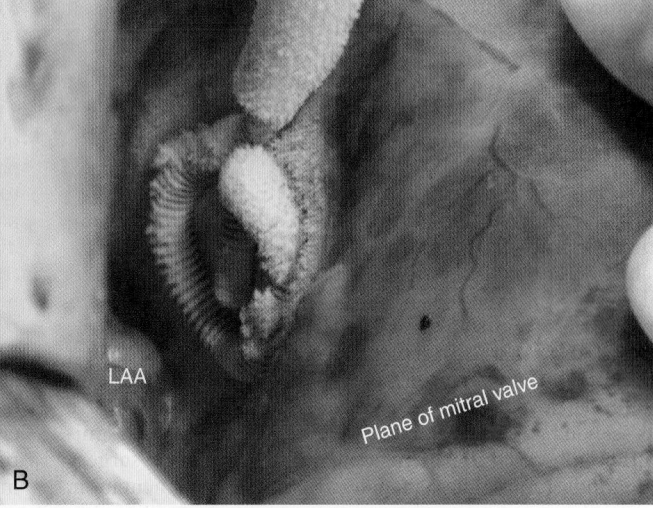

FIGURE 134.6 Two examples of cryothermy application using the Surgifrost Surgical Cryoablation System (Medtronic CryoCath LP, Quebec, Canada). (A) The entire length of the probe (*dotted arrow*) is positioned over the anterior interventricular septum to create a linear lesion. (B) The probe has been coiled to create a circular lesion over the posterolateral left ventricular surface. During cryothermy application, the entire length of the probe, including the insulation sheath, becomes excessively cold, and care has to be taken to avoid contact of the latter with critical cardiac structures. *LAA,* Left atrial appendage; *LV,* left ventricle; *RV,* right ventricle.

On the basis of the surgical VT ablation experience at our center, cryothermy is certainly capable of creating effective lesions.[10,11] However, to create large lesions, the probe needs to be cooled to a temperature of –150° C. This is best achieved in cold and immobile hearts. Thus cold cardioplegia is essential for effective cryothermy in patients undergoing surgical ablation of ventricular arrhythmias.

End Points of Surgical Ablation

The acute end points of surgical VT ablation are determined to a large extent by the mapping strategy used. In cases where the arrhythmia is sustained and mapped during surgical ablation, VT termination and noninducibility should be the end point(s) for procedural success. However, as pointed out earlier, this usually requires a beating heart setup or euthermic cardiac temperatures. In situations where cryothermy is used to create lesions under cold cardioplegia, VT may be impossible to induce or maintain. In these instances, after the lesion set has been completed, the heart is allowed to rewarm; and VT induction can then be attempted by programmed electrical stimulation (PES). In patients with ICDs, PES can be performed in the OR through a device. In subjects without ICDs, this can be accomplished by temporarily suturing an electrode to the cardiac surface. However, PES in the OR can be challenging for several reasons: (1) In patients undergoing additional cardiac procedures (valve, bypass, or VAD placement surgery), this may not be possible to do immediately after the VT ablation; (2) in situations where there is acute decompensation during the surgical procedure, VT induction may not be clinically advisable; (3) other variables (e.g., anesthetic agents, autonomic tone, cardiac filling) can effect arrhythmia induction; (4) lack of a standard 12-lead ECG recording may make it difficult to compare arrhythmia induced in the OR with the clinical arrhythmia; and (5) arrhythmias induced in the OR may be nonspecific. An alternative method to assess ablation efficacy may be to evaluate physical properties of the targeted tissue. As previously discussed, lesions created in the OR by cryothermy are transmural and cause marked induration, which is palpable from both the endocardial and epicardial surfaces (see Fig. 134.5). Effective lesions may also result in alteration in the electrical properties of

the tissue. Thus inability to capture the ablated site at high pacing outputs can serve as an end point for effective lesion creation. In some situations in which lesions are delivered across reentrant channels, one can test the presence of postablation conduction block across the targeted channel.[26] Although whenever possible, arrhythmia induction in the OR should be attempted, we have also found PES beyond the acute phase to be useful for predicting long-term success. We have been able to accomplish PES prior to discharge in at least 50% of surgical VT ablation population.[10,11] We advocate this end point because in a prior study, patients who underwent VT ablation at our center, following acute procedural success (inability to induce VT at the end of the procedure), additional lack of VT induction 48–72 hours after the ablation (by noninvasive programmed stimulation through the ICD) was a strong predictor of long-term VT-free survival.[34]

Postprocedure Arrhythmia Management

Although surgical ablation is successful for treating refractory clinical VT, patients may experience other arrhythmias (e.g., AF, premature ventricular complexes, nonsustained VT) early after the procedure.[35] Thus it is a common practice to maintain these patients on AAD therapy immediately after surgery. In our most recent surgical VT ablation series (21 patients), only one patient who had idiopathic VT originating from the superior basal IVS region was discharged without AADs after successful ablation. The remaining subjects were all prescribed at least one AAD initially, which were subsequently tapered and discontinued in the majority.[10,11] Attempts should be made to modify AAD regimen acutely after the procedure, either by changing patients who are on multiple agents to a single drug or reducing the dose if the patients are only taking one AAD. For patients who have been on extended amiodarone therapy, our practice after successful surgical VT ablation is to switch to another AAD. In patients who have sustained refractory ventricular arrhythmias (not the original clinical VT) early after the surgical ablation, consideration should be given to catheter mapping and ablation. In some instances after surgical ablation, a different VT (previously not seen) can become manifest and this may be amenable to conventional percutaneous ablation.[11] In our experience, early after the surgical

VT ablation (≤1 month), the pericardial space is accessible, and so if indicated, percutaneous epicardial mapping and ablation remain feasible. However, beyond this period, pericardial adhesions may form and then epicardial access can be challenging.

Complications

Surgical VT ablation is a highly invasive procedure. Furthermore, it is usually performed on subjects who are experiencing VT that is refractory to multiple AADs and percutaneous catheter ablation attempts. Frequently, these patients require additional cardiac interventions (e.g., valve replacement or repair, coronary artery bypass grafting, VAD placement) at the time of surgical ablation. These patients also have concomitant heart failure. For all of these reasons, procedure-related complications are common in this group of patients. The majority of adverse events seen in patients undergoing surgical VT ablation are similar to those observed in patients undergoing open-heart surgery for other indications. These include infection, altered mentation, worsening heart failure, prolonged inotropic support, persistent hypoxemia, and arrhythmias.[35] Complications that are specific to the surgical ablation itself are few and are discussed next.

Ventricular Arrhythmias

As previously discussed, surgical VT ablation can sometimes be proarrhythmic and, in rare instances, patients may have worsening ventricular arrhythmias immediately after.[10,11,36] If these are nonsustained and do not cause hemodynamic compromise, then a combination of AADs is sufficient to control them. However, if these arrhythmias become sustained, then patients may need extracorporeal membrane oxygenation support or VAD to maintain end-organ perfusion. In these instances, consideration should also be given to percutaneous catheter ablation and/or additional ablation attempts in the OR.[16] For sustained ventricular arrhythmias that remain refractory to all of these interventions, cardiac transplantation may be the only remaining option. Patients with acute sustained ventricular arrhythmias after surgical VT ablation have the worst prognosis, and early mortality in this group can be as high as approximately 50%.[2,5,10,11]

Worsening Heart Failure

Worsening heart failure is not uncommon after surgical VT ablation for several reasons: a majority of patients undergoing the procedure have baseline LV dysfunction, surgical ablation lesions can worsen LV function, myocardial contractility may be suppressed after cold cardioplegia, etc. In this context, limiting the number of lesions is important to minimize ablation-related worsening of LV function. This is best achieved by targeting critical components of the VT circuit identified by mapping either in the OR or a priori in the EP laboratory. The latter is an effective strategy in patients with nonischemic cardiomyopathy in whom the scar is patchy and not easily identifiable visually during open-heart surgery.[10,11,13,37] The acute mortality in our recent surgical VT ablation experience was 9.5%.[11] Two patients died during the index hospitalization (at 6 and 10 weeks after the surgical ablation): one from progressive heart failure and the other from sepsis. In the remaining 19 patients, the median time from surgery to discharge was 9 days (mean: 21 ± 31 days).[11]

Long-Term Expectations

The most extensive long-term outcome experience of surgical VT ablation is in patients who underwent the procedure 20–30 years earlier for refractory VT in the setting of healed myocardial infarcts.[2,3,7,38,39] The ablation strategy in the majority of these cases comprised aneurysmectomy and subendocardial resection.

More recently, we have used surgical ablation to successfully treat refractory VT in patients with nonischemic cardiomyopathy.[10,11] Although this is a relatively small group of patients, the average postprocedure follow-up duration is sufficiently long (43 ± 31 months; longest patient followed for 7 years). In our series, overall survival was 62% (13 patients were alive). Of the eight patients who died, four died from pump failure, one from refractory VT, two from malignancy, and one from septic shock. One patient who underwent primary surgical ablation during VAD implantation for end-stage cardiomyopathy and VT storm was transplanted after 35 months because of worsening heart failure without VT recurrence. Of the 12 living nontransplanted patients, 6 experienced recurrent VT with 4 becoming VT free on AAD alone, 1 with sympathectomy, and 1 with redo catheter ablation. Overall, a significant reduction was found in VT events, from 6 ± 6 events per patient in the 3 months prior to surgical cryoablation to 1 ± 2.3 events per patient for the remaining duration of the follow-up. Similarly, a significant reduction was found in ICD shocks, from 6.2 ± 4.9 per patient in the 3 months preceding surgical cryoablation to 1.8 ± 2.5 shocks per patient for the remaining follow-up duration following surgical cryoablation ($p < .001$). In another series, the 1-year survival after surgical VT ablation was 80%. However, over a 5-year period, a steady decline in survival led to the death of 25% of subjects at the fifth year.[39] Although these survival data are sobering, they are similar to the 5-year survival data in patients with impaired LV function and heart failure who have undergone open-heart surgery for other indications. Thus surgical VT ablation can improve long-term mortality in an otherwise sick group of patients who may not have survived acutely without this intervention.[7,39]

Future Developments

Despite the overall success of surgical ablation in treating refractory ventricular arrhythmias, the procedure can be challenging. A major limitation of surgical VT ablation remains the inability to induce and map clinical arrhythmias during the procedure. Thus any development that can facilitate ventricular arrhythmia mapping in the OR is highly desirable. A hybrid OR capable of supporting percutaneous interventions and open-heart surgical procedures may help accomplish this. In such a setup, it is conceivable to induce and map the arrhythmia using the same tools as in the EP laboratory (intracardiac multipolar electrode recordings and EAM), albeit with an open heart.[36] Using this approach, the critical parts of the VT circuit and/or site of origin may be better identified. We have been able to accomplish this approach in a few cases at our center (see Fig. 134.4). Development of energy sources and platforms that can create effective lesions without the need for cold cardioplegia is also highly desirable, because that may allow ablation during ongoing arrhythmia and so may provide a more rigorous and easily reproducible end point of arrhythmia termination during lesion creation and/or inability to induce the targeted arrhythmia afterward. Furthermore, this approach may also reduce the complications that are typically associated with "on-pump" open-heart surgery. Another improvement in the surgical ablation technique would be the ability to map and ablate ventricular arrhythmias using a less invasive approach (without median sternotomy). This has been accomplished for AF ablation, which can now be performed by minimally invasive surgery. However, the challenge during ablation of refractory VA remains the need to target areas of the heart that typically require full sternotomy for best visualization. However, certain areas of the heart (inferior IVS regions, anterior LV wall, RV) can be accessed by partial sternotomy. Additional innovations that can allow us to map and successfully ablate VA arising from other cardiac locations using minimally invasive surgical techniques are also desirable because they may help reduce procedure-related morbidity.

Conclusions

Surgical ablation is used to treat ventricular arrhythmias that remain refractory to drugs and percutaneous catheter ablation attempts. The reason for failure of conventional catheter ablation in these instances is because the arrhythmia source or circuits are intramural and cannot be targeted by catheter-based RF energy. In the OR, this is overcome by creating much larger lesions (~60 mm) via median sternotomy under cold cardioplegia using cryothermy. Although this approach is successful for treating refractory ventricular arrhythmias in patients with both ischemic and nonischemic cardiomyopathies, it is highly invasive. A major challenge during surgical ablation is the ability to reproducibly induce and map the clinical arrhythmia. To overcome this, patients can undergo detailed percutaneous arrhythmia mapping a priori in the EP laboratory, during which critical components of the VT circuit and sites of origin can be targeted by RF ablation. These RF lesions, although ineffective, can serve as targets for precise cryoenergy application during the surgical ablation without the need for additional mapping in the OR. Future improvements in the surgical ablation of ventricular arrhythmias include the ability to map the clinical arrhythmia in the OR and to target it effectively using a less invasive approach. Until this is accomplished, surgical ablation will remain the treatment of last resort in the management of ventricular arrhythmias.

REFERENCES

1. Chen WY, Lai ST, Shih CC. Endoaneurysmorrhaphy and cryoablation for post infarction left ventricular aneurysm with ventricular tachycardia. *J Chin Med Assoc.* 2007;70:117–120.
2. Sami M, Chaitman BR, Bourassa MG, et al. Long term follow-up of aneurysmectomy for recurrent ventricular tachycardia or fibrillation. *Am Heart J.* 1978;96:3030–3038.
3. Josephson ME, Harken AH, Horowitz LN. Endocardial excision: a new surgical technique for the treatment of recurrent ventricular tachycardia. *Circulation.* 1979;60:1430–1439.
4. Horowitz LN, Harken AH, Kastor JA, et al. Ventricular resection guided by epicardial and endocardial mapping for treatment of recurrent ventricular tachycardia. *N Engl J Med.* 1980;302:589–593.
5. Wellens F, Geelen P, Demirsoy E, et al. Surgical treatment of tachyarrhythmias due to post infarction left ventricular endoaneurysmorrhaphy and cryoablation. *Eur J Cardiothorac Surg.* 2002;22:771–776.
6. Haines DE, Lerman BB, Kron IL, et al. Surgical ablation of ventricular tachycardia with sequential map-guided subendocardial resection: electrophysiologic assessment and long-term follow-up. *Circulation.* 1988;77:131–141.
7. Matthias Bechtel JF, Tolg R, Graf B, et al. High incidence of sudden death late after anterior aneurysm repair. *Eur J Cardiothorac Surg.* 2004;25:807–811.
8. Aliot EM, Stevenson WG, Almendral-Garrote JM, et al. EHRA/HRS Expert Consensus on Catheter Ablation of Ventricular Arrhythmias: developed in a partnership with the European Heart Rhythm Association (EHRA), a Registered Branch of the European Society of Cardiology (ESC), and the Heart Rhythm Society (HRS); in collaboration with the American College of Cardiology (ACC) and the American Heart Association (AHA). *Heart Rhythm.* 2009;6:886–933.
9. Zipes DP, Camm AJ, Borggrefe M, et al. ACC/AHA/ESC 2006 Guidelines for management of patients with ventricular arrhythmias and the prevention of sudden cardiac death: a report of the American College of Cardiology/American Heart Association Task Force and the European Society of Cardiology Committee for Practice Guidelines (writing committee to develop Guidelines for Management of Patients With Ventricular Arrhythmias and the Prevention of Sudden Cardiac Death): developed in collaboration with the European Heart Rhythm Association and the Heart Rhythm Society. *Circulation.* 2006;114:e385–e484.
10. Anter E, Hutchinson MD, Deo R, et al. Surgical ablation of refractory ventricular tachycardia in patients with non-ischemic cardiomyopathy. *Circ Arrhythm Electrophysiol.* 2011;4:494–500.
11. Betensky B, Zado E, Anter E, et al. Surgical ablation of refractory ventricular tachycardia in patients with non-ischemic cardiomyopathy: ablation strategies and long term outcomes. *Heart Rhythm.* 2015;12:S-28.
12. Bhavani SS, Tchou P, Chung M, et al. Intra-operative electro-anatomical mapping and beating heart ablation of ventricular tachycardia. *Ann Thorac Surg.* 2006;82:1091–1093.
13. Bajan V, Gerstenfeld E, Garcia F, et al. Site specific twelve lead ECG features to identify an epicardial origin for left ventricular tachycardia in the absence of myocardial infarction. *Heart Rhythm.* 2007;4:1403–1410.
14. Haqqani HM, Tschabrunn CM, Tzou WS, et al. Isolated septal substrate for ventricular tachycardia in nonischemic dilated cardiomyopathy: incidence, characterization and implications. *Heart Rhythm.* 2011;8:1169–1176.
15. Zado ES, Santangeli P, Supple G, et al. Surgical cryoablation at the time of LVAD implantation. *Circulation.* 2015;132:A16647.
16. Patel M, Rojas F, Shabari FR, et al. Safety and feasibility of open chest epicardial mapping and ablation of ventricular tachycardia during the period of left ventricular assist device placement. *J Cardiovasc Electrophysiol.* 2016;27:95–101.
17. Mill MR, Wilcox BR, Anderson RH. Surgical anatomy of the heart. In: Cohn LH, ed. *Cardiac Surgery in the Adult.* New York: McGraw-Hill; 2008:29–50.
18. Mihaljevic T, Sayeed MR, Stamou SC, et al. Pathophysiology of aortic valve disease. In: Cohn LH, ed. *Cardiac Surgery in the Adult.* New York: McGraw-Hill; 2008:825–840.
19. Fann JI, Ingels Jr NB, Miller DC. Pathophysiology of mitral valve disease. In: Cohn LH, ed. *Cardiac Surgery in the Adult.* New York: McGraw-Hill; 2008:973–1012.
20. Rubino AS, Onorati F, Serraino GF, et al. Transmitral approach to monopolar radiofrequency ablation of inferior papillary muscle for refractory ischemic ventricular tachycardia. *Tex Heart Inst J.* 2010;37:371–372.
21. Bhawani SS, Tchou P, Saliba W, et al. Surgical options for refractory ventricular tachycardia. *J Card Surg.* 2007;22:533–534.
22. Hammon JW. Extracorporeal circulation: organ damage. In: Cohn LH, ed. *Cardiac Surgery in the Adult.* New York: McGraw-Hill; 2008:389–414.
23. Chitwood WRJ, Rodriguez E. Minimally invasive and robotic mitral valve surgery. In: Cohn LH, ed. *Cardiac Surgery in the Adult.* New York: McGraw-Hill; 2008:1079–1100.
24. Kumar S, Barbhaiya C, Sobieszczyk P, et al. Role of alternative interventional procedures when endo and epicardial catheter ablation attempts for ventricular arrhythmias fail. *Circ Arrhythm Electrophysiol.* 2015;8:606–615.
25. Michowitz Y, Mathuria N, Tung R, et al. Hybrid procedures for epicardial catheter ablation of ventricular tachycardia: value of surgical access. *Heart Rhythm.* 2010;7:1635–1643.
26. Mavroudis C, Deal BJ, Backer CL, et al. Arrhythmia surgery in patients with and without congenital heart disease. *Ann Thorac Surg.* 2008;86:857–868.
27. Van Dessel PF, Van Hemel NM, Van Swieten HA, et al. Successful surgical ablation of sustained ventricular tachycardia associated with mitral valve prolapse guided by a multielectrode basket catheter. *PACE.* 2001;24:1029–1031.
28. Dixit S, Callans DJ. Role of contact and non-contact mapping systems in the treatment of cardiac arrhythmias. *Curr Opin Cardiol.* 2002;17:65–72.
29. Krul SP, Driessen AH, van Bowen WJ, et al. Thoracoscopic video assisted pulmonary vein antrum isolation, ganglionated plexus ablation, and periprocedural confirmation of ablation lesions. First results of hybrid surgical-electrophysiological approach for atrial fibrillation. *Circ Arrhythm Electrophysiol.* 2011;4:262–270.
30. Mesnildrey P, Laborde F, Bruneval P, et al. Therapeutic and prophylactic surgical treatment of ventricular tachycardia by Nd-YAG laser irradiation. In: Fontaine G, Schienman MM, eds. *Ablation in Cardiac Arrhythmias.* Mount Kisco, NY: Futura Publishing; 1987:441–448.
31. Saksena S, Gielchinsky I, Tullo NG. Argon laser ablation of malignant ventricular tachycardia associated with coronary artery disease. *Am J Cardiol.* 1989;64:1298–1304.
32. Thomas SP, Clout R, Deery C, et al. Microwave ablation of myocardial tissue: the effect of element design, tissue coupling, blood flow, power and duration of exposure on lesion size. *J Cardiovasc Electrophysiol.* 1999;10:72–78.
33. Braun MU, Knaut M, Rauwolf T, et al. Microwave ablation of an ischemic sustained ventricular tachycardia during aortocoronary bypass, mitral valve and tricuspid valve surgery guided by a three-dimensional nonfluoroscopic mapping system (CARTO). *J Interv Cardiac Electrophysiol.* 2005;13:243–247.
34. Frankel DS, Mountantonakis SE, Zado ES, et al. Non-invasive programmed ventricular stimulation early after ventricular tachycardia ablation to predict risk of late recurrence. *J Am Coll Cardiol.* 2012;59:1529–1535.
35. Khalpey ZI, Ganim R Bi, Rawn J Di. Postoperative care of cardiac surgery patients. In: Cohn LH, ed. *Cardiac Surgery in the Adult.* New York: McGraw-Hill; 2008:465–486.
36. Eckart RE, Epstein L Mi. Interventional therapy for atrial and ventricular arrhythmias. In: Cohn LH, ed. *Cardiac Surgery in the Adult.* New York: McGraw-Hill; 2008:1357–1374.
37. Hutchinson MD, Gerstenfeld EP, Desjardins B, et al. Endocardial unipolar voltage mapping to detect epicardial ventricular tachycardia substrate in patients with nonischemic left ventricular cardiomyopathy. *Circ Arrhythm Electrophysiol.* 2011;4:49–55.
38. Lindblom D, Albage A, Sartipy U. Surgery for ventricular tachycardia in patients undergoing surgical ventricular restoration. *Multimed Man Cardiothorac Surg.* 2007:1–5.
39. Pirk J, Bytesnik J, Kautzner J, et al. Surgical ablation of ventricular tachycardia guided by mapping in sinus rhythm: long term results. *Eur J Cardiothorac Surg.* 2004;26:323–329.

135 Vagus Nerve Stimulation for the Treatment of Heart Failure

Hani N. Sabbah

Autonomic abnormalities evidenced by sustained sympathetic overdrive and parasympathetic withdrawal are characteristic features of the heart failure (HF) state[1] and have long been recognized as a cause of increased mortality and morbidity in patients with HF.[2,3] In HF, sympathovagal imbalance leads to increased heart rate, excess release of proinflammatory cytokines, dysregulation of nitric oxide (NO) pathways, and arrhythmogenesis, all of which are adverse features that directly or indirectly contribute to worsening HF and death. The increase in heart rate in patients with HF, for instance, is a recognized predictor of mortality and morbidity,[4] while the sustained increase in sympathetic activity contributes to progressive left ventricular (LV) dysfunction and LV remodeling.[5] Pharmacological interventions that reduce heart rate and/or limit sympathetic drive in patients with HF, such as β-blockers and more recently, ivabradine, a specific and selective inhibitor of the cardiac pacemaker current I*f*, have been shown to improve survival, reduce hospitalization, and attenuate progressive LV remodeling.[6,7]

Since the 1990s, emphasis was placed on treating chronic HF (CHF) through suppression of neurohumoral activation, an approach that gave rise to effective drugs such as angiotensin-converting enzyme inhibitors, β-adrenergic receptor blockers, and aldosterone antagonists. More recently, renewed interest has emerged in modulating parasympathetic activity as a therapeutic target for treating CHF. Recognizing that an alteration in the cardiac vagal efferent activity through peripheral cardiac nerve stimulation decreased heart rate and improved ventricular contractile function provided added support to this approach,[8] as did a wealth of other investigations that uncovered the potential merits of electrical cervical vagus nerve stimulation (VNS) in preventing sudden cardiac death (SCD) and improving long-term survival.[9,10]

Effects of Vagus Nerve Stimulation on Left Ventricular Function and Chamber Remodeling in Experimental Heart Failure

While the theoretical and experimental foundations of VNS as a potential therapy for HF existed for decades, only recently have advances in technology and instrumentation allowed for the development of implantable devices that can test the full range of safety and efficacy of this therapeutic approach in animal models of HF.[11,12] One such device is the CardioFit VNS system (BioControl Medical Ltd., Yehud, Israel) (Fig. 135.1). The CardioFit VNS system delivers electrical stimulation via a lead placed surgically around the right cervical vagus nerve and attached to an implantable pulse generator.[11] A second lead is placed in the right ventricle for electrocardiogram (ECG) sensing and heart rate detection. Heart rate detection is used to silence the VNS when heart rate decreases below a preset level so as to avoid the adverse effects of bradycardia. The stimulation lead is a modified bipolar cuff electrode designed to activate vagus cardioinhibitory B fibers while maintaining a large degree of unidirectionality with respect to low-threshold A fibers recruited in the 1–2 mA range.

In dogs with coronary microembolization–induced HF (LV ejection fraction of ~35%), long-term (3 months) VNS monotherapy was shown to significantly improve LV ejection fraction, significantly reduce LV end-systolic and end-diastolic volumes, and significantly increase stroke volume compared with untreated controls (Fig. 135.2).[11,13] The improvement in LV systolic function and prevention of progressive LV dilation were associated with a significant reduction in plasma levels of N-terminal pro-brain natriuretic peptide (nt-pro BNP) compared with controls (see Fig. 135.2). Furthermore, ambulatory ECG Holter monitoring showed reductions in minimum, average, and maximum heart rate by 1, 10, and 28 beats/min, respectively, in VNS-treated dogs compared with changes in heart rate by only 2, 1, and 0.5 beats/min, respectively, in control dogs.[11,13] Long-term VNS in dogs with HF also elicited improvements in indices of LV diastolic function, as evidenced by a decrease in LV end-diastolic pressure, increased deceleration time of rapid mitral inflow velocity, reduced LV end-diastolic circumferential wall stress, and increased peak mitral inflow velocity ratio (PE/PA; see Fig. 135.2).[11,13] Because both heart rate and LV wall stress decrease and because both are

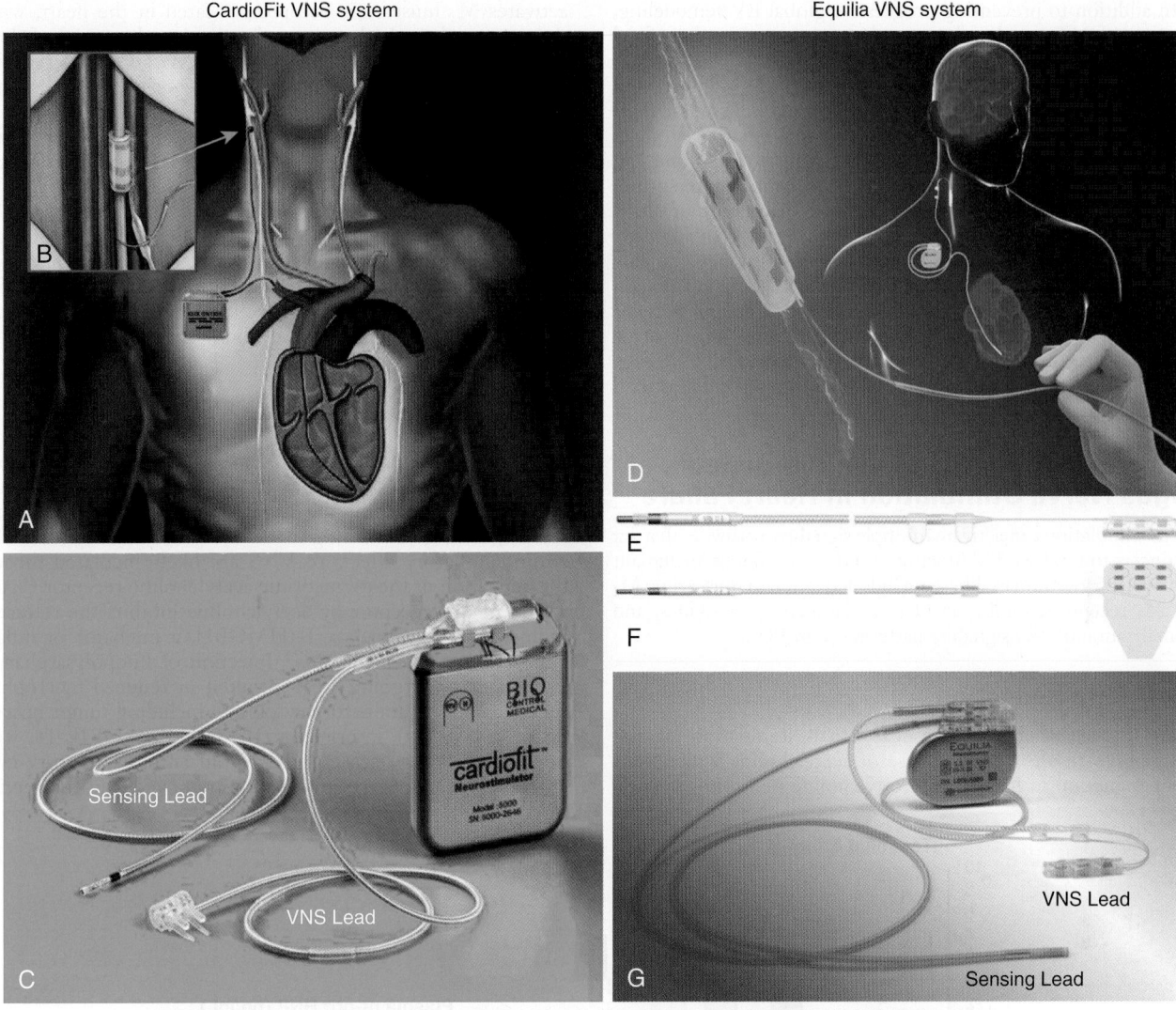

FIGURE 135.1 (A) Depiction of an implanted CardioFit vagus nerve stimulation (*VNS*) device showing the position of VNS lead on the right vagus nerve, (B) inset showing positioning of the CardioFit stimulation lead around the right vagus nerve, and (C) a photograph of the CardioFit VNS implantable neurostimulator, sensing lead, and VNS lead. (D) Depiction of an implanted Equilia EquiCurl VNS device showing the position of VNS lead on the right vagus nerve, depicting in the foreground the retracted EquiCurl stimulation electrode; (E) shows a diagram of the retracted electrode; (F) a diagram of the unfolded electrode; and (G) a photograph of the entire Equilia VNS system, including the implantable neurostimulator, sensing lead, and VNS lead. ([A–C] Modified from Sabbah HN. Electrical vagus nerve stimulation for the treatment of chronic heart failure. *Cleve Clin J Med.* 2011;78;S24-S29. [D–F] Courtesy LivaNova, Houston, TX.)

primary determinants of myocardial oxygen consumption (MVO_2), it is reasonable to conclude that VNS can improve LV function without increasing MVO_2, the latter a desirable feature of therapies that target the HF state. Because VNS and β-blockade both reduce heart rate, VNS stimulation in dogs with HF was also examined using a background therapy with β-blockade.[14] In HF dogs receiving background therapy with metoprolol succinate, the addition of VNS increased LV ejection fraction and decreased LV end-systolic volume compared with dogs treated with metoprolol alone.[14] In these canine studies, a current amplitude of 4–6 mA was used for stimulation and was delivered for approximately 30% of the time.

VNS as a therapy for CHF was also examined in dogs with HF produced by high-rate ventricular pacing using the Cyberonics VNS system (Cyberonics Inc., Houston, TX).[12] Dogs were randomized to control (n = 7) or monotherapy with VNS (n = 8) and followed up for 8 weeks, with measurements made at ~15 minutes after temporarily turning off the ventricular pacemaker.

In these studies, VNS also resulted in significant reductions in LV end-diastolic and end-systolic volumes and an increase in LV ejection fraction compared with controls.[12] The improvement was accompanied by reduced plasma levels of norepinephrine, angiotensin II, and C-reactive protein and increased baroreflex sensitivity. Because rapid pacing was maintained throughout the study, except for short periods of time when measurements were made, one can argue that the benefits of VNS therapy, in this model of HF, were independent of heart rate.[12] Several studies on dogs with microembolization-induced HF, in which VNS was delivered for a long term at stimulation levels that did not acutely decrease heart rate, also showed significant improvements in LV ejection fraction along with reduction in LV size.[15] These studies also showed that improvement in LV function with VNS was also associated with increased protein expression of SERCA-2a and reduced expression of the proapoptotic protein caspase-3 in LV myocardium.[16]

In addition to preventing progressive global LV remodeling, long-term VNS was also shown to have an important beneficial impact on LV structural remodeling at the cellular level. In dogs with coronary microembolization–induced HF, VNS decreased the volume fraction of replacement fibrosis and the volume fraction of interstitial fibrosis.[17] The finding suggests that VNS in HF can limit ongoing loss of functional cardiac units and can limit the accumulation of collagen in the cardiac interstitium and hence the expansion of the extracellular space, both of which favor improved LV systolic and diastolic function.[17] In addition, VNS was shown to decrease oxygen diffusion distance and cardiomyocyte hypertrophy.[17] These alterations at the structural–cellular level can help minimize the adverse effects of hypoxia and the burden of pathological hypertrophy on the failing myocardium. Amelioration of these structural measures by VNS suggests that this form of therapy can also help preserve myocardial structural integrity.

Mechanisms That Underlie the Benefits of Vagus Nerve Stimulation in Heart Failure

Vagus stimulation can activate multiple signaling pathways that act in concert to improve LV function in HF and suppress malignant ventricular arrhythmias. These include activation of muscarinic M_2 and M_3 receptors, inhibition of proinflammatory cytokines, and normalization of NO signaling pathways (Fig. 135.3).

Heart Rate Reduction

There is overwhelming consensus that stimulation of the vagus nerve results in the release of acetylcholine with subsequent reduction in heart rate. Acetylcholine neurotransmission activates M_2 muscarinic receptors located in the heart, where they act to slow the heart rate by slowing the speed of depolarization. M_2 muscarinic receptors act via a Gi-type receptor, which also causes a decrease in cyclic adenosine monophosphate (cAMP) in the cell and inhibits voltage-gated Ca^{2+} channels. In the setting of HF, the reduction in heart rate, elicited by activation of M_2 receptors, mediates an improvement in LV function by reducing cardiac workload through a reduction in MVO_2. The latter restores a better physiological balance between the energy demand and energy supply within the failing myocardium. Therapeutic modalities that reduce heart rate have been shown to improve LV ejection fraction in HF.[4–6,18] Therefore heart rate reduction elicited by VNS or other neuromodulation therapies is likely a major contributor to the benefits derived from this form of therapy.

Proinflammatory Cytokines

Cytokine production by the immune system contributes importantly to both health and disease. The nervous system, via an inflammatory reflex of the vagus nerve, can inhibit cytokine release, thereby preventing tissue injury and cell death.[19,20] The antiinflammatory effects of VNS are likely mediated through the activation of the α7 nicotinic acetylcholine receptor.[21] Activation of this receptor by acetylcholine inhibits the release of high-mobility group box 1 (HMGB1), a mediator of inflammation, from macrophages.[21] Injection of lipopolysaccharides in animals undergoing VNS resulted in reduced macrophage release of proinflammatory cytokines, including tumor necrosis factor-α (TNF-α), interleukin (IL)-6 (IL-6), and IL-18, without affecting the release of IL-10, an antiinflammatory cytokine.[22,23] Vagus nerve transection removed this protection.

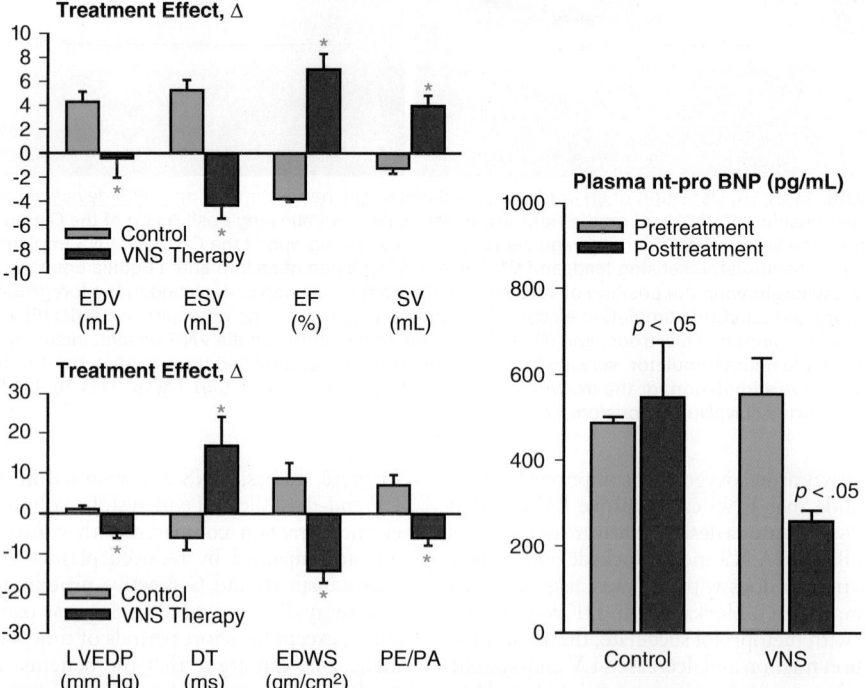

FIGURE 135.2 *Top left,* Change Δ (treatment effect) between pre- and posttreatment of left ventricular (*LV*) end-diastolic volume (*EDV*), end-systolic volume (*ESV*), ejection fraction (*EF*), and stroke volume (*SV*) in untreated control dogs (*blue bars*) and dogs treated for 3 months with vagus nerve stimulation (*VNS*). *, $p < .05$ vs. control. *Bottom left,* Treatment effect, Δ, LV end-diastolic pressure (*EDP*), deceleration time (*DT*), end-diastolic wall stress (*EDWS*), and peak mitral valve inflow velocity ratio (*PE/PA*) in control dogs (*blue bars*) and dogs treated for 3 months with VNS. *, $p < .05$ vs. control. *Right,* Plasma levels of N-terminal pro-brain natriuretic peptide (*nt-pro BNP*) measured before initiating therapy (pretreatment) and 3 months after initiating therapy (posttreatment) in untreated control dogs and dogs treated for 3 months with VNS.

In human macrophage cell cultures, acetylcholine inhibited TNF-α when the cultures were exposed to lipopolysaccharide.[23] Proinflammatory cytokines are significantly elevated in HF and are associated with increased mortality and morbidity. In dogs with microembolization-induced HF, LV tissue levels of TNF-α and IL-6 are elevated compared with LV tissue from normal dogs (Fig. 135.4). Long-term monotherapy with VNS in dogs with HF was shown to significantly reduce plasma circulating levels as well as LV tissue protein levels of TNF-α and IL-6[13,16] (see Fig. 135.4).

Nitric Oxide Signaling

NO is formed by a family of NO synthases (NOS) and is involved in parasympathetic regulation of myocardial contractility. In normal dogs, Hare et al.[24] showed that the inotropic response to dobutamine on cardiac contractility could be attenuated by VNS and that infusion of the NOS inhibitor L-NMMA reduced the impact of vagus nerve inhibition, while infusion of the NOS substrate arginine had the opposite effect. The three isoforms of NOS identified to date are endothelin NOS (eNOS), inducible NOS (iNOS), and neuronal NOS (nNOS). NO produced by eNOS plays an important role in the regulation of cell growth and apoptosis and can enhance myocardial relaxation and regulate contractility.[25,26] Normal levels of eNOS are also important in maintaining normal mitochondrial biogenesis,[27] a process essential for physiological turnover of these energy-producing organelles. In dogs with coronary microembolization–induced HF, mRNA and protein expression of eNOS in the LV myocardium were significantly downregulated compared with normal dogs, and therapy with VNS significantly improved the expression of eNOS[13,16] (see Fig. 135.4). Inducible NOS is upregulated in HF. Overexpression of iNOS in cardiomyocytes of mice has been shown to result in peroxynitrite generation associated with fibrosis, LV hypertrophy, chamber dilation, cardiomyopathic phenotype, heart block, and SCD.[28] An increase in iNOS can also contribute to myocardial dysfunction through suppression of mitochondrial respiration, resulting in reduced steady-state adenosine triphosphate (ATP) levels.[27] Abnormal mitochondrial respiration is a key maladaptation of the failing myocardium. NO produced from iNOS can also inhibit the activity of cytochrome c oxidase (complex IV) by competing with binding sites for oxygen. In dogs with HF, mRNA and protein expression of iNOS in LV myocardium were significantly upregulated compared with normal dogs, and long-term therapy with VNS tended to normalize the expression[13,16] (see Fig. 135.4). nNOS has been shown to be upregulated in rats following myocardial infarctions and in the

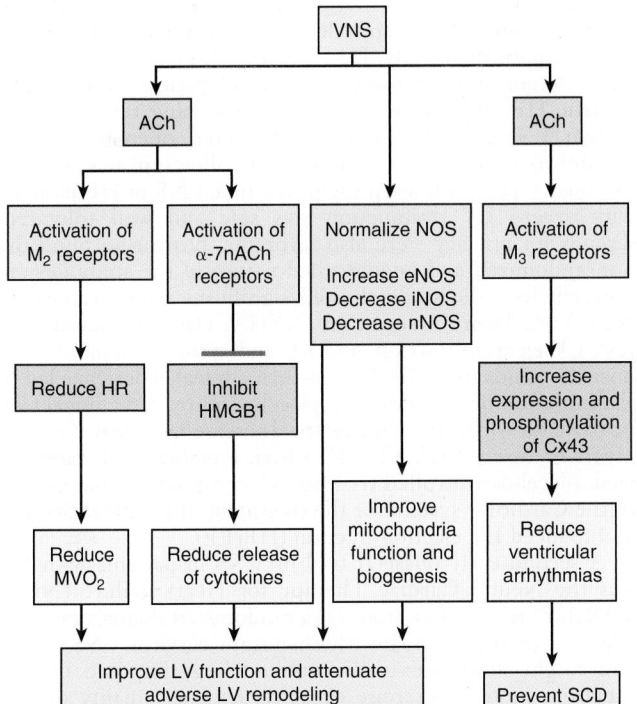

FIGURE 135.3 Diagram depicting potential mechanisms by which vagus nerve stimulation (*VNS*) elicits improvements in left ventricular (*LV*) function and prevents the development of malignant ventricular arrhythmias *ACh*, Acetylcholine; *α-7nACh*, α7 nicotinic acetylcholine receptor; *Cx43*, connexin 43; *e*, endothelial; *HMGB1*, high-mobility group box 1; *HR*, heart rate; *i*, inducible; *M₂*, muscarinic M₂; *M₃*, muscarinic M₃; *MVO₂*, myocardial oxygen consumption; *n*, neuronal; *NOS*, nitric oxide synthase; *SCD*, sudden cardiac death.

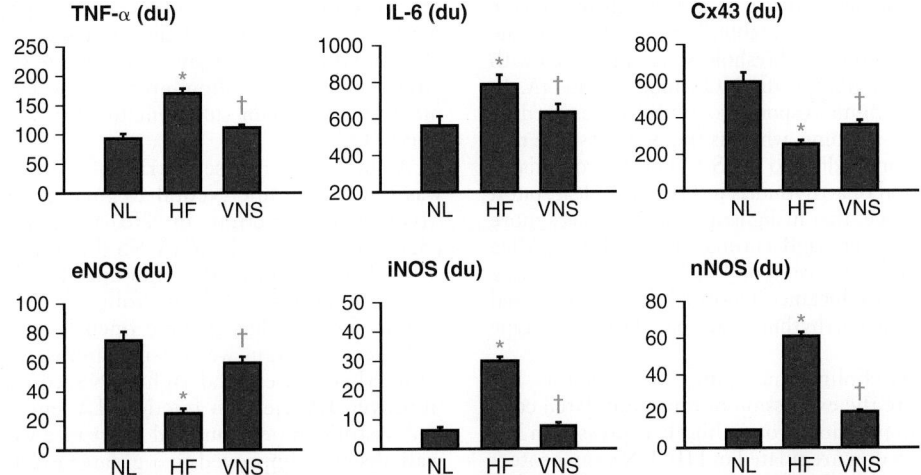

FIGURE 135.4 Bar graphs (mean ± standard error) illustrating the changes in various cytokines, connexins, and nitric oxide synthases in the left ventricular myocardium of normal (*NL*) dogs, dogs with heart failure (*HF*) that were not treated (controls), and dogs with HF treated for 3 months with vagus nerve stimulation (VNS). *, $p < .05$ vs. NL; †, $p < .05$ vs. HF. *Cx43*, connexin 43; *e*, endothelial; *i*, inducible; *IL-6*, interleukin 6; *n*, neuronal; *NOS*, nitric oxide synthase; *TNF-α*, tumor necrosis factor-α.

human failing heart.[29] In rats with HF, inhibition of nNOS led to increased sensitivity of the myocardium to β-adrenergic stimulation and observation, consistent with a role of nNOS in the autocrine regulation of myocardial contractility.[29] In dogs with coronary microembolization–induced HF, mRNA and protein expression of nNOS in LV myocardium were shown to be significantly upregulated compared with normal dogs, and long-term therapy with VNS tended to normalize the expression of nNOS in the failing dog LV myocardium.[13,16]

Vagus Nerve Stimulation and Ventricular Arrhythmias

SCD caused by malignant ventricular arrhythmias, including ventricular tachycardia (VT) and ventricular fibrillation (VF), is a major unresolved clinical problem. The search for a prophylactic treatment for SCD remains important, particularly in patients with HF who are at high risk for arrhythmic death. There is a significant body of evidence from experimental and clinical studies that demonstrate that stimulation of the vagus nerve has an antiarrhythmic action, protecting against induced and spontaneously occurring ventricular arrhythmias.[30-32] Vagus stimulation modulates ventricular arrhythmias by a number of direct and indirect actions, including activation of muscarinic receptors, antagonism of sympathetic actions, heart rate reduction, prolonged action potential duration (APD) and reduced APD dispersion, effects on restitution/refractoriness, and possibly via NO. Infusion of atropine, a nonselective muscarinic receptor antagonist, has been shown to increase the occurrence of induced VF in several studies.[33,34] An obvious consideration when stimulating the vagus nerve is the resulting bradycardia. Some studies suggest that the antiarrhythmic influence of the vagus nerve is reduced when heart rate is controlled.[35] The mechanisms by which a reduction in heart rate could protect from ventricular arrhythmias are not understood but may include rate-dependent alterations in ventricular APD, refractoriness, and dispersion of both factors. Another important concept in the generation of ventricular arrhythmias is that of APD dispersion. APD dispersion is a known mechanism that underlies circus movement reentry around refractory regions. VNS may prevent arrhythmias by antagonizing sympathetic-mediated changes in spatial depolarization. This idea may be particularly relevant in HF where there is increased activation and influence of the sympathetic nervous system. Other studies have suggested that VNS exerts a direct antiarrhythmic action at the ventricle level through the release of NO.[36] In an innervated perfused rabbit heart preparation, the beneficial effects of VNS on VT threshold were eliminated with the administration of the nonspecific NOS inhibitor L-NA. In this study, the antiarrhythmic response to VNS was restored by supplementation with L-arginine, which is the NO substrate that competes with L-NA for binding to NOS.[37] The role of inflammation in the generation of arrhythmias in HF is not clear, but it is recognized, for instance, that malignant arrhythmias are more likely in patients with acute and chronic myocarditis.[38] Mice with HF induced by overexpression of TNF-α exhibited a large number of ion channel conductance abnormalities and increased susceptibility to ventricular arrhythmias compared with wild-type controls.[39]

Activation of acetylcholine muscarinic M_3 receptors has been shown to regulate the expression of phosphorylated connexin 43 (Cx43), a gap junction protein highly expressed in LV tissue and significantly downregulated in HF. VNS can protect the heart from ischemia-induced arrhythmias by preventing a reduction in phosphorylated Cx43.[40] In dogs with coronary microembolization–induced HF, mRNA and protein expression of Cx43 in LV myocardium were shown to be markedly downregulated compared with normal dogs, and long-term therapy with VNS was associated with a significant increase

in the expression of Cx43 in LV myocardium of dogs with HF (see Fig. 135.4).[13,16]

Early Experience of Vagus Nerve Stimulation in Patients With Heart Failure

In patients with HF, reduced vagal activity is associated with increased mortality. Furthermore, vagal withdrawal has also been shown to precede episodes of acute decompensation. In a recently published study, De Ferrari et al. examined the safety and tolerability of chronic VNS in 32 patients with symptomatic HF and severe LV dysfunction using the CardioFit system.[41] The results of this multicenter, open-label phase II clinical trial with 3–6 months of follow-up and with an optional 1-year follow-up suggested that VNS in HF patients with severe LV dysfunction was safe and well tolerated. Trends for efficacy were also favorable, bearing in mind the nonrandomized and uncontrolled nature of the study design. Nevertheless, the study showed significant improvements in New York Heart Association (NYHA) class, 6-minute walk test, LV ejection fraction, and LV end-systolic volume.[41] The positive trends from this first-in-man clinical experience led to the initiation of a randomized placebo-controlled clinical trial in patients with HF, namely the Increase of Vagal Tone in Heart Failure (INOVATE-HF) trial, a pivotal U.S. randomized, placebo-controlled trial, to assess the safety and efficacy of the CardioFit system for the treatment of patients with HF and reduced LV ejection fraction (HFrEF).

A second early phase II trial of VNS in patients with HF was the Neural Cardiac Therapy for Heart Failure (NEC-TAR-HF) trial.[42] The trial was a randomized sham-controlled trial designed to evaluate whether right cervical VNS is safe and might attenuate cardiac remodeling, improve cardiac function, increase exercise capacity, enhance quality of life, and favorably impact circulating biomarkers in patients with symptomatic HFrEF. The trial enrolled 96 patients with HF in Europe in a 2:1 randomization (two treatment patients for each control patient) and patients were followed for 6 months. VNS, as delivered in the NECTAR-HF trial, was safe but failed to demonstrate a significant effect on LV ejection fraction, LV end-systolic dimension, and functional capacity, but the quality of life measures showed significant improvements as evidenced by significant improvements in the Minnesota Living with Heart Failure Questionnaire, NYHA class, and the 36-item short-form survey (SF-36) physical component.[42] A potential limitation of this trial was the low VNS current achieved during the study. The average stimulation amplitude after the 3-month follow-up visit was 1.42 ± 0.80 mA, which may not have been sufficient to activate the necessary vagus nerve B fibers.

A third early phase II trial of VNS in patients with HF was the Autonomic Neural Regulation Therapy to Enhance Myocardial Function in Heart Failure (ANTHEM-HF) trial.[43] The trial evaluated VNS therapy in 60 HFrEF patients with NYHA class II–III randomized to left (n = 31) or right (n = 29) cervical VNS and followed up for 6 months. The results showed that chronic open-loop VNS via the left or right cervical vagus was feasible and well tolerated in patients with HFrEF. Left and right VNS equally and significantly improved LV ejection fraction, LV end-systolic volume, LV end-systolic dimension, and heart rate variability. Six-minute walk distance improved to a greater extent in patients receiving right cervical VNS compared with those receiving left cervical VNS. NYHA class improved in 77% of all patients.[43] In the ANTHEM-HF trial, the average VNS current amplitude was 2.2 ± 0.5 mA and was higher than that used in NECTAR-HF but lower than that used in the clinical pilot study of the CardioFit VNS system.

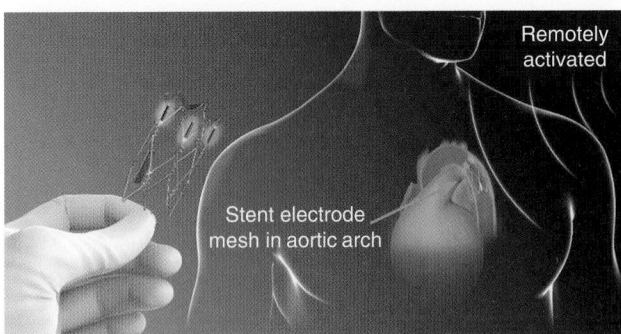

FIGURE 135.5 In the background is a depiction of an implanted Enopace Harmony neuromodulation system with a stent electrode mesh deployed in the upper descending aorta. The *foreground* shows a detailed depiction of the remotely activated stent electrode mesh.

New Approaches and Instrumentation for Neuromodulation in Heart Failure

As new clinical trials are initiated and older trials continue to forge ahead with the aim to evaluate potential clinical benefits of cervical VNS and neuromodulation in general in patients with HF, so do the development of new instrumentation and approaches to better implement this form of therapy. One such new instrumentation is the development of a self-sizing cuff electrode (one size fits all) for direct placement on the cervical vagus nerve. The EquiCurl electrode (see Fig. 135.1) is a component of the new Equilia VNS system developed by LivaNova, Inc. (Houston, TX). Long-term testing of this system in dogs with microembolization-induced CHF showed a significant reduction in heart rate along with significant improvements in LV ejection fraction and LV end-systolic volume. Efforts to surgically remove the electrode off the nerve after long-term implantation (3–4 months) were surprisingly easy compared with other types of fixed rigid cuff or spiral-type cuff electrodes.[44]

To date, many of the approaches to VNS or neuromodulation for patients with HF have required surgical intervention and direct placement of cuff-type electrodes on the cervical vagus nerve. A new percutaneous approach, under development by Enopace Biomedical (Caesarea, Israel), implements neuromodulation for the treatment of HF using a stent-type electrode mesh deployed near the aortic arch (Fig. 135.5). The Enopace Harmony system is designed to be activated remotely to improve ventricular-arterial coupling by activating the aortic afferent fibers that lead into the left vagal trunk. When stimulated by the system, these afferent fibers transmit signals to the brain through neural pathways, which lead to reductions in heart rate, systemic blood pressure, and MVO$_2$ with improvements in LV function.

Approaches to Neuromodulation in Heart Failure Other Than Vagus Nerve Stimulation

The enthusiasm for VNS as a therapeutic target for HF has also given rise to other non-VNS approaches that are being explored

for the treatment of HF, such as baroreflex activation therapy (BAT)[45] and spinal cord stimulation (SCS) therapy.[46] Neuromodulation in patients with HF via SCS therapy was based on the placement of a multiple electrode–tipped lead in the epidural space at approximately the L2/L3 level. In dogs with experimentally induced HF, SCS therapy significantly improved cardiac LV contractile function and decreased ventricular arrhythmias.[46] In a recently completed feasibility study in patients with HFrEF (DEFEAT-HF trial), 6 months of study with SCS therapy failed to provide evidence of a meaningful change in clinical outcome in this patient population.[47] BAT is another form of neuromodulation that is aimed at treating patients with HF. BAT elicits its potential benefits by stimulating the baroreflex nerves through electrical impulses delivered through an electrode placed directly on the carotid sinus.[45] In dogs with coronary microembolization–induced HF, long-term therapy with BAT significantly improved LV function and partially reversed LV remodeling at the global, cellular, and molecular levels.[46] BAT is currently undergoing effectiveness and safety testing in a clinical trial (HOPE4HF) of patients with HFrEF using the *Barostim neo* system (CVRx, Inc.).

Conclusions

In conclusion, preclinical studies conducted to date support the concept that electrical VNS and other electrical neuromodulation approaches, such as SCS therapy and BAT, can favorably modify the underlying pathophysiology of HF. Animal studies have shown that VNS, SCS therapy, and BAT can improve LV function and prevent progressive LV remodeling. VNS can prevent the development of malignant ventricular arrhythmias responsible for SCD. These benefits of neuromodulation arise from multiple mechanisms of action that include reduced heart rate, normalization of sympathetic overdrive, suppression of proinflammatory cytokines, and normalization of NO signaling pathways. While first-in-man studies in patients with HF have shown that VNS is safe, feasible, and well tolerated, most phase II clinical trials conducted to date that use VNS or SCS therapy in patients with HFrEF showed little or no benefit. The negative results may be attributable to variability in the amplitude of the stimulation current used as well as to variability in the design characteristics of VNS leads. Another possibility is the lack of major heart rate reduction in patients with HF who undergo neuromodulation therapy. Heart rate reduction was a major component in every preclinical study conducted to date. Inability to achieve appropriate current amplitudes as well as background therapy in the form of β-blockade may have removed heart rate reduction as a contributing mechanism of action in patients with HFrEF. Full appreciation for the potential effectiveness of electrical neuromodulation as a treatment for patients with HF requires more research targeted toward a better understanding of the mechanisms responsible for the benefits seen in animals with HF and greater knowledge on how to evoke these beneficial mechanisms once translation is made into the clinical arena.

Acknowledgments

This chapter is supported, in part, by research grants from Bio-Control Medical, Ltd., Boston Scientific Corporation, and the National Heart, Lung, and Blood Institute (PO1 HL074237-10).

REFERENCES

1. Olshansky B, Sabbah HN, Hauptman PJ, et al. Parasympathetic nervous system and heart failure: pathophysiology and potential implications for therapy. *Circulation.* 2008;118:863–871.
2. Schwatrz PJ, Vanoli E, Stramba-Badiale M, et al. Autonomic mechanisms and sudden death. New insights from the analysis of baroreceptor reflexes in conscious dogs with and without myocardial infarction. *Circulation.* 1988;78:969–973.
3. Mortara A, La Rovere MT, Pinna GD, et al. Arterial baroreflex modulation of heart rate in chronic heart failure: clinical and hemodynamic correlates and prognostic implications. *Circulation.* 1997;96:3450–3458.
4. Lechat P, Hulot JS, Escolano S, et al. Heart rate and cardiac rhythm relationships with bisoprolol benefit in chronic heart failure in CIBIS II trial. *Circulation.* 2001;103:1428–1433.
5. Sabbah HN, Shimoyama H, Kono T, et al. Effects of long-term monotherapy with enalapril, metoprolol and digoxin on the progression of left ventricular dysfunction and dilation in dogs with reduced ejection fraction. *Circulation.* 1994;89:2852–2859.
6. Swedberg K, Komajda M, Bohm M, et al. Ivabradine and outcomes in chronic heart failure (SHIFT): a randomized placebo-controlled study. *Lancet.* 2010;376:875–885.

7. MERIT-HF Study Group. Effect of metoprolol CR/XL in chronic heart failure: Metoprolol CR/XL Randomised Intervention Trial in Congestive Heart Failure (MERIT-HF). *Lancet.* 1999;353:2001–2007.

8. Harman MA, Reeves TJ. Effects of efferent nerve stimulation on atrial and ventricular function. *Am J Physiol.* 1968;215:1210–1217.

9. Li M, Zheng C, Sato T, et al. Vagal nerve stimulation markedly improves long-term survival after chronic heart failure in rats. *Circulation.* 2004;109:120–124.

10. Zheng C, Li M, Inagaki M, et al. Vagal stimulation markedly suppresses arrhythmias in conscious rats with chronic heart failure after myocardial infarction. *Conf Proc IEEE Eng Med Biol Soc.* 2005;7:7072–7075.

11. Sabbah HN, Ilsar I, Zaretsky A, et al. Vagus nerve stimulation in experimental heart failure. *Heart Fail Rev.* 2011;16:171–178.

12. Zhang Y, Popovic ZB, Bibevski S, et al. Chronic vagus nerve stimulation improves autonomic control and attenuates systemic inflammation and heart failure progression in a canine high-rate pacing model. *Circulation.* 2009;2:692–699.

13. Sabbah HN. Electrical vagus nerve stimulation for the treatment of chronic heart failure. *Cleve Clin J Med.* 2011;78:S24–S29.

14. Sabbah HN, Imai M, Zaretsky A, et al. Therapy with vagus nerve stimulation combined with beta-blockade improves left ventricular function in dogs with heart failure beyond that seen with beta-blockade alone. *Eur J Heart Fail.* 2007;6:114.

15. Sabbah HN, Wang M, Jiang A, et al. Right vagus nerve stimulation improves left ventricular function in dogs with heart failure. *J Am Coll Cardiol.* 2010;55:A16–E151.

16. Ruble SB, Hamann JJ, Gupta RC, et al. Chronic vagal nerve stimulation impacts biomarkers of heart failure in canines. *J Am Coll Cardiol.* 2010;55:A16–E153.

17. Sabbah HN, Sharov VG, Lesch M, et al. Progression of heart failure: a role for interstitial fibrosis. *Mol Cell Biochem.* 1995;147:29–34.

18. Sabbah HN, Wang M, Jiang A, et al. Long-term monotherapy with ivabradine improves left ventricular function and prevents progressive chamber remodeling in dogs with moderate heart failure. *Circulation.* 2009;120:S867.

19. Tracey KJ. Physiology and immunology of the cholinergic antiinflammatory pathway. *J Clin Invest.* 2007;117:289–296.

20. Oke SL, Tracey KJ. From CNI-1493 to the immunological homunculus: physiology of the inflammatory reflex. *J Leukoc Biol.* 2008;83:1–6.

21. Wang H, Liao H, Ochani M, et al. Cholinergic agonists inhibit HMGB1 release and improve survival in experimental sepsis. *Nat Med.* 2004;10:1216–1221.

22. Aukrust P, Gullestad L, Ueland T, et al. Inflammatory and anti-inflammatory cytokines in chronic heart failure: potential therapeutic implications. *Ann Med.* 2005;37:74–85.

23. Shishehbor MH, Alves C, Rajagopal V. Inflammation: implications for understanding the heart-brain connection. *Cleve Clin J Med.* 2007;74:S37–S41.

24. Hare JM, Keaney Jr JF, Balligand JL, et al. Role of nitric oxide in parasympathetic modulation of beta adrenergic myocardial contractility in normal dogs. *J Clin Invest.* 1995;95:360–366.

25. Feng Q, Song W, Lu X, et al. Development of heart failure and congenital septal defects in mice lacking endothelial nitric oxide synthase. *Circulation.* 2002;106:873–879.

26. Kelly RA, Balligand JL, Smith TW. Nitric oxide and cardiac function. *Circ Res.* 1996;79:363–380.

27. Nisoli E, Carruba MO. Nitric oxide and mitochondrial biogenesis. *J Cell Sci.* 2006;119:2855–2862.

28. Mungrue IN, Gros R, You X, et al. Cardiomyocyte overexpression of iNOS in mice results in peroxynitrite generation, heart block and sudden death. *J Clin Invest.* 2002;109:735–743.

29. Bendall JK, Damy T, Ratajczak P, et al. Role of myocardial neuronal nitric oxide synthase-derived nitric oxide in β-adrenergic hyporesponsiveness after myocardial infarction-induced heart failure in rat. *Circulation.* 2004;110:2368–2375.

30. Goldstein RE, Karsh RB, Smith ER, et al. Influence of atropine and of vagally mediated bradycardia on the occurrence of ventricular arrhythmias following acute coronary occlusion in closed-chest dogs. *Circulation.* 1973;47:1180–1190.

31. Schwartz PJ, Billman GE, Stone HL. Autonomic mechanisms in ventricular fibrillation induced by myocardial ischemia during exercise in dogs with healed myocardial infarction. An experimental preparation for sudden cardiac death. *Circulation.* 1984;69:790–800.

32. Kolman B, Verrier R, Lown B. The effect of vagus nerve stimulation upon vulnerability of the canine ventricle: role of sympathetic-parasympathetic interactions. *Circulation.* 1975;52:578–585.

33. De Ferrari GM, Vanoli E, Stramba-Badiale M, et al. Vagal reflexes and survival during acute myocardial ischemia in conscious dogs with healed myocardial infarction. *Am J Physiol.* 1991;61:H63–H69.

34. Kent KM, Smith ER, Redwood DR, Epstein SE. Electrical stability of acutely ischemic myocardium. Influences of heart rate and vagal stimulation. *Circulation.* 1973;47:291–298.

35. Ng GA, Brack KE, Patel VH, et al. Autonomic modulation of electrical restitution, alternans and ventricular fibrillation initiation in the isolated heart. *Cardiovasc Res.* 2007;73:750–760.

36. Brack KE, Coote JH, Ng GA. Vagus nerve stimulation protects against ventricular fibrillation independent of muscarinic receptor activation. *Cardiovasc Res.* 2011;91:437–446.

37. Brack KE, Patel VH, Coote JH, et al. Nitric oxide mediates the vagal protective effect on ventricular fibrillation via effects on action potential duration restitution in the rabbit heart. *J Physiol.* 2007;583:695–704.

38. Corrado D, Basso C, Thiene G. Sudden cardiac death in young people with apparently normal heart. *Cardiovasc Res.* 2001;50:399–408.

39. London B, Baker LC, Lee JS, et al. Calcium-dependent arrhythmias in transgenic mice with heart failure. *Am J Physiol.* 2003;284:H431–H441.

40. Ando M, Katare RG, Katinuma Y, et al. Efferent vagal nerve stimulation protects the heart against ischemia-induced arrhythmias by preserving connexin43 protein. *Circulation.* 2005;112:164–170.

41. De Ferrari GM, Crijns HJGM, Borggrefe M, et al. Chronic vagus nerve stimulation: a new and promising therapeutic approach for chronic heart failure. *Eur Heart J.* 2011;32:847–855.

42. Zannad F, De Ferrari GM, Tuinenburg AE, et al. Chronic vagal stimulation for the treatment of low ejection fraction heart failure: results of the NEural Cardiac TherApy foR Heart Failure (NECTAR-HF) randomized controlled trial. *Eur Heart J.* 2015;36:425–433.

43. Premchand RK, Sharma K, Mittal S, et al. Autonomic regulation therapy via the left or right cervical vagus nerve stimulation in patients with chronic heart failure: results of the ANTHEM-HF trial. *J Cardiac Fail.* 2014;20:808–816.

44. Sabbah HN, Wang MJ, Zhang KF, et al. Right vagus nerve stimulation with a novel self-sizing cuff electrode improves left ventricular function in dogs with heart failure (Abstract). *J Cardiac Fail.* 2015;2:S93.

45. Sabbah HN, Gupta RC, Imai M, et al. Chronic electrical stimulation of the carotid sinus baroreflex improves LV function and promotes reversal of ventricular remodeling in dogs with advanced heart failure. *Circ Heart Fail.* 2011;4:65–70.

46. Lopshire JC, Zhou X, Dusa C, et al. Spinal cord stimulation improves ventricular function and reduces ventricular arrhythmias in a canine postinfarction heart failure model. *Circulation.* 2009;120:286–294.

47. Zipes DP, Neuzil P, Theres H, et al. Determining the feasibility of spinal cord neuromodulation for the treatment of chronic systolic heart failure: the DEFEAT-HF study. *JACC Heart Fail.* 2016;4:129–136.

136 Baroreceptor Stimulation

Gino Seravalle and Guido Grassi

In the last decades, significant evidence has suggested a causative or accessory role of sympathetic nerve activity in the pathogenesis of several cardiovascular diseases.[1] Findings indicate that a sympathoexcitatory state is pronounced in individuals with hypertension and difficult blood pressure (BP) control; obesity; metabolic syndrome; obstructive sleep apnea; altered dipping profile, as in extreme dippers (i.e., individuals who, compared with average daytime BP levels, display reductions in average nighttime systolic and diastolic BP of >20%) or reverse dippers (i.e., those who do not display a reduction at all or display an increase in nocturnal BP); kidney diseases; and congestive heart failure.[1–12] These studies suggest that suppression of sympathetic activity should be one of the major roles of the therapy. With this aim, an intervention that targets the carotid baroreflex has received renewed interest. This chapter will start with an overview of anatomical characteristics and physiological background and then describe the methods to investigate baroreflex sensitivity in the laboratory and daily life, the novel interventional therapies to modulate autonomic tone, and the clinical results obtained with this approach.

Anatomical Aspects

The neural pathways and effector mechanisms involved in the baroreflex control of circulation are summarized in Fig. 136.1. The cell bodies of carotid sinus and aortic arch baroreceptor neurons are located in the petrosal and nodose ganglia, respectively. The corresponding afferent baroreceptor activity is transmitted to the nucleus tractus solitarius (NTS) in the medullary brainstem via carotid sinus and glossopharyngeal nerves and aortic depressor and vagus nerves, respectively. The baroreceptor inputs are integrated and relayed through a network of central nervous system (CNS) neurons that control efferent parasympathetic nerve activity, sympathetic nerve activity, and release of the vasoconstrictor and antidiuretic peptide vasopressin from the posterior pituitary gland.[13]

Receptors are located in the transverse aortic arch (aortic baroreceptors) and carotid sinuses of internal carotid arteries (carotid baroreceptors), known as "arterial baroreceptors," and exert an important regulatory function in the homeostatic control of BP.[13] Arterial baroreceptors are stretch receptors that are stimulated by distortion of the arterial wall during changes not only in the mean BP level but also in the direction and rate of change in BP. Consequently, baroreceptor activity will increase or decrease to a greater extent when the change in BP occurs more rapidly, leading to more effective reflex compensation. Similarly, baroreceptor activity is higher during the systolic phase of the arterial pressure pulse and is lower or absent during the diastolic phase of the arterial pressure pulse. The phasic discharge of afferent activity facilitates reflex inhibition of sympathetic nerve activity.[13] As the arterial baroreflex represents a major inhibiting mechanism of the sympathetic nervous system, it seems rational to assume that an alteration in baroreflex activity is implicated in the pathogenesis of hypertension and other pathophysiological conditions.[1,13]

Methods to Investigate Baroreceptor Activity in Humans and Physiological Background

In humans, stimulation or deactivation of arterial baroreceptors can be achieved by a variety of techniques such as infusion of vasoactive drugs into the systemic circulation (phenylephrine or nitroprusside) or the application of positive or negative pressures by a device positioned over the neck, where carotid arteries and carotid baroreceptors are anatomically located.[13] Using these techniques, it has been possible to show that in physiological conditions in which BP increases, there is a marked deactivation of aortic and carotid baroreceptors. This triggers a reduction in heart rate and an inhibition of sympathetic vasoconstrictor drive. As a net result, BP decreases with a concomitant reduction in cardiac output and peripheral vascular resistance. Conversely, in physiological conditions in which BP decreases, there is a marked stimulation of aortic and carotid baroreceptors. This triggers an increase in heart rate and an enhancement of sympathetic vasoconstrictor tone. As a result, BP increases with a concomitant increase in cardiac output and peripheral vascular resistance.

Other laboratory methods for assessing baroreflex sensitivity are (1) the Valsalva maneuver, (2) head-up tilting and lower body negative pressure application, (3) neck chamber (mentioned earlier), and (4) techniques for analyzing spontaneous baroreflex modulation of heart rate (Box 136.1).

The Valsalva maneuver is a widely used method to explore arterial baroreflex modulation of the heart through quantification of tachycardia and bradycardia, which occur during the initial decrease and subsequent increase in BP, respectively, that follow the maintenance for 15–20 seconds of a constant expiratory pressure of 40 mm Hg.[14,15] This technique is simple and noninvasive, but it triggers alterations in the chemoreceptor and cardiopulmonary receptor activity. The evaluation of baroreflex sensitivity by head-up tilting is quantified by the reflex effects on heart rate and peripheral resistance but not by reflex effects on BP. This method has limited specificity because it produces cardiopulmonary receptor deactivation as a result of reduction in venous return, central blood volume, and vestibular stimulation, which may contribute to cardiovascular adjustment.[13]

A neck chamber consists of a rigid chamber sealed around the subject's neck in which the air pressure is increased or decreased in a graded fashion, resulting in graded and quantifiable reductions or increases in carotid transmural pressure. It allows not only heart rate but also BP modulation by arterial baroreceptors to be investigated. Disadvantages are that only carotid baroreceptor function can be assessed and that the effect of carotid baroreceptor involvement is counteracted by the aortic baroreflex,

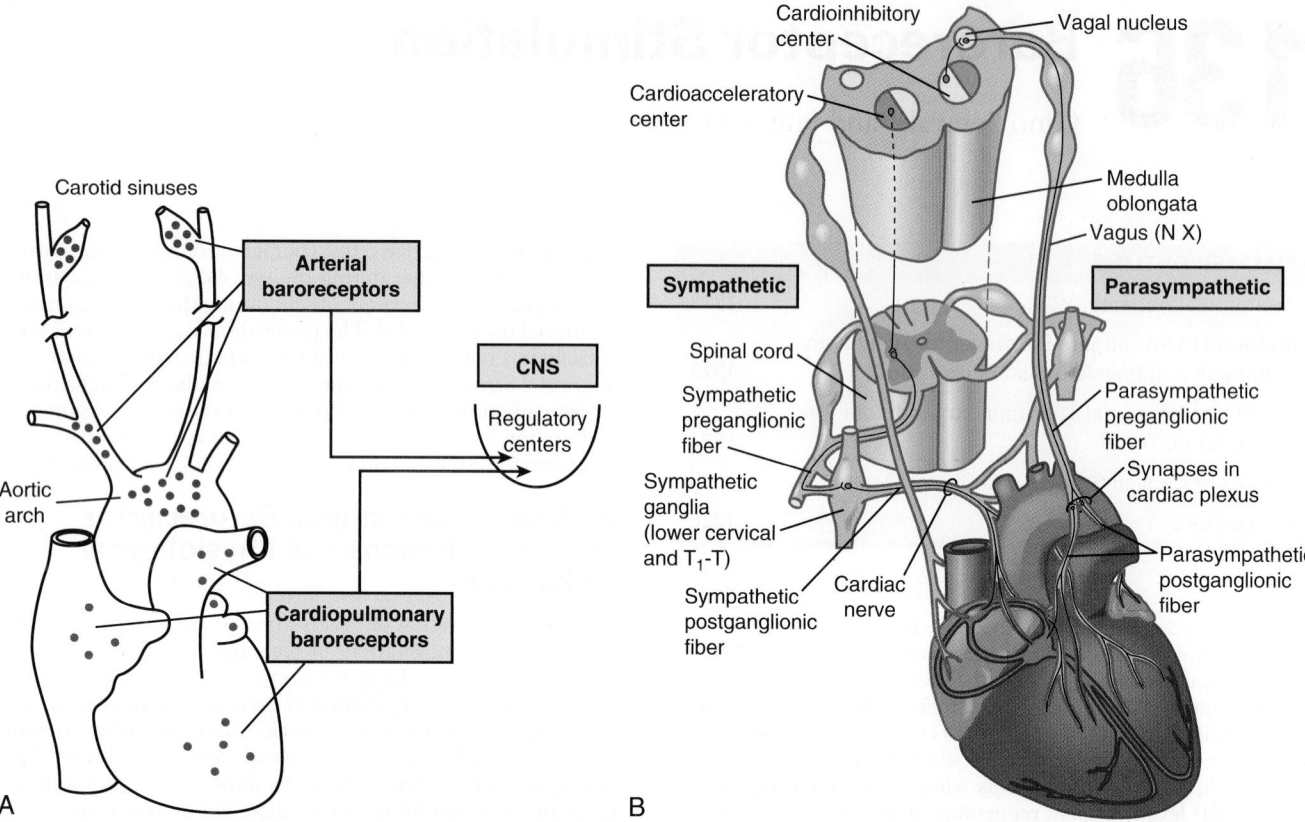

FIGURE 136.1 (A) Location of baroreceptors, and (B) neural pathways that mediate baroreflex responses. *CNS,* Central nervous system.

BOX 136.1   Methods to assess baroreflex function: from laboratory to daily life

- Electrical stimulation of carotid sinus nerves
- Anesthesia of carotid sinus nerves and vagi
- Occlusion of common carotid artery
- Carotid sinus massage
- Valsalva maneuver
- Head-up tilting
- Lower body negative pressure
- Intravenous bolus injection of vasoactive agents with limited effect on the heart
- Intravenous stepwise infusion of vasoactive agents
- Assessment of reflex changes in muscle sympathetic nerve activity induced by blood pressure changes following vasoactive drug infusion
- Neck chamber technique
- Sequence technique
- RR interval SBP cross correlation
- Modulus of RR interval–SBP transfer function at 0.1 Hz
- Squared ratio of RR interval/SBP spectral powers at 0.1 and 0.3 Hz (α coefficient)
- Closed-loop RR interval–SBP transfer function (ARMA modeling)
- Statistical dependence of RR interval on SBP fluctuations

ARMA, Autoregressive moving average; *SBP,* systolic blood pressure.

---

which is deactivated during the BP decrease induced by carotid baroreceptor stimulation and vice versa.[16,17]

Modern techniques for the analysis of the sensitivity of spontaneous baroreflex control of heart rate[18] do not require any external intervention on the subject under evaluation and can be used in resting and dynamic conditions.[19] These indirect methods are all based on the combined computer analysis of spontaneous BP and heart rate fluctuations: the sequence technique,[20,21]

spectral analysis of the alpha coefficient,[22,23] and mathematical models using autoregressive and moving average techniques[24,25] to assess the interactions between systolic BP and RR interval, which occur physiologically in a closed-loop condition.

Novel Interventional Therapies to Modulate the Autonomic Tone

Arterial baroreceptor (particularly, carotid baroreceptor) function is impaired in essential hypertension and several other pathophysiological conditions.[1–13] This baroreceptor dysfunction includes the impairment of baroreceptor modulation of heart rate (which is mediated by vagal fibers) and by an alteration in the baroreceptor control of BP (which is mediated by sympathetic fibers). In the latter case, the baroreceptor alteration is known as "resetting" of the operational set point of the reflex function,[26] i.e., although not primarily altered, baroreceptor control of BP is reset toward more elevated BP levels with an attenuation of its pressor influences and potentiation of the depressor ones. The concept of carotid baroreceptor activation is based on the idea that increases in sympathetic outflow from the carotid sinus to brainstem cardiovascular centers would result in a sustained decrease in BP and heart rate and a "re-reset" in baroreflexes with more easily controlled BP levels.

The first experimental studies[27–29] showed that a significant reduction in BP was achieved in normotensive dogs for periods of up to 90 minutes following direct electrical stimulation of the carotid sinus nerve. Reductions in cardiac output, peripheral resistance, mean arterial pressure, and heart rate were also observed with bilateral electrical stimulation of the carotid sinus nerve in the initial human studies.[30–32] The use of these early devices was not devoid of adverse events (paralysis of the hypoglossal nerve with dysarthria and hemiatrophy of the tongue, blurring of vision and dizziness in the standing position, and perioperative deaths)

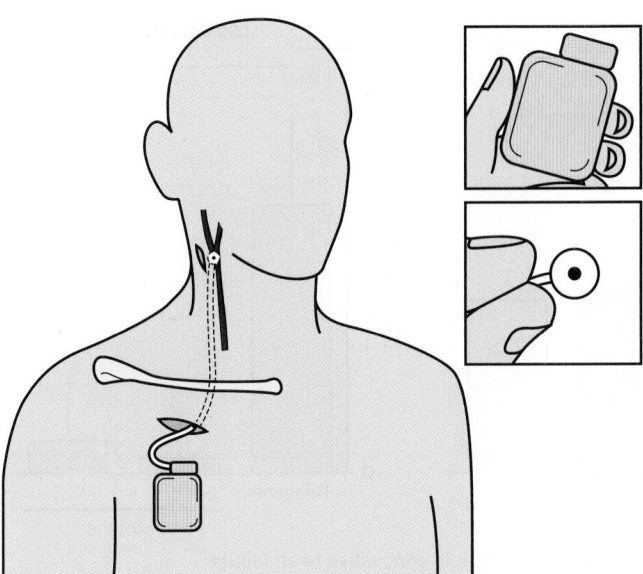

FIGURE 136.2 Schematic diagram of a patient with carotid body stimulation system. The *left image* shows the location of the baroreflex activation lead and implantable pulse generator. *Right images* show the dimension of the second-generation pulse generator Barostim neo *(upper)* and of the single lead *(lower)*.

and technical difficulties (current spread around the inserted electrode with discomfort and pain, difficulties in communication between the external antenna and inserted receiver, nerve damage, stimulation of the nearby chemoreceptor afferents, leading to sympathoexcitation).

It has taken several decades for investigators of baroreflex activation therapy (BAT) to develop a safe medical device capable of producing reliable suppression of sympathetic activity and effective BP reduction by electrical activation of the carotid baroreflex. Recent technological advances have led to the development of implantable baroreflex activation systems based on a pulse generator and electrodes that allow electrical field stimulation of the carotid sinus wall[33,34] (Fig. 136.2). Chronic electrical activation of the carotid baroreflex, known as BAT, has been commercially available and tested in patients with resistant hypertension and heart failure.[35-37] For the traditional Rheos system (CVRx Inc., Minneapolis, MN), the implantation involves surgical exposure of both carotid sinuses and bilateral placement of electrodes around the carotid adventitial surface. The leads are subcutaneously tunneled and connected to an implantable stimulation device placed in a subclavian subcutaneous position on the anterior chest wall. The newer generation (Barostim neo, also from CVRx, Inc.) has only one smaller carotid sinus electrode that delivers less power, enables easier implantation, and has fewer adverse effects.

Results of Clinical Studies and Clinical Trials

Baroreflex Activation Therapy in Hypertension

The clinical experience with modern devices has been collected in a small number of clinical studies and trials. The first data were collected in the Rheos Feasibility Trial that was conducted in 10 patients with resistant hypertension.[38] Following a recovery period of 1 month after implantation, the device was activated and this enabled a marked BP reduction with a maximal response that amounted to 42 and 21 mm Hg for systolic and diastolic BP, respectively. The magnitude of the response was quite stable over the 10-month follow-up (raw data were not included in this first publication). The procedure was uneventful and without significant side effects (two infections at the site of the surgical intervention were successfully treated). This publication was followed

by two other articles that aimed at clarifying the mechanisms through which the procedure reduced BP.[39,40] Both studies confirmed the profound sympathoinhibition triggered by the electrical field stimulation of carotid baroreceptors, the magnitude of which was directly and significantly related to the degree of systolic BP reduction elicited by the intervention. Other effects that have been observed were a small reduction in heart rate, decrease of 20% in plasma renin activity levels, tendency of the low-frequency component of heart rate variability to increase (consistent with an improvement in vagal control of heart rate), and substantially unchanged baroreflex modulation of heart rate assessed via cross-spectral analysis and a sequence technique. The information collected in these earlier studies was supplemented by the results of two recent trials: the Device-Based Therapy in Hypertension Trial (DEBuT-HT)[41] and the Rheos Pivotal Trial.[42] In the 2010 report, of 45 patients enrolled in the DEBuT-HT study, 18 successfully completed the 4-year follow-up.[41] Both systolic and diastolic BPs were significantly lowered by 53 and 30 mm Hg, respectively. These reductions were superimposable on those observed after 3 and 12 months after activation of the device. A reduction of >30 mm Hg in systolic BP was observed in 72% of patients, and 67% of patients had a systolic BP of <140 mm Hg. The reduction in BP was accompanied by a reduction in target organ damage: –24 g/m² in the left ventricular mass index and –1.3 to 1.4 mm in wall thickness. A sustained change in heart rate variability associated with inhibition of sympathetic activity and increase in parasympathetic activity was also observed during chronic baroreceptor stimulation.[40] The Rheos Pivotal Trial,[42] a randomized, double-blind, parallel-design trial, enrolled 265 patients with resistant hypertension and showed decreases in BPs of 26 and 35 mm Hg at 6 and 12 months, respectively. Over 50% of subjects were able to achieve a systolic BP of <140 mm Hg, and safety was confirmed with <9% of subjects experiencing side effects, most related to the surgical or anesthetic procedure.

Additional benefits of BAT have been observed in studies of hypertensive patients with preexisting cardiovascular disease. A study of 12 patients with resistant hypertension who were fitted with the Rheos device did not show impairment in renal function after 1-year follow-up[43]; glomerular filtration rate remained unchanged, while effective plasma flow showed a decrease, thus resulting in a subsequent significant increase in filtration fraction.

The study by Heusser et al.[40] has also shown that acute electrical baroreflex stimulation not only decreased systolic BP but also muscle sympathetic nerve activity, heart rate, and plasma renin concentration. This result is relevant because it shows that the surgical procedure does not impair, either through scarring, inflammation, or direct baroreceptor damage, the ability of the reflex to exert its sympathetic and vasomotor modulation.

To facilitate the operational implantation, the Barostim neo system, a second-generation system, has been developed.[36] The new system consists of one pulse generator, one lead electrode directly sutured to the unilateral carotid sinus, and a laptop computer–based programming system. The carotid sinus electrode serves as the cathode (6 mm in diameter), while the pulse generator acts as the anode. In an open-label, nonrandomized study of 30 patients with resistant hypertension, BP decreased by an average of 26/12 mm Hg during the 6-month follow-up, which was superimposable with that reported in previous studies with the old generation device. The new system not only significantly decreased BP but was also safe, with 97% of patients being event free at 180 days.

Baroreflex Activation Therapy in Heart Failure

Congestive heart failure, a disease with high mortality and increasing prevalence,[44] is characterized by autonomic imbalance, including decreased parasympathetic tone,[45] increased sympathetic tone,[11,12,46] and impaired baroreflex control of sympathetic activity.[12,47] These alterations emerge early in heart failure, evolving

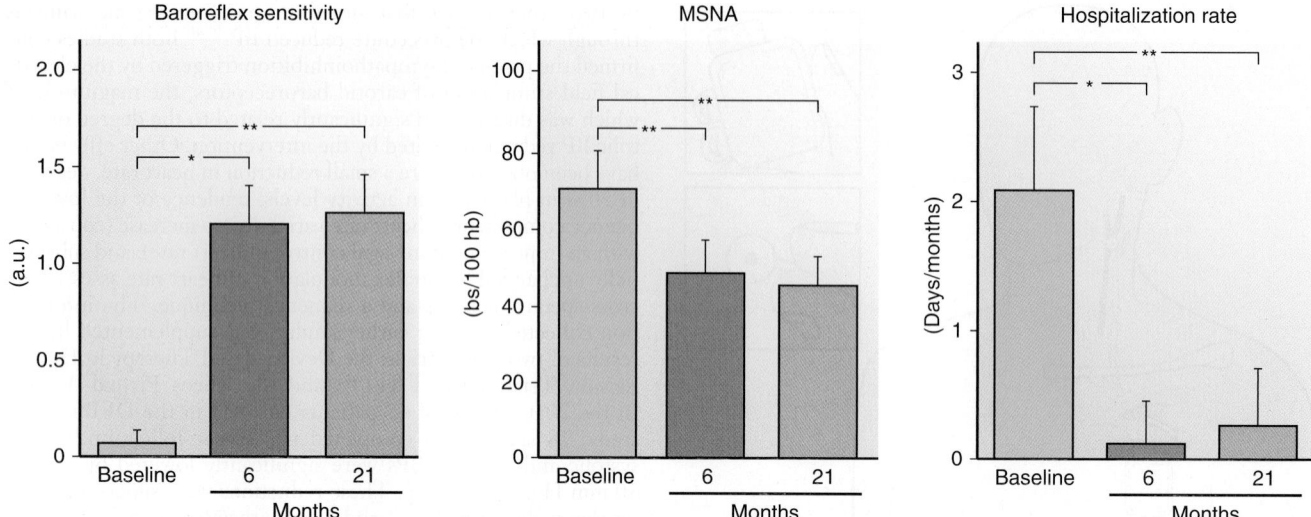

FIGURE 136.3 Effects of chronic (6 and 21.5 months) baroreflex activation in congestive heart failure patients on baroreflex sensitivity (*left*), muscle sympathetic nerve activity (*MSNA; middle*), and hospitalization rate (*right*). Data are expressed as mean ± standard deviation. *Asterisks* (* $p < .05$, ** $p < .01$) refer to the statistical significance versus baseline. (Modified from Gronda E, Seravalle G, Quarti Trevano F, et al. Long-term chronic baroreflex activation: persistent efficacy in patients with heart failure and reduced ejection fraction. *J Hypertens.* 2015;33:1704-1708.)

from the initial compensatory role to disease progression, cardiovascular complications, and death.[46] Pharmacotherapy, attempting to restore the autonomic imbalance with drugs such as β-blockers, angiotensin-converting enzyme inhibitors/angiotensin II receptor blockers, and aldosterone receptor antagonists, improves survival among heart failure patients and is recommended in patients with reduced ejection fraction.[44] However, the daunting prospect of increasing heart failure burden and lack of recent breakthroughs in pharmacotherapy have led to investigations of nonpharmacological approaches that can favorably modulate the autonomic tone.[48] Preliminary data on BAT suggest that beneficial effects of this intervention can extend to heart failure. In a microembolization canine model of heart failure,[49] BAT was able to reduce plasma norepinephrine, increase left ventricular ejection fraction, and decrease susceptibility to induction of life-threatening ventricular arrhythmias. In a rapid pacing model of heart failure, the device reduced left ventricular filling pressure, decreased plasma norepinephrine and angiotensin II, and improved survival.[50] A case report on heart failure with preserved ejection fraction showed favorable cardiac remodeling, increased functional capacity, and reduced burden of medical therapy.[51]

Recently, Gronda et al.[37] have reported the results of a single-center, open-label, single-arm study in 11 patients with left ventricular ejection fraction of ≤40% and New York Heart Association (NYHA) class III heart failure symptoms while on optimal medical therapy who received BAT for 6 months. Results showed for the first time that chronic BAT was associated with significant improvement in baroreflex sensitivity, left ventricular ejection fraction, NYHA class, quality of life, and 6-minute walk distance, along with significant decrease in muscle sympathetic nerve activity (31%). A new report of the same group[52] described observation at 12 and 21.5 months of follow-up. While two patients died because of septic shock and electromechanical dissociation, in the surviving nine patients with heart failure, BAT maintained its beneficial effects over a long term. The sympathetic reduction observed at 6 months was maintained (Fig. 136.3) in association with restored baroreflex sensitivity, improvements in quality of life, 6-minute walk distance, and NYHA class, while the number of days/months in the hospital was significantly reduced.

Extending these findings, the recently reported Barostim HOPE4HF study randomized 146 patients to goal-directed medical therapy alone versus the addition of BAT.[53] There was no standard dosing protocol, with device stimulation intensity increased over a 3-month period unless associated with an excessive reduction in heart rate or BP. At the 6-month follow-up, compared with medical therapy, BAT was associated with modest, but significant, improvement in functional endpoints, reduction in natriuretic peptide concentration, and a trend toward reduction in the number of days of hospitalization. Ongoing studies involving BAT in heart failure include the Rheos Diastolic Heart Failure Trial (available at https://clinicaltrials.gov/ct2/show/NCT00718939) and the Rheos HOPE4HF trial (available at https://clinicaltrials.gov/ct2/show/NCT00957073), both of which are randomized, controlled assessments of BAT in patients with relatively preserved left ventricular ejection fraction, and the XR-1 Randomized Heart Failure Study of 150 NYHA class III heart failure patients with left ventricular ejection fraction of ≤35% (available at https://clinicaltrials.gov/ct2/show/NCT01471860).

Caution should be exercised when examining the ongoing trials of new modalities for heart failure. In addition to the inherent difficulty of ensuring true double-blindness of these interventional and device-based treatment modalities, a major criticism is that most of the studies have used soft endpoints, such as changes in echocardiographic findings or periprocedural safety, rather than hard endpoints, such as cardiovascular mortality or events requiring hospitalization.

Conclusions

Although intriguing, the results obtained via a procedure based on electrical stimulation of carotid baroreceptors for the treatment of resistant hypertension and heart failure leave open a number of clinically relevant questions that call for new investigations. Nevertheless, baroreceptor stimulation provides a new therapeutic option for these conditions and also for other clinical conditions, characterized by marked sympathetic activation, such as renal failure, obesity, and metabolic syndrome.

REFERENCES

1. Grassi G, Mark AL, Esler M. The sympathetic nervous system alterations in human hypertension. *Circ Res.* 2015;116:976–990.
2. Seravalle G, Lonati L, Buzzi S, et al. Sympathetic nerve traffic and baroreflex function in optimal, normal and high-normal blood pressure states. *J Hypertens.* 2015;33:1411–1417.
3. Grassi G, Seravalle G, Bertinieri G, et al. Sympathetic and reflex alterations in systo-diastolic and systolic hypertension of the elderly. *J Hypertens.* 2000;18:587–593.
4. Grassi G, Seravalle G, Brambilla G, et al. Marked sympathetic activation and baroreflex dysfunction in true resistant hypertension. *Int J Cardiol.* 2014;177:1020–1025.
5. Grassi G, Seravalle G, Dell'Oro R, et al. Adrenergic and reflex abnormalities in obesity-related hypertension. *Hypertension.* 2000;36:538–542.
6. Grassi G, Dell'Oro R, Quarti Trevano F, et al. Neuroadrenergic and reflex abnormalities in patients with metabolic syndrome. *Diabetologia.* 2005;48:1359–1365.
7. Somers VK, Dyken ME, Clary MP, et al. Sympathetic neural mechanisms in obstructive sleep apnea. *J Clin Invest.* 1995;96:1897–1904.
8. Grassi G, Seravalle G, Quarti Trevano F, et al. Adrenergic, metabolic, and reflex abnormalities in reverse and extreme dipper hypertensives. *Hypertension.* 2008;52:925–931.
9. Grassi G, Quarti Trevano F, Seravalle G, et al. Early sympathetic activation in the initial stages of chronic renal failure. *Hypertension.* 2011;57:846–851.
10. Hausberg M, Kosch M, Harmelink P, et al. Sympathetic nerve activity in end-stage renal disease. *Circulation.* 2002;106:1974–1979.
11. Hasking GJ, Esler MD, Jennings GL, et al. Norepinephrine spillover to plasma in patients with congestive heart failure: evidence of increased overall and cardiorenal sympathetic nervous activity. *Circulation.* 1986;73:615–621.
12. Grassi G, Seravalle G, Cattaneo BM, et al. Sympathetic activation and loss of reflex sympathetic control in mild congestive heart failure. *Circulation.* 1995;92:3206–3211.
13. Mancia G, Mark AL. Arterial baroreflexes in humans. In: Shepherd JT, Abboud FM, eds. *Handbook of Physiology.* Bethesda, MD: American Physiologic Society; 1983:755–793.
14. Korner PI, Tomkin AM, Uther JB. Reflex and mechanical circulatory effects of graded Valsalva maneuvers in normal man. *J Appl Physiol.* 1976;40:434–440.
15. Korner PI, Tomkin AM, Uther JB. Valsalva constrictor and heart rate reflexes in subjects with essential hypertension and normal blood pressure. *Clin Exp Pharmacol Physiol.* 1979;6:97–110.
16. Eckberg DL, Cavanaugh MS, Mark AL, et al. A simplified neck suction device for activation of carotid baroreceptors. *J Lab Clin Med.* 1975;85:167–173.
17. Ludbrook J, Mancia G, Ferrari A, et al. The variable neck-chamber method for studying the carotid baroreflex in man. *Clin Sci Mol Med.* 1977;53:165–171.
18. Parati G, Di Rienzo M, Castiglioni P, et al. Daily-life baroreflex modulation: new perspectives from computer analysis of blood pressure and heart rate variability. In: Di Rienzo M, Mancia G, Parati G, et al., eds. *Computer Analysis of Cardiovascular Signals.* Amsterdam: IOS Press; 1995:209–218.
19. Iellamo F, Hughson RL, Castrucci F, et al. Evaluation of spontaneous baroreflex modulation of sinus node during isometric exercise in healthy humans. *Am J Physiol.* 1994;267:H994–H1001.

20. Di Rienzo M, Bertinieri G, Mancia G, et al. A new method for evaluating the baroreflex role by a joint pattern analysis of pulse interval and systolic blood pressure series. *Med Biol Eng Comput.* 1985;23:313–314.
21. Parati G, Di Rienzo M, Castiglioni P, et al. Spontaneous baroreflex sensitivity: from the cardiovascular laboratory to patient's bedside. In: Di Rienzo M, Mancia G, Parati G, et al., eds. *Frontiers of Blood Pressure and Heart Rate Analysis.* Amsterdam: IOS Press; 1997:219–240.
22. De Boer RW, Karemaker JM, Strackee J. Haemodynamic fluctuations and baroreflex sensitivity in humans: a beat-to-beat model. *Am J Physiol.* 1987;253:H680–H689.
23. Robbe HWJ, Mulder LJM, Ruddel H, et al. Assessment of baroreceptor reflex sensitivity by means of spectral analysis. *Hypertension.* 1987;10:538–543.
24. Saul JP, Berger RD, Albrecht P, et al. Transfer function analysis of the circulation: unique insights into cardiovascular regulation. *Am J Physiol.* 1991;251:H1231–H1245.
25. Parati G, Saul JP, Di Rienzo M, et al. Spectral analysis of blood pressure and heart rate variability in evaluating cardiovascular regulation. A critical appraisal. *Hypertension.* 1995;25:1276–1286.
26. Mancia G, Ludbrook J, Ferrari A, et al. Baroreceptor reflexes in human hypertension. *Circ Res.* 1978;43:170–177.
27. McCubbin JW, Green JH, Page IH. Baroreceptor function in chronic renal hypertension. *Circ Res.* 1956;4:205–210.
28. Werner HR. The frequency-dependent nature of blood pressure regulation by the carotid sinus studied with an electrical analog. *Circ Res.* 1958;6:35–40.
29. Bilgutay A, Lillehei W. Treatment hypertension with an implantable electronic device. *JAMA.* 1965;191:113–117.
30. Tuckman J, Reich T, Lyon A, et al. Electrical stimulation of the sinus nerves in hypertensive patients—clinical evaluation and physiological studies. *Hypertension.* 1967;194:23–38.
31. Peters T, Koralewski HE, Zerbst F. The principle of electrical carotid sinus nerve stimulation: a nerve pacemaker system for angina pectoris and hypertension therapy. *Ann Biomed Eng.* 1980;8:445–458.
32. Wallin BG, Sundlof G, Delius W. The effect of carotid sinus nerve stimulation on muscle and skin nerve sympathetic activity in man. *Pflugers Arch.* 1975;358:101–110.
33. Lohmeier TE, Iliescu R. Chronic lowering of blood pressure by carotid baroreflex activation. Mechanisms and potential for hypertension therapy. *Hypertension.* 2011;57:880–886.
34. Gassler JP, Bisognano JD. Baroreflex activation therapy in hypertension. *J Hum Hypertens.* 2014;28:469–474.
35. Bakris GL, Nadim MK, Haller H, et al. Baroreflex activation therapy provides durable benefit in patients with resistant hypertension: results of long-term follow-up in the Rheos Pivotal Trial. *J Am Soc Hypertens.* 2012;6:152–158.
36. Hoppe UC, Brandt MC, Wachter R, et al. Minimally invasive system for baroreflex activation therapy chronically lowers blood pressure with pacemaker-like safety profile: results from the Barostim neo trial. *J Am Soc Hypertens.* 2012;6:270–276.
37. Gronda E, Seravalle G, Brambilla G, et al. Chronic baroreceptor activation effects on sympathetic nerve traffic, baroreflex function, and cardiac hemodynamics in heart failure: a proof-of-concept study. *Eur J Heart Fail.* 2014;16:977–983.

38. Illig KA, Levy M, Sanchez L, et al. An implantable carotid sinus stimulator for drug-resistant hypertension: surgical technique and short term outcome from the multicenter phase II Rheos feasibility trial. *J Vasc Surg.* 2006;44:1213–1218.
39. Wustmann K, Kucera JP, Scheffers I, et al. Effects of chronic baroreceptor stimulation on the autonomic cardiovascular regulation in patients with drug-resistant arterial hypertension. *Hypertension.* 2009;54:530–536.
40. Heusser K, Tank J, Engeli S, et al. Carotid baroreceptor stimulation, sympathetic activity, baroreflex function, and blood pressure in hypertensive patients. *Hypertension.* 2010;55:619–626.
41. Kroon A, Schmidli J, Scheffers I, et al. Chronically implanted system: 4-year data of Rheos DEBuT-HT Study in patients with resistant hypertension. *J Hypertens.* 2010;28:e441.
42. Bisognano JD, Bakris G, Nadim MK, et al. Baroreflex activation therapy lowers blood pressure in patients with resistant hypertension: results from the double-blind, randomized, placebo-controlled Rheos Pivotal Trial. *J Am Coll Cardiol.* 2011;58:765–773.
43. Scheffers I, Kroon AA, de Leeuw P. Renal hemodynamic during chronic therapy with electrical stimulation of the carotid sinus in humans. *J Hypertens.* 2008;26:S465.
44. Go AS, Mozaffarian D, Roger VL, et al. American Heart Association Statistics Committee and Stroke Statistics Subcommittee. Heart disease and stroke statistics – 2014 update: a report from the American Heart Association. *Circulation.* 2014;129:e28–e292.
45. Porter TR, Eckberg DL, Fritsch JM, et al. Autonomic pathophysiology in heart failure patients. Sympathetic–cholinergic interrelations. *J Clin Invest.* 1990;85:1362–1371.
46. Cohn JN, Levine TB, Olivari MT, et al. Plasma norepinephrine as a guide to prognosis in patients with chronic congestive heart failure. *N Engl J Med.* 1984;311:819–823.
47. Ferguson DW, Abboud FM, Mark AL. Selective impairment of baroreflex-mediated vasoconstrictor responses in patients with ventricular dysfunction. *Circulation.* 1984;69:451–460.
48. Singh JP, Kandala J, Camm AJ. Non-pharmacological modulation of the autonomic tone to treat heart failure. *Eur Heart J.* 2014;35:77–85.
49. Sabbah HN. Baroreflex activation for the treatment of heart failure. *Curr Cardiol Rep.* 2012;14:326–333.
50. Zucker IH, Hackley JF, Cornish KG, et al. Chronic baroreceptor activation enhances survival in dogs with pacing-induced heart failure. *Hypertension.* 2007;50:904–910.
51. Brandt MC, Madershahian N, Velden R, et al. Baroreflex activation as a novel therapeutic strategy for diastolic heart failure. *Clin Res Cardiol.* 2011;100:249–251.
52. Gronda E, Seravalle G, Quarti Trevano F, et al. Long-term chronic baroreflex activation: persistent efficacy in patients with heart failure and reduced ejection fraction. *J Hypertens.* 2015;33:1704–1708.
53. Abraham WT, Zile MR, Weaver FA, et al. Baroreflex activation therapy for the treatment of heart failure with a reduced ejection fraction. *JACC Heart Fail.* 2015;3:487–496.

137 Spinal Cord Stimulation for Heart Failure and Arrhythmias

Mark J. Shen and Douglas P. Zipes

Background

Heart failure (HF) and many ventricular arrhythmias are associated with cardiac autonomic imbalance—decreased parasympathetic activity[1,2] and hyperactive sympathetic activity.[3–5] While β-blockers remain a cornerstone therapy for both conditions, interventional and device-based therapies, including spinal cord stimulation (SCS), aiming to "rebalance" the autonomic activity have been under investigation as additive therapeutic modalities to reduce the incidence of lethal arrhythmias and to improve heart function and quality of life among patients with HF.[6] The latter is an ever-growing population that continues to burden the public health system.[7]

For many years, SCS has been used clinically to treat chronic pain (approved in the United States) as well as peripheral vascular disease and refractory angina (in Europe). It involves the placement of an epidural stimulation lead with distal poles at the upper thoracic level. The lead is connected to an implanted pulse generator in the paraspinal lumbar region (Fig. 137.1). SCS is typically applied at 90% of the maximum tolerated voltage at a frequency of 50 Hz and a pulse width of 0.2 ms. Various studies have applied different stimulation levels and duty cycles, and these nuances may explain the differential effects and efficacies among studies (see the following text).

How Spinal Cord Stimulation Affects the Cardiac Autonomic Tone

Several studies have sought to delineate the underlying mechanisms of how SCS affects the heart. During cardiac ischemia, the heightened excitability of intrinsic cardiac neurons was found to be suppressed by SCS at the level of T_1–T_2 without affecting other cardiac indices, such as heart rate, aortic pressure, or left ventricular (LV) systolic or diastolic pressures.[8] The authors concluded that SCS may exert its antianginal effects partly by modifying intrinsic cardiac nerve activities. Transection of the subclavian ansae (sympathectomy) eliminated these effects, indicating that the effects of SCS on intrinsic cardiac neurons are mediated by intrathoracic sympathetic nerves. With SCS at the same level, Olgin et al.[9] demonstrated in canines that SCS increased the sinus cycle length and prolonged the atrioventricular (AV) nodal conduction (atrium-to-His interval). These effects were abolished after the transection of the bilateral cervical vagus nerves but not after the transection of the ansae subclaviae, suggesting that the negative chronotropic and dromotropic effects of SCS are vagally mediated. Another study by Bernstein et al.[10] showed that SCS at the T_1–T_5 level prolonged the atrial effective refractory period. Nonetheless, with the same stimulation parameters, SCS at this level was not associated with obvious chronotropic and dromotropic effects. These conflicting results depict complex neural interconnections between the spinal cord and cardiac autonomic system and suggest that SCS delivered over various segments of the spinal cord and/or at various stimulation strengths may preferentially activate certain inputs and modulate cardiac autonomic tone differently.

Preclinical Studies

In the same study by Bernstein et al.[10] with prolongation of atrial effective refractory period, early application of SCS substantially decreased the atrial fibrillation (AF) burden and inducibility by rapid atrial pacing.[10] The broader level of stimulation (T_1–T_5) may create a more balanced autonomic modulation, thereby divorcing SCS from pure vagal effects, which typically shorten the atrial effective refractory period. This echoes the observation that subthreshold cervical vagus nerve stimulation (without noticeable effects on heart rate) significantly reduced AF in a canine study.[11] In another canine study,[12] SCS at the T_1–T_2 level during transient myocardial ischemia caused a marked reduction in combined ventricular tachycardia (VT) and ventricular fibrillation (VF) events from 59% to 23% in dogs with postinfarct HF. Consistent with the aforementioned study by Olgin et al.,[9] this antiarrhythmic effect was associated with a reduction in the sinus rate, prolongation of the PR interval, and lowering of the blood pressure. The antisympathetic properties of SCS were further supported by two canine studies that directly measured the sympathetic nerve activity. In anesthetized dogs, Wang et al. showed that SCS suppressed left stellate ganglion nerve activity during an acute myocardial infarction.[13] Garlie et al. found that in ambulatory dogs following myocardial infarction and tachypacing-induced HF, SCS significantly attenuated the augmented stellate ganglion nerve activity.[14] Histologically, SCS is associated with the reversion of deleterious neuronal remodeling during atrial tachypacing, such as the upregulation of nerve growth factor and downregulation of small conductance calcium-activated potassium channel type 2 in the stellate ganglion and intrinsic cardiac ganglia,[15] which is similar to the effect seen in direct vagus nerve stimulation.[16]

The chronic cardioprotective effect of SCS in HF was best demonstrated in a canine study by Lopshire et al.[17] In this study, canines underwent foam embolization to the left anterior descending coronary artery to induce myocardial infarction followed by ventricular tachypacing for 3 weeks to induce HF. Animals were randomized to four groups: SCS at T_4 delivered at 90% motor threshold, 50 Hz, 0.2-ms pulse width, for 2 hours three times daily; standard medical therapy (carvedilol + ramipril); SCS plus medical therapy; and controls. After 10 weeks, significant decreases in spontaneous and ischemic ventricular arrhythmias, compared with the control group, were noted in animals assigned to the SCS, medical therapy,

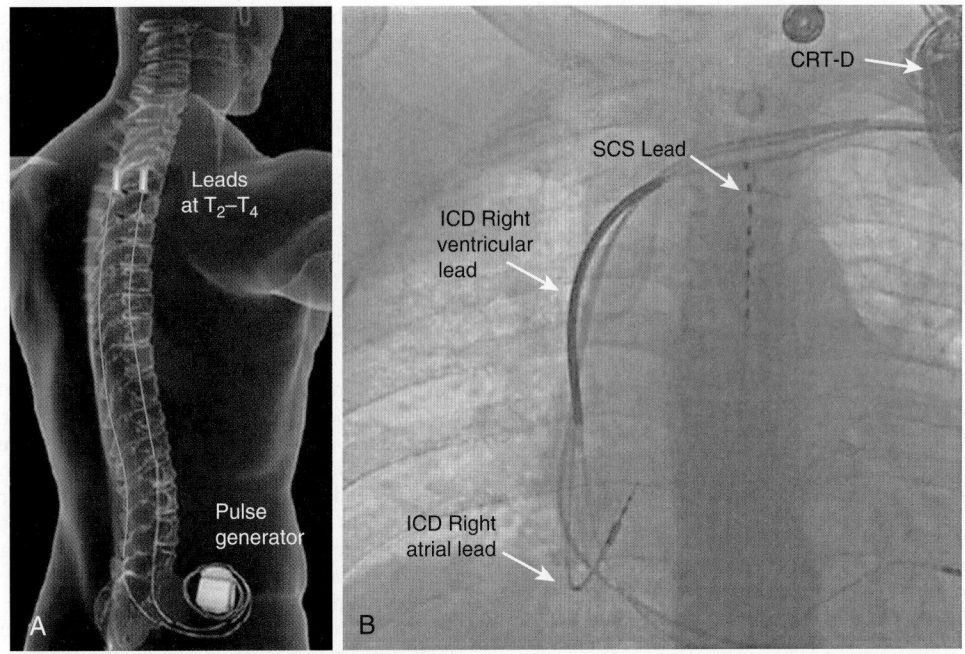

FIGURE 137.1 Spinal cord stimulation (*SCS*). (A) Schematic representation of an SCS system. (B) X-ray image showing the placement of the SCS lead with concurrent cardiac resynchronization therapy-defibrillator (*CRT-D*) device and leads. *ICD*, Implantable cardioverter defibrillator. (From Torre-Amione G, Alo K, Estep JD, et al. Spinal cord stimulation is safe and feasible in patients with advanced heart failure: early clinical experience. *Eur J Heart Fail.* 2014;16:788-795.)

and SCS plus medical therapy groups, with the SCS group showing the greatest decrease in ventricular tachyarrhythmias. Furthermore, clinical HF parameters such as resting heart rate, systolic blood pressures, and oxygen saturation were all significantly improved in dogs receiving SCS. This clinical improvement was accompanied by recovery of LV ejection fraction (LVEF) (from 17% to 52%) (Fig. 137.2) and reversal of LV dilatation. Correspondingly, serum norepinephrine and B-type natriuretic peptide levels were reduced after the completion of treatment interval in dogs receiving SCS compared with the standard medical therapy group or control group. These findings suggest that SCS acts via a discrete mechanism from standard HF medical therapy, which focused on β-blockade and renin-angiotensin-aldosterone axis blockade. A comprehensive neural modulatory effect that involves both extrinsic and intrinsic cardiac nerves is the likely explanation of its particular beneficial efficacy. A subsequent study demonstrated that the greatest effects were achieved with stimulation at the T_1–T_4 level.[18]

Clinical Trials

Based on the promising preclinical data, several clinical studies[19–22] have been performed to test whether SCS is safe and able to improve outcomes in patients with HF or arrhythmias. In a recent case series involving two patients with a high VT/VF burden, administration of SCS chronically for 2 months was associated with a reduction of VT/VF events.[19] With respect to SCS in HF patients, a small, prospective trial that enrolled nine patients with LVEF ≤ 30% and New York Heart Association (NYHA) class III HF symptoms while on optimal medical therapy has been published.[20] During the 7-month follow-up, five patients had improved symptoms by at least one NYHA class and three were unchanged, while no one worsened. Despite the small sample size, this study demonstrated the safety and feasibility of SCS in patients with advanced HF. In particular, SCS did not affect the functions (sensing,

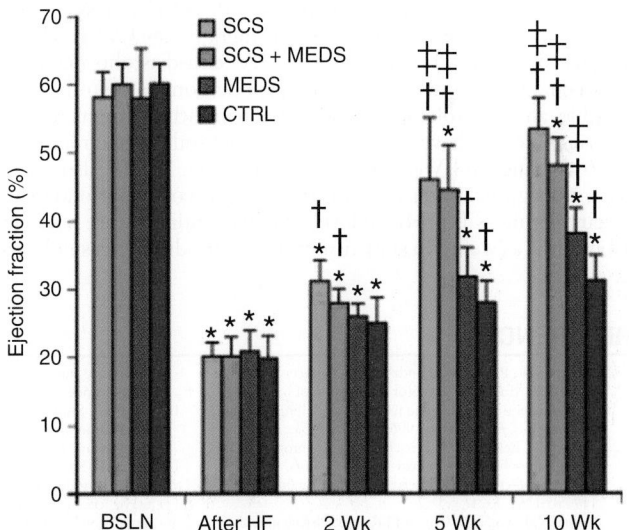

FIGURE 137.2 Spinal cord stimulation (*SCS*) improves left ventricular function in experimental heart failure. *BSLN,* Baseline; *After HF,* after heart failure induction; *2 wk,* after 2 weeks of neuromodulation stage; *5 wk,* after 5 weeks of neuromodulation stage; *10 wk,* after 10 weeks (completion) of neuromodulation stage. * $p < .05$ versus group baseline. † $p < .05$ versus group after heart failure induction, ‡ $p < .05$ versus control group at the same time point. (From Lopshire JC, Zhou X, Dusa C, et al. Spinal cord stimulation improves ventricular function and reduces ventricular arrhythmias in a canine postinfarction heart failure model. *Circulation.* 2009;120:286-294.)

detection, and therapy delivery) of the implantable cardioverter defibrillator (ICD). In another larger, prospective, multicenter trial (SCS HEART study[21]) with 22 patients, SCS was found to be safe, and it improved symptoms, functional status, and LV function and remodeling in patients with severe, symptomatic, systolic HF.

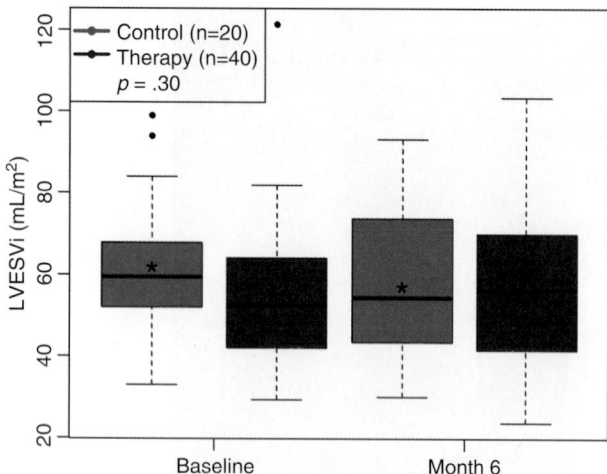

FIGURE 137.3 Spinal cord stimulation (SCS) did not change left ventricular end-systolic volume index (*LVESi*) at 6 months. The dotted lines represent the individual patients, while the solid line represents mean with SCS "off" in *red* and SCS "on" in *blue*. Sixty-two patients completed a 6-month visit, but two echoes were unreadable and excluded, leaving 40 SCS "on" patients and 20 SCS "off" patients contributing to the primary endpoint. (From Zipes DP, Neuzil P, Theres H, et al. Determining the feasibility of spinal cord neuromodulation for the treatment of chronic systolic heart failure: the DEFEAT-HF study. *JACC Heart Fail.* 2016;4:129-136.)

The largest human trial to date is the DEFEAT-HF trial.[22] It was a prospective, multicenter, randomized, placebo-controlled investigation that studied 66 patients with NYHA class III HF symptoms while on optimal medical therapy, an LVEF ≤35%, a QRS duration <120 ms, and an LV end-diastolic diameter between 55 and 80 mm. SCS was again demonstrated to be safe, feasible, and well tolerated; however, at 6 months, patients receiving SCS did not show significant LV structural reverse remodeling (no change in LV end-systolic volume, Fig. 137.3). Also, there were no significant changes in peak oxygen consumption (VO_2) or circulating NT-proBNP levels. Similar findings were noted at 12 months as well. No statistically significant differences in heart rates were observed between control and therapy arms. Among 19 control and 33 therapy patients that had concomitant ICDs with device data available for analysis, no statistically significant differences were observed in treated VT/VF episodes or the rate of nonsustained VT and premature ventricular complexes.

The authors of the latter study concluded that a number of potential reasons may explain the apparent contradictory results between DEFEAT-HF and SCS HEART. First, in DEFEAT-HF, SCS was applied at T_2–T_4 with a single stimulation electrode, whereas in SCS HEART, it was applied at slightly higher level at T_1–T_3 using dual electrodes, with one targeted at the midline and the other left of the midline. Second, an intermittent stimulation cycle (12 hours per day) was used in DEFEAT-HF, while in SCS HEART, stimulation was on with a continuous duty cycle of 24 hours per day, which may be more effective, at least in a porcine model.[23] As observed in preclinical studies, SCS at different levels and/or stimulation parameters might differentially activate cardiac autonomic input, thereby contrasting therapeutic efficacies and clinical outcomes. A third difference is that SCS HEART was a single-arm study without an actual control group and therefore subjected to a placebo effect. Future studies should monitor physiological responses to SCS so that appropriate stimulation parameters can be selected. Duty cycle, frequency, intensity of stimulation, and electrode shape and position can all affect outcomes as seen in the recent cervical vagal stimulation studies that showed no effect in the NECTAR-HF study[24] but an improvement in 6-month LVEF and LV end-systolic volume in the ANTHEM-HF trial.[25]

Conclusions

Despite the promising results of multiple preclinical studies and smaller human trials, the negative results of the DEFEAT-HF are disappointing. As Thomas Huxley famously remarked, "the great tragedy of science is the slaying of a beautiful hypothesis by an ugly fact" (Presidential Address at the British Association in 1870). Given the lack of information regarding what constitutes appropriate stimulation parameters, level of stimulation, and patient selection, it may be premature to conclude that SCS will not have a role in treating patients with systolic HF in the future. Further studies are warranted.

REFERENCES

1. Newton GE, Parker AB, Landzberg JS, Colucci WS, Parker JD. Muscarinic receptor modulation of basal and beta-adrenergic stimulated function of the failing human left ventricle. *J Clin Invest.* 1996;98:2756–2763.
2. Porter TR, Eckberg DL, Fritsch JM, et al. Autonomic pathophysiology in heart failure patients. Sympathetic-cholinergic interrelations. *J Clin Invest.* 1990;85:1362–1371.
3. Cohn JN, Levine TB, Olivari MT, et al. Plasma norepinephrine as a guide to prognosis in patients with chronic congestive heart failure. *N Engl J Med.* 1984;311:819–823.
4. Hasking GJ, Esler MD, Jennings GL, Burton D, Johns JA, Korner PI. Norepinephrine spillover to plasma in patients with congestive heart failure: evidence of increased overall and cardiorenal sympathetic nervous activity. *Circulation.* 1986;73:615–621.
5. Shen MJ, Zipes DP. Role of the autonomic nervous system in modulating cardiac arrhythmias. *Circ Res.* 2014;114:1004–1021.
6. Shen MJ, Zipes DP. Interventional and device-based autonomic modulation in heart failure. *Heart Fail Clin.* 2015;11:337–348.
7. Yancy CW, Jessup M, Bozkurt B, et al. 2013 ACCF/AHA guideline for the management of heart failure: executive summary: a report of the American College of Cardiology Foundation/American Heart Association Task Force on practice guidelines. *Circulation.* 2013;128:1810–1852.
8. Foreman RD, Linderoth B, Ardell JL, et al. Modulation of intrinsic cardiac neurons by spinal cord stimulation: implications for its therapeutic use in angina pectoris. *Cardiovasc Res.* 2000;47:367–375.
9. Olgin JE, Takahashi T, Wilson E, Vereckei A, Steinberg H, Zipes DP. Effects of thoracic spinal cord stimulation

on cardiac autonomic regulation of the sinus and atrioventricular nodes. *J Cardiovasc Electrophysiol.* 2002;13:475–481.
10. Bernstein SA, Wong B, Vasquez C, et al. Spinal cord stimulation protects against atrial fibrillation induced by tachypacing. *Heart Rhythm.* 2012;9:1426–1433. e3.
11. Shen MJ, Shinohara T, Park HW, et al. Continuous low-level vagus nerve stimulation reduces stellate ganglion nerve activity and paroxysmal atrial tachyarrhythmias in ambulatory canines. *Circulation.* 2011;123:2204–2212.
12. Issa ZF, Zhou X, Ujhelyi MR, et al. Thoracic spinal cord stimulation reduces the risk of ischemic ventricular arrhythmias in a postinfarction heart failure canine model. *Circulation.* 2005;111:3217–3220.
13. Wang S, Zhou X, Huang B, et al. Spinal cord stimulation protects against ventricular arrhythmias by suppressing left stellate ganglion neural activity in an acute myocardial infarction canine model. *Heart Rhythm.* 2015;12:1628–1635.
14. Garlie JB, Zhou X, Shen MJ, et al. The increased ambulatory nerve activity and ventricular tachycardia in canine post-infarction heart failure is attenuated by spinal cord stimulation (abstract). *Heart Rhythm.* 2012:PO3–PO112.
15. Wang S, Zhou X, Huang B, et al. Spinal cord stimulation suppresses atrial fibrillation by inhibiting autonomic remodeling. *Heart Rhythm.* 2016;13:274–281.
16. Shen MJ, Hao-Che C, Park HW, et al. Low-level vagus nerve stimulation upregulates small conductance calcium-activated potassium channels in the stellate ganglion. *Heart Rhythm.* 2013;10:910–915.
17. Lopshire JC, Zhou X, Dusa C, et al. Spinal cord stimulation improves ventricular function and reduces ventricular arrhythmias in a canine postinfarction heart failure model. *Circulation.* 2009;120:286–294.

18. Lopshire JC, Zipes DP. Spinal cord stimulation for heart failure: preclinical studies to determine optimal stimulation parameters for clinical efficacy. *J Cardiovasc Transl Res.* 2014;7:321–329.
19. Grimaldi R, de Luca A, Kornet L, Castagno D, Gaita F. Can spinal cord stimulation reduce ventricular arrhythmias? *Heart Rhythm.* 2012;9:1884–1887.
20. Torre-Amione G, Alo K, Estep JD, et al. Spinal cord stimulation is safe and feasible in patients with advanced heart failure: early clinical experience. *Eur J Heart Fail.* 2014;16:788–795.
21. Tse HF, Turner S, Sanders P, et al. Thoracic Spinal Cord Stimulation for Heart Failure as a Restorative Treatment (SCS HEART study): first-in-man experience. *Heart Rhythm.* 2015;12:588–595.
22. Determining the Feasibility of Spinal Cord Neuromodulation for the Treatment of Chronic Heart Failure (DEFEAT-HF) available at http://clinicaltrials.gov/ct2/show/NCT01112579?term=NCT01112579&rank=1; Accessed August 10, 2011.
23. Tse HF, Lie Y, Zuo M, et al. Intermittent versus continuous spinal cord stimulation for treatment of ischemic heart failure. *Eur Heart J.* 2012;33:963–964.
24. Zannad F, De Ferrari GM, Tuinenburg AE, et al. Chronic vagal stimulation for the treatment of low ejection fraction heart failure: results of the NEural Cardiac TherApy foR Heart Failure (NECTAR-HF) randomized controlled trial. *Eur Heart J.* 2015;36:425–433.
25. Premchand RK, Sharma K, Mittal S, et al. Autonomic regulation therapy via left or right cervical vagus nerve stimulation in patients with chronic heart failure: results of the ANTHEM-HF trial. *J Card Fail.* 2014;20:808–816.

138 Renal Sympathetic Denervation

Jacob S. Koruth, Sujata Balulad, and Andre d'Avila

The sympathetic nervous system (SNS) modulates cardiovascular physiology via a complex system of central and peripheral neuroendocrine pathways that link the brain, heart, endothelium, nervous system, and kidneys. Several arrhythmias, such as atrial fibrillation (AF) and ventricular tachycardia/fibrillation (VT/VF), have been demonstrated to be influenced by abnormal autonomic tone.[1-3] The mechanisms by which autonomic activation is arrhythmogenic or antiarrhythmic are complex and different for each specific arrhythmia. However, the identification of specific autonomic triggers for different arrhythmias supports the approach of modulating autonomic activity in an attempt to prevent and treat these arrhythmias. Subsequently, strategies, such as vagal nerve stimulation, carotid baroreceptor stimulation, spinal cord stimulation, ganglionated plexi (GP) ablation, and cardiac sympathetic denervation, were developed and have been demonstrated to have beneficial effects on cardiac arrhythmias.[4]

Among the many inputs to the autonomic nervous system, the renal sympathetic system plays an important and rather unique role. Its influence on the SNS and cardiovascular system has therefore been targeted to beneficially influence cardiac arrhythmias. Renal sympathetic denervation (RSDN) is one such strategy that is achieved by interrupting the afferent and efferent sympathetic signaling between the kidney and the central SNS.

Renal Sympathetic System

The renal SNS consists of a network of postganglionic efferent fibers that run from the hypothalamus to the kidneys. The postganglionic efferent innervation of the kidneys passes from pre- and paravertebral ganglia (T10-L2) along the adventitial surface of the renal arteries. The afferent renal sympathetic nerves emerge mostly from the renal pelvic wall and are activated by stretch and chemoreceptors that can detect ischemia and biochemical changes. The afferent fibers also follow the course of the adventitial wall of the renal artery and make their way to the central autonomic centers via the dorsal root ganglia and to the contralateral kidneys. Stimulation of these nerves has been shown to have several cardiovascular effects (Fig. 138.1). Prominent among these effects is elevation of systemic blood pressure (BP). This occurs via two main mechanisms: (1) stimulation of α-adrenergic receptors that elicit direct vasoconstriction and (2) stimulation of β-adrenergic receptors of the juxtaglomerular apparatus that leads to sodium retention, decreased renal blood flow, and activation of the renin-angiotensin-aldosterone system. On the other hand, signals from sensory renal afferents help to regulate the overall sympathetic tone via modulation of posterior hypothalamic activity, which in turn further sustains renal efferent sympathetic activity.[5] However, the effect of the renal SNS on centrally mediated sympathetic control of the heart is of significant interest in the field of cardiac electrophysiology.

Renal Sympathetic Denervation

RSDN was initially explored as a treatment option for uncontrolled hypertension (HTN) based on the abovementioned pathophysiology and supportive data from experimental models and prior clinical data. The SYMPLICITY HTN (Renal Sympathetic Denervation in Patients with Treatment-Resistant Hypertension) trials recently demonstrated that sympathetic nerve fibers along the renal arterial vasculature could be targeted by percutaneous catheter ablation using a specialized radiofrequency (RF) ablation catheter.[6,7] The first proof-of-concept study in this series, SYMPLICITY HTN-1, was a nonrandomized study of drug-resistant hypertensive patients, and it demonstrated substantial reductions in BP.[8] The long-term follow-up of this trial further demonstrated decreases of 10 mm Hg or more in systolic BP in 69% of patients at 1 month, 85% at 12 months, and 93% at 36 months with good safety. SYMPLICITY HTN-2, a randomized study, subsequently demonstrated that at 6 months, 84% of patients who underwent renal denervation had a reduction in systolic BP of 10 mm Hg or more compared with 35% of controls ($p < .0001$). Finally, SYMPLICITY HTN-3, a larger randomized sham-controlled trial, surprisingly did not meet its primary efficacy endpoint, showing no benefit of RSDN on systolic BP compared with controls.[9] There has been much controversy over the contrasting results of these trials, and a number of possible explanations have been offered as to why SYMPLICITY HTN-3 had negative findings. Inadequate ablation of the renal SNS is one such potential explanation. These potential explanations, an improved understanding of the limitations of the current approach, and availability of newer and potentially more efficacious approaches to RSDN have kept the interest in RSDN alive.[10] One must note that RSDN, besides its demonstrated effect on BP, also led to a reduction in efferent muscle sympathetic nerve activity, a marker of central sympathetic output. On this basis, RSDN and its potential impact on sympathetically modulated cardiac arrhythmias have been evaluated in several studies.

Renal Sympathetic Denervation and Atrial Fibrillation

Conditions associated with increased sympathetic activation, such as HTN, heart failure (HF), and sleep apnea, have been demonstrated to result in structural, neural, and electrophysiological changes within the atria. In addition, autonomic activity has been shown to play a significant role in the initiation of AF and in the creation of an arrhythmogenic atrial substrate.[11-13] The role of autonomic modulation of AF is further supported by preclinical studies. One such important preclinical study used implanted radio transmitters to demonstrate that spontaneous sympathetic (from left stellate ganglion) and parasympathetic (vagus nerve)

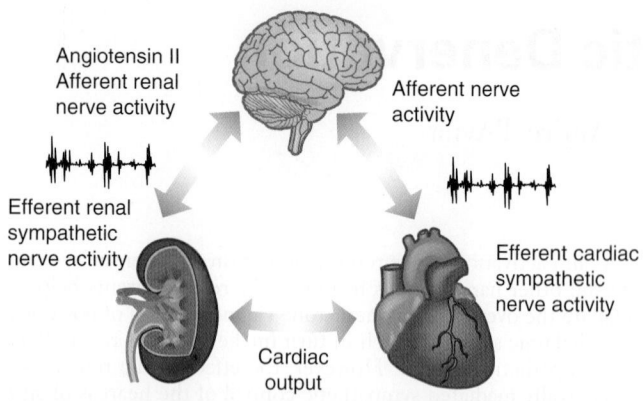

FIGURE 138.1 Summary of the actions of renal sympathetic nerves on cardiac function. Increased sympathetic nerve activity to the kidney has the potential not only to increase cardiac output via increased filling pressure but also to increase renal afferent nerve activity and circulating angiotensin II concentrations, which in turn centrally acts to increase cardiac sympathetic nerve activity. (From Symposium report: Barrett, CJ. Renal sympathetic nerves–what have they got to do with cardiovascular disease? *Exp Physiol.* 2015;100:359-365.)

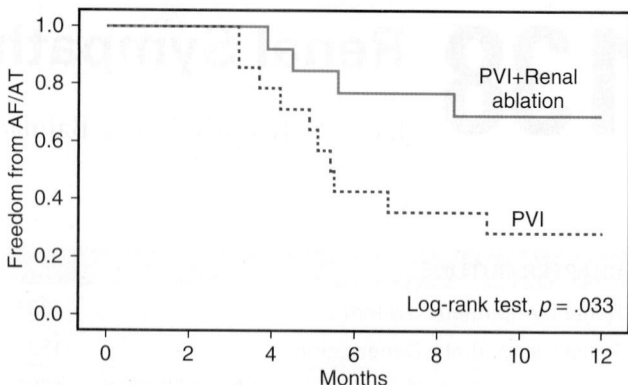

FIGURE 138.2 Incidence of atrial fibrillation (*AF*) recurrences in patients with and without renal artery denervation. The study arm with pulmonary vein isolation (*PVI*) and renal artery ablation had significantly reduced AF recurrence rate over time compared with the control PVI–only group. *AT*, Atrial tachyarrhythmia. (From Pokushalov E, Romanov A, Corbucci G, et al. A randomized comparison of pulmonary vein isolation with versus without concomitant renal artery denervation in patients with refractory symptomatic atrial fibrillation and resistant hypertension. *J Am Coll Cardiol.* 2012;60:1163-1170.)

nerve activity was observed to precede the onset of paroxysmal AF in ambulatory dogs with rapid atrial pacing.[14] Cryoablation of bilateral stellate ganglia and of the superior cardiac branches of the left vagus nerve eliminated all such episodes of paroxysmal AF in these animals. Furthermore, a recent randomized clinical trial compared the efficacy of pulmonary vein isolation (PVI), GP ablation alone, and PVI followed by GP ablation. After 2 years of follow-up, freedom from AF was achieved in 56%, 48%, and 74%, respectively, supporting the role of autonomic modulation via GP ablation. Based on these studies, investigators have explored the effects of RSDN in the management of AF.

Preclinical Data

Several preclinical studies support the role of RSDN in AF. A porcine study by Linz et al. demonstrated that RSDN significantly increased the RR interval and atrioventricular nodal conduction times during sinus rhythm, lowered ventricular rates during AF, and significantly shortened duration of pacing-induced AF episodes.[15] A more recent preclinical study by Linz et al., comparing RSDN against a sham procedure, demonstrated reduced atrial sympathetic nerve sprouting, lower atrial endomysial content, and lower AF complexity in animals with persistent AF, independent of changes in BP.[16] In further support of the role of renal SNS in AF, authors used a porcine model of obstructive sleep apnea to demonstrate that compared with atenolol, RSDN significantly reduced AF inducibility and also attenuated atrial effective refractory period (ERP) shortening to a greater extent than atenolol.[17] In addition, RSDN resulted in the inhibition of spontaneous episodes of AF, AF duration, and spontaneous atrial premature beats. These and many other studies provide the foundation on which investigators have explored the role of RSDN in the management of AF.

Clinical Data

Clinical data concerning the roles of RSDN and AF are limited to a few studies only. Pokushalov and colleagues prospectively randomized patients with symptomatic AF (paroxysmal and persistent) and drug-resistant HTN (systolic BP >160 mm Hg, despite triple drug therapy) to one of the following two arms: PVI only (n = 14) versus PVI with RSDN (n = 13).[18] At the 12-month follow-up, significant reductions in systolic (from 181 to 156 mm Hg;

$p < .001$) and diastolic (from 97 to 87 mm Hg; $p < .001$) BPs were observed in patients treated with PVI and RSDN, without significant changes observed in the PVI only group. In terms of AF, 9 of 13 patients (69%) in the PVI with RSDN group were free of AF, whereas in the PVI-only group, only 4 of 14 patients (29%) were free of AF ($p = .033$) (Fig. 138.2). Subsequently, a separate analysis was performed where data from the aforementioned trial were combined with additional patients (86 patients). A significant difference in freedom from AF was limited to patients with severe HTN (>160/100 mm Hg), and no significant difference was observed in patients with moderate HTN.

Although these studies have significant limitations, they demonstrate that RSDN has the potential to offer incremental control of AF burden in patients with HTN and AF. However, it remains unclear if the mechanism of reduction of AF is mediated by reduced vascular tone and atrial unloading, diminished sympathetic activity, or both. The role of RSDN in non-HTN AF patients, however, is even more uncertain at this time. There are several ongoing/unreported clinical trials that aim to evaluate the safety and effectiveness of RSDN in the treatment of AF, and until the results of these trials are available, the efficacy of this procedure in AF management remains unknown. Some of these trials include A Feasibility Study to Evaluate the Effect of Concomitant Renal Denervation and Cardiac Ablation on AF Recurrence (RDN + AF), Adjunctive Renal Denervation to Modify Hypertension and Sympathetic Tone as Upstream Therapy in the Treatment of Atrial Fibrillation (H-FIB), and Ganglionated Plexi Ablation vs. Renal Denervation in Patients Undergoing Pulmonary Vein Isolation.

Other clinical effects of RSDN on atrial electrical properties have also been clinically described; electrocardiographical analysis of a study that included 136 patients with resistant HTN who underwent RSDN showed a reduction in sinus rate and an increase in the PR interval.[19]

Renal Sympathetic Denervation and Ventricular Arrhythmias

Despite significant advances in the management of ventricular arrhythmias (VAs), considerable challenges remain, given the frequent recurrences of VAs, despite using antiarrhythmic drugs and catheter-based cardiac ablation. The importance of the role of autonomic modulation in the management of VAs is widely

TABLE 138.1 Renal denervation outcomes for ventricular tachyarrhythmias: literature review

AUTHORS	CARDIAC ETIOLOGY	VENTRICULAR ARRHYTHMIA TYPE	FOLLOW-UP	POST-RSDN RECURRENCE/SUCCESS
Ukena et al.[34]	2 patients, HCM/DCM	VT/VF	6 months	1 recurrence at week 4, none after (first patient), and 12 episodes in 24 hours (second), none after
Hoffmann et al.[35]	1 patient, acute ischemia	VT	6 months	6 episodes in first month, none after
Staico et al.[36]	1 patient, DCM	VT	5 months	11 episodes in first month, none after
Remo et al.[37]	4 patients, ICM and DCM	VT	8.75 months	Mean of 2.5 episodes in first 4 months, none after
Scholz et al.[38]	1 patient, DCM	VT	5 months	1 episode in the second month, no further episode after
Hilbert et al.[39]	1 patient, ICM	VT	12 months	2 episodes within first week, none after
Kosiuk et al.[40]	1 patient, ICM	VT	10 months	No episodes
Armaganijan et al.[41]	10 patients, ICM, DCM, and Chagas disease	VT/VF	6 months	Median number of VT/VF episodes decreased from 28.5/20.5 to 1/0 at 1 month and 0/0 at 6 months
Ukena et al.[42]	13 patients, ischemic, DCM	VT/VF	1-13 months	Median number of VT/VF episodes decreased from 21 to 2 at 1 month and 0 at 3 months

DCM, Dilated cardiomyopathy; *HCM,* hypertrophic cardiomyopathy; *ICM,* ischemic cardiomyopathy; *RSDN,* renal sympathetic denervation; *VF,* ventricular fibrillation; *VT,* ventricular tachycardia.

appreciated. Besides preclinical studies in this area, multiple non-randomized clinical reports have demonstrated that autonomic interventions, such as cardiac sympathetic denervation (targeting stellate ganglia) and thoracic epidural anesthesia, have[20] beneficial effects[21] on certain VAs, such as those associated[22,23] with long QT syndrome and catecholaminergic polymorphic ventricular tachycardia. Given the recent recognition that RSDN offers another approach by which we can favorably affect the SNS, investigators have explored its utility in the setting of VA management. Besides potential direct antiarrhythmic effects of RSDN, its potential effects on HF[24] may also play an adjunctive role in VA suppression.

Preclinical Data

Several preclinical studies have examined the effect of RSDN on VAs. This chapter summarizes a few selected studies that demonstrate this. The effects of RSDN on VAs were assessed in a porcine model of myocardial infarction that was induced by ligation of the left anterior descending (LAD) artery.[25] Denervation was surgically performed in the intervention arm, and a sham arm was included. In animals that underwent RSDN, during LAD occlusion, the occurrence of spontaneous premature ventricular contractions (PVCs) was significantly reduced, as was the occurrence of VF. This antiarrhythmic effect was comparable with the effects of β-blockers in the same model.[25] Another canine study examining VAs during myocardial ischemia also demonstrated a reduction in spontaneous VAs.[26] In another study, 19 canines were studied across three arms: a control arm, an HF (rapid ventricular pacing) arm, and an HF and RSD arm.[27] Canines in the HF and RSDN group underwent bilateral catheter–based RSDN. The QT interval, QT dispersion (in sinus), and ventricular ERPs were noted to be longer in the HF arm than in the control and HF + RSDN arms. Occurrences of VAs, provoked by programmed ventricular stimulation, were also reduced in the RSDN arm.

Clinical Data

The first-in-man use of RSDN was performed in two patients who presented with refractory VA storm.[28] The first patient had hypertrophic cardiomyopathy with recurrent monomorphic VT, and the second patient had a history of dilated cardiomyopathy with recurrent polymorphic ventricular tachycardia.

After bilateral RSDN, VAs were reduced immediately in the first patient and after 24 hours in the second patient, followed by adequate control in the months afterward. Multiple other groups have demonstrated efficacy in small series and case reports, as shown in Table 138.1.

As can be inferred from the earlier reports, RSDN may have beneficial effects on VA control; however, the reader must be made aware that to date no large prospective randomized studies have been performed to evaluate the impact of RSDN for the prevention of recurrent VT. Furthermore, confounding interventions performed in some of the reports mentioned here may have resulted in an overestimation of perceived effects of RSDN. A number of ongoing trials, such as REnal SympathetiC denervation to sUpprEss Ventricular Tachyarrhythmias (RES-CUE-VT), REnal Sympathetic dEnervaTion as an adjunct to catheter-based VT ablation (RESET-VT), Renal Denervation in Patient Undergoing VT Ablation: Combined Renal Denervation and VT Ablation vs. Simply VT Ablation (ARDEVAT), will help develop an understanding of the efficacy and safety of this approach.

Percutaneous Techniques for Renal Sympathetic Denervation

The field of sympathetic denervation was initially limited to various surgical approaches that were developed six to seven decades ago for the treatment of severe HTN. However, these approaches[29] were very invasive as they targeted sympathetic structures within the thorax and abdomen and therefore also did not specifically target the renal SNS. Although this approach was soon clinically discontinued, it at the very least laid the foundation on which present-day minimally invasive approaches to renal denervation were developed.

The anatomical proximity of sympathetic nerves along the wall of the renal artery led to the novel concept of achieving denervation by applying RF energy from the luminal aspect of the renal artery using a catheter-based percutaneous approach. The concept was based on the creation of focal thermal injury within the wall of the artery that could damage the renal sympathetic nerve fibers embedded in the adventitia and beyond. By creating multiple such transmural ablation lesions along the course of the artery, it was hoped that the neural plexus that surrounds bilateral renal arteries would be damaged and the sympathetic signaling would be permanently interrupted.

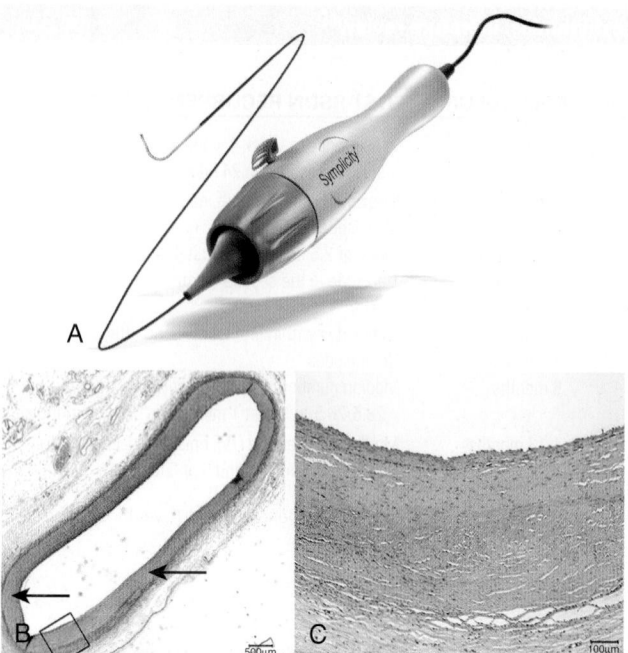

FIGURE 138.3 (A) Symplicity catheter system. (B and C) Six-month histology results showing the most extensive medial injury (up to 25% of the total media affected) that was noted in three sections of treated vessels. Both sections stained with Movat pentachrome. (B) The area of medial injury (*yellow-green*) is located between the *arrows*. (C) A higher magnification of a transmurally affected vessel wall (*rectangular area*) in (A). Sections show minimal intimal thickening and minimal internal elastic lamina injury overlying areas of mild full thickness medial fibrosis (*yellow* [fibrosis] with *green* [proteoglycan deposition]) and adventitial fibrosis (*yellow*). No significant inflammatory cells are present, suggesting that the healing process is complete. (Symplicity photo courtesy Medtronic, Inc.)

The first catheter-based renal denervation procedure for drug-resistant HTN was performed in 2007 using the Symplicity catheter system (Medtronic, Minneapolis, MN). This particular catheter has undergone the most clinical investigation to date compared with other catheters (Fig. 138.3). This catheter delivers low-level RF energy through the wall of the renal artery to achieve renal denervation. The Symplicity catheter is a 6-Fr guide–compatible steerable catheter that delivers unipolar RF to create multiple RF lesions within each renal artery in a helical fashion. The Symplicity generator delivers RF energy via a dynamic algorithm that continually monitors and adjusts the power input, considering impedance and temperature measurements. Numerous other ablation approaches over the past several years have been pursued and are at various development stages. Some examples of other RF-based devices include an ablation catheter with a basket-like deflectable tip that has four electrodes for simultaneous contact and energy delivery to the arterial wall (EnligHTN, multielectrode renal denervation system, St. Jude Medical, Minneapolis, MN). Two other noteworthy RF approaches use a balloon, one with multiple bipolar electrodes on its surface (Vessix Denervation System, Boston Scientific Corp., Natick, MA) and the other with helical electrodes on its outer surface and tip irrigation to reduce heat generation (OneShot, Covidien Inc, Mansfield, MA).

The use of standard electrophysiology RF ablation catheters[30] for RSDN is of particular interest to electrophysiologists. The use of irrigated RF ablation catheters (3.5-mm tip Thermocool catheter, Biosense Webster, Diamond Bar, CA) has been investigated in two studies. The utility of this catheter lies in (1) the familiarity electrophysiologists have with manipulating this catheter and their understanding of RF parameter selection and lesion creation; (2) the presence of saline irrigation that allows for deep lesion creation, reducing luminal thrombus formation, and the possibility of sparing the intimal layer from thermal injury; and (3) using the same catheter for ablating arrhythmia and performing RSDN. Authors have also demonstrated the utility of electroanatomical mapping systems that can allow reduction of fluoroscopic requirements and more importantly annotation of lesion location during the procedure (Fig. 138.4). The workflow described in one report[7] includes using a flexible 45-cm 8-Fr sheath (Arrow International, Inc., Reading, PA) that is advanced over the ablation catheter to engage the renal artery to allow for contrast visualization of the renal artery during catheter manipulation. The ablation catheter was then maneuvered within the renal artery to allow for serial energy delivery in a circumferential, longitudinally staggered manner to minimize the chance of renal artery stenosis. Energy titration was performed using a standard RF generator for cardiac ablation. Power was titrated to achieve a 10%–20% decrease in impedance at each location, with power settings typically varying between 10 and 15 watts. No more than five to seven ablation lesions, lasting 30–90 seconds each, were placed within each renal artery in this particular report. Of note, in this report, although acute procedural adverse events were not noted, nonstenotic luminal irregularities were frequently noted postablation on angiography. These irregularities were treated with intraarterial nitroglycerin, and at the 3-month follow-up, repeat renal angiography demonstrated resolution of these irregularities. However, one must be cautious with the use of these catheters within the narrow confines of the renal artery because small single-center studies do not offer sufficient safety data. It is likely that other renally focused ablation catheters will replace the use of these catheters as they will prove to be more effective and easier to use and possibly safer.

Some of the alternative approaches to RSDN utilize the delivery of ultrasound energy to cause nerve fiber damage. These approaches include the PARADISE system (ReCor Medical Inc., Ronkonkoma, NY) that uses an ultrasonic transducer that is centered within the renal artery lumen. The transducer delivers circumferential energy to ablate nerves. Another approach is to use local directed delivery systems to deliver pharmacological agents that cause nerve damage. An example of such technology is the Bullfrog microinfusion catheter (Mercator MedSystems Inc., San Leandro, CA), which is equipped with a microneedle and protective balloon system. Once the balloon catheter is positioned and inflated within the renal artery, a needle is unsheathed that then penetrates the vessel wall, enabling perivascular delivery of the pharmacological agent.[31]

All of these procedures, given their minimally invasive design, are performed under either deep sedation or general anesthesia. Typically, standard femoral arterial access is obtained, and a pigtail catheter is advanced to the abdominal aorta to perform contrast angiography. This allows the operator to localize and assess renal arteries for accessibility and appropriateness for RSDN. For the anatomy to be appropriate, identifying the take-off of each renal artery from the aorta must be amenable to catheter cannulation, and there must be no significant renal arterial atherosclerosis. Once the anatomy is deemed acceptable, the catheter is advanced under fluoroscopic guidance. The ablation catheter is then maneuvered within the renal artery to allow for energy delivery as required for the technology being used.

As in any percutaneous catheter–based arterial intervention, adverse events can occur. With renal denervation, besides arterial access–related complications, the occurrence of arterial occlusion, either from thermal injury with or without spasm or from arterial dissection, has been described. In case of the renal artery, this may lead to functional impairment of the perfused kidney. In the long term, renal arterial stenosis has been a significant concern, given the lack of understanding and the uncertainty that exists with respect to the long-term consequences of focal thermal injury to the renal arterial system. The promotion of local reactive changes, either proliferative or atherosclerotic, could in theory lead to the development of luminal occlusion down

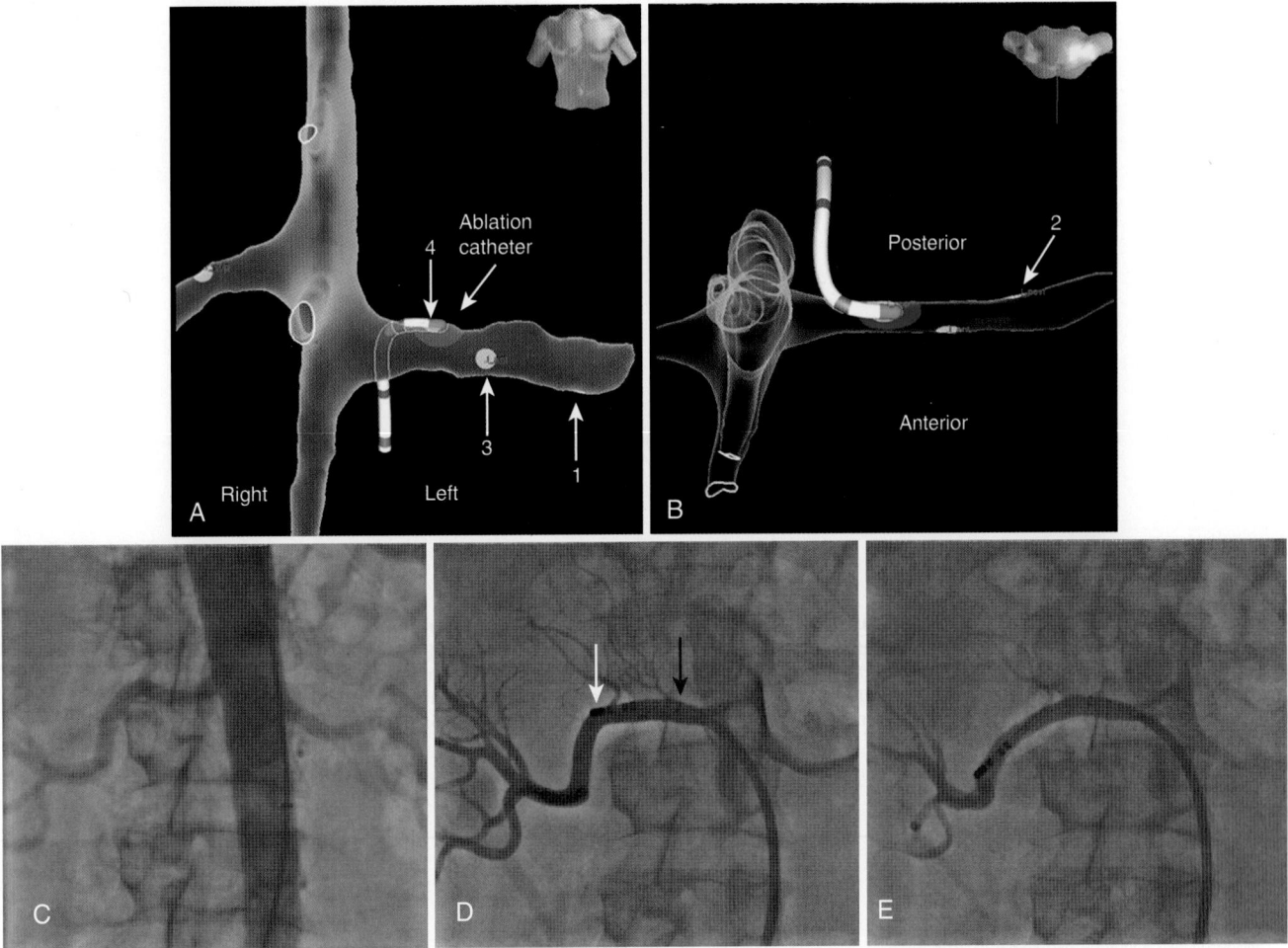

FIGURE 138.4 (A and B) Impedance-based electroanatomical mapping system used to visualize bilateral renal arteries with ablation catheter placed within the left renal artery. (C) Contrast injection into the abdominal aorta identifies the locations and number of renal arteries. (D) With the saline-irrigated radiofrequency ablation catheter (*white arrow* at tip) placed within the right renal artery, the vascular sheath (*black arrow* at tip) is advanced over the catheter into the artery, and contrast is injected to visualize the vessel. (E) Then the catheter is advanced along the superior aspect of the right renal artery to deliver radiofrequency energy at this site. ([A and B] From Miller MA, Gangireddy SR, Dukkipati SR, et al. Renal sympathetic denervation using an electroanatomic mapping system. *J Am Coll Cardiol.* 2014;63:1697.)

the road. Some such adverse events have been described with the Symplicity catheter; however, these events are rare and this particular catheter has been demonstrated to have a good safety profile, as per published data. Some of the many other RSDN technologies that have been developed lack sufficient long-term safety data, whereas some technologies offer approaches that in theory may be safer, given their ability to spare the luminal aspect of the artery, thereby reducing the risk for renal artery stenosis.

Conclusion

In light of the recently published negative SYMPLICITY-HTN 3 trial, several investigators have questioned the overall utility of this procedure as an antihypertensive intervention; this has resulted in significant waning of interest in this procedure. As a consequence, its antiarrhythmic efficacy has also been questioned. While it is apparent that rigorous trial designs are required to truly assess the role of RSDN in arrhythmias, data that exist as of today certainly merit further investigation of the role of RSDN in the field of electrophysiology.

The inability to measure the degree of denervation achieved after RSDN has always been considered to critically limit our understanding of the true potential of RSDN. Reports have raised the possibility that RSDN, as was done in the SYMPLICITY trials, was not optimal[32] (Fig. 138.5). An improved understanding of the location of renal SNS along the renal artery has been proposed; i.e., investigators have proposed that the preferential site of ablation may be more distal, nearer to the arterial branch points, rather than proximally within the main renal artery as was advocated during most of the studies.[33] In addition, it is possible that the RF power used was too low and nerves beyond 2–3 mm from the artery were therefore spared. This further supports the school of thought that considers that we may not have truly performed effective and consistent denervation with the Symplicity catheter system. Another proposed reason for the lack of effect of RSDN for resistant HTN is variability in the role that SNS plays in the pathogenesis of resistant HTN in patients.

All this therefore can be extrapolated to the antiarrhythmic effects of RSDN. As this field continues to evolve and as renal denervation becomes more efficacious, safe, and even quantifiable, its role in the field of electrophysiology will become increasingly clear. In the meantime, ongoing trials examining the effects of RSDN on AF and VA will add to our evolving assessment of the effectiveness of RSDN.

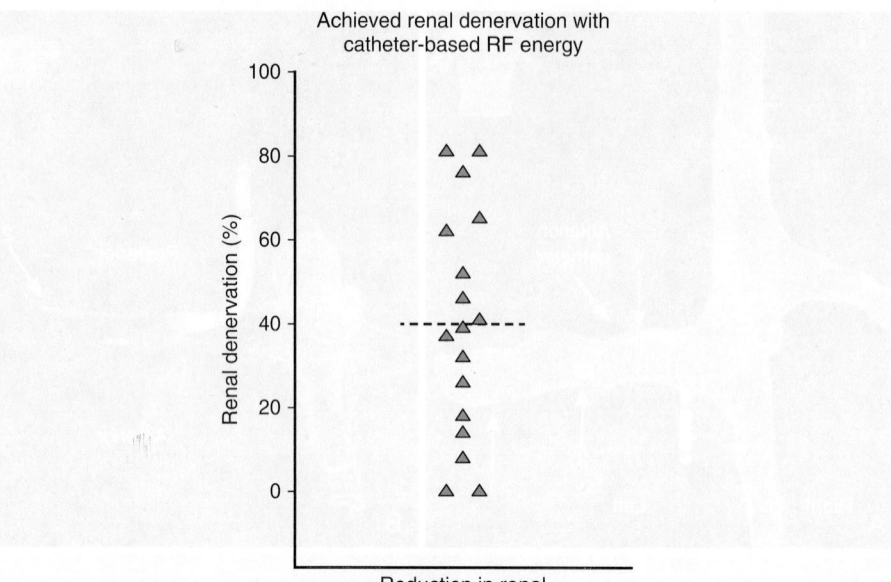

FIGURE 138.5 Renal norepinephrine spillover measurements made before and 30 days after the procedure. The pronounced nonuniformity between patients suggests denervation was incomplete. *RF,* Radiofrequency. (From Esler M. Renal denervation for treatment of drug-resistant hypertension. *Trends Cardiovasc Med.* 2015;25:107-115.)

REFERENCES

1. Brunner-La Rocca HP, Esler MD, Jennings GL, et al. Effect of cardiac sympathetic nervous activity on mode of death in congestive heart failure. *Eur Heart J.* 2001;22:1136–1143.
2. Kaye DM, Lefkovits J, Jennings GL, et al. Adverse consequences of high sympathetic nervous activity in the failing human heart. *J Am Coll Cardiol.* 1995;26:1257–1263.
3. Shen MJ, Zipes DP. Role of the autonomic nervous system in modulating cardiac arrhythmias. *Circ Res.* 2014;114:1004–1021.
4. Hou Y, Zhou Q, Po SS. Neuromodulation for cardiac arrhythmia. *Heart Rhythm.* 2016;13:584–592.
5. Johns EJ, Kopp UC, DiBona GF. Neural control of renal function. *Compr Physiol.* 2011;1:731–767.
6. Esler MD, Krum H, Sobotka PA, et al. Renal sympathetic denervation in patients with treatment-resistant hypertension (the Symplicity HTN-2 trial): a randomised controlled trial. *Lancet.* 2010;376:1903–1909.
7. Ahmed H, Neuzil P, Skoda J, et al. Renal sympathetic denervation using an irrigated radiofrequency ablation catheter for the management of drug-resistant hypertension. *JACC Cardiovasc Interv.* 2012;5:758–765.
8. Simplicity HTN-1 Investigators. Catheter-based renal sympathetic denervation for resistant hypertension: durability of blood pressure reduction out to 24 months. *Hypertension.* 2011;57:911–917.
9. Bhatt DL, Kandzari DE, O'Neill WW, et al. A controlled trial of renal denervation for resistant hypertension. *N Engl J Med.* 2014;370:1393–1401.
10. Reddy VY, Olin JW. Renal denervation for resistant hypertension: not dead yet. *J Am Coll Cardiol.* 2014;64:1088–1091.
11. Ng J, Villuendas R, Cokic I, et al. Autonomic remodeling in the left atrium and pulmonary veins in heart failure: creation of a dynamic substrate for atrial fibrillation. *Circ Arrhythm Electrophysiol.* 2011;4:388–396.
12. Gould PA, Yii M, McLean C, et al. Evidence for increased atrial sympathetic innervation in persistent human atrial fibrillation. *Pacing Clin Electrophysiol.* 2006;29:821–829.
13. Yu L, Scherlag BJ, Sha Y, et al. Interactions between atrial electrical remodeling and autonomic remodeling: how to break the vicious cycle. *Heart Rhythm.* 2012;9:804–809.
14. Dimmer C, Tavernier R, Gjorgov N, et al. Variations of autonomic tone preceding onset of atrial fibrillation after coronary artery bypass grafting. *Am J Cardiol.* 1998;82:22–25.
15. Linz D, Mahfoud F, Schotten U, et al. Renal sympathetic denervation provides ventricular rate control but does not prevent atrial electrical remodeling during atrial fibrillation. *Hypertension.* 2013;61:225–231.

16. Linz D, van Hunnik A, Hohl M, et al. Catheter-based renal denervation reduces atrial nerve sprouting and complexity of atrial fibrillation in goats. *Circ Arrhythm Electrophysiol.* 2015;8:466–474.
17. Linz D, Mahfoud F, Schotten U, et al. Renal sympathetic denervation suppresses postapneic blood pressure rises and atrial fibrillation in a model for sleep apnea. *Hypertension.* 2012;60:172–178.
18. Pokushalov E, Romanov A, Corbucci G, et al. A randomized comparison of pulmonary vein isolation with versus without concomitant renal artery denervation in patients with refractory symptomatic atrial fibrillation and resistant hypertension. *J Am Coll Cardiol.* 2012;60:1163–1170.
19. Ukena C, Mahfoud F, Spies A, et al. Effects of renal sympathetic denervation on heart rate and atrioventricular conduction in patients with resistant hypertension. *Int J Cardiol.* 2013;167:2846–2851.
20. Bourke T, Vaseghi M, Michowitz Y, et al. Neuraxial modulation for refractory ventricular arrhythmias: value of thoracic epidural anesthesia and surgical left cardiac sympathetic denervation. *Circulation.* 2010;121:2255–2262.
21. Vaseghi M, Gima J, Kanaan C, et al. Cardiac sympathetic denervation in patients with refractory ventricular arrhythmias or electrical storm: intermediate and long-term follow-up. *Heart Rhythm.* 2014;11:360–366.
22. Schwartz PJ, Priori SG, Cerrone M, et al. Left cardiac sympathetic denervation in the management of high-risk patients affected by the long-QT syndrome. *Circulation.* 2004;109:1826–1833.
23. Wilde AA, Bhuiyan ZA, Crotti L, et al. Left cardiac sympathetic denervation for catecholaminergic polymorphic ventricular tachycardia. *N Engl J Med.* 2008;358:2024–2029.
24. Davies JE, Manisty CH, Petraco R, et al. First-in-man safety evaluation of renal denervation for chronic systolic heart failure: primary outcome from REACH-Pilot study. *Int J Cardiol.* 2013;162:189–192.
25. Linz D, Wirth K, Ukena C, et al. Renal denervation suppresses ventricular arrhythmias during acute ventricular ischemia in pigs. *Heart Rhythm.* 2013;10:1525–1530.
26. Huang B, Yu L, He B, et al. Renal sympathetic denervation modulates ventricular electrophysiology and has a protective effect on ischaemia-induced ventricular arrhythmia. *Exp Physiol.* 2014;99:1467–1477.
27. Guo Z, Zhao Q, Deng H, et al. Renal sympathetic denervation attenuates the ventricular substrate and electrophysiological remodeling in dogs with pacing-induced heart failure. *Int J Cardiol.* 2014;175:185–186.
28. Ukena C, Bauer A, Mahfoud F, et al. Renal sympathetic denervation for treatment of electrical storm: first-in-man experience. *Clin Res Cardiol.* 2012;101:63–67.

29. Smithwick RH, Thompson JE. Splanchnicectomy for essential hypertension; results in 1,266 cases. *J Am Med Assoc.* 1953;152:1501–1504.
30. Miller MA, Gangireddy SR, Dukkipati SR, et al. Renal sympathetic denervation using an electroanatomic mapping system. *J Am Coll Cardiol.* 2014;63:1697.
31. Saha SP, Ziada KM, Whayne TF. Surgical, interventional, and device innovations in the management of hypertension. *Int J Angiol.* 2015;24:1–10.
32. Esler M. Renal denervation for treatment of drug-resistant hypertension. *Trends Cardiovasc Med.* 2015;25:107–115.
33. Sakakura K, Ladich E, Cheng Q, et al. Anatomic assessment of sympathetic peri-arterial renal nerves in man. *J Am Coll Cardiol.* 2014;64:635–643.
34. Ukena C, Bauer A, Mahfoud F, et al. Renal sympathetic denervation for treatment of ventricular arrhythmia: first-in-man experience. *Clin Res Cardiol.* 2012;101:63–67.
35. Hoffmann BA, Steven D, Willems S, et al. Renal sympathetic denervation as an adjunct to catheter ablation for the treatment of ventricular electrical storm in the setting of acute myocardial infarction. *J Cardiovasc Electrophysiol.* 2013;24:1175–1178.
36. Staico R, Armaganijan L, Moreira D, et al. Renal sympathetic denervation and ventricular arrhythmias: a case of electrical storm with multiple renal arteries. *EuroIntervention.* 2014;10:166.
37. Remo BF, Preminger M, Bradfield J, et al. Safety and efficacy of renal denervation as a novel treatment of ventricular tachycardia storm in patients with cardiomyopathy. *Heart Rhythm.* 2014;11:541–546.
38. Scholz EP, Raake P, Thomas D, et al. Rescue renal sympathetic denervation in a patient with ventricular electrical storm refractory to endo- and epicardial catheter ablation. *Clin Res Cardiol.* 2015;104:79–84.
39. Hilbert S, Rogge C, Papageorgiou P, et al. Successful single-sided renal denervation in drug-resistant hypertension and ventricular tachycardia. *Clin Res Cardiol.* 2015;104:279–281.
40. Kosiuk J, Hilbert S, Pokushalov E, et al. Renal denervation for treatment of cardiac arrhythmias: state of the art and future directions. *J Cardiovasc Electrophysiol.* 2015;26:233–238.
41. Armaganijan LV, Staico R, Moreira DA, et al. 6-Month outcomes in patients with implantable cardioverter-defibrillators undergoing renal sympathetic denervation for the treatment of refractory ventricular arrhythmias. *JACC Cardiovasc Interv.* 2015;8:984–990.
42. Ukena C, Mahfoud F, Ewen S, et al. Renal denervation for treatment of ventricular arrhythmias: data from an International Multicenter Registry. *Clin Res Cardiol.* 2016;105:873–879.

139 Left Atrial Appendage Closure

Mohammad Sarraf, Douglas L. Packer, and David R. Holmes, Jr.

Atrial fibrillation (AF) is the most common persistent arrhythmia in clinical practice.[1] AF carries a 5-fold higher risk for stroke, systemic thromboembolism, and death.[2] The increased thrombogenicity in patients with AF is because of several pathophysiological mechanisms. These mechanisms include abnormal changes in flow that are evident by stasis in the left atrium (LA) and can be seen as spontaneous echo contrast. Furthermore, abnormal changes in the atrial wall, including progressive atrial dilatation, endocardial denudation, and edematous or fibroelastic infiltration of the extracellular matrix, contribute to thrombus formation.[3] Therefore occlusion of the LA appendage (LAA) has the potential for significant change in the strategies for stroke prevention in patients with nonvalvular AF.[4–7] Multiple anecdotal cases[8] (Fig. 139.1) and a series of pathological and echocardiographic studies have documented that the LAA is the nidus for thrombus,[9] resulting in stroke. Nearly 57% of thrombi in patients with rheumatic heart disease and 91% of thrombi in those with nonvalvular AF develop in the LAA.[9] The hypothesis of the link between thrombus in the LAA and subsequent stroke has been substantiated in the randomized PROTECT-AF trial,[5,7] in which LAA occlusion alone was found to be noninferior to anticoagulation for stroke prevention. One should remember that other sources of thromboembolic stroke exist, for example, the LA itself in the setting of significant structural heart disease, complicated patent foramen ovale, left ventricular thrombus, mobile aortic atheroma, and carotid arterial disease. In these latter situations, chronic anticoagulant therapy may be effective for preventing stroke or systemic thromboembolism, but LAA occlusion by itself would have no beneficial effect.

Given the well-known relationship between the increasing incidence of AF and advancing age, the numbers of patients at risk is estimated to increase dramatically.[10–12] Moreover, advanced age is an independent risk factor for major bleeding, which may occur even with a subtherapeutic international normalized ratio (INR).[13] Between 10% and 30% of strokes occur in the setting of diagnosed or undiagnosed AF.

Stroke prevention in the setting of AF has been the focus of intense investigation, resulting in multiple professional societal guidelines[10,12] and the evaluation and testing of risk scores.[14–18] The most common risk score until recently was the CHADS$_2$ score, which combined clinical factors that are useful for predicting the occurrence of stroke. This system has been superseded by CHA$_2$DS$_2$-VASc (Table 139.1).

One of the largest studies that evaluated risk stratification for both ischemic stroke and bleeding included 182,678 patients with AF in the Swedish National Registry.[15] In a subset of 90,490 patients without warfarin throughout follow-up, the rate of stroke, transient ischemic attack (TIA), or peripheral embolization per 100 years at risk when adjusted for aspirin administration ranged from 0.9 to 19.4 using the CHADS$_2$ score and from 0.3 to 20.3 using the CHA$_2$DS$_2$-VASc score (Table 139.2). There was improved predictive performance of the CHA$_2$DS$_2$-VASc score for the composite thromboembolism endpoint. This expanded score appears to be of special importance in patients with lower CHADS$_2$ scores of 0–1, and it is based on an incremental improvement in the predictive value of the added risk factors of age, sex, and presence of vascular disease.[18] In addition, it has important implications for identifying the need for anticoagulant therapy in these groups with the lowest risk.

There has been controversy regarding the specific risk score that identifies a positive benefit or risk for anticoagulation; however, in general, CHADS$_2$ score of ≥2 is an indication.[10,12] It is important to recognize that undertreatment with the occurrence of stroke is generally considered more harmful than overtreatment with potential bleeding.

Conventional therapy has been centered on warfarin,[10,12] with which there are many problems, including absolute or relative contraindications, potential for bleeding, medication interactions, variability in dosing and effect, and the need for chronic intermittent monitoring. Aggregate data show that patients remain in the target INR only 60%–65% of the time.[19] On the other hand, it is estimated that being below the target INR at least 60% of the time may offset the benefit of anticoagulation.[20] To overcome these problems, newer agents have been tested in large randomized trials that involve in aggregate >70,000 patients.[21–29] In general, the new agents have been found to be more effective than warfarin with either somewhat less or similar bleeding risk, without the need for long-term monitoring of INR. One important aspect of all of these new oral anticoagulants (NOACs) is the low absolute risk reduction of NOACs compared with warfarin (Table 139.3). The number needed to treat (NNT) in these studies to prevent cardioembolic phenomena is consistently high. High NNTs in these studies are regardless of the mechanism of action in the coagulation pathway, dose, and frequency of drug administration.[21,23,24,26,29] In addition, when one administers NOACs over time, the cost may have significant economic impact. The economic impact also affects the cost effectiveness of warfarin therapy in the long term. Although warfarin is not an expensive medication, the frequent follow-up of INR over time and potential complications, such as central nervous system (CNS) or non-CNS bleeding, may accrue to an enormous cost burden. The current literature on cost effectiveness of NOACs appears to be in favor of NOACs.[30–32] Yet when these studies are carefully analyzed, many have flaws in the cost-analysis models used.[33] For example, the lack of double blinding of the warfarin arm can simply overestimate the cost by 17% against warfarin when compared with an NOAC.[33]

The role of LAA occlusion must be considered within this context. There are several considerations in this regard:
1. Some patients might have absolute or relative contraindications to both warfarin and new anticoagulant agents.
2. New agents might be associated with somewhat less bleeding, but the slope of the curve is only decreased and bleeding potential still increases over time.
3. The occurrences of gastrointestinal, pulmonary, and other side effects of the new agents are not trivial because they may result in discontinuation of the drug over time. At 2 years, 20%–25% of patients being treated with an NOAC have discontinued medication.

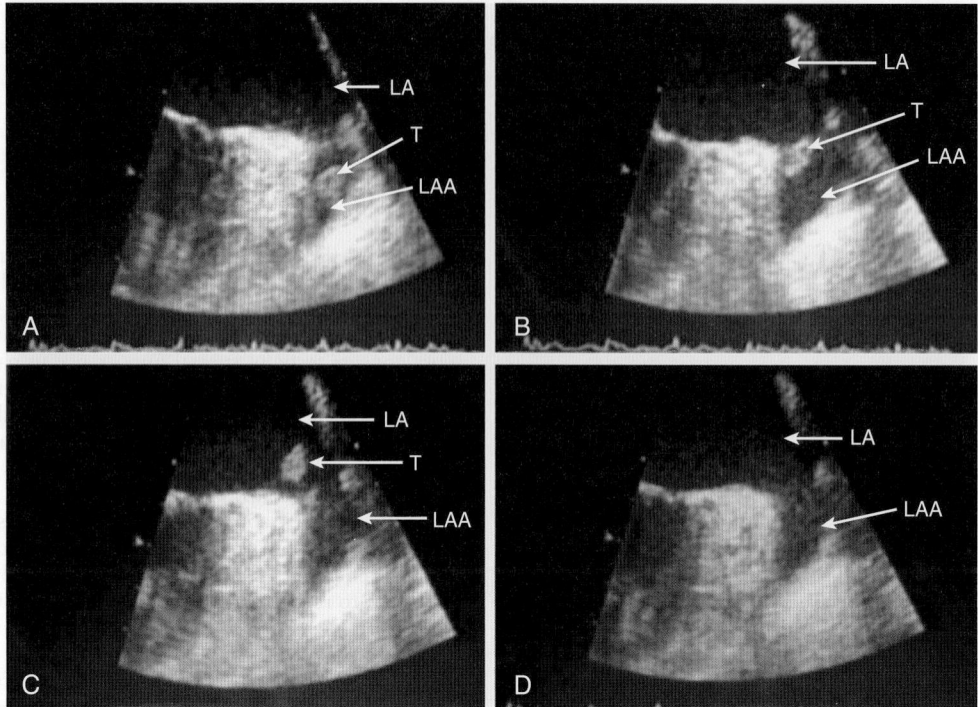

FIGURE 139.1 Disappearance of a left atrial appendage (*LAA*) clot under direct visualization in real time. *LA,* Left atrium; *T,* thrombus. (From Parekh A, Jaladi R, Sharma S, et al. Images in cardiovascular medicine. The case of a disappearing left atrial appendage thrombus: direct visualization of left atrial thrombus migration, captured by echocardiography, in a patient with atrial fibrillation, resulting in a stroke. *Circulation.* 2006;114:e513-e514.)

TABLE 139.1	Predictors of stroke and thromboembolism
RISK FACTORS	**POINTS**
CHADS₂ Score	
Congestive heart failure	1
Hypertension	1
Age >75 years	1
Diabetes mellitus	1
Prior stroke or transient ischemic attack	1
CHA₂DS₂-VASc	
Congestive heart failure	1
Hypertension	1
Age >75 years	2
Diabetes mellitus	1
Prior stroke, transient ischemic attack, or thromboembolism	2
Vascular disease	1
Age between 65 and 74 years	1
Female sex	1

4. In patients with higher CHADS₂ or CHA₂DS₂-VASc scores, even after successful ablation, anticoagulation is recommended.
5. The lifelong need for anticoagulants with the potential for side effects or drug–drug interactions and costs is substantial.
6. A substantial number of patients might develop coronary artery disease over time, requiring additional antiplatelet therapy and thus increasing the risk for bleeding, known to accompany P2Y12 inhibitor therapy. Currently, there are no studies on patients receiving NOACs who require P2Y12 inhibitors.

For these reasons, there has been substantial interest in LAA occlusion. For this approach to be accepted and more widely used, it has to meet several conditions:
1. It must be equally or more effective than alternative anticoagulation in clinical practice for stroke prevention, as demonstrated by large randomized clinical trials. The availability of data from well-executed, adequately powered randomized controlled trials is extremely important in this regard, although only two such trials for one device have been published.
2. The risk-to-benefit ratio must be favorable. This issue is complex because as with any invasive procedure, there will be at least some early procedural risks that are otherwise not present when medication alone is prescribed; with the latter, there may be long-term safety risks from hemorrhage.
3. The procedure must be performable in a substantial percentage of patient candidates.
4. The procedure must be available at a variety of institutions with well-trained specialists.
5. The approach should also be cost effective, without an adverse effect on the quality of life.

If these criteria can be met, LAA occlusion will play a substantial role in stroke prevention in patients with nonvalvular AF who are at increased risk for stroke.

Major bleeding occurs persistently at a rate of about 3% per year among patients taking warfarin.[21,23,24,26] LAA isolation potentially reduces the stroke risk without the ongoing bleeding risks associated with warfarin or NOACs. Furthermore, LAA isolation also eliminates the time in therapeutic range, medications and/or food interactions, management of medications perioperatively, and drug intolerance due to side effects. Most importantly, despite the benefit of NOACs over warfarin, there is a subset of patients who cannot tolerate anticoagulants altogether, such as those with history of CNS bleeding, significant gastrointestinal bleeding, frequent falls, or hemarthrosis.

TABLE 139.2 Stroke or thromboembolism per 100 patient-years at risk in relation to $CHADS_2$ and CHA_2DS_2-VASc scores in 90,490 patients without warfarin throughout follow-up[15]

SCORE	N	ISCHEMIC STROKE		STROKE, TIA, PERIPHERAL EMBOLISM	
		UNADJUSTED FOR ASPIRIN	ADJUSTED FOR ASPIRIN	UNADJUSTED FOR ASPIRIN	ADJUSTED FOR ASPIRIN
$CHADS_2$					
0	13,258	0.6	0.6	0.9	0.9
1	23,041	3.0	3.4	4.3	4.9
2	25,813	4.2	4.7	6.1	6.8
3	15,527	7.1	8.0	9.9	11.1
4	8767	11.1	12.6	14.9	16.8
5	3315	12.5	14.1	16.7	18.9
6	769	13.0	14.6	17.2	19.4
CHA_2DS_2-VASc					
0	5343	0.2	0.2	0.3	0.3
1	6770	0.6	0.6	0.9	1.0
2	11,240	2.2	2.5	2.9	3.3
3	17,689	3.2	3.7	4.6	5.3
4	19,091	4.8	5.5	6.7	7.8
5	14,488	7.2	8.4	10.0	11.7
6	9577	9.7	11.4	13.6	15.9
7	4465	11.2	13.1	15.7	18.4
8	1559	10.8	12.6	15.2	17.9
9	268	12.2	14.4	17.4	20.3
All	90,490	4.5	5.0	6.2	7.0

TIA, Transient ischemic stroke.

TABLE 139.3 Magnitude of new oral anticoagulants on stroke and/or thromboembolism (TE) and number needed to treat (NNT)

STUDY	TREATMENT	STROKE OR TE	NNT
RE-LY[21]	Dabigatran 110 mg twice daily	1.53	625
	Dabigatran 150 mg twice daily	1.11	172
	Warfarin	1.69	
ROCKET-AF[26]	Rivaroxaban	1.7	200
	Warfarin	2.2	
ARISTOTLE[24]	Apixaban	1.27	303
	Warfarin	1.6	
ENGAGE AF-TIMI[48,23]	Edoxaban high dose	1.18	313
	Edoxaban low dose	1.61	—
	Warfarin	1.5	

Left Atrial Appendage Anatomy

The LA is formed from the fusion of the pulmonary venous bud and the primitive muscular LA during the third week of gestation. During this stage, the LAA is formed and ultimately becomes a remnant of the original muscular LA. The smooth wall of the LA is derived from the outgrowing of the pulmonary venous system, while the trabeculated primitive LA persists as the LAA.[34] The LAA is a multilobed tubular structure that lies within the pericardium (Fig. 139.2). It is grossly divided into the ostium, neck, and body (Fig. 139.3). The ostial size and shape are variable. Approximately 70% of ostia are oval shaped.[35] The neck connects the ostium to the body of the LAA and is typically the narrowest part of the LAA.[36] The body is a finger-like multilobed tubular structure, with >80% of LAAs having two or more lobes, and these lobes extend in multiple directions.[37] Recently, the morphology of the LAA has been the focus of investigation for varied risk for

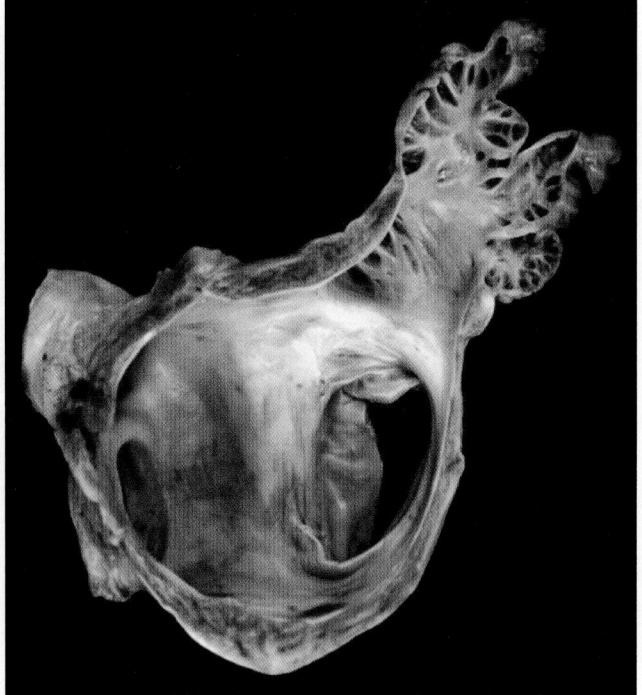

FIGURE 139.2 An autopsy specimen of a left atrial appendage and left atrium (LA) with a sagittal section. The morphology of the LA and the smooth portion of the LA because of outgrowing of the pulmonary venous bud are evident.

thromboembolism in patients with AF. The LAA is classified into various morphologies based on its computed tomography (CT)/magnetic resonance imaging (MRI)–derived shape by Wang and et al.[35] and Di Biase et al.[38] The types are (1) cactus, (2) chicken wing, (3) windsock, and (4) cauliflower (Fig. 139.4 A to D). The

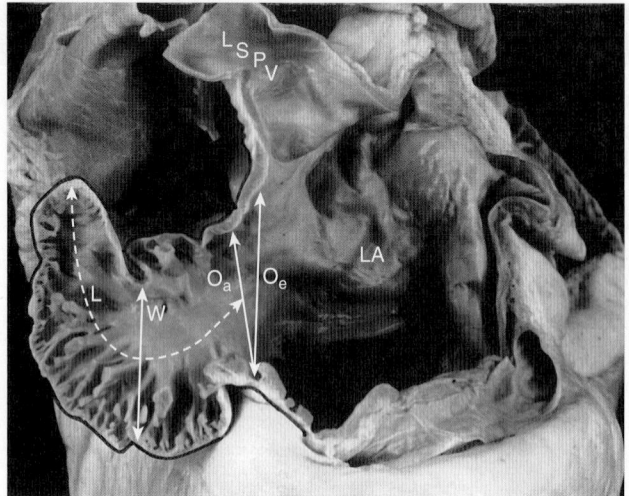

FIGURE 139.3 Measurements of the left atrial appendage (LAA) in a postmortem specimen. It is important to comprehend the curvilinear relationship of the body of the LAA to the left atrium (*LA*). The length (*L*) of the appendage is a curvilinear distance (*dashed line*) from the Oa to the tip of the tail, whereas the maximal width (*W*) is a straight-line measurement. *LSPV*, Left superior pulmonary vein; *Oa*, anatomical orifice; *Oe*, echocardiographic orifice. (From Veinot JP, Harrity PJ, Gentile F, et al. Anatomy of the normal left atrial appendage: a quantitative study of age-related changes in 500 autopsy hearts: implications for echocardiographic examination. *Circulation.* 1997;96:3112-3115.)

chicken wing was the most common type and was present in 48% of the study patients.

The chicken wing LAA morphology has been found to have three times lower risk for stroke compared with non-chicken wing morphology.[38] The increased risk for stroke in non-chicken wing morphology is six times higher, even in patients with CHADS$_2$ scores as low as 0 or 1.[38] Other morphological and anatomical features of the LAA correlate with increased risk for stroke. Larger dimensions and volume of the LAA have been associated with increased risk for stroke.[39] LAA volume of >34 cm^3 has been associated with increased risk for stroke and thromboembolism in a small study.[40]

Imaging of the Left Atrial Appendage

Echocardiographic Assessment

Transesophageal echocardiography (TEE) should be used for a comprehensive approach to the LAA closure procedure to understand the anatomy and function and to help guide the procedure. TEE is of particular importance for patient screening because of the potential presence of LAA thrombus. When LAA thrombus is detected, device placement should not be attempted; in this setting, anticoagulation should be administered for 1–3 months, and repeated TEE should be performed. If there has been resolution of the thrombus at the time of follow-up TEE, then device placement can be performed. The presence of dense, spontaneous echo contrast is also potentially problematic because it has been linked to the development of thrombus, although this is somewhat

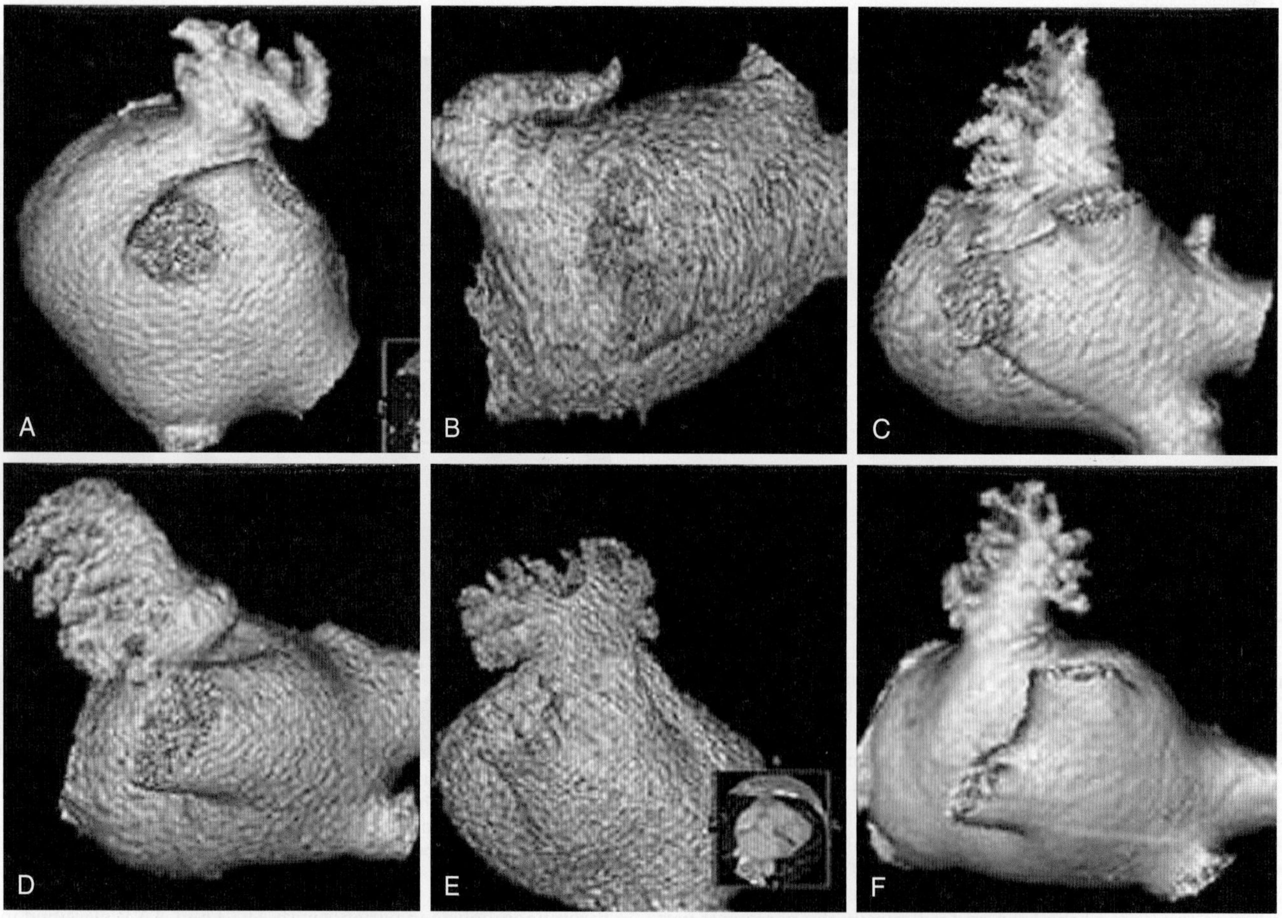

FIGURE 139.4 Assessment of the shape of the left atrial appendage can affect selection of a specific device. Wang et al. have developed a classification scheme based on computed tomographic imaging. The "chicken wing" configuration (A and B) may make it difficult to fully intubate and deliver a device. The other subtypes—windsock (C and D), cauliflower (E), and cactus (F)—can also affect the selection of specific devices.

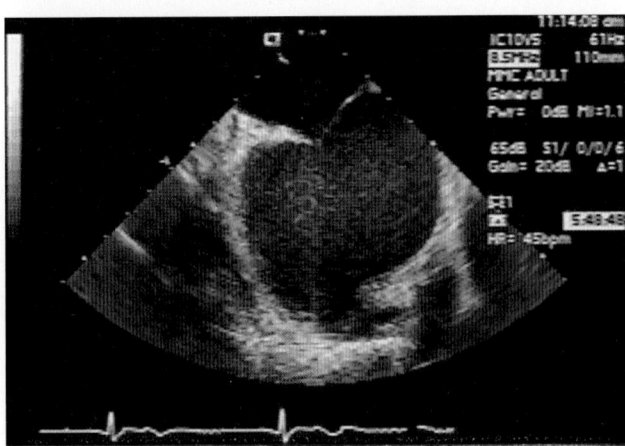

FIGURE 139.5 Optimal positioning of the transseptal needle using an intracardiac echocardiogram during the procedure.

controversial. TEE is also important for assessing the anatomical features of the LAA and its orientation in space. In combination with transthoracic echocardiography (TTE) and cardiac CT scan, TEE is also essential in evaluating the details of other cardiac chambers, specifically evaluating the intraatrial septum and identifying other abnormalities that can either affect the performance of the procedure or increase the potential for other sources of thrombus.

During the procedure, TEE serves several functions. With TEE guidance, the exact location of the interatrial septal puncture can be identified, which is advantageous to optimize the ability to engage the LAA once the transseptal puncture has been performed. The LAA ostium is anatomically located anterolateral and slightly superior in the LA. The ideal trajectory of the delivery system of any LAA closure device is from posterior and inferior. Hence, TEE is an excellent imaging approach for locating the ideal transseptal puncture. Real-time three-dimensional TEE is being used with increasing frequency and helps in overcoming some of the limitations of inadequate spatial resolution and sensitivity seen with two-dimensional TEE. LAA dimensions and geometry can be more accurately assessed with three-dimensional TEE compared with two-dimensional TEE.

Intracardiac echocardiography (ICE) is also used for LAA imaging and has the advantage of avoiding the need for either deep sedation or general anesthesia, which is used for TEE; it also helps to avoid the potential for rare but serious complications seen with TEE (e.g., esophageal trauma). In addition, ICE can be performed by an interventional operator during the procedure, thus avoiding the need for additional physician support, which is needed for TEE. ICE imaging can identify details of the intraatrial septum accurately (Fig. 139.5); it can also be used to guide the placement of the delivery sheath within the LAA. ICE may also be used for measurement of LAA dimensions for device sizing, device placement, as well as residual leak assessment and device stability before final deployment. Although the superior-to-inferior dimensions can be seen from a right atrial (RA) imaging venue, the anterior-to-posterior dimensions are best imaged from a location below the tricuspid valve. It is noteworthy that LAA dimensions obtained by ICE might be different from those obtained by two-dimensional TEE because of the different spatial angulation of the imaging planes.

Computed Tomography

CT allows detailed assessment of LAA dimensions for consideration of device sizing and placement. Of particular importance is that it also allows for assessment of the three-dimensional orientation in space and the relationships among other cardiac structures. Preprocedural CT is part of the routine workup for the evaluation of one specific device (LARIAT, SentreHeart, Inc.,

Palo Alto, CA). If on CT imaging, the tip of the LAA is seen to be oriented extremely superiorly, the procedure is best avoided with this device because of the difficulty with reaching and capturing the tip with the suture device. Although less frequently used, CT can also be performed during follow-up to assess device position and the completeness of exclusion. Recently, there has been a higher tendency to study the LAA with cardiac CT for most devices.

Left Atrial Appendage Closure Techniques

Surgical

Surgical resection of the LAA was proposed in 1949 for patients with AF as a potential therapy to reduce mortality. Over the next five decades, there was tremendous heterogeneity of surgical techniques for LAA closure with few well-conducted clinical studies. The results of surgical LAA closure have remained controversial. Furthermore, the definition of LAA closure has not been previously well described in these studies. A meta-analysis, involving 1400 patients and five clinical trials, appeared to show no clear benefit for surgical exclusion of the LAA; only one showed a benefit, three were neutral, and one demonstrated increased risk from the exclusion itself.[41] Currently, the Left Atrial Appendage Occlusion Study III (LAAOS III) is designed to randomize nearly 4700 patients with AF, undergoing cardiac surgery, to either LAA excision or exclusion versus conventional medical therapy[42] (www .clinicaltrials.gov; NCT01561651). All patients will continue to receive usual antithrombotic therapy. The primary outcome will be the composite of stroke or non-CNS embolization. The specific surgical LAA occlusion technique will be at the individual operator's discretion.

Percutaneous: the Watchman Experience

To date, the Watchman is the only device that has been rigorously studied and investigated in multiple randomized controlled trials and registries. The Watchman device was initially studied in a US and European feasibility trial of 75 patients. During this study, the device underwent a new iteration; nevertheless, 66 patients (88%) had successful LAA closure and 90% of patients were able to discontinue anticoagulation during a mean follow-up of 740 days.[43]

Safety and clinical efficacies have been evaluated in two randomized clinical trials that investigated the noninferiority of the Watchman LAA occluder to warfarin therapy in patients eligible for chronic anticoagulation.[5,44] Both studies were Bayesian and randomized clinical trials, investigating whether LAA occlusion with the Watchman was noninferior to warfarin for the primary efficacy endpoint of stroke, systemic embolism, and cardiovascular or unexplained death.

The PROTECT-AF trial randomized 707 patients with AF and CHADS$_2$ score of ≥1 in a 2:1 ratio to the Watchman versus warfarin therapy, with the combined endpoint of stroke, systemic embolism, and cardiovascular death. The Bayesian hierarchical model allowed for up to 1500 patient-years, although the follow-up later was ongoing for up to 5 years.[45] The patients had to have CHADS$_2$ score of ≥1 to enter the study.

There are several important points to be considered in evaluating this trial:
1. The trial, which included 707 patients who were randomized in a 2:1 device-to-control drug ratio, met the 1-year specified primary noninferiority efficacy endpoint (3.0 vs. 4.9 events per 100 patient-years, respectively, with an RR of 0.62 (95% Bayesian credible interval, 0.3–1.25).
2. There was an early safety hazard in the device limb. The primary safety endpoint occurred significantly more frequently in the device group at 7.4 versus 4.4 events per 100 patient-years. The RR was 1.69, with a 95% Bayesian credible interval

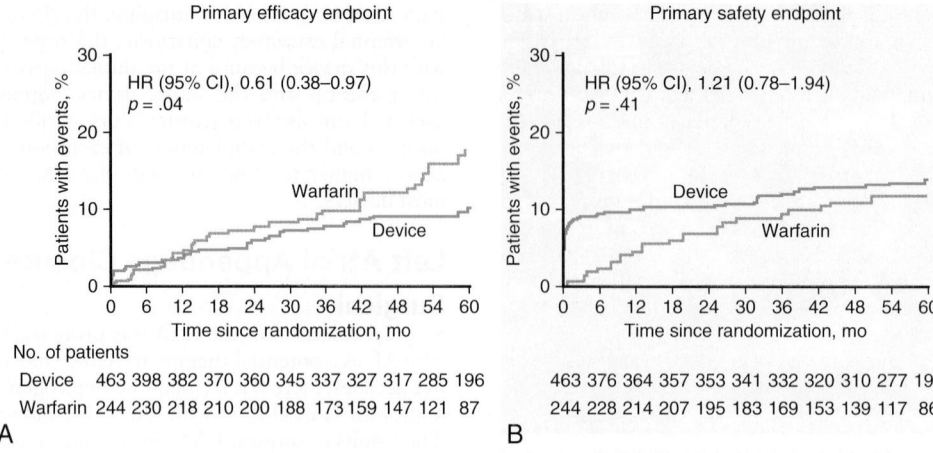

FIGURE 139.6 Long-term clinical and safety outcomes in the PROTECT-AF trial. (A) The primary efficacy outcome of cardiovascular death, stroke, or systemic embolism. The mean follow-up of patients was 3.8 years (2621 patient-years). (B) The primary safety outcome was a composite of major bleeding events and procedure-related complications. Despite the apparent early hazard in the device group, the overall safety was similar in both groups. *CI*, Confidence interval; *HR*, hazard ratio.

of 1.01–3.19. This primary safety endpoint was the result of periprocedural events, which included most commonly 22 pericardial effusions in 4.8% and stroke in 0.9% (typically because of air embolization). In contrast to this early safety device concern, the control group had a high prevalence of major bleeding and hemorrhagic stroke compared with the device group: 4.1% in the control group versus 3.5% with the device and hemorrhagic stroke and 2.5% in the control group versus 0.2% with the device.

3. With expanded operator experience in an expanded continued access protocol, the pericardial effusion rate has diminished significantly to 2.2%, and periprocedural strokes appear to have been eliminated.

4. In the final analysis of the PROTECT-AF trial, at 1588 patient-years follow-up, primary event rates were 3.0% and 4.3% per year in the LAA closure group versus the warfarin group (RR, 0.71; 95% credible interval, 0.44–1.30 per year). When a landmark-type analysis was performed to isolate the risk contribution of LAA closure from the complications of implantation, LAA closure was found to be superior to warfarin.

5. Patients randomized to the device received warfarin for the first 45 days to facilitate endothelialization of the device surface. This dosing potentially exposed patients to bleeding risk in the device group related to the short-term use of warfarin. Device success rate was seen in approximately 95%; furthermore, 95% of patients, randomized to the device, were able to discontinue warfarin.

6. A final issue relates to the completeness of closure.[46,47] In the PROTECT-AF trial, 445 patients with successful device implantation underwent TEE at 45 days. Of these patients, 389 had 12-month studies.[46] Device flow was categorized as no residual flow, minor flow (<1 mm), moderate flow (1–3 mm), or major flow (>3 mm). The prevalence of any flow decreased from 40.9% at 45 days to 33.8% at 6 months and then to 32.1% at 12 months. A moderate leak (1–3 mm) was the most common at all three time points. The primary efficacy event rates, ischemic stroke, and systemic embolism were not different between patients with any residual flow and those with no residual flow. Not all studies have documented a decrease in leak size over time.[47] In a smaller analysis of 58 patients with the Watchman device, a "peridevice gap" was noted in 29.3% at 45 days, but the incidence had increased to 34.5% at 1 year. This issue of incomplete sealing of the LAA has important

implications, particularly in the relationship with subsequent events.

7. A follow-up analysis of 3.8 ± 1.7 years with 2621 patient-years demonstrated a composite efficacy endpoint of 8.4% in the device group compared with 13.9% in the warfarin group (rate ratio, 0.6; 95% confidence interval, 0.41–1.05). These findings met the criteria for both noninferiority (posterior probability, >99.9%) and superiority (posterior probability, >96%) (Fig. 139.6).

Despite the convincing results of the PROTECT-AF trial, a number of cautionary notes were raised. Some of the criticisms were the small sample size, low CHADS$_2$ score, liberal use of anticoagulation in the device group, and relatively short duration of follow-up.[48] These criticisms led to the design and execution of the PREVAIL trial (see later).

The aim of the smaller PREVAIL trial was to confirm procedural safety, particularly among new operators (39%; 25% was required by the study design) and new centers (39%; 20% was required by the study design), as well as further exploring the clinical efficacy of LAA closure with the Watchman device. The PREVAIL trial randomized 407 patients in a 2:1 fashion to the Watchman device (N = 269) or warfarin (N = 138).[44] The eligible patients had a CHADS$_2$ score of ≥2 or CHADS$_2$ score of 1 with one or more high-risk features for stroke or TIA. The following high-risk features were considered: (1) females aged ≥75 years; (2) left ventricular ejection fraction between 30% and 35%; (3) age between 65 and 75 years with diabetes or coronary artery disease; and (4) ≥65 years of age with documented congestive heart failure. The PREVAIL Bayesian statistical design incorporated prior patients from the PROTECT-AF trial and newly randomized patients in the PREVAIL trial, while discounting the contribution of the PROTECT-AF patients. The study had three coprimary endpoints: (1) primary efficacy, a composite of hemorrhagic or ischemic stroke, systemic embolism, and cardiovascular or unexplained death; (2) late-ischemic efficacy (ischemic stroke or systemic embolism) with landmark analysis after 7 days of device deployment; and (3) early safety, a composite of all-cause death, ischemic stroke, systemic embolism, or device-related complications, leading to a surgical or nonsurgical intervention within 7 days of the procedure or during the index hospitalization.

The findings of the PREVAIL trial have a number of important findings that are worthy of further discussion:

1. The Watchman device failed to meet the noninferiority criterion for the primary efficacy endpoint (18-month rate of

stroke, systemic embolism, and cardiovascular or unexplained death), with a mean follow-up of 11.8 ± 5.8 months. The 18-month event rate was 0.064 for the device group and 0.063 for the control group, and the rate ratio was 1.07 with a 95% credible interval of 0.57–1.89. The upper bound of the 95% credible interval for the 18-month rate ratio was 1.75.

2. The late ischemic primary efficacy endpoint (stroke or systemic embolism of >7 days after randomization) met the noninferiority criterion. The device group had a rate of 0.0253, while the control group had a rate of 0.0200 (18-month risk difference, 0.0053; 95% credible interval, –0.0190–0.0273). The upper bound for noninferiority was <0.0275; therefore the study met the noninferiority criteria.

3. The primary safety endpoint was evaluated using a Bayesian model from the previous studies of PROTECT-AF[5] and the Continued Access Registry to PROTECT (CAP) registry.[7] Of 269 patients, only six patients met the criteria for the safety endpoint (2.2%) that was below the upper bound of the credible interval of 2.67%.

4. It is important to recognize that both the PROTECT-AF and PREVAIL trials compared a very particular strategy. All patients who received the Watchman device were on 81 mg of aspirin and warfarin (target INR, 2–3) for 45 days, followed by 81–325 mg of aspirin and 75 mg of clopidogrel daily for 6 months, followed by 81–325 mg of aspirin daily for life. The totality of data from PROTECT-AF and PREVAIL trials confirm the efficacy of the device.

5. The procedural learning curve was carefully examined in this trial. Although the study design mandated 25% new operators and 20% new centers, the study included significantly higher numbers of new operators and centers (39% and 39%, respectively). Nevertheless, there was no reduced successful implantation rate or increased major adverse event rate. This confirms that the implemented training program provided by the sponsors is effective and translatable to real-life practice.

6. The Watchman procedure, similar to any other new technique, has a steep learning curve. Therefore the potential complications related to the procedure should be carefully scrutinized. In the PROTECT-AF trial, the acute safety of the Watchman device was a major concern, especially in the first half of the patients. The rate of safety events in the PROTECT-AF trial was 9.9% in the first half, which precipitously decreased to 4.8% in the second half of enrollment. This experience proved to remain durable in the CAP registry and PREVAIL trial, in which the safety event rates were 4.1% and 4.2%, respectively. From the PROTECT-AF trial to the PREVAIL trial, the rates of cardiac perforations requiring surgery, tamponade, and strokes because of air embolism decreased.

The PROTECT-AF and PREVAIL trials were both designed for patients eligible for anticoagulation. A significant portion of patients with AF are not able to tolerate anticoagulation for a variety of reasons. Some examples include significant gastrointestinal bleeding, intracranial or intraparenchymal hemorrhage, patients with high risk for stroke and concomitant high risk for bleeding, patients who have had a stroke on anticoagulation, and noncompliance.[49] The ASA Plavix Feasibility Study with Watchman Left Atrial Appendage Closure Technology (ASAP) trial was specifically designed for patients with AF who were ineligible for anticoagulation. The study was a prospective, multicenter but nonrandomized study that evaluated the clinical efficacy of the Watchman device in 150 patients. The mean age of the patients was 72.5 years, with mean $CHADS_2$ score of 2.8 ± 1.2 and mean CHA_2DS_2-VASc score of 4.4 ± 1.7. Patients

were followed up for a mean of 14.4 ± 8.6 months. The rate of stroke or systemic embolism was 2.3% per year (four patients) during the follow-up. The rate of ischemic stroke was 1.7% in 100 patient-years, with 0.1% risk for hemorrhagic stroke in 100 patient-years during the same period. The expected rate of stroke was 7.4% on the basis of $CHADS_2$ score. Although this registry study proves that dual antiplatelet therapy is safe and feasible, further studies are required to robustly recommend a dual antiplatelet strategy for patients undergoing this procedure.

The aggregate data on the Watchman device have been recently analyzed in a patient-level meta-analysis, using data from the PROTECT-AF, PREVAIL, CAP, and Continued Access Registry to PREVAIL (CAP2) studies.[50] The meta-analysis includes 2406 patients with 5931 patient-years of follow-up. After a mean follow-up of 2.69 years, patients receiving the Watchman device had significantly less hemorrhagic strokes (0.15 vs. 0.96 events/100 patient-years; hazard ratio [HR], 0.22; p = .004), cardiovascular or unexplained death (1.1 vs. 2.3 events/100 patient-years; HR, 0.48; p = .006), and nonprocedural bleeding (6.0% vs. 11.3%; HR, 0.51; p = .006) compared with warfarin. All-cause stroke and systemic embolism were not different between the groups (1.75 vs. 1.87 events/100 patient-years; HR, 1.02; 95% CI, 0.62–1.7; p = .94). But the rate of ischemic strokes was higher in the Watchman group (1.6 vs. 0.9 and 0.2 vs. 1.0 events/100 patient-years; HR, 1.95 and 0.22, respectively; p = .05 and .004, respectively). This meta-analysis demonstrates that the Watchman device protects patients by excluding the LAA from the systemic circulation as well as by preventing future episodes of bleeding, which ultimately can translate into long-term benefit and improve survival. Because the bleeding risk does not plateau over time and in fact, always increases with age, it is reasonable to suspect that the long-term survival benefit with the Watchman device may accrue over time.

The US Food and Drug Administration (FDA) approved the Watchman device in March 2015 for patients with AF with the following conditions:

"The Watchman should only be used in patients who:

- have atrial fibrillation not related to valvular heart disease
- are at increased risk for a stroke
- are recommended for blood thinning medicines
- are suitable for warfarin (a blood thinner also known as Coumadin)
- have an appropriate reason to seek a non-drug alternative to warfarin"

It is noteworthy that the Watchman device is not intended to replace warfarin or anticoagulation; therefore appropriate patient selection is important.

Conclusion

AF is associated with increased rates of stroke and systemic embolism, and with the aging of the population, the incidence and prevalence of stroke will continue to increase. The risk factors for stroke and bleeding overlap significantly, which makes anticoagulation a less desirable option. Because most of the thromboembolic phenomena in AF occur in the LAA, LAA closure technology remains a viable and attractive option for patients with high risk for bleeding or failed anticoagulation therapy. As the data continue to emerge with the Watchman and other novel devices, this approach will continue to grow. Furthermore, LA procedures, including LAA closure, have a steep learning curve; therefore patient selection for LAA closure must be carefully weighed against potential complications of the procedure as well as device-specific procedures.

REFERENCES

1. Chugh SS, Blackshear JL, Shen WK, et al. Epidemiology and natural history of atrial fibrillation: clinical implications. *J Am Coll Cardiol.* 2001;37:371–378.
2. Wolf PA, Abbott RD, Kannel WB. Atrial fibrillation as an independent risk factor for stroke: the Framingham Study. *Stroke.* 1991;22:983–988.
3. Watson T, Shantsila E, Lip GY. Mechanisms of thrombogenesis in atrial fibrillation: Virchow's triad revisited. *Lancet.* 2009;373:155–166.
4. Bayard YL, Omran H, Neuzil P, et al. PLAATO (Percutaneous Left Atrial Appendage Transcatheter Occlusion) for prevention of cardioembolic stroke in non-anticoagulation eligible atrial fibrillation patients: results from the European PLAATO study. *EuroIntervention.* 2010;6:220–226.
5. Holmes DR, Reddy VY, Turi ZG, et al. Percutaneous closure of the left atrial appendage versus warfarin therapy for prevention of stroke in patients with atrial fibrillation: a randomised non-inferiority trial. *Lancet.* 2009;374:534–542.
6. Park JW, Bethencourt A, Sievert H, et al. Left atrial appendage closure with Amplatzer cardiac plug in atrial fibrillation: initial European experience. *Catheter Cardiovasc Interv.* 2011;77:700–706.
7. Reddy VY, Holmes D, Doshi SK, et al. Safety of percutaneous left atrial appendage closure: results from the Watchman Left Atrial Appendage System for Embolic Protection in Patients with AF (PROTECT AF) clinical trial and the Continued Access Registry. *Circulation.* 2011;123:417–424.
8. Parekh A, Jaladi R, Sharma S, et al. Images in cardiovascular medicine. The case of a disappearing left atrial appendage thrombus: direct visualization of left atrial thrombus migration, captured by echocardiography, in a patient with atrial fibrillation, resulting in a stroke. *Circulation.* 2006;114:e513–e514.
9. Blackshear JL, Odell JA. Appendage obliteration to reduce stroke in cardiac surgical patients with atrial fibrillation. *Ann Thorac Surg.* 1996;61:755–759.
10. European Heart Rhythm Association; European Association for Cardio-Thoracic Surgery, Camm AJ, et al. Guidelines for the management of atrial fibrillation: the Task Force for the Management of Atrial Fibrillation of the European Society of Cardiology (ESC). *Eur Heart J.* 2010;31:2369–2429.
11. Go AS, Hylek EM, Phillips KA, et al. Prevalence of diagnosed atrial fibrillation in adults: national implications for rhythm management and stroke prevention: the AnTicoagulation and Risk Factors in Atrial Fibrillation (ATRIA) Study. *JAMA.* 2001;285:2370–2375.
12. January CT, Wann LS, Alpert JS, et al. 2014 AHA/ACC/HRS guideline for the management of patients with atrial fibrillation: a report of the American College of Cardiology/American Heart Association Task Force on Practice Guidelines and the Heart Rhythm Society. *Circulation.* 2014;130:e199–e267.
13. Smith EE, Rosand J, Knudsen KA, et al. Leukoaraiosis is associated with warfarin-related hemorrhage following ischemic stroke. *Neurology.* 2002;59:193–197.
14. Stroke Risk in Atrial Fibrillation Working Group. Comparison of 12 risk stratification schemes to predict stroke in patients with nonvalvular atrial fibrillation. *Stroke.* 2008;39:1901–1910.
15. Friberg L, Rosenqvist M, Lip GY. Evaluation of risk stratification schemes for ischaemic stroke and bleeding in 182 678 patients with atrial fibrillation: the Swedish Atrial Fibrillation cohort study. *Eur Heart J.* 2012;33:1500–1510.
16. Gage BF, Waterman AD, Shannon W, et al. Validation of clinical classification schemes for predicting stroke: results from the National Registry of Atrial Fibrillation. *JAMA.* 2001;285:2864–2870.
17. Lip GY, Frison L, Halperin JL, et al. Identifying patients at high risk for stroke despite anticoagulation: a comparison of contemporary stroke risk stratification schemes in an anticoagulated atrial fibrillation cohort. *Stroke.* 2010;41:2731–2738.
18. Olesen JB, Torp-Pedersen C, Hansen ML, et al. The value of the CHA2DS2-VASc score for refining stroke risk stratification in patients with atrial fibrillation with a CHADS2 score 0-1: a nationwide cohort study. *Thromb Haemost.* 2012;107:1172–1179.
19. Agarwal S, Hachamovitch R, Menon V. Current trial-associated outcomes with warfarin in prevention of stroke in patients with nonvalvular atrial fibrillation: a meta-analysis. *Arch Intern Med.* 2012;172:623–631. discussion 631–623.
20. Go AS, Hylek EM, Chang Y, et al. Anticoagulation therapy for stroke prevention in atrial fibrillation: how well do randomized trials translate into clinical practice? *JAMA.* 2003;290:2685–2692.
21. Connolly SJ, Ezekowitz MD, Yusuf S, et al. Dabigatran versus warfarin in patients with atrial fibrillation. *N Engl J Med.* 2009;361:1139–1151.
22. Connolly SJ, Pogue J, Hart RG, et al. Effect of clopidogrel added to aspirin in patients with atrial fibrillation. *N Engl J Med.* 2009;360:2066–2078.
23. Giugliano RP, Ruff CT, Braunwald E, et al. Edoxaban versus warfarin in patients with atrial fibrillation. *N Engl J Med.* 2013;369:2093–2104.
24. Granger CB, Alexander JH, McMurray JJ, et al. Apixaban versus warfarin in patients with atrial fibrillation. *N Engl J Med.* 2011;365:981–992.
25. Hylek EM, Go AS, Chang Y, et al. Effect of intensity of oral anticoagulation on stroke severity and mortality in atrial fibrillation. *N Engl J Med.* 2003;349:1019–1026.
26. Patel MR, Mahaffey KW, Garg J, et al. Rivaroxaban versus warfarin in nonvalvular atrial fibrillation. *N Engl J Med.* 2011;365:883–891.
27. Singer DE, Albers GW, Dalen JE, et al. Antithrombotic therapy in atrial fibrillation: American College of Chest Physicians Evidence-Based Clinical Practice Guidelines (8th Edition). *Chest.* 2008;133:546S–592S.
28. Sudlow M, Thomson R, Thwaites B, et al. Prevalence of atrial fibrillation and eligibility for anticoagulants in the community. *Lancet.* 1998;352:1167–1171.
29. Wallentin L, Yusuf S, Ezekowitz MD, et al. Efficacy and safety of dabigatran compared with warfarin at different levels of international normalised ratio control for stroke prevention in atrial fibrillation: an analysis of the RE-LY trial. *Lancet.* 2010;376:975–983.
30. Coyle D, Coyle K, Cameron C, et al. Cost-effectiveness of new oral anticoagulants compared with warfarin in preventing stroke and other cardiovascular events in patients with atrial fibrillation. *Value Health.* 2013;16:498–506.
31. Dorian P, Kongnakorn T, Phatak H, et al. Cost-effectiveness of apixaban vs. current standard of care for stroke prevention in patients with atrial fibrillation. *Eur Heart J.* 2014;35:1897–1906.
32. Kasmeridis C, Apostolakis S, Ehlers L, et al. Cost effectiveness of treatments for stroke prevention in atrial fibrillation: focus on the novel oral anticoagulants. *Pharmacoeconomics.* 2013;31:971–980.
33. Limone BL, Baker WL, Mearns ES, et al. Common flaws exist in published cost-effectiveness models of pharmacologic stroke prevention in atrial fibrillation. *J Clin Epidemiol.* 2014;67:1093–1102.
34. Abdulla R, Blew GA, Holterman MJ. Cardiovascular embryology. *Pediatr Cardiol.* 2004;25:191–200.
35. Wang Y, Di Biase L, Horton RP, et al. Left atrial appendage studied by computed tomography to help planning for appendage closure device placement. *J Cardiovasc Electrophysiol.* 2010;21:973–982.
36. Ho SY, Cabrera JA, Sanchez-Quintana D. Left atrial anatomy revisited. *Circ Arrhythm Electrophysiol.* 2012;5:220–228.
37. Veinot JP, Harrity PJ, Gentile F, et al. Anatomy of the normal left atrial appendage: a quantitative study of age-related changes in 500 autopsy hearts: implications for echocardiographic examination. *Circulation.* 1997;96:3112–3115.
38. Di Biase L, Santangeli P, Anselmino M, et al. Does the left atrial appendage morphology correlate with the risk of stroke in patients with atrial fibrillation? Results from a multicenter study. *J Am Coll Cardiol.* 2012;60:531–538.
39. Beinart R, Heist EK, Newell JB, et al. Left atrial appendage dimensions predict the risk of stroke/TIA in patients with atrial fibrillation. *J Cardiovasc Electrophysiol.* 2011;22:10–15.
40. Burrell LD, Horne BD, Anderson JL, et al. Usefulness of left atrial appendage volume as a predictor of embolic stroke in patients with atrial fibrillation. *Am J Cardiol.* 2013;112:1148–1152.
41. Dawson AG, Asopa S, Dunning J. Should patients undergoing cardiac surgery with atrial fibrillation have left atrial appendage exclusion? *Interact Cardiovasc Thorac Surg.* 2010;10:306–311.
42. Whitlock R, Healey J, Vincent J, et al. Rationale and design of the Left Atrial Appendage Occlusion Study (LAAOS) III. *Ann Cardiothorac Surg.* 2014;3:45–54.
43. Sick PB, Schuler G, Hauptmann KE, et al. Initial worldwide experience with the WATCHMAN left atrial appendage system for stroke prevention in atrial fibrillation. *J Am Coll Cardiol.* 2007;49:1490–1495.
44. Holmes Jr DR, Kar S, Price MJ, et al. Prospective randomized evaluation of the Watchman Left Atrial Appendage Closure device in patients with atrial fibrillation versus long-term warfarin therapy: the PREVAIL trial. *J Am Coll Cardiol.* 2014;64:1–12.
45. Fountain RB, Holmes DR, Chandrasekaran K, et al. The PROTECT AF (WATCHMAN Left Atrial Appendage System for Embolic PROTECTion in Patients with Atrial Fibrillation) trial. *Am Heart J.* 2006;151:956–961.
46. Viles-Gonzalez JF, Kar S, Douglas P, et al. The clinical impact of incomplete left atrial appendage closure with the Watchman Device in patients with atrial fibrillation: a PROTECT AF (Percutaneous Closure of the Left Atrial Appendage Versus Warfarin Therapy for Prevention of Stroke in Patients With Atrial Fibrillation) substudy. *J Am Coll Cardiol.* 2012;59:923–929.
47. Bai R, Horton RP, Di Biase L, et al. Intraprocedural and long-term incomplete occlusion of the left atrial appendage following placement of the WATCHMAN device: a single center experience. *J Cardiovasc Electrophysiol.* 2012;23:455–461.
48. Maisel WH. Left atrial appendage occlusion–closure or just the beginning? *N Engl J Med.* 2009;360:2601–2603.
49. Alli O, Asirvatham S, Holmes Jr DR. Strategies to incorporate left atrial appendage occlusion into clinical practice. *J Am Coll Cardiol.* 2015;65:2337–2344.
50. Holmes Jr DR, Doshi SK, Kar S, et al. Left atrial appendage closure as an alternative to warfarin for stroke prevention in atrial fibrillation: a patient-level meta-analysis. *J Am Coll Cardiol.* 2015;65:2614–2623.

INDEX

Page numbers followed by f indicate figures; b, boxes; t, tables.